D1528783

EDITION 9

SABISTON & SPENCER

SURGERY of the CHEST

Frank W. Sellke, MD
Karl Karlson & Gloria Karlson Professor and Chief of Cardiothoracic Surgery
Warren Alpert Medical School of Brown University and Rhode Island Hospital
Director, Lifespan Cardiovascular Institute
Providence, Rhode Island

Pedro J. del Nido, MD
William E. Ladd Professor of Surgery
Harvard Medical School
Chairman, Department of Cardiac Surgery
Boston Children's Hospital
Boston, Massachusetts

Scott J. Swanson, MD
Director, Minimally Invasive Thoracic Surgery
Brigham and Women's Hospital
Vice Chair, Cancer Affairs
Department of Surgery, Brigham and Women's Hospital
Chief Surgical Officer
Dana-Farber Cancer Institute
Professor of Surgery
Harvard Medical School
Boston, Massachusetts

ELSEVIER

ELSEVIER

1600 John F. Kennedy Blvd.
Ste 1800
Philadelphia, PA 19103-2899

SABISTON & SPENCER SURGERY OF THE CHEST, NINTH EDITION

ISBN: 978-0-323-24126-7

Copyright © 2016, 2010, 2005, 1995, 1990, 1983, 1976, 1969, 1962 by Elsevier, Inc. All rights reserved.

Chapter 50 (Ventricular Mechanics): in the public domain.
Chapter 105 (Segmental Anatomy): Stephen P. Sanders retains copyright of the chapter.

No part of this publication may be reproduced or transmitted in any form or by any means, electronic or mechanical, including photocopying, recording, or any information storage and retrieval system, without permission in writing from the publisher. Details on how to seek permission, further information about the Publisher's permissions policies and our arrangements with organizations such as the Copyright Clearance Center and the Copyright Licensing Agency, can be found at our website: www.elsevier.com/permissions.

This book and the individual contributions contained in it are protected under copyright by the Publisher (other than as may be noted herein).

Notices

Knowledge and best practice in this field are constantly changing. As new research and experience broaden our understanding, changes in research methods, professional practices, or medical treatment may become necessary.

Practitioners and researchers must always rely on their own experience and knowledge in evaluating and using any information, methods, compounds, or experiments described herein. In using such information or methods they should be mindful of their own safety and the safety of others, including parties for whom they have a professional responsibility.

With respect to any drug or pharmaceutical products identified, readers are advised to check the most current information provided (i) on procedures featured or (ii) by the manufacturer of each product to be administered, to verify the recommended dose or formula, the method and duration of administration, and contraindications. It is the responsibility of practitioners, relying on their own experience and knowledge of their patients, to make diagnoses, to determine dosages and the best treatment for each individual patient, and to take all appropriate safety precautions.

To the fullest extent of the law, neither the Publisher nor the authors, contributors, or editors assume any liability for any injury and/or damage to persons or property as a matter of products liability, negligence or otherwise, or from any use or operation of any methods, products, instructions, or ideas contained in the material herein.

1962 copyright renewed 1990 by John H. Gibbon, Jr. All rights reserved.

Library of Congress Cataloging-in-Publication Data

Sabiston & Spencer surgery of the chest / [edited by] Frank W. Sellke, Pedro J. del Nido, Scott J. Swanson.—Ninth edition.
p. ; cm.
Sabiston and Spencer surgery of the chest
Surgery of the chest
Includes bibliographical references and index.
ISBN 978-0-323-24126-7 (hardcover : alk. paper)
I. Sellke, Frank W., editor. II. Del Nido, Pedro J., editor. III. Swanson, Scott J., editor.
IV. Title: Sabiston and Spencer surgery of the chest. V. Title: Surgery of the chest.
[DNLM: 1. Thoracic Surgical Procedures—methods. WF 980]
RD536
617.5′4—dc23

2015020235

Publishing Manager: Michael Houston
Senior Content Development Manager: Maureen Iannuzzi
Senior Content Development Specialist: Joan Ryan
Publishing Services Manager: Catherine Jackson
Project Manager: Rhoda Howell
Design Direction: Maggie Reid

Printed in China

Last digit is the print number: 9 8 7 6 5 4 3 2 1

ELSEVIER Book Aid International
Working together to grow libraries in developing countries
www.elsevier.com • www.bookaid.org

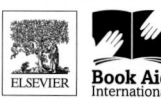

To my wife, Amy, who gives me love, inspiration,
and unwavering support and to our children,
Michelle, Eric, Nicholas, and Amanda.
They provide us with unlimited pleasure.

FWS

To Martha, my loving wife, and to my children,
Alexander and his wife Erika, to Sara, Daniel,
Elizabeth, and to my grandson Matthew who keeps
reminding us of the important things in life.
Thank you.

PJD

To my mother, Anne Parkhurst, and my wife,
Donna, and our children, Whit, Kate, and Maggie:
I am very appreciative and grateful for the guidance,
love, and support; gives meaning to all of what I do.
To my patients: the inspiration to work hard and do
better every day.

SJS

CONTRIBUTORS

Brian G. Abbott, MD
Associate Professor of Medicine
Cardiovascular Institute
Warren Alpert Medical School of Brown University
Providence, Rhode Island

J. Dawn Abbott, MD
Associate Professor of Medicine
Director, Interventional Cardiology
Fellowship Training Program
Warren Alpert Medical School of Brown University
Interventional Cardiologist
Rhode Island Hospital
Providence, Rhode Island

David H. Adams, MD
Professor and Chairman
Department of Cardiovascular Surgery
The Mount Sinai Medical Center
New York, New York

Talal Al-Atassi, MD, CM, MPH
Chief Resident
Division of Cardiac Surgery
University of Ottawa Heart Institute
Ottawa, Ontario, Canada

Ali Al-Dameh, MD
Clinical Fellow in Thoracic Surgery
Brigham and Women's Hospital
Boston, Massachusetts

Mark S. Allen, MD
Professor of Surgery
Thoracic Surgery
Mayo Clinic
Rochester, Minnesota

Nasser K. Altorki, MB, BCh
Professor of Cardiothoracic Surgery
Weill Cornell Medical College
Chief, Division of Thoracic Surgery
Cardiothoracic Surgery
New York Presbyterian Hospital/Weill Cornell Medical College
New York, New York

Jatin Anand, MD
Michael E. DeBakey Department of Surgery
Baylor College of Medicine
Cardiovascular Research
Center for Cardiac Support
Texas Heart Institute
Houston, Texas

Robert H. Anderson, BSc, MD, FRC Path
Emeritus Professor
Institute of Child Health
University College
London, United Kingdom;
Visiting Professor
Division of Pediatric Cardiology
Medical University of South Carolina
Charleston, South Carolina;
Visiting Professor
Institute of Human Genetics
Newcastle University
Newcastle Upon Tyne, United Kingdom

Masaki Anraku, MD, MSc
Assistant Professor
Department of Thoracic Surgery
Graduate School of Medicine
The University of Tokyo
Tokyo, Japan

Anelechi C. Anyanwu, MD
Professor and Vice Chairman
Department of Cardiovascular Surgery
The Mount Sinai Medical Center
New York, New York

Amit Arora, MD
Department of Cardiovascular Surgery
The Mount Sinai Medical Center
New York, New York

Erle H. Austin, III, MD
Professor and Vice Chairman
Department of Cardiovascular and Thoracic Surgery
University of Louisville
Chief, Cardiothoracic Surgery
Kosair Children's Hospital
Louisville, Kentucky

Eric H. Awtry, MD
Associate Professor of Medicine
Boston University School of Medicine
Vice Chair for Clinical Affairs
Division of Cardiology
Boston Medical Center
Boston, Massachusetts

Emile A. Bacha, MD, FACS
Chief, Division of Cardiothoracic and Vascular Surgery
Department of Surgery
Columbia University Medical Center
New York Presbyterian Hospital
New York, New York

Leah M. Backhus, MD
Assistant Professor
Division of Cardiothoracic Surgery
University of Washington
Seattle, Washington

Jayant Bagai, MD
Assistant Professor of Medicine
Division of Cardiovascular Medicine
Vanderbilt University Medical Center
Nashville, Tennessee

Richard Baillot, MD, FRCSC
Institut Universitaire de Cardiologie et de Pneumologie de Québec
Québec City, Québec, Canada

Christopher W. Baird, MD
Assistant Professor of Surgery
Harvard Medical School
Associate in Cardiac Surgery
Boston Children's Hospital
Boston, Massachusetts

David J. Barron, MD, FRCP, FRCS(CT)
Consultant Cardiac Surgeon
Birmingham Children's Hospital
NHS Foundation Trust
Birmingham, United Kingdom

Joseph E. Bavaria, MD
Brooke Roberts/William Maul Measey Professor of Surgery
Vice Chair, Division of Cardiovascular Surgery
Director, Thoracic Aortic Surgery
Department of Surgery
Division of Cardiovascular Surgery
University of Pennsylvania
Hospital of University of Pennsylvania
Philadelphia, Pennsylvania

Jose M. Bernal, MD, PhD
Consultant and Professor of Surgery
Department of Cardiovascular Surgery
Hospital Valdecilla
University of Cantabria
Santander, Spain

Valentino J. Bianco, DO, MPH
Research Fellow, Thoracic Surgery
Department of Cardiothoracic Surgery
University of Pittsburgh School of Medicine
University of Pittsburgh Medical Center
Pittsburgh, Pennsylvania

David P. Bichell, MD
Cornelius Vanderbilt Chair in Surgery
Professor of Surgery
Cardiac Surgery
Vanderbilt University School of Medicine
Nashville, Tennessee

Sigurbjorn Birgisson, MD
Department of Gastroenterology
Digestive Disease Institute
Cleveland Clinic
Cleveland, Ohio

Nick J.R. Blackburn, BSc
Division of Cardiac Surgery
University of Ottawa Heart Institute
Department of Cellular and Molecular Medicine
University of Ottawa
Ottawa, Ontario, Canada

Johannes Bonatti, MD
Chairman, Department of Cardiothoracic Surgery
Cleveland Clinic Abu Dhabi
Abu Dhabi, United Arab Emirates

Munir Boodhwani, MD, MMSc
Associate Professor
Division of Cardiac Surgery
University of Ottawa Heart Institute
Ottawa, Ontario, Canada

Edward L. Bove, MD
Helen F. and Marvin M. Kirsh Professor of Cardiac Surgery
Chair, Department of Cardiac Surgery
Professor of Cardiac Surgery
Professor of Pediatrics and Communicable Disease
University of Michigan
Ann Arbor, Michigan

William J. Brawn, CBE, FRCS, FRACS
Consultant Cardiac Surgeon
Birmingham Children's Hospital
NHS Foundation Trust
Birmingham, United Kingdom

Christian P. Brizard, MD
Associate Professor
University of Melbourne Faculty of Medicine, Dentistry
Health Sciences School of Medicine
Cardiac Surgery Unit
Royal Children's Hospital
Melbourne, Victoria, Australia

Julie A. Brothers, MD
Assistant Professor of Pediatrics
Perelman School of Medicine
University of Pennsylvania
Attending Physician, Cardiology
Medical Director, Coronary Anomaly Management Program
Medical Director, Lipid Heart Clinic
The Children's Hospital of Philadelphia
Philadelphia, Pennsylvania

Lisa M. Brown, MD, MAS
Cardiothoracic Surgery Fellow
Division of Cardiothoracic Surgery
Washington University
St. Louis, Missouri

Ayesha S. Bryant, MD
Assistant Professor of Surgery
Division of Cardiothoracic Surgery
University of Alabama at Birmingham
Birmingham, Alabama

Harold M. Burkhart, MD
Professor of Surgery
Section of Cardiothoracic Surgery
The University of Oklahoma Health Sciences School of Medicine
Director of Pediatric Cardiovascular Surgery
Medical Director of Pediatric Cardiovascular Surgical Services
The Children's Hospital
Oklahoma City, Oklahoma

Christopher A. Caldarone, MD, FRCSC
Cardiovascular Surgery
The Hospital for Sick Children
Toronto, Ontario, Canada

Jeremy W. Cannon, MD, SM, FACS
Lieutenant Colonel, U.S. Air Force
Chief, Trauma and Critical Care
San Antonio Military Medical Center
San Antonio, Texas
Associate Professor of Surgery
Uniformed Services University of the Health Sciences
Bethesda, Maryland

Justine M. Carr, MD
Chief Medical Officer
Steward Health Care System
Senior Director, Department of Clinical Resource Management
Beth Israel Deaconess Medical Center
Boston, Massachusetts

Serenella Castelvecchio, MD
Department of Cardiac Surgery
IRCCS Policlinico San Donato
Milan, Italy

Javier G. Castillo, MD
Department of Cardiovascular Surgery
The Mount Sinai Medical Center
New York, New York

Frank Cecchin, MD
Professor of Pediatrics
Pediatric Cardiology
New York University
New York, New York

Robert J. Cerfolio, MD
Chief of Thoracic Surgery
Professor of Cardiothoracic Surgery
University of Alabama at Birmingham
Birmingham, Alabama

A. Alfred Chahine, MD
Associate Professor of Surgery and Pediatrics
George Washington University School of Medicine
Attending Surgeon
Children's National Medical Center
Chief of Pediatric Surgery
MedStar Georgetown University Hospital
Washington, DC

Elliot L. Chaikof, MD, PhD
Johnson and Johnson Professor of Surgery
Chairman, Roberta and Stephen R. Weiner Department of Surgery
Harvard Medical School
Surgeon-in-Chief
Beth Israel Deaconess Medical Center
Boston, Massachusetts

Vincent Chan, MD, MPH
Assistant Professor
Division of Cardiac Surgery
University of Ottawa Heart Institute
Ottawa, Ontario, Canada

Sunit-Preet Chaudhry, MD
Cardiovascular Institute
Warren Alpert Medical School of Brown University
Providence, Rhode Island

Frederick Y. Chen, MD, PhD
Associate Professor of Cardiac Surgery
Harvard Medical School
Department of Surgery
Division of Cardiac Surgery
Brigham and Women's Hospital
Boston, Massachusetts

Stuart H. Chen, MD
Clinical Fellow in Medicine
Beth Israel Deaconess Medical Center
Boston, Massachusetts

Aaron M. Cheng, MD
Assistant Professor
Division of Cardiothoracic Surgery
University of Washington
Seattle, Washington

Victor Chien, MD
Research Fellow in Surgery
Harvard Medical School
Beth Israel Deaconess Medical Center
Boston, Massachusetts

Alvin J. Chin, MD
Professor of Pediatrics, Emeritus
Perelman School of Medicine
University of Pennsylvania
Philadelphia, Pennsylvania

Cynthia S. Chin, MD
Director of the Women's Cancer Program Services
Thoracic Surgery
White Plains Hospital
White Plains, New York

Peter Chiu, MD
Resident, Department of Cardiothoracic Surgery
Stanford University School of Medicine
Stanford, California

Joseph C. Cleveland, Jr., MD
Professor of Cardiothoracic Surgery
Surgical Director, Cardiac Transplantation and MCS
University of Colorado Anschutz Medical Center
Aurora, Colorado

Lawrence H. Cohn, MD
Hubbard Professor of Cardiac Surgery
Harvard Medical School
Department of Surgery
Division of Cardiac Surgery
Brigham and Women's Hospital
Boston, Massachusetts

William E. Cohn, MD
Professor of Surgery
Michael E. DeBakey Department of Surgery
Baylor College of Medicine
Director, Center for Technology and Innovation
Director, Cullen Cardiovascular Research Laboratory
Texas Heart Institute
Houston, Texas

Yolonda L. Colson, MD, PhD
Professor
Department of Surgery
Harvard Medical School
Brigham and Women's Hospital
Boston, Massachusetts

Wilson S. Colucci, MD
Thomas J. Ryan Professor of Medicine
Professor of Physiology
Boston University School of Medicine
Chief, Section of Cardiovascular Medicine
Co-Director, Cardiovascular Center
Boston Medical Center
Boston, Massachusetts

Andrew C. Cook, PhD
Senior Lecturer
Cardiac Unit
UCL Institute of Cardiovascular Science
Great Ormond Street Hospital
NHS Foundation Trust
London, United Kingdom

Joseph S. Coselli, MD
Professor and Chief
Division of Cardiothoracic Surgery
Michael E. DeBakey Department of Surgery
Baylor College of Medicine
Chief, Section of Adult Cardiac Surgery
The Texas Heart Institute
Houston, Texas

Todd C. Crawford, MD
Division of Thoracic Surgery
The Johns Hopkins Medical Institutions
Baltimore, Maryland

Melissa Culligan, BSN, RN
Department of Thoracic Surgery
University of Pennsylvania Health System–Presbyterian
Philadelphia, Pennsylvania

François Dagenais, MD, FRCSC
Institut Universitaire de Cardiologie et de Pneumologie de Québec
Québec City, Québec, Canada

Ralph J. Damiano, Jr., MD
Evarts A. Graham Professor of Surgery
Chief, Division of Cardiothoracic Surgery
Washington University School of Medicine
Barnes-Jewish Hospital
St. Louis, Missouri

Thomas A. D'Amico, MD
Gary Hock Endowed Professor and Vice Chair of Surgery
Duke University School of Medicine
Chief, Section of General Thoracic Surgery
Program Director, Thoracic Surgery
Duke University Medical Center
Durham, North Carolina

Philippe G. Dartevelle, MD
Head, Service de Chirurgie Thoracique, Vasculaire et Transplantation Cardiopulmonaire
Hôpital Marie Lannelongue
Le Plessis Robinson, France

Tirone E. David, MD
Professor of Surgery
University of Toronto
Attending Surgeon
Peter Munk Cardiac Centre
Toronto General Hospital
Toronto, Ontario, Canada

Jonathan D'Cunha, MD, PhD
Associate Professor of Surgery
Vice Chairman, Academic Affairs and Education
Surgical Director, Lung Transplantation
Associate Program Director, Thoracic Surgery
Department of Cardiothoracic Surgery
University of Pittsburgh
Pittsburgh, Pennsylvania

Kim I. de la Cruz, MD
Assistant Professor of Cardiothoracic Surgery
Michael E. DeBakey Department of Surgery
Baylor College of Medicine
Clinical Staff
The Texas Heart Institute
Houston, Texas

Joseph A. Dearani, MD
Professor of Surgery
Chair, Cardiac Surgery
Division of Cardiovascular Surgery
Mayo Clinic
Rochester, Minnesota

Daniel T. DeArmond, MD
Cardiothoracic Surgery
University of Texas Health Science Center
San Antonio, Texas

Pedro J. del Nido, MD
William E. Ladd Professor of Surgery
Harvard Medical School
Chairman, Department of Cardiac Surgery
Boston Children's Hospital
Boston, Massachusetts

Tom R. DeMeester, MD
Professor and Chairman, Emeritus
Department of Surgery
University of Southern California
Los Angeles, California

Philippe Demers, MD, MSC, FRCSC
Associate Professor of Surgery
Cardiac Surgery
University of Montreal
Cardiovascular Surgeon
Montreal Heart Institute
Montreal, Quebec, Canada

Todd L. Demmy, MD
Chairman, Department of Thoracic Surgery
Roswell Park Cancer Institute
Buffalo, New York

Elisabeth U. Dexter, MD
Assistant Professor of Oncology
Department of Thoracic Surgery
Roswell Park Cancer Institute
Assistant Professor of Surgery
SUNY University at Buffalo
Buffalo, New York

Rajeev Dhupar, MD
Assistant Professor of Surgery
Department of Cardiothoracic Surgery
Division of Thoracic and Foregut Surgery
University of Pittsburgh Medical Center
Pittsburgh, Pennsylvania

James A. DiNardo, MD
Professor of Anesthesia
Boston Children's Hospital
Harvard Medical School
Boston, Massachusetts

Thomas P. Doyle, MD
Associate Professor of Pediatrics
Division of Cardiology
Vanderbilt University School of Medicine
Nashville, Tennessee

Afshin Ehsan, MD
Assistant Professor of Surgery
Brown Alpert Medical School
Rhode Island Hospital
Providence, Rhode Island

Gebrine El Khoury, MD, PhD
Professor
Department of Cardiovascular and Thoracic Surgery
Cliniques Universitaires Saint-Luc
Brussels, Belgium

Ethan R. Ellis, MD
Harvard-Thorndike Electrophysiology Institute
Cardiovascular Division
Harvard Medical School
Beth Israel Deaconess Medical Center
Boston, Massachusetts

Nassrene Y. Elmadhun, MD
Research Fellow
Cardiovascular Research Center
Warren Alpert Medical School
Brown University
Providence, Rhode Island
Surgical Resident
Beth Israel Deaconess Medical Center
Boston, Massachusetts

Sitaram M. Emani, MD
Assistant Professor in Surgery
Harvard Medical School
Assistant in Cardiac Surgery
Surgical Director, Adult Congenital Heart Program
Director, Complex Biventricular Repair Program
Surgical Director, Division of Cardiovascular Critical Care
Boston Children's Hospital
Boston, Massachusetts

Jeremy J. Erasmus, MD
Professor
Department of Diagnostic Imaging
The University of Texas MD Anderson Cancer Center
Houston, Texas

Dario O. Fauza, MD
Associate Professor of Surgery
Harvard Medical School
Associate in Surgery
Boston Children's Hospital
Boston, Massachusetts

Adam S. Fein, MD
Cardiac Services
Beth Israel Deaconess Medical Center
Boston, Massachusetts

Amy G. Fiedler, MD
Clinical Fellow in Surgery
Department of Surgery
Division of Cardiac Surgery
Brigham and Women's Hospital
Boston, Massachusetts

Murilo Foppa, MD, DSc
Department of Medicine
Cardiovascular Division
Harvard-Thorndike Laboratory
Harvard Medical School
Beth Israel Deaconess Medical Center
Boston, Massachusetts;
Division of Cardiology
Hospital de Clinicas de Porto Alegre
Federal University of Rio Grande do Sul
Brazil

Rosario V. Freeman, MD, MS
Medical Director, Echocardiography
Program Director, Cardiology Fellowship Programs
University of Washington
Seattle, Washington

Joseph Friedberg, MD, FACS
Chief of Thoracic Surgery
University of Pennsylvania Health System–Presbyterian
Philadelphia, Pennsylvania

Michael Friscia, MD
Associate, Thoracic and Cardiac Surgery
Geisinger Health System
Danville, Pennsylvania

Francis Fynn-Thompson, MD
Assistant Professor of Surgery
Surgical Director, Heart and Lung Transplantation
Surgical Director, Mechanical Circulatory Support Program
Program Director, Congenital Cardiac Surgery Residency/Fellowship
Department of Cardiac Surgery
Boston Children's Hospital
Harvard Medical School
Boston, Massachusetts

J. William Gaynor, MD
Professor of Surgery
Perelman School of Medicine
University of Pennsylvania
Attending Surgeon
Director, Fetal Neuroprotection and Neuroplasticity Program
Daniel M. Tabas Endowed Chair, Pediatric Cardiothoracic Surgery
The Children's Hospital of Philadelphia
Philadelphia, Pennsylvania

Liang Ge, PhD
Assistant Professor of Surgery
Department of Surgery
University of California, San Francisco School of Medicine
Department of Surgery
San Francisco VA Medical Center
San Francisco, California

Tal Geva, MD
Professor of Pediatrics
Harvard Medical School
Chief, Division of Noninvasive Cardiac Imaging
Senior Associate, Department of Cardiology
Boston Children's Hospital
Boston, Massachusetts

Neil M. Gheewala, MD
Cardiovascular Institute
Warren Alpert Medical School of Brown University
Providence, Rhode Island

A. Marc Gillinov, MD
The Judith Dion Pyle Chair in Heart Valve Research
Department of Thoracic and Cardiovascular Surgery
Cleveland Clinic
Cleveland, Ohio

Donald D. Glower, MD
Professor of Surgery
Department of Surgery
Division of Cardiovascular and Thoracic Surgery
Duke University School of Medicine
Durham, North Carolina

Andrew B. Goldstone, MD
Postdoctoral Research Fellow
Department of Cardiothoracic Surgery
Stanford University School of Medicine
Stanford, California

Shawn S. Groth, MD, MS
Assistant Professor of Surgery
Division of General Thoracic Surgery
Baylor College of Medicine
Houston, Texas

Frederick L. Grover, MD
Professor of Cardiothoracic Surgery
University of Colorado Anschutz Medical Center
Aurora, Colorado

Julius Guccione, PhD
Professor of Surgery
Department of Surgery
University of California, San Francisco School of Medicine
Associate Professor of Surgery
San Francisco VA Medical Center
San Francisco, California

Richard Ha, MD
Clinical Assistant Professor
Surgical Director, Mechanical Circulatory Support Program
Department of Cardiothoracic Surgery
Stanford University School of Medicine
Stanford, California

John W. Hammon, MD
Wake Forest University Baptist Medical Center
Winston-Salem, North Carolina

Jennifer M. Hanna, MD
Resident, General Surgery
Duke University School of Medicine
Durham, North Carolina

David G. Harrison, MD
Betty and Jack Bailey Professor of Medicine and Pharmacology
Director, Division of Clinical Pharmacology
Director, Center for Vascular Biology
Vanderbilt University Medical Center
Nashville, Tennessee

Thomas H. Hauser, MD, MMSc, MPH
Department of Medicine
Cardiovascular Division
Harvard-Thorndike Laboratory
Harvard Medical School
Beth Israel Deaconess Medical Center
Boston, Massachusetts

Matthew C. Henn, MD
Resident, Division of Cardiothoracic Surgery
Washington University School of Medicine
Barnes-Jewish Hospital
St. Louis, Missouri

Jennifer C. Hirsch-Romano, MD
Assistant Professor of Cardiac Surgery
University of Michigan
Ann Arbor, Michigan

Chuong D. Hoang, MD
Assistant Professor
Department of Cardiothoracic Surgery
Division of Thoracic Surgery
Stanford University School of Medicine
Stanford, California

Wayne L. Hofstetter, MD
Professor of Surgery
Director of Esophageal Surgery
Department of Thoracic and Cardiovascular Surgery
The University of Texas MD Anderson Cancer Center
Houston, Texas

Osami Honjo, MD, PhD
Cardiovascular Surgery
The Hospital for Sick Children
Toronto, Ontario, Canada

Tam T. Huynh, MD
Professor
Department of Thoracic and Cardiovascular Surgery
The University of Texas MD Anderson Cancer Center
Houston, Texas

Carlos E. Bravo Iñiguez, MD
Postdoctoral Fellow
Division of Thoracic Surgery
Brigham and Women's Hospital
Harvard Medical School
Boston, Massachusetts

Sebastian Iturra, MD
Structural Heart and Valve Center
Division of Cardiothoracic Surgery
Joseph B. Whitehead Department of Surgery
Emory University School of Medicine
Atlanta, Georgia

Jeffrey P. Jacobs, MD, FACS, FACC, FCCP
Professor of Surgery
Division of Cardiac Surgery
Department of Surgery
Johns Hopkins University
Baltimore, Maryland;
Chief, Division of Cardiovascular Surgery
Director, Andrews/Daicoff Cardiovascular Program
Surgical Director of Heart Transplantation and Extracorporeal Life Support Programs
Johns Hopkins All Children's Heart Institute
All Children's Hospital and Florida Hospital for Children
Saint Petersburg, Tampa, and Orlando, Florida

Marshall L. Jacobs, MD
Division of Cardiac Surgery
Department of Surgery
Johns Hopkins University
Baltimore, Maryland

Michael T. Jaklitsch, MD
Associate Professor
Surgeon, Division of Thoracic Surgery
Brigham & Women's Hospital
Harvard Medical School
Boston, Massachusetts

Stuart W. Jamieson, MB, FRCS
Distinguished Professor of Surgery
Endowed Chair, Division of Cardiothoracic Surgery
University of California, San Diego
San Diego, California

Doraid Jarrar, MD
Thoracic Surgeon
Einstein Healthcare
East Norriton, Pennsylvania

Craig M. Jarrett, MD
Department of Thoracic and Cardiovascular Surgery
Cleveland Clinic
Cleveland, Ohio

David R. Jones, MD
Professor and Chief of Thoracic Surgery
Memorial Sloan-Kettering Cancer Center
New York, New York

Mark E. Josephson, MD
Harvard-Thorndike Electrophysiology Institute, Cardiovascular Division
Harvard Medical School
Beth Israel Deaconess Medical Center
Boston, Massachusetts

Lilian P. Joventino, MD
Wentworth Health Partners Cardiovascular Group
Dover, New Hampshire

Amy L. Juraszek, MD
Associate Professor
Departments of Pediatrics and Pathology
University of Texas Southwestern Medical Center
Dallas, Texas

Stefan S. Kachala, MD
Department of Thoracic and Cardiovascular Surgery
Cleveland Clinic
Cleveland, Ohio

Larry R. Kaiser, MD
Dean and Professor of Surgery
Temple University School of Medicine
President and CEO
Temple University Health System
Sr. Executive Vice President for the Health Sciences
Temple University
Philadelphia, Pennsylvania

Kirk R. Kanter, MD
Professor of Surgery
Pediatric Cardiac Surgery
Emory University School of Medicine
Atlanta, Georgia

John M. Karamichalis, MD
Clinical Instructor in Surgery
Department of Surgery
Division of Pediatric Cardiothoracic Surgery
University of California, San Francisco
San Francisco, California

Aditya K. Kaza, MD
Assistant Professor of Surgery
Harvard Medical School
Associate in Cardiac Surgery
Department of Cardiac Surgery
Boston Children's Hospital
Boston, Massachusetts

Clinton D. Kemp, MD
Division of Thoracic Surgery
The Johns Hopkins Medical Institutions
Baltimore, Maryland

Kemp H. Kernstine, Sr., MD, PhD
Professor and Chief, Division of Thoracic Surgery
Department of Cardiovascular & Thoracic Surgery
University of Texas Southwestern Medical Center
Dallas, Texas

Suresh Keshavamurthy, MD
Cleveland Clinic
Cleveland, Ohio

Shaf Keshavjee, MD, MSc, FRCSC, FACS
Surgeon-in-Chief, University Health Network
James Wallace McCutcheon Chair in Surgery
Professor, Division of Thoracic Surgery
University of Toronto
Toronto, Ontario, Canada

Deborah J. Kozik, DO
Assistant Professor of Surgery
Department of Cardiovascular and Thoracic Surgery
University of Louisville
Cardiothoracic Surgery
Kosair Children's Hospital
Louisville, Kentucky

Roger J. Laham, MD
Associate Professor of Medicine
Harvard Medical School
Research Investigator
CardioVascular Institute
Beth Israel Deaconess Medical Center
Boston, Massachusetts

Michael J. Landzberg, MD
Director, Boston Adult Congenital Heart (BACH) and Pulmonary Hypertension Program
Department of Cardiology
Brigham and Women's Hospital and Boston Children's Hospital
Boston, Massachusetts

Christopher P. Lawrance, MD
Resident, Division of Cardiothoracic Surgery
Washington University School of Medicine
Barnes-Jewish Hospital
St. Louis, Missouri

Lawrence S. Lee, MD
Clinical Fellow in Surgery
Harvard Medical School
Department of Surgery
Division of Cardiac Surgery
Brigham and Women's Hospital
Boston, Massachusetts

Scott A. LeMaire, MD
Professor and Vice Chair for Research
Michael E. DeBakey Department of Surgery
Baylor College of Medicine
Professional Staff, Department of Cardiovascular Surgery
The Texas Heart Institute
Houston, Texas

Sidney Levitsky, MD
David W. and David Cheever Professor of Surgery
Harvard Medical School
Director, Cardiothoracic Surgery Care Group
Senior Vice Chairman, Department of Surgery
Beth Israel Deaconess Medical Center
Boston, Massachusetts

Jerrold H. Levy, MD, FAHA, FCCM
Professor of Anesthesiology
Associate Professor of Surgery
Departments of Anesthesiology, Surgery, and Critical Care
Co-Director, Cardiothoracic ICU
Duke University School of Medicine
Duke University Medical Center
Durham, North Carolina

Philip A. Linden, MD
Associate Professor of Surgery
Case Western Reserve School of Medicine
Chief, Division of Thoracic and Esophageal Surgery
University Hospitals Case Medical Center
Cleveland, Ohio

Michael J. Liptay, MD
The Mary and John Bent Professor and Chairperson
Department of Cardiovascular and Thoracic Surgery
Rush University Medical Center
Chicago, Illinois

Virginia R. Litle, MD, FACS
Associate Professor of Surgery
Department of Surgery
Division of Thoracic Surgery
Boston University School of Medicine
Boston, Massachusetts

Mauro Lo Rito, MD
Cardiovascular Surgery
The Hospital for Sick Children
Toronto, Ontario, Canada

James D. Luketich, MD
Henry T. Bahnson Professor and Chairman
Department of Cardiothoracic Surgery
Chief, Division of Thoracic and Foregut Surgery
University of Pittsburgh School of Medicine
Director, Thoracic Surgical Oncology
Co-Director, Lung Cancer Center
University of Pittsburgh Medical Center
Pittsburgh, Pennsylvania

Bruce W. Lytle, MD
Chairman, Strategic Development and Planning for Cardiovascular Medicine and Surgery
The Heart Hospital Baylor Plano
Plano, Texas

Michael Madani, MD
Professor of Surgery
Chief, Division of Cardiothoracic Surgery
University of California, San Diego
San Diego, California

Feroze Mahmood, MD
Associate Professor of Anaesthesiology
Harvard Medical School
Director, Vascular Anesthesia/Perioperative Echocardiography
Beth Israel Deaconess Medical Center
Harvard Medical Faculty Physicians at Beth Israel Deaconess Medical Center
Boston, Massachusetts

Hari R. Mallidi, MD
Associate Professor of Surgery
Chief, Division of Transplant & Assist Devices
Lester and Sue Smith Endowed Chair in Surgery
Baylor College of Medicine
Houston, Texas

Abeel A. Mangi, MD
Associate Professor of Surgery, Section of Cardiac Surgery
Surgical Director, Center for Advanced Heart Failure, Mechanical Circulatory Support and Heart Transplantation
Surgical Director, Trans-Catheter Therapies
Yale University
New Haven, Connecticut

Warren J. Manning, MD
Departments of Medicine and Radiology
Cardiovascular Division
Harvard-Thorndike Laboratory
Harvard Medical School
Beth Israel Deaconess Medical Center
Boston, Massachusetts

Edith M. Marom, MD
Professor
Department of Diagnostic Imaging
The University of Texas MD Anderson Cancer Center
Houston, Texas

Audrey C. Marshall, MD
Chief, Invasive Cardiology
Boston Children's Hospital
Boston, Massachusetts

Mauricio Perez Martinez, MD
Division of Thoracic Surgery
Brigham and Women's Hospital
Harvard Medical School
Boston, Massachusetts

Christopher E. Mascio, MD
Assistant Professor of Clinical Medicine
Perelman School of Medicine
University of Pennsylvania
Pediatric Cardiothoracic Surgeon
Division of Cardiothoracic Surgery
The Children's Hospital of Philadelphia
Philadelphia, Pennsylvania

David P. Mason, MD
Chief, Thoracic Surgery and Lung Transplantation
Department of Thoracic Surgery
Baylor University Medical Center
Dallas, Texas

Douglas J. Mathisen, MD
Chief of Thoracic Surgery
Massachusetts General Hospital
Boston, Massachusetts

Kenneth L. Mattox, MD, FACS
Professor of Surgery
Division of Cardiothoracic Surgery
Michael E. DeBakey Department of Surgery
Baylor College of Medicine
Houston, Texas

Robina Matyal, MD
Associate Professor of Anaesthesiology
Harvard Medical School
Beth Israel Deaconess Medical Center
Boston, Massachusetts

James D. McCully, PhD
Associate Professor of Surgery
Harvard Medical School
Department of Cardiac Surgery
Boston Children's Hospital
Boston, Massachusetts

Robert J. McKenna, Jr., MD
Director, Thoracic Surgery
Surgery
Cedars-Sinai Medical Center
Los Angeles, California

Ciaran McNamee, MD
Instructor in Surgery
Harvard Medical School
Associate Surgeon
Brigham and Women's Hospital
Boston, Massachusetts

Jeffrey D. McNeil, MD
Colonel, U.S. Air Force
Chief, Cardiothoracic Surgery Service
San Antonio Military Medical Center
San Antonio, Texas
Clinical Assistant Professor, Cardiothoracic Surgery
University of Texas Health Science Center, San Antonio
San Antonio, Texas

Lorenzo Menicanti, MD
Chief of Cardiac Surgery
IRCCS Policlinico San Donato
Milan, Italy

Carlos A. Mestres, MD, PhD, FETCS
Senior Consultant
Department of Cardiovascular Surgery
Hospital Clinico
University of Barcelona
Barcelona, Spain;
Cardiothoracic and Vascular Surgery
Heart and Vascular Institute
Cleveland Clinic Abu Dhabi
Abu Dhabi, United Arab Emirates

Bret A. Mettler, MD
Assistant Professor
Division of Pediatric Cardiac Surgery
Vanderbilt University School of Medicine
Department of Cardiac Surgery
Vanderbilt University Medical Center
Nashville, Tennessee

Bryan Fitch Meyers, MD, MPH
Patrick and Joy Williamson Professor of Surgery
Chief, Thoracic Surgery
Washington University School of Medicine
St. Louis, Missouri

Stephanie Mick, MD
Cardiovascular Surgeon
Department of Thoracic and Cardiovascular Surgery
Cleveland Clinic
Cleveland, Ohio

Tomislav Mihaljevic, MD
Chief of Staff and Chairman of the Heart and Vascular Institute
Cleveland Clinic Abu Dhabi
Abu Dhabi, United Arab Emirates;
Attending Surgeon
Department of Thoracic and Cardiovascular Surgery
Cleveland Clinic
Professor of Surgery
Cleveland Clinic Lerner College of Medicine at Case Western University
Cleveland, Ohio

Carmelo A. Milano, MD
Professor of Surgery
Cardiovascular and Thoracic Surgery
Duke University
Durham, North Carolina

D. Craig Miller, MD
Thelma and Henry Doelger Professor of Cardiovascular Surgery
Department of Cardiovascular Surgery
Stanford University School of Medicine
Department of Cardiothoracic Surgery
Stanford University Medical Center
Stanford, California

Daniel L. Miller, MD, FACS
Clinical Professor of Surgery
Georgia Regents University
Chief, General Thoracic Surgery
WellStar Health System
Mayo Clinic Care Network
Marietta, Georgia

Meagan M. Miller, RN, BSN
Vanderbilt University Medical Center
Nashville, Tennessee

John D. Mitchell, MD
Courtenay C. and Lucy Patten Davis Endowed Chair in Thoracic Surgery
Professor and Chief, Section of General Thoracic Surgery
Division of Cardiothoracic Surgery
University of Colorado School of Medicine
Aurora, Colorado

Mario Montealegre-Gallegos, MD
Department of Anaesthesia
Harvard Medical School
Beth Israel Deaconess Medical Center
Boston, Massachusetts

Neal G. Moores, MD
Department of Thoracic and Cardiovascular Surgery
Cleveland Clinic
Cleveland, Ohio

Charles E. Murphy, MD
Assistant Professor of Surgery
Division of Cardiovascular and Thoracic Surgery
Duke University School of Medicine
Duke University Medical Center
Durham, North Carolina

Raghav A. Murthy, MD
Department of Cardiovascular & Thoracic Surgery
University of Texas Southwestern Medical Center
Dallas, Texas

Sudish C. Murthy, MD, PhD
Section Head, General Thoracic Surgery
Surgical Director, Center for Major Airway Disease
Department of Thoracic and Cardiovascular Surgery
Cleveland Clinic
Cleveland, Ohio

Sacha Mussot, MD
Hôpital Marie Lannelongue
Service de Chirurgie Thoracique, Vasculaire et Transplantation Cardiopulmonaire
Le Plessis Robinson, France

Yoshifumi Naka, MD, PhD
Professor of Surgery
Columbia University College of Physicians and Surgeons
Attending Surgeon
New York–Presbyterian Hospital
New York, New York

Meena Nathan, MD, FRCS
Instructor in Surgery
Harvard Medical School
Staff Cardiac Surgeon
Department of Cardiac Surgery
Boston Children's Hospital
Boston, Massachusetts

Kurt D. Newman, MD
President and Chief Executive Officer
Children's National Medical Center
Washington, DC

Chukwumere Nwogu, MD
Associate Professor
Department of Thoracic Surgery
Roswell Park Cancer Institute
Buffalo, New York

Kirsten C. Odegard, MD
Associate Professor
Department of Anesthesiology, Perioperative and Pain Medicine
Boston Children's Hospital
Boston, Massachusetts

Daniel S. Oh, MD
Assistant Professor of Surgery
Division of Thoracic Surgery
University of Southern California
Los Angeles, California

Richard G. Ohye, MD
Professor of Cardiac Surgery
University of Michigan
Ann Arbor, Michigan

Mark W. Onaitis, MD
Associate Professor of Surgery
Department of Surgery
Division of Cardiovascular and Thoracic Surgery
Duke University School of Medicine
Duke University Medical Center
Durham, North Carolina

Aleksandra Ostojic, MSc
Division of Cardiac Surgery
University of Ottawa Heart Institute
Department of Cellular and Molecular Medicine
University of Ottawa
Ottawa, Ontario, Canada

Harald C. Ott, MD
Division of Thoracic Surgery
Massachusetts General Hospital
Boston, Massachusetts

Maral Ouzounian, MD, PhD
Assistant Professor of Surgery
University of Toronto
Cardiovascular Surgeon
Division of Cardiovascular Surgery
University Health Network
Toronto General Hospital
Toronto, Ontario, Canada

Khurram Owais, MD
Department of Anaesthesia
Harvard Medical School
Beth Israel Deaconess Medical Center
Boston, Massachusetts

Massimo Padalino, MD, PhD
Department of Cardio Thoracic and Vascular Sciences
University Hospital
Padova, Italy

Konstantinos Papadakis, MD
Instructor in Surgery
Harvard Medical School
Department of Surgery
Boston Children's Hospital
Boston, Massachusetts

G. A. Patterson, MD
Evarts A. Graham Professor of Surgery
Chief, Division of Cardiothoracic Surgery
Washington University
St. Louis, Missouri

Edward F. Patz, Jr., MD
Professor
Department of Radiology
Duke University
Durham, North Carolina

Subroto Paul, MD
Associate Professor
Department of Cardiothoracic Surgery
Weill Cornell Medical College
New York, New York

Arjun Pennathur, MD
Sampson Family Endowed Chair in Thoracic Surgical Oncology
Associate Professor of Cardiothoracic Surgery
Department of Cardiothoracic Surgery
University of Pittsburgh School of Medicine
University of Pittsburgh Medical Center
Pittsburgh, Pennsylvania

Yaron Perry, MD
Clinical Associate Professor of Surgery
Case Western Reserve University School of Medicine
Director, Minimally Invasive Esophageal Surgery
University Hospitals Case Medical Center
Cleveland, Ohio

Robert N. Piana, MD
Professor of Medicine
Division of Cardiovascular Medicine
Director, Adult Congenital Interventional Program
Vanderbilt University Medical Center
Nashville, Tennessee

Frank A. Pigula, MD
Associate Professor of Surgery
Harvard Medical School
Senior Associate in Cardiac Surgery
Clinical Director, Cardiac Surgery Program
Director, Neonatal Cardiac Surgery Program
Boston Children's Hospital
Boston, Massachusetts

Duane S. Pinto, MD, MPH
Associate Professor of Medicine
Harvard Medical School
Associate Director, Cardiac Catheterization Laboratory
Beth Israel Deaconess Medical Center
Boston, Massachusetts

Jose L. Pomar, MD, PhD, FETCS
Senior Consultant and Professor of Surgery
Department of Cardiovascular Surgery
Hospital Clinico
University of Barcelona
Barcelona, Spain

Ourania Preventza, MD
Assistant Professor of Cardiothoracic Surgery
Michael E. DeBakey Department of Surgery
Baylor College of Medicine
Clinical Staff
The Texas Heart Institute
Houston, Texas

Bradley Pua, MD
Assistant Professor of Radiology
Weill Cornell Medical College
Program Director, Interventional Radiology Fellowship
Director, Lung Cancer Screening Program
New York Presbyterian Hospital/Weill Cornell Medical Center
New York, New York

Varun Puri, MD
Assistant Professor of Surgery
Division of Cardiothoracic Surgery
Washington University
St. Louis, Missouri

Luis Quinonez, MD
Instructor in Surgery
Harvard Medical School
Assistant in Cardiac Surgery
Department of Cardiac Surgery
Boston Children's Hospital
Boston, Massachusetts

Siva Raja, MD, PhD
Department of Thoracic and Cardiovascular Surgery
Cleveland Clinic
Cleveland, Ohio

Mark Ratcliffe, MD
Professor of Surgery
Department of Surgery
University of California, San Francisco
Chief Surgical Consultant
Sierra Pacific VA Network
San Francisco, California

Michael J. Reardon, MD
Professor of Cardiothoracic Surgery
Allison Family Distinguished Chair of Cardiovascular Research
Houston Methodist DeBakey Heart & Vascular Center
Houston, Texas

John J. Reilly, Jr., MD
Dean
University of Colorado School of Medicine
Vice Chancellor for Health Affairs
University of Colorado
Aurora, Colorado

Karl G. Reyes, MD
Department of Thoracic and Cardiovascular Surgery
Cleveland Clinic
Cleveland, Ohio

Thomas W. Rice, MD
Head, Section of General Thoracic Surgery
Department of Thoracic and Cardiovascular Surgery
Heart and Vascular Institute
Cleveland Clinic
Cleveland, Ohio

Robert C. Robbins, MD
President and Chief Executive Officer
Texas Medical Center
Houston, Texas;
Consulting Professor
Stanford Cardiovascular Institute
Stanford, California

Gaetano Rocco, MD, FRCS(Ed), FECTS
Director, Department of Thoracic Surgery and Oncology
National Cancer Institute, Pascale Foundation
Naples, Italy

Fraser D. Rubens, MD, MSc, FACS, FRCSC
Professor of Surgery
Division of Cardiac Surgery
Residency Program Director
University of Ottawa Heart Institute
Ottawa, Ontario, Canada

Marc Ruel, MD, MPH
Professor and Chair
Division of Cardiac Surgery
University of Ottawa Heart Institute
Ottawa, Ontario, Canada

Valerie W. Rusch, MD
Attending Surgeon, Thoracic Service
Vice Chair for Clinical Research
Miner Family Chair in Intrathoracic Cancers
Department of Surgery
Memorial Sloan-Kettering Cancer Center
New York, New York

Ashraf A. Sabe, MD
Clinical Teaching Fellow, General Surgery
Harvard Medical School
Resident, General Surgery
Beth Israel Deaconess Medical Center
Boston, Massachusetts;
Research Fellow, Cardiothoracic Surgery
Warren Alpert Medical School of Brown University
Providence, Rhode Island

Sameh M. Said, MD
Senior Associate Consultant
Division of Cardiovascular Surgery
Mayo Clinic
Rochester, Minnesota

Pamela P. Samson, MD, MPHS
Resident, Department of Surgery
Washington University and Barnes-Jewish Hospital
St. Louis, Missouri

Stephen P. Sanders, MD
Professor of Pediatrics
Harvard Medical School
Director, Cardiac Registry
Departments of Cardiology, Pathology, Cardiac Surgery
Boston Children's Hospital
Boston, Massachusetts

Eric L. Sarin, MD
Assistant Professor of Surgery
Structural Heart and Valve Center
Division of Cardiothoracic Surgery
Joseph B. Whitehead Department of Surgery
Emory University School of Medicine
Atlanta, Georgia

Hartzell V. Schaff, MD
Professor of Surgery
Mayo Clinic
Rochester, Minnesota

Lara W. Schaheen, MD
Resident, Department of Cardiothoracic Surgery
University of Pittsburgh School of Medicine
Pittsburgh, Pennsylvania

Christopher W. Seder, MD
Assistant Professor of Thoracic and Cardiac Surgery
Rush University Medical Center
Chicago, Illinois

Frank W. Sellke, MD
Karl Karlson & Gloria Karlson Professor and Chief of Cardiothoracic Surgery
Warren Alpert Medical School of Brown University and Rhode Island Hospital
Director, Lifespan Cardiovascular Institute
Providence, Rhode Island

Boris Sepesi, MD
Assistant Professor
Department of Thoracic and Cardiovascular Surgery
Division of Surgery
The University of Texas MD Anderson Cancer Center
Houston, Texas

Rohit Shahani, MD
Cardiothoracic Surgery
Hudson Cardiothoracic Surgeons
Poughkeepsie, New York

Robert C. Shamberger, MD
Robert E. Gross Professor of Surgery
Harvard Medical School
Chief of Surgery
Boston Children's Hospital
Boston, Massachusetts

Oz M. Shapira, MD
Professor and Chairman
Department of Cardiothoracic Surgery
Hebrew University
Hadassah Medical Center
Jerusalem, Israel

Steven S. Shay, MD
Department of Gastroenterology
Digestive Disease Institute
Cleveland Clinic
Cleveland, Ohio

Joseph B. Shrager, MD
Professor, Department of Cardiothoracic Surgery
Chief, Division of Thoracic Surgery
Stanford University School of Medicine
Stanford, California

Ming-Sing Si, MD
Assistant Professor of Cardiac Surgery
University of Michigan
Ann Arbor, Michigan

Steve K. Singh, MD, MSc, FRCSC
Assistant Professor of Surgery
Division of Transplant & Assist Devices
Baylor College of Medicine
Houston, Texas

Peter K. Smith, MD
Professor and Chief, Thoracic Surgery
Duke University
Durham, North Carolina

Neel R. Sodha, MD
Assistant Professor of Surgery
Cardiothoracic Surgery
Warren Alpert Medical School of Brown University
Providence, Rhode Island

R. John Solaro, PhD
Distinguished University Professor and Head
Department of Physiology and Biophysics
University of Illinois at Chicago College of Medicine
Chicago, Illinois

Harmik J. Soukiasian, MD
Associate Director, Thoracic Surgery
Cedars-Sinai Medical Center
Los Angeles, California

David Spurlock, MD
Junior Fellow, Cardiac Surgery
University of Michigan
Ann Arbor, Michigan

Giovanni Stellin, MD
Director of Pediatric and Congenital Cardiac Surgery
Department of Cardio Thoracic and Vascular Sciences
University Hospital
Padova, Italy

Brendon M. Stiles, MD
Associate Professor of Cardiothoracic Surgery
Weill Cornell Medical College
Cardiothoracic Surgery
New York Presbyterian Hospital/Weill Cornell Medical College
New York, New York

Michaela Straznicka, MD
Thoracic Surgeon
Sutter Health Medical Center
Walnut Creek, California

David A. Stump, PhD
Wake Forest University Baptist Medical Center
Winston-Salem, North Carolina

David J. Sugarbaker, MD
Director, The Lung Institute
Chief, Division of Thoracic Surgery
The Olga Keith Wiess Chair of Surgery
Baylor College of Medicine
Houston, Texas

Erik J. Suuronen, PhD
Division of Cardiac Surgery
University of Ottawa Heart Institute
Department of Cellular and Molecular Medicine
University of Ottawa
Ottawa, Ontario, Canada

Lars G. Svensson, MD, PhD
Professor of Surgery, Thoracic and Cardiovascular Surgery
Chairman, Heart and Vascular Institute
Cleveland Clinic
Cleveland, Ohio

Scott J. Swanson, MD
Director, Minimally Invasive Thoracic Surgery
Brigham and Women's Hospital
Vice Chair, Cancer Affairs
Department of Surgery, Brigham and Women's Hospital
Chief Surgical Officer
Dana-Farber Cancer Institute
Professor of Surgery
Harvard Medical School
Boston, Massachusetts

Wilson Y. Szeto, MD
Associate Professor of Surgery
Division of Cardiovascular Surgery
Department of Surgery
University of Pennsylvania
Philadelphia, Pennsylvania

Sharven Taghavi, MD
Resident, Department of Surgery
Temple University
Philadelphia, Pennsylvania

Hiroo Takayama, MD, PhD
Assistant Professor of Surgery
Columbia University College of Physicians and Surgeons
Attending Surgeon
New York–Presbyterian Hospital
New York, New York

Koji Takeda, MD, PhD
Assistant Professor of Surgery
Columbia University College of Physicians and Surgeons
Attending Surgeon
New York–Presbyterian Hospital
New York, New York

Ravi R. Thiagarajan, MBBS, MPH
Senior Associate in Cardiology
Associate Professor of Pediatrics
Boston Children's Hospital
Boston, Massachusetts

Patricia A. Thistlethwaite, MD, PhD
Professor of Surgery
Program Director, Division of Cardiothoracic Surgery
University of California, San Diego
San Diego, California

Vinod H. Thourani, MD
Professor of Surgery
Structural Heart and Valve Center
Division of Cardiothoracic Surgery
Joseph B. Whitehead Department of Surgery
Emory University School of Medicine
Atlanta, Georgia

Hadi D. Toeg, MD, MSc
Surgical Resident
Division of Cardiac Surgery
University of Ottawa Heart Institute
Ottawa, Ontario, Canada

Michael Z. Tong, MD, MBA
Associate Staff, Thoracic and Cardiovascular Surgery
Heart and Vascular Institute
Cleveland Clinic
Cleveland, Ohio

Alexander G. Truesdell, MD
Cardiac and Vascular Interventionalist
PinnacleHealth CardioVascular Institute
Harrisburg, Pennsylvania

Peter I. Tsai, MD, FACS
Assistant Professor of Surgery
Division of Cardiothoracic Surgery
Michael E. DeBakey Department of Surgery
Baylor College of Medicine
Houston, Texas

Harold C. Urschel, Jr., MD†
Professor of Cardiovascular and Thoracic Surgery
University of Texas Southwestern Medical School
Chair, Cardiovascular and Thoracic Surgical Research, Education, and Clinical Excellence
Department of Cardiovascular and Thoracic Surgery
Baylor University Medical Center
Dallas, Texas

†Deceased.

Anne Marie Valente, MD
Associate Professor of Pediatrics and Internal Medicine
Harvard Medical School
Outpatient Director, Boston Adult Congenital Heart Disease and Pulmonary Hypertension Program
Department of Cardiology
Boston Children's Hospital
Department of Medicine
Division of Cardiology
Brigham and Women's Hospital
Boston, Massachusetts

Prashanth Vallabhajosyula, MD, MS
Assistant Professor of Surgery
Division of Cardiovascular Surgery
Department of Surgery
University of Pennsylvania
Philadelphia, Pennsylvania

Jeffrey B. Velotta, MD
Thoracic Surgery
Oakland Medical Center
Oakland, California

Vladimiro Vida, MD, PhD
Department of Cardio Thoracic and Vascular Sciences
University Hospital
Padova, Italy

Gus J. Vlahakes, MD
Professor of Surgery
Harvard Medical School
Massachusetts General Hospital
Boston, Massachusetts

Pierre Voisine, MD, FRCSC
Department of Cardiac Surgery
Institut Universitaire de Cardiologie et de Pneumologie de Québec
Québec City, Québec, Canada

Matthew J. Wall, Jr., MD, FACS
Professor of Surgery
Division of Cardiothoracic Surgery
Michael E. DeBakey Department of Surgery
Baylor College of Medicine
Houston, Texas

Garrett L. Walsh, MD
Professor of Surgery
Department of Thoracic and Cardiovascular Surgery
Division of Surgery
The University of Texas MD Anderson Cancer Center
Houston, Texas

Dustin M. Walters, MD
Division of Cardiothoracic Surgery
University of Washington Medical Center
Seattle, Washington

Benjamin Wei, MD
Assistant Professor of Surgery
Division of Cardiothoracic Surgery
University of Alabama at Birmingham
Birmingham, Alabama

Ian J. Welsby, MB BS
Associate Professor of Anesthesiology
Departments of Anesthesiology, Surgery, and Critical Care
Duke University School of Medicine
Durham, North Carolina

Margaret V. Westfall, PhD
Associate Professor
Department of Cardiac Surgery
University of Michigan School of Medicine
Ann Arbor, Michigan

Daniel C. Wiener, MD
Assistant Professor of Surgery
Harvard Medical School
Thoracic Surgeon
Brigham and Women's Hospital
Boston, Massachusetts

Benson R. Wilcox, MD†
Professor of Surgery
Department of Cardiothoracic Surgery
University of North Carolina at Chapel Hill
University of North Carolina Hospital
Chapel Hill, North Carolina

Judson B. Williams, MD, MHS
Resident, Cardiothoracic Surgery
Duke University
Durham, North Carolina

Jay M. Wilson, MD
Associate Professor of Surgery
Harvard Medical School
Senior Associate in Surgery
Boston Children's Hospital
Boston, Massachusetts

Y. Joseph Woo, MD
Norman E. Shumway Professor and Chair
Department of Cardiothoracic Surgery
Stanford University School of Medicine
Professor, by courtesy, Department of Bioengineering
Stanford University
Stanford, California

Douglas E. Wood, MD
Professor and Chief, Endowed Chair in Lung Cancer Research
Division of Cardiothoracic Surgery
University of Washington
Seattle, Washington

John V. Wylie, Jr., MD
Tufts University School of Medicine
St. Elizabeth's Medical Center
Boston, Massachusetts

Stephen C. Yang, MD
Professor of Surgery
The Johns Hopkins Medical Institutions
Baltimore, Maryland

Sai Yendamuri, MD
Associate Professor
Department of Thoracic Surgery
Roswell Park Cancer Institute
Buffalo, New York

Susan B. Yeon, MD, JD
Department of Medicine
Cardiovascular Division
Harvard-Thorndike Laboratory
Harvard Medical School
Beth Israel Deaconess Medical Center
Boston, Massachusetts;
Deputy Editor
UpToDate
Wolters Kluwer Health
Waltham, Massachusetts

Peter J. Zimetbaum, MD
Associate Professor of Medicine
Harvard Medical School
Cardiac Services
Beth Israel Deaconess Medical Center
Boston, Massachusetts

†Deceased.

PREFACE

Since its beginning as a specialty to treat tuberculosis and empyema, thoracic surgery has undergone constant change. Indeed, much has evolved in the fields of adult and pediatric cardiovascular and thoracic surgery even since our last edition. Our new ninth edition contains the latest information on the diagnosis and treatment of disease of the thorax. Especially in such areas as repair of aortic and mitral valvular disease, intervention for congenital heart disease, minimally invasive thoracic and cardiac surgery, surgical treatment of arrhythmias, and endovascular treatment of aortic disease, the field has markedly transformed. As with the previous editions, many of the same authors were asked to update their chapters, but some chapters have been added or eliminated and many others have been completely rewritten. Often new authors were chosen not based on poorly written previous chapters but to provide a novel perspective. We hope that the ninth edition will be received with the same enthusiasm as the last.

Several years ago, we lost one of the former editors of this textbook and a giant in the field of surgery, Dr. David Sabiston. We are fortunate to still have with us another editor, Dr. Frank Spencer. Dr. Spencer is not only one of the true pioneers in our specialty but a great mentor to many in our field. We are all indebted to both Dr. Sabiston and Dr. Spencer for their innumerable contributions to the field of surgery.

Finally, we would like to thank our families for providing immeasurable support not only for this textbook but for our entire careers.

Frank W. Sellke
Pedro J. del Nido
Scott J. Swanson

CONTENTS

VOLUME ONE

SECTION 1 THORACIC SURGERY

PART H
CHEST WALL, 398

PART I
PLEURA, 461

PART J
DIAPHRAGM, 525

PART K
ESOPHAGUS—BENIGN DISEASE, 574

PART L
ESOPHAGUS—CANCER, 644

PART M
MEDIASTINUM, 697

PART N
THE FUTURE, 751

SECTION 2
ADULT CARDIAC SURGERY

PART A
BASIC SCIENCE, 786

VIDEO CONTENTS

---

[1]From Coselli JS, LeMaire SA: Extent II repair of thoracoabdominal aortic aneurysm secondary to chronic dissection. *Ann Cardiothorac Surg* 1(3):394–397, 2012.
[2]Courtesy Ralph Chitwood, MD, Karen A. Gersch, MD, Michael W. Chu, MD, L. W. Nifong, MD, and Jerome Fuller, MD.
[3]From *Sabiston & Spencer Surgery of the Chest*, ed 8.
[4]From Vassiliades TA: Endoscopic and traditional minimally invasive direct coronary artery bypass. In Sellke FW, editor: *Atlas of cardiac surgical techniques*, Philadelphia, 2009, Elsevier.
[5]Courtesy Keith Horvath, MD.
[6]From Frazier OH: Implantation of the Heart Mate II. In Sellke FW, editor: *Atlas of cardiac surgical techniques*, Philadelphia, 2009, Elsevier.
[7]From Reitz BA, Baumgartner WA, Borkon AM, the American College of Surgeons Video-Based Education Collection.
[8]Courtesy Lorenzo Menicanti, MD, and Marisa Di Donato, MD.

SABISTON & SPENCER

SURGERY *of the* CHEST

PART E

SURGICAL MANAGEMENT OF AORTIC DISEASE

PART OUTLINE

CHAPTER 67

Surgery of the Aortic Root and Ascending Aorta

Tirone E. David

CHAPTER OUTLINE

FUNCTIONAL ANATOMY OF THE AORTIC ROOT

The aortic root is the anatomic segment between the left ventricle and the ascending aorta. It contains the aortic valve and other anatomic elements, which function as a unit. The aortic root has several anatomic components: the subcommissural triangles, the aortic annulus, the aortic cusps, the aortic sinuses or sinuses of Valsalva, and the sinotubular junction.

The subcommissural triangles are part of the left ventricular outflow tract, but they play an important role in the function of the aortic valve. The subcommissural triangles of the noncoronary aortic cusp are fibrous extension of the intervalvular fibrous body and membranous septum, whereas the subcommissural triangle beneath the left and the right aortic cusps is an extension of the muscular interventricular septum (Fig. 67-1). The aortic annulus, a fibrous structure with a scalloped shape, attaches the aortic valve to the left ventricle. It is attached directly to the myocardium in approximately 45% of its circumference, and to fibrous structures in the remaining 55%. Histologic examination of the aortic annulus reveals that the aortic root has a fibrous continuity with the anterior leaflet of the mitral valve and membranous septum, and it is attached to the muscular interventricular septum by fibrous strands (Fig. 67-2). An important structure immediately below the membranous septum is the bundle of His. The atrioventricular node lies in the floor of the right atrium between the tricuspid annulus and the coronary sinus orifice. This node gives origin to the bundle of His, which travels through the right fibrous trigone along the posterior edge of the membranous septum to the muscular interventricular septum. At this point, the bundle of His divides into left and right bundle branches, which run subendocardially along both sides of the interventricular septum.

The normal aortic valve has three cusps. Each cusp has a semilunar shape and has a base and a free margin. The base is attached to the aortic annulus in a crescent fashion. The point at which the free margin of a cusp joins its base is the commissure, and the ridge in the aortic wall that lies immediately above the commissures is the sinotubular junction. The spaces contained between the aortic annulus and the sinotubular junction are the

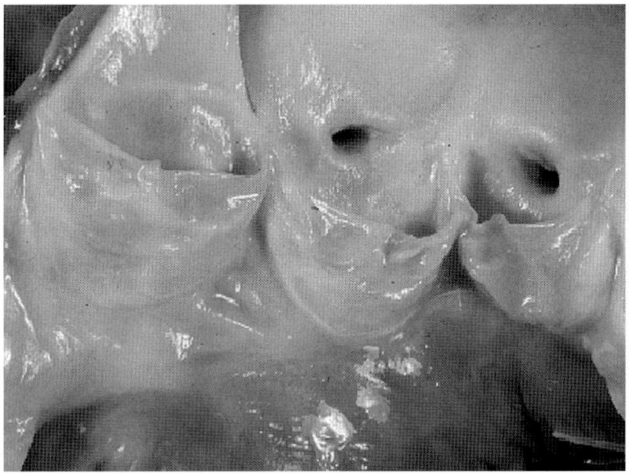

FIGURE 67-1 ■ The inside of the aortic root.

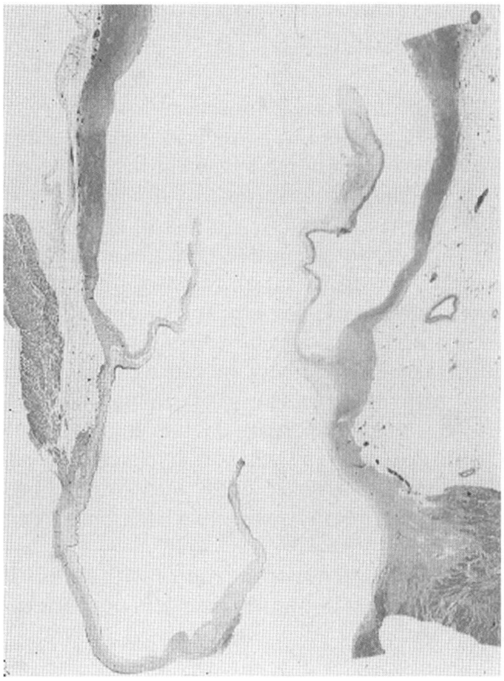

FIGURE 67-2 ■ Microphotograph of the aortic annulus, cusps, and sinuses.

aortic sinuses, or sinuses of Valsalva. There are three cusps and three sinuses: left cusp and sinus, right cusp and sinus, and noncoronary cusp and sinus. The left main coronary artery arises from the left aortic sinus, and the right coronary artery arises from the right aortic sinus.

The normal aortic root has a fairly consistent shape, and the sizes of the cusps, the aortic annulus, the aortic sinuses, and the sinotubular junction are somewhat interdependent.[1-4] Thus, large cusps have a proportionally large annulus, sinus, and sinotubular junction. The three aortic cusps often have different sizes in a person, and the right and noncoronary cusps are usually larger than the left cusp.[3] The same cusp may have different sizes in individuals with the same body surface area.[3,4] There are, however, certain geometric parameters that are fairly constant among the various components of the aortic root, and this knowledge is indispensable to understanding the principles of aortic valve repair or replacement with stentless biological valves.

The free margin of an aortic cusp extends from one of its commissures to the other. The length of the free margin of an aortic cusp is approximately 1.5 times the length of its base (Fig. 67-3). During diastole, the free margins and part of the body of the three cusps touch each other approximately in the center of the aortic root to seal the aortic orifice. Thus, the average length of the free margins of three aortic cusps must exceed the diameter of the sinotubular junction to allow the cusps to coapt centrally and render the aortic valve competent. If a pathologic process causes shortening of the length of the free margin of a cusp, or if the sinotubular junction dilates, the cusps cannot coapt centrally, resulting in aortic insufficiency (Fig. 67-4). If the length of a free margin is elongated, the cusp prolapses, and depending on the degree of prolapse, aortic insufficiency ensues (Fig. 67-5).

The diameter of the aortic annulus is 10% to 20% larger than the diameter of the sinotubular junction of the aortic root in young patients (see Fig. 67-3). As the number of elastic fibers in the arterial wall decreases with age, the sinotubular junction dilates, and its diameter tends to become equal to that of the aortic annulus in older patients.

Dilation of the aortic annulus pulls the belly of the aortic cusps apart, decreasing the coaptation area, and it

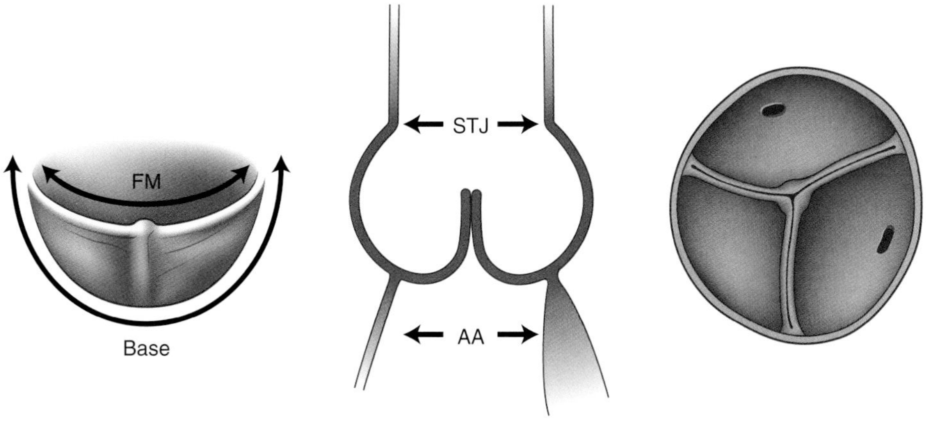

FIGURE 67-3 ■ Geometric relationship between the free margin (FM) and base of the aortic cusps, sinotubular junction (STJ), and aortic annulus (AA).

eventually causes aortic insufficiency (Fig. 67-6). With dilation of the aortic annulus, the subcommissural triangles of the noncoronary cusp tend to become more obtuse as the crescent shape of the aortic annulus along its fibrous insertion flattens (see Fig. 67-6). The subcommissural triangle beneath the right and left cusps does not change much in patients with annuloaortic ectasia, because it is part of the muscular interventricular septum and is not affected by the connective tissue disorder that causes dilation of the fibrous skeleton of the heart.

The aortic sinuses facilitate closure of the aortic valve by creating eddies and currents between the cusps and arterial wall (Fig. 67-7). They also prevent the cusps from occluding the coronary artery orifices during systole, thus guaranteeing myocardial perfusion during the entire cardiac cycle. Isolated dilation of the aortic sinuses does not cause aortic insufficiency.[5]

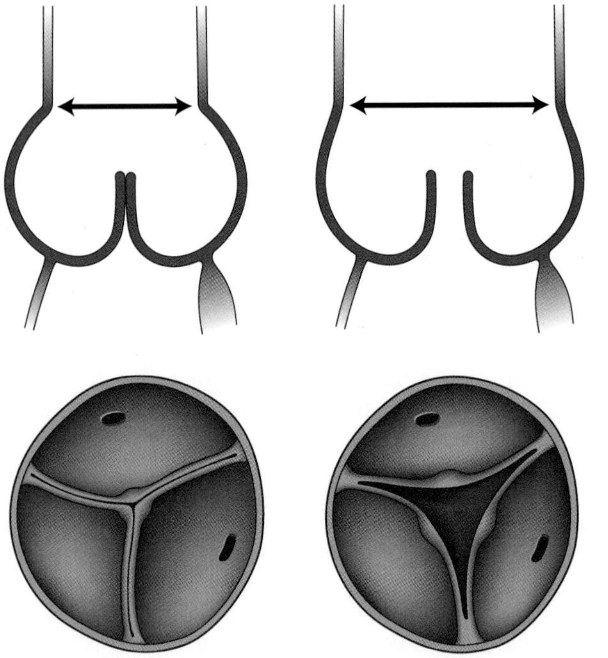

FIGURE 67-4 ■ Dilation of the sinotubular junction causes aortic insufficiency.

The aortic root of young individuals is elastic and very compliant. It expands and contracts during the cardiac cycle. Expansion and contraction of the aortic annulus are heterogeneous, probably because of its attachments to contractile myocardium and to fibrous structures such as the membranous septum and intervalvular fibrous body. On the other hand, the expansion and contraction of the sinotubular junction are more uniform. The aortic root also displays some degree of torsion during isovolumic contraction and ejection of the left ventricle.[6] Compliance decreases with aging because of loss of elastic fibers, and the movements of the aortic annulus, cusps, sinuses, and sinotubular junction also change.

PATHOLOGY OF THE AORTIC ROOT AND ASCENDING AORTA

The wall of the aorta is composed of three layers: intima, media, and adventitia. The intima is a thin layer of ground substance lined by endothelium, and it is easily traumatized. The media is the thickest of the three layers, and it is made of elastic fibers arranged in spiral fashion to increase the tensile strength. The adventitia is a thin, fibrous layer and contains the vasa vasorum, which carries the nutrients to the media. The aorta is highly compliant, and it expands and contracts during the cardiac cycle because of the elastic fibers in the media. Compliance decreases with aging because of fragmentation of the elastic fibers and an increase in the amount of fibrous tissue in the media. Hypertension, hypercholesterolemia, and coronary artery disease cause premature aging of the aorta.[7-9] Exercise seems to protect the elasticity of the aorta.[8]

Degenerative diseases of the media with aneurysm formation are the most common disorders of the aortic root

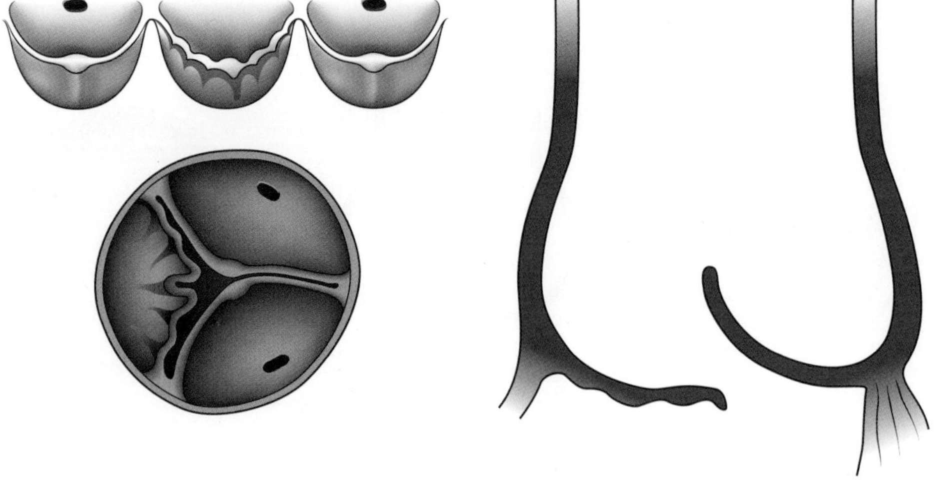

FIGURE 67-5 ■ Elongation of the free margin of an aortic cusp causes prolapse with resulting aortic insufficiency.

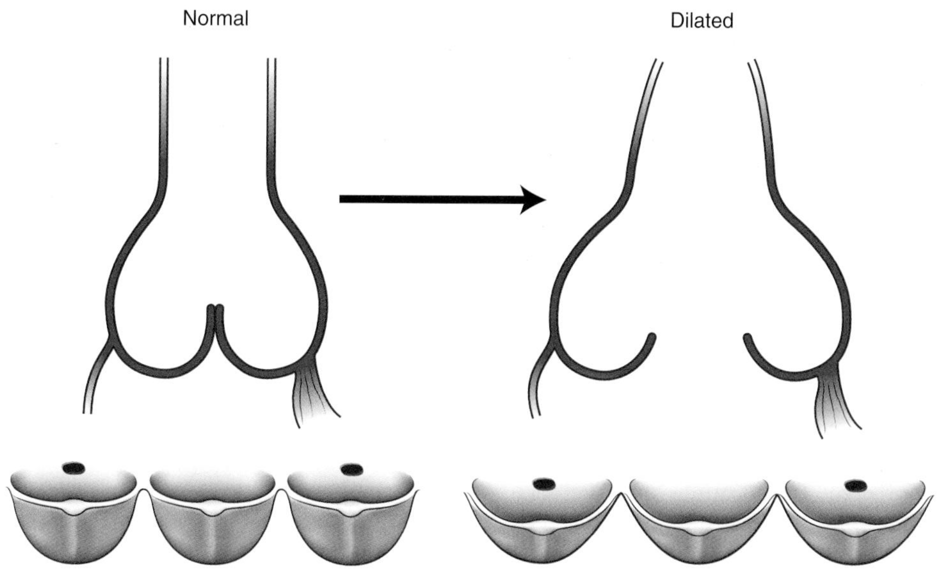

FIGURE 67-6 ■ Dilation of the aortic annulus. The subcommissural triangles of the noncoronary cusp become more obtuse.

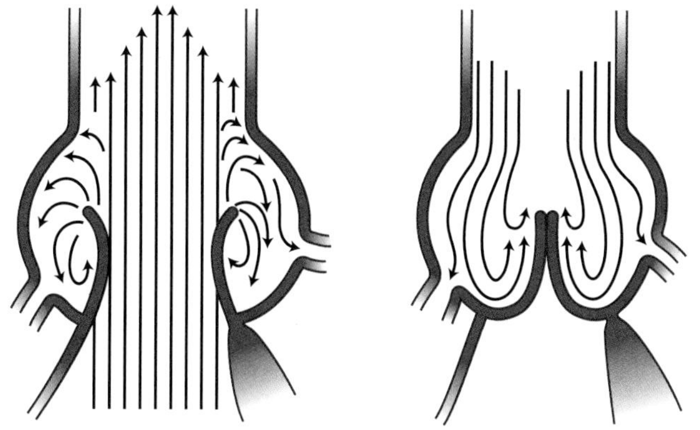

FIGURE 67-7 ■ The aortic sinuses create eddies and currents and facilitate aortic valve closure.

and ascending aorta. A broad spectrum of pathologic and clinical entities is grouped under degenerative disorders, ranging from severe degeneration of the media, which can become clinically important early in life in cases such as Marfan syndrome in children, to cases of the not so important mild dilation of the ascending aorta in older adults. Bicuspid and unicusp aortic valve diseases are often associated with dilation of the aorta. Atherosclerosis, infectious and noninfectious aortitis, and trauma are other pathologic entities with which the cardiac surgeon must be familiar. Primary tumors of the aortic root and ascending aorta are rare. False aneurysms and aortic root abscess are problems commonly encountered in clinical practice.

Degenerative Aneurysms of the Proximal Aorta

Degenerative aneurysms of the thoracic aorta in older patients are often related to risk factors such as smoking, hypertension, and hyperlipidemia. In young patients without risk factors, the explanation for aneurysm formation is on a genetic basis. Genetic aneurysms of the aorta can be classified into three main groups:

1. Inherited syndromes predisposing to early onset of aortic aneurysms, such as Marfan syndrome, Loeys-Dietz syndrome, and aneurysm-osteoarthritis syndrome
2. Familial aneurysms
3. Sporadic aneurysms including young patients without family history of aneurysm

Aneurysms of the proximal aorta are often caused by cystic medial degeneration (cystic medial necrosis). Histologically, necrosis and disappearance of muscle cells in the elastic lamina, and cystic spaces filled with mucoid material are often observed. Although these changes occur more often in the proximal aorta, they can affect any portion or the entire aorta. These changes weaken the arterial wall, which dilates and forms a fusiform aneurysm. The aortic root may be involved in this pathologic process, and in patients with Marfan syndrome, the aneurysm usually begins in the aortic sinuses. Patients with aortic root aneurysms are usually in their second or third decade of life when the diagnosis is made. Other patients have relatively normal aortic roots but develop ascending aortic aneurysms. These patients are usually in their fifth or sixth decade of life. Finally, certain patients have extensive degenerative disease of the entire aorta and develop the so-called mega-aorta syndrome with dilation of the thoracic and abdominal aorta.

Ascending aortic aneurysms tend to increase in size and eventually rupture or cause aortic dissection. The transverse diameter of the aneurysm is the most important predictor of rupture or dissection. In a study by Coady and associates[10] of 370 patients with thoracic aneurysms (201 ascending aortic aneurysms), during a mean follow-up of 29.4 months, the incidence of acute dissection or rupture was 8.8% for aneurysms smaller than 4 cm, 9.5% for aneurysms of 4 to 4.9 cm, 17.8% for 5 to 5.9 cm, and 27.9% for those larger than 6 cm. The median size of the ascending aortic aneurysm at the time of rupture or dissection was 5.9 cm.

The growth rates of thoracic aneurysms are exponential.[10] In the study by Coady and associates,[10] the growth rate ranged from 0.08 cm/yr for small (<4 cm) aneurysms to 0.16 cm/yr for large (8 cm) aneurysms. The growth rates for chronic dissecting aneurysms were much higher than for chronic nondissecting aneurysms. Other studies found greater annual growth rates than did the Coady group.[11,12] In addition, the growth rates for aortic root aneurysms may be different from those of ascending aortic aneurysms.

Most patients with aortic root or ascending aortic aneurysms are asymptomatic, and the aneurysm is usually found during routine chest radiographs, which show a widened mediastinum.[13] Tracheal and esophageal displacement may be observed in the posterolateral view of the chest radiographs. Approximately one third of the patients complain of vague chest pain.[13] In patients with a massive ascending aortic aneurysm, signs of superior vena cava obstruction may be present. If aortic insufficiency is present, there may be cardiac enlargement and the physical findings associated with it. The diagnoses of aortic root and ascending aortic aneurysm can be confirmed with echocardiography.

Transesophageal echocardiography is the best diagnostic tool to study aortic root aneurysm and the mechanism of aortic insufficiency. The echocardiographer should obtain information on each component of the aortic root, and particularly the aortic cusps. The number of cusps, their thickness, the appearance of free margins, and the excursion of each cusp during the cardiac cycle must be observed carefully. The coaptation areas of the cusps should also be investigated in multiple views, and Doppler imaging should be recorded. Information regarding the morphologic features of the aortic sinuses, sinotubular junction, and ascending aorta is also important. The diameters of the aortic annulus, aortic sinuses, sinotubular junction, and ascending aorta should be obtained in multiple views. The lengths of the free margins of the cusps should be estimated if possible. The mechanism of aortic insufficiency can often be determined with transesophageal echocardiography. Dilation of the sinotubular junction is a common cause of aortic insufficiency in patients with ascending aortic aneurysm and normal aortic cusps. Dilation of the aortic annulus and of the sinotubular junction is usually the cause of aortic insufficiency in patients with aortic root aneurysm. Although fenestrations in the cusps are not easily seen with echocardiography, a regurgitant jet in a commissural area is suggestive of fenestration.

Computed tomography (CT) with intravenous contrast enhancement permits accurate evaluation of the extent and size of the aneurysm. Three-dimensional imaging techniques can provide additional information on the extensiveness and type of aneurysm (e.g., fusiform or saccular).

Magnetic resonance imaging (MRI) provides even more information than CT scanning because it visualizes the arterial wall and surrounding structures with greater contrast. In addition, it has been increasingly used in the diagnosis and management of patients with heart diseases.[14] Magnetic resonance angiography is replacing contrast angiography.[15]

Inherited Aneurysms of the Proximal Aorta

Marfan Syndrome

Marfan syndrome is an autosomal dominant, variably penetrant, inherited disorder of the connective tissue in which cardiovascular, skeletal, ocular, and other abnormalities may be present to variable degrees. The prevalence is estimated to be approximately 1 in 5000 individuals. It is caused by mutations in the gene that encodes fibrillin-1 *(FBN1)* on chromosome 15. This is a large gene (approximately 10,000 nucleotides in the messenger RNA), and identification of the mutation is a complex task. More than 1000 mutations in FBN1 have been identified. The phenotype is highly variable because of varying genotype expression.

The clinical features of Marfan syndrome were thought to be caused by weaker connective tissues resulting from defects in FBN1, a glycoprotein and principal component of the extracellular matrix microfibril. This concept was inadequate to explain the overgrowth of long bones, osteopenia, reduced muscular mass and adiposity, and craniofacial abnormalities often seen in Marfan syndrome.[16] Dietz and colleagues[16,17] showed in experimental mice with Marfan syndrome that many findings are the result of abnormal levels of activation of transforming growth factor β (TGF-β), a potent stimulator of inflammation, fibrosis, and activation of certain matrix metalloproteinases, especially matrix metalloproteinases 2 and 9. Excess TGF-β activation in tissues correlates with failure of lung septation, development of a myxomatous mitral valve, and aortic root dilation in mice.[18] This combination of structural microfibril matrix abnormality, dysregulation of matrix homeostasis mediated by excess TGF-β, and abnormal cell–matrix interactions is responsible for the phenotypic features of Marfan syndrome.[16-18] Ongoing destruction of the elastic and collagen lamellae and medial degeneration result in progressive dilation of the aortic root, as well as in a predisposition to aortic dissection from the loss of appropriate medial layer support. Loss of elasticity in the media causes increased aortic stiffness and decreased distensibility.[19]

The main features of Marfan syndrome include disproportionate long bone overgrowth, ectopia lentis and aortic root aneurysm. Diagnosis is not always simple, and a multidisciplinary approach is needed to diagnose and manage patients with this autosomal dominant disorder. In 1996, a panel of experts developed the "Ghent criteria" for the diagnosis of Marfan syndrome.[20] Table 67-1 shows the original Ghent criteria, which contain a set of "major" and "minor" manifestations in various organs including cardiovascular, ocular, skeletal, pulmonary, dura mater, and skin.[20] The presence of major criteria in two separate systems and involvement of a third (minor or major) was needed to establish the diagnosis of Marfan syndrome.[20] Using these criteria, a high proportion of patients diagnosed as Marfan are found to have *FBN1* mutations. However, some manifestations contained in the Ghent criteria are age dependent, and there are patients with skeletal abnormalities and ectopia lentis without aortic root aneurysm, even in the presence of

TABLE 67-1 **Diagnostic Criteria for Marfan Syndrome***

System	Major Criteria	Minor Criteria
Family history	Independent diagnosis in parent, child, sibling	None
Genetics	Mutation in *FBN1*	None
Cardiovascular	Aortic root dilation Dissection of ascending aorta	Mitral valve prolapse Calcification of the mitral valve (age < 40 yr) Dilation of the pulmonary artery Dilation or dissection of the descending aorta
Ocular	Ectopia lentis	Two needed: Flat cornea Myopia Elongated globe
Skeletal	Pectus excavatum needing surgery Pectus carinatum Pes planus Wrist and thumb sign Scoliosis > 20 degrees or spondylolisthesis Arm span–height ratio > 1.05 Protrusio acetabula (radiograph, MRI) Diminished extension elbows (<170 degrees)	Two major or one major and two minor signs: Moderate pectus excavatum High, narrowly arched palate Typical facies Joint hypermobility
Pulmonary	—	Spontaneous pneumothorax Apical bullae
Skin	—	Unexplained stretch marks (striae) Recurrent or incisional hernia
Central nervous	Lumbosacral dural ectasia (CT or MRI)	—

*The presence of major criteria in two separate systems and involvement of a third (minor or major) are needed to establish the diagnosis of Marfan syndrome.
CT, Computed tomography; *MRI*, magnetic resonance imaging.

BOX 67-1 Revised Ghent Criteria for the Diagnosis of Marfan Syndrome

IN THE ABSENCE OF FAMILY HISTORY

1. Aortic root dilation (Z > 2) or dissection and ectopia lentis = Marfan
2. Aortic root dilation (Z > 2) or dissection and FBN1 mutation = Marfan
3. Aortic root dilation (Z > 2) or dissection and systemic score ≥7 points = Marfan
4. Ectopia lentis and FBN1 known to associated aortic root dilation/dissection

IN THE PRESENCE OF FAMILY HISTORY

5. Ectopia lentis and family history of Marfan
6. Systemic score (≥7 points) and family history of Marfan
7. Aortic root dilation (Z ≥ 2 in >20 years of age; Z ≥ 3 in <20 years of age) and family history of Marfan

From Loeys BL, Dietz HC, Braverman AC, et al: The revised nosology for the Marfan syndrome. J Med Genet 47:476–485, 2010.

FBN1 mutations. Experts in this area got together again and developed a "Revised Ghent Nosology for the Marfan Syndrome" (Box 67-1) which emphasizes aortic root aneurysm, ascending aortic dissection and ectopia lentis.[21]

The most common cardiovascular features of Marfan syndrome are aortic root aneurysm and mitral valve prolapse. These anatomic abnormalities may cause aortic rupture, aortic dissection, aortic insufficiency, and mitral insufficiency.

Mitral valve prolapse is age dependent and is more common in women. It is caused by myxomatous degeneration of the mitral valve apparatus, which is present in up to 80% of patients with Marfan syndrome, but only 25% of them develop mitral insufficiency. The posterior mitral annulus is grossly dilated in patients with mitral insufficiency, and it is often displaced posteriorly.[22] The mitral annulus can also become heavily calcified and display a horseshoe appearance on radiographs.

The dilation of the aortic root is often progressive, and the rate of expansion, which varies somewhat, is usually less than 1 or 2 mm/yr. Shores and colleagues[12] randomized 70 patients with Marfan syndrome into propranolol-treated and placebo groups. The growth rates of the aortic root aneurysms in untreated patients were slightly more than three times those of patients who received β-adrenergic blockage. This study has been the scientific basis to treat these patients with a β-blocker agent. Calcium antagonists and angiotension-converting enzymes have also been reported as effective in delaying aortic dilation, but at present, β-blocker remains the drug of choice.[23] A prospective randomized clinical trial showed that losartan is effective in reducing the rate of aortic root dilation in patients with Marfan syndrome, and it reduces the rate of dilation of the arch after aortic root replacement.[24] The combination of losartan with a β-blocker was more effective in preventing dilation of the aortic root than β-blocker alone in a small, randomized trial in children.[25]

Aortic dissection is rare in patients with aortic root aneurysm of less than 50 mm, unless they have a family history of aortic dissection.[26] The dissection in most patients starts at the level of the sinotubular junction (Stanford type A aortic dissection). Surgery of the aortic root is recommended when the transverse diameter of the aortic sinuses reaches 50 mm. In patients with family history of dissection, surgery should be considered when the diameter reaches 45 mm. Without surgery, most patients with Marfan syndrome die in their third decade, from complications of aortic root aneurysm such as rupture, aortic dissection, or aortic insufficiency.[27,28] In approximately 10% of patients, the dissection starts just beyond the left subclavian artery (Stanford type B aortic dissection).

Patients with Marfan syndrome should be followed at regular time intervals. Doppler echocardiography is the best diagnostic tool for monitoring changes in the mitral valve and aortic root. Patients with an aortic root greater than 40 mm should be followed with echocardiographic measurements twice yearly. MRI of the remaining thoracic and abdominal aorta should also be used when indicated.

Pregnancy in women with Marfan syndrome has two potential problems: the risk of having a child who will inherit the disorder and the risk of acute aortic dissection during the third trimester, parturition, or the first postpartum month. Offspring have a 50% risk of inheriting the syndrome. The risk of aortic dissection is less known, but it appears to be low in patients with normal aortic root and cardiac function.[29]

Loeys-Dietz Syndrome

Mutations in the genes encoding TGF-β receptors 1 and 2 have been found in association with a continuum of clinical features. On the mild end is a presentation similar to that of the Marfan syndrome, or familial thoracic aneurysm and dissection,[30,31] and on the severe end, there is a complex phenotype in which aortic dissection or rupture commonly occurs in childhood.[32] This complex phenotype is characterized by the triad of hypertelorism, bifid uvula (or cleft palate), and generalized arterial tortuosity with widespread vascular aneurysm and dissection. This phenotype has been classified as Loeys-Dietz syndrome.[32] Affected patients have a high risk of aortic dissection or rupture at an early age and at relatively small aortic diameters. CT angiograms should be obtained from the head to the pelvis. Surgery is recommended for adults when the aortic root exceeds 4 cm or the descending thoracic aorta exceeds 5 cm. If the craniofacial features are severe in children, surgery is recommended when the aortic root z-score is greater than 3, or when the expansion is greater than 0.5 cm in 1 year.[33]

Ehlers-Danlos Syndrome

The Ehlers-Danlos syndrome encompasses a group of heterogeneous connective tissue disorders that involve the skin and joints and cause hyperelasticity and fragility of the former and hypermobility of the latter. It can also involve the cardiovascular system. Vascular Ehlers-Danlos syndrome is a rare autosomal dominant inherited disorder of the connective tissue resulting from mutation of the *COL3A1* gene encoding type III collagen.[34] Afflicted individuals are prone to serious vascular, intestinal, and obstetric complications. These problems are rare during infancy but occur in up to 25% of affected persons before the age of 20 years and in 80% before the age of 40. Median survival is 48 years. Spontaneous rupture without dissection of large- and medium-caliber arteries, such as the abdominal aorta and its branches, the branches of the aortic arch, and the large arteries of the limbs accounts for most deaths. Intestinal perforation, usually involving the colon, is less often fatal. Pregnancy is a high risk for women with this syndrome. Aortic root dilation was present in 28% in a series of 71 patients with Ehlers-Danlos syndrome.[35] Aortic dissection is uncommon.

As with many rare diseases, delayed or incorrect diagnosis can lead to inadequate or inappropriate management. Diagnosis is based on clinical findings, including specific facial features, thin translucent skin, propensity to bleeding, and rupture of vessels or viscera. Diagnosis can be confirmed by biochemical assays showing qualitative or quantitative abnormalities in type III collagen secretion, or by molecular biology studies demonstrating mutation of the *COL3A1* gene. Varied molecular mechanisms have been observed with different mutations in each family. No correlation has been established between genotype and phenotype. Diagnosis should be suggested in any young person with arterial or visceral rupture or colonic perforation. There is currently no specific treatment for this syndrome.

Bicuspid Aortic Valve Disease

Congenital aortic valve malformations include a phenotypic continuum of unicuspid valves (severe form), the various types of bicuspid aortic valves (moderate form), tricuspid valves (normal), and the rare quadricuspid valves.[36]

Bicuspid aortic valve, the most common of these malformations, occurs in 1% to 2% of the population. Movahed and colleagues[37] recently reviewed 24,265 patients who had echocardiograms performed for various clinical reasons, and 1742 echocardiograms obtained by screening teenage athletes in Southern California, and found a prevalence of bicuspid aortic valves of 0.6% in the large cohort and 0.5% in the smaller one. Males are affected more than females at a ratio of 4:1. There is a relatively high incidence of familial clustering, which suggests an autosomal dominant inheritance with reduced penetrance[38,39]; however, it remains unproved that bicuspid aortic valve is an inherited disorder. Patients with bicuspid aortic valve usually have three aortic sinuses and two cusps of different sizes. The larger cusp, usually the one attached to the interventricular septum, contains a raphe, which probably represents an incomplete commissure. The raphe extends from the mid portion of the cusp to the aortic annulus, and its insertion in the aortic root is at a lower level than the other two commissures. Bicuspid aortic valves with two cusps and two sinuses are uncommon and called "type 0"; the most common type is with one raphe and is called "type 1," and finally with two raphes is "type 2."[40] Types 1 and 2 can be subclassified according to the fused cusps: left-right is the most common form (a raphe in between the left and right cusps). Abnormal origin of the coronary arteries and circumflex artery dominance are common in patients with bicuspid aortic valve.[41]

Normally functioning bicuspid aortic valves may last the patient's lifetime. Others become stenotic by the fourth or fifth decade of life. Aortic insufficiency can also occur, and it is often associated with dilated aortic annulus.[42] It is more common in younger patients, and it results from the prolapse of one cusp, usually the one that contains the raphe.

Both bicuspid and unicuspid aortic valves are often associated with premature degenerative changes in the media of the wall of the aortic root and ascending aorta.[43,44] These patients are at risk of developing chronic degenerative aneurysms of the ascending aorta and type A aortic dissection.[45]

Atherosclerosis

Atherosclerosis of the ascending aorta and transverse arch is a common cause of stroke.[46,47] Sometimes, atherosclerosis can cause extensive calcification of the aortic root, ascending aorta, and transverse arch, which is often associated with coronary artery disease, stenosis of one or both coronary arteries orifices, and aortic valve stenosis. Extensive calcification of the ascending aorta is clinically described as "porcelain" aorta.[48,49] Atherosclerotic aneurysms of the ascending aorta are uncommon; they are more common in the abdominal aorta and to a lesser degree in the descending thoracic aorta. Atherosclerosis often causes irregular and saccular aneurysms of the ascending aorta rather than the more fusiform shape of those caused by degenerative disease of the media.

Infectious Aneurysms

Syphilis was a common cause of aneurysm of the ascending aorta, but it is now rare. The spirochetal infection destroys the muscular and elastic fibers of the media, which are replaced by fibrous and other inflammatory tissues. The ascending aorta is the most common site of involvement, and the aneurysm is usually saccular.[50] The wall of the ascending aorta is frequently calcified. Syphilitic aortitis also causes coronary ostial stenosis and aortic valve insufficiency.[50] Although rare, other bacteria can also cause aneurysm of the ascending aorta.

Aortitis

Various types of aortitis can involve the ascending aorta.[51-56] Giant cell arteritis is among the more common, and it involves medium-sized arteries, but the aorta and its branches are involved in approximately 15% of cases.[55] The etiology of aortitis, also called *temporal arteritis*, is unknown. The characteristic lesion is a granulomatous inflammation of the media of large- and medium-caliber arteries, such as the temporal artery. Narrowing of the aorta is rare. Occasionally, the inflammatory process weakens the aorta, leading to aneurysm formation, aortoannular ectasia, and aortic insufficiency.[54] Patients are usually older than 50 years, with a mean age of 67 years, and most are women. Diagnosis is established by biopsy of the involved artery, usually the temporal artery.

Takayasu arteritis is a chronic inflammatory disease that often involves the aortic arch and its major branches. The pulmonary artery may also be involved. The lesions are purely stenotic in 85% of patients, aneurysmal in 2%, and mixed in 13%.[52,53] Aortic insufficiency occurs in approximately 25% of the cases. It has been classified as type I when the aortic arch is involved, type II when the arch is free of disease but the thoracoabdominal aorta and its branches are affected, type III when both areas are affected, and type IV when the pulmonary artery is involved.[53,56] The etiology is unknown, but it is probably an autoimmune disorder. It occurs worldwide, but most cases are seen in Asia and Africa. The disease affects women more than men at a ratio of 8:1.[51,53] The mean age at the time of the diagnosis is 29 years.

Ankylosing spondylitis, Reiter syndrome, psoriatic arthritis, and polyarteritis nodosa can cause aortic insufficiency because of annuloaortic ectasia. Behçet disease can cause aneurysm of the ascending aorta.

Aortic Dissection

Aortic dissections are discussed in Chapters 70 and 71.

Ascending Aorta Tumors

Primary tumors of the ascending aorta are extremely rare. Most aortic tumors are located in the descending thoracic or abdominal aorta, and they are usually sarcomas.[57,58]

Ascending Aorta Trauma

Nonpenetrating traumatic injuries of the ascending aorta are often fatal and diagnosed at autopsy.[59] The penetrating trauma is usually a bullet or stab wound, and it causes cardiac tamponade when the intrapericardial portion of the aorta is involved. These injuries are frequently fatal.

SURGICAL TREATMENT OF ASCENDING AORTIC ANEURYSM

Although ascending aortic aneurysms may be isolated lesions, more often they are associated with aortic valve disease. Both bicuspid and tricuspid aortic valve diseases may be associated with degenerative aneurysms of the ascending aorta, but bicuspid aortic valve disease appears to be associated with premature degeneration of the media of the aorta.

Ascending aortic aneurysm can cause aortic insufficiency in patients with anatomically normal aortic valve cusps if the sinotubular junction becomes dilated (see Fig. 67-4). These patients can develop symptoms related to the aortic insufficiency, but more often the aneurysm is asymptomatic and is discovered during a routine chest radiograph or echocardiogram as part of the workup for an unrelated problem. Surgery should be considered when the transverse diameter of the ascending aorta exceeds 55 mm.[60] If there is moderate or severe aortic insufficiency, the aortic valve cusps are normal by echocardiography, and the valve is judged to be repairable, then operation is justifiable when the ascending aorta reaches 50 mm in diameter.[61] If the aneurysm is associated with a genetic syndrome, surgery should be considered when the diameter reaches 50 mm.[60] If associated with a normally functioning bicuspid aortic valve, surgery is recommended when the diameter reaches 55 mm.[60a]

Operative Techniques

Surgery for ascending aortic aneurysm is performed using cardiopulmonary bypass, which is established by cannulating the transverse aortic arch, right axillary artery or femoral artery, and the right atrium. In patients with bicuspid aortic valve the aneurysm frequently extends up to the innominate artery and a brief period of circulatory arrest is necessary to resect the proximal arch and perform the distal anastomosis. The proximal anastomosis should be performed at the level of the sinotubular junction. The Dacron graft used to replace the ascending aorta should not be too long or too large. When the ascending aorta expands to develop an aneurysm, it also becomes elongated. Thus, during its replacement, the graft should be much shorter than the aneurysm. In fact, a graft of 4 to 6 cm in length is all that is needed to replace the entire ascending aorta from sinotubular junction to the level of the innominate artery. Longer grafts can kink and cause partial obstruction and even hemolysis. A single graft can be used, but it should be beveled at the distal anastomosis, and its shorter side should be aligned with the medial part of the arch (Fig. 67-8). The diameter of the graft should be between 24 and 32 mm, depending on the patient's body surface area. When the diameter of the graft used is larger than the diameter of the sinotubular junction by more than a couple of millimeters, its caliber should be reduced to that of the sinotubular junction at the level of the anastomosis. This is easily done by plication of that end of the graft. Matching the diameter of the graft to that of the sinotubular junction is important to prevent late development of aortic insufficiency.

If the aortic valve is incompetent but the aortic cusps are normal and the sinotubular junction is dilated, all that is needed to reestablish valve competence is to reduce the

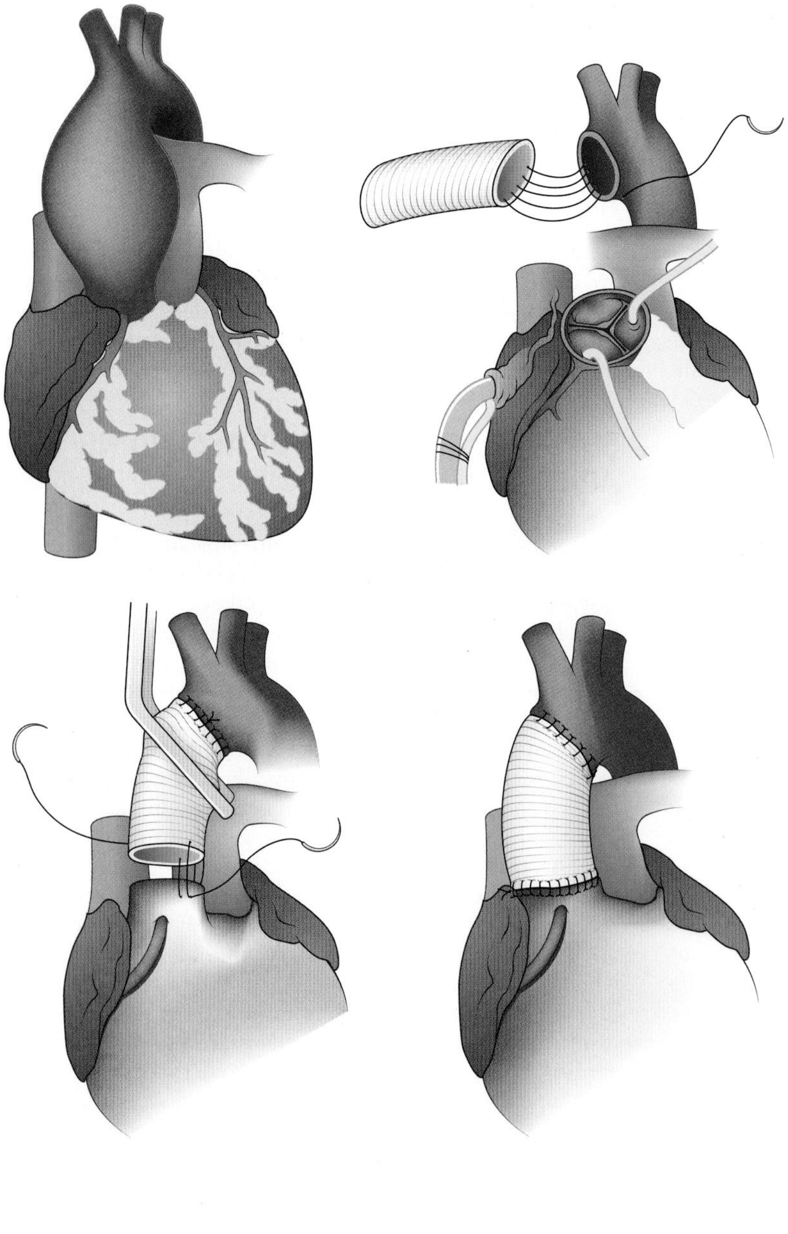

FIGURE 67-8 ■ Replacement of the ascending aorta for aneurysm.

diameter of the sinotubular junction to allow the cusps to coapt again. The ascending aorta is transected 5 mm above the sinotubular junction. All three commissures are pulled upward and approximate to each other until the cusps coapt centrally. The diameter of an imaginary circle that contains all three commissures is the correct diameter of the sinotubular junction. A graft of that diameter is then sutured to the remnants of ascending aorta wall at the level of the sinotubular junction. Because the aortic cusps are frequently of different sizes, the spaces between the commissures should reflect that during performance of the proximal anastomosis. Aortic valve competence can be assessed by injecting cardioplegia solution under pressure in the graft and observing the left ventricle for distention. In our group, we prefer to use two separate segments of grafts when aortic valve repair is necessary and the entire ascending aorta or transverse arch, or both, need replacement. We usually do the distal anastomosis first (under hypothermic circulatory arrest) and work on the aortic valve during rewarming of the patient. The distal and proximal grafts are trimmed and sutured to one another (Fig. 67-9).

If the noncoronary aortic sinus is aneurysmal, it should be replaced along with the ascending aorta. This is accomplished by selecting a graft of an appropriate diameter, as previously described, and then creating a neoaortic sinus in one of its ends. The width of the neoaortic sinus is equal to the distance between the commissures of the cusp, and the height is approximately equal to the diameter of the graft. This neoaortic sinus is sutured directly to the remnant of arterial wall and aortic annulus (Fig. 67-10).

Sometimes one aortic cusp is slightly elongated, and its free margin coapts at a level lower than the other two cusps. The free margin can be shortened by plication of the central portion along the nodule of Arantius (Fig. 67-11). If the free margin is elongated and thinned or has a fenestration near a commissure, it can be reinforced with a double layer of a 6-0 expanded polytetrafluoroethylene suture (Fig. 67-12).

Patients with a normally functioning bicuspid aortic valve, normal aortic root, and ascending aortic aneurysm can be treated with simple replacement of the ascending aorta.

Patients with aortic valve disease that is not amenable to repair and an ascending aortic aneurysm are treated with aortic valve replacement and supracoronary replacement of the ascending aorta. If only the noncoronary aortic sinus is dilated, aortic valve replacement of the ascending aorta with a graft extension into the noncoronary sinus (see Fig. 67-10) is preferable to composite

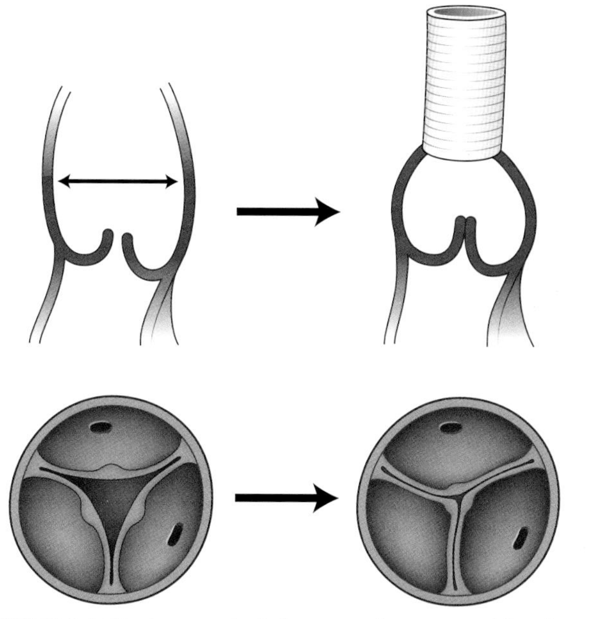

FIGURE 67-9 ■ Replacement of the ascending aorta with adjustment of the diameter of the sinotubular junction.

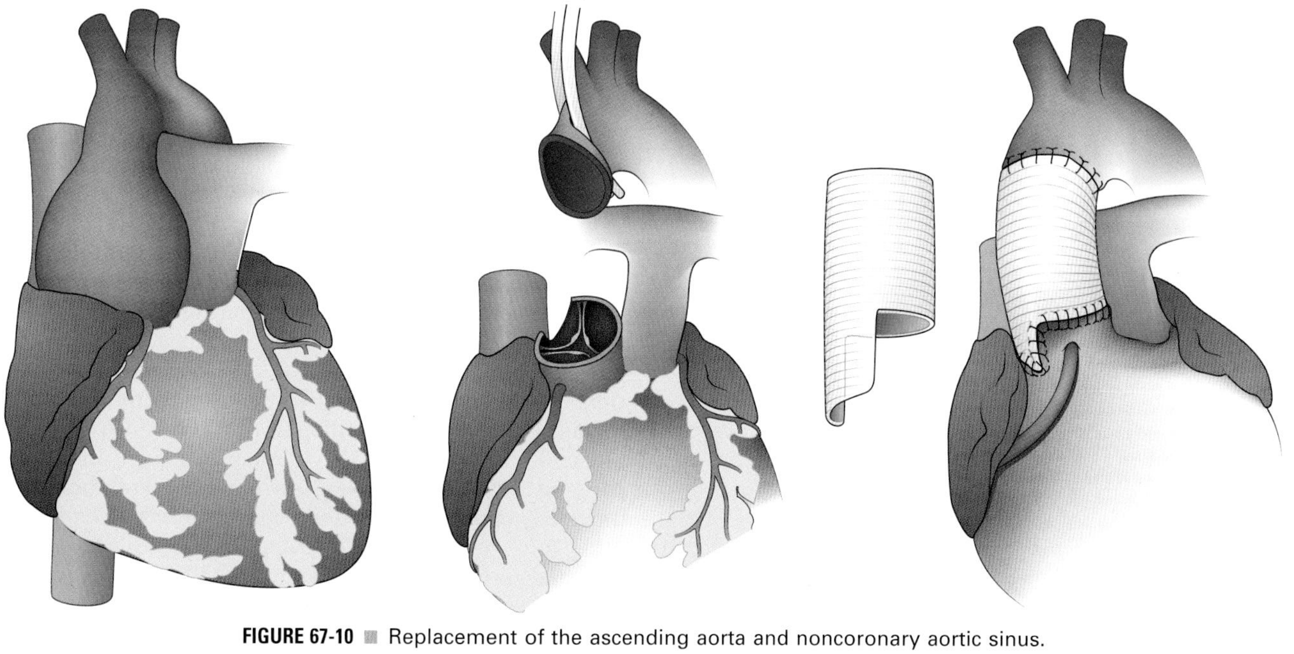

FIGURE 67-10 ■ Replacement of the ascending aorta and noncoronary aortic sinus.

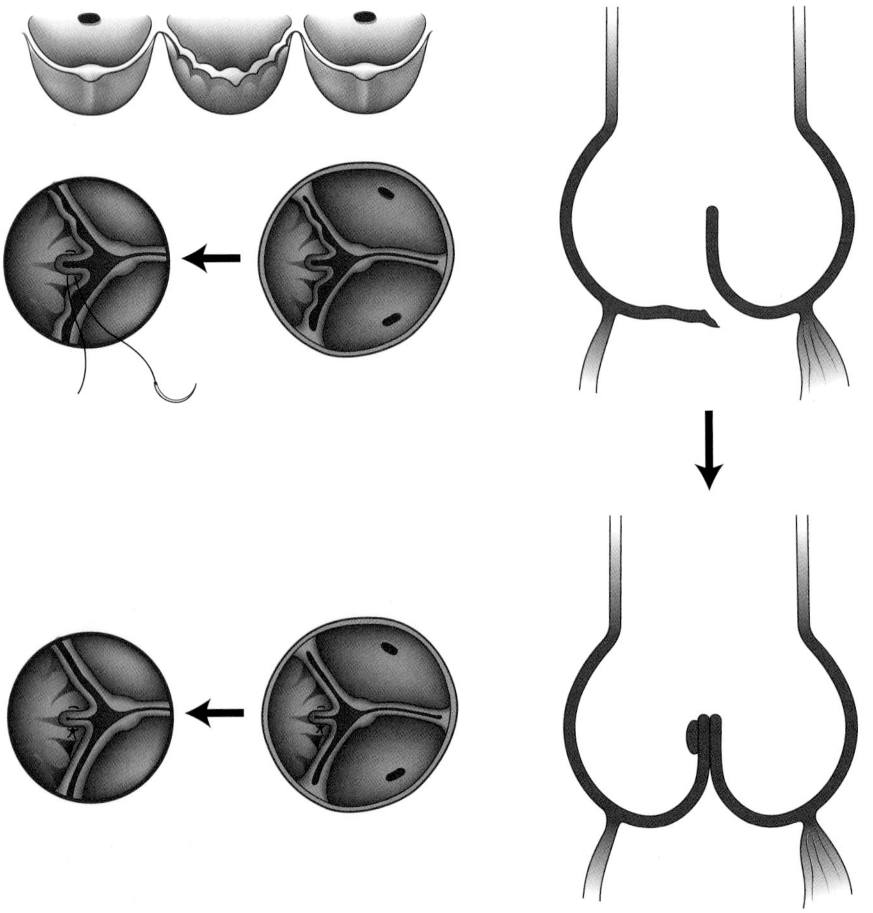

FIGURE 67-11 ■ Repair of aortic cusp prolapse by shortening its free margin.

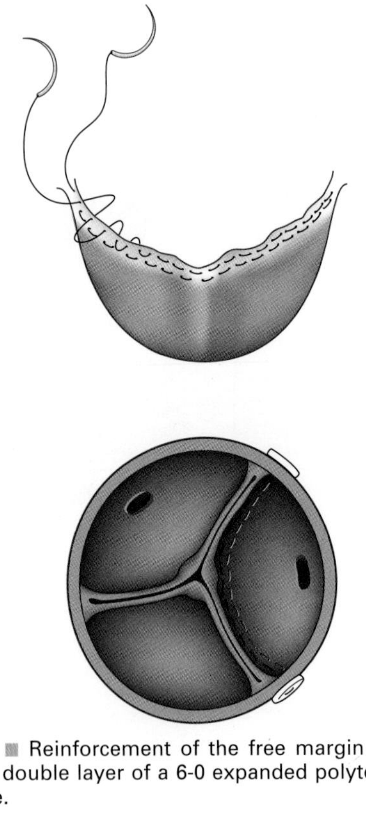

FIGURE 67-12 ■ Reinforcement of the free margin of the aortic cusp with a double layer of a 6-0 expanded polytetrafluoroethylene suture.

replacement of the aortic valve and ascending aorta with reimplantation of the coronary arteries. If two aortic sinuses are dilated, composite replacement of the aortic valve and ascending aorta with reimplantation of the coronary arteries should be performed as described for aortic root aneurysm.

Clinical Outcomes

Isolated replacement of the ascending aorta for chronic aneurysm is uncommon.[61,62] Patients with ascending aortic aneurysm often have aortic insufficiency or aortic valve disease that may also need surgical attention. Whether the operation is performed in isolation or combined with other procedures, the operative mortality for elective surgery is low.[61-64] In our experience with 103 patients who had aortic valve–sparing operations for ascending aortic aneurysm and aortic insufficiency, only one patient died perioperatively.[61] We reviewed our experience with aortic valve replacement and supracoronary replacement of the ascending aorta at Toronto General Hospital during a 12-year interval and identified 132 patients.[64] There were six operative deaths, and the series included acute aortic dissections, acute infective endocarditis, and reoperations.[64] Cohn and colleagues[62] also reported a low operative mortality for replacement of the ascending aorta. The operative mortality for ascending aortic surgery has decreased over the past four decades.[65]

Age, functional class, and associated diseases play an important role in the operative risk.

The long-term survival of our 103 patients who had aortic valve–sparing operations for ascending aortic aneurysm and aortic insufficiency was only 54% at 10 years, but most of them had extensive vascular disease including transverse aortic arch disease or mega-aorta syndrome.[61] Our patients who had aortic valve replacement and supracoronary replacement of the ascending aorta had a 10-year survival of 70%, but they were younger than those who had aortic valve repair and had less extensive vascular disease.[64]

Patients who had replacement of the ascending aorta with or without aortic valve surgery must be evaluated annually with echocardiography to assess the size of the retained aortic root and the function of the aortic valve; they should also have CT scans or MRI of the remaining thoracic and abdominal aorta. Aneurysms of the aortic root, false aneurysms, valve dysfunction, and infections in the graft or aortic valve are problems that can develop and need surgical treatment.[66]

Patients who had aortic valve repair or replacement with bioprosthetic valves do not need anticoagulation if they are in sinus rhythm. Two recent retrospective observational studies in older patients with bioprosthetic aortic valves suggested that anticoagulation during the first 6 months was associated with a survival benefit, but there was a higher risk of bleeding.[67,68] Our clinical experience does not support that, and we continue to recommend aspirin only for these patients.[69] Replacement of the ascending aorta with a tubular Dacron graft appears to have no effect on the durability of bioprosthetic heart valves.[70] Patients with mechanical valves should be anticoagulated with warfarin sodium.

SURGICAL TREATMENT OF AORTIC ROOT ANEURYSMS

Patients with Marfan syndrome and other genetically linked aortic root aneurysm should be considered for surgery when the transverse diameter of the aortic sinuses reaches 50 mm.[66] In Loeys-Dietz syndrome, the threshold is 42 mm.[66] In older patients without a known aortic genetic link, it may be appropriate to wait until the root reaches 55 mm,[66] unless the cusps are normal and an aortic valve sparing is feasible, in which case 50 mm is reasonable. As mentioned before, if there is family history of dissection, surgery should be considered at an earlier stage of dilation of the aortic root.

The aortic cusps are often normal or minimally stretched when the indication for surgery is the diameter of the aortic sinuses and an aortic valve sparing operation should be performed.[66,71] If the cusps are abnormal, composite replacement of the aortic valve and ascending aorta with reimplantation of the coronary arteries should be performed.[72]

Operative Techniques

The two basic types of aortic valve–sparing operations for patients with aortic root aneurysms are remodeling of the aortic root and reimplantation of the aortic valve.[66,71]

Remodeling of the Aortic Root

The aortic root is dissected circumferentially down to the level of the aortic annulus, and the three aortic sinuses are excised, leaving approximately 5 mm of tissue attached to the aortic annulus and around the coronary artery orifices. The three commissures are gently suspended upward and are approximated until the three cusps coapt. The diameter of an imaginary circle that includes all three commissures is approximately the diameter of the tubular Dacron graft to be used for reconstruction of the aortic sinuses (Fig. 67-13). One of the ends of this graft is tailored to create neoaortic sinuses. The widths of the neoaortic sinuses are based on the distance between commissures of each cusp when they are pulled upward to determine the diameter of the graft. The heights of the neoaortic sinuses should be approximately equal to their width. The three commissures are secured on the outside of the graft immediately above the neoaortic sinuses, and the remnants of aortic wall and aortic annulus are sutured to the neoaortic sinuses with a continuous 4-0 polypropylene (see Fig. 67-13). The coronary arteries are reimplanted into their respective sinuses. If an aortic cusp coapts at a level lower than the other two, shortening of the free margin corrects the problem (see Figs. 67-11 and 67-12).

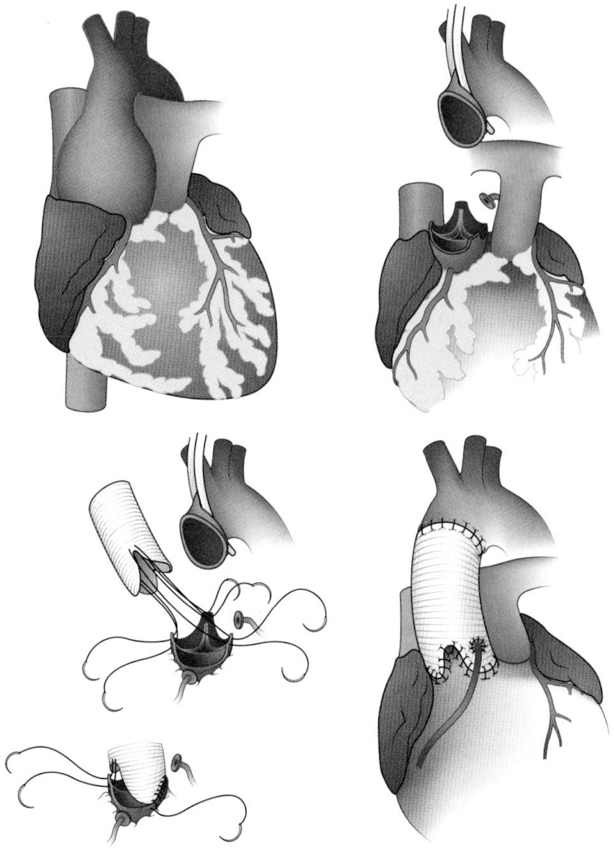

FIGURE 67-13 ■ Aortic valve–sparing operation: remodeling of the aortic root.

Reimplantation of the Aortic Valve

The aortic root is dissected circumferentially to a level immediately below the aortic annulus. This is not possible beneath the commissure between right and noncoronary aortic cusps, and it should be stopped where the right ventricle and atrium are attached to the root. Next, multiple 2-0 or 3-0 polyester sutures with Teflon felt pledgets are passed from the inside to the outside of the left ventricular outflow tract through a single horizontal plane corresponding to the lowest portion of the aortic annulus along its fibrous components and following the scalloped shape of the annulus along its muscular component and slightly less so along the membranous septum to avoid the bundle of His (Fig. 67-14). The diameter of the sinotubular junction is estimated by pulling the three commissures upward until the cusps coapt. A tubular Dacron graft 4 to 6 mm larger than the diameter of the sinotubular junction is selected, and a small triangular excision is made in one of its ends and the remaining portion is plicated in two or three places to reduce its diameter by 2 to 4 mm depending on the diameter of the aortic annulus. Most grafts that we currently use are 28 to 34 mm in diameter, depending on the size of the patient and the aortic cusps. The sutures passed through the left ventricular outflow tract are then passed from the inside to the outside of the tailored end of the graft. If reduction in diameter of the aortic annulus is desirable, it is done beneath the commissures of the noncoronary cusp. This is accomplished by placing the sutures closer in the graft than they are beneath the commissures of the noncoronary cusp. The aortic valve is placed inside the graft and all sutures are tied on the outside. The spatial distribution of these sutures is important to prevent tears or distortion of the aortic annulus. The three commissures are suspended inside the graft and secured to it with 4-0 polypropylene sutures with Teflon felt pledgets. These sutures are then used to secure the aortic annulus and remnants of the aortic sinuses to the graft. The coronary arteries are reimplanted into their respective sinuses. The spaces between commissures are plicated to create a slight bulge in the neoaortic sinuses and to reduce the diameter of the graft to that of the desirable sinotubular junction. Cusp prolapse or reinforcement of the free margin with fine Gore-Tex sutures can be done if needed (see Figs. 67-11 and 67-12).

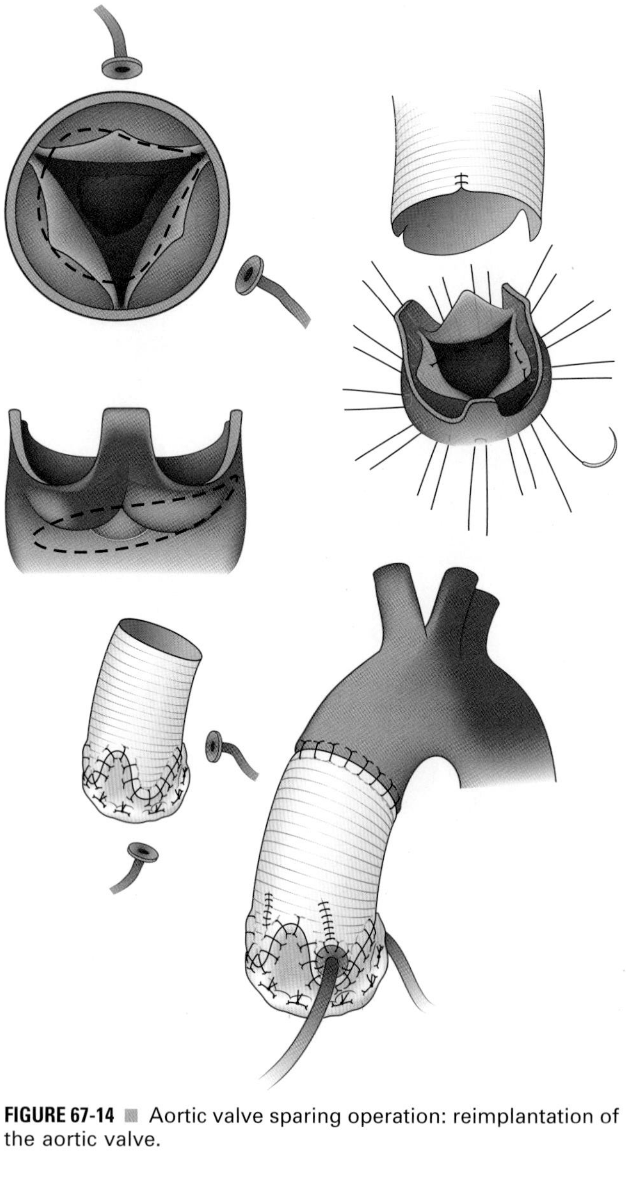

FIGURE 67-14 ■ Aortic valve sparing operation: reimplantation of the aortic valve.

Patients with a normally functioning bicuspid aortic valve and aortic root aneurysm are also candidates for aortic valve–sparing operations.

There is a commercially available Dacron graft with neo-sinuses of Valsalva.[73] Some surgeons who have wide experience with aortic valve sparing procedures have used the "Valsalva graft" for aortic valve reimplantation.[74] We have not used it because we believe that it deforms the aortic annulus, which normally evolves along a single horizontal plane. If the aortic annulus is correctly resuspended into the Valsalva graft, the annulus plane changes from a horizontal to a curved shape. This may compromise the durability of the repair.

Aortic Root Replacement

Replacement of the aortic root is performed when the aortic cusps are abnormal and cannot be safely repaired.[63,64] The aortic cusps are excised and the coronary arteries detached from their sinuses with 5 or 6 mm of aortic sinus wall around them. A valved conduit is then used to replace the aortic root. This conduit can be a commercially available Dacron tube with a mechanical valve already attached to one of its ends. The valved conduit is sutured to the aortic annulus, and the coronary arteries are reimplanted into the graft (Fig. 67-15).

An aortic homograft or a xenograft can also be used for aortic root replacement. It is not wise to use a pulmonary autograft for replacement of the aortic root in patients with aortic root aneurysms, because the pulmonary autograft may become aneurysmal when subjected to systemic pressures. Finally, aortic root replacement also can be performed with a conduit prepared in the operating room. When a stented bioprosthetic valve is desirable, the bioprosthesis and the Dacron tube can be secured to the aortic annulus using the same sutures. Another method is to secure the bioprosthetic valve

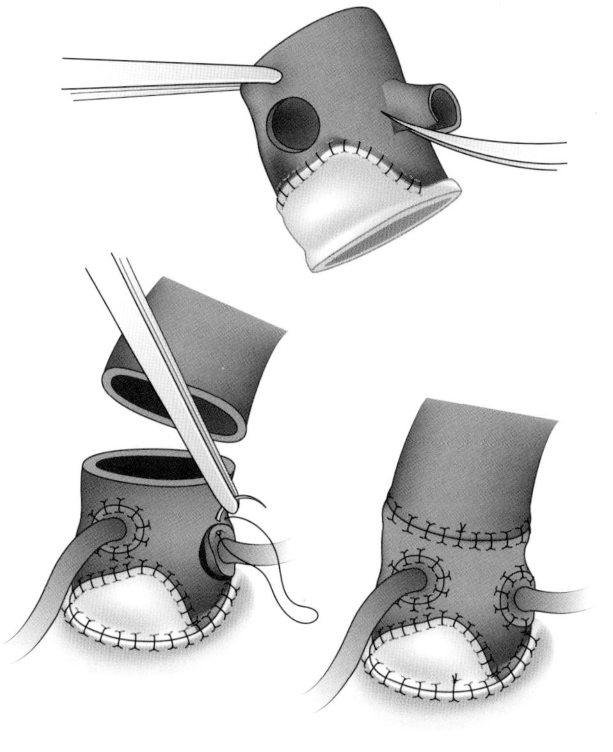

FIGURE 67-15 ■ Composite replacement of the ascending aorta and aortic valve with a stentless porcine aortic root.

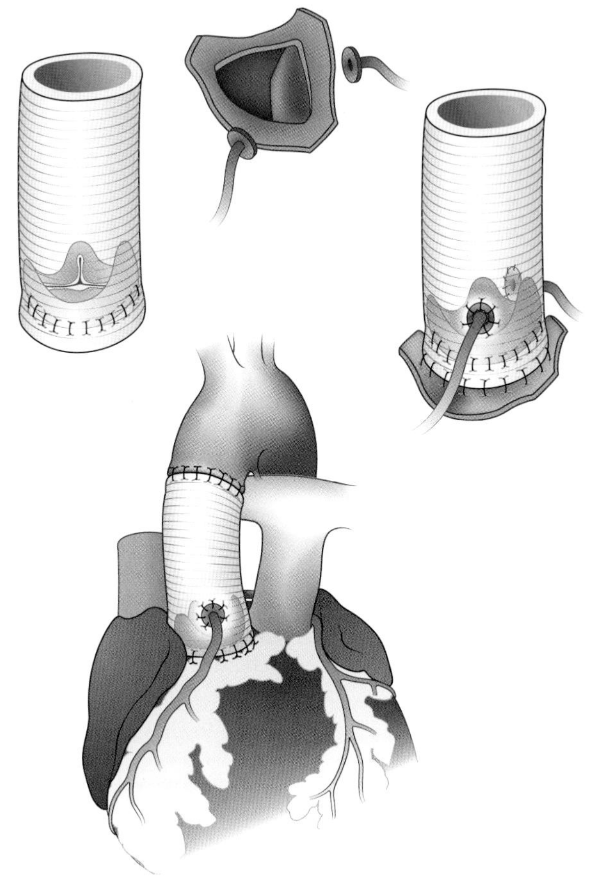

FIGURE 67-16 ■ Composite replacement of the ascending aorta and aortic valve with a bioprosthetic valve.

inside a tubular Dacron graft 1 cm from one of its ends and secure the Dacron graft alone to the annulus (Fig. 67-16). This approach allows aortic valve re-replacement without taking down the original graft or the coronary arteries when the bioprosthetic valve fails. The technique of securing a tubular Dacron graft in the left ventricular outflow tract before implanting a prosthetic valve into it is very useful when there is, for example, a narrow or destroyed aortic annulus resulting from multiple previous operations, calcification, or endocarditis. The Dacron graft can be tailored to conform to the anatomy of the left ventricular outflow tract before it is sutured to it.[75]

In the original description of aortic root replacement by Bentall and DeBono in 1968,[72] the aneurysm was opened and a tubular Teflon graft containing a mechanical valve was sutured to the aortic annulus, to the coronary arteries (by suturing the graft to the aortic sinus wall around their orifices), and to the distal aorta. The aneurysm wall was wrapped around the graft and closed tightly for hemostasis. Pseudoaneurysm formation at the coronary artery and the aortic anastomoses was a complication of this technique.[76] To decompress the space between the graft and aneurysm wall, Cabrol and colleagues[77] described the creation of a shunt between that space and the right atrium. Kouchoukos and coworkers[76] stressed the importance of not wrapping the graft with the aneurysm wall to avoid tension on the anastomoses when accumulation of blood occurs between the aneurysmal wall and the graft. They recommended an open technique in which the coronary arteries are detached from the aortic sinuses and sutured to the tubular Dacron graft.[76] Cabrol and colleagues[78] described another technique whereby the two coronary arteries were connected to each other with a smaller graft and anastomosed side to side with the valved conduit. This technique, however, has not provided long-term results that were as good as direct coronary artery reimplantation.[79]

Clinical Outcomes

Surgery for aortic root aneurysm is associated with low operative mortality and morbidity, particularly when performed electively. In a report of our experience with aortic valve sparing operations, there were only three operative deaths among 220 patients operated for aortic root aneurysms, including 24 with acute type A aortic dissection.[80] Other series showed similarly low operative mortality rates.[74,81-83] Long-term outcomes of aortic valve sparing operations have been excellent.[81-84] We recently reported our experience with aortic valve sparing operations for aortic root aneurysm in 371 patients.[85] Their mean age was 47 ± 15 years, 78% were men, 35.5% had Marfan syndrome, 12% had type A aortic dissection, and 9% had bicuspid aortic valves. Approximately one half of the patients had moderate or severe aortic insufficiency before surgery. The technique of remodeling of the aortic root was used in 75 patients and the reimplantation of the aortic valve in 226. There were 4 operative and 35 late deaths. Patients' survival at 18 years was 76.8% and approximately 10% lower than that of the general population matched for age and gender. Ten patients required reoperation on the aortic valve (5 reimplantation and 5 remodeling) for aortic insufficiency in 8 and infective endocarditis in 2. One valve was re-repaired and 9 replaced; all patients survived reoperation. The freedom from reoperation on the aortic valve at 18 years was 94.8%. Eighteen patients developed moderate or severe aortic insufficiency (12 reimplantation and 6 remodeling). Overall freedom from moderate or severe aortic insufficiency at 18 years was 78% and similar for both types of aortic valve sparing operations. These findings suggest that aortic valve sparing operations provide excellent long-term outcomes, but there is evidence of gradual deterioration in aortic valve function during the first two decades of follow-up. Patients with Marfan syndrome and other inherited aortic root aneurysms seem to have a more stable aortic valve function after reimplantation of the aortic root than after remodeling of the aortic root.[86,87] Kerchove and colleagues[88] have shown that this is also true with incompetent bicuspid aortic valves which frequently have dilated aortic annulus.

The principal cause of early failure after aortic valve sparing operations is technical errors,[89] probably because of unrecognized cusp prolapse after reconstruction of the aortic root.

It remains unknown whether aortic valve sparing operations offer a survival benefit over aortic valve replacement with either biological or mechanical valves. Comparative studies suggest similar outcomes, but most studies contain series with relatively short-term follow-up because aortic valve sparing operations are relatively new in comparison with aortic root replacement.

Aortic root replacement with valved conduit is probably more frequently performed than aortic valve sparing operations during surgical treatment of aortic root aneurysm. In a report by Gott and coworkers[90] on the outcomes of aortic root surgery in patients with Marfan syndrome operated on at 10 experienced surgical centers, the operative mortality was 1.5% among 455 patients who had elective surgery, 2.6% among 117 who had urgent surgery, and 11.7% among 103 who had emergency surgery, mostly for acute aortic dissection. However, in the experience of Gott and colleagues at the Johns Hopkins Hospital,[91] there was no operative death among 235 patients who had elective surgery and only two deaths among 36 who had urgent or emergent surgery. In our personal experience with 105 patients with Marfan syndrome in whom 44 had root replacement and 61 had aortic valve sparing, there was only one operative death, which occurred in a patient who was in preoperative cardiogenic shock because of end-stage aortic insufficiency.[92] Patients with Marfan syndrome are usually young when they require aortic root surgery, which is one reason the operative mortality is low. Surgery in older patients is associated with higher risk.[79,93] Age and clinical presentation are important determinants of outcome.[63,79,93,94] Surgery in patients with acute type A aortic dissection is associated with higher operative and late mortality (see Chapter 70). Overall, the operative mortality for aortic root replacement is around 5% to 10%.[63,64,79,93,94]

The long-term survival after aortic root replacement in patients with Marfan syndrome is very good. Gott and associates[90] reported from multiple institutions that the 10-year survival after aortic root surgery ranged from 60% to 80%, depending on the clinical presentation, but the 10-year survival was 81% in their experience at Johns Hopkins.[91]

An unresolved problem with patients with inherited aortic root aneurysms is the risk of aortic dissection late after repair of the aortic root, regardless of the technique used to repair the aortic root.[74,81,84,90,91,95]

Thromboembolism, hemorrhage, and endocarditis remain problems for patients who have aortic root replacement with mechanical valves,[79,90,92,93] and tissue degeneration and reoperation are problems for those who have a biological aortic valve.[92]

Patients who have aortic root replacement require periodic checkups including a transthoracic echocardiogram and CT scans or MRI of the residual aorta. Patients with Marfan syndrome should receive a β-blocker after repair of the aortic root aneurysm.

Reoperations in the aortic root after replacement with valved conduits can be difficult, but in the hands of experts it can be done with relatively low operative mortality.[75,96,97] When the problem is graft infection, the use of an aortic homograft is believed to offer the patient the best chance of cure.[98,99] We and others have obtained similar results by using an approach of radical resection of infected tissues and reconstruction with synthetic grafts.[100-102]

ROSS PROCEDURE

The Ross procedure is a complex operation whereby the diseased aortic valve is replaced with the patient's own normal pulmonary valve, and a biological valve, usually a pulmonary homograft, is used to replace the pulmonary valve. This operation was first described in the experimental laboratory by Lower and colleagues[103] in 1960 and clinically performed by Ross in 1967.[104] The original technique consisted of implanting the pulmonary autograft inside the aortic root in a subcoronary position. For the next two decades, Donald Ross was practically the only surgeon performing this procedure.[105] Interest in this operation increased after the initial report by Stelzer and colleagues[106] in the late 1980s, who performed it using the technique of aortic root replacement, a more reproducible method.

The Ross procedure is ideal for children because the pulmonary autograft grows with the child.[107] Although the Ross procedure can be used in patients of any age,[108] most surgeons prefer to use it in children and young adults.[109,110] Some surgeons consider it ideal for treating patients with active infective endocarditis.[111] The Ross procedure also has been performed in patients with dilated ascending aorta or even aneurysms.[112] It should not be used in patients with known genetic disorders of the proximal aorta or in patients with connective tissue disorders.

Although the Ross procedure was developed almost five decades ago, it gained popularity only in the 1990s.

According to the Society of Thoracic Surgeons Database, its peak usage in adults was in 1998 with 1.2% of all isolated aortic valve replacements; its use declined steadily to 0.09% in 2010.[113]

Operative Techniques

The three basic methods to transfer the pulmonary autograft into the aortic position are subcoronary implantation, aortic root replacement, and aortic root inclusion.

Subcoronary Implantation

The aortic valve should be exposed through a transverse aortotomy 1 cm above the sinotubular junction. The diseased aortic valve is excised, and all calcified tissues are completely débrided from the aortic annulus, membranous septum, and anterior leaflet of the mitral valve. The diameters of the aortic annulus and sinotubular junction are measured with a metric sizer. The pulmonary artery is opened just before its bifurcation, and the valve cusps are inspected. If the cusps are normal, the pulmonary root is excised. The incision in the right ventricular outflow tract is made along a single horizontal plane approximately 3 mm below the lowest level of the pulmonary annulus. Care must be exercised to prevent damage to the left anterior descending artery and the first septal perforator branch. It is difficult to measure the diameter of the pulmonary annulus because it is entirely attached to distensible muscle, but it can be estimated by measuring the diameter of the sinotubular junction of the pulmonary root. The diameter of the pulmonary annulus is 15% to 20% larger than the diameter of the sinotubular junction. If the diameters of the aortic annulus and sinotubular junction of the two roots are similar, the technique of subcoronary implantation will work well. If there is mismatch in size, an alternative technique should be used, and the difference in diameters should be corrected.[114] When the pulmonary annulus is slightly larger than the aortic annulus, it can be reduced by placing the sutures beneath the subcommissural triangles close together in the left ventricular outflow tract rather than in the pulmonary autograft. The smallest pulmonary sinus (usually the posterior sinus) should be oriented toward the left aortic sinus. The pulmonary autograft is secured to the left ventricular outflow tract and aortic annulus with multiple interrupted 4-0 polyester sutures. All sutures must be distributed precisely along a single horizontal plane at the level where the pulmonary annulus coincides with the level of the aortic annulus. We agree with Yacoub and colleagues,[115] who believe that it is important to excise the muscle beneath the commissures of the pulmonary autograft before implanting it into the left ventricular outflow tract. This makes it easier to place the pulmonary annulus to the same level of slightly below the level of the aortic annulus. One has to be meticulous about the spatial distribution of the three subcommissural spaces and maintenance of the normal scallop-shaped pulmonary annulus. Once the inflow suture line is completed, the three commissures are precisely suspended in the aortic root, and stay sutures through both arterial walls are placed immediately above the commissures. The sinuses of the pulmonary autograft that face the left and right coronary arteries are partially excised and sutured to the aortic sinuses around the coronary artery orifices with a continuous 6-0 or 5-0 polypropylene suture. The sinus of the pulmonary autograft that faces the noncoronary aortic sinus need not be excised, and it is sutured to the aortic root at the level of the sinotubular junction. It is important not to alter the diameter of the sinotubular junction of the pulmonary autograft when it is being sutured to the aortic root or when the aortotomy is closed. The right side of the heart is reconstructed with a pulmonary homograft. This homograft should be larger than the pulmonary autograft. Figure 67-17 illustrates the technique of subcoronary implantation.

Aortic Root Replacement

Aortic root replacement with a pulmonary autograft is performed as described previously for aortic root aneurysm. The aortic valve is excised and so are the sinuses, leaving 5 mm of arterial wall around the coronary artery orifices. The same steps described previously are used to harvest the pulmonary autograft and measure it. If the aortic annulus is larger than the pulmonary annulus, a reduction annuloplasty is necessary. This can be accomplished by closing the subcommissural triangles of the noncoronary sinus of the aortic root (Fig. 67-18). The pulmonary autograft is secured to the left ventricular outflow tract with simple multiple interrupted 4-0 polyester sutures along a single horizontal plane. A strip of Teflon felt in this suture line improves hemostasis and may prevent annular dilation. The coronary arteries are reimplanted into the respective sinuses. The pulmonary autograft is sutured to the ascending aorta. If the ascending aorta is dilated, it may need replacement or plication (Fig. 67-19). A strip of Dacron fabric or Teflon felt along this anastomosis prevents late dilation of the sinotubular junction.[116]

Aortic Root Inclusion

Another method of implanting the pulmonary autograft is the aortic root inclusion technique. The noncoronary aortic sinus should be incised vertically toward the aortic annulus to enhance exposure of the aortic root. The pulmonary autograft is secured to the aortic annulus using the technique described previously. After suturing the pulmonary autograft in the left ventricular outflow tract, the three commissures are pulled gently upward to determine the positions of the right and left coronary artery orifices in the pulmonary autograft. Small openings (5 or 6 mm in diameter) are made in the pulmonary autograft sinuses that correspond to the coronary artery orifices. The arterial wall of the pulmonary sinus is then sutured to the aortic sinus around the coronary artery orifices with a continuous 6-0 polypropylene suture. The three commissures of the pulmonary autograft are also sutured to the aortic wall, and the aortotomy is closed, including the aortic and pulmonary arterial walls. The incision made in the noncoronary sinus of the aortic root should be closed only if there is no bleeding between the two roots and if closure causes no distortion of the pulmonary

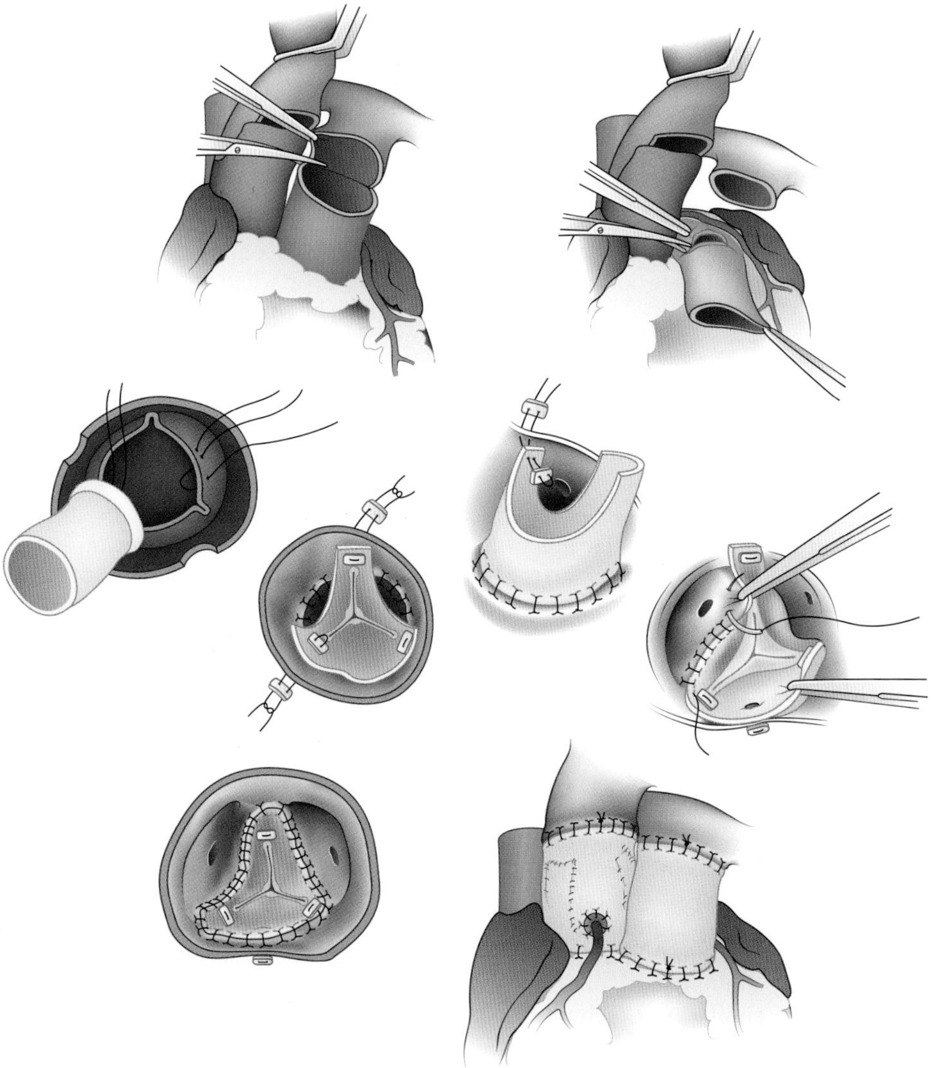

FIGURE 67-17 ■ The Ross procedure: subcoronary implantation.

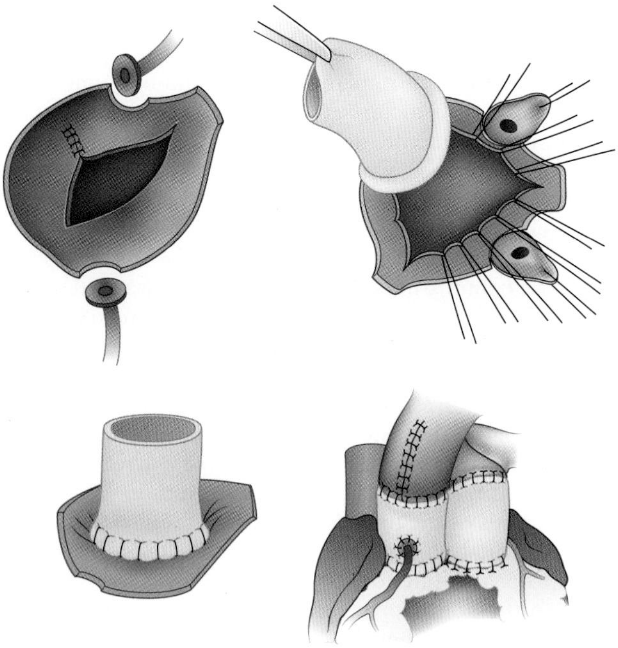

FIGURE 67-18 ■ The Ross procedure: aortic root replacement.

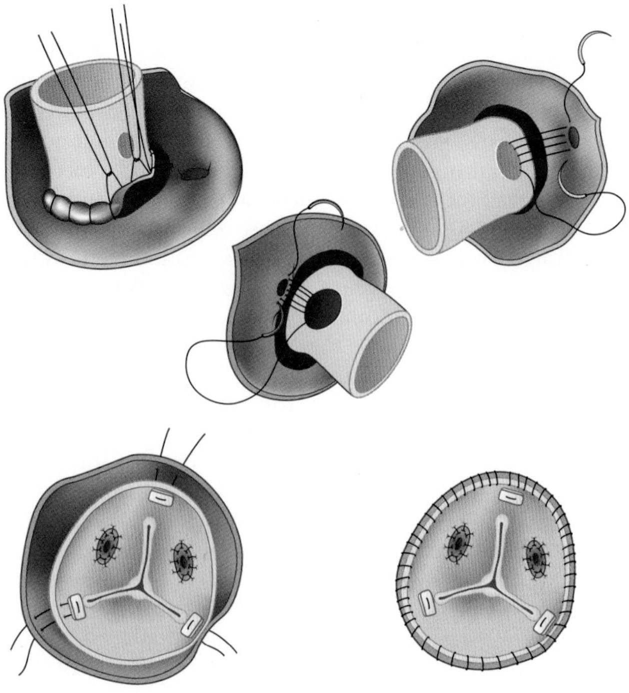

FIGURE 67-19 ■ The Ross procedure: aortic root inclusion.

autograft after unclamping the aorta. Figure 67-19 illustrates the technique of aortic root inclusion.

Clinical Outcomes

Despite its technical complexity, the operative mortality associated with the Ross procedure is reportedly low in centers with large experience.[108-110,117-119] However, in the STS Database the risk adjusted operative mortality for the Ross procedure was higher than for isolated aortic valve replacement in adults.[113] The main problem with the Ross procedure is that it can potentially transform a patient with isolated aortic valve disease to one with both aortic and pulmonary valve disease and even coronary artery disease, because they may undergo reimplantation if the technique of aortic root replacement is used. Early aortic insufficiency is usually due to technical errors.[114] Thromboembolic complications are rare because of the nature of the valves used and the patients' ages. Once the pulmonary autograft is healed in the aortic root, it should not be the source of thrombus. We have documented a few episodes of transient ischemic attacks during the first few weeks after surgery, but seldom after 2 or 3 months. The risk of infective endocarditis is also very low, and when it happens it is usually in the pulmonary homograft.[119] Subaortic false aneurysm is rare, but it may occur during the first postoperative year.[119] Long-term survival after the Ross procedure is excellent and in some series appears to be similar to that of the general population.[117-119]

Patients who had the Ross procedure should have annual Doppler echocardiography to assess the function of the neoaortic valve and pulmonary homograft, and to measure the size of the aortic root. The early development of aortic insufficiency is usually the result of technical problems,[114] and late aortic insufficiency is caused by dilation or degeneration of the pulmonary autograft.[109,110,117-119] Dilation of the aortic root is less common after the subcoronary and aortic root inclusion techniques than after aortic root replacement.[118-119] Preoperative aortic insufficiency and dilated aortic annulus (≥15 mm/m^2) are predictors of aortic insufficiency.[110,118-121] Aneurysms of the sinuses of the pulmonary autograft have been described; if the pulmonary cusps remain normal, an aortic valve sparing operation is feasible.[120,121]

We recently published our experience in a cohort of 212 patients followed prospectively with periodic assessment of valve function, and the freedom from reoperation for any reason in the pulmonary autograft was 93% at 15 years and 81.8% at 20 years.[119] Other investigators have reported similar results[117,118,122] and some reported worse outcomes.[109,110] In series by Mokhles and colleagues,[109] the freedom from reoperation on the pulmonary autograft was 51% at 18 years. The reasons for these differences in failure rates are unclear. Pathology of the aortic valve, patient age, operative technique, and surgeon experience can all play a role.[119]

Many surgeons believe that patients who have aortic root replacement with pulmonary autograft should be treated with a β-blocker or angiotensin-converting enzyme inhibitor, or both, during the first postoperative year to prevent dilation during the adaptation of the graft to systemic pressures, but there are no scientific data to support this treatment.

Another problem with the Ross procedure is dysfunction of the biological valve used to reconstruct the right ventricular outflow tract. A pulmonary homograft is probably the best conduit to use, but it is not free from complications, and a number of patients develop stenosis, insufficiency or both.[109,118-119] In our series, eight patients have required reintervention for a freedom from reoperation of 92.7% at 20 years.[119] When the homograft fails, percutaneous deployment of a stented tissue valve is often feasible, and the results are good.[108]

The usefulness of the Ross procedure remains controversial, but we believe that it is an excellent valve for women during child-bearing years and for young adults who are physically active.

REFERENCES

1. Brewer R, Deck JD, Capati B, et al: The dynamic aortic root: its role in aortic valve function. *J Thorac Cardiovasc Surg* 72:413–417, 1976.
2. Kunzelman KS, Grande J, David TE, et al: Aortic root and valve relationships: impact on surgical repair. *J Thorac Cardiovasc Surg* 107:162–170, 1994.
3. Sands MP, Rittenhouse EA, Mohri H, et al: An anatomical comparison of human, pig, calf and sheep aortic valves. *Ann Thorac Surg* 8:407–414, 1969.
4. Swanson WM, Clark RE: Dimensions and geometric relationships of the human aortic valve as a function of pressure. *Circ Res* 35:871–882, 1974.
5. Furukawa K, Ohteki H, Cao ZL, et al: Does dilatation of the sinotubular junction cause aortic insufficiency? *Ann Thorac Surg* 68:949–953, 1989.
6. Dagum P, Green GR, Nistal FJ, et al: Deformational dynamics of the aortic root: modes and physiologic determinants. *Circulation* 100(Suppl II):II-54–II-62, 1999.
7. Dart AM, Lacombe F, Yeoh JK, et al: Aortic distensibility in patients with isolated hypercholesterolemia, coronary artery disease, or cardiac transplant. *Lancet* 338:270–273, 1991.
8. Mohiaddin RH, Underwood SR, Bogren HG, et al: Regional aortic compliance studied by magnetic resonance imaging: the effects of age, training, and coronary artery disease. *Br Heart J* 62:90–96, 1989.
9. Shimojo M, Tsuda N, Iwasaka T, et al: Age-related changes in aortic elasticity determined by gated radionuclide angiography in patients with systemic hypertension or healed myocardial infarcts and in normal subjects. *Am J Cardiol* 68:950–953, 1991.
10. Coady MA, Rizzo JA, Hammond GL, et al: Surgical intervention criteria for thoracic aortic aneurysms: a study of growth rates and complications. *Ann Thorac Surg* 67:1922–1926, 1999.
11. Hirose Y, Hamada S, Takamiya M, et al: Aortic aneurysms: growth rates measured with CT. *Radiology* 185:249–252, 1992.
12. Shores J, Berger KR, Murphy EA, et al: Progression of aortic dilatation and the benefit of long-term b-adrenergic blockage in Marfan's syndrome. *N Engl J Med* 330:1335–1341, 1994.
13. Pressler V, McNamara JJ: Aneurysm of the thoracic aorta: review of 260 cases. *J Thorac Cardiovasc Surg* 89:50–54, 1985.
14. Paelinck BP, Lasbm HJ, Bax JJ, et al: Assessment of diastolic function by cardiovascular magnetic resonance. *Am Heart J* 144:198–205, 2002.
15. Blankenship J, Iliadis L: Coronary magnetic resonance angiography. *N Engl J Med* 346:1413–1414, 2002.
16. Dietz HC, Loeys BL, Carta L, et al: Recent progress towards a molecular understanding of Marfan syndrome. *Am J Med Genet* 139C:4–9, 2005.
17. Bee KJ, Wilkes D, Devereux RB, et al: Structural and functional genetic disorders of the great vessels and outflow tracts. *Ann N Y Acad Sci* 1085:256–269, 2006.
18. Ng CM, Cheng A, Myers LA, et al: TGF-β-dependent pathogenesis of mitral valve prolapse in a mouse model of Marfan syndrome. *J Clin Invest* 114:1586–1592, 2004.

19. Hirata K, Tripsokiadis F, Sparks E, et al: The Marfan syndrome: abnormal aortic properties. *J Am Coll Cardiol* 18:57–63, 1991.
20. De Paepe A, Devereux RB, Dietz HC, et al: Revised diagnostic criteria for the Marfan syndrome. *Am J Med Genet* 62:417–426, 1996.
21. Loeys BL, Dietz HC, Braverman AC, et al: The revised nosology for the Marfan syndrome. *J Med Genet* 47:476–485, 2010.
22. Hutchins GM, Moore GW, Skoog DK: The association of floppy mitral valve with disjunction of the mitral annulus fibrosus. *N Engl J Med* 14:535–540, 1996.
23. Williams A, Davies S, Stuart AG, et al: Medical treatment of Marfan syndrome: a time for change. *Heart* 94:414–421, 2008.
24. Groenink M, den Hartog AW, Franker R, et al: Losartan reduces aortic dilatation rate in adults with Marfan syndrome: a randomized controlled trial. *Eur Heart J* 2013. [Epub ahead of print].
25. Kim EK, Choi SH, Sung K, et al: Aortic diameter predicts acute type A aortic dissection in patients with Marfan syndrome but not in patients without Marfan syndrome. *J Thorac Cardiovasc Surg* 2013. [Epub ahead of print].
26. Chiu HH, Wu MH, Wang JK, et al: Losartan added to β-blockade therapy for aortic root dilation in Marfan syndrome: a randomized, open-label pilot study. *Mayo Clin Proc* 88:271–276, 2013.
27. Murdoch JL, Walker BA, Halpern BL: Life expectancy and causes of death in the Marfan syndrome. *N Engl J Med* 286:804–808, 1972.
28. Silverman DI, Burton KJ, Gray J: Life expectancy in the Marfan syndrome. *Am J Cardiol* 75:157–160, 1995.
29. Rossiter JP, Morales AJ, Repke JT, et al: A prospective longitudinal evaluation of pregnancy in the Marfan syndrome. *Am J Obstet Gynecol* 173:1599–1604, 1995.
30. Mizuguchi T, Collod-Beroud G, Akiyama T, et al: Heterozygous TGFBR2 mutations in Marfan syndrome. *Nat Genet* 36:855–860, 2004.
31. Pannu H, Fadulu VT, Chang J, et al: Mutations in transforming growth factor-beta receptor type II cause familial thoracic aortic aneurysms and dissections. *Circulation* 112:513–520, 2005.
32. Loeys BL, Chen J, Neptune ER, et al: A syndrome of altered cardiovascular, craniofacial, neurocognitive and skeletal development caused by mutations in TGFBR1 or TGFBR2. *Nat Genet* 37:275–281, 2005.
33. Williams JA, Loeys BL, Nwakanma LU, et al: Early surgical experience with Loeys-Dietz: a new syndrome of aggressive thoracic aortic aneurysm disease. *Ann Thorac Surg* 83:S757–S763, 2007.
34. Germain DP: Clinical and genetic features of vascular Ehlers-Danlos syndrome. *Ann Vasc Surg* 16(3):391–397, 2002.
35. Wenstrup RJ, Meyer RA, Lyle JS, et al: Prevalence of aortic root dilation in the Ehlers-Danlos syndrome. *Genet Med* 4:112–117, 2002.
36. Fernandez MC, Duran AC, Real R, et al: Coronary artery anomalies and aortic valve morphology in the Syrian hamster. *Lab Anim* 34:145–154, 2000.
37. Movahed MR, Hepner AD, Ahmadi-Kashani M: Echocardiographic prevalence of bicuspid aortic valve in the population. *Heart Lung Circ* 15:297–299, 2006.
38. Clementi M, Notari L, Gorghi A, et al: Familial congenital bicuspid aortic valve: a disorder of uncertain inheritance. *Am J Med Genet* 62:336–338, 1996.
39. Huntington K, Hunter AG, Char KL: A prospective study to assess the frequency of familial clustering of congenital bicuspid aortic valve. *J Am Coll Cardiol* 30:1809–1812, 1997.
40. Sievers HH, Schmidtke C: A classification system for the bicuspid aortic valve from 304 surgical specimens. *J Thorac Cardiovasc Surg* 133:1226–1233, 2007.
41. Higgins CB, Wexler L: Reversal of dominance of the coronary arterial system in isolated aortic stenosis and bicuspid aortic valve. *Circulation* 52:292–296, 1975.
42. Sadee A, Becker AE, Verheul HA, et al: Aortic valve regurgitation and the congenitally bicuspid aortic valve: a clinico-pathological correlation. *Br Heart J* 67:439–441, 1992.
43. de Sa M, Moshkovitz Y, Butany J, et al: Histologic abnormalities of the ascending aorta and pulmonary trunk in patient with bicuspid aortic valve disease: clinical relevance to the Ross procedure. *J Thorac Cardiovasc Surg* 118:588–594, 1999.
44. Niwa K, Perloff JK, Bhuta SM, et al: Structural abnormalities of great arterial walls in congenital heart disease: light and electron microscopic analyses. *Circulation* 103:393–400, 2001.
45. Edwards WD, Leaf DS, Edwards JE: Dissecting aortic aneurysm associated with congenital bicuspid aortic valve. *Circulation* 57:1022–1025, 1978.
46. Amarenco P, Cohen A, Tzourio C, et al: Atherosclerotic disease of the aortic arch and the risk of ischemic stroke. *N Engl J Med* 331:1474–1479, 1994.
47. Matsumura Y, Osaki Y, Fukui T, et al: Protruding atherosclerotic aortic plaques and dyslipidaemia: correlation to subtypes of ischaemic stroke. *Eur J Echocardiogr* 3:1–2, 2002.
48. Byrne JG, Aranki SF, Cohn LH: Aortic valve operations under deep hypothermic circulatory arrest for the porcelain aorta: "no touch" technique. *Ann Thorac Surg* 65:1313–1315, 1998.
49. Yasuda T, Kawasuji M, Sakakibara N, et al: Aortic valve replacement for calcified ascending aorta in homozygous familial hypercholesterolemia. *Eur J Cardiothorac Surg* 18:249–250, 2000.
50. Heggtveit HA: Syphilitic aortitis: a clinicopathologic autopsy study of 100 cases, 1950 to 1960. *Circulation* 29:346–352, 1994.
51. Kerr LD, Chang YJ, Spiera H, et al: Occult active giant cell aortitis necessitating surgical repair. *J Thorac Cardiovasc Surg* 120:813–815, 2000.
52. Klein RG, Hunder GG, Stanson AW, et al: Larger artery involvement in giant cell (temporal) arteritis. *Ann Intern Med* 83:806–812, 1975.
53. Lupi-Herrera E, Sanches-Torres G, Marcushamer J, et al: Takayasu's arteritis: clinical study of 107 cases. *Am Heart J* 93:94–103, 1977.
54. Nesi G, Anichini C, Pedemonte E, et al: Giant cell arteritis presenting with annuloaortic ectasia. *Chest* 121:1365–1367, 2002.
55. Rojo-Leyva F, Ratliff NB, Cosgrove DM, 3rd, et al: Study of 52 patients with idiopathic aortitis from a cohort of 1,204 surgical cases. *Arthritis Rheum* 43:901–907, 2000.
56. Ueno A, Awane G, Wakabayachi A: Successfully operated obliterative brachiocephalic arteritis (Takayasu) associated with elongated coarctation. *Jpn Heart* 8:538–544, 1967.
57. Fyfe BS, Quintana CS, Kaneka M, et al: Aortic sarcoma four years after Dacron graft insertion. *Ann Thorac Surg* 58:1752–1754, 1994.
58. Wright EP, Glick AD, Virmani R, et al: Aortic intimal sarcoma with embolic metastases. *Am J Surg Pathol* 9:950–957, 1985.
59. Feczko JD, Lynch L, Pless JE, et al: An autopsy case review of 142 nonpenetrating (blunt) injuries to the aorta. *J Trauma* 33:846–849, 1992.
60. Svensson LG, Adams DH, Bonow RD, et al: Aortic valve and ascending aorta guidelines for management and quality measures: executive summary. *Ann Thorac Surg* 95:1491–1505, 2013.
60a. Nishimura RA, Otto CM, Bonow RO, et al: 2014 AHA/ACC guideline for the management of patients with valvular heart disease: executive summary: a report of the American College of Cardiology/American Heart Association Task Force on Practice Guidelines. *Circulation* 129:2440–2492, 2014.
61. David TE, Feindel CM, Armstrong S, et al: Replacement of the ascending aorta with reduction of the diameter of the sinotubular junction to treat aortic insufficiency in patients with ascending aortic aneurysm. *J Thorac Cardiovasc Surg* 133:414–418, 2007.
62. Cohn LH, Rizzo RJ, Adams DH, et al: Reduced mortality and morbidity for ascending aortic aneurysm resection regardless of cause. *Ann Thorac Surg* 62:463–468, 1996.
63. Kouchoukos NT, Wareing TH, Murphy SF, et al: Sixteen-year experience with aortic root replacement. *Ann Surg* 214:308–320, 1991.
64. Sioris T, David TE, Ivanov J, et al: Clinical outcomes after separate and composite replacement of the aortic valve and ascending aorta. *J Thorac Cardiovasc Surg* 128:260–265, 2004.
65. Lawrie GM, Earle N, DeBakey ME: Long-term fate of the aortic root and aortic valve after ascending aneurysm surgery. *Ann Surg* 217:711–720, 1993.
66. David TE: Remodeling of the aortic root and preservation of the native aortic valve. *Oper Tech Cardiovasc Thorac Surg* 1:44–56, 1996.
67. Brennan JM, Edwards FH, Zhao Y, et al: Early anticoagulation of bioprosthetic aortic valves in older patients. Results from the

Society of Thoracic Surgeons Adult Cardiac Surgery National Database. *J Am Coll Cardiol* 60:971–977, 2012.
68. Merie C, Kober L, Olsen PS, et al: Association of warfarin therapy duration after bioprosthetic aortic valve replacement with risk of mortality, thromboembolic complications, and bleeding. *JAM* 308:2118–2125, 2012.
69. David TE, Armstrong S, Maganti M: Hancock II bioprosthesis for aortic valve replacement: the gold standard of bioprosthetic valves durability? *Ann Thorac Surg* 90:775–781, 2010.
70. Garrido-Olivares L, Maganti M, Armstrong S, et al: Aortic valve replacement with Hancock II bioprothesis with and without replacement of the ascending aorta. *Ann Thorac Surg* 92:541–547, 2011.
71. David TE: Surgery of the aortic valve. *Curr Probl Surg* 36:421–504, 1999.
72. Bentall HH, DeBono A: A technique of complete replacement of the ascending aorta. *Thorax* 23:338–339, 1968.
73. De Paulis R, De Matteis GM, Nardi P, et al: One-year appraisal of a new aortic root conduit with sinuses of Valsalva. *J Thorac Cardiovasc Surg* 123:33–39, 2002.
74. Patel ND, Weiss ES, Alejo DE, et al: Aortic root operations for Marfan syndrome: a comparison of the Bentall and valve-sparing procedures. *Ann Thorac Surg* 85:2003–2010, 2008.
75. Krasopoulos G, David TE, Armstrong S: Custom-tailored valved conduit for complex aortic root disease. *J Thorac Cardiovasc Surg* 135:3–7, 2008.
76. Kouchoukos NT, Marshall WG, Jr, Wedige-Stecher TA: Eleven-year experience with composite graft replacement of the ascending aorta and aortic valve. *J Thorac Cardiovasc Surg* 92:691–705, 1986.
77. Cabrol C, Pavie A, Gandjbakhch I, et al: Complete replacement of the ascending aorta with reimplantation of the coronary arteries: new surgical approach. *J Thorac Cardiovasc Surg* 81:309–315, 1981.
78. Cabrol C, Pavie A, Mesnildrey P, et al: Long-term results with total replacement of the ascending aorta and reimplantation of the coronary arteries. *J Thorac Cardiovasc Surg* 91:17–25, 1986.
79. Bachet K, Termignon JL, Goudot B, et al: Aortic root replacement with a composite graft: factors influencing immediate and long-term results. *Eur J Cardiothorac Surg* 10:207–213, 1996.
80. David TE, Feindel CM, Webb GD, et al: Long-term results of aortic valve-sparing operations for aortic root aneurysm. *J Thorac Cardiovasc Surg* 132:347–354, 2006.
81. Shrestha M, Baraki H, Maeding I, et al: Long-term results after aortic valve-sparing operation (David I). *Eur J Cardiothorac Surg* 41:56–61, 2012.
82. De Paulis R, et al: Use of the Valsalva graft and long-term follow-up. *J Thorac Cardiovasc Surg* 140(Suppl 6):S23–S27, 2012.
83. Yacoub MH, Gehle P, Chandrasekaran V, et al: Late results of a valve-preserving operation in patients with aneurysms of the ascending aorta and root. *J Thorac Cardiovasc Surg* 115:1080–1090, 1998.
84. David TE, Armstrong S, Maganti M, et al: Long-term results of aortic valve-sparing operations in patients with Marfan syndrome. *J Thorac Cardiovasc Surg* 138:859–864, 2009.
85. David TE, Feindel CM, David CM, et al: A quarter of century experience with aortic valve sparing operations. *J Thorac Cardiovasc Surg* 148:872–879, 2015.
86. Hanke T, Charitos EI, Stierle U, et al: Factors associated with the development of aortic valve regurgitation over time after two different techniques of valve-sparing aortic root surgery. *J Thorac Cardiovasc Surg* 137:314–319, 2009.
87. Liu L, Wang W, Wang X, et al: Reimplantation versus remodeling: a meta-analysis. *J Card Surg* 26:82–87, 2011.
88. de Kerchove L, et al: Valve sparing-root replacement with the reimplantation technique to increase the durability of bicuspid aortic valve repair. *J Thorac Cardiovasc Surg* 142:1430–1438, 2011.
89. Oka T, Okita Y, Matsumori M, et al: Aortic regurgitation after valve-sparing aortic root replacement: modes of failure. *Ann Thorac Surg* 92:1639–1644, 2011.
90. Gott VL, Greene PS, Alejo DE, et al: Replacement of the aortic root in patients with Marfan's syndrome. *N Engl J Med* 340:1307–1313, 1999.
91. Gott VL, Cameron DE, Alejo DE, et al: Aortic root replacement in 271 Marfan patients: a 24-year experience. *Ann Thorac Surg* 73:438–443, 2002.
92. de Oliveira NC, David TE, Ivanov J, et al: Results of surgery for aortic root aneurysm in patients with the Marfan syndrome. *J Thorac Cardiovasc Surg* 125:1143–1152, 2003.
93. Mingke D, Dresler C, Stone CD, et al: Composite graft replacement of the aortic root in 335 patients with aneurysm or dissection. *Thorac Cardiovasc Surg* 46:12–19, 1998.
94. Dossche KM, Schepens MA, Morshuis WJ, et al: A 23-year experience with composite valve graft replacement of the aortic root. *Ann Thorac Surg* 67:1070–1077, 1999.
95. Schoenhoff FS, Jungi S, Czerny M, et al: Acute aortic dissection determines the fate of initially untreated aortic segments in Marfan syndrome. *Circulation* 127:1569–1575, 2013.
96. LeMaire SA, DiBardino DJ, Koksoy C, et al: Proximal aortic reoperations in patients with composite valve grafts. *Ann Thorac Surg* 74:S1777–S1780, 2002.
97. Raanani E, David TE, Dellgren G, et al: Redo aortic root replacement: experience with 31 patients. *Ann Thorac Surg* 71:1460–1463, 2001.
98. Lytle BW, Sabik JF, Blackstone EH, et al: Reoperative cryopreserved root and ascending aorta replacement for acute aortic prosthetic valve endocarditis. *Ann Thorac Surg* 74:S1754–S1757, 2002.
99. Vogt PR, Brunner-LaRocca HP, Carrel T, et al: Cryopreserved arterial allografts in the treatment of major vascular infection: a comparison with conventional surgical techniques. *J Thorac Cardiovasc Surg* 116:965–972, 1998.
100. Hagl C, Galla JD, Lansman SL, et al: Replacing the ascending aorta and aortic valve for acute prosthetic valve endocarditis: is using prosthetic material contraindicated? *Ann Thorac Surg* 74:S1781–S1785, 2002.
101. Ralph-Edwards A, David TE, Bos J: Infective endocarditis in patients who had replacement of the aortic root. *Ann Thorac Surg* 35:429–433, 1994.
102. David TE, Regesta T, Gavra G, et al: Surgical treatment of paravalvular abscess: long-term results. *Eur J Cardiothorac Surg* 31:43–48, 2007.
103. Lower RR, Stoffer RC, Shumway NE: Autotransplantation of the pulmonic valve into the aorta. *J Thorac Cardiovasc Surg* 39:680–687, 1960.
104. Ross DN: Replacement of aortic and mitral valves with a pulmonary autograft. *Lancet* 2:956–958, 1967.
105. Matsuki O, Okita Y, Almeida RS, et al: Two decades' experience with aortic valve replacement with pulmonary autograft. *J Thorac Cardiovasc Surg* 95:705–711, 1988.
106. Stelzer P, Jones DJ, Elkins RC: Aortic root replacement with pulmonary autograft. *Circulation* 80(Suppl III):III209–III213, 1988.
107. Elkins RC, Knott-Craig CJ, Ward KE, et al: Pulmonary autograft in children: realized growth potential. *Ann Thorac Surg* 57:1387–1394, 1994.
108. Chemidtke C, Bechtel MF, Noetzold A, et al: Up to seven years experience with the Ross procedure in patients >60 years of age. *J Am Coll Cardiol* 36:1173–1177, 2000.
109. Mokhles MM, Rizopoulos D, Andrinopoulou ER, et al: Autograft and pulmonary allograft performance in the second post-operative decade after the Ross procedure: insights from the Rotterdam Prospective Cohort Study. *Eur Heart J* 33:2213–2224, 2012.
110. Elkins RC, Thompson DM, Lane MM, et al: Ross operation: 16-year experience. *J Thorac Cardiovasc Surg* 136:623–630, 2008.
111. Oswalt JD, Dewan SJ, Mueller MC, et al: Highlights of a ten-year experience with the Ross procedure. *Ann Thorac Surg* 71:S332–S335, 2001.
112. Elkins RC, Lane MM, McCue C: Ross procedure for ascending aortic replacement. *Ann Thorac Surg* 67:1843–1845, 1999.
113. Reece TB, Welke KF, O'Brien S, et al: Rethinking the Ross Procedure in Adults. *Ann Thorac Surg* 2013. [Epub ahead of print].
114. David TE, Omran A, Webb G, et al: Geometric mismatch of the aortic and pulmonary roots causes aortic insufficiency after the Ross procedure. *J Thorac Cardiovasc Surg* 112:1231–1239, 1996.
115. Yacoub MH, Klieverik LM, Melina G, et al: An evaluation of the Ross operation in adults. *J Heart Valve Dis* 15:531–539, 2006.

116. David TE, Omran A, Ivanov J, et al: Dilation of the pulmonary autograft after the Ross procedure. *J Thorac Cardiovasc Surg* 119:210–220, 2000.
117. Weimar T, Charitos EI, Liebrich M, et al: Quo vadis pulmonary autograft—the Ross procedure in its second decade: a single-center experience in 645 patients. *Ann Thorac Surg* 2013. [Epub ahead of print].
118. Skillington PD, Mokhles MM, Takkenberg JJ, et al: Twenty-year analysis of autologous support of the pulmonary autograft in the Ross procedure. *Ann Thorac Surg* 96:823–829, 2013.
119. David TE, David C, Woo A, et al: The Ross procedure: outcomes at 20 years. *J Thorac Cardiovasc Surg* 147:85–93, 2014.
120. Schmidtke C, Stierle U, Sievers HH: Valve-sparing aortic root remodeling for pulmonary autograft aneurysm. *J Heart Valve Dis* 123:437–441, 2002.
121. Sundt TM, Moon MR, Xu R: Reoperation for dilatation of the pulmonary autograft after the Ross procedure. *J Thorac Cardiovasc Surg* 122:1249–1252, 2001.
122. Charitos EI, Stierle U, Hanke T, et al: Long-term results of 203 young and middle-aged patients with more than 10 years of follow-up after the original subcoronary Ross operation. *Ann Thorac Surg* 93:495–502, 2012.

CHAPTER 68

SURGERY OF THE AORTIC ARCH

Michael Z. Tong • Lars G. Svensson

CHAPTER OUTLINE

The history of cardioaortic surgery has been replete with new techniques for ascending and aortic arch repairs since 1956, when Denton Cooley and Michael DeBakey replaced the ascending aorta with a homograft using cardiac bypass.[1,2] In 1957, DeBakey and colleagues first described aortic arch replacement using antegrade brain perfusion.[3] Before this, one of the few successful ascending aortic repairs was reported in 1932 by Blalock, who repaired a stab wound of the ascending aorta caused by an ice pick.[4] By removing the occluding clot, Blalock noted the "bright red blood that shot over the screen at the head of the table on the anesthetist's clothes." Using only nitrous oxide and oxygen for anesthesia in a patient with cardiac tamponade most likely contributed to the hypertension and description of the procedure.

With the advent of cardiopulmonary bypass, many technical problems of aortic arch surgery were largely overcome. In 1950, Bigelow first published the results of his experiments in dogs using deep hypothermia for cardiovascular operations without cardiopulmonary bypass.[4] Nonetheless, it was not until 1963 that Barnard combined deep hypothermia with circulatory arrest and cardiopulmonary bypass for aortic arch operations and dissection.[5] In 1964, Borst reported using deep hypothermia and circulatory arrest to repair an arteriovenous fistula between the innominate vein and the aorta caused by shrapnel.[4] The routine use of deep hypothermia and circulatory arrest did not, however, become popular until 1975, when Griepp reported a series of aortic arch replacements using deep hypothermia and circulatory arrest.[4] In 1983, Borst and colleagues[6,7] and others[8] reported replacing the aortic arch and leaving a tube graft lying free in the descending aorta, which they called the elephant trunk technique. In 1990, Crawford and Svensson[4,9] reported replacement of the entire aorta as a staged procedure using a modified elephant trunk technique. The modification of inverting the graft into the descending aorta while sewing the distal anastomosis resulted in a more secure anastomosis with less risk of bleeding or rupture. Subsequently, in 1993, Svensson and colleagues[4] successfully replaced the entire aorta from the aortic valve to the aortic bifurcation during a single operation using a combined mediastinal and thoracoabdominal incision with deep hypothermia and circulatory arrest.[3]

Aortic arch surgery has become relatively common and safe, with a mortality risk of 2% and a stroke risk of 2%.[10] In 2012, we performed 1282 aorta operations: 1065 on the thoracic aorta and 724 on the ascending aorta and aortic arch. Our approach is discussed later. In this chapter, we discuss the potential causes of aortic arch aneurysms, the association with some pathologic entities, diagnostic workup, brain protection, perfusion methods, different operative approaches, and outcomes after aortic arch surgery.

DEFINITIONS AND CLASSIFICATION

Anatomically, the aortic arch is defined as the segment of aorta between a line at a right angle proximal to the innominate artery origin and extending to a line drawn at a right angle distal to the origin of the left subclavian artery. Aneurysms are irreversible dilations of the aorta exceeding the normal diameter for the age and height of the patient.[4] The exact size at which the aorta is labeled "aneurysmal" varies. Definitions vary from 1.5 times to twice the normal diameter of the aorta. For patients with Marfan syndrome, we suggest that when the cross-sectional area (in square centimeters) divided by the patient's height (in meters) exceeds a ratio of 10, it should be considered significant and an indication that the patient requires surgical repair.[11] Thus, in some respect, the definition of an aneurysm is not absolute but rather refers to the significant dilation of the aorta.

Aneurysms can be divided further into aortic aneurysms without penetration through the aortic adventitia (true aneurysms) and those that penetrate through the adventitia and are contained by the surrounding tissue, which prevents exsanguination of the patient (false aneurysms).[4] In addition, aneurysms are classified according to their likely causes: medial degenerative aneurysms (typically showing loss of elastic tissue); those related to aortic dissection; other disorders of connective tissue, particularly loss of collagen as in Ehlers-Danlos syndrome or loss of elastic tissue as in Marfan syndrome; those associated with blunt trauma; aortitis; primary aortic infections or after previous cardiovascular surgery, especially graft infection in the ascending aorta; and congenital abnormalities.[4]

We prefer the term *medial degenerative aneurysms* to *atherosclerotic aneurysms* simply because not all medial degenerative aneurysms have atherosclerosis.[4] Furthermore, atherosclerosis does not necessarily appear to be the sole causative factor in the development of medial degenerative aneurysms. It appears that atheroma formation, fibrosis, and calcification are results of degeneration that follow the primary injurious event that caused the aneurysm.

Aneurysms can be either fusiform, showing uniform dilation, or saccular in appearance.[4] The three most common sites for saccular aneurysms are on the lesser curve of the aortic arch, on the descending aorta, and opposite the visceral vessels.[4] The saccular aneurysms in the aortic arch are usually related to penetrating ulcers, often with localized dissection or mycotic aneurysm formation.[4] Fusiform aneurysms of the aortic arch are typically associated with dilation of the ascending aorta, particularly when associated with inflammatory aortitis. Medial degenerative aneurysms of the root are known as *annuloaortic ectasia*, a term coined by Cooley.[4] This results in a flasklike or hourglass appearance of the aortic root (Erdheim deformity), which is also associated, in particular, with Marfan syndrome. For example, in patients with Marfan syndrome, initiation of aortic root dilation results early in the annuloaortic ectasia stage, and, if it is not treated, there is subsequent development of aortic root, ascending aorta, and aortic arch aneurysm formation. In fact, at this late stage, aortic dissection often precedes aortic arch aneurysm formation.

The human artery consists of five distinct layers. The first or innermost layer (the endothelial layer, which lies on a basement membrane) is known as the tunica intima. Between the tunica intima and the tunica media is a fenestrated sheath of elastic fibers known as the internal elastic lamina. The tunica media has several layers of elastic-tissue lamellae arranged concentrically along the length of the aorta, and it forms the bulk of the aortic wall. The amount of elastic tissue decreases in amount from the sinotubular ridge as the aorta progresses down to the aortic bifurcation. In the tunica media lie smooth muscle cells and the ground substance of the aorta. The latter consists of proteoglycans. The outer third of the tunica media receives its nutrition from the vasa vasorum, lymphatics, and nerves. On the outside of the tunica media is the external elastic lamina, which separates the media from the adventitia. The tunica adventitia consists of strong, tough layers of collagen and elastic fibers. Because of its strength, this is the critical layer wherein the surgeon must suture the graft placement.[4]

No clear, systematic classification of aortic pathology appears in the literature, and different pathologists have coined various terms. We favor a definition of aortic pathology based on hematoxylin and eosin (H&E) findings and elastic tissue stains. Thus, medial degenerative disease is defined as a loss of elastic fibers, and medial necrosis as a loss of smooth muscle cells. The presence of atherosclerosis superimposed on degenerative disease is described as atherosclerotic with or without calcification. Atheroma is also frequently superimposed. Inflammatory disease is diagnosed when there is evidence of chronic inflammatory cell infiltrates. The intima and adventitia may also show various degrees of hyperplasia.[4]

CAUSATIVE AND PREDISPOSING FACTORS

Congenital Aneurysms

Congenital aneurysms of the aortic arch are extremely rare, although they may be associated with aberrant right subclavian arteries from a Kommerell diverticulum situated in either the distal aortic arch or the proximal descending aorta (Figs. 68-1 and 68-2).[4] Similarly, aneurysms can be associated with one of two types of right-sided congenital arches. For the Felson and Palayew type I right-sided arches, a vascular ring encircles and compresses the esophagus and trachea (Fig. 68-3).[12] The distal arch and descending aorta may be aneurysmal. In patients with type II right-sided arches (Fig. 68-4), the anatomy is basically a mirror image of an aberrant right subclavian artery with a Kommerell diverticulum. Thus, an aberrant left subclavian artery comes off the right-sided descending aorta.[12] More frequently, however, the aortic arch, in association with these two varieties, is hypoplastic unless the hypoplasia is severe enough to cause aortic stenosis, and prestenosis or poststenosis aneurysm formation occurs. Coarctation of the aorta is often associated with a bicuspid valve and an ascending aortic aneurysm, but, if left untreated, it may be associated with aortic arch aneurysm formation. A history of patent ductus arteriosus or ventricular septal defect may also be noted. More rarely, adult patients who have been

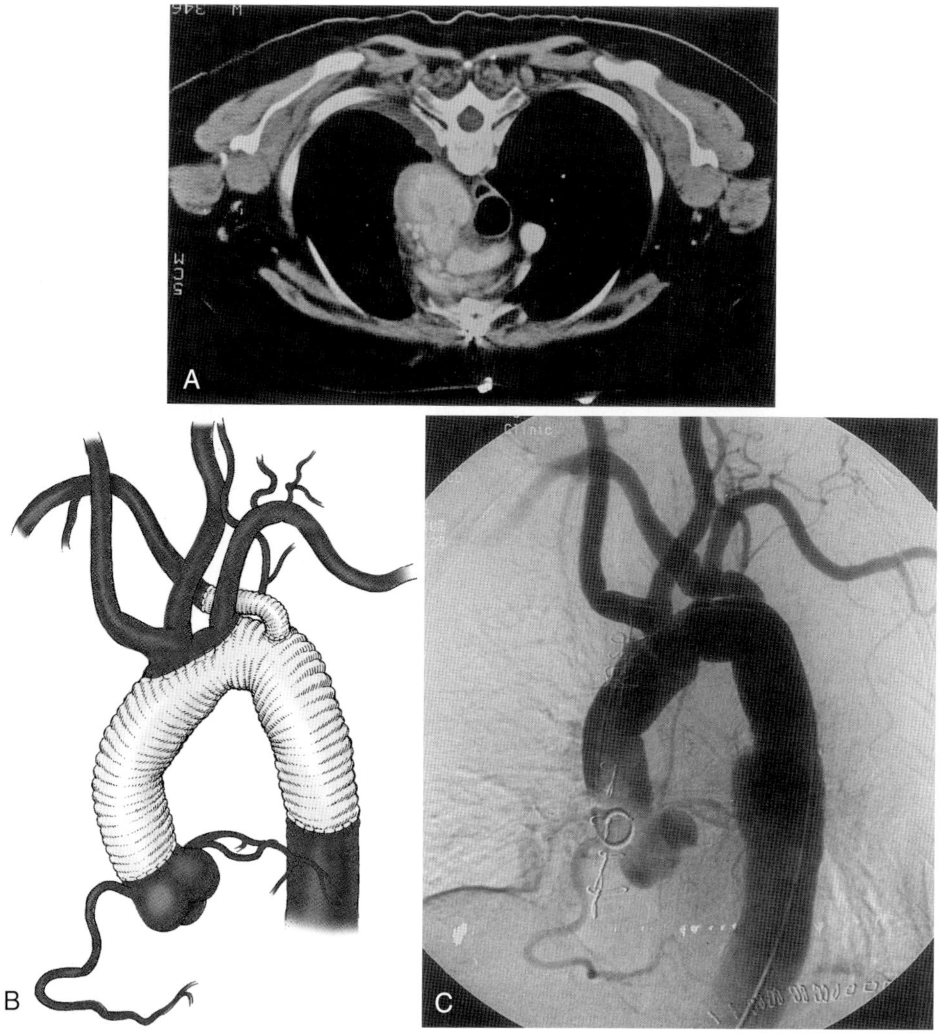

FIGURE 68-1 ■ A, Computed tomography scan of an aortic arch aneurysm associated with an aberrant right subclavian artery that was treated by a modified elephant trunk technique. B, The first stage of the elephant trunk procedure was done with an anastomosis between the left subclavian artery and the aberrant right subclavian artery, and the second stage was performed with an interposition graft to the right subclavian artery. C, Angiogram of the completed repair. Note the tube graft to the right subclavian artery arising from the more distal part of the aortic arch.

previously operated on for an interrupted aortic arch can develop ascending and aortic arch aneurysms.[4]

Medial Degenerative Aneurysms

Medial degenerative aneurysms typically occur in older adult patients who were long-term smokers or have a long history of hypertension. If the smoking history is severe and there is presence of chronic obstructive pulmonary disease (COPD), extensive atheroma formation may also be found in the aneurysms. These types of aneurysms, with extensive atheroma and atherosclerosis formation, typically involve not only the ascending aorta and the aortic arch but also the descending and thoracoabdominal aorta. Coronary artery disease and carotid artery disease are also common associations. When the aorta is inspected, small ulcers are often observed, and these can later form penetrating ulcers that result in dissection in the medial adventitial plane or false aneurysm formation if the adventitia is penetrated.[4] Less typically, medial degenerative aneurysms are associated with systemic inflammatory disease and various types of arthritis or vasculitis (see Vasculitis and Aortitis, later).

Aortic Dissection

The DeBakey and Stanford classifications of aortic dissection differ, and there are also different classes of dissection (Fig. 68-5)[13] regarding replacement of the aortic arch. The class of intimal tear also influences the aortic arch repair technique.[13]

Mycotic Aneurysms

For reasons not entirely clear, true primary mycotic aneurysms of the aorta, as described by Svensson and Crawford,[4] have a tendency to occur either on the lesser curve of the aortic arch, with a variable extent of involvement, or opposite the visceral vessels in the abdomen. It is unclear whether this is related to the structure of the aorta or to the flow patterns that result in turbulence in these areas opposite the branches of the aorta. The typical

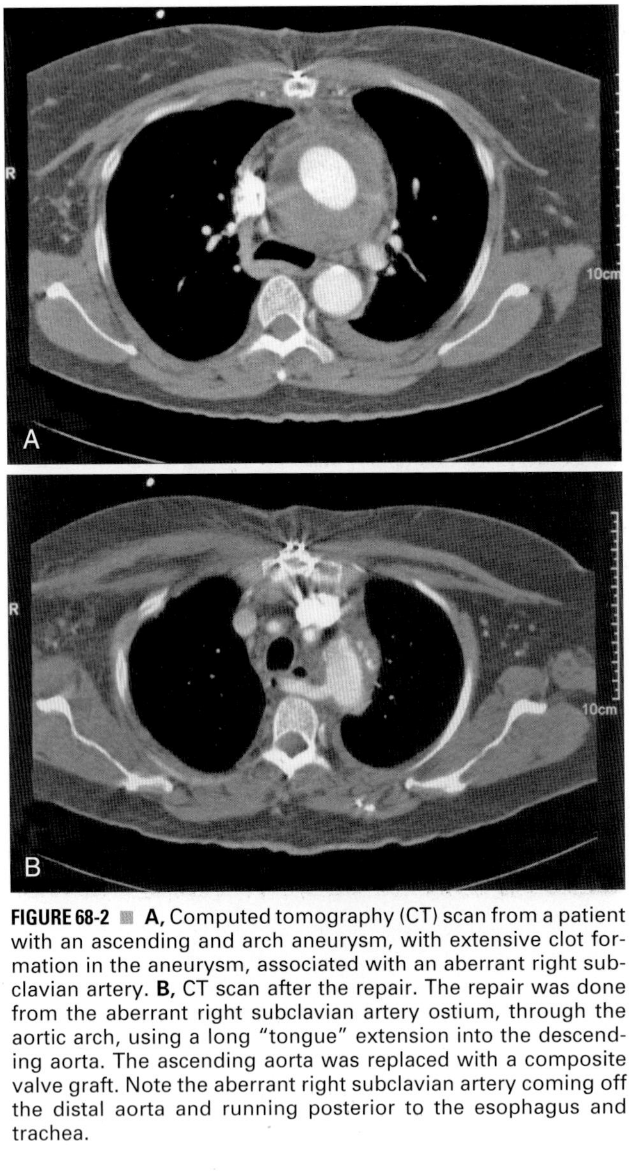

FIGURE 68-2 ■ **A,** Computed tomography (CT) scan from a patient with an ascending and arch aneurysm, with extensive clot formation in the aneurysm, associated with an aberrant right subclavian artery. **B,** CT scan after the repair. The repair was done from the aberrant right subclavian artery ostium, through the aortic arch, using a long "tongue" extension into the descending aorta. The ascending aorta was replaced with a composite valve graft. Note the aberrant right subclavian artery coming off the distal aorta and running posterior to the esophagus and trachea.

infective organisms are *Escherichia coli*, staphylococci, *Salmonella*, and streptococci, including *Streptococcus pneumoniae*. Other strains, however, may sometimes be detected. Some of these may be related to atherosclerotic ulcers, which initially act as a nidus for subsequent infection. Mycotic aneurysms frequently penetrate through the aortic arch wall, resulting in false aneurysms or free rupture. Osler called these aneurysms mycotic because the gray, slimy lining reminded him of fungal growth. Fungal infections in the vessel walls are, on the whole, very rare, except in patients who have had graft-related infections.[4]

Vasculitis and Aortitis

Inflammatory infiltrates of the aorta are not infrequent. In a prospective examination of histologic specimens by both H&E and elastic-tissue stains, inflammatory infiltrates were found in many of the specimens. Although these inflammatory infiltrates consist of various types of leukocytes, often associated with the diseases listed later, an associated systemic illness may be absent. This suggests that the original cause of the aortic injury was unrecognized, subsequently appearing as a medial degenerative aneurysm, with formation of atherosclerosis and calcification. Previous chest radiation for Hodgkin disease or breast malignancies may also be noted in the history. Radiation-induced vasculitis is associated with severe calcification and a porcelain aorta. A stiff left ventricle, scarred right ventricle, and fixed cardiac output increase the risk of surgery.

Inflammatory systemic diseases may result in aneurysms. For example, the development of aortitis is commonly associated with Takayasu disease (nonspecific aortoarteritis) (Fig. 68-6); giant cell arteritis (Horton disease); temporal arteritis; polymyalgia rheumatica; Behçet, Buerger, Logan, Sjögren, Reiter, or Kawasaki disease; relapsing polychondritis; systemic lupus erythematosus (often mycotic); rheumatoid arthritis; sarcoid

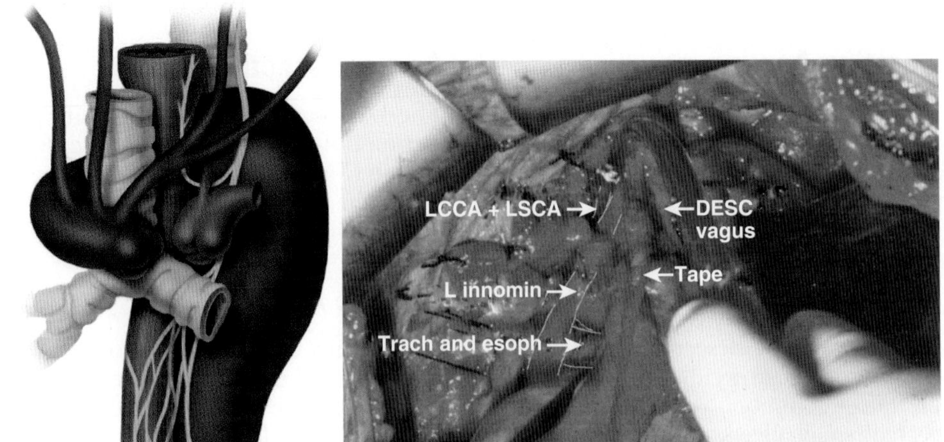

FIGURE 68-3 ■ **A,** Illustration of right-sided aortic arch with vascular ring. **B,** Intraoperative findings. *DESC,* Descending aorta; *esoph,* esophagus; *L innomin,* left innominate artery; *LCAA,* left common carotid artery; *LSCA,* left subclavian artery; *trach,* trachea.

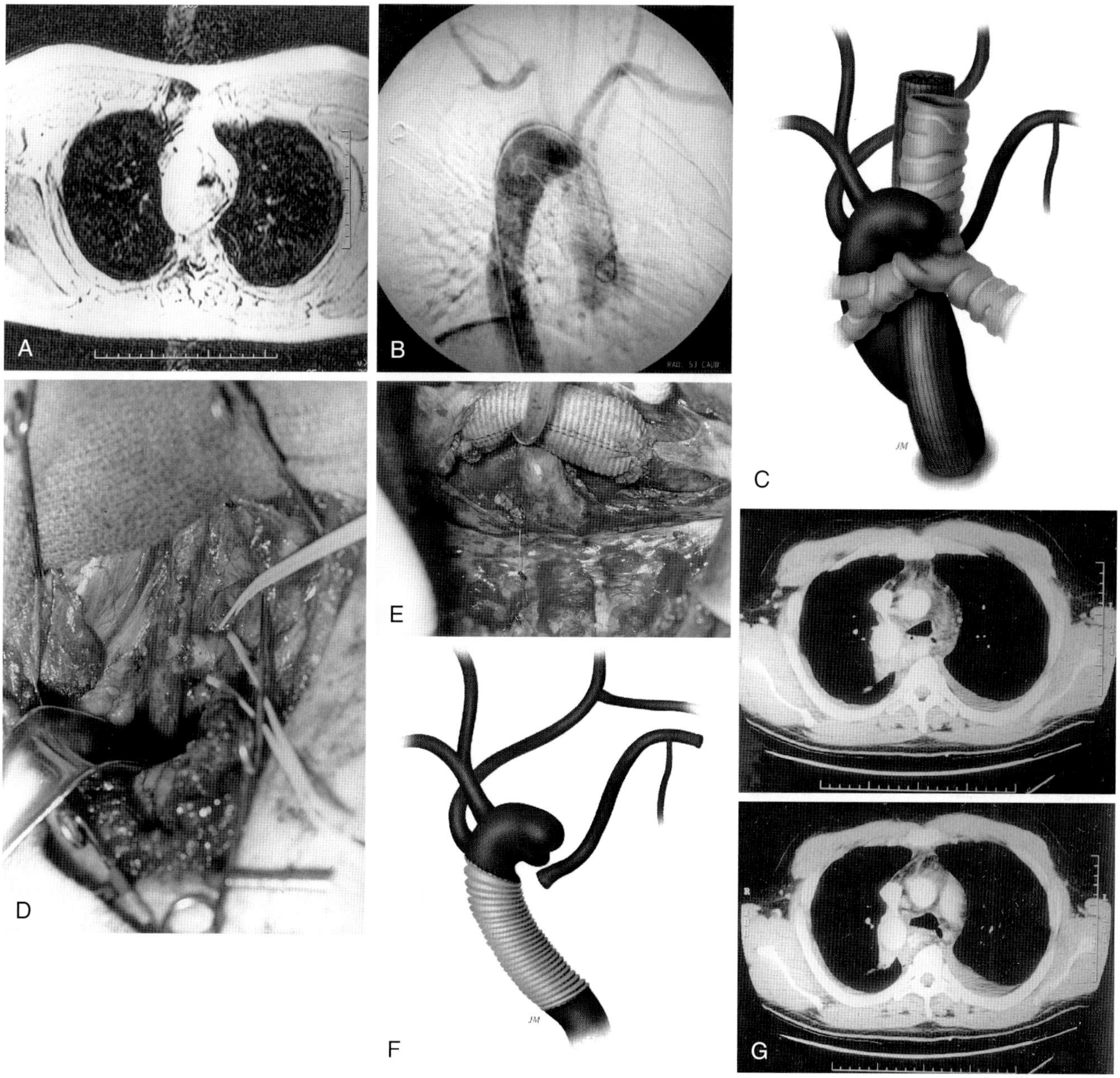

FIGURE 68-4 ■ **A,** Magnetic resonance imaging of a right-sided arch compressing the trachea, bronchus, and esophagus. **B,** Angiogram. **C,** Anatomy illustration. **D,** Left subclavian-to-carotid anastomosis. **E,** Distal arch and descending aorta replacement with Kommerell diverticulum oversewn (a stay suture is attached to the stump). **F,** Illustration of repair. **G,** Postoperative computed tomography scans with tracheal compression relieved.

and ankylosing spondylitis; osteoarthritis of unknown origin; ulcerative colitis; and potentially autoimmune diseases of the thyroid, such as Hashimoto.

Histologically, Takayasu disease has panaortitis, severe intimal hyperplasia, and severe adventitial fibrosis with perivascular inflammation. In contradistinction, giant cell aortitis has inflammatory margins around areas of medial necrosis and inflammation of the media. Fibrosis and intimal hyperplasia are minimal.

Trauma

Ten percent of traumatic lesions of the aorta occur in the aortic arch. The remaining 90% occur in other segments that are discussed in Chapters 69 and 75. The aneurysms are most often related to tears at the hinge point of the aorta during acceleration or deceleration injuries. Thus, the usual sites of primary tears are the origin of either the innominate artery or the subclavian artery (70% to 80%), although the origin of the common carotid artery may also be involved.[4] Although blunt trauma is the most common cause in the United States, traumatic arch injuries are more frequently caused by penetrating injuries from shrapnel or bullets or knife injuries in developing countries. With penetrating lesions, involvement of the trachea, esophagus, venous system, nerves, and vertebral column significantly complicates management.

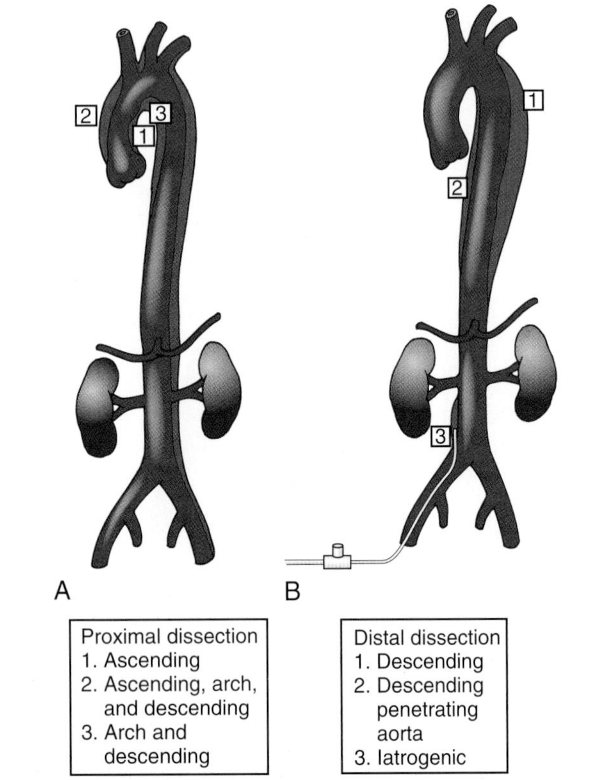

FIGURE 68-5 ■ Aortic dissection classification. **A,** Proximal dissection: (1) involvement of the ascending aorta only; (2) ascending, aortic arch, and descending aorta involvement; and (3) arch and descending involvement. **B,** Distal dissection: (1) involvement of the descending aorta with or without the abdominal aorta; (2) penetrating aortic ulcer with descending dissection; and (3) abdominal dissection (usually iatrogenic).

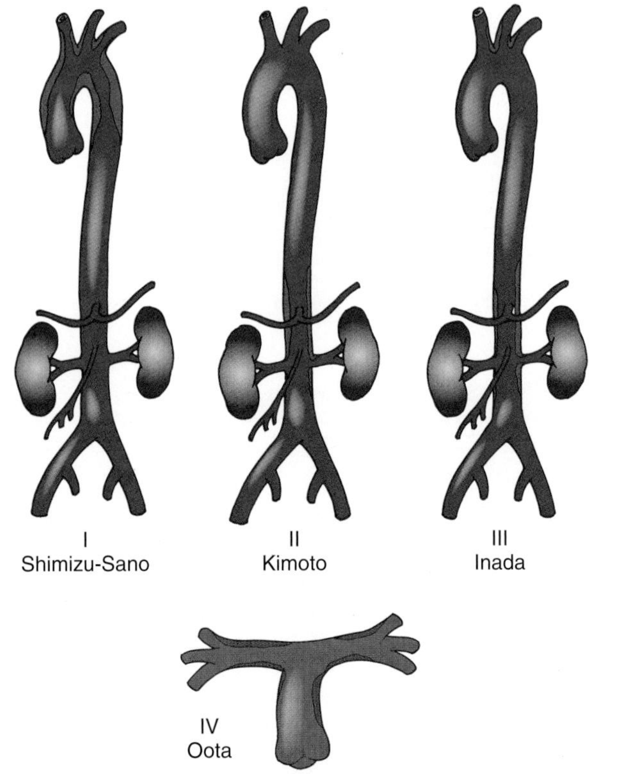

FIGURE 68-6 ■ Classification of Takayasu aortitis. Subtypes and their extents are depicted. (From Svensson LG, Crawford ES: *Cardiovascular and vascular diseases of the aorta,* Philadelphia, 1997, Saunders, pp 42–83.)

Tumors of the Arch

Tumors of the aortic arch are extremely rare, but when they occur they are usually found distal to the subclavian artery. Very rarely have tumors been related to prosthetic grafts.[4]

Reoperations

Patients who have undergone previous cardiovascular surgery may require reoperation either for new aneurysm formation or for false aneurysm formation. Approximately half of all patients undergoing arch operations have had previous cardiovascular surgery. There are two typical scenarios.

The first scenario involves a patient who earlier underwent acute dissection repair and subsequently developed an aortic arch aneurysm because the aorta, weakened from the dissection, had dilated over the course of time. This situation occurs commonly in patients with Marfan syndrome. It is preferable to repair only the ascending aorta at the time of the acute dissection repair,[4,14] first because the first priority is to save the patient's life, and second because trying to repair the aortic arch simultaneously carries a much higher mortality risk.[4,14] Furthermore, the risk of a patient's requiring another operation after acute dissection repair is, in most cases, small.[4,14] It is, however, important that the initial acute dissection repair should be performed with circulatory arrest unless the dissection is a DeBakey type II. This is so that the inside of the aortic arch can be inspected and a more complete hemiarch repair can be performed at the initial operation. A tear in the aortic arch can often be repaired with pledgeted 4-0 Prolene running sutures.[4,14] The use of biological glues may also increase the risk of recurrent aneurysms.

The second scenario for reoperation involves a patient in whom there was progression of the aneurysm formation in the aortic arch after initial ascending aorta repairs, or, at the time of the ascending aorta repair, not enough of a hemiarch was repaired, particularly when circulatory arrest was not performed.

An uncommon group of patients who require reoperations are those who form aneurysms at either the origin of the greater vessels, most typically the innominate artery, or at the site where a Carrel patch of the aorta was used for reattachment of the greater vessels. The site becomes aneurysmal and enlarges. This latter scenario should be watched for particularly in patients with Marfan, Loeys-Dietz, or Ehlers-Danlos syndrome, especially if they have suffered aortic dissection and the aorta is fragile.[4,14,15]

Although aortic graft infections are rare in our experience, such cases are often referred to us. They require extensive débridement and repair, usually with homografts (allografts). Alternatively, if homografts are not available, rifampin-soaked Gelweave grafts can be used. We also like to put in an irrigation system with a Blake drain infusing appropriate antibiotic depending on sensitivity or 5% Betadine in saline at 50 mL/hr over a few days. If there is a cavity, omental or muscle flaps are used to fill the space (Fig. 68-7). Patients are kept on lifelong antibiotics or, for fungal infections, fungal antimicrobials, particularly the newer, less toxic form of amphotericin B. In sick, high-risk patients, conservative approaches with either percutaneous or surgical drainage have also been reported with some success as long as the infection does not involve any suture-line, graft-enteric fistulas or involve invasive gram-negative organisms such as *Pseudomonas* or *Salmonella*.[16,17]

Syndromes Associated with Aortic Arch Pathology

Aneurysms may form in association with genetic diseases such as Marfan syndrome, Ehlers-Danlos syndrome, Erdheim syndrome (annuloaortic ectasia), Noonan syndrome, hereditary polycystic kidney disease, osteogenesis imperfecta, and Turner syndrome.[4]

HISTORY AND PHYSICAL EXAMINATION

When patients have a potential aortic arch aneurysm, neither questioning about symptoms nor physical examination is particularly informative. During the questioning, however, any history of aortic valvular disease associated with aortic root aneurysms needs to be sought, along with any history of neurologic or neurocognitive events. Computed tomography (CT) scans or magnetic resonance imaging (MRI) studies before aortic arch surgery have shown that between 40% and 60% of patients have evidence of brain injury. In a prospective randomized study, 38% of our patients, excluding those who had strokes with residual deficits and those older than 75 years, had a neurocognitive deficit before undergoing aortic arch surgery.[18,19]

If the aortic arch aneurysms are particularly large, hoarseness may develop, particularly if the distal aortic arch is enlarged. The reason is that the left recurrent nerve wraps around the distal aortic arch at the

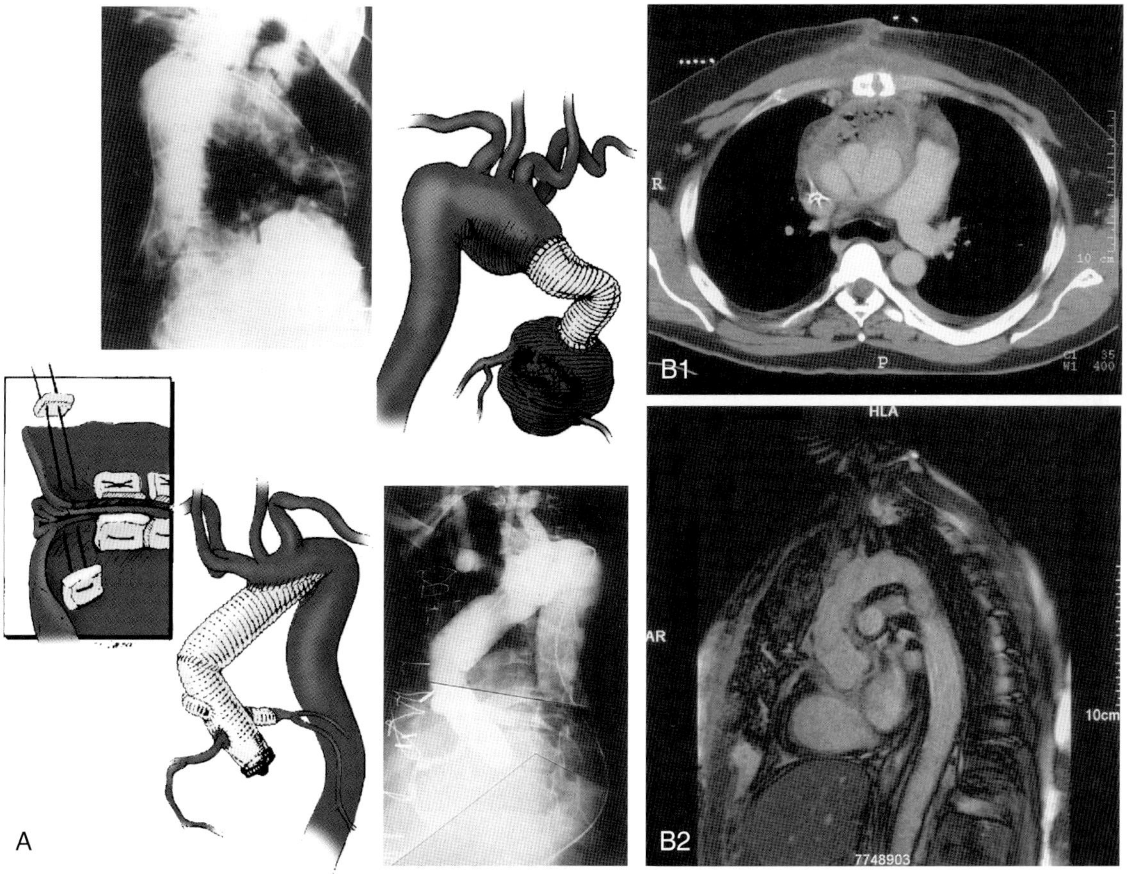

FIGURE 68-7 ■ **A,** An infected ascending aorta graft after initial replacement followed by reoperation with graft insertion (done elsewhere). During the third procedure, a new composite valve graft was inserted. The left main and the right coronary arteries were reattached as buttons, and the hemiarch was replaced with a separate graft. The annulus had to be reconstructed because of extensive annular abscess. Although the organism was *Staphylococcus aureus,* the patient, on suppressive antibiotics, has continued to be free of further infection. An omental flap was swung into the chest to fill dead space. **B1,** Computed tomography scan from a patient who had undergone two previous heart operations, including a composite valve graft insertion that became infected. The patient also underwent a limited sternal débridement elsewhere but later developed an abscess under the skin and associated air in the mediastinum. **B2,** The postoperative magnetic resonance angiogram after the repair. The patient had two allografts (homografts) inserted to replace the aortic root and the aortic arch. In addition, an omental flap was swung into the chest to fill the dead space.

ligamentum arteriosum and can become stretched by the aneurysm. Dysphagia may also occur, but this is more frequent with congenital lesions (see Fig. 68-4). In 1794, Bayford called this "lusoria," referring to the Latin term *lusus naturae* meaning "a freak of nature." This is often described as dysphagia lusoria or arteria lusoria. Dyspnea can also be a symptom when the pulmonary artery or left bronchus is constricted.[4]

Patients may complain of occasional mid-scapular pain if the aneurysms are large, although this is associated more with enlarged descending or thoracoabdominal aorta aneurysms. With aortic dissection or a false aneurysm related to a penetrating ulcer or mycotic aneurysm, severe chest pain may be present. This may be anterior or posterior chest pain with extension into the neck (see Chapters 70 and 71).

On examination, most patients do not have any physical findings specifically related to the aortic arch aneurysm, although, when the aneurysm is large, the anterior chest wall may be pulsatile and, in the worst of circumstances, may have eroded through the sternum or manubrium, particularly if infected. An associated pulsatile mass or a fullness of the neck with a pulsatile mass in the lower neck may be present. Displacement of the arch cranially may result in tortuosity of the carotid arteries. Palpation above the clavicle on the left side, at the thoracic outlet, may reveal a pulsatile mass.

During examination, the patient's arm, neck, and head pulses should be checked, because there may be discrepancies or absent pulses related to aortic dissection or aortitis, particularly giant cell arteritis or Takayasu disease.

Preoperative Studies

In addition to routine laboratory work, preoperative investigations include pulmonary function tests, because many patients may have predisposing factors such as a smoking history, Marfan syndrome with bullae formation, obstructive lesions related to the arch aneurysms (particularly with a congenital aberrant right subclavian artery lesion) (see Fig. 68-2), and right-sided aortic arches (see Fig. 68-3). Some patients are treated for a number of years for asthma because of expiratory wheezes caused by compression of the trachea or bronchi by aneurysms.[4]

Brain MRI or CT should be performed before surgery to detect any asymptomatic infarcts or brain lesions.[20] Most patients undergo carotid ultrasound studies if a history of coronary artery disease, peripheral vascular disease, or left main coronary artery stenosis is present. All patients undergo echocardiography before surgery,[21,22] and, if possible, good views of the ascending aorta and descending aorta are obtained by transesophageal echocardiography to check for atheromatous disease, as this will affect the method of cannulation for arterial inflow. All patients should also undergo cardiac catheterization to identify the presence of any coronary artery disease or valvular heart disease. If time allows, we obtain preoperative neurocognitive test results. Routine 24-hour Holter monitor examinations are included in the preoperative workup because many of these patients have cardiac arrhythmias, most likely related to valvular heart disease, chronic hypertension, coronary artery disease, or displacement of the left ventricle and the heart downward and to the left by the aneurysm. Patients with some syndromes, such as Marfan syndrome, exhibit more frequent prolonged QT intervals. Indeed, some aneurysms enlarge not only in diameter but also in length. Arrhythmias may also be related to abnormal vagal and sympathetic innervation stimulation.

At the time of cardiac catheterization, cardiologists are requested to obtain left anterior-oblique views of the aortic arch with injection of contrast material immediately proximal to the innominate artery. This is one of the best methods for obtaining good views of the aortic arch and determining the extent of the aortic arch repair that is required, including the need for an elephant trunk procedure. In the preoperative workup, before referral, patients have usually undergone contrast CT of the chest or MRI studies. CT three-dimensional reconstruction is also useful for planning.

Aortography is no longer done in all patients because of the time needed for scheduling and because it is invasive and because the dye load, often administered the day before the surgery, could compromise renal function. The operative procedure planned is discussed with the patient. On the basis of preoperative studies, it can usually be accurately predetermined whether a hemiarch, a total arch, or a total arch plus elephant trunk procedure is necessary. Additionally, it can be ascertained whether the greater vessels require bypasses because of stenotic lesions or aneurysmal disease, particularly in association with aortic dissection.

Next, again determined from preoperative studies, a decision is made as to the site of the arterial inflow for the operation. For most patients undergoing aortic arch surgery, the right subclavian artery is preferentially used for arterial inflow. In young patients, however, who need only a hemiarch procedure, particularly for Marfan syndrome, the right femoral artery is most often used. Usually, the left femoral artery is not used in patients with aortic dissection because the dissection typically extends into the left iliac artery and, thus, the femoral artery perfusion cannula may perfuse the false lumen, resulting in a flutter-valve effect and inadequate perfusion. Similarly, the aortic arch is not used because (1) it limits the extent of the repair, (2) the cannula gets in the way of the operation, (3) aortic dissection may be precipitated, and (4) if a graft is inserted, the cannula must be repositioned, either through a side graft or directly into the new aortic graft. Occasionally, the right subclavian artery is dissected and the femoral artery or aorta is used.

CARDIOPULMONARY PERFUSION ASPECTS

When the right subclavian artery is used, the technique is similar to that previously reported and shown in Figure 68-8. In a prospective randomized study, it was thought this would be a useful means for antegrade brain perfusion.[18,19] To do this, the innominate artery, in addition to the common carotid artery, was occluded with a balloon

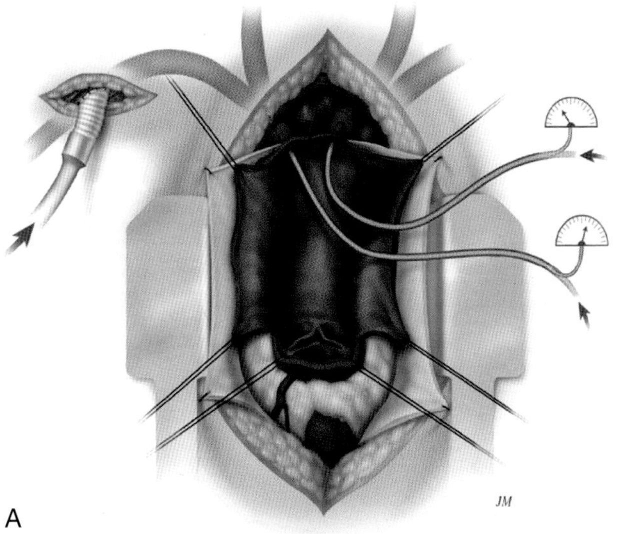

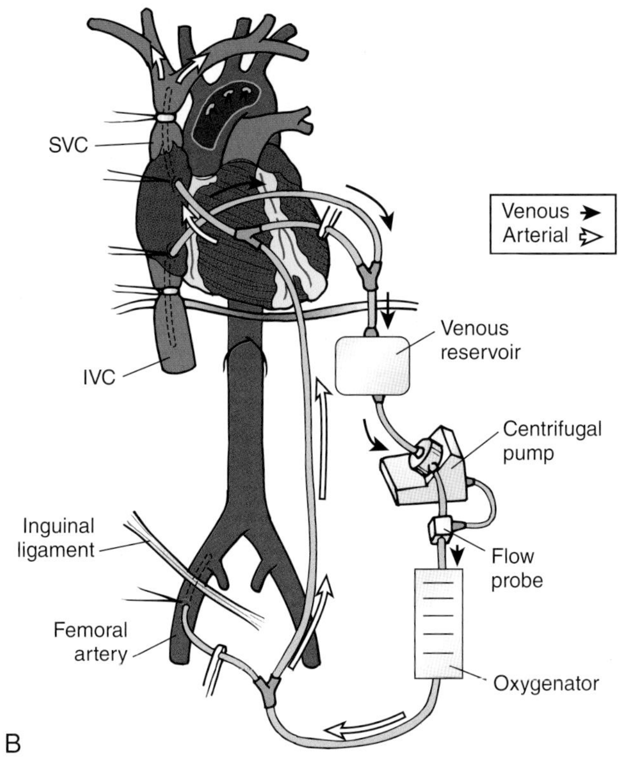

FIGURE 68-8 ■ **A,** Cannulation methods for antegrade brain perfusion with a side graft attached to the right subclavian artery and balloon occlusion catheters in the innominate and common carotid arteries. If a right brachial or radial artery pressure-monitoring cannula has not been inserted, pressures can be monitored in the innominate balloon catheter and, similarly, if perfusion is carried out through the left common carotid cannula, the pressure can also be monitored. **B,** Diagram of the usual setup for retrograde brain perfusion with a cannula in the superior vena cava (SVC) that has been looped with a Y arterial line that can be run through the SVC. *IVC,* Inferior vena cava.

catheter. The balloon catheter in the common carotid artery allowed perfusion of the left side of the brain (see Fig. 68-8). This has proved to be a safe and effective technique.

Our preference is to attach a side graft to the subclavian artery, defined as the part of the artery proximal to the lateral edge of the first rib. The reason for this is that there are fewer branches in this area and the nerve that swings across the artery to the pectoral muscles more distally does not obstruct the view. It does, however, require that the subclavius muscle be divided with electrocautery under the clavicle. Caution should be taken that the vein is not injured during this procedure. To dissect the axillary artery more laterally, care should be taken to retract the nerves out of the way and also to not injure the arterial branches. We have found the safest and best method for obtaining perfusion of the subclavian artery is to attach an 8-mm side graft, end to side. This is sewn into position with a 5-0 Prolene suture, and any leaks are oversewn with 6-0 Prolene. This allows perfusion of the vessel, both proximally and distally, and greater flow rates. Thus, by avoiding direct cannulation of the subclavian artery, there are fewer tears and there is less difficulty in repairing the artery at the end. Also, it circumvents the problem of the cannula's being inserted too far into the subclavian artery, which could result in occlusion of the common carotid artery or inadequate flow if the cannula presses up against the innominate artery wall. In our report on 1336 circulatory arrest patients, use of a side graft in the subclavian artery reduced the risk of stroke by 40%.[23]

An exception to the use of the subclavian artery, however, is that it should be avoided in patients who have had aortic dissection and when the extension of the aortic dissection is noted in the vessel (see Fig. 68-5*A*). In three patients in whom we used the subclavian artery, when dissection was present in the artery, two suffered postoperative strokes, probably from malperfusion related to the dissection. In patients exceeding 250 pounds, a larger 10-mm side-graft is usually used.

The graft is attached after the patient is heparinized, and a basket or coil sucker is placed in the wound to collect any leaking blood or blood that accumulates within the subclavian incision pocket. The graft is carefully de-aired and connected to a three-eighths-inch to quarter-inch perfusion connector that is then connected to the arterial line of the cardiopulmonary bypass machine.

As mentioned, when the femoral artery is used, the right femoral artery is preferable. When the femoral artery is used, care must be taken, as much as possible, to ascertain that there is no atheroma present in the arterial system that may potentially embolize with retrograde pumping through the femoral artery up to the brain. Thus, the femoral artery is avoided in older adult patients and patients with atherosclerotic disease, aneurysms of the descending thoracoabdominal and abdominal aorta, reoperations, DeBakey type I and type III aortic dissections, or extensive aortitis. Similarly, when we plan to use antegrade brain perfusion or the elephant trunk procedure (see Operative Techniques, later) or acute dissection repair, the subclavian artery is the vessel of choice.[10,18,19]

BRAIN PROTECTION

Multiple viewpoints are held about how to best protect the brain during aortic arch surgery. The areas of consideration are the degree of hypothermia at onset of circulatory arrest, either moderate (24° to 28° C) or deep (18° to 20° C); and brain perfusion, either none, retrograde, selective antegrade through right axillary, or bilateral through right axillary and left carotid. The reasoning and some of the research that we have performed resulting in the techniques we recommend are discussed here. In summary, our findings include the following: the subclavian artery is the preferred cannulation site (see earlier discussion) and the femoral artery is less so, deep hypothermia to 20° C is preferable although moderate hypothermia at 28° C with antegrade brain perfusion may be as safe if circulatory arrest times are less than 45 minutes,[24-26] electroencephalogram (EEG) silence is desirable,[24] antegrade or retrograde brain protection should be used although antegrade is preferable for longer circulatory arrest times (exceeding 40 minutes), long cardiopulmonary bypass times are harmful (particularly with inadequate filtration), and excessive rewarming may be harmful.[27-29]

Brain protection will be discussed from three aspects: (1) avoidance of doing harm during aortic arch surgery, (2) prevention of stroke, and (3) prevention of neurocognitive deficits.

Primum non nocere: First Do No Harm

Before the safe use of cardiopulmonary bypass, aortic arch operations were designed to use bypass shunts from the ascending aorta to the greater vessels to avoid using a heart-lung machine. These operations were generally limited to patients who had a normal aortic root and not extensive aneurysms, but the techniques were associated with a high incidence of stroke and death. With the advent of cardiopulmonary bypass, the operations became considerably safer. Nevertheless, attempts by Crawford and coworkers[30] to directly cannulate aortic arch greater vessels for perfusion of the brain during aortic arch operations were associated with a high incidence of stroke—occurring in up to one third of the patients. Their view was that this was related to injury of the greater vessels by balloon catheters and occluding clamps, or by atheroma resulting in stroke. Barnard[5] and Borst and colleagues[6,7] independently pioneered deep hypothermia for arch surgery; however, the technique was popularized by Griepp. Deep hypothermia and circulatory arrest, without perfusion of the greater vessels, thus became popular.[4,10,31,32] Cooley[33] and Livesay emphasized the usefulness of doing an "open" distal anastomosis.

In 1993, we reported a 10% mortality and a 7% stroke rate in a series of 656 patients with deep hypothermia and circulatory arrest alone for aortic arch operations (Fig. 68-9).[34] In this paper, however, we described retrograde brain perfusion (see Fig. 68-8*B*) in 50 patients with initial encouraging results. Our subsequent study in animals also showed promising findings.[4,35] At that time, the consensus was that strokes were related to embolic events or ongoing brain metabolism during deep hypothermia with circulatory arrest. As reports showed increasing success with retrograde perfusion of the heart during cardiac arrest, it was hoped that retrograde brain perfusion might have a protective role. Mills and Ochsner[36] reported using retrograde brain perfusion in a patient in whom air embolization occurred to the brain from the arterial

BRAIN PROTECTION: 656 DHCA

Time (minutes)	Stroke
7–29	4%
30–34	7.5%
45–59	10.7%
60–120	14.6%

Univariate: Age, CVA, CA time, CPB time, +Desc repair
Multivariate: CVA, Desc / TAA / TAAA repair, CPB time (AR)

A

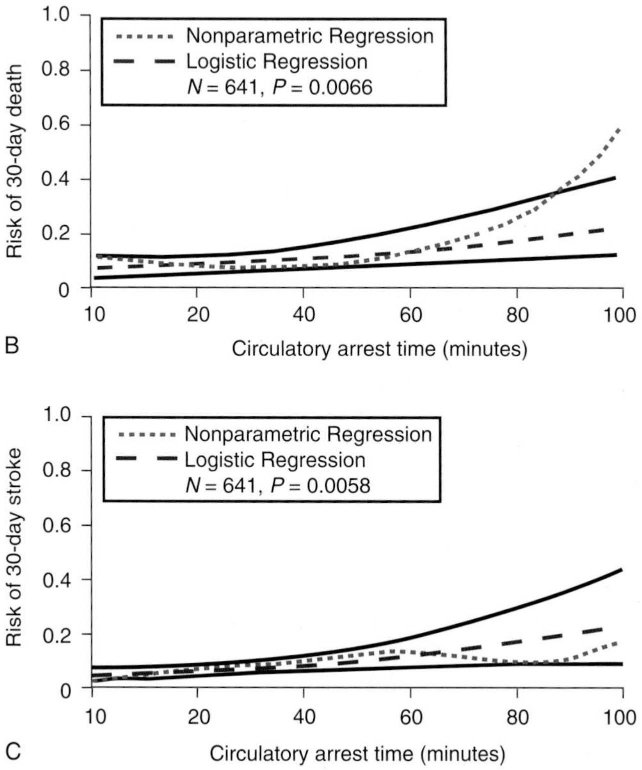

FIGURE 68-9 ■ **A,** Incidence of stroke in 656 patients undergoing deep hypothermia with circulatory arrest according to the length of time of circulatory arrest *(left column).* **B,** Relationship between circulatory arrest time and the risk of 30-day death. Note that after 65 minutes, there is an exponential increase in the risk of death. **C,** Relationship between circulatory arrest time and the risk of 30-day stroke. Note that after 40 minutes, there is an increase in the risk of stroke; however, at 60 minutes, the risk appears to decline. This is a statistical aberration because, after 60 minutes of circulatory arrest, there is a rapid increase in the risk of death and, therefore, patients could not necessarily be assessed for neurologic function. *AAA,* Abdominal aneurysm repair; *AR,* aortic valve regurgitation (in parentheses because aortic valve regurgitation was significantly associated with lower risk); *CA,* circulatory arrest; *CPB,* cardiopulmonary bypass; *CVA,* cerebrovascular accident (history); *+Desc,* with descending aorta repair at the same time; *DHCA,* deep hypothermia and circulatory arrest; *TAA,* thoracoabdominal aneurysm repair.

inflow cannula.[10,29,37] They placed the patient on cardiopulmonary bypass with arterial blood flow into the superior vena cava to try to "retrograde flush-out" air from the arterial system. Subsequently, Lemole reported using retrograde brain perfusion for aortic arch operations.[4] This was later popularized by Ueda.[2,4,20] More recent studies by Griepp's group,[38] Okita and colleagues, and others, however, have indicated that retrograde brain perfusion may also be associated with harmful side effects, including a higher incidence of stroke or neurocognitive deficits and depression.[10,39] It has been speculated that brain edema may be a factor. In our initial use of retrograde brain perfusion, we were careful not to exceed a perfusion pressure of between 25 and 30 cm H_2O, because we knew patients with congestive heart failure could tolerate a central venous pressure at this level. Subsequently, studies suggest that a higher perfusion pressure is needed to obtain any retrograde perfusion of the brain. Furthermore, this group demonstrated that perfusion pressures that exceed 60 cm H_2O resulted in brain edema. Retrospective studies, however, show that in comparison with historical controls, results are improved.[40] There is no doubt that this method is effective in removing embolic material from the aortic arch, including atheromatous emboli. Nevertheless, the technique may be associated with harmful side effects. In our prospective, randomized study from 2000, depression appeared more common in this group of patients, and there appeared to be no neurocognitive benefit over deep hypothermia and circulatory arrest alone. In our more recent prospective, randomized study of 121 patients undergoing total aortic arch replacement in 2012, comparing retrograde and antegrade brain perfusion for total aortic arch replacements, both in conjunction to deep hypothermic circulatory arrest, there was no difference in clinical stroke rates, radiologic evidence of stroke or neuropsychologic decline. The mortality rate of the cohort was 0.8%, and clinically detected stroke occurred at a rate of 0.8%.

Milewski also showed no difference between retrograde brain perfusion/deep hypothermic circulatory arrest and antegrade brain perfusion/moderate hypothermic circulatory arrest in terms of permanent neurologic deficit, temporary neurologic dysfunction, renal failure, or death when the circulatory arrest time is less than 45 min.[41] Likewise, many recent large series and randomized clinical trials have shown the safety of moderate hypothermic circulatory arrest when used with antegrade brain perfusion for circulatory arrest times less than 45 minutes. There are advantages to moderate hypothermia: it avoids the long cooling and rewarming periods, decreases cardiopulmonary bypass times, and avoids the side effects of deep cooling, mainly coagulopathy.[26,42-45] However, should the circulatory arrest times exceed 45 minutes because of technical difficulties or the need to perform individual head vessel anastomosis, at moderate hypothermia there is a risk of systemic ischemic injury, multiple organ failure, and injury to the spinal cord. For this reason and because the procedure is not entirely predictable, we prefer always performing circulatory arrest under deep hypothermia. Finally, for circulatory arrest durations of longer than 45 minutes, bilateral antegrade brain perfusion is advisable.

Prevention of Stroke

As our knowledge of cardiopulmonary pathophysiology improved, it became clear that most strokes after cardiac surgery were related to microemboli. Most of these emboli seem to be the result of atheromatous or calcific debris from the aorta. For most patients undergoing aortic arch surgery, other sources, such as from the left atrium in patients with chronic atrial fibrillation or transiting through an atrial septal defect, are less of a problem. Another potential source of emboli is from the descending aorta or abdominal aorta or iliac and femoral arteries during femoral artery perfusion; hence, we advocate the routine use of cannulating the right axillary artery with an 8 mm graft as our aortic inflow. We prefer the use of an 8 mm graft as opposed to direct cannulation of the axillary because we have previously shown that it decreases the incidence of stroke by 40%.[46] With modern cardiopulmonary bypass techniques, the risk of massive air embolism or pump failure that can result in strokes has been greatly lessened.[4,47] Various techniques have been used to reduce the risk of embolic-related strokes. We have not tested every method, but early on, we established a protocol based on the level of knowledge at the time that we considered of value (Table 68-1). With reference to cardiopulmonary bypass, it appears that the following are beneficial: a centrifugal pump, arterial line filtration (at least 25 μm), leukocyte filtration, closed-bag venous reservoir, cell saver, avoiding pump suction, and reducing cardiopulmonary bypass time. If a leukocyte filter is used, it is important to use immediate preoperative plasmapheresis to remove platelets and clotting factors from the patient, because leukocyte filters tend to remove platelets from the circulation. The platelet-rich plasma is reinfused at the end of the operation. For pH management during cardiopulmonary bypass and circulatory arrest, we favor using the alpha-stat method. In the pediatric age group, there is more convincing evidence that the pH-stat method works better. In adults, however, the alpha-stat method is generally preferred, although no prospective or randomized studies have definitively answered the question of which is best in adults. An advantage with the alpha-stat method is that the lactic acid that accumulates in the brain during circulatory arrest can, to some extent, be buffered by histamine molecules on hemoglobin.[4,10,29,47]

We advise flooding the field with carbon dioxide so any air accumulating in the heart or the field will be displaced.[48] This includes the aortic arch so that when circulation to the brain is restarted, any potentially gaseous material is carbon dioxide rather than air. Carbon dioxide is reabsorbed approximately 25 times faster than air, reducing the risk of microcirculation obstruction related to gaseous material.

In addition to perfusion aspects and the site of cannulation, we recommend packing the patient's head in ice because it reduces the risk that the ambient operating room temperature might raise the temperature of the patient's head during circulatory arrest.

The usage of neuroprotective agents during circulatory arrest remains controversial. Thiopental may be useful by lowering oxygen consumption, although the

TABLE 68-1 **Brain Protection Protocol**

Population	Protective Measures
All patients	Electroencephalogram silence Temperatures less than 20°C Head packed in ice Mannitol prime and after arrest Alpha-stat pH control LeukoGuard filter CO_2 flooding of field Thiopental 5 mg/kg 5 min before arrest Lidocaine 200 mg before arrest Magnesium sulfate 2 g Centrifugal pump Membrane oxygenator Closed-circuit bag venous reservoir Pre-bypass plasmapheresis Routine use of cell saver device
Patients receiving antegrade brain perfusion	Right subclavian and side graft Innominate and carotid balloon occlusion (retrograde cardioplegia balloon occlusion catheter) Pressure maintained at 40-60 mm Hg Sequential removal of catheters as arch anastomosis completed
Patients receiving retrograde brain perfusion	Superior vena cava cannula Snared below azygous vein Flow rate: 300-500 mL/min Pressure: <25-35 mm Hg

evidence on clinical benefit is inconclusive. However, there is suggestion that if thiopental is administered before circulatory arrest, it may replete the cerebral energy state before arrest and prove detrimental.[49] The usage of barbiturates has declined over the years partly because of its unavailability. In a German registry for type A dissection of over 2000 patients, only 48% of patients received a neuroprotective agent such as steroids, mannitol, or barbiturates. The stroke rates were slightly lower in patients receiving steroids versus no agents (7.1% vs. 10.6%), and usage of mannitol led to lower 30-day mortality. These results are observational and have not been shown in prospective studies.[50]

In our randomized clinical trial in 2012 comparing retrograde brain perfusion to antegrade brain perfusion, only 0.8% of patients had clinically evident stroke, but 9% had showed evidence of new MRI or CT infarcts or brain tissue changes, suggesting that many infarcts are clinically silent.[51] In this study, we also gave patients neurocognitive tests preoperatively and 4 to 6 months after the index procedure. For each neurocognitive test, the baseline and follow-up data were used to calculate a test-retest reliability coefficient, a reliable change index (RCI), and associated 90% confidence interval for the RCI. A patient was considered to have declined neurocognitively if he or she had two or more RCIs that fell below the lower 90% confidence limit for the respective, corrected reliable change interval. Surprisingly, there was little correlation between patients who had neurocognitive dysfunction and patients who had new radiologic evidence of stroke. In total, 14% of patients had neurocognitive deficits. Of these patients, only 18% had evidence of infarct on CT or MRI, and 56% of patients with radiologic evidence of stroke had neurocognitive decline. From the remaining 5 patients who had radiologic evidence of stroke without neurocognitive decline, 4 had strokes located in the occipital or cerebellar areas. On multivariate analysis, neither retrograde brain perfusion nor antegrade brain perfusion was an independent predictor of neurocognitive decline, clinical stroke, or radiologic stroke. To summarize, our study showed that clinical exam for neurologic events was insensitive, MRI detects more events, and the most sensitive is neurocognitive examination, which may not detect occipital or cerebellar events.

Prevention of Neurocognitive Deficits

With improved results for aortic arch surgery and fewer complications such as strokes, interest has focused on prevention of postoperative neurocognitive deficits. As mentioned, 38% of patients in our prospective randomized study were found to have, before surgery, neurocognitive deficits.[18,19] The reason is not entirely clear, but it may be related to silent brain injury before surgery. There is also a correlation between neurocognitive deficits and other preoperative factors such as heart failure and New York Heart Association degree of dyspnea.[29] This would be in keeping with the finding that patients who exhibit a greater degree of systemic cardiovascular disease experience more neurocognitive deficits. The possible reasons include inadequate brain perfusion, brain edema, other factors affecting the brain vasculature, general overall poor health, and silent ischemia and white matter injury, as we have documented. Indeed, it is our impression that patients with preoperative neurocognitive deficits do not tolerate deep hypothermia and circulatory arrest well. In a previous study of 656 patients undergoing deep hypothermia and circulatory arrest,[34] older patients did not tolerate circulatory arrest as well as younger patients, putting them more at risk for stroke. The same probably holds true for the risk of neurocognitive deficits, but this has not been formally studied.

The incidence of neurocognitive deficits after cardiac surgery remains controversial.[18,19,28] So much depends on the method of defining when neurocognitive deficits occur. There are many reasons why deficits can occur (e.g., preoperative neurocognitive dysfunction or atherosclerosis of the microvasculature of the brain, similar to that affecting coronary arteries). Some large studies that have examined neurocognitive dysfunction after coronary bypass surgery have used cardiopulmonary bypass pump setups that were out of date. It is also instructive that some studies have shown no differences between off-pump and on-pump incidences of neurocognitive deficits, suggesting that other factors, such as anesthesia management, are important. Studies have also shown no differences between coronary artery bypass surgery and major abdominal aortic surgery. Indeed, there is no difference between percutaneous coronary intervention and coronary bypass operations. Patients who undergo anesthesia often have neurocognitive dysfunction after surgery despite having no obvious risk factors that cause neurologic dysfunction. In our prospective, randomized study, although over 90% of patients had neurocognitive dysfunction 3 to 6 days after surgery, by 2 to 3 weeks only 9% had a new neurocognitive deficit, and by 6 months all had recovered.[18,19] The entire field of neurocognitive dysfunction requires further study to determine when a deficit occurs in an individual patient and what the change in global scores for an entire group of patients means. In our prospective randomized study from 2000 (Fig. 68-10), we found that patients' IQs improved after circulatory arrest over time, which clearly is not likely! The explanation was that the patients underwent repeated IQ testing (four) and learned to do the tests over time. Nevertheless, it was gratifying to note that the patients' IQs did not deteriorate after deep hypothermia and circulatory arrest. Indeed, the practice effect on reported neurocognitive scores is difficult to compensate for. Figure 68-11 shows the serum S-100 protein value changes of each group studied.

There are many reasons for potential neurocognitive dysfunction after surgery. Anesthetic gases and pharmacologic agents, including barbiturates, are factors. Other potential reasons are brain edema and swelling from third-space fluid accumulation. Undoubtedly, chemical and metabolite accumulation also play a role. Microemboli, in the form of small fat globules, or air or carbon dioxide gaseous emboli, may also be a factor.

It was once thought that emboli to the frontal lobes were largely silent and that there was selective streaming of emboli, including platelet aggregates, to the middle cerebral artery, resulting in middle cerebral artery territory infarcts. A study was done using radioactive platelet aggregates in a baboon model to test this theory.[52] We found injection of the platelet aggregates into the left atrium resulted in equal distribution across the brain, including occipital lobes and distribution to the eye, as expected from an anatomic point of view. Injection into the common carotid arteries had a similar effect, although the occipital lobes were spared. Injection into the internal carotid artery did not reveal any preferential streaming into the middle cerebral artery. From this we infer that the emboli to the frontal lobes do cause infarcts of equal frequency, although these may be more silent in the sense that critical motor and sensory functions are not affected. We do, however, believe that these so-called silent infarcts affect neurocognitive function, as expected from a more recent understanding of brain pathophysiology. Some neurocognitive decline after cardiopulmonary bypass may thus be related to microemboli to the frontal lobes and infarction. This is an evolving field, and the correlation between microembolic phenomena and postoperative neurocognitive function needs to be further defined. For example, it is unclear how high-intensity transient Doppler signals, produced by aortic valve prostheses, affect neurocognitive function both early and in the long term. Studies in patients with various types of aortic valve prostheses suggest that many of these are gaseous microemboli, but that they are usually transient and rapidly return into solution without causing permanent brain dysfunction.[10,53]

In our 2000 prospective randomized study, we failed to show any benefit from antegrade or retrograde brain perfusion regarding neurocognitive function when compared with deep hypothermia with circulatory arrest alone. However, the circulatory arrest was relatively short, and for hemiarch repairs, antegrade brain perfusion resulted in significantly longer circulatory arrest time because of the time required to insert the common carotid artery catheter and the innominate artery catheter and then to work around them. For total arch replacement, there were no differences in circulatory arrest times. Retrograde brain perfusion was associated with slightly longer circulatory arrest times compared with circulatory arrest alone, probably because retrograde brain perfusion results in blood

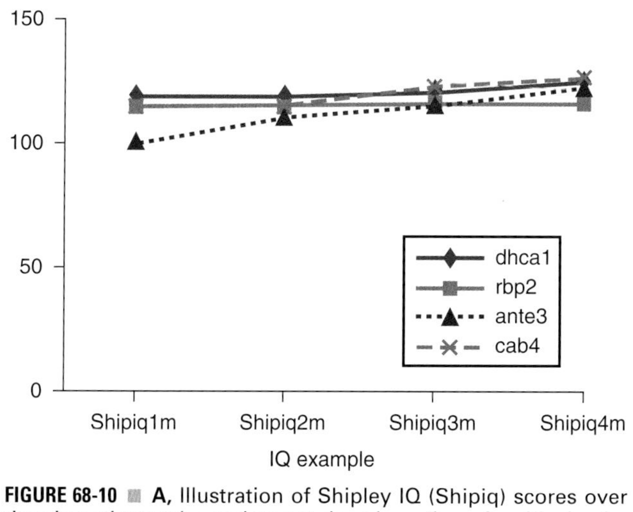

FIGURE 68-10 **A,** Illustration of Shipley IQ (Shipiq) scores over time in patients who underwent deep hypothermia with circulatory arrest (dhca), retrograde brain perfusion (rbp), antegrade brain perfusion (ante), and coronary artery bypass (cab). The first tests were done preoperatively (1m), then 3 to 6 days after surgery (2m), 2 to 3 weeks after surgery (3m), and 6 months after surgery (4m).

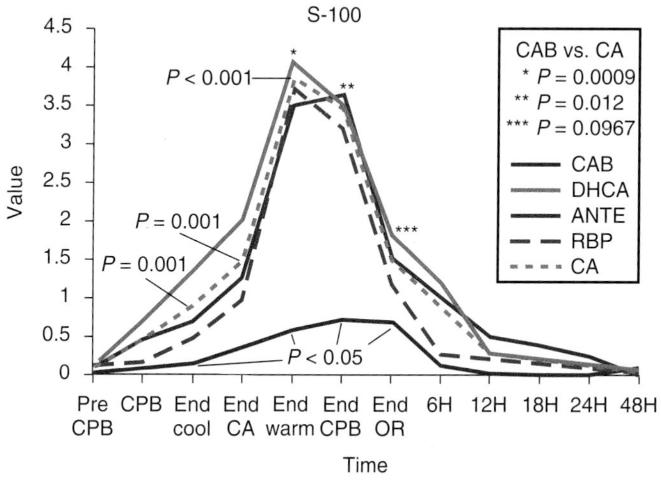

FIGURE 68-11 Relationship of time point during operation to the serum S-100 protein value. Graphed curves: *ANTE,* Antegrade brain perfusion; *CA,* all circulatory arrest patients; *CAB,* coronary artery bypass; *DHCA,* deep hypothermia and circulatory arrest alone; *RBP,* retrograde brain perfusion. On *x*-axis: *CA,* Circulatory arrest; *CPB,* cardiopulmonary bypass; *H,* time after surgery in the intensive care unit; *OR,* operating room.

accumulating in the operative field, which obscures the field when suturing. If we expect atheroma in the aorta at the time of surgery, and if the patient may require endarterectomy, we use antegrade perfusion via the right subclavian artery (as discussed) or retrograde brain perfusion to flush out embolic material.[18,19]

When patients are undergoing total arch replacement and the circulatory arrest time may exceed 30 to 40 minutes, antegrade or retrograde brain perfusion is used for the repair. Data in the pediatric cardiac surgical literature show that, as with pulmonary embolectomy in adults for thrombotic material, circulatory arrest with intermittent periods of brain perfusion followed by circulatory arrest is better than one long period of circulatory arrest. For one patient undergoing a fourth complex cardiac reoperation at deep hypothermia, we were able to successfully protect the brain for more than 90 minutes by running antegrade brain perfusion for 5-minute periods every 30 minutes. He was extubated the day after surgery without a neurologic deficit. We therefore usually run antegrade brain perfusion, if not throughout the period of circulatory arrest for total arches, at least at intermittent intervals when convenient from the point of view of visualizing the field and suturing. The balloon occlusion catheter can easily be led out of the field so that it does not obstruct the view. Because the right subclavian artery is perfused in these patients, once the balloon catheter is withdrawn from the arch, the arch is flushed of any embolic material before anastomosis is completed. If an elephant trunk procedure is being used, a side graft to the elephant trunk is not required for antegrade perfusion, because the right subclavian artery is being perfused. Similarly, in patients undergoing acute dissection repairs, a side graft to the aortic arch is not required because the subclavian artery is being perfused.[1,10,4,18,19]

Fourteen percent of patients have an incomplete circle of Willis; however, extracranial collaterals will still allow the perfusion of the left brain in most of these patients. Although unilateral perfusion is adequate for shorter circulatory arrest times, (<45 min), bilateral perfusion through an additional left carotid cannula would be advisable.[1,4,10,18-20,42,54]

Future research is needed to determine the best perfusion method for brain protection during total arch replacements, including the best temperature.

OPERATIVE TECHNIQUES

The operative procedures for aortic arch replacement are most commonly hemiarch repairs or entire arch repairs, with or without a distal descending elephant trunk procedure.[4] Other unusual types of operations are options in specific situations. To a large extent, the choice of aortic arch procedure is influenced by the proximal aortic root or by the ascending aorta operative technique, whether it is a composite graft, root remodeling, separate valve and graft, valve reimplantation, Ross procedure, or no valve procedure. Also, in choosing a valve type, it is important to consider durability, particularly for biological valves, as a third or fourth operation will be complicated.[53]

Hemiarch Replacement

Hemiarch replacement of the aortic arch is the simplest and quickest operative technique. The anastomosis can be achieved in 5 to 15 minutes depending on the aortic arch pathology. Once the patient has been cooled down and the method of brain protection and perfusion has been decided, the patient's circulation is stopped with the patient in the head-down position. In patients undergoing reoperations, we use one of two approaches: either full median sternotomy or a minimally invasive approach. The ascending aorta is then opened between stay sutures. A decision is made as to whether the aortic arch should be transected for the anastomosis. Briefly, transection of the aorta is indicated for acute aortic dissections in those patients who have had an aortic root procedure in which the aorta has already been transected proximally, and for most patients who need hemiarch replacements. The reason is that it is easier to obtain hemostasis at the distal anastomosis if the aorta was transected, and thus the risk of false aneurysm formation is also less. The transection line usually runs from the proximal base of the innominate artery to the midpoint of the lesser curve of the aortic arch. In patients with acute dissections, it is important to be certain that all layers are transected, and that the adventitia is freed of the posterior-lying pulmonary artery and a bit further cranial to the pulmonary artery to ensure adequate tissue is present for effective suturing. The anastomosis is performed with a running 4-0 or 3-0 Prolene suture, dependent on the pathology. For patients with acute dissections, it is best to use a 4-0 or even 5-0 Prolene. When the anastomosis is near completion, the graft and arch are filled with blood by restarting the arterial flow from the pump. Any potential embolic material is sucked away, and gaseous pockets are evacuated. To further reduce risk of gaseous embolism, carbon dioxide is run into the operative field during the procedure. The anastomosis is completed and the suture is tied down. The patient is rewarmed, and the proximal ascending aorta anastomosis or aortic root procedure is completed.

In patients who have either had aortic root remodeling using techniques described by David and Feindel, Sarsam and Yacoub, or us, or who have a modified valve reimplantation procedure, an interposition graft is usually required between the aortic root graft and the aortic arch.[37,55-57] If, however, the valve remodeling was done while cooling, an interposition graft may not be necessary. However, when the patient has undergone aortic valve replacement only, the hemiarch graft is used to suture the proximal anastomosis immediately above the aortic valve and coronary arteries. When a composite valve graft will be inserted, the proximal anastomosis of the composite valve graft to the aortic valve annulus and the left main coronary artery anastomosis can first be performed while cooling the patient, and the hemiarch anastomosis can be done directly to the composite graft without using an interposition graft, but always being careful to de-air the graft. Alternatively, if the patient cools quickly, a separate hemiarch graft is placed and later anastomosed to the proximal composite valve graft with a graft-to-graft anastomosis while the patient is rewarmed.

In patients who have had a homograft inserted with an aortic root repair, a decision needs to be made as to whether prosthetic polyester graft material should be used for the hemiarch, or whether a homograft (without an aortic valve) (see Fig. 68-7) should be used to bridge the gap between the aortic valve and the homograft. In patients with extensive infection of a previously inserted graft (e.g., a composite graft), we replace the aortic root with a new homograft and use another homograft to bridge the gap between the root homograft and the aortic arch so that there is no prosthetic material other than Prolene suture material (see Fig. 68-7*B*). In most cases, these grafts are wrapped with omentum to further obliterate any dead space. For those patients undergoing reoperations who have extensive scar tissue formation that restricts the ability to transect the proximal and distal aorta, the hemiarch anastomosis may be done inside the aortic arch without transecting the aorta. Rarely, if bleeding cannot be controlled, a Cabrol fistula can be formed from the aneurysm sac to the right atrium or the superior vena cava.

A variation on the hemiarch replacement is a long tongue of the graft used to replace the entire aortic arch, potentially down onto the descending aorta to approximately the middle third of the descending aorta, depending on the size of the aortic arch aneurysm (see Fig. 68-2). When using a long tongue for the total aortic arch replacement and down the descending aorta, there are some points worth noting. First, if the anastomosis is quite far down the descending aorta, parachuting the distal anastomosis makes it easier. Second, the patient should be warned before surgery that hoarseness may occur because the recurrent laryngeal nerve often cannot be preserved where it wraps around the distal aortic arch. Third, hemostasis at the distal anastomosis must be secure before continuing the operation, after doing the arch repair, because obtaining hemostasis is much more difficult once the graft is pressurized and connected proximally. Fourth, the extent distally to which the anastomosis can be performed may be judged, to some extent, by examining the CT scan or the left anterior oblique view of the arch on magnetic resonance angiography or cardiac catheterization. As a rule, an anastomosis can be easily performed no more than a few centimeters beyond the lowest level of the lesser curve of the aortic arch: the larger the aortic arch aneurysm is, the farther down the descending aorta within the descending aorta the anastomosis can be performed. If the anastomosis cannot be performed through the aortic arch, an alternative method should be considered (see Replacement of the Entire Aortic Arch, later). When doing a hemiarch with these long "tongues," care must be taken that the aortic graft not become stenosed or badly kinked. This may obstruct blood flow through the repaired aortic arch, resulting in excessive cardiac afterload. This may progress to either early acute heart failure or later ventricular hypertrophy and congestive heart failure if the gradients are too large.

Replacement of the Entire Aortic Arch

Replacement of the entire aortic arch can be done with or without a distal elephant trunk procedure. The procedures involving an elephant trunk will be discussed first (Fig. 68-12).

Multiple variations of elephant trunk procedures have been used, including hybrid procedures. We have classified them as follows (Fig. 68-13).[58]

- Type I: Classic elephant trunk: ascending tube graft with total arch replacement and elephant trunk anastomosis in classic position distal to left subclavian artery (LSCA)
  - Type Ia: Type I repair with stent graft
- Type II: Ascending aorta tube graft with arch replacement and elephant trunk anastomosis proximal to LSCA
  - Type IIa: Subsequent thoracic stent graft with proximal landing zone covering LSCA and a descending-to-LSCA bypass
- Type III: Elephant trunk placed into large descending aortic aneurysm used as a landing zone for distal thoracic stent graft
- Type IV: Ascending aorta tube graft with classic elephant trunk anastomosis into distal thoracic aneurysm with branched graft for total arch replacement
  - Type IVa: Ascending branched graft for replacement of ascending aorta and arch, with end-to-side elephant trunk in classic position
  - Type IVb: Subsequent thoracic stent graft in type IV repair
- Type V: Ascending aorta tube graft with elephant trunk anastomosis proximal to brachiocephalic artery and a branched graft for total arch replacement
  - Type Va: Type V repair configuration with thoracic stent graft in distal aneurysm

In type I repairs, to shorten the period of circulatory arrest, the elephant trunk and inverted graft should be prepared while the patient is cooled. This is done by first suturing and tying a silk stitch to the end of the graft that will be used for the proximal repair of the ascending aorta. The distal elephant trunk should be approximately 10 to 15 cm in length. If the second stage will be done with stent grafts (type Ia) because of comorbid disease (e.g., chronic pulmonary disease), then metal clips and a loop of wire (pacing) are attached to the distal end. The proximal part with the stitch attached to it is then inverted into the distal elephant trunk. It is important to ensure that the edge of the inversion is at the same level and smooth. If retrograde brain perfusion or circulatory arrest alone is used and the subclavian artery has not been used for arterial inflow, a side graft needs to be attached to the aortic arch and inverted into the distal elephant trunk. This side graft should be attached approximately 2 to 4 cm proximal to the edge of the inverted graft. If the right subclavian artery is used for arterial inflow, there is no need to attach a side graft to the elephant trunk graft.

Once circulatory arrest is established and the patient is in a head-down position, the graft is fed into the descending aorta, ensuring it is neither kinked nor twisted into a spiral. In patients with chronic dissection, the septum or flap should be excised as much as possible so that the graft perfuses both true and false lumens.

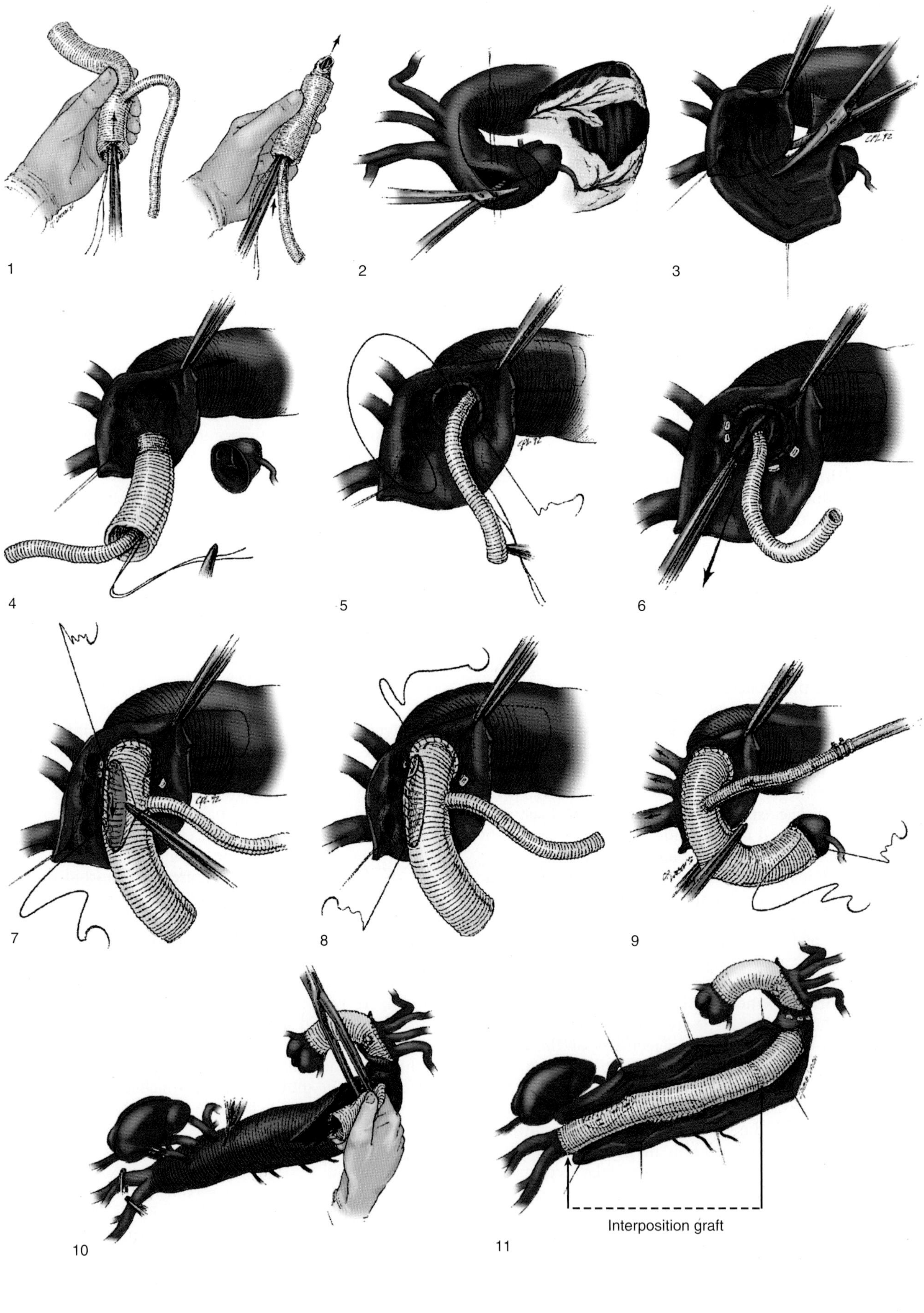
1
2
3
4
5
6
7
8
9
10
11
Interposition graft

Perfusion of either the true or false lumen alone may result in paraplegia or renal failure. It is also important that the elephant trunk not be excessively long. In a previous review of 84 elephant trunk procedures,[9] three patients developed paralysis postoperatively, one with dense paraplegia and the other two with paraparesis from excessively long elephant trunks. Subsequent to shortening the length of the elephant trunk, this has not been a problem. The reason for this appears to be either that the elephant trunk is too long and perfusion of the intercostal arteries is inadequate, or that, as noted at the second-stage procedure, extensive clot formation occurs around the elephant trunk, which can occlude critical intercostals. Because of this clot formation, when using the elephant trunk, patients often require multiple platelet transfusions as the clot builds up around the elephant trunk in the descending aorta.

The elephant trunk graft material should be one of the collagen-coated woven grafts and not a gel-coated graft. The gel of gel-coated grafts is absorbed quickly. At the time of the second-stage operation, bleeding from a proximal elephant trunk can be excessive and potentially uncontrollable because the graft is porous after the gel has been absorbed.

The anastomosis between the inverted edge of the elephant trunk graft and the distal aortic arch beyond the left subclavian artery is then performed. The patient should be warned that hoarseness may occur postoperatively, as this procedure is in the region of the recurrent laryngeal nerve.

Reasons for inverting the graft on itself and placing it in the descending aorta are several.[9] First, the anastomosis is easier to perform, even though it can be difficult to drive the needle through a double layer of graft material. However, with collagen-coated grafts, this is not much of a problem. Second, when the inverted graft is withdrawn from inside the elephant trunk, it has the effect of tightening the anastomosis, improving hemostasis at the distal anastomosis. Third, the larger contact surface area between the graft and aortic wall is increased so that there is less bleeding past the anastomosis. Fourth, if the graft is not inverted, suturing in a tight space between a graft and the aorta in a deep V results more often in the aorta's tearing, with the potential for a disastrous rupture in the postoperative period. This problem of rupture was experienced in the early period of using the elephant trunk technique without inverting it.[9]

One of the problems with elephant trunk procedures is the risk of rupture during the interval between the first operation and the second-stage operation. Rupture of the descending aorta continues to be a potential risk of the elephant trunk procedure during the postoperative period, because the systemic inflammatory response results in release of collagenase and elastinase, which can result in rupture of the aneurysm. Furthermore, the aneurysm may grow in the interim, while the patient is recovering from the first operation. In Safi and colleagues' series from 2001, the interim mortality rate was 3.6%, and 75% of deaths were caused by aneurysm rupture.[59] Because of the interval aneurysm growth and risk of rupture, patients need to be closely followed. If a hybrid second-stage procedure is planned, this can be done at the time of the first stage or before hospital discharge. We reviewed our series of elephant trunk and endovascular completion and demonstrated good early and mid-term results. In the mid to late term, there is a risk of stent migration and endoleak; therefore, lifelong imaging follow-up is required. Alternatively, a stent graft can be inserted antegrade into the elephant trunk to anchor it, or the separate stent graft can be sewn into position in the distal arch; the latter approach, however, has a tendency toward higher complication risk[58,60] (see Frozen Elephant Trunk, below).

A second-stage operation is usually planned after the patient's recovery from respiratory problems related to the first operation, usually 6 weeks to 4 months after the first stage. Alternatively, if the patient is in poor condition after the first operation, including experiencing respiratory problems, we electively proceed to stent grafting the elephant trunk as part of the second-stage procedure, provided that the descending aorta down to the celiac artery can be stented. On occasion, a limited thoracoabdominal incision has been used to place bypasses from the iliac artery to the visceral vessels and, thereafter, a stent graft has been inserted to replace the remaining aorta from the elephant trunk down to the aortic bifurcation or iliac arteries. With the increasing use of thoracoabdominal stents, second-stage stenting with inclusion of the thoracoabdominal aorta is also an option. In patients with acute dissection, total arch replacement is avoided if possible. If total arch replacement must be done, an elephant trunk can be placed in the true lumen in the descending aorta after transecting the aorta beyond the left subclavian artery. Transecting the aorta ensures that all layers are cut and a completely hemostatic suture line is achieved with a rim of Teflon felt around the aorta. The recurrent nerve usually ends up being transected.

FIGURE 68-12 ■ Steps for the elephant trunk procedure technique modified by inverting the graft and placing it in the descending aorta. **(1)** A side graft is sewn to the graft that will be used for the aortic replacement and then the graft is inverted on itself, including the side graft. The distal extent of the elephant trunk should be 10 to 15 cm in length, and a rim of approximately 1 to 2 cm is left between the side graft and the inverted edge turned down for sewing. If the right subclavian artery is used for arterial inflow, the side graft is not necessary. **(2)** When the patient is cold enough, circulation is arrested and the aorta is opened. **(3)** The aorta can be transected to improve exposure, if needed. **(4)** The previously prepared graft is then placed in the descending aorta. **(5)** The distal anastomosis is performed starting at the three-o'clock position as the surgeon looks at the anastomosis. **(6)** The inner inverted tube is then pulled back into the operative field. **(7)** The posterior suture line is performed for the aortic arch. **(8)** The anterior suture line is performed. Once the anastomosis has been completed, arterial inflow is started through the side graft again to perfuse the brain if the right subclavian artery has not been used. **(9)** At the second stage of the operation, the graft is exposed in the aneurysm and clamped. It is not necessary to encircle the aorta to perform this, because the graft is surrounded by clot and can be exposed without much bleeding and then digitally clamped before applying a mechanical clamp. **(10)** The remainder of the aorta is then repaired. **(11)** For thoracoabdominal aneurysms, an interposition graft is necessary to complete the repair.

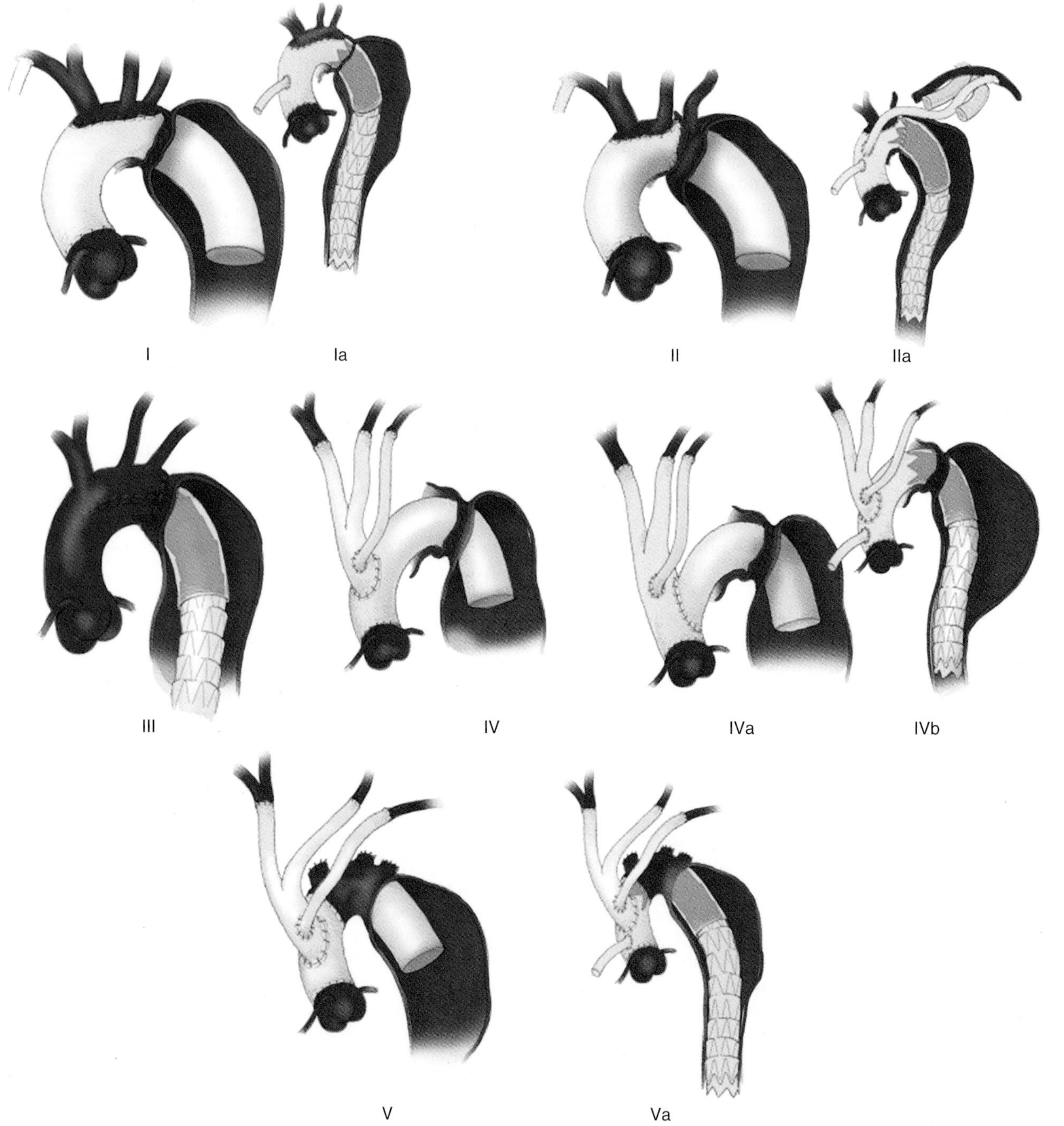

FIGURE 68-13 ■ Classification of anastomotic sites of elephant trunk for repair of thoracic aorta disease. Classic elephant trunk: **(I)** ascending tube graft with total arch replacement and elephant trunk anastomosis in classic position, distal to left subclavian artery (LSCA); **(Ia)** this repair with subsequent stent graft. **(II)** Ascending aorta tube graft with arch replacement and elephant trunk anastomosis proximal to LSCA; **(IIa)** subsequent thoracic stent graft with proximal landing zone covering LSCA, and a descending-to-LSCA bypass. **(III)** Elephant trunk placed into large descending aortic aneurysm to be used as a landing zone for distal thoracic stent graft. **(IV)** Ascending aorta tube graft with classic elephant trunk anastomosis into distal thoracic aneurysm, with branched graft for total arch replacement; **(IVa)** ascending branched graft for replacement of ascending aorta and arch, with end-to-side elephant trunk in classic position; **(IVb)** subsequent thoracic stent graft in type IV repair. **(V)** Ascending aorta tube graft with elephant trunk anastomosis proximal to brachiocephalic artery and a branched graft for total arch replacement; **(Va)** this repair configuration with thoracic stent graft in distal aneurysm.

Type II is the most common alternative elephant anastomosis; using this type, the anastomosis is performed between the common carotid and the left subclavian artery (Fig. 68-14).[61] If the distal aortic arch beyond the left subclavian artery is enlarged and there is no "landing site" for doing the distal anastomosis, then the aortic arch is often more narrow between the left common carotid and left subclavian artery. Thus, doing the anastomosis at this site results in a shorter circulatory arrest period, because the suture line is shorter and exposure is better.

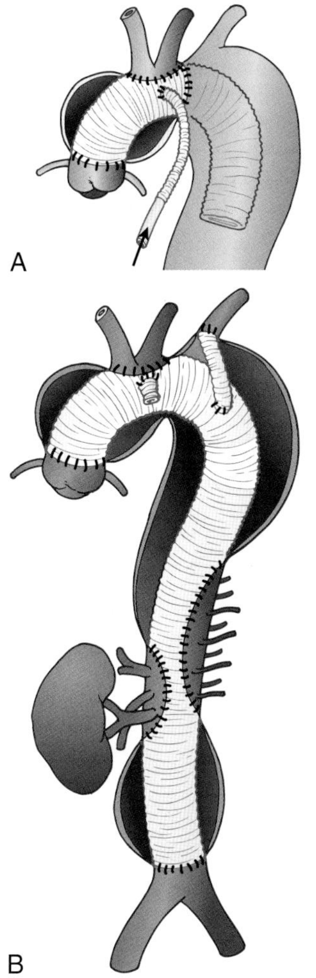

FIGURE 68-14 ■ **A,** Diagram of a modified elephant trunk technique with an anastomosis performed between the left common carotid and left subclavian arteries. **B,** Completion of the second stage of the elephant trunk procedure, with a tube graft to the left subclavian artery.

The downside of doing the anastomosis between the left common carotid and left subclavian arteries is that the left subclavian artery needs to be anastomosed to the elephant trunk during the second-stage operation. This is typically done with an interposition graft. An alternative method is to attach the left subclavian artery to the left carotid artery at the first-stage operation. Another strategy would be to oversew the left subclavian artery and use a sidearm graft through the first or second intercostal space to revascularize the left axillary artery, as described by Baeza and Svensson.[62]

Once the distal anastomosis has been performed, the inner inverted graft is withdrawn and an opening is made opposite the greater vessels. The posterior suture line is performed, followed by the anterior suture line. The graft is flushed, any potential embolic material is removed, and then the graft is clamped. The graft is checked for hemostasis at both the distal anastomosis and the aortic arch. The proximal anastomosis is performed to the ascending aorta, depending on the root technique used.

Increasingly, patients who are referred for descending thoracic or thoracoabdominal operations have severe cardiac disease, either valvular or coronary.[63] If the proximal descending aorta or distal arch is also enlarged, we place a descending thoracic elephant graft with the proximal anastomosis sewn just beyond the left subclavian artery in preparation for the second-stage operation or stent grafting (type III). One reason for this is that the left subclavian artery can also be used. If not, the distal arch could not be clamped at the second operation with a patent left internal mammary artery.

Japanese surgeons, when doing aortic arch replacements, like to use branch grafts to the greater vessels. Branch grafts have a neo-aortic larger graft with four-sided grafts attached end to side, typically 8 or 10 mm in size, or larger. The distal anastomosis is first performed between the neo-aortic graft and the descending aorta, followed by the greater vessel anastomoses. The left subclavian artery and the left common carotid and innominate artery are anastomosed to the branch grafts sequentially. Cannulas in the transected greater vessels are used to maintain antegrade perfusion while these anastomoses are performed. The fourth side graft is used for perfusing the aortic arch and reestablishing blood flow to the greater vessels as they become attached to the branch graft. This approach is not generally favored by most surgeons in Europe and the United States, although there is some virtue to this technique in patients with extensive calcification and atheroma of the aortic arch, when suturing beyond the atheroma and calcification in the greater vessels is required. Disadvantages of this technique are a very long pump time, potential kinking of the graft or side branches, prolonged total body systemic circulatory arrest, and the longer period of nonpulsatile flow to the brain. Indeed, for aortic arch surgery, the pump time is the best predictor of mortality and risk of stroke.[4,34] A method we have used in conjunction with subclavian arterial perfusion is to sew a bifurcated graft to the innominate artery and carotid artery first, and then to do an elephant trunk procedure and left carotid bypass (type IV). These are then connected to the neo-aortic graft. The advantage is that the brain arrest time is 5 to 15 minutes.

A technique that can be used occasionally is to place a bifurcated graft on the anterolateral aspect of the ascending aorta, suturing the other ends of the bifurcated graft to the greater vessels so that the native greater vessel stumps in the aortic arch can be oversewn. A separate graft is used to bypass the left subclavian artery, or a left carotid subclavian bypass can be done. The aortic arch and descending aorta are then addressed with an elephant trunk (type V) or are stented (type Va) as needed, either immediately through a side graft or later. If a stent graft is to be used, a large clip can be placed at the heel of the anastomosis between the graft and the aorta to guide stent placement. The stent graft is oversized by 10% to 20% and placed with a stiff guidewire placed in the left ventricle as a rail. The major advantage of this procedure is that it can often be done without circulatory arrest and sometimes off pump. Lee and coworkers compared the series of arch debranching procedures to standard elephant trunk procedures and found equivalent results with the aortic debranching group needing cardiopulmonary bypass in 68% of patients and circulatory arrest in only

27%.[64] The rates of spinal cord ischemia, stroke, and 30-day mortality were 0%, 11%, and 16%, respectively, for arch debranching and 0%, 10%, and 20%, respectively, for standard elephant trunk.

If the entire thoracic aorta or the entire aorta is going to be replaced through both a mediastinal and a left thoracoabdominal incision, the distal anastomosis in the aortic arch does not need to be done; only the anastomosis to the greater vessels is needed. This operative technique is discussed in Chapter 69. Also, if the descending aorta, arch, and ascending aorta are replaced through a "clam-shell" incision, a distal arch anastomosis is not needed.

If the elephant trunk procedure is not used for the distal anastomosis, the distal anastomosis is performed in the descending aorta with a simple running suture (Fig. 68-15). Usually, the aorta is not transected because of the risk of cutting the recurrent laryngeal nerve. The transition between the aneurysm to the normal aorta usually has fairly tough tissue to suture. As mentioned, if this is within the proximal third of the descending aorta, the anastomosis can be performed without a problem, particularly if the parachuting technique is used. If there is an aberrant right subclavian artery without a Kommerell diverticulum aneurysm, it can be included in the repair (see Fig. 68-2). An alternative is a technique in which the graft is placed in the descending aorta while the anastomosis is performed, and then the inverted graft in the descending aorta is withdrawn for the aortic arch repair.[4]

Other Techniques

In patients with saccular aneurysms with a fairly narrow neck, a patch of graft material can be sewn to the neck in the aortic arch, usually on the lesser curve. One needs to ensure that the edge of the aorta is strong and will hold sutures. This technique is also useful for saccular aneurysms of the proximal descending aorta. However, a decision has to be made as to whether a mediastinal approach or a left thoracotomy is better. When a patch technique

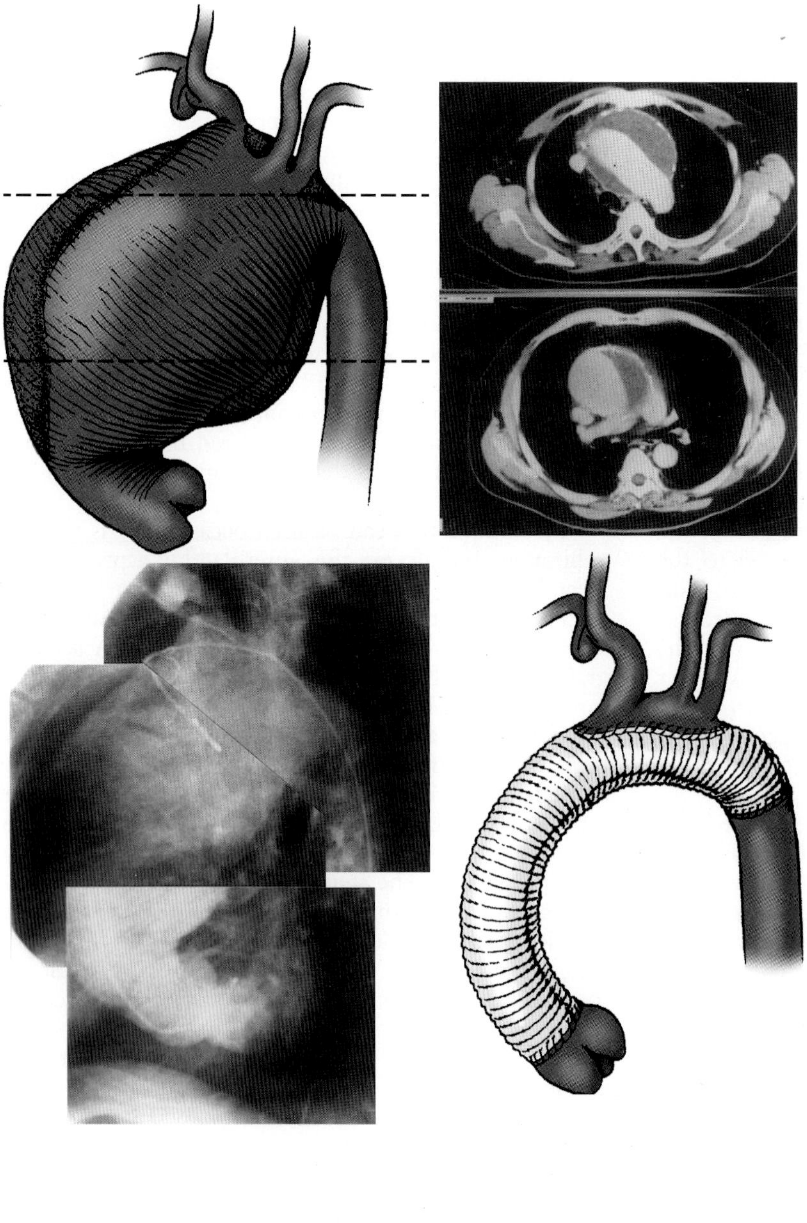

FIGURE 68-15 ■ For this aneurysm involving only the ascending and aortic arch and proximal descending aorta, an elephant trunk procedure was not necessary. Note the extensive clot formation in the aneurysm shown on the computed tomography scan. The arch was repaired by sewing the graft into the proximal descending aorta and then reattaching the greater vessels as a Carrel patch.

is used, because there is usually extensive atheroma, it is advisable to use the right subclavian artery for arterial inflow to ensure that any potential embolic material is not flushed back up into the brain but rather washed into the descending aorta.

Griepp and the Mt. Sinai group have described a technique of suturing a large graft to the greater vessels island and then perfusing this graft from the pump while another graft is used for doing both distal and proximal anastomoses in the aorta.[31,38,65] Finally, an anastomosis between the graft to the greater vessels and the separate aortic arch graft is performed. This technique allows a shorter circulatory arrest to the brain but requires that additional anastomoses be performed.

In patients with extensive atheroma and calcification, endarterectomy of the aortic arch also may be required. In our experience with 45 patients, the results have been surprisingly good when doing endarterectomies at the same time as aneurysm repairs of the aortic arch.[29] When performing endarterectomies of the aortic arch and greater vessels, a meticulous technique must be used to ensure that no embolic material gets into the ostia of the greater vessels. For this reason, we use antegrade brain perfusion and often combine this with retrograde brain perfusion to ensure maximal flushing of the greater vessels while doing these types of repairs.[29]

Another option is using a minimal invasive approach for re-do aortic arch surgery. The advantage of using this method at reoperations is that the rest of the heart and the right atrium do not need to be dissected out. Because the patient has typically undergone a previous aortic root procedure, an elephant trunk procedure can be done distally and the proximal anastomosis performed to the ascending aorta. We have used this method now in 125 patients with a 95% survival rate and a 2.6% stroke incidence.[47,66,67]

We do not use the new biological glues extensively for aortic arch repairs. In our experience, patients who return for reoperations who have had repairs with these glues often have tissue that is extremely thick, hard, and often calcified, making it difficult to work with. In addition, there is the risk in aortic arch surgery that some of the glue may embolize distally; this is particularly the case with the gelatin-resorcinol-formaldehyde (GRF) glues. Infection and false aneurysms also can be problems.

For patients with aneurysms or stenosis of the greater vessels, various operative techniques can be used at the time of aortic arch surgery. Most of these involve placing bypasses from the neo-aortic graft to a more distal normal segment of the greater vessel. Sometimes, if only the origin of the greater vessels of the aortic arch is involved, these procedures can be performed without placing the patient on cardiopulmonary bypass. For example, a side-biting clamp can be placed on the ascending aorta and a bifurcated graft sewn to the ascending aorta. Alternatively, the ascending aorta can be replaced by a tube graft and the bypass graft attached to it. The distal grafts can then be used to bypass the innominate, the common carotid, or the subclavian arteries. Figure 68-16 shows magnetic resonance angiograms of a patient in whom this technique was used to attach the bifurcated graft to the ascending aorta using a side-biting clamp: the two distal grafts were routed through the chest pleural spaces and through the first intercostal space to the bilateral axillary arteries, where anastomoses were performed.[62]

Frozen Elephant Trunk

The frozen elephant trunk technique is a single-stage approach for the repair of arch and thoracic aortic disease where a stent graft is first delivered in the descending aorta either antegrade or retrograde. The distal anastomosis of the aortic arch graft is then sewn on to the distal aortic arch with the suture line incorporating the stent.[68,69] According to European E-vita Open Registry data, the use of the frozen elephant trunk technique for chronic dissection leads to an 80% rate of complete thrombosis in the false lumen.[70,71] In patients with acute type A dissection, the residual dissected descending aorta present in 50% of cases is prone to aneurysmal enlargement, and up to 40% of these patients require reintervention. Roselli and colleagues described a simplified frozen elephant trunk technique to potentially address this issue.[72] A single commercially available thoracic stent graft is delivered antegrade down the descending aorta into the true lumen. The proximal end is then trimmed and sutured into the aortic arch. In this series of 17 patients, no perioperative deaths occurred and 88% of patients had a fully thrombosed false lumen at follow-up. In a large Japanese series of 156 patients, of which 100 had dissection and 56 had aneurysmal disease, the rates for mortality, stroke, and paraplegia were 3.2%, 2.6%, and 2.0%, respectively. At 12 months, the false lumen shrank in 46% of cases and was obliterated in 37% of patients. Whether this improved remodeling of the aorta leads to long-term survival advantage is yet to be demonstrated.

Occasionally, the aortic arch cannot be replaced or operated on. A valved conduit from the left ventricular apex to the descending aorta is one option of treatment in this event (Fig. 68-17).

Finally, as hybrid operating rooms are becoming increasingly common, and with increasing familiarity and comfort with percutaneous and endovascular techniques, an expanding array of complex cases can be addressed with minimally invasive approaches. We recently performed a case where the left common carotid artery and descending aorta were concomitantly stented with a transapical transcatheter aortic valve replacement.

OUTCOMES

In a historical study from 1993 and an analysis of 656 patients who underwent deep hypothermia and circulatory arrest, mostly for aortic arch replacements, the mortality rate was 10% and the stroke rate was 7%.[34] This large study noted that the longer the circulatory arrest was, the greater was the risk of stroke. It is of interest that some patients tolerated circulatory arrest periods of up to 120 minutes without developing frank strokes. In this series of patients, the predictors of stroke by multivariate analysis were history of cerebrovascular disease, previous aortic surgery beyond the left subclavian artery, and cardiopulmonary bypass time ($P < 0.05$).[34]

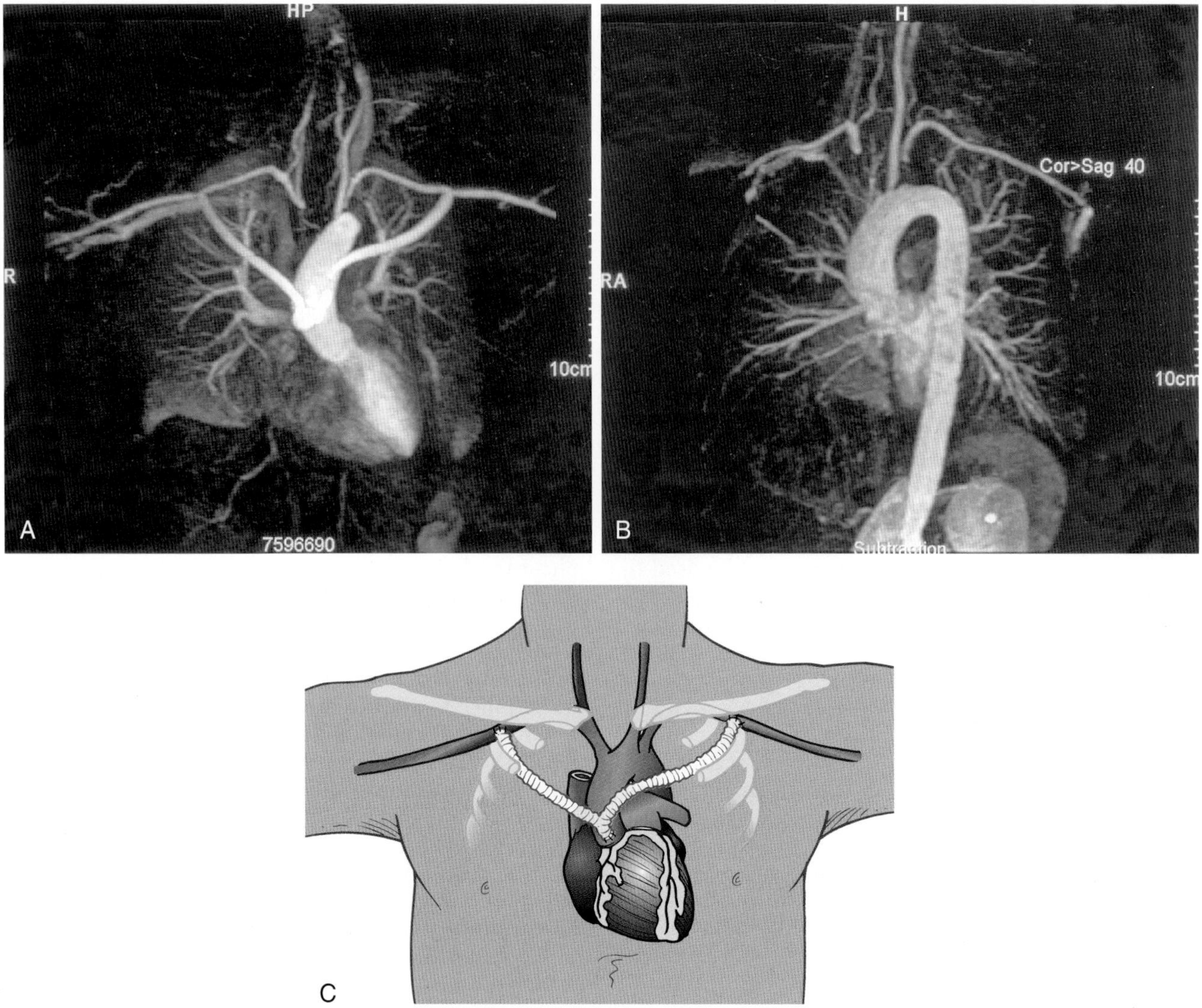

FIGURE 68-16 ■ **A,** Magnetic resonance angiogram (MRA) shows occluded innominate and left subclavian arteries and 50% narrowing of the left common carotid artery. **B,** Postoperative MRA after off-pump insertion of a bifurcated graft from the ascending aorta to both axillary arteries with a transpleural approach. **C,** Diagram of the completed procedure.

Results with aortic arch surgery continue to improve. Safi and colleagues' series from 2001 had a 5.1% 30-day mortality for the first stage, 3.6% interval mortality, and 6.2% 30-day mortality for the second stage. In our series of 526 unselected elephant trunk procedures, the survival rate for the first operation was 92%, with no statistical significant difference between the LCCA-LSCA (left common carotid artery–left subclavian artery) group and the classic group. The overall stroke rate was 8%. The 1-, 4-, and 8-year risk of death before second-stage elephant trunk was 16%, 22%, and 27%, respectively; the larger the descending aorta is, the greater the likelihood is of a second-stage completion.

In a prospective randomized study, we reported a survival rate of 100%, and no patient suffered stroke after aortic arch repairs.[29] Although 91% of patients had a neurocognitive deficit when tested between 3 and 6 days after undergoing aortic arch repairs, by 2 to 3 weeks after surgery, with repeat testing using 51 neurocognitive tests, 9% had a deficit, and by 6 months, all the patients with new neurocognitive deficits had recovered. As mentioned, 38% of patients had had a preoperative deficit. In another analysis, of 403 patients undergoing ascending and aortic arch operations using a protocol to protect the brain as much as possible from strokes and neurocognitive deficits, the survival rate was 98%, stroke rate 2%, and incidence of neurocognitive gross clinical deficits 2.5%.[54] The predictor of death by multivariate analysis was pump time; for stroke it was aorta symptom grade, peripheral vascular disease, and pump time; and for neurocognitive dysfunction, it was New York Heart Association dyspnea class, pump time, arrest time, day extubated, and antegrade perfusion. In our recent randomized clinical trial of 121 patients with aortic arch repairs, only 0.8% had clinically evident stroke, although 9% had radiologic evidence of new stroke and 14% had new onset of neurocognitive dysfunction.[51] These studies emphasize the importance of awareness that patients may have suffered silent strokes and developed neurocognitive deficits before undergoing aortic arch surgery.

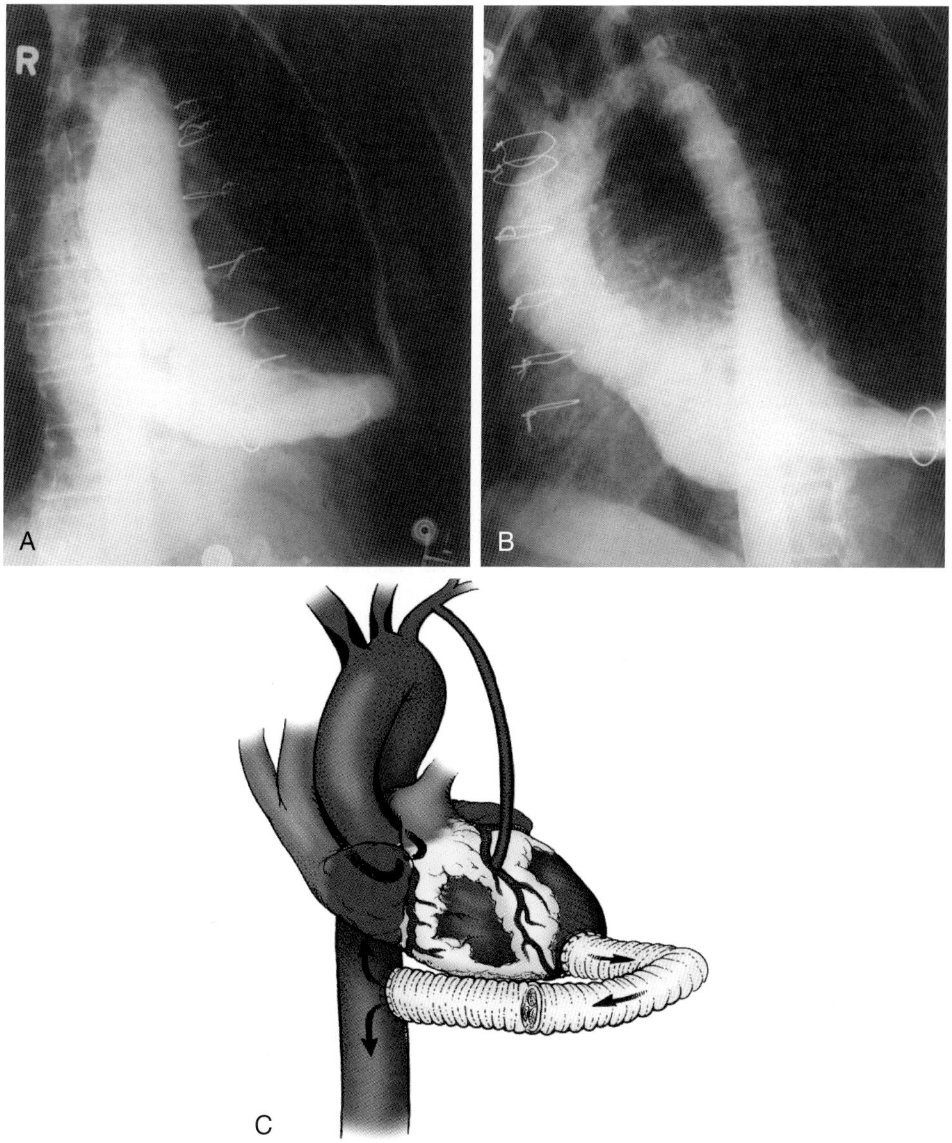

FIGURE 68-17 ■ This patient had undergone previous coronary artery bypass surgery, had systemic lupus and renal disease, was on high-dose steroids, and had heart failure from aortic valve stenosis. There was extensive calcification of the ascending aorta and aortic arch, including modest stenosis of the greater vessels. **A** and **B,** A valved tube graft was placed from the left ventricle apex to the descending aorta. The operation was done without cardiopulmonary bypass. **C,** Diagram of the operative procedure.

SUMMARY

In the past, aortic arch surgery was among the most formidable of cardiovascular operations. With modern techniques, surgery for the aortic arch is considerably safer, and satisfactory results can be achieved in most patients.

REFERENCES

1. Bachet J, Guilmet D, Goudot B, et al: Antegrade cerebral perfusion with cold blood: a 13-year experience. *Ann Thorac Surg* 67:1874–1878, discussion 1891–1894, 1999.
2. Ueda Y, Miki S, Kusuhara K, et al: Deep hypothermic systemic circulatory arrest and continuous retrograde cerebral perfusion for surgery of aortic arch aneurysm. *Eur J Cardiothorac Surg* 6:36–41, discussion 42, 1992.
3. De Bakey ME, Crawford ES, Cooley DA, et al: Successful resection of fusiform aneurysm of aortic arch with replacement by homograft. *Surg Gynecol Obstet* 105:657–664, 1957.
4. Svensson LG, Crawford ES: *Cardiovascular and vascular diseases of the aorta*, Philadelphia, 1997, WB Saunders, pp 42–83.
5. Barnard CN: Surgical treatment of acquired aneurysms of the thoracic aorta. *N Z Med J* 64(Suppl):61–63, 1965.
6. Borst HG, Frank G, Schaps D: Treatment of extensive aortic aneurysms by a new multiple-stage approach. *J Thorac Cardiovasc Surg* 95:11–13, 1988.
7. Borst HG, Walterbusch G, Schaps D: Extensive aortic replacement using "elephant trunk" prosthesis. *Thorac Cardiovasc Surg* 31:37–40, 1983.
8. Heinemann MK, Buehner B, Jurmann MJ, et al: Use of the "elephant trunk technique" in aortic surgery. *Ann Thorac Surg* 60:2–6, discussion 7, 1995.
9. Svensson LG: Rationale and technique for replacement of the ascending aorta, arch, and distal aorta using a modified elephant trunk procedure. *J Card Surg* 7:301–312, 1992.
10. Svensson LG: Antegrade perfusion during suspended animation? *J Thorac Cardiovasc Surg* 124:1068–1070, 2002.
11. Svensson LG, Khitin L: Aortic cross-sectional area/height ratio timing of aortic surgery in asymptomatic patients with Marfan syndrome. *J Thorac Cardiovasc Surg* 123:360–361, 2002.

12. Robinson BL, Nadolny EM, Entrup MH, et al: Management of right-sided aortic arch aneurysms. *Ann Thorac Surg* 72:1764–1765, 2001.
13. Svensson LG, Labib SB, Eisenhauer AC, et al: Intimal tear without hematoma: an important variant of aortic dissection that can elude current imaging techniques. *Circulation* 99:1331–1336, 1999.
14. Svensson LG, Crawford ES: Aortic dissection and aortic aneurysm surgery: clinical observations, experimental investigations, and statistical analyses. Part II. *Curr Probl Surg* 29:913–1057, 1992.
15. Svensson LG, Crawford ES, Coselli JS, et al: Impact of cardiovascular operation on survival in the Marfan patient. *Circulation* 80:I233–I242, 1989.
16. Lawrence PF: Conservative treatment of aortic graft infection. *Semin Vasc Surg* 24:199–204, 2011.
17. Igari K, Kudo T, Toyofuku T, et al: Treatment strategies for aortic and peripheral prosthetic graft infection. *Surg Today* 2013.
18. Svensson LG, Husain A, Penney DL, et al: A prospective randomized study of neurocognitive function and s-100 protein after antegrade or retrograde brain perfusion with hypothermic arrest for aortic surgery. *J Thorac Cardiovasc Surg* 119:163–167, 2000.
19. Svensson LG, Nadolny EM, Penney DL, et al: Prospective randomized neurocognitive and S-100 study of hypothermic circulatory arrest, retrograde brain perfusion, and antegrade brain perfusion for aortic arch operations. *Ann Thorac Surg* 71:1905–1912, 2001.
20. Ueda T, Shimizu H, Ito T, et al: Cerebral complications associated with selective perfusion of the arch vessels. *Ann Thorac Surg* 70:1472–1477, 2000.
21. Cigarroa JE, Isselbacher EM, DeSanctis RW, et al: Diagnostic imaging in the evaluation of suspected aortic dissection. Old standards and new directions. *N Engl J Med* 328:35–43, 1993.
22. Nienaber CA, von Kodolitsch Y, Petersen B, et al: Intramural hemorrhage of the thoracic aorta. Diagnostic and therapeutic implications. *Circulation* 92:1465–1472, 1995.
23. Svensson LG: Invited commentary. *Ann Thorac Surg* 82:80, 2006.
24. Coselli JS, Crawford ES, Beall AC, Jr, et al: Determination of brain temperatures for safe circulatory arrest during cardiovascular operation. *Ann Thorac Surg* 45:638–642, 1988.
25. Iba Y, Minatoya K, Matsuda H, et al: Contemporary open aortic arch repair with selective cerebral perfusion in the era of endovascular aortic repair. *J Thorac Cardiovasc Surg* 145:S72–S77, 2013.
26. Zierer A, El-Sayed Ahmad A, Papadopoulos N, et al: Selective antegrade cerebral perfusion and mild (28 degrees C-30 degrees C) systemic hypothermic circulatory arrest for aortic arch replacement: results from 1002 patients. *J Thorac Cardiovasc Surg* 144: 1042–1049, 2012.
27. Davis EA, Gillinov AM, Cameron DE, et al: Hypothermic circulatory arrest as a surgical adjunct: a 5-year experience with 60 adult patients. *Ann Thorac Surg* 53:402–406, discussion 406–407, 1992.
28. Engelman RM, Pleet AB, Rousou JA, et al: Does cardiopulmonary bypass temperature correlate with postoperative central nervous system dysfunction? *J Card Surg* 10:493–497, 1995.
29. Svensson LG, Nadolny EM, Kimmel WA: Multimodal protocol influence on stroke and neurocognitive deficit prevention after ascending/arch aortic operations. *Ann Thorac Surg* 74:2040–2046, 2002.
30. Crawford ES, Svensson LG, Coselli JS, et al: Surgical treatment of aneurysm and/or dissection of the ascending aorta, transverse aortic arch, and ascending aorta and transverse aortic arch. Factors influencing survival in 717 patients. *J Thorac Cardiovasc Surg* 98:659–673, discussion 673–674, 1989.
31. Ergin MA, Galla JD, Lansmans L, et al: Hypothermic circulatory arrest in operations on the thoracic aorta. Determinants of operative mortality and neurologic outcome. *J Thorac Cardiovasc Surg* 107:788–797, discussion 797–799, 1994.
32. Griepp RB, Ergin MA, McCullough JN, et al: Use of hypothermic circulatory arrest for cerebral protection during aortic surgery. *J Card Surg* 12:312–321, 1997.
33. Cooley DA, Baldwin RT: Technique of open distal anastomosis for repair of descending thoracic aortic aneurysms. *Ann Thorac Surg* 54:932–936, 1992.
34. Svensson LG, Crawford ES, Hess KR, et al: Deep hypothermia with circulatory arrest. Determinants of stroke and early mortality in 656 patients. *J Thorac Cardiovasc Surg* 106:19–28, discussion 28–31, 1993.
35. Safi HJ, Brien HW, Winter JN, et al: Brain protection via cerebral retrograde perfusion during aortic arch aneurysm repair. *Ann Thorac Surg* 56:270–276, 1993.
36. Mills NL, Ochsner JL: Massive air embolism during cardiopulmonary bypass. Causes, prevention, and management. *J Thorac Cardiovasc Surg* 80:708–717, 1980.
37. Svensson LG, Longoria J, Kimmel WA, et al: Management of aortic valve disease during aortic surgery. *Ann Thorac Surg* 69:778–783, discussion 783–784, 2000.
38. Griepp RB, Juvonen T, Griepp EB, et al: Is retrograde cerebral perfusion an effective means of neural support during deep hypothermic circulatory arrest? *Ann Thorac Surg* 64:913–916, 1997.
39. Juvonen T, Weisz DJ, Wolfe D, et al: Can retrograde perfusion mitigate cerebral injury after particulate embolization? A study in a chronic porcine model. *J Thorac Cardiovasc Surg* 115:1142–1159, 1998.
40. Lytle BW, McCarthy PM, Meaney KM, et al: Systemic hypothermia and circulatory arrest combined with arterial perfusion of the superior vena cava. Effective intraoperative cerebral protection. *J Thorac Cardiovasc Surg* 109:738–743, 1995.
41. Milewski RK, Pacini D, Moser GW, et al: Retrograde and antegrade cerebral perfusion: results in short elective arch reconstructive times. *Ann Thorac Surg* 89:1448–1457, 2010.
42. Spielvogel D, Kai M, Tang GH, et al: Selective cerebral perfusion: a review of the evidence. *J Thorac Cardiovasc Surg* 145:S59–S62, 2013.
43. Sugiura T, Imoto K, Uchida K, et al: Comparative study of brain protection in ascending aorta replacement for acute type A aortic dissection: retrograde cerebral perfusion versus selective antegrade cerebral perfusion. *Gen Thorac Cardiovasc Surg* 60:645–648, 2012.
44. Usui A, Miyata H, Ueda Y, et al: Risk-adjusted and case-matched comparative study between antegrade and retrograde cerebral perfusion during aortic arch surgery: based on the Japan Adult Cardiovascular Surgery Database: the Japan Cardiovascular Surgery Database Organization. *Gen Thorac Cardiovasc Surg* 60:132–139, 2012.
45. Williams ML, Ganzel BL, Slater AD, et al: Antegrade versus retrograde cerebral protection in repair of acute ascending aortic dissection. *Am Surg* 78:349–351, 2012.
46. Svensson LG, Blackstone EH, Rajeswaran J, et al: Does the arterial cannulation site for circulatory arrest influence stroke risk? *Ann Thorac Surg* 78:1274–1284, discussion 1274–1284, 2004.
47. Guiraudon GM, Ofiesh JG, Kaushik R: Extended vertical transatrial septal approach to the mitral valve. *Ann Thorac Surg* 52:1058–1060, discussion 1060–1062, 1991.
48. Nadolny EM, Svensson LG: Carbon dioxide field flooding techniques for open heart surgery: monitoring and minimizing potential adverse effects. *Perfusion* 15:151–153, 2000.
49. Al-Hashimi S, Zaman M, Waterworth P, et al: Does the use of thiopental provide added cerebral protection during deep hypothermic circulatory arrest? *Interact Cardiovasc Thorac Surg* 17:392–397, 2013.
50. Kruger T, Hoffmann I, Blettner M, et al: Intraoperative neuroprotective drugs without beneficial effects? Results of the German Registry for Acute Aortic Dissection Type A (GERAADA). *Eur J Cardiothorac Surg* 2013.
51. Svensson LG, Blackstone E, Apperson C, et al: Granularity of neurological assessment after a prospective trial of total aortic arch replacement; *pending publication*.
52. Svensson LG, Robinson MF, Esser J, et al: Influence of anatomic origin on intracranial distribution of micro-emboli in the baboon. *Stroke* 17:1198–1202, 1986.
53. Svensson LG, Blackstone EH, Cosgrove DM, 3rd: Surgical options in young adults with aortic valve disease. *Curr Probl Cardiol* 28:417–480, 2003.
54. Svensson LG: Sizing for modified David's reimplantation procedure. *Ann Thorac Surg* 76:1751–1753, 2003.
55. David TE, Feindel CM: An aortic valve-sparing operation for patients with aortic incompetence and aneurysm of the ascending aorta. *J Thorac Cardiovasc Surg* 103:617–621, discussion 622, 1992.

56. Sarsam MA, Yacoub M: Remodeling of the aortic valve anulus. *J Thorac Cardiovasc Surg* 105:435–438, 1993.
57. Swain JA, McDonald TJ, Jr, Griffith PK, et al: Low-flow hypothermic cardiopulmonary bypass protects the brain. *J Thorac Cardiovasc Surg* 102:76–83, discussion 83–84, 1991.
58. Svensson LG, Rushing GD, Valenzuela ES, et al: Modifications, classification, and outcomes of elephant-trunk procedures. *Ann Thorac Surg* 96:548–558, 2013.
59. Safi HJ, Miller CC, 3rd, Estrera AL, et al: Staged repair of extensive aortic aneurysms: morbidity and mortality in the elephant trunk technique. *Circulation* 104:2938–2942, 2001.
60. Andersen ND, Williams JB, Hanna JM, et al: Results with an algorithmic approach to hybrid repair of the aortic arch. *J Vasc Surg* 57:655–667, discussion 666–667, 2013.
61. Svensson LG, Kaushik SD, Marinko E: Elephant trunk anastomosis between left carotid and subclavian arteries for aneurysmal distal aortic arch. *Ann Thorac Surg* 71:1050–1052, 2001.
62. Baeza CR, Beyer E, Svensson LG: Smoking-related greater vessel stenoses and bilateral axillary artery revascularization. *Ann Thorac Surg* 77:1847, 2004.
63. Svensson LG, Kim KH, Blackstone EH, et al: Elephant trunk procedure: newer indications and uses. *Ann Thorac Surg* 78:109–116, discussion 109–116, 2004.
64. Lee CW, Beaver TM, Klodell CT, Jr, et al: Arch debranching versus elephant trunk procedures for hybrid repair of thoracic aortic pathologies. *Ann Thorac Surg* 91:465–471, 2011.
65. Ergin MA, Uysal S, Reich DL, et al: Temporary neurological dysfunction after deep hypothermic circulatory arrest: a clinical marker of long-term functional deficit. *Ann Thorac Surg* 67:1887–1890, discussion 1891–1894, 1999.
66. Navia JL, Cosgrove DM, 3rd: Minimally invasive mitral valve operations. *Ann Thorac Surg* 62:1542–1544, 1996.
67. Svensson LG: Minimal-access "J" or "j" sternotomy for valvular, aortic, and coronary operations or reoperations. *Ann Thorac Surg* 64:1501–1503, 1997.
68. Karck M, Chavan A, Hagl C, et al: The frozen elephant trunk technique: a new treatment for thoracic aortic aneurysms. *J Thorac Cardiovasc Surg* 125:1550–1553, 2003.
69. Schoenhoff FS, Schmidli J, Eckstein FS, et al: The frozen elephant trunk: an interesting hybrid endovascular-surgical technique to treat complex pathologies of the thoracic aorta. *J Vasc Surg* 45:597–599, 2007.
70. Pacini D, Tsagakis K, Jakob H, et al: The frozen elephant trunk for the treatment of chronic dissection of the thoracic aorta: a multicenter experience. *Ann Thorac Surg* 92:1663–1670, discussion 1670, 2011.
71. Roselli EE, Soltesz EG, Mastracci T, et al: Antegrade delivery of stent grafts to treat complex thoracic aortic disease. *Ann Thorac Surg* 90:539–546, 2010.
72. Roselli EE, Rafael A, Soltesz EG, et al: Simplified frozen elephant trunk repair for acute DeBakey type I dissection. *J Thorac Cardiovasc Surg* 145:S197–S201, 2013.

CHAPTER 69

DESCENDING THORACIC AND THORACOABDOMINAL AORTIC SURGERY

Joseph S. Coselli • Kim I. de la Cruz • Ourania Preventza • Scott A. LeMaire

CHAPTER OUTLINE

INTRODUCTION

Aortic aneurysm is defined as a localized dilation of the aorta that is at least 50% greater than that of nondiseased adjacent aorta. In the distal aorta, namely the descending thoracic and thoracoabdominal aorta, most aneurysms form as a result of nonspecific medial degeneration, expansion related to chronic aortic dissection, or the disease processes of connective tissue disorders. Whereas aortic aneurysms may be either fusiform (a symmetrical dilation of the aorta) or saccular (a localized outpouching of the aorta), saccular aneurysms are uncommon in the distal aorta and tend to be associated with infection. False aneurysms (also called pseudoaneurysms) may occur and are caused by a disruption of the aortic layers that then permits leaking blood to be contained by the outermost layer of the aorta and may additionally involve the periaortic tissue. Under such conditions, the aortic wall may become dilated beyond its capacity to expand and subsequently rupture.

Contemporary surgery involves a balanced approach toward maximizing the patient's long-term benefit by replacing as much diseased aorta as possible with the need to limit aortic resection to reduce ischemic and other operative risk. Our contemporary approach to open surgical repair of the descending thoracic and thoracoabdominal aorta is presented in this chapter.

Developing a Surgical Approach to Repair

The replacement of aneurysmal sections of the distal aorta built on the successful homograft-replacement repairs of aortic coarctation by Gross and others in the mid-1940s.[1,2] In 1950, Swan used a homograft to replace an 8-cm section of the descending thoracic aorta in a teenage patient with a coarctation-related aneurysm.[3] However, it remained unclear how patients with degenerative aneurysm, who were typically far older, would respond to aortic clamping, because they tended to lack the extensive collateral circulation present in patients with congenital coarctation. Soon after Swan's initial repair, Lam and Aram[4] attempted to replace a fusiform aneurysm of the descending thoracic aorta with a homograft. Despite the use of a shunt to maintain distal perfusion and of other adjuncts in use in this era, this repair failed because the patient became septic; the authors speculated that a successful repair may necessitate full aneurysm extirpation. In 1953, DeBakey and Cooley[5] were able to successfully "clamp and sew" a homograft replacement of a very large aneurysm of the descending thoracic aorta that impinged on the celiac axis (this would arguably be considered an extent I thoracoabdominal aortic aneurysm [TAAA] repair today). And in 1955, Etheredge and colleagues[6] reported a successful homograft replacement of a TAAA, and they perfused the distal aorta by using a small temporary shunt. Also in 1955, Rob[7] reported several TAAA repairs performed by using a clamp-and-sew approach.

Over the next decade, the emerging availability of Dacron grafts facilitated the use of an extra-anatomic approach in which the graft would be placed around the aneurysm—before completely resecting it—such that it could be used as a bypass shunt during repair. For TAAAs, these repairs would be done in a bottom-to-top fashion to quickly restore blood flow to the visceral organs. Notably, all early grafts had significant limitations. Early Dacron grafts were extremely porous and readily permitted blood to seep through. Early aortic repairs were associated with high rates of death, paraplegia, and kidney failure.[8]

In 1974, Crawford[9] detailed his experience with 28 TAAA patients. His technique for TAAA repair was vastly different from the established extra-anatomic approach embraced by DeBakey and his contemporaries. By drawing on a variety of techniques devised by others,[10,11] as well as developing new techniques to expedite repair, he achieved an impressive survival rate of 92%. Crawford used an anatomic endoaortic-graft-inclusion technique and chose to avoid full resection of the aneurysm, carefully securing the remaining aortic wall around the replacement graft to reduce bleeding; he used island reattachment strategies to reimplant the visceral vessels and select intercostal arteries to restore perfusion to the viscera and spinal cord. Although Crawford's approach was not immediately adopted, it became the foundation for contemporary surgical approaches to TAAA repair, and his classification[12] of TAAA repairs (Fig. 69-1) remains in use.

Natural History

Whereas the aorta expands very slowly in normal circumstances, the distal aorta tends to grow at a faster rate than the proximal aorta. Documented growth rates for the distal aorta range from 0.1 to 0.3 cm per year; growth rates are further increased in larger diameter aortas (8 cm and larger) and in patients with chronic dissection.[13-15] Elefteriades and his colleagues at Yale[16] identified aortic diameter as a strong predictor of rupture, dissection, and mortality. A critical diameter of 7.0 cm was identified for descending thoracic aortic aneurysms (DTAAs), with a corresponding risk of rupture or dissection of 43%. Saccular aneurysms tend to grow faster and less predictably than do fusiform aneurysms. Although it typically takes years for an aneurysm to reach a diameter-based threshold for repair, many distal aortic aneurysms increase in size and eventually progress to cause serious complications. In addition, as distal aortic aneurysms form, they are commonly lined with substantial amounts of friable, atheromatous plaque and mural thrombus.

CLASSIFICATION BY EXTENT OF REPAIR

Repair of the distal aorta poses substantially different risks than proximal aortic repair. Subsequently, operative strategy and expected outcomes vary with the extent of aortic replacement; generally speaking, risk increases as longer sections of the aorta are replaced. Thus, repair of TAAAs is typically more complicated than repair of DTAAs. Understanding of the extent of aortic involvement is the key to planning an appropriate strategy for operative repair.

Distal aortic disease may be limited to short sections of the descending thoracic aorta, or it may involve long sections of the aorta and necessitate substantial exposure. Aneurysms may begin near the left subclavian artery (LSCA) and extend beyond the level of the diaphragmatic hiatus to include varying segments of the abdominal aorta. DTAAs usually begin just distal to the LSCA and extend toward (but not past) the crura of the diaphragm. Conversely, repair of TAAAs necessitates exposing the aorta above and below the diaphragm and involves incorporating the segment from which the visceral arteries arise into the repair.

The Crawford classification schema[12] conveys useful information about TAAA repair and divides these repairs into four "extents" according to the amount of aorta replaced (see Fig. 69-1). Crawford extent I repairs involve the aorta from just distal to the LSCA to the origins of the celiac axis and superior mesenteric arteries and may also involve the renal arteries; however, these repairs do not extend into the infrarenal aorta. Extent II is the most

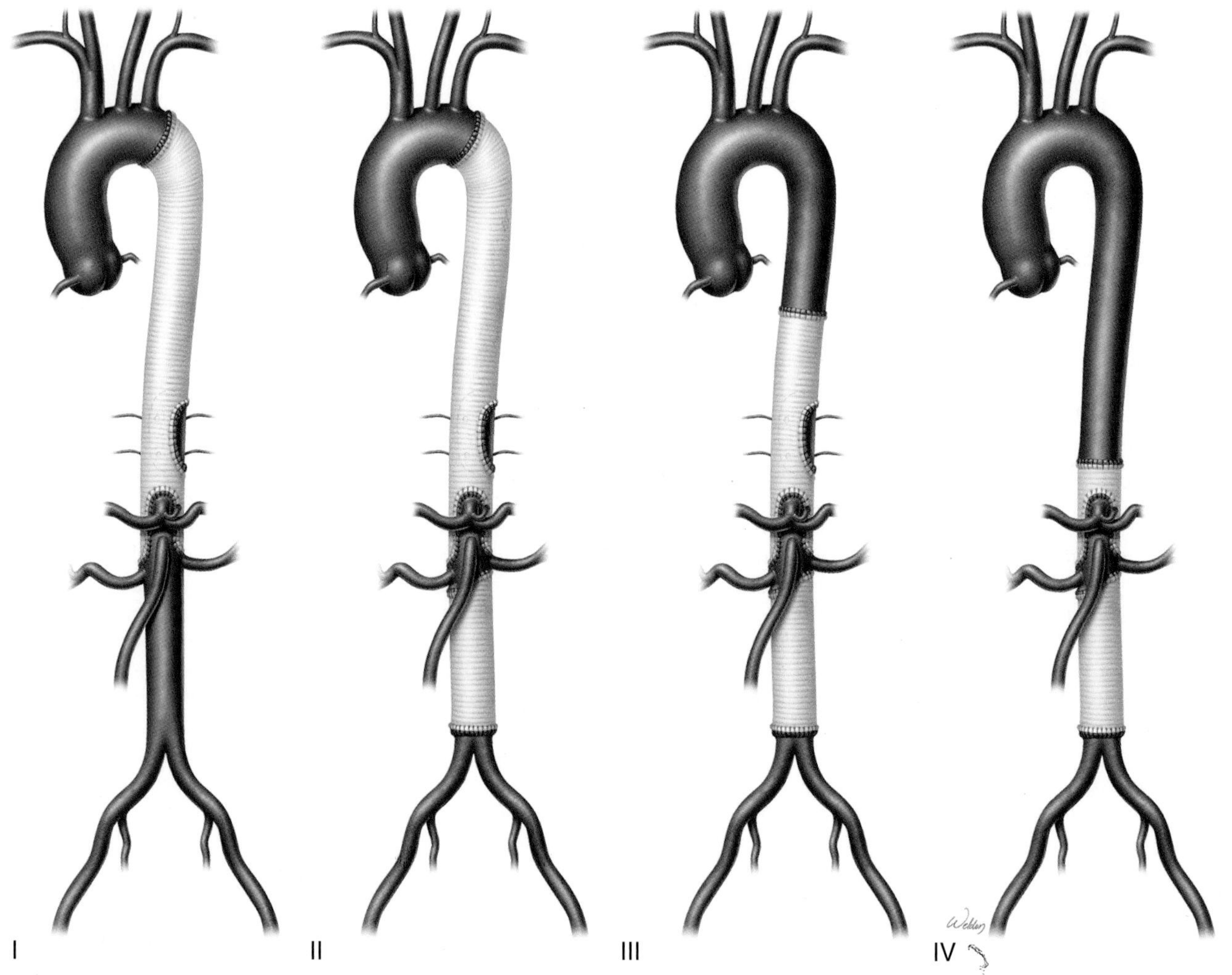

FIGURE 69-1 ■ The Crawford classification system for describing the extent of thoracoabdominal aortic aneurysm repair. (Used with permission of Baylor College of Medicine.)

extensive repair and involves almost the entire distal aorta, from near the LSCA to the infrarenal abdominal aorta, and it often extends to the aortoiliac bifurcation; extent II repairs generally incur the greatest operative risk. Extent III repairs involve the mid-descending thoracic aorta (below the sixth rib) and a variable amount of the abdominal aorta. Extent IV repairs begin within the diaphragmatic hiatus and extend through the abdominal aorta. Although some centers use a modified Crawford classification schema that includes an extent V repair,[17] we do not; extent V repairs tend to fall under the extent III category of repair, and these two types of repair typically have similar outcomes.

CAUSES AND PREDISPOSING FACTORS

Nonspecific Medial Degeneration

Although the underlying mechanisms of aortic disease remain unknown, nonspecific medial degeneration is the most common cause of thoracic aortic aneurysms and dissections. Although the fragmentation of elastic fibers and loss of smooth muscle cells are to be expected in the aging aorta, these processes are accelerated in medial degenerative aortic disease and lead to continual weakening of the aortic wall, aneurysm or dissection formation, and eventual rupture. Although atherosclerosis is often construed as a cause of thoracic aortic aneurysms, it may be merely a concomitant condition rather than a distinct cause of aortic aneurysm.

Chronic Aortic Dissection

Chronic dissection is a common cause of TAAA; consequently, reported rates range from 15% to almost 40% of TAAA repairs.[18,19] Aortic dissection (which is more fully covered in Chapters 70 and 71) usually begins as a tear in the innermost layer of the aortic wall. This tear allows pulsatile blood flow to cause a progressive separation of the medial layers, thereby creating two channels of blood flow within the aorta (Fig. 69-2*A*). This process substantially weakens the outer aortic wall, leading to aortic dilation and eventual aneurysm formation. Chronic dissection in the distal aorta occurs in survivors of acute DeBakey type I and III dissection events. Although it is generally assumed that chronically dissected aortas of either type dilate at similar rates, emerging evidence

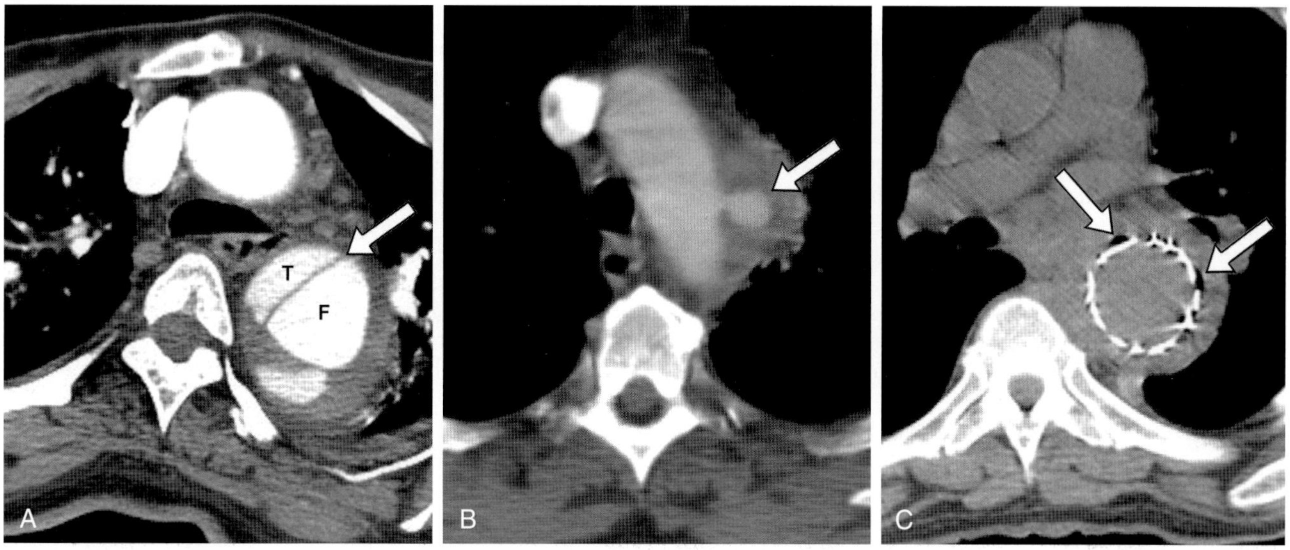

FIGURE 69-2 ■ Computed tomography scans showing key diagnostic findings. **A,** Chronic distal aortic dissection; the dividing septum is relatively straight *(arrow),* and the true (T) and false (F) lumens are indicated. **B,** Mycotic aneurysm, which is saccular in shape *(arrow).* **C,** Infection of an endograft; gas bubbles, indicated by *arrows,* may be seen near the endograft. (Used with permission of Baylor College of Medicine.)

suggests there may be differing rates of expansion between types.[20] Moreover, for incompletely understood reasons, patients with chronic dissection may also develop a superimposed acute dissection; this is a dangerous development, and urgent treatment is warranted.

Connective Tissue and Genetic Disorders

Connective tissue and related genetic disorders occur in 4% to 14% of patients who undergo DTAA or TAAA repair.[19,21-24] These disorders range from the relatively well-established Marfan syndrome (MFS) to lesser known, emerging disorders such as Loeys-Dietz and aneurysms-osteoarthritis syndromes. Of these conditions, MFS is the most common in DTAA and TAAA patients; however, surgeons should be aware of the other, more aggressive disorders so as to best formulate individualized strategies for treatment. Most of these syndromes are suspected on the basis of clinical features or a positive family history; as needed, confirmatory genetic tests should be conducted.

Marfan syndrome is an autosomal dominant genetic disorder that predisposes patients to aortic aneurysm and dissection. Although most patients with MFS have a family history of the disease, a substantial number of patients develop the mutation de novo; numerous mutations in the fibrillin-1 gene have been discovered.[25,26] It was long thought that the presence of abnormal fibrillin in the extracellular matrix reduced the strength of the aortic wall (and thus predisposed the aorta to dilation), but emerging evidence indicates that the abnormal fibrillin alters biomolecular pathways, leading to aberrant signaling of transforming growth factor beta (TGF-β) and a related cascade of events and, ultimately, to degeneration of the aortic wall matrix.[25] The clinical features of MFS usually include a tall and lanky stature with long limbs, eye lens disorders, mitral valve prolapse, joint hypermobility, high palate, and aortic aneurysms in young adults.

Most commonly, MFS affects the proximal aorta, namely the ascending aorta and aortic root. Most patients with MFS who undergo distal aortic aneurysm repair have chronic aortic dissection. Whereas most of these patients are operative survivors of acute DeBakey type I dissection, a substantial number of repairs are done in patients with initially medically managed DeBakey type III aortic dissection.[27]

Loeys-Dietz syndrome is an aggressive aortic disease that tends to affect patients at a much younger age than does MFS.[28] Characterized by widespread systemic arterial tortuosity and aneurysm formation, clinical features include the presence of a bifid uvula or cleft palate and widely spaced eyes (hypertelorism). In the past, many of these patients were identified as having MFS,[29] and like that disorder, this condition is autosomal dominant. However, Loeys-Dietz syndrome is caused by heterozygous mutations in the genes encoding TGF-β receptors I and II.[30] Patients with Loeys-Dietz syndrome require exceedingly careful monitoring because they are predisposed to dissection and rupture at far smaller aortic diameters than are patients with MFS.[31]

Other disorders,[32] such as Ehlers-Danlos syndrome, aneurysms-osteoarthritis syndrome, and nonsyndromic familial aortic aneurysm and dissection, are currently thought to be infrequently encountered in patients who need distal aortic repair. Ehlers-Danlos syndrome comprises a spectrum of disorders of collagen synthesis; the vascular subtype (previously referred to as "type IV") of Ehlers-Danlos syndrome involves a defect in type III collagen synthesis that lends itself to cardiovascular manifestations, chief among which is spontaneous arterial rupture.[33] Poor aortic tissue integrity tends to complicate surgical repair.[34] Recently identified, aneurysms-osteoarthritis syndrome is an autosomal dominant disorder caused by a mutation in the gene responsible for transcribing TGF-β, *SMAD3*.[35] Clinically, this syndrome is reminiscent of Loeys-Dietz syndrome, but, in contrast, these patients also have early-onset osteoarthritis. Of note, these patients have a high incidence of aortic dissection at moderately dilated aortic diameters (4 to 4.5 cm), well below standard thresholds of repair.[36] Several other heritable mutations, affecting families with variable expression, have been documented in the genes for TGF-β receptors, TGF-β_2, β-myosin, SMAD3, and α-smooth muscle cell actin.[37-41] Although familial aortic thoracic aneurysms most commonly affect the proximal aorta, such heritable nonsyndromic disease may present as dissection or aneurysm in the distal aorta.

Aortitis

In rare cases, systemic autoimmune disorders, such as giant cell arteritis, Takayasu arteritis, and Behçet disease, may also lead to aneurysm formation in the distal aorta. A granulomatous inflammation may occur in patients with giant cell arteritis (temporal arteritis) that involves the entire thickness of the aortic wall and thus cause intimal thickening and medial destruction. Although Takayasu arteritis generally produces severe intimal thickening that causes obstructive lesions, it can also lead to aneurysm formation. A more common presentation of aortitis occurs when patients with preexisting degenerative aortic aneurysms then develop localized transmural inflammation. Although the reasons for this inflammation remain unclear, its onset can lead to expansion and further weaken the aortic wall. In addition, fibrosis and an infiltrate of plasma cells, giant cells, and lymphocytes can develop in the affected tissue. In Behçet disease, both arteries and veins are affected, and the disease process involves lymphocytic infiltration of the medial layer, which may progress to aneurysm or pseudoaneurysm formation.

Mycotic Aneurysm

In rare cases, infection of the native aorta precipitates distal aortic aneurysm formation. Such lesions are commonly called *mycotic aneurysms*, even though the responsible pathogens are usually bacteria rather than fungi. Mycotic aneurysms may form as bacteria inoculate healthy aortic tissue, which then contributes to subsequent aneurysm formation, or they may result from the secondary infection of an existing aneurysm. In addition, mycotic aneurysms may be pseudoaneurysms, rather than true aneurysms, and can develop as a late complication of previous iatrogenic aortic injury created during invasive imaging procedures or cardiac or aortic operations (e.g., aortic cannulation sites). Establishing a diagnosis for patients with a mycotic aneurysm can be exceedingly difficult because symptoms can be vague, such as a persistent low-grade fever or unexpected weight loss, and such infection is rare.[42] Further complicating matters, there are a variety of mechanisms by which the source bacteria may infect the aorta; these include vertebral or other abscess, general sepsis or septic emboli, empyema, infected lymph nodes,[43] and other factors that can be difficult to elucidate. Unlike most other distal aortic aneurysms, which tend to be fusiform in shape, mycotic aneurysms are often saccular in shape (see Fig. 69-2*B*) and correspond to localized areas of tissue destruction. Common causative organisms include *Staphylococcus aureus*, *Staphylococcus epidermidis*, *Salmonella*, and *Streptococcus*,[44] and more than one pathogen may be present. Outside the United States, tuberculosis aortitis may present as saccular aneurysm of the thoracoabdominal aorta, and sometimes even as multiple saccular aneurysms.[45] Of note, saccular aneurysms can be unpredictable, are prone to rapid growth rates, and tend to rupture more readily than fusiform aneurysms caused by medial degeneration; when mycotic saccular aneurysm is suspected, urgent evaluation is warranted.[46]

Repair after Previous Open Aortic Repair (Noncongenital)

Over time, late complications of previous distal aortic repair may develop (Fig. 69-3); such complications include pseudoaneurysms and aneurysms that develop around sites of aortic reattachment (e.g., buttons of tissue surrounding reattached visceral or intercostal arteries may later become aneurysmal). In addition, aortic disease may progress such that previously normal sections of the aorta adjacent to the site of a previous repair may later become aneurysmal. Late complications tend to occur more frequently in patients with MFS and other connective tissue disorders and in patients with aortic infection. Overall, distal redo operation (previous open repair of the descending thoracic, thoracoabdominal, or abdominal aorta) rates tend to range from 16% to 27% in reported series of TAAA repairs.[18,19,47,48]

Pseudoaneurysms often represent chronic leaks that are contained by surrounding tissues. The outer wall of a pseudoaneurysm develops from organized thrombus and associated fibrosis. Pseudoaneurysms can arise from primary defects in the aortic wall (such as a leak from a fistula or contained rupture) or from degraded suture lines or graft material (anastomotic leaks were common in the era of silk suture, which readily degraded, and graft infection may also degrade the suture line), from sites of previous cannulation (leaks that occur after cardiovascular surgery), or from a wire penetrating or otherwise damaging the aorta during invasive aortic imaging and testing. Anastomotic pseudoaneurysms can also be caused by tension between the graft and native aortic tissue. With modern suture, graft material, and technique, the incidences of pseudoaneurysm and other late complications have decreased; however, should they occur, urgent evaluation is warranted because they have a tendency toward rupture.

Repair after Previous Endovascular Aortic Repair

In the contemporary era, the use of aortic stent-grafts in the distal aorta is common in patients with aneurysm and dissection (this topic is fully covered in Chapters 70 and 71). Occasionally, patients who have undergone endovascular aortic repair develop problems that necessitate open repair.[49-55] Open aortic repair after endovascular aortic

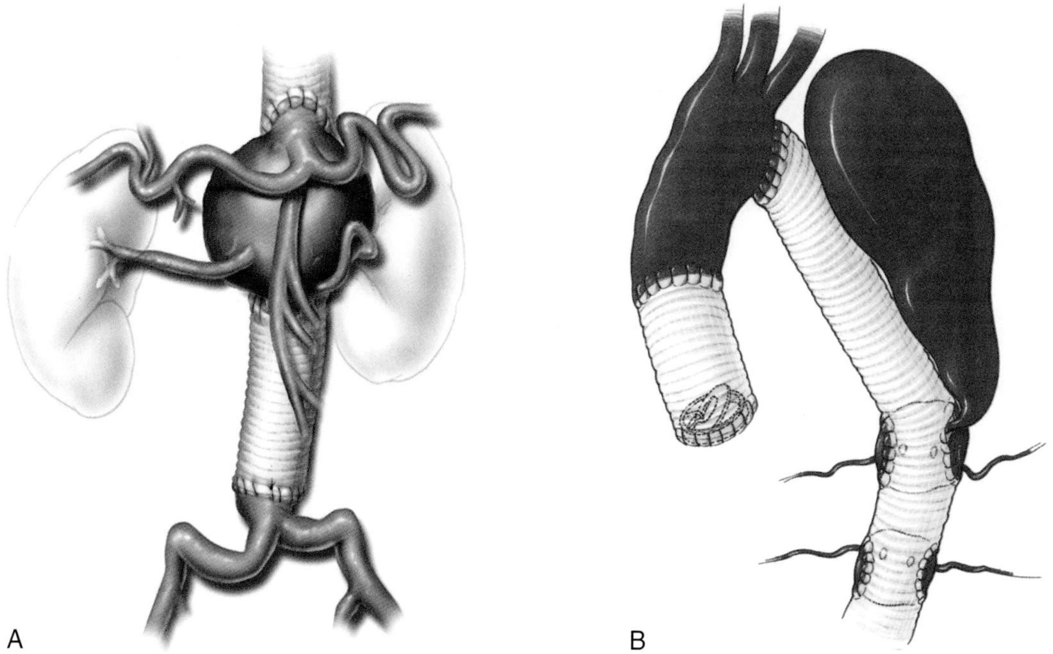

FIGURE 69-3 ■ Illustration showing late complications of open aortic repair. **A,** A visceral patch aneurysm has developed in the residual native aortic tissue. **B,** A pseudoaneurysm has developed near the suture line of an intercostal artery reattachment site.

procedures may be necessary to treat continued dilation of the aorta at or near the stent-graft landing zones, infection of the endograft (see Fig. 69-2*C*), the development of a fistula (Fig. 69-4), stent-graft collapse or migration, or ongoing aneurysm expansion, which may result in rupture. Progressive expansion of the aneurysm may occur because of an inadequate seal between the stent-graft and aorta (type I endoleak), bleeding into the aneurysmal sac from any covered branching artery (type II endoleak), a gap between overlapping stent-grafts (type III endoleak), retrograde perfusion through the false lumen into the aneurysmal sac in patients with extensive aortic dissection, or other causes.

Coarctation in the Adult (Congenital)

Aortic coarctation may occur in patients with bicuspid aortic valve or other congenital heart disease or in patients with Turner syndrome.[56] The typical presentation of aortic coarctation involves a narrowing of a short section of the descending thoracic aorta, located just beyond the LSCA; the quality of aortic tissue in this section is generally poor because it is delicate and friable. Over the past several decades, several open approaches have been used to treat aortic coarctation in early childhood, including subclavian flap repair, patch aortoplasty, and interposition aortic grafting. In adults, open or endovascular repair may be needed to treat previously undiscovered native coarctation or late complications (aneurysm, pseudoaneurysm, or restenosis) of previously repaired coarctation,[57,58] which tend to develop in the first or second decade after initial repair.[59] The ideal repair for discrete and previously unrepaired coarctation in adults is somewhat controversial; current guidelines indicate that either an endovascular or an open repair may be performed.[56]

In rare cases, adults need primary repair for extreme forms of previously untreated coarctation, such as an interrupted or a hypoplastic aortic arch (Fig. 69-5), or a long-segment aortic coarctation (also known as middle aortic syndrome and sometimes seen with rib notching); for these patients, current guidelines recommend open repair (Class I recommendation, level of evidence B). For patients with discrete restenosis after open repair, endovascular repair is recommended unless significant aortopathy is also present (Class I recommendation, level of evidence B).[56] Today, many experienced centers achieve good results by using a variety of approaches to coarctation repair, including open, endovascular, and hybrid techniques.[57,58,60-64]

Patients with aortic coarctation commonly have hypertension, and even with treatment, hypertension remains difficult to control. It is thought that uncontrolled hypertension plays a role in the late development of aneurysms, both in patients with previous aortic repair and in those without. In previously untreated adults, extensive collateral circulation may develop; during open repair, these branching vessels may enhance the risk of operative bleeding, and these vessels are commonly ligated when possible. Patients with long-segment coarctation may be treated with extra-anatomic bypass grafts rather than in situ graft replacement.

INDICATIONS FOR REPAIR

Descending thoracic and thoracoabdominal aortic aneurysms most commonly present in asymptomatic, older patients (60 years of age and older) and are often incidentally discovered through imaging studies ordered to evaluate other, unrelated health problems. In patients

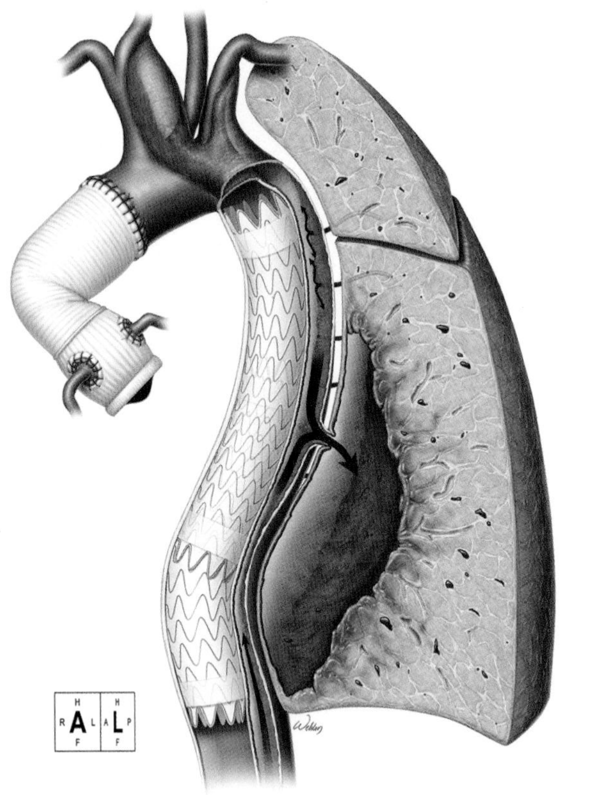

FIGURE 69-4 ■ Illustration showing the development of an aortopulmonary fistula, a rare late complication of thoracic endovascular aortic repair. Here, the stent-graft is shown to be within the true lumen. The distal descending thoracic aorta has ruptured into the lower lobe of the left lung *(arrow)*; the false lumen continued to be perfused from re-entry sites below the distal landing zone of this stent-graft. Blood flow from collateral vessels additionally perfused the false lumen. (From Matos JM, de la Cruz KI, Ouzounian M, et al: Endovascular repair as a bridge to surgical repair of an aortobronchial fistula complicating chronic residual aortic dissection. *Tex Heart Inst J* 41:198–202, 2014, Fig. 5. Reproduced with permission. Copyright the Texas Heart Institute.)

with known risk factors for distal aortic aneurysms (as described in the previous section), imaging studies are used to carefully monitor the aorta until diameter-based thresholds of repair are met or until symptoms develop. Therefore, the management of distal aortic disease is typically dependent on regularly repeated imaging studies and enhanced awareness of emerging symptoms through patient education and optimization efforts (at a minimum, optimization efforts include strict blood pressure control and cessation of smoking).

Diagnostic Imaging Evaluation

Although developing an appropriate distal aortic imaging strategy is somewhat dependent on local expertise and equipment availability, recently efforts have been made to standardize image acquisition and reporting by suggesting specific aortic landmarks to measure (Fig. 69-6); for the distal aorta, these include the isthmus or proximal descending thoracic aorta (2 cm distal to the LSCA), the middle of the descending aorta (between the isthmus and the diaphragm), the aorta at the diaphragm (roughly 2 cm above the celiac axis), and the aorta at the origin of the celiac axis.[43] Aortic imaging reports should clearly state the location of aortic abnormalities (using the previously mentioned locations whenever possible) and report the maximum external aortic diameter (reporting the internal lumen diameter may fail to account for aortic wall inflammation, intraluminal clot, or mural thrombus, or identify both channels in cases of aortic dissection). Any extension of disease into branching vessels, such as is possible with chronic distal aortic dissection and other conditions, should be documented. Evidence of rupture should be reported, as well as any identified calcification or internal filling defects that are consistent with thrombus or atheroma. Ideally, results should be compared with the most recent prior imaging study available; precise measurement is needed because the yearly rate of aortic

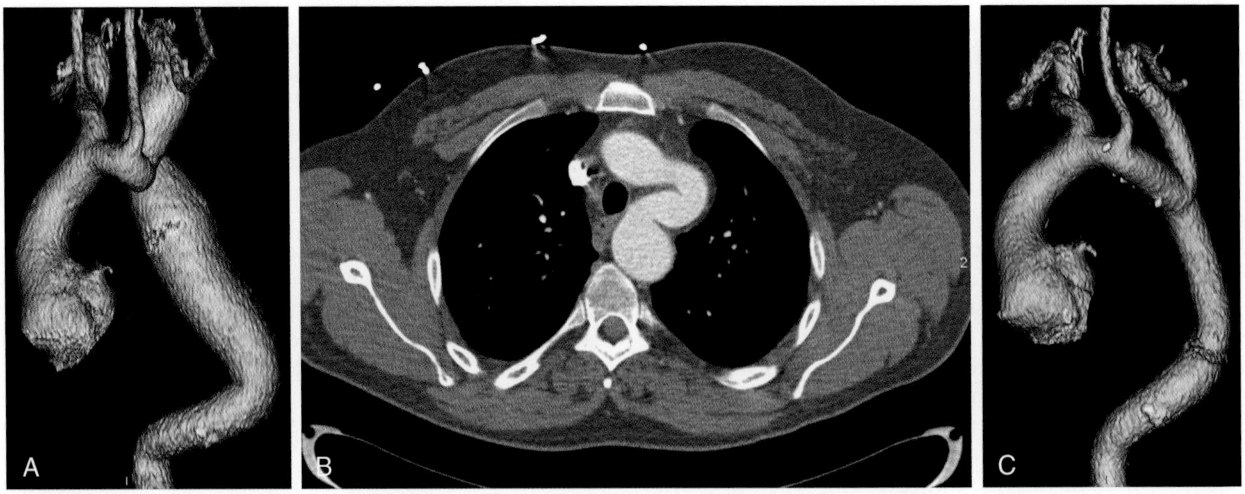

FIGURE 69-5 ■ Computed tomographic angiograms in a patient with bicuspid aortic valve, related proximal and distal aortopathy, and coarctation. **A,** Three-dimensional reconstruction showing coarctation of the descending thoracic aorta. **B,** Axial image showing hypoplasia and tortuosity of the aortic arch. **C,** Post-repair three-dimensional reconstruction showing surgical correction of the aortic arch, descending thoracic aorta, and the left subclavian artery. (From Preventza O, Livesay JJ, Cooley DA, et al: Coarctation-associated aneurysms: a localized disease or diffuse aortopathy. *Ann Thorac Surg* 95:1961–1967, 2013, Fig. 1. Used with permission. Copyright Society of Thoracic Surgeons.)

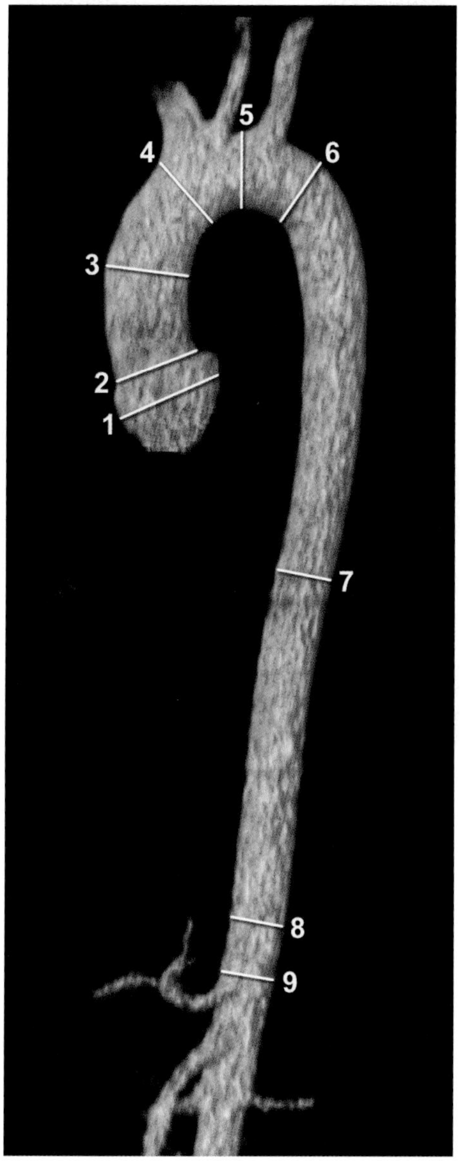

FIGURE 69-6 ■ Current practice guidelines[43] seek to standardize the reporting of aortic diameters by indicating key anatomic locations to be measured. These include (1) the sinuses of Valsalva, (2) the sinotubular junction, (3) the mid-ascending aorta, (4) the proximal aortic arch at the origins of the innominate artery, (5) the mid-aortic arch, which is between the left common carotid and left subclavian arteries, (6) the proximal descending thoracic aorta, which begins at the isthmus (approximately 2 cm distal to the origins of the left subclavian artery), (7) the mid-descending thoracic artery, (8) the aorta at the diaphragm, and (9) the abdominal aorta at the origins of the celiac axis. (Used with permission of Baylor College of Medicine.)

expansion is generally quite small, and thus, detecting a small but abnormal growth rate can be challenging.

Although a routine chest radiograph may suggest an aortic abnormality, the most useful diagnostic imaging modalities include computed tomographic (CT) and magnetic resonance imaging or angiography scans of the chest and abdomen to delineate the extent of aortic and branch-vessel involvement. Since the CT was first reported to identify aortic disease in 1976,[65] it has become widely available and is the most commonly used imaging modality for identifying aortic aneurysms. Information about the aneurysm's location and extent, external diameter, the presence of aortic dissection, the relationship to branching vessels, and anatomic abnormalities are all readily provided by iodinated intravenous contrast-enhanced CT imaging (Fig. 69-7). Such imaging may also aid in determining the presence of aortic infection, because nearby gas bubbles can be readily identified.[42] Benefits of CT imaging include the short time needed to acquire the imaging data, the ability to render three-dimensional imaging, and the ability to provide multiplanar evaluation, as well as locating the presence of any aortic calcification or thrombus. Disadvantages of contrast-enhanced CT scanning include repeated exposure to ionizing radiation and the possibility of contrast-induced allergy or contrast-induced acute renal dysfunction in patients. Whenever possible, surgery is performed at least 1 day after contrast administration to allow time to observe renal function and, if needed, to permit renal function to return to normal.

Although magnetic resonance angiography (MRA) is not used as commonly as CT imaging to detect aortic aneurysm, it produces comparable or better aortic images and does not expose patients to ionizing radiation. It offers excellent visualization of all facets of branching vessels and facilitates the identification of left ventricular dysfunction. Disadvantages of MRA include the generally higher expense, the extended time needed to acquire imaging data (which poses a challenge in the critically ill patient), the suboptimal identification of aortic calcification, and the generation of artifacts created by ferromagnetic materials (such as pacemakers and other implants). In addition, the contrast agent for MRA, gadolinium, is associated with nephrogenic systemic fibrosis in patients with comorbid renal dysfunction.[66,67] In young and otherwise healthy patients, such as those with MFS, MRA may be a valuable supplement to lifelong surveillance imaging because it avoids exposure to radiation. Echocardiography and ultrasonography are not used to evaluate DTAAs because these techniques cannot adequately visualize disease involving this segment.

Diameter-Based Thresholds for Repair

All aneurysms are repaired to prevent fatal rupture. Although replacing the aorta can be life-saving in patients with aortic disease, surgical intervention carries substantial risks for both morbidity and mortality. Because of the inherent risks associated with surgical intervention, surgery is generally indicated only when the risk of rupture or other catastrophic aortic complications exceeds it. Studies of the natural history of distal aortic aneurysms (as described in a previous section) helped to formulate diameter-based thresholds of repair in asymptomatic patients. Current practice guidelines[43] recommend elective open aortic repair in asymptomatic patients when the diameter of a TAAA exceeds 6.0 cm; a lower threshold is recommended if the patient has a connective tissue disorder (Class I recommendation; level of evidence C). In patients with chronic aortic dissection, elective open repair is indicated when the descending thoracic aorta exceeds 5.5 cm (Class I recommendation; level of

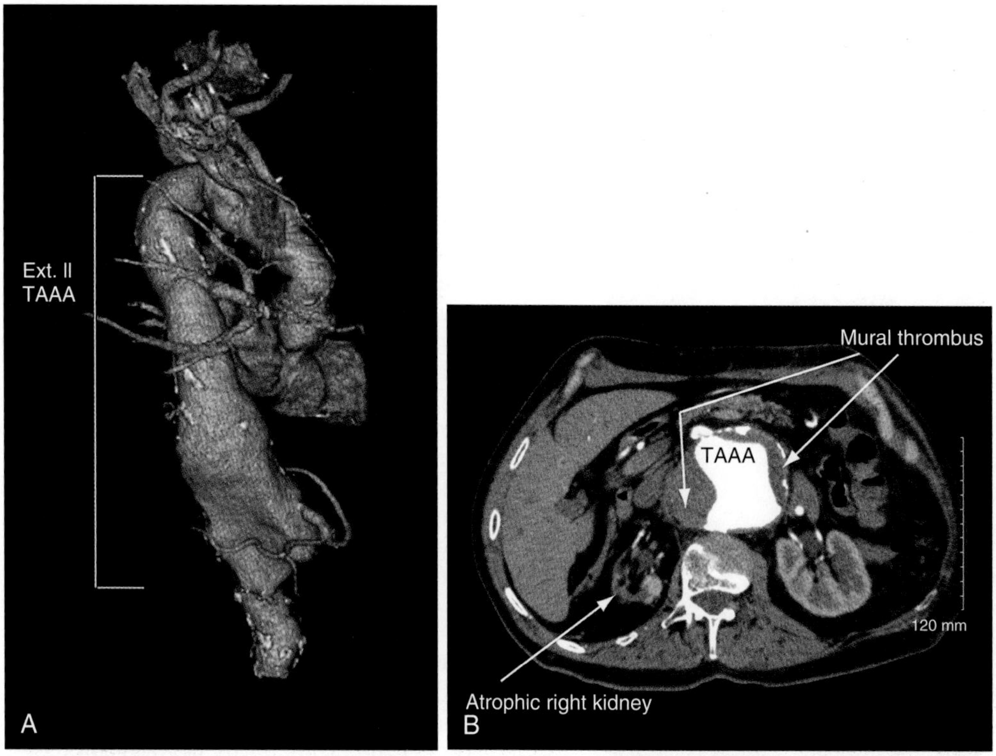

FIGURE 69-7 ■ Three-dimensional reconstruction **(A)** and axial contrast-enhanced computed tomographic image **(B)** of a thoracoabdominal aortic aneurysm (TAAA). Note that the aneurysm is lined with thrombus and that the right kidney is severely atrophic *(arrows)*. (From Vaughn SB, LeMaire SA, Collard CD: Case scenario: anesthetic considerations for thoracoabdominal aortic aneurysm repair. *Anesthesiology* 115:1093–1102, 2011, Fig. 1. Used with permission.)

evidence B). Although not expressly recommended for the distal aorta, elective repair of the proximal aorta is recommended when the rate of dilation exceeds 0.5 cm per year; it is reasonable to follow this recommendation in distal aortic repairs also, because such rapid growth indicates an unstable aneurysm.

Symptoms

When specific symptoms are present, they are usually related to aneurysmal expansion and compression of surrounding structures or to malperfusion related to aortic dissection. The onset of symptoms is usually considered an indication of impending rupture or significant malperfusion and should prompt urgent evaluation. Pain, the most common symptom, may be located in the chest, back, abdomen, or left flank; it may be described as a sharp or stabbing acute pain or as refractory pain. However, pain may be chronic and the cause poorly understood in these typically older patients.

Myriad other symptoms can arise, and whenever possible, a careful medical history should be obtained from each patient. In rare cases, fistulas can develop in patients with distal aortic aneurysm, and unexplained bleeding may be present. Dysphagia can result from compression of the esophagus, whereas coughing, wheezing, or pneumonitis can result from impingement on the trachea or proximal bronchi; hemoptysis may result from erosion into these structures. Hoarseness may result from partial vocal cord paralysis if the recurrent laryngeal nerve is compromised. Pressure from expanding aneurysms can erode spinal bodies (often resulting in pain) or the bowel wall (causing gastrointestinal bleeding). Duodenal obstruction may occur through related compression. In rare cases, jaundice can result from compression of the biliary tract. Compression of the inferior vena cava or iliac vein can result in distal venous stasis and can present as an abdominal bruit, with widened pulse pressure and edema, and may result in heart failure.

Additional symptoms related to embolization, frank rupture, or either acute-onset dissection or expanding chronic dissection can result. Plaque and thrombus may embolize distally, causing occlusion and thrombosis of the visceral, renal, or lower extremity branches and subsequent malperfusion. Shock, refractory hypertension, or rapid aortic expansion may indicate existing or pending rupture; DTAAs tend to rupture into the pleural cavity, often resulting in severe hemorrhagic shock. Spontaneous paraplegia; abdominal pain; cold, blue, or painful extremities; nausea; vomiting; and incontinence or abnormal urination can be signs of malperfusion caused by aortic dissection.

The assessment of possibly aneurysm-related symptoms is essential to developing an appropriate management plan. Patients who develop symptoms undergo surgical repair regardless of aneurysm diameter. The most common indication for emergent repair of a TAAA is aortic rupture or an acute dissection superimposed on an existing chronic dissection; often such dissection rapidly progresses to aortic rupture. Although emergent repair is well understood to carry greater operative risk than does elective repair, any inappropriate delay of repair risks death; appropriate delay includes transfer to an experienced center.

Contraindications to Repair

Contraindications to open repair of the distal aorta are patient-specific and individualized to the experience of each surgeon. In general, patients with limited life expectancy are not candidates for open surgical repair, although aortic repair in survivable forms of cancer may be warranted before its treatment. Although patients at prohibitive risk of open surgical repair are sometimes offered hybrid endovascular repair, such repair in patients with TAAA involves invasive debranching of the visceral arteries and is generally poorly tolerated by patients, except in a handful of centers.[68] Operative risk models for TAAA repair commonly identify advanced age as a predictor of early death[69]; operative results in patients 80 years and older tend to be somewhat poor.[70] In addition, patients should be presented with information regarding the risk of developing life-altering complications such as stroke, renal failure resulting in dialysis dependence, and paraplegia. Other patient-specific comorbid risks include chronic renal insufficiency, chronic obstructive pulmonary disease, heart failure, and coronary artery disease.[71,72]

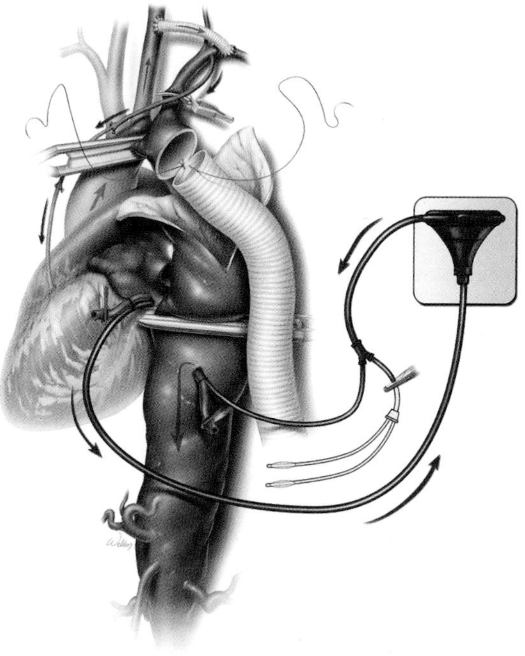

FIGURE 69-8 ■ Drawing of a thoracoabdominal aortic aneurysm repair in a patient with a patent left internal thoracic artery–to–left anterior descending coronary artery graft. The proximal anastomosis is being performed while the aorta is clamped between the left common carotid and subclavian arteries. Myocardial perfusion is maintained through the carotid-subclavian bypass graft. Thus, the potential for causing cardiac ischemia during repair is mitigated. (From Jones MM, Akay M, Murariu D, et al: Safe aortic arch clamping in patients with patent internal thoracic artery grafts. *Ann Thorac Surg* 89:e31–32, 2010, Fig. 2. Used with permission. Copyright Society of Thoracic Surgeons.)

STRATEGY FOR REPAIR

Preoperative Evaluation

Comorbidities that are typically considered predictive of operative risk should be carefully evaluated and modified whenever possible to mitigate risk; similarly, preoperative evaluation of patients' physiologic reserve is critical to obtaining a beneficial outcome. Except in those patients who require emergent repair, all patients should undergo a thorough preoperative evaluation emphasizing cardiac, pulmonary, and renal function, as well as a careful review of imaging studies. As needed, additional studies may be warranted; in patients identified as high risk for carotid artery disease, carotid Doppler ultrasonography is warranted, and potential clotting problems or cirrhosis may be evaluated with coagulation and liver function tests.

Cardiac Function

Patients need significant cardiac reserve to tolerate thoracic aortic clamping. Transthoracic echocardiography and electrocardiography are routinely used to assess cardiac function. Patients with an ejection fraction less than 30% or with symptoms of coronary artery disease should additionally undergo cardiac catheterization or, when necessary, a noninvasive assessment of myocardial perfusion (such as dobutamine echocardiography or a dipyridamole thallium scan). When significant coronary artery disease is identified in an elective surgical candidate, myocardial revascularization is recommended before aortic replacement. Patients who have already undergone coronary artery revascularization should be carefully assessed; if the left internal thoracic artery has been used to revascularize the heart, and if the aortic clamp may need to be placed proximal to the origin of the LSCA (a common placement site for DTAA and extent I and II TAAA repairs), a left carotid–to–subclavian artery bypass (Fig. 69-8) can be performed before aortic replacement to avoid myocardial ischemia.[73]

Pulmonary Function

Sufficient pulmonary function is needed to tolerate the single-lung ventilation that is commonly used in distal aortic repair; pulmonary complications are the most common form of postoperative complication and typically affect 30% or more of patients with distal aortic repair. In most patients, lung function is assessed with pulmonary function studies, including forced expiratory volume in 1 second (FEV_1) and arterial blood gas analysis. All patients with an FEV_1 greater than 1.0 liters and a blood carbon dioxide partial pressure (PCO_2) less than 45 mm Hg are considered satisfactory surgical candidates. Whenever possible, in patients with an FEV_1 less than 1.0 liter or a PCO_2 of greater than 45 mm Hg, pulmonary function is optimized over a period of 1 to 3 months by means of smoking cessation, bronchodilator therapy, weight loss, an appropriate exercise regimen, and pulmonary rehabilitation. Optimizing lung function preoperatively is thought to lessen postoperative pulmonary complications. In addition, diaphragm-sparing techniques may be selectively used in patients with particularly poor pulmonary function.

Renal Function

Preoperative renal dysfunction is an important predictor of early postoperative mortality and morbidity after aortic replacement.[48,71] Unfortunately, CT imaging (which is often used in planning aortic repair) may adversely affect renal function through the necessary use of nephrotoxic contrast agents. In patients with borderline renal function, preventive measures are taken before imaging studies are conducted. A solution of 5% dextrose and Ringer lactate solution with 25 g/liter mannitol and 1 amp/liter sodium bicarbonate may be administered intravenously before image acquisition. In addition, acetylcysteine may be administered before and after such studies to further reduce the risk of contrast-induced nephropathy. When possible, after CT scanning or aortography, surgery is delayed for 24 hours or longer until renal function has returned to baseline.

Evaluation of Imaging Studies

Essential to forming an operative strategy, available imaging studies should be carefully reviewed and, if necessary, additional imaging studies should be obtained to clarify findings. The diameter of the aorta throughout the diseased and nonaneurysmal portions is established. Potential sites for aortic clamping and cannulation are reviewed for calcification, dissection, and mural thrombus. Close attention is paid to anatomic variants, such as a retroaortic left renal vein, as well as any previous use of the left internal thoracic artery to provide coronary revascularization. The locations of particularly large intercostal arteries are noted. Branching vessels, such as the visceral and renal arteries, are carefully assessed for stenotic origins, their spatial orientation relative to each other, and, in cases of chronic aortic dissection, whether blood is supplied by the true lumen, false lumen, or both.

Anesthesia

It is crucial to establish communication among the surgeon, anesthesiologist, and perfusionist during distal aortic repair. Adequate intraoperative monitoring and venous access must be ensured because patient hemodynamics can fluctuate greatly during aortic clamping and unclamping. Patients generally undergo placement of a right radial or brachial arterial line, a pulmonary artery catheter, and a large-bore central venous catheter that permits rapid fluid administration. Whenever blood flow through the LSCA will be compromised by the site of aortic clamping, the arterial catheter is placed in the right radial artery. To monitor temperature, a probe is placed in the patient's nasopharynx.

A method for anesthesia induction is specifically chosen according to each patient's hemodynamics, cardiac contractile function, and whether or not motor-evoked potential monitoring of the spinal cord will be used. Muscle relaxation is typically achieved by using pancuronium bromide. Because the presence of many muscle relaxants will not allow a proper motor-evoked potential response to be generated, shorter acting muscle relaxants are used during intubation and then reversed. A double-lumen endobronchial tube or left mainstem bronchial blockade is used to orotracheally intubate all patients and permit selective deflation of the left lung; this ensures adequate exposure of the descending thoracic aorta and reduces the chance of damage to the lung from handling while the patient is heparinized. If the tracheobronchial anatomy becomes distorted from pressure exerted by a large aneurysm, a standard left-sided double-lumen tube will be difficult to use; in this case, a right-sided tube, placed with fiberoptic guidance, will usually work. In extent IV TAAA repairs, left lung isolation is not as critical to obtaining sufficient exposure.

Attention to volume status by the operative team during aortic replacement is important for avoiding wide fluctuation in blood pressure and, perhaps, distal organ ischemia. Frequent arterial blood gas analysis and close monitoring of serum electrolytes and hematocrit are necessary. To maintain filling pressures, hydration with crystalloid solutions begins at the start of the operation. Mannitol may also be administered at the induction of anesthesia to help maintain diuresis and enhance renal perfusion. Aortic cross-clamp placement causes a large increase in afterload. During aortic cross-clamping, all attempts should be made to keep systemic blood pressure within a normal range and thus avoid hypertension related to clamping. As needed, vasodilating agents such as nitroglycerin, nicardipine, and nitroprusside may be used. When left heart bypass is used as an adjunct, an effective means of blood pressure control in the vessels above the proximal clamp site is to increase flow through the left heart bypass circuit. Blood loss is carefully monitored, and lost blood is replaced. Reinfusion of shed blood recycled from a cell-saving device is useful in decreasing the amount of transfused blood and blood products. During periods when blood loss is extensive (such as when the aorta is being opened), rapid reinfusion permits the use of unwashed, filtered whole blood. Although the meticulous reinfusion of shed blood may at times avoid the need for transfusion, in many cases, fresh-frozen plasma and platelet transfusion are used to restore adequate clotting function and thus facilitate hemostasis.

As repair nears completion, the hypotension that usually occurs when the aortic clamp is removed is avoided or mitigated by discontinuing the use of vasodilating agents shortly before unclamping and also by infusing fluids to account for any volume lost during the repair. Typically, one can achieve hypervolemia with rapid fluid administration just before aortic clamp release. A sodium bicarbonate infusion may be used to treat any acidosis encountered during aortic cross-clamping. Whenever possible, at the conclusion of repair, the double-lumen tube may be exchanged with a single-lumen one; however, this is not always possible at this time because upper airway edema is common, so this exchange is often delayed for several hours.

Positioning

To facilitate adequate exposure, the patient is positioned on a beanbag in a modified right lateral decubitus position with the shoulders at 60 to 80 degrees and the hips flexed to 30 to 40 degrees from horizontal. To maintain the patient's position, the beanbag is suction-deflated and secured as the left arm is elevated and extended at an angle above the shoulders, similar to a freestyle swimming stroke position. Sterile draping should allow access to the entire left chest, abdomen, and both groins. Although removing a rib was common in past eras, we now avoid doing so whenever possible and instead use a table-mounted retractor to provide sufficient exposure during the repair. To reduce the risk of graft and surgical wound infection, we often soak the graft in an antibiotic solution before use; whenever possible, prophylactic broad-spectrum intravenous antibiotics are administered 1 hour before skin incision.

Multimodal Strategy Based on Extent of Repair

Despite the significant innovation that has taken place in the field of aortic surgery over the past 6 decades, successful repair remains challenging; this is largely because aortic clamping causes downstream ischemia, which may adversely affect multiple organs. Although the strategy of repair (Box 69-1) remains largely dictated by the extent of repair, we routinely use moderate heparinization (1 mg/kg), mild passive hypothermia (32-34°C), the aggressive reattachment of segmental arteries (especially those between T8 and L1), sequential aortic clamping when possible, and cold crystalloid renal perfusion whenever the renal ostia are accessible.

Aortic repair has grown to encompass novel adjuncts designed to mitigate specific surgical morbidities, such as the major causes of morbidity and mortality in distal aortic repair—renal ischemia and spinal cord ischemia. The development and use of surgical adjuncts like left heart bypass, visceral perfusion, and cerebrospinal fluid drainage have significantly reduced the mortality and morbidity rates traditionally associated with extensive aortic repair.[74]

BOX 69-1 Current Multimodal Strategy for Surgical Repair of Distal Thoracic Aortic Aneurysms

ALL EXTENTS OF DISTAL AORTIC REPAIR

- Mild passive hypothermia (32-34° C, nasopharyngeal)
- Moderate heparinization (1 mg/kg)
- Aggressive reattachment of intercostal and lumbar arteries (especially between T8 and L1)
- Sequential aortic clamping (when possible)

ALL THORACOABDOMINAL AORTIC REPAIRS

- Cold renal perfusion (4° C) when renal ostia are accessible

CRAWFORD EXTENT I AND II THORACOABDOMINAL AORTIC REPAIRS AND SELECT OTHER REPAIRS

- Cerebrospinal fluid drainage
- Left heart bypass (during proximal anastomosis)
- Selective perfusion of celiac axis and superior mesenteric artery (following completion of left heart bypass)

CERTAIN EXTENSIVE OR HIGHLY COMPLEX AORTIC REPAIRS

- Hypothermic circulatory arrest
- Elephant trunk completion or reversed elephant trunk repair
- Extraction, full salvage, or partial salvage of prior endovascular repair

Left Heart Bypass

Left heart bypass (LHB) is a well-supported strategy to provide distal aortic perfusion and reduce ischemic conditions.[43] We typically reserve LHB for patients undergoing extensive TAAA repairs (extent I and II TAAA repairs), as well as for select patients with poor cardiac function, in whom LHB effectively unloads the left ventricle and improves their ability to tolerate aortic clamping. As the proximal anastomosis is performed, we use a closed-circuit in-line centrifugal pump (without a warming device, oxygenator, or cardiotomy reservoir) to deliver isothermic oxygenated blood distal to the aortic segment being repaired. After heparin is administered (1 mg/kg), cannulas (24 Fr angled-tip cannulas) are placed first in the left inferior pulmonary vein to enter the left atrium and second in the distal descending thoracic aorta or the left femoral artery. Our preferred approach is cannulating the distal descending thoracic aorta a few centimeters proximal to the origin of the celiac axis, because this approach eliminates the need for, and potential risks associated with, femoral artery cannulation. After LHB is initiated (at a modest flow of 500 mL/min), a straight, padded aortic cross-clamp is applied to the aorta at the previously identified proximal site. A second clamp, generally a large Crawford clamp, is then placed across the mid-descending thoracic aorta to isolate the proximal descending segment. With a goal mean arterial pressure of 80 mm Hg, flows of LHB are generally increased to 1.5 to 2.5 liter/min. As mentioned earlier, using LHB allows rapid adjustment of the proximal arterial pressure and minimizes the need for pharmacologic intervention.

Visceral Protection

On completion of the proximal anastomosis, the LHB circuit is generally discontinued; however, typically, the LHB circuit is then converted such that it can be used to provide selective visceral perfusion with minimal added risk. As is the case with LHB, the direct perfusion of visceral arteries is often limited to those patients with extent I or II TAAA repairs. Within the origins of the celiac and superior mesenteric arteries, 9 Fr balloon perfusion catheters are used to perfuse these respective arteries with isothermic oxygenated blood, using a Y-branch off of the arterial return tubing of the LHB circuit. This greatly minimizes the total mesenteric and hepatic ischemic time during these complex aortic repairs. Although evidence supporting this technique is lacking,[43] we believe its potential benefits, such as the reduced risk of postoperative coagulopathy and bacterial translocation from the bowels, outweigh any added risk. Additional techniques to enhance visceral perfusion include endarterectomy of the exposed origins, stenting with balloon-expandable stents, and replacing unsalvageable or widely displaced arteries with branch grafts.

Spinal Cord Protection

During distal aortic replacement, a large number of intercostal and lumbar arteries are sacrificed; this sacrifice is greatest during the most extensive repair (i.e., extent II TAAA repair). This loss of spinal-perfusing arteries (Fig. 69-9) is coupled with substantial fluctuations in blood pressure that are related to aortic clamping and enhances the risk of spinal cord ischemic deficits, namely paraplegia or paraparesis. Thus, in patients who undergo the most extensive distal aortic replacement procedures (extent I and II TAAA repairs), we routinely use cerebrospinal fluid (CSF) drainage. We also use this adjunct in select patients undergoing less extensive repairs if they have previously had portions of their descending thoracic or abdominal aorta replaced. Current guidelines recommend the use of CSF drainage during both open and endovascular repairs in patients at high risk of developing paraplegia (Class I recommendation, level of evidence B).[43] Known risk factors for paraplegia include advanced age, comorbid renal dysfunction, emergency surgery, aortic rupture, acute dissection, extensive repair, and extended duration of surgery, as well as the position of the aortic cross-clamp, prior abdominal aortic surgery, and exclusion of the hypogastric artery.[43]

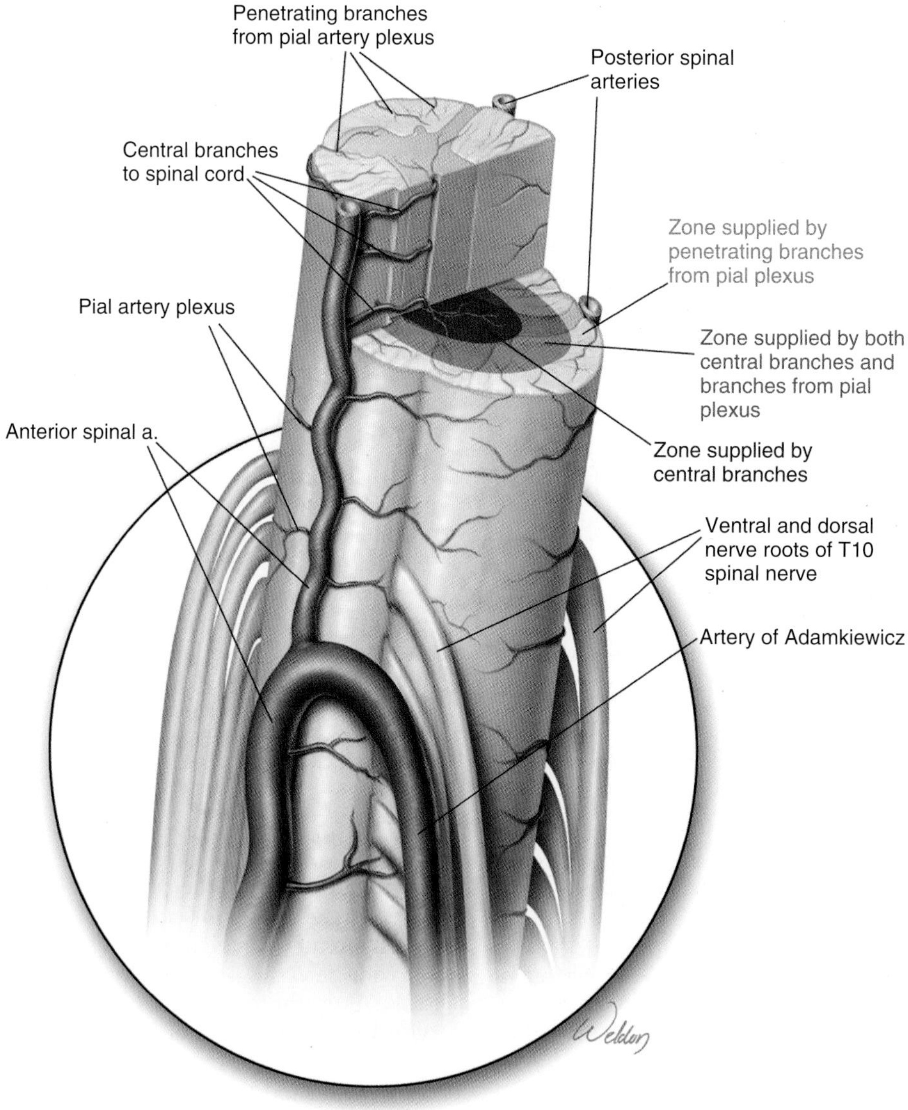

FIGURE 69-9 ■ Illustration showing spinal cord blood supply. A single anterior spinal artery supplies the anterior two thirds of the spinal cord, and two posterior spinal arteries supply the posterior third of the spinal cord. The artery of Adamkiewicz is the largest radicular artery supplying the spinal cord and is considered to play an integral role in preserving spinal cord function. (From Vaughn SB, LeMaire SA, Collard CD: Case scenario: anesthetic considerations for thoracoabdominal aortic aneurysm repair. *Anesthesiology* 115:1093–1102, 2011, Fig. 5. Used with permission.)

CSF drainage enhances spinal perfusion by reducing competing CSF pressure. After induction of anesthesia, an 18-gauge intrathecal catheter is placed through the second or third lumbar space. The catheter permits passive drainage of CSF while allowing the CSF pressure to be carefully monitored during the operation and afterward. During repair, we aim to achieve a target pressure between 8 and 10 mm Hg. The CSF drain is left in place for approximately 48 hours after the aortic repair because spinal cord ischemia may occur immediately or in a delayed fashion postoperatively. Careful postoperative monitoring is necessitated and even brief periods of hypotension should be avoided. The benefits of this CSF drainage in extensive aortic repair have been confirmed in a prospective, randomized trial performed by our group.[75] Significant drawbacks associated with CSF drainage include intracranial bleeding, paraspinal hematoma, and meningitis, all of which can result in death. Less serious complications include a related headache, which is the most common complaint.[76]

In addition, we routinely reattach pairs of large intercostal arteries, particularly if they exhibit minimal backbleeding, to restore spinal cord perfusion. Although some groups routinely use motor-evoked or somatosensory-evoked potentials to monitor the spinal cord throughout the operation, we have not adopted this practice.[77,78] Such approaches monitor spinal cord motor neuron function during aortic replacement to guide the selection of specific intercostal arteries for reattachment. These monitoring techniques also provide general indications to either increase spinal perfusion pressure or increase the rate of CSF drainage. Monitoring motor-evoked potentials requires preserving basal motor function, and thus, as mentioned previously, commonly used anesthetic agents to relax muscle function interfere with testing, so alternate strategies must be used. Additional strategies to preserve spinal cord function include direct epidural infusion of cold perfusate to induce regional spinal hypothermia or reducing spinal metabolism with the use of naloxone and other barbiturate-based agents. However, none of these strategies is as widely used or as highly recommended by current guidelines as is CSF drainage.

Renal Protection

Current guidelines for thoracic aortic repair[43] support both the administration of intraoperative mannitol (Class IIb recommendation, level of evidence C) and direct perfusion of the renal arteries with cold crystalloid or blood (Class IIb recommendation, level of evidence B). We liberally use both of these strategies. Our first randomized clinical trial compared cold crystalloid with isothermic blood and showed that cold renal perfusion mitigates acute renal dysfunction.[79] More recently, our second randomized clinical trial compared cold blood perfusion with cold crystalloid perfusion and found no benefit to using cold blood[80]; therefore, to avoid potential disadvantages associated with using cold blood, we generally use cold crystalloid perfusion. Whenever the renal ostia are accessible, we insert 9 Fr balloon perfusion catheters and use these to deliver 200- to 400-mL boluses of cold (4° C) lactated Ringer solution (prepared with 12.5 g/liter mannitol and 125 mg/liter methylprednisolone) every 15 to 20 minutes. Careful monitoring is needed to ensure that the patient is not overloaded with fluid or overcooled. In patients with a small arterial orifice, branch-vessel dissection, or atherosclerotic occlusive disease, it may be challenging to insert perfusion catheters into the renal arteries. A 6 Fr catheter, rather than the standard 9 Fr catheter, may be used in patients with small renal ostia. Catheters should be used with great care so as to avoid perforating or dissecting the renal arteries; similarly, overexpansion of catheter balloons can rupture these arteries. Similar to its use in visceral arteries, endarterectomy or stenting (or both) may be needed to improve renal perfusion; however, the risk of perforation or rupture is particularly high after endarterectomy. Bleeding related to right renal artery perforation is difficult to identify; the blood flows into the right retroperitoneum. Any unexplained hypovolemia after blood flow is restored to the visceral arteries should prompt a careful evaluation of the mesentery and retroperitoneal anatomy to rule out branch-vessel rupture. If small and readily accessible, the perforation may be sutured; if extensive or multiple perforations are present, a replacement branch graft may be needed.

Hypothermia

Although Kouchoukos and others[81,82] routinely use deep hypothermic circulatory arrest (HCA) during DTA and TAAA repair, we prefer to use mild permissive hypothermia (32° C to 34° C) as our standard approach. Deep HCA (typically conducted between 15° C and 18° C) may introduce risks, namely coagulopathy, cold injury to the lung, retraction injury to a heparinized lung, adult respiratory distress syndrome, and an enhanced risk of stroke. We limit the use of deep HCA to scenarios where aortic clamping would be extremely challenging or generate added risk, such as rupture, aneurysms that are prohibitively large or extend into the distal transverse aortic arch (such as a "mega-aorta"), or prior endovascular repair that hinders clamping. Additional factors that may limit aortic clamping in select patients include severe atherosclerosis or calcification (i.e., porcelain aorta) and large thrombus.

When HCA is necessary, cardiopulmonary bypass is initiated by establishing venous drainage, using a 28 Fr to 32 Fr, long, multiholed cannula inserted into the left femoral vein and positioned in the right atrium. Correct positioning is crucial, and this is verified by transesophageal echocardiography. Vacuum-assisted venous drainage is initiated at flows of 1.8 to 2.4 liter/min/m^2 or 50 mL/min/kg. Although a cannula may be placed in the left atrial appendage or the pulmonary artery to prevent left ventricular distention, we prefer to use an angled cannula (20 Fr or 22 F) that is connected to a Y-branch of the venous line and placed through the inferior pulmonary vein into the left atrium.

The location of the return cannula depends on patient-specific factors. In older patients with severe atherosclerosis or thrombus, a 22 Fr angled cannula is placed in the lower descending thoracic aorta, whereas in younger patients with minimal atherosclerosis, the arterial return cannula is a 20 Fr or 22 Fr straight cannula placed in the left femoral artery. Other return cannulation sites include the left common carotid artery or the left axillary artery. As systemic cooling is initiated, we administer methylprednisolone (5 to 10 mg/kg), sodium thiopental (10 to 15 mg/kg), lidocaine (100 mg), and a short-acting beta blocker for added protection. Circulatory arrest is initiated once the patient has been cooled to electrocerebral silence (usually at a nasopharyngeal temperature of 15° C to 18° C). The aneurysm is then opened, and the proximal anastomosis is constructed. Additional protective adjuncts are not used during repair because the profound systemic hypothermia achieved confers sufficient protection to downstream organs. On completion of the proximal anastomosis, the arterial line is connected to a side branch of the graft; the main graft is then de-aired and clamped distal to the side branch, permitting pump flow to be restored to the upper body, and the remainder of the aortic repair is performed.

OPERATIVE TECHNIQUE

Exposure

DTAAs are repaired through a left thoracotomy made after single right-lung ventilation is initiated (Fig. 69-10). Commonly, this is done by entering through the sixth intercostal space; as needed, the fifth intercostal space may be used to enhance exposure of the distal aortic arch in case of rupture or large aneurysm involving the

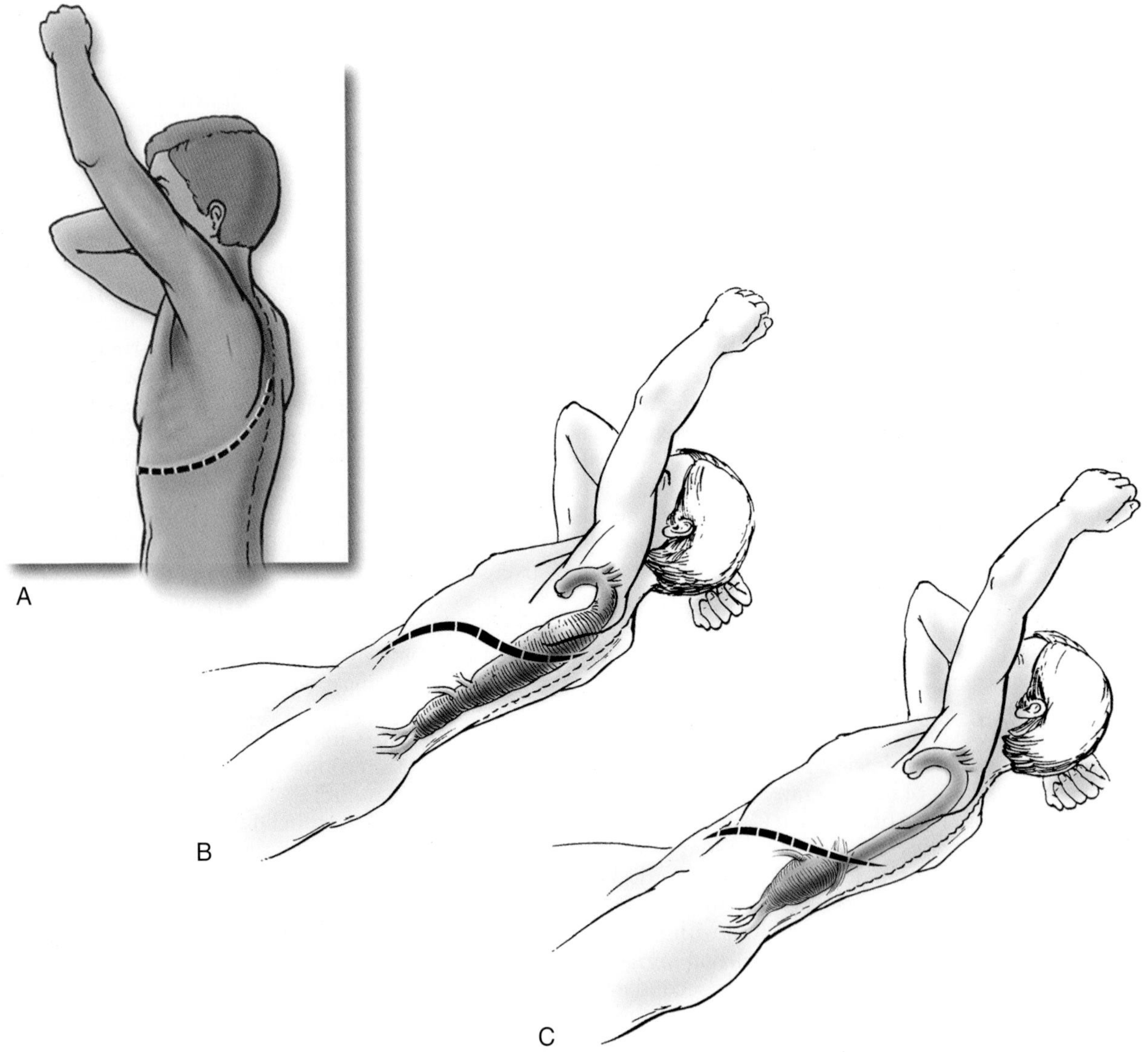

FIGURE 69-10 ■ Approaches to exposure in descending thoracic and thoracoabdominal aortic repairs of different extents. The patient is positioned in a modified right lateral decubitus position that optimizes exposure of the descending thoracic and thoracoabdominal aorta while also facilitating exposure of the femoral arteries, if needed. **A,** A lateral thoracotomy is used for descending thoracic aortic repairs. **B,** For Crawford extent I, II, and III thoracoabdominal aortic repairs, a curvilinear incision is made. **C,** For Crawford extent IV thoracoabdominal aortic repairs, a more linear oblique incision suffices. (Reproduced with permission from Baylor College of Medicine.)

proximal descending thoracic aorta. For extensive repairs, such as extent I and II TAAA repairs, the incision is extended across the costal margin and into the abdomen and commonly terminates at the level of the umbilicus; if further exposure is necessary, this incision may be extended to address iliac artery disease. For the less extensive extent III repair, the seventh or eighth intercostal space is entered, and the incision is then curved into the abdomen. To prevent tissue necrosis, acute angulations near the costal margin should be avoided. For the predominantly abdominal extent IV repair, a straight oblique incision is made through the ninth or tenth interspace to better control the thoracic aorta. As noted previously, we generally do not remove a rib to increase exposure.

For TAAA repairs, we use a transperitoneal approach to perform medial visceral rotation. Equally acceptable, a retroperitoneal approach may be used, but our preference is for a transperitoneal approach because it enables direct evaluation of the bowel and spleen before and after aortic repair. Electrocautery is used to dissect along the line of Toldt, and the diaphragm is divided circumferentially so as to leave a 3- to 4-cm rim of diaphragm along the lateral and posterior chest wall. One or two retraction sutures are placed along the edge of the divided diaphragm on the cardiac side. Exposure generally continues distally into the intra-abdominal aorta and, when necessary, to the aortic bifurcation. The origin of the left renal artery is identified, and all attempts are made to keep the planned aortotomy incision posterior to the left ureter and gonadal vein.

Proximal Anastomosis

For patients undergoing DTAA (Fig. 69-11) or extent I or II TAAA repair (Fig. 69-12; see Video 69-1), the proximal clamp site is typically prepared in the most proximal aspect of the descending thoracic aorta, just distal to the origin of the LSCA. During preparation of the proximal clamp site, the ligamentum arteriosum is often divided, and the vagus and recurrent laryngeal nerves are identified and protected; not infrequently, the vagus and left recurrent laryngeal nerves are adherent to the aortic wall and are at risk of injury. Preserving the left recurrent laryngeal nerve is particularly important in patients with compromised pulmonary function. In cases of postoperative hoarseness, vocal cord paralysis should be suspected; if it is confirmed by endoscopic examination, patients should be offered restorative treatment via direct cord medialization.

If possible, the proximal clamp is placed distal to the LSCA to preserve its contribution to spinal cord flow. As needed, however, the proximal aortic clamp may be positioned between the left common carotid artery and the LSCA (a separate bulldog clamp is applied here; this alternate approach is helpful when there is a large distal arch aneurysm). In extent III TAAAs, the proximal clamp site is prepared more distally, corresponding to a lower incision made through the seventh or eighth intercostal space. For extent IV TAAA repairs, the proximal clamp is placed just superior to the diaphragm, and the proximal anastomosis is typically done end to end at the level of the diaphragm or as a bevel that lies behind the origins of the visceral arteries.

The distal aortic clamp site is often located at the junction of the upper and middle thirds of the descending thoracic aorta and is prepared anterior to the hemiazygos and intercostal veins; a few of these veins may be clipped for safe positioning of the distal clamp. A distal clamp is rarely used during DTAA repair, permitting an open distal anastomosis to suitable aortic tissue; consequently, only the proximal clamp site is prepared.

In extensive distal aortic repair (extents I and II TAAA repairs), LHB is initiated, and the isolated aortic segment is confirmed to be unpressurized. This segment is then opened longitudinally with electrocautery, and the aneurysmal wall edges are retracted with size 0 silk sutures.

As the aorta is opened, it is cleared of any thrombus or debris. Typically, in DTAA and extent I and II TAAA repairs, all upper intercostal arteries are oversewn to prevent back-bleeding, thereby reducing blood loss and "steal" from the spinal cord.

The proximal descending thoracic aorta is then transected 2 to 3 cm from the proximal clamp to prepare a cuff of tissue. This cuff is carefully separated from the underlying esophagus so as not to injure or inadvertently incorporate the esophagus into the proximal anastomosis. Injury to the esophagus during the proximal anastomosis can have catastrophic consequences, including the development of a secondary aortoesophageal fistula.

For all extents of repair, an appropriately sized Dacron graft (commonly 20, 22, or 24 mm in diameter) is selected and is sewn end to end to the proximal aortic cuff with continuous 3-0 polypropylene sutures (finer suture, such as 4-0 polypropylene suture, may be needed in patients with connective tissue disorders or other conditions that make the aortic tissue fragile). Because meticulous suturing is needed to achieve hemostasis, the primary suture line is often reinforced circumferentially with either a second layer of continuous suture or with a series of interrupted pledgeted horizontal mattress sutures. If the proximal aortic clamp has been placed between the LSCA and the left common carotid artery, whenever possible, it is now repositioned onto the graft to allow perfusion of the LSCA, which provides collateral circulation to the spinal cord.

In extensive TAAA repair, after the proximal anastomosis is complete, LHB is slowly discontinued; typically, this circuit is now converted to provide isothermic visceral perfusion to the celiac axis and superior mesenteric artery. The distal aortic clamp is removed, and electrocautery is used to open the thoracoabdominal aorta down to the aortic bifurcation. As the distal aortic segment is prepared, any large pieces of thrombus are removed. In patients with chronic aortic dissection, the septum is excised (this is discussed in greater detail later). As the renal ostia become accessible, cold crystalloid is used to perfuse the left and right renal arteries.

Reattachment Strategies and Other Considerations

As mentioned earlier, we aggressively reattach one or more pairs of intercostal or lumbar arteries (segmental

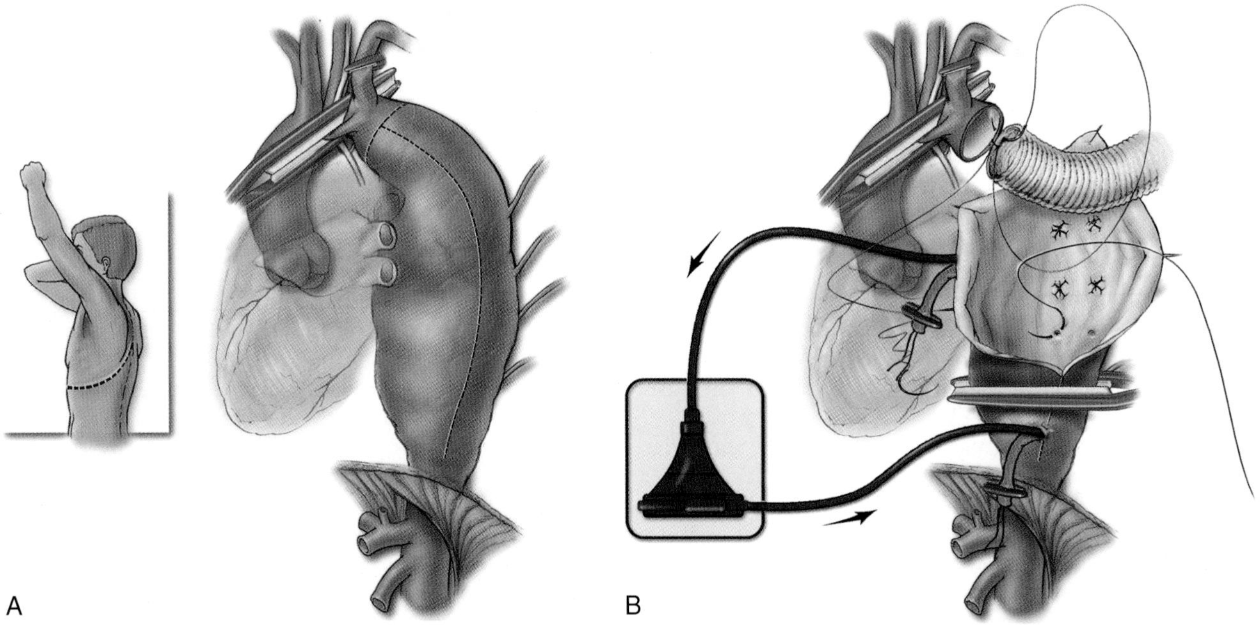

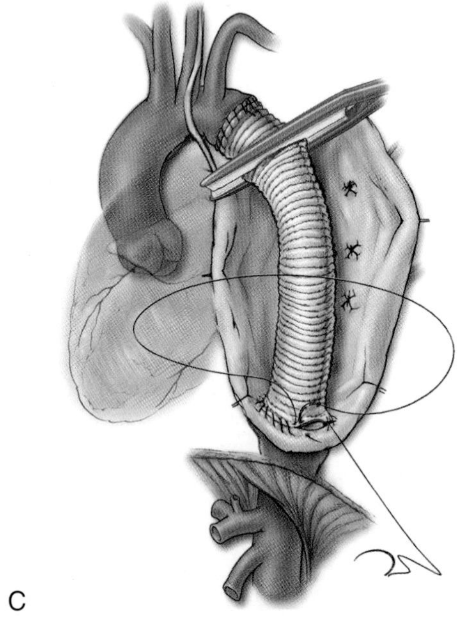

FIGURE 69-11 ■ Illustrations of the clamp-and-sew technique for repair of a descending thoracic aortic aneurysm. **A,** The operation is performed through a thoracotomy *(inset).* Clamps are placed on the aortic arch between the left common carotid and left subclavian arteries and directly on the left subclavian artery. The aorta is opened longitudinally and divided circumferentially a few centimeters beyond the proximal clamp. **B,** After the proximal anastomosis is complete, the aortic clamp is repositioned onto the graft, blood flow is restored to the left subclavian artery, and the remainder of the aneurysm is open longitudinally. An open distal anastomosis completes the repair. **C,** As an alternative to the clamp-and-sew technique, left heart bypass can be used to provide distal aortic perfusion during the repair. (From Coselli JS, LeMaire SA: Descending and thoracoabdominal aortic aneurysms. In Cohn LH, editor: *Cardiac surgery in the adult,* ed 3, New York, 2007, McGraw-Hill, pp 1277–1298, Fig. 54-8. Reproduced with permission.)

arteries) as aortic repair progresses distally; such arteries that are not incorporated into the repair are carefully oversewn to prevent ongoing back-bleeding, which may contribute to spinal cord ischemia. Patent segmental arteries, particularly those between T8 and L1, are carefully inspected. We tend to select segmental arteries that are large and do not exhibit significant back-bleeding, provided that nearby aortic tissue is of suitable quality for anastomosis. Commonly, segmental arteries are reimplanted as a patch by making a small opening in the graft and constructing a side-to-side anastomosis with continuous 3-0 or 4-0 polypropylene suture. Alternatively, a small-diameter interposition graft may be used to incorporate segmental arteries into the repair by end-to-side reattachment. Whenever possible, the proximal aortic clamp is then moved immediately distal to the intercostal patch (see Fig. 69-12*F*) to reperfuse that portion of the spinal cord.

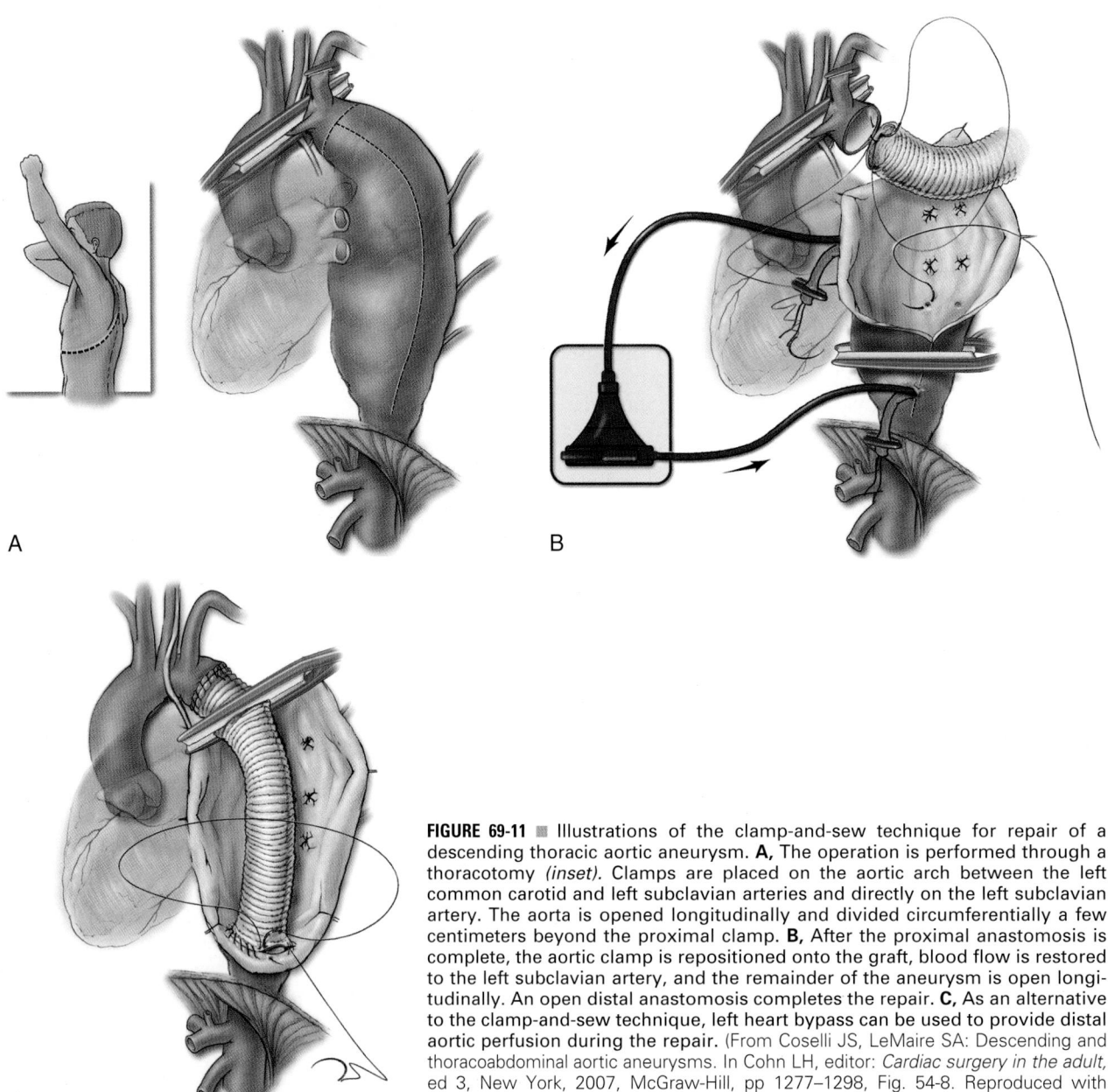

The visceral arteries are incorporated into thoracoabdominal aortic repair in accordance with the extent of repair and taking into account factors such as the age of the patient, the presence or likelihood of connective tissue disease, and whether the origins of the arteries are widely displaced from one another. In addition, any stenosis or other disease involving the visceral arteries may necessitate endarterectomy or stenting to improve circulation before incorporation into the overall aortic repair. In extent I TAAA repairs, the visceral arteries are usually incorporated by surrounding them with a beveled distal anastomosis. Similarly, a beveled approach may be used in the proximal anastomosis of select extent IV TAAA repairs. In older patients with degenerative aortic disease

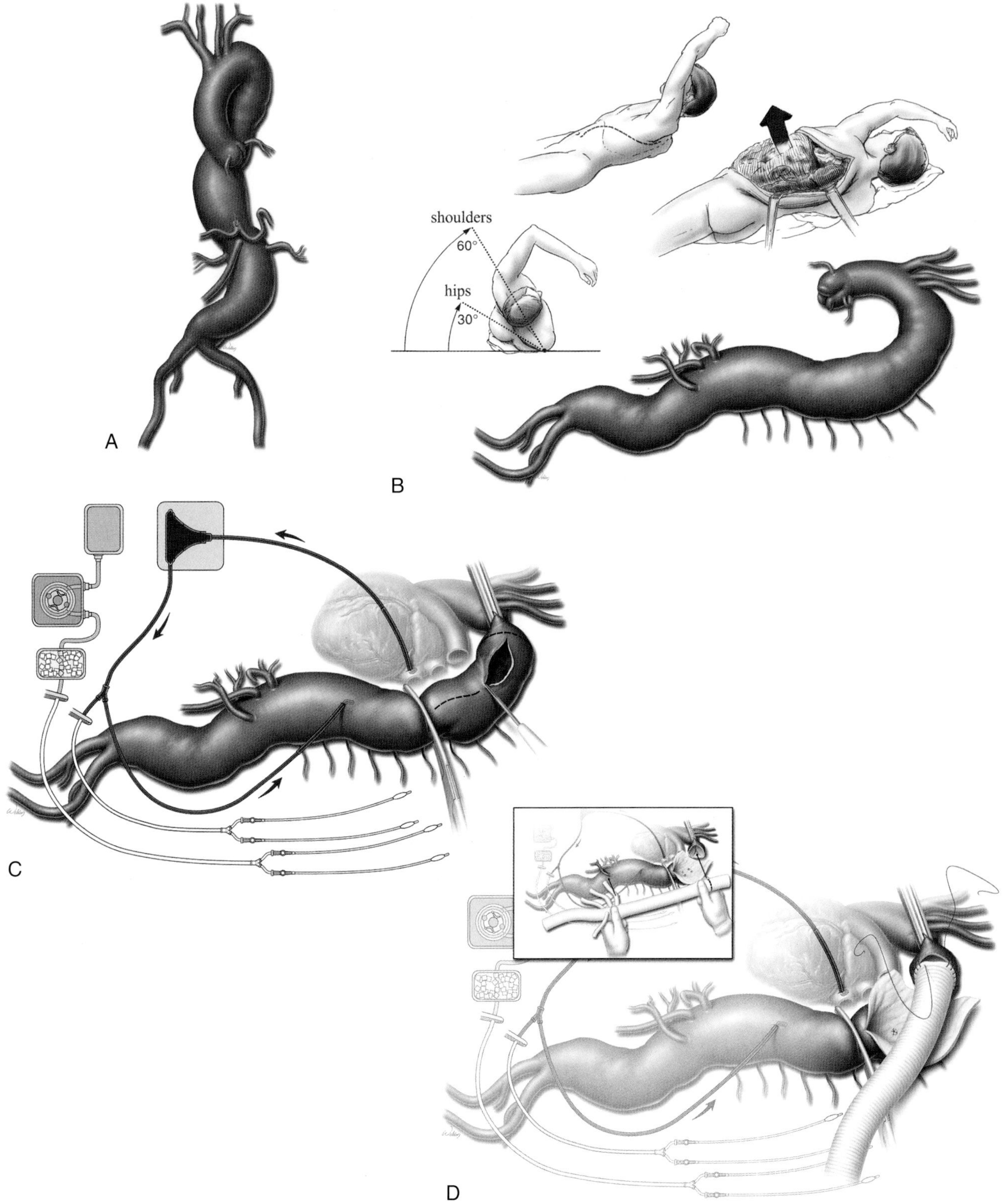

FIGURE 69-12 ■ Illustration of an extent II thoracoabdominal aortic aneurysm repair using a multibranched graft. **A,** A typical patient undergoing such a repair will have an aneurysm extending from the left subclavian artery down to the aortic bifurcation. In this patient, the visceral arteries are widely displaced from each other, making the traditional reattachment approach using a visceral patch difficult. **B,** The chest is entered through the sixth intercostal space. Left medial visceral rotation and circumferential division of the diaphragm enable exposure of the entire thoracoabdominal aorta. The use of table-mounted self-retaining retractors maintains stable exposure throughout the procedure. **C,** Left heart bypass (LHB) is initiated by placing a cannula in the left atrium via a left inferior pulmonary venotomy and then connecting it to the drainage line of the LHB circuit. After LHB flow is initiated, the proximal aortic clamp is placed just distal to the left subclavian artery, and the distal aortic clamp is applied across the mid-descending thoracic aorta. The aortic segment between the two clamps is opened longitudinally by using electrocautery. **D,** After back-bleeding intercostal arteries are ligated, the aorta is transected 2 to 3 cm distal to the aortic clamp and separated from the underlying esophagus. A four-branched aortic graft is tailored by stretching the graft so that it is taut, lining up the origin of the celiac graft with the origin of the left renal artery, and cutting the proximal end of the aortic graft at the point where it reaches the proximal anastomosis site (inset).

Continued

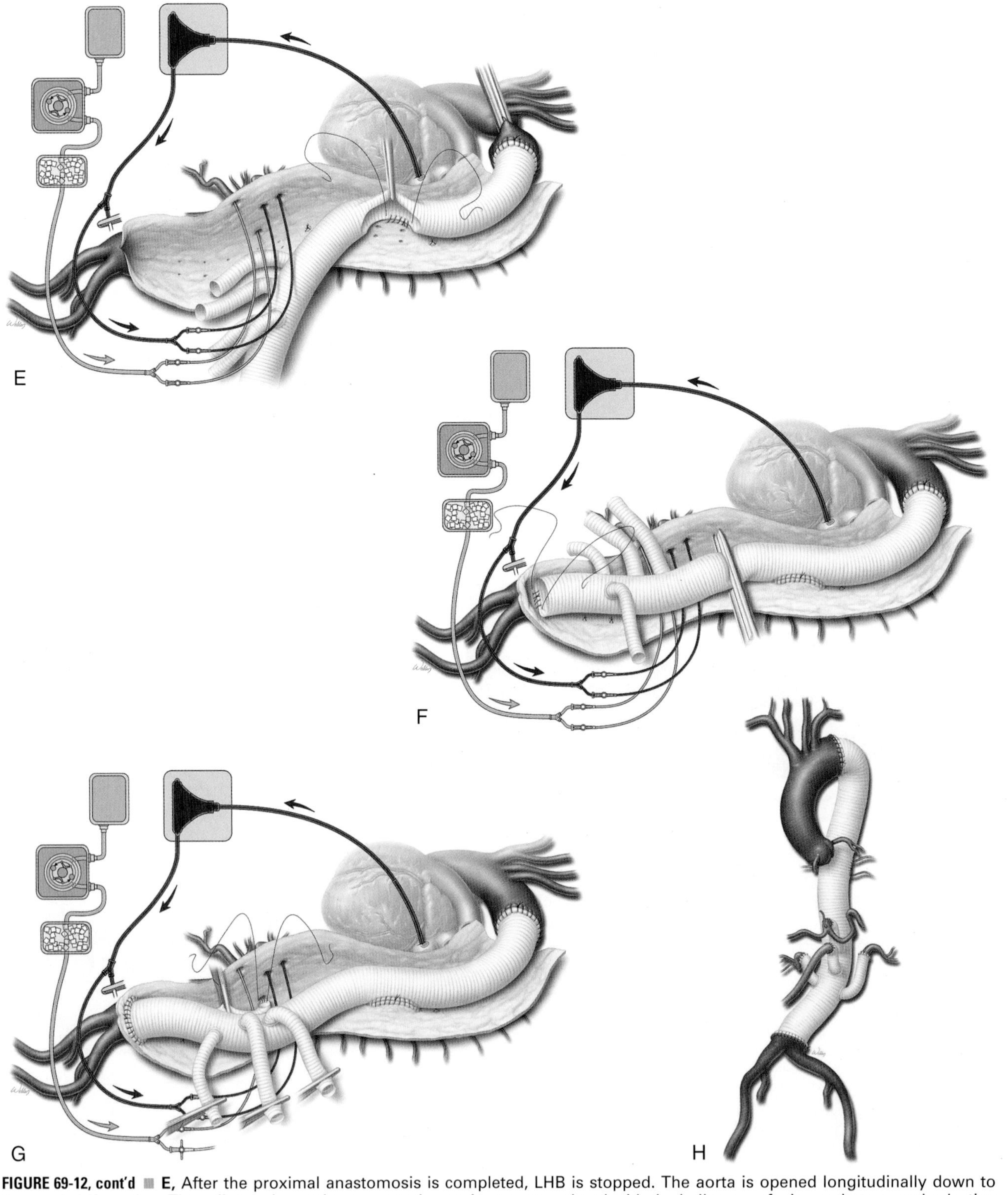

FIGURE 69-12, cont'd ■ **E,** After the proximal anastomosis is completed, LHB is stopped. The aorta is opened longitudinally down to the aortic bifurcation. The celiac and superior mesenteric arteries are cannulated with the balloon perfusion catheters, and selective perfusion is initiated. The renal arteries are similarly cannulated with balloon perfusion catheters to enable intermittent perfusion with cold crystalloid solution. **F,** The aortic cross-clamp is moved down to the aortic graft distal to the intercostal patch. After the graft is trimmed, the distal anastomosis is performed. **G,** The right renal artery is anastomosed. **H,** The completed repair is shown. (Reproduced with permission from Baylor College of Medicine.)

who are free of connective tissue disorders and whose four vessels are in close proximity to one another, the origins of all four arteries may be reattached in one patch to an oval opening in the graft; in such patients, this is the simplest and most expeditious method of reattachment, and there is only a small chance a patch aneurysm will develop in the near future. Typically, in this approach, the anastomosis is made immediately adjacent to the edges of the ostia of the vessels to reduce the amount of native aortic tissue that is incorporated into the repair.

However, for various reasons, some patients need an alternate strategy for reattachment. For example, patients with connective tissue disorders are at high risk for the late development of patch aneurysms if the inherently compromised residual aortic tissue is not minimized through use of an alternate reattachment strategy. In these patients, as well as in those in whom the visceral vessels are otherwise diseased or anatomically displaced, one or more of the visceral arteries can be individually attached with either separate buttons or small-diameter Dacron grafts sewn to the aortic graft, or with a prefabricated, multibranched aortic graft (with four pre-sewn branches). Commonly, when the left renal artery is widely displaced from the other visceral branches because of chronic dissection or extensive aneurysm expansion, it is separately reattached on a button of tissue or with a separate branch graft. In addition, in a younger patient with connective tissue disease, we generally use a multibranched graft to reimplant each vessel separately to effectively minimize native aortic tissue. An advantage of using a multibranched graft is that it permits the distal aortic anastomosis to be performed before the visceral branches are reattached; this restores blood flow to the iliac arteries and provides a needed source of collateral perfusion to the at-risk spinal cord. Although the order of reattachment depends on patient-specific anatomy and baseline renal function, the general order is right renal artery, superior mesenteric artery, celiac axis, and left renal artery.

Chronic aortic dissection is relatively common in patients undergoing TAAA repair. Although the operative approach used in these patients is similar to the one used in patients without chronic dissection, there are some key differences to consider. The dissecting membrane within the aorta is excised to locate all important branch vessels and to clearly identify the true and false lumens. If the dissection extends beyond the ostia of the visceral arteries, there are a couple of options. The false lumen can be obliterated with suture or small-diameter intraluminal stents, or the membrane can be fenestrated. Also, because of asymmetrical expansion, the left renal artery commonly becomes widely displaced; a separate opening in the graft can be used to reattach it as a small button, or it can be replaced with a separate branch graft. Care should be taken when constructing the proximal and distal anastomoses to remove a wedge of the dissecting membrane to facilitate perfusion of both true and false lumens.

Distal Anastomosis

Selecting the location of the distal anastomosis depends on the extent of repair and the degree of dilation of the distal aorta, iliac, and femoral vessels. In patients with chronic dissection, repair is typically limited to those sections with substantial dilation, leaving the residually dissected aortic tissue in place, in the hope of increasing early survival. In DTAA repairs, the graft is typically anastomosed with continuous suture to the distal descending thoracic aorta in an open fashion. In extent I TAAA repairs, the visceral arteries are incorporated into a beveled distal anastomosis. In preparation for the distal anastomosis in extent II-IV repairs, the aortic clamp is moved distal to the site of visceral artery reattachment; this permits visceral-organ reperfusion. The distal anastomosis is then carried out in an open fashion without a clamp (an open-distal technique). If the aorta is of sufficient quality (and without substantial dilation) proximal to the iliac bifurcation, an end-to-end anastomosis is made at this level with continuous suture.

If disease continues beyond the bifurcation, we secure an additional, prefabricated bifurcated abdominal graft to the replacement graft in an end-to-end fashion by using continuous 2-0 or 3-0 polypropylene suture. The limbs of this graft are then anastomosed to the common iliac, external iliac, or common femoral arteries; flow into the internal iliac arteries is preserved whenever possible. As a general guideline, we limit replacement and target a proximal location on each bifurcation that has distal arteries of sufficient quality and caliber. If acute dissection extends beyond the location of the distal anastomosis, the false lumen is obliterated by inclusion within the suture line, effectively directing the blood flow entirely to the true lumen; as mentioned previously, chronic dissections are fenestrated to avoid malperfusion. In addition, as discussed earlier, the use of a four-branched TAAA graft permits the distal aortic anastomosis to be performed before the visceral arteries are reattached, thus facilitating perfusion of the spinal cord.

Elephant Trunk Approaches

Open repairs of extensive aortic aneurysm (i.e., repairs that involve replacing the aorta almost entirely, which are often called "mega-aorta" repairs) require a specialized approach to enable sufficient exposure. Although such repair is performed in a single stage in some centers,[83] in our practice these repairs are usually done in two stages and generally with an elephant trunk approach. Traditional elephant trunk repair, as introduced by Borst[84] and modified by Svensson[85] and others,[86] involves a staged approach in which the proximal aorta is replaced during the first operation and the distal aorta is replaced during the second operation (Fig. 69-13). However, if the distal aorta is at risk of rupture, or if the patient has related symptoms, the distal aorta is replaced in the first operation and the proximal aorta is replaced at a later time. This approach is called the reversed elephant trunk (Fig. 69-14), and we first used this approach almost 2 decades ago.[87]

Traditional elephant trunk repairs involve first replacing the ascending aorta and aortic arch (using a standard island or contemporary Y-graft approach) and incorporating a segment of Dacron graft into the distal anastomosis such that it hangs into the proximal descending thoracic aorta. In the recent past, this was commonly done by using an island patch approach to arch replacement and

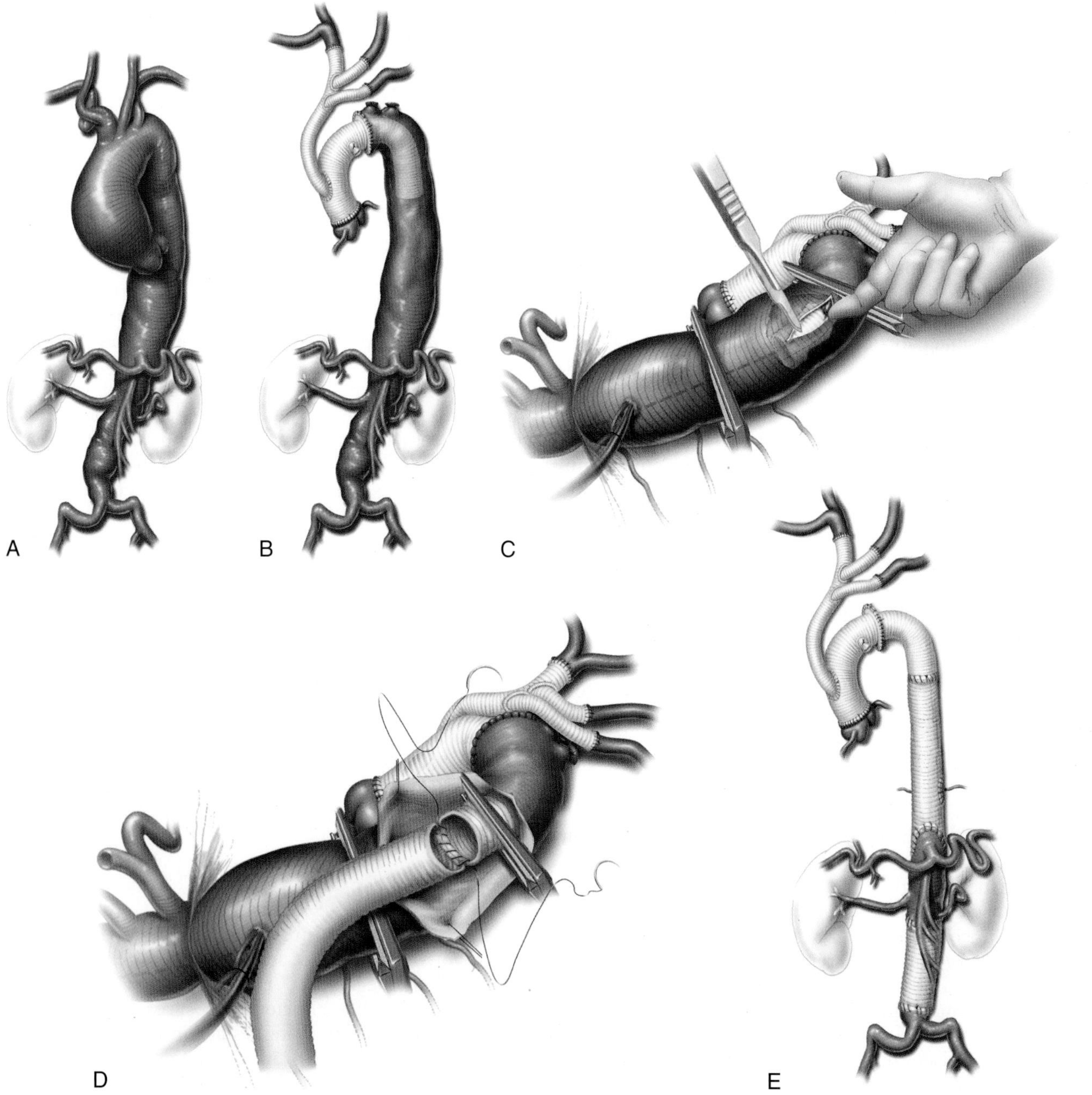

FIGURE 69-13 ■ Illustration of the elephant trunk approach to repair for **(A)** extensive aortic aneurysms that involve the ascending aorta, the aortic arch, and the thoracoabdominal aorta. **B,** During the first-stage procedure, the large aneurysm of the ascending aorta and aortic arch is replaced with a graft, a segment of which (the elephant trunk) is left suspended inside the aneurysmal descending thoracic aortic segment. **C,** This trunk is retrieved during the second-stage procedure and **(D)** used to create the proximal anastomosis. **E,** The completed repair is shown. (Reproduced with permission from Baylor College of Medicine.)

incorporating the trunk (usually ≈10 cm of extra graft material) into the distal anastomosis, which was typically located just beyond the anatomic origins of the LSCA. Contemporary approaches include the use of Y-graft arch debranching techniques[88] with a prefabricated, collared elephant trunk graft; this approach permits the distal anastomosis to be brought proximally—generally in line with the anatomic origins of the innominate artery—and the collar reduces anastomotic tension because the diameter of residual aorta can be matched by trimming the collar. Both of these approaches may be encountered in second-stage repair, and the use of relatively short "trunks" is generally supported in the United States. In Japan, longer elephant trunks have been used, but this appears to increase the risk of paraplegia.[89]

Elephant trunk repairs may be done on a prophylactic basis (such as in the case of patients with distal aortic dilation that does not yet meet a diameter-based threshold for repair) or as part of a planned extensive repair in which the second stage is usually performed within several weeks. During the second-stage completion repair, the elephant trunk greatly facilitates the proximal

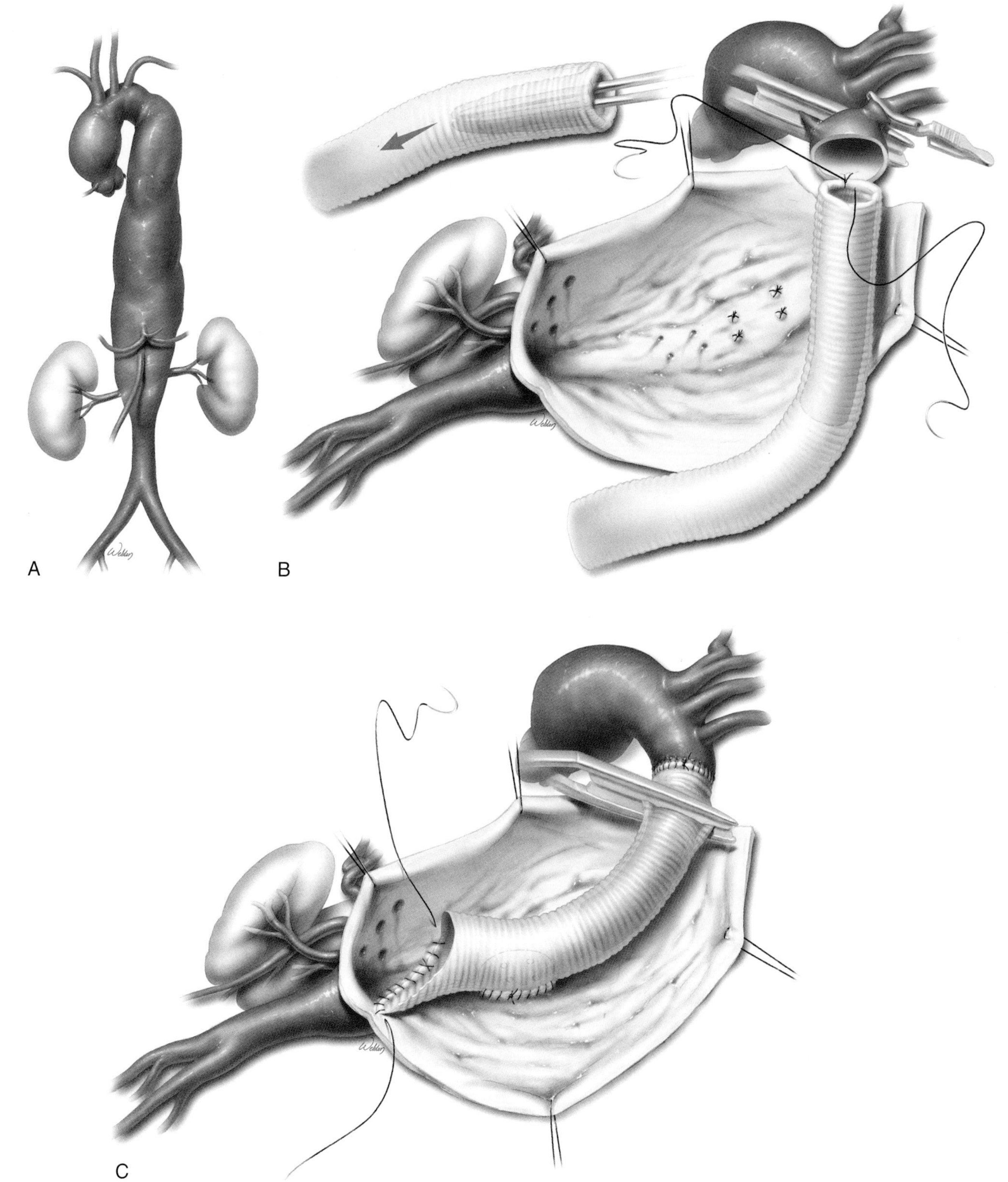

FIGURE 69-14 ■ Illustration of the reversed elephant trunk approach to repair for **(A)** extensive aortic aneurysms that involve the ascending aorta, the aortic arch, and the thoracoabdominal aorta. In this repair, the distal aorta is of greatest concern, so it is repaired first. **B,** During the first-stage procedure, the thoracoabdominal aorta is replaced with a graft whose proximal portion is invaginated. The folded edge is used to create the proximal anastomosis. **C,** After intercostal arteries are reattached, a beveled distal anastomosis is created behind the visceral ostia.

Continued

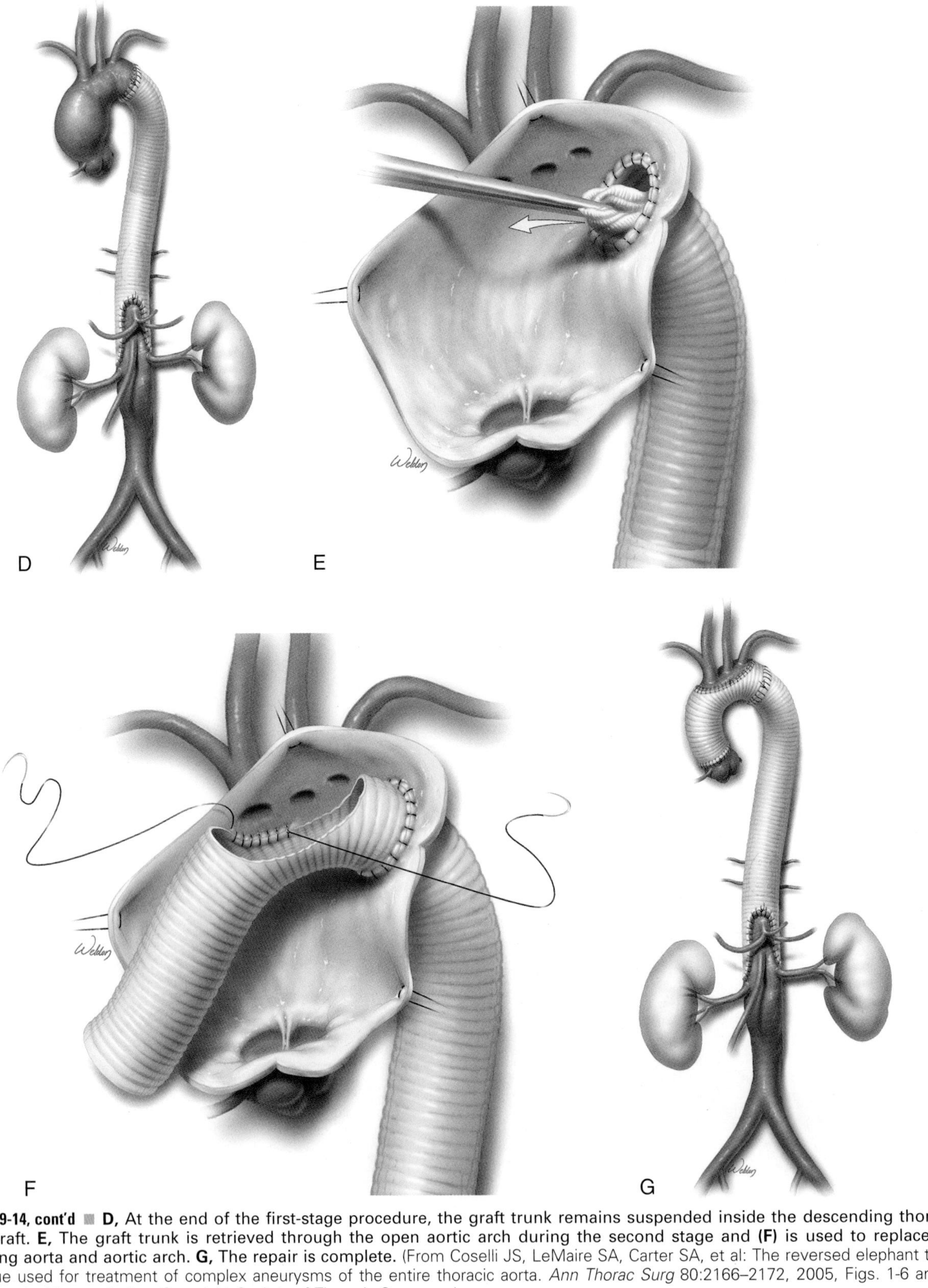

FIGURE 69-14, cont'd ■ **D,** At the end of the first-stage procedure, the graft trunk remains suspended inside the descending thoracic aortic graft. **E,** The graft trunk is retrieved through the open aortic arch during the second stage and **(F)** is used to replace the ascending aorta and aortic arch. **G,** The repair is complete. (From Coselli JS, LeMaire SA, Carter SA, et al: The reversed elephant trunk technique used for treatment of complex aneurysms of the entire thoracic aorta. *Ann Thorac Surg* 80:2166–2172, 2005, Figs. 1-6 and 8. Reproduced with permission. Copyright Society of Thoracic Surgeons.)

anastomosis because it allows direct and secure clamping of the elephant trunk, rather than clamping the replaced arch or proximal descending thoracic aorta, which are often surrounded by dense scar tissue after the initial operation. This is especially helpful when there is a very large aneurysm involving the proximal descending thoracic segment. In patients with DTAA, elephant trunk completion repairs may be done endovascularly rather than by an open approach through a thoracotomy[90,91]; however, this approach necessitates the availability of at least 2 cm of aortic tissue above the celiac axis to use as the distal landing zone for the endograft. Radiographic clips are usually placed on the end of the elephant trunk graft, and these can be used to guide deployment.

In a reversed elephant trunk procedure, the distal aorta is generally determined to be at greater risk of rupture than is the proximal aorta. At the initiation of repair, the graft is invaginated into itself and the proximal anastomosis is constructed between the aorta and the folded edge of the graft. During the second-stage repair of the proximal aorta, the invaginated segment of graft is retrieved and used to replace the aortic arch and ascending aorta. This approach obviates the need to perform a distal anastomosis at the aortic arch.[87,92]

Open Repair after Endovascular Aortic Repair

In several ways, open distal aortic repair after endovascular aortic repair (Fig. 69-15) is similar to the methods described previously, with the extent of repair dictating our standard use of surgical adjuncts. The presence of a stent-graft may limit the surgeon's ability to safely clamp the proximal aorta; when the stent-graft covers a substantial portion of the aortic arch, HCA may be necessary. In patients who present with repair failure after a previous endovascular procedure, a high degree of suspicion regarding endograft infection should be maintained, even in asymptomatic patients; the presence of infection may warrant the use of additional techniques, such as omental wrapping, placing antibiotic-irrigation catheters, and soaking the graft in antibiotics. Occasionally, an extra-anatomic approach may be justified in an infected field. When open repair is performed after previous abdominal aortic endovascular repair, an oblique incision, such as that used for extent IV TAAA repairs, is often used to ensure sufficient exposure of the visceral vessels.

Depending on circumstances, stent-grafts may be fully or partly salvaged (Fig. 69-16) in patients without infection and should be completely removed in patients with infection. The entire stent-graft can be left in place when the new aneurysm results from a progression of adjacent aortic disease rather than a late endovascular failure. Partial salvage may involve leaving a very small portion of the stent-graft proximally if it has been previously sutured directly to the aortic wall (rather than risking further damage by removing it), as is commonly done in the frozen elephant trunk approach, or more commonly, leaving relatively large portions of bifurcated abdominal stent-grafts in place after the main body of the stent-graft

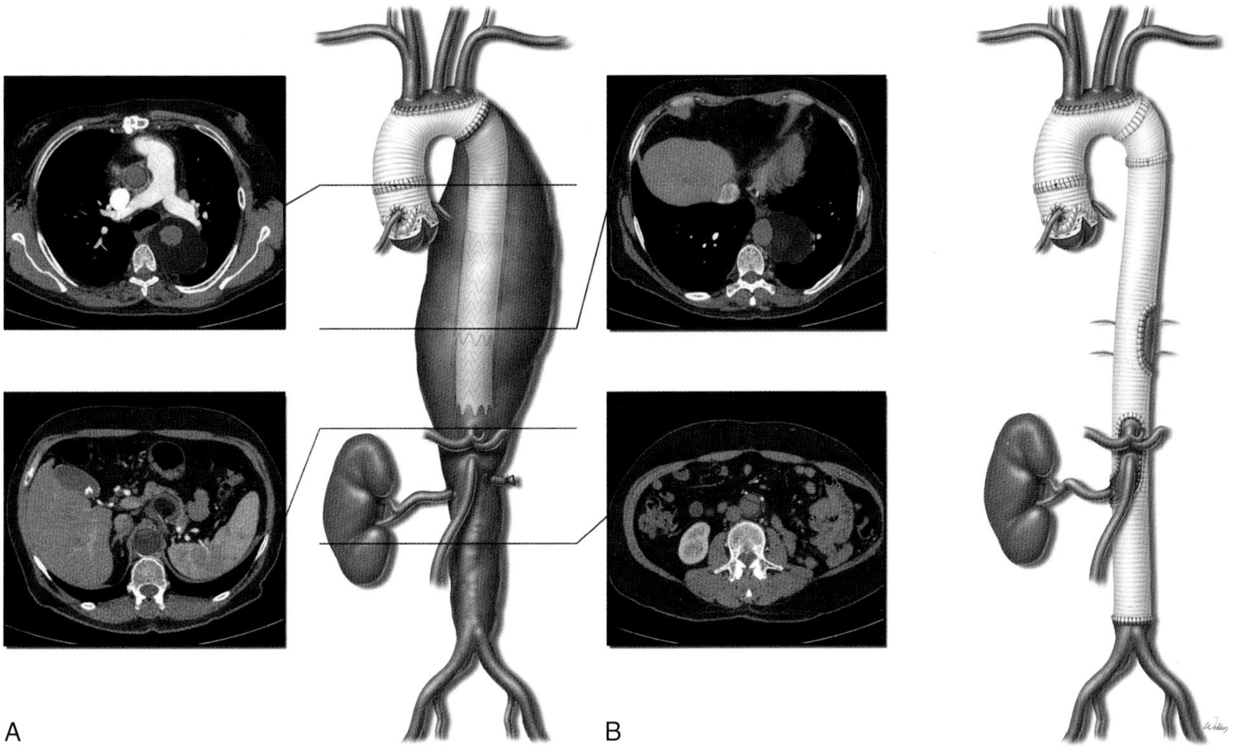

FIGURE 69-15 ■ Preoperative drawing and computed tomography images illustrating **(A)** a thoracoabdominal aortic aneurysm caused by chronic dissection in a patient who previously underwent replacement of the aortic root, ascending aorta, and aortic arch, followed by endovascular repair of the descending thoracic aorta using the elephant trunk graft as the proximal landing zone. **B,** Repair involved complete removal of the stent-graft and extent II graft replacement of the thoracoabdominal aorta. (Used with permission of Baylor College of Medicine.)

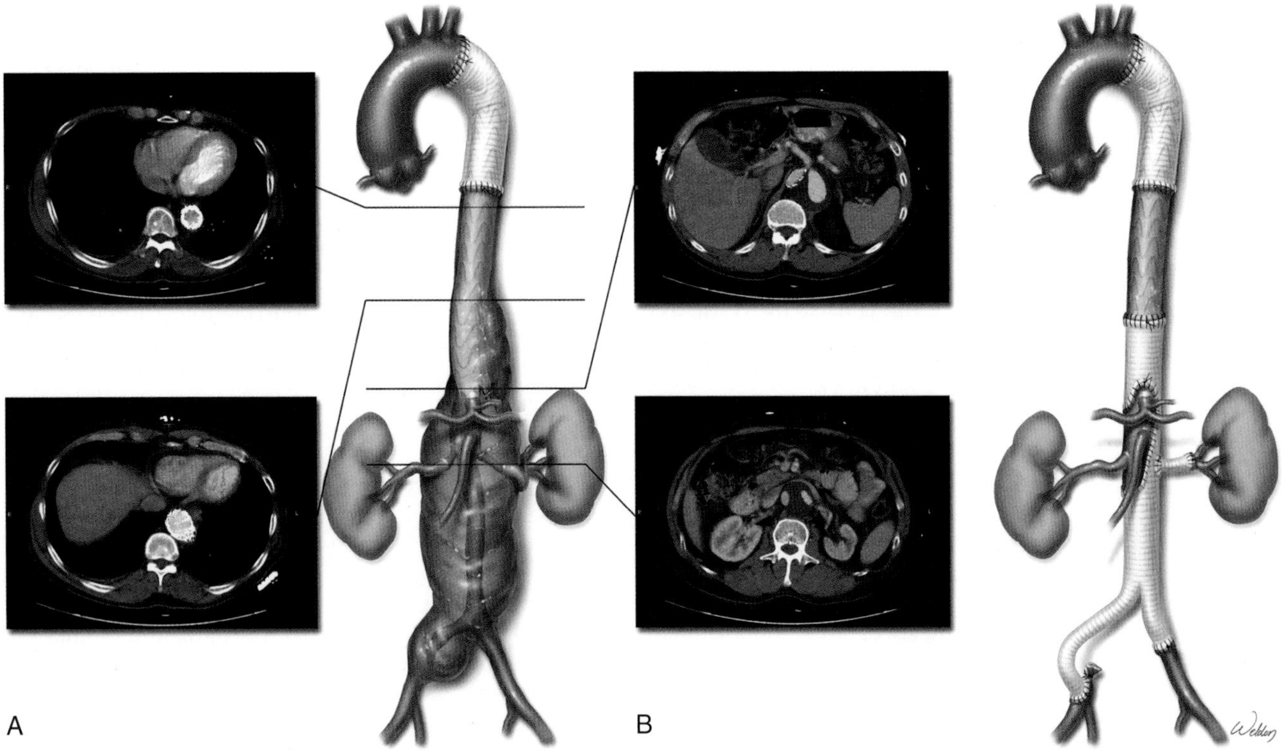

FIGURE 69-16 ■ Preoperative drawing and computed tomography images illustrating **(A)** a thoracoabdominal aortic aneurysm caused by chronic dissection in a patient who previously underwent open graft replacement of the proximal descending thoracic aorta and endovascular repair of the distal descending thoracic aorta. Over time, the aortic disease progressed to include additional segments of the distal aorta. **B,** Repair involved partial removal of the stent-graft and extent III graft replacement of the thoracoabdominal aorta. A portion of the stent-graft was well-adhered to the aortic tissue, which permitted partial salvage of the device. (Used with permission of Baylor College of Medicine.)

is trimmed, particularly if the extension limbs are well adhered. These anastomoses are typically performed end to end and incorporate the endovascular device, the residual aortic wall, and the replacement polyester graft. Ideally, a full thickness of the aortic wall, surrounding and adherent to the stent-graft, is incorporated in the anastomosis to prevent excessive bleeding from needle holes in the endograft material. In cases of infection, a careful inspection of adjacent tissues is warranted, because there is a possibility of concomitant fistulae. An in situ swab or other measures should be used to identify the infecting agent so that an appropriate antibiotic regimen can be implemented.

Closure

On aortic unclamping and repair completion, systemic heparinization is reversed with intravenous protamine sulfate, and the adequacy of renal perfusion is assessed by administering indigo carmine dye. It is crucial to obtain secure hemostasis, so each anastomosis and cannulation site is carefully inspected for bleeding. As needed, anastomoses may be additionally secured by using reinforcing sutures with felt strips or pledgets and by prudent use of surgical adhesives.[93]

To gently rewarm the patient and to further assess hemostasis, the field is irrigated with warm water; if necessary, additional blood products are administered. Sufficient perfusion to the visceral organs, as well as the iliac and femoral arteries, is confirmed. The appearance of the bowel is noted, and the spleen is assessed to ensure that there are no subcapsular hematomas or capsular tears. The residual aneurysmal wall is then wrapped around the aortic graft and secured with continuous suture.

Thoracic drainage tubes are placed within the pleural cavity (anteroapical and posterobasal), and a closed-suction abdominal drain is placed in the retroperitoneum. The diaphragm is reapproximated with a continuous #1 polypropylene suture, and the intercostal space is closed with heavy braided suture and stainless steel wire. Pericostal catheters are placed to allow delivery of local anesthetic postoperatively, and the abdominal fascia, serratus anterior, and latissimus dorsi are then closed with continuous suture.

POSTOPERATIVE MANAGEMENT

Immediate Postoperative Management

A systematic approach to postoperative care is extremely important because operative complications are not uncommon and early correction is the key to minimizing the impact of emerging complications. Laboratory results are carefully reviewed, drains and fluid outputs are carefully assessed, and peripheral pulses are monitored closely.

Ideally, the patient is weaned from the ventilator and extubated within the first 24 to 36 hours after the operation; physical therapy and ambulation are emphasized early in the recovery process.

In the early postoperative period, aortic anastomoses are extremely fragile. Thus, for the first 24 to 48 hours, blood pressure is meticulously kept within a narrow range—mean pressures are maintained between 80 and 90 mm Hg. Typically, this is achieved with nicardipine and intravenous beta antagonists. For patients with particularly fragile aortic tissue, such as patients with connective tissue disorders or acute dissection, the target range for mean pressure may be reduced to 70 to 80 mm Hg. Hypotension is avoided because it can lead to ischemic complications such as delayed paraplegia or paraparesis. Even brief hypertension can disrupt suture lines, leading to severe bleeding and hypotension, or to pseudoaneurysm formation.[94]

When a CSF drain is in place, intrathecal pressure is kept between 10 and 12 mm Hg during the early postoperative period. As necessary, CSF is passively drained. As soon as the patient awakens from anesthesia and before further sedatives are administered, lower extremity movement is assessed; once satisfactory motor function of the legs is confirmed, the CSF pressure target may be increased to 12 to 15 mm Hg. Patients are carefully monitored because delayed paraplegia or paraparesis accounts for roughly half of all spinal cord complications. Often, the CSF drain is stopped for several hours, and if the patient remains neurologically intact, the CSF drain is then removed; this usually takes place within 48 hours. If paraplegia or paraparesis does arise, it is treated aggressively because it can often be fully or partially reversed. If a CSF drain is not in place, one is inserted immediately; the intrathecal pressure is then reduced to less than 10 mm Hg. Additional rescue measures that may be used in conjunction with CSF drainage include optimizing hemodynamics, raising the mean arterial blood pressure to a higher range (85 to 95 mm Hg), administering steroids and osmotic diuretics, correcting anemia, and reducing fever, if present.

As emerging complications arise, corrective measures are immediately taken. Pulmonary complications are relatively common, and affected patients may need to resume ventilator support. Creatinine levels are carefully monitored, and if a significant increase occurs, we increase the patient's blood pressure by adjusting medications to better perfuse the kidneys.

It is crucial to prevent graft infection after aortic replacement, given the associated increased risk of mortality. During surgery, close attention is paid to technique and sterility, and topical antibiotics may be used prophylactically to prepare the graft. Broad-spectrum antibiotics are administered during the early postoperative course until all drains and central venous catheters are removed. After 24 hours, the retroperitoneal closed suction drain may be removed; typically within 72 hours, thoracic drainage tubes are removed provided that drainage is less than 300 mL/day.

In cases of postoperative hoarseness, vocal cord paralysis should be suspected. If it is confirmed by endoscopic examination, patients should be offered restorative treatment with direct cord medialization.

Long-Term Management

Long-term patient education and surveillance protocols are initiated when patients prepare for discharge. Patients should be made aware that they should seek urgent treatment if concerning symptoms develop (such as the sudden onset of pain or any ischemic complications). In addition, patients should be counseled that they remain at risk for subsequent aneurysm formation in any remaining native aortic segments, including reattachment sites, even if they have no connective tissue disorders or other major risk factors for aneurysm development. Furthermore, many of our patients tend to have poorly controlled hypertension, which can contribute to the gradual weakening of suture lines and lead to the development of pseudoaneurysms. In rare cases, aortic replacement grafts become infected, which can also lead to suture-line disruption and pseudoaneurysm formation. We recommend that all patients undergo at least yearly CT imaging of the chest and abdomen. In younger patients, it is reasonable to use magnetic resonance imaging to reduce lifetime radiation exposure. Adequate surveillance imaging is especially important in patients with connective tissue disorders, especially the aggressive forms such as Loeys-Dietz syndrome.

Additional education regarding lifestyle modifications may be warranted. Maintaining a healthy blood pressure, heart rate, and weight is ideal. Patients should be educated regarding the association between smoking and aneurysmal disease. Patients in whom cocaine or methamphetamine use has precipitated dissection are counseled about the importance of cessation of drug abuse. Whereas light aerobic exercise is generally beneficial to overall health, extreme isometric exercise such as weightlifting should be limited. Similarly, although many patients can expect a full return to employment, strenuous manual labor should be avoided.

OUTCOMES

Although it is difficult to predict with certainty the consequences of distal aortic repair for individual patients, distal aortic repair poses the risk of operative death and of life-altering complications such as paraplegia, renal failure necessitating lifelong dialysis, and stroke. In general, advanced age (65 years and older), urgent or emergent repair, rupture, and extensive repair are the most valuable predictors of early death and adverse outcomes.[69,71] Other patient-specific factors that increase operative risk include a history of stroke and poor cardiac, renal, or pulmonary function.[48,71] Whenever possible, elective repair is planned to follow any interventions needed to improve health; in patients with known aortic disease (even those with prior repair), adherence to an imaging-surveillance protocol is crucial to avoiding emergent repair, which more than quadruples the risk of early death and substantially increases the risk of other major complications.[48,71,95]

Without doubt, pulmonary complications are the most common type of complication to arise after distal aortic repair, affecting approximately 30% to 40% of patients.[19,96] Pulmonary complications are highly varied and are, in many ways, largely unavoidable, because single-lung ventilation is typically necessary to provide sufficient surgical exposure. Although the lack of standardization in defining complications makes it difficult to compare complication rates over time, it is generally understood that the outcomes of distal aortic repair are better now than they were in decades past. For example, the risk of developing permanent postoperative paraplegia is now almost half of what it was in the Crawford era,[19,48] and there is much greater awareness of the risk factors related to its development, including delayed-onset paraplegia.[94] In contrast, the risk of developing renal failure necessitating dialysis is only slightly lower now than it was in the Crawford era.[19,48]

TABLE 69-1 **Results of 840 Contemporary (2006-2013) Open Distal Aortic Repairs**

Extent of Repair	*N*	30-Day Deaths	Permanent Paraplegia	Permanent Renal Failure
DTAA	84	3 (4%)	1 (1%)	3 (4%)
Extent I TAAA	192	6 (3%)	2 (1%)	7 (4%)
Extent II TAAA	239	16 (7%)	14 (6%)	23 (10%)
Extent III TAAA	148	7 (5%)	12 (8%)	14 (9%)
Extent IV TAAA	177	7 (4%)	4 (2%)	8 (5%)
Total	840	39 (4.6%)	33 (3.9%)	55 (6.5%)

DTAA, Descending thoracic aortic aneurysm; *TAAA,* thoracoabdominal aortic aneurysm.

Descending Thoracic Aortic Aneurysm Repair

Today, the widespread use of endovascular approaches to aortic repair has reduced the use of open surgical approaches to DTAA repair. In fact, this shift has resulted in a tendency to reserve open surgery for the more complex DTAA repairs (such as those performed in patients with a failed prior endovascular repair or a connective tissue disorder). Contemporary results of open repairs of DTAA indicate that early mortality rates range from 3% to 6%, renal failure rates range from 1% to 8%, and paraplegia rates range from 1% to 5%.[21,24,97-99] Stroke is relatively uncommon after open DTAA repair but may be more likely when HCA is used (2% vs. 3% to 7%, respectively).[21,24,97] Regarding open coarctation-related DTAA repair, experienced centers report excellent outcomes, and results show up to 1% for early mortality and 1% to 3% for renal failure; no paraplegia has been reported.[58,60,61]

Thoracoabdominal Aortic Aneurysm Repair

Volume-based analysis suggests that open TAAA repair is most successful when performed in high-volume centers, whereas operative mortality tends to be excessive when this procedure is performed in low-volume centers.[100] In experienced centers, contemporary outcomes for open TAAA repairs range from 4% to 10% for early mortality, from 4% to 6% for renal failure, and from 2% to 8% for paraplegia.[19,81,101,102] As with open DTAA repair, stroke rates associated with TAAA tend to be relatively low. A recent analysis of National Surgical Quality Improvement Program data found a stroke rate of 2.2%.[96] Not unexpectedly, results vary greatly by the extent of TAAA repair; early mortality ranges from 5% to 8% for extent I repair, from 8% to 9% for extent II, from 7% to 13% for extent III, and from 3% to 6 % for extent IV.[18,19,22,103] Extent II TAAA repairs have been traditionally associated with the highest rates of mortality and morbidity.[95] For patients who undergo complex thoracoabdominal aortic repairs, such as reversed elephant trunk procedures or elephant trunk completion procedures, early mortality rates range from 9% to 16%.[92,104-106] Several centers have reported their experience with open thoracoabdominal aortic repair after endovascular repair. In many reports, these patients' outcomes are not substantially different from those of patients without prior endovascular repair unless infection is present, in which case patients with prior endovascular repair do poorly.[52,54,55] Notably, patients with connective tissue disorders, as well as those with chronic aortic dissection, tend to have better outcomes after distal aortic repair than do other patients, probably because of their younger age, better health, and lower atherosclerotic burden.[107,108]

Previously, we published the results of large series of DTAA and TAAA repairs that were performed over a span of 2 decades.[24,109] In Table 69-1, we present our experience with 840 patients who underwent various extents of DTAA ($n = 84$) and TAAA repair ($n = 756$) over a recent 7-year interval. Overall, the 30-day mortality rate was 4.6%, and operative mortality (as defined by Overman et al[110]) was 7.3%. By extent of repair, 30-day mortality varied from 3% in extent I TAAA repair patients to 7% in extent II TAAA repair patients. Our overall rate of permanent paraplegia was 3.9% and ranged by extent of repair from 1% in DTAA and extent I TAAA repairs to 8% in extent III TAAA repairs. Renal failure necessitating hemodialysis at discharge remains a significant complication, with an overall rate of 6.5%. Similar to other outcomes, the rates of renal failure varied by extent, ranging from 4% in DTAA and extent I TAAA repairs to 10% in extent II TAAA repairs.

Acknowledgments

The authors express gratitude to Stephen N. Palmer, PhD, ELS, of the Texas Heart Institute, and Susan Y. Green, MPH, for editorial assistance, and Scott A. Weldon, MA, CMI, Carol P. Larson, CMI, and Benjamin Y. Cheong, MD, for creating the illustrations and assisting with image selection.

Disclosure

Dr. Coselli serves as a consultant for Vascutek Ltd., a subsidiary of Terumo Corporation, and Medtronic, Inc.;

in addition, he is the principal investigator for ongoing clinical trials for GlaxoSmithKline, WL Gore & Associates, and Medtronic, Inc. Dr. Preventza serves as a consultant for Medtronic, Inc., and has had conference-related travel expenses paid by WL Gore & Associates, and Cook, Inc. Dr. LeMaire serves as a consultant for Medtronic, Inc.

Funding

This work received no external financial support.

REFERENCES

1. Crafoord C, Ejrup B, Gladnikoff H: Coarctation of the aorta. *Thorax* 2:121–152, 1947.
2. Gross RE: Treatment of certain aortic coarctations by homologous grafts; a report of nineteen cases. *Ann Surg* 134:753–768, 1951.
3. Swan H, Maaske C, Johnson M, et al: Arterial homografts. II. Resection of thoracic aortic aneurysm using a stored human arterial transplant. *AMA Arch Surg* 61:732–737, 1950.
4. Lam CR, Aram HH: Resection of the descending thoracic aorta for aneurysm: a report of the use of a homograft in a case and an experimental study. *Ann Surg* 134:743–752, 1951.
5. DeBakey ME, Cooley DA: Successful resection of aneurysm of thoracic aorta and replacement by graft. *JAMA* 152:673–676, 1953.
6. Etheredge SN, Yee J, Smith JV, et al: Successful resection of a large aneurysm of the upper abdominal aorta and replacement with homograft. *Surgery* 38:1071–1081, 1955.
7. Rob C: The surgery of the abdominal aorta and its major branches. *Ann R Coll Surg Engl* 17:307–318, 1955.
8. DeBakey ME, Crawford ES, Garrett HE, et al: Surgical considerations in the treatment of aneurysms of the thoraco-abdominal aorta. *Ann Surg* 162:650–662, 1965.
9. Crawford ES: Thoraco-abdominal and abdominal aortic aneurysms involving renal, superior mesenteric, celiac arteries. *Ann Surg* 179:763–772, 1974.
10. Carrel A, Guthrie C: Resultats du "patching" des arteres. *Comptes Rendus Hebdomadaires des Seances et Memoires* 60:1009–1015, 1906.
11. Javid H, Julian OC, Dye WS, et al: Complications of abdominal aortic grafts. *Arch Surg* 85:650–662, 1962.
12. Crawford ES, Crawford JL, Safi HJ, et al: Thoracoabdominal aortic aneurysms: preoperative and intraoperative factors determining immediate and long-term results of operations in 605 patients. *J Vasc Surg* 3:389–404, 1986.
13. Coady MA, Rizzo JA, Hammond GL, et al: Surgical intervention criteria for thoracic aortic aneurysms: a study of growth rates and complications. *Ann Thorac Surg* 67:1922–1926, discussion 1953–1958, 1999.
14. Coady MA, Rizzo JA, Hammond GL, et al: What is the appropriate size criterion for resection of thoracic aortic aneurysms? *J Thorac Cardiovasc Surg* 113:476–491, discussion 489–491, 1997.
15. Larsen M, Bartnes K, Tsai TT, et al: Extent of preoperative false lumen thrombosis does not influence long-term survival in patients with acute type A aortic dissection. *J Am Heart Assoc* 2:e000112, 2013.
16. Elefteriades JA: Natural history of thoracic aortic aneurysms: indications for surgery, and surgical versus nonsurgical risks. *Ann Thorac Surg* 74:S1877–S1880, discussion S1892–1898, 2002.
17. Safi HJ: How I do it: thoracoabdominal aortic aneurysm graft replacement. *Cardiovasc Surg* 7:607–613, 1999.
18. Conrad MF, Crawford RS, Davison JK, et al: Thoracoabdominal aneurysm repair: a 20-year perspective. *Ann Thorac Surg* 83:S856–S861, discussion S890–S892, 2007.
19. LeMaire SA, Price MD, Green SY, et al: Results of open thoracoabdominal aortic aneurysm repair. *Ann Cardiothorac Surg* 1:286–292, 2012.
20. Schoenhoff FS, Jungi S, Czerny M, et al: Acute aortic dissection determines the fate of initially untreated aortic segments in Marfan syndrome. *Circulation* 127:1569–1575, 2013.
21. Kulik A, Castner CF, Kouchoukos NT: Replacement of the descending thoracic aorta: contemporary outcomes using hypothermic circulatory arrest. *J Thorac Cardiovasc Surg* 139:249–255, 2010.
22. Kulik A, Castner CF, Kouchoukos NT: Outcomes after thoracoabdominal aortic aneurysm repair with hypothermic circulatory arrest. *J Thorac Cardiovasc Surg* 141:953–960, 2011.
23. Conway AM, Sadek M, Lugo J, et al: Outcomes of open surgical repair for chronic type B aortic dissections. *J Vasc Surg* 59:1217–1223, 2014.
24. Coselli JS, LeMaire SA, Conklin LD, et al: Left heart bypass during descending thoracic aortic aneurysm repair does not reduce the incidence of paraplegia. *Ann Thorac Surg* 77:1298–1303, discussion 1303, 2004.
25. Romaniello F, Mazzaglia D, Pellegrino A, et al: Aortopathy in Marfan syndrome: an update. *Cardiovasc Pathol* 23:261–266, 2014.
26. Canadas V, Vilacosta I, Bruna I, et al: Marfan syndrome. Part 1: pathophysiology and diagnosis. *Nat Rev Cardiol* 7:256–265, 2010.
27. Canadas V, Vilacosta I, Bruna I, et al: Marfan syndrome. Part 2: treatment and management of patients. *Nat Rev Cardiol* 7:266–276, 2010.
28. Loeys BL, Schwarze U, Holm T, et al: Aneurysm syndromes caused by mutations in the TGF-beta receptor. *N Engl J Med* 355:788–798, 2006.
29. Schoenhoff FS, Mueller C, Czerny M, et al: Outcome of aortic surgery in patients with Loeys-Dietz syndrome primarily treated as having Marfan syndrome. *Eur J Cardiothorac Surg* 46:444–449, 2014.
30. MacCarrick G, Black JH, 3rd, Bowdin S, et al: Loeys-Dietz syndrome: a primer for diagnosis and management. *Genet Med* 16:576–587, 2014.
31. Williams JA, Loeys BL, Nwakanma LU, et al: Early surgical experience with Loeys-Dietz: a new syndrome of aggressive thoracic aortic aneurysm disease. *Ann Thorac Surg* 83:S757–S763, discussion S785–790, 2007.
32. Cook JR, Carta L, Galatioto J, et al: Cardiovascular manifestations in Marfan syndrome and related diseases; multiple genes causing similar phenotypes. *Clin Genet* 87:11–20, 2015.
33. De Paepe A, Malfait F: The Ehlers-Danlos syndrome, a disorder with many faces. *Clin Genet* 82:1–11, 2012.
34. Bergqvist D, Bjorck M, Wanhainen A: Treatment of vascular Ehlers-Danlos syndrome: a systematic review. *Ann Surg* 258:257–261, 2013.
35. van de Laar IM, Oldenburg RA, Pals G, et al: Mutations in SMAD3 cause a syndromic form of aortic aneurysms and dissections with early-onset osteoarthritis. *Nat Genet* 43:121–126, 2011.
36. van der Linde D, van de Laar IM, Bertoli-Avella AM, et al: Aggressive cardiovascular phenotype of aneurysms-osteoarthritis syndrome caused by pathogenic SMAD3 variants. *J Am Coll Cardiol* 60:397–403, 2012.
37. Guo DC, Papke CL, Tran-Fadulu V, et al: Mutations in smooth muscle alpha-actin (ACTA2) cause coronary artery disease, stroke, and Moyamoya disease, along with thoracic aortic disease. *Am J Hum Genet* 84:617–627, 2009.
38. Boileau C, Guo DC, Hanna N, et al: TGFB2 mutations cause familial thoracic aortic aneurysms and dissections associated with mild systemic features of Marfan syndrome. *Nat Genet* 44:916–921, 2012.
39. Regalado ES, Guo DC, Villamizar C, et al: Exome sequencing identifies SMAD3 mutations as a cause of familial thoracic aortic aneurysm and dissection with intracranial and other arterial aneurysms. *Circ Res* 109:680–686, 2011.
40. Pannu H, Tran-Fadulu V, Papke CL, et al: MYH11 mutations result in a distinct vascular pathology driven by insulin-like growth factor 1 and angiotensin II. *Hum Mol Genet* 16:2453–2462, 2007.
41. Milewicz DM, Chen H, Park E, et al: Reduced penetrance and avriable expressivity of familial thoracic aortic aneurysms/dissections. *Am J Cardiol* 82:474–479, 1998.
42. Raman SP, Fishman EK: Mycotic aneurysms: a critical diagnosis in the emergency setting. *Emerg Radiol* 21:191–196, 2014.
43. Hiratzka LF, Bakris GL, Beckman JA, et al: 2010 ACCF/AHA/AATS/ACR/ASA/SCA/SCAI/SIR/STS/SVM guidelines for the diagnosis and management of patients with thoracic aortic disease: a report of the American College of Cardiology Foundation/American Heart Association Task Force on Practice Guidelines, American Association for Thoracic Surgery, American College of

Radiology, American Stroke Association, Society of Cardiovascular Anesthesiologists, Society for Cardiovascular Angiography and Interventions, Society of Interventional Radiology, Society of Thoracic Surgeons, and Society for Vascular Medicine. *Circulation* 121:e266–e369, 2010.

44. Brown SL, Busuttil RW, Baker JD, et al: Bacteriologic and surgical determinants of survival in patients with mycotic aneurysms. *J Vasc Surg* 1:541–547, 1984.
45. Benjelloun A, Henry M, Ghannam A, et al: Endovascular treatment of a tuberculous thoracoabdominal aneurysm with the Multilayer stent. *J Endovasc Ther* 19:115–120, 2012.
46. Jaffer U, Gibbs R: Mycotic thoracoabdominal aneurysms. *Ann Cardiothorac Surg* 1:417–425, 2012.
47. Lombardi JV, Carpenter JP, Pochettino A, et al: Thoracoabdominal aortic aneurysm repair after prior aortic surgery. *J Vasc Surg* 38:1185–1190, 2003.
48. Svensson LG, Crawford ES, Hess KR, et al: Experience with 1509 patients undergoing thoracoabdominal aortic operations. *J Vasc Surg* 17:357–368, 1993.
49. Geisbusch P, Hoffmann S, Kotelis D, et al: Reinterventions during midterm follow-up after endovascular treatment of thoracic aortic disease. *J Vasc Surg* 53:1528–1533, 2011.
50. Karimi A, Walker KL, Martin TD, et al: Midterm cost and effectiveness of thoracic endovascular aortic repair versus open repair. *Ann Thorac Surg* 93:473–479, 2012.
51. Morales JP, Greenberg RK, Lu Q, et al: Endoleaks following endovascular repair of thoracic aortic aneurysm: etiology and outcomes. *J Endovasc Ther* 15:631–638, 2008.
52. Canaud L, Alric P, Gandet T, et al: Open surgical secondary procedures after thoracic endovascular aortic repair. *Eur J Vasc Endovasc Surg* 46:667–674, 2013.
53. Girdauskas E, Falk V, Kuntze T, et al: Secondary surgical procedures after endovascular stent grafting of the thoracic aorta: successful approaches to a challenging clinical problem. *J Thorac Cardiovasc Surg* 136:1289–1294, 2008.
54. LeMaire SA, Green SY, Kim JH, et al: Thoracic or thoracoabdominal approaches to endovascular device removal and open aortic repair. *Ann Thorac Surg* 93:726–732, discussion 733, 2012.
55. Roselli EE, Abdel-Halim M, Johnston DR, et al: Open aortic repair after prior thoracic endovascular aortic repair. *Ann Thorac Surg* 97:750–756, 2014.
56. Warnes CA, Williams RG, Bashore TM, et al: ACC/AHA 2008 guidelines for the management of adults with congenital heart disease: a report of the American College of Cardiology/American Heart Association Task Force on Practice Guidelines (Writing Committee to Develop Guidelines on the Management of Adults With Congenital Heart Disease). Developed in Collaboration With the American Society of Echocardiography, Heart Rhythm Society, International Society for Adult Congenital Heart Disease, Society for Cardiovascular Angiography and Interventions, and Society of Thoracic Surgeons. *J Am Coll Cardiol* 52:e143–e263, 2008.
57. Webb G: Treatment of coarctation and late complications in the adult. *Semin Thorac Cardiovasc Surg* 17:139–142, 2005.
58. Preventza O, Livesay JJ, Cooley DA, et al: Coarctation-associated aneurysms: a localized disease or diffuse aortopathy. *Ann Thorac Surg* 95:1961–1967, discussion 1967, 2013.
59. Hoffman JL, Gray RG, LuAnn Minich L, et al: Screening for aortic aneurysm after treatment of coarctation. *Pediatr Cardiol* 35:47–52, 2014.
60. Roselli EE, Qureshi A, Idrees J, et al: Open, hybrid, and endovascular treatment for aortic coarctation and postrepair aneurysm in adolescents and adults. *Ann Thorac Surg* 94:751–756, discussion 757–758, 2012.
61. Brown ML, Burkhart HM, Connolly HM, et al: Late outcomes of reintervention on the descending aorta after repair of aortic coarctation. *Circulation* 122:S81–S84, 2010.
62. Gawenda M, Aleksic M, Heckenkamp J, et al: Endovascular repair of aneurysm after previous surgical coarctation repair. *J Thorac Cardiovasc Surg* 130:1039–1043, 2005.
63. Preventza O, Mohammed S, Cheong BY, et al: Endovascular therapy in patients with genetically triggered thoracic aortic disease: applications and short- and mid-term outcomes. *Eur J Cardiothorac Surg* 46:248–253, 2014.
64. Ananiadou OG, Koutsogiannidis C, Ampatzidou F, et al: Aortic root aneurysm in an adult patient with aortic coarctation: a single-stage approach. *Interact Cardiovasc Thorac Surg* 15:534–536, 2012.
65. Axelbaum SP, Schellinger D, Gomes MN, et al: Computed tomographic evaluation of aortic aneurysms. *AJR Am J Roentgenol* 127:75–78, 1976.
66. Ergun I, Keven K, Uruc I, et al: The safety of gadolinium in patients with stage 3 and 4 renal failure. *Nephrol Dial Transplant* 21:697–700, 2006.
67. Shellock FG, Spinazzi A: MRI safety update 2008: part 1, MRI contrast agents and nephrogenic systemic fibrosis. *AJR Am J Roentgenol* 191:1129–1139, 2008.
68. Hughes GC, Andersen ND, Hanna JM, et al: Thoracoabdominal aortic aneurysm: hybrid repair outcomes. *Ann Cardiothorac Surg* 1:311–319, 2012.
69. LeMaire SA, Miller CC, 3rd, Conklin LD, et al: A new predictive model for adverse outcomes after elective thoracoabdominal aortic aneurysm repair. *Ann Thorac Surg* 71:1233–1238, 2001.
70. Aftab M, Songdechakraiwut T, Green SY, et al: Contemporary outcomes of open thoracoabdominal aortic aneurysm repair in octogenarians. *J Thorac Cardiovasc Surg* 18:2014. [Epub ahead of print].
71. Wong DR, Parenti JL, Green SY, et al: Open repair of thoracoabdominal aortic aneurysm in the modern surgical era: contemporary outcomes in 509 patients. *J Am Coll Surg* 212:569–579, discussion 579–581, 2011.
72. Coselli JS, LeMaire SA: Left heart bypass reduces paraplegia rates after thoracoabdominal aortic aneurysm repair. *Ann Thorac Surg* 67:1931–1934, discussion 1953–1958, 1999.
73. Jones MM, Akay M, Murariu D, et al: Safe aortic arch clamping in patients with patent internal thoracic artery grafts. *Ann Thorac Surg* 89:e31–e32, 2010.
74. Black JH, 3rd, Cambria RP: Contemporary results of open surgical repair of descending thoracic aortic aneurysms. *Semin Vasc Surg* 19:11–17, 2006.
75. Coselli JS, LeMaire SA, Koksoy C, et al: Cerebrospinal fluid drainage reduces paraplegia after thoracoabdominal aortic aneurysm repair: results of a randomized clinical trial. *J Vasc Surg* 35:631–639, 2002.
76. Youngblood SC, Tolpin DA, LeMaire SA, et al: Complications of cerebrospinal fluid drainage after thoracic aortic surgery: a review of 504 patients over 5 years. *J Thorac Cardiovasc Surg* 146:166–171, 2013.
77. Jacobs MJ, Mess W, Mochtar B, et al: The value of motor evoked potentials in reducing paraplegia during thoracoabdominal aneurysm repair. *J Vasc Surg* 43:239–246, 2006.
78. Schurink GW, De Haan MW, Peppelenbosch AG, et al: Spinal cord function monitoring during endovascular treatment of thoracoabdominal aneurysms: implications for staged procedures. *J Cardiovasc Surg (Torino)* 54:117–124, 2013.
79. Koksoy C, LeMaire SA, Curling PE, et al: Renal perfusion during thoracoabdominal aortic operations: cold crystalloid is superior to normothermic blood. *Ann Thorac Surg* 73:730–738, 2002.
80. LeMaire SA, Jones MM, Conklin LD, et al: Randomized comparison of cold blood and cold crystalloid renal perfusion for renal protection during thoracoabdominal aortic aneurysm repair. *J Vasc Surg* 49:11–19, discussion 19, 2009.
81. Kouchoukos NT, Kulik A, Castner CF: Outcomes after thoracoabdominal aortic aneurysm repair using hypothermic circulatory arrest. *J Thorac Cardiovasc Surg* 145:S139–S141, 2013.
82. Fehrenbacher JW, Siderys H, Terry C, et al: Early and late results of descending thoracic and thoracoabdominal aortic aneurysm open repair with deep hypothermia and circulatory arrest. *J Thorac Cardiovasc Surg* 140:S154–S160, discussion S185–S190, 2010.
83. Kouchoukos NT: One-stage repair of extensive thoracic aortic disease. *J Thorac Cardiovasc Surg* 140:S150–S153, discussion S185–S190, 2010.
84. Borst HG, Walterbusch G, Schaps D: Extensive aortic replacement using "elephant trunk" prosthesis. *Thorac Cardiovasc Surg* 31:37–40, 1983.
85. Svensson LG: Rationale and technique for replacement of the ascending aorta, arch, and distal aorta using a modified elephant trunk procedure. *J Card Surg* 7:301–312, 1992.
86. Carrel T, Althaus U: Extension of the "elephant trunk" technique in complex aortic pathology: the "bidirectional" option. *Ann Thorac Surg* 63:1755–1758, 1997.

87. Coselli JS, Oberwalder P: Successful repair of mega aorta using reversed elephant trunk procedure. *J Vasc Surg* 27:183–188, 1998.
88. LeMaire SA, Price MD, Parenti JL, et al: Early outcomes after aortic arch replacement by using the Y-graft technique. *Ann Thorac Surg* 91:700–707, discussion 707–708, 2011.
89. Toda K, Taniguchi K, Masai T, et al: Arch aneurysm repair with long elephant trunk: a 10-year experience in 111 patients. *Ann Thorac Surg* 88:16–22, 2009.
90. Fann JI, Dake MD, Semba CP, et al: Endovascular stent-grafting after arch aneurysm repair using the "elephant trunk." *Ann Thorac Surg* 60:1102–1105, 1995.
91. Greenberg RK, Haddad F, Svensson L, et al: Hybrid approaches to thoracic aortic aneurysms: the role of endovascular elephant trunk completion. *Circulation* 112:2619–2626, 2005.
92. Coselli JS, LeMaire SA, Carter SA, et al: The reversed elephant trunk technique used for treatment of complex aneurysms of the entire thoracic aorta. *Ann Thorac Surg* 80:2166–2172, discussion 2172, 2005.
93. Bhamidipati CM, Coselli JS, LeMaire SA: BioGlue in 2011: what is its role in cardiac surgery? *J Extra Corpor Technol* 44:P6–P12, 2012.
94. Wong DR, Coselli JS, Amerman K, et al: Delayed spinal cord deficits after thoracoabdominal aortic aneurysm repair. *Ann Thorac Surg* 83:1345–1355, discussion 1355, 2007.
95. Coselli JS, LeMaire SA, Conklin LD, et al: Morbidity and mortality after extent II thoracoabdominal aortic aneurysm repair. *Ann Thorac Surg* 73:1107–1115, discussion 1115–1116, 2002.
96. Bensley RP, Curran T, Hurks R, et al: Open repair of intact thoracoabdominal aortic aneurysms in the American College of Surgeons National Surgical Quality Improvement Program. *J Vasc Surg* 58:894–900, 2013.
97. Kieffer E, Chiche L, Cluzel P, et al: Open surgical repair of descending thoracic aortic aneurysms in the endovascular era: a 9-year single-center study. *Ann Vasc Surg* 23:60–66, 2009.
98. Patel HJ, Shillingford MS, Mihalik S, et al: Resection of the descending thoracic aorta: outcomes after use of hypothermic circulatory arrest. *Ann Thorac Surg* 82:90–95, discussion 95–96, 2006.
99. Sadek M, Abjigitova D, Pellet Y, et al: Operative outcomes after open repair of descending thoracic aortic aneurysms in the era of endovascular surgery. *Ann Thorac Surg* 97:1562–1567, 2014.
100. Cowan JA, Jr, Dimick JB, Henke PK, et al: Surgical treatment of intact thoracoabdominal aortic aneurysms in the United States: hospital and surgeon volume-related outcomes. *J Vasc Surg* 37:1169–1174, 2003.
101. Di Luozzo G, Geisbusch S, Lin HM, et al: Open repair of descending and thoracoabdominal aortic aneurysms and dissections in patients aged younger than 60 years: superior to endovascular repair? *Ann Thorac Surg* 95:12–19, discussion 19, 2013.
102. Lancaster RT, Conrad MF, Patel VI, et al: Further experience with distal aortic perfusion and motor-evoked potential monitoring in the management of extent I-III thoracoabdominal aortic aneurysms. *J Vasc Surg* 58:283–290, 2013.
103. Patel VI, Ergul E, Conrad MF, et al: Continued favorable results with open surgical repair of type IV thoracoabdominal aortic aneurysms. *J Vasc Surg* 53:1492–1498, 2011.
104. LeMaire SA, Carter SA, Coselli JS: The elephant trunk technique for staged repair of complex aneurysms of the entire thoracic aorta. *Ann Thorac Surg* 81:1561–1569, discussion 1569, 2006.
105. Safi HJ, Miller CC, III, Estrera AL, et al: Staged repair of extensive aortic aneurysms: long-term experience with the elephant trunk technique. *Ann Surg* 240:677–684, 2004.
106. Svensson LG, Kim KH, Blackstone EH, et al: Elephant trunk procedure: newer indications and uses. *Ann Thorac Surg* 78:109–116, discussion 109–116, 2004.
107. Coselli JS, Green SY, Zarda S, et al: Outcomes of open distal aortic aneurysm repair in patients with chronic DeBakey type I dissection. *J Thorac Cardiovasc Surg* 148:2986–2993.e1-2, 2014.
108. Omura A, Tanaka A, Miyahara S, et al: Early and late results of graft replacement for dissecting aneurysm of thoracoabdominal aorta in patients with Marfan syndrome. *Ann Thorac Surg* 94:759–765, 2012.
109. Coselli JS, Bozinovski J, LeMaire SA: Open surgical repair of 2286 thoracoabdominal aortic aneurysms. *Ann Thorac Surg* 83:S862–S864, discussion S890–S892, 2007.
110. Overman DM, Jacobs JP, Prager RL, et al: Report from the Society of Thoracic Surgeons National Database Workforce: clarifying the definition of operative mortality. *World J Pediatr Congenit Heart Surg* 4:10–12, 2013.

CHAPTER 70

TYPE A AORTIC DISSECTION

Philippe Demers • D. Craig Miller

CHAPTER OUTLINE

Acute aortic dissection is one of the most common catastrophes involving the aorta. Dissection of the aorta is characterized by the separation of the aortic media by pulsatile blood, with variable extents of proximal and distal extension along the aorta and its branches. The process of dissection creates a false lumen in the aortic wall that parallels the aortic true lumen. In the majority of cases, a primary intimal tear initiates the dissection and allows blood flow communication between the true and false lumens, which are separated by a dissection flap or septum. Because this acute event is rarely associated with a preexisting aneurysm and the aortic intima (true lumen) is actually smaller than normal, the older term *dissecting aneurysm* is misleading and inappropriate; to be semantically correct, an aortic dissection should be called a *false aneurysm*. A thorough understanding of the pathophysiology of aortic dissection is critical for prompt diagnosis and effective management in the acute setting. On the other hand, aortic dissection in its chronic phase is responsible for a substantial proportion of thoracic aortic disease and aortic rupture due to false aneurysmal degeneration of the false lumen. Numerous advances in diagnostic modalities, medical and surgical treatment, and long-term management have changed the prognosis for patients with this lethal condition. This chapter summarizes current knowledge regarding the diagnosis and treatment of Stanford type A aortic dissection.

HISTORICAL NOTE

The observations by Morgagni in 1761 were followed by multiple early anatomic and postmortem reports describing aortic dissection, including the famous autopsy report on King George II of England in 1776.[1] In 1802, Maunoir, describing this disease, used the term *dissection*.[2] Almost 20 years later, René Laennec coined the term *aneurysme dissequant*, or dissecting aneurysm, believing that this entity represented the early stage of a saccular aneurysm.[3] Later, in 1863, Peacock published a comprehensive review of 80 cases of aortic dissection.[4] Until the last half of the twentieth century, the diagnosis of aortic dissection was almost exclusively an autopsy finding. Antemortem diagnosis was made in only 6 of 300 cases reviewed by Shennan in 1934.[5] The use of contrast angiography for the diagnosis of aortic dissection was reported by Paullin and James.[6] The first attempt to treat this condition was described in 1935 by Gurin and colleagues,[7] who used surgical iliac artery fenestration to relieve lower extremity ischemia. Although quickly abandoned, cellophane wrapping of the dissected aorta was also attempted to prevent rupture.[8] In 1955, DeBakey and associates[9] launched the modern era of surgical management with graft replacement of the dissected aorta. Subsequently, the same group introduced the use of cardiopulmonary bypass during clamping of the descending thoracic aorta.[10] The first large clinical series of patients with an aortic dissection was published in 1958 by Hirst and colleagues[11]; analyzing 505 cases allowed these authors to emphasize the high mortality rate and the glaring rarity of antemortem diagnosis at that time. The modern medical approach to aortic dissection with use of pharmacologic agents to diminish aortic dP/dt (anti-impulse therapy) was introduced by Wheat and associates in 1965.[12] The venerable DeBakey type I, II, III classification of aortic dissection was introduced the same year. The simplified Stanford classification system (type A or type B) based on pathophysiologic characteristics was proposed in 1970 by Daily and colleagues.[13,14] Since then, other important advances have followed, such as less invasive and more accurate diagnostic modalities, improved anesthetic methods, safer extracorporeal perfusion techniques, profound hypothermic circulatory arrest for thoracic aortic arch surgery (introduced by Griepp and coworkers[15] from Stanford in 1975), improved and safer prosthetic vascular grafts, and refinement of cardiovascular surgical techniques.

CLASSIFICATION

It is important to understand and to apply accurately the classification of aortic dissection in order to treat patients most appropriately and to compare rigorously the results of various medical and surgical therapeutic interventions reported from different institutions. Considerable confusion about classifying aortic dissections has arisen in the past. Numerous systems have been proposed, beginning in 1955 with nine categories initially suggested by DeBakey and associates.[9] The more widely used DeBakey type I, type II, and type III three-category classification scheme was introduced in 1965[14]; importantly, DeBakey modified this scheme in 1982[16] to conform with the Stanford A/B functional criteria based on whether the ascending aorta is involved, regardless of the location of the tear and distal extent of dissection. Despite the use of different labels, a consensus has emerged concerning the essential elements of a common functional classification system of aortic dissection. The key point of all classification systems used today is the presence or absence of involvement of the ascending aorta, regardless of the location of the primary intimal tear and irrespective of the antegrade extension of the dissection process.[17] The simplified Stanford classification approach as proposed by Daily and associates[13] in 1970 has gained broad acceptance during the past 44 years. If the dissection involves the ascending aorta, it is a Stanford type A, which corresponds to a DeBakey type I,[16] University of Alabama "ascending,"[18] Massachusetts General Hospital "proximal,"[19] and Najafi "anterior" dissection.[20] Both DeBakey type I and type II dissections involve the ascending aorta; type I extends beyond the innominate artery, whereas type II is confined just to the ascending aorta. If the ascending aorta proximal to the innominate artery is not involved in the process, the dissection is called a Stanford type B, DeBakey type III, descending, distal, or posterior dissection (Fig. 70-1), even though many of these patients have some limited extent of retrograde dissection involvement in the arch, a point that is not broadly appreciated. A subtype of dissection in which the primary intimal tear is in the descending aorta or even farther distal, yet the dissection process propagates in a retrograde fashion to involve the arch and ascending aorta, was originally termed a *DeBakey type III-D* by Reul and colleagues[21] in 1975, but now is simply termed a *retro-A dissection*. Retro-A dissections constitute approximately 6% of all type A dissections,[22] and recently they have been seen more frequently as a complication of stent-graft descending thoracic endovascular aortic repair (TEVAR).

This functional classification approach reflects the pathophysiology of aortic dissection, considering that involvement of the ascending aorta is the principal predictor of the biological behavior of the disease process and the most common fatal complications; moreover, it simplifies diagnosis because it is easier to identify involvement of the ascending aorta accurately than to determine the exact site of the primary intimal tear (or tears) or the extent of propagation of the dissection process. Furthermore, the Stanford classification system facilitates clinical decision making and expedites definitive management. Patients with acute Stanford type A dissections should be treated surgically in essentially all cases; individuals with Stanford type B dissections can be treated with open surgical intervention, with an endovascular TEVAR, or with medical management, depending on the presence or absence of major complications. More specifically, patients with type A dissections require a median sternotomy, total cardiopulmonary bypass (CPB), and

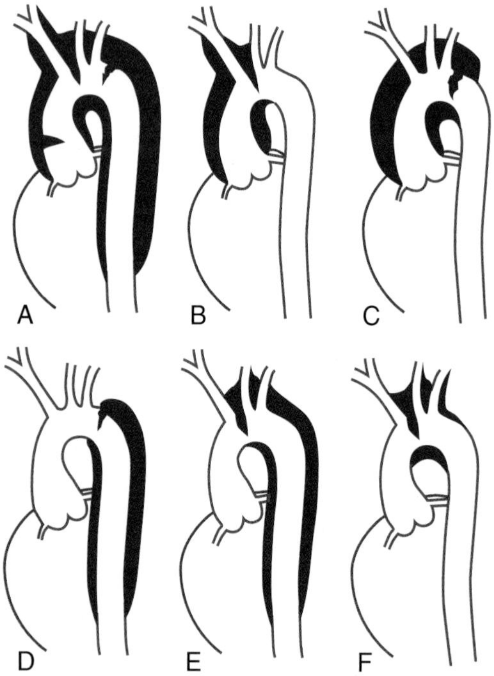

FIGURE 70-1 ■ Schematic illustration of the Stanford classification system of aortic dissections. The three examples in the *top row* are all type A aortic dissections because the ascending aorta is involved. The primary intimal tear can be located in the ascending aorta **(A)**, in the transverse arch **(B)**, or in the descending thoracic aorta **(C)**. This last example is now called a *retro-A dissection* and is equivalent to a type III-D dissection. The dissections in **(D)** and **(E)** are type B dissections; whether the tear is in the descending thoracic aorta or the arch, the ascending aorta is not involved. The last example **(F)** is an isolated arch dissection without retrograde or antegrade propagation; these are rare. (From Miller DC: Surgical management of aortic dissections: indications, perioperative management, and long-term results. In Doroghazi RM, Slater EE, editors: *Aortic dissection*, New York, 1983, McGraw-Hill, p 196.)

profound hypothermic circulatory arrest (PHCA); those with type B dissections are approached surgically using a left posterolateral thoracotomy, total CPB with PHCA, partial CPB, or isolated left heart bypass.

Aortic dissections diagnosed within 14 days of the onset of presenting symptoms are defined as acute; those diagnosed more than 14 days after onset are classified as chronic dissections.[23-25] According to the International Registry of Acute Aortic Dissection (IRAD) investigators,[24] the cumulative mortality after acute type A and type B dissection treated medically reached a plateau after the fourteenth day after presentation, demonstrating the prognostic importance of this venerable but arbitrary 14-day time distinction (Fig. 70-2). DeBakey and colleagues[16] introduced the term *subacute* to describe dissections between 2 weeks and 2 months old, but this distinction has been rarely used; however, the term *subacute* has recently gained popularity because of the use of TEVAR and can mean anything between 2 weeks and 6 or more months. Its use should be rejected because it is ambiguous.

During the past two decades, advances in vascular imaging technology have led to increasing recognition of intramural hematoma (IMH) and penetrating atherosclerotic ulcers (PAUs) as distinct pathologic variants in the spectrum of acute aortic diseases, which can evolve into classic aortic dissection.[26,27] Both are characterized by the absence of the classic intimal flap dividing the aorta into true and false channels. IMH can be caused by an ulcer penetrating into the internal elastic lamina or can occur spontaneously without any intimal disruption. IMH can involve the ascending aorta (type A IMH) as well as the descending aorta (type B IMH). On occasion, IMH can suddenly evolve into classic aortic dissection with blood flow in both lumens,[28] as different phases of a dynamic aortic pathologic process. PAUs occur most commonly in the descending thoracic aorta in older patients. Distinguishing IMH (with or without a PAU) or PAU from classic aortic dissection is critical because the pathophysiologic process, clinical behavior, prognosis, and management of these lesions can differ,[29,30] depending on which segment of the aorta is involved and the patient's symptomatic status.

EPIDEMIOLOGY

Aortic dissection is seen in all age groups, although the majority of the cases occur between the ages of 50 and 69 years. In a series of 464 patients reviewed in the IRAD registry, mean age was 63 years.[24] Two thirds of aortic dissections involve the ascending aorta (Stanford type A) and a third involve the descending aorta (Stanford type B).[24] Typically, patients with type B dissection are older than those with type A dissection.[10,24] Dissection in patients younger than 40 years typically is a type A dissection. According to the IRAD investigators, younger patients with acute aortic dissections are less likely to be hypertensive and are more likely to have Marfan syndrome, bicuspid aortic valve, some other connective tissue disorder, or prior aortic surgery.[31] In all studies, there is a clear male predominance with an estimated male-to-female ratio ranging from 2 : 1 to 3 : 1. Although less frequently affected by acute aortic syndromes, women are older at the time of diagnosis with a mean age of 67 years and have worse outcomes, perhaps due to atypical symptoms and delay in diagnosis.[24,32] Hirst and colleagues[11] found a higher incidence of aortic dissection in African Americans, which might be related more to hypertension than to any intrinsic racial pathologic weakness of the aorta. Similarly, a high prevalence of hypertension may also explain why the incidence of aortic dissection and its variants is higher in Japan and other Asian countries.

The true incidence of aortic dissection is difficult to determine because many patients die without the correct diagnosis being made antemortem.[33] It is not widely appreciated that acute aortic dissection is the most common clinical catastrophe involving the aorta. Moreover, its incidence has been increasing in the industrialized world, in part because of increasing life expectancy and more years exposed to elevated blood pressure. In a 1964 Danish study of 6480 autopsies covering 90% of a regional population, the incidence of acute aortic dissection was 5.2 per million population per year, higher than the incidence of ruptured abdominal aortic aneurysm (3.6 per million population per year) and more than four

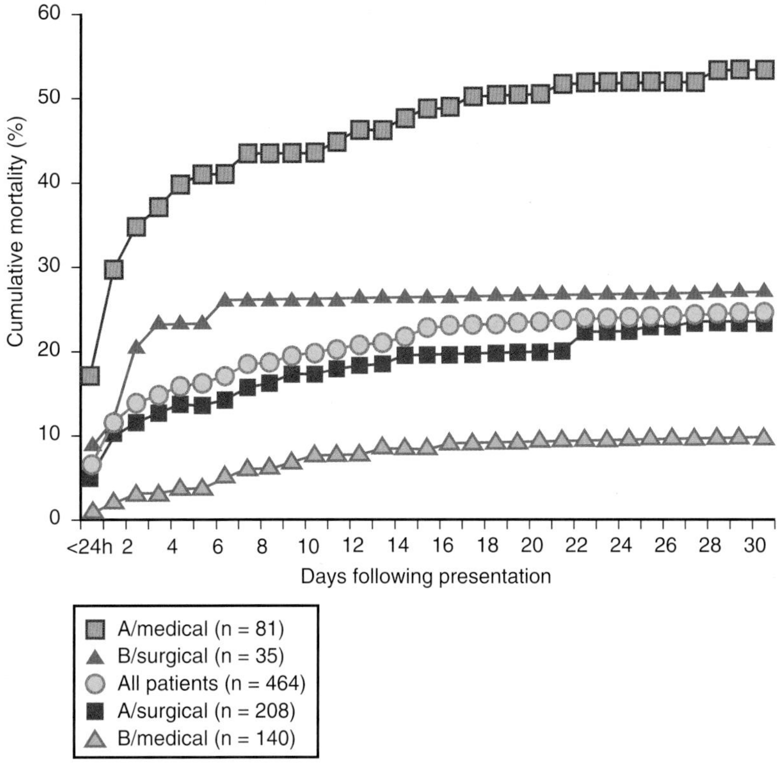

FIGURE 70-2 ■ Thirty-day mortality according to dissection type and management in the International Registry of Acute Aortic Dissection. (From Hagan PG, Nienaber CA, Isselbacher EM, et al: The International Registry of Acute Aortic Dissection [IRAD]: new insights into an old disease. *JAMA* 283:897–903, 2000.)

times the prevalence of ruptured thoracic aortic aneurysm (1.2 per million population per year).[34] In the seminal 1958 pathologic series by Hirst and associates,[11] acute aortic dissection was found in 1% to 2% of autopsies. In the 1970s, it was estimated that the incidence of acute aortic dissection in an urban population containing many African Americans in the southeastern United States might be as high as 10 to 20 cases per million population per year,[35] or approximately 2000 to 4500 new cases each year.[36] According to a review of all thoracic aortic diseases among the residents of Olmsted County, Minnesota, between 1980 and 1994, the annual incidence of acute aortic dissection was estimated at 3.5 per 100,000 person-years.[33] More recently, in a comprehensive review of the entire Swedish national healthcare registry during a 15-year period, it was observed that the incidence of thoracic aortic aneurysm and dissection had increased substantially between 1987 and 2002; specifically, the incidence of thoracic aortic disease rose by 52% in men and by 28% in women during this period to reach 16.3 cases per 100,000 per year and 9.1 cases per 100,000 per year, respectively.[37] In general, these prevalence estimates undoubtedly underestimate the real incidence because they do not capture patients who die suddenly of a complication of aortic dissection and who are presumed to have succumbed to coronary disease or an arrhythmic event in the absence of a postmortem examination; importantly, this was not the case in the report from Sweden, where many dissections were identified only at the time of forensic autopsy, which is still performed almost universally in that country. Most physicians tend to think that ruptured abdominal aortic aneurysms are more common; this misconception comes from the fact that ruptured abdominal aortic aneurysm is diagnosed correctly more often than is acute aortic dissection.

NATURAL HISTORY

According to the historical autopsy analyses, untreated acute aortic dissection is a highly lethal event. In the study by Shennan published in 1934,[5] 40% of patients with dissection involving the ascending aorta died immediately, 70% within the first 24 hours, 94% within the first week, and 100% within 5 weeks. In 1967, Lindsay and Hurst[38] reported that one third of patients sustaining an acute aortic dissection died within 24 hours, 50% within 48 hours, 80% within 7 days, and 95% within the first month. In patients with chronic dissection, only 15% were still alive after 5 years. In patients with dissection involving the descending thoracic aorta (Stanford type B), 25% had died 1 month after onset. Later, Anagnostopoulos and coworkers,[39] in a large collected series of 963 cases of patients not surgically treated with aortic dissection of all types, reported a cumulative mortality of 70% at 1 week and 90% at 3 months, but as in other retrospective investigations the true patient denominator was unknown.

Most patients with untreated acute type A dissection die of intrapericardial rupture culminating in cardiac tamponade; other causes of death include acute aortic valvular regurgitation resulting in left ventricular failure, coronary ostial compromise causing acute myocardial ischemia, occlusion of aortic branches supplying the cerebral or visceral circulation, and free aortic rupture. Patients with untreated acute type B dissection usually die of aortic rupture or of distal end-organ malperfusion (occlusion of major aortic branches resulting in ischemic injury to vital abdominal organs, termed thoracoabdominal malperfusion).[23] In the Stanford experience, lower extremity ischemia at presentation did not significantly increase surgical mortality risk, whereas occlusion of major abdominal tributaries resulting in renal or splanchnic ischemia was associated with very high mortality rates.[40,41]

Only 10% of acute dissections are estimated to "heal" spontaneously, eventually becoming chronic dissections. Distal reentry sites are found in nearly all cases, allowing decompression of the false lumen.[42,43] After acute aortic dissection, the false lumen usually remains patent but may thrombose rarely, depending mainly on the presence, size, and site of distal false lumen reentry sites. When the false lumen remains patent, it is prone to progressive expansion over time, resulting in the formation of a false aneurysm. It is noteworthy that a large fraction of acute serious or fatal dissection complications are caused by a *non-reentering* false lumen, which compromises distal blood flow by extrinsically narrowing or occluding the true lumen.

PREDISPOSING FACTORS

Hypertension

In patients with aortic dissection, the prevalence of hypertension varies between 45% and 80%,[10,23,24,43,44] being highest in patients with acute type B dissection. Untreated hypertension promotes medial smooth muscle cell degeneration and other changes in the aortic wall, which may increase the susceptibility for aortic dissection.[45] Although there is no evidence to suggest that hypertension initiates the actual process, it is a major risk factor.

Connective Tissue Disorders

Heritable connective tissue disorders such as Marfan, Ehlers-Danlos, and Loeys-Dietz syndromes are associated with an increased risk of aortic dissection. The Marfan syndrome is inherited as an autosomal dominant trait and is characterized by mutations of the *FBN1* gene encoding the glycoprotein fibrillin 1, which is a major component of elastic fibers of the extracellular matrix in various organs.[46,47] In addition to cardiovascular manifestations, including mitral valve prolapse, progressive aortic root dilation, aortic valve regurgitation, and aortic dissection, these patients can have several other ocular and musculoskeletal abnormalities. The diagnosis of Marfan syndrome is made according to the revised 2010 Ghent criteria (major and minor), which characterize the involvement of different organ systems, as well as genetic testing identifying a *FBN1* mutation.[48,49] When a patient demonstrates the classic Marfan syndrome phenotype, the diagnosis is rarely in doubt; however, many patients have only some of the characteristic phenotypic features (variable penetrance), including aortic root dilation with or without aortic valve regurgitation, which has been called the *forme fruste* of Marfan syndrome.[46] Aortic-related complications, including acute dissection and rupture, are the leading causes of death in patients with Marfan syndrome. If a patient with Marfan syndrome has a family history of aortic dissection or other aortic catastrophe at an early age, the risk of dissection or rupture is considerably higher.[47,49] The prevalence of Marfan syndrome in patients presenting with acute aortic dissection ranges between 5% and 12%.[10,24,44,50]

Patients with Ehlers-Danlos syndrome, particularly those with type IV (vascular type) Ehlers-Danlos syndrome, which is transmitted in most cases as an autosomal dominant trait, have arterial weakness of all large and muscular arteries; type IV Ehlers-Danlos syndrome is characterized by a procollagen type 3 (COL3A1) abnormality and an increased risk of aortic dissection or spontaneous rupture of peripheral arteries or a hollow abdominal viscus.[51] Aortic rupture has also been reported in patients with Ehlers-Danlos syndrome type I and type VI. Extremely fragile arteries are found in patients with Ehlers-Danlos syndrome, and vascular procedures, including simple arterial puncture and suture repair, can be fraught with devastating complications.[52] The diagnosis of (vascular type) Ehlers-Danlos syndrome is based on genetic testing identifying a mutation in the gene *COL3A1* coding for type III procollagen.[49,53,54]

Loeys-Dietz syndrome is a more recently recognized autosomal dominant connective tissue disorder characterized by premature arterial aneurysms (typically aortic root aneurysm) and aortic dissection along with diffuse peripheral arterial tortuosity. It is caused by heterogeneous mutations in the genes encoding transforming growth factor β receptors 1 and 2 (TGFBR1 and TGFBR2), and the diagnosis is confirmed through identification of these mutations.[49,55] Phenotypic features of Loeys-Dietz syndrome include hypertelorism, bifid uvula or cleft palate or both, hyperlucent skin, and generalized arterial hypertortuosity, especially of the extracranial carotid or iliac arteries. In these patients, the risk of aortic rupture and aortic dissection exceeds that of any other known connective tissue disorders. In addition, aortic rupture and dissection occur at a younger age (even in infants) and at small (almost normal) aortic diameters.

More recently, a genetic basis of nonsyndromic familial thoracic aortic aneurysms and dissection has been defined involving multiple defective genes. Specifically, several gene mutations have been identified causing various defects in cell signaling pathways (TGFBR2 mutations different than in Loeys-Dietz syndrome) and protein synthesis of components in the contractile apparatus of vascular smooth muscle cells (MYH11 and ACTA2 mutations), resulting in thoracic aortic aneurysms and aortic dissection occurring at aortic diameter less than 5 cm.[43,49,56]

Congenital Abnormalities

Congenital heart problems, such as bicuspid aortic valve and coarctation of the aorta, are associated with an increased risk of aortic dissection compared with that in the general population. In an analysis of 186 autopsies of patients who died of type A aortic dissection, it was found that the prevalence of unicuspid or bicuspid aortic valves was 9%.[57] The risk of perioperative and late postoperative dissection is also increased in patients with a bicuspid aortic valve after any type of cardiac surgery, especially in patients with dilation of the ascending aorta.[49,58,59] Aortic dissection predominantly involves the ascending aorta in patients with coarctation and the transverse arch is relatively hypoplastic,[60] and the dissection may not propagate beyond the aortic isthmus. Simultaneous management of an acute type A aortic dissection in patients with uncorrected severe coarctation is challenging and may require modification of the CPB arterial cannulation strategy and occasionally the use of an extra-anatomic thoracic aortic graft to bypass the coarctation.[61,62]

Iatrogenic Injury

Aortic dissection is a rare complication of cardiac catheterization and other percutaneous diagnostic and therapeutic interventional techniques involving manipulation of catheters inside the thoracic aorta.[63] Catheter and guidewire injuries are usually self-limited, localized subintimal dissections that only rarely require surgical intervention. On the other hand, life-threatening iatrogenic dissections can occur during endovascular device deployment (TEVAR or transfemoral percutaneous aortic valve replacement) or open surgical procedures; among 7000 cardiac operations, iatrogenic aortic dissection complicated 0.3% of cases.[64] These can be due to ascending aortic cannulation, retrograde dissection after femoral artery cannulation, aortic cross-clamp or partial occluding clamp injury, and intimal injury at the site of a proximal bypass graft anastomosis.[63,65] The incidence of iatrogenic perioperative type A aortic dissection is higher in patients undergoing off-pump coronary artery bypass grafting, which was attributed to multiple ascending aortic manipulations for construction of the proximal anastomoses.[66]

Pregnancy

In women younger than 40 years, approximately 50% of dissections occur during the third trimester or during labor and delivery; a substantial proportion of these women have connective tissue disorders, such as Marfan syndrome, or a bicuspid aortic valve associated with a dilated tubular segment of the ascending aorta.[67,68] The hemodynamic and hormonal alterations of pregnancy, culminating in the third trimester, are thought to be the causes of dissection in susceptible individuals.

Illicit Drug Related

One of the cardiovascular complications of cocaine use, particularly crack cocaine inhalation, is acute aortic dissection.[69,70] Aortic dissection in this setting occurs presumably as a consequence of abrupt, severe hypertension and catecholamine release, and this diagnosis should be considered in cocaine or methamphetamine abusers presenting with chest pain.

Other Associations

Aortic dissections also occur more frequently than in the general population in patients with autosomal dominant polycystic kidney disease, Turner syndrome, Noonan syndrome, and Alagille syndrome.[49,71] Inflammatory diseases such as Takayasu arteritis, giant cell arteritis, Behçet disease, autoimmune disorders such as systemic lupus erythematous, and infection of the aorta, such as syphilis, have been rarely associated with acute aortic dissection.[42,43,49]

PATHOPHYSIOLOGY AND PATHOLOGIC FINDINGS

Medial Degeneration

In 1929, Erdheim[72] was the first to describe what he called "cystic medial necrosis," a nonspecific pathologic process involving medial smooth muscle cell loss, elastic lamellar disruption, and acid mucopolysaccharide accumulation within the aortic media. This abnormal architecture is believed to lead to changes in the distribution of both circumferential wall stress and shear stress in the aortic media, potentially leading to an intimal tear.[73] The word *cystic* is actually a misnomer, because these medial lesions do not form true cysts (they are not lined by epithelial cells). The term *necrosis* is also incorrect because it is singularly absent. In young patients (particularly those with a heritable connective tissue disorder), the elastic elements of the aortic media are disrupted and disorganized; in older individuals, it is the smooth muscle elements of the aortic media that are abnormal because of aging and hypertension,[74,75] and probably represent changes associated with repeated aortic wall injury and repair. Thus, the well-known moniker "cystic medial necrosis" should be abandoned and replaced by more specific terms relating to alterations of the elastic fibers ("elastic type") and smooth muscle cells ("smooth muscle type") in the media in younger and older patients, respectively. In patients with inherited connective tissue disorders, such as Marfan syndrome, pathologic examination of the aortic wall frequently revealed pronounced medial degeneration, with severe loss of elastic lamellae and accumulation of mucoid substance within the media. These young patients typically have an acute type A dissection. On the other hand, in older individuals, type B dissections are more common and are associated with medial degeneration characterized by loss of smooth muscle cells. It was proposed that the coexistence of activated T lymphocytes and macrophages and markers of apoptotic vascular cell death in the aortic media of patients with aortic dissection may contribute to the two pathways leading to medial degeneration, namely, loss of vascular smooth muscle cells and degradation of the extracellular matrix.[76] Increased contents of collagen types I and III as well as increased activity of connective tissue growth factor have been observed in the media and adventitia of patients with aortic dissection[77]; these phenomena are likely to be responsible for the reduced aortic distensibility and compliance. Another contributing factor to progressive degradation of the extracellular matrix is excessive activation of matrix metalloproteinases, particularly matrix metalloproteinase 9, which are zinc-dependent proteolytic enzymes that can disrupt the balance composition of vascular smooth muscle cells and extracellular matrix proteins.[78] Specific nucleotide polymorphism of the gene encoding matrix metalloproteinase 9, more specifically, the presence of the −8202A/G allele, seems to be associated with an increased risk of aortic dissection.[79]

Primary Intimal Tear

Most authorities believe that the initiating event in aortic dissection is a tear in the intima allowing blood to enter the aortic wall that culminates in progressive separation of the medial layers of the aorta (elastic and circumferential smooth muscle fibers) with propagation of the dissecting hematoma. The primary intimal tear allows communication between the true aortic lumen and the false lumen. Only 2% to 4% of aortic dissections do not have an identifiable primary intimal tear and are usually confined to the descending thoracic aorta.[11] Rarely in patients with connective tissue disorders, a localized intimal disruption can be present without extensive undermining of the intima, pseudoaneurysm development, or any false lumen,[80] what we colloquially call "intimal stretch marks." If they are associated with a localized hematoma within the wall, they have a "mushroom cap" appearance. Whether an intimal tear is the precipitating event in all aortic dissections is still debated.[73] IMH owing to rupture of the vasa vasorum is another potential but infrequent initiating event leading to frank dissection. Rupture of the intima usually happens at points of maximal wall stress along the thoracic aorta. Intimal tears are usually transverse in orientation and typically involve one half to two thirds of the aortic circumference. Infrequently, total disruption of intimal continuity with a complete circumferential tear can lead to intimo-intimal intussusception and mechanical obstruction of blood flow[81] because of gross prolapse of the circumferential intima. In type A dissections, the majority of intimal tears (60% to 70%) are located in the ascending aorta, usually just distal to the sinotubular junction (Fig. 70-3).[11,82,83] In 10% to 20%, the intimal tear is located in the aortic arch, most commonly on the lesser curvature.[84,85] The intimal tear can also originate in the proximal one third of the descending aorta, near the aortic isthmus ("retro-A dissection"). In less than 5% of cases, the intimal tear can be located in the abdominal aorta, and the dissection will either be confined to the abdominal aorta or propagate in a retrograde fashion to involve the ascending thoracic aorta.[86,87]

Propagation and Reentry

Within the aortic wall, the false lumen is situated between the inner two thirds and the outer one third of the aortic media. On pathoanatomic examination, the dissected aorta is a false aneurysm, because the aortic intima containing the true lumen is not dilated and actually is smaller than normal. Once initiated, aortic dissections usually propagate antegrade or "downstream" but may also extend in a retrograde direction. The dissection often proceeds in a spiral fashion down along the aorta. Propagation of the dissection depends on several factors,

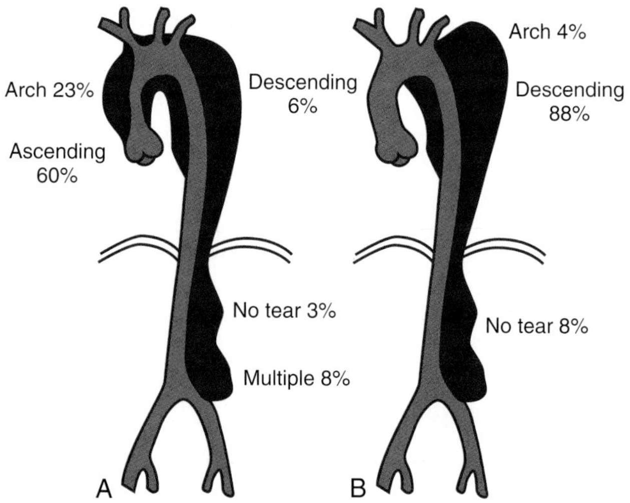

FIGURE 70-3 ■ Location of the primary intimal tear in a series of 168 patients who underwent operative repair of **(A)** acute type A aortic dissection (*n* = 169) and **(B)** acute type B aortic dissection (*n* = 29). (From Lansman SL, McCullough JN, Nguyen KH, et al: Subtypes of acute aortic dissection. *Ann Thorac Surg* 67:1975–1978, 1999.)

including rate of increase of aortic systolic pressure (or aortic dP/dt), magnitude of aortic diastolic elastic recoil and stiffness, mean and peak arterial pressure, and aortic wall integrity and strength.[42,43,88,89] The mainstay of medical treatment of aortic dissection, as described by Wheat and Palmer in 1965, is directed at reducing aortic dP/dt, called *anti-impulse therapy*.[12] In the ascending aorta, the false lumen usually occupies the right anterior portion; in the arch, the false lumen usually is located along the greater curvature and may extend into the innominate, left carotid, or left subclavian arteries. In the descending and abdominal aorta, the false lumen often runs along the anterior and lateral aortic walls, frequently incorporating the take-off of the left renal artery.[11] Distal progression of the dissection may be limited by extensive atherosclerosis or anatomic constraints such as aortic coarctation, infrarenal abdominal aortic aneurysm, or abdominal aortic graft anastomosis.[60] Otherwise, in young individuals the dissection almost always involves the entire thoracic and abdominal aorta and extends into the iliac arteries. Limited Stanford type A, DeBakey type II dissections are rare in our experience. In patients surviving the acute episode, the false lumen usually remains patent but rarely may thrombose spontaneously. The presence of distal reentry sites or fenestrations contributes to persistent patency of the false lumen. Partial or complete thrombosis of the false lumen may allow "healing" of the aorta; conversely, if the false lumen reenters distally and stays patent, it is prone to progressive false aneurysmal enlargement. A patent distal false lumen is observed in up to 90% of patients after surgical repair of acute type A dissections and may portend an adverse prognosis associated with a higher incidence of late "downstream" false aneurysmal degeneration.[90,91] Reentry sites are usually multiple and frequently occur at the ostia of sheared off branches, such as the intercostal, visceral, renal, or iliac arteries. Reentry into the true lumen,

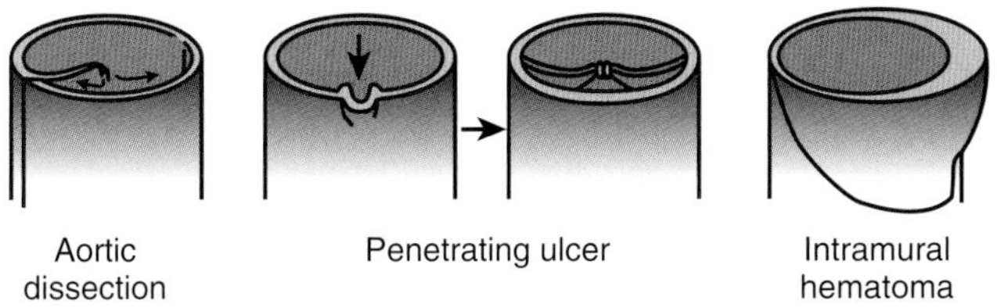

FIGURE 70-4 ■ Schematic illustration of classic aortic dissection with a distinct intimal flap separating the true and false lumens *(left),* penetrating atherosclerotic ulcer with a localized intimal lesion burrowing into the media and leading in some cases to localized dissection *(middle),* and intramural hematoma without intimal lesion *(right).* (From Coady MA, Rizzo JA, Elefteriades JA: Pathologic variants of thoracic aortic dissections. Penetrating atherosclerotic ulcers and intramural hematomas. *Cardiol Clin* 17:637–657, 1999.)

described by Peacock in 1843 as "an imperfect natural cure of the disease,"[1] allows decompression of the false lumen and is the rationale behind surgical and percutaneous flap fenestration techniques.[92,93]

Intramural Hematoma

In 1920, Krukenberg[94] first described aortic IMH as a "dissection without intimal tear." IMH is believed to originate from rupture of the vasa vasorum within the outer third of the media, resulting in the circumferential accumulation of blood (Fig. 70-4), with no apparent intimal defect visualized on imaging studies.[29] IMH can occur spontaneously in predisposed individuals (e.g., older and hypertensive patients) or be a secondary phenomenon after the rupture of an atheromatous plaque through the internal elastic lamina and the formation of a penetrating atherosclerotic ulcer allowing extravasation of blood into the aortic wall (see Fig. 70-4).[27] The natural history of these lesions was not well characterized until the last two decades. The evolution of IMH may either be benign, with a stable clinical course and eventual healing, or a progressive, often fatal disease, with extension, evolution into classic aortic dissection, aneurysmal degeneration, or aortic rupture.[28-30,95] In recent years, it was recognized that IMH involving the ascending (type A IMH) or descending (type B IMH) aorta can occasionally portend a different clinical course from that of classic aortic dissection, especially if it is detected incidentally in asymptomatic patients undergoing cross-sectional imaging. Conversely, patients with acute severe chest pain are more prone to disease progression and aortic rupture, similar to those with full-blown acute dissections, especially in the presence of an associated deep penetrating ulcer.[26,30,95,96] We believe that IMH of the ascending aorta usually has a malignant prognosis almost identical to that of acute type A aortic dissection, and these patients should be treated accordingly.

Aortic Branch Compromise

Peripheral branch vessel ischemia or malperfusion arises when the dissection process compromises blood flow to various aortic tributaries through several mechanisms, including extrinsic compression of the true lumen by the

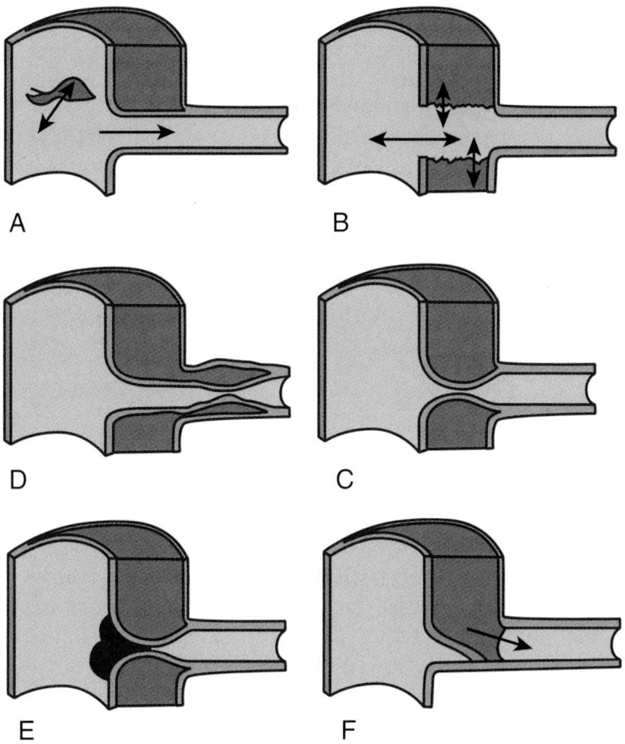

FIGURE 70-5 ■ Examples of branch artery involvement in aortic dissection. Continued adequate perfusion of an aortic tributary is illustrated in **(A)**, **(B)**, and **(F)**; however, perfusion is from the true lumen in **(A)** and **(B)** and through the false lumen in **(F)**. Obstruction of an aortic tributary owing to extrinsic compression is shown in **(C)** and **(D)**, whereas compromise of the ostium of the true lumen with secondary thrombosis is shown in **(E)**. In **(F)**, reentry of the dissection into the branch vessel has created an intimal flap. This can become a permanent situation if the flap heals to the opposite wall of the artery in the chronic phase, thus rendering this branch solely dependent on false lumen perfusion. (From Miller DC: Surgical management of aortic dissections: indications, perioperative management, and long-term results. In Doroghazi RA, Slater EE, editors: *Aortic dissection,* New York, 1983, McGraw-Hill.)

pressurized false lumen (particularly a false lumen that does not reenter), an intimal flap compromising the orifice of the branch artery (Fig. 70-5), and occlusion of the tributary if the dissection continues into the branch because of false lumen extrinsic compression of the true lumen distally. A useful pathophysiologic classification of aortic branch compromise was proposed by Williams and associates[97]: *static obstruction* occurs when the dissection flap extends into a branch vessel, resulting in mechanical compromise of flow; *dynamic obstruction* occurs when the dissection flap narrows the aortic true lumen above the branch because of a large false lumen or when the flap prolapses into the vessel origin. As the dissection progresses in a spiral fashion along the aorta, some aortic branches may be spared and continue to be perfused by the true lumen, whereas other arteries may be perfused exclusively from the false lumen after being sheared off; in this latter scenario, the affected branch subsequently becomes permanently dependent on the false lumen for perfusion. In some cases, compression by the false lumen may almost eliminate the entire aortic true channel (true lumen collapse or true lumen obliteration) with resultant severe distal thoracoabdominal malperfusion.[97,98] The pattern of branch artery involvement and the degree of perfusion compromise determine the clinical presentation, which is enormously variable and often leads to delay before the correct diagnosis is established. Indeed, acute aortic dissection has been called "The Great Masquerader" because the symptoms can mimic those of many other acute illnesses. In the large autopsy series by Hirst and colleagues,[11] the most commonly affected aortic branches were the iliac arteries, followed (in descending order) by the innominate, left common carotid, left subclavian, coronary, renal, superior mesenteric, and celiac axis.

CLINICAL MANIFESTATIONS

Patient Characteristics

Patients with type A dissections are usually younger, including those with Marfan syndrome and other heritable connective tissue disorders or congenital aortic valve disease, whereas type B dissection is usually seen in middle-aged and older men. Either type of dissection can occur in women, usually at an older age, but is exceptionally rare in children and teenagers.[10,24,32,43] Older patients usually have coexisting medical conditions, including hypertension and generalized arteriosclerosis, as well as associated medical comorbidities, such as cerebrovascular, cardiac, pulmonary, and renal disease.

Acute Type A Dissection

Pain

The most common presenting symptom of aortic dissection is severe chest pain, usually originating in the anterior chest or in the interscapular region, which correlates with the location of the dissection. The onset of pain is typically abrupt and most severe at onset, described as sharp or tearing, and it is thought to be due to stretching of the aortic adventitial nerve fibers by the dissection; the pain typically then migrates down the chest and into the abdomen. Persistence of pain suggests continuing expansion within the chest or distal propagation. Differentiation of the chest pain associated with acute aortic dissection from other causes, such as acute myocardial ischemia, pulmonary embolism, or pericarditis, is critical in the initial evaluation of these patients to allow prompt management. The presence of additional clinical findings, such as a diastolic murmur, blood pressure difference between arms or legs, and new neurologic deficit, increase the likelihood of an acute type A aortic dissection in the presence of chest pain.[99] In some patients, the initial pain will disappear either spontaneously or with institution of medical treatment; recurrent pain thereafter is an ominous sign suggesting impending aortic rupture or continuing downstream extension of the dissection.[100] On occasion, acute dissection can be painless. A high clinical index of suspicion is required for patients with aortic dissection as its manifestations can mimic any other acute medical or surgical illness. In an IRAD report, pain of abrupt onset was the presenting symptom in 85% of patients, and the most common site was the chest. It was located anteriorly in 71% of patients with type A dissection, but 47% and 22%, respectively, of these patients reported back pain and abdominal pain.[24,43]

Systemic Manifestations

One third to half of all patients with acute aortic dissection demonstrate signs and symptoms secondary to cardiac and other organ system involvement.* Aortic branch compromise, aortic rupture or leak, and compression of adjacent organs by an expanding false lumen are the most common mechanisms responsible for complications of aortic dissection.

Cardiovascular Manifestations

Patients with acute aortic dissection appear pale and poorly perfused peripherally but generally have elevated blood pressure because of preexisting arterial hypertension, high circulating levels of catecholamines, pain, or renal artery compromise by the dissection. Blood pressure must be recorded in both arms, and a thorough evaluation of peripheral pulses in all four extremities is essential. Hypotension in patients with acute dissection suggests cardiac tamponade[103] or impending rupture; shock is usually due to intrapericardial rupture with tamponade, intrathoracic rupture, or acute left ventricular failure secondary to myocardial ischemia or acute, severe aortic valve regurgitation. Aortic rupture is the most frequent cause of death in the acute setting[11]; the most common site of rupture is near the site of the primary intimal tear.[89] Ascending aortic and arch involvement can rupture into the pericardial cavity or the mediastinum; however, rupture of a more distal thoracic aortic segment is also possible with exsanguination into the left pleural space or rarely the retroperitoneum. Aortic valve regurgitation is present in 20% to 50% of patients with acute type A dissection.[10,23-25,104] Extension of the dissection retrograde into the aortic root with shearing off of one or more aortic valve commissures causes diastolic prolapse of the cusps. A murmur of aortic regurgitation is heard in 25% to 45% of patients and may be associated with an S_3 gallop and pulmonary rales.[24,42] Acute, severe aortic regurgitation leading to left ventricular failure is the second most common cause of death in patients with type A dissection, after aortic rupture. Less commonly, proximal extension of the dissection into the coronary ostia can impair coronary perfusion and cause myocardial ischemia or infarction.[105] In this situation, involvement of the right coronary artery is more common than involvement of the left coronary artery, and the electrocardiographic findings may include changes consistent with acute inferior myocardial infarction. Contained or frank aortic rupture or, more commonly, transudation of fluid from the false lumen through the intact aortic epicardial layer (there is no adventitia because the ascending aorta is an intrapericardial structure) into the pericardial cavity can

*References 10, 24, 42, 43, 99, 101, 102.

lead to pericardial effusion and cardiac tamponade associated with jugular venous distention, Kussmaul sign, paradoxical pulse, or pericardial friction rub. Cardiac tamponade is reported in 10% to 20% of patients with acute type A dissection and mandates emergency surgical intervention.[103] Rarely, the expanding false lumen may compress surrounding structures, such as the pulmonary artery or the superior vena cava, or rupture into one of the cardiac chambers, resulting in an aorto-atrial or aortoventricular fistula.[106,107] Heart block can be seen in cases with involvement of the membranous and interatrial septum by a pressurized dissection-related hematoma.[108]

Peripheral Vascular Complications

Systemic arterial manifestations of aortic dissection are the result of the propagation of the dissection process leading to aortic branch compromise and ischemia or infarction of various end organs. Approximately 30% of patients initially exhibit symptoms related to acute peripheral arterial compromise or will develop such complications.[16,101,102,109,110] Clinical manifestations include coma, stroke, paraplegia, upper or lower extremity ischemia, and anuria or abdominal pain due to renal or mesenteric ischemia.

In a historical review of the Stanford University experience with management of aortic dissection associated with acute peripheral vascular complications by Fann and associates,[102] 85 (31%) of 272 patients (128 acute type A, 40 acute type B dissection) had one or more peripheral arterial manifestations. Among these 168 patients, 4% presented with acute carotid occlusion and stroke, 5% had acute paraplegia secondary to spinal cord ischemia, 33% sustained loss of one or more peripheral pulses, 11% had impaired renal perfusion demonstrated angiographically, and 6% had compromised visceral perfusion by angiography. The prevalence of these complications according to type of dissection and the operative mortality after definitive intrathoracic surgical management are summarized in Table 70-1. Those with advanced intra-abdominal ischemia or infarction had a dismal prognosis, but simple loss of a peripheral pulse did not predict higher mortality or morbidity. In the literature, it is essential to differentiate between visceral (or renal) ischemia defined on a clinical or symptomatic basis (the most important issue) or on an imaging basis, which overestimates the incidence of clinically meaningful complications.

TABLE 70-1 Peripheral Vascular Complications and Associated Operative Mortality Rates Among 128 Patients with Acute Type A Aortic Dissection

Peripheral Vascular Complication	Prevalence *(n)*	Mortality *(n)*
Stroke	6% ± 3% (7)	14% ± 14% (1)
Paraplegia	6% ± 3% (7)	43% ± 19% (3)
Pulse deficit	38% ± 5% (48)	25% ± 6% (12)
Renal ischemia	12% ± 4% (15)	53% ± 13% (8)
Visceral ischemia	6% ± 3% (8)	50% ± 18% (4)

Data from Fann JI, Sarris GE, Mitchell RS, et al: Treatment of patients with aortic dissection presenting with peripheral vascular complications. Ann Surg 212:705–713, 1990.

Acute stroke or transient ischemic attack with hemiplegia is the most common neurologic manifestation. These result from cerebral hypoperfusion secondary to aortic arch involvement or obstruction of the true lumen in a carotid or vertebral artery. Stroke or transient ischemic attack usually occurs in patients with an acute type A dissection, and the reported incidence ranges from 3% to 7% in large series.[16,101,110,111] Beside stroke, altered cerebral perfusion can lead to altered or fluctuating mental status, coma, or syncope in as much as 12% of patients.[24] Extensive dissection can compromise perfusion of the spinal cord by shearing off critical intercostal arteries, thereby interrupting flow to the radicularis magna artery and causing paraplegia or paraparesis in 2% to 6% of cases.[16,101,102] Symptoms related to involvement of peripheral nerves, such as paresthesia and Horner syndrome, are due to peripheral ischemic neuropathy or to direct compression of a nerve by the expanding false lumen. In rare circumstances, stroke, paraplegia, or syncope without chest pain may be the only clinical manifestation of aortic dissection.[24]

The incidence of renal ischemia owing to acute dissection varies from 5% to 25%.[43,101,102,110] This wide variability is probably related to methods of detection (ultrasonography, computed tomography, angiography versus autopsy) more than to true population differences. Whether and how it is defined on a clinical or imaging basis is also of paramount importance. Dissection resulting in renal artery compromise may be asymptomatic and remain undetected unless diagnostic imaging studies are performed, but can be associated with oliguria or anuria and worsening renal function. Other clinical manifestations of impaired renal perfusion include refractory hypertension, flank pain, and hematuria. In contrast to previous reports observing that the left renal artery is more frequently involved,[11] the right renal artery was more often compromised in our experience[102]; nonetheless, the left renal artery is more frequently fed by the aortic false lumen than by the true lumen.

Aortic dissection involving the visceral arteries leads to mesenteric ischemia or infarction, which is a highly lethal complication. Compromised splanchnic perfusion causing clinical events is relatively uncommon, occurring in less than 5% of cases, although autopsy studies suggest that dissection involvement of the celiac or superior mesenteric arteries is present in more than 10% of patients.[11,102] At Stanford, the incidence of angiographically defined visceral ischemia was 6% in patients with acute type A dissection. Visceral ischemia portends a grave prognosis,[101,102] but it can have various clinical presentations ranging from asymptomatic angiographic evidence of visceral hypoperfusion to frank bowel infarction. The cardinal association of abdominal pain out of proportion to the findings on physical examination should lead to prompt consideration of gut ischemia.

Peripheral pulse loss occurs in 30% to 50% of patients with acute type A dissection and 25% of all patients irrespective of dissection type.[102] The clinical course of patients with peripheral limb ischemia is highly variable and dynamic; therefore, frequent comprehensive pulse examinations are important. In the Massachusetts General Hospital experience, one third of these patients experienced either spontaneous resolution of the pulse deficit or a fluctuating clinical picture.[101] This phenomenon is thought to be related to spontaneous reentry of flow into the true lumen from the false lumen when the false lumen earlier was non-reentering and compromising the true lumen by means of extrinsic compression. Alternatively, loss of a peripheral pulse can be asymptomatic, especially in the upper extremities. Rarely, proximal descending thoracic aortic obstruction owing to "true lumen collapse" or dynamic "true lumen obliteration" can cause severe ischemia of the entire lower body.[98]

Chronic Type A Dissection

Patients surviving the initial acute phase of acute dissection, surgically treated or not, will be at risk for development of aortic complications in the chronic phase of the disease. Most patients with chronic type A dissection are asymptomatic until they develop problems related to progressive expansion of the downstream aortic false lumen with aneurysmal degeneration, worsening aortic valve regurgitation, aneurysmal degeneration of preserved sinuses of Valsalva, or false aneurysms from previous surgical graft anastomoses. It has been estimated that up to one fourth of patients will develop downstream false lumen aneurysmal degeneration and require reoperation or interventional reintervention within 10 to 15 years after an acute dissection, emphasizing the importance of indefinite, comprehensive follow-up care and serial imaging studies.[16,90,112-114] Uncommonly, patients who had an asymptomatic acute dissection may present many months to years later with a thoracic aortic false aneurysm discovered incidentally on a chest radiograph or a computed tomographic (CT) scan done for an unrelated problem. Progressive expansion of the false lumen may produce compression, obstruction, or erosion into adjacent mediastinal structures. Therefore, symptoms related to aortic aneurysmal enlargement can include chest pain, dyspnea, wheezing or stridor, hoarseness, dysphagia, superior vena cava syndrome, hemoptysis (aortobronchial or aortopulmonary fistula), and hematemesis (aortoesophageal fistula). Signs and symptoms of heart failure can result if the degree of aortic regurgitation becomes severe. Rarely, late thrombosis of the false lumen can compromise flow in a critical branch perfused solely by the false lumen, resulting in complications such as paraplegia, lower extremity ischemia, new-onset renal failure, refractory arterial hypertension, or abdominal angina (visceral ischemia). Late aortic rupture can occur into the pericardium, bronchi, esophagus, or pleural cavity, causing tamponade or exsanguination. Nonetheless, a large majority of patients with chronic aortic dissection problems remain asymptomatic and are diagnosed incidentally.

DIAGNOSTIC MODALITIES

Prompt and accurate diagnosis of acute aortic dissection is crucial to determine the optimal treatment strategy. The initial diagnostic step is exercising a high degree of clinical suspicion, which is especially important considering that aortic dissection has been referred to as the great clinical masquerader. Historically, aortography was considered the gold standard for the diagnosis of aortic dissections, but major developments in cardiovascular cross-sectional imaging during the past 35 years have greatly expanded the spectrum of less invasive modalities available for evaluation of thoracic aortic disease. Specifically, CT scanning, transesophageal echocardiography (TEE), and magnetic resonance imaging (MRI) can quickly and accurately confirm the diagnosis of aortic dissection. It is rare that one must resort to angiography today, unless a catheter interventional procedure is being performed for malperfusion. In selecting which imaging study is best, the clinician should keep in mind what information is needed most in patients with suspected acute aortic dissection. As a general rule, the best initial diagnostic imaging study is the one that can be performed most rapidly in any particular hospital.[43,44,49,99,115-117] In most medical centers, the procedure of choice is either CT or TEE, which can reliably confirm or rule out the suspected diagnosis quickly. The imaging modality determines conclusively whether the dissection involves the ascending aorta (Stanford type A) or is restricted to the descending thoracic aorta and/or arch (Stanford type B). Determining the severity of aortic valve regurgitation and identification of a large pericardial effusion are also important, which reinforces the clinical utility of TEE.[118] Last, localization of the primary intimal tear, determination of the extent of the dissection process, status of the false lumen (patent, partially thrombosed, or completely thrombosed), and the presence or absence of aortic branch compromise are additional key features that should be identified. Interestingly, in an IRAD report, two thirds of patients with acute aortic dissection required two or more imaging studies before a definitive diagnosis could be made before definitive management was begun.[119]

Although chest radiography is neither sensitive nor specific for the diagnosis of aortic dissection, some findings may be suggestive. Widening of the mediastinal silhouette can be present in up to 50% of cases.[24,99] Other findings can include the displacement of intimal calcification, a localized hump on the ascending aorta or arch, a widening of the aortic knob, a double aortic shadow, and a pleural effusion.[120] Similarly, electrocardiographic findings, such as ST-segment or T-wave changes, are nonspecific, and an abnormal electrocardiogram can be observed in up to two thirds of patients.[24]

Aortography

Historically, after the introduction of retrograde catheter aortography through the femoral artery in 1953 by Seldinger this technique became the diagnostic method of choice for acute dissection of the aorta.[121,122] Diagnosis of aortic dissection relies on the detection of direct or indirect angiographic signs. Direct signs include evidence of a double lumen or an intimal flap; indirect signs are suggestive of acute dissection and include compression of the true lumen by the false lumen, thickening of the aortic wall, aortic regurgitation, ulcer-like projections in the aortic wall, and abnormal position of the guide wire or catheter in the aorta.[115,123] Biplane angiographic imaging of the thoracic aorta is mandatory because single-plane aortography can easily miss the diagnosis. The reported sensitivity and specificity of aortography in the evaluation of aortic dissection range between 80% and 90% and 85% and 95%, respectively.[43,115] An aortic root injection can also detect coexistent coronary artery disease. In emergency situations, selective coronary angiography is not recommended unless the patient has undergone previous coronary bypass grafting or has a compelling clinical history suggesting severe coronary artery disease, because it delays institution of definitive treatment and can be hazardous. Aortography is an invasive technique and requires the use of iodinated contrast agents, which is another reason that catheter aortography is only of historical interest today. Aortography can be time consuming and is not an innocuous technique; moreover, concerns have been raised about the risk of iatrogenic proximal propagation or perforation of the dissection during manipulation of a guide wire or catheter within the aorta.[124]

Computed Tomography

Harris and associates[125] were the first to report on the use of CT scanning in the diagnosis of aortic dissection in 1979. CT scanning is noninvasive, easy, and rapid to perform and can usually be performed without delay in emergency situations because a CT scanner is available near the emergency department in almost all hospitals, large or small. Because of major technological advances, acquisition of a large number of thin-slice images within seconds during one breath hold is now possible to create a CT angiogram (CTA). The newer dual-energy multidetector CT machines substantially also reduce the amount of radiation required. Currently we use a second-generation dual-source scanner with two 128-slice detector systems, 270-ms gantry rotation time, and 75-ms temporal resolution (Siemens FLASH). A third-generation dual-source technology scanner is being installed soon. Furthermore, computer technology allows for complex reconstruction of high-quality CTA two-dimensional data, creating three-dimensional images or four-dimensional "cine" reconstructed video clips. The definitive diagnosis of aortic dissection requires the identification of blood flow in two distinct lumens separated by an intimal flap[115]; ancillary findings include compression of the true lumen by the false lumen, displaced intimal calcification, thrombosed false lumen or IMH, and ulcer-like projection of contrast material within the aortic wall consistent with a penetrating aortic ulcer.[126] A CTA is useful for accurate measurement of the aortic lumen diameters, and it can detect pericardial and pleural effusions; it also provides information about extent of dissection, arch involvement, and perfusion status of all major aortic branches. ECG-gated CTA can also image the coronary arteries adequately if the heart rate is not too high. The CT scan can also rule out other causes of acute chest pain. In the evaluation of patients with suspected aortic dissection, contrast-enhanced CTA has a sensitivity of 82% to 100% and a specificity of 90% to 100%.[†] Disadvantages (beside the requirement for intravenous administration of contrast and use of ionizing radiation) of CT include the occasional inability to localize the primary intimal tear accurately, not being able to determine the severity of aortic regurgitation, and occasional poor visualization of rapidly moving flaps in an acutely dissected aorta because of relatively slow temporal resolution or motion artifacts, which has been minimized with the advent of ECG-gated thin-slice three-dimensional CTA.

Magnetic Resonance Imaging

The initial description of the use of MRI in the diagnosis of acute aortic dissection was made in 1983. MRI also is noninvasive; unlike aortography and CT scanning, MRI does not require the mandatory use of iodinated contrast even though magnetic resonance angiography (MRA) uses intravenous administration of gadolinium. MRI relies on the hydrogen ion concentration of blood and tissues to generate images.[119] MRI can produce high-quality images of the aorta in the transverse, coronal, sagittal, and oblique projections, allowing excellent delineation of the entire aorta, reasonably accurate diameter measurement, and excellent assessment of associated pathoanatomic features (e.g., extent, localization of the primary intimal tear, branch artery involvement, and the presence of a pericardial effusion). Dynamic imaging with ECG-gated sequences and cine MRI modes can provide information about severity of aortic valve regurgitation and flow timing and direction in the aortic false and true lumens.[115,117] In nonemergency situations, phase-contrast MRI has the unique capability to depict time-resolved three-dimensional blood aortic flow patterns as four-dimensional cine video clips. As with CT scanning, the criterion for the diagnosis of acute aortic dissection with MRI is the identification of two lumens with blood flow separated by an intimal flap. Similarly, identification of ancillary findings, as described before for CT imaging, is suggestive but not diagnostic of dissection.[115] Several studies have shown that MRI is associated with sensitivity and specificity rates in the range of 95% to 100%.[‡] Immediate availability of MRA in urgent circumstances is not always present; another shortcoming of MRI is that it cannot be performed safely in patients with implanted pacemakers, defibrillators, or other ferrous metallic devices.[130] In the context of acute aortic dissection, MRI has many other limitations because of the relatively long time necessary for image acquisition and the inability to monitor and to treat severely ill, hemodynamically unstable patients while they are in the magnet. These practical factors make MRI not the first choice in patients with acute aortic dissection.

Echocardiography

Echocardiography is an attractive technique for the evaluation of patients with suspected aortic dissection because

[†]References 43, 44, 49, 115-117, 119, 126-129.
[‡]References 43, 44, 49, 115, 117, 119, 127-129.

it is ubiquitous, noninvasive, and easily performed at the bedside, and it does not necessitate the use of contrast material.[115,117] Initially, only M-mode transthoracic echocardiography was available, but the introduction of two-dimensional echocardiography, color flow Doppler mapping, and now real-time three-dimensional echocardiography greatly improved visualization of the heart and the ascending aorta and permitted accurate assessment of valvular abnormalities and ascending aortic flow patterns.[42,114,131,132] Transthoracic echocardiography only has a limited role because of suboptimal accuracy compared to other modern imaging modalities.[117,127,133] The development of TEE overcame most of the technical limitations of transthoracic echocardiography in the evaluation of aortic dissection. High-resolution imaging of the heart and the thoracic aorta is possible with TEE because of the proximity of the esophagus to the aorta and heart. In addition, TEE provides information about aortic valve function, flow characteristics within the true and false lumens, left ventricular size and systolic function, and other associated cardiac valvular problems. Furthermore, TEE can also image the main left and right coronary arteries to rule out proximal coronary disease or involvement by the dissection. A limitation of TEE with the use of first-generation monoplane probes was limited visualization of the distal portion of the ascending aorta and the proximal arch because of the interposition of the trachea and left bronchus[116]; this limitation is now minimal with the use of multiplane or phased-array TEE probes. TEE can be performed in the emergency department, cardiac care unit, intensive care unit, or operating room with light sedation and topical anesthesia. Ideally, TEE should be performed after a fasting period of 1 hour or more to minimize the risk of aspiration, but in emergency situations this is not usually possible in the emergency diagnosis of acute aortic dissection. Close monitoring of vital signs is important during TEE. Contraindications to TEE include known esophageal disease (e.g., stricture, varices) and possibly severe coagulopathy.[117] In the evaluation of patients with suspected aortic dissection, the most important diagnostic finding is the identification and location of an intimal flap, ideally seen in more than one view, undulating independently from the motion of the aortic wall or other cardiac structures.[115,116,127,132,134] Visualization of different flow patterns in the true and false lumens and extrinsic compression in cases of false lumen thrombosis are other findings that suggest dissection or one of its variants, such as IMH or penetrating atherosclerotic ulcer with or without IMH.[135,136] TEE for assessment of suspected aortic dissection has a sensitivity rate of 97% to 100% and a specificity rate of 68% to 98%.[§] False-positive test results, accounting for the lower specificity, were usually due to reverberation artifacts from surrounding cardiac structures or the aortic wall itself, producing echo images that were misinterpreted as an intimal flap in the ascending aorta.[115,127] M-mode echocardiography can distinguish between a genuine intimal flap in the ascending aorta and reverberation artifact.[134] The main limitations of TEE involve operator experience to interpret the findings accurately and the inability to assess branch vessel involvement (other than the coronary arteries) and extent of the dissection below the celiac axis level.

[§]References 43, 44, 49, 99, 115-117, 119, 127-129, 134, 137, 138.

DIAGNOSTIC STRATEGY AT STANFORD UNIVERSITY AND SPECIAL DIAGNOSTIC CONSIDERATIONS

Stanford Diagnostic Strategy

Transesophageal echocardiography is currently the initial diagnostic procedure of choice for patients with suspected acute type A dissection because of its accuracy, safety, rapidity, and convenience. Patients with clear-cut TEE diagnostic findings are taken directly to the operating room for repair, whereas patients with inconclusive TEE findings require additional diagnostic studies (CTA or possibly MRA). Most patients transferred from outlying hospitals with suspected dissection have usually already undergone a contrast-enhanced CT scan and are taken directly from the helipad to the operating room, where the diagnosis is confirmed with TEE. In patients with symptoms of malperfusion or branch artery compromise, thin-slice gated CT angiography is the preferred diagnostic modality to evaluate both ascending aortic involvement and perfusion of major aortic branches in the chest and the abdomen. If malperfusion persists after proximal aortic repair, another emergency CT scan is performed immediately postoperatively to delineate the mechanism of persistent branch vessel compromise, which will guide appropriate endovascular catheter interventions to restore satisfactory distal perfusion.[41,93,110] On the other hand, CTA or MRA is the best modality today to plan surgical intervention in patients with chronic type A dissection as well as to follow the aorta postoperatively. We prefer CTA preoperatively because it provides more detailed anatomic information for operative planning, but we use MRA liberally for serial surveillance follow-up scanning to minimize cumulative radiation exposure.[49,99]

Intramural Hematoma

Criteria for the diagnosis of IMH involving the ascending aorta are displaced intimal calcification, a crescent-shaped nonopacified area along the aortic wall of more than 5 mm thickness, increased aortic wall diameter, and no evidence of aortic intimal disruption or flap.[135,139] TEE, CTA, and MRA can detect IMH accurately and are capable of assessing progression or regression of the process during follow-up.[140] In this setting, MRI methods can estimate the age of the hematoma on the basis of the degradation of hemoglobin into methemoglobin after the acute event, resulting in high-intensity signals within the aortic wall on both T1- and T2-weighted images.[28]

Coronary Angiography

The need for a selective coronary angiogram before surgical repair of patients with acute aortic dissection is vanishingly rare today and confined solely to special circumstances. The incidence of clinically important coronary artery disease (at least one stenosis ≥50% or left main stenosis ≥75% diameter reduction) in patients with acute type A dissection is between 10% and 35%.[141,142] Ideally, patients in stable condition with an acute type A aortic dissection and a history of chronic angina, myocardial infarction, ischemic heart disease, or coronary artery bypass grafting should undergo coronary angiography preoperatively.[142-144] On the other hand, coronary angiography should not be performed in patients who are unstable, which is frequently the case.[44] The drawbacks of coronary angiography include the obligate delay, technical difficulties, risk, and potential for false-positive findings. The Cleveland Clinic group reported that preoperative coronary angiography before emergency aortic surgery did not reduce perioperative mortality and did not affect the proportion of patients requiring coronary artery bypass grafting at the time of ascending aortic repair because 74% of coronary bypass grafts were performed for coronary dissection and not intrinsic coronary artery disease.[144] An earlier study from the Brigham and Women's Hospital by Rizzo and colleagues[145] indicated that coronary angiography was a surrogate for preoperative delay, which actually increased operative risk.

Biomarkers

The development of a reliable biomarker for the diagnosis of acute aortic dissection, in addition to imaging modalities, would help in the early identification of acute aortic syndromes in patients presenting with acute chest pain. Several such biomarkers have been investigated, such as D-dimer, circulating smooth muscle myosin heavy chain protein, soluble elastin fragments, calponin, and C-reactive protein.[44,146-149] However, there currently is no rapid and reliable biomarker available that has been validated to confirm or to rule out the diagnosis of acute aortic dissection and its variants. More research in this arena is ongoing.

MANAGEMENT

Acute Type A Dissection

The aim of therapy in patients with acute aortic dissection is to prevent death and irreversible end-organ damage. A high clinical index of suspicion is mandatory in patients with suggestive signs and symptoms, followed by prompt confirmation of the diagnosis to determine the optimal management strategy. All patients with acute type A aortic dissections should be considered for emergency surgical repair of the ascending aorta to prevent life-threatening complications such as aortic rupture or tamponade.[‖] Exceptions to early operative intervention in patients with acute type A dissection are few, including those with an irreversible major stroke or deep coma,[10,17,99,111] those with advanced, debilitating systemic diseases that limit life expectancy or preclude meaningful rehabilitation, and perhaps those older than 80 years who have multiple major complications.[151] These relative contraindications, however, have been challenged by some authors.[152-155] For example, according to recent IRAD reports, patients with major brain injury or mesenteric malperfusion should not be denied early surgical intervention because their early and long-term prognosis is significantly improved compared with medical therapy only,[111,155] because a majority of patients with stroke may experience partial or complete neurologic recovery after graft replacement of the ascending aorta. Individuals with paraplegia should also not necessarily be denied emergency operation; however, the chance of recovery of spinal cord function is almost zero. In our opinion, surgical repair of the ascending aorta should precede percutaneous vascular interventions addressing peripheral arterial complications of the dissection because "proximal" or "central" aortic repair will usually obviate the need for such distal revascularization procedures.[102,156] In the Stanford experience focusing on aortic dissection associated with peripheral vascular complications, additional procedures after thoracic aortic repair were necessary in less than 10% of patients.[102] Over the last 15 years, an alternative strategy has been advocated by the University of Michigan group that relies on initial percutaneous catheter interventions (flap fenestration, true lumen bare metal stenting) to restore end-organ perfusion with delayed repair of the ascending aorta after resolution of the malperfusion syndrome.[157,158] This approach is attractive in that it allows immediate reperfusion and stabilizes the patient, and planned operative repair of the ascending aorta can be performed under better circumstances. In addition, if the end-organ ischemia or infarction has already become irreversible at the time of the catheter intervention, these complications are usually fatal, precluding attempting ascending aortic repair. Conversely, according to the limited data available so far, up to 15% of patients treated according to this alternative approach may die of aortic rupture during the stabilization period.

In most centers in North America and Europe, including Stanford, patients with acute type A IMH are managed identically to those with an acute type A aortic dissection because of the high complication risk that patients with acute type A IMH face.[¶] The rationale behind this approach is to prevent aortic rupture and cardiac tamponade as well as to avoid the rapid evolution of IMH into a classic full-blown dissection.** This approach has been challenged by some, particularly in Korea, where intensive medical therapy is advocated for certain patients with uncomplicated acute type A IMH.[159-161] If a patient with acute type A IMH is treated medically, frequent serial imaging studies are mandatory because these patients can progress to overt dissection or aortic rupture within a short time; indeed, most ultimately require surgical intervention within 1 to 2 months.

As soon as the diagnosis of acute type A aortic dissection is suspected, comprehensive monitoring of neurologic status, arterial blood pressure, electrocardiogram,

‖References 14, 16, 17, 20, 23, 24, 35, 38, 40, 42-44, 49, 83, 99, 146, 150.

¶References 26, 28, 43, 44, 49, 95, 99.

**References 26, 28, 30, 95, 135, 140.

urine output, and peripheral pulses is initiated. An arterial line, a central venous catheter, and a urinary catheter should be inserted. Intensive anti-impulse or negative inotropic therapy (lowering mean and diastolic arterial pressure and, more important, aortic dP/dt) is an integral part of the surgical management of patients with acute type A dissection before and after surgical repair to minimize propagation of the dissection, to decrease the risk of aortic rupture, and to control pain.[12] Intravenous antihypertensive and negative inotropic therapy should be started emergently, as soon as acute aortic dissection is suggested, using a beta blocker (e.g., intravenous esmolol, labetalol) initially or, if required, adding a short-acting arteriolar vasodilator, such as sodium nitroprusside.[17,43,44,49,162] Calcium channel antagonists can be used if contraindications to beta blockade exist. Hemodynamic instability suggests free aortic rupture, intrapericardial rupture with tamponade, or acute left ventricular failure secondary to severe aortic valve regurgitation or coronary compromise. In patients with severe hypotension and evidence of tamponade, pericardiocentesis should be attempted to resuscitate the patient only if immediate surgical intervention is not practical, with the goal of aspirating only enough fluid to allow the patient's blood pressure to rise to the lowest acceptable level to minimize the risk of frank aortic rupture (which can occur if the tamponade is completely relieved, causing arterial blood pressure to increase dramatically to high levels).[103]

Surgical Principles

The primary goal of surgical treatment of patients with acute type A dissection is to replace the ascending aorta and proximal arch to prevent aortic rupture or proximal extension of the process with resultant tamponade. The primary intimal tear should be completely resected if it is located in the ascending aorta or the arch. The dissected aortic layers are reconstituted proximally and distally with fine continuous sutures (5-0 Prolene on C1 needle) with or without reinforcement to obliterate the false lumen. Aortic blood flow is redirected into the true aortic lumen distally, increasing the likelihood of reperfusion of aortic branches previously compromised by static or dynamic obstruction. When aortic valve regurgitation is present, aortic valve competence is achieved by reconstruction of the sinuses of Valsalva and aortic root with resuspension of the commissures, which is possible in many cases.[99,104,163] If one or more of the sinuses of Valsalva is severely damaged by the dissection process, the patient has Marfan syndrome or other connective tissue disorder, a large root aneurysm is present, the patient has severe annuloaortic ectasia, or the valve needs to be replaced for other reasons (e.g., severe aortic stenosis), then complete aortic root replacement with reimplantation of the coronary ostia is indicated by use of either a composite valve graft (CVG) or a valve-sparing aortic root replacement technique, as advocated by Yacoub and David.[164-166] In most cases, the noncoronary sinus of Valsalva is the most severely traumatized and can be treacherous to reconstruct satisfactorily; replacement of just the noncoronary sinus and the tubular ascending aorta (a "uni-Yacoub" procedure) is a simple approach that works well in these circumstances. Valve-sparing aortic root replacement using David's reimplantation method might be the ideal technique in the setting of acute aortic dissection in young patients with normal valve leaflets, resulting in complete removal of all diseased tissue, less bleeding, and low incidence of need for late reintervention for aortic root or aortic valve problems.[167] The older technique of separate aortic valve replacement and supracoronary aortic graft replacement is not used frequently any longer in patients with acute type A aortic dissections, but it is appropriate in older patients in whom the sinuses can be salvaged but aortic valve competence is not achievable otherwise.

Technical Considerations

Satisfactory hemostasis remains one of the chief technical challenges surrounding surgical repair of acute type A aortic dissection because of the friable dissected aortic tissue and the coagulopathy that may be present preoperatively. In the past, inclusion-wrap CVG methods (Bentall procedure) and ringed intraluminal grafts were used in an attempt to minimize bleeding; however, these techniques were associated with high failure rates and late problems, including perigraft leakage and false aneurysm formation with the former technique and migration, erosion, and stenosis with the latter.[168,169] Most surgical authorities now believe that replacement of the dissected aorta includes complete transection of the aorta both proximally and distally and use of full-thickness aorta-to-graft anastomoses to minimize the risks of late complications.[170-172] A precise anastomotic technique is critical; deep suture bites should be used, with a continuous 5-0 C1 or 4-0 BB (⅜ circle needles) polypropylene (Prolene, Ethicon, Somerville, NJ). The needle must be advanced carefully on its full curve through the aortic tissue paying particular attention to the needle follow-through to avoid needle hole tears, which can cause troublesome bleeding or anastomotic disruption. If the aortic tissue is highly friable, reinforcement of the dissected aortic layers can be facilitated by reapproximation of the dissection flap to the aortic wall with strips of autologous or bovine pericardium or Teflon felt. European surgeons in the 1980s pioneered the use of gelatin-resorcin-formalin (GRF; "French glue") biological glue to reapproximate the dissected aortic layers which strengthened the aortic tissue to facilitate anastomotic suturing.[173] Despite wide use and good early results in many centers around the world,[174] concerns soon arose about the potential toxicity of the formalin component of GRF glue; late aortic wall necrosis leading to false aneurysm formation or anastomotic dehiscence occurred.[175,176] As an alternative to GRF glue, a tissue adhesive composed of purified bovine serum albumin and 10% glutaraldehyde is currently approved (BioGlue, CryoLife, Inc., Kennesaw, GA) in the United States and can be used if necessary. This surgical adhesive is easy to use, facilitates the aortic repair, and decreases blood loss,[177,178] but it is important to apply BioGlue cautiously. Minimal amounts should be used (just a 2-mm-thick layer extending only 2 cm into the false lumen is recommended), the regions of the coronary ostia must be avoided, and the adhesive should not be applied far downstream where it may inadvertently enter the true lumen through a flap fenestration. Long-term results after the use of BioGlue are not available, but it also can cause necrosis of the delicate aortic wall. We have seen many cases in which the use of a large amount of BioGlue during the acute type A dissection repair later resulted in false aneurysms of the thoracic aorta, graft dehiscence, and full-thickness aortic necrosis 1 to 3 years later. Technical problems seen in earlier years with stiff woven vascular grafts have been eliminated by the advent of soft-woven, double-velour Dacron grafts that are presealed with bovine collagen impregnation (WDV Hemashield, Maquet Corp., Sunnyvale, CA), which are now routinely used for thoracic aortic surgery.[179] Satisfactory woven vascular grafts presealed with other types of biological sealants (e.g., gelatin in the Terumo Vascutek GelWeave grafts; Vascutek Ltd., Renfrewshire, Scotland) are also now available. Prophylactic administration of coagulation components including small, graduated doses of NovaSeven is also practiced today.

During the past two decades, PHCA, now coupled with selective antegrade cerebral perfusion (SACP) using axillary or innominate artery CPB cannulation, has become routine and safe in patients with acute type A dissection.[85,99,180,181] This allows careful inspection of the aortic arch and performance of an open distal aortic anastomosis replacing the bulk of the transverse arch. Careful inspection of the arch minimizes the possibility of leaving unrecognized intimal tears in the arch, which are present in up to 20% to 30% of patients[22,182] and increase the risk of late distal aortic reoperation. Radical "hemiarch" replacement is preferred, sewing obliquely from the ligamentum arteriosum on the lesser curve of the arch to the innominate artery take-off on the greater curve, which eliminates as much dissected aorta as possible. Simply performing an oblique "open" anastomosis in the distal ascending aorta is not recommended. Careful construction of a sound, completely hemostatic distal anastomosis is technically easier in the absence of an aortic cross-clamp, which itself can also traumatize the fragile dissected aortic tissue and tear the intima. An earlier analysis of all acute type A dissection repairs performed with or without PHCA at Stanford using propensity score analysis methodology demonstrated that aortic repair with circulatory arrest was associated with comparable early complication and survival rates.[183] This lack of superiority favoring PHCA was explained by the fact that in cases in the early years of this experience, PHCA was usually resorted to in desperate circumstances (e.g., aortic disruption or uncontrollable bleeding after the initial repair without PHCA). Although the long-term survival and late distal aortic complications were not improved after the use of PHCA in this risk-adjusted analysis, all surgeons at Stanford use PHCA with SACP routinely today in these patients on the basis of the technical advantages and theoretical potential merit of PHCA associated with an open distal aortic anastomosis. Adjunctive and more aggressive treatment of the distal dissected descending thoracic aorta using a "frozen elephant trunk" (FET) graft has recently gained favor in some experienced centers, as described later.

Operative Technique

General anesthesia is induced intravenously. After intubation, anesthesia is maintained with a combination of inhalation agents and short-acting narcotics. An antifibrinolytic agent such as ε aminocaproic acid (Amicar) or tranexamic acid is used routinely to minimize fibrinolytic activity typically observed with CPB and PHCA.[184] Electrocardiography, arterial pulse oximetry, radial and femoral arterial pressure, central venous pressure, bladder (or nasopharyngeal) and tympanic membrane temperatures, and noninvasive near-infrared cerebral oximetry are monitored throughout the operation. TEE is used in all patients to assess the dissected aorta, flow patterns in both the true and false lumens (before, during, and after CPB), aortic valve competency, and left ventricular size and systolic function.

A midline sternotomy incision is used for repair of acute type A dissection. Simultaneous exposure of the right axillary artery is made for arterial CPB cannulation, which is used preferentially in patients with acute type A dissections to provide antegrade blood flow during CPB perfusion and cooling,[49,99,185-187] and then SACP when PHCA is instituted; this technique is safe, is simple to perform, and avoids retrograde femoral arterial perfusion, which can lead to inadvertent false lumen pressurization and thoracoabdominal or cerebral malperfusion as well as cerebral embolization from debris in the abdominal or descending aorta. Subclavian arterial cannulation is performed with a short, 6- or 8-mm knitted double velour (Microvel Hemashield, Maquet Corp., Wayne, NJ) Dacron graft anastomosed end-to-side to the right axillary artery. If the artery is dissected, it is essential to sew the perfusion graft to the true lumen for safe CPB perfusion. A two-stage venous cannula is inserted into the right atrium through the appendage. The typical CPB circuit used for the surgical management of acute type A aortic dissection is illustrated in Figure 70-6. CPB is established slowly with continuous TEE monitoring of the flow pattern within the ascending and descending aorta and arch to detect any evidence of distal malperfusion, which is suspected if the true lumen becomes small or obliterated. If this occurs, direct cannulation of the aortic true lumen in the arch using the Seldinger technique either with TEE guidance[99,188-190] or by passing a longer arterial cannula through the left ventricular apex and across the aortic valve into the true lumen (as originally described by Wada and Kazui in the 1970s for mitral valve surgery through a left thoracotomy).[99,191] One drawback of direct aortic or transapical LV arterial CPB cannulation is that additional steps are necessary to institute SACP when the pump is turned off to do the arch anastomosis; this might explain the high neurologic complication rates seen in Hannover and Essen, Germany, where the direct aortic cannulation technique was popularized. In emergency situations, starting with femoral CPB cannulation is acceptable followed by CPB perfusion from the ascending aortic graft or a side-branch. Alternatively, carotid artery cannulation has been described.[192] A vent is inserted into the left ventricle through the right superior pulmonary vein or directly across the ventricular apex to prevent

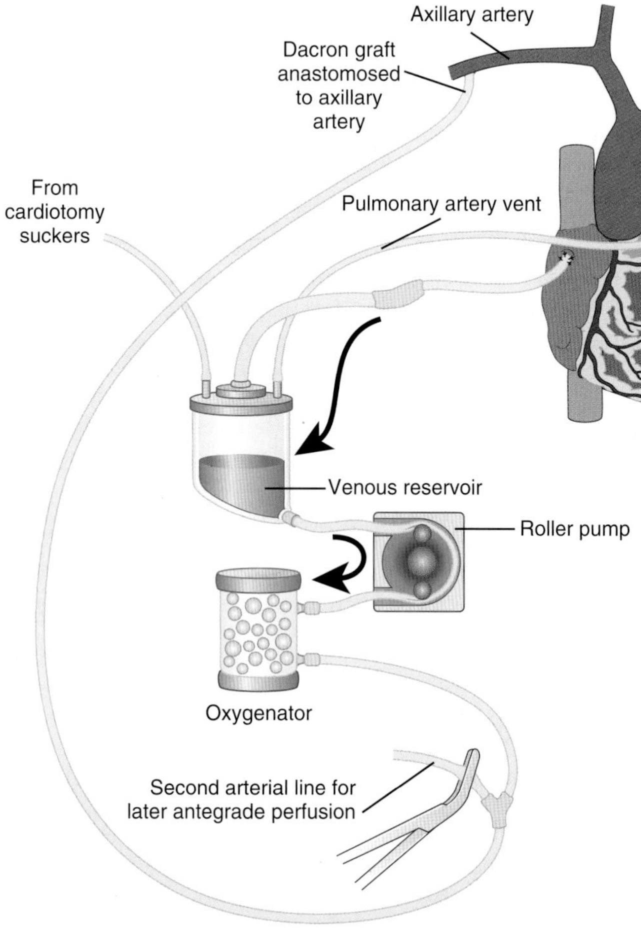

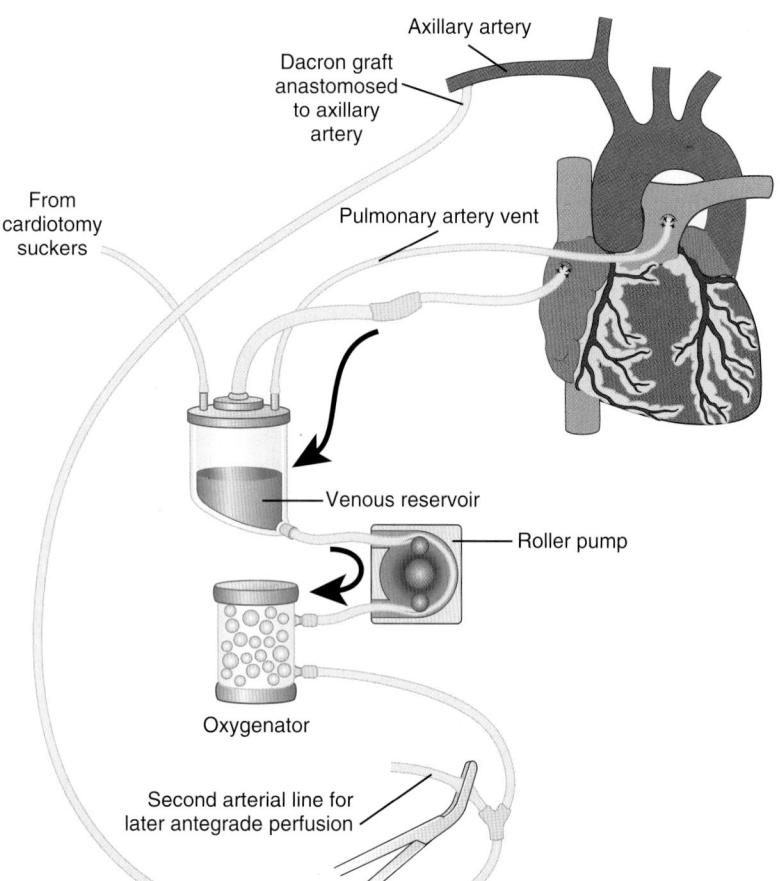

FIGURE 70-6 ■ Schematic of the cardiopulmonary bypass circuit for repair of an acute type A aortic dissection with an open distal anastomosis during a period of hypothermic circulatory arrest and selective antegrade cerebral perfusion. Arterial cannulation is performed with a short 6-mm Dacron graft anastomosed end to side to the right axillary artery.

distention. Systemic cooling is initiated, avoiding gradients of more than 10° C between the patient and the arterial perfusate temperature, and continued for at least 30 minutes or until tympanic temperatures approaches 20° C; bladder temperature is usually in the range of 25° to 28° C. It is important to monitor the tympanic membrane temperatures and cerebral oximetry during cooling and rewarming to detect inadequate or asymmetric cerebral CPB perfusion. If such perfusion occurs, the aorta is examined using TEE to determine why one of the arch branches is not being perfused adequately, and recannulation needs to be considered. In addition, preparations are made in advance to perfuse the left common carotid artery and/or left subclavian artery with balloon-tipped perfusion cannulae when SACP is instituted. During cooling, the aortic root and ascending aorta are carefully dissected away from the right and left atria, right ventricular outflow tract myocardium, pulmonary valve annulus, and main and right pulmonary arteries. The pericardial reflection (or "veil") covering the left main coronary artery, which extends anteriorly and leftward to the pulmonary annulus, must be divided following the right and main pulmonary arteries. The ascending aorta is not clamped during cooling except when unmanageable severe aortic valve insufficiency mandates aortic clamping to prevent left ventricular distention. Dexamethasone (8 to 12 mg) is administered before commencement of CPB to enhance cerebral and spinal cord protection. Mannitol (0.3 to 0.4 g/kg) and furosemide (40 to 80 mg) are given when commencing CPB to minimize ischemic reperfusion injury (hydroxyl and superoxide free radical scavengers). The head is packed in ice. The field is flooded with CO_2 gas. After CPB flow is reduced to 10 mL/kg/min, the cross-clamp is removed, the aorta is opened, and SACP is begun slowly. After confirmation that CPB pump flow is entering the arch from the true lumen of the innominate artery, the innominate artery is clamped, and the back-bleeding down the left common carotid artery and then the left subclavian artery is inspected, indicating patency of the circle of Willis. If the back-bleeding is red and relatively brisk, these two arch branches are sequentially clamped. If the left common carotid artery or subclavian artery back-bleeding is visually judged to be inadequate (trickle back flow or dark blood returning) or asymmetric tympanic membrane temperatures or cerebral oximetry is detected, additional perfusion cannulas can be inserted directly into the left common carotid and/or subclavian arteries. Unilateral SACP is usually adequate in our experience, but it should be noted that Dr. Kazui's original SACP method involved perfusion of all three arch branches at a total flow rate of 10 mL/kg/min.[111] Intermittent retrograde cold blood cardioplegia and topical cooling (Daily Cooling Jacket, Daily Medical Products, Luke Medical, Inc., Plymouth, MN) are used for myocardial protection.

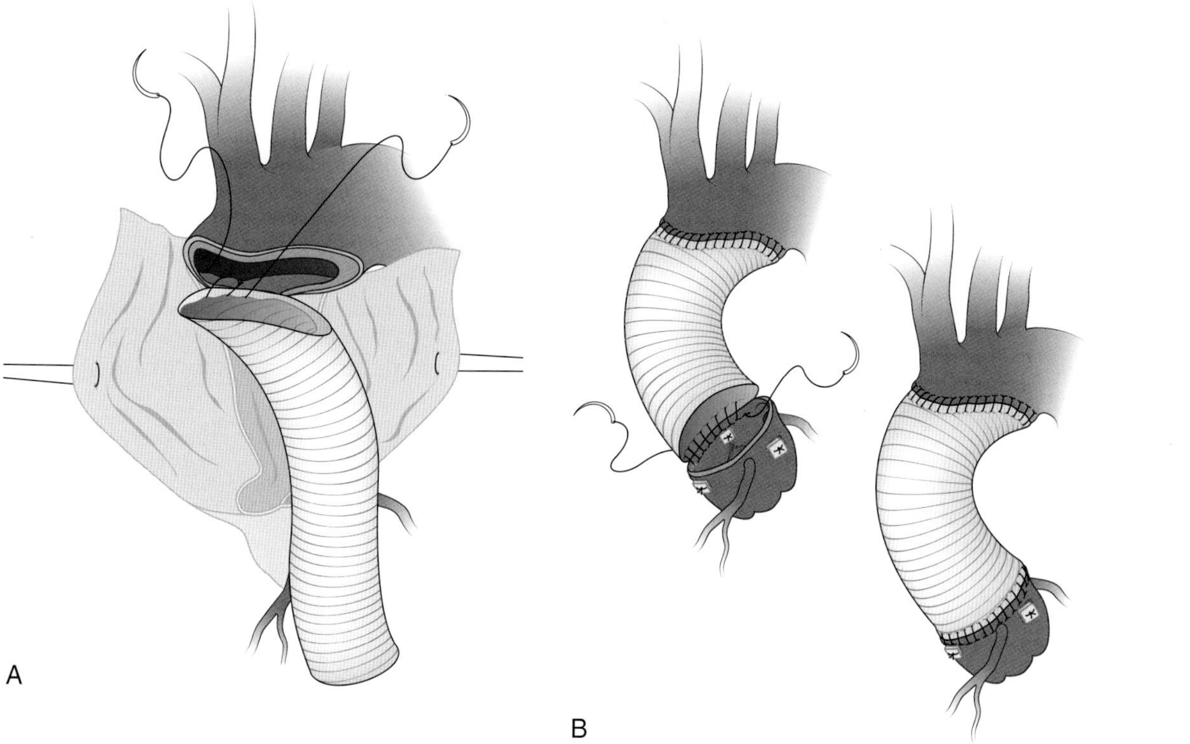

FIGURE 70-7 ■ **A,** An open distal anastomosis is always used to avoid intimal damage with a clamp and to allow inspection of the aortic arch. The aorta is transected immediately proximal to the innominate artery and distally toward the lesser curvature to the level of the left subclavian artery. An appropriately sized graft is beveled and anastomosed with 4-0 polypropylene suture. The Griepp method of rotating the beveled end of the graft 180 degrees such that the "toe" of the graft actually apposes the greater curve of the arch near the innominate artery is used, which tucks the completed graft into the natural curve of the arch and prevents excessive angulation of the graft. Most commonly, the false lumen is obliterated with the anastomotic suture line without reinforcing material. **B,** After aortic root reconstruction and resuspension of the valve commissures, the graft is anastomosed to the reconstructed proximal aortic cuff in an end-to-end fashion with a running 4-0 polypropylene suture.

The ascending aorta is opened to locate the primary intimal tear and to evaluate the aortic valve and sinuses, and then the arch and proximal descending thoracic aorta are inspected. The aortic segment containing the intimal tear is resected, and the aortic arch is trimmed circumferentially in an oblique fashion in preparation for extended hemiarch replacement. Reapproximation of the distal aortic layers is preferentially accomplished as part of the distal anastomotic suture line in the arch; if absolutely necessary, a small amount of tissue adhesive or BioGlue between the dissected layers can be helpful. An end-to-end aortic anastomosis is then carried out with an appropriately sized and beveled woven, double velour Hemashield Dacron graft with a continuous 5-0 C1 or 4-0 BB polypropylene suture (Fig. 70-7*A*). We do not prefer to do so, but suturing two strips of pericardium or Teflon felt (one inside the false lumen and one externally) with a separate 4-0 BB polypropylene suture line to form a solid full-thickness distal aortic cuff can be done to reconstitute very friable aortic layers before the distal arch anastomosis. The counter-intuitive technique pioneered by Dr. Randall Griepp of rotating the beveled distal end of the graft 180 degrees such that the "toe" of the graft actually apposes the greater curve of the arch near the innominate artery is important and always is used, which tucks the completed graft tightly into the natural curve of the arch and prevents the lesser curve of the graft from being too long, which causes excessive angulation of the graft rightward and anteriorly and kinking. When the arch anastomosis is completed, the left subclavian artery, left common carotid artery, and innominate artery clamps are sequentially removed with the patient placed in steep Trendelenburg position, and the arch and great vessels are de-aired using manual massage. CPB flow is resumed in an antegrade fashion using the original axillary artery cannula, and the arch graft is clamped. Flow in the descending aorta is quickly assessed with TEE to ensure that the true lumen has not become obliterated by a pressurized false lumen. After 10 minutes of cold systemic reperfusion, gradual rewarming of the patient to 35° C (bladder) is initiated.

The aortic root and valve are then evaluated and additional intimal tears are excised. If aortic root replacement is not necessary, the ascending aorta is transected immediately above the sinotubular junction. Valvular regurgitation secondary to commissural detachment can be corrected by resuspension of the tops of the commissures at the level of the sinotubular junction using pledgeted 5-0 polypropylene sutures at each commissure to approximate the dissected layers of the sinuses of Valsalva; this technique will result in aortic valve competence in 70% to 80% of patients.[104,163,193] A second woven double velour graft of appropriate diameter is then anastomosed to the reconstructed proximal aortic cuff in an end-to-end fashion with a running 5-0 C1 or 4-0 BB polypropylene suture (see Fig. 70-7*B*). Finally, the two grafts are shortened on reverse bevels such that the lesser curve side is much shorter, and a graft-to-graft anastomosis is constructed using 3-0 RB1 polypropylene. We use two separate grafts to avoid geometric distortion and torqueing the friable aortic anastomoses. A needle vent is inserted in the graft for de-airing, and the cross-clamp is released. TEE rapidly confirms whether the aortic valve is competent, and the anastomoses are inspected. Short-axis TEE views of the aortic root confirm satisfactory main coronary artery perfusion. When the patient is adequately rewarmed, CPB is discontinued, and protamine sulfate is administered after all anastomoses are judged to be technically satisfactory with minimal bleeding. Platelets, fresh-frozen plasma, cryoprecipitate, or small fractionated doses of NovaSeven are administered if diffuse hemorrhage from needle holes, suture lines, and raw surfaces is evident after a normal activated clotting time is achieved. Coagulation abnormalities identified by rotational thromboelastography guides administration of specific coagulation components.[194]

More Radical Management of the Aortic Root

Patients with dissection-related destruction of the aortic root, individuals with Marfan syndrome or other connective tissue disorder (including bicuspid aortic valve), and those with markedly dilated sinuses of Valsalva or annuloaortic ectasia should undergo CVG root replacement or valve-sparing aortic root replacement using the David reimplantation method with complete excision of the sinuses of Valsalva (see Chapter 67), rather than resuspension of the aortic valve and preservation of the sinuses. A conservative approach limited to replacement of just the tubular segment of the ascending aorta in these cases is associated with suboptimal long-term results and a high likelihood of subsequent aortic or aortic valve problems requiring reoperation.[104,171,195] Complete aortic root replacement with a CVG has become more popular over the past decade since it is reliable and no residual dissected or weak sinus tissue remains, but does expose the patient to the consequent cumulative morbidity associated with valve replacement.

Since the noncoronary sinus of Valsalva usually is the one most severely involved by the dissection process, an alternative technique is a "uni-Yacoub" procedure where the entire noncoronary sinus is replaced using a single proximal "U-shaped" tongue fashioned from the aortic graft suturing close to the hinge of the aortic cusp with a fine (5-0 C1) polypropylene suture. Occasionally, even a "bi-Yacoub" procedure—replacing the noncoronary and the right sinuses of Valsalva with right coronary artery reimplantation—can be useful if both sinuses are destroyed. If the aortic valve is markedly abnormal or cannot be repaired in a durable fashion, separate valve and supracoronary aortic graft replacement is a reasonable alternative in certain patients if it is performed according to the tenets of the original Wheat-Shumway-Groves procedure, in which minimal sinus tissue remains above the annulus except for tongues surrounding the left and right coronary ostia.[195] Direct extension of the dissection into the coronary ostia is not common (more often in the right coronary artery), and can be challenging to correct.[105] The flap in the sinus running close to the proximal main coronary ostium can usually be glued together in the proximal aortic reconstruction. On occasion, the safest solution is complete CVG root replacement with reimplantation of reconstituted coronary artery ostia as full-thickness Carrel patches (or buttons) into the graft, either directly or using a short interposition saphenous vein graft as introduced by Zubiate and Kay.[196] Alternative techniques include the Cabrol-II moustache coronary reconstruction with a small synthetic graft[197] and, in exceptional circumstances, suture ligation of the coronary and bypass grafting.[105,198]

Management of the Aortic Arch

In up to approximately 30% of patients, the primary intimal tear is found in the aortic arch, which has historically been associated with a poorer prognosis.[22,84,85,182] Most tears are located on the lesser curve of the arch under the innominate artery, permitting complete resection of the tear using the extended arch technique with a single sigmoid-shaped suture line running from the ligamentum on the lesser curve to the innominate artery on the greater curve. In cases in which the primary intimal tear is located more distally in the arch, on the greater curve in proximity to branch vessels, or when arch rupture or a preexistent arch aneurysm is encountered, total arch replacement is required, but is associated with higher perioperative mortality and morbidity, especially in older and critically ill patients.[84,85,199,200] With a primary tear located in the arch, failure to include the arch in the repair increases the probability of requiring subsequent distal aortic reoperation and reduces long-term survival.[85] Improvements in surgical techniques and brain protection during PHCA and SACP[201] have made concomitant total arch replacement a reasonable and safe option in selected patients when necessary.[99,202] A recent report from the German Registry for Acute Aortic Dissection Type A (GERAADA) evaluating cerebral protection methods in 1558 patients operated between 2006 and 2009 found that the operative mortality and the incidence of permanent neurologic dysfunction were lower using SACP compared with PHCA only, especially for longer circulatory arrest periods that are required for complex arch reconstructions.[201] In these circumstances, total arch replacement is performed using a distal elephant trunk graft technique, which can be a simple downstream FET stent-graft in the aortic true lumen tacked around the left subclavian artery takeoff, as popularized by Pochettino and colleagues[203,204] and Roselli and colleagues[205] (discussed later), or complete arch replacement. Instead of using the original 1982 Borst arch replacement with elephant trunk graft technique, in which the three arch branches were reimplanted en bloc as a single island (see Chapter 68),[206] a multibranched arch graft is used when complete arch replacement is necessary.[207,208]

Distal Frozen Elephant Trunk Graft

The open arch replacement approach enables one to add a downstream surgical elephant trunk graft or a FET stent-graft in the true lumen of the descending aorta, which theoretically will reduce the rate of late false lumen aneurysmal degeneration. Pochettino and Roselli in the United States, Karck, Jakob, Haverich, Mestres, and Di Bartolomeo in Europe, Kazui and others in Japan, and Sun in China have championed this approach,[203,205,209-211] which can be performed by modifying a commercial thoracic aortic stent-graft or using a specially designed commercial device. This downstream adjunctive procedure, however, does increase the chance of spinal cord injury, and may incrementally increase operative mortality risk. In Europe, this is being accomplished using commercial hybrid integrated stent-graft devices such as the Terumo Vascutek Thoraflex multi-branch graft (Vascutek Ltd.) and the Jotec "E-vita open" system (Jotec, Hechingen, Germany), which are specially designed integrated commercial devices that incorporate the arch graft segment and the distal stent-graft.[212] In China, the Cronus FET (MicroPort Medical, Shanghai, China) along with a standard four-branch arch graft have been used extensively by Sun and his group in Beijing.[213] While this approach is gaining popularity, what is not known is which patients are at highest risk for subsequent downstream aortic complications who theoretically would benefit most from this more aggressive adjunctive procedure during the initial operation.[214] Results of future investigations using these devices will help to define who will benefit from this aggressive downstream surgical approach. Ideally, a multicenter, prospective randomized controlled trial will be launched to investigate this question, but securing adequate funding for such a trial has been unsuccessful.

Special Situations

Primary Intimal Tear in the Descending Thoracic Aorta (Retro-A Dissection). In 5% to 10% of cases, acute type A aortic dissection is due to retrograde extension of the dissecting process from a primary intimal tear located in the descending thoracic aorta, a situation that Reul and Cooley in 1975 termed a *DeBakey type III-D dissection*.[17,21] We prefer the simpler term *retro-A dissection*, as introduced by Lansman, Griepp, and the Mount Sinai group.[22] Furthermore, the incidence of retro-A dissections has increased considerably as a devastating complication of endovascular descending aortic stent-grafting (TEVAR). Patients with this subtype of acute type A dissection were thought to have a poor prognosis because of intraoperative complications,[17,22] including hemorrhage from the distal aortic anastomosis, or rupture of the descending aortic false lumen during or after ascending aortic replacement.[22,215] To prevent these complications, single-stage resection of the primary intimal tear in the descending aorta with replacement of the ascending aorta and entire arch through a median sternotomy or left thoracosternotomy incision has been proposed in carefully selected patients with a patent false lumen in the ascending aorta, aortic regurgitation, cardiac tamponade, or marked dilation of the ascending aorta.[215]

In patients in whom the false lumen of the ascending aorta has thrombosed and no dilation of the ascending aorta or aortic regurgitation is present, continuing medical therapy may be reasonable[216,217]; however, our philosophy usually calls for more aggressive surgical treatment, meaning at least graft replacement of the ascending aorta and partial or total arch replacement in younger individuals if they are suitable operative candidates. More recently, TEVAR has been applied in patients with a natural retro-A dissection with favorable midterm results[218,219] as an isolated procedure designed to cover the primary intimal tear in the descending aorta hoping this will accelerate thrombosis of the false lumen in the arch and ascending aorta, or in conjunction with extended surgical replacement of the ascending aorta and arch.[211] Arch replacement plus a distal frozen elephant trunk approach, described above, can also be an option in these circumstances.[203-205,209-215]

Type A Aortic Dissection and Coarctation. Acute aortic dissection in the presence of an untreated aortic coarctation is a rare problem, with few reported cases in adults.[60,62] Simultaneous repair through a median sternotomy incision is advocated by most authors if the patient is young. Retrograde femoral arterial CPB perfusion of the brain through the coarctation is problematic in this situation, with resultant cerebral hypoperfusion; this potential problem is avoided with right axillary artery CPB cannulation coupled with simultaneous femoral CPB perfusion if the obstruction at the coarctation is severe. In addition to standard ascending aortic and arch dissection repair, the coarctation can be treated with a bare metal stent, TEVAR, or an extra-anatomic bypass from the ascending aortic graft to the distal descending aorta, through the posterior pericardium.[61,62]

Postoperative Malperfusion. Diligent surveillance postoperatively is needed to detect persistent or new malperfusion before irreversible infarction of important end organs occurs. Today, most if not all of the persistent or new malperfusion syndromes after surgical repair of aortic dissection can be managed with endovascular techniques, including stent-graft implantation, balloon flap fenestration, and direct stenting of the true lumen of compromised branches.[41,99] Specific management of branch vessel malperfusion is discussed in more detail in Chapters 71 and 72.

Chronic Type A Dissections

Indications for Operative Intervention

Operation for patients with chronic type A dissection is indicated if symptoms occur or if progressive aortic enlargement is present, including symptoms of congestive heart failure or evidence of left ventricular dysfunction or dilation because of severe aortic valvular regurgitation. In asymptomatic patients, surgical intervention is generally recommended when the diameter of the ascending aorta is greater than 55 to 60 mm (50 mm in patients with Marfan syndrome) or if the documented rate of expansion is greater than 5 to 10 mm during 1 year.[49,112,220,221] Dissected thoracic aortas rupture at a smaller size than do degenerative or atherosclerotic thoracic aortic aneurysms.[222] Seasoned surgical judgment is important on an individualized basis. The expected benefits of graft replacement of the aorta in asymptomatic patients must be weighed against the operative risk, taking into account the frequent medical comorbidities these patients have that increase surgical risk or otherwise limit life expectancy; these risk factors, paradoxically, are also the same variables that portend a higher risk of aortic rupture (e.g., Marfan syndrome, other connective tissue disorders, uncontrolled hypertension, increasing age, and chronic obstructive pulmonary disease).[220,221] Expansion of the size of the false lumen in the distal aorta (usually the proximal descending thoracic aorta) after successful proximal aortic repair or local complications of a previous operation (e.g., aortic root aneurysm, anastomotic false aneurysm, worsening aortic regurgitation) are also indications for operation in patients with a chronic type A aortic dissection.[112,223]

Surgical Technique

More extensive resection and more complex aortic reconstruction are generally necessary in patients with chronic type A dissections compared to their acute type A counterparts. Preservation of the aortic valve and sinuses of Valsalva is usually not achievable in these circumstances; if it is possible, the repair may not be durable. Aortic root replacement using a CVG is required in most circumstances. In highly select young patients, the Tirone David reimplantation technique valve-sparing aortic root replacement may be feasible to avoid long-term anticoagulation, but only if minimal scarring is present or if there is not too much deformity and scar around the synthetic material used at a previous operation (see Chapter 67).[164,166] Since large false lumen aneurysmal degeneration frequently exists in the aortic arch and descending thoracic aorta in the setting of chronic type A dissection, total arch replacement with an elephant trunk graft after flap septectomy in the descending thoracic aorta is often necessary to facilitate staged subsequent replacement of the descending thoracic aorta; alternatively, if there are no or few large fenestrations in the dissection flap in the descending aorta, then a stent-graft (TEVAR or FET) deployed antegrade carefully in the true lumen of the descending aorta can result in subsequent false lumen thrombosis proximally, which hopefully progresses caudad over time (see Chapters 68 and 72).[112,206,223-225] Alternatively, a single-stage "arch first" approach using PHCA (with antegrade SACP via the right axillary artery) for patients with chronic type A dissections as pioneered by Kouchoukos using a bilateral anterior thoracotomy or clamshell incision provides excellent long-term durability with reasonable operative mortality and morbidity risks.[226] The most common complication is respiratory insufficiency requiring temporary tracheostomy. This simultaneous approach involves replacement of the transverse arch first under deep hypothermic circulatory arrest to minimize cerebral ischemic time, followed by descending thoracic or thoracoabdominal aortic replacement.[226]

In contrast to patients with acute dissection, perfusion of downstream vital organs may depend solely on a patent false lumen in the chronic phase of dissection; hence, maintaining antegrade flow in both the true and the false lumens can be vital to avoid iatrogenic malperfusion after aortic repair. To achieve this goal, flap septectomy with or without distal flap fenestration is performed to allow blood flow to perfuse both the distal aortic true and false lumens downstream with a short dangling elephant trunk graft in the distal "common chamber" of the descending thoracic aorta or supraceliac abdominal aorta.

RESULTS

Early Survival

Contemporary reports have documented improved surgical outcome in patients with aortic dissection, with perioperative mortality rates decreasing from 30% to 60% in the 1960s to 5% to 25% in the last 2 decades.[††] These lower early mortality rates were attributed to progressive advances in diagnosis and imaging; improved surgical methods, better myocardial protection, more sophisticated CPB techniques; improved perioperative management; and increased surgical experience. Other factors, such as patient referral patterns and patient selection bias, however, must also be considered when comparing retrospective results between various eras and between different institutions. It is sobering to note that the most recent IRAD 2014 report showed that the early mortality rate in surgically treated patients with acute type A dissection was greater than 20% between 1996 and 2013 in 1995 patients collected from 24 centers worldwide.[240] At Stanford University between 1963 and 1992, the overall operative mortality rate was 26% in 174 consecutive patients undergoing surgical repair for acute type A aortic dissection, decreasing from 38% in the 1963-1976 period to 27% in the 1988-1992 period.[10] In this 30-year experience, the independent determinants of early mortality were earlier operative year, older age, hypertension, preoperative cardiac tamponade, and renal dysfunction. More recently, the early mortality rate decreased to 17% in a series of 151 patients presenting with an acute type A aortic dissection operated on between 1993 and 1999 (see Fig. 70-7),[183] consonant with other large contemporary series of surgical treatment of patients with acute type A dissections.[‡‡] In the entire cohort of Stanford patients, the independent risk factors for early death were again earlier operative year, older age, preoperative tamponade, and renal dysfunction. Overall, it appears that patient-specific factors and not treatment strategies (e.g., the use of PHCA) were the main determinants of adverse outcome. The only potentially modifiable factors, moreover, were cardiac tamponade and renal dysfunction, which might theoretically be lower if the diagnosis is made earlier. Interestingly, site of intimal tear, pulmonary disease, and arterial hypertension, which were significant in earlier analyses,[150] did not increase the likelihood of death in the later years of this 37-year series.

These observations parallel findings reported in other contemporary reports from centers with special expertise

[††]References 10, 16, 24, 37, 38, 43, 44, 49, 82-84, 99, 150, 170, 180, 183, 227-239.

[‡‡]References 37, 82, 180, 227-229, 232, 233, 235, 237.

in thoracic aortic surgery. According to older analyses by Crawford and colleagues, earlier operative date, severe symptoms, presence of coronary artery disease, diabetes mellitus, reoperation for bleeding, postoperative stroke, and cardiac complications were independent risk factors for early death after surgical treatment of type A dissection.[84,234] In the Cleveland Clinic experience with 135 acute and 73 chronic type A dissections, independent predictors of early mortality were earlier operative year, hemodynamic instability, not using PHCA, longer PHCA time, need for composite valve graft for aortic root replacement, and concomitant coronary artery bypass grafting.[233] Increasing age, hemodynamic compromise, and absence of hypertension were identified as risk factors for hospital death in the Mount Sinai experience[82]; renal or mesenteric ischemia and preoperative shock predicted early deaths in Kazui's experience in Japan.[229] In a retrospective analysis of a U.S. national administrative database (nationwide inpatient sample [NIS]) including 3013 patients undergoing surgical repair of acute type A aortic dissection between 1995 and 2003 in the United States, the mortality rate was 26% and the only independent determinants of early death were increasing age and operation in a nonacademic hospital.[237] Another analysis of outcomes in 5184 patients operated for acute aortic dissection from 2003 to 2008 in the U.S. NIS database observed an overall mortality rate of 21.6% (19.1% between 2005 and 2008) and found a strong inverse relationship between operative mortality and both surgeon and institutional volume, suggesting that repair of acute aortic dissection may display a volume-outcome relationship similar to what is seen in other cardiovascular surgical diseases.[239] Among 526 patients in IRDA with acute type A dissection enrolled prospectively between 1996 and 2001, predictors of early death were previous aortic valve replacement, migrating chest pain, shock or tamponade at presentation, and preoperative peripheral malperfusion,[236] again emphasizing the importance of patient-specific factors and dissection-related complications in terms of surgical risk.

Finally, perhaps all is not stagnant in this field. In 2014, a report from Duke University demonstrated that these sobering surgical results for acute type A aortic dissection can be improved if a dedicated multidisciplinary thoracic aortic team is implemented.[241] They compared their results over 5-year intervals before (1999-2005) and after (2005-2011) this team was established. In the earlier era, an average of nine acute type A repairs were performed each year by 11 different surgeons. After 2005, an average of 12 cases was done annually, but 97% of them were performed by two specially trained thoracic aortic surgeons. Operative mortality rate fell from 34% to 2.8%, and this translated directly into improved 4- to 5-year survival results. Using the IRAD predicted risk algorithm, the observed-to-expected 30-day mortality ratio fell from 1.26 to 0.15; although the more recent patient substrate was at somewhat lower risk, this is a tremendous achievement. Although an annual acute type A dissection volume of 9 to 12 cannot be considered to be a high-volume institution, one of the NIS studies revealed that only 15 NIS-participating institutions in the United States performed over 10 cases per year, which is an astoundingly low number.[237] Nonetheless, the accompanying editorial declared that ample opportunity clearly exists in the United States and presumably other countries around the world to improve outcomes if health policy regulators and payers enforce strict regionalization of thoracic aortic surgical services such that the vast majority of patients with all types of thoracic aortic disorders—including acute type A dissections—would be cared for in a small number of institutions with greater experience and special expertise.[242] The editorialist opined that in the United States only one thoracic surgical center would be necessary for every 5 to 10 million inhabitants, meaning only 32 or possibly 64 specialized institutions in the United States (out of approximately 1325 hospitals performing more than one thoracic aortic case per year between 1999 and 2010) would be reimbursed for thoracic aortic surgery cases to cover our population of 316 million.[242] This health policy process improvement step is long overdue.

On the other hand, early mortality risk after surgical treatment of patients with chronic type A dissection is generally lower than that for patients with acute dissections. In the 1995 summary of the Stanford 30-year experience, early mortality rate was 17% in 106 patients with chronic type A dissections and only 6% in the subgroup of patients with Marfan syndrome.[10] In an analysis of 690 patients with aortic dissections during a 33-year period, Crawford and colleagues[234] observed a 30-day mortality rate of 12% in patients with chronic type A dissections operated on before 1986 and only 8% in those operated on after 1986. Independent determinants of death were severity of symptoms, previous aortic surgery, concomitant coronary artery disease, use of intra-aortic balloon pump, cardiac complications, and postoperative stroke. Similarly, Sabik and associates[233] from the Cleveland Clinic reported an early mortality rate of 11% in 73 patients with chronic type A dissections treated surgically. More recently, refinements in surgical techniques, including the use of the FET technique or the arch-first technique, have led to improvements in surgical outcomes with reported early mortality rates as low as 4%.[112,223,226]

Late Survival

In DeBakey's seminal 1982 report on long-term results in 527 surgically treated patients with aortic dissection (type A or B, acute or chronic), the overall survival estimates were 57%, 32%, and 5%, after 5, 10, and 20 years, respectively.[16] In patients with type A dissections, 29% of late deaths were attributed to complications related to rupture of the dissected aorta in a remote downstream location, emphasizing the long-term life-threatening nature of aortic dissection and the need for improved long-term imaging surveillance, prophylactic reoperation when indicated, and intensive medical follow-up care.

In the 30-year Stanford experience, the overall survival rates (including hospital deaths) for patients with acute type A dissections at 1, 5, 10, and 15 years were 67%, 55%, 37%, and 24%, respectively.[10] For patients with chronic type A dissections, long-term survival estimates at these same times were, respectively, 76%, 65%, 45%,

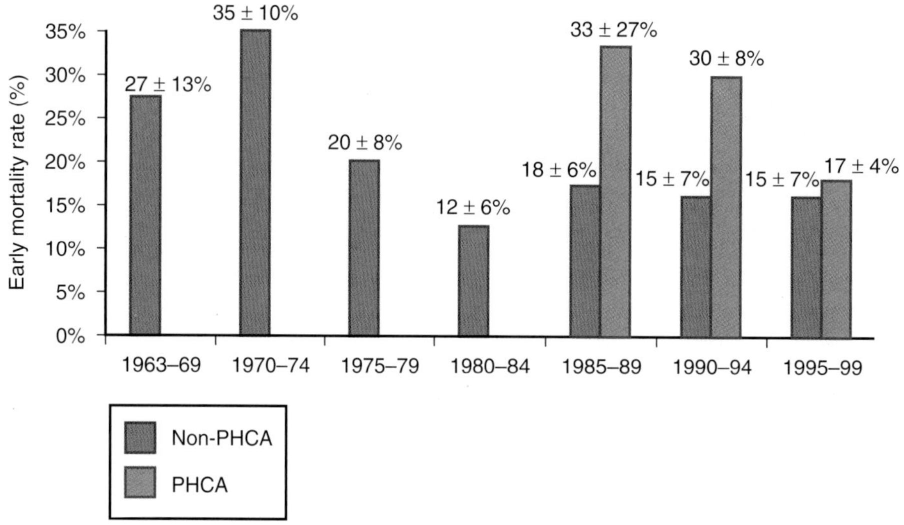

FIGURE 70-8 ■ Operative mortality rates as a function of time for patients with acute type A dissection operated on between 1963 and 1999 at Stanford University and broken down according to treatment method. *Non-PHCA,* No circulatory arrest; *PHCA,* profound hypothermic circulatory arrest. (From Lai DT, Robbins RC, Mitchell RS, et al: Does profound hypothermic circulatory arrest improve survival in patients with acute type A aortic dissection? *Circulation* 106:I218–I228, 2002. Copyright 2002, American Heart Association.)

and 27%. For patients with acute type A dissections, the late survival estimate for discharged patients was 91%, 75%, 51%, and 32% at 1 year, 5 years, 10 years, and 15 years, respectively, compared with 93%, 79%, 54%, and 33% for those with chronic type A dissections. One third of the late deaths were cardiac related, but at least 15% of deaths were due to complications related to the downstream chronic aortic dissection. Multivariable analysis identified older age and previous cardiovascular operation to be significant risk factors for late death; interestingly, previous stroke, remote myocardial infarction, chronic renal dysfunction, and earlier operative date, which were independent predictors of adverse late outcome in the 1985 Stanford analysis,[40] no longer emerged as risk factors in the larger, more recent analysis. In the more recent report from Stanford of patients with surgically treated acute type A dissections, independent determinants of late death were increasing age, previous sternotomy, prior stroke, hypertension, liver disease, tamponade, arch involvement, and earlier year of operation; use of PHCA and resection of the intimal tear were not identified as significant predictors of late death.[183] Actuarial survival after surgical repair of acute and chronic type A aortic dissections in the patients operated on at Stanford University between 1963 and 2000 is shown in Figures 70-8 and 70-9.

In Crawford's 1990 report, survival at 1, 5, and 10 years in patients with proximal dissections (acute or chronic) was 78%, 63%, and 55%, respectively[234]; life expectancy was significantly worse in patients with acute dissections (67% for acute versus 81% for chronic at 1 year, and 51% versus 68% at 5 years). Independent predictors of late death in all patients included severity of symptoms, New York Heart Association (NYHA) functional class, distal extent of resection, unresected residual aneurysm, postoperative complications, and earlier year of operation. In his 1992 updated series focusing only on acute type A aortic dissections,[84] Crawford reported

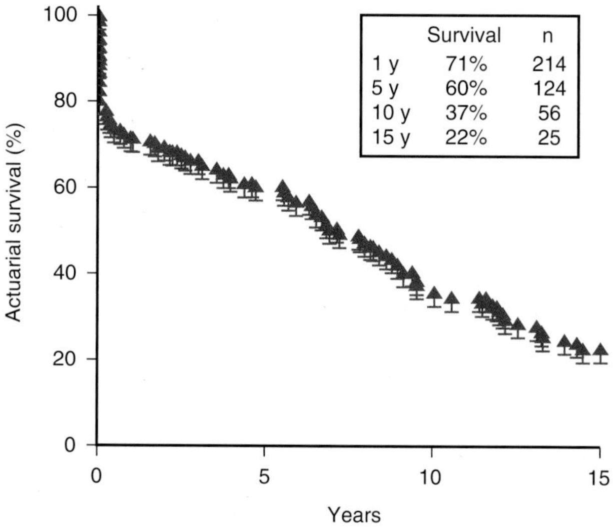

FIGURE 70-9 ■ Actuarial survival after operative repair of acute type A aortic dissection in 323 consecutive patients operated on between 1963 and 2000 at Stanford University Medical Center.

survival estimates at 5, 10, and 20 years after surgical repair of 56%, 46%, and 30%, respectively. Determinants of mortality in this series were earlier year of operation, inclusion of the arch in the repair, NYHA functional class, diabetes, and concomitant coronary artery bypass grafting. In the Cleveland Clinic experience, long-term survival was comparable between those with acute and those with chronic type A dissections; older age, higher blood urea nitrogen concentration, aortic arch replacement, and earlier date of operation were incremental risk factors for late death.[233]

Recent, large single-center and multicenter clinical reports corroborate these results and show only modest improvement in the long-term prognosis after surgical repair of acute type A aortic dissections during the last two decades. In their extensive experience with 315 patients operated on during a period of 27 years, Tan and colleagues from the Netherlands reported survival (of discharged patients only) at 1 year, 10 years, and 20 years of 96%, 68%, and 39%, respectively. In their series, advancing age and renal failure were the only predictors of late death.[242a] In the Mt. Sinai analysis of their contemporary cohort of patients operated on with a standardized surgical approach, Griepp and colleagues reported survival estimates at 1, 5, and 10 years of 91%, 78%, and 66%, respectively, for hospital survivors.[113] Independent risk factors for late mortality were advancing age, neurologic deficit at presentation, and patent false lumen postoperatively. Finally, in the IRAD analysis of long-term survival after acute type A aortic dissection, patients who survived initial surgical repair had 1- and 3-year survival rates of 96% and 89%, respectively.[238] The only significant predictors of late death identified were history of atherosclerosis and previous cardiac surgery. These figures need to be interpreted with caution, however, as the IRAD consortium did not mandate long-term follow-up after initial hospital discharge; late vital status and clinical data were available in approximately half of their patients.

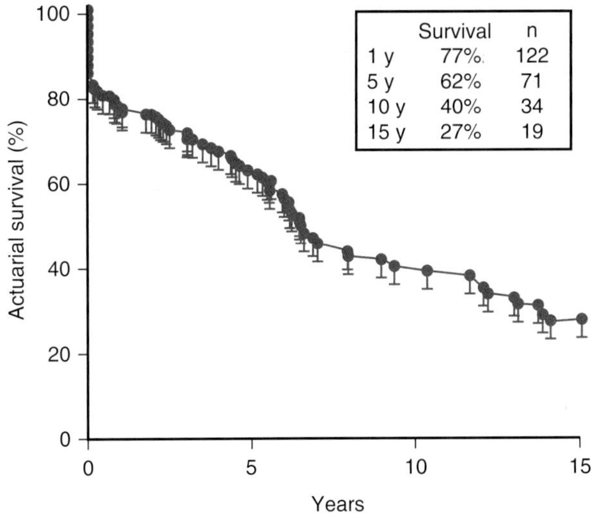

FIGURE 70-10 Actuarial survival after operative repair of chronic type A aortic dissection in 165 consecutive patients operated on between 1964 and 2000 at Stanford University Medical Center.

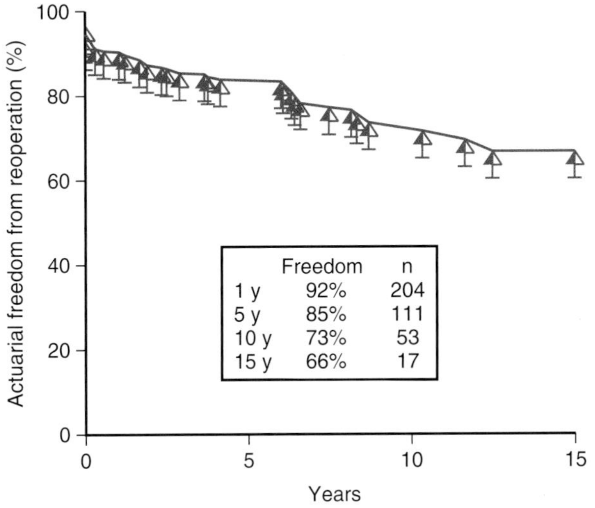

FIGURE 70-11 Actuarial freedom from proximal or distal aortic reoperation after operative repair of acute type A aortic dissection in 323 patients operated on between 1963 and 2000 at Stanford University Medical Center.

Reoperation

After repair of acute type A aortic dissection, growth rates of the arch and thoracoabdominal aorta have been estimated to be 1 to 5 mm per year by several investigators.[113,114] As such, despite successful intervention in the acute or chronic phase of the disease, aneurysmal degeneration of the false lumen in other downstream segments of the aorta can occur in a substantial proportion of patients, which can lead to late aortic rupture and death or require reintervention. As discussed previously, aortic root aneurysm, new or recurrent severe aortic regurgitation, and anastomotic false aneurysm are other indications that require repeat surgical intervention. Late reoperations for aortic dissection can be technically challenging, usually require extensive aortic reconstruction, and frequently involve thoracoabdominal aortic repair which have been considered high-risk procedures, especially in the emergency setting.[10,112,171] More recently, however, reoperative early mortality rates between 4% and 11% have been reported from centers with large experience in thoracic aortic surgery.[113,114,223,226]

In the Stanford 30-year experience, freedom from late reoperation for patients with acute type A dissections at 1, 5, 10, and 15 years was 94%, 83%, 65%, and 65%, respectively.[10] For chronic type A dissections, these freedom estimates were 96%, 88%, 65%, and 52%, respectively. Younger age was the only significant, independent risk factor portending a higher likelihood of reoperation. In the more recent Stanford report focusing on patients with acute type A dissections, male gender, Marfan syndrome, coronary artery disease, peripheral pulse deficit, and arch involvement were associated with a higher likelihood of late distal aortic reintervention.[183] Freedom from proximal or distal aortic reoperations after surgical repair of acute or chronic type A aortic dissections in the patients operated on at Stanford University between 1963 and 2000 is shown in Figures 70-10 through 70-12.

In the Baylor experience, overall freedom from reoperation for patients with all types of dissections was 96%, 91%, and 78% at 1 year, 5 years, and 10 years, respectively.[234] In the Cleveland Clinic series, these respective freedom from reoperation estimates were 98%, 91%, and 85% for patients with type A dissections.[233] On the other hand, freedom from reoperation after repair of acute type A dissection was 66%, 58%, 52%, and 43% at 1 year, 5 years, 10 years, and 15 years, respectively, in the experience of Loisance and colleagues.[243] In the recent report from the Washington University in St. Louis, freedom from reoperation was 74% at 10 years[114]; in the University of Pennsylvania experience from 1993 to 2004,

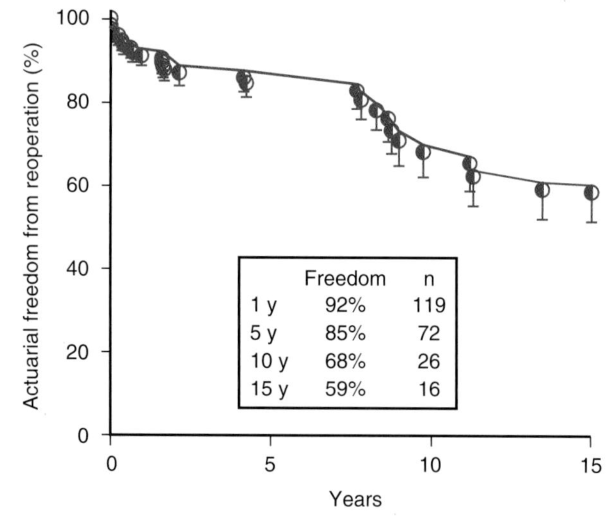

FIGURE 70-12 ■ Actuarial freedom from proximal or distal aortic reoperation after operative repair of chronic type A aortic dissection in 165 patients operated on between 1964 and 2000 at Stanford University Medical Center.

actuarial freedom from any reoperation was 87% at 5 years and 70% at 10 years.[243] Interestingly, using the systematic Mt. Sinai long-term clinical and radiologic follow-up database, the estimated risk of reoperation on the distal aorta was only 16% 10 years after initial surgical repair of acute type A dissection using open arch repair and aggressive resection of the primary intimal tear.[113]

Younger age at the initial operation has been a strong risk factor for late aortic reinterventions.[114,233,243-245] Marfan syndrome has also been associated with a higher risk of recurrent problems in the aortic root as well as the distal thoracic aorta, suggesting that a more radical approach is justified in patients with connective tissue disorders to reduce the incidence of late reoperations.[113,114,228,243-245] More severe aortic valve regurgitation at the time of the initial operation has been identified by different authors to be a risk factor portending a higher probability of proximal reoperation on the aortic root and valve.[243,246] The wisdom of using GRF or fibrin glue to reconstruct the dissected aortic root and distal aorta has also been questioned because of its late complications, including false aneurysms.[175,176,228] Failure to excise the primary intimal tear, leaving behind unresected residual aneurysm at the index operation, and persistent patency of the false lumen have also been linked to a higher incidence of late distal aortic reoperations.[91,114,229,233,243,245]

Concerning both late survival and need for late reoperation, it remains to be determined whether contemporary surgical techniques of total or partial arch replacement using a distal surgical elephant trunk graft in the descending thoracic aorta or a FET in the distal aortic true lumen will be associated with fewer late deaths and reoperations.[203-205,209-215] We must learn which patients with acute type A dissections are at highest risk for untoward late complications such that these more aggressive techniques can then be selectively applied to optimize the risk-to-benefit ratio.

FOLLOW-UP

Close medical follow-up and careful periodic imaging surveillance on a rigorous basis are mandatory for all patients with aortic dissections forever. After operative repair, early postoperative serial CTA or MRI of the thoracic and abdominal aorta is essential to define the baseline pathoanatomy and thereafter to detect dissection complications; these scans should be performed at 3- to 6-month intervals during the first year and then every 12 months indefinitely. A transthoracic echocardiogram should also be performed annually to evaluate the aortic root and aortic valve function. Strict long-term blood pressure control is critical for all these patients, as uncontrolled hypertension in the chronic phase of aortic dissection has been associated with an increase in late aortic complications.[114] A combination of conventional antihypertensive agents and negative inotropic medications, such as oral beta blockers which have been shown to improve late survival in type A aortic dissection, is required and must be continued indefinitely.[247] Antihypertensive drugs such as the angiotensin-converting enzyme inhibitors and angiotensin receptor blockers, which paradoxically increase aortic dP/dt, should be avoided, if at all possible; if severe hypertension requires more aggressive therapy and one of these drugs, it is essential that adequate beta blockade be maintained concomitantly.

REFERENCES

1. Leonard JC: Thomas Bevill Peacock and the early history of dissecting aneurysm. *BMJ* 2:260–262, 1979.
2. Maunoir JP: *Memoires physiologiques et pratiques sur l'aneurysme et la ligature des arteres*, Geneva, 1802, J.J. Paschoud.
3. Laennec RTH: *De l'auscultations mediate, ou traité du diagnostic des maladies des poumons et du coeur, fondé principalement sur ce nouveau moyen d'exploration*, Paris, 1819, Brosson & Chaude.
4. Peacock TB: Report on cases of dissecting aneurysms. *Trans Pathol Soc Lond* 14:87, 1863.
5. Shennan T: *Dissecting aneurysms. Special report Medical Research Council series No. 193*, London, 1934, His Majesty's Stationary Office.
6. Paullin JE, James DF: Dissecting aneurysm of aorta. *Postgrad Med* 4:291, 1948.
7. Gurin D, Bulmer JW, Derby R: Dissecting aneurysm of the aorta: diagnosis and operative relief of acute arterial obstruction due to this cause. *N Y State J Med* 35:1200–1202, 1935.
8. Abbott OA: Clinical experiences with application of polythene cellophane upon aneurysms of thoracic vessels. *J Thorac Surg* 18:435, 1949.
9. DeBakey ME, Cooley D, Creech O, Jr: Surgical considerations of dissecting aneurysm of the aorta. *Ann Surg* 142:586–612, 1955.
10. Fann JI, Smith JA, Miller DC, et al: Surgical management of aortic dissection during a 30-year period. *Circulation* 92(Suppl II):II113–II121, 1995.
11. Hirst AE, Johns VJ, Krime SJ: Dissecting aneurysm of the aorta: a review of 505 cases. *Medicine* 37:217–279, 1958.
12. Wheat MW, Palmer RF, Bantley TD, et al: Treatment of dissecting aneurysms of the aorta without surgery. *J Thorac Cardiovasc Surg* 50:364–373, 1965.
13. Daily PO, Trueblood HW, Stinson EB, et al: Management of acute aortic dissections. *Ann Thorac Surg* 10:237–247, 1970.
14. DeBakey ME, Henry WS, Cooley DA, et al: Surgical management of dissecting aneurysms of the aorta. *J Thorac Cardiovasc Surg* 49:130–149, 1965.
15. Griepp RB, Stinson EB, Hollingsworth JF, et al: Prosthetic replacement of the aortic arch. *J Thorac Cardiovasc Surg* 70:1051–1063, 1975.

16. DeBakey ME, McCollum CH, Crawford ES, et al: Dissection and dissecting aneurysms of the aorta: twenty-year follow-up of five hundred and twenty-seven patients treated surgically. *Surgery* 92:1118–1134, 1982.
17. Miller DC: Surgical management of aortic dissections: indications, perioperative management, and long-term results. In Doroghazi RM, Slater EE, editors: *Aortic dissection*, New York, 1983, McGraw-Hill, pp 193–243.
18. Applebaum A, Karp RB, Kirklin JW: Ascending vs. descending aortic dissections. *Ann Surg* 183:296–300, 1976.
19. Doroghazi RM, Slater EE, DeSanctis RW, et al: Long-term survival of patients with treated aortic dissections. *J Am Coll Cardiol* 3:1026–1034, 1984.
20. Ming RL, Najafi H, Javid H, et al: Acute ascending aortic dissection: surgical management. *Circulation* 64(Suppl II):II231–II234, 1981.
21. Reul GJ, Cooley DA, Hallman GL, et al: Dissecting aneurysm of the descending aorta. Improved surgical results in 91 patients. *Arch Surg* 110:632–640, 1975.
22. Lansman SL, McCullough JN, Nguyen KH, et al: Subtypes of acute aortic dissection. *Ann Thorac Surg* 67:1975–1978, 1999.
23. DeSanctis RW, Doroghazi RM, Austen WG, et al: Aortic dissection. *N Engl J Med* 317:1060–1067, 1987.
24. Hagan PG, Nienaber CA, Isselbacher EM, et al: The International Registry of Acute Aortic Dissection (IRAD). *JAMA* 283:897–903, 2000.
25. Slater EE: Aortic dissection: presentation and diagnosis. In Doroghazi RM, Slater EE, editors: *Aortic dissection*, New York, 1983, McGraw-Hill, pp 61–70.
26. Robbins RC, McManus RP, Mitchell RS, et al: Management of patients with intramural hematoma of the thoracic aorta. *Circulation* 88(Suppl II):II1–II10, 1993.
27. Stanson AW, Kazmier FJ, Hollier LH, et al: Penetrating atherosclerotic ulcers of the thoracic aorta: natural history and clinicopathologic correlations. *Ann Vasc Surg* 1:15–23, 1986.
28. Nienaber CA, von Kodolitsch Y, Petersen B, et al: Intramural hemorrhage of the aorta: diagnostic and clinical implications. *Circulation* 92:1465–1472, 1995.
29. Coady MA, Rizzo JA, Hammond GL, et al: Penetrating ulcer of the thoracic aorta: what is it? How do we recognize it? How do we manage it? *J Vasc Surg* 27:1006–1016, 1998.
30. Ganaha F, Miller DC, Sugimoto K, et al: Prognosis of aortic intramural hematoma with and without penetrating atherosclerotic ulcer. A clinical and radiologic analysis. *Circulation* 106:342–348, 2002.
31. Januzzi JL, Isselbacher EM, Fattori R, et al: Characterizing the young patient with aortic dissection: results from the International Registry of Aortic Dissection. *J Am Coll Cardiol* 43:665–669, 2004.
32. Nienaber CA, Fattori R, Mehta RH, et al: International Registry of Acute Aortic Dissection. Gender-related differences in acute aortic dissection. *Circulation* 109:3014–3021, 2004.
33. Clouse WD, Hallett JW, Schaff HV, et al: Acute aortic dissection: population-based incidence compared with degenerative aortic aneurysm rupture. *Mayo Clin Proc* 79:176–180, 2004.
34. Sorenson HR, Olsen H: Ruptured and dissecting aneurysms of the aorta. incidence and prospects of surgery. *Acta Chir Scand* 128:644, 1964.
35. Pate JW, Richardson RL, Eastridge CE: Acute aortic dissections. *Am Surg* 42:395–404, 1976.
36. Bickerstaff LK, Pairolero PC, Hollier LH, et al: Thoracic aortic aneurysms: a population-based study. *Surgery* 92:1103–1108, 1982.
37. Olssen C, Thelin S, Stahle E, et al: Thoracic aortic aneurysm and dissection. increasing prevalence and improved outcomes reported in a nationwide population-based study of more than 14000 cases from 1987 to 2002. *Circulation* 114:2611–2618, 2006.
38. Lindsay J, Jr, Hurst JW: Clinical features and prognosis in dissecting aneurysms of the aorta: a re-appraisal. *Circulation* 35:880–888, 1967.
39. Anagnostopoulos CE, Prabhakar MJS, Vittle CF: Aortic dissections and dissecting aneurysms. *Am J Cardiol* 30:263–273, 1972.
40. Haverich A, Miller DC, Scott WC, et al: Acute and chronic aortic dissections—determinants of long-term outcome for operative survivors. *Circulation* 72(Suppl II):II22–II34, 1985.
41. Slonim SM, Miller DC, Mitchell RS, et al: Percutaneous balloon fenestration and stenting for life-threatening ischemic complications in patients with acute aortic dissection. *J Thorac Cardiovasc Surg* 117:1118–1126, 1999.
42. DeSanctis RW, Eagle KA: Aortic dissection. *Curr Probl Cardiol* 14:227–278, 1989.
43. Nienaber CA, Powell JT: Management of acute aortic syndromes. *Eur Heart J* 33:26–35, 2012.
44. Tsai TT, Nienaber CA, Eagle KA: Acute aortic syndromes. *Circulation* 112:3802–3813, 2005.
45. Carlson RG, Lillehei CW, Edwards JE: Cystic medial necrosis of the ascending aorta in relation to age and hypertension. *Am J Cardiol* 25:411–415, 1970.
46. Pyeritz RE: The Marfan syndrome. *Annu Rev Med* 51:481–510, 2000.
47. Svensson LG, Crawford ES, Coselli JS, et al: Impact of cardiovascular operation on survival in the Marfan patient. *Circulation* 80(Suppl I):I233–I242, 1989.
48. Loeys BL, Dietz HC, Braverman AC, et al: The revised Ghent nosology for the Marfan syndrome. *J Med Genet* 47:476–485, 2010.
49. Hiratzka LF, Bakris GL, Beckman JA, et al: 2010 ACCF/AHA/AATS/ASA/SCA/SCAI/SIR/ATS/SVM guidelines for the management of patients with thoracic aortic disease: executive summary. A report from the American College of Cardiology Foundation/American Heart Association Task Force on Practice Guidelines, American Association for Thoracic Surgery, American College of Radiology, American Stroke Association, Society of Cardiovascular Anesthesiologists, Society for Cardiovascular Angiography and Interventions, Society of Interventional Radiology, Society of Thoracic Surgeons, and Society for Vascular Medicine. *Circulation* 121:e266–e369, 2010.
50. Januzzi JL, Marayati F, Mehta RH, et al: Comparison of aortic dissection in patients with and without Marfan's syndrome (results from the International Registry of Aortic Dissection). *Am J Cardiol* 94:400–402, 2004.
51. Beighton P, DePaepe A, Danks D, et al: International nosology of heritable disorders of connective tissue, Berlin, 1986. *Am J Med Genet* 29:581–594, 1988.
52. Cikrit DF, Miles JH, Silver D: Spontaneous arterial perforation: the Ehler-Danlos specter. *J Vasc Surg* 8:470–475, 1987.
53. Kontusaari S, Tromp G, Kuivaniemi H, et al: A mutation in the gene for type III procollagen (COL3A1) in a family with aortic aneurysms. *J Clin Invest* 86:1465–1473, 1990.
54. Pepin M, Schwarze U, Superti-Furga A, et al: Clinical and genetic features of Ehlers-Danlos syndrome type IV, the vascular type. *N Engl J Med* 342:673–680, 2000.
55. Loeys BL, Schwarze U, Holm T, et al: Aneurysm syndromes caused by mutations in the TGF-beta receptor. *N Engl J Med* 355:788–798, 2006.
56. Guo DC, Papke CL, Tran-Fadulu V, et al: Mutations in smooth muscle alpha—actin (ACTA2) cause coronary artery disease, stroke, and Moyamoya disease, along with thoracic aortic disease. *Am J Hum Genet* 84:617–627, 2009.
57. Roberts C, Roberts W: Dissection of the aorta associated with congenital malformation of the aortic valve. *J Am Coll Cardiol* 17:712–716, 1991.
58. Muna WF, Spray TL, Morrow AG, et al: Aortic dissection after aortic valve replacement in patients with valvular aortic stenosis. *J Thorac Cardiovasc Surg* 74:65–69, 1977.
59. Pieters F, Widdenshoven J, Gerardy A, et al: Risk of aortic dissection after aortic valve replacement. *Am J Cardiol* 72:1043–1047, 1993.
60. Abbott ME: Coarctation of the aorta of the adult type II. *Am Heart J* 3:574–618, 1928.
61. Connolly HM, Schaff HV, Izhar U, et al: Posterior pericardial ascending-to-descending aortic bypass: an alternative approach for complex coarctation of the aorta. *Circulation* 104(Suppl I):I133–I137, 2001.
62. Svensson LG: Management of acute dissection with coarctation of the aorta in a single operation. *Ann Thorac Surg* 58:241–243, 1994.
63. Januzzi JL, Sabatine MS, Eagle KA, et al: Iatrogenic aortic dissection. *Am J Cardiol* 89:623–625, 2002.

64. Murphy DA, Craver JM, Jones EL, et al: Recognition and management of ascending aortic dissection complicating cardiac surgical operations. *J Thorac Cardiovasc Surg* 85:247–256, 1983.
65. Gillinov AM, Lytle BW, Kaplon RJ, et al: Dissection of the ascending aorta after previous cardiac surgery: differences in presentation and management. *J Thorac Cardiovasc Surg* 117:252–260, 1999.
66. Chavanon O, Carrier M, Cartier R, et al: Increased incidence of acute ascending aortic dissection with off-pump aorto-coronary bypass surgery? *Ann Thorac Surg* 71:117–121, 2001.
67. Schnitker MA, Bayer CA: Dissecting aneurysm of the aorta in young individuals, particularly in association with pregnancy; with report of a case. *Ann Intern Med* 20:486–511, 1944.
68. Immer FF, Bansi AG, Immer-Bansi AS, et al: Aortic dissection and pregnancy: analysis of risk factors and outcomes. *Ann Thorac Surg* 76:309–314, 2003.
69. Eagle KA, Isselbacher EM, DeSanctis RW: Cocaine-related aortic dissection in perspective. *Circulation* 105:1529–1530, 2002.
70. Rushid J, Eisenberg MJ, Topol EJ: Cocaine-induced aortic dissection. *Am Heart J* 132:1301–1304, 1996.
71. Matura LA, Ho VB, Rosing DR, et al: Aortic dilatation and dissection in Turner syndrome. *Circulation* 116:1663–1670, 2007.
72. Erdheim J: Medionecrosis aortae idiopathica cystica. *Virchows Arch Pathol Anat* 276:187–229, 1930.
73. Davies MJ, Treasure T, Richardson PD: The pathogenesis of spontaneous arterial dissection. *Heart* 75:434–435, 1996.
74. Nakashima Y, Kurozumi T, Sueishi K, et al: Dissecting aneurysm: a clinicopathologic and histopathologic study of 111 autopsied cases. *Hum Pathol* 21:291–296, 1990.
75. Nakashima Y, Shiokawa Y, Sueishi K: Alterations of elastic architecture in human aortic dissecting aneurysm. *Lab Invest* 62:751–760, 1990.
76. He R, Guo DC, Estrera EL, et al: Characterization of the inflammatory and apoptotic cells in the aortas of patients with ascending thoracic aortic aneurysms and dissections. *J Thorac Cardiovasc Surg* 131:671–678, 2006.
77. Wang X, LeMaire SA, Chen L, et al: Increased collagen deposition and elevated expression of connective tissue growth factor in human thoracic aortic dissection. *Circulation* 114:I200–I205, 2006.
78. Ishii T, Asuwa N: Collagen and elastin degradation by matrix metalloproteinases and tissue inhibitors of matrix metalloproteinase in aortic dissection. *Hum Pathol* 31:640–646, 2000.
79. Chen L, Wang X, Carter SA, et al: A single nucleotide polymorphism in the matrix metalloproteinase 9 gene (–8202A/G) is associated with thoracic aortic aneurysms and thoracic aortic dissection. *J Thorac Cardiovasc Surg* 131:1045–1052, 2006.
80. Svensson LG, Labib SB, Eisenhauer AC, et al: Intimal tear without hematoma: an important variant of aortic dissection that can elude current imaging techniques. *Circulation* 99:1331–1336, 1999.
81. Symbas PN, Kelly TF, Vlasis SE, et al: Intimo-intimal intussusception and other unusual manifestations of aortic dissection. *J Thorac Cardiovasc Surg* 79:926–932, 1980.
82. Erhlich MP, Ergin MA, McCullough JN, et al: Results of immediate surgical treatment of all acute type A dissections. *Circulation* 102(Suppl III):III248–III252, 2000.
83. Miller DC, Stinson EB, Oyer PE, et al: Operative treatment of aortic dissections. experience with 125 patients over a sixteen-year period. *J Thorac Cardiovasc Surg* 78:365–382, 1979.
84. Crawford ES, Kirklin JW, Naftel DC, et al: Surgery for acute dissection of ascending aorta: should the arch be included? *J Thorac Cardiovasc Surg* 104:46–59, 1992.
85. Yun KL, Glower DD, Miller DC, et al: Aortic dissection resulting from tear of transverse arch: is concomitant arch repair warranted? *J Thorac Cardiovasc Surg* 102:355–368, 1991.
86. Farber A, Wagner WH, Cossman DV, et al: Isolated dissection of the abdominal aorta: clinical presentation and therapeutic options. *J Vasc Surg* 36:205–210, 2002.
87. Roberts CS, Roberts WC: Aortic dissection with the entrance tear in abdominal aorta. *Am Heart J* 121:1834–1835, 1991.
88. Hirst AE, Gore I: Is cystic medionecrosis the cause of dissecting aortic aneurysm? *Am Heart J* 53:915–916, 1976.
89. Roberts WC: Aortic dissection: anatomy, consequences, and cause. *Am Heart J* 101:195–214, 1981.
90. Erbel R, Oelert H, Meyer J, et al: Effect of medical and surgical therapy on aortic dissection evaluated by transesophageal echocardiography: implications for prognosis and therapy. *Circulation* 87:1604–1615, 1993.
91. Ergin MA, Phillips RA, Galla JD, et al: Significance of distal false lumen after type A dissection repair. *Ann Thorac Surg* 57:820–824, 1994.
92. Elefteriades JA, Hammond GL, Gusberg RJ, et al: Fenestration revisited. a safe and effective procedure for descending aortic dissection. *Arch Surg* 125:786–790, 1990.
93. Slonim SM, Nyman URO, Semba CP, et al: Aortic dissection: percutaneous management of ischemic complications with endovascular stents and balloon fenestration. *J Vasc Surg* 23:241–253, 1996.
94. Krukenberg E: Beitrage sur Frage des Aneurysma dissecans. *Beitr Pathol Anat Allg Pathol* 67:329–351, 1920.
95. Evangelista A, Mukherjee D, Mehta RH, et al: Acute intramural hematoma of the aorta. A mystery in evolution. *Circulation* 111:1063–1070, 2005.
96. Tittle SL, Lynch RJ, Cole PE, et al: Midterm follow-up of penetrating ulcer and intramural hematoma of the aorta. *J Thorac Cardiovasc Surg* 123:1051–1059, 2002.
97. Williams DM, Lee DY, Hamilton BH, et al: The dissected aorta: percutaneous treatment of ischemic complications—principles and results. *J Vasc Interv Radiol* 8:605–625, 1997.
98. Slonim SM, Nyman UR, Semba CP, et al: True lumen obliteration in complicated aortic dissection: endovascular treatment. *Radiology* 201:161–166, 1996.
99. Kruger T, Conzelmann LO, Bonser RS, et al: Acute aortic dissection type A. *Br J Surg* 99:1331–1344, 2012.
100. Meszaros I, Morocz J, Szlavi J, et al: Epidemiology and clinicopathology of aortic dissection. *Chest* 117:1271–1278, 2000.
101. Cambria RP, Brewster DC, Gertler J, et al: Vascular complications associated with spontaneous aortic dissection. *J Vasc Surg* 7:199–202, 1988.
102. Fann JI, Sarris GE, Mitchell RS, et al: Treatment of patients with aortic dissection presenting with peripheral vascular complications. *Ann Surg* 212:705–713, 1990.
103. Isselbacher EM, Cigarroa JE, Eagle KA: Cardiac tamponade complicating proximal aortic dissection. is pericardiocentesis harmful? *Circulation* 90:2375–2378, 1994.
104. Lai DT, Miller DC, Mitchell RS, et al: Acute type A aortic dissection complicated by aortic regurgitation: composition valve graft versus separate valve graft versus conservative valve repair. *J Thorac Cardiovasc Surg* 126:1978–1986, 2003.
105. Kawahito K, Adachi H, Murata SI, et al: Coronary malperfusion due to type A aortic dissection: mechanism and surgical management. *Ann Thorac Surg* 76:1471–1476, 2003.
106. Lindsay J, Jr: Aorto-cameral fistula: a rare complication of aortic dissection. *Am Heart J* 126:441–443, 1993.
107. Link MD, Pietrzak MP: Aortic dissection presenting as superior vena cava syndrome. *Am J Emerg Med* 12:326–328, 1994.
108. Yacoub MH, Schottenfeld M, Kittle CF: Hematoma of the interatrial septum with heart block secondary to dissecting aneurysm of the aorta: a clinicopathologic entity. *Circulation* 46:537–545, 1972.
109. Bossone E, Rampoldi V, Nienaber CA, et al: Usefulness of pulse deficit to predict in-hospital complications and mortality in patients with acute type A aortic dissection. *Am J Cardiol* 89:851–855, 2002.
110. Lauterbach SR, Cambria RP, Brewster DC, et al: Contemporary management of aortic branch compromise resulting from acute aortic dissection. *J Vasc Surg* 33:1185–1192, 2001.
111. Fann JI, Sarris GE, Miller DC, et al: Surgical management of acute aortic dissection complicated by a stroke. *Circulation* 80(Suppl I):I257–I263, 1989.
112. Kobuch R, Hilker M, Rupprecht L, et al: Late reoperations after repaired acute type A aortic dissection. *J Thorac Cardiovasc Surg* 144:300–307, 2012.
113. Halstead JC, Meier M, Etz C, et al: The fate of the distal aorta after repair of acute type A aortic dissection. *J Thorac Cardiovasc Surg* 133:127–135, 2007.
114. Zierer A, Voeller RK, Hill KE, et al: Aortic enlargement and late reoperation after repair of acute type A aortic dissection. *Ann Thorac Surg* 84:478–487, 2007.

Aortic branch vessel involvement or thoracoabdominal malperfusion results when the dissection compromises blood flow to important downstream aortic tributaries. As illustrated in Figure 70-4 of Chapter 70, the most common mechanisms producing aortic branch compromise are extrinsic compression of the aortic true lumen by the false lumen and an intimal flap compromising the orifice of the branch artery. As defined by Williams and associates,[49] static branch compromise is extension of the dissection flap into a branch vessel with subsequent mechanical obstruction of flow; conversely, in dynamic branch compromise, the dissection flap prolapses into the vessel origin or the true lumen is narrowed above it because the bulk of flow is in the aortic false lumen. Compression by the large false lumen can thus result in near-obliteration of the true channel (true lumen collapse or "obliteration").[50] With extension of the dissection, some aortic tributaries may be spared and continue to be perfused by the true lumen; others may be perfused exclusively from the false lumen after being sheared off and eventually become permanently dependent on flow from the aortic false lumen. Thus, clinical presentation is dependent on which aortic branches are involved and on the severity of compromised perfusion, which can be variable, thus confounding and delaying the correct diagnosis. Simultaneous occurrence of a variety of acute clinical problems without a readily apparent unifying cause should prompt consideration of acute aortic dissection.

CLINICAL MANIFESTATIONS

Patients with acute type B dissection can present with symptoms and physical findings that suggest almost any other acute medical or surgical disease process.[3,23,32] These numerous, nonspecific manifestations are the main reason that the rapid, correct diagnosis of aortic dissection remains such a formidable clinical challenge.[7,51] Indeed, aortic dissection occurs more frequently than ruptured abdominal aortic aneurysm, but it is diagnosed correctly less frequently antemortem.[3,23]

Most commonly, the clinical hallmark of acute type B aortic dissection is the acute onset of severe, lancinating chest or back pain.[3,5,7,23,32] The initial pain can be in any location, but it usually originates in the interscapular region with later migration to the lower back or abdomen. Pain in acute dissection is thought to be secondary to stretching of the aortic adventitia caused by the dissecting hematoma. Abrupt onset of symptoms and description of sharp, ripping, or tearing pain are also characteristic of acute dissection. Persistence or further migration of pain suggests continuing expansion or distal extension of the dissecting process. In rare cases, acute dissection can be painless; vigilance is essential to recognize other manifestations of aortic dissection in these cases. In a summary from the International Registry of Acute Aortic Dissection (IRAD), 98% of 175 patients with acute type B dissection reported some pain, pain was of sudden onset in 84%, and 63% reported chest pain (anterior in 44%, posterior in 41%) that was significantly different from acute type A dissection (chest pain in 79% and anterior in 71%).[31] Back pain was observed in 64% and abdominal pain in 43% of patients with acute type B dissections, much more frequently than in patients with type A dissection.[31] Moreover, the pain was described as the "worst ever" in 90% of patients, sharp in 68%, and tearing in 52%. Radiating pain was observed in 30% of cases, whereas migration was reported in only 19%.

Despite clinical signs of poor peripheral perfusion, elevated blood pressure is usually observed. In the IRAD report, 70% of patients with acute type B dissection were hypertensive at initial presentation; only 4% were hypotensive and in shock, compared with 25% of patients with acute type A dissection. If the patient is hypotensive, aortic rupture should be suspected. Cardiac tamponade is rare in acute type B dissection; only 2% of patients with acute type B dissection in the 30-year Stanford experience had tamponade, which was thought to be the result of leakage of blood and fluid into the pericardial sac from a large, high-pressure mediastinal hematoma.[30]

The constellation of other symptoms and signs relates largely to which distal aortic branches are involved in the dissection. Approximately 25% of patients present with symptoms related to aortic branch compromise or develop such symptoms early in the course of their illness[52]; alternatively, loss of a peripheral pulse may be clinically asymptomatic. In a review of the Stanford experience with peripheral vascular complications of aortic dissection by Fann and colleagues,[53] 85 (31%) of 272 patients with all types of dissections sustained at least one peripheral vascular complication, whereas 20% of patients with type B dissections had such complications (Fig. 71-2). Of the 85 patients with a vascular complication, 18 individuals (21%) suffered two complications, and 7 (8%) had three or more vascular problems. Among the 40 patients with acute type B dissection, no patient presented with a stroke, 3% had acute paraplegia at presentation, 20% sustained loss of one or more peripheral pulses, 8% had impaired renal perfusion demonstrated angiographically, and 5% had compromised visceral perfusion by angiography. The incidence of these complications with the attendant operative mortality rate after surgical graft replacement of the descending thoracic aorta is summarized in Table 71-1. The distribution of specific sites of peripheral pulse loss in these patients is summarized in Table 71-2. Others authors have reported similar figures, with the prevalence of peripheral vascular manifestations ranging from 10% to 30%.[5,21,52,54,55] As a general rule, morbidity and mortality rates are higher in patients presenting with branch vessel involvement.[29,52]

The clinical course of peripheral limb ischemia can vary; up to one third of patients may experience spontaneous resolution of the peripheral pulse deficit or a fluctuating course, often because of the reentry of flow into the distal true lumen from the false lumen.[54] Stroke and transient ischemic attack can complicate acute type A dissection but are seen only rarely in patients with type B dissections. Neurologic findings can vary from minor sensory deficits to frank paraplegia resulting from spinal cord ischemia caused by interruption of intercostal artery blood supply to peripheral ischemic neuropathy.[32,52] Abdominal pain out of proportion to the physical abdominal findings must be considered potentially to reflect

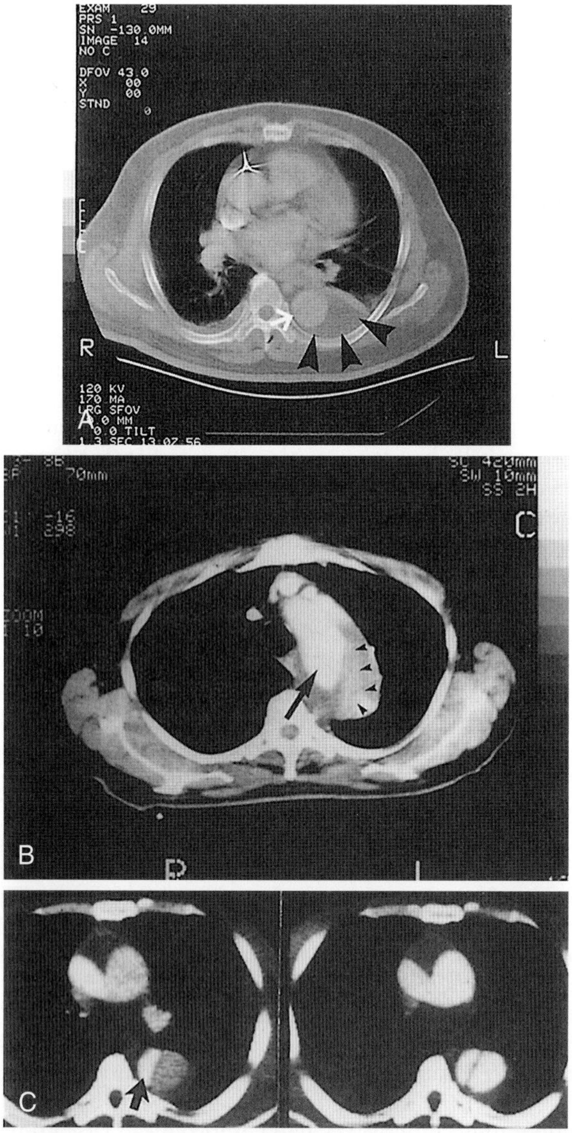

FIGURE 71-2 ■ Examples of diagnostic computed tomography (CT) scans. **A,** The CT scan shows the linear flap *(black lucency, white arrow)* between the two aortic lumens in the descending thoracic aorta that is characteristic of aortic dissection. In addition, a relatively large hematoma surrounding the aorta is seen *(arrowheads),* representing recent hemorrhage contained in the posterior mediastinum. Despite this ominous appearance, this patient did well with medical therapy for more than 1 year until progressive enlargement of a localized false aneurysm prompted referral for operation. **B,** CT scan from a different patient with an acute type B dissection illustrating a false aneurysm involving the distal arch and proximal descending thoracic aorta. The false lumen *(arrowheads)* is partially thrombosed; therefore, it opacifies only faintly compared with the contrast seen in the true lumen *(arrow).* **C,** Although this patient had a type A dissection (note the deformed true lumen in the large ascending aorta), this CT scan demonstrates differential opacification of the true and false lumens in the descending thoracic aorta. The true lumen *(arrow)* is completely opacified in the left panel; later in the cardiac cycle *(right panel),* both true and false lumens are equally opacified. (From Miller DC: Acute dissection of the descending thoracic aorta. *Chest Surg Clin North Am* 2:347–378, 1992.)

TABLE 71-1 Peripheral Vascular Complications and Associated Operative Mortality Rates in a Series of 40 Patients with Complicated Acute Type B Aortic Dissection

Peripheral Vascular Complication	Prevalence *(n)*	Mortality *(n)*
Stroke	0% (0)	—
Paraplegia	3% ± 3% (1)	100% (1)
Pulse loss	20% ± 8% (8)	50% ± 18% (4)
Renal ischemia	8% ± 4% (3)	67% ± 28% (2)
Visceral ischemia	5% ± 3% (2)	50% ± 37% (1)

Data from Fann JI, Sarris GE, Mitchell RS, et al: Treatment of patients with aortic dissection presenting with peripheral vascular complications. Ann Surg 212:705–713, 1990.

TABLE 71-2 Location of Peripheral Pulse Deficits in 56 of 168 Patients with Acute Type A or Type B Aortic Dissection

Location	Type A (*n* = 128)	Type B (*n* = 40)
Right carotid	6	0
Left carotid	6	0
Right arm	25	0
Left arm	10	2
Right leg	21	4
Left leg	14	3
Total	82	9

Data from Fann JI, Sarris GE, Mitchell RS, et al: Treatment of patients with aortic dissection presenting with peripheral vascular complications. Ann Surg 212:705–713, 1990.

mesenteric ischemia or infarction, which must be confirmed or ruled out expeditiously.[54] Oliguria or anuria suggests renal perfusion compromise; flank pain or hematuria caused by renal malperfusion or infarction can mimic symptoms usually associated with ureteral colic or kidney stones.

Physical examination of patients with suspected aortic dissection should include measurement of blood pressure in both upper and lower extremities. A complete evaluation of peripheral pulses is imperative, in addition to a comprehensive motor and sensory neurologic examination. The patient should be reexamined periodically because new vascular or neurologic deficits may come and go. The remainder of the physical examination is often normal.

Most patients with *chronic* type B dissection are asymptomatic. However, progressive enlargement of the aortic false lumen may eventually produce compression, obstruction, or erosion into adjacent thoracic structures, producing symptoms such as chest pain, dyspnea, wheezing, hoarseness, dysphagia, hemoptysis (aortobronchial fistula or erosion into the lung), and hematemesis (aortoesophageal fistula) and symptoms secondary to compromised flow in an important distal aortic branch.

DIAGNOSTIC MODALITIES

Definitive diagnostic procedures should be performed as expeditiously as possible to confirm the diagnosis of acute type B aortic dissection. Before the widespread availability of newer imaging techniques, the diagnosis was generally made by conventional catheter aortography. Today, much better options include multislice computed tomographic angiography (CTA), transesophageal echocardiography (TEE), and magnetic resonance imaging (MRI). Chest radiography is neither sensitive nor specific. The imaging modality chosen should determine the type of dissection and its extent, the site of the primary intimal tear, and the presence or absence of major aortic branch compromise. More than one imaging study may be necessary to confirm the diagnosis or to identify additional pathoanatomic details; in IRAD, multiple imaging studies were needed in 76% of patients, and an average of 2.2 imaging studies were carried out in patients with acute type B dissection before definitive treatment.[31,52]

CT scanning has markedly facilitated the rapid and accurate diagnosis of acute aortic dissection. In most cases, a thin-slice spiral CTA with intravenous administration of contrast material can determine rapidly and noninvasively the dissection type (type A or B), as illustrated in Figure 71-2. The extent of dissection, the perfusion status of individual aortic branches, and the size of the true and false lumens in all aortic segments can also be assessed accurately. Identification of two distinct lumens in the descending thoracic aorta separated by an intimal flap confirms the diagnosis of type B aortic dissection.[56] Other important signs include compression of the true lumen by the false lumen, displaced intimal calcification, thrombosed false lumen, nonopacified crescent-shaped area along the aortic wall (IMH), and ulcer-like projection of contrast material within the aortic wall indicating a PAU.[57] The presence or absence of pericardial or pleural effusions is also defined. The sensitivity and specificity, respectively, of CTA in making the diagnosis of acute type B aortic dissection are between 82% and 100% and 89% and 100%.* In the 1993 study by Nienaber and coworkers[59] that prospectively evaluated noninvasive modalities in 110 patients with suspected acute dissection, the sensitivity and specificity of CT scanning were 96% and 89% in patients with type B dissection; the positive and negative predictive values were 80% and 98%, respectively. A drawback associated with CT scanning is the requirement for administration of intravenous contrast material in patients with impaired renal function.

In most centers worldwide, TEE and/or CTA are the diagnostic modalities of choice in patients with suspected type B aortic dissection, and many patients do not require additional corroborative studies.† TEE is rapid, convenient, and noninvasive and can be performed in the emergency department, in the intensive care unit, or in the operating room with minimal risk. Undesirable blood pressure elevation is a potential risk of TEE, mandating adequate sedation of the patient. Multiplanar, phased array TEE with color flow imaging can accurately demonstrate flow in both aortic channels and the flap separating the true and false lumens; real-time three-dimensional TEE imaging can provide spectacular surface-rendered images. The most important finding is identification of an intimal flap, ideally seen in more than one view, oscillating independently of the motion of the aortic wall.[56,59,61,63] Frequently, the primary intimal tear and secondary fenestrations in the descending thoracic aorta can also be identified. Overall, the sensitivity and specificity of TEE in the evaluation of suspected type B aortic dissection are between 97% and 100% and 94% and 98%, respectively.‡ Limitations of TEE include dependence on an experienced interpretation of the findings and limited capability to assess abdominal branch vessel involvement and extent of the dissection below the diaphragm; if the patient is very small or very thin, as in Japan, the takeoff of the celiac axis, superior mesenteric artery, and occasionally one or both renal arteries can be visualized with TEE.

Currently, MRI does not play a major diagnostic role in patients with acute dissection because these individuals are often critically ill and connected to various monitoring devices, infusion pumps, or respirators.[7,32] In the acute setting, the limited 24-hour availability, the relatively long time necessary for image acquisition, and the limited access to the patient during the procedure make MRI much less practical than other diagnostic modalities. Nevertheless, MRI can delineate noninvasively the entire thoracoabdominal aorta and demonstrate the intimal flap, both aortic channels, and involvement of major aortic branches. As with CTA, the most important criterion for the diagnosis of acute aortic dissection with MRI is the identification of two distinct flow lumens separated by an intimal flap.[56] Many investigators have reported that MRI is associated with high sensitivity and specificity in the evaluation of suspected aortic dissection, both in the range of 95% to 100%.§ For suspected acute type B dissection, Nienaber and coworkers[59] observed that MRI had a sensitivity of 97% and a specificity of 100%. Today, magnetic resonance scans are most useful for serial, long-term follow-up of patients with chronic aortic dissections, including postoperative patients and those initially treated medically.

Contrast aortography historically was the "gold standard" in the diagnosis of aortic dissection (Fig. 71-3).[65] Angiography, however, is invasive, is time-consuming, and necessitates the use of contrast material; moreover, it is not infallible, and the technique carries a risk of morbidity and mortality, but it can provide detailed information about perfusion status of important aortic branches.[32,56,66] Angiographic diagnosis of acute dissection requires identification of a double lumen or an intimal flap; indirect signs that are suggestive of an acute dissection include compression of the true channel by an expanding false lumen, thickening of the aortic wall,

*References 3, 5, 7, 10, 11, 29, and 56-62.
†References 3, 5, 7, 11, 29, 56, 59, and 63.
‡References 3, 5, 7, 11, 29, 56, and 59-63.
§References 3, 5, 7, 11, 29, 56, and 59-64.

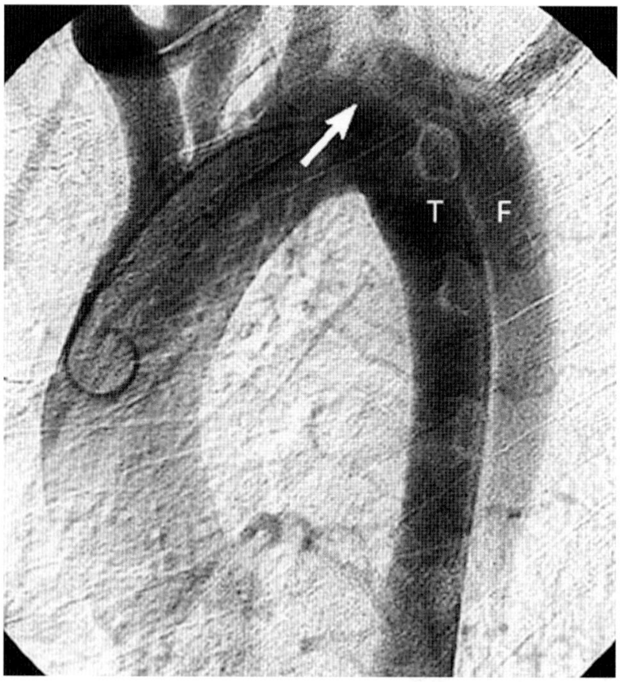

FIGURE 71-3 ■ Aortographic findings in acute type B aortic dissection. The true aortic lumen (T) is extrinsically narrowed by the false lumen (F). The true lumen is characteristically smaller and located medially. Note that the pigtail angiographic catheter has been passed up the true lumen from below. The primary intimal tear *(arrow)* is located just distal to the left subclavian artery.

ulcer-like projection in the aortic wall (in cases of penetrating atherosclerotic ulcer), and abnormal position of the guidewire or catheter in the aorta.[26,27,56,65] Biplane angiographic studies of the thoracic aorta are mandatory because single-plane aortography can miss important findings; false-negative results can also occur when the false lumen is thrombosed and in cases of IMH.[5,27,56] The sensitivity and specificity of aortography in the evaluation of aortic dissection range between 80% and 90% and 85% and 95%, respectively.[5,7,29,56] Currently, aortography is reserved for patients with acute type B dissection presenting with clinical evidence of malperfusion or those with persistent peripheral vascular complications after proximal aortic repair to delineate the mechanism of aortic branch vessel compromise and guide subsequent appropriate endovascular interventions to restore distal perfusion.‖

MANAGEMENT

Strategy

The aim of therapy in patients with aortic dissection is to prevent death and irreversible end-organ damage. As discussed in Chapter 70, almost all patients with acute type A dissection should be considered for emergency surgical repair of the ascending thoracic aorta.[2,3,5,7] In contrast, the optimal treatment strategy for patients

BOX 71-1 Firm or Relative Indications for Surgical or Endovascular Intervention in Patients with Acute Type B Aortic Dissection

Persistent pain
Refractory arterial hypertension
Progression or expansion of dissection
Aortic rupture or impending rupture
Evidence of impaired distal organ perfusion
Sizable localized false aneurysm
Connective tissue disorders (Early surgical intervention to be strongly considered)

with acute type B dissection continues to be debated.¶ In 1965, Wheat and Palmer and colleagues[15] recommended medical "anti-impulse" therapy for acute aortic dissection, and in 1970, Daily and colleagues[20] from Stanford concluded that there was no major difference in early outcome between patients treated medically and those treated surgically. The rationale behind medical management is based on three observations: (1) medical therapy prevents early death in most patients[1,5-7,31,73]; (2) operative mortality for patients with acute type B dissections requiring emergency operations has been relatively high[6,7,31,43]; and (3) long-term outcome has been similar for patients treated medically or surgically.[1-3,6,7,73]

Today, most groups favor a complication-specific approach for patients with acute type B dissections (Box 71-1), reserving surgical or endovascular intervention on the descending aorta for those with rupture, thoracoabdominal malperfusion, impending rupture, or other life-threatening complications. In the past, other "soft" indications included persistent pain and refractory hypertension, but these are too subjective and have been discarded by the FDA in the new registries for TEVAR.[1-7,10,11,70,71] These are clinical indications and do not include offering asymptomatic patients a semi-elective TEVAR simply because it may help promote aortic remodeling over time, as was the case in the INSTEAD trial.[74,75] On the other hand, we and some other groups have advocated consideration of early surgical replacement of the descending aorta for selected patients with acute type B dissections who are young and otherwise good operative candidates, irrespective of the presence or absence of complications; this includes predominantly patients with connective tissue disorders such as Marfan syndrome and Loeys-Dietz syndrome.[7-9,68,76,77] If the operation is successful, these patients theoretically should be at lower risk of sustaining late dissection-related complications or requiring aortic reoperation.

The Stanford aortic dissection classification concept has also been applied to IMH because the prognostic impact of the location and its treatment have been considered comparable to those in patients with a classic aortic dissection.[27,47,78] It is generally accepted that patients with IMH involving the descending thoracic aorta (type B IMH) can usually be successfully managed conservatively with aggressive blood pressure control in

‖References 16, 17, 29, 55, 56, and 67.

¶References 1-10, 17, 18, 20, 32, and 68-72.

the absence of disease progression.** Several groups have reported, however, that the prognosis of markedly symptomatic patients with penetrating ulcers located in the descending thoracic aorta and type B IMH coexistent with a deep PAU was worse than the prognosis of those with classic aortic dissection because of a higher incidence of aortic rupture.[26,27,48] In these cases, early surgical or endovascular treatment should be considered, especially if persistent pain, increasing pleural effusion, and a large, deep PAU are present.

Initial Medical Treatment

As soon as acute aortic dissection is suspected, emergency medical therapy should be initiated and continued while the diagnostic procedures are performed.[5,7,32] The cornerstone of modern medical therapy, as originally described by Wheat and collaborators, is reduction of mean, peak, and diastolic recoil arterial pressure and the rate of rise of arterial pressure or aortic dP/dt (*not* left ventricular dP/dt) to the lowest acceptable level while adequate cerebral, coronary, and renal perfusion is maintained.[5,7,14,15,29] The goals of medical treatment are to relieve pain, to control systemic blood pressure, and to limit extension of the dissection. Reasonable targets are a heart rate less than 60 bpm and a systolic blood pressure between 100 and 120 mm Hg.[10] Intensive, continuous monitoring of the patient in an intensive care unit is important, including electrocardiography and insertion of indwelling radial or femoral arterial and central venous lines. A urinary bladder catheter and a pulse oximeter are used. Intravenous beta blockers (e.g., esmolol, metoprolol, labetalol, propranolol) are administered in small boluses or as a continuous intravenous infusion; if needed, an intravenous vasodilator infusion, most commonly sodium nitroprusside, is then added. Labetalol, an α_1-adrenergic and nonspecific β-adrenergic antagonist, is a good alternative to a combination of agents. Parenteral calcium channel antagonists, such as diltiazem, nifedipine, and nicardipine, that lower arterial blood pressure and left ventricular dP/dt can also be used. It must be remembered that because sodium nitroprusside, angiotensin-converting enzyme inhibitors (e.g., enalapril, lisinopril), and angiotensin receptor blockers are pure arteriolar vasodilators, these agents increase aortic dP/dt; therefore, concomitant administration of a negative inotropic agent is essential. If surgical intervention or percutaneous endovascular treatment is carried out, antihypertensive and negative inotropic therapy is continued during anesthetic induction, intraoperatively, and postoperatively.

Definitive Long-term Medical Management

Whether the patient is initially treated medically or surgically, the intravenous antihypertensive and negative inotropic drugs are gradually transitioned to oral agents during the hospitalization. An oral beta blocker (e.g., labetalol, metoprolol succinate [Toprol-XL], atenolol) or, if a beta blocker is not tolerated, a calcium channel antagonist like verapamil or nicardipine is preferentially used and continued indefinitely, complemented by an oral angiotensin-converting enzyme inhibitor or an angiotensin receptor blocker. Recent data from the IRAD investigators suggest that the use of a calcium channel antagonist at discharge from the hospital was associated with improved long-term survival in patients with type B aortic dissection treated medically.[79] Because it is incorporated into mucopolysaccharides of the media and may weaken the aortic wall,[7] hydralazine should be avoided, as should any drug that increases aortic dP/dt. Conversely, there is some unpublished evidence (Harry C. Dietz, Johns Hopkins University, personal communication) that in genetic mouse models of the Marfan syndrome, hydralazine has salutary effects on aortic wall remodeling.

OPERATIVE APPROACH

Acute Type B Dissections

The goal of surgical treatment of patients with acute type B aortic dissection is graft replacement of a limited segment of the descending thoracic aorta, including the site of the primary intimal tear.[7] At Stanford, after induction of general anesthesia, insertion of a double-lumen endobronchial tube, and usually a lumbar intrathecal catheter for cerebrospinal fluid drainage, patients with acute type B dissections are explored through a left posterolateral thoracotomy.[7,66] Our preference calls for total cardiopulmonary bypass (CPB) by advancing a long right femoral venous catheter into the right atrium from the *right* femoral vein and, if possible, *antegrade* arterial CPB perfusion. This can be accomplished using a short 6-mm vascular graft sewn end to side to the left subclavian or left carotid artery; inserting an arterial cannula into the undissected ascending aorta or arch or into the descending aortic true lumen and advancing it using TEE guidance over a guidewire into the ascending aorta, or into the left ventricular apex and across the aortic valve (Wada and Kazui method of left ventricular apical aortic CPB perfusion); fluoroscopically manipulating a long, small venous cannula (e.g., 15 Fr) over a stiff guidewire up into the undissected ascending aorta or arch via the femoral artery; or, as a last resort, cannulating the femoral artery on the side that is perfused by the aortic true lumen (almost always the one with the reduced or absent pulse).[80,81] On occasion, if a venous cannula cannot be passed from the femoral vein, an angled venous cannula can be placed through the main pulmonary artery into the right ventricle to provide (or to augment) venous CPB return. Moderate systemic hypothermia (bladder temperature, 25° to 28° C; tympanic membrane temperature, 20° to 22° C) is generally used such that an open proximal anastomosis can be performed in the distal arch during a brief period of hypothermic circulatory arrest. After the open proximal anastomosis is completed, reperfusion to the head and heart is then immediately started using a side limb off the aortic graft or inserting a metal right-angle cannula into the proximal graft. Hypothermic circulatory arrest is also used in almost all cases of chronic type B dissections to facilitate

**References 9-10, 24, 27, 29, 30, 47, and 78.

the proximal anastomosis in the arch, allowing the chronic arch flap to be safely excised along with evacuation of any thrombus in the false lumen. The circulatory arrest times are longer and unpredictable in these chronic cases, and having the left carotid artery cannulated for antegrade selective cerebral perfusion can be useful (the Siena technique popularized by Neri and coworkers).[82,83] The patient is placed in a steep Trendelenburg position, and uncontrolled venous retroperfusion backward up the venous cannula at 500 to 1000 mL/min is used during hypothermic circulatory arrest to keep the left side of the heart and ascending aorta free of air. Some of this venous retroperfusion trickles back down into the arch through the arch branches. No preliminary proximal or distal aortic dissection is done, and no aortic cross-clamps are applied either proximally or distally. When the pump is turned down, the proximal aorta is opened and transected after mobilization of the phrenic, vagus, and recurrent laryngeal nerves. In acute type B cases, an open proximal anastomosis is performed with a 4-0 BB 54-inch or 5-0 C1 polypropylene suture incorporating a full-thickness aortic cuff (thereby reapproximating the aortic intima and adventitia and obliterating any proximal false lumen) at the distal arch level. An arterial perfusion cannula is then inserted directly into a single side branch of the aortic graft. After arch de-airing, CPB perfusion to the head and the heart is resumed, with care taken to evacuate any air trapped in the heart or ascending aorta. After 5 to 10 minutes of cold CPB reperfusion, systemic warming is started. Proximal intercostal arteries are oversewn. A conservative segment of descending aorta containing the primary intimal tear and the most severe associated injury is replaced with a woven double velour Dacron Hemashield graft. Continuous 4-0 BB or 4-0 SH-1 polypropylene suture and use of deep suture bites—again, with care to incorporate both aortic layers and to obliterate the false lumen in acute dissection cases—is used for the distal anastomosis.[7] Although we have avoided using Teflon felt for the past 20 years at Stanford, the proximal or distal aorta can be reinforced with strips of Teflon felt or bovine pericardium or, alternatively, by using a small amount of tissue adhesive between the dissected layers, such as BioGlue (CryoLife, Inc., Kennesaw, GA). The proximal cross-clamp is released, air is evacuated, and the anastomoses are checked for hemostasis. After systemic rewarming to a target of 35° to 36° C, CPB is discontinued. Protamine sulfate is administered after all anastomoses are judged to be technically satisfactory with minimal bleeding. Platelets, fresh-frozen plasma, and cryoprecipitate are used if diffuse hemorrhage from suture lines and raw surfaces are evident after a normal activated clotting time is achieved if abnormal coagulation parameters are identified through use of rotational thromboelastography.

Postoperative management of the patient involves intensive monitoring, including serial abdominal, neurologic, and pulse examinations, as well as strict blood pressure control. Cerebrospinal fluid is drained continuously to keep cerebrospinal fluid pressure lower than 10 mm Hg. In patients without spinal cord injury, the drain is removed on the second or third postoperative day. With use of partial CPB (without hypothermic circulatory arrest in that era) and confining the extent of resection to a short aortic segment, the incidence of new postoperative paraplegia in our earlier experience was only 4% in patients with acute type B dissections.[43] We believe that our current method using hypothermic circulatory arrest for an open proximal anastomosis has reduced the incidence of stroke and spinal cord injury.

Management of Peripheral Vascular Complications

The Stanford approach in patients presenting with aortic dissection and ischemic peripheral vascular complications before the advent of endovascular stent grafts (TEVAR) was to proceed initially with surgical repair of the thoracic aorta because central aortic repair usually obviated the need for peripheral revascularization procedures.[7,53] The operative mortality rate for patients with all types of peripheral vascular compromise was no higher than that for those without such complications; however, visceral ischemia and impaired renal perfusion portended a high risk of death. If persistent mesenteric, renal, or limb ischemia was detected after thoracic aortic repair, surgical fenestration of the distal descending thoracic aorta or suprarenal abdominal aorta or direct revascularization was traditionally attempted as a lifesaving maneuver.[7,53,54,84] Today, percutaneous endovascular treatment is the preferred initial intervention in cases of postoperative malperfusion and also in high-risk patients with complicated acute type B dissections (see Chapter 72).[††] Endovascular interventions using bare stents in the collapsed true lumen in the aorta or one of its branches or flap fenestration of the aortic dissection flap (to increase flow in the distal true lumen by decompressing the false lumen) can usually reestablish adequate end-organ perfusion in most cases.[49,85] These endovascular approaches are described in detail in Chapter 72. In the past 2 decades, endovascular stent grafts have been used increasingly in patients with complicated acute type B dissections to cover the primary intimal tear in the thoracic aorta and to restore blood flow in the distal aortic true lumen, which can be "obliterated" or "collapsed"; this successfully relieved distal ischemia in 76% of all compromised aortic branches (and 100% of those with dynamic obstruction).[17,86]

Endovascular Stent Grafts

Since 1996, endovascular stent grafts have been used in selected patients with acute type B aortic dissections at Stanford.[17] The Stanford University and Mie University combined series showed that endovascular stent graft repair in patients with complicated acute type B dissections was associated with an encouraging early mortality rate of only 16%. The long-term effectiveness and durability of this new therapeutic approach, however, remain unknown. In 2008 and 2010, the Society of Thoracic Surgeons and the American Heart Association published practice guidelines for the management of patients with descending thoracic aortic disease. These guidelines include potential indications for endovascular stent graft treatment based on existing observational studies and opinions of experts.[10,11,87] Acute type B aortic dissection

[††]References 10-11, 49, 50, 55, 85, and 86.

with life-threatening complications and acutely symptomatic IMH with or without penetrating ulcer of the descending thoracic aorta were identified as situations in which endovascular stent graft repair seemed justified.[10,87] Endovascular stent graft coverage of the primary intimal tear, however, is more a temporary resuscitation therapy allowing stabilization of very sick patients rather than a curative procedure; late complications and the need for reintervention are not unusual. Nonetheless, emergency stent grafting can be lifesaving in patients with severe malperfusion even though the therapeutic goal is not to eliminate all blood flow from the false lumen, as is the case in treating thoracic aortic aneurysms. Later sequelae of the dissection can be treated definitively with open surgical repair or additional endovascular interventions if necessary when the patient is not in extremis. Rigorous prospective controlled comparison of this interventional stent graft approach with conventional emergency surgical treatment (for complicated type B dissections) or with medical therapy (for uncomplicated type B dissections) is not yet available. One study, the INSTEAD trial, enrolled 140 patients with uncomplicated subacute or chronic (14 to 52 weeks) type B aortic dissections who were randomized to best medical therapy versus stent graft treatment. All-cause mortality at 2 years was higher in the stent graft limb group, but the difference did not reach statistical significance.[74] Additionally, freedom from aorta-related mortality and freedom from progressive aortic disease (a composite endpoint for aortic death, conversion, or additional intervention) was comparable between groups. Despite the absence of clinical benefit, thoracic false lumen thrombosis occurred in 91% of the patients in the stent graft group versus 19% of those receiving medical therapy, a highly significant difference. A recent update of INSTEAD reported significantly lower aorta-related mortality and disease progression (a composite endpoint for conversion, additional intervention, or aortic expansion) at 5 years in the stent graft treatment arm.[75] The ADSORB trial, a second randomized study, compared treatment with a Gore TAG stent graft versus best medical treatment alone in 61 patients with acute (<2 weeks) uncomplicated type B dissections.[88] The study endpoints had to be changed and the trial ended prematurely because of inadequate patient enrollment rates. There were no differences in clinical outcomes, including death, at 1 year, but false lumen thrombosis in the descending thoracic aorta occurred much more frequently in the TEVAR subgroup than in the medically treated subgroup (57% vs. 3%). Endovascular stent graft treatment of aortic dissection is discussed in detail in Chapter 72.

Chronic Type B Dissections

Surgical intervention for patients with chronic type B dissection is considered when they have symptoms related to the dissection (e.g., pain or symptoms secondary to compression of adjacent anatomic structures, renovascular hypertension [with or without renal dysfunction], mesenteric ischemia, claudication) or if documented expansion of the false lumen occurs. Asymptomatic patients with large chronic aortic dissections (exceeding 55 to 60 mm in diameter) are also offered surgical graft replacement if they are reasonable surgical candidates. In addition to maximal aortic diameter and symptoms, consideration of other risk factors that modulate the expected risk of aortic rupture, such as increasing age, connective tissue disorders, uncontrolled hypertension, and chronic obstructive pulmonary disease, is also important to determine the optimal timing for operation and to enhance selection of patients.[89,90]

Open operative surgical graft replacement is conducted similarly to that described before for patients with acute type B aortic dissections, including our CPB perfusion strategy. In these chronic dissection cases, it is even more important whenever feasible to avoid retrograde arterial CPB perfusion from the femoral artery during systemic cooling, as this can blow debris and thrombus from the aortic true or false lumen up into the arch branches and brain or coronary arteries. Furthermore, retrograde femoral arterial CPB perfusion in patients with a chronic dissection is uncontrolled and unpredictable because CPB flow may not necessarily reach all important aortic tributaries, depending on dynamic motion of the dissection flap and local pathoanatomic factors. Deep hypothermic circulatory arrest also makes reattachment of important lower intercostal arteries as Carrel patches safer and helps protect the visceral organs and spinal cord. If the entire thoracoabdominal aorta (Crawford extent II) is being replaced, as is often necessary in young patients with connective tissue disorders and chronic type A or B aortic dissection, we cool the patient to 15° to 20° C (bladder), and CPB rewarming is not begun until all important intercostal arteries have been reimplanted down to the level of the celiac axis. CPB reperfusion is commenced both proximally (with a cannula inserted into a side branch of the proximal graft) and from below with use of either a femoral artery or a cannula in the distal thoracoabdominal aorta graft after completion of the most distal aortic or iliac anastomosis. In chronic dissection cases, we excise the dissection flap in the arch proximally and in the distal descending thoracic aorta. Because the chronic dissection usually extends down into the abdominal aorta, in replacing only the descending thoracic aorta, we frequently use the "elephant trunk" graft technique distally such that if downstream thoracoabdominal aortic replacement should become necessary, the new graft is simply sewn to the dangling elephant trunk graft proximally. It is important in using an elephant trunk graft in patients with aortic dissections to make sure that the dissection flap distally has been excised for a distance exceeding the length of the planned elephant trunk graft to avoid inadvertent trapping of the graft into one lumen or the other.

RESULTS

Comparison of Results of Surgical and Medical Treatment

Historical Perspective

The controversy about the optimal therapy for patients with aortic dissections dates to the 1960s, when DeBakey and colleagues reported results in 179 patients treated surgically with an early mortality rate of 21% and a

5-year survival rate of 50%.[91] DeBakey and colleagues concluded that all patients with aortic dissection should undergo surgical intervention. Importantly, careful inspection of this paper subsequently revealed a skewed patient population; only 38% of the patients had an acute dissection, and most had a DeBakey type III (Stanford type B) dissection. Wheat and Palmer and colleagues[15] then proposed a selective approach to the management of patients with acute dissection, arguing for medical treatment with a combination of agents that decreased arterial blood pressure and also the rate of rise of aortic pressure (aortic dP/dt). In 1970, Daily and colleagues[20] introduced the Stanford type A/B dissection classification system and observed no major difference in early outcome in patients with type B dissections treated medically or surgically. In a 1979 Stanford paper, the early results from 11 studies published in the 1970s were analyzed. The overall mortality rate in this era was 33% in medically treated patients (range, 21% to 67%), and the average operative mortality rate for patients with acute type B dissections treated surgically was 36%.[92] Of course, the patient cohorts differed considerably, which confounded critical comparison of outcomes. Thereafter, the consensus opinion has been that most patients with acute type B dissections should be treated medically, unless life-threatening dissection-related complications are present.[‡‡]

Contemporary Comparative Studies of Surgical versus Medical Treatment

No prospective controlled trials comparing surgical with medical management of patients with acute type B dissections have been carried out; however, comprehensive comparative retrospective analyses, including a 2002 report by Umaña and associates from Stanford, have been published.[1,6,39] Strict interpretation of the results of these two treatment modalities is difficult because of a marked disparity in the clinical characteristics of the medical and surgical cohorts, which created a pronounced selection bias. In most series, patients with uncomplicated acute type B dissections are treated medically, whereas those presenting with life-threatening complications or developing complications while being treated medically are treated with TEVAR.

A 1984 report from the Massachusetts General Hospital concluded that early survival in patients presenting with an acute type B dissection was determined primarily by the number and severity of presenting complications due to the dissection, irrespective of mode of treatment.[39] In the 1989 combined Stanford and Duke University study, 136 patients with acute type B dissections between 1975 and 1988 were treated medically (63%) or surgically (37%); patients treated medically tended to have more comorbidities or renal disease, whereas those in the surgical cohort were more likely to have aortic rupture or arch involvement.[6,71] Sequential analyses were performed to adjust for differences in baseline characteristics to separate patients with acute dissections into three subgroups: all patients (subset I), patients presenting without compelling indications for emergency operation (subset II), and those individuals from subset II who did not have severe comorbidities (subset III). This last cohort represented low-risk, uncomplicated patients who could have been treated either medically or surgically. For all patients, the statistically significant independent determinants of overall mortality were aortic rupture, other dissection-related complications, increasing age, and cardiac disease. Treatment method was not a predictor of outcome in any subset. In the low-risk subset of patients (subset III), moreover, the early mortality rate was similar between the medically and surgically treated patients (16% vs. 9%), as was the long-term survival rate. More recently, a 36-year review of the Stanford experience including 189 patients with acute type B dissections used propensity score analysis to identify subsets of patients treated either medically or surgically who were at similar risks of death. The impact of treatment method on survival, reoperation, and late aortic complications or death was then determined in these more homogeneous samples to neutralize bias.[1] This statistical analysis identified 142 well-matched patients who did not have any compelling emergency surgical indications (111 were treated medically and 31 underwent operation). Long-term survival was similar in the two matched groups. Freedom from aortic reintervention and from late aortic complication or death was also comparable between the medically treated and surgical subsets. In all patients, multivariable analyses did not identify treatment method as a predictor of outcome; instead, patient-related factors and dissection-specific complications determined the prognosis.

Current Results

Early Survival

During the past 30 years, advances in diagnostic imaging modalities, medical critical care, anesthetic expertise, and surgical techniques have allowed clinicians to make the definitive diagnosis more quickly and have improved early survival rate of patients with acute type B aortic dissection treated medically or surgically.[§§] In the 2000 IRAD review of 175 patients with acute type B dissections treated in 12 centers between 1996 and 1998, the 30-day mortality rate was 11% in medically treated patients and 31% in patients who underwent surgery; of course, the two patient cohorts were markedly different.[31] Similarly, in two more recent IRAD reports focusing on a large cohort of patients with acute type B aortic dissection, it was shown that the early mortality rate of patients treated medically was now lower than 10%; those requiring surgical intervention for acute aortic dissection–related complications, including aortic rupture and shock, had an early mortality rate closer to 30%.[98,99] Interestingly, in the small group of patients treated with endovascular TEVAR for complicated aortic dissections, in-hospital complications occurred in 20% (compared

‡‡References 2, 3, 10, 19, 32, 51, 66, 73, and 93-95.

§§References 4, 5, 7, 8, 29, 30, 52, 71, 95-97.

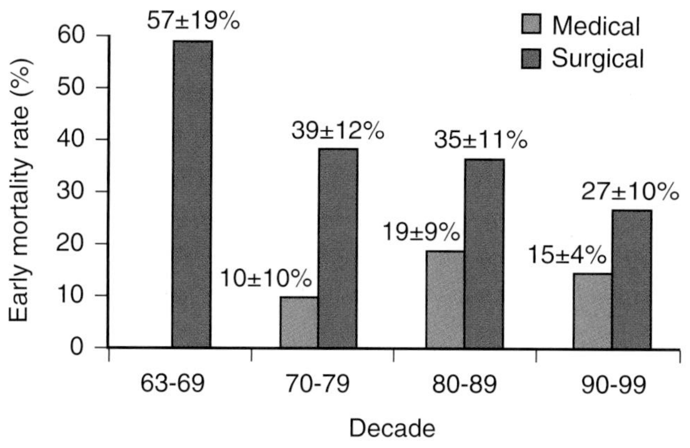

FIGURE 71-4 Early (30-day) mortality rates illustrated as a function of time (decades) and broken down into medical and surgical subgroups in the overall Stanford experience. (From Umaña JP, Lai DT, Mitchell RS, et al: Is medical therapy still the optimal treatment strategy for patients with acute type B aortic dissections? *J Thorac Cardiovasc Surg* 124:896–910, 2002.)

with 40% of the patients treated surgically) and the mortality rate was only 11%, both significantly lower than after surgical treatment.[99] In the 2002 Stanford paper, the early mortality rate for patients treated medically did not change significantly between 1970 and 1999, ranging from 10% to 19% (Fig. 71-4).[1] On the other hand, the early mortality rate for patients treated surgically decreased from 57% in the 1960s to 27% in the 1990s. Other centers with special expertise in thoracic aortic surgery also demonstrated that early mortality rates closer to 20% can be achieved in the current era in selected patients with acute type B dissections.[10,100] In an earlier Stanford investigation, multivariable analysis revealed that the independent determinants of operative risk in patients with type B dissections (acute or chronic) were renal or visceral ischemia, aortic rupture, and older age.[43] Acute type B dissection caused by an intimal tear located in the arch, whether the patient was treated medically or surgically, was associated with high early mortality rates in a subsequent Duke-Stanford cooperative 1989 report.[6] In Crawford's surgical experience, the independent risk factors portending operative death were earlier year of operation, surgery within 24 hours of onset of symptoms, and chronic obstructive pulmonary disease.[95] In the IRAD registry, independent predictors of in-hospital mortality in the overall cohort were hypotension or shock, absence of pain on presentation, and branch vessel involvement; age older than 70 years and hypotension or shock were independent predictors of mortality in the subgroup of patients requiring surgical intervention.[52,98]

Late Survival

In the 36-year overall Stanford experience, actuarial survival for the entire patient cohort was 71%, 60%, 35%, and 17% at 1 year, 5 years, 10 years, and 15 years, respectively.[1] As illustrated in Figure 71-5*A*, there was no significant difference in survival between the medical and surgical patients. Multivariable analyses identified shock, visceral ischemia, arch involvement, aortic rupture, stroke, previous sternotomy, pulmonary disease, and female gender as significant, independent predictors of overall death. In the Baylor series, actuarial survival after surgical repair of type B dissections was 76%, 54%, and 35% at 1 year, 5 years, and 10 years, respectively; independent determinants of late death were earlier year of operation, older age, severe symptoms, higher New York Heart Association functional class, extent of aorta replaced, type of procedure, residual aneurysmal disease, and postoperative complications.[95] More recent midterm data from IRAD indicated that 3-year survival of patients discharged alive from the hospital was 78% for those treated medically, 82% with surgical treatment, and 76% with endovascular techniques (P = NS).[100] Predictors of late death were female gender, prior aortic aneurysm, history of atherosclerosis, in-hospital renal failure, in-hospital pleural effusion, and hypotension or shock during hospitalization.

Congestive heart failure, renal failure, stroke, and cancer accounted for almost 50% of the late deaths in patients with acute type B dissections in the Stanford series, emphasizing the importance of patient-specific factors in determining their long-term prognosis.[1] Rupture of a contiguous or remote segment of the aorta was responsible for 16% of late deaths in this Stanford series, compared with 29% of late deaths in the 20-year long-term follow-up study from DeBakey and coworkers.[21] This sobering figure should be amenable to improvement if more diligent patient follow-up imaging surveillance and medical care are provided.

Aortic Reintervention

The actuarial freedom from late aortic reoperation and late aortic-related complications after treatment of acute type B dissection in the overall Stanford experience is illustrated in Figure 71-5*B-D*. Surprisingly, there was no significant difference in reoperation rate between patients treated medically and those treated surgically.[1] After 5 years, reoperation was necessary in 14% of the medical group and 13% of the surgical patients; at 10 years, reoperation was necessary in 17% of both groups. The only independent predictor of late aortic reoperation was Marfan syndrome, underscoring the fragility of the dissected aorta in these patients. In Crawford's 1990 study analyzing a 33-year experience with surgical management of aortic dissection (type A or B, acute or chronic), 22% of patients required aortic reoperation 10 years later and 88% were free from aortic rupture.[95] Residual aneurysmal disease, no cardioplegia (probably indicative of improved surgical techniques over time), and preoperative New York Heart Association functional class were the determinants of late aortic rupture; a higher likelihood of reoperation was significantly linked to earlier year of operation, previous proximal aortic procedure, aortic cross-clamp time, and more limited surgical procedures that have been abandoned (e.g., primary repair, aortoplasty, patch repair). In a retrospective analysis of 101 patients with uncomplicated acute type B dissections treated medically, Marui and colleagues[70,101] from Japan reported that patent false lumen, aortic diameter exceeding 40 mm, and fusiform dilation of the proximal

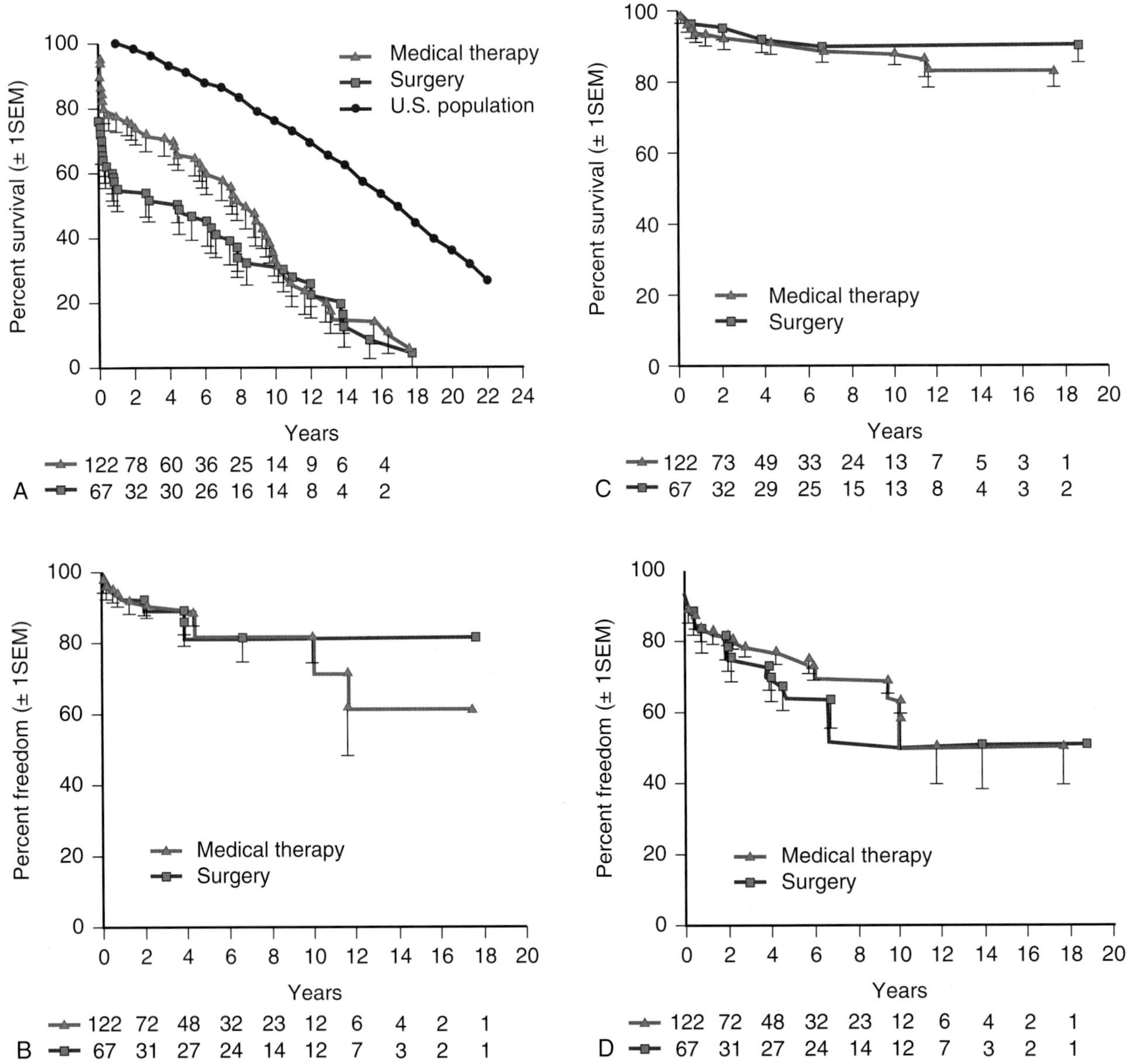

FIGURE 71-5 ■ **A,** Actuarial survival for all patients with acute type B dissections subdivided according to initial treatment method. There was no statistically significant difference in survival between those treated surgically and those treated medically. For perspective, this graph also portrays the survival curve for the age- and gender-matched U.S. population; this indicates that only 35% of patients this age can be expected to be alive 20 years later. **B,** Actuarial freedom from late aortic reoperation (defined as surgical procedures related to the aorta or to complications of the dissection) subdivided according to initial treatment. There was no statistically significant difference between treatment modalities. **C,** Freedom from reoperation for all patients, expressed in actual (or observed cumulative frequency) terms. **D,** Actuarial freedom from late aortic-related complications or death for all 189 patients. (From Umaña JP, Lai DT, Mitchell RS, et al: Is medical therapy still the optimal treatment strategy for patients with acute type B aortic dissections? *J Thorac Cardiovasc Surg* 124:896–910, 2002.)

descending aorta were predictors of late aortic events; these authors recommended that such patients be considered for early surgical intervention.

FOLLOW-UP

In patients with acute type B aortic dissection, whether they were initially treated medically or surgically, an early predischarge CTA or MRI scan is mandatory to rule out early complications and to serve as a baseline reference. During the first few weeks, these patients require close outpatient medical care; attention should be focused on blood pressure control and cerebral, cardiac, and renal function.[7,29] Periodic imaging studies of the entire thoracic and abdominal aorta are essential indefinitely to detect aortic complications, such as aneurysmal degeneration of the downstream aortic false lumen, before rupture or death. Attention should also be paid to the patency of the false lumen because it is now known that partial thrombosis of the false lumen (as opposed to patent false lumen or complete thrombosis of the false lumen) is associated with higher mortality than in patients with a patent false lumen.[102] Our protocol calls for the interval between imaging studies to be lengthened gradually from 3 to 6 months during the first year after the acute event if no worrisome interval changes are detected, then annually thereafter. Lifelong rigorous blood pressure control and negative inotropic therapy are also critically important. In DeBakey and colleagues' 1982 report,[21] late aneurysmal formation occurred in 45% of patients with poor blood pressure control, compared with 17% of those with well-controlled hypertension. A combination of conventional antihypertensive agents and negative inotropic medications is usually required and needs to be continued indefinitely, even in normotensive patients.[79] Improvements in the follow-up management of these patients are still needed because mortality rates after discharge from the hospital are still higher than expected (almost one in four patients dying within the first 3 years), irrespective of initial treatment modality.[1,100]

REFERENCES

1. Umaña JP, Lai DT, Mitchell RS, et al: Is medical therapy still the optimal treatment strategy for patients with acute type B aortic dissections? *J Thorac Cardiovasc Surg* 124:896–910, 2002.
2. Crawford ES: The diagnosis and management of aortic dissection. *JAMA* 264:2537–2541, 1990.
3. Nienaber CA, Powell JT: Management of acute aortic syndromes. *Eur Heart J* 33:26–35, 2012.
4. Elefteriades JA, Lovoulos CJ, Coady MA, et al: Management of descending aortic dissection. *Ann Thorac Surg* 67:2002–2005, 1999.
5. Fann JI, Miller DC: Aortic dissection. *Ann Vasc Surg* 9:311–323, 1995.
6. Glower DD, Fann JI, Speier RH, et al: Comparison of medical and surgical therapy for uncomplicated descending aortic dissection. *Circulation* 82(Suppl IV):39–46, 1990.
7. Miller DC: Acute dissection of the descending thoracic aorta. *Chest Surg Clin North Am* 2:347–378, 1992.
8. Lansman SL, Hagl C, Fink D, et al: Acute type B aortic dissection: surgical therapy. *Ann Thorac Surg* 74:S1833–S1835, 2002.
9. Miller DC: Surgical management of acute aortic dissection: new data. *Semin Thorac Cardiovasc Surg* 3:225–237, 1991.
10. Coady MA, Ikonomidis JS, Cheung AT, et al: Surgical management of descending thoracic aortic disease: open and endovascular approaches: a scientific statement from the American Heart Association. *Circulation* 121:2780–2804, 2010.
11. Hiratzka LF, Bakris GL, Beckman JA, et al: 2010 ACCF/AHA/AATS/ASA/SCA/SCAI/SIR/ATS/SVM guidelines for the management of patients with thoracic aortic disease: executive summary. A report from the American College of Cardiology Foundation/American Heart Association Task Force on Practice Guidelines, American Association for Thoracic Surgery, American College of Radiology, American Stroke Association, Society of Cardiovascular Anesthesiologists, Society for Cardiovascular Angiography and Interventions, Society of Interventional Radiology, Society of Thoracic Surgeons, and Society for Vascular Medicine. *Circulation* e-266–e369, 2010.
12. Gurin D, Bulmer JW, Derby R: Dissecting aneurysm of aorta: diagnosis and operative relief of acute arterial obstruction due to this cause. *N Y State J Med* 35:1200–1202, 1935.
13. DeBakey ME, Cooley D, Creech O, Jr: Surgical considerations of dissecting aneurysm of the aorta. *Ann Surg* 142:586–612, 1955.
14. Cooley DA, DeBakey ME, Morris GC, Jr: Controlled extracorporeal circulation in surgical treatment of aortic aneurysm. *Ann Surg* 146:473, 1957.
15. Wheat MW, Palmer RF, Bantley TD, et al: Treatment of dissecting aneurysms of the aorta without surgery. *J Thorac Cardiovasc Surg* 50:364–373, 1965.
16. Slonim SM, Miller DC, Mitchell RS, et al: Percutaneous balloon fenestrating and stenting for life-threatening ischemic complications in patients with acute aortic dissection. *J Thorac Cardiovasc Surg* 117:1118–1127, 1999.
17. Dake MD, Kato N, Mitchell RS, et al: Endovascular stent-graft placement for the treatment of acute aortic dissection. *N Engl J Med* 340:1546–1552, 1999.
18. Nienaber CA, Fattori R, Lund G, et al: Nonsurgical reconstruction of thoracic aortic dissection by stent-graft placement. *N Engl J Med* 340:1539–1545, 1999.
19. Applebaum A, Karp RB, Kirklin JW: Ascending vs. descending aortic dissections. *Ann Surg* 183:296–300, 1976.
20. Daily PO, Trueblood HW, Stinson EB, et al: Management of acute aortic dissections. *Ann Thorac Surg* 10:237–247, 1970.
21. DeBakey ME, McCollum CH, Crawford ES, et al: Dissection and dissecting aneurysms of the aorta: twenty-year follow-up of five hundred and twenty-seven patients treated surgically. *Surgery* 92:1118–1134, 1982.
22. Ming RL, Najafi H, Javid H, et al: Acute ascending aortic dissection: surgical management. *Circulation* 64(Suppl II):II231–II234, 1981.
23. Slater EE: Aortic dissection: presentation and diagnosis. In Doroghazi RM, Slater EE, editors: *Aortic dissection*, New York, 1983, McGraw-Hill, pp 61–70.
24. Robbins RC, McManus RP, Mitchell RS, et al: Management of patients with intramural hematoma of the thoracic aorta. *Circulation* 88(Suppl II):II1–II10, 1993.
25. Stanson AW, Kazmier FJ, Hollier LH, et al: Penetrating atherosclerotic ulcers of the thoracic aorta: natural history and clinicopathologic correlations. *Ann Vasc Surg* 1:15–23, 1986.
26. Coady MA, Rizzo JA, Hammond GL, et al: Penetrating ulcer of the thoracic aorta: What is it? How do we recognize it? How do we manage it? *J Vasc Surg* 27:1006–1016, 1998.
27. Ganaha F, Miller DC, Sugimoto K, et al: Prognosis of aortic intramural hematoma with and without penetrating atherosclerotic ulcer. A clinical and radiologic analysis. *Circulation* 106:342–348, 2002.
28. Hirst AE, Johns VJ, Krime SJ: Dissecting aneurysm of the aorta: a review of 505 cases. *Medicine* 37:217–279, 1958.
29. Tsai TT, Nienaber CA, Eagle KA: Acute aortic syndromes. *Circulation* 112:3802–3813, 2005.
30. Fann JI, Smith JA, Miller DC, et al: Surgical management of aortic dissection during a 30-year period. *Circulation* 92(Suppl II):II113–II121, 1995.
31. Hagan PG, Nienaber CA, Isselbacher EM, et al: The international registry of acute aortic dissection (IRAD). *JAMA* 283:897–903, 2000.
32. DeSanctis RW, Eagle KA: Aortic dissection. *Curr Probl Cardiol* 14:227–278, 1989.
33. Anagnostopoulos CE, Prabhakar MJS, Vittle CF: Aortic dissections and dissecting aneurysms. *Am J Cardiol* 30:263–273, 1972.
34. Lindsay J, Jr, Hurst JW: Clinical features and prognosis in dissecting aneurysms of the aorta: a re-appraisal. *Circulation* 35:880–888, 1967.
35. Clouse WD, Hallett JW, Schaff HV, et al: Acute aortic dissection: population-based incidence compared with degenerative aortic aneurysm rupture. *Mayo Clin Proc* 79:176–180, 2004.
36. Olssen C, Thelin S, Stahle E, et al: Thoracic aortic aneurysm and dissection. Increasing prevalence and improved outcomes reported in a nationwide population-based study of more than 14000 cases from 1987 to 2002. *Circulation* 114:2611–2618, 2006.
37. Roberts CS, Roberts WC: Aortic dissection with entrance tear in the descending thoracic aorta: analysis of 40 necropsy patients. *Ann Surg* 231:356–368, 1991.
38. Schlatmann TJM, Becker AE: Histologic changes in the normal aging aorta. Implications for dissecting aortic aneurysm. *Am J Cardiol* 39:13–20, 1977.
39. Schlatmann TJM, Becker AE: Pathogenesis of dissecting aneurysm of the aorta. Comparative histopathologic study of significance of medial changes. *Am J Cardiol* 39:21–26, 1977.
40. Larson EW, Edwards WD: Risk factors for aortic dissection: a necropsy study of 161 cases. *Am J Cardiol* 53:849–855, 1984.
41. Hirst AE, Gore I: Is cystic medionecrosis the cause of dissecting aortic aneurysm? *Am Heart J* 53:915–916, 1976.
42. Roberts WC: Aortic dissection: anatomy, consequences, and cause. *Am Heart J* 101:195–214, 1981.
43. Miller DC, Mitchell RS, Oyer PE, et al: Independent determinants of operative mortality for patients with aortic dissections. *Circulation* 70(Suppl I):I153–I164, 1984.
44. Farber A, Wagner WH, Cossman DV, et al: Isolated dissection of the abdominal aorta: clinical presentation and therapeutic options. *J Vasc Surg* 36:205–210, 2002.

45. Trimarchi S, Tsai TT, Eagle KA, et al: Acute abdominal aortic dissection: insight from the International Registry of Acute Aortic Dissection. *J Vasc Surg* 46:913–919, 2007.
46. Evangelista A, Mukherjee D, Mehta RH, et al: Acute intramural hematoma of the aorta. A mystery in evolution. *Circulation* 111:1063–1070, 2005.
47. Cho RK, Stanson AW, Potter DD, et al: Penetrating atherosclerotic ulcer of the descending thoracic aorta and arch. *J Thorac Cardiovasc Surg* 127:1393–1399, 2004.
48. Tittle SL, Lynch RJ, Cole PE, et al: Midterm follow-up of penetrating ulcer and intramural hematoma of the aorta. *J Thorac Cardiovasc Surg* 123:1051–1059, 2002.
49. Williams DM, Lee DY, Hamilton BH, et al: The dissected aorta: percutaneous treatment of ischemic complications—principles and results. *J Vasc Interv Radiol* 8:605–625, 1997.
50. Slonim SM, Nyman UR, Semba CP, et al: True lumen obliteration in complicated aortic dissection: endovascular treatment. *Radiology* 201:161–166, 1996.
51. Miller DC: Acute dissection of the aorta—continuing need for earlier diagnosis and treatment. *Modern Concepts Cardiovasc Dis* 54:51–55, 1985.
52. Suzuki T, Mehta RH, Ince H, et al: Clinical profiles and outcomes of acute type B aortic dissection in the current era: lessons from the International Registry of Acute Aortic Dissection (IRAD). *Circulation* 108:II312–II317, 2003.
53. Fann JI, Sarris GE, Mitchell RS, et al: Treatment of patients with aortic dissection presenting with peripheral vascular complications. *Ann Surg* 212:705–713, 1990.
54. Cambria RP, Brewster DC, Gertler J, et al: Vascular complications associated with spontaneous aortic dissection. *J Vasc Surg* 7:199–202, 1988.
55. Lauterbach SR, Cambria RP, Brewster DC, et al: Contemporary management of aortic branch compromise resulting from acute aortic dissection. *J Vasc Surg* 33:1185–1192, 2001.
56. Cigarroa JE, Isselbacher EM, DeSanctis RW, et al: Diagnostic imaging in the evaluation of suspected aortic dissection. *N Engl J Med* 328:35–43, 1993.
57. Godwin JD, Herfkens RL, Skioldebrand CG, et al: Evaluation of dissections and aneurysms of the thoracic aorta by conventional and dynamic CT scanning. *Radiology* 136:135–139, 1980.
58. Moore AG, Eagle KA, Bruckman D, et al: Choice of computed tomography, transesophageal echocardiography, magnetic resonance imaging, and aortography in acute aortic dissection: International Registry of Acute Aortic Dissection (IRAD). *Am J Cardiol* 89:1235–1238, 2002.
59. Nienaber CA, von Kodolitsch Y, Petersen B, et al: The diagnosis of thoracic aortic dissection by noninvasive imaging procedures. *N Engl J Med* 328:1–9, 1993.
60. Sommer T, Fehske W, Holzknecht N, et al: Aortic dissection: a comparative study of diagnosis with spiral CT, multiplanar transesophageal echocardiography and MR imaging. *Radiology* 199:347–352, 1996.
61. Urban BA, Bluemke DA, Johnson KM, et al: Imaging of thoracic aortic disease. *Cardiol Clin* 17:659–682, 1999.
62. Shiga T, Wajima Z, Apfel CC, et al: Diagnostic accuracy of transesophageal echocardiography, helical computed tomography and magnetic resonance imaging for suspected thoracic aortic dissection. *Arch Intern Med* 166:1350–1356, 2006.
63. Erbel R, Engberding R, Daniel W, et al: Echocardiography in the diagnosis of aortic dissection. *Lancet* 1:457–461, 1989.
64. Nienaber CA, Spielmann RP, von Kodolitsch Y, et al: Diagnosis of thoracic aortic dissection. Magnetic resonance imaging versus transesophageal echocardiography. *Circulation* 85:434–447, 1992.
65. Stein HL, Steinberg I: Selective aortography, the definitive technique for diagnosis of dissecting aneurysm of the aorta. *Am J Roentgenol* 102:333–348, 1968.
66. Miller DC: Surgical treatment of aortic dissections. In Jamieson SW, Shumway NE, editors: *Operative surgery—cardiac surgery*, London, 1986, Butterworth, pp 526–537.
67. Henke PK, Williams DM, Upchurch GR, et al: Acute limb ischemia associated with type B aortic dissection: clinical relevance and therapy. *Surgery* 140:532–540, 2006.
68. Haverich A: Letter to Hans Georg Borst. *J Thorac Cardiovasc Surg* 124:891–893, 2002.
69. Lansman SL, McCullough JN, Nguyen KH, et al: Subtypes of acute aortic dissection. *Ann Thorac Surg* 67:1975–1978, 1999.
70. Marui A, Mochizuki T, Mitsui N, et al: Toward the best treatment of uncomplicated patients with type B acute aortic dissection. A consideration for sound surgical intervention. *Circulation* 100(Suppl II):II275–II280, 1999.
71. Miller DC: The continuing dilemma concerning medical versus surgical management of patients with acute type B dissections. *Semin Thorac Cardiovasc Surg* 5:33–46, 1993.
72. Neya K, Omoto R, Kyo S, et al: Outcome of Stanford type B dissection. *Circulation* 86(Suppl II):II1–II7, 1992.
73. Doroghazi RM, Slater EE, DeSanctis RW, et al: Long-term survival of patients with treated aortic dissections. *J Am Coll Cardiol* 3:1026–1034, 1984.
74. Nienaber CA, Rousseau H, Eggebrecht H, et al: Randomized comparison of strategies for type B aortic dissection: the investigation of stent-grafts in aortic dissection trial. *Circulation* 130:2519–2528, 2009.
75. Nienaber CA, Kische S, Rousseau H, et al: Endovascular repair of type B aortic dissection. Long-term results of the randomized investigation of stent-grafts in aortic dissection trial. *Circ Cardiovasc Interv* 6:407–416, 2013.
76. Lee RS, Fazel S, Schwarze U, et al: Rapid aneurysmal degeneration of a Stanford type B aortic dissection in a patient with Loeys-Dietz syndrome. *J Thorac Cardiovasc Surg* 134:242–243, 2007.
77. Loeys BL, Schwarze U, Holm T, et al: Aneurysm syndromes caused by mutations in the TGF-β receptor. *N Engl J Med* 355:788–798, 2006.
78. Nienaber CA, von Kodolitsch Y, Petersen B, et al: Intramural hemorrhage of the thoracic aorta: diagnostic and therapeutic implications. *Circulation* 92:1465–1472, 1995.
79. Suzuki T, Isselbacher EM, Nienaber CA, et al: Type-selective benefits of medications in treatment of acute aortic dissection (from the International Registry of Acute Aortic Dissection IRAD). *Am J Cardiol* 109:122–127, 2012.
80. Neri E, Massetti M, Barabesi L, et al: Extrathoracic cannulation of the left common carotid artery in thoracic aorta operations through a left thoracotomy: preliminary experience in 26 patients. *J Thorac Cardiovasc Surg* 123:901–910, 2002.
81. Tanaka T, Kawamura T, Ohara K, et al: Transapical aortic perfusion with a double-barreled cannula. *Ann Thorac Surg* 25:209–214, 1978.
82. Crawford ES, Coselli JS, Safi HJ: Partial cardiopulmonary bypass, hypothermic circulatory arrest, and posterolateral exposure for thoracic aneurysm operation. *J Thorac Cardiovasc Surg* 94:824–827, 1987.
83. Kouchoukos NT, Massetti P, Rokkas CK, et al: Safety and efficacy of hypothermic cardiopulmonary bypass and circulatory arrest for operations on the descending thoracic and thoracoabdominal aorta. *Ann Thorac Surg* 72:699–708, 2001.
84. Oderich GS, Panneton JM, Bower TC, et al: Aortic dissection with aortic side branch compromise: impact of malperfusion on patient outcome. *Perspect Vasc Surg Endovasc Ther* 20:190–200, 2008.
85. Slonim SM, Nyman URO, Semba CP, et al: Aortic dissection: percutaneous management of ischemic complications with endovascular stents and balloon fenestration. *J Vasc Surg* 23:241–253, 1996.
86. Dake MD, Semba CP, Razavi MK, et al: Endovascular procedures for the treatment of aortic dissection: techniques and results. *J Cardiovasc Surg* 39(Suppl 1):45–52, 1998.
87. Svensson LG, Kouchoukos NT, Miller DC, et al: Expert consensus document on the treatment of descending thoracic aortic disease using endovascular stent-grafts. *Ann Thorac Surg* 85:S1–S41, 2008.
88. Brunkwall J, Kasprzak P, Verhoeven E, et al and ADSORB Trialists: endovascular repair of acute uncomplicated aortic type B dissection promotes aortic remodelling: 1 year results of the ADSORB Trial. *Eur J Vasc Endovasc Surg* 48:285–291, 2014.
89. Coady MA, Rizzo JA, Hammond GL, et al: What is the appropriate size criterion for resection of thoracic aortic aneurysms? *J Thorac Cardiovasc Surg* 113:476–491, 1997.
90. Juvonen T, Ergin MA, Galla JD, et al: Risk factors for rupture of chronic type B dissections. *J Thorac Cardiovasc Surg* 117:776–786, 1999.

91. DeBakey ME, Henly WS, Cooley DA, et al: Surgical management of dissecting aneurysms of the aorta. *J Thorac Cardiovasc Surg* 49:130–149, 1965.
92. Miller DC, Stinson EB, Oyer PE, et al: Operative treatment of aortic dissections. *J Thorac Cardiovasc Surg* 78:365–382, 1979.
93. Miller DC: Surgical management of aortic dissections: indications, perioperative management, and long-term results. In Doroghazi RM, Slater EE, editors: *Aortic dissection*, New York, 1983, McGraw-Hill, pp 193–243.
94. Reul GJ, Cooley DA, Hallman GL, et al: Dissecting aneurysm of the descending aorta. *Arch Surg* 110:632–640, 1975.
95. Svensson LG, Crawford ES, Hess KR, et al: Dissection of the aorta and dissecting aneurysms: improving early and long-term surgical results. *Circulation* 82(Suppl 4):24–38, 1990.
96. Safi HJ, Estrera AL: Aortic dissection. *Br J Surg* 91:523–525, 2004.
97. Estrera AL, Miller CC, Safi HJ, et al: Outcomes of medical management of acute type B aortic dissection. *Circulation* 114:I384–I389, 2006.
98. Trimarchi S, Nienaber CA, Rampoldi V, et al: Role and results of surgery in acute type B aortic dissection. Insights from the International Registry of Acute Aortic Dissection (IRAD). *Circulation* 114:I357–I364, 2006.
99. Fattori R, Tsai TT, Myrmel T, et al: Complicated acute type B dissection: is surgery still the best option? A report from the International Registry of Acute Aortic Dissection. *JACC Cardiovasc Interv* 1:395–402, 2008.
100. Bozinovski J, Coselli JS: Outcomes and survival in surgical treatment of descending thoracic aorta with acute dissection. *Ann Thorac Surg* 85:965–971, 2008.
101. Tsai TT, Fattori R, Trimarchi S, et al: Long-term survival in patients presenting with type B acute aortic dissection. Insights from the International Registry of Acute Aortic Dissection (IRAD). *Circulation* 114:2226–2231, 2006.
102. Marui A, Mochizuki T, Koyama T, et al: Degree of fusiform dilatation of the proximal descending aorta in type B acute aortic dissection can predict late aortic events. *J Thorac Cardiovasc Surg* 134:1163–1170, 2007.

CHAPTER 72

ENDOVASCULAR THERAPY FOR THE TREATMENT OF THORACIC AORTIC PATHOLOGIES

Prashanth Vallabhajosyula • Wilson Y. Szeto • Joseph E. Bavaria

CHAPTER OUTLINE

The development of thoracic endovascular aortic repair (TEVAR) has dramatically revolutionized the field of cardiovascular surgery. Since Parodi's first description of an intraluminal stent graft device for the treatment of abdominal aortic aneurysms,[1] endovascular device technology has rapidly evolved to treat the multiple pathologies seen in the thoracic aorta. In 1994, Dake first reported the initial Stanford experience with 13 patients undergoing endovascular therapy of descending thoracic aortic aneurysms.[2] Since then, indications involving off-label use have expanded to include the treatment of aortic dissections, traumatic transections, penetrating atherosclerotic ulcers (PAUs), and intramural hematoma (IMH). Currently, there are four stent graft devices approved by the U.S. Food and Drug Administration (FDA) for the treatment of descending thoracic aortic aneurysms. Questions and concerns remain regarding the appropriate timing, indication of intervention, and durability of this fast-evolving technology. TEVAR has gained worldwide acceptance in the treatment of pathologies of the descending thoracic aorta (DTA). In the span of a decade, TEVAR has gained on-label FDA approval for the treatment of thoracic aortic aneurysm, PAU, blunt thoracic aortic injury, and type B aortic dissection. This change attests to the rapid evolution and adoption of this technology in treating thoracic aortic pathology.

As TEVAR technology evolves, recent reports have shed light on the utility of endovascular technology in treating ascending aortic and aortic arch pathology—primarily ascending aortic dissection, ascending aorta IMH/PAU, and aortic arch aneurysms in poor open surgical candidates. With improving technology, it is likely that in the future TEVAR will have a defined role in the treatment of ascending aortic and aortic arch pathology. Currently, it has become the gold standard for treatment of descending thoracic aortic pathologies.

DESCENDING THORACIC AORTIC ANEURYSMS

Natural History and Indications for Intervention

Thoracic aortic aneurysms are abnormal dilation of the aorta, characterized by elastin fragmentation and fibrosis, resulting in medial degeneration of the aortic wall.[3] These age-related changes likely result in the reduction of aortic integrity and strength. As the population ages, the incidence of thoracic aortic aneurysms appears to be increasing. In a recent Swedish study examining the national health care registry from 1987 to 2002, the incidence of thoracic aortic pathology rose by 52% in men and by 28% in women, reaching 16.3 per 100,000 per year and 9.1 per 100,000 per year, respectively. In the same study, the annual incidence of operations performed on the thoracic aorta increased from 0.8 per 100,000 per year in 1987 to 5.6 per 100,000 per year in 2002 for an overall sevenfold increase. In women, the increase was 15-fold, from 0.2 per 100,000 per year in 1987 to 3.0 per 100,000 per year in 2002.[4]

The natural history of thoracoabdominal aortic aneurysms has been examined in large single-institutional series. Characterized by slow growth over time, aortic aneurysmal degeneration is an indolent pathologic process of aortic dilation leading to potential rupture or dissection. The human aorta grows generally at a rate of about 0.07 cm per year in the ascending aorta, and 0.19 cm per year in the descending thoracoabdominal aorta.[5] If dissection is present, the thoracoabdominal aorta may grow at a slightly faster rate of 0.28 cm per year.[6,7]

The major risk in thoracic aortic aneurysms pertains to the catastrophic events of rupture or dissection. The risk of rupture or dissection as a function of maximum aortic diameter has been examined in multiple studies. Clouse and coworkers examined the Olmstead County database and demonstrated that in patients with a maximum aortic diameter measuring 4.0 to 5.9 cm, the risk of rupture was 16% over a period of 5 years. When the maximum aortic diameter is greater than 6.0 cm, the risk of rupture exceeds 30% over the same period of 5 years.[8] The Yale group have also identified "hinge points" of maximum aortic diameter that represent significant increases in the risk for rupture. In the ascending aorta, this "hinge point" appears to be at 6 cm, with a risk of rupture or dissection at 34% over the lifetime of the patients. In the DTA, the "hinge point" appears to be at 7 cm, with a 43% risk of rupture or dissection.[6] The annual risk of rupture or dissection as a function of maximum aortic diameter has also been examined. Davies and coauthors[5] demonstrated that in patients with a maximum aortic diameter of less than 6.0 cm, the yearly rates of rupture, dissection, or death, is less than 8%; however, the annual risk of rupture, dissection, or death dramatically increases to 15.6% when the maximum aortic diameter is greater than or equal to 6.0 cm.

General recommendation for the indication for surgical intervention has been made based on these large institutional population studies. The decision to intervene surgically must be based on a balance between the risk of surgery or intervention (in the case of TEVAR) versus the risk of rupture or dissection with medical management. The general consensus for conventional open repair is to intervene surgically at a diameter of 5.5 cm for the ascending aorta and a diameter of 6.5 cm for the DTA. Certainly, patients with significant family history of aortic disease or connective tissue disorder such as Marfan syndrome may warrant intervention at a lower threshold of aortic diameter. Furthermore, for patients with symptomatic aneurysmal disease, urgent surgical intervention is recommended regardless of size, because symptoms are an early indicator of impending rupture.

In the era of TEVAR, the perceived lower rates of morbidity and mortality have urged the question: Should the threshold for intervention in the DTA be lowered? With a mortality rate of less than 5% with TEVAR in most centers of excellence,[9-12] most patients with a descending thoracic aortic diameter greater than 5.5 cm may be considered for endovascular repair (Fig. 72-1). However, the final decision to intervene must be based on previously established surgical dictum: the risk of rupture must outweigh the risk of surgery, regardless of approach.

Device Development

Since the early devices were first described by the Stanford group in 1994,[2] TEVAR devices have undergone multiple modifications and clinical trials. There are four thoracic endoprostheses currently approved for the treatment of descending thoracic aortic aneurysms. Second- and third-generation devices, as well as disease-specific devices, are currently being investigated.

Gore TAG

The Gore TAG thoracic endoprosthesis (W.L. Gore, Inc., Flagstaff, AZ) was approved by the FDA in March 2005 for the treatment of descending thoracic aortic aneurysms. The first device to be approved, the Gore TAG, is a self-expanding polytetrafluoroethylene endograft comprised of nitinol support. Concern over fracture of the longitudinal support wire led to the revision of the

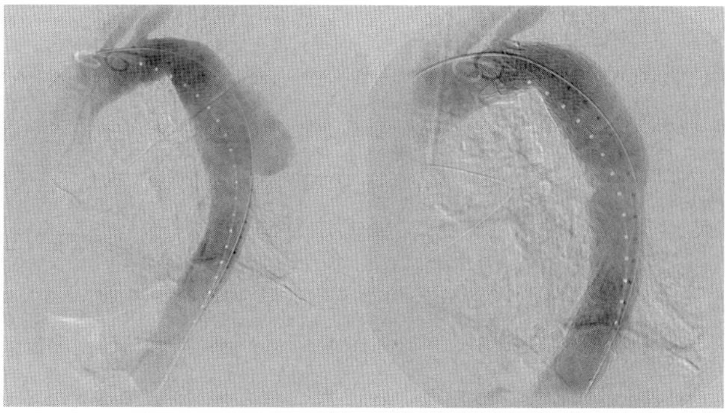

FIGURE 72-1 ■ Angiogram demonstrating endovascular treatment of thoracic aortic aneurysm.

original Gore device to its current Gore TAG endoprosthesis. Unique to this device system is the introducer sheath, which enables the delivery of multiple devices and minimizes traumatic injury to the femoral access vessels. The introducer sheath ranges from an inner diameter of 20 Fr to 24 Fr depending on the size of the Gore TAG devices required for treatment. The Gore TAG endoprosthesis ranges from a minimal diameter of 26 mm to a maximum diameter of 40 mm, with lengths ranging from a minimum of 10 cm to a maximum of 20 cm (Fig. 72-2). The mechanism of deployment involves release of the endograft from a center to peripheral fashion. Thus, precise deployment of the proximal and distal landing zones may be difficult.

In August 2011, Gore Conformable-TAG (C-TAG) device received FDA approval. The C-TAG has essentially replaced the older-generation TAG device. It provides greater flexibility and conformability, with a broad, oversizing window (6%-33%), and is available in straight and tapered forms. The C-TAG is available in a smaller-diameter range than the TAG device (21 mm) and can be placed using an 18 Fr (inner diameter) delivery system. C-TAG is now FDA approved for use in thoracic aortic aneurysm disease, PAU, blunt thoracic aortic injury, and complicated type B dissection.

Medtronic Talent and Valiant Thoracic Endoprosthesis

The Talent Device. Recently approved in June 2008 by the FDA for the treatment of descending thoracic aortic aneurysms, the Talent device is a preloaded stent graft incorporated into a CoilTrac delivery system. It is a stent graft composed of a polyester graft (Dacron) sewn to a self-expanding nitinol wireframe skeleton. Radiopaque markers are sewn to the graft material to aid in visualization during fluoroscopy. The CoilTrac delivery system is a sheathless, push-rod–based delivery system. Preloaded onto an inner catheter, the Talent device is deployed by pulling back an outer catheter, allowing the device to self-expand and contour to the aorta. A balloon may be used to ensure proper apposition of the graft to the aneurysmal aorta after deployment.

The Talent device is designed as a modular system. Forty-seven different configurations ranging from a diameter of 22 to 46 mm and cover lengths from 112 to 116 mm are available. To accommodate the size differences often found between the proximal and distal portions of the aorta in thoracic aneurysms, tapered grafts are available for better aneurysmal conformability and prevention of junctional endoleaks. Four configuration categories are available: proximal main, proximal extension, distal main, and distal extension (Fig. 72-3). The proximal configurations and the distal extension are offered with a bare-spring design (Free-Flo design). The bare-spring design allows for placement of the device crossing the arch vessels proximally and the celiac artery distally for suprasubclavian and infraceliac fixation, respectively.

The Valiant Device. The Valiant device is designed based on the experience with the Talent device. Similar to the Talent device, the Valiant device is also a preloaded stent graft made of the same polyester graft built onto a self-expanding nitinol skeleton. Modification has been made to improve trackability, conformability, and deployment of the Valiant device. First, device lengths have been increased to a maximum of 230 mm (130 mm for Talent). Because the device is a sheathless system, each piece requires an individual deployment through the access vessel, resulting in repeated exchange in the artery. Longer lengths have been designed to minimize device exchange

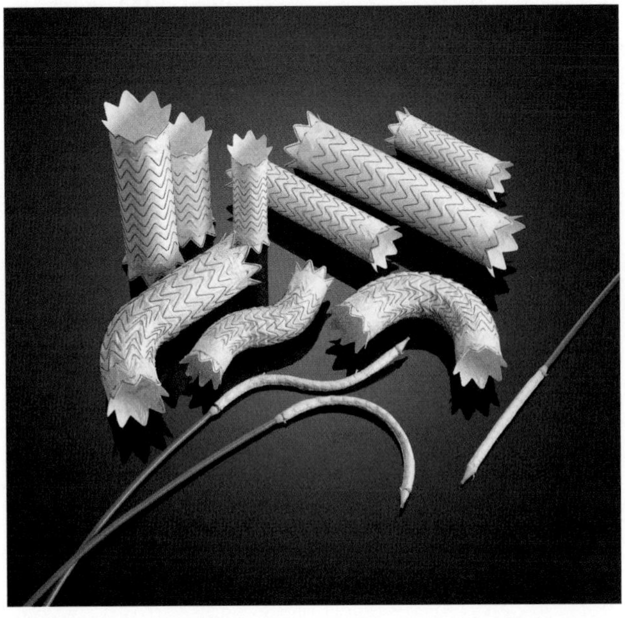

FIGURE 72-2 ■ The Gore TAG thoracic endoprosthesis. (Courtesy W.L. Gore, Inc., Flagstaff, AZ.)

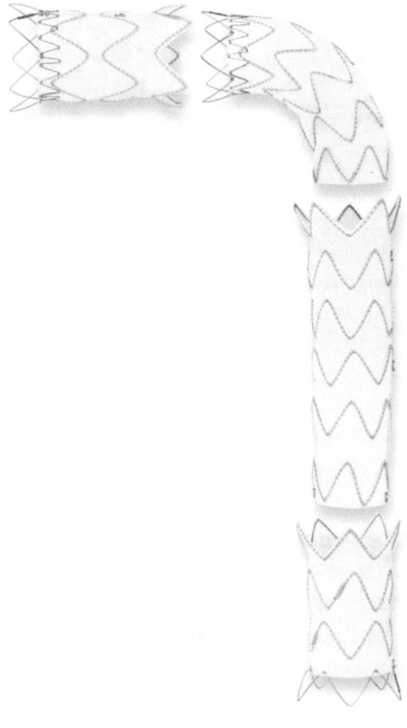

FIGURE 72-3 ■ The Medtronic Talent thoracic endoprosthesis (Medtronic Vascular, Santa Clara, CA).

during deployment. Second, the connecting bar has been removed in the Valiant device for improved conformability, especially in the arch. Third, the number of bare springs at the proximal and distal ends of the device has been increased from 5 to 8 in the Valiant device to improve circumferential force distribution and fixation along the aorta wall. Finally, the Valiant device is introduced in a new delivery system, the Xcelerant Delivery System. First available to physicians in the United States for the AneuRx AAA device, the Xcelerant Delivery System has been modified for the Valiant Device to provide a more comfortable deployment mechanism of the device, especially in tortuous anatomy of the distal arch and thoracic aorta. As opposed to a simple pullback unsheathing mechanism, the deployment of the Xcelerant Delivery System includes a gearing, ratchet-like mechanism in the handle to allow easy deployment. The amount of force required to deploy the device is reduced significantly without compromising the precision of the deployment.

Similar to the Talent device, The Valiant device is a modular design. Eighty-eight different configurations ranging from a diameter of 22 to 46 mm and cover lengths from 110 to 200 mm are available in the Valiant device. Four configurations categories are available: proximal FreeFlo straight component, proximal closed-web straight component, proximal closed-web tapered component, and distal bare-spring straight component. The proximal FreeFlo straight component is designed for the most proximal deployment zone, because the bare springs are designed to allow precise and crossing deployment of the arch vessels. In addition, it is designed as the first piece to be deployed.

In 2012, results of the VALOR II trial were reported for the use of the Valiant endoprosthesis for DTA aneurysm repair.[13] The pivotal trial was conducted at 24 U.S. sites, assessing 30-day and 12-month outcomes. At 30 days, there were rates of 3.1% mortality, 38.1% major adverse events, 0.6% paraplegia, and 2.5% stroke. At 12 months, aneurysm-related mortality was 4%, with a stent migration rate of 2.9% and an endoleak rate of 13%.

Cook Zenith TX2 Thoracic Endoprosthesis. Recently approved in 2008 by the FDA, the Cook Zenith TX2 thoracic endoprosthesis (Cook, Inc., Bloomington, IN) is designed as a modular system with a specific proximal and distal configuration (Fig. 72-4). The graft consists of stainless steel Z-stents with full-thickness polyester fabric. Similar to the Medtronic delivery system, the Zenith TX2 system does not require a delivery sheath, and it is introduced as a preloaded catheter with triggers. The device sheath has a hydrophilic coating and sizes range from 18 to 22 Fr, depending on the diameter of the endoprosthesis. The diameter of the endoprosthesis ranges from 22 to 42 mm and lengths from 120 mm to 207 mm. The two components are designed to be deployed from a proximal to distal direction, and tapered devices are available.

Deployment of the TX2 is achieved through a trigger system to ensure a controlled deployment. Flushed at the proximal end with barbs to prevent migration and endoleak, the device is deployed by an unsheathing mechanism. To minimize the "wind sock" effect during deployment (thus distal migration), the proximal barb component of the device is not released until the graft is deployed and the trigger released. The distal component is deployed in a similar mechanism. However, in addition to barbs, the distal component also has bare springs at its caudal portion. Proximal and distal extensions are available if additional coverage is necessary.

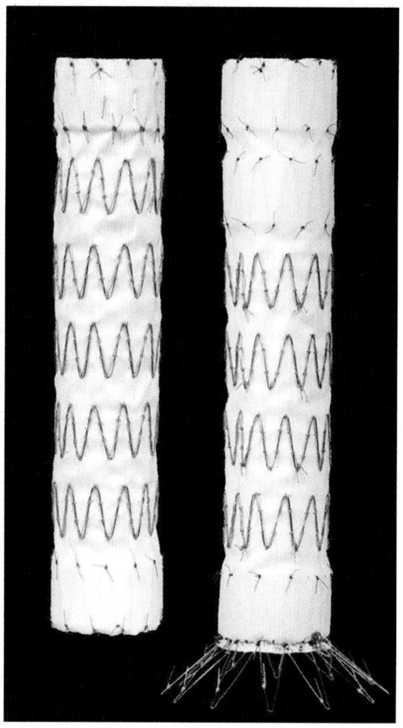

FIGURE 72-4 ■ The Cook ZenithTX2 thoracic endoprosthesis (Cook, Inc., Bloomington, IN).

Bolton Relay Prosthesis. The Bolton Relay graft (Bolton Medical, Inc., Sunrise, FL) is the latest new company to receive FDA approval (in 2012) for TEVAR treatment of DTA aneurysmal pathology. The Relay system features a four-step sheath delivery system for modular delivery (outer diameter 22-26 Fr), with graft lengths ranging from 100 to 250 mm in straight and tapered forms; graft diameters range from 22 to 46 mm, with proximal and distal components. Proximal grafts are available in two types—Relay uncovered graft and Relay NBS covered graft. They feature S-bar (spiral support strut) technology that runs longitudinally along the stent graft, enabling improved support to the entire structure. The Relay system enables proximal capture of stent graft for precise placement, along with a secondary sealing and fixation zone that provides an extra sealing independent of proximal sealing.

Anatomic and Technical Considerations

Anatomic requirements and key technical considerations for successful TEVAR revolve around answering the question of what makes a patient a suitable anatomical candidate for a thoracic aortic stent graft. Initial assessment of a stent graft candidate begins with an extensive preoperative workup and evaluation. Key points of the history and physical examination should include a detailed neurologic and cardiovascular examination. Distal vascular pulses and preoperative neurologic deficiencies must be documented. Previous abdominal, pelvic, and inguinal surgeries should be noted, because these procedures may demand an alternate access route.

Access

Safe vascular access for thoracic aortic device deployment is the key to thoracic aortic stent grafting. The majority of the morbidity and mortality is a direct result of arterial access complications.[9,10,12] Extensive preoperative planning with appropriate imaging is mandatory. The "gold standard" for preoperative evaluation is a computed tomography (CT) angiogram that includes the thorax, abdomen, pelvis, and femoral arteries. Fine-cut helical CT scanning with at minimum 3-mm slices is ideal (Fig. 72-5). In patients who cannot receive a CT with contrast, magnetic resonance angiography is an acceptable substitution.

All the thoracic endovascular devices take a long time to reach the descending aorta, are of large caliber to contain the thoracic aortic endoluminal graft, and are relatively stiff to allow "pushability" through the iliofemoral access points and through the abdominal aorta. The management of the delivery of the thoracic aortic stent graft is often the most challenging aspect of the case. Delivery systems of the three currently FDA-approved thoracic endoprostheses will require arterial access size of a minimum of 7.5 to 8.0 mm. Creation of a conduit to the femoral or iliac artery may be necessary to achieve adequate access. Not only the size of the arterial vessels, but also the anatomy of the iliofemoral and abdominal aorta, must be considered when planning the access route. Excessive tortuosity and atherosclerosis with occlusive disease may provide barriers to safe delivery of the endograft. In approximately 20% of patients, retroperitoneal access to the common iliac arteries will be required owing to issues of femoral or external iliac artery size and/or tortuosity.[14]

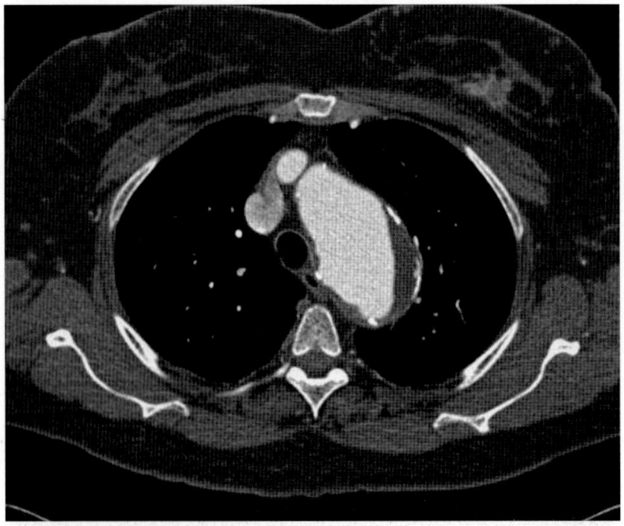

FIGURE 72-5 ■ Computed tomographic angiography of a descending thoracic aortic aneurysm.

Careful review of preoperative studies will indicate which patients will have difficult access. Patients with atherosclerotic occlusive iliac disease may be treated with standard endovascular techniques of balloon angioplasty to reduce the obstruction. Iliac stents should be avoided because of the potential interference of these stents with the thoracic aortic access devices. These procedures on the access vessels should be carried out at least 6 weeks before thoracic aortic stent grafting to allow healing of the iliac arteries post-angioplasty and manipulation. At the completion of the thoracic aortic endografting, iliac stents may be placed if appropriate.

Access to the retroperitoneum allows several options for safe device deployment. The common iliac artery may be used for device deployment. An open surgical conduit can be constructed to allow an end-to-end anastomosis or a side-to-side anastomosis. A 10-mm conduit of synthetic Dacron is commonly used and allows ample size for insertion of all necessary devices. The conduit may be brought through a separate counterincision in the groin to allow better angulation of the relatively long and stiff deployment devices. At the conclusion of the procedure, these conduits may be used to revascularize distal obstructions if needed.

Alternatively, the retroperitoneal iliac vessels, or even the distal aorta, may be accessed using direct sheath insertion. A double purse string of 4-0 Tycron is used to secure the vessel and provide hemostasis with the application of two sets of tourniquets. Direct needle puncture of the artery is followed by dilation and insertion of the device. At completion, the device is removed and the purse string sutures are tied down. Excessive tortuosity of the iliofemoral arteries requires adaptive strategies. The use of external manual manipulation provides a simple method of straightening some of the tortuosity of the aorta and iliac arteries. During fluoroscopy the operator hand can provide gentle force to the tortuous arterial segment to allow straightening and subsequent endovascular access.

In cases of iliac artery tortuosity, advanced endovascular techniques may aid in straightening these segments. The use of stiff wires or buddy wire techniques can provide some degree of straightening of the diseased arteries. In severe cases of tortuosity, brachiofemoral access may be required to perform "body flossing" with an appropriately stiff wire. Typically, a 5 Fr sheath with a long catheter is placed into the aortic arch and then into the descending aorta. A long, stiff wire, such as a 450-cm SS Guidewire (Boston Scientific, Natick, MA), is guided from the brachial artery and retrieved through the femoral artery. Gentle traction on both the brachial and femoral sites will straighten out the tortuosity. Of note, a long catheter must be placed through the brachial artery into the aorta to prevent excessive trauma by the stiff wire along the arch and innominate vessels.

At the completion of the deployment and ballooning of the thoracic stent graft, the entire route of access must be carefully examined to ensure that there has been no injury. The stiff guidewire that was used to position the thoracic endograft should be left in place as the sheaths and remaining endovascular materials are removed. A smaller sheath should be reinserted and a diagnostic

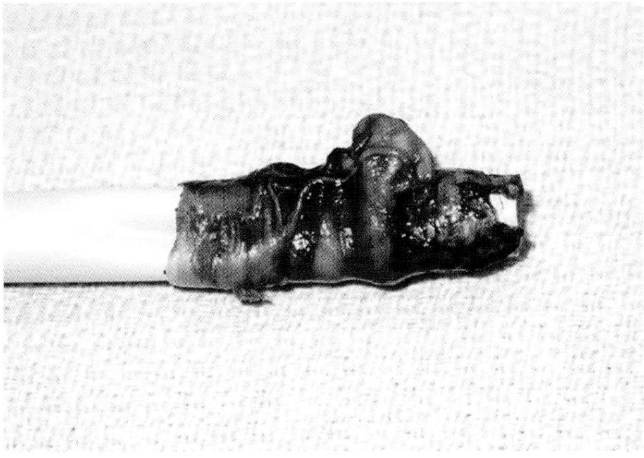

FIGURE 72-6 ■ Iliac artery avulsion after removal of an endovascular delivery system.

aortoiliac arteriogram should be performed to evaluate for thrombus, dissection, or complete avulsion.

The removal of the large sheath, especially when inserted with some force and manipulation, is a particularly dangerous period when injury may occur. There have been numerous reports of successful thoracic endografting with a sheath removed with a complete iliac artery avulsed and attached (Fig. 72-6). At the time of recognition, a stiff wire through this injured artery may be life-saving and allow insertion of an occluding balloon proximally to allow control of a potentially life-threatening bleed. In addition, both blood pressure and heart rate should be carefully monitored during removal and completion of the endovascular procedure for signs of an occult injury.

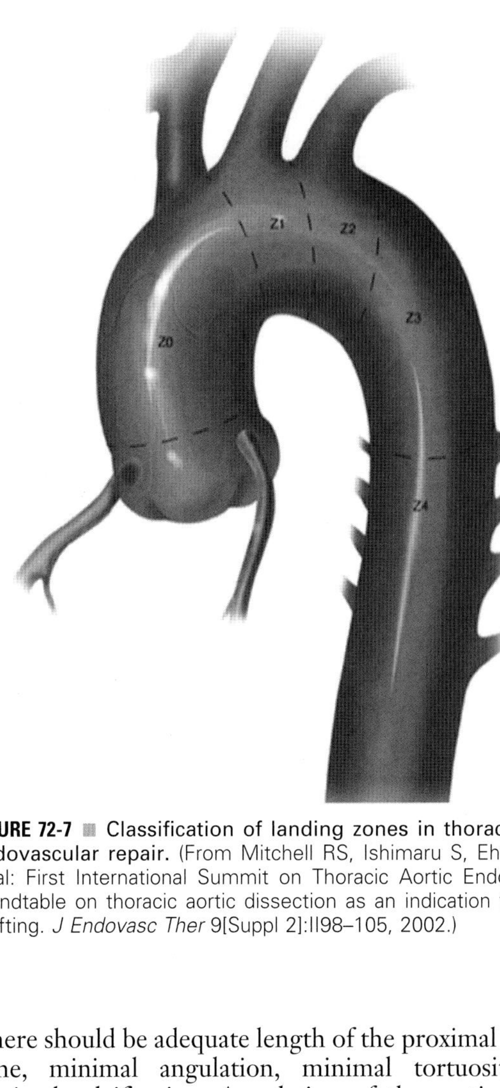

FIGURE 72-7 ■ Classification of landing zones in thoracic aortic endovascular repair. (From Mitchell RS, Ishimaru S, Ehrlich MP, et al: First International Summit on Thoracic Aortic Endografting: roundtable on thoracic aortic dissection as an indication for endografting. *J Endovasc Ther* 9[Suppl 2]:II98–105, 2002.)

Landing Zones

The proximal aorta is divided into landing zones as illustrated in Figure 72-7. Unless revascularization is performed, proximal landing in zones 0 and 1 is unacceptable because of the necessary occlusion of the left common carotid artery in zone 1 and the innominate artery in zone 0. Proximal landing in zone 2 is commonly used with either partial or total occlusion of the left subclavian artery. Zone 3 landing is dependent on the exact anatomical neck at the arch. Proximal landing in zone 3 can lead to angulation of the graft, which provides inadequate sealing of the proximal graft along the lesser arch and "bird beaking" or "stove piping" graft placement, which results in a high incidence of Type II endoleaks. Zone 4 landing is usually straightforward because of the lack of angulation and distance from the arch vessels.

The proximal and distal landing zones must be of an appropriate diameter to allow for stent grafting with available devices. In general, devices should be oversized over the diameter of the landing zone between 15% and 20%, depending on the presenting aortic pathology. As has been discussed, the proximal landing zone of the aorta must be carefully examined on preoperative imaging workup. The goal is to create a good "seal" of 15 to 20 mm between the graft and the aortic wall on a disease-free, nontapered, nonangulated portion of the aorta. There should be adequate length of the proximal landing zone, minimal angulation, minimal tortuosity, and minimal calcification. Angulation of the aortic arch is acceptable if the inner radius is greater than 35 mm and the outer radius is greater than 70 mm. These parameters allow adequate conformation of the aortic stent graft to the arch.

Because zone 2 is often the site of best proximal landing to avoid excessive angulation and tortuosity, the management of the left subclavian artery requires preoperative planning. Some of the possible complications of covering the left subclavian artery include vertebrobasilar artery insufficiency or stroke, left arm ischemia, or ischemia of the heart in patients with a previous left internal mammary artery to left anterior descending coronary artery bypass graft. An evaluation of the right vertebral artery and the adequacy of the circle of Willis is crucial when planning to cover the left subclavian artery. In patients with inadequate collaterals through the circle of Willis, stenotic right vertebral artery, or a dominant left vertebral artery, strong consideration should be made to bypass the left subclavian artery before covering. One option is to transpose the left subclavian artery to the left common carotid artery with oversewing of the proximal left subclavian artery. A second option is to bypass from the left common carotid artery to the left subclavian artery. Either surgical ligation of the proximal left subclavian at the time of bypass or staged-coil embolization of the proximal left subclavian artery at the time of graft delivery may be used. Bypass of the left subclavian artery may be preferable because it avoids any mediastinal dissection and there is no interruption of antegrade flow to the vertebral artery or internal mammary artery branch vessels.[15]

Evaluation of the distal landing zone also requires careful preoperative workup. The distal landing zone should again have 15 to 20 mm of normal aorta with minimal calcification, angulation, and tapering. The celiac artery is the first distal branch vessel that must be avoided. Therefore, the length of the aortic graft must be correctly planned. Enough graft length should cover the aortic pathology while avoiding excessive coverage of the DTA. The goal is to preserve the distal vertebral artery branches and perfusion to the spinal cord.

Results

Multicenter Clinical Trials

The Gore TAG endoprosthesis was approved as a result of the phase 2 U.S. multicenter trial comparing the Gore TAG endoprosthesis (W.L. Gore) to an open surgical control group in the treatment of descending thoracic aortic aneurysms.[9] Between September 1999 and May 2001, 140 patients with descending thoracic aortic aneurysms were enrolled from 17 sites in the United States. All patients were required to have adequate landing zones of at least 2 cm length of nonaneurysmal aorta distal to the left carotid and proximal to the celiac axis. At the same centers, the open surgical control cohort enrolled 94 patients. Forty-four patients were concurrent controls and 50 were historically and retrospectively acquired by selecting the most recent surgical patients in reverse chronological order.

In the endograft group, statistically significant improvement was seen in the 30-day mortality, incidence of postoperative respiratory failure, renal failure, spinal cord ischemia (SCI), mean intensive care unit, and hospital stay. Thirty-day mortality was 2.1% and 11.7% in the Gore TAG group and the open surgical control group, respectively. SCI was 2.9% in the Gore TAG group versus 13.8% in the control group. However, peripheral vascular complications were significantly higher in the endograft group (14% vs. 4% control group).[9]

The mean duration of follow-up was 25.8 months in the endograft group and 24.9 months in the open control group. Kaplan-Meier 2-year survival was similar between the two groups (78% endograft group vs. 76% control). The incidence of endoleak at 1-year and 2-year follow-up was 6% (6/103) and 9% (7/80), respectively. There were no cases of aneurysm rupture in either group. At 2-year follow up, 45% of the endograft group had aneurysmal regression of 5 mm or greater, 42% had no change, and 13% had aneurysmal progression of 5 mm or greater.[9] At 5-year follow-up, all-cause mortality remains similar between the two groups (68% endograft group vs. 67% control). Aneurysm-related mortality was lower in the endograft group (2.8%) when compared with the control group (11.7%).[16]

The Vascular Talent Thoracic Stent Graft System for the Treatment of Thoracic Aortic Aneurysms (VALOR) trial led to the approval of the Talent endoprosthesis for the treatment of thoracic aortic aneurysms. The Medtronic VALOR trial was a prospective, multicenter, nonrandomized, observational trial evaluating the use of the Medtronic Talent thoracic stent graft system in the treatment of thoracic aortic pathology. The study was conducted from 2003 to 2005 and involved 38 sites. A total of 195 patients were enrolled, with 189 patients identified as retrospective open surgical controls. In the Talent group, the 30-day mortality was 2.1%, with an incidence of paraplegia of 1.5% and stroke of 3.6%. One-year mortality was 16.1% with aneurysm-related mortality of 3.1%. When compared with the surgical control group, the Talent arm demonstrated statistically superior outcome in perioperative mortality (2% vs. 8%, $P < 0.01$), 30-day major adverse events (41% vs. 84.4%, $P < 0.001$), and 12-month aneurysm-related mortality (3.1% vs. 11.6%, $P < 0.002$). In 2012, results were reported from the VALOR II trial, which assessed the Valiant stent graft system for degenerative disease of the DTA.[13] It was a prospective, nonrandomized, pivotal trial conducted at 24 U.S. sites enrolling 160 patients. The perioperative mortality rate was 3.1%, stroke rate was 2.5%, and paraplegia/paraparesis rate was 2.5%. At 12 months, endoleak rate was 13%, with 4% aneurysm-related mortality. The Valiant device was statistically noninferior to the Talent graft.

Published in 2008, the international controlled clinical trial of the TX2 device is a nonrandomized, controlled, multicenter, international trial comparing the treatment of thoracic aortic aneurysm with the TX2 endoprosthesis versus open repair. Enrollment began in March 2004 and was completed by July 2006. From 42 institutions, a total of 160 patients were enrolled in the endovascular group and 70 patients in the open group. The 30-day survival rate was noninferior for the TX2 group when compared with the control group (98.1% vs. 94.3%). The 30-day cumulative major morbidity scores were significantly lower in the TX2 group when compared with the control group (1.3 vs. 2.9). Although not statistically significant, the incidence of neurologic complications trended in favor of endovascular repair. The incidence of stroke in the TX2 group was 2.5% at 30 days compared with 8.6% in the control group. The incidence of paraplegia in the TX2 group was 1.3% versus 5.7% in the control group. At 12 months' follow-up, aneurysmal growth was seen in 7.1%, endoleak in 3.9%, and device migration in 2.8%. One-year survival estimated from all-cause mortality was similar between the TX2 group (91.6%) and the control group (85.5%). The 1-year survival estimate from aneurysm-related mortality was also similar between the TX2 group (94.2%) and the open surgical control group (88.2%).[12]

In September 2012, the Bolton Relay thoracic stent with Plus delivery system received FDA approval. Current on-label indications for Relay stent graft use in the United States include thoracic aortic aneurysm and PAU. In a study by the RESTORE investigators[17] (multicenter, prospective European trial), outcomes for Relay stent graft treatment of a variety of thoracic aortic pathologies (aneurysm dissection, PAU, IMH, pseudoaneurysm) were assessed in 304 enrolled patients. Thirty-day mortality was 7.2%, and perioperative stroke and paraplegia rates were 1.6% and 2%, respectively. Two-year freedom from device-related mortality was 95.9%. In a more recent study looking at subgroup analysis in patients treated for traumatic aortic injury, the clinical success with Relay graft was achieved in all 40 cases. Thirty-day mortality was 2.5%, and actuarial 2-year survival was 93.7%.

European Registries

Multicenter experience with TEVAR has also been accumulating in Europe. The Talent Thoracic Registry (TTR) is a database collected from seven European centers. All patients in the registry underwent TEVAR with the Medtronic Talent endoprosthesis between November 1996 and March 2004. The registry involved 457 patients, and the spectrum of pathologies comprised 180 (39.4%) thoracic aortic dissections, 137 (29.9%) atherosclerotic aneurysms, 14 (3%) pseudoaneurysms, 29 (6.35%) penetrating ulcers, 12 (2.6%) IMHs, and 85 (18%) traumatic aneurysms.[11] The in-hospital mortality rate was 5%. Technical failure defined as failure to complete an intended stent graft deployment was 2.2%, with a conversion rate to surgery of 2.2%. The in-hospital complication rate was 12.7% and included stroke (3.7%), paraplegia (1.7%), and vascular access issues (3.3%). The mean follow-up was 24 months with 11 late aneurysm–related deaths. Kaplan-Meier overall survival estimate at 1 year was 90.97% and at 5 years was 77.49%. Freedom from reintervention was 92.45% and 70.0% at 1 and 5 years, respectively.[11]

The results from the European Collaborators on Stent Graft Techniques for Thoracic Aortic Aneurysm and Dissection Repair (EUROSTAR) and United Kingdom Thoracic Endograft Registry were recently published in 2004.[18] This registry included a total of 443 patients (EUROSTAR 340, UK 103) with thoracic aneurysms or dissections in the thoracic aorta who underwent endovascular repair between 1997 and 2003. The patients were recruited from 62 European countries, and the devices deployed included Medtronic Talent, Gore Excluder, and Zenith or Endofit (Endomed). Technical success was achieved in 87% of patients with degenerative aneurysms and 89% with aortic dissection. The 30-day mortality rate in the entire group was 9.3%, with 30-day mortality of 5.3% in the elective aneurysmal group. In the aneurysmal group, neurologic complications included paraplegia (4.0%) and stroke (2.8%). At one-year follow-up, cumulative survival in the degenerative aneurysm group was 80.3%, with 2 (2.1%) aneurysmal-related deaths. The incidence of endoleak at one year was 4.2%, with a reintervention rate of 5.2%.

Complications

Vascular Access

The most common complication associated with TEVAR has been related to vascular access because of the requirement of large-diameter devices. In most series, the access complication rates can be as much as 22.5%.[9-12] Complications include vessel disruption, dissection, frank rupture, pseudoaneurysm, arteriovenous fistula, thrombosis, and distal embolic events. Extensive preoperative planning and decisive intraoperative bailout maneuvers are necessary to minimize potentially lethal vascular access complications.

Endoleak

Endoleak is defined as the presence of persistent blood flow into the aneurysm sac after the deployment of an endovascular aortic stent graft device. In earlier series, TEVAR has been associated with an endoleak incidence of 9.6% to 25.9%.[9-12] Table 72-1 demonstrates the classification of endoleaks associated with endovascular repair of aortic aneurysms.

The presence and the potential development of endoleak during follow-up mandate life-long aortic surveillance with computed tomographic angiography (CTA). Proximal and distal endoleaks (type I) are most commonly the result of inadequate or poor landing zones. Type III, or junctional, endoleaks are likely the result of inadequate overlap of devices, aneurysmal sac expansion, or aortic lengthening over time. In contrast to type II or type IV endoleaks, types I and III endoleaks will likely require further reintervention, either at the time of the primary endografting or at late reintervention during follow-up. Types II and IV endoleaks require strict follow-up and likely will not need further intervention unless symptoms or complications develop.

We recently reviewed the impact of endoleak on our TEVAR experience.[19] Over a 6-year retrospective review period, 105 patients underwent TEVAR with either the Medtronic Talent or the Gore TAG device. Of these 105 patients, 69 patients had sufficient radiographic follow-up to be evaluated. The mean follow-up period was 17.3 months. The total incidence of endoleak was 29%. In these patients, types I, II, and III endoleaks were seen in 40%, 35%, and 20%, respectively. Predictors of endoleaks include more extensive and larger aneurysms at the time of TEVAR, male sex, length of aortic treatment, and increasing number of devices used. The majority of types I and III endoleaks were treated successfully with reintervention, and significant aneurysmal sac regression was seen on follow-up. In contrast, most type II endoleaks were successfully managed with conservative therapy and strict surveillance.

Neurologic Complications

Neurologic complications associated with TEVAR fall within two major areas: stroke and SCI. Stroke is a devastating complication of TEVAR, with an incidence of approximately 3% to 9%.[9-12] The risks for stroke in TEVAR are likely multifactorial. Arch atheroma burden and embolic events are likely significant risk factors, because endovascular placement of thoracic aortic stent graft often requires multiple wire manipulations in the aortic arch. These manipulations may contribute to increased stroke risk by producing distal emboli. Other risk factors for stroke include history of previous stroke

TABLE 72-1 **Classification Scheme for Endoleak and Endotension**

	Description
Endoleaks* **(Type)**	**Source of Perigraft Flow**
I	Attachment site leaks†
A	Proximal end of endograft
B	Distal end of endograft
C	Iliac occluder (plug)
II	Branch leaks‡ (without attachment site connection)
A	Simple or to-and-fro (from only 1 patent branch)
B	Complex or flow-through (with 2 or more patent branches)
III	Graft defect†
A	Junctional leak or modular disconnect
B	Fabric disruption (midgraft hole)
	Minor (<2 mm; e.g., suture holes)
	Major (≥2 mm)
IV	Graft wall (fabric) porosity (<30 days after graft placement)
Endotension§ (Type)	
A	With no endoleak
B	With sealed endoleak (virtual endoleak)
C	With type I or type III leak‖
D	With type II leak‖

*Endoleaks also can be classified on the basis of the time of first detection as: perioperative, within 24 hours of EVAR; early, 1 to 90 days after EVAR; and late, after 90 days. In addition, they can be described as primary, from time of EVAR; secondary, appearing only after not being present at time of EVAR; and delayed, occurring after prior negative computed tomographic scan results. Endoleaks also can be described as persistent, transient or sealed, recurrent, treated successfully, or treated unsuccessfully. Endoleaks and endotension may be associated with AAA enlargement, stability, or shrinkage.

†Some type I and type III leaks also may have patent branches opening from AAA sac and providing outflow for leak.

‡From lumbar, inferior mesenteric, hypogastric, renal, or other arteries.

§Endotension (strict definition) is defined here as increased intrasac pressure after EVAR without visualized endoleak on delayed-contrast computed tomographic scans. In the generic sense, endotension is any elevation of intrasac pressure and occurs with type I, type III, and most type II leaks and endotension in the strict sense.

‖Detectable only on opening aneurysm sac.

From Veith FJ, Baum RA, Ohki T, et al: Nature and significance of endoleaks and endotension: summary of opinions expressed at an international conference. J Vasc Surg 35:1029–1035, 2002.

and grade V atheroma of the aortic arch, and coverage of the left subclavian artery.[20]

SCI resulting in paraplegia is an equally devastating complication of thoracic aortic surgery. Endovascular stent graft repair of isolated descending thoracic aortic aneurysms has a reported SCI frequency that ranges from 3.6% to 12.0%, with approximately two-thirds of these cases being permanent deficits.[21] Endovascular therapy offers several potential advantages in reducing the risk of SCI. These advantages include the avoidance of an aortic crossclamp, fewer episodes of hypotension, less bleeding, and an earlier emergence from general anesthesia to allow detection and treatment of a neurologic deficit. Conversely, stent grafting may have the disadvantages of requiring more extensive aortic coverage to allow adequate sealing between endoluminal graft and aorta, the inability to reimplant intercostal arteries, and injury to iliofemoral vessels that may provide flow to the anterior spinal artery through the hypogastric and pelvic vascular plexus.

Identified risk factors for SCI after thoracic aortic stent grafting include previous abdominal aortic aneurysm repair (AAA), long segment of thoracic aortic stent graft, mobile atheroma, vascular injury, hemorrhage, and hypotension.[21-23] The mechanisms that contribute to SCI are multifactorial. The risk of SCI in patients with previous AAA repair may be explained by the destruction of pelvic and hypogastric arterial collateral to the anterior spinal artery. Extended graft coverage, especially in the levels of T6 to T12, compromises the vertebral levels that supply the anterior spinal artery. Hypotension and hemorrhage contribute by decreasing the perfusion pressure to the spinal cord.

Techniques to reduce the risk of SCI include using lumbar cerebrospinal fluid drains and neurocerebral monitoring. The use of a lumbar cerebrospinal fluid drain has been shown in numerous studies to decrease the risk of SCI in open surgical thoracoabdominal aortic aneurysm repairs and endovascular thoracic aortic aneurysm and dissection stent graft repair.[24,25] The use of neurophysiologic monitoring has been traditionally used to detect intraoperative spinal cord ischemic changes and to allow changes in perfusion management to reverse insults. The use of neurophysiologic monitoring in endovascular treatment of the thoracic aorta has been reported to also allow early detection and intervention to augment spinal cord perfusion pressure to decrease the risk.[26]

AORTIC DISSECTIONS

Although TEVAR for elective repair of descending thoracic aortic aneurysm has been performed worldwide with increasing frequency, it is the potential role of TEVAR in acute thoracic aortic pathologies such as aortic dissections and traumatic aortic injury that has garnered increasing investigation. Through recent surgical advances, morbidity and mortality with conventional surgical repair have been reduced to acceptable perioperative complication rates. However, mortality for emergent thoracic aortic pathologies remains significant. The minimally invasive nature of TEVAR potentially offers a surgical alternative for this group of high-risk patients. The emerging role of TEVAR in acute aortic dissection will be discussed next.

Natural History and Indications for Intervention

In 1650, Sennertus was the first to describe the process of a tear in the intima of the aorta. However, the term *dissection* was not described until 1802, by Manoir. Until this century, aortic dissection was a postmortem diagnosis. Over the centuries, numerous surgical techniques for aortic dissection have been described with limited clinical success. It was not until the 1950s, with the development of cardiopulmonary bypass, that surgical repair of aortic dissection became a clinical success.[27] Over the last 50 years, techniques to repair ascending aortic dissection have been refined, and surgical intervention has become the preferable therapeutic option.

Classification

Aortic dissection is classified based on the location of the primary tear site and dissection flap. Two classification systems currently exist. The DeBakey system classifies dissection based on the location of the dissection and its extension. Type I dissection begins in the ascending aorta and may involve most of the remaining distal aorta, whereas type II dissection involves only the ascending aorta with no extension beyond the aortic arch. Type III dissection begins distal to the left subclavian artery and involves the proximal thoracic aorta (type IIIa) or further to the iliac arteries (type IIIb). In contrast, the Stanford system classifies dissections into two types. Dissection involving the ascending aorta regardless of its extension is classified as type A. Type B dissection begins distal to the left subclavian artery and involves only the DTA.

Aortic dissection has also been classified based on its timing of presentation. Acute dissection has traditionally been classified as presentation within the first two weeks of the initial symptoms, whereas subacute dissection has been classified as presentation between two weeks and two months. Patients with dissections who present after two months after the initial symptoms are classified as chronic dissection.

Indications for Intervention

Surgical treatment of acute proximal aortic dissection (Stanford type A) has been established as the standard of care, demonstrating significant improvement in survival when compared with medical management. In all but the highest-risk patients, the presence of a dissection in the ascending aorta is in itself an indication for surgery. Current series have demonstrated surgical mortality rates ranging from 9% to 25%.[28-35] In contrast, medical therapy is associated with a 1-month mortality rate as high as 60%.[36] Experience with endovascular repair of acute type A aortic dissection remains limited.[37-39] Because of these limitations in the current technology, widespread clinical use has not been adopted. However, future development may result in the application of endovascular technique in the ascending aorta.

The management of acute type B aortic dissection remains less well defined. Traditionally, acute type B dissection without complications (i.e., rupture, malperfusion, hemodynamic instability) has been managed successfully with anti-impulse medical therapy, demonstrating low morbidity and mortality rates. According to the International Registry of Acute Aortic Dissection (IRAD),[36] uncomplicated type B dissection treated with medical therapy is associated with a mortality rate of 10.7%. In contrast, emergent open surgical repair has historically been associated with significantly higher morbidity and mortality.[36]

Although medical therapy of uncomplicated type B dissections is associated with good early outcomes, long-term outcome and survival of patients with type B dissection remain disappointing. As much as 20% of patients with type B dissection develop complications (i.e., rupture, malperfusion) requiring surgical intervention.[36] Actuarial survival for all patients was 71%, 60%, 35%, and 17%, at 1, 5, 10, and 15 years, respectively, regardless of medical versus surgical therapy.[40] In most series, 10-year survival regardless of the mode of therapy is between 40% and 50%.[40-43] Furthermore, there appears to be no difference in the freedom from reoperation and freedom from aortic-related complications between the medical and surgical treatment.[40]

The poor long-term outcome of uncomplicated type B dissection is a result of the predisposition of these patients to develop aneurysmal dilation of the thoracoabdominal aorta.[44] Contemporary series have reported the incidence to be upwards of 80% over a five-year period.[45,46] Subgroup populations of patients with acute type B aortic dissections also appear to be at risk of poor long-term survival. Predictors of increased long-term mortality include persistent patency with partial thrombosis of the false lumen,[44,47-49] false lumen diameter greater than 22 mm at the time of initial presentation,[50] and total aortic diameter greater than 40 mm.[51]

Patients with acute type B aortic dissections who present with life-threatening complications including rupture or malperfusion syndrome remain a challenging group to manage. Historically, conventional open surgical therapy in this group of patients has been associated with significant morbidity and mortality, ranging from 30% to 50%.[52-54] Despite improvement in surgical technique, in-hospital mortality remains significant. In the most recent IRAD review, in-hospital mortality in patients undergoing surgical repair of type B aortic dissection was 29.3%. For patients presenting with malperfusion and rupture, the in-hospital mortality rates were 27.8% and 62.5%, respectively.[54]

An alternative surgical option for both acute uncomplicated and complicated type B aortic dissection remains desirable. Many have examined the role of endovascular technique in the acute type B aortic dissection. In uncomplicated cases, the role of TEVAR remains unclear. For patients with complicated type B dissection, the role of TEVAR has emerged as the gold standard, replacing open surgery as the first-line treatment for complicated type B dissection.

Anatomic and Technical Considerations

Endovascular therapy for acute aortic dissection is technically demanding. Some have argued that the current technology is not ideal and that devices designed specifically for dissection are needed.[55,56] Nonetheless, we emphasize that the complexity involved with endovascular therapy for aortic dissection requires an algorithmic approach that must begin at the primary tear site. Wire access in the true lumen cannot be overemphasized, because deployment of thoracic stent graft devices in the false lumen will have catastrophic consequences. When confirmation of wire access in the true lumen is needed, intravascular ultrasound has proven to be a valuable tool.

The fundamental principles of endovascular treatment of aortic dissection have major conceptual differences from aneurysmal pathology. The primary goal is coverage of the primary tear site, thus expanding the true lumen and initiating thrombosis and obliteration of the false lumen (Fig. 72-8). Often, the tear site is located in close proximity to the left subclavian artery and coverage is necessary. Despite successful thoracic stent graft therapy, persistent patency of the false lumen may occur because of complex reentry points in the distal thoracoabdominal aorta. In contrast to aneurysmal disease, sizing of the endograft devices should be conservative. The endograft devices should be minimally oversized relative to the diameter of the dissected aorta, generally at most 10%. Aggressive ballooning of the landing zones should also be discouraged.

Particularly in cases with malperfusion syndrome (because the goal of therapy is to restore distal perfusion and correct end-organ ischemia), false-lumen patency may persist despite thoracic aortic endografting. The true lumen may continue to be compressed, thereby resulting in continued malperfusion and end-organ ischemia. Called the PETTICOAT (Provisional Extension to Induce Complete Attachment) concept,[57] the principle refers to an algorithmic evaluation and treatment of the thoracoabdominal aorta in type B aortic dissection. After coverage of the primary tear site, the status of the true lumen is assessed. If persistent malperfusion is present, deployment of an additional distal device is performed. This evaluation and treatment algorithm is repeated with each adjunct device until distal malperfusion is corrected. In patients with persistent visceral malperfusion despite coverage of the primary tear site, TEVAR in the distal thoracic aorta with adjunct celiac, superior mesenteric artery, or renal bare metal stents should be considered. Subsequently, persistent lower extremity malperfusion may require infrarenal aortic and iliofemoral adjunct procedures including bare metal stents.

For dissections complicated by rupture, coverage of the primary tear site is equally essential. However, the site of rupture must also be addressed with TEVAR. Because of the extent of the dissection and the potential for perfusion of the false lumen through distal complex reentry sites, often the coverage of the entire thoracic aorta from the left subclavian artery to the celiac artery is required. Failure to recognize this concept may result in continued hemorrhage from the rupture site and potentially death.

Results

Uncomplicated Type B Dissection

The rationale for the use of TEVAR in type B dissections is based on the concept that the obliteration, or thrombosis, of the false lumen with an endograft may result in positive aortic remodeling and thus improvement in long-term outcome and survival. Closure of the primary tear site of a type B dissection should promote decompression of the false lumen, with subsequent reestablishment and stabilization of the true lumen of the aorta.

The first use of TEVAR in type B dissections was reported by Dake and coworkers in 1999. The series involved 19 patients undergoing TEVAR for acute aortic dissections; 15 patients had the diagnosis of acute type B aortic dissections. Complete thrombosis of the thoracic aortic false lumen was achieved in 15 patients (79%), with a 30-day mortality rate of 16%. In the follow-up period of 13 months, there was no death.[58]

Many other investigators have reported favorable short-term results with complete and partial obliteration of the false lumen in type B dissections, demonstrating stabilization of the descending aorta in as much as 75% of patients.[59-65] Kusagawa and coworkers reported a series of 49 patients with type B dissections (32 acute, 17 chronic). The mean follow-up period ranged from 4 months to 6 years. In the acute dissection group, the average false lumen decreased from an average of 16 mm

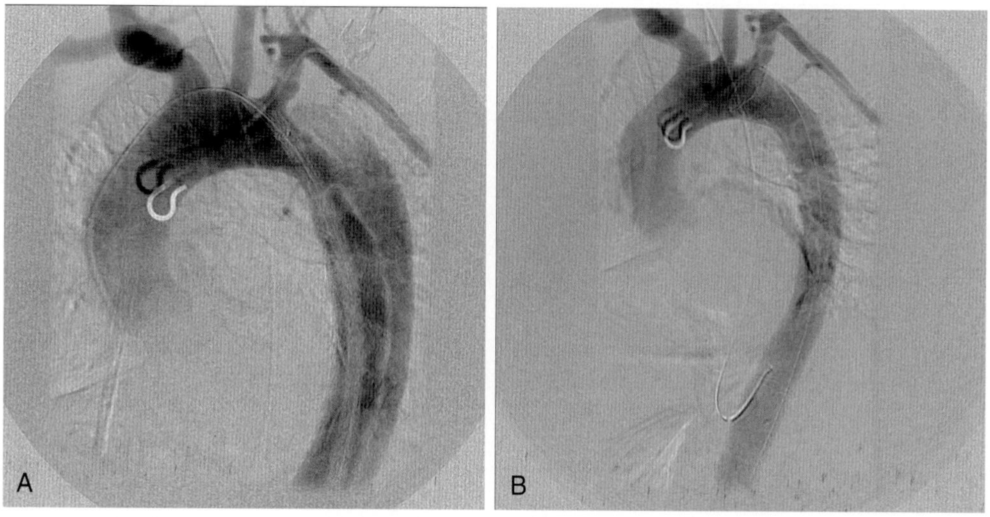

FIGURE 72-8 ■ Angiogram demonstrating endovascular treatment of acute type B aortic dissection. **A**, Positioning of the thoracic endovascular aortic repair (TEVAR) graft in the true lumen of the proximal descending thoracic aorta (DTA) is shown predeployment. **B**, Aortic arch and DTA angiogram post-TEVAR deployment in the true lumen shows loss of filling in the false lumen.

to 3 mm at 2 years after treatment. In 76% of the patients, the false lumen of the thoracic aorta completely disappeared after 2 years. The results were less dramatic in the chronic group.[59]

Dialetto and coworkers reported a series of 56 patients with type B dissections treated either medically (n = 28) or with aortic stent grafts (n = 28). Follow-up ranged from 1 to 61 months, with 100% follow-up. In-hospital mortality was 10.7% with no incidence of spinal cord ischemia. Follow-up CT scans demonstrated complete thrombosis of the false lumen in 75% of patients treated with TEVAR compared with only 10.7% of patients in the medically treated group. Aneurysmal dilation of the descending aorta was seen in only 3.5% of patients treated with TEVAR compared with 28.5% of patients in the medically treated group.[60]

Eggebrecht and coworkers recently reported a meta-analysis of TEVAR for patients with type B dissections. Thirty-nine studies were included, with a total of 609 patients. The mean follow-up period was 19.5 months. The mean procedural success rate was 98.2%, with a complication rate of 11.1%. The rate of neurologic complications was 2.9%, with stroke at 1.9% and paraplegia at 0.8%. Overall, complications were statistically higher in patients with acute type B dissection (21.7%) when compared with chronic type B dissection (9.1%). The 30-day mortality rate in the acute and chronic dissection groups were 9.8% and 3.2%, respectively. False-lumen thrombosis was seen in 75.5% of patients. Late surgical conversion was required in 2.5% of patients. Endovascular reintervention with TEVAR was necessary in 4.6% of patients. Overall survival by Kaplan-Meier analysis was 90.6%, 89.9%, and 88.8% at 6 months, 1 year, and 2 years, respectively.[55]

The role of TEVAR in acute uncomplicated type B aortic dissection was recently examined in the INvestigation of STEnt grafts in patients with type B Aortic Dissection (INSTEAD) trial. It was a multicenter, prospective, randomized trial in Europe designed to compare the outcomes of uncomplicated type B dissections treated by (1) TEVAR (Medtronic Talent device) adjunctive to anti-impulse therapy or (2) anti-impulse therapy alone. The study period was 2 years with the primary outcome measure as all-cause mortality. Secondary outcomes included conversions to TEVAR or surgery, false lumen thrombosis, cardiovascular morbidity, rate of aortic dilation, quality of life, and length of intensive care unit and hospital stay. At 1 year, there was no difference in all-cause mortality between the medical (3%) versus the TEVAR (10%) group.[66] Long-term results of the INSTEAD trial were recently published.[67] Compared with optimal medical management, TEVAR showed an improved risk of all-cause mortality (6.9% vs. 19.3%, $P = 0.13$) and aorta-specific mortality (6.9% vs. 19.3%, $P = 0.04$) at 5 years. Elective TEVAR rendered improved false-lumen thrombosis in 90.6% of cases ($P < 0.001$).

Recently, outcomes with the management of acute uncomplicated type B dissection with best medical therapy versus best medical therapy with Gore TAG stent graft was assessed. This was a prospective randomized trial (ADSORB trial).[68] Sixty-one patients were randomized, of which 80% had DeBakey type IIIB dissection. Although there was no mortality difference at 30 days and 1 year, there was a significantly improved false-lumen thrombosis rate (57% vs. 3%) and false-lumen-diameter reduction ($P < 0.001$) in the best medical therapy + Gore TAG arm. The study concluded that acute uncomplicated type B dissection can be safely treated with stent grafting, with improved aortic remodeling.

In summary, the benefit of TEVAR in acute uncomplicated type B aortic dissection is becoming increasingly evident. Results of TEVAR for the treatment of type B dissection appear promising, demonstrating early evidence of false-lumen thrombosis and aortic remodeling. However, further long-term follow-up data from future trials will be needed before definitive conclusions can be made regarding the impact on aortic remodeling and survival benefit.

Complicated Type B Dissection

Endovascular therapy in the treatment of complicated type B dissections in the acute setting has emerged as a viable surgical alternative, and in some institutions, TEVAR has become the preferred therapy of choice. Duebener and coworkers reported a series of 10 patients with complicated acute type B dissections treated with TEVAR. The mean interval to treatment from the time of diagnosis was 11 hours. Indications for TEVAR were rupture (n = 2), malperfusion (n = 5), rapid aortic expansion (n = 1), and refractory pain (n = 2). The primary tear site was covered in 90% of patients, and the early mortality was 20% (n = 2). The causes of death in the two patients were aortic disruption distal to the stent graft and hemorrhagic shock after surgical fenestration of the abdominal aorta for persistent malperfusion. The duration of follow-up ranged from 1 to 38 months.[69]

Doss and coworkers reported their experience of 54 patients undergoing emergent surgical management of thoracic aortic diseases, with 28 patients undergoing conventional open surgical technique and 26 patients undergoing TEVAR. The mean age of the patients ranged from 28 to 83 years. Of the 54 patients, the indication for intervention was perforated type B dissection in 14 patients. The mortality rate was 17.8% in the conventional surgical group versus 3.8% in the TEVAR group. Paraplegia rates were 3.6% and 0% in the conventional surgical and the TEVAR groups, respectively.[70] The same investigators reported their more recent experience with emergent endovascular treatment of acutely perforated type B dissections. In a series of 11 patients over a 10-month period, 7 patients were treated for ruptured aortic aneurysms and 4 for acutely perforated type B dissections. The average interval from diagnosis to treatment was 28 hours. Technical failure (i.e., access failure) occurred in 2 patients. At a mean follow-up of 12 months, there were no cases of paraplegia, stent migration, or endoleaks.[71]

Nienaber and coworkers[72] reported their experience of 11 patients undergoing emergency TEVAR for acute type B dissections complicated by contained ruptures. Emergency TEVAR was successful with no morbidity and stent-graft–related complications. At a mean follow-up of 15 months, there was no mortality. This was a statistically significant improvement compared with a historic-matched control group of patients undergoing conventional surgical therapy (death, n = 4).[72]

At the University of Pennsylvania, we reviewed our experience with TEVAR for the treatment of acute type B aortic dissection complicated by rupture or malperfusion.[73] In our series from 2004 to 2007, 35 patients with acute type B aortic dissection were treated with TEVAR with a technical success rate of 97.1%. The indications for surgery were rupture in 18 patients and malperfusion in 17 patients. Malperfusion involved the mesenteric and renal vasculature in 5 patients, the lower extremity in 3 patients, and both in 9 patients. In addition to thoracic endograft devices, adjunct stent therapy including infrarenal aortic stents, iliofemoral stents, and celiac/mesenteric stents was required in 12 (34.3%) patients. The rate of renal failure (2.8%), CVA (2.8%), permanent spinal cord ischemia (2.8%), vascular access complications (14.2%), and 30-day mortality (2.8%) compare favorably with conventional open repair. Overall one-year survival was 93.4%. The recent IRAD database demonstrates that conventional open repair for acute type B aortic dissection in the current era is still associated with a significant risk of cerebrovascular accident (9.0%), paraplegia (4.5%), visceral ischemia/infarction (6.8%), and acute renal failure (18.3%), all of which were correlated with postoperative death. The overall in-hospital mortality rate was 29.3%, and for patients undergoing surgery within 48 hours, the in-hospital mortality rate was 39.2%.[54] The dramatic difference in morbidity and mortality between TEVAR and conventional open repair suggests that TEVAR is an effective surgical alternative and supports a new surgical paradigm for the treatment of acute complicated type B aortic dissection. At our institution, TEVAR has emerged as the surgical therapy of choice for the management of acute complicated type B aortic dissection.

PENETRATING ATHEROSCLEROTIC ULCER, INTRAMURAL HEMATOMA, AND BLUNT THORACIC AORTIC INJURY

Historically, PAU with IMH in the DTA has been managed medically. The behavior and clinical management of PAU and IMH in the DTA is not well defined and remains a clinical challenge. Furthermore, the natural history of PAU and IMH remains unclear.[74-76] Cho and coworkers[77] recently reviewed the Mayo Clinic experience with PAU of the DTA over a 25-year period. From 1977 to 2002, 105 patients with PAU of the DTA with (n = 85) and without (n = 20) IMH were included in the study. The medical group included 76 patients and the surgical group included 29 patients. Thirty-day mortality in the medical group was 4% versus 21% in the surgery group ($P < 0.5$). Defined as conversion to surgery or death, failure of medical therapy was predicted by the presence of rupture at presentation and the era of treatment (before 1990). Aortic diameter, ulcer, or extent of hematoma were not risk factors for medical therapy failure or death.[77]

The introduction of TEVAR has prompted investigators to examine the role of this new technology in descending thoracic aortic PAU and IMH. Jin and coworkers[78] reported their experience with TEVAR for PAU in the DTA. In their series of 14 patients, the majority of patients was symptomatic and was treated emergently. Endoleaks were present in two patients at completion angiography. With a mean follow-up period of 17.2 months, coverage of PAU was achieved in all patients, with complete resorption of IMH in 2 patients. One patient died of rupture of pseudoaneurysm at one month after surgery. Other investigators have also reported small series of endovascular aortic stent graft therapy for PAU and IMH.[78-81] Technical success with good short-term follow-up has been demonstrated with low mortality.

In summary, TEVAR for PAU and IMH in the DTA is promising. Endovascular therapy for complicated or symptomatic PAU appears to be indicated. However, more evidence and long-term follow-up are needed to arrive at definitive conclusions. Currently, the TX2, Valiant, and Relay devices have approved on-label indications for PAU treatment in the United States.

Blunt thoracic aortic injury is associated with high mortality, with only 10% of patients arriving to a hospital alive, of which up to 50% die within 24 hours. Endovascular repair of blunt thoracic aortic injury has gained increasing acceptance as the treatment of choice over open surgery. The C-TAG and Valiant endograft devices have received on-label indications by the FDA for the treatment of this condition.

AORTIC ARCH/ASCENDING AORTIC PATHOLOGIES

The introduction of TEVAR has provided an alternative surgical option in patients thought to be at prohibitively high risk for conventional open aortic arch or ascending aortic repair, although the use of endovascular technology in ascending aorta and aortic arch is through off-label use only.

Aortic Arch Endovascular Repair

The arch hybrid repair is essentially a landing zone "0" endovascular repair of the aortic arch and it is guided by two fundamental concepts: (1) brachiocephalic bypass, or revascularization of the great vessels; and (2) construction of optimal proximal and distal landing zones for TEVAR. The arch hybrid repair is especially appealing in patients who are poor candidates for prolonged periods of cardiopulmonary bypass or circulatory arrest—that is, older patients and those with significant comorbidities.

Landing Zones

The principle of anatomic landing zone selection is similar in arch hybrid cases to DTA stent grafting. The hybrid arch concept is an extension of the TEVAR proximal landing zone scheme. Hybrid arch procedures are typically performed with the proximal landing zone in Z0. Therefore, the arch hybrid concept necessitates a

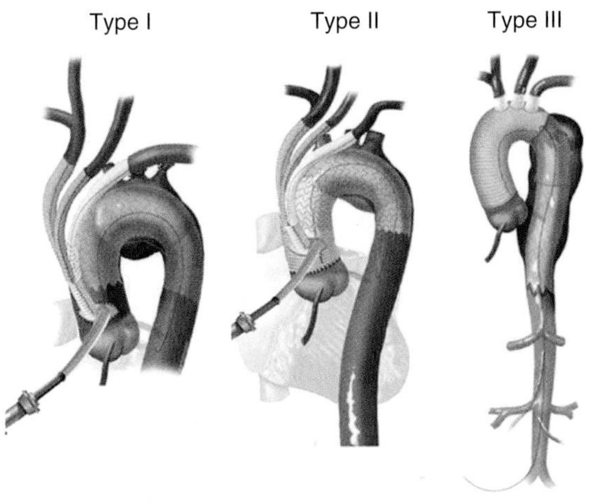

FIGURE 72-9 Arch hybrid classification is shown.

brachiocephalic revascularization procedure to preserve flow through the great vessels.

The hybrid arch repair classification is based on aortic arch aneurysm anatomy and proximal and distal landing zone feasibility. The scheme divides aortic arch aneurysms into three types (Fig. 72-9). The type I arch hybrid is typically done with a classic arch aneurysm, where the ascending and descending thoracic aortas are not aneurysmal or dissected. This anatomy has favorable proximal Z0 and distal Z3/Z4 landing zones, respectively. A type I arch hybrid repair only requires great vessel revascularization with either concomitant antegrade TEVAR stenting or delayed retrograde TEVAR from the iliofemoral vasculature. A type II arch hybrid is an ideal approach in an arch aneurysm without a good Z0 proximal landing zone but has a good distal landing zone in the DTA. Therefore, a type II repair necessitates an open surgical Z0 landing zone reconstruction for proper deployment and seal of the proximal stent graft. Type III arch hybrid repair can be used for even more complex aortopathies such as the mega-aorta syndrome. In this case, the native aorta does not have good proximal or distal landing zones for stent graft deployment. Therefore, a type III repair necessitates an open surgical reconstruction of proximal aorta and arch as a total arch replacement with elephant trunk for stent-graft landing in the DTA. It is important to note that in progression from a type I to a type III arch hybrid repair, the circulatory management options become increasingly complex and therefore must be tailored to patient status and anatomy.

Outcomes

To date there have been no randomized trials evaluating the use of hybrid techniques for the treatment of aortic arch pathology. Several groups have published their single-institution hybrid experience with an in-hospital mortality rate of 0% to 13%, and a permanent stroke rate between 0% and 8%. The incidence of paraplegia was between 0% and 24%.[82]

Two groups reported their outcomes with type I hybrid arch repair. Both groups report a 0% stroke rate and one in-hospital death in a total group of 30 patients.[83,84] Shimamura and colleagues[83] reviewed 126 type II hybrids and reported a total stroke rate of 5.6%, a paraplegia rate of 2.3%, and an in-hospital mortality rate of 3.2%. The largest series of type III hybrids, done by Kawaharada and associates,[84] demonstrated a stroke rate of 3.2%, a paraplegia rate of 0%, and an in-hospital mortality rate of 6.4%.[84] Although the data reported by these studies are encouraging, they remain limited by the small number of patients treated in their retrospective analysis.

A meta-analysis of 15 studies reporting outcomes for arch hybrid procedures revealed an overall 30-day mortality rate of 8.3%, a stroke rate of 4.4%, a paraplegia rate of 3.9%, and an endoleak rate of 9.2%. A total of 463 patients were included in this analysis.[85]

Ascending Aorta Endovascular Repair

TEVAR is not currently indicated for ascending aortic pathology; however, several centers have described their anecdotal experiences with endografting in the ascending aorta.[37,86-88] To date, there have been no clinical trials or large series describing outcomes with TEVAR in the ascending aorta. Kolvenbach and colleagues[89] have described their experience with ascending aorta TEVAR in 11 patients. They report a stroke rate, endoleak rate, and mortality rate of 9%, with a combined mortality and morbidity of 18%. Technical success was achieved in 91% of patients. They concluded that a significant number of their complications were a result of using an endograft that was not designed for unique anatomy of the ascending aorta.

In January 2012, Metcalf and colleagues[88] described the first case of ascending aorta TEVAR with an endograft designed specifically for the ascending aorta. Their group implanted a Zenith Ascending Dissection device (Cook Medical, Bjaeverskov, Denmark) in a 68-year-old man with an acute type A dissection.[88] The patient made an uneventful recovery. Currently, several devices are under development for use in clinical trials evaluating the use of TEVAR in the ascending aorta.

SUMMARY

TEVAR has emerged as a viable surgical alternative to the treatment of thoracic aortic pathology. For the treatment of aneurysmal disease, perioperative morbidity and mortality is favorable when compared with conventional open techniques. Midterm outcome and long-term follow-up demonstrate durable results with long-term survival comparable with conventional open repair. Perhaps it is in the setting of acute aortic syndromes that TEVAR may potentially have its greatest impact. Historically associated with significant morbidity and mortality, acute aortic syndromes including traumatic transection, rupture, pseudoaneurysm, and dissection remain major clinical challenges. Although TEVAR is technically more challenging, its results have been favorable in the treatment of acute aortic dissections.

REFERENCES

1. Parodi JC, Palmaz JC, Barone HD: Transfemoral intraluminal graft implantation for abdominal aortic aneurysms. *Ann Vasc Surg* 5(6):491–499, 1991.
2. Dake MD, Miller DC, Semba CP, et al: Transluminal placement of endovascular stent-grafts for 2he treatment of descending thoracic aortic aneurysms. *N Engl J Med* 331(26):1729–1734, 1994.
3. Schlatmann TJ, Becker AE: Histologic changes in the normal aging aorta: implications for dissecting aortic aneurysm. *Am J Cardiol* 39(1):13–20, 1977.
4. Olsson C, Thelin S, Stahle E, et al: Thoracic aortic aneurysm and dissection: increasing prevalence and improved outcomes reported in a nationwide population-based study of more than 14,000 cases from 1987 to 2002. *Circulation* 114(24):2611–2618, 2006.
5. Davies RR, Goldstein LJ, Coady MA, et al: Yearly rupture or dissection rates for thoracic aortic aneurysms: simple prediction based on size. *Ann Thorac Surg* 73(1):17–27, discussion 27–28, 2002.
6. Coady MA, Rizzo JA, Hammond GL, et al: What is the appropriate size criterion for resection of thoracic aortic aneurysms? *J Thorac Cardiovasc Surg* 113(3):476–491, discussion 489–491, 1997.
7. Svensson LG, Kouchoukos NT, Miller DC, et al: Expert consensus document on the treatment of descending thoracic aortic disease using endovascular stent-grafts. *Ann Thorac Surg* 85(1 Suppl):S1–S41, 2008.
8. Clouse WD, Hallett JW, Jr, Schaff HV, et al: Improved prognosis of thoracic aortic aneurysms: a population-based study. *JAMA* 280(22):1926–1929, 1998.
9. Bavaria JE, Appoo JJ, Makaroun MS, et al: Endovascular stent grafting versus open surgical repair of descending thoracic aortic aneurysms in low-risk patients: a multicenter comparative trial. *J Thorac Cardiovasc Surg* 133(2):369–377, 2007.
10. Fairman RM, Criado F, Farber M, et al: Pivotal results of the Medtronic Vascular Talent Thoracic Stent Graft System: the VALOR trial. *J Vasc Surg* 48(3):546–554, 2008.
11. Fattori R, Nienaber CA, Rousseau H, et al: Results of endovascular repair of the thoracic aorta with the Talent Thoracic stent graft: the Talent Thoracic Retrospective Registry. *J Thorac Cardiovasc Surg* 132(2):332–339, 2006.
12. Matsumura JS, Cambria RP, Dake MD, et al: International controlled clinical trial of thoracic endovascular aneurysm repair with the Zenith TX2 endovascular graft: 1-year results. *J Vasc Surg* 47(2):247–257, discussion 257, 2008.
13. Fairman RM, Tuchek JM, Lee WA, et al: Pivotal results for the Medtronic Valiant Thoracic Stent Graft System in the VALOR II trial. *J Vasc Surg* 56(5):1222–1231, e1, 2012.
14. Czerny M, Fleck T, Zimpfer D, et al: Risk factors of mortality and permanent neurologic injury in patients undergoing ascending aortic and arch repair. *J Thorac Cardiovasc Surg* 126(5):1296–1301, 2003.
15. Woo EY, Carpenter JP, Jackson BM, et al: Left subclavian artery coverage during thoracic endovascular aortic repair: a single-center experience. *J Vasc Surg* 48(3):555–560, 2008.
16. Makaroun MS, Dillavou ED, Wheatley GH, et al: Five-year results of endovascular treatment with the Gore TAG device compared with open repair of thoracic aortic aneurysms. *J Vasc Surg* 47(5):912–918, 2008.
17. Riambau V, Zipfel B, Coppi G, et al: Final operative and midterm results of the European experience in the RELAY Endovascular Registry for Thoracic Disease (RESTORE) study. *J Vasc Surg* 53(3):565–573, 2011.
18. Leurs LJ, Hobo R, Buth J, et al: The multicenter experience with a third-generation endovascular device for abdominal aortic aneurysm repair. A report from the EUROSTAR database. *J Cardiovasc Surg (Torino)* 45(4):293–300, 2004.
19. Parmer SS, Carpenter JP, Stavropoulos SW, et al: Endoleaks after endovascular repair of thoracic aortic aneurysms. *J Vasc Surg* 44(3):447–452, 2006.
20. Gutsche JT, Cheung AT, McGarvey ML, et al: Risk factors for perioperative stroke after thoracic endovascular aortic repair. *Ann Thorac Surg* 84(4):1195–1200, discussion 1200, 2007.
21. Cheung AT, Pochettino A, McGarvey ML, et al: Strategies to manage paraplegia risk after endovascular stent repair of descending thoracic aortic aneurysms. *Ann Thorac Surg* 80(4):1280–1288, discussion 1288–1289, 2005.
22. Gravereaux EC, Faries PL, Burks JA, et al: Risk of spinal cord ischemia after endograft repair of thoracic aortic aneurysms. *J Vasc Surg* 34(6):997–1003, 2001.
23. Greenberg R, Resch T, Nyman U, et al: Endovascular repair of descending thoracic aortic aneurysms: an early experience with intermediate-term follow-up. *J Vasc Surg* 31(1 Pt 1):147–156, 2000.
24. Ortiz-Gomez JR, Gonzalez-Solis FJ, Fernandez-Alonso L, et al: Reversal of acute paraplegia with cerebrospinal fluid drainage after endovascular thoracic aortic aneurysm repair. *Anesthesiology* 95(5):1288–1289, 2001.
25. Coselli JS, Lemaire SA, Koksoy C, et al: Cerebrospinal fluid drainage reduces paraplegia after thoracoabdominal aortic aneurysm repair: results of a randomized clinical trial. *J Vasc Surg* 35(4):631–639, 2002.
26. Bafort C, Astarci P, Goffette P, et al: Predicting spinal cord ischemia before endovascular thoracoabdominal aneurysm repair: monitoring somatosensory evoked potentials. *J Endovasc Ther* 9(3):289–294, 2002.
27. De Bakey ME, Cooley DA, Creech O, Jr: Surgical considerations of dissecting aneurysm of the aorta. *Ann Surg* 142(4):586–610, discussion, 611–612, 1955.
28. Bavaria JE, Brinster DR, Gorman RC, et al: Advances in the treatment of acute type A dissection: an integrated approach. *Ann Thorac Surg* 74(5):S1848–S1852, discussion S1857–S1863, 2002.
29. Ehrlich MP, Ergin MA, McCullough JN, et al: Results of immediate surgical treatment of all acute type A dissections. *Circulation* 102(19 Suppl 3):III248–III252, 2000.
30. Kallenbach K, Oelze T, Salcher R, et al: Evolving strategies for treatment of acute aortic dissection type A. *Circulation* 110(11 Suppl 1):II243–II249, 2004.
31. Tan ME, Dossche KM, Morshuis WJ, et al: Operative risk factors of type A aortic dissection: analysis of 252 consecutive patients. *Cardiovasc Surg* 11(4):277–285, 2003.
32. Lai DT, Miller DC, Mitchell RS, et al: Acute type A aortic dissection complicated by aortic regurgitation: composite valve graft versus separate valve graft versus conservative valve repair. *J Thorac Cardiovasc Surg* 126(6):1978–1986, 2003.
33. Driever R, Botsios S, Schmitz E, et al: Long-term effectiveness of operative procedures for Stanford type A aortic dissections. *Cardiovasc Surg* 11(4):265–272, 2003.
34. Moon MR, Sundt TM, 3rd, Pasque MK, et al: Does the extent of proximal or distal resection influence outcome for type A dissections? *Ann Thorac Surg* 71(4):1244–1249, discussion 1249–1250, 2001.
35. Lansman SL, McCullough JN, Nguyen KH, et al: Subtypes of acute aortic dissection. *Ann Thorac Surg* 67(6):1975–1978, discussion 1979–1980, 1999.
36. Hagan PG, Nienaber CA, Isselbacher EM, et al: The International Registry of Acute Aortic Dissection (IRAD): new insights into an old disease. *JAMA* 283(7):897–903, 2000.
37. Zimpfer D, Czerny M, Kettenbach J, et al: Treatment of acute type A dissection by percutaneous endovascular stent-graft placement. *Ann Thorac Surg* 82:747–749, 2006.
38. Zhang H, Li M, Jin W, et al: Endoluminal and surgical treatment for the management of Stanford Type A aortic dissection. *Eur J Cardiothorac Surg* 26(4):857–859, 2004.
39. Ihnken K, Sze D, Dake MD, et al: Successful treatment of a Stanford type A dissection by percutaneous placement of a covered stent graft in the ascending aorta. *J Thorac Cardiovasc Surg* 127(6):1808–1810, 2004.
40. Umana JP, Lai DT, Mitchell RS, et al: Is medical therapy still the optimal treatment strategy for patients with acute type B aortic dissections? *J Thorac Cardiovasc Surg* 124(5):896–910, 2002.
41. Glower DD, Fann JI, Speier RH, et al: Comparison of medical and surgical therapy for uncomplicated descending aortic dissection. *Circulation* 82(5 Suppl):IV39–IV46, 1990.
42. Gysi J, Schaffner T, Mohacsi P, et al: Early and late outcome of operated and non-operated acute dissection of the descending aorta. *Eur J Cardiothorac Surg* 11(6):1163–1169, discussion 1169–1170, 1997.
43. Safi HJ, Harlin SA, Miller CC, et al: Predictive factors for acute renal failure in thoracic and thoracoabdominal aortic aneurysm surgery. *J Vasc Surg* 24(3):338–344, discussion 344–345, 1996.

44. Yeh CH, Chen MC, Wu YC, et al: Risk factors for descending aortic aneurysm formation in medium-term follow-up of patients with type A aortic dissection. *Chest* 124(3):989–995, 2003.
45. Fann JI, Smith JA, Miller DC, et al: Surgical management of aortic dissection during a 30-year period. *Circulation* 92(9 Suppl):II113–II121, 1995.
46. Juvonen T, Ergin MA, Galla JD, et al: Prospective study of the natural history of thoracic aortic aneurysms. *Ann Thorac Surg* 63(6):1533–1545, 1997.
47. Tsai TT, Evangelista A, Nienaber CA, et al: Partial thrombosis of the false lumen in patients with acute type B aortic dissection. *N Engl J Med* 357(4):349–359, 2007.
48. Akutsu K, Nejima J, Kiuchi K, et al: Effects of the patent false lumen on the long-term outcome of type B acute aortic dissection. *Eur J Cardiothorac Surg* 26(2):359–366, 2004.
49. Ergin MA, Phillips RA, Galla JD, et al: Significance of distal false lumen after type A dissection repair. *Ann Thorac Surg* 57(4):820–824, discussion 825, 1994.
50. Song JM, Kim SD, Kim JH, et al: Long-term predictors of descending aorta aneurismal change in patients with aortic dissection. *J Am Coll Cardiol* 50(8):799–804, 2007.
51. Marui A, Mochizuki T, Koyama T, et al: Degree of fusiform dilatation of the proximal descending aorta in type B acute aortic dissection can predict late aortic events. *J Thorac Cardiovasc Surg* 134(5):1163–1170, 2007.
52. Miller DC, Mitchell RS, Oyer PE, et al: Independent determinants of operative mortality for patients with aortic dissections. *Circulation* 70(3 Pt 2):I153–I164, 1984.
53. Svensson LG, Crawford ES, Hess KR, et al: Dissection of the aorta and dissecting aortic aneurysms. Improving early and long-term surgical results. *Circulation* 82(5 Suppl):IV24–IV38, 1990.
54. Trimarchi S, Nienaber CA, Rampoldi V, et al: Role and results of surgery in acute type B aortic dissection: insights from the International Registry of Acute Aortic Dissection (IRAD). *Circulation* 114(1 Suppl):I357–I364, 2006.
55. Moon MC, Pablo Morales J, Greenberg RK: Complicated acute type B dissection and endovascular repair: indications and pitfalls. *Perspect Vasc Surg Endovasc Ther* 19(2):146–159, 2007.
56. Mossop PJ, McLachlan CS, Amukotuwa SA, et al: Staged endovascular treatment for complicated type B aortic dissection. *Nat Clin Pract Cardiovasc Med* 2(6):316–321, quiz 322, 2005.
57. Nienaber CA, Kische S, Zeller T, et al: Provisional extension to induce complete attachment after stent-graft placement in type B aortic dissection: the PETTICOAT concept. *J Endovasc Ther* 13(6):738–746, 2006.
58. Dake MD, Kato N, Mitchell RS, et al: Endovascular stent-graft placement for the treatment of acute aortic dissection. *N Engl J Med* 340(20):1546–1552, 1999.
59. Kusagawa H, Shimono T, Ishida M, et al: Changes in false lumen after transluminal stent-graft placement in aortic dissections: six years' experience. *Circulation* 111(22):2951–2957, 2005.
60. Dialetto G, Covino FE, Scognamiglio G, et al: Treatment of type B aortic dissection: endoluminal repair or conventional medical therapy? *Eur J Cardiothorac Surg* 27(5):826–830, 2005.
61. Eggebrecht H, Nienaber CA, Neuhauser M, et al: Endovascular stent-graft placement in aortic dissection: a meta-analysis. *Eur Heart J* 27(4):489–498, 2006.
62. Nienaber CA, Fattori R, Lund G, et al: Nonsurgical reconstruction of thoracic aortic dissection by stent-graft placement. *N Engl J Med* 340(20):1539–1545, 1999.
63. Czermak BV, Waldenberger P, Fraedrich G, et al: Treatment of Stanford type B aortic dissection with stent-grafts: preliminary results. *Radiology* 217(2):544–550, 2000.
64. Hausegger KA, Tiesenhausen K, Schedlbauer P, et al: Treatment of acute aortic type B dissection with stent-grafts. *Cardiovasc Intervent Radiol* 24(5):306–312, 2001.
65. Hutschala D, Fleck T, Czerny M, et al: Endoluminal stent-graft placement in patients with acute aortic dissection type B. *Eur J Cardiothorac Surg* 21(6):964–969, 2002.
66. Nienaber CA, Zannetti S, Barbieri B, et al: INvestigation of STEnt grafts in patients with type B Aortic Dissection: design of the INSTEAD trial–a prospective, multicenter, European randomized trial. *Am Heart J* 149(4):592–599, 2005.
67. Nienaber CA, Kische S, Rousseau H, et al: Endovascular repair of type B aortic dissection: long-term results of the randomized investigation of stent grafts in aortic dissection trial. *Circ Cardiovasc Interv* 6(4):407–416, 2013.
68. Brunkwall J, Kasprzak P, Verhoeven E, et al: ADSORB trialists. Endovascular repair of acute uncomplicated aortic type B dissection promotes aortic remodelling: 1 year results of the ADSORB trial. *Eur J Vasc Endovasc Surg* 48(3):285–291, 2014.
69. Duebener LF, Lorenzen P, Richardt G, et al: Emergency endovascular stent-grafting for life-threatening acute type B aortic dissections. *Ann Thorac Surg* 78(4):1261–1266, discussion 1266–1267, 2004.
70. Doss M, Balzer J, Martens S, et al: Surgical versus endovascular treatment of acute thoracic aortic rupture: a single-center experience. *Ann Thorac Surg* 76(5):1465–1469, discussion 1469–1470, 2003.
71. Doss M, Balzer J, Martens S, et al: Emergent endovascular stent grafting for perforated acute type B dissections and ruptured thoracic aortic aneurysms. *Ann Thorac Surg* 76(2):493–498, discussion 497–498, 2003.
72. Nienaber CA, Ince H, Weber F, et al: Emergency stent-graft placement in thoracic aortic dissection and evolving rupture. *J Card Surg* 18(5):464–470, 2003.
73. Szeto WY, McGarvey M, Pochettino A, et al: Results of a new surgical paradigm: endovascular repair for acute complicated type B aortic dissection. *Ann Thorac Surg* 86(1):87–93, discussion 93–94, 2008.
74. Robbins RC, McManus RP, Mitchell RS, et al: Management of patients with intramural hematoma of the thoracic aorta. *Circulation* 88(5 Pt 2):II1–II10, 1993.
75. Vilacosta I, San Roman JA, Ferreiros J, et al: Natural history and serial morphology of aortic intramural hematoma: a novel variant of aortic dissection. *Am Heart J* 134(3):495–507, 1997.
76. Nienaber CA, von Kodolitsch Y, Petersen B, et al: Intramural hemorrhage of the thoracic aorta. Diagnostic and therapeutic implications. *Circulation* 92(6):1465–1472, 1995.
77. Cho KR, Stanson AW, Potter DD, et al: Penetrating atherosclerotic ulcer of the descending thoracic aorta and arch. *J Thorac Cardiovasc Surg* 127(5):1393–1399, discussion 1399–1401, 2004.
78. Jin JL, Huang LJ, Yu FC, et al: [Endovascular stent-graft repair for penetrating atherosclerotic ulcer of the descending aorta]. *Zhonghua Yi Xue Za Zhi* 86(16):1115–1117, 2006.
79. Kaya A, Heijmen RH, Overtoom TT, et al: Thoracic stent grafting for acute aortic pathology. *Ann Thorac Surg* 82(2):560–565, 2006.
80. Raupach J, Lojik M, Beran L, et al: [Penetrating aortic ulcers–case report on endovascular therapy]. *Cas Lek Cesk* 145(5):404–407, discussion 408–409, 2006.
81. Brinster DR, Wheatley GH, 3rd, Williams J, et al: Are penetrating aortic ulcers best treated using an endovascular approach? *Ann Thorac Surg* 82(5):1688–1691, 2006.
82. Saleh HM, Inglese L: Combined surgical and endovascular treatment of arch aneurysms. *J Vasc Surg* 44:460–466, 2006.
83. Shimamura K, Kuratani T, Matsumiya G, et al: Long-term results of the open stent-grafting technique for extended aortic arch disease. *J Thorac Cardiovasc Surg* 135:1261–1269, 2008.
84. Kawaharada N, Kurimoto Y, Ito T, et al: Hybrid treatment for aortic arch and proximal descending thoracic aneurysm: experience with stent grafting for second-stage elephant trunk repair. *Eur J Cardiothorac Surg* 36:956–961, 2009.
85. Koullias GJ, Wheatley GH: State of the art of hybrid procedures for the aortic arch: a meta-analysis. *Ann Thorac Surg* 90:689–697, 2010.
86. Szeto WY, Fairman RM, Acker MA, et al: Emergency endovascular deployment of stent graft in the ascending aorta for contained rupture of innominate artery pseudoaneurysm in a pediatric patient. *Ann Thorac Surg* 81(5):1872–1875, 2006.
87. Szeto WY, Moser WG, Desai ND, et al: Transapical deployment of endovascular thoracic stent graft for an ascending aortic pseudoaneurysm. *Ann Thorac Surg* 89:616–618, 2010.
88. Metcalfe MJ, Karthikesalingam A, Black SA, et al: The first endovascular repair of an acute type A dissection using an endograft designed for the ascending aorta. *J Vasc Surg* 55:220–222, 2012.
89. Kolvenbach RR, Karmeli R, Pinter LS, et al: Endovascular management of ascending aortic pathology. *J Vasc Surg* 53:1431–1438, 2011.

CHAPTER 73

Occlusive Disease of the Brachiocephalic Vessels and Management of Simultaneous Surgical Carotid and Coronary Disease

Maral Ouzounian • Scott A. LeMaire • Joseph S. Coselli*

CHAPTER OUTLINE

Frequently, and in a variety of clinical settings, cardiovascular surgeons encounter occlusive disease involving the branches arising from the aortic arch. As a result of the increasing average life expectancy of human beings, there is a growing subset of older patients who are found to have brachiocephalic occlusive disease incidentally during preoperative evaluation for more routine cardiac surgery. In addition, the widespread use of the internal thoracic artery (ITA) as the conduit of choice for patients with surgically correctable coronary artery disease has created a subset of patients who, postoperatively, are susceptible to coronary ischemia from occlusive disease involving the subclavian vessels, which produces coronary-subclavian steal syndrome.

Although atherosclerosis is the most common cause of brachiocephalic occlusive disease, other, less common causes of aortic branch occlusive disease, such as Takayasu arteritis and radiation-induced arteritis, can also manifest as occlusion of the aortic arch branch vessels that occasionally requires surgical intervention. Regardless of the cause of intrathoracic brachiocephalic occlusive

*Disclosure: Dr. Coselli serves as a consultant for Vascutek Ltd., a subsidiary of Terumo Corporation.

disease, advancements in diagnostic imaging, technical improvements in end-organ protection, the development of endovascular techniques, strategic anesthetic management, and a better understanding of critical care all have enabled cardiovascular surgeons to perform a wide variety of procedures to treat patients with this problem with low operative risk.

Concomitant occlusive disease involving coronary and carotid arteries can pose particular challenges for cardiovascular surgeons, and the ideal treatment strategy for these combined lesions remains controversial. Treatment algorithms for concomitant coronary and carotid occlusive disease have recently expanded with the advent of endovascular techniques. Current strategies for treating patients with this problem include synchronous revascularization, staged procedures, hybrid approaches using endovascular devices, and medical treatment.

OCCLUSIVE DISEASE INVOLVING THE BRACHIOCEPHALIC ARTERIES

Pathophysiology

Atherosclerosis of the aortic arch has been recognized recently as a significant contributor to and an independent predictor of embolic stroke and generalized atherosclerotic disease, and it is the most common cause of intrathoracic brachiocephalic occlusive disease.[1] In addition to its well-known associations with cigarette smoking, peripheral arterial occlusive disease, dyslipidemia, hypertension, male sex, and diabetes mellitus, atheroma has also been associated with elevated levels of fibrinogen and homocysteine.[2,3] Aortic arch atheroma, first seen early in the patient's adult life, is characterized by gradually increasing severity.[4] The progression of aortic arch atheroma to brachiocephalic occlusive disease is influenced directly by the presence of aggravating risk factors.

Two important pathologic sequelae directly related to aortic arch plaques are atheroembolism and thromboembolism.[5] Within the aging aortic arch, a variety of pathophysiologic processes occur: these include calcification, the destruction of smooth muscle and elastic fibers (including the loss of internal elastic lamina), the formation of thrombi, and most importantly, the deposition of atherosclerotic plaques.[6] The vast majority of occlusive lesions of branching vessels of the arch and of the upper-extremity arterial branches are atherosclerotic in origin, and disease often involves multiple vessels.[7-9] In addition, because of the irregular nature of these plaques, embolic phenomena resulting from thrombus deposits—composed of both platelets and fibrin—can occur in nearly a third of such patients. Thrombotic or thromboembolic events predominantly occur in patients with multifocal disease. Embolic phenomena owing to ostial disease of the aortic arch branches are uncommon. A cardiogenic source of embolism must be excluded before emboli can be conclusively attributed to arch branch disease.[10]

Inflammatory disorders, such as Takayasu arteritis or polymyalgia rheumatica, are among the less common causes of arch branch occlusive disease. The prototypic vasculitis syndrome that commonly leads to occlusive disease of the thoracic aorta and its branches is Takayasu arteritis. This disease is characterized by immune-mediated destruction of the medial elastic fibers of the affected vessel, followed by scarring of the media and internal elastic lamina, which causes compensatory intimal proliferation. Takayasu arteritis remains an idiopathic large-vessel vasculitis that generally affects women of reproductive age and predominates in Asians; however, it has been reported in patients of all ethnicities.[11] Cardiac failure and cardiomegaly are usually secondary to hypertension and aortic valvular insufficiency. Approximately 60% of patients with Takayasu arteritis require some form of vascular intervention, most commonly involving the coronary arteries, followed by the carotid and upper-extremity arteries.

Additional disorders that can be causative include arteritis stemming from radioactive therapy (for malignancies of the neck or Hodgkin disease), traumatic injuries (e.g., penetrating missile injuries and blunt deceleration injuries), vasospastic disorders, thoracic outlet syndrome, and possibly connective tissue disorders. Radiation therapy can lead to stenosis of the brachiocephalic vessels and induce unpredictable atherosclerotic changes several years after treatment, ultimately resulting in embolic or diminished-flow phenomena.

Clinical Presentation

Clinical manifestations of brachiocephalic occlusive disease (Fig. 73-1) are predominately related to the degree of luminal encroachment in the primary vessel affected and the extent of collateral disease if multiple vascular beds are compromised. Stenosis of aortic arch branches can have direct ischemia-related consequences or lead to steal syndromes in which increases in blood flow to one region result in ischemia in another. Involvement of the innominate artery can lead to anterior, posterior, or combined cerebral symptoms, depending on the amount of collateral flow from the contralateral side via the circle of Willis and the extent of concomitant subclavian or common carotid artery (CCA) involvement. Isolated right-sided steal syndromes can occur, but only if the disease arises in the right subclavian artery and the innominate is relatively spared. In contrast, involvement of the left subclavian artery can result in either upper-extremity claudication or vertebral steal manifesting as vertebrobasilar symptoms, depending on the exact location of the stenotic lesion.

In general, the clinical presentation of patients with brachiocephalic occlusive disease involves either an acute embolic or a chronic stenotic event. Acute embolic symptoms tend to involve cerebral hemispheric events related to anterior circulation and, similar to carotid bifurcation disease, amaurosis fugax. Less often, emboli can affect the upper extremities, usually evidenced by cold or numb hands or fingers. Commonly, stenotic lesions reduce blood flow to upper extremities (and occasionally to lower extremities) and can result in subclavian steal syndrome. Exercise can induce ischemia and cause hand or arm cramping or fatigue (this process is also known as *claudication*); in time, these symptoms can progress to rest pain and possibly to tissue loss.

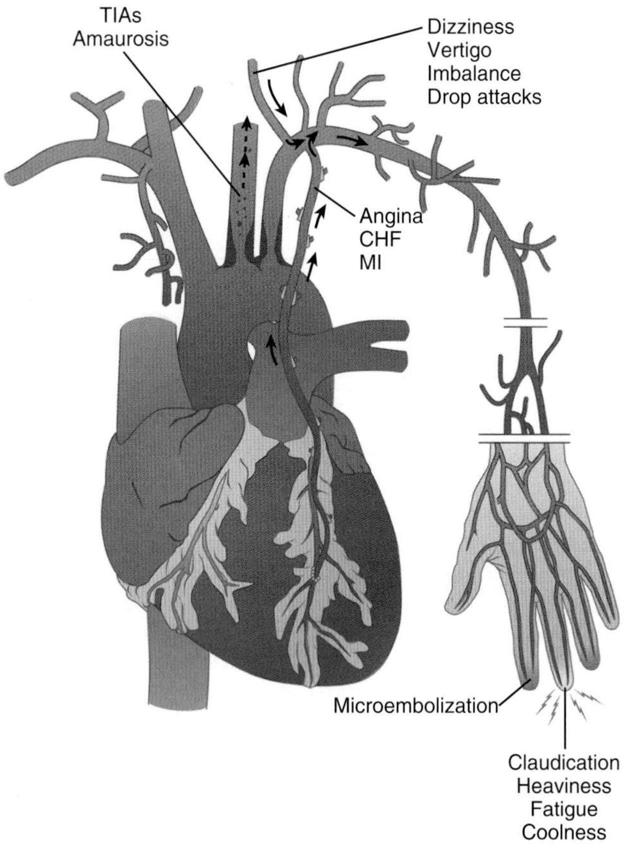

FIGURE 73-1 ■ Common symptoms of occlusive disease involving the brachiocephalic branches. Compromised flow or emboli from common carotid artery lesions can cause a variety of neurologic symptoms, including transient ischemic attacks (TIAs) and amaurosis fugax. Subclavian artery lesions can cause vertebrobasilar insufficiency (including vertebral-subclavian steal), cardiac complications (including angina, myocardial infarction [MI], and congestive heart failure [CHF]) caused by coronary-subclavian steal, and upper-extremity arterial insufficiency or microembolization. (From Takach TJ, Reul GJ Jr, Cooley DA, et al: Myocardial thievery: the coronary-subclavian steal syndrome. *Ann Thorac Surg* 81:386–392, 2006.)

Takayasu arteritis is associated with a broad spectrum of clinical presentations that range from a fairly indolent chronic course to an acute fulminant disease. The initial symptoms most commonly reported by patients are constitutional and include myalgia, arthralgia, and headaches. Vascular symptoms commonly include claudicatory symptoms, carotidynia, and pulseless extremity. The diffuse involvement of major branches of the aorta contributes to an overall diminution of peripheral pulses in these patients, which is why Takayasu arteritis is sometimes referred to as *pulseless disease*. The nonspecific nature of the initial presentation contributes to the delay in the diagnosis of most cases of Takayasu arteritis. The Ueno classification system categorizes the disease into four types according to the extent and location of involvement. Types 1 and 3 are characterized by a disease process that affects the aortic arch and its branches.[12] Stenosis and occlusion are typical of Takayasu arteritis, and the lesions can be either short and segmental or long and diffuse. De novo aneurysms are rare but have been reported in all major branches of the aortic arch.[13,14] Most aneurysms arise from sites of previous anastomoses or surgical repair.[15,16]

The age at presentation for patients with radiation-induced disease primarily depends on the age at which they were exposed to radiation, and is often younger than for those with atherosclerotic occlusive disease. These patients have angiographically atypical lesions that appear diffuse, unlike the focal lesions typical of atherosclerosis.[17] Presentation includes either embolic or flow-limiting symptoms.

Diagnostic Evaluation

Diagnostic imaging, performed after a detailed initial vascular and neurologic examination, plays an important role in determining the appropriate treatment for each patient. A thorough neurologic examination, even in patients with isolated upper-extremity ischemic symptoms, is essential, because such symptoms could potentially be a manifestation of a steal syndrome and concomitant disease elsewhere. Other critical components of a thorough physical examination include measuring the blood pressure in both arms (a systolic difference greater than 20 mm Hg usually suggests proximal occlusive disease) and conducting a detailed pulse examination of the subclavian artery distribution at several locations: the wrist (radial and ulnar arteries), the upper arm and elbow (brachial artery), the armpit (axillary artery), and in the supraclavicular fossa. An absent or weakened pulse found anywhere other than the supraclavicular fossa tends to indicate arterial occlusion. In addition, an Allen test should be performed because the absence of a blush in any section of the hand usually indicates an incomplete palmar arch. Palpation of the infraclavicular and supraclavicular fossae is helpful to identify a subclavian aneurysm or cervical rib. A bruit identified during auscultation of the subclavian artery may indicate thoracic outlet compression of the artery.

The diagnosis of Takayasu arteritis is usually suspected from the patient's history and clinical presentation, and it is supported by the findings of specific serologic tests, tests for inflammatory markers, and angiography.[18] Angiographic studies show a characteristic pattern of stenosis, poststenotic dilation, aneurysm formation, and occlusion with collateral formation. These findings tend to be localized to the aorta and the proximal aspect of its branches.[19,20] Total body arteriography is an important component of the diagnostic workup of these patients to characterize the full extent of the disease and to provide a baseline for future comparison, because these patients require frequent serial imaging and monitoring for the rest of their lives.

Conventional Imaging Modalities

Digital subtraction angiography offers the opportunity for immediate endovascular intervention if a problem is discovered. As with any intravascular manipulation and imaging technique, the risk of embolic stroke always exists, especially in patients with atherosclerotic disease and plaques.[21] The development of high-resolution computed tomographic angiography with reconstructive capabilities has allowed this modality to substitute for digital subtraction angiography in the assessment of the aortic arch branches in specific circumstances. Computed tomography (CT) and magnetic resonance imaging (MRI) provide valuable imaging for assessing the extent of brachiocephalic disease. Contrast-enhanced MRI with reconstruction provides information equivalent to that obtained from conventional CT angiography. Magnetic resonance angiography (MRA), in addition, can yield useful information about occluded vessels reconstituted via collaterals because the imaging process is not contrast dependent. In addition, MRA provides valuable information about factors that affect the risk of embolization and consequent stroke, including the size, extent, and composition of atherosclerotic lesions. We recommend obtaining a preoperative CT angiogram or MRA for all patients who undergo surgical intervention on the branches of the aortic arch; the images serve as a baseline for future comparisons and for assessing the progression of the disease. Lifelong postoperative surveillance imaging and follow-up is an essential component of the care of these patients.[22]

Ultrasonography and Emerging Imaging Modalities

Transthoracic echocardiography, although reliable for assessing the ascending aorta, is not ideal for assessing the arch and its branches because of its shallow depth of penetration and because the overlying ribs obscure these vessels. Similarly, transesophageal echocardiography (TEE) is limited in its ability to image the branches of the aortic arch, primarily because of shadowing from the trachea.[23] Intravascular ultrasonography is an emerging technology that may be useful during endovascular interventions.

The advent of transesophageal magnetic coils has made it possible to perform transesophageal MRI (TEMRI).[24,25] Although TEMRI allows multiplanar reconstruction and provides better quantification of the extent of aortic atherosclerosis, real-time imaging and assessment of plaque mobility are feasible only with the help of TEE. Nonetheless, TEMRI provides a better assessment of the circumferential extent of atherosclerotic involvement than TEE does, and it could become an important option for imaging the supra-aortic great vessels.

Anatomic Considerations in Operative Exposures of Brachiocephalic Vessels

A thorough knowledge of thoracic anatomy is invaluable for the successful exposure of the supra-aortic vessels, and operative success is heavily dependent on good exposure with appropriate proximal and distal control. A median sternotomy provides adequate exposure for all the major arch vessels, including, in most cases, the left subclavian artery. A mini upper sternotomy up to the third or fourth intercostal space provides good exposure for the mid to distal innominate artery. This is useful in situations in which the proximal innominate artery is free of disease and the aorta does not require clamping for proximal control. A Rummel tourniquet can be used for proximal control in these cases; however, this approach can be challenging to use when innominate artery bypass is necessary or when multiple vessels must be addressed. A full sternotomy is preferred in these circumstances. Extending the median sternotomy incision along the anterior border of the right sternocleidomastoid muscle provides adequate exposure of the bifurcation of the innominate artery and the right CCA. The same incision can be extended over the upper border of the right clavicle if exposure of the more distal aspects of the right subclavian artery is required. The right sternoclavicular joint may need to be dislocated to enhance exposure. Extending the median sternotomy along the anterior border of the left sternocleidomastoid enhances exposure for the left CCA.

The posterior location of the left subclavian artery makes exposure more challenging. When a median sternotomy is performed, it may be necessary to extend the incision over the left clavicle and to dislocate the left sternoclavicular joint for adequate exposure of the intrathoracic course of the left subclavian artery. Isolated left subclavian artery disease can be approached easily via a left posterolateral thoracotomy incision through the fourth intercostal space.

Structures that can interfere with exposure, as well as conduit positioning, are the thymic remnant and the left brachiocephalic vein. The thymus can be split longitudinally or even resected to provide adequate exposure. The brachiocephalic vein can be mobilized as far laterally as necessary so that it may be retracted out of the way to provide better exposure of the proximal arch branches. Ligating the vessel is occasionally necessary to enhance exposure of the left subclavian artery and left CCA. Ligation usually has no significant consequences except for transient left upper-extremity venous congestion. Ligating the brachiocephalic vein is not usually required for bypass procedures; bypass grafts can generally be safely tunneled behind the vein. Attention should be paid to the course of the recurrent laryngeal nerves if the dissection is carried out far laterally into the right subclavian artery and when one is gaining proximal control of the left subclavian artery and the subjacent aorta. The phrenic nerve is vulnerable to injury along its course over the anterior scalene muscle when the sternotomy incisions are extended over the clavicle. In addition, excessive traction in these incisions could jeopardize the functional integrity of the brachial plexus, producing undesirable long-term sequelae.

Cerebral protection is of concern in any operative manipulation involving the innominate artery or the CCAs. During the preoperative evaluation, one should thoroughly ascertain the patient's vascular anatomy, including the patency and size of the vertebral arteries and the completeness of the circle of Willis. Caution should be exercised, as usual, during placement of the proximal clamp and selection of the site for the proximal anastomosis to avoid any area on the aorta with atherosclerotic involvement. Epiaortic ultrasound can be helpful in selecting an ideal clamp site. The robust collateral circulation of the cerebral vasculature allows safe clamping of the innominate artery or proximal CCAs, provided there is no diffuse or multivessel involvement. Flow through the left CCA should be ensured while the innominate artery is clamped. Similarly, it may be prudent to monitor a right subclavian arterial line when the left CCA is intervened on to ensure that there is flow through the innominate system. Furthermore, it may be helpful to monitor estimated hemispheric perfusion by using near-infrared spectroscopy to perform transcranial oximetry during innominate or left CCA clamping. The strategy for cerebral protection is more complicated in patients with contralateral carotid occlusion or multivessel disease, which occasionally necessitates the use of intraoperative shunts to ensure cerebral protection.

Surprisingly, postoperative neurologic complications are rare, even in patients with multivessel disease. Unless multivessel disease involving one or both carotids is encountered, electroencephalographic monitoring or shunting is usually unnecessary. Cerebral protection is more challenging in patients with a bovine aortic arch configuration, in whom clamping the innominate artery is not an option because this would compromise blood flow through both CCAs; shunting or temporary bypass conduits are essential in this circumstance.

Treatment

In 1958, DeBakey and colleagues[26] reported a large series of cases that included a direct transthoracic repair of the supra-aortic trunks—a major feat at that time. Surgical treatment was further advanced by Crawford and coworkers[27] with the use of extra-anatomic bypass techniques, which dramatically decreased the mortality associated with these operations from 22% to 5.6%. Currently, extra-anatomic bypass with synthetic grafts is the most common technique for treating these complex lesions (Fig. 73-2). The use of shunting for cerebral protection when necessary and the recognition of high-risk patients who are likely to benefit from cerebral protective measures have dramatically curtailed the adverse neurologic consequences associated with these procedures. Alternative techniques include direct endarterectomy, endovascular stenting, and transposition.[28] In general, direct surgical approaches, such as bypass techniques, are preferred for multivessel and long-segment disease, whereas endovascular techniques are preferred for isolated ostial disease or short-segment disease. Surgical intervention has reportedly produced survival rates of 98% and relieved symptoms in 94% of patients at a mean follow-up of 7.5 years. Crawford and associates[27] reported survival rates of 85% at 5 years, 58% at 10 years, and 25% at 15 years. Hybrid and endovascular approaches have been added recently to the surgeon's armamentarium, and they are gradually becoming the preferred treatment modalities for occlusive disease of the supra-aortic trunks, particularly for older patients with significant comorbidity.[29,30]

Innominate Artery Occlusive Disease

Innominate artery disease is uncommon. It typically involves the ostium or the proximal aspect of the artery and extends along the posterior and lateral walls. Innominate artery occlusion accounts for only 4.7% of cases of

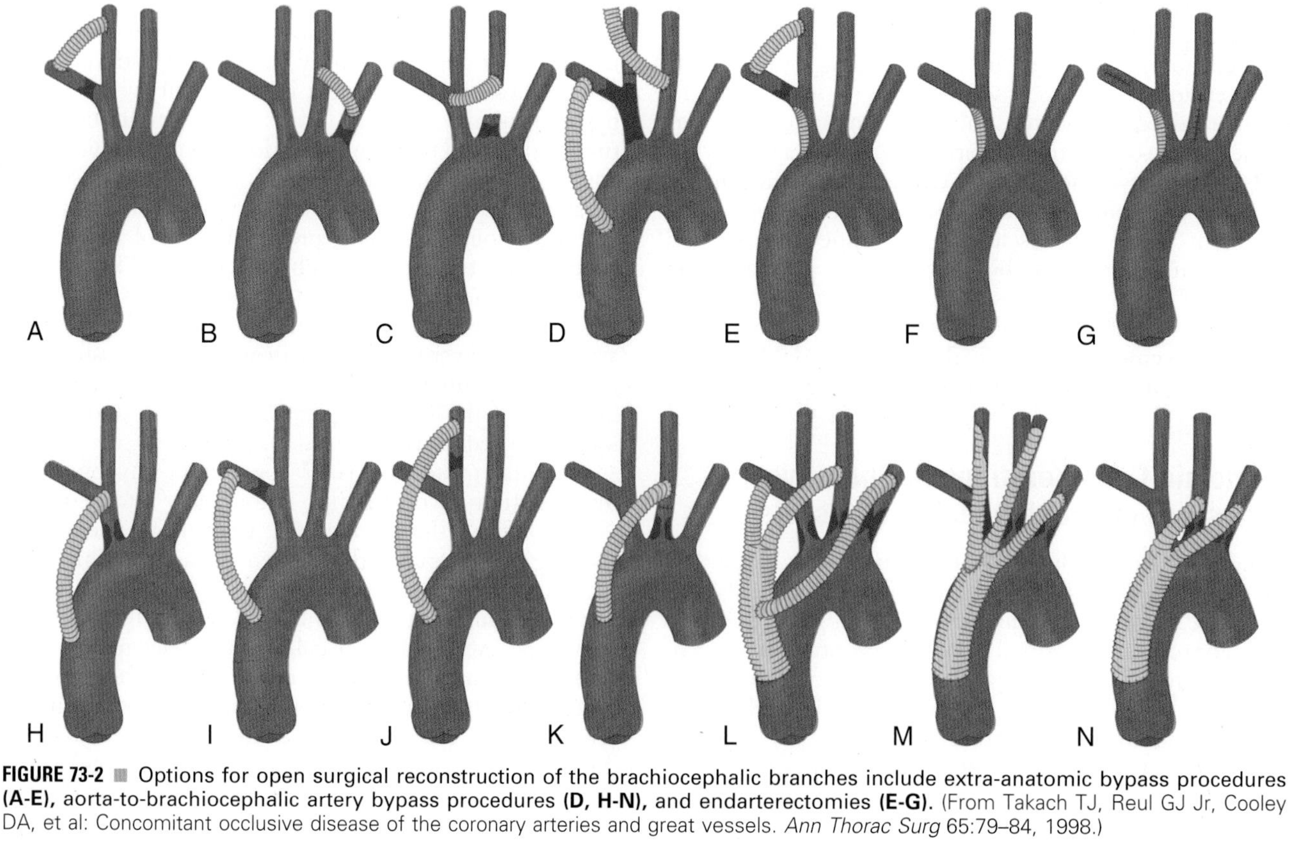

FIGURE 73-2 ■ Options for open surgical reconstruction of the brachiocephalic branches include extra-anatomic bypass procedures **(A-E)**, aorta-to-brachiocephalic artery bypass procedures **(D, H-N)**, and endarterectomies **(E-G)**. (From Takach TJ, Reul GJ Jr, Cooley DA, et al: Concomitant occlusive disease of the coronary arteries and great vessels. *Ann Thorac Surg* 65:79–84, 1998.)

extracranial cerebrovascular disease.[31] In these cases, the innominate artery is seldom the only vessel requiring revascularization.[32] Reul and colleagues[33] found that 60% of patients undergoing revascularization for innominate artery symptoms required intervention in at least one other vessel. Early studies of treatments for innominate atherosclerotic disease favored an extrathoracic approach because of the high morbidity and mortality rates associated with intrathoracic repair.[27] Advances in surgical technique and anesthesia, however, produced equivalent results of either extrathoracic or intrathoracic approaches.[34] Current clinical indications for treating symptomatic stenosis include transient ischemic attacks (TIAs), stroke, vertebrobasilar insufficiency, subclavian steal syndrome, and upper limb ischemia.

In patients with atheroembolic manifestations, direct operative treatment by excluding the embolic source is an essential element of the treatment strategy for symptom relief. Direct repair or bypass using the transthoracic approach is preferred because it produces less morbidity than using the extrathoracic approach, which is reserved for patients in whom transthoracic repair is contraindicated.[35,36] Relative contraindications to intrathoracic revascularization include a heavily diseased or calcified arch, previous thoracic surgery, and advanced age or poor medical condition. Extra-anatomic bypass techniques can be used in cases of primary graft infection, in which one would consider routing the graft well away from the preferred primary route. When revascularization of isolated innominate artery disease is contemplated, two transthoracic options exist: endarterectomy and bypass. Recent advances in endovascular treatment also represent a viable treatment strategy.

Innominate Artery Endarterectomy. Endarterectomy for isolated branch disease is reported to have excellent results.[36] Relative contraindications include inability to clamp the innominate artery, severe arch atherosclerosis, proximal origin of the left CCA (including a common brachiocephalic trunk), and multivessel disease; a bypass procedure may be preferable in these cases. Whenever possible, endarterectomy should be avoided in patients with Takayasu disease or radiation arteritis, because the transmural inflammatory process complicates the creation of an endarterectomy plane. The endarterectomy proceeds as illustrated in Figure 73-3. Performing intraoperative epiaortic ultrasonography before clamping may be of benefit, because most of these patients have aortic arch atherosclerosis. The vessel can be closed primarily or by patch angioplasty if luminal narrowing is of concern. Long-segment endarterectomies reportedly have been accomplished by extending the arteriotomy or performing separate arteriotomies on the branch vessels.[34]

Innominate Artery Bypass. Bypass grafting with synthetic prosthetic graft material has produced excellent results and has become the operative procedure of choice. Although the results are comparable to those of endarterectomy, the technical ease of the operation has led surgeons to favor the bypass approach. Bypass techniques are especially well suited for use in cases of Takayasu arteritis, radiation injury, and recurrent atherosclerotic disease.

During the early phases of the development of arterial replacement surgery, operative techniques involved resecting the primary vessel and then placing an interposition graft; this approach was associated with significant

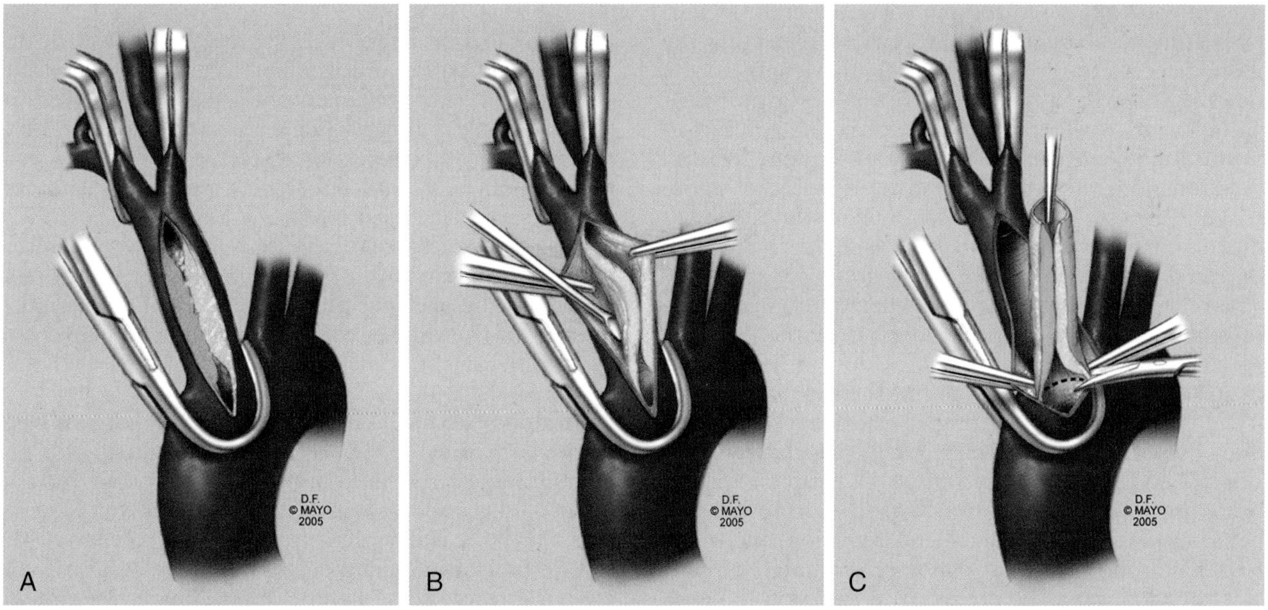

FIGURE 73-3 ■ **A,** After the right common carotid and subclavian arteries are clamped, proximal control of the innominate artery is established with a partial occluding clamp placed on the aortic arch. A longitudinal arteriotomy is created to expose the lesion. **B,** A circumferential endarterectomy plane is developed in the middle of the media. **C,** The endarterectomy is tapered distally to an appropriate endpoint. The lesion is divided proximally *(dashed line)* near the origin of the innominate artery; if the plaque extends into the arch, the intima is secured with tacking sutures to prevent dissection. The arteriotomy can be closed primarily or with a patch. (From Mozes G, Gloviczki P, Huang Y: Atherosclerotic occlusive disease. In Coselli JS, LeMaire SA, editors: *Aortic arch surgery: principles, strategies and outcomes.* West Sussex, United Kingdom, 2008, Wiley-Blackwell, p 311. Copyright Mayo 2005.)

perioperative morbidity and mortality. The introduction of the bypass technique by Crawford and coworkers[37] eliminated unnecessary manipulation and dissection of the diseased native artery while allowing the restoration of antegrade flow in the affected territory. This strategy reduced postoperative morbidity rates and significantly improved results. Late graft patency and patient survival (in those without stroke) appear to be good. Berguer and colleagues[35] reported 10-year estimates of 88% ± 6% and 81% ± 7%, respectively. Concomitant coronary artery disease significantly influences both early and late death rates.

As with endarterectomy, epiaortic ultrasound is often useful in selecting the site of the proximal anastomosis and aortic clamping. Typically, an 8- to 10-mm Dacron graft is used to construct the bypass. When there is multivessel disease, a bifurcated or branched graft can be used. If at all possible, the proximal anastomosis should be constructed toward the right lateral aspect of the ascending aorta to avoid potential compression from the sternum or mediastinal contents. As reported by Crawford and colleagues,[38] the potential complications of such compression include venous compression and tracheal compromise resulting in death. Care should be taken to construct the bevel with the appropriate orientation to prevent kinking of the graft. The distal anastomosis is constructed in an end-to-side fashion unless the innominate artery is suspected to be the source of embolic disease. In that situation, the surgeon should consider excluding the diseased segment and performing the distal anastomosis in an end-to-end fashion.

Appropriate positioning of the graft is essential to avoid kinking or compression of the graft, which is directly responsible for most eventual failures of this operation. Several maneuvers have been described to create adequate space to accommodate the graft, including ligating the brachiocephalic vein and resecting the innominate artery. Properly gauging the length of the graft avoids leaving a redundant portion of the graft that will be prone to either kinking or traversing anterior to the aorta and being compressed by the sternum. To avoid overestimation, the sternal retractor is released before the graft length is determined. Theoretically, single-branch grafts have the advantage of being less bulky than bifurcated grafts. When bifurcated grafts are used, the common trunk should be left longer, which makes the flow more laminar at the bifurcation of the graft by reducing interference from the high flow of the ascending aorta. In certain circumstances, the lack of intrathoracic domain may preclude proper placement of a bypass graft. These circumstances include a mediastinal reoperation, saphenous vein conduits placed in certain locations during previous coronary artery bypass grafting (CABG) operations, extensive periaortic inflammation, and stents inserted during previous endovascular interventions. Endarterectomy may be preferred to bypass techniques in these circumstances.

Innominate Artery Stenting. Endovascular options for innominate artery disease have been expanding in the past decade. Initial reports had important limitations, including small numbers of patients, short follow-up periods, and grouping of the data with data from patients with subclavian artery disease, which tends to skew the results.[31] Only a few studies have examined stenting as a treatment for isolated innominate artery lesions.[39-42] The technical success rate varies from 83% to 96%; stenotic lesions have a higher treatment success rate than total occlusions do. Although early primary and secondary patency rates are excellent (>95% and >98%, respectively, at up to 2 years), long-term data vary, showing primary patency rates around 70%.

The endovascular approach can be antegrade via the common femoral artery, retrograde via the brachial artery, or a hybrid approach through a retrograde cervical cut-down of the CCA. Innominate artery stenting is particularly useful in treating short-segment disease. In contrast, endovascular stenting should be avoided in long-segment occlusion of brachiocephalic vessels or extensive vessel calcifications because it can increase the risk of complications and poor treatment outcomes, including vessel rupture, catheter-induced cerebral embolization, and vessel occlusion.[43,44]

The major advantages of endovascular treatment include a reduction in periprocedural morbidity and mortality; the risk of any neurologic deficit ranges from 2% to 4%, while the risk of minor complications hovers at approximately 6%, and the risk of major complications ranges from 1% to 2%.[39-42] Endovascular approaches also offer the benefits of a less invasive approach, a shorter hospital stay, and greater acceptance by patients. The lack of long-term durability data, however, maintains open operation as the first-line treatment for young, otherwise healthy patients who may derive long-term benefit from an open procedure.

Common Carotid Artery Occlusive Disease

Common carotid artery occlusive diseases are usually due to retropropagation of thrombus secondary to occlusion at the carotid bifurcation; less often, these diseases are due to primary ostial disease. There are several approaches to managing carotid bifurcation disease, and any of the techniques could be expanded to include retrograde endarterectomy via transcervical approaches. In patients with CCA occlusion, two key factors must be ascertained before a transcervical or transthoracic approach can be contemplated: (1) the presence or absence of carotid bifurcation disease and (2) whether there is concomitant involvement of the other major branches of the aortic arch.

Common Carotid Artery Bypass. For patients with isolated proximal CCA occlusion and sparing of the carotid bifurcation, a transcervical approach, such as carotid-subclavian bypass or transposition, can be used (Fig. 73-4). It is essential to ensure the patency of the carotid bifurcation and the absence of any proximal subclavian artery disease before this technique is contemplated. In cases of multivessel disease involving the arch branch vessels or common carotid arteries, a transthoracic approach with direct CCA revascularization should be considered. Transthoracic approaches are used selectively in patients with multivessel disease and extensive proximal CCA disease that spares the carotid bifurcation.

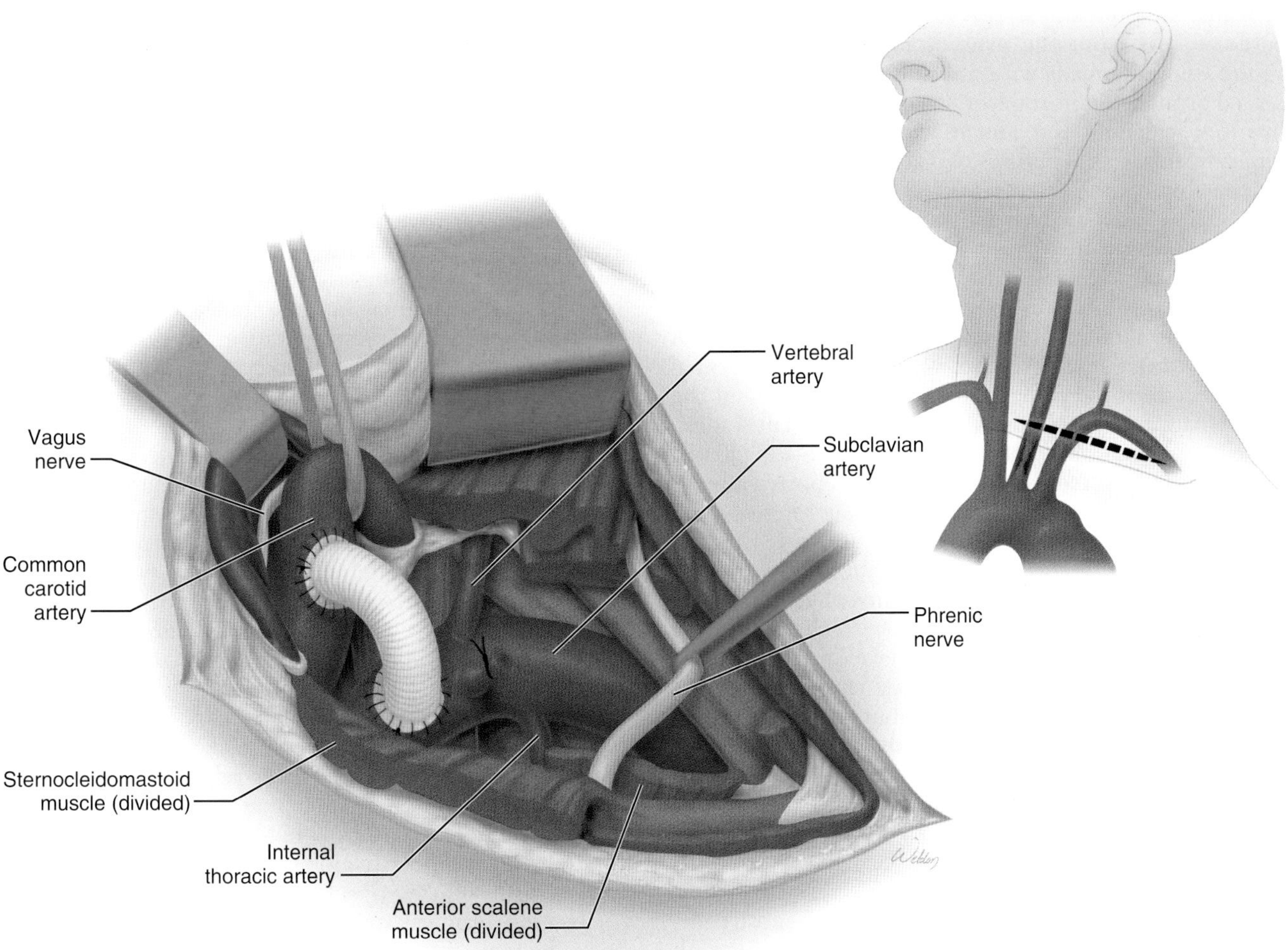

FIGURE 73-4 ■ A left subclavian-to-carotid artery bypass for treatment of common carotid artery stenosis. The procedure is performed through a supraclavicular incision *(inset)* and can be used to treat subclavian artery stenosis. (From Bozinovski J, LeMaire SA, Weldon SA, et al: Hybrid repairs of the aortic arch and proximal descending thoracic aorta. *Op Tech Thorac Cardiovasc Surg* 12:167, 2007, Figure 10. Used with permission. Copyright Elsevier.)

An aorta-to-CCA bypass with a bifurcated tube graft is preferable when both the subclavian and common carotid arteries are involved.

In all cases of CCA reconstruction, preoperative workup should establish the patency of the distal carotid vessels before any operative intervention is undertaken. Most patients who have occluded CCAs also have occluded internal carotid arteries (ICAs). Only rarely, ICA patency exists above a CCA occlusion through collateral flow via the ipsilateral external carotid artery or an aberrant branch of the ICA. Contralateral carotid occlusion, even if asymptomatic, poses a significant additional risk for perioperative stroke in such patients. Although the natural history of asymptomatic proximal CCA occlusion in patients with patent ICAs is unknown, it is likely benign, and surgery is not indicated in these circumstances.[45] Many surgeons might not consider reestablishing flow in patients with chronic asymptomatic total carotid occlusion, because the incidence of stroke is high during reestablishment of flow, and interventions might not necessarily be beneficial in preventing stroke.

Carotid Endarterectomy with Retrograde Stenting of the Innominate or Left Common Carotid Artery. In patients with carotid bifurcation disease with retropropagation of the thrombus or concomitant proximal CCA or innominate artery disease, several authors have proposed performing a concomitant transcervical carotid endarterectomy (CEA) with retrograde endarterectomy or angioplasty and stenting.[46,47] In this treatment approach, CEA is generally done first using local or general anesthesia. Before closing the carotid arteriotomy, the operator inserts a 7-French introducer sheath in retrograde fashion and places a vascular clamp distally to reduce the likelihood of cerebral embolization. After the stent is positioned, the sheath is withdrawn, permitting the arteriotomy incision to be closed. If open exposure of a carotid artery is performed strictly for access to a lesion that involves either the proximal innominate or carotid arteries, an 18-gauge needle and a Bentson wire are often used to cross the lesion, allowing an introducer sheath to be placed and the stent to be positioned. In addition, a stent may be placed in the proximal innominate artery stent via a right carotid cutdown. To close the arteriotomy, a figure-of-eight suture (typically made with 5-0 polypropylene suture) is placed around the introducer sheath. Another approach involves widening the lumen with patch angioplasty; typically, this is used in cases of diseased vessels or simultaneous bifurcation disease.

A recent meta-analysis by Sfyroeras and colleagues[48] used data from the largest collection of patients to undergo hybrid treatment for high-grade tandem stenoses of the carotid bifurcation and either the proximal left CCA or the innominate artery. Thirteen studies, which included a total of 133 patients, were identified (proximal lesions were in the ipsilateral CCA in 85 cases and the innominate artery in 48 cases). In the most recent studies, a primary stenting strategy with balloon-expandable stents was most often used. The authors reported a technical success rate of 97%, with low 30-day rates of mortality (0.7%) and stroke (1.5%). Among the 13 studies, mean follow-up ranged from 12 to 36 months; during this time, 5 patients exhibited symptoms of cerebral ischemia, and 17 patients died. Of the 79 patients who received stents, 3 patients (3.7%) developed restenosis, compared with 7 (14%) of the 50 patients treated with angioplasty alone. The authors attributed the low procedural risk to the distal placement of the clamp on the ICA prior to retrograde angioplasty, which reduces the likelihood of cerebral embolization.

Subclavian Artery Occlusive Disease

The left subclavian artery is the arch vessel most commonly occluded by atherosclerosis, even in patients with multifocal disease. The subclavian artery supplies blood to the arm and to the posterior cerebral and cerebellar circulation. Proximal subclavian artery stenosis can result in symptoms originating from either territory because of competition for flow distribution. In patients who have undergone CABG surgery, the presence of a patent ITA graft to the left anterior descending coronary artery (LAD) adds another potentially competing territory. Proximal subclavian artery occlusive disease has various manifestations, including vertebrobasilar insufficiency from posterior cerebral circulatory compromise or from upper-extremity claudication or ischemia, and recurrent heart failure or angina in patients with left ITA-to-LAD grafts (see Fig. 73-1). Intervention is generally not indicated for isolated asymptomatic subclavian stenosis, because isolated proximal artery stenosis is unlikely to cause stroke if the carotid vessels are patent. However, the likelihood of stroke is greater in patients with multivessel disease; therefore, a complete evaluation of the cerebral vasculature is essential, even in patients with symptoms pertaining to the subclavian territory alone. Isolated subclavian artery symptoms, therefore, do not necessarily indicate isolated subclavian artery disease, and patients with such symptoms may require intervention.

Subclavian Artery Bypass. The aim of any treatment strategy for subclavian artery occlusive disease, be it operative bypass or endovascular stenting, is to restore antegrade flow in both the vertebral and distal subclavian vessels—in essence, to prevent retrograde steal. From an operative perspective, this therapeutic objective can be accomplished with various surgical approaches, which include subclavian-carotid bypass grafting (see Fig. 73-4), subclavian-carotid transposition, vertebral artery transposition to the CCA, and extra-anatomic axillary bypass. In addition, for patients with isolated proximal left subclavian artery occlusive disease, a descending aorta–to–left subclavian artery bypass proximal to the origin of the left vertebral artery may be accomplished with a left thoracotomy approach. These operative strategies have been associated with excellent outcome and a low incidence of symptom recurrence.

Subclavian Artery Stenting. Advancements in endovascular intervention have resulted in remarkable treatment outcomes by providing a less invasive percutaneous approach. Catheter-based primary stenting of the subclavian arteries can be safely performed and produce satisfactory midterm outcomes.[49,50] In one of the largest series of endovascular repairs of occlusive lesions of the subclavian artery, Sixt and colleagues[49] reported on 99 patients treated between 1996 and 2004 with mostly (90%) atherosclerotic lesions. The overall primary success rate was 97% (less for total occlusions; 87%), with no neurologic complications and only two access-related complications. The 1-year primary patency rate was 88% for all 97 patients eligible for follow-up, 79% for the patients treated with angioplasty alone, and 89% for the patients treated with stenting ($P = 0.2$).

Routine primary stenting is recommended in most cases because it achieves longer-lasting patency and greater freedom from symptoms of atheroembolism than balloon angioplasty alone. Balloon-expandable stents exert more radial force than nitinol stents do, and they are useful in ostial subclavian lesions because these lesions are usually calcified. A 1- to 2-mm overhang of the stent into the aortic lumen is desirable for ostial lesions. For postvertebral lesions, self-expanding nitinol stents are preferred to balloon-expandable stents because the nitinol stents are more pliable and less likely to be deformed by extrinsic compression.

In patients with coronary-subclavian steal syndrome (CSS), caution is exercised to prevent inadvertent occlusion of the takeoff of a patent left ITA-to-LAD graft when these stents are deployed. If technically feasible, stents should be deployed in a manner that does not compromise the origins of the ITA and vertebral artery. Dietrich and colleagues[51] have shown that CSS can be treated with angioplasty and stenting; rates were 86% for primary patency and 100% for assisted-primary patency after 29 months of follow-up.

Clinical patency is accomplished in more than 80% of patients at 5-year follow up, and 80% of patients are symptom-free for more than 3 years. Complications related to endovascular interventions include stroke, atheroembolism, dissection, and complications related to the access site, such as bleeding, dissection, pseudoaneurysm, stenosis, and thrombosis. Surgery is now typically considered a second-line intervention to be used when endovascular approaches fail.[52,53]

Multivessel Occlusive Disease

Multivessel involvement is noted in 25% of all cases of intrathoracic aortic arch branch-vessel disease, although reports of some large series note a prevalence in excess of 60%.[7,27,34] Hence, thorough preoperative diagnostic imaging is necessary, even in patients with isolated symptoms involving a single branch territory. Transsternal aortic branch bypass appears to be the procedure best suited to these situations, and it can be carried out in one of two ways: creating multiple grafts from the aorta to individual vessels, or using branched or bifurcated grafts (see Fig. 73-2). Again, it is essential that aortic manipulation be kept to a minimum, because these patients have significant concomitant aortic arch disease; thus, the best approach may be to place a single-trunk tube graft with branches of appropriate size. The operative challenge in this circumstance is ideally positioning the bulky graft and its branches in an already compromised supra-aortic territory. It is important to position the graft along the greater curvature of the aortic arch and to tailor the length to minimize kinking or compression from surrounding structures.

Takayasu Arteritis

The treatment of Takayasu arteritis involves a combination of immunosuppressive therapy and percutaneous or surgical interventions. The first line of medical therapy remains glucocorticoids; antimetabolites are the second-line drugs in unresponsive cases.[54,55] Surgical intervention is indicated in patients with symptomatic stenotic lesions or concomitant aneurysm formation. It is important to determine the prognostic stage—determined by using the Ishikawa criteria, which include existing complications, the pattern of the past clinical course, and the erythrocyte sedimentation rate—when considering surgical intervention.[56] Surgical treatment for patients with Takayasu arteritis might increase survival in those with stage 3 disease, but not in those with stage 1 disease.[56] Thus, conservative treatment is generally suggested for stage 1 or 2 disease, and most surgeons prudently avoid surgical intervention until the disease has reached a chronic fibro-occlusive stage.

In 1951, Shimizu and Sano[57] described surgical treatment for occlusive disease of the aortic arch branches in a patient with Takayasu arteritis. The principles of surgical bypass grafting described in the preceding sections apply to most patients, with a few notable exceptions as described here. Several techniques have been used, including endarterectomy with patch angioplasty, resection with interposition grafting, and bypass techniques. Innominate artery stenosis should be dealt with through distal grafting and not endarterectomy. Panarteritis and fibrosis yield an inconsistent plane for endarterectomy, and the adventitia that reconstitutes the vessel is often affected. Moreover, the stenotic lesions affect long segments of the supra-aortic trunk, making bypass procedures technically more feasible.[58] The disadvantage of bypass procedures, however, is the risk of subsequent pseudoaneurysm formation at the suture lines.

When proximal and distal anastomoses are constructed, sites free of disease should be chosen. Although this practice is not supported by clear scientific evidence, the absence of macroscopic disease is believed by some surgeons to decrease the likelihood of recurrent stenosis or aneurysm formation. Also, most of the involved vessels are surrounded by dense perivascular inflammation, making dissection tedious and potentially dangerous. This problem can be circumvented by planning bypass procedures such that the anastomotic sites are well away from diseased segments. Allowance should be made for progression of the disease, leading to recurrent occlusive disease; therefore, large and generous anastomoses are preferred.[55,59,60] Subsequent aneurysm formation also needs to be considered in surgical treatment of Takayasu arteritis. Hence, the patients require lifelong follow-up with CT, MRI, or Doppler ultrasonography to monitor for the development of aneurysms. Systemic inflammation or steroid administration has little influence on anastomotic aneurysm formation. Anastomotic aneurysms tend to arise after operations for prior aneurysmal lesions and can develop any time after the initial operation. No specific factor, except the presence of an aneurysmal lesion, seems to predict recurrent aneurysm formation. The cumulative incidence of anastomotic aneurysm at 20 years is reported to be nearly 14%.[61]

Although no operative technique has been shown to have significant influence on the postoperative incidence of recurrent disease or aneurysm formation, surgeons prefer to operate on patients with Takayasu arteritis during the quiescent stage of the disease, using felt or bovine pericardial patches and reinforcement sutures to decrease the risk of recurrent aneurysm. Concomitant use of endovascular techniques with medical management has helped to reduce mortality to less than 10% and to improve 10-year graft patency to approximately 70%. Recently, endovascular stenting has been used to treat de novo thoracic aortic aneurysm and stenotic disease secondary to Takayasu arteritis, although the long-term consequences of using this approach remain unknown.[62-64]

CORONARY-SUBCLAVIAN STEAL SYNDROME

When a reversal of flow occurs in a previous ITA coronary bypass, myocardial ischemia can occur and result in CSS syndrome (see Fig. 73-1). The resulting ischemic pain can be confused with exertional chest pain of myocardial origin when patients report chest pain from strenuous upper-extremity activity. Often, CSS syndrome occurs in patients with an ipsilateral ITA coronary conduit and proximal subclavian artery stenosis. However, CSS has been reported in cases of inflammatory arteritis involving the proximal subclavian vessels, hemodialysis fistula in the ipsilateral upper extremity, and specific anomalies of the brachiocephalic arteries (dextro-transposition of the left subclavian artery and pulmonary artery).[65,66]

Clinical manifestations include "silent" ischemia, ischemic cardiomyopathy, generalized heart failure, myocardial infarction (MI), and possibly sudden death. The CSS syndrome can be prevented by identifying patients who have or may be at risk for developing subclavian artery occlusive disease.[67] Steal syndrome and myocardial ischemia can develop if substantial subclavian disease is present but untreated before placement of an ipsilateral ITA coronary conduit.[68] All patients undergoing evaluation before CABG in which the use of ITA grafts is anticipated are examined for ischemia (upper-extremity or cerebrovascular ischemia), bruits (cervical or supraclavicular), and a blood pressure differential of more than 20 mm Hg in the upper extremities. During coronary arteriography, brachiocephalic arteriography should be done in patients with suspected diffuse atherosclerotic vascular disease for better identification of subclavian artery occlusive disease.[69]

In patients with significant brachiocephalic disease who are to undergo CABG surgery, options for preventing CSS include using all-vein conduits, using an ITA conduit once brachiocephalic reconstruction is completed, and using free ITA grafts or radial artery conduits during CABG. In patients who develop CSS after CABG, symptoms can be relieved by aortic-subclavian bypass, carotid-subclavian bypass, transposition of the ITA, or endovascular procedures.[70]

CONCURRENT CAROTID AND CORONARY ARTERY ATHEROSCLEROSIS

Overview

The treatment of patients with multisite arterial disease, specifically those with severe carotid disease who also require CABG, is challenging and controversial.[71-73] The current guidelines suggest that carotid revascularization with CEA or carotid artery stenting (CAS) either before or concurrent with CABG surgery is a reasonable strategy in symptomatic patients with substantial carotid stenosis (>80%; class IIa recommendation, level of evidence C).[74] Furthermore, the safety and efficacy of performing carotid revascularization before or concurrently with surgical coronary revascularization are clear in patients with severe or lesser asymptomatic carotid stenosis (class IIb recommendation, level of evidence C).[74] It is important to note that these guidelines stem from expert consensus and that there is a general lack of evidence to guide clinical choice. Most experts agree that carotid revascularization is indicated if the lesion is symptomatic, bilateral, or both. However, patients in this population most often have unilateral, asymptomatic disease for which carotid revascularization before or at the time of CABG might not improve clinical outcomes when compared with optimal medical therapy and CABG.[75-77]

In patients referred for CABG, the prevalence of ≥50% carotid stenosis was between 10% and 22%, and the prevalence of ≥80% carotid stenosis was between 4% and 10%.[78] The 2011 American CABG guidelines indicate that duplex scanning is a reasonable option in select high-risk patients (patients ≥65 years old and those with left main disease, peripheral artery disease, diabetes, or a history of TIA or stroke, hypertension, or smoking; class IIa, level of evidence C).[79] The 2011 European peripheral artery disease guidelines recommend carotid duplex ultrasonography in older patients (patients ≥70 years of age), as well as patients with a history of cerebrovascular disease, carotid bruit, multivessel coronary artery disease, or peripheral artery disease (class I, level of evidence B).[80]

Stroke is a devastating complication of cardiac surgery and is associated with increased major disability and mortality risk and with healthcare costs. Authors from the Cleveland Clinic reported a stroke rate of 1.6% among 45,432 isolated CABG patients.[81] Patients who had a stroke had significantly higher in-hospital mortality (19% vs. 3.7%), as well as poorer long-term outcomes, compared with propensity-matched patients without a neurologic insult.

Risk Factors for Stroke after Cardiac Surgery

Many patient and surgical factors have been identified as independent predictors of postoperative stroke after cardiac surgery, including clinical characteristics, the anatomic features and symptomatic nature of the carotid disease, atherosclerosis of the ascending aorta and transverse arch, and the type of cardiac surgery (Box 73-1). The multifactorial etiology of perioperative stroke partly explains why the neurologic insult can occur in a delayed fashion and on the contralateral side to the carotid lesion.

In the most comprehensive meta-analysis published to date,[77] 166 studies regarding carotid artery stenosis or occlusion were reviewed. The 30-day incidences of

BOX 73-1 Risk Factors for Stroke after Cardiac Surgery

Clinical Factors

- Increased age
- History of TIA/stroke
- Peripheral vascular disease
- Atrial fibrillation
- Diabetes
- Hypertension
- Heart failure
- Renal failure

Anatomic Factors

- Carotid lesion
  - Degree of stenosis
  - Plaque morphology
  - Progressive stenosis
  - Contralateral stenosis/occlusion
- Atherosclerosis of ascending aorta and transverse arch

Surgical Factors

- Duration of cross-clamp and cardiopulmonary bypass
- On-pump surgery
- Open heart surgery (valve or aortic surgery)
- Redo operation
- Partial clamping of ascending aorta for proximal anastomosis

TIA, Transient ischemic attack

Adapted from Roffi M, Ribichini F, Castriota F, et al: Management of combined severe carotid and coronary artery disease. Curr Cardiol Rep 14:125–134, 2012, with permission.

ipsilateral stroke and of any stroke were only 2.0% and 2.9%, respectively, among patients with unilateral, asymptomatic, 50% to 99% carotid stenosis who underwent isolated cardiac surgery without prophylactic carotid revascularization. In asymptomatic patients, these risks did not increase with stenosis severity. In contrast, patients with a history of stroke, TIA, or severe bilateral carotid disease had markedly increased rates of postoperative death and stroke. Additional subanalysis of 26 published reports with a total of 2531 patients showed that when symptomatic patients were also included, patients with 50% to 99% stenosis or occlusion had a 7.4% stroke risk after cardiac surgery; this risk increased to 9.1% in patients with 80% to 99% stenosis or occlusion. The risk of stroke was 6.5% in patients undergoing cardiac surgery with bilateral, asymptomatic, 50% to 99% stenosis, or 50 to 99% stenosis with contralateral occlusion. The risk of death or stroke in such patients was 9.1%. The importance of neurologic symptoms was also shown in an earlier meta-analysis of patients with carotid stenosis who underwent CABG: patients with previous TIA or stroke had a postoperative stroke rate of 8.5%, compared with 2.2% in asymptomatic patients (odds ratio, 3.6).[82] A few centers have reported no increased stroke by limiting carotid revascularization in CABG patients with asymptomatic carotid stenosis.[83,84] In a large retrospective study of 4335 patients, the risk of perioperative stroke was significantly increased in the synchronous CEA-CABG group compared with the group that underwent CABG alone (15.1% vs. 0%; $P = 0.004$).[85]

It is generally understood that stroke after cardiac surgery among patients with asymptomatic carotid disease is relatively rare. Furthermore, since the early pivotal randomized trials comparing medical therapy to CEA were performed, contemporary optimal medical therapy has improved considerably. Thus, many argue that if such trials were performed with today's optimal medical therapy (e.g., modern antiplatelet, lipid-lowering, antihypertensive regimens), the previously reported benefit of CEA over medical therapy in asymptomatic patients (5% to 6% vs. 11% to 12%, respectively, for a combined death or stroke rate at 5 years) may be less compelling.[86-88] These data call into question the rationale for performing prophylactic carotid revascularization in neurologically asymptomatic patients with unilateral carotid disease. Importantly, among 27,084 patients in the United States who underwent synchronous carotid and coronary revascularization procedures between 2000 and 2004, the vast majority (>95%) had asymptomatic carotid disease.[89]

Surgical Approaches to Concurrent Carotid and Coronary Disease

Strategies to address concomitant, surgically correctable carotid and coronary disease include synchronous CEA and CABG, staged repair with either CEA or CAS followed by CABG, "reverse" staged repair (CABG then CEA or CAS), or no treatment of the carotid disease (CABG alone). The aim of any operative strategy is to minimize the risk of specific major adverse cardiovascular events. The staged and reverse-staged approaches risk between-stage events such as death, stroke, or MI; this is not entirely unexpected, given that patients might have a severe form of coronary artery disease. Although conducting a carotid intervention before CABG has the advantage of lowering the patient's risk of peri-CABG stroke, the risk of acute MI is still high in the timeframe surrounding the carotid intervention and during the interval between the two interventions. Performing CABG before carotid intervention, on the other hand, could be associated with a high stroke rate. The approach must be individualized to the patient at hand, with careful attention to the symptomatic territory and institutional experience with various strategies. Because no randomized trial has yet compared management strategies for carotid disease at the time of cardiac surgery, the interpretation of available data from observational studies has inherent limitations.

Synchronous Carotid Endarterectomy and Coronary Artery Bypass Grafting

Since the introduction of the concept by Bernhard and colleagues[90] in 1972, the combined surgical approach has remained a topic of controversy. In the decade from 1992 to 2002, combined CEA-CABG represented only a small portion (1.1%) of all CABG procedures in the United States.[91] In an excellent review of the literature that summarized outcome data from patients ($n = 11,854$) with carotid and coronary disease who underwent synchronous CEA-CABG, Venkatachalam and colleagues[72] reported an early mortality rate of 5%, a stroke rate of 4%, an MI rate of 3%, and a death, stroke, or MI rate of 10%. Similarly, Timaran and colleagues[89] reported a mortality rate of 5.2%, a stroke rate of 3.9%, and a death or stroke rate of 8.6% among 26,197 patients who underwent combined CEA-CABG.

Using the Nationwide Inpatient Sample (NIS) database, Gopaldas and colleagues[92] compared patients who underwent staged repair (CEA before or after CABG during the same admission but not on the same day; $n = 6152$) with patients who underwent synchronous repair (both procedures on the same day; $n = 16,639$). Patients who underwent synchronous CEA-CABG had an in-hospital mortality rate of 4.5%, a stroke rate of 3.9%, and a death or stroke rate of 7.7%. The staged patients had similar mortality (4.2%) but higher morbidity, including more cardiac, wound, respiratory, and renal complications. Among patients who undergo combined procedures, the stroke rate tends to be highest (>10%) in patients who have contralateral carotid occlusion. The presence of neurologic symptoms significantly increases the risk of postoperative death or stroke after combined carotid interventions and coronary bypass (odds ratio, 4.9; $P < 0.001$).[89]

Staged Approach: Carotid Revascularization Followed by Coronary Artery Bypass Grafting

The staged approach involves operative intervention on the diseased carotid vessels followed by myocardial revascularization, with the obvious theoretical benefit being the reduction of stroke risk during CABG. The risk of MI in the peri-CEA period and during the time interval between the two procedures remains the major drawback of this approach. Takach and colleagues[93] reported a low overall stroke rate of 1.9% with the staged approach. In their series, 512 patients underwent intervention for comorbid carotid and coronary disease over a period of 21 years. Before 1986, the incidence of adverse events was greater in patients who underwent combined procedures than in those who had staged interventions (9.4% vs. 2.6%; $P < 0.01$). However, since 1986, both groups have had similar rates of stroke (1.9% vs. 2.0%), death (3.8% vs. 3.0%), and MI (3.8% vs. 5.0%). In this series, approximately 30% of strokes occurred in the contralateral cerebrovascular territory in both the staged and the simultaneous groups. Hemodynamic instability or arrhythmia accompanied 10 of the 15 strokes that occurred during both the synchronous and the staged procedures. Advances in anesthesia, surgical technique, intraoperative monitoring for cerebral ischemia, and myocardial protection have all improved surgical teams' ability to maintain perioperative hemodynamic stability in patients with combined disease. The improvement in neurologic outcomes that occurred after 1986 in patients who underwent combined procedures in this series was attributed to these advances. The risk of stroke was affected by neither the use of a carotid shunt nor the use of patch closure of the carotid arteriotomy. Operative approach (synchronous or staged) was not a predictor of either stroke or death. The staged approach, however, lengthened hospital stay, increased the cost of hospitalization, and raised the risk of acute ischemia and MI in the interval between the CEA and CABG procedures.

Clearly, preventing stroke in patients with coronary disease is a multifactorial problem. Although carotid bifurcation disease may be a major contributing factor for perioperative stroke, it does not directly explain strokes in the contralateral territory, which occur in approximately one third of patients. More than anything else, the presence of carotid bifurcation disease is a marker for generalized atherosclerosis, which by itself increases the risk of hemorrhage, hemodynamic instability, cardiac failure, and atheroemboli. Also, the fact that adverse outcomes are more frequent in patients who undergo combined or staged procedures than in patients who undergo isolated CABG or CEA suggests that patients with concomitant carotid and coronary disease are at greater risk overall and have a poorer physiologic performance status, possibly secondary to diffuse atherosclerosis.

Reverse Staged Approach: Coronary Artery Bypass Grafting Followed by Carotid Endarterectomy

The advantage of the reverse staged approach is that the risk of MI is minimized by intervention on the coronary vessels before a CEA is performed. Unlike the staged approach, in which the elimination of hemodynamically significant carotid stenosis removes only one of the many potential causes of stroke during CABG, a reverse staged approach essentially eliminates the one major and clearly defined complication of CEA: MI. The meta-analysis by Naylor and colleagues[94] found that perioperative MI rates were lowest after the reverse staged procedure (0.9%; 95% confidence interval [CI], 0.5-1.4) and were highest in patients who underwent staged CEA-CABG (6.5%; 95% CI, 3.2-9.7). However, patients with reverse staged procedures (CABG-CEA) had a higher risk of ipsilateral stroke (5.8%; 95% CI, 0.0-14.3) and of any stroke (6.3%; 95% CI, 1.0-11.7) than patients with other operative approaches (synchronous or staged).

In a recent randomized trial, 185 patients with asymptomatic unilateral carotid stenosis greater than 70% underwent CEA either early (before or concomitantly with CABG; $n = 94$) or late (1 to 3 months after CABG; $n = 91$).[95] All patients had general anesthesia, and CEA routinely involved carotid artery shunting. Although early death rates were similar between groups (1.0% vs. 1.1%; $P = 0.98$), there was a significant difference between groups concerning combined 90-day stroke and death rate; this was substantially lower in the early CEA group (1.0% vs. 8.8%; $P = 0.02$). Furthermore, delayed CEA significantly predicted combined stroke and death at 90 days (odds ratio, 14.2; $P = 0.03$). Thus, it was found that CEA before or concomitantly with CABG surgery greatly lowers the risk of stroke.

Carotid Artery Stenting Followed by Coronary Artery Bypass Grafting

Endovascular approaches have pushed the envelope further amidst the controversy surrounding the treatment of patients with combined coronary and carotid disease.[96] A retrospective study by Timaran and colleagues[89] of NIS data has provided interesting insights into CAS before CABG. During the 5-year period from 2000 through 2004, 27,084 patients underwent carotid revascularization and CABG during the same hospitalization. Of these patients, 96.7% underwent either staged or synchronous CEA-CABG, and only 3.3% underwent CAS-CABG. Patients who underwent CAS-CABG tended to have fewer major adverse events than did those who underwent CEA-CABG. Specifically, CAS-CABG patients had significantly lower incidences of in-hospital stroke (2.4% vs. 3.9%; $P < 0.001$) and combined stroke and death (6.9% vs. 8.6%; $P < 0.001$) than did CEA-CABG patients; however, the incidence of in-hospital death was similar (5.2% vs 5.4%) between the two groups. The study, however, did not include separate comparisons either between CAS-CABG and staged CEA-CABG or between CAS-CABG and synchronous CEA-CABG. Unfortunately, typically reported 30-day data were not available in the NIS dataset, and only in-hospital events were captured; thus, major adverse events could be greater than presented. Ziada and colleagues[97] compared 30-day outcomes between staged CAS-CABG ($n = 56$) and combined CEA-CABG ($n = 112$) groups. Although no significant difference was found for combined death, MI, or stroke ($P = 0.12$), after propensity adjustment, a nearly significant difference was noted for lower stroke or MI rates in the CAS-CABG group.

A prospective, single-center study from Europe examined outcomes in 356 patients who underwent staged CAS followed by CABG.[98] None of the patients had symptoms of carotid disease in the 4 months preceding CAS, and patients with major neurologic deficits, diffuse common carotid disease, chronic total occlusions, and preocclusive or string sign lesions were excluded. Cardiac surgery occurred with a mean delay of 22 days (range, 14 to 30 days). Despite aspirin and clopidogrel being withheld for 5 days before surgery, there were no cases of carotid stent thrombosis. Following CABG, the 30-day cumulative incidence of death, MI, or stroke was 8.7%. At nearly 3 years' follow-up, the authors reported a remarkable neurologic death rate of 1.1% and a major ipsilateral stroke rate of 1.1%.

As reported by Mas and colleagues,[99] in patients with isolated yet symptomatic carotid disease (>60% stenosis), CAS produced outcomes inferior to those of the gold standard treatment, CEA. The trial was stopped prematurely when preliminary analyses showed that the incidence of stroke or death was 3.9% after CEA (95% CI, 2.0-7.2) and 9.6% after CAS (95% CI, 6.4-14.0) and that the 30-day incidence of disabling stroke or death was 1.5% after CEA versus 3.4% after CAS. Likewise, the incidence of perioperative stroke was reported to be fivefold higher in symptomatic patients undergoing CAS-CABG than in symptomatic patients undergoing CEA-CABG. However, Versaci and colleagues[100] have supported the feasibility of sequential hybrid CAS immediately followed by CABG; in their 37 patients, the combined incidence of disabling stroke, MI, or death was 8.1%.

The most comprehensive study comparing the three most common surgical strategies for concomitant carotid and coronary artery disease comes from a retrospective review of 350 patients treated at the Cleveland Clinic from 1997 to 2009.[101] The majority of patients had asymptomatic disease (81%) and underwent CABG with or without concomitant valve surgery (92%); only 8% of these patients had open heart surgery (OHS) that did not involve CABG (e.g., isolated valve or aortic repair). The study compared three groups: combined carotid endarterectomy and OHS under a single anesthetic (combined CEA-OHS; $n = 195$), staged carotid endarterectomy followed by open heart surgery (staged CEA-OHS; $n = 45$), and staged carotid stenting followed by open heart surgery (CAS-OHS; $n = 110$). In staged CEA-OHS, CEA was performed a median of 14 days before OHS, whereas in the staged CAS-OHS group, patients underwent 3 to 4 weeks of antiplatelet therapy (median interval, 47 days) between CAS and CABG. The authors performed a propensity-adjusted analysis examining the early (up to 1 year) and late (beyond 1 year) risks of the composite endpoint (all-cause death, stroke, and MI). In the early phase, the staged CAS-OHS group's risk of adverse events was similar to that of the combined CEA-OHS group, whereas the staged CEA-OHS group had more adverse events, primarily driven by a higher inter-stage MI rate. Early mortality rates were similar among all three treatment strategies. Beyond 1 year, the staged CAS-OHS group experienced fewer adverse events than either the staged CEA-OHS group (adjusted hazard ratio 0.33; $P = 0.01$) or the combined CEA-OHS group (adjusted hazard ratio 0.35; $P = 0.003$) did. This late divergence was largely due to increased all-cause mortality in the staged and combined CEA groups. The systematic analysis of all interstage events and the direct comparison of three treatment strategies with a median follow-up of 3.7 years were the strengths of this study. The findings suggest that for patients who require urgent CABG, combined CEA-CABG is the optimal strategy for revascularization. However, for patients with stable angina who could tolerate a few weeks of dual-antiplatelet therapy, staged CAS-CABG may be advantageous. Staged CEA followed by CABG is associated with increased short-term MI and long-term mortality and may not be the optimal approach.

Synchronous Off-Pump Coronary Artery Bypass Grafting and Carotid Endarterectomy

Off-pump CABG has the potential advantage of reducing aortic manipulation, which is a major risk factor for embolic stroke. However, in the largest reported series ($n = 358$), Mishra and colleagues[61] found no significant difference in major adverse cardiovascular events between conventional CABG and off-pump CABG when CEA was performed simultaneously. The difference between off-pump and conventional CABG in terms of stroke rate and outcomes is a separate issue and is beyond the scope of this chapter. Suffice it to say, there is no evidence that this approach to treating concomitant coronary and carotid disease is superior to others that use cardiopulmonary bypass during CABG.

SUMMARY

The surgeon's approach to concurrent severe carotid and coronary artery disease must be individualized to the patient's anatomy, clinical presentation, and comorbid diseases. The clinical challenge is to balance sufficient repair of multisite arterial disease with minimal adverse outcomes, specifically perioperative MI, stroke, and death, including interstage events for staged procedures. In the absence of large-scale randomized trial data, carefully designed retrospective studies provide the best evidence available to guide clinical decision making. The differences in reported outcomes stem from clinical heterogeneity and differences in study design, comparator groups, surgical era, and analytical methods. Experts agree that when significant symptomatic or bilateral carotid artery stenosis is present, whenever possible, carotid revascularization is generally indicated in patients with planned CABG surgery.[73] Both the mode (CEA vs. CAS) and the timing (before, during, or after CABG) of carotid revascularization depend largely on the patient's symptoms, as well as on institutional experience. Synchronous, staged, and reverse-staged procedures have each been performed with a low incidence of morbidity and mortality. For patients with unilateral asymptomatic carotid artery stenosis, there might not be a benefit to routine carotid intervention as compared with contemporary optimal medical therapy and CABG alone. Further studies are needed to elucidate the roles and timing of CEA, CAS, and optimal medical therapy in the management of patients with concomitant severe carotid and coronary artery disease.

Acknowledgments

The authors wish to thank Scott A. Weldon, MA, CMI, for assisting with the illustrations; Stephen N. Palmer, PhD, ELS, and Susan Y. Green, MPH, for editorial assistance; and Raja R. Gopaldas, MD, and Peter H. Lin, MD, for their substantial contributions to the chapter published in the previous edition of this textbook, on which this updated chapter was based.

REFERENCES

1. Macleod MR, Amarenco P, Davis SM, et al: Atheroma of the aortic arch: an important and poorly recognised factor in the aetiology of stroke. *Lancet Neurol* 3:408–414, 2004.
2. Tribouilloy C, Peltier M, Colas L, et al: Fibrinogen is an independent marker for thoracic aortic atherosclerosis. *Am J Cardiol* 81:321–326, 1998.
3. Tribouilloy CM, Peltier M, Iannetta Peltier MC, et al: Plasma homocysteine and severity of thoracic aortic atherosclerosis. *Chest* 118:1685–1689, 2000.
4. Sen S, Oppenheimer SM, Lima J, et al: Risk factors for progression of aortic atheroma in stroke and transient ischemic attack patients. *Stroke* 33:930–935, 2002.
5. Tunick PA, Kronzon I: Atheromas of the thoracic aorta: clinical and therapeutic update. *J Am Coll Cardiol* 35:545–554, 2000.
6. Mohiuddin I, Silberfein EJ, Peden E: Supra-aortic trunk and upper extremity arterial disease. In Lumsden AB, Lin PH, Bush RL, et al, editors: *Endovascular therapy: principles of peripheral interventions*, Malden, Mass., 2006, Blackwell Futura, pp 88–102.
7. Kieffer E, Sabatier J, Koskas F, et al: Atherosclerotic innominate artery occlusive disease: early and long-term results of surgical reconstruction. *J Vasc Surg* 21:326–336, discussion 336–337, 1995.
8. Rhodes JM, Cherry KJ, Jr, Clark RC, et al: Aortic-origin reconstruction of the great vessels: risk factors of early and late complications. *J Vasc Surg* 31:260–269, 2000.
9. Hass WK, Fields WS, North RR, et al: Joint study of extracranial arterial occlusion. II. Arteriography, techniques, sites, and complications. *JAMA* 203:961–968, 1968.
10. Amarenco P, Cohen A, Tzourio C, et al: Atherosclerotic disease of the aortic arch and the risk of ischemic stroke. *N Engl J Med* 331:1474–1479, 1994.
11. Abularrage CJ, Slidell MB, Sidawy AN, et al: Quality of life of patients with Takayasu's arteritis. *J Vasc Surg* 47:131–136, discussion 136–137, 2008.
12. Ueno A, Awane Y, Wakabayashi A, et al: Successfully operated obliterative brachiocephalic arteritis (Takayasu) associated with the elongated coarctation. *Jpn Heart J* 8:538–544, 1967.
13. Chiou AC, Fantini GA: Subclavian artery aneurysm: an unusual manifestation of Takayasu's arteritis. *Cardiovasc Surg* 7:310–314, 1999.
14. Tabata M, Kitagawa T, Saito T, et al: Extracranial carotid aneurysm in Takayasu's arteritis. *J Vasc Surg* 34:739–742, 2001.
15. Regina G, Fullone M, Testini M, et al: Aneurysms of the supra-aortic trunks in Takayasu's disease: report of two cases. *J Cardiovasc Surg (Torino)* 39:757–760, 1998.
16. Miyata T, Sato O, Koyama H, et al: Long-term survival after surgical treatment of patients with Takayasu's arteritis. *Circulation* 108:1474–1480, 2003.
17. Mathes SJ, Alexander J: Radiation injury. *Surg Oncol Clin N Am* 5:809–824, 1996.
18. Sheikhzadeh A, Tettenborn I, Noohi F, et al: Occlusive thromboaortopathy (Takayasu disease): clinical and angiographic features and a brief review of literature. *Angiology* 53:29–40, 2002.
19. Park JH: Conventional and CT angiographic diagnosis of Takayasu arteritis. *Int J Cardiol* 54(Suppl):S165–S171, 1996.
20. Yamada I, Nakagawa T, Himeno Y, et al: Takayasu arteritis: evaluation of the thoracic aorta with CT angiography. *Radiology* 209:103–109, 1998.
21. Peterson BG, Resnick SA, Morasch MD, et al: Aortic arch vessel stenting: a single-center experience using cerebral protection. *Arch Surg* 141:560–563, discussion 563–564, 2006.
22. Von Tengg-Kobligk H, Weber TF, Rengier F, et al: Imaging modalities for the thoracic aorta. *J Cardiovasc Surg (Torino)* 49:429–447, 2008.
23. Shunk KA, Garot J, Atalar E, et al: Transesophageal magnetic resonance imaging of the aortic arch and descending thoracic aorta in patients with aortic atherosclerosis. *J Am Coll Cardiol* 37:2031–2035, 2001.
24. Chu VF, Chow CM, Stewart J, et al: Transesophageal echocardiography for ascending aortic dissection: is it enough for surgical intervention? *J Card Surg* 13:260–265, 1998.
25. Fayad ZA, Nahar T, Fallon JT, et al: In vivo magnetic resonance evaluation of atherosclerotic plaques in the human thoracic aorta: a comparison with transesophageal echocardiography. *Circulation* 101:2503–2509, 2000.
26. DeBakey ME, Morris GC, Jr, Jordan GL, Jr, et al: Segmental thrombo-obliterative disease of branches of aortic arch: successful surgical treatment. *J Am Med Assoc* 166:998–1003, 1958.
27. Crawford ES, De Bakey ME, Morris GC, Jr, et al: Surgical treatment of occlusion of the innominate, common carotid, and subclavian arteries: a 10 year experience. *Surgery* 65:17–31, 1969.
28. Queral LA, Criado FJ: The treatment of focal aortic arch branch lesions with Palmaz stents. *J Vasc Surg* 23:368–375, 1996.
29. Aiello F, Morrissey NJ: Open and endovascular management of subclavian and innominate arterial pathology. *Semin Vasc Surg* 24:31–35, 2011.
30. Ernemann U, Bender B, Melms A, et al: Current concepts of the interventional treatment of proximal supraaortic vessel stenosis. *Vasa* 41:313–318, 2012.
31. Palchik E, Bakken AM, Wolford HY, et al: Evolving strategies in treatment of isolated symptomatic innominate artery disease. *Vasc Endovascular Surg* 42:440–445, 2008.
32. Cherry KJ: Direct reconstruction of the innominate artery. *Cardiovasc Surg* 10:383–388, 2002.
33. Reul GJ, Jacobs MJ, Gregoric ID, et al: Innominate artery occlusive disease: surgical approach and long-term results. *J Vasc Surg* 14:405–412, 1991.
34. Azakie A, McElhinney DB, Higashima R, et al: Innominate artery reconstruction: over 3 decades of experience. *Ann Surg* 228:402–410, 1998.
35. Berguer R, Morasch MD, Kline RA: Transthoracic repair of innominate and common carotid artery disease: immediate and long-term outcome for 100 consecutive surgical reconstructions. *J Vasc Surg* 27:34–41, discussion 42, 1998.
36. Cherry KJ, Jr, McCullough JL, Hallett JW, Jr, et al: Technical principles of direct innominate artery revascularization: a comparison of endarterectomy and bypass grafts. *J Vasc Surg* 9:718–723, discussion 723–724, 1989.
37. Crawford ES, DeBakey ME, Morris GC, Jr, et al: Thrombo-obliterative disease of the great vessels arising from the aortic arch. *Thorac Cardiovasc Surg* 43:38–53, 1962.
38. Crawford ES, Stowe CL, Powers RW, Jr: Occlusion of the innominate, common carotid, and subclavian arteries: long-term results of surgical treatment. *Surgery* 94:781–791, 1983.
39. Paukovits TM, Lukacs L, Berczi V, et al: Percutaneous endovascular treatment of innominate artery lesions: a single-centre experience on 77 lesions. *Eur J Vasc Endovasc Surg* 40:35–43, 2010.
40. Huttl K, Nemes B, Simonffy A, et al: Angioplasty of the innominate artery in 89 patients: experience over 19 years. *Cardiovasc Intervent Radiol* 25:109–114, 2002.
41. van Hattum ES, de Vries JP, Lalezari F, et al: Angioplasty with or without stent placement in the brachiocephalic artery: feasible and durable? A retrospective cohort study. *J Vasc Interv Radiol* 18:1088–1093, 2007.
42. Mordasini P, Gralla J, Do DD, et al: Percutaneous and open retrograde endovascular stenting of symptomatic high-grade innominate artery stenosis: technique and follow-up. *AJNR Am J Neuroradiol* 32:1726–1731, 2011.
43. Sullivan TM, Gray BH, Bacharach JM, et al: Angioplasty and primary stenting of the subclavian, innominate, and common carotid arteries in 83 patients. *J Vasc Surg* 28:1059–1065, 1998.

44. Hadjipetrou P, Cox S, Piemonte T, et al: Percutaneous revascularization of atherosclerotic obstruction of aortic arch vessels. *J Am Coll Cardiol* 33:1238–1245, 1999.
45. Cull DL, Hansen JC, Taylor SM, et al: Internal carotid artery patency following common carotid artery occlusion: management of the asymptomatic patient. *Ann Vasc Surg* 13:73–76, 1999.
46. Grego F, Frigatti P, Lepidi S, et al: Synchronous carotid endarterectomy and retrograde endovascular treatment of brachiocephalic or common carotid artery stenosis. *Eur J Vasc Endovasc Surg* 26:392–395, 2003.
47. Allie DE, Hebert CJ, Lirtzman MD, et al: Intraoperative innominate and common carotid intervention combined with carotid endarterectomy: a "true" endovascular surgical approach. *J Endovasc Ther* 11:258–262, 2004.
48. Sfyroeras GS, Karathanos C, Antoniou GA, et al: A meta-analysis of combined endarterectomy and proximal balloon angioplasty for tandem disease of the arch vessels and carotid bifurcation. *J Vasc Surg* 54:534–540, 2011.
49. Sixt S, Rastan A, Schwarzwalder U, et al: Results after balloon angioplasty or stenting of atherosclerotic subclavian artery obstruction. *Catheter Cardiovasc Interv* 73:395–403, 2009.
50. Henry M, Henry I, Polydorou A, et al: Percutaneous transluminal angioplasty of the subclavian arteries. *Int Angiol* 26:324–340, 2007.
51. Westerband A, Rodriguez JA, Ramaiah VG, et al: Endovascular therapy in prevention and management of coronary-subclavian steal. *J Vasc Surg* 38:699–703, discussion 704, 2003.
52. Patel SN, White CJ, Collins TJ, et al: Catheter-based treatment of the subclavian and innominate arteries. *Catheter Cardiovasc Interv* 71:963–968, 2008.
53. Miyakoshi A, Hatano T, Tsukahara T, et al: Percutaneous transluminal angioplasty for atherosclerotic stenosis of the subclavian or innominate artery: angiographic and clinical outcomes in 36 patients. *Neurosurg Rev* 35:121–125, discussion 125–126, 2012.
54. Ando M, Sasako Y, Okita Y, et al: Surgical considerations of occlusive lesions associated with Takayasu's arteritis. *Jpn J Thorac Cardiovasc Surg* 48:173–179, 2000.
55. Sparks SR, Chock A, Seslar S, et al: Surgical treatment of Takayasu's arteritis: case report and literature review. *Ann Vasc Surg* 14:125–129, 2000.
56. Ishikawa K, Maetani S: Long-term outcome for 120 Japanese patients with Takayasu's disease: clinical and statistical analyses of related prognostic factors. *Circulation* 90:1855–1860, 1994.
57. Shimizu K, Sano K: Pulseless disease. *J Neuropathol Clin Neurol* 1:37–47, 1951.
58. Duncan JM, Cooley DA: Surgical considerations in aortitis with special emphasis on Takayasu's arteritis. *Tex Heart Inst J* 10:233–247, 1983.
59. Miyata T, Sato O, Deguchi J, et al: Anastomotic aneurysms after surgical treatment of Takayasu's arteritis: a 40-year experience. *J Vasc Surg* 27:438–445, 1998.
60. Robbs JV, Human RR, Rajaruthnam P: Operative treatment of nonspecific aortoarteritis (Takayasu's arteritis). *J Vasc Surg* 3:605–616, 1986.
61. Mishra Y, Wasir H, Kohli V, et al: Concomitant carotid endarterectomy and coronary bypass surgery: outcome of on-pump and off-pump techniques. *Ann Thorac Surg* 78:2037–2042, discussion 2042–2043, 2004.
62. Baril DT, Carroccio A, Palchik E, et al: Endovascular treatment of complicated aortic aneurysms in patients with underlying arteriopathies. *Ann Vasc Surg* 20:464–471, 2006.
63. Tyagi S, Gupta MD, Singh P, et al: Percutaneous revascularization of sole arch artery for severe cerebral ischemia resulting from Takayasu arteritis. *J Vasc Interv Radiol* 19:1699–1703, 2008.
64. Qureshi MA, Martin Z, Greenberg RK: Endovascular management of patients with Takayasu arteritis: stents versus stent grafts. *Semin Vasc Surg* 24:44–52, 2011.
65. Davidson D, Louridas G, Guzman R, et al: Steal syndrome complicating upper extremity hemoaccess procedures: incidence and risk factors. *Can J Surg* 46:408–412, 2003.
66. McMahon CJ, Thompson KS, Kearney DL, et al: Subclavian steal syndrome in anomalous connection of the left subclavian artery to the pulmonary artery in d-transposition of the great arteries. *Pediatr Cardiol* 22:60–62, 2001.
67. Takach TJ, Reul GJ, Cooley DA, et al: Myocardial thievery: the coronary-subclavian steal syndrome. *Ann Thorac Surg* 81:386–392, 2006.
68. Takach TJ, Reul GJ, Gregoric I, et al: Concomitant subclavian and coronary artery disease. *Ann Thorac Surg* 71:187–189, 2001.
69. Marshall WG, Jr, Miller EC, Kouchoukos NT: The coronary-subclavian steal syndrome: report of a case and recommendations for prevention and management. *Ann Thorac Surg* 46:93–96, 1988.
70. Takach TJ, Reul GJ, Duncan JM, et al: Concomitant brachiocephalic and coronary artery disease: outcome and decision analysis. *Ann Thorac Surg* 80:564–569, 2005.
71. Roffi M, Ribichini F, Castriota F, et al: Management of combined severe carotid and coronary artery disease. *Curr Cardiol Rep* 14:125–134, 2012.
72. Venkatachalam S, Gray BH, Mukherjee D, et al: Contemporary management of concomitant carotid and coronary artery disease. *Heart* 97:175–180, 2011.
73. Augoustides JG: Advances in the management of carotid artery disease: focus on recent evidence and guidelines. *J Cardiothorac Vasc Anesth* 26:166–171, 2012.
74. Brott TG, Halperin JL, Abbara S, et al: 2011 ASA/ACCF/AHA/AANN/AANS/ACR/ASNR/CNS/SAIP/SCAI/SIR/SNIS/SVM/SVS guideline on the management of patients with extracranial carotid and vertebral artery disease. A report of the American College of Cardiology Foundation/American Heart Association Task Force on Practice Guidelines, and the American Stroke Association, American Association of Neuroscience Nurses, American Association of Neurological Surgeons, American College of Radiology, American Society of Neuroradiology, Congress of Neurological Surgeons, Society of Atherosclerosis Imaging and Prevention, Society for Cardiovascular Angiography and Interventions, Society of Interventional Radiology, Society of NeuroInterventional Surgery, Society for Vascular Medicine, and Society for Vascular Surgery. *Circulation* 124:e54–e130, 2011.
75. Mahmoudi M, Hill PC, Xue Z, et al: Patients with severe asymptomatic carotid artery stenosis do not have a higher risk of stroke and mortality after coronary artery bypass surgery. *Stroke* 42:2801–2805, 2011.
76. Baiou D, Karageorge A, Spyt T, et al: Patients undergoing cardiac surgery with asymptomatic unilateral carotid stenoses have a low risk of peri-operative stroke. *Eur J Vasc Endovasc Surg* 38:556–559, 2009.
77. Naylor AR, Bown MJ: Stroke after cardiac surgery and its association with asymptomatic carotid disease: an updated systematic review and meta-analysis. *Eur J Vasc Endovasc Surg* 41:607–624, 2011.
78. Aboyans V, Lacroix P: Indications for carotid screening in patients with coronary artery disease. *Presse Med* 38:977–986, 2009.
79. Hillis LD, Smith PK, Anderson JL, et al: 2011 ACCF/AHA Guideline for Coronary Artery Bypass Graft Surgery: a report of the American College of Cardiology Foundation/American Heart Association Task Force on Practice Guidelines. *Circulation* 124:e652–e735, 2011.
80. Tendera M, Aboyans V, Bartelink ML, et al: ESC Guidelines on the diagnosis and treatment of peripheral artery diseases: document covering atherosclerotic disease of extracranial carotid and vertebral, mesenteric, renal, upper and lower extremity arteries: the Task Force on the Diagnosis and Treatment of Peripheral Artery Diseases of the European Society of Cardiology (ESC). *Eur Heart J* 32:2851–2906, 2011.
81. Tarakji KG, Sabik JF, III, Bhudia SK, et al: Temporal onset, risk factors, and outcomes associated with stroke after coronary artery bypass grafting. *JAMA* 305:381–390, 2011.
82. Naylor AR, Mehta Z, Rothwell PM, et al: Carotid artery disease and stroke during coronary artery bypass: a critical review of the literature. *Eur J Vasc Endovasc Surg* 23:283–294, 2002.
83. Ghosh J, Murray D, Khwaja N, et al: The influence of asymptomatic significant carotid disease on mortality and morbidity in patients undergoing coronary artery bypass surgery. *Eur J Vasc Endovasc Surg* 29:88–90, 2005.
84. Naylor AR: The importance of initiating "best medical therapy" and intervening as soon as possible in patients with symptomatic carotid artery disease: time for a radical rethink of practice. *J Cardiovasc Surg (Torino)* 50:773–782, 2009.
85. Li Y, Walicki D, Mathiesen C, et al: Strokes after cardiac surgery and relationship to carotid stenosis. *Arch Neurol* 66:1091–1096, 2009.

86. Endarterectomy for asymptomatic carotid artery stenosis. Executive Committee for the Asymptomatic Carotid Atherosclerosis Study. *JAMA* 273:1421–1428, 1995.
87. Halliday A, Mansfield A, Marro J, et al: Prevention of disabling and fatal strokes by successful carotid endarterectomy in patients without recent neurological symptoms: randomised controlled trial. *Lancet* 363:1491–1502, 2004.
88. Mahmud E, Reeves R: Carotid revascularization before open heart surgery: the data-driven treatment strategy. *J Am Coll Cardiol* 62:1957–1959, 2013.
89. Timaran CH, Rosero EB, Smith ST, et al: Trends and outcomes of concurrent carotid revascularization and coronary bypass. *J Vasc Surg* 48:355–360, discussion 360–361, 2008.
90. Bernhard VM, Johnson WD, Peterson JJ: Carotid artery stenosis: association with surgery for coronary artery disease. *Arch Surg* 105:837–840, 1972.
91. Dubinsky RM, Lai SM: Mortality from combined carotid endarterectomy and coronary artery bypass surgery in the US. *Neurology* 68:195–197, 2007.
92. Gopaldas RR, Chu D, Dao TK, et al: Staged versus synchronous carotid endarterectomy and coronary artery bypass grafting: analysis of 10-year nationwide outcomes. *Ann Thorac Surg* 91:1323–1329, discussion 1329, 2011.
93. Takach TJ, Reul GJ, Jr, Cooley DA, et al: Is an integrated approach warranted for concomitant carotid and coronary artery disease? *Ann Thorac Surg* 64:16–22, 1997.
94. Naylor AR, Cuffe RL, Rothwell PM, et al: A systematic review of outcomes following staged and synchronous carotid endarterectomy and coronary artery bypass. *Eur J Vasc Endovasc Surg* 25:380–389, 2003.
95. Illuminati G, Ricco JB, Calio F, et al: Short-term results of a randomized trial examining timing of carotid endarterectomy in patients with severe asymptomatic unilateral carotid stenosis undergoing coronary artery bypass grafting. *J Vasc Surg* 54:993–999, discussion 998–999, 2011.
96. Yadav JS, Wholey MH, Kuntz RE, et al: Protected carotid-artery stenting versus endarterectomy in high-risk patients. *N Engl J Med* 351:1493–1501, 2004.
97. Ziada KM, Yadav JS, Mukherjee D, et al: Comparison of results of carotid stenting followed by open heart surgery versus combined carotid endarterectomy and open heart surgery (coronary bypass with or without another procedure). *Am J Cardiol* 96:519–523, 2005.
98. Van der Heyden J, Suttorp MJ, Bal ET, et al: Staged carotid angioplasty and stenting followed by cardiac surgery in patients with severe asymptomatic carotid artery stenosis: early and long-term results. *Circulation* 116:2036–2042, 2007.
99. Mas JL, Chatellier G, Beyssen B, et al: Endarterectomy versus stenting in patients with symptomatic severe carotid stenosis. *N Engl J Med* 355:1660–1671, 2006.
100. Versaci F, Del Giudice C, Scafuri A, et al: Sequential hybrid carotid and coronary artery revascularization: immediate and mid-term results. *Ann Thorac Surg* 84:1508–1513, discussion 1513–1514, 2007.
101. Shishehbor MH, Venkatachalam S, Sun Z, et al: A direct comparison of early and late outcomes with three approaches to carotid revascularization and open heart surgery. *J Am Coll Cardiol* 62:1948–1956, 2013.

CHAPTER 74

Percutaneous Intervention on Abdominal Aortic and Peripheral Vascular Disease

Victor Chien • Elliot L. Chaikof

CHAPTER OUTLINE

Peripheral arterial occlusive disease (PAD) is a major cause of disability, loss of work, and lifestyle changes. The natural history of PAD is often characterized by slow progression in symptoms over time.[1-5] However, 70% of patients will remain stable or improve over time, approximately 30% will require an intervention, and 10% will require amputation.[6] Limb loss is the tragic final outcome of PAD and is associated with a significant degree of disability and a poor overall prognosis.[7] The aging of the population, continued tobacco abuse, high-fat diets, sedentary lifestyles, and rising prevalence of obesity parallel the increasing prevalence of PAD. The prevalence of PAD in the general population is 3% to 10%, and it is 15% to 20% among patients older than 70 years.[8] This prevalence probably underestimates the true burden of disease, however, as PAD may be asymptomatic. Because of the rising prevalence of PAD, many cardiovascular specialists have adopted a strategy of "global vascular management" for their patients. In this strategy, the evaluation, care, and intervention plan is more comprehensive in its scope, and it includes the management of vascular disease in all of its manifestations and anatomic locations. This chapter reviews the general aspects of peripheral vascular disease, with particular emphasis on the angiographic and percutaneous interventions after medical evaluation.

PERIPHERAL ANGIOGRAPHY

Indications

The purpose of peripheral angiography is to define the vascular anatomy and to identify significant arterial narrowing that requires revascularization (either percutaneous or surgical). As with any invasive diagnostic test, the risk-benefit ratio should be evaluated before angiography to identify patients who might fully benefit from imaging.[9-11]

Lower extremity claudication is classified according to the level of debilitation or restriction of activities. It is important to select the appropriate patient for angiography, given that the morbidity from vascular access might be particularly high among patients with PAD. The most commonly used clinical grading system for PAD is the Rutherford-Becker scale, a 7-point scale from 0, which denotes asymptomatic disease, to 6, which denotes major tissue loss (Table 74-1). In general, patients with Rutherford scale 2 and higher and noninvasive studies that demonstrate evidence of significant disease are likely to benefit from angiography and revascularization. Any patient with symptomatically limiting lower extremity claudication should undergo angiography to fully define the anatomy with a consideration toward revascularization.

TABLE 74-1 **Rutherford Scale**

Grade	Category	Clinical Description	Objective Criteria
0	0	Asymptomatic	Normal treadmill test
	1	Mild claudication	Ankle pressure after exercise <50 mm Hg but >25 mm Hg less than brachial
I	2	Moderate claudication	More moderate symptoms
	3	Severe claudication	Does not complete treadmill test Ankle pressure after exercise <50 mm Hg
II	4	Ischemic rest pain	Resting ankle pressure <60 mm Hg Decreased pulse volume recording
	5	Minor tissue loss Nonhealing ulcers	Resting ankle pressure <40 mm Hg Pulse volume recording moderately decreased
III	6	Major tissue loss Loss above the metatarsal limb no longer salvageable	As noted in category 5

Angiography is indicated in patients with threat of limb loss owing to acute thromboembolism. Patients with acute onset of a cool, pulseless extremity after catheterization or trauma require angiography to define the anatomy and site of occlusion in addition to allowing the direct infusion of intra-arterial fibrinolytic therapy or mechanical or rheolytic thrombectomy if necessary.[12-17]

Angiography may be warranted among patients with an abdominal aortic aneurysm or thoracic aneurysm to fully delineate the anatomy, particularly if endovascular repair is considered. However, given current noninvasive imaging techniques, such as magnetic resonance angiography and computed tomographic angiography, it is unlikely that invasive angiography is necessary to define anatomy among patients who are at low surgical risk, in whom an open repair may be most beneficial. Only if invasive angiography answers a particular question (e.g., the angle of the aneurysm neck) that cannot adequately be answered with noninvasive imaging should peripheral catheterization be pursued.

Magnetic resonance angiography may also be useful in the evaluation of coarctation of the aorta. When angiography is needed, anteroposterior (AP) and lateral images are the most useful for patients with coarctation who have not been operated on. Angiography usually confirms the anatomic coarctation, invariably seen just distal to the origin of the left subclavian artery. Further, if the head and neck vessels are imaged with the thoracic aorta, an idea of collateral flows can be inferred as well (i.e., carotid or mammary).

Invasive renal angiography is indicated in patients who have evidence of significant stenosis on noninvasive testing, such as magnetic resonance angiography and Doppler ultrasonography. Other indications include new uncontrolled hypertension in patients younger than 30 years or older than 55 years, refractory hypertension, rising creatinine concentration (specifically after the institution of angiotensin-converting enzyme inhibitor therapy), or unexplained acute pulmonary edema.[18] The prevalence of renovascular hypertension may be as high as 5% in the general population and 30% among patients with coronary artery disease or other PAD.

Because of the multiple-source blood supply to the upper extremity, which is derived principally from the subclavian and vertebral arteries, upper extremity claudication is rare. Upper extremity claudication symptoms include an inability to perform activities with the affected limb, such as combing hair, brushing teeth, or repeated lifting. Another constellation of symptoms indicating obstructive disease in the upper extremity may come from significant obstruction in the posterior circulation. In this situation, there is a reversal of flow from the vertebral artery in a patient with disease in the ipsilateral vertebral artery, leading to dizziness or difficulties with gait.[19-22] Among patients who have undergone coronary artery bypass graft surgery with use of the internal mammary artery, persistent angina and anterior ischemia on noninvasive testing may suggest left subclavian stenosis as the cause of coronary ischemia.[21,23-27] Therefore, any patient with symptoms of upper extremity claudication, anterior ischemia after coronary artery bypass grafting with the use of the left internal mammary artery, or posterior circulation events and a difference in upper extremity blood pressures should be evaluated for the possibility of subclavian stenosis and undergo evaluation, including angiography.

A critical stenosis of one or both carotid arteries on noninvasive imaging or evidence of transient ischemic attack or stroke and a critical stenosis identified on noninvasive testing is an indication for invasive carotid or cerebral angiography.

Contraindications

The principal contraindications to peripheral angiography are bleeding diathesis, renal failure (true or impending), fever, ongoing infection, and severe anemia (Box 74-1).

Complications

Complications of invasive peripheral angiography primarily involve vascular access site complications, catheter manipulation within atherosclerotic vessels, emboli, clot formation, stroke, myocardial infarction, worsening renal function, or congestive heart failure (Box 74-2). A particularly devastating complication of catheter manipulation within the arterial tree is an atheroembolic event. In its most severe form to the lower extremities, it may cause loss of limb or digits. Likewise, emboli to the renal

BOX 74-1 Relative Contraindications to Catheterization and Angiography

- Bleeding diathesis or inability to take aspirin or adenosine diphosphate inhibitor
- Concurrent febrile illness
- Severe renal insufficiency or anuria without dialysis planned
- Severe allergy to contrast agents
- Severe hypokalemia or digitalis toxicity
- Severe hypertension or ongoing unstable coronary syndrome

BOX 74-2 Possible Complications of Peripheral Catheterization

- Vascular access dissection or perforation: 0.1%-0.2%
- Bleeding or hematoma: 1.5%-2.0%
- Allergic reaction: 0.5%-2.0%
- Vasovagal events: 1.0%-2.0%
- Death: 0.1%-0.2%

circulation can lead to acute renal decompensation or failure requiring dialysis.[28-30] Pseudoaneurysm or vascular access complications can be as high as 3% in patients with severe peripheral occlusive disease.[31,32]

General Considerations

There are several important differences in imaging of peripheral vascular structures and coronary arteries. Peripheral angiography commonly uses a larger image intensifier field (14 inches [36 cm]) to encompass larger regions of interest. Digital (not film-based) angiography allows online display of acquired images as well as advanced processing techniques to enhance brightness, contrast, or shift of underlying bone structures to enhance the final image (Fig. 74-1). Frequently, digital subtraction angiography is used. With this imaging method, a baseline background image, referred to as a mask, is obtained immediately before injection of contrast material to digitally subtract bone, calcifications, air, or soft tissues from the final image, leading to the best image quality with the most definition of vascular anatomy. Another advantage of digital subtraction angiography is that it can reduce the volume of contrast material and imaging acquisition time required.

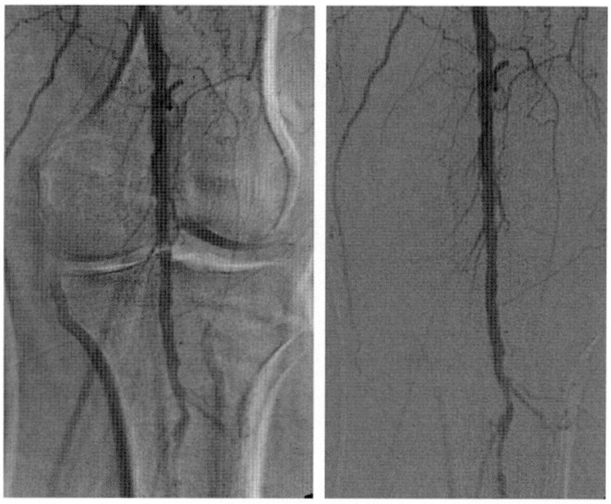

FIGURE 74-1 ■ Digital subtraction angiogram of the popliteal artery with moderate motion of the patient confounding the popliteal evaluation and after "shifting" of the image to re-mask the underlying bone structures for direct angiographic evaluation of the anatomy.

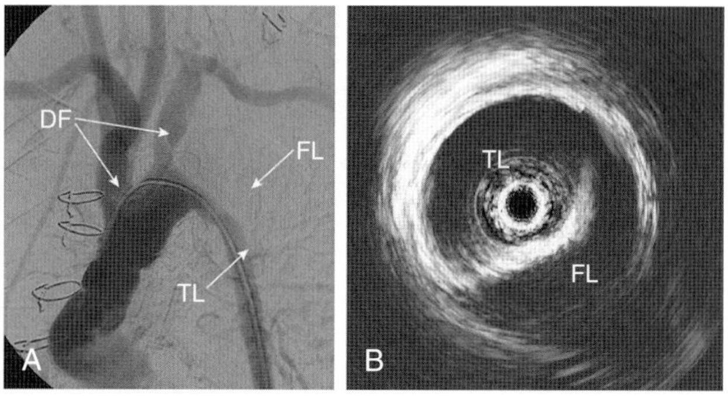

FIGURE 74-2 ■ **(A)** Angiogram and **(B)** intravascular ultrasound image of a patient with type A dissection of the aortic arch. The false lumen (FL) and true lumen (TL) are evident in the intravascular ultrasound image. The *arrows* on the angiogram correlate with the site of the intravascular ultrasound image. *DF,* Dissection flap.

SPECIFIC ANATOMIC IMAGING

Thoracic Aorta

Thoracic aortography is used to define the anatomic relation of the aortic arch and the great vessels, to determine the diameter of the thoracic aorta, to obtain evidence of dissection (Fig. 74-2), and to evaluate for trauma or other vascular injuries. The optimal view of the aortic arch is obtained in the left anterior oblique projection at 30 to 40 degrees oblique. The injection of 30 to 40 mL of contrast material at 20 to 30 mL/sec generally opacifies the vessels for adequate imaging. If digital subtraction angiography is used, the patient should be instructed to hold his or her breath to avoid artifacts caused by motion or breathing. The three principal vessels originating from the arch are (1) the brachiocephalic (innominate), leading ultimately to the right subclavian and right carotid arteries; (2) the left common carotid; and (3) the left subclavian artery (Fig. 74-3). The most common normal variant of this anatomy is the so-called bovine arch, in which the left common carotid artery originates from the brachiocephalic trunk. This normal variant occurs in approximately 10% of patients.[32]

Abdominal Aorta

The abdominal aorta should be angiographically imaged for evaluation of abdominal aortic aneurysm, dissection, lower extremity claudication, mesenteric ischemia, and renovascular disease. The abdominal aorta begins at the level of the diaphragm. The principal vessels are, in descending order, (1) the celiac artery at the level of L1,

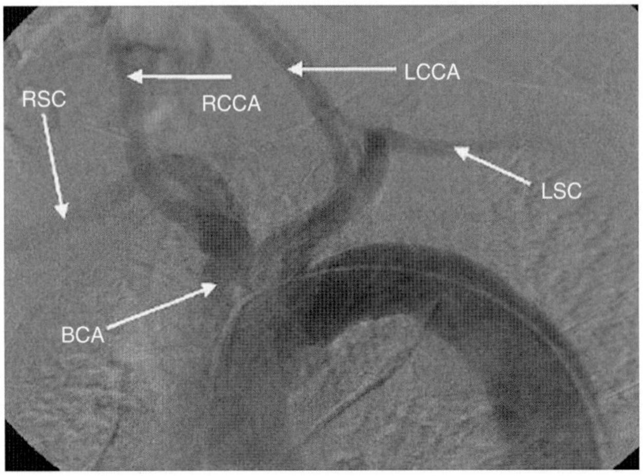

FIGURE 74-3 ■ Digital subtraction angiography of the thoracic arch and great vessels. *BCA,* Brachiocephalic artery; *LCCA,* left common carotid artery; *LSC,* left subclavian artery; *RCCA,* right common carotid artery; *RSC,* right subclavian artery.

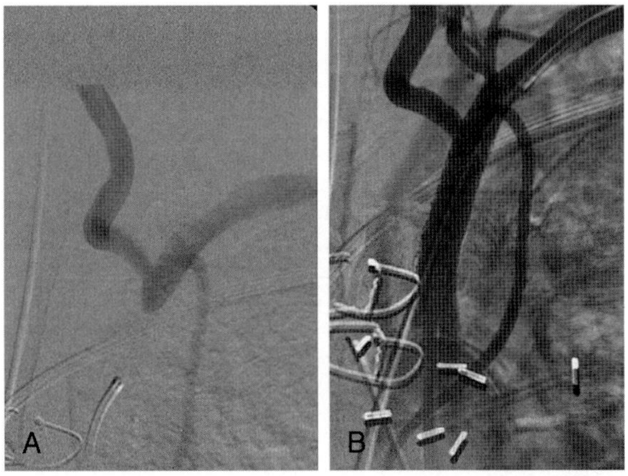

FIGURE 74-5 ■ Digital subtraction angiography of the left subclavian artery before and after intervention. **A,** The left subclavian artery is occluded. **B,** After crossing the left subclavian artery in a retrograde fashion from the left brachial artery, the subclavian is stented, with the final angiographic result noted.

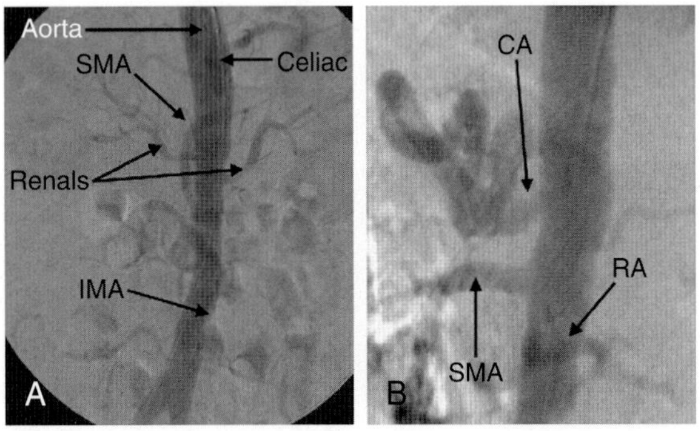

FIGURE 74-4 ■ **A,** Anteroposterior view of digital subtraction angiography of the abdominal aorta and major branches. **B,** Lateral digital subtraction angiography of the abdominal aorta and major branches. *CA,* Celiac artery; *IMA,* inferior mesenteric artery; *RA,* renal artery; *SMA,* superior mesenteric artery.

(2) the superior mesenteric artery at the level of L2-3, (3) the renal arteries at the level of L2-3 just caudal to the superior mesenteric artery, and (4) the inferior mesenteric artery at the level of L4. The abdominal aorta terminates at the bifurcation and the origin of the iliac arteries.

In general, 20 to 40 mL of contrast material injected at 15 to 30 mL/sec will adequately opacify the vessels to define the anatomy. Again, as in the thoracic aorta, it is critical to fully opacify the lumen and the vessels of interest. AP and lateral images (Fig. 74-4) of the abdominal aorta are usually sufficient to delineate all anatomic areas of interest in the abdominal aorta and mesenteric vessels. If selected conduits require further visualization, a soft-tipped catheter can provide selective angiography without requiring large loads of contrast material to fully define the anatomy.

Head and Neck Angiography

The three primary branches emanating from the aortic arch are the brachiocephalic, left common carotid, and left subclavian arteries. The right subclavian and carotid arteries are the terminal branches of the brachiocephalic trunk. The most common variant of this anatomy is the bovine arch, in which the left carotid and brachiocephalic share a common origin.[32]

Subclavian artery disease, stenosis, and occlusion are common.[33] Symptoms are rare because of the dual supply of blood to the upper extremity through the subclavian and vertebral arteries. Upper extremity claudication is rare but is manifested by upper extremity discomfort while engaging in activity with the upper extremity or in activities of daily living. More commonly, subclavian stenosis or occlusion is manifested by either posterior circulation symptoms, such as dizziness and gait instability, which are rare, or anterior ischemia (coronary steal syndrome) in the patient who has been treated with left internal mammary artery coronary bypass grafting (Fig. 74-5).[23-27,34]

Subclavian artery angiography is optimally performed with both AP and ipsilateral oblique views. Selective angiography can be performed with any straight or slightly angulated catheters. As in the thoracic aorta, nonselective angiography, in general, requires 30 to 40 mL of contrast material injected at 20 to 30 mL/sec to adequately opacify all vessels in the arch. The vessels are usually accessed with the use of the guide wire as a rail, and then the catheter is advanced over the wire. Access to the brachiocephalic, carotid, and subclavian arteries usually requires a counterclockwise movement of the catheter in the ascending aorta for it to engage the vessel of interest. The J-wire is then advanced into the vessel, and ultimately the catheter is advanced over the wire. Once the wire has been removed and the catheter has been flushed, angiography can be performed safely. There is usually some shoulder and neck discomfort with moderate injections of contrast material, and the patient should be forewarned of a sensation of warmth that will follow injections. Discomfort can be minimized, if necessary, with the use of half-diluted contrast material. Excessively vigorous injections should be avoided to prevent subintimal injection or dye staining into the intima of the subclavian artery.

Atherosclerosis of the subclavian artery is generally proximal at the origin or within the first few millimeters from the aortic origin. The origin of the inferior mesenteric artery is usually spared of atherosclerosis. The origin of the vertebral artery may be involved with atherosclerotic disease, but the need for intervention is low because of the dual blood supply to the posterior circulation that arises from both the contralateral vertebral and ipsilateral carotid arteries with an intact intracerebral circulation.

The carotid arteries generally bifurcate at the level of the fourth cervical vertebra into the internal and external carotid arteries (Fig. 74-6*A*). The internal carotid usually has no major branches and becomes tortuous below the petrous bone, the so-called carotid siphon. Once the vessel enters the petrous bone, it is considered the intracranial internal carotid artery. On exiting the petrous bone, the internal carotid artery bifurcates early into the anterior and middle cerebral arteries. The external carotid artery has several branches that supply the face.

Carotid atherosclerosis is common.[35,36] Intervention in the internal carotid artery is performed either percutaneously or surgically. Annually, there are 600,000 strokes in the United States, of which 500,000 are first attacks and 160,000 are fatal. Cerebral occlusive disease encompasses stroke, transient ischemic attack, and posterior circulation (vertebral-basilar) events. Several studies have evaluated the efficacy of various revascularization strategies in preventing future events.[37-39] The National Heart, Lung, and Blood Institute's Atherosclerosis Risk in Communities study[40] reported that 83% of all strokes were ischemic, 40% were lacunar, and 14% were thromboembolic. Most patients with extracranial carotid artery disease are asymptomatic.

Risk factors for the presence and progression of carotid artery disease are similar to those of coronary artery disease and include diabetes mellitus, hypertension, hyperlipidemia, and family history. A bruit can aid in identifying patients with carotid stenoses, but the presence of a bruit is neither sensitive nor specific for the detection of clinically meaningful carotid stenosis. For example, in one study,[41] only 37% of 330 patients referred to a neurology clinic with a cervical bruit had a high-grade carotid artery lesion noted with duplex imaging. A carotid bruit may be associated with subsequent risk of stroke, as the Framingham Heart Study demonstrated that asymptomatic patients with a carotid bruit have twice the risk of stroke.[42] In addition, a bruit can be a marker of more general cardiovascular risk.[43] In asymptomatic patients, risk of stroke was 2.5% if the stenosis was more than 75%. The risk was higher for patients with symptoms (3.3%).[44-46]

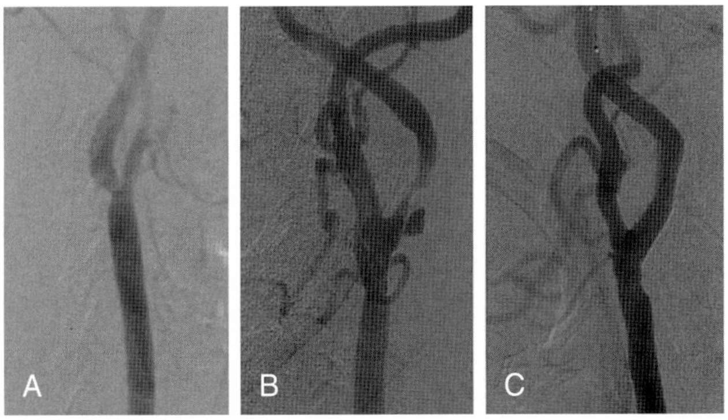

FIGURE 74-6 ■ **A,** Angiogram of a normal carotid and its bifurcation. **B,** Abnormality on an angiogram with an ulcerated left internal carotid artery in a patient several weeks after a transient ischemic attack. **C,** Final angiogram after angioplasty and stenting.

Angiography of the carotid artery is generally performed in the AP and lateral views. Selective angiography should be performed with care to ensure adequate position of the catheter and distance from the bifurcation.

Renal Vascular Imaging

The prevalence of renovascular disease can be as high as 50% in patients with coronary artery disease or other PAD.[47,48] Renovascular disease is a cause of secondary hypertension in 0.5% to 5% of the general population.[49,50] Whereas other noninvasive and functional studies such as Doppler ultrasonography, captopril nuclear studies, and magnetic resonance angiography remain useful screening tools, contrast angiography remains the gold standard. The renal arteries have a posterior takeoff from the abdominal aorta. Injection of 15 to 20 mL of contrast material at 30 mL/sec should opacify the intended vessels adequately. An improvement in blood pressure control is one goal of percutaneous revascularization of renal arteries.[51-53] Another potential benefit of renal artery revascularization is preservation of renal function.[48,54-56]

Lower Extremity Angiography

Iliac Vessels

The iliac vessels originate at the termination of the abdominal aorta, usually at the L4-5 level. They remain retroperitoneal throughout their course until they cross the inguinal ligament and become the common femoral artery. The principal bifurcation in the iliac artery is the terminal bifurcation of the common iliac into the internal and external iliac arteries (Fig. 74-7).

Angiography of the iliac arteries is best achieved in the AP and oblique positions (left anterior oblique for the right internal iliac and right anterior oblique for the left internal iliac). The imaging catheter is positioned just above the aortic bifurcation to allow the best opacification of the iliac arteries. In general, 15 to 30 mL of contrast material injected at 20 to 30 mL/sec is sufficient to provide adequate opacification.

In patients with lower extremity claudication, noninvasive testing with ankle-brachial indices by duplex and Doppler imaging is critical. Evaluation with and without exercise, either 5 minutes at 1.5 miles per hour or 40 calf raises is often necessary to provoke symptoms and, more important, to determine the level of stenosis.[57] Doppler imaging is vital in the evaluation of the lower extremities. Normal flow patterns are triphasic or biphasic (Fig. 74-8). When a critical lesion is present, the waveform becomes

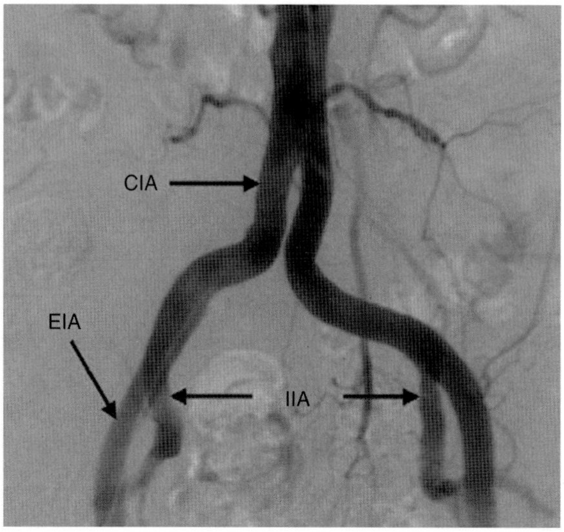

FIGURE 74-7 ■ Digital subtraction angiography in the anteroposterior projection of the terminal abdominal aortic bifurcation. *CIA,* Common iliac artery; *EIA,* external iliac artery; *IIA,* internal iliac artery.

monophasic. Furthermore, during exertion, resting triphasic and biphasic waveforms become monophasic distal to a critical stenosis. The location of the transition in the waveform pattern indicates the level of critical disease and can allow more directed and focused lower extremity angiography. Because the lower extremity arterial tree is relatively superficial, the anatomy can occasionally be directly visualized noninvasively with duplex imaging. Therefore, in some cases, the level and extent of disease may be delineated without vascular access.

Angiographic Technique

Lower extremity angiography can be performed in many ways. There has been an increase in the use of digital angiography and bolus-chase techniques, in which the table stops at various points of the run to mask the image, then returns to the same location and follows the original bolus of contrast material throughout the course. These methods allow a single injection of contrast material and delineation of the anatomy without the need for multiple

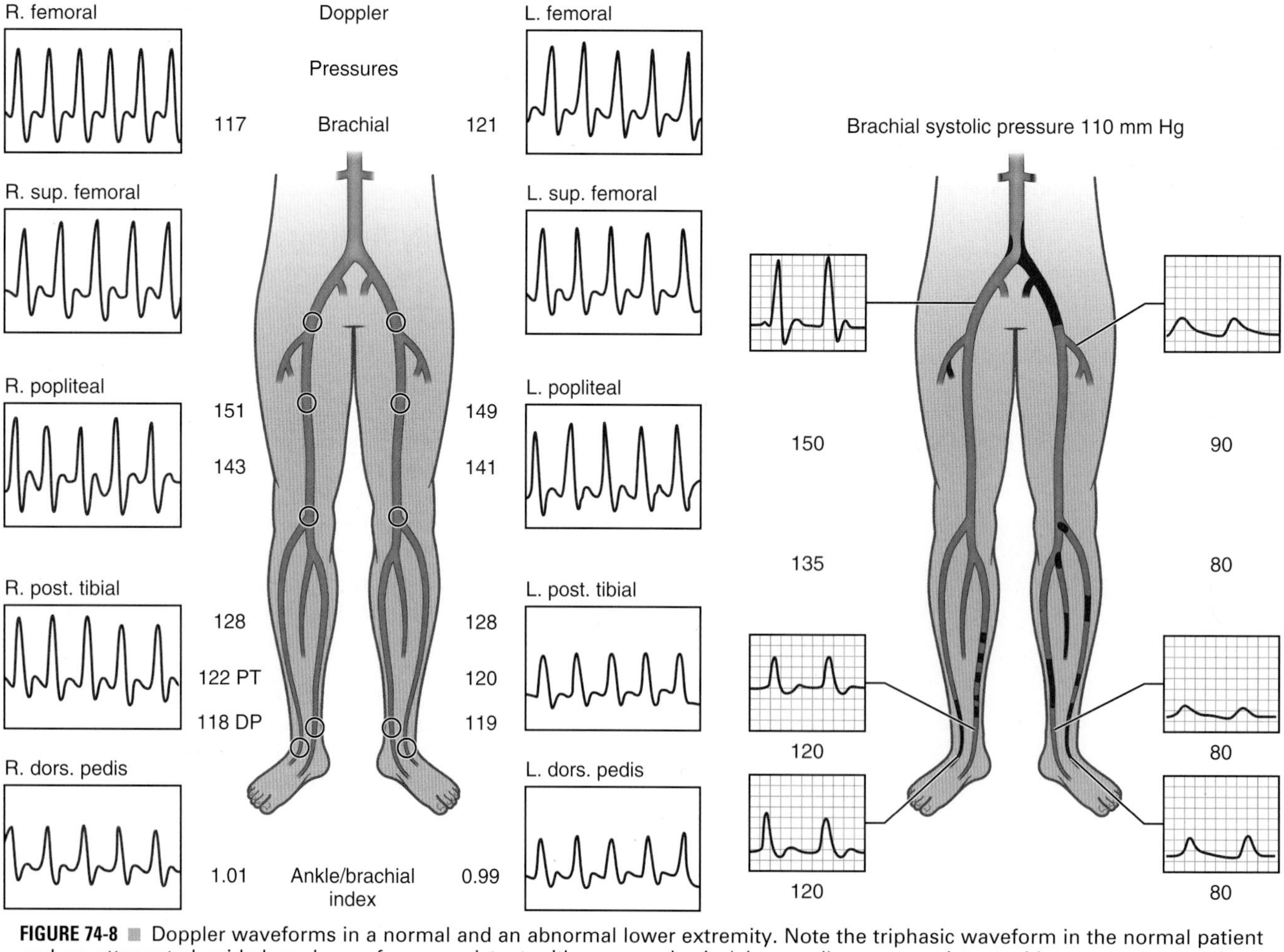

FIGURE 74-8 ■ Doppler waveforms in a normal and an abnormal lower extremity. Note the triphasic waveform in the normal patient and an attenuated, wide-based waveform consistent with a monophasic (abnormal) wave consistent with upstream stenosis or occlusion. *L,* Left; *R,* right.

injections. The principal problem with this technique occurs when there is significant motion of the patient from the mask to the contrast bolus-chase and the images are out of register and of poor quality. Small motion from the patient may be digitally shifted in the final angiogram without much difficulty to remove the underlying bone structures and to enhance the final angiographic image (see Fig. 74-1). In general, volumes of contrast material for the lower extremity bolus-chase technique range from 30 to 40 mL at 8 to 10 mL/sec. Other techniques include static images and older cut-film changers. In the static image technique, a focal area is evaluated with a single bolus injection of contrast material of 15 to 30 mL at 8 to 10 mL/sec or by hand injection.

One unique aspect of peripheral angiography is the antegrade puncture of the femoral artery. The common femoral artery is entered as with standard retrograde access, but it is entered in the antegrade direction (in the direction of blood flow to the leg). The entry is less steep (≈45 degrees) but should enter the common femoral artery over the femoral head and below the inguinal ligament. This access allows direct intervention for the infrainguinal vessels.

Infrainguinal Vessels

The arterial tree below the inguinal ligament begins with the common femoral artery. This vessel bifurcates early, at the level of the femoral head, into the profunda femoral artery and the superficial femoral artery (Fig. 74-9*A*). The superficial femoral artery is the principal vessel supplying the lower extremity. It courses anteriorly through the proximal 60% of its length and then begins to course posteriorly, entering the adductor canal (Hunter canal), a musculofascial canal bounded by the sartorius muscle anteriorly, the vastus medialis muscle laterally, and the adductor longus and magnus muscles posteriorly. This canal exits posteriorly, and the artery becomes the popliteal artery as it exits. The popliteal artery then terminates at the level of the tibial plateau into the anterior tibial artery and tibial-peroneal trunk vessels. The tibial-peroneal trunk then terminally bifurcates into the posterior tibial artery and the peroneal artery (see Fig. 74-9*B*). The posterior tibial and anterior tibial arteries usually are the principal vessels supplying the foot. The posterior tibial artery supplies the medial and lateral plantar vessels, and the anterior tibial artery supplies the dorsalis pedal artery. The distal plantar arteries, along with the dorsalis pedal artery, often communicate to form the plantar arch of the foot.

PERCUTANEOUS INTERVENTION

Thoracic and Abdominal Aorta

Intervention to the thoracic and abdominal aorta is usually performed for dissection, coarctation, or aneurysm and is discussed in full detail elsewhere in this text. Percutaneous intervention with stenting has become the primary method of correction of coarctation.[58-70] Success rates for percutaneous interventions are 70% to 80% with a reduction of peak gradient less than 20 mm Hg. Most of the patients are seen within a pediatric population, and as such, adult disease is rarely seen as native coarctation. Percutaneous intervention to postoperative coarctation is feasible and limits the risk of a second open procedure (Fig. 74-10).[60]

In general, there is a greater degree of atherosclerosis in the aorta after it crosses the diaphragm into the abdomen. The consequence of this is either lower extremity claudication or mesenteric ischemia. As disease in the abdominal aorta can lead to lower extremity claudication, it is a possible site of angioplasty and stent implantation

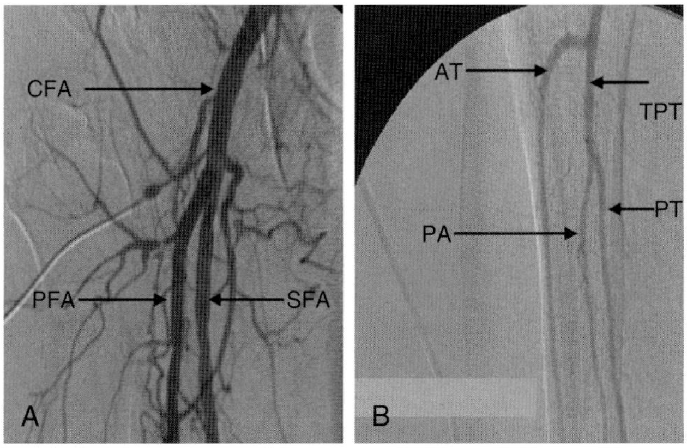

FIGURE 74-9 ■ **A,** Digital subtraction angiography in the anteroposterior projection of the right common femoral artery. **B,** Infrapopliteal digital subtraction angiography in the anteroposterior projection. *AT,* Anterior tibial artery; *CFA,* common femoral artery; *PA,* peroneal artery; *PFA,* profunda femoral artery; *PT,* posterior tibial artery; *SFA,* superficial femoral artery; *TPT,* tibial-peroneal trunk.

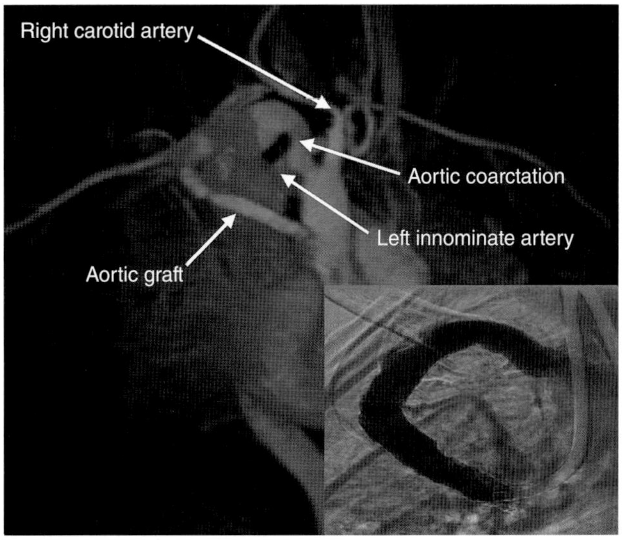

FIGURE 74-10 ■ Magnetic resonance angiographic anteroposterior view of hypoplastic aortic arch with a coarctation. The anatomy of this right-sided arch is as shown with the initial takeoff of the right carotid, then right subclavian (not shown), followed by left brachiocephalic off the descending aorta with intervening aortic-aortic graft. *Inset:* Completed stenting to the aortic-aortic graft.

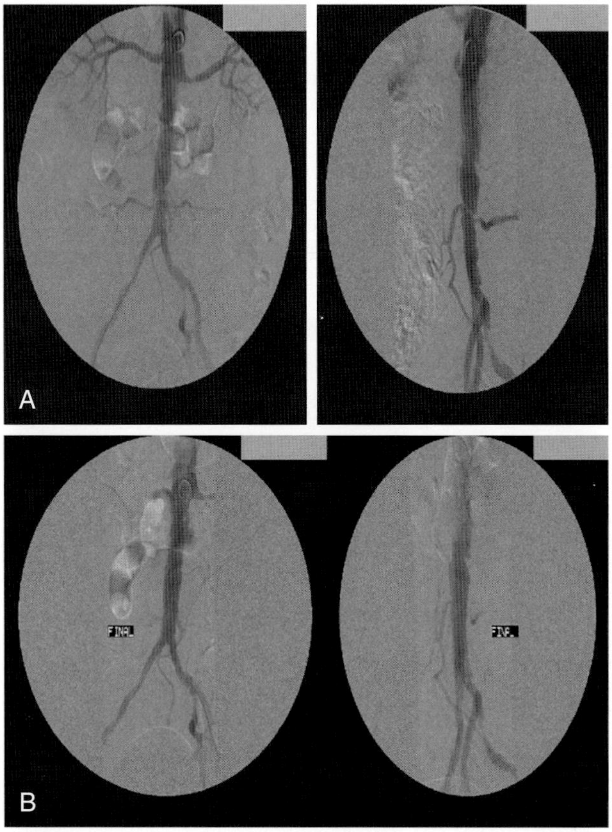

FIGURE 74-11 ■ **A,** Anteroposterior and lateral digital subtraction angiograms of the distal abdominal aorta showing a distal lesion at the level of the inferior mesenteric artery. **B,** A widely patent vessel shown after angioplasty and stenting of the distal abdominal aorta.

(Fig. 74-11). Here, it is important to determine the significance of the lesion and the possibility of intervention. Once the characteristics of the lesion are defined and percutaneous intervention is pursued, the key element is to gain access in each femoral artery. One access point will serve as the primary intervention for the aorta, and the other will then cross the aortic stent, with further intervention to the iliac arteries performed in a "kissing" manner (see Fig. 74-11).

Mesenteric ischemia is somewhat uncommon, given the redundant blood supply to the intestine. If mesenteric ischemia is suspected and revascularization is warranted, a percutaneous procedure may afford less risk to the patient than that from an open surgical procedure. Stenting of the mesenteric vessels is performed usually from the common femoral artery. The long-term restenosis rate is approximately 10% to 15% after several years. Care should be taken in advancing the catheter or other devices through the lesion, because distal embolization can lead to further acute mesenteric ischemia.

Head and Neck Vessels

Whereas some patients have significant stenoses without any signs or symptoms, those patients who are symptomatic face a higher risk of future events.[37,38] The North American Symptomatic Carotid Endarterectomy Trial (NASCET) demonstrated that among patients with stroke, the incidence of recurrent ipsilateral stroke at 2 years was 26% for medical therapy as opposed to 9% with carotid endarterectomy (CEA) among patients with a lesion of more than 70% noted by angiography.[37] Similarly, the European Carotid Surgery Trial (ECST) demonstrated that in symptomatic patients with all levels of stenosis, patients treated with medical therapy had a 17% rate of stroke compared with 2.8% with surgical revascularization.[38] Thus, in symptomatic patients with high-grade stenoses (>70%), CEA appears to be beneficial.

Percutaneous transluminal angioplasty with stenting of the extracranial carotid artery has been performed for more than two decades (see Fig. 74-6*B* and *C*).[71] The Global Utilization Report demonstrated the following incidence rates at 30 days: transient ischemic attack, 2.6%; minor stroke, 2.5%; major stroke, 1.4%; and mortality, 0.8%.[71] The Carotid and Vertebral Artery Transluminal Angioplasty Study (CAVATAS) compared, in a nonrandomized trial, carotid percutaneous transluminal angioplasty and stenting with CEA.[72] Overall, the combined stroke and mortality rate was similar between groups, at 10% and 9.9% by 30 days. At 3 years, outcomes remained similar.[73-75]

There have been two major trials comparing percutaneous techniques with CEA among high-risk[76] and average-risk patients.[77] The Stenting and Angioplasty with Protection in Patients at High Risk for Endarterectomy (SAPPHIRE) study was the first large-scale randomized trial comparing CEA with carotid artery stenting (CAS) with the use of distal protection devices.[76] SAPPHIRE was designed to test the hypothesis that CAS was not inferior to CEA. High-risk patients were defined as those with clinically significant cardiac disease, severe pulmonary disease, contralateral carotid occlusion or laryngeal nerve palsy, previous radical neck surgery, recurrent stenosis after CEA, or age greater than 80 years. Patients with symptomatic carotid artery disease required a stenosis of at least 50%, and those presenting with asymptomatic carotid disease required stenosis of at least 80%. The surgeons and the interventionists were compelled to agree that the patient was a suitable candidate for either procedure. The primary outcome was a composite of death, stroke, or myocardial infarction within 30 days or death or ipsilateral stroke between 30 days and 1 year. The primary endpoint occurred in 12.2% of patients who underwent CAS and 20.1% of patients who underwent CEA, which demonstrated noninferiority and nearly reached criteria for superiority ($P = 0.053$). Long-term efficacy and safety were evaluated at 3 years with a composite endpoint of death, stroke, or myocardial infarction in 24.6% of patients in the CAS group and 26.9% of patients in the CEA group—a nonsignificant difference.[78]

Several randomized trials have challenged these results. In an attempt to extend the use of CAS to symptomatic patients of average surgical risk, the EVA-3S (Endarterectomy versus Angioplasty in Patients with Symptomatic Severe Carotid Stenosis) and SPACE (Stent-Supported Percutaneous Angioplasty of the Carotid Artery versus Endarterectomy) trials were undertaken.[77,79]

To be enrolled in EVA-3S, patients had to have had a transient ischemic attack or stroke within the previous 120 days and an ipsilateral carotid stenosis of 60% to 99%.[77] The primary endpoint was the composite of stroke or death within 30 days after the procedure. The trial was ended prematurely after the enrollment of 527 patients because of safety concerns. Patients who underwent CAS had a 9.6% incidence of the primary endpoint, significantly higher than for patients who underwent CEA (3.9%). A major criticism of the trial was the lack of use of distal protection devices early in the trial, although the incidence of stroke even with the use of protection later in the trial was relatively high (7.9%) and still higher than the incidence among patients undergoing CEA. Furthermore, the use of several distal embolic devices with limited user experience was another significant criticism.

SPACE enrolled 1200 patients with a moderate stroke or transient ischemic attack within the previous 180 days.[79] The primary outcome—ipsilateral ischemic stroke or death through 30 days—was reached by 6.84% of patients in the CAS group and 6.34% of those in the CEA group, a difference that did not reach statistical significance for noninferiority. A major criticism of this trial was that distal protection devices were not mandated.[80] Furthermore, operators had limited experience with CAS.

Percutaneous outcomes can be improved with the use of distal protection devices (Fig. 74-12), such as the balloon occlusion GuardWire (PercuSurge, Sunnyvale, Calif.), the filter device AngioGuard (Cordis, Warren, N.J.), or the EPI filter (EPI, Inc., Boston, Mass.). Such distal protection devices have been shown to capture distal emboli that can be liberated with catheter manipulation, balloon inflations, or stenting in the carotid arteries (Fig. 74-13). The major difference is that the balloon occlusion device interrupts flow distally, whereas the filter devices allow flow to continue but capture the debris.

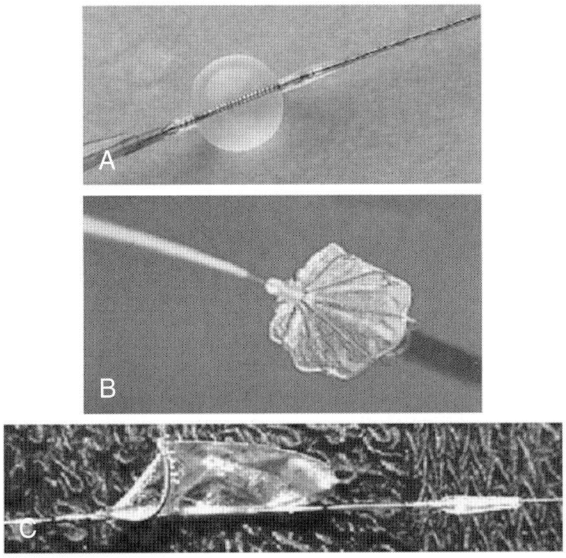

FIGURE 74-12 ■ Distal protection devices. **A,** GuardWire (PercuSurge, Inc., Sunnyvale, Calif.). **B,** AngioGuard (Cordis, Warren, N.J.). **C,** EPI filter (EPI, Inc., Boston, Mass.).

The more recently completed CREST (Carotid Revascularization Endarterectomy versus Stenting Trial) trial was a large-scale randomized trial comparing traditional CEA with CAS with concurrent use of distal protection devices.[81] The multicenter trial enrolled 2502 patients to assess CAS and CEA for both symptomatic and asymptomatic patients. Symptomatic patients were defined as those that had a transient ischemic attack, amaurosis fugax, or minor nondisabling stroke in the distribution of the study artery within 180 days of randomization, as well as stenosis of the carotid artery greater than 50% by angiography, greater than 70% by ultrasound, or greater than 70% by computed tomographic or magnetic resonance angiography if ultrasound was 50% to 69%. Asymptomatic patients were defined as having carotid stenosis of greater than 60% by angiography, greater than 70% by ultrasound, or greater than 80% by computed tomographic or magnetic resonance angiography if ultrasound was 50% to 69%. Patients with previous disabling stroke or chronic atrial fibrillation were excluded. Results suggested similar short-term and longer-term outcomes between CAS and CEA; however, there was higher stroke risk with CAS and higher myocardial infarction risk with CEA.

Renal Arteries

There are three major clinical trials evaluating the role of renal artery angioplasty or stent implantation among patients with documented renal artery stenosis and difficult-to-control hypertension.

Van Jaarsveld and colleagues[53] compared angioplasty alone with medical therapy in the control of hypertension in 106 patients with renal artery stenosis. Inclusion criteria included diastolic blood pressure of 95 mm Hg or higher despite the use of at least two antihypertensive agents, serum creatinine concentration of 1.7 mg/dL or less, and stenosis of 50% or more. More than 40% of patients in the drug therapy group underwent angioplasty in the 12-month follow-up period. Mean blood pressure did not differ significantly between the groups. At 3 months, patients in the angioplasty group were taking significantly fewer antihypertensive drugs, but this difference was not significant at 12 months. More patients in

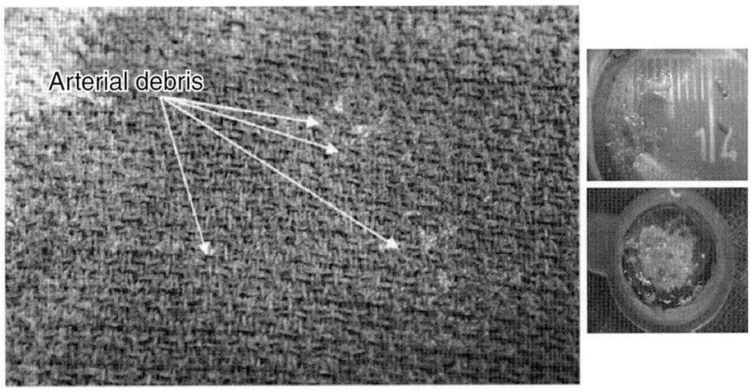

FIGURE 74-13 ■ Distal macroscopic emboli captured with the GuardWire in an ulcerated left internal carotid lesion after predilation with angioplasty before stenting.

the angioplasty group had better blood pressure control, defined as a decrease of 10 mm Hg or more in diastolic blood pressure with no change in medications or a decrease in the number of drugs with no change in diastolic blood pressure. Median serum creatinine concentration was lower in the angioplasty group at 3 months but was not significantly different at 12 months. Major criticisms of the trial include its relatively short follow-up period and the high degree of crossover from the medical therapy group to the angioplasty group, thus limiting the true comparison of the treatment strategies. In addition, although a 50% stenosis was used as an inclusion criterion, pressure gradients across stenotic lesions in the renal vasculature may be more predictive of the pathologic effect of renal artery stenosis than the degree of angiographic stenosis.

A smaller prior study demonstrated a significant reduction in blood pressure compared with medical therapy for bilateral renal artery stenosis but not for unilateral stenosis,[82] whereas a third study reported a decrease in the number of drugs needed to control hypertension.[83]

Recent efforts have focused on the development of risk stratification tools to identify patients who would benefit from intervention. A normal resistive index (<80) is associated with a benefit from revascularization, whereas an index greater than 80 is not associated with a benefit from revascularization.[55] Although assessment of the pressure gradient is critical in selecting appropriate patients for revascularization, the presence of a catheter in a diseased ostium can falsely elevate the gradient. Figure 74-14 shows a technique to ensure that the pressure gradient is not falsely elevated. As illustrated, when a catheter is placed across a lesion and the pressure difference is measured with the central aortic pressure, the small catheter contributes significantly to the overall gradient, which falsely elevates the true gradient as measured with a pressure wire alone. In this way, more physiologic gradients are measured and may help in revascularizing more appropriate lesions in the renal vasculature.

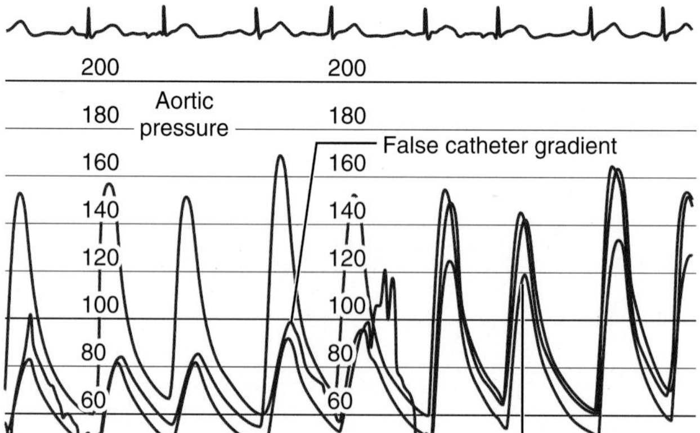

FIGURE 74-14 Pressure measurements across a renal artery lesion with use of a 4 Fr multipurpose catheter and a 0.014-inch PressureWire (St. Jude Medical, Inc., St. Paul, MN) revealing a "false" gradient and a more physiologic gradient after the catheter is removed from the lesion.

The recently completed Cardiovascular Outcomes in Renal Atherosclerotic Lesions (CORAL) trial enrolled 947 patients with atherosclerotic renal artery stenosis and either systolic hypertension while taking two or more antihypertensive drugs or chronic kidney disease. Patients were treated with either medical therapy and renal artery stenting or medical therapy alone. Median follow-up was 43 months. Participants were followed for the occurrence of adverse cardiovascular and renal events with a composite endpoint of death from cardiovascular or renal causes, myocardial infarction, stroke, hospitalization for congestive heart failure, progressive renal insufficiency, or the need for renal replacement therapy. Prior randomized studies, such as the Angioplasty and Stenting for Renal Artery Lesions (ASTRAL) trial[84] and the Stent Placement and Blood Pressure and Lipid-Lowering for the Prevention of Progression of Renal Dysfunction Caused by Atherosclerotic Ostial Stenosis of the Renal Artery (STAR) trial,[85] assessed the effect of stenting on kidney function and showed no significant difference, but both have been criticized for enrolling participants without clinically significant stenosis. Furthermore, neither of these studies was specifically designed to detect a benefit with regard to the incidence of clinical events. Nonetheless, the primary conclusion of the CORAL trial suggests that renal artery stenting did not confer a significant benefit with respect to the prevention of clinical events when added to comprehensive, multifactorial medical therapy in people with atherosclerotic renal artery stenosis and hypertension or chronic kidney disease.

Lower Extremity

Iliac Vessels

Once a lesion is identified on angiography, its functional significance and suitability for intervention can be further assessed with pressure wire measurements. A mean gradient greater than 10 mm Hg at rest or after induction of hyperemia following vasodilation (nitroglycerin or papaverine) is considered significant. The presence of symptoms, abnormal results of noninvasive studies, a significant stenosis on angiography, and a gradient of this magnitude indicate that the lesion is likely to merit revascularization.

Various revascularization techniques are available. Intravascular stenting has been associated with improved long-term patency compared with conventional balloon angioplasty,[8,86-90] and clinical outcomes after stent placement appear to be similar to long-term outcomes after vascular surgery.[32,91,92] Results from the STAG (Stents versus Angioplasty for the Treatment of Iliac Artery Occlusions) trial[93] was inconclusive regarding a difference in 1-year patency, although a reduction in perioperative complications with primary stenting versus angioplasty was observed. There are multiple stents currently approved for this location, including the Palmaz stent, Boston Scientific Express stent, and SMART stent. Recent studies continue to explore the efficacy of primary stenting for aortoiliac disease.

The advent and evolution of endovascular techniques has led to the use of an endovascular approach to revascularization in this region when necessary, as with extensive or complex aortoiliac occlusive disease. The multicenter Covered Versus Balloon Expandable Stent Trial[94] recently suggested that covered stents can provide increased freedom from stenosis compared with bare metal stents at 12 and 18 months; this remains an area that bears further attention, and it will be addressed in the proposed Dutch Iliac Stent (DISCOVER) trial: covered balloon-expandable versus uncovered balloon-expandable stents in the common iliac artery.[95]

Infrainguinal Vessels

Percutaneous interventions to the infrainguinal vessels are acutely successful in most patients, but balloon angioplasty alone remains associated with poor long-term patency.[8,96-98] Stenting of the superficial femoral artery was not associated with improved patency in two small trials,[99,100] but the introduction of nitinol stents has led to a significant reduction in restenosis and a significant improvement in walking distance compared with balloon angioplasty with provisional stent implantation in patients with infrainguinal disease.[101,102] Schillinger and coworkers[101] randomized 104 patients with severe claudication or chronic limb ischemia (Rutherford stages 3 to 5), a stenosis of 50% or more, a target lesion length of 3 cm or more, and at least one patent tibioperoneal runoff vessel to balloon angioplasty with provisional stent implantation for residual stenosis of 30% or more or the presence of flow-limiting dissection versus routine nitinol stent implantation. Average lesion length was approximately 13 cm, and 32% of patients in the angioplasty group underwent secondary stent implantation after failed angioplasty. Restenosis, defined as a stenosis of more than 50% on duplex ultrasonography, occurred in 37% of patients in the stent group and 63% of patients in the angioplasty group at 1 year. In addition, patients in the routine stent group were able to walk significantly farther on a treadmill at 6 and 12 months, and the ankle-brachial index was significantly better in the routine stent group at 12 months. The difference in restenosis rate remained significant at 2 years, although reintervention rates and clinical benefit were not significantly different (37.0% among patients undergoing balloon angioplasty and 53.8% among patients who underwent stent implantation; $P = 0.14$).[102]

These results were not reproduced in a larger trial of patients with somewhat shorter lesions (1-10 cm to be enrolled; mean lesion length, 4.5 cm).[103] Restenosis rates at 12 months were 38.6% in the angioplasty group and 31.7% in the routine stent group, a nonsignificant difference.

In general, lesions in the superficial femoral artery are best treated percutaneously if the lesion is focal and less than 10 cm.[104-106] As the lesion length increases, there is an increase in restenosis after angioplasty alone and, thus, stenting has become the default therapy for these lesion lengths.[97,104-107] Of particular interest is the use of covered stents, such as the Viabahn stent (W.L. Gore & Associates, Newark, DE). This stent, approved by the U.S. Food and Drug Administration, has a technical success rate greater than 90%. Long-term efficacy was demonstrated by Saxon and coworkers,[108] who randomized 200 patients with lesions of 13 cm or shorter to Viabahn stent implantation or angioplasty alone. At 12 months, patency rates were 65% in the stent group and 40% in the angioplasty group. Assisted primary vessel patency at 4 years has been reported to be 82%.[109] In a 3-year follow-up to the RESILIENT (Randomized Study Comparing the Edwards Self-Expanding LifeStent versus Angioplasty-alone In LEsions INvolving The SFA and/or Proximal Popliteal Artery) trial,[110,111] the authors sought to evaluate late outcomes of primary nitinol stenting for the treatment of femoropopliteal lesions up to 15 cm long. Nitinol stents were found to have superior short-term patency when compared to balloon angioplasty with 12-month freedom from target lesion revascularization at 87% for the stent group compared with 45% for the angioplasty group ($P < 0.0001$) and no difference in survival at 3 years (90% vs. 92%; $P = 0.71$) or major adverse events (75% vs. 75%; $P = 0.98$). Though Duplex ultrasound was not mandated after the first year of the study, freedom from target lesion revascularization at 3 years was significantly better in the stent group (76% vs. 42%; $P < 0.0001$), as was clinical success (63% vs. 18%; $P < 0.0001$). A recent study exploring the efficacy of primary stenting compared with percutaneous transluminal angiography with provisional stenting in popliteal artery lesions suggested equivalent 1-year patency.[111]

In addition to traditional angioplasty and stent implantation, a number of alternative devices have been used to treat infrainguinal vessels, including atherectomy devices (both directional and rotational), atheroablative devices (e.g., laser), and specialized balloon catheters such as cryoplasty and drug-coated balloons.

The atheroablative technologies include the directional atherectomy catheters. This type of intervention, which was initially designed for use in the coronary circulation, has found a resurgence in the peripheral vasculature. Recently, the SilverHawk device from FoxHollow Technologies (Redwood City, Calif.) has been used in a nonrandomized registry of 84 patients.[112] De novo lesions had an 84% patency rate at 12 months and 73% patency at 18 months. Target vessel revascularization was required in 16% of lesions at 12 months.

Excimer laser technology can be used in many different anatomic locations and scenarios, including in-stent restenosis, and it can be used for patients with complex lesions as an adjunctive agent before stent implantation.[113,114] Cryoplasty is another possible option that has had acute and short-term success in registry studies,[115] although more rigorous evaluation with randomized clinical trials in longer lesions remains to be performed.

In superficial femoral artery lesions of moderate length, the use of a paclitaxel-coated balloon can also reduce the incidence of target vessel revascularization.[116,117] With percutaneous intervention of the infrapopliteal arteries, patency is more difficult to maintain, given the small diameter of the vessels and their dynamic properties at the level of the lower extremity. Research continues with the goal of further elucidating optimal endovascular treatment in the infrainguinal vasculature based on lesion type and location, patient characteristics, and advances in endovascular technology.

REFERENCES

1. Second European Consensus: Document on chronic critical leg ischemia. *Circulation* 84:IV1–IV26, 1991.
2. Criqui MH, Langer RD, Fronek A, et al: Mortality over a period of 10 years in patients with peripheral arterial disease. *N Engl J Med* 326:381–386, 1992.
3. Pentecost MJ, Criqui MH, Dorros G, et al: Guidelines for peripheral percutaneous transluminal angioplasty of the abdominal aorta and lower extremity vessels. A statement for health professionals from a Special Writing Group of the Councils on Cardiovascular Radiology, Arteriosclerosis, Cardio-Thoracic and Vascular Surgery, Clinical Cardiology, and Epidemiology and Prevention, the American Heart Association. *J Vasc Interv Radiol* 14:S495–S515, 2003.
4. Smith GD, Shipley MJ, Rose G: Intermittent claudication, heart disease risk factors, and mortality. The Whitehall Study. *Circulation* 82:1925–1931, 1990.
5. Weitz JI, Byrne J, Clagett GP, et al: Diagnosis and treatment of chronic arterial insufficiency of the lower extremities: a critical review. *Circulation* 94:3026–3049, 1996.
6. Dormandy J, Heeck L, Vig S: The natural history of claudication: risk to life and limb. *Semin Vasc Surg* 12:123–137, 1999.
7. Dormandy J, Heeck L, Vig S: Major amputations: clinical patterns and predictors. *Semin Vasc Surg* 12:154–161, 1999.
8. Norgren L, Hiatt WR, Dormandy JA, et al: Inter-society consensus for the management of peripheral arterial disease (TASC II). *J Vasc Surg* 45(Suppl S):S5–S67, 2007.
9. Guidelines for coronary angiography. A report of the American College of Cardiology/American Heart Association Task Force on Assessment of diagnostic and therapeutic cardiovascular procedures (subcommittee on coronary angiography). *Circulation* 76:963A–977A, 1987.
10. Cohn PF, Goldberg S: Cardiac catheterization and coronary angiography. In Cohn PF, editor: *Diagnosis and therapy of coronary artery disease*, Boston, 1985, Martinus Nijhoff, p 219.
11. Grossman W: Cardiac catheterization, angiography and intervention. In Baim DS, Grossman W, editors: *Cardiac catheterization, angiography and intervention*, Philadelphia, 2000, Lippincott Williams & Wilkins, p 6.
12. Thrombolysis in the management of lower limb peripheral arterial occlusion—a consensus document. Working Party on Thrombolysis in the Management of Limb Ischemia. *Am J Cardiol* 81:207–218, 1998.
13. Baguneid M, Dodd D, Fulford P, et al: Management of acute nontraumatic upper limb ischemia. *Angiology* 50:715–720, 1999.
14. Hall TB, Matson M, Belli AM: Thrombolysis in the peripheral vascular system. *Eur Radiol* 11:439–445, 2001.
15. Kasirajan K, Gray B, Beavers FP, et al: Rheolytic thrombectomy in the management of acute and subacute limb-threatening ischemia. *J Vasc Interv Radiol* 12:413–421, 2001.
16. Korn P, Khilnani NM, Fellers JC, et al: Thrombolysis for native arterial occlusions of the lower extremities: clinical outcome and cost. *J Vasc Surg* 33:1148–1157, 2001.
17. Ouriel K, Veith FJ, Sasahara AA: A comparison of recombinant urokinase with vascular surgery as initial treatment for acute arterial occlusion of the legs. Thrombolysis or Peripheral Arterial Surgery (TOPAS) Investigators. *N Engl J Med* 338:1105–1111, 1998.
18. White CJ, Jaff MR, Haskal ZJ, et al: Indications for renal arteriography at the time of coronary arteriography: a science advisory from the American Heart Association Committee on Diagnostic and Interventional Cardiac Catheterization, Council on Clinical Cardiology, and the Councils on Cardiovascular Radiology and Intervention and on Kidney in Cardiovascular Disease. *Circulation* 114:1892–1895, 2006.
19. Azakie A, McElhinney DB, Dowd CF, et al: Percutaneous stenting for symptomatic stenosis of aberrant right subclavian artery. *J Vasc Surg* 27:756–758, 1998.
20. Chang JB, Stein TA, Liu JP, et al: Long-term results with axillo-axillary bypass grafts for symptomatic subclavian artery insufficiency. *J Vasc Surg* 25:173–178, 1997.
21. Schwend RB, Hambsch K, Baker L, et al: Carotid steal syndrome: a case study. *J Neuroimaging* 5:195–197, 1995.
22. Tan TY, Lien LM, Schminke U, et al: Hemodynamic effects of innominate artery occlusive disease on anterior cerebral artery. *J Neuroimaging* 12:59–62, 2002.
23. Scali ST, Chang CK, Pape SG, et al: Subclavian revasularization in the age of thoracic endovascular aortic repair and comparison of outcomes in patients with occlusive disease. *J Vasc Surg* 58:901–909, 2013.
24. Diethrich EB, Cozacov JC: Subclavian stent implantation to alleviate coronary steal through a patent internal mammary artery graft. *J Endovasc Surg* 2:77–80, 1995.
25. Fisher CM: A new vascular syndrome—"the subclavian steal." *N Engl J Med* 265:912, 1961.
26. Stagg SJ, 3rd, Abben RP, Chaisson GA, et al: Management of the coronary-subclavian steal syndrome with balloon angioplasty. A case report and review of the literature. *Angiology* 45:725–731, 1994.
27. Van Son JA, Aengevaeren WR, Skotnicki SH, et al: Diagnosis and management of the coronary-subclavian steal syndrome. *Eur J Cardiothorac Surg* 3:565–567, 1989.
28. Haas M, Spargo BH, Wit EJ, et al: Etiologies and outcome of acute renal insufficiency in older adults: a renal biopsy study of 259 cases. *Am J Kidney Dis* 35:433–447, 2000.
29. Kolh PH, Torchiana DF, Buckley MJ: Atheroembolization in cardiac surgery. The need for preoperative diagnosis. *J Cardiovasc Surg (Torino)* 40:77–81, 1999.
30. Vassalotti JA, Delgado FA, Whelton A: Atheroembolic renal disease. *Am J Ther* 3:544–549, 1996.
31. Braunwald E, Gorlin R, McIntosh HD, et al: Cooperative study on cardiac catheterization. Summary. *Circulation* 37:III93–III101, 1968.
32. Kadir S: Regional anatomy of the thoracic aorta. In Kadir S, editor: *Atlas of normal and variant angiographic anatomy*, Philadelphia, 1991, WB Saunders.
33. Kandarpa K, Becker GJ, Hunink MG, et al: Transcatheter interventions for the treatment of peripheral atherosclerotic lesions: part I. *J Vasc Interv Radiol* 12:683–695, 2001.
34. Brown AH: Coronary steal by internal mammary graft with subclavian stenosis. *J Thorac Cardiovasc Surg* 73:690–693, 1977.
35. Dormandy J, Heeck L, Vig S: Lower-extremity arteriosclerosis as a reflection of a systemic process: implications for concomitant coronary and carotid disease. *Semin Vasc Surg* 12:118–122, 1999.
36. Mukherjee D, Yadav JS: Carotid and cerebrovascular disease. *Cardiol Rev* 8:322–332, 2000.
37. North American Symptomatic Carotid Endarterectomy Trial Collaborators: Beneficial effect of carotid endarterectomy in symptomatic patients with high-grade carotid stenosis. *N Engl J Med* 325:445–453, 1991.
38. MRC European Carotid Surgery Trial. Interim results for symptomatic patients with severe (70-99%) or with mild (0-29%) carotid stenosis. European Carotid Surgery Trialists' Collaborative Group. *Lancet* 337:1235–1243, 1991.
39. Endarterectomy for asymptomatic carotid artery stenosis. Executive Committee for the Asymptomatic Carotid Atherosclerosis Study. *JAMA* 273:1421–1428, 1995.
40. Rosamond WD, Folsom AR, Chambless LE, et al: Stroke incidence and survival among middle-aged adults: 9-year follow-up of the Atherosclerosis Risk in Communities (ARIC) cohort. *Stroke* 30:736–743, 1999.
41. Davies KN, Humphrey PR: Do carotid bruits predict disease of the internal carotid arteries? *Postgrad Med J* 70:433–435, 1994.
42. Wolf PA, Kannel WB, Sorlie P, et al: Asymptomatic carotid bruit and risk of stroke. The Framingham study. *JAMA* 245:1442–1445, 1981.
43. Pickett CA, Jackson JL, Hemann BA, et al: Carotid bruits as a prognostic indicator of cardiovascular death and myocardial infarction: a meta-analysis. *Lancet* 371:1587–1594, 2008.
44. Allaqaband S, Tumuluri RJ, Goel AK, et al: Diagnosis and management of carotid artery disease: the role of carotid artery stenting. *Curr Probl Cardiol* 26:499–555, 2001.
45. Norris JW, Zhu CZ, Bornstein NM, et al: Vascular risks of asymptomatic carotid stenosis. *Stroke* 22:1485–1490, 1991.
46. Sacco RL: Identifying patient populations at high risk for stroke. *Neurology* 51:S27–S30, 1998.

47. Hansen KJ: Prevalence of ischemic nephropathy in the atherosclerotic population. *Am J Kidney Dis* 24:615–621, 1994.
48. Safian RD, Textor SC: Renal-artery stenosis. *N Engl J Med* 344:431–442, 2001.
49. Derkx FH, Schalekamp MA: Renal artery stenosis and hypertension. *Lancet* 344:237–239, 1994.
50. Rimmer JM, Gennari FJ: Atherosclerotic renovascular disease and progressive renal failure. *Ann Intern Med* 118:712–719, 1993.
51. Bush RL, Najibi S, MacDonald MJ, et al: Endovascular revascularization of renal artery stenosis: technical and clinical results. *J Vasc Surg* 33:1041–1049, 2001.
52. Dorros G, Jaff M, Mathiak L, et al: Four-year follow-up of Palmaz-Schatz stent revascularization as treatment for atherosclerotic renal artery stenosis. *Circulation* 98:642–647, 1998.
53. Van Jaarsveld BC, Krijnen P, Pieterman H, et al: The effect of balloon angioplasty on hypertension in atherosclerotic renal-artery stenosis. Dutch Renal Artery Stenosis Intervention Cooperative Study Group. *N Engl J Med* 342:1007–1014, 2000.
54. Harden PN, MacLeod MJ, Rodger RS, et al: Effect of renal-artery stenting on progression of renovascular renal failure. *Lancet* 349:1133–1136, 1997.
55. Radermacher J, Chavan A, Bleck J, et al: Use of Doppler ultrasonography to predict the outcome of therapy for renal-artery stenosis. *N Engl J Med* 344:410–417, 2001.
56. Watson PS, Hadjipetrou P, Cox SV, et al: Effect of renal artery stenting on renal function and size in patients with atherosclerotic renovascular disease. *Circulation* 102:1671–1677, 2000.
57. McPhail IR, Spittell PC, Weston SA, et al: Intermittent claudication: an objective office-based assessment. *J Am Coll Cardiol* 37:1381–1385, 2001.
58. de Giovanni JV: Covered stents in the treatment of aortic coarctation. *J Interv Cardiol* 14:187–190, 2001.
59. Duke C, Qureshi SA: Aortic coarctation and recoarctation: to stent or not to stent? *J Interv Cardiol* 14:283–298, 2001.
60. Garcia LA, Carrozza JP, Jr: Percutaneous revascularization of surgically corrected coarctation with graft restenosis. *J Invasive Cardiol* 14:400–403, 2002.
61. Gibbs JL: Treatment options for coarctation of the aorta. *Heart* 84:11–13, 2000.
62. Hamdan MA, Maheshwari S, Fahey JT, et al: Endovascular stents for coarctation of the aorta: initial results and intermediate-term follow-up. *J Am Coll Cardiol* 38:1518–1523, 2001.
63. Harrison DA, McLaughlin PR, Lazzam C, et al: Endovascular stents in the management of coarctation of the aorta in the adolescent and adult: one year follow up. *Heart* 85:561–566, 2001.
64. Hornung TS, Benson LN, McLaughlin PR: Interventions for aortic coarctation. *Cardiol Rev* 10:139–148, 2002.
65. Keith DS, Markey B, Schiedler M: Successful long-term stenting of an atypical descending aortic coarctation. *J Vasc Surg* 35:166–167, 2002.
66. Koerselman J, de Vries H, Jaarsma W, et al: Balloon angioplasty of coarctation of the aorta: a safe alternative for surgery in adults: immediate and mid-term results. *Catheter Cardiovasc Interv* 50:28–33, 2000.
67. Magee AG, Blauth CI, Qureshi SA: Interventional and surgical management of aortic stenosis and coarctation. *Ann Thorac Surg* 71:713–715, 2001.
68. Rao PS: Which aortic coarctations should we balloon-dilate? *Am Heart J* 117:987–989, 1989.
69. Recto MR, Elbl F, Austin E: Use of the new IntraStent for treatment of transverse arch hypoplasia/coarctation of the aorta. *Catheter Cardiovasc Interv* 53:499–503, 2001.
70. Tynan M, Finley JP, Fontes V, et al: Balloon angioplasty for the treatment of native coarctation: results of Valvuloplasty and Angioplasty of Congenital Anomalies Registry. *Am J Cardiol* 65:790–792, 1990.
71. Wholey MH, Wholey M, Mathias K, et al: Global experience in cervical carotid artery stent placement. *Catheter Cardiovasc Interv* 50:160–167, 2000.
72. Coward LJ, McCabe DJ, Ederle J, et al: Long-term outcome after angioplasty and stenting for symptomatic vertebral artery stenosis compared with medical treatment in the Carotid and Vertebral Artery Transluminal Angioplasty Study (CAVATAS): a randomized trial. *Stroke* 38:1526–1530, 2007.
73. Golledge J, Mitchell A, Greenhalgh RM, et al: Systematic comparison of the early outcome of angioplasty and endarterectomy for symptomatic carotid artery disease. *Stroke* 31:1439–1443, 2000.
74. Ramee SR, Dawson R, McKinley KL, et al: Provisional stenting for symptomatic intracranial stenosis using a multidisciplinary approach: acute results, unexpected benefit, and one-year outcome. *Catheter Cardiovasc Interv* 52:457–467, 2001.
75. Yadav JS, Roubin GS, Iyer S, et al: Elective stenting of the extracranial carotid arteries. *Circulation* 95:376–381, 1997.
76. Yadav JS, Wholey MH, Kuntz RE, et al: Protected carotid-artery stenting versus endarterectomy in high-risk patients. *N Engl J Med* 351:1493–1501, 2004.
77. Mas JL, Chatellier G, Beyssen B, et al: Endarterectomy versus stenting in patients with symptomatic severe carotid stenosis. *N Engl J Med* 355:1660–1671, 2006.
78. Gurm HS, Yadav JS, Fayad P, et al: Long-term results of carotid stenting versus endarterectomy in high-risk patients. *N Engl J Med* 358:1572–1579, 2008.
79. Ringleb PA, Allenberg J, Bruckmann H, et al: 30 day results from the SPACE trial of stent-protected angioplasty versus carotid endarterectomy in symptomatic patients: a randomised non-inferiority trial. *Lancet* 368:1239–1247, 2006.
80. Naylor AR: SPACE: not the final frontier. *Lancet* 368:1215–1216, 2006.
81. Brott TG, Hobson RW, 2nd, Howard G, et al; CREST Investigators: Stenting versus endarterectomy for treatment of carotid-artery stenosis. *N Engl J Med* 363(1):11–23, 2010.
82. Webster J, Marshall F, Abdalla M, et al: Randomised comparison of percutaneous angioplasty vs continued medical therapy for hypertensive patients with atheromatous renal artery stenosis. Scottish and Newcastle Renal Artery Stenosis Collaborative Group. *J Hum Hypertens* 12:329–335, 1998.
83. Plouin PF, Chatellier G, Darne B, et al: Blood pressure outcome of angioplasty in atherosclerotic renal artery stenosis: a randomized trial. Essai Multicentrique Medicaments vs Angioplastie (EMMA) Study Group. *Hypertension* 31:823–829, 1998.
84. The ASTRAL Investigators: Revascularization versus medical therapy for renal-artery stenosis. *N Engl J Med* 361:1953–1962, 2009.
85. Cooper CJ, Murphy TP, Cutlip DE, et al; CORAL Investigators: Stenting and medical therapy for atherosclerotic renal-artery stenosis. *N Engl J Med* 370(1):13–22, 2014.
86. Henry M, Amor M, Ethevenot G, et al: Palmaz stent placement in iliac and femoropopliteal arteries: primary and secondary patency in 310 patients with 2-4-year follow-up. *Radiology* 197:167–174, 1995.
87. Murphy TP, Webb MS, Lambiase RE, et al: Percutaneous revascularization of complex iliac artery stenoses and occlusions with use of Wallstents: three-year experience. *J Vasc Interv Radiol* 7:21–27, 1996.
88. Tetteroo E, van der Graaf Y, Bosch JL, et al: Randomised comparison of primary stent placement versus primary angioplasty followed by selective stent placement in patients with iliac-artery occlusive disease. Dutch Iliac Stent Trial Study Group. *Lancet* 351:1153–1159, 1998.
89. Vorwerk D, Bucker A, Alzen G, et al: Chronic venous occlusions in haemodialysis shunts: efficacy of percutaneous treatment. *Nephrol Dial Transplant* 10:1869–1873, 1995.
90. Wolf YG, Schatz RA, Knowles HJ, et al: Initial experience with the Palmaz stent for aortoiliac stenoses. *Ann Vasc Surg* 7:254–261, 1993.
91. Bonn J: Percutaneous vascular intervention: value of hemodynamic measurements. *Radiology* 201:18–20, 1996.
92. Tetteroo E, Haaring C, van der Graaf Y, et al: Intraarterial pressure gradients after randomized angioplasty or stenting of iliac artery lesions. Dutch Iliac Stent Trial Study Group. *Cardiovasc Intervent Radiol* 19:411–417, 1996.
93. Goode SD, Cleveland TJ, Gaines PA; STAG trial collaborators: Randomized clinical trial of stents versus angioplasty for the treatment of iliac artery occlusions (STAG trial). *Br J Surg* 100(9):1148–1153, 2013.
94. Mwipatayi BP, Thomas S, Wong J, et al: A comparison of covered vs bare expandable stents for the treatment of aortoiliac occlusive disease. *J Vasc Surg* 54:1561–1570, 2012.

95. Bekken JA, Vos JA, Aarts RA, et al: DISCOVER: Dutch Iliac Stent trial: COVERed balloon-expandable versus uncovered balloon-expandable stents in the common iliac artery: study protocol for a randomized controlled trial. *Trials* 13:215, 2012.
96. Matsi PJ, Manninen HI, Vanninen RL, et al: Femoropopliteal angioplasty in patients with claudication: primary and secondary patency in 140 limbs with 1-3-year follow-up. *Radiology* 191:727–733, 1994.
97. Murray JG, Apthorp LA, Wilkins RA: Long-segment (> or = 10 cm) femoropopliteal angioplasty: improved technical success and long-term patency. *Radiology* 195:158–162, 1995.
98. Dormandy JA, Rutherford RB: Management of peripheral arterial disease (PAD). TASC Working Group. TransAtlantic Inter-Society Consensus (TASC). *J Vasc Surg* 31:S1–S296, 2000.
99. Gray BH, Olin JW: Limitations of percutaneous transluminal angioplasty with stenting for femoropopliteal arterial occlusive disease. *Semin Vasc Surg* 10:8–16, 1997.
100. Gray BH, Sullivan TM, Childs MB, et al: High incidence of restenosis/reocclusion of stents in the percutaneous treatment of long-segment superficial femoral artery disease after suboptimal angioplasty. *J Vasc Surg* 25:74–83, 1997.
101. Schillinger M, Sabeti S, Loewe C, et al: Balloon angioplasty versus implantation of nitinol stents in the superficial femoral artery. *N Engl J Med* 354:1879–1888, 2006.
102. Schillinger M, Sabeti S, Dick P, et al: Sustained benefit at 2 years of primary femoropopliteal stenting compared with balloon angioplasty with optional stenting. *Circulation* 115:2745–2749, 2007.
103. Krankenberg H, Schluter M, Steinkamp HJ, et al: Nitinol stent implantation versus percutaneous transluminal angioplasty in superficial femoral artery lesions up to 10 cm in length: the Femoral Artery Stenting Trial (FAST). *Circulation* 116:285–292, 2007.
104. Gallino A, Mahler F, Probst P, et al: Percutaneous transluminal angioplasty of the arteries of the lower limbs: a 5 year follow-up. *Circulation* 70:619–623, 1984.
105. Johnston KW: Femoral and popliteal arteries: reanalysis of results of balloon angioplasty. *Radiology* 183:767–771, 1992.
106. Krepel VM, van Andel GJ, van Erp WF, et al: Percutaneous transluminal angioplasty of the femoropopliteal artery: initial and long-term results. *Radiology* 156:325–328, 1985.
107. Currie IC, Wakeley CJ, Cole SE, et al: Femoropopliteal angioplasty for severe limb ischaemia. *Br J Surg* 81:191–193, 1994.
108. Saxon RR, Dake MD, Volgelzang RL, et al: Randomized, multicenter study comparing expanded polytetrafluoroethylene–covered endoprosthesis placement with percutaneous transluminal angioplasty in the treatment of superficial femoral artery occlusive disease. *J Vasc Interv Radiol* 19:823–832, 2008.
109. Saxon RR, Coffman JM, Gooding JM, et al: Long-term patency and clinical outcome of the Viabahn stent-graft for femoropopliteal artery obstructions. *J Vasc Interv Radiol* 18:1341–1349, quiz 1350, 2007.
110. Laird JR1, Katzen BT, Scheinert D, et al: RESILIENT Investigators: Nitinol stent implantation versus balloon angioplasty for lesions in the superficial femoral artery and proximal popliteal artery: twelve-month results from the RESILIENT randomized trial. *Circ Cardiovasc Interv* 3(3):267–276, 2010.
111. Laird JR, Katzen BT, Scheinert D, et al: RESILIENT Investigators: nitinol stent implantation vs. balloon angioplasty for lesions in the superficial femoral and proximal popliteal arteries of patients with claudication: three-year follow-up from the RESILIENT randomized trial. *J Endovasc Ther* 19(1):1–9, 2012.
112. Zeller T, Rastan A, Sixt S, et al: Long-term results after directional atherectomy of femoro-popliteal lesions. *J Am Coll Cardiol* 48:1573–1578, 2006.
113. Laird JR, Zeller T, Gray BH, et al: Limb salvage following laser-assisted angioplasty for critical limb ischemia: results of the LACI multicenter trial. *J Endovasc Ther* 13:1–11, 2006.
114. Tan JW, Yeo KK, Laird JR: Excimer laser assisted angioplasty for complex infrainguinal peripheral artery disease: a 2008 update. *J Cardiovasc Surg (Torino)* 49:329–340, 2008.
115. Das T, McNamara T, Gray B, et al: Cryoplasty therapy for limb salvage in patients with critical limb ischemia. *J Endovasc Ther* 14:753–762, 2007.
116. Tepe G, Zeller T, Albrecht T, et al: Local delivery of paclitaxel to inhibit restenosis during angioplasty of the leg. *N Engl J Med* 358:689–699, 2008.
117. Liistro F, Porto I, Angioli P, et al: Drug-eluting balloon in peripheral intervention for below the knee angioplasty evaluation (DEBATE-BTK): a randomized trial in diabetic patients with critical limb ischemia. *Circulation* 128:615–621, 2013.

CHAPTER 75

INJURY TO THE HEART AND GREAT VESSELS

Peter I. Tsai • Matthew J. Wall, Jr. • Kenneth L. Mattox

CHAPTER OUTLINE

The heart is a vital organ, with its arch vessels encased in the chest cavity and protected by the manubrium, sternum, and rib cage. Injury to this organ can come from blunt trauma, which includes blunt cardiac injury, more commonly referred to as cardiac contusion, coronary artery injury, atrial/ventricular/valvular rupture, and aortic or arch vessel rupture. Injury can also result from penetrating trauma, with the right ventricle being most commonly injured, and ventricular septal defect being the most common intracardiac injury.

BLUNT CARDIAC INJURY

Historical Perspective

The first recorded cardiac chamber rupture and myocardial contusion were reported after autopsy findings as early as 1679 by Borch (as reported by Osborn[1]) and in 1764 by Akenside,[2] respectively. In 1868, 76 cases reported by Fischer[3] described 7 myocardial contusions and 69 traumatic ruptures. Experimental animal work and clinical autopsies by Bright and Beck[4] have demonstrated that substantially severe forces are responsible for an entire range of cardiac trauma, whereas enormous force is required to rupture the heart. It is also observed that recovery is the general rule, and rupture is the exception. In 1958, a hallmark study by Parmley and colleagues[5] of a large series of autopsy cases in the Armed Forces Institute of Pathology demonstrated that blunt traumatic heart injury had a 0.1% incidence, with the majority being isolated chamber ruptures (right then left ventricle, followed by right and left atria in decreasing order of occurrence) and some associated with combined aortic ruptures. Myocardial contusion or blunt cardiac injury, although rare, is the most common injury, whereas chamber or aortic rupture is usually fatal.

Mechanism, Pathophysiology, and Incidence

Mechanisms responsible for blunt cardiac injuries can occur from any deliverance of kinetic energy such as blast effect; direct crushing forces through the sternum or rib cage, which can also cause compression of heart against the vertebral column; and traction and torsion from deceleration forces owing to high-speed vehicular collisions and falls from great heights. A sudden rise of blood pressure from compression of the chest can injure the cardiac valves, cause a tear in the ventricular wall or septum, or result in chamber rupture.

These forces result in a continuous spectrum of cardiac injury, ranging from simple contusion to fatal cardiac chamber rupture, including *comotio cordis*, described as sudden cardiac arrest resultant from a sternal blow.[6] Myocardial contusion, characterized by patchy areas of muscle necrosis and hemorrhagic infiltrate, can also impair ventricular contraction and lead to arrhythmia.

The true incidence of blunt cardiac injury remains expectedly difficult to measure, because the autopsy cases of fatal cardiac chamber rupture do not account for the majority of the blunt trauma cases, which go on to recover.

Clinical Presentation

The rupture of a cardiac chamber, coronary artery, or major intrapericardial vein or artery is usually fatal because of acute tamponade. The few patients who survive do so only because of tears in a cavity under low pressure.[7-9] Myocardial contusion induces cardiac failure and arrhythmia that improve with time.[10] Injury to a coronary artery can lead to immediate or delayed myocardial infarction with spasm or dissection of arterial wall.[11] Valvular tears resulting in aortic or mitral insufficiency can develop into cardiac failure within a few weeks, whereas tricuspid insufficiency can appear only after several years.[12-14]

Diagnosis

Paramount to an accurate diagnosis is the awareness from the history and physical findings of pain and tenderness over the anterior chest wall (which may be indistinguishable from a classic myocardial infarction), evidence of contusion, ecchymosis, anterior rib fractures, or flail chest.[15] Many patients, however, do not exhibit characteristic symptoms.[10,16] The presence of complex arrhythmias, subtle findings of a precordial thrill, or presence of a murmur may be all that is present at exam. Cardiac injury can also be reflected with hemodynamic instability marked by refractory hypotension and elevated venous pressure (external jugular vein distention may be absent in cases of severe blood loss) in the presence of cardiogenic shock.

Electrocardiography

Serial 12-lead electrocardiography has traditionally been used to screen patients to detect conduction disturbances resulting from blunt injury; however, there is no pathognomonic finding that can reliably establish the diagnosis of blunt cardiac injury.[15] Abnormalities range from sinus tachycardia, the most commonly encountered arrhythmia, to supraventricular arrhythmias, such as atrial flutter and atrial fibrillation, ventricular tachycardia, premature ventricular contractions, ventricular fibrillation, right bundle branch block with first-degree heart block or hemiblock, third degree heart block, and T-wave or ST-segment abnormalities.[15] The presence of a normal electrocardiography in a patient who is hemodynamically stable warrants no further investigation.

Cardiac Enzymes and Troponins

The measurement of creatine phosphokinase with myocardial band has been shown to be unreliable,[10,16-18] except for more specific muscle proteins including troponin (cTnT and cTnI).[19,20] Combined abnormalities in electrocardiography and serial cTnI levels have been promising in showing increased sensitivity (62% if both positive) and specificity (100% if both negative),[21] although another study has shown otherwise.[22]

Admission electrocardiography and serial troponin levels should be obtained in patients suspected of blunt cardiac injury and followed by transthoracic echocardiography if clinically significant arrhythmias arise.

Two-Dimensional Transthoracic and Transesophageal Echocardiography

Bedside echocardiography has become an important diagnostic tool in trauma patients, detecting abnormalities in the heart (ventricular dyskinesia and valvular dysfunction), thoracic aorta, and presence of pericardial fluid.[15,23-25] Patients are selected for this modality of examination after demonstration of abnormal electrocardiography and cardiac troponins.

Transthoracic echocardiography cannot be performed in 25% to 30% patients limited by chest wall edema, fractured ribs, and flail chest, whereas transesophageal echocardiography—a more useful adjunct in elucidating periaortic hematoma and other cardiac injuries—is limited by expertise and frequent requirement of intubation, and it cannot be performed in patients with facial or cervical trauma.[23,24]

Radionuclide Scans

Technetium-99m pyrophosphate, thallium 201, single photon emission computed tomography (SPECT), and multiple gated acquisition scans (MUGA), all use the concept of radioactive substances binding to injured or infarcted sites in the myocardium. However, all have been abandoned secondary to low sensitivity and specificity in the detection of blunt cardiac injury.[15]

Spectrum of Blunt Cardiac Injury: Assessment and Management

Pericardial Injury

Blunt rupture of the pericardium can occur from a direct forceful impact to transmitted force from sudden increased intra-abdominal pressure. Left pericardial tears parallel to the phrenic nerve are most common, followed by diaphragmatic, and right and mediastinal tears.[7] The heart might eviscerate into the abdominal cavity or herniate through the pericardial sac with torsion of the great vessels. Patients who are stable are worked up and diagnosed with chest radiography, sonography, or computed tomography. Patients who are hemodynamically compromised clinically are treated with immediate surgical intervention (ER thoracotomy), at which time diagnosis is made and the heart is placed back into the pericardial sac, with closure of pericardium, with or without a Gore-Tex patch, to achieve a tension-free repair.

Valvular, Papillary Muscle, Chordae Tendinea, and Septal Injury

Rarely, valvular injuries occur, with the aortic valve being most commonly affected, followed by the mitral valve. Rapid displacement of blood secondary to crushing or compressive forces applied to the thoracic cage during ventricular diastole can lacerate cardiac valve leaflets (most common in the left coronary cusp, followed by the noncoronary cusp), papillary muscles, or chordae tendinea leading to valvular insufficiency.[5] The classic signs of valvular insufficiency (new murmur, thrill or left ventricular dysfunction with cardiogenic shock, and associated pulmonary edema) may not be immediately recognized, secondary to other concomitant life-threatening injuries. In patients in stable condition, such findings should prompt further diagnostic studies, depending on the clinical status of the patient and prompt repair or replacement as necessary. Septal rupture is also uncommon, and prompt repair is necessary if the patient is symptomatic from significant left-to-right shunt resulting in pulmonary over circulation and right heart dysfunction.

Blunt Coronary Artery Injury

Injuries of the coronary arteries are extremely rare. The proximal right coronary and, more commonly, the left anterior descending artery (because of the location relative to the sternum) become injured with direct compression of sternum to coronary vessel or stretching of the vessel secondary to cardiac torsion, leading to thrombosis or intimal disruption. The result is no different than an acute myocardial infarction. Long-term sequelae of these injuries can also lead to ventricular aneurysm and eventual rupture, ventricular failure, production of emboli, or malignant arrhythmia.[5]

Cardiac Chamber Rupture

Cardiac chamber rupture is relatively uncommon, and only a small percentage of patients survive to reach the hospital.[7,26,27] Several mechanisms for blunt cardiac rupture have been postulated,[7] including direct precordial impacts, compression of heart between sternum and vertebral body, transmission of pressure via abdomen into the venous return rupturing particularly the atria, acceleration/deceleration injuries leading to tears of the heart at the attachment sites to the great vessels, blast effects, and concussive blows thought to be fatal secondary to the production of malignant arrhythmias. Patients usually have persistent hypotension with evidence of pericardial tamponade. Diagnosis of widened mediastinum on chest radiograph or evidence of pericardial fluid from sonographic examination requires prompt intervention in the form of a subxyphoid window. For patients with cardiopulmonary arrest, emergency department (ED) thoracotomy may be the only chance, although the survival rate is dismal.

Myocardial Contusion

The terms *myocardial contusion* and *concussion* should be eliminated in favor of terminology that more precisely describes the injury.[28]

- Blunt chest injury with electrocardiographic abnormality
- Blunt chest injury with free wall cardiac rupture
- Blunt chest injury with cardiac valve tear
- Blunt chest injury with septal defect
- Blunt chest injury with abnormal cardiac enzymes

We recommend that asymptomatic patients with anterior chest wall injuries not be admitted to the surgical intensive care unit for continuous electrocardiographic monitoring and serial determination of CPK-MB levels or be subjected to further cardiac imaging.

Conclusion

When blunt cardiac injury is suggested secondary to a good history and physical examination, further diagnostic testing with electrocardiographic monitoring and serial enzyme measurements should follow. Sonographic examination can elucidate the presence of pericardial fluid or cardiac or valvular dysfunction that might require prompt surgical intervention.

PENETRATING CARDIAC INJURY

Historical Perspective

In the past, cardiac injury has always resulted in death, as described in the death of Sarpedon from an impalement of a lance to the heart in *The Iliad*.[29]

In 1761, Morgagni[30] described the compressive effects of blood on the heart. Larrey[31,32] was credited for pioneering the technique of pericardial window. Duval[33] first described the median sternotomy incision, whereas Spangaro[34] first described the left anterolateral thoracotomy incision in 1906. In 1926, Beck described the Triad physiology of cardiac tamponade, and later described the repair technique of placing mattress sutures under the coronary vessels to spare ligation.[35,36]

In 1946, Harken[37] described the removal of foreign bodies adjacent to the heart and great vessels. Beal[38-41] first described ED thoracotomy and, along with Cooley,[40] reported the potential benefits for cardiopulmonary bypass in the management of selected intracardiac injuries. Mattox[42-44] further refined and championed ED thoracotomy and cardiorrhaphy, including emergency cardiopulmonary bypass by surgeons.

Incidence

Penetrating cardiac injuries are uncommon and are usually seen only in busy urban trauma centers. The true incidence is difficult to ascertain, as the numbers fluctuate with influence of violent crimes involving firearms or penetrating objects. In 1989, Mattox[45] reported on a 30-year experience at Ben Taub Hospital in Houston, Texas, of 539 cardiac injuries. Asensio[46,47] reported a total of 165 cardiac injuries within a 3-year period at LAC/USC Medical Center in Los Angeles, California. Other major trauma centers reported significantly fewer injuries,[48] which again indicates the rarity.

Etiology

In the civilian arena, the majority of penetrating cardiac injuries results from gunshot wounds and stab wounds, with shotgun and impalement injuries accounting for a small percentage.

In the military arena, most soldiers do not survive the high-velocity automatic rifles encountered in battle. The majority of these patients have sustained injuries from fragments of grenades or shrapnel. Dominguez[49] described such injuries over a 6-month period in a small series in Baghdad, Iraq.

Clinical Presentation

Most cardiac injuries related to stab wounds are logically based on the trajectory of the insult. This is not so with gunshot wounds, which can injure the heart from precordial and extra-precordial entrance sites.[50] Hirshberg[51] described 26% associated cardiac injuries in 82 patients presenting with combined thoracoabdominal injuries, whereas Asensio and colleagues[52] reported 44% incidence of associated penetrating cardiac injuries in his series of 73 patients who sustained thoracoabdominal injuries.

Frank penetrating injuries to the cardiac chambers can lead to acute cardiac tamponade and death, or, similarly, hemorrhage through the lacerated pericardium into the hemithorax, with death as well. Patients that survive such injuries with intact pericardium to prevent fatal exsanguinating hemorrhage, allowing them to reach the trauma center alive, have varying degrees of hemodynamic instability[46,47] secondary to pericardial tamponade. Interestingly, the Beck triad or Kussmaul sign is present in only 10% of patients[50] with pericardial tamponade.

Moreno and colleagues,[53] in a retrospective study of 100 patients with penetrating cardiac injuries, reported higher survival (77% vs. 11%) in patients with pericardial tamponade, and that right-side chamber injuries confer a higher survival of 79% versus 28% for left-side chamber injuries. Clarke and colleagues,[54] in a prospective review of 1862 patients over a 3-year period, demonstrated that penetrating thoracic trauma has a high mortality rate of 30% for stab wounds and 52% for gunshot wounds.

Diagnosis

Penetrating injuries, whether by stab wounds or gunshot wounds, should be highly suggestive of potential cardiac injuries. Hemodynamically stable patients still require routine chest radiography, and a widened mediastinum should elicit caution for further workup. Sonography can determine the presence of pericardial fluid, which is supported by a physical examination that might detect the Beck triad or Kussmaul sign. Evidence of direct trajectory, where the heart is in the path, should require preparation for emergent bedside anterolateral thoracotomy should the patient acutely decompensate clinically.

Subxyphoid Pericardial Window

The reliability of this technique has been proved valuable in ascertaining penetrating cardiac injury.[55,56] In addition, a transdiaphragmatic pericardial window[57] has been effectively described in cases of patients sustaining combined thoracoabdominal injuries and cardiac injury needing to be investigated. This technique is also valuable when two-dimensional echocardiography (applied in focused abdominal sonography in trauma) is not available.

Two-Dimensional Echocardiography

Echocardiography has become the gold standard in diagnosis and evaluation of patients with penetrating thoracic injury. It is fast, painless, reproducible, and easily repeated.[50,57,58] The procedure has 96% accuracy and 97% specificity.[59] Furthermore, it can be used to delineate intramyocardial foreign bodies versus missiles located within the cardiac chamber.[60,61]

Management

In patients with penetrating cardiac injury, the majority would have a fatal outcome, no matter the prehospital intervention. In the select group that is still stable enough for transport to the trauma center, time is of utmost importance. This prehospital course is marked by certain surrogate parameters for either improved or dire prognosis.

Under no circumstances should emergency medical personnel delay transport by inserting intravenous lines; this should occur during transport. Concomitant notification of the trauma center to activate the trauma team is also of paramount importance.[50] Gervin and Fisher[62] demonstrated a survival advantage if transport to the trauma center was within 9 minutes, whereas all patients with transport time greater than 25 minutes died. Mattox and Feliciano[63] found no survivors in 100 patients who received external cardiac compression for more than 3 minutes in the prehospital period. Lorenz and colleagues[64] noted better survival if patients had systolic blood pressures of 60 mm Hg or greater in the field and upon arrival in the ED. Durham and colleagues[65] linked prehospital intubation to better tolerance and successful prolongation with prehospital cardiopulmonary resuscitation of less than 5 minutes.

Upon arrival to the ED, the trauma team should be ready to perform advanced trauma life support protocol.[66] Patients are usually hemodynamically stable at presentation, allowing for expedited yet detailed workup. Another group will be unstable but respond to fluid resuscitation, allowing time to proceed to the operating room for life-saving surgery. The last group will go into cardiopulmonary arrest requiring ED thoracotomy.[46,47,50,67] ED thoracotomy, if performed under strict indications for cardiac injuries, has been shown to improve survival rate as much as 31%.[68] However, patients sustaining multiple cardiac or great vessel gunshot wounds were nearly unsalvageable with ED thoracotomy.[69]

Techniques for Cardiac Injury Repair

Incisions

Median sternotomy, as well as the anterolateral thoracotomy, are the two main incisions of choice. The former is acceptable in patients who are treated for penetrating low anterior chest injuries and who arrive in some degree of hemodynamic instability, but are stable enough for sonographic and chest radiography workup for occult cardiac injuries. The latter is the incision of choice in the management of patients who arrive in extremis. This incision is also used in the ED for emergent resuscitative purposes.[46,47,50,67,70] The anterolateral thoracotomy can also be extended into the right chest to provide for optimal exposure of the mediastinum and both hemithoracic cavities as necessary.

Adjunct Maneuvers

Exposure of the heart to repair posterior injuries can be accomplished a number of ways. The first step is to place the patient in acute Trendelenburg position, which will optimize the following described strategies for further exposure of the posterior side of the heart. Pledgeted sutures can be placed on the apex of the heart with the sutures cut long, to retract the apex slowly and superiorly to gain access to the posterior injury. A Satinsky clamp can also be used on the right ventricular angle to achieve the same exposure.[71] Sequential placement of folded wet towels behind the heart will gradually lift the heart without causing it to go into arrhythmia and will provide exposure to the posterior injury as well. Stabilizing devices can also be used to provide exposure and steady placement of repair stitches on laceration injuries to the heart without causing further tearing.

Total inflow occlusion of the heart can be performed by placing clamps on the intrapericardial location to isolate and repair injuries at the level of atriocaval junction. The heart will frequently fibrillate, requiring paddle defibrillation and pharmacologic intervention.[50,70]

Repair of Atrial Injuries

Right atrial injuries can usually be controlled with a Satinsky clamp followed by repair using 4-0 nonpledgeted polypropylene monofilament sutures. The atrium is thin walled and easily torn; therefore, caution and gentle traction aid in repair without further tearing.

Repair of Ventricular Injuries

Blast injuries resulting from gunshots, unlike a stab incision to the ventricle, can make the epicardium and myocardium more friable and unforgiving with standard suture repair. Coupled with high-pressured bleeding, particularly from a left ventricle injury and tachycardia, the repair can be challenging; 2-0, 3-0, or 4-0 polypropylene with pledgeted sutures should be used and placed in a horizontal mattress fashion. Commercial brand fibrin sealant can be used to reinforce the suture line if necessary.

Coronary Artery Injuries

Direct coronary artery injury can be challenging to repair. Proximal injuries require bypass, especially if there is gross evidence of cardiac ventricular dysfunction. Distal coronary artery injuries, particularly the distal third of the vessel being injured or lacerated, might not require bypass if the heart remains without ventricular dysfunction and tolerates ligation.

Pericoronary artery injuries to the heart with significant bleeding can be managed with horizontal mattress sutures underneath the coronary vessel for safe repair, taking care not to narrow or occlude the coronary artery in the process.[50,67,72]

Complex and Combined Injuries

Complex and combined injuries can be defined as penetrating cardiac injury in addition to associated thoracic, thoracic-vascular, neck, abdominal, abdominal-vascular, or peripheral vascular injuries. Priority should be given to treatment of injury with the greatest risk of blood loss or being life-threatening.[50,67,73-75]

Wall and colleagues[76] described complex cardiac injuries as those beyond lacerations of the myocardium. These injuries often include concomitant coronary artery injuries, cardiac valvular injuries, intracardiac fistulas, and ventricular false aneurysms and coronary sinus injuries. These injuries can be addressed by the cardiac surgeon once the other life-threatening injuries are temporized and addressed.

Conclusion

Penetrating cardiac injury should prompt a comprehensive workup, with a sonographic examination being useful to diagnose the presence of pericardial fluid. Workup can be more extensive in a hemodynamically stable patient with computed tomography (CT) studies. Anterolateral thoracotomy can be used in the emergent setting to cross-clamp the descending aorta and to perform necessary cardiac repairs. Median sternotomy can be used in a patient in stable condition with identified cardiac injuries repaired.

THORACIC AORTA AND ARCH VESSEL INJURIES

Mechanisms and Types of Injury

Penetrating trauma to the thoracic aorta or its arch vessels can lead to immediate exsanguination or a pattern of injury, much like blunt trauma to the vessels, which can include pseudoaneurysm, partial transection with resultant intimal flap, intimal dissection, thrombosis, and propagation.

Blunt trauma is more interesting from the standpoint that different forces can create injury to the thoracic aorta and its arch vessels. Traction and deceleration forces are classic mechanisms of injury to the thoracic vessels. Vertical deceleration can acutely strain the ascending aorta and innominate artery, as the heart is being displaced caudally and into the left pleural cavity by its natural lay in the mediastinum.[77,78] Horizontal deceleration acutely strains the aortic isthmus,[77] whereas sudden extension of the neck or traction at the shoulder will stretch and strain the arch vessels to produce a spectrum of injuries to the vessels including intimal tear, disruption of the media, and complete rupture of the arterial wall.[77,78] These injuries may again lead to intimal dissection, thrombosis, and propagation or development of pseudoaneurysm.

Natural History

Vessel injuries that involve mural hematoma or limited intimal flap have a benign course and frequently resolve with time.[79] However, pseudoaneurysms, including small ones, have an insidious course; they tend to expand, compress surrounding structures, and fistulize to surrounding organs, with eventual rupture.[78,79]

Arch vessel injuries from penetrating or blunt trauma with partial transection bleed and are contained by the local tissues.[80,81] Avulsions of the arch vessel at the takeoff from the arch can bleed into the pericardial or pleural cavity. Acute occlusion of the subclavian artery rarely leads to limb ischemia because of the rich collateral network; however, acute occlusion of the common carotid artery can result in brain ischemia.[82,83]

Free rupture of the thoracic aorta by penetrating or blunt trauma leads to immediate death in 75% to 90% of cases. Of the few who survive with containment of pseudoaneurysm by the parietal pleura, statistically 8% to 13% will rupture within the first hour of admission, 30% will rupture within 24 hours, and 50% will rupture within 1 week.[84,85]

Diagnosis

A good history and physical examination will capture many of the injuries of the thoracic vessels. A high-speed head-on collision, fall from great height, ejection from a vehicle, death of another person in the same motor vehicle crash, presence of a seatbelt sign—all should alert one to the possibility of deceleration injury to the thoracic vessels. Penetrating trauma to the base of the neck and chest cavity will lead to the suggestion of injury to the vessels from its trajectory. Gunshot wounds should lead one to suspect any type of injury, which is possible from the ricochet of the bullet on entrance into the chest cavity.

Clinical presentation of arch vessel injury can include cervical or supraclavicular hematoma, bruit, or diminished peripheral pulse.[80] An aortic isthmus injury can produce decreased blood pressure in the left arm, although this occurs in only 5% of patients.[86,87] Brachial plexus injury is usually associated with subclavian artery injury as well.[81,82] Coma or hemistroke can occur with common carotid injury.[80,82,84]

Radiographic studies should begin with chest radiography, which in the presence of an injury would typically show a widened mediastinum, blunting of the aortic-knob, and enlargement of paratracheal stripe.[86] Helical CT can detect arterial lesions and has excellent accuracy.[88] The gold standard is aortic angiography, which provides imaging of the entire thoracic aorta and arch vessels, but this takes time and requires a patient in relatively stable condition.[87] Transesophageal echocardiography can evaluate the aortic isthmus effectively, but it is less effective in evaluating the distal ascending aorta or arch vessels secondary to interference of the respiratory tract.[89] There has been a shift in widespread use of CT angiography, and almost complete elimination of aortography and transesophageal echocardiography over the last 10 years.[90]

Assessment and Management

With a normal chest radiograph, the risk of thoracic aortic injury is low; however, if given the history of great fall or deceleration accident, a CT scan would be appropriate. Normal CT results almost certainly rule out injury to the aorta and obviate the need for further investigation. If the mediastinum is enlarged, then the diagnosis of thoracic vessel injury should be determined by angiography because both CT and transesophageal echocardiography can miss certain vascular injuries, especially the arch vessels.[89]

Medical treatment especially aimed at treatment of suspected or identified aortic tear should address prevention of hypertension and pain. Short-acting β-blockers reduce blood pressure, the force of arterial upstroke, and heart rate, with good effect on reducing stress (anti-impulse) on the aortic wall.[84,91]

Surgery is indicated for repair of most diagnosed thoracic artery lesions.[87,92] Arch vessels can usually be repaired without circulatory support or arterial shunting. Repair of the aortic isthmus can be done with or without partial circulatory support.[85] Repair of the ascending aorta and arch usually necessitates full circulatory support with extracorporeal circulation, and possibly with hypothermic circulatory arrest.[93]

Ascending Aorta and Arch Vessel Injuries

Injuries to ascending aorta or to arch vessels are best repaired by the cardiac surgeon for definitive repair. Isolated ascending aortic injury can be repaired with cardiopulmonary bypass and graft interposition to replace the area of injury. Care should be taken to address intimal dissection—the dissection plane should be obliterated with a combination of felt pledgets and bioglue.

Arch injury can also require circulatory arrest with isolated right subclavian artery (advantage of antegrade cerebral perfusion) or femoral artery cannulation with femoral–atrial venous cannulation bypass to repair the injury with interposition graft successfully.

Descending Thoracic Aortic Injuries

The approach is optimized with a left thoracotomy incision. Identification of the left subclavian artery, left recurrent laryngeal nerve, and left common carotid artery is prudent to allow for safe proximal aortic control, as the aortic clamp is placed between the left common carotid artery and left subclavian artery, avoiding injury to the recurrent laryngeal nerve. Distal aortic control requires a clamp to be placed distal to the area of injury.

Left heart bypass or clamp-and-sew technique can be used to repair the injury, usually with an interposition graft versus primary repair of the injured descending aorta; this carries a significant risk of spinal cord ischemic injury as well.

Recent improvements in technology have allowed the placement of an aortic endograft stent across the injury, which significantly decreases the risk of spinal cord ischemia.[94] However, long-term follow-up needs to be performed and outcome assessed in the otherwise young, healthy population with descending aortic injury that would have undergone an open repair.

Innominate and Arch Vessel Injuries

The approach to innominate or arch vessel injury is via median sternotomy with or without cardiopulmonary bypass. Debranching repair can be performed with partial aortic cross-clamp to isolate the base of the arch vessel, which can then be divided, with the base oversewn. The distal arch vessel can then be sewn to an interposition graft that is reattached to the ascending aorta with partial aortic cross-clamp as well.

Conclusion

Blunt or penetrating injuries to the chest may involve the thoracic aorta and great vessels. Successful repair is determined by complete proximal and distal control of the injury with or without cardiopulmonary bypass. Interposition graft is usually used, although primary repair is equally optimal if the tissue reapproximates well. Intimal dissection should be checked during repair and then treated. Aortic endograft stent repair is gaining notice, and it should be part of the armamentarium of the surgeon.

REFERENCES

1. Osborn LR: Findings in 262 fatal accidents. *Lancet* 2:277, 1943.
2. Akenside M: An account of a blow upon the heart and its effects. *Philosophical Transact* 53:353, 1764.
3. Fischer G: Die wunden des herzens und des herzbeutels. *Arch Klin Chir* 9:571, 1868.
4. Bright EF, Beck CS: Nonpenetrating wound of the heart: a clinical and experimental study. *Am Heart J* 10:293, 1935.
5. Parmley LF, Manion WC, Mattingly TW: Nonpenetrating traumatic injury of the heart. *Circulation* 18:371, 1958.
6. Asensio JA, Garcia-Nunez LM, Petrone P: *Trauma of the heart*, ed 6, Trauma, 2008, McGraw-Hill Publishing, chapter 28.
7. Fulda G, Brathwaite CEM, Rodriguez A, et al: Blunt traumatic rupture of the heart and pericardium: a ten-year experience(1979-1989). *J Trauma* 31:167–173, 1991.
8. Kato K, Kushimoto S, Mashiko K, et al: Blunt traumatic rupture of the heart: an experience in Tokyo. *J Trauma* 36:859–864, 1994.
9. Baumgartel ED: Cardiac rupture from blunt trauma with atrial septal defect. *Arch Surg* 127:347–348, 1992.
10. Baxter BT, Moore EE, Moore FA, et al: A plea for sensible management of myocardial contusion. *Am J Surg* 158:557–562, 1989.
11. Neiman J, Hui WKK: Posteromedial papillary muscle rupture as a result of right coronary artery occlusion after blunt chest injury. *Am Heart J* 123:1694–1699, 1992.
12. Pretre R, Faidutti B: Surgical management of aortic valve injury following nonpenetrating trauma. *Ann Thorac Surg* 56:1426–1431, 1993.
13. Shammas NW, Kaul S, Stuhlmuller JE, et al: Traumatic mitral insufficiency complicating blunt chest trauma treated medically: a case report and review. *Crit Care Med* 20:1064–1068, 1992.
14. van Son JAM, Danielson GK, Schaff HV, et al: Traumatic tricuspid valve insufficiency: experience in thirteen patients. *J Thorac Cardiovasc Surg* 108:893–898, 1994.
15. Newman PG, Feliciano DV: Blunt cardiac injury. *New Horizons* 7:26, 1999.
16. Cachecho R, Grindlinger GA, Lee VW: The clinical significance of myocardial contusion. *J Trauma* 33:68–73, 1992.
17. Biffl WL, Moore FA, Moore EE, et al: Cardiac enzymes are irrelevant in the patient with suspected myocardial contusion. *Am J Surg* 169:523, 1994.
18. Frazee RC, Mucha P, Jr, Farnell MB, et al: Objective evaluation of blunt cardiac trauma. *J Trauma* 226:510, 1986.
19. Katus HA, Remppis A, Neumann FJ, et al: Diagnostic efficiency of troponin T measurements in acute myocardial infarction. *Circulation* 83:902, 1991.
20. Adams JE, III, Davilla-Roman VG, Bassey PQ, et al: Improved detection of cardiac contusion with cardiac troponin I. *Am Heart J* 131:308, 1996.
21. Salim A, Velmahos GC, Jindal A, et al: Clinically significant blunt cardiac trauma. Role of serum troponin levels combined with electrocardiographic findings. *J Trauma* 50:237, 2001.
22. Bertinchant JP, Polge A, Mohty D, et al: Evaluation of incidence, clinical significance and prognostic value of circulating cardiac troponin I and T elevation in hemodynamically stable patients with suspected myocardial contusion after blunt chest trauma. *J Trauma* 48:924, 2000.
23. Karalis DG, Victor MF, Davis GA, et al: The role of echocardiography in blunt chest trauma: a transthoracic and transesophageal echocardiographic study. *J Trauma* 36:53–58, 1994.
24. Catoire P, Orliaguet G, Liu N, et al: Systematic transesophageal echocardiography for detection of mediastinal lesions in patients with multiple injuries. *J Trauma* 38:96–102, 1995.
25. Smith MD, Cassidy JM, Souther S, et al: transesophageal echocardiography in the diagnosis of traumatic rupture of the aorta. *N Eng J Med* 332:356–362, 1995.
26. Perchinsky MJ, Long WB, Hill JG: Blunt cardiac rupture. The Emanuel trauma center experience. *Arch Surg* 130:852, 1995.
27. Turk EE, Tsokos M: Blunt cardiac trauma caused by fatal falls from height: an autopsy-based assessment of the injury pattern. *J Trauma* 57:301, 2004.
28. Mattox KL, Flint LM, Carrico CT, et al: Blunt cardiac injury. *J Trauma* 33:649–650, 1992.
29. Homer: *The Iliad, vol XIII, line 442*, New York, 1992, McMillan & Co, p 259. Translated by Lang, Leaf and Myers.
30. Morgagni JB: De sedibus et causes morborum. *Lipsiae sumptibus Leopoldii vossiim* 1829. As quoted by Beck CS. Wounds of the heart: the technique of suture. *Arch Surg* 13:205, 1926.
31. Larrey DJ: Memoires de chirurgie militaire. *BullSci Med* 6:284, 1819.
32. Larrey DJ: Memoires de chirurgie militaire. *Chirurgie* 2:303, 1829.
33. Duval P: Le incision median thoraco-laparotomie. *Bull Mem Soc Chir Paris* 33:15, 1907. As quoted by Ballana C. Bradshaw Lecture: The surgery of the heart. *Lancet* CXCVIII:73, 1920.
34. Spangaro S: Sulla tecnica da seguirenegli interventi chirurgici er ferrite del cuore e su di un nuovo processo di toracotomia. *Clin Chir* 14:227, 1906. As quoted by Beck CS. Wounds of the heart: the technique of suture. *Arch Surg* 13:205, 1926.
35. Beck CS: Wounds of the heart: the technique of suture. *Arch Surg* 13:205, 1926.
36. Beck CS: Further observations on stab wounds of the heart. *Ann Surg* 115:698, 1942.
37. Harken DE: Foreign bodies in, and in relation to the thoracic blood vessels and heart. *Surg Gynecol Obstet* 14:117, 1946.

38. Beall AC, Dietrich EB, Crawford HW: Surgical management of penetrating cardiac injuries. *Am J Surg* 112:686, 1966.
39. Beall AC, Gasior RM, Bricker DL: Gunshot wounds of the heart. Changing patterns of surgical management. *Ann Thorac Surg* 11:523, 1971.
40. Beall AC, Morris GC, Cooley DA: Temporary cardiopulmonary bypass in the management of penetrating wounds of the heart. *Surgery* 52:330, 1962.
41. Beall AC, Oschner JL, Morris GC, et al: Penetrating wounds of the heart. *J Trauma* 1:195, 1961.
42. Mattox KL, Espada R, Beall AC, et al: Performing thoracotomy in the emergency center. *J Am Coll Emerg Phys* 3:13, 1974.
43. Mattox KL, Beall AC, Jordan GL, et al: Cardiorrhaphy in the emergency center. *J Am Coll Emerg Phys* 68:886, 1974.
44. Mattox KL, Limacher MC, Feliciano DR, et al: Cardiac evaluation following heart injury. *J Trauma* 25:758, 1985.
45. Mattox KL, Feliciano DV, Buurch J, et al: Five thousand seven hundred sixty cardiovascular injuries in 4459 patients. Epidemiologic evolution 1958 to 1987. *Ann Surg* 210:698, 1989.
46. Asensio JA, Murray J, Demetriades D, et al: Penetrating cardiac injuries; Prospective one year preliminary report: an analysis of variables predicting outcome. *J Am Coll Surg* 186:24, 1998.
47. Asensio JA, Berne JD, Demetriades D, et al: One hundred and five penetrating cardiac injuries. A two year prospective evaluation. *J Trauma* 44:1073, 1998.
48. Pereira BM, Nogueira VB, Calderan TR, et al: Penetrating cardiac trauma: 20-y experience from a university teaching hospital. *J Surg Res* 183:792, 2013.
49. Dominguez F, Beekley AC, Huffer LL, et al: High-velocity penetrating thoracic trauma with suspected cardiac involvement in a combat support hospital. *Gen Thorac Cardiovasc Surg* 59:547, 2011.
50. Asensio JA, Stewart BM, Murray JA, et al: Penetrating cardiac injuries. *Surg Clin North Am* 76:685, 1996.
51. Hirshberg A, Wall MJ, Allen MK, et al: Double jeopardy: thoracoabdominal injuries requiring surgical intervention in both chest and abdomen. *J Trauma* 39:225, 1995.
52. Asensio JA, Arroyo H, Jr, Veloz W, et al: Penetrating thoracoabdominal injuries: ongoing dilemma—which cavity and when? *World J Surg* 26:539, 2002.
53. Moreno C, Moore EE, Majure JA, et al: Pericardial tamponade, a critical determinant for survival following penetrating cardiac wounds. *J Trauma* 26:821, 1986.
54. Clarke DL, Quazi MA, Reddy K, et al: Emergency operation for penetrating thoracic trauma in a metropolitan surgical service in South Africa. *J Thorac and Cardiovasc Surg* 142:563, 2011.
55. Duncan A, Scalea TM, Sclafani S, et al: Evaluation of occult cardiac injuries using subxyphoid pericardial window. *J Trauma* 29:955, 1989.
56. Andrade-Alegre R, Mon L: Subxyphoid pericardial window in the diagnosis of penetrating cardiac trauma. *Ann Thorac Surg* 58:1139, 1994.
57. Garrison RN, Richardson JD, Fry DE: Diagnostic transdiaphragmatic pericardiotomy in thoracoabdominal trauma. *J Trauma* 22:147, 1982.
58. Rozycki GS, Feliciano DV, Oschner MG, et al: The role of surgeon-performed ultrasound in patients with possible penetrating cardiac wounds: a prospective multi-center study. *J Trauma* 45:190, 1998.
59. Jimenez E, Martin M, Krukenkamp I, et al: Subxyphoid pericardiotomy versus echocardiography; a prospective evaluation of the diagnosis of occult penetrating cardiac injury. *Surgery* 108:676, 1990.
60. Hassett A, Moran J, Sabiston DC, et al: Utility of echocardiography in the management of patients with penetrating missile wounds of the heart. *Am J Cardiol* 7:1151, 1987.
61. Robison RJ, Brown JW, Caldwell R, et al: Management of asymptomatic intracardiac missiles using echocardiography. *J Trauma* 28:1402, 1988.
62. Gervin AS, Fisher RP: The importance of prompt transport in salvage of patients with penetrating heart wounds. *J Trauma* 22:443, 1982.
63. Mattox KL, Feliciano DV: Role of external cardiac compression in truncal trauma. *J Trauma* 22:934, 1982.
64. Lorenz PH, Steinmetz B, Lieberman J, et al: Emergency thoracotomy: survival correlates with physiologic status. *J Trauma* 32:780, 1992.
65. Durham LA, Richardson RJ, Wall MJ, et al: Emergency center thoracotomy: impact of prehospital resuscitation. *J Trauma* 32:775, 1992.
66. Advanced Trauma Life Support Manual: Chicago, Illinois, 2008, Committee on Trauma-American College of Surgeons, ed 8.
67. Asensio JA, Petrone P, Costa D, et al: An evidenced-based critical appraisal of emergency department thoracotomy. *Evid Based Surg* 1:11, 2003.
68. Asensio JA, Wall MJ, Jr, Minei J, et al: Working group, ad hoc subcommittee on outcomes. American College of Surgeons-committee on Trauma. Practice management guidelines for emergency department thoracotomy. *J Am Coll Surg* 13:303, 2001.
69. Seamon MJ, Shiroff AM, Franco M, et al: Emergency department thoracotomy for penetrating injuries of the heart and great vessels: an appraisal of 283 consecutive cases from two urban trauma centers. *J Trauma* 67:1250, 2009.
70. Asensio JA, Hanpeter D, Demetriades D, et al: *The futility of the liberal utilization of emergency department thoracotomy. A prospective study. Proceedings of the American Association for the Surgery of Trauma, 58th Annual Meeting*, Baltimore, MD, 1998, p 210.
71. Grabowski MW, Buckman RF, Goldberg A, et al: Clamp control of the right ventricle angle to facilitate exposure and repair of cardiac wounds. *Am J Surg* 170:399, 1995.
72. Espada R, Wisennand HH, Mattox KL, et al: Surgical management of penetrating injuries to the coronary arteries. *Surgery* 78:755–760, 1975.
73. Thourani VH, Feliciano DV, Cooper WA, et al: Penetrating cardiac trauma at an urban trauma center: a 22-year perspective. *Am Surg* 65:811, 1999.
74. Gonzalez RP, Luterman A: Reviewer summary of "Rhee PM, Foy H, Kaufman C, et al: Penetrating cardiac injuries: a population based study. J Trauma 45:366, 1998." *Curr Surg* 58:173, 2001.
75. Gonzalez RP, Luterman A: Reviewer summary of "Thourani VH, Feliciano DV, Cooper WA, et al: Penetrating cardiac trauma at an urban center; a 22-year perspective. Am Surg 65:811, 1999." *Curr Surg* 58:177, 2001.
76. Wall MJ, Jr, Mattox KL, Chen C, et al: Acute management of complex cardiac injuries. *J Trauma* 42:905, 1997.
77. Williams JS, Graff JA, Uku JM, et al: Aortic injury in vehicular trauma. *Ann Thorac Surg* 57:726–730, 1994.
78. Pretre R, LaHarpe R, Cheretakis K, et al: Blunt injury to the ascending aorta: three patterns of presentation. *Surgery* 119:603–610, 1996.
79. Frykberg ER, Crump JM, Dennis JW, et al: Nonoperative observation of clinically occult arterial injuries: a prospective evaluation. *Surgery* 109:85–96, 1991.
80. Castagna J, Nelson RJ: Blunt injuries to branches of the aortic arch. *J Thorac Cardiovas Surg* 69:521–532, 1975.
81. Johnson SF, Johnson SB, Strodel WE, et al: Brachial plexus injury: association with subclavian and axillary vascular trauma. *J Trauma* 31:1546–1550, 1991.
82. George SM, Jr, Croce MA, Fabian TC, et al: Cervicothoracic arterial injuries: recommendations for diagnosis and management. *World J Surg* 15:134–140, 1991.
83. Cogbill TH, Moore EE, Meissner M, et al: The spectrum of blunt injury to the carotid artery: a multi-center perspective. *J Trauma* 37:473–479, 1994.
84. Pate JW, Fabian TC, Walker W: Traumatic rupture of the aortic isthmus: an emergency? *World J Surg* 19:119–126, 1995.
85. von Oppell UO, Dunne TT, De Groot MK, et al: Traumatic aortic rupture: twenty-year meta-analysis of mortality and risk of paraplegia. *Ann Thorac Surg* 58:585–593, 1994.
86. Kram HB, Wohlmuth DA, Appel PL, et al: Clinical and radiographic indications for aortography in blunt chest trauma. *J Vasc Surg* 6:168–176, 1987.
87. Cowley RA, Turney SZ, Hakins JR, et al: Rupture of thoracic aorta caused by blunt trauma: a fifteen-year experience. *J Thorac Cardiovasc Surg* 100:652–660, 1990.
88. Gavant ML, Menke PG, Fabian T, et al: Blunt traumatic aortic rupture; detection with helical CT of the chest. *Radiology* 197:125–133, 1995.
89. Smith DC, Bansal RC: Transesophageal echocardiography in the diagnosis of traumatic rupture of the aorta. *N Eng J Med* 333:457–458, 1995.

90. Demetriades D, Velmahos GC, Scalea TM, et al: Diagnosis and treatment of blunt thoracic aortic injuries: changing perspectives. *J Trauma* 64:1415–1418, 2008.
91. Maggisano R, Nathens A, Alexandrova NA, et al: Traumatic rupture of the thoracic aorta: should one always operate immediately? *Ann Vasc Surg* 9:44–52, 1995.
92. Mattox KL: Approaches to trauma involving the major vessels of the thorax. *Surg Clin North Am* 69:77–91, 1989.
93. Peltz M, Douglass DS, Meyer DM, et al: Hypothermic circulatory arrest for repair of injuries of the thoracic aorta and great vessels. *Interact Cardiovasc Thorac Surg* 5:560–565, 2006.
94. Martinelli O, Malaj A, Gossetti B, et al: Outcomes in the emergency endovascular repair of blunt thoracic aortic injuries. *J Vasc Surg* 58:832, 2013.

PART F

SURGICAL MANAGEMENT OF VALVULAR HEART DISEASE

PART OUTLINE

CHAPTER 76

VALVE REPLACEMENT THERAPY: HISTORY, VALVE TYPES, AND OPTIONS

Afshin Ehsan • Gus J. Vlahakes

CHAPTER OUTLINE

THE IDEAL VALVE

Many acceptable substitutes exist today for the replacement of diseased human heart valves. The ideal valvular prosthesis as described by Harken[1] remains the gold standard of cardiac surgery. According to Harken this valve would be durable, with a longevity approaching that of a native valve, thrombogenicity would not be a factor, and therefore no need for supplemental anticoagulation would exist. In addition, this valve would have no inherent gradient, thus allowing unimpeded outflow, and could be implanted with ease while being readily available. Lastly, the valve could grow commensurate with that of the recipient. While the technology of valve prostheses has evolved considerably over the past six decades, this lofty goal has yet to be met.

HISTORY

The first human heart valve operation was a digital valvotomy of a stenotic aortic valve performed by Tuffier in 1914. Cutler, Souttar, Brock, Swan, and Harken refined valvotomies and commissurotomies in the ensuing decades; however, the limited success of these techniques brought to light the need for an effective means of replacing the entire valve. The first step in the evolution of this technology came in 1950 when Hufnagel developed a ball valve that he placed in the descending thoracic aorta of a patient with severe aortic insufficiency.[2] In 1956, Murray implanted an aortic homograft in the descending thoracic aorta of a patient with severe aortic insufficiency.[3] The introduction of cardiopulmonary bypass opened the era of implanting valve prostheses in their native positions. In 1960, Braunwald and Harken successfully replaced the mitral and aortic valves using valves made of polyurethane.[4] In 1961 Albert Starr, a surgeon, and Lowell Edwards, an engineer, developed a caged ball valve that resulted in acceptable long-term survival.[5] Despite their success, the high profile of caged ball valves made implantation in patients with small ventricles and small aortic roots difficult. These valves also had inherently high gradients along with less favorable thromboembolic profiles, making them less desirable as new prostheses were introduced. Edwards Lifesciences (Irvine, CA) discontinued production of the Starr-Edwards valve in 2007.

The next generation of valve prosthesis used a tilting disc that would pivot into an open and close position according to the flow of blood across the valve. Wada was the first to introduce these tilting disc valves in 1966.[6] The Lillehei-Kaster valve, introduced in 1967, was a hingeless valve with a freely rotating pivoting disc retained by struts. Björk, working with Shiley Laboratories, developed a similar version of a hingeless pivoting disc valve in 1969. Although the hemodynamic profile was improved relative to the caged ball valves, these early pivoting valves were subject to occasional thrombosis. The 60-degree convexoconcave Björk-Shiley valve was prone to catastrophic structural failure secondary to fracture of its welded struts, allowing escape of the occluder disc.[7]

Seeking to improve on the durability and thrombogenicity problems of these early pivoting disc valves, Hall, Woien, Kaster, and the Medtronic Corporation (Minneapolis, MN) introduced the Medtronic-Hall valve in

1977. The valve housing was constructed from one piece of titanium alloy with no introduced welds or bends. The round central disc was made from tungsten-impregnated graphite with a pyrolytic carbon coating, and it had a central hole that allowed the disc to be retained by a curved central guide strut that was part of the housing. Valve washing was improved by a relatively larger minor orifice and a disc that lifted out of the housing and rotated with opening. It had a moderately high profile in the open position and a low transvalvular gradient. Occluder impingement was possible because its position at the equator of the valve housing made it susceptible to obstruction from retained valve elements, sutures cut too long, or pannus. Loss of structural integrity, however, was never reported. The valve could be rotated after implantation to achieve the desired orientation. Several studies reported a low incidence of valve-related morbidity and mortality.[8,9] Svennevig and colleagues reported a 25-year experience of 816 patients that underwent an aortic valve replacement using the Medtronic-Hall valve.[10] Linearized rates of thrombotic complications, warfarin-related bleeding, and endocarditis were 1.5%, 0.7%, and 0.16% per patient-year, respectively. Valve thrombosis was seen in only four patients. Seventy-nine percent of the patients were in New York Heart Association classes I or II. Despite these outcomes, Medtronic discontinued manufacturing the valve in September of 2009, removing the last of the tilting disc prosthesis available for clinical use.

The next step in the evolution of valve prostheses came in 1977 when St. Jude Medical (Minneapolis, MN) introduced a bileaflet mechanical valve.[11] The design has undergone several refinements since its introduction. Its advantage over the caged ball valves or the tilting disc valves are its greater effective orifice area and therefore improved gradients, along with reduced thrombogenicity.

In light of the thrombogenic potential of mechanical valves and the need for lifelong anticoagulation, development of tissue-based valves was undertaken in parallel with mechanical prosthesis. In 1962, Ross reported the use of aortic homografts for aortic valve replacement (AVR) and subsequently developed the Ross procedure, which uses a pulmonary autograft for replacement of the aortic valve.[12] In 1969, Carpentier and Hancock developed the first porcine xenografts,[13] and Ionescu developed the first glutaraldehyde-preserved bovine pericardial valve in 1971.[14] Limited long-term durability secondary to leaflet calcification and subsequent valve failure plagued the early generation of bioprostheses. Significant progress has been made in improving the durability of these valves through improved fixation strategies and overall valve design. State-of-the-art anticalcification methods are now being used in an effort to improve valve longevity. Given the inherent gradients with stented bioprostheses, stentless xenografts were introduced in 1986, and they have remained an effective option for a tissue-based prosthesis.[15]

MORBIDITY AND MORTALITY GUIDELINES FOR VALVE OPERATIONS

Clinical studies are crucial for determining outcomes after cardiac valve operations and precise definitions of outcomes are critical in comparing valve prostheses. To address this need, the councils of the Society of Thoracic Surgeons (STS) and the American Association of Thoracic Surgery (AATS) formulated the Ad Hoc Liaison Committee for Standardizing Definitions of Prosthetic Heart Valve Morbidity. The initial report of this committee was issued in 1988[16] with an update in 1996.[17] The report strictly defines types of morbidity and mortality that can occur after valvular surgery. An understanding of these definitions is crucial for interpreting studies dealing with valvular prostheses.

The guidelines distinguish two types of mortality: hospital mortality and 30-day mortality. *Hospital mortality* refers to death occurring at any time before discharge during a patient's initial hospitalization. Thirty-day mortality, also referred to as *operative mortality*, is death that occurs at any time or place within 30 days of the procedure. There are several precise definitions of valve-related morbidity. *Structural valve deterioration* (SVD) refers to "any change in function of an operated valve resulting from an intrinsic abnormality of the valve that causes stenosis or regurgitation."[17] It includes "changes intrinsic to the valve, such as wear, fracture, poppet escape, calcification, leaflet tear, stent creep and suture line disruption of components ... of an operated valve."[17] Thrombotic or infectious causes of valve dysfunction are not included.

Nonstructural dysfunction includes nonthrombotic and noninfectious causes of valvular stenosis or regurgitation that are not intrinsic to the valve itself. "Examples ... include entrapment by pannus, tissue, or suture; paravalvular leak; inappropriate sizing or positioning; residual leak or obstruction from valve implantation or repair; and clinically important hemolytic anemia."[17] Morbid events are often reported as the composite linearized rate, or the number of events divided by the number of patient-years of follow-up (events/patient-years). The composite linearized rate for nonstructural dysfunction of the commonly available mechanical valves is 0.2 to 0.8 (events/patient-years) for the aortic position and 0.3 to 1.4 (events/patient-years) for the mitral position.[9] Valve thrombosis is defined as thrombus in or about the valve that is not associated with infection and that interferes with valve function or obstructs blood flow through the valve. The composite linearized rate of thrombosis of mechanical valves is 0 to 0.2 (events/patient-years) in the aortic position and 0.4 to 0.8 (events/patient-years) for the mitral position.[9]

Embolism refers to any embolic event not associated with endocarditis that occurs after the immediate perioperative period and after the emergence from anesthesia. Embolic events are further delineated into neurologic events and peripheral embolic events. The composite linearized rate of thromboembolism ranges from 1.4 to 2.5 (events/patient-years) for the aortic position and 1.8 to 3.6 (events/patient-years) for the mitral position.[9]

A bleeding event refers to any clinically significant bleed requiring hospitalization or transfusion or causing death. A patient does not have to be taking an anticoagulant to sustain a bleeding event. Composite linearized rates vary from 0.8 to 2.5 (events/patient-years) for the aortic position and 1.2 to 2.2 (events/patient-years) for the mitral position.[9]

Endocarditis involving an operated valve is designated operated valvular endocarditis. "Morbidity associated with active infection, such as valve-thrombosis, thrombotic embolus, bleeding event, or paravalvular leak, is included under this category and is not included in other categories of morbidity."[17] Composite linearized rates for prosthetic valve endocarditis range from 0.4 to 0.7 (events/patient-years) for both the aortic and mitral positions.

Consequences of morbid events are also defined by the guidelines. A reoperation is any operation on "a previously operated valve."[17] The composite linearized rate for reoperation ranges from 0.3 to 1.8 (events/patient-years) for the aortic position and 0.6 to 1.6 (events/patient-years) for the mitral position.[9]

Valve-related mortality is any death after a valve operation caused by a morbid event that is not related to progressive heart failure in patients with functioning valves. Unexplained deaths are just that, and they should be listed as such. Cardiac deaths include valve-related deaths, sudden deaths, and non–valve-related cardiac deaths. *Total deaths* refer to any and all deaths after a valve operation. *Permanent valve-related impairment* refers to any "permanent neurologic or functions deficit" caused by a morbid event.[17]

PROSTHETIC HEART VALVES

The following section lists and describes prosthetic heart valves available worldwide. The valves are grouped according to their structural type (i.e., mechanical vs. bioprosthetic), manufacturer, and design specifications. The order in which they appear in no way delineates a preference by the authors. For a summary of clinically available valves, implantation positions, and sizes please see Tables 76-1 and 76-2.

Mechanical Valves

Bileaflet Prostheses

Medtronic. The Medtronic Open Pivot Mechanical Heart Valve (Fig. 76-1*A*) is a bileaflet valve that was originally developed and owned by ATS Medical, Inc. (Minneapolis, MN). The valve is made of a solid pyrolytic carbon orifice and a titanium strengthening band that provides it with added durability. Its unique design eliminates shallow recesses in the hinge area where clots may form. These design features lead to a continuous gentle flow of blood across the valve, resulting in low levels of clotting while helping to prevent damage to blood cells. Furthermore, with the Open Pivot design, the unimpeded flow of blood provides for a continuous passive washing of the valve. Within the Open Pivot Series, there are three subtypes, each geared toward different potential clinical needs. The AP360 is an aortic valve prosthesis with a supra-annular flanged cuff configuration designed for added flexibility and conformability, and it is available in sizes from 16 to 26 mm. The AP valve has a supra-annular compact cuff configuration for ease of suturing and overall conformability. The valve can be placed in either the

TABLE 76-1 **Mechanical Valve Choices**

Valve Type	Manufacturer	Name	Position	Available Sizes (mm)
Bileaflet	Medtronic	Open Pivot AP360	Aortic	16-26
		Open Pivot AP	Aortic	16-26
			Mitral	16-26
		Open Pivot Standard	Aortic	19-31
			Mitral	25-33
	St. Jude Medical	Masters	Aortic	19-31
			Mitral	19-33
		Masters HP	Aortic	17-27
			Mitral	17-27
		Regent	Aortic	19-27
	Sorin Group	Bicarbon Fitline*	Aortic	19-31
			Mitral	19-33
		Bicarbon Overline*	Aortic	16-24
		Bicarbon Slimline*	Aortic	17-27
		Carbomedics Top Hat	Aortic	19-27
		Carbomedics OptiForm	Mitral	23-33
		Carbomedics Reduced	Aortic	19-29
		Carbomedics Standard	Aortic	19-31
			Mitral	21-33
		Carbomedics Standard Pediatrics	Aortic	16-18
			Mitral	16, 18, 21
		Carbomedics Orbis*	Aortic	19-31
			Mitral	21-33
	On-X	Standard Sewing Ring	Aortic	19-27/29
			Mitral	23-31/33
		Conform-X Sewing Ring	Aortic	19-27/29
			Mitral	25/33
		Anatomic Sewing Ring	Aortic	19-27/29

*Available only outside the United States.

TABLE 76-2 **Bioprosthetic Valve Choices**

Valve Type	Manufacturer	Name	Position	Available Sizes (mm)
Stented porcine	Medtronic	Hancock II	Aortic	21-29
			Mitral	25-33
		Hancock II Ultra	Aortic	21-29
		Mosaic	Aortic	19-29
			Mitral	25-33
		Mosaic Ultra	Aortic	19-29
	Edwards Lifesciences	Carpentier-Edwards Standard Porcine (2625 and 6625)	Aortic	19-31
			Mitral	25-33
		Carpentier-Edwards S.A.V. Porcine (2650)	Aortic	19-31*
			Mitral†	25-33
		Carpentier-Edwards Duraflex Low Pressure Porcine‡ (6625LP)	Mitral	27-35
		Carpentier-Edwards Duraflex Low Pressure Porcine with Extended Sewing Ring‡ (6625-ESR-LP)	Mitral	27-35
	St. Jude Medical	Epic	Aortic	21-29
			Mitral	25-33
		Epic Supra	Aortic	19-27
		Biocor	Aortic	21-29
			Mitral	25-33
		Biocor Supra	Aortic	19-27
Stented bovine pericardial	Edwards Lifesciences	Carpentier-Edwards PERIMOUNT (2700 and 2700TFX)	Aortic	19-29
		Carpentier-Edwards PERIMOUNT RSR (2800 and 2800TFX)	Aortic	19-29
		Carpentier-Edwards PERIMOUNT Plus (6900P and 6900PTFX)	Mitral	25-33
		Carpentier-Edwards PERIMOUNT Magna (3000 and 3000TFX)	Aortic	19-29
		Carpentier-Edwards PERIMOUNT Magna Ease (3300TFX, 7300TFX)	Aortic	19-29
			Mitral	25-33
	Sorin Group	Mitroflow	Aortic	19-29
		Soprano Armonia†	Aortic	19-33
		Pericarbon More†	Mitral	19-33
	St. Jude Medical	Trifecta	Aortic	19-29
Stentless	Medtronic	Freestyle	Aortic	19-29
		3f	Aortic	19-29
	Sorin Group	Pericarbon Freedom†	Aortic	15-29
		Freedom Solo†	Aortic	19-27
	Edwards Lifesciences	Prima Plus	Aortic	21-29
Sutureless bovine pericardial	Medtronic	3f Enable†	Aortic	19-29
	Sorin Group	Perceval S†	Aortic	S, M, L, XL
	Edwards Lifesciences	Edwards Intuity†	Aortic	19-27
Transcatheter	Edwards Lifesciences	Sapien	Aortic	23, 26
		Sapien XT	Aortic	23, 26, 29
	Medtronic	CoreValve	Aortic	23, 26, 29, 31
	St. Jude Medical	Portico†	Aortic	25

*Sizes 19, 29, and 31 available only outside the United States.
†Available only outside the United States.
‡Available only in the United States.
RSR, Reduced sewing ring.

aortic or mitral position and is also available in sizes from 16 to 26 mm. The Standard valve is designed for intra-annular placement and has a generous and compliant cuff. The valve is available in sizes from 19 to 31 mm in the aortic position and 25 to 33 mm in the mitral position. All the Open Pivot valves are rotatable in situ.

Several studies have demonstrated good hemodynamics and an overall low complication rate with these valves.[18-21] Bernet and colleagues[22] reported their outcomes for a series of 1161 patients that received either the SJM valve or the Open Pivot Mechanical Valve. Cumulative survival and freedom from valve-related mortality at 10 years for the SJM valve and Open Pivot Mechanical Valve were 66% ± 3% versus 68% ± 5% (P = 0.84) and 96% ± 1% versus 97% ± 1% (P = 0.36), respectively. No structural valve failure was encountered for both valve types. The linearized rates for valve-related adverse events for the SJM valve and Open Pivot Mechanical Valve were, respectively: thromboembolism, 0.9% and 1.1% per patient-year; major bleeding requiring transfusion, 0.3% and 0.5% per patient-year; prosthetic endocarditis, 0.03% and 0.1% per patient-year; paravalvular leak, 0.1% and 0.6% per patient-year.[22]

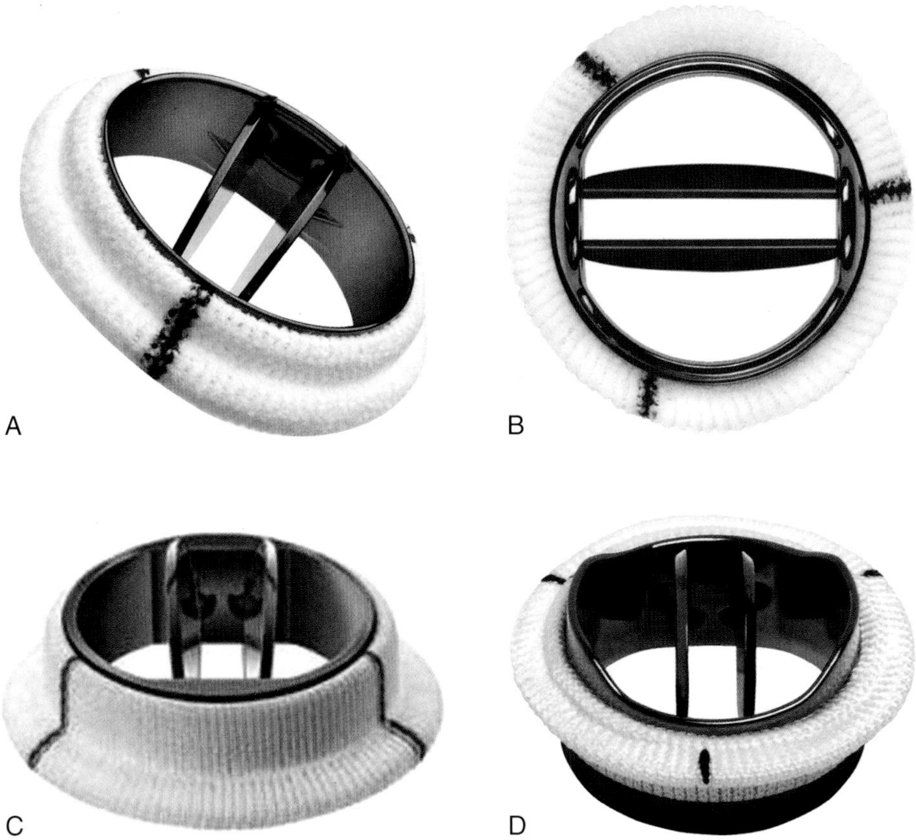

FIGURE 76-1 ■ Mechanical bileaflet valves. **A,** Open Pivot Mechanical Valve. **B,** The Regent mechanical valve. **C,** The Top Hat mechanical valve. **D,** The On-X Heart Valve. (**A,** Courtesy Medtronic, Inc., Minneapolis, MN. **B,** Courtesy St. Jude Medical, Inc., Minneapolis, MN. **C,** Courtesy Sorin Group, Inc., Milan, Italy. **D,** Courtesy On-X Life Technologies, Inc., Austin, TX.)

St. Jude Medical. The St. Jude Medical (SJM) Standard valve prosthesis was approved by the U.S. Food and Drug Administration (FDA) in 1977, and more than 2.3 million valves have been implanted worldwide. The SJM leaflets and ring orifice are constructed with pyrolytic carbon and are highly durable. The 85-degree leaflet opening angle provides improved laminar flow and reduces turbulence. The Hemodynamic Plus (HP) series was developed to address the inherent gradient in smaller valves and the potential for patient–prosthesis mismatch. With the small annulus in mind, the sewing cuff was reduced and redesigned to allow supra-annular placement of the valve, leading to an increased effective orifice area (EOA). The Masters Series was later introduced, providing the ability to rotate the valve to the desired orientation after implantation. The Standard and HP valves are offered only within the Masters Series. The available Standard valve sizes are 19 to 31 mm for the aortic position and 19 to 33 mm for the mitral position, whereas the available HP valve sizes are 17 to 27 mm for both the aortic and mitral positions. The Regent valve (see Fig. 76-1*B*) is the most recent evolution of the bileaflet design, developed to improve hemodynamic performance. In addition to a supra-annular cuff, the carbon rim was shifted to the supra-annular position. As with the Masters Series it is fully rotatable as well. This redesign allows the valve to achieve an increased EOA and an up to 84% orifice-to-annulus ratio. The Regent valve is available only for the aortic position and for sizes ranging from 19 to 27 mm.

Several reports have documented the outcomes of the various valve series produced by SJM.[22-27] Tool and colleagues[28] reported their 25-year experience in which 946 valve recipients were followed prospectively at 12-month intervals from 1979 to 2007. The series included implants using all SJM designs, with the original Standard valve being the most widely used. Among aortic valve recipients, 25-year freedom from reoperation, thromboembolism, bleeding, and endocarditis was 90% ± 2%, 69% ± 5%, 67% ± 3%, and 92% ± 3%, respectively. Among mitral valve recipients, 25-year freedom from reoperation, thromboembolism, bleeding, and endocarditis was 81% ± 10%, 52% ± 8%, 64% ± 6%, and 97% ± 1%, respectively. Freedom from valve-related mortality was 66% ± 8% and 87 ± 3% for aortic and mitral valve replacement (MVR), respectively.[28]

Head-to-head comparisons between the standard and HP designs have also been reported. Vitale and colleagues[29] reported results from the Multicenter Study Group for the SJM HP aortic valve prosthesis. This prospective randomized study included 140 patients with 21- and 23-mm–annulus diameters and who received either the SJM Standard valve or the HP valve. Postoperatively and at 6 months, echocardiographic hemodynamic variables such as ejection fraction, cardiac output, peak gradient, mean gradient, EOA, indexed EOA (iEOA), and performance index were calculated. Decreased peak and mean gradients and increased EOA, iEOA, and performance indexes were found for the HP valve. The authors concluded that use of the HP valve allows implantation of smaller prostheses without patient–prosthesis mismatch (PPM) and with avoidance of the additional morbidity associated with root enlargement procedures.[29] Ismeno and colleagues[30] similarly reported their results comparing the 19-mm standard and HP valve in the aortic position after 5 years. Those who received the HP valve had statistically better hemodynamics with lower peak and mean gradients and larger EOAs. There was no difference, however, in terms of 5-year survival, late complications, or left ventricular mass reduction between the two groups.[30]

The Regent valve has also demonstrated good in vivo hemodynamics and clinical outcomes. Bach and colleagues[31] reported the results of a multicenter study from North America and Europe of 361 patients that underwent aortic valve replacement using the Regent valve. The mean gradient at 6 months was 9.7 ± 5.3 mm Hg for the 19-mm valve, with the larger valves having progressively lower gradients. The iEOA was equal to or greater than 1.0 cm^2/m^2 for all valve sizes and left ventricular mass index decreased significantly between early postoperative (165.9 ± 57.1 g/m^2) and 6-month follow-up (137.9 ± 41.0 g/m^2; $P < 0.0001$).[31]

Sorin Group. The Sorin Group (Milan, Italy) manufactures two mechanical valve series: the Bicarbon Product Line, developed internally by Sorin, and the CarboMedics Product Line, acquired through the purchase of Sulzer CarboMedics. Within each series there are multiple subtypes geared toward a variety of clinical needs. As a whole, the mechanical valves in their catalog are bileaflet. For Bicarbon, the leaflets are constructed from pyrolytic carbon deposited on a graphite substrate and a housing made of titanium alloy treated with a proprietary Carbofilm coating for enhanced hemo-biocompatibility. For the Carbomedics valve the leaflets are constructed from pyrolytic carbon deposited on a graphite substrate, like those of the Bicarbon valve. The housing of the Carbomedics valve is fabricated from nonsubstrated pure pyrolytic carbon reinforced with a titanium reinforcing ring.

The Bicarbon series features the Fitline valve, which is designed for intra-annular implantation and is available for both aortic and mitral valve replacement. It will fit annular sizes of 19 to 31 mm for the aortic position and 19 to 33 mm for the mitral position. The Bicarbon Overline maintains the same design as the Fitline while improving hemodynamics through its supra-annular seating and 100% orifice-to-annulus ratio. These design features make the valve suitable for small annuli and create the potential benefit of decreasing the need for annulus enlargement. The Overline valve is available only for the aortic position and for 16- to 24-mm sizes. The Bicarbon Slimline is designed for partial supra-annular seating and therefore improved hemodynamics, while maintaining the same design features as the Fitline. The Slimline valve is available only for the aortic position and for sizes from 17 to 27 mm. All the Bicarbon valves are rotatable in situ and are available only outside the United States.

The CarboMedics mechanical valve series has six different valve designs within its portfolio. The Top Hat valve (see Fig. 76-1*C*) is designed for supra-annular implantation in the aortic position. By virtue of the design, the valve has no ventricular protrusions and leaves no valve components in the annulus. In turn, this design allows for improved seating in a smaller annulus with the advantage of reducing the need for a root enlargement along with a potential 100% orifice to annulus match. The Top Hat is available for sizes ranging from 19 to 27 mm. The OptiForm valve has a symmetrical cuff design that allows the valve to be placed in a supra-annular, intra-annular or subannular position simply by varying suture entry and exit sites. This valve is available for the mitral position only and for sizes from 23 to 33 mm. The Reduced Series valve is an intra-annular valve and was designed primarily for a smaller annulus and root size. The small external diameter and the smaller, pliable cork-shaped sewing cuff allows for improved seating and once again provides the potential advantage of reducing the need for root enlargement. This valve is available for the aortic position only and for sizes from 19 to 29 mm. The Standard valve offers a generous sewing cuff and is available for the aortic and mitral position. Its low-profile pivot design reduces the risk of coronary obstruction for aortic valve replacements and limits protrusion into the atrium for mitral valve replacements, thus reducing potential thrombus formation. The valve is available in sizes from 19 to 31 mm in the aortic position and 21 to 33 mm in the mitral position. The Standard Pediatric valve was designed for small adults or pediatric patients and is available for both the aortic and mitral position. The placement of the aortic valve can be supra- or intra-annular, and the valve available in sizes from 16 to 18 mm. The mitral valve is available in 16 and 18 mm for either supra- or intra-annular placement, while a 21-mm valve is designed for intra-annular placement only. The Orbis valve, available only outside the United States, has a multipurpose cuff design that allows for a variety of implantation techniques. This valve is offered for both aortic and mitral valve replacement and will fit sizes from 19- to 31-mm in the aortic position and 21- to 33-mm in the mitral position. All CarboMedics valves are rotatable in situ.

A number of reports have been published demonstrating good clinical outcomes using the Bicarbon and CarboMedics Series.[32,33] The specific types of Bicarbon or CarboMedics valves used, however, are not detailed in these reports. Azarnoush and colleagues[34] reported the 15-year clinical outcomes of the Sorin Bicarbon prosthesis from a multicenter European study where 1704 patients received aortic valve replacement, mitral valve replacement, or both. Actuarial freedom from valve-related deaths at 15 years was 76.4%, and actuarial freedom from thromboembolism, hemorrhage, and endocarditis at 15 years was 88.8%, 77.5%, and 96.8%, respectively. No cases of structural failure were observed.[34] Bouchard and colleagues[35] reported their 20-year experience with 3297 patients who received a CarboMedics valve as an aortic valve replacement or mitral valve replacement. At 20 years, freedom from valve-related mortality for AVR and MVR was 78.3% and 74.6%, respectively. Freedom from thromboembolic events, reoperation, and bleeding were 91.6%, 89.2%, and 89.5% for AVR and 88.5%, 80.3%, and 88% for MVR, respectively. Freedom from endocarditis was 97.3% for both AVR and MVR.[35] In a direct comparison, Bryan and colleagues[24] reported the 10-year follow-up of their prospective randomized trial where 485 patients received either the CarboMedics valve or the SJM mechanical valve in either the aortic position, mitral position or both. Freedom at 10 years from valve-related mortality was 95.0% in the CarboMedics group and 93.0% in the SJM group. Linearized rates per patient-year were 1.1% in the CarboMedics group and 0.8% in the SJM group for thromboembolism; 2.3% in the CarboMedics group and 3.2% in the SJM group for bleeding events; and 0.72% in the CarboMedics group and 0.47% in the SJM group for nonstructural valve dysfunction.[24]

On-X Life Technologies. The On-X Heart Valve (On-X Life Technologies, Austin, TX; see Fig. 75-1*D*) is a bileaflet valve constructed completely of pyrolytic carbon. The manufacturer claims that the lack of silicon doping in the valve's carbon construction potentially decreases its thrombogenicity. Its design includes a tall, flared inlet that increases the orifice area and decreases the ability of retained valve tissue to interfere with opening and closing. In addition, the stasis-free pivot design allows the valve to wash itself, and the 90-degree leaflet opening provides improved laminar flow and reduced turbulence. The On-X Heart Valve is available for both aortic and mitral valve replacement. There are three different sewing rings available, each catered to a particular clinical setting. The valve construct within the three sewing rings is the same. The Standard ring is available in sizes from 19 to 27/29 mm in the aortic position and 23 to 31/33 mm in the mitral position. The Conform X model provides a more flexible sewing ring and is available in sizes from 19 to 27/29 mm in the aortic position, whereas for the mitral position it offers one size that is intended to fit an annular size ranging from 25 to 33 mm. The Anatomic sewing ring is designed to fit the contours of the aortic valve annulus and is available in sizes ranging from 19 to 27/29 mm.

Under FDA investigational device exemption, the Prospective Randomized On-X Anticoagulation Clinical Trial (PROACT) has been testing the safety of less aggressive anticoagulation than recommended by the American College of Cardiology and American Heart Association guidelines after implantation of the On-X valve. In the first limb of the PROACT, Puskas and colleagues[36] reported their results of 375 patients with elevated risk factors for thromboembolism who underwent an aortic valve replacement. While receiving 81 mg of aspirin daily, patients received either low-dose warfarin with a target international normalized ratio (INR) of 1.5 to 2 or standard warfarin dosing targeting an INR of 2 to 3. The mean INR was 2.50 ± 0.63 for the control group and 1.89 ± 0.49 for the low dose group ($P < 0.0001$). The low-dose group experienced significantly lower major (1.48% vs. 3.26% per patient-year; $P = 0.047$) and minor (1.32% vs. 3.41% per patient-year; $P = 0.021$) bleeding rates. The incidence of stroke, transient ischemic attack, total neurologic events, and all-cause mortality were similar between the two groups.[36] Enrollment for the low-risk aortic and mitral valve replacement arm of the PROACT was completed in 2013.

Bioprosthetic Valves

The inherent clinical benefit of bioprosthetic valves lies with the patient's ability to avoid life-long anticoagulation. Long-term durability, however, remains the Achilles heel of these valves. During the years since the first valve replacement with a porcine xenograft was reported by Binet and colleagues,[37] tissue fixation methods have concentrated on improving durability. First-generation bioprosthetic valves were treated with high-pressure (60 to 80 mm Hg) glutaraldehyde fixation; however, it soon became evident that this process led to calcification of the xenograft tissue.[13] The pathophysiology of calcification is not well understood, but it is believed to be related partly to the affinity of calcium for aldehyde groups that are generated by glutaraldehyde along with the affinity of calcium for collagen in the extracellular matrix of the cells exposed to glutaraldehyde.[38] Damage caused by shear stress–induced turbulence is also a contributing factor leading to calcification.[39] Amino oleic acid treatment of tissue valves has been shown to prevent calcium from binding to collagen.[40] Low-pressure and zero-pressure glutaraldehyde fixations have been shown to maintain a more natural collagen alignment and are currently part of the strategies used for bioprosthetic valves. More recently, valve manufacturers have developed proprietary anticalcification strategies for bioprosthetic valves; however, the true efficacy of these treatments has yet to be determined.

Stented Porcine Bioprostheses

Medtronic. The Hancock II is a porcine bioprosthesis that has a record for safety and durability greater than 25 years. The valve is available in sizes ranging from 21 to 29 mm in the aortic position and 25 to 33 mm in the mitral position. The Hancock II Ultra features a reduced sewing cuff designed specifically for supra-annular implantation in a small aortic root, and it is available in sizes ranging from 21 to 29 mm. The valves are treated with sodium dodecyl sulfate (T6), which removes phospholipids in an effort to reduce calcification. A modified fixation process minimizes the septal muscle shelf, thus leading to a larger orifice area and subsequent better hemodynamics. The Cinch Implant System pulls the stent posts centrally and therefore serves as an automated deflection system to assist with suture tying; it further facilitates aortic valve insertion, particularly through a tight sinotubular space, and helps to prevent suture "looping" around stent posts for mitral valve replacement. Several reports have demonstrated good long-term outcomes with the Hancock II.[41,42] Valfre and colleagues[43] reported their experience of 517 patients who received the valve in the aortic or mitral positions. Late freedom from reoperation was 85.5% and 79.3% at 15 and 20 years, respectively, in the AVR population, whereas in the MVR population it was 73.3% and 52.8%, respectively.[43]

The Mosaic valve (Fig. 76-2*A*) is the next generation of porcine bioprosthesis developed by Medtronic. The valve undergoes zero-pressure glutaraldehyde fixation to maintain collagen crimp morphology and leaflet flexibility. The valve also undergoes anticalcification treatment with alpha-amino oleic acid in an effort to reduce leaflet calcification. It has a low-profile semiflexible stent, and its porcine root is predilated in an attempt to maximize valve orifice area. The valve is available in sizes ranging from 19 to 29 mm in the aortic position and 25 to 33 mm in the mitral position. The Mosaic Ultra has a reduced scalloped sewing cuff that conforms to the aortic annulus for complete supra-annular placement and is available in sizes from 19 to 29 mm. The Cinch Implant System is also available for the Mosaic and Mosaic Ultra. Once again multiple groups have reported good durability and safety using this valve.[44-47] Twelve-year data on 1029 patients receiving either an AVR or MVR was reported by Jamieson and colleagues.[46] Freedoms from valve-related mortality were 87.1% ± 3.1% for AVR and 82.5% ± 7.7% for MVR, whereas freedoms from reoperation were 84.0% ± 3.3% for AVR and 82.5% ± 7.5% for MVR. Lastly, freedoms from structural valve deterioration by explant reoperation at 12 years for AVR were 93.3% ± 2.6% for patients at least 60 years old and 75.9% ± 9.3% for patients younger than 60 years. The 15-year compendium of the same cohort published by Medtronic demonstrates continued durability and good clinical outcomes.

Edwards Lifesciences. The Carpentier-Edwards standard porcine valve (see Fig. 76-2*B*) is a stented bioprosthesis that was introduced in 1975. The leaflets are fixed with glutaraldehyde at moderate pressure (60 mm Hg) and mounted on a flexible cobalt-chromium alloy stent. The septal muscle shelf is sewn onto the stent to prevent obstruction of the valve inlet orifice. In addition, the leaflets receive the proprietary XenoLogiX treatment, which is designed to reduce calcification by extracting up to 95% of leaflet membrane phospholipids. The valve is available for both the aortic (model 2625) and mitral (model 6625) positions, in sizes ranging from 19 to 31 mm and 25 to 33 mm, respectively. The Carpentier-Edwards S.A.V. valve (CE-SAV; model 2650) is the next-generation porcine bioprosthesis that was introduced in 1982 to improve valve durability and transvalvular gradients observed with the Standard design. The valve is constructed using the same flexible cobalt-chromium alloy stent and XenoLogiX-treated leaflets. The glutaraldehyde fixation process, however, was reduced from moderate to low pressure (2 mm Hg). It features a low-profile design to prevent coronary obstruction in the aortic position and to decrease protrusion into the left ventricular outflow tract in the mitral position. The aortic prosthesis is designed for supra-annular placement to improve transvalvular gradients and EOA, and it has a scalloped contour for better anatomic fit. The aortic valve is available in sizes ranging from 19 to 31 mm; however, the 19, 29, and 31 mm sizes are available only outside the United States. The mitral prosthesis (model 6650) is available in sizes ranging from 25 to 33 mm and is available only outside the United States.

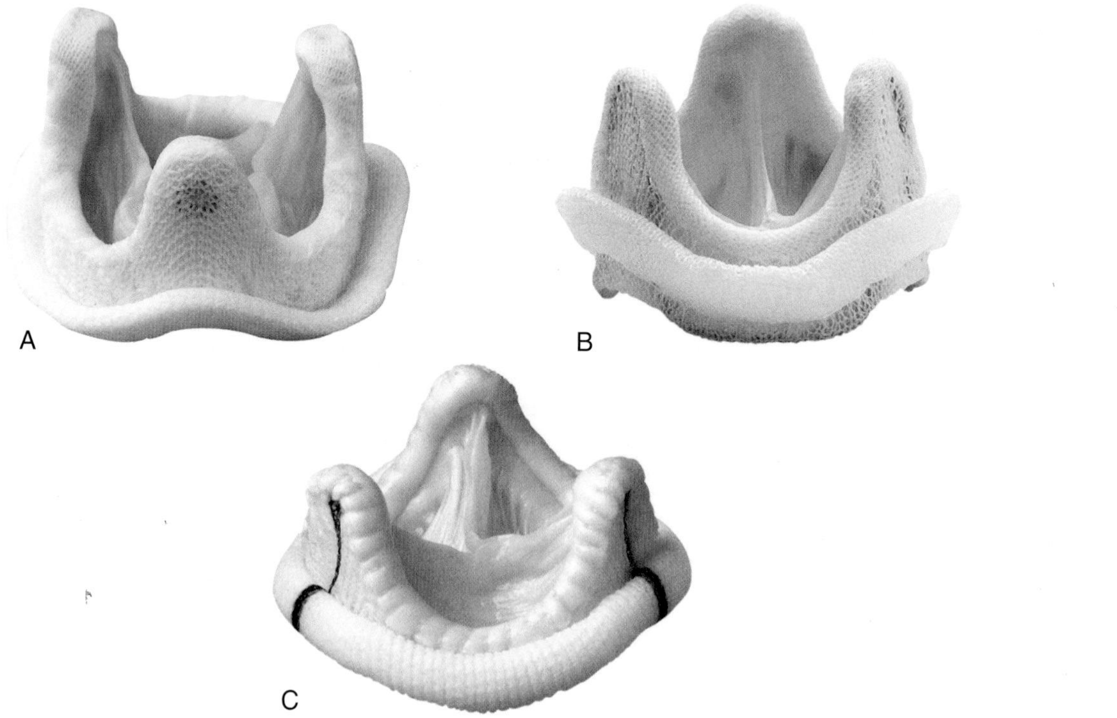

FIGURE 76-2 ■ Stented porcine valves. **A,** Mosaic Bioprosthesis. **B,** The Carpentier-Edwards Standard porcine valve. **C,** The Epic porcine valve. (**A,** Courtesy Medtronic, Inc., Minneapolis, MN. **B,** Courtesy Edwards Lifesciences Corp., Irvine, CA. **C,** Courtesy St. Jude Medical, Inc., Minneapolis, MN.)

The Carpentier-Edwards Duraflex low-pressure mitral porcine valve (model 6625LP) has all the same structural and design features as the CE-SAV mitral valve, and it is available only in the United States. The extended sewing ring model (model 6625-ESR-LP) is designed to offer greater ease of implantation when a larger suture surface is required. This valve is available in sizes ranging from 27 to 35 mm.

Jamieson and colleagues[48] reported their 20-year experience with the CE-SAV, which included 1823 patients who underwent AVR. Overall actual freedom from reoperation at 18 years was 85.0% ± 1.2%. Furthermore, the actual freedom from structural valve deterioration at 18 years was 86.4% ± 1.2% overall; 90.5% ± 1.8% for age 61 to 70 years; and 98.2% ± 0.6% for age greater than 70 years.[48] The only long-term study that evaluated the performance of the porcine mitral valve was by Corbineau and colleagues,[49] using the Standard valve. Of 139 patients who received the prosthesis, 30 demonstrated structural valve deterioration, with a mean time to onset of 9.0 ± 2.7 years. Although structural valve deterioration was independent of age, the frequency of deterioration was higher in younger recipients. After the age of 65 years, the frequency of structural valve deterioration was no longer variable.[49]

St. Jude Medical. The Biocor valve is a stented porcine bioprosthesis with 20 years of established clinical experience.[50,51] The valve was acquired by SJM in 1996 and approved by the FDA in 2005. It is available for the aortic and mitral positions in sizes ranging from 21 to 29 mm and 25 to 33 mm, respectively. The design features a flexible stent that adapts easily to the annulus and provides greater ease for knot tying. In addition, its low profile minimizes aortic wall protrusion and reduces left ventricular outflow tract obstruction in the mitral position. The Biocor Supra is designed for supra-annular implantation in the aortic position with the intention of providing better hemodynamics, and it is available in sizes ranging from 19 to 27 mm. The Epic (see Fig. 76-2*C*) and Epic Supra series use the same valve design as Biocor with the added benefit of receiving the Linx AC Technology, a patented, proprietary anticalcification treatment, designed to improve long-term performance and valve durability. The Epic series was approved by the FDA in 2007, and it is available for the same valve positions and sizes as the Biocor series.

Mykén and colleagues reported their 20-year data of 1712 patients who received the Biocor valve in either the aortic or mitral position. Actuarial freedom from reoperation because of structural valve deterioration was 61.1% ± 8.5% and 79.3% ± 6.0% after aortic valve replacement and mitral valve replacement, respectively.[51] The results of the FDA regulatory investigation of Epic valve were reported by Jamieson and colleagues,[52] in which 761 patients received the Epic valve in the aortic position, the mitral position, or both. The actuarial freedom from reoperation at 4 years, because of structural valve deterioration for AVR for age 60 years or less, was 93.3% ± 6.4%; for ages 61 to 70 years, 98.1% ± 1.9%; and for older than 70 years, 100% ($P = 0.0006$ for >70 vs. ≤60 years). There were no events of structural deterioration with mitral valve replacement. The actuarial freedom from major thromboembolism for all patients at 4 years was 93.6% ± 1.0%.[52]

Stented Bovine Pericardial Bioprostheses

Edwards Lifesciences. The Carpentier-Edwards PERIMOUNT valves are stented bovine pericardial bioprostheses with up to 25 years of demonstrated clinical durability. All PERIMOUNT valves feature a flexible cobalt-chromium alloy stent designed to absorb energy during the cardiac cycle, with three independent symmetrical pericardial leaflets mounted beneath the stent. The leaflets undergo a proprietary stress-free fixation, and they are meticulously matched for thickness and elasticity. The aortic heart valve series consists of the 2700 model, which undergoes XenoLogiX anticalcification treatment, and the 2700TFX model, which undergoes the ThermaFix process, a next generation anticalcification treatment that cross-links unstable glutaraldehyde moieties, in addition to reducing membrane phospholipids. The reduced sewing ring aortic heart valve series consists of the 2800 model and the 2800TFX model. Models 2900 and 2900TFX, available only outside the United States, are identical to models 2800 and 2800TFX, respectively. This series features a reduction in the sewing ring size by 2 to 3 mm, depending on the valve size, and it is designed to facilitate implantation into a smaller aortic root. The two models are distinguished by their anticalcification treatments, with the 2800 receiving the XenoLogiX treatment and the 2800TFX undergoing the ThermaFix process. The Magna aortic heart valve series (3000 and 3000TFX models) further improved the valve design by positioning the stent on top of the sewing ring rather than occupying space within the ring, effectively increasing the EOA and therefore improving valve hemodynamics. Once again, the two models differ only in their anticalcification strategies. Lastly, the Magna Ease aortic heart valve series (3300TFX model) features the same stent placement above the sewing ring, but with a lowered stent base that reduces the overall profile of the valve (Fig. 76-3*A*). The lower profile maximizes coronary ostia clearance and ease of aortotomy closure. This is the only valve series that is exclusively treated with the ThermaFix anticalcification process. All aortic models are available in sizes ranging from 19 to 29 mm.

A number of reports have documented the long-term safety and durability of the PERIMOUNT valve in the aortic position.[53,54] Vakil and colleagues[55] reported the rate of structural valve deterioration, as well as the risk factors influencing this phenomenon for 12,569 patients over a 20-year period. Actuarial rates of explantation for SVD at 10 and 20 years were 2% and 15%, respectively. Younger age ($P < 0.0001$) and higher total cholesterol ($P = 0.002$) were associated with increased risk of explantation for SVD. Smaller valve sizes alone were not associated with increased risk for valvular deterioration; however, higher postoperative peak and mean gradients were significant predictors of SVD ($P < 0.0001$).[55]

The mitral heart valve series features the same design and structural elements as the aortic series. The 6900P model (PERIMOUNT Plus mitral heart valve) and the

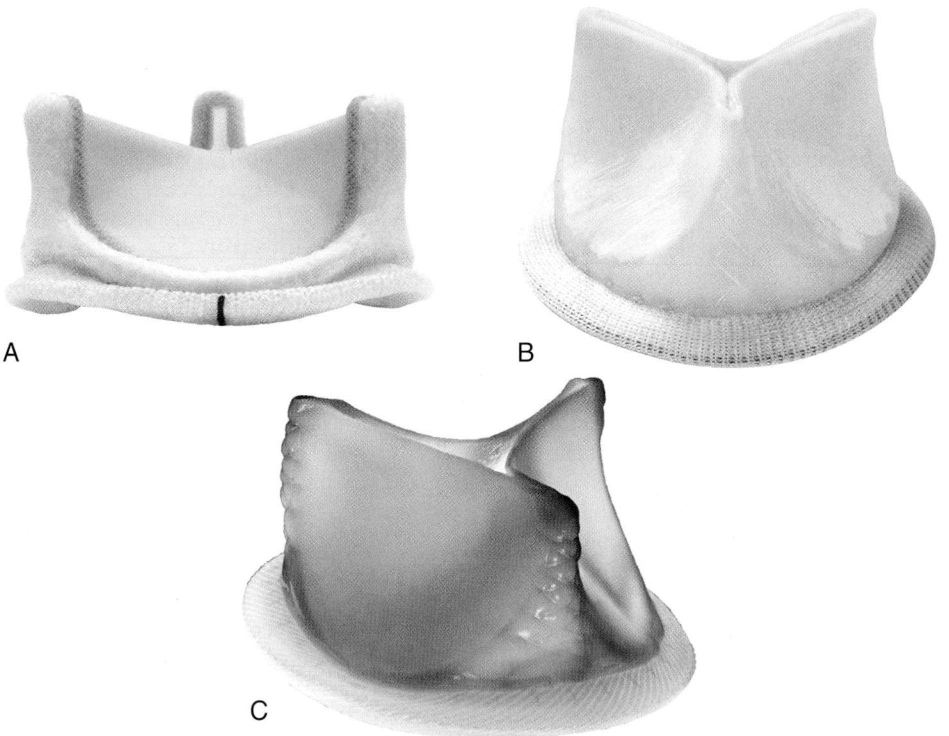

FIGURE 76-3 ■ Stented bovine pericardial valves. **A,** The Carpentier-Edwards PERIMOUNT valve. **B,** The Mitroflow valve. **C,** The Trifecta valve. (**A,** Courtesy Edwards Lifesciences Corp., Irvine, CA. **B,** Courtesy Sorin Group, Inc., Milan, Italy. **C,** Courtesy St. Jude Medical, Inc., Minneapolis, MN.)

6900PTFX model differ only in the anticalcification strategies they receive. The Magna Mitral Ease valve (7300TFX) design modifications feature an asymmetric and widened sewing cuff designed to increase the effective suture area and to enhance coaptation between the anterior and posterior aspects of the native mitral annulus. The low-profile design limits projection into the left ventricular outflow tract, and the anatomic sewing ring is designed to tilt the valve away from the left ventricular free wall to reduce the risk of left ventricular free wall abrasion. The Magna Mitral Ease valve exclusively receives the ThermaFix anticalcification treatment. The entire mitral PERIMOUNT valve portfolio includes the Tricentrix holder system, which is intended to prevent inadvertent looping of valve sutures around the stent posts during surgical implantation. All PERIMOUNT mitral valve prostheses are available in sizes ranging from 25 to 33 mm.

Bourguignon and colleagues reported their 20-year outcomes of the PERIMOUNT valve placed in the mitral position in 404 patients. Actuarial freedom from explant because of structural valve deterioration at 20 years was 40.5% ± 8.0% (1.9% per valve-year). Competing risk analysis demonstrated an actual risk of explant caused by structural valve dysfunction at 20 years of 25.5% ± 2.9%. Rates of valve failure were inversely correlated with recipient age, and the expected valve durability was 16.6 years for the entire cohort (11.4, 16.6, and 19.4 years for the patients younger than 60 years, between 60 and 70 years, and older than 70 years, respectively). Actuarial freedom from thromboembolism was 83.9% ± 7.6% (0.5% per valve-year), freedom from hemorrhage was 80.2% ± 10.8% (0.7% per valve-year), freedom from endocarditis was 94.8% ± 1.4% (0.4% per valve-year), and freedom from structural valve dysfunction was 23.7% ± 6.9% (2.3% per valve-year).[56]

Sorin Group. The Mitroflow valve (see Fig. 76-3*B*) is a stented bovine pericardial bioprosthesis designed for supra-annular implantation in the aortic position. The valve has been available worldwide, except in the United States, since 1982. The current model was introduced in 1991 and was approved by the FDA in 2007.[57] The valve design features a single pericardial sheet that is mounted around the stent posts, giving it a cylindrical wide leaflet opening for improved hemodynamics. The valve is constructed on a flexible polymer stent that couples maximal flow area with structural strength and resistance to permanent deformation. Its small sewing ring and low profile are designed to ease implantation. The leaflets undergo phospholipid reduction treatment (PRT), a proprietary anticalcification strategy recently approved in the United States. The valve is available in sizes from 19 to 29 mm.

The ISTHMUS investigators reported their results of a multicenter experience with Mitroflow over a 20-year period in which 1591 patients underwent an AVR. Reoperation was required in 96 patients (5.9%), of whom 59 patients (3.7%) had repeated surgery for structural valve degeneration. The actuarial freedom from prosthetic valve degeneration at 18 years was 65.5% (78% in patients older than 70 years) with a linearized rate of 1.4 patients per year (0.8 patients per year in patients older than 70 years). At 18 years, freedom from embolism was 82% (0.9 patients per year), freedom from valve endocarditis was 89% (0.6 patients per year) and freedom from bleeding episodes was 95% (0.2 patients per year), respectively.[58]

The Soprano Armonia valve is a stented bovine pericardial bioprosthesis designed for supra-annular implantation in the aortic position. It features a soft and easy-fitting sewing ring treated with Carbofilm coating for enhanced hemo-biocompatibility along with a low profile and scalloped stent. The leaflets have a double-sheet design intended to avoid contact between the pericardium and synthetic material. The tissue undergoes postfixation detoxification with homocysteic acid, which neutralizes residues of unbound aldehyde groups, aimed at improving performance in terms of durability, safety, and biocompatibility. The valve is available in sizes ranging from 19 to 33 mm and is clinically approved for use outside the United States only. Fischlein and colleagues[59] reported the European multicenter study using the Soprano valve in 501 patients at 1 year. Freedom from valve-related death was 98.6%, and actuarial freedoms from thromboembolism, bleeding, endocarditis, and paravalvular leak were 97.1%, 98.9%, 99.1%, and 99.6%, respectively. No events of thrombosis and SVD were observed. They also demonstrated a significant reduction in left ventricular mass, from 211 ± 78.5 g at 1 month to 185 ± 64.7 g at 12 months ($P < 0.0001$).[59]

The Pericarbon More valve is a stented bovine pericardial bioprosthesis designed for placement in the mitral position only. In addition to all the design features and treatments of the Soprano, it has the addition of an anti-looping protection system. The valve is available in sizes ranging from 19 to 33 mm and is clinically approved for use outside the United States only. The largest series using the valve in the mitral position was reported by Caimmi and colleagues.[60] At a single institution, 78 patients underwent an MVR by the same surgeon using the 29-mm valve. At 12 years, valve-related survival rate was 93.1% ± 3.0% while freedom from embolic events was 83.0% ± 4.5% and freedom from endocarditis was 98.7% ± 1.3%. The freedom from primary tissue failure was 56.8% ± 6.6% with an 86.3% ± 7.5% rate in patients older than 60 years and a 36.8% ± 8.2% rate in younger patients.[60]

St. Jude Medical. The Trifecta valve (see Fig. 76-3*C*) is a stented bovine pericardial bioprosthesis designed for supra-annular implantation in the aortic position that was approved by the FDA in 2011. The valve stent is made from fatigue-resistant, high-strength titanium, designed to reduce stress on the leaflets during the cardiac cycle. The stent posts are covered by porcine pericardium to provide tissue-to-tissue contact between the valve leaflets and stent to reduce leaflet abrasion and potential valve deterioration. The leaflets are from a single sheet of bovine pericardium that is externally mounted to optimize coaptation and maximize flow. Proper leaflet shaping and coaptation are achieved through a proprietary tissue leaflet fixation process. Lastly, the leaflets are treated with the Linx AC Technology aimed toward anticalcification. The valve is available in sizes ranging from 19 to 29 mm.

Results from the global, multicenter, prospective clinical study for Trifecta, in which 1014 patients received implants at 31 centers, were reported by Bavaria and colleagues.[61] Overall freedom from valve explant was 99.4% at 2 years. At the time of discharge, average mean gradients ranged from 9.3 to 4.1 mm Hg for valve sizes ranging 19 to 29 mm, respectively. There were 27 early thromboembolic events, including 8 (0.8%) strokes, 17 (1.7%) reversible neurologic events, and 2 (0.2%) systemic embolic events. There were no instances of early valve thrombosis, endocarditis, or clinically significant hemolysis. Lastly, there were five late valve explants, including one for structural deterioration and four for endocarditis.[61]

Stentless Bioprostheses

The first use of a xenograft stentless valve for aortic valve replacement was in 1986.[15] Because these prostheses have no rigid metal stent, there is little or no inherent gradient across the valve. These valves are supported by the aortic root of the patient once they are implanted by the subcoronary or inclusion cylinder technique. Certain stentless valves can also be implanted as stand-alone aortic root replacement prosthesis, similar to that of a homograft. Implantation of these valves, however, is more complex and often associated with longer cross-clamp times. These issues, along with the evolution of stented bioprostheses toward decreasing transvalvular gradients, have reduced the popularity of stentless valves in recent years.

Medtronic. The Freestyle valve (Fig. 76-4*A*) is a stentless porcine bioprosthesis with up to 15 years of demonstrated clinical durability. The valve is a full porcine root that undergoes a proprietary physiologic fixation process that is designed to retain the valve's natural anatomical shape along with alpha-amino oleic acid anticalcification treatment. It can be used as a freestanding aortic root prosthesis, or it can be trimmed and implanted with a subcoronary technique. The valve is available in sizes ranging from 19 to 29 mm. Bach and colleagues[62] reported their long-term outcomes of a multicenter cohort from North America and Europe where 725 patients were followed for up to 15 years. Freedom from valve-related death at 10 and 15 years was 94.9% ± 1.5% and 92.7% ± 3.5%. Freedom from explant owing to structural valve deterioration was 96.5% ± 1.3% and 83.3% ± 4.8% at 10 and 15 years, respectively. Increased age was associated with a lower risk of reoperation and explant caused by structural valve deterioration.[62]

The 3f (form follows function) valve is a stentless bioprosthesis made from three equal equine pericardial leaflets that undergo zero pressure fixation. Its tubular design was aimed to mimic the physiological function of the native aortic valve as closely as possible. The valve is affixed both to the annulus and with sutures at the commissural posts, creating greater valve flexibility and thus facilitating implantation. Given its unique design, the point of maximal stress on the valve is shifted from the commissure to the semilunar "belly" of leaflet. The valve is available in sizes ranging from 19 to 29 mm. Linneweber and colleagues[63] reported a 5-year follow-up of 123 patients receiving the 3f valve. There was no severe

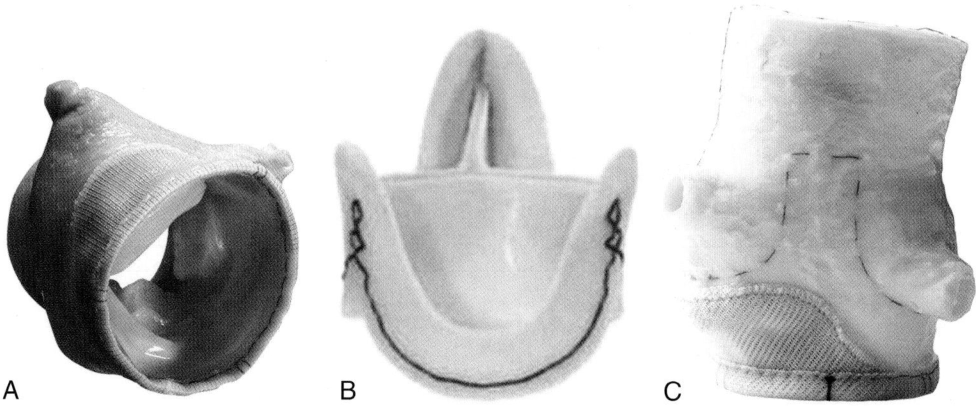

FIGURE 76-4 ■ Stentless valves. **A,** Freestyle Aortic Root Bioprostheses. **B,** The Freedom Solo valve. **C,** The Prima Plus valve. (**A,** Courtesy Medtronic, Inc., Minneapolis, MN. **B,** Courtesy Sorin Group, Inc., Milan, Italy. **C,** Courtesy Edwards Lifesciences Corp., Irvine, CA.)

structural or nonstructural valve dysfunction identified. Freedom from endocarditis was 100%, and there was minimal paravalvular regurgitation detected in four patients. Collectively, this resulted in a 100% freedom from reoperation. Freedom from severe adverse events was 89%, which included one permanent and three transient neuroembolic events. The mean transvalvular gradients remained low, and the ventricular mass was significantly improved.[63]

Sorin Group. The Pericarbon Freedom is a stentless bovine pericardial bioprosthesis that undergoes the manufacturer's postfixation detoxification treatment; it is stored in an aldehyde-free solution, thus eliminating the need for rinsing before implantation. It can be used as a freestanding aortic root prosthesis, or it can be trimmed and implanted with a subcoronary technique. The valve is available in sizes ranging from 15 to 29 mm, and is clinically approved for use outside the United States only. Milano and colleagues[64] reported 10-year outcomes for 85 patients who received the Pericarbon Freedom valve. Actuarial freedom from structural valve deterioration was 96% ± 3%. Two patients required reoperation because of SVD, one for endocarditis and one for dilation of the sinotubular junction, resulting in an actuarial freedom from reoperation of 93% ± 4%. Left ventricular mass index decreased from 213 ± 51 gm/m^2 to 157 ± 436 gm/m^2 ($P < 0.001$).[64]

The Freedom Solo (see Fig. 76-4*B*) is a next-generation stentless bovine pericardial bioprosthesis, designed for supra-annular seating aimed at establishing a 100% orifice-to-annulus ratio. The valve is designed for subcoronary implantation only and is available in sizes ranging from 19 to 27 mm. It is currently available only outside the United States, but it is expected to receive FDA approval in the near future. A number of reports have demonstrated low transvalvular gradients after implantation and associated regression of left ventricular mass within several months; however, long-term data on the durability of the valve are not available.[65,66] There have also been several reports of severe but transient thrombocytopenia in patients that receive the valve, relative to other available options.[67,68] The etiology of the thrombocytopenia is unknown.

Edwards Lifesciences. The Edwards Prima Plus valve (see Fig. 76-4*C*) is a stentless porcine bioprosthesis that undergoes low-pressure fixation and receives XenoLogiX anticalcification treatment. A woven polyester cloth is sewn to the annulus to provide additional support to the first suture line. It can be implanted as a full root replacement or trimmed and placed using a subcoronary technique; however, the approved indication in the United States is for the subcoronary implantation only. The valve is available in sizes ranging from 21 to 29 mm. Auriemma and colleagues[69] reported their 10-year outcomes in 318 patients who received the Edwards Prima Plus valve. Actuarial freedom from valve reoperation and structural valve deterioration at 10 years were 100% and 64%, respectively. Actuarial freedom from embolic events and endocarditis at 10 years were 84% and 81%, respectively.[69]

Sutureless Valves

Sutureless prosthetic heart valves were initially developed in the 1960s to facilitate valve implantation while reducing ischemic and procedural times. These valves were abandoned, however, because of multiple complications such as paravalvular leaks and valve-related thromboembolic events.[70] The rapid development of transcatheter technology has fueled a reemergence of the sutureless strategy, once again in an effort to reduce the morbidity and mortality of patients requiring valve replacement. The acceleration of the surgical procedure has the potential to reduce the adverse outcomes seen in higher-risk patients and in those requiring complex multivalve or combined valve and coronary procedures.[71]

Medtronic. The 3f Enable (Fig. 76-5*A*) is a sutureless bioprosthesis constructed with the 3f stentless valve placed over a self-expanding nitinol frame. The inflow flange is covered with polyester fabric and is scalloped to conform to the aortic annulus. Implantation requires a

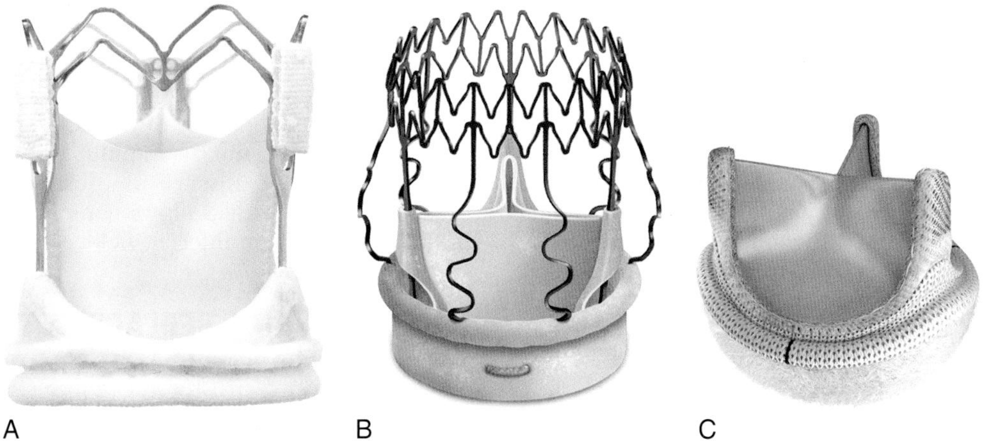

FIGURE 76-5 ■ Sutureless valves. **A,** The 3f Enable valve. **B,** The Perceval S valve. **C,** The Intuity valve. (**A,** Courtesy Medtronic, Inc., Minneapolis, MN. **B,** Courtesy Sorin Group, Inc., Milan, Italy. **C,** Courtesy Edwards Lifesciences Corp., Irvine, CA.)

transverse aortotomy at least 2 cm above the sinotubular junction. As with traditional sutured valves, the leaflets must be excised followed by meticulous débridement of the annulus. A single guiding suture is placed in the nadir of the noncoronary sinus, and the valve commissures need to be aligned to the native valve commissures. The chronic outward force of the nitinol, along with the polyester flange, ensure fixation of the valve and minimize the potential for paravalvular leaks.[71] The valve is contraindicated in bicuspid aortic valves along with irregular or heavily calcified valves. It received CE Mark approval in 2009 and is currently awaiting FDA approval. The valve is available in sizes ranging from 19 to 29 mm. A number of groups have reported their outcomes with the 3f Enable.[72,73] Eichstaedt and colleagues[73] reported their single-center experience of 120 patients with up to 18 months of follow-up. In a population of patients with a mean Society of Thoracic Surgeons risk score of 14.8%, the 30-day mortality was 6.7% overall and 1.4% in standalone procedures. Mean and peak transvalvular gradients were 9 mm Hg (4 to 13 mm Hg) and 14 mm Hg (8 to 22 mmHg) at discharge, respectively. In 8 patients (6.7%), permanent pacemaker implantation was necessary. No thromboembolic or bleeding events related to the bioprosthesis were observed.[73]

Sorin Group. The Perceval S (see Fig. 76-5*B*) is a stentless, bovine pericardial bioprosthesis attached to a self-expandable nitinol anchoring device, which has the dual role of supporting the valve and providing fixation to the implantation site. The anchoring device is characterized by two ring segments (outflow and inflow ring), three commissural elements supporting the valve, and three pairs of sinusoidal elements providing fixation in the sinuses of Valsalva. The anchoring device is treated with the manufacturer's proprietary Carbofilm coating. In addition to the double-sheet pericardial design, there is a pericardial sealing collar designed to encourage adaptation to the aortic annulus and prevention of paravalvular leaks. The proximal aortotomy should be 3 to 3.5 cm above the valve annulus or 0.5 to 1 cm above the sinotubular junction. The leaflets must be excised; however, the annulus does not require decalcification. Only eccentric and bulky intra-annular calcium needs to be removed. Guiding sutures are then placed 2 to 3 mm below the nadir of each sinus, maintaining 120 degrees equidistance between each suture. In correspondence to each valve sinus, a buttonhole is provided on the inflow ring, through which the guiding sutures are passed. Before implantation, the prosthesis diameter is reduced to a suitable size and then loaded on the holder. After in situ positioning, the valve is released in two steps. First the inflow ring at the level of the annulus and, when proper positioning is verified, the complete prosthesis is released. Following implantation, a postdilation balloon catheter is inflated inside the prosthesis at the inflow level to improve apposition by modeling the inflow ring on the annulus.[71] The valve is available in small (S), medium (M), large (L), and extra-large (XL) sizes. The valve received CE Mark approval in 2011, and it is expected to receive FDA approval shortly.

Several reports have demonstrated the safety and efficacy of the valve.[74,75] Rubino and colleagues[76] reported a multicenter European cohort of 314 patients who underwent AVR using the Perceval S as a standalone procedure or combined with surgical revascularization. The valve was successfully implanted in 99.4% of cases, whereas two patients were converted to a traditional AVR because of severe paravalvular leak. In-hospital mortality was 3.2% and was lower in isolated AVR compared with a combined procedure (1.4% vs. 7.4%; $P = 0.005$). Six patients (1.9%) experienced perioperative stroke, five (1.6%) needed renal replacement therapy, and 25 (8.0%) required pacemaker implantation. Octogenarians and younger patients experienced similar in-hospital outcomes. At 2 years, overall survival was 84.1% ± 4.2%, whereas freedom from valve-related death was 97.9% ± 1.3%. Freedom from stroke was 98.9% ± 0.8%, freedom from endocarditis was 99.1% ± 0.6%, and freedom from reoperation on the aortic valve was 98.5% ± 0.9%. Once again, no differences were observed in octogenarians compared with the younger population.[76]

Edwards Lifesciences. The Edwards Intuity (see Fig. 76-5*C*) is a stentless bovine pericardial bioprosthesis that uses the PERIMOUNT design with a proprietary balloon-expandable subannular stainless steel frame. The leaflets receive the manufacturer's ThermaFix anticalcification treatment, and the frame is covered with a broad polyester sealing cloth that is expanded slightly below the native aortic valve annulus. Implantation is performed after a traditional aortotomy and excision of the leaflets. Decalcification of the annulus should be performed to where the inner surface of the annulus is smooth. Guiding sutures are placed through the annulus at the nadirs of each sinus and are later secured to the valve. The Intuity received CE Mark approval in 2012, and it is currently being trialed in the United States for future FDA approval. The valve is available in sizes ranging from 19 to 27 mm. The Surgical Treatment of Aortic Stenosis With a Next Generation Surgical Aortic Valve (TRITON) trial reported the 1-year outcomes of 152 patients who underwent AVR using the Edwards Intuity valve. Implantation was successful in 96.1% of patients (146/152), whereas early valve-related mortality was 1.4% and cumulative survival was 92.5% at a mean follow-up of 9.8 ± 5.1 months. Independent core laboratory-adjudicated mean effective orifice area and aortic valve pressure gradient were 1.7 ± 0.2 cm^2 and 8.8 ± 3.0 mm Hg at 3 months, and 1.7 ± 0.2 cm^2 and 8.4 ± 3.4 mm Hg at 1 year, respectively.[77]

Transcatheter Valves

Transcatheter valves have created a paradigm shift in the approach to treating valvular heart disease. With the approval of the Edwards Sapien aortic valve and the Medtronic CoreValve, a new generation of valvular therapy was introduced. Approved for nonoperative and high-risk surgical patients with aortic stenosis, these valves have demonstrated significant benefits over medical therapy and comparable outcomes to traditional surgical aortic valve replacement.[78-80] SJM has received CE Mark approval for the Portico aortic valve, which is being trialed in the United States for future FDA approval. Transcatheter approaches to mitral, tricuspid, and pulmonary valve replacements are being developed as well, and will likely be clinically available in the near future. As this technology evolves, it will likely reshape the indications for surgical valve replacement while further improving the care of patients with valvular heart disease. A more detailed review of transcatheter valve therapies is presented in Chapter 79.

Homograft Valve Replacement

Homograft valves are harvested from cadaveric donors and cryopreserved until they are ready for use. They are commonly used in congenital cardiac surgery for reconstruction of complex great vessel and semilunar valve anomalies. Currently, the primary indication for a homograft in adult cardiac surgery is as a full root replacement for complicated native aortic valve endocarditis[81] or infected composite aortic root grafts. Initially there was optimism that homograft valves would offer improved durability over conventional bioprosthesis; however, studies have shown that modern biologic valves are equal if not greater in durability.[82] Subcoronary and inclusion techniques for implantation were initially described, but these approaches have fallen out of favor. For effective treatment of endocarditis, all infected tissue has to be radically débrided. To that end, the mitral valve curtain and attached septal muscle of the homograft can help in reconstructing the mitral annulus and left ventricular outflow tract. The absence of prosthetic material can offer an advantage that allows complex reconstructions in the presence of an infected field.

CHOICE OF VALVE REPLACEMENT

The choice of valve prosthesis can be a challenging decision faced by both the surgeon and patient. The first and most important step in the process is choosing between a mechanical and bioprosthetic valve. Important factors to consider are the patient's age, life expectancy, preference, indications or contraindications to anticoagulation, and comorbidities. The 2006 American College of Cardiology/American Heart Association (ACC/AHA) and 2007 European guidelines reduced the weight placed on the patient's age and gave greater emphasis to patient preference.[83,84] The most recent ACC/AHA guidelines further emphasize that the choice of prosthetic valve type should be a shared decision-making process that accounts for the patient's values and preferences, with full disclosure of the indications for and risks of anticoagulant therapy and the potential need for reoperation. A bioprosthetic valve is believed to be reasonable in patients older than 70 years and recommended in patients of any age for whom anticoagulant therapy is contraindicated, cannot be managed appropriately, or is not desired. Either a bioprosthetic or mechanical valve is considered reasonable in patients between 60 and 70 years old, and a mechanical prosthesis is reasonable for AVR or MVR in patients younger than 60 years who do not have a contraindication to anticoagulation (Table 76-3).[85]

Another important factor in the selection process is choosing a valve that provides optimal hemodynamic performance. The performance of the valve is determined by the size of the prosthesis that can fit the patient's annulus and by the total cross-sectional area of that prosthesis, or the EOA of the valve, that is available for blood flow. PPM occurs when the EOA of the implanted valve is too small relative to the patient's body surface area. The most widely accepted measure of PPM is the iEOA. In the aortic position, an iEOA greater than 0.85 cm^2/m^2 is considered acceptable. Moderate PPM occurs when the iEOA is between 0.85 and 0.65 cm^2/m^2, whereas severe PPM occurs when the iEOA is less than 0.65 cm^2/m^2. Several reports have demonstrated that PPM after AVR is associated with less improvement in symptoms and functional class, impaired exercise tolerance, less regression of left ventricular hypertrophy, less improvement in coronary flow reserve, more adverse cardiac events, and increased short- and long-term mortality. Moreover, the effect of PPM is more pronounced in younger patients and in those with depressed left ventricular function.[86]

It is important to understand that there are significant discrepancies between the actual dimensions of a valve prosthesis and the labeled prosthesis size when

TABLE 76-3 Summary of Recommendations for Prosthetic Valve Choice from 2014 AHA/ACC Guidelines

Recommendations	COR	LOE
Choice of valve intervention and prosthetic valve type should be a shared decision process.	I	C
A bioprosthesis is recommended in patients of any age for whom anticoagulant therapy is contraindicated, cannot be managed appropriately, or is not desired.	I	C
A mechanical prosthesis is reasonable for AVR or MVR in patients younger than 60 years who do not have a contraindication to anticoagulation.	IIa	B
A bioprosthesis is reasonable in patients older than 70 years.	IIa	B
Either a bioprosthetic or mechanical valve is reasonable in patients between 60 and 70 years old.	IIa	B
Replacement of the aortic valve by a pulmonary autograft (the Ross procedure), when performed by an experienced surgeon, may be considered in young patients when VKA anticoagulation is contraindicated or undesirable.	IIb	C

AVR, Aortic valve replacement; *COR,* class of recommendation; *LOE,* level of evidence; *MVR,* mitral valve replacement; *VKA,* vitamin K antagonist.

(From Nishimura RA, Otto CM, Bonow RO, et al: 2014 AHA/ACC Guideline for the Management of Patients with Valvular Heart Disease: a report of the American College of Cardiology/American Heart Association Task Force on Practice Guidelines. Circulation 129:e521–643, 2014.)

comparing different models. Therefore, one must be cautious when evaluating the hemodynamic performance of different prosthesis models on the basis of the labeled size. A particular annulus can accommodate a size 21 valve from one manufacturer, whereas the same annulus can accommodate only a size 19 valve from an alternate manufacturer. In general, newer-generation valves have superior performance over older devices, and mechanical prostheses are better when compared with stented bioprostheses. A recent meta-analysis showed that stentless valves provide larger EOAs, reduced transprosthetic gradients, and greater left ventricular mass regression when compared with stented bioprostheses, but at the expense of prolonged cardiopulmonary bypass times. In the end, the choice of valve prosthesis is a multifactorial decision that should be individualized to the needs of each patient, with the intention of achieving an optimal hemodynamic and clinical outcome.[86]

REFERENCES

1. Harken DE: Heart valves: ten commandments and still counting. *Ann Thorac Surg* 48(3 Suppl):S18–S19, 1989.
2. Hufnagel CA, et al: Surgical correction of aortic insufficiency. *Surgery* 35(5):673–683, 1954.
3. Clarke DR: Value, viability, and valves. *J Thorac Cardiovasc Surg* 124(1):1–6, 2002.
4. Edmunds LH, Jr: Evolution of prosthetic heart valves. *Am Heart J* 141(5):849–855, 2001.
5. Starr A, Edwards ML: Mitral replacement: clinical experience with a ball-valve prosthesis. *Ann Surg* 154:726–740, 1961.
6. Wada J, Komatsu S: [Implantation of heart valve prosthesis and its problems. The Wada hingeless valve]. *Saishin Igaku* 23(1):111–120, 1968.
7. Bjork VO, Lindblom D: The Monostrut Bjork-Shiley heart valve. *J Am Coll Cardiol* 6(5):1142–1148, 1985.
8. Butchart EG, et al: Twenty years' experience with the Medtronic Hall valve. *J Thorac Cardiovasc Surg* 121(6):1090–1100, 2001.
9. Akins CW: Long-term results with the Medtronic-Hall valvular prosthesis. *Ann Thorac Surg* 61(3):806–813, 1996.
10. Svennevig JL, Abdelnoor M, Nitter-Hauge S: Twenty-five-year experience with the Medtronic-Hall valve prosthesis in the aortic position: a follow-up cohort study of 816 consecutive patients. *Circulation* 116(16):1795–1800, 2007.
11. Emery RW, et al: A new cardiac valve prosthesis: in vitro results. *Trans Am Soc Artif Intern Organs* 24:550–556, 1978.
12. Gunning AJ: Ross' first homograft replacement of the aortic valve. *Ann Thorac Surg* 54(4):809–810, 1992.
13. Carpentier A, et al: Biological factors affecting long-term results of valvular heterografts. *J Thorac Cardiovasc Surg* 58(4):467–483, 1969.
14. Ionescu MI, et al: Heart valve replacement with the Ionescu-Shiley pericardial xenograft. *J Thorac Cardiovasc Surg* 73(1):31–42, 1977.
15. David TE, Pollick C, Bos J: Aortic valve replacement with stentless porcine aortic bioprosthesis. *J Thorac Cardiovasc Surg* 99(1):113–118, 1990.
16. Clark RE, et al: Guidelines for reporting morbidity and mortality after cardiac valvular operations. *Eur J Cardiothorac Surg* 2(5):293–295, 1988.
17. Edmunds LH, Jr, et al: Guidelines for reporting morbidity and mortality after cardiac valvular operations. Ad Hoc Liaison Committee for Standardizing Definitions of Prosthetic Heart Valve Morbidity of The American Association for Thoracic Surgery and The Society of Thoracic Surgeons. *J Thorac Cardiovasc Surg* 112(3):708–711, 1996.
18. Kelly SG, et al: A three-dimensional analysis of flow in the pivot regions of an ATS bileaflet valve. *Int J Artif Organs* 22(11):754–763, 1999.
19. Emery RW, et al: Five-year follow up of the ATS mechanical heart valve. *J Heart Valve Dis* 13(2):231–238, 2004.
20. Van Nooten GJ, et al: Fifteen years' single-center experience with the ATS bileaflet valve. *J Heart Valve Dis* 18(4):444–452, 2009.
21. Villemot JP, et al: Nine-year routine clinical experience of aortic valve replacement with ATS mechanical valves. *J Heart Valve Dis* 17(6):648–656, 2008.
22. Bernet FH, et al: Single-center outcome analysis of 1,161 patients with St. Jude medical and ATS open pivot mechanical heart valves. *J Heart Valve Dis* 16(2):151–158, 2007.
23. Lund O, et al: Standard aortic St. Jude valve at 18 years: performance profile and determinants of outcome. *Ann Thorac Surg* 69(5):1459–1465, 2000.
24. Bryan AJ, et al: Prospective randomized comparison of CarboMedics and St. Jude Medical bileaflet mechanical heart valve prostheses: ten-year follow-up. *J Thorac Cardiovasc Surg* 133(3):614–622, 2007.
25. Lehmann S, et al: Eight-year follow-up after prospectively randomized implantation of different mechanical aortic valves. *Clin Res Cardiol* 97(6):376–382, 2008.
26. Van Nooten GJ, et al: Twenty years' single-center experience with mechanical heart valves: a critical review of anticoagulation policy. *J Heart Valve Dis* 21(1):88–98, 2012.
27. Emery RW, et al: The St. Jude Medical cardiac valve prosthesis: a 25-year experience with single valve replacement. *Ann Thorac Surg* 79(3):776–782, discussion 782–783, 2005.
28. Toole JM, et al: Twenty-five year experience with the St. Jude medical mechanical valve prosthesis. *Ann Thorac Surg* 89(5):1402–1409, 2010.
29. Vitale N, et al: Clinical evaluation of St Jude Medical Hemodynamic Plus versus standard aortic valve prostheses: the Italian multicenter, prospective, randomized study. *J Thorac Cardiovasc Surg* 122(4):691–698, 2001.
30. Ismeno G, et al: Standard versus hemodynamic plus 19-mm St Jude Medical aortic valves. *J Thorac Cardiovasc Surg* 121(4):723–728, 2001.
31. Bach DS, et al: Hemodynamics and early clinical performance of the St. Jude Medical Regent mechanical aortic valve. *Ann Thorac Surg* 74(6):2003–2009, discussion 2009, 2002.
32. Soga Y, et al: Up to 8-year follow-up of valve replacement with carbomedics valve. *Ann Thorac Surg* 73(2):474–479, 2002.

33. Fiane AE, Geiran OR, Svennevig JL: Up to eight years' follow-up of 997 patients receiving the CarboMedics prosthetic heart valve. *Ann Thorac Surg* 66(2):443–448, 1998.
34. Azarnoush K, Laborde F, de Riberolles C: The Sorin Bicarbon over 15 years clinical outcomes: multicentre experience in 1704 patients. *Eur J Cardiothorac Surg* 38(6):759–766, 2010.
35. Bouchard D, et al: Twenty-year experience with the CarboMedics mechanical valve prosthesis. *Ann Thorac Surg* 97:816–823, 2014.
36. Puskas J, et al: Reduced anticoagulation after mechanical aortic valve replacement: interim results from the Prospective Randomized On-X Valve Anticoagulation Clinical Trial randomized Food and Drug Administration investigational device exemption trial. *J Thorac Cardiovasc Surg* 147(4):1202–1210, 2014.
37. Binet JP, et al: Heterologous aortic valve transplantation. *Lancet* 2(7425):1275, 1965.
38. Gong G, et al: Aldehyde tanning: the villain in bioprosthetic calcification. *Eur J Cardiothorac Surg* 5(6):288–299, discussion 293, 1991.
39. Thubrikar MJ, et al: Role of mechanical stress in calcification of aortic bioprosthetic valves. *J Thorac Cardiovasc Surg* 86(1):115–125, 1983.
40. Girardot MN, Torrianni M, Girardot JM: Effect of AOA on glutaraldehyde-fixed bioprosthetic heart valve cusps and walls: binding and calcification studies. *Int J Artif Organs* 17(2):76–82, 1994.
41. Borger MA, et al: Twenty-year results of the Hancock II bioprosthesis. *J Heart Valve Dis* 15(1):49–55, discussion 55–56, 2006.
42. David TE, Armstrong S, Maganti M: Hancock II bioprosthesis for aortic valve replacement: the gold standard of bioprosthetic valves durability? *Ann Thorac Surg* 90(3):775–781, 2010.
43. Valfre C, et al: The fate of Hancock II porcine valve recipients 25 years after implant. *Eur J Cardiothorac Surg* 38(2):141–146, 2010.
44. Fradet G, et al: The mosaic valve clinical performance at seven years: results from a multicenter prospective clinical trial. *J Heart Valve Dis* 13(2):239–246, discussion 246–247, 2004.
45. Riess FC, et al: Clinical results of the Medtronic Mosaic porcine bioprosthesis up to 13 years. *Eur J Cardiothorac Surg* 37(1):145–153, 2010.
46. Jamieson WR, et al: Medtronic Mosaic porcine bioprosthesis: assessment of 12-year performance. *J Thorac Cardiovasc Surg* 142(2):302–307, e2, 2011.
47. Anselmi A, et al: Long-term results of the Medtronic Mosaic porcine bioprosthesis in the aortic position. *J Thorac Cardiovasc Surg* 147:1884–1891, 2014.
48. Jamieson WR, et al: Carpentier-Edwards supra-annular aortic porcine bioprosthesis: clinical performance over 20 years. *J Thorac Cardiovasc Surg* 130(4):994–1000, 2005.
49. Corbineau H, et al: Structural durability in Carpentier Edwards Standard bioprosthesis in the mitral position: a 20-year experience. *J Heart Valve Dis* 10(4):443–448, 2001.
50. Eichinger WB, et al: Twenty-year experience with the St. Jude medical Biocor bioprosthesis in the aortic position. *Ann Thorac Surg* 86(4):1204–1210, 2008.
51. Mykén PS, Bech-Hansen O: A 20-year experience of 1712 patients with the Biocor porcine bioprosthesis. *J Thorac Cardiovasc Surg* 137(1):76–81, 2009.
52. Jamieson WR, et al: St Jude Medical Epic porcine bioprosthesis: results of the regulatory evaluation. *J Thorac Cardiovasc Surg* 141(6):1449–1454, e2, 2011.
53. Banbury MK, et al: Hemodynamic stability during 17 years of the Carpentier-Edwards aortic pericardial bioprosthesis. *Ann Thorac Surg* 73(5):1460–1465, 2002.
54. Dellgren G, et al: Late hemodynamic and clinical outcomes of aortic valve replacement with the Carpentier-Edwards Perimount pericardial bioprosthesis. *J Thorac Cardiovasc Surg* 124(1):146–154, 2002.
55. Vakil N, et al: Factors influencing structural valve deterioration of aortic prostheses: implications for valve choice and medical management, in 50th Annual Meeting of the Society of Thoracic Surgeons, Orlando, FL, 2014.
56. Bourguignon T, et al: Very Late outcomes for mitral valve replacement with the Carpentier-Edwards pericardial bioprosthesis: 25-year follow-up of 450 implantations, in AATS Mitral Valve Conclave, New York, NY, 2013.
57. Jamieson WR, et al: Mitroflow aortic pericardial bioprosthesis—clinical performance. *Eur J Cardiothorac Surg* 36(5):818–824, 2009.
58. ISTHMUS Investigators, et al: The Italian study on the Mitroflow postoperative results (ISTHMUS): a 20-year, multicentre evaluation of Mitroflow pericardial bioprosthesis. *Eur J Cardiothorac Surg* 39(1):18–26, discussion 26, 2011.
59. Fischlein T, et al: European multicenter study with the Soprano valve for aortic valve replacement: one-year clinical experience and hemodynamic data. *J Heart Valve Dis* 20(6):695–703, 2011.
60. Caimmi PP, et al: Twelve-year follow up with the Sorin Pericarbon bioprosthesis in the mitral position. *J Heart Valve Dis* 7(4):400–406, 1998.
61. Bavaria JE, et al: The St Jude Medical Trifecta aortic pericardial valve: results from a global, multicenter, prospective clinical study. *J Thorac Cardiovasc Surg* 147(2):590–597, 2014.
62. Bach DS, Kon ND: Long-term clinical outcomes 15 years after aortic valve replacement with the Freestyle stentless aortic bioprosthesis. *Ann Thorac Surg* 97(2):544–551, 2014.
63. Linneweber J, et al: Clinical experience with the ATS 3F stentless aortic bioprosthesis: five years' follow up. *J Heart Valve Dis* 19(6):772–777, 2010.
64. Milano AD, et al: The Sorin freedom stentless pericardial valve: clinical and echocardiographic performance at 10 years. *Int J Artif Organs* 35(7):481–488, 2012.
65. Repossini A, et al: Early clinical and haemodynamic results after aortic valve replacement with the Freedom SOLO bioprosthesis (experience of Italian multicenter study). *Eur J Cardiothorac Surg* 41(5):1104–1110, 2012.
66. Iliopoulos DC, et al: Single-center experience using the Freedom SOLO aortic bioprosthesis. *J Thorac Cardiovasc Surg* 146(1):96–102, 2013.
67. Pozzoli A, et al: Severe thrombocytopenia and its clinical impact after implant of the stentless Freedom Solo bioprosthesis. *Ann Thorac Surg* 96(5):1581–1586, 2013.
68. Piccardo A, et al: Thrombocytopenia after aortic valve replacement with freedom solo bioprosthesis: a propensity study. *Ann Thorac Surg* 89(5):1425–1430, 2010.
69. Auriemma S, et al: Long-term results of aortic valve replacement with Edwards Prima Plus stentless bioprosthesis: eleven years' follow up. *J Heart Valve Dis* 15(5):691–695, discussion 695, 2006.
70. Magovern GJ, Cromie HW: Sutureless prosthetic heart valves. *J Thorac Cardiovasc Surg* 46:726–736, 1963.
71. Carrell T, Englberger L, Stalder M: Recent developments for surgical aortic valve replacement: the concept of sutureless valve technology. *Open Journal of Cardiology* 4(1), 2013.
72. Concistre G, et al: Short-term follow up with the 3f Enable aortic bioprosthesis: clinical and echocardiographic results. *J Heart Valve Dis* 22(6):817–823, 2013.
73. Eichstaedt HC, et al: Early single-center experience in sutureless aortic valve implantation in 120 patients. *J Thorac Cardiovasc Surg* 147(1):370–375, 2014.
74. Folliguet TA, et al: Sutureless perceval aortic valve replacement: results of two European centers. *Ann Thorac Surg* 93(5):1483–1488, 2012.
75. Santarpino G, et al: The Perceval S aortic valve has the potential of shortening surgical time: does it also result in improved outcome? *Ann Thorac Surg* 96(1):77–81, discussion 81–82, 2013.
76. Rubino A, et al: Surgical aortic valve replacement with sutureless valve: a multicenter study, in AATS annual meeting, Toronto, ON, Canada, 2014.
77. Kocher AA, et al: One-year outcomes of the Surgical Treatment of Aortic Stenosis With a Next Generation Surgical Aortic Valve (TRITON) trial: a prospective multicenter study of rapid-deployment aortic valve replacement with the EDWARDS INTUITY Valve System. *J Thorac Cardiovasc Surg* 145(1):110–115, discussion 115–116, 2013.
78. Leon MB, et al: Transcatheter aortic-valve implantation for aortic stenosis in patients who cannot undergo surgery. *N Engl J Med* 363(17):1597–1607, 2010.
79. Smith CR, et al: Transcatheter versus surgical aortic-valve replacement in high-risk patients. *N Engl J Med* 364(23):2187–2198, 2011.
80. Adams DH, et al: Transcatheter Aortic-Valve Replacement with a Self-Expanding Prosthesis. *N Engl J Med* 371(10):967, 2014.
81. Lytle BW, et al: Reoperative cryopreserved root and ascending aorta replacement for acute aortic prosthetic valve endocarditis. *Ann Thorac Surg* 74(5):S1754–S1757, discussion S1792–S1799, 2002.

82. Smedira NG, et al: Are allografts the biologic valve of choice for aortic valve replacement in nonelderly patients? Comparison of explantation for structural valve deterioration of allograft and pericardial prostheses. *J Thorac Cardiovasc Surg* 131(3):558–564, e4, 2006.
83. Bonow RO, et al: ACC/AHA 2006 guidelines for the management of patients with valvular heart disease: a report of the American College of Cardiology/American Heart Association Task Force on Practice Guidelines (writing committee to revise the 1998 Guidelines for the Management of Patients With Valvular Heart Disease): developed in collaboration with the Society of Cardiovascular Anesthesiologists: endorsed by the Society for Cardiovascular Angiography and Interventions and the Society of Thoracic Surgeons. *Circulation* 114(5):e84–e231, 2006.
84. Vahanian A, et al: Guidelines on the management of valvular heart disease: the Task Force on the Management of Valvular Heart Disease of the European Society of Cardiology. *Eur Heart J* 28(2):230–268, 2007.
85. Nishimura RA, et al: 2014 AHA/ACC Guideline for the Management of Patients With Valvular Heart Disease: a report of the American College of Cardiology/American Heart Association Task Force on Practice Guidelines. *Circulation* 129(23):e521–e643, 2014.
86. Pibarot P, Dumesnil JG: Prosthetic heart valves: selection of the optimal prosthesis and long-term management. *Circulation* 119(7): 1034–1048, 2009.

CHAPTER 77

SURGICAL TREATMENT OF AORTIC VALVE DISEASE

Talal Al-Atassi • Gebrine El Khoury • Munir Boodhwani

CHAPTER OUTLINE

FUNCTIONAL ANATOMY OF THE AORTIC VALVE

The aortic valve is the last of four cardiac valves through which the blood is pumped before it goes to the rest of the body. It separates the left ventricular outflow tract from the aorta. Its main function is to prevent backward blood flow from the aorta to the left ventricle, while allowing the blood to flow forward during systole with minimal resistance. The normal aortic valve has three semilunar cusps (tricuspid): the left coronary, the right coronary, and the noncoronary cusps. Each cusp is attached below one of the three sinuses of Valsalva, which are slight dilations of the aorta associated with each cusp. These sinuses end at the sinotubular junction, which is the narrowest part of the aortic root. The fibrous skeleton supports the aortic valve and is continuous with the anterior leaflet of the mitral valve.

AORTIC STENOSIS

Epidemiology and Etiology

Isolated aortic stenosis (AS) is more common in men than in women and is found in 2% of people 65 years of age and older. The most common causes of AS include age-related calcific degeneration, bicuspid aortic valve, and rheumatic aortic valve. The distribution of these causes varies across age groups and geographic regions. Age-related degeneration is the most common cause of AS in patients older than 70 years. In contrast, bicuspid aortic valve calcification accounts for most surgical cases in patients younger than 70 years.

Pathophysiology

No appreciable gradient exists across the normal aortic valve during systole. In AS, gradual obstruction of the left ventricular outflow leads to an increased left ventricular afterload and left ventricular wall stress, elevated left ventricular systolic and diastolic pressures, decreased aortic pressure, and prolonged left ventricular ejection time. Over time, this results in compensatory concentric left ventricular hypertrophy (LVH) to maintain ejection fraction. In patients with chronic severe AS, this compensatory mechanism may become insufficient, leading to gradual dilation and thinning of the left ventricle, and result in a decrease in ejection fraction and in congestive heart failure.

Myocardial oxygen supply and demand is also altered in AS. LVH, increased systolic pressure, and prolonged ejection time result in increased myocardial oxygen demand. Increased diastolic pressure and prolonged systolic ejection time result in decreased diastolic and myocardial perfusion time and hence myocardial oxygen supply. The alteration in myocardial oxygen supply and demand is the underlying mechanism behind myocardial ischemia in patients with AS, even in the absence of coronary artery disease.

TABLE 77-1 Severity of Aortic Stenosis According to Echocardiographic Criteria

Parameter	Mild	Moderate	Severe
Aortic valve area (cm^2)	1.6-2.5	1.1-1.5	≤1.0
Mean pressure gradient (mm Hg)	<20	20-39	≥40
Aortic jet velocity (m/sec)	2.0-2.9	3.0-3.9	≥4.0

From Nishimura RA, Otto CM, Bonow RO, et al: 2014 AHA/ACC guideline for the management of patients with valvular heart disease: a report of the American College of Cardiology/American Heart Association Task Force on Practice Guidelines. Circulation 129:e521–643, 2014.

Clinical Features

The classic symptoms of AS are angina, exertional syncope, and symptoms of congestive heart failure such as shortness of breath. The mechanisms for angina and congestive heart failure are explained in the previous section. The mechanism for syncope is likely related to the blunting of exercise-induced augmentation in stroke volume as a result of outflow obstruction coupled with exercise-induced peripheral vasodilation. These changes cause a drop in systemic blood pressure leading to cerebral hypoperfusion and syncope.

The classic physical finding is a crescendo-decrescendo systolic ejection murmur heard best at the second right intercostal space, which may variably radiate to the carotid arteries. A palpable thrill may be present in severe cases of AS. Palpation of the arterial pulse may reveal a weak and delayed pulse known as *pulsus parvus et tardus*.

Diagnosis and Grading

Two-dimensional transthoracic echocardiography is the most common modality for the diagnosis and grading of AS (Table 77-1). In most patients, this modality can reliably establish aortic jet velocity, aortic valve peak and mean gradients, and aortic valve area.

Natural History

Without intervention, symptomatic AS has dismal outcomes. Multiple studies consistently reported survivals of 3 years for angina and syncope and 1.5 to 2 years for dyspnea and heart failure.[2] These findings have driven recommendations for early surgical intervention in patients with symptomatic AS. One third of asymptomatic patients with severe AS will become symptomatic in 2 years with an estimated cardiac death of less than 1% each year to 5% each year.[3] Patients with higher grades of AS severity seem to progress at a faster rate than lower grades of AS. After AS becomes moderate, aortic valve area decreases on average by 0.1 cm^2 per year, the pressure gradient across the valve rises on average by 7 mm Hg per year, and the jet velocity increases by 0.3 m/sec per year.[4-7]

Indications for Surgery

The class I recommendations for aortic valve replacement (AVR) in patients with AS according to the American College of Cardiology (ACC) and the American Heart Association (AHA)[1] are the following:

1. Symptomatic patients with severe AS
2. Patients with severe AS undergoing concomitant coronary artery bypass graft (CABG) surgery, heart valve surgery, or aortic surgery
3. Patients with severe AS and left ventricular systolic dysfunction (ejection fraction < 50%)

The class IIa recommendations[1] for AVR are the following:

1. Asymptomatic patients with very severe AS (aortic jet velocity ≥ 5.0 m/sec or mean pressure gradient ≥ 60 mm Hg) and low surgical risk
2. Apparently asymptomatic patients with severe AS and an exercise test demonstrating decreased exercise tolerance or a fall in systolic blood pressure
3. Symptomatic patients with low-flow/low-gradient severe AS with reduced LVEF (resting valve area ≤ 1.0 cm^2, aortic jet velocity < 4.0 m/sec or mean pressure gradient < 40 mm Hg, LVEF < 50%, and low-dose dobutamine stress study showing an aortic jet velocity ≥ 4.0 m/sec mean pressure gradient ≥ 40 mm Hg with a valve area ≤ 1.0 cm^2)
4. Symptomatic patients with low-flow/low-gradient severe AS with an LVEF ≥ 50%, a calcified aortic valve with significantly reduced leaflet motion, and a valve area ≤ 1.0 cm^2 only if clinical, hemodynamic, and anatomic data support valve obstruction as the most likely cause of symptoms and data recorded when the patient is normotensive (systolic blood pressure < 140 mm Hg) indicate an aortic jet velocity < 4.0 m/sec or mean pressure gradient < 40 mm Hg, and a stroke volume index < 35 mL/m^2, and an indexed valve area ≤ 0.6 cm^2/m^2.
5. Patients with moderate AS who are undergoing cardiac surgery for another indication.

The class IIb recommendation[1] for AVR is the following:

1. Asymptomatic patients with severe AS if the patient is at low surgical risk and serial testing shows an increase in aortic velocity of ≥ 0.3 m/sec per year.

AORTIC REGURGITATION

Isolated aortic regurgitation is the primary lesion for patients undergoing AVR in only a minority of patients (≈10% to 15%). Aortic valve repair is emerging as an attractive alternative to replacement in selected patients with aortic regurgitation. The details of epidemiology, pathophysiology, diagnosis, and treatment of aortic regurgitation are reviewed in the chapter on aortic valve repair.

AORTIC VALVE REPLACEMENT

Operative Techniques

The traditional and most common approach for an AVR is through a median sternotomy. After exposure of the heart, the patient is heparinized and cannulated. An aortic cannula is placed in the distal ascending aorta, and a two-staged venous cannula is placed in the right atrium. Aortic calcification may preclude safe ascending aortic cannulation, and alternative arterial cannulation, including femoral or axillary cannulation, may be considered. Deep hypothermia and circulatory arrest for management of the heavily calcified ascending aorta have been used, but they carry a significant risk of stroke. Alternate venous cannulation may be used if required for other concomitant procedures. Antegrade cardioplegia is typically used. However, retrograde cardioplegia delivery through the coronary sinus may be useful in the setting of severe aortic regurgitation, coronary disease, or LVH to supplement myocardial protection. A vent is placed through the right superior pulmonary vein. Following initiation of cardiopulmonary bypass and cardioplegic arrest, additional cardioplegia doses may be delivered in a retrograde fashion or directly through the coronary ostia. Patients with AS often have ventricular hypertrophy and may require larger cardioplegia volumes.

The aortotomy is started anteriorly and may be performed in a transverse fashion (in a plane parallel to and approximately 1 cm above the sinotubular junction) or may be an oblique one (starting with a transverse incision above the right coronary, but extending through the sinotubular junction and into the noncoronary sinus). Sufficient distance should be maintained from the right coronary artery to prevent injury during closure.

Retraction sutures are placed in the aortic wall above each commissure, and the distal aorta is retracted cephalad to facilitate exposure (Fig. 77-1). Valve excision is performed one cusp at a time, starting at the commissure between the right and noncoronary cusps and excising the right coronary cusp (Fig. 77-2). Next, the left coronary cusp is excised starting at the commissure between the left and right coronary cusps. The noncoronary cusp is then excised starting at the commissure between the left and noncoronary cusps. Use of a #11 blade for leaflet excision can permit complete decalcification by cutting around rather than through the calcified regions. Alternatively, after the valve is excised, débridement of calcium from the annulus is performed using forceps and rongeur. After satisfactory decalcification, the aortic root, ascending aorta, and left ventricle are irrigated to remove all free calcium deposits. During irrigation, care should be taken to prevent embolization of calcific debris into the coronary ostia.

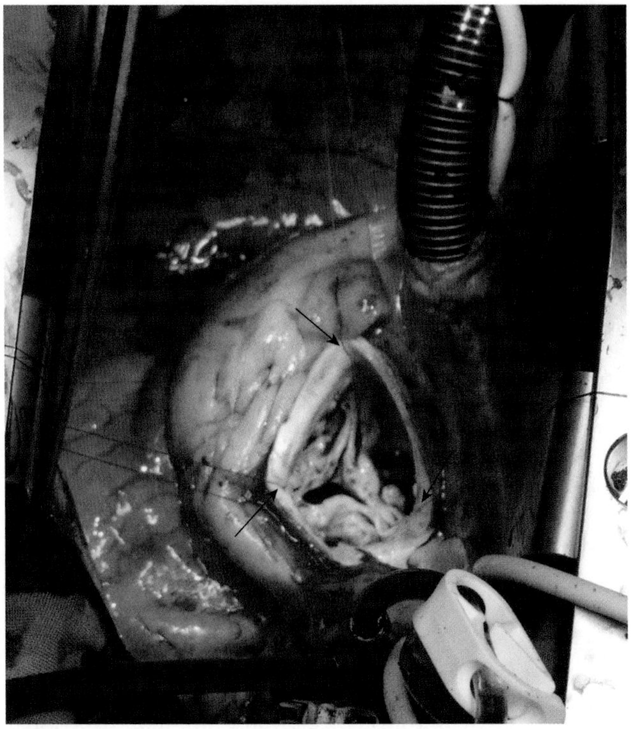

FIGURE 77-1 ■ Aortic valve exposure through a transverse aortotomy aided by three commissural sutures *(arrows)* and a suture retracting the distal portion of the ascending aorta cephalad.

Sizing may be performed before or after leaflet excision. In nondilated aortic roots, the sinotubular junction is typically the limiting factor in choosing the largest possible valve. The annulus is measured using commercial valve sizers, and an appropriate-sized valve is used (Fig. 77-3). If the annulus is too small, aortic root enlargement techniques may have to be performed (see next section).

There are two techniques to implant the valve: the continuous and the interrupted suture techniques. The continuous suture technique has fewer knots, which may save time and minimize foreign material left behind. Larger prosthesis may be implanted, as there is less "purse-stringing" effect on the tissues of the aortic root. However, this technique may be problematic if the aortic annulus is fragile or heavily calcified, or if there is suture dehiscence or breakage. The interrupted suture technique (Fig. 77-4) without the use of pledgets is our standard for implantation because it provides the maximum strength for prosthetic attachment, minimizes foreign material, allows placement of the largest possible

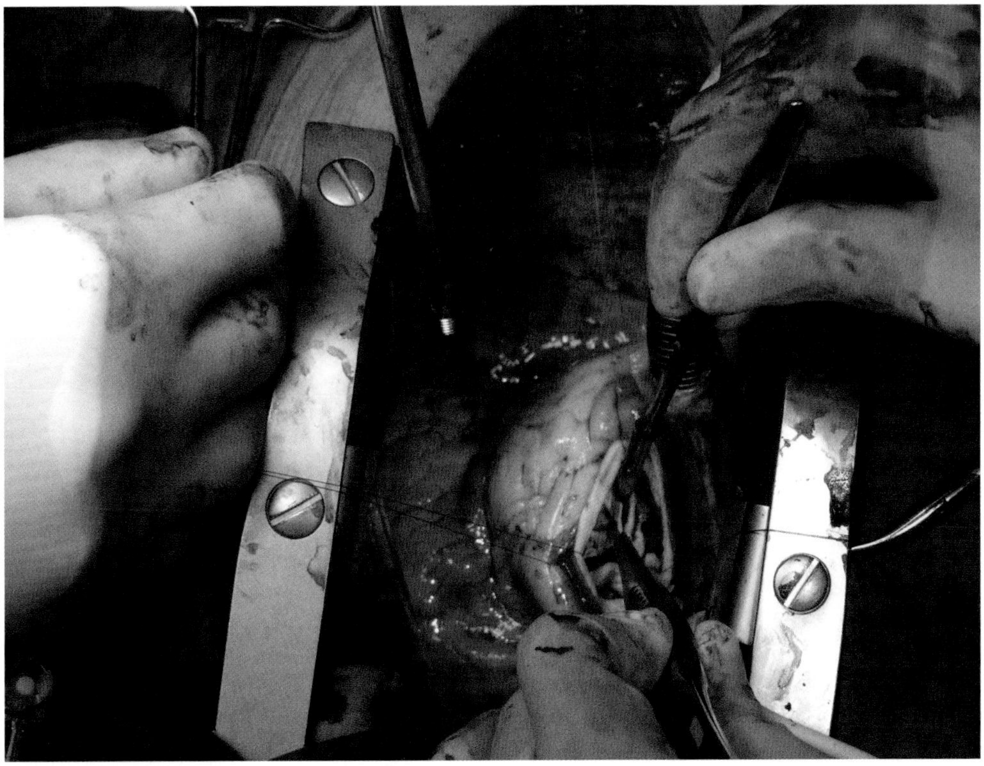

FIGURE 77-2 ■ Sharp excision of the aortic valve is performed using a #11 blade, starting with the right coronary cusp.

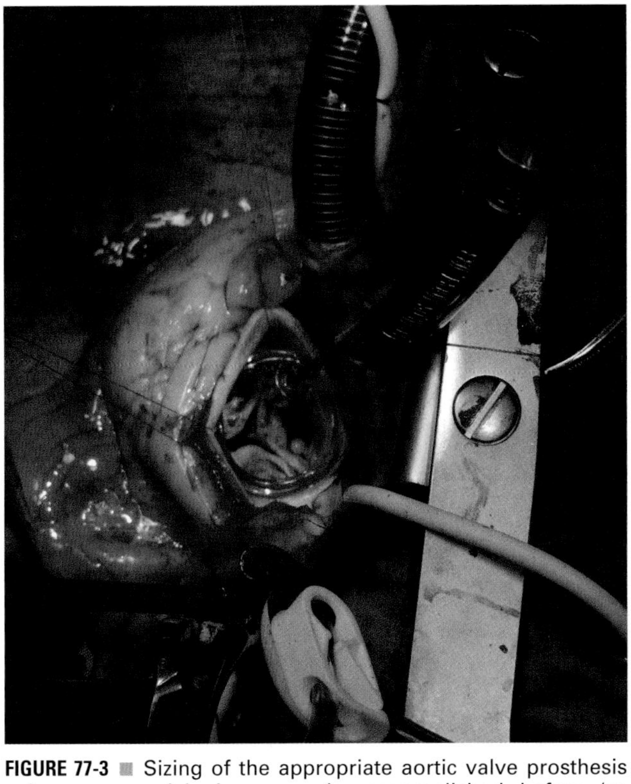

FIGURE 77-3 ■ Sizing of the appropriate aortic valve prosthesis using commercial sizers can be accomplished before (as depicted in this picture) or after valve excision.

prosthesis, and has low risk of paravalvular leak. Alternately colored, double-needle, 2-0 nonabsorbable, braided sutures are passed through the sewing ring of the prosthetic valve, and then through the native aortic annulus, from the ventricular to the aortic side, starting with the left coronary region, followed by the right coronary region, and then the noncoronary region (see Figs. 77-4 and 77-5). The sutures alternate in color (green and white) to simplify identification. Pledgets may be used if the aortic annulus is particularly fragile. The pledgets, using a horizontal mattress technique, are placed below the annulus, allowing the valve to sit above the annulus. The sutures are then passed through the sewing ring of the prosthetic valve, with attention paid to symmetrical spacing around the prosthetic valve. Alternatively, the needles are passed from above to below the annulus, placing the pledgets above and the valve below the annulus. Supra-annular positioning of the valve allows for a larger valve to be used. Great care must be exercised and judicious needle bites taken between the noncoronary and right coronary annuli and near the left coronary annulus because deep bites in these areas may cause heart block and left coronary artery injury, respectively.

After the valve is parachuted down (Fig. 77-6), all the sutures are then tied systematically starting with the left coronary cusp, followed by the right coronary cusp, and finally the noncoronary cusp (Fig. 77-7). The aortotomy is then closed in two layers using two running double-needle polypropylene sutures (Fig. 77-8). If the aortic tissue is thin and friable, Teflon felt or autologous pericardial strips may be used to reinforce the closure.

After the aortotomy is closed, de-airing maneuvers are performed. The aortic root vent is turned on, volume is

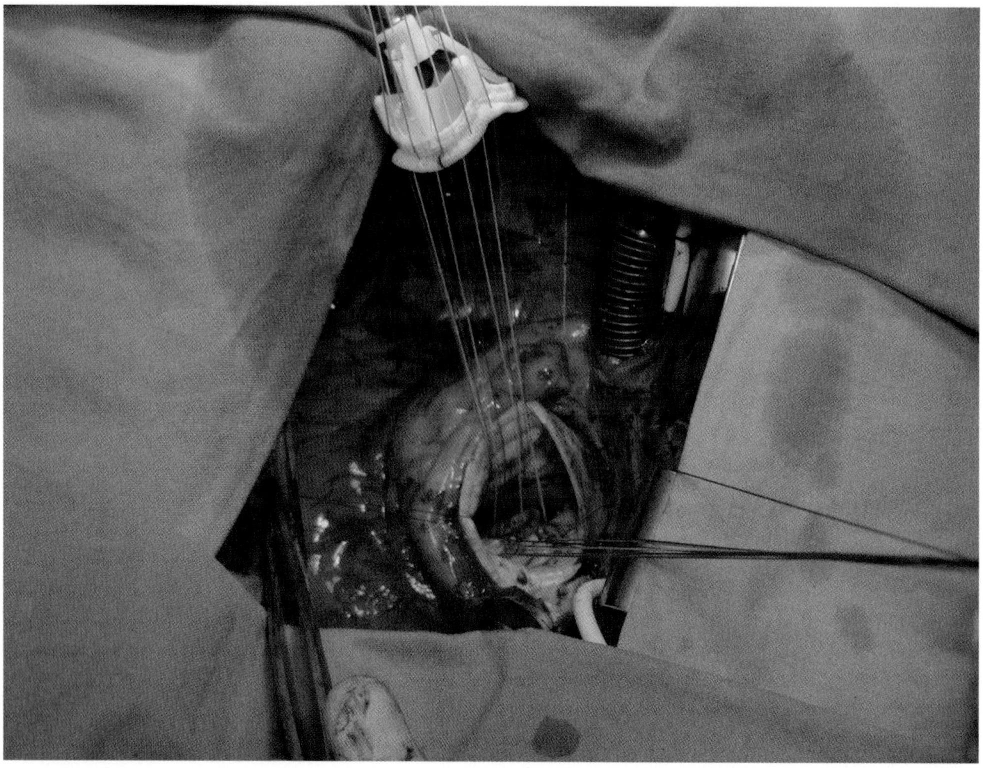

FIGURE 77-4 ■ Alternating green and white valve sutures are systematically passed through the aortic valve annulus and then through the sewing ring of the prosthetic valve traveling from the commissure between the left and right coronary cusps to the commissure between the left coronary and noncoronary cusps.

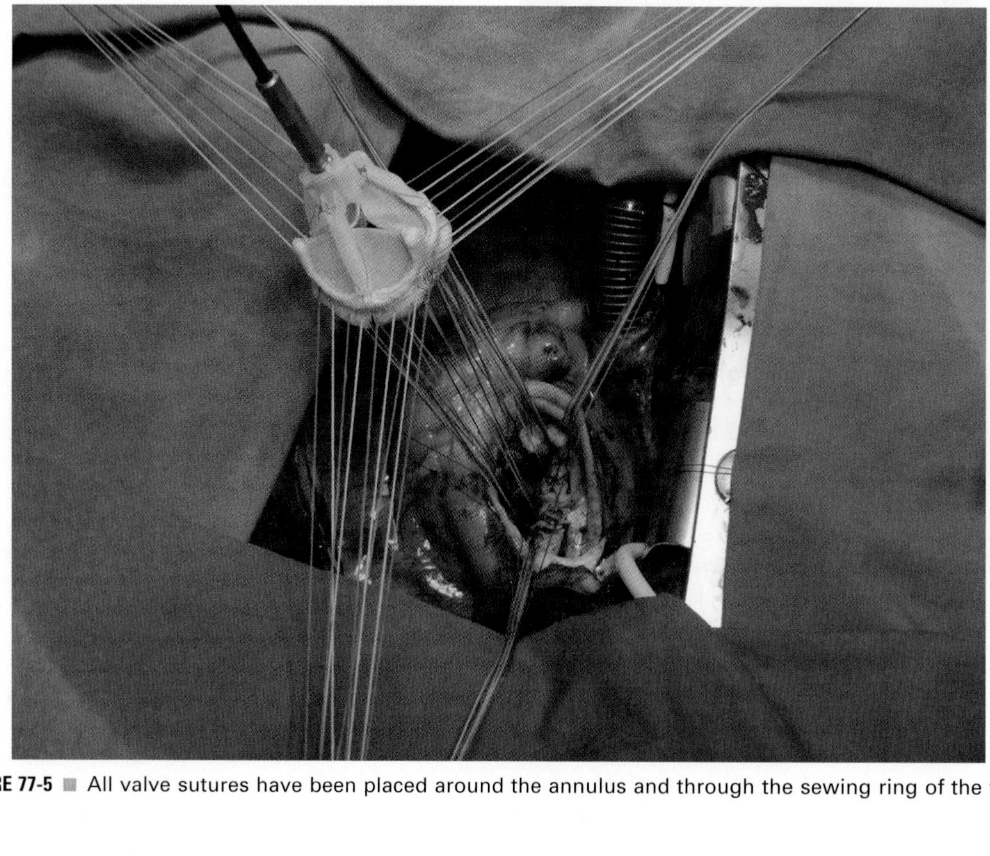

FIGURE 77-5 ■ All valve sutures have been placed around the annulus and through the sewing ring of the valve.

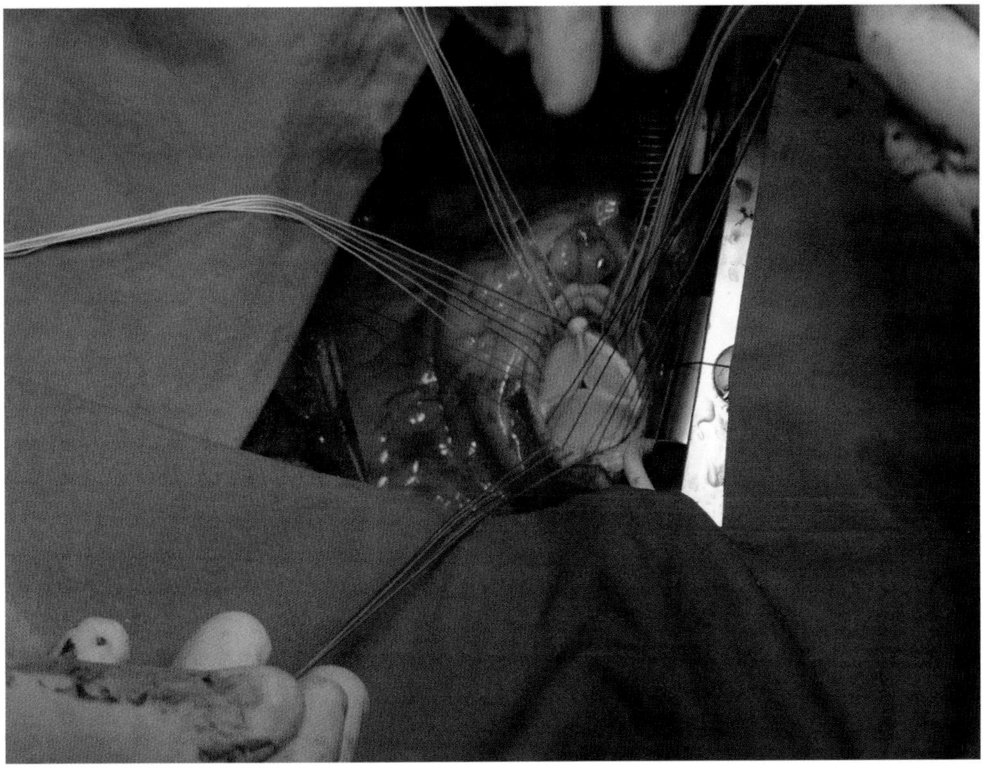

FIGURE 77-6 ■ The prosthetic valve is parachuted down into position by the surgeon who holds one set of valve sutures and the prosthetic valve along with the valve holder. The assistant holds the other two sets of valve sutures. The surgeon and assistant pull on the valve sutures while the surgeon parachutes the valve down into position.

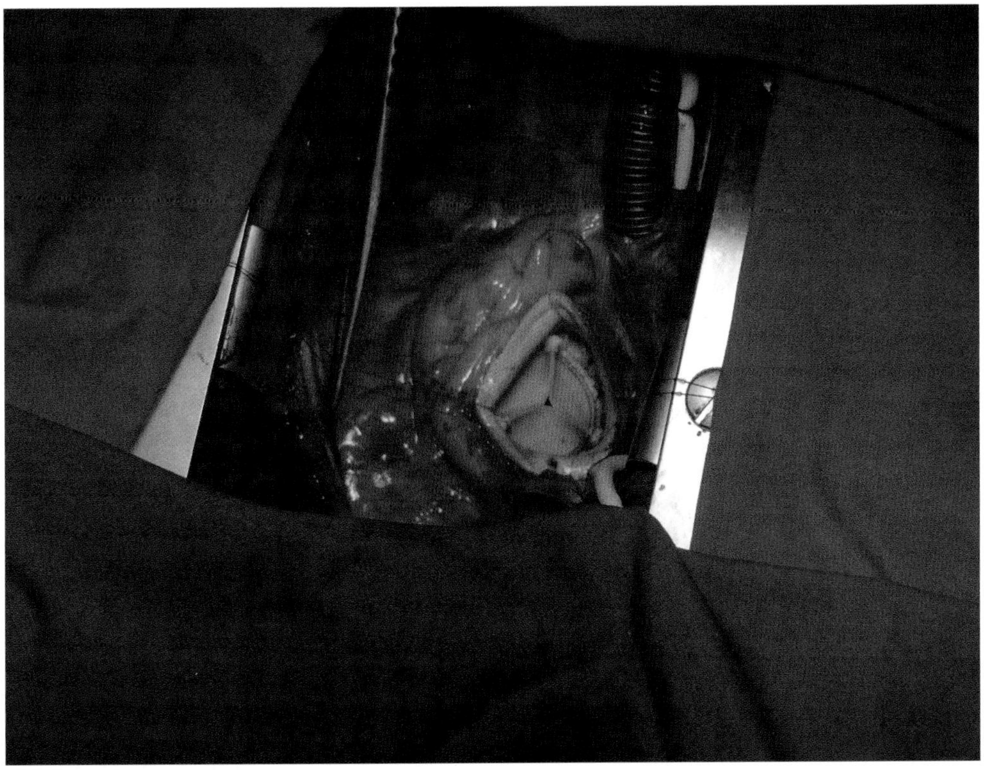

FIGURE 77-7 ■ Picture of prosthetic aortic valve in position after tying all valve sutures systematically beginning with the left coronary cusp, followed by the right coronary cusp, and then the noncoronary cusp.

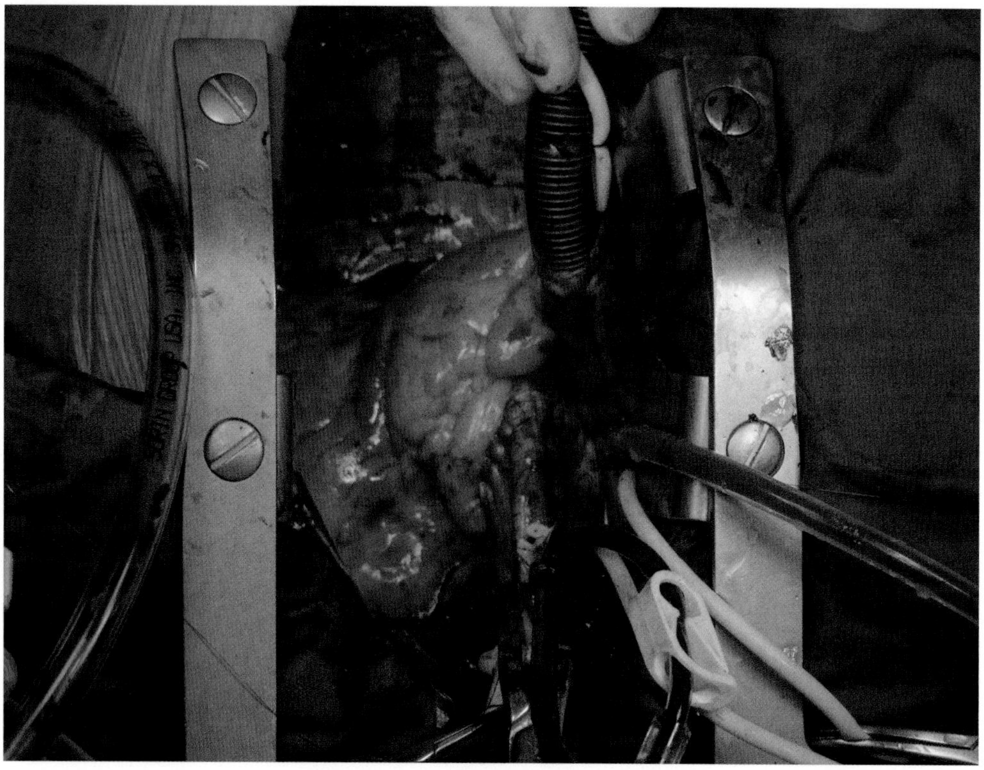

FIGURE 77-8 ■ Closure of the aortotomy can be performed using a one- (depicted in picture) or two-layer technique.

added to the heart, the pulmonary vent is temporarily turned off, the lungs are ventilated, and the left ventricle is gently massaged to displace the intracardiac air into the aortic root vent. After placing the patient in Trendelenburg position, the aortic cross-clamp is removed and the pulmonary vent resumed.

Using transesophageal echocardiography (TEE), paravalvular leak is ruled out, hemodynamic performance of the valve is assessed, and any remaining intracavitary air is detected and removed using additional de-airing maneuvers such as digitally tapping areas found to have a collection of air on TEE or allowing the heart to eject with the aortic root vent on suction. Alternatively, a needle can be used to aspirate the air through the left ventricular apex. All patients undergoing an AVR should receive both atrial and ventricular temporary pacing wires, as there is higher risk of atrioventricular blocks and other arrhythmias following this surgery. The patient is weaned from cardiopulmonary bypass, heparin is reversed with protamine, the cannulae are removed, and the incisions are closed in the usual fashion.

Aortic Root Enlargement

In patients with a small aortic annulus, implanting a small stented bioprosthetic valve or a mechanical valve may leave residual gradient across the aortic valve. Forcing a small prosthetic valve may result in perivalvular leak or disruption of the aorta or left ventricle. Ideally, the patient with a small aortic annulus should be identified preoperatively for optimal planning. However, in some cases precise sizing can only be achieved intraoperatively. If there is a concern about the possibility of prosthesis-patient mismatch (see later), a root enlargement procedure may be performed. Alternatively, stentless tissue valves or mechanical valves, which have larger effective orifice areas, may be used.

Three different aortic root enlargement techniques have been described. Posterior enlargement of the aortic root (Fig. 77-9) is performed by either the Nicks-Nunez[8] or the Rittenhouse-Manouguian[9] technique, whereas anterior enlargement is performed using the Konno-Rastan[10,11] aortoventriculoplasty technique.

Nicks-Nunez Technique

The Nicks-Nunez method (Fig. 77-10) of aortic root enlargement involves a vertical incision through the commissure between the left coronary and noncoronary cusp and extending down in the interleaflet triangle, followed by patch reconstruction of the aortic root. This method can enlarge the aortic root by 2-3 mm. If larger enlargement is needed, the incision must be extended beyond the interleaflet triangle into the anterior leaflet of the mitral valve and the left atrial roof. After making the incision, either an autologous pericardium or a prosthetic patch is fashioned into a diamond shape. One end of the patch is sewed onto the deep end of the enlarging incision at the level of the aortic-mitral continuity if the incision stopped at the interleaflet triangle. Interrupted pledgeted horizontal mattress sutures are used at the interleaflet triangle and the needles are passed through the sewing ring of the prosthetic valve. The rest of the valve sutures are placed through the aortic annulus as described above.

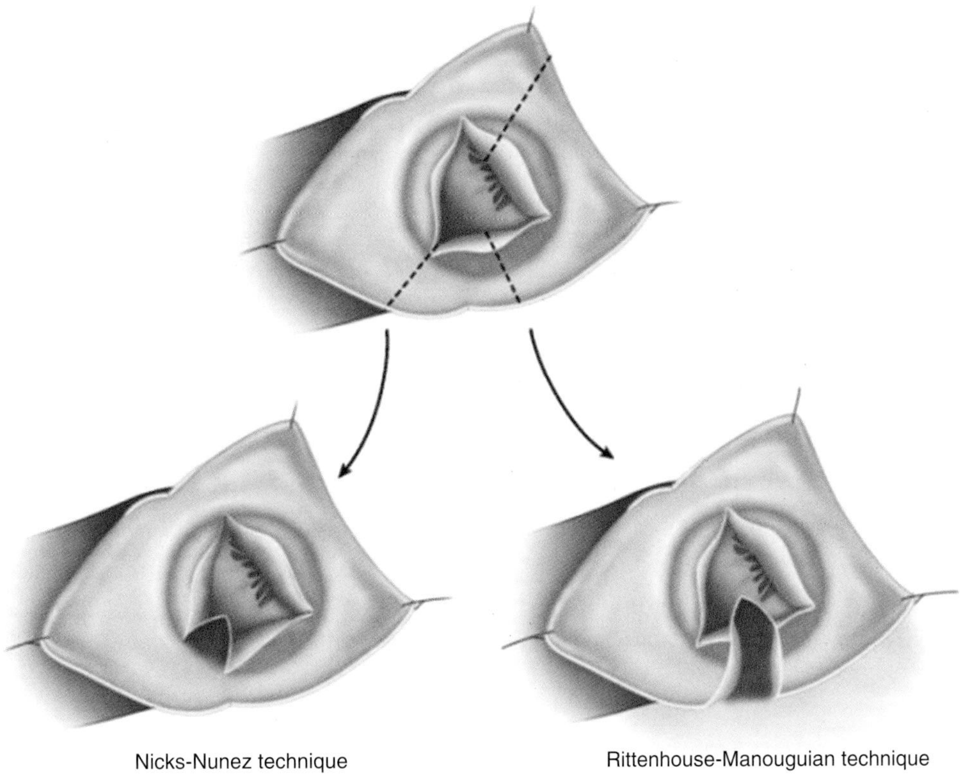

FIGURE 77-9 ■ Posterior enlargement of the aortic root using either the Nicks-Nunez or the Rittenhouse-Manouguian technique.

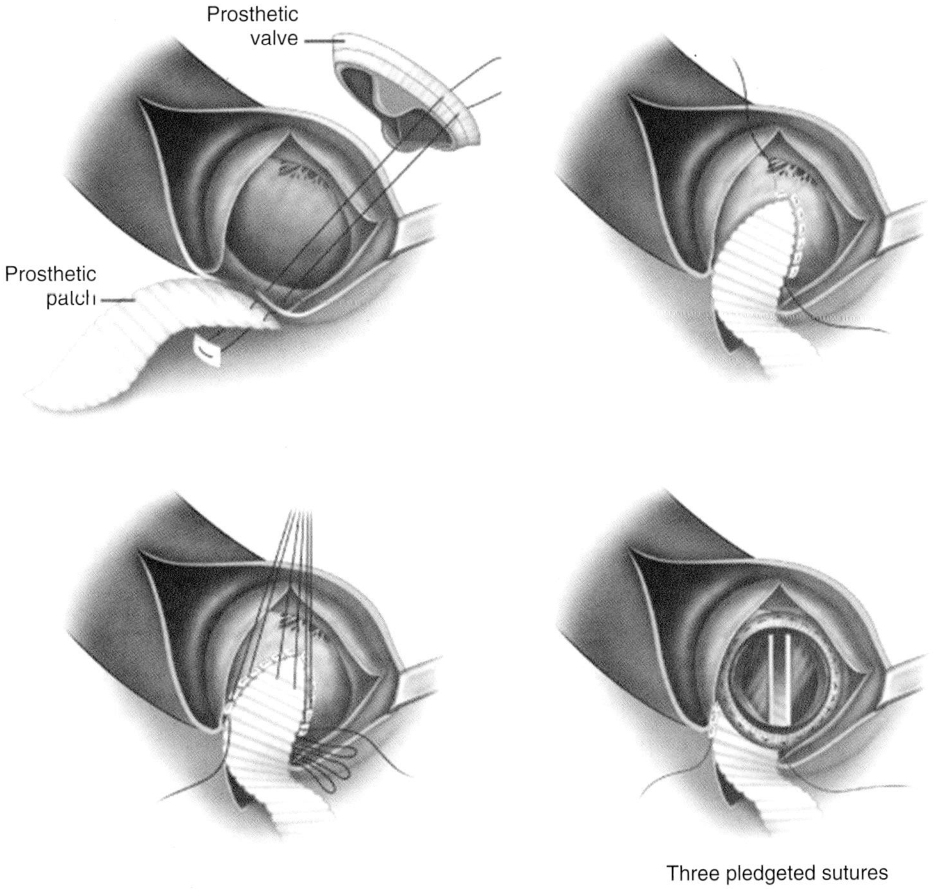

FIGURE 77-10 ■ A diamond-shaped patch of autologous pericardium or prosthetic material is fashioned. One end of the patch is inserted into the distal end of the enlargement using interrupted sutures with pledgets. At the level of the aortic annulus the sutures are passed through the sewing ring of the prosthetic valve. The remainder of the valve sutures are placed through the aortic annulus in a standard fashion.

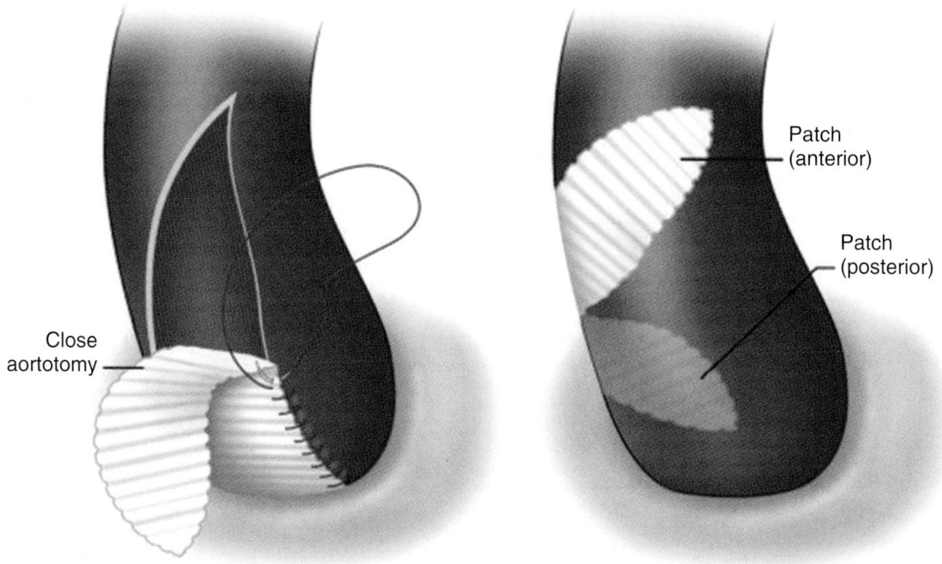

FIGURE 77-11 ■ The diamond patch is then tailored for closure of the aortotomy. If a transverse aortotomy is used, then the patch is transected at the level of the transverse aortotomy and incorporated as part of the anastomosis of the aortic root to the ascending aorta.

If the enlarging incision was extended onto the anterior leaflet of the mitral valve and the left atrium, the diamond-shaped patch is similarly first sewed at the deepest end of the incision, repairing the mitral leaflet. Interrupted sutures without pledgets are used for the mitral leaflet portion. At the level of the annulus, interrupted pledgeted horizontal mattress sutures are passed through the annulus, then the patch, and lastly into the sewing ring of the prosthetic valve. After the valve is tied down, the remaining proximal end of the patch is tailored to close the aortotomy if an oblique incision is used (Fig. 77-11), or cut flat at the level of the transverse aortotomy and incorporated into the anastomosis of the ascending aorta to the aortic root.

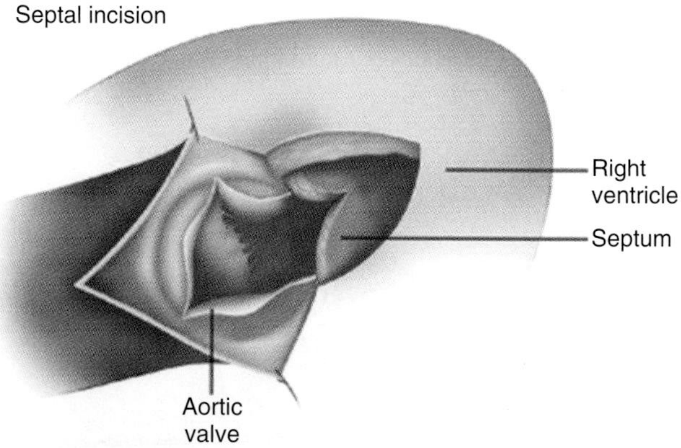

FIGURE 77-12 ■ In the Konno-Rastan method of aortic root enlargement, an incision is made through the right coronary region of the aortic annulus, near the commissure between the left and right coronary cusps. The incision is carried further into the interventricular septum, and a similar incision is made on the right ventricular free wall.

Rittenhouse-Manouguian Technique

The Rittenhouse-Manouguian method of aortic root enlargement involves a vertical incision through the middle of the noncoronary sinus extending through the annulus and into the anterior leaflet of the mitral valve. After the incision is made, the patch reconstruction is similar to the Nick-Nunez technique described in the previous paragraph.

Konno-Rastan Technique

The Konno-Rastan method of aortic root enlargement is an anterior root enlargement technique, or aortoventriculoplasty, whereby a vertical aortotomy is extended into the right coronary sinus left of the right coronary artery, through the aortic annulus near the commissure between the right and left coronary cusps, and into the interventricular septum. A second incision is performed on the right ventricular free wall (Fig. 77-12). After the two incisions are made, a diamond- and a triangle-shaped patch are fashioned. One end of the diamond patch is sewed to the deep end of the incision in a continuous fashion to repair the interventricular septum up to the level of the aortic annulus (Fig. 77-13). Then the base of the triangular patch is attached using interrupted pledgeted mattress sutures to the diamond patch at the level of the annulus. The same sutures are also passed through the sewing ring of the prosthetic valve (Fig. 77-14). The rest of the valve sutures are placed through the valve annulus as described above. The triangular patch is then folded to cover the right ventricular outflow tract defect and sewed using continuous running suture. Finally, the left ventricular outflow tract patch is used to close the vertical aortotomy using continuous suture technique (Fig. 77-15).

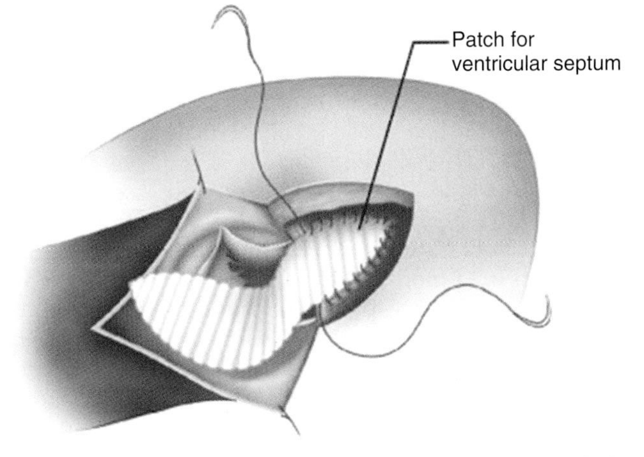

FIGURE 77-13 ■ One end of a diamond patch is sewed to the deep end of the incision in a continuous fashion to repair the interventricular septum up to the level of the aortic annulus.

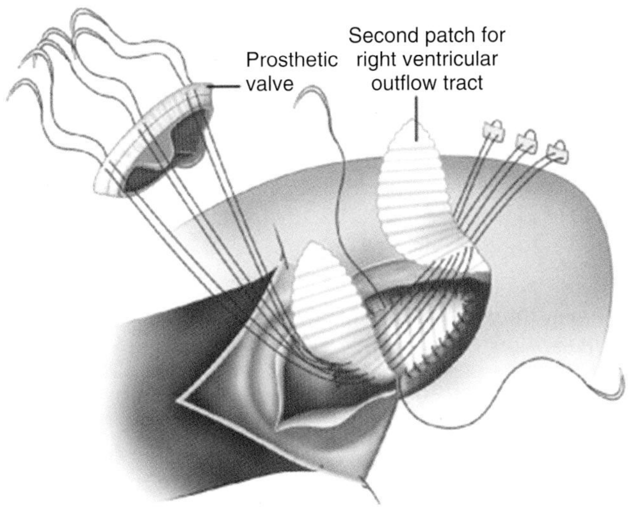

FIGURE 77-14 ■ The base of a triangular patch is attached using interrupted pledgeted mattress sutures to the diamond patch at the level of the annulus. The same sutures are also passed through the sewing ring of the prosthetic valve.

SPECIAL CONSIDERATIONS OF POSTOPERATIVE CARE

Postoperative care after AVR is similar to that of other types of cardiac surgery in most regards. However, one important factor to consider is that patients with AS commonly present with LVH, causing decreased left ventricular compliance. Reduction in compliance that occurs during cardiac surgery exacerbates the situation. Therefore, the left ventricle is highly dependent on higher than usual preload for sufficient filling. To that end, filling pressures (central venous pressure) should be kept between 15 and 18 mm Hg with intravenous volume infusions, rather than the usually accepted 8 to 10 mm Hg pressures. Atrial fibrillation, with consequent loss of atrial contractility, is less tolerated in these patients because they are losing up to 20% of their ventricular filling. Rhythm control strategies may be more beneficial in these patients.

OUTCOMES

Early Mortality

Early mortality after AVR is most commonly related to acute cardiac failure, neurologic complications, hemorrhage, and infection. The Society of Thoracic Surgeons (STS) National Database reports a 3.2% 30-day mortality for isolated AVR.[12] When adding CABG, mortality rises to 5.6%.[13] Although, in the past, isolated reoperative AVR increased the risk of early mortality,[14,15] it does not appear to do so in the current era.[14] Early mortality has improved with time and continues to do so. In the 1990s early mortality for isolated AVR was approximately 4.3%[15] compared with the more contemporary 3.2%.[12] Similarly, the early mortality of combined AVR and CABG improved significantly with time from 8.0%[15] to 5.6%.[13] Double valve surgery, including an AVR and either mitral valve or tricuspid valve replacement, raises the operative mortality to 11% to 14%.[16] Triple valve

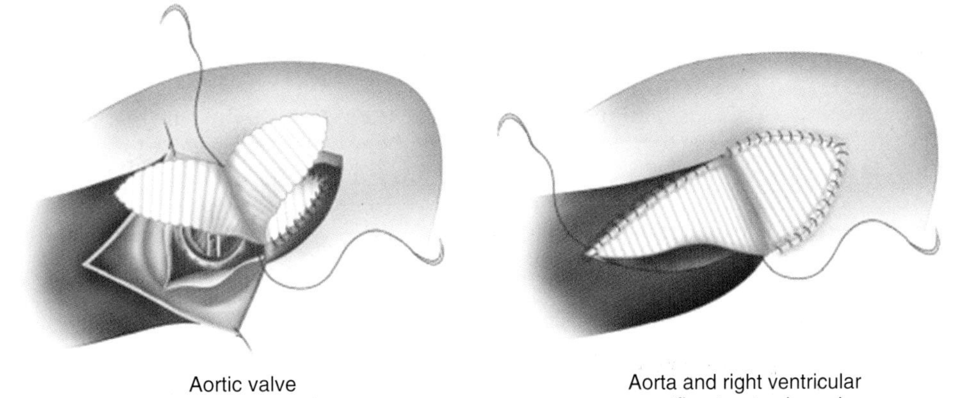

FIGURE 77-15 ■ The triangular patch is then folded to cover the right ventricular outflow tract defect and sewed using continuous running suture. The left ventricular outflow tract patch is finally used to close the vertical aortotomy using continuous suture technique.

surgery, including AVR, mitral valve replacement, and tricuspid valve replacement, raises the operative mortality rate to higher than 15%.[16] Risk factors for early mortality include increasing age, higher New York Heart Association (NYHA) functional class, LVH, left ventricular enlargement, presence of aortic regurgitation, renal dysfunction, severe chronic obstructive pulmonary disease (COPD), multiple reoperations, and concomitant CABG or heart valve surgery.[17-21]

Long-Term Survival

Late mortality can be divided into valve-related mortality and non–valve-related cardiac mortality. The former includes deaths caused by structural valve deterioration, nonstructural valve dysfunction, valve thromboembolism, bleeding, valve endocarditis, death related to a reoperation on an operated valve, or sudden and unexpected death in a patient with an operated valve. Non–valve-related mortality comprises other cardiac causes of death, such as progressive heart failure in a patient with a well-functioning prosthetic valve.[22] The latter makes up 63% of all deaths in patients with mechanical valves and 59% of all deaths in patients with bioprosthetic valves at 15 years.[23] Although there does not appear to be a survival difference between patients with bioprosthetic and mechanical aortic valves at 10 years,[24] structural bioprosthetic valve deterioration leads to a survival benefit for patients with mechanical valves at 15 years follow-up.[23] In contrast, other research has shown that even at 15, 20, and 25 years, there is no survival difference between patients who receive bioprosthetic versus mechanical valves in the aortic position.[15,21] Risk factors for late mortality include increasing age, higher NYHA functional class, LVH, left ventricular enlargement, left ventricular dysfunction, increased left atrial size, functional mitral regurgitation, atrial fibrillation, ventricular arrhythmia, renal dysfunction, diabetes mellitus, peripheral arterial disease, female gender, smoking, severe COPD, multiple cardiac reoperations, and concomitant CABG or heart valve surgery.[17-21,25-27]

Early Complications

Neurologic Complications

The joint Society of Thoracic Surgeons/American Association for Thoracic Surgery (STS/AATS) panel subclassified cerebral embolic events into transient ischemic attacks (TIAs), which are fully reversible neurologic events lasting less than 24 hours; reversible ischemic neurologic deficit, which are fully reversible neurologic events lasting between 24 hours and 3 weeks; and strokes, which are nonreversible neurologic deficits lasting longer than 3 weeks.[22] The rate of stroke for isolated AVR, according to the STS database, is 1.5%.[12] In high-risk (STS predicted risk of mortality > 10%) and older patients (>80 years old), the risk of stroke rises to between 2% and 4.4%.[28-31] The addition of CABG to the AVR also raises the risk to between 4.9% and 5.8%.[32,33] Risk factors for early postoperative stroke include low LVEF (<40%), ascending aortic calcification, older than 70 years, female sex, diabetes mellitus, bypass time greater than 120 minutes, a history of stroke, carotid artery disease, and walking less than 300 meters during a 6-minute walk test.[34-41] The annual rate of late stroke is 1.3% and 1.4% for bioprosthetic and mechanical valves, respectively. Risk factors for late stroke include female sex, older than 75 years, atrial fibrillation, current or previous smoking, diabetes mellitus, and carotid artery disease.[42,43] Most postoperative strokes (55% to 76%) occur within the first 24 to 48 hours after surgery, but the high-risk period likely lasts for 3 months after surgery.[38,44-47] Postoperative stroke is a significant predictor of mortality, raising the mortality rate to 31% for those with early stroke (<24 h) and 14% for those with late stroke (>24 h) compared with the baseline 4.6% mortality rate in one study.[38] Although early strokes seem to be related to the operation, late strokes are more influenced by patient- and disease-related factors.[47]

Approximately one third of patients who have undergone cardiac surgery experience postoperative delirium.[48] Preexisting organic mental disorders, significant prior alcohol consumption, advanced age, intracranial cerebral artery disease, and longer cardiopulmonary bypass time are risk factors for postoperative delirium.[48,49] Perioperative medications such as opiates and sedatives are known contributors as well.[49]

In one study, postoperative neurocognitive deficits detected on neuropsychiatric testing were identified in 38% of patients at discharge and 19% of patients at 3 months. These changes were not associated with clinically important differences in outcome or in quality of life.[50]

Heart Block and Permanent Pacemaker Implantation

Atrioventricular node block occurs more frequently after heart valve surgery compared with other types of cardiac surgery, with 3% to 8% of patients requiring permanent pacemaker insertion.[30,51,52] It is rather a unique feature of valve surgery, and it is because of the close proximity of the conduction system to the aortic valve in the area of the membranous septum. Judicious decalcification must be exercised and shallower needle bites must be taken at the level of the commissure between the noncoronary and right coronary cusps. Heart block may be transient because of edema of the tissues around the conduction system. However, if a patient remains pacer-dependent 7 to 10 days postoperatively, we recommend a permanent pacemaker insertion. Predictors of complete heart block and permanent pacemaker insertion include preoperative first-degree atrioventricular block or bundle branch block, postoperative cardiac arrest, combined aortic and mitral valve surgery, and infective endocarditis.[52] The type of aortic valve prosthesis used was not an important predictor in one study.[52]

Late Complications

Thromboembolism, Anticoagulation, and Bleeding Complications

Beyond the 3-month period after surgery when the risk of thromboembolism and bleeding is highest, the risk of thromboembolism is approximately constant. The overall linearized rate of thromboembolism for mechanical aortic valves is quoted as 2 per 100 patient-years and approximately half of that for bioprosthetic aortic valves, according to one report.[53] In another report, the rates of thromboembolism are similar among various mechanical valves, ranging between 1.16% and 1.33%,[54] with one report quoting a lower rate for the On-X bileaflet mechanical valve (On-X Life Technologies Inc., Austin, TX) at 0.6% per year.[55] The rates are also comparable among different stented bioprosthetic valves, ranging between 0.78% and 1.22% per year.[54] However, the rate is much lower for allografts with a median of 0.23% per year.[54] Bleeding rates from anticoagulation appear to be independent of the prosthesis and range from 1% to 2% per year in a recent report.[54] Fluctuations in the international normalized ratio (INR) seem to be an important risk factor for both thromboembolic and bleeding events.[56,57] Therefore, close monitoring of the INR to minimize fluctuations may be important to prevent these complications.[57] New point-of-care home testing may aid in achieving this goal.[58] Anticoagulation with a minimum target INR of 2.0 to 3.0 for low-risk patients and valves with low thrombogenicity (bileaflet valves) is recommended for mechanical AVR.[59-61] However, interim results from the first limb of the Prospective Randomized On-X Anticoagulation Clinical Trial (PROACT) suggest that INR may be safely maintained between 1.5 and 2.0 with lower risk of bleeding and without a significant increase in thromboembolism.[62] The target INR should be 2.5 to 3.5 for patients at high risk for thromboembolism or who receive mechanical valves with high thrombogenicity (disc valves). For bioprosthetic AVR, the bulk of the evidence favors no anticoagulation in patients at low risk for thromboembolism because antiplatelet therapy suffices in this patient population.[46,63-70] The recommendations are shifting from anticoagulation in the first 3 months followed by antiplatelet therapy thereafter in low-risk patients to only antiplatelet therapy right after surgery.[59-61] Patients at high risk for thromboembolism should have a different consideration and anticoagulation may be warranted in this group.

Prosthesis thrombosis is a serious but rare complication of AVR that occurs in less than 0.2% of cases per year.[71] It is more common in mechanical valves. Although often ineffective, thrombolysis may be attempted in patients with heart failure caused by valve dysfunction and who are considered too high risk for surgery.[72] Surgical thrombectomy or re-replacement of the prosthetic valve is usually required and is associated with a high mortality rate of 10% to 15%.[71,72]

Prosthetic Valve Endocarditis

Prosthetic valve endocarditis (PVE) is a serious complication of AVR and is divided into early PVE if it occurs less than 60 days post implantation and late PVE if it occurs more than 60 days post implantation. The rate of PVE is approximately 0.5% to 1% per year, with a slightly higher rate in the first 6 to 12 months compared to less than 12 months.[73-76] Early PVE is usually a result of perioperative seeding of the prosthetic valve either intraoperatively or from wound infections or indwelling intravascular catheters postoperatively. Late PVE usually results from noncardiac sources of bacteremia or sometimes from insidious infections with less virulent organisms introduced perioperatively. The microbiological profile of early PVE includes *Staphylococcus aureus*, *S. epidermidis*, gram-negative bacteria, and fungal infections. For late PVE, the microbiological profile resembles that of native endocarditis and includes *Streptococcus* and *Staphylococcus* species. Patients presenting with fever after an AVR should be thoroughly investigated for PVE. Serial blood cultures and transthoracic or transesophageal echocardiography are important components of the diagnostic workup. Surgical indications for the management of PVE include early PVE, valve dysfunction including dehiscence or paravalvular leak, associated heart failure, presence of new conduction defect, abscess, aneurysm or fistula, persistent bacteremia despite maximum and appropriate medical therapy, vegetations larger than 10 mm in size, systemic embolization, all fungal infections, and virulent strains of *S. aureus*, *Serratia marcescens*, and *Pseudomonas aeruginosa*. The timing of surgery has been an area of debate. Sterilization of the valve is ideal before reoperation and is more likely if the vegetation is limited to the leaflets without annular involvement. Strokes from septic emboli are a common occurrence in patients with PVE, and differentiating ischemic stroke from hemorrhagic stroke is important because the former does not adversely affect outcome after reoperation whereas the latter does.[77] Computed tomography is an important modality in patients with neurologic signs or symptoms of stroke. The outcome following PVE is poor. Early PVE is associated with 30% to 80% mortality, whereas late PVE is associated with 20% to 40% mortality.[78]

Structural Valve Deterioration and Freedom from Reoperation

In the quest for the ideal valve, new valves are constantly being introduced to the market after testing and short-term clinical trials, making the choice between different valves for AVR a challenge. An in-depth discussion of the different valve types is found in Chapter 76. We limit the discussion in this section to structural valve deterioration (SVD) and freedom from reoperation of mechanical and bioprosthetic valves in the aortic position. Third-generation bileaflet mechanical valves have high structural integrity, and SVD is not observed or reported in several large series totaling more than 50,000 patient-years of follow-up.[79-82] The durability of these valves is excellent, resulting in a freedom from reoperation of approximately 94% at 10 years[82] and in one report up to 98% at 25 years after surgery.[79,83]

Glutaraldehyde-treated biological valves are subject to degenerative changes and calcification with time. Therapies to mitigate these processes help to slow down SVD and include using compounds such as surfactants, alpha oleic acid, and ethanol. The use of bioprosthetic valves has increased dramatically over the past couple of decades, increasing from 42% in 1996 to 82% in 2011.[84] Although the risk of thromboembolism and anticoagulation-related bleeding events is lower in bioprosthetic valves, the concern about higher rates of SVD and perhaps higher rates of PVE remains.[83] Surgeons must therefore balance between the risks and benefits of various valve choices. There is no convincing evidence to suggest that various second-generation pericardial and porcine bioprostheses differ in longevity; therefore, choice of the valve should depend on surgeon comfort and institutional preferences. Age is an important contributing factor to SVD in patients with bioprosthetic valves. Younger patients seem to have an accelerated rate of SVD probably as a result of a combination of factors, such as calcium metabolism and hemodynamics. In all series, patients older than 70 years have a greater than 90% freedom from reoperation at 15 to 25 years. This rate falls slowly in patients 60 to 70 years old, and precipitously in patients younger than 60 years.[85-96] Actuarial freedom from reoperation in these studies probably overestimates the rate of SVD compared with actual freedom. In a recent report, the reoperation rate was 4% at 25 years after bioprosthetic AVR, with 2.6% due to SVD.[88]

Paravalvular Leak and Hemolysis

The continuous suture technique of aortic valve implantation was traditionally thought to be a risk factor for paravalvular leak compared with an interrupted suture technique. However, recent reports show no difference in the rate of paravalvular leak between the two suture techniques.[97-99] In the absence of infection, important paravalvular leak in mechanical or bioprosthetic aortic valves is uncommon, although minor leaks may occur.[100] A contemporary report quotes a 0.01% annual rate.[79] If a paravalvular leak occurs, it can usually be detected in the first few months after surgery.[73] There may be an anatomic predisposition in the area extending from the right and noncoronary commissure to one third the distance along the right coronary cusp in one direction and two thirds the distance along the noncoronary cusp in the other direction.[101] Minor hemolysis may be managed conservatively, whereas clinically significant hemolysis requires surgical intervention.

Symptomatic Relief

Most surviving patients experience significant functional improvement after an AVR, with 70% to 90% of patients in NYHA functional classes II through IV becoming class I.[102] Even 10 years after surgery, 90% of patients remain in NYHA class I or II.

Left Ventricular Remodeling

Increased left ventricular mass (LVM) is a common occurrence later in patients with aortic valve disease, either through concentric LVH in AS or through left ventricular dilation and eccentric hypertrophy in aortic regurgitation. Increased LVM is a strong negative prognostic factor in aortic valve disease.[103,104] AVR relieves the left ventricular pressure and volume overload in AS and aortic regurgitation, allowing the left ventricular myocardium to remodel and the LVM to regress. Left ventricular remodeling occurs in the first 18 months after surgery but can last up to 5 years.[105-107] However, in patients with decreased left ventricular contractility, signifying late-stage aortic valve disease, or reduced exercise capacity preoperatively, remodeling may fail to occur.[106,108-111] Myocardial gene expression of microRNA-133a (miR-133a) is currently being explored as a potential predictor of left ventricular remodeling in patients with AS, with several reports demonstrating promising results.[112-114] Further research may clarify the role of miR-133a in AVR decision making, especially in asymptomatic patients with signs of LVH. The presence of prosthesis-patient mismatch may also hinder LVM regression, as discussed in the next subsection.

Prosthesis-Patient Mismatch

The theoretical goal of an AVR is to reduce the pressure and volume overload on the left ventricle. Although transprosthetic gradients postoperatively should be minimal to allow left ventricular remodeling, high gradients are occasionally seen despite an appropriately functioning valve. The persistence of left ventricular outflow obstruction postoperatively is termed *prosthesis-patient mismatch* (PPM).[115,116] The parameter that most consistently correlates with postoperative transprosthetic gradients is the effective orifice area (EOA) indexed to the patient's body surface area or, indexed effective orifice area (IEOA).[116] The EOA is measured by echocardiography using the continuity equation or by cardiac catheterization using the Gorlin formula. An IEOA of 0.65 to 0.85 cm^2/m^2 is generally defined as moderate PPM, and less than 0.65 cm^2/m^2 is defined as severe PPM. The prevalence of moderate PPM ranges from 20% to 70% and severe PPM ranges from 2% to 11%.[115] The significance of PPM is a controversial topic and may depend on the definition of PPM used in various studies. Some studies have shown that PPM does not influence mid-term and long-term survival or left ventricular mass at mid-term follow-up.[18,117,118] In contrast, other groups have shown that PPM after AVR is associated with less improvement in functional status, less regression of LVH, higher risk of congestive heart failure, and increased long-term mortality.[119-123] Patients with left ventricular dysfunction, including low-gradient AS, and younger patients (<60 years) who may be more active are particularly susceptible to PPM.[119,124-127] Several options exist if a surgeon anticipates PPM in a large patient with a small aortic annulus. In young active patients or patients with left ventricular dysfunction (ejection fraction < 50%) choosing prosthetic valves with larger IEOAs according to manufacturer-available user-friendly charts is one option. Aortic root enlargement is another method to allow for the implantation of larger prosthetic valve sizes. However, in older and sedentary patients, the extra risk in performing aortic root enlargement may not be worth the benefit of the extra valve size, and a certain amount of PPM may need to be accepted.[128]

REFERENCES

1. Nishimura RA, Otto CM, Bonow RO, et al: 2014 AHA/ACC guideline for the management of patients with valvular heart

disease: a report of the American College of Cardiology/American Heart Association Task Force on Practice Guidelines. *Circulation* 129:e521–e643, 2014.
2. Ross J, Jr, Braunwald E: Aortic stenosis. *Circulation* 38:61–67, 1968.
3. Dal-Bianco JP, Khandheria BK, Mookadam F, et al: Management of asymptomatic severe aortic stenosis. *J Am Coll Cardiol* 52:1279–1292, 2008.
4. Brener SJ, Duffy CI, Thomas JD, et al: Progression of aortic stenosis in 394 patients: relation to changes in myocardial and mitral valve dysfunction. *J Am Coll Cardiol* 25:305–310, 1995.
5. Faggiano P, Ghizzoni G, Sorgato A, et al: Rate of progression of valvular aortic stenosis in adults. *Am J Cardiol* 70:229–233, 1992.
6. Otto CM, Burwash IG, Legget ME, et al: Prospective study of asymptomatic valvular aortic stenosis. Clinical, echocardiographic, and exercise predictors of outcome. *Circulation* 95:2262–2270, 1997.
7. Roger VL, Tajik AJ, Bailey KR, et al: Progression of aortic stenosis in adults: new appraisal using Doppler echocardiography. *Am Heart J* 119:331–338, 1990.
8. Nicks R, Cartmill T, Bernstein L: Hypoplasia of the aortic root. The problem of aortic valve replacement. *Thorax* 25:339–346, 1970.
9. Manouguian S, Seybold-Epting W: Patch enlargement of the aortic valve ring by extending the aortic incision into the anterior mitral leaflet. New operative technique. *J Thorac Cardiovasc Surg* 78:402–412, 1979.
10. Rastan H, Koncz J: Aortoventriculoplasty: a new technique for the treatment of left ventricular outflow tract obstruction. *J Thorac Cardiovasc Surg* 71:920–927, 1976.
11. Konno S, Imai Y, Iida Y, et al: A new method for prosthetic valve replacement in congenital aortic stenosis associated with hypoplasia of the aortic valve ring. *J Thorac Cardiovasc Surg* 70:909–917, 1975.
12. O'Brien SM, Shahian DM, Filardo G, et al: The Society of Thoracic Surgeons 2008 cardiac surgery risk models: Part 2—isolated valve surgery. *Ann Thorac Surg* 88:S23–S42, 2009.
13. Shahian DM, O'Brien SM, Filardo G, et al: The Society of Thoracic Surgeons 2008 cardiac surgery risk models: Part 3—valve plus coronary artery bypass grafting surgery. *Ann Thorac Surg* 88: S43–S62, 2009.
14. LaPar DJ, Yang Z, Stukenborg GJ, et al: Outcomes of reoperative aortic valve replacement after previous sternotomy. *J Thorac Cardiovasc Surg* 139:263–272, 2010.
15. Jamieson WR, Edwards FH, Schwartz M, et al: Risk stratification for cardiac valve replacement. National cardiac surgery database. Database committee of the Society of Thoracic Surgeons. *Ann Thorac Surg* 67:943–951, 1999.
16. Rankin JS, Hammill BG, Ferguson TB, Jr, et al: Determinants of operative mortality in valvular heart surgery. *J Thorac Cardiovasc Surg* 131:547–557, 2006.
17. Beach JM, Mihaljevic T, Rajeswaran J, et al: Ventricular hypertrophy and left atrial dilatation persist and are associated with reduced survival after valve replacement for aortic stenosis. *J Thorac Cardiovasc Surg* 147:362–369.e8, 2014.
18. Blackstone EH, Cosgrove DM, Jamieson WR, et al: Prosthesis size and long-term survival after aortic valve replacement. *J Thorac Cardiovasc Surg* 126:783–796, 2003.
19. Di Eusanio M, Fortuna D, De Palma R, et al: Aortic valve replacement: results and predictors of mortality from a contemporary series of 2256 patients. *J Thorac Cardiovasc Surg* 141:940–947, 2011.
20. Mihaljevic T, Nowicki ER, Rajeswaran J, et al: Survival after valve replacement for aortic stenosis: implications for decision making. *J Thorac Cardiovasc Surg* 135:1270–1278, discussion 1278–1279, 2008.
21. Ruel M, Chan V, Bedard P, et al: Very long-term survival implications of heart valve replacement with tissue versus mechanical prostheses in adults <60 years of age. *Circulation* 116:I294–I300, 2007.
22. Edmunds LH, Jr, Clark RE, Cohn LH, et al: Guidelines for reporting morbidity and mortality after cardiac valvular operations. *Eur J Cardiothorac Surg* 10:812–816, 1996.
23. Hammermeister K, Sethi GK, Henderson WG, et al: Outcomes 15 years after valve replacement with a mechanical versus a bioprosthetic valve: final report of the veterans affairs randomized trial. *J Am Coll Cardiol* 36:1152–1158, 2000.
24. Hammermeister KE, Sethi GK, Henderson WG, et al: A comparison of outcomes in men 11 years after heart-valve replacement with a mechanical valve or bioprosthesis. Veterans affairs cooperative study on valvular heart disease. *N Engl J Med* 328:1289–1296, 1993.
25. Casaclang-Verzosa G, Malouf JF, Scott CG, et al: Does left atrial size predict mortality in asymptomatic patients with severe aortic stenosis? *Echocardiography* 27:105–109, 2010.
26. Klodas E, Enriquez-Sarano M, Tajik AJ, et al: Surgery for aortic regurgitation in women. Contrasting indications and outcomes compared with men. *Circulation* 94:2472–2478, 1996.
27. Kvidal P, Bergstrom R, Horte LG, et al: Observed and relative survival after aortic valve replacement. *J Am Coll Cardiol* 35:747–756, 2000.
28. ElBardissi AW, Shekar P, Couper GS, et al: Minimally invasive aortic valve replacement in octogenarian, high-risk, transcatheter aortic valve implantation candidates. *J Thorac Cardiovasc Surg* 141:328–335, 2011.
29. Ferrari E, Tozzi P, Hurni M, et al: Primary isolated aortic valve surgery in octogenarians. *Eur J Cardiothorac Surg* 38:128–133, 2010.
30. Thourani VH, Ailawadi G, Szeto WY, et al: Outcomes of surgical aortic valve replacement in high-risk patients: a multiinstitutional study. *Ann Thorac Surg* 91:49–55, discussion 55–56, 2011.
31. Thourani VH, Myung R, Kilgo P, et al: Long-term outcomes after isolated aortic valve replacement in octogenarians: a modern perspective. *Ann Thorac Surg* 86:1458–1464, discussion 1464–1465, 2008.
32. Alexander KP, Anstrom KJ, Muhlbaier LH, et al: Outcomes of cardiac surgery in patients > or = 80 years: results from the national cardiovascular network. *J Am Coll Cardiol* 35:731–738, 2000.
33. Calvo D, Lozano I, Llosa JC, et al: Aortic valve replacement in octogenarians with severe aortic stenosis. Experience in a series of consecutive patients at a single center. *Rev Esp Cardiol* 60:720–726, 2007.
34. Boeken U, Litmathe J, Feindt P, et al: Neurological complications after cardiac surgery: risk factors and correlation to the surgical procedure. *Thorac Cardiovasc Surg* 53:33–36, 2005.
35. Chikwe J, Croft LB, Goldstone AB, et al: Comparison of the results of aortic valve replacement with or without concomitant coronary artery bypass grafting in patients with left ventricular ejection fraction < or = 30% versus patients with ejection fraction >30%. *Am J Cardiol* 104:1717–1721, 2009.
36. Craver JM, Weintraub WS, Jones EL, et al: Predictors of mortality, complications, and length of stay in aortic valve replacement for aortic stenosis. *Circulation* 78:I85–I90, 1988.
37. de Arenaza DP, Pepper J, Lees B, et al: Preoperative 6-minute walk test adds prognostic information to euroscore in patients undergoing aortic valve replacement. *Heart* 96:113–117, 2010.
38. Filsoufi F, Rahmanian PB, Castillo JG, et al: Incidence, imaging analysis, and early and late outcomes of stroke after cardiac valve operation. *Am J Cardiol* 101:1472–1478, 2008.
39. Gillinov AM, Lytle BW, Hoang V, et al: The atherosclerotic aorta at aortic valve replacement: surgical strategies and results. *J Thorac Cardiovasc Surg* 120:957–963, 2000.
40. Girardi LN, Krieger KH, Mack CA, et al: No-clamp technique for valve repair or replacement in patients with a porcelain aorta. *Ann Thorac Surg* 80:1688–1692, 2005.
41. Sharony R, Grossi EA, Saunders PC, et al: Aortic valve replacement in patients with impaired ventricular function. *Ann Thorac Surg* 75:1808–1814, 2003.
42. Gulbins H, Florath I, Ennker J: Cerebrovascular events after stentless aortic valve replacement during a 9-year follow-up period. *Ann Thorac Surg* 86:769–773, 2008.
43. Ruel M, Masters RG, Rubens FD, et al: Late incidence and determinants of stroke after aortic and mitral valve replacement. *Ann Thorac Surg* 78:77–83, discussion 83–84, 2004.
44. Al-Atassi T, Lam K, Forgie M, et al: Cerebral microembolization after bioprosthetic aortic valve replacement: comparison of warfarin plus aspirin versus aspirin only. *Circulation* 126:S239–S244, 2012.

45. Li Y, Walicki D, Mathiesen C, et al: Strokes after cardiac surgery and relationship to carotid stenosis. *Arch Neurol* 66:1091–1096, 2009.
46. Sundt TM, Zehr KJ, Dearani JA, et al: Is early anticoagulation with warfarin necessary after bioprosthetic aortic valve replacement? *J Thorac Cardiovasc Surg* 129:1024–1031, 2005.
47. Miller DC, Blackstone EH, Mack MJ, et al: Transcatheter (TAVR) versus surgical (AVR) aortic valve replacement: occurrence, hazard, risk factors, and consequences of neurologic events in the partner trial. *J Thorac Cardiovasc Surg* 143:832–843, e813, 2012.
48. Guenther U, Theuerkauf N, Frommann I, et al: Predisposing and precipitating factors of delirium after cardiac surgery: a prospective observational cohort study. *Ann Surg* 257:1160–1167, 2013.
49. Smith LW, Dimsdale JE: Postcardiotomy delirium: conclusions after 25 years? *Am J Psychiatry* 146:452–458, 1989.
50. Toeg HD, Nathan H, Rubens F, et al: Clinical impact of neurocognitive deficits after cardiac surgery. *J Thorac Cardiovasc Surg* 145:1545–1549, 2013.
51. Baraki H, Al Ahmad A, Jeng-Singh S, et al: Pacemaker dependency after isolated aortic valve replacement: do conductance disorders recover over time? *Interact Cardiovasc Thorac Surg* 16:476–481, 2013.
52. Huynh H, Dalloul G, Ghanbari H, et al: Permanent pacemaker implantation following aortic valve replacement: current prevalence and clinical predictors. *Pacing Clin Electrophysiol* 32:1520–1525, 2009.
53. Edmunds LH, Jr: Thrombotic and bleeding complications of prosthetic heart valves. *Ann Thorac Surg* 44:430–445, 1987.
54. Grunkemeier GL, Li HH, Naftel DC, et al: Long-term performance of heart valve prostheses. *Curr Probl Cardiol* 25:73–154, 2000.
55. Chambers JB, Pomar JL, Mestres CA, et al: Clinical event rates with the on-x bileaflet mechanical heart valve: a multicenter experience with follow-up to 12 years. *J Thorac Cardiovasc Surg* 145: 420–424, 2013.
56. Bourguignon T, Bergoend E, Mirza A, et al: Risk factors for valve-related complications after mechanical heart valve replacement in 505 patients with long-term follow up. *J Heart Valve Dis* 20:673–680, 2011.
57. Rhie S, Choi JY, Jang IS, et al: Relationship between the occurrence of thromboembolism and INR measurement interval in low intensity anticoagulation after aortic mechanical valve replacement. *Korean J Thorac Cardiovasc Surg* 44:220–224, 2011.
58. Koertke H, Minami K, Boethig D, et al: Inr self-management permits lower anticoagulation levels after mechanical heart valve replacement. *Circulation* 108(Suppl 1):II75–II78, 2003.
59. Bonow RO, Carabello BA, Chatterjee K, et al: 2008 focused update incorporated into the acc/aha 2006 guidelines for the management of patients with valvular heart disease: a report of the American College of Cardiology/American Heart Association task force on practice guidelines (writing committee to revise the 1998 guidelines for the management of patients with valvular heart disease). Endorsed by the society of cardiovascular anesthesiologists, society for cardiovascular angiography and interventions, and Society of Thoracic Surgeons. *J Am Coll Cardiol* 52:e1–e142, 2008.
60. Joint Task Force on the Management of Valvular Heart Disease of the European Society of C, European Association for Cardio-Thoracic S, Vahanian A, Alfieri O, Andreotti F, et al: Guidelines on the management of valvular heart disease (version 2012). *Eur Heart J* 33:2451–2496, 2012.
61. Whitlock RP, Sun JC, Fremes SE, et al: Antithrombotic and thrombolytic therapy for valvular disease: antithrombotic therapy and prevention of thrombosis, 9th ed: American college of chest physicians evidence-based clinical practice guidelines. *Chest* 141: e576S–600S, 2012.
62. Puskas J, Gerdisch M, Nichols D, et al: Reduced anticoagulation after mechanical aortic valve replacement: interim results from the prospective randomized on-X valve anticoagulation clinical trial randomized Food and Drug Administration investigational device exemption trial. *J Thorac Cardiovasc Surg* 147:1202–1211, 2014.
63. Aramendi JI, Mestres CA, Martinez-Leon J, et al: Triflusal versus oral anticoagulation for primary prevention of thromboembolism after bioprosthetic valve replacement (TRAC): prospective, randomized, co-operative trial. *Eur J Cardiothorac Surg* 27:854–860, 2005.
64. Blair KL, Hatton AC, White WD, et al: Comparison of anticoagulation regimens after Carpentier-Edwards aortic or mitral valve replacement. *Circulation* 90:II214–II219, 1994.
65. Colli A, Mestres CA, Castella M, et al: Comparing warfarin to aspirin (WoA) after aortic valve replacement with the St. Jude medical epic heart valve bioprosthesis: results of the WoA Epic pilot trial. *J Heart Valve Dis* 16:667–671, 2007.
66. ElBardissi AW, DiBardino DJ, Chen FY, et al: Is early antithrombotic therapy necessary in patients with bioprosthetic aortic valves in normal sinus rhythm? *J Thorac Cardiovasc Surg* 139:1137–1145, 2010.
67. Gherli T, Colli A, Fragnito C, et al: Comparing warfarin with aspirin after biological aortic valve replacement: a prospective study. *Circulation* 110:496–500, 2004.
68. Moinuddeen K, Quin J, Shaw R, et al: Anticoagulation is unnecessary after biological aortic valve replacement. *Circulation* 98:II95–II98, discussion II98–II99, 1998.
69. Orszulak TA, Schaff HV, Mullany CJ, et al: Risk of thromboembolism with the aortic Carpentier-Edwards bioprosthesis. *Ann Thorac Surg* 59:462–468, 1995.
70. Colli A, Verhoye JP, Heijmen R, et al: Low-dose acetyl salicylic acid versus oral anticoagulation after bioprosthetic aortic valve replacement. Final report of the action registry. *Int J Cardiol* 168:1229–1236, 2013.
71. Lengyel M, Vandor L: The role of thrombolysis in the management of left-sided prosthetic valve thrombosis: a study of 85 cases diagnosed by transesophageal echocardiography. *J Heart Valve Dis* 10:636–649, 2001.
72. Lengyel M, Fuster V, Keltai M, et al: Guidelines for management of left-sided prosthetic valve thrombosis: a role for thrombolytic therapy. Consensus conference on prosthetic valve thrombosis. *J Am Coll Cardiol* 30:1521–1526, 1997.
73. Blackstone EH, Kirklin JW: Death and other time-related events after valve replacement. *Circulation* 72:753–767, 1985.
74. Gordon SM, Serkey JM, Longworth DL, et al: Early onset prosthetic valve endocarditis: the Cleveland Clinic experience 1992–1997. *Ann Thorac Surg* 69:1388–1392, 2000.
75. Ivert TS, Dismukes WE, Cobbs CG, et al: Prosthetic valve endocarditis. *Circulation* 69:223–232, 1984.
76. Wang A, Athan E, Pappas PA, et al: Contemporary clinical profile and outcome of prosthetic valve endocarditis. *JAMA* 297:1354–1361, 2007.
77. Prendergast BD, Tornos P: Surgery for infective endocarditis: who and when? *Circulation* 121:1141–1152, 2010.
78. David TE, Ivanov J, Armstrong S, et al: Late results of heart valve replacement with the Hancock II bioprosthesis. *J Thorac Cardiovasc Surg* 121:268–277, 2001.
79. Emery RW, Krogh CC, Arom KV, et al: The St. Jude medical cardiac valve prosthesis: a 25-year experience with single valve replacement. *Ann Thorac Surg* 79:776–782, discussion 782–783, 2005.
80. Ikonomidis JS, Kratz JM, Crumbley AJ, 3rd, et al: Twenty-year experience with the St. Jude medical mechanical valve prosthesis. *J Thorac Cardiovasc Surg* 126:2022–2031, 2003.
81. Khan SS, Trento A, DeRobertis M, et al: Twenty-year comparison of tissue and mechanical valve replacement. *J Thorac Cardiovasc Surg* 122:257–269, 2001.
82. Bouhout I, Stevens LM, Mazine A, et al: Long-term outcomes after elective isolated mechanical aortic valve replacement in young adults. *J Thorac Cardiovasc Surg* 148:1341–1346.e1, 2014.
83. Brennan JM, Edwards FH, Zhao Y, et al: Long-term safety and effectiveness of mechanical versus biologic aortic valve prostheses in older patients: results from the Society of Thoracic Surgeons Adult Cardiac Surgery National Database. *Circulation* 127:1647–1655, 2013.
84. Brown JM, O'Brien SM, Wu C, et al: Isolated aortic valve replacement in North America comprising 108,687 patients in 10 years: changes in risks, valve types, and outcomes in the Society of Thoracic Surgeons National Database. *J Thorac Cardiovasc Surg* 137:82–90, 2009.
85. Aupart MR, Mirza A, Meurisse YA, et al: Perimount pericardial bioprosthesis for aortic calcified stenosis: 18-year experience with

1133 patients. *J Heart Valve Dis* 15:768–775, discussion 775–776, 2006.
86. David TE, Armstrong S, Maganti M: Hancock II bioprosthesis for aortic valve replacement: the gold standard of bioprosthetic valves durability? *Ann Thorac Surg* 90:775–781, 2010.
87. Eichinger WB, Hettich IM, Ruzicka DJ, et al: Twenty-year experience with the St. Jude medical biocor bioprosthesis in the aortic position. *Ann Thorac Surg* 86:1204–1210, 2008.
88. Forcillo J, Pellerin M, Perrault LP, et al: Carpentier-Edwards pericardial valve in the aortic position: 25-years experience. *Ann Thorac Surg* 96:486–493, 2013.
89. Investigators I: The Italian study on the mitroflow postoperative results (isthmus): a 20-year, multicentre evaluation of mitroflow pericardial bioprosthesis. *Eur J Cardiothorac Surg* 39:18–26, discussion 26, 2011.
90. Jamieson WR, Burr LH, Miyagishima RT, et al: Carpentier-Edwards supra-annular aortic porcine bioprosthesis: clinical performance over 20 years. *J Thorac Cardiovasc Surg* 130:994–1000, 2005.
91. Jamieson WR, Germann E, Aupart MR, et al: 15-year comparison of supra-annular porcine and perimount aortic bioprostheses. *Asian Cardiovasc Thorac Ann* 14:200–205, 2006.
92. McClure RS, Narayanasamy N, Wiegerinck E, et al: Late outcomes for aortic valve replacement with the Carpentier-Edwards pericardial bioprosthesis: up to 17-year follow-up in 1,000 patients. *Ann Thorac Surg* 89:1410–1416, 2010.
93. Myken PS, Bech-Hansen O: A 20-year experience of 1712 patients with the biocor porcine bioprosthesis. *J Thorac Cardiovasc Surg* 137:76–81, 2009.
94. Prasongsukarn K, Jamieson WR, Lichtenstein SV: Performance of bioprostheses and mechanical prostheses in age group 61–70 years. *J Heart Valve Dis* 14:501–508, 510–511; discussion 509, 2005.
95. Valfre C, Ius P, Minniti G, et al: The fate of hancock ii porcine valve recipients 25 years after implant. *Eur J Cardiothorac Surg* 38:141–146, 2010.
96. Yankah CA, Pasic M, Musci M, et al: Aortic valve replacement with the mitroflow pericardial bioprosthesis: durability results up to 21 years. *J Thorac Cardiovasc Surg* 136:688–696, 2008.
97. Choi JB, Kim JH, Park HK, et al: Aortic valve replacement using continuous suture technique in patients with aortic valve disease. *Korean J Thorac Cardiovasc Surg* 46:249–255, 2013.
98. Qicai H, Zili C, Zhengfu H, et al: Continuous-suture technique in aortic valve replacement. *J Card Surg* 21:178–181, 2006.
99. Watanabe G, Ushijima T, Tomita S, et al: Revival of continuous suture technique in aortic valve replacement in patient with aortic valve stenosis: a novel modified technique. *Innovations* 6:311–315, 2011.
100. Jacobs ML, Fowler BN, Vezeridis MP, et al: Aortic valve replacement: a 9-year experience. *Ann Thorac Surg* 30:439–447, 1980.
101. De Cicco G, Lorusso R, Colli A, et al: Aortic valve periprosthetic leakage: anatomic observations and surgical results. *Ann Thorac Surg* 79:1480–1485, 2005.
102. Carr-White GS, Kilner PJ, Hon JK, et al: Incidence, location, pathology, and significance of pulmonary homograft stenosis after the ross operation. *Circulation* 104:I16–I20, 2001.
103. Haider AW, Larson MG, Benjamin EJ, et al: Increased left ventricular mass and hypertrophy are associated with increased risk for sudden death. *J Am Coll Cardiol* 32:1454–1459, 1998.
104. Levy D, Garrison RJ, Savage DD, et al: Prognostic implications of echocardiographically determined left ventricular mass in the Framingham heart study. *N Engl J Med* 322:1561–1566, 1990.
105. Christakis GT, Joyner CD, Morgan CD, et al: Left ventricular mass regression early after aortic valve replacement. *Ann Thorac Surg* 62:1084–1089, 1996.
106. Kennedy JW, Doces J, Stewart DK: Left ventricular function before and following aortic valve replacement. *Circulation* 56:944–950, 1977.
107. Kuhl HP, Franke A, Puschmann D, et al: Regression of left ventricular mass one year after aortic valve replacement for pure severe aortic stenosis. *Am J Cardiol* 89:408–413, 2002.
108. Carabello BA, Green LH, Grossman W, et al: Hemodynamic determinants of prognosis of aortic valve replacement in critical aortic stenosis and advanced congestive heart failure. *Circulation* 62:42–48, 1980.
109. Hwang MH, Hammermeister KE, Oprian C, et al: Preoperative identification of patients likely to have left ventricular dysfunction after aortic valve replacement. Participants in the veterans administration cooperative study on valvular heart disease. *Circulation* 80:I65–I76, 1989.
110. Schwarz F, Flameng W, Thormann J, et al: Recovery from myocardial failure after aortic valve replacement. *J Thorac Cardiovasc Surg* 75:854–864, 1978.
111. Bonow RO, Borer JS, Rosing DR, et al: Preoperative exercise capacity in symptomatic patients with aortic regurgitation as a predictor of postoperative left ventricular function and long-term prognosis. *Circulation* 62:1280–1290, 1980.
112. Garcia R, Villar AV, Cobo M, et al: Circulating levels of mir-133a predict the regression potential of left ventricular hypertrophy after valve replacement surgery in patients with aortic stenosis. *J Am Heart Assoc* 2:e000211, 2013.
113. Villar AV, Garcia R, Merino D, et al: Myocardial and circulating levels of microrna-21 reflect left ventricular fibrosis in aortic stenosis patients. *Int J Cardiol* 167:2875–2881, 2013.
114. Villar AV, Merino D, Wenner M, et al: Myocardial gene expression of microrna-133a and myosin heavy and light chains, in conjunction with clinical parameters, predict regression of left ventricular hypertrophy after valve replacement in patients with aortic stenosis. *Heart* 97:1132–1137, 2011.
115. Pibarot P, Dumesnil JG: Prosthesis-patient mismatch: definition, clinical impact, and prevention. *Heart* 92:1022–1029, 2006.
116. Pibarot P, Dumesnil JG, Cartier PC, et al: Patient-prosthesis mismatch can be predicted at the time of operation. *Ann Thorac Surg* 71:S265–S268, 2001.
117. Hanayama N, Christakis GT, Mallidi HR, et al: Patient prosthesis mismatch is rare after aortic valve replacement: valve size may be irrelevant. *Ann Thorac Surg* 73:1822–1829, discussion 1829, 2002.
118. Medalion B, Blackstone EH, Lytle BW, et al: Aortic valve replacement: is valve size important? *J Thorac Cardiovasc Surg* 119:963–974, 2000.
119. Blais C, Dumesnil JG, Baillot R, et al: Impact of valve prosthesis-patient mismatch on short-term mortality after aortic valve replacement. *Circulation* 108:983–988, 2003.
120. Pibarot P, Dumesnil JG, Lemieux M, et al: Impact of prosthesis-patient mismatch on hemodynamic and symptomatic status, morbidity and mortality after aortic valve replacement with a bioprosthetic heart valve. *J Heart Valve Dis* 7:211–218, 1998.
121. Rao V, Jamieson WR, Ivanov J, et al: Prosthesis-patient mismatch affects survival after aortic valve replacement. *Circulation* 102:III5–III9, 2000.
122. Ruel M, Rubens FD, Masters RG, et al: Late incidence and predictors of persistent or recurrent heart failure in patients with mitral prosthetic valves. *J Thorac Cardiovasc Surg* 128:278–283, 2004.
123. Tasca G, Brunelli F, Cirillo M, et al: Impact of valve prosthesis-patient mismatch on left ventricular mass regression following aortic valve replacement. *Ann Thorac Surg* 79:505–510, 2005.
124. Kulik A, Burwash IG, Kapila V, et al: Long-term outcomes after valve replacement for low-gradient aortic stenosis: impact of prosthesis-patient mismatch. *Circulation* 114:I553–I558, 2006.
125. Moon MR, Pasque MK, Munfakh NA, et al: Prosthesis-patient mismatch after aortic valve replacement: impact of age and body size on late survival. *Ann Thorac Surg* 81:481–488, discussion 489, 2006.
126. Price J, Lapierre H, Ressler L, et al: Prosthesis-patient mismatch is less frequent and more clinically indolent in patients operated for aortic insufficiency. *J Thorac Cardiovasc Surg* 138:639–645, 2009.
127. Ruel M, Al-Faleh H, Kulik A, et al: Prosthesis-patient mismatch after aortic valve replacement predominantly affects patients with preexisting left ventricular dysfunction: effect on survival, freedom from heart failure, and left ventricular mass regression. *J Thorac Cardiovasc Surg* 131:1036–1044, 2006.
128. Kulik A, Al-Saigh M, Chan V, et al: Enlargement of the small aortic root during aortic valve replacement: is there a benefit? *Ann Thorac Surg* 85:94–100, 2008.

CHAPTER 78

AORTIC VALVE REPAIR

Munir Boodhwani • Gebrine El Khoury

CHAPTER OUTLINE

Aortic valve replacement remains the gold standard for the treatment of severe aortic valve disease. However, valve repair is emerging as a feasible and attractive alternative to valve replacement in selected patients. Valve repair can reduce or eliminate the risks of prosthesis-related complications including thromboembolism, endocarditis, anticoagulant-related hemorrhage, and reoperation owing to structural valve deterioration among others. Analogous to the mitral valve, a reconstructive approach to the aortic valve requires a thorough and detailed understanding of three-dimensional valve anatomy, valve function, assessment and classification of pathologic lesions, and treatment of all affected components of the valve. In this chapter, we review the key features of aortic valve insufficiency, aortic valve and root anatomy, an approach to valve assessment and lesion classification, and a demonstration of commonly used reparative techniques for aortic valve repair. Furthermore, we review the outcomes of aortic valve repair in unselected cohorts and in distinct subsets of patients undergoing aortic valve preservation and repair.

AORTIC REGURGITATION

Epidemiology and Etiology

The causes of aortic regurgitation (AR) are numerous and can be attributed to a disturbance in any of the components of the functional unit of the aortic valve (e.g., cusps, sinuses of Valsalva, sinotubular junction, ventriculoaortic junction). In general, the causes can be divided into those that affect the valve cusps (e.g., calcific degeneration, congenitally bicuspid valve, infective endocarditis, rheumatic disease, myxomatous degeneration) and those that affect the aortic root (e.g., aortic dissection, aortitis of various etiologies such as syphilis, connective tissue disorders such as Marfan syndrome).

Pathophysiology

The pathophysiology of AR is dependent on the acuity of onset and duration of the disease process. In acute AR, typically caused by aortic dissection, infective endocarditis, trauma, or valve prosthesis failure, there is a sudden increase in left ventricular end-diastolic volume because of the regurgitation. Since the left ventricle has limited compliance and does not have time to adapt, the left ventricular end-diastolic pressure (LVEDP) rises rapidly.

In chronic AR, there is a slow and insidious progression of left ventricular (LV) dilation and eccentric hypertrophy because of an increase in left ventricular end-diastolic volume, LVEDP, and wall stress. Dilation of the LV, while maintaining normal systolic function, increases total stroke volume and maintains forward flow.[1] This increase in stroke volume coupled with an increase in LVEDP is associated with the wide pulse pressure typical of chronic AR. Eventually, the hypertrophic response is exhausted, and LVEF drops as afterload increases, leading to heart failure and its associated clinical presentation.[2,3]

Clinical Features

Patients with acute AR usually exhibit sudden or rapidly progressive cardiovascular collapse, which can be life threatening if not addressed promptly. They often exhibit ischemic symptoms because of the decrease in coronary blood flow and increased myocardial oxygen demand. In contrast, patients with chronic AR are asymptomatic for a long period of time because of the compensatory LV changes discussed earlier. Once the compensatory response is exhausted, the patients start having heart failure symptoms such as exertional dyspnea, orthopnea, and paroxysmal nocturnal dyspnea. Patients may also feel palpitations and angina.

The classic murmur of AR is an early diastolic, blowing, decrescendo murmur heard best at the level of the diaphragm at the left sternal border while the patient is sitting, leaning forward, and in deep exhalation. It may become holodiastolic in severe AR, and isometric exercises tend to accentuate the murmur. Classic signs of widened pulse pressure may also be found, including Corrigan or water-hammer pulse, De Musset sign (bobbing of the head with heart beats), Quincke pulse (pulsations of the lip and fingers), Traube sign (pistol shot sounds over the femoral artery), and Müller sign (pulsations of the uvula).

Diagnostic Criteria

Transthoracic echocardiography with Doppler color-flow is the most useful tool for the diagnosis of AR.[4] The jet width and vena contracta width on Doppler color-flow are used to qualitatively assess the severity of AR, whereas the regurgitant volume, regurgitant fraction, and regurgitant orifice area are used for the quantitative assessment.

Indications for Surgery

Decision making for surgical intervention for aortic valve surgery needs to incorporate the natural history of medically managed disease, the risks associated with surgical intervention, and longer-term risks that might accrue related to prosthetic valve implantation. The class I recommendations for aortic valve intervention in patients with AR according to the 2014 American College of Cardiology and the American Heart Association[5] are the following: symptomatic patients with chronic severe AR, asymptomatic patients with chronic severe AR and LV dysfunction (ejection fraction < 50%) at rest, and patients with chronic severe AR who are undergoing concomitant coronary artery bypass grafting, aortic surgery, or other heart valve surgery.

The class IIa recommendation is for patients with asymptomatic AR and normal LV systolic function (ejection fraction > 50%) but with severe LV dilation (end-systolic diameter > 50 mm). The class IIb recommendation is for patients with moderate AR who are undergoing coronary artery bypass grafting, aortic surgery, or other heart valve surgery. Aortic valve intervention may also be reasonable in asymptomatic patients with chronic severe AR, normal LV systolic function, and severe LV dilation (end-diastolic diameter > 65 mm) if the operative risk is low. Other considerations can include evidence of progressive LV dilation, declining exercise tolerance, or abnormal hemodynamic response to exercise.

However, aortic valve repair carries a similar, if not lower, risk of perioperative complication with a low risk of valve-related events over time. Similar to mitral valve repair for mitral regurgitation,[6] there is some suggestion that aortic valve intervention should be considered earlier in patients in whom aortic valve repair is likely.[7]

Another broad category of patients who undergo aortic valve preservation and repair are those with primary aortic pathology involving the aortic root and/or the ascending aorta and varying degrees of associated aortic valvular disease. In these patients, the primary indication for intervention is driven by aortic size, discussed in the American,[8] European,[9] and Canadian Guidelines.[10]

From a technical perspective, all patients with primary aortic insufficiency are potentially candidates for repair. However, the success of aortic valve repair is determined largely by the quality of cusp tissue available. Thus, patients with significant leaflet calcification, destruction owing to active endocarditis, or rheumatic involvement are least likely to undergo successful and durable aortic valve repair.[11] In contrast, repair has been shown to have good results in patients with bicuspid[12,13] (and in smaller series, unicuspid,[14] and quadricuspid[15]) aortic valves, despite the abnormalities in cusp anatomy. An important limitation to the universal application of aortic valve repair techniques is the lack of surgical expertise and experience in this field; however, this is changing rapidly with increasing interest in aortic valve repair. Patients who are candidates for repair should be referred to centers with appropriate expertise.

AORTIC VALVE ANATOMY AND FUNCTION

The anatomy of the aortic valve and root is familiar to cardiac surgeons.[16] However, there are some features outlined here that are particularly relevant to aortic valve preserving and repair surgery.[17] Like the mitral valve,

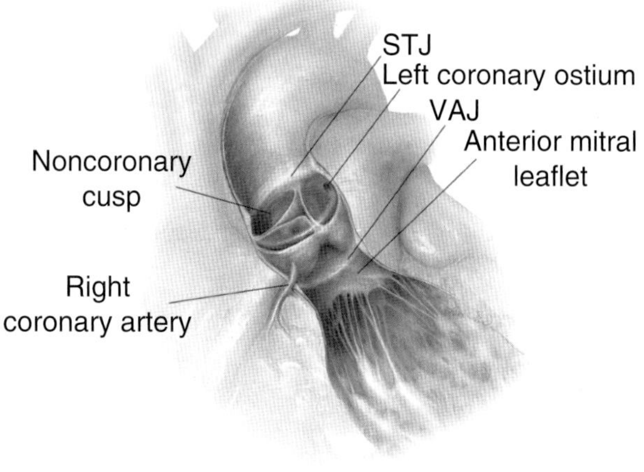

FIGURE 78-1 ■ Anatomy of the aortic valve and the functional aortic annulus. *STJ,* Sinotubular junction; *VAJ,* ventriculo-aortic junction.

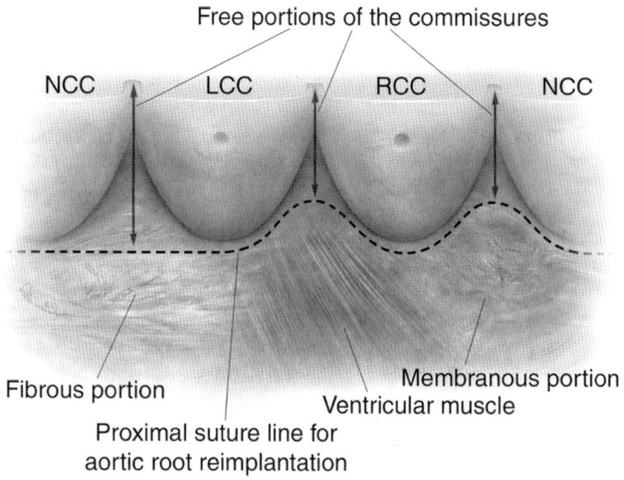

FIGURE 78-2 ■ Anatomy of the subvalvular region of the aortic valve. The dotted line marks the limits of external dissection of the aortic root and the proximal suture line for a valve-sparing root replacement procedure using the reimplantation technique. *LCC,* Left coronary cusp; *NCC,* noncoronary cusp; *RCC,* right coronary cusp.

aortic valve function involves an important interaction between the valve annulus and leaflets. Importantly, however, the annulus of the aortic valve is not a single structure but rather consists of three different components—namely, the sinotubular junction, the ventriculoaortic junction, and the anatomic crown-shaped annulus, which serves as the insertion point of the aortic valve cusps[18] (Fig. 78-1). These components work together to facilitate normal valve function and together are termed the *functional aortic annulus*. The aortic valve leaflets insert into the aortic annulus proximally at the ventriculo-aortic junction (VAJ) and distally at the sinotubular junction (STJ). In a normal aortic valve, the cusps coapt at the center of the aortic valve orifice with a coaptation height that is approximately at the mid-level between the VAJ and the STJ. The height of the sinuses of Valsalva (from the VAJ to the STJ) corresponds to the external diameter of the STJ, which can be useful to size prostheses for aortic root replacement and to assess cusp geometry after aortic valve repair.

As a functional entity, the aortic valve consists of the functional aortic annulus (FAA), and the valve cusps. The integrity of these two functional components is the basis for good valvular function, and alteration in one of these components is frequently associated with alteration in the other. Thus, a fundamental principle in aortic valve repair is that lesions of the cusps and the FAA should both be addressed at the time of valve repair.

The anatomy of the subvalvular region of the aortic valve and its surrounding structures also has important implications for aortic valve repair[19] (Fig. 78-2). An important observation is that external dissection of the aortic root from its surrounding structures is limited by the membranous septum (at the junction of the noncoronary [NC] and right coronary [RC] cusps) and by ventricular muscle (at the junction of the left coronary [LC] and RC cusps), whereas at all other points, external dissection down to the level of the anatomic valve annulus is possible and necessary when valve-sparing root replacement is performed using the reimplantation technique. Thus, the proximal suture line for the aortic valve reimplantation procedure follows these external limitations in a curvilinear fashion.

CLASSIFICATION OF AORTIC INSUFFICIENCY

Until recently, a major limitation to the more generalized application of aortic valve repair techniques was the absence of a common framework for valve assessment to help guide the approach to valve repair. Important lessons in this regard can be learned from the development of mitral valve repair. The Carpentier classification[20] of mitral valve insufficiency was responsible, in large part, for the development and generalized dissemination of repair techniques for the mitral valve because it provided a common language for cardiologists, anesthesiologists, and surgeons to communicate about disease mechanisms and pathology. Key characteristics of that classification system were that it encompassed the entire spectrum of disease, it clarified and provided insight into the mechanism of insufficiency, it could be consistently applied using different assessment modalities (i.e., echocardiography and surgical assessment), it guided the repair techniques, and it provided a framework for the assessment of long-term outcome for differing mitral valve pathologies.

Over the past decade, a similar classification of aortic valve insufficiency has been developed with the above characteristics in mind[11] (Fig. 78-3). This classification centers on the idea that the aortic valve, much like the mitral valve, consists of two major components: the aortic annulus and the valve leaflets. Contrary to the mitral valve, however, the annulus of the aortic valve is not a single anatomic structure. The functional aortic annulus consists of two separate components, namely the ventriculoaortic junction and the sinotubular junction. As in Carpentier's classification of mitral valve disease,

AI Class	Type I Normal cusp motion with FAA dilation or cusp perforation				Type II Cusp prolapse	Type III Cusp restriction
	Ia	Ib	Ic	Id		
Mechanism	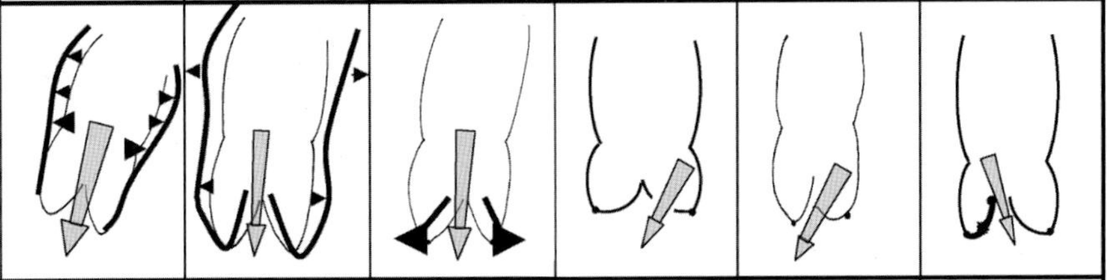					
Repair Techniques (Primary)	STJ remodeling *Ascending aortic graft*	Aortic valve sparing: *Reimplantation or Remodeling with SCA*	SCA	Patch repair *Autologous or bovine pericardium*	Prolapse repair *Free margin plication* *Triangular resection* *Free margin resuspension*	Leaflet repair *Shaving* *Decalcification* *Patch*
(Secondary)	SCA		STJ annuloplasty	SCA	SCA	SCA

FIGURE 78-3 ■ Repair-oriented classification of aortic insufficiency. *FAA,* Functional aortic annulus; *SCA,* subcommissural annuloplasty; *STJ,* sinotubular junction.

regurgitation associated with normal leaflet motion is designated as type I. This is largely due to lesions of the functional aortic annulus with type 1a aortic insufficiency (AI) owing to sinotubular junction enlargement and dilation of the ascending aorta, type Ib owing to dilation of the sinuses of Valsalva and the sinotubular junction, type Ic owing to dilation of the ventriculoaortic junction, and lastly type 1d owing to cusp perforation without a primary functional aortic annulus lesion. Type II AI is due to leaflet prolapse secondary to excessive cusp tissue or due to commissural disruption. Type III AI is due to leaflet restriction, which can be found in bicuspid, degenerative, or rheumatic valvular disease because of calcification, thickening, and fibrosis of the aortic valve leaflets.

Patients can exhibit either single or multiple lesions contributing to their aortic insufficiency. For example, patients with isolated type Ib AI (owing to dilation of the sinuses of Valsalva) are expected to have a central regurgitant jet. Thus, the presence of a sinus of Valsalva aneurysm with an eccentric AI jet suggests concomitant leaflet prolapse (type II) or restriction (type III). Further assessment of leaflet anatomy can help to better delineate the different mechanisms contributing to AI. Once the mechanism of AI is well understood, the classification system can help to guide the surgeon in the choice of surgical techniques for correction of the pathology.

SURGICAL TECHNIQUES

Exposure and Assessment

Aortic valve repair procedures are generally performed through a median sternotomy. Arterial cannulation is performed distal to any diseased aortic segments, typically in the distal ascending aorta or aortic arch. Alternatively, axillary artery cannulation may be performed in the setting of aortic arch pathology. A single, two-stage venous cannula is inserted through the right atrial appendage unless alternative cannulation strategies are required to treat coexisting pathology. After cardioplegia, a transverse aortotomy is performed approximately 1 cm above the sinotubular junction starting above the NC sinus and the posterior 2 to 3 cm of aortic wall is left intact. The distal aorta is retracted cephalad. Full-thickness 4-0 polypropylene traction sutures are placed at the three commissures and retracted using clamps, but not tied, to permit a dynamic assessment of valve anatomy. Axial traction is applied (perpendicular to the level of the annular plane) on the commissural traction sutures. This maneuver demonstrates physiologic aortic valve closure position, and the area and height of coaptation is observed. Leaflets are inspected to assess mobility, restriction, calcification, and prolapse. A prolapsing cusp will exhibit a transverse fibrous band at this time, which is also visible on echocardiography[17] (Fig. 78-4).

Interventions on the Aortic Root and Annulus

Type 1 lesions are most frequently due to dilation of the various components of the functional aortic annulus; they can occur in isolation or in association with cusp disease. A type 1a lesion occurs because of a supracoronary ascending aortic aneurysm with concomitant dilation of the STJ. This is corrected by replacing the ascending aorta and remodeling the STJ using a Dacron tube graft. When significant associated AI is present, subcommissural annuloplasty is also performed. Aneurysms of the aortic root (type 1b) are frequently associated with

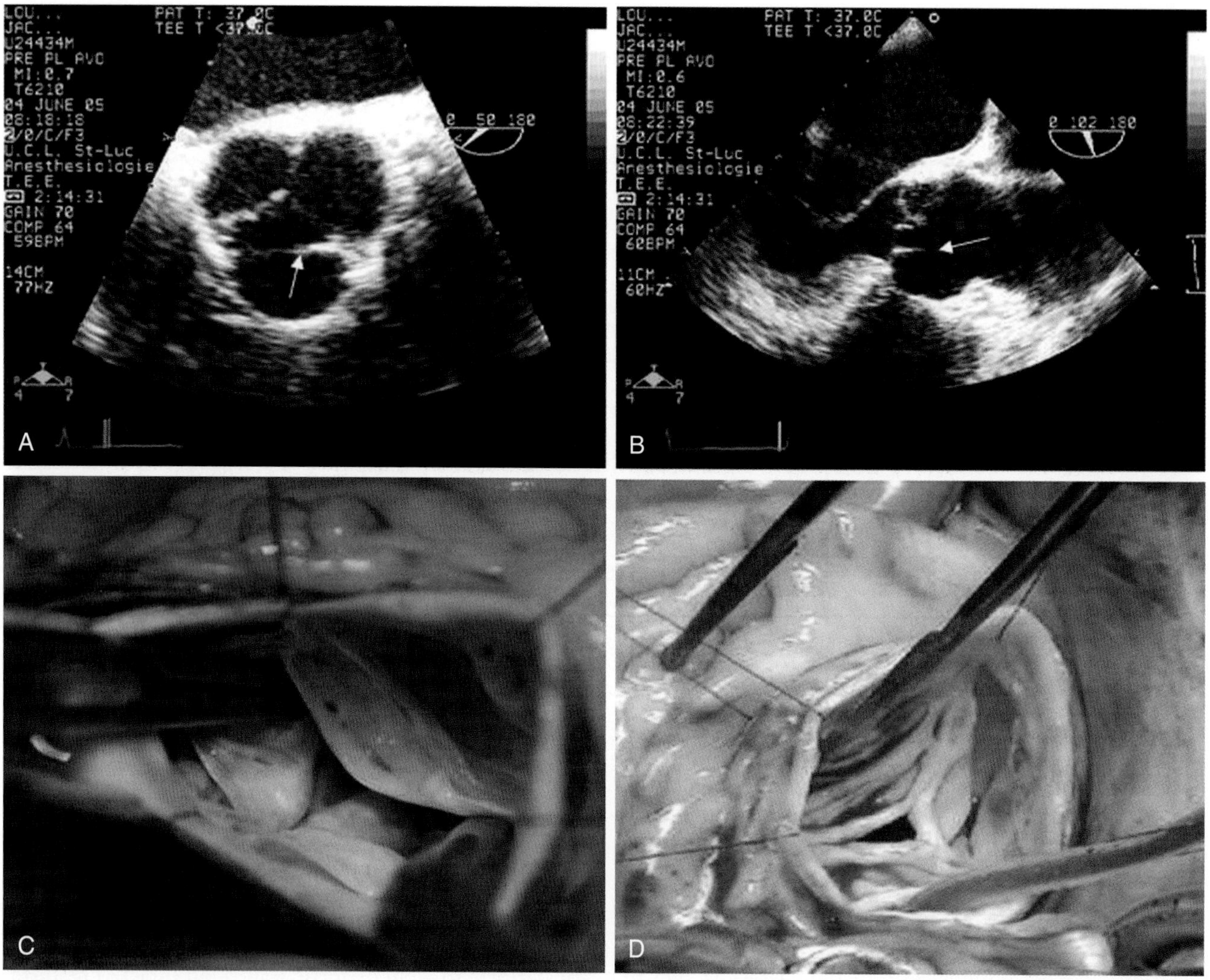

FIGURE 78-4 ■ **A** and **B,** A transverse fibrous band is typically visible on echocardiography *(arrow)* and surgical inspection **(C, D)** in the setting cusp prolapse in trileaflet aortic valves and may help in the detection and localization of cusp prolapse.

dilation of the STJ and the VAJ. These aneurysms are treated using valve-sparing root replacement, preferentially using the reimplantation technique[21] because it provides better stabilization of the VAJ. Aortic root remodeling[22] can also be used to treat aneurysms of the aortic root, and it is particularly useful when only one or two sinuses are involved or in patients in whom there is no risk of ongoing VAJ dilation.

Subcommissural Annuloplasty

Subcommissural annuloplasty is typically performed at midcommissural height, except at the NC/RC commissure, where it should be performed higher to avoid the membranous septum and conduction tissue (Fig. 78-5). Care should also be taken in this area during tying of the suture, to avoid a tear in the septum. At the other two commissures, the subcommissural annuloplasty can be performed at a lower level if a greater increase in the coaptation surface is desired. A subcommissural annuloplasty reduces the width of the interleaflet triangle, improves cusp coaptation, and can help to stabilize the

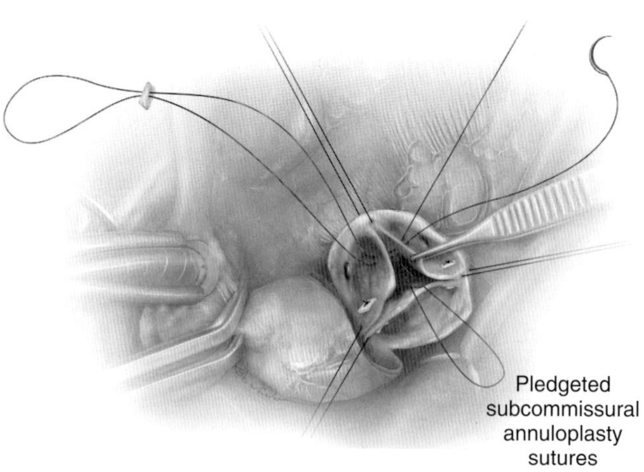

FIGURE 78-5 ■ Subcommissural annuloplasty.

ventriculoaortic junction. In the setting of a bicuspid aortic valve, however, subcommissural is not always sufficient for the prevention of future VAJ dilation.[49]

Valve-Sparing Root Replacement: Reimplantation Technique

A valve-sparing root replacement using the reimplantation technique provides the most stable form of functional aortic annuloplasty. In addition to being used in patients with aortic root aneurysms, this technique can also facilitate aortic valve repair in patients with moderate root dilation in the setting of bicuspid aortic valves. Originally pioneered by David and colleagues, multiple modifications of this procedure have been reported. The important steps of this procedure are described below.[23]

Aortic Root Preparation. The key principle is to dissect the aortic root externally as low as possible, given the natural anatomic limitations (i.e., where the root inserts into ventricular muscle). The root dissection is started along the NC sinus and continued towards the LC/NC commissure. In this area, the subannular region of the aortic valve is fibrous and dissection can therefore be carried to below the level of insertion of the leaflets. Moving toward the RC/NC commissure and along the right sinus and the RC/LC commissure, the dissection is limited by nonfibrous portions of the annulus (Fig. 78-6). The sinuses of Valsalva are then resected leaving approximately 5 mm of aortic wall attached and the coronary buttons are harvested.

Prosthesis Sizing. The three commissural traction sutures are pulled perpendicular to the annular plane with a slight inward motion to ensure good leaflet coaptation. When the leaflets are coapting adequately, a Hagar dilator is used to size the circle that includes the three commissures, and a graft 4 mm larger is chosen as this graft will sit outside the commissural posts. An alternative approach to prosthesis sizing takes advantage of the principle that in a normally functioning aortic valve, the height of the commissure (measured from the base of the interleaflet triangle to the top of the commissure) is equal to external diameter of the sinotubular junction[24] (Fig. 78-7). Although various components of the aortic root and the functional aortic annulus may dilate in the setting of root aneurysms, the height of the commissure remains relatively constant. The height of the commissure is most

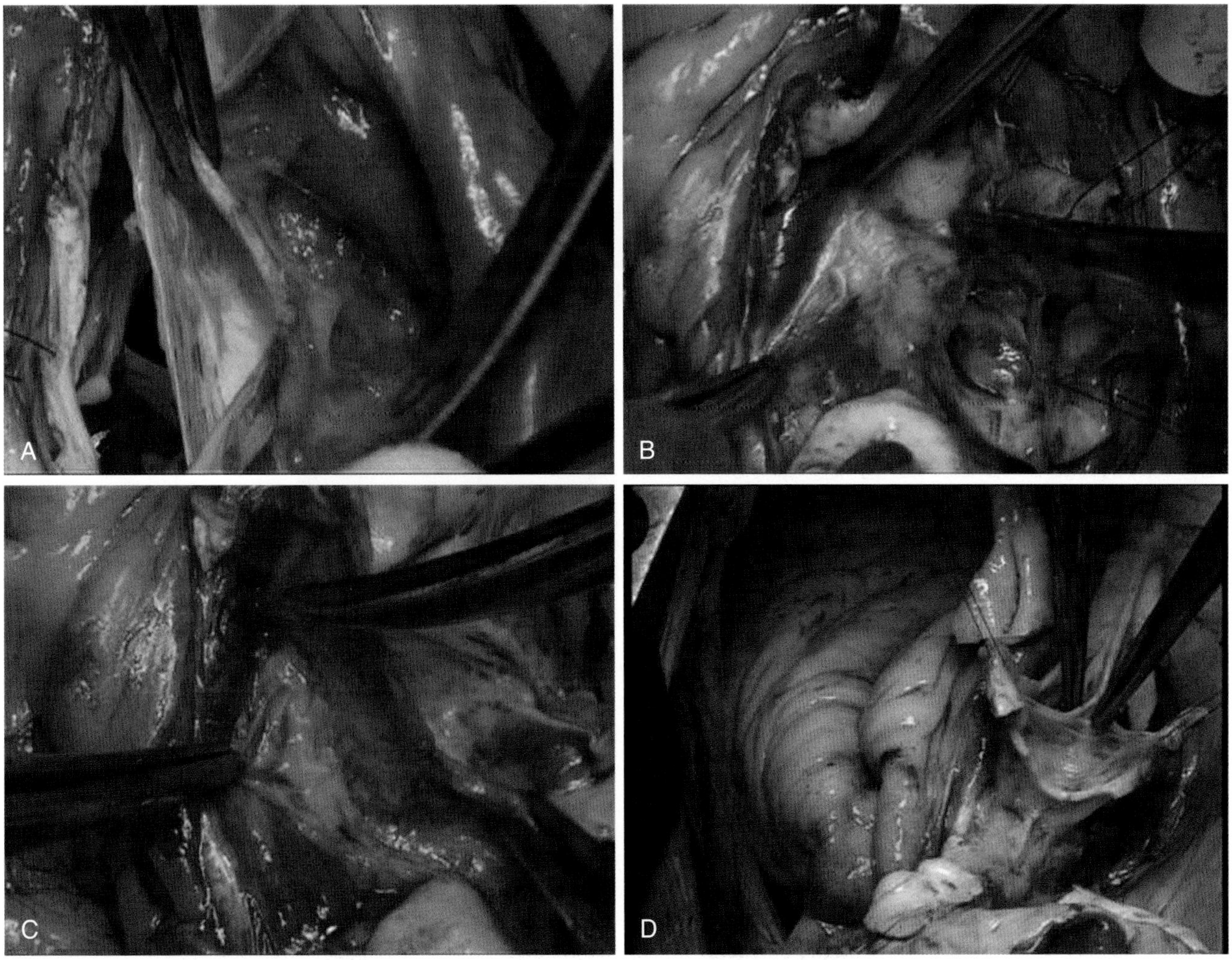

FIGURE 78-6 ■ External dissection for a valve-sparing root replacement procedure using the reimplantation technique.

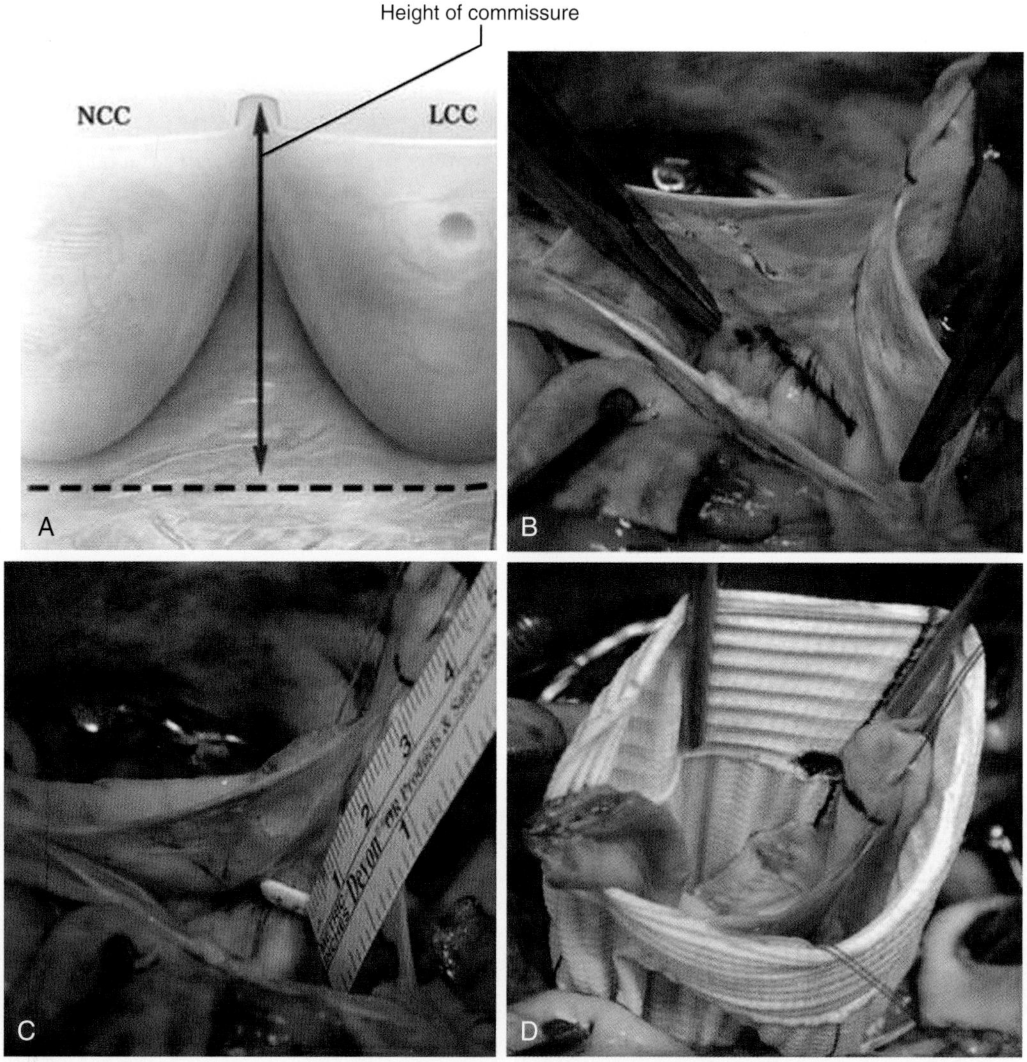

FIGURE 78-7 ■ A novel method for prosthesis sizing when using the reimplantation technique. *LCC,* Left coronary cusp; *NCC,* noncoronary cusp.

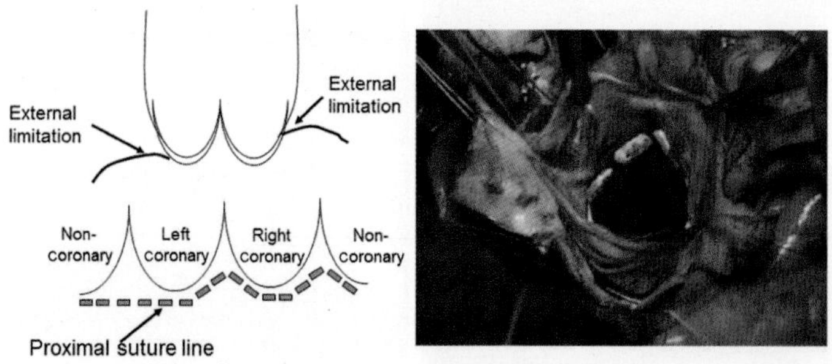

FIGURE 78-8 ■ Proximal suture line for a valve-sparing root replacement procedure using the reimplantation technique.

easily measured at the NC/LC commissure by first drawing a connecting line between the nadirs of the two adjacent cusps (base of interleaflet triangle) and measuring the distance between this line and the top of the commissure. This height corresponds to the diameter of the graft chosen.

Proximal Suture Line. 2-0 Tycron sutures with pledgets are passed from inside to outside the aorta with the pledgets on the inside, starting from the NC/LC commissure and moving clockwise. Along the fibrous portion of the aortic annulus, these sutures are inserted along the horizontal plane formed by the base of the inter-leaflet triangles. Importantly, however, along the nonfibrous portions of the annulus where the external dissection of the aortic root is limited by muscle, these sutures are inserted along the lowest portion of the freely dissected aortic root, making the proximal suture line slightly higher at the RC/NC and RC/LC commissures compared with the LC/NC commissure (Fig. 78-8).

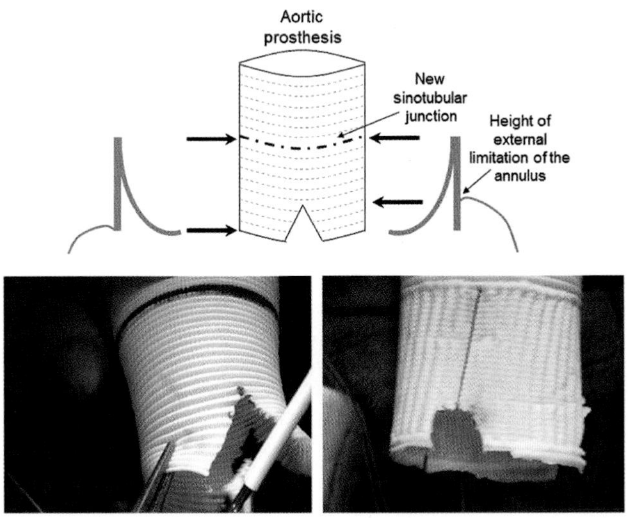

FIGURE 78-9 ■ Tailoring of the prosthesis for the reimplantation technique.

Prosthesis Preparation and Fixation. A Dacron prosthesis with or without built-in neoaortic sinuses can be used. The three commissures are attached to the prosthesis along the same plane—the new sinotubular junction. Because of external limitations of root dissection, the graft has to be tailored. First, the distance from the base of the interleaflet triangle to the top of the commissure is measured at the LC/NC commissure and marked on the graft. Next, at the RC/NC and RC/LC commissures, the distance from the proximal suture to the top of the commissure is measured and used to determine the amount of graft material that needs to be trimmed (Fig. 78-9). The pledgeted sutures are then passed through the base of the prosthesis, respecting the spaces between sutures and the curvilinear contour of the suture line. The commissural traction sutures are pulled up together while tying down the prosthesis to ensure appropriate seating around the aortic annulus.

Valve Reimplantation. The commissures are reimplanted first using 4-0 polypropylene sutures while pulling up on the prosthesis and the native commissure and then tied into place. This running suture line is performed in small regular steps passing the suture from outside the prosthesis to inside and through the aortic wall, staying close to the annulus, and then back out of the prosthesis.

Leaflet Assessment and Repair. After valve reimplantation, it is critical to reexamine the leaflets for any unmasked prolapse, symmetry, and the height and depth of coaptation. Prolapse can be repaired using a variety of techniques described later. Cardioplegia is administered through the distal end of the graft with partial clamping to distend the new aortic root and to assess root pressure and signs of LV dilation. A limited echocardiographic view can be obtained at this time. The cardioplegia solution is then slowly aspirated out of the prosthesis without distorting the leaflets. This gives another visual assessment of the aortic valve in its physiologic closed state as well as the area and height of coaptation. Coronary ostia are then reimplanted on the graft, and the distal anastomosis is performed at the level of normal aorta.

Alternative Approaches to Aortic Valve Annuloplasty

The reimplantation technique provides the most stable form of annuloplasty of the aortic valve and allows the surgeon to modulate a variety of parameters, including the VAJ, STJ, and cusp and commissural orientation; however, it involves extensive dissection of the aortic valve, root, and surrounding structures, and it necessitates reimplantation of the coronary ostia. In patients with normal-sized aortic roots and dilation of the VAJ, use of the reimplantation procedure for annuloplasty is controversial and can expose the patients to unnecessary risk. Therefore, alternative approaches to annuloplasty of the aortic valve, without root replacement, are currently under development and in various stages of evaluation. External annuloplasty is the most frequently used option using a flexible ring.[25] This option is typically used as an adjunct to the remodeling technique for aortic root replacement to provide more VAJ support, but in theory can be used in isolation as well. An important limitation to the external annuloplasty is the inability to place the external ring at the level of the true VAJ because of the limits of external dissection. To overcome this limitation, a number of different internal annuloplasty systems are currently being developed.[26,27] A suture-based internal VAJ annuloplasty using a large-caliber PTFE suture has also been proposed. However, results of these techniques on long-term valve function are lacking.

Cusp Repair Techniques

Cusp prolapse is the most frequently encountered lesion and is associated with excess length of the free margin, which can be corrected using either central free margin plication or free margin resuspension. When a single cusp is prolapsing, the two nonprolapsing cusps serve as the reference and are used to estimate the required reduction in the free margin length. When two cusps are prolapsing, the third nonprolapsing cusp is used as a reference to indicate the desired height of coaptation. In the rare instance that all the cusps are prolapsing, the goal is to achieve a cusp coaptation height at the midlevel of the sinuses of Valsalva. Alternatively, calipers that permit measurement of effective cusp height can be used.[28]

Free Margin Plication

The technique for central free margin plication has been described previously[29] (Fig. 78-10). A 7-0 polypropylene suture is passed through the center of the two nonprolapsing reference cusps, and gentle axial traction is applied. The prolapsing cusp is gently pulled parallel to the reference cusp, and a 6-0 polypropylene suture is passed through the prolapsing cusp, from the aortic to ventricular side, at the point at which it meets the center of the reference cusp. Next, the direction of traction on the prolapsing cusp is reversed, and the same suture is passed from the ventricular to the aortic side of the cusp

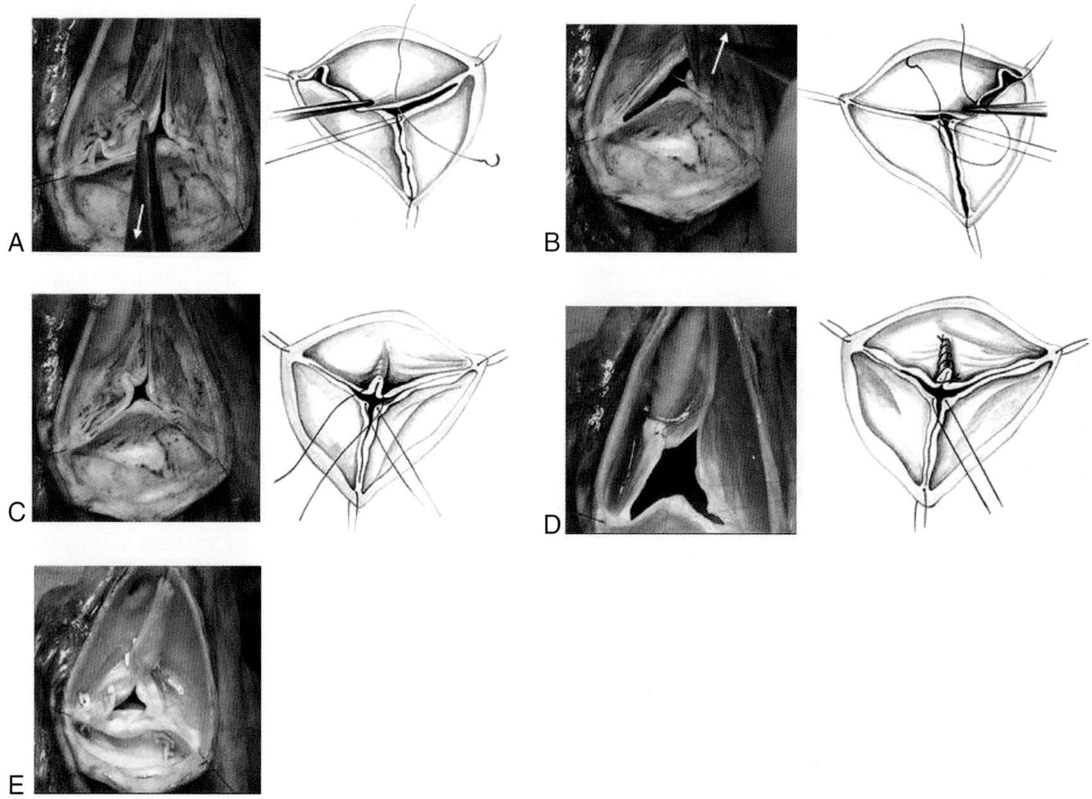

FIGURE 78-10 ■ Free margin plication technique for the correction of cusp prolapse.

where it meets the middle of the reference cusp. The length of cusp free margin between the two ends of this 6-0 suture represents the quantity of excess free margin, which is then plicated by tying this suture with the excess tissue on the aortic side.

The plication is extended by 5 to 10 mm onto the body of the aortic cusp by adding interrupted or running locked 6-0 polypropylene sutures. If there is significant excessive tissue, it can be shaved off using a scalpel or scissors, keeping sufficient tissue to bring the edges together.

Free Margin Resuspension

Excess length of the cusp free margin can also be corrected using resuspension with polytetrafluoroethylene (PTFE) suture[30,31] (Fig. 78-11). A 7-0 polypropylene suture is first passed through the center (nodule of Arantius) of the two nonprolapsing cusps, which serves as a reference. A 7-0 PTFE suture is passed twice at the top of the commissure. Next, one arm of the suture is passed over the length of the free margin in a running fashion. The suture is locked at the other commissure. A second 7-0 PTFE is then passed in the same fashion along the cusp free margin. The length of the free margin is reduced by applying gentle traction on each branch of the PTFE sutures and applying opposite resistance with a forceps at the middle of the free margin. This maneuver is used to plicate and shorten the free margin until it reaches the same length as the adjacent reference cusp free margin. The same maneuver is applied for the second half of the free margin. This two-step technique for free margin resuspension allows symmetric and homogenous shortening. When the appropriate amount of free margin shortening is achieved, the two suture ends at each commissure are tied.

This technique can be used in isolation or in combination with other cusp repair techniques, and it is particularly useful in the setting of a fragile free margin with multiple fenestrations or to homogenize the free margin when a pericardial patch is used for cusp augmentation.

Cusp Shaving, Resection, and Patch Use

In contrast to cusp prolapse, management of restrictive cusp pathology owing to localized calcification, inflammatory or rheumatic disease, or bicuspid valve with restrictive raphe (discussed later) can be more challenging. Localized shaving and decalcification of the cusp can be performed, while leaving the cusp surface intact, to improve mobility. When this is not possible or in the setting of endocarditis, localized resection can be performed with the placement of patch material for cusp restoration. The presence of restrictive disease and the use of a patch have both been associated with reduced repair durability.[13,32] In contrast, pericardial patch closure of fenestrations has been suggested to have acceptable outcomes.[33] The use of newer biomaterials is currently being explored and may help to overcome this limitation.[34]

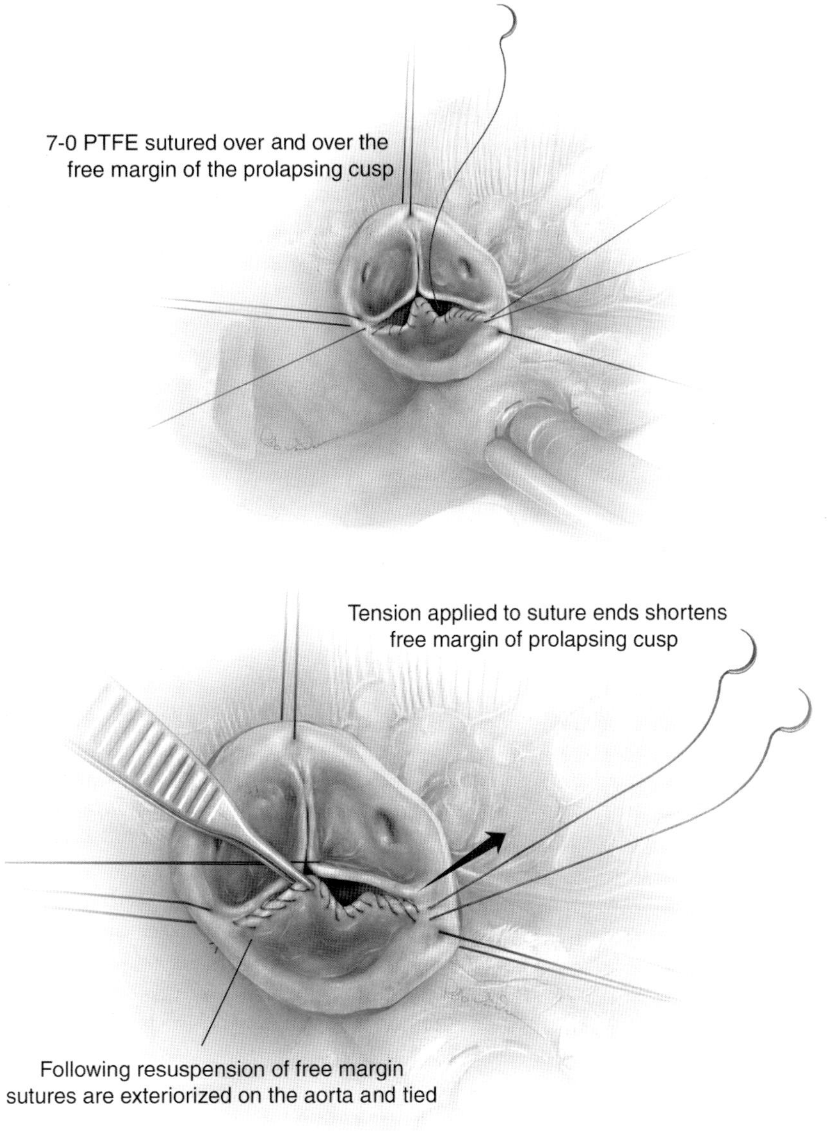
7-0 PTFE sutured over and over the
free margin of the prolapsing cusp
Tension applied to suture ends shortens
free margin of prolapsing cusp
Following resuspension of free margin
sutures are exteriorized on the aorta and tied

FIGURE 78-11 Free margin resuspension technique using polytetrafluoroethylene (PTFE; Gore-Tex) suture for cusp prolapse correction.

Bicuspid Aortic Valve Repair

Bicuspid aortic valve disease affects not only the valve cusps, but also the functional aortic annulus. Bicuspid aortic valve can be divided into two general types[13, 35] (Fig. 78-12). Type 0 bicuspid aortic valves do not contain a median raphe, have two symmetric aortic sinuses, two commissures, and a symmetric base of leaflet implantation of the two cusps. This configuration is present in a minority of cases. The mechanism of AI in this setting is usually cusp prolapse of one or both cusps because of the presence of excess cusp tissue.

Type 1 bicuspid aortic valves, which are significantly more prevalent, have a median raphe on the conjoint cusp and an asymmetric distribution of the aortic sinuses, with a large aortic sinus accompanying a large nonconjoint cusp and two smaller cusps fused together with a median raphe. The raphe often attaches to the cusp base in the form of a "pseudocommissure," which has a height less than that of the true commissures. The raphe may be restrictive, fibrotic, calcified, or prolapsing. Furthermore, the base of leaflet implantation is typically larger (i.e., occupying a greater proportion of valve circumference) and higher on the conjoint cusp compared to the nonconjoint cusp. The mechanisms of AI in type 1 valves can be due to a rigid and restrictive raphe associated with small fused cusps resulting in a triangular coaptation defect. Alternatively, the raphe may be short and nonrestrictive with well-developed cusps and associated prolapse of the conjoint cusp. Bicuspid valve anatomy can be anywhere along a spectrum between type 0 and type 1. The general algorithm for the repair of bicuspid aortic valves is presented in Figure 78-13.

In type 0 valves, the degree of prolapse is assessed by comparing the prolapsing cusp to the nonprolapsing cusp, similar to trileaflet valves. If both cusps are prolapsing, the goal is to restore the height of coaptation to the midpoint of the sinuses of Valsalva. This can be performed using free

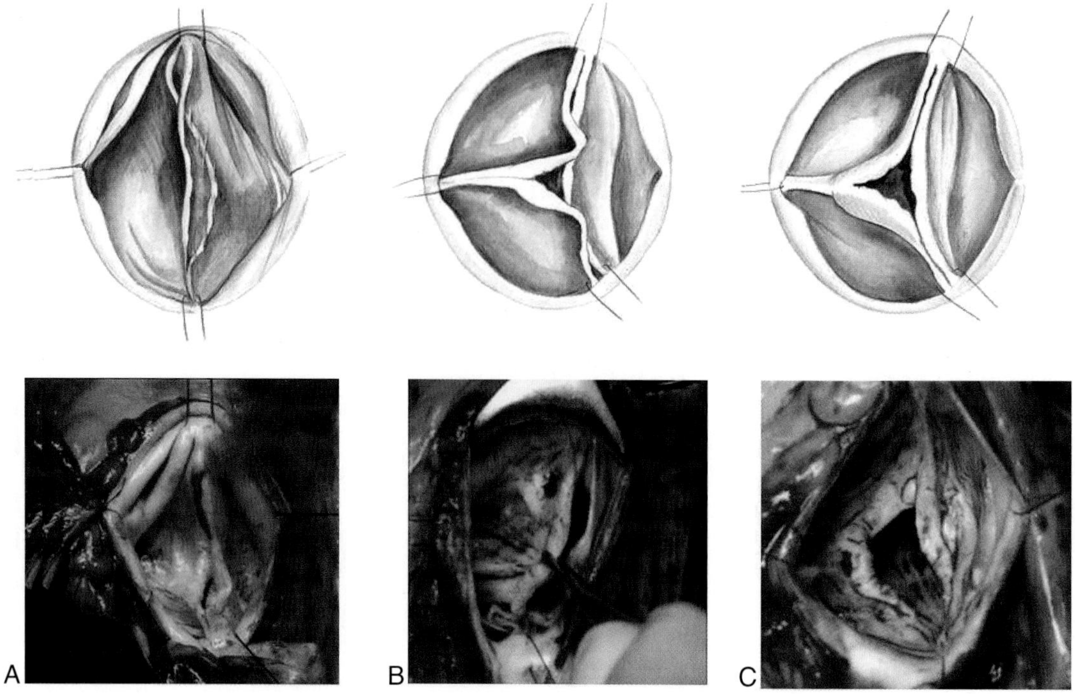

FIGURE 78-12 ■ Cusp anatomy in bicuspid aortic valves.

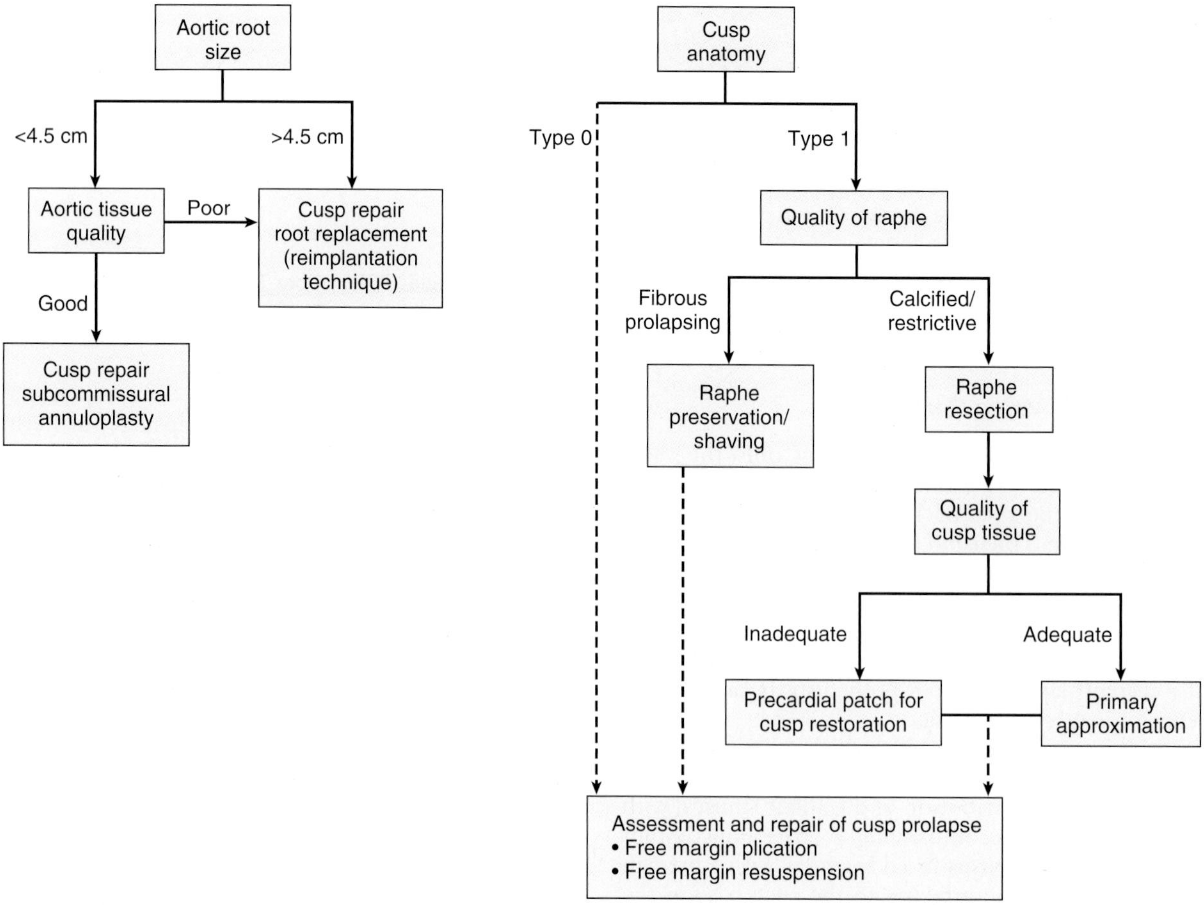

FIGURE 78-13 ■ Algorithm for annulus and cusp management in bicuspid aortic valve repair.

margin plication, free margin resuspension with 7-0 PTFE suture, or both as previously described for trileaflet valves. Thickened, fibrotic areas of the leaflet (typically central aspect of the free margin) are shaved, and localized decalcification is performed if calcium is present.

In type 1 valves, the median raphe is addressed first. If the raphe is relatively mobile and only mildly thickened and fibrosed, it is preserved and shaved using a combination of a scalpel and scissors (Fig. 78-14). When a severely restrictive or calcified raphe is present, a parsimonious triangular resection of this tissue is performed (Fig. 78-15). Next, the quantity of remaining cusp tissue is assessed by putting the two arms of a 6-0 polypropylene suture on the free margin of the conjoint cusp, on either side of the resected raphe. At this point, lack of cusp restriction and good valve opening are signs of the presence of adequate cusp tissue. The leaflet edges are reapproximated primarily when adequate cusp tissue is present using running locked or interrupted 6-0 polypropylene sutures. In the absence of adequate tissue, a triangular autologous treated or bovine pericardial patch is used for cusp restoration (Fig. 78-16).

Next, the free margins of both cusps are compared for the presence of any prolapse, which is corrected using free margin plication or resuspension with PTFE.

Unicuspid and Quadricuspid Aortic Valves

Unicuspid and quadricuspid are rare variants of aortic valve anatomy, and both can manifest with either valve

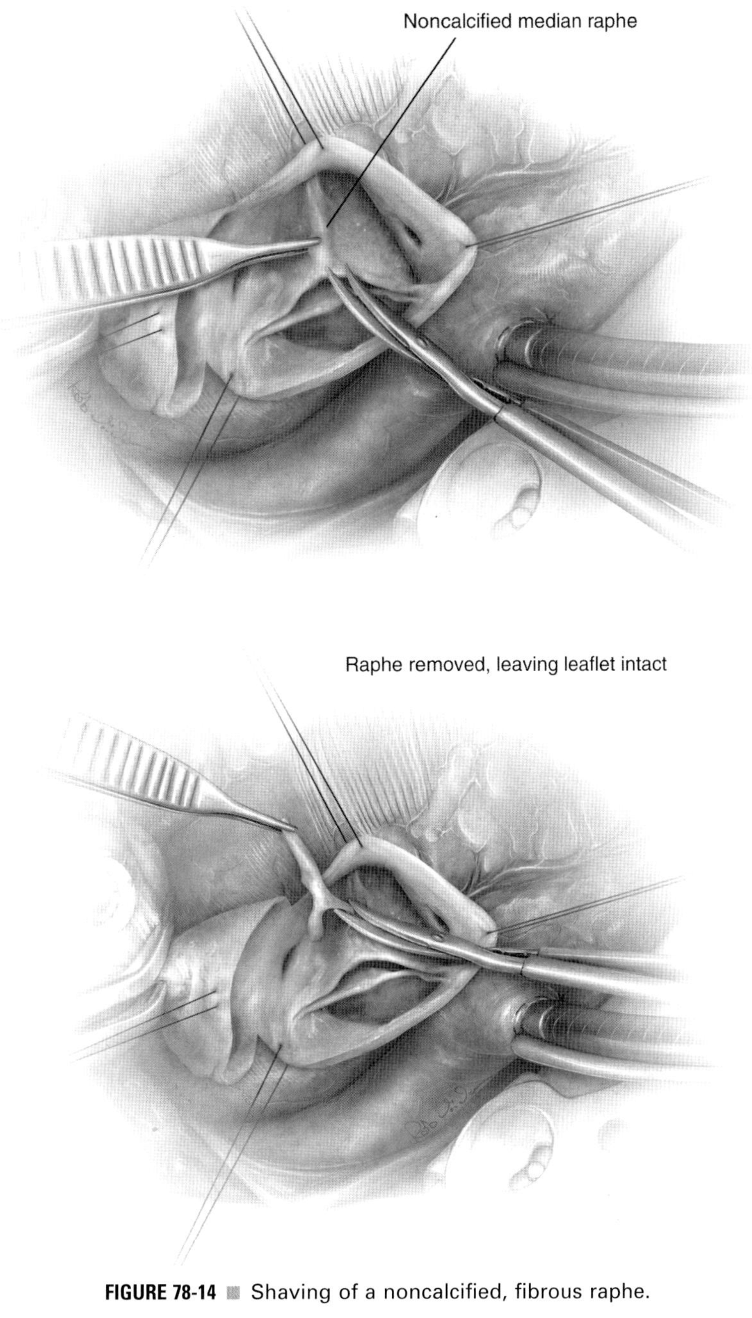

FIGURE 78-14 ■ Shaving of a noncalcified, fibrous raphe.

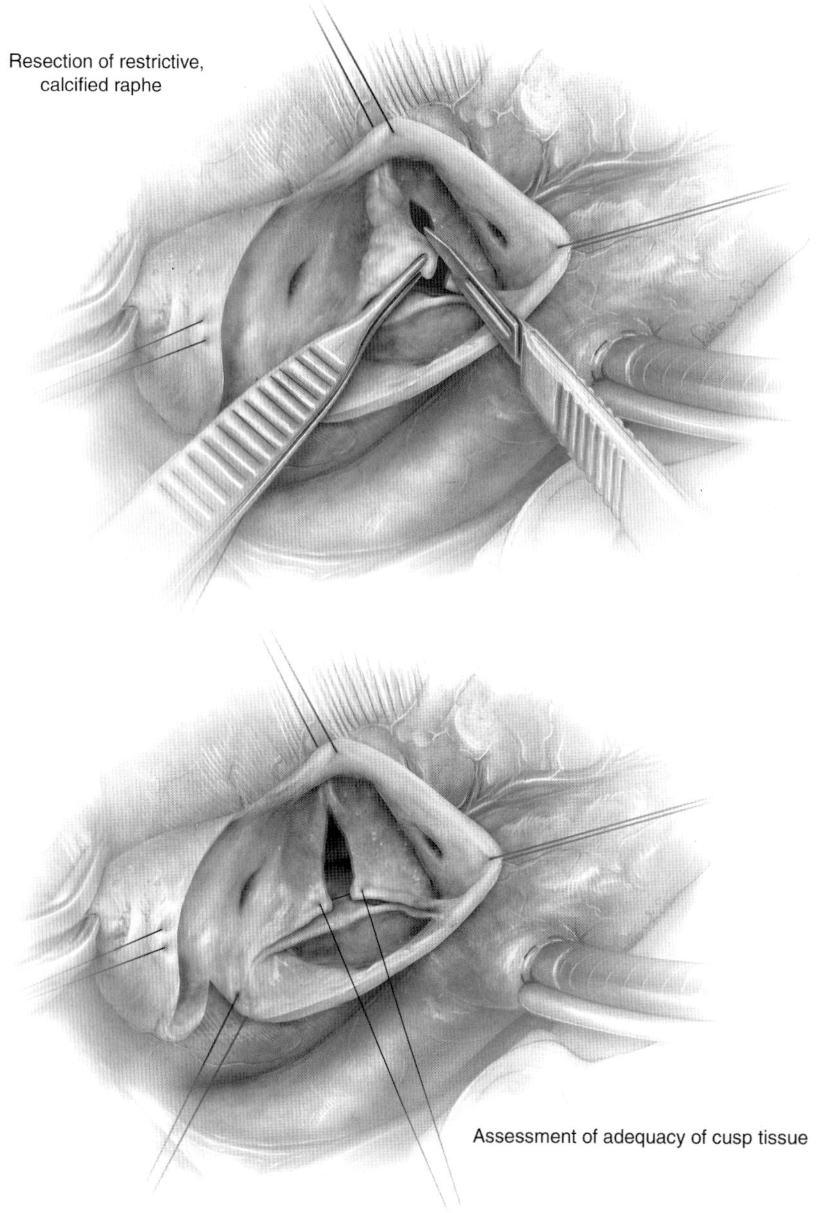

FIGURE 78-15 ■ Resection of a restrictive or calcified raphe *(top)* and assessment of the quantity of available tissue *(bottom)*.

stenosis or insufficiency. The most common approach to the repair of the regurgitant unicuspid valve involves bicuspidization by creating a neocommissure using a pericardial patch. Techniques using a single or double patch have been described.[32,36] These repairs are typically performed in the pediatric or young adult population, and long-term data on valve durability are lacking.

Quadricuspid aortic valves can have a variety of different orientations and may also be associated with aortopathy. Typically, one of the cusps has an additional attachment to the aortic wall and a raphe-like structure that causes cusp restriction. Repair is typically achieved by tricuspidizing the valve by taking down this attachment and raphe and by repairing the affected cusp. Small case series using this technique have shown good early results, but long-term data are lacking.[15,37,38]

INTRAOPERATIVE ECHOCARDIOGRAPHY

In addition to providing important information regarding valve anatomy and mechanism of valve dysfunction, postrepair transesophageal echocardiography is mandatory in patients undergoing aortic valve repair.[39] More than trivial to mild residual aortic insufficiency (particularly eccentric jets), coaptation height below the aortic annulus, and coaptation length less than 5 mm have been shown to be important predictors of late repair failure and warrant aortic valve reexploration.[40]

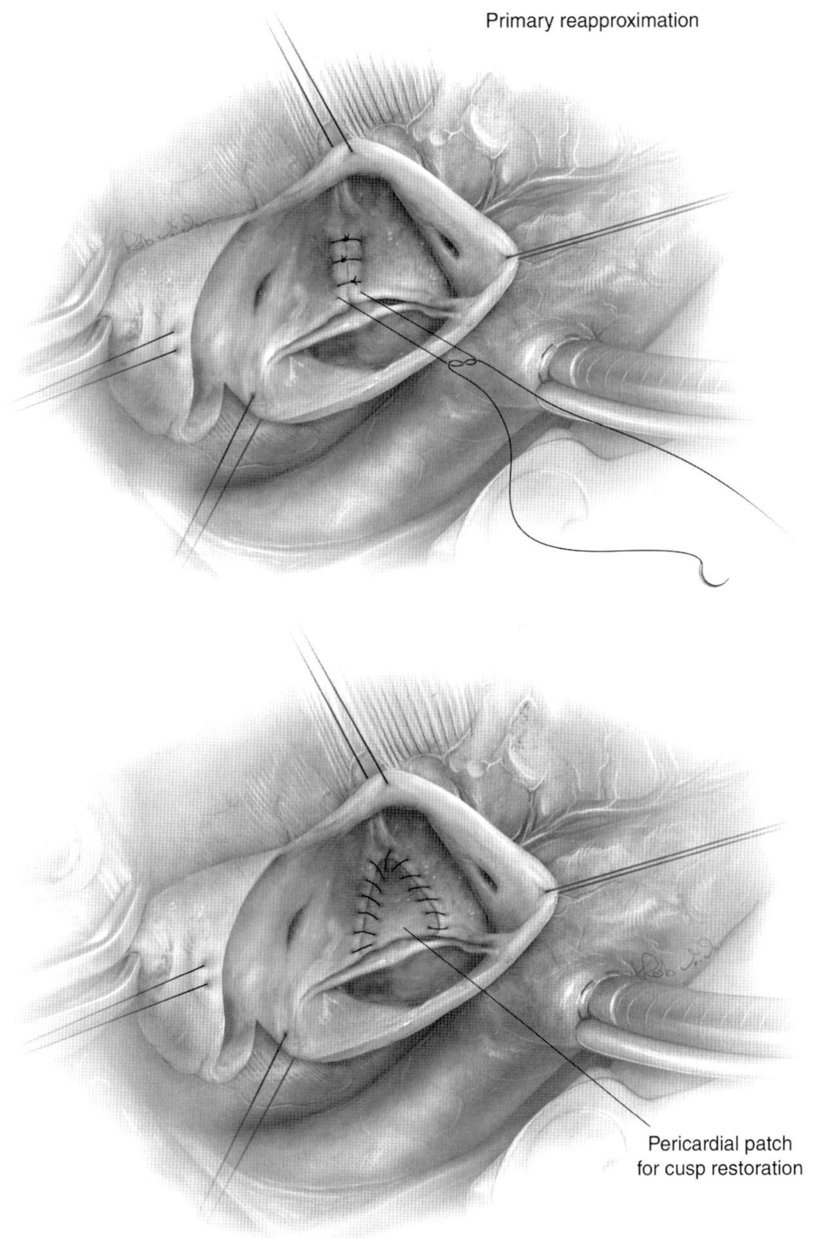

FIGURE 78-16 ■ Primary reapproximation *(top)* or use of pericardial patch for cusp restoration *(bottom)*.

OUTCOMES

There are no randomized controlled trials comparing the outcomes of aortic valve repair versus replacement. Data on the durability of aortic valve repair techniques are currently limited to single-center series that are small to moderate in size, with a mean follow-up time of 5 to 10 years. However, data up to 18 to 20 years are emerging in certain subgroups. Important outcome variables include early mortality and morbidity, late freedom from reoperation and recurrent aortic valve insufficiency or stenosis, and the incidence of valve related complications of thromboembolism, bleeding, and endocarditis.

Overall

There are few studies reporting the outcome of unselected patients referred for aortic valve repair surgery. The success rate of valve preservation and repair in this context is rarely reported. Patients with aortic valve repair are typically a heterogenous group representing the spectrum from young patients with congenital valve disease to older patients with degenerative aortic aneurysms and concomitant AI. As such, outcomes are frequently reported for specific subsets of patients undergoing aortic valve repair.

In a study examining the role of AI classification on surgical techniques and outcome, we evaluated 264 unselected patients undergoing aortic valve repair (mean age, 54 ± 16 years; 80% male).[11] Approximately two thirds of patients were identified as having a single lesion causing AI. Two lesions were identified in 30% and three in 6% of patients. Fifty percent of lesions were type I (normal leaflet motion with FAA dilation or cusp perforation), 35% were type II (leaflet prolapse), and 15% were type III (leaflet restriction). The most common set of multiple lesions were prolapse of aortic valve leaflet in combination with type Ia (STJ dilation) or type Ib (aortic root aneurysm) disease. The classification of AI correctly predicted the surgical technique used in the vast majority of patients (82% to 100%). Overall survival in this cohort was 95% ± 3% at 5 years and 87% ± 8% at 8 years. Freedom from cardiac death was 95% ± 5% at 8 years. Freedom from aortic valve reoperation and replacement at 8 years was 91% ± 5% and 93% ± 4%, respectively. Importantly, classification of AI was also predictive of late outcome with patients with type III (restrictive cusp disease) demonstrating increased late aortic valve reoperation and recurrent AI (Fig. 78-17).

A recent meta-analysis examined the outcome of aortic valve preservation and repair in acute type A dissection and found good valve durability, low risk of valve-related complications, but a significant attrition of patients over time (4.7% per year).[41]

Valve-Sparing Aortic Replacement

Outcomes following valve-sparing aortic root replacement have been reported by a number of groups. Results from large cohorts of patients performed in centers with experience with this technique generally show similar outcomes. David and colleagues[42] were pioneers of the reimplantation technique and reported their experience in 289 patients, 228 of which underwent the reimplantation technique and 61 underwent the remodeling technique.[43,44] Early mortality was 1.7%, and 12-year survival was 83%. Late freedom from reoperation at 12 years was 90% with the remodeling technique and 97% with the reimplantation technique (P = 0.09). Freedom from recurrent AI at 12 years was 83% after remodeling and 91% after reimplantation (P = 0.035). The authors concluded that the reimplantation technique provides more durable outcome.

Schafers and colleagues reported the outcome of the remodeling approach in 274 patients and found that early mortality was 3.6%, freedom from reoperation was 96% at 10 years and freedom from recurrent AI was 87% at 10 years.[45]

Our group has reported outcomes in 164 consecutive patients who underwent valve-sparing aortic root replacement (74% reimplantation, 26% remodeling) specifically examining the effect of presence of preoperative aortic insufficiency on late outcome.[46] Severe preoperative AI was present in 57% of patients. In this cohort, early mortality was 0.6% and late survival was 88% at 8 years. Freedom from reoperation was 90% at 8 years, and freedom from recurrent AI was 90% at 5 years; both were independent of preoperative AI severity.

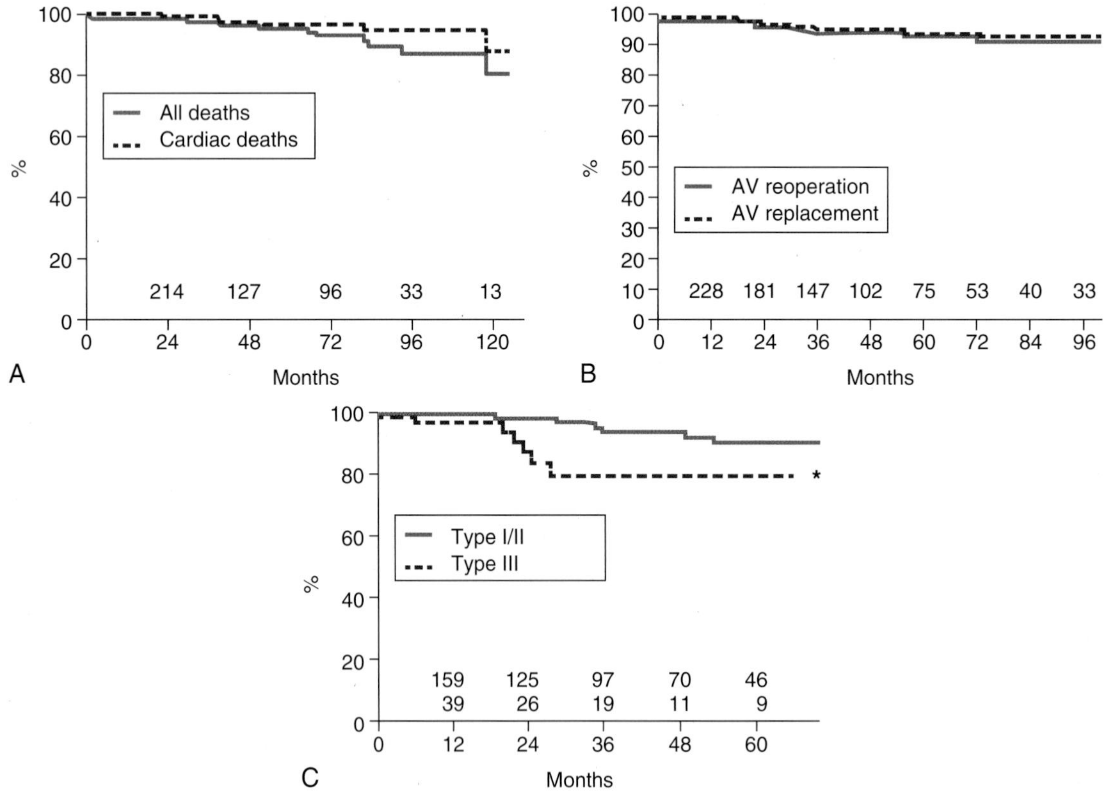

FIGURE 78-17 Survival **(A)** and freedom **(B)** from aortic valve (AV) reoperation or replacement in an unselected cohort of patients undergoing aortic valve repair. **C,** Recurrence of aortic insufficiency (AI) according to lesion type shows increased AI recurrence in patients with type III disease.

Bicuspid Aortic Valve Repair

Unlike the results of valve-sparing aortic root replacement, results of bicuspid aortic valve repair reported in the literature have been highly variable between groups. These differences are largely due to the heterogeneity in the surgical techniques used, particularly the degree of annular stabilization. Schafers and colleagues[47] performed bicuspid aortic valve repair in 174 patients and found that freedom from reoperation was 97% at 5 years in those undergoing the remodeling approach but only 53% in those not undergoing root replacement.[47] A more recent update of their experience in 316 patients showed a 10-year survival of 92% and a 10-year freedom from reoperation of 81%. Absence of root replacement and a number of anatomic features of the bicuspid valve, including commissural orientation and VAJ diameter, were predictors of repair failure.[12] Alsoufi and colleagues[48] reported outcome following bicuspid aortic valve repair in 71 patients. Despite low early and late mortality, freedom from reoperation and recurrent AI at 8 years were 82% and 44%, respectively.

In our cohort of 122 patients undergoing bicuspid aortic valve repair (mean age, 44 years; 80% male, 57% with associated aortic dilation), there was no early mortality and late survival was 97% at 8 years.[13] Freedom from late aortic valve reoperation was 98% and 87% at 5 and 8 years, respectively, and freedom from recurrent AI was 94% at 5 years. In our experience, root replacement led to a more durable outcome compared with subcommissural annuloplasty alone (Fig. 78-18). A follow-up study was performed comparing patients undergoing valve-sparing root replacement using the reimplantation technique to all other forms of annular stabilization. Patients were matched for root and annular size and severity of preoperative AI. We found that patients undergoing the reimplantation technique had significantly lower rates of reoperation and recurrent AI.[49] This confirms the notion that the VAJ in patients with bicuspid aortic valve disease may continue to dilate over time and may cause repair failure.

Trileaflet Aortic Valve Repair

Different techniques can be used to correct cusp prolapse in trileaflet aortic valves. Free margin plication and free margin resuspension are the most commonly used techniques. Studies comparing the two techniques

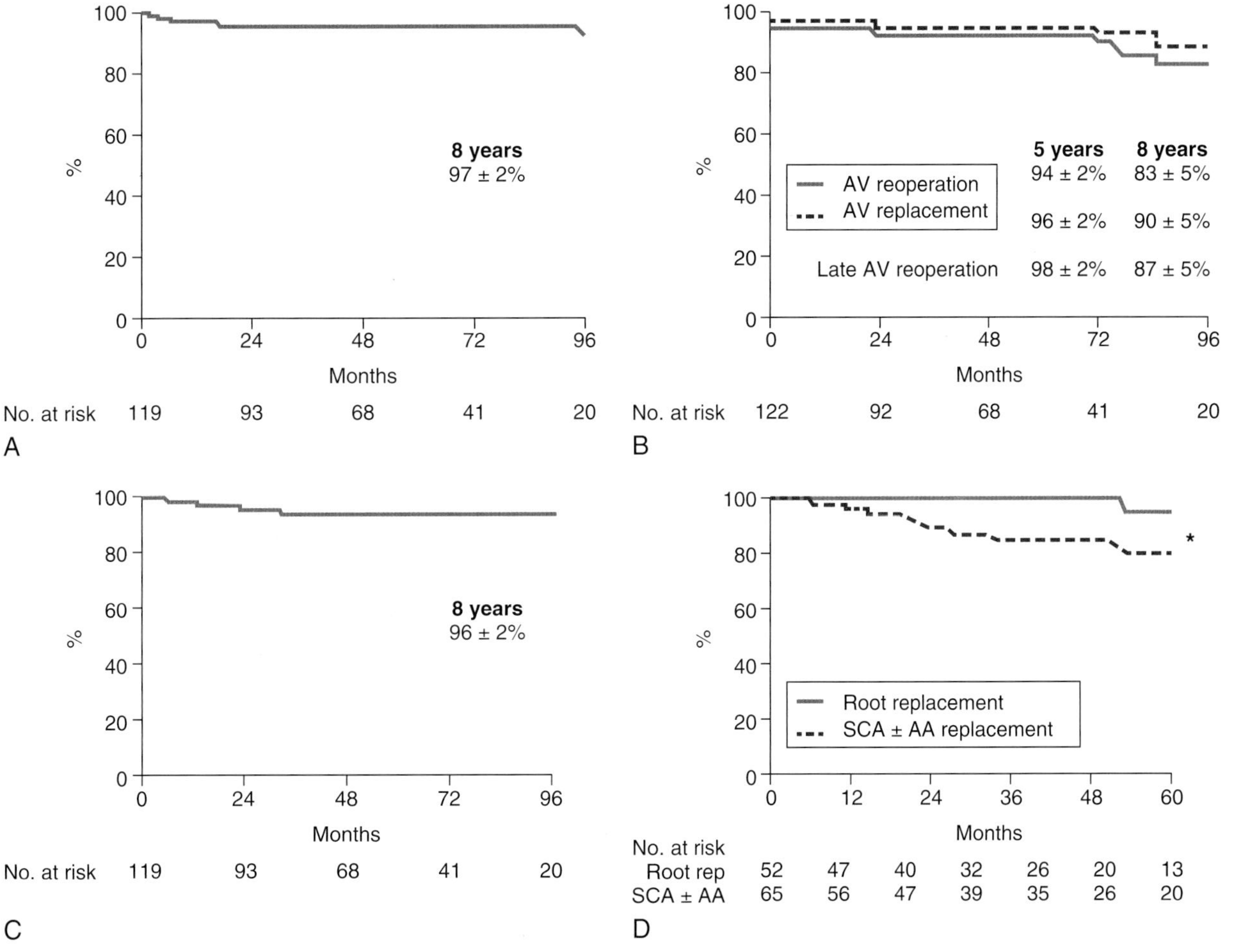

FIGURE 78-18 Survival **(A)** and freedom **(B)** from aortic valve (AV) reoperation or replacement, and **(C)** freedom from thromboembolism and bleeding in patients undergoing bicuspid aortic valve repair. **D,** Patients undergoing valve-sparing aortic root replacement had a higher freedom from recurrent aortic insufficiency than those undergoing subcommissural annuloplasty (SCA) with or without supracoronary ascending aortic (AA) replacement.

demonstrate equivalent durability in terms of freedom from reoperation or recurrent AI.[31,50] Another important question in the repair of trileaflet aortic valves is the appropriate detection and localization of cusp prolapse. We examined echocardiographic and intraoperative features that could predict the need for cusp prolapse repair in trileaflet aortic valves with or without aortic root pathology. We found that the presence of a preoperative eccentric AI jet, regardless of severity, and the presence of a transverse fibrous band (see Fig. 78-4) were most useful in the detection and correct localization of cusp prolapse.[17]

Valve-Related Complications

A consistent finding across all longitudinal studies of aortic valve repair outcome is the low incidence of valve-related events. For prosthetic aortic valve replacements, the rate of thromboembolic events is typically between 1% and 2% per year.[51,52] For patients with mechanical aortic valves, the rate of anticoagulant related hemorrhage is also 1% to 2% per year. Furthermore, valve thrombosis and prosthetic valve endocarditis are infrequent but devastating complications. In contrast, the combined rate of thromboembolism, bleeding events, and endocarditis following aortic valve repair has been reported in several studies to be less than 0.5% per year.[11,13,53] This is particularly attractive for young patients who continue to accrue the risk of valve-related events over time.

CONCLUSION

Over the past two decades, important advances have been made in the field of aortic valve repair. These advances include a better understanding of the functional anatomy of the aortic valve, the development of a repair-oriented classification system for aortic insufficiency, the application of valve-sparing techniques to the preservation and repair of regurgitant aortic valves, and the development of cusp repair techniques. New data are available indicating the durability of aortic valve repair up to 10 years. Additional long-term studies and studies comparing aortic valve repair to replacement are needed to better define the role of aortic valve repair in patients with aortic insufficiency.

REFERENCES

1. Mann T, McLaurin L, Grossman W, et al: Assessing the hemodynamic severity of acute aortic regurgitation due to infective endocarditis. *N Engl J Med* 293(3):108–113, 1975.
2. Gaasch WH: Left ventricular radius to wall thickness ratio. *Am J Cardiol* 43(6):1189–1194, 1979.
3. Ross J, Jr: Afterload mismatch in aortic and mitral valve disease: implications for surgical therapy. *J Am Coll Cardiol* 5(4):811–826, 1985.
4. Enriquez-Sarano M, Bailey KR, Seward JB, et al: Quantitative Doppler assessment of valvular regurgitation. *Circulation* 87(3):841–848, 1993.
5. Nishimura RA, Otto CM, Bonow RO, et al: 2014 AHA/ACC guideline for the management of patients with valvular heart disease: a report of the American College of Cardiology/American Heart Association Task Force on Practice Guidelines. *J Thorac Cardiovasc Surg* 148(1):e1–e132, 2014.
6. Gillinov AM, Mihaljevic T, Blackstone EH, et al: Should patients with severe degenerative mitral regurgitation delay surgery until symptoms develop? *Ann Thorac Surg* 90(2):481–488, 2010.
7. Sharma V, Suri RM, Dearani JA, et al: Expanding relevance of aortic valve repair-is earlier operation indicated? *J Thorac Cardiovasc Surg* 147(1):100–107, 2013.
8. Hiratzka LF, Bakris GL, Beckman JA, et al: 2010 ACCF/AHA/AATS/ACR/ASA/SCA/SCAI/SIR/STS/SVM guidelines for the diagnosis and management of patients with Thoracic Aortic Disease: a report of the American College of Cardiology Foundation/American Heart Association Task Force on Practice Guidelines, American Association for Thoracic Surgery, American College of Radiology, American Stroke Association, Society of Cardiovascular Anesthesiologists, Society for Cardiovascular Angiography and Interventions, Society of Interventional Radiology, Society of Thoracic Surgeons, and Society for Vascular Medicine. *Circulation* 121(13):e266–e369, 2010.
9. Erbel R, Aboyans V, Boileau C, et al: 2014 ESC Guidelines on the diagnosis and treatment of aortic diseases: document covering acute and chronic aortic diseases of the thoracic and abdominal aorta of the adult. The Task Force for the Diagnosis and Treatment of Aortic Diseases of the European Society of Cardiology (ESC). *Eur Heart J* 35(41):2873–2926, 2014.
10. Boodhwani M, Andelfinger G, Leipsic J, et al: Canadian Cardiovascular Society position statement on the management of thoracic aortic disease. *Can J Cardiol* 30(6):577–589, 2014.
11. Boodhwani M, de Kerchove L, Glineur D, et al: Repair-oriented classification of aortic insufficiency: impact on surgical techniques and clinical outcomes. *J Thorac Cardiovasc Surg* 137(2):286–294, 2009.
12. Aicher D, Kunihara T, Abou Issa O, et al: Valve configuration determines long-term results after repair of the bicuspid aortic valve. *Circulation* 123(2):178–185, 2011.
13. Boodhwani M, de Kerchove L, Glineur D, et al: Repair of regurgitant bicuspid aortic valves: a systematic approach. *J Thorac Cardiovasc Surg* 140(2):276–284, 2010.
14. Schafers HJ, Aicher D, Riodionycheva S, et al: Bicuspidization of the unicuspid aortic valve: a new reconstructive approach. *Ann Thorac Surg* 85(6):2012–2018, 2008.
15. Jeanmart H, de Kerchove L, El Bitar F, et al: Tricuspidation of quadricuspid aortic valve: case reports. *J Heart Valve Dis* 16(2):148–150, 2007.
16. Anderson RH: Clinical anatomy of the aortic root. *Heart* 84(6):670–673, 2000.
17. Boodhwani M, de Kerchove L, Watremez C, et al: Assessment and repair of aortic valve cusp prolapse: implications for valve-sparing procedures. *J Thorac Cardiovasc Surg* 141(4):917–925, 2011.
18. Underwood MJ, El Khoury G, Deronck D, et al: The aortic root: structure, function, and surgical reconstruction. *Heart* 83(4):376–380, 2000.
19. Boodhwani M, El Khoury G: Aortic valve repair. *Operative techniques in thoracic and cardiovascular surgery* 14(4):266–280, 2009.
20. Carpentier A: Cardiac valve surgery—the "French correction." *J Thorac Cardiovasc Surg* 86(3):323–337, 1983.
21. David TE, Feindel CM: An aortic valve-sparing operation for patients with aortic incompetence and aneurysm of the ascending aorta. *J Thorac Cardiovasc Surg* 103(4):617–621, discussion 622, 1992.
22. Yacoub MH, Gehle P, Chandrasekaran V, et al: Late results of a valve-preserving operation in patients with aneurysms of the ascending aorta and root. *J Thorac Cardiovasc Surg* 115(5):1080–1090, 1998.
23. Boodhwani M, de Kerchove L, El Khoury G: Aortic root replacement using the reimplantation technique: tips and tricks. *Interact Cardiovasc Thorac Surg* 8(5):584–586, 2009.
24. de Kerchove L, Boodhwani M, Glineur D, et al: A new simple and objective method for graft sizing in valve-sparing root replacement using the reimplantation technique. *Ann Thorac Surg* 92(2):749–751, 2011.
25. Lansac E, Di Centa I, Bonnet N, et al: Gandjbakhch I. Aortic prosthetic ring annuloplasty: a useful adjunct to a standardized aortic valve-sparing procedure? *Eur J Cardiothorac Surg* 29(4):537–544, 2006.
26. Mazzitelli D, Nobauer C, Rankin JS, et al: Early results after implantation of a new geometric annuloplasty ring for aortic valve repair. *Ann Thorac Surg* 95(1):94–97, 2013.

27. Scharfschwerdt M, Pawlik M, Sievers HH, et al: In vitro investigation of aortic valve annuloplasty using prosthetic ring devices. *Eur J Cardiothorac Surg* 40(5):1127–1130, 2011.
28. Schafers HJ, Schmied W, Marom G, et al: Cusp height in aortic valves. *J Thorac Cardiovasc Surg* 146(2):269–274, 2013.
29. Boodhwani M, de Kerchove L, Glineur D, et al: A simple method for the quantification and correction of aortic cusp prolapse by means of free margin plication. *J Thorac Cardiovasc Surg* 139(4):1075–1077, 2010.
30. David TE, Armstrong S: Aortic cusp repair with Gore-Tex sutures during aortic valve-sparing operations. *J Thorac Cardiovasc Surg* 139:1340–1342, 2010.
31. de Kerchove L, Boodhwani M, Glineur D, et al: Cusp prolapse repair in trileaflet aortic valves: free margin plication and free margin resuspension techniques. *Ann Thorac Surg* 88(2):455–461, discussion 461, 2009.
32. Mosala Nezhad Z, de Kerchove L, Hechadi J, et al: Aortic valve repair with patch in non-rheumatic disease: indication, techniques and durability. *Eur J Cardiothorac Surg* 46(6):997–1005, 2014.
33. Schafers HJ, Langer F, Glombitza P, et al: Aortic valve reconstruction in myxomatous degeneration of aortic valves: are fenestrations a risk factor for repair failure? *J Thorac Cardiovasc Surg* 139(3):660–664, 2010.
34. Toeg HD, Abessi O, Al-Atassi T, et al: Finding the ideal biomaterial for aortic valve repair with ex vivo porcine left heart simulator and finite element modeling. *J Thorac Cardiovasc Surg* 148(4):1739–1745, 2014.
35. Sievers HH, Schmidtke C: A classification system for the bicuspid aortic valve from 304 surgical specimens. *J Thorac Cardiovasc Surg* 133(5):1226–1233, 2007.
36. Aicher D, Schafers HJ: Bicuspidization of the regurgitant unicuspid aortic valve. *Multimed Man Cardiothorac Surg* 2010(324): mmcts.2009.004069, 2010.
37. Elmistekawy EM, Malas T, Hynes M, et al: Repair of quadricuspid aortic valve associated with ascending aorta dilatation. *J Heart Valve Dis* 21(6):740–742, 2012.
38. Schmidt KI, Jeserich M, Aicher D, et al: Tricuspidization of the quadricuspid aortic valve. *Ann Thorac Surg* 85(3):1087–1089, 2008.
39. Van Dyck MJ, Watremez C, Boodhwani M, et al: Transesophageal echocardiographic evaluation during aortic valve repair surgery. *Anesth Analg* 111:59–70, 2010.
40. le Polain de Waroux JB, Pouleur AC, Robert A, et al: Mechanisms of recurrent aortic regurgitation after aortic valve repair: predictive value of intraoperative transesophageal echocardiography. *JACC Cardiovasc Imaging* 2(8):931–939, 2009.
41. Saczkowski R, Malas T, Mesana T, et al: Aortic valve preservation and repair in acute Type A aortic dissection. *Eur J Cardiothorac Surg* 45(6):e220–e226, 2014.
42. David TE, Maganti M, Armstrong S: Aortic root aneurysm: principles of repair and long-term follow-up. *J Thorac Cardiovasc Surg* 140(6 Suppl):S14–S19, discussion S45–51, 2010.
43. David TE, Feindel CM, Webb GD, et al: Aortic valve preservation in patients with aortic root aneurysm: results of the reimplantation technique. *Ann Thorac Surg* 83(2):S732–S735, discussion S785–790, 2007.
44. David TE, Feindel CM, Webb GD, et al: Long-term results of aortic valve-sparing operations for aortic root aneurysm. *J Thorac Cardiovasc Surg* 132(2):347–354, 2006.
45. Aicher D, Langer F, Lausberg H, et al: Aortic root remodeling: ten-year experience with 274 patients. *J Thorac Cardiovasc Surg* 134(4):909–915, 2007.
46. de Kerchove L, Boodhwani M, Glineur D, et al: Effects of preoperative aortic insufficiency on outcome after aortic valve-sparing surgery. *Circulation* 120(11 Suppl):S120–S126, 2009.
47. Schafers HJ, Aicher D, Langer F, et al: Preservation of the bicuspid aortic valve. *Ann Thorac Surg* 83(2):S740–S745, discussion S785–790, 2007.
48. Alsoufi B, Borger MA, Armstrong S, et al: Results of valve preservation and repair for bicuspid aortic valve insufficiency. *J Heart Valve Dis* 14(6):752–758, discussion 758–759, 2005.
49. Navarra E, El Khoury G, Glineur D, et al: Effect of annulus dimension and annuloplasty on bicuspid aortic valve repair. *Eur J Cardiothorac Surg* 44(2):316–322, discussion 322–313, 2013.
50. de Kerchove L, Glineur D, Poncelet A, et al: Repair of aortic leaflet prolapse: a ten-year experience. *Eur J Cardiothorac Surg* 34(4):785–791, 2008.
51. Peterseim DS, Cen YY, Cheruvu S, et al: Long-term outcome after biologic versus mechanical aortic valve replacement in 841 patients. *J Thorac Cardiovasc Surg* 117(5):890–897, 1999.
52. Ruel M, Masters RG, Rubens FD, et al: Late incidence and determinants of stroke after aortic and mitral valve replacement. *Ann Thorac Surg* 78(1):77–83, discussion 83–84, 2004.
53. Aicher D, Fries R, Rodionycheva S, et al: Aortic valve repair leads to a low incidence of valve-related complications. *Eur J Cardiothorac Surg* 37(1):127–132, 2010.

CHAPTER 79

Transcatheter Aortic Valve Replacement

Vinod H. Thourani • Sebastian Iturra • Eric L. Sarin

CHAPTER OUTLINE

INTRODUCTION

Aortic stenosis is the most frequent acquired valve disease in older adult patients; consequently, the number of patients requiring treatment increases as the population ages. Current U.S. Census predictions indicate that by 2050 the number of citizens 85 years and older will reach 17.9 million and the number of citizens 65 years and older will reach 83.7 million.[1] Historically, aortic stenosis was treated with surgical aortic valve replacement (SAVR) using cardiopulmonary bypass via either a median sternotomy or minimally invasive techniques. These techniques have produced durable results with low morbidity and acceptable long-term survival rates.[2-5] However, as the older adult population expands, more patients are developing aortic stenosis and multiple medical comorbidities that increase their operative risk. Despite several series demonstrating good clinical outcomes following SAVR in older adult patients,[2,4,6] many physicians are reluctant to recommend surgery for high surgical risk patients with comorbidities. At least 30% of patients with severe symptomatic aortic stenosis are not treated with SAVR because of reluctance by referring physicians, patients, or patients' families.[6] In an attempt to mitigate risk in this frail, older adult population, transcatheter strategies for aortic valve replacement have been developed.[7] In 2002, Cribier performed the first transcatheter aortic valve replacement (TAVR) through an antegrade approach using the femoral vein and a transseptal puncture technique due to advanced peripheral artery disease in an inoperable patient with severe aortic disease.[8] In the subsequent decade, it is estimated that more than 60,000 TAVRs were performed worldwide.[9] The techniques for TAVR have evolved and are currently being performed via retrograde transfemoral (TF), left ventricular transapical (TA), transascending aortic (TAo), transsubclavian (TS), and transcarotid (TC) approaches. This chapter focuses on the indications, preoperative evaluation, operative technique, outcomes, complications, and future of TAVR.

INDICATIONS

The classic indications for an isolated SAVR are symptomatic patients with severe aortic stenosis on transthoracic echocardiography (TTE), defined as a peak aortic-jet velocity (V_{max}) of at least 4.0 m/sec or mean aortic-valve gradient 40 mm Hg or higher.[10] Typically the aortic valve area (AVA) is 1.0 cm^2 or less or an AVA index (AVAi) 0.6 cm^2 or less, but it can be larger secondary to mixed aortic stenosis/aortic regurgitation. The most common symptoms include exertional dyspnea or decreased exercise tolerance, angina, or syncope. In those with symptomatic but low-flow or low-gradient aortic stenosis with a reduced left ventricular ejection fraction, a dobutamine stress echocardiography can be used to ascertain the severity of the valve stenosis. In those patients who are asymptomatic, yet with very severe aortic stenosis ($V_{max} \geq 5.0$ m/sec or mean aortic-valve gradient $\geq$ 60 mm Hg), valve replacement is recommended.[10] Currently in the United States, TAVR is indicated in those patients with a life expectancy exceeding 1 year and severe aortic stenosis who are considered either high risk or inoperative by a multidisciplinary heart team, including those with expertise in cardiac surgery, invasive cardiology, echocardiography, cardiac anesthesia, and imaging specialties. Generally, high-risk patients are considered those defined by a Society of Thoracic Surgeons (STS) predicted risk score of mortality (PROM) of 8% or higher or by the presence of coexisting conditions that would be associated with a predicted risk of death by 30 days after surgery of at least 15%.[11] Outside the United States, the indications for TAVR are quite varied and are dependent on the institutional and geographic conditions.

PREOPERATIVE EVALUATION AND PLANNING

Patient selection is the key to successful TAVR. The methods of assessment of surgical risk vary but typically include the logistic EuroSCORE and/or the STS risk model. A logistic EuroSCORE higher than 20% and STS score higher than 8% expected mortality is generally accepted as high risk for surgery. Patients with limited life expectancy (<1 year), advanced chronic kidney disease (creatinine > 3.0), preoperative hemodialysis, advanced neurologic disease, and bicuspid aortic valves have been excluded from trials, and experience in these populations is limited but growing.

Pre-TAVR evaluation should seek to answer several questions, including (1) severity of aortic stenosis; (2) ileofemoral vessel size, calcification, and tortuosity; (3) anatomic details of the aortic valve leaflets; (4) annulus, sinotubular, and sinus of Valsalva dimensions; (5) ventricular viability; and (6) extent of coronary artery disease. A combination of imaging techniques may be used to answer these questions. At our institution, to discern these aspects a left heart catheterization, high-definition computed tomography (CT) of the chest, abdomen, and pelvis, and TTE or transesophageal echocardiography (TEE) are used to assess each patient prior to TAVR. Furthermore, objective frailty testing, pulmonary function tests, and carotid duplex ultrasound are performed to assess lung function and carotid stenosis. Severe, hemodynamically significant carotid lesions should be treated prior to TAVR.

Aortic Valve Assessment

A complete echocardiographic assessment is required to assess the aortic valve, most commonly using a TTE. From the parasternal long-axis view, the right and noncoronary cusps are identified, and the annulus is measured between the insertion points of the leaflets (Fig. 79-1). Accurate measurement is essential because this is what determines the size of the valve selected. If calcification, body habitus, or other factors preclude the accurate measurement of the annulus, a TEE ought to be performed. The right and noncoronary artery cusps are identified from the long-axis view at 120 degrees. Measurements of the sinus of Valsalva and sinotubular junction are also obtained from this view. The failure to properly size the annulus may result in a valve too small for the annulus with subsequent perivalvular leak or embolization, whereas a valve too big for the annulus may result in aortic dissection or annular damage. A TEE with three-dimensional reconstruction (Fig. 79-2) can be helpful in determining aortic annulus area and perimeter, which is

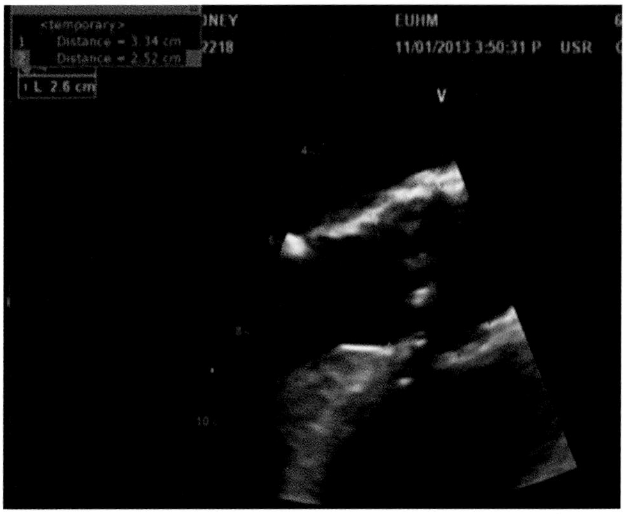

FIGURE 79-1 ■ Transthoracic echocardiogram. Parasternal long-axis view measuring the left ventricular outflow tract.

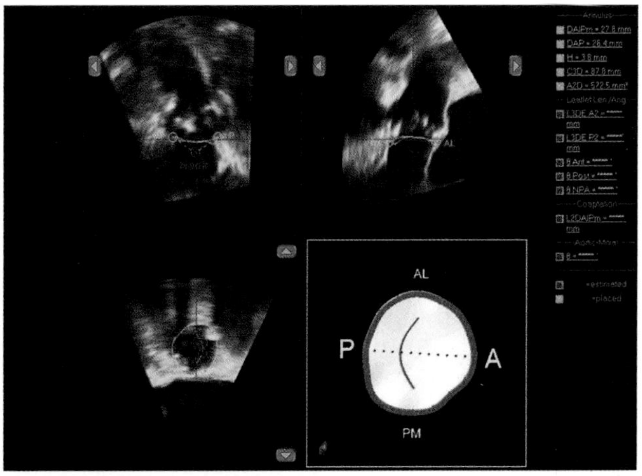

FIGURE 79-2 ■ Transesophageal echocardiogram with three-dimensional reconstruction measuring the aortic annulus area.

particularly useful in patients that were not able to get a three-dimensional CT reconstruction. Sizing of the annulus with supravalvular aortography during balloon aortic valvuloplasty (BAV) may provide additional information when the aortic annulus remains questionable.

All patients should have a CT scan from the aortic valve to the femoral arterial bifurcation. A gated, contrast CT will allow three-dimensional reconstruction, which will show in detail the aortic root anatomy, including the annular, sinotubular, and sinus of Valsalva dimensions, as well as coronary heights above the annulus (Fig. 79-3). Measurement of the annular area or perimeter have supplanted two-dimensional echocardiography in sizing for the appropriate TAVR device and are now the standard of care for assessment of implant size. Each vendor has a sizing chart corresponding to the annular area or perimeter. In those with chronic kidney disease, a three-dimensional TEE as aforementioned is performed to calculate the aortic annulus area and perimeter. This same CT will also delineate aortobifemoral anatomy, details of arterial vessel diameter, and tortuosity and calcification (Fig. 79-4). In those with chronic kidney disease, a noncontrast CT and an invasive lower extremity angiogram provide complementary information, allowing for calibrated measurements of arterial diameters and easy detection of very focal stenosis and tortuosity.

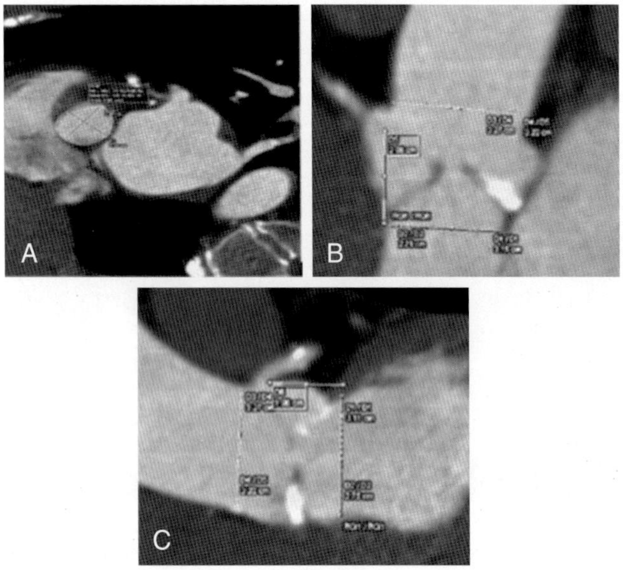

FIGURE 79-3 ■ Cardiac contrast computed tomography with three-dimensional reconstruction measuring the aortic annulus area. **A-C,** Multiple views on computed tomography of the aortic annulus that are required for evaluation of the aortic valve for preoperative TAVR planning.

Lower Extremity Assessment

Assessment of the lower extremities begins with either a CT scan or lower extremity angiography at the time of cardiac catheterization. Calcification of the large iliac arteries is common but generally does not prevent a femoral artery approach unless the calcification is circumferential and limiting in size. However, calcification in the smaller common femoral arteries is more problematic and may preclude the safe placement of TF systems and should be performed using alternative access techniques. Tortuosity, particularly in the external iliac artery, may complicate the advancement of the sheath. Consequently, moderate calcification in tortuous external iliac arteries (which tend to dive deep into the pelvis) may increase the likelihood of major vascular complications (Fig. 79-5). Tortuous vessels free of significant calcium are often compliant and can usually be straightened by a stiff guidewire. Figure 79-6 is a CT scan representation of severe iliac calcification precluding TF-TAVR.

Other Comorbidity Assessment

Patients with severe coronary artery disease and significant lesions that are amenable to percutaneous coronary intervention can undergo implantation of a bare-metal or drug-eluting stent prior to TAVR. Another potential concern is that the valve may displace a leaflet and cover a coronary ostium when deployed. A sinus of Valsalva that is narrow, a shallow sinus of Valsalva (within 5 mm of the annulus size), a short distance between the annulus and the coronary ostia (<10 mm), and bulky leaflet calcification can increase the risk for coronary obstruction. A sinus of Valsalva greater than 27 mm should accommodate smaller valves, whereas a sinus greater than 29 mm is adequate for all devices.

Alternative Access Considerations

Patients whose preoperative imaging study shows that a TF-TAVR is not advisable need to be evaluated for

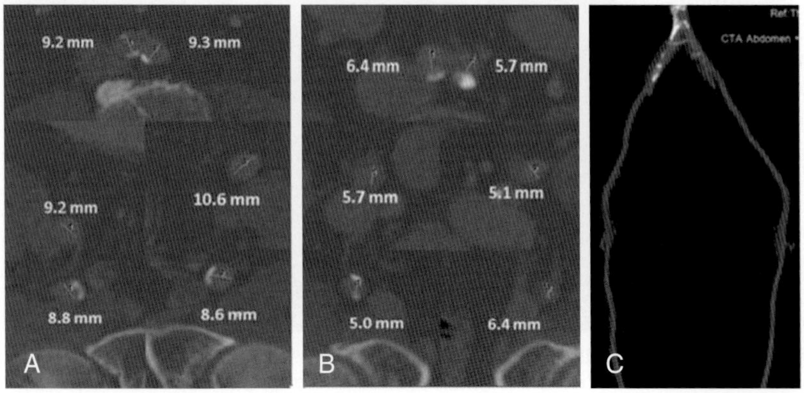

FIGURE 79-4 ■ Contrast computed tomography with three-dimensional reconstruction evaluating the aortoiliac/femoral anatomy. **A,** Anatomy adequate for most transfemoral TAVR valves. **B,** Anatomy not adequate for most transfemoral TAVR valves. **C,** Three-dimensional reconstruction of the iliac and femoral arteries.

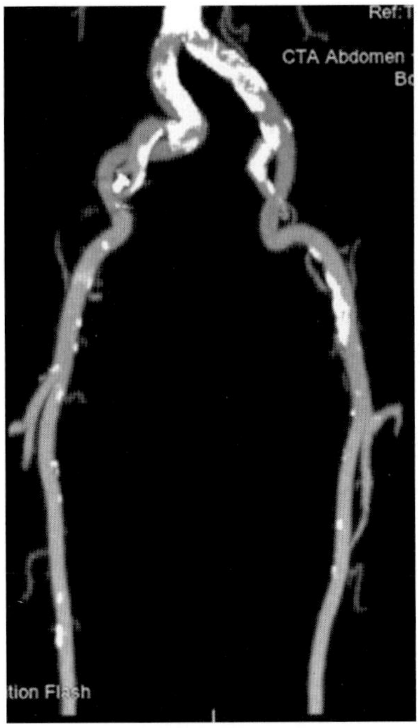

FIGURE 79-5 ■ Contrast computed tomography with three-dimensional reconstruction with significant tortuosity of iliac vessels.

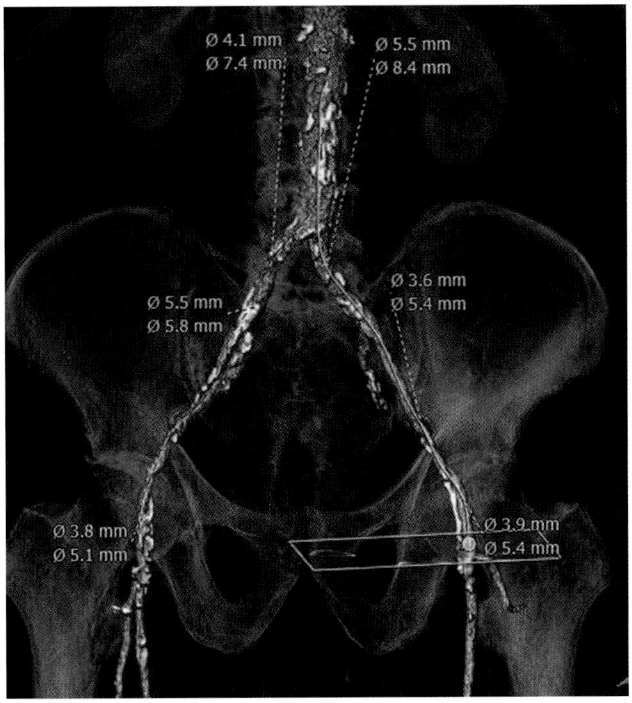

FIGURE 79-6 ■ Contrast computed tomography with three-dimensional reconstruction showing severe iliac-femoral calcifications.

alternative access techniques. A TA approach, via an anterior left mini-thoracotomy, has traditionally been used as the alternative in these patients. However, this approach comes with additional challenges and a different risk set compared with TF-TAVR and may not be appropriate for all patients, particularly those with significant parenchymal lung disease or low ejection fraction secondary to

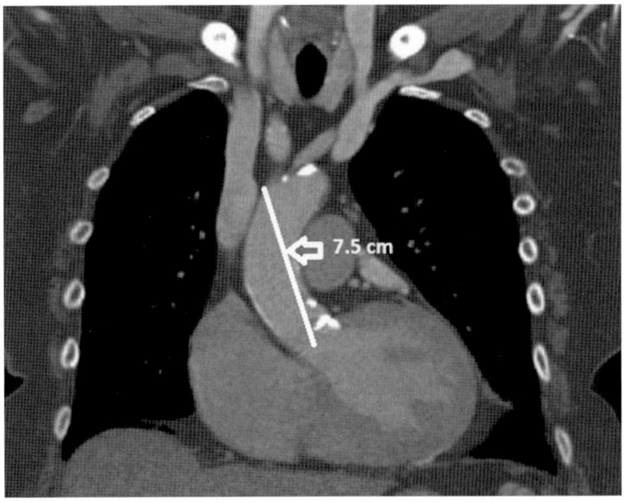

FIGURE 79-7 ■ Contrast computed tomography with three-dimensional reconstruction to evaluate ascending aorta.

the direct cannulation of the left ventricle.[12] TAo is a feasible alternative approach for a TAVR in patients who have not had a previous sternotomy. It is important to evaluate the degree of ascending and aortic arch calcification and the distance from the cannulation (>7 cm) site and the aortic root to ensure adequate deployment of the valve (Fig. 79-7). The transcarotid approach has been used successfully in patients who are not candidates for TF, TA, or TAo.[13]

OPERATIVE TECHNIQUES

Transfemoral TAVR

The TF approach is the least invasive of all TAVR techniques and is the initial procedure of choice by most operators. A 6 Fr sheath is placed in the artery and vein on the nonimplant side. A pigtail catheter is advanced to the aortic valve and aortography is performed to confirm the correct valve plane for valve placement. Through the femoral vein, a temporary pacemaker is advanced to the right ventricular apex for purposes of rapid ventricular pacing. Maintaining consistent pacing capture is essential to safe TAVR. To gain stability and facilitate adequate contact of the pacemaker with the right ventricular myocardium, an 8 Fr Mullins sheath is advanced into the right atrium.

Alignment of the three cusps of the aortic valve is performed via ascending aortic root angiography. This can be performed with the angled pigtail catheter in the right coronary cusp or via power injection with the catheter in the aortic root. The proper aortic plane is identified when all three cusps are visualized at an equal height (Fig. 79-8).

Access to the femoral artery on the implant side is performed using a microneedle under vascular road mapping. The tract is dilated with a 7 Fr sheath and the artery is preclosed with two Perclose devices. Alternatively, a surgical cutdown to obtain femoral access can be performed to insert the sheath. The dilators are placed

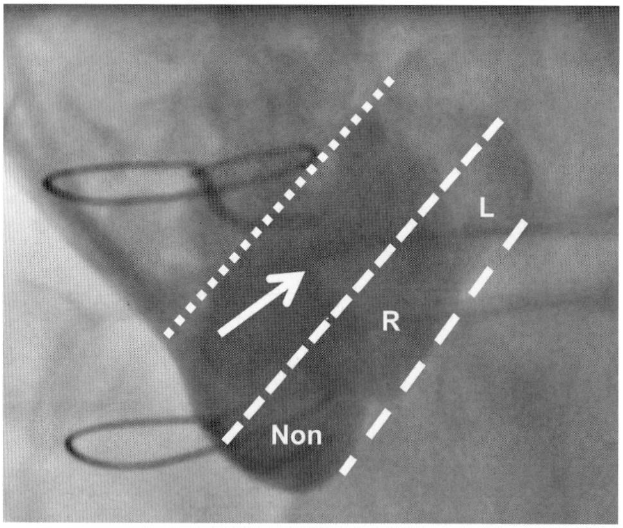

FIGURE 79-8 ■ Aortic root angiogram. Alignment of all three coronary cusps. *L,* Left coronary cusp; *Non,* noncoronary cusp; *R,* right coronary cusp.

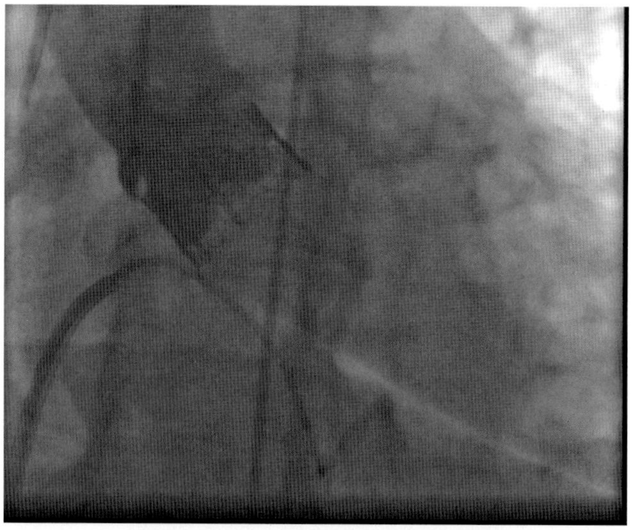

FIGURE 79-9 ■ Fluoroscopy of position of the SAPIEN valve in relation to the aortic annulus and coronary arteries.

and the appropriate sheath is inserted. The patient is heparinized to an activated clotting time (ACT) of longer than 250 seconds. Excessive force should not be applied when passing the dilators to avoid vascular complications during insertion and removal. Next the aortic valve is crossed with an Amplatz left-1 (AL1) catheter. A straight-tipped guidewire or hydrophilic wire is used to cross the aortic valve and advanced into the ventricle. This is exchanged for a 260-cm long, 0.035-inch diameter Amplatz Extra Stiff J guidewire, which has an exaggerated pigtail bend at the proximal end. A BAV is performed under rapid ventricular pacing (generally 180 to 220 beats/min) using a Z-Med 20- or 23-mm balloon catheter.

The appropriate valve delivery system is inserted and advanced to the aortic annulus. Difficulty crossing the aortic valve can occur because the stiff wire can bias to the greater aortic curvature and become lodged in a commissure. Gentle pulling of the wire will allow the delivery system to centralize and cross the valve easier. Excessive force should not be used when crossing because dissection of the aorta can occur. Once the valve has crossed the native valve, the system should not be advanced further because perforation of the left ventricular apex by the nosecone is possible. The proper positioning of the valve is guided by fluoroscopy and echocardiography. The SAPIEN valve, a balloon-expandable valve, is ideally positioned so that its upper margin covers the aortic leaflet tips and the ventricular end covers the aortic annulus or below (Fig. 79-9). When the device is appropriately positioned, the implanting physician should coordinate a long cine-fluoroscopic run with rapid pacing and inflation/deflation of the delivery balloon. We advocate a slow inflation to ensure proper valve position. The balloon should be at maximal inflation for 4 seconds before deflation. It is important that pacing begins before balloon inflation and continues until the balloon is almost completely deflated. Successful rapid pacing with 1:1 ventricular capture at 180 to 220 beats/min lowers the blood pressure below 60 mm Hg and prevents forceful contractions that may move the balloon catheter.

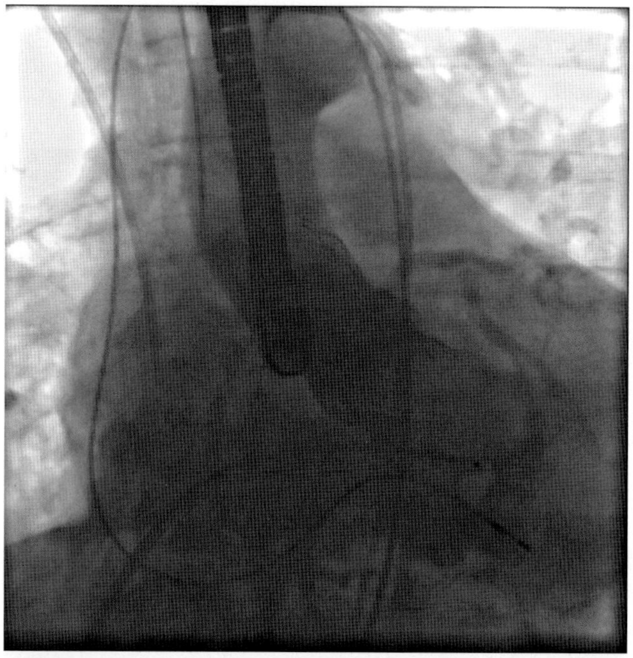

FIGURE 79-10 ■ Fluoroscopy of position of the CoreValve in relation to the aortic annulus.

The CoreValve, a self-expanding aortic valve, is positioned by determining its three-tiered design in relationship with the aortic annulus. The inflow portion of the valve is ideally placed 6 mm (one diamond segment of the stent frame) below the point of leaflet attachment. Thus, the portion of the valve with high radial force sits firmly in the annulus, but not so low as to compress the adjacent cardiac conduction system (Fig. 79-10). The uppermost part of the CoreValve rests in the ascending aorta, parallel to the direction of blood flow. The CoreValve system does not commonly require rapid ventricular pacing during deployment.

Following deployment of the aortic valve, proper positioning is assessed with echocardiography. Patency of the coronary arteries is checked, and proper positioning of the device confirmed, with aortography. A valve too low in the ventricle may necessitate the placement of a second valve. Placing the valve too high in the annulus might result in embolization of the device into the ascending aorta or occlusion of the coronary arteries. A trace or mild amount of perivalvular leak is expected after TAVR. If there is more than mild leak around a correctly positioned valve, post-deployment balloon dilation using the balloon on the delivery catheter can further expand the valve and improve the insufficiency.

Transapical TAVR

The transapical TAVR is the second most common TAVR technique and thus far has been used primarily with a balloon-expandable valve. In those patients with severe peripheral vascular disease, the TA approach is an expeditious procedure. This technique is the only antegrade of all approaches with very low stroke rates and the least amount of postoperative paravalvular leaks. Furthermore, the TA procedure is best in those with a prior sternotomy or porcelain aorta. The most serious complication includes left ventricular bleeding, but this is not common. The only relative contraindications to the TA procedure are severe chronic obstructive pulmonary disease (COPD) with a forced expiratory volume (FEV_1) predicted less than 30% or an ejection fraction less than 20%.

The patient is placed supine on the operating room table and femoral artery and vein access is achieved. A femoral transvenous pacer is placed in the right ventricle and a pigtail catheter is placed in the aortic root via the femoral artery. A 4- to 5-cm anterolateral thoracotomy is made in the fifth or sixth intercostal space to expose the left ventricle. Two apical pledgeted 3-0 Prolene purse-string sutures are placed just cephalad to the apex lateral to the left anterior descending artery. The purse-string sutures into the myocardium should be deep stitches but not transmural (Fig. 79-11).

Fluoroscopy is used to position the aortic root and annulus perpendicular to each other, and to align all three aortic cusps in the same plane in a similar fashion as in the TF approach. The left ventricle cavity is accessed with a needle, and a 0.035-inch wire is passed into the left ventricle, across the aortic valve, and into the ascending aorta. The wire is maintained in the ascending aorta and not allowed to pass into the right carotid artery. A 7 Fr catheter is placed through the left ventricle apex and across the aortic valve. The 0.035-inch wire is manipulated into the descending aorta using a right Judkins catheter. The 0.035-inch wire is exchanged for a stiff wire (Amplatz Super Stiff; Boston Scientific, Natick, MA) and left in the abdominal aorta. The 7 Fr catheter is exchanged for the appropriate sized delivery sheath, which is positioned 4 cm inside the left ventricle. A BAV is performed with or without rapid ventricular pacing. The balloon is removed and the valve is placed through the left ventricular delivery sheath and positioned across the valve. Positioning, deployment, and post-assessment of the valve are similar to that as aforementioned in the TF-TAVR section. After adequate evaluation, all catheters and wires are removed and the apex sutures are tied down under rapid ventricular pacing. Protamine is administered. If possible, the pericardium is closed over the left ventricular apex surgical site, and a small flexible chest tube is placed in the left pleural space.

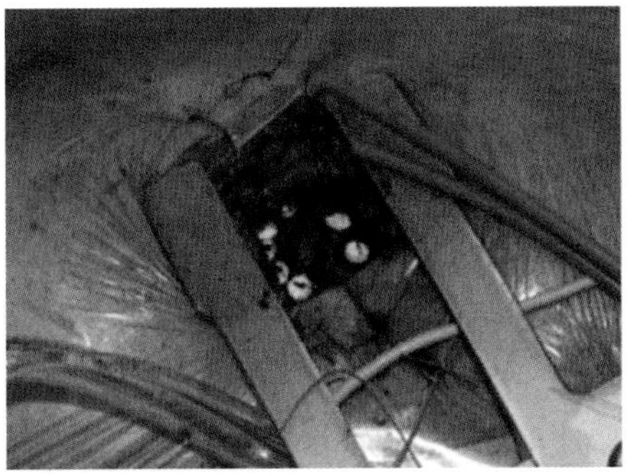

FIGURE 79-11 ■ Transapical transcatheter aortic valve replacement approach. Left thoracotomy with exposure of the apex of the heart with two purse-string sutures.

Transaortic TAVR

The TAo approach is the third most common TAVR technique and is used in those with balloon- or self-expanding valves. The TAo approach has several theoretical and practical advantages, including avoiding a thoracotomy in patients with poor respiratory function, less postoperative pain, and faster recovery. In addition, the direct aortic cannulation, a procedure with which most cardiac surgeons are comfortable, potentially allows for a more hemostatic closure than in a patient with a fragile left ventricular apex. However, although the TAo approach offers several advantages, it is not appropriate for all patients. TAo-TAVR is contraindicated in patients with porcelain aorta. There are also additional technical challenges when considering the TAo approach in patients with previous sternotomies, prior left internal mammary artery (LIMA) grafts that overlay the aorta, or otherwise hostile mediastinum (e.g., patients with a history of cobalt radiation).

The patient is placed supine on the operating room table with the lower neck exposed to allow for the counter-incision for the delivery sheath. An angled pigtail catheter is placed in the aortic root and a femoral transvenous pacer is placed in the right ventricle. The CT can provide the adequate information of the relationship of the distal ascending aorta to the sternum, the extension of calcification, and the distance from the site of cannulation to the aortic root. This distance should be ideally greater than 7 cm to allow enough space between the delivery system and the free inflation of the balloon during the valve implantation (see Fig. 79-7).

A 5- to 6-cm sternotomy incision is made below the suprasternal notch extending below the angle of Louis at the second intercostal space. A mini-sternotomy is performed using a standard saw, dividing the sternum down to the second intercostal space, where the "J" is completed with a transverse sternotomy. The distal ascending aorta is exposed and two aortic purse-string sutures are placed at the base of the innominate artery. The patient is heparinized to maintain an ACT greater than 250 seconds. A counter-incision is made in the lower neck through which an 18-gauge needle with a 0.035-inch soft guidewire is passed and used to puncture the aorta through the purse-string sutures (Fig. 79-12). The needle is exchanged for a 7 Fr sheath, and a multipurpose catheter with a straight soft wire is used to cross the valve. This is exchanged for a 260-cm, 0.035-inch Amplatz Extra Stiff J guidewire, which has an exaggerated pigtail bend at the proximal end. The appropriate sheath is placed into the aorta to 2 to 4 cm. A BAV is performed under rapid ventricular pacing. The balloon is removed and the TAVR valve is placed through the delivery sheath and positioned across the stenotic valve. Positioning, deployment, and post-assessment of the valve are similar to that as aforementioned in the TF-TAVR section. After adequate evaluation, all catheters and wires are removed and the aortic sutures are tied down under rapid ventricular pacing. Protamine is administered and generally the pericardium is left open. A small flexible chest tube is placed in the mediastinum and generally the pleural spaces are not opened.

Subclavian TAVR

The transsubclavian approach is the fourth most common TAVR technique and is used primarily in those with a self-expanding valve. Approaching TAVR from the axillary artery presents a few distinct advantages when compared with the other alternative access routes. It remains less invasive compared with the TA or TAo approach because it does not require thoracotomy or limited sternotomy. This makes it appealing for the older, debilitated patient in whom the transfemoral approach is limited by anatomy. Furthermore, in cases of aortic calcification, which would limit the TAo approach, or severe left ventricular or pulmonary dysfunction, which would limit the TA approach, the axillary access route is potentially preferable.

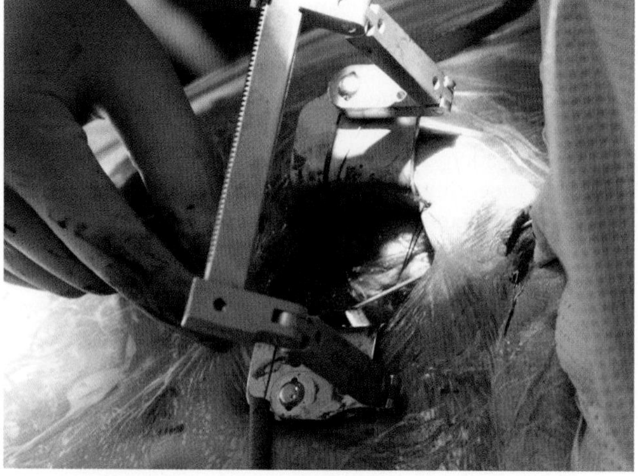

FIGURE 79-12 ■ Transaortic transcatheter aortic valve replacement approach.

Standard femoral artery and vein access is obtained as aforementioned. Surgical cutdown for the left axillary artery is familiar to most cardiac surgeons because it is routinely used as an arterial inflow cannulation site, particularly in the setting of aortic surgery. An oblique incision is made in the deltopectoral groove. The first portion of the axillary artery can be exposed with lateral retraction of the pectoralis minor. Division of the head of pectoralis minor can be performed with minimal morbidity if necessary to obtain optimum exposure. Great care is taken to avoid injury to the medial and lateral cords of the brachial plexus, as they often travel in close association with the artery, particularly in its second portion. The patient is heparinized to maintain an ACT greater than 250 seconds. Use of a synthetic graft in an end-to-side orientation, which is then cannulated with the delivery sheath, is favored by some, whereas others use direct access via a purse-string suture. Using the Seldinger technique, the access site is dilated to accommodate the appropriate caliber delivery sheath for the chosen device. This is advanced over a stiff wire, using fluoroscopic guidance with the tip of the sheath left at the origin of the innominate artery when approached from the left. When approaching from the right, the concern for potential occlusion of the right common carotid artery has led some high-volume centers to position the sheath tip at the origin of the right subclavian artery. Once the sheath is appropriately placed, TAVR deployment proceeds using the usual protocol of the transaortic TAVR. At the conclusion of the procedure, following removal of the delivery sheath, vascular control of the access site is obtained and selective angiography can be used to confirm vessel integrity at the access site.

Transcarotid TAVR

For patients who are not candidates for TF-, TA-, or TAo-TAVR and who have a common carotid artery diameter larger than 8 mm without evidence of stenosis, the TC approach to TAVR can be used.[13] A 6 Fr sheath is placed in the femoral artery through which an angled pigtail catheter is used for ascending aortography. In the contralateral femoral artery, a 16 Fr Fem-Flex II cannula (Edwards Lifesciences, Irvine, CA) is placed percutaneously. This cannula is connected to perfusion tubing and a 14/15 Sundt carotid bypass shunt (Covidien, Mansfield, MA) (Fig. 79-13). A pacing catheter is placed via the femoral vein. The right common carotid artery is exposed

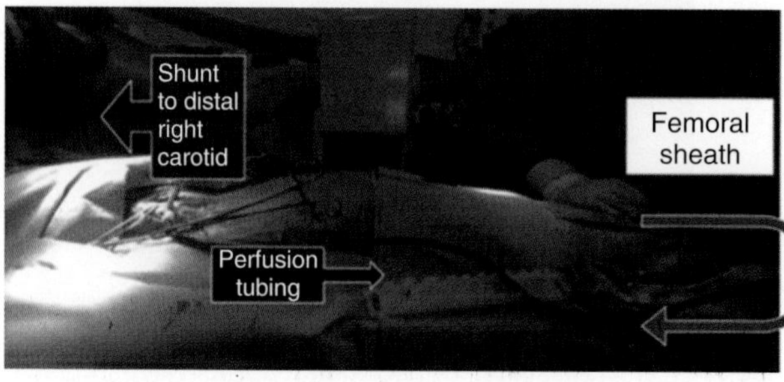

FIGURE 79-13 ■ Transcarotid transcatheter aortic valve replacement approach with visualization of the femoral-carotid shunt.

and after proximal cross-clamping of the common carotid artery, it is opened longitudinally for 2.5 cm. The de-aired bypass shunt is placed in the distal carotid arteriotomy to maintain cerebral perfusion. Cerebral oximetry from the left and right hemispheres is monitored throughout the procedure. Through the proximal arteriotomy, a 0.035-inch J-tipped wire and 7 Fr introducer are placed in the ascending aorta. A multipurpose catheter is then inserted into the ascending aorta and a straight wire is used to cross the native aortic valve. The straight wire is exchanged for an Amplatz Extra Stiff wire, and a Retroflex sheath is introduced into the ascending aorta. Similar to the transfemoral TAVR, a BAV followed by the placement of a valve is performed. Finally, the wires, catheters, and sheath are removed, and the carotid artery is repaired with a bovine pericardial patch.

RESULTS

SAPIEN Valve

The Placement of Aortic Transcatheter Valves (PARTNER) trial was a landmark and the first randomized study that demonstrated the superiority of TAVR over medical therapy in inoperable patients[11,14] and the noninferiority of TAVR versus SAVR in high-risk surgical candidates using the balloon-expandable SAPIEN valve.[15,16] Based on the 1-year outcomes from PARTNER, the SAPIEN valve was approved by the U.S. Food and Drug Administration for use in patients who are not candidates or are at high risk for SAVR.

The results of the randomized, multicenter U.S. PARTNER trial in patients too high-risk for surgery have been published by Leon and colleagues. In this report of 179 patients, the procedural success rate was 96.6%. The AVA and mean gradients across the aortic valve were significantly improved to 1.5 ± 0.5 cm^2 and 11.1 ± 6.9 mm Hg at 1-year follow-up (preprocedure AVA 0.6 ± 0.2 cm^2 and mean gradient 44.5 ± 15.7 mm Hg; $P < 0.001$). Mortality was 5.0% and 30.7% at 30 days and 1 year, respectively, following TAVR, establishing its superiority to medical therapy (1-year mortality 49.7%; $P < 0.001$).[11]

An evaluation of the STS adult cardiac surgery database notes that approximately 6% to 7% of patients presenting for surgical AVR in North America are considered at high risk with an STS score of 8% or higher.[3,4] At a minimum, this represents a large number of patients who now will have an option for TAVR or SAVR. It is estimated that approximately 30% to 38% of high-risk, older adult patients are not receiving SAVR despite echocardiographic evidence of severe aortic stenosis.[6,17] The PARTNER trial represents the first randomized trial comparing TAVR with SAVR in high-risk patients. Many physicians have noted that the results may be skewed secondary to the surgical procedure being performed in select university settings. In a multi-institutional study, 159 patients undergoing isolated, primary SAVR with an average STS PROM of 16% ± 7% had a 3-year survival of 57% and a median survival of 3.7 years.[18] In a real-world analysis of the STS database, Brennan and coworkers noted a median survival of 2.5 to 2.7 years in high-risk patients (STS ≥ 10%) undergoing SAVR.[4] Similarly, the SAVR group in the current series has a 55.8% survival at 3 years and a median survival of 3.4 years.

A report by Thourani and colleagues represents the largest series and the first long-term analysis using fully adjudicated outcomes in randomized high-risk patients with aortic stenosis undergoing TAVR with a balloon-expandable valve or surgery (PARTNER trial).[19] At a minimum of 3 years, there was no difference in all-cause and cardiovascular mortality rates between the TAVR and SAVR groups (Fig. 79-14). Strokes were similar between the groups at 3 years, despite increased periprocedural neurologic events in TAVR patients. There was no late (after 30 days) stroke hazard in TAVR compared with SAVR. At 3 years, TAVR hemodynamic performance was maintained with valve gradients and AVAs similar to those of SAVR (Fig. 79-15). In both groups,

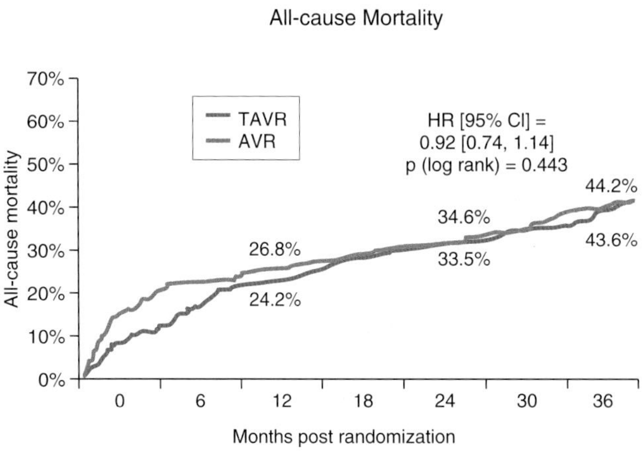

Numbers at risk						
TAVR	298	262	243	228	210	188
AVR	351	236	224	209	191	168

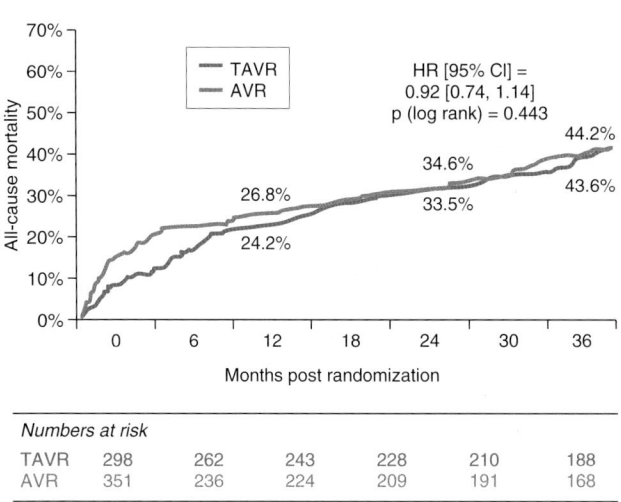

FIGURE 79-14 PARTNER trial 3-year analysis: all-cause mortality. *AVR,* Aortic valve replacement; *CI,* confidence interval; *HR,* hazard ratio; *TAVR,* transcatheter aortic valve replacement.

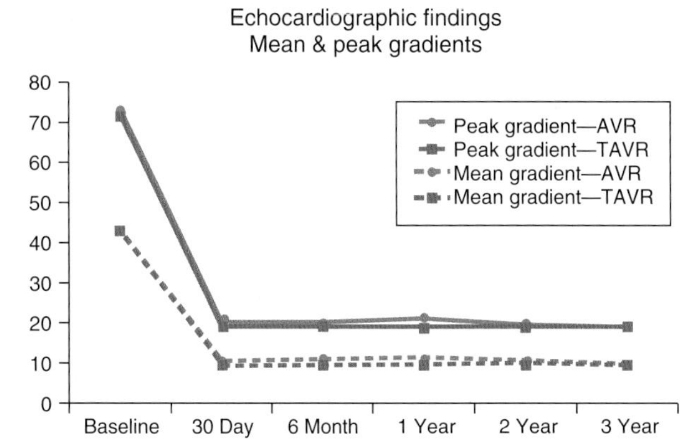

Number of echos						
TAVR	310	277	233	219	155	88
AVR	299	230	169	158	123	72

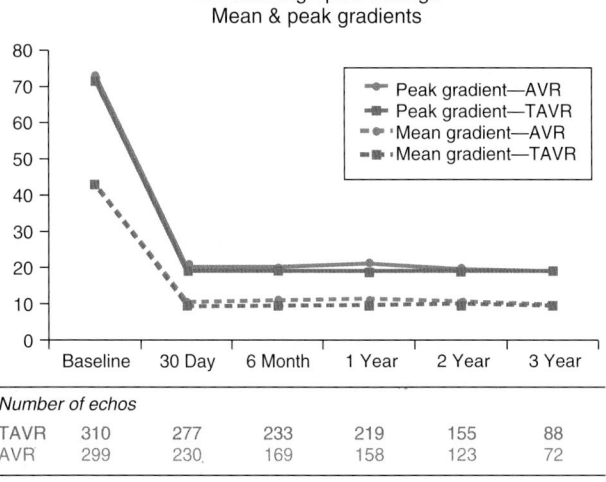

FIGURE 79-15 PARTNER trial 3-year analysis: hemodynamic valve performance by echocardiography. *AVR,* Aortic valve replacement; *TAVR,* transcatheter aortic valve replacement.

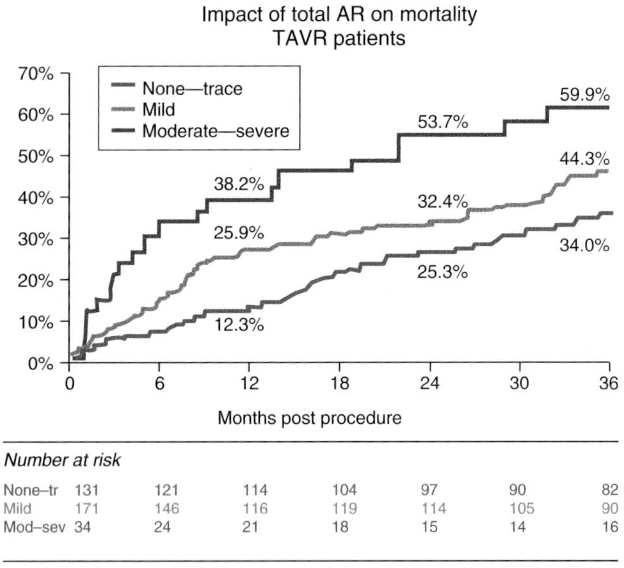

FIGURE 79-16 ■ PARTNER trial 3-year analysis: impact of aortic regurgitation (AR) on mortality. *TAVR,* Transcatheter aortic valve replacement.

structural valve deterioration was not apparent at the 3-year follow-up. Postprocedural paravalvular aortic regurgitation was frequent after TAVR without important changes during the 3-year follow-up (Fig. 79-16). Of note, and as has been previously reported, even mild postprocedural aortic regurgitation (paravalvular leak [PVL] and total aortic regurgitation) was associated with increased subsequent mortality.[16]

Other reports have noted the mid- and long-term TAVR survival rates in Gurvitch and colleagues' study of 70 patients (mean STS score 9.6% and EuroSCORE 31.7%) who underwent successful TAVR with a balloon-expandable valve and who survived 30 days and were followed for a minimum of 3 years.[20] The authors noted a survival at 2 and 3 years of 74% and 61%, respectively.[20] Correspondingly, the PARTNER series of 348 TAVR patients (mean STS PROM 11.8%) had a 66.5% survival at 2 years and 56.4% survival at 3 years. Similar to the PARTNER series, Gurvitch and colleagues noted no cases of structural valvular deterioration, and only one patient (1.5%) in their series underwent reoperation secondary to endocarditis. In a retrospective, single-center European analysis, Bleiziffer and colleagues reviewed outcomes in 227 patients undergoing TAVR with both balloon-expandable and self-expanding valves for at least 2 years follow-up. In their series, the mean STS PROM was 7% and EuroSCORE 21%, possibly representing a lower risk patient population. They noted a 2-year survival of 66.4%.[21] In the multicenter UK TAVI Registry of 870 patients undergoing balloon-expandable and self-expanding valve implantation, Moat and colleagues noted a 73.7% all-cause survival at 2 years.[22] This figure compares favorably to the 66.5% survival at 2 years in the PARTNER series. However, the UK registry data may not represent a high-risk patient population, with only an average logistic EuroSCORE of 18%.

CoreValve

An early, pioneering series from Grube and colleagues established the self-expanding CoreValve as a viable treatment option for severe aortic stenosis in patients at high risk for morbidity or mortality related to operative intervention (SAVR). Of 25 consecutive patients receiving the CoreValve, 21 (84%) patients were designated procedural successes, and there was a 20% overall mortality.[23] With progressive refinements in technique and device iterations, procedural success improved and the 30-day mortality decreased to 12%. Based on the positive results of these studies and others,[24,25] CE mark designation for the self-expanding valve was obtained in April 2007.

In the year following obtaining CE mark, 646 patients treated with CoreValve were followed in a multicenter registry. Procedural success was achieved in 97% of patients with a procedural mortality of 1.5%. The incidence of vascular access complications was 1.9% and the 30-day mortality was 8%. A total of 60 patients (9.3%) required placement of a permanent pacemaker. Approximately 70% of the patients had residual aortic insufficiency of grade 1 or 2.[26]

The introduction of CoreValve to the United States began with a multicenter randomized trial that began in late 2010. The Medtronic CoreValve U.S. pivotal trial adopted a similar trial design to that of the PARTNER trial by targeting aortic stenosis patients at high risk or extreme risk for traditional SAVR. The extreme risk group did not require randomization because the previous findings from the PARTNER study demonstrated a clear survival benefit for TAVR compared with medical therapy. Popma and colleagues reported on 489 patients with a mean STS risk score of 10.3% and mean age of 83 years. The noted all-cause death was 8.4% at 30 days and 24.3% at 1 year. Major stroke was noted at 2.3% at 30 days and 4.3% at 1 year. Major or life-threatening bleeding was noted in 36.7% and the need for permanent pacemaker was 21.6%. The percentage of patients with moderate or severe PVL at discharge was 10.5%. Interestingly, the investigators noted that the severity of PVL diminished over time. In fact, 80% of the patients who had moderate PVL 1 month and survived to 1 year had a reduction in PVL severity.[27]

In a follow-up study, Adams and associates reported on 795 high-risk patients randomized to either SAVR or TAVR with severe aortic stenosis.[28] The mean STS risk score was approximately 7.4% and represented a less sick group than the PARTNER high-risk study, which had a mean STS score of 11.8%.[15] The primary endpoint of all-cause mortality at 1 year illustrated a statistically significant difference between the two groups. Patients undergoing TAVR had a lower all-cause mortality at 1 year (14.2% vs. 19.1%; $P = 0.04$). Permanent pacemaker implantation was higher for CoreValve recipients at 30 days (19.8% vs. 7.1%; $P < 0.001$) and again at 1 year (22.3% vs. 11.3%; $P < 0.001$). Once again, investigators noticed an improvement in paravalvular regurgitation over time. In fact, most of the patients with moderate or severe paravalvular regurgitation at discharge had improved by 1 year to mild or better. Overall the study represents the first prospectively randomized comparison demonstrating improved survival at 1 year for TAVR compared with SAVR.

The early challenges related to pacemaker implants and PVL have been demonstrated by others. The UK TAVI Registry reported prospectively collected data on TAVR patients implanted up until December 2009.[22] Of the 452 CoreValve implants included in the study, 17.3% had moderate to severe aortic insufficiency compared with 9.6% of SAPIEN implants (P = 0.001). Furthermore, 24.4% required permanent pacemaker implantation compared with 7.4% of SAPIEN implants (P < 0.001). Procedural success was still excellent (98.2%) and 30-day mortality remained acceptable at 5.8%. In the only randomized trial comparing the transfemoral balloon-expandable (SAPIEN XT) and self-expanding (CoreValve) valves, Abdel-Wahab and colleagues randomized 240 patients to receive one of the two valves.[29] They noted a significantly lower frequency of residual aortic regurgitation based on intraoperative angiography (41% vs. 18%; P < 0.001) and less frequent need for implanting more than one valve in the SAPIEN patients. Cardiovascular and overall mortality at 30 days was similar in both groups. They also noted that the need for a permanent pacemaker was significantly lower in the SAPIEN valve group (17% vs. 38%; P = 0.001).

In general, when compared with SAVR, TAVR has been shown in high-risk surgical patient populations to have similar mid-term mortality.[15,16,19,30,31] An important observation of the aforementioned studies is that despite the relief of aortic stenosis, this high-risk patient cohort continues to have a progressive mortality rate reaching approximately 40% to 45% at 3 years. Although this may be secondary to the inherent comorbidities and age of this patient population, it remains incumbent for health care providers to redefine the most appropriate patients for any therapy or TAVR or SAVR.

TAVR in Patients with Prior SAVR

Tissue prostheses carry a low risk of thromboembolic events (between 0.5% and 1% risk per year without anticoagulation) but have a higher chance of valvular degeneration, requiring the potential need of a repeat surgical intervention at 10 to 15 years from implantation.

Fundamental types of information to determine are the valve type, valve size, and technical technique used in the primary valve surgery. There are numerous types of bioprostheses valves implanted in the aortic position. This could be xenografts (most frequently obtained from bovine pericardial or the porcine aortic valve or root) or homografts. Bioprostheses can also be divided into stented and stentless valves. For each surgical valve to be treated, it requires understanding of the structural and fluoroscopic characteristics for an accurate positioning of the valve in valve (V-in-V). When planning for the adequate sizing for the V-in-V, the important measurement is the true inner diameter of the valve. Other relevant measures include post and leaflet heights, the position of the valves within the aortic root and the relationship with the coronary ostia, and the presence of coronary bypasses.[32]

The complications resulting from TAVR in patients with prior SAVR differ from those of standard TAVR. Because the V-in-V is deployed in a fixed structure, it is less frequent to have annular rupture, bleeding complications, paravalvular regurgitation, and new events of conduction abnormalities. There is, however, an increased incidence of valve malpositioning (especially in previous aortic root replacement or stentless valves secondary to the absence of fluoroscopic markers), coronary obstruction (mainly secondary to the displaced leaflets of the failing prosthesis against the coronary ostia), and increase of postoperative aortic prosthesis gradients secondary to underexpansion of the transcatheter valve in a nonexpandable failing prosthesis ring.[33]

SPECIFIC PATIENT COMORBIDITIES

With increasing awareness of less invasive techniques available for the treatment of high-risk patients with severe aortic stenosis, there remains controversy over the appropriate therapy regarding SAVR or TAVR. Although this decision may be difficult when based solely on the STS predicted risk of mortality, a more realistic decision-making tool includes the identification of specific patient subgroups that may benefit preferentially from TAVR or SAVR.

Gender

To date, there remains a paucity of studies investigating the impact of gender-related differences following TAVR or SAVR.[34-37] In an analysis of patients from the PARTNER trial by Williams and coworkers, there was reduced procedural mortality in females undergoing TAVR compared with SAVR (6.8% vs. 13.1%; P = 0.07).[35] At 2 years, all-cause mortality was significantly lower in females undergoing TAVR (28.2% vs. 38.2%; P = 0.049). These investigators also noted that the differences in the reduced late mortality were predominantly in the transfemoral cohort (23.4% vs. 36.9%; P = 0.02), whereas there was a less striking benefit in the transapical cohort (37.3% vs. 41.7%; P = 0.62). Although procedural mortality also favored TAVR over SAVR in males (6.0% vs. 12.1%; P = 0.03), there was no benefit in all-cause mortality at 2 years in the TAVR group (37.7% vs. 32.3%; P = 0.42). Moreover, there was no reduction in 2-year mortality in either the transfemoral (P = 0.86) or the transapical arms (P = 0.21) in males.[35] It is plausible that these results suggest that TAVR and, when feasible, the transfemoral route might be the preferred treatment option for older women with symptomatic severe aortic stenosis.

Diabetes Mellitus

Another high-risk patient population presenting with severe aortic stenosis are those with preoperative diabetes mellitus. In 1391 patients undergoing isolated SAVR, Halkos and his colleagues at Emory reported significantly reduced 10-year survival in patients with diabetes (40.5%) compared with those without diabetes (71.2%; P <

0.001).[38] Only one report thus far has compared outcomes in high-risk diabetic patients undergoing TAVR (n = 145) and SAVR (n = 130). From a post hoc analysis of the PARTNER trial, Lindman and colleagues noted all-cause mortality at 1 year was 18.0% in TAVR patients and 27.4% in the surgical group (P = 0.04).[39] In contrast, there was no significant difference in 1-year mortality in nondiabetic patients between groups (P = 0.48). These data suggest that TAVR may be the preferred treatment approach for patients with aortic stenosis and diabetes who are at high risk for surgery.

Mitral Regurgitation

The presence of moderate or severe mitral regurgitation (MR) with concomitant aortic stenosis represents a difficult and common patient population. Following isolated SAVR,[40] but not TAVR,[41,42] preoperative moderate or severe MR has been associated with worse early and late survival. In a post hoc analysis of the PARTNER trial comparing SAVR and TAVR in those with concomitant MR, Barbanti and coworkers showed that similar changes in left ventricular remodeling and improvement in left ventricular function occur following relief of the aortic stenosis by either SAVR or TAVR.[42] Correspondingly, improvements in symptoms and functional class were found with both procedures, regardless of the severity of MR. However, in those undergoing SAVR, all-cause mortality at 2 years was higher in those with preoperative moderate or severe MR compared with those with mild or less MR (49.8% vs. 28.1%; P = 0.04). In contrast, MR severity at baseline did not affect mortality in TAVR patients (37.0% vs. 32.7%; P = 0.58). Unfortunately, current studies have not differentiated the impact of TAVR route (i.e., TF, TA, TAo) on long-term outcomes in this patient population. In select high-risk patients with nondegenerative moderate to severe MR and concomitant severe aortic stenosis, it may be reasonable to consider TAVR as a less invasive mode of therapy.

Renal Dysfunction

A strong association exists between aortic stenosis and renal dysfunction with up to 75% of patients having mild, moderate, or severe renal dysfunction.[43] We and others have shown that preoperatively impaired renal function represents a strong independent predictor of adverse short- and long-term outcomes in SAVR and TAVR patients.[43,44] Recently, Nguyen and colleagues from Emory University compared renal dysfunction within SAVR (n = 1336) and TAVR (n = 343) patients. They noted an in-hospital mortality in TAVR patients for mild, moderate, and severe renal dysfunction of 3.8%, 2.9%, and 4.4% (P = 0.89), respectively. On the contrary, in the SAVR group, worsening renal function was associated with a stepwise increase in short-term mortality, at 2.6%, 4.1%, and 8.9% for mild, moderate, and severe renal dysfunction, respectively. Furthermore, worsening renal function was strongly associated with increased mid- and long-term mortality in the SAVR group, whereas Kaplan-Meier survival estimates for TAVR stratified by renal function do not demonstrate this relationship. In all patients, the adjusted odds ratio for death was 0.47 when comparing TAVR with SAVR.[45] In SAVR patients, the adjusted odds ratio for death was 2.6 when comparing severe/dialysis with normal patients. In TAVR patients, the odds ratio was 1.01 when comparing severe/dialysis with normal patients. Although more research and analysis is needed to elucidate the preferential benefit of TAVR in patients with renal dysfunction, it is possible that TAVR mitigates the effect of moderate and severe renal dysfunction on short- and mid-term survival.

COMPLICATIONS

Although TAVR was designed to be a less invasive form of aortic valve replacement for high-risk patients, it still carries many of the same potential complications for open, traditional aortic valve replacement. The Valve Academic Research Consortium-2 (VARC-2) has standardized the endpoint definitions for studies evaluating the use of TAVR, which will lead to improved comparability and interpretability of the study results.[46] Denoted in this section are the most common complications associated with TAVR.

Acute Hypotension

Acute hypotension during TAVR is not uncommon and may be due to acute aortic insufficiency, left ventricular dysfunction (caused by "stunning" with rapid pacing, ostial coronary occlusion, or other factors), pericardial effusion (typically from right ventricular perforation by the pacing wire or aortic root trauma), arrhythmia, peripheral vascular injury, a "suicide ventricle" (hyperdynamic intraventricular obstruction after unloading by BAV or TAVR), or other factors. Treatment of acute hypotension is dictated by its causes. In the absence of an anesthesiologist, operator-administered boluses of intra-aortic, intraventricular, or intravenous epinephrine or norepinephrine are immediately deliverable and effective temporizing measures. The suicide ventricle, although uncommon, is suggested by high residual gradients, especially dynamic obstruction (worse after a premature beat); can be identified echocardiographically; and is important to differentiate from other causes of acute heart failure: it will be aggravated by diuresis and positive inotropes but can be effectively treated with volume, vasoconstrictors, and negative inotropes.

Stroke

In addition to mortality, one of the most devastating consequences following aortic valve replacement is a new postoperative permanent stroke. Following SAVR in high-risk surgical patients, stroke rates have been reported between 3% and 5%.[4,5,15,18] The incidence of cerebrovascular events (transient ischemic event or a stroke) during the 30-day period after TAVR ranges from 3% to 7%.[47] Approximately 50% to 70% of these events occur during, or within 24 hours of, the procedure. In the PARTNER study, an analysis of 30-day and 1-year outcomes, there was an increased periprocedural stroke following TAVR when compared with SAVR.[15,48] However, at 2 years and in a more recent study of the PARTNER patients by Thourani and coworkers, there does not appear to be any evidence of a continued increased stroke at the 2- and 3-year follow-up in TAVR patients.[16,19] In an analysis of the PARTNER trial by Dewey and colleagues, the authors noted improvement in the periprocedural stroke rate from 6.7% in the premarket approval TA-TAVR ($N = 104$) when compared with 2.2% in the nonrandomized continued access TA-TAVR group ($N = 975$).[49] In a recent meta-analysis, Eggebrecht and associates have shown an overall 30-day stroke/TIA rate was 3.3 ± 1.8% with most being major strokes (2.9 ± 1.8%).[50]

Stroke in association with TAVR can occur because of atheroembolism, thromboembolism, cardiogenic shock during the procedure, preexisting cerebral vascular disease, or interaction of these factors. However, catheter manipulation in the ascending aorta is the most likely cause of most strokes observed with TAVR. Predictors of neurologic events were balloon post dilation, valve embolization, and new onset of atrial fibrillation.[51] Major, ischemic stroke may be treated by catheter-based, mechanical embolic retrieval where available. Thrombolysis may also be considered, although the expected benefit may be reduced (particularly with atheroembolism); bleeding risk is typically high because of patient age and morbidity as well as the arteriotomies created for TAVR (if recent). Clinical studies evaluating the most appropriate anticoagulation regimen are also forthcoming.

One of the most recent aspects of stroke prevention includes new cerebroembolic protection devices, which are actively being evaluated and have shown promise in the reduction of embolic debris during TAVR.[52-54] These devices can be categorized in two broad categories: (1) deflectors, which prevent passage of emboli to the cerebrovascular system by redirecting them to the lower half of the body, and (2) retrieval devices, which capture and collect emboli for removal from the systemic circulation.

Among the deflector devices, the Embrella Embolic Deflector (Edwards Lifesciences) and the Triguard (Keystone Heart, Ltd.) have the largest clinical experience to date (Fig. 79-17). Both devices use a nitinol frame that is positioned across the origin of the great vessels in the aortic arch. The Embrella device uses a polyurethane membrane with pore size of 100 μm to selectively deflect emboli. The Triguard is a nitinol mesh with a pore size of 140 μm. The Embrella uses a right radial or brachial approach for deployment, whereas the Triguard is delivered via the femoral artery and covers the entire arch, including the left subclavian artery.

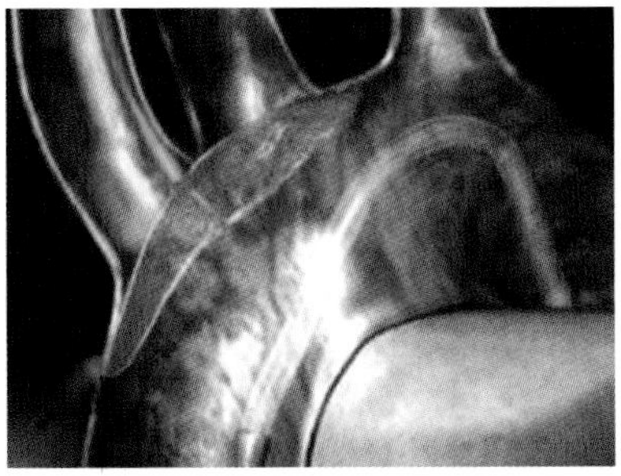

FIGURE 79-17 ■ Embrella Embolic Deflector (Edwards Lifesciences).

The retrieval system with the most clinical experience to date is the Montage Dual Filter (Claret Medical, Inc.) (Fig. 79-18). The system uses right upper extremity access to place two conical filters with 140-μm polyurethane membranes in the brachiocephalic and left common carotid arteries. At the completion of the procedure, the filters are withdrawn and captured debris is removed from the circulation. A first-in-human series was reported in 2012 detailing use in 40 patients. The series included two generations of the device with improvements in proper placement for the second generation (87%) compared with the first generation device (60%).[53] Macroscopic debris was removed from 19 (54%) patients treated; one minor stroke (at 30 days) and two major strokes (at 4 hours, at 27 days) were observed.

Acute Kidney Disease

Significant acute kidney injury (AKI) after TAVR has been reported to be 8%, being an independent predictor of mortality.[55] The origin of AKI is likely to be multifactorial, involving predisposing conditions such as diabetes mellitus, chronic kidney disease, or peripheral vascular disease, and procedure-related events such as aortic plaque embolism in the renal arteries and hypoperfusion during rapid ventricular pacing. The use of the TA approach has been reported to be an independent predictor of AKI in several studies, probably reflecting underlying comorbidities that predispose these patients to such a complication.

Vascular Complications

Vascular injury at the access site is the most frequent problem with transfemoral TAVR. Major vascular complications occurred in 15% of patients within 30 days of TF-TAVR in the PARTNER trial and were associated

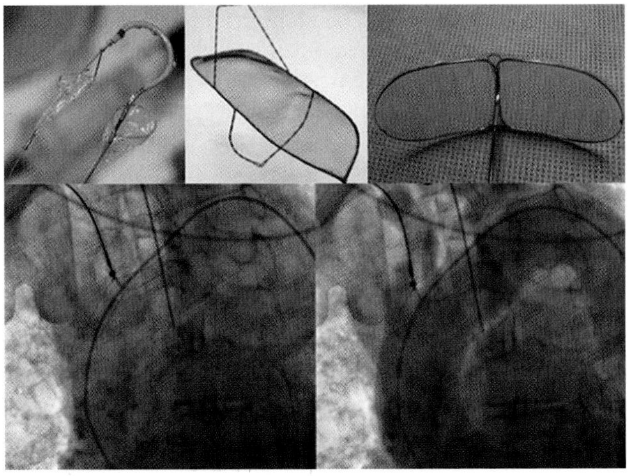

FIGURE 79-18 ■ Montage Dual Filter (Claret Medical, Inc.).

with significantly higher rates of 30-day and 1-year mortality.[11] Vascular access site complications are mainly related to the large caliber sheaths used to deliver the valve. The first generation of sheaths (22 to 25 Fr, corresponding to an outer diameter of 9 to 10 mm) was associated with high rates of vascular complications. However, with growing operator experience, improved patient screening and selection, and the smaller diameter of the newer generation of sheaths (18 or 19 Fr, corresponding to an outer diameter of 7.2 to 7.5 mm), the incidence of vascular complication has significantly decreased over time. Within the next few years, we would expect vascular injuries to be below 5%.

Other major vascular complications include thoracic aortic dissection; rupture of the aortic annulus; distal embolization (noncerebral) from a vascular source, requiring surgery or resulting in amputation or irreversible end-organ damage; access-site or access-related injury leading to death, the need for blood transfusion (>4 units), unplanned percutaneous or surgical intervention, or irreversible end-organ damage.[46]

Aortoiliac avulsion or perforation may be suspected during arterial dilation and insertion of the delivery sheath, but it may not be clinically manifest until removal of the delivery sheath. If perforation is identified at sheath removal, the sheath should be immediately reinserted (with dilator in place) to help tamponade the bleeding while preparation for more definitive treatment is made. Depending on the site and severity of injury, an aortic occlusion balloon such as the Coda balloon (Cook Medical, Bloomington, Illinois) may be inserted from the contralateral arterial access site. Prolonged balloon tamponade using peripheral angioplasty balloons may be helpful for iliac or femoral perforation, and deployment of covered stents may seal the perforation. Iliofemoral dissection is usually retrograde and does not limit flow, but severe dissections may be flow-limiting or even occlusive. Flow-limiting dissections should be treated with endovascular or surgical repair. Suture-mediated, severe stenosis of the common femoral artery at the access site often responds to gentle balloon dilation, which does not need to completely eliminate the narrowing to be successful: mild to moderate residual narrowing is rarely symptomatic.

Aortic annulus rupture, a rare occurrence, is associated with high mortality. Independent predictors of this complication include valve oversizing and the presence of moderate or severe calcification in the left ventricular outflow tract. [56] It may present subtly with thickening of the interatrial septum on echocardiography and subsequent development of pericardial effusion. Effusion may be treated with pericardiocentesis, and surgical repair may be considered. Immediate treatment with protamine and blood pressure control are recommended for conservative management.

In the meta-analysis by Genereux and colleagues, the overall incidence of bleeding was 41% (life-threatening, 16%).[57] Life-threatening bleeding is associated with a 6 to 9 times increase in 30-day mortality after TAVR and was an independent predictor of 1-year mortality. The TA route for TAVR has consistently been reported as an independent predictor of life-threatening bleeding.[58]

Aortic Insufficiency

Acute, moderate, or severe prosthetic aortic regurgitation after TAVR will be paravalvular, transvalvular, or mixed. The 2- and 3-year follow-up of the PARTNER trial using the balloon-expandable valves resulted in significantly worse PVL than SAVR with more than 50% of TAVR patients experiencing at least mild PVL.[16,19,59] There has been much focus on the effect of aortic regurgitation on survival following TAVR. A number of studies have identified aortic regurgitation higher than grade 2+ to be an independent predictor of short- and long-term mortality.[60] The direct causal relationship between PVL and mortality still needs to be determined, as does the significant heterogeneity in the assessment of PVL; thus far controversy regarding the use of echocardiography or magnetic resonance imaging continues.[61] The use of cross-sectional CT has improved the accuracy of aortic annular sizing for TAVR and has led to the overall reduction of PVL, displacing two-dimensional TTE as the gold standard for TAVR valve selection.[62]

Acute transvalvular regurgitation may occur as a result of incomplete valve closure when the valve is deployed in the setting of systemic arterial hypotension and this improves when the blood pressure is increased. The valve also may simply require a brief period of time (minutes) to "warm up" and achieve full leaflet mobility. A third scenario for transvalvular aortic regurgitation is that it may be caused by an overhanging native aortic leaflet, which can prevent closure of the TAVR valve leaflets. In this case, the operator can attempt to close the TAVR valve leaflets by placing an angled-pigtail catheter in each aortic cusp. If this is unsuccessful, another TAVR valve should be deployed just aortic to the initial TAVR valve to adequately displace the native aortic leaflets.

The more common scenario includes that of the paravalvular aortic leak. For patients with more than mild PVL noted during the procedure, the position of the transcatheter heart valve should be assessed. If the valve is malpositioned, a second valve may be implanted in the first valve. However, if the valve is well positioned, dilating the stent-valve with a balloon catheter may expand the valve and fill the annulus more completely. Chronic, moderate, or severe paravalvular aortic regurgitation after TAVR may be treated percutaneously by implantation of a second valve or by implantation of one or more vascular plugs.

Valve Embolization

Valve embolization is most commonly caused by loss of capture during rapid ventricular pacing (leading to ejection of the incompletely deployed valve from the annulus), but it also may be caused by malpositioning or, in rare cases, choosing a valve too small for the annulus. Embolization is best avoided by confirmation of stable pacing and by careful valve positioning prior to and during slow, controlled deployment. In the event of aortic movement during deployment, the valve may be immediately pushed back into the annulus if the deploying operator has maintained pressure on the inflation syringe (to hold the no-longer-crimped valve on the partially inflated balloon) without further inflation or deflation. If the valve cannot be pushed back across the annulus, then it may be pulled into the arch (and ideally into the descending aorta) before being deployed. If the deployment balloon has been deflated, the valve will be loose on the wire and should be recaptured with the balloon and deployed in a safe location, either just distal to the left subclavian artery or immediately proximal to the common iliac bifurcation. Wire position across the valve must be maintained to prevent the valve from turning and obstructing the aorta. After the embolized valve is secured, a second valve may be implanted in the annulus to complete the TAVR. Valve embolization into the left ventricle is less common and almost always requires surgical intervention.

Coronary Occlusion

Myocardial infarction is a rare yet catastrophic complication during TAVR and occurs in less than 1% of patients.[11,63] Acute, aorto-ostial coronary occlusion may be treated effectively with immediate percutaneous coronary intervention (PCI) or emergent peripheral cardiopulmonary bypass followed by PCI. Left main coronary artery occlusion is most likely, although right coronary artery obstruction has also been described. Most commonly, patients experience acute hemodynamic compromise with ST-segment elevation suggesting acute myocardial infarct. Percutaneous intervention can be facilitated in high-risk cases by placing a 0.014-inch coronary interventional wire and/or balloon into the coronary artery at risk prior to deployment of the new valve (Fig. 79-19). Prevention remains the mainstay of treatment for this dreadful complication. Coronary artery orifice less than 12 mm as determined by a high-definition CT scan should prompt concern. In such scenarios, performing a BAV with a concomitant root angiogram may discern the potential for main coronary artery occlusion.

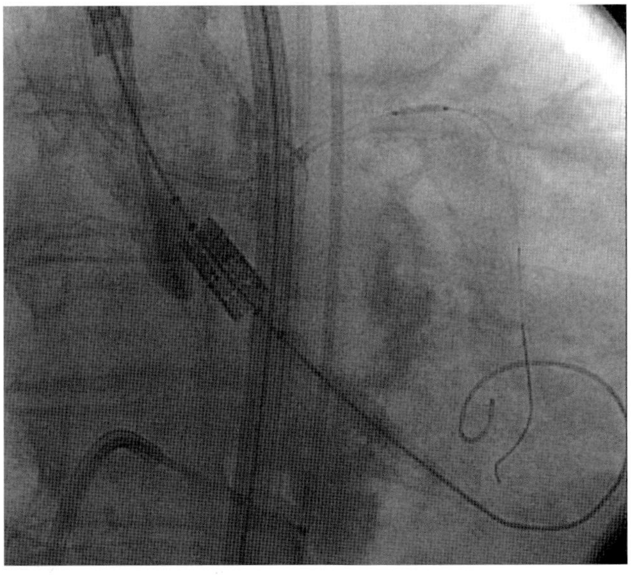

FIGURE 79-19 ■ Left main coronary wire during valve-in-valve deployment.

Conduction Abnormalities

Transcatheter aortic valves intentionally oversize the aortic annulus and are partially placed in a subannular position, bringing them into proximity with the cardiac conduction system as it enters the ventricular septum. The need for a pacemaker post TAVR is infrequent with the Edwards-SAPIEN valve reported at 3.4% in the randomized PARTNER US trial.[11,15] There remains an important difference in the need for permanent pacemakers after TAVR between the balloon-expandable (6.5%) and self-expanding valves (25.8%).[64,65]

Complete heart block following TAVR is immediately treated by backup pacing from the temporary pacing wire. The bradyarrhythmia may be transient and the temporary wire may be left in place until the question of need for permanent pacing has been elucidated.

New left bundle branch block (LBBB) occurred in 121 of 1151 (10.5%) patients and persisted in more than half at 6 months to 1 year according to the PARTNER trial data.[66] New LBBB was not associated with significant differences in 1-year mortality, cardiovascular mortality, repeat hospitalization, stroke, or myocardial infarction. However, it was associated with increased permanent pacemaker implantation during hospitalization (8.3 vs. 2.8%, $P < 0.005$) and from discharge to 1 year (4.7 vs. 1.5%; $P < 0.01$). The ejection fraction failed to improve after TAVR in patients with new LBBB and remained lower at 6 months to 1 year (52.8 vs. 58.1%; $P < 0.001$).[66]

Uncommon Complications

Other uncommon complications reported include tamponade and mitral valve injury. Tamponade can result from cardiac perforation in the right ventricle during placement of the pacemaker and the left ventricle by the stiff wire used for the BAV and TAVR. Large inspiratory drops in systemic arterial pressure (pulsus paradoxus) suggest a hemodynamically significant effusion, which can be confirmed with echocardiography. Treatment with pericardiocentesis is reasonable because the bleeding into the pericardium is often self-limited. If blood loss is substantial, blood may be autotransfused from the pericardium into a systemic vein while preparation is made for surgical exploration. The site of perforation may not be identifiable at surgery.

The mitral valve, including the chordae, may be damaged by guidewires in the left ventricle. Furthermore, the anterior leaflet of the mitral valve can be impinged on by a transcatheter heart valve placed too low in the ventricle. If severe mitral valve damage has occurred, operative interventions are the treatment of choice. Luckily, this is an extremely rare complication.

FUTURE DIRECTIONS

Catheter-based treatment options for patients with structural heart disease are rapidly improving with experience. Although the first randomized trials in North America have only recently been completed, the next generation of TAVR valves has grown immensely around the world.

Devices have been developed to decrease the known TAVR complications, including PVL and embolization. Technology now allows device repositionability and redeployment. The lower profile sheaths and valves will allow more transfemoral access and potentially reduce the need for alternative access devices. Lastly, the use of TAVR in intermediate-risk patients is forthcoming with the completion of the randomized PARTNER 2 intermediate trial with the SAPIEN XT valve and the ongoing SURTAVI trial with the CoreValve system.

REFERENCES

1. United States Population Projections: 2000 to 2050. http://www.census.gov/population/projections/data/national/2012.html.
2. Thourani VH, Myung R, Kilgo P, et al: Long-term outcomes after isolated aortic valve replacement in octogenarians: a modern perspective. *Ann Thorac Surg* 86:1458–1464, 2008.
3. Thourani VH, Suri R, Gunter RL, et al: Contemporary real-world outcomes of surgical aortic valve replacement in 141,905 low-, intermediate, and high-risk patients. *Ann Thorac Surg* 99:55–61, 2015.
4. Brennan JM, Edwards FH, Zhao Y, et al: Developing Evidence to Inform Decisions About Effectiveness–Aortic Valve Replacement (DEcIDE AVR) Research Team. Long-term survival after aortic valve replacement among high-risk elderly patients in the United States: insights from the Society of Thoracic Surgeons Adult Cardiac Surgery Database, 1991 to 2007. *Circulation* 126:1621–1629, 2012.
5. Brown JM, O'Brien SM, Wu CW, et al: Isolated aortic valve replacement in North America comprising 108,687 patients in 10 years: changes in risks, valve types, and outcomes in the Society of Thoracic Surgeons National Database. *J Thorac Cardiovasc Surg* 137:82–90, 2009.
6. Iung B, Cachier A, Baron G, et al: Decision-making in elderly patients with severe aortic stenosis: why are so many denied surgery? *Eur Heart J* 26:2714–2720, 2005.
7. Anderson HR, Knudsen LL, Hasenkam JM: Transluminal implantation of artificial heart valves. Description of a new expandable aortic valve and initial results with implantation by catheter technique in closed chest pigs. *Eur Heart J* 13:704–708, 1992.
8. Cribier A, Eltchaninoff H, Bash A, et al: Percutaneous transcatheter implantation of an aortic valve prosthesis for calcific aortic stenosis: first human case description. *Circulation* 106:3006–3008, 2002.
9. Mack MJ, Holmes DR, Webb J, et al: Patient selection for transcatheter aortic valve replacement. *J Am Coll Cardiol* 62(Suppl S):S1–S10, 2013.
10. Nishimura RA, Otto CM, Bonow RO, et al: 2014 AHA/ACC guideline for the management of patients with valvular heart disease: executive summary: a report of the American College of Cardiology/American Heart Association task force on practice guidelines. *J Am Coll Cardiol* 63:2438–2488, 2014.
11. Leon MB, Smith CR, Mack M, et al: Transcatheter aortic valve implantation for aortic stenosis in patients who cannot undergo surgery. *N Engl J Med* 363:1597–1607, 2010.
12. Thourani VH, Gunter RL, Neravetla S, et al: Use of transaortic, transapical and trans carotid transcatheter aortic valve replacement in inoperable patients. *Ann Thorac Surg* 96:1349–1357, 2013.
13. Guyton RA, Block PC, Thourani VH, et al: Carotid artery access for transcatheter aortic valve replacement. *Catheter Cardiovasc Interv* 82:E583–E586, 2013.
14. Makkar RR, Fontanta GP, Jilaihawi H, et al: Transcatheter aortic-valve replacement for inoperable severe aortic stenosis. *N Engl J Med* 366:1696–1704, 2012.
15. Smith CR, Leon MB, Mack M, et al: Transcatheter versus surgical aortic valve replacement in high-risk patients. *N Engl J Med* 364:2187–2198, 2011.
16. Kodali SK, Williams MR, Smith CR, et al: Two-year outcomes after transcatheter or surgical aortic valve replacement. *N Engl J Med* 366:1686–1695, 2012.
17. Bach DS, Cimino N, Deeb GM: Unoperated patients with severe aortic stenosis. *J Am Coll Cardiol* 50:2018–2019, 2007.
18. Thourani VH, Ailawadi G, Szeto WY, et al: Outcomes of surgical aortic valve replacement in high-risk patients: a multiinstitutional study. *Ann Thorac Surg* 91:49–55, 2011.
19. Thourani VH, Babaliaros V, Kodali S, et al: Three-year outcomes from the PARTNER trial in high-risk patients with aortic stenosis treated with transcatheter or surgical aortic valve replacement. *Circulation* 2014. submitted.
20. Gurvitch R, Wood DA, Tay EL, et al: Transcatheter aortic valve implantation: durability of clinical and hemodynamic outcomes beyond 3 years in a large patient cohort. *Circulation* 122:1319–1327, 2010.
21. Bleiziffer S, Mazzitelli D, Opitz A, et al: Beyond the short-term: clinical outcome and valve performance 2 years after transcatheter aortic valve implantation in 227 patients. *J Thorac Cardiovasc Surg* 143:310–317, 2012.
22. Moat NE, Ludman P, de Belder MA, et al: Long-term outcomes after transcatheter aortic valve implantation in high-risk patients with severe aortic stenosis: the U.K. TAVI (United Kingdom transcatheter aortic valve implantation) registry. *J Am Coll Cardiol* 58:2130–2138, 2011.
23. Grube E, Laborde JC, Gerckens U, et al: Percutaneous implantation of the CoreValve self-expanding valve prosthesis in high-risk patients with aortic valve disease: the Siegburg first-in-man study. *Circulation* 114:1616–1624, 2006.
24. Tamburino C, Capodanno D, Mule M, et al: Procedural success and 30-day clinical outcomes after percutaneous aortic valve replacement using current third-generation self-expanding CoreValve prosthesis. *J Invasive Cardiol* 21:93–98, 2009.
25. Grube E, Schuler G, Buellesfeld L, et al: Percutaneous aortic valve replacement for severe aortic stenosis in high-risk patients using the second- and current third-generation self-expanding CoreValve prosthesis: device success and 30-day clinical outcome. *J Am Coll Cardiol* 50:69–76, 2007.
26. Piazza N, Grube E, Gerckens U, et al: Procedural and 30-day outcomes following transcatheter aortic valve implantation using the third generation (18 Fr) CoreValve revalving system: results from the multicentre, expanded evaluation registry 1-year following CE mark approval. *EuroIntervention* 4:242–249, 2008.
27. Popma JJ, Adams DH, Reardon MJ, et al: Transcatheter aortic valve replacement using a self-expanding bioprosthesis in patients with severe aortic stenosis at extreme risk of surgery. *J Am Coll Cardiol* 63:1972–1981, 2014.
28. Adams DH, Popma JJ, Reardon MJ, et al: Transcatheter aortic-valve replacement with a self-expanding prosthesis. *N Engl J Med* 370:1790–1798, 2014.
29. Abdel-Wahab M, Mehilli J, Frerker C, et al: Comparison of balloon-expandable vs self-expandable valves in patients undergoing transcatheter aortic valve replacement: the CHOICE randomized clinical trial. *JAMA* 311:1503–1514, 2014.
30. Conradi L, Seiffert M, Treede H, et al: Transcatheter aortic valve implantation versus surgical aortic valve replacement: a propensity score analysis in patients at high surgical risk. *J Thorac Cardiovasc Surg* 143:64–71, 2011.
31. Panchal HB, Ladia V, Desai S, et al: A meta-analysis of mortality and major adverse cardiovascular and cerebrovascular events following transcatheter aortic valve implantation versus surgical aortic valve replacement for severe aortic stenosis. *Am J Cardiol* 112:850–860, 2013.
32. Dvir D, Barbanti M, Tan J, et al: Transcatheter aortic valve-in-valve implantation for patients with degenerative surgical bioprosthetic valves. *Curr Probl Cardiol* 39:7–27, 2014.
33. Dvir D, Webb J, Brecker S, et al: Transcatheter aortic valve replacement for degenerative bioprosthetic surgical valves: results from the global valve-in-valve registry. *Circulation* 126:2335–2344, 2012.
34. Onorati F, D'Errigo P, Barbanti M, et al: Different impact of sex on baseline characteristics and major periprocedural outcomes of transcatheter and surgical aortic valve interventions: results of the multicenter Italian OBSERVANT Registry. *J Thorac Cardiovasc Surg* 147:1529–1539, 2013.
35. Willliams M, Kodali SK, Hahn RT, et al: Sex-related differences in outcomes following transcatheter or surgical aortic valve replacement in patients with severe aortic stenosis: insights from the PARTNER trial. *J Am Coll Cardiol* 63:1522–1528, 2014.

36. Humphries KH, Toggweiler S, Rodés-Cabau J, et al: Sex differences in mortality after transcatheter aortic valve replacement for severe aortic stenosis. *J Am Coll Cardiol* 60:882–886, 2012.
37. Buja P, Napodano M, Tamburino C, et al: Comparison of variables in men versus women undergoing transcatheter aortic valve implantation for severe aortic stenosis (from Italian Multicenter CoreValve registry). *Am J Cardiol* 111:88–93, 2013.
38. Halkos ME, Kilgo P, Lattouf OM, et al: The effect of diabetes mellitus on in-hospital and long-term outcomes after heart valve operations. *Ann Thorac Surg* 90:124–130, 2010.
39. Lindman BR, Pibarot P, Arnold SV, et al: Transcatheter versus surgical aortic valve replacement in patients with diabetes and severe aortic stenosis at high risk for surgery: an analysis of the PARTNER trial. *J Am Coll Cardiol* 63:1090–1099, 2014.
40. Harling L, Saso S, Jarral OA, et al: Aortic valve replacement for aortic stenosis in patients with concomitant mitral regurgitation: should the mitral valve be dealt with? *Eur J Cardiothorac Surg* 40:1087–1096, 2011.
41. D'Onofrio A, Gasparetto V, Napodano M, et al: Impact of preoperative mitral valve regurgitation on outcomes after transcatheter aortic valve implantation. *Eur J Cardiothorac Surg* 41:1271–1276, 2012.
42. Barbanti M, Webb JG, Hahn RT, et al: Impact of preoperative moderate/severe mitral regurgitation on 2-year outcome after transcatheter and surgical aortic valve replacement: insight from the placement of aortic transcatheter valve (PARTNER) trial cohort A. *Circulation* 128:2276–2284, 2013.
43. Thourani VH, Keeling WB, Sarin EL, et al: Impact of preoperative renal dysfunction on long-term survival for patients undergoing aortic valve replacement. *Ann Thorac Surg* 91:1798–1806, 2011.
44. Sinning JM, Ghanem A, Steinhäuser H, et al: Renal function as predictor of mortality in patients after percutaneous transcatheter aortic valve implantation. *JACC Cardiovasc Interv* 3:1141–1149, 2010.
45. Nguyen TC, Babaliaros VC, Razavi SA, et al: Impact of varying degrees of renal dysfunction on transcatheter and surgical aortic valve replacement. *J Thorac Cardiovasc Surg* 146:1399–1406, 2013.
46. Kappetein AP, Head SJ, Genereux P, et al: Updated standardized endpoint definitions for transcatheter aortic valve implantation: the Valve Academic Research Consortium-2 consensus document (VARC-2). *Eur J Cardiothorac Surg* 42:S45–S60, 2012.
47. Martin T, Schymik G, Walther T, et al: Thirty-day results of the SAPIEN aortic bioprosthesis European outcome (SOURCE) registry: a European registry of transcatheter aortic valve implantation using the Edwards SAPIEN valve. *Circulation* 122:62–69, 2010.
48. Miller DC, Blackstone EH, Mack MJ, et al: Transcatheter (TAVR) versus surgical (AVR) aortic valve replacement: occurrence, hazard, risk factors, and consequences of neurologic events in the PARTNER trial. *J Thorac Cardiovasc Surg* 143:832–843, 2012.
49. Dewey TM, Bowers B, Thourani VH, et al: Transapical aortic valve replacement for severe aortic stenosis: results from the nonrandomized continued access cohort of the PARTNER trial. *Ann Thorac Surg* 96:2083–2089, 2013.
50. Eggebrecht H, Schmermund A, Voigtländer T, et al: Risk of stroke after transcatheter aortic valve implantation (TAVI): a meta-analysis of 10,037 published patients. *EuroIntervention* 8:129–138, 2012.
51. Nombela-Franco L, Webb JG, de Jaegere PP, et al: Timing, predictive factors, and prognostic value of cerebrovascular events in a large cohort of patients undergoing transcatheter aortic valve implantation. *Circulation* 126:3041–3053, 2012.
52. Van Mieghem NM, Schipper ME, Ladich E, et al: Histopathology of embolic debris captured during transcatheter aortic valve replacement. *Circulation* 127:2194–2201, 2013.
53. Naber CK, Ghanem A, Abizaid AA, et al: First-in-man use of a novel embolic protection device for patients undergoing transcatheter aortic valve implantation. *EuroIntervention* 8:43–50, 2012.
54. Nietlispach F, Wijesinghe N, Gurvitch R, et al: An embolic deflection device for aortic valve interventions. *JACC Cardiovasc Interv* 3:1133–1138, 2010.
55. Genereux P, Kodali SK, Green P, et al: Incidence and effect of acute kidney injury after transcatheter aortic valve replacement using the new valve academic research consortium criteria. *Am J Cardiol* 111:100–105, 2013.
56. Barbanti M, Yang TH, Cabau R, et al: Anatomical and procedural features associated with aortic root rupture during balloon-expandable transcatheter aortic valve replacement. *Circulation* 128:244–253, 2013.
57. Genereux P, Head SJ, Van Mieghem N, et al: Clinical outcomes after transcatheter aortic valve replacement using valve academic research consortium definitions: a weighted meta-analysis of 3,519 patients from 16 studies. *J Am Coll Cardiol* 59:2317–2326, 2012.
58. Borz B, Durand E, Godin M, et al: Incidence, predictors and impact of bleeding after transcatheter aortic valve implantation using the balloon-expandable Edwards prosthesis. *Heart* 99:860–865, 2013.
59. Leon MV, Gada H, Fontana GP: Challenges and future opportunities for transcatheter aortic valve therapy. *Prog Cardiovasc Dis* 56:635–645, 2014.
60. Genereux P, Head SJ, Hahn R, et al: Paravalvular leak after transcatheter aortic valve replacement. *J Am Coll Cardiol* 61:1125–1136, 2013.
61. Hahn RT: Use of imaging for procedural guidance during transcatheter aortic valve replacement. *Curr Opin Cardiol* 28:512–517, 2013.
62. Jilaihawi H, Kashif M, Fontana G, et al: Cross-sectional computed tomographic assessment improves accuracy of aortic annular sizing for transcatheter aortic valve replacement and reduces the incidence of paravalvular aortic regurgitation. *J Am Coll Cardiol* 59:1275–1286, 2012.
63. Ribeiro HB, Webb JG, Makkar RR, et al: Predictive factors, management and clinical outcomes of coronary obstruction following transcatheter aortic valve implantation: insights from a large multicenter registry. *J Am Coll Cardiol* 62:1552–1562, 2013.
64. Erkapic C, De Rosa S, Kelava A, et al: Risk for permanent pacemaker after transcatheter aortic valve implantation: a comprehensive analysis of the literature. *J Cardiovasc Electrophysiol* 23:391–397, 2012.
65. Leon MV, Gada H, Fontana GP: Challenges and future opportunities for transcatheter aortic valve therapy. *Prog Cardiovasc Dis* 56:635–645, 2014.
66. Nazif TM, Williams MR, Hahn RT, et al: Clinical implications of new-onset left bundle branch block after transcatheter aortic valve replacement: analysis of the PARTNER experience. *Eur Heart J* 35:1599–1607, 2013.

CHAPTER 80

Surgical Treatment of the Mitral Valve

Andrew B. Goldstone • Y. Joseph Woo

CHAPTER OUTLINE

ANATOMY

The mitral valve apparatus is composed of the mitral annulus, leaflets, chordae tendineae, papillary muscles, and the left ventricular lateral wall (Fig. 80-1). Chordae tendineae and papillary muscles comprise the subvalvular apparatus.

Annulus

The right fibrous trigone is a dense fibrous area of continuity between the annuli of the mitral, tricuspid, and noncoronary cusp of the aortic valve, as well as the membranous interventricular septum. The left fibrous trigone forms the leftmost border of fibrous continuity between the aortic and mitral valves. The mitral valve leaflets are attached to an ovoid ring, or annulus of fibrous tissue, that extends from the right and left fibrous trigones to form the junction between the left atrium and ventricle. In three-dimensional space, the annulus maintains a hyperbolic paraboloid shape (saddle shape).[1] The mid-anterior and mid-posterior annular segments are highest (farthest away from the ventricular apex), whereas the anterolateral and posteromedial commissures are lowest. The mitral annulus is thinnest at the insertion site of the posterior leaflet. As this segment is not attached to any rigid cardiac structures, it is the most mobile throughout the cardiac cycle and is the most prone to annular dilation.

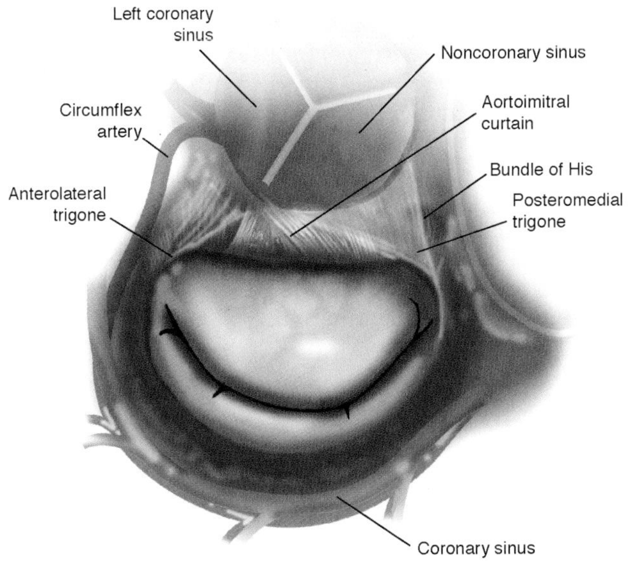

FIGURE 80-1 ■ Surgical anatomy of the mitral valve and other important neighboring structures.

Leaflets

The mitral valve has two major leaflets: the larger anterior (aortic) leaflet and the smaller posterior (mural) leaflet. The anterior leaflet is semicircular and is attached to one third of the annular circumference. The leaflet free edge does not have indentations. The anterior leaflet defines the boundary between the inflow and outflow tracts of the left ventricle. The posterior leaflet is quadrangular and is attached to two thirds of the annular circumference. The leaflet typically contains three or more scallops separated by fetal clefts or subcommissures, which develop to variable degrees in each individual.[2]

The subcommissures of the posterior leaflet permit further division of the mitral valve into eight segments (Fig. 80-2). The three posterior leaflet scallops are anatomically termed *anterolateral* (P1), *middle* (P2), and *posteromedial* (P3) segments. The three corresponding segments of the anterior leaflet are the anterior segment (A1), middle segment (A2), and posterior segment (A3). The anterolateral and posteromedial commissures comprise the remaining two segments. The posteromedial and anterolateral commissures are identified by the axis of the corresponding papillary muscles and the commissural chordae. The distance between the free edge of the commissures and the annulus is approximately 8 mm. As such, during open commissurotomy it is important to maintain this distance to reduce the risk of leaflet tearing and subsequent mitral regurgitation.

The atrial surface of the leaflets is divided into two zones: a marginal rough zone and central smooth zone. The rough zone is the coaptation surface of the valve and is the insertion site of most of the chordae tendineae.

Chordae Tendineae

The chordae tendineae are collagenous leaflet extensions connecting the papillary muscles and the ventricular side of the leaflets (Fig. 80-3). Chordae are classified based on

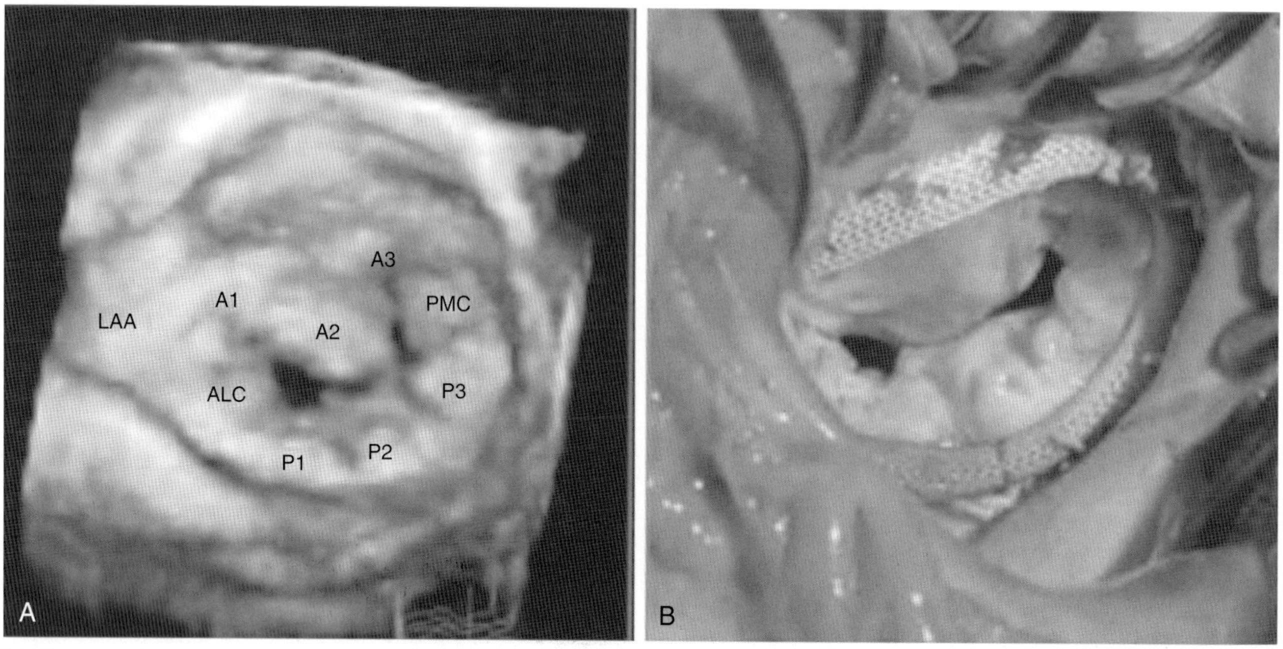

FIGURE 80-2 ■ Segmental anatomy of the mitral valve from the surgical view is demonstrated **(A)** grossly and **(B)** with three-dimensional transesophageal echocardiography. (Modified from Debonnaire P, Palmen M, Marsan NA, et al: Contemporary imaging of normal mitral valve anatomy and function. *Curr Opin Cardiol* 27:457, 2012.)

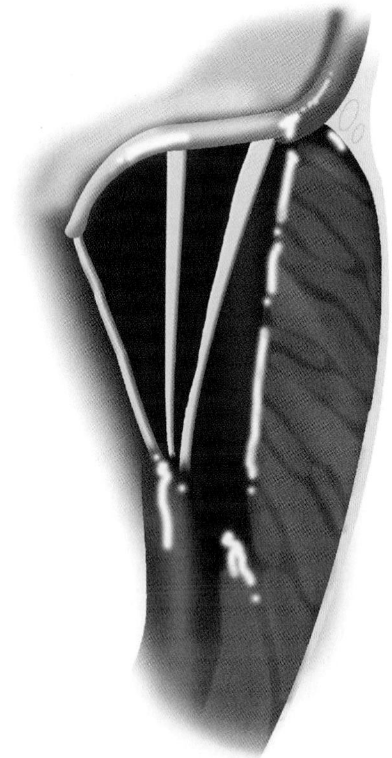

FIGURE 80-3 ■ Subvalvular apparatus. Primary chordae are attached to the free margin of the leaflet, secondary chordae are attached to the ventricular surface of the leaflet body, and tertiary chordae are attached to the ventricular surface of the leaflet base.

the site of insertion on the leaflet. Primary chordae insert on the leaflet free margin and act to prevent leaflet prolapse. Secondary chordae insert on the ventricular surface of the leaflets and reduce excess tension on the leaflet tissue. Tertiary chordae connect the leaflet base to the mitral annulus and surrounding myocardium. Tertiary chordae are limited to the posterior leaflet of the mitral valve. Often, the diameter of the chordae increases from the leaflet edge to the annulus.

Papillary Muscles and Left Ventricular Wall

Two papillary muscles arise between the middle and apical thirds of the left ventricle. The anterolateral papillary muscle is typically composed of one muscle body while the posteromedial papillary muscle usually arises from two muscle bodies. Each papillary muscle supplies chordae to both leaflets. The anterolateral papillary muscle receives blood from both the left anterior descending artery as well as a diagonal or obtuse marginal branch of the circumflex artery. However, the posteromedial papillary muscle receives blood from only one source: either the circumflex or right coronary artery. Consequently, the posteromedial papillary muscle is more sensitive to myocardial ischemia than the anterolateral papillary muscle. As the lateral wall of the left ventricle supports the base of the papillary muscles, it may also be considered part of the mitral valve apparatus. In fact, the left ventricular lateral wall is integral in the pathogenesis of ischemic mitral regurgitation.

MITRAL STENOSIS

Pathophysiology

In non-diseased adult human hearts, the normal mitral valve area is 4 to 6 cm^2. Once the mitral valve orifice narrows to less than 2.5 cm^2, a pressure gradient is necessary to generate blood flow from the left atrium into the

TABLE 80-1 **Classification of Mitral Stenosis Severity**

Findings	Mild	Moderate	Severe
Specific			
Valve area (cm^2)	>1.5	1.0-1.5	<1.0
Supportive			
Mean gradient (mm Hg)*	<5	5-10	>10
Pulmonary artery pressure (mm Hg)	<30	30-50	>50

*At heart rates between 60 and 80 beats/min and in sinus rhythm.
From Baumgartner H, Hung J, Bermejo J, et al: Echocardiographic assessment of valve stenosis: EAE/ASE recommendations for clinical practice. J Am Soc Echocardiogr 22:17, 2009.

left ventricle. Based on a semi-quantitative grading system, mitral stenosis is typically classified as mild if the valve area is >1.5 cm^2, moderate when the valve area is between 1.0 and 1.5 cm^2, and severe when the valve area is <1.0 cm^2 or the mean transvalvular pressure gradient exceeds 10 mm Hg (Table 80-1). However, it should be noted that the definition of *severe mitral stenosis* used by the American College of Cardiology/American Heart Association (ACC/AHA) is based on the severity at which symptoms occur as well as the severity at which intervention will improve symptoms (in essence, "severe" in professional society guidelines should be read as "significant").[3] Thus, in the 2014 iteration of the ACC/AHA guidelines, a mitral valve area of 1.5 cm^2 or less and a mean transvalvular gradient between 5 and 10 mm Hg is considered severe.

The transvalvular gradient results in elevated left atrial and pulmonary venous pressures. Over time, pulmonary artery hypertension develops from a combination of compensatory arterial vasoconstriction, intimal hypertrophy of the pulmonary arterioles and obliterative change, and passive retrograde transmission of the elevated pulmonary venous pressure. Pulmonary edema results when pulmonary venous pressure exceeds plasma oncotic pressure. At rest, mitral stenosis is often asymptomatic; however, any increase in flow across the mitral valve or decrease in duration of diastole results in an increase in the transvalvular pressure gradient. Consequently, dyspnea is typically precipitated by exercise, stress, infection, pregnancy, or rapid atrial fibrillation.

As pulmonary artery pressures rise, both right ventricular end-diastolic pressure and volume increase, resulting in right ventricular dilation and tricuspid regurgitation. Because left ventricular inflow is restricted, left ventricular chamber size or end-diastolic volume is normal or less than normal, and end-diastolic pressure is generally low. Although most patients with mitral stenosis have normal left ventricular dimensions and systolic function, ejection fraction is significantly reduced in a small proportion of patients (generally older adults).[4] These patients often have severe segmental wall contraction abnormalities of the posterobasal or anterolateral segments likely from papillary muscle fibrosis and immobilization.[4,5] Diffuse hypokinesis has also been described and is likely due to a chronic low cardiac output state.

Etiology

Although the prevalence of rheumatic disease has markedly decreased in recent decades, particularly in developed nations, it remains the predominant cause of mitral stenosis in the United States and worldwide.[6] However, only half to two thirds of patients report a definite history of rheumatic fever, with at least a 2:1 female-to-male predominance. Rheumatic valve disease is generally acquired before age 20, and becomes clinically evident one to three decades later.[7] Nonrheumatic etiologies of mitral stenosis include severe mitral annular calcification (common in older people), congenital mitral valve deformities, carcinoid syndrome, systemic lupus, neoplasm, and prosthetic valve calcification.

Rheumatic heart disease is an insidious fibrotic process that affects all segments of the mitral apparatus, as well as other valves. Mimicry between group A streptococcal antigens and epitopes found on human tissue stimulate autoimmune mediated damage to cardiac tissue.[6] The mitral valve is the most commonly affected (isolated mitral stenosis is found in 40% of patients), followed by concomitant aortic and mitral valve disease, and least frequently isolated aortic valve disease. Early valvular lesions include: (1) leaflet thickening; (2) chordal thickening, fusion, and shortening; and (3) commissural fusion (Fig. 80-4). Progressive valvulopathy produces a characteristic "fish mouth" single central opening, with restricted leaflet motion during systole and diastole. Chordal thickening and fusion can create a dense fibrotic subvalvular mass that can further obstruct forward flow. Calcification, particularly at the commissural edges and occasionally extending posteriorly into the annulus and subvalvular apparatus, is common late in the disease process and in older patients. These lesions, especially chordal fusion and shortening, often reduce leaflet coaptation by restricting leaflet mobility and thereby yield concomitant mitral regurgitation.

Clinical Characteristics and Diagnosis

The diagnosis of mitral stenosis can be based on medical history, physical examination, electrocardiography, chest radiography, echocardiography, and invasive hemodynamics. As explained previously, patients are most often women and are frequently asymptomatic, although symptoms can include fatigue, dyspnea, hemoptysis (from rupture of dilated bronchial veins), new onset atrial fibrillation, or systemic thromboembolism.

Patients with chronic severe mitral stenosis are often cachectic because of longstanding low cardiac output. In the absence of left ventricular dysfunction, peripheral pulses are normal and the apical impulse is in the standard position on chest palpation. A right ventricular parasternal heave is present in the setting of pulmonary hypertension. Auscultatory findings include a loud S_1, an opening snap, and a diastolic murmur. The diastolic murmur is a low-pitched rumble best heard at the apex. The early diastolic opening snap is generated by sudden tensing of the pliable leaflets during valve opening and is absent later in the disease when the leaflets are immobile. The electrocardiogram may be normal but often

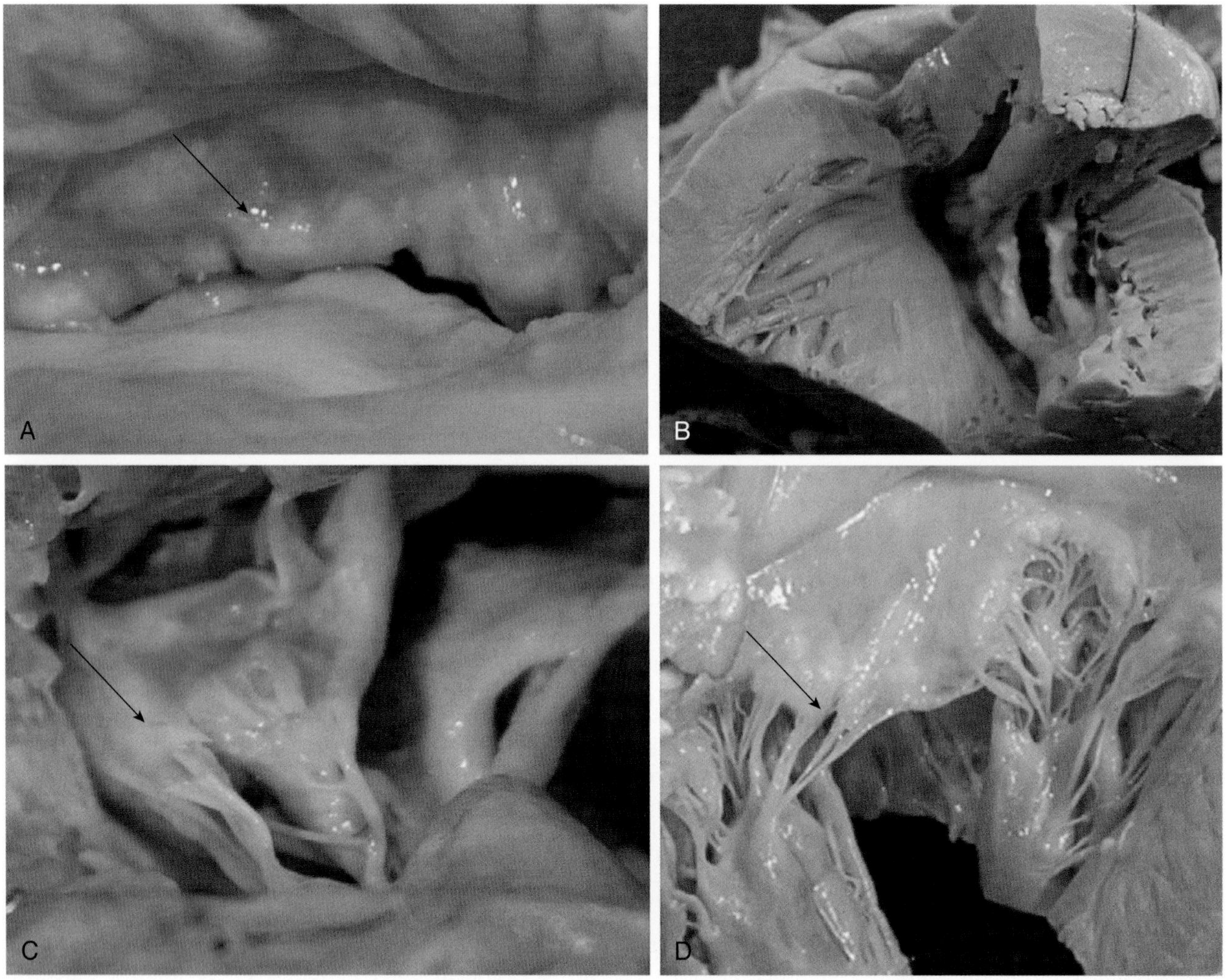

FIGURE 80-4 ■ Pathologic changes of the mitral valve in mitral stenosis. Thickened, rigid, nodular appearance of the mitral valve leaflets as viewed from the atria **(A)** and ventricle **(B)**. The commissures are calcified and fused, thereby creating the characteristic "fish mouth"–shaped valve. **B** and **C,** The subvalvular apparatus is thickened, fused, and shortened. **D,** Healthy mitral valve leaflets. (From Chandrashekar Y, Westaby S, Narula J: Mitral stenosis. *Lancet* 374:1273, 2009.)

demonstrates P-wave abnormalities indicative of left atrial enlargement (biphasic P-wave in lead V_1; or broad, notched P-wave in lead II), atrial fibrillation, or right ventricular hypertrophy (right-axis deviation and a tall R-wave in lead V_1). The chest radiograph may be normal; however, a large left atrium is frequently seen. In patients with severe mitral stenosis and pulmonary hypertension, the right atrium and ventricle may also be enlarged.

Echocardiography has become the principle diagnostic method for assessing mitral valve disease. Echocardiography permits evaluation of the morphology, mobility, and extent of calcification of the mitral leaflets, commissures, and subvalvular apparatus. In addition, the severity of mitral stenosis can be assessed by measuring the mitral valve area, the transmitral gradient, left atrial size, and the pulmonary artery pressures (see Table 80-1). Transthoracic echocardiography also provides a noninvasive evaluation of other valves, as well as right and left ventricular function. Echocardiographic characteristics of the mitral valve apparatus are used to determine candidacy for percutaneous balloon valvuloplasty.

Left-sided heart catheterization is not usually necessary for diagnosis of mitral stenosis, but it can be useful when there is a discrepancy between data from noninvasive assessments. In patients that meet criteria for surgical intervention, cardiac catheterization should be performed to ascertain whether coronary artery disease is present. Right-sided heart catheterization is performed to measure the severity of pulmonary hypertension, and it can be used to determine reversibility after administration of pulmonary vasodilators.

Natural History

Although the average age of index cases of rheumatic fever is approximately 12 years, symptoms do not generally become apparent until 30 years of age.[7] Once symptoms develop, progression to incapacitating disability occurs over approximately 10 years, and those with more severe symptoms have poorer prognoses (Fig. 80-5).[8] As such, the development of symptoms is integral in the treatment decision-making process. In surgically

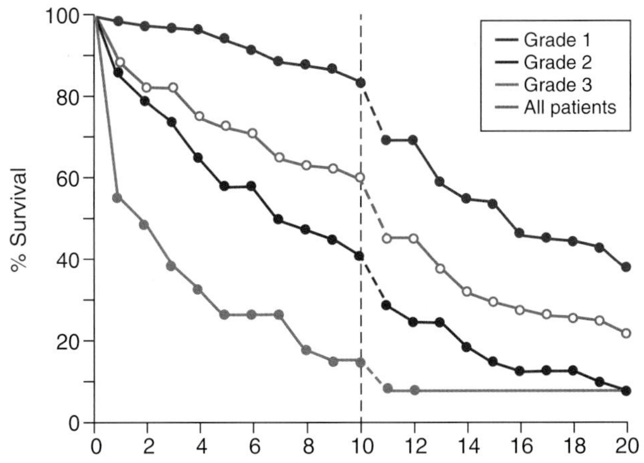

FIGURE 80-5 Survival of patients with surgically untreated mitral stenosis stratified by symptom severity at initial evaluation. *Grade 1,* Asymptomatic; *Grade 2,* mild symptoms; *Grade 3,* moderate or moderately severe symptoms. (From Rowe JC, Bland EF, Sprague HB, et al: The course of mitral stenosis without surgery: ten- and twenty-year perspectives. *Ann Intern Med* 52:741–749, 1960.)

untreated patients with mitral stenosis, the average age of death is between 40 and 50 years.[8,9]

Various sequelae often develop during the course of surgically untreated mitral stenosis that shorten the interval between symptom onset and death. Left atrial hypertension ultimately distorts atrial cardiomyocyte architecture and predisposes patients to atrial fibrillation. The onset of atrial fibrillation often initiates symptoms because patients with mitral stenosis rely heavily on atrial contraction for ventricular filling, and rapid heart rates reduce the duration of diastole. Consequently, cardiac output declines and left atrial pressure rises. In fact, atrial fibrillation incrementally increases the risk of death in patients with surgically untreated mitral stenosis; 20-year survival was 10% in patients with atrial fibrillation compared with 29% in those in sinus rhythm.[10]

Systemic thromboembolism also significantly alters the course of the disease, particularly when it results in stroke. Although most emboli originate in the left atrial appendage or left atrium, atrial fibrillation is not prerequisite for thrombus formation in surgically untreated mitral stenosis. Overall, arterial thromboembolization occurs in at least 10% of surgically untreated patients with mitral stenosis.[11]

Pulmonary hemorrhage infrequently can develop in even mildly symptomatic patients, but the risk remits after surgical correction of the stenotic valve. Finally, infective endocarditis is uncommon in patients with mitral stenosis.

It is important to emphasize that these data and complicating events correspond to medically treated and surgically untreated patients with mitral stenosis. In fact, progression from initial symptoms to death was likely much shorter before medical therapies such as diuretics were developed. Similarly, surgical treatment has significantly altered the disease course. The increased life expectancy of such patients after surgical correction of mitral stenosis has resulted in the manifestation of late significant rheumatic aortic valve disease and late secondary tricuspid regurgitation.

Indications for Surgery

Untreated mitral stenosis is associated with a poor prognosis once severe symptoms occur.[12] Percutaneous balloon mitral commissurotomy is the first-line therapy for mitral stenosis in patients with favorable anatomy. This procedure is indicated in symptomatic patients (stage D) with isolated severe mitral stenosis (mitral valve area $\leq$1.5 cm^2; Fig. 80-6).[3] Left atrial thrombus and greater than mild mitral regurgitation are contraindications to balloon commissurotomy. Percutaneous balloon commissurotomy may also be appropriate in asymptomatic patients with severe mitral stenosis (valve area <1.0 cm^2) and in those with severe mitral stenosis and new onset atrial fibrillation. Finally, balloon commissurotomy can be considered in symptomatic individuals with mitral valve area greater than 1.5 cm^2 if there is hemodynamic evidence of significant mitral stenosis with exercise (e.g., pulmonary capillary wedge pressure > 25 mm Hg). The Wilkins scoring system grades mitral valve morphology by use of echocardiography (Table 80-2). Four characteristics, graded on a scale from 0 to 4, are assessed: leaflet mobility, leaflet thickening, valve calcification, and extent of subvalvular disease. A total score greater than 8 is predictive of low success with percutaneous balloon mitral commissurotomy.[13,14] Percutaneous balloon commissurotomy is associated with recurrent mitral stenosis, especially in patients undergoing repeat procedures for recurrence, as well as iatrogenic mitral regurgitation, particularly in patients with high Wilkins scores.[14]

Mitral valve surgery is an established therapy for mitral stenosis that predates balloon commissurotomy. Surgical options include commissurotomy (either closed or open, the latter permitting more extensive surgery under direct visualization) or mitral valve replacement. Because of the insidious nature of mitral stenosis and evidence that mitral stenosis does not have longstanding detrimental effects on the left ventricle, surgery should be delayed until the patient has severe, limiting symptoms (New York Heart Association [NYHA] class III or IV).[3] Thus, mitral valve surgery is indicated in severely symptomatic patients (NYHA class III or IV) with severe mitral stenosis (mitral valve area $\leq$ 1.5 cm^2) who are not high risk for surgery and who are not candidates for or who have failed previous percutaneous balloon mitral commissurotomy (see Fig. 80-6).[3] Concomitant mitral valve surgery is also recommended in patients with severe mitral stenosis undergoing cardiac surgery for other primary indications.

MITRAL REGURGITATION

Pathophysiology

Mitral regurgitation, the retrograde ejection of blood from the left ventricle into the left atrium during systole, may be acute, chronic and compensated, or chronic and

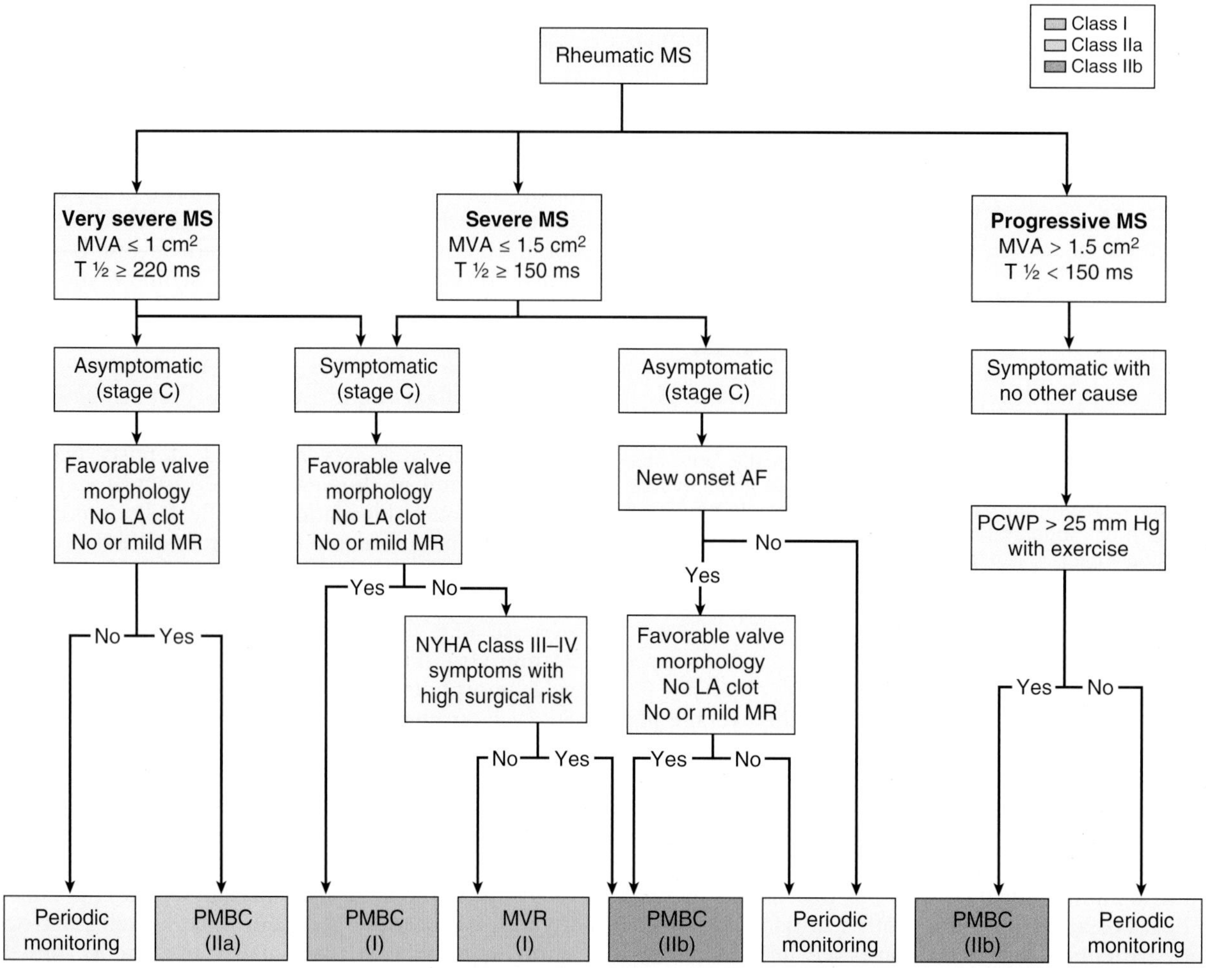

FIGURE 80-6 ■ Indications for intervention for mitral stenosis. *AF,* Atrial fibrillation; *LA,* left atrial; *MR,* mitral regurgitation; *MS,* mitral stenosis; *MVA,* mitral valve area; *MVR,* mitral valve surgery (repair or replacement); *NYHA,* New York Heart Association; *PCWP,* pulmonary capillary wedge pressure; *PMBC,* percutaneous mitral balloon commissurotomy; *T ½*, pressure half-time. (From Nishimura RA, Otto CM, Bonow RO, et al: 2014 AHA/ACC Guideline for the Management of Patients with Valvular Heart Disease: a report of the American College of Cardiology/American Heart Association Task Force on Practice Guidelines. *Circulation* 129:e554, 2014.)

TABLE 80-2 **Assessment of the Mitral Valve with the Wilkins Score**

Grade	Mobility	Thickening	Calcification	Subvalvular Thickening
1	Highly mobile valve with only leaflet tips restricted	Minimal leaflet thickening (4-5 mm)	Single area of increased echo brightness	Minimal thickening just below the mitral leaflets
2	Leaflet mid and base portions have normal mobility	Midleaflets normal, considerable marginal thickening (5-8 mm)	Scattered areas of brightness confined to leaflet margins	Thickening of chordal structures extending to one-third the chordal length
3	Valve continues to move forward in diastole, mainly from the base	Entire leaflet thickened (5-8 mm)	Brightness extends into mid-portion of leaflets	Thickening extended to distal third of the chords
4	No or minimal forward movement of the leaflets in diastole	Considerable thickening of entire leaflet (>8-10 mm)	Extensive brightness throughout much of the leaflet tissue	Extensive thickening and shortening of all chordal structures that extends to the papillary muscles

Total score is the sum of the four items and ranges between 4 and 16.

Modified from Baumgartner H, Hung J, Bermejo J, et al: Echocardiographic assessment of valve stenosis: EAE/ASE recommendations for clinical practice. J Am Soc Echocardiogr 22:14, 2009.

decompensated. The new low resistance, regurgitant pathway results in volume overload of the left ventricle at end diastole (increased preload) as well as in a reduction of afterload.[15] Subsequently, a larger volume of blood is ejected from the left ventricle with each contraction. However, the effective forward stroke volume and cardiac output actually decrease because a proportion of the blood volume is ejected retrograde into the left atrium. Volume overload in the left atrium increases left atrial pressure from a normal level of approximately 10 mm Hg to as high as 25 mm Hg. The increased preload ultimately induces ventricular remodeling through eccentric hypertrophy and dilation.[15] A larger ventricular cavity allows for an increase in total stroke volume, thereby maintaining forward stroke volume at near normal levels. This is chronic compensated mitral regurgitation.

Because the annulus is continuous with the left ventricle, annular dilation results from ventricular enlargement. The normal ratio between the anteroposterior and transverse diameters of the mitral annulus is 3:4 in systole. In chronic mitral regurgitation, this ratio is inverted, impairing proper leaflet coaptation and generating regurgitant flow even in the absence of leaflet prolapse. Annular dilation affects the posterior annulus to a greater extent than the anterior annulus.

Similar to ventricular compensation via enlargement, the left atrium dilates to accommodate the volume overload at lower filling pressures.[15] Atrial enlargement increases the risk of atrial arrhythmias, such as atrial fibrillation and consequent mural thrombi from stasis. When mitral regurgitation develops suddenly from chordal rupture, papillary muscle infarction, or leaflet perforation, there is inadequate time for left atrial and ventricular compensation. Thus, patients with acute mitral regurgitation typically present in a state of acute pulmonary edema and cardiogenic shock.

Ultimately, volume overload and eccentric ventricular hypertrophy impair ventricular performance and prevent effective ventricular contraction; this is chronic decompensated mitral regurgitation. Stroke volume and cardiac output decline as blood preferentially flows retrograde into the lower resistance pathway. Consequently, the pressure in the left atrium and pulmonary vasculature increases. Untreated decompensated mitral regurgitation progresses to irreversible pulmonary hypertension, pulmonary edema, and congestive heart failure. The presence of left ventricular dysfunction portends a worse prognosis regardless of the treatment modality. Although ventricular reverse remodeling can follow surgical correction of mitral regurgitation, it remains evident that normalization of cardiac dimensions is less likely or impossible once the ventricle has enlarged to a certain extent.[16]

Functional Classification

A thorough description of valve disease should incorporate the pathophysiologic triad first proposed by Carpentier (Table 80-3).[17] The triad includes etiology (cause of the disease), valve lesions (structural changes resulting from the disease process), and leaflet dysfunction (alterations in leaflet motion resulting from the structural lesion). This classification scheme is emphasized because prognosis is etiology dependent, treatment strategy is determined by the type of valve dysfunction, and different surgical techniques are selected for specific valve lesions.

TABLE 80-3 **Pathophysiologic Triad of Mitral Regurgitation**

Dysfunction	Lesions	Etiology
Type I		
Normal leaflet motion	Annular dilation	Ischemic cardiomyopathy Dilated cardiomyopathy Permanent atrial fibrillation
	Leaflet perforation	Endocarditis
Type II		
Increased leaflet motion above annular plane (leaflet prolapse)	Chordal elongation or rupture	Degenerative disease Fibroelastic deficiency Barlow's disease Marfan syndrome Endocarditis Rheumatic Trauma
	Papillary muscle elongation or rupture	Ischemic cardiomyopathy Barlow's disease (elongation)
Type IIIa		
Restricted leaflet motion (systole and diastole)	Leaflet thickening or retraction Chordal thickening, retraction, or fusion Commissural fusion	Rheumatic disease Carcinoid heart disease Mitral annular calcification
Type IIIb		
Restricted leaflet motion (systole only)	Papillary muscle displacement Leaflet tethering	Ischemic cardiomyopathy Dilated cardiomyopathy Submitral ventricular aneurysm

The mechanism of mitral regurgitation can be categorized using Carpentier's functional classification (Fig. 80-7).[17] The classification system is compartmentalized according to variations in leaflet motion. In type I dysfunction, leaflet motion is normal and a central mitral regurgitation jet is generated by annular dilation or leaflet perforation. Type II dysfunction describes leaflet prolapse, where the free margin of one or both leaflets rises above the annular plane in systole. Such leaflet dysfunction is most commonly due to chordal elongation or rupture, followed by papillary muscle elongation and rupture. In type III dysfunction leaflet motion is restricted. Leaflet motion restricted during both diastole and systole is classified as type IIIa. Lesions commonly associated with rheumatic valvulitis are most often responsible for type IIIa dysfunction, including (1) leaflet thickening and retraction; (2) chordal thickening, shortening, or fusion; and (3) commissural fusion. As such, coexistent mitral stenosis is not uncommon in the setting of type IIIa mitral regurgitation. Type IIIb dysfunction describes leaflet motion restricted only during systole. Such dysfunction is the result of left ventricular dilation and subsequent leaflet tethering from papillary muscle displacement.

Etiology

Degenerative Disease

Systolic prolapse of a mitral valve leaflet is a relatively common and complex disease process. When severe, mitral prolapse begets significant mitral regurgitation, albeit infrequently (about 10% of patients).[18] Nevertheless, degenerative mitral valve disease is the most common cause of isolated mitral regurgitation in the United States.[19,20] Pathologic examination of degenerative mitral valves reveals mitral leaflet redundancy and myxomatous leaflet thickening that typically result from collagen replacement by acid mucopolysaccharides.[21] Mutual support is lost as redundant and elongated leaflets improperly coapt during systole. Consequently, the leaflets extend into the left atrium and the valve is rendered regurgitant. Simultaneously, chordae are placed under abnormal strain. The chordae elongate and may ultimately rupture, generating more regurgitation. Annular dilation and calcification can also arise to varying extents and further contribute to the complexity of the mitral valve dysfunction.

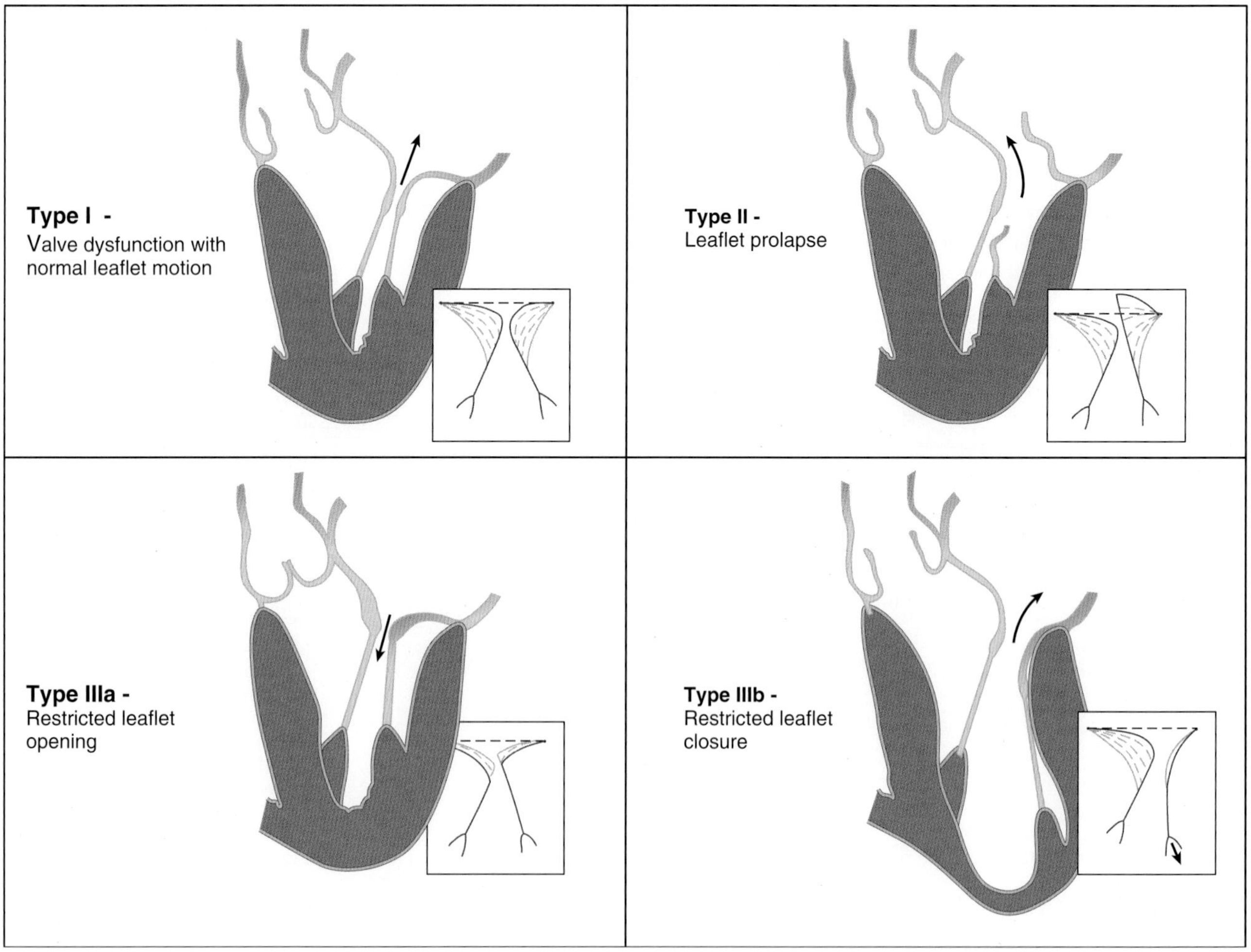

FIGURE 80-7 ■ Carpentier's functional classification of mitral regurgitation: *Type I,* normal leaflet motion; *Type II,* increased leaflet motion resulting in prolapse; *Type III,* restricted leaflet motion; *IIIa,* during diastole and systole; *IIIb,* during systole only. The *arrow* demonstrates the direction of regurgitant flow in types I, II, and IIIb. In type IIIa, the *arrow* demonstrates the frequent association with coexistent mitral stenosis. (From Carpentier A, Adams DH, Filsoufi F: *Carpentier's reconstructive valve surgery,* St. Louis, 2010, Elsevier.)

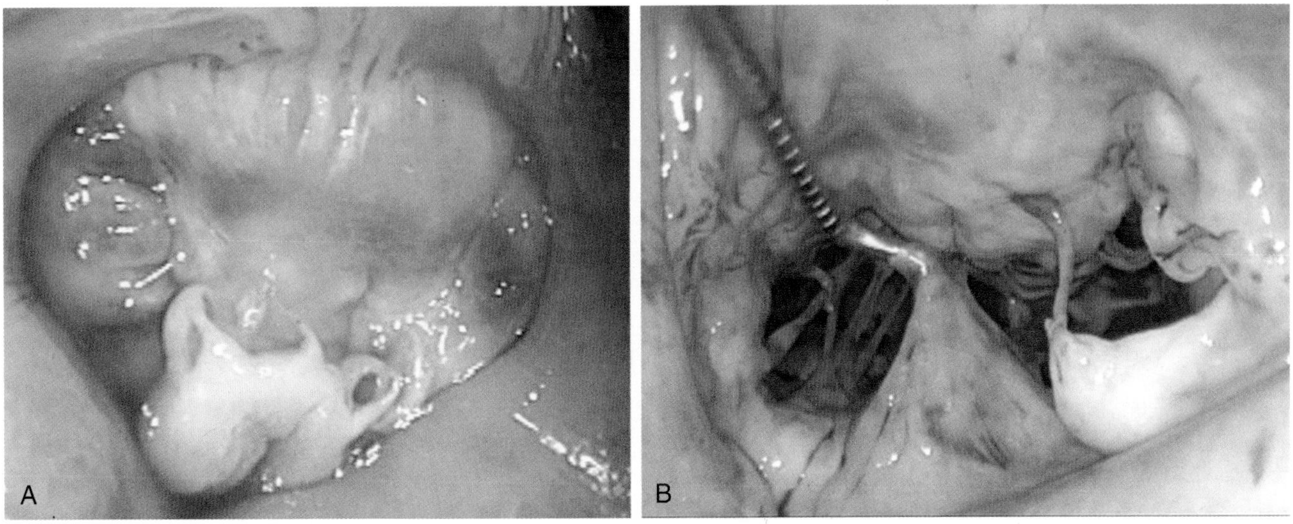

FIGURE 80-8 ■ Surgical lesions in fibroelastic deficiency. **A,** Prolapse of P2 owing to multiple ruptured chordae; the leaflet tissue is thickened compared with other segments. Note the translucency of the anterior leaflet, and normal height and thickness of P1 and P3, in contrast to findings in Barlow's disease (see Fig. 80-9). **B,** Prolapse of P3 with ruptured chord. Note that P3 is thickened, but P2 and P1 are thin and of normal height. (From Anyanwu AC, Adams DH: Etiologic classification of degenerative mitral valve disease: Barlow's disease and fibroelastic deficiency. *Semin Thorac Cardiovasc Surg* 19:94, 2007.)

The spectrum of degenerative mitral valve disease is often subclassified into fibroelastic deficiency and Barlow's disease.[22] In fibroelastic deficiency, or idiopathic chordal rupture, a considerable portion of leaflet tissue is unaffected by the myxomatous transformation (Fig. 80-8).[23] Typically, regurgitation is caused by rupture of a single chord that supports the posteromedial portion of the posterior leaflet (P2). Following rupture, the less supported leaflet segment becomes redundant and flail. More extensive posterior chordal rupture may sometimes occur. Patients with fibroelastic deficiency are characteristically older with a short history of mitral regurgitation.

On the opposite end of the degenerative mitral valve disease spectrum, Barlow's disease presents early in life, and most patients have a long history of a systolic murmur. Barlow's disease is characterized by extensive excess leaflet tissue in a dilated annulus (Fig. 80-9).[21,22] Leaflet tissue is thickened, and there is marked redundancy in multiple segments. In addition, chordae and occasionally papillary muscles are thickened and elongated. Regurgitation is complex and secondary to multisegment leaflet prolapse. Forme fruste valves share morphologic features of Barlow's disease and fibroelastic deficiency: multisegment thickening and prolapse within a smaller valve.

Rheumatic Disease

Progressive leaflet thickening and retraction, as well as chordal shortening and fusion from chronic valvulitis restrict leaflet motion during both diastole and systole, thereby rendering the valve regurgitant (see Fig. 80-4). The anterior leaflet is typically less thickened, and particularly in younger patients, elongated major chordae may allow regurgitation from anterior leaflet prolapse.[24] Annular dilation from extensive myocarditis may cause transient mitral regurgitation in the acute rheumatic process. This mitral regurgitation can spontaneously regress after remission of the pancarditic acute rheumatic process.

Mitral Annular Calcification

Annular calcification is most often seen in older people.[25] Although it can occur without apparent disease of the leaflets or chordae, it may be more common in patients with myxomatous degeneration of the mitral leaflets. Calcifying disease of the annulus is a degenerative process that usually involves the posterior circumference of the annulus more than other portions.[25,26] Annular calcification can extend into the adjacent myocardium of the left ventricle, and it yields mitral regurgitation through restricted motion of the posterior leaflet. Such calcification can substantially complicate mitral repair or replacement.[25,27]

Infective Endocarditis

Endocarditis is a relatively uncommon cause of isolated mitral regurgitation compared with the frequency in which it is accountable for aortic regurgitation. Mitral valve endocarditis typically occurs in patients with an already structurally abnormal valve because of underlying degenerative or rheumatic valve disease. However, several virulent organisms, such as *Staphylococcus aureus*, may infect nondiseased valves.[28] *Staphylococci* and *Streptococci* now account for 80% of cases of endocarditis.[28,29] Upon infection of a normal or abnormal mitral valve, mitral regurgitation can result from destruction of leaflet cusps, chordae, or both. Because of their spatial interrelatedness, aortic valve endocarditis may directly extend to the mitral valve as vegetations may drop down onto and infect the central portion of the anterior leaflet of the mitral valve (Fig. 80-10).[30]

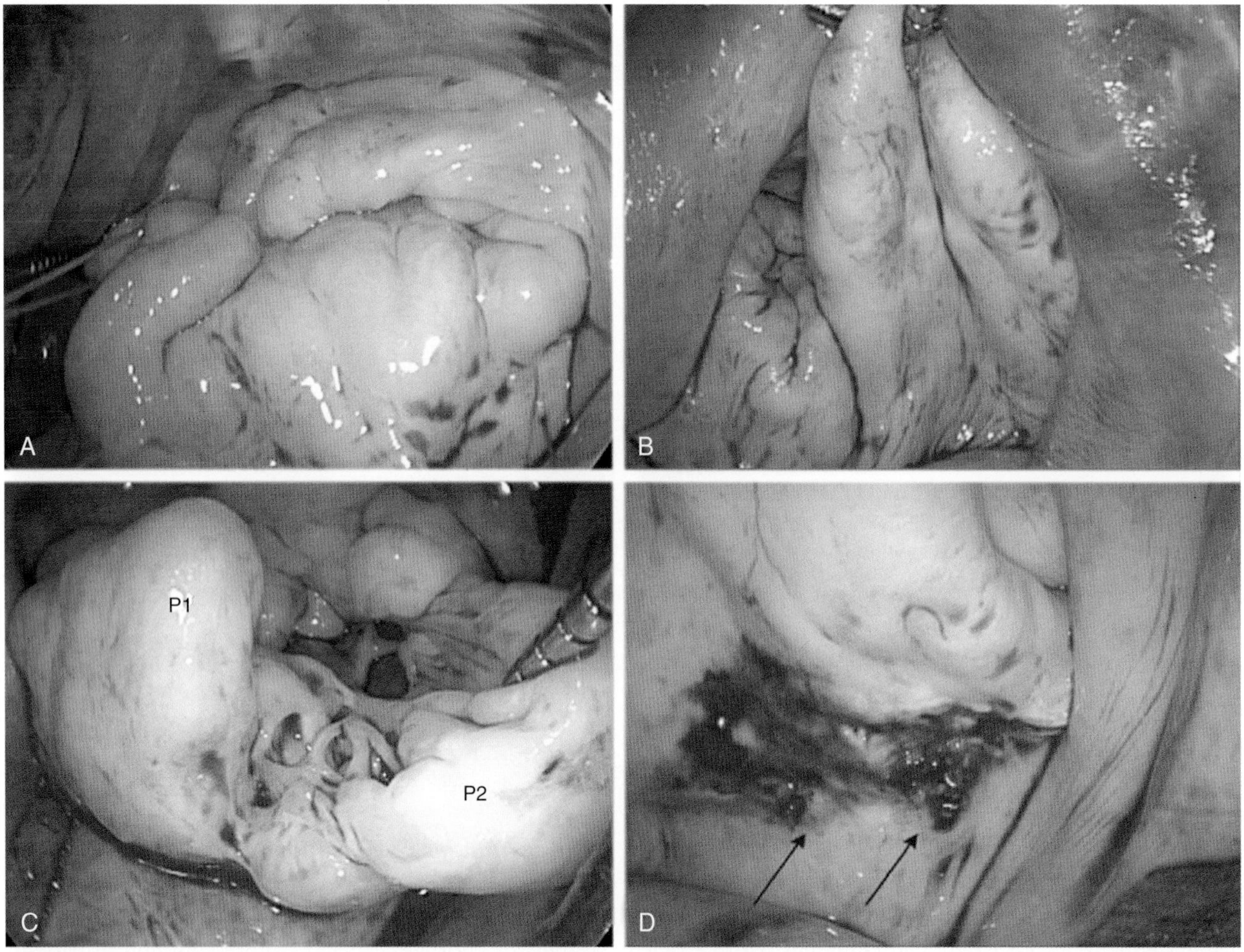

FIGURE 80-9 ■ Surgical lesions in Barlow's disease. **A,** Large valve with redundant, thick, bulky leaflets. **B,** Tall, posterior leaflet with tip rising to anterior annulus. **C,** Calcified anterior papillary muscle with fused, matted chords restricting the P1/P2 junction. **D,** Atrialization of the base of the posterior leaflet. Note the blurring of the atrial-leaflet junction with fissures and microthrombi *(arrows).* (From Anyanwu AC, Adams DH: Etiologic classification of degenerative mitral valve disease: Barlow's disease and fibroelastic deficiency. *Semin Thorac Cardiovasc Surg* 19:93, 2007.)

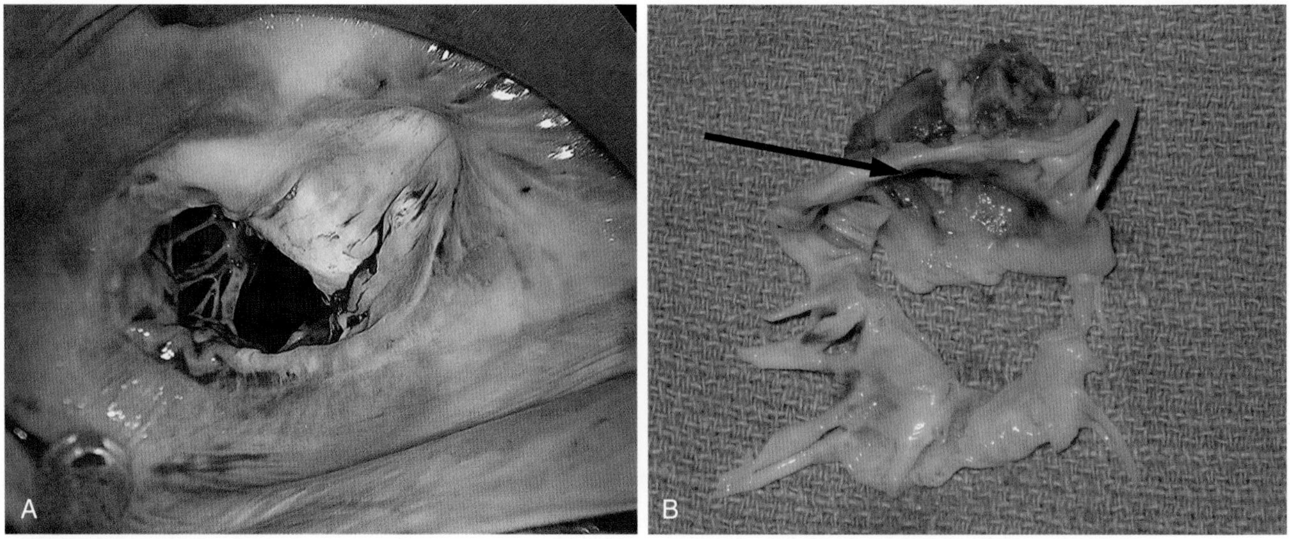

FIGURE 80-10 ■ Surgical lesions in ischemic cardiomyopathy and infective endocarditis. **A,** A dilated annulus with severe posterior leaflet tethering is characteristic of ischemic mitral regurgitation. **B,** Perforation *(arrow)* of the anterior leaflet of the mitral valve secondary to infective endocarditis.

Ischemic Cardiomyopathy

Left ventricular remodeling after myocardial infarction results in a conversion of the ventricular shape from ellipsoidal to spherical. Consequently, the papillary muscles are displaced, leading to restriction or tethering of posterior leaflet motion during systole (see Fig. 80-10).[31,32] Leaflet coaptation surface area is compromised, resulting in mitral regurgitation. Furthermore, because of structural continuity between the ventricle and annulus, ventricular dilation leads to annular dilation that may exacerbate mitral regurgitation. Acute mitral regurgitation can result from ischemic papillary muscle dysfunction or rupture.[33] Occasionally, the papillary muscle will not rupture, but will become fibrotic and subsequently elongate, leading to leaflet prolapse.

Dilated Cardiomyopathy and Submitral Left Ventricular Aneurysms

The etiology of this disease is frequently idiopathic; however, known causes include chronic atrial fibrillation, myocarditis, excessive alcohol consumption, and immunologic abnormalities. Similar to ischemic cardiomyopathy, the natural history of the disease is often complicated by functional mitral regurgitation secondary to ventricular remodeling.

Submitral ventricular aneurysms can also result in mitral regurgitation. Such an aneurysm is not due to myocardial ischemia, and it occurs almost exclusively in Africa.[34] The aneurysm is generally situated directly beneath the posterior mitral leaflet; therefore, mitral regurgitation develops from aneurysmal distortion of the posterior leaflet.[34,35]

Clinical Characteristics and Diagnosis

Chronic

Patients with chronic mitral regurgitation are often asymptomatic for years. During this time, left ventricular size can gradually increase and myocardial contractility declines. Ultimately, patients develop exercise intolerance and symptoms consistent with pulmonary venous hypertension. Fluid retention, chronic cardiac failure, and occasionally cardiac cachexia are representative of longstanding untreated disease. Coexistent secondary tricuspid regurgitation is frequently apparent at such late stages of the disease.[36]

Similar to mitral stenosis, significant mitral regurgitation can generally be diagnosed on the basis of history, physical examination, electrocardiogram, and chest radiograph. On auscultation, a classic pansystolic murmur is appreciable, loudest at the apex, and radiates to the left axilla. However, murmurs may be heard in the parasternal aortic area or infrascapular–posterior cervical area in the setting of eccentric jets from posterior leaflet or anterior leaflet prolapse, respectively. An S_3 may be present because of augmented transmitral flow from volume overload and left ventricular dilation. In addition, lateral displacement of the left ventricular apical impulse from ventricular dilation and parasternal lift from elevated pulmonary arterial pressures indicate more severe disease.

The electrocardiogram may remain unremarkable despite severe mitral regurgitation; however, evidence of ventricular hypertrophy or left atrial enlargement may also be present. Chest radiography in severe chronic mitral regurgitation may demonstrate left atrial and ventricular dilation (typically greater than in patients with mitral stenosis), and prominent pulmonary vasculature suggests the presence of pulmonary hypertension.

Two-dimensional echocardiography via transthoracic and transesophageal approaches delineate the mechanism and severity of mitral regurgitation (Table 80-4; Fig. 80-11). Echocardiography can also be used to assess left ventricular dimensions and global and regional contractility. Three-dimensional echocardiographic imaging techniques clearly identify leaflet pathology and specific areas of regurgitation within the mitral valve.[37] Novel magnetic resonance imaging techniques also accurately characterize anatomic and functional details of mitral valve dysfunction.

Mitral regurgitation can be characterized by left ventriculography. Leaflet prolapse can be visualized, and the degree of regurgitation can be estimated. Quantitative ventriculography permits calculation of regurgitant flow and left ventricular stroke volume, and forward flow can be assessed through measurement of cardiac output.[38] Furthermore, left heart catheterization is particularly useful to discern the extent of coronary artery disease, if present.

Acute

Mitral regurgitation can develop acutely because of chordal rupture or infective endocarditis or early in the evolution of acute myocardial infarction. Symptoms and signs are consistent with acute elevation of pulmonary venous pressures and low cardiac output. On auscultation, the murmur of mitral regurgitation is often midsystolic and higher pitched compared with the classic pansystolic murmur of chronic mitral regurgitation. The left atrium and left ventricle are normal in size because of inadequate time for compensation through dilation. Because of acute elevation of pulmonary venous pressure, significant pulmonary edema is often noted on chest radiography.

Natural History

Defining the natural history of mitral regurgitation is problematic because the disease etiology varies, age at onset varies, mitral regurgitation may not worsen for many years, and left ventricular function declines at different rates. It is important to note that left ventricular contractility is not truly assessed by ejection fraction. In fact, in the setting of mitral regurgitation, ventricular contractility often declines despite normal systolic function (ejection fraction) because part of the stroke volume is ejected retrograde into the low pressure left atrium. Ejection fraction does not actually decrease until later in the disease process. Patients with mitral regurgitation can

TABLE 80-4 Specific and Supportive Signs and Quantitative Parameters in Grading Mitral Regurgitation Severity

	Mild	Moderate		Severe
Specific Signs of Severity	Small central jet <4 cm^2 or <20% of LA area* Vena contracta width <0.3 cm No or minimal flow convergence†	Signs of MR > mild present, but no criteria for severe MR		Vena contracta width ≥0.7 cm with large central MR jet (area >40% of LA) or with a wall-impinging jet of any size, swirling in LA* Large flow convergence† Systolic reversal in pulmonary veins Prominent flail MV leaflet or ruptured papillary muscle
Supportive Signs of Severity	Systolic dominant flow in pulmonary veins A-wave dominant mitral inflow‡ Soft density, parabolic CW Doppler MR signal Normal LV size§	Intermediate signs and findings		Dense, triangular CW Doppler MR jet E-wave dominant mitral inflow (E>1.2 m/sec)‡ Enlarged LV and LA size‖ (particularly when LV function is normal)
Quantitative Parameters¶				
R Vol (mL/beat)	<30	30-44	45-59	≥60
RF (%)	<30	30-39	40-49	≥50
EROA (cm^2)	<0.20	0.20-0.29	0.30-0.39	≥0.40

*At a Nyquist limit of 50-60 cm/sec.
†Minimal and large flow convergence radius <0.4 cm and ≤0.9 cm for central jets, respectively, with a baseline shift at a Nyquist of 40 cm/sec. Cutoffs for eccentric jets are higher and should be angle corrected.
‡Usually above 50 years of age or in conditions of impaired relaxation, in the absence of mitral stenosis or other causes of elevated LA pressure.
§LV size applied only to chronic lesions.
‖In the absence of other etiologies of LV and LA dilation and acute MR.
¶Quantitative parameters can help to subclassify the moderate regurgitation group into mild-to-moderate and moderate-to-severe as shown.
CW, Continuous wave; *EROA,* effective regurgitant orifice area; *LA,* left atrium; *LV,* left ventricle; *MR,* mitral regurgitation; *MV,* mitral valve; *R Vol,* regurgitant volume; *RF,* regurgitant fraction.
From Zoghbi WA, Enriquez-Sarano M, Foster E, et al: Recommendations for evaluation of the severity of native valvular regurgitation with two-dimensional and Doppler echocardiography. J Am Soc Echocardiogr 16:777–802, 2003.

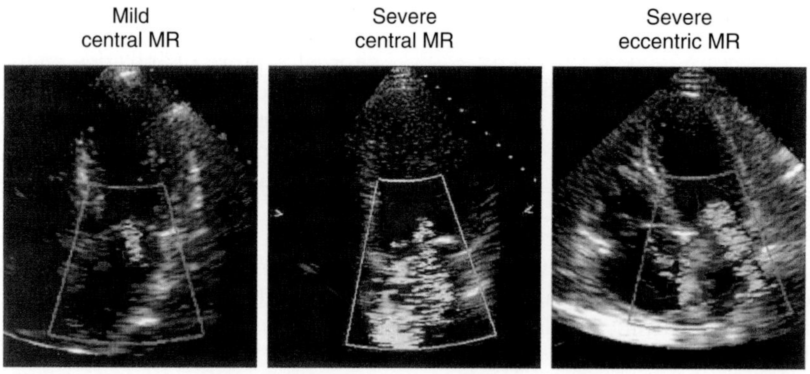

FIGURE 80-11 ■ Examples of color flow recordings of different mitral regurgitation (MR) lesions from the apical window. The case of mild regurgitation has no flow convergence and a small regurgitant jet area, in contrast to that of severe central MR, which shows a prominent flow convergence and large regurgitant jet area. The example with severe eccentric MR has a small jet area impinging on the wall of the left atrium but a large flow convergence and a wide vena contracta. (From Zoghbi WA, Enriquez-Sarano M, Foster E, et al: Recommendations for evaluation of the severity of native valvular regurgitation with two-dimensional and Doppler echocardiography. *J Am Soc Echocardiogr* 16:784, 2003.)

also develop secondary tricuspid regurgitation, which also affects natural history.[36]

Degenerative Disease

Degenerative disease, the most common organic mitral valve disease in the United States, occurs in approximately 2% to 3% of adults.[19,20] However, many patients do not progress to developing significant regurgitation requiring intervention. In fact, severe mitral regurgitation requiring valve repair or replacement is uncommon before the age of 50. Although the prevalence increases steeply thereafter, persons with mitral valve prolapse who reach age 70 still only have about a 5% chance of requiring mitral valve surgery.[39] Nevertheless, once significant mitral regurgitation develops, the disease progresses similarly to those with ruptured chordae and flail leaflets.

Once a diagnosis of flail leaflet is made, medical management typically is inadequate in improving patient symptoms and survival. Patients with surgically untreated mitral regurgitation because of flail leaflet have mortality rates significantly higher than expected (6.3% yearly).[40] Severe symptoms portend a worse prognosis as patients even transiently in NYHA class III or IV have much higher mortality rates (34% yearly), although the rate is notable even among those in NYHA class I or II (4% yearly).[40,41] Essentially, surgery is almost unavoidable within 10 years after the diagnosis and is associated with an improved prognosis in patients with degenerative disease.

Ischemic Cardiomyopathy

The natural history of ischemic mitral regurgitation is covered in Chapter 92. Because ischemic mitral regurgitation is a manifestation of a ventricular disease, it is not surprising that these patients typically have a significantly worse survival than those with degenerative disease.

Rheumatic Disease

Patients with surgically untreated but significant rheumatic mitral regurgitation demonstrate survival similar to those with rheumatic mitral stenosis.[9,42] Likewise, the survival curves are considerably shorter in particular geographic areas and in certain races: 5-year survival after initial evaluation for rheumatic mitral regurgitation in the United States was 80% compared with 46% in Venezuela.[42]

Infective Endocarditis

Infection of a previously mildly abnormal mitral valve can generate acute mitral regurgitation. The natural history of such a condition is similar to that of mitral regurgitation caused by chordal rupture. However, the early mortality is significantly higher as death can occur from overwhelming infection and sepsis.

Indications for Surgery

Intervention for patients with primary mitral regurgitation consists of either surgical mitral valve repair or replacement. Mitral valve repair is preferred over replacement if a successful and durable repair can be achieved. Reparability is dependent on valve morphology and surgeon expertise.[3]

Acute severe mitral regurgitation is an indication for urgent surgery. The indications for surgery in chronic severe mitral regurgitation have evolved during the last decade to reflect incremental improvements in the safety and efficacy of mitral valve repair as well as a better understanding of long-term outcomes in surgically untreated patients. Recommendations by the ACC/AHA for surgical intervention are predicated on symptoms, left ventricular dysfunction, atrial fibrillation, pulmonary hypertension, and valve reparability (Fig. 80-12).[3]

Symptoms

The onset of symptoms that results from severe mitral regurgitation worsens prognosis even when left ventricular function appears to be normal. This negative prognostic effect extends even to mild symptoms.[43] Thus, an increasing number of clinicians advocate operating earlier in less-symptomatic patients because NYHA functional class has been shown to be an independent predictor of postoperative mortality and left ventricular dysfunction.[44] Postoperative long-term survival is higher in patients in NYHA class I or II before surgery compared with those in class III or IV, (at 10 years, 76% vs. 48%), and operative mortality is lower (0.5% vs. 5.4%; Fig. 80-13).[43]

Left Ventricular Dysfunction and Enlargement

Preoperative left ventricular dysfunction, as assessed by ejection fraction and end-systolic dimension, is one of the strongest predictors of survival, postoperative ventricular function, and functional status after surgery for chronic primary mitral regurgitation.[43,45-48] Specifically, it has been reported that when the ejection fraction falls below 60%, mortality increases precipitously and prompt surgical referral is critical to outcome (Fig. 80-14).[45] Thus, the goal of therapy in mitral regurgitation is to correct it before the onset of left ventricular systolic dysfunction and the subsequent adverse effect on patient outcomes. Ideally, mitral valve surgery should be performed when the patient's left ventricle approaches but has not yet reached the parameters that indicate systolic dysfunction (left ventricular ejection fraction [LVEF] $\leq$ 60% or left ventricular end-systolic dimension [LVESD] $\geq$ 40 mm), even if the patient is asymptomatic.[3] Because symptoms do not always coincide with left ventricular dysfunction, imaging surveillance is used to plan surgery before ventricular function has severely deteriorated. Further delay, even though symptoms are absent, will lead to greater left ventricular dysfunction and an even worse prognosis. Although it is inadvisable to allow patients' left ventricular function to deteriorate beyond the benchmarks of an LVEF $\leq$ 60% and/or LVESD $\geq$ 40 mm, some recovery of left ventricular function can still occur even if these thresholds have been crossed.

Atrial Fibrillation and Pulmonary Hypertension

In nonrheumatic mitral regurgitation, the onset of atrial fibrillation is in part due to enlarging left atrial size, and its presence worsens surgical outcome.[40,49-51] Furthermore, the longer atrial fibrillation is present, the more likely it is to persist despite intervention. Therefore, it may be reasonable to restore mitral competence by low-risk repair with the hope that the ensuing reduction in left atrial size will help restore and maintain sinus rhythm. The ACC/AHA guidelines advocate surgery in asymptomatic patients with severe mitral regurgitation and new onset atrial fibrillation.[3] However, restoration of sinus rhythm following valve surgery is uncertain, and concomitant surgical ablation of atrial fibrillation should be

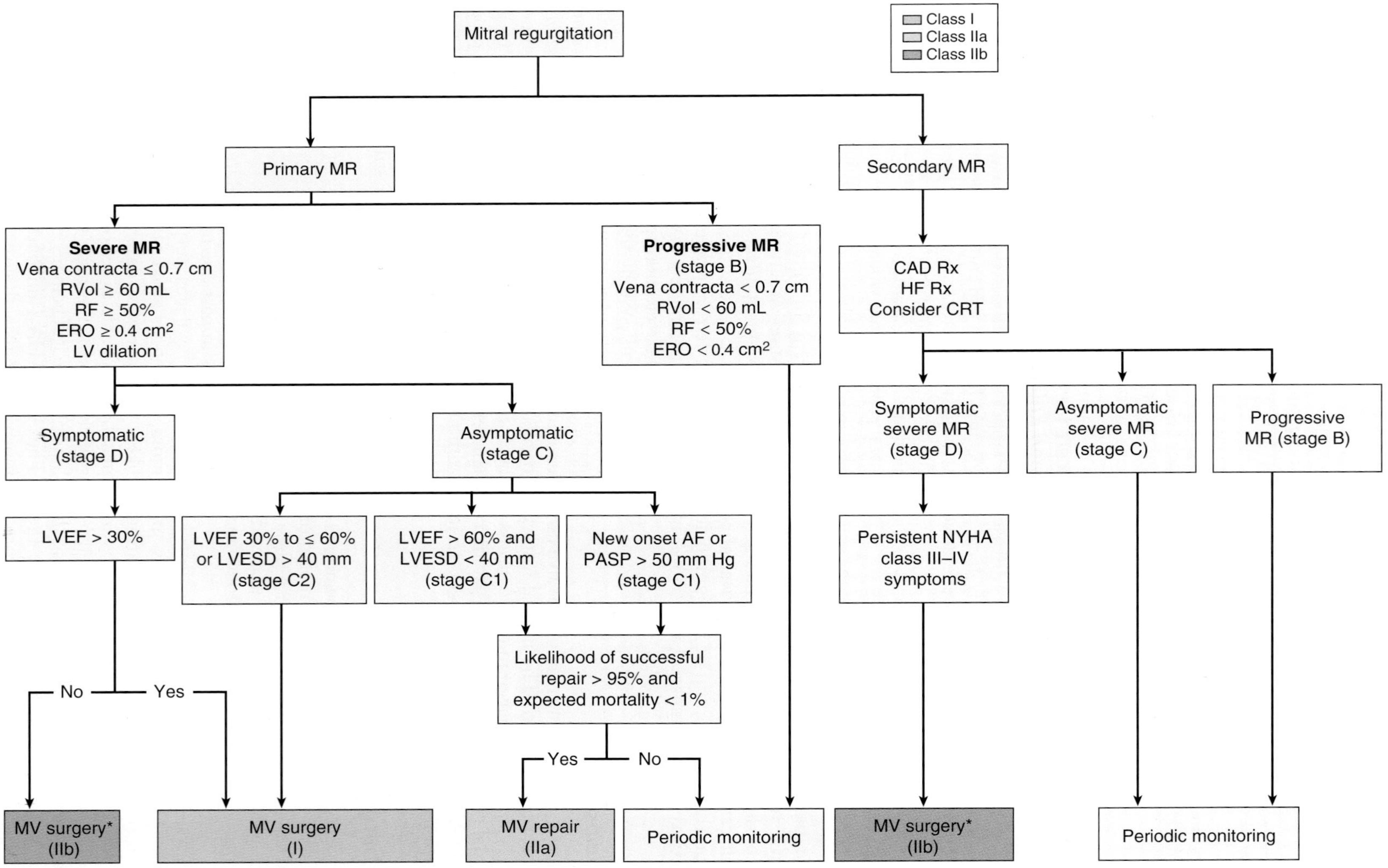

FIGURE 80-12 ■ Indications for surgery for mitral regurgitation. *AF,* Atrial fibrillation; *CAD,* coronary artery disease; *CRT,* cardiac resynchronization therapy; *ERO,* effective regurgitant orifice; *HF,* heart failure; *LV,* left ventricular; *LVEF,* left ventricular ejection fraction; *LVESD,* left ventricular end-systolic dimension; *MR,* mitral regurgitation; *MV,* mitral valve; *MVR,* mitral valve replacement; *NYHA,* New York Heart Association; *PASP,* pulmonary artery systolic pressure; *RF,* regurgitant fraction; *RVol,* regurgitant volume; *Rx,* therapy. *Mitral valve repair is preferred over MVR when possible. (From Nishimura RA, Otto CM, Bonow RO, et al: 2014 AHA/ACC Guideline for the Management of Patients with Valvular Heart Disease: a report of the American College of Cardiology/American Heart Association Task Force on Practice Guidelines. *Circulation* 129:e569, 2014.)

a standard adjunct to patients with a history atrial arrhythmia. This strategy does not apply to rheumatic mitral regurgitation, in which active atrial inflammation can make restoration of sinus rhythm less likely and valve scarring reduces the likelihood of a successful repair. The presence of resting pulmonary arterial hypertension caused by mitral regurgitation is associated with poorer operative and long-term survival after valve surgery.[46,52,53] Thus, it is reasonable to consider surgery in these asymptomatic patients if resting pulmonary artery systolic pressure exceeds 50 mm Hg and if there is a high likelihood of a successful and durable repair.[3]

Reparability

Mitral valve repair is preferred over replacement if a successful and durable repair can be achieved. Mitral valve repair is performed at a lower operative mortality rate than replacement. Although no randomized trials exist for degenerative mitral valve disease, nearly every clinical report has demonstrated that operative risk for repair is approximately half that of replacement. Valve repair not only avoids the risks inherent to prosthetic heart valves, but it better preserves left ventricular function by preserving the subvalvular apparatus. In the case of posterior leaflet prolapse, repair has become sufficiently standardized so that repair is the standard of care. The ACC/AHA guidelines recommend that a successful repair rate of 90% or greater be the expectation of every cardiac surgeon who performs mitral valve procedures.[3] Because the probability of successful mitral valve repair is strongly influenced by surgeon-specific mitral procedure volume,[54] it is recommended that more complex valves be referred to heart teams with particular expertise in this area.[3]

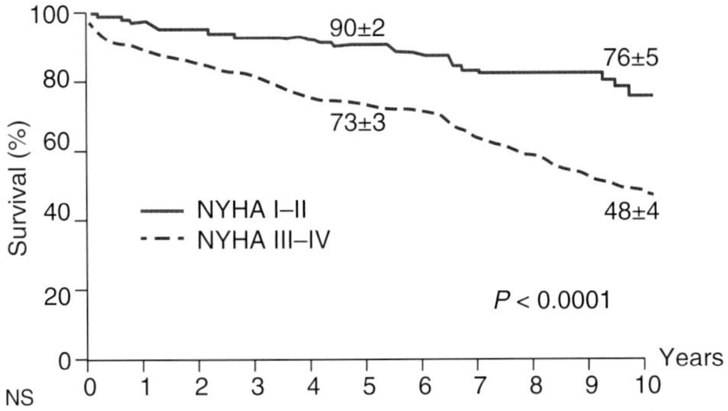

NS	0	1	2	3	4	5	6	7	8	9	10
I–II	199	192	187	184	181	169	125	95	63	42	34
III–IV	279	249	236	227	211	201	174	133	103	74	51

FIGURE 80-13 ■ Overall postoperative survival compared between patients in New York Heart Association (NYHA) class I or II and patients in class III or IV. Numbers at bottom indicate patients at risk. (From Tribouilloy CM, Enriquez-Sarano M, Schaff HV, et al: Impact of preoperative symptoms on survival after surgical correction of organic mitral regurgitation: rationale for optimizing surgical indications. *Circulation* 99:402, 1999.)

SURGERY

Anesthesia and Monitoring

Standard monitoring lines are used if the procedure is performed through a median sternotomy. A pulmonary artery catheter should be placed in cases of complex mitral valve surgery and multivalve surgery, as well as in high-risk operative candidates. Carbon dioxide insufflation is routinely used to facilitate deairing and reduce the risk of air embolism following aortic cross-clamp removal. A thorough transesophageal echocardiography study should routinely be performed before the initiation of cardiopulmonary bypass to characterize the mechanism and severity of mitral regurgitation, as well as other valve lesions. Transesophageal echocardiography also permits assessment of left ventricular function, quality of the repair, and extent of deairing. External defibrillator and cardioversion pads are placed in patients undergoing reoperative surgery.

If a right minithoracotomy is planned, the anesthesiologist should place a double-lumen endotracheal tube to permit left lung ventilation and right lung deflation.

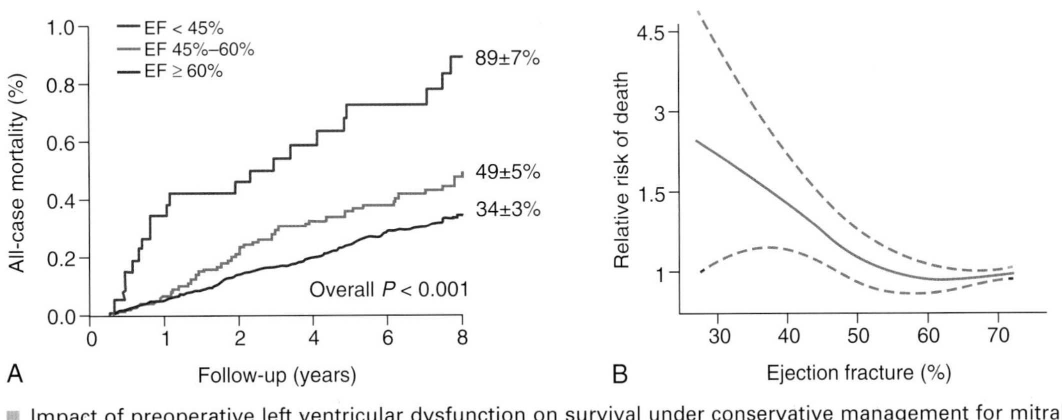

FIGURE 80-14 ■ Impact of preoperative left ventricular dysfunction on survival under conservative management for mitral regurgitation. **A,** All-cause mortality stratified by ejection fraction (EF). **B,** Association between EF and the risk of all-cause death under conservative management. Hazard ratio *(solid line)* and 95% confidence intervals *(dashed lines)* were estimated in a Cox multivariable model with ejection fraction represented as a spline function and adjusted for sex, comorbidity index, symptoms, and coronary artery disease. (Modified from Tribouilloy C, Rusinaru D, Grigioni F, et al: Long-term mortality associated with left ventricular dysfunction in mitral regurgitation due to flail leaflets: a multicenter analysis. *Circ Cardiovasc Imaging* 7:366, 2014.)

External defibrillator pads are placed under the right scapula and over the left anterolateral chest. If an endoaortic balloon occlusion catheter will be used, bilateral radial arterial lines can be placed to facilitate rapid detection of balloon distal migration and innominate artery obstruction. Inadvertent balloon migration is not uncommon, and vascular injuries including aortic dissection have contributed to decreased utilization of this approach. Our institution prefers a transthoracic Chitwood aortic cross clamp and standard antegrade cardioplegia, retrograde cardioplegia, and right superior pulmonary vein venting cannulae placed across the chest wall or directly through the working incision. Thoracic epidural placement is not commonly used, because pain is reportedly mild after minithoracotomy incisions, particularly if rib spreading is avoided.

Surgical Approaches

Median Sternotomy

Median sternotomy is the most common surgical approach in mitral valve surgery.[55] Because it provides excellent access to all cardiac structures, it remains the surgical approach of choice in patients undergoing multivalve (other than concomitant mitral and tricuspid valve surgery) or combined mitral and coronary bypass grafting surgery. If a median sternotomy is the planned approach for mediastinal entry, then a Sarns 6-mm cannula is placed in the ascending aorta for arterial cannulation. 24 Fr superior vena cava and 28 Fr inferior vena cava metal tip cannulae are preferentially used for bicaval cannulation to maximize exposure and access to the mitral valve via Sondergaard's groove.

Minimally Invasive Approaches

Over the past 20 years, the increasing popularity of less invasive procedures has affected nearly every surgical specialty, including cardiac surgery. Advancements in imaging, surgical instrumentation, and robotic technology have enabled surgeons to perform complex cardiac surgical procedures through small incisions, often eliminating the need for sternotomy or cardiopulmonary bypass.[56-59] In addition to benefits of improved cosmesis, minimally invasive mitral valve surgery was pioneered with the intent of reducing morbidity, postoperative pain, blood loss, hospital length of stay, and time to return to normal activity.[60-63]

Although initial reports of less invasive mitral valve surgery used parasternal[61,64] or lower hemisternotomy[65] approaches for mediastinal access, the right anterolateral minithoracotomy has become the minimally invasive approach of choice for correcting mitral valve disease (Fig. 80-15).[63,66,67] Compared with lower partial sternotomy, this approach provides a more en face view of the mitral valve and avoids surgery in the xiphisternal region, the area most prone to wound breakdown and infection following sternotomy. The right thoracotomy approach is considerably more resistant to infection because of overlying pectoralis muscle and soft tissue to seal the surgical site.[68] Robotic and port access mitral valve surgery are thus performed through a 3- to 4-cm incision in the inframammary crease in female patients and just above the nipple in male patients, and the thoracic cavity is entered through the third or fourth interspace. Additional sub-centimeter ports facilitate introduction of a camera, left atrial retractor, suction, and in the case of robotic surgery, working arms (Fig. 80-16). Peripheral cannulation for cardiopulmonary bypass via the femoral arterial and venous vessels as well as the internal jugular vein facilitates smaller working incisions and less clutter of the surgical field. However, the ascending aorta and right atrium can be cannulated directly with the Seldinger technique if a contraindication precludes direct femoral cannulation. Aortic cross-clamping is achieved with a transthoracic Chitwood clamp or endovascularly with an endoaortic balloon occlusion device. Although beating- or fibrillating-heart strategies are used in some centers, concerns for higher stroke rates have led many surgeons to advocate using these techniques with caution.[55,69] However, this risk is confounded by the nature of the patient for which these strategies must be used, such as patients with prior cardiac surgery, aortic pathology contraindicating cross-clamp application, or severe ventricular dysfunction. As robotic and thoracoscopic port access approaches facilitate all standard resectional and nonresectional valve repair techniques, the procedure of mitral valve repair is akin to the operation performed through conventional sternotomy.[58,70-72]

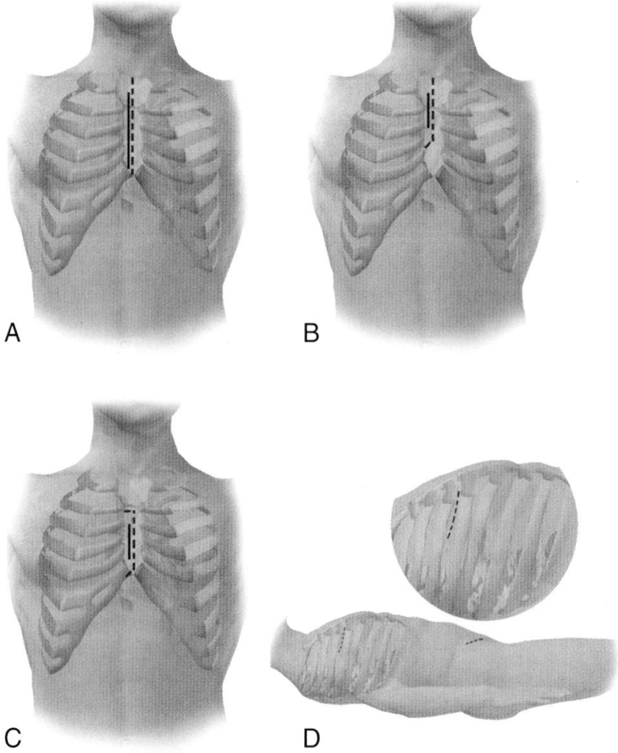

FIGURE 80-15 ■ Surgical incisions. **A,** Conventional median sternotomy. **B,** Upper hemisternotomy. **C,** Lower hemisternotomy. **D,** Right minithoracotomy and groin incision for peripheral cannulation. Solid line represents skin incision and dotted line represents sternotomy.

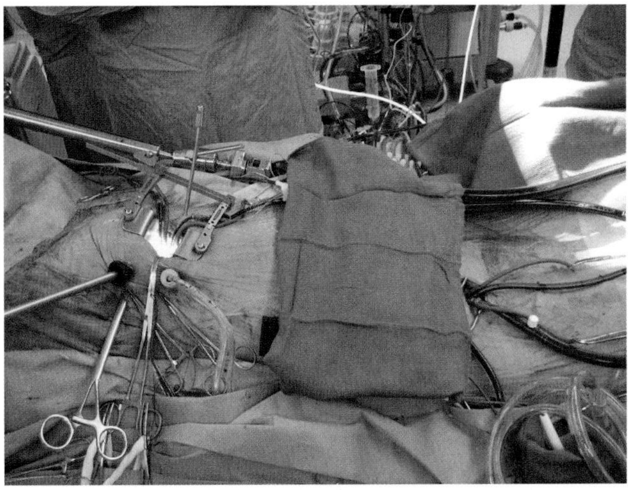

FIGURE 80-16 ■ Exposure and cannulation technique for minimally invasive mitral valve surgery via right anterolateral minithoracotomy. (From Goldstone AB, Woo YJ: Minimally invasive surgical treatment of valvular heart disease. *Semin Thorac Cardiovasc Surg* 26:37, 2014.)

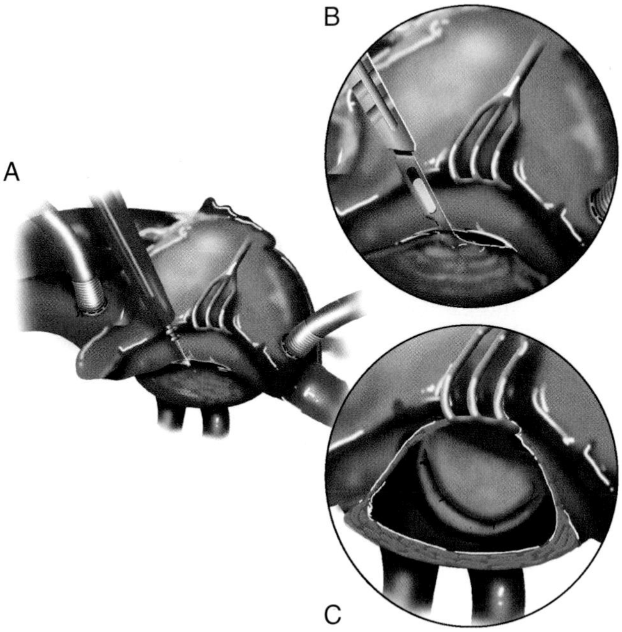

FIGURE 80-17 ■ Interatrial exposure of the mitral valve. **A,** Interatrial groove is dissected to fossa ovalis to expose roof of left atrium. **B,** Left atrium is incised and extended toward the superior and inferior vena cavae. **C,** Anterior retraction of the left atrium to expose the mitral valve.

Myocardial Management

Cardioplegic arrest is the most commonly used myocardial protection strategy during mitral valve surgery. Alternative techniques, such as beating heart and ventricular fibrillatory arrest, are occasionally used in select patients. Cardioplegic arrest uses cold blood high-potassium cardioplegia solution delivered via intermittent antegrade or combined antegrade and retrograde infusion. Further myocardial protection can be achieved with moderate systemic hypothermia and local hypothermia with topical ice.

Alternative protection strategies should be considered in certain clinical scenarios, such as in patients with severely depressed left ventricular function (beating heart) and severe atherosclerotic disease of the ascending aorta (beating heart or ventricular fibrillatory arrest). These alternative protection strategies are also useful in reoperative mitral valve surgery, when it may be difficult to cross-clamp the ascending aorta and when patent bypass grafts dissuade reoperative median sternotomy.

Operative Sequence in Context of Concomitant Procedures

When performing concomitant procedures, mitral valve surgery is typically performed at a specific juncture in the operation to accommodate anatomic constraints, facilitate operative flow, and avoid potential injury. Examples best illustrate these principles. When performing concomitant coronary bypass, the distal anastomoses are completed before mitral valve intervention. This avoids manipulation and anterior displacement of the heart after placement of a mitral prosthesis, which may beget posterior ventricular wall injury. When performing concomitant aortic valve replacement, the aortic valve leaflets are first resected and the annulus is débrided to avoid potential cutting of mitral annular sutures. The mitral procedure is performed before the aortic valve replacement because the aortic valve prosthesis distorts and obscures the anterior mitral annulus, particularly at the anterolateral commissure. When performing concomitant tricuspid valve surgery, a trans-septal approach is most efficient, and the mitral valve operation is conducted first. The interatrial septum is closed and the tricuspid annuloplasty can then be performed with the cross-clamp removed.

Exposure of the Mitral Valve

Excellent exposure of the mitral valve is essential before any mitral valve intervention. Various techniques have been described, including the interatrial approach through Sondergaard's (or Waterston's) groove, the right atrial trans-septal approach, and the left atrial dome approach.

Interatrial Approach through Sondergaard's Groove

The interatrial approach through Sondergaard's groove is the most commonly employed approach for mitral valve exposure (Fig. 80-17). First, the fatty tissue just anterior to the right superior and right inferior pulmonary veins is dissected, essentially separating the right atrium from the anterior surface of the left atrium. It is important to start this incision on the actual body of the left atrium to avoid any potential involvement of the pulmonary venous ostia. If this incision is extended too medially, the right atrium can be entered accidentally. This issue can be addressed easily with caval tapes or vacuum assisted venous return. Generally, it is not necessary to add additional time to close the inadvertent right atriotomy separately because it can be incorporated in the left atriotomy closure at completion of the mitral operation. If extensive exposure is necessary, the posterior aspect of the superior vena cava can be dissected from the left atrium to free additional portions of the roof of the left atrium for atriotomy.

Right Atrial Trans-septal Approach

In this approach, bicaval cannulation and caval snaring with tapes are generally helpful. The right atriotomy is initiated and extended posteriorly toward the left atrium (Fig. 80-18). The interatrial septum and fossa ovalis are visualized, and an incision is made in the most posterior aspect toward the patient's right (near the pulmonary veins). Thus, sufficient septal tissue remains not only for retraction of the left atrial roof for exposure of the mitral valve, but also for closure of the atrial septum at the end of the procedure. The septal incision is carried inferiorly down to the end of the fossa ovalis. An incision carried any further will essentially become an extended right atriotomy below the inferior vena cava and should be avoided. Superiorly, the incision is extended beyond the fossa ovalis onto the more muscular portion between the left and right atria near the superior vena cava inlet. Anterior retraction on this left atrial septum results in excellent visualization of the mitral valve because the trans-septal incision is closer to the mitral valve than a standard left atriotomy incision. This incision is particularly useful in the setting of biatrial enlargement often seen in mitral stenosis, as well as in reoperative scenarios in which a previous interatrial groove left atriotomy was performed. It is also a useful approach in patients who have had prior aortic valve replacement, as exposure of the anterolateral commissure can be difficult in this setting. A variation of this trans-septal incision is the extended trans-septal approach whereby the upper portion of the trans-septal incision is extended over the dome of the left atrium.[73] This incision provides outstanding exposure, but is more challenging to properly reapproximate.

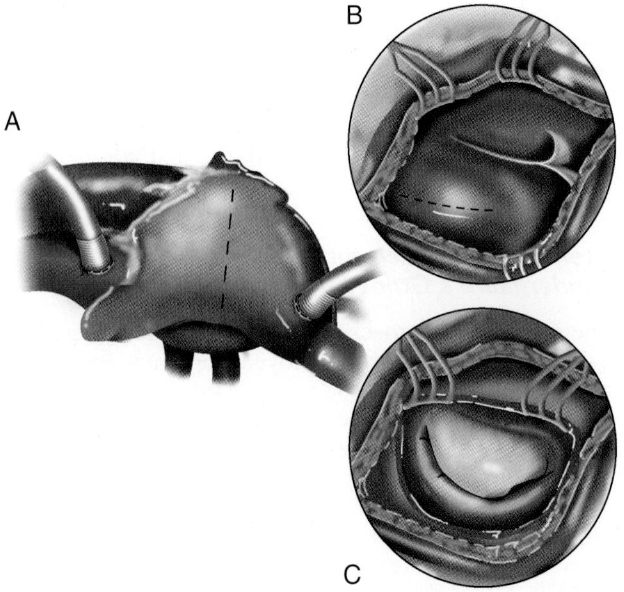

FIGURE 80-18 ■ Trans-septal exposure of the mitral valve. **A,** The right atrium is incised and extended posteriorly. **B,** The septum is incised and extended inferiorly down to the end of the fossa ovalis. **C,** Anterior retraction of the septum exposes the mitral valve.

Left Atrial Dome Approach

Another less used atriotomy is the isolated left atrial dome approach whereby the roof of the left atrium, in between the aorta and superior vena cava, is incised and retracted. Overall, this incision is smaller given space constraints; however, the direct view of the mitral valve is outstanding. Particular care should be taken during closure of this atrial incision, because bleeding from this incision can be somewhat difficult to repair after weaning from cardiopulmonary bypass, because the incision is obscured by the fully distended aorta and superior vena cava. In most of the aforementioned approaches to the mitral valve, a left atrial vent placed via the right superior pulmonary vein can be positioned with the tip in the left inferior pulmonary vein. An additional suction catheter can be placed from the pericardium into the right inferior pulmonary vein. Typically, one or both of these suction catheters will maintain a completely bloodless operative field and allow perfect visualization of the mitral valve. Two extremely rare and unusual approaches to the mitral valve include a transventricular approach performed in the setting of a left ventricular aneurysm repair[74] and a transaortic approach performed in the setting of aorto-mitral endocarditis.[75]

Open Commissurotomy

Mitral commissurotomy is indicated in patients with pure mitral stenosis with commissural fusion and preserved leaflet mobility (Fig. 80-19). After left atriotomy, the mitral valve is examined to determine suitability for commissurotomy, and a decision must be made regarding whether the leaflets will be sufficiently pliable after commissurotomy to open adequately at a low left atrial pressure. Ideal valves lack chordal fusion and are not calcified; however, mitral commissurotomy can be performed with acceptable results in less than ideally suited valves.[76] Yet, advanced commissural calcification, subvalvular fusion, and leaflet retraction may be better treated with valve replacement.

Advanced rheumatic changes can complicate identification of the true commissure locations. Retraction of a stay suture placed in the midportion of the anterior leaflet free edge and another placed similarly in the posterior leaflet helps to identify the commissural groove. Commissurotomy is initiated with sharp dissection along this groove toward the annulus and then toward the center of the valve orifice. It is important to leave a 3-mm ridge of tissue at the commissure to prevent iatrogenic mitral regurgitation. In general, chordae are often more fused beneath the posteromedial commissure. When fused chordae are encountered, they should be fenestrated by removing a triangular wedge of tissue. The incision can be extended to divide the papillary muscle longitudinally

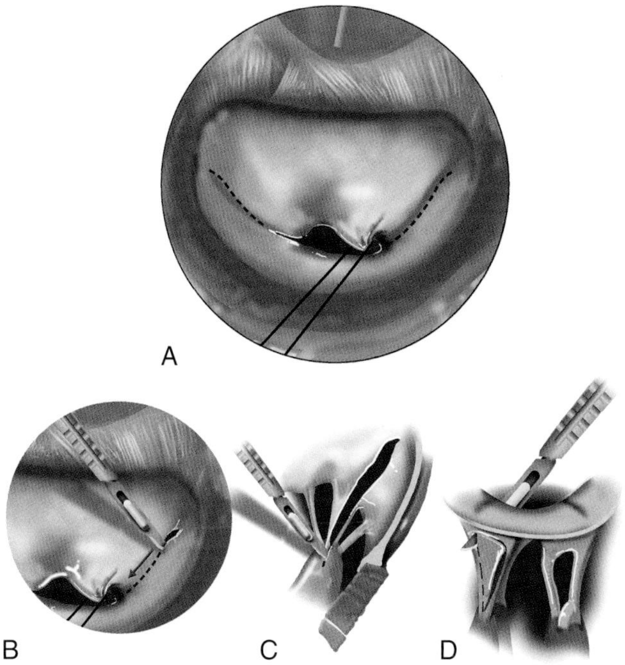

FIGURE 80-19 ■ Open mitral commissurotomy. **A,** Traction on the anterior leaflet delineates the true commissure between the anterior and posterior leaflet. **B,** The fused commissure is incised sharply and extended toward the valve orifice. **C,** The papillary muscle may be split to improve leaflet mobility. **D,** A triangular wedge is removed to fenestrate fused chordae.

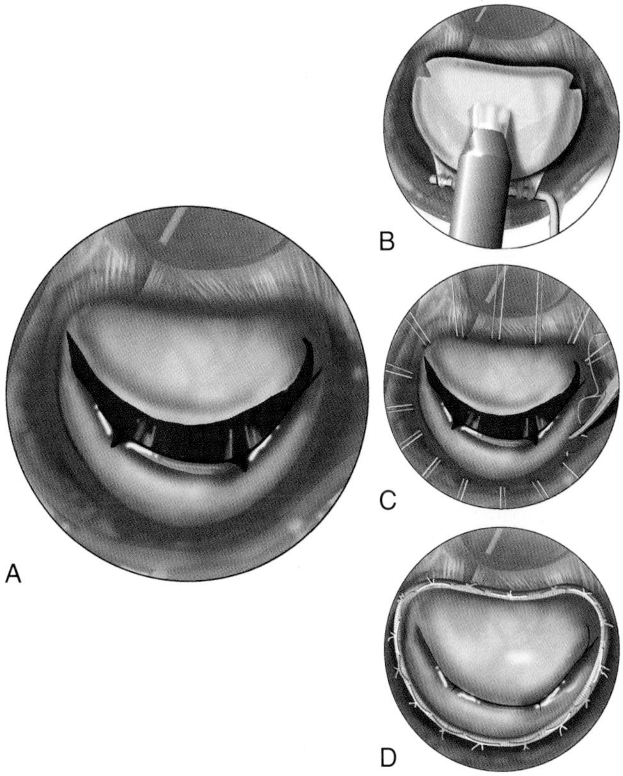

FIGURE 80-20 ■ Remodeling annuloplasty ring implantation. **A,** Dilated annulus with leaflet malcoaptation. **B,** Ring selection is based on measurements of the intercommissural distance and the height of the anterior leaflet. **C,** Sutures are placed circumferentially around the annulus and through the ring. **D,** The annuloplasty ring restores the normal physiologic size ratio and shape of the annulus.

to improve mobility. Finally, localized calcium deposits can be removed from the leaflets with a rongeur forceps.

Mitral Valve Repair

Mitral valve repair is the procedure of choice for correcting severe mitral regurgitation.[3] Although techniques for repair are numerous, all valve repairs should aim to restore a large surface of leaflet coaptation, preserve leaflet mobility, and restore physiologic annular geometry with a remodeling annuloplasty.[17] Regardless of the techniques being used, a systematic approach to reconstructive surgery should be used that includes a determination of the mechanism of mitral regurgitation via imaging and valve analysis, application of appropriate repair techniques depending on the culprit lesions, and assessment of the repair quality by pressurized saline testing and echocardiography.

Fundamentals of Reconstructive Surgery

Valve Analysis. The mitral valve apparatus should first be carefully examined to confirm the mechanism of regurgitation, evaluate the feasibility of repair, and plan the technical operation. The mitral annulus is inspected to determine the extent of dilation. Segmental valve analysis with a nerve hook can identify areas of leaflet prolapse or restriction.[77] It should be noted that prolapse of P1 is less common, and the free margin of other valve segments can be compared with P1 to determine severity of prolapse.

Remodeling Ring Annuloplasty. Regardless of the etiology of valve disease, all patients with chronic mitral regurgitation demonstrate some degree of annular dilation and benefit from a remodeling annuloplasty. As discussed previously, the annulus is weakest along the mural segments and thus typically dilates in the anteroposterior dimension. A remodeling ring annuloplasty restores the normal physiologic size ratio and shape of the annulus, and it improves the surface area of leaflet coaptation. In addition, it improves the longevity of the repair by preventing late annular dilation. Although annular support can be achieved with a posterior band or incomplete ring, the ends of this band must be properly secured in the medial and lateral fibrous trigones to prevent late posteriorly directed annular migration and recurrent mitral regurgitation. Thus, a complete ring with full anterior anchoring typically will more assuredly produce annular remodeling. In most scenarios, annuloplasty sutures are placed first and retracted under tension to improve exposure of the mitral leaflets. Leaflet repair is then conducted (specific techniques to follow; categorized by leaflet pathology), and ring sizing and implantation are performed.

Appropriate ring sizing is based on the intercommissural distance and the surface area of the anterior leaflet (Fig. 80-20). There is usually a strong correlation between the intercommissural distance and the height of the anterior leaflet. However, if the free edge of the anterior leaflet extends 2 to 4 mm beyond the inferior edge of the selected sizer, a ring that is one size larger should be selected to prevent the risk of systolic anterior motion of the anterior mitral valve leaflet.[78] Ring sizing also depends on the leaflet repair technique and the amount of functional posterior leaflet tissue that remains. For example, the ring may need to be sized to the mitral orifice area when repairs with artificial neochordae are used.

Simple sutures should be placed circumferentially around the mitral valve and into the mitral annulus (see Fig. 80-20). When placing sutures within the anterior annulus, care should be taken to avoid inadvertent injury to the aortic valve leaflets by taking shallower bites. Similar care should be taken when placing sutures in the area of the anterolateral commissure to avoid iatrogenic injury to the circumflex coronary artery and aortic leaflets. Exposure of the anterolateral trigone region can be improved by exerting traction on the adjacent suture in the posterior annulus. Stretching the commissure in this fashion facilitates proper suture placement. Sutures are then passed through the selected annuloplasty ring. Since the intercommissural distance is equivalent on the anterior annulus and the ring, sutures should be placed evenly through their corresponding places on the ring. However, as the posterior annulus is usually dilated, the spaces of the sutures within the annulus should be greater than their respective spacing on the ring. The ring is then seated to conform the annulus to the shape and size of the prosthetic ring.

Assessment of Repair. The quality of the repair should be evaluated with a saline test after completion of the leaflet repair and again after ring implantation, but before tying the annuloplasty ring sutures so that the surgeon is still free to make additional changes at each stage if corrections are necessary. While the aortic root is vented, saline is injected into the ventricular cavity to prevent air embolism into the coronary arteries. Once air is removed, the aortic root vent is clamped and saline is injected again into the ventricle at a higher pressure. A symmetrical line of coaptation, parallel to the posterior part of the remodeling ring and at a reasonable distance from the left ventricular outflow tract, indicates a successful repair. Asymmetric coaptation lines reveal residual leaflet prolapse or restriction that requires correction prior to separation from cardiopulmonary bypass. A supplemental "ink test" can be performed to further assess the quality of the repair. The valve closure line is traced with a marking pen after pressurizing the ventricle with saline. Saline is aspirated and the leaflet margins are surveyed. Ideal coaptation depth ranges from 4 to 10 mm. A depth less than 4 mm should be corrected by resection of restrictive secondary chordae, cleft closure, or downsizing the annuloplasty ring because shorter coaptation depths suggest limited repair durability. In contrast, depths greater than 10 mm are worrisome for resultant systolic anterior motion, which may warrant further reduction of the height of the posterior leaflet. All valve repairs should be interrogated thoroughly with transesophageal echocardiography after separation from cardiopulmonary bypass.

Valve Repair in Type I Dysfunction

Mitral regurgitation due to type I dysfunction may be due to two aforementioned lesions. Annular dilation is the most common cause, which should be corrected with a complete rigid or semirigid remodeling annuloplasty (see Fig. 80-19).[79] Type I valve regurgitation may also be secondary to leaflet perforation, commonly seen in infective endocarditis. The management of patching such a lesion is described in further detail later (see Considerations in Endocarditis).

Valve Repair in Type II Dysfunction

Posterior Leaflet Prolapse. Resection of the prolapsed area or segment has been the conventional technique for repair of posterior leaflet prolapse. However, various nonresecting leaflet repair techniques aimed at preservation of leaflet tissue are well described and increasingly are being adopted.

Quadrangular Resection with or without Sliding Plasty and Triangular Resection. Regardless of the technique chosen, initial placement of annuloplasty sutures helps lift and expose the valve to facilitate repair. When performing the conventional quadrangular resection (Fig. 80-21), stay sutures are placed around normal chordae to delineate the prolapsed area. The prolapsed segment is excised with perpendicular incisions from the leaflet margin toward the annulus to remove a quadrangular section of leaflet tissue. Plication sutures are placed along the posterior annulus in the area of resection. The free edges of the resection gap are then reapproximated with interrupted polypropylene suture to restore leaflet continuity. When the area of prolapse is less extensive, the prolapsing area can be excised with a triangular resection (Fig. 80-22). The free edges of the resection are then reapproximated with polypropylene suture.

In the setting of excessive posterior leaflet tissue, such as in Barlow's disease, it is critical to reduce the height of the posterior leaflet to avoid systolic anterior motion.[80] Thus, a sliding leaflet plasty technique is performed after initial quadrangular resection (Fig. 80-23). The P1 and P3 segments are detached from the annulus and the gap between the two scallops is then closed with interrupted sutures, taking narrower bites near the free margin and wider bites closer to the annulus. A sliding plasty may also be necessary when a large portion of the posterior leaflet is removed. Interrupted annular plication sutures also facilitate leaflet reapproximation after sliding plasty. However, note that plication of a large segment of the posterior annulus must be avoided because the circumflex artery may kink.

Posterior Ventricular Anchoring Neochordal Remodeling Repair. Minor drawbacks continue to accompany resectional approaches to mitral repair, including irreversibility of leaflet resection, time-consuming leaflet reapproximation with sliding annuloplasty, monoleaflet function, risk for postrepair systolic anterior motion, and potential for dynamic mitral stenosis. Such disadvantages have led to nonresectional paradigms of valve repair, the majority of which are centered on artificial chordal replacement (see Artificial Neochordae Section). After

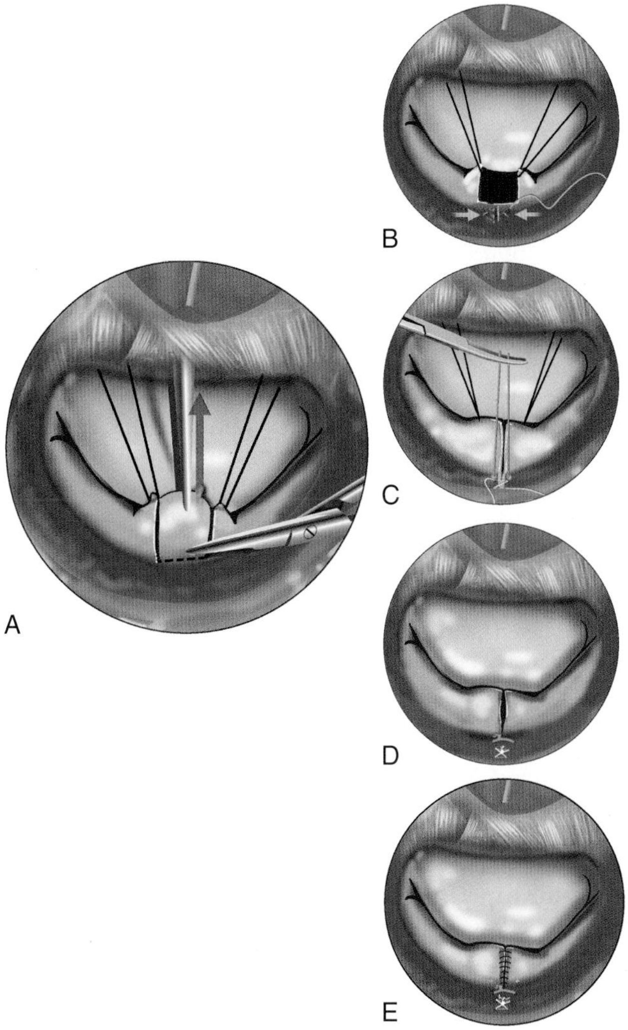

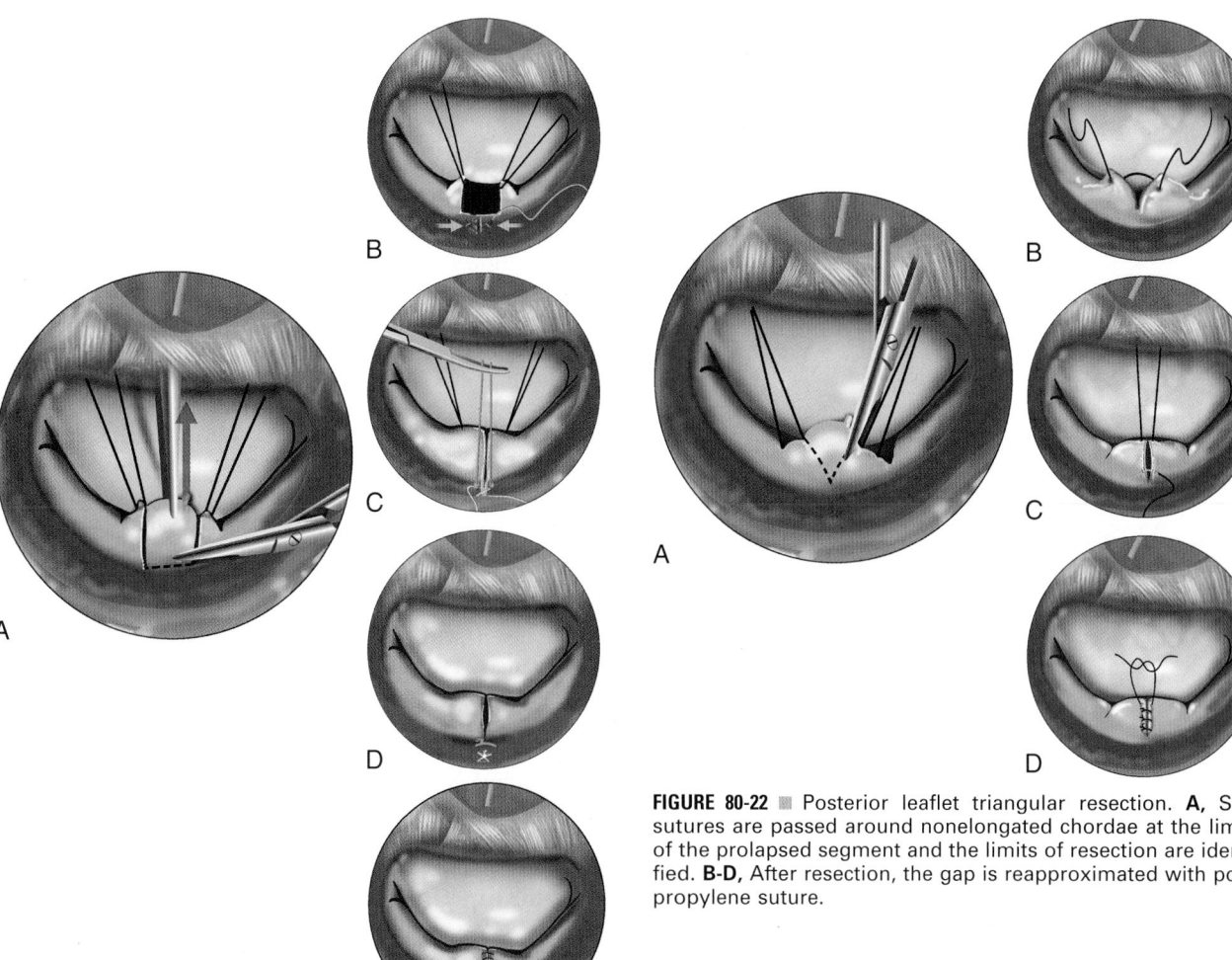

FIGURE 80-21 ■ Posterior leaflet quadrangular resection with annular plication. **A,** The limits of the resection are identified and a quadrangular segment of leaflet tissue is removed. **B-D,** Interrupted annular plication sutures are placed to facilitate gap closure. **E,** The residual defect between P1 and P3 is closed.

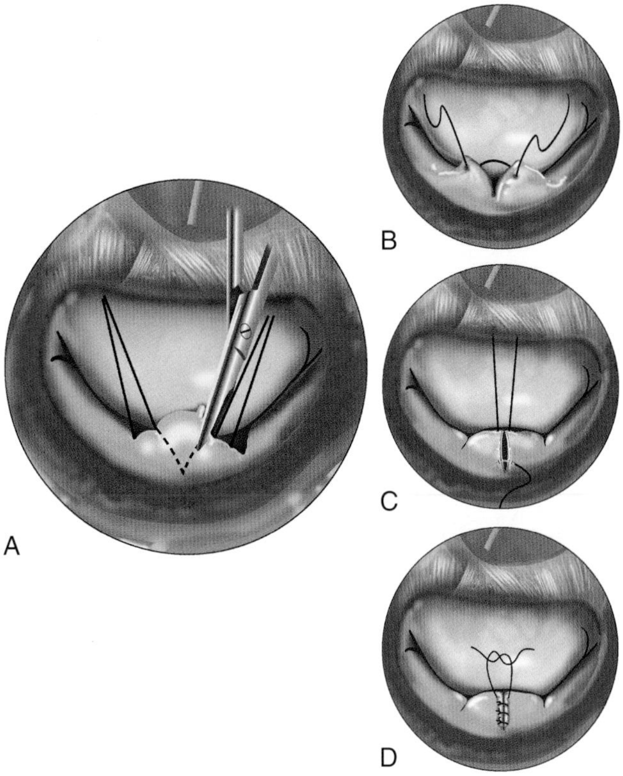

FIGURE 80-22 ■ Posterior leaflet triangular resection. **A,** Stay sutures are passed around nonelongated chordae at the limits of the prolapsed segment and the limits of resection are identified. **B-D,** After resection, the gap is reapproximated with polypropylene suture.

less successful attempts with different tissue, Frater and colleagues[81] described the utility of polytetrafluoroethylene (PTFE) for chordal replacement in the setting of diseased or ruptured chordae. Numerous modifications to artificial chordal replacement are well described, including the loop,[82] loop-in-loop,[83] haircut,[84] and butterfly techniques.[85] Although neochordal construction circumvents many of the drawbacks of leaflet resection, precise sizing is challenging and maintenance of excess leaflet tissue may risk systolic anterior motion of the mitral valve.

In an effort to develop a mitral valve repair technique that avoids the potential disadvantages of leaflet resection and artificial chordal replacement, while simultaneously facilitating port access approaches by reducing leaflet manipulation and simplifying suture management, we implemented a strategy based on a modified leaflet plication repair.[86] Single suture imbrication of excess prolapsing leaflet tissue onto the noncoaptation ventricular side of the leaflet effectively creates a smooth coaptation surface without residual prolapse. This technique, however, carries a theoretical risk of basing the repair on potentially diseased native chordae and the potential for the mobile posterior leaflet to advance anteriorly, risking systolic anterior motion. Therefore, we addressed these concerns by further modifying our technique such that a single PTFE suture is used to anchor, support, and remodel the posterior leaflet posteriorly (Fig. 80-24).[72]

The prolapsed segment is grasped and retracted into the atrium to expose the left ventricular endomyocardium directly below the leaflet. A CV5 PTFE suture is passed into the myocardium approximately 3 to 4 mm deep and loosely tied. The needles are then passed through the margin of the diseased segment at a width of approximately half of the size of the prolapsed region. An inversion plasty is then performed by grasping the leading edge of the diseased segment and inverting it into the left ventricle. The near-apposing leaflet folds are then approximated in a double running fashion with the same PTFE suture that was used to anchor the prolapsed segment. If necessary, additional tissue can be imbricated into the left ventricle using the second half of the PTFE suture.

Posterior ventricular anchoring is not necessary for repair of all cases of posterior leaflet prolapse. If the burden of excess leaflet tissue is not alarming for systolic anterior motion and the subvalvular apparatus does not appear severely diseased, then an isolated inversion plasty may be successfully performed. However, in the setting

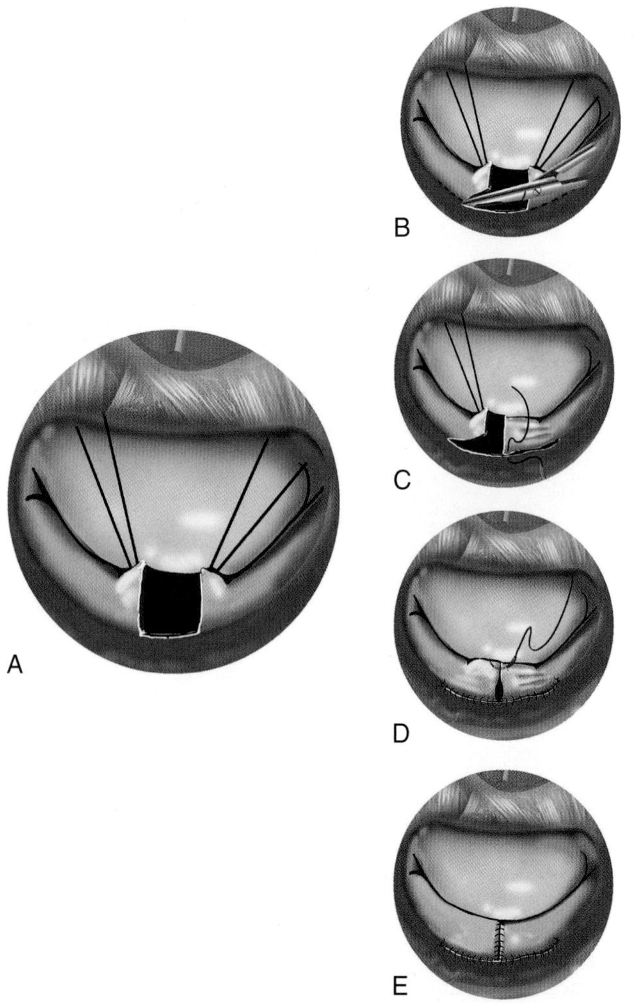

FIGURE 80-23 ■ Posterior leaflet sliding plasty. **A,** After quadrangular resection, the gap between the leaflets is too large to permit direct reapproximation. **B,** P1 and P3 are partially detached from the annulus to permit translocation medially. **C,** P1 and P3 are then reapproximated to the annulus, with greater travel along the annulus than along the leaflet to permit medial translocation. **D** and **E,** The now apposed leaflet remnants are reapproximated with polypropylene suture.

of billowing excess leaflet tissue, multiple torn chordae, or severely elongated chordae, it is prudent to perform a posterior ventricular anchoring repair. This repair minimizes risk for systolic anterior motion and helps to buttress a repair that otherwise would be based on diseased native chordae.

It should be noted that several of the following techniques described for repair of anterior leaflet prolapse can be used on the posterior leaflet, particularly in valves with insufficient leaflet tissue.

Anterior Leaflet Prolapse. Several techniques have been described to correct anterior leaflet prolapse. It is our preference to use chordal techniques instead of resection or papillary muscle techniques. However, these additional repair techniques can maximize the probability of repair.

Triangular Resection. Limited prolapse of the anterior leaflet with excess tissue can be treated with a narrow triangular resection of the prolapsed area. The free edges are then reapproximated with polypropylene suture.[88] Of note, large resections of the anterior leaflet greatly reduce coaptation area and increase risk for failure. As such, resections of the anterior leaflet should be small (no greater than 10% of the leaflet surface area).

Chordal Transposition. In the absence of normal secondary anterior leaflet chordae, a posterior leaflet chordal transposition may be performed (Fig. 80-25). This procedure is predicated on the presence of normal marginal posterior leaflet chordae opposite the segment of anterior leaflet prolapse. The segment of the posterior leaflet facing the area of anterior leaflet prolapse is identified. A 3-mm-wide strip of posterior leaflet tissue along the leaflet margin is mobilized with supporting chordae. The width of the strip should approximate the width of the prolapsing area. The papillary muscle to which the chordae are attached is mobilized toward the area of anterior leaflet prolapse by splitting. The posterior leaflet strip is then attached to the free edge of the prolapsing segment. The defect at the posterior leaflet donor site is then closed with interrupted polypropylene sutures.[78] The primary advantage of this technique is that the difficulty surrounding artificial chordoplasty relating to papillary muscle fixation, neochordal length measurement, and tying is eliminated.

Artificial Neochordae. Artificial chordoplasty is particularly useful when the number of normal chordae is inadequate. The primary difficulty surrounding artificial chordoplasty is adjusting the distance between the tip of the papillary muscle and the prolapsing leaflet edge to the precise length needed. Furthermore, fixing the PTFE suture at the correct length is challenging because the slippery nature of PTFE suture causes knots to slide significantly. Lastly, with suboptimal exposure, visualization of and chordal implantation into the papillary muscles can be challenging. In fact, a multitude of techniques has been proposed to tackle these obstacles.[78,82,89,90]

In the majority of patients, an adjacent normal, nonprolapsing segment of either the anterior or posterior leaflet provides a reference point for the correct plane of leaflet apposition. The appropriate distance is measured between the correct plane of apposition of a nonprolapsing segment and its corresponding papillary muscle with a measuring device or echocardiography. In the "loop" technique (Fig. 80-26),[82] using a caliper or measuring device as a template, a PTFE neochord loop is fashioned to this premeasured length by tying a knot over a pledget at the required distance. Each end of the suture is passed again through the pledget twice to stabilize the knot position. The needles are then passed anterior to posterior on the respective papillary muscle and tied over a second pledget. A correct, premeasured PTFE loop is thus secured to the papillary muscle. An additional PTFE suture is then used to fix the premeasured PTFE loop to the prolapsing segment of the mitral leaflet, preferably with the knot facing the ventricular surface. Similar to chordal transfer, multiple artificial neochordae may be required for larger areas of leaflet prolapse, and it is essential that no portion of the leaflet margin greater than 4 mm be left unsupported.[78]

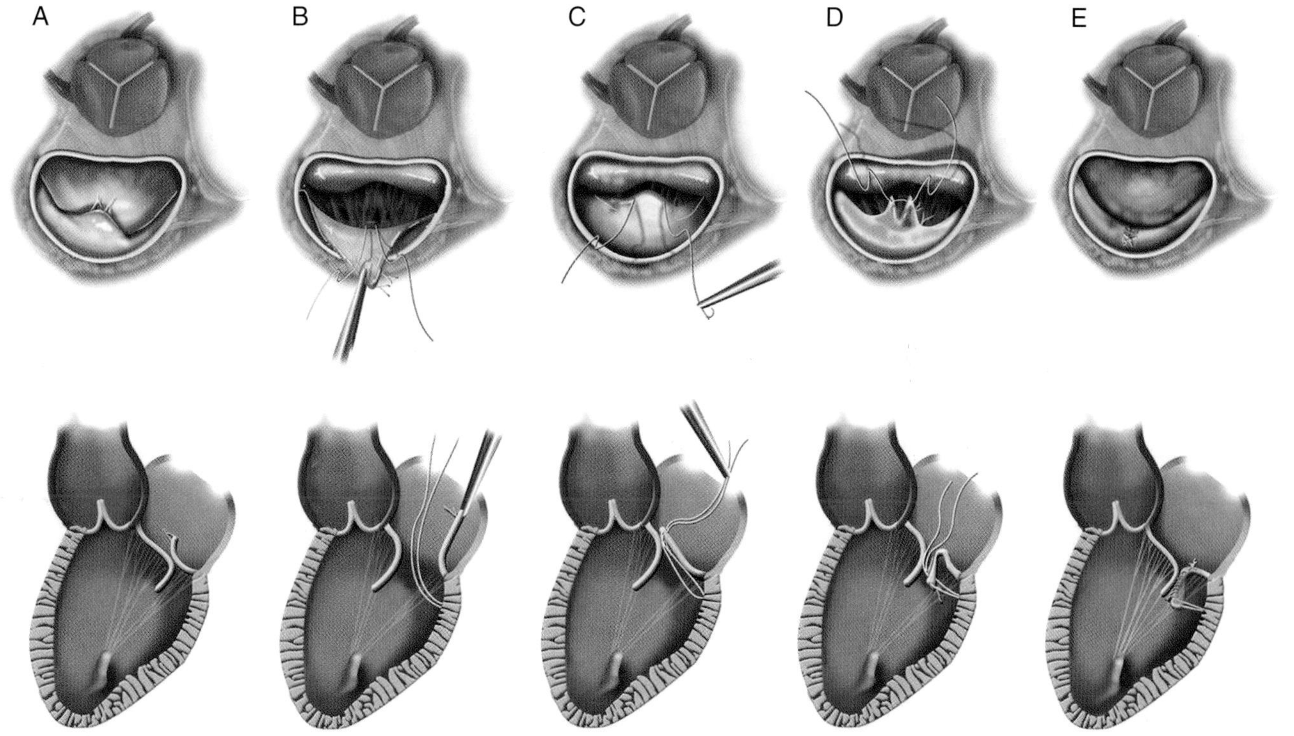

FIGURE 80-24 ■ Posterior ventricular anchoring neochordal repair. **A,** Short- and long-axis drawings depicting degenerative mitral valve disease with posterior leaflet prolapse/flail due to ruptured chordae. **B,** The prolapsed segment is retracted into the left atrium to expose the posterior ventricular wall just beneath the leaflet, and an anchoring CV5 PTFE suture is placed. **C,** The suture is loosely tied and the ends brought through the leading edge of the prolapsed segment. **D,** The margin of the prolapsed segment is inverted into the left ventricle, generating two near-apposing radial folds that are then sutured together. **E,** This eliminates prolapse, yielding a smooth broad coaptation surface. (From Woo YJ, MacArthur JW: Posterior ventricular anchoring neochordal repair of degenerative mitral regurgitation efficiently remodels and repositions posterior leaflet prolapse. *Eur J Cardiothorac Surg* 44:487, 2013.)

Alternatively, a PTFE suture can be passed through the papillary muscle and then through the free margin of the prolapsing segment. Following implantation of the annuloplasty ring, the PTFE suture is tied in the setting of a pressurized ventricle. The knot can then be secured at the appropriate level, where coaptation is restored and the visualized regurgitant flow is eliminated. This freehand technique is more versatile and less complex, but it requires a degree of judgment and skill for determining the proper chord length and for tying without slipping the knot, thereby overly shortening the neochord.

Double Orifice Edge-to-Edge Repair. Alfieri's edge-to-edge technique effectively creates a double orifice mitral valve and may be used to correct posterior, anterior, or bileaflet prolapse (Fig. 80-27).[91] The prolapsing portion of a leaflet is first identified and then resuspended to the corresponding margin of the opposing leaflet with a figure-of-eight polypropylene suture. The depth of each bite from the leaflet free edge depends on the extent of the leaflet redundancy. For example, in Barlow's disease the desired depth is at least 1 cm, which simultaneously decreases the leaflet height to prevent systolic anterior motion of the mitral valve. When leaflet tissue is thin, additional mattress sutures reinforced with pericardial pledgets can be used to support the suture line. If the prolapsing or flail segment does not involve A2 or P2, the valve will be rendered asymmetric with this repair and the size of the two orifices will differ. The overall mitral valve area is assessed by direct inspection; however, when in doubt, Hegar dilators can be inserted into each orifice. A total valve area greater than 2.5 cm^2 is acceptable for average-size patients.[92]

Commissural Prolapse. Commissural prolapse is effectively treated with resection of the prolapsed area and sliding plasty of the adjacent paracommissural segments (e.g., A1 and P1 sliding plasty for anterolateral commissural prolapse). Additional inverting sutures should be placed in the neocommissure to prevent residual regurgitation. Oftentimes, however, less extensive commissural prolapse can be corrected with a simple inverting suture between the lateral most paracommissural segments. Infrequently, a patient will have commissural prolapse secondary to rupture of a two-headed papillary muscle. In this situation, the prolapse can be corrected with reattachment to the remaining papillary muscle. Furthermore, papillary muscle sliding plasty and shortening are useful options for the correction of extensive commissural and paracommissural prolapse.

Valve Repair in Type IIIa Dysfunction

Repair of type IIIa dysfunction must address leaflet immobility and restriction. Leaflet immobility is primarily related to commissural and chordal fusion. These lesions should be addressed with commissurotomy and chordal fenestration as described previously (see Fig. 80-19).

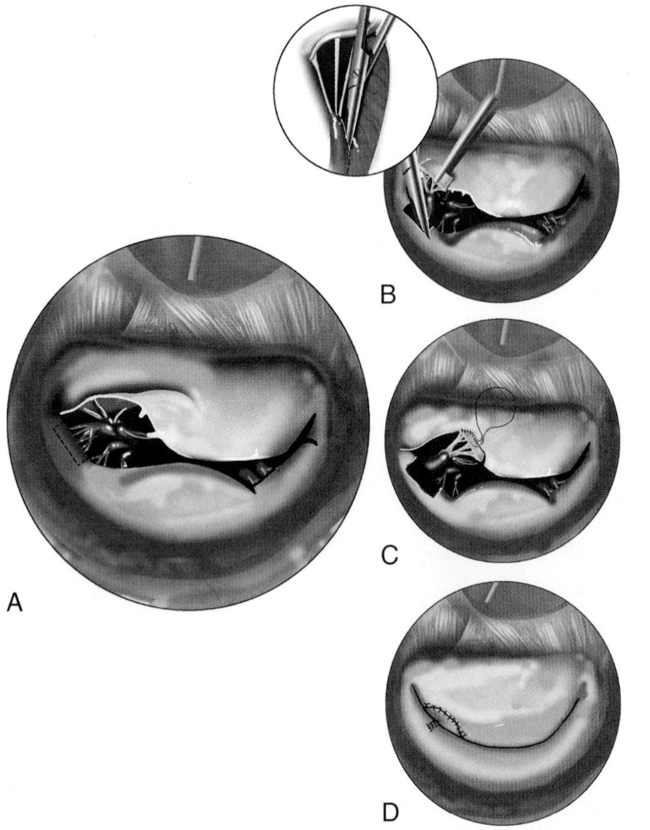

FIGURE 80-25 ■ Chordal transposition. **A,** The segment of the posterior leaflet facing the area of anterior leaflet prolapse is identified. **B,** A strip of posterior leaflet margin tissue is mobilized with its supporting chordae. The corresponding papillary muscle may be split to facilitate transposition. **C,** The posterior leaflet strip is attached to the margin of the prolapsed area on the anterior leaflet. **D,** The residual defect in the posterior leaflet is closed.

The diastolic restriction of leaflet motion characteristic of type IIIa dysfunction can be corrected with leaflet augmentation (Fig. 80-28). For posterior leaflet augmentation, a transverse incision is made 5 mm from the posterior annulus. This incision facilitates excision of fibrotic secondary chordae, but care should be taken to preserve marginal chordae. Autologous or glutaraldehyde-fixed bovine pericardium is then constructed into an elliptical patch. The patch should be sized to increase the height of the posterior leaflet to 15 to 20 mm, leaving a 2-mm margin on the patch for the suture line. The patch is sewn posteriorly from the midline to the annulus and then anteriorly to the leaflet tissue. To account for the new posterior leaflet size, an annuloplasty ring should be chosen that is one size larger than that recommended by standard sizing techniques. The anterior leaflet can also be augmented in a similar fashion; however, a vertical leaflet incision is commonly used.[78] The patch is sized to the natural gap created by the leaflet incision. Because the anterior leaflet is augmented, an annuloplasty ring should be chosen that is the true size of the new anterior leaflet.

Valve Repair in Type IIIb Dysfunction

Remodeling annuloplasty with an undersized ring is the standard technique to repair type IIIb dysfunction (see Fig. 80-20).[79] However, the insertion of an undersized prosthetic ring in a severely dilated annulus can cause excessive tension on the sutures, thereby predisposing to ring dehiscence. One can safeguard against this complication by placing multiple sutures around the annulus that overlap. In ischemic mitral regurgitation, this overlapping is particularly important in the area of the posteromedial commissure and P3 segment. In select

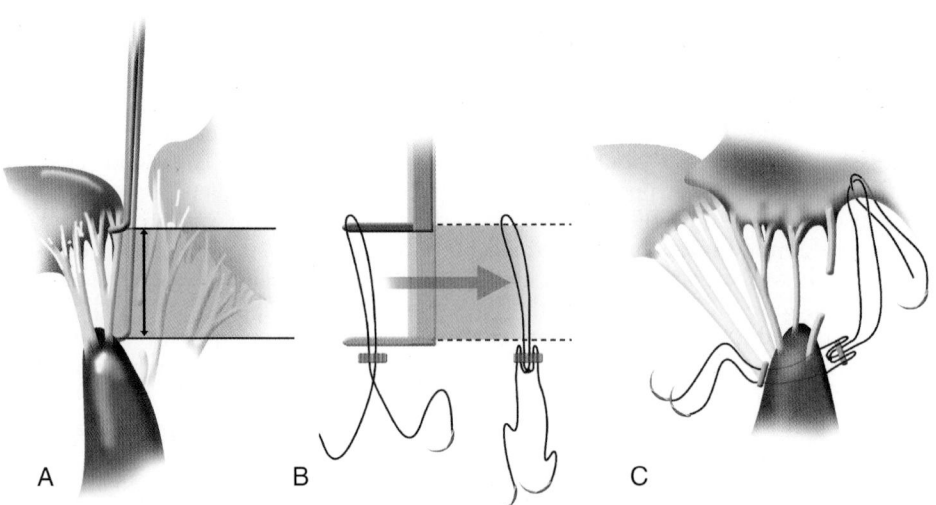

FIGURE 80-26 ■ Artificial chordoplasty using the "loop" technique. **A,** The correct plane of apposition of a nonprolapsing segment and its corresponding papillary muscle with a measuring device. **B,** A polytetrafluoroethylene (PTFE) loop is fashioned to this premeasured length by tying a knot over a pledget at the required distance. **C,** The needles are then passed anterior to posterior on the respective papillary muscle and tied over a second pledget. An additional PTFE suture is then used to fix the premeasured PTFE loop to the prolapsing segment of the mitral leaflet.

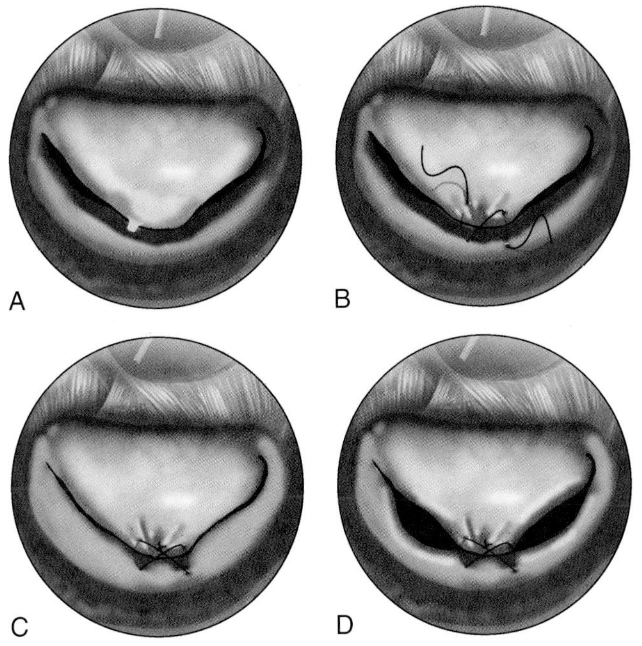

FIGURE 80-27 ■ Double orifice edge-to-edge repair. **A** and **B,** A polypropylene stitch is passed in a figure-of-eight fashion through the midportion of the prolapsing segment (in this case A2) and its opposing nonprolapsing segment (in this case P2) to create a double orifice. **C,** During systole, the valve is no longer regurgitant. **D,** During diastole, the double orifice permits ventricular filling.

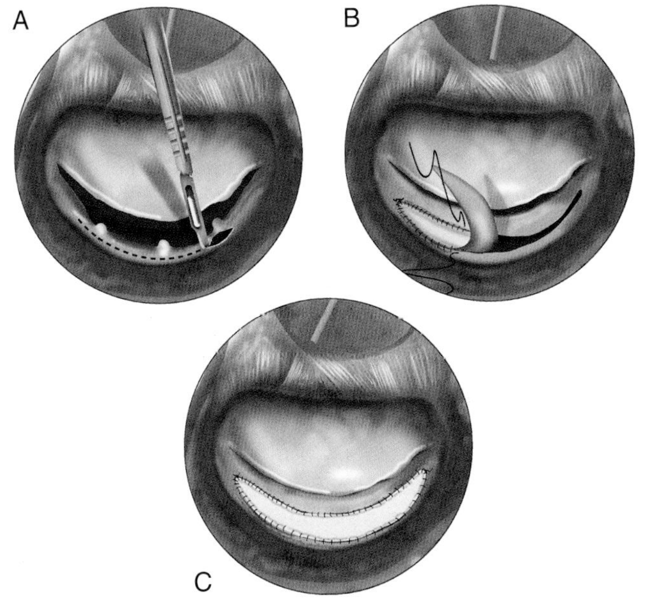

FIGURE 80-28 ■ Pericardial patch leaflet augmentation. **A,** A transverse incision is made in the posterior leaflet 5 mm from the annulus. Fibrotic secondary chordae can be excised through the leaflet incision. **B** and **C,** Pericardium is fashioned into an elliptical patch to increase the posterior leaflet height to 15 to 20 mm. The patch is sewn posteriorly to the annulus and then anteriorly to the leaflet tissue.

patients, posterior leaflet patch augmentation and resection of secondary chordae may be necessary to ensure a more durable repair.

Annular Decalcification and Annular Reconstruction

Annular calcification complicates mitral valve surgery. The risks of atrioventricular disruption, paravalvular leak, and valve dehiscence are all increased in this setting. In general, débridement of calcific foci is obligatory before valve repair or replacement. Annular decalcification is executed by separation of the leaflet from the annulus and en bloc removal of calcium deposits.[25,93,94] Often, annular reconstruction is required to repair localized atrioventricular disruption following calcium excision. Similarly, débridement of annular abscesses in the treatment of infective endocarditis may necessitate annular reconstruction.

David and colleagues[95-97] and Carpentier and colleagues[25] have described different techniques for mitral annular reconstruction. In David's technique, mitral annular reconstruction is conducted using autologous or glutaraldehyde-fixed bovine pericardium. The posterior annulus is reconstructed with a semicircular pericardial patch. The patch is usually 2 cm wide but must be wide enough to cover the defect. One of the margins of this strip is sutured to the smooth endocardium of the inflow of the left ventricle, and the other margin is sutured to the posterior left atrial wall with a continuous 3-0 polypropylene suture. The detached posterior leaflet is then reattached to the pericardial patch at the level of the original annulus. In patients with complete destruction of the annulus, a circumferential patch is tailored for annular reconstruction. An annuloplasty ring is then secured to the pericardial patch. Similar techniques use felt.[94]

In Carpentier's technique (Fig. 80-29), the mitral annulus is reconstructed with figure-of-eight atrioventricular mattress sutures to minimize use of foreign material. Braided 2-0 suture is first passed through the atrial edge and then through the ventricular edge, avoiding injury to the circumflex vessels. The suture is passed again in the same fashion and then upward through the atrial tissue to maintain all suture on the atrial side. Ventricular passes should be at least 1 cm wide and involve one third of the thickness of the ventricle to incorporate any fibrous tissue possible. Closure of the atrioventricular junction is facilitated by downward displacement of the atrial edge with forceps. Not only do the figure-of-eight sutures reduce the size of the annulus, but they also displace the surrounding fat and circumflex vessels away from the reconstructed annulus. The free ends of the figure-of-eight mattress sutures are maintained for later insertion of a remodeling annuloplasty ring. The neoatrioventricular junction is further buttressed with a running polyester suture along the line of closure.

Considerations in Endocarditis

The primary goal of any surgery for endocarditis is complete débridement of all infected and necrotic tissue. The

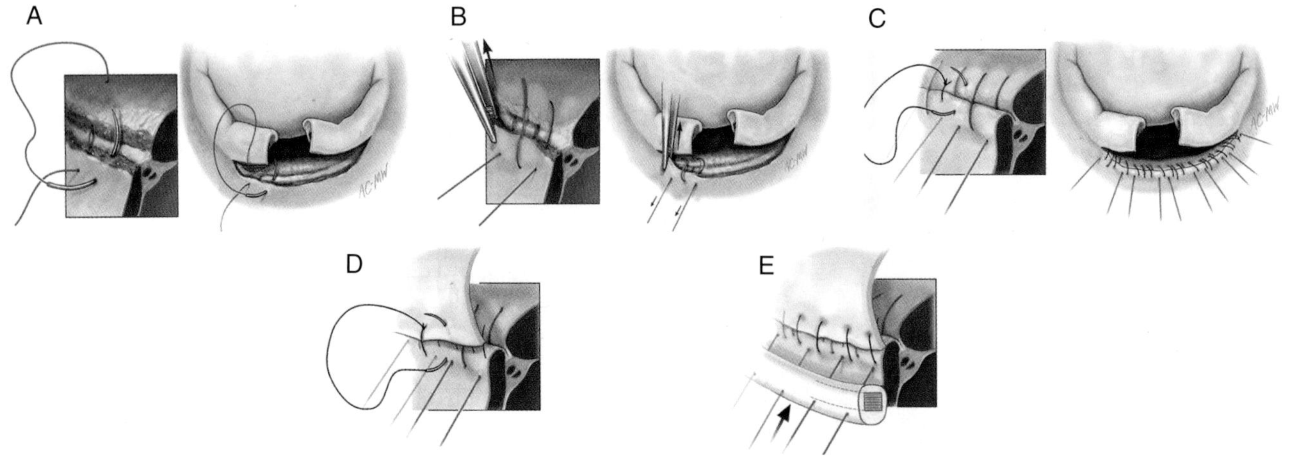

FIGURE 80-29 ■ Annular reconstruction using Carpentier's technique. **A,** Annular débridement results in a defect necessitating reconstruction. A braided 2-0 suture is first passed through the atrial edge and then through the ventricular edge of the defect. **B,** The suture is passed again in the same fashion and then upward through the atrial tissue. Closure of the atrioventricular junction is facilitated by downward displacement of the atrial edge with forceps. **C,** A running suture line further strengthens the neoatrioventricular junction. **D,** The posterior leaflet is reattached to the reconstructed annulus with a running suture. **E,** The free ends of the figure-of-eight mattress sutures are used for annuloplasty ring insertion. (From Carpentier A, Adams DH, Filsoufi F: *Carpentier's reconstructive valve surgery,* St. Louis, 2010, Elsevier.)

feasibility of mitral valve repair depends on the extent of normal tissue remaining after débridement. Extensive leaflet involvement or subvalvular destruction precludes valve repair. However, valve repair is achievable in a majority of cases provided sufficient tissue remains for reconstruction.[98-101] Mitral regurgitation resulting from localized leaflet perforation (typically the anterior leaflet) is amenable to patch repair with autologous pericardium. To address more extensive valve destruction, surgical reconstruction should integrate the many aforementioned techniques in a lesion-specific approach. Although the implantation of a prosthetic ring remains controversial, in the setting of a dilated annulus, a remodeling annuloplasty ring should be implanted routinely.

Systolic Anterior Motion of the Anterior Leaflet

Systolic anterior motion of the mitral valve is a complication after valve repair that results from a discrepancy between the amount of leaflet tissue and the mitral valve orifice area (Fig. 80-30).[102] Effectively, the plane of coaptation is displaced too anteriorly. It is most frequently observed after valve reconstruction when there is excess posterior leaflet tissue and/or an inappropriately undersized annuloplasty ring. It can also result when there is excess anterior mobility of the posterior leaflet, which can occur when artificial chordae are too long. Consequently, the anterior leaflet is displaced toward the left ventricular outflow tract causing both obstruction and late systolic mitral regurgitation. In most instances, systolic anterior motion of the anterior leaflet may be treated nonoperatively. Ventricular underfilling is corrected by increasing preload with volume, raising afterload with pure alpha agonists, and slowing the heart rate to increase diastolic duration. Ventricular hypercontractility is addressed by suspending administration of inotropes. In addition, in the setting of asynchrony, ventricular filling is augmented by atrioventricular pacing. With these maneuvers, most postrepair systolic anterior motion will resolve, and moderate residual ventriculoaortic gradients (<30 mm Hg) usually normalize in weeks to months from left ventricular outflow tract remodeling.[103]

When systolic anterior motion is irreversible, the repair must be re-addressed, and various measures are enacted depending on the causative factor. Chordal length is corrected if believed to be too long. If the posterior leaflet is too tall, excess posterior leaflet tissue is removed with an ovoid leaflet resection at the base of the posterior leaflet. Thus, the height of the posterior leaflet is reduced and the coaptation zone is moved posteriorly. A posterior anchoring neochord can also be inserted. If systolic anterior motion is due to an undersized annuloplasty ring, the ring should be replaced with a larger ring that is appropriately sized to the anterior leaflet.[104]

Mitral Valve Replacement

Mitral valve replacement should be performed in patients in whom mitral valve repair is not suitable (e.g., extensive valve destruction from endocarditis, severe leaflet calcification and fibrosis from rheumatic heart disease, or select patients with ischemic cardiomyopathy).[79] When possible, chordal-sparing mitral valve replacement is the preferred technique because left ventricular function is better preserved (Fig. 80-31).[105,106]

Typically, the posterior leaflet is left intact and the tissue is used to better support valve replacement sutures. In addition, this strategy automatically preserves the posterior subvalvular apparatus. In contrast, the anterior leaflet must be transferred if it is to be retained. Otherwise, it will be displaced into the left ventricular outflow tract by the valve prosthesis and obstruct outflow. In certain settings (e.g., highly fibrotic, stenotic valve) the anterior leaflet may need to be completely resected. However, whenever possible, the anterior leaflet and its

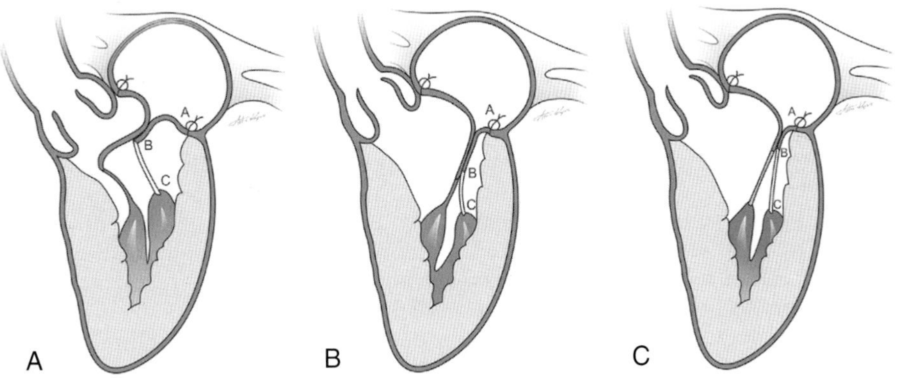

FIGURE 80-30 ■ Systolic anterior motion of the mitral valve and the issue of excess tissue. **A,** Dynamic left ventricular outflow tract obstruction from anterior displacement of the zone of coaptation. **B,** Correction by bringing the coaptation zone posteriorly using shorter artificial chordae. **C,** Correction by moving the coaptation zone posteriorly with a sliding plasty to lower the height of the posterior leaflet. *AB,* Height of the posterior leaflet; *B,* free margin of the posterior leaflet; *BC,* length of the chordae. (From Perier P, Hohenberger W, Lakew F, et al: Toward a new paradigm for the reconstruction of posterior leaflet prolapse: midterm results of the "respect rather than resect" approach. *Ann Thorac Surg* 86:722, 2008.)

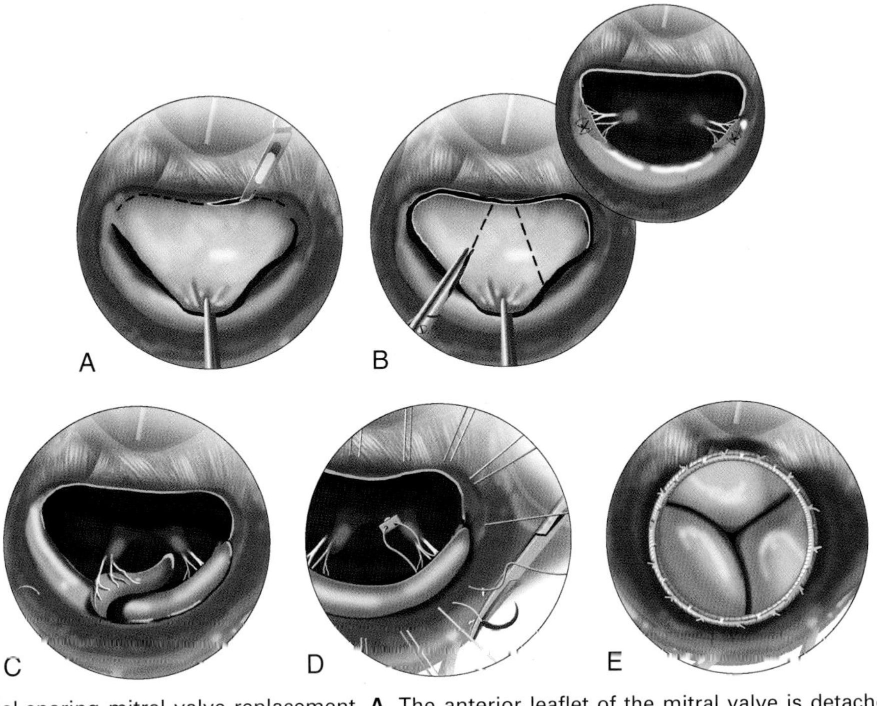

FIGURE 80-31 ■ Chordal-sparing mitral valve replacement. **A,** The anterior leaflet of the mitral valve is detached from the annulus from commissure to commissure. The anterior leaflet chordae can then be spared in two ways: **(B)** excision of the central portion of the leaflet and tacking the remaining segments to their respective 3- and 9-o'clock positions, or **(C)** direct attachment of the anterior leaflet to the posterior annulus from the 5- to 7-o'clock positions. **D,** Horizontal mattress sutures are placed circumferentially around the annulus (supra-annular, noneverting suture placement shown). **E,** Sutures are passed through the sewing ring of the mitral prosthesis and the valve is secured in position.

chordal apparatus should be preserved. The anterior leaflet is incised in a circumferential manner approximately 3 to 4 mm from the mitral valve annulus, and it is detached from commissure to commissure. The chordae to the anterior leaflet can then be preserved in two different manners. One approach is to excise the central portion of the anterior leaflet (which does not contain chordal attachments) and then suture the remaining anterior leaflet segments at their respective 3- and 9-o'clock positions. Alternatively, the detached anterior leaflet can be attached directly to the posterior annulus, from the 5- to 7-o'clock positions (see Fig. 80-31). In addition to simplicity and rapidity, this technique offers the additional advantage of buttressing the valve replacement sutures in the posterior annulus, which often is extensively calcified. Thus, the anterior leaflet can effectively double as a broad biologic pledget.

Horizontal mattress mitral valve replacement sutures are placed circumferentially around the annulus in an everting (intra-annular) or noneverting (supra-annular) fashion (see Fig. 80-31). By surrounding the prosthetic valve sewing ring with everted native mitral valve tissue, the intra-annular technique minimizes any possibility of a paravalvular leak. This technique is especially well suited for mechanical valve replacement because it avoids the possibility of leaflet tissue interfering with the hinge mechanism or the leaflet closure edge of a bileaflet mechanical valve. The disadvantage of the intra-annular technique is that smaller valve prostheses will be implanted compared with prostheses placed using a supra-annular technique. A supra-annular technique facilitates the implantation of much larger prostheses, particularly when using a bioprosthetic valve, because the entire sewing ring is secured in the left atrium rather than within the annulus. This supra-annular location also moves more of the valve out of the left ventricular outflow tract and into the atrium. Disadvantages include difficulty visualizing and properly seating pledgets on the ventricular side of the anterior annulus. Hence, sealing the valve sewing ring down onto the annulus when tying the valve sutures is purely by feel as opposed to direct visualization.

If the anterior annulus is exposed suboptimally, it is helpful to begin the leaflet incision but not completely detach the anterior leaflet from the annulus. The leaflet can then be used as a handle. Applying posterior tension on the partially divided leaflet will bring the anterior annulus further into view and facilitate placement of a mitral valve replacement suture. Once the suture is placed, the anterior mitral leaflet incision can be extended in either direction toward the commissures to allow stepwise placement of the remaining mitral valve replacement sutures in the anterior annulus.

Prosthesis Orientation

With a bioprosthetic valve, the three commissures should be oriented at approximately the 1-, 5-, and 9-o'clock positions, and ideally more toward the 1:30, 5:30, and 9:30 positions. This avoids inadvertent placement of a strut directly in the middle of the left ventricular outflow tract (which rests primarily in between the 10- and 1-o'clock positions). This positioning is slightly less important when using a supra-annular technique, because seating the valve above the annulus results in less valve in the left ventricular outflow tract. Orientation of a bileaflet mechanical valve is not as critical given the relatively low profile of the contemporary hinge guards. However, it is ideal to orient the leaflets in the horizontal plane to ensure that the valve guard is not near the left ventricular outflow tract. Far more important than hinge orientation is confirmation that both leaflets move uninterrupted, and that there is no subvalvular tissue interfering with proper valve closure. If interference is encountered, rotating the valve within the housing can be performed easily using the valve holder. Rotation will usually address the issue by repositioning the closing mechanism away from the area of tissue impingement. If interference persists, the culprit tissue can be resected through the valve or retracted away from the valve with a nonpledgeted suture.

A catheter or vent may be placed through the mitral prosthesis to provide left ventricular decompression by maintaining the mitral prosthetic valve incompetent. The atriotomy is then closed in standard fashion.

Prosthesis Selection

Important considerations in prosthesis selection include the requirement of permanent anticoagulation, durability, and, of course, patient preference. Because of the limited durability of bioprosthetic valves (particularly in younger individuals), recipient age and life expectancy help to guide professional society recommendations. In patients without a contraindication to anticoagulation, the ACC and AHA recommend a mechanical prosthesis for those younger than 60 years, a biologic prosthesis for those over age 70 years, and either prosthesis for those between 60 and 70 years.[3] Finally, patients that have contraindications to permanent anticoagulation should receive a biologic prosthesis.

In general, patients younger than 60 years of age at the time of prosthesis implantation have a higher incidence of primary structural valve degeneration and a reoperation rate as high as 40% in patients 50 years of age, 55% in patients 40 years of age, 75% in patients 30 years of age, and 90% in patients 20 years of age.[3] Anticoagulation with warfarin carries an acceptable risk in those younger than 60 years, especially in compliant patients who are carefully monitored. Thus, the balance between durability and risk of thromboembolism or bleeding may favor mechanical prosthesis implantation in those younger than 60 years.[3]

The likelihood of structural valve degeneration 15 to 20 years after biologic prosthesis implantation in patients older than 70 years is approximately 10%.[3] In addition, older patients are at higher risk of bleeding complications from permanent anticoagulation. Because the expected number of remaining life years at 70 years of age in men and women is 13.6 and 15.9 years, respectively, the durability of biologic prostheses typically exceeds life expectancy. Therefore, it is reasonable to implant a biologic prosthesis in those older than 70 years to avoid risks of anticoagulation.[3]

These recommendations are not absolute and are certainly subject to patient preference. Younger patients might not want to make the lifestyle modifications necessary for permanent anticoagulation. In addition, younger women may prefer a biologic prosthesis to facilitate safer pregnancy. With transcatheter mitral valve replacement technology on the horizon, some younger patients may prefer a bioprosthesis with the prospect of rescue valve-in-valve therapy in the future. Thus, prosthesis selection must be individualized to each patient.

RESULTS

There is an increasing need to minimize adverse outcomes in patients with mitral valve disease, particularly given new professional society guidelines advocating surgery in asymptomatic adults. Operative mortality was the principle outcome measure in the early era of mitral valve surgery. However, as current hospital mortality after valve surgery approaches zero, additional performance variables such as long-term survival, functional status, and reintervention rates have become increasingly important in evaluating modern surgical treatments of mitral valve disease.

Commissurotomy for Mitral Stenosis

Early Mortality and Late Survival

Although mortality in the early experience with closed mitral commissurotomy was high, contemporary outcomes of mortality after either closed or open commissurotomy are low and similar (less than 0.5%).[76,107] However, in most institutions, percutaneous balloon commissurotomy has essentially replaced surgical commissurotomy for mitral stenosis. Procedural mortality is near zero, and risk of complications such as severe mitral regurgitation or bleeding requiring urgent operation is low. Furthermore, midterm survival in patients with a good hemodynamic result is satisfactory.

Closed, open, and balloon mitral commissurotomy are not curative procedures. As such, survival increasingly deviates from that of an age-, gender-, and ethnicity-matched population over time (Fig. 80-32).[76,108,109] It should be noted that death typically results from thromboembolism or reoperation and mitral valve replacement, as opposed to consequences of recurrent or residual mitral stenosis or regurgitation.

Morphologic risk factors identified in the aforementioned scoring systems to assess candidacy for balloon commissurotomy likewise impact the risk of recurrent disease and symptoms. As these risk factors also predict need for reintervention, which is typically valve replacement, it is not surprising that morphologic characteristics also predict survival trends. Survival after redo mitral commissurotomy is also acceptable, with 10- and 15-year survival rates of 83% and 63% being reported. However, 31% of hospital survivors required yet another intervention (typically valve replacement), within an average of 8 years.[110]

Functional Status

In appropriately selected patients, successful commissurotomy significantly improves cardiovascular symptom burden. In fact, greater than 90% of patients are in NYHA functional class I or II within the first 2 years after surgery.[109,111,112] Symptom burden is directly related to mitral valve orifice area. Initial relief of symptoms is due to the large increase in mitral valve area afforded by commissurotomy. Various reports demonstrate valve area increases by an average of 0.9 to 2.6 cm^2 after commissurotomy,[113,114] with open commissurotomy and balloon valvotomy demonstrating superior results compared with those of closed commissurotomy (Fig. 80-33).[109,115] However, functional status gradually declines from the continued valvulopathic process with resultant reduction in mitral valve orifice area, regardless of whether rheumatic fever reoccurs (Fig. 80-34).[116] This phenomenon is evidenced by the correlation between late postoperative mean mitral orifice area and functional class: 2.0 cm^2 in patients in class I, 1.7 cm^2 in class II, and 1.6 cm^2 in class III.[117] Risk factors for poor functional status after mitral commissurotomy include older age, higher preoperative functional class, and greater degrees of valve calcification and leaflet immobility.[76]

Mitral Regurgitation after Commissurotomy

Mitral regurgitation is a clear risk of any commissurotomy procedure. Rates of immediate postprocedure mitral regurgitation vary with type of commissurotomy and are lowest for open commissurotomy (2% to 5% for open,[109] 10% for closed,[76] and 10% for percutaneous balloon[118]). Although emergency operation for new mitral regurgitation after commissurotomy is rare, surgery may be necessary within a few months. In addition, severity of mitral regurgitation affects the need for mitral valve replacement and survival, with mild mitral regurgitation demonstrating a minimal effect while more severe grades adversely affect both.[76]

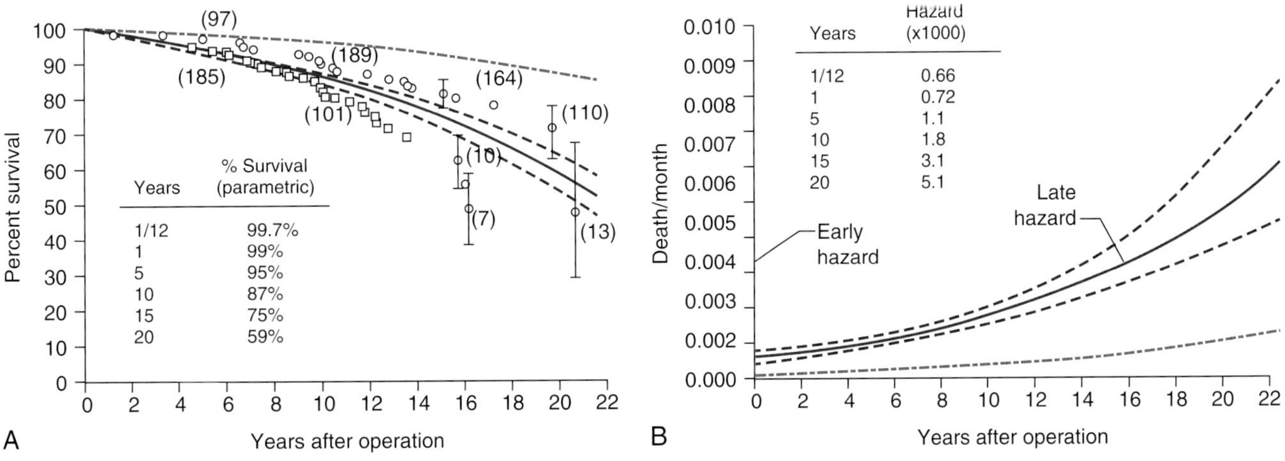

FIGURE 80-32 ■ Survival after surgical mitral commissurotomy. **A,** Actuarial survival analysis with circles representing individual deaths. **B,** Parametric analysis demonstrating the hazard of death after commissurotomy. *Dashed dot lines* represent an age-, gender-, and race-matched U.S. population. (From Hickey MS, Blackstone EH, Kirklin JW, et al: Outcome probabilities and life history after surgical mitral commissurotomy: implications for balloon commissurotomy. *J Am Coll Cardiol* 17:31, 1991.)

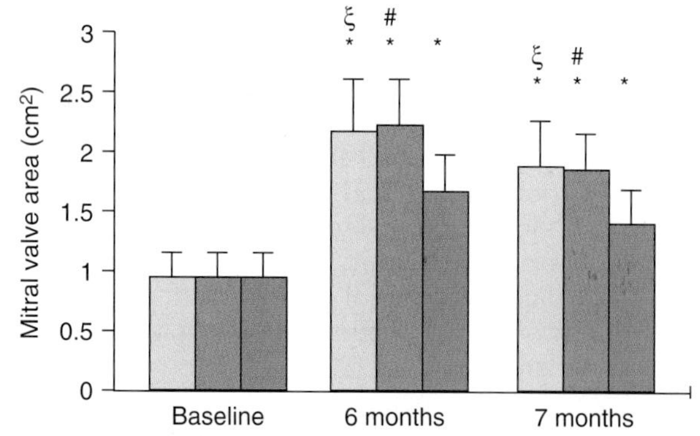

FIGURE 80-33 Mitral valve area after percutaneous balloon *(yellow)*, open *(red)*, and closed *(blue)* commissurotomy. *$P < 0.001$ compared with baseline. $^{\xi,\#}P < 0.001$ compared with closed commissurotomy. (From Ben Farhat M, Ayari F, Maatouk F, et al: Percutaneous balloon versus surgical closed and open mitral commissurotomy: seven-year follow-up results of a randomized trial. *Circulation* 97:248, 1998.)

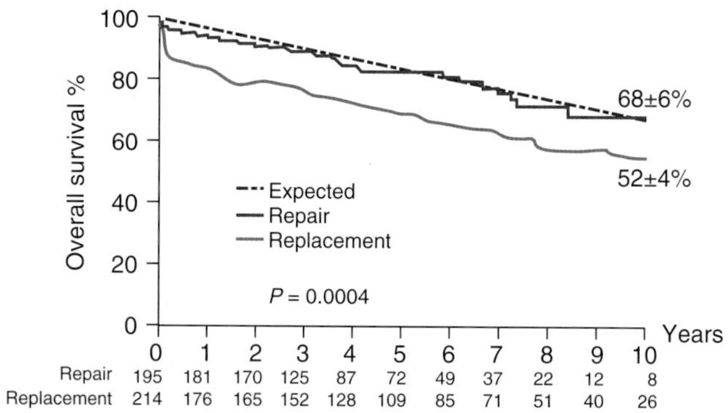

FIGURE 80-35 Comparison of overall survival after mitral valve repair or replacement. The *purple dashed dot line* represents expected survival of the general population, which is similar to survival after valve repair. (From Enriquez-Sarano M, Schaff HV, Orszulak TA, et al: Valve repair improves the outcome of surgery for mitral regurgitation. A multivariate analysis. *Circulation* 91:1022–1028, 1995.)

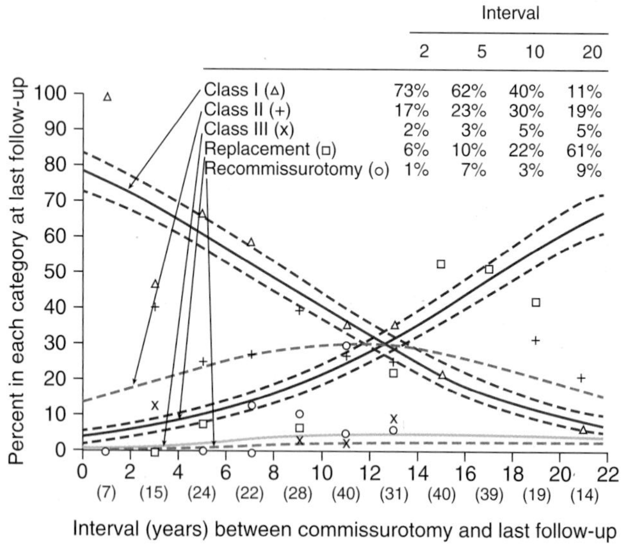

FIGURE 80-34 Functional status after surgical commissurotomy in relation to time since the initial surgery. Note the declining percentage of patients in New York Heart Association class I. In addition, the percentage of patients undergoing mitral valve replacement greatly increases over time. Numbers in parentheses along the *x*-axis are numbers of patients at each follow-up interval. (From Hickey MS, Blackstone EH, Kirklin JW, et al: Outcome probabilities and life history after surgical mitral commissurotomy: implications for balloon commissurotomy. *J Am Coll Cardiol* 17:34, 1991.)

Reintervention

Because mitral commissurotomy is not a curative procedure, most patients that undergo this procedure require subsequent procedures at some time postoperatively. Most often the subsequent procedure is a mitral valve replacement because worsening leaflet mobility and calcification, as well as progressive subvalvular pathology preclude successful redo commissurotomy. After surgical commissurotomy, valve replacement is performed in approximately 20% of patients within 10 years and 50% within 20 years (see Fig. 80-34).[76] Similar results are noted in the current era of percutaneous balloon valvotomy, with 60% of patients undergoing repeat intervention within 20 years of the index procedure (76% valve replacement and 24% repeat balloon valvotomy).[119] Risk factors for mitral valve replacement after commissurotomy include smaller precommissurotomy valve area, greater leaflet immobility and calcification, greater postprocedure mitral regurgitation, and older age.[76,119]

Valve Repair for Mitral Regurgitation

Early Mortality and Late Survival

Hospital mortality after isolated mitral valve repair for nonischemic mitral regurgitation is very low. In an analysis of more than 40,000 patients in the Society ofThoracic Surgeons Adult Cardiac Surgery Database, hospital mortality was 1.4% for patients who underwent isolated mitral valve repair between 2007 and 2010.[120] Furthermore, reference centers have reported hospital mortality rates after mitral valve repair that approach zero.[63,65,121-125]

Survival over time, inclusive of hospital mortality, of patients with mitral regurgitation who undergo mitral valve repair with or without concomitant procedures is generally better than that of patients undergoing replacement (with the exception of ischemic mitral regurgitation[79]). Contemporary survival data are similar across most centers, with 10-year survival after repair ranging from 68% to 94%,[63,65,122,126-129] and 20-year survival approaching 50%.[126,127,130] Variability in survival between reports and improved survival after repair compared with replacement is only partly attributed to the difference in baseline risk profiles of each study population. In the Mayo Clinic experience,[128,129] operative mortality was 2.6% for mitral repair compared to 10.3% for replacement ($P = 0.002$), and after valve repair late survival (in operative survivors) at 10 years was 69% compared to 58% after replacement ($P = 0.018$). Furthermore, late survival after valve repair did not differ from the expected survival of the general population (Fig. 80-35); however, the two groups differed in their degree of preoperative heart failure and incidence of atrial arrhythmias. To mitigate treatment allocation bias, a number of recent studies have used propensity-score matching to compare outcomes of mitral valve repair and replacement, all of which corroborate the survival advantage conferred by mitral repair, including in the elderly.[131-134]

Congestive heart failure owing to left ventricular dysfunction is the most common cause of late death after mitral valve repair, and it is best predicted by preoperative left ventricular dysfunction.[135] Many other variables, such as preoperative symptom burden, cause of valve disease (Fig. 80-36), and age also significantly affect survival.[13,130,136,137]

Functional Status

After mitral valve repair, symptoms typically resolve and functional capacity is excellent; greater than 90% of surviving patients are reported to be in NYHA functional class I or II 20 years after surgery.[126,127,137]

Left Ventricular Dysfunction and Remodeling

Beneficial responses of left ventricular performance to mitral valve repair are largely dependent on proper timing of surgery.[16,45,135,138] In general, mitral valve repair leads to decreased left ventricular strain, regression of left ventricular mass, and decreased left ventricular volume.[138-140] In fact, in many patients preoperative left ventricular function is preserved. However, even patients with "normal" systolic function preoperatively (ejection fraction > 60%) may develop postoperative left ventricular dysfunction. Quintana and colleagues[141] noted that 18.4% of patients had a postrepair ejection fraction of less than 50% despite having "normal" preoperative ventricular function. This ventricular dysfunction failed to recover over 15 years postoperatively in two thirds of those individuals and conferred a 70% increase in the hazard of late death. Similar to other indices of remodeling, ventricular performance is better preserved or improved after mitral valve repair when left ventricular dilation is less severe preoperatively.[16,139,141] This evidence strongly supports earlier intervention in asymptomatic patients with progressive left ventricular enlargement.

Residual and Recurrent Mitral Regurgitation

Failure after repair can be classified into three groups: immediate failure (intraoperatively), early failure (<2 years), and late failure (>2 years). Immediate and early failures are typically related to technique, whereas late failure generally is due to continued progression of the valvulopathic process. Analyses of reoperation for failure of mitral valve repair suggest that repair failures are often procedure-related in degenerative disease (usually immediate and early failure) and valve-related in rheumatic disease (usually late failure).[142-145]

The majority of patients have no residual mitral regurgitation immediately after mitral valve repair. In fact, large series from multiple centers report that only 5% of patients demonstrate mild mitral regurgitation prior to hospital discharge, with the remainder having trace or undetectable regurgitation.[63,146] Intraoperative valve assessment is critical to detect immediate failure. Such failures often are due to suture dehiscence, interscallop leakage, systolic anterior motion of the anterior leaflet, or inadequate surface of coaptation. An unsatisfactory immediate result should prompt re-exploration of the mitral valve and a repeated attempt at effective correction, because residual mitral regurgitation at the end of surgery is directly associated with a high reoperation rate (Fig. 80-37).[125,129,147,148]

Early failure is defined as new mitral regurgitation after an initially successful repair. Primary causes include absence of a remodeling annuloplasty ring, ring dehiscence from improper sizing or inadequate suture placement, rupture of repaired chordae, or suture line dehiscence on leaflet tissue. Late failure results from progression of underlying disease and typically manifests as new segmental prolapse in patients with degenerative disease or worsening valve and subvalvular fibrosis in patients with rheumatic disease.

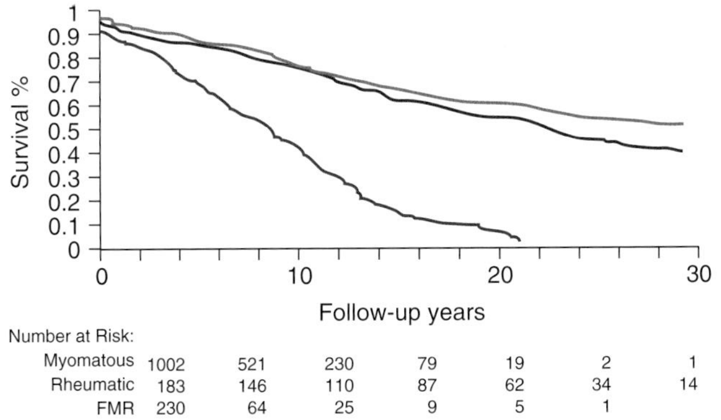

FIGURE 80-36 Overall survival after mitral valve repair stratified by etiology of mitral valve regurgitation. Lines: *green,* degenerative mitral valve disease; *red,* rheumatic valve disease; *blue,* ischemic/nonischemic functional mitral valve disease. *FMR,* Functional mitral regurgitation. (From DiBardino DJ, ElBardissi AW, McClure RS, et al: Four decades of experience with mitral valve repair: analysis of differential indications, technical evolution, and long-term outcome. *J Thorac Cardiovasc Surg* 139:79, 2010.)

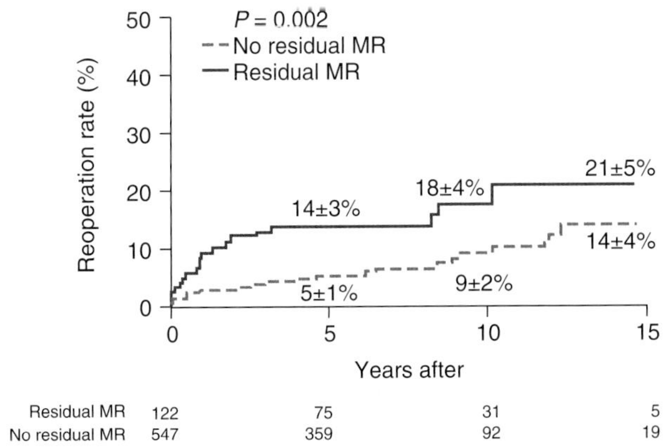

FIGURE 80-37 Reoperation rate after mitral valve repair stratified by the presence of residual mitral regurgitation immediately after repair. *MR,* Mitral regurgitation. (From Mohty D, Orszulak TA, Schaff HV, et al: Very long-term survival and durability of mitral valve repair for mitral valve prolapse. *Circulation* 104:I1–17, 2001.)

Although reoperation rate may underestimate the prevalence of late significant regurgitation, the excellent durability of mitral repair is supported by reports of freedom from reoperation ranging between 80% and 96% at 10- to 20-year follow-up.[121,125-127,130,149] Although there does not appear to be a definitive relationship between repair technique and recurrent regurgitation, repair failure is clearly influenced by disease etiology and valve lesion (Fig. 80-38). After repair of mitral regurgitation owing to degenerative or rheumatic disease, 20-year freedom from reoperation was 82% and 34%, respectively ($P < 0.001$).[130] In contrast, greater than 30% of patients randomized to mitral repair with ischemic mitral regurgitation in a multicenter trial demonstrated moderate or severe recurrent regurgitation in just 1 year.[79]

Traditionally, categorization of mitral valves by location of leaflet prolapse (posterior, anterior, or bileaflet) is of prognostic consequence as a number of series document lower repair rates and inferior repair durability for isolated anterior or bileaflet prolapse.[130,150-153] However, durable repair of anterior leaflet prolapse has improved in the current era, and some report equivalent durability compared to that of posterior leaflet repair.[154,155] With respect to repair techniques, for complex repairs and those involving the anterior leaflet, chordal replacement is superior to chordal shortening.[156] Yet, a randomized trial of the most common techniques for posterior leaflet prolapse did not reveal an appreciable difference in repair durability between leaflet resection and artificial chordoplasty.[157]

Thromboembolic Events

Late thromboembolic complications are uncommon after mitral valve repair, although such patients are rarely anticoagulated for the long term. After an initial high hazard of thromboembolism in the perioperative period, the linearized rates of thromboembolic and bleeding events are as low as 0.2% and 0.1% per patient-year, respectively, over a 20-year period.[126] David and colleagues[127] found nearly 90% freedom from thromboembolism within the first 10 years after repair, and greater than 80% freedom after 20 years from the index repair.

Systolic Anterior Motion of the Anterior Leaflet

Systolic anterior motion of the mitral valve is noted immediately postrepair in 5% to 10% of patients with mitral valve prolapse.[158-160] As previously mentioned, this complication that results from anterior displacement of the coaptation zone is limited to patients with degenerative mitral valve disease.[102] However, the incidence of systolic anterior motion appears to have decreased given mechanistic insight and the advent of novel nonresectional leaflet remodeling techniques.[71,72,161,162] It is important to note that most cases of systolic anterior motion do not require surgical intervention. Grossi and colleagues[158] identified systolic anterior motion in 6.4% of mitral valve repair patients intraoperatively, but all patients were treated medically and gradients resolved in every patient within 1 year.

Infective Endocarditis

Infective endocarditis is extremely rare after mitral valve repair as opposed to replacement. Long-term retrospective studies confirm the low risk of postrepair endocarditis, with 10- to 20-year rates of freedom from endocarditis approaching 100%.[127,137]

Reoperation

The hazard function of reoperation after mitral valve repair is low and constant, without the rising late hazard phase observed with bioprosthetic valve implantation (Fig. 80-39).[137] As previously discussed, durability of mitral valve repair is excellent, with freedom from reoperation ranging between 80% and 96% 10- to 20-years after surgery.[121,125-127,130] Etiology of mitral valve disease, location of leaflet prolapse (posterior vs. anterior), and residual regurgitation at the completion of the initial procedure are the greatest risk factors for recurrent mitral regurgitation and reoperation. However, the type of repair technique appears to have no effect on the prevalence of reoperation.[157] A handful of series have examined reoperations after mitral valve repair. Anyanwu and

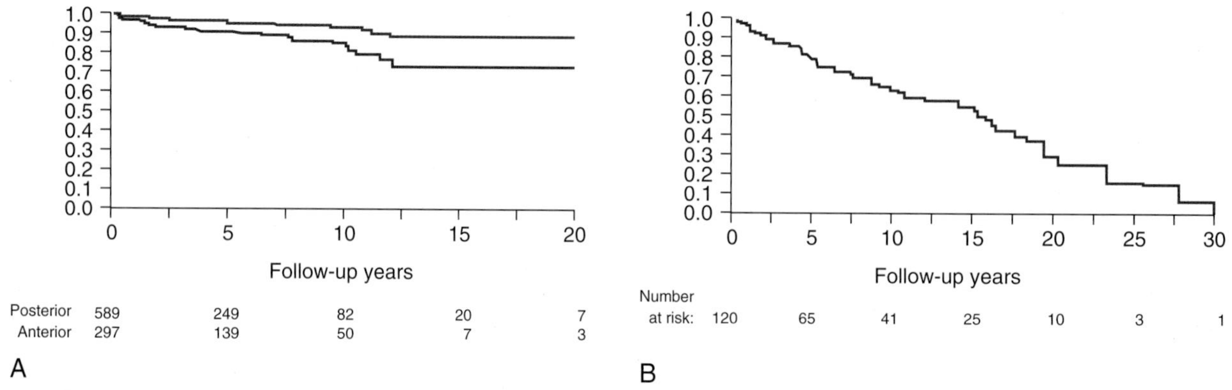

FIGURE 80-38 Reoperation after mitral valve repair for **(A)** degenerative mitral valve disease stratified by location of leaflet prolapse (posterior, *blue line;* anterior, *red line*) and **(B)** rheumatic mitral valve disease. (From DiBardino DJ, ElBardissi AW, McClure RS, et al: Four decades of experience with mitral valve repair: analysis of differential indications, technical evolution, and long-term outcome. *J Thorac Cardiovasc Surg* 139:79–80, 2010.)

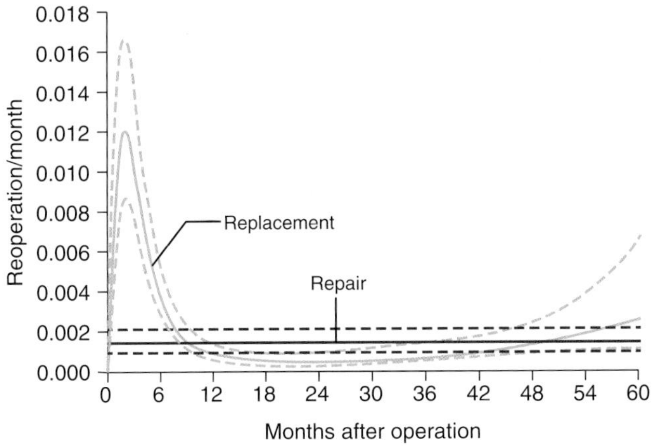

FIGURE 80-39 Hazard functions for mitral valve reoperation in patients with mitral regurgitation who underwent mitral valve repair or replacement. (From Sand ME, Naftel DC, Blackstone EH, et al: A comparison of repair and replacement for mitral valve incompetence. *J Thorac Cardiovasc Surg* 94:208–219, 1987.)

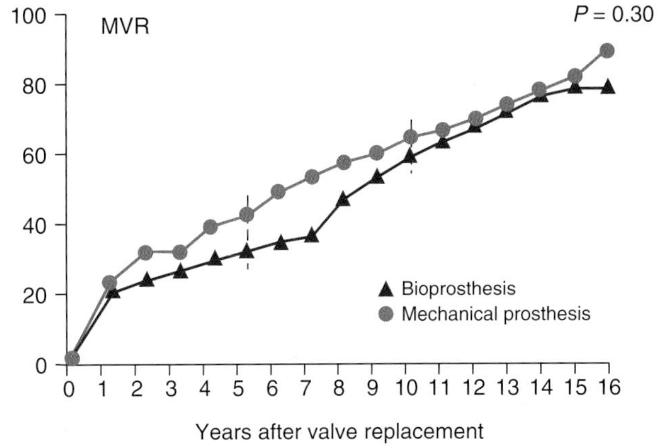

FIGURE 80-40 All-cause mortality after mitral valve replacement (MVR) stratified by prosthesis type (biologic versus mechanical) up to 16 years postoperatively. (From Hammermeister K, Sethi GK, Henderson WG, et al: Outcomes 15 years after valve replacement with a mechanical versus a bioprosthetic valve: final report of the Veterans Affairs randomized trial. *J Am Coll Cardiol* 36:1152–1158, 2000.)

colleagues[145] noted that mode of failure was attributable to progression of original disease in 36%, technical failure in 38%, and new disease in 26% of patients. Feasibility of valve re-repair depends on the primary etiology of valve disease and is successfully accomplished in 36% to 85% of patients.[144,145,163,164] The advantages of mitral repair over replacement appear to persist during reoperation. In an analysis of the Mayo Clinic's experience of reoperative mitral valve surgery, mitral re-repair independently improved survival compared to replacement.[144]

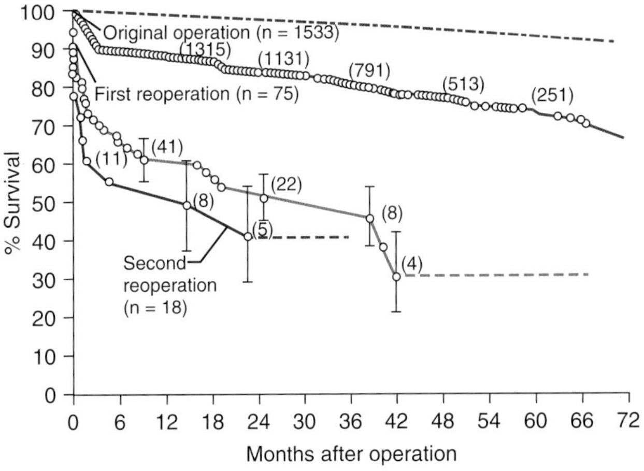

FIGURE 80-41 Actuarial survival after primary valve replacement, first reoperative valve replacement, and second reoperative valve replacement. The *purple dashed dot line* represents survival for an age-, sex-, and race-matched general population. (From Blackstone EH, Kirklin JW: Death and other time-related events after valve replacement. *Circulation* 72:755, 1985.)

Mitral Valve Replacement

Early Mortality and Late Survival

Hospital mortality after isolated mitral valve replacement for mitral valve disease ranges between 2% and 7% in a number of series.[79,131,165-168] A recent examination of 24,404 patients from the Society of Thoracic Surgeons Adult Cardiac Surgery Database revealed a hospital mortality of 3.8% following valve replacement for any etiology of mitral valve disease.[169] However, in older adults (>65 years) who are eligible for Medicare, operative mortality after isolated mitral valve replacement is higher (8.9%).[170]

Ten-year survival after mitral valve replacement is generally between 50% and 60%, and long-term survival is independent of prosthesis type chosen (mechanical or biologic; Fig. 80-40).[168,171-175] Concomitant procedures, such as coronary bypass or tricuspid annuloplasty, decrease long-term survival compared with that of isolated mitral valve replacement.[137,165,176] However, it should be noted that published results of mitral valve replacement have improved,[177,178] likely from the adoption of chordal sparing valve replacement. Preservation of papillary muscles and normal ventricular geometry minimize risk of midventricular rupture[179] and aid in maintenance of early postoperative cardiac output.[180]

Early and late survival after reoperative mitral valve replacement is less than after the index mitral valve replacement (Fig. 80-41).[175,181] This is likely a result of increased technical difficulty inherent to cardiac reoperation, greater functional disability in reoperative patients, and the fact that prosthetic valve endocarditis is a common indication for reoperation. In the current era, however, hospital mortality after reoperative mitral valve replacement has significantly decreased to under 10%.[182,183]

The most common cause of early and late death after mitral valve replacement is cardiac failure. Modes of late death in operative survivors not owing to cardiac failure include thromboembolism, anticoagulant precipitated hemorrhage, and endocarditis. Unlike patients with acquired aortic valve disease, lethal arrhythmias rarely cause sudden death in patients after mitral valve replacement. Risk factors for premature death include older age (particularly >75 years), left ventricular enlargement and dysfunction, left atrial enlargement, ischemic cardiomyopathy, significant tricuspid valve disease, severe preoperative functional disability, and failure to preserve the subvalvular apparatus during replacement.[182]

Functional Status

In most patients (>90%), symptoms improve to NYHA functional class II or better. However, patients with more severe chronic disability preoperatively are less likely to gain as much functional improvement. In fact, only half of patients with chronic severe preoperative disability return to NYHA class I after surgery, thereby suggesting that such patients probably harbor a secondary irreversible ventricular cardiomyopathy.

Left Ventricular Dysfunction and Remodeling

In the current era, beneficial responses of ventricular performance are similar to that of repair, though less significant, and largely depend on timing of surgery. Historically, after valve replacement for chronic mitral regurgitation, ejection fraction is at least transiently lower than preoperative values.[184] Although slightly reduced, ejection fraction typically remains within the range of normal when preoperative left ventricular dilation is limited (end-systolic dimension < 5 cm or end-diastolic dimension < 7 cm). When preoperative left ventricular enlargement is severe (end-systolic dimension > 5 cm or end-diastolic dimension > 7 cm), ejection fraction is significantly reduced postoperatively and in some patients may decline even further over time.[184] Ventricular performance and remodeling were significantly improved with the advent of chordal sparing mitral valve replacement. Maintenance of valvular-ventricular interaction preserves systolic performance and leads to beneficial reductions in left ventricular volume and wall stress.[105,185-187] This has translated into improved survival and global left ventricular function at early and later time points.[188,189]

Thromboembolic Events

Thromboembolism is one of the more common complications of mitral prostheses, but the incidence is somewhat less in patients with biologic valves (Table 80-5).[190] The incidence of thromboembolism in currently available bileaflet and tilting-disk valves is 1.5% to 2.0% per patient-year. Risk is higher in patients with a large left atrium, intra-atrial clot, or chronic atrial fibrillation. Maintenance of life-long therapeutic anticoagulation, typically with warfarin, is the most important factor influencing the rate of thromboembolism in patients with a mechanical mitral prosthesis. Alternatively, warfarin therapy for 3 months postoperatively and aspirin indefinitely are as effective as long-term warfarin therapy in patients with a biologic mitral prosthesis.[190]

Acute Valve Thrombosis

Acute thrombosis of a mitral prosthesis occurs more frequently with a mechanical device than a biologic valve.[190]

TABLE 80-5 Incidence of Thromboembolism and Hemorrhagic Events from Anticoagulation for Currently Available Mitral Valve Prostheses

Valve	Thromboembolism (%/pt-year)	Anticoagulant Hemorrhage (%/pt-year)
Mechanical Prostheses		
Starr-Edwards[230-232]	1.3-6.6	0.6-3.7
Medtronic Hall[233-235]	1.8-4.2	1.4-3.2
Omniscience[236-239]	0.4-2.5	0.0-2.7
St. Jude[240-243]	0.7-3.0	0.3-2.7
Carbomedics[244-247]	0.5-4.6	0.0-2.8
ATS[248,249]	0.5-3.0	0.0-2.3
On-X[250-252]	1.5-1.8	0.0-3.1
Biologic Prostheses		
Hancock standard[253,254]	1.1-2.4	0.4-1.0
Hancock II[255]	1.7	1.1
Carpentier Edwards porcine[253,256,257]	0.8-2.4	0.7-1.2
Carpentier Edwards pericardial[258,259]	0.6-1.7	0.3-1.2
Mosaic[260,261]	0.2-1.4	0.9-2.0
Biocor[262,263]	1.8-2.1	1.1

This complication occurs almost exclusively in the setting of suboptimal anticoagulation. Patients usually present acutely and report a short duration of symptoms (1 to 3 days). Echocardiography is diagnostic, but fluoroscopy may also reveal the diagnosis with evidence of restricted leaflet movement. If the patient is not in cardiogenic shock, acute thrombotic occlusion can be treated with thrombolytic agents.[191,192] Hemodynamic instability warrants emergency operation, and surgical thrombectomy typically achieves a good result.[193]

Hemorrhagic Events from Anticoagulation

Hemorrhage from anticoagulation usually occurs in the gastrointestinal, urogenital, and central nervous systems, and severity is proportional to the INR. The linearized rate of important hemorrhage has declined, and a recent meta-analysis reported rates of 1% to 2% per year (see Table 80-5).[194] This improvement has coincided with hemodynamic improvements of mitral valve prostheses (Table 80-6) that permit less intense anticoagulation goals (INR required for ball-and-cage valves was 3.5 to 4.5 compared to 2.5 to 3.5 for current mechanical prostheses).

Structural Valve Degeneration

Structural valve degeneration is the principle complication of biologic prostheses in the mitral position. In fact, prosthesis failure accounts for at least two thirds of reoperations in patients with biologic valves.[195] This complication is uncommon in the first 5 years after valve

TABLE 80-6 In Vivo Hemodynamics of Currently Available Prostheses for Mitral Valve Replacement

	Effective Orifice Area (cm²)					Mean Diastolic Transmitral Gradient (mm Hg)				
Valve	**25 mm**	**27 mm**	**29 mm**	**31 mm**	**33 mm**	**25 mm**	**27 mm**	**29 mm**	**31 mm**	**33 mm**
Mechanical Prostheses										
Starr-Edwards[264,265]		1.4	1.4	1.9			6.3-8.0	6.7-10.0	5.0	
Medtronic Hall[266,267]						4.0	3.0-4.3	2.7-3.1	2.0-2.9	2.7
Omniscience[236,268,269]	1.7	1.9	1.6-2.2	1.9-2.0	2.0	4.3-9.0	3.6-6.0	3.5-5.1	2.0-6.0	4
St. Jude[267,270,271]	2.6	2.5	2.1-2.4	2.8	3.1	3.0	3.3	1.9-3.8	1.5-1.8	1.6-2.5
Carbomedics[272,273]		2.1-2.9	2.1-3.0	1.8-3.0		5.3	3.9-4.9	3.3-4.6	3.3-4.6	4.9
Bjork-Shiley[274]	2.3	1.8		2.5		2.3-7.0	2.0-6.0		2.3-4.0	
ATS[271,275,276]	2.3	2.6-3.0	2.0-2.7	2.0	2.0	7.8	6.0	6.0	4.0	3.0
Biologic Prostheses										
Hancock standard[277,278]		1.3-1.5	1.0-2.5	1.0-1.8			7.0-12.0	5.0-7.6	5.0-7.4	
Carpentier Edwards porcine[279-281]		1.7	2.2-3.0	2.5-3.2			6.5-7.0	2.0-7.4	2.6-5.3	
Carpentier Edwards pericardial[258]	2.6	2.7	2.6	3.1		4.1	3.0	3.0	3.0	3.1
Mosaic[260,261]	1.6-2.6	1.5-1.7	1.8	1.7-2.1	1.9	4.6-5.7	3.8-4.6	4.4	2.7-3.7	3.4
Biocor[263]			3.1	3.3	3.6			6.7	6.2	5.4
Standard Values										
Normal			4-6					0		
Severe stenosis			<1					>12		
Desired value			>1.5					<10		

TABLE 80-7 Freedom from Structural Valve Degeneration Stratified by Biologic Prosthesis and Age

		Time Since Primary Mitral Valve Replacement			
Valve	**Age at Implant (yr)**	**5 years**	**10 years**	**15 years**	**20 years**
Hancock standard[254]	≤40		68%		
	41-69		84%		
	≥70		84%		
Hancock II[197,282]	<65			76%	27%
	≥65			89%	59%
Carpentier Edwards porcine[283]	≤35	79%	51%	0%	
	36-50	99%	64%	10%	
	51-64	98%	73%	26%	
	65-69	98%	67%	40%	
	≥70	100%	92%	75%	
Carpentier Edwards pericardial[259,284]	≤60	100%	78%		
	61-70	100%	89%		
	>70	100%	100%		
Biocor[263,285]	≤50		100%	71%	
	51-60		100%	90%	
	≥61		100%	100%	

replacement, but begins to increase thereafter with 15-year freedom from structural valve degeneration in earlier biologic valves nearing 40%.[195-197] Rates of biologic valve failure are higher in the mitral position than in the aortic position, and they are significantly higher in younger individuals (<65 years; Table 80-7).[196] Modes of failure include leaflet tear causing prosthetic mitral regurgitation or leaflet calcification causing prosthetic mitral stenosis. The incidence of structural valve degeneration approaches zero for bileaflet, tilting-disk, and ball-and-cage mechanical valves. Mechanical valve dysfunction owing to chronic ingrowth of tissue and impairment of the closure mechanism is observed infrequently.

Periprosthetic Leakage

Periprosthetic leakage is an uncommon complication following mitral valve replacement that is generally caused by technical errors. In the current era, the incidence of periprosthetic leakage approaches zero in uninfected patients.[198] Preoperative infective endocarditis and mitral annular calcification increase the risk of this complication. It can cause refractory hemolytic anemia in contrast to the milder hemolysis observed with some mechanical prostheses, particularly tilting-disk valves.[199] Surgery is indicated in all symptomatic patients and in those with minimal symptoms that require transfusion.[200] Alternatively, off-label application of transcatheter septal defect closure devices for these leaks has been successful.

Prosthetic Valve Endocarditis

Prosthetic mitral valve endocarditis is significantly less common than prosthetic valve endocarditis in the aortic position.[201] However, it remains a serious complication that results in the death of more than half of those affected.[198,202] Prosthetic valve endocarditis that occurs within 6 months of the primary operation is usually due to contamination in the operating theater. Endocarditis that arises later is generally the result of a new bacteremia.

Prosthetic mitral valve endocarditis that occurs early after surgery greatly increases the risk of dehiscence and death. Broad-spectrum antibiotic therapy should be initiated until sensitivities are identified. In most cases, early prosthetic valve replacement is required. Reoperation should only be deferred if there is a superb response to antibiotic therapy without evidence of peripheral embolization or periprosthetic leakage. Yet, the patient must be followed closely to allow for reoperation if clinical status declines. A similar management strategy applies to prosthetic valve endocarditis that presents over 6 months after surgery. These patients have a better likelihood of responding to medical management compared with those who develop endocarditis earlier. However, medical management is less effective when the culprit organism is more virulent, such as *Staphylococcus*.

Reoperation

Reoperation after mitral valve replacement generally is due to periprosthetic leakage and/or infective endocarditis, as well as structural valve degeneration in the case of biologic prostheses. Actuarial freedom from reoperation 5 and 10 years after valve replacement is approximately 95% and 70% to 85%, respectively. However, the hazard functions for reoperation differ greatly between mechanical and biologic prostheses. Because of structural degeneration, biologic prostheses demonstrate a late rise in risk of reoperation (Fig. 80-42).[175] After reoperation, risk of death and reoperation are higher than after the primary operation, and increase with each successive reoperation (see Fig. 80-41).[175]

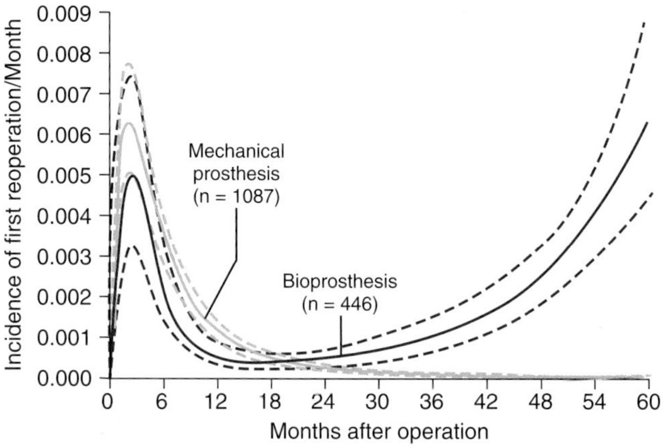

FIGURE 80-42 Hazard of reoperation after mitral valve replacement with a mechanical or biologic prosthesis. While both prosthesis types demonstrate early peaking phases, the hazard function for biologic prostheses also has a late rising phase due to structural valve degeneration. (From Blackstone EH, Kirklin JW: Death and other time-related events after valve replacement. *Circulation* 72:760, 1985.)

Minimally Invasive Mitral Valve Surgery

A minimally invasive approach to valve surgery must permit performance of a procedure equal or superior to that of the reference standard median sternotomy approach. Therefore, minimally invasive mitral valve surgery must be as safe, effective, and durable as the traditional "open" approach. In addition to benefits of improved cosmesis, minimally invasive mitral valve surgery was pioneered with the intent of reducing morbidity, postoperative pain, blood loss, hospital length of stay, and time to return to normal activity.

Early Mortality and Late Survival

To date, no comparison study has shown a significant difference in operative mortality when comparing minimally invasive mitral valve surgery to that through median sternotomy.[63,122,203-207] Although reports of initial experiences with port access mitral valve surgery documented mortality rates near 10%,[208] recent studies reproducibly demonstrate mortality rates less than 1%, particularly in the case of degenerative mitral valve disease.[63,122,124,203] Intermediate and long-term results are also encouraging. Propensity score matched comparisons of minimally invasive and sternotomy approaches to mitral valve surgery reveal similar survival up to a decade after surgery.[63,122,204] In an analysis of 402 well-matched patient pairs at the University of Pennsylvania with mitral regurgitation of any etiology, the 1-, 5-, and 9-year survival was 96%, 96%, and 96%, respectively, after minimally invasive mitral valve repair, and 97%, 92%, and 89%, respectively, following the conventional approach (P = 0.8; Fig. 80-43).[63]

Residual and Recurrent Mitral Regurgitation

Operative approach does not appear to have a significant effect on the likelihood of successful mitral valve repair, with near 100% repair rates achieved for degenerative mitral valve disease through minithoracotomy.[63] Durability of the repair is also similar regardless of operative approach. Svensson and colleagues[122] found that the return of 3+ to 4+ mitral regurgitation after repair at 1 and 5 years were 4% and 5% after minimally invasive surgery, and 6% and 7% after conventional surgery, respectively ($P > 0.1$).[122]

Postoperative Bleeding and Transfusion

Reductions in postoperative bleeding and transfusion requirements after minimally invasive mitral valve surgery are likely due to smaller incisions and less extensive

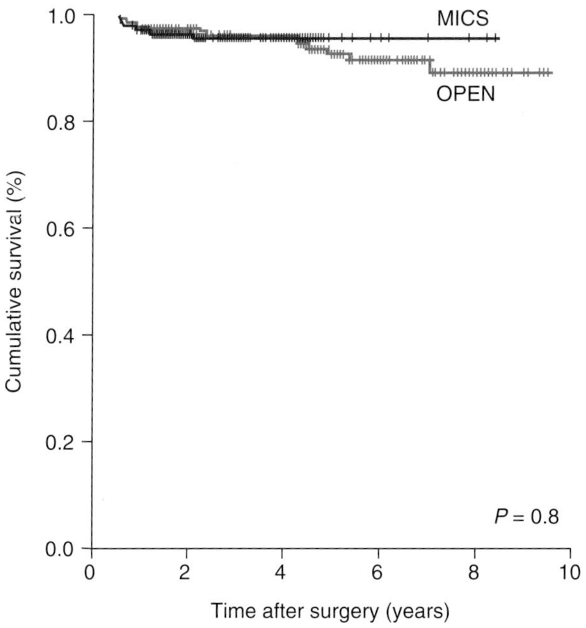

FIGURE 80-43 Actuarial survival after mitral valve repair performed via conventional sternotomy or minithoracotomy in a propensity score-matched cohort. *MICS,* Minithoracotomy approach; *OPEN,* median sternotomy approach. (From Goldstone AB, Atluri P, Szeto WY, et al: Minimally invasive approach provides at least equivalent results for surgical correction of mitral regurgitation: a propensity-matched comparison. *J Thorac Cardiovasc Surg* 145:753, 2013.)

mediastinal dissection.* In a propensity score–matched comparison, Svensson and colleagues documented significantly less mediastinal drainage in patients who underwent mitral valve surgery via partial lower sternotomy.[122] Others have also demonstrated significant associations between less invasive mitral valve surgery and reduced bleeding and transfusion (12% vs. 20% of patients transfused, $P = 0.04$).[63] Finally, three separate meta-analyses reported significant reductions in postoperative bleeding and transfusion requirements when surgery was performed via right minithoracotomy or partial lower sternotomy.[206,207,213] As blood transfusion is associated with an increase in crude risk of major infection, reduction in transfusion requirement may improve both resource utilization and care quality.[214]

Pulmonary Function

The benefit of minimally invasive approaches to mitral valve surgery on pulmonary function remains uncertain. A number of studies, including meta-analyses, documented reductions in the duration of mechanical ventilation when minimally invasive approaches were utilized.† Furthermore, in a study from a mitral valve reference center, a significantly higher proportion of patients were extubated in the operating room (18% vs. 6%; $P < 0.0001$) and postoperative FEV1 was higher.[122] Yet, other experienced centers have not shown such a benefit.[63,205]

*References 61, 63, 67, 68, 122, 205, 209-212.
†References 67, 124, 205, 207, 210, 213, 215.

It remains undetermined whether expedited extubation is actually a consequence of enhanced preservation of mechanical chest wall functionality and pain control, or whether different management protocols drive the divergence in duration of mechanical ventilatory support.

Length of Stay

Less invasive platforms for mitral valve surgery also have been advantageous in terms of shortening intensive care unit (ICU) and hospital length of stay.‡ In fact, more than half of the studies identified in a meta-analysis by Modi and colleagues[206] reported significant reductions in the length of hospital stay. Although the overall meta-analysis failed to demonstrate a significant reduction in length of hospital stay, a recent meta-analysis that focused on surgery mainly via minithoracotomy documented significantly shorter ICU and hospital stays (approximately 1 day shorter) in patients that underwent less invasive mitral valve surgery.[207] This benefit has also been observed in higher risk patient populations, including older people[218] and obese people.[219]

Postoperative Pain and Cosmetic Benefits

Outcomes such as postoperative pain and scar cosmesis are difficult to interpret secondary to their inherent subjectivity. In a survey of 187 patients who underwent thoracoscopic assisted mitral valve repair, 93% of patients were highly satisfied with the procedure and reported mild or no postoperative pain, and 99% of patients believed that their scar was aesthetically pleasing.[220] Vleissis and Bolling[221] used patients as their own controls when they interviewed 22 patients who underwent reoperative mitral valve surgery via minithoracotomy after previous median sternotomy. All patients in the study believed that their recovery was more rapid and less painful than after their original sternotomy. A more quantitative evaluation of procedural success is time to return to normal activity. A handful of experienced centers have documented that patients return to normal activity an average of 5 weeks earlier after less invasive mitral valve surgery than after mitral valve surgery via median sternotomy.[61,215]

Cost

In the current era of health care reform and economics, procedural cost and resource utilization have become increasingly important. Prior to cost analysis studies, hospital and ICU length of stay were used as surrogate measures of procedural cost. Subsequently, multiple groups have equated shorter hospital stays after less invasive mitral valve surgery to cost savings ranging from 7% to 34%.[61,64,67] Further economic benefit may stem from lower rehabilitation requirements and lower rates of early rehospitaliztion.[61,63] In an in-depth economic analysis of cost differences between minimally invasive and sternotomy approaches to mitral valve surgery, Iribarne and

‡References 67, 204, 210, 212, 216, 217.

colleagues[222] concluded that minimally invasive mitral valve surgery was both cost effective and cost saving; minimally invasive operations were associated with average savings of greater than $9000 per patient.

Robotic Technology

It is important to note that robot-assisted port access mitral valve surgery has become increasingly adopted at certain reference centers. Initial experience with robotic technology has been favorable.[66,223,224] Experienced robotic surgeons have demonstrated that the standard surgical mitral repair techniques are replicated with robot assistance and allow for safe and effective repair of all types of leaflet prolapse.[66,223] In addition to the benefit of reduced ICU and hospital stays, postoperative survival and durability of mitral valve repair have consistently and reproducibly been comparable to that of the reference standard approach, median sternotomy.[66,223]

Risks

Despite the many benefits of minimally invasive mitral valve surgery, meta-analyses demonstrate that patients may incur an increased 30-day risk of stroke (relative risk [RR], 1.79; 95% confidence interval [CI], 1.35-2.38), aortic dissection/injury (RR, 5.68; 95% CI, 1.23-26.17), and groin infection (RR, 5.62; 95% CI, 1.26-25.13).[207]

Learning Curve

Although there is a growing demand for minimally invasive mitral valve surgery, its adoption has not been as widespread as expected. In an analysis of the Society of Thoracic Surgeons Adult Cardiac Surgery Database, Gammie and colleagues[55] found that among centers that perform less invasive valve surgery, the median number of minimally invasive mitral valve surgeries performed was only 3, and robotic surgery was only performed in 7.2% of database contributing institutions.[55] The limited adoption of less invasive mitral valve surgery is likely in part a consequence of the steep learning curve associated with these platforms, particularly robotic cardiac surgery. Chitwood and colleagues[225] demonstrated that rates of repair failure fell from 7% to 4.5% after the first 100 robotic mitral valve procedures. Suri and colleagues[226] noted significant reductions in operative times following the first 50 robotic cases. Most recently, Holzhey and colleagues[227] analyzed 3895 mitral valve surgeries performed via right minithoracotomy by 17 surgeons. With the aid of cumulative sum sequential probability analysis, they concluded that the typical number of operations to overcome the minimally invasive learning curve was between 75 and 125. In addition, more than one minimally invasive operation per week was necessary to sustain acceptable results.[227] Thus, a true learning curve exists for minimally invasive surgery of the mitral valve, and given the heterogeneity of individual learning curves, good mentoring in the initial phase is critical. However, as minimally invasive surgeons must perform the same technical operation through smaller incisions, aptitude in mitral valve surgery via the conventional approach is recommended before transitioning to endoscopic platforms.

Percutaneous Technology

Catheter-based cardiovascular interventions have proven particularly effective in the treatment of coronary artery

Subgroup	Percutaneous repair	Surgery	*P* value for interaction
	no. of events/total no. (%)		
All patients	100/181 (55)	65/89 (73)	
Sex			0.97
Male	63/114 (55)	43/59 (73)	
Female	37/67 (55)	22/30 (73)	
Age			0.009
≥70 yr	52/86 (60)	23/38 (61)	
<70 yr	48/95 (51)	42/51 (82)	
MR			
Functional	26/48 (54)	12/24 (50)	0.02
Degenerative	74/133 (56)	53/65 (82)	
LVEF			0.06
<60%	35/68 (51)	15/28 (54)	
≥60%	64/111 (58)	50/61 (82)	

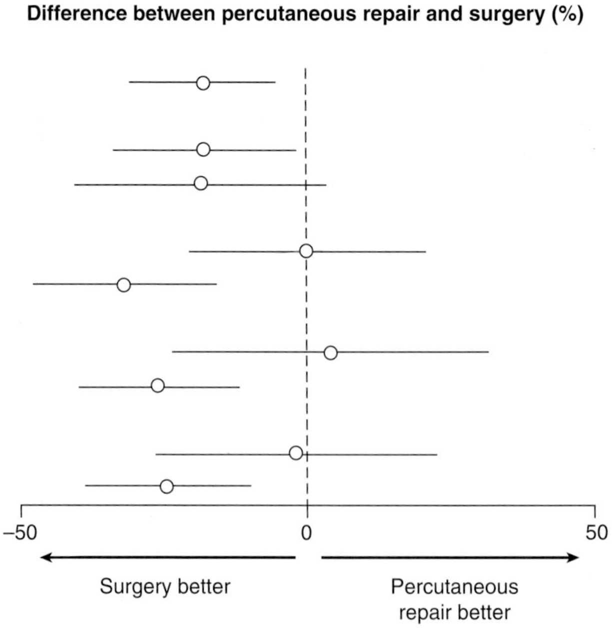

FIGURE 80-44 ■ Differences in rates of freedom from death, mitral valve surgery, or 3+ to 4+ mitral regurgitation between patients who underwent percutaneous repair or conventional mitral valve surgery. Also shown are subgroup analyses for the study cohort. *LVEF,* Left ventricular ejection fraction; *MR,* mitral regurgitation. (From Feldman T, Foster E, Glower DD, et al: Percutaneous repair or surgery for mitral regurgitation. *N Engl J Med* 364:1404, 2011.)

disease. Recently, there has been rapid adoption and implementation of percutaneous treatments for structural heart disease, specifically transcatheter aortic valve replacement. Efforts to recreate the complex surgical techniques of mitral valve repair with catheter-based technologies, however, have been less successful. Alfieri's edge-to-edge technique[91] effectively constructs a double-orifice mitral valve by affixing the anterior and posterior leaflets, but in the contemporary era of mitral valve repair, is generally used as a secondary repair modality. The MitraClip (Abbott Vascular, Abbott Park, IL) replicates the edge-to-edge repair, and is the first catheter-based mitral valve repair system approved for use in the United States. However, initial experience with the device demonstrated poor early and late correction of mitral regurgitation in clinical trials.[228,229] A phase III comparison of the MitraClip with conventional mitral valve surgery, the EVEREST II trial revealed similar safety outcomes between approaches, but the benefit of reduced blood transfusion requirements was offset by limitations of procedural efficacy (Fig. 80-44).[228] Twenty percent of patients randomized to the MitraClip required salvage with mitral valve surgery due to significant residual mitral regurgitation at 1 year,[228] and approximately 25% needed reoperation at 4 years.[229] Regrettably, salvage mitral valve repair was not possible in nearly half of cases, presumably from physiologic leaflet scarring in response to the clip.[229] Thus, the MitraClip should be reserved for inoperable or prohibitively high-risk patients, as "clip first" strategies may ultimately prevent subsequent mitral valve repair in a significant proportion of patients who may have truly benefitted from the reference standard operation. Additional transcatheter therapies are in earlier stages of development, and they reduce mitral regurgitation via annular reduction or neochordal implantation. As is evident in conventional mitral valve repair, perhaps the most effective and durable transcatheter repair strategy will use more than one repair technique and will be tailored to the cause of the mitral regurgitation. Transcatheter mitral valve replacement devices are likewise in early stages of development and investigation.

REFERENCES

1. Levine RA, Triulzi MO, Harrigan P, et al: The relationship of mitral annular shape to the diagnosis of mitral valve prolapse. *Circulation* 75:756–767, 1987.
2. Ranganathan N, Lam JH, Wigle ED, et al: Morphology of the human mitral valve. II. The value leaflets. *Circulation* 41:459–467, 1970.
3. Nishimura RA, Otto CM, Bonow RO, et al: 2014 AHA/ACC Guideline for the Management of Patients With Valvular Heart Disease: a report of the American College of Cardiology/American Heart Association Task Force on Practice Guidelines. *Circulation* 129:e521–e643, 2014.
4. Bolen JL, Lopes MG, Harrison DC, et al: Analysis of left ventricular function in response to afterload changes in patients with mitral stenosis. *Circulation* 52:894–900, 1975.
5. Curry GC, Elliott LP, Ramsey HW: Quantitative left ventricular angiocardiographic findings in mitral stenosis. Detailed analysis of the anterolateral wall of the left ventricle. *Am J Cardiol* 29:621–627, 1972.
6. Marijon E, Mirabel M, Celermajer DS, et al: Rheumatic heart disease. *Lancet* 379:953–964, 2012.
7. Bland EF, Duckett Jones T: Rheumatic fever and rheumatic heart disease; a twenty year report on 1000 patients followed since childhood. *Circulation* 4:836–843, 1951.
8. Rowe JC, Bland EF, Sprague HB, et al: The course of mitral stenosis without surgery: ten- and twenty-year perspectives. *Ann Intern Med* 52:741–749, 1960.
9. Rapaport E: Natural history of aortic and mitral valve disease. *Am J Cardiol* 35:221–227, 1975.
10. Olesen KH: The natural history of 271 patients with mitral stenosis under medical treatment. *Br Heart J* 24:349–357, 1962.
11. Selzer A, Cohn KE: Natural history of mitral stenosis: a review. *Circulation* 45:878–890, 1972.
12. Chandrashekhar Y, Westaby S, Narula J: Mitral stenosis. *Lancet* 374:1271–1283, 2009.
13. Wilkins GT, Weyman AE, Abascal VM, et al: Percutaneous balloon dilatation of the mitral valve: an analysis of echocardiographic variables related to outcome and the mechanism of dilatation. *Br Heart J* 60:299–308, 1988.
14. Abascal VM, Wilkins GT, O'Shea JP, et al: Prediction of successful outcome in 130 patients undergoing percutaneous balloon mitral valvotomy. *Circulation* 82:448–456, 1990.
15. Braunwald E: Mitral regurgitation: physiologic, clinical and surgical considerations. *N Engl J Med* 281:425–433, 1969.
16. Athanasopoulos LV, McGurk S, Khalpey Z, et al: Usefulness of preoperative cardiac dimensions to predict success of reverse cardiac remodeling in patients undergoing repair for mitral valve prolapse. *Am J Cardiol* 113:1006–1010, 2014.
17. Carpentier A: Cardiac valve surgery—the "French correction." *J Thorac Cardiovasc Surg* 86:323–337, 1983.
18. Mills P, Rose J, Hollingsworth J, et al: Long-term prognosis of mitral-valve prolapse. *N Engl J Med* 297:13–18, 1977.
19. Freed LA, Levy D, Levine RA, et al: Prevalence and clinical outcome of mitral-valve prolapse. *N Engl J Med* 341:1–7, 1999.
20. Devereux RB, Jones EC, Roman MJ, et al: Prevalence and correlates of mitral valve prolapse in a population-based sample of American Indians: the Strong Heart Study. *Am J Med* 111:679–685, 2001.
21. Fornes P, Heudes D, Fuzellier JF, et al: Correlation between clinical and histologic patterns of degenerative mitral valve insufficiency: a histomorphometric study of 130 excised segments. *Cardiovasc Pathol* 8:81–92, 1999.
22. Anyanwu AC, Adams DH: Etiologic classification of degenerative mitral valve disease: Barlow's disease and fibroelastic deficiency. *Semin Thorac Cardiovasc Surg* 19:90–96, 2007.
23. Jeresaty RM, Edwards JE, Chawla SK: Mitral valve prolapse and ruptured chordae tendineae. *Am J Cardiol* 55:138–142, 1985.
24. Chauvaud S, Fuzellier JF, Berrebi A, et al: Long-term (29 years) results of reconstructive surgery in rheumatic mitral valve insufficiency. *Circulation* 104:I12–I15, 2001.
25. Carpentier AF, Pellerin M, Fuzellier JF, et al: Extensive calcification of the mitral valve anulus: pathology and surgical management. *J Thorac Cardiovasc Surg* 111:718–729, discussion 729–730, 1996.
26. Korn D, Desanctis RW, Sell S: Massive calcification of the mitral annulus. A clinicopathological study of fourteen cases. *N Engl J Med* 267:900–909, 1962.
27. el Asmar B, Acker M, Couetil JP, et al: Mitral valve repair in the extensively calcified mitral valve annulus. *Ann Thorac Surg* 52:66–69, 1991.
28. Duval X, Delahaye F, Alla F, et al: Temporal trends in infective endocarditis in the context of prophylaxis guideline modifications: three successive population-based surveys. *J Am Coll Cardiol* 59:1968–1976, 2012.
29. Selton-Suty C, Celard M, Le Moing V, et al: Preeminence of Staphylococcus aureus in infective endocarditis: a 1-year population-based survey. *Clin Infect Dis* 54:1230–1239, 2012.
30. Gillinov AM, Diaz R, Blackstone EH, et al: Double valve endocarditis. *Ann Thorac Surg* 71:1874–1879, 2001.
31. Llaneras MR, Nance ML, Streicher JT, et al: Pathogenesis of ischemic mitral insufficiency. *J Thorac Cardiovasc Surg* 105:439–442, discussion 442–443, 1993.
32. Gorman RC, McCaughan JS, Ratcliffe MB, et al: Pathogenesis of acute ischemic mitral regurgitation in three dimensions. *J Thorac Cardiovasc Surg* 109:684–693, 1995.
33. Gorman JH, 3rd, Gorman RC, Jackson BM, et al: Distortions of the mitral valve in acute ischemic mitral regurgitation. *Ann Thorac Surg* 64:1026–1031, 1997.

34. Antunes MJ: Submitral left ventricular aneurysms. Correction by a new transatrial approach. *J Thorac Cardiovasc Surg* 94:241–245, 1987.
35. Ruiz D, Domingo P, Canals E, et al: Annular submitral left ventricular aneurysm. *Eur Heart J* 13:424–425, 1992.
36. Goldstone AB, Howard JL, Cohen JE, et al: Natural history of coexistent tricuspid regurgitation in patients with degenerative mitral valve disease: implications for future guidelines. *J Thorac Cardiovasc Surg* 148:2802–2809, 2014.
37. Chikwe J, Adams DH, Su KN, et al: Can three-dimensional echocardiography accurately predict complexity of mitral valve repair? *Eur J Cardiothorac Surg* 41:518–524, 2012.
38. Rackley CE, Hood WP, Jr: Quantitative angiographic evaluation and pathophysiologic mechanisms in valvular heart disease. *Prog Cardiovasc Dis* 15:427–447, 1973.
39. Wilcken DE, Hickey AJ: Lifetime risk for patients with mitral valve prolapse of developing severe valve regurgitation requiring surgery. *Circulation* 78:10–14, 1988.
40. Ling LH, Enriquez-Sarano M, Seward JB, et al: Clinical outcome of mitral regurgitation due to flail leaflet. *N Engl J Med* 335:1417–1423, 1996.
41. Enriquez-Sarano M, Avierinos JF, Messika-Zeitoun D, et al: Quantitative determinants of the outcome of asymptomatic mitral regurgitation. *N Engl J Med* 352:875–883, 2005.
42. Munoz S, Gallardo J, Diaz-Gorrin JR, et al: Influence of surgery on the natural history of rheumatic mitral and aortic valve disease. *Am J Cardiol* 35:234–242, 1975.
43. Tribouilloy CM, Enriquez-Sarano M, Schaff HV, et al: Impact of preoperative symptoms on survival after surgical correction of organic mitral regurgitation: rationale for optimizing surgical indications. *Circulation* 99:400–405, 1999.
44. Suri RM, Vanoverschelde JL, Grigioni F, et al: Association between early surgical intervention vs watchful waiting and outcomes for mitral regurgitation due to flail mitral valve leaflets. *JAMA* 310:609–616, 2013.
45. Tribouilloy C, Rusinaru D, Grigioni F, et al: Long-term mortality associated with left ventricular dysfunction in mitral regurgitation due to flail leaflets: a multicenter analysis. *Circ Cardiovasc Imaging* 7:363–370, 2014.
46. Crawford MH, Souchek J, Oprian CA, et al: Determinants of survival and left ventricular performance after mitral valve replacement. Department of Veterans Affairs Cooperative Study on Valvular Heart Disease. *Circulation* 81:1173–1181, 1990.
47. Enriquez-Sarano M, Tajik AJ, Schaff HV, et al: Echocardiographic prediction of left ventricular function after correction of mitral regurgitation: results and clinical implications. *J Am Coll Cardiol* 24:1536–1543, 1994.
48. Enriquez-Sarano M, Tajik AJ, Schaff HV, et al: Echocardiographic prediction of survival after surgical correction of organic mitral regurgitation. *Circulation* 90:830–837, 1994.
49. Sherrid MV, Clark RD, Cohn K: Echocardiographic analysis of left atrial size before and after operation in mitral valve disease. *Am J Cardiol* 43:171–178, 1979.
50. Kang DH, Kim JH, Rim JH, et al: Comparison of early surgery versus conventional treatment in asymptomatic severe mitral regurgitation. *Circulation* 119:797–804, 2009.
51. Ngaage DL, Schaff HV, Mullany CJ, et al: Influence of preoperative atrial fibrillation on late results of mitral repair: is concomitant ablation justified? *Ann Thorac Surg* 84:434–442, discussion 442–443, 2007.
52. Nashef SA, Roques F, Michel P, et al: European system for cardiac operative risk evaluation (EuroSCORE). *Eur J Cardiothorac Surg* 16:9–13, 1999.
53. Goldstone AB, Chikwe J, Pinney SP, et al: Incidence, epidemiology, and prognosis of residual pulmonary hypertension after mitral valve repair for degenerative mitral regurgitation. *Am J Cardiol* 107:755–760, 2011.
54. Bolling SF, Li S, O'Brien SM, et al: Predictors of mitral valve repair: clinical and surgeon factors. *Ann Thorac Surg* 90:1904–1911, discussion 1912, 2010.
55. Gammie JS, Zhao Y, Peterson ED, et al: J. Maxwell Chamberlain Memorial Paper for adult cardiac surgery. Less-invasive mitral valve operations: trends and outcomes from the Society of Thoracic Surgeons Adult Cardiac Surgery Database. *Ann Thorac Surg* 90:1401–1408, 1410.e1, discussion 1408–1410, 2010.
56. Woo YJ, Seeburger J, Mohr FW: Minimally invasive valve surgery. *Semin Thorac Cardiovasc Surg* 19:289–298, 2007.
57. Schmitto JD, Mokashi SA, Cohn LH: Minimally-invasive valve surgery. *J Am Coll Cardiol* 56:455–462, 2010.
58. Woo YJ: Minimally invasive valve surgery. *Surg Clin North Am* 89:923–949, x, 2009.
59. Padala M, Jimenez JH, Yoganathan AP, et al: Transapical beating heart cardioscopy technique for off-pump visualization of heart valves. *J Thorac Cardiovasc Surg* 144:231–234, 2012.
60. Cosgrove DM, 3rd, Sabik JF, Navia JL: Minimally invasive valve operations. *Ann Thorac Surg* 65:1535–1538, discussion 1538–1539, 1998.
61. Cohn LH, Adams DH, Couper GS, et al: Minimally invasive cardiac valve surgery improves patient satisfaction while reducing costs of cardiac valve replacement and repair. *Ann Surg* 226:421–426, discussion 427–428, 1997.
62. Goldstone AB, Joseph Woo Y: Minimally invasive surgical treatment of valvular heart disease. *Semin Thorac Cardiovasc Surg* 26:36–43, 2014.
63. Goldstone AB, Atluri P, Szeto WY, et al: Minimally invasive approach provides at least equivalent results for surgical correction of mitral regurgitation: a propensity-matched comparison. *J Thorac Cardiovasc Surg* 145:748–756, 2013.
64. Navia JL, Cosgrove DM, 3rd: Minimally invasive mitral valve operations. *Ann Thorac Surg* 62:1542–1544, 1996.
65. McClure RS, Athanasopoulos LV, McGurk S, et al: One thousand minimally invasive mitral valve operations: early outcomes, late outcomes, and echocardiographic follow-up. *J Thorac Cardiovasc Surg* 145:1199–1206, 2013.
66. Suri RM, Burkhart HM, Daly RC, et al: Robotic mitral valve repair for all prolapse subsets using techniques identical to open valvuloplasty: establishing the benchmark against which percutaneous interventions should be judged. *J Thorac Cardiovasc Surg* 142:970–979, 2011.
67. Chitwood WR, Jr, Wixon CL, Elbeery JR, et al: Video-assisted minimally invasive mitral valve surgery. *J Thorac Cardiovasc Surg* 114:773–780, discussion 780–782, 1997.
68. Grossi EA, Galloway AC, Ribakove GH, et al: Impact of minimally invasive valvular heart surgery: a case-control study. *Ann Thorac Surg* 71:807–810, 2001.
69. Suri RM, Thalji NM: Minimally invasive heart valve surgery: how and why in 2012. *Curr Cardiol Rep* 14:171–179, 2012.
70. Atluri P, Woo YJ, Goldstone AB, et al: Minimally invasive mitral valve surgery can be performed with optimal outcomes in the presence of left ventricular dysfunction. *Ann Thorac Surg* 96:1596–1602, 2013.
71. MacArthur JW, Jr, Cohen JE, Goldstone AB, et al: Nonresectional single-suture leaflet remodeling for degenerative mitral regurgitation facilitates minimally invasive mitral valve repair. *Ann Thorac Surg* 96:1603–1606, 2013.
72. Woo YJ, MacArthur JW, Jr: Posterior ventricular anchoring neochordal repair of degenerative mitral regurgitation efficiently remodels and repositions posterior leaflet prolapse. *Eur J Cardiothorac Surg* 44:485–489, discussion 489, 2013.
73. Deloche A, Acar C, Jebara V, et al: Biatrial transseptal approach in case of difficult exposure to the mitral valve. *Ann Thorac Surg* 50:318–319, 1990.
74. Kaczorowski DJ, Blank M, Woo YJ: Intracardiac exposure for transventricular mitral valve ring annuloplasty repair during Dor ventriculoplasty. *J Heart Lung Transplant* 31:1236–1238, 2012.
75. Frederick JR, Woo YJ: Transaortic mitral valve replacement. *Ann Thorac Surg* 94:302–304, 2012.
76. Hickey MS, Blackstone EH, Kirklin JW, et al: Outcome probabilities and life history after surgical mitral commissurotomy: implications for balloon commissurotomy. *J Am Coll Cardiol* 17:29–42, 1991.
77. Carpentier AF, Lessana A, Relland JY, et al: The "physio-ring": an advanced concept in mitral valve annuloplasty. *Ann Thorac Surg* 60:1177–1185, discussion 1185–1186, 1995.
78. Carpentier A, Adams DH, Filsoufi F: Valve exposure, intraoperative valve analysis, and reconstruction. In *Carpentier's reconstructive valve surgery*, St. Louis, 2010, Saunders, pp 55–63.
79. Acker MA, Parides MK, Perrault LP, et al: Mitral-valve repair versus replacement for severe ischemic mitral regurgitation. *N Engl J Med* 370:23–32, 2014.

80. Jebara VA, Mihaileanu S, Acar C, et al: Left ventricular outflow tract obstruction after mitral valve repair. Results of the sliding leaflet technique. *Circulation* 88:II30–II34, 1993.
81. Frater RW, Vetter HO, Zussa C, et al: Chordal replacement in mitral valve repair. *Circulation* 82:IV125–IV130, 1990.
82. von Oppell UO, Mohr FW: Chordal replacement for both minimally invasive and conventional mitral valve surgery using premeasured Gore-Tex loops. *Ann Thorac Surg* 70:2166–2168, 2000.
83. Okamoto K, Yozu R, Kudo M: Loop-in-loop technique in mitral valve repair via minithoracotomy. *Ann Thorac Surg* 93:1329–1330, 2012.
84. Chu MW, Gersch KA, Rodriguez E, et al: Robotic "haircut" mitral valve repair: posterior leaflet-plasty. *Ann Thorac Surg* 85:1460–1462, 2008.
85. Asai T, Kinoshita T, Hosoba S, et al: Butterfly resection is safe and avoids systolic anterior motion in posterior leaflet prolapse repair. *Ann Thorac Surg* 92:2097–2102, discussion 2102–2103, 2011.
86. Woo YJ, MacArthur JW, Jr: Simplified nonresectional leaflet remodeling mitral valve repair for degenerative mitral regurgitation. *J Thorac Cardiovasc Surg* 143:749–753, 2012.
87. Reference deleted in page proofs.
88. Saunders PC, Grossi EA, Schwartz CF, et al: Anterior leaflet resection of the mitral valve. *Semin Thorac Cardiovasc Surg* 16:188–193, 2004.
89. Adams DH, Kadner A, Chen RH: Artificial mitral valve chordae replacement made simple. *Ann Thorac Surg* 71:1377–1378, discussion 1378–1379, 2001.
90. Kobayashi J, Sasako Y, Bando K, et al: Ten-year experience of chordal replacement with expanded polytetrafluoroethylene in mitral valve repair. *Circulation* 102:III30–III34, 2000.
91. Alfieri O, Maisano F, De Bonis M, et al: The double-orifice technique in mitral valve repair: a simple solution for complex problems. *J Thorac Cardiovasc Surg* 122:674–681, 2001.
92. De Bonis M, Lapenna E, Lorusso R, et al: Very long-term results (up to 17 years) with the double-orifice mitral valve repair combined with ring annuloplasty for degenerative mitral regurgitation. *J Thorac Cardiovasc Surg* 144:1019–1024, 2012.
93. Bichell DP, Adams DH, Aranki SF, et al: Repair of mitral regurgitation from myxomatous degeneration in the patient with a severely calcified posterior annulus. *J Card Surg* 10:281–284, 1995.
94. Hussain ST, Idrees J, Brozzi NA, et al: Use of annulus washer after debridement: a new mitral valve replacement technique for patients with severe mitral annular calcification. *J Thorac Cardiovasc Surg* 145:1672–1674, 2013.
95. David TE, Kuo J, Armstrong S: Aortic and mitral valve replacement with reconstruction of the intervalvular fibrous body. *J Thorac Cardiovasc Surg* 114:766–771, discussion 771–772, 1997.
96. David TE, Feindel CM: Reconstruction of the mitral anulus. *Circulation* 76:III102–III107, 1987.
97. David TE, Feindel CM, Armstrong S, et al: Reconstruction of the mitral anulus. A ten-year experience. *J Thorac Cardiovasc Surg* 110:1323–1332, 1995.
98. Dreyfus G, Serraf A, Jebara VA, et al: Valve repair in acute endocarditis. *Ann Thorac Surg* 49:706–711, discussion 712–713, 1990.
99. Hendren WG, Morris AS, Rosenkranz ER, et al: Mitral valve repair for bacterial endocarditis. *J Thorac Cardiovasc Surg* 103:124–128, discussion 128–129, 1992.
100. Muehrcke DD, Cosgrove DM, 3rd, Lytle BW, et al: Is there an advantage to repairing infected mitral valves? *Ann Thorac Surg* 63:1718–1724, 1997.
101. Zegdi R, Debieche M, Latremouille C, et al: Long-term results of mitral valve repair in active endocarditis. *Circulation* 111:2532–2536, 2005.
102. Mihaileanu S, Marino JP, Chauvaud S, et al: Left ventricular outflow obstruction after mitral valve repair (Carpentier's technique). Proposed mechanisms of disease. *Circulation* 78:I78–I184, 1988.
103. Brown ML, Abel MD, Click RL, et al: Systolic anterior motion after mitral valve repair: is surgical intervention necessary? *J Thorac Cardiovasc Surg* 133:136–143, 2007.
104. Adams DH, Anyanwu AC, Rahmanian PB, et al: Large annuloplasty rings facilitate mitral valve repair in Barlow's disease. *Ann Thorac Surg* 82:2096–2100, discussion 2101, 2006.
105. Yun KL, Sintek CF, Miller DC, et al: Randomized trial comparing partial versus complete chordal-sparing mitral valve replacement: effects on left ventricular volume and function. *J Thorac Cardiovasc Surg* 123:707–714, 2002.
106. Yun KL, Sintek CF, Miller DC, et al: Randomized trial of partial versus complete chordal preservation methods of mitral valve replacement: a preliminary report. *Circulation* 100:II90–II94, 1999.
107. Ravkilde JL, Hansen PS: Late results following closed mitral valvotomy in isolated mitral valve stenosis: analysis of thirty-five years of follow-up in 240 patients using Cox regression. *Thorac Cardiovasc Surg* 39:133–139, 1991.
108. Cohn LH, Allred EN, Cohn LA, et al: Long-term results of open mitral valve reconstruction for mitral stenosis. *Am J Cardiol* 55:731–734, 1985.
109. Smith WM, Neutze JM, Barratt-Boyes BG, et al: Open mitral valvotomy. Effect of preoperative factors on result. *J Thorac Cardiovasc Surg* 82:738–751, 1981.
110. Peper WA, Lytle BW, Cosgrove DM, et al: Repeat mitral commissurotomy: long-term results. *Circulation* 76:III97–III101, 1987.
111. Housman LB, Bonchek L, Lambert L, et al: Prognosis of patients after open mitral commissurotomy. Actuarial analysis of late results in 100 patients. *J Thorac Cardiovasc Surg* 73:742–745, 1977.
112. Gross RI, Cunningham JN, Jr, Snively SL, et al: Long-term results of open radical mitral commissurotomy: ten year follow-up study of 202 patients. *Am J Cardiol* 47:821–825, 1981.
113. Nakano S, Kawashima Y, Hirose H, et al: Reconsiderations of indications for open mitral commissurotomy based on pathologic features of the stenosed mitral valve. A fourteen-year follow-up study in 347 consecutive patients. *J Thorac Cardiovasc Surg* 94:336–342, 1987.
114. Feigenbaum H, Linback RE, Nasser WK: Hemodynamic studies before and after instrumental mitral commissurotomy. A reappraisal of the pathophysiology of mitral stenosis and the efficacy of mitral valvotomy. *Circulation* 38:261–276, 1968.
115. Ben Farhat M, Ayari M, Maatouk F, et al: Percutaneous balloon versus surgical closed and open mitral commissurotomy: seven-year follow-up results of a randomized trial. *Circulation* 97:245–250, 1998.
116. Essop R, Rothlisberger C, Dullabh A, et al: Can the long-term outcomes of percutaneous balloon mitral valvotomy and surgical commissurotomy be expected to be similar? *J Heart Valve Dis* 4:446–452, 1995.
117. Breyer RH, Mills SA, Hudspeth AS, et al: Open mitral commissurotomy: long-term results with echocardiographic correlation. *J Cardiovasc Surg (Torino)* 26:46–52, 1985.
118. Abascal VM, Wilkins GT, Choong CY, et al: Mitral regurgitation after percutaneous balloon mitral valvuloplasty in adults: evaluation by pulsed Doppler echocardiography. *J Am Coll Cardiol* 11:257–263, 1988.
119. Bouleti C, Iung B, Himbert D, et al: Reinterventions after percutaneous mitral commissurotomy during long-term follow-up, up to 20 years: the role of repeat percutaneous mitral commissurotomy. *Eur Heart J* 34:1923–1930, 2013.
120. Chatterjee S, Rankin JS, Gammie JS, et al: Isolated mitral valve surgery risk in 77,836 patients from the Society of Thoracic Surgeons database. *Ann Thorac Surg* 96:1587–1594, discussion 1594–1595, 2013.
121. Gillinov AM, Cosgrove DM, Blackstone EH, et al: Durability of mitral valve repair for degenerative disease. *J Thorac Cardiovasc Surg* 116:734–743, 1998.
122. Svensson LG, Atik FA, Cosgrove DM, et al: Minimally invasive versus conventional mitral valve surgery: a propensity-matched comparison. *J Thorac Cardiovasc Surg* 139:926–932, e921–922, 2010.
123. Weiner MM, Hofer I, Lin HM, et al: Relationship among surgical volume, repair quality, and perioperative outcomes for repair of mitral insufficiency in a mitral valve reference center. *J Thorac Cardiovasc Surg* 148:2021–2026, 2014.
124. Suri RM, Schaff HV, Meyer SR, et al: Thoracoscopic versus open mitral valve repair: a propensity score analysis of early outcomes. *Ann Thorac Surg* 88:1185–1190, 2009.

125. De Bonis M, Lapenna E, Taramasso M, et al: Very long-term durability of the edge-to-edge repair for isolated anterior mitral leaflet prolapse: up to 21 years of clinical and echocardiographic results. *J Thorac Cardiovasc Surg* 148:2027–2032, 2014.
126. Braunberger E, Deloche A, Berrebi A, et al: Very long-term results (more than 20 years) of valve repair with carpentier's techniques in nonrheumatic mitral valve insufficiency. *Circulation* 104:I8–I11, 2001.
127. David TE, Armstrong S, McCrindle BW, et al: Late outcomes of mitral valve repair for mitral regurgitation due to degenerative disease. *Circulation* 127:1485–1492, 2013.
128. Enriquez-Sarano M, Schaff HV, Orszulak TA, et al: Valve repair improves the outcome of surgery for mitral regurgitation. A multivariate analysis. *Circulation* 91:1022–1028, 1995.
129. Mohty D, Orszulak TA, Schaff HV, et al: Very long-term survival and durability of mitral valve repair for mitral valve prolapse. *Circulation* 104:I1–I7, 2001.
130. DiBardino DJ, ElBardissi AW, McClure RS, et al: Four decades of experience with mitral valve repair: analysis of differential indications, technical evolution, and long-term outcome. *J Thorac Cardiovasc Surg* 139:76–83, discussion 83–84, 2010.
131. Gillinov AM, Blackstone EH, Nowicki ER, et al: Valve repair versus valve replacement for degenerative mitral valve disease. *J Thorac Cardiovasc Surg* 135:885–893, 893 e881–882, 2008.
132. Gaur P, Kaneko T, McGurk S, et al: Mitral valve repair versus replacement in the elderly: short-term and long-term outcomes. *J Thorac Cardiovasc Surg* 148:1400–1406, 2014.
133. Chikwe J, Goldstone AB, Passage J, et al: A propensity score-adjusted retrospective comparison of early and mid-term results of mitral valve repair versus replacement in octogenarians. *Eur Heart J* 32:618–626, 2011.
134. Gillinov AM, Faber C, Houghtaling PL, et al: Repair versus replacement for degenerative mitral valve disease with coexisting ischemic heart disease. *J Thorac Cardiovasc Surg* 125:1350–1362, 2003.
135. Enriquez-Sarano M, Schaff HV, Orszulak TA, et al: Congestive heart failure after surgical correction of mitral regurgitation. A long-term study. *Circulation* 92:2496–2503, 1995.
136. Mohty D, Enriquez-Sarano M: The long-term outcome of mitral valve repair for mitral valve prolapse. *Curr Cardiol Rep* 4:104–110, 2002.
137. Sand ME, Naftel DC, Blackstone EH, et al: A comparison of repair and replacement for mitral valve incompetence. *J Thorac Cardiovasc Surg* 94:208–219, 1987.
138. Stulak JM, Suri RM, Dearani JA, et al: Does early surgical intervention improve left ventricular mass regression after mitral valve repair for leaflet prolapse? *J Thorac Cardiovasc Surg* 141:122–129, 2011.
139. Senechal M, MacHaalany J, Bertrand OF, et al: Predictors of left ventricular remodeling after surgical repair or replacement for pure severe mitral regurgitation caused by leaflet prolapse. *Am J Cardiol* 112:567–573, 2013.
140. Gaasch WH, Zile MR: Left ventricular function after surgical correction of chronic mitral regurgitation. *Eur Heart J* 12(Suppl B):48–51, 1991.
141. Quintana E, Suri RM, Thalji NM, et al: Left ventricular dysfunction after mitral valve repair-the fallacy of "normal" preoperative myocardial function. *J Thorac Cardiovasc Surg* 148:2752–2760, 2014.
142. Gillinov AM, Cosgrove DM, Lytle BW, et al: Reoperation for failure of mitral valve repair. *J Thorac Cardiovasc Surg* 113:467–473, discussion 473–475, 1997.
143. Cerfolio RJ, Orzulak TA, Pluth JR, et al: Reoperation after valve repair for mitral regurgitation: early and intermediate results. *J Thorac Cardiovasc Surg* 111:1177–1183, discussion 1183–1184, 1996.
144. Suri RM, Schaff HV, Dearani JA, et al: Recurrent mitral regurgitation after repair: should the mitral valve be re-repaired? *J Thorac Cardiovasc Surg* 132:1390–1397, 2006.
145. Anyanwu AC, Itagaki S, Varghese R, et al: Re-repair of the mitral valve as a primary strategy for early and late failures of mitral valve repair. *Eur J Cardiothorac Surg* 45:352–357, discussion 357–358, 2014.
146. Castillo JG, Anyanwu AC, Fuster V, et al: A near 100% repair rate for mitral valve prolapse is achievable in a reference center: implications for future guidelines. *J Thorac Cardiovasc Surg* 144:308–312, 2012.
147. Fix J, Isada L, Cosgrove D, et al: Do patients with less than 'echo-perfect' results from mitral valve repair by intraoperative echocardiography have a different outcome? *Circulation* 88:II39–II48, 1993.
148. Saiki Y, Kasegawa H, Kawase M, et al: Intraoperative TEE during mitral valve repair: does it predict early and late postoperative mitral valve dysfunction? *Ann Thorac Surg* 66:1277–1281, 1998.
149. Badhwar V, Peterson ED, Jacobs JP, et al: Longitudinal outcome of isolated mitral repair in older patients: results from 14,604 procedures performed from 1991 to 2007. *Ann Thorac Surg* 94:1870–1877, discussion 1877–1879, 2012.
150. Gillinov AM, Blackstone EH, Alaulaqi A, et al: Outcomes after repair of the anterior mitral leaflet for degenerative disease. *Ann Thorac Surg* 86:708–717, discussion 708–717, 2008.
151. Adams DH, Rosenhek R, Falk V: Degenerative mitral valve regurgitation: best practice revolution. *Eur Heart J* 31:1958–1966, 2010.
152. Castillo JG, Anyanwu AC, El-Eshmawi A, et al: All anterior and bileaflet mitral valve prolapses are repairable in the modern era of reconstructive surgery. *Eur J Cardiothorac Surg* 45:139–145, discussion 145, 2014.
153. Suri RM, Schaff HV, Dearani JA, et al: Survival advantage and improved durability of mitral repair for leaflet prolapse subsets in the current era. *Ann Thorac Surg* 82:819–826, 2006.
154. Lawrie GM, Earle EA, Earle N: Intermediate-term results of a nonresectional dynamic repair technique in 662 patients with mitral valve prolapse and mitral regurgitation. *J Thorac Cardiovasc Surg* 141:368–376, 2011.
155. Orszulak TA, Schaff HV, Danielson GK, et al: Mitral regurgitation due to ruptured chordae tendineae. Early and late results of valve repair. *J Thorac Cardiovasc Surg* 89:491–498, 1985.
156. Phillips MR, Daly RC, Schaff HV, et al: Repair of anterior leaflet mitral valve prolapse: chordal replacement versus chordal shortening. *Ann Thorac Surg* 69:25–29, 2000.
157. Falk V, Seeburger J, Czesla M, et al: How does the use of polytetrafluoroethylene neochordae for posterior mitral valve prolapse (loop technique) compare with leaflet resection? A prospective randomized trial. *J Thorac Cardiovasc Surg* 136:1205, discussion 1205–1206, 2008.
158. Grossi EA, Galloway AC, Parish MA, et al: Experience with twenty-eight cases of systolic anterior motion after mitral valve reconstruction by the Carpentier technique. *J Thorac Cardiovasc Surg* 103:466–470, 1992.
159. Galler M, Kronzon I, Slater J, et al: Long-term follow-up after mitral valve reconstruction: incidence of postoperative left ventricular outflow obstruction. *Circulation* 74:I99–I103, 1986.
160. Varghese R, Itagaki S, Anyanwu AC, et al: Predicting systolic anterior motion after mitral valve reconstruction: using intraoperative transoesophageal echocardiography to identify those at greatest risk. *Eur J Cardiothorac Surg* 45:132–137, discussion 137–138, 2014.
161. Grossi EA, Steinberg BM, LeBoutillier M, 3rd, et al: Decreasing incidence of systolic anterior motion after mitral valve reconstruction. *Circulation* 90:II195–II197, 1994.
162. Abicht TO, Andrei AC, Kruse J, et al: A simple approach to mitral valve repair: posterior leaflet height adjustment using a partial fold of the free edge. *J Thorac Cardiovasc Surg* 148:2780–2786, 2014.
163. Dumont E, Gillinov AM, Blackstone EH, et al: Reoperation after mitral valve repair for degenerative disease. *Ann Thorac Surg* 84:444–450, discussion 450, 2007.
164. Zegdi R, Sleilaty G, Latremouille C, et al: Reoperation for failure of mitral valve repair in degenerative disease: a single-center experience. *Ann Thorac Surg* 86:1480–1484, 2008.
165. Thourani VH, Weintraub WS, Craver JM, et al: Influence of concomitant CABG and urgent/emergent status on mitral valve replacement surgery. *Ann Thorac Surg* 70:778–783, discussion 783–784, 2000.
166. Chan V, Ahrari A, Ruel M, et al: Perioperative deaths after mitral valve operations may be overestimated by contemporary risk models. *Ann Thorac Surg* 98:605–610, 2014.

167. Ozdemir AC, Emrecan B, Baltalarli A: Bileaflet versus posterior-leaflet-only preservation in mitral valve replacement. *Tex Heart Inst J* 41:165–169, 2014.
168. Toole JM, Stroud MR, Kratz JM, et al: Twenty-five year experience with the St. Jude medical mechanical valve prosthesis. *Ann Thorac Surg* 89:1402–1409, 2010.
169. Gammie JS, Sheng S, Griffith BP, et al: Trends in mitral valve surgery in the United States: results from the Society of Thoracic Surgeons Adult Cardiac Surgery Database. *Ann Thorac Surg* 87:1431–1437, discussion 1437–1439, 2009.
170. Vassileva CM, Mishkel G, McNeely C, et al: Long-term survival of patients undergoing mitral valve repair and replacement: a longitudinal analysis of Medicare fee-for-service beneficiaries. *Circulation* 127:1870–1876, 2013.
171. Grossi EA, Galloway AC, Miller JS, et al: Valve repair versus replacement for mitral insufficiency: when is a mechanical valve still indicated? *J Thorac Cardiovasc Surg* 115:389–394, discussion 394–396, 1998.
172. Hammermeister K, Sethi GK, Henderson WG, et al: Outcomes 15 years after valve replacement with a mechanical versus a bioprosthetic valve: final report of the Veterans Affairs randomized trial. *J Am Coll Cardiol* 36:1152–1158, 2000.
173. Sidhu P, O'Kane H, Ali N, et al: Mechanical or bioprosthetic valves in the elderly: a 20-year comparison. *Ann Thorac Surg* 71:S257–S260, 2001.
174. Badhwar V, Ofenloch JC, Rovin JD, et al: Noninferiority of closely monitored mechanical valves to bioprostheses overshadowed by early mortality benefit in younger patients. *Ann Thorac Surg* 93:748–753, 2012.
175. Blackstone EH, Kirklin JW: Death and other time-related events after valve replacement. *Circulation* 72:753–767, 1985.
176. Thourani VH, Weintraub WS, Guyton RA, et al: Outcomes and long-term survival for patients undergoing mitral valve repair versus replacement: effect of age and concomitant coronary artery bypass grafting. *Circulation* 108:298–304, 2003.
177. Birkmeyer NJ, Marrin CA, Morton JR, et al: Decreasing mortality for aortic and mitral valve surgery in Northern New England. Northern New England Cardiovascular Disease Study Group. *Ann Thorac Surg* 70:432–437, 2000.
178. Dodson JA, Wang Y, Desai MM, et al: Outcomes for mitral valve surgery among Medicare fee-for-service beneficiaries, 1999 to 2008. *Circ Cardiovasc Qual Outcomes* 5:298–307, 2012.
179. Spencer FC, Galloway AC, Colvin SB: A clinical evaluation of the hypothesis that rupture of the left ventricle following mitral valve replacement can be prevented by preservation of the chordae of the mural leaflet. *Ann Surg* 202:673–680, 1985.
180. Okita Y, Miki S, Ueda Y, et al: Left ventricular function after mitral valve replacement with or without chordal preservation. *J Heart Valve Dis* 4(Suppl 2):S181–S192, discussion S192–193, 1995.
181. Kaneko T, Aranki S, Javed Q, et al: Mechanical versus bioprosthetic mitral valve replacement in patients <65 years old. *J Thorac Cardiovasc Surg* 147:117–126, 2014.
182. Borger MA, Yau TM, Rao V, et al: Reoperative mitral valve replacement: importance of preservation of the subvalvular apparatus. *Ann Thorac Surg* 74:1482–1487, 2002.
183. Cohn LH, Aranki SF, Rizzo RJ, et al: Decrease in operative risk of reoperative valve surgery. *Ann Thorac Surg* 56:15–20, discussion 20–21, 1993.
184. Schuler G, Peterson KL, Johnson A, et al: Temporal response of left ventricular performance to mitral valve surgery. *Circulation* 59:1218–1231, 1979.
185. Hansen DE, Cahill PD, DeCampli WM, et al: Valvular-ventricular interaction: importance of the mitral apparatus in canine left ventricular systolic performance. *Circulation* 73:1310–1320, 1986.
186. Rozich JD, Carabello BA, Usher BW, et al: Mitral valve replacement with and without chordal preservation in patients with chronic mitral regurgitation. Mechanisms for differences in postoperative ejection performance. *Circulation* 86:1718–1726, 1992.
187. Smerup M, Funder J, Nyboe C, et al: Strut chordal-sparing mitral valve replacement preserves long-term left ventricular shape and function in pigs. *J Thorac Cardiovasc Surg* 130:1675–1682, 2005.
188. David TE, Burns RJ, Bacchus CM, et al: Mitral valve replacement for mitral regurgitation with and without preservation of chordae tendineae. *J Thorac Cardiovasc Surg* 88:718–725, 1984.
189. Miki S, Kusuhara K, Ueda Y, et al: Mitral valve replacement with preservation of chordae tendineae and papillary muscles. *Ann Thorac Surg* 45:28–34, 1988.
190. Edmunds LH, Jr: Thrombotic and bleeding complications of prosthetic heart valves. *Ann Thorac Surg* 44:430–445, 1987.
191. Silber H, Khan SS, Matloff JM, et al: The St. Jude valve. Thrombolysis as the first line of therapy for cardiac valve thrombosis. *Circulation* 87:30–37, 1993.
192. Manteiga R, Carlos Souto J, Altes A, et al: Short-course thrombolysis as the first line of therapy for cardiac valve thrombosis. *J Thorac Cardiovasc Surg* 115:780–784, 1998.
193. Durrleman N, Pellerin M, Bouchard D, et al: Prosthetic valve thrombosis: twenty-year experience at the Montreal Heart Institute. *J Thorac Cardiovasc Surg* 127:1388–1392, 2004.
194. Grunkemeier GL, Li HH, Naftel DC, et al: Long-term performance of heart valve prostheses. *Curr Probl Cardiol* 25:73–154, 2000.
195. Bernal JM, Rabasa JM, Cagigas JC, et al: Valve-related complications with the Hancock I porcine bioprosthesis. A twelve- to fourteen-year follow-up study. *J Thorac Cardiovasc Surg* 101:871–880, 1991.
196. Corbineau H, Du Haut Cilly FB, Langanay T, et al: Structural durability in Carpentier Edwards Standard bioprosthesis in the mitral position: a 20-year experience. *J Heart Valve Dis* 10:443–448, 2001.
197. Borger MA, Ivanov J, Armstrong S, et al: Twenty-year results of the Hancock II bioprosthesis. *J Heart Valve Dis* 15:49–55, discussion 55–56, 2006.
198. Dhasmana JP, Blackstone EH, Kirklin JW, et al: Factors associated with periprosthetic leakage following primary mitral valve replacement: with special consideration of the suture technique. *Ann Thorac Surg* 35:170–178, 1983.
199. Ahmad R, Manohitharajah SM, Deverall PB, et al: Chronic hemolysis following mitral valve replacement. A comparative study of the Bjork-Shiley, composite-seat Starr-Edwards, and frame-mounted aortic homograft valves. *J Thorac Cardiovasc Surg* 71:212–217, 1976.
200. Genoni M, Franzen D, Vogt P, et al: Paravalvular leakage after mitral valve replacement: improved long-term survival with aggressive surgery? *Eur J Cardiothorac Surg* 17:14–19, 2000.
201. Baumgartner WA, Miller DC, Reitz BA, et al: Surgical treatment of prosthetic valve endocarditis. *Ann Thorac Surg* 35:87–104, 1983.
202. Ivert TS, Dismukes WE, Cobbs CG, et al: Prosthetic valve endocarditis. *Circulation* 69:223–232, 1984.
203. Grossi EA, LaPietra A, Ribakove GH, et al: Minimally invasive versus sternotomy approaches for mitral reconstruction: comparison of intermediate-term results. *J Thorac Cardiovasc Surg* 121:708–713, 2001.
204. Iribarne A, Russo MJ, Easterwood R, et al: Minimally invasive versus sternotomy approach for mitral valve surgery: a propensity analysis. *Ann Thorac Surg* 90:1471–1477, discussion 1477–1478, 2010.
205. Dogan S, Aybek T, Risteski PS, et al: Minimally invasive port access versus conventional mitral valve surgery: prospective randomized study. *Ann Thorac Surg* 79:492–498, 2005.
206. Modi P, Hassan A, Chitwood WR, Jr: Minimally invasive mitral valve surgery: a systematic review and meta-analysis. *Eur J Cardiothorac Surg* 34:943–952, 2008.
207. Cheng DC, Martin J, Lal A, et al: Minimally invasive versus conventional open mitral valve surgery: a meta-analysis and systematic review. *Innovations (Phila)* 6:84–103, 2011.
208. Mohr FW, Falk V, Diegeler A, et al: Minimally invasive port-access mitral valve surgery. *J Thorac Cardiovasc Surg* 115:567–574, discussion 574–576, 1998.
209. Grossi EA, Galloway AC, Ribakove GH, et al: Minimally invasive port access surgery reduces operative morbidity for valve replacement in the elderly. *Heart Surg Forum* 2:212–215, 1999.
210. Bolotin G, Kypson AP, Reade CC, et al: Should a video-assisted mini-thoracotomy be the approach of choice for reoperative mitral valve surgery? *J Heart Valve Dis* 13:155–158, discussion 158, 2004.
211. Felger JE, Chitwood WR, Jr, Nifong LW, et al: Evolution of mitral valve surgery: toward a totally endoscopic approach. *Ann Thorac Surg* 72:1203–1208, discussion 1208–1209, 2001.

212. Woo YJ, Nacke EA: Robotic minimally invasive mitral valve reconstruction yields less blood product transfusion and shorter length of stay. *Surgery* 140:263–267, 2006.
213. Richardson L, Richardson M, Hunter S: Is a port-access mitral valve repair superior to the sternotomy approach in accelerating postoperative recovery? *Interact Cardiovasc Thorac Surg* 7:678–683, 2008.
214. Horvath KA, Acker MA, Chang H, et al: Blood transfusion and infection after cardiac surgery. *Ann Thorac Surg* 95:2194–2201, 2013.
215. Glower DD, Landolfo KP, Clements F, et al: Mitral valve operation via Port Access versus median sternotomy. *Eur J Cardiothorac Surg* 14(Suppl 1):S143–S147, 1998.
216. Walther T, Falk V, Metz S, et al: Pain and quality of life after minimally invasive versus conventional cardiac surgery. *Ann Thorac Surg* 67:1643–1647, 1999.
217. Mihaljevic T, Cohn LH, Unic D, et al: One thousand minimally invasive valve operations: early and late results. *Ann Surg* 240:529–534, discussion 534, 2004.
218. Iribarne A, Easterwood R, Russo MJ, et al: Comparative effectiveness of minimally invasive versus traditional sternotomy mitral valve surgery in elderly patients. *J Thorac Cardiovasc Surg* 143:S86–S90, 2012.
219. Santana O, Reyna J, Grana R, et al: Outcomes of minimally invasive valve surgery versus standard sternotomy in obese patients undergoing isolated valve surgery. *Ann Thorac Surg* 91:406–410, 2011.
220. Casselman FP, Van Slycke S, Dom H, et al: Endoscopic mitral valve repair: feasible, reproducible, and durable. *J Thorac Cardiovasc Surg* 125:273–282, 2003.
221. Vleissis AA, Bolling SF: Mini-reoperative mitral valve surgery. *J Card Surg* 13:468–470, 1998.
222. Iribarne A, Easterwood R, Russo MJ, et al: A minimally invasive approach is more cost-effective than a traditional sternotomy approach for mitral valve surgery. *J Thorac Cardiovasc Surg* 142:1507–1514, 2011.
223. Mihaljevic T, Jarrett CM, Gillinov AM, et al: Robotic repair of posterior mitral valve prolapse versus conventional approaches: potential realized. *J Thorac Cardiovasc Surg* 141:72–80, e71–74, 2011.
224. Nifong LW, Rodriguez E, Chitwood WR, Jr: 540 consecutive robotic mitral valve repairs including concomitant atrial fibrillation cryoablation. *Ann Thorac Surg* 94:38–42, discussion 43, 2012.
225. Chitwood WR, Jr, Rodriguez E, Chu MW, et al: Robotic mitral valve repairs in 300 patients: a single-center experience. *J Thorac Cardiovasc Surg* 136:436–441, 2008.
226. Suri RM, Burkhart HM, Rehfeldt KH, et al: Robotic mitral valve repair for all categories of leaflet prolapse: improving patient appeal and advancing standard of care. *Mayo Clin Proc* 86:838–844, 2011.
227. Holzhey DM, Seeburger J, Misfeld M, et al: Learning minimally invasive mitral valve surgery: a cumulative sum sequential probability analysis of 3895 operations from a single high-volume center. *Circulation* 128:483–491, 2013.
228. Feldman T, Foster E, Glower DD, et al: Percutaneous repair or surgery for mitral regurgitation. *N Engl J Med* 364:1395–1406, 2011.
229. Mauri L, Foster E, Glower DD, et al: 4-year results of a randomized controlled trial of percutaneous repair versus surgery for mitral regurgitation. *J Am Coll Cardiol* 62:317–328, 2013.
230. Miller DC, Oyer PE, Stinson EB, et al: Ten to fifteen year reassessment of the performance characteristics of the Starr-Edwards Model 6120 mitral valve prosthesis. *J Thorac Cardiovasc Surg* 85:1–20, 1983.
231. Agathos EA, Starr A: Mitral valve replacement. *Curr Probl Surg* 30:481–592, 1993.
232. Godje OL, Fischlein T, Adelhard K, et al: Thirty-year results of Starr-Edwards prostheses in the aortic and mitral position. *Ann Thorac Surg* 63:613–619, 1997.
233. Akins CW: Mechanical cardiac valvular prostheses. *Ann Thorac Surg* 52:161–172, 1991.
234. Antunes MJ, Wessels A, Sadowski RG, et al: Medtronic Hall valve replacement in a third-world population group. A review of the performance of 1000 prostheses. *J Thorac Cardiovasc Surg* 95:980–993, 1988.
235. Butchart EG, Li HH, Payne N, et al: Twenty years' experience with the Medtronic Hall valve. *J Thorac Cardiovasc Surg* 121:1090–1100, 2001.
236. di Summa M, Poletti G, Brero L, et al: Long-term outcome after valve replacement with the omnicarbon prosthesis. *J Heart Valve Dis* 11:517–523, 2002.
237. Akalin H, Corapcioglu ET, Ozyurda U, et al: Clinical evaluation of the Omniscience cardiac valve prosthesis. Follow-up of up to 6 years. *J Thorac Cardiovasc Surg* 103:259–266, 1992.
238. Damle A, Coles J, Teijeira J, et al: A six-year study of the Omniscience valve in four Canadian centers. *Ann Thorac Surg* 43:513–521, 1987.
239. Otaki M, Kitamura N: Six years' experience with the Omnicarbon valve prosthesis. *Cardiovasc Surg* 1:594–598, 1993.
240. Remadi JP, Baron O, Roussel C, et al: Isolated mitral valve replacement with St. Jude medical prosthesis: long-term results: a follow-up of 19 years. *Circulation* 103:1542–1545, 2001.
241. Kratz JM, Crawford FA, Jr, Sade RM, et al: St. Jude prosthesis for aortic and mitral valve replacement: a ten-year experience. *Ann Thorac Surg* 56:462–468, 1993.
242. Emery RW, Krogh CC, Arom KV, et al: The St. Jude Medical cardiac valve prosthesis: a 25-year experience with single valve replacement. *Ann Thorac Surg* 79:776–782, discussion 782–783, 2005.
243. Aoyagi S, Oryoji A, Nishi Y, et al: Long-term results of valve replacement with the St. Jude Medical valve. *J Thorac Cardiovasc Surg* 108:1021–1029, 1994.
244. Wu Y, Gao G, Mody S, et al: Update of the Providence Health System experience with the CarboMedics prosthesis. *J Heart Valve Dis* 15:414–420, 2006.
245. Jamieson WR, Fradet GJ, Miyagishima RT, et al: CarboMedics mechanical prosthesis: performance at eight years. *J Heart Valve Dis* 9:678–687, 2000.
246. de Luca L, Vitale N, Giannolo B, et al: Mid-term follow-up after heart valve replacement with CarboMedics bileaflet prostheses. *J Thorac Cardiovasc Surg* 106:1158–1165, 1993.
247. Nistal JF, Hurle A, Revuelta JM, et al: Clinical experience with the CarboMedics valve: early results with a new bileaflet mechanical prosthesis. *J Thorac Cardiovasc Surg* 112:59–68, 1996.
248. Emery RW, Krogh CC, Jones DJ, et al: Five-year follow up of the ATS mechanical heart valve. *J Heart Valve Dis* 13:231–238, 2004.
249. Stefanidis C, Nana AM, De Canniere D, et al: 10-year experience with the ATS mechanical valve in the mitral position. *Ann Thorac Surg* 79:1934–1938, 2005.
250. Puskas J, Gerdisch M, Nichols D, et al: Reduced anticoagulation after mechanical aortic valve replacement: interim results from the prospective randomized on-X valve anticoagulation clinical trial randomized Food and Drug Administration investigational device exemption trial. *J Thorac Cardiovasc Surg* 147:1202–1210, discussion 1210–1211, 2014.
251. Laczkovics A, Heidt M, Oelert H, et al: Early clinical experience with the On-X prosthetic heart valve. *J Heart Valve Dis* 10:94–99, 2001.
252. McNicholas KW, Ivey TD, Metras J, et al: North American multicenter experience with the On-X prosthetic heart valve. *J Heart Valve Dis* 15:73–78, discussion 79, 2006.
253. Perier P, Deloche A, Chauvaud S, et al: A 10-year comparison of mitral valve replacement with Carpentier-Edwards and Hancock porcine bioprostheses. *Ann Thorac Surg* 48:54–59, 1989.
254. Cohn LH, Collins JJ, Jr, DiSesa VJ, et al: Fifteen-year experience with 1678 Hancock porcine bioprosthetic heart valve replacements. *Ann Surg* 210:435–442, discussion 442–443, 1989.
255. Rizzoli G, Bottio T, Thiene G, et al: Long-term durability of the Hancock II porcine bioprosthesis. *J Thorac Cardiovasc Surg* 126:66–74, 2003.
256. Jamieson WR, Munro AI, Miyagishima RT, et al: The Carpentier-Edwards supra-annular porcine bioprosthesis: new generation low pressure glutaraldehyde fixed prosthesis. *J Card Surg* 3:507–521, 1988.
257. Akins CW, Carroll DL, Buckley MJ, et al: Late results with Carpentier-Edwards porcine bioprosthesis. *Circulation* 82:IV65–IV74, 1990.
258. Aupart MR, Neville PH, Hammami S, et al: Carpentier-Edwards pericardial valves in the mitral position: ten-year follow-up. *J Thorac Cardiovasc Surg* 113:492–498, 1997.

259. Poirer NC, Pelletier LC, Pellerin M, et al: 15-year experience with the Carpentier-Edwards pericardial bioprosthesis. *Ann Thorac Surg* 66:S57–S61, 1998.
260. Fradet GJ, Bleese N, Burgess J, et al: Mosaic valve international clinical trial: early performance results. *Ann Thorac Surg* 71:S273–S277, 2001.
261. Thomson DJ, Jamieson WR, Dumesnil JG, et al: Medtronic Mosaic porcine bioprosthesis: midterm investigational trial results. *Ann Thorac Surg* 71:S269–S272, 2001.
262. Myken PS: Seventeen-year experience with the St. Jude medical biocor porcine bioprosthesis. *J Heart Valve Dis* 14:486–492, 2005.
263. Rizzoli G, Bottio T, Vida V, et al: Intermediate results of isolated mitral valve replacement with a Biocor porcine valve. *J Thorac Cardiovasc Surg* 129:322–329, 2005.
264. Pyle RB, Mayer JE, Jr, Lindsay WG, et al: Hemodynamic evaluation of Lillehei-Kaiser and Starr-Edwards prosthesis. *Ann Thorac Surg* 26:336–343, 1978.
265. Sala A, Schoevaerdts JC, Jaumin P, et al: Review of 387 isolated mitral valve replacements by the Model 6120 Starr-Edwards prosthesis. *J Thorac Cardiovasc Surg* 84:744–750, 1982.
266. Hall KV, Nitter-Hauge S, Abdelnoor M: Seven and one-half years' experience with the Medtronic-Hall valve. *J Am Coll Cardiol* 6:1417–1421, 1985.
267. Fiore AC, Barner HB, Swartz MT, et al: Mitral valve replacement: randomized trial of St. Jude and Medtronic Hall prostheses. *Ann Thorac Surg* 66:707–712, discussion 712–713, 1998.
268. Messner-Pellenc P, Wittenberg O, Leclercq F, et al: Doppler echocardiographic evaluation of the Omnicarbon cardiac valve prostheses. *J Cardiovasc Surg (Torino)* 34:195–202, 1993.
269. Fehske W, Kessel D, Kirchhoff PG, et al: Echocardiographic profile of the normally functioning Omnicarbon valve. *J Heart Valve Dis* 3:263–274, 1994.
270. Chaux A, Gray RJ, Matloff JM, et al: An appreciation of the new St. Jude valvular prosthesis. *J Thorac Cardiovasc Surg* 81:202–211, 1981.
271. Hasegawa M: Clinical evaluation of ATS prosthetic valve by doppler echocardiography: comparison with St. Jude Medical (SJM) valve. *Ann Thorac Cardiovasc Surg* 6:247–251, 2000.
272. Chambers J, Cross J, Deverall P, et al: Echocardiographic description of the CarboMedics bileaflet prosthetic heart valve. *J Am Coll Cardiol* 21:398–405, 1993.
273. Carrier M, Pellerin M, Basmadjian A, et al: Fifteen years of clinical and echocardiographic follow up with the carbomedics heart valve. *J Heart Valve Dis* 15:67–72, discussion 72, 2006.
274. Aris A, Padro JM, Camara ML, et al: Clinical and hemodynamic results of cardiac valve replacement with the Monostrut Bjork-Shiley prosthesis. *J Thorac Cardiovasc Surg* 95:423–431, 1988.
275. Emery RW, Petersen RJ, Kersten TE, et al: The initial United States experience with the ATS mechanical cardiac valve prosthesis. *Heart Surg Forum* 4:346–352, discussion 352–353, 2001.
276. Westaby S, Van Nooten G, Sharif H, et al: Valve replacement with the ATS open pivot bileaflet prosthesis. *Eur J Cardiothorac Surg* 10:660–665, 1996.
277. Khuri SF, Folland ED, Sethi GK, et al: Six month postoperative hemodynamics of the Hancock heterograft and the Bjork-Shiley prosthesis: results of a Veterans Administration cooperative prospective randomized trial. *J Am Coll Cardiol* 12:8–18, 1988.
278. Johnson AD, Daily PO, Peterson KL, et al: Functional evaluation of the porcine heterograft in the mitral position. *Circulation* 52:I40–I48, 1975.
279. Pelletier C, Chaitman BR, Baillot R, et al: Clinical and hemodynamic results with the Carpentier-Edwards porcine bioprosthesis. *Ann Thorac Surg* 34:612–624, 1982.
280. Levine FH, Carter JE, Buckley MJ, et al: Hemodynamic evaluation of Hancock and Carpentier-Edwards bioprostheses. *Circulation* 64:II192–II195, 1981.
281. Chaitman BR, Bonan R, Lepage G, et al: Hemodynamic evaluation of the Carpentier-Edwards porcine xenograft. *Circulation* 60:1170–1182, 1979.
282. David TE, Ivanov J, Armstrong S, et al: Late results of heart valve replacement with the Hancock II bioprosthesis. *J Thorac Cardiovasc Surg* 121:268–277, 2001.
283. Jamieson WR, Munro AI, Miyagishima RT, et al: Carpentier-Edwards standard porcine bioprosthesis: clinical performance to seventeen years. *Ann Thorac Surg* 60:999–1006, discussion 1007, 1995.
284. Marchand M, Aupart M, Norton R, et al: Twelve-year experience with Carpentier-Edwards PERIMOUNT pericardial valve in the mitral position: a multicenter study. *J Heart Valve Dis* 7:292–298, 1998.
285. Myken P, Bech-Hanssen O, Phipps B, et al: Fifteen years follow up with the St. Jude Medical Biocor porcine bioprosthesis. *J Heart Valve Dis* 9:415–422, 2000.

CHAPTER 81

SURGICAL TREATMENT OF TRICUSPID VALVE DISEASES

Carlos A. Mestres • Jose M. Bernal • Jose L. Pomar

CHAPTER OUTLINE

The tricuspid valve is often ignored by cardiologists and surgeons because of its unique characteristics. It is frequently called "The Forgotten Valve," and there still is scant information regarding the effects of tricuspid valve diseases on the prognosis of cardiac patients.[1,2] With the exception of infective endocarditis, primary isolated lesions of the tricuspid valve are rare. There are just a few reports on isolated congenital, rheumatic, tumoral, or ischemic diseases. Frequently, the prominent effect of other valve diseases minimizes its importance. Located at the entrance of the heart, the tricuspid valve, when diseased, produces symptoms that are primarily extracardiac and often silent. The behavior of the tricuspid valve is closely related to the function of the right ventricle; in most cases, tricuspid regurgitation is secondary to right ventricular failure. It follows the dictates of the mitral valve; resolution of the mitral valve problem is often followed by improvement in the degree of tricuspid regurgitation. As the right heart is a low-pressure system, it is difficult to evaluate its preoperative importance and to assess the value of different surgical techniques. These characteristics often lead cardiologists and surgeons to ignore the tricuspid valve. However, the developments in diagnostic tools, and echocardiography in particular, have increased the awareness of this valve, which has been called the "Cinderella" of all cardiac valves.[3]

SURGICAL ANATOMY

Situated at the base of the heart, the tricuspid valve separates the right atrium from the right ventricle.

Traditionally, it has been accepted that the tricuspid valve consists of three very thin leaflets attached to the tricuspid valve annulus.

Tricuspid Valve Annulus

Whereas the base of the anterior and posterior leaflets is attached to the free wall of the right ventricle, the septal leaflet is inserted into the base of the interventricular septum. This line of leaflet attachment, known as the tricuspid valve annulus, is more a landmark than an actual fibrous ring. This absence of an encircling fibrotic structure explains the large changes in the tricuspid valve orifice during the cardiac cycle and its easy dilation in disease. The mobility and size of the tricuspid valve orifice are dependent on the transversely oriented myocardial fibers that surround the atrioventricular valves according to the breaking studies on anatomy and function by Torrent-Guasp and colleagues[4] and Buckberg and colleagues[5] over the past 15 years.[5] Tsakiris and associates[6] found in a canine model that the size of the tricuspid valve orifice changed continuously during the cardiac cycle. The orifice area contracted (from its maximal diastolic size) by 20% to 30%. Tei and associates[7] confirmed these findings in humans with echocardiography. Hiro and colleagues[8] and Jouan and colleagues,[9] working with Duran, analyzed an ovine model for the changes in the normal tricuspid valve orifice during the cardiac cycle as detected by the changes in distance between ultrasound crystals placed around the line of insertion of the leaflets (Fig. 81-1). The tricuspid valve orifice area expands and contracts twice during the cardiac cycle. Orifice contraction begins during the isovolumic relaxation phase of the cardiac cycle and continues through the first half of diastole. Starting with the beginning of isovolumic contraction, a second contraction occurs during ejection, which reduces the tricuspid valve orifice to its minimum area. This contraction corresponds to closure of the valve completed at the end of isovolumic contraction.

The reduction in orifice perimeter is not uniform. The segment of the annulus corresponding to the septal leaflet shortens by 12%, the anterior segment by 15%, and the posterior segment by 17%.[8] The dilation of the annulus occurs in the anterior and posterior segments, and the dilation of the septal segment is restricted because of the relationship with the cardiac fibrous skeleton.[10] This narrowing of the tricuspid valve orifice is due not only to contraction of its perimeter but, more important, to changes in the shape of the annulus. During contraction, the orifice becomes more elliptical because of displacement of the anteroposterior commissure toward the septum and the bulging of the septum. As in the mitral valve, the "annulus" is not in a single plane. In fact, the tricuspid valve annulus is saddle shaped, with its horn or pommel corresponding to the area of the anteroseptal commissure and its cantle to the midpoint of the base of the posterior leaflet (Fig. 81-2). This saddle shape or hyperbolic paraboloid, well known to architects as an ideal design to reduce building tension, has been shown in the mitral valve to significantly reduce peak leaflet stress.[11] Furthermore, the increase in the saddle shape during contraction has a "folding" and reducing effect on

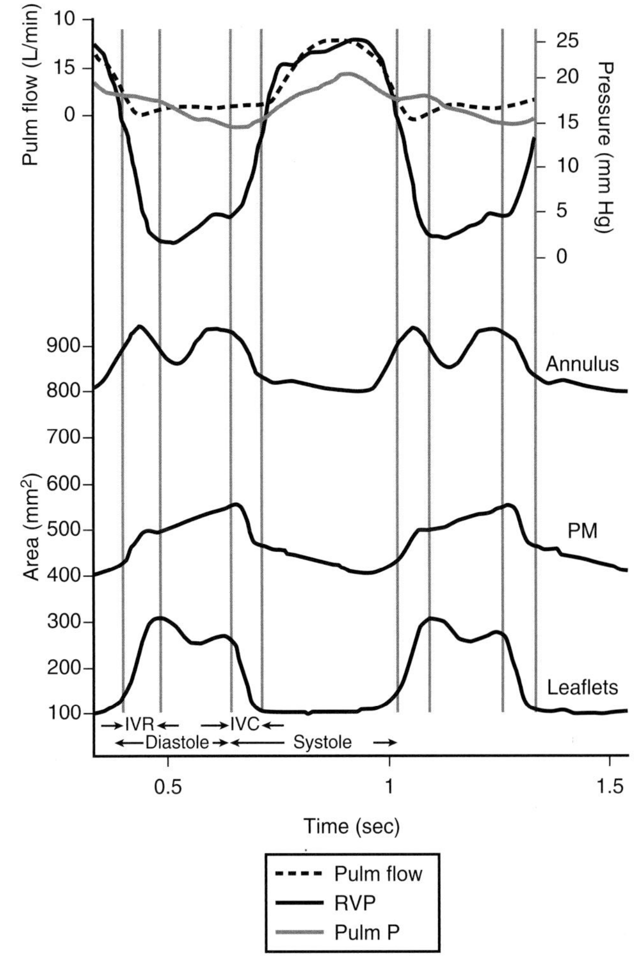

FIGURE 81-1 Changes in the normal tricuspid valve during the cardiac cycle. *Top,* Pressure curves of blood flow in the pulmonary artery (Pulm flow), the right ventricle (RVP), and the pulmonary artery (Pulm P). *Bottom,* Changes in the areas delineated by the ultrasound transducers placed around the tricuspid annulus (Annulus), the tips of the three papillary muscles (PM), and the free edges of the three leaflets (Leaflets) during two cardiac cycles. These recordings allowed the cardiac cycle to be split into diastole, systole, isovolumic contraction (IVC), and isovolumic relaxation (IVR). (Reproduced with permission from Jouan J, Pagel MR, Hiro ME, et al: Further information from a sonometric study of the normal tricuspid valve annulus in sheep: geometric changes during the cardiac cycle. *J Heart Valve Dis* 16:511–518, 2007.)

the normal tricuspid valve orifice. In cases of tricuspid regurgitation, besides an increase of tricuspid valve annulus area, there is an increase in planarity or flattening of the normal annulus, which induces leaflet tethering.[12] Rigid structures, such as stented prostheses and rigid annuloplasty rings, destroy this configuration and are likely to have a negative impact on the function of the right ventricle.

Leaflets

Although the number of tricuspid valve leaflets varies according to author,[13,14] it is generally accepted that the tricuspid valve consists of three leaflets. These three leaflets are known as *anterior, septal,* and *posterior,* and they

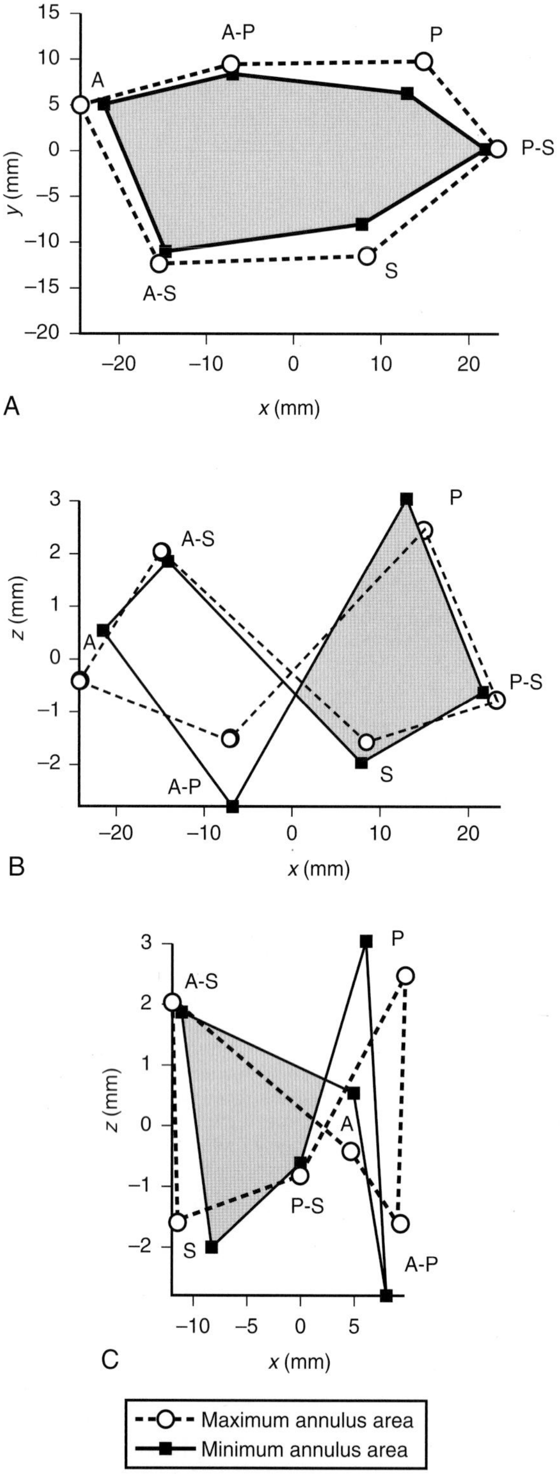

FIGURE 81-2 Geometric changes of the normal tricuspid valve annulus during the cardiac cycle. Orthogonal representations of the tricuspid valve annulus at maximum *(dotted line)* and minimum *(continuous line)* area during the cardiac cycle. *Circles* and *squares* represent the location of transducers at the midpoint of the bases of the anterior (A), posterior (P), and septal (S) leaflets and at the anteroposterior (A-P), anteroseptal (A-S), and posteroseptal (P-S) commissures. Two relative maxima can be noted in the *x-z* **(B)** and *y-z* **(C)** planes. P and A-S represent the pommel and the cantle of the tricuspid valve's saddle shape. The representation of the *x-y* plane is shown in **A.** (Reproduced with permission from Jouan J, Pagel MR, Hiro ME, et al: Further information from a sonometric study of the normal tricuspid valve annulus in sheep: geometric changes during the cardiac cycle. *J Heart Valve Dis* 16:511–518, 2007.)

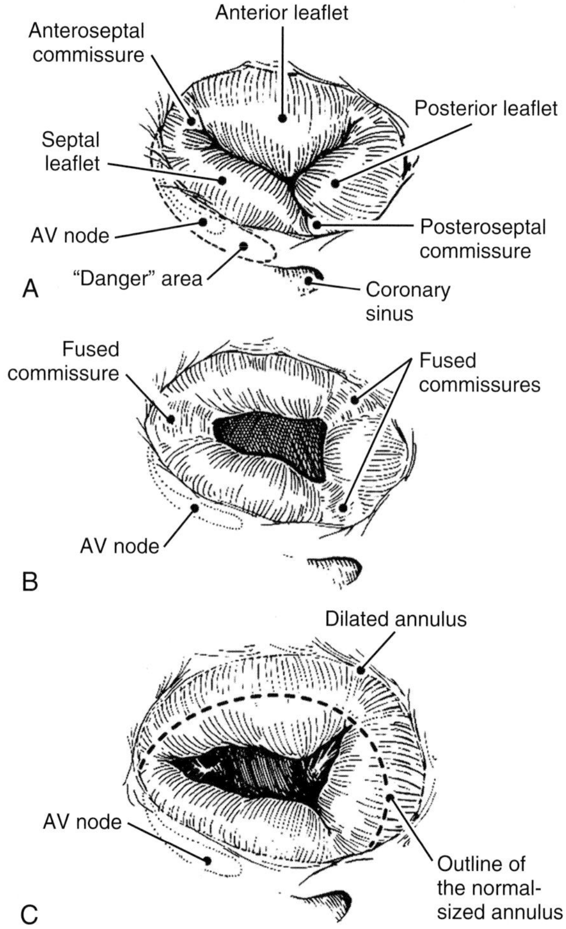

FIGURE 81-3 Atrial view of the normal **(A)**, stenotic **(B)**, and insufficient **(C)** tricuspid valve. *AV*, Atrioventricular. (Reproduced with permission from Duran CMG: Duran ring annuloplasty of the tricuspid valve. *Oper Tech Thorac Cardiovasc Surg* 8:201–212, 2003.)

are separated by three clefts or commissures named *anteroseptal*, *anteromedial*, and *posteroseptal* (Fig. 81-3*A*). These clefts do not reach the annulus but delineate small "commissural leaflets." This is an important surgical point because in cases of fused commissures, their incision should not extend all the way to the annulus; doing so destroys the commissural leaflets. The largest leaflet is the anterior, followed by the posterior, with the septal being the smallest. The excursion of each leaflet (defined as the angle between leaflet free edge and the plane of the annulus) is different.[9] The excursion of the septal leaflet is significantly smaller than that of the other leaflets. This normal, smaller septal excursion might explain the finding at surgery of a septal leaflet plastered against the septum. This finding, often seen in cases of functional regurgitation, is a sign of severity and is a predictor of a poor result after repair.

Chordae Tendineae and Papillary Muscles

The leaflets are held down by marginal and basal chords that arise from three papillary muscle groups. The marginal chords are inserted into the leaflets free margin, and the basal chords are inserted into the ventricular surface of the leaflets. Elongation or rupture of the marginal chords results in leaflet prolapse. The basal chords of the tricuspid valve, although far less prominent than the mitral valve basal chords, probably play a similar role in maintaining valvular and ventricular geometry. In most tricuspid valve cases, three papillary muscle groups are found and can be identified as anterior, posterior, and septal. Whereas the anterior and posterior muscles are virtually always present, the septal muscle might be absent in 20% of patients. The anterior papillary muscle is the longest; it most often has a single head and sustains the largest number of chordae.[15,16] Elegant anatomic studies by Victor and Nayak in hearts harvested at random confirm that every heart has a unique chordal configuration.[17]

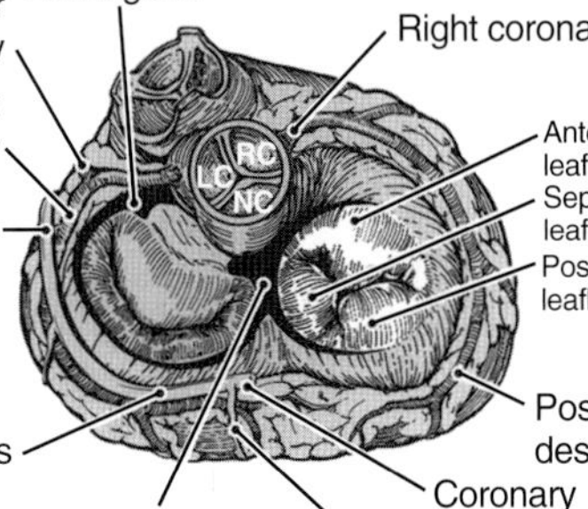

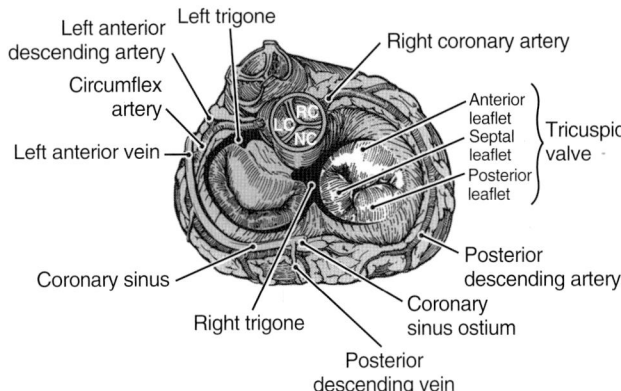

FIGURE 81-4 Base of the heart showing the anatomic relationships of the tricuspid valve. (Reproduced with permission from Duran CMG: Duran ring annuloplasty of the tricuspid valve. *Oper Tech Thorac Cardiovasc Surg* 8:201–212, 2003.)

Terminology

New surgical techniques demand deeper knowledge of the anatomy of the region and, consequently, more precise terminology. A common set of anatomic definitions is needed to report precise preoperative and postoperative echocardiographic information important to both the echocardiographer and the surgeon. Aiming to standardize all anatomic findings, Kumar and colleagues[18] developed a detailed tricuspid valve terminology that parallels previously described mitral valve nomenclature. Although it is based on a surgical, atrial view of the valve, their terminology encompasses all three elements of the tricuspid valve apparatus (i.e., leaflets, chords, and papillary muscles).[16]

This alphanumeric system is based on the three papillary muscle groups as defined by the numerals 1 for the anteroseptal, 2 for the posteroseptal, and 3 for the anteroposterior groups of muscles. Each leaflet is identified with the initial letter of its traditional name: *S*, septal; *A*, anterior; and *P*, posterior. Because the lesion does not often affect the whole leaflet or is limited to the chordae, each leaflet is divided into two areas identified by the papillary origin of the corresponding chords. For instance, the septal leaflet (S) is divided into two halves (S1 and S2), identified by the chords that originate from the anteroseptal papillary muscle[4] or the chords that originate from the posteroseptal papillary muscle.[6] The commissures (C) are identified by their papillary origin (1, 2, or 3) as C1, C2, and C3. All chords are identified by their papillary origin and leaflet insertion.

Although it is initially confusing, this nomenclature makes it possible to pinpoint the exact location of a lesion and to describe the surgical maneuvers applied. Its use is particularly significant for reporting of chordal disease and chordal replacement.

Anatomic Relationships

The area corresponding to the anteroseptal commissure is close to the aortic root noncoronary sinus of Valsalva (Fig. 81-4). This fact has important surgical implications because placement of anchoring sutures for a tricuspid valve prosthetic device can be difficult at this level if a stented aortic prosthesis is already present. When a concomitant aortic valve replacement is planned, it is preferable to place the tricuspid valve sutures before undertaking the aortic valve replacement, because tears at this level can be difficult to repair. Of course, the experience and expertise of the operating surgeon finally dictates the operative procedure.

The right coronary artery and sinus run parallel to the segment of the annulus corresponding to the right ventricular free wall. Despite this proximity, injury to these vascular structures in performing a valve replacement or annuloplasty is extremely rare. The ostium of the coronary sinus is situated above the posteroseptal commissure. Because of its distance from the conducting system (close to the right trigone), it is safe to place a pursestring suture around the ostium of the coronary sinus to hold a retrograde cardioplegia cannula. This simple anchoring technique described by Martinez-Leon and colleagues[19] more than 25 years ago allows for a reliable positioning of the retrograde cannula.

PATHOPHYSIOLOGY

Tricuspid valve lesions have traditionally been classified into two groups: organic and functional. These classifications have an important effect on both the type of surgery performed and its long-term results. Organic lesions are those in which the valve apparatus is macroscopically abnormal (see Fig. 81-3*B*). Functional lesions are those in which regurgitation occurs in the presence of an apparently normal tricuspid valve apparatus (see Fig. 81-3*C*).

A different classification, proposed by Carpentier[20] in relation to the pathology of the mitral valve, distinguishes three main types of disease according to the mobility of the tricuspid valve leaflets: type I, normal leaflet motion with annular dilation; type II, increased leaflet motion owing to leaflet prolapse that is secondary to chordal rupture or elongation; and type III, reduced leaflet motion due to leaflet thickening, fused commissures, or leaflet tethering.

BOX 81-1 Causes of Organic Tricuspid Valve Disease

Infective endocarditis
Rheumatic fever
Degenerative (myxomatous)
Traumatic damage
Postinfarction damage
Carcinoid
Appetite-suppressant drugs
Endocardial fibroelastosis
Lupus erythematosus
Tumors (myxoma)
Mediastinal fibrosis

Organic Tricuspid Valve Disease

A variety of etiologic factors can induce organic regurgitation, but still today the most frequent cause of organic tricuspid valve disease in urban populations is infective endocarditis (Box 81-1). Tricuspid valve endocarditis used to be relatively rare, with an incidence of only 5% to 10% of patients with infective endocarditis; however, its frequency dramatically increased with the spread of intravenous drug abuse,[21,22] with a peak incidence until early in the beginning of the twenty-first century.[23] In this population, the tricuspid valve usually has no preexisting pathologic change. The lesions vary from isolated vegetations to total destruction of the valve, including the annulus. *Staphylococcus aureus* remains the most common organism found in drug addicts, followed by gram-negative organisms and *Candida* species. Fungal infections are also increasing because of longer periods of invasive monitoring of patients with multiorgan failure in intensive care units.[24]

In the so-called developing world, rheumatic fever is the primary cause of organic valvular heart disease. Typical lesions show varying degrees of leaflet thickening and (most often) commissural fusion. In severe cases, the thickened leaflets become diaphragm-like, with a central circular orifice (see Fig. 81-3*B*). The subvalvular apparatus is seldom affected, and calcifications are rare. Although tricuspid valve stenosis is the classic lesion, predominant insufficiency is just as common. In a series of 253 patients with rheumatic heart disease who underwent tricuspid valve surgery, Prabhakar and colleagues[25] found that organic involvement was present in 45% of the cases and that 45% of them also had annulus dilation. In a classic study of 100 postmortem hearts with rheumatic disease, Gross and Friedberg[26] found microscopic evidence of inflammation in the annulus of all four valves (in the acute rheumatic attack). Rheumatic tricuspid valve disease is always associated with rheumatic mitral valve or mitral-aortic valve lesions. The incidence of chronic rheumatic tricuspid valve disease associated with rheumatic mitral valve disease varies widely, from 6% in an echocardiographic study[27] to 33% in an anatomic series[28] and 11% in the series of Prabhakar and colleagues[25] of 1052 patients undergoing rheumatic valvular surgery. In a Mayo Clinic surgical pathology study of excised tricuspid valves at the time of valve replacement,[29] postinflammatory etiology was responsible for 53% of the 363 valves studied. However, this frequency had diminished from 79% during the period from 1963 to 1967 to 24% during 1983 through 1987, reflecting the reduction in the incidence of rheumatic fever in the United States as it happened across Europe. Out of these regions, rheumatic heart disease is still a major epidemiologic problem. Leaflet tears and total or partial avulsion of a papillary muscle head occur after closed chest trauma. They are occasionally diagnosed at surgery and only classified postoperatively as traumatic by the patient, who recalls an old accident when prompted by the surgeon.[30-32] As imaging has greatly improved in the past two decades, traumatic tricuspid regurgitation is better diagnosed and characterized.[33-34]

An occasional cause of traumatic tricuspid regurgitation is that induced by the bioptome during a right myocardial biopsy in transplanted patients. Leaflet tears or chordal avulsion results in severe regurgitation that may require urgent surgery.[35-37]

Degenerative tricuspid regurgitation associated with mitral valve prolapse is being increasingly observed. This double valve lesion is particularly frequent in Marfan syndrome as a manifestation of a fibrillopathy that also involves the aortic valve and ascending aorta. The reported frequency of tricuspid valve involvement among patients with mitral valve myxomatous disease ranges between 21% and 52% at all ages.[12,38-40] Less common causes include organic tricuspid valve lesions secondary to carcinoid syndrome and appetite-suppressant drugs.[41-43] In both cases, the leaflets are encased by a fibrous sheath that reduces their mobility, resulting in stenotic and regurgitant lesions. Other rare causes are listed in Box 81-1.[44-53]

Functional Tricuspid Regurgitation

Functional tricuspid insufficiency is understood to be exclusively due to annulus dilation and dysfunction (see Fig. 81-3*C*). The leaflets, chords, and papillary muscles are otherwise normal. Because of the lack of an anatomic fibrous annulus, the tricuspid valve annulus follows the dilation of the right ventricle. The total perimeter of the normal annulus is approximately 100 to 120 mm. In cases of functional tricuspid regurgitation, the circumference of the annulus can reach 150 to 170 mm.[54-55] This annulus dilation is nonhomogeneous. In a postmortem study that included normal controls and hearts with rheumatic or myxomatous tricuspid valve disease, Carpentier and colleagues[56] showed that the anterior and posterior segments of the annulus dilated far more than the septal portion of the annulus (Fig. 81-5). This report, 40 years ago, formed the basis for all annuloplasties that selectively reduce the whole annulus except at the level of the septum. The role of the papillary muscles in this setting is debatable, although it can be considered a correctable influencing factor.[57]

In congestive heart failure, functional tricuspid regurgitation is a predictor of poor survival[58] and may be an independent risk factor for the development of cardiac cachexia and protein-losing enteropathy.[59] Cardiac cachexia continues to be a major risk factor in valvular

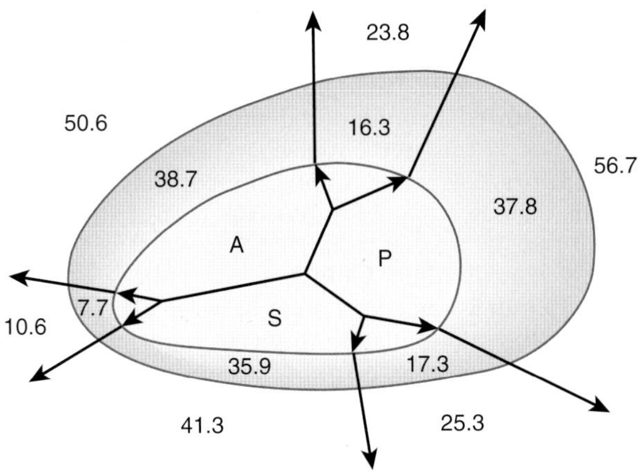

FIGURE 81-5 ■ Diagram of the tricuspid valve annulus showing the normal *(inner ellipse)* and myxomatous *(outer ellipse)* valve in centimeters. A, anterior leaflet; P, posterior leaflet; S, septal leaflet. (From Carpentier A, Deloche A, Hanania G, et al: Surgical management of acquired tricuspid valve disease. *J Thorac Cardiovasc Surg* 67:55, 1974, with permission from Excerpta Medica, Inc.)

surgery of any origin.[60] Koelling and colleagues[61] studied a total of 1436 patients with left ventricular systolic dysfunction (ejection fraction < 35%). Mitral regurgitation was moderate in 30% and severe in 19% of patients. Moderate tricuspid regurgitation was present in 23% and severe in 12% of patients. Patients with severe mitral regurgitation were more likely also to have tricuspid regurgitation. The association is clear and it is confirmed that the severity of tricuspid regurgitation is related to the degree of congestive heart failure.[62]

Advances in echocardiography have revealed another subvalvular mechanism that applies to both mitral and tricuspid functional regurgitations. Originally observed in functional ischemic mitral regurgitations, this mechanism also applies to the ischemic tricuspid valve and most probably to all functional insufficiencies.[57] Right or left ventricular remodeling induces a lateral displacement of one or more papillary muscles that apically pulls through the basal chords the body of the corresponding leaflet. The leaflet becomes tethered down, losing its coaptation.[12,63] Tethering in tricuspid valve regurgitation can currently be treated with valve augmentation.[64,65]

Functional tricuspid regurgitation is an expression of right ventricular failure with a generalized distortion of ventricular geometry. Although annuloplasty can reduce or abolish functional tricuspid regurgitation by reducing the dilated annulus, it does not address the altered subvalvular geometry. Atrioventricular valve regurgitation is therefore influenced by extravalvular factors. Surgery addresses the myocardial component and is aimed at correcting the geometric distortion.[66]

Right ventricular failure and subsequent functional regurgitation are to play a role in the current era of transcatheter valves. If transcatheter valves aim at reducing surgical risks in patients who are deemed inoperable or carrying a risk which is considered too high, the technology and technique should be able to offer better outcomes. In transcatheter repair of mitral regurgitation using the Mitra-Clip (Abbott Vascular, Abbott Park, IL), outcomes are influenced by the residual baseline degree of tricuspid regurgitation. This has been pointed out recently by Ohno and colleagues,[67] confirming that 30-day primary safety endpoint was impaired in the GRASP Registry (Getting Reduction of Mitral Insufficiency by Percutaneous Clip Implantation) patients with moderate or severe residual tricuspid endocarditis. Valve regurgitation negatively influenced death and rehospitalization for congestive heart failure at 12 postoperative months; this is in contradistinction with the results after mitral valve surgery. After mitral valve repair or replacement, the risk of progression of tricuspid regurgitation is low, between 3% and 6% up to 5 years postoperatively. The rationale behind a timely operation on the mitral valve encompasses, too, a reduction in progression of tricuspid regurgitation over time.

DIAGNOSIS

The symptoms of the patient with tricuspid valve disease tend to be minimal and overshadowed by the more apparent left-sided symptoms. Because the tricuspid valve is situated at the entrance of the heart, its symptoms are extracardiac. With the exception of advanced cardiomyopathy, it is now uncommon to encounter a patient with the classic symptoms of venous engorgement, such as peripheral edema, hepatomegaly, and ascites. Tricuspid valve disease is mostly silent; the patient mostly complains of asthenia.

The clinical diagnosis of tricuspid valve disease has always been considered difficult. Before the advent of two-dimensional echocardiography[68] and its application in the operating room through transesophageal probe,[69] the surgeon used to explore the tricuspid valve digitally through the right atrium and decide whether to treat or to ignore the lesion according to the intensity of the regurgitant jet. This was a common practice three decades ago. This method has been completely abandoned because of its subjectivity and the inability to detect moderate degrees of insufficiency. Right-sided heart catheterization and ventriculography, which were considered the gold standards for the study of all cardiac valves,[70] have been superseded by two-dimensional color Doppler echocardiography. Because of its noninvasiveness, reliability, and visual impact, two-dimensional Doppler echocardiography is the best tool for determination of the presence, degree, and etiology of tricuspid valve disease. Although transesophageal echocardiography provides invaluable anatomic information at the time of surgery, transthoracic echocardiography remains the most important examination regarding the tricuspid valve. Besides the better window obtained with transthoracic echocardiography, the main reason for its superiority lies in the notorious temporal variability in the degree of tricuspid regurgitation. This is particularly important in functional insufficiencies, in which changes in blood volume secondary to diuretic administration or vascular tone under general anesthesia can severely reduce the degree of regurgitation. Lack of awareness of these facts and exclusive reliance on intraoperative transesophageal echocardiographic examination often result in ignoring significant regurgitations. The advent of three-dimensional echocardiography is changing the perception of the estimates in tricuspid valve disease, with the understanding of the superiority of two-dimensional echocardiography.

From a surgical point of view, the essential preoperative information includes the following: whether the patient has tricuspid valve disease and whether it is organic, functional, or mixed; quantification of the degree of regurgitation and the direction of the regurgitant jet; pulmonary artery peak and mean pressures; presence and quantification of transvalvular pressure gradients; maximum and minimum tricuspid valve annulus diameter and its systolic shortening; anatomic features of the valve (i.e., leaflet thickness, mobility, billowing of the leaflet body, location of the prolapsing free edge toward the right atrium); and absence of a patent foramen ovale. It is imperative to be aware that underestimation and overestimation of the regurgitant jet area are possible because of changes in gain, filter settings, angle, and distance of the transducer. Experience is required to gain a three-dimensional concept of the direction, location, size, and number of regurgitant jets as the tricuspid annulus is a dynamic multiplanar structure with regional changes.[71,72] Color Doppler study can even discover minimal regurgitations in 60% to 100% of the normal population, as documented by Yoshida and colleagues[73] in normal subjects to set the basis for current understanding. The so-called physiologic regurgitations are useful to evaluate right ventricular and pulmonary pressures.[74] Contrast echocardiography is a reliable method for detecting tricuspid regurgitation[75-77] and a patent foramen ovale.

Semiquantitative evaluation of the severity of tricuspid regurgitation is based on the degree of penetration of the regurgitant jet into the right atrium. A jet that penetrates 2 cm into the right atrium indicates mild regurgitation. A jet that penetrates 3 to 5 cm is considered moderate regurgitation; if it is accompanied by systolic flow reversal of hepatic or caval veins, it is considered severe regurgitation. A more quantitative assessment of the degree of tricuspid regurgitation is performed by the orifice flow acceleration proximal isovelocity surface area radius method. A radius of 1 to 4 mm indicates mild regurgitation; 5 to 8 mm indicates moderate regurgitation; and greater than 9 mm indicates severe regurgitation.[78-80] These methods are considered essential in the evaluation of mitral regurgitation, particularly in the intraoperative evaluation of residual regurgitations after repair, and have the same value in the tricuspid valve. Accuracy in determining the actual degree of tricuspid regurgitation is a crucial point in the surgical decision-making process.

Knowledge of the tricuspid valve annulus diameter is important for the surgeon, but its echocardiographic measurement is difficult because the annulus is not circular. As stated, it is a dynamic multiplanar structure with changing regional behavior as clearly depicted by Owais and colleagues.[72] Small variations in the orientation of the ultrasound beam can provide radically different measurements. The search has been ongoing for a "critical annulus diameter" beyond which the tricuspid valve should not be ignored by the surgeon. Thirty years ago, Ubago and colleagues[55] suggested 27 mm/m^2 as the "critical diameter" above which functional regurgitation always appeared (Fig. 81-6). Using transthoracic echocardiographic examination of 11 consecutive patients with severe clinical tricuspid regurgitation, Come and Riley[81] reported a nonindexed mean diastolic annulus diameter of 51 mm in the four-chamber view and 54 mm in the short-axis view. Among 15 controls, the mean annulus diameter was 34 mm in the four-chamber view and 33 mm in the short-axis view in what is almost a classical contribution. Goldman and colleagues[75] suggested 30 mm as the cutoff point between absent or mild regurgitation and moderate to severe regurgitation.

A cutoff point must be found beyond which an annuloplasty will fail. Fukuda and associates[82] in a preoperative and postoperative echocardiographic study of 216 patients with functional tricuspid regurgitation, found that age, tethering height (distance between annulus plane and leaflet coaptation point), and severity of regurgitation were independent parameters predicting residual regurgitation. Preoperative annulus dimension was not associated with outcome of tricuspid valve annuloplasty. In practical terms, it is safe to consider a nonindexed annulus size beyond 40 mm an indication for surgery. When echocardiographic data are not available or are considered unreliable, Dreyfus and colleagues[83] suggested using a ruler to measure the maximal stretched orifice from the anteroseptal to anteroposterior commissures. Patients with a dimension greater than or equal to 70 mm (circumference ± 140 mm, diameter ± 44 mm) should undergo annuloplasty. All of this forms the basis for the indication for annuloplasty despite some inaccuracy according to the differences among operators.[84]

Preoperative differentiation between organic and functional tricuspid valve disease is also possible and important. Transvalvular gradients, leaflet irregularities, thickening, and doming are clear indications of organic disease. Transvalvular gradients calculated with continuous wave Doppler echocardiography have been shown to correlate well with cardiac catheterization when catheterization was widely used until echocardiography became an established and preferred diagnostic tool.[85] The normal mean gradient is less than 2 mm Hg, and the end-diastolic gradient is nearly zero. Significant stenosis of the tricuspid valve may be present with a mean gradient of 3 to 5 mm Hg and an end-diastolic gradient of 1 to 3 mm Hg.[78] Annulus dilation is most often present in both organic and functional lesions, but it is larger in functional regurgitation.[54,80]

Three-dimensional echocardiography, although preferred for the assessment of the mitral valve, has expanded knowledge of the geometric changes in the normal and diseased tricuspid valve. It is already providing invaluable information on the annulopapillary complex in any valve condition. Accurate assessment is required.[12,86-88]

INDICATIONS FOR SURGERY

The current consensus is that most diseased tricuspid valves can be repaired easily. Severe lesions are usually treated, but real or erroneously labeled "moderate" lesions are ignored. The problem in the past used to be often related to the absence of a detailed preoperative

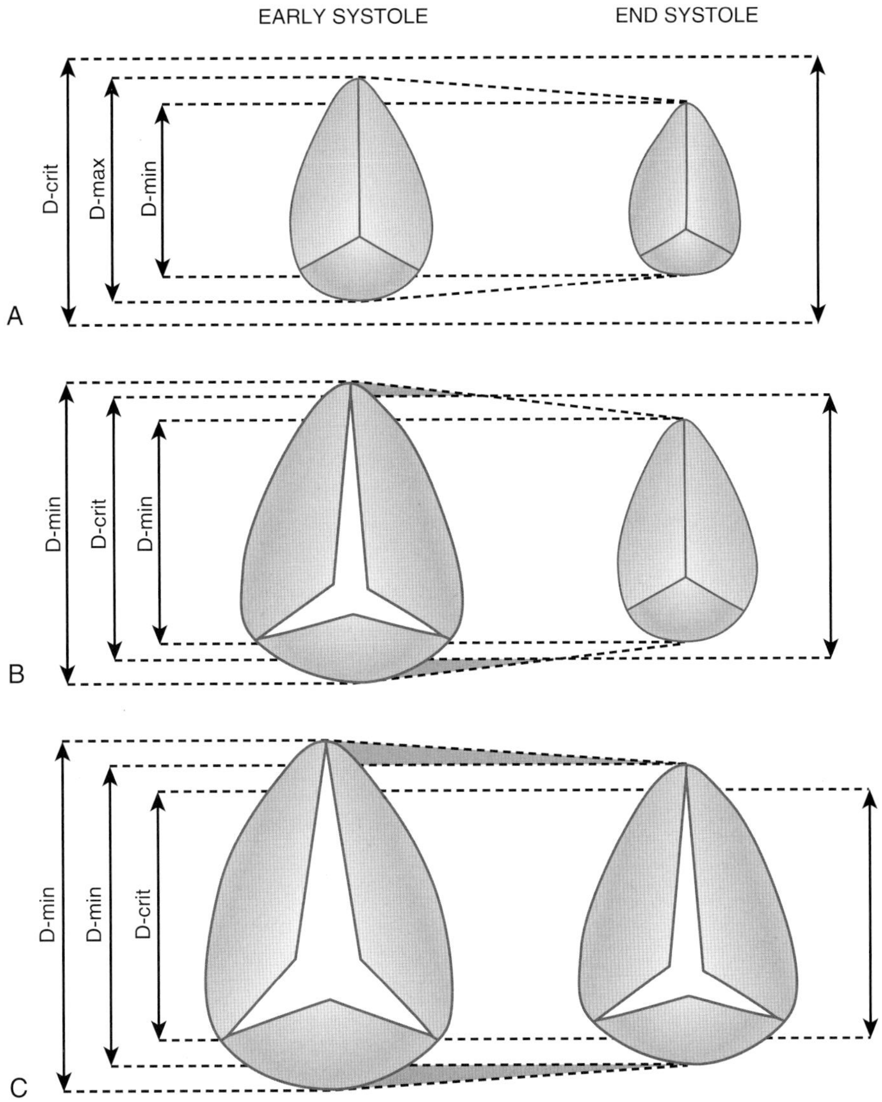

FIGURE 81-6 Diagram of the tricuspid valve. **A,** Patients without regurgitation. Both maximal early systolic (D-max) and minimal late end-systolic (D-min) diameters are below the critical diameter (D-crit) of 27 mm/m^2. **B,** Patients with mild regurgitation. D-max is larger, but D-min is smaller than D-crit. No cusp apposition occurs during early and mid systole. **C,** Patients with severe regurgitation. D-max and D-min are above D-crit. Pansystolic regurgitation. (From Ubago JL, Figueroa A, Ochoteco A, et al: Analysis of the amount of tricuspid valvular annular dilatation required to produce functional tricuspid regurgitation. *Am J Cardiol* 52:157, 1983, with permission from Excerpta Medica, Inc.)

search for tricuspid valve disease. Intraoperative decision making is unreliable unless the lesion is severe. Preoperative transthoracic echocardiography specifically interrogating the tricuspid valve is an absolute requirement. Current trends in three-dimensional echocardiography result in additional preoperative information per the changing behavior of the tricuspid annulus, which is useful in surgical planning.[89] The value of intraoperative transesophageal echocardiography cannot be neglected.

Can Tricuspid Valve Disease Be Ignored?

In the early phases of valve surgery, the current knowledge indicated that tricuspid regurgitation in the setting of stenotic valve disease could be solved after mitral valve replacement.[90] This conservative approach was based on the assumption of postoperative regression of pulmonary hypertension, which would reduce the tricuspid regurgitation. However, early reports like that of Duran and colleagues[91] stressed the effect of residual tricuspid regurgitation on outcomes and warned on the need for early repair of mitral lesions and tricuspid organic disease, when analyzing 150 patients with mitral valve repair and concomitant tricuspid valve disease. Almost 40 years later, there is agreement that residual noncorrected tricuspid regurgitation is associated with suboptimal or poor outcomes.[92-95] These patients with residual uncorrected regurgitation remain at high risk of cardiac death over the follow-up. Reoperative tricuspid patients requiring valve replacement are clinically in poor condition and increased pulmonary hypertension.[92,95]

Specific Surgical Indications

The severity of the lesion and its reparability are major drivers for the indication for surgery. As stated, the preoperative clinical condition plays a role in the outcomes, too. Severe lesions demand surgical correction regardless of whether repair or replacement will be performed. Moderate lesions should be treated if repair is expected. This principle emphasizes the importance of a precise and accurate preoperative diagnosis. The advances in imaging have allowed better understanding of tricuspid disease and better surgical planning.

Tricuspid Valve Disease Associated with Left-Sided Valvular Lesions

Previous discussion and accumulated data over time support that tricuspid valve disease associated with left-sided valvular lesions should not be ignored, even if it is mild to moderate (≥2+). It should be treated at the time of the surgery for the other valves.[92,93,95]

Organic Lesions

Organic lesions should always be treated.[91,96] In cases of rheumatic multivalvular disease, ignoring the tricuspid valve lesion on the basis of the small gradient present before surgery is dangerous, because it is likely to become significant postoperatively. This is due to the increase in cardiac output after repair of the left-sided lesions. In addition, the persistence of right ventricular preload will further affect the right ventricle and promote further functional regurgitation.

Traumatic Insufficiencies

Traumatic tricuspid insufficiency of any origin has been increasingly diagnosed because of the development in imaging techniques. This can be due to blunt trauma, defibrillator leads, or endomyocardial biopsies among other causes. Traumatic insufficiencies are virtually always amenable to repair. More than 200 brief reports on traumatic tricuspid regurgitation are currently available, and the vast majority report repairs. In chronic cases, the common finding is a leaflet prolapse because of a fibrotic and elongated papillary muscle head. Repair by plication of the elongated head is not technically complex and is usually successful. Acute tears of a leaflet and avulsion of a chord are treated by resection of the unsupported area with reapproximation of its edges followed by selective reduction of the annulus with an annuloplasty. Polytetrafluoroethylene neochords, following experiences in the mitral valve, have also been attempted in addition to regular repair techniques.[97]

Infective Endocarditis

Right-sided infective endocarditis represents less than 10% of the cases of endocarditis.[98] Surgery for tricuspid valve is usually not the first option in the setting of infective endocarditis, as more than 95% of the cases are cured with antibiotic therapy. However, in patients with persistent bacteremia or septic shock, septic pulmonary emboli must be operated. The changing spectrum of the complications of the disease take into account a more aggressive disease.[99] The rate of successful repair is directly related to the degree of valve destruction. Localized lesion may be easily repaired; a destroyed valve requires replacement.

Functional Tricuspid Regurgitation

Functional tricuspid regurgitation must be treated surgically. The initial conduct dictates repair. The current accumulated information confirms the need for surgery in this setting.[96] It is clear now that residual tricuspid regurgitation is likely to progress over time, as it has been discussed extensively in the literature and previously in this chapter. Tricuspid annuloplasty, per se, is not an incremental risk factor for mortality and can be performed with the heart beating, according to the experience of the surgeon. Despite the ongoing discussions on whether mild to moderate functional regurgitation needs repair, it sounds appropriate today to perform annuloplasty, especially if there is increased pulmonary artery resistance.[96,100,101] A maximum valve diameter greater than 40 mm is also an additional indication for repair.

Functional Tricuspid Regurgitation after Heart Transplantation

A special subset of patients with functional tricuspid insufficiency are those with regurgitation that appears after heart transplantation. Possible causes of tricuspid regurgitation after transplantation include distortion of tricuspid valve annulus geometry because of the right atrial anastomosis.[102] It has been shown that the change in surgical technique from biatrial to bicaval anastomosis significantly reduces the incidence of immediate regurgitations, size mismatch of the donor heart, and the pericardial cavity.[103,104] The bicaval technique results in less tricuspid regurgitation early after transplantation, although long-term outcomes do not show differences in functional capacity in relation with the technique. Patients with moderate or severe tricuspid regurgitation at discharge have an increased mortality during the first five postoperative years.[105]

Congestive Heart Failure Secondary to Ischemic or Idiopathic Cardiomyopathy with Mitral Valve Regurgitation

Congestive heart failure secondary to ischemic or idiopathic cardiomyopathy with mitral regurgitation is currently treated by "overcorrection" with an "undersizing" ring annuloplasty.[106,107] This has proved to be effective in improving clinical condition. Tricuspid valve annuloplasty should be added because tricuspid regurgitation is frequently present. It also avoids the progression of annular dilation. Uncorrected tricuspid regurgitation in patients with cardiomyopathy and mitral regurgitation have worse outcomes. As De Bonis and colleagues[108] demonstrated in an elegant contribution with a somewhat large cohort of 91 patients, tricuspid regurgitation develops because of progression of the disease or failure of repair. Like in other conditions, the degree of residual tricuspid regurgitation and preoperative right ventricular dysfunction are the predictors for late tricuspid regurgitation. This, therefore, supports an aggressive management of tricuspid regurgitation in this setting.

TRICUSPID VALVE SURGERY

Reconstructive techniques and valve prostheses used in the tricuspid valve are similar to those designed for the mitral position. The evolution of the surgery for atrioventricular valves in the past four decades has mostly relied on the Carpentier[20,109] and Duran[110,111] techniques as a reference for repair. Replacement devices have been designed for atrioventricular valves with no specific design differences.

Surgical Approaches to the Tricuspid Valve

The approach to the tricuspid valve is easy because of its anatomic location. It can be visualized through a midsternotomy or a right thoracotomy. Unless an isolated tricuspid valve lesion is contemplated, the type of thoracotomy and incision are dictated by the concomitant surgery on the other valves. A standard or a minimally invasive approach can be used safely.[112] To establish cardiopulmonary bypass, separate superior and inferior caval and ascending aorta cannulations are used. The right atrial incision is started close to the appendage and directed toward the posterior aspect of the atrium between the right inferior pulmonary vein and the inferior vena cava (Fig. 81-7). This incision minimizes the problem when an accidental tear of the lower extremity of the incision occurs from excessive retraction. The tricuspid valve surgery can be performed easily in the beating heart; however, a number of surgeons prefer cardioplegic arrest. If retrograde cardioplegia is planned, the coronary sinus is located above the posteroseptal commissure and directly cannulated. To ensure maximal distribution of cardioplegia to the whole heart, a pursestring is placed around the coronary ostium. After the retrograde cannula is in place, the pursestring is tightened, the balloon is inflated, and the catheter is pulled outward until it is arrested by the pursestring. This is an old but simple and effective technique to secure the catheter.[19,113]

In recent years, the principles of a percutaneous approach to the cardiac valves have been applied to the tricuspid valve. It is likely that percutaneous tricuspid valve repair will become widespread because of the accessibility of the valve and the low-pressure environment of the right heart. There is no preferred approach when simultaneous mitral valve surgery is required. A separate biatrial approach is popular, but transeptal approach from the inferior edge of the fossa ovalis or the most complex transatrial septal incision was described by Guiraudon and colleagues.[114]

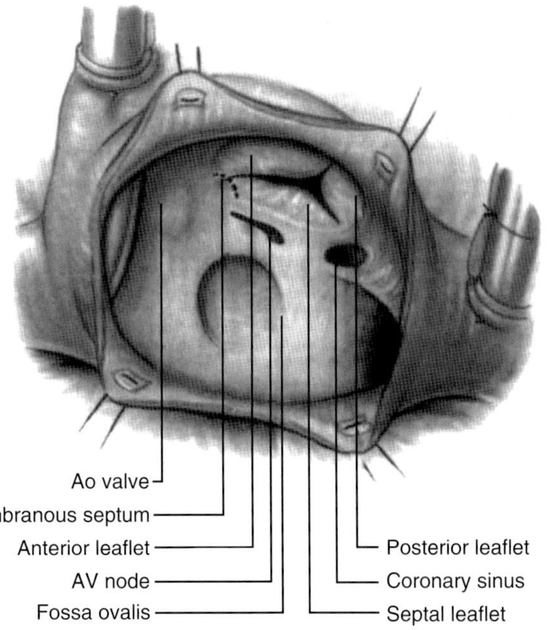

FIGURE 81-7 ■ Surgical view of the tricuspid valve through a standard right atriotomy. The "danger" area corresponding to the atrioventricular (AV) node is located near the anterior half of the base of the septal leaflet. *Ao,* Aortic. (Reproduced with permission from Duran CMG: Reoperations on the mitral and tricuspid valves. In Sabiston DC Jr, Stark J, Pacifico A, et al, editors: *Reoperations in cardiac surgery,* New York, 1989, Springer-Verlag, p 346.)

Tricuspid Valve Commissurotomy

The first closed tricuspid valve commissurotomy was performed in 1952 by Charles Bailey.[115] Cardiopulmonary bypass brought more precise techniques like open commissurotomy. Percutaneous balloon dilation has replaced closed commissurotomy, which is based on the principle of splitting the commissures through the distending pressure exercised on the leaflets, although the experience in the tricuspid valve is scant.[116,117] Tricuspid valve balloon dilation is currently reserved for a small number of patients for whom its minimal invasiveness compensates for its mediocre results. In addition, the low pressure in the right cavities minimizes the importance of the frequent residual gradients and iatrogenic regurgitations. Most tricuspid valve lesions are treated surgically in the setting of advanced mitral valve problems that demand surgery.

In performing an open tricuspid valve commissurotomy, the valve should be inspected carefully because, in severe cases, it can appear as a diaphragm with a central circular orifice and fibrotic edges (see Fig. 81-3B). In these extreme cases, it is difficult to identify the commissures. The subvalvular apparatus is often fairly intact; therefore, a conservative procedure is still possible, although the result may be suboptimal. Valve hooks are placed on either side of the commissure to explore the "fan" chordae always present at the commissures. The incision must ensure that its two edges are supported by chordae. It is often easier to start the incision 4 to 5 mm from the annulus rather than at the edge of the fused

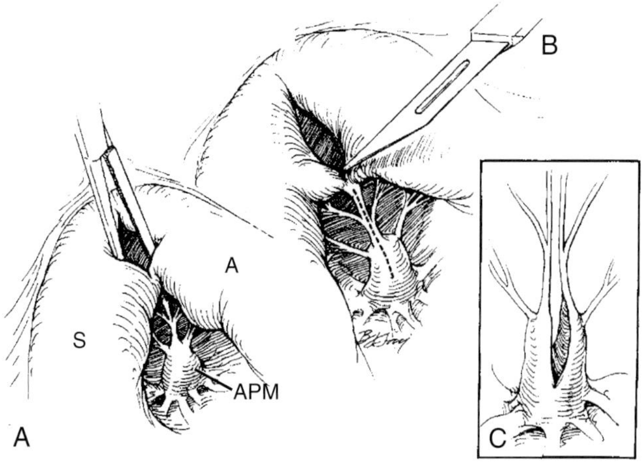

FIGURE 81-8 ■ Tricuspid valve commissurotomy. **A,** Opening of the commissure. **B,** Splitting of fused chordae and papillary muscle. **C,** Split papillary muscle. The anteroseptal commissure is opened distal to the free edge to identify the fused chords. *A,* Anterior leaflet; *APM,* anterior papillary muscle; *S,* septal leaflet. (From Revuelta JM, Garcia-Rinaldi R, Duran CMG: Tricuspid commissurotomy. *Ann Thorac Surg* 39:5:489–491, 1985, with permission from the Society of Thoracic Surgeons.)

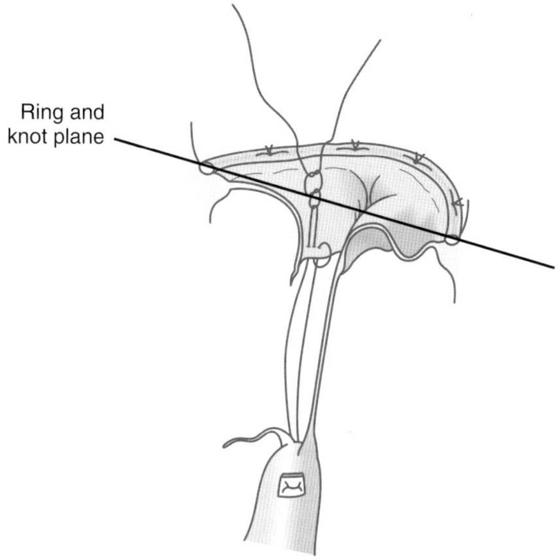

FIGURE 81-9 ■ A simple method to determine the correct length of an artificial neochord. The double-ended suture is anchored to the papillary muscle and passed through the leaflet edge, but not tied. After ring annuloplasty, the suture is tied at the level of the annulus (i.e., the level of the annuloplasty). (Reproduced with permission from Duran CMG, Pekar F: Techniques for ensuring the correct length of new mitral chords. *J Heart Valve Dis* 108:727–735, 1994.)

leaflets (Fig. 81-8). A better view of the chords will direct the incision toward the free edge. In most cases, two fanlike, thin chords are fused. This incision is then prolonged apically into the papillary muscle for at least 1 cm. The purpose of this essential maneuver is to slow the ongoing fibrotic process and to increase leaflet mobility. At present, these severe forms of commissural fusion are rare in the Western world. Lesser degrees of fusion are frequently present and missed unless the valve is carefully inspected. Often only one or two commissures are affected; the anteroseptal commissure is the most frequently fused. In most cases, a tricuspid annuloplasty must accompany the commissurotomy because of a lack of leaflet tissue or because annular dilation is also present.

Repair Maneuvers

Because most tricuspid valve regurgitations are functional, repair maneuvers other than annuloplasty are less often needed than in mitral valve repair. In acute infective endocarditis, the vegetations must be excised. The vegetation is resected a few millimeters beyond its base in the leaflet. This resection should be in healthy tissue, which is easily identified because of its normal coloration compared with the reddish color of the inflamed area. A triangular resection with its base at the free edge of the leaflet is the best solution. The gap is closed with 5-0 polypropylene sutures. Unless this resection is small, an annuloplasty must follow. Leaflet perforations present in healed endocarditis can be closed with sutures or, if extensive, with a patch of glutaraldehyde-treated autologous pericardium. Fresh autologous pericardium should not be used because it will undergo progressive fibrous retraction. Important tissue destructions can be reconstructed with pericardium supported by polytetrafluroethylene neochords.[97]

Chordal replacement is not as popular as in the case of the mitral valve. Although papillary muscle and leaflet anchoring of the neochord is not a problem, determination of its appropriate length remains intuitive and based on personal experience, which is globally limited when it comes to the tricuspid valve. Following numerous in vitro approaches to this problem, an easy and simple technique was developed by Duran and Pekar.[118] A double-ended, 5-0 Gore-Tex (W. L. Gore and Associates, Flagstaff, AZ) suture is anchored to the papillary muscle and the free edge of the prolapsing leaflet (Fig. 81-9) but not tied. After the annuloplasty ring is placed, the two arms of the Gore-Tex suture are tied at the level of the plane of the annuloplasty. Most failures are due to overcorrection, resulting in a neochord that is too short. To simplify this maneuver, the ring holder incorporates two "guide sutures" that traverse the valve orifice at the level of the annuloplasty. After the ring is in place but still attached to the holder, each arm of the artificial chord is passed on either side of the guiding suture and tied (Fig. 81-10) and the holder is removed. In some cases, a patient may need several neochords arising from the same papillary muscle. Implantation of a new neochord is difficult across the annuloplasty. In these cases, a neopapillary muscle is constructed (Fig. 81-11). A loop of approximately 5 mm is made with a double-ended 2-0 Gore-Tex suture. Each arm of the suture is then anchored to the papillary muscle and secured over pledgets. New artificial chords can then be passed easily through the loop (Fig. 81-12). Because of their simplicity, these techniques have transformed mitral and tricuspid valve repair. The edge-to-edge technique, originally described by Alfieri and his group for mitral valve prolapse,[119] has also been applied to the tricuspid valve[120] to configure a double orifice valve. Leaflet suture approximation techniques including the clover technique have been used on a restricted basis.[121]

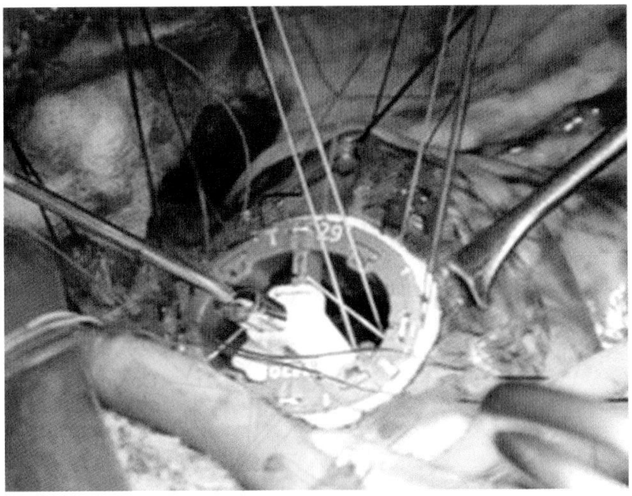

FIGURE 81-10 Intraoperative view: determination of the correct length of the neochord. The annuloplasty ring is already anchored, but the holder is still in place. Each arm of the neochord is placed on either side of the guide and tied at that level. The holder is then removed.

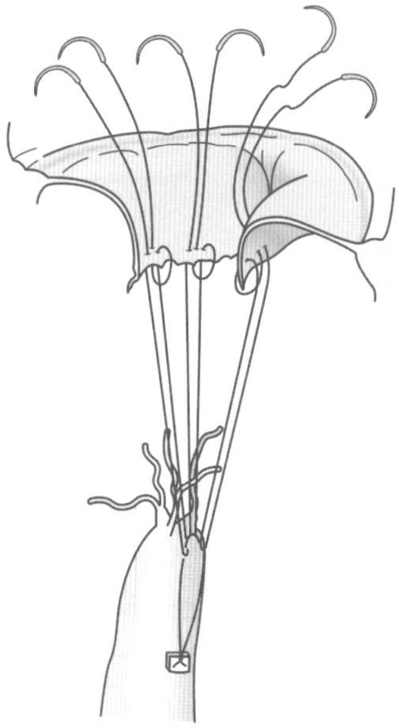

FIGURE 81-12 Multiple neochords anchored by the neopapillary muscle. One loop can sustain all chords corresponding to one papillary muscle. If there is a need to anchor neochords sustained by other papillary muscles, a separate loop must be constructed.

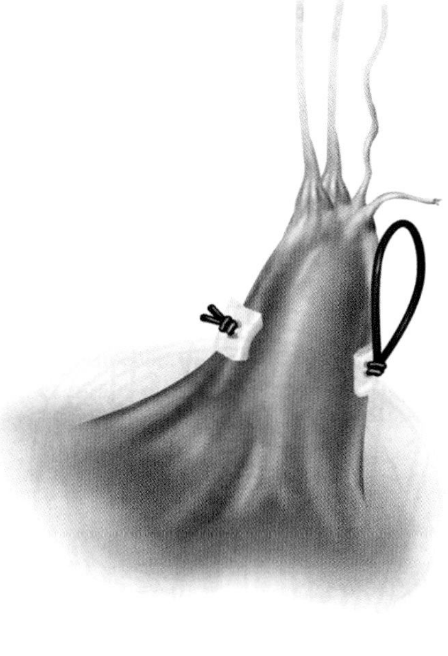

FIGURE 81-11 Neopapillary muscle loop. A 5-mm loop is constructed with 2-0 double-ended Gore-Tex. Each suture's arm is anchored to the medial aspect of the patient's papillary muscle. A number of neochords are passed through the loop.

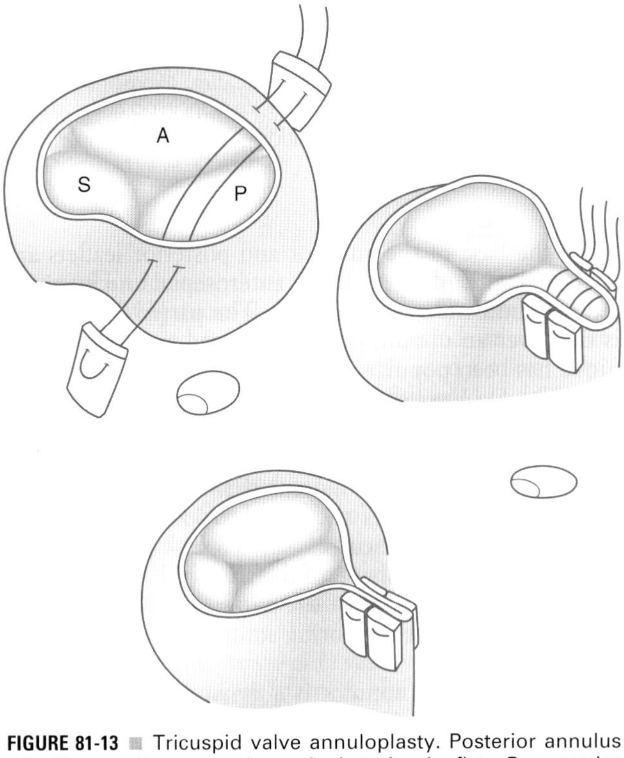

FIGURE 81-13 Tricuspid valve annuloplasty. Posterior annulus plication or Kay procedure. *A,* Anterior leaflet; *P,* posterior leaflet; *S,* septal leaflet. (From Boyd AD, Engelman RM, Isom OW, et al: Tricuspid annuloplasty. Five and one-half years' experience with 78 patients. *J Thorac Cardiovasc Surg* 68:347, 1974, with permission from Excerpta Medica, Inc.)

Tricuspid Valve Annuloplasty

The principle behind tricuspid valve annuloplasty is to selectively reduce the perimeter of the tricuspid valve annulus and, consequently, the size of the tricuspid valve orifice. The lack of leaflet coaptation is compensated by the induced smaller tricuspid valve orifice. The earliest annuloplasties consisted of plication of the annulus at the level of the base of the posterior leaflet. This approach, borrowed from the early mitral valve annuloplasties, was described by Wooler and colleagues[122] and Kay and colleagues[123] (Fig. 81-13). Both have been abandoned because of the difficulty in determining the amount of plication necessary and the lack of support for the remaining annulus. Cabrol[124] and De Vega[125] independently described a partial encircling suture to narrow the annulus. The extremities of a double suture that runs

avoiding myocardial tissue. These riff sutures not only increase the holding power of the stitches but also maintain the continuity between the annulus and papillary muscles, which have been shown in the mitral valve to be essential to ventricular function. The controversy on whether a mechanical or a tissue valve is preferable in the tricuspid position is still active and proponents define the need for anticoagulation and good right ventricular function as preoperative indicators for such an implant.[136]

RESULTS

Annuloplasty

The review of the literature has regularly shown inconsistent results. As the tricuspid valve is a low-pressure system, different degrees of incompetence can be acceptable and well tolerated despite suboptimal results. This was highlighted by Duran and colleagues three decades ago in their elegant review of a series of 150 patients with mitral and tricuspid regurgitation who had preoperative and postoperative hemodynamic evaluations at different intervals extending up to 5 years.[91] All patients had mitral valve repair, and 119 had concomitant tricuspid valve repair; in 31 cases, the tricuspid valve lesion was ignored by the surgeon. Independently of whether the tricuspid valve repair was categorized as "good," "bad," or "ignored," 97% of those with a good mitral valve repair were in functional class I or class II. The quality of the mitral valve repair determined the postoperative cardiac index. At that time and because of these data, strongly emphasizing the need for an early repair of left-sided lesions, these authors were able to conclude that functional TI could be ignored only in patients with predictable and significant reduction in pulmonary vascular resistances and that organic disease of the tricuspid valve must be repaired.

During the 1980s, the superiority of repair over replacement became clearly established. It was shown that repair was possible in most cases including organic lesions. The experience of Prabhakar and colleagues[25] with the repair of rheumatic organic lesions with over 90% of patients with satisfactory functional results was encouraging at that time. The absence of valve thrombosis, the unnecessary permanent anticoagulation, and a low reoperation rate have reduced valve replacement to the exceptional case in the case of degenerative or functional disease.[137,138] The experience of Duran with 306 patients, 92 with proactive tricuspid valve surgery generally indicated in healthier patients yielded in-hospital mortality of 7.5% and actuarial survival rate of 77% at 48 months.[110] This relatively low survival at an interval shorter than 5 years indicated that these tricuspid patients were in worse condition than expected. The selection process at that time was negatively influenced by the lack of good imaging of the tricuspid valve preoperatively, intraoperatively, and postoperatively.

These findings favored a more aggressive surgical attitude toward the tricuspid valve, and consequently, earlier indications extended into the lower-risk patients. This attitude has been documented over time with different devices for tricuspid annuloplasty. The recent experience of Ratschiller and colleagues[139] is confirmation, although the follow-up for specific devices is still short. The experience over four decades with different techniques of annuloplasty with or without rings or bands confirms that, over time, residual stenosis and regurgitation can become a problem that was documented when early studies showed significant gradients in 50% of patients with a De Vega annular reduction and residual or recurrent regurgitation in 41%.[140] The same occurred with the early types of ring, the Carpentier-Edwards rigid ring (Edwards Lifesciences, Irvine, CA; 48% significant gradients, 31% residual or recurrent regurgitation) when analyzed in early studies[141] and the Duran flexible ring (Medtronic, Inc., Minneapolis, MN; 31% significant gradients, 30% residual or recurrent regurgitation).[54] Technical failures over time, such as ring fracture, were not common although documented.[142] Late factors for ring annuloplasty failure were studied by McCarthy and colleagues[143] in a large series of 790 patients with functional tricuspid insufficiency; residual or recurrent significant regurgitation graded as 3+ to 4+ was detected in 32% of the patients with the Peri-Guard band (Synovis Life Technologies, St. Paul, MN), 28% with the De Vega suture, 18% with the Cosgrove-Edwards band, and 17% with the Carpentier-Edwards rigid ring. On the other hand, tricuspid regurgitation can develop after successful mitral valve repair for functional ischemic regurgitation, as shown by Matsunaga and colleagues.[144] Almost 50% of patients had significant tricuspid regurgitation at the latest follow-up control after myocardial revascularization and reduction mitral annuloplasty.[144] These results suggested that tricuspid valve reduction annuloplasty might not consistently protect against recurrent functional regurgitation. Functional regurgitation of the atrioventricular valves continues to be a problem, the reason being, as it is currently well known, that cardiomyopathy-induced ischemic disease leads to changes in the right and left ventricular geometry. It is unlikely that the myocardial component can be corrected by any type of prosthetic annuloplasty device of any configuration.[2] Additional controversy between rigid rings and flexible bands is still active. The lack of controlled studies aiming to shed some light is still a limitation; however, a recent best-evidence topic suggests that although there is relatively less risk of ring dehiscence or fracture in the flexible group, with the rigid ring there is a trend toward a more sustainable and stable postoperative regurgitation.[145]

Tricuspid Valve Replacement

Almost 60 years is the interval between the earliest documentation of experimental tricuspid valve replacement and today.[146] It would not be fair to state that things have not changed much when discussing the fate of right atrioventricular valve and orifice in the adult. Cardiac surgery has evolved in a way in which, from a primitive surgical conduct, the current trends are signaling toward a global reduction in the access to the heart following the call of technology.[147] However, the replacement of the tricuspid valve continues to be a challenge for the physicians and surgeons. As it is clear, the preoperative condition of the patient with tricuspid valve disease dictates outcomes, and these patients usually arrive late and in bad shape predominantly because of right heart failure. Some predictors for failure of repair have been identified in recent years,[83,148] and the ability of surgeons to achieve a satisfactory anatomic and functional result have rendered tricuspid valve replacement an uncommon operation when compared with mitral or aortic valve replacement in the adult setting.

A number of problems with tricuspid valve replacement are notorious. Despite acceptable results in some series with different types of replacement devices over time,[149-151] prosthetic valve dysfunction is a well-recognized condition that carries risk of morbidity and mortality in otherwise usually sick patients.[152] Current data have not been able to show the superiority of a specific prosthetic device.[153] Speculation about outcomes related to specific factors like gender,[154] among others, has not been confirmed due to the lack of robust data over time.

As tricuspid valve repair is achievable in a large proportion of patients, the published series of tricuspid valve replacement include reduced numbers.[153] Follow-up has always been a problem in medicine, and it is a key tool to assess the effectiveness of any procedure. There is not an agreed definition of what *long-term* means, and it usually remains a subjective interpretation of time frames depending on what the author wants to report. In cardiothoracic surgery, there has always been an interest in reporting over time. As we enter the sixth decade of valve replacement,[155] we are in a position to analyze actual long-term results of procedures performed by our predecessors. This is the case in valve surgery, which is why we are in need of studies that span a long time, diluting the improvements that have occurred in cardiac surgery. Reports with long follow-up, over two decades, include very different tricuspid valve pathologic processes and often include reoperations.[156] Furthermore, only severe tricuspid valve lesions are treated in poor-risk and evolved patients. Moderate lesions are rarely treated with replacement in current times. The reported hospital mortalities varied between 15% and 25%[156-160] and have not substantially improved in the past 20 years. When isolated tricuspid valve replacement was reported, the hospital mortality went up to 39% in the series of Poveda and colleagues,[161] which included patients operated on between 1974 and 1993. When the replacement was subsequent to previous open heart surgery, Hornick and associates[162] reported a hospital mortality of 50% in patients operated on between 1985 and 1993. A more recent experience of 34 patients undergoing isolated tricuspid valve surgery after prior left-sided heart surgery between 1980 and 1997 showed a hospital mortality of 8.8%.[163] However, at 5 years, the event-free actuarial survival was only 41%. Predictors of poor outcome were the age of the patient, number of previous surgeries, preoperative functional class, congestive heart failure, and pulmonary artery pressure.[161,162] The published late mortalities were close to 50%[157-159] with survivals of 70% at 3 years for Sanfelippo and colleagues,[164] 47% at 10 years for Thorburn and colleagues,[165] and 41% at 8 years for Kratz and colleagues.[166] In most series that stretch back to the 1970s, insignificant differences in the overall results are found between mechanical and tissue prostheses for tricuspid valve replacement. Recent series, with or without comparison with tricuspid valve repair, confirm the knowledge that tricuspid valve replacement is associated with long-term cardiac death and valve-related events.[167-169]

Standard bioprostheses in the mitral and aortic positions are known to fail because of leaflet tears and calcification, with an incidence of about 25% at 10 years after implantation. There is currently important accumulated information supporting that specific model and tissues have good behavior beyond two decades. Bourguignon and colleagues[170] have recently shown that the actual risk of explant at 20 years of the Carpentier-Edwards pericardial xenograft is 25.5% in a series of over 400 patients followed up to 25 years. Good results have also been reported for other bioprosthesis like the Hancock II, with 20-year freedom from reoperation at 41.4% in mitral patients younger and 61.9% in patients older than 60 years. These can be considered good results.[171]

However, such complications are rare in the low-pressure pulmonary and tricuspid positions in the adult and children.[172] Ohata and colleagues[173] reported a comparative study of patients with the Carpentier-Edwards pericardial xenograft in the mitral and in the tricuspid positions. The actuarial freedom from structural deterioration and reoperation at 13 years was 78% for the mitral valve versus 100% for the tricuspid valve. Although these findings would favor the tissue valve, several studies do not show significant differences between mechanical valves and bioprostheses. Carrier and associates[174] in 2003 reported a series of 97 patients with tricuspid valve replacement who were observed for up to 25 years. The overall hospital mortality was 17.5%. Because of their acknowledged preference for the bioprostheses, the authors compared two unequal groups of 81 patients with bioprostheses versus 15 patients with a mechanical valve operated on between 1977 and 2002. No significant differences were found in survival and reoperation rates between the groups. The 5-year actuarial survival was 56% in the bioprosthesis group and 60% in the mechanical group. The freedom from reoperation at 5 years was 97% and 91%, respectively. Describing 435 patients in the U.K. Heart Valve Registry, Ratnatunga and colleagues[175] showed similar survival and reoperation rates of patients with biological and mechanical prostheses. Kaplan and associates[176] also reported similar results among 122 patients averaging 35 years of age at the time of tricuspid valve replacement. Although prosthetic thrombosis and pulmonary embolism occurred in 10 patients, the authors recommended the use of low-profile, bileaflet prostheses. Still, the decision regarding the implantation of a mechanical or tissue valve in the tricuspid position has to be individualized. Songur and colleagues[153] did not find statistically significant differences over the long-term in their series of 132 patients—one of the largest series. The problem of mechanical valve thrombosis was highlighted by Kawano and colleagues,[177] who reported thrombosis in 6 of 23 patients with a St. Jude Medical valve in their contribution of the year 2000.

Historical series had a proportion of patients dying in whom the actual cause of death was unknown. This might have been due to the lack of postmortem examinations, thus leaving doubts regarding eventual thrombosis.[149] Although thrombosis of a bioprosthesis in the tricuspid position is rare, fibrous pannus formation occurs more often. It leads to progressive stenosis requiring reoperation. Kawachi and associates[178] reported a small series of 23 patients who underwent tricuspid valve replacement with a standard Hancock bioprosthesis. All patients were observed for up to 16 years. The actuarial freedom from structural degeneration was 94% at 10 years. This also occurred in mechanical valves, but only brief reports have been made available.[179] The evolution of imaging techniques has allowed for better visualization of the atrial and ventricular aspects of the valves, thus providing better chances of accurate diagnosis. Three-dimensional echocardiography and more recently multidetector computed tomography have improved our ability to assess atrioventricular prosthetic heart valves.[180]

It is difficult to confirm at this point in time if tissue valves are superior to mechanical valves for tricuspid valve replacement. The fact is that there are no large series supporting the superiority of one over the other. The series of Songur includes 123 patients and is one of the largest published recently.[153] Hemodynamics alone might not be the problem.[181] The danger of thrombosis and the need for a stringent anticoagulation regimen when a mechanical valve is used versus the satisfactory performance of tissue valves tilt the balance toward the bioprostheses. History describes our inability to appropriately address atrioventricular valve replacement and especially in the tricuspid position there is a need for more anatomic and, consequently, more physiologic new tricuspid valve prostheses. The underlying message is that patients requiring tricuspid valve replacement are in poor condition preoperatively, and this is the major driver for increased risk and mortality.

KNOWLEDGE AND EVIDENCE

Knowledge

It is clear that the controversy still exists. After many years of experience with the surgical treatment of tricuspid valve diseases, some topics still are difficult to handle. The type of disease is a key component in the discussion. In Westernized countries, functional tricuspid regurgitation seems to be the most frequent diagnosis[100] with valvular regurgitation mostly developing after left-sided valve procedure. The question is whether the degree of regurgitation matters[182] or whether the effect on myocardial function will affect survival.[183] Kammerlander and colleagues[184] recently analyzed a series of 91 patients who underwent left-sided surgery and found that although late survival was worse in patients with tricuspid regurgitation, right ventricular dysfunction was associated with survival in these patients. Hyllén and colleagues[185] focused on the role of pulmonary hypertension as part of the disease complex also showing poor right ventricular function.

This confirms the need for further study and reinforces our thinking that tricuspid regurgitation of any origin is detrimental to the right ventricle. It is of interest to notice that this also applies to any nonvalvular procedure as well. Transventricular pacing is becoming also a matter of discussion in current times when all types of intracardiac devices for the treatment of malignant arrhythmias and heart failure are implanted in escalating proportions under an increasing number of more or less powerful indications.[186] The effect of regurgitation after single or multiple lead implantation across the tricuspid valve is definitely not known, and more information is needed to update current knowledge.[187,188]

Organic disease is still a significant problem in non-Westernized countries, and it continues to contribute to the burden of valve disease[189] and cannot be neglected. Once again, the lack of large series may preclude drawing conclusions, but current knowledge indicates that the problem continues to be the worse profile of patients with long-standing tricuspid regurgitation in patients with rheumatic heart disease. Rodríguez-Capitán and colleagues[190] have recently pointed out the problem in another important series of patients with rheumatic involvement. Rheumatic disease involves all valve structures, which is the reason repair rates are much lower than in functional disease. In Westernized countries the incidence of organic disease may be estimated around 15% for patients[191] requiring surgery although some series may show higher incidence.[190] As the results of tricuspid surgery are usually less predictable than its mitral counterpart, there are still gaps between the problem, the proposals, the solutions, and the outcomes. In its elegant contribution, Gonzalez-Santos and Arnaiz-Garcia[191] have briefly and thoughtfully addressed the problem.

The indications for surgery of tricuspid regurgitation are becoming clear when it comes to the recommendations. The accumulation of information has led to modifications of Practice Guidelines in the past 5 years; however, in the case of tricuspid surgery, we are still missing well-designed controlled studies. Most of the information comes from observational studies, short series, and expert opinion. Current guidelines show some differences, and the most recent confirm that for both primary and functional tricuspid regurgitation in patients requiring left-sided valve surgery, tricuspid surgery is a must as expressed with class I recommendation.[192,193] The remaining indications still remain in the IIa level.

Finally, from the methodology standpoint, the lack of prospective controlled studies still makes the decision-making process somewhat uncomfortable. It is not that we may not have the ideal tools for analysis, it is the fact that the tricuspid valve has consistently been neglected by many in the community since the days of Braunwald's contribution[90]; this is easily represented by literature data. As we have already pointed out, a quick search through the United States National Library of Medicine using the terms *aortic valve*, *mitral valve*, and *tricuspid valve* yielded the following number of articles with these terms in the title: 13,608 (44.8%), 14,134 (46.6%), and 2625 (8.6%), respectively. When the search was limited to the twenty-first century, the observed results were

5. Buckberg GD, Hoffman JI, Coghlan HC, et al: Ventricular structure-function relations in health and disease: part II. Clinical considerations. *Eur J Cardiothorac Surg* 47:778–787, 2015.
6. Tsakiris AG, Mair DD, Seki S, et al: Motion of the tricuspid valve annulus in anesthetized intact dogs. *Circulation Res* 36:43–48, 1975.
7. Tei C, Pilgrim JF, Shah PM, et al: The tricuspid valve annulus: study in size and motion in normal subjects and in patients with tricuspid regurgitation. *Circulation* 66:665–671, 1982.
8. Hiro ME, Jouan J, Pagel MR, et al: Sonometric study of the normal tricuspid valve annulus in sheep. *J Heart Valve Dis* 13:452–460, 2004.
9. Jouan J, Pagel MR, Hiro ME, et al: Further information from a sonometric study of the normal tricuspid valve annulus in sheep: geometric changes during the cardiac cycle. *J Heart Valve Dis* 16:511–518, 2007.
10. De Bonis M, Taramasso M, Lapenna E, et al: Management of tricuspid regurgitation. *F1000Prime Rep* 6:58, 2014.
11. Salgo IS, Gorman IIIJH, Gorman RC, et al: Effect of annular shape on leaflet curvature in reducing mitral leaflet stress. *Circulation* 106:711–717, 2002.
12. Ton-Nu TT, Levine RA, Handschumacher MD, et al: Geometric determinants of functional tricuspid regurgitation. Insights from 3-dimensional echocardiography. *Circulation* 114:143–149, 2006.
13. Victor S, Nayak VM: The tricuspid valve is bicuspid. *J Heart Valve Dis* 3:27–36, 1994.
14. Victor S, Nayak VM, Raveen R, et al: Bicuspid evolution of the arterial and venous atrioventricular valves. *J Heart Valve Dis* 4:78–87, 1995.
15. Nigri GR, Di Dio LJA, Baptista CAC: Papillary muscles and tendinous chords of the right ventricle of the human heart: morphologic characteristics. *Surg Radiol Anat* 23:45–49, 2001.
16. Joudinaud TM, Flecher EM, Duran CMG: Functional terminology for the tricuspid valve. *J Heart Valve Dis* 15:382–388, 2006.
17. Victor S, Nayak VM: Variations in the papillary muscles of the normal mitral valve and their surgical relevance. *J Card Surg* 10:597–607, 1995.
18. Kumar N, Kumar M, Duran CMG: A revised terminology for recording surgical findings of the mitral valve. *J Heart Valve Dis* 4:70–75, 1995.
19. Martinez-Leon J, Carbonell C, Ortega J: A new technical approach for retrograde administration of cardioplegic solutions. *Thorac Cardiovasc Surg* 37:372–373, 1989.
20. Carpentier A: Cardiac valve surgery—the French correction. *J Thorac Cardiovasc Surg* 88:323–327, 1983.
21. Pomar JL, Mestres CA: Tricuspid valve replacement using a mitral homograft. Surgical technique and initial results. *J Heart Valve Dis* 2:125–128, 1993.
22. Mestres CA, Miro JM, Pare JC, et al: Six-year experience with cryopreserved mitral homografts in the treatment of tricuspid valve endocarditis in HIV-infected drug addicts. *J Heart Valve Dis* 8:575–577, 1999.
23. Mestres CA, Miro JM, Pare JC, and The Grupo de Trabajo de la Endocarditis Infecciosa del Hospital Clinic de Barcelona: Organization and functioning of a multidisciplinary team for the diagnosis and treatment of infective endocarditis: a 30-year perspective (1985-2014). *Rev Esp Cardiol* 2015. (In press).
24. Miró JM, Moreno A, Mestres CA: Infective endocarditis in intravenous drug abusers. *Curr Infect Dis Rep* 5:307–316, 2003.
25. Prabhakar G, Kumar N, Gometza B, et al: Surgery for organic rheumatic disease of the tricuspid valve. *J Heart Valve Dis* 2:561–566, 1993.
26. Gross L, Friedberg CK: Lesions of cardiac valve rings in rheumatic fever. *Am J Pathol* 12:469, 1936.
27. Daniels SJ, Mintz GS, Kotler MN: Rheumatic tricuspid valve disease: two dimensional echocardiographic, hemodynamic, and angiographic correlations. *Am J Cardiol* 51:492–496, 1983.
28. Carrel T, Schaffner A, Vogt P, et al: Endocarditis in intravenous drug addicts and HIV-infected patients: possibility and limitations of surgical treatment. *J Heart Valve Dis* 2:140–1487, 1993.
29. Hauck AJ, Freeman DP, Ackerman DP, et al: Surgical pathology of the tricuspid valve: a study of 363 cases spanning 25 years. *Mayo Clin Proc* 63:851–853, 1988.
30. Hashiro Y, Sugimoto S, Takagi N, et al: Native valve salvage for post-traumatic tricuspid regurgitation. *J Heart Valve Dis* 10:275–278, 2001.
31. van Son JA, Danielson GK, Schaff HV, et al: Traumatic tricuspid insufficiency. Experience in 13 patients. *J Thorac Cardiovasc Surg* 108:893–898, 1994.
32. Almeida M, Canada M, Neves J, et al: Longstanding traumatic tricuspid regurgitation with severe right ventricular failure. *J Heart Valve Dis* 6:642–646, 1997.
33. Looi JL, Lee AP, Wong RH, et al: 3D echocardiography for traumatic tricuspid regurgitation. *JACC Cardiovasc Imaging* 5:1285–1287, 2012.
34. Stankovic I, Daraban AM, Jasaityte R, et al: Incremental value of the en face view of the tricuspid valve by two-dimensional and three-dimensional echocardiography for accurate identification of tricuspid valve leaflets. *J Am Soc Echocardiogr* 27:376–384, 2014.
35. Yankah AC, Musci M, Weng Y, et al: Tricuspid valve dysfunction after orthotopic cardiac transplantation. *Eur J Cardiothorac Surg* 17:343–348, 2000.
36. Fiorelli AI, Coelho GH, Aiello VD, et al: Tricuspid valve injury after heart transplantation due to endomyocardial biopsy: an analysis of 3550 biopsies. *Transplant Proc* 44:2479–2482, 2012.
37. Jang SY, Cho Y, Song JH, et al: Complication rate of transfemoral endomyocardial biopsy with fluoroscopic and two dimensional echocardiographic guidance: a 10-year experience of 228 consecutive procedures. *J Korean Med Sci* 28:1323–1328, 2013.
38. Ogawa S, Hayashi J, Sasaki H, et al: Evaluation of combined valvular prolapse syndrome by two-dimensional echocardiography. *Circulation* 65:174–180, 1982.
39. Chen CC, Morganroth J, Mardelli TJ, et al: Tricuspid regurgitation in tricuspid valve prolapse demonstrated with contrast cross-sectional echocardiography. *Am J Cardiol* 46:983–987, 1980.
40. Ozdemir O, Olgunturk R, Kula S, et al: Echocardiographic findings in children with Marfan syndrome. *Cardiovasc J Afr* 22:245–248, 2011.
41. Mabvuure N, Cumberworth A, Hindocha S: In patients with carcinoid syndrome undergoing valve replacement: will a biological valve have acceptable durability? *Interact Cardiovasc Thorac Surg* 15:467–471, 2012.
42. Connolly HM, Crary JL, McGoon MD, et al: Valvular tricuspid disease associated with fenfluramine-phentermine. *N Engl J Med* 337:581–588, 1997.
43. Surapaneni P, Vinales KL, Najib MQ, et al: Valvular heart disease with the use of fenfluramine-phentermine. *Tex Heart Inst J* 38:581–583, 2011.
44. Ootaki Y, Yamaguchi M, Yoshimura N, et al: Congenital heart disease with hypereosinophilic syndrome. *Pediatr Cardiol* 24:608–610, 2003.
45. De Cock C, Lemaitre J, Deuvaert FE: Löeffler endomyocarditis: a clinical presentation as right ventricular tumor. *J Heart Valve Dis* 7:668–671, 1998.
46. Metzler B, Günther E, Perier P, et al: Löffler's parietal fibroplastic endocarditis. Echocardiographic course over 5 years]. *Dtsch Med Wochenschr* 122:182–187, 1997.
47. San José A, Bosch JA, Candell J, et al: Cardiac and hematological involvement in idiopathic hypereosinophilic syndrome. Study of 12 cases. *Med Clin (Barc)* 98:161–165, 1992.
48. Harley JB, McIntosh CL, Kirklin JJ, et al: Atrioventricular valve replacement in the idiopathic hypereosinophilic syndrome. *Am J Med* 73:77–78, 1982.
49. Knight CJ, Sutton GC: Complete heart block and severe tricuspid regurgitation after radiotherapy. Case report and review of the literature. *Chest* 108:1748–1751, 1995.
50. Crestanello JA, McGregor CG, Danielson GK, et al: Mitral and tricuspid valve repair in patients with previous mediastinal radiation therapy. *Ann Thorac Surg* 78:826–831, 2004.
51. Lauper J, Frand M, Milo S: Valve replacement for severe tricuspid regurgitation caused by Libman-Sacks endocarditis. *Br Heart J* 48:294–297, 1982.
52. Eiken PW, Edwards WD, Tazelaar HD, et al: Surgical pathology of nonbacterial thrombotic endocarditis in 30 patients, 1985-2000. *Mayo Clin Proc* 76:1204–1212, 2001.
53. Moyssakis I, Tektonidou MG, Vasilliou VA, et al: Libman-Sacks endocarditis in systemic lupus erythematosus: prevalence, associations, and evolution. *Am J Med* 120:636–642, 2007.
54. Waller BF, Moriarty AT, Eble JN, et al: Etiology of pure tricuspid regurgitation based on annulus circumference and leaflet area: analysis of 45 necropsy patients with clinical and morphologic

evidence of pure tricuspid regurgitation. *Am J Cardiol* 7:1063–1074, 1986.
55. Ubago JL, Figueroa A, Ochoteco A, et al: Analysis of the amount of tricuspid valve annular dilatation required to produce functional tricuspid regurgitation. *Am J Cardiol* 52:155–158, 1983.
56. Carpentier A, Deloche A, Hanania G, et al: Surgical management of acquired tricuspid valve disease. *J Thorac Cardiovasc Surg* 67:53–65, 1974.
57. Lohchab SS, Chahal AK, Agrawal N: Papillary muscle approximation to septum for functional tricuspid regurgitation. *Asian Cardiovasc Thorac Ann* 2015. [Epub ahead of print].
58. Hung J, Koelling T, Semigran MJ, et al: Usefulness of echocardiographic determined tricuspid regurgitation in predicting event-free survival in severe heart failure secondary to idiopathic-dilated cardiomyopathy or ischemic cardiomyopathy. *Am J Cardiol* 82:1301–1303, 1998.
59. Ajayi AA, Adigun AQ, Ojofeitimi EO, et al: Anthropometric evaluation of cachexia in chronic congestive heart failure: the role of tricuspid regurgitation. *Int J Cardiol* 71:79–84, 1999.
60. Tepsuwan T, Schuarattanapong S, Woragidpoonpol S, et al: Incidence and impact of cardiac cachexia in valvular surgery. *Asian Cardiovasc Thorac Ann* 17:617–621, 2009.
61. Koelling TM, Aaronson KD, Cody RJ, et al: Prognostic significance of mitral regurgitation and tricuspid regurgitation in patients with left ventricular systolic dysfunction. *Am Heart J* 144:524–529, 2002.
62. Otsuji Y, Handschumacher MD, Schwammenthal E, et al: Insights from three dimensional echocardiography into the mechanisms of functional mitral regurgitation: direct in vivo demonstration of altered leaflet tethering geometry. *Circulation* 96:1999–2008, 1997.
63. Neuhold S, Huelsmann M, Pernicka E, et al: Impact of tricuspid regurgitation on survival in patients with chronic heart failure: unexpected findings of a long-term observational study. *Eur Heart J* 34:844–852, 2013.
64. Myers PO, Kalangos A: Patch augmentation for tricuspid valve tethering. *J Card Surg* 28:730, 2013.
65. Quarti A, Iezzi F, Soura E, et al: Anterior and posterior leaflets augmentation to treat tricuspid valve regurgitation. *J Card Surg* 2014. [Epub ahead of print].
66. Hung J, Chaput M, Guerrero JL, et al: Persistent reduction of ischemic mitral regurgitation by papillary muscle repositioning: structural stabilization of the papillary muscle–ventricular wall complex. *Circulation* 116(Suppl 11):I259–I1263, 2007.
67. Ohno Y, Attizzani GF, Capodanno D, et al: Association of tricuspid regurgitation with clinical and echocardiographic outcomes after percutaneous mitral valve repair with the MitraClip system: 30-day and 12-month follow-up from the GRASP Registry. *Eur Heart J Cardiovasc Imaging* 15:1246–1255, 2014.
68. Brubakk OA, Angelsen BAJ, Hatle L: Diagnosis of valvular heart disease using transcutaneous Doppler ultrasound. *Cardiovasc Res* 11:461–469, 1977.
69. Guéret P, Diebold B, Peronneau P, et al: Clinical application of echocardiography using a transesophageal approach. *Arch Mal Coeur Vaiss* 82:585–592, 1989.
70. Ubago JL, Figueroa A, Ochoteco A, et al: A new method of right ventriculography for diagnosing tricuspid valve insufficiency. *Rev Esp Cardiol* 34:227–230, 1981.
71. Child JS: Improved guides to tricuspid valve repair: two-dimensional echocardiographic analysis of tricuspid annulus function and color flow imaging of severity of tricuspid regurgitation. *J Am Coll Cardiol* 14:1275–1277, 1989.
72. Owais K, Taylor CE, Jiang L, et al: Tricuspid annulus: a three-dimensional deconstruction and reconstruction. *Ann Thorac Surg* 98:1536–1542, 2014.
73. Yoshida K, Yoshikawa J, Shakudo M, et al: Color Doppler evaluation of valvular regurgitation in normal subjects. *Circulation* 78:840–847, 1988.
74. Bossone E, Rubenfire M, Bach DS, et al: Range of tricuspid regurgitation velocity at rest and during exercise in normal adult men: implications for the diagnosis of pulmonary hypertension. *J Am Coll Cardiol* 33:1662–1666, 1999.
75. Goldman ME, Guarino T, Fuster V, et al: The necessity for tricuspid valve repair can be determined intraoperatively by two-dimensional echocardiography. *J Thorac Cardiovasc Surg* 94:542–950, 1987.
76. Byrd BF, 3rd, O'Kelly BF, Schiller NB: Contrast echocardiography enhances tricuspid but not mitral regurgitation. *Clin Cardiol* 14(11 Suppl 5):V10–V14, 1991.
77. Lopes LR, Loureiro MJ, Miranda R, et al: The usefulness of contrast during exercise echocardiography for the assessment of systolic pulmonary pressure. *Cardiovasc Ultrasound* 6:51, 2008.
78. Shah PM, Raney AA: Tricuspid valve disease. *Curr Probl Cardiol* 33:47–84, 2008.
79. Lancellotti P, Tribouilloy C, Hagendorff A, et al: Recommendations for the echocardiographic assessment of native valvular regurgitation: an executive summary from the European Association of Cardiovascular Imaging. *Eur Heart J Cardiovasc Imaging* 14:611–644, 2013.
80. Hahn RT, Abraham T, Adams MS, et al: Guidelines for performing a comprehensive transesophageal echocardiographic examination: recommendations from the American Society of Echocardiography and the Society of Cardiovascular Anesthesiologists. *J Am Soc Echocardiogr* 26:921–964, 2013.
81. Come PC, Riley MF: Tricuspid anular dilatation and failure of tricuspid leaflet coaptation in tricuspid regurgitation. *Am J Cardiol* 55:599–601, 1985.
82. Fukuda S, Song JM, Gillinov M, et al: Tricuspid valve tethering predicts residual tricuspid regurgitation after tricuspid annuloplasty. *Circulation* 111:975–979, 2005.
83. Dreyfus GD, Corbi PJ, Chan KM, et al: Secondary tricuspid regurgitation or dilatation: which should be the criteria for surgical repair? *Ann Thorac Surg* 79:127–132, 2005.
84. Raja SG, Dreyfus GD: Basis for intervention on functional tricuspid regurgitation. *Semin Thorac Cardiovasc Surg* 22:79–83, 2010.
85. Ubago JL, Figueroa A, Colman T, et al: Hemodynamic diagnosis of organic disease in the tricuspid valve. *Rev Esp Cardiol* 33:515–523, 1980.
86. Fukuda S, Saracino G, Matsumura Y, et al: Three-dimensional geometry of the tricuspid annulus in healthy subjects and in patients with functional tricuspid regurgitation a real time 3-dimensional echocardiographic study. *Circulation* 114(Suppl I):I492–I498, 2006.
87. Shiota T: Role of modern 3D echocardiography in valvular heart disease. *Korean J Intern Med* 29:685–702, 2014.
88. Sungur A, Hsiung MC, Meggo Quiroz LD, et al: The advantages of live/real time three-dimensional transesophageal echocardiography in the assessment of tricuspid valve infective endocarditis. *Echocardiography* 31:1293–1309, 2014.
89. Miglioranza MH, Mihăilă S, Muraru D, et al: Dynamic changes in tricuspid annular diameter measurement in relation to the echocardiographic view and timing during the cardiac cycle. *J Am Soc Echocardiogr* 28:226–235, 2015.
90. Braunwald NS, Ross J, Morrow AG: Conservative management of tricuspid regurgitation in patients undergoing mitral valve replacement. *Circulation* 35(Suppl 4):163–169, 1967.
91. Duran CMG, Pomar JL, Colman T, et al: Is tricuspid valve repair necessary? *J Thorac Cardiovasc Surg* 80:849–860, 1980.
92. Bernal JM, Morales D, Revuelta C, et al: Reoperations after tricuspid valve repair. *J Thorac Cardiovasc Surg* 130:498–503, 2005.
93. Mestres CA, Fita G, Parra VM, et al: Tricuspid valve surgery. *HSR Proc Intensive Care Cardiovasc Anesth* 4:261–267, 2012.
94. Pfannmüller B, Moz M, Misfeld M, et al: Isolated tricuspid valve surgery in patients with previous cardiac surgery. *J Thorac Cardiovasc Surg* 146:841–847, 2013.
95. Buzzatti N, Iaci G, Taramasso M, et al: Long-term outcomes of tricuspid valve replacement after previous left-side heart surgery. *Eur J Cardiothorac Surg* 46:713–719, 2014.
96. Shinn SH, Schaff HV: Evidence-based surgical management of acquired tricuspid valve disease. *Nat Rev Cardiol* 10:190–203, 2013.
97. García-Rinaldi R: Tricuspid anterior leaflet replacement with autologous pericardium and polytetrafluoroethylene chordae, followed by edge-to-edge repair. *Tex Heart Inst J* 34:310–312, 2007.
98. Ortiz C, López J, García H, et al: Clinical classification and prognosis of isolated right-sided infective endocarditis. *Medicine (Baltimore)* 93(27):e137, 2014.
99. Yuan SM: Right-sided infective endocarditis: recent epidemiologic changes. *Int J Clin Exp Med.* 7:199–218, 2014.
100. Bellavia D, Pentiricci S, Senni M, et al: Update on tricuspid regurgitation. *G Ital Cardiol (Rome)* 15:418–429, 2014.

101. Goldstone AB, Howard JL, Cohen JE, et al: Natural history of coexistent tricuspid regurgitation in patients with degenerative mitral valve disease: implications for future guidelines. *J Thorac Cardiovasc Surg* 148:2802–2809, 2014.
102. Angermann CE, Spes CH, Tammen A, et al: Anatomic characteristics and valvular function of the transplanted heart: transthoracic versus transesophageal echocardiographic findings. *J Heart Transplant* 9:331–338, 1990.
103. Berger Y, Har Zahav Y, Kassif Y, et al: Tricuspid valve regurgitation after orthotopic heart transplantation: prevalence and etiology. *J Transplant* 120702:2012, 2012.
104. Wartig M, Tesan S, Gäbel J, et al: Tricuspid regurgitation influences outcome after heart transplantation. *J Heart Lung Transplant* 33:829–835, 2014.
105. Czer LS, Cohen MH, Gallagher SP, et al: Exercise performance comparison of bicaval and biatrial orthotopic heart transplant recipients. *Transplant Proc* 43:3857–3862, 2011.
106. De Bonis M, Taramasso M, Verzini A, et al: Long-term results of mitral repair for functional mitral regurgitation in idiopathic dilated cardiomyopathy. *Eur J Cardiothorac Surg* 42:640–646, 2012.
107. Bolling SF: Mitral repair for functional mitral regurgitation in idiopathic dilated cardiomyopathy: a good operation done well may help. *Eur J Cardiothorac Surg* 42:646–647, 2012.
108. De Bonis M, Lapenna E, Sorrentino F, et al: Evolution of tricuspid regurgitation after mitral valve repair for functional mitral regurgitation in dilated cardiomyopathy. *Eur J Cardiothorac Surg* 33:600–606, 2008.
109. Carpentier A: La valvuloplasty reconstitutive. Une nouvelle technique de valvuloplastie mitrale. *Presse Med* 7:251–253, 1969.
110. Duran CMG, Ubago JL: Clinical and hemodynamic performance of a totally flexible prosthetic ring for atrioventricular valve reconstruction. *Ann Thorac Cardiovasc Surg* 22:458–463, 1976.
111. Durán CM, Pomar JL, Cucchiara G: A flexible ring for atrioventricular heart valve reconstruction. *J Cardiovasc Surg (Torino)* 19:417–420, 1978.
112. Pfannmueller B, Verevkin A, Borger MA, et al: Role of tricuspid valve repair for moderate tricuspid regurgitation during minimally invasive mitral valve surgery. *Thorac Cardiovasc Surg* 61:386–391, 2013.
113. Martinez-Leon J, Carbonell-Canti C, Ortega-Serrano J: Myocardial protection by retrograde cardioplegic perfusion in the presence of acute coronary artery obstruction. An experimental study. *Scand J Thorac Cardiovasc Surg* 26:207–212, 1992.
114. Guiraudon GM, Ofiesh AG, Kushk R: Extended vertical transatrial septal approach to the mitral valve. *Ann Thorac Surg* 53:1058–1062, 1991.
115. Bailey CP: Tricuspid stenosis. In Bailey CP, editor: *Surgery of the heart*, Philadelphia, 1955, Lea & Febiger, pp 846–861.
116. Al Zaibag M, Ribeiro P, Al Kasab S: Percutaneous balloon valvotomy in tricuspid stenosis. *Br Heart J* 57:51–53, 1987.
117. Michiels V, Delabays A, Eeckhout E: Percutaneous balloon valvotomy for the treatment of pacemaker lead-induced tricuspid stenosis. *Heart* 100:352, 2014.
118. Duran CMG, Pekar F: Techniques for ensuring the correct length of new mitral chords. *J Heart Valve Dis* 108:727–735, 1994.
119. Alfieri O, Maisano F: An effective technique to correct anterior mitral leaflet prolapse. *J Card Surg* 14:468–470, 1999.
120. Cui YC, Li JH, Zhang C, et al: Utilization of the edge-to-edge valve plasty technique to correct severe tricuspid regurgitation in patients with congenital heart disease. *J Card Surg* 24:727–731, 2009.
121. Lapenna E, De Bonis M, Verzini A, et al: The clover technique for the treatment of complex tricuspid valve insufficiency: midterm clinical and echocardiographic results in 66 patients. *Eur J Cardiothorac Surg* 37:1297–1303, 2010.
122. Wooler GH, Nixon PG, Grimshaw VA, et al: Experiences with the repair of the mitral valve in mitral incompetence. *Thorax* 17:49–57, 1962.
123. Kay JH, Maselli-Campagna G, Tsuji KK: Surgical treatment of tricuspid insufficiency. *Ann Surg* 162:53–58, 1965.
124. Cabrol C: Valvular annuloplasty. A new method. *Nouv Presse Med* 1:1366, 1972.
125. De Vega NG: La anuloplastia selective, regulable y permanente. *Rev Esp Cardiol* 25:555–560, 1972.
126. Kumar AS: The world view on De Vega annuloplasty. *Cir Cardiov* 19:357–360, 2012.
127. Parolari A, Barili F, Pilozzi A, et al: Ring or suture annuloplasty for tricuspid regurgitation? A meta-analysis review. *Ann Thorac Surg* 98:2255–2563, 2014.
128. Duran CMG: Duran ring annuloplasty of the tricuspid valve. *Oper Tech Thorac Cardiovasc Surg* 8:201–212, 2003.
129. Cosgrove DM, Arcidi JM, Rodriguez L, et al: Initial experience with the Cosgrove- Edwards annuloplasty system. *Ann Thorac Surg* 60:499–504, 1995.
130. Lansac E, Lim KH, Shomura Y, et al: Dynamic balance of the aortomitral junction. *J Thorac Cardiovasc Surg* 123:911–918, 2002.
131. Arbulu A, Holmes RJ: Surgical treatment of intractable right-sided infective endocarditis in drug addicts: 25 years' experience. *J Heart Valve Dis* 2:129–137, 1993.
132. Robicsek F: Cardiac valve transplantation. *Acta Med Hung* 1–2:81–91, 1954.
133. Hubka M, Siska K, Brozman M, et al: Replacement of the mitral and tricuspid valves by mitral homografts. *J Thorac Cardiovasc Surg* 51:195–294, 1966.
134. di Summa M, Donegani E, Zattera GF, et al: Successful orthotopic transplantation of a fresh tricuspid valve homograft in a human. *Ann Thorac Surg* 56:1407–1408, 1993.
135. Campelos P, Encalada JF, Ramírez J, et al: An old mitral homograft in the tricuspid position. *J Heart Valve Dis* 22:732–734, 2013.
136. Said SM, Burkhart HM, Schaff HV, et al: When should a mechanical tricuspid valve replacement be considered? *J Thorac Cardiovasc Surg* 148:603–608, 2014.
137. Zientara A, Genoni M, Graves K, et al: Tricuspid valve repair for the poor right ventricle: tricuspid valve repair in patients with mild-to-moderate tricuspid regurgitation undergoing mitral valve repair improves in-hospital outcome. *Thorac Cardiovasc Surg* 2015. [Epub ahead of print].
138. Murashita T, Okada Y, Kanemitsu H, et al: Long-term outcomes of tricuspid annuloplasty for functional tricuspid regurgitation associated with degenerative mitral regurgitation: suture annuloplasty versus ring annuloplasty using a flexible band. *Ann Thorac Cardiovasc Surg* 20:1026–1033, 2014.
139. Ratschiller T, Guenther T, Guenzinger R, et al: Early experiences with a new three-dimensional annuloplasty ring for the treatment of functional tricuspid regurgitation. *Ann Thorac Surg* 98:2039–2044, 2014.
140. Haerten K, Seipel L, Loogen F, et al: Hemodynamic studies after de Vega's tricuspid annuloplasty. *Circulation* 58(3 Pt 2):I28–I33, 1978.
141. Hanania G, Sellier P, Deloche A, et al: Mid-term results of Carpentier's reconstructive tricuspid annuloplasty. Apropos of 25 cases with postoperative catheterization. *Arch Mal Coeur Vaiss* 67:895–909, 1974.
142. Galiñanes M, Duarte J, de Caleya DF, et al: Fracture of the Carpentier-Edwards ring in tricuspid position: a report of three cases. *Ann Thorac Surg* 42:74–76, 1986.
143. McCarthy PM, Bhudia SK, Rajeswaran J, et al: Tricuspid valve repair: durability and risk factors for failure. *Thorac Cardiovasc Surg* 127:674–685, 2004.
144. Matsunaga A, Duran CMG: Progression of tricuspid regurgitation after repaired functional ischemic mitral regurgitation. *Circulation* 112(Suppl 9):I453–I457, 2005.
145. Zhu TY, Wang JG, Meng X: Is a rigid tricuspid annuloplasty ring superior to a flexible band when correcting secondary tricuspid regurgitation? *Interact Cardiovasc Thorac Surg* 17:1009–1014, 2013.
146. Pollock AV, Thomas V: Replacement of a tricuspid valve cusp by a homologous cusp in dogs. *Surg Gynecol Obstet* 103:731–735, 1956.
147. Ricci D, Boffini M, Barbero C, et al: Minimally invasive tricuspid valve surgery in patients at high risk. *J Thorac Cardiovasc Surg* 147:996–1001, 2014.
148. Dreyfus GD, Chan KM: Functional tricuspid regurgitation: a more complex entity than it appears. *Heart* 95:868–869, 2009.
149. Mestres CA, Igual A, Murtra M: The Björk-Shiley tilting disc valve in the tricuspid position. 10-year experience. *Scand J Thorac Cardiovasc Surg* 17:197–199, 1983.
150. Kawachi Y, Tominaga R, Hisahara M, et al: Excellent durability of the Hancock porcine bioprosthesis in the tricuspid position. A

sixteen-year follow-up study. *J Thorac Cardiovasc Surg* 104:1561–1566, 1992.
151. Kawano H, Oda T, Fukunaga S, et al: Tricuspid valve replacement with the St. Jude Medical valve: 19 years of experience. *Eur J Cardiothorac Surg* 18:565–569, 2000.
152. Jegaden O, Perinetti M, Barthelet M, et al: Clinical and hemodynamic prognosis after tricuspid valve replacement with bioprosthesis. *Arch Mal Coeur Vaiss* 85:1413–1418, 1992.
153. Songur CM, Simsek E, Ozen A, et al: Long term results comparing mechanical and biological prostheses in the tricuspid valve position: which valve types are better - mechanical or biological prostheses? *Heart Lung Circ* 23:1175–1178, 2014.
154. Leviner DB, Medalion B, Baruch I, et al: Tricuspid valve replacement: the effect of gender on operative results. *J Heart Valve Dis* 23:209–215, 2014.
155. Starr A, Edwards ML: Mitral replacement: clinical experience with ball-valve prosthesis. Starr A, Edwards ML. *Ann Surg* 154:726–740, 1961.
156. Iscan ZH, Vural KM, Bahar I, et al: What to expect after tricuspid valve replacement? Long-term results. *Eur J Cardiothorac Surg* 32:296–300, 2007.
157. Carrier M, Heber Y, Pellerin M, et al: Tricuspid valve replacement: an analysis of 25 years of experience at a single center. *Ann Thorac Surg* 75:47–50, 2003.
158. McGrath LB, Gonzalez-Lavin L, Bailey BM, et al: Tricuspid valve operations in 530 patients. Twenty-five-year assessment of early and late phase events. *J Thorac Cardiovasc Surg* 99:124–133, 1990.
159. Munro AI, Jamieson WRE, Tyers GFO, et al: Tricuspid valve replacement: porcine bioprosthesis and mechanical prosthesis. *Ann Thorac Surg* 59:S470–S471, 1995.
160. Nakano K, Eishi K, Kosakai Y, et al: Ten-year experience with the Carpentier-Edwards pericardial xenograft in the tricuspid position. *J Thorac Cardiovasc Surg* 111:605–612, 1996.
161. Poveda JJ, Bernal JM, Matorras P, et al: Tricuspid valve replacement in rheumatic disease: preoperative predictors of hospital mortality. *J Heart Valve Dis* 5:26–30, 1996.
162. Hornick P, Harris PA, Taylor KM: Tricuspid valve replacement subsequent to previous open heart surgery. *J Heart Valve Dis* 5:20–25, 1996.
163. Staab ME, Nishimura RA, Dearani JA: Isolated tricuspid valve surgery for severe tricuspid regurgitation following prior left heart surgery: analysis of outcome in 34 patients. *J Heart Valve Dis* 6:567–574, 1999.
164. Sanfelippo PM, Giuliani ER, Danielson GK, et al: Tricuspid valve prosthetic replacement. *J Thorac Cardiovasc Surg* 71:445–446, 1976.
165. Thorburn CW, Morgan JJ, Shanahan MX, et al: Long-term results of tricuspid valve replacement and the problem of tricuspid valve thrombosis. *Am J Cardiol* 51:1128–1132, 1983.
166. Kratz JM, Crawford FA, Stoud MR, et al: Trends and results in tricuspid surgery. *Chest* 88:837–840, 1985.
167. Bernal JM, Morales D, Revuelta C, et al: Reoperations after tricuspid valve repair. *J Thorac Cardiovasc Surg* 130:498–503, 2005.
168. Bernal JM, Pontón A, Diez B, et al: Surgery for rheumatic tricuspid valve disease: a 30-year experience. *J Thorac Cardiovasc Surg* 136:476–481, 2008.
169. Hwang HY, Kim KH, Kim KB, et al: Treatment for severe functional tricuspid regurgitation: annuloplasty versus valve replacement. *Eur J Cardiothorac Surg* 46:e21–e27, 2014.
170. Bourguignon T, Bouquiaux-Stablo AL, Loardi C, et al: Very late outcomes for mitral valve replacement with the Carpentier-Edwards pericardial bioprosthesis: 25-year follow-up of 450 implantations. *J Thorac Cardiovasc Surg* 148:2004–2011, 2014.
171. Valfrè C, Ius P, Minniti G, et al: The fate of Hancock II porcine valve recipients 25 years after implant. *Eur J Cardiothorac Surg* 38:141–146, 2010.
172. Fleming WH, Sarafian LB, Moulton AL, et al: Valve replacement in the right side of the heart in children: long-term follow-up. *Ann Thorac Surg* 48:404–408, 1989.
173. Ohata T, Kigawa I, Tohda E, et al: Comparison of durability of bioprosthesis in tricuspid and mitral position. *Ann Thorac Surg* 71:S240–S243, 2001.
174. Carrier M, Heber Y, Pellerin M, et al: Tricuspid valve replacement: an analysis of 25 years of experience at a single center. *Ann Thorac Surg* 75:47–50, 2003.
175. Ratnatunga CP, Edwards MD, Dore CJ, et al: Tricuspid valve replacement: UK heart valve registry mid-term results comparing mechanical and biological prosthesis. *Ann Thorac Surg* 66:1940–1947, 1998.
176. Kaplan M, Kut MS, Demirtas MM, et al: Prosthetic replacement of tricuspid valve: bioprosthesis or mechanical? *Ann Thorac Surg* 73:467–473, 2002.
177. Kawano H, Oda T, Fukunaga S, et al: Tricuspid valve replacement with the St. Jude Medical valve. *Eur J Cardiothoracic Surg* 18:565–569, 2000.
178. Kawachi Y, Tominaga R, Hisahara M, et al: Excellent durability of the Hancock porcine bioprosthesis in the tricuspid position. *J Thorac Cardiovasc Surg* 104:1561–1566, 1992.
179. Abad C, Barriuso C, Pomar JL, et al: Dysfunction of a Duromedics valve in the tricuspid position. Case report. *J Cardiovasc Surg (Torino)* 31:47–49, 1990.
180. Habets J, Symersky P, van Herwerden LA, et al: Prosthetic heart valve assessment with multidetector-row CT: imaging characteristics of 91 valves in 83 patients. *Eur Radiol* 21:1390–1396, 2011.
181. Altaani HA, Jaber S: Tricuspid Valve Replacement, Mechanical vs. Biological Valve, Which Is Better? *Int Cardiovasc Res J* 77:71–74, 2013.
182. Bolling SF: Tricuspid regurgitation after left heart surgery: does it matter? *J Am Coll Cardiol* 64:2643–2644, 2014.
183. Agricola E, Stella S, Gullace M, et al: Impact of functional tricuspid regurgitation on heart failure and death in patients with functional mitral regurgitation and left ventricular dysfunction. *Eur J Heart Fail* 14:902–908, 2012.
184. Kammerlander AA, Marzluf BA, Graf A, et al: Right ventricular dysfunction, but not tricuspid regurgitation, is associated with outcome late after left heart valve procedure. *J Am Coll Cardiol* 64:2633–2642, 2014.
185. Hyllén S, Nozohoor S, Ingvarsson A, et al: Right ventricular performance after valve repair for chronic degenerative mitral regurgitation. *Ann Thorac Surg* 98:2023–2030, 2014.
186. Al-Khatib SM, Hellkamp A, Curtis J, et al: Non-evidence-based ICD implantations in the United States. *JAMA* 305:43–49, 2011.
187. Najib MQ, Vittala SS, Challa S, et al: Predictors of severe tricuspid regurgitation in patients with permanent pacemaker or automatic implantable cardioverter-defibrillator leads. *Tex Heart Inst J* 40:529–533, 2013.
188. Baquero GA, Luck J, Naccarelli GV, et al: Tricuspid valve incompetence following implantation of ventricular leads. *Curr Heart Fail Rep* 12:150–157, 2015.
189. Manjunath CN, Srinivas P, Ravindranath KS, et al: Incidence and patterns of valvular heart disease in a tertiary care high-volume cardiac center: a single center experience. *Indian Heart J* 66:320–326, 2014.
190. Rodríguez-Capitán J, Gómez-Doblas JJ, Fernández-López L, et al: Short- and long-term outcomes of surgery for severe tricuspid regurgitation. *Rev Esp Cardiol (Engl Ed)* 66:629–635, 2013.
191. Gonzalez-Santos JM, Arnaiz-Garcia ME: Correcting tricuspid regurgitation: an unresolved issue. *Rev Esp Cardiol (Engl Ed)* 66:609–612, 2013.
192. Bonow RO, Carabello BA, Chatterjee K, et al: 2008 Focused update incorporated into the ACC/AHA 2006 Guidelines for the management of patients with valvular heart disease: a report of the American College of Cardiology/American Heart Association Task Force on Practice Guidelines. *Circulation* 118:e523–e661, 2008.
193. Joint Task Force on the management of valvular heart disease of The European Society of Cardiology (ESC) and The European Association for Cardio-Thoracic Surgery, (EACTS): Guidelines on the management of valvular heart disease (version, 2012). *Eur Heart J* 33:2451–2456, 2012.
194. Bernal JM, Mestres CA: Surgical treatment of organic and functional tricuspid valve disease. *Rev Esp Cardiol (Engl Ed)* 66:1006, 2013.
195. Rivera R, Duran E, Ajuria M: Carpentier's flexible ring versus De Vega's annuloplasty. A prospective randomized study. *J Thorac Cardiovasc Surg* 89:196–203, 1985.
196. Roshanali F, Saidi B, Mandegar MH, et al: Echocardiographic approach to the decision-making process for tricuspid valve repair. *J Thorac Cardiovasc Surg* 139:1483–1487, 2010.

197. Khorsandi M, Banerjee A, Singh H, et al: Is a tricuspid annuloplasty ring significantly better than a De Vega's annuloplasty stitch when repairing severe tricuspid regurgitation? *Interact Cardiovasc Thorac Surg* 15:129–135, 2012.
198. De Vega NG: Yesterday's future: the gap between where we are now and where we were supposed to be. *Eur J Cardiothorac Surg* 43:66, 2013.
199. Guenther T, Mazzitelli D, Noebauer C, et al: Tricuspid valve repair: is ring annuloplasty superior? *Eur J Cardiothorac Surg* 43:58–65, 2013.
200. Yilmaz O, Suri RM, Dearani JA, et al: Functional tricuspid regurgitation at the time of mitral valve repair for degenerative leaflet prolapse: the case for a selective approach. *J Thorac Cardiovasc Surg* 142:608–613, 2011.
201. Pfannmüller B, Davierwala P, Hirnle G, et al: Concomitant tricuspid valve repair in patients with minimally invasive mitral valve surgery. *Ann Cardiothorac Surg* 2:758–764, 2013.
202. Merk DR, Lehmann S, Holzhey DM, et al: Minimal invasive aortic valve replacement surgery is associated with improved survival: a propensity-matched comparison. *Eur J Cardiothorac Surg* 47:11–17, discussion 17, 2015.
203. Mohr FW: Decade in review–valvular disease: current perspectives on treatment of valvular heart disease. *Nat Rev Cardiol* 11:637–638, 2014.
204. Schnittger I, Appleton CP, Hatle LK, et al: Diastolic mitral and tricuspid regurgitation by Doppler echocardiography in patients with atrioventricular block: new insight into the mechanism of atrioventricular valve closure. *J Am Coll Cardiol* 11:83–88, 1988.
205. Skyaerpe T, Hatle L: Diagnosis of tricuspid regurgitation. Sensitivity of Doppler ultrasound compared with contrast echocardiography. *Eur Heart J* 6:429–436, 1985.
206. Chambers JB, Monaghan MJ, Jackson G: Echocardiography. *BMJ* 297:1071–1076, 1988.
207. Mestres CA, Fita G, Azqueta M, et al: Role of echocardiogram in decision making for surgery of endocarditis. *Curr Infect Dis Rep* 12:321–328, 2010.
208. Eidet J, Dahle G, Bugge JF, et al: Transcatheter aortic valve implantation and intraoperative left ventricular function: a myocardial tissue Doppler imaging study. *J Cardiothorac Vasc Anesth* 29:115–120, 2015.
209. Essandoh M, Portillo J, Zuleta-Alarcon A, et al: Elevated transaortic valvular gradients after combined aortic valve and mitral valve replacement: an intraoperative dilemma. *Semin Cardiothorac Vasc Anesth* 19:61–65, 2015.
210. Lang RM, Badano LP, Mor-Avi V, et al: Recommendations for cardiac chamber quantification by echocardiography in adults: an update from the american society of echocardiography and the European association of cardiovascular imaging. *J Am Soc Echocardiogr* 28:1–39, 2015.
211. Voigt JU, Pedrizzetti G, Lysyansky P, et al: Definitions for a common standard for 2D speckle tracking echocardiography: consensus document of the EACVI/ASE/Industry Task Force to standardize deformation imaging. *J Am Soc Echocardiogr* 28:183–193, 2015.
212. Miglioranza MH, Mihaila S, Muraru D, et al: Variability of tricuspid annulus diameter measurement in healthy volunteers. *JACC Cardiovasc Imaging* 2014. [Epub ahead of print].
213. Pica S, Ghio S, Tonti G, et al: Analyses of longitudinal and of transverse right ventricular function provide different clinical information in patients with pulmonary hypertension. *Ultrasound Med Biol* 40:1096–1103, 2014.
214. De Bonis M, Lapenna E, Taramasso M, et al: Mid-term results of tricuspid annuloplasty with a three-dimensional remodelling ring. *J Card Surg* 27:288–294, 2012.
215. Yoda M, Tanabe H, Kadoma Y, et al: Mid-term results of tricuspid annuloplasty using the MC3 ring for secondary tricuspid valve regurgitation. *Interact Cardiovasc Thorac Surg* 13:7–10, 2011.
216. Jeong DS, Kim KH: Tricuspid annuloplasty using the MC3 ring for functional tricuspid regurgitation. *Circ J* 74:278–283, 2010.
217. Duran CM, Balasundaram SG, Bianchi S, et al: The vanishing tricuspid annuloplasty. A new concept. *J Thorac Cardiovasc Surg* 104:796–801, 1992.
218. Duran CM, Kumar N, Prabhakar G, et al: Vanishing De Vega annuloplasty for functional tricuspid regurgitation. *J Thorac Cardiovasc Surg* 106:609–613, 1993.
219. Kalangos A, Sierra J, Vala D, et al: Annuloplasty for valve repair with a new biodegradable ring: an experimental study. *J Heart Valve Dis* 15:783–790, 2006.
220. Myers PO, Kalangos A: Valve repair using biodegradable ring annuloplasty: from bench to long-term clinical results. *Heart Lung Vessel* 5:213–218, 2013.
221. Myers PO, Cikirikcioglu M, Kalangos A: Biodegradable materials for surgical management of infective endocarditis: new solution or a dead end street? *BMC Surg* 14:48, 2014.
222. Mrowczynski W, Mrozinski B, Kalangos A, et al: A biodegradable ring enables growth of the native tricuspid annulus. *J Heart Valve Dis* 20:205–215, 2011.
223. Panos A, Myers PO, Kalangos A: Thoracoscopic and robotic tricuspid valve annuloplasty with a biodegradable ring: an initial experience. *J Heart Valve Dis* 19:201–205, 2010.
224. Kalfa D, Bel A, Chen-Tournoux A, et al: A polydioxanone electrospun valved patch to replace the right ventricular outflow tract in a growing lamb model. *Biomaterials* 31:4056–4063, 2010.
225. DeMaria AN: Structural heart disease? *J Am Coll Cardiol* 63:603–604, 2014.
226. Attubato MJ, Stroh JA, Bach RG, et al: Percutaneous double-balloon valvuloplasty of porcine bioprosthetic valves in the tricuspid position. *Int J Cardiol* 20:133–137, 1988.
227. Slama MS, Drieu LH, Malergue MC, et al: Percutaneous double balloon valvuloplasty for stenosis of porcine bioprostheses in the tricuspid valve position: a report of 2 cases. *Cathet Cardiovasc Diagn* 20:202–204, 1990.
228. Hon JK, Cheung A, Ye J, et al: Transatrial transcatheter tricuspid valve-in-valve implantation of balloon expandable bioprosthesis. *Ann Thorac Surg* 90:1696–1697, 2010.
229. Roberts PA, Boudjemline Y, Cheatham JP, et al: Percutaneous tricuspid valve replacement in congenital and acquired heart disease. *Int J Cardiol* 142:e45–e47, 2010.
230. Jux C, Akintuerk H, Schranz D: Two Melodies in concert: transcatheter double-valve replacement. *Circ Cardiovasc Int* 4:615–620, 2011.
231. Filsoof DM, Snipelisky DF, Shapiro BP: Use of a melody pulmonary valve in transcatheter valve-in-valve replacement for tricuspid valve bioprosthesis degeneration. *Tex Heart Inst J* 41:511–513, 2014.
232. Sevimli S, Aksakal E, Tanboga IH, et al: Percutaneous valve-in-valve transcatheter tricuspid valve replacement with simultaneous paravalvular leak closure in a patient with refractory right heart failure. *JACC Cardiovasc Interv* 7:e79–e80, 2014.
233. Mortazavi A, Reul RM, Cannizzaro L, et al: Transvenous transcatheter valve-in-valve implantation after bioprosthetic tricuspid valve failure. *Tex Heart Inst J* 41:507–510, 2014.
234. Tzifa A, Momenah T, Al Sahari A, et al: Transcatheter valve-in-valve implantation in the tricuspid position. *EuroIntervention* 10:995–999, 2014.
235. Petit CJ, Justino H, Ing FF: Melody valve implantation in the pulmonary and tricuspid position. *Eurointervention* 8:628–633, 2012.
236. Hoendermis ES, Douglas YL, van den Heuvel AF: Percutaneous Edwards SAPIEN valve implantation in the tricuspid position: case report and review of literature. *Catheter Cardiovasc Interv* 82:428–435, 2013.
237. Bhamidipati CM, Scott Lim D, Ragosta M, et al: Percutaneous transjugular implantation of MELODY valve into tricuspid bioprosthesis. *JACC Cardiovasc Interv* 6:598–605, 2013.
238. Reddy G, Ahmed M, Alli O: Percutaneous valvuloplasty for severe bioprosthetic tricuspid valve stenosis in the setting of infective endocarditis. *Korean Circ J* 43:273–276, 2013.
239. Dahle G, Rein KA, Bapat V: Concomitant transatrial valve-in-valve in pulmonal and tricuspid position. *Ann Thorac Surg* 98:1826–1827, 2014.
240. Hermsen JL, Permut LC, McQuinn TC, et al: Tricuspid valve replacement with a melody stented bovine jugular vein conduit. *Ann Thorac Surg* 98:1826–1827, 2014.
241. Godart F, Baruteau AE, Petit J, et al: Transcatheter tricuspid valve implantation: a multicentre French study. *Eurointervention* 10:995–999, 2014.
242. Cullen MW, Cabalka AK, Alli OO, et al: Transvenous, antegrade Melody valve-in-valve implantation for bioprosthetic mitral and

tricuspid valve dysfunction: a case series in children and adults. *Catheter Cardiovasc Interv* 82:E944–E946, 2013.
243. Hasan BS, McElhinney DB, Brown DW, et al: Short-term performance of the transcatheter Melody valve in high-pressure hemodynamic environments in the pulmonary and systemic circulations. *J Am Coll Cardiol* 58:117–122, 2011.
244. Whisenant B, Jones K, Miller D, et al: Thrombosis following mitral and tricuspid valve-in-valve replacement. *J Thorac Cardiovasc Surg* 149:e26–e29, 2015.
245. Bentham J, Qureshi S, Eicken A, et al: Early percutaneous valve failure within bioprosthetic tricuspid tissue valve replacements. *J Am Soc Echocardiogr* 25:383–392, 2012.
246. Latib A, Naim C, De Bonis M, et al: TAVR-associated prosthetic valve infective endocarditis: results of a large, multicenter registry. *J Am Coll Cardiol* 64:2176–2178, 2014.
247. Latib A, Naim C, De Bonis M, et al: TAVR-associated prosthetic valve infective endocarditis: results of a large, multicenter registry. *J Am Coll Cardiol* 64:2176–2178, 2014.
248. Pericas JM, Llopis J, Cervera C, et al the Hospital Clinic Endocarditis Study Group: Infective endocarditis in patients with an implanted transcatheter aortic valve: clinical characteristics and outcome of a new entity. *J Infect* 2015. [Epub ahead of print].
249. Jeevanandam V, Russell H, Mather P, et al: Donor tricuspid annuloplasty during orthotopic heart transplantation: long-term results of a prospective controlled study. *Ann Thorac Surg* 82:2089–2095, 2006.
250. Fiorelli AI, Oliveira JL, Santos RH, et al: Can tricuspid annuloplasty of the donor heart reduce valve insufficiency following cardiac transplantation with bicaval anastomosis? *Heart Surg Forum* 13:E168–E171, 2010.
251. Vahanian A, Alfieri O, Andreotti F, et al: Guidelines on the management of valvular heart disease (version 2012): the Joint Task Force on the Management of Valvular Heart Disease of the European Society of Cardiology (ESC) and the European Association for Cardio-Thoracic Surgery (EACTS). *Eur J Cardiothorac Surg* 42:S1–S44, 2012.
252. Benedetto U, Melina G, Angeloni E, et al: Prophylactic tricuspid annuloplasty in patients with dilated tricuspid annulus undergoing mitral valve surgery. *J Thorac Cardiovasc Surg* 143:632–638, 2012.
253. Zhu TY, Meng X, Han J, et al: An alternative intraoperative method based on annular circumference for the decision-making of prophylactic tricuspid annuloplasty. *J Heart Valve Dis* 23:370–376, 2014.
254. Teman NR, Huffman LC, Krajacic M, et al: Prophylactic" tricuspid repair for functional tricuspid regurgitation. *Ann Thorac Surg* 97:1520–1524, 2014.
255. Zhu TY, Min XP, Zhang HB, et al: Preoperative risk factors for residual tricuspid regurgitation after isolated left-sided valve surgery: a systematic review and meta-analysis. *Cardiology* 129:242–249, 2014.
256. Boudjemline Y, Agnoletti G, Bonnet D, et al: Steps toward the percutaneous replacement of atrioventricular valves an experimental study. *Cathet Cardiovasc Diagn* 28:142–148, 1993.
257. Bai Y, Chen HY, Zong GJ, et al: Percutaneous establishment of tricuspid regurgitation: an experimental model for transcatheter tricuspid valve replacement. *Eur Heart J* 31:1274–1281, 2010.
258. Bai Y, Zong GJ, Wang HR, et al: An integrated pericardial valved stent special for percutaneous tricuspid implantation: an animal feasibility study. *J Am Coll Cardiol* 46:360–365, 2005.
259. Lauten A, Figulla HR, Willich C, et al: Percutaneous caval stent valve implantation: investigation of an interventional approach for treatment of tricuspid regurgitation. *J Surg Res* 160:215–221, 2010.
260. Akinosoglou K, Apostolakis E, Marangos M, et al: Native valve right sided infective endocarditis. *Eur J Intern Med* 24:510–519, 2013.
261. Gerdisch MW, Boyd WD, Harlan JL, et al: Early experience treating tricuspid valve endocarditis with a novel extracellular matrix cylinder reconstruction. *J Thorac Cardiovasc Surg* 148:3042–3048, 2014.
262. Toyoda Y, Kashem MA, Hisamoto K, et al: Tricuspid valve reconstruction with the extracellular matrix tube technique: a word of caution. *J Thorac Cardiovasc Surg* 148:e141–e143, 2014.
263. Bajona P, Salizzoni S, Vandenberghe S, et al: "The Balloon Plug Concept" for Tricuspid Valve Repair: Ex Vivo Proof of Concept. *Innovations (Phila)* 10:27–32, 2015.

CHAPTER 82

Native and Prosthetic Valve Endocarditis

Amy G. Fiedler • Lawrence S. Lee • Frederick Y. Chen • Lawrence H. Cohn

CHAPTER OUTLINE

Endocarditis of a patient's native heart valve is defined as *native valve endocarditis* (NVE), and endocarditis of a prosthetic device is termed *prosthetic valve endocarditis* (PVE). The incidence of NVE in developed countries is approximately 1.7 to 7.0 cases out of 100,000 persons per year and is highest in older adults.[1-3] NVE typically affects the left heart, with right heart involvement observed in only 5% to 10%.[3,4] Whereas the overall incidence of NVE and PVE has remained consistent over the past several decades, the causes and risk factors for both NVE and PVE have changed in recent years from rheumatic heart disease to degenerative valve disease, intravenous drug use, intravascular devices, and nosocomial infections predominating.

NATIVE VALVE ENDOCARDITIS

Pathology

Two conditions must be present for the development of almost all cases of NVE: endocardial injury causing a disruption of the valvular endocardial surface, and subsequent infiltration of the injured site by bloodborne microorganisms, typically bacteria.[5] Endocardial trauma results from degenerative calcific changes, rheumatic disease, mitral valve prolapse, regurgitant jet flow, congenital abnormalities (e.g., bicuspid aortic valve), or iatrogenic causes (e.g., cardiac catheterization). Endocardial injury results in the deposition of platelet-fibrin products, which then serve as a nidus for the attachment of microorganisms. Organisms that cause NVE enter the bloodstream through compromise of the skin, mucosal surfaces, or other sites of focal infection. Common causes for bacteremia or fungemia that predispose to NVE include intravenous drug use, indwelling catheters, debilitated condition, medical procedures, and even simple events such as tooth brushing and mastication.[5-7]

In all cases of NVE, complications and symptoms of the infection may be divided into two categories. Systemic manifestations of the disease result from sepsis and embolic phenomena, such as stroke, kidney failure, or fever. In addition, there are sequelae that are the direct results of infection and the location of the infection with respect to any critical myocardial anatomy.

In native *aortic* valve endocarditis, infection may spread into the aortic annulus, destroy the aortic valve, or result in paravalvular abscess formation. Conduction system pathology may result, including heart block, depending on the extent of the infection. Other complications include cardiac fistulas, coronary and systemic embolization of vegetations, stroke, cerebral infarction, and mycotic aneurysms. Large aortic valve vegetations can prolapse into the left ventricular cavity, contact the anterior leaflet of the mitral valve, and cause subsequent double-valve endocarditis. Typically, aortic insufficiency results from aortic valve endocarditis. Untreated cases can lead to destruction of the fibrous trigones and the tissue between the anterior mitral leaflet and the aorta. Heart failure may occur because of volume overload secondary to aortic insufficiency. Fistulas between the aorta and right atrium are also possible.

The most common site of vegetations in native *mitral* valve endocarditis is the mitral valve leaflet near the annulus on the atrial side. Vegetations may be located anywhere on the leaflets or the chordae, and they may occur on the ventricular side as well. Vegetations and debris may destroy part of the ventricular tissue. Complications include invasion into the atrioventricular (AV) groove proper and abscess formation, with severe cases leading to separation at the AV junction and complete destruction of the fibrous skeleton surrounding the valve.

Native *tricuspid* valve endocarditis usually affects the free margins of the leaflets with relatively infrequent involvement of the annular tissue. Complications of tricuspid NVE include cardiac and pulmonary sequelae as a consequence of valve destruction and embolism. Tricuspid regurgitation with chamber dilation and right heart failure can result, and local extension can cause abscess and fistula formation. Septic pulmonary emboli lead to pulmonary infarction, pulmonary abscess, empyema, and, in rare cases, mycotic aneurysms of the pulmonary arteries.

Microbiology

Endocarditis is caused principally by staphylococci and streptococci. The most common agents are *Staphylococcus aureus* (32%), viridans group streptococci (18%), enterococci (11%), coagulase-negative staphylococci (11%), and *Streptococcus bovis* (7%).[8,9] Gram-negative bacteria can also cause NVE and are classified into either the HACEK group (fastidious gram-negative bacilli, including *Haemophilus aphrophilus*, *Actinobacillus actinomycetemcomitans*, *Cardiobacterium hominis*, *Eikenella corrodens*, and *Kingella kingae*) or non-HACEK group, with each accounting for approximately 2% of all cases. These organisms require a prolonged incubation period before growth and are often resistant to many antibiotics. Fungal NVE, usually caused by *Candida albicans* or *Aspergillus fumigatus*, is rare but can lead to devastating complications.[10,11]

The microbiology of NVE differs somewhat depending on specific individual risk factors and demographics. For example, viridans group streptococci is more prevalent in community-acquired endocarditis, whereas the more virulent *S. aureus* is more common in nosocomial cases.[1-3,8] NVE of the right heart is predominantly a disease of intravenous drug users, and in this population native tricuspid valve endocarditis caused by *S. aureus* is the predominant form of the disease.[4]

Approximately 2% to 7% of NVE cases are deemed "culture-negative endocarditis" when no microorganisms can be cultured from the blood or tissue samples.[12-15] This occurs more frequently in developing countries, where fastidious or rare organisms are more likely to cause human infection. The most common reasons for culture-negative endocarditis in developed countries are administration of antimicrobial agents before cultures are taken, inadequate microbiological techniques, and infection with highly fastidious bacteria or nonbacterial pathogens (e.g., fungi). In all cases of culture-negative NVE, it is important to ascertain the absence of any underlying undiscovered infection and to initiate aggressive empiric treatment despite the negative culture data.

Diagnosis

Clinical Presentation

The onset of NVE usually begins with fever and malaise. Common physical examination findings include a new heart murmur or change to an existing heart murmur, petechiae, splenomegaly, clubbing of the digits, splinter hemorrhages, Osler nodes, Janeway lesions, and Roth spots. The latter two are found almost exclusively in acute endocarditis when overwhelming signs of sepsis are displayed early in the clinical course. The virulence of the offending organism affects the severity of symptoms seen, with less virulent organisms such as viridans group streptococcus causing a subacute, protracted clinical course that often can be cured with antibiotics alone.

Laboratory findings include moderate leukocytosis, anemia without reticulocytosis, and hematuria. Blood cultures must be drawn from separate sites and usually help clinicians identify the infective organisms in cases of bacterial NVE. Cultures should be drawn before antibiotics are started.

Imaging Studies

Doppler echocardiography is the single most useful diagnostic modality for documenting endocarditis.[16-19] Transesophageal echocardiography is the preferred study, with a sensitivity and specificity of 95% and 90%, respectively.[20] Transthoracic echocardiography is less sensitive for endocarditis but can be used when transesophageal studies are not feasible. Echocardiography can be used to identify vegetations, paravalvular leaks, abscesses, and fistulas. Patients with NVE and concern for metastatic or embolic disease should undergo further imaging with computed tomography (CT) scans of the abdomen and/or head as appropriate. Embolic involvement of the brain can also be investigated with magnetic resonance imaging (MRI).[21]

Duke Criteria

The diagnosis of endocarditis is based on a combination of clinical findings rather than a single test result. Several classification systems for the diagnosis of endocarditis have been published, but the most commonly used is the Duke system.[22] First described by Duke University researchers in 1994, this system uses both clinical and pathologic criteria to confirm or reject the diagnosis of infective endocarditis. There are two groups of criteria: "major" (positive blood cultures, positive echocardiographic findings) and "minor" (fever, predisposing conditions, vascular phenomena, immunologic phenomena, equivocal microbiological findings). Based on the number of criteria met, cases are classified into three diagnostic categories: low clinical likelihood of endocarditis, possible endocarditis, and definite endocarditis. Definite endocarditis is diagnosed by documentation of two major criteria, of one major and three minor criteria, or of five minor criteria. Cases are considered possible endocarditis when either one major and one minor criterion or three minor criteria are identified. Most authorities accept a recently modified version of the Duke criteria, as shown in Table 82-1.[23]

Management

Aggressive antibiotic therapy is the first and most important intervention in all cases of NVE. Antibiotics should

then migrate to the new device. Risk factors associated with early PVE include but are not limited to infective endocarditis of the native valve, history of intravenous drug abuse, male gender, and a long cardiopulmonary bypass time.[81]

Late PVE is classified as PVE occurring more than 12 months after valve placement. The offending organisms and pathogenesis of late PVE more closely resemble what has been described in NVE.[82] The most common scenario of late PVE involves a transient bacteremia that occurs as a result of direct organism inoculation into the bloodstream, which then localizes onto the prosthetic valve. Dental procedures are a common culprit for bacterial inoculation.

The most common organism responsible for early PVE is *Staphylococcus epidermidis*. Late PVE microorganisms tend to be more similar to those encountered in NVE, such as viridans group streptococci and *S. aureus*.

The clinical signs and symptomatology associated with PVE are similar to those encountered with NVE. The important distinguishing factor between the two is that cardiac complications, such as new and changing murmurs as a result of a paravalvular leak secondary to valve ring dehiscence, and conduction defects from abscess extension into the intraventricular septum are more prevalent in PVE and require urgent if not emergent surgical intervention.

Diagnostic confusion may arise in the immediate postoperative period. Blood cultures that demonstrate staphylococci and yeast likely represent true PVE. Gram-negative bacteremia in an early postoperative patient is statistically more likely to be a result of an indwelling catheter infection, not PVE. In patients with late PVE caused by staphylococci or streptococci, blood cultures are consistently positive if the patient has not been on antimicrobial therapy.

If cardiac complications such as a new or changing murmur arise, indicating the possibility of a paravalvular leak or ring dehiscence, urgent if not emergent operative débridement and replacement are advised. Treatment strategies from an antimicrobial perspective are somewhat more aggressive in PVE than NVE. Therapy should be chosen and tailored based on the identification and susceptibilities of the specific microorganism. If an organism is yet to be identified, vancomycin and gentamicin should be instituted empirically to cover *S. epidermidis*, *S. aureus*, and streptococci. The choice of antibiotics should also consider pathogens standardly encountered at the given hospital. Patients with PVE should be treated for 6 to 8 weeks in most cases, whether or not the valve is removed. If microorganisms are isolated at the time of valve replacement, an additional 6 to 8 weeks of therapy beginning at the time of organism isolation should be instituted.[84]

SUMMARY

NVE and PVE remain significant causes of morbidity and mortality, although recent developments in antimicrobial agents, diagnostic tools, and surgical techniques have improved the prognosis for patients affected by these diseases. Early detection combined with aggressive antibiotic therapy and early surgical intervention can successfully treat most cases of NVE and PVE. Notable challenges for the cardiac surgeon include the determination of the appropriate timing of operation, removal of all infected tissue, and restoration of physiologic valve function, but sound clinical judgment and meticulous surgical technique can allow for safe and effective surgery.

REFERENCES

1. Karchmer AW: Infective endocarditis. In Fauci AS, Braunwald E, Kasper DL, et al, editors: *Harrison's principles of internal medicine*, ed 17, New York, NY, 2008, McGraw-Hill Medical, pp 789–798.
2. Moreillon P, Que YA: Infective endocarditis. *Lancet* 363:144, 2004.
3. Hoen B, Alla F, Selton-Suty C, et al: Changing profile of infective endocarditis: results of a 1-year survey in France. *JAMA* 288:75, 2002.
4. Moss R, Munt B: Injection drug use and right sided endocarditis. *Heart* 89:577–581, 2003.
5. David TE: Surgical treatment of aortic valve endocarditis. In Cohn LH, editor: *Cardiac surgery in the adult*, ed 3, New York, NY, 2008, McGraw-Hill Medical, pp 949–953.
6. McKinsey DS, Ratts TE, Bisno AL: Underlying cardiac lesions in adults with infective endocarditis. The changing spectrum. *Am J Med* 82:681, 1987.
7. Weinstein L, Schlesinger JJ: Pathoanatomic, pathophysiologic and clinical correlations in endocarditis (second of two parts). *N Engl J Med* 291:1122, 1974.
8. Fowler VG, Miro JM, Hoen B, et al: Staphylococcus aureus endocarditis: a consequence of medical progress. *JAMA* 293(24):3012–3021, 2005.
9. Quagliarello V: Infective endocarditis: global, regional, and future perspectives. *JAMA* 293:3061, 2005.
10. Ellis ME, Al-Abdely H, Sandridge A, et al: Fungal endocarditis: evidence in the world literature, 1965-1995. *Clin Infect Dis* 32(1):50–62, 2001.
11. Pierrotti LC, Baddour LM: Fungal endocarditis, 1995-2000. *Chest* 122(1):302–310, 2002.
12. Lamas CC, Eykyn SJ: Blood culture negative endocarditis: analysis of 63 cases presenting over 25 years. *Heart* 89:258, 2003.
13. Tariq M, Alam M, Munir G, et al: Infective endocarditis: a five-year experience at a tertiary care hospital in Pakistan. *Int J Infect Dis* 8(3):163–170, 2004.
14. Mylonakis E, Calderwood SB: Infective endocarditis in adults. *N Engl J Med* 345:1318, 2001.
15. Werner M, Andersson R, Olaison L, et al: A clinical study of culture-negative endocarditis. *Medicine (Baltimore)* 82:263, 2003.
16. Buda AJ, Zotx RJ, Lemire MS, et al: Prognostic significance of vegetations detected by two-dimensional echocardiography in infective endocarditis. *Am Heart J* 112:1291, 1986.
17. Lowry RW, Zoghbi WA, Baker WB, et al: Clinical impact of transesophageal echocardiography in the diagnosis and management of infective endocarditis. *Am J Cardiol* 73:1089, 1994.
18. DiSalvo G, Habib G, Pergola V, et al: Echocardiography predicts embolic events in infective endocarditis. *J Am Coll Cardiol* 15:1069, 2001.
19. Daniel WG, Mugge A, Martin RP, et al: Improvement in the diagnosis of abscesses associated with endocarditis by transesophageal echocardiography. *N Engl J Med* 324:795, 1991.
20. Daniel WG, Mugge A, Grote J, et al: Comparison of transthoracic and transesophageal echocardiography for detection of abnormalities of prosthetic and bioprosthetic valves in the mitral and aortic positions. *Am J Cardiol* 71:210, 1993.
21. Stamou SC, Petterson G, Gillinov AM: Surgical treatment of mitral valve endocarditis. In Cohn LH, editor: *Cardiac surgery in the adult*, ed 3, New York, NY, 2008, McGraw-Hill Medical, pp 1069–1077.
22. Durack DT, Lukes AS, Bright DK: New criteria for diagnosis of infective endocarditis: utilization of specific echocardiographic findings. Duke Endocarditis Service. *Am J Med* 96:200, 1994.
23. Li JS, Sexton DJ, Mick N, et al: Proposed modifications to the Duke criteria for the diagnosis of infective endocarditis. *Clin Infect Dis* 30:633, 2000.

24. Bauernschmitt R, Jakob HG, Vahl C-F, et al: Operation for infective endocarditis: results after implantation of mechanical valves. *Ann Thorac Surg* 65:359, 1998.
25. Middlemost S, Wisenbaugh T, Meyerowitz C, et al: A case for early surgery in native left-sided endocarditis complicated by heart failure: results in 203 patients. *J Am Coll Cardiol* 18:663, 1991.
26. Habib G, Avierinos JF, Thuny F: Aortic valve endocarditis: is there an optimal surgical timing? *Curr Opin Cardiol* 22:77, 2007.
27. Bonow RO, Carabello BA, Chatterjee K, et al: ACC/AHA 2006 guidelines for the management of patients with valvular heart disease. A report of the American College of Cardiology/American Heart Association Task Force on Practice Guidelines (Writing committee to revise the 1998 guidelines for the management of patients with valvular heart disease). *J Am Coll Cardiol* 48:e1, 2006.
28. Davenport J, Hart RG: Prosthetic valve endocarditis 1976-1987: antibiotics, anticoagulation, and stroke. *Stroke* 21:993, 1990.
29. Ting W, Silverman N, Levistky S: Valve replacement in patients with endocarditis and cerebral septic emboli. *Ann Thorac Surg* 51:18, 1991.
30. Matsushita K, Kuriyama Y, Sawada T, et al: Hemorrhagic and ischemic cerebrovascular complications of active infective endocarditis of native valve. *Eur Neurol* 33:267, 1993.
31. Gillinov AM, Shah RV, Curtis WE, et al: Valve replacement in patients with endocarditis and acute neurologic deficit. *Ann Thorac Surg* 61:1125, 1996.
32. Eishi K, Kawazoe K, Kuriyama Y, et al: Surgical management of infective endocarditis associated with cerebral complications. Multi-center retrospective study in Japan. *J Thorac Cardiovasc Surg* 110:1745, 1995.
33. Moon MR, Miller DC, Moore KA, et al: Treatment of endocarditis with valve replacement: the question of tissue versus mechanical prosthesis. *Ann Thorac Surg* 71:1164, 2001.
34. David TE, Komeda M, Brofman PR: Surgical treatment of aortic root abscess. *Circulation* 80(Suppl 1):269, 1989.
35. d'Udekem Y, David TE, Feindel CM, et al: Long-term results of operation for paravalvular abscess. *Ann Thorac Surg* 62:48, 1996.
36. Jault F, Gandjbakhch I, Chastre JC, et al: Prosthetic valve endocarditis with ring abscesses: surgical management and long-term results. *J Thorac Cardiovasc Surg* 105:1106, 1993.
37. Fiore AC, Ivey TD, McKeown PP, et al: Patch closure of aortic annulus mycotic aneurysm. *Ann Thorac Surg* 42:372, 1986.
38. Glazier JJ, Verwilghen J, Donaldson RM, et al: Treatment of complicated prosthetic aortic valve endocarditis with annular abscess formation by homograft root replacement. *J Am Coll Cardiol* 17:1177, 1991.
39. Yankah AC, pasic M, Klose H, et al: Homograft reconstruction of the aortic root for endocarditis with periannular abscess: a 17-year study. *Eur J Cardiothorac Surg* 28:69, 2005.
40. Dossche KM, Defauw JJ, Ernst SM, et al: Allograft aortic root replacement in prosthetic aortic valve endocarditis: a review of 32 patients. *Ann Thorac Surg* 63:1644, 1997.
41. Knosalla C, Weng Y, Yankah AC, et al: Surgical treatment of active infective aortic valve endocarditis with associated periannular abscess—11 year results. *Eur Heart J* 21:421, 2000.
42. David TE, Kuo J, Armstrong S: Aortic and mitral valve replacement with reconstruction of the intervalvular fibrous body. *J Thorac Cardiovasc Surg* 114:766, 1997.
43. David TE, Feindel CM, Armstrong S, et al: Reconstruction of the mitral annulus: a ten-year experience. *J Thorac Cardiovasc Surg* 110:1323, 1995.
44. Obadia JF, Raisky O, Sebbag L, et al: Monobloc aorto-mitral homograft as a treatment of complex cases of endocarditis. *J Thorac Cardiovasc Surg* 121:584, 2001.
45. Lytle BW, Priest BP, Taylor PC, et al: Surgical treatment of prosthetic valve endocarditis. *J Thorac Cardiovasc Surg* 111:198, 1996.
46. Lytle BW: Prosthetic valve endocarditis. In Vlessis AA, Bolling SF, editors: *Endocarditis: a multidisciplinary approach to modern treatment*, Armonk, NY, 1999, Future Publishing, p 344.
47. Gillinov AM, Diz R, Blackstone EH, et al: Double valve endocarditis. *Ann Thorac Surg* 71:1874, 2001.
48. D'Udekem Y, David TE, Feindel CM, et al: Long-term results of surgery for active infective endocarditis. *Eur J Cardiothorac Surg* 11:46, 1997.
49. Alexiou C, Langley SM, Stafford H, et al: Surgery for active culture-positive endocarditis: determinants of early and late outcome. *Ann Thorac Surg* 69:1448, 2000.
50. Cachera JP, Loisance D, Mourtada A, et al: Surgical techniques for treatment of bacterial endocarditis of the mitral valve. *J Card Surg* 2:265, 1987.
51. David TE, Feindel CM: Reconstruction of the mitral anulus. *Circulation* 76:III102–III107, 1987.
52. Carpentier AF, Pellerin M, Fuzellier JF, et al: Extensive calcification of the mitral valve anulus: pathology and surgical management. *J Thorac Cardiovasc Surg* 111(4):718–729, 1996.
53. Gardner TJ, Spray TL: *Operative cardiac surgery*, ed 5, London, 2004, Arnold Publishers.
54. David TE, Gavra G, Feindel CM, et al: Surgical treatment of active infective endocarditis: a continued challenge. *J Thorac Cardiovasc Surg* 133:144, 2007.
55. Moon MR, Miller DC, Moore KA, et al: Treatment of endocarditis with valve replacement: the question of tissue versus mechanical prosthesis. *Ann Thorac Surg* 71:1164–1171, 2001.
56. Dreyfus G, Serraf A, Jebara VA, et al: Valve repair in acute endocarditis. *Ann Thorac Surg* 49:706, 1990.
57. Hendren WG, Morris AS, Rosenkranz ER, et al: Mitral valve repair for bacterial endocarditis. *J Thorac Cardiovasc Surg* 103:124, 1992.
58. Mihaljevic T, Paul S, Leacche M, et al: Tailored surgical therapy for acute native mitral valve endocarditis. *J Heart Valve Dis* 13:210–216, 2004.
59. Muehrcke DD, Cosgrove DM, 3rd, Lytle BW, et al: Is there an advantage to repairing infected mitral valves? *Ann Thorac Surg* 63:1718, 1997.
60. Ruttmann E, Legit C, Poelzl G, et al: Mitral valve repair provides improved outcome over replacement in active infective endocarditis. *J Thorac Cardiovasc Surg* 130:765, 2005.
61. Aranki SF, Adams DH, Rizzo RJ, et al: Determinants of early mortality and late survival in mitral valve endocarditis. *Circulation* 92(Suppl 9):II143–II149, 1995.
62. Karavas AN, Filsoufi F, Mihaljevic T, et al: Risk factors and management of endocarditis after mitral valve repair. *J Heart Valve Dis* 11(5):660–664, 2002.
63. Arbulu A, Holmes RJ, Asfaw I: Surgical treatment of intractable right-sided infective endocarditis in drug addicts: 25 years experience. *J Heart Valve Dis* 2:129–137, 1993.
64. Arbulu A, Asfaw I: Tricuspid valvulectomy without prosthetic replacement: ten years of clinical experience. *J Thorac Cardiovasc Surg* 82:684–689, 1981.
65. Robin E, Thomas NW, Arbulu A, et al: Hemodynamic consequences of total removal of the tricuspid valve without prosthetic replacement. *Am J Cardiol* 35:481–486, 1975.
66. Carrier M, Heber Y, Pellerin M, et al: Tricuspid valve replacement: an analysis of 25 years of experience at a single center. *Ann Thorac Surg* 75:47–50, 2003.
67. Kaplan M, Kut MS, Demirtas MM, et al: Prosthetic replacement of tricuspid valve: bioprosthesis or mechanical? *Ann Thorac Surg* 73:467–473, 2001.
68. Ratnatunga CP, Edwards MD, Dore CJ, et al: Tricuspid valve replacement: UK heart valve registry mid-term results comparing mechanical and biological prosthesis. *Ann Thorac Surg* 66:1940–1947, 1998.
69. Yee ES, Ullyot DJ: Reparative approach for right-sided endocarditis. Operative considerations and results of valvuloplasty. *J Thorac Cardiovasc Surg* 96:133–140, 1988.
70. Stern HJ, Sisto DA, Strom JA, et al: Immediate tricuspid valve replacement for endocarditis. Indications and results. *J Thorac Cardiovasc Surg* 91:163–167, 1986.
71. Wilcox BR, Murray GF, Starek PJ: The long-term outlook for valve replacement in active endocarditis. *J Thorac Cardiovasc Surg* 74:860–863, 1977.
72. Mestres CA, Castella M, Moreno A, et al: Cryopreserved mitral homograft in the tricuspid position for infective endocarditis: a valve that can be repaired in the long-term (13 years). *J Heart Valve Dis* 15:389–391, 2006.
73. Couetil JP, Argyriadis PG, Shafy A, et al: Partial replacement of the tricuspid valve by mitral homografts in acute endocarditis. *Ann Thorac Surg* 73:1808–1812, 2002.

74. Lange R, De Simone R, Bauernschmitt R, et al: Tricuspid valve reconstruction, a treatment option in acute endocarditis. *Eur J Cardiothorac Surg* 10:320–326, 1996.
75. Bortolotti U, Tursi V, Fasoli G, et al: Tricuspid valve endocarditis: repair with the use of artificial chordae. *J Heart Valve Dis* 2:567–570, 1993.
76. Kay JH, Maselli-Campagna G, Tsuji KK: Surgical treatment of tricuspid insufficiency. *Ann Surg* 162:53–58, 1965.
77. d'Udekem Y, Sluysmans T, Rubay JE: Tricuspid valve repair for tricuspid valve endocarditis after Fallot repair. *Ann Thorac Surg* 63:830–832, 1997.
78. Yee ES, Ullyot DJ: Reparative approach for right-sided endocarditis. Operative considerations and results of valvuloplasty. *J Thorac Cardiovasc Surg* 96:133–140, 1988.
79. Gottardi R, Bialy J, Devyatko E, et al: Midterm follow-up of tricuspid valve reconstruction due to active infective endocarditis. *Ann Thorac Surg* 84(6):1943–1948, 2007.
80. Muscia M, Siniawskia H, Pasic M, et al: Surgical treatment of right-sided active infective endocarditis with or without involvement of the left heart: 20-year single center experience. *Eur J Cardiothorac Surg* 32(1):118–125, 2007.
81. Ivert TSA, Dismukes WE, Cobbs CG, et al: Prosthetic valve endocarditis. *Circulation* 69:223, 1984.
82. Karchmer AW, Dismukes WE, Buckley MJ, et al: Late prosthetic valve endocarditis: clinical features influencing therapy. *Am J Med* 64:199, 1978.
83. Fang G, Keys TF, Gentry LO, et al: Prosthetic valve endocarditis resulting from nosocomial bactermia. *Ann Intern Med* 119:560, 1993.
84. Mayer KH, Schoenbaum SC: Evaluation and management of prosthetic valve endocarditis. *Prog Cardiovasc Dis* 25:43, 1982.

CHAPTER 83

Anticoagulation, Thrombosis, and Thromboembolism of Prosthetic Cardiac Valves

Joseph C. Cleveland, Jr. • Frederick L. Grover

CHAPTER OUTLINE

ARTIFICIAL SURFACES, COAGULATION CASCADES, THROMBOSIS, AND LYSIS

Intravascular placement of a foreign body with its nonendothelial surface activates the clotting mechanism, leading to thrombus formation. The exposure of blood to the synthetic surface leads rapidly to deposition of a fine layer of plasma components, mostly protein, followed by platelet deposition. The intrinsic coagulation cascade is initiated along with the extrinsic coagulation cascade: the inflammatory response, including leukocyte activation; the complement system; and fibrinolysis.

Fibrinogen is one of the major plasma proteins, often the first that is deposited on these artificial surfaces. Once the layer of fibrinogen is absorbed onto the surface, platelets can adhere to the fibrinogen. Although surfaces vary greatly in their tendency to promote thrombosis, the reactivity of most materials to blood can be significantly increased if they are first exposed to fibrinogen.[1] Other proteins also are deposited, including fibronectin (a surface protein of many cells), von Willebrand factor (a glycoprotein essential for the adhesion of platelets to subendothelial tissue), thrombospondin (a platelet protein secreted by activated platelets), and factor XII (Hageman factor, the primary activator of the intrinsic coagulation system).

Once platelets attach to the protein layer and spread out on the artificial surface, materials present in the platelet intracellular granules are secreted, including β-thromboglobulin, which inhibits prostacyclin production; platelet factor 4, which neutralizes heparin sulfate in the endothelium; and serotonin, adenosine triphosphate (ATP), and adenosine diphosphate (ADP). Synthesis of prostaglandins E and F is evident as well, suggesting that endoperoxide metabolism has taken place along with formation of thromboxane A2 from platelet arachidonic acid. Serotonin, thromboxane A2, and endoperoxide are potent vasoconstrictors and platelet stimulatory factors.[2] Finally, platelet aggregation follows platelet adhesion, probably by ADP and serotonin secretion from the adherent platelets. Fibrinogen and thromboxane A2 are key in this step.

The coagulation cascade is initiated either by reaction of plasma proteins with the artificial surface to form enzymatically active components such as factor XII (intrinsic system) or by introduction of thromboplastin through exposure of subendothelial tissue to the surface (extrinsic system). Figure 83-1 is a schematic diagram of the clotting cascade. Activation of factors XIIa and XIa initiates the intrinsic system, leading to activated factor Xa. Platelets provide the phospholipid surface for this reaction. Activated factor XIIa also initiates the kininogen-kallikrein system, and kallikrein provides positive feedback for the contact activation. Kallikrein cleaves factor XII to convert it to factor XIIa, thereby accelerating contact activation. Bradykinin is also released when kallikrein cleaves high-molecular-weight kininogen. Activated high-molecular-weight kininogen can then bind more prekallikrein and factor XI to the activating surface,

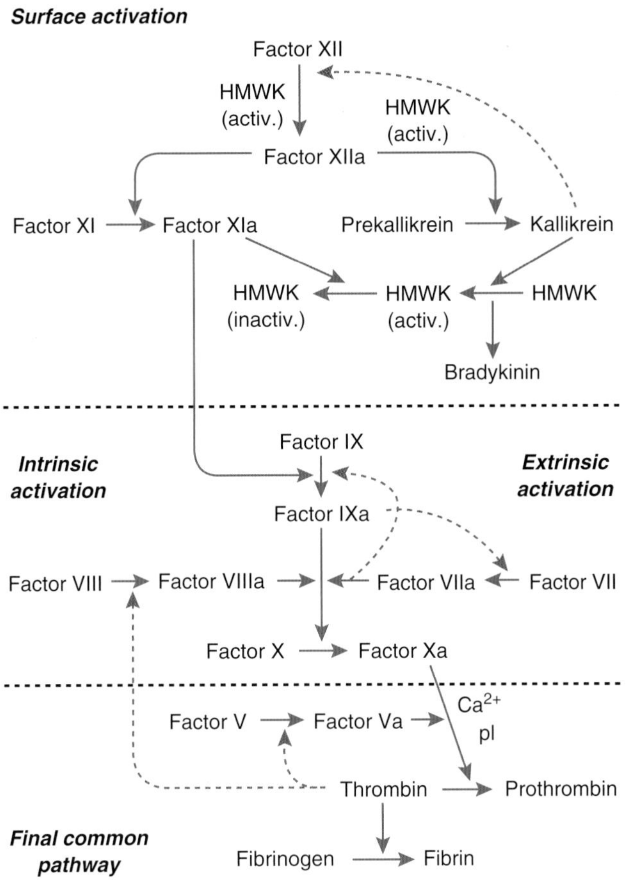

FIGURE 83-1 The coagulation cascade from surface activation to the final common pathway. *HMWK,* High-molecular-weight kininogen; *pl,* phospholipid. (From Ware JA, Lewis J, Salzman EW: Antithrombotic therapy. In Rutherford RB, editor: *Vascular surgery,* ed 3, Philadelphia, 1989, Saunders.)

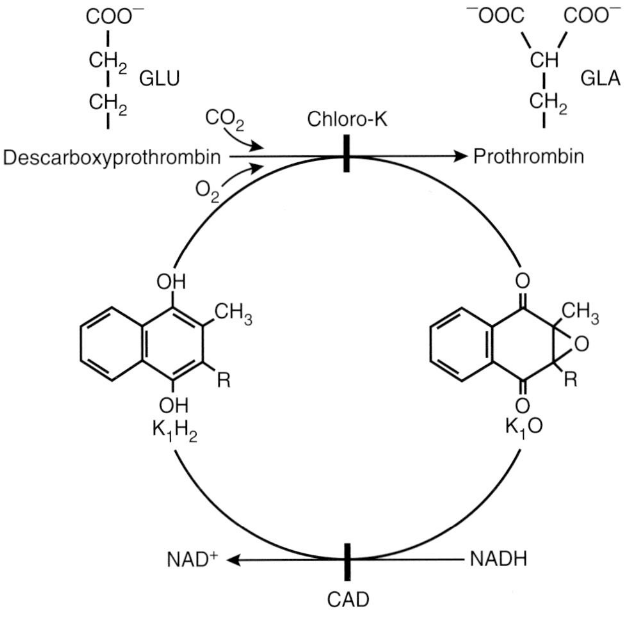

FIGURE 83-2 The vitamin K cycle in the formation of the vitamin K–dependent clotting factors. Vitamin K enters the body and is reduced to vitamin K_1H_2. K_1H_2 and carboxylase convert vitamin K–dependent clotting factor precursor proteins into active factors; epoxidase converts vitamin K_1H_2 to vitamin K_1–epoxide (K_1O). Reduced vitamin K_1H_2 is regenerated by reduced nicotinamide adenine dinucleotide (NADH) and is the warfarin-sensitive step. *CAD,* Coumarin-type anticoagulant drugs. (From O'Reilly RA: Therapeutic modalities for thrombotic disorders: vitamin K antagonists. In Coleman RW, Hirsh J, Marder VJ, et al, editors: *Hemostasis and thrombosis: basic principles and clinical practice,* ed 2, Philadelphia, 1987, Lippincott Williams & Wilkins.)

which further increases the reaction. In the final common pathway, prothrombin is converted to thrombin, and fibrinogen is converted to fibrin. Thrombin recruits more platelets, creating more adhesion and aggregation. A fibrin platelet clot is formed, and thrombosis occurs.

Activation of the clotting cascade on the surface of an artificial device occurs similarly whether it is on the cardiac valve, cardiopulmonary bypass system, vascular graft, extracorporeal membrane oxygenation (ECMO) circuit, mechanical assist device, or vascular catheter. It will produce thrombus formation, and macroscopic and microscopic platelet-fibrin emboli occur commonly as well. Factor XII, kallikrein, and plasmin activate the complement system and activate neutrophils, and kinin formation mediates vasodilation, vascular permeability, and white blood cell migration. Normally, a delicate balance is maintained between these two systems so that uncontrolled clotting or hemorrhage does not occur. The coagulation cascade is initiated, and factor XII and kallikrein initiate clot lysis with conversion of plasminogen to plasmin. Antiplasmins in the circulating blood, particularly α_2-antiplasmin, rapidly neutralize most of the circulating plasmin; however, plasmin also is incorporated into the clot during clot formation. The fibrin meshwork protects plasmin from antiplasmin once the plasmin is activated to plasmin, allowing fibrin degradation in the clot. In fact, many natural inhibitors offset activated procoagulant protein. Protein C, heparin, antithrombin III, protein S, thrombomodulin, prostacyclin, and plasmin all counter steps in the coagulation cascade.[3]

ANTICOAGULATION THERAPY

Clinically useful drugs that block the clotting cascade fall into the following primary groups: orally administered vitamin K antagonists; natural anticoagulants, such as the heparin–antithrombin III system; direct thrombin inhibitors, antiplatelet drugs, factor Xa inhibitors; and fibrinolytic agents.

Warfarin sodium remains the most popular orally administered vitamin K antagonist used today in the United States. It blocks the formation of the four vitamin K–dependent clotting factors (prothrombin and factors VII, IX, and X), creating a buildup of their precursors. Warfarin sodium blocks the vitamin K cycle at the regeneration of reduced vitamin K, which is the active form of vitamin K (Fig. 83-2).

Heparin's anticoagulant effect is fairly complex and not completely understood. Heparin sulfate is a glycosaminoglycan that binds to antithrombin III and activates this serine protease inhibitor. Heparin and antithrombin III occur naturally in humans, are secreted by endothelial cells, and are required to produce their anticoagulant effect. Antithrombin III binds to thrombin and blocks the enzymes of the intrinsic coagulation cascade, including thrombin and factors IXa, Xa, XIa, and XIIa. Both unfractionated heparin and low-molecular-weight heparins work via the previously mentioned mechanisms.

Direct thrombin inhibitors and factor Xa inhibitors have emerged as alternative agents to warfarin for oral anticoagulation. Dabigatran is an orally administered direct thrombin inhibitor, whereas rivaroxaban and apixaban are factor Xa inhibitors. Dabigatran received U.S. Food and Drug Administration (FDA) approval for prevention and treatment of venous thromboembolic disease and treatment of nonvalvular atrial fibrillation based primarily on data from the RE-LY trial.[4] Several intravenous direct thrombin inhibitors exist, including lepirudin, desirudin, argatroban, and bivalirudin. These agents are used primarily as alternatives to heparin when heparin-induced thrombocytopenia is suspected or confirmed with appropriate diagnostic studies.

Rivaroxaban is an orally administered competitive, direct factor Xa inhibitor. Noteworthy is that this agent is contraindicated in patients with creatinine clearance of less than 15 mL/min or patients on hemodialysis. Rivaroxaban was studied in the ROCKET-AF trial and found to be non-inferior to warfarin in the prevention of stroke in patients with atrial fibrillation.[5] This agent also was studied for prevention of venous thromboembolism (VTE) during orthopedic surgery and showed efficacy.[6]

The various antiplatelet drugs have different mechanisms of action, making them more or less useful as therapeutic anticoagulation agents. Figure 83-3 is a schematic diagram of the actions of antiplatelet drugs. Aspirin inhibits platelet aggregation by irreversible acetylation of platelet cyclooxygenase, hence blocking the synthesis of prostaglandins and thromboxane A2. Aspirin prolongs the bleeding time, although variable responses to aspirin's anticoagulant effect exist. Aspirin inhibits platelet aggregation for the life span of the platelet, which is typically 7 to 10 days.

Four adenosine diphosphate P2Y12 (ADP PY212) receptor antagonists are FDA approved. These agents reduce platelet aggregation mediated by the binding of fibrinogen to activated glycoprotein (GP) IIb/IIIa receptors on platelets. The thienopyridines are in widespread use as potent antiplatelet agents and are typically used in dual antiplatelet therapy following percutaneous coronary intervention. Clopidogrel in vitro does not affect platelet aggregation. However, in vivo, clopidogrel is metabolized by the liver to several active metabolites—with these metabolites irreversibly inhibiting the $P2Y_{12}$ platelet receptor. Clopidogrel supplanted ticlopidine principally because ticlopidine is associated with aplastic anemia and thrombotic thrombocytopenic purpura.[7] The thienopyridine prasugrel converts to active metabolites more efficiently than does clopidogrel; as such, the bleeding risk with this agent is increased compared with other agents in this class. Lastly, ticagrelor is a novel thienopyridine that directly antagonizes the P2Y12 receptor. This drug is also reversible in its inhibition of the receptor. However, it requires twice-daily dosing in contrast with the other thienopyridines. It is presently a Class I recommendation to discontinue all P2Y12 inhibitors before cardiac surgery. The exact duration in days of discontinuation cannot be specified as the safe interval between discontinuation and cardiac surgery is unknown.[8] In general, the range for cessation is between 3 and 7 days.

Dipyridamole is a reversible platelet agent, a weak vasodilator, and a weak inhibitor of the enzyme phosphodiesterase, which degrades cyclic adenosine monophosphate (cAMP) to 5′-AMP. With this block, more cAMP is available to inhibit platelet aggregation. Sulfinpyrazone appears to reversibly block platelet prostaglandin synthesis and is another fairly weak anticoagulant. At clinical dosages, neither dipyridamole nor sulfinpyrazone prolongs the bleeding time.

Finally, fibrinolytic therapy has a small but definite place in the management of thrombosis of artificial devices. Streptokinase and urokinase act similarly and induce rapid thrombolysis by activating plasminogen and subsequently forming plasmin. Plasmin causes degradation of the fibrin, reducing thrombus size. Unfortunately, streptokinase and urokinase also induce a generalized plasma proteolytic state as well as local fibrin degradation in the thrombus, and this can lead to uncontrolled hemorrhage. Newer agents (second-generation plasminogen activators) such as recombinant tissue plasminogen activator were developed to prevent induction of this generalized plasma proteolytic state by making these agents fibrin specific. However, this function appears to depend on the dose, and clinical use has not confirmed the decrease in potential for hemorrhage that was hoped for with these drugs.

COMPLICATIONS OF ANTICOAGULATION

Warfarin Sodium

Bleeding is the most common and most significant complication encountered with the use of warfarin, and therefore close monitoring of the prothrombin time is mandatory. Excessive amounts of warfarin that increase the prothrombin time beyond 2.5 times control and the international normalized ratio (INR) above 5 will increase bleeding complications four to eight times. The gastrointestinal tract is the site of most bleeding complications and is often associated with preexisting disease states, such as peptic ulcer, gastritis, genitourinary lesions, cancer, and hypertension. Indeed, based on the increase in dispensed prescription for warfarin rising by 45% from 1998 to 2004, warfarin is now among the top 10 drugs in the United States with the highest number of serious adverse event reports. Data submitted to the FDA and from a study auditing U.S. death certificates suggest that major bleed frequencies for warfarin are as high as 10% to 16%.[9]

Another significant complication of initial warfarin therapy is skin necrosis. This is secondary to a temporary hypercoagulable state induced in the capillaries when the concentration of protein C (a natural vitamin K–dependent and warfarin sodium–sensitive anticoagulant that circulates in the blood) falls before warfarin's

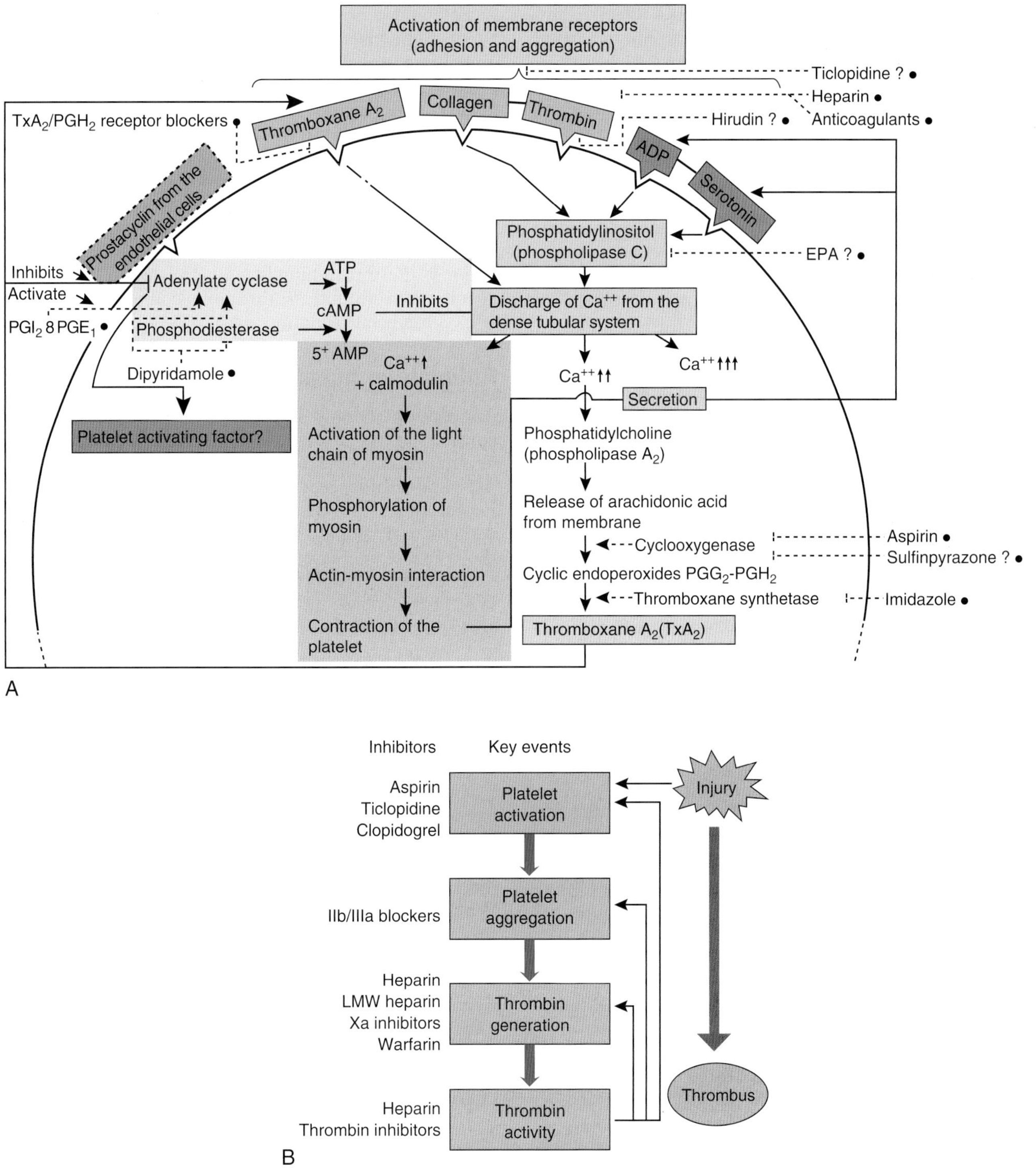

FIGURE 83-3 ■ **A,** Presumed sites of action of various platelet inhibitors. Cyclic adenosine monophosphate (cAMP) inhibits calcium (Ca) mobilization from the dense tubular system. *Circles* indicate a platelet inhibitor drug. *Dashed lines* indicate the presumed site of action of the drug. **B,** Key events in thrombosis formation and inhibitors that can prevent specific steps in the process. *ATP,* Adenosine triphosphate; *EPA,* eicosapentaenoic acid; *LMW,* low molecular weight; *PG,* prostaglandin. (**A,** From Stein B, Fuster V, Israel DH, et al: Platelet inhibitor agents in cardiovascular disease: an update. *J Am Coll Cardiol* 14:813–836, 1989. Reprinted with permission of the American College of Cardiology. **B,** Reprinted with permission from the Institute for Continuing Healthcare Education: *The rationale for extended antithrombotic therapy for patients with post-acute coronary syndromes.*)

inhibition of factors II, IX, and X becomes effective and the desired hypocoagulable state occurs. The activated form of protein C is a powerful inactivator of factors V and VIII. Why this is limited to the skin is unknown.[10] When warfarin is used in pregnant women, it can cause embryopathy in 4% to 8% of fetuses exposed in the first trimester, and exposure to warfarin in the second and third trimesters causes central nervous system abnormalities in 3% of pregnancies. Finally, prematurity, fetal hemorrhage, and stillbirth are increased in infants exposed to warfarin.[11,12] For these reasons, bioprostheses or allografts should be placed, when possible, in women of childbearing age.

Heparin Sulfate System

Again, the most common complication of heparin therapy is bleeding. Hemorrhagic complications occur in 10% to 20% of patients with normal hemostasis and in up to 50% of patients with thrombocytopenia or uremia.[13] Thrombocytopenia has been reported in up to 31% of patients and can cause significant morbidity and mortality when it is associated with platelet clumping and thrombosis. Heparin-induced thrombocytopenia (HIT) has become an increasingly recognized and important clinicopathologic syndrome. The frequency of HIT among patients exposed to heparin is highly variable and related to the type of heparin, the patient population, the duration of heparin exposure, and the patient's sex.[14] The immunoglobulin G antibodies form a complex against platelet factor 4/heparin, which binds to the platelet Fc receptor, leading to platelet aggregation and release of prothrombotic microparticles. Cardiac surgery patients are prone to formation of anti–platelet factor 4/heparin antibodies. Accordingly, if the platelet count falls by more than 50% between postoperative days 5 and 14, investigation for HIT antibodies should occur. If HIT is suspected or diagnosed, a direct thrombin inhibitor (lepirudin, bivalirudin, or argatroban) should be initiated and continued until the platelet count normalizes. It is imperative that all sources of heparin be stopped if HIT is suspected. This includes removal of a pulmonary artery catheter if it is heparin coated. If further anticoagulation becomes necessary, such as cardiac reoperation, the surgeon can wait for the antibodies to become undetectable and reuse heparin.[15] However, this may take up to 40 days. Another alternative is to use nonheparin anticoagulants such as danaparoid sodium, lepirudin, and argatroban.[16] Platelet inhibition with glycoprotein IIb/IIIa antagonists followed by unfractionated heparins has also been used successfully.[17]

Fractions of heparin that display this effect have the least anticoagulant activity, so the use of low-molecular-weight heparin with high anticoagulant effect and low ability to lead to platelet clumping has become clinically more important.

Direct Thrombin Inhibitors and Factor Xa Inhibitors

Given the widespread adoption of orally available thrombin and Xa inhibitors, clinicians will encounter minor and occasionally serious, life-threatening bleeding from these agents. The bleeding rates with dabigatran, rivaroxaban, and apixaban reported by various trials are generally 4% to 14%. Management of minor bleeding from these agents usually includes cessation of the agent. The period of time required for cessation of these agents before major procedures is unknown, but a minimum of 5 to 7 days without the drug before a cardiac operation seems prudent. The management of severe, life-threatening bleeding from these agents is challenging because no direct reversal agents are available. In general, to stop major or life-threatening bleeding related to one of these agents, nonactivated prothrombin complex concentrate (PCC) has been recommended.[18]

Antiplatelet Agents

Antiplatelet therapy is the mainstay of treatment for coronary artery disease. In some cases, patients require urgent cardiac operations while on these medications. Aspirin does not seem to confer an unduly increased risk for bleeding. The data for clopidogrel suggest that for patients undergoing cardiac surgery within 5 days from the last dose, increased bleeding can be anticipated.[19]

The data regarding the newer P2Y12 agents and bleeding after coronary artery bypass graft (CABG) are still emerging. The TRITON-TIMI 38 trial examined prasugrel in comparison with clopidogrel for acute coronary syndromes. Although only 437 patients of 13,608 in this study underwent CABG after receiving either prasugrel or clopidogrel, the rates of minor and major bleeding with prasugrel were 14.1% versus 4.5% in the clopidogrel group.[20] Based on these data, it would be prudent to wait 7 days before embarking on a cardiac operation after the last dose of prasugrel if possible. If unable to wait, it is suggested that platelet transfusions can be effective in dealing with bleeding if there has been at least 12 hours between the last dose of prasugrel and the platelet transfusions.[21] With regard to ticagrelor and bleeding after cardiac surgery, there are insufficient data to base firm decisions. There are little data supporting management of post-CABG bleeding with this agent. It would seem prudent to wait a minimum of 5 days before undergoing cardiac surgical procedures in this group. The latest Society of Thoracic Surgeons Guideline Statement regarding this subject gives credence to the idea of testing platelet inhibition rather than waiting an arbitrary amount of time.[8]

PROSTHETIC HEART VALVES

Edmunds and coworkers[22,23] and Cohn[24] have detailed the need for standardized reporting of thrombotic complications, including uniform definitions; stratification of the data to include the severity of the event, including death; and careful, complete long-term follow-up. Without this standardization, it is difficult to make accurate statements about results, complications, and appropriate anticoagulation therapy. Similarly, it is difficult to compare valves placed in the 1960s and 1970s and their associated complications with valves placed in later decades and their complications.

Through the years, bioengineering advances have led to fewer thrombogenic materials, such as carbon Pyrolite for the St. Jude valve, and a better mechanical valve design has decreased the incidence of valve thrombosis and thromboembolism through greater central flow characteristics. However, more effective anticoagulation has been the most important factor for the decreased incidence of thrombosis in the 1980s and 1990s compared with the 1960s and 1970s, particularly with mechanical valves. Bioprosthetic valves have less inherent thrombogenicity, but this is a result of better central flow characteristics, flexible leaflets, and sinusoidal washout rather than true thromboresistance of the preserved tissue.[25] At present, stented porcine xenograft valves and pericardial valves are in use as tissue bioprostheses. The major problem with the pericardial xenograft valves was their durability; both valves developed tearing of the cusps secondary to stress after only a few years of use. The pericardial valves used today are much better and tend to fail by calcification.[26]

Most prosthetic valves have a sewing ring that is covered with a Dacron or Teflon cloth. When this is exposed to the blood, an adherent layer of thrombus is laid down and serves as a blood-compatible coating. It is initially thin and delicate but later becomes invaded by well-vascularized fibrous tissue. This resists further formation of thrombus. However, if the flow pattern is abnormal, this tissue ingrowth can creep into the orifice from below the valve–sewing ring, forming an obstructive pannus. Finally, allograft aortic valves and pulmonary valved conduits have almost normal platelet survival time and do not form thrombi.

Prosthetic and Mechanical Heart Valves and Thromboembolism

Determining the risk of thromboembolism for patients who undergo mechanical valve replacement is subject to various complex patient- and prosthesis-related factors. A few general principles apply, however. Data from early small case series in which patients were followed who had contraindications to vitamin K antagonists support major thromboembolism rates of 4.0 per 100 patient-years to more than 8.6 per 100 patient-years for total embolic rates.[27] The data regarding optimal INR targets for mechanical aortic and mitral valves were derived from retrospective observational studies.[28] In general, mechanical valves in the mitral position have roughly 1.5 to 2 times the thromboembolic risk over mechanical valves in the aortic position. Both the American College of Cardiology/American Heart Association (ACC/AHA) and the European Society of Cardiology maintain guideline-supported recommendations for target INR with both mechanical and bioprosthetic valves.[29,30]

The incidence of all thrombotic complications, including thromboembolic events, for a mechanical aortic prosthesis is approximately 1% to 2% per patient-year, whereas the rate for bioprosthetic valves in the aortic position is approximately half that of the mechanical prostheses.[3] The risk of bleeding complication is, however, generally accepted to be higher for mechanical valves in the aortic position versus bioprosthetic valves because of the use of warfarin anticoagulation. In the two large randomized trials that compared outcomes for patients with either a mechanical or porcine heart valve, both the Edinburgh Heart Trial and the Veterans Affairs Cooperative Trial showed a higher rate of bleeding with mechanical valves.[31,32]

Bioprosthetic Valves and Thromboembolism

The rate of thromboembolic events for patients with bioprosthetic valves is thought to be highest during the first 90 days after implantation. Specifically, this rate is highest for the first 10 days after aortic valve implantation for the aortic position in patients without warfarin anticoagulation. The thromboembolic rate for a bioprosthetic valve is also high for the mitral position in patients without anticoagulation for days 1 through 10 and for days 11 through 90.[33] Based on these data, it became common practice for patients who received either an aortic or a mitral bioprosthesis to receive 3 months of vitamin K antagonist anticoagulation.

This practice of routinely anticoagulating bioprosthetic valves in the aortic position has been revisited. ElBardissi and colleagues studied 861 patients who underwent bioprosthetic aortic valve replacement. Of these 861 patients, 133 patients (15%) received warfarin anticoagulation and 782 (85%) did not. No difference in thromboembolic events was found between the two groups.[34] However, a large Danish registry study recently established a very high thromboembolic rate for patients without warfarin anticoagulation: 7.00 per 100 patient-years versus 2.69 per 100 patient-years in patients treated with warfarin anticoagulation for the first 90 days after bioprosthetic aortic valve replacement.[35] Based on current evidence-based guidelines, the 2014 ACC/AHA guidelines suggest that it is a Class IIb recommendation for warfarin administration for 3 months following implantation of a bioprosthetic valve in the aortic position. It should be noted that it remains a IIa recommendation regarding warfarin administration for patients who receive bioprosthetic valves in the mitral position.[29]

Hammermeister and the Veterans Affairs Cooperative Study on Valvular Heart Disease[32] concluded that after 15 years, the rates of survival for patients receiving a mechanical aortic valve replacement were higher than those for patients receiving a bioprosthetic aortic valve replacement. For patients receiving mitral valve replacement, there were no differences in survival rates between patients receiving mechanical valves and those receiving tissue valves. The improved survival rate in the mechanical aortic valve replacement group was offset by a higher rate of bleeding. Structural failure, however, was observed only with the bioprosthetic valves, and bleeding complications were statistically more frequent among patients who received mechanical valves. Hammond and associates,[36] in a study of 1012 adult patients who underwent placement of either a mechanical valve or a bioprosthesis with a follow-up of 4814 patient-years, found little direct evidence to strongly support the generalized use of one type of valve over another.

Unfortunately, bioprostheses have a very high failure rate in children, probably because of accelerated calcium metabolism, and there is currently a renewed interest in the use of both fresh and commercially available frozen allograft valves for children and young adults to prevent anticoagulation. The risk of thrombotic or thromboembolic events with use of allograft aortic valves in the subcoronary position, as a free-sewn graft or by root replacement in which a cylinder including the valve is placed by the technique of Ross,[37] is almost zero without anticoagulation. Matsuki and coworkers[38] reported on 555 consecutive hospital survivors who underwent isolated aortic valve replacement with a free-sewn allograft. The incidence of thromboembolism was 0.034% per patient-year, or 1 patient of the 555 studied. Results with the aortic root replacement in 108 patients described by Okita and associates[39] showed no incidence of thromboembolism in 180 patient-years of follow-up. Penta and colleagues[40] similarly found no incidence of thrombosis or thromboemboli in 140 consecutive patients who underwent homograft replacement of the aortic valve and were observed for a minimum of 10 years. Many of these valves were either fresh or antibiotic-preserved valves. O'Brien and associates[41] reported on a comparison of aortic valve replacements with viable cryopreserved and fresh allograft valves. The freedom from thromboembolism for both groups was 97% at 10 years and 96% at 15 years; the reoperation rate for valve failure was much higher in the group that received the fresh valves. O'Brien initially believed that cryopreserved valves were superior because fibroblastic cell viability is preserved, providing durability. However, recent developments have pointed toward an immunologic basis for valve deterioration with live cells.

The fate of the aortic valve or pulmonary valve used as a conduit to reconstruct the right ventricular outflow tract is not as clear. Bull and associates[42] described 249 patients who received extracardiac conduits in the right side of the heart. Of the 173 patients who survived 30 days, 72 underwent placement of xenograft conduits of various types, and 4 underwent placement of valveless tubes. The complication and reoperation rates for both valved conduit groups were similar. Calcification of the allograft tube occurred commonly, but the obstruction tended to be at the proximal portion of the conduit where Dacron extensions, which are circumferential, were commonly placed. The development of the neointimal peel in this position led to the obstruction in more than two thirds of patients.

If a noncircumferential proximal hood is used, thrombus and neointimal peel formation is minimal, and obstruction is markedly decreased. Livi and associates[43] have shown that the valve of choice for right ventricular outflow tract reconstruction is, in fact, the pulmonary allograft rather than the aortic allograft. Finally, Matsuki and associates[44] have used the pulmonary autograft valve (the patient's own pulmonary valve) to replace the aortic valve with excellent results (Ross procedure). However, this procedure requires the reconstruction of the right ventricular outflow tract with a pulmonary or aortic allograft, essentially giving the patient disease of two valves rather than the one-valve disease the patient had originally. Despite this, Matsuki and associates[44] have shown excellent results with this technique. Finally, the Contegra bovine valved jugular vein seems to be a good alternative for pediatric right ventricular outflow tract reconstruction.

Several general rules make some clinically applicable sense out of these sometimes conflicting data. For children, aortic valve replacement should be carried out either with a mechanical valve, such as the St. Jude bileaflet valve, or with the pulmonary autograft technique to replace the aortic valve as described by Ross in 1967.[45] This has become the method of choice for aortic valve replacement in children. For mitral valve replacement in children, mechanical valves are required, and these patients should undergo full anticoagulation with warfarin and aspirin. Xenograft bioprostheses should not be used because of the rapid calcification and degeneration that occur with these valves in children. Similar guidelines should be followed for young adults. For women who are of childbearing age or wish to have children, mechanical valves should be strongly discouraged. The complications of anticoagulation, particularly with warfarin sodium and heparin, place the young woman and unborn child at too great a risk. For non-childbearing women and for men younger than 60 years, individual differences in the patients and their desired lifestyle after valve replacement should be strongly considered in choosing the valve. Finally, probably for patients older than 60 years but definitely for those older than 70 years, the use of xenograft bioprostheses (stented or stentless) should be strongly considered in view of the decreased degeneration rate of these valves in older patients and the higher risk of anticoagulation in this population of patients. Guideline-supported recommendations regarding choice of mechanical or bioprosthetic valves support a patient-centered approach to discussing the risks and benefits of prosthetic valve options.[29]

Management of Prosthetic Valve Thrombosis

All prosthetic valves, including bioprostheses, can develop thrombotic occlusion, but the incidence is higher for the mechanical valve, specifically the caged ball valve and the tilting disc valve. The thrombosis is usually more acute, manifesting as "sudden" valve dysfunction with clinical shock, pulmonary edema, and loss of valve click sounds in mechanical valves and muffled sounds in bioprostheses. The diagnosis is made by fluoroscopy or two-dimensional transthoracic echocardiography, or both. Mortality is high without either fibrinolytic therapy or reoperation. The incidence of this complication is less than 0.3 per 100 patient-years, except for the Omniscience tilting disc valve placed in the mitral position, which has a significantly higher incidence of thrombosis.[3]

With regard to management of a suspected thrombosis of a left-sided prosthetic heart valve, determination of whether the thrombus is obstructive based on imaging studies is the initial priority. If the thrombus is obstructive and the patient is critically ill, then surgical replacement of the prosthesis is warranted unless the patient is deemed too high risk for operation because of comorbid conditions. It is arguably difficult to determine which patient or subset of patients is too high risk, because the operative mortality rate approaches 15% and all cases of prosthetic valve thrombosis are therefore "high risk." Based on the limited data set, the following therapeutic strategies are suggested: thrombolysis is reserved as the initial strategy for patients in NYHA Class I/II heart failure, if surgery is not available (e.g., patient is in a location without cardiac surgery and too unstable to transport), the patient refuses surgery, or if the thrombus is nonobstructive and small (<0.8 cm^2). Almost all right-sided prosthetic valve thromboses can be treated with lytic therapy initially, and surgery used if thrombolysis is unsuccessful.[46]

REFERENCES

1. Salzman EW, Merrill EW: Interaction of blood, with artificial surfaces. In Coleman RW, Hirsh J, Marder VJ, et al, editors: *Hemostasis and thrombosis*, Philadelphia, 1987, Lippincott.
2. Mehta P, Mehta J: Effects of aspirin in arterial thrombosis: why don't animals behave the way humans do? *J Am Coll Cardiol* 21:511, 1993.
3. Edmunds LH: Thrombotic and bleeding complications of prosthetic heart valves. *Ann Thorac Surg* 44:430, 1987.
4. Healey JS, Eikelboom J, Douketis J, et al: Periprocedural bleeding and thromboembolic events with dabigatran compared with warfarin: results from the Randomized Evaluation of Long-Term Anticoagulation Therapy (RE-LY) randomized trial. *Circulation* 126:343–348, 2012.
5. Patel MR, Mahaffey KW, Garg J, et al: Rivaroxaban versus warfarin in nonvalvular atrial fibrillation. *N Engl J Med* 365:883–891, 2011.
6. King CS, Holley AB, Moores LK: Moving toward a more ideal anticoagulant. *Chest* 143:1106–1116, 2013.
7. Bennett C, Davidson C, Raisch D, et al: Thrombotic thrombocytopenic purpura associated with ticlopidine in the setting of coronary artery stents and stroke prevention. *Arch Intern Med* 159:2524–2528, 1999.
8. Ferraris VA, Saha SP, Oestreich JH, et al: Update to the Society of Thoracic Surgeons Guideline on the use of antiplatelet drugs in patients having cardiac and noncardiac operations. *Ann Thorac Surg* 94:1761–1781, 2012.
9. Wysowski DK, Nourjah P, Swartz L: Bleeding complications with warfarin use. A prevalent adverse effect resulting in regulatory action. *Arch Intern Med* 167:1414–1419, 2007.
10. Crouse LH, Comp PC: The regulation of hemostasis: the protein C system. *N Engl J Med* 314:1298, 1986.
11. Iturbe-Alessio I, Fonseca M, Mutchinik O, et al: Risks of anticoagulant therapy in pregnant women with artificial heart valves. *N Engl J Med* 315:1390, 1986.
12. Lutz DJ, Noller KL, Spittell JA, et al: Pregnancy and its complications following cardiac valve prostheses. *Am J Obstet Gynecol* 131:460, 1978.
13. Ware JA, Lewis J, Salzman EW: Antithrombic therapy. In Rutherford RB, editor: *Vascular surgery*, Philadelphia, 1989, WB Saunders.
14. Warkentin TE, Greinacher A, Koster A, et al: Treatment and prevention of heparin-induced thrombocytopenia. *Chest* 133:340S–380S, 2008.
15. Potzsch B, Klovekorn WP, Madlener K: Use of heparin-induced thrombocytopenia. *N Engl J Med* 343:515, 2000.
16. Furukawa K, Ohteki H, Hirahara K, et al: The use of argatroban as an anticoagulant for cardiopulmonary bypass in cardiac operations. *J Thorac Cardiovasc Surg* 122:1255–1256, 2001.
17. Koster A, Meyer O, Fischer T, et al: One-year experience with the platelet glycoprotein IIb/IIIa antagonist tirofiban and heparin during cardiopulmonary bypass in patients with heparin-induced thrombocytopenia type II. *J Thorac Cardiovasc Surg* 122:1254–1255, 2001.
18. Yates S, Sarode R: Novel thrombin and factor Xa inhibitors: challenges to reversal of their anticoagulation effects. *Curr Opin Hematol* 20:552–557, 2013.
19. Yusuf S, Zhao F, Mehta SR, et al: Effects of clopidogrel in addition to aspirin in patients with acute coronary syndromes without ST-segment elevation. *N Engl J Med* 345:494–502, 2001.
20. Wiviott SD, Braunwald E, McCabe CH, et al: Prasugrel versus clopidogrel in patients with acute coronary syndromes. *N Engl J Med* 357:2001–2015, 2007.
21. Fitchett D, Mazer CD, Eikelboom J, et al: Antiplatelet therapy and cardiac surgery: review of recent evidence and clinical implications. *Can J Cardiol* 29:1042–1047, 2013.
22. Edmunds LH, Clark RE, Cohn LH, et al: Guidelines for reporting morbidity and mortality after cardiac valvular operations. *J Thorac Cardiovasc Surg* 112:708, 1996.
23. Edmunds LH, Clark RE, Cohn LH, et al: Guidelines for reporting morbidity and mortality after cardiac valvular operations. *J Thorac Cardiovasc Surg* 96:351, 1988.
24. Cohn LH: Statistical treatment of valve surgery outcomes: an influence on the evaluation of devices as well as practice. *J Am Coll Cardiol* 15:574, 1990.
25. Magilligan DJ, Jr, Oyama C, Klein S, et al: Platelet adherence to bioprosthetic cardiac valves. *Am J Cardiol* 53:945, 1984.
26. Banbury MK, Cosgrove IIIDM, Lytle BW, et al: Long-term results of the Carpentier-Edwards pericardial aortic valve: a 12-year follow-up. *Ann Thorac Surg* 66:573–576, 1998.
27. Cannegeiter SC, Rosendaal FR, Briet E: Thromboembolic and bleeding complications in patients with mechanical heart valve prosthesis. *Circulation* 89:635–641, 1994.
28. Cannegeiter SC, Rosendaal FR, Wintzen AR, et al: Optimal oral anticoagulant therapy in patients with mechanical heart valves. *N Engl J Med* 333:11–17, 1995.
29. Nishimura RA, Otto CM, Bonow RO, et al: 2014 AHA/ACC guideline for the management of patients with valvular heart disease: executive summary: a report of the American College of Cardiology/American Heart Association Task Force on Practice Guidelines. *J Am Coll Cardiol* 63:2438–2488, 2014.
30. Vahanian A, Alfieri O, Andreotti F, et al: Guidelines on the management of valvular heart disease (version 2012). The joint task force on the management of valvular heart disease of the European society of cardiology (ESC) and the European association of cardiothoracic surgery (EACTS). *Eur Heart J* 33:2451–2496, 2012.
31. Bloomfield P, Wheatley DJ, Prescott RJ, et al: Twelve-year comparison of a Bjork-Shiley mechanical heart valve with porcine bioprosthesis. *N Engl J Med* 324:573–579, 1991.
32. Hammermeister KE, Sethi GK, Henderson WC, et al: Outcomes 15 years after valve replacement with a mechanical versus bioprosthetic valve: final report of the Veterans Affairs randomized trial. *J Am Coll Cardiol* 36:1152–1158, 2000.
33. Heras M, Chesebro JH, Fuster V, et al: High risk of thromboemboli early after bioprosthetic cardiac valve replacement. *J Am Coll Cardiol* 25:1111–1119, 1995.
34. ElBardissi AW, DiBardino DJ, Chen FY, et al: Is early antithrombotic therapy necessary in patients with bioprosthetic aortic valves in normal sinus rhythm? *J Thorac Cardiovasc Surg* 139:1137–1145, 2010.
35. Merie C, Kober L, Olson PS, et al: Association of warfarin therapy duration after bioprosthetic aortic valve replacement with risk of mortality, thromboembolic complications, and bleeding. *JAMA* 308:2118–2125, 2012.
36. Hammond GL, Geha AS, Kopf GS, et al: Biological versus mechanical valves. *J Thorac Cardiovasc Surg* 93:182, 1987.
37. Sommerville J, Ross D: Homograft replacement of the aortic root with reimplantation of the coronary arteries. *Br Heart J* 47:473, 1982.
38. Matsuki O, Robles A, Gibbs S, et al: Long-term performance of 555 aortic homografts in the aortic position. *Ann Thorac Surg* 46:187–191, 1988.
39. Okita Y, Franciosi G, Matsuki O, et al: Early and late results of aortic root replacement with antibiotic sterilized aortic homograft. *J Thorac Cardiovasc Surg* 95:696, 1988.
40. Penta A, Qureshi S, Radley-Smith R, et al: Patient status 10 or more years after "fresh" homograft replacement of the aortic valve. *Circulation* 70(Suppl I):182, 1984.
41. O'Brien MF, Stafford EG, Gardner MAH, et al: A comparison of aortic valve replacement with viable cryopreserved and fresh

allograft valves with a note on chromosome studies. *J Thorac Cardiovasc Surg* 94:812, 1987.

42. Bull C, Horvath P, Merrill W, et al: Evaluation of long term results of homograft and heterograft valves in extracardiac conduits. *J Thorac Cardiovasc Surg* 94:12, 1987.
43. Livi U, Abdulla AK, Parker R, et al: Viability and morphology of aortic and pulmonary homografts. A comparative study. *J Thorac Cardiovasc Surg* 93:755, 1987.
44. Matsuki O, Okita Y, Almoida RS, et al: Two decades experience with aortic valve replacement with pulmonary autograft. *J Thorac Cardiovasc Surg* 95:705, 1988.
45. Ross DN: Replacement of aortic and mitral valves with a pulmonary autograft. *Lancet* 2:956, 1967.
46. Huang G, Schaff HV, Sundt TM, et al: Treatment of obstructed thrombosed prosthetic heart valve. *J Am Coll Cardiol* 62:1731–1736, 2013.

CHAPTER 84

Robotic and Minimally Invasive Mitral Valve Surgery

Craig M. Jarrett • A. Marc Gillinov • Tomislav Mihaljevic

CHAPTER OUTLINE

Cardiac surgery has traditionally been performed through a complete median sternotomy, which provides generous operative exposure to all structures in and around the heart. With this approach, complex cardiovascular procedures can be performed safely and effectively. Reductions in incision size and tissue manipulation became possible with the advent of closed-chest cardiopulmonary techniques and advances in instrumentation. Improvements in intracardiac visualization and robotic telemanipulation have pushed the bounds even further.

Today, robotic cardiac surgery, particularly valve surgery, has become standard practice for some surgeons. In this chapter, we describe our experience with robotic mitral valve surgery and other minimally invasive approaches. A number of future systems and novel visualization techniques that might enhance future robotic systems are outlined as well.

ROBOTIC SYSTEMS

Three-dimensional vision and seven degrees of freedom are optimal to manipulate and freely orient objects in a three-dimensional space, such as a body cavity. Consequently, standard endoscopic surgery with only two-dimensional vision and four degrees of freedom reduces accuracy, efficiency, and dexterity of movement. Human motor skill, specifically eye-hand coordination, deteriorates with the indirect observation and manipulation of instruments and tissues in endoscopic surgery. In addition, instrument shaft shear, or drag, necessitates higher manipulation forces by the surgeon, leading to hand muscle fatigue. The surgeon must reverse hand motions in endoscopic surgery because the fixed entry point (fulcrum effect), such as a trocar, makes it a motor skill set that is nonintuitive to learn. Computer-enhanced systems have been developed to overcome these and other limitations. Through telemanipulation, the surgeon operates from a console with a three-dimensional view of the operative field. The surgeon's movements are reproduced in a scaled proportion by instruments mounted on robotic arms inserted through the chest wall. The robotic arms and "micro-wrist" instruments mimic the human arm and wrist with seven full degrees of freedom. For cardiac surgery, a robotic telemanipulation system, the da Vinci Surgical System (Intuitive Surgical, Inc., Sunnyvale, CA), is currently available, with two different versions.

The da Vinci *S* Surgical System has three components: a surgeon console, a patient-side cart, and a vision cart. The surgeon console is separated physically from the patient and allows the surgeon to sit ergonomically with his or her head positioned in a three-dimensional vision system, arms at the side, and hands beneath the vision system. This natural eye-hand-instrument alignment replicates the experience of open surgery. The surgeon's analog finger and wrist movements, along with any tremor, are converted to digital signals by sensors in the console. The movements are scaled, whereby movements of the surgeon at the console are larger than movements of the instruments in the patient. The tremors are filtered and smoothed, which removes inherent human tremor with a frequency of 8 to 10 Hertz. This motion scaling and tremor suppression enhance precision at the tissue level. A clutching mechanism at the console, which temporarily disconnects the surgeon's and instruments' movements, enables readjustment of hand positions to maintain optimal ergonomics. The surgeon's movements are transferred to the patient cart digitally, where the instruments move synchronously through one of the four independent effector arms. For cardiac surgery, the arms are used to control the camera, the surgeon's left and right hands, and the atrial retractor. The vision cart houses the image-processing equipment and a large viewing monitor, which provides the operating room team, including the patient-side assistant, a view of the operative field. The three-dimensional vision system facilitates natural depth perception with high-power magnification (10×) via both 0-degree and 30-degree endoscopes.

The da Vinci *Si* Surgical System, the most recent version, incorporates dual-console capability, enhanced three-dimensional 1080i high-definition visualization, an updated user interface, and improved operating room integration. The dual-console feature supports training and collaboration by allowing two surgeons to sit at separate consoles and easily and quickly take control of the instruments at any time during surgery. Three-dimensional high-definition visualization with capability of 10× magnification increases viewing resolution, providing improved clarity and detail of the anatomic structures. The updated user interface with easy-to-use touchscreen controls simplifies intraoperative system and vision adjustments. Addressing the increasing trend toward operating room integration, vision system components traditionally housed in the vision cart can be installed on an operating room boom, and a multiple-input display allows viewing of up to three video sources, such as the operative field, ultrasound, and electrocardiogram (ECG), at one time.

EVOLUTION OF ROBOTIC CARDIAC SURGERY

Initially, advances in minimally invasive surgery were based on modifications of previously used approaches performed under direct vision. Mini-sternotomies, partial sternotomies, parasternal approaches, and mini-thoracotomies simply reduced the size of the incisions and the degree of tissue manipulation.[1-4] Advances in cannulation methods and video-optics opened the door for totally endoscopic robotic surgery.

The introduction of Port-Access technology (Cardiovations, Inc., Ethicon, Somerville, NJ) in 1996 combined a minimally invasive surgical approach (nonsternotomy) with total cardiopulmonary bypass and an arrested heart.[5,6] The system provides extrathoracic cardiopulmonary bypass with a specialized set of endovascular cannulas and catheters to provide antegrade or retrograde cardioplegic arrest, and ventricular decompression. Encouraging results confirmed the feasibility and safety of these techniques and paved the way for the development of less invasive operations. Advances in video-optics started a wave of new endoscopic approaches in general, urologic, gynecologic, and orthopedic surgery. Video assistance in cardiac surgery was first used for closed chest internal mammary artery harvests and congenital heart operations.[7-9] In 1996, Carpentier and colleagues performed the first video-assisted mitral valve repair using ventricular fibrillation via a mini-thoracotomy.[10] Soon thereafter, Chitwood and coworkers performed a video-assisted mitral valve replacement using a microincision, percutaneous transthoracic aortic clamp, and retrograde cardioplegia.[11]

Cardiac surgery entered the robotic age in 1997 when Mohr first used the AESOP (Intuitive Surgical, Inc., Sunnyvale, CA) voice-activated camera robotic arm in mitral valve surgery. In addition to freeing up the surgeon's hands during surgery, this device allowed for better valve and subvalvular visualization with even smaller incisions.[12] In 1998, Chitwood performed the first video-directed mitral operation in the United States, using the voice-controlled AESOP 3000 robotic arm and a Vista three-dimensional camera (Vista Cardiothoracic Systems, Inc., Westborough, MA).[11] The combination of robotic camera control and three-dimensional visualization was an essential step toward the totally endoscopic mitral operations performed today. The first mitral valve repair using an early prototype (the da Vinci articulated intracardiac wrist robotic device) of the present da Vinci robot was done by Carpentier and colleagues in 1998.[13] The first complete repair in North America using the da Vinci system was performed by Chitwood and colleagues in 2000.[14] A 4-cm incision was used for assistant access, but advancements in three-dimensional video and robotic instrumentation progressed to a point where totally endoscopic procedures were feasible. Lange and coworkers performed the first totally endoscopic mitral valve repair using only 1-cm ports with the da Vinci in 2000.[15]

In contrast to mitral valve surgery, closed-chest (nonsternotomy) coronary artery bypass surgery could be performed only after the robotic telemanipulation system had been developed. Technically complex maneuvers, such as coronary anastomosis, could not be done with conventional thoracoscopic instruments because dexterity was lacking. Freedom of movement with the "endowrist" instruments, where additional articulation occurs within the patient near the tip of the instrument, was critical in achieving this goal. Early reports of success originated from several centers that were pioneering the effort.[15-18] Although robotic coronary surgery has gained less traction than mitral surgery, today it can be performed safely with reproducible results at dedicated centers.[19,20]

CLINICAL APPLICATIONS AND PATIENT SELECTION

The da Vinci robot is used for mitral valve repair and single-vessel coronary artery bypass. It is less frequently used for mitral valve commissurotomy and tricuspid valve repair. In our experience, patients are offered robotic mitral valve surgery if they meet strict criteria (Box 84-1). Patients who have coronary artery disease or other valvular disease that would warrant surgery are excluded. Although tricuspid valve repair and coronary artery bypass graft surgery can be done using a robotic approach, the port placement and patient positioning are different. Mild aortic regurgitation (1+) or greater is also a contraindication because of the inability to reliably arrest the heart with retrograde cardioplegia alone. Patients with a prior sternotomy or right thoracotomy, or who have

BOX 84-1 Robotic Mitral Surgery Exclusion Criteria

- Coronary artery disease or other valvular disease requiring surgery
- Mild (1+) aortic regurgitation or greater
- Prior sternotomy or right thoracotomy
- Significant chest wall deformity that would limit access
- Severely calcified mitral valve annulus
- Aortic, iliac, or femoral atherosclerosis greater than minimal, or femoral vessels less than 7 mm (consider axillary artery cannulation)

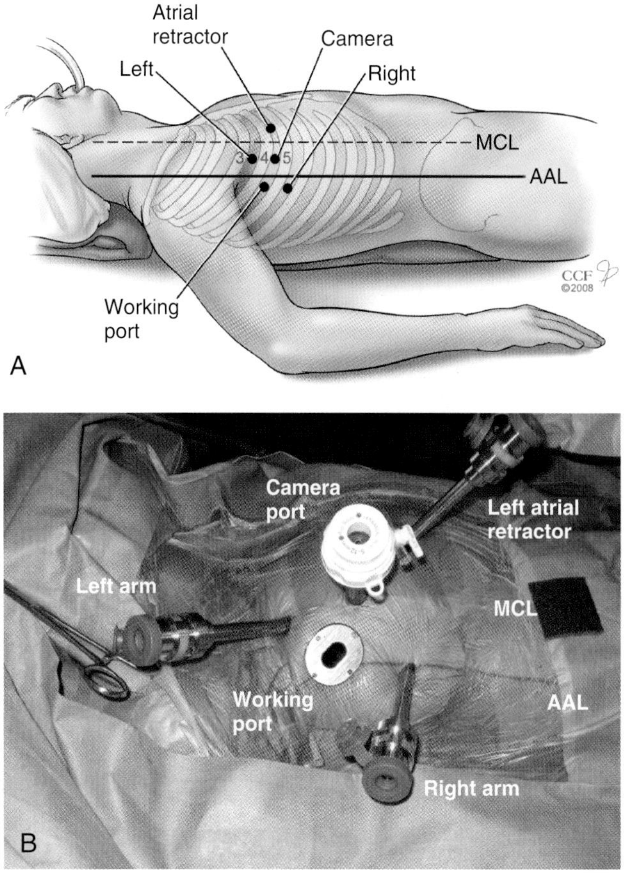

FIGURE 84-1 Schematic **(A)** and photograph **(B)** of port placement for robotic mitral valve surgery. *AAL,* Anterior axillary line; *MCL,* midclavicular line.

significant chest wall deformities that would limit access, are also excluded in our current practice, although there is some early experience with operations on such patients at other centers. Patients with a severely calcified mitral annulus are not candidates because decalcification requires further refinement of instruments and a more reliable means of evacuating any calcium that falls into the ventricle. Lastly, aortic, iliac, or femoral atherosclerosis greater than minimal, and femoral vessel diameter less than 7 mm, are relative contraindications; however, in such cases axillary perfusion may be substituted for femoral artery perfusion.

SURGICAL TECHNIQUES

After induction of general anesthesia, the patient is intubated with a double-lumen endotracheal tube, and a transesophageal echocardiography (TEE) probe is placed. A retrograde coronary sinus catheter is placed via the internal jugular vein and positioned under echocardiographic guidance. Bilateral arterial lines are placed if endoaortic balloon technology is to be used for aortic occlusion and cardioplegia delivery. The patient is positioned with the right chest elevated 30 degrees with a roll caudal to the right scapula and arms tucked at the patient's side.

Subsequent steps should follow a well-defined order to minimize unnecessary morbidity if patient factors preclude a robotic approach and the approach needs to be converted. The femoral vessels are exposed through a small skin incision superior and parallel to the inguinal crease. Once the vessels are deemed appropriate for cannulation (size at least 7 mm and free of atherosclerosis), single left-lung ventilation is established and the robotic ports incisions are made. First, the camera port is placed in the fourth intercostal space 2 to 3 cm lateral to the midclavicular line, and a 30-degree, three-dimensional, high-definition camera is inserted. After inspecting the intrathoracic anatomy and planning the port placement for optimal visualization and repair of the valve, a 2-cm working port is made in the same interspace 2 to 3 cm lateral to the camera port. The left robotic arm port is placed in the third intercostal space 2 to 3 cm medial to the anterior axillary line. The right robotic arm port is placed in the fifth or sixth intercostal space just lateral to the anterior axillary line. The left atrial retractor port is placed through the fourth or fifth intercostal space just medial to the midclavicular line (Fig. 84-1).

A femoral venous cannula (22 or 25 Fr, Edwards Lifesciences, Irvine, CA) is positioned in the superior vena cava (SVC) under echocardiographic guidance, and in most cases a separate SVC cannula (17 Fr) is placed via the internal jugular vein over a wire. Arterial cannulation (19 or 21 Fr) is accomplished via the femoral artery (Fig. 84-2). Cardiopulmonary bypass is established at moderate hypothermia (32° C) and the pericardium is incised 2 to 3 cm anterior to the right phrenic nerve. In patients with a normal sized aorta (less than 4 cm), no evidence of atherosclerosis, and no aortic regurgitation, an aortic endoballoon is used for antegrade cardioplegia. Correct positioning is ensured by TEE and monitoring of bilateral upper extremity pressures. If an endoballoon is contraindicated, a separate antegrade cardioplegia catheter is inserted in the proximal aorta and a transthoracic aortic cross-clamp is positioned in the third intercostal space in the midaxillary line (Fig. 84-3). After cardioplegic arrest, a 3- to 4-cm left atriotomy is made medial to the right superior pulmonary vein, the atrial retractor is inserted in the atrium, and the atriotomy is extended to allow complete exposure of the mitral valve.

The surgeon performs the surgery at the console while the patient-side assistant changes instruments, changes supplies, and retrieves operative materials. Close

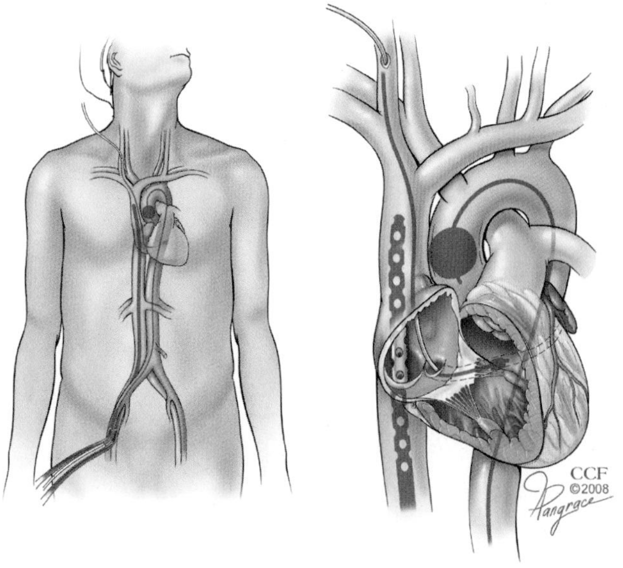

FIGURE 84-2 ■ Overview of cannulation showing femoral venous and arterial cannulas, retrograde coronary sinus catheter, and endoballoon.

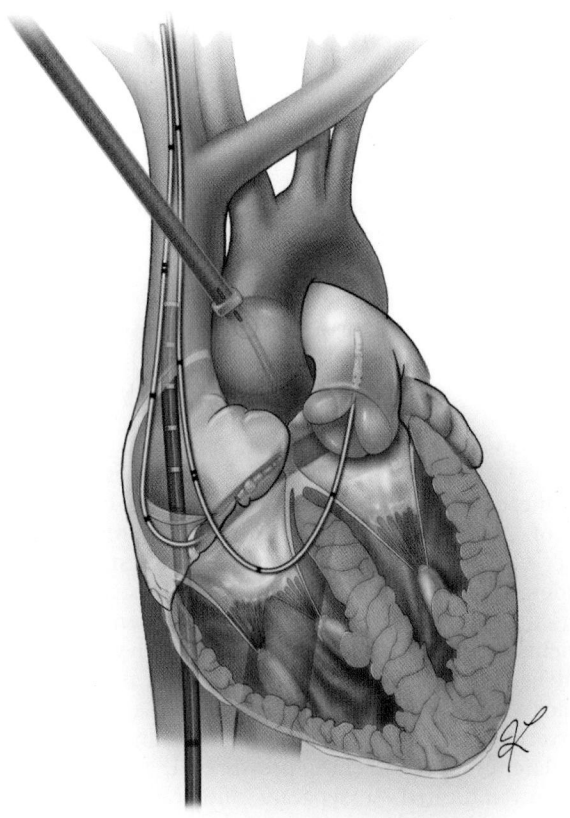

FIGURE 84-3 ■ Transthoracic aortic cross-clamp and direct antegrade cardioplegia catheter.

inspection of the valve will determine what type of repair is required—leaflet resection and artificial chordae are the two most common techniques used to correct leaflet prolapse. Insertion of a partial flexible annuloplasty band using the running technique supports the repair and

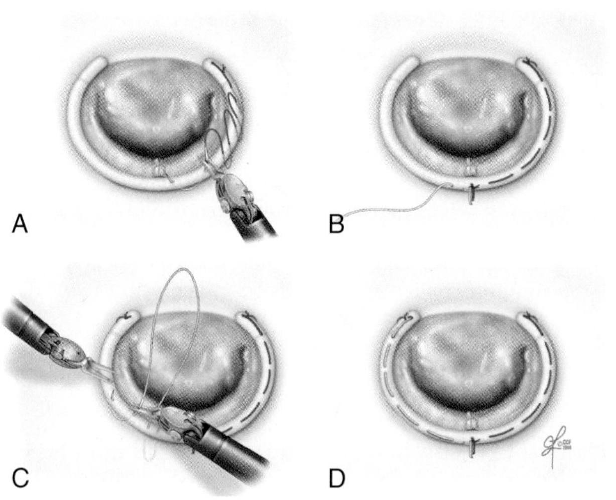

FIGURE 84-4 ■ Schematic diagram of running annuloplasty suture technique using a partial flexible band. **A,** First suture is tied at right trigone and run clockwise to mid-portion of annulus. **B,** Second suture is tied at mid-portion of annulus and tails are tied to first suture. **C,** Second suture is run clockwise to left trigone. **D,** Third suture is tied at left trigone and tails are tied to second suture.

provides annular reduction (Fig. 84-4).[21] Sutures to complete the repair are tied intracorporeally and retrieved by the patient-side assistant. Competency of the valve is tested by administration of antegrade cardioplegia and saline insufflation. The left atrium is closed using a running polytetrafluoroethylene (PTFE) suture. The robotic arms are removed, and standard de-airing and weaning procedures are performed under TEE. All patients have a transthoracic echocardiogram before discharge.

CLINICAL OUTCOMES

The world experience of robotic mitral valve surgery to date is mostly a collection of retrospective case series. Currently, only one large study exists that compares robotic mitral valve repair with alternative approaches. Nevertheless, surgical results thus far have been encouraging, and short-term outcomes appear similar to outcomes for repair using conventional approaches.

In 2000, Chitwood and colleagues completed the first phase I robotic mitral valve repair trial, which consisted of 10 patients.[22] The average total arrest time and total operating room time were 150 minutes and 4.8 hours, respectively. There were no device-related complications and there was one reoperation for bleeding. Average postoperative length of stay was 4 days, and mitral regurgitation was trace or less for all patients at 3-month follow up. Based on these results, an extension of the trial was granted and subsequently reported in 2003 on 38 patients.[23] In this study, total operating room time decreased from 5.1 hours in the first group of 19 patients to 4.4 hours in the second group of 19 patients. Both cross-clamp and bypass times decreased significantly with experience as well. One patient underwent replacement for failed repair.

Mohr and coworkers described their initial experience in 2001 in 17 patients who underwent robotic mitral valve repair.[24] Conversion to an alternative approach was necessary in 3 of the 17 cases (17.6%). The average cross-clamp time was 89 ± 18 minutes. Intraoperative mitral regurgitation was trace or less in all but one patient who underwent an immediate endoscopic valve replacement. Another patient had postoperative failure before discharge and required replacement.

A multicenter phase II clinical trial involving 112 patients at 10 institutions was published in 2005.[21] Total robot, aortic cross-clamp, and cardiopulmonary bypass times were 77.9 ± 0.3 minutes, 2.1 ± 0.1 hours, and 2.8 ± 0.1 hours, respectively. At 1-month echocardiographic follow-up, 9 patients (8%) had 2+ mitral regurgitation, and 6 (5.4%) of these had reoperations (5 replacements and 1 repair). There were no deaths, strokes, or device-related complications.

In 2006, Murphy and colleagues published their results of 127 robotic mitral valve operations.[25] Six of the 127 cases (4.7%) were converted to another approach. Of the 121 robotic surgeries, mitral valve repair was completed in 114 patients (94.2%), with the remaining 7 undergoing replacement. Mean aortic occlusion time (with endoaortic balloon) was 102 ± 28 minutes, and mean cardiopulmonary bypass time was 131 ± 34 minutes. Two patients (1.7%) required reoperation on the mitral valve, and there was one hospital death (0.8%). Echocardiographic follow-up was completed in 98 patients with a mean follow-up of 8.4 ± 8.1 months. Mitral regurgitation of trace or less was seen in 95 patients (96.9%).

Our initial results at Cleveland Clinic were published in early 2011.[26] From January 2006 to January 2009, 759 patients with degenerative mitral valve disease and posterior leaflet prolapse underwent primary isolated mitral valve surgery by complete sternotomy (n = 114), partial sternotomy (n = 270), right mini-anterolateral thoracotomy (n = 114), or a robotic approach (n = 261). Outcomes were compared on an intent-to-treat basis using propensity-score matching. Mitral valve repair was achieved in all patients except 1 patient in the complete sternotomy group. In matched groups, median cardiopulmonary bypass time was 42 minutes longer for robotic than complete sternotomy, 39 minutes longer than partial sternotomy, and 11 minutes longer than right mini-anterolateral thoracotomy ($P < 0.0001$); median myocardial ischemic time was 26 minutes longer than complete sternotomy and partial sternotomy, and 16 minutes longer than right mini-anterolateral thoracotomy ($P < 0.0001$). Quality of mitral valve repair was similar among matched groups (P = 0.6, 0.2, and 0.1, respectively). There were no in-hospital deaths. Neurologic, pulmonary, and renal complications were similar among groups ($P > 0.1$). The robotic group had the lowest occurrences of atrial fibrillation and pleural effusion, contributing to the shortest hospital stay (median 4.2 days), 1.0, 1.6, and 0.9 days shorter than for complete sternotomy, partial sternotomy, and right mini-anterolateral thoracotomy (all $P < 0.001$), respectively.

An early major concern of robotic mitral valve surgery has been the ability to perform complex repairs, such as anterior leaflet of bileaflet repair. Although we began our experience by focusing primarily on posterior leaflet prolapse, we now feel confident with the robotic approach in patients with anterior or bileaflet prolapse as well. In addition, robotic surgery is offered to patients with mitral valve regurgitation and atrial fibrillation or tricuspid regurgitation.

LIMITATIONS

A significant limitation of contemporary robotic systems is the lack of haptics or tactile feedback. Haptics do for touch what computer graphics do for vision. Although the optics and vision systems have continued to improve dramatically, tactile feedback to the surgeon does not yet exist in robotic surgery. In conventional surgery, almost everything a surgeon does relates to force feedback. The response of tissues to manipulation and the forces applied and given back to the surgeon are essential to identifying pathologic areas, assessing tissue boundaries, and determining the quality of an operation. Currently, surgeons performing robotic surgery assess the force applied to tissue by what they see—how tight tissue appears, how sharp tissue contours are, how subtle color changes are, and so forth. Improving tactile feedback is critical to the continued evolution of robotic technology in minimally invasive surgery.

Another limitation to greater adoption of robotic cardiac surgery is the capital investment required. The cost of $1.5 million to $2 million per system (depending on the model, features, service contracts, etc.) plus a per-case cost and additional annual service agreements place it beyond the reach of many institutions. Taking into account these costs, a number of studies have shown higher in-hospital costs for robotic cardiac surgery; this may be shortsighted. In our experience, the per-case cost of robotic surgery is similar to that of conventional surgery when economic outcomes beyond hospital discharge are taken into account.

Longer operative times necessary for robotic mitral valve repair have in part slowed its adoption, although whether or not these longer times affect clinical outcomes remains to be determined. In addition to the setup time for robotic cardiac surgery, a significant portion of time is dedicated to placement of the annuloplasty ring, which is usually anchored with individual mattress sutures that require time-consuming instrument tying. Alternative methods of securing the annuloplasty band, such as a running suture technique or the use of nitinol U-clips (Medtronic, Minneapolis, MN) have shortened operative times and lessened the technical burden of tying a large number of knots endoscopically. In a 2010 report from our institution, a cohort of patients in whom the annuloplasty rings were secured with interrupted sutures (n = 50) was compared with a cohort of patients in whom the annuloplasty rings were secured with a running technique (n = 50).[21] Median total procedure (wheels in to wheels out), cardiopulmonary bypass, and aortic occlusion times were significantly decreased by 38, 32, and 19 minutes ($P < 0.01$ in all), respectively, in the running annuloplasty cohort without sacrificing short-term outcomes. In 2007, investigators at Eastern Carolina University reported on a cohort of patients in whom U-clips were used ($n = 50$) in comparison with a cohort of patients in whom conventional sutures were used ($n = 72$).[27] Cardiopulmonary bypass, aortic occlusion, and annuloplasty band placement times were shorter in the U-clip cohort (U-clips versus sutures: 144 ± 50 minutes versus 169 ± 35 minutes, 105 ± 30 minutes versus 132 ± 29 minutes, and 26 ± 5 minutes versus 40 ± 10 minutes, respectively, $P < 0.01$ for all).

Robotic coronary artery bypass surgery continues to be a challenging procedure. The most significant limitation to the success and adoption of robotic bypass surgery is the inability to consistently reproduce a high-quality anastomosis in a timely fashion. Using conventional suture and tying knots adds a significant amount of time to the procedure. Nitinol U-clips (Coalescent Surgical, Inc., Sunnyvale, CA) have been used successfully as an alternative to sutured anastomosis with excellent short-term and mid-term graft patency.[22,23] Additional alternative methods of creating vascular anastomoses, such as glue or connecting devices, may avert the need to use conventional sutured techniques.[25,28]

OTHER MINIMALLY INVASIVE APPROACHES

In addition to the robotic approach, many minimally invasive approaches have been described for mitral valve surgery, including the partial sternotomy and right thoracotomy. Common variations of the partial sternotomy include a right-sided partial sternotomy, an upper J incision, a right parasternal incision, and a lower half ministernotomy (T incision).[1,3,4,17,19,20] Investigators at our institution pioneered the partial upper sternotomy with J incision. Initial results using this approach and an extended transseptal incision were favorable. In our initial experience of 462 cases published in 1999, conversion to a complete sternotomy was necessary in 3%, and there were low rates of wound infection (0.2%), low transfusion requirements, and excellent cosmesis.[2] In a 2010 report of 590 well-matched patient pairs who underwent conventional minimally invasive surgery versus complete sternotomy, there were cosmetic, blood product use, respiratory, and pain advantages in the minimally invasive cohort with no apparent detriments.[6] Conventional minimally invasive approaches have since continued to demonstrate improved outcomes and economic benefits over similar surgeries performed through complete sternotomies.[3] Given these advantages, mortality and morbidity for robotic and percutaneous mitral valve procedures should be compared with those of conventional minimally invasive approaches rather than with the complete sternotomy.

FUTURE SYSTEMS AND NOVEL VISUALIZATION TECHNIQUES

Technologic advances in cardiac surgery are occurring at a rapid pace. Robotic cardiac surgery has become commonplace for some surgeons. Future incremental modifications and improvements of current systems and instruments undoubtedly will occur. In addition, novel technology will be developed that will radically change the current paradigm of robotic cardiac surgery and robotic cardiac surgery training.

Current robotic systems are large, take up a lot of space in the operating room, and are cumbersome to move. As technology develops, systems will become smaller, have lower profiles, and be more mobile. Port sizes for the camera and working arms will become even smaller. Further miniaturization may allow for the development of surgical micro-robots, magnetically controlled devices that can be navigated remotely, ingestible cameras, and implantable sensors. Research is currently under way to develop wireless imaging and task-assisting robots that can be placed inside the abdominal cavity during surgery.[15] In addition, investigators at Carnegie Mellon University have described a mobile robotic device that can adhere to the epicardium and navigate to any location in a porcine beating heart model.[29]

Improving surgical dexterity with haptic feedback is essential to the continued evolution of cardiac surgery, and haptics in robotic surgery is an area of active research. Researchers at Pennsylvania State and Millersville Universities developed a haptic suture simulator that gives a realistic feeling when handling and suturing tissue.[7] In this simulator, artificial skin deforms relative to the pressure applied to a network of masses and springs through the surgical tool. Specialized software calculates contact forces in the tissue and returns the appropriate forces to the user to simulate the impact of pushing, pulling, cutting, and suturing the skin and underlying tissue. Technology like this could eventually be applied to robotic surgery and allow the surgeon to "feel" the tissue through the robotic arms. The lack of force feedback in current systems makes it possible for the surgeon to inadvertently apply excessive force to the tissue and cause tissue damage. By incorporating haptic feedback into future systems, surgeons will gain a more precise and realistic feel of how tissue is responding to the forces generated by the robotic end-effectors.

Further advancements in visualization will continue to push the field of robotic cardiac surgery forward. In contrast to conventional surgery, the robotic surgeon looks through a vision system rather than directly at the operative field. The three-dimensional display, high definition, and up to 10× magnification of the system augment the surgeon's visualization of important structures. In addition, this artificial visualization offers some unique opportunities, such as image stabilization and image overlay. Currently, creation of small-vessel anastomoses on the beating heart is challenging with the robot. Image stabilization systems using a virtual motion compensation scheme are under development with the goal of rendering a motion-stabilized view of the area of interest.[12] Image overlay with the robotic instruments is another unique concept with the robot. Three-dimensional modeling and reconstruction from computed tomography (CT), magnetic resonance imaging (MRI), or ultrasound superimposed with the robotic instruments could provide real-time data acquisition of pathologic characteristics or repair quality. For example, investigators at the University of Western Ontario used real-time three-dimensional echocardiography as the sole guiding method for atrial septal defect closure in porcine hearts.[11] When compared with conventional two-dimensional echocardiography, task completion times were improved by as much as 70%. Investigators at our institution have demonstrated direct endoscopy-guided mitral and tricuspid valve repair in an open-chest, beating-heart bovine model.[30,31] Using this technique, investigators showed the technical feasibility of beating-heart valve surgery under direct endoscopic imaging. Although the study was performed under open-chest conditions, it is a first step toward closed-chest intracardiac surgery using direct endoscopic visualization. Someday the robotic cardiac surgeon may be able to switch the display and use an alternative imaging source in place of, or in conjunction with, the three-dimensional display to perform beating-heart intracardiac operations.

The future of robotic cardiac surgery is bright. Although years away from full development, it is conceivable that one day a system will exist that will perform fully robotic or automated cardiac surgery. In this scenario, the surgeon will enter all preoperative imaging data on a patient, perform the operation on a virtual simulator, and then transfer the simulation to a robotic telemanipulation system that will perform the operation flawlessly. In addition, a scenario where the operation is planned by software and then performed by a robotic system is imaginable. Although scenarios such as these are years away, existing work has clearly laid the groundwork for automated cardiac surgery.

CONCLUSION

A renaissance in cardiac surgery is under way. Robotic technology is now well established in cardiac surgery and has become standard practice for some surgeons. The success of robotic cardiac surgery is largely the result of advancements in cannulation methods, video optics, instrumentation, and training methods. The development of extrathoracic cardiopulmonary bypass with specialized endovascular cannulas and catheters has allowed for adequate antegrade and retrograde cardioplegic arrest, and ventricular decompression. Enhanced three-dimensional high-definition visualization with the capability of 10× magnification has provided improved clarity and detail of the anastomotic structures. Seven degrees of freedom with the "endo-wrist" instruments, where additional articulation occurs near the tip of the instrument, was critical in improving dexterity in tight spaces. Lastly, the dual-console capability in the newest system allows two surgeons to sit at separate consoles and easily and quickly take control of the instruments at any time during surgery, a situation that helps in training.

Numerous developments must be made in robotic cardiac surgery to increase adoption of robotic technology for coronary revascularization. The creation of robotic coronary vascular anastomoses on a beating heart is technically challenging with current technology, and the inability to consistently reproduce high-quality anastomoses remains a limiting factor in adoption. Improved stabilization devices, automated vascular anastomotic devices, and the ability to reach all areas of a beating, full heart in a closed chest environment needs to be developed for robotic revascularization surgery to reach its full potential.

Similar to other technologic advances in surgery, robotic cardiac surgery is an evolutionary process. Even the greatest skeptics must concede that substantial progress has been made. In the present era, robotic mitral valve repair has safety and short-term effectiveness profiles similar to those of conventional surgery and has the additional benefits of shorter lengths of stay and faster return to work. Despite enthusiasm, caution cannot be overemphasized because long-term durability of repair has yet to be determined. Any new technology, approach, or technique, including robotic cardiac surgery, must be critically compared with traditional operations, which continue to exhibit long-term success and ever-decreasing rates of morbidity and mortality.

REFERENCES

1. Cosgrove DM, 3rd, Sabik JF, Navia JL: Minimally invasive valve operations. *Ann Thorac Surg* 65(6):1535–1538, discussion 1538–1539, 1998.
2. Gillinov AM, Cosgrove DM: Minimally invasive mitral valve surgery: mini-sternotomy with extended transseptal approach. *Semin Thorac Cardiovasc Surg* 11(3):206–211, 1999.
3. Cohn LH, Adams DH, Couper GS, et al: Minimally invasive cardiac valve surgery improves patient satisfaction while reducing costs of cardiac valve replacement and repair. *Ann Surg* 226(4):421–426, discussion 427–428, 1997.
4. Doty DB, DiRusso GB, Doty JR: Full-spectrum cardiac surgery through a minimal incision: mini-sternotomy (lower half) technique. *Ann Thorac Surg* 65(2):573–577, 1998.
5. Zenati MA: Robotic heart surgery. *Cardiol Rev* 9(5):287–294, 2001.
6. Svensson LG, Atik FA, Cosgrove DM, et al: Minimally invasive versus conventional mitral valve surgery: a propensity-matched comparison. *J Thorac Cardiovasc Surg* 139(4):926–932 e1–2, 2010.
7. Webster RW, Zimmerman DI, Mohler BJ, et al: A prototype haptic suturing simulator. *Stud Health Technol Inform* 81:567–569, 2001.
8. Burke RP, Wernovsky G, van der Velde M, et al: Video-assisted thoracoscopic surgery for congenital heart disease. *J Thorac Cardiovasc Surg* 109(3):499–507, discussion 508, 1995.
9. Nataf P, Lima L, Regan M, et al: Minimally invasive coronary surgery with thoracoscopic internal mammary artery dissection: surgical technique. *J Card Surg* 11(4):288–292, 1996.
10. Carpentier A, Loulmet D, Carpentier A, et al: [Open heart operation under videosurgery and minithoracotomy. First case (mitral valvuloplasty) operated with success]. *Comptes rendus de l'Academie des sciences Serie III, Sciences de la vie* 319(3):219–223, 1996.
11. Chitwood WR, Jr, Elbeery JR, Chapman WH, et al: Video-assisted minimally invasive mitral valve surgery: the "micro-mitral" operation. *J Thorac Cardiovasc Surg* 113(2):413–414, 1997.
12. Falk V, Walther T, Autschbach R, et al: Robot-assisted minimally invasive solo mitral valve operation. *J Thorac Cardiovasc Surg* 115(2):470–471, 1998.
13. Carpentier A, Loulmet D, Aupecle B, et al: [Computer assisted open heart surgery. First case operated on with success]. *Comptes rendus de l'Academie des sciences Serie III, Sciences de la vie* 321(5):437–442, 1998.
14. Chitwood WR, Jr, Nifong LW, Elbeery JE, et al: Robotic mitral valve repair: trapezoidal resection and prosthetic annuloplasty with the da vinci surgical system. *J Thorac Cardiovasc Surg* 120(6):1171–1172, 2000.
15. Mehmanesh H, Henze R, Lange R: Totally endoscopic mitral valve repair. *J Thorac Cardiovasc Surg* 123(1):96–97, 2002.
16. Damiano RJ, Jr, Ehrman WJ, Ducko CT, et al: Initial United States clinical trial of robotically assisted endoscopic coronary artery bypass grafting. *J Thorac Cardiovasc Surg* 119(1):77–82, 2000.

17. Kasegawa H, Shimokawa T, Matsushita Y, et al: Right-sided partial sternotomy for minimally invasive valve operation: "open door method." *Ann Thorac Surg* 65(2):569–570, 1998.
18. Reichenspurner H, Boehm DH, Gulbins H, et al: Robotically assisted endoscopic coronary artery bypass procedures without cardiopulmonary bypass. *J Thorac Cardiovasc Surg* 118(5):960–961, 1999.
19. Svensson LG, D'Agostino RS: "J" incision minimal-access valve operations. *Ann Thorac Surg* 66(3):1110–1112, 1998.
20. Svensson LG: Minimal-access "J" or "j" sternotomy for valvular, aortic, and coronary operations or reoperations. *Ann Thorac Surg* 64(5):1501–1503, 1997.
21. Nifong LW, Chitwood WR, Pappas PS, et al: Robotic mitral valve surgery: a United States multicenter trial. *J Thorac Cardiovasc Surg* 129(6):1395–1404, 2005.
22. Kypson AP, Nifong LW, Chitwood WR, Jr: Robotic mitral valve surgery. *Semin Thorac Cardiovasc Surg* 15(2):121–129, 2003.
23. Nifong LW, Chu VF, Bailey BM, et al: Robotic mitral valve repair: experience with the da Vinci system. *Ann Thorac Surg* 75(2):438–442, discussion 443, 2003.
24. Mohr FW, Falk V, Diegeler A, et al: Computer-enhanced "robotic" cardiac surgery: experience in 148 patients. *J Thorac Cardiovasc Surg* 121(5):842–853, 2001.
25. Murphy DA, Miller JS, Langford DA, et al: Endoscopic robotic mitral valve surgery. *J Thorac Cardiovasc Surg* 132(4):776–781, 2006.
26. Mihaljevic T, Jarrett CM, Gillinov AM, et al: Robotic repair of posterior mitral valve prolapse versus conventional approaches: potential realized. *J Thorac Cardiovasc Surg* 141(1):72–80.e1–4, 2011.
27. Cook RC, Nifong LW, Enterkin JE, et al: Significant reduction in annuloplasty operative time with the use of nitinol clips in robotically assisted mitral valve repair. *J Thorac Cardiovasc Surg* 133(5):1264–1267, 2007.
28. Jacobs S, Holzhey D, Stein H, et al: Catheter-based endoscopic bypass grafting: an experimental feasibility study. *Ann Thorac Surg* 84(5):1724–1727, 2007.
29. Patronik NA, Zenati MA, Riviere CN: Preliminary evaluation of a mobile robotic device for navigation and intervention on the beating heart. *Comput Aided Surg* 10(4):225–232, 2005.
30. Horai T, Fukamachi K, Fumoto H, et al: Direct endoscopy-guided mitral valve repair in the beating heart: an acute animal study. *Innovations (Philadelphia, Pa)* 6(2):122–125, 2011.
31. Shiose A, Takaseya T, Fumoto H, et al: Cardioscopy-guided surgery: intracardiac mitral and tricuspid valve repair under direct visualization in the beating heart. *J Thorac Cardiovasc Surg* 142(1):199–202, 2011.

PART **G**

MANAGEMENT OF CARDIAC ARRHYTHMIAS

PART OUTLINE

CHAPTER 85

Cardiac Devices for the Treatment of Bradyarrhythmias and Tachyarrhythmias

Adam S. Fein • Lilian P. Joventino • Peter J. Zimetbaum

CHAPTER OUTLINE

HISTORICAL PERSPECTIVE AND OVERVIEW

Paul Zoll developed the first transcutaneous electronic pacemaker in 1952 for the treatment of life-threatening bradycardia.[1] The first internal pacemaker was implanted in 1958 for the treatment of complete heart block[2] and in the management of Stokes-Adams seizures.[3] Early pacemaker models were simple, fixed-rate devices. Thoracic surgeons performed most early implants by placing epimyocardial leads directly on the exposed heart; these leads were connected to an abdominally implanted pulse generator. Modern pacemakers have sophisticated microprocessors that apply diagnostic and therapeutic algorithms, which have dramatically increased their versatility.

The development of the implantable cardioverter-defibrillator (ICD) was pioneered by Michel Mirowski.[4-6] The initial purpose of the ICD was to provide immediate, automatic defibrillation to ambulatory patients who were victims of a lethal ventricular arrhythmia. Mirowski performed the first human ICD implantation in 1980.[6] First-generation ICDs were composed of large generators (>200 cm^3 volume) implanted in an abdominal pocket with epicardial defibrillator patches. Whereas these early ICDs were capable of only high-energy shocks, current ICDs are small (<40 cm^3 volume), yet they contain all the advanced pacing functions of modern pacemakers as well as complex tachycardia treatment options (Figs. 85-1 and 85-2). Despite their diminutive size, newer ICDs have become progressively superior in their sensing, diagnosis, and treatment of arrhythmias. Since the late 1990s, ICDs have emerged as the single most effective lifesaving intervention in the prevention of sudden cardiac death.[7-11]

With increased sophistication and miniaturization of pulse generators and the development of the much simpler and safer transvenous approach for implantation of cardiac devices, indications for cardiac pacing as well as for ICDs have dramatically expanded.[12,13] In addition, the U.S. Food and Drug Administration (FDA) approved the totally subcutaneous ICD in September 2012. It is estimated that approximately 400,000 devices are implanted each year in the United States, and there are more than 3 million patients with implanted cardiac devices currently.

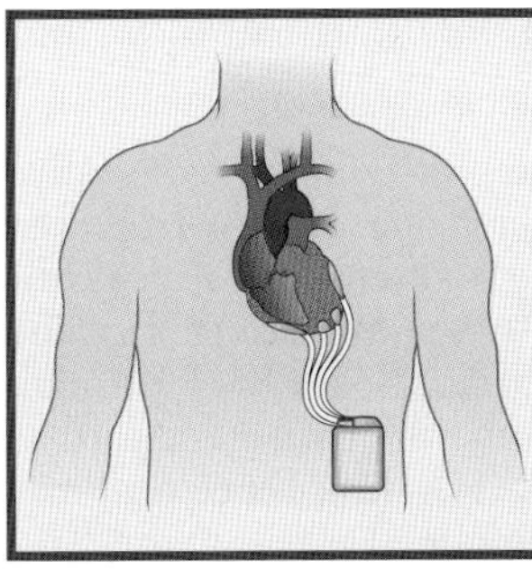

• Large devices—Abdominal site
• First human implants
• Thoracotomy, multiple incisions
• General anesthesia
• Long hospital stays
• Complications from major surgery
• Perioperative mortality up to 9%
• Nonprogrammable therapy
• High-energy shock only
• Device longevity ~1.5 years
• Fewer than 1000 implants per year

FIGURE 85-1 ■ Implantable cardioverter-defibrillators in 1980. (Courtesy Medtronic, Inc., Minneapolis, MN.)

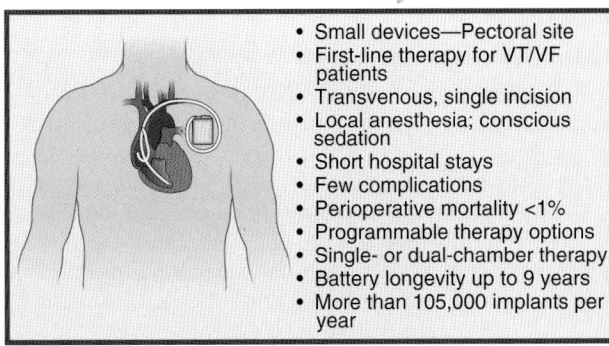

The remainder of this chapter focuses on the description, implantation techniques, indications, and complications of current implantable cardiac pacemakers and defibrillators.

INDICATIONS FOR IMPLANTATION OF CARDIAC DEVICES

The American College of Cardiology/American Heart Association/Heart Rhythm Society (ACC/AHA/HRS) guidelines for device-based therapy of cardiac rhythm abnormalities were updated in 2012.[14]

Temporary Pacemakers

Indications

Placement of a temporary pacemaker is indicated whenever hemodynamic compromise is present because of a bradyarrhythmia. Temporary pacemakers should also be placed prophylactically if a high risk for development of hemodynamically untolerated bradycardia is present. Specific guidelines for placement of temporary pacemakers in the setting of acute myocardial infarction exist.[15] Temporary transvenous pacing is indicated in symptomatic sinus bradycardia, sinus pauses of more than 3 seconds, or sinus bradycardia with a heart rate below 40 beats/minute associated with hypotension or hemodynamic compromise, and if unresponsive to a maximum dose (2 mg) of intravenous atropine. Other class I indications for temporary transvenous pacing in acute myocardial infarction include ventricular asystole, alternating left and right bundle branch block, recurrent polymorphic ventricular tachycardia with a heart rate less than 60 beats/minute and prolonged QT, and new bundle branch block or fascicular block and right bundle branch block in the setting of Möbitz II second-degree atrioventricular (AV) block.[15]

Venous Access

Table 85-1 summarizes the different sites that can be used for insertion of a temporary pacemaker.[16] The particular patient and the advantages and disadvantages of each site are important factors in the decision of which site to use.

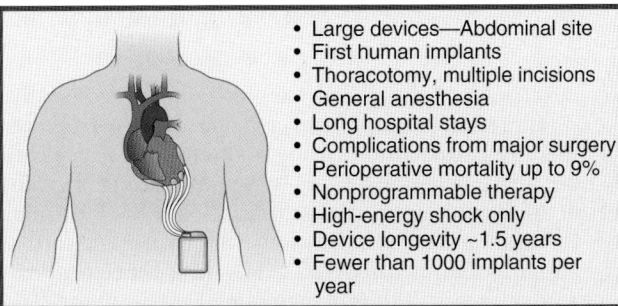

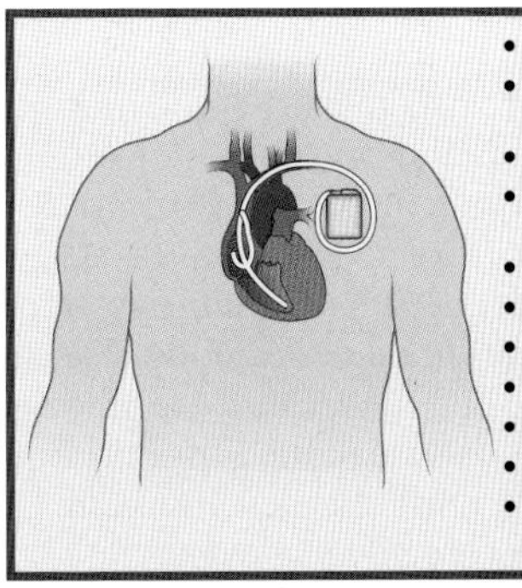

• Small devices—Pectoral site
• First-line therapy for VT/VF patients
• Transvenous, single incision
• Local anesthesia; conscious sedation
• Short hospital stays
• Few complications
• Perioperative mortality <1%
• Programmable therapy options
• Single- or dual-chamber therapy
• Battery longevity up to 9 years
• More than 105,000 implants per year

FIGURE 85-2 ■ Implantable cardioverter-defibrillators today. *VT/VF*, Ventricular tachycardia/ventricular flutter. (Courtesy Medtronic, Inc., Minneapolis, MN.)

TABLE 85-1 Sites for Placement of a Temporary Pacemaker

Site	Advantages	Disadvantages
Femoral vein	Easy access	Leg must remain immobilized High infection risk Fluoroscopy required for proper placement Patient must lie flat
Internal jugular vein	Good site for pacer placement (right better than left)	Risk of pneumothorax, inadvertent carotid artery puncture Patient must lie flat for access; Trendelenburg position preferred to avoid air embolism
Subclavian vein	Good site for pacer placement (left better than right)	Risk of pneumothorax, hemothorax with inadvertent subclavian artery puncture Patient must lie flat for access; Trendelenburg position preferred to avoid air embolism
Antecubital vein (basilic, median basilic, or cephalic)	Access is low risk Good site for pacer placement (left better than right)	Risk of dislodgement; arm must remain immobilized Basilic or median basilic preferred (cephalic has tortuous course to central veins) Fluoroscopy required for pacer placement

From Baim DS, Grossman W, editors: Grossman's cardiac catheterization, angiography, and intervention, ed 6, Philadelphia, 2000, Lippincott Williams & Wilkins.

For example, the internal jugular and subclavian veins may be chosen when need for stability and longer pacing requirement is anticipated. If a permanent pacemaker will be required in the future, the temporary pacemaker should be placed through a vein remote from the preferred site for permanent pacemaker implantation. Use of the antecubital veins minimizes bleeding in the coagulopathic patient. However, the risk of cardiac perforation or lead dislodgement is higher if the arm is not kept fully immobilized.

Permanent Pacemakers

Indications

Justifications for permanent pacemaker implantation include alleviation of symptoms and prevention of subsequent morbidity or mortality as a direct result of bradycardia. Bradycardia can result from a variety of disorders of the sinus node, the AV node, the His-Purkinje system, or a combination of these. Sinus node or AV node disease is often not life-threatening but may cause significant symptoms. On the other hand, disease of the His-Purkinje system may be asymptomatic until the development of AV block and its associated severe adverse events.

Symptoms from bradycardia generally result from inadequate cardiac output. Such symptoms may be vague and include fatigue, decreased exercise tolerance, dyspnea on exertion, lightheadedness, dizziness, congestive heart failure, presyncope, and syncope. Patient-triggered ambulatory cardiac monitoring is often helpful in establishing that such nonspecific symptoms are in fact the result of symptomatic bradycardia. Boxes 85-1 through 85-12 summarize the indications for permanent cardiac pacing published by the ACC/AHA Task Force on Practice Guidelines in 2008 and maintained as part of the 2012 focused update.[12,14]

BOX 85-1 Recommendations for Permanent Pacing in Sinus Node Dysfunction

CLASS I

1. Permanent pacemaker implantation is indicated for sinus node dysfunction (SND) with documented symptomatic bradycardia, including frequent sinus pauses that produce symptoms. *(Level of Evidence: C)*
2. Permanent pacemaker implantation is indicated for symptomatic chronotropic incompetence. *(Level of Evidence: C)*
3. Permanent pacemaker implantation is indicated for symptomatic sinus bradycardia that results from required drug therapy for medical conditions. *(Level of Evidence: C)*

CLASS IIA

1. Permanent pacemaker implantation is reasonable for SND with heart rate less than 40 beats per minute (bpm) when a clear association between significant symptoms consistent with bradycardia and the actual presence of bradycardia has not been documented. *(Level of Evidence: C)*
2. Permanent pacemaker implantation is reasonable for syncope of unexplained origin when clinically significant abnormalities of sinus node function are discovered or provoked in electrophysiologic studies. *(Level of Evidence: C)*

CLASS IIB

1. Permanent pacemaker implantation may be considered in minimally symptomatic patients with chronic heart rate less than 40 bpm while awake. *(Level of Evidence: C)*

CLASS III

1. Permanent pacemaker implantation is not indicated for SND in asymptomatic patients. *(Level of Evidence: C)*
2. Permanent pacemaker implantation is not indicated for SND in patients for whom the symptoms suggestive of bradycardia have been clearly documented to occur in the absence of bradycardia. *(Level of Evidence: C)*
3. Permanent pacemaker implantation is not indicated for SND with symptomatic bradycardia due to nonessential drug therapy. *(Level of Evidence: C)*

From Epstein AE, DiMarco JP, Ellenbogen KA, et al: ACC/AHA/HRS 2008 Guidelines for device-based therapy of cardiac rhythm abnormalities: a report of the American College of Cardiology/American Heart Association Task Force on Practice Guidelines (Writing Committee to Revise the ACC/AHA/NASPE 2002 Guideline Update for Implantation of Cardiac Pacemakers and Antiarrhythmia Devices) developed in collaboration with the American Association for Thoracic Surgery and Society of Thoracic Surgeons. J Am Coll Cardiol 51:e1–e62, 2008.

Text continued on p. 1491

BOX 85-2 Recommendations for Acquired Atrioventricular Block in Adults

CLASS I

1. Permanent pacemaker implantation is indicated for third-degree and advanced second-degree atrioventricular (AV) block at any anatomic level associated with bradycardia with symptoms (including heart failure) or ventricular arrhythmias presumed to be due to AV block. *(Level of Evidence: C)*
2. Permanent pacemaker implantation is indicated for third-degree and advanced second-degree AV block at any anatomic level associated with arrhythmias and other medical conditions that require drug therapy that results in symptomatic bradycardia. *(Level of Evidence: C)*
3. Permanent pacemaker implantation is indicated for third-degree and advanced second-degree AV block at any anatomic level in awake, symptom-free patients in sinus rhythm, with documented periods of asystole greater than or equal to 3.0 seconds or any escape rate less than 40 beats per minute (bpm), or with an escape rhythm that is below the AV node. *(Level of Evidence: C)*
4. Permanent pacemaker implantation is indicated for third-degree and advanced second-degree AV block at any anatomic level in awake, symptom-free patients with atrial fibrillation (AF) and bradycardia with 1 or more pauses of at least 5 seconds or longer. *(Level of Evidence: C)*
5. Permanent pacemaker implantation is indicated for third-degree and advanced second-degree AV block at any anatomic level after catheter ablation of the AV junction. *(Level of Evidence: C)*
6. Permanent pacemaker implantation is indicated for third-degree and advanced second-degree AV block at any anatomic level associated with postoperative AV block at any anatomic level associated with postoperative AV block that is not expected to resolve after cardiac surgery. *(Level of Evidence: C)*
7. Permanent pacemaker implantation is indicated for third-degree and advanced second-degree AV block at any anatomic level associated with neuromuscular diseases with AV block, such as myotonic muscular dystrophy, Kearns-Sayre syndrome, Erb dystrophy (limb-girdle muscular dystrophy), and peroneal muscular atrophy, with or without symptoms. *(Level of Evidence: B)*
8. Permanent pacemaker implantation is indicated for second-degree AV block with associated symptomatic bradycardia regardless of type or site of block. *(Level of Evidence: B)*
9. Permanent pacemaker implantation is indicated for asymptomatic persistent third-degree AV block at any anatomic site with average awake ventricular rates of 40 bpm or faster if cardiomegaly or left ventricular (LV) dysfunction is present or if the site of block is below the AV node. *(Level of Evidence: B)*
10. Permanent pacemaker implantation is indicated for second- or third-degree AV block during exercise in the absence of myocardial ischemia. *(Level of Evidence: C)*

CLASS IIA

1. Permanent pacemaker implantation is reasonable for persistent third-degree AV block with an escape rate greater than 40 bpm in asymptomatic adult patients without cardiomegaly. *(Level of Evidence: C)*
2. Permanent pacemaker implantation is reasonable for asymptomatic second-degree AV block at intra- or infra-His levels found at electrophysiologic study. *(Level of Evidence: B)*
3. Permanent pacemaker implantation is reasonable for first- or second-degree AV block with symptoms similar to those of pacemaker syndrome or hemodynamic compromise. *(Level of Evidence: B)*
4. Permanent pacemaker implantation is reasonable for asymptomatic type II second-degree AV block with a narrow QRS. When type II second-degree AV block occurs with a wide QRS, including isolated right bundle branch block, pacing becomes a class I recommendation. (See Section 2.1.3, "Chronic Bifascicular Block.") *(Level of Evidence: B)*

CLASS IIB

1. Permanent pacemaker implantation may be considered for neuromuscular disease such as myotonic muscular dystrophy. Erb dystrophy (limb-girdle muscular dystrophy), and peroneal muscular atrophy with any degree of AV block (including first-degree AV block), with or without symptoms, because there may be unpredictable progression of AV conduction disease. *(Level of Evidence: B)*
2. Permanent pacemaker implantation may be considered for AV block in the setting of drug use and/or drug toxicity when the block is expected to recur even after the drug is withdrawn. *(Level of Evidence: B)*

CLASS III

1. Permanent pacemaker implantation is not indicated for asymptomatic first-degree AV block. (See Section 2.1.3, "Chronic Bifascicular Block.") *(Level of Evidence: B)*
2. Permanent pacemaker implantation is not indicated for asymptomatic type I second-degree AV block at the supra-His (AV node) level or that which is not known to be intra or infra or infra-Hisian. *(Level of Evidence: C)*
3. Permanent pacemaker implantation is not indicated for AV block that is expected to resolve and is unlikely to recur (e.g., drug toxicity, Lyme disease, or transient increases in vagal tone or during hypoxia in sleep apnea syndrome in the absence of symptoms). *(Level of Evidence: B)*

From Epstein AE, DiMarco JP, Ellenbogen KA, et al: ACC/AHA/HRS 2008 Guidelines for device-based therapy of cardiac rhythm abnormalities: a report of the American College of Cardiology/American Heart Association Task Force on Practice Guidelines (Writing Committee to Revise the ACC/AHA/NASPE 2002 Guideline Update for Implantation of Cardiac Pacemakers and Antiarrhythmia Devices) developed in collaboration with the American Association for Thoracic Surgery and Society of Thoracic Surgeons. J Am Coll Cardiol 51:e1–e62, 2008.

BOX 85-3 Recommendations for Permanent Pacing in Chronic Bifascicular Block

Class I

1. Permanent pacemaker implantation is indicated for advanced second-degree atrioventricular (AV) block or intermittent third-degree AV block. *(Level of Evidence: B)*
2. Permanent pacemaker implantation is indicated for type II second-degree AV block. *(Level of Evidence: B)*
3. Permanent pacemaker implantation is indicated for alternating bundle branch block. *(Level of Evidence: C)*

Class IIa

1. Permanent pacemaker implantation is reasonable for syncope not demonstrated to be due to AV block when other likely causes have been excluded, specifically ventricular tachycardia (VT). *(Level of Evidence: B)*
2. Permanent pacemaker implantation is reasonable for an incidental finding at electrophysiologic study of a markedly prolonged HV interval (greater than or equal to 100 milliseconds) in asymptomatic patients. *(Level of Evidence: B)*
3. Permanent pacemaker implantation is reasonable for an incidental finding at electrophysiologic study of pacing-induced infra-His block that is not physiologic. *(Level of Evidence: B)*

Class IIb

1. Permanent pacemaker implantation may be considered in the setting of neuromuscular diseases such as myotonic muscular dystrophy, Erb dystrophy (limb-girdle muscular dystrophy), and peroneal muscular atrophy with bifascicular block or any fascicular block, with or without symptoms. *(Level of Evidence: C)*

Class III

1. Permanent pacemaker implantation is not indicated for fascicular block without AV block or symptoms. *(Level of Evidence: B)*
2. Permanent pacemaker implantation is not indicated for fascicular block with first-degree AV block without symptoms. *(Level of Evidence: B)*

From Epstein AE, DiMarco JP, Ellenbogen KA, et al: ACC/AHA/HRS 2008 Guidelines for device-based therapy of cardiac rhythm abnormalities: a report of the American College of Cardiology/American Heart Association Task Force on Practice Guidelines (Writing Committee to Revise the ACC/AHA/NASPE 2002 Guideline Update for Implantation of Cardiac Pacemakers and Antiarrhythmia Devices) developed in collaboration with the American Association for Thoracic Surgery and Society of Thoracic Surgeons. J Am Coll Cardiol 51:e1–e62, 2008.

BOX 85-4 Recommendations for Permanent Pacing after the Acute Phase of Myocardial Infarction

Class I

1. Permanent ventricular pacing is indicated for persistent second-degree atrioventricular (AV) block in the His-Purkinje system with alternating bundle branch block or third-degree AV block within or below the His-Purkinje system after ST-segment elevation myocardial infarction (MI). *(Level of Evidence: B)*
2. Permanent ventricular pacing is indicated for transient advanced second- or third-degree infranodal AV block and associated bundle branch block. If the site of block is uncertain, an electrophysiologic study may be necessary. *(Level of Evidence: B)*
3. Permanent ventricular pacing is indicated for persistent and symptomatic second- or third-degree AV block. *(Level of Evidence: C)*

Class IIb

1. Permanent ventricular pacing may be considered for persistent second- or third-degree AV block at the AV node level, even in the absence of symptoms. *(Level of Evidence: B)*

Class III

1. Permanent ventricular pacing is not indicated for transient AV block in the absence of intraventricular conduction defects. *(Level of Evidence: B)*
2. Permanent ventricular pacing is not indicated for transient AV block in the presence of isolated left anterior fascicular block. *(Level of Evidence: B)*
3. Permanent ventricular pacing is not indicated for new bundle branch block or fascicular block in the absence of AV block. *(Level of Evidence: B)*
4. Permanent ventricular pacing is not indicated for persistent asymptomatic first-degree AV block in the presence of bundle branch or fascicular block. *(Level of Evidence: B)*

From Epstein AE, DiMarco JP, Ellenbogen KA, et al: ACC/AHA/HRS 2008 Guidelines for device-based therapy of cardiac rhythm abnormalities: a report of the American College of Cardiology/American Heart Association Task Force on Practice Guidelines (Writing Committee to Revise the ACC/AHA/NASPE 2002 Guideline Update for Implantation of Cardiac Pacemakers and Antiarrhythmia Devices) developed in collaboration with the American Association for Thoracic Surgery and Society of Thoracic Surgeons. J Am Coll Cardiol 51:e1–e62, 2008.

BOX 85-5 Recommendations for Permanent Pacing in Hypersensitive Carotid Sinus Syndrome and Neurocardiogenic Syncope

Class I

1. Permanent pacing is indicated for recurrent syncope caused by spontaneously occurring carotid sinus stimulation and carotid sinus pressure that induces ventricular asystole of more than 3 seconds. *(Level of Evidence: C)*

Class IIa

1. Permanent pacing is reasonable for syncope without clear, provocative events and with a hypersensitive cardioinhibitory response of 3 seconds or longer. *(Level of Evidence: C)*

Class IIb

1. Permanent pacing may be considered for significantly symptomatic neurocardiogenic syncope associated with bradycardia documented spontaneously or at the time of tilt-table testing. *(Level of Evidence: B)*

Class III

1. Permanent pacing is not indicated for a hypersensitive cardioinhibitory response to carotid sinus stimulation without symptoms or with vague symptoms. *(Level of Evidence: C)*
2. Permanent pacing is not indicated for situational vasovagal syncope in which avoidance behavior is effective and preferred. *(Level of Evidence: C)*

From Epstein AE, DiMarco JP, Ellenbogen KA, et al: ACC/AHA/HRS 2008 Guidelines for device-based therapy of cardiac rhythm abnormalities: a report of the American College of Cardiology/American Heart Association Task Force on Practice Guidelines (Writing Committee to Revise the ACC/AHA/NASPE 2002 Guideline Update for Implantation of Cardiac Pacemakers and Antiarrhythmia Devices) developed in collaboration with the American Association for Thoracic Surgery and Society of Thoracic Surgeons. J Am Coll Cardiol 51:e1–e62, 2008.

BOX 85-6 Recommendations for Pacing after Cardiac Transplantation

CLASS I

1. Permanent pacing is indicated for persistent inappropriate or symptomatic bradycardia not expected to resolve and for other class I indications for permanent pacing. *(Level of Evidence: C)*

CLASS IIB

1. Permanent pacing may be considered when relative bradycardia is prolonged or recurrent, which limits rehabilitation or discharge after postoperative recovery from cardiac transplantation. *(Level of Evidence: C)*
2. Permanent pacing may be considered for syncope after cardiac transplantation even when bradyarrhythmia has not been documented. *(Level of Evidence: C)*

From Epstein AE, DiMarco JP, Ellenbogen KA, et al: ACC/AHA/HRS 2008 Guidelines for device-based therapy of cardiac rhythm abnormalities: a report of the American College of Cardiology/American Heart Association Task Force on Practice Guidelines (Writing Committee to Revise the ACC/AHA/NASPE 2002 Guideline Update for Implantation of Cardiac Pacemakers and Antiarrhythmia Devices) developed in collaboration with the American Association for Thoracic Surgery and Society of Thoracic Surgeons. J Am Coll Cardiol 51:e1–e62, 2008.

BOX 85-7 Recommendations for Permanent Pacemakers that Automatically Detect and Pace to Terminate Tachycardias

CLASS IIA

1. Permanent pacing is reasonable for symptomatic recurrent supraventricular tachycardia (SVT) that is reproducibly terminated by pacing when catheter ablation and/or drugs fail to control the arrhythmia or produce intolerable side effects. *(Level of Evidence: C)*

CLASS III

1. Permanent pacing is not indicated in the presence of an accessory pathway that has the capacity for rapid anterograde conduction. *(Level of Evidence: C)*

From Epstein AE, DiMarco JP, Ellenbogen KA, et al: ACC/AHA/HRS 2008 Guidelines for device-based therapy of cardiac rhythm abnormalities: a report of the American College of Cardiology/American Heart Association Task Force on Practice Guidelines (Writing Committee to Revise the ACC/AHA/NASPE 2002 Guideline Update for Implantation of Cardiac Pacemakers and Antiarrhythmia Devices) developed in collaboration with the American Association for Thoracic Surgery and Society of Thoracic Surgeons. J Am Coll Cardiol 51:e1–e62, 2008.

BOX 85-8 Recommendations for Pacing to Prevent Tachycardia

CLASS I

1. Permanent pacing is indicated for sustained pause-dependent ventricular tachycardia (VT), with or without QT prolongation. *(Level of Evidence: C)*

CLASS IIA

1. Permanent pacing is reasonable for high-risk patients with congenital long-QT syndrome. *(Level of Evidence: C)*

CLASS IIB

1. Permanent pacing may be considered for prevention of symptomatic, drug-refractory, recurrent atrial fibrillation (AF) in patients with coexisting sinus node dysfunction (SND). *(Level of Evidence: B)*

CLASS III

1. Permanent pacing is not indicated for frequent or complex ventricular ectopic activity without sustained VT in the absence of the long-QT syndrome. *(Level of Evidence: C)*
2. Permanent pacing is not indicated for torsade de pointes VT due to reversible causes. *(Level of Evidence: A)*

From Epstein AE, DiMarco JP, Ellenbogen KA, et al: ACC/AHA/HRS 2008 Guidelines for device-based therapy of cardiac rhythm abnormalities: a report of the American College of Cardiology/American Heart Association Task Force on Practice Guidelines (Writing Committee to Revise the ACC/AHA/NASPE 2002 Guideline Update for Implantation of Cardiac Pacemakers and Antiarrhythmia Devices) developed in collaboration with the American Association for Thoracic Surgery and Society of Thoracic Surgeons. J Am Coll Cardiol 51:e1–e62, 2008.

BOX 85-9 Recommendation for Pacing to Prevent Atrial Fibrillation

CLASS III

1. Permanent pacing is not indicated for the prevention of atrial fibrillation (AF) in patients without any other indication for pacemaker implantation. *(Level of Evidence: B)*

From Epstein AE, DiMarco JP, Ellenbogen KA, et al: ACC/AHA/HRS 2008 Guidelines for device-based therapy of cardiac rhythm abnormalities: a report of the American College of Cardiology/American Heart Association Task Force on Practice Guidelines (Writing Committee to Revise the ACC/AHA/NASPE 2002 Guideline Update for Implantation of Cardiac Pacemakers and Antiarrhythmia Devices) developed in collaboration with the American Association for Thoracic Surgery and Society of Thoracic Surgeons. J Am Coll Cardiol 51:e1–e62, 2008.

BOX 85-10 Recommendations for Cardiac Resynchronization Therapy in Patients with Severe Systolic Heart Failure

Class I

1. Cardiac resynchronization therapy (CRT) is indicated for patients who have left ventricular ejection fraction (LVEF) less than or equal to 35%, sinus rhythm, left bundle branch block (LBBB) with a QRS duration greater than or equal to 150 msec, and New York Heart Association (NYHA) class II, III, or ambulatory IV symptoms on optimal recommended medical therapy. *(Level of Evidence: A for NYHA class III/IV; Level of Evidence: B for NYHA class II)*

Class IIa

1. CRT can be useful for patients who have LVEF less than or equal to 35%, sinus rhythm, LBBB with a QRS duration 120 to 149 msec, and NYHA class II, III, or ambulatory IV symptoms on optimal recommended medical therapy. *(Level of Evidence: B)*
2. CRT can be useful for patients who have LVEF less than or equal to 35%, sinus rhythm, a non-LBBB pattern with a QRS duration greater than or equal to 150 msec, and NYHA class III/ambulatory class IV symptoms on optimal recommended medical therapy. *(Level of Evidence: A)*
3. CRT can be useful in patients with atrial fibrillation and LVEF less than or equal to 35% on guideline-directed medical therapy (GDMT) if (a) the patient requires ventricular pacing or otherwise meets CRT criteria and (b) atrioventricular (AV) nodal ablation or pharmacologic rate control will allow near 100% ventricular pacing with CRT. *(Level of Evidence: B)*
4. CRT can be useful for patients on GDMT who have LVEF less than or equal to 35% and are undergoing new or replacement device placement with anticipated requirement for significant (>40%) ventricular pacing. *(Level of Evidence: C)*

Class IIb

1. CRT may be considered for patients who have LVEF less than or equal to 30%, ischemic etiology of heart failure, sinus rhythm, LBBB with a QRS duration of greater than or equal to 150 msec, and NYHA class I symptoms on optimal medical therapy. *(Level of Evidence: C)*
2. CRT may be considered for patients who have LVEF less than or equal to 35%, sinus rhythm, a non-LBBB pattern with QRS duration 120 to 149 msec, and NYHA class III/ambulatory class IV on optimal medical therapy *(Level of Evidence: B)*
3. CRT may be considered for patients who have LVEF less than or equal to 35%, sinus rhythm, a non-LBBB pattern with a QRS duration greater than or equal to 150 msec, and NYHA class II symptoms on optimal medical therapy. *(Level of Evidence: B)*

Class III

1. CRT is not recommended for patients with NYHA class I or II symptoms and non-LBBB pattern with QRS duration less than 150 msec. *(Level of Evidence: B)*
2. CRT is not indicated for patients whose comorbidities and/or frailty limit survival with good functional capacity to less than 1 year. *(Level of Evidence: C)*

From Epstein AE, DiMarco JP, Ellenbogen KA, et al: ACC/AHA/HRS 2008 Guidelines for device-based therapy of cardiac rhythm abnormalities: a report of the American College of Cardiology/American Heart Association Task Force on Practice Guidelines (Writing Committee to Revise the ACC/AHA/NASPE 2002 Guideline Update for Implantation of Cardiac Pacemakers and Antiarrhythmia Devices) developed in collaboration with the American Association for Thoracic Surgery and Society of Thoracic Surgeons. J Am Coll Cardiol 51:e1–e62, 2008.

BOX 85-11 Recommendations for Pacing in Patients with Hypertrophic Cardiomyopathy

Class I

1. Permanent pacing is indicated for sinus node dysfunction (SND) or atrioventricular (AV) block in patients with hypertrophic cardiomyopathy (HCM) as described previously (see Section 2.1.1, "Sinus Node Dysfunction," and Section 2.1.2, "Acquired Atrioventricular Block in Adults"). *(Level of Evidence: C)*

Class IIb

1. Permanent pacing may be considered in medically refractory symptomatic patients with HCM and significant resting or provoked LV outflow tract obstruction. *(Level of Evidence: A)* As for class I indications, when risk factors for sudden cardiac death (SCD) are present, consider a DDD implantable cardioverter-defibrillator (ICD) (see Section 3, "Indications for Implantable Cardioverter-Defibrillator Therapy").

Class III

1. Permanent pacemaker implantation is not indicated for patients who are asymptomatic or whose symptoms are medically controlled. *(Level of Evidence: C)*
2. Permanent pacemaker implantation is not indicated for symptomatic patients without evidence of LV outflow tract obstruction. *(Level of Evidence: C)*

From Epstein AE, DiMarco JP, Ellenbogen KA, et al: ACC/AHA/HRS 2008 Guidelines for device-based therapy of cardiac rhythm abnormalities: a report of the American College of Cardiology/American Heart Association Task Force on Practice Guidelines (Writing Committee to Revise the ACC/AHA/NASPE 2002 Guideline Update for Implantation of Cardiac Pacemakers and Antiarrhythmia Devices) developed in collaboration with the American Association for Thoracic Surgery and Society of Thoracic Surgeons. J Am Coll Cardiol 51:e1–e62, 2008.

BOX 85-12 Recommendations for Permanent Pacing in Children, Adolescents, and Patients with Congenital Heart Disease

Class I

1. Permanent pacemaker implantation is indicated for advanced second- or third-degree atrioventricular (AV) block associated with symptomatic bradycardia, ventricular dysfunction, or low cardiac output. *(Level of Evidence: C)*
2. Permanent pacemaker implantation is indicated for sinus node dysfunction (SND) with correlation of symptoms during age-inappropriate bradycardia. The definition of bradycardia varies with the patient's age and expected heart rate. *(Level of Evidence: B)*
3. Permanent pacemaker implantation is indicated for postoperative advanced second- or third-degree AV block that is not expected to resolve or that persists at least 7 days after cardiac surgery. *(Level of Evidence: B)*
4. Permanent pacemaker implantation is indicated for congenital third-degree AV block with a wide QRS escape rhythm, complex ventricular ectopy, or ventricular dysfunction. *(Level of Evidence: B)*
5. Permanent pacemaker implantation is indicated for congenital third-degree AV block in the infant with a ventricular rate less than 55 bpm or with congenital heart disease and a ventricular rate less than 70 bpm. *(Level of Evidence: C)*

Class IIa

1. Permanent pacemaker implantation is reasonable for patients with congenital heart disease and sinus bradycardia for the prevention of recurrent episodes of intra-atrial reentrant tachycardia; SND may be intrinsic or secondary to antiarrhythmic treatment. *(Level of Evidence: C)*
2. Permanent pacemaker implantation is reasonable for congenital third-degree AV block beyond the first year of life with an average heart rate less than 50 bpm, abrupt pauses in ventricular rate that are 2 or 3 times the basic cycle length, or associated with symptoms due to chronotropic incompetence. *(Level of Evidence: B)*
3. Permanent pacemaker implantation is reasonable for sinus bradycardia with complex congenital heart disease with a resting heart rate less than 40 bpm or pauses in ventricular rate longer than 3 seconds. *(Level of Evidence: C)*
4. Permanent pacemaker implantation is reasonable for patients with congenital heart disease and impaired hemodynamics due to sinus bradycardia or loss of AV synchrony. *(Level of Evidence: C)*
5. Permanent pacemaker implantation is reasonable for unexplained syncope in the patient with prior congenital heart surgery complicated by transient complete heart block with residual fascicular block after a careful evaluation to exclude other causes of syncope. *(Level of Evidence: B)*

Class IIb

1. Permanent pacemaker implantation may be considered for transient postoperative third-degree AV block that reverts to sinus rhythm with residual bifascicular block. *(Level of Evidence: C)*
2. Permanent pacemaker implantation may be considered for congenital third-degree AV block in asymptomatic children or adolescents with an acceptable rate, a narrow QRS complex, and normal ventricular function. *(Level of Evidence: B)*
3. Permanent pacemaker implantation may be considered for asymptomatic sinus bradycardia after biventricular repair of congenital heart disease with a resting heart rate less than 40 bpm or pauses in ventricular rate longer than 3 seconds. *(Level of Evidence: C)*

Class III

1. Permanent pacemaker implantation is not indicated for transient postoperative AV block with return of normal AV conduction in the otherwise asymptomatic patient. *(Level of Evidence: B)*
2. Permanent pacemaker implantation is not indicated for asymptomatic bifascicular block with or without first-degree AV block after surgery for congenital heart disease in the absence of prior transient complete AV block. *(Level of Evidence: C)*
3. Permanent pacemaker implantation is not indicated for asymptomatic type I second-degree AV block. *(Level of Evidence: C)*
4. Permanent pacemaker implantation is not indicated for asymptomatic sinus bradycardia with the longest relative risk interval less than 3 seconds and a minimum heart rate more than 40 bpm. *(Level of Evidence: C)*

From Epstein AE, DiMarco JP, Ellenbogen KA, et al: ACC/AHA/HRS 2008 Guidelines for device-based therapy of cardiac rhythm abnormalities: a report of the American College of Cardiology/American Heart Association Task Force on Practice Guidelines (Writing Committee to Revise the ACC/AHA/NASPE 2002 Guideline Update for Implantation of Cardiac Pacemakers and Antiarrhythmia Devices) developed in collaboration with the American Association for Thoracic Surgery and Society of Thoracic Surgeons. J Am Coll Cardiol 51:e1–e62, 2008.

Cardiac Resynchronization Therapy (or Biventricular Pacing) for the Treatment of Congestive Heart Failure

The 2012 guidelines updated the formal recommendations (see Box 85-10) for cardiac resynchronization therapy (CRT), or biventricular pacing, as an adjunctive treatment for patients with advanced congestive heart failure.[14] Over the past decade, CRT has emerged as a proven therapy for patients with congestive heart failure (New York Heart Association [NYHA] class >II) caused by systolic dysfunction (left ventricular ejection fraction ≤ 35%) with intraventricular conduction delay, generally of the left bundle branch block type. Patients with QRS duration of more than 150 msec have the strongest clinical response to CRT. There is currently no established role for the use of echocardiographic evidence of mechanical dyssynchrony to select patients for CRT. The 2012 guidelines reflected the growing body of evidence that CRT therapy may benefit patients with milder NYHA I and II symptoms in the setting of pronounced intraventricular conduction delay over 150 msec.[17,18] Intraventricular conduction delay is present in a large proportion of patients with heart failure, and it is frequently accompanied by mechanical dyssynchrony. Patients who have benefited from biventricular pacing can have systolic dysfunction as a result of either coronary or noncoronary cardiomyopathies. The therapeutic intent is to improve the mechanical efficiency of the heart by simultaneously activating both ventricles with the use of an implantable pacemaker or pacemaker-defibrillator system. Approximately two thirds of patients who are treated with CRT derive clinical benefit that can be demonstrated by improvement in functional status, quality-of-life scores, and objective measures of exercise capacity, as well as decreases in mortality rate and number of heart failure hospitalizations. In addition, the degree of mitral regurgitation frequently present in the patients treated with CRT often improves, as does left ventricular ejection fraction, with biventricular pacing.

Simultaneous pacing of both ventricles is achieved by pacing the right ventricle from a standard transvenous right ventricular apical lead while the left ventricle is paced by a transvenously placed coronary sinus lead. The preferred location for the coronary sinus lead is within the posterolateral coronary sinus vein, where the activation delay is generally most pronounced because of dyschronous activation in the setting of the baseline left bundle branch block type of intraventricular conduction delay. Figure 85-3 illustrates typical lead positions for a biventricular pacing system.

Contraindications

Active infection is a contraindication to placement of permanent pacemaker systems. If the need for pacing is urgent, a temporary transvenous pacemaker should be used. In patients with recurrent or protracted infectious illnesses, temporary placement of a standard (screw-in) pacemaker lead is suggested. The proximal end of the lead is externalized and connected to an external pulse generator, and a sterile dressing is placed over the entry site. Such temporary systems may be left in place for weeks and may serve as a bridge to implantation of a permanent pacemaker. Alternatively, an epicardial pacing system can be implanted.

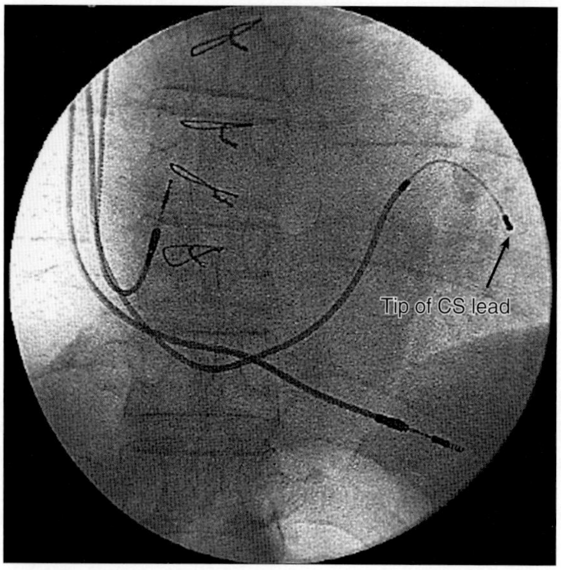

FIGURE 85-3 ■ Fluoroscopic view of a biventricular pacing device. The tip of the coronary sinus (CS) lead is seen within the posterolateral coronary sinus vein.

Implantable Cardioverter-Defibrillators

Indications

Current ACC/AHA/HRS practice guidelines for ICD therapy are listed in Boxes 85-13 and 85-14.[14]

A class I indication for ICD therapy is present for patients who survived a cardiac arrest caused by ventricular fibrillation (VF) or hemodynamically significant ventricular tachycardia (VT) not thought to be due to reversible causes. Other class I indications for ICD therapy include spontaneous VT in patients with structural heart disease and syncope of undetermined causes with clinically significant VT or VF induced at electrophysiology study.[14]

Several other class I indications for ICD therapy now exist to include the patient population studied in three large clinical trials: MUSTT,[8] MADIT II,[10] and SCD-HeFT.[11] ICD therapy is indicated for patients with left ventricular ejection fraction below 35% (as a result of previous myocardial infarction, who are at least 40 days post myocardial infarction or as a result of nonischemic cardiomyopathy) with functional status consistent with NYHA class II or class III.[11] Class I indication for ICD therapy also exists for patients with left ventricular ejection fraction below 30% as a result of previous myocardial infarction (at least 40 days old) who have NYHA class I functional status.[10] In addition, ICD therapy is indicated in patients with left ventricular ejection fraction below 40% as a result of previous myocardial infarction who have nonsustained VT and inducible VT or VF at electrophysiology study.[8]

Other high-risk conditions where ICD therapy is a IIa indication—including arrhythmogenic right ventricular dysplasia/cardiomyopathy (ARVD/C), hypertrophic cardiomyopathy, long QT syndrome, and Brugada syndrome—have been addressed in the 2012 societal guidelines (see Box 85-13).

In September 2012, the FDA approved the totally subcutaneous ICD for the treatment of life-threatening ventricular tachyarrhythmias in patients who do not have symptomatic bradycardia, incessant VT, or spontaneous, frequently recurring VT that is reliably terminated with antitachycardia pacing. These devices hold the promise of lifesaving defibrillation without some of the known problems of transvenous systems, including limited vascular access, transvenous lead durability, hazardous lead extractions, and risks of bloodstream infections. There are no current societal guidelines for which patients should be considered for the S-ICD system.

Contraindications to Implantable Cardioverter-Defibrillator Therapy

If VT/VF is a result of a reversible cause such as acute myocardial infarction or serious electrolyte derangements, ICD implantation is not indicated. An ICD is not

BOX 85-13 Recommendations for Implantable Cardioverter-Defibrillators

CLASS I

1. Implantable cardioverter-defibrillator (ICD) therapy is indicated in patients who are survivors of cardiac arrest due to ventricular fibrillation (VF) or hemodynamically unstable sustained ventricular tachycardia (VT) after evaluation to define the cause of the event and to exclude any completely reversible causes. *(Level of Evidence: A)*
2. ICD therapy is indicated in patients with structural heart disease and spontaneous sustained VT, whether hemodynamically stable or unstable. *(Level of Evidence: B)*
3. ICD therapy is indicated in patients with syncope of undetermined origin with clinically relevant, hemodynamically significant sustained VT or VF induced at electrophysiologic study. *(Level of Evidence: B)*
4. ICD therapy is indicated in patients with left ventricular ejection fraction (LVEF) less than 35% due to prior myocardial infarction (MI) who are at least 40 days post MI and are in New York Heart Association (NYHA) functional class II or III. *(Level of Evidence: A)*
5. ICD therapy is indicated in patients with nonischemic dilated cardiomyopathy (DCM) who have an LVEF less than or equal to 35% and who are in NYHA functional class II or III. *(Level of Evidence: B)*
6. ICD therapy is indicated in patients with LV dysfunction due to prior MI who are at least 40 days post MI, have an LVEF less than 30%, and are in NYHA functional class I. *(Level of Evidence: A)*
7. ICD therapy is indicated in patients with nonsustained VT due to prior MI, LVEF less than 40%, and inducible VF or sustained VT at electrophysiologic study. *(Level of Evidence: B)*

CLASS IIA

1. ICD implantation is reasonable for patients with unexplained syncope, significant left ventricular (LV) dysfunction, and nonischemic DCM. *(Level of Evidence: C)*
2. ICD implantation is reasonable for patients with sustained VT and normal or near-normal ventricular function. *(Level of Evidence: C)*
3. ICD implantation is reasonable for patients with HCM who have one or more major risk factors for sudden cardiac death (SCD). *(Level of Evidence: C)*
4. ICD implantation is reasonable for the prevention of SCD in patients with arrhythmogenic right ventricular dysplasia/cardiomyopathy (ARVD/C) who have one or more risk factors for SCD. *(Level of Evidence: C)*
5. ICD implantation is reasonable to reduce SCD in patients with long-QT syndrome who are experiencing syncope and/or VT while receiving beta blockers. *(Level of Evidence: B)*
6. ICD implantation is reasonable for nonhospitalized patients awaiting transplantation. *(Level of Evidence: C)*
7. ICD implantation is reasonable for patients with Brugada syndrome who have had syncope. *(Level of Evidence: C)*
8. ICD implantation is reasonable for patients with Brugada syndrome who have documented VT that has not resulted in cardiac arrest. *(Level of Evidence: C)*
9. ICD implantation is reasonable for patients with catecholaminergic polymorphic VT who have syncope and/or documented sustained VT while receiving beta blocker. *(Level of Evidence: C)*
10. ICD implantation is reasonable for patients with cardiac sarcoidosis, giant cell myocarditis, or Chagas disease. *(Level of Evidence: C)*

CLASS IIB

1. ICD therapy may be considered in patients with nonischemic heart disease who have an LVEF of less than or equal to 35% and who are in NYHA functional class I. *(Level of Evidence: C)*
2. ICD therapy may be considered for patients with long-QT syndrome and risk factors for SCD. *(Level of Evidence: B)*
3. ICD therapy may be considered in patients with syncope and advanced structural heart disease in whom thorough invasive and noninvasive investigations have failed to define a cause. *(Level of Evidence: C)*
4. ICD therapy may be considered in patients with a familial cardiomyopathy associated with sudden death. *(Level of Evidence: C)*
5. ICD therapy may be considered in patients with LV noncompaction. *(Level of Evidence: C)*

CLASS III

1. ICD therapy is not indicated for patients who do not have a reasonable expectation of survival with an acceptable functional status for at least 1 year, even if they meet ICD implantation criteria specified in the class I, IIa, and IIb recommendations above. *(Level of Evidence: C)*
2. ICD therapy is not indicated for patients with incessant VT or VF. *(Level of Evidence: C)*
3. ICD therapy is not indicated in patients with significant psychiatric illnesses that may be aggravated by device implantation or that may preclude systematic follow-up. *(Level of Evidence: C)*
4. ICD therapy is not indicated for NYHA class IV patients with drug-refractory congestive heart failure who are not candidates for cardiac transplantation or CRT-D. *(Level of Evidence: C)*
5. ICD therapy is not indicated for syncope of undetermined cause in a patient without inducible ventricular tachyarrhythmias and without structural heart disease. *(Level of Evidence: C)*
6. ICD therapy is not indicated when VF or VT is amenable to surgical or catheter ablation (e.g., atrial arrhythmias associated with the Wolff-Parkinson-White syndrome, right ventricular (RV) or LV outflow tract VT, idiopathic VT, or fascicular VT in the absence of structural heart disease). *(Level of Evidence: C)*
7. ICD therapy is not indicated for patients with ventricular tachyarrhythmias due to a completely reversible disorder in the absence of structural heart disease (e.g., electrolyte imbalance, drugs, or trauma). *(Level of Evidence: B)*

From Epstein AE, DiMarco JP, Ellenbogen KA, et al: ACC/AHA/HRS 2008 Guidelines for device-based therapy of cardiac rhythm abnormalities: a report of the American College of Cardiology/American Heart Association Task Force on Practice Guidelines (Writing Committee to Revise the ACC/AHA/NASPE 2002 Guideline Update for Implantation of Cardiac Pacemakers and Antiarrhythmia Devices) developed in collaboration with the American Association for Thoracic Surgery and Society of Thoracic Surgeons. J Am Coll Cardiol 51:e1–e62, 2008.

BOX 85-14 Recommendations for Implantable Cardioverter-Defibrillators in Pediatric Patients and Patients with Congenital Heart Disease

Class I

1. Implantable cardioverter-defibrillator (ICD) implantation is indicated in the survivor of cardiac arrest after evaluation to define the cause of the event and to exclude any reversible causes. *(Level of Evidence: B)*
2. ICD implantation is indicated for patients with symptomatic sustained ventricular tachycardia (VT) in association with congenital heart disease who have undergone hemodynamic and electrophysiologic evaluation. Catheter ablation or surgical repair may offer possible alternatives in carefully selected patients. *(Level of Evidence: C)*

Class IIa

1. ICD implantation is reasonable for patients with congenital heart disease with recurrent syncope of undetermined origin in the presence of either ventricular dysfunction or inducible ventricular arrhythmias at electrophysiologic study. *(Level of Evidence: B)*

Class IIb

1. ICD implantation may be considered for patients with recurrent syncope associated with complex congenital heart disease and advanced systemic ventricular dysfunction when thorough invasive and noninvasive investigations have failed to define a cause. *(Level of Evidence: C)*

Class III

1. All class III recommendations found in Section 3, "Indications for Implantable Cardioverter-Defibrillator Therapy," apply to pediatric patients and patients with congenital heart disease, and ICD implantation is not indicated in these patient populations. *(Level of Evidence: C)*

From Epstein AE, DiMarco JP, Ellenbogen KA, et al: ACC/AHA/HRS 2008 Guidelines for device-based therapy of cardiac rhythm abnormalities: a report of the American College of Cardiology/American Heart Association Task Force on Practice Guidelines (Writing Committee to Revise the ACC/AHA/NASPE 2002 Guideline Update for Implantation of Cardiac Pacemakers and Antiarrhythmia Devices) developed in collaboration with the American Association for Thoracic Surgery and Society of Thoracic Surgeons. J Am Coll Cardiol 51:e1–e62, 2008.

recommended for patients who have a terminal illness and whose life expectancy with an acceptable functional status is less than 12 months.[14] Patients who have severe psychiatric disorders whose illness may be exacerbated by ICD shocks or whose illness may preclude proper ICD follow-up may not be appropriate candidates for ICD implantation. In addition, incessant VT/VF that is refractory to medications is also considered a contraindication to ICD implantation until the arrhythmia is controlled by surgical or catheter ablation.

Similar to implantation of permanent pacemakers, ICD implantation is not recommended in patients with active ongoing infection. Patients with infectious issues who have an indication for ICD therapy can undergo telemetry monitoring in an acute care or rehabilitation facility until their infection is cleared. Alternatively, a wearable external automated defibrillator is now available for patients who are at high risk for sudden cardiac death as a bridge to permanent ICD therapy. This product is manufactured by ZOLL Medical Corporation (Pittsburgh, PA) and was approved by the FDA in 2002.

BASIC CONCEPTS OF PACING AND ANTITACHYCARDIA THERAPY

Permanent Pacemakers

Pulse Generator

Despite the many variations and designs of modern pacemakers, basic components are similar and include power source (battery), circuitry (output, sensing, telemetry, microprocessor, and memory), metal shell (can), ceramic feedthrough (a piece of wire surrounded by glass or sapphire) to provide an electric connection through the can, outlets through which pacing leads are connected to the header of the pacemaker, and sensors.[20] Most pacemaker batteries since 1975 are lithium iodide based. Lithium-based batteries have an ideal energy density that has allowed newer pacemakers to be of small volume yet to possess longer battery life. In addition, as opposed to the original mercury-zinc cells, which develop a sudden decrease in voltage shortly before battery depletion, lithium iodide cells have a predictable and gradual decrease in battery voltage as they approach depletion.[19]

At the beginning of life, the lithium iodide battery has a voltage output of approximately 2.8 V. The initial decay is slow until the battery approaches depletion, at which time the battery voltage decays more rapidly. When the battery voltage reaches 2.0 to 2.4 V, the elective replacement indicator is triggered, which may precipitate a change in pacing mode (such as dual-chamber to single-chamber pacing), rate response to nonrate response, or a change in magnet rate behavior.[20] Once the elective replacement indicator is triggered, the device has approximately 3 to 6 months before it reaches its end of useful life.

The pulse generator is connected with up to three pacing leads and subsequently implanted into a subcutaneous or submuscular pocket (see implantation techniques). The leads are placed under fluoroscopic guidance at standard right atrial, right ventricular, or in the coronary sinus (for left ventricular pacing) locations. The generator is programmed to sense and pace according to a chosen mode that addresses the individual patient's needs.

Pacemaker Leads

Pacing leads are the direct connection between the pulse generator and the myocardium. The distal end of pacing leads consists of one or two exposed metal electrodes that are linked to the pulse generator by insulated wires.

Leads may be unipolar or bipolar; these distinctions apply to both sensing and pacing functions. Unipolar leads have a single electrode incorporated into the lead (typically the cathode) and the other electrode (typically the anode) incorporated into the generator. Bipolar leads have both electrodes (the anode and the cathode) incorporated into the distal end of the lead. The difference in electrical potential sensed or created (to produce a pacing stimulus) by a bipolar lead occurs over a few millimeters; the difference in a unipolar lead spans the distance between the tip of the lead and the pulse generator across the chest. Bipolar leads possess significant advantages over their unipolar counterparts: no sensing of musculoskeletal potentials that may inappropriately inhibit pacing, less chance of "cross-talk" between the two leads of dual-chamber devices, less chance of interference with an ICD (ICDs should not be used in conjunction with unipolar leads), and less chance of pacing skeletal muscle. In addition, most generators are compatible with unipolar pacing through a bipolar lead if needed as a result of lead damage or high pacing thresholds.

Leads have fixation mechanisms that may be passive (e.g., tines, talons, and fins) or active (e.g., helical screws), both of which are depicted in Figure 85-4. Passive-fixation leads acquire stability by becoming entrapped in myocardial trabeculations. Active-fixation leads have distal screws that are deployed and penetrate the myocardial wall. Active mechanisms carry a lower risk of dislodgement and provide greater versatility in the choice of implantation sites, because their stability does not depend on the presence of trabeculations. However, active-fixation leads generate a more extensive inflammatory response, which may lead to acute rises in pacing threshold after implantation. Steroid-eluting leads are now available to address the problem of acute rise in capture threshold. Such leads have a reservoir of steroid near the electrode that flows through the porous electrode into the myocardium, thereby reducing the inflammatory response and the rise in pacing threshold.[20-22]

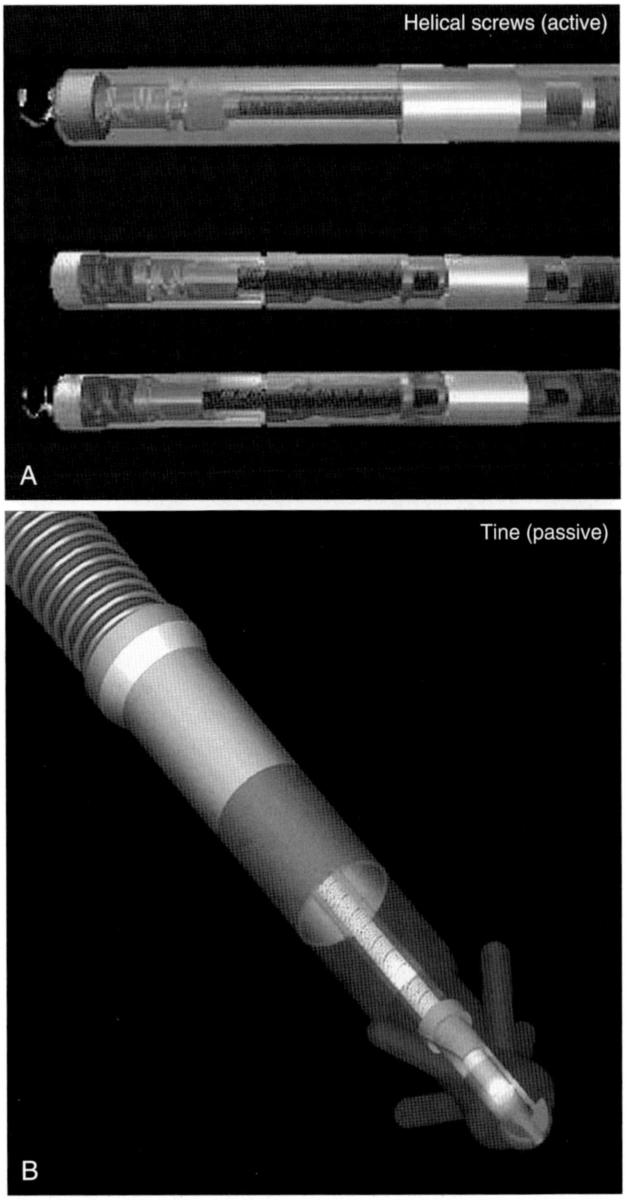

FIGURE 85-4 ■ Fixation mechanisms of pacing leads. **A,** Active fixation (screw) mechanism. **B,** Passive fixation (tines) mechanism. (Courtesy Medtronic, Inc., Minneapolis, MN.)

Pacing

Effective cardiac pacing requires the timed introduction of an electrical impulse, which depolarizes nearby myocardium, leading to propagation of an activation wave front. The term *capture* is used to indicate that successful pacing has occurred.[16] The minimum amount of energy required to produce successful myocardial depolarization and pacing is called the stimulation (or pacing) threshold. The pacing energy threshold is a function of the voltage (denoted in volts) delivered by each electrical impulse and the time duration over which the impulse is delivered (pulse width, denoted in milliseconds). For chronic pacing leads, pacing output is conventionally programmed at twofold the value of the pacing threshold voltage or threefold pacing threshold pulse width, considered the safety margin.

Sensing

Sensing is required for the pacemaker to coordinate pacing with any intrinsic electrical cardiac activity. The earliest pacemakers were not able to sense and paced only in VOO mode (see "Basic Pacing Modes," later). Pacing leads have a recording electrode and an indifferent electrode. As a wave of depolarization approaches the recording electrode and then proceeds away from it, it creates what is called an intrinsic deflection, which is the transition from the approaching to the receding deflection. The slope of the intrinsic deflection is called the slew rate. The pacemaker system has an amplifier that increases the signal from the recording electrode and a band pass filter to delete signals with frequencies too high or too low to represent an intrinsic deflection. The electrogram is "sensed" when the amplitude of the filtered signal exceeds the programmed sensing threshold. When sensing occurs, the programmed timing circuits of the pulse generator are reset. In general, a twofold to threefold sensing safety margin is also incorporated in the pacemaker programming. This allows for reliable sensing of activated myocardium but reduces the incidence of far-field oversensing.

Note that pacing intervals and cycle lengths are expressed in milliseconds, and pacing rates are denoted in beats per minute or pulses per minute. Rate and cycle lengths are inversely related and easily converted into one another: rate in beats per minute (or pulses per minute) may be obtained by dividing 60,000 by the cycle length in milliseconds; conversely, cycle length in milliseconds may be determined by dividing 60,000 by the rate in beats per minute (or pulses per minute).

Basic Pacing Modes

A generic pacemaker code allows the uniform functional classification of all pacing systems.

The first three letters are the most widely used and refer to the pacing and sensing functions of the pacemaker.[24] The first position denotes the cardiac chambers that may be *paced*, that is, the atrium (A), ventricle (V), both (D), or none (O). The second position refers to the chambers being *sensed*. The third position is used to indicate the *response the pacemaker has to sensing*, or the action performed by the pacemaker in response to sensing of intrinsic electrical activity. The response to sensing events by the pacemaker may be triggered (T), inhibited (I), both (D), or none (O). In a triggered mode, a sensed event leads to delivery of a pacing stimulus. The triggered mode is used to prevent inappropriate inhibition by an incorrectly sensed event, such as skeletal muscle myopotentials. This function can be lifesaving in patients who are pacemaker dependent. The inhibited mode leads to inhibition of stimulus delivery in the designated chamber after sensing of intrinsic electrical activity. When the sensing response is dual (i.e., triggered and inhibited), pacing in the ventricle or atrium does not occur for a programmable time after intrinsic ventricular activity is sensed (i.e., pacing is inhibited). In addition, when the sensing response is dual, sensing of intrinsic atrial activity leads to inhibition of an atrial pacing stimulus, but it results in triggering of a ventricular pacing stimulus after the programmed AV delay.

The fourth position of the generic pacemaker code denotes the *programmability or rate modulation*. The possible functions at this position include simple programmable (P), multiprogrammable (M), communicating (C), rate modulation (R), or none (O).[24] Simple programmable suggests that the programmability of the pacemaker is limited to certain parameters; multiprogrammable pacemakers are able to program a large number of parameters. The communicating function refers to the ability to exchange signals between the pacemaker and a pacemaker programming device. Rate modulation is the most commonly denoted function in the fourth position. It denotes the capability of the pacemaker to adjust the pacing rate according to a sensor device. Pacemaker manufacturers have designed a variety of sensors that attempt to match the individual's physical activity or metabolic demands by responding to different sources, such as motion, temperature, and chest wall impedance (as an estimate of minute ventilation).

The fifth position in the pacemaker code relates to *antitachycardia therapies:* antitachycardia pacing (P), shock (S), dual (D, shock and pacing), or none (O).[23] Since the advent of ICDs, the fifth position is not generally used in referring to pacing systems.

As a result of emerging data that suggest an increased risk of heart failure hospitalization in patients with high burden of right ventricular pacing, algorithms designed to minimize right ventricular pacing have recently become available in pacemakers and defibrillators.[24-26] Such algorithms provide pacing in AAI mode but will mode switch to DDD whenever necessary if high-grade AV block occurs. If the AV block is transient, the pacing mode will switch back to AAI. Table 85-2 summarizes the most commonly used pacing modes, including advantages and disadvantages of each one as well as their clinical applications.[23] See Figure 85-5 for an example of DDD pacing mode on a 12-lead electrocardiogram.

Implantable Cardioverter-Defibrillators

The guidelines for implantation of ICDs are reviewed earlier in this chapter. Despite the ongoing advancement in the development of today's defibrillators, their primary

TABLE 85-2 **Commonly Encountered Pacing Modes**

Mode	Advantages	Disadvantages	Clinical Uses
AAI(R)	Requires only a single lead Simple	Slow ventricular rates may develop if atrioventricular (AV) block occurs	Sinus node dysfunction without AV node dysfunction
VVI(R)	Requires only a single lead Simple	During pacing, AV synchrony is not preserved	AV block in a patient with atrial fibrillation
DDD(R)	AV synchrony is maintained for patients with sinus node and AV node disease	Requires two leads More complex	Bradycardia caused by sinus node disease or AV node disease
VDD(R)	AV synchrony is maintained for patients with AV node disease One specially designed lead can be used	AV synchrony is lost if the patient develops sinus bradycardia	Bradycardia caused by AV node disease
DDI(R)	AV synchrony is maintained during atrial pacing	AV synchrony is not maintained during atrial sensing	For patients with bradycardia and intermittent atrial tachycardias Not used as a stand-alone pacing mode but as a mode-switching pacing mode

From Wang PJ, et al: Modes of pacemaker function. In Kusumoto FM, Goldschlager NF, editors: Cardiac pacing for the clinician, Philadelphia, 2001, Lippincott Williams & Wilkins, pp 63–90.

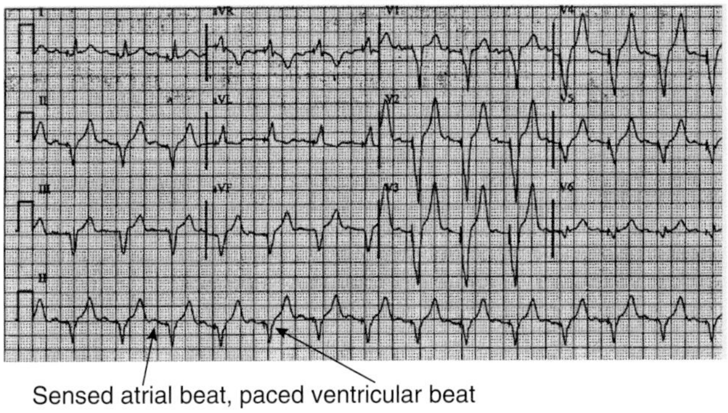

FIGURE 85-5 ■ Example of DDD pacing mode on a 12-lead electrocardiogram.

goal remains to deliver rapid and effective treatment of ventricular tachyarrhythmias.

Pulse Generator

Most ICD generators are currently implanted in the pectoral region. The pulse generator is composed of a lithium/silver vanadium oxide battery and a capacitor. Whereas in 1989, generator volumes exceeded 200 cm^3, current generators are less than 40 cm^3.[27] Progressively smaller ICD generators have become viable as a result of continued progress in battery and capacitor technology. Essential functions that must be reliably performed by the ICD generator include monitoring of cardiac electrical activity through sense amplifiers, analysis of waveforms for the proper diagnosis of arrhythmias, and delivery of appropriate therapy. The lifetime of the battery depends on the battery capacity, and it is inversely related to the number of shocks and to the percentage of time spent in monitoring and pacing.

In addition to the battery and capacitor, the generator houses the operational circuitry of the device, which is composed of low-power circuits (sensing, pacing, amplifiers, microprocessors) and high-power charging and output circuits.[27]

Leads

Early defibrillators used high-voltage epicardial (or pericardial) electrode patches for defibrillation. These electrode patches were also responsible for sensing, but frequent problems caused by oversensing prompted the use of a separate sensing lead (epicardial or endocardial). With the development of transvenous defibrillators, electrode patches are now only rarely used.

Currently used endocardial leads are made of high-voltage conductors. At least one conductor is used as the defibrillation coil, which is generally found near the tip of the lead and placed along the posterior right ventricular wall. Some leads have two conductors (or two shocking coils). In such dual-coil leads, the distal coil is in the right ventricle and the proximal coil resides anywhere between the subclavian vein, superior vena cava, and right atrium. Separate single-coil leads may instead be implanted in the right ventricle, superior vena cava, coronary sinus, or a combination of these sites; subcutaneous tissue arrays may also be used. Leads placed in the right ventricle are required to exhibit sensing and pacing capabilities, whereas such functions are not necessary in leads placed in the superior vena cava or coronary sinus.

In general, defibrillation with use of the pulse generator as one of the electrodes can be achieved by lower energies than defibrillation with a combination of leads. The defibrillation threshold (DFT) is the "lowest clinically obtained energy that can achieve defibrillation."[16] A combination of any three electrodes may be used, instead of two, in an attempt to lower the DFT.

Endocardial ICD leads perform sensing through a distal electrode at the tip of the lead. The same electrode may also be used for pacing. Unipolar ICD leads (normally placed in the superior vena cava or coronary sinus) have a single high-voltage coil used for defibrillation and are not able to pace or sense. Bipolar ICD leads have two conductors, one of which is used for defibrillation and the other for sensing. Such leads sense intrinsic electrical activity between the tip of the lead and anywhere along the extent of the shocking coil (integrated bipolar sensing). In contrast to true bipolar sensing, integrated bipolar sensing more often leads to oversensing because of noise and far-field artifact as well as to undersensing after high-voltage defibrillation.[27] Newer defibrillator leads perform true bipolar sensing between the distal tip of the lead and a ring located approximately 1 cm proximal from the tip. Most recently, "quadripolar" leads are now available that perform true bipolar sensing (between the tip of the lead and the ring, as described earlier) and also incorporate two defibrillation coils. In the subcutaneous ICD system, a subcutaneous electrode with a defibrillation coil is tunneled in the skin parallel to the left sternum.

Tachyarrhythmia Detection

Detection of tachyarrhythmias occurs when the device analyzes recent cycle lengths and R-wave morphologies to classify rhythms and to determine appropriate programmed therapy.[27] Because some arrhythmias are unsustained, ICDs must effectively be able to detect the arrhythmia, confirm it before delivering therapy, and redetect the arrhythmia if the delivered therapy was unsuccessful. Current devices may be set to have multiple zones of detection (e.g., VT, fast VT, and VF zones) for which specific therapies can be individually programmed (tiered therapy).

Although arrhythmia detection by current ICDs is reliable, inappropriate shocks may still occur even if the device is functioning properly. Such unnecessary shocks most commonly occur in the setting of atrial fibrillation (or other supraventricular tachycardia) or sinus tachycardia if the ventricular rate falls into one of the detection zones.[28] Newer and more sophisticated devices have built-in algorithms or additional detection parameters designed to prevent inappropriate shocks by increasing the specificity of VT detection. For safety reasons, these algorithms are available only in the lowest VT rate cutoff zones and include sudden onset and rate stability criteria as well as a criterion based on electrogram morphology.

Tachyarrhythmia Therapy

Current devices can deliver a range of programmable therapies: high-energy defibrillation shocks, low-energy synchronized cardioversion, and antitachycardia pacing (ATP).

High-Energy Defibrillation. As previously described, the DFT is the lowest clinically obtained energy that can accomplish defibrillation. The patient's autonomic and metabolic state may alter the DFT such that an energy output previously able to achieve defibrillation at a particular time may fail at others. Therefore, after the DFT is determined, a safety margin of at least 7 to 10 J is recommended between the maximum output of the device and the DFT. Figure 85-6 depicts an episode of successful defibrillation of VF by a high-energy therapy delivered by an ICD.

Antiarrhythmic drugs may alter the DFT. Amiodarone commonly raises the DFT, whereas sotalol lowers it.[29,30] Procainamide and quinidine do not appear to affect DFT.[31] Physicians can consider DFT testing 3 months after initiation of amiodarone to confirm an acceptable safety margin between the DFT and the programmed high-energy defibrillation output.

Low-Energy Synchronized Cardioversions. Low-energy synchronized cardioversions can be delivered faster (shorter charging time) than high-energy defibrillation and may save device battery. Unlike VF, some VT can be terminated with very low energy therapies, which may cause less discomfort to the patient. Disadvantages of low-energy synchronized shocks include acceleration of VT to VF, which may delay definitive therapy.

Antitachycardia Pacing. Multiple extra stimuli (with or without addition of premature stimuli to a train of extra stimuli) delivered during tachycardia may interact with the tachycardia circuit and thereby terminate it. ATP can be programmed in today's ICDs, and it is widely used as initial therapy for VT. Similar to low-energy synchronized cardioversions, ATP carries the risk of accelerating VT to VF, in which case a high-voltage shock could be delivered to terminate VF. Advantages of ATP as initial therapy for VT include faster delivery time, less discomfort to the patient, and sparing of device battery (if successful). Figure 85-7 shows an example of successful termination of VT by ATP; Figure 85-8 depicts a failed ATP attempt to terminate VT.

PREOPERATIVE EVALUATION BEFORE IMPLANTATION OF CARDIAC DEVICES

Clinical Considerations

A careful history and physical examination should be performed, with focus on the assessment of prior injury or disease within the planned region for device implantation. A history of prior shoulder or chest injury, surgery,

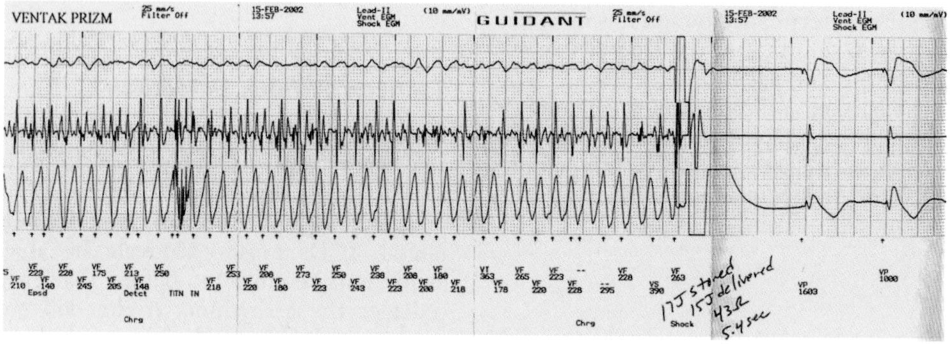

FIGURE 85-6 ■ High-energy defibrillation of ventricular fibrillation.

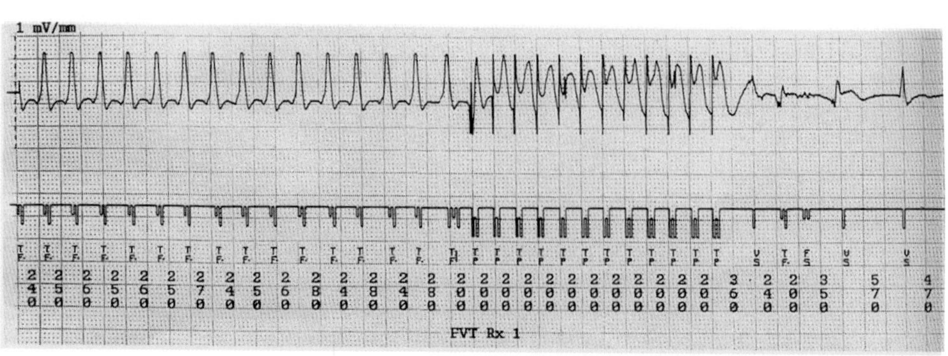

FIGURE 85-7 ■ Electrograms of antitachycardia pacing–induced termination of ventricular tachycardia stored by implantable cardioverter-defibrillator; 250 msec = 240 beats/min. *FVT,* Fast ventricular tachycardia.

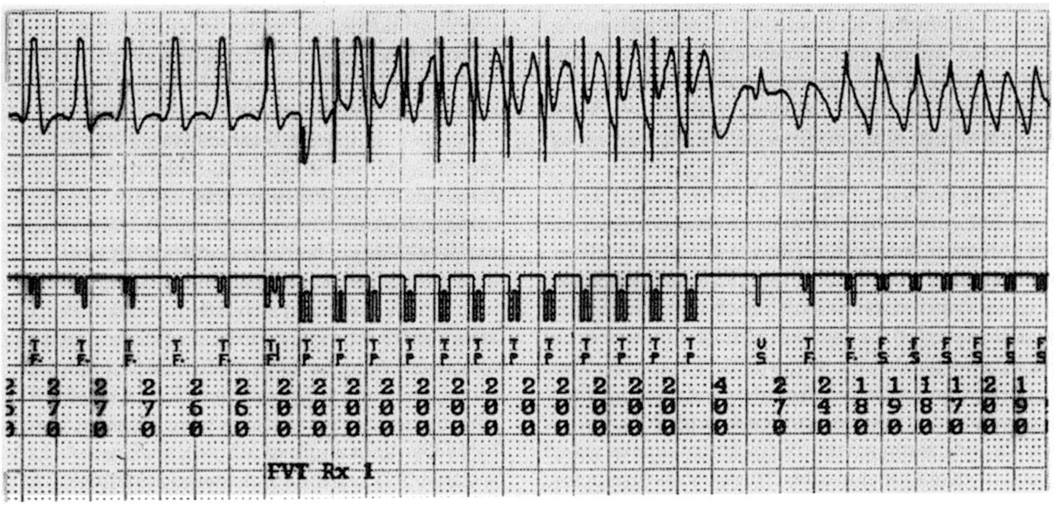

FIGURE 85-8 Failed attempt by antitachycardia pacing to terminate ventricular tachycardia. *FVT,* Fast ventricular tachycardia.

or radiation therapy may alert the implanting physician of the potential for abnormal venous drainage, which may increase the technical complexity of the implantation. Allergies to medications (including antibiotics, local anesthetic, and intravenous narcotics and benzodiazepines used for conscious sedation) and intravenous contrast material occasionally used for venography should be identified and recorded. It is especially important to recognize and appropriately treat signs and symptoms of active infection before implantation of a permanent cardiac device. Prophylactic antibiotics are administered immediately before and for 72 hours after device implantation. Another essential consideration is the patient's respiratory status. Device implantations generally require that the patient lie flat for the duration of the procedure (up to 2 to 3 hours). Therefore, oxygenation and volume status should be optimized before implantation.

Patients being treated with warfarin or any of the novel oral anticoagulants may remain on anticoagulation therapy during their device implantation. In our institution, it is generally required that the International Normalized Ratio (INR) be less than 3.5 before implantation. We avoid the use of injectable low-molecular-weight heparin or unfractionated heparin bridging around the time of device implantation, because we believe this is associated with greater rates of pocket hematomas.

STANDARD TRANSVENOUS TECHNIQUES FOR IMPLANTATION OF CARDIAC DEVICES

Temporary Transvenous Pacemakers

Percutaneous venous access may be obtained through the internal jugular, subclavian, femoral, or antecubital veins. A lock-down sheath should be introduced in the vein for better lead stability. Fluoroscopy should always be used to guide lead placement when the femoral and antecubital veins are used. The pacing catheter should be advanced to the right ventricle with care to avoid excessive force that could result in cardiac perforation. The ideal position for the catheter tip is the distal right ventricular septum or inferoapex. The right ventricular free wall and outflow tract should be avoided because of the risk of catheter-induced ectopy and decreased lead stability. After placement of the lead, the sensing and pacing thresholds should be determined. An R wave of 5 mV or more and a pacing threshold of 1 mA or less are adequate. After acceptable placement of the lead has occurred, the sheath should be locked down around the lead. The sheath should then be sutured and the lead secured to the adjacent skin and covered with a dry sterile dressing. A postprocedure chest radiograph should be obtained to confirm lead position and to rule out pneumothorax. At least twice daily, sensing and pacing thresholds should be assessed.

If fluoroscopy is not available, a balloon-tipped catheter should be introduced through the internal jugular or subclavian veins. The distal electrode tip (generally negatively charged) should be connected to one of the precordial leads of a 12-lead electrocardiogram (generally V_1). The limb leads (e.g., lead II) should be recorded and the intracardiac electrogram should be monitored as the balloon-tipped pacing catheter is slowly introduced. When the distal electrode on the tip of the catheter reaches the right atrium, a large atrial electrogram (corresponding to the P wave seen on the limb leads) followed by a smaller ventricular electrogram (corresponding to the QRS on the surface electrocardiogram) should be noted. As the catheter is advanced into the right ventricle, the ventricular electrogram grows larger and the atrial signal becomes smaller. Once the tip of the pacing catheter comes in contact with the myocardium, an injury current (reminiscent of ST elevation) will be recorded immediately after the ventricular electrogram, and the catheter should not be advanced farther. After the pacing catheter is positioned and secured, a 12-lead electrocardiogram should always be obtained to corroborate, on the basis of the morphology of the paced QRS complexes, proper positioning of the catheter.

When asystole (or severe bradycardia) is present, the pacing electrode tips (distal and proximal) should be connected to an active pacing box (or generator) programmed to pace in VVI mode. Paced QRS complexes should emerge once contact of the catheter tip to myocardium occurs.

When temporary atrial (instead of ventricular) or AV sequential pacing is required, a temporary pacing catheter/lead can be placed in the right atrium (active-fixation lead) or in the coronary sinus. The atrial pacing threshold is generally higher in the coronary sinus than in the right atrium.

Duration of temporary pacing should be limited to less than 72 hours to minimize the risk of infection, cardiac perforation, and lead dislodgement. Active-fixation leads connected to an externalized pacemaker generator may be left in place for longer periods.

Permanent Pacemakers

Most permanent transvenous pacemakers are placed in the right or left pectoral region through the cephalic, axillary, or subclavian veins. A peripheral intravenous catheter should be placed on the upper extremity ipsilateral to the planned implant in case venography is necessary to define the anatomy or availability of access. Unless the patient is left-handed or the left side is inaccessible, the left pectoral region is preferable because of greater simplicity of lead placement and manipulation. Prophylactic antibiotics should be administered as described earlier, and the pectoral region should be prepared and draped in sterile fashion.

Cephalic Vein (Cutdown) Approach

Local anesthetic is delivered to the pectoral region. An oblique incision is made over the deltopectoral groove and extended inward by use of blunt dissection. Alternatively, a horizontal incision 2 cm below the clavicle (with its lateral border extending over the deltopectoral groove) may be chosen. The cephalic vein runs in the deltopectoral groove, which can be identified by the presence of a fatty streak between the pectoralis and deltoid muscles. Once the cephalic vein is identified, it should be dissected free from the surrounding fat and connective tissue. Figure 85-9 illustrates the anatomic location of the subclavian, axillary, and cephalic veins.

A 0 silk suture is placed around the vein (but not tied) proximally and another one distally, and a 5 French (Fr) dilator is placed in the vein. Under fluoroscopic guidance, a guidewire is introduced into the 5 Fr dilator and advanced to the inferior vena cava through the subclavian vein, the superior vena cava, the right atrium, and into the inferior vena cava; the 5 Fr dilator is then removed. Venography may be necessary through the 5 Fr introducer or a peripheral line to establish patency of the vessels or to define the venous anatomy if difficulty in advancing the wire is encountered.

Axillary Vein Approach

The axillary vein can be cannulated through the same cutdown location in the deltopectoral region. The axillary vein is accessed through a single wall puncture technique by landmarks or direct visualization through venography.

Subclavian Vein Approach

The subclavian vein may also be accessed by a single wall puncture technique. The subclavian vein approach is generally the least desirable because of the risk of pneumothorax and the potential risk of crush injury to the pacing leads as they pass between the clavicle and first rib.

Technique

Regardless of the vein used for access, a guidewire is advanced to the inferior vena cava under fluoroscopic

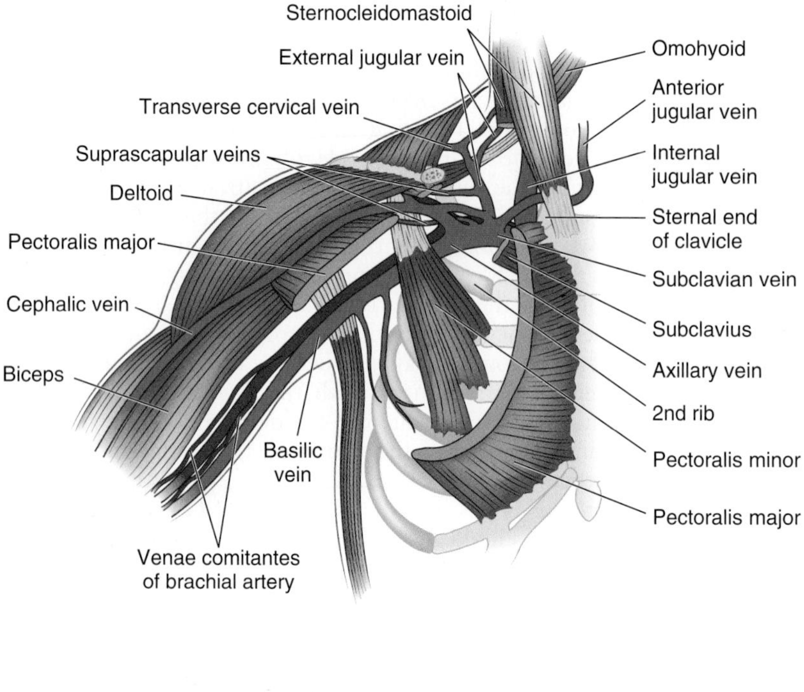

FIGURE 85-9 ■ Anatomic illustration of the subclavian, axillary, and cephalic veins. (Modified from Agur AMR, Lee MJ: Upper limb. In *Grant's atlas of anatomy,* ed 10, Philadelphia, 1999, Lippincott Williams & Wilkins.)

guidance. Once venous access has been secured and the guidewire positioned, sheaths (or introducers) are used for sequential placement of atrial and ventricular leads. While a lead is being placed through the sheath, the patient should be instructed to transiently refrain from talking or breathing to avoid complication by air embolus through the introducer sheath. The fluoroscopic view for optimal placement of the right ventricle lead is generally obtained from the right anterior oblique position. This view allows proper visualization of the full length of the right ventricle (foreshortened in the anteroposterior view). Adequate lead position along the right ventricular inferoseptum and apex should also be confirmed in the left anterior oblique view. Ventricular ectopy may occur during lead placement, but it is generally transient. If there is persistent VT, the lead should be repositioned. If VT continues despite lead repositioning, the rhythm should be terminated by ATP or defibrillation.

Ventricular sensing and pacing thresholds should be checked, and the QRS morphology in lead V_1 should be assessed to confirm that pacing originates from the right ventricle (left bundle branch block morphology should be present in lead V_1). When a right bundle branch block morphology is present in lead V_1, pacing from the left ventricular endocardium (through an atrial or ventricular septal defect), from the coronary sinus, or from the left ventricular epicardium (as a result of cardiac perforation) should be suspected. On occasion, a right bundle branch block morphology will be seen with pacing from the right ventricular septum.

The atrial lead is generally placed in the right atrial appendage if it is present. Use of a curled wire stylet will enable positioning in the right atrial appendage. However, any location in the right atrium is acceptable if it is stable, provided no excessive sensing of the ventricular electrogram is present.

Once acceptable positions for both leads have been obtained, lead stability should be confirmed during coughing and deep breathing exercises. Lead locations should be confirmed from the right anterior oblique and left anterior oblique views. High-output pacing should be performed from both leads to rule out diaphragmatic capture during pacing. Stylets and guidewire should be removed, and proper amount of slack in each lead should be ensured fluoroscopically. After optimal lead positions are confirmed, the leads should be secured to the pectoralis muscle with nonabsorbable suture tied around anchoring sleeves. Final sensing and pacing thresholds should be checked after the leads have been sutured to the pectoralis fascia.

After the leads are secured, local anesthesia is administered to the subcutaneous tissues medial to the deltopectoral groove to create a subcutaneous (or submuscular) pocket for the device generator. The pocket is created by blunt dissection and copiously irrigated. The leads are then connected to the pulse generator according to the indicated positions. The leads are coiled under the generator, and the entire system is implanted into the pocket. Proper sensing and pacing by the device should be confirmed.

The subcutaneous tissues are closed with absorbable suture, and the skin is closed with a subcuticular layer of absorbable suture or staples. A dry sterile dressing should be placed over the wound.

Implantation of single-chamber devices is done by the same technique except for placement of the second lead. Figure 85-10 depicts a chest radiograph with the expected lead position for a single-chamber transvenous pacemaker.

As discussed previously, the biventricular pacing of both left and right ventricles is appropriate in a particular heart failure patient population. The left ventricle is paced through a passive pacing lead that is advanced through the coronary sinus into a posterolateral vein. If an implanting physician is unable to achieve an optimal location for coronary sinus pacing, an epicardial lead can be placed surgically.

Implantable Cardioverter-Defibrillators

Surgical techniques to implant epicardial patches used in early ICDs are not discussed in this chapter. Instead, this chapter concentrates on the transvenous implantation of current cardioverter-defibrillators.

The left pectoral region is preferred for most ICD implants, whether the patient is right- or left-handed. The coil configuration obtained with a left-sided implant allows a more effective field orientation for defibrillation, when one of the shocking electrodes lies within the pulse generator. The technique used to place modern transvenous ICDs is the same as the technique described to implant transvenous permanent pacemakers (see earlier), although the first transvenous ICDs required abdominal pulse generators because of their large size (transvenous leads were tunneled subcutaneously to the abdomen, where the generator was implanted). Also, subcutaneous patches or arrays were often necessary in early ICDs to achieve acceptable DFT. In Figure 85-11, a postprocedure chest radiograph confirms appropriate lead positions in a dual-chamber transvenous ICD.

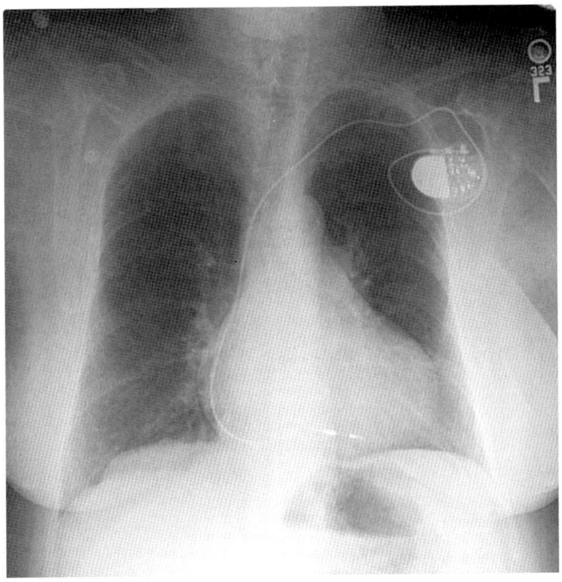

FIGURE 85-1 ■ Posteroanterior chest radiograph showing appropriate lead position for a single-chamber transvenous pacemaker.

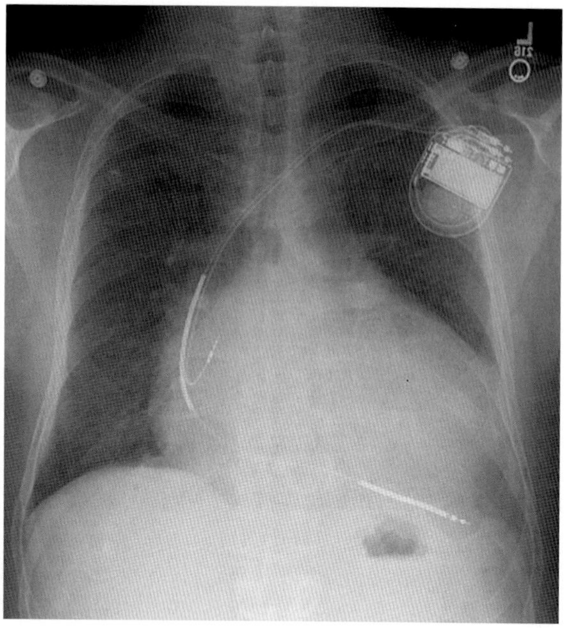

FIGURE 85-11 ■ Posteroanterior chest radiograph showing appropriate lead positions for a dual-chamber transvenous implantable cardioverter-defibrillator.

Recently, the use of a fully subcutaneous ICD has become an option in a selected patient population. In this system, the pulse generator is placed within a pocket created between the fourth and fifth intercostal spaces at the midaxillary line. An electrode is positioned through two subcutaneous tunnels, extending from the pocket to a small xiphoid incision and from the xiphoid to a superior sternal incision.

Defibrillation Threshold Testing

The procedure for any ICD implant can include defibrillation testing to determine the DFT. The prevailing rationale for the routine evaluation of DFTs has been to ensure appropriate sensing of ventricular fibrillation, system integrity, and effective defibrillation. Defibrillation testing is generally performed before wound closure, after the leads are connected to the pulse generator and after the system is implanted into the pocket.

The programmer is used to communicate with the device through a sterile wand placed over the pocket. Recently, wireless devices are available that can communicate with the programmer without physical contact once initial connection with the generator has been established. Before VF induction and ICD testing, some operators deliver a low-energy synchronized shock to allow confirmation of intact connections by checking the high-voltage lead impedance. External defibrillation hands-off pads are also placed and connected to an external biphasic defibrillator in the event of device failure to terminate VF. Testing is generally performed at the least sensitive device setting for detection of VF to ensure an adequate safety margin. After successful testing, the device is programmed at the most sensitive setting for VF detection. VF is most commonly induced by timed T-wave shocks or by rapid-burst ventricular pacing at 50 Hz.

At our institution, initial testing is performed with a selected energy (10 J lower than the maximum device output) that allows an adequate safety margin between the tested energy and the maximum device output (margin-verification protocol). A second shock with a lower energy is often performed. Before testing, we generally set the second device therapy as a maximum output shock, which is delivered if the first tested energy fails and after VF is redetected. If a high-output shock through the device fails to terminate VF, a 360-J biphasic shock is externally delivered.

Normally, a 5-minute "rest" period is provided between each induction of VF. Other important parameters evaluated during ICD testing include the high-voltage lead impedance and the charge time for delivery of high-voltage therapies. If an adequate DFT is not obtained during testing, addition of extra defibrillation coils (including subcutaneous arrays or patches), reversal of shock polarity, or repositioning of the right ventricle lead may be necessary. A 7- to 10-J safety margin should be incorporated in the final therapy programming of the device. After an acceptable DFT is obtained, the wound is closed as described previously.

Contemporary ICD systems using active cans, pectoralis pulse generators, biphasic waveforms, and intravascular high-voltage leads have considerably lowered the incidence of elevated DFTs. The reliability of current ICD systems has led to recent literature reevaluating the necessity for routine DFT testing at ICD implantation.[32-34] As such, observational studies have noted an elimination of DFT testing in one third of initial implants and two thirds of replacements. A study estimates that 5-year survival is expected to be higher in patients who undergo DFT testing at implantation only if the annual risk of a lethal arrhythmia (or the risk of a narrow safety margin) is at least 5%.[32] At our institution, we no longer perform routine DFT testing at the time of device implantation or generator change.

POSTIMPLANTATION CARE OF TRANSVENOUS CARDIAC DEVICES

Patients undergoing implantation of electrophysiologic cardiac devices should be observed overnight in the hospital. Continuous telemetry monitoring should be performed during this time to allow early diagnosis and treatment of lead malfunction or dislodgement (the most common complication in the early postoperative period). Bed rest is recommended overnight, and the arm ipsilateral to the implant is placed in a sling for 24 hours. The patient is allowed to move that arm after 24 hours, but lifting of objects weighing more than 5 to 10 pounds and raising the arm above shoulder level should be avoided for 6 weeks after the procedure. A posteroanterior and lateral chest radiograph should be obtained on the morning after implantation to assess adequate lead and generator positions. If the subclavian vein was used for venous access, a portable chest radiograph is required immediately after implantation to rule out pneumothorax. Anticoagulation with intravenous heparin or low-molecular-weight heparin should be avoided for at least the first 8 hours after implantation. We recommend the continuation of oral anticoagulation of patients through their device implantation if they are already on blood-thinning medication. The use of prophylactic antibiotics should be prescribed as described previously.

The device should be interrogated on the day after implantation to ensure proper device function and to fine-tune the device programming if necessary. The wound should be kept dry for at least 3 days after implantation. A follow-up appointment should be scheduled within 7 to 10 days of discharge for wound check and device reinterrogation. Marked changes in lead impedance and in pacing and sensing thresholds would be identified at that time and could indicate lead dislodgement or malfunction.

COMPLICATIONS OF IMPLANTABLE CARDIAC DEVICES

Serious complications of device implantation occur in less than 2% of patients undergoing the procedure. Procedural complications may be classified as early, which may include intraoperative, perioperative (within 24 hours), or postoperative complications (after 24 hours but within 30 days of the procedure), or late, occurring after 30 days from the procedure.

Examples of early complications are outlined in Box 85-15 and include bleeding, vascular injury, infection, pneumothorax, hemothorax, air embolus, cardiac perforation or tamponade, rhythm abnormalities, deep venous thrombosis, pulmonary embolism, lead dislodgement, lead fracture or damage, and pocket hematoma. Late complications are also listed in Box 85-15 and may include lead fracture or insulation break, lead dislodgement, pocket skin erosion, infection, migration of generator possibly leading to lead twisting and fracture, and deep venous thrombosis or scarring. Figure 85-12 shows an example of skin erosion with subsequent infection of a device pocket.

BOX 85-15 Early and Late Complications of Implantable Cardiac Devices

EARLY

- Bleeding
- Infection
- Pneumothorax, hemothorax
- Cardiac perforation
- Superior vena cava perforation
- Lead migration or dislodgement (2%)
- Air embolus
- Venous thrombosis
- Atrial tachyarrhythmias
- Ventricular tachycardia
- Atrioventricular (AV) block by contact injury to the conduction system
- Pocket hematoma

LATE

- Infection of device pocket or leads (2.7%)
- Pocket erosion, wound breakdown
- Lead fracture, insulation damage (0.2%)
- Venous thrombosis
- Chronic pain
- Tricuspid regurgitation
- Left ventricular dysfunction
- Migration of pulse generator
- Twisting or fracture of leads due to manipulation of generator (twiddler syndrome)

EXTRACTION OF CHRONIC LEADS USED IN TRANSVENOUS CARDIAC DEVICES

Overview

Since the introduction of transvenous pacing electrodes in 1958 by Furman and Schwedel,[3] techniques to safely remove such leads have been developed and perfected. Earlier techniques focused on the simple use of traction, which can be done safely and without the assistance of specially designed tools only in recently implanted leads (generally, implants less than 1 year old) that have not developed significant fibrosis. For more chronic leads, complications preclude the use of simple traction, and surgical approaches that require sternotomy or thoracotomy were initially the only viable options. Since the mid-1980s,[35-38] safer transvenous methods for chronic lead extraction have been developed.

Official definitions and guidelines for the practice of transvenously placed lead extractions were published in 2000, and subsequently updated in 2009.[39,40] The term *lead extraction* is reserved only for the removal of a lead that requires specialized equipment (laser sheath, traction devices, electrosurgical sheaths, rotational threaded tip sheaths, or telescoping sheaths) or from a route other than the implant vein and of any lead implanted for more than 1 year. A complete summary of indications for lead extraction is provided in Box 85-16. Class I indications include serious illness caused by an infected lead, clinical need for a new transvenous cardiac device when all usable veins are obstructed, and malfunctioning, fractured, or

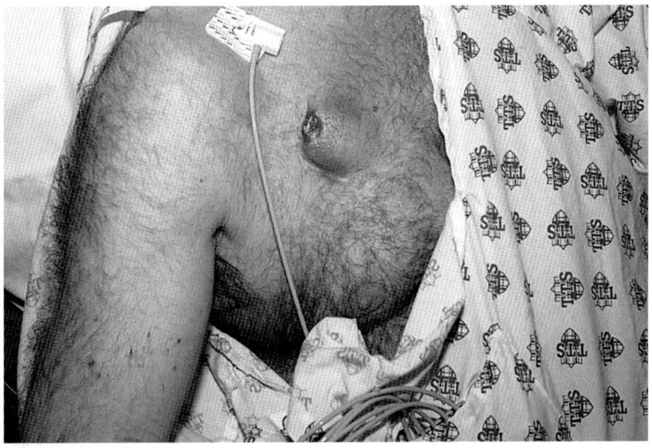

FIGURE 85-12 ■ Example of skin erosion and subsequent infection of device pocket. (Courtesy Medtronic, Inc., Minneapolis, MN.)

BOX 85-16 Indications for Lead Removal/Extraction by Transvenous Techniques

INFECTION

Class I

1. Definite system infection, as evidenced by valvular endocarditis, lead endocarditis, or sepsis
2. Pocket infection as evidenced by pocket abscess, device erosion, skin adherence, or chronic draining sinus
3. Valvular endocarditis without definite involvement of the lead(s) and/or device
4. Occult gram-p2ositive bacteremia (not contaminant)

Class IIa

1. Persistent occult gram-negative bacteremia

Class III

1. Not indicated for a superficial or incisional infection without involvement of the device and/or leads
2. Not indicated to treat chronic bacteremia due to a source other than the cardiovascular implantable electronic device (CIED), when long-term suppressive antibiotics are required

CHRONIC PAIN

Class IIa

1. Severe chronic pain, at the device or lead insertion site, that causes significant discomfort for the patient

THROMBOSIS AND VENOUS STENOSIS

Class I

1. Significant thromboembolic events associated with thrombus on a lead or a lead fragment
2. Bilateral subclavian vein or superior vena cava (SVC) occlusion precluding implantation of a needed transvenous lead
3. SVC stenosis or occlusion with limiting symptoms
4. Ipsilateral venous occlusion preventing access to the venous circulation for required placement of an additional lead when there is a contraindication for using the contralateral side (e.g., contralateral AV fistula, shunt or vascular access port, mastectomy)

Class IIa

1. Ipsilateral venous occlusion preventing access to the venous circulation for required placement of an additional lead, when there is no contraindication for using the contralateral side

FUNCTIONAL AND NONFUNCTIONAL LEADS

Class I

1. Life-threatening arrhythmias secondary to retained leads
2. Lead design failure that poses an immediate threat to the patient if left in place
3. Leads that interfere with the treatment of a malignancy (radiation/reconstructive surgery)

Class IIa

1. Nonfunctional leads that due to design failure pose a threat to the patient that is not immediate or imminent if left in place
2. Nonfunctional lead removal to avoid more than four leads on one side or more than five leads through the SVC
3. Nonfunctional lead removal is reasonable in patients that require specific needed imaging techniques and cannot be imaged due to the presence of the device

Class IIb

1. Functioning leads that due to design failure pose a potential future threat to the patient if left in place
2. Functional leads not being used
3. To permit the implantation of a magnetic resonance imaging (MRI)–compatible system
4. At the time of an indicated device implantation in patients with nonfunctional leads

Class III

1. Not indicated if patient has a life expectancy of less than 1 year
2. Not indicated in patients with known anomalous placement of leads through structures other than normal venous and cardiac structures unless clinical situation compelling

From Love CJ, Wilkoff BL, Byrd CL, et al: Recommendations for extraction of chronically implanted transvenous pacing and defibrillator leads: indications, facilities, training. North American Society of Pacing and Electrophysiology Lead Extraction Conference Faculty. Pacing Clin Electrophysiol 23(4 Pt 1):544–551, 2000.

suboptimally positioned leads that pose danger to the patient. Relative contraindications to transvenous lead extraction include lead calcification (detected on radiography) involving the right atrium or the superior vena cava, unavailability of suitable equipment, patient's clinical condition that precludes emergent thoracotomy or less than 1 year survival, or lead placement through unusual routes (e.g., subclavian artery, pericardial space). Because of the potentially serious complications of transvenous lead extractions, physicians properly trained in these techniques and adequately equipped institutions are absolute requirements for the performance of lead extractions.

Data from the U.S. Extraction Database for intravascular extraction of infected or problematic pacemaker leads from January 1994 to April 1996 were published in 1999.[41] In this series, the success rate was 93% for complete removal of the leads and 5% for partial removal of the leads; 2% failed. Major complications occurred in 1.4% of patients (<1% in centers that performed >300 extractions) and minor complications in 1.7% of patients. Major complications occurred more frequently in women. Predictors of incomplete lead removal or failure included longer implant duration, less experienced operators, ventricular lead location, noninfected leads, and younger age of the patient. Reports using the more modern laser lead extraction technique involving 2561 pacing and defibrillator leads in 1684 patients at 89 sites describe a procedural success rate of 90% with a major complication rate of 1.9% with an in-hospital death rate of 0.8%.[42]

Tools Used in Chronic Lead Transvenous Extractions

Angiographic Catheters, Snares, Forceps, and Locking Stylets

Angiographic catheters that are commonly used to assist in lead extractions include the angled pigtail catheter, the Judkins right coronary catheter, the multipurpose coronary catheter, and the Amplatz catheter. These catheters are used in combination with common guidewires or tip-deflecting guidewires that loop around or hook onto the pacemaker lead to retrieve it. This approach may also be used to retrieve loose lead ends or free-floating lead remnants. Other tools used include the basket retriever catheter, the Dotter intravascular retriever (helical loop basket) that gets irreversibly entrapped in the lead, and the Dormia basket.

Different types of snares are also available and are used in conjunction with catheters and guidewires to recover and to extract chronic pacemaker leads. Examples of snares include the Curry snare (used to form a wire-loop system), the Amplatz gooseneck snare (loop at a right angle to the guidewire), and the Needle's Eye snare created by Cook Vascular, Inc. (consisting of a hoop-shaped loop and a locking slide threader), which provides a reversible system able to release the seized object. Cook Vascular, Inc., has also developed a "locking stylet" that is efficient in seizing and holding the lead while preventing the lead from stretching or uncoiling as it is being retrieved.[43]

Forceps (grasping forceps, alligator forceps, and myocardial bicep forceps) have also been used for lead extractions. This stylet intensifies the tensile power of the lead and directs the extraction force to the tip of the lead. The locking system is engaged and released by counterclockwise and clockwise rotation, respectively.

Byrd Dilator Sheaths

These sheaths were marketed by Cook Vascular, Inc., and may be used to assist with extractions performed through the implant vein. They consist of telescoping stainless steel sheaths with metal dilators that are advanced over the lead to sever through the thick fibrous adhesions found at the venous entry site and distal ends of chronic leads. Once entrance to the vein is attained, the metal dilators are exchanged for telescoping flexible plastic sheaths that are able to negotiate the turns.

Excimer Laser Sheaths

Excimer laser sheaths were developed by Charles Byrd and are used in association with the Spectranetics CVX-300 excimer laser system.[43] The laser sheath contains a ring of optical fibers at its distal tip able to emit pulses of ultraviolet light that destroy the surrounding fibrous tissues around the lead. Mild countertraction and counterpressure activate the laser. An advantage of the laser system is that tissue vaporization is achieved, as opposed to blunt tissue dissection and shredding. One disadvantage is that the system is not effective against calcifications, which are often encountered around older leads.

Electrosurgical Dissection Systems

The most recent advancement in lead extraction equipment includes the electrosurgical dissection system developed by Cook Vascular, Inc. Such systems use radiofrequency energy (instead of laser or blunt dissection) to destroy the fibrous endovascular adhesions that anchor device leads to venous walls. The most recent radiofrequency-based system has a dual electrode scheme that performs a bipolar dissection while also functioning as a mechanical dissection sheath. The tip electrode spacing is such that it effectively localizes the disruptive energies to the specific regions interfering with extraction of the lead, as opposed to circumferentially obliterating the endovascular border.

Techniques of Chronic Lead Transvenous Extractions

Transvenous lead extractions should preferably be performed in a setting appropriate for emergent thoracotomy; a cardiothoracic surgeon should be promptly available. Before any transvenous extraction of chronic pacemaker leads, the patient should be prepared in advance for potential thoracotomy. Intra-arterial blood pressure monitoring is recommended. Transthoracic and transesophageal echocardiography and a pericardiocentesis tray should be readily accessible to allow expeditious diagnosis and treatment of possible complications. A temporary pacing wire should be placed through the femoral vein if the patient is pacemaker dependent.

Extraction through the Implant Vein

The generator should be removed and the leads completely freed from adhesions and sutures and dissected down to the venous entry site. If the patient is pacemaker dependent, a temporary pacing wire (normally introduced through the femoral vein) should have been placed ahead of time. The proximal end of the lead, which includes the connector pin, should be cut, and 1 cm of the lead inner coil should be exposed. A coil expander is used to remove any wire burs and to ensure patency of the lead lumen. A locking stylet should then be advanced into the lead inner coil until it reaches the distal tip of the lead. The locking mechanism is activated, and the outer lead insulation should be secured with a tie before introduction of the sheaths. If simple traction is not sufficient to free the lead from the myocardium once the locking stylet is in place, sheaths should be introduced to disrupt fibrous adhesions or scarring. Telescoping stainless steel sheaths (or other available sheaths, including excimer laser sheaths and, most recently, electrosurgical dissection sheaths) should be advanced over the lead down to the venous entry site, where they disrupt the scar tissue surrounding the lead. The sheaths should be advanced down under fluoroscopic guidance to the distal tip of the lead as continuous traction is placed on the locking stylet system. The lead tip may then be pulled free by counterpressure and countertraction, and the entire lead is extracted. If this method is unsuccessful, another technique (e.g., extraction through the femoral vein) may be used.

Extraction through the Femoral Vein

The femoral vein approach is the preferred technique to extract lead remnants or broken or cut leads that are free-floating in the venous system, heart, or pulmonary artery.[43] It may also be used as a primary approach for transvenous extraction of permanent leads, especially if there is concern for pushing infected debris from the original entry site into the circulation. This approach engages angiographic catheters such as the angled pigtail catheter or a variety of snares (see earlier for different types of available snares) to grasp loose lead ends or the deflecting wire and Dotter retriever if no freed ends are available. Traction is applied to pull the lead (or lead remnants) from the heart, and the lead is then withdrawn from the body through the femoral vein sheath.

Complications

Serious complications may occur as a result of transvenous lead extractions. Complications may be intraoperative, perioperative (events that occur or are diagnosed within 24 hours after the procedure), postoperative (events that occur or are diagnosed after 24 hours but within 30 days of the procedure), or late (events that occur or are diagnosed more than 30 days after the procedure date). Box 85-17 summarizes major and minor complications related to transvenous lead extractions.

BOX 85-17 Major and Minor Complications Related to Transvenous Lead Extractions

Major Complications

- Death
- Cardiac avulsion or tear requiring thoracotomy, pericardiocentesis, chest tube, or surgical repair
- Vascular avulsion or tear requiring thoracotomy, pericardiocentesis, chest tube, or surgical repair
- Hemothorax or severe bleeding from any source requiring transfusion
- Pneumothorax requiring chest tube drainage
- Pulmonary embolism requiring surgical intervention
- Respiratory arrest
- Septic shock
- Stroke

Minor Complications

- Pericardial effusion not requiring pericardiocentesis or surgical intervention
- Hemodynamically significant air embolism
- Pulmonary embolism not requiring intervention
- Vascular repair near the implant site or venous entry site
- Arrhythmia requiring cardioversion
- Hematoma at the pocket requiring drainage
- Arm swelling or thrombosis of implant veins resulting in medical intervention
- Sepsis in a previously nonseptic patient with infection
- Pacing system–related infection of a previously noninfected site

Observation

- Transient hypotension that responds to fluids or minor pharmacologic intervention
- Nonsignificant air embolism
- Small pneumothorax not requiring intervention
- Ectopy not requiring cardioversion
- Arm swelling or thrombosis of implant veins without need for medical intervention
- Pain at cutdown site
- Myocardial avulsion without sequelae
- Migrated lead fragment without sequelae

From Love CJ, Wilkoff BL, Byrd CL, et al: Recommendations for extraction of chronically implanted transvenous pacing and defibrillator leads: indications, facilities, training. North American Society of Pacing and Electrophysiology Lead Extraction Conference Faculty. Pacing Clin Electrophysiol 23(4 Pt 1):544–551, 2000.

MANAGEMENT OF CARDIAC DEVICES DURING AND AFTER SURGERY

Pacemakers

Application of a magnet over a pacemaker inhibits all sensing function of the pacemaker. The previously programmed pacing mode is subsequently transiently changed to DOO, VOO, or AOO until the magnet is removed. The magnet pacing rate varies according to the pacemaker manufacturer. The magnet may be used prophylactically before surgical procedures to avoid inappropriate sensing by the pacer as a result of noise artifact created by cautery. Other procedures during which there is a risk of inhibition of the pacer by inappropriate sensing of noise include electroconvulsive therapy, extracorporeal shockwave lithotripsy, and occasionally electric cardioversions.

Implantable Cardioverter-Defibrillators

Unlike standard pacemakers, defibrillators with backup pacing and pacemaker-defibrillators do not have their sensing function inhibited by a magnet. The magnet does, however, inhibit delivery of any antitachycardia therapy, such as ATP or high-energy defibrillation. Magnet inhibition of antitachycardia therapies prevents delivery of inappropriate ICD therapies during cautery or other procedures that could produce noise erroneously sensed by the lead as VT or VF. Although a magnet is applied to an ICD, causing inhibition of the programmed ICD therapies, the patient should be treated like any patient who does not have an ICD in the event that a tachyarrhythmia occurs. Alternatively, cautery (or other problematic procedures) may be transiently halted and the magnet removed from the ICD to allow implementation and delivery of programmed ICD therapies.

In addition, if a patient is pacemaker dependent, the pacing mode of the ICD should be reprogrammed to DOO, VOO, or AOO (as clinically indicated) before anticipated cautery. Alternatively, a temporary pacing wire should be placed to avoid inappropriate sensing of noise and subsequent inappropriate inhibition of the pacing function of the ICD. Such inappropriate inhibition of pacing in a pacemaker-dependent patient could be catastrophic if it is not anticipated. After the procedure, the initial ICD parameters should be restored. In general, even if no reprogramming is necessary, ICDs should be interrogated after surgery or a magnet applied to confirm proper functioning and parameter settings.

Of note, some ICD generators are part of a magnet reed switch manufacturer recall and thus have their magnet function permanently turned off. For such generators, ICD therapies should be turned off before surgery expected to require cautery and turned back on after the procedure.

REFERENCES

1. Zoll PM: Resuscitation of the heart in ventricular standstill by external electric stimulation. *N Engl J Med* 247:768–771, 1952.
2. Chardack WM, Gage AA, Greatbatch W: A transistorized, self-contained, implantable pacemaker for the long-term correction of complete heart block. *Surgery* 48:643–654, 1960.
3. Furman S, Schwedel JB: An intracardiac pacemaker for Stokes-Adams seizures. *N Engl J Med* 261:943–948, 1959.
4. Mirowski M: The automatic implantable cardioverter-defibrillator: an overview. *J Am Coll Cardiol* 6:461–466, 1985.
5. Mirowski M, Mower MM, Staewen WS, et al: Standby automatic defibrillator. An approach to prevention of sudden coronary death. *Arch Intern Med* 126:158–161, 1970.
6. Mirowski M, Reid PR, Mower MM, et al: Termination of malignant ventricular arrhythmias with an implanted automatic defibrillator in human beings. *N Engl J Med* 303:322–324, 1980.
7. A comparison of antiarrhythmic-drug therapy with implantable defibrillators in patients resuscitated from near-fatal ventricular arrhythmias. The antiarrhythmics versus implantable defibrillators (avid) investigators. *N Engl J Med* 337:1576–1583, 1997.
8. Buxton AE, Lee KL, Fisher JD, et al: A randomized study of the prevention of sudden death in patients with coronary artery disease. Multicenter unsustained tachycardia trial investigators. *N Engl J Med* 341:1882–1890, 1999.
9. Moss AJ, Hall WJ, Cannom DS, et al: Improved survival with an implanted defibrillator in patients with coronary disease at high risk for ventricular arrhythmia. Multicenter automatic defibrillator implantation trial investigators. *N Engl J Med* 335:1933–1940, 1996.
10. Moss AJ, Zareba W, Hall WJ, et al: Prophylactic implantation of a defibrillator in patients with myocardial infarction and reduced ejection fraction. *N Engl J Med* 346:877–883, 2002.
11. Bardy GH, Lee KL, Mark DB, et al: Amiodarone or an implantable cardioverter-defibrillator for congestive heart failure. *N Engl J Med* 352:225–237, 2005.
12. Epstein AE, DiMarco JP, Ellenbogen KA, et al: ACC/AHA/HRS 2008 guidelines for device-based therapy of cardiac rhythm abnormalities: a report of the American College of Cardiology/American Heart Association Task Force on Practice Guidelines (Writing Committee to revise the ACC/AHA/NASPE 2002 guideline update for implantation of cardiac pacemakers and antiarrhythmia devices) developed in collaboration with the American Association for Thoracic Surgery and Society of Thoracic Surgeons. *J Am Coll Cardiol* 51:e1–e62, 2008.
13. Gregoratos G, Abrams J, Epstein AE, et al: ACC/AHA/NASPE 2002 guideline update for implantation of cardiac pacemakers and antiarrhythmia devices–summary article: a report of the American College of Cardiology/American Heart Association task force on practice guidelines (ACC/AHA/NASPE committee to update the 1998 pacemaker guidelines). *J Am Coll Cardiol* 40:1703–1719, 2002.
14. Tracy CM, Epstein AE, Darbar D, et al: 2012 ACCF/AHA/HRS focused update of the 2008 guidelines for device-based therapy of cardiac rhythm abnormalities: a report of the American College of Cardiology Foundation/American Heart Association task force on practice guidelines. *J Am Coll Cardiol* 60:1297–1313, 2012.
15. Antman EM, Anbe DT, Armstrong PW, et al: ACC/AHA guidelines for the management of patients with ST-elevation myocardial infarction–executive summary: a report of the American College of Cardiology/American Heart Association task force on practice guidelines (writing committee to revise the 1999 guidelines for the management of patients with acute myocardial infarction). *Circulation* 110:588–636, 2004.
16. Smith TWC, Epstein LM: Implantable devices for the treatment of cardiac arrhythmia. In Grossman WBD, editor: *Grossman's cardiac catheterization, angiography, and intervention*, Philadelphia, 2000, Lippincott Williams & Wilkins, pp 489–543.
17. Moss AJ, Hall WJ, Cannom DS, et al: Cardiac-resynchronization therapy for the prevention of heart-failure events. *N Engl J Med* 361:1329–1338, 2009.
18. Tang AS, Wells GA, Talajic M, et al: Cardiac-resynchronization therapy for mild-to-moderate heart failure. *N Engl J Med* 363:2385–2395, 2010.
19. Sanders R: The pulse generator. In Kusumoto FM, Goldschlager NF, editors: *Cardiac pacing for the clinician*, Philadelphia, 2001, Lippincott Williams & Wilkins, pp 41–62.
20. Kruse IM, Terpstra B: Acute and long-term atrial and ventricular stimulation thresholds with a steroid-eluting electrode. *Pacing Clin Electrophysiol* 8:45–49, 1985.
21. Mond H, Stokes K, Helland J, et al: The porous titanium steroid eluting electrode: a double blind study assessing the stimulation threshold effects of steroid. *Pacing Clin Electrophysiol* 11:214–219, 1988.
22. Pirzada FA, Moschitto LJ, Diorio D: Clinical experience with steroid-eluting unipolar electrodes. *Pacing Clin Electrophysiol* 11:1739–1744, 1988.
23. Wang PJ, et al: Modes of pacemaker function. In Kusumoto FM, Goldschlager NF, editors: *Cardiac pacing for the clinician*, Philadelphia, 2001, Lippincott Williams & Wilkins, pp 63–90.
24. Sweeney MO, Ellenbogen KA, Casavant D, et al: Multicenter, prospective, randomized safety and efficacy study of a new atrial-based managed ventricular pacing mode (MVP) in dual chamber ICDs. *J Cardiovasc Electrophysiol* 16:811–817, 2005.
25. Wilkoff BL, Cook JR, Epstein AE, et al: Dual-chamber pacing or ventricular backup pacing in patients with an implantable defibrillator: the dual chamber and VVI implantable defibrillator (DAVID) trial. *JAMA* 288:3115–3123, 2002.
26. Lamas GA, Lee K, Sweeney M, et al: The MOde Selection Trial (MOST) in sinus node dysfunction: design, rationale, and baseline characteristics of the first 1000 patients. *Am Heart J* 140:541–551, 2000.
27. Chen J, et al: Defibrillator function and implantation. In Kusumoto FM, Goldschlager NF, editors: *Cardiac pacing for the clinician*, Philadelphia, 2001, Lippincott Williams & Wilkins, pp 426–452.
28. Grimm W, Flores BF, Marchlinski FE: Electrocardiographically documented unnecessary, spontaneous shocks in 241 patients with implantable cardioverter defibrillators. *Pacing Clin Electrophysiol* 15:1667–1673, 1992.
29. Guarnieri T, Levine JH, Veltri EP, et al: Success of chronic defibrillation and the role of antiarrhythmic drugs with the automatic implantable cardioverter/defibrillator. *Am J Cardiol* 60:1061–1064, 1987.
30. Movsowitz C, Marchlinski FE: Interactions between implantable cardioverter-defibrillators and class iii agents. *Am J Cardiol* 82:41I–48I, 1998.
31. Deeb GM, Hardesty RL, Griffith BP, et al: The effects of cardiovascular drugs on the defibrillation threshold and the pathological effects on the heart using an automatic implantable defibrillator. *Ann Thorac Surg* 35:361–366, 1983.
32. Gula LJ, Massel D, Krahn AD, et al: Is defibrillation testing still necessary? A decision analysis and markov model. *J Cardiovasc Electrophysiol* 19:400–405, 2008.
33. Strickberger SA, Klein GJ: Is defibrillation testing required for defibrillator implantation? *J Am Coll Cardiol* 44:88–91, 2004.
34. Viskin S, Rosso R: The top 10 reasons to avoid defibrillation threshold testing during icd implantation. *Heart Rhythm* 5:391–393, 2008.
35. Byrd CL, Schwartz SJ, Hedin N: Intravascular techniques for extraction of permanent pacemaker leads. *J Thorac Cardiovasc Surg* 101:989–997, 1991.

36. Byrd CL, Schwartz SJ, Hedin NB, et al: Intravascular lead extraction using locking stylets and sheaths. *Pacing Clin Electrophysiol* 13:1871–1875, 1990.
37. Byrd CL, Schwartz SJ, Hedin NB: Lead extraction: techniques and indications. In Barold SS, Mugica J, editors: *New perspectives in cardiac pacing*, Mount Kisco, NY, 1993, Futura Publishing, pp 29–55.
38. Goode LB, Byrd CL, Wilkoff BL, et al: Development of a new technique for explantation of chronic transvenous pacemaker leads: five initial case studies. *Biomed Instrum Technol* 25:50–53, 1991.
39. Love CJ, Wilkoff BL, Byrd CL, et al: Recommendations for extraction of chronically implanted transvenous pacing and defibrillator leads: indications, facilities, training. North American Society of Pacing and Electrophysiology lead extraction conference faculty. *Pacing Clin Electrophysiol* 23:544–551, 2000.
40. Wilkoff BL, Love CJ, Byrd CL, et al: Transvenous lead extraction: Heart Rhythm Society expert consensus on facilities, training, indications, and patient management: this document was endorsed by the American Heart Association (AHA). *Heart Rhythm* 6:1085–1104, 2009.
41. Byrd CL, Wilkoff BL, Love CJ, et al: Intravascular extraction of problematic or infected permanent pacemaker leads: 1994-1996. U.S. Extraction database, med institute. *Pacing Clin Electrophysiol* 22:1348–1357, 1999.
42. Byrd CL, Wilkoff BL, Love CJ, et al: Clinical study of the laser sheath for lead extraction: the total experience in the United States. *Pacing Clin Electrophysiol* 25:804–808, 2002.
43. Belott PH: Endocardial lead extraction. In Kusumoto FM, Goldschlager NF, editors: *Cardiac pacing for the clinician*, Philadelphia, 2001, Lippincott Williams & Wilkins, pp 162–192.

CHAPTER 86

CATHETER ABLATION OF ARRHYTHMIAS

Ethan R. Ellis • John V. Wylie, Jr. • Mark E. Josephson

CHAPTER OUTLINE

Over the past 40 years, cardiac electrophysiology has progressed from an esoteric field dedicated to understanding arrhythmia mechanisms to an indispensable modality in the diagnosis and treatment of cardiac arrhythmias. Electrophysiology therapeutics first began with cardiac surgery for the treatment of arrhythmias. After it became clear that invasive surgical strategies could cure arrhythmias, methods for delivery of energy through catheter-based techniques were developed. The advent of catheter ablation has revolutionized the management of patients with tachyarrhythmias. Radiofrequency current has become the energy source of choice for catheter ablation and has made it the first-line therapy for the treatment of many tachycardias.

PROCEDURAL TECHNIQUE AND THE ELECTROPHYSIOLOGY STUDY

The electrophysiology study (EPS) is an indispensable prelude to catheter ablation allowing for the identification of tachycardia mechanism and the most appropriate site for energy delivery. The EPS involves placing electrode catheters in various chambers of the heart for recording, stimulation, mapping, and ablation. Femoral veins and arteries are the most common sites of vascular access used for EPS. Less commonly used sites include the antecubital fossa, subclavian, and jugular veins. Adequate local anesthesia is administered before vascular puncture. A 0.035-inch short J guidewire is placed via the percutaneous Seldinger technique into the femoral vein or artery just below the inguinal ligament. Additional wires, up to three in a single vein, are placed 5 to 10 mm caudal to the first wire. Double- and triple-headed vascular access devices that can accommodate two or three catheters through a single access sheath are commercially available and are used in some laboratories. Hemostatic sheaths (size 6 Fr to 11 Fr) are placed over the guidewires, up to three in a single vein. If more than three catheters are required, another vein is used, typically the contralateral femoral vein.

For His bundle recordings, the femoral approach allows superior catheter stability. However, catheterization of the coronary sinus (CS) is more readily accomplished via the internal jugular, left subclavian, or left antecubital veins. The lateral antecubital veins that drain into the cephalic vein are avoided because of the right angle at which they enter the axillary vein, making catheter manipulation more difficult. These nonfemoral sites are usually reserved for patients with inaccessible femoral access or difficult CS cannulation despite attempting via the femoral approach with a steerable catheter, but in some laboratories, CS cannulation is routinely performed via the left subclavian vein or right internal jugular vein. Although accessing the CS through a femoral vein is generally more difficult, in experienced hands it can be readily accomplished either via a direct approach, often facilitated by bending the catheter in the hepatic vein to achieve a greater posterior angulation, using a steerable catheter, or more indirectly by forming a catheter loop within the right atrium.

The catheters used in an EPS are either steerable or nonsteerable woven Dacron or synthetic catheters containing electrodes that can be manipulated under fluoroscopy in the cardiac chambers. Nonsteerable catheters are available in a variety of electrode configurations and preformed curves, but the most common catheters have either 4 or 10 electrodes for pacing and sensing. Steerable catheters have internal tension wires that allow the tip to be deflected up to 180 degrees or more by manipulating a control at the handle. Diagnostic steerable catheters may contain up to 20 electrodes. Catheters used for radiofrequency ablation are all steerable and generally consist of a 3.5- to 10-mm electrode used for ablation and three proximal recording electrodes. A diagnostic EPS typically requires at least three catheter locations: in the high right atrium near the sinus node, at His bundle area across the superior tricuspid valve, and at the right ventricular apex. Depending on the type of study, additional catheters may be placed in the right ventricular outflow tract, CS, anterolateral right atrium, interatrial septum, left atrium, pulmonary veins, and left ventricle.

Accessing the left ventricular cavity is accomplished either via the mitral valve from transseptal left atrial catheterization or via retrograde aortic approach through the arterial system, typically the femoral artery. Although left ventricular catheterization is not a routine part of a diagnostic EPS, it may have importance in patients with ventricular tachycardia and accessory pathway–mediated tachycardia (atrioventricular reciprocating tachycardia). Detailed catheter mapping of the left ventricular endocardium may also have benefit in defining the myocardial substrate in patients with ventricular arrhythmias, depressed ventricular function, history of myocardial infarction, and congestive heart failure.

CARDIAC MAPPING TECHNIQUES

Understanding the mechanism of arrhythmia is vital, before targeting with ablation, to maximize the success of the procedure. Understanding the arrhythmia mechanism can often be achieved with EPS but can be further refined with the use of cardiac mapping techniques. Cardiac mapping allows the identification of temporal and special relationships of electrical potentials during atrial and ventricular arrhythmias. The focus of cardiac mapping is generally to identify the origin of a focal arrhythmia or a site of critical conduction for a reentrant arrhythmia. The most common approaches to mapping are simple activation mapping, pace mapping, and electroanatomic activation mapping.

Electrograms acquired during mapping techniques are either bipolar or unipolar. Bipolar electrograms reveal the local electrical activity of the heart between two designated electrodes on the catheter. This typically is over an interelectrode spacing ranging from 1 to 10 mm. Unipolar electrograms reveal the local electrical activity at a single catheter point (usually the distal tip) relative to an electrode placed at a distance from the heart. The advantages of using unipolar mapping are that it gives a more precise measure of local activation and it provides information about the direction of impulse propagation. The advantages of using bipolar mapping include superior signal-to-noise ratio and less contribution from distant electrical activity ("far-field" activity). Frequently, accurate mapping involves using both bipolar and unipolar electrograms at different points of the study.

Simple activation mapping is achieved by moving a single roving mapping catheter to various points of interest during an arrhythmia, spontaneous or induced, while measuring local activation times relative to a fiducial marker at a second site, such as the onset of the P wave or QRS complex or a stable intracardiac electrogram. Depending on the arrhythmia mechanism, the area of earliest activation is often a reasonable target for ablation of the arrhythmia.

Pace mapping is a mapping technique that can be used when the patient is not in the arrhythmia.[1] It is often used in conjunction with activation mapping as a second confirmatory test to determine the accuracy of the selected site for ablation, but it can be used as a stand-alone mapping technique if the documented clinical arrhythmia cannot be induced during EPS or is not hemodynamically tolerated. Pace mapping entails pacing the suspected target area for ablation at a rate similar to the clinical arrhythmia, and comparing the 12-lead electrocardiogram (ECG) to the ECG of the arrhythmia. A good pace map will have an exact match in 12 out of 12 leads; however, this is often difficult to achieve. When only minor differences in the ECG configuration and amplitude are noted, the spatial resolution of pace mapping can be as good as 5 mm. However, if only assessing for major differences in the 12-lead ECGs, special resolution may be as poor as 15 mm.[2] In addition to the 12-lead ECG, pace mapping also compares the intracardiac activation sequence seen on the electrophysiology catheters with the sequence observed during the arrhythmia if present or inducible.

Electroanatomic activation mapping relies on the use of specialized three-dimensional electroanatomic systems to assist with intracardiac mapping. The use of these systems can greatly reduce the amount of fluoroscopy time required for a procedure. Most commonly used are the CARTO 3 system (Biosense Webster) and the EnSite NavX system (St. Jude Medical) although the technology of cardiac mapping continues to evolve and newer mapping systems are currently in development. The CARTO 3 mapping system allows three-dimensional electroanatomic mapping using a low-intensity magnetic field and current-based visualization data to provide localization of multiple catheter tips and curves. The system can visualize up to five catheters with and without magnetic sensors but requires the use of compatible Biosense Webster catheters with magnetic sensors for electroanatomic mapping. Biosense Webster mapping catheters have miniature magnetic field sensors at the tip of the catheters, which can determine the location and orientation of the catheter within the magnetic field. With this information, one can create a three-dimensional reconstruction of cardiac chamber geometry. Isochromes of electrical activity can then be overlaid onto this geometry to help define reentrant circuits as well as localize the origin of focal arrhythmias. Additionally, voltage mapping can be performed in sinus rhythm to better delineate the underlying myocardial substrate in any chamber in question. The system has been shown to be highly accurate and reproducible in vitro and in vivo.[3]

The EnSite NavX mapping system also allows for three-dimensional localization of an intracardiac catheter through the use of three pairs of skin patches that send three independent, alternating, low-power currents through a patient's chest, each with a slightly different frequency. These currents can then be used to calculate different levels of impedances in all three planes corresponding to specific anatomic locations within the chest. Mapping catheter electrodes can then be used to measure different levels of impedance corresponding to specific locations in the heart as they are manipulated within the cardiac chambers. Using these calculated impedance coordinates, the system allows for real-time visualization of the position and motion of up to 64 different electrodes on the ablation catheter as well as other standard intracardiac catheters.[4] Like CARTO 3, EnSite NavX can create three-dimensional geography of cardiac chambers and superimpose activation isochromes while mapping an arrhythmia or voltage measurements taken during sinus rhythm. However, unlike the CARTO 3 system, the EnSite NavX system does not require proprietary catheters for localization and mapping. EnSite also offers a noncontact mapping option using a 64-pole balloon catheter that generates mathematically derived electrograms and places them on a map of a cardiac chamber defined by a second, roving contact catheter.[5,6]

CATHETER ABLATION

Catheter-based ablation techniques have been so successful in treating a variety of arrhythmias that they have virtually replaced surgical approaches. In catheter-based ablation, energy is delivered to a precise area of the heart. This is most often performed on the endocardial surface of the heart, although epicardial ablation is possible percutaneously via the subxiphoid approach and is performed routinely at many centers.[7,8] After mapping techniques are used to identify the area or areas to be targeted for ablation, an ablation catheter is positioned in the desired location and connected to an energy source. Radiofrequency (RF) energy is the modality most commonly used clinically, having replaced direct current (DC) ablation because of superior safety and efficacy. Freezing the target area of the heart through a catheter-based cryoablation system is another method that can be used and is most commonly used in pediatric patients and in ablations performed adjacent to the intrinsic conduction system although cryoablation for atrial fibrillation using a cryoballoon catheter is becoming more common.

RF current is typically delivered in a unipolar configuration from the distal tip of the ablation catheter to a cutaneous grounding patch. The energy is generated as an alternating current with a frequency of 300 to 750 kHz.[9] These frequencies produce effective heating with negligible muscle stimulation. During RF ablation, the electrical energy is converted to thermal energy by resistive heating. Most of the heating is concentrated at the tip of the catheter secondary to the small surface area of the tip relative to the cutaneous patch. The heat that is generated is transferred to the adjacent cardiac tissue primarily by conduction and to a lesser extent by radiation, which decreases by the fourth power of the distance from the catheter tip. At steady state the RF lesion size is proportional to the temperature measured at the tissue-catheter interface, as well as proportional to the RF power amplitude.[10]

RF ablation results in thermal injury with coagulation necrosis when tissue heating exceeds approximately 50° C for at least 10 seconds.[9-12] As heat is produced at the catheter-myocardial interface, the impedance drops. A drop of 5 to 10 Ω is a sign of conductive heating to the adjacent tissue. The time to electrophysiologic effect after onset of RF current delivery is often shorter than one would anticipate for a pure thermal mechanism based on the documented rate of tissue temperature rise contiguous to the electrode. This raises the possibility that there is a contribution of a direct electrical effect in addition to the thermal effect of RF.

RF lesion size and power delivery are limited by tissue heating at the catheter-tissue interface on the endocardium. Newer ablation systems use external or internal saline irrigation to cool the catheter tip, which allows greater power delivery and the creation of deeper and larger lesions.[13] The formation of coagulum may also be decreased with these systems. The catheters typically infuse saline either in a closed system running to the catheter tip or in an open system in which saline flows out small holes at the catheter tip at 17 to 30 mL/min during ablation, similar to irrigated surgical RF ablation devices. Externally irrigated ablation catheters have become the most common catheter used for ablation procedures for the treatment of ventricular tachycardia and atrial fibrillation.[14,15]

Cryoablation has been used in the surgical treatment of arrhythmias for more than 20 years. Near-transmural lesions can be produced intraoperatively at temperatures of −60° C in the presence of cold cardioplegia. The blood pool presents catheter-based cryoablation systems with a major impediment in achieving adequate temperature. However, a catheter-based closed coolant system has been developed and is in clinical use. The major advantage is the ability to induce a nonpermanent change in tissue conduction, referred to as "ice mapping," followed by a permanent lesion if the ice mapping reveals a desirable location. This method has been used surgically with temperatures of approximately 0° C producing transient loss of electrical function and −60° C producing irreversible damage.[16] A percutaneous approach is complicated by the warming effect of the circulating blood pool, and mean temperatures of −27° C were needed to achieve transient altering of electrical function.[17] However, the temperature required for irreversible damage was similar to that needed in surgery (−58° C). Cryoablation catheters are most commonly used in the pediatric population and in ablations performed near the intrinsic conduction system where the risk of developing complete heart block is elevated. More recently, a cryoablation balloon has been developed which is capable of delivering a circumferential cryoablation lesion at the antrum of the pulmonary veins. This technology has been shown to reduce procedure times for pulmonary vein isolation with similar efficacy and adverse events compared with standard RF ablation.[18-20]

SPECIFIC ARRHYTHMIAS

Atrioventricular Nodal Reentrant Tachycardia

Atrioventricular nodal reentrant tachycardia (AVNRT) is the most common form of supraventricular tachycardia.[21,22] Medically, this arrhythmia is often treated with atrioventricular (AV) nodal blocking agents as well as occasionally with antiarrhythmic agents. The ability to cure this arrhythmia with a safe, well tolerated, and highly efficacious catheter ablation has made this a viable option for first-line therapy of AVNRT.[23]

The AV node lies within the triangle of Koch, an area confined by the septal leaflet of the tricuspid valve inferiorly, the tendon of Todaro superiorly, and the CS os posteriorly.[24] In 1956, Moe and colleagues described physiologic evidence for a dual AV nodal pathway system.[25] These pathways were termed "slow" and "fast" based on their conduction time. However, there are no specific anatomic pathways that have been described that correlate with the fast and slow pathways. The functional dissociation of AV conduction into fast and slow pathways provides the substrate most often associated with AVNRT. The fast pathway normally lies at the apex of the triangle of Koch and the slow pathway at the base, near the CS os. However, there is often heterogeneity of atrial activation and these locations are not universal.

"Typical" or "common" AVNRT is usually initiated when a premature atrial impulse blocks in the fast pathway, conducts antegrade over the slow pathway, and then reenters the fast pathway in the retrograde direction (Fig. 86-1). This "slow-fast" AVNRT is responsible for approximately 90% of cases. The "atypical" or "uncommon" form of AVNRT uses the slow pathway retrograde and fast pathway anterograde. Uncommonly, two relatively slow pathways constitute the reentry circuit ("slow-slow"). Although the terms "slow-fast," "fast-slow," and "slow-slow" are commonly used, attempting to classify all AVNRT into these groups is overly simplistic and incomplete given the complexity of AV nodal physiology and the lack of true discrete pathways in its structure.

Initial catheter ablation of AVNRT targeted the fast pathway region in the anterior interatrial septum.[26] Ablation at the apex of the triangle of Koch in the region of the fast pathway was more than 90% successful, but it carried an unacceptably high risk of AV block (5% to 10%). Ablation of the slow pathway[27] is accomplished via a posterior approach, with the ablation catheter initially positioned near the CS os, at the base of the triangle of Koch (see Fig. 86-1). RF current in the slow pathway region is often accompanied by transient accelerated junctional rhythm with rapid retrograde atrial conduction. This rhythm serves as a marker of a potentially successful ablation. However, rapid junctional tachycardia can be a marker for complete heart block, and ablation should be halted if it is seen.[28] Energy delivery should also be stopped if AV block or junctional rhythm with retrograde block is seen. Ablation is performed under continuous fluoroscopic monitoring or three-dimensional electroanatomic mapping to ensure catheter stability. In approximately 40% of cases, dual pathways are still present after ablation, but sustained ANVRT cannot be induced. Single AV nodal complexes ("echo beats") are observed in three fourths of these patients with dual pathways post ablation, with block always occurring antegradely in the slow pathway. The success rate using a slow

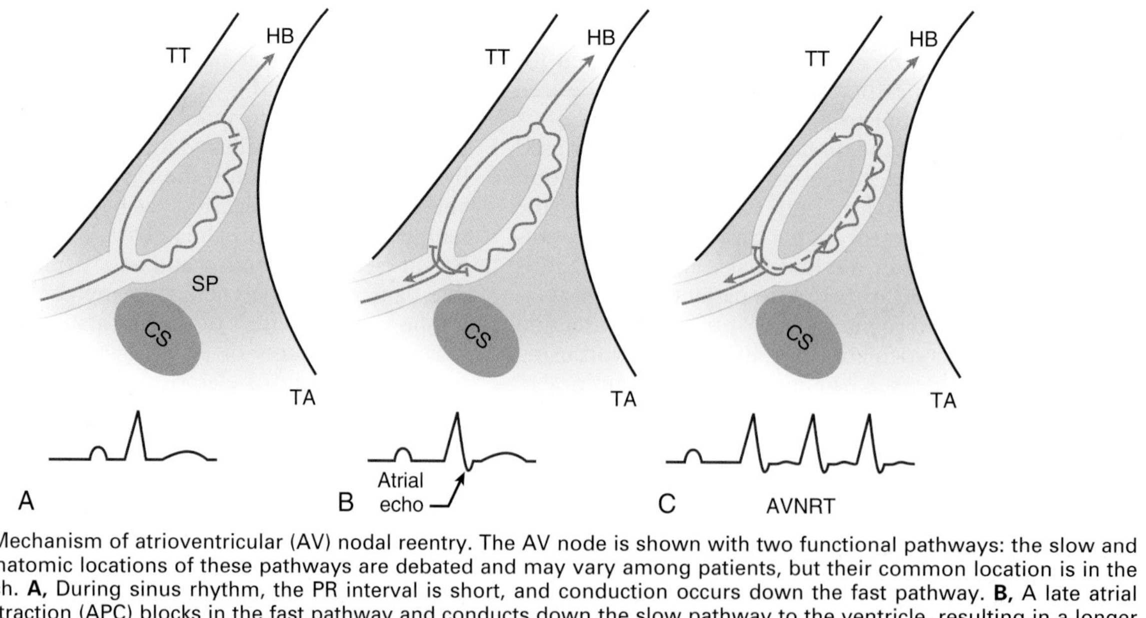

FIGURE 86-1 ■ Mechanism of atrioventricular (AV) nodal reentry. The AV node is shown with two functional pathways: the slow and the fast. The anatomic locations of these pathways are debated and may vary among patients, but their common location is in the triangle of Koch. **A,** During sinus rhythm, the PR interval is short, and conduction occurs down the fast pathway. **B,** A late atrial premature contraction (APC) blocks in the fast pathway and conducts down the slow pathway to the ventricle, resulting in a longer PR interval. The fast pathway recovers the ability to conduct, and retrograde conduction occurs up to the atrium, resulting in an AV nodal echo beat. The slow pathway is refractory, however, so tachycardia does not occur. **C,** A critically timed APC causes more delay in the slow pathway, allowing retrograde conduction up the fast pathway and sequential activation over the slow pathway to initiate typical AV nodal reentrant tachycardia (AVNRT). *CS,* Coronary sinus; *HB,* His bundle; *SP,* slow pathway; *TA,* tricuspid annulus; *TT,* tendon of Todaro.

pathway approach is in excess of 95%.[29] Slow pathway ablation is preferred to fast pathway because of the equivalent success rate and the much lower risk of complete heart block (1% to 2%).

Atrial Tachycardia

Atrial tachycardias in patients who have never had an ablation or cardiac surgery are usually focal arrhythmias originating in the left or right atria with rates of 100 to 220 beats/min. The mechanism of atrial tachycardias may be automatic or triggered from focal sites or may be microreentrant involving a small area of atrial myocardium. Atrial tachycardias that are incessant and are caused by abnormal automaticity or triggered activity are most amenable to ablation and tend to be resistant to drug therapy.[30] Microreentrant atrial tachycardias are frequently easily managed pharmacologically, making ablation second-line therapy. Macroreentrant atrial tachycardias are commonly seen after atrial fibrillation ablation procedures or after cardiac surgeries using atriotomies. These macroreentrant arrhythmias are more common in such scenarios because scarring from previous procedures provides areas of functional block and slow conduction necessary for the initiation of reentry.

Incessant focal atrial tachycardias can occur from various locations in the heart but seem to have a propensity for the crista terminalis, both atrial appendages, the CS, the regions of the mitral and tricuspid annuli, and the pulmonary veins. It is unclear why these structures are prone to develop these rhythms. It has been postulated that regions such as the crista terminalis are sources of automatic atrial tachycardias because of relatively poor cell-to-cell coupling.[31] Fractionated electrograms at successful ablation sites may be markers of a nonuniform anisotropic substrate because of poor coupling that allows focal automaticity to occur. In adults, atrial tachycardia foci are somewhat more common in the right atrium, and multiple foci are present in 10% to 15% of patients.

Because most incessant atrial tachycardias are focal in origin, the goal of catheter mapping is to find the earliest site of activation (Fig. 86-2). If the tachycardia is not incessant, catecholamine infusion, such as isoproterenol 1 to 10 μg/min IV or atropine 0.5 to 1.0 mg IV, may be necessary to induce sustained arrhythmia. The initial localization of the arrhythmia focus is made by analysis of the P wave morphology and axis. Catheter mapping is then performed by identifying the site of earliest atrial activation relative to the onset of the P wave. Three-dimensional electroanatomic mapping systems (described earlier) are often used to aid in mapping the atrial activation sequence during tachycardia (Fig. 86-3). Once the catheter is positioned at what appears to be the earliest site of atrial activation, further evidence that it is the correct site of origin can be obtained by pace mapping. In this setting, pace mapping involves pacing at the earliest intracardiac site and comparing the resultant paced P wave morphology with the tachycardia P wave morphology, as well as comparing the sequence of intracardiac atrial activation during pacing and during the tachycardia.[32] Pacing with higher output at the proposed site of ablation also helps confirm minimal risk of injury to the surrounding extracardiac structures. This is particularly important in the right atrium with the proximity of the phrenic nerve; however, left phrenic nerve damage has also been reported with ablation in the left atrium.[33] Pacing that results in diaphragmatic stimulation would preclude ablation at that site.

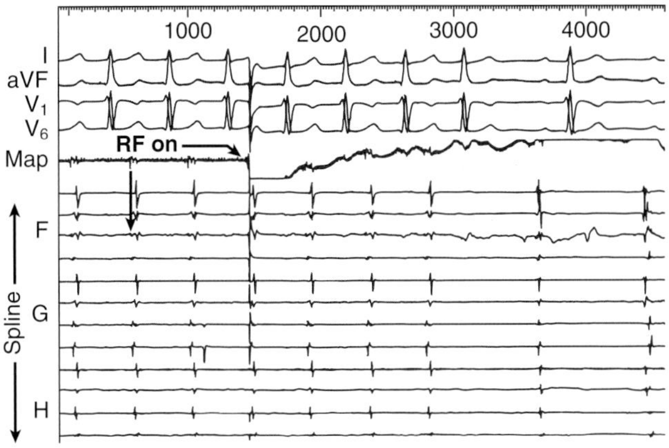

FIGURE 86-2 ■ Ablation of atrial tachycardia. Atrial tachycardia is present. The ablation/mapping catheter is placed at the earliest electrogram recorded on a 64-pole basket catheter *(vertical arrow).* Radiofrequency (RF) energy delivered at this site terminates the tachycardia. Surface electrocardiograph leads I, aVF, V_1, and V_6 are shown. *Map* is the ablation catheter signal, and the letters F, G, and H refer to electrodes on the 64-pole basket catheter.

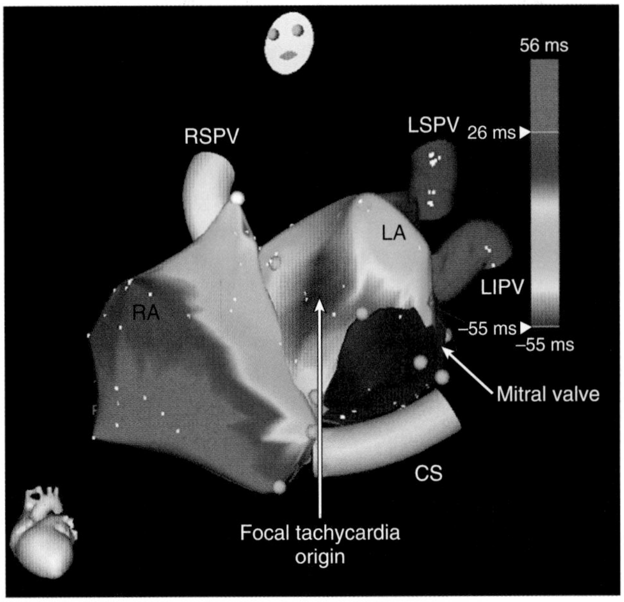

FIGURE 86-3 ■ Three-dimensional electroanatomic activation map depicting a focal atrial tachycardia. Maps of the right atrium (RA) and left atrium (LA) were created using point-by-point mapping with the CARTO system (see text). The *color scale* at the upper right represents the intracardiac activation timing at each point relative to a fixed reference in the coronary sinus. *Red areas* are earlier and *purple areas* are activated latest. Mapping of both the right and the left atrium revealed that the tachycardia was a focal atrial tachycardia originating anterior in the left atrium, near the aortic valve–mitral valve continuity. Ablation at this site successfully terminated the tachycardia. *CS,* Coronary sinus; *LIPV,* left inferior pulmonary vein; *LSPV,* left superior pulmonary vein; *RSPV,* right superior pulmonary vein.

The success rate of atrial tachycardia ablation is variable. For incessant tachyarrhythmias, the success rate approaches 90%, although the recurrence rate may be as high as 25%.[32,34-36] Because the arrhythmia may not be reliably present or inducible at EPS (factors such as conscious sedation may serve to make them less inducible), a true success rate on an intention-to-treat basis is lower than 90%.

Sinoatrial node reentrant tachycardia represents a distinct entity within the category of atrial tachycardias. Criteria for the diagnosis are consistent atrial activation sequence and P wave morphology in sinus rhythm and tachycardia, consistent initiation and termination with programmed electrical stimulation, and termination of tachycardia with vagal maneuvers or with adenosine.[37-39] Catheter ablation can be accomplished with good results and a paucity of complications, typically by ablating in the high posterolateral region of the right atrium at the "tail" of the sinus node.[40] Macroreentrant atrial tachycardias most often arise from the left atrium although they can also be seen in the right atrium. In the right atrium, the most common boundaries used for reentry aside from the cavotricuspid isthmus (discussed in detail in the atrial flutter section) include the CS ostium, the fossa ovalis, or scars from prior surgical incisions. In the left atrium, many left atrial tachycardias circulate around the mitral annulus with the pulmonary veins and the fossa ovalis as posterior boundaries.[41] Scars from prior surgical or ablation procedures can also provide obstacles that lead to atrial tachycardias with large excitable gaps. In macroreentrant atrial tachycardias, electroanatomic mapping systems are often used to identify the macroreentrant circuit, anatomic or functional barriers used by the arrhythmia, gaps in regions of scar, and areas of slow conduction. Successful ablation of macroreentrant arrhythmias may be focal if targeting critical areas of slow conduction or gaps along areas of scar. However, in the case of large anatomic barriers or scars, lines of RF lesions may be required to connect anatomic barriers or scars to one another to interrupt the reentrant circuit.[42]

Atrial Flutter

Atrial flutter is a rapid atrial arrhythmia with a rate faster than 220 beats/min. Typical isthmus-dependent atrial flutter is a macroreentrant circuit involving the right atrium. The posterior barrier of the circuit is formed by the crista terminalis and its continuation as the eustachian ridge.[43] The anterior barrier in typical flutter is the tricuspid annulus.[44] Typical atrial flutter is either counterclockwise or clockwise, depending on the direction of rotation in the frontal plane around the tricuspid annulus. Although counterclockwise flutter is the more common clinical entity, clockwise flutter can be initiated in most patients with typical atrial flutter.[45]

The 12-lead ECG can give clues to the mechanism of the atrial flutter but sometimes can be ambiguous or misleading. Counterclockwise flutter is characterized by a predominantly negative, sawtooth-like atrial pattern in the inferior leads, with positive atrial deflections in lead V_1 and negative deflections in lead V_6. Clockwise flutter is characterized by a predominantly positive, notched atrial pattern in the inferior lead, with negative atrial deflections in lead V_1 and positive deflections in lead V_6.

The term *atypical atrial flutter* is generally used to describe an arrhythmia with flutter waves on the 12-lead ECG felt to be inconsistent with an isthmus dependent arrhythmia. However, as noted earlier, the 12-lead ECG can be misleading in the case of atrial flutter, and it is not uncommon to identify an arrhythmia as isthmus-dependent atrial flutter at the time of EPS that terminates with ablation in the cavotricuspid isthmus, despite a 12-lead ECG inconsistent with the classic 12-lead ECG findings described earlier. If an atrial flutter is shown to be non-isthmus dependent, despite the lack of an obvious isoelectric interval on 12-lead ECG, a more appropriate classification would be macroreentrant atrial tachycardia. Further complicating matters, other macroreentrant right atrial tachycardias may have an appearance consistent with typical atrial flutter on surface ECG but may not rely on the cavotricuspid isthmus for reentry. For example, a reentrant circuit around the CS os (termed *intraisthmus reentry*) may have a 12-lead ECG appearance consistent with typical atrial flutter, but it requires a more medial cavotricuspid isthmus ablation beginning anterior to the CS os to facilitate termination.

In a catheter ablation procedure for typical atrial flutter, multielectrode catheters are placed in the CS and in the anterolateral right atrium, around a portion of the tricuspid annulus anterior to the crista terminalis. The catheter around the tricuspid annulus can help determine the direction of rotation, with atrial activation craniocaudal in counterclockwise flutter and caudocranial in clockwise flutter.

Catheter ablation of atrial flutter is dependent on the ability to interrupt the macroreentrant circuit at a critical narrow portion between barriers to conduction, termed the *isthmus*. In both counterclockwise and clockwise flutter, the isthmus targeted for ablation lies anterior to the inferior vena cava (IVC) and eustachian ridge, and posterior to the tricuspid annulus. During flutter, this isthmus is a zone of slow conduction.[46] Pacing from within this area slightly faster than the tachycardia will help demonstrate if the flutter uses this critical isthmus (i.e., isthmus dependent). If pacing in the isthmus at a rate slightly faster than the tachycardia entrains the tachycardia without alteration of the surface ECG flutter wave morphology and the local post-pacing interval equals the tachycardia cycle length, the tachycardia can be termed *isthmus dependent*. This pacing maneuver proves that the isthmus is a part of the atrial flutter circuit and that ablation in this area will effectively terminate the tachycardia.

Ablation of isthmus-dependent atrial flutter consists of creating a line of block across the right atrial cavotricuspid isthmus. Although this has been described for connecting the CS os to the tricuspid annulus, this approach can be prone to failure because of slow conduction through the eustachian ridge, which is not necessarily a fixed obstacle that produces block.[47] This can lead to a lower loop of reentry around the IVC, which meets the flutter loop going around the tricuspid annulus in a figure-of-eight manner.[48] Ablation between the tricuspid annulus and the IVC will eliminate lower loop reentry as well as isthmus-dependent flutter and is the preferred ablation method.

Ablation is usually performed during atrial flutter. If flutter is not present at baseline, it can be induced with one or two atrial extrastimuli and/or rapid atrial pacing in 90% of atrial flutter patients and 95% of patients with isthmus-dependent flutter.[42] Ablation can also be performed during pacing from the CS if the patient is not in atrial flutter at the time of the procedure. In patients in flutter, the arrhythmia is typically terminated during RF application in the isthmus; however, termination does not necessarily mean that the line of block is complete. Lack of complete isthmus block has been described in over 50% of cases when RF energy terminates flutter.[31] To increase the success of the procedure, bidirectional block must be demonstrated.[49-51] This is demonstrated by pacing the CS catheter, which is medial to the line of isthmus block. When the ablation line is complete, there is no clockwise propagation through the isthmus, and activation is around the tricuspid annulus in a counterclockwise direction. This is seen on the tricuspid annulus catheter as craniocaudal activation during CS pacing. To verify the bidirectional nature of the block, pacing is performed from the lateral tricuspid annulus, lateral to the line of isthmus block. If the line of block is complete, there is no counterclockwise propagation through the isthmus, and activation is around the tricuspid annulus in a clockwise direction. In addition to bidirectional block, at the conclusion of the procedure, split atrial potentials (>100 ms apart) or absence of atrial potentials (electrograms <0.05 mV) may be seen along the ablation line. If bidirectional block is demonstrated, the incidence of atrial flutter recurrence is less than 10%.[42]

Accessory Pathway–Mediated Tachycardia

Accessory AV connections ("accessory pathways," "bypass tracts") are part of a group of physiologic connections producing preexcitation syndromes. This group includes AV connections and nodoventricular, nodofascicular, atriofascicular, and fasciculoventricular connections.[52-54] These pathways appear to represent developmental abnormalities, and it is not surprising that multiple types of accessory pathways may exist in any one patient. AV connections are responsible for the classic Wolff-Parkinson-White syndrome, which is defined as preexcitation seen on an ECG and the presence of an arrhythmia. These connections can conduct antegradely, leading to a preexcited ECG, whereas some may be "concealed" and only conduct retrogradely, from the ventricle to the atrium.

The clinical tachycardia most frequently associated with accessory AV pathways is atrioventricular reciprocating tachycardia (AVRT, or "circus movement tachycardia"). AVRT can be either orthodromic or antidromic. Orthodromic tachycardia results from antegrade conduction down the AV node and retrograde conduction up the accessory pathway. Antidromic tachycardia uses the same circuit but in the opposite direction.

The initial step in an ablation procedure is careful inspection of the 12-lead ECG. Determining the site of an accessory pathway requires either manifest preexcitation (i.e., presence of a delta wave) on the ECG or visible retrograde P waves during orthodromic AVRT. Although complex schema have been proposed, a simpler approach is most prudent because of variability in degree of preexcitation, variability in precordial lead placement, and variations in body shape/size, heart size, and position in the chest.[55-58] This approach divides the location of accessory pathways into five regions: anteroseptal, right free wall, posteroseptal, left posterior free wall, and left lateral free wall. Full description of our approach to localizing pathways based on 12-lead ECG is well described elsewhere[42] and is summarized in Table 86-1. Newer anatomic designations of accessory pathway locations are also provided in this table.[59]

TABLE 86-1 Localizing Accessory Pathways Using ECG Criteria

AP Location (Anatomic Description)	ECG Characteristics of Delta Wave
Left lateral *Posterior**	Negative delta waves in leads I and aVL, and positive in inferior leads and precordial leads
Left posterior free wall *Inferoposterior*	Positive delta waves in lead I, negative in inferior leads, and positive in right precordial leads
Posteroseptal *Inferoparaseptal*	Positive delta wave in leads I and aVL and negative in inferior leads (although lead II may be isoelectric or biphasic, the more negative the more leftward the location)
Right free wall *Anterior*	Negative delta waves in leads V_1 and V_2, positive in I and II, and slightly negative in III
Anteroseptal *Superoparaseptal*	Positive delta wave in lead I, positive in inferior leads (with lead II greater than III), and precordial leads with primarily negative or biphasic delta waves

*Newer anatomic descriptions for accessory pathway locations are in italics.
AP, Accessory pathway; *ECG*, electrocardiogram.

In the past, cardiac surgery was the only option for definitive treatment of accessory pathway–mediated tachycardias, but catheter ablation has replaced surgery as the preferred therapy over the past 20 years. In a catheter ablation procedure, a CS catheter is advanced to the anterolateral mitral annulus to permit mapping of all left-sided pathways except possibly the most anterolateral pathways, and additional catheters are placed in the right atrium and ventricle and adjacent to the His bundle.

Left-sided accessory pathways can use either a transseptal approach or a retrograde aortic approach. Atrial pacing is performed to elicit maximal preexcitation, and the location of the earliest ventricular activation along the CS is noted as the ventricular insertion of the pathway. To identify the atrial insertion, retrograde conduction over the pathway is mapped during ventricular pacing or, preferably, during circus movement tachycardia (to ensure no contribution of retrograde AV nodal conduction), with the site of earliest atrial activation identifying the atrial insertion. It is important to identify both atrial and ventricular insertions of any accessory pathway when possible, given that slanted pathways are common and ablation at an insertion site may not adequately target the pathway itself. In the setting of concealed pathways, only the atrial insertion can be mapped, although other maneuvers can be used to assess for the presence of a slanted pathway.[42] If retrograde conduction over the pathway is intermittent or tenuous during the resting sedated state of EPS, isoproterenol can be administered. This can also facilitate initiation of circus movement tachycardia. If rapid retrograde conduction over the AV node during ventricular pacing makes localization difficult, verapamil can be administered to facilitate conduction over the pathway.

After mapping of the accessory pathway, a steerable ablation catheter is then advanced to a position near the accessory pathway. The ventricular insertion of the pathway is best approached via the retrograde aortic approach, whereas the transseptal approach allows easiest access to the atrial insertion site. Success rates of initial attempts at ablation appear to be similar in either approach.[60] Ablation should target the area between the atrial and ventricular insertions when both can be identified, which is generally near the site of the earliest ventricular activation in manifest pathways and the earliest atrial activation in concealed pathways as the shortest AV and ventriculoatrial (VA) intervals may not be the best target for ablation in slanted pathways. Electrograms recorded at insertion sites of pathways are often fractionated, and occasionally a bypass tract potential can be recorded.

Factors that predict a successful ablation site for a pathway include a stable electrogram, catheter stability and catheter motion in conjunction with the CS catheter, presence of an accessory pathway potential, catheter position at the shortest recorded AV interval (or shortest VA interval if concealed), and activation of the local ventricular electrogram before the onset of the QRS if it is a manifest pathway.

The mapping of right-sided pathways uses similar principles to those used for left-sided pathways. An atrial approach is most commonly used for right-sided accessory pathways. Right atrial pathway ablation can be more complicated because of (1) the presence of a "sack" of atrial myocardium folding over the tricuspid AV ring, which makes catheter manipulation more difficult; (2) possible circumferential tricuspid pathway location versus only approximately 75% of the mitral annulus because of lack of pathways in the region of aortomitral continuity; and (3) lack of an AV groove reference catheter. A multipolar halo catheter can be positioned around the tricuspid annulus to serve as an AV groove reference, but positioning may not always be accurate as it can be difficult to place in a true annular position. When endocardial ablation fails to eliminate accessory pathway conduction, epicardial mapping and ablation can be performed with percutaneous access to the pericardial space.[61] In this procedure, via a subxiphoid approach, a standard sheath is advanced over a wire into the pericardial space and an ablation catheter is manipulated under fluoroscopic guidance for epicardial mapping.[62]

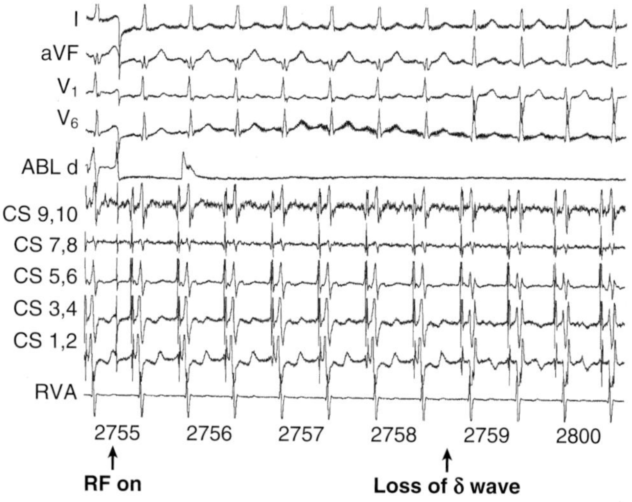

FIGURE 86-4 ■ Ablation in Wolff-Parkinson-White syndrome. Electrocardiogram leads I, aVF, V_1, and V_6 and proximal (CS 9,10) to distal (CS 1,2), and RV apical (RVA) recordings are shown. The bypass tract is a left posterior bypass tract. Radiofrequency (RF) energy produces loss of the delta (δ) wave in 4 seconds (see text).

Coronary angiography is usually required before ablation to ensure ablation is not performed over large epicardial arteries. Pericardial scarring often prohibits this approach in patients who have had cardiac surgery.

After adequately localizing the accessory pathway, RF current is delivered through the distal electrode of the ablation catheter. Successful ablation typically results in loss of accessory pathway conduction within 10 seconds (Fig. 86-4). The patient is then monitored for at least 20 minutes to watch for resumption of accessory pathway conduction, often in the presence of isoproterenol given intravenously. The success rate for catheter ablation of all accessory pathways is greater than 90%.[63]

Reentrant Ventricular Tachycardia and Structural Heart Disease

Most sustained monomorphic ventricular tachycardia (VT) seen clinically is in patients with coronary artery disease and is most frequently the result of scarred myocardial substrate from a prior myocardial infarction (MI). In this setting, the primary mechanism for VT is reentry. Reentrant circuits are prone to develop secondary to fibrosis from the prior infarction causing disruptions in cellular coupling leading to abnormal paths of conduction as well as zones of slow conduction. Surgical subendocardial resection of these areas has proven curative in selected patients. With the advent of catheter ablation, surgical ablation for VT fell out of favor because of unacceptably high morbidity and mortality rates.[64-67] However, these high mortality rates are from surgical series in the 1980s, and one might expect these numbers to be lower today with improved myocardial preservation techniques and additional methods to facilitate the procedure. Thus, surgical therapy for ventricular arrhythmias, particularly in conjunction with coronary artery bypass grafting surgery, is almost certainly an underused procedure today. Nevertheless, catheter-based VT ablation has supplanted surgical treatment in most cases.

Patients with structural heart disease but no known coronary artery disease or prior MI (such as arrhythmogenic right ventricular cardiomyopathy, hypertrophic cardiomyopathy, or non–infarct-related cardiomyopathy) can also present with sustained monomorphic VT related to reentry. As is the case with prior MI, the pathophysiology is generally related to underlying scar and fibrosis. For the purposes of this section, we focus on mapping and ablation of sustained monomorphic VT in the setting of infarct-related cardiomyopathy. However, the approach to mapping and ablation of non–infarct-related VT is generally similar although the most common areas of fibrosis tend to be different, being more often perivalvular or epicardial.

Approximately 95% of patients with a prior MI who present with sustained monomorphic VT will be able to have the clinical arrhythmia induced at EPS. Ideally, to be considered for ablation, the VT should be hemodynamically tolerated, which allows for careful ventricular mapping during the arrhythmia. Substrate mapping during sinus rhythm can identify scarred arrhythmogenic substrate in patients with hemodynamically untolerated VT or in patients in whom VT cannot be induced, which can then be modified with ablation. However, activation and entrainment mapping techniques require hemodynamically tolerated inducible VT. If the rapid rate of a VT is contributing to hemodynamic compromise, administration of agents such as procainamide can slow the VT enough to allow for adequate mapping during VT. Alternatively, vasopressors such as dopamine, norepinephrine, or phenylephrine may be administered to support the patient's blood pressure during an otherwise untolerated VT. A newer alternative involves use of a percutaneous ventricular assist device (pVAD) to maintain adequate perfusion in the setting of rapid VTs or advanced cardiomyopathy. The disadvantages of this strategy are complications inherent in the use of a highly invasive pVAD. However, the potential advantage is that it may allow for induction and mapping of VT, which would be suitable only for a substrate ablation in other circumstances. Further studies are required to determine whether this more invasive strategy translates to improved procedural success rates.[68,69]

The "site of origin" of the VT is essentially the source of electrical activity producing the VT QRS. Although this is a discrete site in automatic and triggered rhythms, post-MI VT is typically a reentrant rhythm. During reentrant VT, the arrhythmia circuit involves normal myocardium and a protected "isthmus" of scarred myocardial tissue. Because of myocardial scarring and fibrosis, electrical conduction through the isthmus is slow, forming the diastolic interval in the tachycardia circuit.[70] This isthmus is identified as an area of low voltage on electroanatomic mapping with fractionated electrograms and diastolic potentials seen during tachycardia. The site of origin represents the exit site from the diastolic pathway to the myocardium giving rise to the QRS. The initial step in localization of the VT is examination of the ECG.[71-73] Approximately 59% of VTs can be localized with 93% accuracy. Left bundle branch block VT morphology can be more accurately localized than can right bundle branch block morphology, and VT from a prior inferior MI can be more easily localized than VT from a prior anterior MI.[42,71,72]

During EPS, once the clinical VT has been induced, an ablation catheter is advanced into the left ventricle after heparinization to an activated clotting time (ACT) of greater than 250 seconds. Either a transseptal or a retrograde aortic approach can be used. Further mapping of the VT is then performed by examination of the electrograms obtained during the VT, as well as their response to pacing during the VT. Stevenson and colleagues have devised a scheme to help understand the various components of the reentry circuit, including the central common pathway or protected isthmus of myocardium that is the target site for ablation.[70]

Regardless of the approach to localizing the protected isthmus, the three major steps are as follows:

1. Activation mapping, consisting of finding the site of early activation closest to mid-diastole. These electrograms frequently are low-amplitude fractionated potentials.
2. Demonstration that this diastolic electrogram has a fixed relationship to the subsequent QRS despite pacing-induced oscillations in the VT cycle length.
3. Performing entrainment mapping to demonstrate an entrained QRS morphology identical to the VT morphology ("concealed entrainment"), with an activation pattern during pacing and after cessation of pacing proving that the site in question is part of the reentry circuit.

If all three criteria are met, there is a greater than 95% chance of terminating the VT with ablation at a single site in the protected isthmus (Fig. 86-5).[74]

Entrainment mapping consists of ventricular pacing at a cycle length slightly shorter than the VT cycle length and seeing if the three previously listed criteria are met.[70,74-78] Pace mapping, as described earlier for atrial tachycardia, is another method for localizing the VT circuit. In this technique, pacing is performed from candidate sites in the ventricle, and the 12-lead ECG is compared with the VT ECG. An identical match in all 12 leads is considered an ideal pace map. We do not advocate using pace mapping as a primary mapping modality for post-MI VT, however. A pace map that appears similar to the VT would only identify the exit point for the critical isthmus and may be distant from the common pathway ablation target. In addition, pacing during sinus rhythm activates the myocardium in both directions from a protected isthmus, whereas the QRS during reentrant VT is the result of unidirectional activation of the myocardium by the cyclical depolarization front.

When the clinical VT cannot be hemodynamically tolerated after being induced during EPS, consideration can be given to mapping and ablation during sinus rhythm. This technique is known as "substrate ablation" and is similar in principle to the intraoperative surgical ablation techniques used in some centers. Low-amplitude fractionated electrograms and late potentials have been demonstrated in areas of infarction using standard catheter techniques during sinus rhythm.[79] One study showed

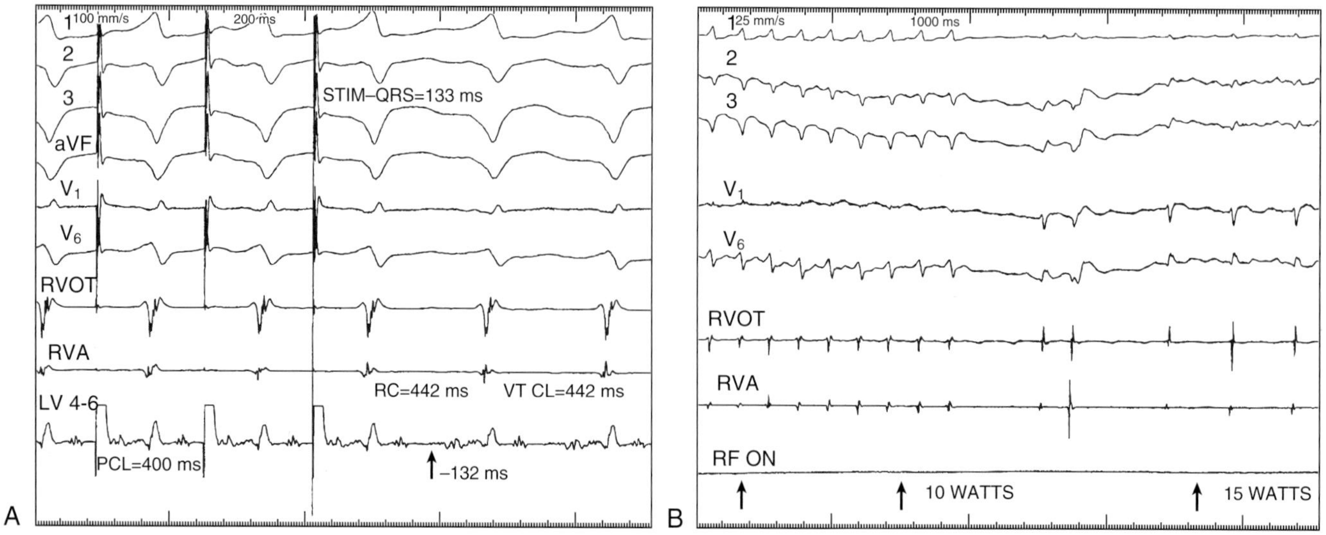

FIGURE 86-5 ■ Mapping and ablation of ventricular tachycardia (VT). **A,** Electrocardiogram leads 1, 2, 3, aVF, V_1, and V_5 are shown during VT with electrograms from the right ventricular outflow tract (RVOT), the right ventricular apex (RVA), and the site of the earliest activity in the left ventricle (LV 4-6). Entrainment of VT from LV 4-6 produces a QRS identical to VT, a stimulus (STIM)-QRS identical to the electrogram to QRS *(arrow).* **B,** Radiofrequency (RF) application at this site terminates VT. *CL,* Cycle length; *PCL,* paced cycle length; *RC,* return cycle.

that although no specific electrogram characteristic could predict a VT site of origin with adequate specificity, 86% of VTs arose from areas with these abnormal electrograms. Another study showed that the number of abnormal electrograms in cardiac arrest patients (who more often have ventricular fibrillation or polymorphic VT) was smaller compared with the number of patients with sustained monomorphic VT.[80] Standard catheter techniques do not allow for precise three-dimensional localization of the abnormal electrograms. Endocardial voltage mapping using an electroanatomic mapping system such as CARTO (see earlier) in a chronic infarct model has been shown to more accurately delineate infarcted myocardium than can pathology.[81,82] Clinically, voltage mapping is used to guide endocardial VT ablation by identifying areas of scar and potential areas of protected isthmuses.[81] Using bipolar voltage mapping, normal endocardial bipolar electrogram voltage using electroanatomic mapping is defined at more than 1.5 mV, based on mapping of controls, and scar is defined as areas with low voltage, less than 0.5 mV. Linear ablation lesions are extended from areas of dense scar to areas of normal voltage myocardium or to anatomic boundaries such as the mitral valve, resulting in a 75% success rate in patients with drug refractory VT that was not hemodynamically tolerated during EPS (Fig. 86-6). A randomized trial showed that prophylactic substrate catheter ablation in patients with a history of VT or ventricular fibrillation was able to reduce the number of implantable cardioverter-defibrillator (ICD) shocks received by patients who had undergone ablation.[83] Although ICDs reduce mortality from ventricular arrhythmias, shocks are uncomfortable and are associated with increased subsequent mortality,[84] and therefore catheter ablation is often considered in patients with ICDs who have received shocks for VT.

Although less commonly performed than endocardial ablation, epicardial ablation of VT is possible both surgically and percutaneously via a subxiphoid approach for access of the pericardial space, often in conjunction with endocardial ablation. This approach is most often used for cardiomyopathies associated with VT of an epicardial origin (non–infarct-related cardiomyopathy, Chagas disease, etc.) or in patients who have refractory VT despite previous endocardial ablation attempts. In some

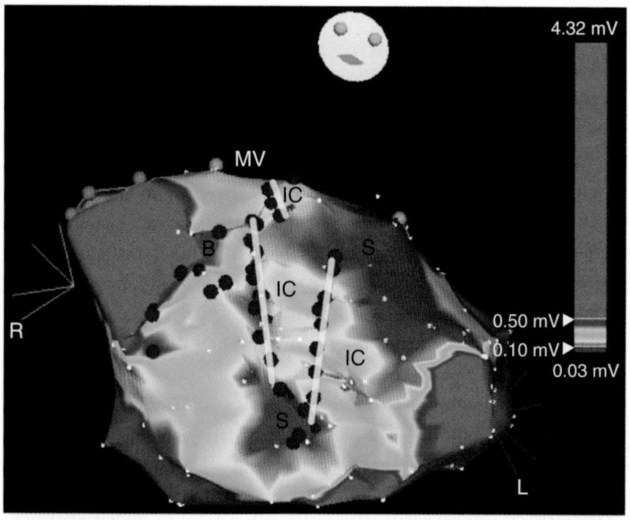

FIGURE 86-6 ■ Substrate ablation of ventricular tachycardia. A three-dimensional electroanatomic CARTO map of the left ventricle is shown in a modified right anterior oblique orientation. The mitral valve (MV) and the septum and part of the anterior and inferior walls are shown. The colors represent electrogram voltage, shown on the scale *(right)* in a range from 0.1 mV to 0.5 mV. *Purple areas* are relatively normal myocardium, *red areas* represent dense scar (S), and between them are areas of viable myocardium with scar. Conduction is slow through these areas, and isthmus channels (IC) can be identified. *Red dots* represent ablation sites. Note that ablation lines *(white lines)* extend from areas of scar across the isthmus channel to adjacent areas of scar and from areas of scar to the mitral valve. Additional ablations were also created in the border zone (B) at areas with fractionated electrograms (see text). *L,* Left; *R,* right.

centers, epicardial ablation is used as a first-line ablation strategy for patients with VT.[85] Once epicardial access has been obtained, the process of mapping and ablation of VT is similar to that of the endocardial approach. However, catheter manipulation can be more challenging in the epicardium, and coronary angiography before the delivery of RF energy is important to ensure the ablation catheter is a safe distance from the large epicardial coronary arteries. In patients status post coronary artery bypass grafting, localization of bypass grafts is important in order to avoid laceration of grafts during catheter manipulation. Furthermore, in any patients with a history of prior open heart surgery, epicardial scarring and pericardial adhesions can make catheter manipulation in the epicardial space difficult if not impossible. Of note, epicardial ablation has also been used for arrhythmias other than VT, including inappropriate sinus tachycardia, refractory atrial arrhythmias despite previous endocardial ablation, and accessory pathways inaccessible from an endocardial approach.[8]

Idiopathic Ventricular Tachycardia

VT occurs most often in patients with underlying structural heart disease. VT is also seen in patients without known structural heart disease; this is known as idiopathic VT. The most common type of idiopathic VT is caused by triggered activity from delayed afterdepolarizations. It is typically catecholamine dependent, frequently brought on by exertion or emotional stress, and can be terminated by vagal maneuvers, adenosine, calcium channel blockers, or sodium channel blockers. The term *idiopathic VT* is a misnomer because patients with underlying structural disease can also have triggered, focal VTs arising from similar locations and behaving in similar ways to VTs seen in patients without structural disease. With this understanding, it is more appropriate to characterize all VTs based on tachycardia mechanism in addition to underlying substrate.[85a] For the purposes of this section, we focus on the approach to triggered, focal VTs in patients without underlying structural disease, most commonly referred to as idiopathic VT. These tachycardias most commonly arise from the right ventricular outflow tract (RVOT),[86,87] coronary cusps, left ventricular outflow tract (LVOT),[88,89] and mitral annulus,[90] but have also been reported at other sites in the left and right ventricles.

The characteristic ECG for RVOT VT is a left bundle, inferior axis, with either a right or left axis depending on the location in the outflow tract. For LVOT/coronary cusp VT, the ECG typically has a small r wave in V_1 with early development of a large R wave in the right precordial leads and an inferior axis. These VTs often require catecholamine infusion during EPS for induction. The approach to mapping and ablation for both RVOT and LVOT/coronary cusp VTs is similar.[91-94] Activation mapping using both bipolar and unipolar electrograms followed by confirmatory pace mapping is the most reliable method for localizing the focal source of these tachycardias. An electroanatomic mapping system is often used to track the timing of catheter points to locate the earliest electrogram relative to the surface ECG and guide ablation. In the absence of structural heart disease, pace mapping for focal idiopathic VT is a viable modality for localizing the site of origin, unlike in post-MI VT.[95] Ablation is performed at the earliest identifiable site of ventricular activation or at the site with a pace map identical to that of the clinical tachycardia.

A second and less common variety of idiopathic VT arises from the left ventricle, is reentrant, and is verapamil sensitive.[93,94,96] The characteristic ECG is right bundle, superior axis, which can be left superior if it is coming from the posterior third of the septum or right superior if it is coming from the apical third. Opinions regarding the optimal approach to ablation vary, but activation mapping of the site of earliest ventricular activation along the septum, followed by pace mapping, is generally a reasonable approach. Some authors advocate targeting presystolic Purkinje potentials or mid-diastolic potentials.[97,98] Electroanatomic activation mapping and identification of the earliest retrograde Purkinje potentials has also been used to guide ablation.[99] Entrainment mapping has been reported but is difficult to achieve. Ablation for this type of VT should use as many mapping modalities as possible, with consideration of the Purkinje spike, concealed entrainment if attainable, activation mapping, and confirmatory pace mapping.

Atrial Fibrillation

Atrial fibrillation (AF) is the most common arrhythmia encountered in clinical practice. Catheter ablation for treatment of AF was previously limited to ablation of the AV junction combined with pacemaker implantation in patients refractory to, or intolerant of, pharmacologic therapy. Over the past 15 years, catheter ablation has become a common strategy for decreasing the burden of AF in patients refractory to medical therapy, through elimination of AF triggers and modification of the atrial substrate responsible for the maintenance of AF.

Atrioventricular Junction Ablation

Ablation of the AV junction was the first use of catheter ablation and used DC energy; however, RF energy is superior and is now used for this procedure.[100,101] This procedure is indicated for patients who have been unable to tolerate medical therapy for AF or in whom it has been ineffective and requires pacemaker implantation before ablation. To perform AV junction ablation, an ablation catheter is advanced beyond the superior aspect of the tricuspid valve, along the ventricular septum, until the maximum amplitude His bundle recording is observed. The catheter is then withdrawn 1 to 2 cm until a large atrial electrogram and occasionally a very small His bundle recording is seen. Ablation is performed in this region until AV block is achieved. This technique targets the distal portion of the AV node and allows for an intact junctional escape pacemaker to persist and provide backup heart rate in the case of pacemaker failure. Occasionally this approach fails and despite ablation of the distal AV node, rapid conduction persists. In these cases, ablation is performed over the His bundle region. In up to 10% of cases, ablation of the His bundle from the left side is required to achieve effective AV block.[102] After ablation, the patient is commonly monitored in the electrophysiology laboratory during isoproterenol infusion to assess for resumption of conduction. The success rate of this procedure for achieving AV block has been reported to be 97.4%.[29]

Ablation of the AV junction has been associated with an increased risk of sudden cardiac death, thought to be caused by polymorphic VT related to electrical instability and changes in repolarization caused by the sudden change in heart rate and myocardial activation sequence.[103-105] These changes may be manifest as QT prolongation and torsades de pointes. As a result, after AV junction ablation, the pacemaker is initially programmed to a lower pacing rate of 80 to 90 beats/min, which is then slowly decreased over several months at follow-up visits.

Catheter Ablation of Atrial Fibrillation

The role of catheter ablation of AF in the management of patients with AF continues to evolve. Haissaguerre and coworkers observed that focal triggers originating in the pulmonary veins may initiate AF; this led to a new catheter-based approach to the treatment of AF.[106] Early procedures used focused catheter ablation of ectopic foci found in pulmonary veins and had limited success. Researchers then proceeded to perform extensive ablation in the pulmonary veins, but this was complicated by pulmonary vein stenosis caused by scarring of the proximal veins.[107] Since that time, multiple newer techniques for isolating the pulmonary veins have been used.

Segmental ostial pulmonary vein isolation is based on the principle that pulmonary vein triggers initiate AF in the left atrium. Ablation is performed around the ostium of each pulmonary vein until conduction block at the left atrium-pulmonary vein border is achieved. The goal of this method is to electrically isolate each vein, thus preventing pulmonary vein triggers from reaching the left atrium to initiate and perpetuate AF.[108,109] More recently, circumferential left atrial (LA) ablation and wide-area left atrial catheter ablation (WACA) have been used for the treatment of AF. This strategy uses creation of ablation lines that encircle the ostia of all four pulmonary veins, usually in two pairs, one around the left pulmonary veins and one around the right pulmonary veins. These ablation lesions are generally driven by anatomic landmarks and do not require detailed mapping of focal electrical connections between the pulmonary veins and the left atrium, which can simplify the procedure although a greater number of ablation lesions is usually required, resulting in longer procedural times. WACA results in more extensive ablation across a wider area of the left atrium compared with segmental ostial pulmonary vein isolation (PVI), which may provide additional means of preventing AF recurrence including autonomic denervation,[110] elimination of AF triggers outside of the pulmonary veins,[111] and modification of the LA substrate that may facilitate perpetuation of AF.[112] In conjunction with ablation around the pulmonary veins, additional ablation lines may be created connecting ablation lines to one another or to anatomic landmarks, such as the mitral annulus. These additional lines are intended to interrupt potential macroreentrant circuits that could otherwise lead to LA tachycardias.

Small randomized studies that compared segmental ostial PVI with circumferential LA ablation yielded conflicting results. One study found that rates of recurrent symptomatic paroxysmal AF were higher in the segmental ostial PVI group, whereas another study reported that symptomatic recurrences and atrial arrhythmias seen on ambulatory monitoring were significantly greater in the circumferential ablation group.[113,114] Unfortunately the two studies are not directly comparable because of differences between patient populations and study design. Currently, most physicians believe that a circumferential or WACA approach is superior to a segmental ostial approach. However, there continue to be wide variations in practice patterns. An expert consensus statement recommends that electrical isolation should be the goal of ablation around the pulmonary veins.[115] Electrophysiologic criteria for ablation success vary, but the most rigorous operators aim for elimination of electrical signals at the site of ablation and elimination of electrical conduction into the pulmonary veins from the left atrium (entrance block) and from the pulmonary veins to the left atrium (exit block).

Beyond electrical isolation of the pulmonary veins, additional focal ablation in the atria at a variety of different locations has become increasingly popular. It has been postulated that nonpulmonary venous structures entering the atria are alternative triggers of AF, and ablation of regions around the superior vena cava, ligament of Marshall, and CS are performed by many operators as adjunctive therapy to PVI.[116] Complex fractionated atrial electrograms (CFAEs) have also been a target of ablation and extensive research. CFAEs are found mostly in areas of slow conduction and it has been postulated that they may be important components of the substrate that allows maintenance of AF. One study reported a high percentage of freedom from arrhythmia following CFAE ablation without PVI in paroxysmal AF patients.[112] Beyond the CFAE debate, controversy also remains regarding the benefits of LA substrate modification with additional ablation lines beyond those created to isolate the pulmonary veins. The argument for the creation of additional lines is that RF lesions may create reentrant circuits. LA tachycardias appear to be more common after circumferential PVI as opposed to segmental ostial PVI, which may add weight to this argument because wider ablation lesions may facilitate development of macroreentry.[113] However, an argument against the creation of additional lines is that LA tachycardia following PVI is often treated successfully with reisolation of the pulmonary veins without additional linear ablation lesions.[117,118]

In practice, AF ablation is now often performed using a stepwise technique.[119] Ablation around the pulmonary veins is first performed with the goal of electrical isolation of the veins. Although this technique is often adequate in patients with paroxysmal AF, patients with persistent or chronic AF often require further ablation. Guided by inducibility of AF and conversion of AF during ablation, additional linear lesions may be created. If the patient continues to have inducible AF or remains in AF, some physicians choose to ablate areas of the left atrium exhibiting CFAEs during LA mapping.[112,119]

Because catheter ablation of AF is invasive and has procedural risks, it is generally reserved for patients who do not respond to medical therapy with antiarrhythmic drugs.[120] With the low efficacy of medications and the high success rates of catheter ablation in experienced centers, this procedure is occasionally considered first-line therapy for patients who do not wish to take antiarrhythmic medication. A meta-analysis has demonstrated that the efficacy of catheter ablation is significantly greater than the efficacy of medical therapy.[121] Reported success rates vary widely, ranging from 42% to 88% for patients with paroxysmal AF in studies with adequate follow-up available.[113,122-124] Success rates for patients with persistent AF are much lower, reported at approximately 50% in most studies, and a recent study of long-standing persistent AF suggested a single procedure success rate as low as 20%.[125] The complication rate for this procedure is as high as 6%, with tamponade, pulmonary vein stenosis, stroke, and access site complications being the most common adverse outcomes.[123] The reasons for this relatively high complication rate include the use of multiple catheters, the transseptal puncture procedure, the need for high-intensity systemic anticoagulation, and the manipulation of catheters and creation of ablation lesions in the left atrium. The most recent American College of Cardiology/American Heart Association/Heart Rhythm Society (ACC/AHA/HRS) guidelines on the management of patients with AF make a strong recommendation for RF ablation for patients with symptomatic paroxysmal AF who have failed treatment with an antiarrhythmic drug and a weak recommendation for RF ablation for patients with symptomatic, persistent AF. They make a very weak recommendation for RF ablation for patients with symptomatic paroxysmal AF and significant LA dilation or significant left ventricular dysfunction.[120]

Although specific techniques vary, most operators place standard electrophysiology catheters in the CS and right atrium. Transseptal puncture is then performed. This is accomplished using the standard technique developed 50 years ago.[126] A long sheath with an inner dilator designed for transseptal access is advanced to the right atrium and placed in the fossa ovalis. Location is confirmed using fluoroscopic landmarks, intracardiac ultrasound, and/or injection of a small amount of contrast dye to "stain" the septum (Fig. 86-7). When location at the fossa ovalis is confirmed, a long needle is advanced from the tip of the dilator until the septum is punctured. Entry into the LA is confirmed by injection of microbubbles seen on intracardiac ultrasound, injection of dye under fluoroscopy, advancement of a wire into the LA or pulmonary vein, and/or direct pressure measurement. Once LA access is achieved with one or two sheaths, an ablation catheter and circular mapping ("lasso") catheter are placed in the left atrium. Systemic anticoagulation with IV heparin is administered throughout LA access with activated clotting times kept between 250 and 400 seconds.

Once LA access is obtained, mapping of the left atrium and pulmonary veins is performed using a three-dimensional electroanatomic mapping system. Recent advances in this technology have allowed the integration of previously acquired computed tomography or magnetic resonance imaging images or real-time tomographic fluoroscopy or intracardiac ultrasound images of the left atrium into the mapping system (Fig. 86-8). Ablation is then performed as described earlier. Manual catheter manipulation remains the most common method, but newer technologies allowing remote magnetic catheter guidance or robotic catheter guidance have been developed and are in limited clinical use.[127-129] These technologies show promise for reducing radiation exposure to patient and operator and possibly increasing the safety of the procedure.

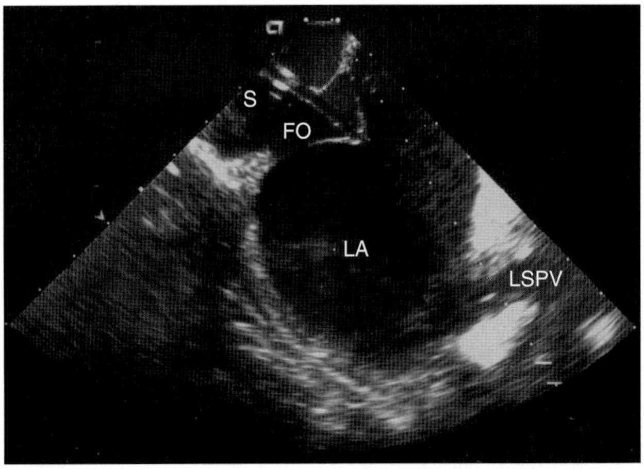

FIGURE 86-7 ■ Intracardiac ultrasound image of transseptal catheterization. The transseptal sheath (S), fossa ovalis (FO), left atrium (LA), and left superior pulmonary vein (LSPV) ostium are shown. The typical "tenting" of the fossa ovalis by the transseptal needle advanced through the sheath confirms appropriate positioning of the needle for puncture of the fossa ovalis.

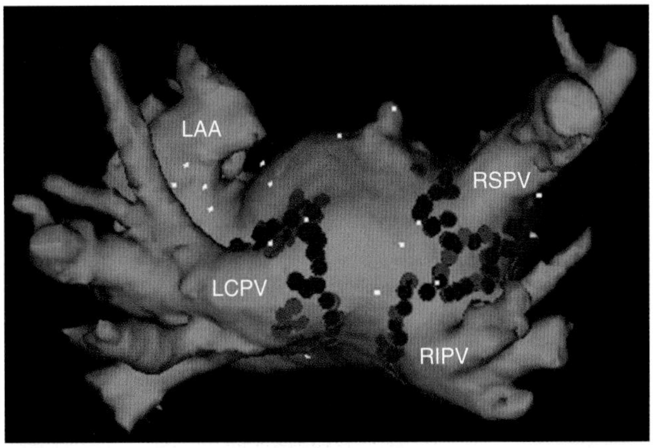

FIGURE 86-8 ■ Three-dimensional electroanatomic map of the left atrium showing integrated information from intracardiac mapping and a previously acquired computed tomography image (CartoMerge, Biosense Webster, Inc.). This patient has a left common pulmonary vein (LCPV) that gives rise to superior and inferior branches, and separate right-sided pulmonary veins. The *red and gray circles* indicate sites of ablation performed in a circumferential pattern around the pulmonary veins. Bidirectional electrical isolation of all pulmonary veins without additional ablation lines was performed in this patient. *LAA,* Left atrial appendage; *RIPV,* right inferior pulmonary vein; *RSPV,* right superior pulmonary vein.

Cryoballoon Ablation of Atrial Fibrillation

As mentioned previously, a cryoballoon catheter has been specifically designed for the treatment of AF and is now in use worldwide. The goal of cryoablation for AF using the cryoballoon is electrical isolation of the pulmonary veins. In comparison to RF therapies for AF, cryoballoon functions most like circumferential pulmonary vein isolation: after balloon deployment, cryothermal energy is delivered at the pulmonary vein antrum but does not target other areas beyond the pulmonary veins. To facilitate cryoballoon ablation, a transseptal catheterization is performed using the technique described earlier. After obtaining LA access, a standard transseptal sheath must be upsized to a specialized 12 Fr steerable sheath designed specifically to deliver the cryoballoon, available in two different sizes. Just as with RF ablation, systemic anticoagulation with IV heparin is administered throughout LA access with activated clotting times kept between 250 and 400 seconds. Through the transseptal sheath, the cryoballoon is advanced to the LA and a specialized circumferential mapping ("lasso") catheter is advanced through the cryoballoon and into the targeted pulmonary vein. The cryoballoon is then inflated in the LA and advanced over the lasso catheter until it is positioned into the antrum of the pulmonary vein. Contrast dye is then injected into the pulmonary vein distal to the cryoballoon under fluoroscopy to assess for occlusion. Color Doppler on intracardiac ultrasound is now widely used to assess for pulmonary vein occlusion. Complete occlusion is considered a surrogate for circumferential contact with the cryoballoon. Cryothermal energy is then delivered through the cryoballoon, generally in two applications. Entrance and exit block is then assessed in the same manner as described earlier. Additional cryoballoon applications can be applied as needed. The process is repeated for all major pulmonary veins. If isolation cannot be achieved with the cryoballoon alone, focal ablations can be performed as needed with a cryoablation catheter or standard RF catheter.

The major advantages of cryoballoon ablation for AF are a decrease in procedure time and reduced risk of complications related to RF energy, specifically thrombus formation at the site of lesion creation and cardiac perforation caused by excessive heating or catheter-related trauma. Theoretically, the cryoballoon ablation is also less complex and less dependent on operator dexterity, which is required to create contiguous curvilinear lesions with focal RF ablation. Centers with extensive cryoballoon experience have reported a progressive decline in procedural times, which are generally shorter than average procedural times for RF ablation.[19] Efficacy of cryoballoon ablation for paroxysmal AF has been shown to be similar to results reported for standard RF ablation in nonrandomized and randomized trials.[18,20,130] For patients with persistent AF, cryoballoon ablation alone has yielded low 1-year procedural success rates, likely related to the knowledge that patients with persistent and permanent AF may require more extensive atrial ablation beyond the pulmonary vein antra to adequately modify their substrate for AF. Combined approaches using cryoballoon ablation and RF ablation for creation of linear ablation lesions have reported better results in such patients.[131]

Complications of cryoballoon ablation appear to differ slightly from those of standard RF ablation. Tamponade and atrioesophageal fistulas have been reported less frequently in cryoballoon ablation. However, phrenic nerve paralysis has been reported with a significantly higher frequency compared with RF ablation, although for most patients, phrenic nerve paralysis is temporary and short-lived.[19,20] Because of the frequency of this complication, routine use of high output phrenic nerve pacing in the superior vena cava with palpation of the diaphragm during energy application in the right pulmonary veins is routine practice. Pulmonary vein stenosis has also been reported with cryoballoon ablation although most patients were asymptomatic and stenosis was discovered as a result of aggressive postprocedure screening.[20]

The optimal therapy for AF remains unclear and must be tailored to each patient. Structural heart disease, sleep apnea, aging, and fibrosis all make catheter ablation less likely to be successful. Combination therapy with antiarrhythmic drugs is often required. Many patients with long-standing AF, severe valvular disease, or severely dilated atria have a very low likelihood of success with catheter ablation, and in these patients a strategy of rate control of AF without aggressive attempts to restore sinus rhythm is often indicated. However, many other patients with AF benefit from pulmonary vein isolation with RF energy, cryoballoon ablation, or a combination of the two, and the use of these modalities has become widespread.

REFERENCES

1. Josephson ME, Waxman HL, Cain ME, et al: Ventricular activation during ventricular endocardial pacing. II. Role of pace-mapping to localize origin of ventricular tachycardia. *Am J Cardiol* 50:11–22, 1982.
2. Kadish AH, Childs K, Schmaltz S, et al: Differences in QRS configuration during unipolar pacing from adjacent sites: implications for the spatial resolution of pace-mapping. *J Am Coll Cardiol* 17:143–151, 1991.
3. Gepstein L, Hayam G, Ben-Haim SA: A novel method for non-fluoroscopic catheter-based electroanatomical mapping of the heart. In vitro and in vivo accuracy results. *Circulation* 95:1611–1622, 1997.
4. Packer DL: Three-dimensional mapping in interventional electrophysiology: techniques and technology. *J Cardiovasc Electrophysiol* 16:1110–1116, 2005.
5. Strickberger SA, Knight BP, Michaud GF, et al: Mapping and ablation of ventricular tachycardia guided by virtual electrograms using a noncontact, computerized mapping system. *J Am Coll Cardiol* 35:414–421, 2000.
6. Gornick CC, Adler SW, Pederson B, et al: Validation of a new noncontact catheter system for electroanatomic mapping of left ventricular endocardium. *Circulation* 99:829–835, 1999.
7. Sosa E, Scanavacca M: Epicardial mapping and ablation techniques to control ventricular tachycardia. *J Cardiovasc Electrophysiol* 16:449–452, 2005.
8. Schweikert RA, Saliba WI, Tomassoni G, et al: Percutaneous pericardial instrumentation for endo-epicardial mapping of previously failed ablations. *Circulation* 108:1329–1335, 2003.
9. Huang SK, Graham AR, Lee MA, et al: Comparison of catheter ablation using radiofrequency versus direct current energy: biophysical, electrophysiologic and pathologic observations. *J Am Coll Cardiol* 18:1091–1097, 1991.
10. Haines DE, Watson DD: Tissue heating during radiofrequency catheter ablation: a thermodynamic model and observations in isolated perfused and superfused canine right ventricular free wall. *Pacing Clin Electrophysiol* 12:962–976, 1989.

11. Haines DE: The biophysics of radiofrequency catheter ablation in the heart: the importance of temperature monitoring. *Pacing Clin Electrophysiol* 16:586–591, 1993.
12. Langberg JJ, Gallagher M, Strickberger SA, et al: Temperature-guided radiofrequency catheter ablation with very large distal electrodes. *Circulation* 88:245–249, 1993.
13. Nakagawa H, Yamanashi WS, Pitha JV, et al: Comparison of in vivo tissue temperature profile and lesion geometry for radiofrequency ablation with a saline-irrigated electrode versus temperature control in a canine thigh muscle preparation. *Circulation* 91:2264–2273, 1995.
14. Macle L, Jais P, Weerasooriya R, et al: Irrigated-tip catheter ablation of pulmonary veins for treatment of atrial fibrillation. *J Cardiovasc Electrophysiol* 13:1067–1073, 2002.
15. Reddy VY, Neuzil P, Taborsky M, et al: Short-term results of substrate mapping and radiofrequency ablation of ischemic ventricular tachycardia using a saline-irrigated catheter. *J Am Coll Cardiol* 41:2228–2236, 2003.
16. Harrison L, Gallagher JJ, Kasell J, et al: Cryosurgical ablation of the A-V node-His bundle: a new method for producing A-V block. *Circulation* 55:463–470, 1977.
17. Dubuc M, Khairy P, Rodriguez-Santiago A, et al: Catheter cryoablation of the atrioventricular node in patients with atrial fibrillation: a novel technology for ablation of cardiac arrhythmias. *J Cardiovasc Electrophysiol* 12:439–444, 2001.
18. Linhart M, Bellmann B, Mittmann-Braun E, et al: Comparison of cryoballoon and radiofrequency ablation of pulmonary veins in 40 patients with paroxysmal atrial fibrillation: a case-control study. *J Cardiovasc Electrophysiol* 20:1343–1348, 2009.
19. Andrade JG, Khairy P, Guerra PG, et al: Efficacy and safety of cryoballoon ablation for atrial fibrillation: a systematic review of published studies. *Heart Rhythm* 8:1444–1451, 2011.
20. Packer DL, Kowal RC, Wheelan KR, et al: Cryoballoon ablation of pulmonary veins for paroxysmal atrial fibrillation: first results of the North American Arctic Front (STOP AF) pivotal trial. *J Am Coll Cardiol* 61:1713–1723, 2013.
21. Josephson ME: Paroxysmal supraventricular tachycardia: an electrophysiologic approach. *Am J Cardiol* 41:1123–1126, 1978.
22. Wu D, Denes P, Amat-y-Leon F, et al: Clinical, electrocardiographic and electrophysiologic observations in patients with paroxysmal supraventricular tachycardia. *Am J Cardiol* 41:1045–1051, 1978.
23. Prystowsky EN: Atrioventricular node reentry: physiology and radiofrequency ablation. *Pacing Clin Electrophysiol* 20:552–571, 1997.
24. Koch W: Ueber das ultimem moriens des menslichen herzens. *Beitr Pathol Anat Allg Pathol* 42:203, 1907.
25. Moe GK, Preston JB, Burlington H: Physiologic evidence for a dual A-V transmission system. *Circ Res* 4:357–375, 1956.
26. Lee MA, Morady F, Kadish A, et al: Catheter modification of the atrioventricular junction with radiofrequency energy for control of atrioventricular nodal reentry tachycardia. *Circulation* 83:827–835, 1991.
27. Jackman WM, Beckman KJ, McClelland JH, et al: Treatment of supraventricular tachycardia due to atrioventricular nodal reentry, by radiofrequency catheter ablation of slow-pathway conduction. *N Engl J Med* 327:313–318, 1992.
28. Lipscomb KJ, Zaidi AM, Fitzpatrick AP, et al: Slow pathway modification for atrioventricular node re-entrant tachycardia: fast junctional tachycardia predicts adverse prognosis. *Heart* 85:44–47, 2001.
29. Scheinman MM, Huang S: The 1998 NASPE prospective catheter ablation registry. *Pacing Clin Electrophysiol* 23:1020–1028, 2000.
30. Gillette PC, Garson A, Jr: Electrophysiologic and pharmacologic characteristics of automatic ectopic atrial tachycardia. *Circulation* 56:571–575, 1977.
31. Lesh M, Kalman J, Olgin J: An electrophysiologic approach to catheter ablation of atrial flutter and tachycardia: from mechanism to practice. In Singer I, editor: *Interventional electrophysiology*, Baltimore, 1997, Williams and Wilkins.
32. Tracy CM, Swartz JF, Fletcher RD, et al: Radiofrequency catheter ablation of ectopic atrial tachycardia using paced activation sequence mapping. *J Am Coll Cardiol* 21:910–917, 1993.
33. Rumbak MJ, Chokshi SK, Abel N, et al: Left phrenic nerve paresis complicating catheter radiofrequency ablation for Wolff-Parkinson-White syndrome. *Am Heart J* 132:1281–1285, 1996.
34. Kay GN, Chong F, Epstein AE, et al: Radiofrequency ablation for treatment of primary atrial tachycardias. *J Am Coll Cardiol* 21:901–909, 1993.
35. Lesh MD, Van Hare GF, Epstein LM, et al: Radiofrequency catheter ablation of atrial arrhythmias. Results and mechanisms. *Circulation* 89:1074–1089, 1994.
36. Kalman JM, Olgin JE, Karch MR, et al: "Cristal tachycardias": origin of right atrial tachycardias from the crista terminalis identified by intracardiac echocardiography. *J Am Coll Cardiol* 31:451–459, 1998.
37. Weisfogel GM, Batsford WP, Paulay KL, et al: Sinus node re-entrant tachycardia in man. *Am Heart J* 90:295–304, 1975.
38. Narula OS: Sinus node re-entry: a mechanism for supraventricular tachycardia. *Circulation* 50:1114–1128, 1974.
39. Griffith MJ, Garratt CJ, Ward DE, et al: The effects of adenosine on sinus node reentrant tachycardia. *Clin Cardiol* 12:409–411, 1989.
40. Sanders WE, Jr, Sorrentino RA, Greenfield RA, et al: Catheter ablation of sinoatrial node reentrant tachycardia. *J Am Coll Cardiol* 23:926–934, 1994.
41. Jais P, Shah DC, Haissaguerre M, et al: Mapping and ablation of left atrial flutters. *Circulation* 101:2928–2934, 2000.
42. Josephson ME. *Clinical cardiac electrophysiology: techniques and interpretations*, ed 3, Philadelphia, 2002, Lippincott Williams & Wilkins.
43. Olgin JE, Kalman JM, Fitzpatrick AP, et al: Role of right atrial endocardial structures as barriers to conduction during human type I atrial flutter. Activation and entrainment mapping guided by intracardiac echocardiography. *Circulation* 92:1839–1848, 1995.
44. Kalman JM, Olgin JE, Saxon LA, et al: Activation and entrainment mapping defines the tricuspid annulus as the anterior barrier in typical atrial flutter. *Circulation* 94:398–406, 1996.
45. Kalman JM, Olgin JE, Saxon LA, et al: Electrocardiographic and electrophysiologic characterization of atypical atrial flutter in man: use of activation and entrainment mapping and implications for catheter ablation. *J Cardiovasc Electrophysiol* 8:121–144, 1997.
46. Olshansky B, Okumura K, Hess PG, et al: Demonstration of an area of slow conduction in human atrial flutter. *J Am Coll Cardiol* 16:1639–1648, 1990.
47. Nakagawa H, Lazzara R, Khastgir T, et al: Role of the tricuspid annulus and the eustachian valve/ridge on atrial flutter. Relevance to catheter ablation of the septal isthmus and a new technique for rapid identification of ablation success. *Circulation* 94:407–424, 1996.
48. Cheng J, Cabeen WR, Jr, Scheinman MM: Right atrial flutter due to lower loop reentry: mechanism and anatomic substrates. *Circulation* 99:1700–1705, 1999.
49. Poty H, Saoudi N, Nair M, et al: Radiofrequency catheter ablation of atrial flutter. Further insights into the various types of isthmus block: application to ablation during sinus rhythm. *Circulation* 94:3204–3213, 1996.
50. Schwartzman D, Callans DJ, Gottlieb CD, et al: Conduction block in the inferior vena caval-tricuspid valve isthmus: association with outcome of radiofrequency ablation of type I atrial flutter. *J Am Coll Cardiol* 28:1519–1531, 1996.
51. Cosio FG, Arribas F, Lopez-Gil M, et al: Radiofrequency ablation of atrial flutter. *J Cardiovasc Electrophysiol* 7:60–70, 1996.
52. Wood F, Wolferth G, Geckler G: Histologic demonstration of accessory muscular connections between auricle and ventricle in a case of short PR interval and prolonged QRS complex. *Am Heart J* 25:454, 1943.
53. James TN: Morphology of the human atrioventricular node, with remarks pertinent to its electrophysiology. *Am Heart J* 62:756–771, 1961.
54. Mahaim I: Kent's fibers and the A-V paraspecific conduction through the upper connections of the bundle of His-Tawara. *Am Heart J* 33:651–653, 1947.
55. Arruda MS, McClelland JH, Wang X, et al: Development and validation of an ECG algorithm for identifying accessory pathway ablation site in Wolff-Parkinson-White syndrome. *J Cardiovasc Electrophysiol* 9:2–12, 1998.
56. Fitzpatrick AP, Gonzales RP, Lesh MD, et al: New algorithm for the localization of accessory atrioventricular connections using a baseline electrocardiogram. *J Am Coll Cardiol* 23:107–116, 1994.

57. Tai CT, Chen SA, Chiang CE, et al: Electrocardiographic and electrophysiologic characteristics of anteroseptal, midseptal, and para-Hisian accessory pathways. Implication for radiofrequency catheter ablation. *Chest* 109:730–740, 1996.
58. Chiang CE, Chen SA, Teo WS, et al: An accurate stepwise electrocardiographic algorithm for localization of accessory pathways in patients with Wolff-Parkinson-White syndrome from a comprehensive analysis of delta waves and R/S ratio during sinus rhythm. *Am J Cardiol* 76:40–46, 1995.
59. Cosio FG, Anderson RH, Kuck KH, et al: Living anatomy of the atrioventricular junctions. A guide to electrophysiologic mapping. A Consensus Statement from the Cardiac Nomenclature Study Group, Working Group of Arrhythmias, European Society of Cardiology, and the Task Force on Cardiac Nomenclature from NASPE. *Circulation* 100:e31–e37, 1999.
60. Lesh MD, Van Hare GF, Scheinman MM, et al: Comparison of the retrograde and transseptal methods for ablation of left free wall accessory pathways. *J Am Coll Cardiol* 22:542–549, 1993.
61. Valderrabano M, Cesario DA, Ji S, et al: Percutaneous epicardial mapping during ablation of difficult accessory pathways as an alternative to cardiac surgery. *Heart Rhythm* 1:311–316, 2004.
62. Sosa E, Scanavacca M, d'Avila A, et al: Nonsurgical transthoracic epicardial catheter ablation to treat recurrent ventricular tachycardia occurring late after myocardial infarction. *J Am Coll Cardiol* 35:1442–1449, 2000.
63. Calkins H, Yong P, Miller JM, et al: Catheter ablation of accessory pathways, atrioventricular nodal reentrant tachycardia, and the atrioventricular junction: final results of a prospective, multicenter clinical trial. The Atakr Multicenter Investigators Group. *Circulation* 99:262–270, 1999.
64. Miller JM, Kienzle MG, Harken AH, et al: Subendocardial resection for ventricular tachycardia: predictors of surgical success. *Circulation* 70:624–631, 1984.
65. Garan H, Nguyen K, McGovern B, et al: Perioperative and long-term results after electrophysiologically directed ventricular surgery for recurrent ventricular tachycardia. *J Am Coll Cardiol* 8:201–209, 1986.
66. Haines DE, Lerman BB, Kron IL, et al: Surgical ablation of ventricular tachycardia with sequential map-guided subendocardial resection: electrophysiologic assessment and long-term follow-up. *Circulation* 77:131–141, 1988.
67. Horowitz LN, Harken AH, Kastor JA, et al: Ventricular resection guided by epicardial and endocardial mapping for treatment of recurrent ventricular tachycardia. *N Engl J Med* 302:589–593, 1980.
68. Miller MA, Dukkipati SR, Mittnacht AJ, et al: Activation and entrainment mapping of hemodynamically unstable ventricular tachycardia using a percutaneous left ventricular assist device. *J Am Coll Cardiol* 58:1363–1371, 2011.
69. Miller MA, Dukkipati SR, Koruth JS, et al: How to perform ventricular tachycardia ablation with a percutaneous left ventricular assist device. *Heart Rhythm* 9:1168–1176, 2012.
70. Stevenson WG, Khan H, Sager P, et al: Identification of reentry circuit sites during catheter mapping and radiofrequency ablation of ventricular tachycardia late after myocardial infarction. *Circulation* 88:1647–1670, 1993.
71. Josephson ME, Horowitz LN, Waxman HL, et al: Sustained ventricular tachycardia: role of the 12-lead electrocardiogram in localizing site of origin. *Circulation* 64:257–272, 1981.
72. Miller JM, Marchlinski FE, Buxton AE, et al: Relationship between the 12-lead electrocardiogram during ventricular tachycardia and endocardial site of origin in patients with coronary artery disease. *Circulation* 77:759–766, 1988.
73. Kuchar DL, Ruskin JN, Garan H: Electrocardiographic localization of the site of origin of ventricular tachycardia in patients with prior myocardial infarction. *J Am Coll Cardiol* 13:893–903, 1989.
74. El-Shalakany A, Hadjis T, Papageorgiou P, et al: Entrainment/mapping criteria for the prediction of termination of ventricular tachycardia by single radiofrequency lesion in patients with coronary artery disease. *Circulation* 99:2283–2289, 1999.
75. Stevenson WG, Sager PT, Friedman PL: Entrainment techniques for mapping atrial and ventricular tachycardias. *J Cardiovasc Electrophysiol* 6:201–216, 1995.
76. Stevenson WG, Friedman PL, Sager PT, et al: Exploring postinfarction reentrant ventricular tachycardia with entrainment mapping. *J Am Coll Cardiol* 29:1180–1189, 1997.
77. Khan HH, Stevenson WG: Activation times in and adjacent to reentry circuits during entrainment: implications for mapping ventricular tachycardia. *Am Heart J* 127:833–842, 1994.
78. Nitta T, Schuessler RB, Mitsuno M, et al: Return cycle mapping after entrainment of ventricular tachycardia. *Circulation* 97:1164–1175, 1998.
79. Vassallo JA, Cassidy D, Simson MB, et al: Relation of late potentials to site of origin of ventricular tachycardia associated with coronary heart disease. *Am J Cardiol* 55:985–989, 1985.
80. Cassidy DM, Vassallo JA, Miller JM, et al: Endocardial catheter mapping in patients in sinus rhythm: relationship to underlying heart disease and ventricular arrhythmias. *Circulation* 73:645–652, 1986.
81. Marchlinski FE, Callans DJ, Gottlieb CD, et al: Linear ablation lesions for control of unmappable ventricular tachycardia in patients with ischemic and nonischemic cardiomyopathy. *Circulation* 101:1288–1296, 2000.
82. Wrobleski D, Houghtaling C, Josephson ME, et al: Use of electrogram characteristics during sinus rhythm to delineate the endocardial scar in a porcine model of healed myocardial infarction. *J Cardiovasc Electrophysiol* 14:524–529, 2003.
83. Reddy VY, Reynolds MR, Neuzil P, et al: Prophylactic catheter ablation for the prevention of defibrillator therapy. *N Engl J Med* 357:2657–2665, 2007.
84. Poole JE, Johnson GW, Hellkamp AS, et al: Prognostic importance of defibrillator shocks in patients with heart failure. *N Engl J Med* 359:1009–1017, 2008.
85. Della Bella P, Brugada J, Zeppenfeld K, et al: Epicardial ablation for ventricular tachycardia: a European multicenter study. *Circ Arrhythm Electrophysiol* 4:653–659, 2011.
85a. Ellis ER, Shvilkin A, Josephson ME: Nonreentrant ventricular arrhythmias in patients with structural heart disease unrelated to abnormal myocardial substrate. *Heart Rhythm* 11(6):946–952, 2014.
86. Movsowitz C, Schwartzman D, Callans DJ, et al: Idiopathic right ventricular outflow tract tachycardia: narrowing the anatomic location for successful ablation. *Am Heart J* 131:930–936, 1996.
87. Buxton AE, Waxman HL, Marchlinski FE, et al: Right ventricular tachycardia: clinical and electrophysiologic characteristics. *Circulation* 68:917–927, 1983.
88. Callans DJ, Menz V, Schwartzman D, et al: Repetitive monomorphic tachycardia from the left ventricular outflow tract: electrocardiographic patterns consistent with a left ventricular site of origin. *J Am Coll Cardiol* 29:1023–1027, 1997.
89. Yamada T, McElderry HT, Doppalapudi H, et al: Idiopathic ventricular arrhythmias originating from the aortic root prevalence, electrocardiographic and electrophysiologic characteristics, and results of radiofrequency catheter ablation. *J Am Coll Cardiol* 52:139–147, 2008.
90. Tada H, Ito S, Naito S, et al: Idiopathic ventricular arrhythmia arising from the mitral annulus: a distinct subgroup of idiopathic ventricular arrhythmias. *J Am Coll Cardiol* 45:877–886, 2005.
91. Varma N, Josephson ME: Therapy of "idiopathic" ventricular tachycardia. *J Cardiovasc Electrophysiol* 8:104–116, 1997.
92. Kamakura S, Shimizu W, Matsuo K, et al: Localization of optimal ablation site of idiopathic ventricular tachycardia from right and left ventricular outflow tract by body surface ECG. *Circulation* 98:1525–1533, 1998.
93. Coggins DL, Lee RJ, Sweeney J, et al: Radiofrequency catheter ablation as a cure for idiopathic tachycardia of both left and right ventricular origin. *J Am Coll Cardiol* 23:1333–1341, 1994.
94. Klein LS, Shih HT, Hackett FK, et al: Radiofrequency catheter ablation of ventricular tachycardia in patients without structural heart disease. *Circulation* 85:1666–1674, 1992.
95. Gerstenfeld EP, Dixit S, Callans DJ, et al: Quantitative comparison of spontaneous and paced 12-lead electrocardiogram during right ventricular outflow tract ventricular tachycardia. *J Am Coll Cardiol* 41:2046–2053, 2003.
96. Belhassen B, Rotmensch HH, Laniado S: Response of recurrent sustained ventricular tachycardia to verapamil. *Br Heart J* 46:679–682, 1981.
97. Nakagawa H, Beckman KJ, McClelland JH, et al: Radiofrequency catheter ablation of idiopathic left ventricular tachycardia guided by a Purkinje potential. *Circulation* 88:2607–2617, 1993.
98. Nogami A: Purkinje-related arrhythmias part I: monomorphic ventricular tachycardias. *Pacing Clin Electrophysiol* 34(5):624–650, 2011.

99. Ouyang F, Cappato R, Ernst S, et al: Electroanatomic substrate of idiopathic left ventricular tachycardia: unidirectional block and macroreentry within the Purkinje network. *Circulation* 105:462–469, 2002.
100. Scheinman MM, Morady F, Hess DS, et al: Catheter-induced ablation of the atrioventricular junction to control refractory supraventricular arrhythmias. *JAMA* 248:851–855, 1982.
101. Morady F, Calkins H, Langberg JJ, et al: A prospective randomized comparison of direct current and radiofrequency ablation of the atrioventricular junction. *J Am Coll Cardiol* 21:102–109, 1993.
102. Kalbfleisch SJ, Williamson B, Man KC, et al: A randomized comparison of the right- and left-sided approaches to ablation of the atrioventricular junction. *Am J Cardiol* 72:1406–1410, 1993.
103. Dizon J, Blitzer M, Rubin D, et al: Time dependent changes in duration of ventricular repolarization after AV node ablation: insights into the possible mechanism of postprocedural sudden death. *Pacing Clin Electrophysiol* 23:1539–1544, 2000.
104. Geelen P, Brugada J, Andries E, et al: Ventricular fibrillation and sudden death after radiofrequency catheter ablation of the atrioventricular junction. *Pacing Clin Electrophysiol* 20:343–348, 1997.
105. Nowinski K, Gadler F, Jensen-Urstad M, et al: Transient proarrhythmic state following atrioventricular junction radiofrequency ablation: pathophysiologic mechanisms and recommendations for management. *Am J Med* 113:596–602, 2002.
106. Haissaguerre M, Jais P, Shah DC, et al: Spontaneous initiation of atrial fibrillation by ectopic beats originating in the pulmonary veins. *N Engl J Med* 339:659–666, 1998.
107. Robbins IM, Colvin EV, Doyle TP, et al: Pulmonary vein stenosis after catheter ablation of atrial fibrillation. *Circulation* 98:1769–1775, 1998.
108. Essebag V, Wylie JV, Jr, Reynolds MR, et al: Bi-directional electrical pulmonary vein isolation as an endpoint for ablation of paroxysmal atrial fibrillation. *J Interv Card Electrophysiol* 17:111–117, 2006.
109. Verma A, Marrouche NF, Natale A: Pulmonary vein antrum isolation: intracardiac echocardiography-guided technique. *J Cardiovasc Electrophysiol* 15:1335–1340, 2004.
110. Pappone C, Santinelli V, Manguso F, et al: Pulmonary vein denervation enhances long-term benefit after circumferential ablation for paroxysmal atrial fibrillation. *Circulation* 109:327–334, 2004.
111. Lin WS, Tai CT, Hsieh MH, et al: Catheter ablation of paroxysmal atrial fibrillation initiated by non-pulmonary vein ectopy. *Circulation* 107:3176–3183, 2003.
112. Nademanee K, McKenzie J, Kosar E, et al: A new approach for catheter ablation of atrial fibrillation: mapping of the electrophysiologic substrate. *J Am Coll Cardiol* 43:2044–2053, 2004.
113. Karch MR, Zrenner B, Deisenhofer I, et al: Freedom from atrial tachyarrhythmias after catheter ablation of atrial fibrillation: a randomized comparison between 2 current ablation strategies. *Circulation* 111:2875–2880, 2005.
114. Oral H, Scharf C, Chugh A, et al: Catheter ablation for paroxysmal atrial fibrillation: segmental pulmonary vein ostial ablation versus left atrial ablation. *Circulation* 108:2355–2360, 2003.
115. Calkins H, Brugada J, Packer DL, et al: HRS/EHRA/ECAS expert Consensus Statement on catheter and surgical ablation of atrial fibrillation: recommendations for personnel, policy, procedures and follow-up. A report of the Heart Rhythm Society (HRS) Task Force on catheter and surgical ablation of atrial fibrillation. *Heart Rhythm* 4:816–861, 2007.
116. Arruda M, Natale A: The adjunctive role of nonpulmonary venous ablation in the cure of atrial fibrillation. *J Cardiovasc Electrophysiol* 17(Suppl 3):S37–S43, 2006.
117. Gerstenfeld EP, Callans DJ, Dixit S, et al: Mechanisms of organized left atrial tachycardias occurring after pulmonary vein isolation. *Circulation* 110:1351–1357, 2004.
118. Cummings JE, Schweikert R, Saliba W, et al: Left atrial flutter following pulmonary vein antrum isolation with radiofrequency energy: linear lesions or repeat isolation. *J Cardiovasc Electrophysiol* 16:293–297, 2005.
119. Takahashi Y, Jais P, Hocini M, et al: Shortening of fibrillatory cycle length in the pulmonary vein during vagal excitation. *J Am Coll Cardiol* 47:774–780, 2006.
120. Wann LS, Curtis AB, Ellenbogen KA, et al: Management of patients with atrial fibrillation (compilation of 2006 ACCF/AHA/ESC and 2011 ACCF/AHA/HRS recommendations): a report of the American College of Cardiology/American Heart Association Task Force on practice guidelines. *Circulation* 127:1916–1926, 2013.
121. Noheria A, Kumar A, Wylie JV, Jr, et al: Catheter ablation vs antiarrhythmic drug therapy for atrial fibrillation: a systematic review. *Arch Intern Med* 168:581–586, 2008.
122. Wazni OM, Marrouche NF, Martin DO, et al: Radiofrequency ablation vs antiarrhythmic drugs as first-line treatment of symptomatic atrial fibrillation: a randomized trial. *JAMA* 293:2634–2640, 2005.
123. Cappato R, Calkins H, Chen SA, et al: Worldwide survey on the methods, efficacy, and safety of catheter ablation for human atrial fibrillation. *Circulation* 111:1100–1105, 2005.
124. Essebag V, Baldessin F, Reynolds MR, et al: Non-inducibility post-pulmonary vein isolation achieving exit block predicts freedom from atrial fibrillation. *Eur Heart J* 26:2550–2555, 2005.
125. Tilz RR, Rillig A, Thum AM, et al: Catheter ablation of long-standing persistent atrial fibrillation: 5-year outcomes of the Hamburg Sequential Ablation Strategy. *J Am Coll Cardiol* 60:1921–1929, 2012.
126. Brockenbrough EC, Braunwald E, Ross J, Jr: Transseptal left heart catheterization. A review of 450 studies and description of an improved technic. *Circulation* 25:15–21, 1962.
127. Pappone C, Vicedomini G, Manguso F, et al: Robotic magnetic navigation for atrial fibrillation ablation. *J Am Coll Cardiol* 47:1390–1400, 2006.
128. Saliba W, Reddy VY, Wazni O, et al: Atrial fibrillation ablation using a robotic catheter remote control system: initial human experience and long-term follow-up results. *J Am Coll Cardiol* 51:2407–2411, 2008.
129. Pappone C, Augello G, Gugliotta F, et al: Robotic and magnetic navigation for atrial fibrillation ablation. How and why? *Expert Rev Med Devices* 4:885–894, 2007.
130. Kojodjojo P, O'Neill MD, Lim PB, et al: Pulmonary venous isolation by antral ablation with a large cryoballoon for treatment of paroxysmal and persistent atrial fibrillation: medium-term outcomes and non-randomised comparison with pulmonary venous isolation by radiofrequency ablation. *Heart* 96:1379–1384, 2010.
131. Mansour M, Forleo GB, Pappalardo A, et al: Combined use of cryoballoon and focal open-irrigation radiofrequency ablation for treatment of persistent atrial fibrillation: results from a pilot study. *Heart Rhythm* 7:452–458, 2010.

CHAPTER 87

SURGICAL TREATMENT OF CARDIAC ARRHYTHMIAS

Christopher P. Lawrance • Matthew C. Henn • Ralph J. Damiano, Jr.

CHAPTER OUTLINE

Current nonpharmacologic treatments for cardiac arrhythmias include catheter ablation, implantation of pacemakers and cardioverter-defibrillator devices, and surgery. These modalities can be used to treat essentially all supraventricular and ventricular tachyarrhythmias. Although the indications for surgical intervention have narrowed, surgery remains an important treatment option, especially for the most common of all arrhythmias, atrial fibrillation.

ATRIAL FIBRILLATION

Background

Atrial fibrillation (AF) is present in up to 2% of the general population and in approximately 10% of patients older than 60 years, making it the most common form of sustained cardiac arrhythmia.[1-5] From 1993 to 2007 the prevalence in Medicare patients 65 years and older has increased 5% each year both because of our aging population and for other reasons that remain poorly defined.[6] Consequently, there has been a 66% increase in hospital admissions for AF over the past 20 years. It is estimated that AF will affect up to 12 million people in the United States by the year 2050.[7] Its financial burden is significant, with a global annual cost of $8705 per patient annually, and $6 billion in the United States alone.[8] Although AF is frequently considered to be an innocuous arrhythmia, it can be associated with significant morbidity and mortality because of its three detrimental sequelae: (1) palpitations, which cause the patient discomfort and anxiety; (2) loss of synchronous atrioventricular contraction, which compromises cardiac hemodynamics, resulting in varying degrees of ventricular dysfunction; and (3) stasis of blood flow in the left atrium, which can result in thromboembolism and stroke.[9-13] Separate from the direct cardiac effects, the most feared complications of AF stem from the development of thrombus in the left atrium. These thrombi can embolize and lead to myocardial infarction, acute mesenteric ischemia, and stroke. Stroke, in particular, is three to five times more likely to occur in patients with AF when compared to patients in sinus rhythm.[14] Conversely, 20% to 30% of all acute stroke patients are found to be in AF.[15-17] Antiarrhythmic medications have largely been unsuccessful thus far, with most series showing the efficacy of antiarrhythmic medications to be less than 50%.[18-20] Antithrombotic drugs for AF carry with them various complications, including an annual risk of major bleeding up to 3%, rising even higher in older adults.[17,21,22] AF also independently increases mortality rates. Using data from the Framingham Heart Study, Benjamin and coworkers established the risk factor–adjusted odds ratio for death in men and women with AF as 1.5 and 1.9, respectively.[23]

Classification of Atrial Fibrillation

AF can be classified in various ways, but the classification system published jointly by the American Heart Association, the American College of Cardiology, and the Heart Rhythm Society is the most widely used.[24] This system defines AF as either paroxysmal or persistent. When a patient has had two or more episodes, AF is considered recurrent. If recurrent AF terminates spontaneously, it is designated paroxysmal, but if it is sustained beyond 7 days, it is termed persistent. Termination by pharmacologic therapy or electrical cardioversion before expected spontaneous termination does not change the designation *persistent*. In a recent consensus statement sponsored by the Heart Rhythm Society, the definition of *permanent* was changed to include only cases in which cardioversion has failed, clarifying that patients with long-standing AF might still be cured by intervention. In those cases, *permanent* has been replaced with the term *long-standing AF* when the duration is more than 1 year.[25]

Electrophysiology of Atrial Fibrillation

AF is characterized by the irregular activation of the atria and an accompanying irregular ventricular response. Activation of the atria during AF can exhibit two different patterns. One pattern consists of a stable source, either a focal trigger or a small reentrant circuit, with fibrillatory conduction away from the source. The other pattern is characterized by multiple changing sources or reentrant circuits. The specific mechanism may change over time in a particular patient. Work from our laboratory obtained from patients undergoing intraoperative mapping before arrhythmia surgery revealed that the source of AF was not stable in almost half of the patients, even moving from one atrium to the other.[26]

Four substrates determine whether AF is initiated and sustained: (1) a trigger, usually a premature depolarization or runs of focal ectopic depolarizations; (2) the refractory period of the atria and its magnitude and spatial distribution; (3) the conduction velocity and its magnitude and anisotropic spread; and (4) the geometry or anatomy, both macroscopic and microscopic. Whatever the pathologic process (e.g., valvular disease, heart failure, ischemia, tachycardia, pericarditis, or inflammation) is, the changes that occur affect one or more of these four factors.[27]

The surgical treatment of AF is directed at alteration of the geometry and anatomy needed to support AF. Non-reentrant mechanisms, such as abnormal automaticity and triggered activity, are important for the generation of premature beats, which act as a trigger for reentry but may also be involved in maintaining AF. The premature beats interact with the underlying distribution of refractory periods. As the distribution becomes more inhomogeneous, unidirectional block can occur. This is a necessary condition for the initiation of reentry. When unidirectional block occurs, a reentrant arrhythmia will occur only if a critical mass of tissue is present. The critical mass is determined by the tissue geometry, the magnitude of refractory periods, and the conduction velocity. The amount of tissue required to support a reentrant circuit is defined by the equation $WL = CV \times RP$ (wavelength = conduction velocity × refractory period). If either CV or RP decreases, the amount of tissue needed to sustain AF decreases, and the probability of a patient's having an arrhythmia increases.[28] Interventional approaches attempt to alter one of these substrates. However, any treatment strategy has the potential to affect the other substrates that cause AF. For example, incisions or ablations not only affect conduction, but they also alter the geometry of the atria, decrease viable myocardial mass, and can denervate regions of the atria, which alters refractory periods.[28]

A great deal of emphasis has been placed on the role of the pulmonary veins in the triggering of AF. Paroxysmal AF often originates in the pulmonary veins.[29] In humans, the anatomy of the pulmonary veins is variable, with electrically excitable cardiac muscle extending 1 to 4 cm beyond the ostium of the veins.[30] Developmental biological studies suggest that pacemaker tissue may be present in the pulmonary veins.[31] Another potential mechanism of focal activation is afterdepolarization.[32] Intraoperative mapping studies have shown ectopic atrial beats originating from the region of the pulmonary veins.[27] Biatrial mapping studies by Schmitt and coworkers[33] have shown that the premature beats that trigger AF were located in the pulmonary veins 53% of the time and in the posterior atrium in another 29% of cases.

Successful cure of AF is achieved in some patients by the isolation of the pulmonary veins.[29] Furthermore, if triggers of AF were outside the pulmonary veins but other substrates that sustain AF were within the veins, AF would be prevented with pulmonary vein isolation. The failure to cure AF by isolating only the pulmonary veins in some patients, especially those with long-standing AF, suggests that other anatomic triggers or more complicated mechanisms may be involved in these cases. Using intraoperative mapping in patients with mitral valve disease, Nitta and colleagues[34] determined that atrial focal activation is one mechanism of AF. Caution should be taken in interpreting various interventional studies, whether catheter ablation or surgery, as to whether they imply an underlying mechanism involved in a patient's AF. Most intraoperative and catheter mapping systems do not have the spatial resolution within the pulmonary veins to separate reentrant from non-reentrant mechanisms. Therefore, even though "focal" fibrillation may be reported from investigational mapping, this does not rule out reentry as a mechanism underlying the arrhythmia. Claims of cure by pulmonary vein isolation alone must be tempered by the knowledge that the "pulmonary vein isolation" intervention actually incorporates much more than just the pulmonary veins. Commonly, the pulmonary veins, the adjacent atrial muscle, and the muscle in the oblique sinus between the veins are ablated during catheter-based pulmonary vein isolation. This area is more than one third of the left atrium. This large area of ablation substantially reduces the critical mass needed to sustain AF and may incorporate other non–pulmonary vein substrates of AF.

The definitions of paroxysmal, persistent, and long-standing AF do not imply a specific mechanism. Even though clinical results have shown that pulmonary vein isolation is effective 70% to 80% of the time in paroxysmal AF, it is clear that the pulmonary veins are not the only substrate driving AF 20% to 30% of the time.[26] Similarly, in persistent AF, pulmonary vein isolation alone is successful in only a small number of patients.[25] Human mapping data from our laboratory did not show any significant difference in mechanism between paroxysmal and persistent AF.[26] Current diagnostic technologies rarely allow a preoperative delineation of mechanism. However, electrophysiologic studies may allow physicians to identify triggers of AF in some patients.[26] Because AF is a complex arrhythmia, mapping requires a high density of closely placed electrodes as well as a sophisticated mapping and signal processing system to define the particular mechanism in an individual patient. In our experience, intraoperative mapping has not been useful in providing real-time information during surgery. The analysis of this complex arrhythmia is time-consuming and difficult. Therefore, the traditional surgical algorithm of obtaining preoperative or intraoperative mapping data and using this information to guide the specific surgical technique, as was done with arrhythmias such as Wolff-Parkinson-White syndrome, has not been feasible for AF. Mapping techniques are currently being developed that may allow interventionalists to customize the lesion set to the specific underlying mechanism.[26,34-36]

One particularly promising technique is electrocardiographic imaging.[37] This technology allows AF to be mapped noninvasively in the awake patient by recording signals from the body surface and solving the inverse equation. This would delineate the mechanism before the proposed intervention and may allow physicians to triage patients to the most effective procedure.

Medical Treatment

Results with medical therapy alone for AF have been disappointing. Antiarrhythmic drugs have had limited long-term efficacy in converting AF to normal sinus rhythm and have significant and sometimes fatal side effects.[38-43] The goal of pharmacotherapy is therefore often shifted from *rhythm* to *rate* control, which involves slowing the ventricular response rate to AF, thus avoiding the development of rate-related cardiomyopathy and symptoms such as palpitations. The Atrial Fibrillation Follow-up Investigation of Rhythm Management (AFFIRM) study[44,45] showed that management with rhythm control did not have any survival benefit over a rate control strategy in anticoagulated patients with AF.[46,47] Furthermore, rate control strategy may potentially have advantages over rhythm control, such as a lower risk for adverse side effects.[46]

Rate control alone clearly has disadvantages. Although the ventricular response rate can often be controlled pharmacologically, the atria are still in fibrillation. With persistent AF, two of the three detrimental sequelae associated with AF persist. In patients with baseline cardiac dysfunction, the absence of atrial "kick" often can result in worsening symptoms of congestive heart failure. Most important, patients with AF are at risk for developing thromboembolism, requiring indefinite anticoagulation with warfarin or one of the newer anticoagulants, such as dabigatran, rivaroxaban, or apixaban.[48] The use of warfarin is associated with a major complication rate of approximately 2% per year.[49-51] Although these newer anticoagulants decrease the risk of intracerebral hemorrhage without the need for routine coagulation monitoring, they have the same effectiveness as warfarin in the reduction of thromboembolism.[48]

Despite the results from the AFFIRM trial supporting no difference in long-term outcome between rhythm and rate control, there are many clinically meaningful advantages of being in normal sinus rhythm. These advantages include increased exercise tolerance, no need for anticoagulation, decreased palpitations, and prevention of atrial remodeling.[45,52] Most important, when time-dependent variables were evaluated in the AFFIRM trial, the presence of sinus rhythm was associated with a significantly decreased risk of death (hazard ratio = 0.53; $P < 0.0001$).[53] Thus, the AFFIRM trial demonstrated that antiarrhythmic drugs are detrimental and that normal sinus rhythm is beneficial in this population of patients, suggesting a role for nonpharmacologic restoration of sinus rhythm.

Historical Aspects of Surgery for Atrial Fibrillation

Because of the inadequacy of medical therapy for AF, several procedures were developed in the 1980s aimed at treatment of AF. Most of these were abandoned because of their inability to eliminate all three of the detrimental sequelae associated with AF.[54-56] Nevertheless, they helped physicians gain fundamental knowledge about the mechanism of AF and laid a foundation for the development of the Cox-Maze procedure and its subsequent iterations. The Cox-Maze procedure is recognized today as the gold standard for surgical cure of AF. The next section briefly describes these various surgical procedures developed in an attempt to cure AF.

Left Atrial Isolation Procedure. In 1980, Dr. James L. Cox and his group developed the left atrial isolation procedure, which confined AF to the left atrium, thus restoring the remainder of the heart to normal sinus rhythm.[56] This procedure had the advantage of restoring normal atrioventricular rhythm without requiring a permanent pacemaker. Because the sinoatrial node, atrioventricular node, and internodal conduction pathways are located in the right atrium and interatrial septum, the left atrial isolation procedure did not interfere with normal atrioventricular conduction.

Electrical isolation of the left atrium also unexpectedly restored normal cardiac hemodynamics. This occurred because the right atrium and the right ventricle contracted in synchrony after the procedure, providing a normal right-sided cardiac output that was then delivered to the left side of the heart. Although the left atrium was isolated, the left ventricle adapted immediately to the normal right-sided cardiac output and delivered a normal forward cardiac output.

By confining AF to the left atrium only, the left atrial isolation procedure eliminated two of the three detrimental sequelae of AF: irregular heartbeat and compromised cardiac hemodynamics. However, because the electrically isolated left atrium remained in AF, this procedure did not eliminate the risk of thromboembolism. It also did not address patients in whom the AF originated in the right atrium.

Catheter Ablation of the Atrioventricular Node–His Bundle Complex. In 1982, Scheinman and colleagues[57] described the catheter fulguration of the His bundle, which controlled the irregular cardiac rhythm associated with AF and other refractory supraventricular arrhythmias. Similar to the left atrial isolation procedure, this procedure electrically isolated the arrhythmia to the atria. However, ablation of the His bundle necessitated implanting a permanent ventricular pacemaker to restore normal ventricular rhythm.

Unfortunately, His bundle ablation eliminated only the irregular heart beat. Both atria still remained in fibrillation, and the vulnerability to thromboembolism was unaffected. Atrioventricular contraction remained desynchronized, compromising cardiac hemodynamics. Despite its drawbacks, this remains a common treatment for medically refractory AF in patients not considered good candidates for a more curative interventional procedure.

Corridor Procedure. In 1985, Guiraudon and associates[58] introduced the corridor procedure for the treatment of AF. This was an operation that isolated a strip of atrial septum harboring both the sinoatrial node and the atrioventricular node, thereby allowing the sinoatrial node to drive the ventricles. This procedure corrected the irregular heart beat associated with AF, but both atria either remained in fibrillation or developed their own asynchronous intrinsic rhythm because they were isolated from the septal "corridor." The atria were also isolated from their respective ventricles, thereby precluding the possibility of atrioventricular synchrony. The corridor procedure was abandoned because neither the hemodynamic compromise nor the risk of thromboembolism associated with AF was addressed.

Atrial Transection Procedure. All three surgical procedures developed in the early 1980s had attempted to isolate and to confine AF to a certain region of the atria, stopping it from propagating its effects to the ventricles. None of these procedures was targeted to cure AF.

In 1985, Cox's group described for the first time a series of experiments that attempted to cure AF in a canine model.[59] After a number of experiments, it was found that a single long incision across both atria and down into the septum cured AF. This "atrial transection" procedure prevented the induction and maintenance of AF or atrial flutter in canines.[60] Unfortunately, this procedure was not successful in its clinical application.

Development of the Cox-Maze Procedure

The first successful curative surgical procedure for the treatment of AF was introduced clinically in 1987 by the team led by Dr. James L. Cox at Washington University in St. Louis.[60-62] The Cox-Maze procedure was designed to interrupt the macro-reentrant circuits that were thought to be responsible for AF, thereby precluding the ability of the atrium to flutter or fibrillate (Fig. 87-1). In contrast to previous procedures, the Maze procedure successfully restored both atrioventricular synchrony and a regular heart beat, thus decreasing the risk of thromboembolism and stroke.[63] The operation involved creating myriad incisions across both the right and left atria. The surgical incisions were placed so that the sinoatrial node could "drive" the propagation of the sinus impulse throughout both atria. It also allowed all of the atrial myocardium to be activated, resulting in preservation of atrial transport function in most patients.[64]

After almost a decade of basic research, the Maze I procedure was introduced in 1987, only to be soon modified to become the Maze II procedure because of late chronotropic incompetence and a high incidence of pacemaker implantations. The Maze II procedure, however, proved to be too technically difficult to perform. It was therefore further modified and renamed the Maze III procedure (Fig. 87-2).[65,66]

During the 1990s, the Cox-Maze III procedure became the gold standard for the surgical treatment of AF. In a long-term study of patients who had the Cox-Maze procedure, 97% of the patients at late follow-up were free of AF.[67] Similar results have been reproduced by other institutions around the world.[68-70]

Surgical Ablation Technology

Despite its proven efficacy, the Cox-Maze III procedure did not gain widespread acceptance. Few cardiac surgeons were willing to add the procedure to coronary revascularization or valve procedures because of its complexity and technical difficulty. In an attempt to simplify the operation, groups around the world have replaced the incisions of the traditional cut-and-sew Cox-Maze III procedure with linear lines of ablation.[71] These linear lines of ablation have been created by use of a variety of energy sources, including radiofrequency energy, microwave, cryoablation, laser, and high-frequency ultrasound.

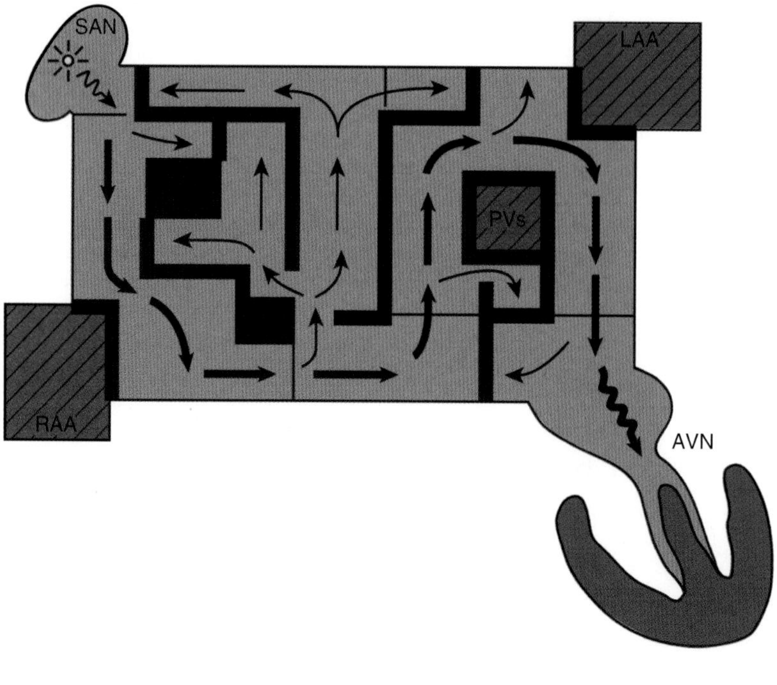

FIGURE 87-1 ■ Original conceptual design of the Cox-Maze procedure for atrial fibrillation. Both atrial appendages were excised, and the pulmonary veins were isolated. *AVN,* Atrioventricular node; *LAA,* left atrial appendage; *PVs,* pulmonary veins; *RAA,* right atrial appendage; *SAN,* sinoatrial node. (From Cox JL, Canavan TE, Schuessler RB, et al: The surgical treatment of atrial fibrillation. II. Intraoperative electrophysiologic mapping and description of the electrophysiologic basis of atrial flutter and atrial fibrillation. *J Thorac Cardiovasc Surg* 101:406–426, 1991.)

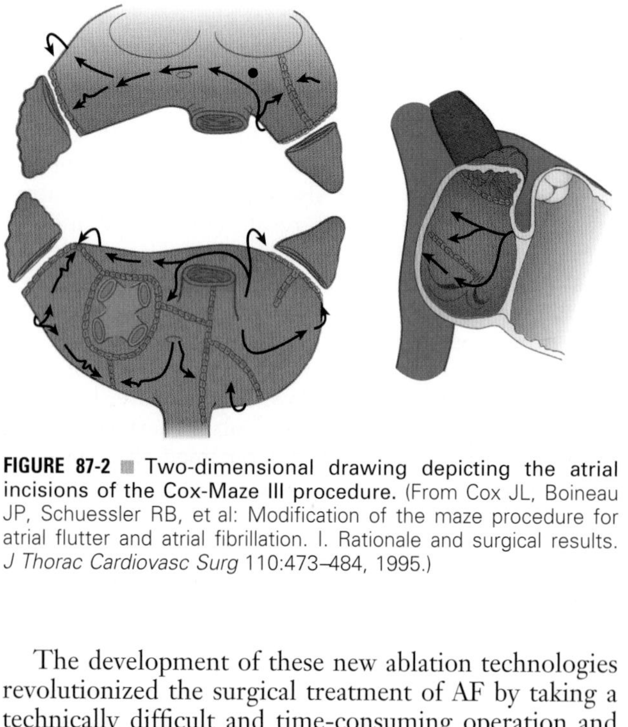

FIGURE 87-2 ■ Two-dimensional drawing depicting the atrial incisions of the Cox-Maze III procedure. (From Cox JL, Boineau JP, Schuessler RB, et al: Modification of the maze procedure for atrial flutter and atrial fibrillation. I. Rationale and surgical results. *J Thorac Cardiovasc Surg* 110:473–484, 1995.)

The development of these new ablation technologies revolutionized the surgical treatment of AF by taking a technically difficult and time-consuming operation and making it relatively easy for most cardiac surgeons to perform. Whereas very few patients (<1%) with AF undergoing cardiac surgery before 2000 underwent a Cox-Maze procedure, a study has shown that more than 40% of patients with AF undergoing cardiac surgery had a concomitant ablation procedure in 2006.[72,73] Another advantage of ablation technologies is that they have facilitated the development of less invasive operations. A minimally invasive beating heart procedure with high efficacy is the ultimate goal of these efforts. With the availability of easy-to-use ablation devices, numerous groups around the world have introduced new procedures for AF involving more limited sets of atrial lesions. Some groups are currently performing only the left atrial lesions, whereas others are advocating pulmonary vein isolation alone. Results with these more limited procedures are discussed in a later section.

For ablation technology to reliably replace the incisions in AF surgery, it must meet several criteria. Foremost, it must reliably produce bidirectional conduction block. This is the mechanism by which incisions prevent AF: by blocking macro-reentrant or micro-reentrant circuits, by isolating trigger foci, or by reducing atrial contiguous mass. To do this with certainty, an ablation device must have the capability to reliably make transmural lesions from either the epicardial or the endocardial surface. Experimental work from our laboratory has shown that even gaps as small as 1 mm in ablation lines can conduct fibrillatory wavefronts.[74]

The second crucial characteristic of an ablation device is safety. This requires a precise definition of dose-response curves to limit excessive or inadequate ablation. The surgeon must have knowledge of the effect of the specific ablation technology on surrounding vital cardiac structures, such as the coronary sinus, coronary arteries, and valves. Third, a device should make AF surgery simpler and require less time for it to be performed. This requires features such as rapidity of lesion formation, simplicity of use, and adequacy of length and flexibility. Finally, the device ideally should be adaptable to a minimally invasive approach. This would require the ability to insert the device through small incisions or ports. It would also be beneficial for the device to be capable of creating epicardial transmural lesions on the beating heart.

The current ablation technologies with their advantages and disadvantages are briefly described in this section. At present, there are no microwave, ultrasound, or laser ablation devices on the market and these energy sources are not discussed. There is still no perfect ablation device. As new devices are introduced in the future, it will be imperative to rigorously examine the effects of the new technology on atrial hemodynamics and electrophysiology.

Radiofrequency Energy

Radiofrequency (RF) energy has been used for cardiac ablation for many years in the electrophysiology laboratory.[75] It also was one of the first energy sources to be used in the operating room. RF energy can be delivered by either unipolar or bipolar electrodes, and the electrodes can be either dry or irrigated.

There have been numerous unipolar RF devices available for ablation. Estech (San Ramon, CA) has marketed several devices, both dry and irrigated unipolar catheters that are segmented and flexible. These devices can create variable lesion lengths of 10 to 95 mm. The electrodes can be individually selected and temperature controlled. Later iterations have included suction stabilization. The devices are targeted for use in the minimally invasive setting, but they have yet to approach the same degree of transmurality that has been achieved with bipolar RF clamps. Both Medtronic and Estech have developed irrigated unipolar RF devices that are used to make point-by-point ablations by dragging the device across tissue to make a linear lesion.

Bipolar RF is similar to unipolar energy except that two electrodes, instead of one, are used to focus the path of energy. This allows faster ablation (usually less than 20 seconds) while focusing destruction to tissue that is within the clamp. With bipolar devices, the electrodes are clamped over the targeted atrial tissue. The first bipolar RF device was introduced by AtriCure, Inc. The Isolator was a specially designed clamp with 1-mm-wide, 5-cm-long electrodes embedded in the jaws of the clamp. The device was unique in that it had an algorithm created to provide a real-time measurement of lesion transmurality. The conductance between the electrodes was measured during ablation. When the conductance dropped to a stable minimum level, this correlated well both experimentally and clinically to histologically transmural lesions.[76-78] More recent iterations have introduced more uniform clamp strength and a dual electrode design to achieve wider and more consistent lesions.

Other RF ablation devices have been released.[79,80] The Cobra Adhere and Cobra Adhere XL (Estech, San Ramon, CA) devices are streamlined with suction stabilization for use in minimally invasive procedures, such as port access and thoracoscopic approaches. The Cobra Fusion (Estech, San Ramon, CA) includes suction stabilization and has a unique electrode configuration to allow both unipolar and bipolar RF ablation.[81] The Medtronic bipolar devices, the Cardioblate BP2 and Cardioblate LP, have an irrigated, flexible jaw along with an articulating head, with 7-cm-long electrodes. These devices have an algorithm to predict transmurality of lesions that has been shown to be effective in experimental and clinical settings.[82,83]

RF energy uses an alternating current in the range of 100 to 1000 kHz. This frequency is high enough to prevent rapid myocardial depolarization and the induction of ventricular fibrillation, yet low enough to avoid tissue vaporization and perforation. Resistive heating occurs only within a narrow rim of tissue in direct contact with the electrode, usually less than 1 mm. The deeper tissue heating occurs by passive conduction. With unipolar catheters, the energy is dispersed between the electrode tip and an indifferent electrode, usually the grounding pad applied to the patient. In the bipolar clamp devices, alternating current is generated between two closely approximated electrodes, which results in a more focused ablation. The lesion size depends on the electrode-tissue contact area, the interface temperature, the current and voltage (power), and the duration of delivery. The depth of the lesion can be limited by char formation at the tissue-electrode interface because of the high temperatures (>100° C). To resolve this problem, irrigated catheters have been developed; this reduces char formation by keeping temperatures cooler at the tissue interface. These irrigated catheters have been shown to create larger volume lesions than those created by the dry RF devices.[84,85]

Dose-response curves for unipolar RF have been described.[86-88] Although unipolar RF has been shown to create transmural lesions on the arrested heart in animals with sufficiently long ablation times (60 to 120 seconds), this has not been the case in humans. In one study, after 2-minute endocardial ablations during mitral valve surgery, only 20% of the in vivo lesions were transmural.[87] Epicardial ablation has been even more difficult. Animal studies have consistently shown that unipolar RF is incapable of creating epicardial transmural lesions on the beating heart.[88,89] Another study in humans resulted in only 7% of lesions being transmural despite electrode temperatures of up to 90° C.[90] The Cobra Adhere is an epicardial suction-stabilized unipolar RF ablation device. Despite the proposed advantages of epicardial ablation, the Cobra Adhere demonstrated only 40% full-thickness ablation of sectioned ablations after a 2-minute ablation period in animal testing. In particular, the device showed difficulty creating full-thickness lesions in atrial tissue thicker than 3 mm.[91] Bipolar RF ablation, on the other hand, has been shown to be capable of creating reliable transmural lesions on the beating heart in animals with average ablation times between 5 and 10 seconds.[76,77,92] Newer devices such as the Cobra Fusion have included a combination of both unipolar and bipolar ablation along with the use of proprietary impedance algorithms to determine the amount of time necessary for ablation. Similar animal studies have shown the Cobra Fusion to create transmural lesions in 94% of sectioned lesions.[81]

Because RF ablation is a well-developed technology, much is known about its safety profile. Clinical complications of unipolar RF devices have been described, including coronary artery injuries, cerebrovascular accidents, and the devastating complication of esophageal perforation leading to atrioesophageal fistula.[93-96] Use of the bipolar RF devices has eliminated virtually all the collateral damage seen with the unipolar devices, and there have been no clinical complications reported in the literature. Unfortunately, at this time bipolar devices have the drawback of requiring that the tissue be clamped in the jaws of the device to consistently make transmural lesions. This has limited the potential lesion set, particularly on the beating heart through a minimally invasive epicardial approach, and has required the use of adjunctive unipolar technology to create a complete Cox-Maze lesion set.

Cryoablation

Currently two commercially available sources of cryothermal energy are available. One technology uses nitrous oxide and is manufactured by AtriCure (Cincinnati, OH). The nitrous oxide devices use both rigid reusable and flexible disposable electrodes. More recently, devices using argon were introduced. The technology is now distributed by Medtronic (Minneapolis, MN). This device originally consisted of a disposable flexible catheter that had a 6-cm ablation probe. Newer iterations have included a 10-cm ablation electrode with the addition of a removable clamp. At 1 atmosphere of pressure, nitrous oxide is capable of cooling tissue to –89.5° C; argon has a minimum temperature of –185.7° C.

The size and depth of cryolesions are determined by numerous factors, including probe temperature, tissue temperature, probe size, duration and number of ablations, and the liquid used as the cooling agent.[97] With conventional nitrous oxide, 2- to 3-minute ablations have been shown to reliably create transmural lesions on both the right and the left atrium. Because of the heat sink provided by circulating endocardial blood, epicardial cryolesions on the beating heart have not been uniformly transmural.[98] In one study, investigators were able to create transmural lesions 62% of the time around the pulmonary veins, and two of eight ablations (25%) on the left atrial appendage were transmural.[98] However, in another study of cryoablation on the beating heart, consistent transmural lesions were created on tissue up to 7 mm thick.[99] Ablations were performed around the pulmonary veins, and acute electrical isolation was achieved in 13 of 13 animals. Although histologic analysis revealed 89% of sections achieved transmural lesions, none of the box lesions around the pulmonary veins was completely transmural, again emphasizing the drawbacks of cryoablation on the beating heart.

Because of its ease of use and safety profile, cryoablation remains popular for the treatment of AF. A European randomized trial comparing mitral valve surgery alone with mitral valve surgery with left atrial ablations found an increase in cure for AF in the cryoablation group (freedom from AF at 12 months: 43% vs. 73%).[100]

Cryoablation has the benefit of preserving the fibrous skeleton of the heart, making this an ideal choice for ablation near valvular tissue. Nitrous oxide cryoablation has had extensive clinical use and has had an excellent safety profile. Although cryothermal energy appears to have no permanent effects on valvular tissue or the coronary sinus, experimental studies have shown late intimal hyperplasia of coronary arteries, and these structures should be avoided.[101-104] Doll and colleagues[98] were able to create mild esophageal lesions with epicardial cryoablation in seven of eight cases.

Cryoablation is unique among the currently available ablation technologies in that it destroys tissue by freezing rather than by heating. The important advantage is its ability to preserve tissue architecture. The potential disadvantages of cryoablation technology include the relatively long time necessary to create a lesion (1 to 3 minutes) and the difficulty in creating lesions on the beating heart. Furthermore, if blood is frozen during epicardial ablation on the beating heart, it coagulates, creating a potential risk of thromboembolism.

Surgical Indications for Treatment of Atrial Fibrillation

The principal indication for surgery for AF is intolerance of the arrhythmia in patients for whom medical management has failed. Patients with paroxysmal atrial flutter or fibrillation are often more symptomatic than those with persistent or long-standing AF. Major symptoms include dyspnea on exertion, easy fatigability, lethargy, palpitations, and general sense of unease. Before surgery, all patients should have a trial of medical management.

The Heart Rhythm Society created a task force to evaluate indications for catheter and for surgical ablation of AF.[25,105] The recommendations were developed in partnership with the European Heart Rhythm Association, the European Cardiac Arrhythmia Society, the American College of Cardiology, the American Heart Association, and the Society of Thoracic Surgeons. The task force recommended that programs involved in the stand-alone surgical treatment of AF should develop a team approach to these patients, including electrophysiologists and surgeons, to ensure appropriate patient selection. The consensus of the task force was that the following were appropriate indications for surgical ablation of AF: (1) symptomatic AF patients undergoing other cardiac surgical procedures and (2) selected asymptomatic AF patients undergoing cardiac surgery in whom the ablation can be performed with minimal risk. Stand-alone AF surgery should be considered for symptomatic AF patients who have failed medical management and either prefer a surgical approach, have failed one or more attempts at catheter ablation, or are not candidates for catheter ablation.[25,105]

Other patients who should be considered for surgery include those who have developed a contraindication to warfarin or who have had a stroke while adequately anticoagulated. The Cox-Maze procedure significantly reduces the risk of stroke in these patients. Approximately 20% of patients who had the original cut-and-sew procedure at our institution had experienced at least one episode of cerebral thromboembolism that resulted in a temporary or permanent neurologic deficit before having the Cox-Maze procedure; less than 2% of patients (6 of 389) had a late neurologic event after surgery (mean follow-up of 6.6 years).[106]

Surgical Technique: Cox-Maze Procedure

The final version of the standard cut-and-sew technique to cure AF was the Cox-Maze III procedure.[60,107-109] However, few cardiac surgeons performed this operation because of its technical complexity. Most centers have replaced most surgical incisions with linear lines of ablation created by various energy sources. At Washington

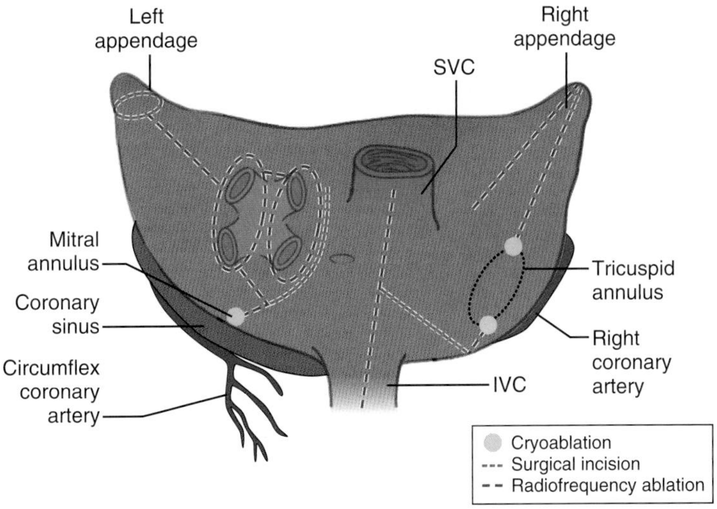

FIGURE 87-3 ■ Cox-Maze IV procedure lesion set. Modifications included independent isolation of pulmonary veins with connecting lesions and no atrial septal incision (originally used for exposure). *IVC,* Inferior vena cava; *SVC,* superior vena cava.

University, bipolar RF energy and cryoenergy have been used successfully to replace most surgical incisions of the Cox-Maze III procedure. Our current procedure incorporates most of the lesions of the Cox-Maze III procedure and has been named the Cox-Maze IV (Fig. 87-3).[110] Our clinical data have shown that this modified operation has significantly shortened the operative time while maintaining the high success rate of the traditional cut-and-sew Cox-Maze III procedure.[111]

Bipolar RF ablation was chosen for the Cox-Maze IV procedure for several reasons. First, the device allows the on-line determination of lesion transmurality by measuring the conductance between the two electrodes.[76,77,87] Second, the bipolar RF device has short ablation times, with 5- to 6-cm-long transmural ablations performed in 5 to 15 seconds. Third, the lesions are narrow (2 to 3 mm in width), and tissue injury is confined to within the clamp. This eliminates the possibility of unwanted collateral injury.[94,112-114]

The Cox-Maze IV procedure has three parts: (1) bilateral pulmonary vein isolation, (2) the right atrial lesion set, and (3) the left atrial lesion set with left atrial excision. The operation is often combined with other procedures and is performed through a sternotomy or a minimally invasive (4- to 5-cm) right mini-thoracotomy. The operation is performed using either central or femoral cannulation for cardiopulmonary bypass depending on the operative approach being a sternotomy or mini-thoracotomy, respectively. The standard sternotomy approach is described in the following paragraphs. The mini-thoracotomy approach was previously described by our group.[115] All patients receive an intraoperative transesophageal echocardiogram to rule out the presence of left atrial clot and are electrically cardioverted followed by amiodarone infusion if found to be in AF at the time of surgery. It should be noted that each RF ablation line is created by performing two or three ablations with the clamp to ensure transmurality.

Pulmonary Vein Isolation

With the patient in a supine position through a median sternotomy, a pericardial cradle is created, and the patient is centrally cannulated. Normothermic cardiopulmonary bypass is initiated. Both the right (Fig. 87-4) and the left (Fig. 87-5) pulmonary veins are bluntly dissected at their confluences and surrounded with umbilical tapes. If the patient is in AF, he or she is cardioverted at this point. The bipolar RF clamp is passed around the pulmonary veins on each side. Typically three ablations are performed to isolate as large an atrial cuff around the pulmonary veins as possible. Exit block is confirmed by attempting to pace from each pulmonary vein.

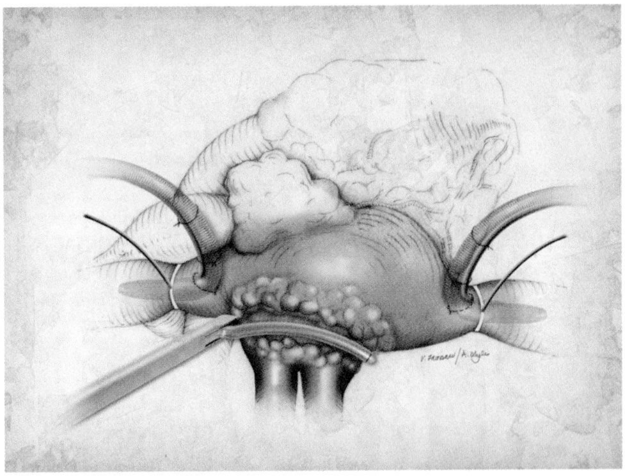

FIGURE 87-4 ■ Right pulmonary vein isolation during Cox-Maze IV procedure. The bipolar radiofrequency device is placed around the right pulmonary veins. The device is clamped on the cuff of atrial tissue surrounding the pulmonary veins.

Right Atrial Lesion Set

The patient is cooled to 34° C. On the beating heart, a pursestring suture wide enough to accommodate one jaw of the bipolar RF clamp is made at the base of the right atrial appendage. Through this pursestring, an ablation line is created along the free wall of the right atrium down toward the junction of the right atrium and

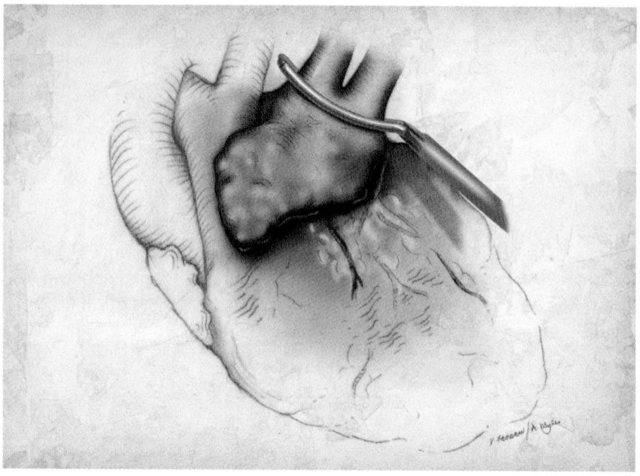

FIGURE 87-5 ■ Left pulmonary vein isolation during Cox-Maze IV procedure. The bipolar radiofrequency device is placed around the left pulmonary veins. The device is clamped on the cuff of atrial tissue surrounding the pulmonary veins. (Modified with permission from AtriCure.)

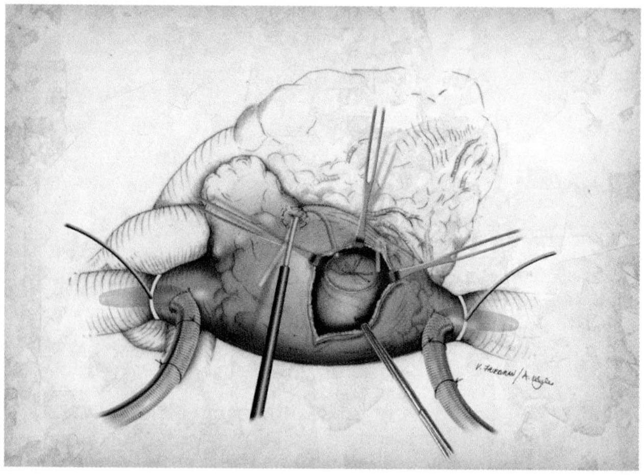

FIGURE 87-7 ■ Endocardial cryoablation through the right atrial pursestring suture to the 10-o'clock position of the tricuspid using a 3-cm linear cryoprobe. (Modified with permission from AtriCure.)

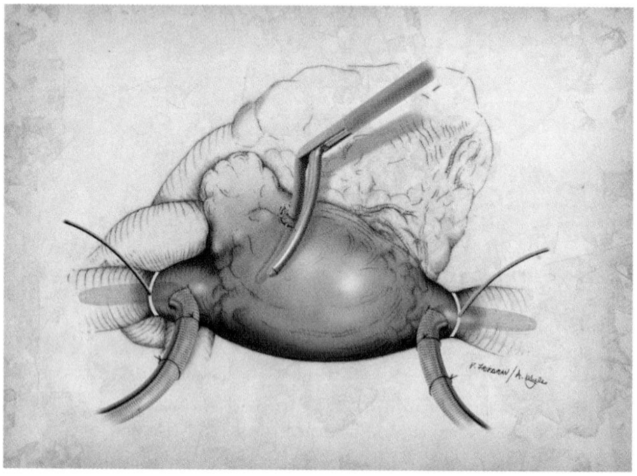

FIGURE 87-6 ■ The right atrial free wall ablation. The bipolar radiofrequency clamp is placed through a pursestring suture in the base of the right atrial appendage and is carried down perpendicularly toward the superior vena cava. (Modified with permission from AtriCure.)

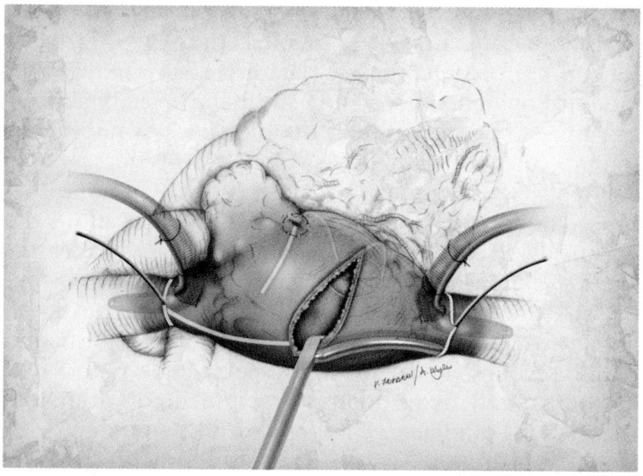

FIGURE 87-8 ■ Bipolar radiofrequency ablation along the superior vena cava and inferior vena cava through the right atriotomy, completing the right atrial lesion set. (Modified with permission from AtriCure.)

superior vena cava (Fig. 87-6). A vertical atriotomy is performed from the intra-atrial septum toward the atrioventricular groove, along the free wall of the right atrium at least 2 cm away from the previous RF ablation (Fig. 87-7). Cryoablation is then used for reasons mentioned previously in this chapter because of its ability to ablate without damaging valvular tissue. From the superior aspect of this atriotomy, a 3-cm linear cryoprobe is used to create an endocardial ablation down to the 2-o'clock position of the tricuspid valve. The cryoprobe is then placed through the pursestring suture at the base of the right atrial appendage, and a second linear endocardial ablation is created down toward the 10-o'clock position of the tricuspid valve. A final bipolar RF ablation line is created along the superior vena cava and down the inferior vena cava (Fig. 87-8).

Left Atrial Lesion Set

The aorta is cross-clamped and cold blood cardioplegia is administered. While the patient is under cardioplegic arrest, the left atrial appendage is amputated. Through this incision, one jaw of the RF ablation clamp is inserted and an ablation line is created to the superior left pulmonary vein. The left atrial appendage is oversewn in two layers. A standard left atriotomy is performed, which can be extended superiorly onto the dome of the left atrium and inferiorly around the orifice of the right inferior pulmonary vein. Two separate bipolar RF ablation lines are then created from both the superior and the inferior aspects of the atriotomy incision to the origin of the left superior and inferior pulmonary veins, respectively, thus completing the "box lesion" (Fig. 87-9). A final bipolar RF ablation line is created from the inferior aspect of the

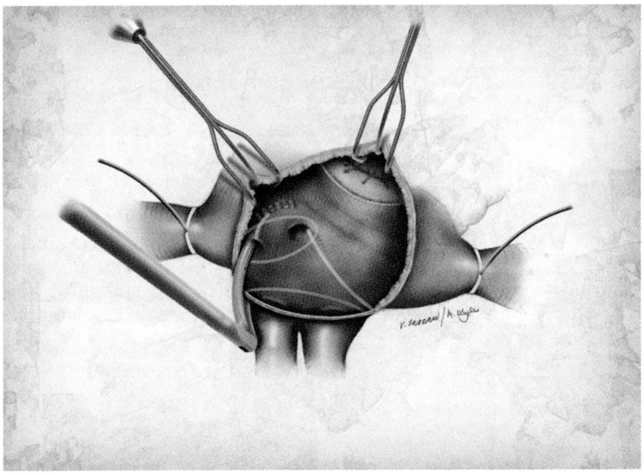

FIGURE 87-9 ■ Completion of left atrial "box lesion" after creating a bipolar radiofrequency ablation line through the amputated atrial appendage to the left superior pulmonary vein and left atriotomy. (Modified with permission from AtriCure.)

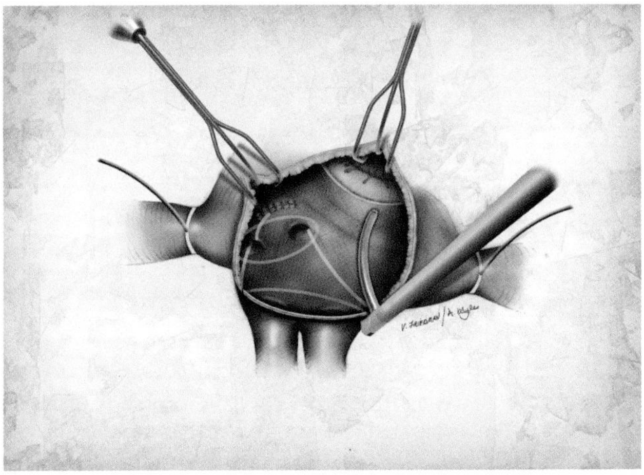

FIGURE 87-10 ■ Bipolar radiofrequency ablation across the floor of the left atrium from the inferior aspect of the atriotomy to the mitral annulus. (Modified with permission from AtriCure.)

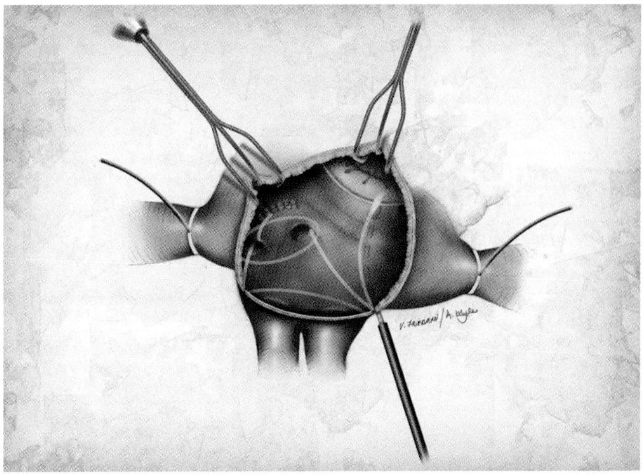

FIGURE 87-11 ■ Epicardial cryoablation over the coronary sinus completing the left atrial isthmus line. Note that this figure does not show simultaneous endocardial ablation over the mitral annulus, which is typically performed. (Modified with permission from AtriCure.)

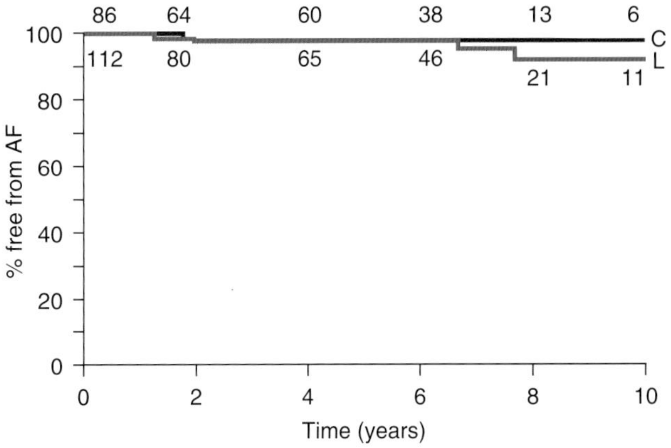

FIGURE 87-12 ■ Kaplan-Meier analysis of freedom from recurrent atrial fibrillation. The numbers on each line indicate the number of patients at risk. There was no difference in the long-term estimate of freedom from atrial fibrillation between the lone Cox-Maze procedure (L) group and the concomitant (C) group ($P = 0.64$). *AF,* Atrial fibrillation. (From Prasad SM, Maniar HS, Camillo CJ, et al: The Cox Maze III procedure for atrial fibrillation: long-term efficacy in patients undergoing lone versus concomitant procedures. *J Thorac Cardiovasc Surg* 126:1822–1828, 2003.)

atriotomy, across the floor of the left atrium, down to the mitral valve annulus (Fig. 87-10). This ablation line should cross the coronary sinus ideally in the space between the circumflex and right coronary circulations. If the patient has a left dominant circulation, this lesion can be created surgically to identify and spare the circumflex artery, although this is rarely needed. The end of this RF ablation line is marked with methylene blue. This ablation line is connected to the mitral valve annulus by performing an endocardial cryoablation, which overlaps onto the posterior leaflet of the mitral valve. A second epicardial cryoablation is performed simultaneously over the coronary sinus with a linear cryoprobe to complete the left atrial isthmus ablation. This should directly oppose the endocardial cryoablation (Fig. 87-11).

Surgical Results: Cox-Maze Procedure

The long-term results of the Cox-Maze III procedure have been excellent. In our series of 198 consecutive patients undergoing surgery, 97% of patients at a mean follow-up of 5.4 years were free from symptomatic AF (Fig. 87-12). There was no difference in cure rates between patients undergoing a lone versus a concomitant procedure. The cure rates off antiarrhythmic medications were 80% and 73%, respectively, in patients undergoing lone and concomitant Cox-Maze procedures at late follow-up.[116]

Our results using bipolar RF ablation (Cox-Maze IV) have been similarly encouraging. In a prospective, single-center trial from our institution, 91% of patients at 6 months of follow-up were free from AF. The operative mortality was 0%.[92] More recently, we prospectively evaluated 100 consecutive patients and demonstrated postoperative freedom from AF at 93%, 90%, and 90% at 6, 12, and 24 months, respectively.[117] A multicenter

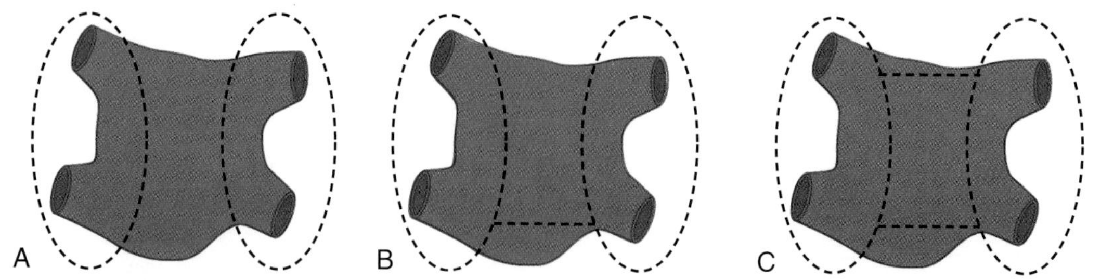

FIGURE 87-13 ■ Pulmonary vein isolation methods. **A,** Left and right pulmonary veins are isolated separately. **B,** Left and right pulmonary veins are isolated separately and then connected with an additional lesion. **C,** Left and right pulmonary veins are isolated separately and connected inferiorly and superiorly, also referred to as a *box lesion.*

trial of the same technology had similar results.[118] At 6 months, 96% of patients were in normal sinus rhythm, and there was no operative mortality in this group of 30 patients.[63] The modifications with use of bipolar RF have shortened the operation considerably while decreasing the major complication rate. The mean cross-clamp time for patients undergoing a lone Cox-Maze III procedure was 92 ± 26 minutes compared with 41 ± 13 minutes with the Cox-Maze IV.[119] The same study demonstrated a major complication rate of 10% in the Cox-Maze III, which was significantly higher than the Cox-Maze IV cohort ($P = 0.004$). Two-year freedom from AF off antiarrhythmics using Holter monitoring was 84%, which was similar to previous reports of the Cox-Maze III documenting an 80% freedom from AF off antiarrhythmics using symptomatic reporting.[119]

The Cox-Maze IV procedure involves a lesion set around all the pulmonary veins, isolating the entire posterior left atrium by creating a "box" or by a simple connecting lesion between the pulmonary veins with a single ablation (Fig. 87-13). Our group demonstrated that isolation of the entire posterior left atrium by the creation of a box lesion had a significantly lower incidence of early atrial tachyarrhythmias, a higher freedom from AF recurrence at 1 and 3 months, and lower use of antiarrhythmic drugs at 3 and 6 months.[120] Furthermore, patients receiving a complete box lesion set had significantly higher freedom from AF and freedom from AF off antiarrhythmic drugs at 1 year compared with patients receiving a non-box ablation set (Fig. 87-14).[117]

The Cox-Maze procedure has also been effective at decreasing the risk of late stroke in this high-risk population of patients. In a report from our institution, 57 of 389 patients (14%) had experienced a neurologic event before surgery. Despite the inherently high risk of stroke in these patients, there were only six neurologic events during long-term follow-up (mean, 6.6 ± 5.0). The long-term stroke rate after the Cox-Maze procedure has been 0.2% per year despite the fact that the majority of patients were able to discontinue anticoagulation.[106]

In a series from Japan, the Cox-Maze procedure was found to significantly decrease the incidence of late stroke, even in those patients already receiving anticoagulation for mechanical mitral valves. Patients with chronic AF who had a concomitant Cox-Maze procedure with their mitral valve replacement were 99% stroke free at a follow-up of 8 years, whereas the group with

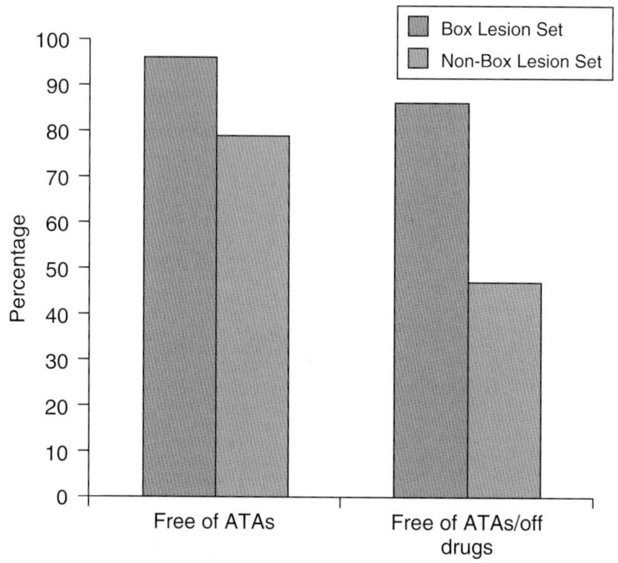

FIGURE 87-14 ■ Freedom from atrial fibrillation on and off antiarrhythmic (ATA) drugs; comparison of box and non-box lesion sets at 12 months. (From Weimar T, Bailey MS, Watanabe Y, et al: The Cox-Maze IV procedure for lone atrial fibrillation: a single center experience in 100 consecutive patients. *J Interv Card Electrophysiol* 31:47–54, 2011.)

mitral valve replacement alone had only an 89% freedom from stroke.[121]

Surgical Technique: Other Atrial Fibrillation Procedures

A number of more limited surgical procedures have been proposed for the cure of AF. These procedures generally fall into two groups. The first group comprises those that incorporate only left atrial lesions, and the second group consists of procedures involving pulmonary vein isolation alone with or without ganglion ablation. The left atrial lesion set generally involves pulmonary vein isolation (either as a box or separately with a connecting lesion) and a lesion to the mitral annulus as well as removal of the left atrial appendage. These lesions have been created with many different energy sources, including unipolar and bipolar RF, cryoablation, and microwave.[93,122-130] The specific technique often depends on the type of device used and has most often been performed on cardiopulmonary bypass.

A number of surgeons have published reports on the technique of pulmonary vein isolation alone for AF.[131-134] This limited lesion set can be done separately, with a connecting lesion, or as a box lesion (see Fig. 87-13). Various devices have been used to create these lesions, including RF, cryoablation, microwave energy, high-frequency ultrasound, and laser. Pulmonary vein isolation alone is attractive because it can be done without the use of cardiopulmonary bypass and often in a minimally invasive setting. Some investigators have proposed isolation of the pulmonary veins and also ablation of the ganglionic plexi.[135-137]

Pruitt and colleagues[138] reported on a minimally invasive technique used on 100 patients. The procedure was accomplished thoracoscopically without cardiopulmonary bypass through use of a unipolar microwave catheter. Wolf and coworkers[131] published a report on a similar technique of bilateral video-assisted thoracoscopic off-pump epicardial pulmonary vein isolation using a bipolar RF clamp. This procedure was performed with two 10-mm ports and one 5- or 6-cm working incision on each side of the thorax. The right-sided pulmonary veins were first isolated while the patient was left side down, and then the patient was repositioned with the opposite side up for the left-sided lesions, including the division of the ligament of Marshall. Finally, the left atrial appendage was resected with an endoscopic stapling device.

A modified version of this approach has been practiced by our group. After double-lumen endotracheal tube intubation, appropriate central venous access, and monitoring (including transesophageal echocardiography to evaluate for left atrial thrombus), the patient is placed left side down with the right arm positioned to expose the right axilla. The third or fourth intercostal space, midaxillary line, scapula, and xiphoid are marked, and the right side of the chest is prepared and draped from the spine to the sternum. A 10- or 12-mm port is placed in the sixth intercostal space approximately 2 cm anterior to the midaxillary line, typically at the level of the xiphoid (Fig. 87-15). Carbon dioxide is insufflated to flood the air space. A 30-degree scope is used to visualize the location of the incision, which is made in the third or fourth intercostal space. A 5-cm muscle-sparing incision is made in the auscultatory triangle. Caution must be exercised in retracting the posterior fat pad to avoid injury to the nerve, artery, and vein located therein. A soft tissue retractor is placed, and the lung is retracted to visualize the right phrenic nerve.

The pericardium is opened anterior and parallel to the phrenic nerve to expose the atriocaval junction. The heart is exposed inferiorly to the diaphragm. Pericardial stay sutures in the lateral edges are anchored posteriorly through the skin. The space between the right pulmonary artery and the right superior pulmonary vein is dissected bluntly. A second 10-mm port is created for direct placement of a specially designed dissector (GlidePath, AtriCure). The dissector is introduced lateral to the inferior vena cava and advanced into the oblique sinus and swept medially behind the right pulmonary veins. The superior vena cava is retracted medially to expose the right pulmonary artery. The dissector hinge is engaged, which advances the tip into the space between the right superior pulmonary vein and the right pulmonary artery. The dissector is articulated in the opposite direction and removed after grasping the GlidePath hood to allow guidance of the bipolar RF clamp into the same space. The plastic hood is attached to the bipolar RF clamp (Isolator, AtriCure), and the clamp is closed and inserted into the chest through the same port site. The clamp is then opened and advanced to position the jaws around the pulmonary veins, being guided by the previously placed plastic GlidePath hood. We routinely establish baseline pacing thresholds from each of the pulmonary veins before ablation. Two ablations are performed, the second after a small advancement of the clamp onto the atrium. Each ablation is made after assurance that the clamp is on the atrial cuff and not the pulmonary veins proper.

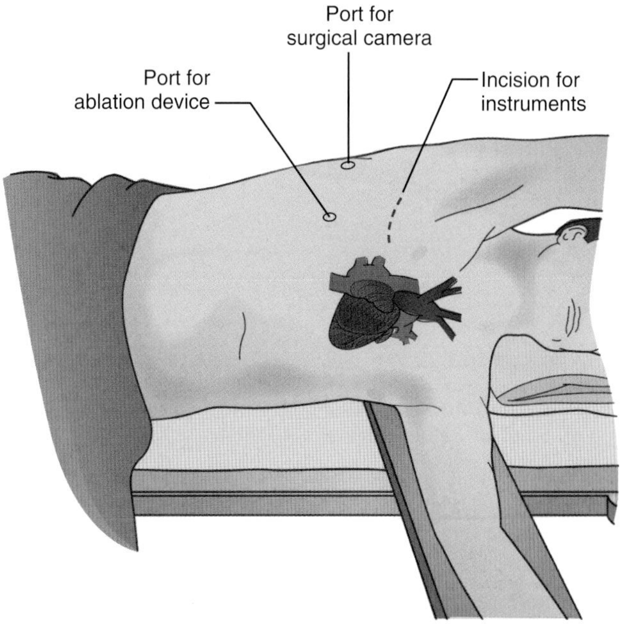

FIGURE 87-15 ■ Incision and port sites for minimally invasive pulmonary vein isolation procedure.

After ablation, conduction block is confirmed by pacing from each of the pulmonary veins. Additional ablations are created until conduction block is achieved. The clamp is removed, the pericardium is reapproximated, an appropriate drain is placed, and the wound is closed.

The patient is then repositioned with the left side up. The left arm is supported superiorly to expose the axilla. A 10-mm port is placed in the sixth intercostal space in the midaxillary line (slightly more posterior than the port on the right side), and a working incision is made in the third intercostal space under direct visualization. The pericardium is initially opened posterior to the phrenic nerve to expose the left pulmonary artery and then widely opened for device access, with caution exercised to preserve the phrenic nerve. Pericardial stay sutures are placed posteriorly and brought through the skin. The ligament of Marshall is divided by electrocautery, and the space between the left pulmonary artery and left superior pulmonary vein is bluntly dissected. The dissector is introduced through a second 10-mm port placed posterior to the first port. The dissector is positioned into the

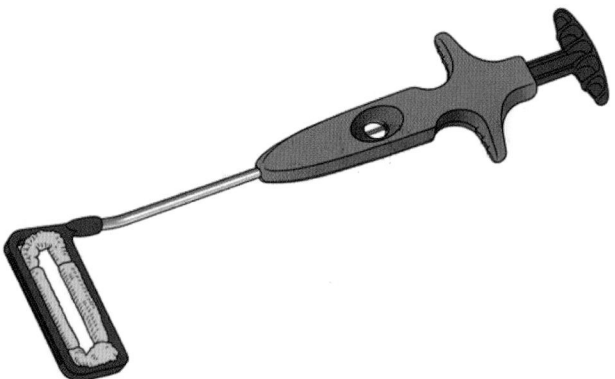

FIGURE 87-16 ■ AtriClip device. (From Emmert MY, Puippe G, Baumüller S, et al: Safe, effective and durable epicardial left atrial appendage clip occlusion in patients with atrial fibrillation undergoing cardiac surgery: first long-term results from a prospective device trial. *Eur J Cardiothorac Surg* 45:126–131, 2014.)

space below the left inferior pulmonary vein and then articulated to swing the tip into the space between the left superior pulmonary vein and the left pulmonary artery. The clamp is similarly brought into the same space by guidance with the plastic hood as on the right side. Ablation of the pulmonary veins is done after baseline pacing thresholds are recorded, with confirmation of conduction block after ablation.

The left atrial appendage is then removed for the reduction of thromboembolic risk. This is done using an atraumatic clip (AtriClip, AtriCure) (Fig. 87-16). This is potentially safer than using a stapler and has better outcomes in terms of completely excluding the left atrial appendage. A multicenter feasibility study demonstrated no adverse events related to the device, and 60 of 61 patients (98.4%) had successful left atrial appendage exclusion, based on results of computed tomography angiography or transesophageal echocardiography, at 3 months.[139] In a study prospectively evaluating the long-term safety and efficacy of the AtriClip, serial computed tomographic scans showed stable clip positioning without left atrial appendage reperfusion with a follow-up of 3.5 ± 0.5 years. In addition, at 36 months follow-up, no intracardiac thrombi or embolic strokes had occurred.[140]

The pericardium is reapproximated with a drain placed, and the left-sided wounds are closed. Patients typically stay in the hospital for 2 or 3 days for drain removal and arrhythmia monitoring.

Surgical Results: Other Atrial Fibrillation Procedures

The performance of only a left atrial lesion set for the treatment of AF is supported by studies showing that most paroxysmal AF originates from around the pulmonary veins and posterior left atrium.[29,33] However, the surgical treatment of AF by a left atrial lesion set alone has had lower success rates than with the biatrial Cox-Maze lesion set. Intraoperative mapping studies of patients undergoing surgical treatment of AF showed a distinct region of stable dominant frequency, which is indicative of the area of origin of the arrhythmia, in the left atrium only 30% of the time. The dominant frequency was located in the right atrium 12% of the time. Most important, the location of dominant frequency moved during the recording period in almost half of the patients.[26] Therefore, it is not surprising that interventions with limited lesion sets, particularly pulmonary vein isolation alone, do not have the same results as the complete Cox-Maze lesion set.

Surgical pulmonary vein isolation has been shown to be superior to catheter ablation in patients with left atrial dilation and hypertension or where previous catheter ablation has failed. The FAST trial was a multicenter randomized trial that compared 63 patients who received linear antral pulmonary vein isolation by way of catheter ablation and 61 patients who received bipolar RF pulmonary vein isolation and ganglionated plexi ablation. At 1 year, freedom from left atrial arrhythmias greater than 30 seconds evaluated by a 7-day Holter was 66% for surgical ablation and 37% for catheter ablation ($P = 0.002$).[141]

A well-known complication of performing only the left atrial lesions is postoperative atrial flutter. In a group of 50 patients described by Golovchiner and colleagues from Tel Aviv, 13% of patients experienced postoperative atrial flutter at a follow-up of only 15 months. Left atrial flutter was present in four of six.[142] In a series from Japan, 5 of 24 patients (21%) experienced recurrent atrial flutter or tachycardia after a left-sided procedure with follow-up of 36.9 ± 14.1 months.[129]

The results with left atrial ablation sets have been variable (cure rates 21% to 95%) and are dependent on the precise lesion set, technology used, and patient population. A randomized trial conducted with patients undergoing mitral valve surgery evaluated whether addition of RF ablation on the left atrium was different from mitral valve surgery alone.[143] Of 101 patients randomized to undergo mitral valve surgery with or without RF ablation, 99 patients eventually met criteria; 45 were evaluated who had RF ablation versus 44 who had valve surgery alone ($P < 0.001$). At 12 months of follow-up, 44% of those undergoing concomitant RF ablation were in sinus rhythm compared with only 5% of those who had mitral valve surgery alone. Although this was significantly better than no ablation at all, this success rate was much lower than has been reported with the Cox-Maze procedure in patients with mitral valve disease.[144]

In a meta-analysis of surgical ablative treatments for AF, Barnett and Ad[145] evaluated 69 studies to assess differences in survival and freedom from AF. These studies included multiple types of energy devices and interventions for lone AF as well as concomitant procedures. Compared with control patients, those undergoing surgical ablation had significantly greater freedom from AF at 2 years (84 ± 6% vs. 40 ± 22%, $P = 0.001$); freedom from AF at 2 years was also significantly better in patients who had biatrial ablations (86 ± 5% vs. 75 ± 2%, $P = 0.001$). These results support a strategy of doing a more complete ablation set (biatrial) when possible, but a more limited lesion set is superior to no intervention for patients with AF.

The results of pulmonary vein isolation alone have been better in patients who have lone AF than in those undergoing concomitant cardiac surgery. In the series by

Wolf and coworkers,[131] 27 patients with AF (18 paroxysmal, 4 persistent, and 5 permanent) underwent video-assisted bilateral pulmonary vein isolation and left atrial appendage exclusion for AF; 91% of patients were free from AF without antiarrhythmias postoperatively. In a more recent series with longer follow-up, Edgerton and coworkers[146] described 57 patients with AF undergoing pulmonary vein isolation plus ablation of the ganglionic plexi. Most patients were observed with prolonged monitoring. In 39 patients with paroxysmal AF, the freedom from AF at 6 months was 82%, and antiarrhythmic medications were discontinued in 74%. In patients with persistent and long-standing AF, the success rate at 6 months was only 56%, and antiarrhythmic medications were discontinued in only 39%.

McClelland and colleagues[135] described 21 patients undergoing pulmonary vein isolation with ganglionic plexi ablation. Procedural success was defined as freedom from AF and drugs at 1 year. In patients with paroxysmal or persistent AF, 88% of patients had a successful procedure. However, in patients with long-standing AF, only 25% had a successful outcome with pulmonary vein isolation alone.[136] In our pulmonary vein isolation experience at Washington University with 43 patients, we have had similar results. Patients have been observed with 24-hour Holter monitoring at 3, 6, and 12 months. Our mean follow-up was 24 ± 37 months. In patients with lone paroxysmal AF, the cure rate was 78%, with 67% both free from AF and off antiarrhythmic drugs. However, in patients with persistent or long-standing AF, the cure rate has been only 38%.

The results with endoscopic microwave pulmonary vein isolation have been worse. This is likely because this technology is not capable of creating reliable transmural lesions on the beating heart.[147] In a group of 50 patients of whom the majority had paroxysmal AF, less than half of the patients were free from AF or reintervention at a mean follow-up of only 7.6 months.[148] In a follow-up report that included 100 patients, the late results were even worse. Only 42% of patients were in sinus rhythm at last follow-up. Although totally thoracoscopic surgical ablation with the microwave device was technically feasible, the clinical results were poor, with no demonstrated electrical isolation of the pulmonary veins and poor long-term cure of AF.[142] Because of these poor results, microwave ablation technology is no longer available.

In our experience, the results with pulmonary vein isolation have been worse in patients undergoing concomitant cardiac procedures than in those undergoing AF intervention alone. At Washington University, 23 patients with AF (12 with paroxysmal AF, 11 with permanent AF) underwent pulmonary vein isolation during concomitant mitral valve surgery or coronary revascularization. The average duration of AF in 12 patients was 6.7 ± 14.2 years. At a mean follow-up of 57 ± 37 months, only 50% of patients were free from AF.[120]

In a series reported by Gaita and colleagues,[122] 105 patients undergoing AF and valve surgery were randomly assigned to three groups: left atrial ablation by two different patterns or pulmonary vein isolation alone. The freedom from AF at last follow-up was only 29% in the pulmonary vein isolation group versus 76% in those who had more extensive left atrial lesions. In another series, a group of 101 patients underwent pulmonary vein isolation with cryoablation in addition to mitral valve surgery; the freedom from AF at last follow-up was only 53%.[149] Only 25% of patients were able to maintain sinus rhythm without antiarrhythmic drugs. In a study from Japan, 66 patients with chronic AF and mitral valve disease underwent pulmonary vein cryoablation. Normal sinus rhythm was seen in only 61% of patients at late follow-up, and antiarrhythmic drugs were discontinued in 17% of patients.[132] These reports of pulmonary vein isolation compare unfavorably with the more than 80% freedom from AF at late follow-up seen in mitral valve patients undergoing the Cox-Maze IV procedure at our institution.[150] However, a limited lesion set may have merit in selected patients, as reported results are better than no intervention at all. Certainly, there are groups of patients who are cured with these methods; continued investigation is needed to identify which factors ultimately determine efficacy in each particular group of patients.

Future Surgical Treatments for Atrial Fibrillation

As surgical techniques and technology have advanced, there has been an increasing trend toward the creation of minimally invasive approaches. Increasingly, groups including our own, are performing ablations through smaller incisions with the aid of thoracoscopic video assistance in properly selected patients. Several groups have started performing epicardial ablations with the aid of suction-based RF and cryoablation probes that can be placed through thoracoscopic ports. Historically, these probes do not achieve the same degree of transmurality achieved with bipolar RF clamps. Others have attempted to solve this problem using a "hybrid" approach, which uses a combination of endocardial catheter ablations and epicardial ablations with either bipolar RF clamps and/or unipolar RF devices.[151,152] This approach can be performed in a single stage or as a dual-stage procedure in which the epicardial ablation is performed first, followed at an interval of time by the endocardial catheter ablation. Both the lesion sets and the approaches using a hybrid method vary greatly from institution to institution, and studies evaluating the hybrid procedure generally have a small number of patients. Although these minimally invasive epicardial and hybrid approaches have yet to match the long-term efficacy of the Cox-Maze IV, they hold promise and require continued clinical investigation to determine their precise role. The ideal surgical treatment for AF would consist of a patient-tailored lesion set using devices that consistently achieve 100% transmurality through a minimally invasive approach without the need for cardiopulmonary bypass. However, further development in ablation technology and improvements in preoperative diagnostic tests to better determine the mechanisms of AF in each particular patient are desperately needed.

Conclusions

The introduction of ablation devices has revolutionized the surgical treatment of AF, making these curative procedures available to a wider population of patients. Whereas there have been few randomized trials comparing the different surgical procedures, conclusions can be drawn from the numerous retrospective series that are available after almost 3 decades of surgical experience. In patients with AF undergoing mitral valve procedures, it is recommended that at least a left atrial Cox-Maze lesion set be performed. This adds only 10 to 15 minutes to the cross-clamp time and cures the majority of patients. At our institution, we prefer a biatrial Cox-Maze IV in these patients because success rates of more than 90% have been reproducible in this population of patients. [144,150]

In patients undergoing coronary artery bypass grafting, the high success rate of the Cox-Maze lesion set has been documented by our group.[153] In patients with AF having on-pump coronary bypass grafting, it is recommended that a full biatrial lesion set be performed. However, there have been no randomized comparisons of lesion sets in this population. In patients with AF undergoing off-pump coronary bypass grafting, our policy had been to perform pulmonary vein isolation with removal of the left atrial appendage. However, poor results in patients with long-standing AF led us to abandon this approach in that group.

In patients with lone AF, pulmonary vein isolation alone has had good early results in patients with paroxysmal AF. At our institution, this procedure is performed in patients who have paroxysmal AF and a left atrial size of 4 cm or less. In patients with large atria, we prefer a full Cox-Maze lesion set because of the high incidence of non–pulmonary vein triggers in this population.[154]

In patients with persistent or long-standing AF, our policy has been to perform a full biatrial Cox-Maze procedure on cardiopulmonary bypass. This is because of the poor results that have been obtained both by us and others with pulmonary vein isolation alone. With the full Cox-Maze IV procedure, success rates in patients with persistent or long-standing AF have been 91% at 1 year, with all antiarrhythmic drugs discontinued in 76% of patients.[150] There has been no difference in our success rates with use of the full lesion set in comparing patients with paroxysmal AF and those with persistent, long-standing AF.

INAPPROPRIATE SINUS TACHYCARDIA

Background and Indications

Inappropriate sinus tachycardia is a rare disorder that is characterized by an abnormally elevated heart rate at rest and an exaggerated rate response with physical activity. To be considered for interventional therapy, a patient's symptoms need to be refractory to dietary modification and medical management. Inappropriate sinus tachycardia was originally described in 1979, but it has only recently been accepted as a medical condition. Patients suffering from this debilitating condition are typically young women. Inappropriate sinus tachycardia is thought to be the result of enhanced automaticity of the sinoatrial node or hypersensitivity to β-adrenergic stimulation. The sinus node impulse may have a multifocal origin, and early activation sites can shift within the sinus node complex in response to autonomic influences. The first-line treatment is medical therapy with beta blockers or calcium channel blockers.

In patients for whom medical management fails, catheter or surgical ablation is the next therapeutic option. The efficacy of catheter ablation remains controversial. Reported series are small, and there have been a high percentage of failures at long-term follow-up.[155,156] This has led many centers to abandon a catheter-based approach. Results with surgical intervention have been better but still leave room for improvement.

Surgical Technique: Superior Right Atrial Isolation

At our center, 10 consecutive patients with inappropriate sinus tachycardia have undergone surgery for this arrhythmia. The first seven patients underwent median sternotomy with cardiopulmonary bypass to ablate or to isolate the sinoatrial node; in the last three patients, a minimally invasive technique developed at our institution was performed.[157] In these latter patients, the sinoatrial node was isolated by bipolar RF ablation through a small inframammary incision, without the use of cardiopulmonary bypass (Fig. 87-17). Isolation and ablation of the sinoatrial node are done through a right 6-cm minithoracotomy. Intraoperatively, intravenous isoproterenol is administered to create sinus tachycardia with rates of 150 to 180 beats per minute. A large cuff of right atrium adjoining the junction of the superior vena cava is isolated from the body of the right atrium with a bipolar RF ablation device. Three sequential circumferential ablations are performed, and isolation is confirmed with pacing and by observing a significant blunting in response to intravenous administration of isoproterenol. Bipolar pacing above and below the ablation line confirms that the sinoatrial node and surrounding atrium are isolated from the remainder of the heart.

Surgical Results

Two reports with traditional cardiopulmonary bypass demonstrated complications requiring pacemaker placement

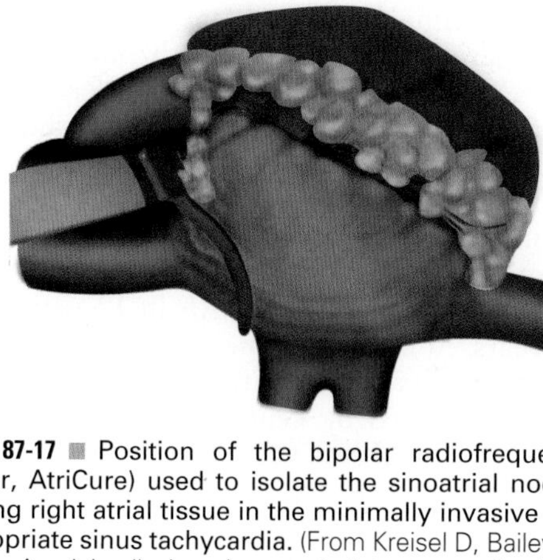

FIGURE 87-17 ■ Position of the bipolar radiofrequency clamp (Isolator, AtriCure) used to isolate the sinoatrial node and surrounding right atrial tissue in the minimally invasive ablation for inappropriate sinus tachycardia. (From Kreisel D, Bailey M, Lindsay B, et al: A minimally invasive surgical treatment for inappropriate sinus tachycardia. *J Thorac Cardiovasc Surg* 130(2):598–599, 2005.)

and development of new supraventricular tachycardia from ectopic foci.[158,159] In our experience, after a mean follow-up of 7.1 ± 5.7 years, there was no evidence of inappropriate sinus tachycardia recurrence; however, four patients required pacemaker implantation for symptomatic bradycardia and a single patient developed ectopic atrial tachycardia. One patient still experienced palpitations. Four patients experienced complete relief from their cardiac symptoms.[157]

Conclusions

Surgical isolation of the sinoatrial node for medically refractory inappropriate sinus tachycardia has acceptable long-term success in preventing recurrence. However, more than half of patients have required pacemaker implantation or have had recurrent symptoms. Less invasive surgical techniques make this a more attractive option for patients with inappropriate sinus tachycardia who have failed medical therapy.

VENTRICULAR TACHYCARDIA

Background

The success of implantable cardioverter-defibrillators (ICDs) and catheter ablation has dramatically diminished the referral of patients with ventricular arrhythmias (ventricular tachycardia) for surgery. However, it is critical that surgeons understand the historically important role of surgery and the present indications for surgical management of ventricular tachycardia. Although ICDs have improved survival by preventing sudden death, they fail to treat the underlying arrhythmogenic substrate. The frequent discharges can impair quality of life.[160] In addition, a population of patients surviving myocardial infarction with ventricular aneurysms, akinetic segments, and ischemic cardiomyopathies develop ventricular arrhythmias and require surgical intervention for treatment of congestive heart failure or coronary artery disease. These patients greatly benefit from concomitant surgery for their ventricular tachycardia.

Historical Aspects of Surgery for Ventricular Tachycardia

In 1961, Estes and Izlar described some patients who underwent successful treatment of ventricular tachycardia with surgical sympathectomy. In the late 1960s, it became apparent that myocardial ischemia initiated many ventricular arrhythmias and that they were related to areas of infarction and scar.[161] Two surgical approaches were developed to address this problem: infarctectomy and coronary artery bypass grafting (CABG).[162,163] Unfortunately, these initial approaches for the surgical treatment of ventricular tachycardia had high mortality rates and relatively poor long-term success. They failed because they were not based on an understanding of the mechanisms involved in ischemic ventricular tachycardia.[164]

Improved understanding of these mechanisms during the 1970s led to new surgical approaches. Wellens and others introduced cardiac mapping techniques that for the first time were able to precisely identify myocardial activation during dysrhythmias.[165-168] Ventricular tachycardia was found to be a reentrant arrhythmia, able to be initiated in the electrophysiology laboratory. It became apparent that ventricular tachycardia often arose from the border zone between infarcted and normal myocardium and that the reentrant circuit was often subendocardial in origin.[169-173] This led to surgical techniques that were guided by both preoperative and intraoperative electrophysiologic studies.

The first directed surgical cure of refractory ventricular tachycardia was reported in 1975.[167] The patient was a 54-year-old man who presented with refractory ventricular tachycardia after two myocardial infarctions. Epicardial mapping was used to localize the site of earliest epicardial activity to the margin of the aneurysm. Subsequent resection of this area abolished the ventricular tachycardia. In 1978, Guiraudon introduced the encircling endocardial ventriculotomy, an operation designed to isolate the entire border zone from normal myocardium.[174] A near-transmural incision was made from the endocardial surface of the left ventricle down to the epicardial surface (Fig. 87-18). Although this technique met with clinical success, it caused significant ventricular dysfunction. In 1979, Harken and colleagues[175] from the University of Pennsylvania introduced a new technique involving endomyocardial resection directed by intraoperative mapping in 12 patients. They reported 1 operative mortality, with the remaining 11 patients having no recurrent arrhythmias at 1 year. In 1982, Moran[176] modified the endomyocardial resection with an extended resection of all visible scar, which obviated the need for intraoperative mapping (Fig. 87-19). These new procedures resulted in operative mortalities of between 10% and 20%. The success rates improved in some series to

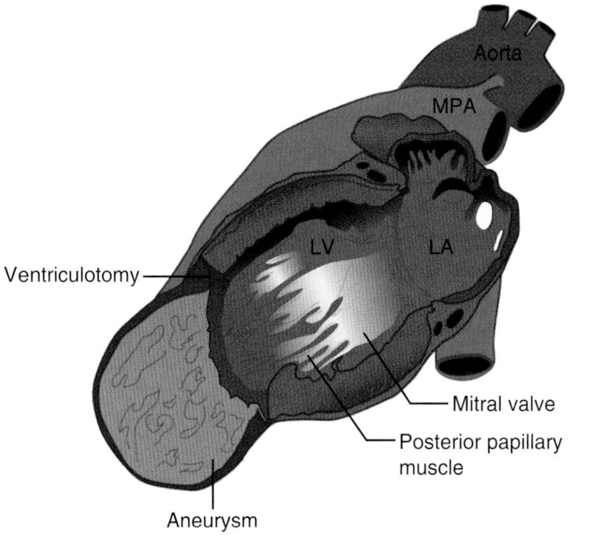

FIGURE 87-18 ■ Encircling endocardial ventriculotomy. *LA,* Left atrium; *LV,* left ventricle; *MPA,* main pulmonary artery. (From Guiraudon G, Fontaine G, Frank R, et al: Encircling endocardial ventriculotomy: a new surgical treatment for life-threatening ventricular tachycardias resistant to medical treatment following myocardial infarction. *Ann Thorac Surg* 26:438–444, 1978.)

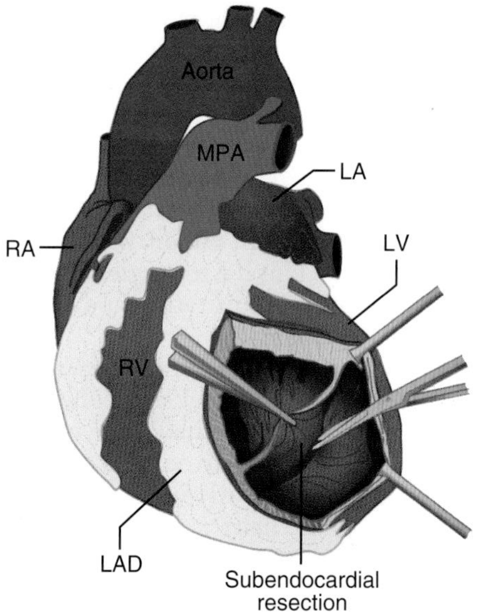

FIGURE 87-19 ■ Endocardial resection procedure. *LA,* Left atrium; *LAD,* left anterior descending coronary artery; *LV,* left ventricle; *MPA,* main pulmonary artery; *RA,* right atrium; *RV,* right ventricle. (From Moran JM, Kehoe RF, Loeb JM, et al: Extended endocardial resection for the treatment of ventricular tachycardia and ventricular fibrillation. *Ann Thorac Surg* 34:538–552, 1982.)

more than 70%, and 5-year survival was approximately 60%.[177-181] Subsequently, surgical experience revealed that intraoperative mapping was not necessary to achieve good results if an extended endomyocardial resection was performed. When examining approximately 500 patients having either map-guided or non-guided extended resections, Hargrove and Miller[182] determined that the number of patients whose arrhythmias are inducible at the postoperative electrophysiologic study was not significantly different between groups.

With the introduction of the ICD into clinical practice, referrals of patients for ventricular tachycardia surgery decreased markedly. With a new generation of electrophysiologists and cardiac surgeons who are largely unfamiliar with ventricular tachycardia surgery, many physicians now overlook the role that surgery continues to play in selected patients. The following two subsections discuss indications and techniques for the surgical treatment of ventricular tachycardia in the ICD era.

Surgical Indications for Ventricular Tachycardia

A number of important points need to be emphasized about surgical options for ventricular tachycardia. First, surgical mortality in the ICD era has been significantly lower than that historically reported in the early clinical experience with direct ventricular tachycardia surgery. This is because high-risk patients (i.e., poor left ventricular function, no discrete aneurysm, polymorphic ventricular tachycardia) are no longer referred for surgery but are preferentially treated with ICDs. In a series of patients reported from the University of Virginia and from our institution, the hospital mortality rate was 4.9% and surgical success rates were above 90%.[183]

From 1988 to 2008, the Washington University experience included 74 patients.[184] During the last 10 years of this study period, 11 patients underwent direct ventricular tachycardia surgery with no operative mortality. During this time, the median hospital length of stay was 11 days. Seventy-three percent of patients (8 of 11) had no recurrence of their ventricular tachycardia at a mean follow-up of 5.8 years, and there were no late deaths in this group because of the liberal use of adjunctive ICD therapy. The overall survival of the group during the 20-year study period was excellent, with a 5-year survival of 65%. Thus, in properly selected patients, a low operative mortality rate can be expected, with good late results.

A second important point and an advantage of surgery is that the underlying left ventricular dysfunction can be addressed. This is not the case with catheter ablation, which eliminates only the arrhythmogenic substrate. Furthermore, coronary bypass grafting, left ventricular reconstruction or remodeling, and mitral valve repair can have a significant impact on late survival in appropriate patients.[185,186] In patients who are referred for surgery for left ventricular dysfunction, it is critical that these patients be offered a concomitant procedure to treat the ventricular tachycardia, when indicated, because of the excellent success rates of preventing recurrent ventricular tachycardia.[185,186] Surgery can improve the patient's quality of life by decreasing the number of defibrillator shocks.

Finally, ventricular tachycardia surgery can play a role in patients who are receiving frequent discharges from their device. Quality of life of these patients is poor.[160,187] In patients who have failed catheter ablation or are poor candidates for this procedure, surgery can play an important role if the patients have an appropriate substrate. The different procedures for ventricular tachycardia are discussed in the following section.

Surgical Techniques for Ventricular Tachycardia

Revascularization

Surgical coronary revascularization (CABG) alone has not been highly effective at treating ventricular tachycardia.[188-190] However, evidence suggests that when ischemia is the primary trigger for ventricular arrhythmias, CABG can alter the arrhythmic substrate in selected patients to reduce ventricular arrhythmias.[191,192] Several groups have documented that 40% to 60% of patients undergoing CABG with a preoperative clinical history of ventricular arrhythmias or fibrillation had no inducible ventricular arrhythmias at postoperative electrophysiologic testing.[189,190] Lee and colleagues demonstrated that only 25% of patients after CABG and ICD implantation for preoperative ventricular arrhythmias had inducible arrhythmias postoperatively.[193] However, in most patients with chronic ischemic ventricular tachycardia, the results of CABG have been too unpredictable, and most patients require concomitant ICD therapy. In patients with poor left ventricular function, ICDs play a role even when those patients have no history of ventricular tachycardia. The Multicenter Automatic Defibrillator Implantation

Trial II (MADIT II) found that prophylactic ICD implantation improved survival in patients with prior myocardial infarction and poor left ventricular function (left ventricular ejection fraction < 0.30).[194]

In patients with ischemic ventricular tachycardia, the only candidates for CABG alone are patients who have significant coronary artery disease, who have no ventricular dilation or aneurysm, and who suffer from documented exercise- or ischemia-induced ventricular arrhythmias. Postoperative exercise testing and electrophysiologic studies are used to determine whether implantation of an ICD is warranted.

Endocardial Resection

The resection of all visible endocardial scar, a procedure introduced by Harken in 1979, has become the gold standard and the most commonly performed operation for ventricular tachycardia.[175] The amount of ventricular tissue involved or its location near the posterior papillary muscle may limit a complete resection. In these cases, alternative ablation techniques are used either adjunctively or as the sole therapy. Although groups have reported use of energy sources such as laser, RF ablation, and microwave, the most commonly used and well-studied ablation technique is cryoablation. Popularized in the 1980s, the cryoablation probe is applied to the scar and typically cooled to −60° C for 2 or 3 minutes, resulting in lesions 2 to 3 cm in depth.

Although intraoperative mapping has yielded a wealth of information into the mechanisms of ventricular arrhythmias, its clinical practicality and questionable added efficacy to ventricular tachycardia surgery have prevented its widespread adoption. Virtually all surgeons have adopted a technique of resecting all visible endocardial scars without the use of intraoperative mapping.

A retrospective review of 74 patients who underwent an endocardial resection procedure (ERP) with adjunctive cryotherapy for ventricular arrhythmias from 1986 to 2007 was performed at Barnes-Jewish Hospital at Washington University in St. Louis. The mean age was 57 ± 14 years, and 81% of patients were male. One quarter of patients were in New York Heart Association class III or class IV heart failure, and the mean left ventricular ejection fraction was 34% ± 9%. Ninety-two percent of patients underwent ERP with a concomitant procedure, and 8% underwent ERP alone. The spectrum of procedures included ERP plus left ventricular aneurysm repair (26%), ERP plus CABG (5%), ERP plus CABG plus left ventricular aneurysm repair (46%), and ERP plus left ventricular aneurysm plus other cardiac procedure (15%). The overall operative mortality rate was 15%, with a median intensive care unit length of stay of 4 days and a median hospital length of stay of 12 days. As stated previously, there was no operative mortality during the last 10 years of our experience. Late follow-up was completed in 89% of patients. A Kaplan-Meier survival analysis was performed, and absolute survival for all patients in this series was 74% at 1 year and 65% at 5 years. Eighty-eight percent of the cases were performed during the first decade (1986 to 1996) and the remaining cases during the next decade (1997 to 2007), reflecting the diminishing role of surgical management in this disease. Since 2007, only three additional ERPs have been performed (Fig. 87-20).

Left Ventricular Reconstruction

In 1985, Vincent Dor described a surgical technique to restore the dilated left ventricle in patients with ischemic cardiomyopathy or ventricular aneurysms to its normal elliptical shape by reducing the volume of the ventricle.[195,196] The Dor procedure uses an endoventricular circular patch to reduce ventricular volume, which subsequently reduces wall tension and ischemia. Good surgical candidates for left ventricular reconstruction typically present with heart failure (left ventricular ejection fraction < 40%), coronary artery disease, large areas of myocardial akinesis (ventricular dilation), or a

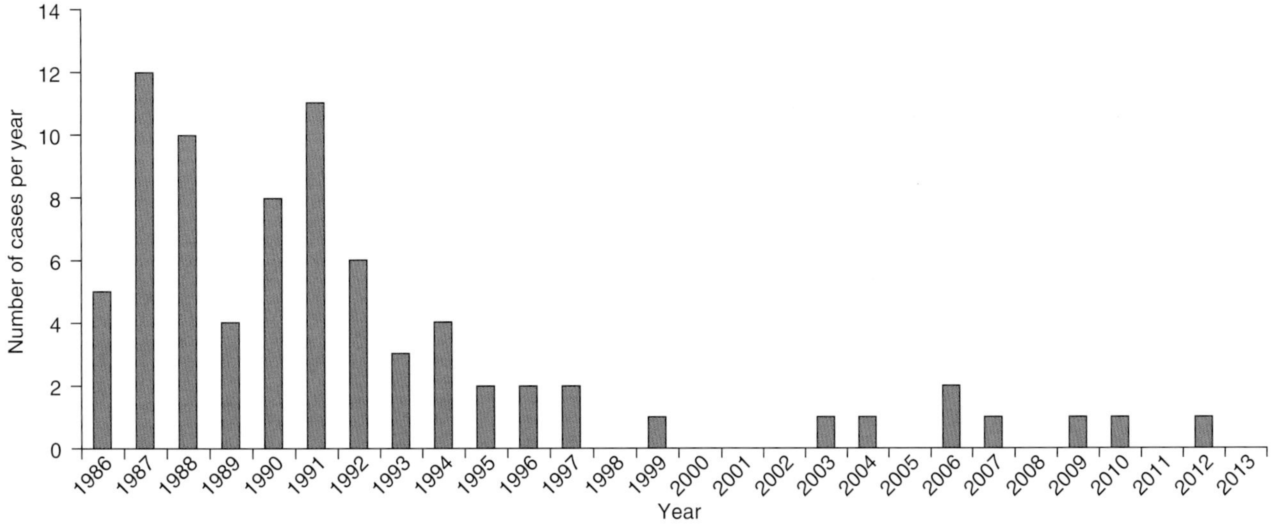

FIGURE 87-20 ■ Washington University School of Medicine/Barnes-Jewish Hospital experience with ventricular tachycardia surgery.

left ventricular aneurysm. These patients commonly have associated ventricular arrhythmias. Currently, Dor emphasizes the importance of complete revascularization (CABG), repair of any mitral disease, and endocardial resection with cryoablation at the same setting. A more complete description of the Dor procedure and its modifications, including technical considerations, can be found in Chapter 100.

In 2004, Maxey and colleagues demonstrated that the Dor procedure restores the left ventricle's geometry, resulting in a mean ejection fraction increase of 12.5%.[197] Ventricular function continues to improve during the patient's lifetime. The RESTORE group experience examined a registry of 1198 postinfarction patients between 1998 and 2003 who underwent left ventricular restoration and found that 5-year freedom from hospital readmission for congestive heart failure was 78%. In addition, 67% of patients were assigned to class III or class IV preoperatively; 85% were assigned to class I or class II postoperatively.[185]

Several groups have demonstrated that the triggers for ventricular arrhythmias occur at the scar border zone in patients with ischemic cardiomyopathy.[165-168] Thus, the Dor procedure addresses ventricular arrhythmias by removing the anatomic substrate during resection of the postinfarction scar or aneurysm. In 1994, Dor and associates[196] reported a 90% freedom from inducible ventricular tachycardia at 1 year after endocardial resection and left ventricle reconstruction in 106 patients. In 2004, Mickleborough and colleagues reported long-term outcomes after left ventricular reconstruction and coronary revascularization for patients with hypokinesis or akinesis and coronary artery disease with poor left ventricular function. Results demonstrated that operative survivors had freedom from ventricular tachycardia and sudden death at 1 year, 5 years, and 10 years of 99%, 97%, and 94%, respectively.[198]

In spite of the excellent results previously mentioned, the efficacy of left ventricular restoration alone for the treatment of ventricular tachycardia has been controversial. The Cleveland Clinic experience illustrated the relative lack of efficacy of the Dor procedure alone without endocardial resection surgery.[199] In this series, 48 of 113 patients (42%) who had a postoperative electrophysiology study had inducible ventricular tachycardia after the Dor procedure. Furthermore, in patients with an ICD, 15% had either sudden cardiac death or appropriate shocks. With early electrophysiology study, ICD implantation, or both, the overall incidence of sudden cardiac death was less than 1%. In 2004, DiDonato and associates demonstrated in 382 patients that left ventricular restoration with endocardial resection reduced the inducible ventricular tachycardia from 41% to 8%, suggesting that many patients may not need a postoperative ICD.[186]

Because of the high lethality of ventricular tachyarrhythmias in patients in whom surgery is not curative, it is generally recommended that all patients after the Dor procedure undergo electrophysiology study or implantation of an ICD if they have had a history of ventricular arrhythmias or inducible ventricular tachycardia preoperatively.

Cardiac Assist Devices and Heart Transplantation

In rare cases, patients present with uncontrolled ventricular arrhythmias refractory to conventional surgical, ICD, or medical therapy. Typically, these patients have an end-stage cardiomyopathy resulting in incessant ventricular tachycardia. If the patients are not amenable to conventional cardiac revascularization or other procedures, these malignant arrhythmias may be effectively palliated with a cardiac assist device, either as a bridge to transplantation or as destination therapy.[200-202] The cardiac assist device effectively reduces myocardial oxygen demand and can decrease the incidence of ischemia-induced arrhythmias.[203]

Conclusions

ICDs and catheter ablation have significantly reduced the role of surgery in the treatment of ventricular arrhythmias. When indicated, however, current surgical techniques can be quite successful. The surgical approach should be individualized to each patient. The current indications for surgery include the following: (1) In patients who have ischemic ventricular tachycardia requiring revascularization and who have poor left ventricular function and no significant wall thinning, the recommended treatment is CABG and ICD placement. If significant wall thinning or a discrete aneurysm is present, ventricular remodeling, extended endomyocardial resection, and cryoablation should be performed. (2) Surgery for ventricular tachycardia should be considered for patients suffering from frequent ICD discharges that are poorly tolerated and have an amenable anatomic substrate. In the presence of frequent ICD shocks with a discrete left ventricular aneurysm or wall thinning, ventricular remodeling, extended endomyocardial resection, and cryoablation should be considered.

REFERENCES

1. Go AS, Mozaffarian D, Roger VL, et al: Heart disease and stroke statistics–2013 update: a report from the American Heart Association. *Circulation* 127:e6–e245, 2013.
2. Lloyd-Jones DM, Wang TJ, Leip EP, et al: Lifetime risk for development of atrial fibrillation: the Framingham Heart Study. *Circulation* 110:1042–1046, 2004.
3. Chugh SS, Blackshear JL, Shen WK, et al: Epidemiology and natural history of atrial fibrillation: clinical implications. *J Am Coll Cardiol* 37:371–378, 2001.
4. Feinberg WM, Blackshear JL, Laupacis A, et al: Prevalence, age distribution, and gender of patients with atrial fibrillation. Analysis and implications. *Arch Intern Med* 155:469–473, 1995.
5. Go AS, Hylek EM, Phillips KA, et al: Prevalence of diagnosed atrial fibrillation in adults: national implications for rhythm management and stroke prevention: the AnTicoagulation and Risk Factors in Atrial Fibrillation (ATRIA) Study. *JAMA* 285:2370–2375, 2001.
6. Piccini JP, Hammill BG, Sinner MF, et al: Incidence and prevalence of atrial fibrillation and associated mortality among Medicare beneficiaries, 1993-2007. *Circ Cardiovasc Qual Outcomes* 5:85–93, 2012.
7. Miyasaka Y, Barnes ME, Gersh BJ, et al: Secular trends in incidence of atrial fibrillation in Olmsted County, Minnesota, 1980 to 2000, and implications on the projections for future prevalence. *Circulation* 114:119–125, 2006.
8. Kim MH, Johnston SS, Chu BC, et al: Estimation of total incremental health care costs in patients with atrial fibrillation in the United States. *Circ Cardiovasc Qual Outcomes* 4:313–320, 2011.

9. Benjamin EJ, Levy D, Vaziri SM, et al: Independent risk factors for atrial fibrillation in a population-based cohort. The Framingham Heart Study. *JAMA* 271:840–844, 1994.
10. Wolf PA, Benjamin EJ, Belanger AJ, et al: Secular trends in the prevalence of atrial fibrillation: the Framingham Study. *Am Heart J* 131:790–795, 1996.
11. Cairns JA: Stroke prevention in atrial fibrillation trial. *Circulation* 84:933–935, 1991.
12. Hart RG, Halperin JL, Pearce LA, et al: Lessons from the Stroke Prevention in Atrial Fibrillation trials. *Ann Intern Med* 138:831–838, 2003.
13. Sherman DG, Kim SG, Boop BS, et al: Occurrence and characteristics of stroke events in the Atrial Fibrillation Follow-up Investigation of Sinus Rhythm Management (AFFIRM) study. *Arch Intern Med* 165:1185–1191, 2005.
14. Wolf PA, Abbott RD, Kannel WB: Atrial fibrillation as an independent risk factor for stroke: the Framingham Study. *Stroke* 22:983–988, 1991.
15. Wazni OM, Marrouche NF, Martin DO, et al: Radiofrequency ablation vs antiarrhythmic drugs as first-line treatment of symptomatic atrial fibrillation: a randomized trial. *JAMA* 293:2634–2640, 2005.
16. Channer KS: Current management of symptomatic atrial fibrillation. *Drugs* 61:1425–1437, 2001.
17. Ezekowitz MD, Levine JA: Preventing stroke in patients with atrial fibrillation. *JAMA* 281:1830–1835, 1999.
18. Glader EL, Stegmayr B, Norrving B, et al: Large variations in the use of oral anticoagulants in stroke patients with atrial fibrillation: a Swedish national perspective. *J Intern Med* 255:22–32, 2004.
19. Steger C, Pratter A, Martinek-Bregel M, et al: Stroke patients with atrial fibrillation have a worse prognosis than patients without: data from the Austrian Stroke registry. *Eur Heart J* 25:1734–1740, 2004.
20. Risk factors for stroke and efficacy of antithrombotic therapy in atrial fibrillation. Analysis of pooled data from five randomized controlled trials. *Arch Intern Med* 154:1449–1457, 1994.
21. Hylek EM, Evans-Molina C, Shea C, et al: Major hemorrhage and tolerability of warfarin in the first year of therapy among elderly patients with atrial fibrillation. *Circulation* 115:2689–2696, 2007.
22. Marinigh R, Lip GY, Fiotti N, et al: Age as a risk factor for stroke in atrial fibrillation patients implications for thromboprophylaxis: implications for thromboprophylaxis. *J Am Coll Cardiol* 56:827–837, 2010.
23. Benjamin EJ, Wolf PA, D'Agostino RB, et al: Impact of atrial fibrillation on the risk of death: the Framingham Heart Study. *Circulation* 98:946–952, 1998.
24. January CT, Wann LS, Alpert JS, et al: 2014 AHA/ACC/HRS guideline for the management of patients with atrial fibrillation: executive summary: a report of the American College of Cardiology/American Heart Association Task Force on practice guidelines and the Heart Rhythm Society. *Circulation* 130(23):2071–2104, 2014.
25. Calkins H, Brugada J, Packer DL, et al: HRS/EHRA/ECAS expert consensus statement on catheter and surgical ablation of atrial fibrillation: recommendations for personnel, policy, procedures and follow-up. A report of the Heart Rhythm Society (HRS) Task Force on Catheter and Surgical Ablation of Atrial Fibrillation developed in partnership with the European Heart Rhythm Association (EHRA) and the European Cardiac Arrhythmia Society (ECAS); in collaboration with the American College of Cardiology (ACC), American Heart Association (AHA), and the Society of Thoracic Surgeons (STS). Endorsed and approved by the governing bodies of the American College of Cardiology, the American Heart Association, the European Cardiac Arrhythmia Society, the European Heart Rhythm Association, the Society of Thoracic Surgeons, and the Heart Rhythm Society. *Europace* 9:335–379, 2007.
26. Schuessler RB, Kay MW, Melby SJ, et al: Spatial and temporal stability of the dominant frequency of activation in human atrial fibrillation. *J Electrocardiol* 39:S7–S12, 2006.
27. Boineau JP, Schuessler RB, Canavan TE, et al: The human atrial pacemaker complex. *J Electrocardiol* 22(Suppl):189–197, 1989.
28. Byrd GD, Prasad SM, Ripplinger CM, et al: Importance of geometry and refractory period in sustaining atrial fibrillation: testing the critical mass hypothesis. *Circulation* 112:I7–I13, 2005.
29. Haissaguerre M, Jais P, Shah DC, et al: Spontaneous initiation of atrial fibrillation by ectopic beats originating in the pulmonary veins. *New Engl J Med* 339:659–666, 1998.
30. Spach MS, Barr RC, Jewett PH: Spread of excitation from the atrium into thoracic veins in human beings and dogs. *Am J Cardiol* 30:844–854, 1972.
31. Blom NA, Gittenberger-de Groot AC, DeRuiter MC, et al: Development of the cardiac conduction tissue in human embryos using HNK-1 antigen expression: possible relevance for understanding of abnormal atrial automaticity. *Circulation* 99:800–806, 1999.
32. Chen YJ, Chen SA, Chang MS, et al: Arrhythmogenic activity of cardiac muscle in pulmonary veins of the dog: implication for the genesis of atrial fibrillation. *Cardiovasc Res* 48:265–273, 2000.
33. Schmitt C, Ndrepepa G, Weber S, et al: Biatrial multisite mapping of atrial premature complexes triggering onset of atrial fibrillation. *Am J Cardiol* 89:1381–1387, 2002.
34. Nitta T, Ishii Y, Miyagi Y, et al: Concurrent multiple left atrial focal activations with fibrillatory conduction and right atrial focal or reentrant activation as the mechanism in atrial fibrillation. *J Thorac Cardiov Sur* 127:770–778, 2004.
35. Nitta T, Ohmori H, Sakamoto S, et al: Map-guided surgery for atrial fibrillation. *J Thorac Cardiov Sur* 129:291–299, 2005.
36. Schuessler RB: Do we need a map to get through the maze? *J Thorac Cardiov Sur* 127:627–628, 2004.
37. Ghosh S, Avari JN, Rhee EK, et al: Hypertrophic cardiomyopathy with preexcitation: insights from noninvasive electrocardiographic imaging (ECGI) and catheter mapping. *J Cardiovasc Electr* 19:1215–1217, 2008.
38. Golzari H, Cebul RD, Bahler RC: Atrial fibrillation: restoration and maintenance of sinus rhythm and indications for anticoagulation therapy. *Ann Intern Med* 125:311–323, 1996.
39. Fang MC, Stafford RS, Ruskin JN, et al: National trends in antiarrhythmic and antithrombotic medication use in atrial fibrillation. *Arch Intern Med* 164:55–60, 2004.
40. Wijffels MC, Crijns HJ: Recent advances in drug therapy for atrial fibrillation. *J Cardiovasc Electr* 14:S40–S47, 2003.
41. Miller MR, McNamara RL, Segal JB, et al: Efficacy of agents for pharmacologic conversion of atrial fibrillation and subsequent maintenance of sinus rhythm: a meta-analysis of clinical trials. *J Fam Practice* 49:1033–1046, 2000.
42. Fuster V, Ryden LE, Asinger RW, et al: ACC/AHA/ESC guidelines for the management of patients with atrial fibrillation: executive summary. A Report of the American College of Cardiology/American Heart Association Task Force on Practice Guidelines and the European Society of Cardiology Committee for Practice Guidelines and Policy Conferences (Committee to Develop Guidelines for the Management of Patients With Atrial Fibrillation): developed in Collaboration With the North American Society of Pacing and Electrophysiology. *J Am Coll Cardiol* 38:1231–1266, 2001.
43. Boriani G, Diemberger I, Biffi M, et al: Pharmacological cardioversion of atrial fibrillation: current management and treatment options. *Drugs* 64:2741–2762, 2004.
44. The Planning and Steering Committees of the AFFIRM study for the NHLBI AFFIRM investigators: atrial fibrillation follow-up investigation of rhythm management—the AFFIRM study design. *Am J Cardiol* 79:1198–1202, 1997.
45. Waldo AL: Management of atrial fibrillation: the need for AFFIRMative action. AFFIRM investigators. Atrial Fibrillation Follow-up Investigation of Rhythm Management. *Am J Cardiol* 84:698–700, 1999.
46. Wyse DG, Waldo AL, DiMarco JP, et al: A comparison of rate control and rhythm control in patients with atrial fibrillation. *New Engl J Med* 347:1825–1833, 2002.
47. Van Gelder IC, Hagens VE, Bosker HA, et al: A comparison of rate control and rhythm control in patients with recurrent persistent atrial fibrillation. *New Engl J Med* 347:1834–1840, 2002.
48. Gomez-Outes A, Terleira-Fernandez AI, Calvo-Rojas G, et al: Dabigatran, rivaroxaban, or apixaban versus warfarin in patients with nonvalvular atrial fibrillation: a systematic review and meta-analysis of subgroups. *Thrombosis* 2013:640723, 2013.
49. DiMarco JP, Flaker G, Waldo AL, et al: Factors affecting bleeding risk during anticoagulant therapy in patients with atrial fibrillation: observations from the Atrial Fibrillation Follow-up Investigation of Rhythm Management (AFFIRM) study. *Am Heart J* 149:650–656, 2005.

50. Copland M, Walker ID, Tait RC: Oral anticoagulation and hemorrhagic complications in an elderly population with atrial fibrillation. *Arch Intern Med* 161:2125–2128, 2001.
51. Levine MN, Raskob G, Landefeld S, et al: Hemorrhagic complications of anticoagulant treatment. *Chest* 119:108S–121S, 2001.
52. Investigators AFADS: Maintenance of sinus rhythm in patients with atrial fibrillation: an AFFIRM substudy of the first antiarrhythmic drug. *J Am Coll Cardiol* 42:20–29, 2003.
53. Corley SD, Epstein AE, DiMarco JP, et al: Relationships between sinus rhythm, treatment, and survival in the Atrial Fibrillation Follow-Up Investigation of Rhythm Management (AFFIRM) Study. *Circulation* 109:1509–1513, 2004.
54. Defauw JJ, Guiraudon GM, van Hemel NM, et al: Surgical therapy of paroxysmal atrial fibrillation with the "corridor" operation. *Ann Thorac Surg* 53:564–570, discussion 71, 1992.
55. Guiraudon GM, Klein GJ, Sharma AD, et al: Surgical alternatives for supraventricular tachycardias. *Am J Cardiol* 64:92J–96J, 1989.
56. Williams JM, Ungerleider RM, Lofland GK, et al: Left atrial isolation: new technique for the treatment of supraventricular arrhythmias. *J Thorac Cardiov Sur* 80:373–380, 1980.
57. Scheinman MM, Morady F, Hess DS, et al: Catheter-induced ablation of the atrioventricular junction to control refractory supraventricular arrhythmias. *JAMA* 248:851–855, 1982.
58. Guiraudon GM, Campbell CS, Jones DL, et al: Combined sinoatrial node atrioventricular node isolation: a surgical alternative to His bundle ablation in patients with atrial fibrillation. *Circulation* 72:220, 1985.
59. Smith PK, Holman WL, Cox JL: Surgical treatment of supraventricular tachyarrhythmias. *Surgical Clin N Am* 65:553–570, 1985.
60. Cox JL: The surgical treatment of atrial fibrillation. IV. Surgical technique. *J Thorac Cardiov Sur* 101:584–592, 1991.
61. Cox JL, Schuessler RB, D'Agostino HJ, Jr, et al: The surgical treatment of atrial fibrillation. III. Development of a definitive surgical procedure. *J Thorac Cardiov Sur* 101:569–583, 1991.
62. Cox JL, Canavan TE, Schuessler RB, et al: The surgical treatment of atrial fibrillation. II. Intraoperative electrophysiologic mapping and description of the electrophysiologic basis of atrial flutter and atrial fibrillation. *J Thorac Cardiov Sur* 101:406–426, 1991.
63. Cox JL, Ad N, Palazzo T: Impact of the maze procedure on the stroke rate in patients with atrial fibrillation. *J Thorac Cardiov Sur* 118:833–840, 1999.
64. Feinberg MS, Waggoner AD, Kater KM, et al: Restoration of atrial function after the maze procedure for patients with atrial fibrillation. Assessment by Doppler echocardiography. *Circulation* 90:II285–II292, 1994.
65. Cox JL, Boineau JP, Schuessler RB, et al: Modification of the maze procedure for atrial flutter and atrial fibrillation. I. Rationale and surgical results. *J Thorac Cardiov Sur* 110:473–484, 1995.
66. JL C: The minimally invasive Maze-III procedure. *Oper Tech Thorac Cardiovasc Surg* 5:79, 2000.
67. Prasad SM, Maniar HS, Camillo CJ, et al: The Cox Maze III procedure for atrial fibrillation long-term efficacy in patients undergoing lone versus concomitant procedures. *J Thorac Cardiov Sur* 126:1822–1828, 2003.
68. McCarthy PM, Gillinov AM, Castle L, et al: The Cox-Maze procedure: the Cleveland Clinic experience. *Semin Thorac Cardiovasc Surg* 12:25–29, 2000.
69. Raanani E, Albage A, David TE, et al: The efficacy of the Cox/maze procedure combined with mitral valve surgery: a matched control study. *Eur J Cardio-Thorac* 19:438–442, 2001.
70. Schaff HV, Dearani JA, Daly RC, et al: Cox-Maze procedure for atrial fibrillation: Mayo Clinic experience. *Semin Thorac Cardiovasc Surg* 12:30–37, 2000.
71. Khargi K, Hutten BA, Lemke B, et al: Surgical treatment of atrial fibrillation; a systematic review. *Eur J Cardio-Thorac* 27:258–265, 2005.
72. Gammie JS, Haddad M, Milford-Beland S, et al: Atrial fibrillation correction surgery: lessons from the Society of Thoracic Surgeons National Cardiac Database. *Ann Thorac Surg* 85:909–914, 2008.
73. Ad N, Suri RM, Gammie JS, et al: Surgical ablation of atrial fibrillation trends and outcomes in North America. *J Thorac Cardiov Sur* 144:1051–1060, 2012.
74. Melby SJ, Lee AM, Schuessler R, et al: The effect of residual gaps in ablation lines for the treatment of atrial fibrillation. *Heart Rhythm* 2:S15, 2005.
75. Viola N, Williams MR, Oz MC, et al: The technology in use for the surgical ablation of atrial fibrillation. *Semin Thorac Cardiovasc Surg* 14:198–205, 2002.
76. Prasad SM, Maniar HS, Schuessler RB, et al: Chronic transmural atrial ablation by using bipolar radiofrequency energy on the beating heart. *J Thorac Cardiov Sur* 124:708–713, 2002.
77. Prasad SM, Maniar HS, Diodato MD, et al: Physiological consequences of bipolar radiofrequency energy on the atria and pulmonary veins: a chronic animal study. *Ann Thorac Surg* 76:836–841, discussion 41–42, 2003.
78. Gaynor SL, Ishii Y, Diodato MD, et al: Successful performance of Cox-Maze procedure on beating heart using bipolar radiofrequency ablation: a feasibility study in animals. *Ann Thorac Surg* 78:1671–1677, 2004.
79. Demazumder D, Mirotznik MS, Schwartzman D: Biophysics of radiofrequency ablation using an irrigated electrode. *J Interv Card Electr* 5:377–389, 2001.
80. Ruchat P, Schlaepfer J, Delabays A, et al: Left atrial radiofrequency compartmentalization for chronic atrial fibrillation during heart surgery. *Thorac Cardiov Surg* 50:155–159, 2002.
81. Saint LL, Lawrance CP, Okada S, et al: Performance of a novel bipolar/monopolar radiofrequency ablation device on the beating heart in an acute porcine model. *Innovations* 8:276–283, 2013.
82. Melby SJ, Gaynor SL, Lubahn JG, et al: Efficacy and safety of right and left atrial ablations on the beating heart with irrigated bipolar radiofrequency energy: a long-term animal study. *J Thorac Cardiov Sur* 132:853–860, 2006.
83. Hamner CE, Potter DD, Jr, Cho KR, et al: Irrigated radiofrequency ablation with transmurality feedback reliably produces Cox Maze lesions in vivo. *Ann Thorac Surg* 80:2263–2270, 2005.
84. Khargi K, Deneke T, Haardt H, et al: Saline-irrigated, cooled-tip radiofrequency ablation is an effective technique to perform the maze procedure. *Ann Thorac Surg* 72:S1090–S1095, 2001.
85. Nakagawa H, Wittkampf FH, Yamanashi WS, et al: Inverse relationship between electrode size and lesion size during radiofrequency ablation with active electrode cooling. *Circulation* 98:458–465, 1998.
86. Kress DC, Krum D, Chekanov V, et al: Validation of a left atrial lesion pattern for intraoperative ablation of atrial fibrillation. *Ann Thorac Surg* 73:1160–1168, 2002.
87. Santiago T, Melo JQ, Gouveia RH, et al: Intra-atrial temperatures in radiofrequency endocardial ablation: histologic evaluation of lesions. *Ann Thorac Surg* 75:1495–1501, 2003.
88. Thomas SP, Guy DJ, Boyd AC, et al: Comparison of epicardial and endocardial linear ablation using handheld probes. *Ann Thorac Surg* 75:543–548, 2003.
89. Hoenicke EM, Strange RG, Patel H, et al: Initial experience with epicardial radiofrequency ablation catheter in an ovine model: moving towards an endoscopic Maze procedure. *Surg Forum* 51:79–82, 2000.
90. Santiago T, Melo J, Gouveia RH, et al: Epicardial radiofrequency applications: in vitro and in vivo studies on human atrial myocardium. *Eur J Cardio-Thorac* 24:481–486, discussion 6, 2003.
91. Schuessler RB, Lee AM, Melby SJ, et al: Animal studies of epicardial atrial ablation. *Heart Rhythm* 6:S41–S45, 2009.
92. Gaynor SL, Diodato MD, Prasad SM, et al: A prospective, single-center clinical trial of a modified Cox Maze procedure with bipolar radiofrequency ablation. *J Thorac Cardiov Sur* 128:535–542, 2004.
93. Kottkamp H, Hindricks G, Autschbach R, et al: Specific linear left atrial lesions in atrial fibrillation: intraoperative radiofrequency ablation using minimally invasive surgical techniques. *J Am Coll Cardiol* 40:475–480, 2002.
94. Gillinov AM, Pettersson G, Rice TW: Esophageal injury during radiofrequency ablation for atrial fibrillation. *J Thorac Cardiov Sur* 122:1239–1240, 2001.
95. Laczkovics A, Khargi K, Deneke T: Esophageal perforation during left atrial radiofrequency ablation. *J Thorac Cardiov Sur* 126:2119–2120, author reply 20, 2003.
96. Demaria RG, Page P, Leung TK, et al: Surgical radiofrequency ablation induces coronary endothelial dysfunction in porcine coronary arteries. *Eur Journal Cardio-Thorac* 23:277–282, 2003.
97. Lustgarten DL, Keane D, Ruskin J: Cryothermal ablation: mechanism of tissue injury and current experience in the treatment of tachyarrhythmias. *Prog Cardiovasc Dis* 41:481–498, 1999.

98. Doll N, Kornherr P, Aupperle H, et al: Epicardial treatment of atrial fibrillation using cryoablation in an acute off-pump sheep model. *Thorac Cardiov Surg* 51:267–273, 2003.
99. Masroor S, Jahnke ME, Carlisle A, et al: Endocardial hypothermia and pulmonary vein isolation with epicardial cryoablation in a porcine beating-heart model. *J Thorac Cardiov Sur* 135:1327–1333, 2008.
100. Blomstrom-Lundqvist C, Johansson B, Berglin E, et al: A randomized double-blind study of epicardial left atrial cryoablation for permanent atrial fibrillation in patients undergoing mitral valve surgery: the SWEDish Multicentre Atrial Fibrillation study (SWEDMAF). *Eur Heart J* 28:2902–2908, 2007.
101. Watanabe H, Hayashi J, Aizawa Y: Myocardial infarction after cryoablation surgery for Wolff-Parkinson-White syndrome. *Jpn J Thorac Cardiovasc Surg* 50:210–212, 2002.
102. Mikat EM, Hackel DB, Harrison L, et al: Reaction of the myocardium and coronary arteries to cryosurgery. *Lab Invest* 37:632–641, 1977.
103. Manasse E, Colombo P, Roncalli M, et al: Myocardial acute and chronic histological modifications induced by cryoablation. *Eur J Cardio-Thorac* 17:339–340, 2000.
104. Holman WL, Ikeshita M, Ungerleider RM, et al: Cryosurgery for cardiac arrhythmias: acute and chronic effects on coronary arteries. *Am J Cardiol* 51:149–155, 1983.
105. Calkins H, Kuck KH, Cappato R, et al: 2012 HRS/EHRA/ECAS expert consensus statement on catheter and surgical ablation of atrial fibrillation: recommendations for patient selection, procedural techniques, patient management and follow-up, definitions, endpoints, and research trial design: a report of the Heart Rhythm Society (HRS) Task Force on Catheter and Surgical Ablation of Atrial Fibrillation. Developed in partnership with the European Heart Rhythm Association (EHRA), a registered branch of the European Society of Cardiology (ESC) and the European Cardiac Arrhythmia Society (ECAS); and in collaboration with the American College of Cardiology (ACC), American Heart Association (AHA), the Asia Pacific Heart Rhythm Society (APHRS), and the Society of Thoracic Surgeons (STS). Endorsed by the governing bodies of the American College of Cardiology Foundation, the American Heart Association, the European Cardiac Arrhythmia Society, the European Heart Rhythm Association, the Society of Thoracic Surgeons, the Asia Pacific Heart Rhythm Society, and the Heart Rhythm Society. *Heart Rhythm* 9:632–696, e21, 2012.
106. Pet M, Robertson JO, Bailey M, et al: The impact of CHADS2 score on late stroke after the Cox Maze procedure. *J Thorac Cardiov Sur* 146:85–89, 2013.
107. Cox JL, Boineau JP, Schuessler RB, et al: Operations for atrial fibrillation. *Clin Cardiol* 14:827–834, 1991.
108. Cox JL, Boineau JP, Schuessler RB, et al: Successful surgical treatment of atrial fibrillation. Review and clinical update. *JAMA* 266:1976–1980, 1991.
109. Cox JL, Schuessler RB, Boineau JP: The development of the Maze procedure for the treatment of atrial fibrillation. *Semin Thorac Cardiovasc Surg* 12:2–14, 2000.
110. Damiano RJ, Gaynor SL: Atrial fibrillation ablation during mitral valve surgery using the AtriCure device. *Oper Tech Thorac Cardiovasc Surg* 9:2–14, 2004.
111. Lall SC, Melby SJ, Voeller RK, et al: The effect of ablation technology on surgical outcomes after the Cox-Maze procedure: a propensity analysis. *J Thorac Cardiov Sur* 133:389–396, 2007.
112. Doll N, Borger MA, Fabricius A, et al: Esophageal perforation during left atrial radiofrequency ablation: is the risk too high? *J Thorac Cardiov Sur* 125:836–842, 2003.
113. Sonmez B, Demirsoy E, Yagan N, et al: A fatal complication due to radiofrequency ablation for atrial fibrillation: atrio-esophageal fistula. *Ann Thorac Surg* 76:281–283, 2003.
114. Fayad G, Modine T, Le Tourneau T, et al: Circumflex artery stenosis induced by intraoperative radiofrequency ablation. *Ann Thorac Surg* 76:1291–1293, 2003.
115. Saint LL, Lawrance CP, Leidenfrost JE, et al: How I do it: minimally invasive Cox-Maze IV procedure. *Ann Cardiothorac Surg* 2014.
116. Prasad SM, Maniar HS, Camillo CJ, et al: The Cox Maze III procedure for atrial fibrillation: long-term efficacy in patients undergoing lone versus concomitant procedures. *J Thorac Cardiov Sur* 126:1822–1828, 2003.
117. Weimar T, Bailey MS, Watanabe Y, et al: The Cox-Maze IV procedure for lone atrial fibrillation: a single center experience in 100 consecutive patients. *J Interv Card Electrophysiol* 31:47–54, 2011.
118. Mokadam NA, McCarthy PM, Gillinov AM, et al: A prospective multicenter trial of bipolar radiofrequency ablation for atrial fibrillation: early results. *Ann Thorac Surg* 78:1665–1670, 2004.
119. Weimar T, Schena S, Bailey MS, et al: The Cox-Maze procedure for lone atrial fibrillation: a single-center experience over 2 decades. *Circ Arrhythmia Electrophysiol* 5:8–14, 2012.
120. Voeller RK, Bailey MS, Zierer A, et al: Isolating the entire posterior left atrium improves surgical outcomes after the Cox Maze procedure. *J Thorac Cardiov Sur* 135:870–877, 2008.
121. Bando K, Kobayashi J, Hirata M, et al: Early and late stroke after mitral valve replacement with a mechanical prosthesis: risk factor analysis of a 24-year experience. *J Thorac Cardiov Sur* 126:358–364, 2003.
122. Gaita F, Riccardi R, Caponi D, et al: Linear cryoablation of the left atrium versus pulmonary vein cryoisolation in patients with permanent atrial fibrillation and valvular heart disease: correlation of electroanatomic mapping and long-term clinical results. *Circulation* 111:136–142, 2005.
123. Fasol R, Meinhart J, Binder T: A modified and simplified radiofrequency ablation in patients with mitral valve disease. *J Thorac Cardiov Sur* 129:215–217, 2005.
124. Sie HT, Beukema WP, Misier AR, et al: Radiofrequency modified maze in patients with atrial fibrillation undergoing concomitant cardiac surgery. *J Thorac Cardiov Sur* 122:249–256, 2001.
125. Deneke T, Khargi K, Grewe PH, et al: Efficacy of an additional MAZE procedure using cooled-tip radiofrequency ablation in patients with chronic atrial fibrillation and mitral valve disease. A randomized, prospective trial. *Eur Heart J* 23:558–566, 2002.
126. Benussi S, Nascimbene S, Agricola E, et al: Surgical ablation of atrial fibrillation using the epicardial radiofrequency approach: mid-term results and risk analysis. *Ann Thorac Surg* 74:1050–1056, discussion 7, 2002.
127. Knaut M, Spitzer SG, Karolyi L, et al: Intraoperative microwave ablation for curative treatment of atrial fibrillation in open heart surgery—the MICRO-STAF and MICRO-PASS pilot trial. MICROwave Application in Surgical treatment of Atrial Fibrillation. MICROwave Application for the Treatment of Atrial Fibrillation in Bypass-Surgery. *Thorac Cardiov Surg* 47(Suppl 3):379–384, 1999.
128. Schuetz A, Schulze CJ, Sarvanakis KK, et al: Surgical treatment of permanent atrial fibrillation using microwave energy ablation: a prospective randomized clinical trial. *Eur J Cardio-Thorac* 24:475–480, discussion 80, 2003.
129. Imai K, Sueda T, Orihashi K, et al: Clinical analysis of results of a simple left atrial procedure for chronic atrial fibrillation. *Ann Thorac Surg* 71:577–581, 2001.
130. Kondo N, Takahashi K, Minakawa M, et al: Left atrial maze procedure: a useful addition to other corrective operations. *Ann Thorac Surg* 75:1490–1494, 2003.
131. Wolf RK, Schneeberger EW, Osterday R, et al: Video-assisted bilateral pulmonary vein isolation and left atrial appendage exclusion for atrial fibrillation. *J Thorac Cardiov Sur* 130:797–802, 2005.
132. Tada H, Ito S, Naito S, et al: Long-term results of cryoablation with a new cryoprobe to eliminate chronic atrial fibrillation associated with mitral valve disease. *Pacing Clin Electrophysiol* 28(Suppl 1):S73–S77, 2005.
133. Geidel S, Lass M, Boczor S, et al: Monopolar and bipolar radiofrequency ablation surgery: 3-year experience in 90 patients with permanent atrial fibrillation. *Heart Surg Forum* 7:E398–E402, 2004.
134. Salenger R, Lahey SJ, Saltman AE: The completely endoscopic treatment of atrial fibrillation: report on the first 14 patients with early results. *Heart Surg Forum* 7:E555–E558, 2004.
135. McClelland JH, Duke D, Reddy R: Preliminary results of a limited thoracotomy: new approach to treat atrial fibrillation. *J Cardiovasc Electr* 18:1289–1295, 2007.
136. Doll N, Pritzwald-Stegmann P, Czesla M, et al: Ablation of ganglionic plexi during combined surgery for atrial fibrillation. *Ann Thorac Surg* 86:1659–1663, 2008.
137. Mehall JR, Kohut RM, Jr, Schneeberger EW, et al: Intraoperative epicardial electrophysiologic mapping and isolation of autonomic ganglionic plexi. *Ann Thorac Surg* 83:538–541, 2007.

138. Pruitt JC, Lazzara RR, Ebra G: Minimally invasive surgical ablation of atrial fibrillation: the thoracoscopic box lesion approach. *J Interv Card Electr* 20:83–87, 2007.
139. Ailawadi G, Gerdisch MW, Harvey RL, et al: Exclusion of the left atrial appendage with a novel device: early results of a multicenter trial. *J Thorac Cardiov Sur* 142:1002–1009, 9 e1, 2011.
140. Emmert MY, Puippe G, Baumüller S, et al: Safe, effective and durable epicardial left atrial appendage clip occlusion in patients with atrial fibrillation undergoing cardiac surgery: first long-term results from a prospective device trial. *Eur J Cardiothorac Surg* 45:126–131, 2014.
141. Boersma LV, Castella M, van Boven W, et al: Atrial fibrillation catheter ablation versus surgical ablation treatment (FAST): a 2-center randomized clinical trial. *Circulation* 125:23–30, 2012.
142. Golovchiner G, Mazur A, Kogan A, et al: Atrial flutter after surgical radiofrequency ablation of the left atrium for atrial fibrillation. *Ann Thorac Surg* 79:108–112, 2005.
143. Doukas G, Samani NJ, Alexiou C, et al: Left atrial radiofrequency ablation during mitral valve surgery for continuous atrial fibrillation: a randomized controlled trial. *JAMA* 294:2323–2329, 2005.
144. Saint LL, Damiano RJ, Jr, Cuculich PS, et al: Incremental risk of the Cox-Maze IV procedure for patients with atrial fibrillation undergoing mitral valve surgery. *J Thorac Cardiov Sur* 146:1072–1077, 2013.
145. Barnett SD, Ad N: Surgical ablation as treatment for the elimination of atrial fibrillation: a meta-analysis. *J Thorac Cardiov Sur* 131:1029–1035, 2006.
146. Edgerton JR, Jackman WM, Mack MJ: Minimally invasive pulmonary vein isolation and partial autonomic denervation for surgical treatment of atrial fibrillation. *J Interv Card Electr* 20:89–93, 2007.
147. Melby SJ, Zierer A, Kaiser SP, et al: Epicardial microwave ablation on the beating heart for atrial fibrillation: the dependency of lesion depth on cardiac output. *J Thorac Cardiov Sur* 132:355–360, 2006.
148. Pruitt JC, Lazzara RR, Dworkin GH, et al: Totally endoscopic ablation of lone atrial fibrillation: initial clinical experience. *Ann Thorac Surg* 81:1325–1330, discussion 30–31, 2006.
149. Isobe N, Taniguchi K, Oshima S, et al: Left atrial appendage outflow velocity is superior to conventional criteria for predicting of maintenance of sinus rhythm after simple cryoablation of pulmonary vein orifices. *Circ J* 69:446–451, 2005.
150. Saint LL, Bailey MS, Prasad S, et al: Cox-Maze IV results for patients with lone atrial fibrillation versus concomitant mitral disease. *Ann Thorac Surg* 93:789–794, discussion 94–95, 2012.
151. Pison L, La Meir M, van Opstal J, et al: Hybrid thoracoscopic surgical and transvenous catheter ablation of atrial fibrillation. *J Am Coll Cardiol* 60:54–61, 2012.
152. Mahapatra S, LaPar DJ, Kamath S, et al: Initial experience of sequential surgical epicardial-catheter endocardial ablation for persistent and long-standing persistent atrial fibrillation with long-term follow-up. *Ann Thorac Surg* 91:1890–1898, 2011.
153. Damiano RJ, Jr, Gaynor SL, Bailey M, et al: The long-term outcome of patients with coronary disease and atrial fibrillation undergoing the Cox Maze procedure. *J Thorac Cardiov Sur* 126:2016–2021, 2003.
154. Lee SH, Tai CT, Hsieh MH, et al: Predictors of non-pulmonary vein ectopic beats initiating paroxysmal atrial fibrillation: implication for catheter ablation. *J Am Coll Cardiol* 46:1054–1059, 2005.
155. Lee SH, Cheng JJ, Kuan P, et al: Radiofrequency catheter modification of sinus node for inappropriate sinus tachycardia: a case report. *Zhonghua Yi Xue Za Zhi (Taipei)* 60:117–123, 1997.
156. Man KC, Knight B, Tse HF, et al: Radiofrequency catheter ablation of inappropriate sinus tachycardia guided by activation mapping. *J Am Coll Cardiol* 35:451–457, 2000.
157. Melby SJ, Kreisel D, Lindsay BD, et al: Surgical treatment for inappropriate sinus tachycardia. *Heart Rhythm* 2:S198, 2005.
158. Hendry PJ, Packer DL, Anstadt MP, et al: Surgical treatment of automatic atrial tachycardias. *Ann Thorac Surg* 49:253–259, discussion 9–60, 1990.
159. Esmailzadeh B, Bernat R, Winkler K, et al: Surgical excision of the sinus node in a patient with inappropriate sinus tachycardia. *J Thorac Cardiov Sur* 114:861–864, 1997.
160. Godemann F, Butter C, Lampe F, et al: Panic disorders and agoraphobia: side effects of treatment with an implantable cardioverter/defibrillator. *Clin Cardiol* 27:321–326, 2004.
161. Estes EH, Jr, Izlar HL, Jr: Recurrent ventricular tachycardia. A case successfully treated by bilateral cardiac sympathectomy. *Am J Med* 31:493–497, 1961.
162. Ecker RR, Mullins CB, Grammer JC, et al: Control of intractable ventricular tachycardia by coronary revascularization. *Circulation* 44:666–670, 1971.
163. Heimbecker RO, Lemire G, Chen C: Surgery for massive myocardial infarction. An experimental study of emergency infarctectomy with a preliminary report on the clinical application. *Circulation* 37:II3–II11, 1968.
164. Ungerleider RM, Holman WL, Stanley TE, 3rd, et al: Encircling endocardial ventriculotomy for refractory ischemic ventricular tachycardia. I. Electrophysiological effects. *J Thorac Cardiov Sur* 83:840–849, 1982.
165. Wellens HJ, Schuilenburg RM, Durrer D: Electrical stimulation of the heart in patients with ventricular tachycardia. *Circulation* 46:216–226, 1972.
166. Josephson ME, Horowitz LN, Farshidi A, et al: Recurrent sustained ventricular tachycardia. 2. Endocardial mapping. *Circulation* 57:440–447, 1978.
167. Gallagher JJ, Oldham HN, Wallace AG, et al: Ventricular aneurysm with ventricular tachycardia. Report of a case with epicardial mapping and successful resection. *Am J Cardiol* 35:696–700, 1975.
168. Wittig JH, Boineau JP: Surgical treatment of ventricular arrhythmias using epicardial, transmural, and endocardial mapping. *Ann Thorac Surg* 20:117–126, 1975.
169. Cox JL, McLaughlin VW, Flowers NC, et al: The ischemic zone surrounding acute myocardial infarction. Its morphology as detected by dehydrogenase staining. *Am Heart J* 76:650–659, 1968.
170. Fenoglio JJ, Jr, Pham TD, Harken AH, et al: Recurrent sustained ventricular tachycardia: structure and ultrastructure of subendocardial regions in which tachycardia originates. *Circulation* 68:518–533, 1983.
171. Scherlag BJ, el-Sherif N, Hope R, et al: Characterization and localization of ventricular arrhythmias resulting from myocardial ischemia and infarction. *Circ Res* 35:372–383, 1974.
172. Gardner PI, Ursell PC, Fenoglio JJ, Jr, et al: Electrophysiologic and anatomic basis for fractionated electrograms recorded from healed myocardial infarcts. *Circulation* 72:596–611, 1985.
173. Dillon SM, Allessie MA, Ursell PC, et al: Influences of anisotropic tissue structure on reentrant circuits in the epicardial border zone of subacute canine infarcts. *Circ Res* 63:182–206, 1988.
174. Guiraudon G, Fontaine G, Frank R, et al: Encircling endocardial ventriculotomy: a new surgical treatment for life-threatening ventricular tachycardias resistant to medical treatment following myocardial infarction. *Ann Thorac Surg* 26:438–444, 1978.
175. Harken AH, Josephson ME, Horowitz LN: Surgical endocardial resection for the treatment of malignant ventricular tachycardia. *Ann Surg* 190:456–460, 1979.
176. Moran JM, Kehoe RF, Loeb JM, et al: Extended endocardial resection for the treatment of ventricular tachycardia and ventricular fibrillation. *Ann Thorac Surg* 34:538–552, 1982.
177. McGiffin DC, Kirklin JK, Plumb VJ, et al: Relief of life-threatening ventricular tachycardia and survival after direct operations. *Circulation* 76:V93–V103, 1987.
178. Swerdlow CD, Mason JW, Stinson EB, et al: Results of operations for ventricular tachycardia in 105 patients. *J Thorac Cardiov Sur* 92:105–113, 1986.
179. Moran JM, Kehoe RF, Loeb JM, et al: Operative therapy of malignant ventricular rhythm disturbances. *Ann Surg* 198:479–486, 1983.
180. Kron IL, Lerman BB, Nolan SP, et al: Sequential endocardial resection for the surgical treatment of refractory ventricular tachycardia. *J Thorac Cardiov Sur* 94:843–847, 1987.
181. Ferguson TB, Jr, Smith JM, Cox JL, et al: Direct operation versus ICD therapy for ischemic ventricular tachycardia. *Ann Thorac Surg* 58:1291–1296, 1994.
182. Hargrove WC, Miller JM: *Endocardial ablation for ischemic ventricular tachycardia*, Philadelphia, 1989, Hanley & Belfus.
183. Johnson D, Cox J: *Ventricular arrhythmias*, London, 1999, Mosby International.
184. Moraca RJ, Bailey MS, Damiano RJ: *Ventricular arrhythmias and sudden cardiac death*, Malden, MA, 2008, Blackwell Publishing.

185. Athanasuleas CL, Buckberg GD, Stanley AW, et al: Surgical ventricular restoration: the RESTORE Group experience. *Heart Fail Rev* 9:287–297, 2004.
186. DiDonato M, Sabatier M, Dor V, et al: Ventricular arrhythmias after LV remodelling: surgical ventricular restoration or ICD? *Heart Fail Rev* 9:299–306, discussion 47–51, 2004.
187. Wallace RL, Sears SF, Jr, Lewis TS, et al: Predictors of quality of life in long-term recipients of implantable cardioverter defibrillators. *J Cardiopulm Rehabil* 22:278–281, 2002.
188. Bigger JT, Jr: Prophylactic use of implanted cardiac defibrillators in patients at high risk for ventricular arrhythmias after coronary-artery bypass graft surgery. Coronary Artery Bypass Graft (CABG) Patch Trial Investigators. *New Engl J Med* 337:1569–1575, 1997.
189. Garan H, Ruskin JN, DiMarco JP, et al: Electrophysiologic studies before and after myocardial revascularization in patients with life-threatening ventricular arrhythmias. *Am J Cardiol* 51:519–524, 1983.
190. Manolis AS, Rastegar H, Estes NA, 3rd: Effects of coronary artery bypass grafting on ventricular arrhythmias: results with electrophysiological testing and long-term follow-up. *Pacing Clin Electrophysiol* 16:984–991, 1993.
191. Can L, Kayikcioglu M, Halil H, et al: The effect of myocardial surgical revascularization on left ventricular late potentials. *Ann Noninvasive Electrocardiol* 6:84–91, 2001.
192. Takami Y, Ina H: Quantitative improvement in signal-averaged electrocardiography after coronary artery bypass grafting. *Circ J* 67:146–148, 2003.
193. Lee JH, Folsom DL, Biblo LA, et al: Combined internal cardioverter-defibrillator implantation and myocardial revascularization for ischemic ventricular arrhythmias: optimal cost-effective strategy. *Cardiovasc Surg* 3:393–397, 1995.
194. Moss AJ, Daubert J, Zareba W: MADIT-II: clinical implications. *Card Electrophysiol Rev* 6:463–465, 2002.
195. Dor V, Saab M, Coste P, et al: Left ventricular aneurysm: a new surgical approach. *Thorac Cardiov Surg* 37:11–19, 1989.
196. Dor V, Sabatier M, Montiglio F, et al: Results of nonguided subtotal endocardiectomy associated with left ventricular reconstruction in patients with ischemic ventricular arrhythmias. *J Thorac Cardiov Sur* 107:1301–1307, discussion 7–8, 1994.
197. Maxey TS, Reece TB, Ellman PI, et al: Coronary artery bypass with ventricular restoration is superior to coronary artery bypass alone in patients with ischemic cardiomyopathy. *J Thorac Cardiov Sur* 127:428–434, 2004.
198. Mickleborough LL, Merchant N, Ivanov J, et al: Left ventricular reconstruction: early and late results. *J Thorac Cardiov Sur* 128:27–37, 2004.
199. O'Neill JO, Starling RC, Khaykin Y, et al: Residual high incidence of ventricular arrhythmias after left ventricular reconstructive surgery. *J Thorac Cardiov Sur* 130:1250–1256, 2005.
200. Fasseas P, Kutalek SP, Samuels FL, et al: Ventricular assist device support for management of sustained ventricular arrhythmias. *Tex Heart Inst J* 29:33–36, 2002.
201. Kulick DM, Bolman RM, 3rd, Salerno CT, et al: Management of recurrent ventricular tachycardia with ventricular assist device placement. *Ann Thorac Surg* 66:571–573, 1998.
202. Ziv O, Dizon J, Thosani A, et al: Effects of left ventricular assist device therapy on ventricular arrhythmias. *J Am Coll Cardiol* 45:1428–1434, 2005.
203. Wadia Y, Delgado RM, 3rd, Odegaard P, et al: Jarvik 2000 Flow-Maker axial-flow left ventricular assist device support for management of refractory ventricular arrhythmias. *Congestive Heart Fail* 10:195–196, 2004.

PART H

SURGICAL MANAGEMENT OF CORONARY ARTERY DISEASE AND ITS COMPLICATIONS

PART OUTLINE

CHAPTER 88

Coronary Artery Bypass Grafting

Talal Al-Atassi • Hadi D. Toeg • Vincent Chan • Marc Ruel

CHAPTER OUTLINE

Coronary artery bypass grafting (CABG) is among the most important surgical procedures in the history of medicine. Arguably, no other operation has prolonged more lives, provided more symptom relief, and been more thoroughly investigated. CABG has been the most common procedure of adult cardiac surgery, but its future is increasingly threatened by medical and percutaneous alternatives. However, CABG is evolving with less invasive options, better postoperative care, and refined medical adjuncts. This treatment strategy remains the most durable means of revascularization for patients with coronary artery disease (CAD) and even more so for patients with diabetes and multivessel CAD. This chapter outlines the history, anatomic considerations, indications, techniques, postoperative care, and results of the modern CABG procedure. Other, complementary chapters in this book cover cardiac anatomy, the coronary circulation, cardiopulmonary bypass, myocardial protection, bypass conduits, off-pump grafting techniques, reoperations, combined procedures, and general postoperative care.

BACKGROUND

History

The initial development of CABG is credited to Dr. Alexis Carrel, who more than a century ago understood the association between angina pectoris and coronary stenosis.[1] In a canine model, Carrel anastomosed a carotid artery segment between the descending thoracic aorta and the left coronary artery. Carrel received the Nobel Prize in Physiology and Medicine for this work in 1912 (Fig. 88-1).[1] Despite this major advance in medical science, the lack of technology to support the heart remained a major hurdle toward the clinical implementation of Carrel's techniques. That surgical roadblock persisted for several decades, until Carrel collaborated with aviator Charles Lindbergh in the 1930s in hopes of developing the world's first heart-lung machine.[2] Although unsuccessful, their work added to the medical knowledge of the time.

In the late 1940s, Montreal surgeon Arthur Vineberg began implanting the left internal thoracic artery (LITA) onto the anterior myocardial territory in patients with severe angina.[3] The Vineberg procedure met with variable success, although many patients experienced symptomatic improvement.[4] In 1958, Johns Hopkins–trained William Longmire reported on his series of five patients treated with coronary artery endarterectomy, without the use of cardiopulmonary bypass (CPB).[5] Longmire was likely the first to perform a direct internal thoracic artery (ITA) to coronary artery anastomosis as a consequence of damage to the right coronary artery during one of his endarterectomy procedures.[6]

At approximately the same time, a number of surgeons across the globe were reporting their early experiences with CABG. In 1962, Sabiston performed the first planned saphenous vein bypass operation at Duke University.[7] In 1964, Kolessov grafted the LITA to the left anterior descending (LAD) artery, without CPB,[8] and DeBakey and Garrett reported aortocoronary saphenous vein grafting (SVG).[9] The world's first CABG program started 3 years later in Cleveland, as Favaloro and Effler began to routinely use reversed saphenous veins for aortocoronary grafting.[10] LITA grafting to the LAD was introduced in the Western world by Green in 1968,[11] sequential grafting by Flemma in 1971,[12] bilateral internal thoracic grafting by Kay in 1972,[13] and the use of radial artery grafts described by Carpentier in 1973 and revived by Acar in 1989.[14,15]

In the 1970s CABG flourished as the sole therapy for CAD. Several randomized trials—namely, the Coronary Artery Surgery Study (CASS),[16] the Veterans Administration Coronary Artery Bypass Trial,[17] and the European Coronary Artery Bypass Trial[18]—were conducted and would lay the foundation for surgical indications. In the modern era of CABG surgery, the prototypical patient is older, has significantly more comorbidities, and is more likely to have undergone percutaneous coronary intervention (PCI) with a drug-eluting stent.[19] However, several multicenter studies comparing CABG with current stent therapy—namely, the Synergy between Percutaneous Coronary Intervention with Taxus and Cardiac Surgery (SYNTAX),[20] Future Revascularization Evaluation in Patients with Diabetes Mellitus: Optimal Management of Multivessel Disease (FREEDOM),[21] and Coronary Artery Revascularization in Diabetes (CARDia)[22] trials—have clearly demonstrated the superiority of CABG when specific patient characteristics, such as diabetes, and coronary anatomy, such as involvement of all three coronary vessels, are taken into account.

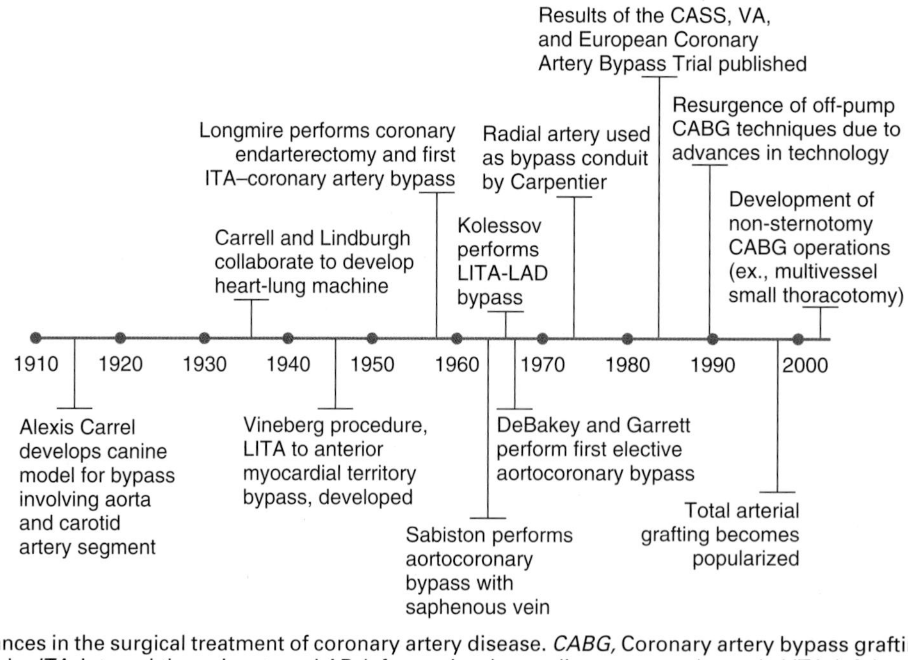

FIGURE 88-1 ■ Advances in the surgical treatment of coronary artery disease. *CABG,* Coronary artery bypass grafting; *CASS,* Coronary Artery Surgery Study; *ITA,* internal thoracic artery; *LAD,* left anterior descending coronary (artery); *LITA,* left internal thoracic artery; *VA,* Veterans Administration Coronary Artery Bypass Surgery Cooperative Study.

Anatomic Considerations

Coronary artery anatomy and size vary widely among individuals. In the absence of CAD, coronary perfusion matches myocardial demand because capillary oxygen extraction is relatively fixed.[23] During exercise, coronary perfusion increases three- to fourfold as a result of vasodilation of coronary arteries and arterioles and from recruitment of additional capillaries.[24]

In the setting of symptomatic CAD, compensatory physiologic processes are insufficient to provide adequate myocardial perfusion. The effect is either *supply ischemia*, responsible for myocardial infarction (MI) and most episodes of unstable angina, or *demand ischemia*, where coronary blood flow is insufficient during periods of increased myocardial demands from exercise, tachycardia, fever, hypertension, or emotional distress.[25] Basal arteriogenesis and collateral formation may be enhanced when new coronary flow patterns and subclinical ischemia develop, but their extent largely depends on the time course of CAD development and is governed by genetic and environmental factors. It is the magnitude of arterial collateralization, of *de novo* arteriolar and capillary development, and dynamic vascular responses that determine the degree of ischemia experienced by a patient. Furthermore, the size and function of the subtended myocardial territory at risk (demand) dictates the degree of ischemia and risk of heart failure in patients with obstructive CAD (supply).

Depending on referral patterns, 40% to 60% of patients who undergo coronary angiography have significant disease involving all three coronary arteries, and 10% to 20% of those patients have stenosis of the left mainstem.[26] In patients with single- or double-vessel disease, the most frequently stenosed coronary artery is the right, followed closely by the LAD and least frequently by the circumflex. In some patients, atherosclerosis may be mimicked by myocardial bridging of a coronary artery, which involves a segment of coronary artery completely surrounded by myocardium. Myocardial bridging can result in cardiac ischemia although traditional noninvasive tests are often negative.[27]

Myocardial hypoperfusion leads to one of four pathophysiologic consequences: stunned myocardium (reversible myocardial dysfunction despite normal/near normal coronary blood flow), hibernating myocardium (reversible myocardial dysfunction with reduced coronary blood flow), nontransmural scar tissue, or transmural scar tissue (irreversible typically nonviable myocardial dysfunction). Patients who describe ischemia on exertion will typically exhibit viable (stunned or hibernating) myocardium, whereas those who describe heart failure symptoms may suffer from irreversible myocardial dysfunction. In addition to clinical evaluation, several contemporary imaging modalities with relatively good sensitivity and specificity are used to further delineate and quantify the proportion of viable myocardium, the most common being nuclear imaging with positron emission tomography (PET) (evaluating viability with glucose uptake of ^{18}F-fluorodeoxyglucose [FDG]), single photon emission computed tomography (SPECT) (with thallium or technetium radiotracer), dobutamine stress echocardiography (with contrast agents), and dobutamine stress cardiac magnetic resonance imaging (MRI). With PET, stunned myocardium appears as a hypocontractile segment with normal perfusion and glucose uptake at rest, and hibernating myocardium as a territory with decreased perfusion but preserved glucose uptake.[28] Scar tissue, unlikely to benefit from CABG, exhibits both reduced perfusion and glucose uptake, with a milder reduction in nontransmural scars and a severe reduction in transmural scars.

In addition to assessment of angiographically defined stenosis and myocardial viability, technologic advances in interventional cardiology have led to quantitative measurement of coronary blood flow across lesions, and ultra-refined topographic imaging of coronary lesions.[29,30] Fractional flow reserve values of less than 0.8 (considered significant flow limiting CAD as measured by flow across coronary lesions) has altered management strategies in patients with borderline angiographic CAD resulting in less graft anastomosis at CABG and thus, less on-pump surgery.[31,32] Alternatively, intravenous ultrasound (IVUS) and optical coherence tomography has improved the resolution and sensitivity of identifying obstructive CAD not traditionally seen on standard angiography.[31,33] In summary, imaging modalities such as coronary angiography (standard and CT) are obligate adjuncts in defining anatomic coronary artery stenosis and can be further characterized by functional studies such as PET viability, fractional flow reserve, or IVUS. These functional preoperative imaging studies help the cardiac surgeon in determining whether the patient meets indications for CABG and predict the degree of improvement after surgery and outcomes in general.

INDICATIONS FOR OPERATION

The indications for CABG described in this section are based on the 2011 American College of Cardiology/American Heart Association (ACC/AHA) guidelines.[34] These updated guidelines include several contemporary multicenter randomized controlled trials comparing CABG to PCI with either first- or second-generation drug-eluting stents, which have become the treatment of choice for PCI.[35,36] In contrast, previous recommendations were mostly based on historical trials comparing either bare-metal stents or angioplasty alone with CABG.[37-40] With the advancement of less thrombotic stents (i.e., everolimus-eluting stents),[41] minimally invasive CABG options or hybrid operations, and better medical treatment for CAD, it is no surprise that indications for surgical revascularization will be further refined, driven by the constant need to improve patient outcomes.

The pivotal SYNTAX trial randomized 1800 patients with left main or triple-vessel disease to undergo either CABG or PCI (drug-eluting stents).[20] The extent of CAD was determined using the SYNTAX score based on severity, location, and extent of coronary stenosis. A low SYNTAX score was defined as less than 22, intermediate as 23 to 32, and high as 33 and above. At 12 months, major adverse cardiac and cerebrovascular events (MACCEs) were significantly higher in the PCI group compared with CABG patients (17.8% vs. 12.4%; $P = 0.002$). This was mostly accounted for, after post hoc analysis, in patients with higher SYNTAX scores (≥33).[20] At 3 years, patients with triple-vessel disease and low to intermediate SYNTAX scores (≤32) had lower rates of MACCE compared with PCI ($P < 0.004$), whereas patients with left main CAD and SYNTAX scores 33 and higher had lower incidence of MACCE compared with PCI ($P = 0.003$).[42] Furthermore, because patients with diabetes had higher rates of revascularization in the PCI group compared with CABG, the FREEDOM trial[21] was conducted to determine whether current PCI therapy (with second-generation drug-eluting stents) or CABG is superior for diabetic patients with multivessel CAD. This randomized controlled trial demonstrated CABG to be superior over PCI in diabetic patients with lower 5-year rates of death and MI; however, stroke rates were slightly higher in CABG patients. Thus, based on the aforementioned historical and latest studies along with the updated ACC/AHA guidelines, the following sections provide detailed anatomic and clinical scenarios for CABG indications.

Clinical Scenarios and CABG Indications

Stable Ischemic Heart Disease

The indications for CABG in the setting of asymptomatic, mild angina, or chronic stable angina are based on the observed survival advantage of CABG over nonsurgical therapy (Table 88-1).[34,39] Class I indications include the use of CABG to treat significant left main disease (≥50%), left main equivalent disease (i.e., proximal stenosis of at least 70% of the proximal LAD and circumflex), triple-vessel disease (especially in patients with left ventricular ejection fraction [LVEF] <50% and/or in whom a large area of myocardial ischemia exists), and proximal LAD disease combined with an LVEF between 35% and 50%.[34] CABG is also indicated for patients with proximal LAD disease without left ventricular dysfunction, and may be indicated for patients with single- or double-vessel disease not involving the proximal LAD (class IIa).[43] Finally, CABG or PCI is indicated in patients with at least one significant coronary artery stenosis with unacceptable angina despite optimal medical therapy (class I) (Table 88-2).[39,44-46] Recent large studies have demonstrated that stable anginal patients treated with either optimal medical therapy or PCI (± CABG) had no significant survival benefit.[44,47-50] Thus, although these updated guidelines provide a treatment algorithm for CAD patients, the ultimate decision regarding revascularization options should be made between the expert clinician and the well-informed patient.

TABLE 88-1 **Class I and IIa Indications for CABG Surgery**

COR	LOE	Clinical or Anatomic Setting
I	A	One or more significant (>70%) coronary artery stenoses amenable to revascularization and unacceptable angina despite best medical therapy *(consider PCI as alternative)*
I	B	Unprotected left main disease (>50%)
I	B	Triple-vessel disease with or without proximal LAD artery disease
I	B	Survivors of sudden cardiac death with ischemia-mediated ventricular tachycardia
I	B	Double-vessel disease with proximal LAD artery disease
I	B	Emergency CABG after failed PCI in presence of ongoing ischemia or threatened occlusion with substantial myocardium at risk (without impaired coagulation and without a previous sternotomy); surgical repair of a postinfarction mechanical complication (i.e., septal or free wall rupture)
I	B	Emergency CABG in patients with cardiogenic shock, suitable for CABG irrespective of time interval from MI to onset of shock and time from MI to CABG.
I	C	Patients undergoing noncoronary cardiac surgery with left main disease (>50%) or any other CAD (>70%)
I	C	Heart team approach recommended for unprotected left main disease or complex CAD
IIa	B	CABG over PCI in patients with complex triple-vessel CAD (i.e., SYNTAX > 22)
IIa	B	Double-vessel disease without proximal LAD disease with extensive ischemia
IIa	B	Single-vessel proximal LAD disease with LITA for long-term benefit
IIa	B	CAD with left ventricular ejection fraction 35% to 50%
IIa	B	Hybrid (LITA to LAD artery CABG + PCI for non-LAD arteries) for limitation for CABG (unsuitable conduits) or unfavorable LAD artery for PCI

CABG, Coronary artery bypass grafting; *CAD,* coronary artery disease; *COR,* class of recommendation; *LAD,* left anterior descending; *LITA,* left internal thoracic artery; *LOE,* level of evidence; *MI,* myocardial infarction; *PCI,* percutaneous coronary intervention.

Derived from 2011 AHA/ACC guidelines for CABG.[43]

Acute Coronary Syndromes

Unstable Angina/Non–ST-Segment Elevation Myocardial Infarction. The indication for CABG in patients with unstable angina or non–ST-segment elevation myocardial infarction (NSTEMI) is anatomically identical to that in patients with stable ischemic heart disease.[43] This includes patients with significant left main or left main equivalent disease, patients with triple-vessel disease, and patients with ongoing ischemia not responsive to maximal nonsurgical therapy or failed/unfavorable PCI (see Table 88-1). The major difference between anatomically similar patients presenting with unstable angina or NSTEMI compared with stable CAD is that achieving revascularization in an acute coronary syndrome, a potentially life-threatening scenario, creates a stronger motive in preventing death.[51-53] The indication for CABG in this setting is further strengthened by the acuity of presentation, degree of ischemia, and benefit of full revascularization.

ST-Segment Elevation (Q Wave) Myocardial Infarction. Primary PCIs and intravenous thrombolytic therapy have supplanted CABG as the first line of therapy

TABLE 88-2 **Pertinent History and Physical Examination Elements for CABG**

Preoperative Assessment	Possible Implications	Management
History		
Symptoms		
SHORTNESS OF BREATH		
Orthopnea	Left ventricular dysfunction; right ventricular dysfunction; valve disease	Warrants echocardiography to determine cardiac anatomy
Aggravated with activity	Cardiac ischemia	May warrant more urgent surgery depending on severity of symptoms
Chest pain	Cardiac ischemia	
Poor sleep quality/snoring	Sleep apnea	Alert anesthesiologist of possible airway difficulty; arrange for CPAP postoperatively
Claudication	Peripheral vascular disease	Assess peripheral and central pulses; brachial-ankle index, echocardiography to assess ascending aortic calcification
Postprandial pain	Mesenteric angina	Imaging to determine disease in celiac-mesenteric axis; contraindicates gastroepiploic artery use
Past Medical History		
Diabetes mellitus	Poor wound healing; difficult glycemic control perioperatively	Consider skeletonized harvesting for bilateral internal thoracic arteries
Previous sternal irradiation	Internal thoracic artery damage	May contraindicate use of internal thoracic artery
Previous TIA/amaurosis fugax/stroke	Atherosclerotic disease involving arch vessels	Warrants carotid duplex examination and echocardiography; possible need for CT or MRI angiogram to elucidate disease extent
Raynaud phenomenon	Compromised flow in upper extremity precluding radial artery use	May warrant Doppler examination of the forearm; contraindicates radial artery use in most cases
Past Surgical History		
Lower extremity vein stripping	Lack of greater saphenous vein	Choose alternative conduits
Abdominal laparotomy	Possible contraindication to gastroepiploic artery use	Choose alternative conduits
Medications		
Chronic steroid use	Poor wound healing postoperatively; consider steroid withdrawal postoperatively; difficult glycemic control perioperatively	May contraindicate use of bilateral internal thoracic artery use; ensure postoperative steroid administration and glycemic control
Physical		
Asymmetric brachial blood pressure	Atherosclerotic disease involving arch vessels	Warrants carotid and subclavian duplex examination; contraindicates use of pedicled internal thoracic artery grafts on the ipsilateral side of subclavian stenosis
Increased JVP/peripheral edema	Left ventricular dysfunction; valve disease	Warrants echocardiography to determine cardiac anatomy
Auscultation		
Increased P2	Pulmonary hypertension	Warrants echocardiography to determine cardiac anatomy ± CT chest
Murmur	Concomitant valve disease	
Clubbing	Bronchiectasis; chronic pulmonary hypertension; lung malignancy	Chest radiograph; echocardiography to determine cardiac anatomy

CABG, Coronary artery bypass grafting; *CPAP,* continuous positive airway pressure; *CT,* computed tomography; *JVP,* jugular venous pressure; *MRI,* magnetic resonance imaging; *TIA,* transient ischemic attack.

for patients in the acute period of ST-segment elevation myocardial infarction (STEMI).[54] As a consequence, ongoing ischemia or cardiogenic shock despite maximal nonsurgical therapy, including intra-aortic balloon pump counterpulsation, currently constitute the main indications for emergency CABG in acute STEMI patients (see Table 88-1).[34] Other indications for emergency CABG in the setting of STEMI include failed PCI or thrombolysis and demonstration of a large myocardial territory at risk, in combination with an unsuitable anatomy for PCI, left main coronary stenosis, left ventricular failure with severe coronary stenosis outside the initial infarct area, significant valve disease, life-threatening ventricular arrhythmias believed to be ischemic in origin (left main or triple-vessel CAD), or a mechanical complication of MI such as severe mitral insufficiency, left ventricular wall rupture, or ventricular septal rupture.[34]

The timing of CABG after an acute coronary syndrome is controversial. Although early surgery may limit the expansion of the infarct, it runs the risk of reperfusion injury that may lead to a hemorrhagic infarct and scar development. In some cases, such as ongoing ischemia and mechanical complications, CABG cannot be delayed and the availability of mechanical support becomes very important. However, data from the New York State

Cardiac Surgery Registry showed that CABG within 6 hours of a nontransmural infarct or within 3 days of a transmural infarct was independently associated with in-hospital mortality. Therefore, CABG should be delayed for at least 6 hours after a nontransmural infarct and 3 days after a transmural infarct when no clear indication for immediate CABG is present.[55,56]

Spontaneous Coronary Artery Dissection. One rare form of acute coronary syndrome is spontaneous coronary artery dissection (SCAD), which affects 0.1% to 4% of patients with acute coronary syndromes.[57] SCAD is a nontraumatic, noniatrogenic separation of the coronary arterial wall by intramural hemorrhage leading to compression of the lumen with intramural hematoma. Typical patients presenting with SCAD include females younger than 50 years without traditional cardiovascular risk factors. Causes of SCAD include pregnancy, connective tissue disorders, systemic inflammatory conditions, coronary artery spasm, and precipitating stress events (intense exercise, emotional stress, labor, or cocaine).[58] Whereas the mainstay of treatment for stable SCAD patients entails beta blockers and antiplatelets, PCI or surgical revascularization should be considered in patients who have ongoing chest pain, show evidence of ischemia, or are hemodynamically unstable despite maximal medical therapy. Specific indications for CABG follow similar anatomic considerations (i.e., left main, left main equivalent, or triple-vessel disease).[58,59]

Concomitant Noncoronary Cardiac Surgery

Patients undergoing other forms of cardiac surgery such as valvular repair, where coronary angiography demonstrates either a 50% luminal diameter narrowing of the left main artery or a more than 70% narrowing of any other epicardial coronary artery, should undergo concomitant CABG (class I; evidence C). Furthermore, the LITA is a reasonable conduit choice for bypassing the LAD artery (class IIa), and other conduits, mostly vein grafts, can be used to bypass moderately diseased coronary arteries (>50% narrowing) (class IIa).[34]

Left Ventricular Dysfunction and Heart Failure

CABG is indicated in patients with left ventricular dysfunction (LVEF 35% to 50%; class IIa and LVEF < 35%; class IIb) and left main or left main equivalent disease, and also in the setting of proximal LAD stenosis with double- or triple-vessel disease.[60-62] Despite the increased risk of left ventricular dysfunction on perioperative mortality, the long-term results of CABG in patients with mild to moderate left ventricular dysfunction appear favorable.[61-63] It is important to note that patients who have poor left ventricular function and/or congestive heart failure (CHF) symptoms must be evaluated for valvular disease and for objective evidence of hibernating myocardium with a perfusion scan. Despite historical studies demonstrating better outcomes with mild to moderate left ventricular dysfunction, results in patients with advanced left ventricular dysfunction (LVEF < 35%) treated with CABG are more controversial. The Surgical Treatment for Ischemic Heart Failure (STITCH) trial enrolled patients with an LVEF less than 35% with or without myocardial viability.[64] The primary endpoint of all-cause mortality did not differ in surgically versus medically treated patients at 5 years follow-up. However, several combined secondary endpoints, including death from any cause and heart failure–related hospitalization, were significantly lower in CABG patients. Thus, in efforts to discriminate a difference in survival, the study will be followed for an additional 5 years.

Life-Threatening Ventricular Arrhythmias and Sudden Cardiac Death

Data describing the benefit of CABG as a treatment for ventricular arrhythmias originate from studies involving survivors of out-of-hospital cardiac arrest. CABG is more effective in treating ventricular fibrillation than ventricular tachycardia, as the latter originates from myocardial scar formation. CABG is also particularly useful in the setting of exercise-induced ventricular arrhythmias,[65,66] and it has been shown to suppress ventricular arrhythmias in the setting of left main or triple-vessel disease. Alternatively, CABG should not be performed on patients with ventricular tachycardia or evidence of scar. All patients should undergo consultation with an electrophysiology specialist for consideration of insertion of an implantable cardioverter-defibrillator (ICD). Patients with depressed left ventricular function, older age, female sex, and extended CPB runs are more prone to developing life-threatening arrhythmias such that temporary mechanical circulatory support may be justified.[67,68]

Failed Percutaneous Coronary Intervention

Because of improved PCI techniques, stent technologies, and antiplatelet options, failed PCI requiring emergency CABG is rare, with an incidence of 0.4% to 0.8%.[69,70] Broad indications for CABG after failed PCI include an acute closure of a coronary vessel (or threatened), vessel dissection, perforation, or malfunction of the PCI equipment (i.e., fractured guidewire). Most patients who undergo emergency CABG exhibit an evolving STEMI, triple-vessel disease, left main disease, cardiogenic shock, or a type C coronary arterial lesion (defined as a lesion with any of the following: diffuse lesion [>2 cm length], inability to protect major side branch, excessive tortuosity, degenerated vein grafts, or total occlusions more than 3 months old).[69,70] As expected, patients who undergo emergency CABG have increased perioperative morbidity and mortality rates. Independent predictors of worse outcomes include advanced age, depressed left ventricular function, cardiogenic shock, absence of angiographic collaterals, and a prolonged time delay for transfer to the operating room.[71,72] However, if complete revascularization can be achieved without protracted delay, the long-term outcomes in emergency CABG patients after failed PCI mirror those of elective CABG patients.[70,73-75] Finally, an off-pump CABG approach for patients in whom PCI failed may be associated with less bleeding requiring reoperation, less renal failure, and less intra-aortic balloon pump usage.[76,77]

Previous Coronary Artery Bypass Grafting

Operative risk associated with reoperative CABG is greater than that for the primary operation because of the fact that on reentry there may be damage to patent grafts or other cardiac structures, such as the right ventricle or innominate vein. Coronary identification at reoperation is also more difficult. Given the increased risk, the indications for reoperative CABG largely depend on the degree of symptoms, size of the myocardial territory at risk, concomitant valvular disease, and suitability for PCI.[78] Current guidelines advocate first, PCI in previous CABG patients refractory to medical therapy (class IIa), followed by redo CABG if disabling angina refractory to maximal medical therapy and PCI occurs (class IIb).[79] Despite the increased risk, advances in current surgical techniques have significantly narrowed the perioperative risk gap between reoperative and primary CABG with studies demonstrating similar long-term outcomes between redo and primary CABG.

In summary, patients undergoing intervention for CAD should be assessed on a case-by-case basis. After clinical, social, and anatomic patient characteristics are taken into account, the use of a heart team is recommended when the choice of revascularization is not apparent. The heart team may take advantage of a hybrid coronary revascularization strategy by performing LITA to LAD artery grafting and PCI of one or more non-LAD arteries. This approach is reasonable in patients with either limitations to traditional CABG (lack of suitable graft conduits, severely calcified aorta) or an unfavorable LAD artery for PCI (tortuous vessel or chronically occluded artery).[34]

SURGICAL TECHNIQUE

Preoperative Preparation

In most cases, patients are referred to cardiac surgery for CABG with the diagnosis of myocardial ischemia confirmed via noninvasive testing, coronary angiography, or both. Despite this, a detailed and focused history, physical examination (including determining the functional status of the patient), and review of all tests should be performed to confirm the surgical indication, determine the operative risk, and allow for optimal surgical planning (see Table 88-2).

History and Physical Examination

Attention must be given to a possible misdiagnosis (especially when symptoms appear out of proportion to the angiographic severity of the coronary stenoses), to comorbid conditions, and to the availability of conduits for revascularization. For example, patients with predominant symptoms of dyspnea may have concomitant valvular disease, cardiomyopathy, or pulmonary hypertension that was missed during preoperative evaluation. On physical examination, this can be determined by the presence of a murmur, an accentuated P2 indicating pulmonary hypertension, signs of cardiomegaly, and subtle cyanosis or clubbing. Symptoms and signs of CHF should be elicited, because the coexistence of CHF may impact preoperative testing, perioperative medical management, intraoperative planning (with respect, in some cases, to the choice of myocardial protection strategy and the selection of conduits), and short- and long-term prognosis after operation.[80] Patients with previous mediastinal irradiation should undergo preoperative echocardiography to rule out valve disease, pulmonary function testing, computed tomography (CT) of the chest to assess the degree of aortic calcification, and carotid duplex examination. Patients with a history of peptic ulcer disease should be identified and the use of perioperative nonsteroidal anti-inflammatory agents avoided.

The peripheral vascular examination is of utmost importance. Brachial blood pressure should be measured in both arms to determine hemodynamically significant subclavian artery stenosis. A difference of systolic blood pressure more than 20 mm Hg warrants Doppler examination and may necessitate the use of a free ITA graft or alternate conduit if a subclavian stenosis is confirmed.[81] The lower extremities should be examined for the presence of varicose veins and incisions from previous saphenectomy or peripheral vascular procedures. The patient should also be asked whether sclerotherapy was ever performed. Lower extremity arterial disease is associated with a relative mortality risk of approximately fivefold, regardless of the presence of symptoms.[82] These patients have the highest incidence of aortic calcification and perioperative stroke, and particular attention must be given to the ascending aorta when assessing the preoperative chest x-ray and reviewing the coronary angiogram.[83] In cases where a suspicion exists, CT of the chest is indicated. Documentation of peripheral pulses is important if intra-aortic balloon counterpulsation is to be considered and provides a rapid, albeit imperfect, baseline assessment for subsequent comparison if late hemodynamic compromise or tamponade is suspected after the patient has left the intensive care unit.

Absolute contraindications to the use of an ITA include previous damage from penetrating trauma or surgery and documentation of the artery as a major source of collateral perfusion to the mesenteric circulation in cases of chronic aortic thrombosis or to a lower extremity in patients with Leriche syndrome (unless lower extremity revascularization is performed concomitantly).[84,85] Patients on chronic hemodialysis should have a free rather than an in situ ITA graft performed on the side of their arteriovenous fistula.[86] Severe obesity, chronic obstructive pulmonary disease (COPD), and diabetes may contraindicate the use of bilateral ITAs, but this is controversial and ultimately depends on individual preferences.[87] Although conventionally believed to be a relative contraindication to ITA use,[88] previous thoracic irradiation appears to confer no overt histologic changes relative to nonirradiated controls.[89] Long-term patency data, however, are scarce; therefore, use of ITA grafts in patients with previous mediastinal irradiation must be evaluated on a case-by-case basis.

Previous upper abdominal surgery or symptoms suggestive of mesenteric angina contraindicate the use of a gastroepiploic artery. Radial artery harvest is avoided in patients with Raynaud syndrome or on the same side in patients who have had recent radial arterial puncture at the time of preoperative coronary catheterization. We prefer to also avoid it, in a side-specific manner, in patients with carpal tunnel syndrome or with a history of previous penetrating trauma involving the wrist or forearm. It is important to both feel for an ulnar pulse and perform the Allen test, using a cutoff of 3 seconds, which has a 100% sensitivity for inadequate collateral hand circulation.[90] The former is important because, in rare cases, the ulnar artery may sometimes be congenitally absent with an otherwise normal Allen test.[91]

Asymptomatic carotid bruits have unreliable predictive accuracy,[92] but their presence warrants carotid duplex examination if CABG can be performed on an elective basis.[93] Perioperative stroke risk is less than 2% in patients with carotid stenoses less than 50%, 10% when stenoses are 50% to 80%, and 11% to 19% in patients with stenoses of more than 80%.[94] A history of transient ischemic attack or stroke warrants a carotid duplex examination to rule out a carotid stenosis and an echocardiogram to rule out a cardiac embolic source or a patent foramen ovale. If no source is found and symptoms suggestive of vertebrobasilar insufficiency are elicited, MRI angiography of the arch vessels should be performed. Patients who had a recent stroke should ideally delay CABG for a minimum of 4 weeks to limit the risk of further neurologic damage. Combined CABG and carotid endarterectomy is controversial although data suggest that the development of postoperative stroke is related to surgical technique and patient factors rather than operative strategy.[95] Recent trends suggest that carotid artery angioplasty and stenting with concomitant CABG is emerging as an alternative to combined CABG and carotid endarterectomy.[96] Preoperative documentation of hemodynamically significant carotid stenoses allows for risk stratification, consideration of a staged procedure preceded by carotid endarterectomy, selection of special intraoperative monitoring, and optimization of blood pressure management perioperatively.

Medications

Aspirin and cardiac medications are continued up to the time of operation, with the exception of digoxin, which is discontinued one day prior to surgery. Warfarin is stopped several days (>5) before surgery in orally anticoagulated elective patients, who are started on low-molecular weight heparin when their international normalized ratio (INR) becomes 2.0 or less; emergent cases are reversed with fresh-frozen plasma, Octaplex, and intravenous vitamin K. Management of the ADP-dependent platelet inhibitors clopidogrel and ticagrelor[97] varies according to personal preferences; our preferred approach in stable patients is to stop the medication 1 week prior to operation with a minimum of 5 days.[43,97] Furthermore, prasugrel is typically withheld for at least 7 days before elective CABG. With patients with drug-eluting stents that are within a year of insertion and who will not have their stented coronary segment(s) bypassed, we prefer to keep them on clopidogrel right up to the day of operation. Patients who have been started on an ACE inhibitor prior to surgical referral should have postoperative serial serum creatinine assessments. If progressive elevation is noted (>25% of baseline), the ACE inhibitor should be stopped to allow the serum creatinine levels to normalize prior to operation.

Laboratory Tests

Complete blood counts, serum chemistries, liver function tests, coagulogram, electrocardiogram (ECG), chest x-ray, and urinalysis are routinely performed. Particular attention is given to a low platelet count (suggestive of possible heparin-induced thrombocytopenia in patients on heparin), an elevated serum creatinine (a strong predictor of increased operative mortality), and the presence of vascular calcification on the chest x-ray. Anterior Q waves with poor R wave progression on the ECG are indicative of transmural myocardial scarring and may warrant echocardiography or preoperative viability testing. Most patients will have undergone preoperative nuclear scintigrams and echocardiography. These are reviewed to determine the functional significance of borderline coronary stenoses and to provide an assessment of valve function, left ventricular systolic wall motion, diastolic function, and right ventricular contractility.

A major improvement in the preoperative evaluation in patients with poor left ventricular function and CHF has been the scintigraphic assessment of myocardial viability. Viability is best assessed with PET; recovery of regional and global left ventricular function after surgical revascularization is correlated with a higher preoperative blood flow and glucose uptake, indicative of less tissue fibrosis and a higher fraction of viable cardiomyocytes in the dysfunctional area (Fig. 88-2).[98] Results are best if both hibernating myocardium and angina symptoms are present and attributed to a myocardial territory subtended by a graftable vessel with significant proximal stenosis; conversely, patients with no viability, no angina symptoms, and diffuse CAD are less likely to derive a survival benefit compared with medical therapy after CABG. If PET is not available, dobutamine stress echocardiography or MRI may be used to identify reversible myocardial dysfunction; although not as sensitive as PET, dobutamine wall-motion indices are specific in predicting postoperative improvement.[99]

Coronary Angiogram

Coronary angiography is still the fundamental diagnostic tool for describing the surgical anatomy of CAD. As a general rule, vessels 1.5 mm or larger with ≥50% to 70% stenosis should be grafted. Consideration is given to smaller vessels if no other target is found in a coronary distribution where myocardial ischemia has been demonstrated on noninvasive testing. With modern techniques of CPB and myocardial protection, incomplete revascularization is rarely justifiable because of its known deleterious effects on short- and long-term outcomes.[100] Failure to bypass a functionally significant and stenosed coronary artery should therefore be exceptional and result from severe comorbidities, from nongraftability, from diffuse

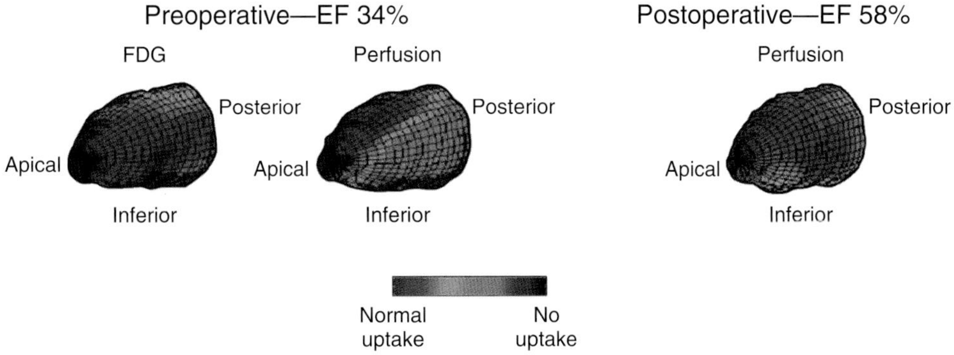

FIGURE 88-2 Myocardial viability assessment. This patient with congestive heart failure symptoms and inferior wall akinesis was evaluated prior to coronary artery bypass grafting (CABG) with ^{18}F-fluorodeoxyglucose (FDG) positron emission tomography and perfusion scintigraphy. Depressed ejection fraction (EF), viable myocytes (indicated by the normal FDG uptake), and the presence of a large posteroinferior perfusion defect were identified preoperatively. After CABG, the perfusion defect disappeared and the EF normalized. (Courtesy Robert S. Beanlands MD, Chief of Cardiology, University of Ottawa Heart Institute).

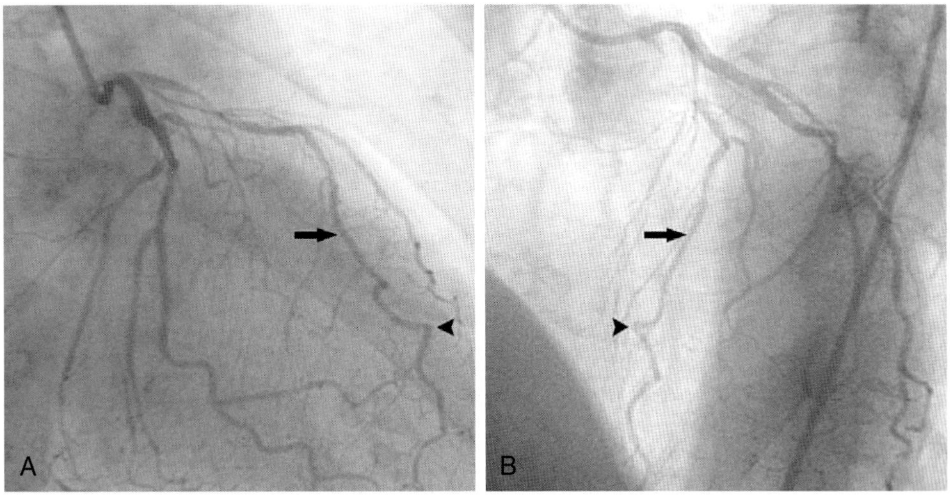

FIGURE 88-3 Intramyocardial left anterior descending artery (LAD). The LAD goes downward *(arrows)* and, after several centimeters, upward on the angiogram *(arrowheads)*. **A,** Right anterior oblique projection. **B,** Left anterior oblique projection.

aortic and branches calcification with inability to perform Y- or T-grafting, from conduit shortage, or from significant, unexpected intraoperative problems.

An intramyocardial LAD can be a vexing problem. Because LITA-LAD grafting provides a significant survival benefit in CABG patients,[101] the failure to graft a stenosed LAD because of its intramyocardial location is clearly suboptimal. However, the situation can be identified preoperatively by seeing the vessel going downward and, after several centimeters, upward on the angiogram or by noticing that the LAD goes straight down to the apex without any curve (Fig. 88-3). Epicardial Doppler or retrograde probing of the LAD after performing a minute arteriotomy at its apical portion (or alternatively on a minor diagonal branch) can be used intraoperatively to identify the LAD at its proximal or mid portion.

Conduit Selection

Internal Thoracic Artery Grafts

The ITA is the preferred conduit for CABG and provides short- and long-term survival benefits in all patient subgroups, including those 75 years of age and older.[101-105] The steps in preparing the ITA conduit are described in Figure 88-4. Use of the LITA to graft the LAD (or a main target vessel on the left coronary circulation if the LAD is free of disease) should be performed except in rare circumstances such as preexisting or iatrogenic damage to the LITA, poor flow from severe spasm or dissection, significant ipsilateral subclavian stenosis, demonstrated involvement of the LITA in providing collateral supply to the lower extremity, mediastinal irradiation (if other arterial conduits are available), and emergency CABG with cardiogenic shock.

Bilateral ITAs should be used whenever possible, as this is associated with lower reoperation rates, lower late PCI rates, and possible long-term survival benefits.[106-110] Possible contraindications to the use of bilateral ITAs include emergency operation, insulin-dependent diabetes mellitus, obesity, and severe COPD for which the patient requires oral or intravenous glucocorticoid therapy. After decades of debate, use of bilateral ITAs appears not to increase the incidence of deep sternal wound infection except in emergent cases, in patients older than 70 years, and in patients with type I diabetes.[109,111,112]

Skeletonization of an ITA involves dissection of the ITA without the accompanying periarterial venous and

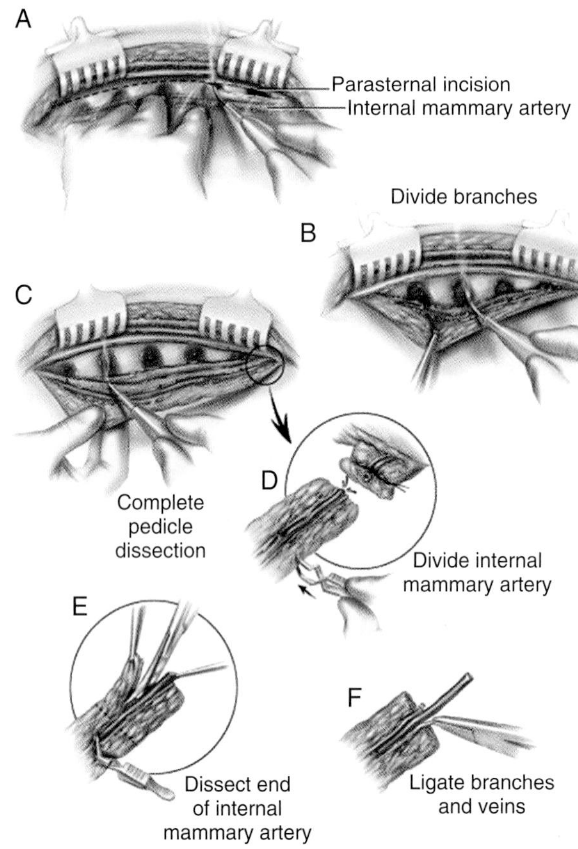

FIGURE 88-4 ■ Preparation of the internal thoracic artery. **A,** After exposure of the posterior surface of the sternum and ribs, electrocautery is used to make an incision along the entire length of the sternum, medial to the internal thoracic artery (ITA). **B,** Cautious tension is applied posteriorly to expose the ITA branches, which are clipped and divided. Blunt dissection is used to mobilize the pedicle in areas with no branches. **C,** After all the branches are clipped, an incision is made lateral to the pedicle to free it from the chest wall along its entire length. **D,** After administration of heparin, the pedicle is divided and the distal end is ligated. Forceful blood flow should be expected from the proximal end. A vascular clamp is applied to the proximal pedicle to control blood flow. **E,** The distal end of the arterial conduit is dissected free from the surrounding venae comitantes and tissue, and **F,** the venae comitantes are clipped. (Adapted from Doty DB, Doty JR, editors: *Cardiac surgery operative technique,* ed 2, Philadelphia, 2012, Saunders, p 409, Figure 36-6.)

fascial tissue. Given that the ITA is a delicate structure, meticulous attention must be paid to avoid artery damage, dissection, or both. Data support the notion that skeletonized ITA use does not impact long-term survival or graft patency, while decreasing sternal wound complications.[109,113-118] The benefits in vascularity are correlated with decreased sensory deficits to the precordium.[119] Patients older than 75 years also appear to benefit from the sternal vascularity benefits of skeletonized ITA use.[102] Excellent results have been reported with the use of skeletonized bilateral ITAs in diabetic patients, and yet some studies showed obese diabetic women had an increased incidence of deep sternal wound infection.[120,121] Other studies, however, found no association between skeletonized bilateral ITA harvesting in diabetic patients and sternal wound infection.[122]

Whether a free or pedicled ITA graft is performed makes little difference with respect to patency and endothelial function, provided that a flawless anastomotic technique is used.[123,124] It is more important to avoid short conduit length, which may invariably lead to angle distortion and resultant compromise in flow and patency. A pedicled ITA graft that appears too short is better cut proximally and repositioned onto the aorta or onto another ITA than left under tension.

In some patients, ITA flow may be very low (i.e., less than 20 mL/min) prior to construction of the anastomosis. This may be because of spasm, small size, or intraoperative injury such as an intimal dissection. If an area of injury is suspected, the ITA should be either converted to a free graft (if long enough) or transected a few millimeters above and below the injury site, the two stumps beveled, and an end-to-end anastomosis performed with 8-0 polypropylene. If no injury is apparent, the ITA in most cases may still be used for grafting, as this does not appear to result in an increased incidence of angiographic string sign or graft occlusion at 1 year postoperatively.[125] Unrecognized ITA intimal dissections in some cases may spontaneously heal with anticoagulation, antiplatelet therapy, and vasodilators alone.[126]

Radial Artery Grafts

Controversy exists regarding the benefit of the radial artery as an alternative to the saphenous vein. More than five randomized controlled trials to date have compared the use of the radial artery with the saphenous vein as a conduit for CABG.[127-134] At 1 year, the radial artery has been found to be equivalent to the saphenous vein in terms of angiographically determined patency.[127,131,132] At 5 years, however, the radial artery appears to offer either slightly superior or similar patency rates compared with saphenous vein grafts.[130,132,135] In patients older than 70 years at the time of operation, the use of the radial artery was associated with improved survival at 6 years.[128] Predictors of lower radial artery graft patency rates when compared with vein grafts include female patients and patients with peripheral vascular disease.[136] Although radial grafts are highly versatile and can be used for virtually any type of grafting configuration (e.g., aortocoronary, Y, or T), they should not be used to graft coronaries with less than 70% stenosis because of reduced patency and vulnerability for competitive flow physiology.[137,138]

Intraoperatively, the radial artery may be treated immediately following harvest with a blood/phenoxybenzamine flush (100 mg of phenoxybenzamine mixed in 50 mL of heparinized blood) and left soaking in this mixture for 5 to 30 minutes. Phenoxybenzamine, a noncompetitive α_1-antagonist agent, is nontoxic for endothelial cells and highly effective in preventing acute spasm of the radial artery.[139,140] In one larger study, phenoxybenzamine was shown to reduce the incidence of perioperative myocardial injury and adverse cardiac events.[141] Alternatively, nitroglycerin can be used to dilate the radial artery prior to grafting. The steps in preparing the radial artery conduit are described in Figure 88-5.

Radial artery harvest is contraindicated in the presence of insufficient collateral supply to the hand or Raynaud

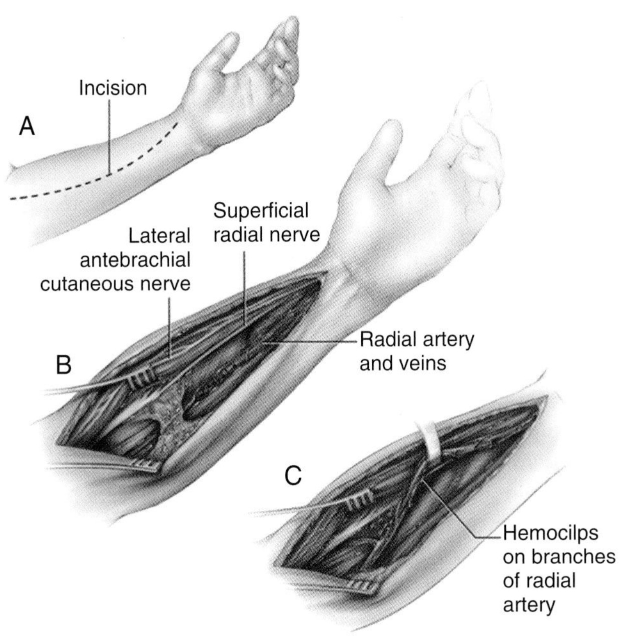

FIGURE 88-5 Open radial artery harvest. **A,** An incision is made in the forearm following the brachioradialis muscle belly. As the dissection is carried deeper, the lateral antebrachial cutaneous nerve will lie lateral to the dissection plane along with the brachioradialis muscle. **B,** The deep fascia of the forearm is opened, exposing the radial artery and veins. The superficial radial nerve also lies lateral to the dissection. **C,** The radial artery and veins are mobilized by clipping branches and using blunt dissection of nonvascular tissue. A vessel loop is used to retract the conduit, avoiding excessive manipulation of the radial artery, which may induce spasm. The dissection is carried out proximally to the recurrent radial artery branch and distally to the fascia enclosing the tendons of the wrist. (Adapted from Doty DB, Doty JR, editors: *Cardiac surgery operative technique,* ed 2, Philadelphia, 2012, Saunders, p 417, Figure 36-9.)

syndrome, in patients with high manual demands such as professional musicians, in the very elderly (who have a high prevalence of radial arteriosclerosis and are unlikely to derive a survival benefit from its preferential use over a vein graft), during emergency operations, and in patients who are likely to require postoperative vasopressors, such as those with very poor left ventricular function. Radial artery use should be expressly discussed during informed patient consent, as the incidence of neurologic complications is approximately 30% and most often consists of decreased thumb strength and sensation abnormality.[142] Diabetes, peripheral vascular disease, elevated creatinine levels, and smoking are associated with an increased incidence of these complications, which resolve with time in most patients.[143]

In efforts to minimize radial artery graft spasm, the predominant cause of early graft failure, the radial artery can be harvested with surrounding perivascular tissues, thereby using an atraumatic "no-touch" technique. Next, replacing mechanical dilation of the free radial artery, pharmacologic dilation with papaverine (or phenoxybenzamine) may enhance nitric oxide production, resulting in decreased endothelial dysfunction. Finally, postoperative radial artery spasm prevention can be considered with either calcium channel blockers or nitrates.[144] Despite little evidence-based literature advocating calcium channel blocker therapy for the prevention of radial artery graft vasospasm, more than 90% of Canadian surgical centers report routine use of calcium channel blocker prophylaxis lasting from several weeks to 6 months.[15,145-147]

Endoscopic radial artery harvest gained popularity in the past decade because it provides better cosmesis and less pain compared with open harvesting.[148] Unlike the concern with regard to patency reported in endoscopic vein harvesting, mid-term patency using endoscopic radial artery harvesting seems equivalent to open harvesting.[149]

Gastroepiploic Artery Grafts

The gastroepiploic artery is a conduit with a higher propensity for intraoperative problems and a lower postoperative patency than the radial artery. Excellent results have been reported by several groups who have developed an expertise with its routine use with 4- to 5-year patency rates of 86% to 90%.[87,150-152] To date, there has been one randomized controlled trial comparing the use of the gastroepiploic artery with use of the saphenous vein graft.[153-155] At 6-month angiographic follow-up, there appeared to be no differences in patency between conduits,[153] although it appeared the patency of the gastroepiploic artery was more influenced by competitive coronary flow.[154] Despite these encouraging results, several factors make it a difficult conduit to systematically recommend: harvest elicits spasm, kinking and torsion may go unrecognized, and anastomotic problems are more likely the result of the small size of the vessel. One study has suggested that use of the gastroepiploic artery to graft coronaries with only moderate proximal stenosis (70% to 80%) or with poor runoff should be avoided, because this results in decreased patency,[156] whereas another study has suggested that its use as a free graft is also associated with a lower patency than the in situ configuration.[157] Based on this evidence, alternative arterial conduits, or possibly saphenous vein conduits, should be exhausted before considering use of the gastroepiploic artery as the conduit of choice for primary revascularization. Moreover, a recent review emphasized that compared with vein graft patency rates, gastroepiploic artery patency rates were inferior during right coronary artery grafting.[158]

Saphenous Vein Grafts

Because of their lower short- and long-term patency compared with ITAs, saphenous veins have not been the conduit of choice for CABG for approximately 20 years.[101] Nevertheless, saphenous veins are the most often used and remain useful in several situations. They constitute the most readily available CABG conduit, provide immediate and reliable coronary flow with a low propensity for spasm or severe compromise during low-output states, and constitute a time-honored means of coronary revascularization during emergency procedures or in patients with severe comorbidity and limited life expectancy in whom procedural simplicity, expeditiousness, and reliability are most desirable. Furthermore, current-era

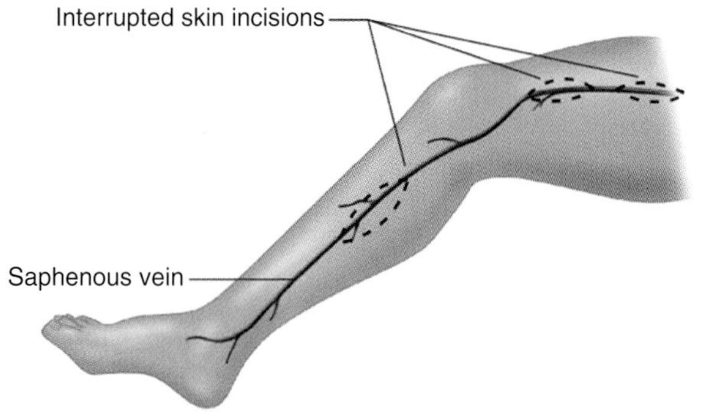

FIGURE 88-6 ■ Interrupted skin incisions to harvest the greater saphenous vein. Compared with a long leg incision, skip incisions provide more cosmesis and lower infection rates while allowing for a direct-vision harvest of the vein. (From Sellke F, Ruel M, editors: *Atlas of cardiac surgical techniques,* Philadelphia, 2009, Saunders.)

antiplatelet and cholesterol medical therapy may improve saphenous vein graft patency beyond that reported in initial CABG series.[28,159,160] Several groups have demonstrated saphenous vein graft patency rates surpassing radial artery patency rates especially when conduits are grafted to moderately diseased arteries[161-163]; furthermore, a recent meta-analysis demonstrated higher side-to-side sequential vein graft patency compared with single vein grafts.[164]

A variety of minimally invasive techniques are widely available for retrieval of the saphenous vein. The spectrum of techniques range from skip incisions (Fig. 88-6) to the use of commercially available endoscopic systems.[165,166] These techniques have been shown to improve patient quality of life and lower harvest site infections.[167,168] On the opposite end of the spectrum, some centers have advocated the use of pedicled saphenous veins to improve on conduit patency and reduce venospasm.[169] Results from three small randomized controlled trials comparing the no-touch saphenous vein harvesting to conventional harvesting demonstrated superior patency rates at mid-term (18 months) and long-term (8.5 years) follow-up along with improved endothelial integrity.[169-172] With more centers performing this technique, further investigation is needed to elucidate the best method for vein harvesting.

Similar to the radial artery, endoscopic vein harvesting was met with enthusiasm a decade ago as studies showed improved cosmesis and lower infection rates compared with open harvesting.[173,174] However, excitement was tempered by a large study reporting lower patency rates and higher rates of death, MI, or repeat revascularization at 3 years compared with open harvesting.[175]

Other Conduits

The lesser saphenous vein, inferior epigastric artery, and right gastroepiploic artery are three alternative autologous conduits. They are rarely needed for primary revascularization, but they may be useful in patients lacking conduit options. Finally, in rare circumstances, cadaveric cryopreserved saphenous veins, bovine chemically treated ITAs, or expanded polytetrafluoroethylene grafts can be used.

Operative Preparation

Intraoperative preparation by the anesthesiologist includes upper extremity peripheral intravenous and arterial access (contralateral to the side of radial artery harvest), induction of general anesthesia, endotracheal intubation, central venous access, and occasionally placement of a pulmonary artery catheter. Intravenous antibiotics with gram-positive coverage are administered 30 to 60 minutes prior to the skin incision. Perioperative antibiotic regimens vary on institutional practices, but often include cefuroxime (1.5 g intravenously [IV] every 12 hours) or cefazolin (1 to 2 g IV every 8 hours for 48 hours); in patients with penicillin allergy, vancomycin (1 g IV every 12 hours) is continued for at least two doses until lines and tubes are removed.[176] A nasogastric tube and transesophageal echocardiography probe, if available, are advanced in the esophagus. Baseline measurements of filling pressures, cardiac output, valvular and ventricular function, arterial blood gases, activated clotting time, hematocrit level, and electrolyte levels are obtained prior to the surgical incision.

The patient is prepared and draped, and a limited midline skin incision is made from the manubrium of the sternum to the xiphoid process. If use of a gastroepiploic artery is planned, the median sternotomy skin incision is carried 2 to 3 inches below the xiphoid. Median sternotomy is performed through this incision by slightly mobilizing the subcutaneous fat in the upper portion of the wound away from the pectoralis muscle while an assistant retracts it superiorly and by proceeding from bottom to top of the sternum with the saw. The assistant then starts harvesting the radial artery, saphenous vein, or both. Meticulous hemostasis is ensured at all stages (unless the patient is acutely ischemic or hemodynamically unstable), because this prevents continuous oozing during the remainder of the operation, minimizes the use of the cardiotomy suction with its potential detrimental effects, prevents coagulopathy, and effectively saves time before closure. Our preference is to open the pericardium before harvesting the ITAs, because this does not lengthen the procedure. In addition, this allows not only digital assessment of the aorta and the performance of epiaortic scanning early in the operation (with the planning of alternate cannulation sites and no-touch Y arterial grafting if significant aortic disease is unveiled), but also the identification of target vessels, the estimation of needed conduit length, and the expeditious cannulation if sudden hemodynamic collapse occurs. Epiaortic scanning is useful as a routine adjunct and can detect ascending aortic atherosclerosis in up to 30% of patients undergoing isolated CABG.[177] Contemporary guidelines recommend intraoperative transesophageal or epiaortic scanning of the aorta to detect nonpalpable plaque (class I, evidence B) and reduce the cerebral embolic load (class IIa, evidence B) in patients at high risk of experiencing a perioperative neurologic event.[178] If epiaortic scanning is unavailable, the incidence of perioperative CVA after CABG can still be minimized by routine preoperative carotid screening, intraoperative transesophageal echocardiography, and a tailored approach to revascularization, thereby avoiding manipulation of the diseased aorta. This includes the use of alternate cannulation sites, fibrillatory arrest, and off-pump revascularization techniques; in a series of more than 6000 CABG patients in whom this approach was used, Trick and coworkers reported a stroke incidence of less than 1%, even in high-risk patients.[179]

The ITAs are harvested and are transected distally only after systemic administration of heparin. There are two ways to perform this while minimizing bleeding during harvest of the second ITA: either a partial dose of heparin (e.g., 5000 to 10,000 units) is given at the completion and prior to transaction of the first ITA (with a completion dose administered prior to transaction of the second ITA), or both ITAs are transected at the same time after the second ITA has been harvested and the full dose of heparin given.

Cardiopulmonary Bypass and Cardioplegia

CPB is established with ascending aortic cannulation, right atrial venous cannula drainage, mild hypothermia (32° to 34° C), and alpha-stat pH management. Venting is performed via the proximal ascending aorta by using the antegrade cardioplegia delivery catheter, often at a site to be used later for a proximal anastomosis. Antegrade intermittent cold blood cardioplegia provides adequate myocardial protection for most primary revascularization cases; consideration is given to a combination of antegrade and retrograde routes in severely ischemic patients or when the LAD is obstructed or severely stenotic.[180] Topical cooling makes little difference on myocardial temperature and outcome when combined with antegrade cold blood cardioplegia and has been associated with an increased incidence of postoperative hemidiaphragmatic paresis and pleural effusions.[181]

Intraoperative transcranial Doppler scanning of the middle cerebral arteries, if available, constitutes a useful adjunct during CPB cases. In our experience, it has helped design minor but effective modifications in cannulation, perfusion, clamping, and venting techniques that have minimized the frequency and overall number of high-intensity transient signals.[182] Use of the cardiotomy suction is best avoided because of its potentiation of clotting activation, micelle formation, and microembolism during perfusion. It can be replaced by a cell-saver device during routine cases. Moderate hypothermia and slow rewarming as well as meticulous control of blood glucose levels can also help decrease the incidence of postoperative neurocognitive deficits.[183,184]

Special Situations

Diffuse Aortic Disease. One of the most formidable technical obstacles that can be encountered during CABG is diffuse disease of the aorta and its branches. Manipulation of a diseased aortic segment may lead to embolization and constitutes the most important risk factor for stroke after CABG.[185] If the aortic disease is focal and does not involve the distal third of the ascending aorta, the area can usually be avoided during cannulation, clamping, and construction of proximal anastomoses (under single cross-clamping). Multifocal disease, diffuse disease, or disease involving the distal third of the ascending aorta, however, mandates the use of femoral or axillary artery cannulation; the relocation of proximal anastomoses to the proximal ascending aorta, brachiocephalic artery, or descending aorta; the use of hypothermic fibrillation or hypothermic circulatory arrest; and, in some cases, ascending aortic replacement. Fortunately, widespread familiarity with off-pump and Y-grafting techniques has significantly increased the options for managing patients with diffuse aortic disease. In most cases of diffuse aortic disease, an off-pump aortic no-touch CABG operation with bilateral pedicled ITAs or Y or T arterial graft configuration can be performed with acceptably low risk, provided the patient is hemodynamically stable and not acutely ischemic.[186] If refractory hemodynamic instability develops, the patient must be managed with cannulation of the axillary or femoral artery,[187] establishment of CPB, hypothermic fibrillatory arrest during performance of distal anastomoses, and construction of the proximal anastomoses to the innominate artery or to a disease-free area of the ascending aorta using a special, local-control device[188] or during a short period of hypothermic circulatory arrest.[83]

Preoperative Cardiogenic Shock. Preoperative cardiogenic shock requires immediate establishment of CPB, performed either via femoral cannulation or sternotomy depending on patient characteristics (such as redo operation or a history of previous aortobifemoral grafting) and the surgeon's preferences. If time and hemodynamic status allow, patients should have an intra-aortic balloon counterpulsation pump inserted preoperatively or stabilized with a nondurable percutaneous mechanical circulatory support device such as the Impella 2.5 or 5.0 (Abiomed, Danvers, MA).[189,190] Combined antegrade and retrograde cardioplegia delivery with warm induction and warm reperfusion techniques can have a net benefit in those patients. Although consideration is given to the use of one ITA graft if the patient is hemodynamically stable, the use of an all–saphenous vein operation is appropriate because of high immediate myocardial demands and anticipated need for postoperative inotropes.[191] Revascularization involves the performance of at least one graft to each ischemic myocardial territory.

Medication-Related Coagulation Impairment. Whether the use of antifibrinolytics is mandated in routine CABG cases remains controversial. Recently, the serine protease inhibitor aprotinin has come under scrutiny. Previous reports had suggested that aprotinin may adversely impact renal, myocardial, cerebral, and pulmonary function.[192-195] In an observational trial involving 3876 patients, Mangano and colleagues found that aprotinin use was associated with an increase in overall mortality at 5 years.[192] Following publication of this study, use of aprotinin dropped precipitously, although some studies have suggested that patients undergoing off-pump CABG may in fact benefit from aprotinin use.[196,197]

Advances in antiplatelet therapy have revolutionized the management of patients with CAD; however, the antiplatelet effects can also impact postoperative hemostasis.[198] Transfusions of platelets, fresh-frozen plasma, and cryoprecipitate may therefore be needed in these patients. Patients on abciximab may benefit from the routine administration of a single platelet transfusion after protamine administration; this approach appears to decrease the rate of reexploration for bleeding.[199]

Previous Tracheostomy. The presence of a tracheal stoma in patients with previous total laryngectomy who require cardiac operations is associated with an increased risk of wound complications, mediastinitis, tracheal injury, or stoma necrosis when a full sternotomy is used. In these patients, a manubrium-sparing sternotomy can be used, where the upper edge of the sternotomy does not extend beyond the top of the third rib. Slow progressive opening of the retractor allows for the operation to be conducted successfully while minimizing the possibility of manubrial fracture, bleeding, and patient discomfort. An alternative approach is to incise the sternum transversely at the second intercostal space and complete the median sternotomy longitudinally down to the xiphoid process.[200]

Distal Anastomoses

Construction of distal coronary anastomoses begins once the first dose of cardioplegia has been delivered. With current methods of myocardial protection and considering the increased prevalence of diffuse CAD in CABG patients, there is little justification for performing proximal anastomoses first during on-pump CABG. Proximal anastomoses are constructed either sequentially (each distal followed by its proximal under single cross-clamping) or all at once after completion of distal anastomoses. One exception to this approach is during performance of arterial Y- or T-grafting, because the surgeon may complete all proximal conduit anastomoses onto one to two pedicled ITAs prior to the establishment of CPB; this strategy minimizes unnecessary CPB time and allows for the assessment of free flow in each ramus of the configuration prior to distal grafting.

Although the order of revascularization is not of critical importance during on-pump CABG, the first graft performed is usually that to the inferior circulation, followed by the lateral wall, the diagonal system, and the LAD artery. Vessels that are completely occluded and for which a free graft is planned may benefit from construction of the distal anastomosis early in the revascularization sequence to improve cardioplegic delivery to the subtended myocardium.

Many conduit-graft configurations are possible, and the choice is based on the needs of the patient. The pedicled LITA is usually grafted to the LAD, although the pedicled right internal thoracic artery (RITA) can also be used with success and placed in the superior mediastinum to decrease the risk of injury during subsequent sternotomy. The next preferred conduit (i.e., the second ITA, followed by the radial, gastroepiploic artery, and saphenous vein) is kept for the target vessel in decreasing order of anatomic importance. Poor-quality, diffusely diseased coronary arteries do not necessarily only deserve a vein graft, as the short- and long-term patency of an ITA or radial graft to a diffusely stenotic vessel may be considerably better. Conduit length problems resulting in inappropriate anastomotic tension are almost always solvable by the use of arterial Y-grafts, which are avoided with saphenous veins because differences in conduit size can result in unpredictable flow patterns.

Exposure of the main coronary branches is not problematic during on-pump CABG. The inferior wall may be exposed by packing a small sponge against the inferior vena cava at the right inferior aspect of the oblique sinus. The lateral wall may be exposed by gently twisting and folding the heart on itself in the long axis and placing a sponge underneath to expose the marginal branches. The anterior wall is exposed by a single sponge under the left ventricle.

The most proximal disease-free portion of the coronary artery to be grafted (i.e., immediately after the most distal involvement) is selected for the anastomosis. The epicardium is incised over the area of the coronary artery with a no. 15 blade or a special rounded blade. The anterior surface of the artery is cleared by gentle transverse brushing with the scalpel. Even with cardioplegia, careful inspection of the artery will reveal a thin central line that is red or translucent, indicating the lumen. The anterior wall of the artery is opened longitudinally over this line by caressing gently with the scalpel so as to not damage the posterior wall. Administration of a small amount of cardioplegia to distend the coronary artery lumen may be useful during this step, especially for small (≤ 1 mm) vessels. Occasionally, when the anterior wall of the artery cannot be placed under proper tension, it may be opened by stabbing it with a sharp-pointed scalpel. The blade must enter the artery obliquely and superficially, so as to not penetrate the posterior wall. The incision is enlarged with angled scissors to a length of 4 to 6 mm for end-to-side anastomoses, and 3 to 5 mm for side-to-side anastomoses. The epicardial incision is extended beyond each angle of the arteriotomy to facilitate the anastomosis. The artery may be sized and proximal, and distal patency can be assessed by passing measuring probes into it. Aortic root venting is used only as necessary so as to not introduce an excessive amount of air into the ascending aorta. The distal end of the conduit is incised longitudinally for approximately 20% longer than the coronary arteriotomy; this in conjunction with slightly further spacing of suture bites on the conduit than on the coronary enables the desirable "cobra head" appearance (Fig. 88-7).

Many anastomotic techniques exist, each with advantages and disadvantages. For the sake of reliability under all circumstances, each surgeon should probably limit himself or herself to one main anastomotic technique that is perfectly mastered and can be used with all conduit types, for end-to-side as well as side-to-side anastomoses, and during on-pump as well as off-pump CABG. General principles include the use of 7-0 or 8-0 polypropylene, the use of a no-touch technique in which the intima of the coronary and the conduit are never grabbed, and compulsive attention to the geometric distribution of sutures as the anastomosis is performed, because an

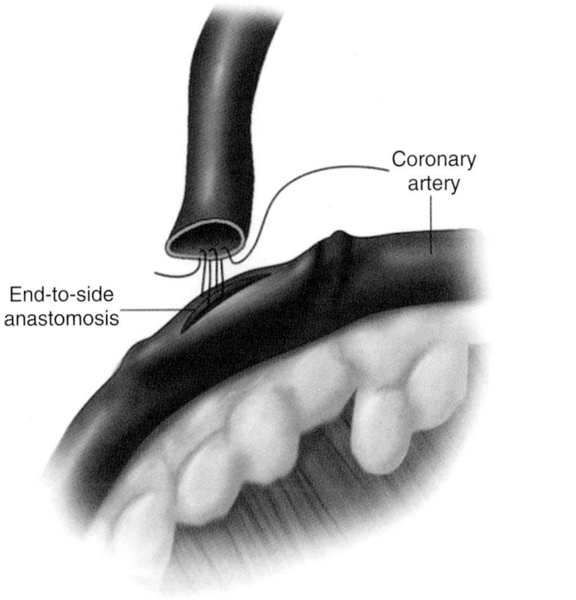

FIGURE 88-7 ■ End-to-side distal anastomosis. After incising the epicardium over the selected coronary artery using a no. 15 blade, an arteriotomy is performed to match the end of the graft. The graft is anastomosed onto the coronary artery using a running 7-0 polypropylene suture. Constant attention is given to the overall anastomosis geometry. (From Sellke F, Ruel M, editors: *Atlas of cardiac surgical techniques,* Philadelphia, 2009, Saunders.)

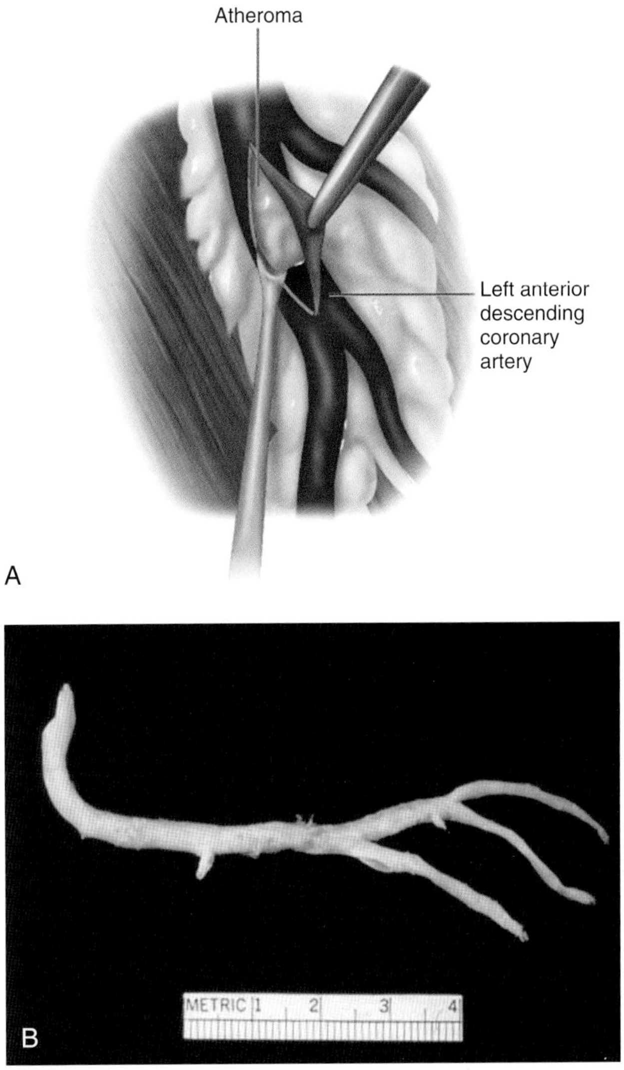

FIGURE 88-8 ■ Coronary endarterectomy. **A,** Representative illustration of a large atheroma removed from the left anterior descending artery. **B,** Specimen removed from a completely occluded right coronary artery and subsequently bypassed with a saphenous vein graft. (Courtesy Dr. John Veinot, Department of Pathology, Ottawa Hospital, Ottawa, Ontario, Canada.)

otherwise adequate but deformed anastomosis may be nonfunctional or prone to thrombosis. Another principle we enforce is that no impediment to native coronary flow should result from construction of an anastomosis, therefore mandating flawless patency at both anastomotic angles so that if for some reason the conduit becomes nonfunctional, native coronary flow will at least be the same as if a bypass graft had not been performed onto this coronary artery.

We prefer to use sequential grafts within a single coronary distribution only (e.g., for two marginal branches of the circumflex system), to avoid possible flow diversion from one myocardial territory to another. Other groups have reported good results using a T-graft configuration that may bridge two or even three myocardial territories.[186,201] In general, sequential grafts allow for a greater number of arterial anastomoses and, with vein grafts, contribute to an increased long-term patency.[163,201] Transverse sequential side-to-side anastomoses may be used for saphenous vein grafts with excellent patency rates[164] but are relatively contraindicated with arterial grafts. Perfect orientation of the sequential arterial anastomoses with respect to each other and avoidance of tension or excessive redundancy on the conduit are crucial. Because of the potential to jeopardize revascularization of two or more vessels, any sequential graft that might appear technically unsatisfactory is best redone or replaced with individual grafts.

Coronary Endarterectomy

Coronary endarterectomy is a technique that preceded the invention of CABG.[5] It is now reserved for select cases of severe diffuse disease where no anastomotic site can be found on a coronary artery that supplies an ischemic and viable myocardial territory (Fig. 88-8). This procedure should not be used because of technical failure to find the true lumen, such as occurs when a diffusely diseased vessel is mistakenly opened into a lateral plaque. Arteries that can be seen on coronary angiography do have a lumen, which can be found despite poor target site selection or extraluminal opening by carefully extending the arteriotomy proximally and distally into the true lumen and performing a long patch angioplasty by using the conduit as an onlay patch. Endarterectomy should also only be used on vessels with high-grade stenoses (>80%). Endarterectomy is combined with an onlay patch angioplasty of the endarterectomized vessel, and a bypass graft is performed using the same conduit. When reserved for carefully selected situations, coronary endarterectomy has been associated with a rate of perioperative MI of 5% or less, a graft–coronary axis patency of 72% at 30 months, and a good functional outcome that can approach outcomes seen in non-endarterectomized patients.[202-204]

Sutureless Distal Coronary Connectors

Significant advances have been made with automated coronary connectors and self-closing U-clip distal anastomotic devices. Preliminary reports on the use of these devices in humans describe geometrically adequate anastomoses, excellent immediate graft flows, and good patency at 3- and 6-month angiographic follow-up.[205-207]

Proximal Anastomoses

Most proximal anastomoses are made on the ascending aorta, but alternative sites such as the brachiocephalic artery, axillary artery, and descending aorta can be used in special situations. Y- and T-grafting involves constructing the inflow anastomosis of a free arterial graft to an in situ arterial conduit, using either an end-to-side or a side-to-side configuration. General principles of proximal anastomosis construction include insurance of a perfect graft lie (i.e., without torsion, tension, or excessive redundancy) and the minimization of aortic manipulations.

Although preferences vary, the use of a side-biting tangential clamp is best avoided because of its association with increased cerebral microembolic load and S-100 release during CABG.[208] In our experience, several techniques can be used to reduce this embolic load to levels equal or below that of single aortic cross-clamp proximal techniques. These consist of (1) using a tangential side-biting clamp only in the presence of a nondiseased ascending aorta (Fig. 88-9), (2) releasing the cross-clamp and applying the side clamp while the pump is momentarily stopped, (3) irrigating the inside of the aorta after punch holes are made, (4) completely displacing air prior to tying the last proximal anastomosis either by saline instillation or by removal of the bulldog clamp on one of the anastomosed free arterial grafts, which backfills the aorta with blood, and (5) releasing the clamp while the pump is momentarily stopped.

To perform a proximal anastomosis a longitudinal slit, approximately 3 mm in length, is made with a no. 11 blade at the chosen site(s) in the aorta. A punch of either 4.0 (for free arterial grafts) or 4.5 mm (for saphenous vein grafts) in diameter is slipped completely and freely into the aorta through each slit and closed so as to punch out a circular piece of aorta at each site (see Fig. 88-9). Each conduit is irrigated intraluminally and its orientation determined under direct vision, measured so as to not prove too short or redundant once the heart fills (pinching of the venous line to fill the right heart is useful in evaluating this), occluded with a light bulldog clamp, spatulated at its proximal end to a perimeter approximately 20% longer than the aortic punch hole, and connected to the aorta using 6-0 polypropylene. If an arterial conduit appears too short, either it is anastomosed in an end-to-end fashion onto a short segment of saphenous vein, which is itself anastomosed to the aorta, or the arterial graft is anastomosed side-to-side (as a Y-graft) onto another arterial graft.

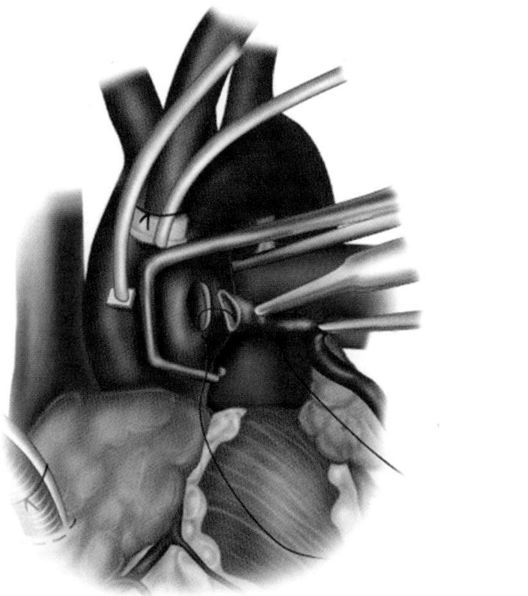

FIGURE 88-9 ■ Proximal anastomosis using a side-biting clamp. With the use of a side-biting clamp and after a small (4- to 4.5-mm) aortotomy is performed, the proximal anastomosis is accomplished with a running 6-0 polypropylene suture. (From Sellke F, Ruel M, editors: *Atlas of cardiac surgical techniques*, Philadelphia, 2009, Saunders.)

Sutureless Proximal Coronary Connectors

Commercially available automated proximal aortic connectors have been used successfully by a growing number of groups with good patency rates; however, a prospective randomized controlled trial is needed to explore some concerns regarding early graft closure.[209-213] Advantages of these connectors include the avoidance of aortic manipulations (except at the anastomotic site) and ease of use, especially for off-pump or robotic-assisted procedures.

Intraoperative Graft Assessment

The high prevalence of small and diffusely diseased target vessels in CABG patients and the increasingly challenging surgical techniques used (such as complex arterial grafting and off-pump procedures) may justify routine graft validation in the operating room. One practice, although subjective, is to gently probe each anastomosis at critical points during construction to ensure proximal, distal, and conduit patency, and rule out a purse-string effect that may insidiously occur if too large or too few bites are taken around the anastomosis, if its geometric configuration is imperfect, or if the assistant pulls excessively on the suture when "following."

The most widely used modality of objective graft assessment is transit-time flow measurement (TTFM). With this tool, a diastolic-to-systolic perfusion pattern of at least 2 : 1 for grafts constructed to vessels overlying the left ventricle (such as the LAD and circumflex branches) and a pulsatility index less than 3 are a good predictor of patency, whereas low absolute flow values can be the result of arterial spasm without anastomotic error.[214,215] Unfortunately, specific cut-off recommendations for graft revision have not been clarified and TTFM remains imperfect in detecting less than critical stenosis on the graft or at the anastomosis, regardless of the adjunctive use of spectral or fast Fourier transformation analysis.[216] Other modalities such as high-frequency epicardial echocardiography and power Doppler imaging have been described, but experience is still limited.[217] Thermal imaging has limited image resolution and is largely unsuitable for off-pump or minimally invasive surgery.[218]

Intraoperative fluorescent cardiac imaging is clinically safe and may prove clinically useful.[219] This modality uses a 0.5-mL injection of indocyanine green and a portable imaging device to visualize coronary anatomy and grafts during conventional CABG, off-pump coronary artery bypass (OPCAB), or minimally invasive direct coronary artery bypass (MIDCAB). Graft and coronary visualization is very good, but anastomotic resolution needs improvement and overlying fat or muscle can artificially obscure the penetration and detection of indocyanine green (ICG) fluorescence. The modality works best with skeletonized arterial grafts and saphenous vein grafts.

Routine intraoperative completion angiography in the setting of a hybrid operating room has shown, in one study, that up to 12% of bypass grafts may have important angiographic defects that need to be addressed intraoperatively.[220] Further studies are needed to clarify the role of completion angiography in hybrid revascularization.

Weaning from Cardiopulmonary Bypass

Once the proximal anastomoses are completed, each vein graft is de-aired with a 27-gauge needle prior to release of the bulldog clamp. Graft conduits are examined for adequateness of lie and hemostasis at each anastomotic site and side branch while the mean arterial pressure is increased to at least 70 mm of Hg. Distal anastomotic jet bleeding is repaired with a single stitch of 7-0 Prolene; if the toe or heel is involved, repair may compromise the anastomosis, and consideration is given to preparing cardioplegia and reapplying the cross-clamp to redo the anastomosis. It is preferable to spend 10 to 15 extra minutes in redoing an anastomosis that has a significant leak at or near the angle than repairing it with a potential for distortion or occlusion. The epicardium may be used to cover and repair small lateral anastomotic leaks but should not be used near an anastomotic angle.

Preparation of the patient for weaning from CPB involves a routine but thorough assessment of the cardiac, pulmonary, and metabolic systems. The chosen temperature for weaning, a point of current controversy, is reached by slowly rewarming the patient and avoiding hyperthermia.[183,221] Hematocrit level and metabolic and electrolyte balance are checked and corrected as necessary. The trachea is suctioned and the lungs are reexpanded by hand under direct vision and mechanically ventilated with 100% O_2. Respiratory monitors and alarms are reactivated. The pleural spaces are checked for the presence of fluid or pneumothorax. Atrial and ventricular epicardial pacing wires are affixed onto the heart and exteriorized on the chest, and heart rhythm and rate are optimized by using synchronized cardioversion or pacing as necessary. Sinus rhythm or atrial pacing at 75 to 95 beats per minute is ideal for weaning, although patients with significant diastolic dysfunction from left ventricular hypertrophy or with incomplete revascularization may benefit from a slower atrial rate in conjunction with a slightly prolonged atrioventricular interval. The ECG is examined for ST-segment changes suggestive of ischemia; if ischemia is present, reassessment and reconstruction of a graft must be considered.

The perfusionist progressively clamps the venous line to provide preload to the ejecting right ventricle, which in turn results in left ventricular preload. Afterload is managed by the anesthesiologist by using either an alpha-agonist agent such as phenylephrine or, in some cases, a direct vasodilator such as nitroprusside. Contractility is assessed by observing left and right ventricular contraction and the evolution of pulmonary arterial pressures during the weaning process, which are reflective of ventricular function, except in cases of pulmonary vascular hypertension. Several adjuncts may be used when weaning is difficult. First, each of the previously described steps is rechecked and corrected as necessary while CPB support is reestablished and a period of reperfusion on the empty beating heart is reinitiated. Second, consideration is given to ischemia or intracoronary air while grafts are reassessed. Third, inotropic support and intra-aortic balloon pump (IABP) are used as necessary. Inotropic and IABP use in nonemergency patients with good left ventricular function preoperatively is abnormal and warrants questioning the adequacy of revascularization (i.e., nonfunctional grafts, plaque or cholesterol embolism during the construction of anastomoses, grafting of wrong coronary vessels or even a coronary vein), and justifies a low threshold for redoing or adding one or several grafts. Further attempts at weaning from CPB are taken after reconsidering the previously mentioned points. If weaning is still unsuccessful after many attempts and clearly related to poor contractility, consideration is given to the use of extracorporeal membrane oxygenation or mechanical ventricular support as a bridge to recovery.

Once the patient is satisfactorily weaned from CPB, the venous cannula is removed and the atrial purse-string suture snared but not tied. The venous line is then sumped with normal saline to return blood to the heart-lung machine reservoir. The aortic line is checked for air that may have migrated from the left ventricle during cardiac ejection, and the perfusionist transfuses aliquots of remaining pump blood according to the directives of the surgeon and anesthesiologist. Excessive right ventricular distention and pulmonary diastolic venous hypertension of more than 22 to 25 mm of Hg are avoided. If these develop and mean arterial pressure is satisfactory, IV nitroglycerine is used as a preload reducer and pulmonary venodilator.

Protamine is administered once stable hemodynamics is achieved and when reestablishment of CPB for support or technical reasons is unlikely to be needed. Chest tubes are inserted in the posterior pericardium, in the anterior mediastinum, and into each pleural cavity entered. Care is taken at ensuring that chest tubes do not lie in proximity to a graft once the chest is closed: not only could they mechanically compress the graft and lead to distortion and thrombosis, but they may also result in damage if the graft is entrapped into a side-hole of the tube during suction.

After administration of the first dose of protamine, the aortic cannula is removed from the ascending aorta in case of hemodynamic collapse caused by an adverse protamine reaction. Cannulation purse-string sutures are securely tied and reinforced with pledgeted stitches as needed. Hemostasis is checked at each anastomotic site, along each conduit, at all cannulation sites, and on the chest wall. If, despite these measures, blood accumulation is still noted in the pericardium, the left atrial appendage is examined for possible damage caused by the cardiotomy suction during CPB. Radio-opaque markers are left around proximal vein graft anastomoses. The pericardium is partially reapproximated over the anterior left ventricle but not closed to avoid adverse hemodynamic effects. Routine closure of the sternotomy incision concludes the operation.

SPECIAL FEATURES OF POSTOPERATIVE CARE

Early Postoperative Period

Despite unclear evidence, patients with a radial, gastroepiploic, or inferior epigastric artery graft are started on intravenous nitroglycerine or calcium channel blockers as soon as arterial blood pressure parameters allow. Nitroglycerine has been shown to be more effective, less costly, and safer (with a lower incidence of bradycardia and negative inotropy) than intravenous diltiazem.[222] Aspirin (650 mg) is given via suppository within 6 hours of operation and subsequently by mouth at a dose of 100 to 325 mg per day (class I).[34,223,224] Patients treated concomitantly with clopidogrel are given a slightly lower aspirin dose (81 mg), although no evidence exists for this practice. It is a reasonable alternative to give clopidogrel (75 mg once daily) to patients who cannot tolerate aspirin (class IIa).[43] Most patients are extubated within 4 to 6 hours of CABG and discharged from the intensive care unit on the following morning (postoperative day 1). Chest tubes are removed when draining less than 100 mL per 12 hours, when no air leaks, and if the chest x-ray shows no significant residual effusion. Most patients experience surprisingly little postoperative pain, which is managed initially with intravenous narcotics and subsequently with oral codeine or hydromorphone. A short course of nonsteroidal anti-inflammatory drugs is added as an adjuvant in patients with normal renal function and without a history of peptic ulcer or CHF. Beta blockers and other antihypertensive medications are usually restarted at half-dose on the morning following the operation and progressively titrated back to the preoperative dose prior to hospital discharge. Mild to moderate dose statin therapy is now recommended in all patients undergoing CABG, whereas higher doses of statins may be required to achieve at least a 30% reduction in serum LDL levels. Optimizing glucose control prior to and after surgery with either oral agents or intravenous insulin has reduced the incidence of adverse clinical outcomes. Patients with moderate left ventricular dysfunction (LVEF between 30% and 50%) and normal renal function are started on angiotensin-converting enzyme (ACE) inhibitors or angiotensin receptor blockers (ARBs) regardless of symptoms.[225] Our practice is to also start patients with radial or gastroepiploic grafts on daily amlodipine, which is more effective than diltiazem and more specific to the arterial vasculature than nifedipine.[145,226] Atrial fibrillation prophylaxis varies according to personal surgeon and center preferences[227]; our approach consists in maximizing the use of beta blockers early postoperatively. The recent 2011 ACC/AHA guidelines recommend prompt (<24 hours) administration of oral beta blockers to all patients without contraindication to reduce the incidence of postoperative atrial fibrillation (class I).[34] Moreover, prophylactic regimens based on the administration of sotalol, amiodarone, and intravenous magnesium have been shown to be effective, although cost-effectiveness remains controversial.[228-230] Patients are discharged home at a median of 5 days postoperatively and in some cases as early as the third postoperative day.

Late Postoperative Period

During the first 3 to 4 weeks after CABG, patients commonly have a poor appetite, insomnia, tiredness, lack of sexual desire, mild neurocognitive deficits, and depressed mood. These phenomena are related to the postoperative state and prove to be transient for most patients; reassurance from the surgeon is often all that is needed. Patients are encouraged to walk progressively as part of convalescence; from a minimum distance of 120 m when discharged from the hospital, patients should progressively increase their daily walking to 1 hour or more by the end of the first postoperative month. Lifting is limited to 3 kg during the first postoperative month, 10 kg during the second month, and 30 kg or less until 6 months after the operation. Structured cardiac rehabilitation programs are a useful adjunct, and patients are encouraged to join as soon as discharged from the hospital. Patients who have a normal convalescence can usually resume driving within 3 weeks of operation and return to work within 2 to 3 months. Patients who have a special occupation in which recurrent cardiac events could put the lives of others at risk (such as bus drivers and pilots) should undergo noninvasive cardiac testing to rule out ischemia prior to resuming work. Despite the invasiveness of CABG, studies looking at the quality of life in patients who participated in the SYNTAX and FREEDOM trials have revealed that quality of life in CABG patients surpasses that of PCI patients after only 6 months.[231,232]

CABG represents only one of many treatment interventions for patients with CAD, as coronary disease continues to progress. Secondary prevention is essential after CABG: aspirin must be continued, smoking must never be resumed, second-hand smoke must be avoided, exercise must be encouraged, obesity if present must be addressed, lipid profile optimized, and hypertension and diabetes strictly controlled. These factors have a significant impact on the progression of saphenous vein graft atherosclerosis and, by extension, can also benefit arterial grafts.[233,234]

Beta blockers are progressively weaned 6 months following uncomplicated CABG in patients with no arrhythmias, no angina, normal ventricular function, and in whom other medications are used for antihypertensive therapy. Amlodipine is discontinued after 1 year in patients with radial or gastroepiploic grafts.[235] Patients with moderate left ventricular dysfunction (LVEF < 40%) should be initiated or continued on ACE inhibitors or ARBs indefinitely, because this is associated with a reduced incidence of cardiac death, acute MI, and clinical heart failure.[34,225]

RESULTS

Morbidity

The most common complications of CABG are postoperative bleeding, low cardiac output syndrome, MI, neurologic events, renal dysfunction, atrial arrhythmias, and sternal wound infections. Other complications are discussed in detail elsewhere in the book. The definition, incidence, prevention, and treatment of these complications are discussed here.

Postoperative Bleeding and Transfusion

Bleeding after CABG can be attributed to surgical and/or medical causes. Reexploration to control hemorrhage occurs in 2% to 6% of CABG cases[236] and carries a 4.5-fold higher risk of mortality.[237] Predisposing factors for postoperative bleeding and transfusion include advanced age, female gender, lower body weight, preoperative cardiogenic shock, anemia, renal dysfunction (especially dialysis-dependent patients), peripheral vascular disease, poor nutritional status, recent thrombolytic therapy, nonelective cases, repeat operations, and longer CPB times.[237-239] Although this practice is not based on evidence, most surgeons use some variation of the following protocol to guide reexploration: (1) blood drainage from the chest tube more than 400 mL in the first hour after surgery, (2) more than 300 mL/hour in the first 2 hours, (3) more than 200 mL/hour in the first 3 hours, (4) more than 100 mL/hour in the first 4 hours, (5) sudden massive bleeding, (6) signs of cardiac tamponade, and (7) excessive bleeding despite correction of coagulopathy. Surgical causes of bleeding in CABG are usually cannulation purse-string leak, graft anastomosis leak, or bleeding from an ITA branch of stumps.

The medical causes of bleeding can include one or more of the following: depletion of coagulation factors by dilution, activation, and consumption as a result of CPB; quantitative and qualitative platelet abnormalities caused by preoperative antiplatelet medications or renal dysfunction, and the direct effect of CPB; hypothermia, which can impair thromboxane synthesis and suppress platelet aggregation; and residual heparin leading to rebound heparin effect.

Strategies to prevent excessive bleeding after CABG include meticulous surgical technique and hemostasis, prevention or reversal of intraoperative hemodilution, prompt reversal of hypothermia, detection and treatment of residual heparin effect with protamine, blood pressure control, administration of antifibrinolytics, and the use of recombinant activated factor VIIa in severe situations. The latter has been increasingly used in cardiac surgery, but the possibility of bypass graft thrombosis caused by a hypercoagulable milieu remains a theoretical concern.[240,241]

The incidence of transfusion during primary on-pump CABG ranges from near 0% up to 50% with most centers transfusing approximately 20% of patients.[238] Institution-specific guidelines dictate transfusion thresholds. Preoperative anemia is one of the most important predictors of blood transfusion.[242] Studies have shown that both preoperative anemia and perioperative blood transfusions are risk factors for mortality and morbidity including acute kidney injury, wound infections, prolonged ventilation, pulmonary problems, and longer length of stay.[243-250] In a large contemporary study of 182,599 patients in the Society of Thoracic Surgery (STS) database,[250] preoperative anemia (hematocrit <33%) had a significant impact on perioperative morbidity and mortality compared to patients with preoperative hematocrit levels higher than 42%. In this study, each 5-point decrease in preoperative hematocrit was associated with 8% higher odds of death, 22% higher odds of postoperative renal failure, and a 10% increase in the risk of deep sternal wound infection. Perioperative blood transfusion was 88.5% in the anemia group compared to 32.5% in the groups with hematocrit levels higher than 42%. Karkouti and associates addressed preoperative anemia with prophylactic transfusion in a pilot trial[251] and found it did not improve outcomes. This was likely because of the risks of transfusion, which can cancel out the beneficial effects of treating the anemia. Therefore, alternatives to transfusion, such as detecting and managing preoperative anemia from a cause-based approach, must be sought.

Low Cardiac Output Syndrome

Low cardiac output syndrome (LCOS) after CABG is generally defined and accepted as requirement of inotropic medications or IABP insertion to keep systolic blood pressure higher than 90 mm Hg and cardiac index (CI) of more than 2.2 L/min/m^2 despite optimization of preload, afterload, electrolytes, and blood gas abnormalities for 30 minutes after surgery.[252] It occurs in 4% to 14% of isolated CABG cases and carries a 10- to 17-fold increase in mortality and significant increase in morbidity.[252-254] Predictors of LCOS include advanced age (>70), female gender, diabetes mellitus, left main and triple-vessel CAD, low ejection fraction (<50%), redo or emergency surgery, recent MI, incomplete revascularization, long CPB time, and poor intraoperative myocardial protection.[252-254] Management of LCOS involves thorough assessment of potential causes directed at the modification of correctable causes, such as immediate cardiac and graft catheterization and return to the operating room if necessary. Initially, preload and afterload should be optimized with appropriate volume infusions and blood pressure control. Contractility may be supported with appropriate inotropic medications. Treating electrolyte and blood gas abnormalities is essential. Hypothermia, if present, must be addressed. An ECG and cardiac enzyme levels must be part of the evaluation to rule out myocardial ischemia or infarction as a culprit. An urgent bedside echocardiogram may be warranted to rule out cardiac tamponade and detect regional wall motion abnormalities if LCOS does not resolve promptly. Evidence supports prophylactic IABP insertion in patients identified preoperatively as at high risk for LCOS.[255-257] However, IABP may also be inserted postoperatively. In some cases, open chest management may be required for 24 to 48 hours after surgery.[258]

Perioperative Myocardial Infarction

Perioperative MI occurs in 2% to 10% of first-time CABG cases, depending on the institutional or study definition,[20,21,259] and carries a higher risk of mortality, morbidity, and reduced long-term quality of life.[260-262] It may be secondary to graft-related problems or native coronary artery problems. Graft-related problems include kinking and overstretching of the grafts, acute occlusion, technical anastomotic stenosis, or conduit spasm. Causes related to the native circulation include inadequate myocardial protection, incomplete revascularization, and coronary embolization. Insertion of an IABP may be required in these circumstances to minimize myocardial ischemia. Although some elevations in cardiac enzymes are ubiquitous after surgery, elevations in the creatine kinase–myocardial bound (CK-MB) and troponin-I beyond five times the upper normal limit defines a perioperative MI,[263] especially when accompanied by new Q waves or new left bundle branch block on ECG,[264] or new regional wall motion abnormalities on transesophageal echocardiography (TEE).[265] In a study of 4000 patients by Brener and colleagues,[266] elevations of cardiac enzymes above 10 times the upper normal limit was associated with a 30% decrease in survival at 3 years. Inotropes, vasopressors, and the use of an IABP may be helpful in unstable patients; however, cardiac catheterization or reexploration may be needed despite other measures.

Neurologic Events

Neurologic deficit after CABG can be divided into two types: type 1 deficits, which represent major, focal neurologic deficits, stupor, and coma; and type 2 deficits, which are characterized by global deterioration of intellectual function or memory.[267] Both types of deficits are likely to be the result of one or a combination of the following: cerebral emboli, hypoperfusion, or inflammation related to CPB. Type I deficits are associated with up to 25% risk of mortality.[268,269] The incidence of stroke after CABG is between 1.4% and 3.8%.[270,271] More than half of these occur after surgery, with the remaining occurring intraoperatively.[272,273] Half of postoperative strokes take place in the first 24 hours after surgery.[270] Stroke after CABG carries a mortality of up to 17%, with early (<24 hours) strokes carrying a threefold higher risk of dying compared with late (>24 hours) strokes.[270] Predictors of stroke include advanced age (>70 years), female sex, previous stroke, CHF, atrial fibrillation, diabetes mellitus, hypertension, peripheral vascular disease (including carotid artery disease), renal failure, atherosclerotic aortic disease, and perioperative hypotension or the use of an IABP.[270,274,275] Although multiple randomized trials did not demonstrate lower prevalence of neurologic injury in off-pump compared with on-pump CABG,[276-278] one study demonstrated that operative or off-pump techniques that avoided aortic manipulation were associated with fewer intraoperative strokes, which suggests a greater role of aortic manipulation causing stroke compared with CPB exposure.[273] A recent meta-analysis also suggested a significant 30% reduction of stroke in off-pump (1.4%) compared with on-pump CABG (2.1%).[279]

Type 2 deficits are more difficult to detect and characterize. Delirium occurs in 3% to 50% of patients after CABG, depending on the definition.[280] It is generally accepted as a transient disturbance of cognitive function that varies in severity and fluctuates temporally. In addition to causing distress to the patient's family and the health care team, delirium seems to carry long-term consequences such as an increase in mortality.[281,282] Risk factors of delirium include previous stroke, history of substance abuse, age older than 65 years, perioperative blood transfusion, and perioperative hypotension.[283] Off-pump CABG and preoperative statins may reduce the incidence of postoperative delirium in some cases.[284,285] Postoperative cognitive dysfunction is common after CABG with an incidence of 30% to 80% at discharge and 20% to 40% six months to 1 year after surgery.[286,287] It often is difficult to detect, and specialized, targeted testing is needed to reveal the deficits. Despite their common occurrence, they do not seem to be associated with negative long-term consequences.[288-290]

Postoperative Renal Dysfunction

Postoperative renal dysfunction (PRD) is a serious complication of CABG occurring in 7.7% of patients in a large multicenter study, of whom 1.4% required dialysis.[291] The risk of mortality increases from a baseline of 0.9% to 19% in patients with PRD, and to 63% in patients requiring dialysis. Other studies confirmed these findings[292] with one study demonstrating an increased 90-day mortality even with a 50% rise in postoperative creatinine.[293] Furthermore, other groups have shown that PRD is associated with increased rates of cardiovascular events, including the long-term risk of heart failure.[294,295] Risk factors for PRD, most of which are nonmodifiable, include age older than 70 years, diabetes mellitus, chronic kidney disease, CHF, reoperation, prolonged CPB times, preoperative anemia, perioperative transfusion, and LCOS.[243,250,291,292] Some propose a more accurate evaluation of renal function through the addition of glomerular filtration rate to serum creatinine after demonstrating the association of occult renal impairment on early and late mortality and cardiovascular events.[296] Although off-pump CABG may be associated with a lower incidence of PRD,[297] this remains controversial, as some randomized trials have not shown this advantage.[278,298]

Recombinant human B-type natriuretic peptide given as an infusion during CPB has been evaluated in a randomized trial of 272 patients undergoing CABG.[299] Patients receiving the infusion had a significantly lower peak increase in serum creatinine, greater urine output in the initial 24 hours after surgery, shorter length of hospital stay, and lower 180-day mortality. Other studies evaluating human atrial natriuretic peptide have shown similar promising results.[300,301] Further research will clarify the role of this strategy in protecting the kidneys after cardiac surgery.

Atrial Fibrillation

Postoperative atrial fibrillation (POAF) develops in 20% to 40% of patients undergoing CABG, with a peak incidence on the second and third postoperative days.[302-304] It is usually transient and most patients return to sinus rhythm within 2 to 3 days of treatment. However, patients with preoperative atrial fibrillation are unlikely to return to sinus rhythm. The underlying mechanism is not fully understood and is likely multifactorial. A combination of pericardial inflammation, excessive catecholamine production, postoperative autonomic imbalance, interstitial mobilization, volume overload, and alterations in the neurohumoral environment likely contributes to the development of POAF.[305,306] POAF is associated with a two- to threefold increase in the risk of stroke, increased length of stay, increased cost, and increased mortality.[302,303,307-309] Predictors for development of atrial fibrillation include advanced age, male sex, smoking, prolonged cross-clamp time, COPD, chronic renal disease, valvular heart disease, atrial enlargement, obesity, prior pericarditis, and withdrawal of beta blockers.[304,306,310-312]

Treatment of POAF[313-315] begins with correcting electrolyte imbalances, hypoxia, and acidosis. Patients in volume overload may benefit from diuresis when stable hemodynamically. In hemodynamically unstable patients, electrical synchronized cardioversion should be performed. In stable patients, rate or pharmacologic rhythm control strategies should be attempted. Commonly used rate control medications include beta blockers, calcium channel blockers, and digoxin. The latter can be helpful in patients with a depressed left ventricle. Amiodarone is a commonly used medication for pharmacologic rhythm control. Consideration for anticoagulation should be given in patients who remain in atrial fibrillation for 48 hours weighing in the risks of bleeding and thromboembolism.

A recent synthesis from the Cochrane Collaboration, in addition to other reports, looking at preventive strategies for POAF found that beta blockers, sotalol, amiodarone, atrial pacing postoperatively, magnesium, and posterior pericardiotomy reduce the incidence of POAF with variable effectiveness.[316,317] A recent meta-analysis provides evidence to suggest that preoperative omega-3 supplementation may also decrease the incidence of POAF.[318]

Sternal Wound Infections

Sternal wound infections (SWIs) can be divided into two types: superficial sternal wound infections (SSWIs) and deep sternal wound infections (DSWIs). The former involves the skin, subcutaneous tissue, and pectoralis fascia and is recognized clinically as the presence of erythema, drainage, fever, or all of these symptoms. The diagnosis of DSWI requires the presence of one of the following: positive culture from mediastinal fluid or tissue; observable mediastinitis during surgery; presence of chest pain, sternal instability, or high-grade fever; and either purulent drainage from the mediastinum or positive blood cultures.[319] The incidence of SWI is reported to be 0.47% to 8.0% and carries a mortality rate of 0.5% to 9.1%, whereas the incidence of DSWI is 0.22% to 1.97% with a mortality rate of 1.0% to 36%.[320-322]

Microbiologically, *Staphylococcus aureus* and coagulase-negative staphylococci are the most common isolated pathogens.[323] Reported risk factors for DSWI include advanced age, male sex, COPD, obesity, diabetes mellitus, smoking history, steroid use, renal insufficiency, nonelective surgery, repeat operations, long operative times, reexploration for bleeding, use of bone wax, perioperative transfusion, prolonged hospital stay (>5 days), and the use of bilateral ITAs.[250,320,324-326] In a recent meta-analysis on this topic,[327] Saso and coworkers concluded that skeletonization of the ITA decreases the risk of all SWIs by 60%, especially in patients with diabetes mellitus, and the advantage is maintained in bilateral ITA harvesting. This is likely because of improved chest perfusion with the skeletonization technique.[119] Important steps to prevent SWIs include preoperative showers with chlorhexidine gluconate, prophylactic intranasal mupirocin, hair clipping instead of shaving, intravenous prophylactic antibiotics before skin incision, aggressive perioperative glucose control, skeletonization of the ITA especially when bilateral ITAs are used in obese patients with diabetes or COPD, and strict adherence to sterility.[328-331] Although SSWIs may be treated conservatively with antibiotics in most cases, DSWIs commonly require reexploration and débridement of necrotic tissue in the operating room with some cases requiring early vascularized muscle flap coverage.

Mortality

The overall operative mortality of CABG (defined as all in-hospital deaths and all out-of-hospital deaths occurring within 30 days of the procedure) across North American centers that are part of the Society of Thoracic Surgeons database is 3.0%, an improvement since 1990 despite an increase in the mean age of patients (65.1 years), the mean priority status, and the prevalence of comorbid conditions.[332] In the 19,016 patients of the Northern New England Cardiovascular Disease Study Group who received a LITA during CABG, the overall 30-day mortality was 2.4%.[333] In two contemporary randomized trials, the SYNTAX trial[20] and the FREEDOM trial,[21] the operative mortalities for CABG patients were 3.5% and 1.7%, respectively. These figures are similar to those reported in several other studies.[111,334]

Predictors of 30-day mortality include high priority of operation, advanced age, female gender, diabetes mellitus, poor left ventricular function (especially in the presence of CHF symptoms), high creatinine level, peripheral vascular disease, pulmonary disease, and left main CAD.[335] Patients who are younger than 65 and presenting with normal left ventricular function and receiving elective CABG have a 30-day mortality of less than 1%.[267]

Long-term survival of patients after CABG may depend on the characteristics of the population studied, on the geographic location of the cohort, and on the surgical era, with the impact of secondary prevention programs and arterial revascularization techniques. Most long-term data, however, come from patients who had surgery in the 1970s and 1980s. Long-term vital data of patients enrolled in the CASS registry[336] (who underwent surgery between 1974 and 1979) have shown that survival after CABG in all patients is 96% at 1 year, 90% at 5 years, 74% at 10 years, and 56% at 15 years. Of particular interest in this report, in which arterial grafting was used in only 13% of patients, is that the survival of patients 65 to 70 years or older exceeded that of a matched U.S. population. Sergeant and colleagues[337] reported on 9600 consecutive CABG patients operated on between 1971 and 1993 and found that survival after CABG was 98% at 30 days, 92% at 5 years, 81% at 10 years, 66% at 15 years, and 51% at 20 years. In the final 10-year follow-up of the Bypass Angioplasty Revascularization Investigation (BARI) trial[338] of 914 patients who were randomly assigned to CABG, the survival was 89% at 5 years and 74% at 10 years. The APPROACH registry[339] is a large clinical data collection and outcome monitoring initiative that captured all patients undergoing cardiac catheterization and revascularization in the province of Alberta, Canada, between 1995 and 2000. In 15,392 patients younger than 70 years of age examined in this registry, 4-year adjusted actuarial survival rates for CABG, PCI, and medical therapy were 95.0%, 93.8%, and 90.5%, respectively. Survival rates decreased to 87.3%, 83.9%, and 79.1% for patients 70 to 79 years of age after CABG, PCI, and medical therapy, respectively, and to 77.4%, 71.6%, and 60.3% for patients 80 years of age or older. The SYNTAX trial 5-year follow-up[340] reported an all-cause mortality of 11.4% at 5 years for the whole CABG cohort.

Despite the possibility of confounding by indication, evidence suggests that the use of bilateral over single ITA may be associated with improved long-term survival after CABG. Lytle and colleagues reported a risk-adjusted survival of 94%, 84%, and 67% at 5, 10, and 15 postoperative years in 2000 patients who received bilateral ITAs versus 92%, 79%, and 64% in 8100 patients who had a single ITA; an even greater reduction was observed with respect to reoperation rates.[106] Other authors also found that single ITA grafting was a predictor of mortality, late MI, or late reoperation when compared with bilateral ITA grafting (RR = 1.3 [1.1 to 1.6]).[341,342] A contemporary propensity-matched study demonstrated that bilateral ITAs provided enhanced long-term survival compared with single ITA in patients with normal and reduced LVEF, without increased operative morbidity and mortality.[343] In a meta-analysis of available observational studies, Taggart and colleagues found that the use of bilateral versus single ITA resulted in a hazard ratio for death of 0.81 (95% CI: 0.70, 0.94).[344] The benefits of bilateral ITA grafting have also been suggested in the diabetic population.[345]

Freedom from Cardiac Events

Fundamentally, CABG is performed for two reasons: to improve survival or to alleviate symptoms of angina and prevent nonfatal outcomes such as MI, CHF, and hospitalization. Unfortunately, long-term studies rarely used arterial grafts and lacked structured secondary prevention after CABG. Sergeant and coworkers[346] found that the freedom rate from return of angina was 94%, 82%, 61%, and 38% at 1, 5, 10, and 15 years, and that secondary prevention and management of noncardiac comorbidity had the most impact on delaying the return of angina. Freedom from MI was 97%, 94%, 86%, 73%, and 56% at 30 days, 5, 10, 15, and 20 years. Freedom from coronary reintervention, whether PCI or CABG, was 99.7%, 97%, 89%, 72%, and 48% at 30 days, 5, 10, 15, and 20 years. In the BARI trial,[338] freedom from angina was 84% at 5 and 10 years. The freedom from coronary reintervention was 80% at 10 years. In the Arterial Revascularization Therapies Study (ARTS) randomized trial,[347] the rates of MI and reintervention at 5 years were 6.4% and 8.8%, respectively. Patients with diabetes mellitus (smaller number) had worse outcomes: their 5-year rates of MI and reintervention were 7.3% and 10.4% compared with 6.3% and 8.4% in patients without diabetes. Arterial grafting probably leads to even better results: in a series of 256 patients[348] with triple-vessel disease who received three arterial grafts, the rates for freedom from MI and angina were 97.3% and 85.7 % at 7 years, respectively. The SYNTAX trial[340] enrolled 1800 patients with triple-vessel or left main CAD across 85 centers. At 5 years, the rates of MI and reintervention were 3.8% and 6.7%, respectively.

Left Ventricular Function

Myocardial ischemia may cause a wide spectrum of myocardial states ranging from viable and functioning, to hibernating, stunned, or scarred and dysfunctional myocardium. The myocardial state and the amount of muscle involved dictates left ventricular function. One of the greatest survival benefits after CABG is in patients with triple-vessel or left main CAD and depressed left ventricular function.[60,267] If patients exhibit depressed left ventricular function caused by stunned or hibernating myocardium, CABG improves EF by 5% to 18%.[349,350] These improvements in systolic function appear as early as 2 weeks and endure up to 10 years after surgery, given no cardiovascular events during that time.[159,351,352] Lack of improvements or deterioration over time is usually related to either incomplete revascularization or graft occlusion. Bax and associates used echocardiography to examine the time course of contractile recovery in stunned and hibernating myocardial PET segments after CABG, and found that 61% of the stunned segments had improved at 3 months, and an additional 9% had improved at 14 months. In contrast, hibernating myocardium segments showed contractile improvement at 3 months in 31% of patients, with a further improvement at 14 months in an additional 61%.[159] Left ventricular diastolic function seems to improve immediately after surgery.[353] Survival of patients with very low LVEF (<20%) range from 59% to 73% at 5 years, with

TABLE 88-3 Reported Conduit Patency in CABG

	Percentage Patency Based on Duration of Angiographic Follow-up		
Conduit	**1**	**5**	**Late**
Saphenous vein graft	84.6%[128] 81%*[376,425,426] 95% at 6 months[153] 94% at 1 yr[377]	75%*%*[376,425,426] 81%[378] 86.4%[130]	15 yr: 50%*[376,425,426]
Internal thoracic artery	98.7%[427]		7 yr: 94%[428] 11 yr: 88%[429-432] 10-20 yr: 90%-95%[384]
Radial artery	91.8%[127]	96% at 4 yr[390] 98.3%[130] 92.5%[391]	7 yr: 92.5%[391]
Gastroepiploic artery	91% at 6 months[153]	84%[150] 63%[156] 86%[151,393,394]	70%[151,393,394]

*Patency results published from series in pre-statin and pre-aspirin era.
CABG, Coronary artery bypass grafting.

significant improvements in heart failure and angina class observed among survivors.[349,352,354-357]

A recent anterior MI with residual wall-motion anomaly is associated with an intramural thrombus in 31% of patients.[358] In contrast, this is much less frequent after an inferior or lateral MI. For these reasons, patients with a recent anterior MI (including a perioperative MI) and significant residual anterior or apical wall-motion abnormality should be anticoagulated for 3 to 6 months after CABG.[359]

Functional Status and Quality of Life

Quality of life after CABG markedly improves in most patients and may correspond to that of a matched control population.[360-362] Predictors of suboptimal or worsening quality of life include female sex, low socioeconomic status, smoking, diabetes mellitus, hypertension, low ejection fraction, recurrent angina, and nonenrollment into a cardiac rehabilitation program.[361,363-365] Improvements in quality of life can be observed at 3 months after surgery, and these improvements seem to endure at least up to 12 years after surgery.[306,364-366] Although advanced age (octa- and nonagenarians) does not preclude improvements in quality of life, they are less pronounced in this group and may not last in the long term.[366-368] In contrast to the overall improvement in quality of life and functional status, persistent sexual problems are relatively common after CABG and are most prevalent in men, diabetics, patients with hyperlipidemia, and those with preoperative sexual problems.[369,370] However, men's sexual satisfaction improved, whereas the women's satisfaction decreased 8 years after surgery.[369] Twelve years after CABG, patients had similar improvements in quality of life whether they had on-pump or off-pump CABG.[371] Contemporary data reveal that quality of life in CABG patients may surpass that of PCI patients as early as 6 months after the intervention.[231,232]

Graft Patency

In comparison with other forms of revascularization such as PCI, OPCAB, MIDCAB, transmyocardial revascularization, or angiogenic therapy, on-pump CABG has a significant advantage in that its long-term procedural outcome has been well characterized. Multiple long-term angiographic studies have described the patency rates of different types of grafts and risk factors associated with their premature closure (Table 88-3). Early closure (i.e., within 2 to 3 months) of any type of graft is usually because of thrombosis, which develops as a result of hemodynamic factors related to poor graft outflow or technical errors.[372] Once the early postoperative period is over, vein grafts start developing a disease complex of their own, namely intimal hyperplasia, which is noted in most grafts as early as 1 month after operation[372,373] and to which the ITA appears immune.[374] This process results in a diffuse concentric reduction in vein graft diameter on angiography, which usually matches that of the native coronary vessel by 1 year after implantation. Intimal hyperplasia can be most significant at suture lines and can lead to anastomotic stenosis in up to 20% of vein grafts. The radial and gastroepiploic arteries have a decreased susceptibility to significant intimal hyperplasia compared with vein grafts, which may translate into better long-term freedom from atherosclerosis and patency considering that intimal hyperplasia usually corresponds to sites that later develop graft atherosclerosis.[375] Graft atherosclerosis may be observed in vein grafts as early as 3 to 4 years after operation and has a predilection for areas of intimal hyperplasia. It is characterized by a noncapsulated lipid-rich core that is much more friable than native coronary atherosclerosis.

Saphenous Vein Grafts

The early patency rate of saphenous vein grafts improved markedly in the post-aspirin and post-statin era, with long-term patency data not as extensively characterized as older studies in the pre-aspirin and pre-statin era. Fitzgibbon and associates[376] found that vein graft patency was 88% early postoperatively, 81% at 1 year, 75% at 5 years, and 50% at 15 years; when stenosed grafts were excluded, the proportion of nondiseased grafts decreased to 40% at 12.5 years. This corresponded to a vein graft occlusion rate of 2.1% per year after the initial postoperative period. In the current era, vein graft patency has been found to be greater than 95% at 1 year[377] and 81% to 86% at 5 years.[130,378] The way SVG is handled may influence its patency; one study suggested a 94% patency rate at 3 years in no-touch saphenous veins.[170,379] Some studies demonstrated a higher patency rate in sequential vein grafts compared to individual ones with up to 76% at 7.5 years for sequential vein grafts and 64.5% for individual vein grafts.[164,380] This is probably a result of higher graft flow as a consequence of improved distal runoff, which may reduce intimal hyperplasia formation. However, another recent trial showed the opposite conclusion, with SVG to multiple distal targets showing higher failure rates at 1 year.[381] Although postoperative aspirin is the standard of care, adding clopidogrel to aspirin did not provide increased vein graft patency or reduce the frequency of adverse cardiovascular events.[377,382]

Internal Thoracic Artery Grafts

Late attrition rates of ITA bypass grafts are low because of the fact that ITA grafts rarely develop significant intimal hyperplasia or late atherosclerosis. Furthermore, the ITA has a potential to grow up to 1.4 times its original size to match the diameter of the coronary artery to which it is anastomosed.[383] Improved pharmacologic therapy and structured secondary prevention programs have improved patency rates in the current era. A 2003 report from the Cleveland Clinic demonstrated a 90% to 95% patency rate of the left ITA anastomosed to the LAD 10 to 20 years after surgery.[384] Free ITA grafts likely have comparable patency rates as compared with pedicled ITA grafts, provided that a flawless anastomotic technique is used.[385] Some studies report[386-389] similar patency rates of the RITA compared with the LITA, whether anastomosed to the LAD, circumflex, or right coronary artery, with some suggesting that flow through the RITA may be even greater because of handedness.[119] Tatoulis and colleagues[387] reported a hierarchy of patency of the RITA depending on the coronary territory grafted (highest patency rates to the LAD and lowest to the right coronary territory). The same authors reported a RITA to LAD patency rate of 95% at 10 years and 90% at 15 years, RITA to circumflex artery patency rate of 91% at 10 years, and RITA to RCA patency rate of 84% at 10 years. They conclude that RITA patency rates are equivalent to LITA for identical territories and are always better than radial arteries and saphenous vein grafts.

Radial Artery Grafts

Acar and coworkers,[15] who are responsible for the revival of the radial artery as a bypass conduit, reported a patency of 83% at 5.6 years in 50 of 910 patients who received a radial artery. Iaco and associates[390] reported a 96% 4-year patency in selected patients, with no difference in patency whether the radial was anastomosed to the aorta or to the ITA as a Y-graft. Collins and colleagues[130] reported radial artery patency of 98.3% based on angiographic data from the RSVP randomized controlled trial. Tatoulis and coworkers[391] reported 92.5% patency at 5 and at 7 years. Similar to the RITA, they also showed a hierarchy of patency depending on the coronary territory grafted (highest to the LAD and lowest to the right coronary). Other authors have shown that moderate severity of native target stenosis (70% or less) and grafting to the right coronary artery were associated with lower patency rates and when the radial artery is used in a composite T-graft configuration.[137] Comparing the mid-term (3-year) angiographic outcomes of the radial artery to those of the saphenous vein, a recent meta-analysis of randomized controlled trials revealed a superior complete graft patency of the radial artery compared with the saphenous vein (88.6% vs. 75.8%; $P = 0.005$), although the radial artery was associated with more string signs.[392]

Gastroepiploic Artery Grafts

Late results regarding patency of the gastroepiploic artery as a bypass graft are not as favorable as those of the ITA and radial artery. The 5-year angiographic patency was reported by Hirose and colleagues to be 84%,[150] and 86% at 5 years and 70% at 10 years by Suma and associates.[151,393,394] Factors associated with premature graft closure include technical anastomotic factors and anastomosis to a less critically stenosed coronary artery in a significant proportion of cases. There has been one randomized controlled trial to date comparing the use of the gastroepiploic artery versus the saphenous vein graft.[153] At 6-month angiographic follow-up, there were no differences in patency between conduits, although it appears that gastroepiploic artery patency is more influenced by competitive coronary flow.[154]

CABG versus PCI

A detailed analysis comparing the outcomes following CABG and PCI is beyond the scope of this chapter. No doubt, the benefits of both treatment modalities will evolve along with advances in technology and improvements in conjunctive care. Although initially believed to rid in-stent stenosis, drug-eluting stents have been found to be associated with late stent thrombosis.[395]

At present, 26 randomized clinical trials have compared CABG with PCI (Table 88-4),[20-22,351,396-417] with most of these studies releasing subgroup analyses and subsequent longer-term follow-up data. Many of these trials were underpowered to show a significant difference in early survival between PCI and CABG. Most of these trials excluded patients with diabetes, poor left ventricular function, and multivessel disease including left main and proximal LAD disease, for which CABG has been shown to be beneficial. However, the most recent trials began including and addressing these patient populations. Another consideration is that because of strict inclusion and exclusion criteria, only approximately 5% of screened patients were enrolled, which has an impact on the external validity of these trials. For trials that presented follow-up data on an original study cohort, no adjustment in the alpha level was made for repeated

TABLE 88-4 **Randomized Controlled Trials Comparing PCI and CABG**

Trial Name Study Dates	Stent Use/ DES %	Centers/Patient Number	DM %	LVEF < 50%	3VD	Follow-up Duration (Years)	Author Conclusions	Remarks
Left Main Disease								
PRECOMBAT[417] 2004-2009	Yes	13/600	32%	Mean 61%	41%	2	PCI noninferior to CABG with respect to MACCE.	Noninferiority margin was wide.
Boudriot[416] 2003-2009	Yes	4/201	36%	Median 65%	14%	1	PCI inferior to CABG at 12 months for unprotected left main disease.	
LE MANS[398] 2001-2004	Yes/35%	7/105	18%	19%	67%	1	LVEF increase at 1 year in PCI group only.	Actual change in LVEF minimal (3.3 ± 6.7 vs. 0.8 ± 0.8).
Proximal LAD								
Lausanne[402] 1989-1993	No	1/134	18%		0%	5	No difference in terms of survival or MACE at 2 years. At 5 years, the incidence of non–Q wave MI and need for repeat procedures was higher in the PTCA group.	
Leipzig[400] 1997-2001	Yes/0%	1/120	30%		0%	0.5	No difference in terms of survival or MACE; although CABG was superior in terms of angina relief and need for repeat procedures.	CABG performed via MIDCAB.
Groningen[401] 1997-1999	Yes	1/102	13%		0%	3	Trend toward improvement in MACE-free survival with CABG; CABG superior in angina relief.	CABG performed via OPCAB.
MASS[406] 1988-1991	No	1/214	17%	0%	0%	3	Survival and MACE similar between PCI and CABG at 3 years.	
SIMA[404]	Yes	6/123	11%	0%		10	CABG superior to PCI regarding the primary composite end of all-cause mortality, MI, and the need for additional revascularization.	
Multivessel Disease								
FREEDOM[21] 2005-2010	Yes/100%	140/1900	100%	2.5% EF < 40%	83%	5	For patients with diabetes and multivessel disease, CABG is superior to PCI. CABG has significantly lower rates of death and MI at 5 years compared with PCI.	
CARDia[22] 2002-2007	Yes/69%	24/510	100%	28% (65% had EF)	62%	1	Trial did not show PCI to be noninferior to CABG in diabetic patients at 1 year.	
SYNTAX[20,340] 2005-2007	Yes/100%	85/1800	35%	1.9% EF < 30%		5	CABG had lower MACCE rates at 1, 3, and 5 years. CABG remains the standard of care for patients with triple-vessel disease or with left main disease and complex lesions. For patients with less complex lesions and left main disease PCI is an acceptable alternative.	
ARTS[412] 1997-1998		68/1205	17%	0%	32%	5	At 5 years, no difference in mortality between PCI and CABG; MACCE was higher with PCI.	
ARTS II[433]		606 with DES; compared with ARTS I cohort of 1205	26%		55%	1	DES results in decrease in frequency of repeat procedures with no change in survival or MACE.	

Continued

TABLE 88-4 Randomized Controlled Trials Comparing PCI and CABG—cont'd

Trial Name Study Dates	Stent Use/ DES %	Centers/Patient Number	DM %	LVEF < 50%	3VD	Follow-up Duration (Years)	Author Conclusions	Remarks
AWESOME[411] 1995-2000	No	16/454 (only 142 randomized)	37%	45%	68%	3	No difference between CABG and PCI in terms of survival or MACE.	
BARI[351,434] 1988-1991	No	18/1792	24%	0%	41%	10	CABG superior in terms of survival, angina relief and need for repeat revascularization at 5 years. At 10 years, survival benefit only remained for patients with DM.	
CABRI[397]	No	26/1054	0%	12%	40%	4	No difference between CABG and PCI in terms of MACE or survival.	
EAST[407] 1987-1990	No	1/392	23%		40%	8	No difference between CABG and PCI in terms of the primary composite endpoint of death, Q wave MI, and a large ischemic defect identified on thallium scanning at 3 years. No difference was observed in terms of survival at 8 years.	CABG superior in terms of angina relief and angiographically determined revascularization at 3 years.
ERACI[409] 1988-1990	No	1/127	11%	0%	45%	3	CABG offered greater freedom from cardiac events and greater angina relief compared with PCI.	
ERACI II[408] 1996-1998	Yes/0%	7/450	17%		56%	1	PCI superior to CABG in terms of survival.	
ERACI III[410] 1996-1998 & 2002-2004	Yes/33%	7/675	18%	50%		1	DES more prone to late stent thrombosis than BMS although no difference in survival was observed.	
GABI[405] 1986-1991	No	8/359	10%		18%	1	CABG superior to PCI in terms of angina relief and need for repeat procedures; not survival.	
GABI II[435]	Yes	8/313				1	No difference between CABG and PCI conducted.	Used a historical surgical cohort.
MASS II[39] 1995-2000	Yes	2/611	29%		58%	5	CABG superior to PCI with regard to the primary composite endpoint of death, Q wave MI, refractory angina requiring revascularization.	
RITA[396]	No	16/1011	6%		12%	6.5	No difference between CABG and PCI in regard to survival or MACE.	
SOS[436,437] 1996-1999	Yes/0%	53/988	14%		42%	6	CABG superior to PCI in terms of survival and need for repeat revascularization.	
Toulouse[399]	No	1/1152	14%		29%	5	CABG superior to PCI in terms of survival, angina relief, and need for repeat procedures.	

BMS, Bare-metal stent; *CABG*, coronary artery bypass grafting; *DES*, drug-eluting stent; *DM*, diabetes mellitus; *LVEF*, left ventricular ejection fraction; *MACCE*, major adverse cardiac and cerebrovascular event; *MACE*, major adverse cardiac event; *MI*, myocardial infarction; *MIDCAB*, minimally invasive direct coronary artery bypass; *OPCAB*, off-pump coronary artery bypass; *PCI*, percutaneous coronary intervention; *PTCA*, percutaneous transluminal coronary angioplasty; *3VD*, triple-vessel disease.

statistical tests. Considering these limitations, a variety of conclusions can be drawn:

1. Although limited data exist comparing unprotected left main stenting (UPLMS) and CABG, UPLMS appears safe in a select patient population. Mid- and long-term results are yet to be established.
2. In the setting of proximal LAD disease, PCI is associated with an increase in the need for repeat revascularization. CABG appears superior in terms of angina relief. Although survival appears similar between CABG and PCI at intermediate follow-up, survival appears superior with CABG in the long term.
3. In patients with triple-vessel disease, CABG provides a survival advantage compared to PCI in patients with intermediate and high baseline SYNTAX scores. CABG is superior to PCI in terms of major adverse cardiac and cerebrovascular events in patients with complex coronary lesions.
4. Diabetic patients derive a survival benefit from CABG, which is maintained over the long term. CABG also reduces the rates of MI compared with PCI.
5. Drug-eluting stents decreased the need for repeat revascularization procedures relative to bare-metal stents; late stent thrombosis with drug-eluting stents does not significantly impact survival compared with bare-metal stents over the long term.

Two contemporary randomized trials were recently completed and contributed further to our understanding of the benefit of PCI with drug-eluting stent versus CABG.[20,21] The SYNTAX trial[20] enrolled 1800 patients with triple-vessel or left main CAD across 85 centers. The primary endpoint of major adverse cardiac or cerebrovascular events at 1 year was higher in the PCI compared with the CABG group (17.8% vs. 12.4%; P = 0.002), which was mostly driven by repeat revascularization. The rates of death and MI were similar between the two groups at 1 year, but stroke rates were significantly higher in the CABG group. After 5 years of follow-up, CABG remained superior with regard to the primary outcome. Although the rates of all-cause mortality and stroke were similar between the two groups, the rates of MI, the combination of death or stroke or MI, and cardiac death were all significantly higher in the PCI group. In subgroup analysis, these findings hold true in patients with triple-vessel disease or left main coronary disease and complex lesions (high or intermediate SYNTAX scores for triple-vessel disease and high SYNTAX scores for left main coronary disease). For patients with less complex lesions (low SYNTAX scores for triple-vessel disease and intermediate or low SYNTAX scores for left main coronary disease), PCI may be an acceptable alternative. In triple-vessel disease, the benefit of CABG over PCI with regard to cardiac death was almost twofold (P = 0.0008 for intermediate SYNTAX score and P = 0.0005 for high SYNTAX score).[340]

The FREEDOM trial[20,21] enrolled 1900 patients with diabetes and multivessel coronary disease across 140 centers. CABG was superior to PCI in that it significantly reduced the rates of death from any cause and MI at 5 years at the cost of significantly higher stroke rates in the CABG group. The conclusions did not change across prespecified subgroups including low, intermediate, and high SYNTAX scores, LVEF <40% and ≥40%.

Although randomization protects against confounding and selection bias, the main problem with randomized studies of CABG versus PCI is generalizability as a result of their nonrepresentativeness and the small proportion of the screened patients who are actually enrolled. The results of seven large registries are more useful for looking at the comparative *effectiveness* of CABG versus PCI in a particular population setting. These registries are the New York State PCI and CABG registries,[418] which compared more than 60,000 patients; the Alberta Provincial Project for Outcomes Assessment in Coronary Heart Disease (APPROACH) registry,[339] which examined approximately 16,000 patients after CABG or PCI; the Northern New England Cardiovascular Disease Study Group Registry,[419] which examined 2766 patients with diabetes; the Duke registry,[420] which examined approximately 7000 patients who underwent CABG versus PCI; the DELTA registry,[421] a multicenter registry evaluating left main coronary artery treatment with PCI versus CABG in 2,775 patients; the CREDO-Kyoto PCI/CABG registry cohort 2, a Japanese registry[422] of approximately 16,000 patients with first coronary revascularization; and the CUSTOMIZE registry,[423] which examined approximately 900 patients undergoing PCI versus CABG in unprotected left main disease. Because these studies are observational, the possibility of selection bias (confounding by indication) remains despite accounting for simple confounding via multivariable analyses. Nevertheless, the results of these studies are worth examining and can be summarized as follows:

1. Stenting unprotected left main CAD may be an option in low and intermediate SYNTAX scores and in older adult patients (>75 years old), with the greater risk of repeat revascularization. In high SYNTAX score lesions, CABG remains the gold standard.
2. Three, four-, and five-year risk-adjusted survival after CABG is superior to PCI for patients with triple-vessel disease in all study participants (regardless of diabetic status or left ventricular function).
3. Patients with high-grade proximal LAD stenosis benefit from CABG over PCI.
4. Superiority of CABG over PCI in diabetic patients is confirmed.
5. There might be an increased benefit of choosing CABG over PCI in older adults; in any case, older adult patients may benefit the most from revascularization over medical therapy for CAD.
6. CABG is superior to PCI with drug-eluting stents in terms of survival, angina relief, and need for repeat procedures.[424]

CONCLUSION

Coronary artery bypass grafting remains the most durable method of coronary revascularization available today. Its future is exciting and should be directed at further development and research to evaluate the role of routine complete arterial grafting, minimally invasive techniques, hybrid coronary revascularization strategies, secondary prevention programs, and adjunct pharmacotherapeutic strategies in achieving the ultimate goal of cardiac surgeons: making CABG a near-zero risk, infallible, and permanent method of coronary revascularization.

REFERENCES

1. Carrel A: On the experimental surgery of the thoracic aorta and the heart. *Ann Surg* 52:83, 1910.
2. Lindbergh C: An apparatus for the culture of whole organs. *J Exp Med* 62:409–431, 1935.
3. Vineberg A: Development of an anastomosis between the coronary vessels and a transplanted internal mammary artery. *Can Med Assoc J* 55:1946.
4. Ochsner J, Moseley P, Mills N, et al: Long-term follow-up of internal mammary artery myocardial implantation. *Ann Thorac Surg* 23:1977.
5. Longmire W, Cannon J, Kattus AA: Direct-vision coronary endarterectomy for angina pectoris. *N Engl J Med* 259:259, 1958.
6. Schumacker H: *The evolution of cardiac surgery*, Bloomington, 1992, Indiana University Press.
7. Mueller RL, Rosengart TK, Isom OW: The history of surgery for ischemic heart disease. *Ann Thorac Surg* 63:869–878, 1997.
8. Kolesov V, Potashov L: Surgery of coronary arteries. *Eksp Khir Anesteziol* 10:3, 1965.
9. Garrett H, Dennis E, DeBakey M: Aortocoronary bypass with saphenous vein graft. Seven-year follow up. *JAMA* 223:792–794, 1973.
10. Favaloro RG: Saphenous vein graft in the surgical treatment of coronary artery disease: operative technique. *J Thorac Cardiovasc Surg* 58:178, 1969.
11. Green GE, Spencer FC, Tice DA, et al: Arterial and venous microsurgical bypass grafts for coronary artery disease. *J Thorac Cardiovasc Surg* 60:491–503, 1970.
12. Flemma RJ, Johnson WD, Lepley D, Jr, et al: Simultaneous valve replacement and aorta-to-coronary saphenous vein bypass. *Ann Thorac Surg* 12:163–170, 1971.
13. Suzuki A, Kay EB, Hardy JD: Direct anastomosis of the bilateral internal mammary artery to the distal coronary artery, without a magnifier, for severe diffuse coronary atherosclerosis. *Circulation* 48:III190–III197, 1973.
14. Carpentier A, Guermonprez JL, Deloche A, et al: The aorta-to-coronary radial artery bypass graft. A technique avoiding pathological changes in grafts. *Ann Thorac Surg* 16:111–121, 1973.
15. Acar C, Jebara VA, Portoghese M, et al: Revival of the radial artery for coronary artery bypass grafting. *Ann Thorac Surg* 54:652–659, discussion 659–660, 1992.
16. Coronary. artery surgery study (CASS): A randomized trial of coronary artery bypass surgery. Survival data. *Circulation* 68:939–950, 1983.
17. Eleven-year survival in the veterans administration randomized trial of coronary bypass surgery for stable angina. The veterans administration coronary artery bypass surgery cooperative study group. *N Engl J Med* 311:1333–1339, 1984.
18. Varnauskas E: Twelve-year follow-up of survival in the randomized European coronary surgery study. *N Engl J Med* 319:332–337, 1988.
19. Ko W, Tranbaugh R, Marmur JD, et al: Myocardial revascularization in New York State: variations in the PCI-to-CABG ratio and their implications. *J Am Heart Assoc* 1:e001446, 2012.
20. Serruys PW, Morice MC, Kappetein AP, et al: Percutaneous coronary intervention versus coronary-artery bypass grafting for severe coronary artery disease. *N Engl J Med* 360:961–972, 2009.
21. Farkouh ME, Domanski M, Sleeper LA, et al: Strategies for multivessel revascularization in patients with diabetes. *N Engl J Med* 367:2375–2384, 2012.
22. Kapur A, Hall RJ, Malik IS, et al: Randomized comparison of percutaneous coronary intervention with coronary artery bypass grafting in diabetic patients. 1-year results of the cardia (coronary artery revascularization in diabetes) trial, *J Am Coll Cardiol* 55:432–440, 2010.
23. Duncker DJ, Bache RJ: Regulation of coronary vasomotor tone under normal conditions and during acute myocardial hypoperfusion. *Pharmacol Ther* 86:87–110, 2000.
24. Duncker DJ, Bache RJ: Regulation of coronary blood flow during exercise. *Physiol Rev* 88:1009–1086, 2008.
25. Ganz P, Ganz W: Coronary blood flow and myocardial ischemia. In Braunwald E, Zipes DP, Libby P, editors: *Heart disease*, Philadelphia, 2001, W.B. Saunders Company, pp 1087–1113.
26. Arques S, Ambrosi P, Gelisse R, et al: Prevalence of angiographic coronary artery disease in patients hospitalized for acute diastolic heart failure without clinical and electrocardiographic evidence of myocardial ischemia on admission. *Am J Cardiol* 94:133–135, 2004.
27. Schwarz ER, Gupta R, Haager PK, et al: Myocardial bridging in absence of coronary artery disease: proposal of a new classification based on clinical-angiographic data and long-term follow-up. *Cardiology* 112:13–21, 2008.
28. Schelbert HR: Measurements of myocardial metabolism in patients with ischemic heart disease. *Am J Cardiol* 82:61K–67K, 1998.
29. Stankovic G, Dobric M: Intravascular ultrasound and fractional flow reserve in assessment of the intermediate coronary stenosis: what you see is not what you get. *J Am Coll Cardiol* 61:924–925, 2013.
30. Ben-Dor I, Torguson R, Deksissa T, et al: Intravascular ultrasound lumen area parameters for assessment of physiological ischemia by fractional flow reserve in intermediate coronary artery stenosis. *Cardiovasc Revasc Med* 13:177–182, 2012.
31. Waksman R, Legutko J, Singh J, et al: First: fractional flow reserve and intravascular ultrasound relationship study. *J Am Coll Cardiol* 61:917–923, 2013.
32. Toth G, De Bruyne B, Casselman F, et al: Fractional flow reserve-guided versus angiography-guided coronary artery bypass graft surgery. *Circulation* 128:1405–1411, 2013.
33. Bezerra HG, Attizzani GF, Sirbu V, et al: Optical coherence tomography versus intravascular ultrasound to evaluate coronary artery disease and percutaneous coronary intervention. *JACC Cardiovasc Interv* 6:228–236, 2013.
34. Hillis LD, Smith PK, Anderson JL, et al: 2011 ACCF/AHA guideline for coronary artery bypass graft surgery: a report of the American College of Cardiology Foundation/American Heart Association Task Force on practice guidelines. *Circulation* 124:e652–e735, 2011.
35. Levine GN, Bates ER, Blankenship JC, et al: 2011 ACCF/AHA/SCAI guideline for percutaneous coronary intervention: a report of the American College of Cardiology Foundation/American Heart Association task force on practice guidelines and the society for cardiovascular angiography and interventions. *Catheter Cardiovasc Interv* 82:E266–E355, 2013.
36. Levine GN, Bates ER, Blankenship JC, et al: 2011 ACCF/AHA/SCAI guideline for percutaneous coronary intervention: a report of the American College of Cardiology Foundation/American Heart Association task force on practice guidelines and the society for cardiovascular angiography and interventions. *Circulation* 124:e574–e651, 2011.
37. Daemen J, Boersma E, Flather M, et al: Long-term safety and efficacy of percutaneous coronary intervention with stenting and coronary artery bypass surgery for multivessel coronary artery disease: a meta-analysis with 5-year patient-level data from the arts, ERACI-II, MASS-II, and SOS trials. *Circulation* 118:1146–1154, 2008.
38. Berreklouw E: Bypass angioplasty revascularization investigation. *N Engl J Med* 336:136, author reply 137–138, 1997.
39. Hueb W, Soares PR, Gersh BJ, et al: The medicine, angioplasty, or surgery study (MASS-II): a randomized, controlled clinical trial of three therapeutic strategies for multivessel coronary artery disease: one-year results. *J Am Coll Cardiol* 43:1743–1751, 2004.
40. Morrison DA, Sethi G, Sacks J, et al; Angina With Extremely Serious Operative Mortality E: Percutaneous coronary intervention versus coronary artery bypass graft surgery for patients with medically refractory myocardial ischemia and risk factors for adverse outcomes with bypass: a multicenter, randomized trial. Investigators of the department of veterans affairs cooperative study #385, the angina with extremely serious operative mortality evaluation (AWESOME). *J Am Coll Cardiol* 38:143–149, 2001.

41. Palmerini T, Biondi-Zoccai G, Della Riva D, et al: Stent thrombosis with drug-eluting and bare-metal stents: evidence from a comprehensive network meta-analysis. *Lancet* 379:1393–1402, 2012.
42. Kappetein AP, Feldman TE, Mack MJ, et al: Comparison of coronary bypass surgery with drug-eluting stenting for the treatment of left main and/or three-vessel disease: 3-year follow-up of the syntax trial. *Eur Heart J* 32:2125–2134, 2011.
43. Hillis LD, Smith PK, Anderson JL, et al: 2011 ACCF/AHA guideline for coronary artery bypass graft surgery: executive summary: a report of the American College of Cardiology Foundation/American Heart Association Task Force on Practice Guidelines. *Circulation* 124:2610–2642, 2011.
44. Boden WE, O'Rourke RA, Teo KK, et al: Optimal medical therapy with or without pci for stable coronary disease. *N Engl J Med* 356:1503–1516, 2007.
45. Wijeysundera HC, Nallamothu BK, Krumholz HM, et al: Meta-analysis: effects of percutaneous coronary intervention versus medical therapy on angina relief. *Ann Intern Med* 152:370–379, 2010.
46. Weintraub WS, Spertus JA, Kolm P, et al: Effect of PCI on quality of life in patients with stable coronary disease. *N Engl J Med* 359:677–687, 2008.
47. Group BDS, Frye RL, August P, et al: A randomized trial of therapies for type 2 diabetes and coronary artery disease. *N Engl J Med* 360:2503–2515, 2009.
48. Trikalinos TA, Alsheikh-Ali AA, Tatsioni A, et al: Percutaneous coronary interventions for non-acute coronary artery disease: a quantitative 20-year synopsis and a network meta-analysis. *Lancet* 373:911–918, 2009.
49. Cecil WT, Kasteridis P, Barnes JW, Jr, et al: A meta-analysis update: percutaneous coronary interventions. *Am J Manag Care* 14:521–528, 2008.
50. Katritsis DG, Ioannidis JPA: Percutaneous coronary intervention versus conservative therapy in nonacute coronary artery disease: a meta-analysis. *Circulation* 111:2906–2912, 2005.
51. Choudhry NK, Singh JM, Barolet A, et al: How should patients with unstable angina and non-ST-segment elevation myocardial infarction be managed? A meta-analysis of randomized trials. *Am J Med* 118:465–474, 2005.
52. Fox KAA, Poole-Wilson PA, Henderson RA, et al; Randomized Intervention Trial of unstable Angina I: Interventional versus conservative treatment for patients with unstable angina or non-ST-elevation myocardial infarction: the British Heart Foundation RITA 3 randomised trial. Randomized intervention trial of unstable angina. *Lancet* 360:743–751, 2002.
53. Fox KAA, Clayton TC, Damman P, et al: Long-term outcome of a routine versus selective invasive strategy in patients with non-st-segment elevation acute coronary syndrome a meta-analysis of individual patient data. *J Am Coll Cardiol* 55:2435–2445, 2010.
54. Le. May MR, So DY, Dionne R, et al: A citywide protocol for primary PCI in ST-segment elevation myocardial infarction. *N Engl J Med* 358:231–240, 2008.
55. Lee DC, Oz MC, Weinberg AD, et al: Optimal timing of revascularization: transmural versus nontransmural acute myocardial infarction. *Ann Thorac Surg* 71:1197–1202, discussion 1202–1204, 2001.
56. Lee DC, Oz MC, Weinberg AD, et al: Appropriate timing of surgical intervention after transmural acute myocardial infarction. *J Thorac Cardiovasc Surg* 125:115–119, discussion 119–120, 2003.
57. Mortensen KH, Thuesen L, Kristensen IB, et al: Spontaneous coronary artery dissection: a western Denmark heart registry study. *Catheter Cardiovasc Interv* 74:710–717, 2009.
58. Kumasawa J, Kurita N, Fukuhara S: Comparative effectiveness of multivessel coronary artery bypass graft surgery and multivessel percutaneous coronary intervention. *Ann Intern Med* 159:435, 2013.
59. Ebersberger U, Lewis AJ, Flowers BA, et al: Spontaneous multivessel coronary artery dissection causing massive myocardial infarction. *J Am Coll Cardiol* 61:589, 2013.
60. Yusuf S, Zucker D, Peduzzi P, et al: Effect of coronary artery bypass graft surgery on survival: overview of 10-year results from randomised trials by the coronary artery bypass graft surgery trialists collaboration. *Lancet* 344:563–570, 1994.
61. Phillips HR, O'Connor CM, Rogers J: Revascularization for heart failure. *Am Heart J* 153:65–73, 2007.
62. Tsuyuki RT, Shrive FM, Galbraith PD, et al: Revascularization in patients with heart failure. *CMAJ* 175:361–365, 2006.
63. O'Connor CM, Velazquez EJ, Gardner LH, et al: Comparison of coronary artery bypass grafting versus medical therapy on long-term outcome in patients with ischemic cardiomyopathy (a 25-year experience from the duke cardiovascular disease databank). *Am J Cardiol* 90:101–107, 2002.
64. Bonow RO, Maurer G, Lee KL, et al: Myocardial viability and survival in ischemic left ventricular dysfunction. *N Engl J Med* 364:1617–1625, 2011.
65. Autschbach R, Falk V, Gonska BD, et al: The effect of coronary bypass graft surgery for the prevention of sudden cardiac death: recurrent episodes after ICD implantation and review of literature. *Pacing Clin Electrophysiol* 17:552–558, 1994.
66. Daoud EG, Niebauer M, Kou WH, et al: Incidence of implantable defibrillator discharges after coronary revascularization in survivors of ischemic sudden cardiac death. *Am Heart J* 130:277–280, 1995.
67. Budeus M, Feindt P, Gams E, et al: Risk factors of ventricular tachyarrhythmias after coronary artery bypass grafting. *Int J Cardiol* 113:201–208, 2006.
68. Yeung-Lai-Wah JA, Qi A, McNeill E, et al: New-onset sustained ventricular tachycardia and fibrillation early after cardiac operations. *Ann Thorac Surg* 77:2083–2088, 2004.
69. Ting HH, Raveendran G, Lennon RJ, et al: A total of 1,007 percutaneous coronary interventions without onsite cardiac surgery: acute and long-term outcomes. *J Am Coll Cardiol* 47:1713–1721, 2006.
70. Roy P, de Labriolle A, Hanna N, et al: Requirement for emergent coronary artery bypass surgery following percutaneous coronary intervention in the stent era. *Am J Cardiol* 103:950–953, 2009.
71. Wang N, Gundry SR, Van Arsdell G, et al: Percutaneous transluminal coronary angioplasty failures in patients with multivessel disease. Is there an increased risk? *J Thorac Cardiovasc Surg* 110:214–221, discussion 221–223, 1995.
72. Hake U, Iversen S, Jakob HG, et al: Influence of incremental preoperative risk factors on the perioperative outcome of patients undergoing emergency versus urgent coronary artery bypass grafting. *Eur J Cardiothorac Surg* 3:162–168, 1989.
73. Ladowski JS, Dillon TA, Deschner WP, et al: Durability of emergency coronary artery bypass for complications of failed angioplasty. *Cardiovasc Surg* 4:23–27, 1996.
74. Barakate MS, Bannon PG, Hughes CF, et al: Emergency surgery after unsuccessful coronary angioplasty: a review of 15 years' experience. *Ann Thorac Surg* 75:1400–1405, 2003.
75. Berger PB, Stensrud PE, Daly RC, et al: Time to reperfusion and other procedural characteristics of emergency coronary artery bypass surgery after unsuccessful coronary angioplasty. *Am J Cardiol* 76:565–569, 1995.
76. Stamou SC, Hill PC, Haile E, et al: Clinical outcomes of nonelective coronary revascularization with and without cardiopulmonary bypass. *J Thorac Cardiovasc Surg* 131:28–33, 2006.
77. Karthik S, Musleh G, Grayson AD, et al: Effect of avoiding cardiopulmonary bypass in non-elective coronary artery bypass surgery: a propensity score analysis. *Eur J Cardiothorac Surg* 24:66–71, 2003.
78. Sabik JF, 3rd, Blackstone EH, Houghtaling PL, et al: Is reoperation still a risk factor in coronary artery bypass surgery? *Ann Thorac Surg* 80:1719–1727, 2005.
79. Weintraub WS, Jones EL, Morris DC, et al: Outcome of reoperative coronary bypass surgery versus coronary angioplasty after previous bypass surgery. *Circulation* 95:868–877, 1997.
80. Filsoufi F, Rahmanian PB, Castillo JG, et al: Results and predictors of early and late outcome of coronary artery bypass grafting in patients with severely depressed left ventricular function. *Ann Thorac Surg* 84:808–816, 2007.
81. Hennen B, Markwirth T, Scheller B, et al: Impaired flow in left internal mammary artery grafts due to subclavian artery stenosis. *Ann Thorac Surg* 72:917–919, 2001.
82. Burek KA, Sutton-Tyrrell K, Brooks MM, et al: Prognostic importance of lower extremity arterial disease in patients undergoing coronary revascularization in the bypass angioplasty

revascularization investigation (BARI). *J Am Coll Cardiol* 34:716–721, 1999.
83. Leyh RG, Bartels C, Notzold A, et al: Management of porcelain aorta during coronary artery bypass grafting. *Ann Thorac Surg* 67:986–988, 1999.
84. Arnold JR, Greenberg JD, Clements S: Internal mammary artery perfusing the Leriche's syndrome. *Ann Thorac Surg* 69:1244–1246, 2000.
85. Hayashida N, Kai E, Enomoto N, et al: Internal thoracic artery as a collateral source to the ischemic lower extremity. *Eur J Cardiothorac Surg* 18:613–616, 2000.
86. Crowley SD, Butterly DW, Peter RH, et al: Coronary steal from a left internal mammary artery coronary bypass graft by a left upper extremity arteriovenous hemodialysis fistula. *Am J Kidney Dis* 40:852–855, 2002.
87. Nishida H, Tomizawa Y, Endo M, et al: Coronary artery bypass with only in situ bilateral internal thoracic arteries and right gastroepiploic artery. *Circulation* 104:I76–I80, 2001.
88. Handa N, McGregor CG, Danielson GK, et al: Coronary artery bypass grafting in patients with previous mediastinal radiation therapy. *J Thorac Cardiovasc Surg* 117:1136–1142, 1999.
89. Gansera B, Schmidtler F, Angelis I, et al: Quality of internal thoracic artery grafts after mediastinal irradiation. *Ann Thorac Surg* 84:1479–1484, 2007.
90. Jarvis MA, Jarvis CL, Jones PR, et al: Reliability of Allen's test in selection of patients for radial artery harvest. *Ann Thorac Surg* 70:1362–1365, 2000.
91. Nunoo-Mensah J: An unexpected complication after harvesting of the radial artery for coronary artery bypass grafting. *Ann Thorac Surg* 66:929–931, 1998.
92. Sauve JS, Thorpe KE, Sackett DL, et al: Can bruits distinguish high-grade from moderate symptomatic carotid stenosis? The North American symptomatic carotid endarterectomy trial. *Ann Intern Med* 120:633–637, 1994.
93. Mickleborough LL, Walker PM, Takagi Y, et al: Risk factors for stroke in patients undergoing coronary artery bypass grafting. *J Thorac Cardiovasc Surg* 112:1250–1258, discussion 1258–1259, 1996.
94. Salasidis GC, Latter DA, Steinmetz OK, et al: Carotid artery duplex scanning in preoperative assessment for coronary artery revascularization: the association between peripheral vascular disease, carotid artery stenosis, and stroke. *J Vasc Surg* 21:154–160, discussion 161–162, 1995.
95. Estes JM, Khabbaz KR, Barnatan M, et al: Outcome after combined carotid endarterectomy and coronary artery bypass is related to patient selection. *J Vasc Surg* 33:1179–1184, 2001.
96. Timaran CH, Rosero EB, Smith ST, et al: Trends and outcomes of concurrent carotid revascularization and coronary bypass. *J Vasc Surg* 48:355–360, discussion 360–361, 2008.
97. Held C, Asenblad N, Bassand JP, et al: Ticagrelor versus clopidogrel in patients with acute coronary syndromes undergoing coronary artery bypass surgery: results from the PLATO (platelet inhibition and patient outcomes) trial. *J Am Coll Cardiol* 57:672–684, 2011.
98. Depre C, Vanoverschelde JL, Gerber B, et al: Correlation of functional recovery with myocardial blood flow, glucose uptake, and morphologic features in patients with chronic left ventricular ischemic dysfunction undergoing coronary artery bypass grafting. *J Thorac Cardiovasc Surg* 113:371–378, 1997.
99. La. Canna G, Alfieri O, Giubbini R, et al: Echocardiography during infusion of dobutamine for identification of reversibly dysfunction in patients with chronic coronary artery disease. *J Am Coll Cardiol* 23:617–626, 1994.
100. Scott R, Blackstone EH, McCarthy PM, et al: Isolated bypass grafting of the left internal thoracic artery to the left anterior descending coronary artery: late consequences of incomplete revascularization. *J Thorac Cardiovasc Surg* 120:173–184, 2000.
101. Loop FD, Lytle BW, Cosgrove DM, et al: Influence of the internal-mammary-artery graft on 10-year survival and other cardiac events. *N Engl J Med* 314:1–6, 1986.
102. Ferguson TB, Jr, Coombs LP, Peterson ED: Internal thoracic artery grafting in the elderly patient undergoing coronary artery bypass grafting: room for process improvement? *J Thorac Cardiovasc Surg* 123:869–880, 2002.
103. Puskas JD, Sadiq A, Vassiliades TA, et al: Bilateral internal thoracic artery grafting is associated with significantly improved long-term survival, even among diabetic patients. *Ann Thorac Surg* 94:710–715, discussion 715–716, 2012.
104. Kato Y, Shibata T, Takanashi S, et al: Results of long segmental reconstruction of left anterior descending artery using left internal thoracic artery. *Ann Thorac Surg* 93:1195–1200, 2012.
105. Buxton BF, Hayward PA: The art of arterial revascularization-total arterial revascularization in patients with triple vessel coronary artery disease. *Ann Cardiothorac Surg* 2:543–551, 2013.
106. Lytle BW, Blackstone EH, Loop FD, et al: Two internal thoracic artery grafts are better than one. *J Thorac Cardiovasc Surg* 117:855–872, 1999.
107. Kurlansky PA, Traad EA, Dorman MJ, et al: Thirty-year follow-up defines survival benefit for second internal mammary artery in propensity-matched groups. *Ann Thorac Surg* 90:101–108, 2010.
108. Lytle BW, Blackstone EH, Sabik JF, et al: The effect of bilateral internal thoracic artery grafting on survival during 20 postoperative years. *Ann Thorac Surg* 78:2005–2012, discussion 2012–2014, 2004.
109. Medalion B, Mohr R, Frid O, et al: Should bilateral internal thoracic artery grafting be used in elderly patients undergoing coronary artery bypass grafting? *Circulation* 127:2186–2193, 2013.
110. Puskas JD, Sadiq A, Vassiliades TA, et al: Bilateral internal thoracic artery grafting is associated with significantly improved long-term survival, even among diabetic patients. *Ann Thorac Surg* 94:710–715, discussion 715–716, 2012.
111. Ioannidis JP, Galanos O, Katritsis D, et al: Early mortality and morbidity of bilateral versus single internal thoracic artery revascularization: propensity and risk modeling. *J Am Coll Cardiol* 37:521–528, 2001.
112. Nakano J, Okabayashi H, Hanyu M, et al: Risk factors for wound infection after off-pump coronary artery bypass grafting: should bilateral internal thoracic arteries be harvested in patients with diabetes? *J Thorac Cardiovasc Surg* 135:540–545, 2008.
113. Pevni D, Uretzky G, Mohr A, et al: Routine use of bilateral skeletonized internal thoracic artery grafting: long-term results. *Circulation* 118:705–712, 2008.
114. Dai C, Lu Z, Zhu H, et al: Bilateral internal mammary artery grafting and risk of sternal wound infection: evidence from observational studies. *Ann Thorac Surg* 95:1938–1945, 2013.
115. Deo SV, Shah IK, Dunlay SM, et al: Bilateral internal thoracic artery harvest and deep sternal wound infection in diabetic patients. *Ann Thorac Surg* 95:862–869, 2013.
116. Itagaki S, Cavallaro P, Adams DH, et al: Bilateral internal mammary artery grafts, mortality and morbidity: an analysis of 1 526 360 coronary bypass operations. *Heart* 99:849–853, 2013.
117. Kramer A, Mohr R, Lev-Ran O, et al: Midterm results of routine bilateral internal thoracic artery grafting. *Heart Surg Forum* 6:348–352, 2003.
118. Sauvage LR, Rosenfeld JG, Roby PV, et al: Internal thoracic artery grafts for the entire heart at a mean of 12 years. *Ann Thorac Surg* 75:501–504, 2003.
119. Boodhwani M, Lam BK, Nathan HJ, et al: Skeletonized internal thoracic artery harvest reduces pain and dysesthesia and improves sternal perfusion after coronary artery bypass surgery: a randomized, double-blind, within-patient comparison. *Circulation* 114:766–773, 2006.
120. Hirotani T, Kameda T, Kumamoto T, et al: Effects of coronary artery bypass grafting using internal mammary arteries for diabetic patients. *J Am Coll Cardiol* 34:532–538, 1999.
121. Matsa M, Paz Y, Gurevitch J, et al: Bilateral skeletonized internal thoracic artery grafts in patients with diabetes mellitus. *J Thorac Cardiovasc Surg* 121:668–674, 2001.
122. Hemo E, Mohr R, Uretzky G, et al: Long-term outcomes of patients with diabetes receiving bilateral internal thoracic artery grafts. *J Thorac Cardiovasc Surg* 146:586–592, 2013.
123. Kushwaha SS, Bustami M, Tadjkarimi S, et al: Late endothelial function of free and pedicled internal mammary artery grafts. *J Thorac Cardiovasc Surg* 110:453–462, 1995.
124. Tashiro T, Nakamura K, Sukehiro S, et al: Midterm results of free internal thoracic artery grafting for myocardial revascularization. *Ann Thorac Surg* 65:951–954, 1998.
125. Hata M, Shiono M, Orime Y, et al: Clinical results of coronary artery bypass grafting with use of the internal thoracic artery

under low free flow conditions. *J Thorac Cardiovasc Surg* 119:125–129, 2000.
126. Mochizuki Y, Okamura Y, Iida H, et al: Healing of the intimal dissection of the internal thoracic artery graft. *Ann Thorac Surg* 67:541–543, 1999.
127. Desai ND, Cohen EA, Naylor CD, et al: A randomized comparison of radial-artery and saphenous-vein coronary bypass grafts. *N Engl J Med* 351:2302–2309, 2004.
128. Hayward PA, Hare DL, Gordon I, et al: Effect of radial artery or saphenous vein conduit for the second graft on 6-year clinical outcome after coronary artery bypass grafting. Results of a randomised trial. *Eur J Cardiothorac Surg* 34:113–117, 2008.
129. Buxton BF, Raman JS, Ruengsakulrach P, et al: Radial artery patency and clinical outcomes: five-year interim results of a randomized trial. *J Thorac Cardiovasc Surg* 125:1363–1371, 2003.
130. Collins P, Webb CM, Chong CF, et al; Radial Artery Versus Saphenous Vein Patency Trial I: Radial artery versus saphenous vein patency randomized trial: five-year angiographic follow-up. *Circulation* 117:2859–2864, 2008.
131. Athanasiou T, Saso S, Rao C, et al: Radial artery versus saphenous vein conduits for coronary artery bypass surgery: forty years of competition–which conduit offers better patency? A systematic review and meta-analysis. *Eur J Cardiothorac Surg* 40:208–220, 2011.
132. Benedetto U, Angeloni E, Refice S, et al: Radial artery versus saphenous vein graft patency: meta-analysis of randomized controlled trials. *J Thorac Cardiovasc Surg* 139:229–231, 2010.
133. Damgaard S, Wetterslev J, Lund JT, et al: One-year results of total arterial revascularization vs. Conventional coronary surgery: carrpo trial. *Eur Heart J* 30:1005–1011, 2009.
134. Goldman S, Sethi GK, Holman W, et al: Radial artery grafts vs saphenous vein grafts in coronary artery bypass surgery: a randomized trial. *JAMA* 305:167–174, 2011.
135. Hayward PA, Gordon IR, Hare DL, et al: Comparable patencies of the radial artery and right internal thoracic artery or saphenous vein beyond 5 years: results from the radial artery patency and clinical outcomes trial. *J Thorac Cardiovasc Surg* 139:60–65, discussion 65–67, 2010.
136. Khot UN, Friedman DT, Pettersson G, et al: Radial artery bypass grafts have an increased occurrence of angiographically severe stenosis and occlusion compared with left internal mammary arteries and saphenous vein grafts. *Circulation* 109:2086–2091, 2004.
137. Maniar HS, Sundt TM, Barner HB, et al: Effect of target stenosis and location on radial artery graft patency. *J Thorac Cardiovasc Surg* 123:45–52, 2002.
138. Moran SV, Baeza R, Guarda E, et al: Predictors of radial artery patency for coronary bypass operations. *Ann Thorac Surg* 72:1552–1556, 2001.
139. Dipp MA, Nye PC, Taggart DP: Phenoxybenzamine is more effective and less harmful than papaverine in the prevention of radial artery vasospasm. *Eur J Cardiothorac Surg* 19:482–486, 2001.
140. Velez DA, Morris CD, Muraki S, et al: Brief pretreatment of radial artery conduits with phenoxybenzamine prevents vasoconstriction long term. *Ann Thorac Surg* 72:1977–1984, 2001.
141. Kulik A, Rubens FD, Gunning D, et al: Radial artery graft treatment with phenoxybenzamine is clinically safe and may reduce perioperative myocardial injury. *Ann Thorac Surg* 83:502–509, 2007.
142. Denton TA, Trento L, Cohen M, et al: Radial artery harvesting for coronary bypass operations: neurologic complications and their potential mechanisms. *J Thorac Cardiovasc Surg* 121:951–956, 2001.
143. Anyanwu AC, Saeed I, Bustami M, et al: Does routine use of the radial artery increase complexity or morbidity of coronary bypass surgery? *Ann Thorac Surg* 71:555–559, discussion 559–560, 2001.
144. Verma S, Szmitko PE, Weisel RD, et al: Should radial arteries be used routinely for coronary artery bypass grafting? *Circulation* 110:e40–e46, 2004.
145. Cable DG, Caccitolo JA, Pearson PJ, et al: New approaches to prevention and treatment of radial artery graft vasospasm. *Circulation* 98:II15–II21, discussion II21–II22, 1998.
146. Myers MG, Fremes SE: Prevention of radial artery graft spasm: a survey of Canadian surgical centres. *Can J Cardiol* 19:677–681, 2003.
147. van Son JA, Smedts F: Revival of the radial artery for coronary artery bypass grafting: l'histoire se repete. *Ann Thorac Surg* 55:1596–1598, 1993.
148. Navia JL, Brozzi N, Chiu J, et al: Endoscopic versus open radial artery harvesting for coronary artery bypass grafting. *Scand Cardiovasc J* 45:279–285, 2011.
149. Dimitrova KR, Hoffman DM, Geller CM, et al: Endoscopic radial artery harvest produces equivalent and excellent midterm patency compared with open harvest. *Innovations* 5:265–269, 2010.
150. Hirose H, Amano A, Takanashi S, et al: Coronary artery bypass grafting using the gastroepiploic artery in 1,000 patients. *Ann Thorac Surg* 73:1371–1379, 2002.
151. Suma H, Tanabe H, Yamada J, et al: Midterm results for use of the skeletonized gastroepiploic artery graft in coronary artery bypass. *Circ J* 71:1503–1505, 2007.
152. Voutilainen S, Verkkala K, Jarvinen A, et al: Angiographic 5-year follow-up study of right gastroepiploic artery grafts. *Ann Thorac Surg* 62:501–505, 1996.
153. Glineur D, Hanet C, Poncelet A, et al: Comparison of saphenous vein graft versus right gastroepiploic artery to revascularize the right coronary artery: a prospective randomized clinical, functional, and angiographic midterm evaluation. *J Thorac Cardiovasc Surg* 136:482–488, 2008.
154. Glineur D, D'Hoore W, El Khoury G, et al: Angiographic predictors of 6-month patency of bypass grafts implanted to the right coronary artery a prospective randomized comparison of gastroepiploic artery and saphenous vein grafts. *J Am Coll Cardiol* 51:120–125, 2008.
155. Glineur D, D'Hoore W, de Kerchove L, et al: Angiographic predictors of 3-year patency of bypass grafts implanted on the right coronary artery system: a prospective randomized comparison of gastroepiploic artery, saphenous vein, and right internal thoracic artery grafts. *J Thorac Cardiovasc Surg* 142:980–988, 2011.
156. Suma H, Isomura T, Horii T, et al: Late angiographic result of using the right gastroepiploic artery as a graft. *J Thorac Cardiovasc Surg* 120:496–498, 2000.
157. Mills NL, Everson CT: Right gastroepiploic artery: a third arterial conduit for coronary artery bypass. *Ann Thorac Surg* 47:706–711, 1989.
158. Mukherjee D, Cheriyan J, Kourliouros A, et al: How does the right gastroepiploic artery compare with the saphenous vein for revascularization of the right coronary artery? *Interact Cardiovasc Thorac Surg* 15:888–892, 2012.
159. Bax JJ, Visser FC, Poldermans D, et al: Time course of functional recovery of stunned and hibernating segments after surgical revascularization. *Circulation* 104:I314–I318, 2001.
160. Maes A, Flameng W, Nuyts J, et al: Histological alterations in chronically hypoperfused myocardium. Correlation with pet findings. *Circulation* 90:735–745, 1994.
161. Christenson JT, Schmuziger M: Sequential venous bypass grafts: results 10 years later. *Ann Thorac Surg* 63:371–376, 1997.
162. Gao C, Wang M, Wang G, et al: Patency of sequential and individual saphenous vein grafts after off-pump coronary artery bypass grafting. *J Card Surg* 25:633–637, 2010.
163. Vural KM, Sener E, Tasdemir O: Long-term patency of sequential and individual saphenous vein coronary bypass grafts. *Eur J Cardiothorac Surg* 19:140–144, 2001.
164. Li J, Liu Y, Zheng J, et al: The patency of sequential and individual vein coronary bypass grafts: a systematic review. *Ann Thorac Surg* 92:1292–1298, 2011.
165. Black EA, Campbell RK, Channon KM, et al: Minimally invasive vein harvesting significantly reduces pain and wound morbidity. *Eur J Cardiothorac Surg* 22:381–386, 2002.
166. Aziz O, Athanasiou T, Darzi A: Minimally invasive conduit harvesting: a systematic review. *Eur J Cardiothorac Surg* 29:324–333, 2006.
167. Rao C, Aziz O, Deeba S, et al: Is minimally invasive harvesting of the great saphenous vein for coronary artery bypass surgery a cost-effective technique? *J Thorac Cardiovasc Surg* 135:809–815, 2008.
168. Krishnamoorthy B, Critchley WR, Glover AT, et al: A randomized study comparing three groups of vein harvesting methods for

coronary artery bypass grafting: endoscopic harvest versus standard bridging and open techniques. *Interact Cardiovasc Thorac Surg* 15:224–228, 2012.

169. Souza DS, Johansson B, Bojo L, et al: Harvesting the saphenous vein with surrounding tissue for CABG provides long-term graft patency comparable to the left internal thoracic artery: results of a randomized longitudinal trial. *J Thorac Cardiovasc Surg* 132:373–378, 2006.
170. Dreifaldt M, Souza DS, Loesch A, et al: The "no-touch" harvesting technique for vein grafts in coronary artery bypass surgery preserves an intact vasa vasorum. *J Thorac Cardiovasc Surg* 141:145–150, 2011.
171. Johansson BL, Souza DS, Bodin L, et al: Slower progression of atherosclerosis in vein grafts harvested with "no touch" technique compared with conventional harvesting technique in coronary artery bypass grafting: an angiographic and intravascular ultrasound study. *Eur J Cardiothorac Surg* 38:414–419, 2010.
172. Rueda F, Souza D, Lima Rde C, et al: Novel no-touch technique of harvesting the saphenous vein for coronary artery bypass grafting. *Arq Bras Cardiol* 90:356–362, 2008.
173. Andreasen JJ, Nekrasas V, Dethlefsen C: Endoscopic vs open saphenous vein harvest for coronary artery bypass grafting: a prospective randomized trial. *Eur J Cardiothorac Surg* 34:384–389, 2008.
174. Kiaii B, Moon BC, Massel D, et al: A prospective randomized trial of endoscopic versus conventional harvesting of the saphenous vein in coronary artery bypass surgery. *J Thorac Cardiovasc Surg* 123:204–212, 2002.
175. Lopes RD, Hafley GE, Allen KB, et al: Endoscopic versus open vein-graft harvesting in coronary-artery bypass surgery. *N Engl J Med* 361:235–244, 2009.
176. Saginur R, Croteau D, Bergeron MG: Comparative efficacy of teicoplanin and cefazolin for cardiac operation prophylaxis in 3027 patients. The ESPRIT group. *J Thorac Cardiovasc Surg* 120:1120–1130, 2000.
177. Sylivris S, Calafiore P, Matalanis G, et al: The intraoperative assessment of ascending aortic atheroma: epiaortic imaging is superior to both transesophageal echocardiography and direct palpation. *J Cardiothorac Vasc Anesth* 11:704–707, 1997.
178. Shann KG, Likosky DS, Murkin JM, et al: An evidence-based review of the practice of cardiopulmonary bypass in adults: a focus on neurologic injury, glycemic control, hemodilution, and the inflammatory response. *J Thorac Cardiovasc Surg* 132:283–290, 2006.
179. Trick WE, Scheckler WE, Tokars JI, et al: Modifiable risk factors associated with deep sternal site infection after coronary artery bypass grafting. *J Thorac Cardiovasc Surg* 119:108–114, 2000.
180. Quintilio C, Voci P, Bilotta F, et al: Risk factors of incomplete distribution of cardioplegic solution during coronary artery grafting. *J Thorac Cardiovasc Surg* 109:439–447, 1995.
181. Nikas DJ, Ramadan FM, Elefteriades JA: Topical hypothermia: ineffective and deleterious as adjunct to cardioplegia for myocardial protection. *Ann Thorac Surg* 65:28–31, 1998.
182. Rodriguez RA, Giachino A, Hosking M, et al: Transcranial doppler characteristics of different embolic materials during in vivo testing. *J Neuroimaging* 12:259–266, 2002.
183. Nathan HJ, Wells GA, Munson JL, et al: Neuroprotective effect of mild hypothermia in patients undergoing coronary artery surgery with cardiopulmonary bypass: a randomized trial. *Circulation* 104:I85–I91, 2001.
184. Boodhwani M, Rubens F, Wozny D, et al: Effects of sustained mild hypothermia on neurocognitive function after coronary artery bypass surgery: a randomized, double-blind study. *J Thorac Cardiovasc Surg* 134:1443–1450, discussion 1451–1452, 2007.
185. Roach GW, Kanchuger M, Mangano CM, et al: Adverse cerebral outcomes after coronary bypass surgery. Multicenter study of perioperative ischemia research group and the ischemia research and education foundation investigators. *N Engl J Med* 335:1857–1863, 1996.
186. Wendler O, Hennen B, Markwirth T, et al: T grafts with the right internal thoracic artery to left internal thoracic artery versus the left internal thoracic artery and radial artery: flow dynamics in the internal thoracic artery main stem. *J Thorac Cardiovasc Surg* 118:841–848, 1999.
187. Sabik JF, Lytle BW, McCarthy PM, et al: Axillary artery: an alternative site of arterial cannulation for patients with extensive aortic and peripheral vascular disease. *J Thorac Cardiovasc Surg* 109:885–890, discussion 890–891, 1995.
188. Akpinar B, Guden M, Sagbas E, et al: Clinical experience with the Novare Enclose II manual proximal anastomotic device during off-pump coronary artery surgery. *Eur J Cardiothorac Surg* 27:1070–1073, 2005.
189. Ferguson JJ, 3rd, Cohen M, Freedman RJ, Jr, et al: The current practice of intra-aortic balloon counterpulsation: results from the benchmark registry. *J Am Coll Cardiol* 38:1456–1462, 2001.
190. Cheng JM, den Uil CA, Hoeks SE, et al: Percutaneous left ventricular assist devices vs. Intra-aortic balloon pump counterpulsation for treatment of cardiogenic shock: a meta-analysis of controlled trials. *Eur Heart J* 30:2102–2108, 2009.
191. Spence PA, Montgomery WD, Santamore WP: High flow demand on small arterial coronary bypass conduits promotes graft spasm. *J Thorac Cardiovasc Surg* 110:952–962, 1995.
192. Mangano DT, Miao Y, Vuylsteke A, et al: Mortality associated with aprotinin during 5 years following coronary artery bypass graft surgery. *JAMA* 297:471–479, 2007.
193. Mangano DT, Tudor IC, Dietzel C: The risk associated with aprotinin in cardiac surgery. *N Engl J Med* 354:353–365, 2006.
194. Karkouti K, Beattie W, KM D: Blood conservation and transfusion alternatives. *Transfusion* 46:327–338, 2006.
195. Cooper JR, Jr, Abrams J, Frazier OH, et al: Fatal pulmonary microthrombi during surgical therapy for end-stage heart failure: possible association with antifibrinolytic therapy. *J Thorac Cardiovasc Surg* 131:963–968, 2006.
196. Grant MC, Kon Z, Joshi A, et al: Is aprotinin safe to use in a cohort at increased risk for thrombotic events: results from a randomized, prospective trial in off-pump coronary artery bypass. *Ann Thorac Surg* 86:815–822, discussion 815–822, 2008.
197. Bittner HB, Lemke J, Lange M, et al: The impact of aprotinin on blood loss and blood transfusion in off-pump coronary artery bypass grafting. *Ann Thorac Surg* 85:1662–1668, 2008.
198. Chu MW, Wilson SR, Novick RJ, et al: Does clopidogrel increase blood loss following coronary artery bypass surgery? *Ann Thorac Surg* 78:1536–1541, 2004.
199. Lincoff AM, LeNarz LA, Despotis GJ, et al: Abciximab and bleeding during coronary surgery: results from the EPILOG and EPISTENT trials. Improve long-term outcome with abciximab GP IIb/IIIa blockade. Evaluation of platelet iib/iiia inhibition in stenting. *Ann Thorac Surg* 70:516–526, 2000.
200. Legarra JJ, Sarralde JA, Lopez Coronado JL, et al: Surgical approach for cardiac surgery in a patient with tracheostoma. *Eur J Cardiothorac Surg* 14:338–339, 1998.
201. Calafiore AM, Contini M, Vitolla G, et al: Bilateral internal thoracic artery grafting: long-term clinical and angiographic results of in situ versus y grafts. *J Thorac Cardiovasc Surg* 120:990–996, 2000.
202. Ruel MA, Wang F, Bourke ME, et al: Is tranexamic acid safe in patients undergoing coronary endarterectomy? *Ann Thorac Surg* 71:1508–1511, 2001.
203. Marinelli G, Chiappini B, Di Eusanio M, et al: Bypass grafting with coronary endarterectomy: immediate and long-term results. *J Thorac Cardiovasc Surg* 124:553–560, 2002.
204. Binsalamah ZM, Al-Sarraf N, Chaturvedi RK, et al: Mid-term outcome and angiographic follow-up of endarterectomy of the left anterior descending artery in patients undergoing coronary artery bypass surgery. *J Card Surg* 2013.
205. Eckstein FS, Bonilla LF, Englberger L, et al: First clinical results with a new mechanical connector for distal coronary artery anastomoses in cabg. *Circulation* 106:I1–I4, 2002.
206. Casselman FP, Meco M, Dom H, et al: Multivessel distal sutureless off-pump coronary artery bypass grafting procedure using magnetic connectors. *Ann Thorac Surg* 78:e38–e40, 2004.
207. Wippermann J, Konstas C, Wahlers T, et al: Feasibility study of sutureless distal coronary anastomoses with degradable y-shunt and tissue adhesives in a porcine off-pump model. *Interact Cardiovasc Thorac Surg* 5:676–679, 2006.
208. Dar MI, Gillott T, Ciulli F, et al: Single aortic cross-clamp technique reduces s-100 release after coronary artery surgery. *Ann Thorac Surg* 71:794–796, 2001.

209. Eckstein FS, Bonilla LF, Englberger L, et al: The st jude medical symmetry aortic connector system for proximal vein graft anastomoses in coronary artery bypass grafting. *J Thorac Cardiovasc Surg* 123:777–782, 2002.
210. Eckstein FS, Bonilla LF, Englberger L, et al: Minimizing aortic manipulation during opcab using the symmetry aortic connector system for proximal vein graft anastomoses. *Ann Thorac Surg* 72:S995–S998, 2001.
211. Cline SL, Guduvalli A, Kalaria VG: Early ostial saphenous vein graft stenosis associated with the use of symmetry sutureless aortic proximal anastomosis device: successful percutaneous revascularization. *Catheter Cardiovasc Interv* 62:203–208, 2004.
212. Katariya K, Yassin S, Tehrani HY, et al: Initial experience with sutureless proximal anastomoses performed with a mechanical connector leading to clampless off-pump coronary artery bypass surgery. *Ann Thorac Surg* 77:563–567, discussion 567–568, 2004.
213. Puehler T, Fraund-Cremer S, Cremer J, et al: Successful six-year follow-up of a sutureless device for proximal anastomoses in a severely calcified ascending aorta. *Interact Cardiovasc Thorac Surg* 7:670–672, 2008.
214. D'Ancona G, Karamanoukian HL, Ricci M, et al: Graft revision after transit time flow measurement in off-pump coronary artery bypass grafting. *Eur J Cardiothorac Surg* 17:287–293, 2000.
215. Shin H, Yozu R, Mitsumaru A, et al: Intraoperative assessment of coronary artery bypass graft: transit-time flowmetry versus angiography. *Ann Thorac Surg* 72:1562–1565, 2001.
216. Takami Y, Ina H: Relation of intraoperative flow measurement with postoperative quantitative angiographic assessment of coronary artery bypass grafting. *Ann Thorac Surg* 72:1270–1274, 2001.
217. Suematsu Y, Takamoto S, Ohtsuka T: Intraoperative echocardiographic imaging of coronary arteries and graft anastomoses during coronary artery bypass grafting without cardiopulmonary bypass. *J Thorac Cardiovasc Surg* 122:1147–1154, 2001.
218. Mohr FW, Falk V: As originally published in 1989: thermal coronary angiography: a method for assessing graft patency and coronary anatomy in coronary bypass surgery. Updated in 1997. *Ann Thorac Surg* 63:1506–1507, 1997.
219. Desai ND, Miwa S, Kodama D, et al: A randomized comparison of intraoperative indocyanine green angiography and transit-time flow measurement to detect technical errors in coronary bypass grafts. *J Thorac Cardiovasc Surg* 132:585–594, 2006.
220. Zhao DX, Leacche M, Balaguer JM, et al: Routine intraoperative completion angiography after coronary artery bypass grafting and 1-stop hybrid revascularization results from a fully integrated hybrid catheterization laboratory/operating room. *J Am Coll Cardiol* 53:232–241, 2009.
221. Nathan HJ, Munson J, Wells G, et al: The management of temperature during cardiopulmonary bypass: effect on neuropsychological outcome. *J Card Surg* 10:481–487, 1995.
222. Shapira OM, Alkon JD, Macron DS, et al: Nitroglycerin is preferable to diltiazem for prevention of coronary bypass conduit spasm. *Ann Thorac Surg* 70:883–888, discussion 888–889, 2000.
223. Mangano DT: Aspirin and mortality from coronary bypass surgery. *N Engl J Med* 347:1309–1317, 2002.
224. Goldman S, Copeland J, Moritz T, et al: Starting aspirin therapy after operation. Effects on early graft patency. Department of veterans affairs cooperative study group. *Circulation* 84:520–526, 1991.
225. Kjoller-Hansen L, Steffensen R, Grande P: The angiotensin-converting enzyme inhibition post revascularization study (APRES). *J Am Coll Cardiol* 35:881–888, 2000.
226. Bond BR, Zellner JL, Dorman BH, et al: Differential effects of calcium channel antagonists in the amelioration of radial artery vasospasm. *Ann Thorac Surg* 69:1035–1040, discussion 1040–1041, 2000.
227. Price J, Tee R, Lam B-K, et al: Current use of prophylactic strategies for postoperative atrial fibrillation: a survey of Canadian cardiac surgeons. *Ann Thorac Surg* 88:106–110, 2009.
228. Mahoney EM, Thompson TD, Veledar E, et al: Cost-effectiveness of targeting patients undergoing cardiac surgery for therapy with intravenous amiodarone to prevent atrial fibrillation. *J Am Coll Cardiol* 40:737–745, 2002.
229. Lee SH, Chang CM, Lu MJ, et al: Intravenous amiodarone for prevention of atrial fibrillation after coronary artery bypass grafting. *Ann Thorac Surg* 70:157–161, 2000.
230. Evrard P, Gonzalez M, Jamart J, et al: Prophylaxis of supraventricular and ventricular arrhythmias after coronary artery bypass grafting with low-dose sotalol. *Ann Thorac Surg* 70:151–156, 2000.
231. Abdallah MS, Wang K, Magnuson EA, et al: Quality of life after PCI vs CABG among patients with diabetes and multivessel coronary artery disease: a randomized clinical trial. *JAMA* 310:1581–1590, 2013.
232. Cohen DJ, Van Hout B, Serruys PW, et al; Synergy between PCIwT, Cardiac Surgery I: Quality of life after PCI with drug-eluting stents or coronary-artery bypass surgery. *N Engl J Med* 364:1016–1026, 2011.
233. Campeau L, Hunninghake DB, Knatterud GL, et al: Aggressive cholesterol lowering delays saphenous vein graft atherosclerosis in women, the elderly, and patients with associated risk factors. NHLBI post coronary artery bypass graft clinical trial. Post CABG trial investigators. *Circulation* 99:3241–3247, 1999.
234. Domanski MJ, Borkowf CB, Campeau L, et al: Prognostic factors for atherosclerosis progression in saphenous vein grafts: the post-coronary artery bypass graft (post-CABG) trial. Post-CABG trial investigators. *J Am Coll Cardiol* 36:1877–1883, 2000.
235. Gaudino M, Glieca F, Luciani N, et al: Clinical and angiographic effects of chronic calcium channel blocker therapy continued beyond first postoperative year in patients with radial artery grafts: results of a prospective randomized investigation. *Circulation* 104:I64–I67, 2001.
236. Karthik S, Grayson AD, McCarron EE, et al: Reexploration for bleeding after coronary artery bypass surgery: risk factors, outcomes, and the effect of time delay. *Ann Thorac Surg* 78:527–534, discussion 534, 2004.
237. Mehta RH, Sheng S, O'Brien SM, et al; Society of Thoracic Surgeons National Cardiac Surgery Database I: Reoperation for bleeding in patients undergoing coronary artery bypass surgery: incidence, risk factors, time trends, and outcomes. *Circ Cardiovasc Qual Outcomes* 2:583–590, 2009.
238. Karkouti K, Cohen MM, McCluskey SA, et al: A multivariable model for predicting the need for blood transfusion in patients undergoing first-time elective coronary bypass graft surgery. *Transfusion* 41:1193–1203, 2001.
239. Ruel MA, Rubens FD: Non-pharmacological strategies for blood conservation in cardiac surgery. *Can J Anaesth* 48:S13–S23, 2001.
240. Aggarwal A, Malkovska V, Catlett JP, et al: Recombinant activated factor vii (rfviia) as salvage treatment for intractable hemorrhage. *Thromb J* 2:9, 2004.
241. Karkouti K, Beattie WS, Wijeysundera DN, et al: Recombinant factor VIIa for intractable blood loss after cardiac surgery: a propensity score-matched case-control analysis. *Transfusion* 45:26–34, 2005.
242. Khanna MP, Hebert PC, Fergusson DA: Review of the clinical practice literature on patient characteristics associated with perioperative allogeneic red blood cell transfusion. *Transfus Med Rev* 17:110–119, 2003.
243. Elmistekawy E, Rubens F, Hudson C, et al: Preoperative anaemia is a risk factor for mortality and morbidity following aortic valve surgery. *Eur J Cardiothorac Surg* 2013.
244. Karkouti K, Wijeysundera DN, Beattie WS, et al; Reducing Bleeding in Cardiac Surgery I: Risk associated with preoperative anemia in cardiac surgery: a multicenter cohort study. *Circulation* 117:478–484, 2008.
245. Koch C, Li L, Figueroa P, et al: Transfusion and pulmonary morbidity after cardiac surgery. *Ann Thorac Surg* 88:1410–1418, 2009.
246. Koch CG, Li L, Duncan AI, et al: Morbidity and mortality risk associated with red blood cell and blood-component transfusion in isolated coronary artery bypass grafting. *Crit Care Med* 34:1608–1616, 2006.
247. Koch CG, Li L, Duncan AI, et al: Transfusion in coronary artery bypass grafting is associated with reduced long-term survival. *Ann Thorac Surg* 81:1650–1657, 2006.
248. Loor G, Rajeswaran J, Li L, et al: The least of 3 evils: exposure to red blood cell transfusion, anemia, or both? *J Thorac Cardiovasc Surg* 2013.
249. Ranucci M, Conti D, Castelvecchio S, et al: Hematocrit on cardiopulmonary bypass and outcome after coronary surgery in non-transfused patients. *Ann Thorac Surg* 89:11–17, 2010.
250. Williams ML, He X, Rankin JS, et al: Preoperative hematocrit is a powerful predictor of adverse outcomes in coronary artery

bypass graft surgery: a report from the society of thoracic surgeons adult cardiac surgery database. *Ann Thorac Surg* 2013.

251. Karkouti K, Wijeysundera DN, Yau TM, et al: Advance targeted transfusion in anemic cardiac surgical patients for kidney protection: an unblinded randomized pilot clinical trial. *Anesthesiology* 116:613–621, 2012.
252. Rao V, Ivanov J, Weisel RD, et al: Predictors of low cardiac output syndrome after coronary artery bypass. *J Thorac Cardiovasc Surg* 112:38–51, 1996.
253. Algarni KD, Maganti M, Yau TM: Predictors of low cardiac output syndrome after isolated coronary artery bypass surgery: trends over 20 years. *Ann Thorac Surg* 92:1678–1684, 2011.
254. Sa MP, Nogueira JR, Ferraz PE, et al: Risk factors for low cardiac output syndrome after coronary artery bypass grafting surgery. *Rev Bras Cir Cardiovasc* 27:217–223, 2012.
255. Dyub AM, Whitlock RP, Abouzahr LL, et al: Preoperative intra-aortic balloon pump in patients undergoing coronary bypass surgery: a systematic review and meta-analysis. *J Card Surg* 23: 79–86, 2008.
256. Miceli A, Fiorani B, Danesi TH, et al: Prophylactic intra-aortic balloon pump in high-risk patients undergoing coronary artery bypass grafting: a propensity score analysis. *Interact Cardiovasc Thorac Surg* 9:291–294, 2009.
257. Sa MP, Ferraz PE, Escobar RR, et al: Prophylactic intra-aortic balloon pump in high-risk patients undergoing coronary artery bypass surgery: a meta-analysis of randomized controlled trials. *Coron Artery Dis* 23:480–486, 2012.
258. Anderson CA, Filsoufi F, Aklog L, et al: Liberal use of delayed sternal closure for postcardiotomy hemodynamic instability. *Ann Thorac Surg* 73:1484–1488, 2002.
259. Yau JM, Alexander JH, Hafley G, et al: Impact of perioperative myocardial infarction on angiographic and clinical outcomes following coronary artery bypass grafting (from project of ex-vivo vein graft engineering via transfection [prevent] iv). *Am J Cardiol* 102:546–551, 2008.
260. Hashemzadeh K, Dehdilani M: Postoperative cardiac troponin I is an independent predictor of in-hospital death after coronary artery bypass grafting. *J Cardiovasc Surg (Torino)* 50:403–409, 2009.
261. Jarvinen O, Julkunen J, Saarinen T, et al: Perioperative myocardial infarction has negative impact on health-related quality of life following coronary artery bypass graft surgery. *Eur J Cardiothorac Surg* 26:621–627, 2004.
262. Klatte K, Chaitman BR, Theroux P, et al: Increased mortality after coronary artery bypass graft surgery is associated with increased levels of postoperative creatine kinase-myocardial band isoenzyme release: results from the guardian trial. *J Am Coll Cardiol* 38:1070–1077, 2001.
263. Thygesen K, Alpert JS, White HD, et al: ACCF/AHA/WHF Task Force for the Redefinition of Myocardial Infarction. Universal definition of myocardial infarction. *J Am Coll Cardiol* 50:2173–2195, 2007.
264. Crescenzi G, Bove T, Pappalardo F, et al: Clinical significance of a new Q wave after cardiac surgery. *Eur J Cardiothorac Surg* 25:1001–1005, 2004.
265. Thielmann M, Massoudy P, Schmermund A, et al: Diagnostic discrimination between graft-related and non-graft-related perioperative myocardial infarction with cardiac troponin i after coronary artery bypass surgery. *Eur Heart J* 26:2440–2447, 2005.
266. Brener SJ, Lytle BW, Schneider JP, et al: Association between CK-MB elevation after percutaneous or surgical revascularization and three-year mortality. *J Am Coll Cardiol* 40:1961–1967, 2002.
267. Eagle KA, Guyton RA, Davidoff R, et al: ACC/AHA guidelines for coronary artery bypass graft surgery: a report of the American College of Cardiology/American Heart Association task force on practice guidelines (committee to revise the 1991 guidelines for coronary artery bypass graft surgery). American College of Cardiology/American Heart Association. *J Am Coll Cardiol* 34:1262–1347, 1999.
268. Dacey LJ, Likosky DS, Leavitt BJ, et al; Northern New England Cardiovascular Disease Study G: Perioperative stroke and long-term survival after coronary bypass graft surgery. *Ann Thorac Surg* 79:532–536, discussion 537, 2005.
269. John R, Choudhri AF, Weinberg AD, et al: Multicenter review of preoperative risk factors for stroke after coronary artery bypass grafting. *Ann Thorac Surg* 69:30–35, discussion 35–36, 2000.
270. Filsoufi F, Rahmanian PB, Castillo JG, et al: Incidence, topography, predictors and long-term survival after stroke in patients undergoing coronary artery bypass grafting. *Ann Thorac Surg* 85:862–870, 2008.
271. Selim M: Perioperative stroke. *N Engl J Med* 356:706–713, 2007.
272. Nishiyama K, Horiguchi M, Shizuta S, et al: Temporal pattern of strokes after on-pump and off-pump coronary artery bypass graft surgery. *Ann Thorac Surg* 87:1839–1844, 2009.
273. Tarakji KG, Sabik JF, 3rd, Bhudia SK, et al: Temporal onset, risk factors, and outcomes associated with stroke after coronary artery bypass grafting. *JAMA* 305:381–390, 2011.
274. Likosky DS, Marrin CA, Caplan LR, et al; Northern New England Cardiovascular Disease Study G: Determination of etiologic mechanisms of strokes secondary to coronary artery bypass graft surgery. *Stroke* 34:2830–2834, 2003.
275. Merie C, Kober L, Olsen PS, et al: Risk of stroke after coronary artery bypass grafting: effect of age and comorbidities. *Stroke* 43:38–43, 2012.
276. Puskas JD, Williams WH, Duke PG, et al: Off-pump coronary artery bypass grafting provides complete revascularization with reduced myocardial injury, transfusion requirements, and length of stay: a prospective randomized comparison of two hundred unselected patients undergoing off-pump versus conventional coronary artery bypass grafting. *J Thorac Cardiovasc Surg* 125:797–808, 2003.
277. Shroyer AL, Grover FL, Hattler B, et al; Veterans Affairs Randomized On/Off Bypass Study G: On-pump versus off-pump coronary-artery bypass surgery. *N Engl J Med* 361:1827–1837, 2009.
278. van Dijk D, Nierich AP, Jansen EW, et al; Octopus Study G: Early outcome after off-pump versus on-pump coronary bypass surgery: results from a randomized study. *Circulation* 104:1761–1766, 2001.
279. Afilalo J, Rasti M, Ohayon SM, et al: Off-pump vs. On-pump coronary artery bypass surgery: an updated meta-analysis and meta-regression of randomized trials. *Eur Heart J* 33:1257–1267, 2012.
280. Koster S, Hensens AG, van der Palen J: The long-term cognitive and functional outcomes of postoperative delirium after cardiac surgery. *Ann Thorac Surg* 87:1469–1474, 2009.
281. Gottesman RF, Grega MA, Bailey MM, et al: Delirium after coronary artery bypass graft surgery and late mortality. *Ann Neurol* 67:338–344, 2010.
282. Martin BJ, Buth KJ, Arora RC, et al: Delirium: a cause for concern beyond the immediate postoperative period. *Ann Thorac Surg* 93:1114–1120, 2012.
283. Koster S, Oosterveld FG, Hensens AG, et al: Delirium after cardiac surgery and predictive validity of a risk checklist. *Ann Thorac Surg* 86:1883–1887, 2008.
284. Bucerius J, Gummert JF, Borger MA, et al: Predictors of delirium after cardiac surgery delirium: effect of beating-heart (off-pump) surgery. *J Thorac Cardiovasc Surg* 127:57–64, 2004.
285. Katznelson R, Djaiani GN, Borger MA, et al: Preoperative use of statins is associated with reduced early delirium rates after cardiac surgery. *Anesthesiology* 110:67–73, 2009.
286. Newman MF, Kirchner JL, Phillips-Bute B, et al; Neurological Outcome Research G, the Cardiothoracic Anesthesiology Research Endeavors I: Longitudinal assessment of neurocognitive function after coronary-artery bypass surgery. *N Engl J Med* 344:395–402, 2001.
287. van Dijk D, Keizer AM, Diephuis JC, et al: Neurocognitive dysfunction after coronary artery bypass surgery: a systematic review. *J Thorac Cardiovasc Surg* 120:632–639, 2000.
288. Evered L, Scott DA, Silbert B, et al: Postoperative cognitive dysfunction is independent of type of surgery and anesthetic. *Anesth Analg* 112:1179–1185, 2011.
289. Selnes OA, Gottesman RF, Grega MA, et al: Cognitive and neurologic outcomes after coronary-artery bypass surgery. *N Engl J Med* 366:250–257, 2012.
290. Toeg HD, Nathan H, Rubens F, et al: Clinical impact of neurocognitive deficits after cardiac surgery. *J Thorac Cardiovasc Surg* 145:1545–1549, 2013.

291. Mangano CM, Diamondstone LS, Ramsay JG, et al: Renal dysfunction after myocardial revascularization: risk factors, adverse outcomes, and hospital resource utilization. The multicenter study of perioperative ischemia research group. *Ann Intern Med* 128:194–203, 1998.
292. Chertow GM, Levy EM, Hammermeister KE, et al: Independent association between acute renal failure and mortality following cardiac surgery. *Am J Med* 104:343–348, 1998.
293. Brown JR, Cochran RP, Dacey LJ, et al; Northern New England Cardiovascular Disease Study G: Perioperative increases in serum creatinine are predictive of increased 90-day mortality after coronary artery bypass graft surgery. *Circulation* 114:I409–I413, 2006.
294. Holzmann MJ, Gardell C, Jeppsson A, et al: Renal dysfunction and long-term risk of heart failure after coronary artery bypass grafting. *Am Heart J* 166:142–149, 2013.
295. Holzmann MJ, Sartipy U: Relation between preoperative renal dysfunction and cardiovascular events (stroke, myocardial infarction, or heart failure or death) within three months of isolated coronary artery bypass grafting. *Am J Cardiol* 112:1342–1346, 2013.
296. Marui A, Okabayashi H, Komiya T, et al: Impact of occult renal impairment on early and late outcomes following coronary artery bypass grafting. *Interact Cardiovasc Thorac Surg* 17:638–643, 2013.
297. Ascione R, Nason G, Al-Ruzzeh S, et al: Coronary revascularization with or without cardiopulmonary bypass in patients with preoperative nondialysis-dependent renal insufficiency. *Ann Thorac Surg* 72:2020–2025, 2001.
298. Bull DA, Neumayer LA, Stringham JC, et al: Coronary artery bypass grafting with cardiopulmonary bypass versus off-pump cardiopulmonary bypass grafting: does eliminating the pump reduce morbidity and cost? *Ann Thorac Surg* 71:170–173, discussion 173–175, 2001.
299. Mentzer RM, Jr, Oz MC, Sladen RN, et al: Effects of perioperative nesiritide in patients with left ventricular dysfunction undergoing cardiac surgery: the NAPA trial. *J Am Coll Cardiol* 49:716–726, 2007.
300. Sezai A, Hata M, Niino T, et al: Influence of continuous infusion of low-dose human atrial natriuretic peptide on renal function during cardiac surgery: a randomized controlled study. *J Am Coll Cardiol* 54:1058–1064, 2009.
301. Sezai A, Nakata K, Iida M, et al: Results of low-dose carperitide infusion in high-risk patients undergoing coronary artery bypass grafting. *Ann Thorac Surg* 96:119–126, 2013.
302. Bramer S, van Straten AH, Soliman Hamad MA, et al: The impact of new-onset postoperative atrial fibrillation on mortality after coronary artery bypass grafting. *Ann Thorac Surg* 90:443–449, 2010.
303. Horwich P, Buth KJ, Legare JF: New onset postoperative atrial fibrillation is associated with a long-term risk for stroke and death following cardiac surgery. *J Card Surg* 28:8–13, 2013.
304. Thoren E, Hellgren L, Jideus L, et al: Prediction of postoperative atrial fibrillation in a large coronary artery bypass grafting cohort. *Interact Cardiovasc Thorac Surg* 14:588–593, 2012.
305. Echahidi N, Pibarot P, O'Hara G, et al: Mechanisms, prevention, and treatment of atrial fibrillation after cardiac surgery. *J Am Coll Cardiol* 51:793–801, 2008.
306. Hogue CW, Jr, Creswell LL, Gutterman DD, et al; American College of Chest P: Epidemiology, mechanisms, and risks: American College of Chest Physicians guidelines for the prevention and management of postoperative atrial fibrillation after cardiac surgery. *Chest* 128:9S–16S, 2005.
307. El-Chami MF, Kilgo P, Thourani V, et al: New-onset atrial fibrillation predicts long-term mortality after coronary artery bypass graft. *J Am Coll Cardiol* 55:1370–1376, 2010.
308. Filardo G, Hamilton C, Hebeler RF, Jr, et al: New-onset postoperative atrial fibrillation after isolated coronary artery bypass graft surgery and long-term survival. *Circ Cardiovasc Qual Outcomes* 2:164–169, 2009.
309. Kim MH, Deeb GM, Morady F, et al: Effect of postoperative atrial fibrillation on length of stay after cardiac surgery (the postoperative atrial fibrillation in cardiac surgery study [PACS(2)]. *Am J Cardiol* 87:881–885, 2001.
310. Her AY, Kim JY, Kim YH, et al: Left atrial strain assessed by speckle tracking imaging is related to new-onset atrial fibrillation after coronary artery bypass grafting. *Can J Cardiol* 29:377–383, 2013.
311. Mathew JP, Fontes ML, Tudor IC, et al; Investigators of the Ischemia R, Education F, Multicenter Study of Perioperative Ischemia Research G: A multicenter risk index for atrial fibrillation after cardiac surgery. *JAMA* 291:1720–1729, 2004.
312. Nardi F, Diena M, Caimmi PP, et al: Relationship between left atrial volume and atrial fibrillation following coronary artery bypass grafting. *J Card Surg* 27:128–135, 2012.
313. Maisel WH, Epstein AE, American College of Chest P: The role of cardiac pacing: American College of Chest Physicians guidelines for the prevention and management of postoperative atrial fibrillation after cardiac surgery. *Chest* 128:36S–38S, 2005.
314. Martinez EA, Bass EB, Zimetbaum P, et al; American College of Chest P: Pharmacologic control of rhythm: American College of Chest Physicians guidelines for the prevention and management of postoperative atrial fibrillation after cardiac surgery. *Chest* 128:48S–55S, 2005.
315. Martinez EA, Epstein AE, Bass EB, et al; American College of Chest P: Pharmacologic control of ventricular rate: American College of Chest Physicians guidelines for the prevention and management of postoperative atrial fibrillation after cardiac surgery. *Chest* 128:56S–60S, 2005.
316. Arsenault KA, Yusuf AM, Crystal E, et al: Interventions for preventing post-operative atrial fibrillation in patients undergoing heart surgery. *Cochrane Database Syst Rev* (1):CD003611, 2013.
317. Piccini JP, Zhao Y, Steinberg BA, et al: Comparative effectiveness of pharmacotherapies for prevention of atrial fibrillation following coronary artery bypass surgery. *Am J Cardiol* 112:954–960, 2013.
318. Costanzo S, di Niro V, Di Castelnuovo A, et al: Prevention of postoperative atrial fibrillation in open heart surgery patients by preoperative supplementation of n-3 polyunsaturated fatty acids: an updated meta-analysis. *J Thorac Cardiovasc Surg* 146:906–911, 2013.
319. Garner JS, Jarvis WR, Emori TG, et al: CDC definitions for nosocomial infections, 1988. *Am J Infect Control* 16:128–140, 1988.
320. Cayci C, Russo M, Cheema FH, et al: Risk analysis of deep sternal wound infections and their impact on long-term survival: a propensity analysis. *Ann Plast Surg* 61:294–301, 2008.
321. Patel NV, Woznick AR, Welsh KS, et al: Predictors of mortality after muscle flap advancement for deep sternal wound infections. *Plast Reconstr Surg* 123:132–138, 2009.
322. Toumpoulis IK, Anagnostopoulos CE, Derose JJ, Jr, et al: The impact of deep sternal wound infection on long-term survival after coronary artery bypass grafting. *Chest* 127:464–471, 2005.
323. Ridderstolpe L, Gill H, Granfeldt H, et al: Superficial and deep sternal wound complications: incidence, risk factors and mortality. *Eur J Cardiothorac Surg* 20:1168–1175, 2001.
324. Braxton JH, Marrin CA, McGrath PD, et al: 10-year follow-up of patients with and without mediastinitis. *Semin Thorac Cardiovasc Surg* 16:70–76, 2004.
325. Centofanti P, Savia F, La Torre M, et al: A prospective study of prevalence of 60-days postoperative wound infections after cardiac surgery. An updated risk factor analysis. *J Cardiovasc Surg (Torino)* 48:641–646, 2007.
326. Eklund AM, Lyytikainen O, Klemets P, et al: Mediastinitis after more than 10,000 cardiac surgical procedures. *Ann Thorac Surg* 82:1784–1789, 2006.
327. Saso S, James D, Vecht JA, et al: Effect of skeletonization of the internal thoracic artery for coronary revascularization on the incidence of sternal wound infection. *Ann Thorac Surg* 89:661–670, 2010.
328. Edwards FH, Engelman RM, Houck P, et al; Society of Thoracic S: The Society of Thoracic Surgeons practice guideline series: antibiotic prophylaxis in cardiac surgery, Part I: duration. *Ann Thorac Surg* 81:397–404, 2006.
329. Engelman R, Shahian D, Shemin R, et al; Workforce on Evidence-Based Medicine SoTS: The Society of Thoracic Surgeons practice guideline series: antibiotic prophylaxis in cardiac surgery, PART II: antibiotic choice. *Ann Thorac Surg* 83:1569–1576, 2007.
330. Furnary AP, Gao G, Grunkemeier GL, et al: Continuous insulin infusion reduces mortality in patients with diabetes undergoing coronary artery bypass grafting. *J Thorac Cardiovasc Surg* 125:1007–1021, 2003.
331. Lazar HL, McDonnell M, Chipkin SR, et al; Society of Thoracic Surgeons Blood Glucose Guideline Task F: The Society of Thoracic Surgeons practice guideline series: blood glucose

management during adult cardiac surgery. *Ann Thorac Surg* 87:663–669, 2009.
332. Ferguson TB, Jr, Hammill BG, Peterson ED, et al; Committee STSND: A decade of change—risk profiles and outcomes for isolated coronary artery bypass grafting procedures, 1990-1999: a report from the STS national database committee and the Duke Clinical Research Institute. Society of Thoracic Surgeons. *Ann Thorac Surg* 73:480–489, discussion 489–490, 2002.
333. Leavitt BJ, O'Connor GT, Olmstead EM, et al: Use of the internal mammary artery graft and in-hospital mortality and other adverse outcomes associated with coronary artery bypass surgery. *Circulation* 103:507–512, 2001.
334. Ghali WA, Rothwell DM, Quan H, et al: A Canadian comparison of data sources for coronary artery bypass surgery outcome "report cards." *Am Heart J* 140:402–408, 2000.
335. Argenziano M, Spotnitz HM, Whang W, et al: Risk stratification for coronary bypass surgery in patients with left ventricular dysfunction: analysis of the coronary artery bypass grafting patch trial database. *Circulation* 100:II119–II124, 1999.
336. Myers WO, Blackstone EH, Davis K, et al: Cass registry long term surgical survival. Coronary Artery Surgery Study. *J Am Coll Cardiol* 33:488–498, 1999.
337. Sergeant P, Blackstone E, Meyns B: Validation and interdependence with patient-variables of the influence of procedural variables on early and late survival after CABG. K.U. Leuven coronary surgery program. *Eur J Cardiothorac Surg* 12:1–19, 1997.
338. Investigators B: The final 10-year follow-up results from the BARI randomized trial. *J Am Coll Cardiol* 49:1600–1606, 2007.
339. Graham MM, Ghali WA, Faris PD, et al; Alberta Provincial Project for Outcomes Assessment in Coronary Heart Disease I: Survival after coronary revascularization in the elderly. *Circulation* 105:2378–2384, 2002.
340. Mohr FW, Morice MC, Kappetein AP, et al: Coronary artery bypass graft surgery versus percutaneous coronary intervention in patients with three-vessel disease and left main coronary disease: 5-year follow-up of the randomised, clinical syntax trial. *Lancet* 381:629–638, 2013.
341. Buxton BF, Komeda M, Fuller JA, et al: Bilateral internal thoracic artery grafting may improve outcome of coronary artery surgery. Risk-adjusted survival. *Circulation* 98:II1–II6, 1998.
342. Endo M, Nishida H, Tomizawa Y, et al: Benefit of bilateral over single internal mammary artery grafts for multiple coronary artery bypass grafting. *Circulation* 104:2164–2170, 2001.
343. Galbut DL, Kurlansky PA, Traad EA, et al: Bilateral internal thoracic artery grafting improves long-term survival in patients with reduced ejection fraction: a propensity-matched study with 30-year follow-up. *J Thorac Cardiovasc Surg* 143:844–853 e844, 2012.
344. Taggart DP, D'Amico R, Altman DG: Effect of arterial revascularisation on survival: a systematic review of studies comparing bilateral and single internal mammary arteries. *Lancet* 358:870–875, 2001.
345. Lev-Ran O, Paz Y, Pevni D, et al: Bilateral internal thoracic artery grafting: midterm results of composite versus in situ crossover graft. *Ann Thorac Surg* 74:704–710, discussion 710–711, 2002.
346. Sergeant P, Blackstone E, Meyns B: Is return of angina after coronary artery bypass grafting immutable, can it be delayed, and is it important? *J Thorac Cardiovasc Surg* 116:440–453, 1998.
347. Serruys PW, Ong AT, van Herwerden LA, et al: Five-year outcomes after coronary stenting versus bypass surgery for the treatment of multivessel disease: the final analysis of the Arterial Revascularization Therapies Study (ARTS) randomized trial. *J Am Coll Cardiol* 46:575–581, 2005.
348. Bergsma TM, Grandjean JG, Voors AA, et al: Low recurrence of angina pectoris after coronary artery bypass graft surgery with bilateral internal thoracic and right gastroepiploic arteries. *Circulation* 97:2402–2405, 1998.
349. Carr JA, Haithcock BE, Paone G, et al: Long-term outcome after coronary artery bypass grafting in patients with severe left ventricular dysfunction. *Ann Thorac Surg* 74:1531–1536, 2002.
350. Lorusso R, La Canna G, Ceconi C, et al: Long-term results of coronary artery bypass grafting procedure in the presence of left ventricular dysfunction and hibernating myocardium. *Eur J Cardiothorac Surg* 20:937–948, 2001.
351. Comparison of coronary bypass surgery with angioplasty in patients with multivessel disease. The bypass angioplasty revascularization investigation (BARI) investigators. *N Engl J Med* 335:217–225, 1996.
352. Garzillo CL, Hueb W, Gersh BJ, et al: Long-term analysis of left ventricular ejection fraction in patients with stable multivessel coronary disease undergoing medicine, angioplasty or surgery: 10-year follow-up of the MASS II trial. *Eur Heart J* 34:3370–3377, 2013.
353. Diller GP, Wasan BS, Kyriacou A, et al: Effect of coronary artery bypass surgery on myocardial function as assessed by tissue Doppler echocardiography. *Eur J Cardiothorac Surg* 34:995–999, 2008.
354. Bouchart F, Tabley A, Litzler PY, et al: Myocardial revascularization in patients with severe ischemic left ventricular dysfunction. Long term follow-up in 141 patients. *Eur J Cardiothorac Surg* 20:1157–1162, 2001.
355. Kaul TK, Agnihotri AK, Fields BL, et al: Coronary artery bypass grafting in patients with an ejection fraction of twenty percent or less. *J Thorac Cardiovasc Surg* 111:1001–1012, 1996.
356. Mickleborough LL, Carson S, Tamariz M, et al: Results of revascularization in patients with severe left ventricular dysfunction. *J Thorac Cardiovasc Surg* 119:550–557, 2000.
357. Yoo JS, Kim JB, Jung SH, et al: Coronary artery bypass grafting in patients with left ventricular dysfunction: predictors of long-term survival and impact of surgical strategies. *Int J Cardiol* 2013.
358. Keren A, Goldberg S, Gottlieb S, et al: Natural history of left ventricular thrombi: their appearance and resolution in the post-hospitalization period of acute myocardial infarction. *J Am Coll Cardiol* 15:790–800, 1990.
359. Johannessen KA, Nordrehaug JE, von der Lippe G: Left ventricular thrombi after short-term high-dose anticoagulants in acute myocardial infarction. *Eur Heart J* 8:975–980, 1987.
360. Kurlansky PA, Traad EA, Galbut DL, et al: Coronary bypass surgery in women: a long-term comparative study of quality of life after bilateral internal mammary artery grafting in men and women. *Ann Thorac Surg* 74:1517–1525, 2002.
361. Lindsay GM, Hanlon P, Smith LN, et al: Assessment of changes in general health status using the short-form 36 questionnaire 1 year following coronary artery bypass grafting. *Eur J Cardiothorac Surg* 18:557–564, 2000.
362. Stoll C, Schelling G, Goetz AE, et al: Health-related quality of life and post-traumatic stress disorder in patients after cardiac surgery and intensive care treatment. *J Thorac Cardiovasc Surg* 120:505–512, 2000.
363. Simchen E, Galai N, Braun D, et al: Sociodemographic and clinical factors associated with low quality of life one year after coronary bypass operations: the Israeli Coronary Artery Bypass study (ISCAB). *J Thorac Cardiovasc Surg* 121:909–919, 2001.
364. Peric V, Borzanovic M, Stolic R, et al: Predictors of worsening of patients' quality of life six months after coronary artery bypass surgery. *J Card Surg* 23:648–654, 2008.
365. Herlitz J, Brandrup-Wognsen G, Caidahl K, et al: Improvement and factors associated with improvement in quality of life during 10 years after coronary artery bypass grafting. *Coron Artery Dis* 14:509–517, 2003.
366. Loponen P, Luther M, Wistbacka JO, et al: Quality of life during 18 months after coronary artery bypass grafting. *Eur J Cardiothorac Surg* 32:77–82, 2007.
367. Caceres M, Cheng W, De Robertis M, et al: Survival and quality of life for nonagenarians after cardiac surgery. *Ann Thorac Surg* 95:1598–1602, 2013.
368. Jarvinen O, Saarinen T, Julkunen J, et al: Changes in health-related quality of life and functional capacity following coronary artery bypass graft surgery. *Eur J Cardiothorac Surg* 24:750–756, 2003.
369. Lukkarinen H, Lukkarinen O: Sexual satisfaction among patients after coronary bypass surgery or percutaneous transluminal angioplasty: eight-year follow-up. *Heart Lung* 36:262–269, 2007.
370. Sjoland H, Caidahl K, Wiklund I, et al: Impact of coronary artery bypass grafting on various aspects of quality of life. *Eur J Cardiothorac Surg* 12:612–619, 1997.
371. Järvinen O, Hokkanen M, Huhtala H: Quality of life 12 years after on-pump and off-pump coronary artery bypass grafting. *Coron Artery Dis* 24(8):663–668, 2013.
372. Harskamp RE, Lopes RD, Baisden CE, et al: Saphenous vein graft failure after coronary artery bypass surgery: pathophysiology, management, and future directions. *Ann Surg* 257:824–833, 2013.

373. Thatte HS, Khuri SF: The coronary artery bypass conduit: I. Intraoperative endothelial injury and its implication on graft patency. *Ann Thorac Surg* 72:S2245–S2252, discussion S2267–S2270, 2001.
374. Ojha M, Leask RL, Johnston KW, et al: Histology and morphology of 59 internal thoracic artery grafts and their distal anastomoses. *Ann Thorac Surg* 70:1338–1344, 2000.
375. Ruengsakulrach P, Sinclair R, Komeda M, et al: Comparative histopathology of radial artery versus internal thoracic artery and risk factors for development of intimal hyperplasia and atherosclerosis. *Circulation* 100:II139–II144, 1999.
376. Fitzgibbon GM, Kafka HP, Leach AJ, et al: Coronary bypass graft fate and patient outcome: angiographic follow-up of 5,065 grafts related to survival and reoperation in 1,388 patients during 25 years. *J Am Coll Cardiol* 28:616–626, 1996.
377. Kulik A, Le May MR, Voisine P, et al: Aspirin plus clopidogrel versus aspirin alone after coronary artery bypass grafting: the Clopidogrel After Surgery for Coronary Artery Disease (CASCADE) trial. *Circulation* 122:2680–2687, 2010.
378. Deb S, Cohen EA, Singh SK, et al: Radial artery and saphenous vein patency more than 5 years after coronary artery bypass surgery: results from RAPS (Radial Artery Patency Study). *J Am Coll Cardiol* 60:28–35, 2012.
379. Dreifaldt M, Mannion JD, Bodin L, et al: The no-touch saphenous vein as the preferred second conduit for coronary artery bypass grafting. *Ann Thorac Surg* 96:105–111, 2013.
380. Dion R, Glineur D, Derouck D, et al: Complementary saphenous grafting: long-term follow-up. *J Thorac Cardiovasc Surg* 122:296–304, 2001.
381. Mehta RH, Ferguson TB, Lopes RD, et al; Project of Ex-vivo Vein Graft Engineering via Transfection IVI: Saphenous vein grafts with multiple versus single distal targets in patients undergoing coronary artery bypass surgery: one-year graft failure and five-year outcomes from the Project of Ex-vivo Vein Graft Engineering via Transfection (PREVENT) IV trial. *Circulation* 124: 280–288, 2011.
382. Gao C, Ren C, Li D, et al: Clopidogrel and aspirin versus clopidogrel alone on graft patency after coronary artery bypass grafting. *Ann Thorac Surg* 88:59–62, 2009.
383. Nakayama Y, Sakata R, Ura M: Growth potential of left internal thoracic artery grafts: analysis of angiographic findings. *Ann Thorac Surg* 71:142–147, 2001.
384. Sabik JF, 3rd, Lytle BW, Blackstone EH, et al: Does competitive flow reduce internal thoracic artery graft patency? *Ann Thorac Surg* 76:1490–1496, discussion 1497, 2003.
385. Yoshizumi T, Ito T, Maekawa A, et al: Is the mid-term outcome of free right internal thoracic artery with a proximal anastomosis modification inferior to in situ right internal thoracic artery? *Gen Thorac Cardiovasc Surg* 60:480–488, 2012.
386. Al-Ruzzeh S, George S, Bustami M, et al: Early clinical and angiographic outcome of the pedicled right internal thoracic artery graft to the left anterior descending artery. *Ann Thorac Surg* 73:1431–1435, 2002.
387. Tatoulis J, Buxton BF, Fuller JA: The right internal thoracic artery: the forgotten conduit–5,766 patients and 991 angiograms. *Ann Thorac Surg* 92:9–15, discussion 15–17, 2011.
388. Ura M, Sakata R, Nakayama Y, et al: Analysis by early angiography of right internal thoracic artery grafting via the transverse sinus: predictors of graft failure. *Circulation* 101:640–646, 2000.
389. Ura M, Sakata R, Nakayama Y, et al: Technical aspects and outcome of in situ right internal thoracic artery grafting to the major branches of the circumflex artery via the transverse sinus. *Ann Thorac Surg* 71:1485–1490, 2001.
390. Iaco AL, Teodori G, Di Giammarco G, et al: Radial artery for myocardial revascularization: long-term clinical and angiographic results. *Ann Thorac Surg* 72:464–468, discussion 468–469, 2001.
391. Tatoulis J, Buxton BF, Fuller JA, et al: Long-term patency of 1108 radial arterial-coronary angiograms over 10 years. *Ann Thorac Surg* 88:23–29, discussion 29–30, 2009.
392. Cao C, Ang SC, Wolak K, et al: A meta-analysis of randomized controlled trials on mid-term angiographic outcomes for radial artery versus saphenous vein in coronary artery bypass graft surgery. *Ann Cardiothorac Surg* 2:401–407, 2013.
393. Suma H, Tanabe H, Takahashi A, et al: Twenty years experience with the gastroepiploic artery graft for cabg. *Circulation* 116:I188–I191, 2007.
394. Suma H: Gastroepiploic artery graft in coronary artery bypass grafting. *Ann Cardiothorac Surg* 2:493–498, 2013.
395. Pfisterer M, Brunner-La Rocca HP, Buser PT, et al: Late clinical events after clopidogrel discontinuation may limit the benefit of drug-eluting stents: an observational study of drug-eluting versus bare-metal stents. *J Am Coll Cardiol* 48:2584–2591, 2006.
396. Coronary angioplasty versus coronary artery bypass surgery: the Randomized Intervention Treatment of Angina (RITA) trial. *Lancet* 341:573–580, 1993.
397. First-year results of CABRI (Coronary Angioplasty versus Bypass Revascularisation Investigation). CABRI trial participants. *Lancet* 346:1179–1184, 1995.
398. Buszman PE, Kiesz SR, Bochenek A, et al: Acute and late outcomes of unprotected left main stenting in comparison with surgical revascularization. *J Am Coll Cardiol* 51:538–545, 2008.
399. Carrie D, Elbaz M, Puel J, et al: Five-year outcome after coronary angioplasty versus bypass surgery in multivessel coronary artery disease: results from the French monocentric study. *Circulation* 96:II-1-6, 1997.
400. Diegeler A, Thiele H, Falk V, et al: Comparison of stenting with minimally invasive bypass surgery for stenosis of the left anterior descending coronary artery. *N Engl J Med* 347:561–566, 2002.
401. Drenth DJ, Veeger NJ, Winter JB, et al: A prospective randomized trial comparing stenting with off-pump coronary surgery for high-grade stenosis in the proximal left anterior descending coronary artery: three-year follow-up. *J Am Coll Cardiol* 40:1955–1960, 2002.
402. Goy JJ, Eeckhout E, Burnand B, et al: Coronary angioplasty versus left internal mammary artery grafting for isolated proximal left anterior descending artery stenosis. *Lancet* 343:1449–1453, 1994.
403. Goy JJ, Kaufmann U, Goy-Eggenberger D, et al: A prospective randomized trial comparing stenting to internal mammary artery grafting for proximal, isolated de novo left anterior coronary artery stenosis: the SIMA trial. Stenting vs internal mammary artery. *Mayo Clin Proc* 75:1116–1123, 2000.
404. Goy JJ, Kaufmann U, Hurni M, et al: 10-year follow-up of a prospective randomized trial comparing bare-metal stenting with internal mammary artery grafting for proximal, isolated de novo left anterior coronary artery stenosis the SIMA (Stenting versus Internal Mammary Artery grafting) trial. *J Am Coll Cardiol* 52:815–817, 2008.
405. Hamm CW, Reimers J, Ischinger T, et al: A randomized study of coronary angioplasty compared with bypass surgery in patients with symptomatic multivessel coronary disease. German angioplasty bypass surgery investigation (GABI). *N Engl J Med* 331:1037–1043, 1994.
406. Hueb WA, Bellotti G, de Oliveira SA, et al: The Medicine, Angioplasty or Surgery Study (MASS): a prospective, randomized trial of medical therapy, balloon angioplasty or bypass surgery for single proximal left anterior descending artery stenoses. *J Am Coll Cardiol* 26:1600–1605, 1995.
407. King SB, 3rd, Lembo NJ, Weintraub WS, et al: A randomized trial comparing coronary angioplasty with coronary bypass surgery. Emory Angioplasty versus Surgery Trial (EAST). *N Engl J Med* 331:1044–1050, 1994.
408. Rodriguez A, Bernardi V, Navia J, et al: Argentine randomized study: coronary angioplasty with stenting versus coronary bypass surgery in patients with multiple-vessel disease (ERACI II): 30-day and one-year follow-up results. ERACI II investigators. *J Am Coll Cardiol* 37:51–58, 2001.
409. Rodriguez A, Boullon F, Perez-Balino N, et al: Argentine randomized trial of percutaneous transluminal coronary angioplasty versus coronary artery bypass surgery in multivessel disease (ERACI): in-hospital results and 1-year follow-up. ERACI group. *J Am Coll Cardiol* 22:1060–1067, 1993.
410. Rodriguez AE, Maree AO, Mieres J, et al: Late loss of early benefit from drug-eluting stents when compared with bare-metal stents and coronary artery bypass surgery: 3 years follow-up of the ERACI III registry. *Eur Heart J* 28:2118–2125, 2007.
411. Sedlis SP, Morrison DA, Lorin JD, et al; Investigators of the Dept. of Veterans Affairs Cooperative Study AWESOME:

Percutaneous coronary intervention versus coronary bypass graft surgery for diabetic patients with unstable angina and risk factors for adverse outcomes with bypass: outcome of diabetic patients in the AWESOME randomized trial and registry. *J Am Coll Cardiol* 40:1555–1566, 2002.

412. Serruys PW, Unger F, Sousa JE, et al; Arterial Revascularization Therapies Study G: Comparison of coronary-artery bypass surgery and stenting for the treatment of multivessel disease. *N Engl J Med* 344:1117–1124, 2001.
413. So SI: Coronary artery bypass surgery versus percutaneous coronary intervention with stent implantation in patients with multivessel coronary artery disease (the stent or surgery trial): a randomised controlled trial. *Lancet* 360:965–970, 2002.
414. Baldus S, Koster R, Kuchler R, et al: percutaneous revascularization of multivessel coronary disease using stents—a multicenter, prospective study. *Dtsch Med Wochenschr* 127:547–552, 2002.
415. Serruys PW, Ong AT, Morice MC, et al: Arterial revascularisation therapies study part II—sirolimus-eluting stents for the treatment of patients with multivessel de novo coronary artery lesions. *EuroIntervention* 1:147–156, 2005.
416. Boudriot E, Thiele H, Walther T, et al: Randomized comparison of percutaneous coronary intervention with sirolimus-eluting stents versus coronary artery bypass grafting in unprotected left main stem stenosis. *J Am Coll Cardiol* 57:538–545, 2011.
417. Park SJ, Kim YH, Park DW, et al: Randomized trial of stents versus bypass surgery for left main coronary artery disease. *N Engl J Med* 364:1718–1727, 2011.
418. Hannan EL, Racz MJ, McCallister BD, et al: A comparison of three-year survival after coronary artery bypass graft surgery and percutaneous transluminal coronary angioplasty. *J Am Coll Cardiol* 33:63–72, 1999.
419. Niles NW, McGrath PD, Malenka D, et al; Northern New England Cardiovascular Disease Study G: Survival of patients with diabetes and multivessel coronary artery disease after surgical or percutaneous coronary revascularization: results of a large regional prospective study. Northern New England Cardiovascular Disease Study Group. *J Am Coll Cardiol* 37:1008–1015, 2001.
420. Jones RH, Kesler K, Phillips HR, 3rd, et al: Long-term survival benefits of coronary artery bypass grafting and percutaneous transluminal angioplasty in patients with coronary artery disease. *J Thorac Cardiovasc Surg* 111:1013–1025, 1996.
421. Chieffo A, Meliga E, Latib A, et al: Drug-eluting stent for left main coronary artery disease. The delta registry: a multicenter registry evaluating percutaneous coronary intervention versus coronary artery bypass grafting for left main treatment. *JACC Cardiovasc Interv* 5:718–727, 2012.
422. Shiomi H, Morimoto T, Hayano M, et al: Comparison of long-term outcome after percutaneous coronary intervention versus coronary artery bypass grafting in patients with unprotected left main coronary artery disease (from the CREDO-Kyoto PCI/CABG Registry Cohort-2). *Am J Cardiol* 110:924–932, 2012.
423. Capodanno D, Caggegi A, Capranzano P, et al: Comparative one-year effectiveness of percutaneous coronary intervention versus coronary artery bypass grafting in patients <75 versus ≥75 years with unprotected left main disease (from the customize registry). *Am J Cardiol* 110:1452–1458, 2012.
424. Hannan EL, Wu C, Walford G, et al: Drug-eluting stents vs. coronary-artery bypass grafting in multivessel coronary disease. *N Engl J Med* 358:331–341, 2008.
425. FitzGibbon GM, Leach AJ, Kafka HP, et al: Coronary bypass graft fate: long-term angiographic study. *J Am Coll Cardiol* 17:1075–1080, 1991.
426. FitzGibbon GM, Burton JR, Leach AJ: Coronary bypass graft fate: angiographic grading of 1400 consecutive grafts early after operation and of 1132 after one year. *Circulation* 57:1070–1074, 1978.
427. Berger PB, Alderman EL, Nadel A, et al: Frequency of early occlusion and stenosis in a left internal mammary artery to left anterior descending artery bypass graft after surgery through a median sternotomy on conventional bypass: benchmark for minimally invasive direct coronary artery bypass. *Circulation* 100:2353–2358, 1999.
428. Lytle BW, Loop FD, Cosgrove DM, et al: Long-term (5 to 12 years) serial studies of internal mammary artery and saphenous vein coronary bypass grafts. *J Thorac Cardiovasc Surg* 89:248–258, 1985.
429. Grondin CM, Campeau L, Lesperance J, et al: Comparison of late changes in internal mammary artery and saphenous vein grafts in two consecutive series of patients 10 years after operation. *Circulation* 70:I208–I212, 1984.
430. Fiore AC, Naunheim KS, Dean P, et al: Results of internal thoracic artery grafting over 15 years: single versus double grafts. *Ann Thorac Surg* 49:202–208, discussion 208–209, 1990.
431. Mack MJ, Osborne JA, Shennib H: Arterial graft patency in coronary artery bypass grafting: what do we really know? *Ann Thorac Surg* 66:1055–1059, 1998.
432. Manninen HI, Jaakkola P, Suhonen M, et al: Angiographic predictors of graft patency and disease progression after coronary artery bypass grafting with arterial and venous grafts. *Ann Thorac Surg* 66:1289–1294, 1998.
433. Serruys P, Ong M, Morice M, et al: Arterial revascularization therapies study part II—sirolimus-eluting stents for treatment of patients with multivessel de novo coronary lesion. *EuroIntervention* 1:147–156, 2005.
434. BARI Investigators: The final 10-year follow-up results from the BARI randomized trial. *J Am Coll Cardiol* 49:1600–1606, 2007.
435. Dietz U, Baldus S, Rupprecht HJ, et al: Angiographic outcome in multivessel disease (GABI II study) using new coronary device interventions and comparison with GABI I trial results. *Cardiology* 102:24–31, 2004.
436. Coronary artery bypass surgery versus percutaneous coronary intervention with stent implantation in patients with multivessel coronary artery disease (the stent or surgery trial): a randomised controlled trial. *Lancet* 360:965–970, 2002.
437. Booth J, Clayton T, Pepper J, et al: Randomized, controlled trial of coronary artery bypass surgery versus percutaneous coronary intervention in patients with multivessel coronary artery disease: six-year follow-up from the Stent Or Surgery trial (SOS). *Circulation* 118:381–388, 2008.

CHAPTER 89

OFF-PUMP CORONARY ARTERY BYPASS GRAFTING AND TRANSMYOCARDIAL LASER REVASCULARIZATION

Jatin Anand • Ashraf A. Sabe • William E. Cohn

CHAPTER OUTLINE

In 1967, Sabiston and colleagues reported the first clinically successful coronary artery bypass graft (CABG) operation. Other early pioneers include Favaloro, who is credited with popularizing the use of autogenous saphenous vein, and Kolesov, who performed the first mammary artery to coronary artery anastomosis. Over the next several years, centers around the world began performing CABG procedures in large numbers. Subsequent refinements in cardiopulmonary bypass (CPB), the introduction of cardioplegia, the growing acceptance of the left internal mammary artery graft, and the development of the intra-aortic balloon pump (IABP) resulted in continued improvements in outcomes after CABG. By the early 1990s, more than 350,000 CABG procedures were being performed each year in the United States alone, with routine application in octogenarians, patients with severely impaired ventricular function, and patients with serious noncardiac morbidities.

As results continued to improve, and as mortality and major morbidity rates in the 2% range became commonplace, many surgeons turned their efforts toward decreasing the invasiveness of CABG and exploring alternative strategies of revascularization. Over the past several years, this effort has produced a number of new technologies, techniques, and variations on traditional CABG—all intended to avoid CPB, minimize aortic manipulation, improve graft patency, and reduce the trauma of surgical access. These variations include multivessel CABG without CPB, single-vessel CABG without CPB via a left mini-thoracotomy, videoscopic single-vessel CABG using surgical robotics, and multivessel CABG via a left mini-thoracotomy using peripheral cannulation and CPB. Other new procedures include transmyocardial revascularization, reoperative CABG through alternative incisions, and grafting strategies and devices that minimize or eliminate aortic manipulation, facilitate construction of the distal anastomosis, and perhaps improve long-term graft patency. This chapter describes these developments, discusses their relative merits, and summarizes current clinical results.

CARDIOPULMONARY BYPASS

The development of the heart-lung machine by Gibbon and its early application by Kirklin initiated the era of open heart surgery, which eventually made CABG possible. CPB and the subsequent introduction of cardioplegia provided a motionless, blood-free surgical field, which enabled the precision and reproducibility necessary for direct coronary anastomosis. Despite the obvious benefits of CPB, however, there is an increasing awareness of its potential deleterious effects. As the formed elements of the blood contact the various components of the heart-lung machine, the blood elements are activated, resulting in a number of hematologic and ultimately systemic changes. Typical sequelae include activation of complement, release of endotoxin, activation of leukocytes, increased expression of adhesion molecules, and release of inflammatory mediators, including cytokines, arachidonic acid metabolites, free radicals, and other components.[1] These sequelae occasionally manifest as coagulopathy, third-space fluid retention, and subtle end-organ dysfunction, including neurocognitive changes. The magnitude of this systemic inflammatory response is generally modest but can be quite severe, especially when the CPB time is prolonged. Furthermore, a small percentage of patients with preoperative end-organ dysfunction sustain significant morbidity when subjected to even a moderate systemic inflammatory response.

Ongoing efforts have been directed at reducing the magnitude of the systemic inflammatory response associated with CPB. These efforts include decreasing the surface area and modifying the surface composition of the CPB circuit to minimize surface activation, reducing hemodilution by decreasing the volume of crystalloid prime needed to institute CPB, avoiding the use of a cardiotomy sucker, and pretreating patients with various anti-inflammatory medications, such as aprotinin.[2] Despite progress in these areas, performing CABG without CPB remains attractive.

MULTIVESSEL OFF-PUMP CORONARY ARTERY BYPASS

Off-pump coronary artery bypass (OPCAB) grafting is as old as coronary surgery itself. Large case series dating back to the 1970s document its feasibility.[3-5] Nevertheless, OPCAB only recently gained widespread acceptance and entered the mainstream of clinical practice, propelled by a greater awareness of the potential morbidity of CPB and aortic manipulation and facilitated by improvements in surgical tools and techniques. OPCAB is part of the procedural armamentarium of a growing proportion of surgeons worldwide, and it can be performed in virtually any patient requiring coronary revascularization.

The introduction of self-retaining coronary stabilizers and the development of techniques for their use are key factors that have led to resurgent interest in OPCAB. When properly used, coronary stabilizers provide a relatively motionless and blood-free field, similar to that provided by CPB. The subsequent introduction of self-retaining cardiac positioning devices and the evolution of surgical techniques for rotating the heart enabled precise anastomoses to be constructed on the inferior, posterior, and lateral walls of the beating heart while maintaining adequate hemodynamic values without CPB.

Self-Retaining Coronary Stabilizers

A number of coronary artery stabilizers are available for clinical use. Current stabilizers can be categorized as compression, suction, or capture devices, depending on their design. When used properly, each type provides excellent immobility.

Compression-type stabilizers are generally two-pronged forks that are placed lightly on the epicardial surface so that the prongs are parallel to, and flanking, the coronary artery at the intended anastomotic site. The undersurface of the prongs provides traction to avoid slippage. The fork is attached to the retractor via an articulating arm and can be locked tightly in position once the desired position has been achieved. Generally, the best stability occurs when only light downward force is exerted on the surface of the heart. Paradoxically, an increase in motion occurs when excessive downward force is applied. One should use the exposure techniques described later in this chapter to present the target artery before positioning the stabilizer rather than relying on the stabilizer to retract the heart. Compression-type stabilizers are advantageous in that they may be set up quickly and simply and have an extremely low profile that allows unrestricted access to the coronary artery. For some aspects of the heart, however, compression stabilizers may require slightly more downward pressure to avoid slippage (Fig. 89-1).

Suction-type stabilizers also are generally two-pronged forks attached to the retractor by means of an articulating arm. These stabilizers, however, are constructed with a series of ports on the undersurface of the prongs, which are connected by sterile tubing to a −100 to −300 mm Hg wall-suction unit. The epicardium and epicardial fat that

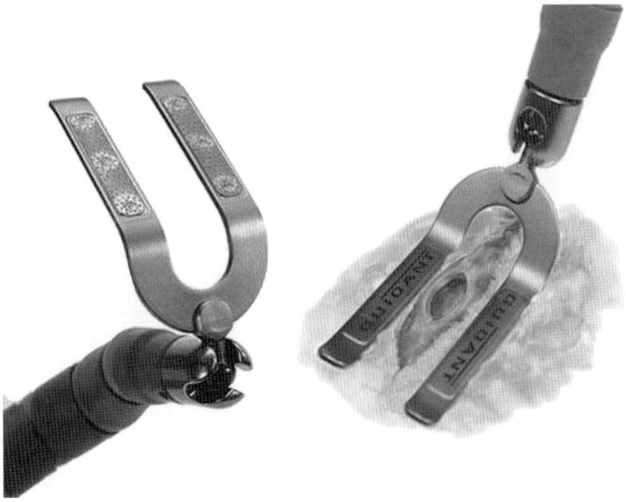

FIGURE 89-1 ■ Compression-type stabilizers generally have a low profile and a textured bottom surface that improves their ability to grip the epicardium.

flank the vessel are sucked into these ports, allowing the stabilizer to grip the surface of the heart. Thus, less downward force is required at the anastomotic site. Suction stabilizers are set up quickly but require a regulated vacuum line. They have the added advantage of providing traction and countertraction of the fat surrounding the coronary artery, so they are well suited for arteries deep within the fat. Suction stabilizers tend to have a slightly higher profile than compression types, but access to the coronary artery is not generally problematic (Fig. 89-2).

Capture-type stabilizers are usually fenestrated platforms that frame the intended anastomotic site. Silicone elastic tapes are passed deep under the coronary and locked to the platform under tension, pulling the epicardium up against the platform's undersurface (Fig. 89-3*A*). Like suction, this effect reduces the demand for downward force to prevent slippage. Capture stabilizers, by virtue of their circumferential effect, provide superior anastomotic stability.[6] Additionally, the silicone elastic tapes compress the coronary against the platform's posterior aspect, providing integrated biplane coronary occlusion (see Fig. 89-3*B*). Capture stabilizers are arguably more complex to position, however, and require proper spacing and alignment of the silicone elastic tapes to ensure adequate hemostasis. Furthermore, because of their larger size, they may not be well suited for use during construction of tightly spaced sequential anastomoses.

Preventing Hemodynamic Compromise during Multivessel OPCAB

One of the greatest challenges of the early OPCAB procedures was to maintain hemodynamic stability while grafting coronaries on the lateral and posterolateral aspects of the heart. This challenge was greatest in patients with poor ventricular function and marginally compensated ischemia. The problem has been largely eliminated by advances in surgical technique, including placement of deep pericardial retraction sutures, right vertical pericardiotomy and pleurotomy, and right hemisternal elevation, as well as the introduction of cardiac positioning devices and advances in anesthetic management. To understand how these tools and techniques minimize the adverse effects of cardiac manipulation, it is important to understand the causes of potential hemodynamic compromise during OPCAB.

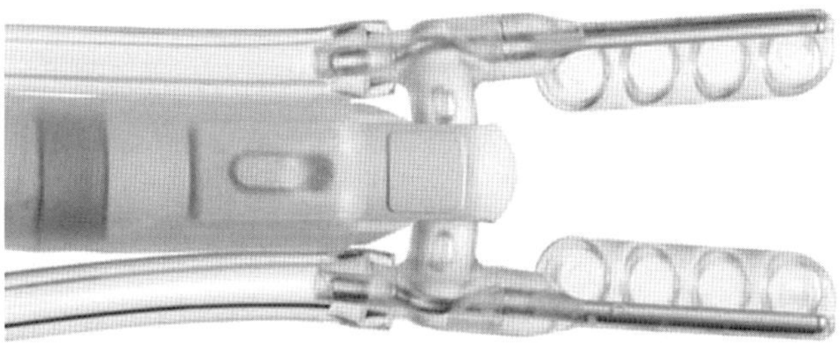

FIGURE 89-2 ■ Suction-type stabilizers use a series of suction cups to grip the epicardium. Although they have a slightly higher profile than compression-type stabilizers, they often require less downward force than compressive footplates.

Left Ventricular Compromise

When a coronary stabilizer is positioned by using excessive downward force, the stabilized aspect of the heart is constrained, leading to diastolic dysfunction and a decreased left ventricular end-diastolic volume (LVEDV), stroke volume, and cardiac output.[7] Whereas volume loading and Trendelenburg positioning attenuate these effects by elevating left ventricular (LV) filling pressures, recourse to these methods carries a risk of exacerbating intraoperative third-space fluid sequestration and associated morbidity. Similarly, the use of short-acting α-adrenergic agents can effectively maintain perfusion pressure in this setting, but they may be associated with an increased risk of perioperative mesenteric ischemia.[8] β-Adrenergic agents should similarly be avoided in the setting of yet-to-be-grafted coronary arteries. There are also anecdotal reports of severe mitral regurgitation during exposure of the lateral wall, possibly related to deformation of subvalvular structures in combination with coronary insufficiency. Exposure techniques that minimize or eliminate LV deformation are therefore desirable.

Right Ventricular Compromise

Exposure of the lateral LV wall displaces the heart toward the right, compressing the right ventricle against the pericardium and right side of the sternum. The relatively low pressure in the right ventricle makes that chamber

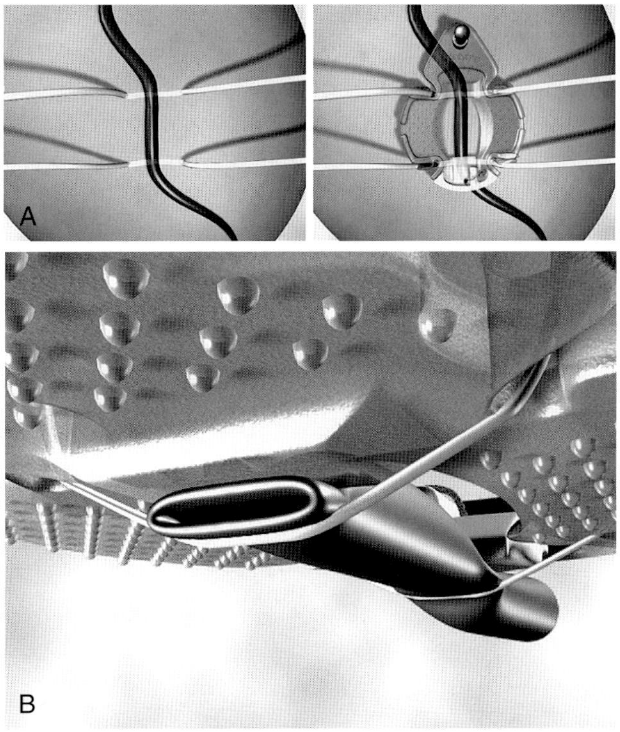

FIGURE 89-3 ■ Capture-type stabilizers use silicone elastic tapes to ensure tight apposition of the textured surface of the footplate and the epicardial surface. This arrangement results in integrated coronary compression. **A,** The surgeon's view of a coronary vessel in a capture-type stabilizer demonstrating spacing of the silicone elastic tapes. **B,** Simulated view of the coronary vessel segment from the underside of the stabilizer.

particularly vulnerable to deformation and reduction of the right ventricular end-diastolic volume (RVEDV).[9,10] The decreased right ventricular (RV) stroke volume leads to poor LV filling and a decrease in cardiac output. Volume loading and use of the Trendelenburg position can compensate for this effect, as noted in the previous paragraph, but not without potential risk. RV compromise is thought to be the dominant cause in many cases of hemodynamic instability that occurs during exposure of the lateral wall. Various groups have proposed the use of RV assistance as palliation for RV compromise during multivessel OPCAB.[11,12] Clearly, however, exposure techniques that minimize RV deformation are desirable.

Myocardial Ischemia

Intraoperative myocardial ischemia, secondary to decompensated coronary disease, transient coronary snaring during grafting, or poor perfusion pressure during heart manipulation, is another mechanism that leads to hemodynamic instability. This complication is best prevented by close communication with the anesthesiologist, a revascularization strategy that minimizes myocardial ischemia, and exposure techniques that maintain hemodynamic stability. Whereas each patient should be managed on an individual basis, useful axioms exist. Patients with significant left main stenosis and marginally compensated ischemia may benefit from completion of the left internal mammary artery (LIMA) to left anterior descending (LAD) graft before manipulation of the heart. Similarly, initial revascularization of occluded, collateralized coronary arteries should be carried out before one transiently occludes the vessels that supply collaterals to those arteries. Selective use of intracoronary shunts, aortocoronary shunts, or assisted coronary perfusion devices[13] can be essential when grafting a moderately stenosed right coronary artery (RCA) proximal to the origin of the posterior descending branch, or when grafting the proximal portion of a moderately stenosed LAD (Fig. 89-4). The judicious use of an intra-aortic balloon pump can occasionally prove invaluable.[14]

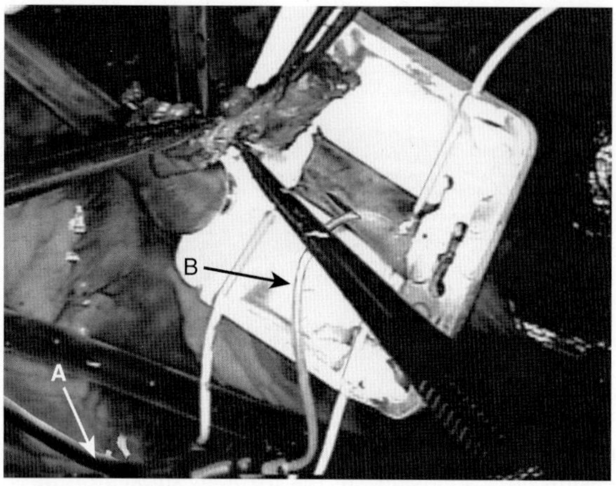

FIGURE 89-4 ■ A small, flexible, olive-tipped shunt inserted in the distal coronary artery *(B)* is attached to a short extension of IV tubing connected to a small cannula in the ascending aorta *(A)* to provide uninterrupted blood flow to the distal coronary bed while the anastomosis is constructed.

Exposure Techniques

Depending on the size and shape of the heart and the dimensions of the chest cavity, visualization of the proximal obtuse marginal and posterolateral branches of the circumflex system may be obstructed by the left hemisternum. Although intuitive attempts at improving exposure may involve applying additional rightward force to that aspect of the heart with the stabilizer, this maneuver frequently leads to hemodynamic compromise and paradoxically poor stabilization. Maximal access and stability at the anastomotic site with minimal compromise of cardiac performance is most readily achieved when the stabilizer is applied with little or no pressure; thus, this device should be used only to stabilize the anastomotic field rather than to assist in retracting the heart. In many patients with relatively normal hearts and readily accessible coronaries, little attention to exposure techniques is required. In contrast, during multivessel OPCAB on patients with large, poorly contracting hearts, attention to these techniques is essential. In these patients, exposure of the lateral cardiac wall is best achieved with deep pericardial sutures, a right pleurotomy and pericardiotomy, right hemisternal elevation, or apical suction devices, as described next.

Deep Pericardial Sutures

One of the most important advances in exposure techniques for OPCAB is the use of deep pericardial sutures. First described by Lima,[15] these sutures, when placed under tension, create a ridge of pericardium that supports the base of the lateral left ventricle adjacent to the atrioventricular groove and allows the heart to be rotated rightward to assume an "apex up" position (Fig. 89-5). In this subluxed position, the apex of the heart points toward the ceiling and protrudes through the sternotomy incision, often above the plane of the sternal retractor. This generally allows adequate exposure of the lateral and inferior aspects of the left ventricle before the coronary stabilizer is applied.

Placement of deep pericardial sutures may vary among surgeons and according to the patient's anatomy. Generally, one or two 2-0 silk sutures are placed in the

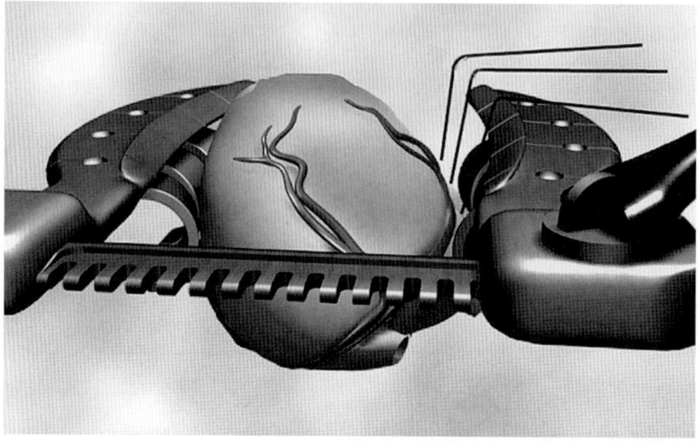

FIGURE 89-5 ■ Deep pericardial sutures secured under tension deliver the heart into an "apex up" position that provides adequate exposure of the lateral wall in many patients.

pericardium posterior to the left phrenic nerve and immediately anterior to one or both left pulmonary veins; one suture is placed deep in the oblique sinus behind the left atrium, and one is placed to the left and posterior to the inferior vena cava (Fig. 89-6). Care must be taken to avoid injury to underlying structures, such as the esophagus and lung.[16] The suture in the oblique sinus is particularly important for obtaining good exposure of the lateral wall near the base of the heart. One commonly used technique consists of placing a single deep pericardial suture in this location, then using that suture to secure the midpoint of a 50-cm gauze strip deep in the oblique sinus. Subsequent traction on the two ends of the strip can be adjusted to optimize exposure of different surfaces of the heart.

Regardless of the technique used, deep pericardial traction sutures generally allow presentation of the lateral, inferior, and even posterior wall of the heart with little change in LV geometry or LVEDV, providing adequate access for multivessel CABG while maintaining hemodynamic stability. In some patients, however, some or all additional maneuvers discussed in the following paragraphs are necessary to accomplish this aim.

Right Pleurotomy and Right Vertical Pericardiotomy

A right pleurotomy and right vertical pericardiotomy are helpful technical adjuncts when lateral wall exposure is difficult. Human pericardium is quite flexible but very inelastic. This inelasticity accounts for the profound hemodynamic effects caused by acute tamponade despite a relatively small volume of intrapericardial fluid. The posterior pericardium, right lateral pericardium, and diaphragmatic pericardium constitute a fixed-volume cusp or pocket. It is into this pocket that the right ventricle is compressed during extreme rightward rotation of the heart. In effect, pressure on the left ventricle results in RV tamponade. Opening the right pleura widely and incising the pericardium will vent the pocket, allowing the heart to herniate into the right pleural space while maintaining the RVEDV.

A right lateral pericardiotomy can be performed by making a right vertical incision that extends from the cut edge of the initial anterior pericardiotomy, 2 cm cephalad and parallel to the diaphragm, down to the level of the inferior vena cava, with care to avoid injuring the right phrenic nerve (Fig. 89-7). The 2-cm rim of pericardium on the diaphragm facilitates closure of the pericardiotomy once grafting is complete. Caution should be exercised in measuring right-sided grafts, as closure of the lateral pericardial incision may affect how they lie. Many surgeons advise closing the lateral pericardiotomy before constructing the proximal anastomosis of a right-sided graft to ensure a tension-free non-kinking graft. In some circumstances, one may also benefit from removing the right pericardiophrenic fat pad, which can be large, and decreasing the tidal volume to provide additional room for the easily deformed right ventricle. These techniques offer some benefit in almost all patients but are extremely valuable in obtaining lateral-wall access in patients with enlarged hearts and marginal hemodynamic stability.

Some surgeons skilled at performing the OPCAB procedure avoid a right pleurotomy and lateral pericardiotomy. These surgeons contend that incising the lateral pericardium and entering an additional body cavity is inconsistent with the objective of decreased invasiveness. Many patients can indeed be treated successfully without this maneuver. In our opinion, however, it facilitates the reproducible performance of a precise anastomosis during multivessel OPCAB. Furthermore, a right pleurotomy neither leaves a scar nor is associated with significant morbidity or additional length of hospital stay.

Right Hemisternal Elevation

In conjunction with the techniques described earlier, asymmetrical right hemisternal elevation can further improve lateral wall exposure. Once the right pericardium and pleura are incised, the right half of the sternum and right blade of the retractor limit rightward displacement of the subluxed apex of the heart. By elevating these structures, the surgeon can cause the apex to clear the posterior aspect of the chest wall. This allows the entire

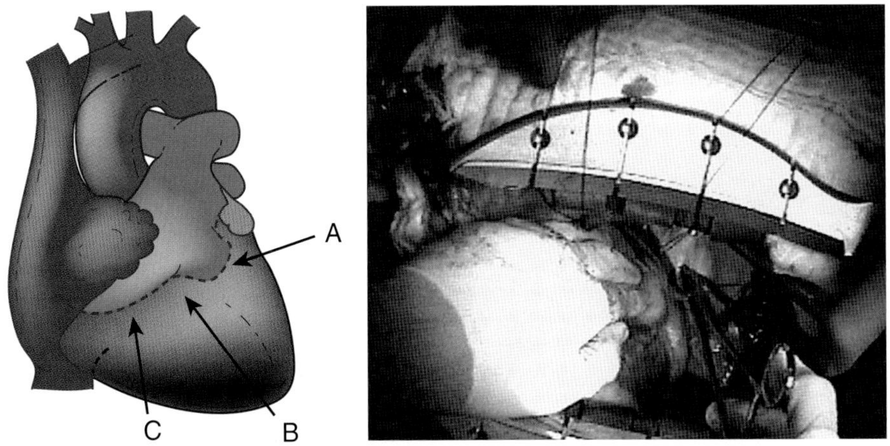

FIGURE 89-6 ■ The diagram shows the approximate locations for the deep pericardial sutures. Most surgeons agree that the suture at *B* is of greatest importance for lateral wall exposure. The photograph shows operative exposure for placement of the deep pericardial sutures, with the heart reflected up and to the right.

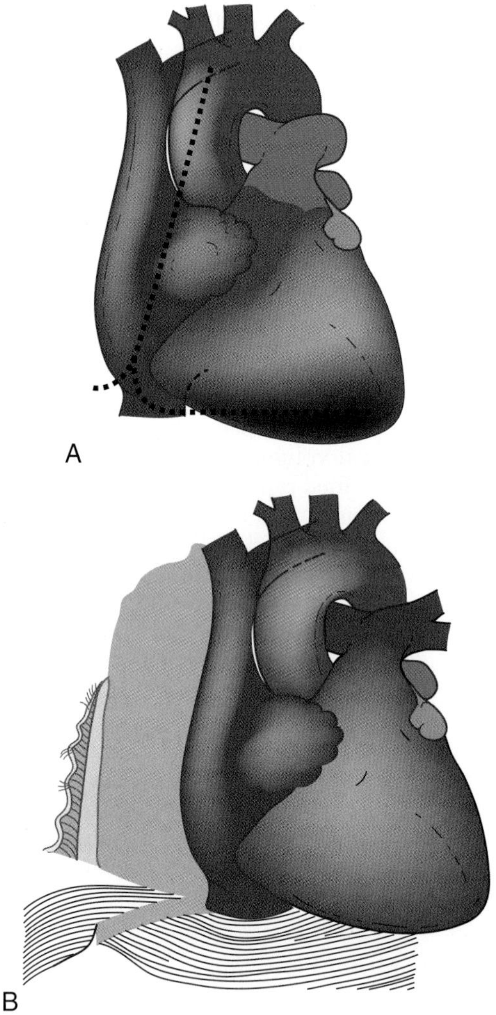

FIGURE 89-7 ■ **A,** An L-shaped pericardiotomy is created to the right of midline with the horizontal component extending to the cardiac apex. The right pleural space is opened widely and the right pericardium is excised almost to the inferior vena cava with care to avoid the right phrenic nerve. **B,** These incisions will vent the pocket, allowing the heart to herniate into the right pleural space to minimize hemodynamic compromise.

heart to rotate into the right pleural space with little change in LV and RV geometry and RVEDV (Fig. 89-8). As a result, the proximal obtuse marginal and posterolateral branches are brought toward the center of the operative field and into the surgeon's view.

Right hemisternal elevation is best carried out as the sternotomy incision is being performed. If anterior traction is applied on the right-sided chest wall when the retractor is first spread, costal microfractures that inevitably form during sternal opening will occur predominantly in the right-sided ribs. The resulting increase in flexibility of the right-sided chest wall will subsequently prevent the need for exaggerated tilting of the sternal retractor, which is often required to overcome the tendency of the left-sided chest wall to rise after internal mammary artery harvest. The diaphragmatic insertion on the inferior aspect of the right hemisternum can also be released to facilitate right hemisternal elevation and create additional room for displacement of the cardiac apex into the right pleural space.

Apical Suction Devices

Self-retaining apical suction retractors have been added to the operative armamentarium of OPCAB surgeons. These tools are used to position the heart for exposure of its lateral and posterior surfaces with little impact on hemodynamic values. The retractors generally consist of a suction cup mounted at the end of an articulating arm that can be locked in position relative to the retractor (Fig. 89-9). The suction cup is placed at or near the apex of the heart and is held in position by a vacuum (300 mm Hg). Pulling the apex away from the base and pivoting the cardiac axis can achieve excellent exposure with little impact on LV geometry and the LVEDV. Although use of these devices adds to the expense of OPCAB, their easy affixation and rapid set-up make them an attractive adjunct for use in challenging cases. In many OPCAB centers, apical suction retractors, in conjunction with a right pleurotomy, vertical pericardiotomy, and sternal tilt, are used in most cases (Fig. 89-10).

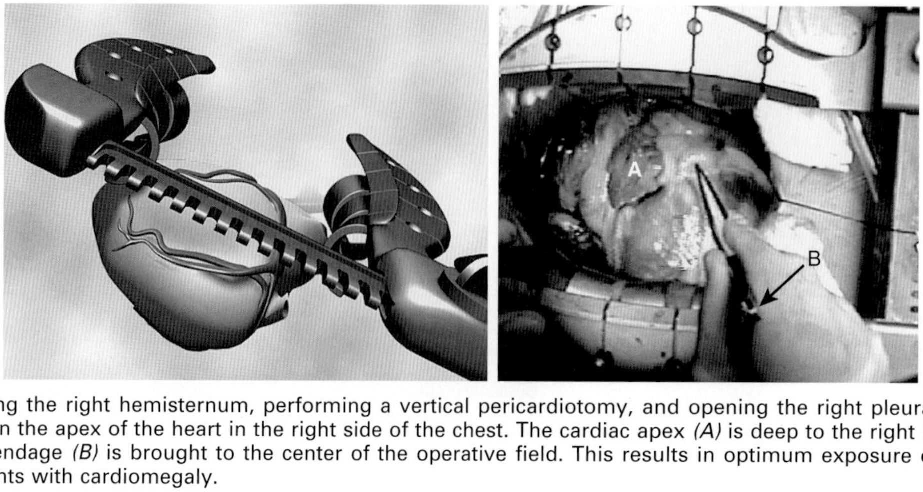

FIGURE 89-8 ■ Tilting the right hemisternum, performing a vertical pericardiotomy, and opening the right pleura often allows the surgeon to position the apex of the heart in the right side of the chest. The cardiac apex *(A)* is deep to the right hemisternum, and the left atrial appendage *(B)* is brought to the center of the operative field. This results in optimum exposure of the lateral wall, especially in patients with cardiomegaly.

Results after OPCAB

The relative merit of OPCAB versus CABG with CPB remains unclear. Few topics in cardiac surgery have given rise to more debate. Since the 1990s, when interest in OPCAB was renewed, researchers have attempted to clarify the ideal role of this treatment modality. Early reports from retrospective, nonrandomized, multicenter series showed lower death and stroke rates, less need for IABP use and postoperative transfusion, and a shorter ventilator time and length of hospital stay for OPCAB than for contemporaneous conventional CABG performed at the same institutions[17-24] or recorded in national databases.[25,26]

These encouraging results led to a number of early prospective, randomized trials, many of which showed no difference between OPCAB and CABG with CPB with regard to mortality, myocardial infarction, or coronary reintervention.[27-31] Early meta-analyses[32,33] and systematic reviews[34] confirmed these results. For years, the use of OPCAB continued to increase. One national, multicenter, observational study showed a peak in 2003, almost one quarter of cases being performed off pump.[35] Increasing interest and ongoing international debate continued to drive intense clinical investigation.

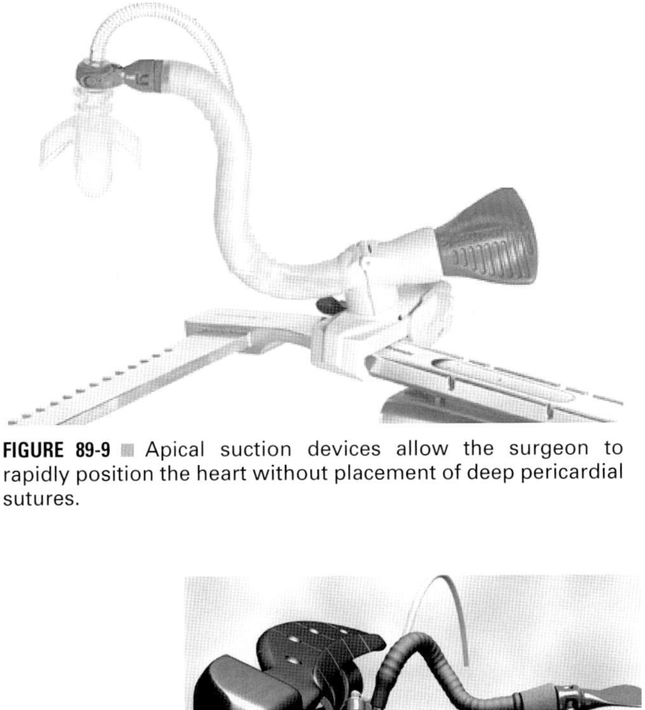

FIGURE 89-9 Apical suction devices allow the surgeon to rapidly position the heart without placement of deep pericardial sutures.

In 2009, the Veterans Affairs Randomized On/Off Bypass (ROOBY) trial investigators reported the first large, multicenter, prospectively randomized study.[36] More than 2000 patients were enrolled, and the results sparked intense debate. Patients undergoing OPCAB had a significantly higher rate of the composite endpoint, including all-cause mortality, nonfatal infarction, and repeat revascularization procedures at 1 year. Closer analysis of the follow-up angiography data revealed that OPCAB resulted in lower rates of FitzGibbon A patency and of effective revascularization.[37] Furthermore, ineffective revascularization was associated with significantly higher rates of adverse cardiac events.

Shortly after the ROOBY trial results were published, several worldwide groups of investigators began to report their own findings. The German Off-Pump Coronary Artery Bypass Grafting in Elderly Patients (GOPCABE) study was another prospective, large-cohort, multicenter trial that focused on patients 75 years of age and older.[38] Again, more than 2000 subjects were randomized to undergo either OPCAB or CABG with CPB. The investigators reported no significant difference in the composite or individual outcomes of death, stroke, infarction, or new renal-replacement therapy at 30 days or at 1 year.

These trials were subjected to intense debate and criticism. Objectors noted that the trials had enrolled too few patients, thereby lacking sufficient statistical power to detect differences in certain clinical endpoints. The technical expertise of the surgeons who performed OPCAB in these trials was also brought into question. To address these potential limitations, Canadian investigators reported initial data from their multicenter, prospective trial, which randomized almost twice the number of patients to undergo OPCAB or CABG with CPB.

The CABG Off or On Pump Revascularization Study (CORONARY) was more effectively powered than previous trials, and participating surgeons were required to have at least 2 years of experience involving more than 100 procedures performed. At 30 days and 1 year, the CORONARY trial showed no significant differences in the rate of primary composite outcome or its individual components, which included death, nonfatal stroke, nonfatal myocardial infarction, or new renal failure requiring dialysis 30 days after randomization.[39,40] The OPCAB

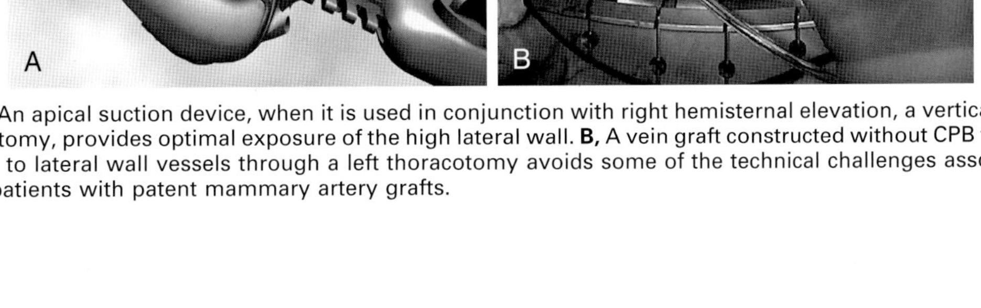

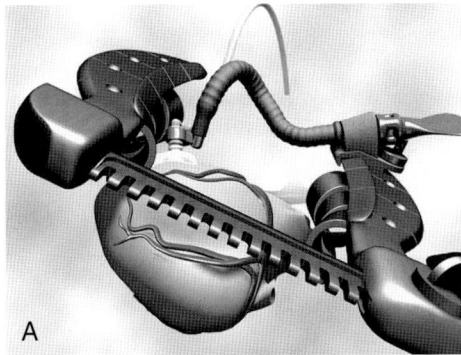

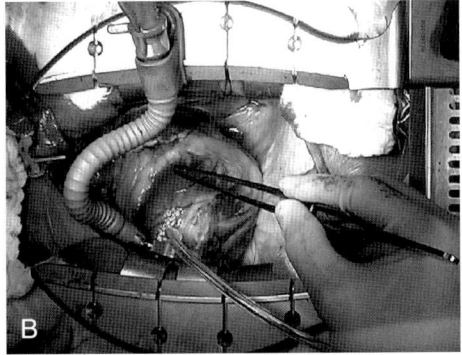

FIGURE 89-10 **A,** An apical suction device, when it is used in conjunction with right hemisternal elevation, a vertical pericardiotomy, and a right pleurotomy, provides optimal exposure of the high lateral wall. **B,** A vein graft constructed without CPB from the descending thoracic aorta to lateral wall vessels through a left thoracotomy avoids some of the technical challenges associated with reoperative CABG in patients with patent mammary artery grafts.

patients had shorter operations and ventilator times, fewer blood-product transfusions, fewer repeat operations for bleeding, and lower rates of respiratory complications and acute kidney injury. However, fewer bypass grafts were completed in the OPCAB group, and the rates of incomplete revascularization were higher. Similar findings regarding fewer numbers of grafts and lower rates of revascularization have been reported in other trials, and these factors are thought to contribute to the inferior long-term outcomes of OPCAB.[41] Five-year follow-up data from the CORONARY trial are anticipated and should provide further evidence for the appropriate use of OPCAB in multivessel CAD.

Although the debate continues, there is still compelling evidence that OPCAB is associated with decreased operative risk in some high-risk groups,[17,42,43] including older patients, those with a reduced ejection fraction, and those with renal failure.[44-47] Several reports have documented that OPCAB is associated with a decreased risk in reoperative patients as well.[48-51]

Because reoperative OPCAB can be performed frequently without dissecting out the ascending aorta or manipulating diseased grafts, it is an attractive approach. However, many surgeons consider the presence of heavily diseased but patent vein grafts a contraindication to OPCAB because of the risk of atheromatous embolization down the grafts while the heart is being repositioned. A tailored left thoracotomy approach has been reported for reoperative grafting of the lateral wall in patients with patent LIMA-to-LAD grafts. Using this exposure, the surgeon can readily construct a graft from the descending thoracic aorta to lateral wall branches while avoiding the technical challenges associated with LIMA-graft mobilization. Long-term patency data are not available for this type of graft. Similarly, lower sternotomy and upper abdominal incisions have been described for constructing grafts to the inferior wall with the right gastroepiploic artery.[52,53]

Although no consensus as yet exists, it is generally agreed that a well-performed OPCAB procedure is superior to a poorly performed conventional CABG operation and vice versa. Furthermore, there are many patients in whom OPCAB would be technically difficult or inadvisable (because of a deep intramuscular LAD, small diffusely diseased coronaries, need for an extensive endarterectomy, or active ischemia associated with hemodynamic compromise); there are also many patients for whom conventional CABG would pose an unnecessary risk (because of an atheromatous ascending aorta or a systemic disease process that might be exacerbated by CPB). Familiarity with the tools and techniques outlined here and the ability to perform OPCAB when necessary are valuable resources for practicing cardiac surgeons.

Minimizing Aortic Manipulation

Most surgeons agree that OPCAB is ideally suited for revascularization in patients with significant atheroma or calcification of the ascending aorta. In this setting, free grafts constructed from either the right internal mammary artery or the right radial artery can be attached to the side of the in situ LIMA, as described initially by Tector and colleagues,[54] and used to perform multivessel OPCAB without manipulating the aorta. Occasionally, the innominate artery can be used as a site for a proximal anastomosis if that artery is free of atheromatous plaque.

Alternatively, free grafts can be attached to a small disease-free area of the aorta with an automated anastomotic device (AAD), which obviates the need for a partial-occlusion clamp (Fig. 89-11). In 2008, the Food and Drug Administration (FDA) cleared these devices for sale in the United States. Although a previous AAD for constructing a clampless proximal anastomosis was approved for U.S. sale in 2001, it was subsequently withdrawn from the market when longer term data suggested that it was associated with decreased graft patency. In contrast, the latest iteration of an AAD for proximal use seems to be associated with equal or improved long-term graft patency when compared to a hand-sewn technique.[55] Although it is compelling to hope that AADs will improve outcomes by decreasing aortic manipulation, this has yet to be demonstrated in a case-control study. It is clear, however, that the current device allows a widely patent proximal anastomosis to be rapidly constructed without a partial-occlusion aortic clamp; moreover, the AAD can be readily used in patients who have areas of ascending aortic plaque that would make application of a partial-occlusion clamp unwise. The ultimate role of proximal AADs in the evolution of CABG surgery will depend on a number of issues, not least of which are economic ones.

Since 2002, several tools have been available that facilitate construction of a hand-sewn proximal anastomosis between a free graft and the ascending aorta without requiring a traditional partial-occlusion clamp.[56-59] Although slightly more labor intensive to use than loading and deploying a proximal AAD, these aortotomy occlusion tools permit construction of a tailored, hand-sewn anastomosis and accommodate a wider range of potential conduits, including radial and free-mammary grafts. These tools require a greater degree of technical facility than does a partial-occlusion clamp, but they decrease aortic manipulation and, like AADs, can be used when aortic plaque would make applying a partial-occlusion clamp ill advised. Using a combination of palpation and epiaortic ultrasonography, the surgeon can frequently identify an appropriate dime-sized area of relatively normal aorta where the occlusion device can be deployed. Although devices of this sort have been shown to liberate fewer gaseous and particulate emboli than do partial-occlusion clamps,[60] there are no compelling data to show that aortotomy occlusion tools are associated with improved outcomes. Nevertheless, these tools allow OPCAB to be readily performed while avoiding the hazards of cannulation and cross-clamping of the diseased ascending aorta.

Neurocognitive Dysfunction after OPCAB

Numerous published reports have described the new onset of subtle neurocognitive dysfunction (NCD) in some patients after CABG. Depending on the sensitivity of the tests used, the incidence has been reported to be

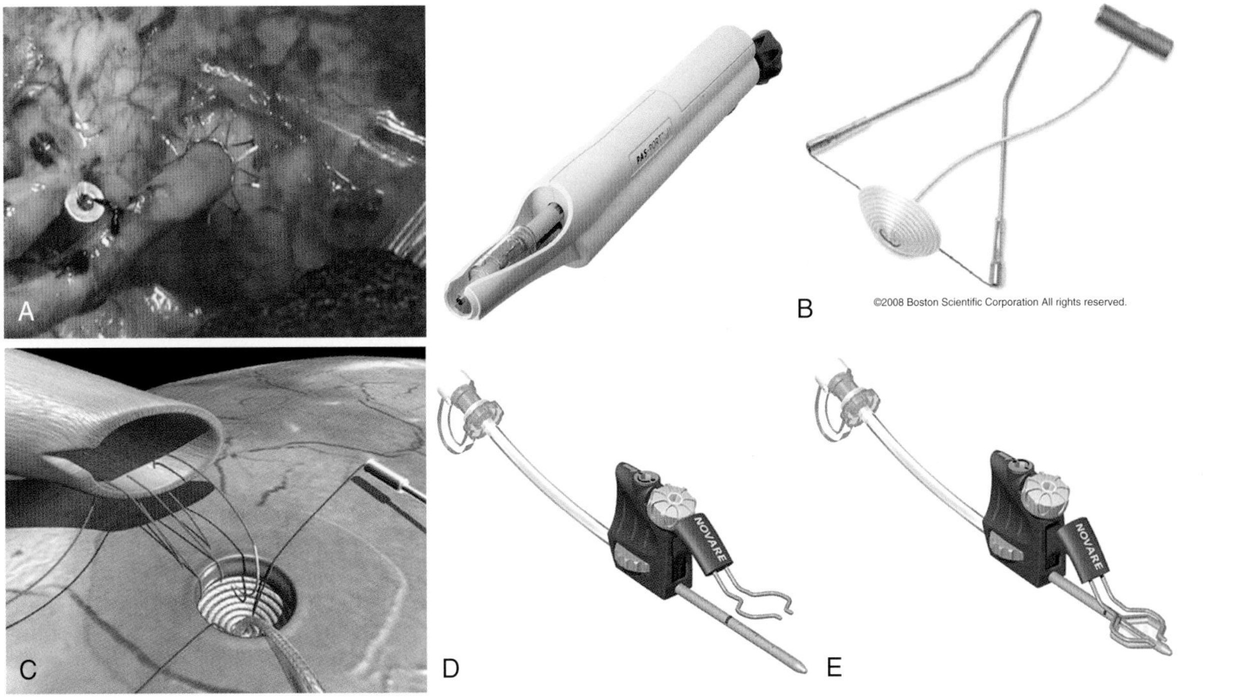

FIGURE 89-11 ■ **A,** An automated device for performing the proximal anastomosis between the ascending aorta and the saphenous vein without a partial-occlusion clamp was approved for clinical use in 2008 after demonstration of intermediate patency equivalent to hand-sewn anastomosis. **B-E,** Tools that facilitate construction of the proximal graft-to-aorta anastomosis without a cross-clamp and automated anastomotic couplers may have an impact on the incidence of neurocognitive deficit after CABG.

5% to 60%. Specific deficits include short-term memory loss, reduced ability to perform simple calculations, and disturbances in personality and mood.[61-63] Many CPB-related factors, including a systemic inflammatory response, alterations in cerebral blood flow, and microemboli—either arising from the CPB circuit or related to cannulation and cross-clamping—have been implicated.[63,64] Several groups have reported that OPCAB is associated with a significantly milder systemic inflammatory response.[44,65,66] The magnitude of the response, however, has not been shown to correlate with the severity of NCD in individual patients.[1] Furthermore, although a few studies have shown that, compared to conventional CABG with CPB, OPCAB is associated with a reduced incidence of NCD,[64,67,68] most studies have shown no significant difference.[31,69-71]

This failure of OPCAB to favorably impact postoperative NCD has been largely attributed to the partial-occluding aortic clamp and to microemboli liberated during its application and removal. Although OPCAB obviates the need to place a perfusion catheter for CPB or a cross-clamp for cardiac arrest, the side-biting partial-occlusion clamp, routinely used at many centers during construction of proximal anastomoses, arguably is equally traumatic.[72] Avoidance of aortic manipulation by using composite grafts arising from the in situ LIMA and OPCAB has been shown to be an important factor in avoiding postoperative stroke.[73,74] A number of new devices recently introduced into clinical practice (see earlier) allow proximal anastomoses to be constructed off-pump without application of a partial-occlusion clamp (see Fig. 89-11). The impact these devices will have on NCD after OPCAB is yet to be determined.

LIMITED-ACCESS CORONARY ARTERY BYPASS

Additional efforts to minimize the invasiveness of CABG have focused on decreasing the trauma of surgical access. Although a median sternotomy is relatively well tolerated, patients must refrain from heavy lifting for 2 to 3 months to allow reunion of the sternum. The incidence of wound complications is low, but sternal wound infections can be life-threatening and generally require repeat operation. Moreover, the musculoskeletal trauma involved in spreading the sternal halves is associated with a small degree of systemic inflammatory response that is synergistic with CPB in causing morbidity.[75,76] Avoiding a sternotomy is, therefore, an attractive idea.

Minimally Invasive Direct Coronary Artery Bypass (MIDCAB)

In 1995, Benetti and coworkers introduced the MIDCAB procedure,[77] which was rapidly adopted by multiple centers in the United States and Europe.[78,79] The procedure is performed through a 7-cm anterior lateral thoracotomy, usually in the fifth intercostal space, and generally consists of a single-vessel off-pump procedure using the LIMA to bypass the LAD. Many early series yielded satisfactory results, including a substantially shorter length of stay than for standard CABG, as well as decreased resource utilization, a reduced requirement for transfusion, and excellent graft patency.[78-81] Other reports suggested a reduced incidence of postoperative atrial fibrillation,[82] but this finding has been refuted.[14,83] Despite initial enthusiasm, traditional MIDCAB with LIMA harvest under direct vision is currently performed in large numbers in only a few U.S. centers. This decreased utilization is due in part to the technical hurdles involved in harvesting the LIMA under direct visualization through a small anterior lateral thoracotomy.

Several early reports documented successful results with endoscopic LIMA harvest.[84,85] At many U.S. centers, however, surgeons chose to mobilize the LIMA by using direct visualization through a small thoracotomy to avoid the learning curve associated with videoscopic instrumentation and visualization. Direct harvest is often technically demanding and occasionally results in a LIMA graft of inadequate length. In addition, the vigorous chest-wall retraction required for LIMA exposure results in significant early postoperative pain. Nevertheless, several groups skilled in MIDCAB continue to perform the procedure in large numbers and report excellent results.[81,86,87]

Hybrid MIDCAB Approach

Several reports have documented the successful application of a hybrid strategy in which a LIMA-to-LAD bypass (MIDCAB) is combined with catheter-based interventions on the circumflex artery and RCA for treating multivessel disease. In one multicenter series, videoscopic mobilization of the LIMA was performed with the aid of a voice-actuated robotic arm used to manipulate the scope (Fig. 89-12).[88] In this series, the pericardium was opened by using videoscopic techniques before the thoracotomy was performed. In many patients, this facilitated accurate placement of the chest-wall incision, allowing the anastomosis between the LIMA and LAD to be constructed without a rib spreader; only soft tissue retractors and a specially designed bed-mounted stabilizer were used to expose the anastomotic site through the natural intercostal space (Fig. 89-13).[89] This approach significantly reduced postoperative pain. This experience generated resurgent interest in the MIDCAB procedure at many centers.

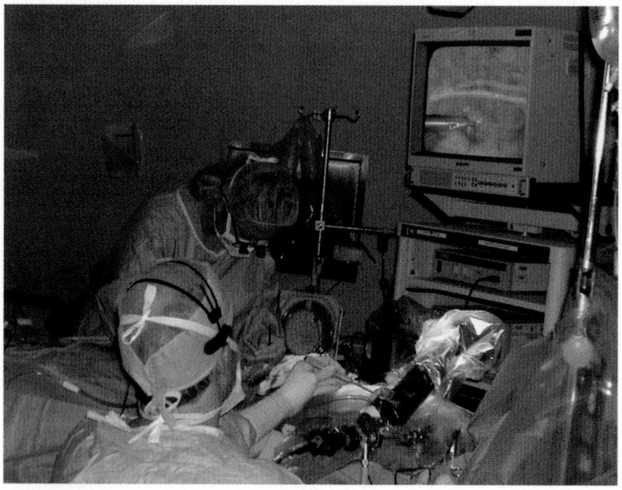

FIGURE 89-12 ■ Videoscopic mobilization of the left internal mammary artery may have a role in the continued evolution of less invasive CABG.

Completely Endoscopic Robotic-Assisted CABG

The literature describes a growing number of series involving completely closed-chest videoscopic LIMA-to-LAD procedures using surgical robots to mobilize the LIMA and to perform the sutured anastomosis, both with CPB[90,91] and without CPB.[90,92,93] The robots allow the surgeon to manipulate fully articulating videoscopic instruments by way of master-slave servos and microprocessor control. These instruments allow multiple degrees of freedom and can precisely emulate the surgeon's movements. An easy-to-use control environment, high-resolution displays that provide realistic three-dimensional stereopsis, and high magnification, as well as tremor filtering and motion-scaling options, offer the potential for superhuman precision. This precision compensates somewhat for the absence of tactile feedback. Although the concept is extremely exciting, the routine use of surgical robotics in CABG surgery does not seem imminent. The robots are expensive, and the learning curve for robotic totally endoscopic CABG (TECAB), especially if performed without CPB, is challenging. Surgeons skilled in the procedure can successfully perform only approximately one in three off-pump TECABs in carefully selected patients, resorting to a small MIDCAB incision to perform the anastomosis in the remainder. Future refinements in surgical robotic tools and techniques,

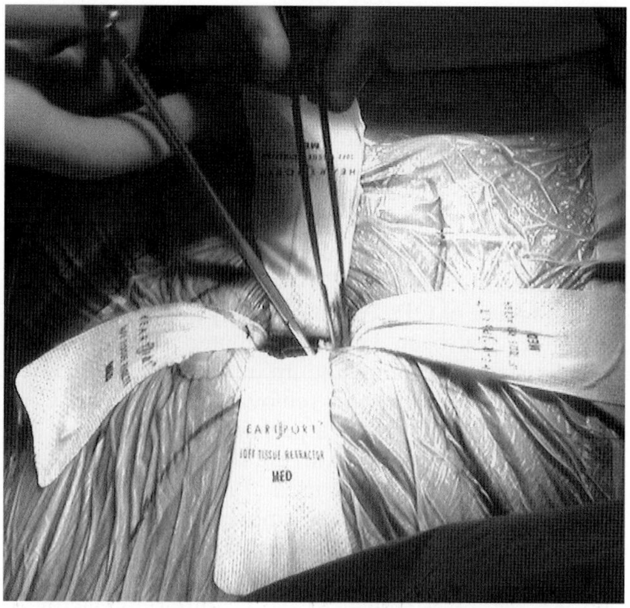

FIGURE 89-13 ■ In one type of less invasive bypass, accurate placement of the chest wall incision often allows the anastomosis between the left internal mammary artery and the left anterior descending artery to be constructed through the natural interspace without placement of a rib spreader.

improvements in automated distal anastomotic devices, and other advances may help determine the ultimate utility of robotics in CABG procedures.

Port-Access CABG

In 1996, Heartport introduced port-access cardiac surgery as a means of decreasing the trauma of surgical access. This strategy uses specialized catheters that are inserted into the femoral artery and vein and allow institution of CPB, balloon endoclamping of the ascending aorta, administration of antegrade cardioplegia, and venting of the ascending aorta. Additional catheters introduced percutaneously into the left jugular vein allow delivery of retrograde cardioplegia into the coronary sinus and venting of the pulmonary artery. A small chest incision can then be tailored for the desired procedure. In the late 1990s, several series of multivessel CABG operations performed through small fifth-intercostal-space thoracotomies were published that showed acceptable results from use of port access for institution of CPB,[94-96] but this procedure is not widely used. Decreased enthusiasm is partly due to challenges associated with graft length and lie. Nevertheless, port access has remained an essential component of TECAB in several small series, and it remains an enabling technique in limited-access mitral procedures and atrial-septal defect repair. Advances in surgical robotics and automated distal anastomosis may have an impact on the ultimate role of port-access technology in the evolution of limited-access CABG.

TRANSMYOCARDIAL LASER REVASCULARIZATION

Transmyocardial revascularization (TMR) is an alternative surgical therapy for the treatment of severe coronary artery disease. Currently reserved for patients refractory to medical management, TMR is indicated when complete revascularization cannot be achieved with conventional percutaneous or surgical techniques. In an open TMR procedure, revascularization is achieved with a hand-held laser device that delivers thermal energy to the ventricle, creating 1-mm channels through vaporized myocardium with the aim to improve blood flow.

The efficacy of TMR in relieving symptoms of angina is well documented, and this procedure is no longer considered experimental.[97,98] Initial positive results led to the approval of TMR by the Food and Drug Administration in 1998, and at least 20,000 procedures, in isolation or combined with CABG, have been performed in the United States.[99] To date, there remains a lack of long-term, randomized clinical data showing the superiority of isolated TMR over its use as an adjunctive therapy. Indications and long-term benefits remain in question, but ongoing investigations are helping to clarify the ideal use of this technology.

Operative Procedure

Open TMR is performed under general anesthesia and involves the direct application of laser energy to the epicardial surface of the heart. Preoperative preparation includes chest roentgenography, echocardiography, and a nuclear perfusion scan or dobutamine stress echocardiogram to document hibernating myocardium, as scar tissue does not benefit from TMR.

All patients require intraoperative monitoring with continuous electrocardiography, a Swan-Ganz catheter, an arterial pressure line, and transesophageal echocardiography. A double-lumen endotracheal tube is used to isolate the left lung; this facilitates the procedure in patients who have had previous cardiac surgery and may have pleural or mediastinal adhesions. Skin preparation includes the groin, in case the need arises for IABP insertion. CPB and systemic anticoagulation are not required.

In isolation, TMR can be performed through a left anterior thoracotomy in the fifth intercostal space. After a retractor has been inserted to separate the ribs, the pericardium is opened and the epicardial surface of the heart exposed, with care to avoid previous bypass grafts. Starting near the cardiac base, channels are created in approximately 1-cm increments in a linear fashion, working inferiorly and moving superiorly toward the anterior surface of the heart. This technique prevents expected mild TMR-related bleeding from obstructing the progression of the operation. The number of channels created depends on the size of the ischemic area and of the heart itself. Care must be taken to avoid thinned and dilated myocardium.

TMR is performed with a carbon dioxide (CO_2) or a holmium:yttrium-argon-garnet (Ho:YAG) laser. Both types of lasers rely on thermal energy. The CO_2 laser beam is transmitted through a series of mirrors and lenses, whereas the Ho:YAG laser relies on an optical fiber. The CO_2 device delivers up to 1000 watts of energy, creating 1-mm channels with a 20- to 30-J pulse. By synchronizing the firing of the CO_2 laser with the R wave on the electrocardiogram, one can potentially avoid ventricular arrhythmias. A transmural channel is created by a single 40-msec pulse, which is confirmed on transesophageal echocardiography by the appearance of characteristic changes caused by laser energy dissipating into the blood within the ventricle.

The Ho:YAG laser differs in its method of creating transmyocardial channels. An optical fiber must physically puncture the epicardium before the laser is deployed. The Ho:YAG laser requires 20 to 30 pulses at 2 J to create a single channel, and the pulses are not synchronized to the electrocardiogram, so the arrhythmogenic potential is greater than with the CO_2 laser. The optical fiber must be manually advanced, and successful creation of a transmural channel does not require transesophageal echocardiographic confirmation. After completion of TMR, a chest tube is inserted and the thoracotomy closed. The patient is transferred to the intensive care unit for monitoring.

Clinical Results

Since the first clinical use of open TMR by Mirhoseini and colleagues[100] in 1983, subsequent data have consistently shown a clear and substantial reduction in angina pectoris.[101] In multicenter studies comparing TMR to optimal medical therapy, most TMR patients had at least a two-class reduction in their Canadian Heart Association angina status. Long-term follow-up data have confirmed the persistent relief of symptoms, as well as a possible increase in survival.[102-104] Combined with CABG in selected patients who have limited options for revascularization therapies, TMR may improve long-term symptomatic relief and does not appear to increase the risk of procedure-related adverse events.[103,105] TMR has also been used as an adjunct to stem cell therapy, and initial data have been encouraging.[106,107]

Mechanism

The mechanism by which TMR provides symptomatic relief remains unclear, but three potential contributing effects are recognized: direct perfusion through the channels created by TMR; inflammatory effects resulting in angiogenesis; and sympathetic denervation. Originally, TMR was presumed to provide its benefit via perfusion of the created channels, ultimately affecting nearby capillaries within the myocardium. However, inconsistent reports documenting the long-term patency of these channels have given rise to substantial debate.[108-112] Although some positron emission tomography/computed tomography studies have shown evidence of sympathetic denervation,[113] it is difficult to isolate afferent sympathetic nerve fibers, and this mechanism of benefit remains theoretical. Moreover, neovascularization of the myocardium as a nonspecific response to myocardial injury has been demonstrated in previous studies, which have shown upregulation of molecular factors of angiogenesis, such as vascular endothelial growth factor, platelet-derived endothelial growth factor, and fibroblast growth factor.[114-116] Ongoing research will ultimately help define the role of TMR in clinical practice; meanwhile, this procedure remains a useful tool in the cardiac surgeon's armamentarium.

CONCLUSION

Advances in surgical tools and techniques have given rise to a number of new options in the surgical management of coronary artery disease. Although additional data may be required before the relative merits of these options can be characterized, it is clear that this flexibility will better allow the surgeon to tailor the operative approach to fit the patient. This is especially important given the increased age and comorbidity of patients referred for coronary bypass.

REFERENCES

1. Wan S, LeClerc JL, Vincent JL: Inflammatory response to cardiopulmonary bypass: mechanisms involved and possible therapeutic strategies. *Chest* 112:676–692, 1997.
2. Landis RC, Asimakopoulos G, Poullis M, et al: The antithrombotic and antiinflammatory mechanisms of action of aprotinin. *Ann Thorac Surg* 72:2169–2175, 2001.
3. Ankeny JL: Editorial: To use or not to use the pump oxygenator in coronary bypass operations. *Ann Thorac Surg* 19:108–109, 1975.
4. Laborde F, Abdelmeguid I, Piwnica A: Aortocoronary bypass without extracorporeal circulation: why and when? *Eur J Cardiothorac Surg* 3:152–154, discussion 154–155, 1989.
5. Trapp WG, Bisarya R: Placement of coronary artery bypass graft without pump oxygenator. *Ann Thorac Surg* 19:1–9, 1975.
6. Detter C, Deuse T, Christ F, et al: Comparison of two stabilizer concepts for off-pump coronary artery bypass grafting. *Ann Thorac Surg* 74:497–501, 2002.
7. Biswas S, Clements F, Diodato L, et al: Changes in systolic and diastolic function during multivessel off-pump coronary bypass grafting. *Eur J Cardiothorac Surg* 20:913–917, 2001.
8. Reilly PM, Wilkins KB, Fuh KC, et al: The mesenteric hemodynamic response to circulatory shock: an overview. *Shock* 15:329–343, 2001.
9. Gründeman PF, Borst C, Verlaan CW, et al: Exposure of circumflex branches in the tilted, beating porcine heart: echocardiographic evidence of right ventricular deformation and the effect of right or left heart bypass. *J Thorac Cardiovasc Surg* 118:316–323, 1999.
10. Mathison M, Edgerton JR, Horswell JL, et al: Analysis of hemodynamic changes during beating heart surgical procedures. *Ann Thorac Surg* 70:1355–1360, discussion 1360–1361, 2000.
11. Lima LE, Jatene F, Buffolo E, et al: A multicenter initial clinical experience with right heart support and beating heart coronary surgery. *Heart Surg Forum* 4:60–64, 2001.
12. Sharony R, Autschbach R, Porat E, et al: Right heart support during off-pump coronary artery bypass surgery—a multi-center study. *Heart Surg Forum* 5:13–16, 2002.
13. Guyton RA, Thourani VH, Puskas JD, et al: Perfusion-assisted direct coronary artery bypass: selective graft perfusion in off-pump cases. *Ann Thorac Surg* 69:171–175, 2000.
14. Hravnak M, Hoffman LA, Saul MI, et al: Atrial fibrillation: prevalence after minimally invasive direct and standard coronary artery bypass. *Ann Thorac Surg* 71:1491–1495, 2001.
15. Lima R. Revascularizacion a o da artèria circunflexa sem auxilio da CEC. XII encontro dos discipulos do dr. EJ Zerbini. Curitiba, Parana, Brasil. Sociedade dos discipulos do dr. EJ Zerbini. 1995: 6b.
16. Yokoyama T, Baumgartner FJ, Gheissari A, et al: Off-pump versus on-pump coronary bypass in high-risk subgroups. *Ann Thorac Surg* 70:1546–1550, 2000.
17. Arom KV, Flavin TF, Emery RW, et al: Safety and efficacy of off-pump coronary artery bypass grafting. *Ann Thorac Surg* 69:704–710, 2000.
18. Calafiore AM, Di Mauro M, Contini M, et al: Myocardial revascularization with and without cardiopulmonary bypass in multivessel disease: impact of the strategy on early outcome. *Ann Thorac Surg* 72:456–462, discussion 462–463, 2001.
19. Cartier R, Brann S, Dagenais F, et al: Systematic off-pump coronary artery revascularization in multivessel disease: experience of three hundred cases. *J Thorac Cardiovasc Surg* 119:221–229, 2000.
20. Czerny M, Baumer H, Kilo J, et al: Complete revascularization in coronary artery bypass grafting with and without cardiopulmonary bypass. *Ann Thorac Surg* 71:165–169, 2001.
21. Hart JC, Spooner TH, Pym J, et al: A review of 1,582 consecutive Octopus off-pump coronary bypass patients. *Ann Thorac Surg* 70:1017–1020, 2000.
22. Hernandez F, Cohn WE, Baribeau YR, et al: In-hospital outcomes of off-pump versus on-pump coronary artery bypass procedures: a multicenter experience. *Ann Thorac Surg* 72:1528–1533, discussion 1533–1534, 2001.
23. Magee MJ, Dewey TM, Acuff T, et al: Influence of diabetes on mortality and morbidity: off-pump coronary artery bypass grafting versus coronary artery bypass grafting with cardiopulmonary bypass. *Ann Thorac Surg* 72:776–780, discussion 780–781, 2001.
24. Puskas JD, Thourani VH, Marshall JJ, et al: Clinical outcomes, angiographic patency, and resource utilization in 200 consecutive off-pump coronary bypass patients. *Ann Thorac Surg* 71:1477–1483, discussion 1483–1484, 2001.
25. Cleveland JC, Jr, Shroyer AL, Chen AY, et al: Off-pump coronary artery bypass grafting decreases risk-adjusted mortality and morbidity. *Ann Thorac Surg* 72:1282–1288, discussion 1288–1289, 2001.
26. Plomondon ME, Cleveland JC, Jr, Ludwig ST, et al: Off-pump coronary artery bypass is associated with improved risk-adjusted outcomes. *Ann Thorac Surg* 72:114–119, 2001.
27. Angelini GD, Culliford L, Smith DK, et al: Effects of on- and off-pump coronary artery surgery on graft patency, survival, and health-related quality of life: long-term follow-up of 2

randomized controlled trials. *J Thorac Cardiovasc Surg* 137:295–303, e295, 2009.
28. Hueb W, Lopes NH, Pereira AC, et al: Five-year follow-up of a randomized comparison between off-pump and on-pump stable multivessel coronary artery bypass grafting. The MASS III Trial. *Circulation* 122:S48–S52, 2010.
29. Karolak W, Hirsch G, Buth K, et al: Medium-term outcomes of coronary artery bypass graft surgery on pump versus off pump: results from a randomized controlled trial. *Am Heart J* 153:689–695, 2007.
30. Sousa Uva M, Cavaco S, Oliveira AG, et al: Early graft patency after off-pump and on-pump coronary bypass surgery: a prospective randomized study. *Eur Heart J* 31:2492–2499, 2010.
31. van Dijk D, Spoor M, Hijman R, et al: Cognitive and cardiac outcomes 5 years after off-pump vs on-pump coronary artery bypass graft surgery. *JAMA* 297:701–708, 2007.
32. Parolari A, Alamanni F, Cannata A, et al: Off-pump versus on-pump coronary artery bypass: meta-analysis of currently available randomized trials. *Ann Thorac Surg* 76:37–40, 2003.
33. van der Heijden GJMG, Nathoe HM, Jansen EWL, et al: Meta-analysis on the effect of off-pump coronary bypass surgery. *Eur J Cardiothorac Surg* 26(1):81–84, 2004.
34. Møller CH, Penninga L, Wetterslev J, et al: Off-pump versus on-pump coronary artery bypass grafting for ischaemic heart disease. *Cochrane Database Syst Rev* 3:CD007224, 2012.
35. Bakaeen FG, Kelly RF, Chu D, et al: Trends over time in the relative use and associated mortality of on-pump and off-pump coronary artery bypass grafting in the Veterans Affairs system. *JAMA Surg* 148:1031–1036, 2013.
36. Shroyer AL, Grover FL, Hattler B, et al: On-pump versus off-pump coronary-artery bypass surgery. *N Engl J Med* 361:1827–1837, 2009.
37. Hattler B, Messenger JC, Shroyer AL, et al: Off-pump coronary artery bypass surgery is associated with worse arterial and saphenous vein graft patency and less effective revascularization: results from the Veterans Affairs Randomized On/Off Bypass (ROOBY) trial. *Circulation* 125:2827–2835, 2012.
38. Diegeler A, Börgermann J, Kappert U, et al: Off-pump versus on-pump coronary-artery bypass grafting in elderly patients. *N Engl J Med* 368:1189–1198, 2013.
39. Lamy A, Devereaux PJ, Prabhakaran D, et al: Off-pump or on-pump coronary-artery bypass grafting at 30 days. *N Engl J Med* 366:1489–1497, 2012.
40. Lamy A, Devereaux PJ, Prabhakaran D, et al: Effects of off-pump and on-pump coronary-artery bypass grafting at 1 year. *N Engl J Med* 368:1179–1188, 2013.
41. Omer S, Cornwell LD, Rosengart TK, et al: Completeness of coronary revascularization and survival: impact of age and off-pump surgery. *J Thorac Cardiovasc Surg* 148:1307–1315.e1, 2014.
42. Marui A, Okabayashi H, Komiya T, et al: Benefits of off-pump coronary artery bypass grafting in high-risk patients. *Circulation* 126:S151–S157, 2012.
43. Stamou SC, Corso PJ: Coronary revascularization without cardiopulmonary bypass in high-risk patients: a route to the future. *Ann Thorac Surg* 71:1056–1061, 2001.
44. Arom KV, Flavin TF, Emery RW, et al: Is low ejection fraction safe for off-pump coronary bypass operation? *Ann Thorac Surg* 70:1021–1025, 2000.
45. Koutlas TC, Elbeery JR, Williams JM, et al: Myocardial revascularization in the elderly using beating heart coronary artery bypass surgery. *Ann Thorac Surg* 69:1042–1047, 2000.
46. Sajja LR, Mannam G, Chakravarthi RM, et al: Coronary artery bypass grafting with or without cardiopulmonary bypass in patients with preoperative non-dialysis dependent renal insufficiency: a randomized study. *J Thorac Cardiovasc Surg* 133:378–388, 2007.
47. Stamou SC, Dangas G, Dullum MK, et al: Beating heart surgery in octogenarians: perioperative outcome and comparison with younger age groups. *Ann Thorac Surg* 69:1140–1145, 2000.
48. Kara I, Cakalagaoglu C, Ay Y, et al: Reoperative coronary artery bypass surgery: the role of on-pump and off-pump techniques on factors affecting hospital mortality and morbidity. *Ann Thorac Cardiovasc Surg* 19:435–440, 2013.
49. Stamou SC, Pfister AJ, Dullum MK, et al: Late outcome of reoperative coronary revascularization on the beating heart. *Heart Surg Forum* 4:69–73, 2001.
50. Trehan N, Mishra YK, Malhotra R, et al: Off-pump redo coronary artery bypass grafting. *Ann Thorac Surg* 70:1026–1029, 2000.
51. Usta E, Elkrinawi R, Ursulescu A, et al: Clinical outcome and quality of life after reoperative CABG: off-pump versus on-pump—observational pilot study. *J Cardiothorac Surg* 8:66, 2013.
52. Abraham R, Ricci M, Salerno T, et al: A minimally invasive alternative approach for reoperative grafting of the right coronary artery. *J Card Surg* 17:289–291, 2002.
53. Fonger JD, Doty JR, Salazar JD, et al: Initial experience with MIDCAB grafting using the gastroepiploic artery. *Ann Thorac Surg* 68:431–436, 1999.
54. Tector AJ, Amundsen S, Schmahl TM, et al: Total revascularization with T grafts. *Ann Thorac Surg* 57:33–38, discussion 39, 1994.
55. Puskas JD, Halkos ME, Balkhy H, et al: Evaluation of the PAS-Port Proximal Anastomosis System in coronary artery bypass surgery (the EPIC trial). *J Thorac Cardiovasc Surg* 138:125–132, 2009.
56. El Zayat H, Puskas JD, Hwang S, et al: Avoiding the clamp during off-pump coronary artery bypass reduces cerebral embolic events: results of a prospective randomized trial. *Interact Cardiovasc Thorac Surg* 14:12–16, 2012.
57. Emmert MY, Seifert B, Wilhelm M, et al: Aortic no-touch technique makes the difference in off-pump coronary artery bypass grafting. *J Thorac Cardiovasc Surg* 142:1499–1506, 2011.
58. Seto Y, Yokoyama H, Takase S, et al: The results of the enclose II proximal anastomotic device in 178 off-pump coronary artery bypass surgeries. *Innovations (Phila)* 7:242–246, 2012.
59. Thourani VH, Razavi SA, Nguyen TC, et al: Incidence of Postoperative Stroke Using the Heartstring Device in 1,380 Coronary Artery Bypass Graft Patients With Mild to Severe Atherosclerosis of the Ascending Aorta. *Ann Thorac Surg* 97(6):2066–2072, 2014.
60. Eldaif SM, Thourani VH, Puskas JD: Cerebral emboli generation during off-pump coronary artery bypass grafting with a clampless device versus partial clamping of the ascending aorta. *Innovations (Phila)* 5:7–11, 2010.
61. Clark RE, Brillman J, Davis DA, et al: Microemboli during coronary artery bypass grafting. Genesis and effect on outcome. *J Thorac Cardiovasc Surg* 109:249–257, discussion 257–258, 1995.
62. Sotaniemi KA, Mononen H, Hokkanen TE: Long-term cerebral outcome after open-heart surgery. A five-year neuropsychological follow-up study. *Stroke* 17:410–416, 1986.
63. Stump DA, Rogers AT, Hammon JW, et al: Cerebral emboli and cognitive outcome after cardiac surgery. *J Cardiothorac Vasc Anesth* 10:113–118, quiz 118–119, 1996.
64. Diegeler A, Hirsch R, Schneider F, et al: Neuromonitoring and neurocognitive outcome in off-pump versus conventional coronary bypass operation. *Ann Thorac Surg* 69:1162–1166, 2000.
65. Matata BM, Sosnowski AW, Galiñanes M: Off-pump bypass graft operation significantly reduces oxidative stress and inflammation. *Ann Thorac Surg* 69:785–791, 2000.
66. Okubo N, Hatori N, Ochi M, et al: Comparison of m-RNA expression for inflammatory mediators in leukocytes between on-pump and off-pump coronary artery bypass grafting. *Ann Thorac Cardiovasc Surg* 9:43–49, 2003.
67. Puskas JD, Stringer A, Hwang SN, et al: Neurocognitive and neuroanatomic changes after off-pump versus on-pump coronary artery bypass grafting: long-term follow-up of a randomized trial. *J Thorac Cardiovasc Surg* 141:1116–1127, 2011.
68. Zamvar V, Williams D, Hall J, et al: Assessment of neurocognitive impairment after off-pump and on-pump techniques for coronary artery bypass graft surgery: prospective randomised controlled trial. *BMJ* 325:1268, 2002.
69. Jensen BO, Hughes P, Rasmussen LS, et al: Cognitive outcomes in elderly high-risk patients after off-pump versus conventional coronary artery bypass grafting: a randomized trial. *Circulation* 113:2790–2795, 2006.
70. Taggart DP, Browne SM, Halligan PW, et al: Is cardiopulmonary bypass still the cause of cognitive dysfunction after cardiac operations? *J Thorac Cardiovasc Surg* 118:414–420, discussion 420–421, 1999.
71. Tully PJ, Baker RA: Current readings: neurocognitive impairment and clinical implications after cardiac surgery. *Semin Thorac Cardiovasc Surg* 25:237–244, 2013.
72. Edelman JJ, Yan TD, Bannon PG, et al: Coronary artery bypass grafting with and without manipulation of the ascending aorta—a meta-analysis. *Heart Lung Circ* 20:318–324, 2011.

73. Chavanon O, Durand M, Hacini R, et al: Coronary artery bypass grafting with left internal mammary artery and right gastroepiploic artery, with and without bypass. *Ann Thorac Surg* 73:499–504, 2002.
74. Kobayashi J, Tagusari O, Bando K, et al: Total arterial off-pump coronary revascularization with only internal thoracic artery and composite radial artery grafts. *Heart Surg Forum* 6:30–37, 2002.
75. Gu YJ, Mariani MA, Boonstra PW, et al: Complement activation in coronary artery bypass grafting patients without cardiopulmonary bypass: the role of tissue injury by surgical incision. *Chest* 116:892–898, 1999.
76. Gu YJ, Mariani MA, van Oeveren W, et al: Reduction of the inflammatory response in patients undergoing minimally invasive coronary artery bypass grafting. *Ann Thorac Surg* 65:420–424, 1998.
77. Benetti FJ, Ballester C, Sani G, et al: Video assisted coronary bypass surgery. *J Card Surg* 10:620–625, 1995.
78. Greenspun HG, Adourian UA, Fonger JD, et al: Minimally invasive direct coronary artery bypass (MIDCAB): surgical techniques and anesthetic considerations. *J Cardiothorac Vasc Anesth* 10:507–509, 1996.
79. Subramanian VA, McCabe JC, Geller CM: Minimally invasive direct coronary artery bypass grafting: two-year clinical experience. *Ann Thorac Surg* 64:1648–1653, discussion 1654–1655, 1997.
80. Detter C, Reichenspurner H, Boehm DH, et al: Minimally invasive direct coronary artery bypass grafting (MIDCAB) and off-pump coronary artery bypass grafting (OPCAB): two techniques for beating heart surgery. *Heart Surg Forum* 5:157–162, 2002.
81. Subramanian VA, Patel NU: Current status of MIDCAB procedure. *Curr Opin Cardiol* 16:268–270, 2001.
82. d'Amato TA, Savage EB, Wiechmann RJ, et al: Reduced incidence of atrial fibrillation with minimally invasive direct coronary artery bypass. *Ann Thorac Surg* 70:2013–2016, 2000.
83. Cohn WE, Sirois CA, Johnson RG: Atrial fibrillation after minimally invasive coronary artery bypass grafting: a retrospective, matched study. *J Thorac Cardiovasc Surg* 117:298–301, 1999.
84. Duhaylongsod FG, Mayfield WR, Wolf RK: Thoracoscopic harvest of the internal thoracic artery: a multicenter experience in 218 cases. *Ann Thorac Surg* 66:1012–1017, 1998.
85. Nataf P, Al-Attar N, Ramadan R, et al: Thoracoscopic IMA takedown. *J Card Surg* 15:278–282, 2000.
86. Mehran R, Dangas G, Stamou SC, et al: One-year clinical outcome after minimally invasive direct coronary artery bypass. *Circulation* 102:2799–2802, 2000.
87. Vassiliades TA, Jr, Rogers EW, Nielsen JL, et al: Minimally invasive direct coronary artery bypass grafting: intermediate-term results. *Ann Thorac Surg* 70:1063–1065, 2000.
88. Stahl KD, Boyd WD, Vassiliades TA, et al: Hybrid robotic coronary artery surgery and angioplasty in multivessel coronary artery disease. *Ann Thorac Surg* 74:S1358–S1362, 2002.
89. Vassiliades TA, Jr: Atraumatic coronary artery bypass (ACAB): techniques and outcome. *Heart Surg Forum* 4:331–334, 2001.
90. Detter C, Boehm DH, Reichenspurner H, et al: Robotically-assisted coronary artery surgery with and without cardiopulmonary bypass—from first clinical use to endoscopic operation. *Med Sci Monit* 8:MT118–MT123, 2002.
91. Falk V, Diegeler A, Walther T, et al: Total endoscopic computer enhanced coronary artery bypass grafting. *Eur J Cardiothorac Surg* 17:38–45, 2000.
92. Boehm DH, Reichenspurner H, Detter C, et al: Clinical use of a computer-enhanced surgical robotic system for endoscopic coronary artery bypass grafting on the beating heart. *Thorac Cardiovasc Surg* 48:198–202, 2000.
93. Mohr FW, Falk V, Diegeler A, et al: Computer-enhanced "robotic" cardiac surgery: experience in 148 patients. *J Thorac Cardiovasc Surg* 121:842–853, 2001.
94. Groh MA, Sutherland SE, Burton HG, 3rd, et al: Port-access coronary artery bypass grafting: technique and comparative results. *Ann Thorac Surg* 68:1506–1508, 1999.
95. Grossi EA, Groh MA, Lefrak EA, et al: Results of a prospective multicenter study on port-access coronary bypass grafting. *Ann Thorac Surg* 68:1475–1477, 1999.
96. Reichenspurner H, Gulielmos V, Wunderlich J, et al: Port-access coronary artery bypass grafting with the use of cardiopulmonary bypass and cardioplegic arrest. *Ann Thorac Surg* 65:413–419, 1998.
97. Briones E, Lacalle JR, Marin I: Transmyocardial laser revascularization versus medical therapy for refractory angina. *Cochrane Database Syst Rev* (1):CD003712, 2009.
98. Liao L, Sarria-Santamera A, Matchar DB, et al: Meta-analysis of survival and relief of angina pectoris after transmyocardial revascularization. *Am J Cardiol* 95:1243–1245, 2005.
99. Society of Thoracic Surgeons. Adult Cardiac Surgery Database, Executive Summary, 10 Years. Available at http://www.sts.org/sites/default/files/documents/2ndHarvestExecutiveSummary.pdf. Accessed May 27, 2014.
100. Mirhoseini M, Fisher JC, Cayton M: Myocardial revascularization by laser: a clinical report. *Lasers Surg Med* 3:241–245, 1983.
101. Horvath KA, Aranki SF, Cohn LH, et al: Sustained angina relief 5 years after transmyocardial laser revascularization with a CO(2) laser. *Circulation* 104:I81–I84, 2001.
102. Aaberge L, Rootwelt K, Blomhoff S, et al: Continued symptomatic improvement three to five years after transmyocardial revascularization with CO(2) laser: a late clinical follow-up of the Norwegian Randomized trial with transmyocardial revascularization. *J Am Coll Cardiol* 39:1588–1593, 2002.
103. Allen KB, Dowling RD, Angell WW, et al: Transmyocardial revascularization: 5-year follow-up of a prospective, randomized multicenter trial. *Ann Thorac Surg* 77:1228–1234, 2004.
104. Spertus JA, Jones PG, Coen M, et al: Transmyocardial CO(2) laser revascularization improves symptoms, function, and quality of life: 12-month results from a randomized controlled trial. *Am J Med* 111:341–348, 2001.
105. Frazier OH, Tuzun E, Eichstadt H, et al: Transmyocardial laser revascularization as an adjunct to coronary artery bypass grafting: a randomized, multicenter study with 4-year follow-up. *Tex Heart Inst J* 31:231–239, 2004.
106. Konstanty-Kalandyk J, Piątek J, Miszalski-Jamka T, et al: The combined use of transmyocardial laser revascularisation and intramyocardial injection of bone-marrow derived stem cells in patients with end-stage coronary artery disease: one year follow-up. *Kardiol Pol* 71:485–492, 2013.
107. Shahzad U, Li G, Zhang Y, et al: Transmyocardial revascularization induces mesenchymal stem cell engraftment in infarcted hearts. *Ann Thorac Surg* 94:556–562, 2012.
108. Burkhoff D, Fisher PE, Apfelbaum M, et al: Histologic appearance of transmyocardial laser channels after 4 1/2 weeks. *Ann Thorac Surg* 61:1532–1534, discussion 1534–1535, 1996.
109. Cooley DA, Frazier OH, Kadipasaoglu KA, et al: Transmyocardial laser revascularization. Anatomic evidence of long-term channel patency. *Tex Heart Inst J* 21:220–224, 1994.
110. Gassler N, Wintzer HO, Stubbe HM, et al: Transmyocardial laser revascularization. Histological features in human nonresponder myocardium. *Circulation* 95:371–375, 1997.
111. Krabatsch T, Schäper F, Leder C, et al: Histological findings after transmyocardial laser revascularization. *J Card Surg* 11:326–331, 1996.
112. Ozaki S, Meyns B, Racz R, et al: Effect of transmyocardial laser revascularization on chronic ischemic hearts in sheep. *Eur J Cardiothorac Surg* 18:404–410, 2000.
113. Al-Sheikh T, Allen KB, Straka SP, et al: Cardiac sympathetic denervation after transmyocardial laser revascularization. *Circulation* 100:135–140, 1999.
114. Fuchs S, Baffour R, Vodovotz Y, et al: Laser myocardial revascularization modulates expression of angiogenic, neuronal, and inflammatory cytokines in a porcine model of chronic myocardial ischemia. *J Card Surg* 17:413–424, 2002.
115. Hamman BL, White CH, Cheung EHK, et al: Transmyocardial laser revascularization causes sustained VEGF secretion. *Semin Thorac Cardiovasc Surg* 18:43–45, 2006.
116. Li W, Chiba Y, Kimura T, et al: Transmyocardial laser revascularization induced angiogenesis correlated with the expression of matrix metalloproteinases and platelet-derived endothelial cell growth factor. *Eur J Cardiothorac Surg* 19:156–163, 2001.

CHAPTER 90

ROBOTIC AND ALTERNATIVE APPROACHES TO CORONARY ARTERY BYPASS GRAFTING

Stephanie Mick • Suresh Keshavamurthy • Tomislav Mihaljevic • Johannes Bonatti

CHAPTER OUTLINE

ROBOTIC AND ALTERNATIVE APPROACHES TO CORONARY ARTERY BYPASS GRAFTING

The standard approach for coronary artery bypass grafting (CABG) is median sternotomy using cardiopulmonary bypass. However, less invasive approaches, including off-pump CABG and smaller access surgeries with or without robotic assistance, have been developed. This chapter describes less invasive methods of coronary revascularization along with their associated outcomes, with emphasis on robotic CABG. Hybrid coronary revascularization techniques are also considered.

MINIMALLY INVASIVE SURGICAL CORONARY REVASCULARIZATION

Many alternatives to surgical coronary revascularization have been developed in the form of modifications to conventional CABG. These alternatives come under the broad rubric *minimally invasive coronary revascularization.*

It should be noted that when used in the realm of cardiac surgery, this description "minimally invasive" carries more possible meanings than in other surgical specialties. In contrast to other surgical disciplines where the degree of invasiveness of a procedure is primarily defined by the size of access incisions, in cardiac surgery at least two forms of invasion can be altered. The trauma of physical access can be changed by the use of smaller incisions that involve less (or no) sternal splitting. The physiologic invasiveness can be altered by performing procedures off pump, that is, without the use of cardiopulmonary bypass and cardioplegic arrest. This at least theoretically modifies the degree of physiologic perturbation produced in performing the intervention.

The face of surgical coronary revascularization has been changed by innovations in both of these areas and inventions like the octopus stabilizer, spreaders for mini-thoracotomy approaches, devices for local coronary artery occlusion and shunting, the CO_2 mister-blower, long-shafted thoracoscopic instrumentation, robotic devices, and minimally invasive extracorporeal circulation have led to a completely different appearance of coronary surgery. Because off-pump coronary artery bypass (OPCAB) grafting is covered in Chapter 89, it will not be covered in depth here; rather, this chapter describes techniques of surgical revascularization using access incisions other than conventional median sternotomy, with or without the use of cardiopulmonary bypass. The degree of revascularization possible with each intervention is discussed as well as some of the literature on the clinical outcomes associated with these approaches, with emphasis on robotically assisted approaches.

Minimally Invasive Direct Coronary Bypass

A minimally invasive direct coronary bypass (MIDCAB) operation (also referred to as single-vessel small thoracotomy direct-vision bypass grafting [SVST]) is a procedure using an anterior, medially placed, mini-thoracotomy incision. The incision is used for both direct-vision left internal mammary artery (LIMA) harvest and creation of an anastomosis of the LIMA to a coronary artery.[1] It is performed off pump and requires the use of a stabilizer placed either directly through the operative incision or through a separate port incision.

Because of the limited access to the lateral and posterior surfaces of the beating heart during this procedure, coronary revascularization using MIDCAB is generally limited to the bypass of the left anterior descending (LAD) artery or its diagonal branches. To allow for takedown of the internal mammary artery (IMA) through this incision, specially designed retractors are available. (In the early development of MIDCAB, rib disarticulation or removal of cartilage was carried out.) The MIDCAB, therefore, essentially amounts to a one-vessel OPCAB to the LAD or its diagonal branches through a small thoracotomy.

Having originally been described in 1965 by Kolessov, the MIDCAB procedure was reintroduced in the mid-1990s. The procedure was adopted at many U.S. and European centers after its reintroduction, and many early series demonstrated decreased hospital lengths of stay relative to conventional CABG, decreased utilization of resources, earlier return to full activity, reduced transfusion requirement, and excellent graft patency.[2] When compared to a single-vessel OPCAB, data are limited; however, small studies suggested that durations of mechanical ventilation and total hospital stay were decreased with use of MIDCAB.[3]

The main downside of this procedure is challenging early postoperative control of pain caused by the chest wall retraction involved in LIMA harvest.[1] Even with the smaller incision, the difficulties with postoperative pain may have contributed to the decrease in popularity of this procedure after its original introduction. Nevertheless, several centers skilled in this approach continue to perform it in large numbers and report excellent results.

For example, in one recent European report, Holzhey and coworkers reported their experience with 1768 MIDCABs between 1996 and 2009.[4] This Leipzig group reported a 1.75% rate of conversion to sternotomy, 0.8% postoperative mortality rate, and 0.4% perioperative stroke rate. Routine postoperative angiograms showed 95.5% early graft patency, with a short-term target vessel reintervention rate of 3.3%. MIDCAB procedures have also been used successfully in the reoperative arena[5] with some evidence of decreased operative mortality. The general acceptance of MIDCAB is low, and despite initial enthusiasm, several centers have abandoned the procedure. The significant learning curve for an individual surgeon to reach stable results (additionally requiring continuously high case loads to sustain surgeon skill[4,6]) and less than optimal graft patency at some centers are probably the main causes for this phenomenon.

Preoperative Considerations

All patients should undergo the complete preoperative workup that is standard for open CABG. The patient's body mass index and body habitus are of worthy of note; obesity is a relative contraindication for MIDCAB because the pressure placed on the wound edges by the retractor during LIMA takedown may cause tissue necrosis and predispose the patient to wound infection. For similar reasons, female patients with large breasts may be at increased risk for wound-related complications.[7] With regard to preoperative imaging, preoperative assessment of heart position relative to the interspaces on chest x-ray may be helpful in the planning of the access incision.

Technical Details

The patient is positioned supine with the left side up. Optimally single-lung ventilation is used; however, this is not absolutely necessary. If single-lung ventilation is not used, reduction in tidal volume and packing of the lung away from the field can be used. A left submammary incision in the mid-clavicular line in either the fourth or fifth interspace is used[8,9] (Fig. 90-1). Review of the heart position relative to the interspaces on preoperative chest x-ray can be helpful in the planning of the access incision. It should be noted that the incision is the lower limit of LIMA takedown; the chest wall caudal to the incision cannot be visualized. Therefore, some physicians preferentially take the fourth interspace approach to obtain maximal conduit length.[8] This consideration is important in the case of a distal LAD lesion. Some reports have described extensions of the LIMA by a segment of an

robotic endostabilizer brought in through a subcostal port inserted two fingerbreadths left lateral to the xiphoid angle. This subcostal port is docked to the fourth arm of the robotic system.

The endostabilizer can be used for exposure of the circumflex coronary artery system. The operator should steer the endostabilizer gently over the left ventricle. The lateral wall can be lifted and the obtuse marginal branches accessed. In BH-TECAB, this maneuver can lead to hemodynamic compromise and ischemic changes. A supportive cardiopulmonary bypass run should be used to obviate this problem.

The right coronary artery system may also be accessed from the patient's left side. In this case, the endostabilizer is inserted through the left instrument port (change to a 12-mm port is necessary) and the left robotic instrument is inserted through the subcostal port. The acute margin can be lifted so that the posterior descending artery and the posterolateral branch are easily visible and accessible for anastomosis. It should be noted that thus far, this technique has been performed only on the arrested heart. It is important to take care not to injure the right ventricular epimyocardium with the endostabilizer during these maneuvers.

Once the target coronary artery is properly located and exposed, a robotic DeBakey forceps on the left and robotic Pott scissors on the right are used to incise the epicardium. At first, this can be challenging because of the lack of tactile feedback that is part and parcel to robotic work, and care must be used.

The target vessel is then incised using robotic DeBakey forceps on the left and robotic lancet beaver knife on the right, and the arteriotomy is extended with a robotic Pott's scissors (Fig. 90-6). The LIMA is prepared (Fig. 90-7). Bilateral robotic black diamond microforceps are used as needle drivers, and a 7-cm 7-0 double-armed polypropylene suture is used as suturing material. The first stitch is inside-out on the coronary artery, forming the first bite of the first stitch of the back wall of the anastomosis close to the toe. This needle is then "parked" at a distance from the anastomosis in the epicardium, and the anastomosis is continued with the other arm of the stitch, suturing the whole back wall going inside-out on the graft and outside-in on the target vessel (Fig. 90-8). The first three stitches are placed, and the graft is brought toward the coronary artery wall in typical parachute technique. The operator pulls gently on both suture ends frequently to ensure adequate suture tension. Suturing then continues around the heel of the anastomosis, again suturing the graft inside-out and the target vessel in an outside-in fashion (Fig. 90-9). The needle is then parked in the epicardium and the previously used needle is used to suture the toe and rest of the anterior wall of the anastomosis (Fig. 90-10).

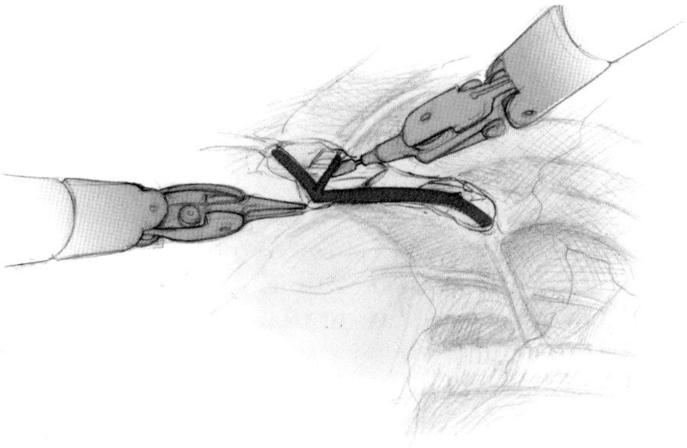

FIGURE 90-6 ■ Robotic left internal mammary artery (LIMA) takedown. (Reprinted with the permission of the Cleveland Clinic Center for Medical Art & Photography © 2014. All rights reserved.)

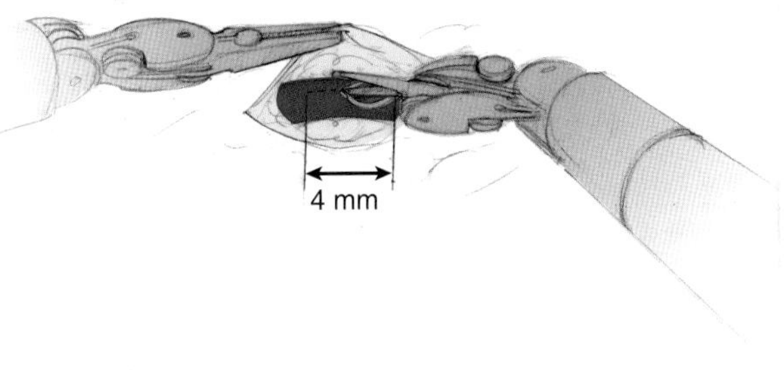

FIGURE 90-7 ■ Exposure of the left anterior descending artery and completion of a 4-mm arteriotomy. (Reprinted with the permission of the Cleveland Clinic Center for Medical Art & Photography © 2014. All rights reserved.)

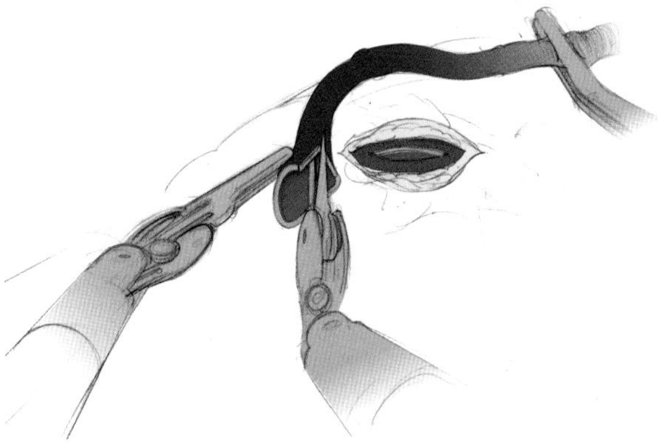

FIGURE 90-8 ■ Preparation of the conduit for grafting. (Reprinted with the permission of the Cleveland Clinic Center for Medical Art & Photography © 2014. All rights reserved.)

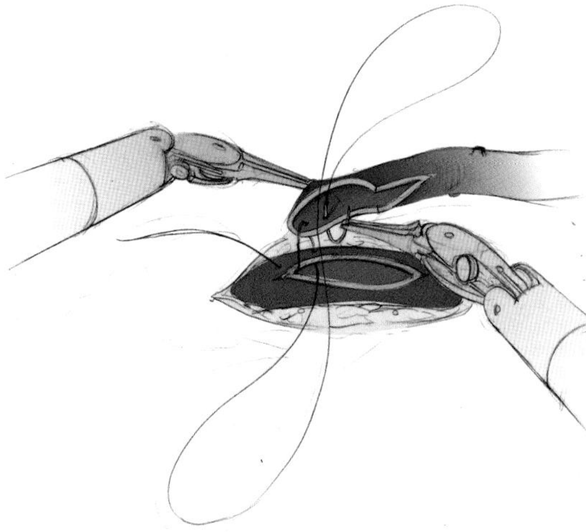

FIGURE 90-9 ■ Technique of anastomosis starting at the "toe." Note inside-out bites on both the coronary artery and the conduit. (Reprinted with the permission of the Cleveland Clinic Center for Medical Art & Photography © 2014. All rights reserved.)

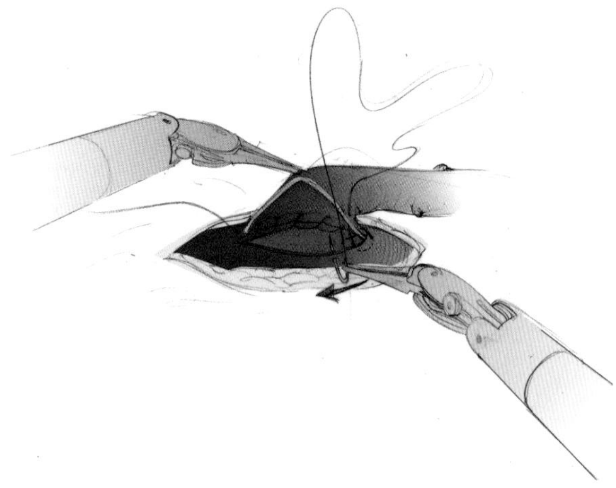

FIGURE 90-10 ■ Progression of totally endoscopic coronary artery bypass (TECAB) anastomosis. Note completion of the "heel" and the direction of suturing. (Reprinted with the permission of the Cleveland Clinic Center for Medical Art & Photography © 2014. All rights reserved.)

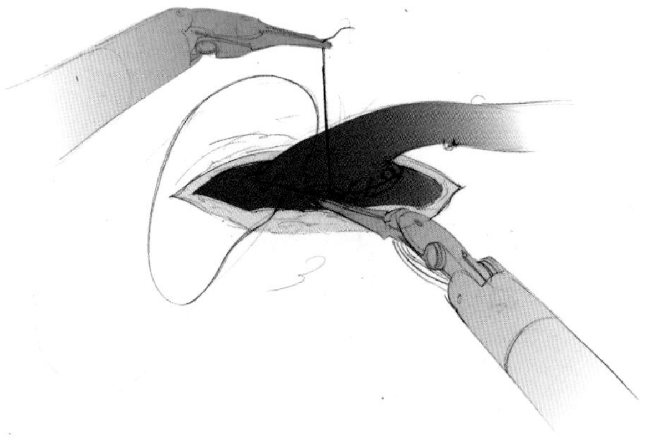

FIGURE 90-11 ■ Completed anastomosis. Note last few bites using the first needle that had previously been "parked." (Reprinted with the permission of the Cleveland Clinic Center for Medical Art & Photography © 2014. All rights reserved.)

Points on Anastomotic Creation in Arrested Heart TECAB

The coronary artery should be incised with antegrade cardioplegia running to fill the vessel and reduce the risk of back wall injury. Use of Silastic vessel occluding loops can be very helpful in cases of target vessel backflow that prevents a clear view of the anastomotic interior. Gentle probing maneuvers at the toe and heel before completion of the anastomosis can be performed safely (Fig. 90-11). All foreign material should be removed from the chest before the aortic endoballoon is deflated. The heart can become hyperdynamic later, and these maneuvers will be difficult.

Points on Anastomotic Creation in Beating Heart TECAB

Vessel-occluding Silastic tapes should be placed both proximally and distally to the anastomotic site although usually only the proximal one needs to be occluded. An intraluminal shunt is then inserted into the distal target vessel and advanced into the proximal target vessel. The general suturing pattern is the same as in AH-TECAB; however, all stitches have to be carried out with an extra degree of gentleness to avoid injury to the target vessel wall. The magnified bouncing operative field is challenging until experience has been gained by the surgeon.

Multivessel TECAB

Multivessel TECAB may be achieved using bilateral in situ mammary artery grafts, sequential grafting, or Y-grafts constructed with the contralateral IMA or radial artery. Use of an endoscopically harvested vein graft with proximal anastomosis creation to the left axillary artery has been described.[30]

Post-Anastomosis Procedures

After completion of the anastomosis, the bulldog clamp on the graft is removed and the anastomosis is inspected. In the robotic setting with high magnification, repair sutures can be placed with excellent visualization if needed. The endostabilizer is removed from the chest and an endoscopic transit time flow probe is brought in for intraoperative flow measurements. Once adequate pump function without signs of myocardial ischemia is ensured, protamine is administered. A tracheal suction tube is brought in through the parasternal assistance port, and residual blood is evacuated from the pleural space. The thoracic cavity is thoroughly inspected and hemostasis is obtained. The robotic system is undocked but all ports are left in place, to be removed under direct videoscopic vision tableside. A chest tube is inserted through the camera porthole with the left lung inflated so as to avoid injuries to the graft during tube insertion.

Postoperative Considerations

Postoperative treatment after TECAB follows the general principles applied in open coronary bypass surgery. Some specifics, however, need to be taken into consideration. Currently no temporary pacing wires that can be placed endoscopically exist; other methods of temporary pacing (e.g., endovenous or transthoracic) are used if necessary. Special attention (neurovascular checks) should be paid to peripheral pulses following cannulation in AH-TECAB. Because of double-lumen tube intubation and single-lung ventilation, respiratory compromise can occur, and the postoperative chest x-ray may show increased rates of atelectasis compared with open surgery and is to be expected. The camera port site is usually the most painful site until the chest tube is removed, and additional pain control is necessary until that time. No sternal precautions are required. In the case of BH-TECAB, we recommend initiation of both aspirin and clopidogrel 6 hours following surgery (or once chest tube drainage is minimal), in keeping with the data suggesting that the use of dual antiplatelet therapy reduces the risk of perioperative myocardial infarction and graft occlusion in off-pump revascularization procedures.[16]

HYBRID CORONARY REVASCULARIZATION

Introduction and Definition

Hybrid coronary revascularization (HCR) combines surgical and catheter-based therapies for the treatment of coronary artery disease. Usually, a LIMA graft to the LAD is placed in concert with PCI of non-LAD targets. Generally, the LIMA to LAD graft is performed using a minimally invasive technique (e.g., MIDCAB or TECAB, described in the earlier sections of this chapter). The hybrid concept can be extended to the treatment of combined coronary and valve diseases, such as a minimally invasive valve surgical procedure combined with PCI to coronary lesions with the intention, for example, of converting a high-risk valve/CABG into a lower risk minimally invasive valve procedure, but these applications are not discussed here.

Rationale and Background

The hybrid approach attempts to "bring the best of two worlds" of cardiac surgery and interventional cardiology together by combining the most effective treatment strategies from the two disciplines for the treatment of multivessel coronary artery disease.

It has been well shown that the LIMA to LAD graft is the most effective and durable option for anterior wall revascularization, primarily because of its resistance to thrombosis and atherosclerosis. The LAD supplies the largest area of myocardium (including the anterior wall and septum) of any of the coronary arteries, and the LIMA to LAD graft is known to improve survival, with 5-year patency rates between 92% and 95% and 10-year patency rates between 95% and 98%.[31] Such proof is lacking for PCI of the LAD. On the contrary, PCI with drug-eluting stents (DESs) offers equal if not better revascularization durability compared with vein and radial artery grafts. One-year saphenous vein graft (SVG) failure rates range between 7% and 30%; 40% to 50% of SVGs will fail or become atherosclerotic by 15 years.[31]

With these factors in mind and in the context of the developing minimally invasive surgical procedures (most particularly suited to the LIMA to LAD anastomosis, such as MIDCAB and TECAB), interest in the potential advantages of hybrid approaches grew beginning in the late 1990s and continuing over the first decade of 2000. Angelini and colleagues reported the first series of six patients, treated with a MIDCAB LIMA to LAD and PTCA or PTCA and stent in 1996. A decade later, a multicenter international trial on the feasibility of coronary hybrid procedures showed the basic feasibility of combining robotic TECAB and PCI.[32] Twenty-seven patients requiring double-vessel revascularization were treated with TECAB LIMA-LAD, and PCI to non-LAD targets (bare-metal stent [BMS] or DES). Three-month follow-up angiography showed an excellent LIMA-LAD patency of 96.3% but a lower than expected PCI patency of 66.7%. No deaths or strokes were observed. One patient suffered a perioperative myocardial infarction. The early reintervention rate, primarily as a result of stent failures, was 29.3%.

Technical and Timing Issues of Hybrid Interventions

Hybrid procedures generally involve a MIDCAB or TECAB surgical procedure for creation of the LIMA to LAD anastomosis along with catheter-based PCI intervention(s). The timing of the surgical procedure in relation to the percutaneous intervention has been a subject of some discussion.

By their nature, all hybrid procedures are staged; only the duration of the staging period and the order in which the procedures are performed can be varied. Two-staged hybrid procedures are those in which PCI and CABG are performed in separate operative locations. The two procedures can be separated by hours, days, or weeks. One-stop procedures are performed in one setting, and the procedures are separated by minutes.[33] In a two-stage hybrid procedure, either the surgical procedure or the percutaneous intervention can be performed first. In a one-stop or simultaneous procedure, the surgical intervention is generally performed first.

The advantages and disadvantages of each approach are discussed next. Each has its theoretical relative merits and drawbacks. At present, there are no data to support any of the approaches above the others; clinicians must weigh the relative merits of each strategy in the context of their practice setting and the clinical scenarios they encounter.

Percutaneous Intervention prior to Surgical Intervention

Performing the percutaneous revascularization before surgical revascularization is associated with several potential advantages. First, the revascularization of the non-LAD targets provides collateral circulation and decreases the risk of ischemia if LAD occlusion is used in the beating heart surgical approach. Second, it allows the interventionalist the opportunity for aggressive multivessel revascularization knowing that if a complication occurs or PCI is not successful, a conventional CABG can be performed at a later time. Most patients who are treated with a "PCI first" approach undergo an acute percutaneous intervention of the culprit lesion for acute coronary syndrome, and the LIMA to LAD graft is placed using a less invasive approach at a later time point.

This approach is associated with a number of disadvantages. It necessitates performing PCI in a setting in which no protection is afforded by a LIMA to LAD graft. Also, unless a third procedure (completion angiogram) is performed after the surgical procedure, no mid-term angiographic imaging of the LIMA-LAD graft is afforded by this sequence of procedures. Most important, the risk of stent thrombosis and need for antiplatelet agents following PCI necessitates either performing the minimally invasive surgical revascularization on clopidogrel (which has been associated with a slightly increased risk of bleeding[1]) or maintaining hospital patients on eptifibatide

(Integrilin; Schering-Plough, Kenilworth, NJ) until their surgical intervention.[1,33]

Surgical Intervention prior to Percutaneous Intervention

Performing PCI after LIMA-LAD grafting makes it possible to avoid antiplatelet-related bleeding complications during the surgical procedure; antiplatelet therapy can be started after surgery and continued long term, in keeping with current recommendations following stent implantation. In addition, the percutaneous interventions can be performed with the protection afforded by the surgical revascularization, allowing interventionalists to more safely approach, for example, left main or diagonal bifurcation lesions.[1] A final benefit to this approach is that it allows for the LIMA-LAD anastomosis to be angiographically evaluated at the time of PCI. However, if there is a complication or failure of the PCI, a second, higher risk operation needs to be performed. This should be a rare occurrence, however, because the incidence of emergent CABG following PCI is less than 1%.[1] Given these considerations, most cardiologists and surgeons who perform two-staged hybrid procedures have adopted this strategy.

At present, the optimal duration of time between the two interventions is unclear. Patients should at least be able to tolerate lying flat on the angiography table, which, because of postoperative respiratory compromise, could take several days. It also seems reasonable to delay PCI until the inflammatory milieu that exists immediately after surgery resolves. This usually requires 3 to 5 days, but patients may need 7 to 10 days of mental and physical recovery following surgery. Ideally, PCI would be performed at the index hospitalization so that the patient would not be discharged without being fully revascularized, but economic issues can make this problematic if long postsurgical recovery periods are required.[1]

Simultaneous Procedures

Two-staged procedures involve two teams, logistical challenges, the costs associated with two separate procedures, and possible hospitalization between the procedures. In addition, many patients would simply prefer not to undergo two separate interventions.[33] In centers with hybrid operating rooms where both percutaneous and surgical procedures can be performed, a one-stop procedure can be performed.

In this approach, there is superb monitoring throughout the procedure under general anesthesia, any complications encountered can be resolved in one setting, and a completion angiogram can be done to evaluate the LIMA-LAD graft. Complete revascularization is accomplished before leaving the operating suite, and the patient experiences the emotional and psychological benefit of a complete "fix" in one anesthetic setting.[1] Potential drawbacks include the need for specialized hybrid facilities, increased operative times, and higher cost with inadequate hospital reimbursement. Concerns about performing PCI in the inflammatory milieu created by the surgical bypass have been raised, and bleeding risk remains a concern because full antiplatelet therapy and incomplete (or no) heparin reversal are practiced after the combined procedure. At this point, the data regarding the effect of clopidogrel on bleeding in patients undergoing hybrid procedure are mixed (with some reporting increased bleeding and others reporting no such increase[34-36]), and the effects of protamine reversal on stent patency are unknown.

The timing of PCI related to TECAB in a hybrid procedure was recently investigated by Srivastava and colleagues.[37] The group retrospectively reviewed 238 patients submitted to hybrid treatment over a 10-year period. Most patients (73%) underwent TECAB before PCI. Overall, the authors observed no drastic impact of PCI timing on outcomes, but patients submitted to PCI before or at the same time as TECAB experienced shorter intensive care unit and hospital lengths of stay in comparison with patients who had surgery first. The authors concluded that timing of interventions can be individually tailored to patients' needs.

Current State of Hybrid Revascularization and Recent Information

At the time of this publication, experience with this technique remains limited. No prospective randomized trials on hybrid revascularization have been published, and only three series with triple-digit numbers of patients have been reported.[38]

The small amount of data available on the subject show a low mortality rate (up to 2%) and a low overall morbidity rate (average of ≈4.7% in hospital morbidity across all studies), with shorter hospital and intensive care unit stays than would be expected with conventional CABG.[33] Immediate LIMA to LAD patency rates range from 92% to 100%.[33] With respect to restenosis rates, the data are mixed. Earlier series, which made use of BMSs or angioplasty without stenting, revealed higher 6-month stent restenosis rates so that in the entire experience thus far, these rates range from 2.3% to 23%, with an average of 11% across all of the literature.[33] However, in one series in which only DESs were used in procedures combining MIDCAB and PCI, 97% 1-year patency rates were reported.[36]

In the largest reported series of robotically assisted hybrid coronary interventions on 226 patients with 5-year follow-up, a 1.3% hospital mortality rate, average hospital stay of 6 days, and a 92.9% 5-year survival rate were found. Five-year freedom from major adverse cardiac and cerebral events was 75.2% and reintervention rates were 2.7% with respect to bypass grafts and 14.2% with respect to PCI targets.[38]

Given the limited data available to evaluate hybrid revascularization, as well as the evolving nature of both minimally invasive surgical approaches and percutaneous therapies, generalized statements regarding outcomes are difficult to make at this time. Additional studies are needed to fully evaluate this approach.

REFERENCES

1. DeRose JJ: Current state of integrated "hybrid" coronary revascularization. *Semin Thorac Cardiovasc Surg* 21(3):229–236, 2009.
2. Sellke FW, Chu LM, Cohn WE: Current state of surgical myocardial revascularization. *Circ J* 74(6):1031–1037, 2010.
3. Karpuzoglu OE, Ozay B, Sener T, et al: Comparison of minimally invasive direct coronary artery bypass and off-pump coronary artery bypass in single vessel disease. *Heart Surg Forum* 12(1):E39–E43, 2009.
4. Holzhey DM, Cornely JP, Rastan AJ, et al: Review of a 13-year single-center experience with minimally invasive direct coronary artery bypass as the primary surgical treatment of coronary artery disease. *Heart Surg Forum* 15(2):E61–E68, 2012.
5. Jacobs S, Holzhey D, Walther T, et al: Redo minimally invasive direct coronary artery bypass grafting. *Ann Thorac Surg* 80(4):1336–1339, 2005.
6. Holzhey DM, Jacobs S, Mochalski M, et al: Seven-year follow-up after minimally invasive direct coronary artery bypass: experience with more than 1300 patients. *Ann Thorac Surg* 83(1):108–114, 2007.
7. Reddy RC: Minimally invasive direct coronary artery bypass: technical considerations. *Semin Thorac Cardiovasc Surg* 23(3):216–219, 2011.
8. Itagaki S, Reddy RC: Options for left internal mammary harvest in minimal access coronary surgery. *J Thorac Dis* 5(Suppl 6):S638–S640, 2013.
9. Subramanian VA: Clinical experience with minimally invasive reoperative coronary bypass surgery. *Eur J Cardiothorac Surg* 10(12):1058–1062, discussion 1062–1063, 1996.
10. Calafiore AM, Teodori G, Di Giammarco G, et al: Left internal mammary elongation with inferior epigastric artery in minimally invasive coronary surgery. *Eur J Cardiothorac Surg* 12(3):393–396, discussion 397–398, 1997.
11. Deo SV, Dunlay SM, Shah IK, et al: Dual anti-platelet therapy after coronary artery bypass grafting: is there any benefit? A systematic review and meta-analysis. *J Card Surg* 28(2):109–116, 2013.
12. Vassiliades TA, Jr, Reddy VS, Puskas JD, et al: Long-term results of the endoscopic atraumatic coronary artery bypass. *Ann Thorac Surg* 83(3):979–984, discussion 984–985, 2007.
13. Vassiliades TA, Jr: Technical aids to performing thoracoscopic robotically-assisted internal mammary artery harvesting. *Heart Surg Forum* 5(2):119–124, 2002.
14. Sellke F, Ruel M: *Atlas of cardiac surgical techniques*, Philadelphia, 2010, Elsevier.
15. Hrapkowicz T, Bisleri G: Endoscopic harvesting of the left internal mammary artery. *Ann Cardiothorac Surg* 2(4):565–569, 2013.
16. Currie ME, Romsa J, Fox SA, et al: Long-term angiographic follow-up of robotic-assisted coronary artery revascularization. *Ann Thorac Surg* 93(5):1426–1431, 2012.
17. Weerasinghe A, Bahrami T: Bilateral MIDCAB for triple vessel coronary disease. *Interact Cardiovasc Thorac Surg* 4(6):523–525, 2005.
18. McGinn JT, Jr, Usman S, Lapierre H, et al: Minimally invasive coronary artery bypass grafting: dual-center experience in 450 consecutive patients. *Circulation* 120(11 Suppl):S78–S84, 2009.
19. Guida MC, Pecora G, Bacalao A, et al: Multivessel revascularization on the beating heart by anterolateral left thoracotomy. *Ann Thorac Surg* 81(6):2142–2146, 2006.
20. Lapierre H, Chan V, Ruel M: Off-pump coronary surgery through mini-incisions: is it reasonable? *Curr Opin Cardiol* 21(6):578–583, 2006.
21. Ruel M, Une D, Bonatti J, et al: Minimally invasive coronary artery bypass grafting: is it time for the robot? *Curr Opin Cardiol* 28(6):639–645, 2013.
22. Lapierre H, Chan V, Sohmer B, et al: Minimally invasive coronary artery bypass grafting via a small thoracotomy versus off-pump: a case-matched study. *Eur J Cardiothorac Surg* 40(4):804–810, 2011.
23. Ruel M, Shariff MA, Lapierre H, et al: Results of the minimally invasive coronary artery bypass grafting angiographic patency study. *J Thorac Cardiovasc Surg* 147(1):203–208, 2014.
24. Robicsek F: Robotic cardiac surgery: time told! *J Thorac Cardiovasc Surg* 135(2):243–246, 2008.
25. Modi P, Rodriguez E, Chitwood WR, Jr: Robot-assisted cardiac surgery. *Interact Cardiovasc Thorac Surg* 9(3):500–505, 2009.
26. Martens TP, Argenziano M, Oz MC: New technology for surgical coronary revascularization. *Circulation* 114(6):606–614, 2006.
26a. Loulmet D, Carpentier A, d'Attellis N, et al: Endoscopic coronary artery bypass grafting with the aid of robotic assisted instruments. *J Thorac Cardiovasc Surg* 118:4–10, 1999.
27. Rehman A, Garcia J, Deshpande S, et al: Totally endoscopic coronary artery bypass grafting is feasible in morbidly obese patients. *Heart Surg Forum* 12(3):E134–E136, 2009.
28. Seco M, Edelman JJ, Yan TD, et al: Systematic review of robotic-assisted, totally endoscopic coronary artery bypass grafting. *Ann Cardiothorac Surg* 2(4):408–418, 2013.
29. Bonatti J, Lehr EJ, Schachner T, et al: Robotic total endoscopic double-vessel coronary artery bypass grafting–state of procedure development. *J Thorac Cardiovasc Surg* 144(5):1061–1066, 2012.
30. Bonatti J, Lee JD, Bonaros N, et al: Robotic totally endoscopic multivessel coronary artery bypass grafting: procedure development, challenges, results. *Innovations (Phila)* 7(1):3–8, 2012.
31. Popma JJ, Nathan S, Hagberg RC, et al: Hybrid myocardial revascularization: an integrated approach to coronary revascularization. *Catheter Cardiovasc Interv* 75(Suppl 1):S28–S34, 2010.
32. Katz MR, Van Praet F, de Canniere D, et al: Integrated coronary revascularization: percutaneous coronary intervention plus robotic totally endoscopic coronary artery bypass. *Circulation* 114(1 Suppl):I473–I476, 2006.
33. Byrne JG, Leacche M, Vaughan DE, et al: Hybrid cardiovascular procedures. *JACC Cardiovasc Interv* 1(5):459–468, 2008.
34. Byrne JG, Leacche M, Unic D, et al: Staged initial percutaneous coronary intervention followed by valve surgery ("hybrid approach") for patients with complex coronary and valve disease. *J Am Coll Cardiol* 45(1):14–18, 2005.
35. Bonatti J, Schachner T, Bonaros N, et al: Simultaneous hybrid coronary revascularization using totally endoscopic left internal mammary artery bypass grafting and placement of rapamycin eluting stents in the same interventional session. The COMBINATION pilot study. *Cardiology* 110(2):92–95, 2008.
36. Kon ZN, Brown EN, Tran R, et al: Simultaneous hybrid coronary revascularization reduces postoperative morbidity compared with results from conventional off-pump coronary artery bypass. *J Thorac Cardiovasc Surg* 135(2):367–375, 2008.
37. Srivastava MC, Vesely MR, Lee JD, et al: Robotically assisted hybrid coronary revascularization: does sequence of intervention matter? *Innovations (Phila)* 8(3):177–183, 2013.
38. Bonatti JO, Zimrin D, Lehr EJ, et al: Hybrid coronary revascularization using robotic totally endoscopic surgery: perioperative outcomes and 5-year results. *Ann Thorac Surg* 94(6):1920–1926, discussion 1926, 2012.

CHAPTER 91

Re-do Coronary Artery Bypass Surgery

Bruce W. Lytle

CHAPTER OUTLINE

Reoperations present coronary surgeons with their greatest challenges. Patients undergoing reoperation for bypass grafting are different from those who undergo primary surgery. In addition to the risks of a repeated median sternotomy, their coronary artery and noncardiac atherosclerosis is more advanced, noncardiac comorbidities are more common, ventricular function is more likely to be abnormal, and the vascular pathologic processes that jeopardize myocardium are distinct and varied.[1-4] All these issues present specific technical challenges.

In addition to the technical difficulties presented by reoperations, decision making is not perfectly straightforward. No major randomized trials have studied patients with prior bypass surgery. In only a few situations do observational studies indicate that reoperative coronary surgery improves prognosis.[5] For many patients, percutaneous intervention is an appealing prospect, but unfortunately the results of percutaneous treatment of patients with prior surgery have been suboptimal even in the era of drug-coated stents.[6-8]

The reasons that patients need coronary reoperations have their anatomic bases in an ineffective first operation, bypass graft failure (early or late), progression of atherosclerosis in native coronary arteries, failure of interventional procedures, and combinations of these problems. The relative contributions of these factors have changed with the evolution of bypass surgery and with the evolution of alternative treatments for coronary atherosclerosis. Today, early vein graft failure, although not rare, is rarely an indication for early reoperation. First, percutaneous interventions are usually available to treat symptomatic patients who experience vein graft failure. Second, as long as an internal thoracic artery (ITA) to left anterior descending (LAD) graft is functioning, sufficient indications for early reoperation are rarely present even if other grafts are imperfect. Early reoperations are usually indicated only in the situation of both ITA and vein graft failure. Late reoperations are usually indicated by a combination of progression of native vessel atherosclerosis and vein graft failure, usually based on the occurrence of vein graft atherosclerosis.

The pathologic changes of vein grafts are important, not only as causes of reoperations but also as causes of events associated with medical or interventional treatment.[9,10] Early vein graft occlusion is usually associated with intimal disruption and thrombosis. Within 2 to 3 months of surgery, a proliferative intimal fibroplasia develops in most vein grafts. This concentric, diffuse, cellular lesion becomes more fibrous with time, possibly as an adaptive response to arterialization. It usually does not cause stenosis or occlusion. The most recent data indicate an occlusion rate of 6.2% at 1 year after operation. In that study, the use of statins and beta blockers were associated with a decreased risk of intimal fibroplasia (defined by interventional ultrasound) and graft occlusion.[11] Within a few years of operation, lipid deposition can occur in association with intimal fibroplasia, and the resulting lesion is termed *vein graft atherosclerosis*. The fully developed lesion of vein graft atherosclerosis is different from native vessel atherosclerosis. Vein graft atherosclerosis is superficial, nonencapsulated, diffuse, and concentric. It is an extremely friable lesion and is much more prone to embolization than is native vessel atherosclerosis. In addition, clinical studies appear to show that it is more consistently progressive than is true of native vessel atherosclerosis, as vein graft stenoses caused by vein graft atherosclerosis predict a high level of clinical events. Patients with coronary risk factors such as hyperlipidemia and diabetes appeared to experience an increased incidence of vein graft atherosclerosis and graft failure.[12] There is now evidence that treatment with platelet inhibitors and statins decreases the rate of late vein graft failure. However, even with these measures, vein graft atherosclerosis has not been eliminated.

ITA grafts rarely develop atherosclerosis, and the patency rate of ITA grafts, particularly to the LAD coronary artery, exceeds that of vein grafts.[12] The use of ITA to LAD grafts at primary operations clearly decreases the risk of reoperation during the first 10 postoperative years, and the use of both ITA grafts further decreases the risk of reoperation (Fig. 91-1).[4,13,14] Furthermore, although patent ITA grafts present technical challenges at reoperation, atherosclerotic embolization is not as high a risk as it is for patients with patent but atherosclerotic vein grafts.

For patients undergoing primary bypass surgery, the likelihood of undergoing a reoperation will depend on the length of their life, the severity of the atherogenic diathesis, the effectiveness of the treatment of that diathesis, the details of the primary operation, the alternative therapies available, and the physician's and patient's preferences. A review of patients undergoing primary bypass surgery at the Cleveland Clinic between 1971 and 1974 documented a 25% chance of reoperation by 20 postoperative years.[15] Today we would expect that figure

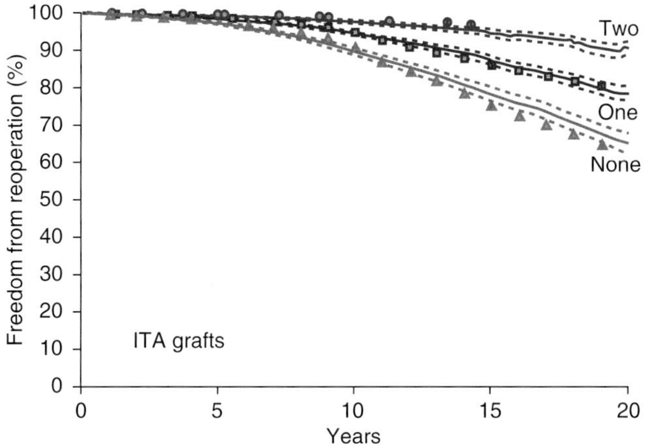

FIGURE 91-1 ■ Predicted freedom from reintervention after primary isolated coronary artery bypass graft stratified by single, double, or no internal thoracic artery (ITA) grafting at primary operation. *Solid lines* represent parametric estimates enclosed within *dashed* 68% confidence limits (±1 SE). (Reprinted with permission from Sabik JF III, Blackstone EH, Gillinov AM, et al: Influence of patient characteristics and arterial grafts on freedom from coronary reoperation. *J Thorac Cardiovasc Surg* 131:90–98, 2006.)

to be much less as the number of isolated coronary reoperations performed has declined. The Society of Thoracic Surgeons database noted 16,091 isolated coronary reoperations reported in 1998, compared with 8820 in 2000 and 5734 in 2009.[16] The reasons for this decline probably include the increased use of ITA grafts at primary operation, better risk factor control producing less progressive vein graft atherosclerosis, and the use of stents to treat vein graft lesions.

INDICATIONS FOR CORONARY REOPERATIONS

The randomized trials of bypass surgery versus medical management or percutaneous coronary intervention did not include patients with previous surgery. Furthermore, patients with previous surgery are extremely heterogeneous, their vascular pathologic processes being multiple and their extent of revascularization not always falling into the categories of single-, double-, and triple-vessel disease. In particular, vein graft atherosclerosis is a more progressive vascular disease, and the presence of vein graft atherosclerosis predicts a particularly unfavorable clinical outcome without repeated surgery. Thus, there is relatively little clarity in terms of the indications for reoperation. Observational studies, however, have provided some important information.

- Early stenoses in vein grafts (<5 years after operation) do not predict unfavorable outcomes if patients are not highly symptomatic.[5,10] Therefore, an early stenosis in a vein graft is not necessarily an indication for either reoperation or reintervention.
- Patients with early stenoses in vein grafts who are highly symptomatic often exhibit marked improvement after reoperation.[5]
- Late (>5 years after operation) stenoses in vein grafts do predict adverse outcomes when patients are managed medically, particularly if the stenotic vein graft subtends the LAD coronary artery or if multiple vein grafts are involved.[5,10]
- Late stenoses in vein grafts are more consistently progressive than native vessel stenoses are.[10]
- Reoperation can improve the survival rate of patients with late stenoses in vein grafts, particularly if that late stenosis involves a vein graft subtending the LAD coronary artery (Fig. 91-2).[5]
- Patients with late stenoses in vein grafts who do have significant symptoms can usually experience improved symptoms after reoperation.[5]
- Patients with a patent and effective ITA-to-LAD graft who are not highly symptomatic have not been shown to have an improved survival rate with reoperation.[5]

As has been true of patients undergoing primary bypass surgery, functional studies could add to the accuracy of identifying patients who are likely to have unfavorable outcomes without reoperation. Patients who demonstrate ischemia and an impaired exercise capacity are at greater risk for death and cardiac events without reoperation than are those with negative or only mildly positive stress test results.[17]

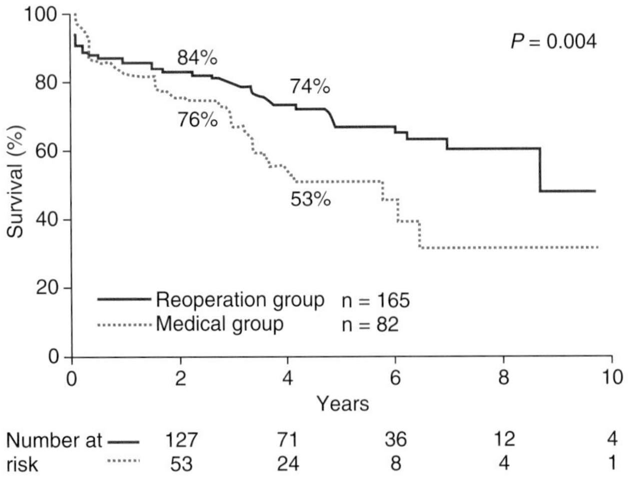

FIGURE 91-2 Comparison of late survival rates for patients with late stenoses of more than 50% in vein grafts subtending the left anterior descending coronary artery shows a distinct survival advantage for patients undergoing reoperation. (Reprinted with permission from Lytle BW, Loop FD, Taylor PC, et al: The effect of coronary reoperation on the survival of patients with stenoses in saphenous vein bypass grafts to coronary arteries. *J Thorac Cardiovasc Surg* 105:605–612, 1993.)

SUMMARY OF CURRENT INDICATIONS FOR TREATMENT OF PATIENTS WITH PREVIOUS BYPASS SURGERY

In the absence of contraindications, all patients with previous bypass surgery should be treated with platelet inhibitors, statin-type drugs, and control of risk factors including hypertension, diabetes, and hyperlipidemia. The indications for more invasive treatment are related to symptom relief and, in some circumstances, improvement of prognosis.

Significant late stenoses in multiple vein grafts or in a vein graft to the LAD coronary artery predict an unfavorable prognosis that can be improved by reoperation; therefore, they constitute a strong indication for repeated surgery. The indications for reoperation in these anatomic situations are particularly strong when they are associated with abnormal left ventricular function, a positive stress test result, and a clear demonstration of myocardium in jeopardy. The presence of multivessel disease jeopardized by native vessel lesions and vein graft disease that includes a proximal LAD lesion also seems to constitute an indication for reoperation for improvement of prognosis. There has not yet been a clear demonstration that reoperation improves the survival rate of patients who have a patent, effective ITA-LAD graft. Severe symptoms of angina combined with severe stenoses in native coronary arteries or grafts subtending areas of viable myocardium constitute good indications for surgery for the purpose of symptom relief.

The availability of percutaneous coronary treatments can be an advantage in the symptomatic treatment of patients with previous bypass surgery. Native vessel disease in particular, when accessible, can be effectively treated with stenting, and in the current era of drug-coated stents, it is often effective. The treatment of vein graft disease with percutaneous intervention has, unfortunately, not been effective in the long term even with the use of drug-coated stents.[8,18-20] However, despite those issues, it is still reasonable to use stenting for treatment of symptomatic vein graft disease when large amounts of myocardium are not jeopardized and symptom relief is the goal. There is no evidence that the treatment of vein graft disease with percutaneous intervention achieves any improvement in prognosis in any situation.

Comparisons of surgical and percutaneous treatments for heterogeneous groups of patients with previous bypass surgery have shown roughly equivalent outcomes. However, these studies have been small in number and have not separated patients into subsets based on the vascular pathologic process needing to be treated and prognostic subgroups based on coronary and vein graft anatomy. Therefore, the relative use of reoperation and percutaneous coronary treatment for the anatomic treatment of patients with previous bypass surgery will depend on multiple factors, including the vascular pathologic process producing the ischemia, the general health of the patient and specific contraindications to surgery, the function of the left ventricle, the area of myocardium in jeopardy, and the experience of the surgical and interventional teams.

TECHNICAL ASPECTS OF CORONARY REOPERATIONS

Reoperations are more difficult than primary operations. Some of that difficulty relates to similar but more extreme pathologic processes that are encountered at reoperation, whereas some problems are unique to reoperations. Potential technical problems during coronary reoperations include sternal reentry, aortic atherosclerosis, atherosclerotic vein grafts, patent arterial bypass grafts, diffuse native coronary artery disease, lack of bypass conduits, locating coronary arteries, and myocardial protection. The most common cause of in-hospital death after coronary reoperation is perioperative myocardial infarction. Those myocardial infarctions are often anatomically based; their causes include injury to bypass grafts, atherosclerotic embolization from vein grafts or from the aorta, myocardial devascularization after graft removal, hypoperfusion through new grafts, incomplete revascularization, early graft occlusion, air embolization, technical error, and inadequate myocardial protection. The planning for reoperation and the intraoperative conduct of the procedure must be designed to avoid these anatomic causes of perioperative myocardial infarction.

PREOPERATIVE ASSESSMENT

The first step in reoperative coronary surgery is a complete coronary angiogram that delineates native coronary and graft anatomy. That step is not as easy as it sounds. If bypass grafts are not demonstrated by a preoperative coronary angiogram, it may be that those grafts are occluded, but it is also possible that the angiographer failed to inject them. A copy of the previous operative note can be important in describing the location of bypass grafts, and it can be helpful to examine old angiograms to identify important coronary arteries and to help understand the previous operative notes. Coronary arteries do not disappear, and a large vessel that was present previously must be accounted for on the current angiogram.

To accomplish symptom relief and improvement of prognosis, there must be a match between graftable coronary arteries and viable myocardium. It is important to establish the state of the myocardium preoperatively by thallium scanning, positron emission tomography, stress echocardiography, or magnetic resonance imaging. Bypass grafts performed to nonviable myocardium do not improve prognosis.

It is important to know which bypass graft conduits will be available. Doppler studies can be used to establish ITA patency, but if the goal of the operation is to use one or both ITAs to bypass important coronary vessels, then it is best to establish their patency with angiography. Venous Doppler studies can be used to assess the presence of greater and lesser saphenous vein grafts, and arterial Doppler studies can assess radial artery status.

Based on studies of intraoperative events, their implication, and the likelihood of rescue once adverse events have occurred, we perform preoperative computed tomographic scanning for all patients undergoing reoperation at the Cleveland Clinic.[21]

MEDIAN STERNOTOMY, CONDUIT PREPARATION, AND CANNULATION

A median sternotomy is the best incision for most coronary reoperations. If computed tomographic scanning demonstrates an increased risk of sternal reentry—those situations including right ventricular enlargement, a patent vein graft to the right coronary artery, an in situ right ITA graft to a left coronary vessel, an in situ left ITA graft that is directly beneath the sternum, aortic enlargement, multiple previous operations, and an injury during a previous sternal incision—we obtain arterial and venous access before reopening the sternotomy (Fig. 91-3). In addition, we prepare the radial artery and saphenous vein segments that are going to be used for bypass grafting before that sternotomy. In difficult situations, cardiopulmonary bypass can be established before a sternotomy is performed, but that is not our usual strategy. We prefer to avoid full heparinization before the dissection and before preparation of the right internal mammary artery. We commonly cut the sternal wires anteriorly but leave them intact posteriorly, and an oscillating saw is used to divide the anterior table of the sternum (see Fig. 91-3). Once that is accomplished, ventilation is stopped, the assistants elevate each side of the sternum with retractors, and the posterior table is divided. We then remove

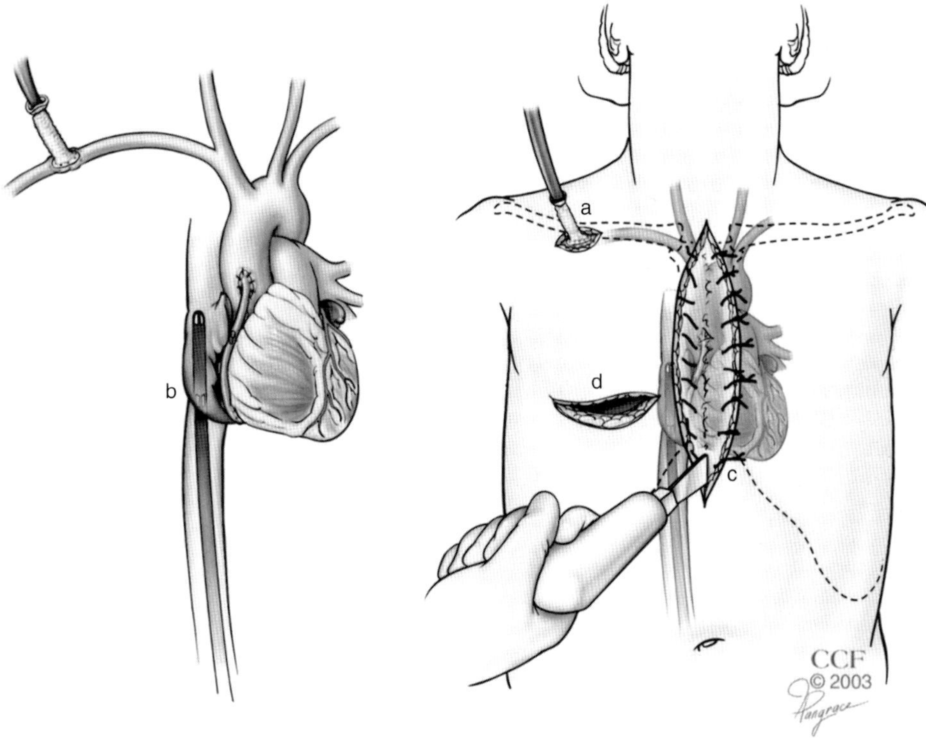

FIGURE 91-3 ■ Strategies for safe sternal reentry during coronary reoperations include *(a)* axillary artery cannulation for arterial access, *(b)* femoral venous cannulation to allow institution of cardiopulmonary bypass and to avoid manipulation of an atherosclerotic saphenous vein graft to the right coronary artery, *(c)* leaving the sternal wires intact posteriorly and using an oscillating saw to reopen the sternum, and *(d)* a small anterior right thoracotomy to allow safe separation of the right ventricle from the sternum. (Reprinted with the permission of the Cleveland Clinic Center for Medical Art & Photography © 2009. All rights reserved.)

the wires once the sternum has been completely divided, because they serve to protect underlying structures. In difficult situations, a small anterolateral right thoracotomy can be performed to facilitate dissection of the heart or the aorta away from the sternum (see Fig. 91-3).

Once the sternum is opened, adhesions are lysed starting at the diaphragmatic level, extending the dissection into the thoracic cavities in a cranial direction. Working from the level of the diaphragm in the cranial direction is the safest approach to avoid graft injury. Superiorly, the innominate vein is freed from the sternum on both sides to prevent a stretch injury. Once the sternum is dissected away from the mediastinal structures, the ITAs are prepared. If there is a patent left ITA graft in place, it is separated from the chest wall. The risk of injury to a patent left ITA graft is established by the location in which the graft is placed at the time of the primary operation. At primary operations, the pericardium should be divided posteriorly and the left ITA is allowed to run posterior into the pericardium. In this location, it is out of danger at reoperation.

Intraoperative echocardiography is used to examine the function of the aortic and mitral valves, intraoperative left ventricular function, and extent of atherosclerosis of the ascending aorta and aortic arch. In the presence of ascending aorta atherosclerosis or lack of room on the ascending aorta, alternative arterial cannulation sites include the axillary artery and the femoral artery. However, for patients undergoing reoperation, the extent of the atherosclerosis really means that the iliofemoral vessels are not ideal for cannulation, and the axillary artery is the preferred site (see Fig. 91-3).

It is important to avoid manipulation of atherosclerotic vein grafts during the dissection of the heart; doing so can result in the embolization of atherosclerotic debris into the distal coronary system and the occurrence of myocardial infarction. This is a specific danger during reoperation, and although a true "no-touch" technique may be difficult to achieve, manipulation of grafts should be minimized.[1,22,23] To avoid manipulation of an atherosclerotic vein graft to the right coronary artery, it is sometimes wise to cannulate the right atrium through the femoral vein (see Fig. 91-3). When atherosclerotic right-sided grafts are absent, we usually use a two-stage venous cannula through the right atrium into the inferior vena cava for venous cannulation.

When a patent left ITA graft is present, we try to isolate it so that it can be occluded with an atraumatic clamp. This is an aid in myocardial protection as long as we can deliver retrograde cardioplegia. When the location of a patent left ITA graft is not clear, the tissue between the aorta and the left lung is isolated by dissecting posteriorly on the medial aspect of the left lung and on the left lateral aspect of the aorta. We then use an atraumatic clamp across that tissue, which usually includes the left ITA graft.

Once arterial and venous cannulation has been accomplished, we can begin cardiopulmonary bypass and place a retrograde coronary sinus cardioplegia cannula through the right atrium into the coronary sinus. The temperature is then cooled to 34° C, and the aorta is cross-clamped and antegrade cardioplegia is given, followed by retrograde cardioplegia. Adequacy of the delivery of retrograde cardioplegia is assessed by the pressure in the coronary sinus, the rate of cooling of the heart, and the degree of distention of the cardiac veins. If retrograde cardioplegia delivery is effective, it is used throughout the rest of the case.[22] The dissection of the left ventricle is accomplished once the heart has been arrested. This strategy leads to an accurate dissection that is atraumatic to the epicardium and decreases the bleeding as well as the amount of manipulation of any atherosclerotic vein grafts. Furthermore, it aids in the identification and isolation of a patent ITA graft. If we are unable to isolate the ITA graft before aortic cross-clamping, we dissect along the diaphragm to the left side of the apical portion of the LAD coronary artery and then continue proximally to the left of the patent ITA graft. That graft will be included in the strip of pericardium, and it can be clamped.

If it is impossible or dangerous to dissect out and control the left ITA graft, we then decrease the systemic temperature usually to 20° C to achieve cardiac arrest and myocardial protection. We believe, however, that this strategy is inferior to being able to occlude the ITA graft and give retrograde cardioplegia. A study comparing these strategies did not show different outcomes although operative mortality rates were 7% to 8% in both groups.[24]

Once the heart has been arrested and dissected out, the coronary vessels that are to be grafted are identified. Again, it is important to have a previous operative note and a clear coronary angiogram to help identify these vessels. Previously constructed bypass grafts can be tracked to their point of insertion, which often helps identify vessels, particularly those that are intramyocardial. Intramyocardial vessels often provide the best sites for anastomoses as they have less atherosclerosis than epicardial vessels.

STENOTIC VEIN GRAFTS AND GRAFTING PATTERNS

The management of atherosclerotic but patent or stenotic vein grafts is a major issue during reoperation. Ideally, any atherosclerotic vein graft should be replaced at a reoperation to prevent atherosclerotic embolization at the time of surgery or late progression and graft failure thereafter. However, graft replacement might not be possible because of the lack of bypass conduits. If patent or stenotic saphenous vein grafts (not totally occluded) are removed at the time of operation, it is important to replace them with grafts of equal size and flow to avoid hypoperfusion.[25] That usually means replacing stenotic vein grafts with other vein grafts. If only arterial grafts are available, it is usually the best idea to add an arterial graft to the coronary artery and leave the vein graft intact. A concern about the second strategy is that persistent flow through the old saphenous vein graft might create enough competitive flow to produce an atretic arterial graft. That usually does not occur if the vein graft has a stenosis of more than 50%.

When arterial grafts are available, they can often be used effectively during reoperation.[1] If the left ITA has not been previously used, it usually functions well as an in situ graft. The right ITA is more difficult to use as an in situ graft at reoperation because of limitations in its length, and in most instances it is better used as a "free" graft with a proximal anastomosis to the aorta, a new left ITA graft, or a previously constructed left ITA graft. If there is a previously constructed left ITA graft that is patent, it has often increased in size and is capable of providing good inflow (Fig. 91-4). The use of a patent left ITA graft for a proximal right ITA graft site allows the length of the right ITA to be maximized. Short segments of the left ITA or other arterial grafts can be used to bridge distal LAD stenoses (see Fig. 91-4).

In constructing proximal anastomoses of arterial grafts to the aorta, we try to use the hood of a new or an old vein graft as the anastomotic site, because a direct arterial graft anastomosis to the thickened reoperative aorta can be difficult.

Alternative arterial bypass grafts, such as the radial artery, the gastroepiploic artery, and the inferior epigastric artery, can also have roles during reoperations. The radial artery is a large vessel that can be used as a single graft from the aorta to almost any coronary artery and sometimes as a sequential graft. Early (<5 years) patency studies show a favorable patency rate for radial artery grafts, but only time will tell their ultimate usefulness. The inferior epigastric artery is not a long vessel, but it can be helpful during reoperations as a composite graft. The gastroepiploic artery as an in situ graft can be useful for grafting the posterior descending branch of the right coronary artery or the distal anterior descending coronary artery.

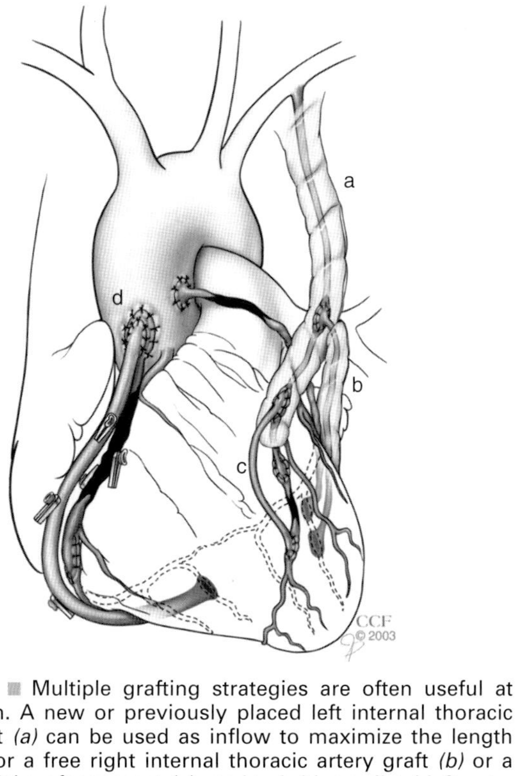

FIGURE 91-4 ■ Multiple grafting strategies are often useful at reoperation. A new or previously placed left internal thoracic artery graft *(a)* can be used as inflow to maximize the length available for a free right internal thoracic artery graft *(b)* or a small arterial graft segment *(c)* used to bridge a distal left anterior descending stenosis. The hood of a previously placed vein graft *(d)* is often the best location for a new arterial free graft or a vein graft. (Reprinted with the permission of the Cleveland Clinic Center for Medical Art & Photography © 2009. All rights reserved.)

DIFFERENTLY INVASIVE STRATEGIES FOR REOPERATIVE CORONARY SURGERY

Although most reoperations are best performed through a median sternotomy because of the need to reach multiple regions of the heart, alternative reoperative strategies can provide an advantage in specific situations. Substantial proportions of primary operations are performed without the use of cardiopulmonary bypass, and this off-pump approach is appropriate for some reoperations. A disadvantage of reoperative off-pump surgery lies in the danger of manipulating patent but atherosclerotic vein grafts during dissection of the heart and causing embolization of atherosclerotic debris into coronary arteries. If all grafts are occluded, this is not a risk.

Target vessel revascularization strategies in which limited areas are approached through alternative incisions and off-pump surgery is performed may be effective because the extensive epicardial dissection that can cause embolization is not needed. An increasingly common operation is to graft the circumflex coronary artery through a left thoracotomy with either a radial artery or saphenous vein graft anastomosed to the descending thoracic aorta or subclavian artery and then to the circumflex artery, usually using an off-pump strategy (Fig. 91-5). This approach avoids the risk of damaging a patent left ITA-LAD graft and avoids cardiopulmonary bypass. The disadvantages of this strategy are that intramyocardial circumflex vessels can be difficult to locate, the descending aorta may be atherosclerotic and a difficult site for a proximal anastomosis, and it makes use of the right ITA difficult. When the left ITA is patent to the LAD coronary artery and there is a major circumflex branch available for grafting, it is usually our intent to use the right

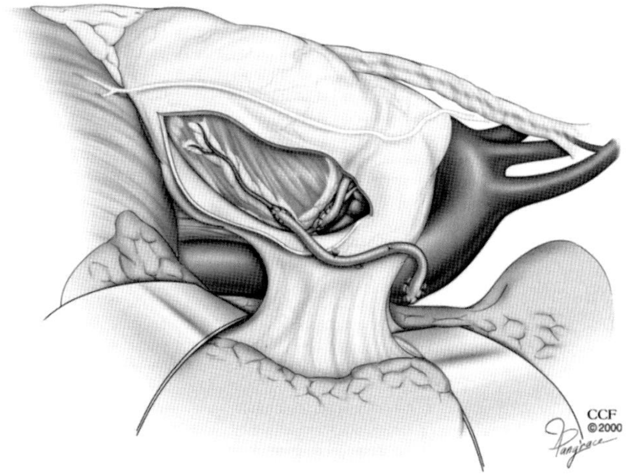

FIGURE 91-5 ■ A left thoracotomy can be used for an off-pump anastomosis of a radial artery or vein graft to the circumflex coronary artery. (Reprinted with the permission of the Cleveland Clinic Center for Medical Art & Photography © 2009. All rights reserved.)

ITA to graft that circumflex vessel, thus maximizing long-term benefit.

The gastroepiploic artery can be used as an in situ graft to graft the posterior descending branch of the right coronary artery through the diaphragm with a small distal sternotomy or transdiaphragmatic approach or the anterior descending coronary artery through a distal sternotomy or small left thoracotomy. The left ITA can be used to graft the anterior descending coronary artery through a small left thoracotomy (minimally invasive direct coronary artery bypass), and the right ITA can be used to graft the anterior descending artery as an in situ graft through a repeated median sternotomy. These strategies can be useful in specific situations in which the goal is limited revascularization. However, most patients who are reoperative candidates need multiple grafts to multiple vessels.

RESULTS OF CORONARY REOPERATIONS

Coronary reoperations have been associated with higher risks of death and in-hospital complications than primary coronary surgery has.[1,3,16,23,26-29] Some of the mortality risk appears to be associated with the technical difficulty of the reoperative situation and some with the higher-risk characteristics of reoperative candidates. Studies from institutions with a high level of experience with reoperation have shown that when patient-related characteristics are adjusted for the reoperative situation itself, risk does not appear to be increased, at least in more recent years.[26-27] On the other hand, studies of broader databases, such as the New York State database, show that reoperation still persists as a specific risk factor in coronary surgery.[3] Coronary reoperations are difficult, and it is possible that patients undergoing these procedures at institutions with a high level of experience have better outcomes and that the specific risks of reoperation can be ameliorated with experience.

A query of the Society of Thoracic Surgeons database, which is probably most reflective of widespread practice, shows a decrease in the mortality risk of coronary reoperations from 6.1% in 1998 (542 deaths of 8820 patients) to 4.6% (261 deaths of 5734 patients) in 2009.[16] It is important to note that the absolute numbers of reoperations have decreased, while the proportion classed as urgent increased during that time interval. It is likely that patient selection and acuity classification changed during that interval. The acuity of the operation has always played a defining role in the prediction of hospital mortality and still does. In the Cleveland Clinic series, the risk of hospital mortality for isolated reoperative bypass surgery was 1.7% in 1998 (5 of 291), 1.5% in 2007 (1 of 67), and 1.5% (22 of 1505) during those years cumulatively, whereas urgent reoperations carried a risk of 3.7% (15 of 401) overall. Thus, in any setting, reoperations in situations of increased acuity generate increased risk.

Other factors that increase the risk of coronary reoperations include advanced age, left ventricular dysfunction, and renal failure. In the past, some of the factors specifically associated with the reoperative situation, including patent ITA grafts and atherosclerotic vein grafts, have been associated with increased risk; however, with the passage of time, the effects of those variables have either decreased or been eliminated. Presumably that has resulted from increased experience and the technical modifications of reoperations, such as the use of retrograde cardioplegia (a factor specifically associated with decreased mortality), minimal manipulation of vein grafts, alternative cannulation sites, and the many other technical modifications used to deal with the reoperative situation.

The late results of reoperation are not as favorable as those after primary procedures. Realistically, reoperations do not make patients as "perfect" as primary operations often do. Few reoperative candidates undergo true complete revascularization, and most have severe native coronary artery disease at the time of their reoperation. It is not surprising, therefore, that anginal symptoms are more common after reoperation than they are after primary bypass surgery. Follow-up of our series of reoperative patients at a mean interval of 72 months after operation showed that 64% of patients were classified as New York Heart Association functional class I, meaning that more than one third had some symptoms.[28] It is true that few patients had severe symptoms, but some angina was present in about one third of patients. Other institutions have also noted a high level of angina recurrence after reoperation.

The late survival rates after reoperation are not as good as those documented after primary surgery. Weintraub and colleagues from Emory University documented a 55% 10-year survival rate and more recently noted diabetes to be a specific risk factor decreasing the late survival rate after both reoperation and percutaneous coronary treatment for patients who have had previous bypass surgery.[2,29] The increased prevalence of diabetes, left ventricular dysfunction, and advanced age in the reoperative population can be expected to correlate with a decrease in late overall survival rates.

MULTIPLE CORONARY REOPERATIONS

Patients with more than one previous bypass operation present incremental problems. A lack of bypass conduits is common, and virtually all patients have highly diffuse native vessel disease. Hospital risks have been increased for patients undergoing third or fourth procedures. In our early experience, we noted an 8% mortality rate of third operations, although more recently the risks for patients younger than 70 years have decreased to 1% to 2%.[30] Likewise, the long-term survival rate is not as favorable, although in our most recent follow-up, 84% of patients with multiple previous operations were alive at 5 years and 66% at 10 years after operation.

COMPLEMENTARY END-STAGE REVASCULARIZATION PROCEDURES

Substantial investigations have been directed toward indirect revascularization strategies that might apply to patients with coronary atherosclerosis so diffuse that neither bypass grafting nor percutaneous coronary treatment will result in complete or effective revascularization. Most patients judged as candidates for these strategies have had previous bypass surgery.

Transmyocardial laser revascularization (TMLR) has been shown with randomized (although not blinded) trials to improve the symptom status of patients receiving only TMLR or TMLR in combination with bypass grafting. We rarely use TMLR in isolation, but we do use it in combination with bypass grafting during reoperation.

THE FUTURE OF CORONARY REOPERATIONS

A huge wave of patients needing coronary reoperations, once feared, has not materialized. However, recurrent ischemic syndromes after bypass surgery are common and are related to time. Despite advances in pharmacologic and interventional therapies for coronary atherosclerosis, many patients still require reoperation, and they present coronary surgeons with their most difficult challenges.

REFERENCES

1. Lytle BW, McElroy D, McCarthy PM, et al: The influence of arterial coronary bypass grafts on the mortality of coronary reoperations. *J Thorac Cardiovasc Surg* 107:675–683, 1994.
2. Cole JH, Jones EL, Craver JM, et al: Outcomes of repeat revascularization in diabetic patients with prior coronary surgery. *J Am Coll Cardiol* 40:1968–1975, 2002.
3. Hannan EL, Wu C, Bennett EV, et al: Risk stratification of in-hospital mortality for coronary artery bypass graft surgery. *J Am Coll Cardiol* 47:661–668, 2006.
4. Sabik JF, III, Blackstone EH, Gillinov AM, et al: Occurrence and risk factors for reintervention after coronary artery bypass grafting. *Circulation* 114(Suppl I):I454–I460, 2006.
5. Lytle BW, Loop FD, Taylor PC, et al: The effect of coronary reoperation on the survival of patients with stenoses in saphenous vein bypass grafts to coronary arteries. *J Thorac Cardiovasc Surg* 105:605–614, 1993.
6. Bourassa MG, Detre KM, Johnston JM, et al, for the Investigators of the NHLBI Dynamic Registry: Effect of prior revascularization on outcome following percutaneous coronary intervention. NHLBI Dynamic Registry. *Eur Heart J* 23:1546–1555, 2002.
7. Brener SJ, Lytle BW, Casserly IP, et al: Predictors of revascularization method and long-term outcome of percutaneous coronary intervention or repeat coronary bypass surgery in patients with multivessel coronary disease and previous coronary bypass surgery. *Eur Heart J* 27:413–418, 2006.
8. Pucelikova T, Mehran R, Kirtane AJ, et al: Short- and long-term outcomes after stent-assisted percutaneous treatment of saphenous vein grafts in the drug-eluting stent era. *Am J Cardiol* 101:63–68, 2008.
9. Bourassa MG, Campeau L, Lesperance J: Changes in grafts and in coronary arteries after coronary bypass surgery. *Cardiovasc Clin* 21:83–100, 1991.
10. Lytle BW, Loop FD, Taylor PC, et al: Vein graft disease: the clinical impact of stenoses in saphenous vein bypass grafts to coronary arteries. *J Thorac Cardiovasc Surg* 103:831–840, 1992.
11. Une D, Kulik A, Voisine P, et al: Correlates of saphenous vein graft hyperplasia and occlusion one year after coronary artery bypass operating: analysis from the CASCADE randomized trial. *Circulation* 128:S213–S218, 2013.
12. Lytle BW, Loop FD, Cosgrove DM, et al: Long-term (5-12 years) serial studies of internal mammary artery and saphenous vein coronary bypass grafts. *J Thorac Cardiovasc Surg* 89:248–258, 1985.
13. Loop FD, Lytle BW, Cosgrove DM, et al: Influence of the internal mammary artery graft on 10-year survival and other cardiac events. *N Engl J Med* 314:1–6, 1986.
14. Lytle BW, Blackstone EH, Loop FD, et al: Two internal thoracic artery grafts are better than one. *J Thorac Cardiovasc Surg* 117:855–872, 1999.
15. Cosgrove DM, Loop FD, Lytle BW, et al: Predictors of reoperation after myocardial revascularization. *J Thorac Cardiovasc Surg* 92:811–821, 1986.
16. Ghanta RK, Kaneko T, Gammie VS, et al: Evolving trends of reoperative coronary artery bypass grafting: an analysis of the Society of Thoracic Surgeons Adult Cardiac Surgery Database. *J Thorac Cardiovasc Surg* 145:364–372, 2013.
17. Lauer MS, Lytle B, Pashkow F, et al: Prediction of death and myocardial infarction by screening exercise-thallium testing after coronary-artery-bypass grafting. *Lancet* 351:615–622, 1998.
18. Ellis SG, Brener SJ, DeLuca S, et al: Late myocardial ischemic events after saphenous vein graft intervention—importance of initially "nonsignificant" vein graft lesions. *Am J Cardiol* 79:1460–1464, 1997.
19. Mehta RH, Honeycutt E, Peterson ED, et al: Impact of internal mammary artery conduit on long-term outcomes after percutaneous intervention of saphenous vein graft. *Circulation* 114(Suppl I):I396–I401, 2006.
20. Brener SJ, Ellis SG, Apperson-Hansen C, et al: Comparison of stenting and balloon angioplasty for narrowings in aortocoronary saphenous vein conduits in place for more than five years. *Am J Cardiol* 79:13–18, 1997.
21. Kamdar AR, Meadows TA, Roselli EE, et al: Multidetector computed tomographic angiography in planning of reoperative cardiothoracic surgery. *Ann Thorac Surg* 85:1239–1246, 2008.
22. Borger MA, Rao V, Weisel RD, et al: Reoperative coronary bypass surgery: effect of patent grafts and retrograde cardioplegia. *J Thorac Cardiovasc Surg* 121:83–90, 2001.
23. Perrault L, Carrier M, Cartier R, et al: Morbidity and mortality of reoperation for coronary artery bypass grafting: significance of atheromatous vein grafts. *Can J Cardiol* 7:427–430, 1991.
24. Smith RL, Ellman PI, Thompson PE, et al: Do you need to clamp a patent left internal thoracic artery—left anterior descending graft is reoperative cardiac surgery? *Ann Thorac Surg* 87:742–747, 2009.
25. Navia D, Cosgrove DM, Lytle BW, et al: Is the internal thoracic artery the conduit of choice to replace a stenotic vein graft? *Ann Thorac Surg* 57:40–44, 1994.
26. Sabik JF, III, Blackstone EH, Houghtaling PL, et al: Is reoperation still a risk factor in coronary artery bypass surgery? *Ann Thorac Surg* 80:1719–1727, 2005.
27. Yau TM, Borger MA, Weisel RD, et al: The changing pattern of reoperative coronary surgery: trends in 1230 consecutive reoperations. *J Thorac Cardiovasc Surg* 120:156–163, 2000.
28. Lytle BW, Loop FD, Cosgrove DM, et al: Fifteen hundred coronary reoperations: results and determinants of early and late survival. *J Thorac Cardiovasc Surg* 93:847–859, 1987.
29. Weintraub WS, Jones EL, Craver JM, et al: In-hospital and long-term outcome after reoperative coronary artery bypass surgery. *Circulation* 92(Suppl II):II50–II57, 1995.
30. Lytle BW, Navia JL, Taylor PC, et al: Third coronary artery bypass operations: risks and costs. *Ann Thorac Surg* 64:1287–1295, 1997.

CHAPTER 92

Ischemic Mitral Regurgitation

Anelechi C. Anyanwu • Javier G. Castillo • Amit Arora • David H. Adams

CHAPTER OUTLINE

Significant advances have been made in the treatment of ischemic cardiomyopathy; however the presence of mitral regurgitation in this population continues to be a significant risk factor for mortality.[1] This chapter addresses the current concepts regarding the pathophysiology, decision making, and treatment of ischemic mitral regurgitation.

DEFINITION

Carpentier's pathophysiologic triad[2] is our preferred approach for defining ischemic mitral regurgitation. Most of the clinical literature on ischemic mitral regurgitation remains difficult to interpret because imprecise definitions are often applied, which leads to marked heterogeneity within and between patient populations. A precise and uniform definition of ischemic mitral regurgitation is critical to the presentation of a relatively homogeneous group of patients for analysis and treatment.[3] A strict definition of ischemic regurgitation according to the pathophysiologic triad typically requires the following:

- The *etiology* in this process is ischemic heart disease. This typically requires demonstration of coronary artery atherosclerosis *and* evidence of prior myocardial infarction with regional or global dysfunction or dilation of the left ventricle.
- The primary *lesion* causing regurgitation seen on echocardiography is tethering of the valve leaflets.
- The primary resulting valve *dysfunction* is mitral regurgitation caused by restriction of leaflet motion, which occurs mainly in systole (Carpentier's type IIIB dysfunction).

Although annular dilation often coexists in chronic ischemic regurgitation, this is usually the secondary, rather than primary, lesion. Ischemic mitral regurgitation with normal unrestricted leaflet motion (Carpentier type I dysfunction) can occur in the setting of a basal infarction, but such cases are infrequent. The infrequently encountered scenario where an infarcted papillary muscle elongates to cause leaflet prolapse (Carpentier type II dysfunction) is a rare form of ischemic mitral regurgitation and is considered briefly at the end of this chapter. When prolapse is seen in patients with ischemic heart disease, the more likely explanation is degenerative, rather than ischemic, etiology. A true type IIIA dysfunction (leaflet restriction in both systole and diastole) is not seen in ischemic mitral regurgitation. If a chronic type II or IIIB dysfunction is seen in a patient with ischemic heart disease, the surgeon must consider nonischemic etiologies: this distinction is important, because the therapy for ischemic mitral regurgitation—a downsized annuloplasty—can be potentially harmful if applied to patients with a type II or IIIA dysfunction if they are misclassified as having ischemic mitral regurgitation (Fig. 92-1).

	Type I	Type II	Type IIIB
	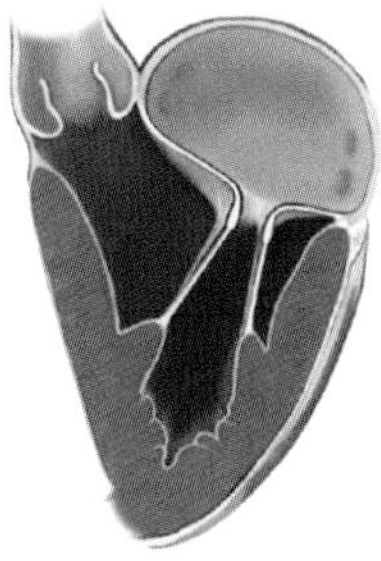	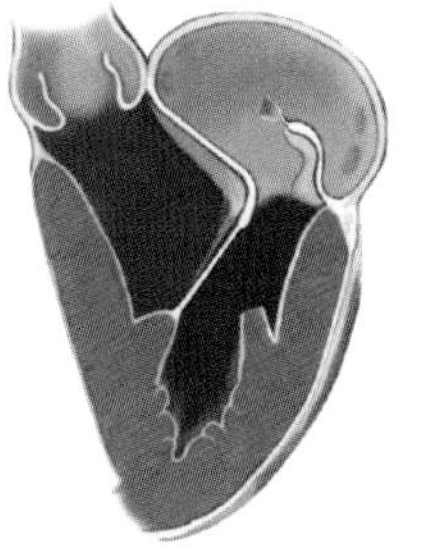	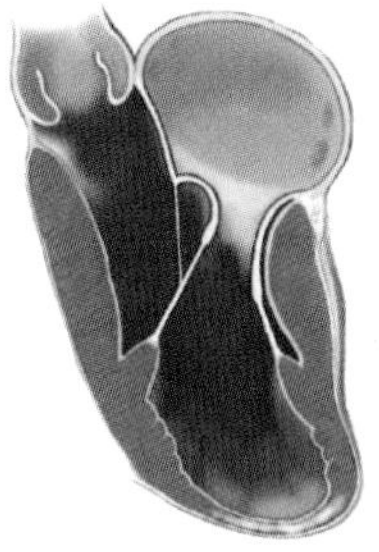
Mechanism	Annular dilation	Leaflet prolapse	Leaflet restriction in systole
Prevalence	Common	Uncommon in acute settings due to early PCI, very rare in chronic scenarios	Most common
Common lesions	Circumferential annular dilation, posterior greater than anterior	Acute papillary muscle rupture (commonly the posterolateral papillary muscle due to single blood supply) or elongation of the papillary muscle due to chronic ischemia	Posterior leaflet restriction and tethering secondary to lateral displacement of the papillary muscles from ventricular remodeling
Surgical techniques	Restrictive ring annuloplasty	Mitral valve replacement Restrictive ring annuloplasty Papillary muscle reattachment (acute) Papillary muscle shortening (chronic) Leaflet resuspension with neochordae	Restrictive rigid ring annuloplasty Mitral valve replacement (severe) Leaflet patch augmentation Chordal cutting (secondary chords) Leaflet resuspension with neochordae (after resection of marginal chords in severe settings) Relocation of papillary muscles

FIGURE 92-1 ■ Carpentier's functional classification in ischemic mitral regurgitation (MR). Type I has normal leaflet motion, and MR is based on annular dilation. Type II dysfunction implies excess leaflet motion with the free edge of the leaflets above the annular plane during systole, which can occur because of papillary muscle rupture (acute infarction) or papillary muscle elongation (chronic). Type IIIB is the most common form of ischemic MR; it results from restricted leaflet motion during systole secondary apical and lateral papillary muscle displacement. *PCI,* Percutaneous coronary intervention.

The majority of patients with ischemic mitral regurgitation have so-called functional ischemic mitral regurgitation from IIIB dysfunction without any leaflet or subvalvular lesions (leaflet tethering occurring because of papillary muscle displacement). Although the term *functional* mitral regurgitation is commonly used to refer to mitral regurgitation without "organic" lesions of the mitral valve, its use should be discouraged, because it is an imprecise term and lacks the mechanistic and therapeutic correlates of the Carpentier functional classification. Furthermore, although it is often assumed that the valve apparatus is normal in functional regurgitation, pathologic studies have shown that these leaflets are thinned out with altered collagen composition compared with autopsy controls.[4] Secondary mitral valve regurgitation is a more appropriate term because it differentiates mitral regurgitation due to secondary ventricular process, from that due to primary pathology of the valve leaflets or subvalvular apparatus.

A documented clinical history of a myocardial infarction (MI) is not mandatory for the diagnosis of ischemic mitral regurgitation. Although a prior MI is almost always present in these patients, it may be silent in many patients, especially in those with diabetes. In addition, the spectrum of ischemic mitral regurgitation likely includes a small number of patients with large areas of ischemic hibernating myocardium (without substantial infarction), causing papillary muscle displacement and type IIIB mitral regurgitation. However, for practical purposes, in this chapter we will assume (unless otherwise stated) that all patients have infarction-induced ventricular remodeling, as true ischemic mitral regurgitation without underlying infarction is not rare.

The optimal way to evaluate ischemic mitral regurgitation is by semiquantitative or quantitative assessment, preferably by transthoracic echocardiography performed while the patient is awake and not actively ischemic. General anesthesia and even the light sedation required for transesophageal echocardiography (TEE) can unload the ventricle and lead to underestimation of the degree of mitral regurgitation.[5] In addition, the potential unloading effects of inotropes, vasodilators, and intra-aortic balloon pump can affect the degree of regurgitation. During the past two decades, state-of-the-art techniques for quantifying mitral regurgitation by echocardiography have emerged, and they are particularly useful for patients with ischemic regurgitation. The recommended method to measure the degree of the mitral regurgitation quantitatively is to calculate the regurgitant volume and the effective regurgitant orifice using the flow-convergence proximal isovelocity surface area method. These calculations along with evaluating for hemodynamic consequences of the regurgitation most accurately define the severity of the mitral regurgitation.[6] The Mayo group has suggested that the thresholds for defining significant mitral regurgitation should be lower (regurgitant volume, ≥30 mL; effective regurgitant orifice area, ≥20 mm^2) in secondary (functional) mitral regurgitation than in primary (organic) mitral regurgitation, given its effect on survival in this group.[7] Cine ventriculography has been superseded by echocardiography for diagnosis and grading of ischemic mitral regurgitation. The absence of mitral regurgitation on ventriculography should not be regarded as sufficient to exclude ischemic mitral regurgitation. This is increasingly important in the current era, as many interventionists have moved toward a low-volume injection technique for ventriculography, which is suboptimal for assessing mitral regurgitation.[8]

CLINICAL PRESENTATION

Ischemic mitral regurgitation has traditionally been characterized as acute or chronic. Rarely, some patients develop acute mitral regurgitation during bouts of ischemia; this type disappears with the revascularization or resolution of the ischemia and is not considered in this chapter. Acute mitral regurgitation as a result of papillary muscle rupture after acute myocardial infarction is discussed at the end of this chapter. The vast majority of patients with ischemic regurgitation have a specific propensity to mitral regurgitation because of effects of prior myocardial infarction, effects that are generally permanent and chronic unless they are ameliorated surgically. In many patients, ischemic mitral regurgitation is asymptomatic and is an incidental finding at echocardiography. When regurgitation is severe or long-standing, or when the degree of accompanying left ventricular dysfunction is severe, patients present with symptoms and signs of heart failure.

Patients with type IIIB ischemic mitral regurgitation typically present with one of two clinical scenarios (Fig. 92-2). The first scenario is a patient with symptomatic multivessel coronary artery disease, with or without associated congestive heart failure symptoms, who is referred for surgical or percutaneous revascularization and who is typically noted to have mild to moderate mitral regurgitation on preoperative or intraoperative imaging. The other scenario is a patient with moderate to severe mitral regurgitation and primarily congestive heart failure symptoms, who is referred for mitral valve surgery and who has significant coronary artery disease. Increasingly, patients in the latter group have undergone prior percutaneous or surgical revascularization. Associated coronary artery disease typically involves more than one vessel, but ischemic mitral regurgitation can also occur in the setting of single-vessel disease.

PATHOPHYSIOLOGY

Normal mitral valve function involves a complex, three-dimensional interaction among the leaflets, the annulus, the subvalvular apparatus, and the left ventricle. The mechanism by which myocardial ischemia and infarction perturb this carefully orchestrated process has been the focus of intensive laboratory investigation. Several groups have carefully analyzed the geometric mechanisms of ischemic mitral regurgitation in large animal models using biplane fluoroscopy, sonomicrometry, and two- and three-dimensional echocardiography. Although these studies have several limitations, they provide significant insight into the pathophysiology of ischemic mitral regurgitation and potential treatment modalities.

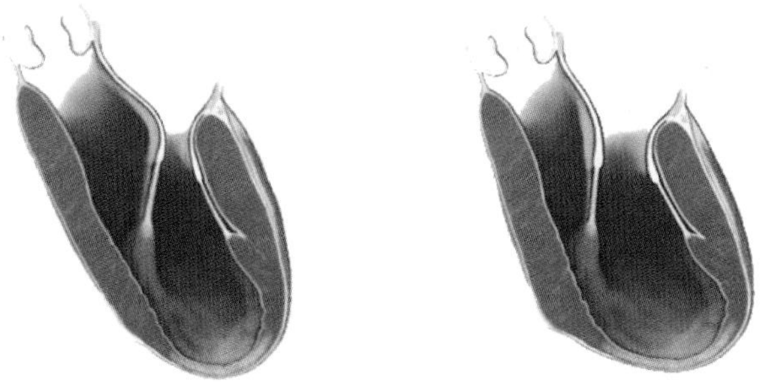

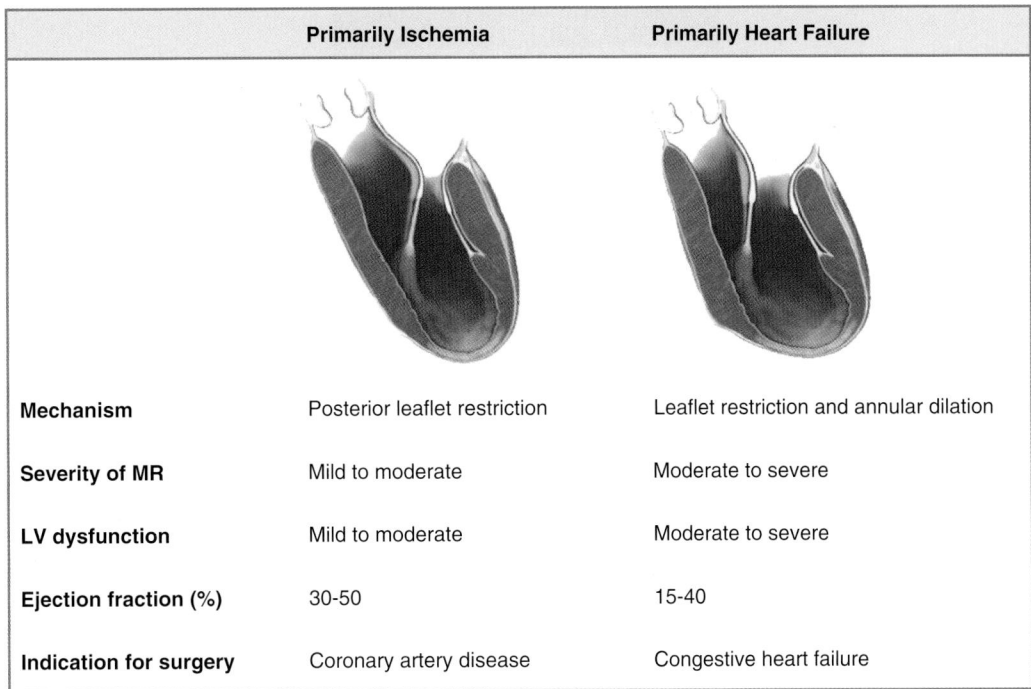

	Primarily Ischemia	Primarily Heart Failure
Mechanism	Posterior leaflet restriction	Leaflet restriction and annular dilation
Severity of MR	Mild to moderate	Moderate to severe
LV dysfunction	Mild to moderate	Moderate to severe
Ejection fraction (%)	30-50	15-40
Indication for surgery	Coronary artery disease	Congestive heart failure

FIGURE 92-2 The two most common and relatively distinct clinical scenarios for patients with ischemic mitral regurgitation. Most patients have primarily ischemic symptoms, and they are noted on evaluation for coronary bypass surgery to have mild to moderate mitral regurgitation. A significant minority, however, primarily have symptoms of congestive heart failure and are noted on evaluation for mitral valve surgery to have significant coronary artery disease. Patients in the latter group tend to have worse left ventricular function. *LV,* Left ventricular; *MR,* mitral regurgitation.

The key pathophysiologic components of types I and IIIB ischemic mitral regurgitation include annular changes (dilation, distortion), subvalvular changes (papillary muscle displacement), and ventricular changes (dilation with increased sphericity, and wall motion abnormalities). Figure 92-3 provides an overview of how these components interact to result in poor leaflet coaptation, which is the final common pathway for all types of mitral regurgitation.

Specific Geometric Abnormalities

Annular

Although annular dilation is a common finding in clinical cases of chronic ischemic mitral regurgitation, the degree of dilation is often not severe and does not necessarily correlate with the degree of mitral regurgitation. Dilation of the annulus causes the leaflets to pull apart and hinders adequate leaflet coaptation. Although the posterior portion of the annulus is far more affected by ventricular or atrial enlargement, the anterior annulus has been shown to dilate as well.[7,9-11] This concept has been demonstrated in both pathologic and imaging studies,[11,12] which showed that although annular dilation is predominant in the region of the posterior commissure, it is often asymmetrically present throughout the annulus as well. Along with dilation, the annulus also flattens, losing its saddle shape, in ischemic mitral disease.[10,12] The degree of annular dilation might not be a fundamental component of ischemic mitral regurgitation pathophysiology. Green and colleagues[8] showed that in an acute sheep model, moderate degrees of annular dilation do not necessarily lead to ischemic mitral regurgitation. Timek and coworkers[13] noted that the mild degrees of annular dilation that they observed during acute occlusion of the left anterior descending or distal left circumflex did not result in ischemic mitral regurgitation. This study, and several others from the same group, noted the critical role of the septolateral (SL) annular dimension in the pathophysiology and treatment of ischemic mitral regurgitation. The SL dimension—also referred to as the anteroposterior (AP) dimension—is the vertical or short axis of the annular ellipse that extends from the middle of the anterior annulus to the middle of the posterior annulus. The horizontal or long axis of the ellipse is referred to as the *commissure-commissure* (CC) dimension. Studies have shown that in the sheep acute ischemia model, an increase in mitral annular area causes mitral regurgitation only to the extent that it increases the SL dimension. Furthermore, these researchers also demonstrated the importance of the SL dimension by using a cinching device to diminish this dimension abolishing ischemic mitral regurgitation in sheep independent of overall annular circumference.[14,15] Although the CC dimension does not usually increase significantly with ischemia,[12-15] it has been shown to change proportionally with the change in the posterior annulus.[9,11,16] This disproportionate posterior annular dilation accounts for the more significant increase in the SL dimension. In severe cases of ischemic mitral regurgitation, the SL dimension can approach the CC dimension, which results in a circular annulus rather than the normal ellipse.

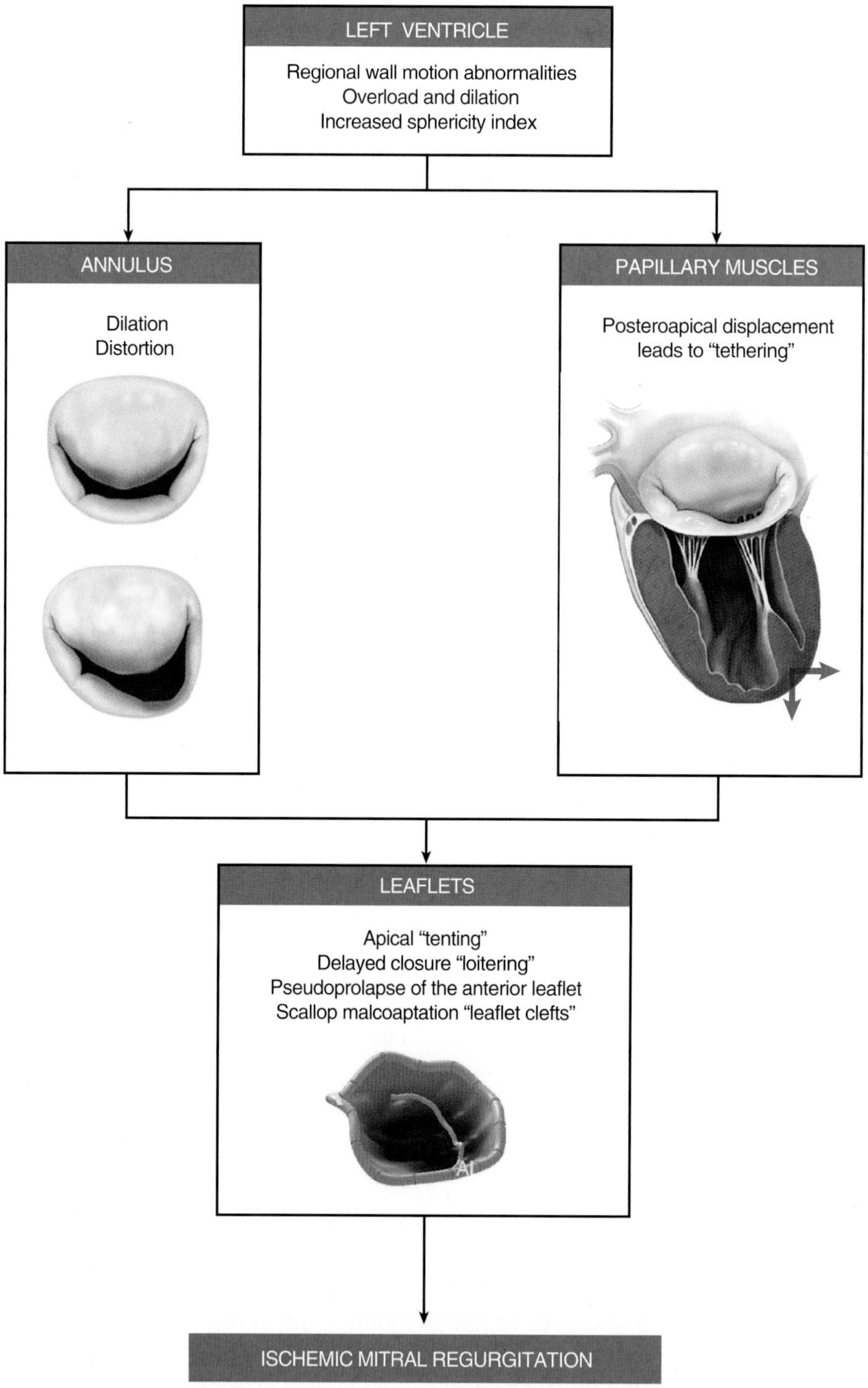

FIGURE 92-3 ■ Pathophysiology of ischemic mitral regurgitation. The interaction among the left ventricle, the papillary muscles, the annulus, and the leaflets leads to poor leaflet coaptation as the final common pathway to mitral regurgitation. The posteroapical displacement of the papillary muscles away from each other *(arrows)* results in ischemic mitral regurgitation.

Subvalvular

Papillary muscle displacement also plays a critical role in the pathophysiology of ischemic mitral regurgitation. It is important to distinguish this from papillary muscle dysfunction (decreased or discoordinated papillary muscle systolic shortening), which had previously been thought to be the primary mechanism for ischemic mitral regurgitation. In fact, papillary muscle dysfunction does not necessarily result in ischemic mitral regurgitation. Timek and coworkers[17] showed that the decreased shortening of one or both papillary muscles did not correlate with ischemic mitral regurgitation in the sheep. On the contrary, Messas and colleagues[18] demonstrated a paradoxical decrease in ischemic mitral regurgitation with papillary muscle dysfunction.

The primary alteration in papillary muscle geometry leading to ischemic mitral regurgitation is papillary muscle displacement. The pattern of displacement is actually fairly complex and cannot simply be described as apical tethering. The papillary muscle tips are displaced away from the midseptal (anterior) annulus (i.e., posterolaterally, apically, and away from each other). The tethering distance has been shown experimentally to correlate with the severity of ischemic mitral regurgitation.[13,17,19] Experimental studies suggest that although displacement of both papillary muscles is probably necessary to induce ischemic mitral regurgitation, displacement of the posteromedial papillary muscle group usually predominates.

Left Ventricular

The initiating insult in ischemic mitral regurgitation is ventricular, specifically myocardial ischemia or infarction with remodeling that leads to regional annular and subvalvular distortion and ultimately poor leaflet coaptation. The independent contribution of global ventricular size and shape to the pathophysiology of ischemic mitral regurgitation is less clear. In an echocardiographic study of 102 patients, Kumanohoso and coworkers[20] showed that in comparison to those with anterior infarctions, patients with inferior infarctions had a higher incidence of ischemic mitral regurgitation despite less severe left ventricular dilation and dysfunction; this was directly attributed to more severe posteromedial papillary muscle tethering in the inferior infarction group. Experimental data, however, suggest that regional left ventricular dysfunction does not lead to ischemic mitral regurgitation without some degree of left ventricular dilation.

It appears that the left ventricular sphericity is more important than the actual ventricular volumes or ejection fraction in the pathophysiology of ischemic mitral regurgitation. Using three-dimensional echocardiography, several groups have shown that the mechanism of regurgitation differs according to the region of infarction. Watanabe and colleagues,[21] for example, found that tethering was more localized and predominant in the medial posterior leaflet in patients with inferior infarction, compared with more widespread tethering of both leaflets in anterior infarction (Fig. 92-4).[21] This observation confirms the critical role of regional ventricular geometry and function in the pathophysiology of ischemic mitral regurgitation and helps to explain why some patients with only mildly impaired global ventricular function have severe ischemic mitral regurgitation. Song and colleagues[22] found that an inferior infarction coexisting with an anterior wall infarct led to a more severe regurgitation, independent of ventricular volume. These observations suggest that geometry of the valve apparatus may be a more important determinant of regurgitation than left ventricular volume or ejection fraction. It is possible, therefore, to have severe ischemic mitral regurgitation in the setting of relatively preserved ventricular function. Tethering is more symmetrical in patients with coexisting inferior and anterior infarction.[22]

Leaflet Dysfunction

Papillary muscle tethering leads to apical tenting of the leaflets (restriction of the motion of the free margins of the leaflets), which prevents the free margins of the leaflets from rising to the plane of the annulus to coapt with one another. Tethering of the secondary chordae can result in an *effet de mouette* deformation of the body of the leaflet, which further impairs coaptation. Leaflet tethering is typically asymmetric in ischemic mitral regurgitation. The posteromedial side of the valve (A3 and P3) has more pronounced restriction when compared with the anterolateral side (A1 and P1).[23,24] Malcoaptation of the scallops of the posterior leaflet from papillary muscle tethering has also been implicated in the pathogenesis of ischemic mitral regurgitation.[25]

THERAPEUTIC TARGETS IN ISCHEMIC MITRAL REGURGITATION

Being essentially a ventricular disease caused by coronary stenosis, with effects on the papillary muscle, cords, and leaflet coaptation, ischemic mitral regurgitation lends itself to several therapeutic targets.

Coronary Artery Disease

Coronary artery revascularization is necessary to recruit any hibernating myocardium and thus improve ventricular function. Revascularization can also help to limit future adverse remodeling resulting from continuing ischemia or new infarction. Revascularization alone is not, however, reliable as sole therapy for ischemic mitral regurgitation as the principal cause of the regurgitation, leaflet tethering caused by regional infarction, cannot generally be reversed by revascularization. Correcting ischemia alone has not been reliable at treating the valvular dysfunction, and leaves patients with residual regurgitation and higher rates of worsening regurgitation.[26,27]

Mitral Annulus

The mitral annulus has been the principal target of surgical therapy for ischemic mitral regurgitation. Bolling and colleagues[28,29] first popularized downsized annuloplasty to address secondary mitral regurgitation owing to cardiomyopathy in the 1990s. In this group's initial experience, flexible band annuloplasty was used; however, recent data support the use of complete rigid or semirigid downsized annuloplasty in ischemic disease.[30-32] The restrictive (or downsized or undersized) annuloplasty partly addresses the pathophysiologic derangements seen in ischemic mitral regurgitation. The annuloplasty corrects circumferential annular dilation, whereas downsizing aims to correct the septolateral displacement and thus reduces the tethering distance. Complete rigid or semirigid rings are preferred, as they ensure that the valve remains fixed in the new reduced SL dimension. Asymmetrical rings may be helpful in addressing the asymmetrical tenting seen in inferior infarction. Incomplete annuloplasty with flexible bands may not adequately reduce the SL dimension.

The differences in tethering between anterior and inferior infarctions raises question as to whether characteristics of annuloplasty rings should differ depending on

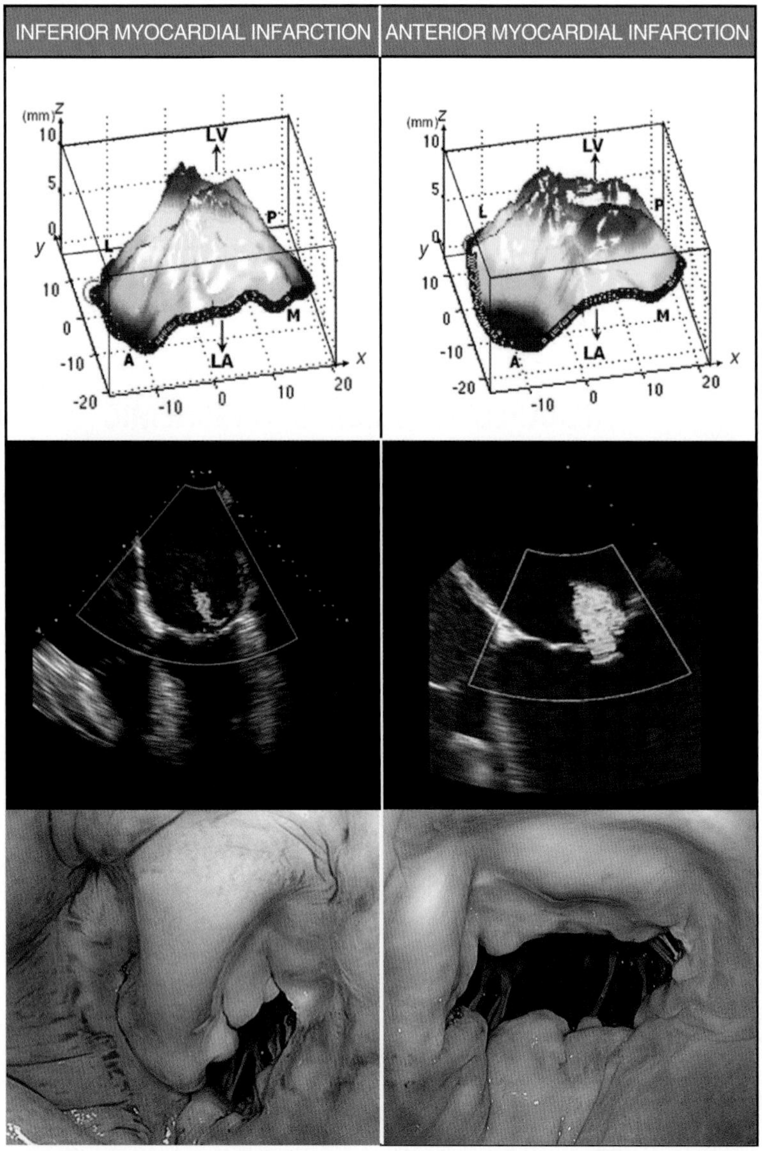

FIGURE 92-4 ■ Tenting and tethering of mitral leaflets into the left ventricle (LV) in patients with ischemic mitral regurgitation. Areas of greatest displacement are shown in *red*. For patients with inferior infarction, tenting of leaflet is more localized with less bulging. For patients with anterior infarction, mitral valve leaflets are widely tethered and bulge toward the LV. The tethered leaflet area is smaller in inferior than in anterior myocardial infarction. *A,* Anterior; *L,* lateral; *LA,* left atrium; *M,* medial; *P,* posterior. (Top panels adapted with permission from Watanabe N, Ogasawara Y, Yamaura Y, et al: Geometric differences of the mitral valve tenting between anterior and inferior myocardial infarction with significant ischemic mitral regurgitation: quantitation by novel software system with transthoracic real-time three-dimensional echocardiography. *J Am Soc Echocardiogr* 19:71–75, 2006.)

location of infarction. Lack of emphasis of the annuloplasty on areas of greatest tethering may be responsible for some recurrences after surgical repair. Better understanding of three-dimensional annular geometry can lead to the development of annuloplasty techniques that are tailored to the individual patient based on specific annular geometry and tenting distribution.

Subvalvular Apparatus

Subvalvular approaches aim to reduce leaflet tethering and thus allow better leaflet coaptation. Two broad approaches exist. First, tethering can be ameliorated by division of secondary chordae (Fig. 92-5).[33] Restrictive primary chords can also be divided and replaced with artificial chordae. Second, the tethering distance between the papillary muscle heads and the annular plane can be reduced by using external or internal devices. Several techniques have been developed that relocate the papillary muscles so that they are closer to the annulus (i.e., less displaced), thereby reducing the leaflet tethering.

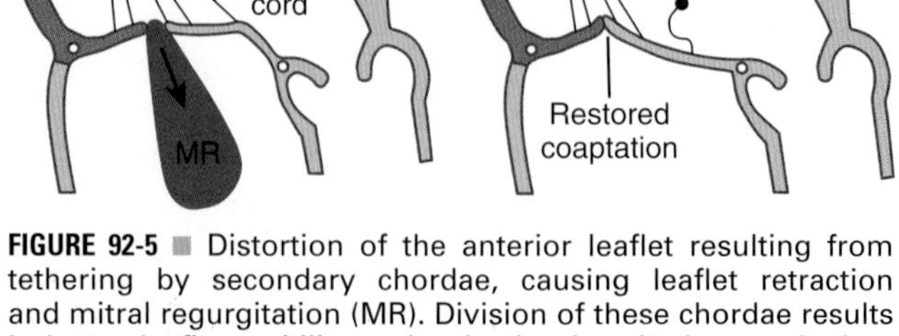

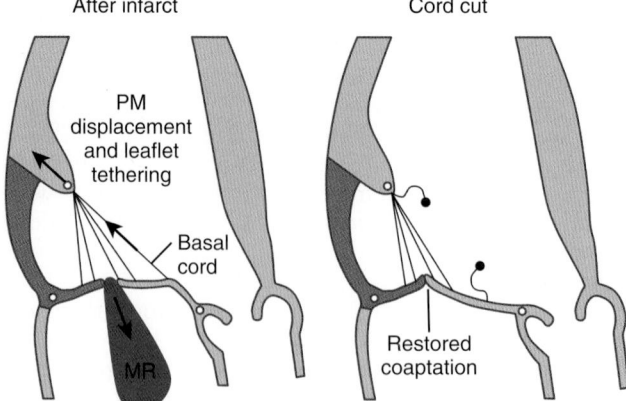

FIGURE 92-5 ■ Distortion of the anterior leaflet resulting from tethering by secondary chordae, causing leaflet retraction and mitral regurgitation (MR). Division of these chordae results in better leaflet mobility and reduction in mitral regurgitation. *PM,* Papillary muscle. (Reprinted with permission from Messas E, Guerrero JL, Handschumacher MD, et al: Chordal cutting: a new therapeutic approach for ischemic mitral regurgitation. *Circulation* 104:1958–1963, 2001.)

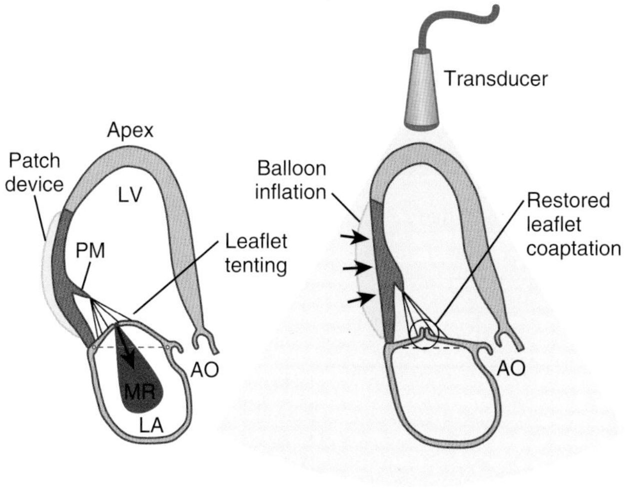

FIGURE 92-6 ■ Patch placement and balloon inflation over infarct region *(black)* to reposition displaced papillary muscle (PM) toward anterior annulus and relieve tethering and mitral regurgitation (MR) under ultrasound guidance in a beating heart. *AO,* Aorta; *LA,* left atrium; *LV,* left ventricle. (Modified with permission from Hung J, Guerrero JL, Handschumacher MD, et al: Reverse ventricular remodeling reduces ischemic mitral regurgitation: echo-guided device application in the beating heart. *Circulation* 106:2594–2600, 2002.)

External devices designed to reduce tethering by displacing infarcted ventricle have also been investigated. Hung and colleagues[34,35] used animal studies to evaluate an external device that works by displacing the infarcted ventricular wall that supported the tethered papillary muscle toward the mitral annulus. Use of this device should reduce tethering and resultant regurgitation (Fig. 92-6).[34,35]

Leaflets

Because the leaflets are not directly involved in the causation of ischemic mitral regurgitation, there is limited scope for surgical intervention on the leaflets. Clefts tend to open up with leaflet tethering, and they may be closed at the time of mitral valve repair. The edge-to-edge leaflet technique has been proposed as an adjunct to annuloplasty,[36] but alone it is not as effective a treatment for ischemic mitral regurgitation compared with annuloplasty.[37] The edge-to-edge approach, however, is increasingly used with the percutaneous clip technique in patients who are not surgical candidates. There have been techniques for patch augmentation of both the anterior and posterior leaflet with acceptable early results; however, they may be technically challenging.[38]

Left Ventricle

Operations to restore left ventricular geometry can reduce papillary muscle displacement and result in reduction of mitral regurgitation. This could be achieved by ventricular remodeling procedures (such as the Dor operation) or by localized plication of a lateral wall infarct. Approaches that halt the process of continued ventricular remodeling can improve durability of ischemic mitral valve repair by limiting further papillary muscle displacement. For example, external ventricular restraint devices wrapped round the ventricle at the time of mitral valve repair have been shown to limit future dilation of the left ventricle[39]; this eliminates one of the key pathophysiologic mechanisms for recurrent regurgitation after mitral annuloplasty (progressive ventricular remodeling). Injection of polymers into infarcted tissue has been explored experimentally by Hung and colleagues,[40] who demonstrated that polymer injection supported the infarcted ventricle and stabilized the papillary muscles, thereby resulting in acute reverse remodeling of the ventricle and reduction in papillary muscle displacement and decrease in mitral regurgitation. Finally, injection of myoblasts or stem cells into infarcted tissue is another potential use of the left ventricle as a target, as this could theoretically reduce mitral regurgitation by restoring ventricular function and therefore reducing tethering.[41]

The Coapsys device (Myocor, Inc., Maple Grove, MN) was an external compression device, placed without cardiopulmonary bypass, with an intracavitary cord that reshapes the left ventricle. By reshaping the ventricle, Coapsys compressed the mitral annulus and subvalvular apparatus and has been shown to decrease ischemic mitral regurgitation in animal studies.[42] The RESTOR-MV trial randomized 149 patients with ischemic mitral regurgitation to CABG and conventional on-pump mitral valve repair or CABG with off-pump Coapsys implantation, and it found better survival and fewer adverse events in the Coapsys arm compared with standard surgical repair.[43] Unfortunately, the RESTOR-MV study was closed prematurely because of corporate financial issues, and the device did not achieve clinical approval, but the study is a useful demonstration that ventricular reshaping may be effective in ischemic mitral regurgitation.

PREOPERATIVE DECISION MAKING

Preoperative decision making in ischemic mitral regurgitation is complex and challenging. The clinical literature is often contradictory, making it difficult to synthesize and distill the information into concrete and practical clinical recommendations. Many factors must be considered in decision making, including the specific clinical scenario, the negative effects of ischemic mitral regurgitation on medium-term survival, the challenge of the intraoperative assessment of mitral regurgitation severity, the effects of coronary artery bypass grafting (CABG) alone on mitral regurgitation severity, the effects of CABG with or without mitral surgery on survival and late functional status, the additional operative risk of mitral valve surgery at the time of CABG, and the choice of valve repair versus replacement. We believe that the cumulative evidence and experience about these various issues are coalescing into a set of principles that can guide modern surgical decision making for the treatment of this disease (Fig. 92-7).

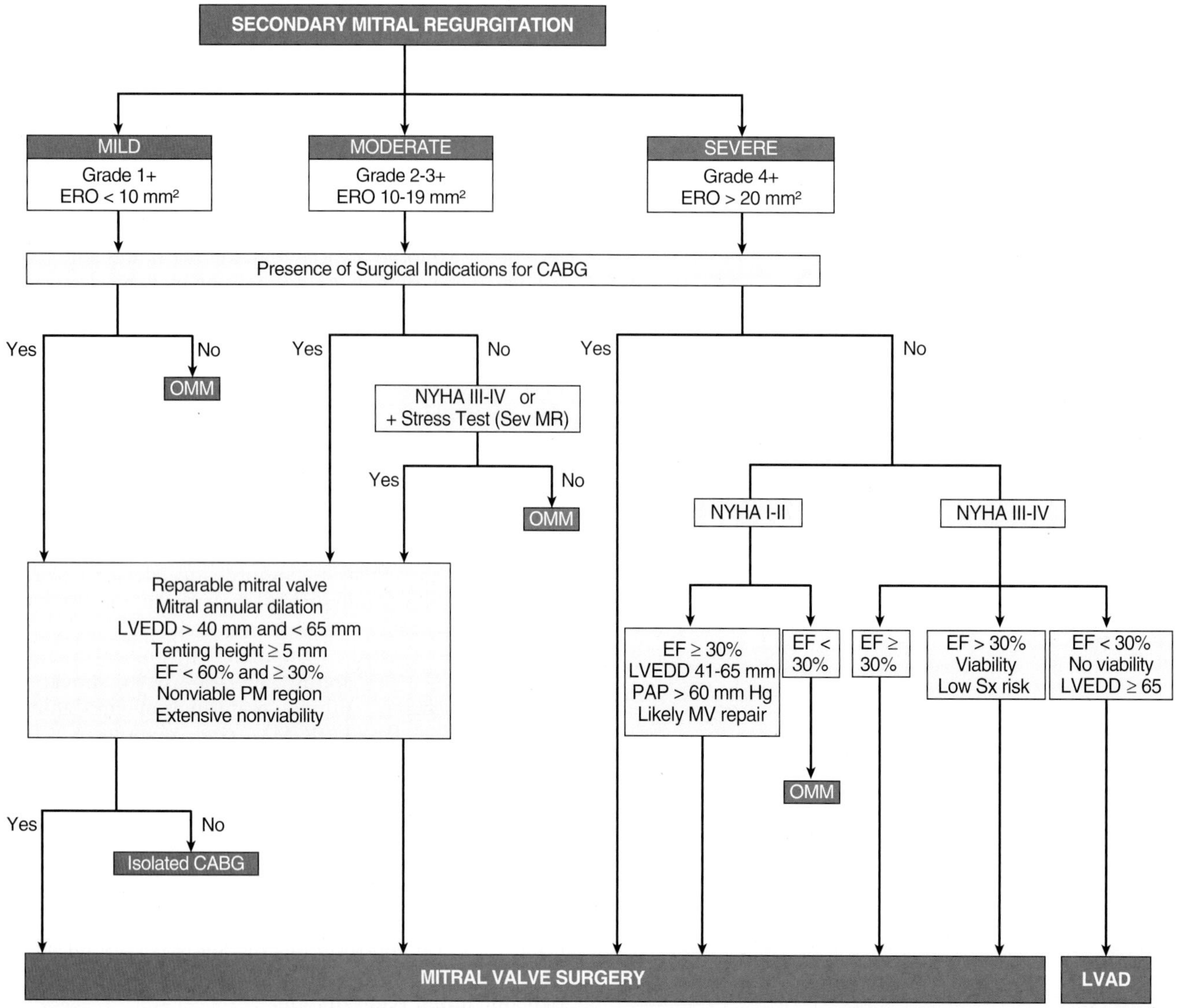

FIGURE 92-7 ■ Decision making algorithm for surgery in patients with secondary mitral regurgitation. *CABG,* Coronary artery bypass grafting; *EF,* ejection fraction; *ERO,* effective regurgitant orifice; *LVAD,* left ventricular assist device; *LVEDD,* left ventricular end-diastolic diameter; *MR,* mitral regurgitation; *NYHA,* New York Heart Association functional class; *OMM,* optimal medical management including cardiac resynchronization therapy; *PAP,* pulmonary artery pressure; *PM,* papillary muscle; *Sx,* surgical. (Modified with permission from Crestanello JA: Surgical approach to mitral regurgitation in chronic heart failure: when is it an option? *Curr Heart Fail Rep* 9:40–50, 2012.)

Decision Making in Specific Clinical Scenarios

Severe Ischemic Mitral Regurgitation with Congestive Heart Failure

Patients with severe mitral regurgitation, symptoms of congestive heart failure, or worsening left ventricular function are referred primarily for mitral valve surgery (as opposed to referred for coronary revascularization). The preoperative coronary angiogram typically shows significant coronary artery disease that may or may not have been symptomatic with angina. Patients may have undergone prior surgical or percutaneous revascularization. These patients typically have evidence of prior myocardial infarction and moderate or severe left ventricular dysfunction. They can be viewed as ischemic cardiomyopathy with associated mitral regurgitation.

It must be stressed that in all these patients the initial therapy is guideline directed heart failure medical management. Medical therapy aims to maintain euvolemia and to reduce cardiac preload and afterload thereby optimizing cardiac performance. In many patients, medical management will result in reduction of severity of regurgitation, with varying degrees of symptom improvement.[44] Medical therapy includes maximally tolerated doses of diuretics, angiotensin converting enzyme inhibitors or angiotensin receptor antagonists, aldosterone antagonists, and beta blockers, especially carvedilol. Cardiac resynchronization therapy (CRT) with biventricular pacing should be used in patients with severe ischemic mitral regurgitation who show evidence of dyssynchrony.

Responders to CRT have been shown to have significant reduction in severity of secondary mitral regurgitation.[45-47] Consideration for mitral valve surgery for severe ischemic regurgitation in the heart failure patient without primary indication for CABG should, therefore, be undertaken only after confirmation that medical therapy is optimal and CRT has been attempted or is not indicated. In general, surgical therapies are not considered, even if regurgitation remains severe on medical therapy, unless symptoms remain severe (New York Heart Association [NYHA] class III or IV). In selected low-risk patients, however, mitral valve surgery can be considered in NYHA II patients where the ventricle is not severely dysfunctional or remodeled with the hope that intervention can delay or prevent further negative remodeling. (Although there is no direct evidence to support this, randomized trials seem to show reverse left ventricular remodeling at 12 months in patients with moderate mitral regurgitation who undergo mitral valve repair.[48])

Patients who remain severely symptomatic (NYHA III or IV) despite medical therapy, and who have an ejection fraction over 30%, should be offered mitral valve surgery as the risk is acceptable (provided no major comorbidity) and patients can expect substantial improvement in symptoms. If the ejection fraction is particularly low (<30%), the decision to operate, in the absence of documented ischemia, is similar to the decision that needs to be made for patients with mitral regurgitation as a result of nonischemic cardiomyopathy. Patients with severe ischemic mitral regurgitation with symptoms of congestive heart failure or worsening left ventricular function (or both) can undergo combined mitral valve surgery and CABG as long as the expected operative morbidity and mortality is not prohibitive. For patients who survive and recover from surgery, the expected benefit of surgery would be better control of heart failure with likely improvement of symptoms. However, there is no clear evidence that life expectancy is improved by mitral valve repair in the setting of left ventricular dysfunction, and indeed some data suggest the contrary.[49] For this reason, advanced therapies for cardiac replacement (transplantation and left ventricular assist device implantation) have been used increasingly as options for treating ischemic mitral regurgitation in the severely dysfunctional and remodeled left ventricle (left ventricular end-diastolic diameter [LVEDD] > 65 mm), particularly where there is limited viability. Young patients with ischemic mitral regurgitation and severe left ventricular dysfunction, with NYHA class III or IV heart failure, should be screened to determine whether they meet indications and criteria for heart transplantation before undertaking mitral valve surgery. Some patients with advanced ischemic cardiomyopathy and ischemic mitral regurgitation, who are not candidates for transplantation, may be suitable for destination left ventricular assist device as an alternative to high risk mitral valve surgery.[50]

An increasingly common scenario is severe mitral regurgitation seen in patients who have undergone prior CABG. Often, this regurgitation had not been addressed at the CABG procedure and has since progressed. These patients present unique challenge because reoperation in the presence of patent coronary bypass grafts may increase operative risk. Thoughtful consideration for appropriate patient selection and operative strategy is warranted.[51] Reoperative surgery to address ischemic mitral regurgitation is generally recommended only when quality of life is greatly impaired, despite optimal medical therapy (NYHA III or IV).

Mild or Moderate Ischemic Mitral Regurgitation in Patients Undergoing Coronary Artery Bypass Grafting

The other common clinical scenario is that of a patient with symptomatic coronary artery disease who is referred for CABG and who is noted to have mild or moderate mitral regurgitation on preoperative or intraoperative echocardiography. Although the patient may have shortness of breath—as an angina equivalent or symptoms or signs of congestive heart failure (sometimes recognized in retrospect)—myocardial ischemia (an acute coronary syndrome or chronic stable angina) usually dominates the clinical picture and is the primary indication for surgical intervention.

Mild mitral regurgitation usually does not need to be addressed at the time of revascularization.[52-54] If there are indications that the mild regurgitation might not run a benign course (e.g., left ventricular enlargement, substantial infarction or nonviability, pulmonary hypertension, excessive leaflet tenting), then it should be managed as moderate regurgitation.

Although most surgeons agree that severe mitral regurgitation should be corrected at the time of CABG, irrespective of the presenting symptoms, the optimal management of moderate ischemic mitral regurgitation remains controversial. One school of thought favors an aggressive repair strategy for moderate regurgitation, and another is more conservative.

Those favoring a conservative approach argue as follows:

1. Revascularizing ischemic areas will improve regional wall motion and reduce the mitral regurgitation.[55,56] This benefit of CABG on ischemic mitral regurgitation is seen most in patients who have viable myocardium in the area of revascularization and in patients who do not have dyssynchrony of the papillary muscles.[57]
2. Some historical studies suggested that performing CABG alone does not have a negative effect on long-term survival or functional status, even if some residual mitral regurgitation persists.[58-60]
3. Mitral valve surgery adds significantly to the operative risk of CABG, with several historical and contemporary series reporting operative mortalities in excess of 10% with combined procedures.[28,47,61-65]
4. Patients with moderate ischemic mitral regurgitation tend to have relatively small left atria, thereby making mitral valve exposure and repair more difficult.[53]
5. Mitral valve replacement, if it is necessary, carries the potential burden of prosthesis-related morbidity.

Many other surgeons, however, advocate the more liberal application of mitral valve surgery in patients with moderate ischemic mitral regurgitation undergoing CABG, arguing the following:

1. Chronic ischemic mitral regurgitation is a dynamic condition that is highly dependent on preload and afterload. The preoperative echocardiogram merely represents a brief snapshot of the severity of mitral regurgitation at the time of the study. The fact that many patients with "moderate" mitral regurgitation, or less, present with symptoms of congestive heart failure or enlarged left atria suggests that they probably have frequent episodes of more severe mitral regurgitation.
2. CABG alone does not correct moderate ischemic mitral regurgitation in many patients, especially those with scarring from myocardial infarction and those with annular and ventricular dilation. Patients who do not have viable or hibernating myocardium are less likely to benefit from revascularization alone.[26,66]
3. Significant residual ischemic mitral regurgitation can, according to several studies, result in late symptoms and decreased long-term survival (discussed later).
4. Mitral annuloplasty is usually technically feasible, and almost always corrects moderate ischemic mitral regurgitation, thereby making mitral valve replacement usually unnecessary (unless the specific preference of the surgeon).[26]
5. The high operative mortality for combined mitral valve surgery and CABG reported in the literature is outdated and reflects a significant number of patients undergoing mitral valve replacement. Mitral valve repair in the modern era can be performed at the time of CABG, with an operative mortality as low as 2% to 4%.[67-70]
6. Leaving significant residual mitral regurgitation exposes the patient to a potential need for reoperative mitral valve surgery in the presence of patent coronary grafts, which carries substantial operative risk.[51]

Two randomized studies have evaluated the role for mitral valve annuloplasty in moderate ischemic mitral regurgitation. Fattouch and colleagues[53] randomized 102 patients to CABG alone or CABG with mitral annuloplasty. This study demonstrated an improvement in NYHA class and a reversal in left ventricular remodeling with the addition of mitral annuloplasty to CABG, but it did not demonstrate a survival advantage.[53] More recently the RIME investigators randomized 73 patients undergoing CABG with moderate ischemic mitral regurgitation to CABG alone or CABG and mitral annuloplasty. Compared with patients who had CABG alone, at 12 months patients who had a concurrent mitral valve annuloplasty had superior functional status measured by both the NYHA class and by peak oxygen consumption. Left ventricular reverse remodeling was also greater in patients who had concurrent mitral valve repair.[48]

The summation of best available evidence is in favor of intervening on moderate degrees of regurgitation at the time of CABG,[71] mainly because of benefit in long-term functional status and left ventricular reverse remodeling. Concurrent mitral annuloplasty should therefore be considered in all patients having coronary artery bypass surgery who have documented moderate or greater mitral regurgitation, unless specific operative or patient-related factors suggest a need for a limited or expeditious operation, or if there is strong basis to believe the mitral regurgitation can reverse with revascularization alone (e.g., good global ventricular function with extensive viability and limited infarction). The recommended surgical intervention for moderate ischemic regurgitation is mitral annuloplasty, as this has been demonstrated in randomized trials to be effective (compared with CABG alone). The efficacy and safety of mitral valve replacement has not been evaluated in the setting of moderate mitral valve regurgitation.

OUTCOMES

There is a growing body of evidence about the negative effects of even modest degrees of ischemic mitral regurgitation on medium-term survival. The modest prognosis of patients with ischemic mitral regurgitation has been documented in a variety of clinical settings, with 3-year survival rates typically being in the range of 50% to 75%, depending on the severity of mitral regurgitation and other patient characteristics.

Effect of Ischemic Mitral Regurgitation on Survival after Myocardial Infarction

Several studies have documented the strong negative effect of mitral regurgitation on survival and occurrence of heart failure after acute myocardial infarction. In their analysis of a subgroup of 727 patients with acute myocardial infarction from the Survival and Ventricular Enlargement (SAVE) trial, Lamas and colleagues[72] found that even mild mitral regurgitation at the time of presentation was an independent predictor of mortality (relative risk, 2.0), and that this effect could not be attributed to differences in left ventricular function. This finding was reaffirmed in a more recent multicenter retrospective review by Rossi and colleagues (Fig. 92-8).[1] Grigioni and coworkers[7] found a direct correlation between survival and the severity of mitral regurgitation using quantitative echocardiography done within 6 weeks of myocardial infarction. Aronson and coworkers[73] showed similar results reporting on 1190 post-acute myocardial infarction patients with ischemic mitral regurgitation. Within 3 years, 30% of those with moderate or severe regurgitation were hospitalized for heart failure, compared with 5% for those without regurgitation (Fig. 92-9). The 3-year mortality was higher in those with moderate or severe regurgitation (35%) when compared to those without regurgitation (8%; hazard ratio, 5.5). Even mild regurgitation was a risk factor for medium-term mortality (hazard ratio, 2.0). The association between ischemic mitral regurgitation after myocardial infarction and increased mortality and heart failure symptoms is independent of left ventricular function.

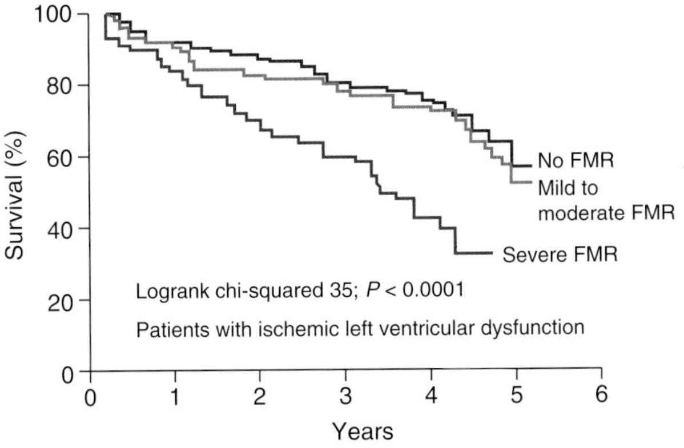

FIGURE 92-8 Midterm effect of functional or secondary mitral regurgitation (FMR) after myocardial infarction. Kaplan-Meier plots showing time to all-cause mortality alone in patients with ischemic left ventricular dysfunction. (Adapted with permission from Rossi A, Dini FL, Faggiano P, et al: Independent prognostic value of functional mitral regurgitation in patients with heart failure. A quantitative analysis of 1256 patients with ischaemic and non-ischaemic dilated cardiomyopathy. *Heart* 97:1675–1680, 2011.)

Effect of Ischemic Mitral Regurgitation on Survival after Percutaneous Coronary Intervention

Pastorius and colleagues[74] examined long-term outcomes in 711 patients with moderate or greater mitral regurgitation at the time of percutaneous coronary intervention (PCI). They found that the presence of moderate or severe mitral regurgitation at that time was associated with a 5-year survival rate of 57%, compared with 97% for those without regurgitation (Fig. 92-10).[74]

Even mild regurgitation was associated with reduced survival (5-year survival rate, 83%). These data corroborate the historical series from Ellis and colleagues,[75] who demonstrated that patients with moderate to severe mitral regurgitation and ejection fraction less than 40% had a 50% mortality at 3 years despite successful PCI. Kang and colleagues examined a prospective database of 185 patients with significant ischemic mitral regurgitation who underwent surgical CABG (with or without mitral annuloplasty) or PCI. This group showed a longer event-free survival with CABG and mitral annuloplasty compared with PCI (with no mitral valve intervention).[76] Other data from nonsurgical series also show that uncorrected regurgitation is associated with a poorer long-term survival.[7] PCI alone should therefore not be considered definitive therapy for patients needing coronary artery disease who have ischemic mitral regurgitation; in patients whose surgical risk is not excessive, the presence of mitral regurgitation should generally be an indication for surgical rather than percutaneous revascularization, provided the surgeon plans to address the mitral insufficiency.

Effect of Ischemic Mitral Regurgitation on Survival after Coronary Artery Bypass Grafting

Two historical studies from the 1980s suggested that preoperative mitral regurgitation is an independent risk factor for late death in patients undergoing CABG.[77,78] Uncorrected mitral regurgitation was an independent risk factor for late death, with a relative risk of 1.5 for each grade of mitral regurgitation. Subsequent studies have demonstrated that CABG alone does not seem to alter the natural history in patients with ischemic mitral regurgitation.[26,79,80] The detrimental effect on survival of residual regurgitation after CABG, however, seems to be small if global left ventricular function is normal; therefore, it is not unreasonable to apply CABG alone in patients with good ventricular function and moderate

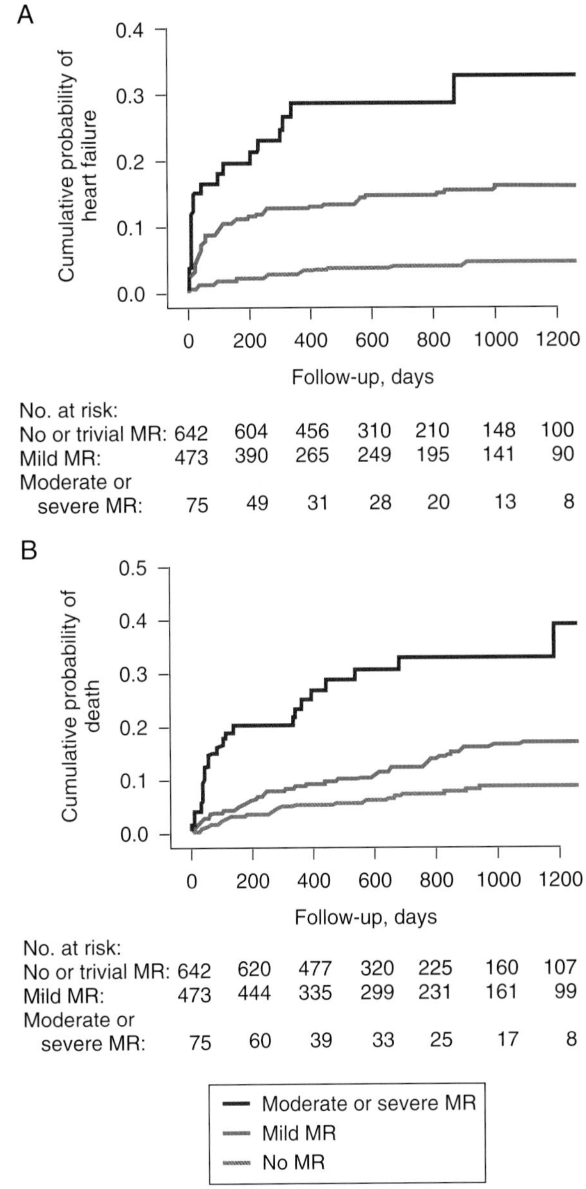

FIGURE 92-9 Short-term effect of ischemic mitral regurgitation (MR) after myocardial infarction. **A,** Cumulative incidence of hospitalization for heart failure treatment. **B,** Cumulative incidence of death. Even patients with mild mitral regurgitation had worse outcomes. (Modified with permission from Aronson D, Goldsher N, Zukermann R, et al: Ischemic mitral regurgitation and risk of heart failure after myocardial infarction. *Arch Intern Med* 166:2362–2368, 2006.)

ischemic regurgitation.[81] However, with depressed left ventricular function, studies consistently demonstrate worse survival and quality of life after CABG alone in patients with regurgitation and a severely depressed ventricular function.[82-85] The best available evidence suggests that coronary artery bypass surgery alone does not eliminate the adverse effects of ischemic mitral regurgitation.[71]

Coronary Artery Bypass Grafting Alone or with Mitral Valve Intervention

Some have suggested[85a] that ischemic mitral regurgitation is merely a marker for severe underlying ischemic heart disease and not a direct cause of late death. The body of evidence supporting a direct effect of ischemic mitral regurgitation on late survival is strong. It is particularly compelling because, in many studies, ischemic mitral regurgitation was a predictor of late mortality independent of the usual risk factors (e.g., age, ejection fraction, functional class), which argues against it simply being a confounding variable.

Although the strong effect of ischemic mitral regurgitation on survival supports mitral valve intervention in many patients with ischemic mitral regurgitation, the decision about whether to intervene in a specific patient can be complex and must take into account multiple factors, including the specific clinical presentation, the presence of comorbid conditions, and the expected operative morbidity and mortality. For purposes of surgical decision making, it is useful to separately consider the two most common clinical scenarios, as noted earlier. Although the detrimental effects of ischemic mitral regurgitation are well known, it is not certain that eliminating mitral regurgitation at the time of CABG improves long-term survival.[81]

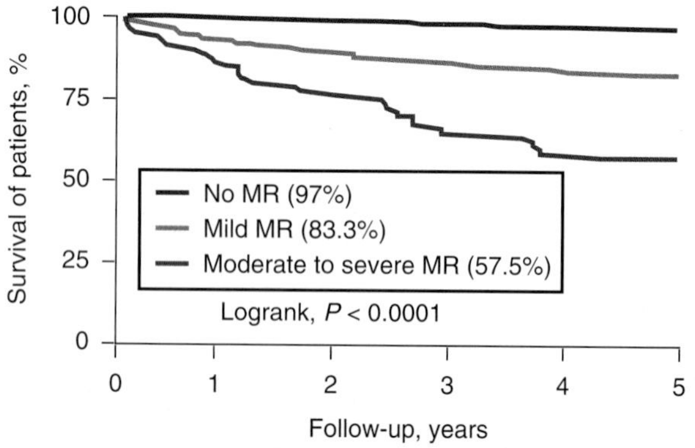

FIGURE 92-10 ■ Influence of severity of mitral regurgitation (MR) on survival after percutaneous coronary revascularization. Presence of moderate or severe MR was associated with substantially poorer 5-year survival. (Reprinted with permission from Pastorius CA, Henry TD, Harris KM: Long-term outcomes of patients with mitral regurgitation undergoing percutaneous coronary intervention. *Am J Cardiol* 100:1218–1223, 2007.)

The severity of mitral regurgitation is of paramount importance when deciding whether to intervene in ischemic mitral regurgitation at the time of CABG. As noted earlier, the evaluation of mitral regurgitation severity should be based on a transthoracic echocardiogram performed in an awake patient. The downgrading of mitral regurgitation by intraoperative TEE has been well documented in the literature. Aklog and colleagues[26] showed that 90% of the patients with moderate mitral regurgitation on preoperative echocardiogram had their mitral regurgitation downgraded to mild or less at intraoperative TEE. In nearly one third of these patients, there was no detectable mitral regurgitation on intraoperative TEE (Fig. 92-11). Bach and coworkers[5] compared preoperative TEE in patients under intravenous conscious sedation with intraoperative TEE in patients under general anesthesia; they noted a significant decrease in the size of the regurgitant jet in patients with "functional" mitral regurgitation, but not in those with flail leaflets. Grewal and colleagues[86] performed a similar study limited to patients with moderate or severe mitral regurgitation. Half of their patients were downgraded at least one grade, and this effect was again limited to those with functional mitral regurgitation.

The mechanism underlying this phenomenon is almost certainly the unloading effect of general anesthesia, which results in arterial vasodilation and venous vasodilation and decreases afterload and preload, respectively. Although the effects of afterload on mitral regurgitation are generally well recognized, the effects of preload are underappreciated and may in fact be more important. Increased preload results in left atrial, left ventricular, and annular dilation (which can increase leaflet separation)

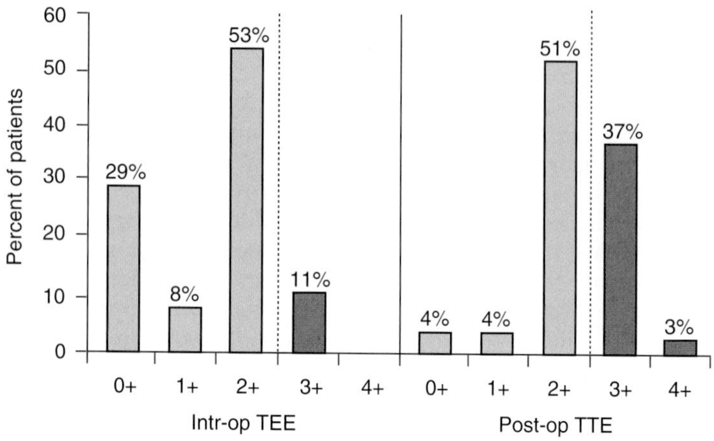

FIGURE 92-11 ■ The effect of coronary artery bypass grafting alone on patients with moderate (3+) ischemic mitral regurgitation (MR). Nearly 90% of patients were downgraded to 2+ MR or less on intraoperative (Intr-op) transesophageal echocardiography (TEE), which indicates that preoperative quantification of MR grade is critical. Although some patients had improvement in MR grade with coronary artery bypass grafting alone, 40% were left with 3 to 4+ MR and only in less than 10% was the MR completely corrected to 0 to 1+. *Post-op,* Postoperative; *TTE,* transthoracic echocardiography. (Adapted with permission from Aklog L, Filsoufi F, Flores KQ: Does coronary artery bypass grafting alone correct moderate ischemic mitral regurgitation? *Circulation* 104: I68–I75, 2001.)

decrease leaflet coaptation and worsen mitral regurgitation severity. Grewal and coworkers[86] documented that decreased end-diastolic and end-systolic volumes in patients under general anesthesia support the role of altered loading conditions in this phenomenon.

Although these findings support careful preoperative echocardiography in patients scheduled for CABG with suspected mitral regurgitation, they do not diminish the importance and utility of intraoperative TEE in this setting.[87] On the contrary, TEE can provide important detailed anatomic information. In addition, intraoperative TEE with provocative testing to increase both preload and afterload may clarify the physiologic importance of the mitral regurgitation and assist with intraoperative decision making if the preoperative assessment is equivocal or unavailable. However, basing the decision not to intervene on (1) a downgraded intraoperative TEE without provocative testing or (2) the residual mitral regurgitation severity on TEE after the bypass graft is performed should be strongly discouraged.

Inadequacy of Coronary Artery Bypass Grafting Alone for Ischemic Mitral Regurgitation

Although earlier data were contradictory, with some studies suggesting that revascularization leads to resolution of ischemic mitral regurgitation[88,89] and others suggesting that regurgitation usually persists or worsens,[90,91] most authorities agree that resolution of mitral regurgitation does not predictably occur after coronary artery bypass surgery. Summation of the current literature seems to suggest that although CABG alone can sometimes decrease mitral regurgitation severity (particularly in patients with mild ischemic mitral regurgitation and poor left ventricular function), revascularization has an inconsistent and relatively weak effect on moderate ischemic mitral regurgitation, leaving many patients with moderate or greater mitral regurgitation.

A landmark study in 2001[26] was notable for challenging the notion that CABG alone was adequate for ischemic mitral regurgitation. One hundred and thirty-six patients with moderate ischemic mitral regurgitation underwent CABG alone. Among the 68 patients who underwent early postoperative transthoracic echocardiography (see Fig. 92-11), 40% showed no improvement and were left with moderate or severe residual mitral regurgitation. Approximately 50% of patients had some improvement and were left with mild mitral regurgitation. Only a few remaining patients (<10%) had significant improvement, with no more than trace (0 to 1+) mitral regurgitation. The study concluded that CABG alone was not the optimal therapy for many patients with moderate ischemic mitral regurgitation. This study was more recently corroborated by two randomized control trials.[10,53]

Although CABG alone might not correct ischemic mitral regurgitation, skeptics have argued that residual mitral regurgitation after CABG alone does not itself have an adverse effect on late functional status or survival. The Emory group followed a cohort of 58 patients undergoing CABG alone for moderate mitral regurgitation between 1977 and 1983, and in their most recent update,[60] 5- and 10-year actuarial survival rates were nearly identical to those of a control group of patients without preoperative mitral regurgitation and who underwent CABG during the same time period. Their patients, however, differ from the patients with typical ischemic mitral regurgitation in most modern series. Specifically, they were relatively young (mean age, 63 years) with normal left ventricular function (mean ejection fraction, 53%) and little or no congestive heart failure (10% in NYHA class III or IV), and nearly a quarter of their patients had nonischemic etiologies such as leaflet prolapse and rheumatic heart disease. However, two large studies from the same era found that mitral regurgitation was an independent risk factor for late death in patients undergoing CABG.[77,78] The authors recommended the more liberal application of concomitant mitral valve repair for moderate and severe mitral regurgitation.

There is limited information in the literature about the late functional status of patients undergoing CABG alone for moderate ischemic mitral regurgitation. The Emory study reported a trend toward more class III and IV angina (29% vs. 6%) and congestive heart failure (14% vs. 6%) as compared with the case-matched controls. These findings suggest that even if the significant rate of residual mitral regurgitation after CABG alone does not result in decreased long-term survival, it can adversely affect long-term functional status and quality of life. Concomitant mitral valve repair may therefore be justified (if it can be performed with relatively low operative risk) to improve long-term functional status independent of effect on survival.

The inadequacy of CABG alone is further supported by various epidemiologic studies that demonstrate that revascularization by either PCI or CABG is still associated with persistent regurgitation and reduced medium-term survival despite revascularization.[7,26,77-80]

Effect of Mitral Valve Surgery on Natural History of Ischemic Mitral Regurgitation

There are no randomized trials comparing CABG alone to CABG and mitral valve surgery in the context of severe ischemic mitral regurgitation (the only trials conducted have been for moderate regurgitation). Studies that have attempted direct comparison of these groups are limited, because undocumented patient and surgical factors, or surgeon preferences and bias, often influence the decision to repair or not repair these valves, making it difficult to directly compare groups.[92] The Cleveland group, using propensity matching to partly balance for selection bias, demonstrated equivalent results with CABG alone compared with CABG and mitral valve repair[81]; that study is, however, of limited applicability to current patient cohorts, as many of the surgical procedures undertaken (notably, use of pericardium and flexible bands) have since been superseded and are no longer recommended by most authorities for treatment of ischemic mitral regurgitation. There are numerous reports in the literature on the outcome of mitral valve repair for ischemic mitral regurgitation. These reports are mixed, with some suggesting it is an effective therapy and others suggesting otherwise. Some reports from the 2000s suggest that mitral valve repair is ineffective for ischemic regurgitation, because many patients were observed to have recurrent regurgitation early after surgery.[93-95] There are, however, flaws in these studies, which we have discussed elsewhere.[3] Notably, the surgical techniques were inconsistent, inadequate, or historical; the follow-up was often incomplete; cohorts were heterogeneous; and the methodologic and statistical approaches were sometimes inappropriate (Table 92-1). These limitations make it impossible to draw reliable conclusions from these studies about the efficacy of mitral valve annuloplasty.

Recent papers continue to add to the controversy over whether mitral valve repair is effective for ischemic mitral regurgitation. Although several studies have reported disappointing outcomes with mitral valve repair,[96] most studies remain limited by critical flaws, thus preventing robust extrapolation.[97] Common to those studies suggesting ineffectiveness of mitral valve repair is the absence of systematic use of a restrictive annuloplasty using a complete rigid or semirigid ring, as varying proportions of patients in these studies received incomplete flexible rings or pericardium for annuloplasty, which are not recommended for ischemic mitral regurgitation. These flaws can be observed in most studies in the current surgical literature that demonstrate lack of effectiveness of annuloplasty, compared with CABG, in ischemic mitral regurgitation.[97]

Excellent Midterm Results with Downsized Annuloplasty

The Leiden group has been notable in their work on systematic downsized annuloplasty to treat functional mitral regurgitation.[66] In a report of 100 consecutive patients who underwent a mitral valve repair for ischemic mitral regurgitation using a semirigid Carpentier Edwards Physio ring annuloplasty (Edwards Lifesciences LLC, Irvine, CA) downsized by two sizes,[98] echocardiography at mean follow-up of 4.3 years showed that 85% had zero or mild regurgitation, and the 5-year survival rate was 71%. They observed superior outcomes when the preoperative LVEDD was 65 mm or less (Fig. 92-12). This group has also observed sustained reduction in left ventricular end-diastolic diameter at midterm follow-up for patients with LVEDD less than 65 mm at the time of repair.[99]

The Leiden experience[66,98] has several notable factors that differentiate it from the reports that suggest poor or limited efficacy of annuloplasty for ischemic mitral regurgitation.[62,65,81,93-96] The immediate postsurgical results suggest that the mitral valve repair was effective because no patients had residual regurgitation leaving the operating room; the patients were all operated in a more recent

TABLE 92-1 Recent Studies Suggesting Limited Efficacy of Restrictive Annuloplasty in Ischemic Mitral Regurgitation

Reference	Main Result	Conclusion	Limitations
Crabtree and colleagues[62]	52% survival at 5 years, 28% moderate or severe MR at latest TTE	Questions the benefit of adding annuloplasty to CABG	Use of inadequate technique: 44% of patients received an incomplete (posterior) annuloplasty with a flexible band. Such bands have limited efficacy, as they do not address tethering and dilation in anterior annulus Echo follow-up available for only 57%
Gelsomino and colleagues[95]	Reverse remodeling seen in only 41% of patients	Annuloplasty + CABG is ineffective in a large percentage of patients	Suboptimal early results: 7% repair failure or residual MR rate Limited revascularization approach: Average of two bypasses per patient suggests incomplete revascularization
Mihaljevic and colleagues[81]	CABG + annuloplasty did not improve long-term functional status or survival compared with CABG alone	Annuloplasty is insufficient to improve long-term clinical outcomes	Historical cohort: Patient inclusion began in 1991, so does not fully reflect recent advances in surgery (e.g., downsized annuloplasty); the current therapy for ischemic regurgitation became routine only in the late 1990s. Unusually high survival rate in CABG-only group: 5-yr survival of 75% not typical in most surgical series Ineffective technique: 15% of propensity-matched patients had annuloplasty with pericardial strips, a technique shown to be ineffective with unacceptably high recurrent MR rate Inadequate technique: 59% of patients received flexible posterior bands, which do not address anterior tethering and dilation.

Adapted from Anyanwu AC, Adams DH: Ischemic mitral regurgitation: recent advances. Curr Treat Options Cardiovasc Med 10:529–537, 2008.

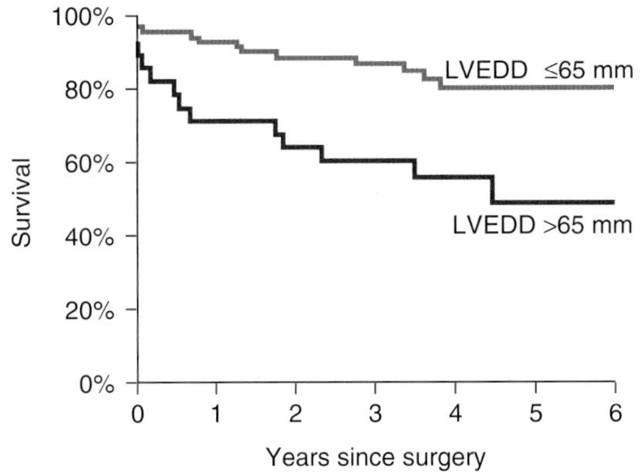

Patients at risk							
LVEDD ≤65	72	67	64	46	31	21	8
LVEDD >65	28	20	18	14	9	6	3

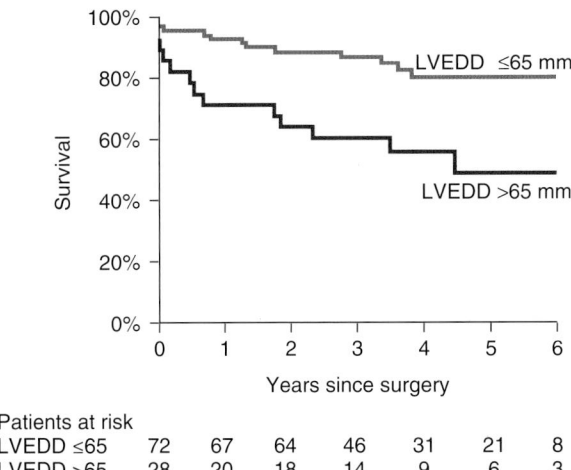

FIGURE 92-12 ■ Actuarial survival rates for two different preoperative left ventricular end-diastolic diameter (LVEDD) cohorts after restrictive annuloplasty, comparing LVEDD greater than 65 mm and LVEDD 65 mm or less (hazard ratio, 3.4; 95% confidence interval, 1.5-7.4; $P = 0.002$). (Adapted with permission from Braun J, van de Veire NR, Klautz RJ, et al: Restrictive mitral annuloplasty cures ischemic mitral regurgitation and heart failure. *Ann Thorac Surg* 85:430–436, 2008.)

era (2000 or after); the annuloplasty was standardized across all patients and always complete, semirigid, and downsized; and echocardiographic follow-up was systematic. Another more contemporary report from Gazoni and colleagues[69] supports the findings of the Leiden group: in a series of 105 ischemic repairs, a 5-year survival of 84% was observed with a low (6.3%) incidence of recurrent regurgitation on medium-term (>12 months) echocardiography. Geidel and colleagues,[70] also using predominantly remodeling annuloplasty, were also able to demonstrate excellent medium-term results with restrictive annuloplasty.

Although no good randomized clinical trial has been performed that demonstrates the superiority of complete rigid ring or semirigid annuloplasty over flexible annuloplasty, there is mounting evidence showing significantly improved rates of recurrent regurgitation with minimal incidence of postoperative mitral stenosis in patients receiving complete rings.[31,32]

Residual Mitral Regurgitation after Ischemic Mitral Valve Repair

Surgical Techniques and Incidence of Residual Mitral Regurgitation

Surgical technique and patient selection are probably the principal determinants of residual mitral regurgitation. With appropriate technique, residual regurgitation (defined as regurgitation other than trivial or mild on leaving the operating room or on predischarge echocardiography) should be infrequent (<5%) after ischemic mitral repair. Clinical and experimental evidence suggest that any technique other than a complete rigid or semirigid ring is prone to a high incidence of residual regurgitation.[93]

Suture annuloplasty has a particularly high incidence of residual mitral regurgitation when applied to patients with ischemic mitral regurgitation. Hausmann and coworkers[63] reported a 28% incidence of residual mitral regurgitation of at least 2+ with this technique. Von Oppell and colleagues[47] had a 13% incidence of moderate mitral regurgitation in a series in which most patients underwent suture annuloplasty. Czer and coworkers[100] found that suture annuloplasty failed to decrease mitral regurgitation severity by two grades in 33% of patients. Grossi and coworkers[101] noted a significant survival benefit (hazard ratio, 0.29) for ring annuloplasty over suture annuloplasty, with a 5-year survival rate of 74.3% compared with 52.7%, respectively ($P = 0.06$). Although appropriately applied suture annuloplasty can eliminate mitral regurgitation in the short term and it preserves annular contraction, as is well demonstrated in animal studies,[102,103] these repairs do not seem to be consistently effective and durable in the clinical setting.[99] Though few groups continue to experience satisfactory results with suture annuloplasty,[104] most surgeons have abandoned the suture method in favor of the more predictable results with ring annuloplasty.

Annuloplasty using a pericardial band has also been shown to be less effective than prosthetic ring annuloplasty, with more than 30% of patients having persisting grade 3+ or 4+ mitral regurgitation after repair.[93] The prosthetic ring or band annuloplasty has better results than other techniques, with many groups reporting residual regurgitation rates of less than 10%.

Partial posterior ring annuloplasty has been used in the past because of ease of implantation, especially when there is difficulty exposing the anterior annulus. However, most surgeons prefer a complete ring annuloplasty to address the anterior annulus, which has been shown to dilate in functional mitral regurgitation.[11] The initial studies reported by Bolling and colleagues[29] described excellent results with a downsized annuloplasty using a flexible ring in ischemic mitral regurgitation. Since those studies, an advantage has been shown using rigid or semirigid ring annuloplasty in this disease process. Tahta and coworkers[95] showed a 29% (2+ regurgitation or greater) recurrence of mitral regurgitation in 100 patients who underwent CABG and annuloplasty with a flexible Duran ring at 3-year follow-up. This was a considerably higher rate than that seen in series of rigid or semirigid annuloplasty.[98] Silberman and colleagues[31] retrospectively compared flexible to semirigid annuloplasty systems. They showed improved hemodynamics, greater reduction in recurrent mitral regurgitation, and a decreased incidence of recurrent regurgitation with the semirigid annuloplasty technique.[31] Kwon and colleagues[30] retrospectively showed an advantage with complete ring annuloplasty when compared with a partial annuloplasty in functional mitral regurgitation (majority of patients were ischemic). Nonflexible rings have been shown to provide better durability in functional disease.[32]

Downsizing of prosthetic annuloplasty seems vital in achieving a zero or near zero rate of residual regurgitation. Bolling and colleagues[29] were the first to popularize the downsized annuloplasty. They achieved no residual mitral regurgitation in 46 patients undergoing an annuloplasty alone at the time of CABG, despite using a flexible rather than a rigid annuloplasty. The Leiden group more recently demonstrated zero residual regurgitation rates with the downsized annuloplasty.[66]

Possible Mechanisms of Residual Mitral Regurgitation

A flexible reduction annuloplasty device, such as the Cosgrove-Edwards (Edwards Lifesciences) band or the Duran (Medtronic, Minneapolis, MN) ring, seeks to improve leaflet coaptation by simply decreasing the annular circumference, which indirectly brings the leaflets together. A rigid or semirigid remodeling annuloplasty ring such as the Carpentier-Edwards Classic (Edwards Lifesciences) is designed not only to decrease the annular circumference but, in addition, remodel the systolic annulus back into a kidney shape. This should, in theory, decrease the SL dimension to a greater degree than would a flexible annuloplasty of the same size. This should, in turn, lead to a larger surface of coaptation and less mitral regurgitation. The difference between reduction and remodeling annuloplasty in patients with type IIIB mitral regurgitation is illustrated in Figure 92-13.

Inadequate downsizing or inappropriate sizing may be a potential explanation for residual regurgitation. A true sized annuloplasty will diminish the mitral regurgitation, but the zone of coaptation might not be sufficient. It has been suggested that the durability of repair is less if the length of the coaptation zone is less than 8 mm. Calafiore and coworkers[105] and Yiu and coworkers[106] have provided evidence that the coaptation depth is important in patients with "functional" mitral regurgitation in the setting of nonischemic cardiomyopathy. Nagasaki and colleagues[107] compared ischemic and nonischemic cardiomyopathy and found that the coaptation depth was the main determinant of severity of regurgitation in the ischemic patients. With appropriate downsizing, the AP dimension is aggressively reduced to bring the restricted posterior leaflet close enough to the anterior leaflet to allow adequate coaptation. Series in which there has been systematic downsizing, especially with a rigid or semirigid ring, report better freedom from recurrent or residual regurgitation compared with series in which there has not been significant downsizing (Fig. 92-14).

Patient Factors Associated with Residual Regurgitation

Patient factors can predispose to residual regurgitation. There are several identified echocardiographic predictors of failure of repair (Box 92-1); these are mainly markers

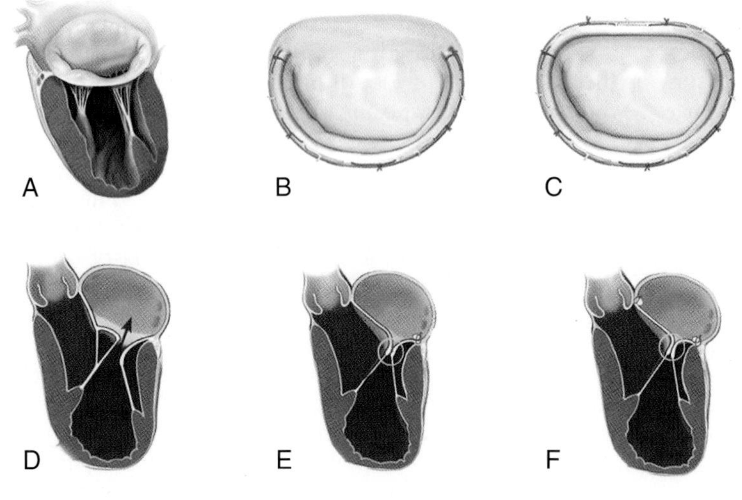

FIGURE 92-13 ■ Unrepaired annulus **(A)** of a patient with type IIIB mitral regurgitation leading to leaflet tethering. **D,** Flexible partial-reduction annuloplasty band **(B)** can reliably reduce the posterior annulus to a specific size, but the degree to which it remodels the annulus and restores coaptation depends on the relative degrees of annular dilation and posterior leaflet restriction. **E,** Downsized remodeling annuloplasty ring **(C)** predictably fixes the anteroposterior dimension, which should result in a larger surface of coaptation **(F)**.

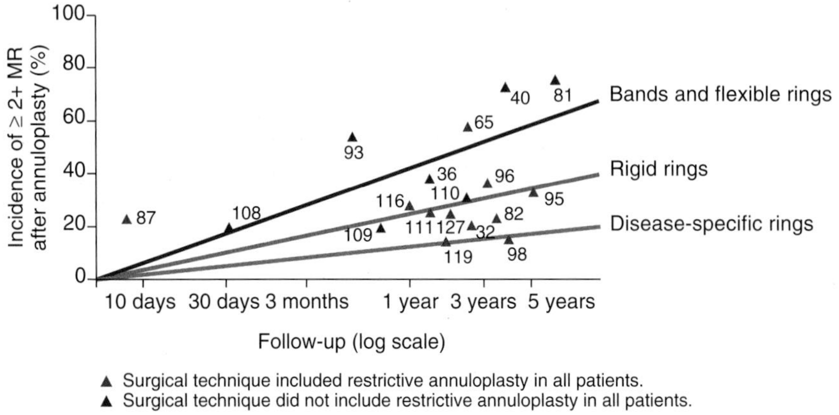

FIGURE 92-14 ■ Incidence of recurrent ≥2+ mitral regurgitation (MR) reported in the literature as a function of time after mitral valve annuloplasty.

BOX 92-1 Predictors of Recurrent Mitral Regurgitation after Mitral Valve Annuloplasty in Patients with Ischemic Mitral Regurgitation

TTE

Indicators of Severe Mitral Valve Tenting

- Systolic tenting area ≥ 2.5 cm^2
- Systolic tenting height ≥ 10 mm
- Posterior mitral leaflet angle ≥ 54 degrees
- Distal anterior mitral leaflet angle ≥ 19 degrees
- Posterior mitral leaflet angle ≥ 45 degrees
- Anterior mitral leaflet tethering angle ≥ 39.5 degrees
- MR jet direction: central or complex

Indicators of Advanced LV Remodeling

- LVESD > 51 mm
- LVEDD > 65 mm
- LVESV ≥ 145 mL
- Interpapillary muscle distance > 20 mm
- Systolic sphericity index ≥ 0.7

Other

- Myocardial performance index ≥ 0.9
- Wall motion score index ≥ 1.5
- Diastolic LV function: restrictive filling

TEE

- Mitral annular diameter in diastole > 3.7 cm
- Tethering area > 1.6 cm^2
- MR severity > 3.5

SURGICAL

- Use of flexible ring
- Use of incomplete ring
- Inadequate ring sizing
- Length of leaflet coaptation < 1.9 mm/m^2 or < 8 mm
- Residual mitral regurgitation

POSTOPERATIVE

- Absence of early LV remodeling (decrease of LVESV < 15%)
- Residual MR at discharge

LV, Left ventricle; *LVEDD,* left ventricle end-diastolic diameter; *LVESD,* left ventricle end-systolic diameter; *LVESV,* left ventricle end-systolic volume; *MR,* mitral regurgitation; *TEE,* transesophageal echocardiography; *TTE,* transthoracic echocardiography.

Adapted from Crestanello JA: Surgical approach to mitral regurgitation in chronic heart failure: when is it an option? Curr Heart Fail Rep 9:40–50, 2012.

of extreme left ventricular remodeling and/or severe valve tethering.[108] A missed primary lesion can be the cause of residual regurgitation,[109] such as regurgitation through a prominent cleft that is exaggerated after adequate loading of the ventricle is achieved.[110] This can be avoided by assuring an adequate zone of coaptation and by closing significant clefts.[111] Occasionally, residual regurgitation could be due to a coexisting nonischemic etiology, such as degenerative prolapse, calcification, or rheumatic changes.

Incremental Operative Risk of Mitral Valve Surgery (versus Coronary Artery Bypass Grafting Alone) in Ischemic Mitral Regurgitation

A critical piece of information that a surgeon must consider when contemplating concomitant mitral valve surgery for ischemic mitral regurgitation is the additive operative risk of intervening on the mitral valve. A low operative risk would justify a more aggressive approach, given the potential benefit on late outcomes that we have outlined. A high incremental risk would justify a more conservative approach, although it should be kept in mind that the benefit of mitral valve surgery may also be greatest in certain high-risk patient groups (e.g., NYHA classes III and IV heart failure). Leaving the operating room with significant mitral regurgitation can also be most detrimental to the postoperative course of the sicker high-risk patients with poor ventricular function and more comorbidity.

The operative risk for patients undergoing surgery for ischemic mitral regurgitation depends on a number of preoperative factors, most notably age, left ventricular dysfunction, and other cardiac surgical risk factors. Because patient characteristics vary widely among different clinical series, it is difficult to precisely quantify the additional operative risk of mitral valve surgery in a given patient with ischemic mitral regurgitation. Extrapolation from the clinical literature is also challenging, because uniform definitions of ischemic mitral regurgitation have not been used. Some studies include patients with ruptured papillary muscles or with chronic ischemic type II dysfunction, and even degenerative patients with incidental coronary artery disease in cohorts of ischemic mitral regurgitation.

Several historical series have, however, suggested that the presence of ischemic mitral regurgitation does appear to increase the operative risk of CABG alone.* The 3% to 12% mortality rates seen in these studies are higher than those of most contemporary CABG series (generally around 2%).

Although the reported operative mortality for mitral valve replacement at the time of CABG has remained relatively high, the outcomes for mitral valve repair appear to be improving over time, with more recent series reporting operative mortalities of less than 5%.[67,69,112]

Mitral Valve Repair versus Replacement for Ischemic Mitral Regurgitation

Although mitral valve repair for ischemic mitral regurgitation carries some of the same obvious benefits over replacement that it does for other etiologies (avoiding prosthetic valve–related complications), the higher incidence of repair failure and lower event-free survival with ischemic disease (compared with degenerative and rheumatic cohorts), makes the benefit of repair over replacement less certain when compared with other etiologies.

*References 26, 55, 56, 89, 91, 92.

For this reason, several authors have questioned whether the more effective (in terms of cure of regurgitation) valve replacement should be the preferred option to mitral valve repair (with less certainty of stable long-term freedom from regurgitation), with the hypothesis that the benefits of a more durable fix for the regurgitation would outweigh the incremental risks of a valve replacement. Although valve replacement would yield more durable elimination of regurgitation, there is a higher risk of surgical mortality, late mortality, valve-related morbidity and mortality, and a lesser degree of reverse remodeling with valve replacement.[113-115] Historically, the poor results of mitral valve replacement in the setting of advanced ischemic or nonischemic cardiomyopathy led to most surgeons abandoning valve replacement in this setting during the 1980s and 1990s. However, some surgeons later adopted mitral valve replacement, with complete chordal and leaflet preservation, as primary therapy for ischemic mitral regurgitation and reported early results similar to those seen with mitral valve repair.[116]

Several observational studies have addressed this dilemma. Gillinov and colleagues[114] retrospectively analyzed outcomes after repair (remodeling annuloplasty was used in one third of patients, with the remainder receiving a partial flexible band or pericardium for annuloplasty) or replacement in patients with ischemic mitral regurgitation and found that although there was a survival benefit seen with valve repair (5-year survival repair 58% versus 36% for replacement), the highest-risk patients had similar survival rates. The benefit of repair over replacement was diminished in patients with lateral wall motion abnormalities and complex regurgitant jets. This suggested that in some high-risk patients with ischemic mitral regurgitation, a chordal-sparing valve replacement may be an acceptable alternative to repair. Grossi and coworkers[117] found better early survival (odds ratio, 0.43), complication-free late survival (odds ratio, 0.5), and a trend toward better overall survival with valve repair.

Most recently, the Cardiothoracic Surgical Trials Network[118] conducted a multicenter randomized study enrolling patients with severe ischemic mitral regurgitation to undergo mitral valve annuloplasty or valve replacement (Fig. 92-15). The randomized trial identified no difference in survival, left ventricular remodeling, or quality of life measures at 12 months. However, the group did see a higher occurrence of recurrent mitral regurgitation at 12 months (32.6% with repair, 2.3% with replacement). The authors, however, do not explicitly recommend either valve replacement or repair as the preferred therapy for ischemic regurgitation, and they note that the higher incidence of regurgitation with repair needs to be balanced against (long-term) adverse effects of a prosthetic valve (these were not analyzed in this study). The high rate of recurrence in the repair group is concerning, however, and further analysis will be required to understand the reasons behind such high failure rate (relative to some contemporary series which show much lower early recurrence rate) and to identify surgical and patient predictors of failure.

In another recent analysis, Lorusso and colleagues[119] reported results of the Italian, multicenter, retrospective study of ischemic mitral regurgitation patients with a reduced ejection fraction. This high risk population was shown to have no benefit with mitral valve repair and, once again, a higher rate of recurrent regurgitation with repair.[119]

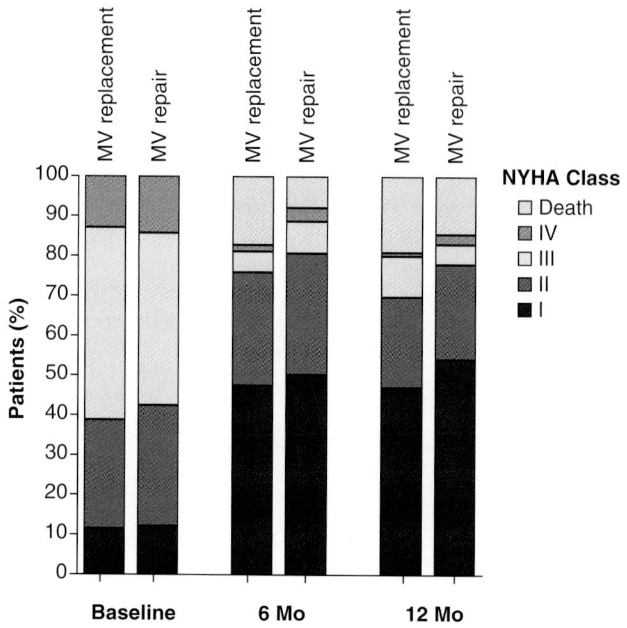

FIGURE 92-15 ■ Rates of New York Heart Association (NYHA) class and death at baseline, 6 months, and 12 months. *MV*, Mitral valve. (Adapted with permission from Acker MA, Parides MK, Perrault LP: Mitral-valve repair versus replacement for severe ischemic mitral regurgitation. *N Engl J Med* 370:23–32, 2014.)

The majority of mitral valve replacements have traditionally been biologic because of the perceived short life expectancy with these patients.[120] As medical therapy has improved, biologic valve degeneration has been seen with patients who initially underwent an operation for ischemic mitral regurgitation. These high-risk patients may then require a reoperation or reintervention that would entail a higher operative risk than the initial operation.

The decision regarding mitral valve repair or replacement is best made in consideration of individual patient characteristics. Patients with ischemic regurgitation who have echocardiographic findings that increase the risk of recurrent mitral regurgitation or repair failure should be considered for mitral valve replacement. Patients with moderate regurgitation and those with severe regurgitation who have minimal predictors of failure (see Box 92-1) are likely to have durable results with a repair. Patients who have unsatisfactory results with repair on intraoperative TEE should be considered for a second bypass run and valve replacement, because it is well documented that patients with residual regurgitation have poor long-term outcomes.

Overall Recommendations for Ischemic Mitral Regurgitation during Coronary Artery Bypass Grafting

Although most surgeons agree that severe mitral regurgitation should be corrected at the time of CABG, there is no consensus on the management of mild to moderate ischemic mitral regurgitation at the time of CABG. A preponderance of evidence seems to support a more liberal application of concomitant mitral valve surgery, which can be summarized in the following recommendations.

1. All patients referred for CABG with suspected ischemic mitral regurgitation should undergo careful preoperative transthoracic echocardiography, preferably with quantitative assessment of mitral regurgitation severity while they are not actively ischemic. Those without complete preoperative assessment should undergo careful intraoperative TEE assessment of their mitral valves to determine whether there is an anatomic substrate for ischemic mitral regurgitation. If intraoperative echocardiography shows less mitral regurgitation than expected on the basis of the clinical picture, the patient should receive provocative testing of the degree of mitral regurgitation
2. Patients with severe ischemic mitral regurgitation should undergo concomitant mitral valve repair. Mitral valve replacement is a reasonable option depending on surgeon preference and expected likelihood of repair durability.
3. Patients with moderate ischemic mitral regurgitation should undergo concomitant mitral valve repair unless preoperative or intraoperative factors suggest that the additional operative morbidity and mortality would be prohibitive (e.g., extensive mitral annular calcification or a strong indication for performing the CABG off pump, such as a heavily diseased ascending aorta).
4. Patients with mild ischemic mitral regurgitation may undergo concomitant mitral valve repair (with caveat similar to that for moderate regurgitation) if history or evaluation is suggestive of periods of greater severity of mitral regurgitation than has been documented. Pointers that suggest the mitral regurgitation may be more severe than appreciated include symptoms of congestive heart failure, enlarged left atrium, enlarged or dysfunctional left ventricle, pulmonary hypertension, and atrial fibrillation. In addition, anatomic findings present on intraoperative TEE should also be considered (e.g., minimal surface of coaptation, severe leaflet tenting coaptation depth, significant annular dilation).

SURGICAL PRINCIPLES

Basic Principles

The basic principles of mitral valve repair for ischemic mitral regurgitation are not fundamentally different from those for degenerative disease. A successful outcome depends on the following:

- Careful review of the preoperative echocardiogram, with particular attention paid to the mechanism of mitral regurgitation, the direction of the mitral regurgitation jets, and specific anatomic abnormalities (e.g., calcification, thickening)
- Good visualization of the entire valve
- Careful segmental valve analysis to confirm the mechanism of mitral regurgitation
- Meticulous suture placement and ring sizing
- Consideration of adjunctive technique, as appropriate

Annuloplasty: Underlying Principles

The significant effects of even mild degrees of ischemic mitral regurgitation on survival should challenge surgeons to make every effort to minimize residual mitral regurgitation after mitral annuloplasty. Careful consideration should be given to choice of annuloplasty method.

The literature does not, in our opinion, support a role for suture or pericardial annuloplasty in this disease. As mentioned previously, the rates of residual mitral regurgitation for these techniques are relatively high. Although the three-dimensional dynamic nature of mitral annulus and its contribution to ventricular function have been well documented, it is unclear what role this plays in pathologic conditions such as ischemic mitral regurgitation. Some laboratory studies suggest that planar fixation of the annulus with a nonflexible ring impairs left ventricular function, whereas others dispute this.[28] We suspect, however, that there is a critical role for annular remodeling, specifically in the SL (or AP) dimension in patients with Carpentier-type IIIB dysfunction. As described earlier, a large body of data has been accumulated from several laboratories that describe the mechanisms that contribute to ischemic mitral regurgitation. Several of these studies emphasize the importance of the increased SL dimension in pathophysiology of ischemic mitral regurgitation. It seems, therefore, that the need to remodel the annulus (with a remodeling rigid or semirigid ring) far outweighs any benefit of preserving annular motion.

As illustrated in Figure 92-16, a reduction annuloplasty will, to some degree, decrease the SL dimension, improve leaflet coaptation, and correct mitral regurgitation. The extent to which it accomplishes this, however, probably depends on whether the annular dilation or posterior leaflet restriction is the dominant mechanism of mitral regurgitation. If there is predominant annular dilation (type I dysfunction), a flexible band is not an unreasonable option. However, for most patients, where valve tethering is dominant, a complete downsized rigid or semirigid ring should be used for ischemic mitral valve repair.

Asymmetric rings designed specifically for the treatment of ischemic mitral regurgitation can be utilized. For example, the Carpentier-McCarthy-Adams IMR ETlogix ring (Edwards Lifesciences, Irvine CA; see Fig. 92-16) has a decreased AP diameter (i.e., is predownsized); and is asymmetrical, with a narrower dimension at P2-P3, and it has a slight dip at P2-P3 to accommodate the greater posterior leaflet restriction in this region.[121]

Valve Exposure

The most common approach to patients with ischemic mitral regurgitation is a full sternotomy with cannulation of the ascending aorta and both venae cava. After completion of bypass grafting, as appropriate, the mitral valve

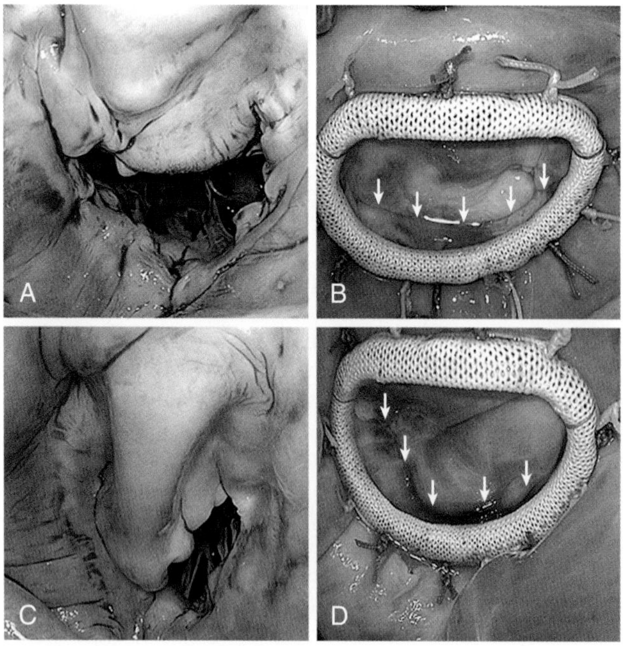

FIGURE 92-16 ■ Symmetrical **(A** and **B)** and asymmetrical **(C** and **D)** patterns of ischemic mitral regurgitation. Note the difference of coaptation lines *(white arrows)* after remodeling annuloplasty.

can be exposed either via the interatrial groove or trans-septally. Patients with ischemic mitral regurgitation may have a small left atrial cavity, depending on the acuity of presentation. Despite this, however, excellent exposure of the valve can be obtained with a standard mitral valve retractor system if certain principles are followed. The interatrial approach is most commonly used, and particular attention should be paid to the following: (1) complete dissection of the interatrial groove before atriotomy and (2) posterior extension of the inferior aspect of the atriotomy, with partial detachment of the right lower pulmonary vein. The trans-septal approach may be useful in the setting of a small left atrium or when an aortic prosthesis is present. A thoracotomy approach can be considered in reoperative setting and in primary cases that do not require concurrent CABG (if coronary arteries have been previously stented).

Valve Analysis

Before segmental valve analysis, it may be helpful to place an exposure suture in the posterior annulus at the junction between P1 and P2 to bring the valve apparatus anterior and lateral. Using two hooks, it is then possible to confirm the pathognomonic findings of secondary mitral regurgitation (i.e., posterior or bileaflet tethering, caused by papillary muscle displacement, with otherwise normal leaflets and no evidence of prolapse or fixed restriction; Fig. 92-17*A*). Associated annular dilation is also commonly present.

Suture Placement

For implanting an annuloplasty ring, 2-0 braided polyester sutures are most commonly used. Because of the potential for increased tension in the setting of type IIIB dysfunction with associated annular dilation, it is preferable to place the sutures close together along the annulus. We prefer to use crossover sutures (see Fig. 92-17*B*) to help accommodate and distribute the excessive tension that a restrictive annuloplasty can impose on the annulus. Using the crossover technique, ring dehiscence is rare. The full curve of the needle should be used to encourage deep, wide placement of individual sutures along the annulus. The anterior commissure is usually the most difficult area to expose, and it is usually approached last, after the placement of sutures along the septal, medial, and lateral portions of the annulus to place tension on prior sutures to expose this area of the annulus.

Sizing and Implantation

After sutures are placed around the annulus, standard ring sizers are used to select the appropriate ring. Placing gentle traction on marginal cords in the A2 portion of the anterior leaflet with a hook allows the height and surface area of the anterior leaflet to be measured. An additional measurement to consider is the intercommissural distance.

Because leaflet restriction in ischemic mitral regurgitation results in less leaflet tissue available for coaptation, it is necessary to downsize the complete remodeling ring by one or two sizes to ensure an adequate surface of coaptation after annuloplasty. Systolic anterior motion is almost unknown, despite aggressive downsizing, because the restricted posterior leaflet cannot displace the anterior leaflet into the outflow tract. After a ring is selected (typically a size between 24 and 28 mm), the interrupted sutures are passed through it, with respect paid to the associated geometry of the annulus, crossing over on the prosthetic ring where sutures have been crossed on the annulus. The individual sutures are then tied, thus securing the ring to the annulus.

After the downsized remodeling annuloplasty is completed, a saline test is used to confirm the line of coaptation along the margin of the leaflets. The ink test confirms an adequate surface of coaptation.[122] The typical appearance of a completed downsized remodeling annuloplasty is shown in Figure 92-16. Nearly the entire orifice is occupied by the anterior leaflet, thereby allowing the entire restricted posterior leaflet to contribute to coaptation.

Adjunctive Procedures

Although the routine use of a remodeling annuloplasty and more aggressive downsizing is likely to minimize the incidence of residual mitral regurgitation after CABG and annuloplasty to well less than 10%, there may be a small group of patients for whom annuloplasty alone is insufficient to correct the mitral regurgitation. A number of adjunctive techniques, applied with the restrictive annuloplasty, can help to eliminate or reduce residual regurgitation in such patients. Some physicians advocate routine use of adjunctive techniques in an expectation that they will yield a more durable repair; however, systematic application of adjunctive techniques has yet to be

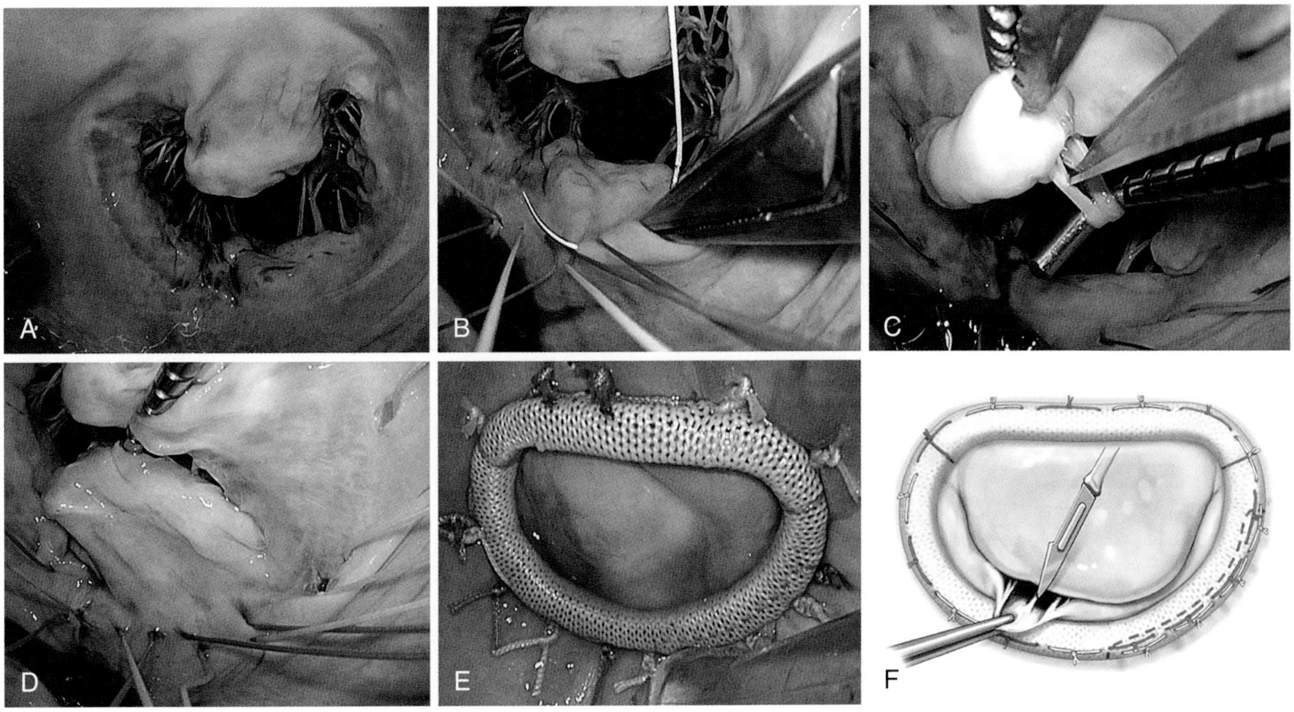

FIGURE 92-17 ■ Surgical approach to ischemic mitral regurgitation in a patient with severe annular dilation symmetric leaflet tethering. **A,** After annular sizing primarily based on the surface area and height of the anterior leaflet, annular sutures are placed. Sutures at the position of the anterior commissure and trigon are placed last, taking advantage of previously placed sutures to expose the area. **B,** Interlocking sutures can be placed along P3 to reinforce the annuloplasty. **C,** Adjunctive techniques in addition to downsized rigid ring annuloplasty include cutting secondary chords to the anterior leaflet. **D,** Closure of leaflet clefts or indentations should be part of the surgical routine when attempting repair to avoid residual leaks because of the lack of tissue. **E,** A full remodeling Carpentier-McCarthy-Adams INR Etlogix ring is placed (disease-specific ring). **F,** Cutting secondary chords of the posterior leaflet can be an option after full repair in patients with generous posterior leaflet tissue.

shown to improve any of the key long-term outcomes (i.e., survival, heart failure, freedom from recurrent regurgitation).

Papillary Muscle Repositioning

Displacement of the papillary muscles is a key component in the pathophysiology of ischemic mitral regurgitation and, in theory, if the distance of displacement is reduced, then mitral regurgitation should be reduced or eliminated because of less leaflet tethering. Reduction in papillary muscle displacement can be achieved by various methods. Kron and coworkers[123] initially treated ischemic mitral regurgitation with papillary muscle repositioning using a pledgeted suture attached from the posterior papillary head to the annulus (Fig. 92-18). Rama and colleagues[124] described suturing the posterior to anterior muscle with autologous pericardial pledgets, whereas Hvass and associates[125] and Ito and coworkers[126] used a polytetrafluoroethylene tube to construct a sling around the base of the papillary muscles (see Fig. 92-18). Several variations of these procedures have been described, including some that allow physiologic adjustment of tethering distance on the beating heart.[127] Although several groups report promising midterm results, it has not been demonstrated that any papillary repositioning techniques result in clinical benefit compared with annuloplasty alone.

Secondary Chordae Cutting

Levine and Schwammenthal demonstrated in animal models that division of secondary mitral valve chordae reduces the degree of tethering in ischemic mitral regurgitation.[128] Borger and colleagues[129] reported on a series of 43 patients in whom a downsized annuloplasty was supplemented with dividing secondary chords to the restricted segments of the anterior leaflet, posterior leaflet, and commissures (see Fig. 92-17*C* and *F*). They compared these patients to 49 historical and concurrent controls who underwent annuloplasty alone. The authors observed less leaflet tenting and a lower incidence of early recurrent regurgitation in the chordal-cutting group. Application of the chordal-cutting technique was, however, limited to a few surgeons; therefore, differences in surgical skill or expertise may have contributed to the superior outcomes in the chordal-cutting subgroup. The annuloplasty-only group had a higher than expected incidence of early recurrent regurgitation—37% versus 15% in the chordal-cutting group—suggesting technical factors related to inadequate technique could have contributed to worse results in the controls. Chordal cutting can be performed through an aortotomy[130] and can achieve better reduction in anterior leaflet tenting. Some questions have been raised as to potential deleterious effects of chordal cutting on left ventricular function, but these have yet to be determined.

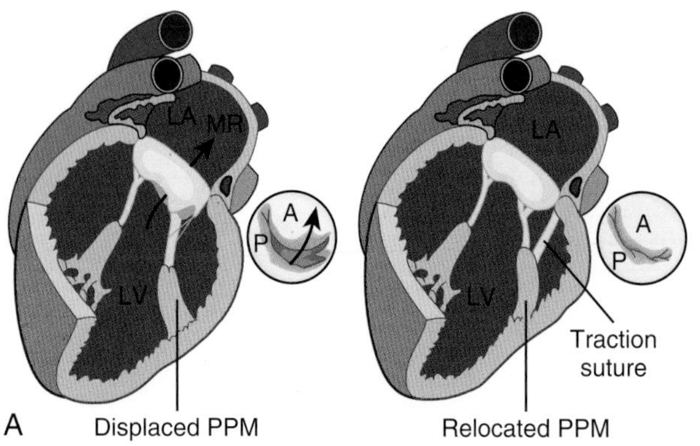

A

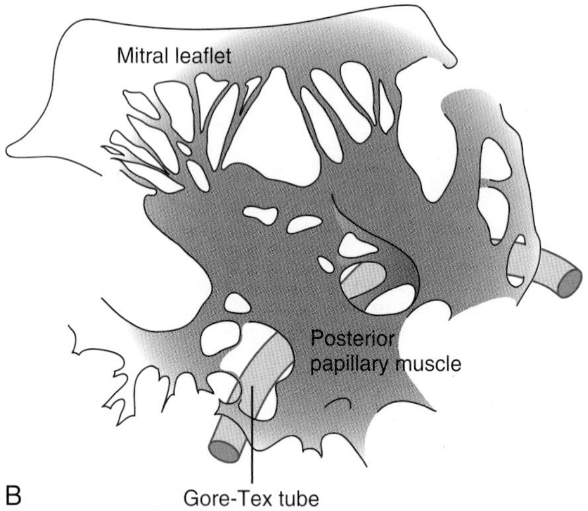

B

FIGURE 92-18 ■ Approaches to papillary muscle repositioning. **A,** Apical displacement of the posterior papillary muscle (PPM) causing tethering of both leaflets at the medial commissure, producing mitral regurgitation (MR; *left*). Placement of a traction suture relocates the tip of the PPM closer to the annulus, permitting better leaflet coaptation *(right)*. **B,** A sling placed around the base of both papillary muscles and tightened reduces displacement of both muscles and thereby also reduces leaflet tethering. *A,* Anterior mitral leaflet; *LA,* left atrium; *LV,* left ventricle; *P,* posterior mitral leaflet. (Modified with permission from Kron IL, Green GR, Cope JT: Surgical relocation of the posterior papillary muscle in chronic ischemic mitral regurgitation. *Ann Thorac Surg* 74:600–601, 2002; and from Hvass U, Tapia M, Baron F, et al: Papillary muscle sling: a new functional approach to mitral repair in patients with ischemic left ventricular dysfunction and functional mitral regurgitation. *Ann Thorac Surg* 75:809–811, 2003.)

Other Approaches

Poor coaptation of the scallops of the posterior leaflet can occur with leaflet restriction; deep indentations or clefts (P1/P2 or P2/P3; see Fig. 92-17*D*) should be closed, particularly if a corresponding jet is noted on saline testing. Posterior leaflet patch extension (Fig. 92-19), especially over the P3 scallop, has been used in patients with severe posterior leaflet restriction.[131] Although the edge-to-edge technique is used as an adjunct by some groups,[36,132] laboratory and clinical data do not provide strong support for its use in surgical repair. Experimental animal work shows that the edge-to-edge repair does not alter the annular, subvalvular, or leaflet geometric alterations seen in the disease. In vitro laboratory studies suggest that although the edge-to-edge repair can partially reduce regurgitation caused by annular dilation, it is not effective in correcting type IIIB dysfunction associated with papillary muscle displacement.[133] Edge-to-edge repair as an adjunct to annuloplasty can exaggerate the risk of mitral stenosis when performed in the context of a downsized annuloplasty. Finally, some surgeons have attempted ventricular solutions to ischemic mitral regurgitation, including plication of left ventricular infarct scar or external device application.[134]

Is Restrictive Annuloplasty Harmful?

Restrictive annuloplasty, the mainstay of current therapy for ischemic mitral regurgitation, invariably results in a valve orifice that is smaller than would be expected for that particular valve, and it also fixes the annulus in a nonphysiologic shape and position. The size 24- to 28-mm rings that are typically used in this disease would be considered small for other pathologies. In theory, therefore, there is a risk of over-narrowing the orifice, resulting in functional mitral stenosis. One clinical study supports this theory. Magne and coworkers[135] compared 24 patients who underwent successful restrictive annuloplasty with 20 controls who had ischemic heart disease but no mitral regurgitation. They used dobutamine stress echocardiography to evaluate transvalvular gradients and functional capacity.[135] Compared with controls, patients who had restrictive annuloplasty had higher gradients at rest (13 vs. 4 mm Hg) and stress (19 vs. 6 mm Hg). They noted that the systolic pulmonary artery pressures rose to 58 mm Hg with stress in patients with restrictive annuloplasty (compared with 38 mm Hg in controls). The indexed orifice valve area at peak stress was 1.0 cm^2/m^2 for the restrictive annuloplasty group (compared with 2.4 cm^2/m^2 in control).[135] These data suggest that restrictive annuloplasty could induce some degree of functional mitral stenosis. The authors, though, did not correlate their findings with symptoms or survival, so it is not clear whether the observed hemodynamics have a bearing on clinical outcome. This study, however, has several limitations that limit the reliability of its findings,[136] and indeed other studies that have included systematic echocardiography did not observe functional stenosis.[98] Animal studies highlight other potentially deleterious effects of restrictive annuloplasty, such as inhibition of basal wall thickening[137] and abolishing of normal annular and leaflet dynamic motion,[103] but the effects of these changes have not been studied in a clinical setting.

Percutaneous Approaches

Because of the relatively high operative risk and uncertain benefit of mitral valve repair in patients with advanced cardiomyopathy and severe ischemic mitral regurgitation, there has been a surging interest in development of percutaneous approaches to treating ischemic mitral valve regurgitation. Attempts at percutaneous therapy for ischemic mitral regurgitation have largely been directed at either annuloplasty or edge-to-edge approaches.

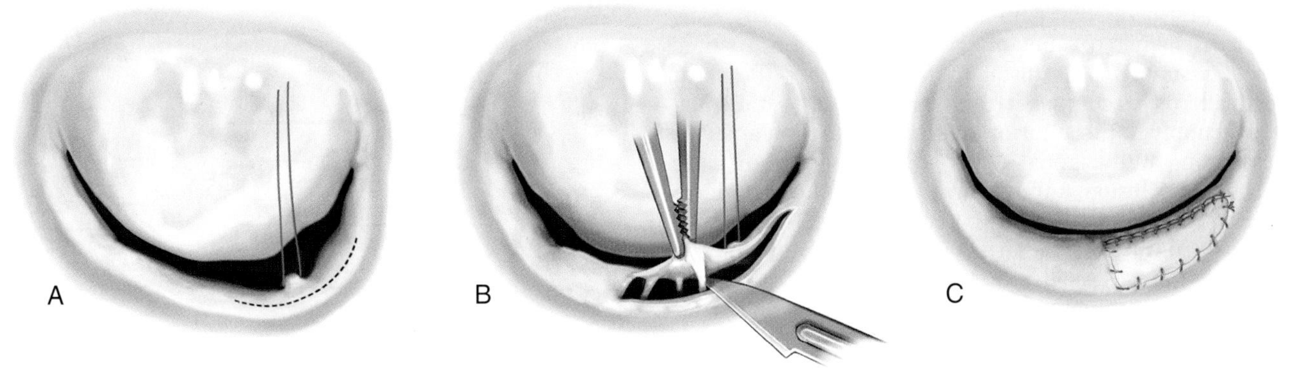

FIGURE 92-19 ■ Posterior leaflet extension with a glutaraldehyde-fixed pericardial patch in patients with ischemic mitral regurgitation. The patch is sutured to the edge of the posterior leaflet defect and the posterior mitral annulus with a running 5-0 polytetrafluoroethylene suture.

Annuloplasty has been fraught with various technical problems, and it is not adequately developed for reproducible and effective application. In a multicenter study of 43 patients with secondary mitral regurgitation, while it was technically feasible to deploy an annuloplasty device in 30 patients, no significant changes were noted in severity of mitral regurgitation, ventricular volumes, or quality of life.[138] The most used percutaneous device in functional ischemic regurgitation is the MitraClip (Abbott Vascular, Santa Clara, CA), which is a cloth-covered cobalt-chromium device that permanently clips the anterior and posterior leaflets, thereby performing a percutaneous edge-to-edge repair. Studies have demonstrated that the MitraClip can reduce severity of secondary mitral regurgitation in patients with end-stage heart failure with most patients reported to have improved symptoms, reduction in left ventricular size and moderate or less regurgitation at short-term follow-up.[139,140] The MitraClip, however, does not eliminate regurgitation in many patients (this is expected as has been demonstrated in surgical studies of edge-to-edge), and up to half the patients remain with residual mild or moderate regurgitation. It is not known whether residual regurgitation will have similar long-term negative prognostic effect in patients undergoing percutaneous therapy, as is the case with residual regurgitation after surgical repair. However, considering the severe symptomatic nature of these patients, the rationale for accepting the less perfect edge-to-edge results is that any reduction in mitral valve regurgitation may be worthwhile and potentially beneficial (the same would not hold for surgical repair because the high risk would not justify an incomplete repair). The MitraClip should, however, be reserved for patients who cannot have surgical repair, as the results of ischemic mitral regurgitation repair are superior with surgery than with the MitraClip in terms of long-term freedom from regurgitation and the early survival is similar with both approaches.[139] Of note, it has not been objectively demonstrated that the reduction in mitral regurgitation grade seen with the MitraClip affects either survival or quality of life compared with optimal guideline-directed medical therapy in patients with advanced heart failure; this is currently the subject of a multicenter randomized trial, Clinical Outcomes Assessment of the MitraClip Percutaneous Therapy for Extremely High-Surgical-Risk Patients (COAPT), which should report in 2016 to 2018. It is possible that some of the presumed benefit of clip therapy arises from factors such as closer medical supervision and management, patient selection, and placebo effect. Of note, a recent systematic review of 16 studies reporting data on 2980 patients showed that despite a low procedural mortality (4.5% at 30 days), high-risk patients who had successful MitraClip repair still had high early mortality (16.4% at 310 days).[141] A single center report of 109 patients with functional regurgitation reported a 3-year survival of 74.5%.[142] It therefore is not clear whether the percutaneous edge-to-edge approach alters the natural history of these patients, as midterm results do not seem to be substantially different from historical controls. Until additional data emerge, therefore, the MitraClip is not considered for primary treatment of severe ischemic mitral regurgitation, except for symptomatic relief in select patients with severe advanced heart failure symptoms who have failed medical therapy and who are not candidates for mitral valve surgery because of excessive risk or presumed futility.

TYPE II ISCHEMIC MITRAL REGURGITATION

Patients with type II (mitral valve prolapse) ischemic mitral valve regurgitation are infrequently encountered in modern clinical practice. Type II ischemic regurgitation can be separated further into acute ischemic mitral valve regurgitation because of papillary muscle rupture or chronic ischemic mitral valve regurgitation secondary to papillary muscle elongation or rupture.

Acute Papillary Muscle Rupture

Historically, acute papillary muscle rupture was observed in up to 5% of patients with transmural myocardial infarction. However, the incidence of acute papillary muscle rupture, and other mechanical complications of acute myocardial infarction, has reduced remarkably in the era of early reperfusion postmyocardial infarction.[143]

The posterior-medial papillary muscle is more susceptible to ischemia because of its dependence on a single vascular supply via a distal branch of either the right coronary or circumflex artery in contrast to the dual blood supply to the anterior muscle from the left anterior descending and diagonal systems. In the setting of acute coronary occlusion, a transmural papillary muscle infarction could potentially lead to muscle necrosis with subsequent rupture of the trunk or one or more of the papillary heads. Usually, the timing of rupture is about 1 week after the initial infarct. Because of the evolution of medical and interventional reperfusion strategies, acute papillary muscle rupture is rare. It must still be considered in the setting of a new systolic murmur and hemodynamic collapse, typically cardiogenic shock, occurring in the first several days after myocardial infarction. Echocardiography is the mainstay for distinguishing the condition from acute ventricular septal defect, free-wall ventricular rupture, or global myocardial dysfunction, which can all produce a similar picture in the setting of transmural myocardial infarction. Lack of a step up in venous oxygen saturation also distinguishes this condition from an acute ventricular septal defect. Once the diagnosis is made, hemodynamic stabilization is usually facilitated by placement of an intra-aortic balloon pump. Surgery should not be delayed, except to optimize hemodynamics and invasive monitoring, because the mainstay of therapy is to correct the embarrassment of massive acute mitral valve regurgitation.

Mitral valve repair with reimplantation of the papillary muscle either into an adjacent nonischemic head or the ventricle can be done, but it is rarely undertaken. One must ensure that the infarcted head itself can hold sutures, usually placed at the insertion of the chordae, and that the reimplantation occurs into an area of viable tissue. Replacement of the chordal apparatus with polytetrafluoroethylene is also feasible, albeit with little known about long-term results in this setting. By far the most common treatment for acute papillary muscle rupture due to myocardial infarction is an expeditious mitral valve replacement. Coronary revascularization is undertaken at the same setting. Surgery carries a high hospital mortality of around 20% in most series.[144-146] Because the burden of coronary disease is low, patients with this condition who survive the initial insult actually have better long-term survival compared with patients with type IIIB ischemic mitral valve regurgitation with long-standing ventricular remodeling and who undergo mitral valve surgery.

The Mayo group[145] analyzed long-term outcomes of 54 patients who had surgery (valve replacement, 41; valve repair, 13) for papillary muscle rupture between 1980 and 2000. As expected, 90% involved the posterior papillary muscle. The overall operative mortality was 18.5%, with most deaths occurring because of low cardiac output or ventricular rupture. Although mitral valve repair was associated with a lower mortality (7.7% vs. 22% for replacement; $P = 0.21$), most repairs were done in the recent era, in which improved outcomes were observed (operative mortality post-1990 was 10%). Patients who had concurrent CABG also had a lower operative mortality. Once patients survived hospitalization, midterm survival was reasonable, with 52% alive and free from heart failure at 5 years (Fig. 92-20). Six patients developed moderate or greater mitral regurgitation in the follow-up period—four after valve repair, and two after valve replacement.

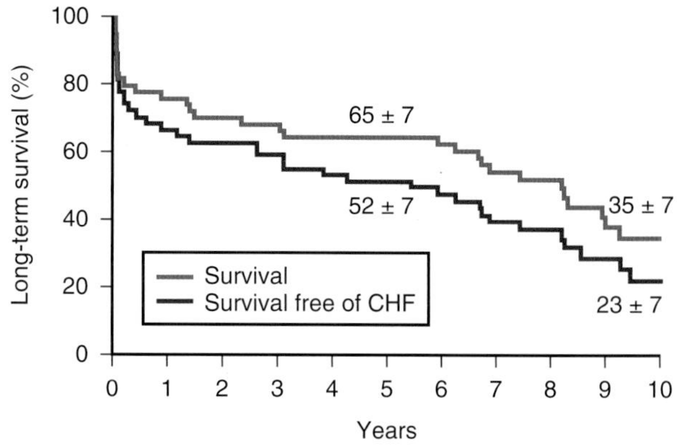

FIGURE 92-20 Overall (including operative mortality) long-term survival *(green line)* and long-term survival free of congestive heart failure (CHF; *red line*) after surgery for postinfarct papillary muscle rupture. Numbers indicate the 5- and 10-year survival (± standard error). (Reproduced with permission from Russo A, Suri RM, Grigioni F, et al: Clinical outcome after surgical correction of mitral regurgitation due to papillary muscle rupture. *Circulation* 118:1528–1534, 2008.)

Chronic Type II Ischemic Mitral Regurgitation

Perhaps even rarer than acute papillary muscle rupture in ischemic mitral valve regurgitation is the occurrence of leaflet prolapse because of elongation, thinning, and fibrosis or rupture of a chronically infarcted papillary muscle. It is usually misdiagnosed preoperatively as degenerative valve disease with chordal elongation with concomitant coronary artery disease. Valve analysis in the operating room generally reveals a fibrotic and thinned-out papillary muscle with normal chords and prolapse of the affected segment owing to elongation of the muscle. The nonprolapsing segments often show a type IIIB restriction. In terms of treatment, chronic type II ischemic regurgitation can usually be treated with valve repair. This lesion condition can be treated like chordal rupture or elongation, as seen in degenerative disease, and it is amenable to a variety of repair techniques. PTFE chordal replacement, chordal transfer, and limited resection and papillary transposition are among repair techniques that can be used to treat this condition. A downsized annuloplasty can also be performed in view of the ischemic etiology and associated type IIIB dysfunction.

Jouan and colleagues[147] reported a series of 44 patients who had surgery for ischemic mitral valve prolapse, of which 66% had chronic mitral regurgitation (more than 60 days after myocardial infarction), whereas the others were operated within 60 days of myocardial infarction. This series included four emergent surgeries. Interestingly, isolated chordal rupture owing to chordal infarction was the postulated mechanism of regurgitation in six patients. The remainders were due to papillary muscle elongation (36%) or rupture (50%). Most of the papillary

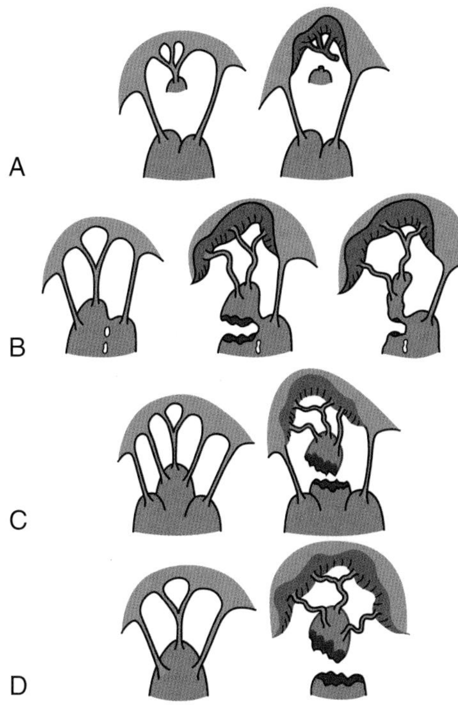

FIGURE 92-21 Classification of papillary muscle rupture according to Jouan and colleagues.[147] **A–C,** Partial rupture, typically present in subacute or chronic fashion. **D,** Classic papillary muscle rupture. Mechanisms of ischemic mitral valve prolapse are shown. **A,** Necrosis of a separate commissural head (inserted close to the annulus) with rupture of the anchorage of the commissural chord. **B,** Necrosis of a single head papillary muscle subdivided in multiple heads with partial rupture. **C,** Necrosis of a fenestrated papillary muscle with detachment of its main insertion: "incomplete" rupture. With time, incomplete rupture mimics papillary muscle elongation. **D,** Single papillary muscle with complete and total rupture.

muscle ruptures were partial or incomplete, thus explaining the subacute or chronic presentation (Fig. 92-21), in contrast to the more dramatic presentation of total rupture (see Fig. 92-21). In addition, all patients had a component of type I or IIIB dysfunction. Mitral valve repair was performed in all but 2 patients. The 5-year survival was 68%, which is comparable to that in type IIIB dysfunction. Repair in the context of ischemic prolapse is expectedly less durable than for prolapse because of degenerative disease, as evident in the 10% actuarial reoperation rate and 30% recurrent moderate or greater mitral regurgitation rate at 5 years, because of greater propensity to recurrence of regurgitation from ongoing ventricular remodeling and from failure of papillary muscle suture techniques when used.

REFERENCES

1. Rossi A, Dini FL, Faggiano P, et al: Independent prognostic value of functional mitral regurgitation in patients with heart failure. A quantitative analysis of 1256 patients with ischaemic and non-ischaemic dilated cardiomyopathy. *Heart* 97:1675–1680, 2011.
2. Carpentier A: Cardiac valve surgery–the "French correction." *J Thorac Cardiovasc Surg* 86:323–337, 1983.
3. Adams DH, Anyanwu A: Pitfalls and limitations in measuring and interpreting the outcomes of mitral valve repair. *J Thorac Cardiovasc Surg* 131:523–529, 2006.
4. Grande-Allen KJ, Barber JE, Klatka KM, et al: Mitral valve stiffening in end-stage heart failure: evidence of an organic contribution to functional mitral regurgitation. *J Thorac Cardiovasc Surg* 130:783–790, 2005.
5. Bach DS, Deeb GM, Bolling SF: Accuracy of intraoperative transesophageal echocardiography for estimating the severity of functional mitral regurgitation. *Am J Cardiol* 76:508–512, 1995.
6. Zoghbi WA, Enriquez-Sarano M, Foster E, et al, American Society of E: Recommendations for evaluation of the severity of native valvular regurgitation with two-dimensional and doppler echocardiography. *J Am Soc Echocardiogr* 16:777–802, 2003.
7. Grigioni F, Enriquez-Sarano M, Zehr KJ, et al: Ischemic mitral regurgitation: long-term outcome and prognostic implications with quantitative Doppler assessment. *Circulation* 103:1759–1764, 2001.
8. Green GR, Dagum P, Glasson JR, et al: Mitral annular dilatation and papillary muscle dislocation without mitral regurgitation in sheep. *Circulation* 100:II95–II102, 1999.
9. Ahmad RM, Gillinov AM, McCarthy PM, et al: Annular geometry and motion in human ischemic mitral regurgitation: novel assessment with three-dimensional echocardiography and computer reconstruction. *Ann Thorac Surg* 78:2063–2068, discussion 2068, 2004.
10. Chan KM, Amirak E, Zakkar M, et al: Ischemic mitral regurgitation: in search of the best treatment for a common condition. *Prog Cardiovasc Dis* 51:460–471, 2009.
11. Hueb AC, Jatene FB, Moreira LF, et al: Ventricular remodeling and mitral valve modifications in dilated cardiomyopathy: new insights from anatomic study. *J Thorac Cardiovasc Surg* 124:1216–1224, 2002.
12. Kaji S, Nasu M, Yamamuro A, et al: Annular geometry in patients with chronic ischemic mitral regurgitation: three-dimensional magnetic resonance imaging study. *Circulation* 112:I409–I414, 2005.
13. Timek TA, Lai DT, Tibayan F, et al: Annular versus subvalvular approaches to acute ischemic mitral regurgitation. *Circulation* 106:I27–I32, 2002.
14. Timek TA, Lai DT, Liang D, et al: Effects of paracommissural septal-lateral annular cinching on acute ischemic mitral regurgitation. *Circulation* 110:II79–II84, 2004.
15. Timek TA, Lai DT, Tibayan F, et al: Septal-lateral annular cinching abolishes acute ischemic mitral regurgitation. *J Thorac Cardiovasc Surg* 123:881–888, 2002.
16. McCarthy PM: Does the intertrigonal distance dilate? Never say never. *J Thorac Cardiovasc Surg* 124:1078–1079, 2002.
17. Timek TA, Lai DT, Tibayan F, et al: Ischemia in three left ventricular regions: insights into the pathogenesis of acute ischemic mitral regurgitation. *J Thorac Cardiovasc Surg* 125:559–569, 2003.
18. Messas E, Guerrero JL, Handschumacher MD, et al: Chordal cutting: a new therapeutic approach for ischemic mitral regurgitation. *Circulation* 104:1958–1963, 2001.
19. Dagum P, Timek TA, Green GR, et al: Coordinate-free analysis of mitral valve dynamics in normal and ischemic hearts. *Circulation* 102:III62–III69, 2000.
20. Kumanohoso T, Otsuji Y, Yoshifuku S, et al: Mechanism of higher incidence of ischemic mitral regurgitation in patients with inferior myocardial infarction: quantitative analysis of left ventricular and mitral valve geometry in 103 patients with prior myocardial infarction. *J Thorac Cardiovasc Surg* 125:135–143, 2003.
21. Watanabe N, Ogasawara Y, Yamaura Y, et al: Geometric differences of the mitral valve tenting between anterior and inferior myocardial infarction with significant ischemic mitral regurgitation: quantitation by novel software system with transthoracic real-time three-dimensional echocardiography. *J Am Soc Echocardiogr* 19:71–75, 2006.
22. Song JM, Qin JX, Kongsaerepong V, et al: Determinants of ischemic mitral regurgitation in patients with chronic anterior wall myocardial infarction: a real time three-dimensional echocardiography study. *Echocardiography* 23:650–657, 2006.
23. Filsoufi F, Rahmanian PB, Anyanwu A, et al: Physiologic basis for the surgical treatment of ischemic mitral regurgitation. *Am Heart Hosp J* 4:261–268, 2006.
24. Kwan J, Shiota T, Agler DA, et al: Real-time three-dimensional echocardiography s. Geometric differences of the mitral apparatus between ischemic and dilated cardiomyopathy with significant

mitral regurgitation: real-time three-dimensional echocardiography study. *Circulation* 107:1135–1140, 2003.
25. Lai DT, Tibayan FA, Myrmel T, et al: Mechanistic insights into posterior mitral leaflet inter-scallop malcoaptation during acute ischemic mitral regurgitation. *Circulation* 106:I40–I45, 2002.
26. Aklog L, Filsoufi F, Flores KQ, et al: Does coronary artery bypass grafting alone correct moderate ischemic mitral regurgitation? *Circulation* 104:I68–I75, 2001.
27. Grossi EA, Woo YJ, Patel N, et al: Outcomes of coronary artery bypass grafting and reduction annuloplasty for functional ischemic mitral regurgitation: a prospective multicenter study (randomized evaluation of a surgical treatment for off-pump repair of the mitral valve). *J Thorac Cardiovasc Surg* 141:91–97, 2011.
28. Bolling SF, Deeb GM, Bach DS: Mitral valve reconstruction in elderly, ischemic patients. *Chest* 109:35–40, 1996.
29. Bolling SF, Pagani FD, Deeb GM, et al: Intermediate-term outcome of mitral reconstruction in cardiomyopathy. *J Thorac Cardiovasc Surg* 115:381–386, discussion 387–388, 1998.
30. Kwon MH, Lee LS, Cevasco M, et al: Recurrence of mitral regurgitation after partial versus complete mitral valve ring annuloplasty for functional mitral regurgitation. *J Thorac Cardiovasc Surg* 146:616–622, 2013.
31. Silberman S, Klutstein MW, Sabag T, et al: Repair of ischemic mitral regurgitation: comparison between flexible and rigid annuloplasty rings. *Ann Thorac Surg* 87:1721–1726, discussion 1726–1727, 2009.
32. Spoor MT, Geltz A, Bolling SF: Flexible versus nonflexible mitral valve rings for congestive heart failure: differential durability of repair. *Circulation* 114:I67–I71, 2006.
33. Messas E, Pouzet B, Touchot B, et al: Efficacy of chordal cutting to relieve chronic persistent ischemic mitral regurgitation. *Circulation* 108(Suppl 1):II111–II115, 2003.
34. Hung J, Chaput M, Guerrero JL, et al: Persistent reduction of ischemic mitral regurgitation by papillary muscle repositioning: structural stabilization of the papillary muscle-ventricular wall complex. *Circulation* 116:I259–I263, 2007.
35. Hung J, Guerrero JL, Handschumacher MD, et al: Reverse ventricular remodeling reduces ischemic mitral regurgitation: echo-guided device application in the beating heart. *Circulation* 106:2594–2600, 2002.
36. De Bonis M, Lapenna E, La Canna G, et al: Mitral valve repair for functional mitral regurgitation in end-stage dilated cardiomyopathy: role of the "edge-to-edge" technique. *Circulation* 112: I402–I408, 2005.
37. Timek TA, Nielsen SL, Lai DT, et al: Edge-to-edge mitral valve repair without ring annuloplasty for acute ischemic mitral regurgitation. *Circulation* 108(Suppl 1):II122–II127, 2003.
38. Kincaid EH, Riley RD, Hines MH, et al: Anterior leaflet augmentation for ischemic mitral regurgitation. *Ann Thorac Surg* 78:564–568, discussion 568, 2004.
39. Acker MA: Clinical results with the acorn cardiac restraint device with and without mitral valve surgery. *Semin Thorac Cardiovasc Surg* 17:361–363, 2005.
40. Hung J, Solis J, Guerrero JL, et al: A novel approach for reducing ischemic mitral regurgitation by injection of a polymer to reverse remodel and reposition displaced papillary muscles. *Circulation* 118:S263–S269, 2008.
41. Messas E, Bel A, Morichetti MC, et al: Autologous myoblast transplantation for chronic ischemic mitral regurgitation. *J Am Coll Cardiol* 47:2086–2093, 2006.
42. Inoue M, McCarthy PM, Popovic ZB, et al: The coapsys device to treat functional mitral regurgitation: in vivo long-term canine study. *J Thorac Cardiovasc Surg* 127:1068–1076, discussion 1076–1077, 2004.
43. Grossi EA, Patel N, Woo YJ, et al: Outcomes of the RESTOR-MV Trial (Randomized Evaluation of a Surgical Treatment for Off-Pump Repair of the Mitral Valve). *J Am Coll Cardiol* 56:1984–1993, 2010.
44. Yancy CW, Jessup M, Bozkurt B, et al: 2013 ACCF/AHA guideline for the management of heart failure: executive summary: a report of the American College of Cardiology Foundation/American Heart Association task force on practice guidelines. *Circulation* 128:1810–1852, 2013.
45. Di Biase L, Auricchio A, Mohanty P, et al: Impact of cardiac resynchronization therapy on the severity of mitral regurgitation. *Europace* 13:829–838, 2011.
46. Onishi T, Onishi T, Marek JJ, et al: Mechanistic features associated with improvement in mitral regurgitation after cardiac resynchronization therapy and their relation to long-term patient outcome. *Circ Heart Fail* 6:685–693, 2013.
47. von Oppell UO, Stemmet F, Brink J, et al: Ischemic mitral valve repair surgery. *J Heart Valve Dis* 9:64–73, discussion 73–74, 2000.
48. Chan KM, Punjabi PP, Flather M, et al: Coronary artery bypass surgery with or without mitral valve annuloplasty in moderate functional ischemic mitral regurgitation: final results of the Randomized Ischemic Mitral Evaluation (RIME) trial. *Circulation* 126:2502–2510, 2012.
49. Wu AH, Aaronson KD, Bolling SF, et al: Impact of mitral valve annuloplasty on mortality risk in patients with mitral regurgitation and left ventricular systolic dysfunction. *J Am Coll Cardiol* 45:381–387, 2005.
50. Maltais S, Tchantchaleishvili V, Schaff HV, et al: Management of severe ischemic cardiomyopathy: left ventricular assist device as destination therapy versus conventional bypass and mitral valve surgery. *J Thorac Cardiovasc Surg* 147:1246–1250, 2014.
51. Byrne JG, Aranki SF, Adams DH, et al: Mitral valve surgery after previous cabg with functioning ima grafts. *Ann Thorac Surg* 68:2243–2247, 1999.
52. Crestanello JA: Surgical approach to mitral regurgitation in chronic heart failure: when is it an option? *Curr Heart Fail Rep* 9:40–50, 2012.
53. Fattouch K, Guccione F, Sampognaro R, et al: Point: efficacy of adding mitral valve restrictive annuloplasty to coronary artery bypass grafting in patients with moderate ischemic mitral valve regurgitation: a randomized trial. *J Thorac Cardiovasc Surg* 138:278–285, 2009.
54. Lancellotti P, Marwick T, Pierard LA: How to manage ischaemic mitral regurgitation. *Heart* 94:1497–1502, 2008.
55. Christenson JT, Simonet F, Bloch A, et al: Should a mild to moderate ischemic mitral valve regurgitation in patients with poor left ventricular function be repaired or not? *J Heart Valve Dis* 4:484–488, discussion 488–489, 1995.
56. Christenson JT, Simonet F, Maurice J, et al: Mitral regurgitation in patients with coronary artery disease and low left ventricular ejection fractions. How should it be treated? *Tex Heart Inst J* 22:243–249, 1995.
57. Penicka M, Linkova H, Lang O, et al: Predictors of improvement of unrepaired moderate ischemic mitral regurgitation in patients undergoing elective isolated coronary artery bypass graft surgery. *Circulation* 120:1474–1481, 2009.
58. Arcidi JM, Jr, Hebeler RF, Craver JM, et al: Treatment of moderate mitral regurgitation and coronary disease by coronary bypass alone. *J Thorac Cardiovasc Surg* 95:951–959, 1988.
59. Connolly MW, Gelbfish JS, Jacobowitz IJ, et al: Surgical results for mitral regurgitation from coronary artery disease. *J Thorac Cardiovasc Surg* 91:379–388, 1986.
60. Duarte IG, Shen Y, MacDonald MJ, et al: Treatment of moderate mitral regurgitation and coronary disease by coronary bypass alone: late results. *Ann Thorac Surg* 68:426–430, 1999.
61. Chen FY, Adams DH, Aranki SF, et al: Mitral valve repair in cardiomyopathy. *Circulation* 98:II124–II127, 1998.
62. Crabtree TD, Bailey MS, Moon MR, et al: Recurrent mitral regurgitation and risk factors for early and late mortality after mitral valve repair for functional ischemic mitral regurgitation. *Ann Thorac Surg* 85:1537–1542, discussion 1542–1543, 2008.
63. Hausmann H, Siniawski H, Hetzer R: Mitral valve reconstruction and replacement for ischemic mitral insufficiency: seven years' follow up. *J Heart Valve Dis* 8:536–542, 1999.
64. Ruvolo G, Speziale G, Bianchini R, et al: Combined coronary bypass grafting and mitral valve surgery: early and late results. *Thorac Cardiovasc Surg* 43:90–93, 1995.
65. Serri K, Bouchard D, Demers P, et al: Is a good perioperative echocardiographic result predictive of durability in ischemic mitral valve repair? *J Thorac Cardiovasc Surg* 131:565–573, e562, 2006.
66. Bax JJ, Braun J, Somer ST, et al: Restrictive annuloplasty and coronary revascularization in ischemic mitral regurgitation results

in reverse left ventricular remodeling. *Circulation* 110:II103–II108, 2004.
67. Daimon M, Fukuda S, Adams DH, et al: Mitral valve repair with Carpentier-McCarthy-Adams IMR ETlogix annuloplasty ring for ischemic mitral regurgitation: early echocardiographic results from a multi-center study. *Circulation* 114:I588–I593, 2006.
68. Gangemi JJ, Tribble CG, Ross SD, et al: Does the additive risk of mitral valve repair in patients with ischemic cardiomyopathy prohibit surgical intervention? *Ann Surg* 231:710–714, 2000.
69. Gazoni LM, Kern JA, Swenson BR, et al: A change in perspective: results for ischemic mitral valve repair are similar to mitral valve repair for degenerative disease. *Ann Thorac Surg* 84:750–757, discussion 758, 2007.
70. Geidel S, Lass M, Krause K, et al: Early and late results of restrictive mitral valve annuloplasty in 121 patients with cardiomyopathy and chronic mitral regurgitation. *Thorac Cardiovasc Surg* 56:262–268, 2008.
71. Raja SG, Berg GA: Moderate ischemic mitral regurgitation: to treat or not to treat? *J Card Surg* 22:362–369, 2007.
72. Lamas GA, Mitchell GF, Flaker GC, et al: Clinical significance of mitral regurgitation after acute myocardial infarction. Survival and ventricular enlargement investigators. *Circulation* 96:827–833, 1997.
73. Aronson D, Goldsher N, Zukermann R, et al: Ischemic mitral regurgitation and risk of heart failure after myocardial infarction. *Arch Intern Med* 166:2362–2368, 2006.
74. Pastorius CA, Henry TD, Harris KM: Long-term outcomes of patients with mitral regurgitation undergoing percutaneous coronary intervention. *Am J Cardiol* 100:1218–1223, 2007.
75. Ellis SG, Whitlow PL, Raymond RE, et al: Impact of mitral regurgitation on long-term survival after percutaneous coronary intervention. *Am J Cardiol* 89:315–318, 2002.
76. Kang DH, Sun BJ, Kim DH, et al: Percutaneous versus surgical revascularization in patients with ischemic mitral regurgitation. *Circulation* 124:S156–S162, 2011.
77. Adler DS, Goldman L, O'Neil A, et al: Long-term survival of more than 2,000 patients after coronary artery bypass grafting. *Am J Cardiol* 58:195–202, 1986.
78. Hickey MS, Smith LR, Muhlbaier LH, et al: Current prognosis of ischemic mitral regurgitation. Implications for future management. *Circulation* 78:I51–I59, 1988.
79. Campwala SZ, Bansal RC, Wang N, et al: Factors affecting regression of mitral regurgitation following isolated coronary artery bypass surgery. *Eur J Cardiothorac Surg* 28:783–787, 2005.
80. Harris KM, Sundt TM, 3rd, Aeppli D, et al: Can late survival of patients with moderate ischemic mitral regurgitation be impacted by intervention on the valve? *Ann Thorac Surg* 74:1468–1475, 2002.
81. Mihaljevic T, Lam BK, Rajeswaran J, et al: Impact of mitral valve annuloplasty combined with revascularization in patients with functional ischemic mitral regurgitation. *J Am Coll Cardiol* 49:2191–2201, 2007.
82. Calafiore AM, Mazzei V, Iaco AL, et al: Impact of ischemic mitral regurgitation on long-term outcome of patients with ejection fraction above 0.30 undergoing first isolated myocardial revascularization. *Ann Thorac Surg* 86:458–464, discussion 464–465, 2008.
83. Di Mauro M, Di Giammarco G, Vitolla G, et al: Impact of no-to-moderate mitral regurgitation on late results after isolated coronary artery bypass grafting in patients with ischemic cardiomyopathy. *Ann Thorac Surg* 81:2128–2134, 2006.
84. Fattouch K, Sampognaro R, Speziale G, et al: Impact of moderate ischemic mitral regurgitation after isolated coronary artery bypass grafting. *Ann Thorac Surg* 90:1187–1194, 2010.
85. Schroder JN, Williams ML, Hata JA, et al: Impact of mitral valve regurgitation evaluated by intraoperative transesophageal echocardiography on long-term outcomes after coronary artery bypass grafting. *Circulation* 112:I293–I298, 2005.
85a. Guy TS, IV, Moainie SL, Gorman JH, III, et al: Prevention of ischemic mitral regurgitation does not influence the outcome of remodeling after posterolateral myocardial infarction. *J Am Coll Cardiol* 43:377–383, 2004.
86. Grewal KS, Malkowski MJ, Piracha AR, et al: Effect of general anesthesia on the severity of mitral regurgitation by transesophageal echocardiography. *Am J Cardiol* 85:199–203, 2000.
87. Magne J, Pibarot P, Dagenais F, et al: Preoperative posterior leaflet angle accurately predicts outcome after restrictive mitral valve annuloplasty for ischemic mitral regurgitation. *Circulation* 115:782–791, 2007.
88. Balu V, Hershowitz S, Zaki Masud AR, et al: Mitral regurgitation in coronary artery disease. *Chest* 81:550–555, 1982.
89. Tolis GA, Jr, Korkolis DP, Kopf GS, et al: Revascularization alone (without mitral valve repair) suffices in patients with advanced ischemic cardiomyopathy and mild-to-moderate mitral regurgitation. *Ann Thorac Surg* 74:1476–1480, discussion 1480–1481, 2002.
90. Kim YH, Czer LS, Soukiasian HJ, et al: Ischemic mitral regurgitation: revascularization alone versus revascularization and mitral valve repair. *Ann Thorac Surg* 79:1895–1901, 2005.
91. Ryden T, Bech-Hanssen O, Brandrup-Wognsen G, et al: The importance of grade 2 ischemic mitral regurgitation in coronary artery bypass grafting. *Eur J Cardiothorac Surg* 20:276–281, 2001.
92. Prifti E, Bonacchi M, Frati G, et al: Ischemic mitral valve regurgitation grade II-III: correction in patients with impaired left ventricular function undergoing simultaneous coronary revascularization. *J Heart Valve Dis* 10:754–762, 2001.
93. McGee EC, Gillinov AM, Blackstone EH, et al: Recurrent mitral regurgitation after annuloplasty for functional ischemic mitral regurgitation. *J Thorac Cardiovasc Surg* 128:916–924, 2004.
94. Seipelt RG, Schoendube FA, Vazquez-Jimenez JF, et al: Combined mitral valve and coronary artery surgery: ischemic versus non-ischemic mitral valve disease. *Eur J Cardiothorac Surg* 20:270–275, 2001.
95. Tahta SA, Oury JH, Maxwell JM, et al: Outcome after mitral valve repair for functional ischemic mitral regurgitation. *J Heart Valve Dis* 11:11–18, discussion 18–19, 2002.
96. Gelsomino S, Lorusso R, Capecchi I, et al: Left ventricular reverse remodeling after undersized mitral ring annuloplasty in patients with ischemic regurgitation. *Ann Thorac Surg* 85:1319–1330, 2008.
97. Anyanwu AC, Adams DH: Ischemic mitral regurgitation: recent advances. *Curr Treat Options Cardiovasc Med* 10:529–537, 2008.
98. Braun J, van de Veire NR, Klautz RJ, et al: Restrictive mitral annuloplasty cures ischemic mitral regurgitation and heart failure. *Ann Thorac Surg* 85:430–436, discussion 436–437, 2008.
99. ten Brinke EA, Klautz RJ, Tulner SA, et al: Clinical and functional effects of restrictive mitral annuloplasty at midterm follow-up in heart failure patients. *Ann Thorac Surg* 90:1913–1920, 2010.
100. Czer LS, Maurer G, Bolger AF, et al: Revascularization alone or combined with suture annuloplasty for ischemic mitral regurgitation. Evaluation by color doppler echocardiography. *Tex Heart Inst J* 23:270–278, 1996.
101. Grossi EA, Bizekis CS, LaPietra A, et al: Late results of isolated mitral annuloplasty for "functional" ischemic mitral insufficiency. *J Card Surg* 16:328–332, 2001.
102. Tibayan FA, Rodriguez F, Langer F, et al: Mitral suture annuloplasty corrects both annular and subvalvular geometry in acute ischemic mitral regurgitation. *J Heart Valve Dis* 13:414–420, 2004.
103. Tibayan FA, Rodriguez F, Liang D, et al: Paneth suture annuloplasty abolishes acute ischemic mitral regurgitation but preserves annular and leaflet dynamics. *Circulation* 108(Suppl 1):II128–II133, 2003.
104. Mikuckaite L, Vaskelyte J, Radauskaite G, et al: Left ventricular remodeling following ischemic mitral valve repair: predictive factors. *Scand Cardiovasc J* 43:57–62, 2009.
105. Calafiore AM, Mauro MD, Gallina S, et al: Surgical treatment of mitral valve regurgitation in dilated cardiomyopathy. *Heart Surg Forum* 7:21–25, 2004.
106. Yiu SF, Enriquez-Sarano M, Tribouilloy C, et al: Determinants of the degree of functional mitral regurgitation in patients with systolic left ventricular dysfunction: a quantitative clinical study. *Circulation* 102:1400–1406, 2000.
107. Nagasaki M, Nishimura S, Ohtaki E, et al: The echocardiographic determinants of functional mitral regurgitation differ in ischemic and non-ischemic cardiomyopathy. *Int J Cardiol* 108:171–176, 2006.
108. Zhu F, Otsuji Y, Yotsumoto G, et al: Mechanism of persistent ischemic mitral regurgitation after annuloplasty: importance of augmented posterior mitral leaflet tethering. *Circulation* 112:I396–I401, 2005.
109. Kongsaerepong V, Shiota M, Gillinov AM, et al: Echocardiographic predictors of successful versus unsuccessful mitral valve repair in ischemic mitral regurgitation. *Am J Cardiol* 98:504–508, 2006.

110. Kuwahara E, Otsuji Y, Iguro Y, et al: Mechanism of recurrent/persistent ischemic/functional mitral regurgitation in the chronic phase after surgical annuloplasty: importance of augmented posterior leaflet tethering. *Circulation* 114:I529–I534, 2006.
111. Roshanali F, Mandegar MH, Yousefnia MA, et al: A prospective study of predicting factors in ischemic mitral regurgitation recurrence after ring annuloplasty. *Ann Thorac Surg* 84:745–749, 2007.
112. Glower DD, Tuttle RH, Shaw LK, et al: Patient survival characteristics after routine mitral valve repair for ischemic mitral regurgitation. *J Thorac Cardiovasc Surg* 129:860–868, 2005.
113. Al-Radi OO, Austin PC, Tu JV, et al: Mitral repair versus replacement for ischemic mitral regurgitation. *Ann Thorac Surg* 79:1260–1267, discussion 1260–1267, 2005.
114. Gillinov AM, Wierup PN, Blackstone EH, et al: Is repair preferable to replacement for ischemic mitral regurgitation? *J Thorac Cardiovasc Surg* 122:1125–1141, 2001.
115. Micovic S, Milacic P, Otasevic P, et al: Comparison of valve annuloplasty and replacement for ischemic mitral valve incompetence. *Heart Surg Forum* 11:E340–E345, 2008.
116. Morishita A, Shimakura T, Nonoyama M, et al: Mitral valve replacement in ischemic mitral regurgitation. Preservation of both anterior and posterior mitral leaflets. *J Cardiovasc Surg (Torino)* 43:147–152, 2002.
117. Grossi EA, Goldberg JD, LaPietra A, et al: Ischemic mitral valve reconstruction and replacement: comparison of long-term survival and complications. *J Thorac Cardiovasc Surg* 122:1107–1124, 2001.
118. Acker MA, Parides MK, Perrault LP, et al: Mitral-valve repair versus replacement for severe ischemic mitral regurgitation. *N Engl J Med* 370:23–32, 2014.
119. Lorusso R, Gelsomino S, Vizzardi E, et al: Mitral valve repair or replacement for ischemic mitral regurgitation? The Italian Study on the Treatment of Ischemic Mitral Regurgitation (ISTIMIR). *J Thorac Cardiovasc Surg* 145:128–139, discussion 137–138, 2013.
120. Gillinov AM: Is ischemic mitral regurgitation an indication for surgical repair or replacement? *Heart Fail Rev* 11:231–239, 2006.
121. Filsoufi F, Castillo JG, Rahmanian PB, et al: Remodeling annuloplasty using a prosthetic ring designed for correcting type-IIIb ischemic mitral regurgitation. *Rev Esp Cardiol* 60:1151–1158, 2007.
122. Anyanwu AC, Adams DH: The intraoperative "ink test": a novel assessment tool in mitral valve repair. *J Thorac Cardiovasc Surg* 133:1635–1636, 2007.
123. Kron IL, Green GR, Cope JT: Surgical relocation of the posterior papillary muscle in chronic ischemic mitral regurgitation. *Ann Thorac Surg* 74:600–601, 2002.
124. Rama A, Nappi F, Praschker BG, et al: Papillary muscle approximation for ischemic mitral valve regurgitation. *J Card Surg* 23:733–735, 2008.
125. Hvass U, Tapia M, Baron F, et al: Papillary muscle sling: a new functional approach to mitral repair in patients with ischemic left ventricular dysfunction and functional mitral regurgitation. *Ann Thorac Surg* 75:809–811, 2003.
126. Ito H, Yamamoto K, Hiraiwa T: Mitral valve repair with papillary muscle sling for functional mitral regurgitation: application of double mitral ring concept in a case of ischemic cardiomyopathy and a case of idiopathic dilated cardiomyopathy. *Gen Thorac Cardiovasc Surg* 55:297–301, 2007.
127. Langer F, Kunihara T, Hell K, et al: RING+STRING: successful repair technique for ischemic mitral regurgitation with severe leaflet tethering. *Circulation* 120:S85–S91, 2009.
128. Levine RA, Schwammenthal E: Ischemic mitral regurgitation on the threshold of a solution: from paradoxes to unifying concepts. *Circulation* 112:745–758, 2005.
129. Borger MA, Murphy PM, Alam A, et al: Initial results of the chordal-cutting operation for ischemic mitral regurgitation. *J Thorac Cardiovasc Surg* 133:1483–1492, 2007.
130. Fayad G, Marechaux S, Modine T, et al: Chordal cutting via aortotomy in ischemic mitral regurgitation: surgical and echocardiographic study. *J Card Surg* 23:52–57, 2008.
131. Rendon F, Aramendi JI, Rodrigo D, et al: Patch enlargement of the posterior mitral leaflet in ischemic regurgitation. *Asian Cardiovasc Thorac Ann* 10:248–250, 2002.
132. Bhudia SK, McCarthy PM, Smedira NG, et al: Edge-to-edge (alfieri) mitral repair: results in diverse clinical settings. *Ann Thorac Surg* 77:1598–1606, 2004.
133. Croft LR, Jimenez JH, Gorman RC, et al: Efficacy of the edge-to-edge repair in the setting of a dilated ventricle: an in vitro study. *Ann Thorac Surg* 84:1578–1584, 2007.
134. Ramadan R, Al-Attar N, Mohammadi S, et al: Left ventricular infarct plication restores mitral function in chronic ischemic mitral regurgitation. *J Thorac Cardiovasc Surg* 129:440–442, 2005.
135. Magne J, Senechal M, Mathieu P, et al: Restrictive annuloplasty for ischemic mitral regurgitation may induce functional mitral stenosis. *J Am Coll Cardiol* 51:1692–1701, 2008.
136. Marwick TH: Restrictive annuloplasty for ischemic mitral regurgitation: too little or too much? *J Am Coll Cardiol* 51:1702–1703, 2008.
137. Cheng A, Nguyen TC, Malinowski M, et al: Undersized mitral annuloplasty inhibits left ventricular basal wall thickening but does not affect equatorial wall cardiac strains. *J Heart Valve Dis* 16:349–358, 2007.
138. Machaalany J, Bilodeau L, Hoffmann R, et al: Treatment of functional mitral valve regurgitation with the permanent percutaneous transvenous mitral annuloplasty system: results of the multicenter international percutaneous transvenous mitral annuloplasty system to reduce mitral valve regurgitation in patients with heart failure trial. *Am Heart J* 165:761–769, 2013.
139. Conradi L, Treede H, Rudolph V, et al: Surgical or percutaneous mitral valve repair for secondary mitral regurgitation: comparison of patient characteristics and clinical outcomes. *Eur J Cardiothorac Surg* 44:490–496, discussion 496, 2013.
140. Glower DD, Kar S, Trento A, et al: Percutaneous mitral valve repair for mitral regurgitation in high-risk patients: results of the Everest II study. *J Am Coll Cardiol* 64:172–181, 2014.
141. Vakil K, Roukoz H, Sarraf M, et al: Safety and efficacy of the MitraClip® system for severe mitral regurgitation: a systematic review. *Catheter Cardiovasc Interv* 84:129–136, 2014.
142. Taramasso M, Maisano F, Latib A, et al: Clinical outcomes of MitraClip for the treatment of functional mitral regurgitation. *EuroIntervention* 2014.
143. Gueret P, Khalife K, Jobic Y, et al: Echocardiographic assessment of the incidence of mechanical complications during the early phase of myocardial infarction in the reperfusion era: a French multicentre prospective registry. *Arch Cardiovasc Dis* 101:41–47, 2008.
144. Chen Q, Darlymple-Hay MJ, Alexiou C, et al: Mitral valve surgery for acute papillary muscle rupture following myocardial infarction. *J Heart Valve Dis* 11:27–31, 2002.
145. Russo A, Suri RM, Grigioni F, et al: Clinical outcome after surgical correction of mitral regurgitation due to papillary muscle rupture. *Circulation* 118:1528–1534, 2008.
146. Tavakoli R, Weber A, Vogt P, et al: Surgical management of acute mitral valve regurgitation due to post-infarction papillary muscle rupture. *J Heart Valve Dis* 11:20–25, discussion 26, 2002.
147. Jouan J, Tapia M, C Cook R, et al: Ischemic mitral valve prolapse: mechanisms and implications for valve repair. *Eur J Cardiothorac Surg* 26:1112–1117, 2004.

CHAPTER 93

Postinfarction Ventricular Septal Defect and Ventricular Rupture

Sharven Taghavi • Abeel A. Mangi

CHAPTER OUTLINE

Disruption of the ventricular septum after myocardial infarction is an infrequent event after a full-thickness myocardial infarction. The resulting clinical syndrome can range from an asymptomatic murmur to an extensive left-to-right intracardiac shunt with resulting heart failure and shock. The first approaches to surgical management emphasized delayed repair, which allowed time for fibrosis to occur so that tissue quality at the defect margins was more substantial.[1,2] Modern approaches recognize that potentially salvageable patients deteriorate during this period of delay. Thus, early surgical intervention is now the accepted treatment.[3]

HISTORICAL PERSPECTIVE

Postinfarction ventricular septal defect (VSD) was first recognized by Latham at autopsy in 1845.[4] The first antemortem diagnosis was made in 1923.[5] In 1956, Cooley accomplished the first successful surgical repair in a patient who had survived several weeks after septal perforation.[6] Most patients in the early era were brought to operation a month or longer after surviving acute infarction with the belief that organization of the tissues surrounding the defect would allow a more secure closure.[1,2] Subsequently, improvements in myocardial protection, the design and refinement of surgical techniques, improved prosthetic materials, and the widespread use of cardiac ultrasonography to permit the earlier diagnosis of VSD have all contributed to making earlier successful repair of this entity a possibility.[7]

INCIDENCE AND DEMOGRAPHICS

Postinfarction VSD complicates 1% to 2% of myocardial infarctions, but it accounts for 5% of deaths after myocardial infarction.[8,9] The incidence appears to be declining because of aggressive pharmacologic and interventional management of acute myocardial infarction and better treatment of postinfarction hypertension.[10-12] Postinfarction VSDs occur more frequently in males (male-to-female ratio, 3:2), reflecting the higher incidence of coronary artery disease in men. The average age is 62 years (range, 44 to 81 years). Septal rupture occurs most often after the first acute myocardial infarction.[13]

ETIOLOGY AND PATHOGENESIS

Angiographic evaluation of patients with postinfarction VSD most often reveals a completely occluded culprit coronary artery.[6] Nearly two thirds of patients have single-vessel disease.[14] There is usually somewhat less extensive disease in other vessels, and less collateralization.[15] Postinfarction VSDs are located most commonly (i.e., in ≈60% of cases) in the anteroapical septum as a result of full-thickness anterior infarction secondary to occlusion of the left anterior descending artery. Twenty percent to 40% of patients with postinfarction VSD have rupture of the posterior septum because of inferoseptal infarction secondary to occlusion of a dominant right or a dominant circumflex coronary artery (Fig. 93-1).[16] Simple rupture, consisting of a direct through-and-through defect, tends to be more common and is usually located anteriorly. Complex rupture with a more serpiginous tract is less common and is usually located inferiorly. Although a single VSD develops in most patients, 5% to 11% of patients may have multiple septal defects.

The myocardial infarction that sets the backdrop for a postinfarction VSD tends to be extensive and has been reported to involve 26% of the free wall on average, compared with only 15% in noncomplicated acute myocardial infarctions.[8] Postinfarction VSD usually develops two to four days after acute myocardial infarction, but it has been reported as early as a few hours after acute myocardial infarction and up to two weeks later.[8,17,18] This time course correlates with histologic findings that show extensive distribution of necrotic myocardium at this time, with relatively sparse vasculogenesis, angiogenesis, or formation of fibrous connective tissue.[19,20] It has been hypothesized that "slippage" of myocytes during infarct expansion may allow blood to dissect through the necrotic myocardium, where it can enter the right ventricle (or the pericardial space in the setting of rupture of the free wall).[21,22] Similarly, autodigestion of necrotic myocardium may allow fissures to form, through which blood can subsequently dissect.[23]

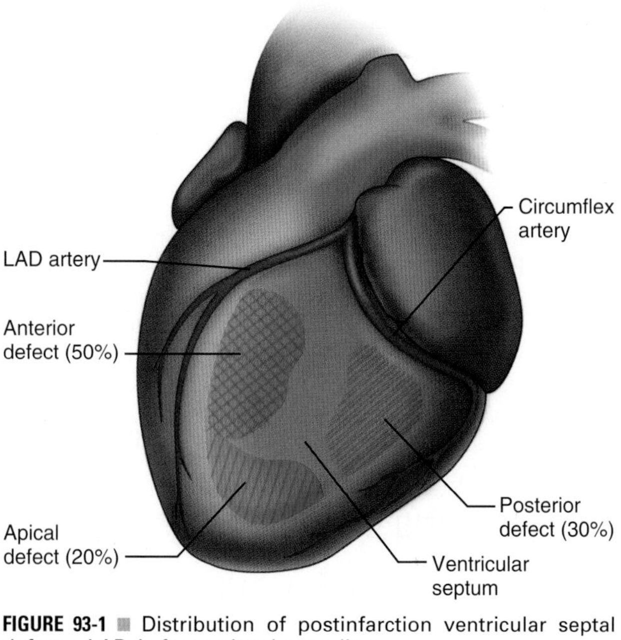

FIGURE 93-1 Distribution of postinfarction ventricular septal defects. *LAD,* Left anterior descending.

Left-ventricular free-wall rupture can occur in 4% to 8% of myocardial infarctions[24,25] and is responsible for 15% of deaths after acute myocardial infarction.[26] Free-wall rupture typically occurs one to four days after infarction and is easily diagnosed with echocardiogram.[24] Acute rupture is almost always fatal; however, some patients with subacute rupture can be saved, but they require emergent surgical intervention.[24,26]

PATHOPHYSIOLOGY

The primary determinant of outcome after postinfarction rupture of the ventricular septum is the development of heart failure (left, right, or biventricular), which is a function of both the size of the defect and the magnitude of the myocardial infarction. Left-sided heart failure tends to predominate in anterior VSDs, and right-sided failure predominates in posterior VSDs.[27-29] The extent of heart failure often cannot be explained solely by postinfarction failure of the ventricle.[30] With the opening of a defect in the ventricular septum, a proportion of each left ventricular ejection is diverted from the systemic circulation across the septum into the right ventricle, thereby both compromising forward systemic cardiac output and overloading the pulmonary circulation. The resulting cardiogenic shock can lead to end-organ malperfusion and organ failure, which may be irreversible and fatal. In addition, the normally compliant right ventricle may demonstrate severe diastolic failure after a prolonged left-to-right shunt. The resulting escalation in right ventricular (RV) diastolic pressures can ultimately result in flow reversal across the septum when RV end-diastolic pressures exceed left ventricular end-diastolic pressures[31] and compound the situation further with systemic hypoxia.

NATURAL HISTORY

Without surgical intervention, one-quarter of patients with postinfarction VSD die within 24 hours. Half will succumb to their illness within the first week, nearly two-thirds will die within two weeks, three-quarters will die within a month, and only 7% will survive longer than one year.[13,32,33] These data have been confirmed in the recent SHOCK (SHould we emergently revascularize Occluded Coronaries in cardiogenic shocK) multicenter trial, in which subgroup analysis of patients who had postinfarction VSD was performed. A total of 55 patients with postinfarction VSD were enrolled in the study a median of 16 hours after infarction and went into shock 7.3 hours thereafter. Of the 24 patients treated medically, only one survived (survival rate, 4%). Of the 31 patients who underwent operation to repair the VSD, 21 underwent concomitant coronary artery bypass grafting. Of these, only six survived (survival rate, 19%). The difference between the groups was statistically significant.[34]

The historical practice of waiting weeks after postinfarction rupture of the ventricular septum selected out patients with lesser pathology and a relatively mild hemodynamic insult.[28,35,36] It is clear that attempting to defer early operation in the hopes of maintaining hemodynamic stability deprives many patients of a chance for a successful outcome before irreversible end-organ damage supervenes.[37,38]

CLINICAL PRESENTATION, PREOPERATIVE MANAGEMENT, AND RISK STRATIFICATION

Presentation

Typically, patients with postinfarction VSD present several days after a myocardial infarction with a harsh new holosystolic murmur that may radiate to the axilla.[18] In more than half of patients, this is associated with recurrent chest pain.[8] Clinical signs are generally those of right-sided heart failure, and pulmonary edema is rare. The electrocardiographic findings in these patients are the changes seen in antecedent anterior, septal, inferior, or posterior infarction. As much as one third of patients may develop transient atrioventricular conduction block that precedes rupture. Chest roentgenogram is generally nonspecific. Unfortunately, there is no reliable predictor of impending rupture.

This clinical syndrome may resemble acute mitral regurgitation secondary to rupture of a papillary muscle. In fact, both entities may coexist and sometimes can be distinguished only by imaging techniques. On physical examination, the murmur associated with postinfarction VSD is more prominent at the left lateral sternal border, is loud, and is associated with a thrill in more than half of patients. In addition, septal rupture is more commonly associated with anterior infarcts and conduction anomalies, whereas papillary muscle rupture is usually associated with posterior infarction and no conduction anomalies. If the patient is deemed salvageable, immediate placement of intra-aortic balloon pump and early operation are the management strategy of choice.

Diagnosis

The classic technique for distinguishing between acute papillary muscle rupture and postinfarction VSD has been right heart catheterization, during which a greater than 9% step-up in the oxygen saturation between the right atrium and the pulmonary artery is diagnostic of VSD in the appropriate clinical setting.[28] Additional findings, such as an elevated pulmonary-to-systemic flow ratio, which can range from 1.4:1 to 8:1, also verify the presence of the VSD and roughly correlate with size.[39] Neither of these techniques accurately localizes the defect. Color-flow Doppler echocardiography can show the size and location of the defect, determine ventricular function, assess pulmonary artery and RV pressures, and exclude concomitant mitral valve disease with sensitivity and specificity approaching 100%.[40-43]

Indications for Operation and Preoperative Management

Because the natural history of untreated postinfarction VSD is dismal, the diagnosis of this entity suffices as an indication for operation.[38] Patients in cardiogenic shock represent a surgical emergency. Sometimes patients are already in established multisystem organ failure. These patients are unlikely to survive emergent repair and may benefit from a mechanical bridge (e.g., intra-aortic balloon counterpulsation or ventricular assist device) for salvage before corrective surgery. Patients in an intermediate status between shock and stable condition need to have surgical repair within 12 to 24 hours after appropriate preoperative evaluations are completed. A small percentage of patients (<5%) who are completely stable with no clinical compromise can undergo repair on a semi-elective basis.

Preoperative management is directed toward maintaining hemodynamic stability and preventing end-organ damage. Specifically, therapy should be targeted toward reducing systemic vascular resistance (thereby reducing left-to-right shunting), maintaining cardiac output and peripheral perfusion, and maintaining or improving coronary blood flow. All three of these objectives can be accomplished by intra-aortic balloon counterpulsation[44-46] or with directed pharmacologic therapy.

Predictors of Risk

Patients with postinfarction VSD comprise a heterogeneous group in which both extremes of risk (i.e., very low risk and very high risk) are possible. For the nonemergent, stable patients, excellent results can be achieved, probability of survival to discharge from the hospital is high, and long-term survival is comparable with that in common cardiac operations. Conversely, patients in extremis tend to have dismal outcomes (Table 93-1).

In various studies, clinical variables have been used to identify the high-risk patient. In several studies, the use of an intra-aortic balloon pump was correlated with increased early mortality[47]; presumably, its use was seen as a marker for disease severity. Other groups have demonstrated that posterior location of the septal rupture is associated with an increased operative mortality,[28,31,48,49] which may be because the repair is more technically difficult, because the risk of mitral regurgitation is increased, or because RV failure is associated with an RV infarction. Proximal VSDs (closer to the atrioventricular groove) have also been shown to strongly predict early mortality, presumably because they are associated with the largest infarctions.[50]

TABLE 93-1 **Preoperative Predictors of Death after Surgical Repair of Postinfarction VSD**

Variable	Predictor of Early Death	Predictor of Late Death
Need for preoperative catecholamines	$P = 0.001$	$P =$ NS
Emergent operation	$P < 0.0001$	$P =$ NS
Anterior VSD	$P = 0.04$	$P =$ NS
Age > 65 years	$P = 0.009$	$P =$ NS
Right-sided heart failure	$P = 0.01$	$P = 0.005$
Elevation in blood urea nitrogen	$P = 0.02$	$P =$ NS
Elevation of serum creatinine	$P =$ NS	$P < 0.05$
Previous myocardial infarction	$P =$ NS	$P < 0.05$
Presence of left main coronary disease	$P =$ NS	$P < 0.05$

VSD, Ventral septal defect.

OPERATIVE MANAGEMENT

General Principles

Cardiopulmonary bypass is established with bicaval venous drainage and cannulation of the ascending aorta. The patient is cooled, and cardiac standstill is achieved with blood cardioplegia via the antegrade and retrograde routes. A variety of alternative strategies for myocardial protection are practiced at Massachusetts General Hospital, including continuous warm-blood cardioplegia, fibrillatory arrest, and cold-blood cardioplegia.[51-54] If myocardial revascularization is to be performed, it should be done before opening the ventricle, to optimize myocardial protection. The general principles of this operation include meticulous attention to myocardial protection, a transinfarct approach to the VSD, thorough trimming of the left ventricular margins of the defect, conservative trimming of the right ventricular margin, close inspection of the papillary muscles and mitral apparatus, a tension-free repair, placement of the patch on the endocardial surface, and buttressing of the repair with Teflon felt to prevent sutures from cutting through the friable muscle.

Infarctectomy

Apical Amputation

The technique of apical amputation was first described by Daggett.[3] An incision is made through the infarcted apex of the left ventricle. Débridement of the necrotic myocardium back to healthy muscle results in amputation of the apex of the heart, including the left ventricle, right ventricle, and septum. The remaining apical portions are then reapproximated to the apical septum using a row of interrupted mattress sutures of 0 Tevdek passed sequentially through a buttressing strip of Teflon felt, the left ventricular wall, a second strip of felt, the septum, a third strip of felt, the right ventricular wall, and a fourth strip of felt. After all of these sutures have been tied, the closure is reinforced with an additional running suture.

Free-Wall Rupture

There have been numerous surgical techniques described for repair of free-wall rupture. Many have advocated closing the defect with infarctectomy and prosthetic patch repair while the patient is on cardiopulmonary bypass.[55-58] The use of cardiopulmonary bypass is fraught with difficulty because of the systemic heparinization causing continuous oozing of blood through necrotic myocardium.[55] For this reason, many clinicians have advocated repair without extracorporeal bypass using an epicardial patch.[59-61] More recently, the use of a prosthetic patch with surgical glue has been advocated for patients without blowout rupture. The advantage of this technique is that it allows for a simple and expedited repair.[62]

Anterior Septal Rupture

These defects are approached via a left ventriculotomy through the infarct. If the defect is small, it can be closed by plication with primary closure.[63] Most defects are larger and require closure with a Dacron prosthetic patch after débridement of necrotic myocardium. This operation is performed by placing a series of pledgeted interrupted mattress sutures around the perimeter of the defect. Sutures are passed through the septum from right to left along the posterior rim, and they are passed from the epicardium to the endocardium along the anterior rim. Once all the sutures are laid, the patch is inserted and all sutures are pledgeted again and then tied. The edges of the ventriculotomy are then reapproximated in a double-layer closure that is buttressed with Teflon felt or glutaraldehyde-preserved bovine pericardium (Fig. 93-2).

Posteroinferior Septal Rupture

Posterior VSD poses the greatest technical challenge (Fig. 93-3). Simple plication has an extremely high failure rate, and the procedure is often complicated by a reopening of the defect or by catastrophic disruption of the infarctectomy closure. Use of the following technique has been associated with improved operative results. After the establishment of cardiopulmonary bypass, the left heart is vented via the right superior pulmonary vein. The heart is then delivered from the pericardial well as for bypass to the posterior descending coronary artery. The infarct may include both ventricles or may be limited to the left ventricle only. The left ventricle is opened in standard fashion and infarctectomy is performed. The mitral apparatus is inspected, and mitral valve replacement is performed only in the setting of frank papillary muscle infarct. This is performed through a separate left atriotomy. The left ventricle needs to be aggressively débrided, but right ventricular débridement can be limited to only as much tissue as is needed to visualize the VSD. If the posterior septum has simply separated from the free wall, it can be reapproximated primarily in

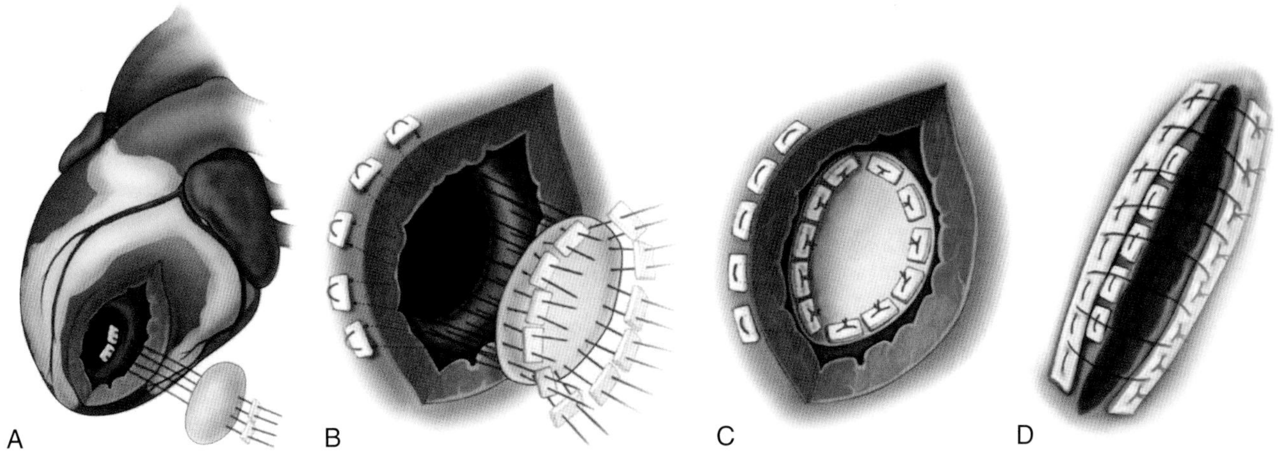

FIGURE 93-2 ■ Technique of repair of anterior postinfarction ventricular septal defect by infarctectomy and patch repair.

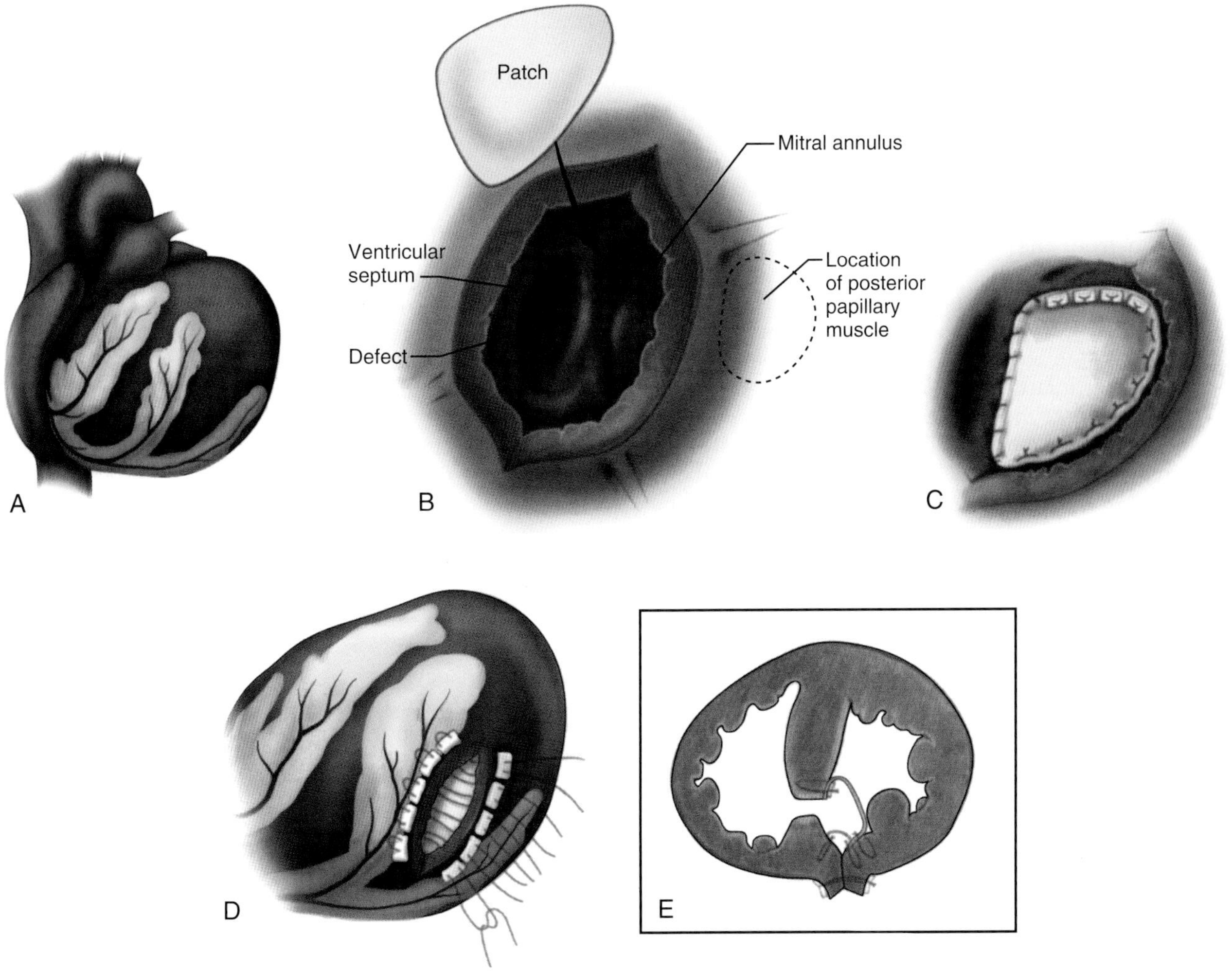

FIGURE 93-3 ■ Technique of repair of posterior postinfarction ventricular septal defect by infarctectomy and patch repair.

a double-layered buttressed closure. Larger defects require patch closure as described earlier. The only difference is that sutures are placed from the right side of the septum and from the epicardial side of the right ventricular free wall. The most important aspect of this operation is to perform a separate patch closure of the infarctectomy, because primary closure of this large tissue defect with its friable edges under tension has historically resulted in catastrophic disruption. We use a Hemashield Dacron graft (Boston Scientific, Natick, MA) for this purpose and pass sutures through the patch, which is seated on the epicardial surface of the heart, and then through the margin of the infarctectomy, from the endocardium to the epicardium. Using an appropriately sized patch can result in restoration of normal ventricular geometry.

Infarct Exclusion with Endocardial Patch Repair

The technique of infarct exclusion with endocardial patch repair emphasizes the importance of restoring normal ventricular geometry as an attempt to preserve or restore ventricular function.[52,53,63-65] The operative strategy is an extrapolation of the technique of Dor and colleagues, ventricular endoaneurysmorrhaphy[66]—which involves intracavitary placement of an endocardial patch to exclude both the septal defect and the infarcted myocardium from the high-pressure zone of the ventricle—while maintaining ventricular geometry, which theoretically enhances ventricular function. Other theoretical benefits of this approach include avoiding resection of the myocardium (which could further compromise ventricular function), and avoiding a suture line in friable muscle (to diminish postoperative bleeding and disruption of the repair).

David and coworkers[27] pioneered this technique, which involves exposing the interventricular septum via a left ventriculotomy through the infarcted anterior wall 1 to 2 cm from the left anterior descending coronary artery. Stay sutures are placed in the ventricular wall to aid in exposure of the septal defect. These authors used a glutaraldehyde-fixed bovine pericardial patch for the repair. The patch is tailored to the endocardial shape of the ventricular infarction (generally about 4 × 6 cm) and is then sutured to healthy muscle (on the endocardial surface) surrounding the septal defect with a continuous 3-0 polypropylene suture. The repair is then carried onto the noninfarcted endocardium of the anterolateral ventricular wall with stitches that are approximately 5 to 7 mm deep and 4 to 5 mm apart. The ventriculotomy is then closed over the patch in two layers and is buttressed with two strips of glutaraldehyde-fixed bovine pericardium. In the case of a posterior septal defect, exposure is achieved via a posterior ventriculotomy with the heart elevated as for bypass grafting to the posterior descending artery.

The repair commences with anchoring of the patch to the fibrous annulus of the mitral valve with a 3-0 continuous polypropylene suture starting at a point corresponding to the posteromedial papillary muscle and moving medially toward the septum until the noninfarcted endocardium is reached. The stitch is then transitioned onto the septal endocardium using the technique described earlier. In this area of the repair, the suture should be reinforced with interrupted, pledgeted sutures. The lateral edge of the patch is sutured to the posterior left ventricle along a line corresponding to the medial margin of the base of the posteromedial papillary muscle. These need to be full-thickness stitches, and they should be buttressed with epicardial bovine pericardium or Teflon felt. Again, the ventriculotomy is closed in two layers of full-thickness sutures buttressed with bovine pericardium or Teflon felt.

Intraoperative Management

Coronary Artery Disease

For patients with postinfarction VSD, the value of preoperative coronary artery angiography and coronary revascularization is controversial. Many of these patients have multivessel coronary disease, and bypassing significantly diseased vessels may increase both early and long-term survival.[27,28,35,64,67,68] Our approach is to perform catheterization when the clinical scenario permits, and to perform concomitant revascularization when indicated. The arguments against simultaneous revascularization are that (1) it provides no additional benefit[69-71] and (2) it subjects patients to preoperative left-side-of-the-heart catheterization, a time-consuming and potentially dangerous procedure. However, one study has found that concomitant revascularization with VSD repair improves early and long-term survival.[72] Other groups have proposed selective left heart catheterization and revascularization[7,73]—avoiding it in patients when a postinfarction VSD is thought to be the result of their first infarction—provided there is no history of angina and no electrocardiographic evidence of previous or ongoing ischemia in another territory.

Weaning from Cardiopulmonary Bypass

We have found routine intraoperative use of a transesophageal echocardiogram to be invaluable for assessing ventricular function, dimensions, residual shunt, and mitral regurgitation when weaning from bypass. For left heart dysfunction, we favor the use of intra-aortic balloon counterpulsation and the use of one of the phosphodiesterase inhibitors, such as milrinone, in the postoperative setting. Strategies to ameliorate right heart failure aim to limit right ventricular afterload while maintaining systemic blood pressure. This can be achieved by right-sided administration of prostaglandin E_1 (0.5 to 2.0 mg/min) with left-sided administration (via a left atrial line) of norepinephrine.[74] Finally, inhaled nitric oxide (20 to 80 ppm) selectively dilates the pulmonary circuit and may be efficacious in ameliorating right heart failure.[75] An inability to wean a patient from cardiopulmonary bypass is unusual if the repair has been successful. If there exists the inability to wean from cardiopulmonary bypass, institution of mechanical assist (left ventricular assist device, right ventricular assist device, or extracorporeal membrane oxygenation) may be considered.

Bleeding

When repairing postinfarction VSD, we generally use antifibrinolytic therapy with either aprotinin or ε-aminocaproic acid before commencing cardiopulmonary bypass. Other maneuvers to avoid postpump suture-line bleeding include application of fibrin sealants to the proposed suture line before repair[76] and the use of biological glues after surgical repair.[77] As a last-resort measure, Baldwin and Cooley[78] have used placement of a left ventricular assist device solely as an adjunct to the repair of friable or damaged myocardium to decrease left ventricular distention, thereby controlling bleeding.

Percutaneous Closure

Successful transcatheter closure of postinfarction ventricular septal rupture, or closure of residual defects after repair, has been reported with increasing frequency. Early experience was with the CardioSEAL device (Nitinol Medical Technologies, Boston, MA), a nitinol double-umbrella prosthesis, which is a transvenous clamshell device.[79] Use of other catheter devices has also been attempted, including the Amplatzer septal occluder and the Rashkind double umbrella.[37,80]

The Amplatzer VSD device allows closure of muscular and membranous VSDs, and it can be used for larger postinfarction defects. In a series of seven patients treated with the Amplatzer, the size of the device ranged from 12 to 24 mm, and there was only one death.[81] The use of such devices in an overall treatment strategy is unclear because data suggest that the devices have a high early failure rate. The most attractive role has been its use in the unstable surgical patient, but data on outcomes in this group are difficult to evaluate and not yet well characterized. Catheter approaches appear to be most effective for treating recurrent or residual defects, and we preferentially use them for these conditions.[82]

Delayed Repair

Sometimes a patient presents with evidence of severe end-organ dysfunction. As was discussed earlier, the risk of repair may be prohibitive in these patients, and consideration should be given to delayed repair. Placement of a ventricular assist device for a defined period of time has the theoretical advantage of allowing reversal of end-organ dysfunction, allowing maturation of the infarct and leading to firmer tissue that could make the closure less prone to technical failure, and permitting recovery of the stunned and energy-depleted myocardium. In our limited experience, this strategy has promise and merits further evaluation. Biventricular support is necessary if instituting left ventricular support results in right-to-left shunting.[83]

Role of Ventricular Assist Devices

In selected patients, there may be a role for temporary mechanical heart support. The successful use of ventricular assist devices with staged repair of ventricular septal rupture has been described.[84-86] Mechanical support may aid in reversing end-organ dysfunction, providing time for maturation of the infarct and leading to firmer tissue. Caution is required, however, because of the potential for high right-to-left shunting across the ventricular septum, which was reported to cause hypoxic brain injury in a patient with postinfarction VSD who was placed on a Heart-Mate left ventricular support device.[83] It is preferable that biventricular support be considered when using mechanical assistance in these patients. In addition to shunting, embolization of necrotic debris is possible, with the potential to cause obstruction in support devices.[87]

Postoperative Management

The postoperative care of these patients is similar to that of other patients undergoing extensive intracardiac operations. Early postoperative diuresis is important to decrease the arterial–alveolar gradient induced by the increased extravascular pulmonary fluid associated with cardiopulmonary bypass. A continuous furosemide drip may sometimes be needed. If the patient suffers from renal dysfunction, we favor early institution of continuous venovenous hemofiltration. Intractable postoperative ventricular arrhythmias are treated with intravenous amiodarone.[88]

OUTCOMES

Operative Mortality

Operative mortality (death before discharge or within 30 days of operation) ranges from 30% to 50% (see Table 93-1). David and colleagues[27] reported outstanding results with the infarct exclusion technique, with only a 19% early mortality rate. Regardless of technique, the most common cause of death after repair of a postinfarction VSD is low cardiac output (52%). Technical failures such as recurrent or residual VSD are the second most common causes of death (22%). Other causes of death include sepsis (17%), recurrent infarction (9%), cerebrovascular complications (4%), and intractable ventricular arrhythmias.

Long-Term Results

Most series report 5-year actuarial survival between 40% and 60% (Table 93-2).[28,89-96] In the Massachusetts General Hospital experience, hospital survivors demonstrated 1-, 5-, and 10-year survival rates of 91%, 70%, and 37%, respectively (Fig. 93-4); 75% reported New York Heart Association (NYHA) class I functional status and 12.5% reported class II functional status after surgery.[10] These favorable results have also been reported by other groups. Gaudiani and coworkers reported an 88% 5-year survival

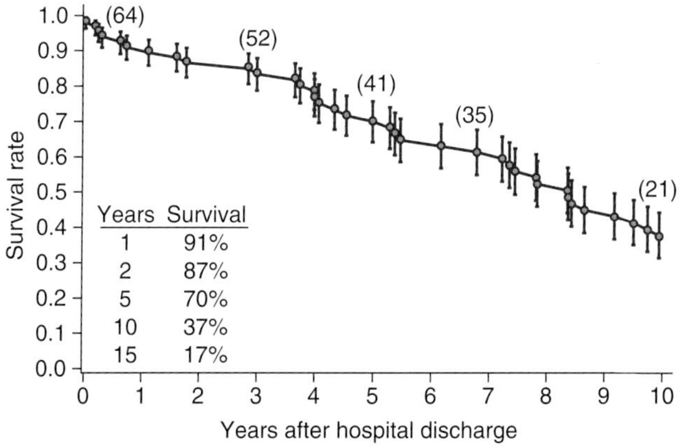

FIGURE 93-4 ■ Postdischarge survival rates after repair of postinfarction ventricular septal defect: The Massachusetts General Hospital experience.

TABLE 93-2 **Recent Clinical Experience* with Surgical Repair of Postinfarction Ventricular Septal Defect**

Institution	City	Year	Patients *(N)*	Hospital Mortality (%)	5-year Survival (%)
Massachusetts General Hospital[1]	Boston	2002	114	37	45
University Hospital[63]	Zurich	2000	54	26	52†
Glenfield General Hospital[27]	Leicester	2000	117	37 (30-day)	46
The Toronto Hospital[24]	Toronto	1998	52	19	65†
Southhampton General[20]	Southampton	1998	179	27	49
MidAmerica Heart Institute[46]	Kansas City	1997	76	41	41
Green Lane Hospital[31]	Auckland	1995	35	31 (30-day)	60†
Hôpital Cardiologique du Haut-Lévèque[28]	Bordeaux	1991	62	38	44
CHU Henri Mondor[53]	Créteil	1991	66	45	44

*Series with fewer than 25 patients and no 5-year follow-up were excluded.
†Value estimated from published graphic or tabular data.

rate, with 74% of survivors in NYHA functional class I.[67] David and colleagues reported a 66% 6-year survival,[27] and Davies and associates reported a 5-year survival rate of 69%.[73]

Recurrent Septal Defects

In 10% to 25% of patients, recurrent or residual VSD may develop,[23] which could result from the reopening of a closed defect, the presence of an overlooked defect, or the development of a new defect in the early postoperative period. Small defects that occur as a result of leaks around the patch are usually asymptomatic and can be controlled with diuretic therapy. Larger defects or those causing symptoms or heart failure should be closed. These attempts may be made first in the catheterization laboratory.

SUMMARY

Although the prevalence of postinfarction VSDs has decreased with modern management of acute myocardial infarction, patients who do come to surgical attention are older and sicker and have complex comorbidities. Surgery is complex and relatively infrequent, and although the results are far better than if the patient had received no treatment at all, morbidity and mortality rates remain high. The use of predictive statistical models can assist us further in helping determine which patients should come to operation early, which patients would be better off temporized with the use of an assist device, and which patients should be turned down or treated percutaneously.

REFERENCES

1. Daicoff AR, Rhodes ML: Surgical repair of ventricular septal rupture and ventricular aneurysms. *JAMA* 203:457, 1968.
2. Dobell ARC, Scott HJ, Cronin RFP, et al: Surgical closure of interventricular septal perforation complicating acute myocardial infarction. *J Thorac Cardiovasc Surg* 43:803, 1962.
3. Daggett WM: Postinfarction VSD repair: retrospective thoughts and historical perspective. *Ann Thorac Surg* 50:1006, 1990.
4. Latham PM: *Lectures on subjects connected with clinical medicine comprising diseases of the heart*, London, 1845, Longman. Rees.
5. Brunn F: Diagnostik der erworbenen rupture der kammerscheidewand des herzens. *Wien Arch Inn Med* 53:140, 1934.
6. Cooley DA, Belmonte BA, Zeis LB, et al: Surgical repair of ruptured interventricular septum following acute myocardial infarction. *Surgery* 41:930, 1957.
7. Skillington PD, Davies RH, Luff AJ, et al: Surgical treatment for infarct-related VSDs. *J Thorac Cardiovasc Surg* 99:798, 1990.
8. Hutchins GM: Rupture of the interventricular septum complicating myocardial infarction: pathologic analysis of 10 patients with clinically diagnosed perforation. *Am Heart J* 97:165, 1979.
9. Lundeberg S, Sodestrom J: Perforation of the interventricular septum in myocardial infarction: a study based on autopsy material. *Acta Med Scand* 172:413, 1962.
10. Daggett WM, Buckley MJ, Akins CW, et al: Improved results of surgical management of postinfarction VSD. *Ann Surg* 196:269, 1982.
11. Figueras J, Alcalde O, Barrabes J, et al: Changes in hospital mortality rates in 425 patients with acute ST-elevation myocardial infarction and cardiac rupture over a 30-year period. *Circulation* 118:2783–2789, 2008.
12. Bueno H, Martinez-Selles M, Perez-David E, et al: Effect of thrombolytic therapy on the risk of cardiac rupture and mortality in older patients with first acute myocardial infarction. *Eur Heart J* 26:1705–1711, 2005.
13. Sanders RJ, Kern WH, Blount SG: Perforation of the interventricular septum complicating myocardial infarction. *Am Heart J* 51:736, 1956.
14. Hill JD, Lary D, Keith WJ, et al: Acquired ventricular septal defects. Evolution of an operation, surgical technique, and results. *J Thorac Cardiovasc Surg* 70:440, 1975.
15. Miller S, Dinsmore RE, Greene RE, et al: Coronary, ventricular and pulmonary abnormalities associated with rupture of the interventricular septum complicating myocardial infarction. *AJR Am J Roentgenol* 131:571, 1978.
16. Swithingbank JM: Perforation of the interventricular septum in myocardial infarction. *Br Heart J* 21:562, 1959.
17. Kitamura S, Mendez A, Kay JH: VSD following myocardial infarction: experience with repair through a left ventriculotomy and review of the literature. *J Thorac Cardiovasc Surg* 61:186, 1971.
18. Selzer A, Gerbode F, Keith WJ: Clinical, hemodynamic and surgical considerations of rupture of the ventricular septum after myocardial infarction. *Am Heart J* 78:598, 1969.
19. Mallory GK, White PD, Salcedo-Salgar J: The speed of healing of myocardial infarction: a study of the pathologic anatomy in seventy cases. *Am Heart J* 18:647, 1939.
20. Silver MD, Butany J, Chiasson DA: The pathology of myocardial infarction and its mechanical complications. In David TE, editor: *Mechanical complications of myocardial infarction*, Austin, 1993, RG Landes.
21. David TE: Surgery for postinfarction VSDs. In David TE, editor: *Mechanical complications of myocardial infarction*, Austin, 1993, RG Landes.

22. Weisman HF, Healy B: Myocardial infarct expansion, infarct extension and reinfarction: pathophysiologic concepts. *Prog Cardiovasc Dis* 30:73, 1987.
23. Beranek JT: Hyaline degeneration of the myocardium is implicated in the pathogenesis of postinfarction heart rupture. *Cor Notes* 9:3, 1994.
24. Sutherland FW, Guell FJ, Pathi VL, et al: Postinfarction ventricular free wall rupture: strategies for diagnosis and treatment. *Ann Thorac Surg* 61:1281–1285, 1996.
25. Bates RJ, Beutler S, Resnekov L, et al: Cardiac rupture—challenge in diagnosis and management. *Am J Cardiol* 40:429–437, 1977.
26. Reardon MJ, Carr CL, Diamond A, et al: Ischemic left ventricular free wall rupture: prediction, diagnosis, and treatment. *Ann Thorac Surg* 64:1509–1513, 1997.
27. David TE, Dale L, Sun Z: Postinfarction ventricular septal rupture: repair by endocardial patch with infarct exclusion. *J Thorac Cardiovasc Surg* 110:1315, 1995.
28. Deville C, Fontan F, Chevalier JM, et al: Surgery of post-infarction ventricular septal defect: risk factors for hospital death and long-term results. *Eur J Cardiothorac Surg* 5:167, 1991.
29. Fanapazir L, Bray CL, Dark JF: Right ventricular dysfunction and surgical outcome in postinfarction VSD. *Eur J Cardiothorac Surg* 4:155, 1983.
30. Radford MJ, Johnson RA, Daggett WM, et al: VSD following myocardial infarction: factors affecting survival. *Clin Res* 26:262A, 1978.
31. Anderson DR, Adams S, Bhat A, et al: Postinfarction VSD. The importance of site of infarction and cardiogenic shock on outcome. *Eur J Cardiothorac Surg* 3:554, 1989.
32. Berger TJ, Blackstone EH, Kirklin JW: Postinfarction VSD. In Barratt-Boyes BG, Kirklin JW, editors: *Cardiac surgery*, New York, 1993, Churchill Livingstone.
33. Omayada A, Queen FB: Spontaneous rupture of the interventricular septum following acute myocardial infarction with some clinicopathologic observations on survival in five cases. Personal communication.
34. Menon V, Webb J, Hillis D, et al: Outcome and profile of ventricular septal rupture with cardiogenic shock after myocardial infarction: a report from the SHOCK registry. *J Am Coll Cardiol* 36:1010, 2000.
35. Daggett WM, Guyton RA, Nundth ED, et al: Surgery for post-myocardial infarct VSDs. *Ann Surg* 186:260, 1977.
36. Kay HRL: In discussion of Daggett WM: surgical management of VSDs complicating myocardial infarction. *World J Surg* 2:753, 1978.
37. Blanche C, Khan SS, Matloff JM, et al: Results of early repair of ventricular septal defect after an acute myocardial infarction. *J Thorac Cardiovasc Surg* 104:961, 1992.
38. Heitmiller R, Jacobs ML, Daggett WM: Surgical management of postinfarction ventricular septal rupture. *Ann Thorac Surg* 41:683, 1986.
39. Heiffila J, Kareojosa M: Ruptured interventricular septum complicating acute myocardial infarction. *Chest* 66:675, 1974.
40. Buckley MJ, Mudth ED, Daggett WM, et al: Surgical therapy for early complications of myocardial infarction. *Surgery* 70:814, 1971.
41. Fortin DF, Sheikh KH, Kisslo J: The utility of echocardiography in the diagnostic strategy of postinfarction ventricular septal rupture: a comparison of two-dimensional versus Doppler color flow imaging. *Am Heart J* 121:25, 1991.
42. Harrison MR, MacPhail B, Gurley JC, et al: Usefulness of color Doppler flow imaging to distinguish VSD from acute mitral regurgitation complicating acute myocardial infarction. *Am J Cardiol* 64:697, 1989.
43. Smyllie JH, Sutherland GR, Geuskens R, et al: Doppler color flow mapping in the diagnosis of ventricular septal rupture and acute mitral regurgitation after myocardial infarction. *J Am Coll Cardiol* 15:1455, 1990.
44. Gold HK, Leinbach RC, Sanders CA, et al: Intra-aortic balloon pumping for VSD complicating acute myocardial infarction. *Circulation* 47:1191, 1973.
45. Monatoya A: Ventricular septal rupture secondary to acute myocardial infarction. In Pifarre R, editor: *Cardiac surgery: acute myocardial infarction and its complications*, Philadelphia, 1992, Hanley and Belfus.
46. Scanlon PJ, Monatoya A, Johnson SA: Urgent surgery for ventricular septal rupture complicating myocardial infarction. *Circulation* 72(Suppl 2):185, 1985.
47. Agnihotri AK, Daggett WM, Torchiana DF, et al: Surgical repair of postinfarction VSD: an analysis of risk. In preparation.
48. Cummings RG, Reimer KA, Catliff R, et al: Quantitative analysis of right and left ventricular infarction in the presence of postinfarction VSD. *Circulation* 77:33, 1988.
49. Moore CA, Nygaard TW, Kaiser DL, et al: Postinfarction ventricular septal rupture: the importance of location of infarction and right ventricular function in determining survival. *Circulation* 74:45, 1986.
50. Cox FF, Morshuis WJ, Plokker HWT, et al: Early mortality after surgical repair of post-infarction ventricular septal rupture: importance of rupture location. *Ann Thorac Surg* 61(6):1752–1757, 1996.
51. Daggett WM, Randolph JD, Jacobs ML, et al: The superiority of cold oxygenated dilute blood cardioplegia. *Ann Thorac Surg* 43:397, 1987.
52. David TE: Surgical treatment of postinfarction ventricular septal rupture. *Australas J Card Thorac Surg* 1:7, 1991.
53. Hendren WG, O'Keefe DD, Geffin GA, et al: Maximal oxygenation of dilute blood cardioplegia solution. *Ann Thorac Surg* 58:1558, 1994.
54. Weisel RD: Myocardial protection during surgery for mechanical complications of myocardial infarction. In David TE, editor: *Mechanical complications of myocardial infarction*, Austin, 1993, RG Landes.
55. Bolooki H: Emergency cardiac procedures in patients in cardiogenic shock due to complications of coronary artery disease. *Circulation* 79(6 Pt 2):I137–I148, 1989.
56. Kendall RW, DeWood MA: Postinfarction cardiac rupture: surgical success and review of the literature. *Ann Thorac Surg* 25:311–315, 1978.
57. Levett JM, Southgate TJ, Jose AB, et al: Technique for repair of left ventricular free wall rupture. *Ann Thorac Surg* 46:248–249, 1988.
58. Pretre R, Benedikt P, Turina MI: Experience with postinfarction left ventricular free wall rupture. *Ann Thorac Surg* 69:1342–1569, 2000.
59. Padro JM, Mesa JM, Silvestre J, et al: Subacute cardiac rupture: repair with a sutureless technique. *Ann Thorac Surg* 55(1):20–23, 1993.
60. McMullan MH, Maples MD, Kilgore TLJ, et al: Surgical experience with left ventricular free wall rupture. *Ann Thorac Surg* 71:1894–1898, 2001.
61. Iemura J, Oku H, Otaki M, et al: Surgical strategy for left ventricular free wall rupture after acute myocardial infarction. *Ann Thorac Surg* 71:201–204, 2001.
62. Canovas S, Lim E, Dalmau M, et al: Midterm clinical and echocardiographic results with patch glue repair of left ventricular free wall rupture. *Circulation* 108:IL237–IL240, 2003.
63. Shumaker H: Suggestions concerning operative management of postinfarction VSDs. *J Thorac Cardiovasc Surg* 64:452, 1972.
64. Alvarez JM, Brady PW, Ross DE: Technical improvements in the repair of acute postinfarction ventricular septal rupture. *J Card Surg* 7:198, 1992.
65. Teoh KH, Christakis GT, Weisel RD, et al: Accelerated myocardial metabolic recovery with terminal warm blood cardioplegia. *J Thorac Cardiovasc Surg* 91:888, 1986.
66. Dor V, Saab M, Coste P, et al: Left ventricular aneurysm: a new surgical approach. *Thorac Cardiovasc Surg* 37:11, 1989.
67. Gaudiani VA, Miller DC, Oyer PE, et al: Post-infarction VSD: an argument for early operation. *Surgery* 89:48, 1981.
68. Komeda M, Fremes SE, David TE: Surgical repair of the postinfarction VSD. *Circulation* 82(Suppl 4):243, 1990.
69. Kaplan MA, Harris CN, Kay JH, et al: Postinfarctional septal rupture: clinical approach and surgical results. *Chest* 69:734, 1976.
70. Matsui K, Kay JH, Mendez M, et al: Ventricular septal rupture secondary to myocardial infarction: clinical approach and surgical results. *JAMA* 245:1537, 1981.
71. Pang P, Sin Y, Lim C, et al: Outcome and survival analysis of surgical repair of post-infarction ventricular septal rupture. *J Cardiothorac Surg* 8:44, 2013.
72. Lundblad R, Abdelnoor M, Geiran OR, et al: Surgical repair of postinfarction ventricular septal rupture: risk factors of early and late death. *J Thorac Cardiovasc Surg* 137:862–868, 2009.

73. Davies RH, Dawkins KD, Skillington PD, et al: Late functional results after surgical closure of acquired VSD. *J Thorac Cardiovasc Surg* 106:592, 1992.
74. D'Ambra MN, LaRaia PJ, Philbin DM, et al: Prostaglandin E_1. A new therapy for refractory right heart failure and pulmonary hypertension after mitral valve replacement. *J Thorac Cardiovasc Surg* 89:567, 1985.
75. Rich GF, Murphy GD, Jr, Roos CM, et al: Inhaled nitric oxide: selective pulmonary vasodilatation in cardiac surgical patients. *Anesthesiology* 78:1028, 1993.
76. Seguin JR, Frapier JM, Colson P, et al: Fibrin sealant for early repair of acquired VSD. *J Thorac Cardiovasc Surg* 104:748, 1992.
77. Fabiani J-N, Jebara VA, Deloche A, et al: Use of surgical glue without replacement in the treatment of type A aortic dissection. *Circulation* 80:264, 1989.
78. Baldwin RT, Cooley DA: Mechanical support for intraventricular decompression in repair of left ventricular disruption. *Ann Thorac Surg* 54:176, 1992.
79. Landzberg MJ, Lock JE: Transcatheter management of ventricular septal rupture after myocardial infarction. *Semin Thorac Cardiovasc Surg* 10:128–132, 1998.
80. Jones MT, Schofield PM, Dark JF: Surgical repair of acquired VSD: determinants of early and late outcome. *J Thorac Cardiovasc Surg* 93:680, 1987.
81. Szkutnik M, Bialkowski J, Kusa J, et al: Postinfarction ventricular septal defect closure with Amplatzer occluders. *Eur J Cardiothorac Surg* 23:323, 2003.
82. Maree A, Jneid H, Palacios I: Percutaneous closure of a postinfarction ventricular septal defect that recurred after surgical repair. *Eur Heart J* 27:1626, 2006.
83. Kshettry V, Salerno C, Bank A: Risk of left ventricular assist device as a bridge to heart transplant following postinfarction ventricular septal rupture. *J Card Surg* 12:93–97, 1997.
84. Aliabadi D, Roland C, Pett S, et al: Percutaneous cardiopulmonary support for the management of catastrophic mechanical complications of acute myocardial infarction. *Cathet Cardiovasc Diagn* 37:223, 1996.
85. Pitsis A, Kelpis T, Visouli A, et al: Left ventricular assist device as a bridge to surgery in postinfarction septal defect. *J Thorac Cardiovasc Surg* 135:951–952, 2008.
86. Conradi L, Treede H, Brickwedel J, et al: Use of initial biventricular mechanical support in a case of postinfarction ventricular septal rupture as a bridge to surgery. *Ann Thorac Surg* 87:e37–e39, 2009.
87. Meyns B, Vanermen H, Vanhaecke J, et al: Hemopump fails as bridge to transplantation in postinfarction ventricular septal defect. *J Heart Lung Transplant* 13:1133, 1994.
88. Saksena S, Rothbart ST, Shah Y: Clinical efficacy and electropharmacology of continuous intravenous amiodarone infusion and chronic oral amiodarone in refractory ventricular tachycardia. *Am J Cardiol* 54:347, 1984.
89. Agnihotri AK, Madsen J, Daggett WM: Unpublished data from Massachusetts General Hospital experience.
90. Pretre R, Ye Q, Grünefelfder J, et al: Role of myocardial revascularization in postinfarction ventricular septal rupture. *Ann Thorac Surg* 69:51–55, 2000.
91. Deja MA, Szostek J, Widenka K, et al: Post infarction VSD—can we do better? *Eur J Cardiothorac Surg* 18:194–201, 2000.
92. David TE, Armstrong S: Surgical repair of postinfarction VSD by infarct exclusion. *Semin Thorac Cardiovasc Surg* 10(2):105–110, 1998.
93. Dalrymple-Hay MJR, Monro JL, Livesey SA, et al: Postinfarction ventricular septal rupture: the Wessex experience. *Semin Thorac Cardiovasc Surg* 10(2):111–116, 1998.
94. Killen DA, Piehler JM, Borkon AM, et al: Early repair of postinfarction ventricular septal rupture. *Ann Thorac Surg* 63:138–142, 1997.
95. Ellis CJ, Parkinson GF, Jaffe WM, et al: Good long-term outcome following surgical repair of post-infarction VSD. *Aust N Z J Med* 25:330–336, 1995.
96. Loisance DY, Lordez JM, Deleuze PH, et al: Acute postinfarction septal rupture: long-term results. *Ann Thorac Surg* 52:474–478, 1991.

CHAPTER 94

NONATHEROSCLEROTIC CORONARY ARTERY DISEASE

Neel R. Sodha • Roger J. Laham • Frank W. Sellke

CHAPTER OUTLINE

Greater than 95% of patients with myocardial ischemia will have underlying atherosclerotic coronary artery disease as the etiology, with the remaining 5% possessing a range of congenital and acquired lesions. Although these lesions are rare individually, clinicians will inevitably encounter some form of nonatherosclerotic coronary artery disease in their practice.

These disorders can be broadly classified as congenital or acquired. Congenital coronary anomalies occur secondary to atresia, an abnormal origin, or abnormal drainage. Acquired disorders can be secondary to mechanical injury to the coronary artery or result from progressive occlusive disease unrelated to atherosclerosis. Diagnosis may be difficult because these disorders may be asymptomatic or may occur in patient populations in which cardiovascular disease is unsuspected. Given the rarity of certain types of these disorders, management recommendations may be based on limited series or expert opinion.

CORONARY ARTERY ANOMALIES

Anomalous Aortic Origin of Coronary Arteries

Approximately one third of all coronary artery anomalies are an anomalous aortic origin. Although multiple variations have been reported, with each of the three major coronary arteries arising from any of the three sinuses of Valsalva, most are benign. The exceptions to this include the right coronary artery arising from the left aortic sinus, and the left main coronary artery arising from the right aortic sinus, both of which are associated with a risk of sudden death.[1,2]

The incidence of sudden death associated with a left main coronary artery arising from the right sinus of Valsalva has been reported to be as high as 57% and is most commonly seen with exercise.[3] When symptomatic, patients will present with angina, myocardial infarction, congestive heart failure, or syncope. From its origin in the right sinus of Valsalva, the left main coronary artery may pass anterior to the pulmonary artery, posterior to the aorta, between the great vessels, or through the conal septum. This anatomic position is believed to result in ischemia because of acute angulation resulting in a narrowed coronary orifice, compression of the artery from the adjacent great vessels, and compression by the intercoronary commissure.[3,4]

The incidence of sudden death from the right coronary artery arising from the left sinus of Valsalva has been reported to be as high as 25% and, as with the left main coronary artery arising from the right sinus, is often exercise related.[3,5] When symptomatic, patients will present with angina, myocardial infarction, conduction disturbances, or syncope. The risk of ischemia is felt to result from ostial obstruction or arterial compression by the aortic root during diastole.[4]

The most common variation in anomalous aortic origin of the coronaries is a circumflex arising from the right sinus of Valsalva, or from the right coronary artery (Fig. 94-1). This condition in general does not manifest with symptoms and is diagnosed incidentally. Because the risk of sudden death is minimal, intervention is not needed.

For all anomalous aortic origins of the coronaries, angiography is needed to delineate anatomy and for surgical planning. In the presence of symptoms, surgery is indicated for all patients. For an anomalous left main coronary artery originating from the right sinus of Valsalva, coronary unroofing is recommended regardless of the presence of symptoms and should be performed urgently if symptoms are present. For patients with an anomalous right coronary artery from the left sinus of Valsalva (Fig. 94-2), surgery should be performed for symptoms, but there remains debate about surgery for the asymptomatic patient.[4] Surgical options include unroofing of the coronary with intimal tacking,[6] aortic reanastomosis, or patch arterioplasty. Proximal ligation of the anomalous coronary with distal bypass grafting is also used but is limited by durability of bypass grafts.[4]

Coronary unroofing with intimal tacking is the currently favored method for correcting an anomalous aortic origin of the left main coronary artery or right coronary artery from the contralateral sinus. After cardiopulmonary bypass grafting is begun, care must be taken when dissecting the aorta from the main pulmonary artery because the aberrant artery may be injured during this dissection. After establishment of cardioplegic arrest, an oblique aortotomy is generally used, but a "hockey-stick" (vertical followed by oblique) aortotomy may be used if there is uncertainty about the course of the aberrant artery to avoid injury. Upon identifying the abnormal origin, a coronary probe is placed in the artery to confirm its course. With the probe in the arterial lumen, the artery is unroofed, using the probe to prevent inadvertent back wall injury. The edges of the unroofed segment are then tacked to the aortic wall with interrupted fine polypropylene suture, thereby creating a new ostium in a more anatomic position (Fig. 94-3).

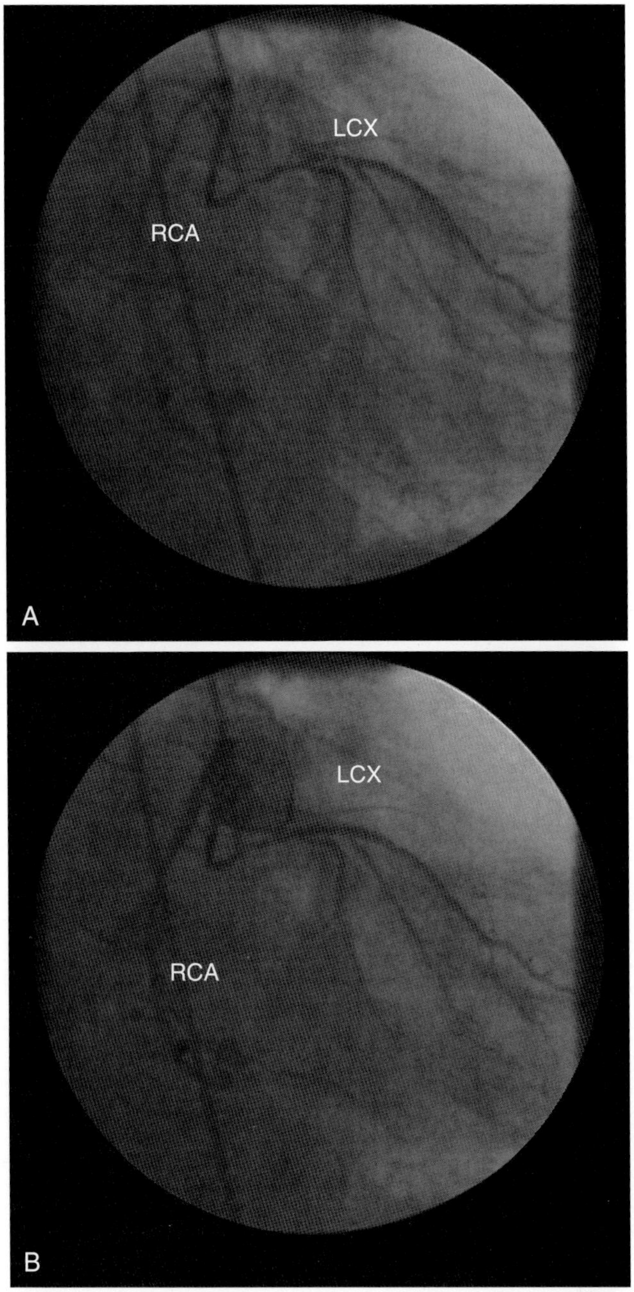

FIGURE 94-1 ■ Anomalous origin of the left circumflex (LCX) from the right coronary artery (RCA) in **(A)** the shallow right anterior oblique, and **(B)** the right anterior oblique projections.

Anomalous Pulmonary Origin of Coronary Arteries

Anomalous Left Main Coronary Artery from the Pulmonary Artery

Anomalous left main coronary artery from the pulmonary artery (ALCAPA) has an incidence of 0.25% to 0.5% and remains one of the most common etiologies of myocardial ischemia in pediatric patients.[7] Symptoms will generally present during infancy unless patients have extensive collateralization from the right coronary artery, in which case symptoms may not present until adulthood. Because they are dependent upon time of diagnosis, symptoms may be related to angina pectoris or heart failure if extensive myocardial infarction has occurred. Diagnosis can be made with echocardiography

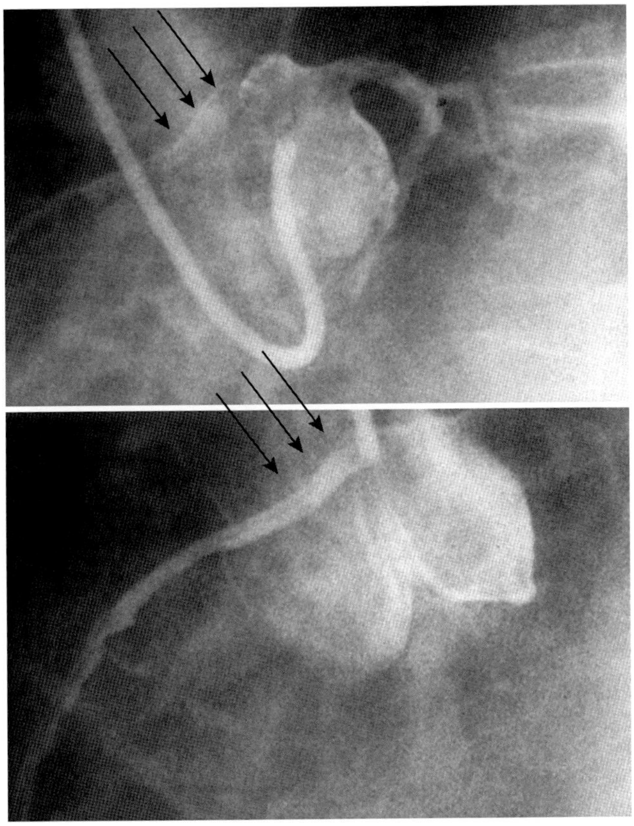

FIGURE 94-2 ■ Anomalous origin of the right coronary artery *(arrows)* from the left cusp high in the aorta above the left main origin.

with color flow, and if the diagnosis remains in question, magnetic resonance angiography or computed tomographic angiography can be used. Once diagnosis is established, surgical correction should be undertaken because of the risk for infarction and sudden death.[8] The currently favored surgical approach to correction is that described by Neches,[9] in which a cuff of pulmonary artery is taken around the coronary and used to reimplant the coronary artery to the aorta. If the anomalous coronary has previously been ligated, or if it cannot be sufficiently mobilized for reimplantation, bypass grafting may be undertaken. Although a certain degree of mitral regurgitation may be present from the prior ischemia, or the ventricular wall may be aneurysmal from prior infarction, most clinicians do not advocate valve repair or aneurysm resection at the time of revascularization because functional improvement is usually seen.[4]

Other Anomalous Pulmonary Origins of Coronary Arteries

As described before, ALCAPA is the most common anomalous pulmonary origin of a coronary artery, with the remainder designated as anomalous pulmonary origins of coronary arteries (APOCA). Anomalous right coronary artery from the pulmonary artery is found in 0.002% of the population and is most commonly discovered before the age of 18.[10] The additional types of APOCA reported include anomalous origin of the circumflex coronary artery from the pulmonary artery and anomalous origin of the right and left coronaries from the pulmonary artery, the latter of which is fatal in the neonatal period. Although patients will commonly present with an asymptomatic murmur, symptoms secondary to myocardial ischemia and heart failure have also been reported.[4] Diagnosis can be made with echocardiography. When the diagnosis is made, most clinicians

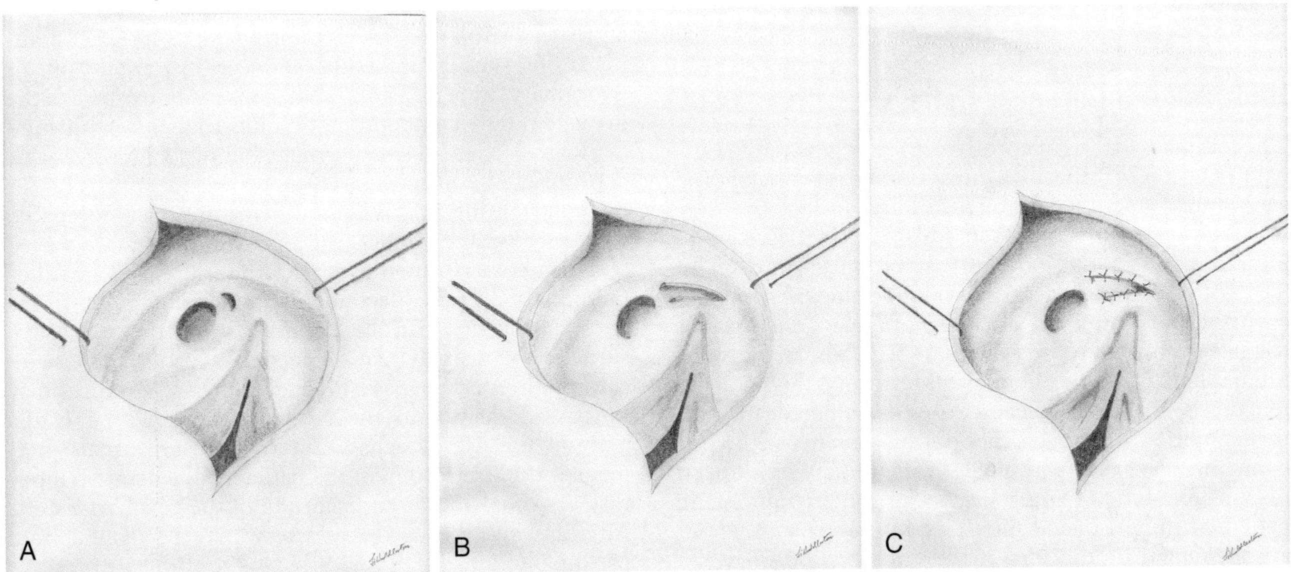

FIGURE 94-3 ■ Anomalous origin of the right coronary artery from the left cusp **(A)** as seen after aortotomy, **(B)** unroofing of the anomalous coronary artery, and **(C)** edge plication for creation of a "neo" ostium. (Courtesy Stephen J. Huddleston, MD, PhD.)

advocate aortic reimplantation of the anomalous coronary because of the risk of sudden death if left uncorrected.[4,10]

Single Coronary Artery

Single coronary artery is an extremely rare coronary anomaly, with an incidence ranging from 0.002% to 0.06%, and is associated with other congenital heart defects in as much as 40% of patients.[11-13] The anomaly can be classified into three types: type 1 describes a single artery supplying the entire heart, type 2 describes a single artery that divides into a right and left coronary artery, and type 3 covers all other variations. Patients will present either with symptoms related to concomitant congenital defects or with angina. Diagnosis is made with coronary angiography. Although some patients will remain asymptomatic, sudden death has been reported secondary to compression between the great vessels, and concerns over angulation and accelerated atherosclerosis have been reported.[13] Percutaneous coronary intervention and coronary artery bypass grafting have been used successfully for the treatment of patients with ischemic symptoms, although no guidelines exist for intervention in asymptomatic patients.[4]

Left Main Coronary Artery Atresia

Congenital atresia of the left main coronary artery is quite rare, with only limited case reports found in the literature. The anomaly may present in infancy with rhythm disturbances, syncope, or sudden death, whereas if there is sufficient collateralization from the right coronary artery, patients may not present until adulthood, at which time ischemic symptoms will manifest. Diagnosis is made with echocardiography and coronary angiography, which allow for differentiation from a single coronary artery and ALCAPA. Surgery is recommended at the time of diagnosis and may consist of distal revascularization with coronary artery bypass grafting[14] or reattaching the proximal left main coronary artery to the aortic sinuses.[15]

High Takeoff Coronary Ostia

The left main and right coronary arteries generally originate from their respective sinuses of Valsalva below the sinotubular junction. Although the incidence varies significantly between series, the coronary arteries may be located significantly above the sinotubular junction in 0.01% to 0.8% of patients.[16,17] The origin will generally occur within 1 to 2 cm of the sinotubular junction but has been reported to be as high as 5 cm above the sinotubular junction. The clinical significance of this anomaly remains controversial because cases of sudden death with this condition have been reported in patients with concomitant coronary pathology, which may have been responsible for the mortality.[17] In the asymptomatic patient with an isolated high takeoff coronary in whom an incidental finding is made, observation may be warranted.

Coronary Artery Fistula

Coronary artery fistulae may be congenital or acquired, with an incidence ranging from 0.2% to 0.85%.[18] The fistulae consist of a direct precapillary communication between a major coronary artery and a cardiac chamber, a major vessel, or a vein. When drainage occurs into a cardiac chamber, the term *coronary-cameral fistula* may be used. Currently, approximately two thirds of coronary artery fistulae are congenital and may be associated with additional congenital heart defects in one third of patients.[19] These are thought to develop because of the persistence of sinusoidal connections between the lumens of the tubular heart in early development.[20] Acquired fistulae may develop after trauma, coronary angiography or other catheter-based intervention, myocardial biopsy, vasculitis, or cardiac surgery. Most commonly, fistulae will be single in approximately 80% of cases, with multiple fistulae occurring in 10% to 15% of patients, and dual right-left coronary fistulae occurring in less than 10% of patients.[20] The left anterior descending and right coronary arteries are the most common sites of origin for fistulae, with the circumflex being an infrequent site.[4] Drainage runs into the low-pressure right heart or pulmonary artery in greater than 90% of cases but may rarely run into the left atrium or ventricle. Fistulae may be classified as type A or type B based on the system proposed by Sakakibara and colleagues.[21] In type A fistulae, the coronary artery proximal to the fistula site is dilated, whereas in type B, the coronary is dilated over its entire length, terminating in the right heart. This distinction is of significance clinically because type A fistulae may be ligated on the epicardial surface of the heart, whereas type B should be ligated intracamerally. If fistulae are large, symptoms may appear during childhood, with angina and dyspnea being the most common complaints. Echocardiography is able to identify a fistula, but catheterization is required for surgical planning and obtaining hemodynamic measurements. Although fistulae rarely close spontaneously, intervention (catheter-based or surgical) is favored by most clinicians in younger patients, even if they are asymptomatic, to prevent complications such as ischemia, endocarditis, aneurysm, or pulmonary hypertension.[4] No consensus exists for the management of asymptomatic older patients with incidentally discovered small fistulae, but observation may be appropriate.[22] Successful catheter-based interventions include stenting or coiling and have not been compared with surgical techniques. Surgical techniques are varied and may be performed with or without the use of cardiopulmonary bypass (dependent upon technique). If the coronary artery can be mobilized on the epicardial surface, the fistula may be ligated without the use of cardiopulmonary bypass. Pledgeted mattress sutures may be passed deep into the artery to occlude the fistula without the use of bypass. Internal closure can be performed via arteriotomy if the patient can tolerate temporary proximal and distal occlusion of the coronary artery. Alternatively, the coronary artery may be ligated both proximally and distally with bypass grafting to preserve distal perfusion. Closure can be performed from within the draining chamber with a purse-string suture or patch, both of which require cardiopulmonary bypass.[20]

Muscle Bridge

The "epicardial" coronary arteries are normally located superficially on the epicardial surface of the heart, but in certain patients they may course through the myocardium for varying lengths, with the overlying muscle termed a *bridge*. Although there exists debate regarding the contribution of muscle bridges to myocardial ischemia,[23] multiple reports demonstrate ischemia secondary to systolic narrowing of the coronary artery from the overlying muscle.[24] In addition to the direct mechanical effects of the bridge, there may be some increase in progression of atherosclerosis proximal to the bridge, which may also contribute to ischemia. The incidence of muscle bridging varies tremendously, from 0.5% to 85%, and is dependent upon the type of study done (angiography versus computed tomography versus autopsy),[4,24] but muscle bridging with arterial compression is seen in only approximately 0.5% of patients undergoing coronary angiography for evaluation of chest pain.[24] If muscle bridging is suspected, coronary angiography with intravascular ultrasonography should be used to confirm the diagnosis (Fig. 94-4). Although some degree of vessel compression is likely benign, reduction of the coronary diameter by greater than 70% during systole and 35% during diastole suggests significant coronary compression.[25] Medical management remains the first-line treatment for symptomatic muscle bridging and consists primarily of beta blockade. Via reducing heart rate and prolonging diastole, beta blockers are able to reduce compression and improve flow.[26] Calcium channel blockers and nitrates may also provide some relief if vasospasm is a concern.[24] For symptoms refractory to medical management, percutaneous coronary intervention with stenting or surgery may be offered. Coronary stenting with drug-eluting stents has demonstrated favorable midterm results, but long-term data are pending.[24] Surgical options for failure of medical management include supra-arterial myotomy or coronary artery bypass grafting. Supra-arterial myotomy has yielded good long-term results, but care must be taken to avoid entry into the right ventricle, which may be vulnerable during unroofing.[27] As an alternative to myotomy, coronary artery bypass distal to the muscle bridge may also be considered for patients with atherosclerotic disease proximal to the bridge and in patients with a thick muscle bridge, because this may increase the risk of inadvertent coronary injury or ventricular entry.

Coronary Aneurysms (Coronary Artery Ectasia and Dilating Coronary Atherosclerosis)

Aneurysms of the coronary artery, defined as a diameter 1.5 times the adjacent normal coronary artery, have been reported to occur in 1.5% to 4.9% of the population.[28,29] Aneurysms are most commonly secondary to underlying atherosclerotic disease but may be congenital or occur secondary to infection, inflammatory disease/vasculitis, or trauma (including iatrogenic trauma after percutaneous intervention). Morphologically, the aneurysms are termed *saccular* or *fusiform*, the latter of which are more commonly seen in patients with atherosclerotic disease. Although fusiform aneurysms are more common, the saccular type is more prone to complications such as rupture or thrombosis. Approximately 50% of coronary artery aneurysms are found in the right coronary artery, with approximately 25% to 50% found in the left anterior descending or left circumflex arteries, and fewer than 10% are found in the left main coronary artery.[29,30] Diagnosis is generally made during evaluation for ischemic complaints. Although echocardiography may demonstrate the aneurysm, coronary angiography remains the definitive diagnostic modality. There is currently no consensus for the treatment of coronary artery aneurysms among medical management, percutaneous intervention with covered stents, and coronary artery bypass grafting. Medical management entails therapy for the underlying pathology (standard management of atherosclerotic coronary disease, clearance of infection, and immunosuppression in the case of vasculitis). Use of statins to inhibit matrix metalloproteinase activity and use of angiotensin II receptor blockers to inhibit transforming growth factor–beta have been tried as adjunct therapy to standard medical management, but no data exist regarding their benefit.[31] Larger aneurysms may benefit from antiplatelet therapy or formal anticoagulation to reduce the risk of thrombosis and embolization, although size criteria and

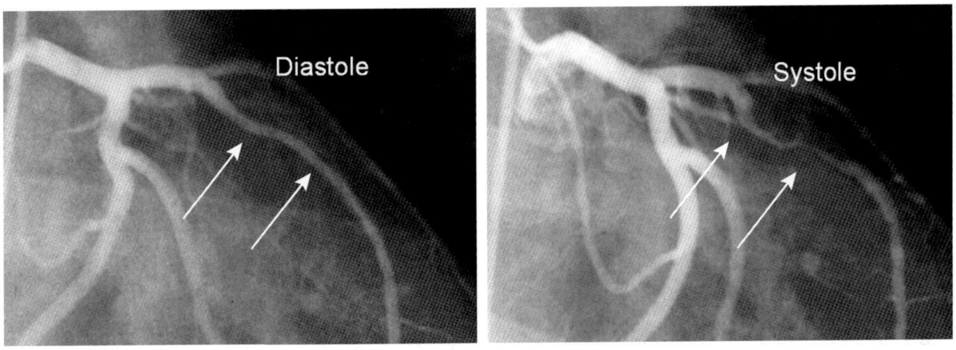

FIGURE 94-4 ■ Muscle bridge *(arrows)* causing compression during systole.

level of anticoagulation have not yet been determined.[32] The successful use of covered stents has been reported (Fig. 94-5), but concerns persist about the risk of stent thrombosis.[31] Indications for surgical intervention include standard indications for coronary artery bypass grafting, aneurysms near large-branch bifurcations, distal embolization with resulting myocardial ischemia, progressive enlargement, left main coronary artery aneurysms, and size threefold the normal coronary diameter.[33,34] Methods for the repair of saccular aneurysms include lateral aneurysmorrhaphy, endarterectomy, and thrombectomy. Fusiform aneurysms are surgically managed with conventional distal bypass grafting and aneurysm ligation.

MECHANICAL INJURY TO THE CORONARY ARTERY

Coronary Artery Embolization

The coronary arteries are partially protected from embolic occlusion by the acute angulation of the coronary ostia relative to aortic outflow and by protection from the aortic valve leaflets during systole. Coronary embolization may be iatrogenically induced during catheter-based interventions (transcatheter aortic valve replacement, coronary angiography) or during cardiac surgery (dislodged thrombus, vegetation, calcium, fat, or

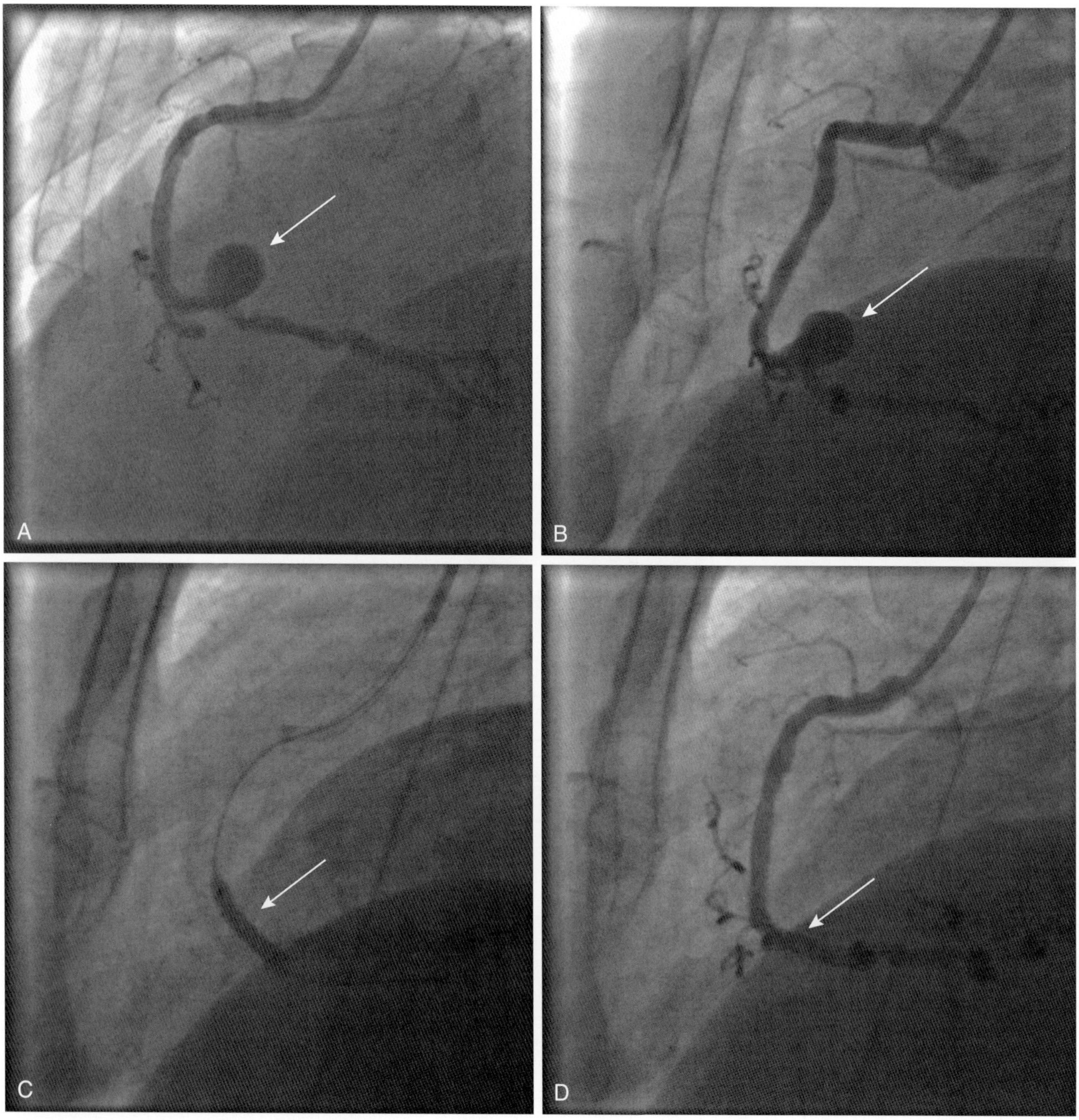

FIGURE 94-5 ■ Right coronary artery pseudoaneurysm *(arrow)* in **(A)** the right anterior oblique projection and **(B)** the left lateral projection. **(C)** Deployment of a balloon-expandable, covered stent with **(D)** aneurysm exclusion.

adhesive/hemostatic compounds). Noniatrogenic causes of coronary embolization include intracardiac or valvular thrombus, tumor, vegetation secondary to endocarditis, or paradoxical emboli in the presence of right-to-left shunting. The clinical consequences of coronary embolization are based on size and location. Most commonly, the left anterior descending coronary artery is affected.[35] Larger emboli may result in significant myocardial ischemia and require intervention. Coronary angiography will often demonstrate an abrupt cut-off point to contrast flow. Percutaneous attempts to restore flow are the mainstay of therapy during diagnostic angiography with bypass surgery or embolectomy reserved for patients in whom percutaneous attempts are unsuccessful with ongoing significant ischemia. For patients who have coronary embolization during surgery, which is identified in the operating room, attempts at clearance via administration of retrograde flushing via the coronary sinus, embolectomy, or bypass graft may be attempted to relieve ischemia.

Coronary Artery Dissection

Coronary artery dissection is defined as separation of the media of the coronary artery with or without an intimal tear. The resulting hemorrhage in the coronary arterial wall can result in luminal narrowing and subsequent ischemia. A dissection is termed *primary* when it occurs spontaneously, or *secondary* when it is caused by an aortic dissection, trauma, or iatrogenic intervention.[36] The dissection can be graded into types A through F based on a National Heart, Lung and Blood Institute classification system.[37] Type A includes radiolucent areas within the coronary artery during contrast injection, which do not persist after the clearance of dye. Type B dissections appear as a double lumen separated by a radiolucent area, which resolves after clearance of dye. Type C appears as contrast outside of the coronary lumen, with persistence after dye clearance. Type D appears as a spiral lesion with persistence of contrast dye. Type E appears as persistent filling defects, and type F appears as total vessel occlusion without antegrade flow.

Spontaneous Coronary Artery Dissection

The reported incidence of spontaneous coronary artery dissection varies widely from 0.2% to 1.1% in patients undergoing coronary angiography.[36,38] The mean age at presentation ranges from 30 to 45 years old, with greater than two thirds of patients being women. Notably, approximately one third of female patients will present in the peripartum period. The left anterior descending coronary artery is most frequently dissected in women, and the right coronary artery in men.[39] The underlying etiology may be related to atherosclerosis, peripartum vascular changes, connective tissue disorders, or vasculitis. The diagnosis is most commonly made with conventional coronary angiography with or without the use of intravascular ultrasonography or optical coherence tomography, although computed tomographic angiography is becoming more widely used for diagnosis and follow-up.[40] Although no specific guidelines exist for the management of spontaneous coronary artery dissection, medical management (e.g., antithrombotic therapy, anti-ischemic therapy with beta blockers and nitrates), percutaneous coronary intervention, and coronary artery bypass grafting have all been used. In hemodynamically stable patients with no evidence of ongoing ischemia, medical management may be considered.[36] In patients with ischemia, the decision to perform percutaneous intervention versus coronary artery bypass grafting should be based on anatomy. Single-vessel dissections may be managed with stenting, if possible. Left main coronary artery and multivessel dissections, as well as failed percutaneous intervention cases, should be managed with conventional coronary artery bypass grafting.[36,38]

Coronary Artery Trauma

Blunt Trauma

Coronary injury secondary to blunt trauma is rare, accounting for less than 2% of injuries in patients presenting after blunt chest injury.[41] The mechanism of injury may be secondary to aortic dissection with retrograde involvement of the coronary ostia, proximal coronary avulsion (partial or complete) from the aortic root, or intimal injury with resulting coronary dissection or thrombosis. The left anterior descending and right coronary arteries are the most commonly injured. Clinical manifestations are generally immediate with resulting hemodynamic compromise from myocardial ischemia or tamponade, but some injuries may result in delayed thrombosis with late presentation. In clinically unstable patients with bleeding, immediate exploration is warranted with concomitant coronary artery bypass if the injury is proximal, whereas in patients without bleeding, coronary angiography with intervention may be done.[42,43]

Penetrating Trauma

Owing to their anatomic location, the left anterior descending and right coronary arteries are the most commonly injured after penetrating chest trauma. The immediate clinical manifestation is generally pericardial tamponade. Penetrating injury with hemodynamic compromise or evidence of pericardial fluid will mandate operative exploration. Small coronary artery branches and the distal third of large epicardial coronary arteries may be ligated without inducing significant ventricular dysfunction, but postoperative arrhythmias may occur as a result of focal infarction. For more proximal coronary arterial injuries, intracoronary shunts may be used to gain temporary control of bleeding. Because many penetrating injuries are anterior, off-pump coronary artery bypass techniques with limited heparinization may be done to primarily repair, vein-patch repair, or perform bypass grafting. Standard on-pump techniques can be used as well if exposure is poor or ventricular function is compromised.[42,43]

Iatrogenic Coronary Artery Trauma

Coronary artery dissection or thrombosis is exceedingly rare after coronary angiography, with rates of less than

0.01%.[44] These complications can often be managed percutaneously with intracoronary stenting but may require emergent coronary artery bypass grafting if there is resulting ischemia. During cardiac surgery, coronary injuries such as dissection may occur secondary to coronary intubation with handheld cardioplegia cannulae, or use of intracoronary probes. Inadvertent coronary ligation secondary to misplaced sutures during repair of ventricular injuries can occur. Often these injuries will manifest as ventricular dysfunction during separation from cardiopulmonary bypass and necessitate distal bypass grafting.

PROGRESSIVE NONATHEROSCLEROTIC CORONARY OCCLUSIVE DISEASE

Coronary Artery Vasculitis

Polyarteritis Nodosa

Polyarteritis nodosa is a systemic necrotizing vasculitis affecting medium and small arteries. The overall incidence of polyarteritis nodosa is low, with estimates between 0.4 and 2 per million per year.[45] The vasculitis most commonly affects the kidneys, gastrointestinal tract, skin, joints, and muscles, with symptomatic coronary involvement reported less frequently. The average age of symptom onset ranges from 30 to 50 years, with a predominance in males. Coronary involvement can result in premature atherosclerosis, coronary aneurysm, dissection, or thrombosis.[46] Medical management of the vasculitis centers on immunosuppression with glucocorticoids and antiplatelet therapy with aspirin. For patients in whom coronary complications develop, the role of surgery versus percutaneous coronary intervention remains to be defined. Most reports indicate that patients are treated with percutaneous intervention initially, with surgery as an option if the former fails. Coronary artery bypass grafting in this patient population is complicated by immunosuppression and concerns with healing, operating during active inflammation, and selection of an appropriate conduit, given concerns of internal mammary artery involvement in some cases of polyarteritis nodosa.[47,48] Given the generally young age at presentation, some clinicians recommend preoperative imaging of the internal mammary arteries and subsequent use as a conduit if suitable, but they favor avoiding the radial artery as a conduit because of the risk of disease involvement.[47]

Systemic Lupus Erythematosus

Systemic lupus erythematosus (SLE) is an immune-mediated inflammatory disease with primarily musculoskeletal and mucocutaneous inflammation and predominance in females. When matched against controls with similar risk factors for coronary artery disease, patients with SLE have a threefold higher risk of subclinical coronary artery disease and present at earlier ages, which may be attributable to chronic inflammation, a prothrombotic state, or chronic use of corticosteroids.[49] When myocardial ischemia is suspected, coronary angiography should be undertaken, with indications for percutaneous intervention versus coronary artery bypass grafting remaining the same as for patients without SLE. If coronary artery bypass grafting is planned, perioperative consideration of concomitant valvular disease and hypercoagulability should be made. Valvular heart disease is the most common cardiac abnormality seen in patients with SLE, with an incidence of 13% to 100% found in autopsy studies, and is a leading cause of morbidity.[50] Left-sided valve involvement predominates, and all patients should undergo preoperative echocardiography before revascularization to aid in surgical planning.[49] Limited case series have reported on the success of coronary artery bypass grafting in patients with SLE and have noted no inflammatory involvement of the left internal mammary artery on pathology specimens, suggesting its suitability for conduit use.[51,52]

Wegener Granulomatosis

Wegener granulomatosis is a necrotizing vasculitis affecting medium and small vessels, most commonly in the respiratory tract and kidneys. Coronary involvement most commonly manifests as arteritis,[53] but clinically significant coronary arterial involvement is extremely rare.[54]

Takayasu Disease

Takayasu arteritis is predominantly a disease found in young Asian women between 10 and 50 years of age and in which the vasculitis affects the aorta and its major branches. The incidence of coronary arterial involvement complicating the arteritis has been reported to be approximately 10%.[55] Proximal coronary arterial involvement is common, increasing the risk for severe myocardial ischemia.[56] Reports of percutaneous management of coronary arterial disease have met with limited long-term success,[57] but use of drug-eluting stents may provide some increase in long-term patency.[58] Given the limited data on long-term patency rates with percutaneous intervention, and the incidence of left main coronary arterial involvement, coronary artery bypass grafting is often considered a potential initial treatment option. Undertaking coronary artery bypass grafting is complicated by the chronic inflammation of the entire aortic wall, which can lead to morbidity from manipulation, clamping, and creation of proximal anastomoses, as well as subclavian arterial involvement, which can limit usability of the internal mammary arteries.[59] Successful series have reported using an off-pump technique limiting aortic manipulation and using other arterial conduits such as the gastroepiploic artery.[59] If the clinical situation allows, surgery should be delayed until inflammation can be controlled with immunosuppressive agents by following serological inflammatory markers. Postoperatively, patients require close long-term follow-up because of the risk of anastomotic aneurysm formation.[60]

Mucocutaneous Lymph Node Syndrome (Kawasaki Disease)

Initially described in 1967, mucocutaneous lymph node syndrome, otherwise known as Kawasaki disease, is a systemic vasculitis most commonly seen in children that can lead to coronary artery aneurysm formation (Fig. 94-6), thrombosis, or stenosis from scarring. In Japan, the incidence is as high as 175 per 100,000, whereas in the United States, the incidence is 19 per 100,000.[61] Although aneurysms may form in as much as 20% of patients, surgery is relatively uncommon because aneurysms may regress over time.[62] In Japan, coronary artery bypass grafting is performed in 0.3% to 0.5% of patients diagnosed with Kawasaki disease.[63,64] The left main coronary artery is the most frequently involved, followed by the left anterior descending artery, the right coronary artery, and the left circumflex artery.[65] Aneurysm formation may occur within the 6 to 8 weeks after onset of symptoms, and as much as 50% of cases will resolve within 5 years with appropriate medical management, with less than 5% progressing to chronic obstructive coronary artery disease.[61] When intervention is required for ischemia or large aneurysm size, coronary artery bypass grafting is favored over percutaneous coronary intervention because of the long-term patency issues with percutaneous intervention,[66] and the use of internal mammary artery grafts are favored because of their long-term patency.[63]

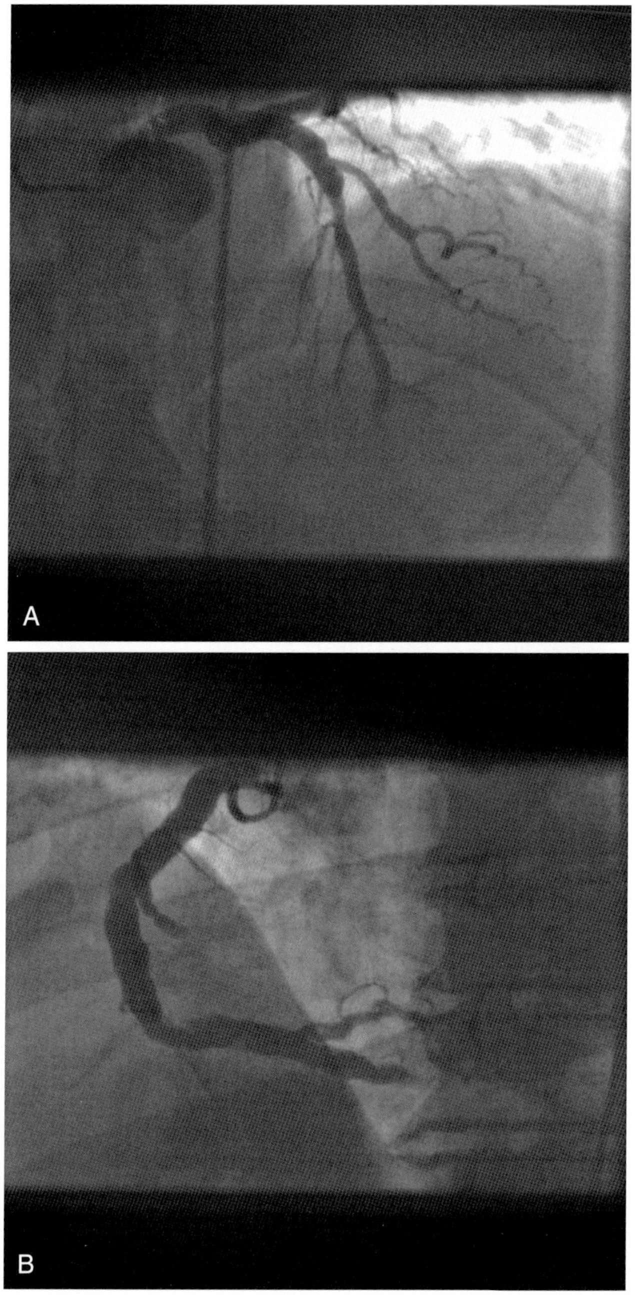

FIGURE 94-6 ■ Coronary dilation in Kawasaki disease seen in **(A)** the left coronary system and **(B)** the right coronary system.

Intimal Proliferation and Fibrosis

Fibrous hyperplasia of the coronary arteries is extremely rare, with only limited case reports published. Disease is most often limited to the intima. Although there is a predominance in females, the etiology remains unknown but is thought to be secondary to genetic, hormonal, or mechanical factors. Fibrous hyperplasia of the coronary arteries can result in sudden death thought to be secondary to arrhythmia.[67]

Ionizing Radiation

Thoracic irradiation is commonly used for the treatment of Hodgkin disease, breast cancer, and certain lung cancers. Patients with a history of thoracic irradiation are at higher risk for the development of atherosclerotic and nonatherosclerotic coronary stenosis secondary to endothelial injury at the time of treatment, and subsequent development of plaques, which may be limited to the intima and independent of cholesterol deposition.[68,69] These patients may present at younger ages, often in the second and third decade after treatment. Indications for revascularization in this patient subset are the same as for other patients with obstructive coronary artery disease, but several considerations should be made before percutaneous intervention or coronary artery bypass grafting is considered. Although data are limited for drug-eluting stents, bare metal stenting and balloon angioplasty have been associated with significantly higher rates of restenosis relative to patients without a history of irradiation.[70] If surgery is planned, consideration should be given to radiation-induced damage to the skin, which may impair healing; mediastinal fibrosis, which may add difficulty to sternal entry; concomitant pericardial disease, which may add difficulty in identifying epicardial coronary arterial targets; and radiation injury to the internal mammary artery, which may preclude its use as a conduit.[69]

Cardiac Transplantation

Cardiac allograft coronary disease secondary to vasculopathy is the leading cause of late mortality in transplant recipients, with greater than 40% of recipients demonstrating coronary disease 8 years after transplantation.[71] Angina is absent secondary to denervation during implantation; therefore, screening is essential for detection. Current screening protocols use coronary angiography with intravascular ultrasonography to establish diagnosis.[72] The vasculopathy often results in diffuse disease limiting the role for intervention, but in selected cases percutaneous coronary intervention and coronary artery bypass grafting have been used successfully, but survival benefits remain to be proven.[73] Retransplantation remains the only definitive treatment for chronic allograft vasculopathy.[72]

Extrinsic Coronary Artery Compression

Compression of the epicardial coronary arteries from adjacent structures, tumor, or abscess may result in myocardial ischemia. The most common adjacent structures to cause extrinsic compression are the pulmonary artery in the setting of pulmonary hypertension, and aortic root/sinus of Valsalva aneurysms. Symptoms will most commonly be angina-related. Contrast-enhanced computed tomography of the chest can raise the clinical suspicion of extrinsic coronary artery compression, but coronary catheterization with intravascular ultrasonography has been advocated as the gold standard for diagnosis.[74] Aneurysm repair and abscess drainage are indicated in the setting of aneurysms and infection, respectively, whereas in the setting of coronary compression secondary to pulmonary arterial hypertension, management options include coronary stenting or bypass grafting.

SUBSTANCE ABUSE

Chest pain has been reported in as much as 40% of patients who present to the emergency department after cocaine use.[75] A small subset of these patients, ranging from 0.7% to 6%, will have myocardial ischemia and/or infarction.[76,77] The etiology of the ischemia is multifactorial, secondary to increases in myocardial oxygen demand, vasoconstriction, and increased propensity for thrombosis.[78] Beyond the acute complications of cocaine use, studies suggest that cocaine users do not have an increased propensity of angiographically significant coronary artery disease when adjustments are made for other atherosclerotic risk factors.[79]

Initial treatment of patients with suspected cocaine-induced ischemia should be similar to all patients with myocardial ischemia. For patients undergoing percutaneous coronary intervention, consideration should be given to the use of bare metal stents over drug-eluting stents secondary to concerns over compliance with antiplatelet agents.[78] Although there are no specific guidelines for surgical management of cocaine-associated and/or -induced myocardial infarction, coronary artery bypass grafting should be considered in cases of multivessel disease, coronary dissection, or coronary thrombosis not amenable to treatment with percutaneous intervention.

REFERENCES

1. Davis JA, Cecchin F, Jones TK, et al: Major coronary artery anomalies in a pediatric population: incidence and clinical importance. *J Am Coll Cardiol* 37(2):593–597, 2001.
2. Eckart RE, Scoville SL, Campbell CL, et al: Sudden death in young adults: a 25-year review of autopsies in military recruits. *Ann Intern Med* 141(11):829–834, 2004.
3. Taylor AJ, Rogan KM, Virmani R: Sudden cardiac death associated with isolated congenital coronary artery anomalies. *J Am Coll Cardiol* 20(3):640–647, 1992.
4. Mavroudis C, Dodge-Khatami A, Stewart RD, et al: An overview of surgery options for congenital coronary artery anomalies. *Future Cardiol* 6(5):627–645, 2010.
5. Roberts WC, Siegel RJ, Zipes DP: Origin of the right coronary artery from the left sinus of valsalva and its functional consequences: analysis of 10 necropsy patients. *Am J Cardiol* 49(4):863–868, 1982.
6. Mustafa I, Gula G, Radley-Smith R, et al: Anomalous origin of the left coronary artery from the anterior aortic sinus: a potential cause of sudden death. Anatomic characterization and surgical treatment. *J Thorac Cardiovasc Surg* 82(2):297–300, 1981.
7. Dodge-Khatami A, Mavroudis C, Backer CL: Anomalous origin of the left coronary artery from the pulmonary artery: collective review of surgical therapy. *Ann Thorac Surg* 74(3):946–955, 2002.
8. Wesselhoeft H, Fawcett JS, Johnson AL: Anomalous origin of the left coronary artery from the pulmonary trunk. Its clinical spectrum, pathology, and pathophysiology, based on a review of 140 cases with seven further cases. *Circulation* 38(2):403–425, 1968.
9. Neches WH, Mathews RA, Park SC, et al: Anomalous origin of the left coronary artery from the pulmonary artery. A new method of surgical repair. *Circulation* 50(3):582–587, 1974.
10. Williams IA, Gersony WM, Hellenbrand WE: Anomalous right coronary artery arising from the pulmonary artery: a report of 7 cases and a review of the literature. *Am Heart J* 152(5):1004 e1009–e1017, 2006.
11. Yamanaka O, Hobbs RE: Coronary artery anomalies in 126,595 patients undergoing coronary arteriography. *Cathet Cardiovasc Diagn* 21(1):28–40, 1990.
12. Desmet W, Vanhaecke J, Vrolix M, et al: Isolated single coronary artery: a review of 50,000 consecutive coronary angiographies. *Eur Heart J* 13(12):1637–1640, 1992.
13. Sharbaugh AH, White RS: Single coronary artery. Analysis of the anatomic variation, clinical importance, and report of five cases. *JAMA* 230(2):243–246, 1974.
14. Fortune RL, Baron PJ, Fitzgerald JW: Atresia of the left main coronary artery: repair with left internal mammary artery bypass. *J Thorac Cardiovasc Surg* 94(1):150–151, 1987.
15. Gay F, Vouhe P, Lecompte Y, et al: Atresia of the left coronary ostium. Repair in a 2-month-old infant. *Arch Mal Coeur Vaiss* 82(5):807–810, 1989.
16. Muriago M, Sheppard MN, Ho SY, et al: Location of the coronary arterial orifices in the normal heart. *Clin Anat* 10(5):297–302, 1997.
17. Rosenthal RL, Carrothers IA, Schussler JM: Benign or malignant anomaly? Very high takeoff of the left main coronary artery above the left coronary sinus. *Tex Heart Inst J* 39(4):538–541, 2012.
18. Gowda RM, Vasavada BC, Khan IA: Coronary artery fistulas: clinical and therapeutic considerations. *Int J Cardiol* 107(1):7–10, 2006.
19. Fernandes ED, Kadivar H, Hallman GL, et al: Congenital malformations of the coronary arteries: the Texas Heart Institute experience. *Ann Thorac Surg* 54(4):732–740, 1992.
20. Mangukia CV: Coronary artery fistula. *Ann Thorac Surg* 93(6):2084–2092, 2012.
21. Sakakibara S, Yokoyama M, Takao A, et al: Coronary arteriovenous fistula. Nine operated cases. *Am Heart J* 72(3):307–314, 1966.
22. Kamiya H, Yasuda T, Nagamine H, et al: Surgical treatment of congenital coronary artery fistulas: 27 years' experience and a review of the literature. *J Card Surg* 17(2):173–177, 2002.
23. Angelini P, Trivellato M, Donis J, et al: Myocardial bridges: a review. *Prog Cardiovasc Dis* 26(1):75–88, 1983.
24. Ishikawa Y, Kawawa Y, Kohda E, et al: Significance of the anatomical properties of a myocardial bridge in coronary heart disease. *Circ J* 75(7):1559–1566, 2011.
25. Bourassa MG, Butnaru A, Lesperance J, et al: Symptomatic myocardial bridges: overview of ischemic mechanisms and current diagnostic and treatment strategies. *J Am Coll Cardiol* 41(3):351–359, 2003.
26. Nair CK, Dang B, Heintz MH, et al: Myocardial bridges: effect of propranolol on systolic compression. *Can J Cardiol* 2(4):218–221, 1986.
27. Downar J, Williams WG, McDonald C, et al: Outcomes after "unroofing" of a myocardial bridge of the left anterior descending coronary artery in children with hypertrophic cardiomyopathy. *Pediatr Cardiol* 25(4):390–393, 2004.
28. Glickel SZ, Maggs PR, Ellis FH, Jr: Coronary artery aneurysm. *Ann Thorac Surg* 25(4):372–376, 1978.
29. Swaye PS, Fisher LD, Litwin P, et al: Aneurysmal coronary artery disease. *Circulation* 67(1):134–138, 1983.
30. Hartnell GG, Parnell BM, Pridie RB: Coronary artery ectasia. Its prevalence and clinical significance in 4993 patients. *Br Heart J* 54(4):392–395, 1985.

31. Zeb M, McKenzie DB, Scott PA, et al: Treatment of coronary aneurysms with covered stents: a review with illustrated case. *J Invasive Cardiol* 24(9):465–469, 2012.
32. Baman TS, Cole JH, Devireddy CM, et al: Risk factors and outcomes in patients with coronary artery aneurysms. *Am J Cardiol* 93(12):1549–1551, 2004.
33. Lima B, Varma SK, Lowe JE: Nonsurgical management of left main coronary artery aneurysms: report of 2 cases and review of the literature. *Tex Heart Inst J* 33(3):376–379, 2006.
34. Nichols L, Lagana S, Parwani A: Coronary artery aneurysm: a review and hypothesis regarding etiology. *Arch Pathol Lab Med* 132(5):823–828, 2008.
35. Reynolds HR: Myocardial infarction without obstructive coronary artery disease. *Curr Opin Cardiol* 27(6):655–660, 2012.
36. Vrints CJ: Spontaneous coronary artery dissection. *Heart* 96(10):801–808, 2010.
37. Huber MS, Mooney JF, Madison J, et al: Use of a morphologic classification to predict clinical outcome after dissection from coronary angioplasty. *Am J Cardiol* 68(5):467–471, 1991.
38. Glamore MJ, Garcia-Covarrubias L, Harrison LH, Jr, et al: Spontaneous coronary artery dissection. *J Card Surg* 27(1):56–59, 2012.
39. Thompson EA, Ferraris S, Gress T, et al: Gender differences and predictors of mortality in spontaneous coronary artery dissection: a review of reported cases. *J Invasive Cardiol* 17(1):59–61, 2005.
40. Satoda M, Takagi K, Uesugi M, et al: Acute myocardial infarction caused by spontaneous postpartum coronary artery dissection. *Nat Clin Pract Cardiovasc Med* 4(12):688–692, 2007.
41. Pretre R, Chilcott M: Blunt trauma to the heart and great vessels. *N Engl J Med* 336(9):626–632, 1997.
42. Embrey R: Cardiac trauma. *Thorac Surg Clin* 17(1):87–93, vii, 2007.
43. Cook CC, Gleason TG: Great vessel and cardiac trauma. *Surg Clin North Am* 89(4):797–820, viii, 2009.
44. Kennedy JW: Complications associated with cardiac catheterization and angiography. *Cathet Cardiovasc Diagn* 8(1):5–11, 1982.
45. Mukhtyar C, Brogan P, Luqmani R: Cardiovascular involvement in primary systemic vasculitis. *Best Pract Res Clin Rheumatol* 23(3):419–428, 2009.
46. Kastner D, Gaffney M, Tak T: Polyarteritis nodosa and myocardial infarction. *Can J Cardiol* 16(4):515–518, 2000.
47. Yanagawa B, Kumar P, Tsuneyoshi H, et al: Coronary artery bypass in the context of polyarteritis nodosa. *Ann Thorac Surg* 89(2):623–625, 2010.
48. Trueb RM, Scheidegger EP, Pericin M, et al: Periarteritis nodosa presenting as a breast lesion: report of a case and review of the literature. *Br J Dermatol* 141(6):1117–1121, 1999.
49. Roldan CA: Valvular and coronary heart disease in systemic inflammatory diseases: systemic disorders in heart disease. *Heart* 94(8):1089–1101, 2008.
50. Roldan CA, Shively BK, Crawford MH: An echocardiographic study of valvular heart disease associated with systemic lupus erythematosus. *N Engl J Med* 335(19):1424–1430, 1996.
51. Ura M, Sakata R, Nakayama Y, et al: Coronary artery bypass grafting in patients with systemic lupus erythematosus. *Eur J Cardiothorac Surg* 15(5):697–701, 1999.
52. Bozbuga N, Erentug V, Kaya E, et al: Coronary artery bypass grafting in patients with systemic lupus erythematosus. *J Card Surg* 19(5):471–472, 2004.
53. Morelli S, Gurgo Di Castelmenardo AM, Conti F, et al: Cardiac involvement in patients with Wegener's granulomatosis. *Rheumatol Int* 19(6):209–212, 2000.
54. Kane GC, Keogh KA: Involvement of the heart by small and medium vessel vasculitis. *Curr Opin Rheumatol* 21(1):29–34, 2009.
55. Rav-Acha M, Plot L, Peled N, et al: Coronary involvement in Takayasu's arteritis. *Autoimmun Rev* 6(8):566–571, 2007.
56. Lupi-Herrera E, Sanchez-Torres G, Marcushamer J, et al: Takayasu's arteritis. Clinical study of 107 cases. *Am Heart J* 93(1):94–103, 1977.
57. Fava MP, Foradori GB, Garcia CB, et al: Percutaneous transluminal angioplasty in patients with Takayasu arteritis: five-year experience. *J Vasc Interv Radiol* 4(5):649–652, 1993.
58. Lee HK, Namgung J, Choi WH, et al: Stenting of the left main coronary artery in a patient with Takayasu's arteritis. *Korean Circ J* 41(1):34–37, 2011.
59. Na KJ, Lee KH, Oh SJ, et al: Anaortic off-pump coronary artery bypass grafting in patients with Takayasu's arteritis. *Korean J Thorac Cardiovasc Surg* 46(4):274–278, 2013.
60. Perera AH, Mason JC, Wolfe JH: Takayasu arteritis: criteria for surgical intervention should not be ignored. *Int J Vasc Med* 2013:618910, 2013.
61. Guo HW, Chang Q, Xu JP, et al: Coronary artery bypass grafting for Kawasaki disease. *Chin Med J* 123(12):1533–1536, 2010.
62. Verma S, Dasarathan C, Premsekar R, et al: Off-pump coronary bypass grafting for Kawasaki disease. *Ann Pediatr Cardiol* 3(2):190–192, 2010.
63. Tsuda E, Kitamura S: National survey of coronary artery bypass grafting for coronary stenosis caused by Kawasaki disease in Japan. *Circulation* 110(11 Suppl 1):II61–II66, 2004.
64. Tsuda E: Coronary artery bypass grafting for coronary artery stenosis caused by Kawasaki disease. *Expert Rev Cardiovasc Ther* 7(5):533–539, 2009.
65. Tatara K, Kusakawa S: Long-term prognosis of giant coronary aneurysm in Kawasaki disease: an angiographic study. *J Pediatr* 111(5):705–710, 1987.
66. Muta H, Ishii M: Percutaneous coronary intervention versus coronary artery bypass grafting for stenotic lesions after Kawasaki disease. *J Pediatr* 157(1):120–126, 2010.
67. Curca G, Sarbu N, Dermengiu D, et al: Coronary fibromuscular dysplasia and sudden death—case report and review of the literature. *Rom J Leg Med* 3:165–172, 2009.
68. Grollier G, Commeau P, Mercier V, et al: Post-radiotherapeutic left main coronary ostial stenosis: clinical and histological study. *Eur Heart J* 9(5):567–570, 1988.
69. Jaworski C, Mariani JA, Wheeler G, et al: Cardiac complications of thoracic irradiation. *J Am Coll Cardiol* 61(23):2319–2328, 2013.
70. Schomig K, Ndrepepa G, Mehilli J, et al: Thoracic radiotherapy in patients with lymphoma and restenosis after coronary stent placement. *Catheter Cardiovasc Interv* 70(3):359–365, 2007.
71. Taylor DO, Edwards LB, Boucek MM, et al: Registry of the International Society for Heart and Lung Transplantation: twenty-third official adult heart transplantation report—2006. *J Heart Lung Transplant* 25(8):869–879, 2006.
72. Schmauss D, Weis M: Cardiac allograft vasculopathy: recent developments. *Circulation* 117(16):2131–2141, 2008.
73. Prada-Delgado O, Estevez-Loureiro R, Lopez-Sainz A, et al: Percutaneous coronary interventions and bypass surgery in patients with cardiac allograft vasculopathy: a single-center experience. *Transplant Proc* 44(9):2657–2659, 2012.
74. Lee MS, Oyama J, Bhatia R, et al: Left main coronary artery compression from pulmonary artery enlargement due to pulmonary hypertension: a contemporary review and argument for percutaneous revascularization. *Catheter Cardiovasc Interv* 76(4):543–550, 2010.
75. Brody SL, Slovis CM, Wrenn KD: Cocaine-related medical problems: consecutive series of 233 patients. *Am J Med* 88(4):325–331, 1990.
76. Weber JE, Chudnofsky CR, Boczar M, et al: Cocaine-associated chest pain: how common is myocardial infarction? *Acad Emerg Med* 7(8):873–877, 2000.
77. Feldman JA, Fish SS, Beshansky JR, et al: Acute cardiac ischemia in patients with cocaine-associated complaints: results of a multicenter trial. *Ann Emerg Med* 36(5):469–476, 2000.
78. McCord J, Jneid H, Hollander JE, et al: Management of cocaine-associated chest pain and myocardial infarction: a scientific statement from the American Heart Association Acute Cardiac Care Committee of the Council on Clinical Cardiology. *Circulation* 117(14):1897–1907, 2008.
79. Patel AD, Sola S, Caneer P, et al: Cocaine use in an urban medical population and the development of angiographically significant coronary artery disease. *Prev Cardiol* 9(3):144–147, 2006.

PART I

SURGICAL MANAGEMENT OF HEART FAILURE

PART OUTLINE

CHAPTER 95

PERICARDIUM AND CONSTRICTIVE PERICARDITIS

Donald D. Glower

CHAPTER OUTLINE

THE PERICARDIUM

History

The earliest descriptions of the pericardium date back to Hippocrates (460 to 377 BC).[1] Galen (AD 129 to 210) described the protective function of the pericardium and also reported a pericardial effusion in animals. Avenzoar (1091 to 1162) described pericarditis,[2] and Vesalius (1514 to 1564) carefully documented the anatomy of the pericardium. Jean Riolan (1649) suggested treating pericarditis with trephination of the sternum, and a case of hemopericardium was reported by William Harvey (1649). The conditions of cardiac tamponade and constrictive pericarditis were described by Richard Lower (1669), John Mayow (1674), and Morgagni (1756). The pathophysiology of constrictive pericarditis was further clarified by Cheevers in 1842.

Kussmaul (1873) noted the association between constrictive pericarditis and decreased intensity of the peripheral pulse (now termed pulsus paradoxus). Kussmaul also described inspiratory jugular venous distention, now termed *Kussmaul sign* (as opposed to *normal inspiratory jugular venous collapse*). Pick (1896) reported three patients with constrictive pericarditis and hepatic cirrhosis (a condition now known as *Pick cirrhosis*).

The first successful pericardiotomy was performed by Romero in 1819, and the first pericardiocentesis was performed by Franz Schuh in 1840. Pericardial resection for constrictive pericarditis was proposed by Weill (1895) and Delorme (1898), with pericardiectomy ultimately performed by Rehn (1913) and Sauerbruch (1925). Early surgical treatment of constrictive pericarditis in the United States was reported by Beck (1930), Churchill (1936), and Blalock (1937). Radical pericardiectomy, including excision of thickened epicardium when necessary, was advocated by Holman (1955).

Anatomy

The pericardium is a fibrous sac surrounding the heart and mediastinal great vessels. The outer wall of the pericardial sac consists of an outer fibrosa and an inner serosa.[3] Histologically, the fibrosa is fibro-collagenous tissue with elastic fibers oriented along the lines of stress, and the pericardial serosa is composed of mesothelial cells with microvilli and an underlying basal lamina.[3]

This outer pericardial sac folds onto the heart and great vessels, where the epicardium and outer adventitial layer of the heart and great vessels constitute the visceral lining of the pericardial sac. Laterally, the pericardium forms the medial walls of the pleural spaces. Inferiorly, the pericardium is the superior surface of the central tendon of the diaphragm, and, superiorly, the pericardium blends with the deep cervical fascia. Anteriorly, the pericardium is loosely joined to the xiphoid process and the sternal manubrium by ligamentous structures. Posteriorly and superiorly, the pericardium envelops the great vessels, the venae cavae, and the pulmonary veins. The posterior pericardial space has two developmental recesses: the transverse sinus separating the great vessels from the pulmonary veins and the oblique sinus separating the left and right pulmonary veins (Fig. 95-1).[3]

The arterial blood supply and venous drainage of the pericardium come from the pericardiophrenic branches of the internal mammary vessels bilaterally. The lymphatic drainage of the visceral pericardium is the tracheal and bronchial lymph chain, and the parietal pericardium shares lymphatic drainage with the sternum, diaphragm, and mid mediastinum. The pericardium is innervated from the phrenic nerves, with some vagal innervation via the esophageal plexus.[3]

The pericardium normally contains 15 to 35 mL of serous fluid. Pericardial fluid is a transudate containing less protein but more albumin than serum; therefore, pericardial fluid has a lower osmolality than does plasma.[3]

Normal Physiology

The pericardium and pericardial fluid minimize friction and energy loss during cardiac motion. While doing so, the normal pericardium and its external attachments maintain cardiac position within the mediastinum in the presence of gravitational or other forces that could impair cardiac filling or function. The pericardium also serves as a barrier, protecting the heart from inflammation or malignancy in adjacent structures.

The normal pericardium has mechanoreceptors connected to phrenic nerve and vagal nerve afferents, which (with stimulation) lower blood pressure, slow heart rate, and contract the spleen in dogs. Pericardial fluid contains prostacyclin, which can affect coronary artery vasomotor tone, and it has fibrinolytic properties that can lyse intrapericardial clot.

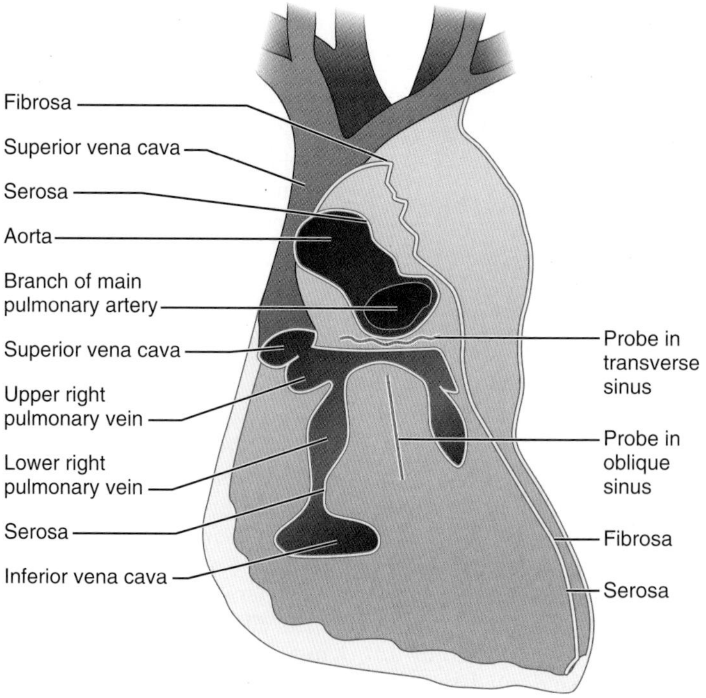

FIGURE 95-1 ■ Anatomy of the posterior pericardial reflections. Note the transverse sinus and the oblique sinus. (From Spodick DH: *The pericardium,* New York, 1997, Marcel Dekker.)

At rest, the normal pericardium probably has little restraining effect on cardiac systolic or diastolic function.[4] However, under conditions of acute cardiac dilation, the normal pericardium probably increases diastolic stiffness and limits diastolic filling of the left and right ventricles.[5] Under normal conditions, relatively little interaction between the left and right ventricles is mediated by the pericardium.[6]

Normal pericardial pressure at end expiration is −2 mm Hg. Like pleural pressure, pericardial pressure decreases during inspiration and increases during expiration. As a result, inspiration normally decreases left ventricular stroke volume and decreases aortic blood pressure by less than 10 mm Hg. The mechanisms for these effects do not require an intact pericardium and are similar to the mechanisms of pulsus paradoxus (see later).

Pathophysiology

Pericardial Effusion

Pericardial effusion (>50 to 100 mL) is the simple result of more fluid transuding into the pericardial space than is resorbed. Pericardial effusions requiring drainage typically contain 500 to 700 mL of fluid. Eventually, pericardial pressure rises high enough that resorption matches fluid production. Sustained increases in pericardial pressure over time cause the pericardial sac to stretch (because of material plasticity, or creep) with slippage of pericardial collagen fibers and pericardial thinning. Causes of increased pericardial fluid production include inflammation or infection of the pericardium. Decreased pericardial fluid resorption can result from venous hypertension or lymphatic obstruction. If pericardial effusion increases pericardial pressure sufficiently, cardiac tamponade and pulsus paradoxus can result (see later).

Cardiac Tamponade

Cardiac tamponade has been defined as hemodynamically significant cardiac compression from accumulating pericardial contents that evoke and defeat compensatory mechanisms.[3] Cardiac tamponade can result from pericardial fluid, pus, blood, air, or tumor. In a normal pericardium, approximately 200 mL of acute pericardial fluid accumulation can produce tamponade, but larger volumes may be required in chronically enlarged pericardial sacs.

The initial effect of cardiac tamponade is decreased venous return to the right heart resulting from a direct pressure effect and from effectively decreased right atrial and right ventricular diastolic compliance. Decreased right ventricular filling decreases stroke volume and thus cardiac output. Pulmonary venous return to the left heart is decreased by increased left atrial pressure and by decreased right ventricular output. Central venous pressures of 14 to 30 mm Hg are typically associated with cardiac tamponade in euvolemic individuals, and lower venous pressures can occur with cardiac tamponade if hypovolemia is also present.

Left ventricular diastolic compliance and diastolic filling are also impaired by cardiac tamponade. Increased diastolic right ventricular pressure relative to left ventricular diastolic pressure can shift the interventricular septum leftward, thus decreasing preload of the interventricular septum and effectively decreasing left ventricular contractility. By combining these mechanisms, inspiration with cardiac tamponade can decrease systolic blood pressure by greater than 10 mm Hg (see Pulsus Paradoxus, next). Eventually, arterial hypotension and increased intrapericardial pressure can decrease coronary perfusion sufficiently to decrease cardiac contractility caused by global cardiac ischemia.

Diagnostic signs of cardiac tamponade are listed in Box 95-1.

BOX 95-1 Diagnostic Signs of Cardiac Tamponade

PHYSICAL EXAMINATION

- Pulsus paradoxus

PULMONARY ARTERY CATHETER FINDINGS

- Central venous pressure > 14 mm Hg
- Near equalization of central venous, pulmonary artery, and capillary wedge pressures in diastole
- Decreased cardiac output

ECHOCARDIOGRAPHY

- Right atrial compression
- Right ventricular diastolic collapse
- Inferior vena caval dilation
- Inspiratory shift of interventricular septum leftward
- Inspiratory flow velocities: ↑ tricuspid and pulmonic, ↓ mitral and aortic

Pulsus Paradoxus

Cardiac tamponade is associated with pulsus paradoxus, which is defined as a fall in systolic blood pressure of greater than 10 mm Hg with inspiration. Pulsus paradoxus is thus an exaggeration of the normal inspiratory decrease in systolic blood pressure because of the same mechanisms (see Normal Physiology, earlier). Although pulsus paradoxus is characteristic of cardiac tamponade, pulsus paradoxus can also be seen in chronic obstructive pulmonary disease, pulmonary embolism, obesity, right heart failure, and ascites, where it occurs by the same mechanisms.[6] Pulsus paradoxus may be absent in cardiac tamponade with severe left ventricular dysfunction, atrial septal defect, severe aortic regurgitation, or positive pressure breathing.[3] Proposed mechanisms of pulsus paradoxus include the following:

- Pooling of blood in the lungs during inspiration
- Increased right ventricular filling during inspiration resulting from lower right ventricular pressure (in turn, right ventricular distention may shift the interventricular septum leftward, thus decreasing septal muscle preload and decreasing left ventricular stroke volume)[7]
- Increased left ventricular afterload (aortic pressure minus pericardial pressure), which decreases left ventricular stroke work[8]

Constrictive Pericarditis

Constrictive pericarditis results when the volume of the pericardial sac itself is sufficiently reduced relative to cardiac volume that cardiac filling is impaired. In constrictive pericarditis, pericardial fluid is generally absent or of normal volume. The wall of the pericardial sac is usually thickened in constrictive pericarditis and may be 3 to 20 mm thick, as opposed to the 1- to 2-mm thickness of normal pericardium (Box 95-2).

Unlike cardiac tamponade, constrictive pericarditis impairs cardiac filling only in late diastole. Thus, early diastolic filling of the right ventricle occurs briefly in constrictive pericarditis until the ventricle suddenly reaches the rigid constraint of the pericardium. The result is the pathognomonic "square root" sign in the right and left ventricular diastolic filling pressure waveforms (Fig. 95-2).

Similarly, in constrictive pericarditis, the central venous pressure tracing has a prominent *y* descent that corresponds to the initial dip of the square root sign of the right and left ventricular tracings. This *y* descent normally results from "diastolic collapse" of the normal venous pressure as rapid atrial filling occurs, and the *y* descent is exaggerated by constrictive pericarditis. Constrictive pericarditis impairs reservoir function and contractile function of the left atrium.[9] Constrictive pericarditis also selectively impairs contractile function in the left and right ventricular free walls relative to that of the interventricular septum on magnetic resonance imaging.[10]

Constrictive pericarditis is associated with inspiratory jugular venous distention (Kussmaul sign; see Fig. 95-2), which is less frequent in cardiac tamponade. Kussmaul sign can also occur in right ventricular failure, restrictive cardiomyopathy, cor pulmonale, and acute pulmonary embolism.

BOX 95-2 Diagnostic Signs of Constrictive Pericarditis

Physical Examination

- Kussmaul sign

Pulmonary Artery Catheter Findings

- Central venous pressure > 14 mm Hg
- Near equalization of central venous, pulmonary artery, and capillary wedge pressures in diastole
- Decreased cardiac output
- Square root sign in right and left ventricular pressure tracings
- Prominent *y* descent in central venous pressure tracing

Echocardiography, Computed Tomography, or Magnetic Resonance Imaging

- Impaired right and left ventricular free wall strains relative to septal strain
- Pericardial thickening
- Right ventricular diastolic collapse
- Minimal pericardial fluid

Chronic elevation of venous pressures in constrictive pericarditis can result in hepatic congestion, cardiac cirrhosis, protein-losing enteropathy, and nephrotic syndrome. Chronically, constrictive pericarditis alters the neurohormonal axis with elevations of serum norepinephrine, renin, aldosterone, cortisol, growth hormone, and atrial natriuretic peptide.[11]

The differential diagnosis of constrictive pericarditis consists primarily of restrictive cardiomyopathy, which can occur simultaneously with constrictive pericarditis.[5,12] Characteristic histology on myocardial biopsy, pulmonary capillary wedge pressure greater than 5 mm Hg greater than central venous pressure, slower early diastolic filling, and impaired left ventricular systolic function all favor restrictive cardiomyopathy over constrictive pericarditis. Acute volume loading of 500 mL during right heart catheterization accentuates the right-sided pressure findings of constrictive pericarditis and produces smaller changes in restrictive cardiomyopathy.

Diagnosis of Pericardial Disease

History and Symptoms

The presenting symptoms of pericardial disease can include fever, malaise, chest discomfort, shortness of breath, pedal edema, and abdominal distention. Medical history may reveal prior chest trauma, chest irradiation, or exposure to infectious agents such as *Mycobacterium tuberculosis*. The time course of pericardial disease is described as *acute* (<3 months), *chronic* (>3 months), or *recurrent*.[5]

Physical Examination

Physical examination of the patient with pericardial disease may reveal findings of fever, tachycardia, or tachypnea. The peripheral arterial pulse may paradoxically diminish during inspiration (pulsus paradoxus). Inspiratory jugular venous distention may be present (Kussmaul sign). Chest examination may show dullness at the lung bases, muffled cardiac sounds, and a pericardial rub or pericardial knock. A prominent S_3 gallop may be present in constrictive pericarditis. Abdominal examination may demonstrate hepatomegaly or ascites, and pedal edema may be present. The extremities may be cool and constricted in tamponade.

Chest Radiograph

The chest radiograph may show cardiomegaly in pericardial effusion. Pericardial calcification can accompany constrictive pericarditis. Pleural effusion may be present in pericardial effusion, pericardial tamponade, and constrictive pericarditis. Chest radiography may also demonstrate pneumopericardium or mediastinal mass resulting from pericardial cyst.

Electrocardiogram

Pericardial disease can be associated with atrial fibrillation, and the electrocardiogram (ECG) may show

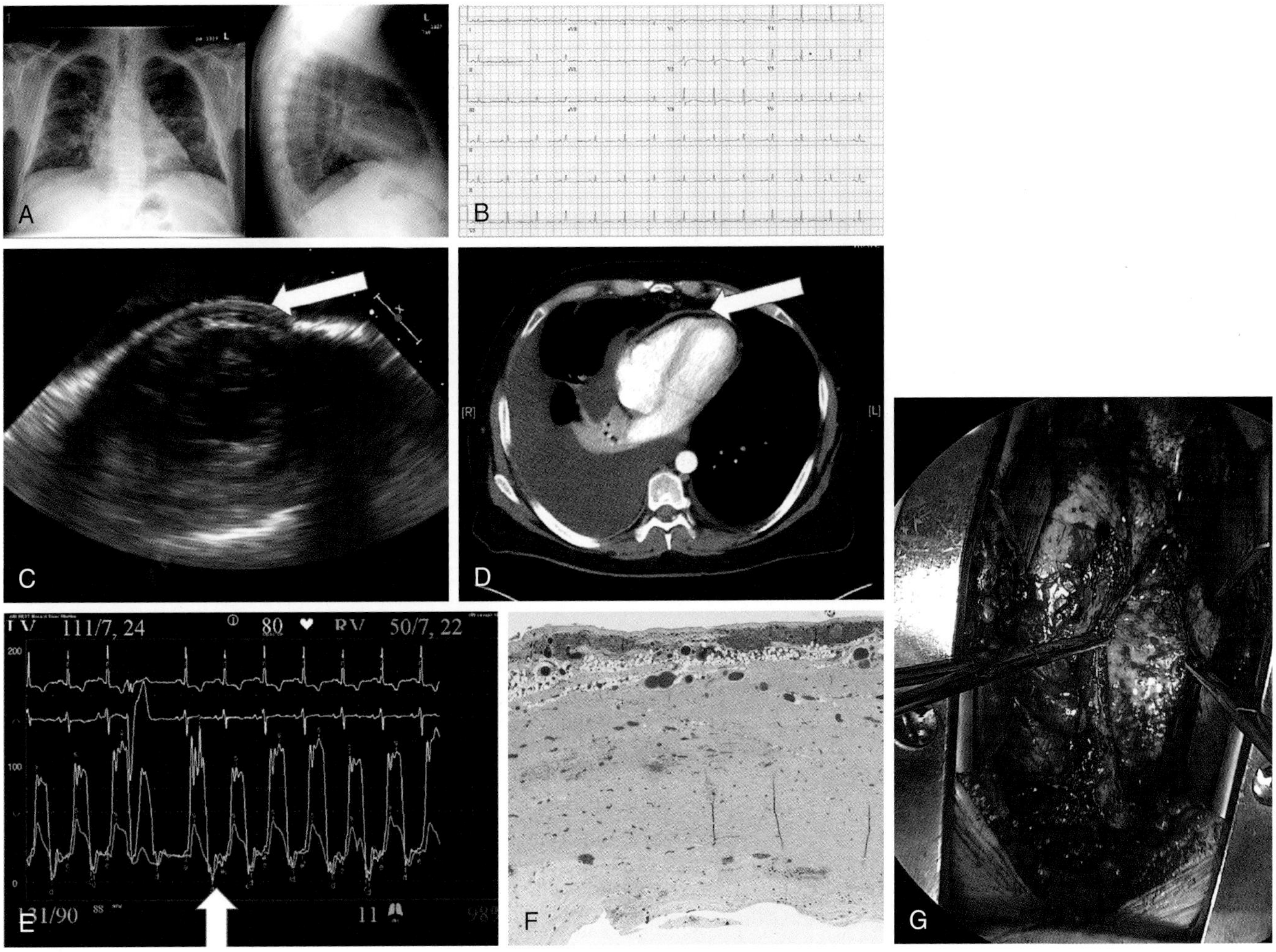

FIGURE 95-2 ■ This patient has constrictive pericarditis. **A,** Chest radiograph with cardiomegaly. **B,** Electrocardiogram with low voltage. **C,** Echocardiogram with pericardial thickening *(arrow).* **D,** Computed tomographic image showing pericardial thickening *(arrow).* **E,** Simultaneous right ventricular *(green)* and left ventricular *(yellow)* pressure tracings with "square root sign" *(arrow)* and equalization of diastolic right and left ventricular pressures. **F,** Histology of resected pericardium with marked fibrous thickening and inflammation of the parietal surface *(top of picture).* **G,** Intraoperative finding of thickened pericardium grasped in clamps.

diminished QRS voltage (see Fig. 95-2). The four stages of ECG changes in acute pericarditis are as follows:

- Stage I—ST elevation in all leads except AVR and V_1
- Stage II—Normal ST segments, but T wave flattening
- Stage III—T wave inversion without Q waves or loss of R wave voltage
- Stage IV—Normalization of T wave

Echocardiography

Echocardiography can easily detect loculated or generalized pericardial effusion. An echo-free pericardial space of less than 10 mm is termed a *small effusion,* whereas circumferential spaces of 10 to 20 mm and greater than 20 mm are considered moderate and large pericardial effusions, respectively.[5,13] The echocardiogram can also be used to diagnose intrapericardial masses, pericardial cysts, pericardial calcification or thickening, or associated cardiac disease. The echocardiogram can be diagnostic of cardiac tamponade with findings of end-diastolic right atrial collapse, diastolic right ventricular collapse, and inspiratory interventricular septal shift leftward with increased tricuspid and pulmonic flow velocities and decreased mitral and aortic flow velocities, and dilation of the inferior vena cava (Fig. 95-3).[13,14]

Computed Tomography

Computed tomography (CT) can demonstrate pericardial effusion, pericardial calcification and thickening, intrapericardial masses, and pericardial cysts (see Fig. 95-2). CT may be more sensitive than magnetic resonance imaging (MRI) in detecting calcification, but it has the disadvantages of requiring intravenous contrast injection and having more motion artifact.[15]

Magnetic Resonance Imaging

MRI can demonstrate pericardial effusion, pericardial thickening, intrapericardial masses, pericardial cysts, and

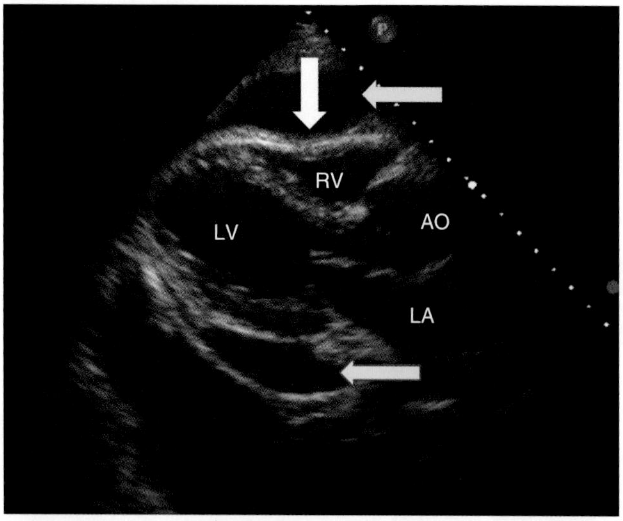

FIGURE 95-3 ■ Two-dimensional echocardiogram (parasternal long-axis view) showing pericardial effusion *(yellow arrows)* and cardiac tamponade with collapse of the right ventricle (RV) at end-diastole *(white arrow)*. *AO*, Aorta; *LA*, left atrium; *LV*, left ventricle.

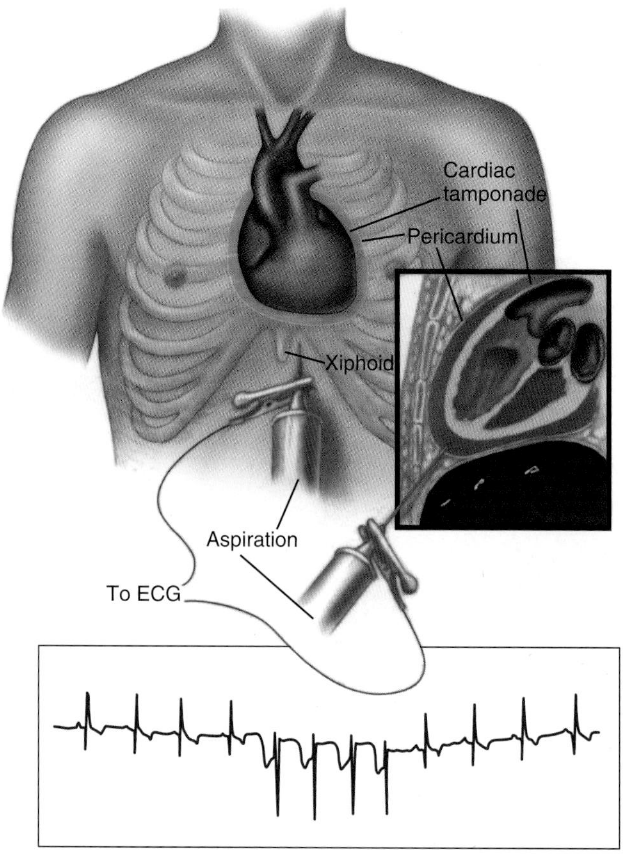

FIGURE 95-4 ■ Technique of subxiphoid pericardiocentesis with electrocardiographic monitoring. Note negative QRS deflection indicating myocardial contact. *ECG*, Electrocardiogram.

even intracardiac disease.[16] Relative to CT, MRI has the advantages of not requiring intravenous contrast injection and of having less motion artifact. MRI may be less sensitive than CT for detecting pericardial calcification. Newer MRI techniques can differentiate restrictive cardiomyopathy from constrictive pericarditis using speckle tracking to compare ventricular free wall strain relative to interventricular septal strain.[10] Pericardial constriction is associated with smaller right ventricular volume and reduced mean trans-tricuspid E:A wave ratios.[17]

Cardiac Catheterization

Cardiac fluoroscopy can demonstrate pericardial calcification or abnormally prominent swinging motion of the left ventricle over the cardiac cycle in pericardial effusion. Right heart catheterization can be diagnostic of cardiac tamponade or pericardial constriction (see earlier; see Fig. 95-2). Both tamponade and constriction show equalization and elevation of diastolic pressures in all four chambers of the heart. Physiologic tamponade or constriction with right atrial mean pressure less than 14 mm Hg is unusual. Constriction may be differentiated from tamponade or restrictive cardiomyopathy by the square root sign in the right and left ventricular tracings (see Fig. 95-2), and the findings of cardiac constriction are accentuated by acute 500-mL volume challenge (see Constrictive Pericarditis, earlier). Given the noninvasive alternative imaging techniques available today, cardiac catheterization may be reserved for patients where clinical and noninvasive imaging data are inconclusive.[18]

Pericardiocentesis

Pericardiocentesis is a means to treat cardiac tamponade rapidly, to prevent tamponade in large effusions, and to obtain pericardial fluid for diagnosis. Contraindications include aortic dissection, coagulopathy, small or loculated effusions, traumatic hemopericardium, and nonviral infectious pericarditis. Pericardiocentesis is generally performed with the patient supine and with local anesthesia. A long, pericardial needle is inserted into the patient's pericardial space left of the xiphoid, inferior to the left costal margin (Fig. 95-4). The needle is advanced toward the patient's left mid scapula while maintaining aspiration pressure on the needle. Cardiac puncture can be avoided by a combination of echocardiography and monitoring an ECG obtained by an electrode attached to the needle. The needle is withdrawn if the ECG shows sudden negative deflection of the QRS complex, indicating contact with the myocardium.

Once the pericardial space is entered, the needle can be exchanged over a wire for a blunt pericardial catheter. The blunt pericardial catheter can be left in the pericardial space for several days to decrease the rate of recurrent effusion (e.g., from 55% to 24%).[19] Pericardial fluid can be sent to the laboratory for cell count and differential, cytology (possibly including tumor markers), culture (including bacterial, fungal, and mycobacterial), and biochemical examination (e.g., polymerase chain reaction for tuberculosis, pH, specific gravity, lactic dehydrogenase, protein content).[3] Peripheral blood can be sent to the laboratory for leukocyte count and erythrocyte sedimentation rate, and for C-reactive protein, serum lactate dehydrogenase, and cardiac isoenzyme values.[5]

Pericardiocentesis is rapid and relatively safe, and it requires little anesthesia. Complication rates vary from 5% to 50% and are increased in smaller effusions, when echocardiographic guidance is not used, and in the presence of coagulopathy.[19] Pericardiocentesis is less effective and less diagnostic in hemopericardium with clot, or in effusion with thick exudate. Most authors believe that pericardiocentesis is optimally used in patients with large anterior effusions and either with tamponade (therapeutic) or a probable infectious or tuberculous etiology (diagnostic).[19] The rate of recurrent effusion and tamponade after successful pericardiocentesis is high (approximately 55%).[19] The incidence of recurrent effusion or tamponade may be decreased by pericardial catheter drainage for 2 to 5 days or surgical drainage.

Pericardial Biopsy

Pericardial biopsy can be performed percutaneously with a pericardioscope or surgically (see Pericardial Surgical Procedures, later).[20] Percutaneous pericardial biopsy is performed by dilating a pericardiocentesis needle track to accept an introducer sheath. A bioptome can then be placed through the introducer using echocardiographic guidance to obtain pericardial biopsy.[21] The value and safety of percutaneous pericardial biopsy have not been established.

Pericardial tissue can be examined to diagnose pericarditis, and together with pericardiocentesis it can demonstrate the cause of pericarditis in 30% to 50% of patients. Pericardial tissue may be sent for hematoxylin-eosin and Gram stains, polymerase chain reaction analysis for tuberculosis, and cultures for bacteria, fungus, and tuberculosis. Special stains can be used to detect certain forms of malignancy.

NONCONSTRICTIVE PERICARDITIS

Diagnosis

Using European Society of Cardiology guidelines, pericarditis has been classified as dry, effusive, effusive-constrictive, and constrictive.[5] The diagnosis of pericarditis requires the pathologic demonstration of pericardial inflammation, scarring, or thickening. Thus certain diagnosis of pericarditis requires pericardial biopsy, generally with surgery to create a subxiphoid or transthoracic pericardial window. The diagnosis of pericarditis can, however, be strongly supported by findings of pericardial effusion or pericardial thickening on echocardiography, CT, or MRI. The diagnosis of pericardial effusion requires only an imaging study demonstrating more fluid than normal (>50 to 100 mL) in the pericardial space.

Etiology and Treatment

Pericardial effusion and pericarditis have a wide variety of causes (Table 95-1).[5,22,23] Medical treatment for pericardial effusion should target the etiology of the effusion. Surgical treatment involves either pericardiocentesis or the creation of a subxiphoid pericardial window or a transpleural pericardial window. Pericardiocentesis or pericardial biopsy can be indicated to determine the cause of the pericarditis and thus define the medical therapy. In a hemodynamically unstable patient, pericardiocentesis is also indicated to treat pericardial tamponade acutely and to achieve hemodynamic stability. Pericardiocentesis can be as effective as pericardial window in achieving diagnosis and draining the pericardial effusion,[24] but pericardiocentesis is more likely than pericardial window to require recurrent treatment for recurrent pericardial symptoms.[19,23,24]

Pericardial window is indicated in any patient with symptomatic pericardial effusion or in whom the cause cannot otherwise be defined. A subxiphoid pericardial window procedure can be performed using local anesthesia; therefore, it is preferable in patients in hemodynamically unstable condition because of tamponade but in whom pericardiocentesis is deemed impractical or unsafe. The transpleural pericardial window is preferable in patients with a good long-term prognosis because of a lower likelihood of recurrent pericardial effusion.[25] Pericardiectomy can improve relapse rate without significant increase in mortality for patients with chronic relapsing pericarditis.[26]

TABLE 95-1 **Frequency of Effusion and Constriction in Pericarditis**

Etiology	Effusion (%)	Constriction (%)
Idiopathic	7-30	50-70
Viral	5-25	0
Bacterial	5-10	0-5
Tuberculous	5-10	15
Autoimmune	5-15	1
Type 2 immune or postoperative	5-25	5-60
Malignant	20-50	0
Traumatic or radiation	5-15	9-20
Metabolic or uremic	10-15	0
Surrounding structures	5	1

Idiopathic Pericarditis

Idiopathic pericarditis is the diagnosis for 3% to 50% of all patients with pericardial effusion or pericarditis. Management is symptomatic, as it is for viral pericarditis. Symptoms of low-grade pain and fever can be treated with anti-inflammatory agents such as ibuprofen (300 to 800 mg every 6 to 8 hours for days to weeks) along with antiulcer agents. Colchicine 0.5 mg bid for 3 months in addition to ibuprofen or aspirin has been shown in a randomized trial to reduce symptoms, readmission, and hospitalization.[22,27] More severe or refractory symptoms may respond to prednisone, beginning with 1 to 1.5 mg/kg per day and tapering over the 1- to 3-month course.[5] Other causes such as infection or uremia need to be excluded before starting steroids. Intrapericardial steroids may be beneficial.[5] Pericarditis can produce atrial fibrillation, which may also require treatment. Outcome from acute pericarditis is good, with the most common complication being recurrent pericarditis.[27] Complete pericardiectomy can significantly improve freedom from relapse relative to medical therapy in patients failing medical therapy including steroids.[26]

Infectious Pericarditis

At least 50% of infectious pericarditis is thought to be viral. The viruses associated with pericarditis include coxsackievirus, cytomegalovirus, echovirus, Epstein-Barr virus, varicella, parvovirus, human immunodeficiency virus, and herpes simplex.[5] Viral pericarditis is a clinical diagnosis that is frequently made with the assistance of viral serologies. It is often accompanied by myocarditis, which can be documented on myocardial biopsy or indirectly suggested by acute deterioration of ventricular function. Like idiopathic pericarditis, it is usually self-limited. Pericardiocentesis or surgical pericardial drainage with biopsy is performed as needed for diagnosis or treatment of symptoms.

Nonviral infectious pericarditis is usually fatal if untreated, and it has a mortality of 8% to 40% in treated patients.[5] The most common bacterial organisms causing pericarditis are *Staphylococcus*, *Streptococcus*, and gram-negative organisms in adults and *Haemophilus* or *Staphylococcus* in children. Bacterial pericarditis can occur from bacteremia or from contiguous spread from bacterial infection in the thoracic cavity. Symptoms of fever and chest pain are common. Diagnosis relies on culture or histologic examination of pericardial fluid obtained by either pericardiocentesis or open pericardial drainage.

Bacterial pericarditis requires both appropriate antibiotic treatment and either acute or chronic pericardial drainage. Bacterial pericarditis may respond to a one-time pericardial drainage, with systemic antibiotic therapy for less virulent organisms such as *Streptococcus*. Pericardiectomy may be necessary if initial drainage fails, especially in organisms such as *Haemophilus*.[19] Constrictive pericarditis can develop at a rate of 5% per year after bacterial pericarditis.[22] Fungal and staphylococcal pericarditis respond better to more chronic drainage of the pericardium by the subxiphoid or transthoracic approach.

Tuberculous pericarditis can appear with effusion or constriction, or both. Acute tuberculous pericarditis is best treated with intermittent pericardiocentesis. Tube drainage of tuberculous pericarditis is to be avoided to prevent chronic draining sinuses along the tube track. Pericardiectomy or open pericardial drainage (preferably after 1 week of chemotherapy) may be necessary if initial drainage fails, and pericardial constriction results in approximately half of patients with tuberculous pericarditis.[28] Amebic or echinococcal pericarditis can require pericardiocentesis or tube drainage depending on the thickness and degree of loculation.[29]

Autoimmune Pericarditis

Connective tissue or inflammatory diseases such as rheumatoid arthritis, lupus, and systemic sclerosis can produce pericarditis in a minority of patients. The underlying condition should be treated if possible, and pericardiocentesis and pericardial window are reserved for symptoms refractory to medical treatment or when needed to make a diagnosis.

Type 2 Immune and Postoperative Pericarditis

Type 2 immune pericarditis can occur 5 to 14 days after cardiac injury or operation. Only 10% of patients undergoing cardiac operation have clinically significant postoperative pericarditis, and symptoms are usually self-limited, resolving after 3 to 4 weeks. Intraoperative use of bioabsorbable films may diminish pericardial scarring without the pericardial capsule formation associated with nonabsorbable pericardial substitute material.[30] Treatment is similar to that given for idiopathic pericarditis.

Malignant Pericarditis

Malignant involvement of the pericardium is generally metastatic and occurs in approximately 10% to 35% of patients with noncardiac neoplasm. The most common tumors that involve the pericardium are lung (38%), breast (29%), and lymphoma (7%), with 26% being other tumors.[31-33] Primary malignancies of the pericardium are rare and include mesothelioma (50%), sarcoma, and malignant teratoma. Malignancy of the pericardium generally manifests as cardiac tamponade resulting from malignant pericardial effusion. Pericardial constriction resulting from malignancy is infrequent. Once pericardial effusion is demonstrated by an imaging study, the diagnosis of malignant pericardial effusion can be made by cytologic examination of pericardial effusion in 20% to 30% of cases. Pericardial biopsy doubles the diagnostic yield of pericardiocentesis alone. Pericardiocentesis has had some success, followed by sclerotherapy and also percutaneous balloon pericardiotomy.[5] The longevity of patients with malignant pericarditis is sufficiently low that subxiphoid drainage and transthoracic drainage have similar success rates.[34] Median survival for malignant pericardial effusion requiring surgical intervention is less than 6 to 12 months.[23,35] Rarely, good long-term results can be obtained with complete excision of localized primary tumors of the pericardium

Traumatic and Radiation-Induced Pericarditis

Only a small fraction of patients receiving mediastinal irradiation develop clinically significant pericarditis. Early pericarditis within 1 to 3 months of initiating mediastinal irradiation is generally self-limited and can be treated symptomatically, as idiopathic pericarditis is treated. Treatment with pericardiocentesis or pericardial window should be reserved for significant refractory symptoms or concern about other causes. A small number of patients may develop constrictive pericarditis, usually 5 to 20 years after irradiation.

Traumatic pericarditis along with hemopericardium and tamponade can result from cardiac intervention such as cardiac catheterization, coronary angioplasty, myocardial biopsy, and balloon valvuloplasty. Pericardiocentesis alone is usually effective if the puncture is isolated to the atria.[5]

Metabolic and Uremic Pericarditis

Metabolic causes of pericarditis include uremia, myxedema, Addison disease, diabetic ketoacidosis, and cholesterol pericarditis. Uremic pericarditis occurs in 20% of patients receiving hemodialysis and in 50% of patients with severe untreated renal disease. Patients may have chronic pericardial thickening that classically looks “shaggy.” Other dialysis patients have less pericardial thickening and significant pericardial effusions because of chronic volume overload.[5] Therapy for uremic pericarditis is focused on treating tamponade. Intensive hemodialysis may avert tamponade in patients with uremic pericarditis, but pericardial tamponade is most effectively treated by pericardial drainage. Tamponade may respond to pericardiocentesis initially, but the incidence of recurrent tamponade in uremic pericardial effusion is highest with pericardiocentesis alone, better with subxiphoid pericardial window, and lowest with transthoracic pericardial window.[19]

Pericarditis from Surrounding Structures

Pericarditis can develop after acute myocardial infarction (Dressler syndrome), aortic dissection, pneumonia, pulmonary infarction, and esophageal disease. Other causes must be excluded. Treatment is focused on the underlying pathology, with care needed to prevent tamponade resulting from myocardial or aortic rupture in patients with larger effusions.[5]

Chylopericardium

Chylopericardium can be idiopathic or follow thoracic surgery. It can be treated with pericardiocentesis or, if recurrent, with subxiphoid or transthoracic pericardial window with or without low thoracic duct ligation.[3]

Hemopericardium

Hemopericardium can result from trauma, recent mediastinal operation, coagulopathy, cardiac perforation owing to instrumentation, cardiac rupture, or aortic rupture. Acute hemopericardium resulting in cardiac tamponade requires emergent treatment (see Cardiac Tamponade, later). In the absence of cardiac tamponade, the treatment of hemopericardium depends on the underlying disease process. Hemopericardium caused by percutaneous cardiac (especially atrial) puncture in the catheterization laboratory can generally be remedied by placing a pigtail catheter in the pericardial space, reversing anticoagulation, aspirating frequently with the pigtail catheter, and watching for cessation of bleeding.

Hemopericardium caused by surgical diseases such as acute aortic dissection, cardiac or aortic rupture, or penetrating trauma is best treated by tube drainage of the pericardium after surgically correcting the source of the bleeding. Hemopericardium caused by blunt trauma or coagulopathy may require surgical drainage by either the subxiphoid or the transthoracic approach to prevent acute tamponade and late pericardial constriction.

Pneumopericardium

Pneumopericardium is a rare condition that most commonly results from severe chest trauma with associated lung injury, or from spontaneous dissection of air from a ruptured bleb in neonates on positive-pressure ventilation.[36] Symptoms are unusual, although tamponade occurs in 37% of patients. Treatment focuses on the underlying disease. Pericardiocentesis or pericardial tube drainage can be effective in patients with tamponade. Mortality is high (58%) because of underlying disease.

CARDIAC TAMPONADE

Etiology

A common cause of acute pericardial tamponade is hemopericardium after recent mediastinal surgery or percutaneous cardiac instrumentation. Other causes include pneumopericardium and hemopericardium resulting from coagulopathy. Approximately half of patients with chronic pericardial effusion present with cardiac tamponade. Malignant effusion and uremic pericarditis are common causes of chronic cardiac tamponade (see Table 95-1).

Diagnosis

Physical examination may show pulsus paradoxus and jugular venous distention. Cardiac tamponade can be diagnosed using right heart catheterization or echocardiography (see Table 95-1). For right heart catheterization, cardiac output is typically reduced with elevation of central venous pressure of at least 14 mm Hg, and with equalization of the central venous pressure, pulmonary artery diastolic pressure, and capillary wedge pressure. Echocardiography will show the pericardial space distended with fluid, with right atrial compression or diastolic right ventricular collapse (or both), and inspiratory interventricular septal shift leftward with increased tricuspid and pulmonic flow velocities and decreased mitral and aortic flow velocities (see Fig. 95-3).[13] Although 80% of patients have pericardial effusions on echocardiography in the first 3 weeks after heart surgery, a moderate or large pericardial effusion has been associated with a 75% likelihood of developing tamponade.[37]

Treatment

Cardiac tamponade resulting from hemopericardium within several days after a surgical procedure is almost always managed by returning to the operating room once coagulopathy is corrected. Back in the operating room, the hemopericardium should be evacuated (generally through the original surgical incision) and drains should be left in the pericardial space.

In the absence of a recent cardiac surgical procedure, patients with cardiac tamponade and hemodynamic compromise can usually be stabilized with emergent pericardiocentesis. Depending on the cause of the tamponade, a single pericardiocentesis may be all that is needed.

Otherwise, a pigtail catheter may be left in the pericardium for up to 48 hours, or more definitive pericardial drainage by the subxiphoid or transpleural window may be desirable.

Subxiphoid pericardial window is ideal for many patients with tamponade, because local anesthesia can be used to avoid the hemodynamic embarrassment of general anesthesia in an unstable patient. Transpleural approaches are less suitable for the unstable patient because of intolerance of one-lung anesthesia or pleural insufflation of carbon dioxide. In patients for whom transpleural pericardial window has advantages, an initial pericardiocentesis should be done to relieve tamponade before anesthetic induction for transpleural drainage. Paradoxic hemodynamic instability after relieving pericardial tamponade is associated with poor long-term survival and may be due to underlying ventricular dysfunction.[31]

CONSTRICTIVE PERICARDITIS

Etiology

The most common etiology of constrictive pericarditis in Western countries is idiopathic, with prior cardiac operation and mediastinal irradiation also being common (see Table 95-1).[38-40] As in earlier decades in the West, tuberculosis in developing countries today is the leading cause of constrictive pericarditis.[41] Pericardial closure at the time of routine cardiac operation can induce some degree of immediate pericardial constriction and decreased cardiac index,[42] and it probably increases the small but real incidence of late constrictive pericarditis. Although routine pericardial closure at the time of cardiac operation can decrease the risk of sternal reentry, some authors have recommended avoiding pericardial closure in patients with ventricular dysfunction, risk of tamponade, or older age when there is a low likelihood of reoperation.[42]

Diagnosis

Physical examination may show jugular venous distention and Kussmaul sign. Pericardial thickening with minimal pericardial fluid on echocardiography, CT, or MRI is present in 85% of patients.[12-14] Pericardial thickening supports the diagnosis, but the pericardium might not be thickened in 15% to 18% of patients with constriction (see Fig. 95-2). Diagnosis of constrictive pericarditis requires demonstration of the right heart hemodynamics typical of constriction (see Fig. 95-2). The findings at right heart catheterization include decreased cardiac output, equalization of diastolic right-sided pressures, and the characteristic square root sign with a steep *y* descent in right and left ventricular diastolic pressure tracings (see Box 95-2 and Fig. 95-2). Detection of these findings can be augmented with a 500-mL volume challenge at the time of right heart catheterization.

Treatment

The treatment for pericardial constriction is pericardiectomy (see Pericardiectomy, later). Patients should be referred before onset of class IV symptoms to minimize postoperative mortality and low cardiac output.[38] Approximately 20% of patients with constriction have at least moderate tricuspid regurgitation, which in turn is associated with worse 5-year survival (47% vs. 87%). Significant tricuspid regurgitation in patients undergoing pericardiectomy should prompt consideration of tricuspid operation.[43] Rarely, the underlying cause also requires treatment, such as for tuberculous pericarditis.[41] Perioperative mortality can be significantly increased with a Class B or C Child-Pugh score.[44] Long-term survival in selected patients without myocardial involvement can approach that of the general population.[39,40,45]

PERICARDIAL CYSTS AND DIVERTICULA

Pericardial cysts and diverticula are usually congenital and occasionally inflammatory in origin, and they represent 10% to 20% of all mediastinal masses.[46,47] Pericardial cysts and diverticula have a fibrous wall lined with mesothelium, whereas bronchial cysts have bronchial epithelium. Pericardial cysts occur more often in men than in women. Most pericardial cysts and diverticula appear as asymptomatic masses on chest radiography, and one third of patients present with chest pain. Pericardial cysts are found at the right costophrenic angle in 77%, at the left costophrenic angle in 22%, and in other areas (posterior mediastinum, hilar region, right paratracheal region, or aortic arch) in 8%.[46-48] Pericardial diverticula communicate with the pericardium and comprise 20% of combined pericardial cysts and diverticula.[48] Cysts or diverticula found to have low fluid density on CT or MRI need no further workup. Masses with a density higher than that of transudate may need further workup to exclude other pericardial masses (Fig. 95-5). Cysts or diverticula that need to be removed to exclude malignancy can be approached thoracoscopically or via thoracotomy. Even when malignancy is unlikely, some authors have recommended excision of most pericardial cysts to prevent complications of rupture, cardiac compression, or tracheal compression.[47,48] Percutaneous cyst aspiration and chemical sclerosis may also be feasible and are preferable to surgery for echinococcal cysts.[5]

PERICARDIAL TUMORS

Most pericardial tumors appear with malignant pericardial effusions resulting from malignant metastases from lung, breast, or lymphoma (see Malignant Pericarditis, earlier). Primary pericardial tumors include lipoma, hemangioma, lymphangioma, leiomyoma, neurofibroma, heterotopic thymus or thyroid, teratoma, mesothelioma, thymoma, liposarcoma, angiosarcoma, and synovial sarcoma. Half of all primary pericardial malignancies are mesotheliomas, with angiosarcoma being the next most common primary malignancy. The differential diagnosis includes pericardial cysts and pericardial diverticula (see earlier), which can often be distinguished with CT or MRI.[33]

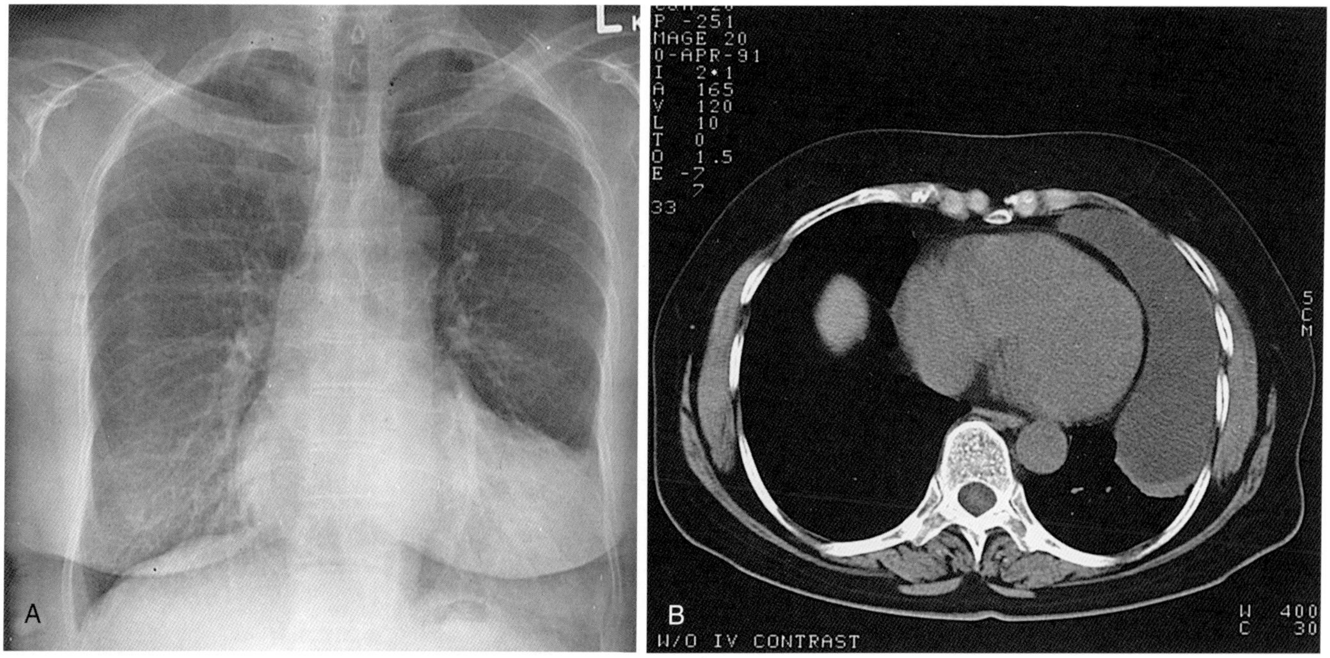

FIGURE 95-5 ■ **A,** Chest radiograph of a patient with a large left-sided pericardial cyst. **B,** Computed tomographic scan of the same patient showing the pericardial cyst extending into the left hemithorax.

Once identified, primary pericardial tumors should be removed if possible. Depending on location and size, either median sternotomy, thoracotomy, or thoracoscopy can be used to approach primary pericardial tumors. Prognosis depends on tumor type and extent. Lipomas, leiomyomas, and heterotopic tissue are generally resectable and have an excellent prognosis. Mesotheliomas almost always spread to contiguous structures in the pericardium, adjacent pleura, and occasionally mediastinal lymph nodes. Mesotheliomas are rarely resectable, and no treatment has been shown to be effective. Survival with pericardial mesothelioma may be 40% at 6 months.[46]

PERICARDIAL DEFECTS

Congenital defects of the pericardium are rare, occurring in 1 in 10,000 autopsies, with a 5 : 1 male-to-female predominance.[47] Approximately 30% of patients with pericardial defects have associated cardiac or pulmonary anomalies. The mean age at diagnosis is 20 years. Complete absence of the pericardium is rare but generally asymptomatic.

Partial pericardial defects are left sided in 70% of cases, and they can produce symptoms by compressing the left atrial appendage, allowing cardiac herniation, or even compressing coronary arteries.[49] Partial pericardial defect can have some risk of death from cardiac herniation, coronary compression, or traumatic aortic dissection.[5] One third of patients are asymptomatic and are detected by abnormal chest radiograph. Symptoms of partial pericardial defect include sharp, fleeting chest pain that is often positional.[50] Other symptoms include dyspnea, sweating, syncope, and circulatory collapse.

When there is complete or partial absence of the pericardium, the chest radiograph is always abnormal, with rotation and leftward displacement of the heart placing the right heart border over the spine. CT and MRI can similarly show displacement and rotation of the heart into the left chest. The presence of a tongue of lung between the pulmonary artery and the aorta is pathognomonic for congenital absence of pericardium.[50]

Complete pericardial absence requires no treatment.[50] Partial left pericardial defects not overlying the left ventricle may be observed if asymptomatic. Patients with symptoms or partial pericardial defects overlying the left ventricle should be treated surgically to prevent cardiac herniation or compression. Surgical approaches include either sternotomy or thoracoscopy to perform pericardiectomy, repair the pericardial defect with a patch, or amputate the left atrial appendage.[49]

Pericardial rupture can occur as the result of blunt trauma, and it is associated with cardiac injury, cardiac rupture, and cardiac tamponade.[51] Pericardial rupture should be repaired to prevent cardiac herniation, but only after associated cardiac injuries are repaired. Mortality is greater than 50%.[5]

PERICARDIAL SURGICAL PROCEDURES

Subxiphoid Pericardial Window

For patients requiring more extensive pericardial drainage than is possible through pericardiocentesis, the subxiphoid pericardial window is an excellent option that minimizes morbidity, especially in patients who are hemodynamically compromised by cardiac tamponade. The subxiphoid pericardial window provides excellent drainage of the pericardial space, allows placement of large-bore pericardial tubes, and potentially drains the right pleural space. An additional advantage is that the

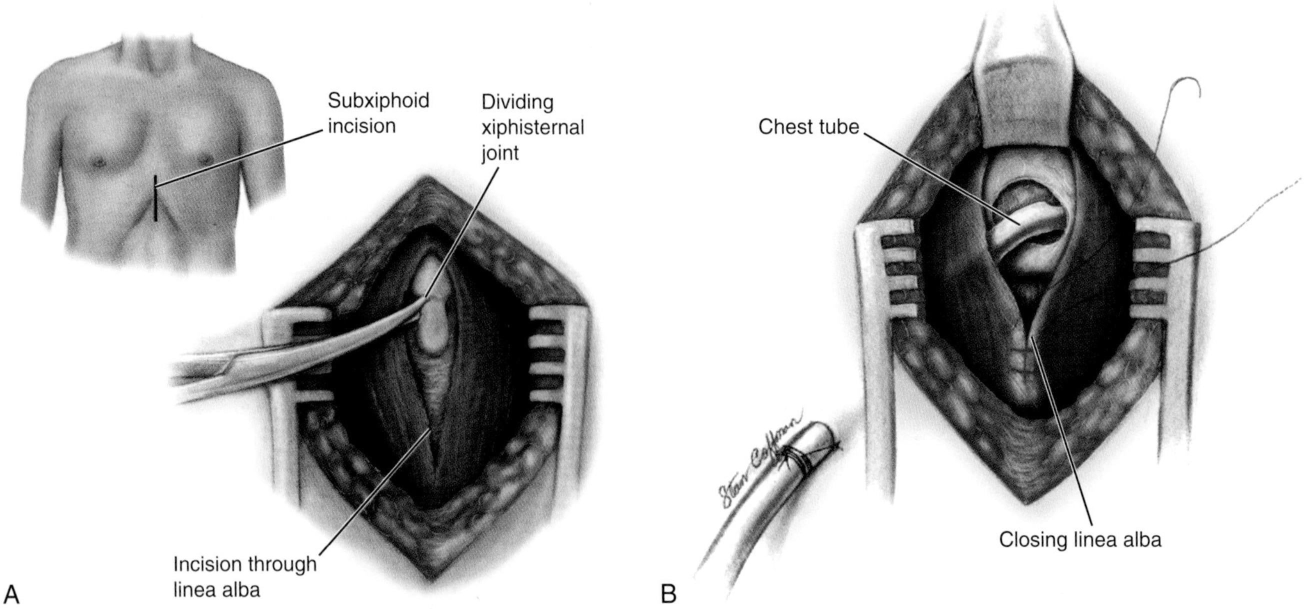

FIGURE 95-6 Technique of subxiphoid pericardial window. **A,** A 7-cm subxiphoid incision is made, the linea alba is opened, and the xiphoid process is excised. **B,** A 2 × 2-cm opening is made in the pericardium, and a tube drain is placed in the pericardial space. (From Glower DD: Pericardial window. In Sabiston DC Jr, editor: *Atlas of cardiothoracic surgery,* Philadelphia, 1995, WB Saunders.)

subxiphoid pericardial window can be created with either local or general anesthesia. Local anesthesia is preferable for patients who are hemodynamically compromised by pericardial tamponade.

After either anesthesia is established, a 6- to 12-cm incision is made in the midline from the cephalad end of the xiphoid to 1 to 2 cm inferior to the xiphoid (Fig. 95-6). The linea alba is divided at the midline, and the xiphoid process is either removed or retracted. With sharp and blunt dissection continuing superiorly and to the patient's left, the pericardium is identified using upward retraction on the sternum and costal cartilages as necessary. Identification of the pericardium can be confirmed by needle aspiration of the pericardium to obtain fluid before making the incision into the pericardial space. When the pericardium is identified, a 4-cm–diameter piece of anterior pericardium is excised. The pericardium and pericardial fluid may be sent for histology and culture. Optionally, the pericardial window can be opened into the right pleural space to drain any right pleural effusion. An angled chest tube can then be placed on the diaphragm in the pericardial space, and an additional chest tube could be placed in the right pleural space. Chest tubes should be brought through the rectus muscle lateral to the incision. The linea alba and remaining incision are then closed.

The mortality directly related to subxiphoid pericardial window is 1% or less, and survival is limited by the underlying disease (50% to 60% survival at 1 year).[23,24,31] The effectiveness in treating tamponade is nearly 100%, and the diagnostic yield is 40% to 80%.[24,31] Recurrent effusion or constriction can occur in 9% to 25% of patients,[23] and it may be more likely after transthoracic pericardial resection for patients with benign disease.[23]

Pericardioscopy

Pericardioscopy has been performed with general anesthesia using the same technique as subxiphoid pericardial window described earlier. Once the pericardial window has been created, a flexible scope is introduced into the pericardial space.[20] The pericardial space is inspected for gross diagnostic purposes, and endoscopically guided biopsy specimens can be obtained. Pericardioscopy combined with pericardiocentesis and subxiphoid pericardial window has been reported to provide a specific diagnosis in 64% of cases, significantly greater than with pericardiocentesis or pericardial window alone.

Transpleural Pericardial Window

A left thoracotomy is generally used to treat hemodynamically stable patients with pericardial effusion and with good long-term prognosis. Thoracotomy may be desired if simultaneous lung biopsy is needed, and chronic pericardial drainage may be more effective than subxiphoid approaches in nonmalignant pericarditis. Thoracotomy is relatively contraindicated in patients with purulent pericarditis to avoid contamination of the pleural space.

A left thoracotomy (as opposed to right thoracotomy) is generally preferred for open transpleural pericardial window because more pericardium is accessible from the left. The patient is placed supine with the left side elevated 30 degrees. General anesthesia is standard, and left lung isolation is optional with either a dual-lumen endotracheal tube or an endobronchial blocker. A 5- to 12-cm submammary incision is made, and the fifth or fourth intercostal space is entered. The lung is retracted

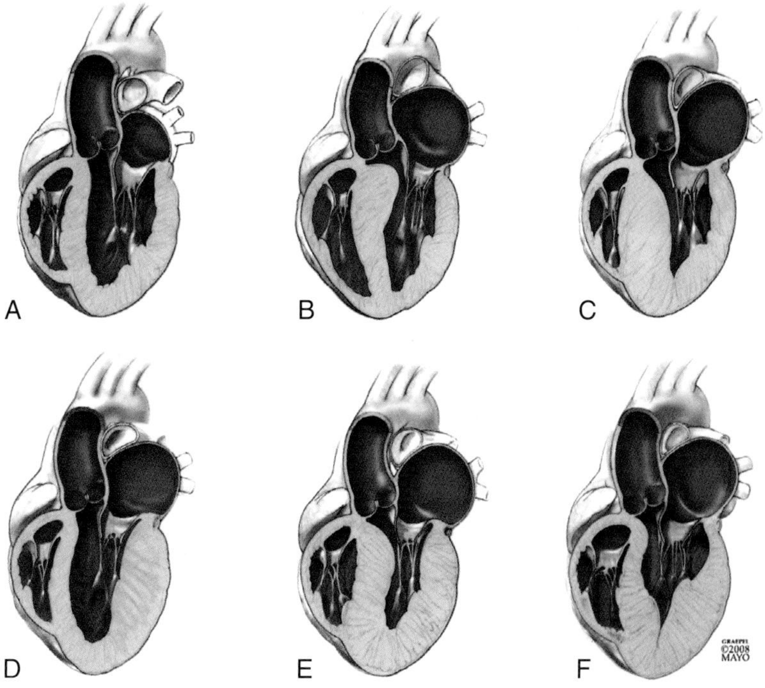

FIGURE 96-1 ■ Morphologic subtypes of hypertrophic cardiomyopathy. Hypertrophy may be localized to the basal septum, as in **B**; diffuse, as in **E**; or predominantly apical, as in **F**. Normal ventricular morphology is shown in **A**. (Adapted and used with permission of Mayo Foundation for Medical Education and Research.)

is debatable, and proposed mechanisms include the Venturi (pull) effect[35,36] and a drag (push) effect.[37,38]

Anomalies of papillary muscles are present in 15% to 20% of patients with HCM who undergo myectomy.[39] These abnormalities include anomalous papillary muscles, direct insertion of papillary muscles into the anterior mitral valve leaflet (Fig. 96-2), fusion of the papillary muscle to the ventricular septum or LV free wall, and accessory muscles and accessory anomalous chordae (false cords). In most cases, these abnormalities do not complicate myectomy or contribute to outflow tract obstruction; however, in some patients, anomalous papillary muscles, especially those that insert directly into the anterior leaflet, can contribute to outflow tract obstruction.[40]

Right Ventricle

Right ventricular wall thickening has been documented in approximately one third of patients with HCM, and 10% have extreme right ventricular wall hypertrophy (≥10 mm).[41] Right ventricular hypertrophy, however, rarely leads to fibrosis as evidenced by hyperenhancement on magnetic resonance imaging, and right ventricular outflow tract obstruction caused by infundibular narrowing is uncommon[42,43] and mainly limited to cases of HCM manifested in children and young adults.[44] Right ventricular hypertrophy also occurs as a result of pulmonary hypertension from elevated LV end-diastolic pressure. Indeed, among patients referred for septal myectomy, pulmonary hypertension (right ventricular systolic pressure ≥ 35 mm Hg) was present in approximately half of the patients and severe pulmonary hypertension (right ventricular systolic pressure ≥ 50 mm Hg) was seen in 17% of patients.[45])

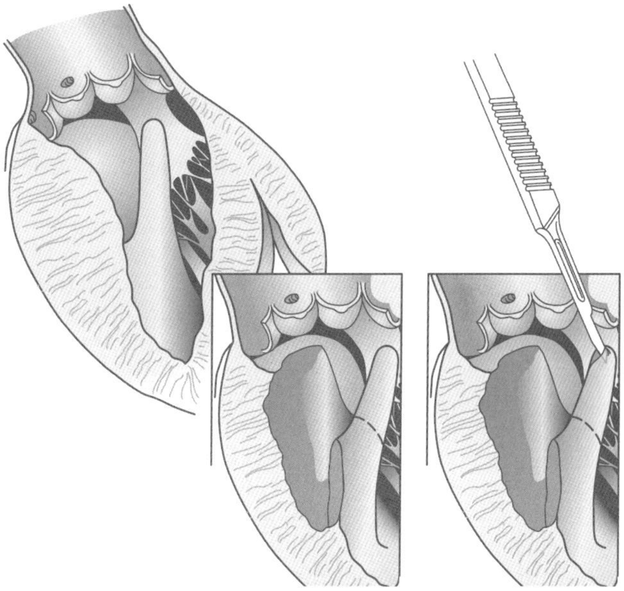

FIGURE 96-2 ■ Anomalous papillary muscles may insert directly into the anterior mitral leaflet and contribute to outflow obstruction. When the anomalous muscle does not support the free edge of the valve, it can be excised. (Adapted and used with permission of Mayo Foundation for Medical Education and Research.)

Aortic Valve

In contrast to congenital membranous subaortic stenosis,[46] LVOT obstruction in patients with HCM does not directly affect the aortic valve. Aortic valve regurgitation has been observed after transaortic myectomy as a result of iatrogenic injury.[47]

Coronary Arteries

Coronary arteries are larger than normal in patients with HCM, and basal coronary flow is increased in the resting state. Coronary flow reserve, however, is decreased in symptomatic patients with HCM compared with controls, and phasic flow is abnormal with a greater amount of flow during diastole, the presence of flow reversal in systole, and a more rapid deceleration of diastolic blood flow compared with normal patients. Decreased flow reserve is associated with a reduction in coronary resistance, suggesting that the mechanism is not a result of narrowing of intramyocardial small arteries or compression of the microcirculation; indeed, the reduction in coronary flow reserve in patients with HCM may be the result of almost maximal vasodilation of the microcirculation in the basal state. It has been speculated that compression of the microcirculation during systole may be the cause of flow reversal in patients with HCM and the inverse correlation between systolic flow and septal thickness; total coronary blood flow in patients with HCM, however, is preserved and even increased under resting conditions.

Atherosclerotic coronary artery disease is present in approximately 5% to 15% of patients with HCM, depending on the population studied. At the Mayo Clinic, significant coronary artery disease was detected in half of patients who were selected for coronary angiography, and disease was severe in 26%.[48] Survival of HCM patients with obstructive coronary artery disease is reduced compared with that of HCM patients without coronary artery disease, and survival is also poorer than that of patients without HCM who have comparable coronary artery disease and normal ventricular function.

Muscle bridging of the left anterior descending coronary artery (LAD) is not uncommon, occurring in 15% of patients with HCM undergoing coronary angiography at our clinic.[49] It is unclear whether bridging of the LAD plays a pathophysiologic role in the disease and associated symptoms of angina. However, for adult patients, risk of death and, in particular, of sudden cardiac death is not increased among patients with HCM with myocardial bridging. In contrast, Yetman and coworkers[50] reported that among children with HCM, systolic compression of LAD was present in 285 cases and was associated with a greater incidence of chest pain (60% vs. 19%; $P = 0.04$), cardiac arrest with subsequent resuscitation (50% vs. 4%; $P = 0.004$), and ventricular tachycardia (80% vs. 8%; $P < 0.001$). Myocardial ischemia was postulated to be the cause of this poor outcome.

Histopathology

Myocardial Fiber Disarray

A characteristic histologic feature of HCM is myocardial fiber disarray, which consists of short runs of severely hypertrophied fibers interspersed by connective tissue. Myocytes show large, bizarre nuclei with degenerating muscle fibers and fibrosis. It is the disorganized whirling of muscle fibers that is characteristic of HCM. Myocardial disarray is present in the ventricular septum and in the LV free wall, but it is not pathognomonic for HCM. Fiber disarray may be present in myocardium in any conditions in which there is pressure overload, but the proportion of myocardial disarray is much greater in HCM.[51,52]

Myocyte disarray has been associated with systolic dysfunction, ventricular dilation, and congestive heart failure.[53] It may also be a substrate for ventricular arrhythmias. Disarray has also been greatest in hearts with only a mild degree of LV hypertrophy or with absence of a subaortic mitral valve contact lesion, but there seems to be no direct relationship between myocyte disarray and fibrosis or small vessel disease.[54]

Interstitial Fibrosis

Interstitial fibrosis is an important histologic feature that is present in variable degrees in the ventricle of patients with HCM.[55,56] It is important not only as a mechanism of diastolic dysfunction but also because fibrosis detected by magnetic resonance imaging has been associated with arrhythmogenesis and risk of sudden cardiac death.[57,58]

Differential Diagnosis

Other diseases may mimic HCM. Cardiac amyloidosis is an infiltrative disorder of the myocardium that typically produces diastolic dysfunction. Up to 30% of patients with cardiac amyloidosis have prominent subaortic thickening that produces LVOT obstruction. The clinical features and hemodynamics of patients with cardiac amyloidosis are similar to those of patients with LVOT obstruction caused by HCM. The finding of LV granular speckling on echocardiography should raise the suspicion of cardiac amyloid, especially if atrial wall thickness is increased.[59] Newer techniques of strain and strain rate imaging from speckle tracking may improve discrimination of cardiac amyloidosis from HCM.[60]

Amyloid deposits may be identified incidentally in myectomy specimens of patients with typical features of obstructive HCM, and the mid-term postoperative survival of such patients is similar to that of an age- and sex-matched HCM population without amyloidosis undergoing septal myectomy. In these patients the most common subtype is senile amyloid, which has a good prognosis and rarely leads to multisystem involvement.

Patients with Fabry's disease may present with ventricular hypertrophy and dynamic LVOT obstruction. The mechanism of cardiac hypertrophy is different from that in other infiltrative cardiomyopathies in that it is secondary to increased cardiac muscle mass and infiltration of glycosphingolipids. The disorder caused by α-galactosidase A deficiency can be treated by enzyme replacement therapy, but ventricular hypertrophy and LVOT obstruction may persist and septal myectomy can relieve cardiac-related symptoms.[5]

GENETICS

HCM has a prevalence of 0.2% for phenotypically expressed disease.[61] Approximately 60% to 80% of cases are familial, and the remainder result from de novo mutations.[62] HCM is genetically diverse, involving sarcomeric and nonsarcomeric proteins, and hundreds of mutations in more than 15 genes have been identified; indeed, double and compound heterozygosity and homozygosity have been reported.[63]

Most patients with familial disease have mutations in three protein-encoding genes, β-myosin heavy chain *(MYH7)* in 35% to 50%, myosin-binding protein C *(MYBPC3)* in 15% to 25%, and cardiac troponin T type 2 *(TNNT2)* in 15% to 20%. In current practice, the clinical value of genetic testing is uncertain. Van Driest and colleagues[64] reported that gene-positive status did not correlate with family history of sudden cardiac death, need for myectomy, or anatomic subtype. Furthermore, specific mutations in HCM are rare; in one study, less than 2% of 293 unrelated patients had putative benign mutations, but serious clinical events developed in these patients, including sudden cardiac death, need for surgical myectomy, and cardiac transplantation.[65]

Other studies suggest that certain mutations are associated with poor prognosis. For example, certain mutations in *TNNT2*, β-tropomyosin *(TPM1)*, and *MYH7* may confer increased risk of sudden cardiac death. Olivotto and coworkers reported that identification of myofilament-positive patients through genetic testing predicted a fourfold increase in the risk of the combined endpoint of cardiovascular death, nonfatal stroke, or progression to New York Heart Association (NYHA) class III or class IV symptoms.[66] Mutations were associated with more severe systolic and diastolic LV dysfunction, and adverse clinical events occurred irrespective of whether the involved myofilament was thin, intermediate, or thick.

A potential benefit of genetic analysis is the preclinical diagnosis in patients with a family history of sudden cardiac death or in those carrying a "malignant" mutation that predisposes them to a severe phenotype. Also, it may be useful to know the precise genetic defect in HCM among asymptomatic family members who carry the mutation and might be at risk of sudden cardiac death.

In addition to variability in clinical course and risk of sudden cardiac death, the phenotype of HCM shows considerable diversity in the severity and distribution of hypertrophy (asymmetrical, concentric, apical), penetrance, and age at onset. This variability may be explained partially by patients who are compound heterozygotes and by the coexistence of other diseases that predispose to hypertrophy.

PATHOPHYSIOLOGY

Diastolic Dysfunction

Diastolic dysfunction with elevation of the LV end-diastolic pressure is the principal pathophysiologic finding in HCM. The resulting increase in left atrial and pulmonary venous pressures accounts for the common symptoms of effort dyspnea and limited aerobic capacity. With worsening diastolic function, LV filling becomes more dependent on atrial contraction, and occurrence of atrial arrhythmias, especially atrial fibrillation, can cause an acute and profound decrease in cardiac output and worsening of symptoms.[67]

Abnormal myocardial relaxation has been observed in patients with HCM before the development of symptoms. The increased chamber stiffness results primarily from increased wall thickness, but there are other factors of surgical importance that aggravate intrinsic diastolic dysfunction related to LV hypertrophy.

LVOT obstruction has a direct effect of increasing end-diastolic pressure and an indirect effect through the often associated mitral regurgitation. Thus, whereas surgical myectomy has a minimal immediate effect on overall LV mass, symptoms related to diastolic dysfunction are immediately improved when outflow gradients and mitral regurgitation are relieved. A secondary effect of septal myectomy on diastolic function is regression of hypertrophy, as discussed later.

In some patients, concentric ventricular hypertrophy is so severe that muscle mass encroaches on the ventricular cavity and reduces normal cavity size. This is particularly striking in patients with the apical form of HCM, in which the distal third to distal half of the left ventricle may be obliterated (during diastole and systole) by muscle. Surgical remodeling by apical myectomy may increase end-diastolic volume and thus improve diastolic function.

Left Ventricular Outflow Obstruction

Surgical treatment of HCM consists primarily of relief of LVOT obstruction. As discussed before, obstruction results from dynamic narrowing of the subaortic area, which in turn is caused by protrusion of the hypertrophied septum in apposition with the anterior leaflet of the mitral valve. Previously, there was debate on the importance of outflow tract obstruction as a mechanism for symptoms in patients with HCM because of the lability of the finding and the question of catheter entrapment when gradients were measured by invasive catheterization.[68] It is now recognized that outflow obstruction is much more common than previously thought, correlates importantly with development of symptoms, and may negatively influence long-term survival.

Maron and colleagues documented resting outflow tract gradients of 50 mm Hg or greater in 37% of 320 patients with HCM and, more important, found exercise-induced gradients (mean 80 ± 43 mm Hg) in an additional 106 patients; thus, as many as 70% of patients with HCM who come to clinical evaluation will have significant outflow tract obstruction.[69] Another important finding in this study was the relative unreliability of the Valsalva maneuver (sensitivity 40%) compared with exercise Doppler echocardiography in detecting these dynamic gradients. Latent obstruction can also be documented during hemodynamic catheterization by isoproterenol challenge, and the technique may be useful in patients who are unable to exercise or in patients in whom reliable Doppler echocardiographic signals cannot be measured.[70]

Mitral Valve Regurgitation

Accelerated blood flow near the hypertrophied basal septum pushes the mitral leaflet at the same time that there may be "suction" forces that contribute to the systolic anterior motion of the mitral valve. Thus, leaflet coaptation is reduced, producing variable degrees of posteriorly directed mitral regurgitation. If the mitral regurgitant jet is directed anteriorly, primary mitral valve disease such as a flail or prolapsing segment should be suspected. As is true with outflow gradients, the degree of mitral regurgitation is often dynamic. Symptomatic patients with moderate or severe degrees of mitral regurgitation associated with HOCM are excellent candidates for operation because the mitral regurgitation and associated symptoms (dyspnea and fatigability) are almost always abolished or significantly improved with adequate septal myectomy.

Intrinsic mitral valve disease may contribute to valvular regurgitation in patients with HOCM. Rupture of chordae with resultant leaflet prolapse can precipitate congestive heart failure, and hemodynamics may worsen if HCM is not recognized and patients are managed medically with afterload reduction.[71]

CLINICAL PRESENTATION AND DIAGNOSTIC CRITERIA

Symptoms

Although some children and adolescents present with cardiac limitations, most patients remain asymptomatic until young adulthood or middle age. The onset of symptoms parallels development of outflow tract obstruction, and limitation is gradual, manifested first by fatigability and then by effort dyspnea, angina, and syncope or presyncope. As discussed previously, dyspnea is caused by LV diastolic dysfunction and variable degrees of mitral regurgitation. Autonomic dysfunction, which is present in approximately 25% of patients with HCM, may also contribute to poor exercise capacity; it is manifested by a failure to increase systolic blood pressure by 20 mm Hg during exercise or an actual decline in blood pressure during exertion.

Although obstructive coronary artery disease may coexist, angina is most likely explained by the combination of increased LV wall thickness (increased myocardial oxygen demand) and decreased capillary network (decreased myocardial oxygen supply) in addition to provoking factors such as increased heart rate and increased afterload.

Signs

In HCM patients without obstruction, clinical findings are those of LV hypertrophy. For patients with obstruction, it is important to differentiate dynamic obstruction from fixed obstruction as occurs with valvular aortic stenosis or congenital membranous subaortic stenosis. Auscultation in patients with HOCM reveals the classic crescendo-decrescendo murmur heard best near the left sternal border, which peaks in mid to late systole and usually ends before the second heart sound. The murmur can radiate across the precordium, but in contrast to valvular aortic stenosis, radiation to the carotid arteries is uncommon. Mitral regurgitation may produce a separate holosystolic murmur audible at the apex. With dynamic outflow obstruction, the carotid pulsation is brisk and bifid. If there is severe hypertrophy, a fourth heart sound may be heard.

Dynamic auscultation can differentiate the murmur of HCM from that of valvular aortic stenosis and mitral regurgitation. Maneuvers such as the Valsalva or stand-squat-stand, which decrease the LV volume, will increase the dynamic gradient and the intensity of the murmur. Other maneuvers to change the intensity of the murmur include leg raising to increase preload and the inhalation of amyl nitrate to decrease afterload and increase heart rate.

Electrocardiography and Chest Radiography

In HCM with obstruction, the electrocardiogram characteristically shows LV hypertrophy with a strain pattern, and Q waves may be present. Electrocardiographic evidence of left atrial enlargement is common, as is a bundle branch block pattern (especially after myectomy). After alcohol septal ablation, a right bundle branch block is commonly observed. With the apical form of HCM, the electrocardiogram shows a distinctive pattern of diffuse symmetrical T wave inversions across the precordium.

Most patients with HCM have normal sinus rhythm, but continuous monitoring will show a high incidence of supraventricular tachycardia (46%), premature ventricular contractions (43%), and nonsustained ventricular tachycardia (26%).[72] Atrial fibrillation develops in up to a quarter of patients, and onset of atrial fibrillation often precipitates symptoms because of loss of atrial contraction and impaired filling of the left ventricle.

Findings on chest radiography are those of LV hypertrophy and pulmonary venous congestion, and enlargement of the pulmonary artery may be apparent in patients with congestive heart failure.

Echocardiography

Two-dimensional and Doppler echocardiography is the essential tool for the diagnosis of HCM, providing information on ventricular morphology, hemodynamics, and valve function. The most common pattern of hypertrophy is diffuse involvement of the ventricular septum. In patients with HCM, average maximal LV wall thickness is 20 to 22 mm, and in 5% to 10% of patients, LV wall thickness is dramatically increased, measuring 30 to 50 mm.[72] Morphology of the septum appears to vary according to age, and older patients with HCM often demonstrate a sigmoid configuration.[73]

The echocardiographic findings of increased wall thickness should prompt a search for other causes, including systemic hypertension (especially in patients on dialysis); valvular aortic stenosis; and infiltrative and glycogen storage diseases, such as cardiac amyloidosis, Fabry's disease, and Friedreich's ataxia.

On continuous wave Doppler echocardiography, LVOT obstruction is seen as a high-velocity, late-peaking, "dagger-shaped" signal. In patients with low velocity at rest (<3 m/sec), maneuvers such as the Valsalva, inhalation of amyl nitrate, and exercise may demonstrate latent obstruction. Presence and severity of mitral regurgitation can be determined by Doppler color flow imaging. It is important to differentiate the true outflow tract velocity from the mitral regurgitation jet.

Mitral regurgitation that results from systolic anterior motion is eccentric and directed posterolaterally during late systole. A centrally directed jet should suggest a primary leaflet abnormality contributing to valve leakage. Preoperative transesophageal echocardiography is unnecessary in most patients, but intraoperative transesophageal echocardiography is critically important for assessing results of myectomy.[74]

Cardiac Magnetic Resonance Imaging

Cardiac magnetic resonance imaging is useful in identifying regions of LV hypertrophy not easily recognized by echocardiography, specifically the anterolateral free wall and the apical area.[75] In addition, magnetic resonance imaging can detect presence and severity of myocardial fibrosis, which appears to be an important risk factor for subsequent ventricular arrhythmias and sudden cardiac death.[76,77]

Invasive Catheterization

In current practice, cardiac catheterization is rarely necessary for the diagnosis of HCM. Coronary angiography is indicated for patients with symptoms of angina and for patients at risk for coronary artery disease (strong family history, abnormal lipids, older age) who undergo myectomy. A hemodynamic study with isoproterenol provocation can be useful in identifying patients with labile obstruction gradients that cannot be elicited during echocardiography.[70]

NATURAL HISTORY

Symptom Course

The clinical course of HCM is highly variable, and some patients remain free of symptoms and cardiac limitation. In many patients, however, onset of symptoms is associated with development of LVOT obstruction, and it is not clear what causes this in adult patients who have had no gradients until the fourth, fifth, or sixth decade of life. Onset of atrial fibrillation can also precipitate symptoms and predispose to systemic embolism, which occurs in 6% of patients.[78] Atrial fibrillation is noted in 30% of older patients with HCM.

Infective endocarditis may occur with HCM, and the reported incidence is 1.4 cases per 1000 person-years. The important feature is that in virtually all cases of endocarditis, there is LVOT obstruction. Indeed, among HCM patients with obstruction, the incidence of endocarditis is 3.8 per 1000 person-years, or a 4% likelihood for development of this complication during 10 years.[79]

Survival

In the general population, survival of patients with HCM is similar to that of individuals without disease, and early reports of high mortality in HCM may be explained by excess numbers of high-risk patients included in studies from tertiary referral centers.[80-82] More recent data indicate that the annual mortality rate of patients with HCM is approximately 1%, but there are several important subgroups that have a higher risk of cardiac death; indeed, HCM is the most common cause of sudden death among young athletes.[7,83,84]

Obstructed versus Nonobstructed Hypertrophic Cardiomyopathy

Until recently, there was uncertainty and debate about the influence of LVOT obstruction on survival of patients with HCM. Convincing studies by Maron and colleagues,[85] Autore and associates,[86] and Elliott and coworkers[87] have demonstrated a strong correlation between resting outflow gradients and late risk of death. In a longitudinal study of 1101 patients with HCM, Maron and colleagues reported that patients with outflow tract obstruction (a basal gradient of at least 30 mm Hg) had a risk of death from HCM or symptom progression that was more than four times that observed among patients without obstruction (Fig. 96-3). The association of outflow tract obstruction on limiting symptoms and death was independent of other clinical variables. Of note, patients with obstruction and mild symptoms (NYHA class II) were more likely to have progression to severe symptoms or to die of heart failure than were asymptomatic patients with cardiomyopathy (Fig. 96-4).[85]

An important clinical question is whether prognosis of asymptomatic HOCM patients with high gradients can be improved by septal reduction. Elliott and coworkers

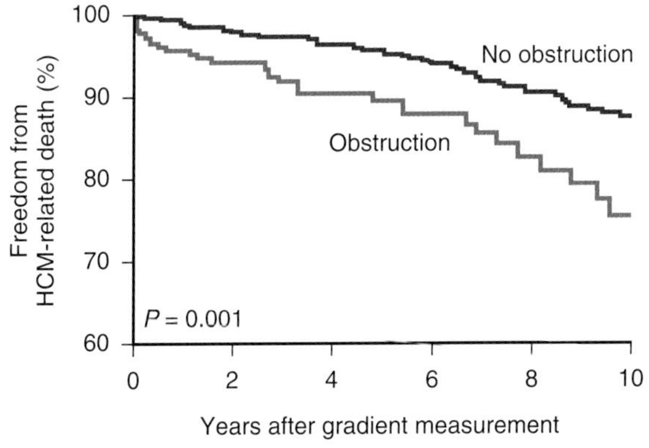

FIGURE 96-3 Survival of patients with hypertrophic cardiomyopathy (HCM) with and without obstruction (≥30 mm Hg). This analysis includes only deaths related to HCM. (From Maron MS, Olivotto I, Betocchi S, et al: Effect of left ventricular outflow tract obstruction on clinical outcome in hypertrophic cardiomyopathy. *N Engl J Med* 348:295–303, 2003.)

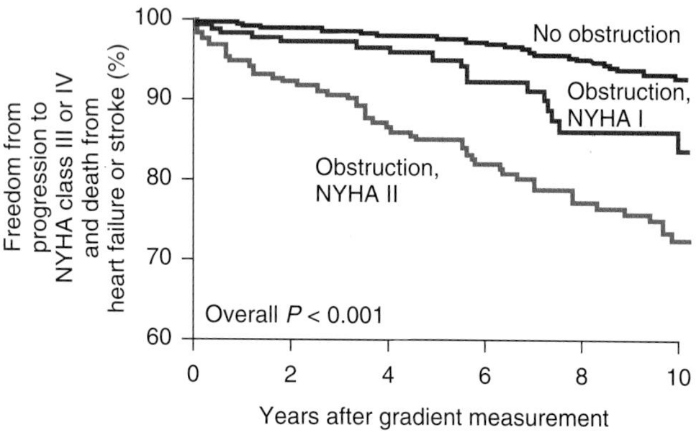

FIGURE 96-4 Probability of progression to severe heart failure, death, or stroke in patients without obstruction and in patients with outflow tract obstruction stratified by presence or absence of symptoms. *NYHA,* New York Heart Association. (From Maron MS, Olivotto I, Betocchi S, et al: Effect of left ventricular outflow tract obstruction on clinical outcome in hypertrophic cardiomyopathy. *N Engl J Med* 348:295–303, 2003.)

reported that risk of sudden death is relatively low (<0.4% per year) in asymptomatic patients with LVOT obstruction and none of the recognized risk factors for sudden cardiac death, but their study demonstrated reduced survival among patients with LVOT obstruction and nonsustained ventricular tachycardia, abnormal exercise blood pressure response, family history of premature sudden death, unexplained syncope, or severe LV hypertrophy.

The prognosis of patients with latent obstruction is less clear, but a study by Vaglio and colleagues[88] suggests that the clinical course is similar to that of patients with resting obstruction. In their series, one quarter of patients required invasive therapy for relief of symptoms, and annual mortality was 2%, a rate higher than that reported for patients with HCM and no LVOT obstruction.

Use of Implantable Cardioverter-Defibrillator

Sudden cardiac death is a special concern in HCM, and there is debate about the appropriate use of implantable cardioverter-defibrillators (ICDs) for primary and secondary prevention of sudden cardiac death. In addition to prior cardiac arrest, clinical variables that appear to identify patients at increased risk of arrhythmic events (major risk factors) include nonsustained ventricular tachycardia, massive ventricular hypertrophy (wall thickness > 30 mm), hypotensive response to exercise, family history of sudden cardiac death, and unexplained syncope.[89] Other findings, such as myocardial bridging in young patients, apical aneurysms, or myocardial fibrosis detected by cardiac magnetic resonance imaging, may also increase risk of sudden death.

Consensus among experts[90] is that an ICD is strongly warranted for secondary prevention of sudden cardiac death in patients with prior cardiac arrest or sustained and spontaneously occurring ventricular tachycardia and should be considered in patients with multiple clinical risk factors and in selected patients with a single major risk factor, such as a history of sudden cardiac death in a close relative. For patients who need ICD implantation and are referred for septal myectomy, we prefer to delay device implantation until the third or fourth day postoperatively to avoid the potential for lead dislocation if the ICD is placed immediately preoperatively.

SURGICAL TREATMENT

Indications for Operation

Septal myectomy is, in general, reserved for patients who continue to have limiting symptoms despite medical treatment. Pharmacologic therapy usually begins with β-adrenergic blocking agents, which have a negative inotropic effect and may mitigate latent outflow gradients provoked with exercise. Beta blockers are less effective in reducing resting gradients. The calcium antagonist verapamil has been used for patients with nonobstructive and obstructive HCM. The drug may improve ventricular relaxation and decreased LV contractility, but hemodynamic and electrophysiologic side effects limit long-term use. Disopyramide has negative inotropic effects and is a type Ia antiarrhythmic agent that can improve symptoms by reducing resting gradients. However, this drug also has side effects, including dry mouth and eyes, constipation, and difficulty in micturition. In addition, it increases atrioventricular nodal conduction and thus may increase ventricular rate in patients with atrial fibrillation. Although medications may ameliorate symptoms, drug therapy does not appear to decrease the probability of sudden death. In a study of 173 patients who were taking amiodarone, beta blockers, verapamil, or sotalol for treatment of symptoms, there was no difference in sudden death mortality compared with patients who were receiving no pharmacologic therapy.[91] Thus, ICDs remain the primary therapy for prevention of sudden death in high-risk HOCM patients.

Technique of Operation

Operation is performed through a median sternotomy, and normothermic cardiopulmonary bypass is established in the standard fashion by use of a single, two-staged venous cannula. The aorta is cross-clamped, and cold blood cardioplegia (1000 to 1200 mL) is infused through the aortic needle vent to arrest the heart. Adequate exposure of the subaortic septum is critically important, and several maneuvers facilitate the operation. First, pericardial sutures are used only on the right side to elevate the pericardium toward the surgeon. Next, an oblique aortotomy is made slightly closer to the sinotubular ridge than is usual for aortic valve replacement, and the incision is carried through the midpoint of the noncoronary aortic sinus of Valsalva to a level approximately 1 cm above the valve annulus. The edge of the proximal aorta is held out of the way with small stay sutures, and a cardiotomy sucker is placed through the aortic valve and used to depress the anterior leaflet of the mitral valve to protect it from injury. The right aortic valve cusp is collapsed against the sinus wall, where it will usually stay. A sponge stick is used to depress the right ventricle and to rotate the septum posteriorly, orienting the LV outflow anteriorly (Fig. 96-5).

A standard no. 10 scalpel blade is used for myectomy; incision in the septum begins just to the right of the nadir of the right aortic sinus (Fig. 96-6). The incision in the septum is made upward and then leftward over to the anterior leaflet of the mitral valve. Scissors are used to complete excision of this initial portion of myocardium. The area of septal excision is then deepened and lengthened toward the apex of the heart, and the hypertrophied septum must be excised beyond endocardial scar (Figs. 96-7 and 96-8). Trabeculations are excised, and the myectomy site is further enlarged with the use of pituitary rongeurs. Adequate septal myectomy usually yields 3 to 12 g of muscle. Use of the sponge stick to depress the heart posteriorly will improve exposure of the distal extent of the myectomy. The aortotomy is closed, and the operation proceeds as usual.

This technique for more extended myectomy[92] differs from the standard Morrow operation,[32] in which parallel incisions create a trough in the septum that extends up to 3 cm from the aortic valve; wider excision of muscle in the immediate subaortic area improves exposure of the distal extent of the hypertrophied septum, and excision

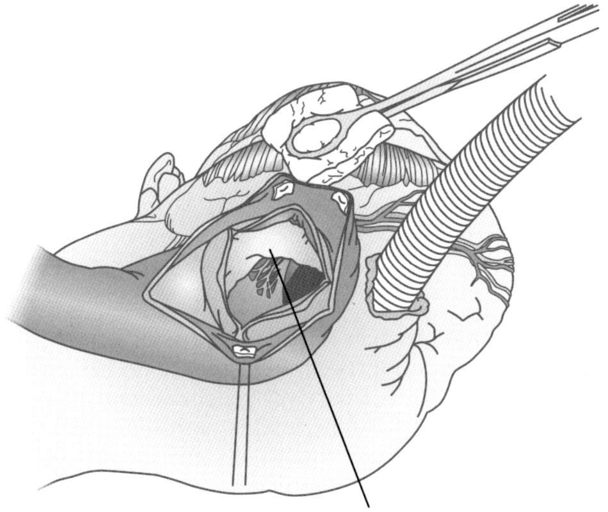

FIGURE 96-5 The subaortic septum is exposed through an oblique aortotomy extended to the base of the noncoronary sinus. The surgeon's view of the septum is improved by depressing and rotating the ventricle posteriorly with a sponge forceps. (Adapted and used with permission of Mayo Foundation for Medical Education and Research.)

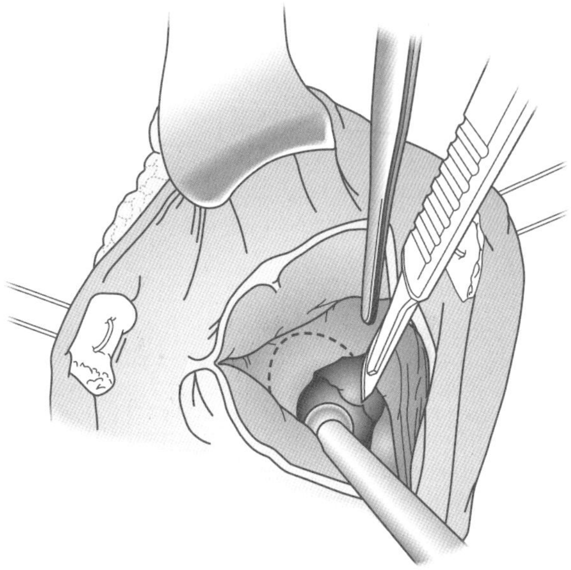

FIGURE 96-6 Septal excision begins just to the right of the nadir of the right aortic sinus and extends leftward toward the anterior leaflet of the mitral valve. After the initial specimen is removed, the area of septal excision should be carried toward the apex of the heart well past the endocardial scar. A wider proximal area of excision improves exposure of the more distal extent of septectomy. (Adapted and used with permission of Mayo Foundation for Medical Education and Research.)

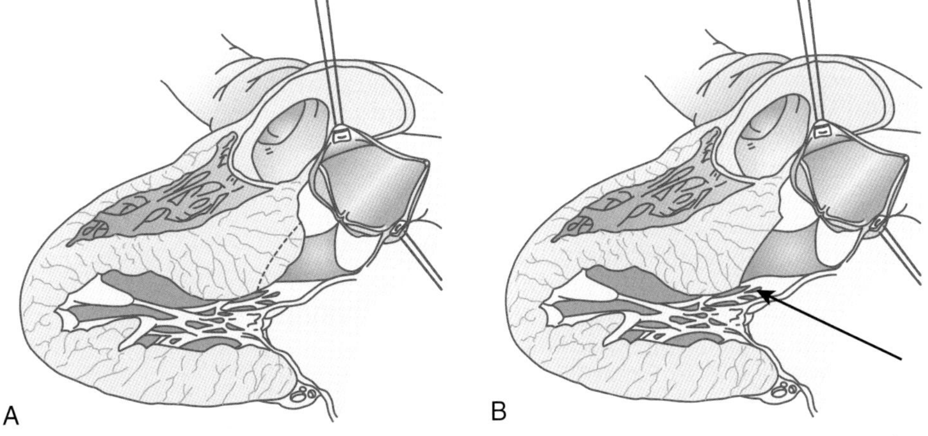

FIGURE 96-7 **A,** A common error in performing septal myectomy is inadequate length (toward the apex) of muscle excision. The bulging septum may appear to be in the immediate subaortic position after initial aortotomy, but if only this portion of the enlarged septum is removed, there may be residual obstruction, as seen by the *arrow* in **B.** (Adapted and used with permission of Mayo Foundation for Medical Education and Research.)

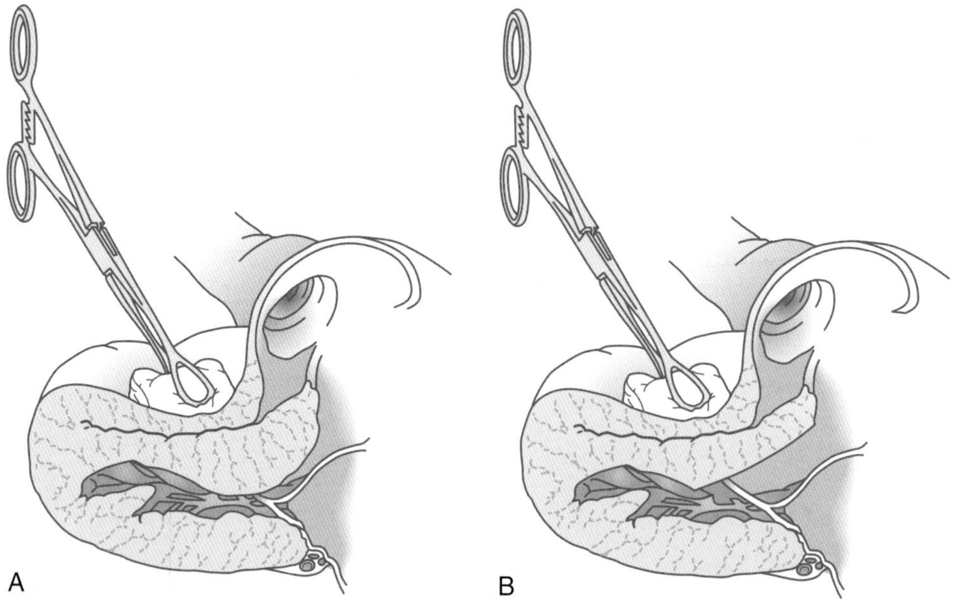

FIGURE 96-8 ■ **A,** Rotation of the ventricle posteriorly improves exposure of the septum and allows the surgeon access to the distal extent of the abstracting segment **(B).** (Adapted and used with permission of Mayo Foundation for Medical Education and Research.)

extends up to 7 cm from the aortic valve. Inadequate myectomy results more often from failure to excise sufficient length of the septum (toward the apex) than from inadequate depth of excision. The methods described have proved adequate for all patients with subaortic obstruction, and maneuvers such as anterior leaflet plication are unnecessary and potentially harmful. Mitral valve replacement is reserved for patients with intrinsic leaflet abnormalities that cannot be repaired. To confirm complete relief of the LVOT obstruction, we routinely measure simultaneous aortic and LV pressure by direct needle puncture before and after myectomy.[93] If the resting LVOT gradient is diminished by effects of anesthesia, premature ventricular beats are induced by stimulating the ventricle to elicit the dynamic gradient produced by the Brockenbrough phenomenon; the post-extrasystolic contraction is more forceful because of increased contractility and decreased afterload. The same maneuver is then repeated after myectomy. Transesophageal echocardiography is routinely used.[74] Intraoperative transesophageal echocardiography can identify residual mitral valve regurgitation, systolic anterior motion, and any septal defects created by excision of septal muscle.

Unroofing of coronary artery bridging is performed in selected cases, particularly young patients and those who have angina preoperatively. After identification of the coronary artery distal to the intramyocardial segment, the anterior surface of the vessel is exposed by sharp dissection that is continued proximally until the LAD reemerges onto the epicardium. The divided myocardium over the artery is usually 3 to 5 mm thick. If the course of the artery is so deep that trabeculations of the right ventricular cavity are entered, pledgeted sutures placed deep into the coronary artery repair the opening into the ventricle. We have combined unroofing of myocardial bridging of the LAD with extended septal myectomy in more than 36 patients with satisfactory outcomes. Angina is improved, but there is no evidence to suggest that there is a survival benefit secondary to the procedure. Thus, in adult patients, unroofing of a myocardial bridge portion should be considered when a patient undergoes myectomy and has a history of angina.[94]

Postoperative Care

Care of patients after myectomy is similar to care of patients who have had valve replacement for aortic stenosis. Systemic vascular resistance should be maintained at or above the normal range so that LV diastolic filling pressure and coronary perfusion pressure are maintained in the hypertrophied ventricles. Vasodilators are avoided, and continuous infusions of phenylephrine or vasopressin may be useful. It is important to maintain atrioventricular synchrony to maximize LV filling, and atrial pacing is often used. The day after operation, we restart beta-blocking medications at half the preoperative dose but do not routinely restart calcium channel blockers or disopyramide. Atrial fibrillation can be especially deleterious to cardiac output and blood pressure, and early electrical cardioversion may be necessary.

OUTCOMES

Early Results

Mortality

Risk of hospital death after isolated septal myectomy for HOCM is low: less than 1% in experienced centers (Fig. 96-9). Surgical risk may be higher among very elderly patients (particularly those with severe disabling symptoms associated with pulmonary hypertension), patients with prior myectomy, or those requiring concomitant procedures.

Morbidity

Complications such as complete heart block requiring permanent pacemaker and iatrogenic ventricular septal perforation have become uncommon (≤1% to 2%).[90] Partial or complete left bundle branch block is a frequent finding after surgical myectomy but is not associated with adverse sequelae. However, if the patient has complete right bundle branch block preoperatively, interruption of the left bundle after myectomy increases risk of complete heart block. This is particularly important in patients who have had alcohol septal ablation before operation. ElBardissi and coworkers[95] reported that risk of postoperative pacemaker insertion was 36% in patients who had alcohol septal ablation before myectomy compared with 3% for those without prior intervention.

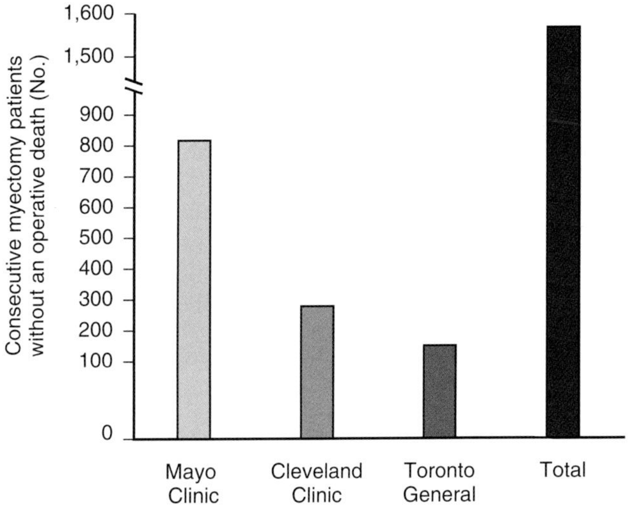

FIGURE 96-9 ■ Operative risk of isolated septal myectomy for hypertrophic cardiomyopathy is less than 1% and approaches zero in centers with broad experience with the procedure. (From Maron BJ: Surgical myectomy remains the primary treatment option for severely symptomatic patients with obstructive hypertrophic cardiomyopathy. *Circulation* 116:196–206, 2007.)

Late Results

Symptom Relief

Improvement in symptoms and exercise capacity after myectomy is highly predictable and durable; more than 90% of severely symptomatic patients have improvement of two or more function classes. Indeed, as illustrated in Figure 96-10, relief of outflow gradients by myectomy is equally effective in improving limitation caused by dyspnea, angina, or syncope.[96] Importantly, symptomatic benefit of myectomy is directly related to reducing the basal outflow gradient and mitral regurgitation and restoring normal LV systolic and end-diastolic pressures (in more than 90% of patients), which in turn may also favorably influence LV diastolic filling and myocardial ischemia. Relief of the gradient may decrease left atrial size and the subsequent risk for development of atrial fibrillation.

The outcome of patients with latent LVOT obstruction preoperatively is especially instructive. Often operation is withheld in these symptomatic patients because the resting LVOT gradient is less than 30 mm Hg, and

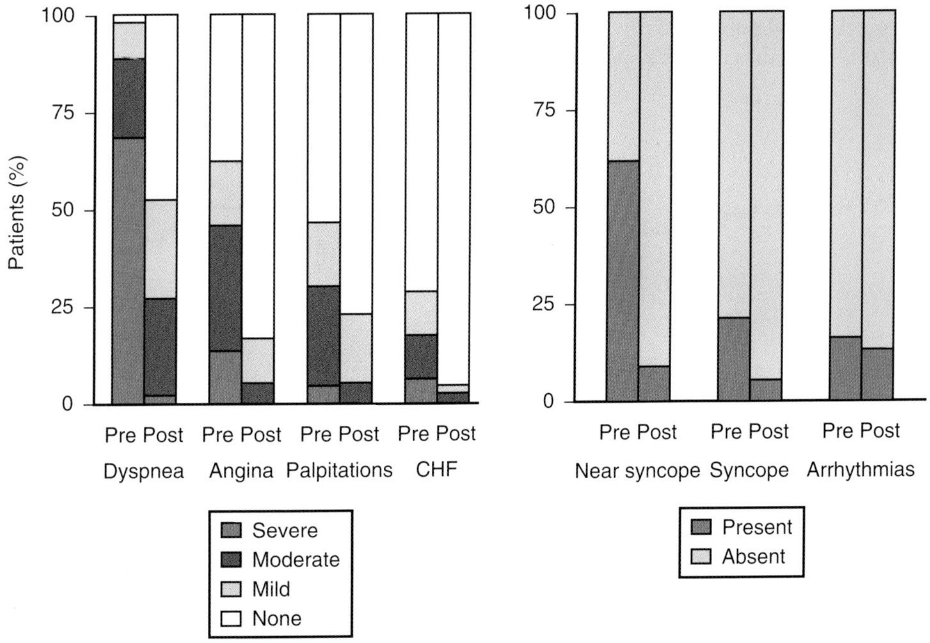

FIGURE 96-10 ■ Symptomatic status of patients with hypertrophic obstructive cardiomyopathy before (Pre) and after (Post) septal myectomy. Relief of obstruction improves angina, dyspnea, and syncope or presyncope. *CHF,* Congestive heart failure. (From McCully RB, Nishimura RA, Tajik AJ, et al: Extent of clinical improvement after surgical treatment of hypertrophic obstructive cardiomyopathy. *Circulation* 94:467–471, 1996.)

disability is presumed to be caused by diastolic dysfunction. But provocative maneuvers frequently elicit higher gradients and systolic anterior motion (SAM)–related mitral regurgitation that correlate with symptoms. Indeed, in our surgical practice, 30% of patients undergoing septal myectomy have latent obstruction with resting gradients less than 30 mm Hg, and postoperatively, NYHA functional class improves dramatically and to a similar extent as seen in patients with high resting LVOT gradients.[97]

Late recurrence of large resting LV outflow gradients is very uncommon after successful myectomy in either adults or children with HOCM, and this is in contrast to patients who have surgery for relief of congenital membranous subaortic stenosis.[46] The most common causes of recurrent symptoms and obstruction are limited myectomy at the initial operation, midventricular obstruction, and anomalies of papillary muscles. Most often, inadequate myectomy at initial operation is a result of failure to extend the myectomy far enough toward the apex of the heart.[98]

SURVIVAL

Septal myectomy is usually performed for relief of symptoms, but there is evidence that operation may improve survival of patients with HOCM. In a report by Ommen and coworkers,[99] late survival of 289 patients with HOCM undergoing septal myectomy was 98%, 96%, and 83% 1 year, 5 years, and 10 years postoperatively, and these survival rates were similar to those of an age- and sex-matched U.S. population and to those of HCM patients without obstruction (Fig. 96-11). In the same study, myectomy patients had superior survival free from all-cause mortality ($P < 0.001$), HCM-related mortality ($P < 0.001$), and sudden cardiac death ($P = 0.003$) compared with those of nonsurgical HCM patients with obstruction (Fig. 96-12), and on multivariable analysis, performance of myectomy had a strong, independent association with survival (hazard ratio, 0.43; $P < 0.001$).

Studies also suggest mechanisms whereby relief of LVOT gradients might improve survival. The extent of LV hypertrophy is an important determinant of survival in patients with HCM,[100] and successful myectomy results in some regression of LV hypertrophy.[101,102] Thus, patients with the obstructive form of HCM may have an additive burden of ventricular hypertrophy caused by pressure overload that is relieved by successful myectomy. It is interesting to note that whereas extent of LV hypertrophy is a risk factor for death in natural history studies of HCM, following myectomy, degree of hypertrophy preoperatively does not predict outcome.[103]

Additional insights on improved survival of myectomy patients come from McLeod and associates,[104] who reviewed patients with HCM who had received ICDs. During follow-up (median, 4.5 years), 12 patients (17%) in the nonmyectomy group and only one patient (2%) in the myectomy group had appropriate ICD discharges (Fig. 96-13). The average annualized event rate was 4.3% per year in the nonmyectomy group compared with 0.24% per year after myectomy ($P = 0.004$). Thus, surgical myectomy and relief of outflow gradient is associated with a marked reduction in the incidence of appropriate ICD discharges and risk of sudden cardiac death.

The potential benefit of septal myectomy on patient survival is supported also by postoperative outcome of patients who present with syncope. The presence of syncope despite medical therapy in patients with HCM is considered an indication for surgical myectomy, and Orme and associates[104a] documented that at median follow-up of approximately 5 years, the recurrence rate of syncopy in myectomy patients was 11% compared to 40% in a medically treated group matched for other risk factors. Further, the 10-year survival rate was greater for patients who had undergone surgical myectomy than for the medically treated patients (82% vs. 69%).

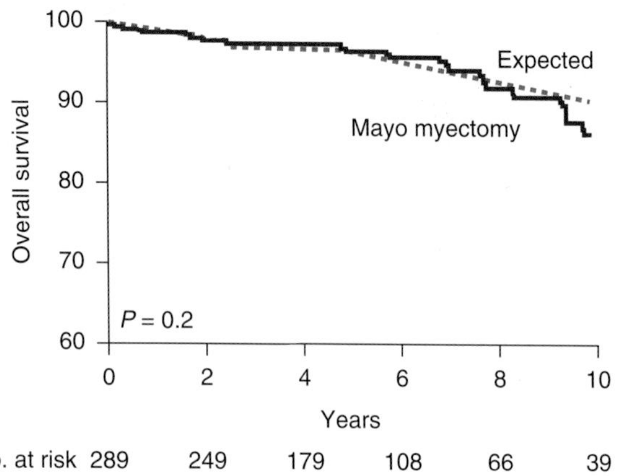

FIGURE 96-11 ■ Survival of patients with hypertrophic obstructive cardiomyopathy after septal myectomy is similar to that of an age- and gender-matched population. (From Ommen SR, Maron BJ, Olivotto I, et al: Long-term effects of surgical septal myectomy on survival in patients with obstructive hypertrophic cardiomyopathy. *J Am Coll Cardiol* 46:470–476, 2005.)

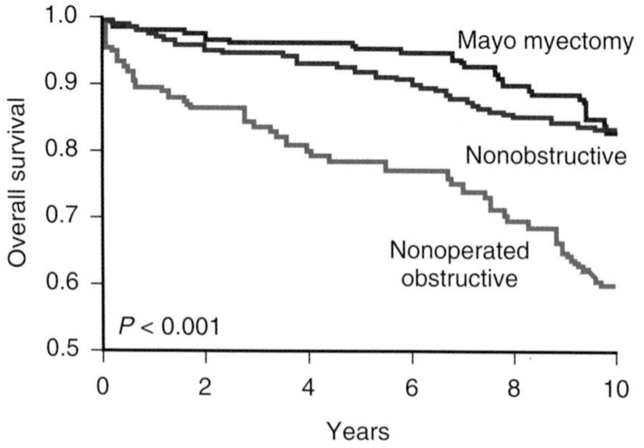

FIGURE 96-12 ■ Survival free from all-cause mortality in three hypertrophic cardiomyopathy patient subgroups: Mayo Clinic surgical myectomy ($n = 289$), nonoperated with obstruction ($n = 228$), and nonobstructive ($n = 820$). Myectomy versus nonoperated obstructive hypertrophic cardiomyopathy, $P < 0.001$; myectomy versus nonobstructive hypertrophic cardiomyopathy, $P = 0.8$. (From Ommen SR, Maron BJ, Olivotto I, et al: Long-term effects of surgical septal myectomy on survival in patients with obstructive hypertrophic cardiomyopathy. *J Am Coll Cardiol* 46:470–476, 2005.)

COMPARISON TO SEPTAL ARTERY ABLATION

Septal reduction can be achieved by selective infarction of septal branches of the LAD, and the advantages of avoiding surgical incision and hospitalization are obvious. In a review of alcohol septal ablation from 42 published studies (2959 patients), resting LVOT gradient decreased from 65 mm Hg to 16 mm Hg ($P < 0.001$), basal septal diameter reduced from 21 mm to 14 mm ($P < 0.001$), and hospital mortality was 1.5%.[105] However, the incidence of complete heart block requiring permanent pacemaker was 11%, and other important complications included coronary dissection (1.8%), pericardial effusion (0.6%), ventricular fibrillation (2.2%), stroke (1.1%), new right bundle branch block (46%), and new left bundle branch block (6.5%). Also, symptoms persisted in 11% of patients, re-do alcohol ablation was required in 6.6%, and surgical myectomy was necessary in 2.0%. Thus, whereas this procedure is less invasive, it is not without significant morbidity and mortality.

Because of unfavorable coronary anatomy, some patients with HOCM are not candidates for alcohol septal ablation.[106] Also, concern has been raised about the potential long-term risk of sudden death related to arrhythmogenic substrate from the resulting septal scar. Cardiac magnetic resonance imaging demonstrates that in most patients, alcohol septal ablation causes transmural tissue necrosis, located more inferiorly in the basal septum than myectomy; the infarct usually extends into the right ventricular side of the septum and sometimes spares the basal septum, leading to residual gradients at follow-up (Fig. 96-14).[107] In a nonrandomized comparative study, Sorajja and colleagues[108] reported that in-hospital complication rate is higher with ablation than with myectomy, and that in patients 65 years of age or younger, symptom relief is better after myectomy.

Thus, alcohol septal ablation is an option for patients who may have increased risk for operation, but septal

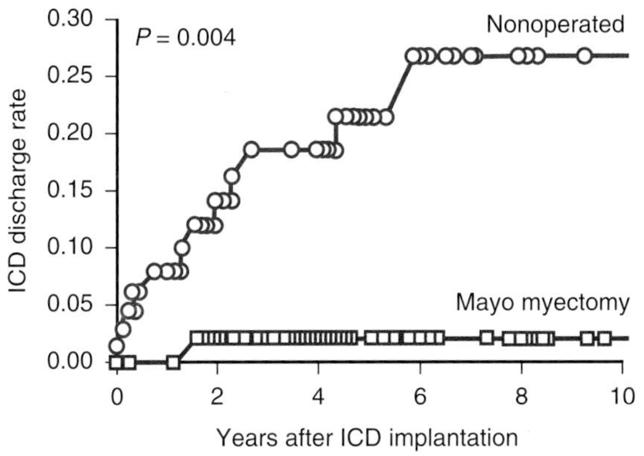

FIGURE 96-13 Implantable cardioverter-defibrillator (ICD) discharge rates among patients with hypertrophic cardiomyopathy who had septal myectomy compared with nonmyectomy patients. Average annualized ICD discharge rates of 0.24% in the myectomy group compared with 4.3% in the nonmyectomy group ($P = 0.004$). (From McLeod CJ, Ommen SR, Ackerman MJ, et al: Surgical septal myectomy decreases the risk for appropriate implantable cardioverter defibrillator discharge in obstructive hypertrophic cardiomyopathy. *Eur Heart J* 28:2583–2588, 2007.)

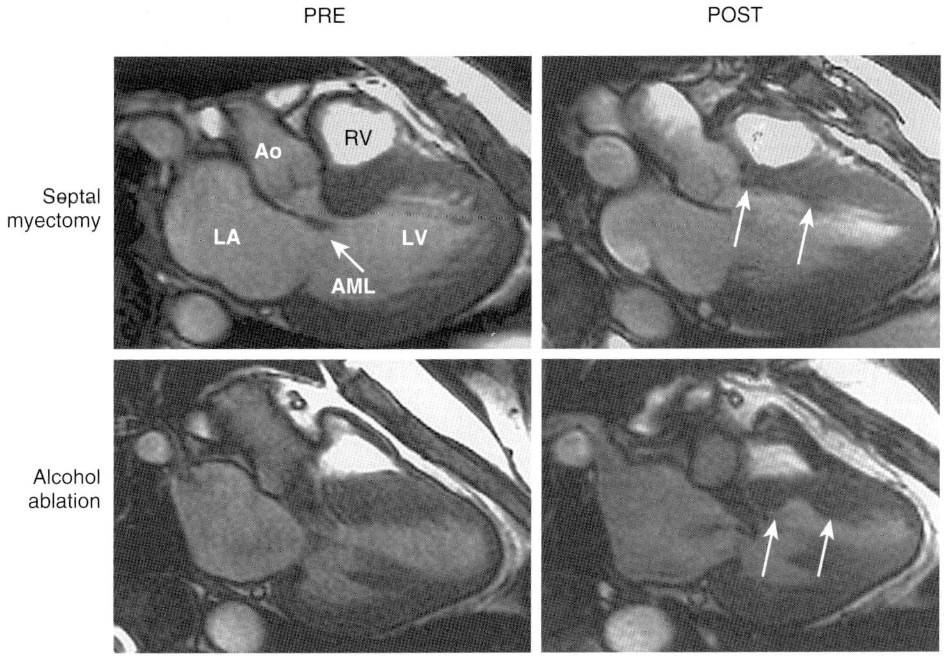

FIGURE 96-14 Cardiac magnetic resonance image after septal myectomy versus septal ablation. *Top panels,* Long-axis views before (Pre) and after (Post) septal myectomy. The portion of basal septum evident in this plane, projecting into the left ventricular (LV) outflow tract, has been excised at myectomy *(arrows)*. *Bottom panels,* Long-axis views before *(left)* and 5 months after *(right)* septal ablation. Ablation has spared the most proximal portion of basal septum. *AML,* Anterior mitral leaflet; *Ao,* aorta; *LA,* left atrium; *RV,* right ventricle. (From Valeti US, Nishimura RA, Holmes DR, et al: Comparison of surgical septal myectomy and alcohol septal ablation with cardiac magnetic resonance imaging in patients with hypertrophic obstructive cardiomyopathy. *J Am Coll Cardiol* 49:350–357, 2007.)

myectomy remains the gold standard for patients with HCM and severe LV outflow obstruction who are refractory to maximal medical therapy.[61,90]

SPECIAL SUBGROUPS

The preceding discussion has focused on surgical treatment of patients with HCM and subaortic obstruction, and, whereas these patients constitute most of the patients considered for surgical treatment, other HCM patients with different ventricular morphology and pathophysiology may benefit from operation. Midventricular obstruction in HCM is less common than subaortic obstruction, has a different pathophysiologic mechanism, and, in untreated patients, may have a worse prognosis.[109] Unlike subaortic obstruction, related to systolic anterior motion of the mitral valve, midventricular obstruction is caused by systolic narrowing of the mid ventricle with apposition of the septum and papillary muscles. Secondary mitral valve regurgitation is uncommon and is not a part of the pathophysiology of symptoms such as dyspnea, but patients with HCM and midventricular obstruction may develop apical pouches/aneurysms that can lead to ventricular arrhythmias or thromboembolism.[110,111]

The decision for myectomy in patients with midventricular obstruction is often confounded by uncertainty whether limiting symptoms are due to the intraventricular gradient or to diastolic dysfunction (or both). Also, there is a wide spectrum of phenotypes, and some patients will have both subaortic obstruction (with systolic anterior motion of the mitral leaflets) and midventricular obstruction.

In our experience, midventricular obstruction is most easily exposed through a transapical incision, and the contact lesion that is uniformly present guides excision of the septum.[112] Among 51 patients having operation for HCM with midventricular obstruction, a transapical approach was used in 32 patients and a combined transapical and transaortic approach was used in 19 patients. In 13 patients, an apical aneurysm or pouch was repaired at the time of midventricular myectomy. No early deaths or complications related to the apical incision have resulted.

REFERENCES

1. Maron BJ, Gardin JM, Flack JM, et al: Prevalence of hypertrophic cardiomyopathy in a general population of young adults. Echocardiographic analysis of 4111 subjects in the CARDIA Study. Coronary Artery Risk Development in (Young) Adults. *Circulation* 92:785–789, 1995.
2. Maron BJ, Spirito P, Roman MJ, et al: Prevalence of hypertrophic cardiomyopathy in a population-based sample of American Indians aged 51 to 77 years (the Strong Heart Study). Prevalence of hypertrophic cardiomyopathy in a population-based sample of American Indians aged 51 to 77 years (the Strong Heart Study). *Am J Cardiol* 93:1510–1514, 2004.
3. Richardson P, McKenna W, Bristow M, et al: Report of the 1995 World Health Organization/International Society and Federation of Cardiology Task Force on the Definition and Classification of cardiomyopathies. *Circulation* 93:841–842, 1996.
4. van Son JA, Schaff HV, Danielson GK, et al: Surgical treatment of discrete and tunnel subaortic stenosis. Late survival and risk of reoperation. *Circulation* 88:II159–II169, 1993.
5. Kunkala MR, Schaff HV, Nishimura RA, et al: Transapical approach to myectomy for midventricular obstruction in hypertrophic cardiomyopathy. *Ann Thorac Surg* 96(2):564–570, 2013.
6. Minami Y, Kajimoto K, Terajima Y, et al: Clinical implications of midventricular obstruction in patients with hypertrophic cardiomyopathy. *J Am Coll Cardiol* 57(23):2346–2355, 2011.
7. Maron MS, Olivotto I, Zenovich AG, et al: Hypertrophic cardiomyopathy is predominantly a disease of left ventricular outflow tract obstruction. *Circulation* 114:2232–2239, 2006.
8. Teare D: Asymmetrical hypertrophy of the heart in young adults. *Br Heart J* 20:1–8, 1958.
9. Hollman A, Goodwin JF, Teare D, et al: A family with obstructive cardiomyopathy. *Br Heart J* 22:449–456, 1960.
10. Brock R: Functional obstruction of the left ventricle (acquired aortic subvalvar stenosis). *Guys Hosp Rep* 106:221–238, 1957.
11. Bercu B, Diettert G, Danforth W, et al: Pseudoaortic stenosis produced by ventricular hypertrophy. *Am J Med* 25:814–818, 1958.
12. Braunwald E, Maron BJ: Eugene Braunwald, MD and the early years of hypertrophic cardiomyopathy: a conversation with Dr. Barry J. Maron. *Am J Cardiol* 109(11):1539–1544, 2012.
13. Brent LB, Aburano A, Fisher DL, et al: Familial muscular subaortic stenosis: an unrecognized form of "idiopathic heart diseases," with clinical and autopsy observations. *Circulation* 21:167–180, 1960.
14. Goodwin JF: Cardiac function in primary myocardial disorder—I. *Br Med J* 1:1527–1533, 1964.
15. Braunwald E, Lambrew CT, Rockoff SD, et al: Idiopathic hypertrophic subaortic stenosis. I. A description of the disease based upon an analysis of 64 patients. *Circulation* 30(Suppl 4):3–119, 1964.
16. Henry WL, Clark CE, Epstein SE: Asymmetric septal hypertrophy (ASH): the unifying link in the IHSS disease spectrum. Observations regarding its pathogenesis, pathophysiology, and course. *Circulation* 47:827–832, 1973.
17. Henry WL, Clark CE, Epstein SE: Asymmetric septal hypertrophy. Echocardiographic identification of the pathognomonic anatomic abnormality of IHSS. *Circulation* 47:225–233, 1973.
18. Brock R: Functional obstruction of the left ventricle (acquired aortic subvalvar stenosis). *Guys Hosp Rep* 108:126–143, 1959.
19. Kirklin JW, Ellis FH, Jr: Surgical relief of diffuse subvalvular aortic stenosis. *Circulation* 24:739–742, 1961.
20. Goodwin JF, Hollman A, Cleland WP, et al: Obstructive cardiomyopathy simulating aortic stenosis. *Br Heart J* 22:403–414, 1960.
21. Morrow AG, Brockenbrough EC: Surgical treatment of idiopathic hypertrophic subaortic stenosis: technic and hemodynamic results of subaortic ventriculomyotomy. *Ann Surg* 154:181–189, 1961.
22. Wigle ED, Heimbecker RO, Gunton RW: Idiopathic ventricular septal hypertrophy causing muscular subaortic stenosis. *Circulation* 26:325–340, 1962.
23. Agnew TM, Barratt-Boyes BG, Brandt PW, et al: Surgical resection in idiopathic hypertrophic subaortic stenosis with a combined approach through aorta and left ventricle. *J Thorac Cardiovasc Surg* 74:307–316, 1977.
24. Dobell AR, Scott HJ: Hypertrophic subaortic stenosis: evolution of a surgical technique. *J Thorac Cardiovasc Surg* 47:26–39, 1964.
25. Lillehei CW, Levy MJ: Transatrial exposure for correction of subaortic stenosis. A new approach. *JAMA* 186:8–13, 1963.
26. Swan H: Subaortic muscular stenosis: a new surgical technique for repair. *J Thorac Cardiovasc Surg* 47:681–684, 1964.
27. Julian OC, Dye WS, Javid H, et al: Apical left ventriculotomy in subaortic stenosis due to a fibromuscular hypertrophy. *Circulation* 31(Suppl 1):44–56, 1965.
28. Harken DE: Discussion. *J Thorac Cardiovasc Surg* 47:33, 1964.
29. Cooley DA, Bloodwell RD, Hallman GL, et al: Surgical treatment of muscular subaortic stenosis. Results from septectomy in twenty-six patients. *Circulation* 35(Suppl 4):I124–I132, 1967.
30. Cooley DA, Wukasch DC, Leachman RD: Mitral valve replacement for idiopathic hypertrophic subaortic stenosis. Results in 27 patients. *J Cardiovasc Surg (Torino)* 17(5):380–387, 1976.
31. Dembitsky WP, Weldon CS: Clinical experience with the use of a valve-bearing conduit to construct a second left ventricular

outflow tract in cases of unresectable intra-ventricular obstruction. *Ann Surg* 184:317–323, 1976.
32. Morrow AG: Hypertrophic subaortic stenosis. Operative methods utilized to relieve left ventricular outflow obstruction. *J Thorac Cardiovasc Surg* 76:423–430, 1978.
33. Grigg LE, Wigle ED, Williams WG, et al: Transesophageal Doppler echocardiography in obstructive hypertrophic cardiomyopathy: clarification of pathophysiology and importance in intraoperative decision making. *J Am Coll Cardiol* 20:42–52, 1992.
34. Maron MS, Olivotto I, Harrigan C, et al: Mitral valve abnormalities identified by cardiovascular magnetic resonance represent a primary phenotypic expression of hypertrophic cardiomyopathy. *Circulation* 124(1):40–47, 2011.
35. Wigle ED, Rakowski H, Kimball BP, et al: Hypertrophic cardiomyopathy. Clinical spectrum and treatment. *Circulation* 92:1680–1692, 1995.
36. Cape EG, Simons D, Jimoh A, et al: Chordal geometry determines the shape and extent of systolic anterior mitral motion: in vitro studies. *J Am Coll Cardiol* 13:1438–1448, 1989.
37. Sherrid MV, Chu CK, Delia E, et al: An echocardiographic study of the fluid mechanics of obstruction in hypertrophic cardiomyopathy. *J Am Coll Cardiol* 22:816–825, 1993.
38. Sherrid MV, Gunsburg DZ, Moldenhauer S: Systolic anterior motion begins at low left ventricular outflow tract velocity in obstructive hypertrophic cardiomyopathy. *J Am Coll Cardiol* 36:1344–1354, 2000.
39. Minakata K, Dearani JA, Nishimura RA, et al: Extended septal myectomy for hypertrophic obstructive cardiomyopathy with anomalous mitral papillary muscles or chordae. *J Thorac Cardiovasc Surg* 127:481–489, 2004.
40. Klues HG, Roberts WC, Maron BJ: Anomalous insertion of papillary muscle directly into anterior mitral leaflet in hypertrophic cardiomyopathy. Significance in producing left ventricular outflow obstruction. *Circulation* 84:1188–1197, 1991.
41. Maron MS, Hauser TH, Dubrow E, et al: Right ventricular involvement in hypertrophic cardiomyopathy. *Am J Cardiol* 100:1293–1298, 2007.
42. Falcone DM, Moore D, Lambert EC: Idiopathic hypertrophic cardiomyopathy involving the right ventricle. *Am J Cardiol* 19: 735–740, 1967.
43. Lockhart A, Charpentier A, Bourdarias JP, et al: Right ventricular involvement in obstructive cardiomyopathies: hemodynamic studies in 13 cases. *Br Heart J* 28:122–123, 1966.
44. Maron BJ, McIntosh CL, Klues HG, et al: Morphologic basis for obstruction to right ventricular outflow in hypertrophic cardiomyopathy. *Am J Cardiol* 71:1089–1094, 1993.
45. Geske JB, Konecny T, Ommen SR, et al: Surgical myectomy improves pulmonary hypertension in obstructive hypertrophic cardiomyopathy. *Eur Heart J* 35:2032–2039, 2014.
46. van Son JA, Schaff HV, Danielson GK, et al: Surgical treatment of discrete and tunnel subaortic stenosis. Late survival and risk of reoperation. *Circulation* 88:II159–II169, 1993.
47. Sasson Z, Prieur T, Skrobik Y, et al: Aortic regurgitation: a common complication after surgery for hypertrophic obstructive cardiomyopathy. *J Am Coll Cardiol* 13:63–67, 1989.
48. Sorajja P, Ommen SR, Nishimura RA, et al: Adverse prognosis of patients with hypertrophic cardiomyopathy who have epicardial coronary artery disease. *Circulation* 108:2342–2348, 2003.
49. Sorajja P, Ommen SR, Nishimura RA, et al: Myocardial bridging in adult patients with hypertrophic cardiomyopathy. *J Am Coll Cardiol* 42:889–894, 2003.
50. Yetman AT, McCrindle BW, MacDonald C, et al: Myocardial bridging in children with hypertrophic cardiomyopathy—a risk factor for sudden death. *N Engl J Med* 339:1201–1209, 1998.
51. Maron BJ, Roberts WC: Hypertrophic cardiomyopathy and cardiac muscle cell disorganization revisited: relation between the two and significance. *Am Heart J* 102:95–110, 1981.
52. Maron BJ, Anan TJ, Roberts WC: Quantitative analysis of the distribution of cardiac muscle cell disorganization in the left ventricular wall of patients with hypertrophic cardiomyopathy. *Circulation* 63:882–894, 1981.
53. Morimoto S, Sekiguchi M, Hiramitsu S, et al: Contribution of cardiac muscle cell disorganization to the clinical features of hypertrophic cardiomyopathy. *Heart Vessels* 15:149–158, 2000.
54. Varnava AM, Elliott PM, Sharma S, et al: Hypertrophic cardiomyopathy: the interrelation of disarray, fibrosis, and small vessel disease. *Heart* 84:476–482, 2000.
55. St. John Sutton MG, Lie JT, Anderson KR, et al: Histopathological specificity of hypertrophic obstructive cardiomyopathy. Myocardial fibre disarray and myocardial fibrosis. *Br Heart J* 44: 433–443, 1980.
56. Tanaka H, Fujiwara H, Onodera T, et al: Quantitative analysis of myocardial fibrosis in normals, hypertensive hearts, and hypertrophic cardiomyopathy. *Br Heart J* 55:575–581, 1986.
57. Moon C, McKenna WJ, McCrohon JA, et al: Toward clinical risk assessment in hypertrophic cardiomyopathy with gadolinium cardiovascular magnetic resonance. *J Am Coll Cardiol* 41:1561–1567, 2003.
58. Adabag AS, Maron BJ, Appelbaum E, et al: Occurrence and frequency of arrhythmias in hypertrophic cardiomyopathy in relation to delayed enhancement on cardiovascular magnetic resonance. *J Am Coll Cardiol* 51:1369–1374, 2008.
59. Tsang W, Lang RM: Echocardiographic evaluation of cardiac amyloid. *Curr Cardiol Rep* 12(3):272–276, 2010.
60. Banypersad SM, Moon JC, Whelan C, et al: Updates in cardiac amyloidosis: a review. *J Am Heart Assoc* 1(2):e000364, 2012.
61. Maron BJ, Maron MS: Hypertrophic cardiomyopathy. *Lancet* 381:242–255, 2013.
62. Marian AJ, Roberts R: The molecular genetic basis for hypertrophic cardiomyopathy. *J Mol Cell Cardiol* 33:655–670, 2001.
63. Richard P, Charron P, Carrier L, et al: Hypertrophic cardiomyopathy: distribution of disease genes, spectrum of mutations, and implications for a molecular diagnostic strategy. *Circulation* 107:2227–2232, 2003.
64. Van Driest SL, Ommen SR, Tajik AJ, et al: Yield of genetic testing in hypertrophic cardiomyopathy. *Mayo Clin Proc* 80:739–744, 2005.
65. Van Driest SL, Ackerman MJ, Ommen SR, et al: Prevalence and severity of "benign" mutations in the beta-myosin heavy chain, cardiac troponin T, and alpha-tropomyosin genes in hypertrophic cardiomyopathy. *Circulation* 106:3085–3090, 2002.
66. Olivotto I, Girolami F, Ackerman MJ, et al: Myofilament protein gene mutation screening and outcome of patients with hypertrophic cardiomyopathy. *Mayo Clin Proc* 83:630–638, 2008.
67. Glancy DL, O'Brien KP, Gold HK, et al: Atrial fibrillation in patients with idiopathic hypertrophic subaortic stenosis. *Br Heart J* 32:652–659, 1970.
68. Criley JM, Siegel RJ: Has "obstruction" hindered our understanding of hypertrophic cardiomyopathy? *Circulation* 72:1148–1154, 1985.
69. Maron MS, Olivotto I, Zenovich AG, et al: Hypertrophic cardiomyopathy is predominantly a disease of left ventricular outflow tract obstruction. *Circulation* 114:2232–2239, 2006.
70. Elesber A, Nishimura RA, Rihal CS, et al: Utility of isoproterenol to provoke outflow tract gradients in patients with hypertrophic cardiomyopathy. *Am J Cardiol* 101:516–520, 2008.
71. Zhu WX, Oh JK, Kopecky SL, et al: Mitral regurgitation due to ruptured chordae tendineae in patients with hypertrophic obstructive cardiomyopathy. *J Am Coll Cardiol* 20:242–247, 1992.
72. Ommen SR, Nishimura RA: Hypertrophic cardiomyopathy. *Curr Probl Cardiol* 29:239–291, 2004.
73. Lever HM, Karam RF, Currie PJ, et al: Hypertrophic cardiomyopathy in the elderly. Distinctions from the young based on cardiac shape. *Circulation* 79:580–589, 1989.
74. Ommen SR, Park SH, Click RL, et al: Impact of intraoperative transesophageal echocardiography in the surgical management of hypertrophic cardiomyopathy. *Am J Cardiol* 90:1022–1024, 2002.
75. Rickers C, Wilke NM, Jerosch-Herold M, et al: Utility of cardiac magnetic resonance imaging in the diagnosis of hypertrophic cardiomyopathy. *Circulation* 112:855–861, 2005.
76. Moon JC, McKenna WJ, McCrohon JA, et al: Toward clinical risk assessment in hypertrophic cardiomyopathy with gadolinium cardiovascular magnetic resonance. *J Am Coll Cardiol* 41:1561–1567, 2003.
77. Adabag AS, Maron BJ, Appelbaum E, et al: Occurrence and frequency of arrhythmias in hypertrophic cardiomyopathy in relation to delayed enhancement on cardiovascular magnetic resonance. *J Am Coll Cardiol* 51:1369–1374, 2008.

78. Maron BJ, Olivotto I, Bellone P, et al: Clinical profile of stroke in 900 patients with hypertrophic cardiomyopathy. *J Am Coll Cardiol* 39:301–307, 2002.
79. Spirito P, Rapezzi C, Bellone P, et al: Infective endocarditis in hypertrophic cardiomyopathy: prevalence, incidence, and indications for antibiotic prophylaxis. *Circulation* 99:2132–2137, 1999.
80. McKenna WJ, Franklin RC, Nihoyannopoulos P, et al: Arrhythmia and prognosis in infants, children and adolescents with hypertrophic cardiomyopathy. *J Am Coll Cardiol* 11:147–153, 1988.
81. McKenna W, Deanfield J, Faruqui A, et al: Prognosis in hypertrophic cardiomyopathy: role of age and clinical, electrocardiographic and hemodynamic features. *Am J Cardiol* 47:532–538, 1981.
82. Cannan CR, Reeder GS, Bailey KR, et al: Natural history of hypertrophic cardiomyopathy. A population-based study, 1976 through 1990. *Circulation* 92:2488–2495, 1995.
83. Maron BJ, Roberts WC, Epstein SE: Sudden death in hypertrophic cardiomyopathy: a profile of 78 patients. *Circulation* 65:1388–1394, 1982.
84. Maron BJ, Epstein SE, Roberts WC: Causes of sudden death in competitive athletes. *J Am Coll Cardiol* 7:204–214, 1986.
85. Maron MS, Olivotto I, Betocchi S, et al: Effect of left ventricular outflow tract obstruction on clinical outcome in hypertrophic cardiomyopathy. *N Engl J Med* 348:295–303, 2003.
86. Autore C, Bernarbò P, Barillà CS, et al: The prognostic importance of left ventricular outflow obstruction in hypertrophic cardiomyopathy varies in relation to the severity of symptoms. *J Am Coll Cardiol* 45:1076–1080, 2005.
87. Elliott PM, Gimeno JR, Tomé MT, et al: Left ventricular outflow tract obstruction and sudden death risk in patients with hypertrophic cardiomyopathy. *Eur Heart J* 27:1933–1941, 2006.
88. Vaglio JC, Jr, Ommen SR, Nishimura RA, et al: Clinical characteristics and outcomes of patients with hypertrophic cardiomyopathy with latent obstruction. *Am Heart J* 156:342–347, 2008.
89. O'Mahony C, Elliott PM: Prevention of sudden death in hypertrophic cardiomyopathy. *Heart* 100:254–260, 2014.
90. Gersh BJ, Maron BJ, Bonow RO, et al: ACCF/AHA guideline for the diagnosis and treatment of hypertrophic cardiomyopathy: a report of the American College of Cardiology Foundation/American Heart Association Task Force on Practice Guidelines. *J Thorac Cardiovasc Surg* 142(6):e153–e203, 2011.
91. Melacini P, Maron BJ, Bobbo F, et al: Evidence that pharmacological strategies lack efficacy for the prevention of sudden death in hypertrophic cardiomyopathy. *Heart* 93:708–710, 2007.
92. Messmer BJ: Extended myectomy for hypertrophic obstructive cardiomyopathy. *Ann Thorac Surg* 58:575–577, 1994.
93. Ashikhmina EA, Schaff HV, Ommen SR, et al: Intraoperative direct measurement of left ventricular outflow tract gradients to guide surgical myectomy for hypertrophic cardiomyopathy. *J Thorac Cardiovasc Surg* 142(1):53–59, 2011.
94. Kunkala MR, Schaff HV, Burkhart H, et al: Outcome of repair of myocardial bridging at the time of septal myectomy. *Ann Thorac Surg* 97(1):118–123, 2014.
95. ElBardissi AW, Dearani JA, Nishimura RA, et al: Septal myectomy after previous septal artery ablation in hypertrophic cardiomyopathy. *Mayo Clin Proc* 82:1516–1522, 2007.
96. McCully RB, Nishimura RA, Tajik AJ, et al: Extent of clinical improvement after surgical treatment of hypertrophic obstructive cardiomyopathy. *Circulation* 94:467–471, 1996.
97. Schaff HV, Dearani JA, Ommen SR, et al: Expanding the indications for septal myectomy in patients with hypertrophic cardiomyopathy: results of operation in patients with latent obstruction. *J Thorac Cardiovasc Surg* 143(2):303–309, 2012.
98. Cho YH, Quintana E, Schaff HV, et al: Residual and recurrent gradients after septal myectomy for hypertrophic cardiomyopathy—Mechanisms of obstruction and outcomes of reoperation. *J Thorac Cardiovasc Surg* in press.
99. Ommen SR, Maron BJ, Olivotto I, et al: Long-term effects of surgical septal myectomy on survival in patients with obstructive hypertrophic cardiomyopathy. *J Am Coll Cardiol* 46:470–476, 2005.
100. Spirito P, Bellone P, Harris KM, et al: Magnitude of left ventricular hypertrophy predicts the risk of sudden death in hypertrophic cardiomyopathy. *N Engl J Med* 342:1778–1785, 2000.
101. Deb SJ, Schaff HV, Dearani JA, et al: Septal myectomy results in regression of left ventricular hypertrophy in patients with hypertrophic obstructive cardiomyopathy. *Ann Thorac Surg* 78:2118–2122, 2004.
102. Monteiro PF, Ommen SR, Gersh BJ, et al: Effects of surgical septal myectomy on left ventricular wall thickness and diastolic filling. *Am J Cardiol* 100:1776–1778, 2007.
103. Brown ML, Schaff HV, Dearani JA, et al: Relationship between left ventricular mass, wall thickness, and survival after subaortic septal myectomy for hypertrophic obstructive cardiomyopathy. *J Thorac Cardiovasc Surg* 141(2):439–443, 2011.
104. McLeod CJ, Ommen SR, Ackerman MJ, et al: Surgical septal myectomy decreases the risk for appropriate implantable cardioverter defibrillator discharge in obstructive hypertrophic cardiomyopathy [see comment]. *Eur Heart J* 28:2583–2588, 2007.
104a. Orme NM, Sorajja P, Dearani JA, et al: Comparison of surgical septal myectomy to medical therapy alone in patients with hypertrophic cardiomyopathy and syncope. *Am J Cardiol* 111:388–392, 2013.
105. Alam M, Dokainish H, Lakkis N: Alcohol septal ablation for hypertrophic obstructive cardiomyopathy: a systematic review of published studies. *J Interv Cardiol* 19:319–327, 2005.
106. Singh M, Edwards WD, Holmes DR, Jr, et al: Anatomy of the first septal perforating artery: a study with implications for ablation therapy for hypertrophic cardiomyopathy. *Mayo Clin Proc* 76:799–802, 2001.
107. Valeti US, Nishimura RA, Holmes DR, et al: Comparison of surgical septal myectomy and alcohol septal ablation with cardiac magnetic resonance imaging in patients with hypertrophic obstructive cardiomyopathy. *J Am Coll Cardiol* 49:350–357, 2007.
108. Sorajja P, Valeti U, Nishimura RA, et al: Outcome of alcohol septal ablation for obstructive hypertrophic cardiomyopathy. *Circulation* 118:131–139, 2008.
109. Minami Y, Kajimoto K, Terajima Y, et al: Clinical implications of midventricular obstruction in patients with hypertrophic cardiomyopathy. *J Am Coll Cardiol* 57:2346–2355, 2011.
110. Maron MS, Finley JJ, Bos JM, et al: Prevalence, clinical significance, and natural history of left ventricular apical aneurysms in hypertrophic cardiomyopathy. *Circulation* 118:1541–1549, 2008.
111. Shah DK, Schaff HV, Abel MD, et al: Ventricular tachycardia in hypertrophic cardiomyopathy with apical aneurysm. *Ann Thorac Surg* 91(4):1263–1265, 2011.
112. Said SM, Schaff HV, Abel MD, et al: Transapical approach for apical myectomy and relief of midventricular obstruction in hypertrophic cardiomyopathy. *J Card Surg* 27(4):443–448, 2012.

CHAPTER 97

Left Ventricular Assist Devices and Total Artificial Heart

Koji Takeda • Hiroo Takayama • Yoshifumi Naka

CHAPTER OUTLINE

Mechanical circulatory support (MCS) has become the standard of care for patients with refractory, end-stage heart failure.[1-7] A landmark trial in MCS demonstrated the superiority of a left ventricular assist device (LVAD) over optimal medical therapy with respect to improving survival and quality of life in this subgroup of patients.[1] Over the past decade, there has been a significant evolution in MCS device-related technologies. Devices have undergone substantial modifications in an effort to improve survival while on support, increase durability, and limit device-related infections, device thrombosis, device malfunction, and perioperative bleeding.[3-5] With improvements in device design yielding devices that can be implanted as destination therapy, the number of durable LVAD implants has dramatically increased in the United States every year (Fig. 97-1).[6]

Current MCS devices can be divided into the following subcategories on the basis of their features:

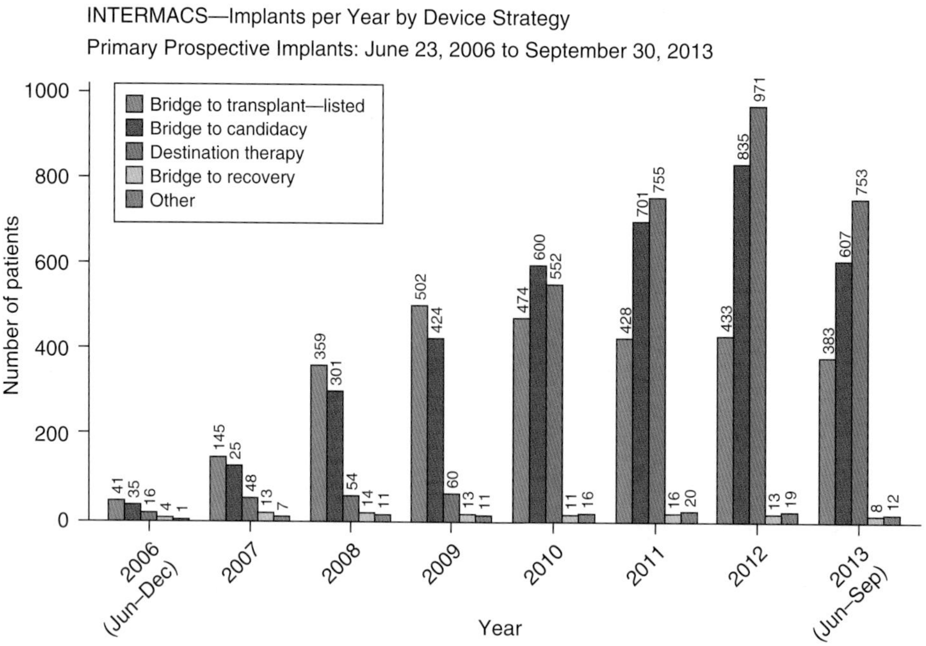

FIGURE 97-1 ■ Number of durable mechanical circulatory support device implants per year by device strategy. (Reproduced with permission from INTERMACS, *Quarterly Statistical Report,* 3rd quarter, 2013.)

short-term versus long-term devices, paracorporeal versus intracorporeal devices, pulsatile versus continuous flow devices, full versus partial support devices, and assist devices versus complete heart replacement (i.e., total artificial heart [TAH]). The indications for implantation of a mechanical device have expanded over time to include acute cardiogenic shock, bridge to transplant (BTT), bridge to candidate (BTC), and destination therapy (DT).[1,3,6,7] This chapter presents a complete overview of MCS, including a historical perspective, indications for MCS, important factors related to patient selection, types of devices, results using MCS, surgical technique, postoperative management, and complications that occur with MCS.

HISTORICAL PERSPECTIVE

Dr. Michael DeBakey implanted the first mechanical assist device in 1963 in a patient with postcardiotomy shock after an aortic valve replacement. With growing interest in MCS, the Artificial Heart Program was founded in 1964. In 1966, DeBakey reported the first successful bridging to recovery with a ventricular assist device (VAD), also in a patient with postcardiotomy shock. The duration of support in this patient was 10 days.

In 1970, the Artificial Heart Program evolved into the Medical Devices Applications Branch of the National Heart and Lung Institute, with the primary focus of developing short- and long-term VADs as well as a TAH for heart replacement therapy. Dr. Denton Cooley reported the first successful bridging to transplant using MCS in 1978. In 1980, the currently named National Heart Lung and Blood Institute (NHLBI) accepted proposals by Abiomed, Baxter, Thermo Cardiosystems, and Thoratec to develop VADs and the TAH. The first successful implantation of a heart replacement therapy, a TAH with the Jarvik-7-100, was reported in 1984. However, this device was removed from clinical practice in 1991 because of a relatively high incidence of device-related complications, such as thromboembolic events and infection.

With concurrent advancements in assist device technology, the U.S. Food and Drug Administration (FDA) approved the use of a mechanical assist device as a BTT in 1994—the first of which was HeartMate (Thoratec Corp., Pleasanton, CA), developed by Thermo Cardiosystems. It soon became clear to the cardiac surgery community that implantation of LVADs could salvage patients who were otherwise nonsalvageable and could also improve the quality of life of patients with advanced heart failure.

A major victory for MCS came in 2001 with the results of the REMATCH trial.[1] This prospective, randomized trial of patients with end-stage heart failure who were not eligible for transplantation demonstrated a significant survival advantage for patients who underwent implantation of a mechanical assist device as compared with those receiving optimal medical therapy. The study, however, also highlighted various complications of mechanical support, such as bleeding, infection, stroke, device malfunction, and development of right heart failure, which became a primary focus for device companies and engineers in subsequent years.

The emergence of newer generation VADs with a continuous flow pump driven by a rotary pump represented a further step in this field. A randomized trial demonstrated that a continuous flow pump significantly improved 2-year survival and device-related morbidity as compared with a pulsatile device.[3] Since the approval of the continuous flow VADs for both transplant-eligible

(BTT) and transplant-ineligible patients (DT), the number of patients receiving MCS device therapy has been growing rapidly.

As VAD therapy entered the mainstream, INTERMACS (Interagency Registry for Mechanically Assisted Circulatory Support)—a national registry for patients who are receiving MCS devices—was established in 2006. This registry was devised as a joint effort of the NHLBI, the Centers for Medicare and Medicaid Services (CMS), the FDA, clinicians, scientists, and industry representatives in conjunction with the University of Alabama at Birmingham and the United Network for Organ Sharing (UNOS). Analysis of the data collected is expected to facilitate further improvements in patient evaluation and management.

IMPLANT STRATEGIES FOR MECHANICAL CIRCULATORY SUPPORT

When considering MCS placement, five broad indications can be defined with regard to the clinical intent at the time of implantation. Complex decisions about candidacy for each strategy should be made by an experienced, multidisciplinary team including surgeons and cardiologists. This process is particularly important in ensuring appropriate selection of the patient, timing for device placement, and device to use.

Bridge to Transplant

BTT is a strategy for patients actively listed for heart transplant who would not survive or would develop end-organ dysfunction as a result of low cardiac output before an organ becomes available. While the patient remains on the waiting list, insertion of a durable LVAD can improve survival, functional status, and quality of life.

Destination Therapy

DT is a strategy for patients requiring long-term, lifelong circulatory support who are not eligible for heart transplant because of relative or absolute contraindications.

Bridge to Candidacy

MCS may be used for patients who are not currently listed for heart transplant, with no absolute or a permanent contraindication to transplant. MCS may allow these patients to be eligible for transplant by improving their end-organ function and nutrition, decreasing pulmonary vascular resistance, as well as resolution of comorbidities or lifestyle-related problems (e.g., weight loss, smoking cessation).

Bridge to Decision

In circumstances when a patient is in acute cardiogenic shock, it may not be possible to determine the candidacy for transplant, long-term VADs or myocardial recovery. Additionally, the patient may or may not have multisystem organ failure, and the patient's neurologic status may or may not be known. A short-term MCS may be used to stabilize the patient's condition and to assess reversibility, as a bridge to more definitive therapies. The next step can be planned while the patient is on the MCS.

Bridge to Recovery

MCS may be used as a temporary circulatory support to unload the ventricle. During this time, MCS use may enhance myocardial recovery from an acute injury enough to wean off the device without the need for transplant.

PATIENT SELECTION

Careful patient selection—a critical element in achieving good clinical results with MCS—requires the evaluation of heart failure severity and the assessment of operative risk and comorbidities.

Common indicators of advanced heart failure for referral for MCS include New York Heart Association (NYHA) class IIIb-IV symptoms, frequent rehospitalizations for heart failure, or unresponsiveness to medical therapies (including neurohormonal antagonists and diuretics), recurrent/refractory ventricular tachyarrhythmia, inotrope dependence, unresponsiveness to cardiac resynchronization therapy, end-organ dysfunction as a result of low cardiac output, peak oxygen consumption less than 14 mL/kg/min, or 6-minute walk distance less than 300 m.[8] The Seattle Heart Failure Model can be used to estimate a heart failure patient's expected mortality in the next 1 to 2 years and identify patients who might benefit from LVAD support.[9]

The INTERMACS registry classifies heart failure patients into seven clinical profiles based on their signs and symptoms (Table 97-1). These profiles also help to define illness acuity and severity and to assess the operative risk.[6] The INTERMACS data showed that the proportion of patients in progressive cardiac decompensation (level 2) or cardiogenic shock (level 1) at the time of implantation of a durable LVAD has decreased from approximately 64% before 2011 to slightly less than 54% in 2012. This is because the patients in INTERMACS levels 1 and 2 have a 5% to 8% decrease in 1-year survival rate compared with patients in other INTERMACS levels (Fig. 97-2). Generally, for patients in INTERMACS level 1, placement of a durable VAD is not recommended because these patients are often compromised by end-organ damage, uncertain neurologic status, infection, or major coagulopathy. Therefore, short-term MCS should be applied in these patients as a bridge to decision (BTD) or recovery. Conversely, patients in INTERMACS level 6 or 7 (NYHA class III) are, in general, considered "too well" for MCS placement. Currently, patients in INTERMACS levels 2, 3, or 4 are likely to be appropriate candidates for a durable LVAD implantation.

It is also important to identify those patients with significant right ventricular (RV) dysfunction before LVAD implantation, because RV failure after LVAD implantation can be a fatal complication.[10-13] The implantation of an LVAD can decrease RV afterload by reducing

TABLE 97-1 **INTERMACS Profile Descriptions**

Profile 1: Critical Cardiogenic Shock
Patients with life-threatening hypotension despite rapidly escalating inotropic support, critical organ hypoperfusion, often confirmed by worsening acidosis and/or lactate levels. "Crash and burn."
Profile 2: Progressive Decline
Patient with declining function despite intravenous inotropic support; may be manifest by worsening renal function, nutritional depletion, inability to restore volume balance. "Sliding on inotropes." Also describes declining status in patients unable to tolerate inotropic therapy.
Profile 3: Stable But Inotrope Dependent
Patient with stable blood pressure, organ function, nutrition, and symptoms on continuous intravenous inotropic support (or a temporary circulatory support device or both) but demonstrating repeated failure to wean from support due to recurrent symptomatic hypotension or renal dysfunction. "Dependent stability."
Profile 4: Resting Symptoms
Patient can be stabilized close to normal volume status but experiences daily symptoms of congestion at rest or during ADLs. Doses of diuretics generally fluctuate at very high levels. More intensive management and surveillance strategies should be considered, which may in some cases reveal poor compliance that would compromise outcomes with any therapy. Some patients may shuttle between 4 and 5.
Profile 5: Exertion Intolerant
Comfortable at rest and with ADLs but unable to engage in any other activity, living predominantly within the house. Patients are comfortable at rest without congestive symptoms but may have underlying refractory elevated volume status, often with renal dysfunction. If underlying nutritional status and organ function are marginal, patient may be more at risk than INTERMACS 4 and require definitive intervention.
Profile 6: Exertion Limited
Patient without evidence of fluid overload is comfortable at rest and with ADLs and minor activities outside the home but fatigues after the first few minutes of any meaningful activity. Attribution to cardiac limitation requires careful measurement of peak oxygen consumption, in some cases with hemodynamic monitoring to confirm severity of cardiac impairment. "Walking wounded."
Profile 7: Advanced NYHA III
A placeholder for more precise specification in future, this level includes patients who are without current or recent episodes of unstable fluid balance, living comfortably with meaningful activity limited to mild physical exertion.

ADLs, Activities of daily living; *NYHA,* New York Heart Association.

Reproduced with permission from Stevenson LW, Pagani FD, Young JB, et al: INTERMACS profiles of advanced heart failure: the current picture. J Heart Lung Transplant 28(6):535–541, 2009.

pulmonary artery pressures. However, at the same time, increasing cardiac output with an LVAD support may increase systemic venous return to a diseased RV that may not be able to accommodate the additional volume. Furthermore, LV pressure unloading by an LVAD can cause the interventricular septum to shift leftward, leading to geometric changes in the RV that reduce RV function, exacerbating tricuspid regurgitation. The presence of depressed RV myocardial function can be determined from preoperative hemodynamic indices, including central venous pressure, pulmonary artery pressure, cardiac output, transpulmonary pressure gradient, pulmonary vascular resistance, and RV stroke work index (RVSWI).[10-13] The RVSWI can be calculated using the following formula: (mean pulmonary artery pressure − mean central venous pressure) × stroke volume ÷ body surface area. Patients with high pulmonary artery pressure and normal central venous pressure (high RVSWI) are at lower risk of postoperative RV failure because the RV is able to generate sufficient pressure. A preoperative echocardiographic assessment of RV function is also important. Attention should be paid to RV dilation, contractility, and degree of tricuspid regurgitation. Numerous studies have attempted to identify the risk factors for the development of RV failure after LVAD placement. The most recent study demonstrated that preoperative predictors of RV failure after implantation of a contemporary continuous flow LVAD included central venous pressure/pulmonary capillary wedge pressure ratio of greater than 0.63, need for preoperative ventilator support, and blood urea nitrogen level greater than 39 mg/dL.[12] Univariate predictors also included RVSWI less than 300 mm Hg × mL/m^2, central venous pressure greater than 15 mm Hg, and elevated white blood cell count. For patients at a significantly high risk of RV failure, planned biventricular assist device placement should be indicated.[14]

Pulmonary hypertension with an elevated pulmonary vascular resistance (>5 wood units) should not be considered an absolute contraindication to MCS. Modern selective pulmonary vasodilators such as sildenafil can reduce pulmonary pressures. In addition, patients who undergo LVAD implantation usually have improved pulmonary vascular resistance.[15,16] The LVAD can be considered as a BTC in possible transplant candidates with fixed pulmonary hypertension.

Contraindications for device implantation include irreversible end-organ failure, particularly renal failure and hepatic failure, which are uniformly independent predictors of poor outcome.[6,17-21] Severe, unrecoverable neurologic injury is also a contraindication for device implantation. Systemic sepsis poses a significant risk to patients undergoing LVAD implantation because it can cause a profound refractory vasodilatory state or lead to an increased incidence of device-related infections, such as device endocarditis.[22,23]

In the pulsatile flow era, numerous studies have identified independent predictors of adverse outcome.[21,24-26] The common denominator among these independent predictors of mortality is end-organ failure, such as respiratory failure requiring mechanical ventilation, renal failure requiring dialysis, ischemic hepatitis with markedly elevated transaminases, and diffuse coagulopathy resulting from malfunctioning clotting mechanisms. In the revised Columbia screening scale, the following clinical factors were identified as preoperative independent predictors of adverse outcome: mechanical ventilation, prior cardiotomy, prior LVAD implantation, central

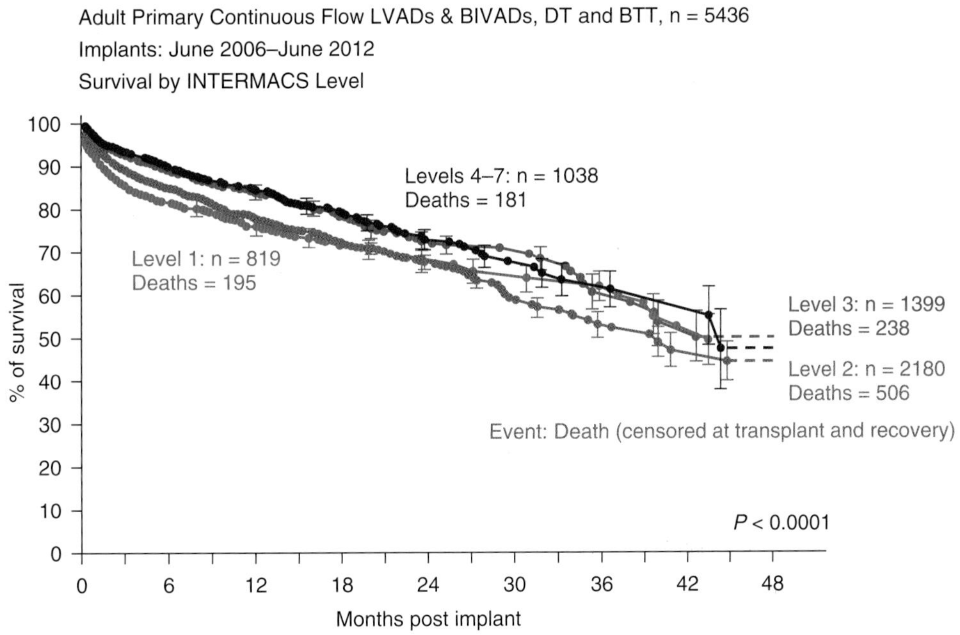

FIGURE 97-2 Survival after durable mechanical circulatory support device implantation by INTERMACS level. *BiVAD,* Biventricular assist device; *BTT,* bridge to transplant; *DT,* destination therapy; *LVAD,* left ventricular assist device. (Reproduced with permission from Kirklin JK, Naftel DC, Kormos RL, et al: Fifth INTERMACS annual report: risk factor analysis from more than 6,000 mechanical circulatory support patients. *J Heart Lung Transplant* 32:141–156, 2013.)

venous pressure of greater than 15 mm Hg, and prothrombin time of longer than 16 sec.[15] Each factor was given a statistically weighted score, with a score of higher than 5 being associated with a 46% mortality rate and a score of 5 or lower being associated with a 12% mortality rate.

In the continuous flow era, from the analysis of 1122 patients receiving the HeartMate II as a BTT or DT, preoperative predictors of 90-day mortality were older patients, greater degree of hypoalbuminemia, renal dysfunction (higher creatinine), coagulopathy (higher INR), and implant surgery at less experienced centers. Based on the calculated risk score from these factors, mortality rates in the low, medium, and high-risk score groups were 4%, 16%, and 29%, respectively.[27] From the INTERMACS registry data, risk factors for mortality included older age, INTERMACS level 1 and 2, DT, renal dysfunction, RV dysfunction, and surgical complexity.[6]

Poor preoperative hepatic function has also been demonstrated to be an independent predictor of mortality after LVAD implantation.[17,21,24,26] Decreased hepatic synthetic function increases the chance of developing a diffuse coagulopathy intraoperatively and postoperatively, which can cause RV failure secondary to increased transfusion requirements of blood products. The Model of End-stage Liver Disease (MELD) score calculated based on serum bilirubin, creatinine, and INR values is reported to be useful in identifying LVAD candidates at high risk for perioperative bleeding and mortality.[28,29] Optimization of hemodynamics with reduction of central venous pressure and improvement of cardiac output should be pursued before LVAD implantation to improve hepatic congestion and increase hepatic blood flow.

Severe renal dysfunction was associated with a major reduction in early survival after durable VAD implantation.[6,18,20,21,26,27] The incremental effect of worsening renal dysfunction was shown by assigning "moderate" renal dysfunction to patients with a creatinine level greater than 2 mg/dL or blood urea nitrogen level greater than 60 mg/dL, and "severe" renal dysfunction to patients requiring dialysis near the time of device implantation.[6] Although renal dysfunction caused by low cardiac output or renal vein congestion generally improves after MCS placement, caution should be paid in a patient with severe intrinsic renal disease such as chronic hypertension or diabetes mellitus. Patients with end-stage renal disease requiring dialysis should not be considered for durable LVAD implantation, because of their increased risk of infection.

Preoperative nutrition status assessment is also important.[30] Patients with cardiac cachexia are predisposed to poor healing, impaired immunity, and infection, which are generally associated with high mortality.[26,27] In contrast, obesity is not a contraindication to using a continuous flow LVAD, although patients with a body mass index higher than 35 kg/m^2 are not eligible for heart transplant.[31] These devices can provide sufficient cardiac output support to meet the metabolic demands of obese patients.[32,33]

To assess the patient's ability to understand VAD care, an investigation of prior psychiatric disorders, history of drug and alcohol abuse, compliance, and cognitive function needs to be conducted. Furthermore, adequate family/caregiver, financial, and environmental support are additional factors for determining potential LVAD candidates.[34]

Although it is important not to delay durable VAD implantation to the point of significant end-organ dysfunction, it is beneficial to optimize a relatively stable patient preoperatively. This may include hemodynamics optimization with diuretics, inotropes, short-term MCS (coagulopathy correction) with vitamin K, platelets, or fresh-frozen plasma, and nutrition management. With appropriate patient selection and timing of LVAD implantation, it is possible to achieve excellent results with relatively low associated morbidity and mortality.

TYPES OF DEVICES

Short-Term Mechanical Circulatory Support

Recent innovation of continuous flow technology contributes to the development of various types of short-term MCS, which can be distinguished by the method of placement (i.e., percutaneous or surgical). The current options for percutaneous circulatory support include intra-aortic balloon pump (IABP), extracorporeal membrane oxygenation (ECMO), the Impella, and TandemHeart. Surgical options include the CentriMag (Thoratec, Pleasanton, CA) ventricular support system. Each of these devices is designed for short-term use.

Percutaneous Devices for Short-Term Mechanical Support

Intra-Aortic Balloon Pump. Insertion of an IABP was first reported by Kantrowitz in 1968. It has since become one of the most common forms of mechanical support for the failing heart. It is commonly used for high-risk percutaneous coronary intervention (PCI), acute cardiogenic shock after myocardial infarction (MI), complications after MI such as a ruptured papillary muscle, cardiotomy shock, and preoperative optimization of an MI patient who is awaiting coronary artery bypass grafting (CABG).[35] Its mechanism of action involves inflation of the balloon in the descending aorta during diastole, which reduces afterload, increases coronary artery perfusion and pressure, improves myocardial oxygen supply, and decreases myocardial oxygen demand.[36] Counterpulsation can be synchronized with either an electrocardiogram or an arterial waveform. Vascular complications of the IABP include femoral artery rupture, pseudoaneurysm, descending aortic dissection, as well as distal ischemia as a result of impedance of forward flow.[37]

Extracorporeal Membrane Oxygenation. For patients in circulatory and respiratory failure, ECMO is a viable option. This system uses a centrifugal pump with an oxygenator and a heat exchanger in the circuit, yielding complete cardiopulmonary bypass. A venovenous ECMO is used for respiratory failure with preserved native heart function. To support the failing heart, a venoarterial (VA) ECMO is required (Fig. 97-3). A VA-ECMO system can provide full circulatory support with over 4.5 liter/min flow and rapidly improve tissue oxygenation. The major advantage of this system is the quick and easy percutaneous insertion of inflow and outflow cannulas—generally via the femoral artery and vein. Major disadvantages include infection, bleeding, and complications related to vascular access. Most survival data reported with ECMO have been in the pediatric literature.[38] The Extracorporeal Life Support Organization (ELSO) registry has accumulated data on more than 50,000 ECMO cases from more than 220 ECMO centers worldwide, including approximately 2300 cases of adult cardiac failure. In 2012, ELSO reported a survival to discharge rate of 39% for adult cardiac failure.[39] No meta-analyses of ECMO or randomized control trials with a mortality endpoint have been published. However, the ECMO system is likely to have the greatest potential for wider clinical use as a short-term MCS in cases such as cardiogenic shock.

TandemHeart. The TandemHeart (CardiacAssist, Inc., Pittsburgh, PA) is another percutaneously inserted device that uses a centrifugal pump. Two cannulas are inserted percutaneously with inflow from the left atrium—via a trans-septal puncture from a catheter entering from the femoral vein to the inferior vena cava to the right atrium and left atrium, and across the interatrial septum—and outflow into the femoral artery (Fig. 97-4). The pump can deliver flow rates up to 5.0 liter/min at a maximum speed of 7500 rpm. The initial clinical experience with this device for patients with high-risk PCI and post-MI cardiogenic shock has been favorable compared with

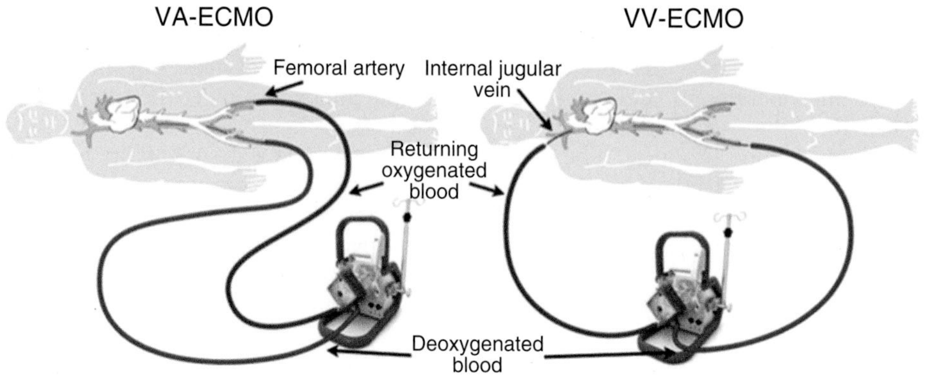

FIGURE 97-3 ■ Extracorporeal membrane oxygenation. *ECMO,* Extracorporeal membrane oxygenation; *VA,* venoarterial; *VV,* venovenous. (Reproduced with permission from Cove ME, MacLaren G: Clinical review: mechanical circulatory support for cardiogenic shock complicating acute myocardial infarction. *Crit Care* 14(5):235, 2010.)

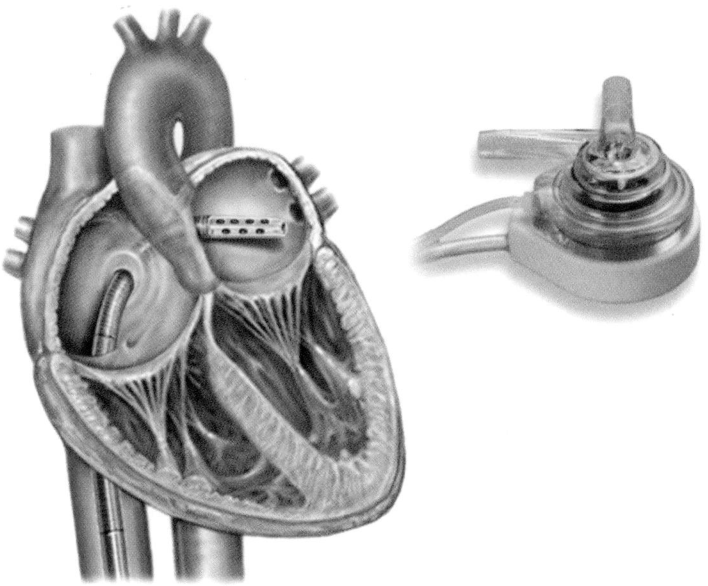

FIGURE 97-4 ■ TandemHeart. (Reproduced with permission from CardiacAssist, Inc.)

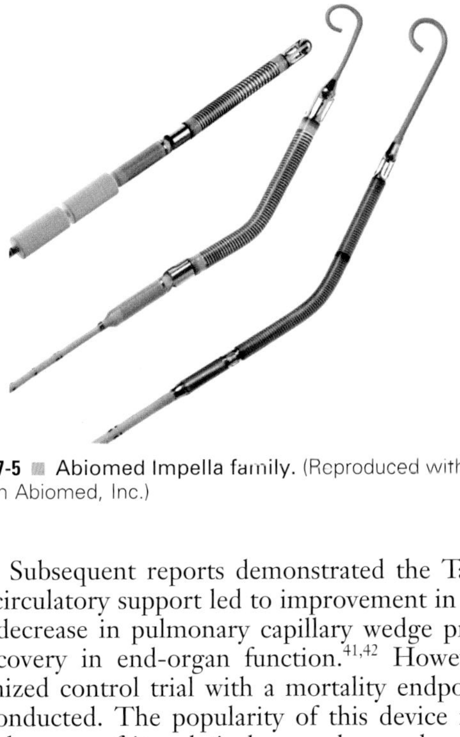

FIGURE 97-5 ■ Abiomed Impella family. (Reproduced with permission from Abiomed, Inc.)

IABP.[40] Subsequent reports demonstrated the TandemHeart circulatory support led to improvement in cardiac index, decrease in pulmonary capillary wedge pressure, and recovery in end-organ function.[41,42] However, no randomized control trial with a mortality endpoint has been conducted. The popularity of this device may be limited because of its relatively complex mode of insertion requiring trans-septal puncture.

Abiomed Impella. The Impella is an intravascular microaxial rotary pump that can be inserted across the aortic valve to provide forward blood flow from the left ventricle into the ascending aorta. The family of the Impella system includes 2.5, CP, 5.0, LD, and RP (Fig. 97-5).

The Abiomed Impella 5.0/LD—providing flow up to 5 liter/min—is inserted by a cardiac surgeon into the ascending aorta or a peripheral artery, such as the femoral or axillary artery. It is used for acute cardiogenic shock or postcardiotomy shock. Preliminary reports demonstrated a better survival benefit with implantation of the Impella than with an IABP for patients with postcardiotomy shock.[43] A subsequent multicenter prospective trial demonstrated that the use of the Impella 5.0/LD in patients with postcardiotomy shock yielded favorable outcomes.[44]

The Impella 2.5 is a minimally invasive cardiac assist device that is usually inserted by an interventional cardiologist percutaneously through the femoral artery up the descending aorta, across the aortic arch, down the ascending aorta, and across the aortic valve into the left ventricle. This is generally performed under either echocardiographic or fluoroscopic guidance. This device can provide flow up to 2.5 liter/min, giving partial circulatory support, and is relatively easy to implant. Clinical trials, focusing on high-risk PCI and acute MI cases,[45-47] have suggested that the Impella 2.5 may provide superior hemodynamic support compared with the IABP. However, similarly to the ECMO and TandemHeart, no conclusive data with mortality as an endpoint are available for the Impella pump family.[48]

The Impella CP has recently become clinically available in the United States. With a maximal flow of 3.5 liter/min, it may overcome the flow limitations of the Impella 2.5.

The Impella RP is specifically designed for RV support and is currently undergoing a clinical trial.

HeartMate Percutaneous Heart Pump. The HeartMate PHP (percutaneous heart pump; Thoratec, Pleasanton, CA) is an investigational device with a catheter-based axial flow pump (Fig. 97-6). Its collapsible elastomeric impeller and nitinol cannula allow for percutaneous insertion. The system can generate 4 to 5 liter/min of flow. It successfully completed the first-in-man phase in 2013 for adjunctive hemodynamic support during a high-risk PCI, with clinical trials planned for 2014.

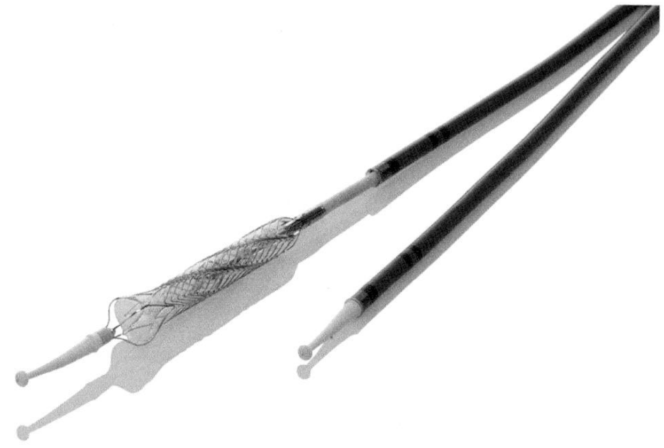

FIGURE 97-6 ■ HeartMate PHP (percutaneous heart pump). In development; not approved for clinical use. (Reproduced with permission from Thoratec Corp.)

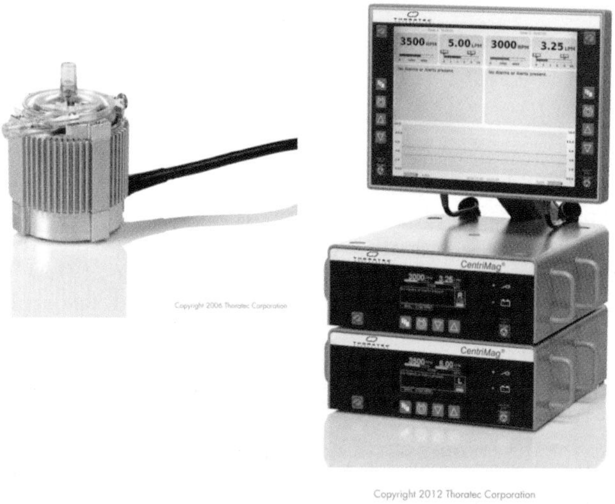

FIGURE 97-7 ■ CentriMag. (Reproduced with permission from Thoratec Corp.)

Surgical Devices for Short-Term Mechanical Support

Abiomed BVS 5000 and AB5000. The Abiomed BVS 5000 is a dual-chambered, pneumatically driven, extracorporeal pump that can be used for short-term support as a univentricular or biventricular assist device. The device is capable of flowing up to 6 liter/min. Many series have reported acceptable results with this device.[49,50]

The Abiomed AB5000—the next-generation device after the BVS 5000—is fully automated and has a vacuum-assisted console. Advantages of this device over its predecessor include allowing patients to be more mobile and extending the duration of device support.

CentriMag. The CentriMag blood pump (Thoratec, Pleasanton, CA) is an extracorporeal centrifugal pump that is FDA approved for up to 6 hours of support time, operating without mechanical bearings or seals.[50-52] The system combines the drive, magnetic bearing, and the rotor function into a single unit (Fig. 97-7). The rotor is magnetically levitated, which enables the device to rotate without friction or wear, and eliminates heat production. This serves to minimize trauma to the blood and avoids mechanical failure. Because the rotor surface is uniformly washed, blood stagnation and turbulence in the pump are minimized. Hemolysis is reduced because the mechanical gaps in the pump are wider than 0.6 mm, reducing shear forces. The device can produce flows of up to 10 liter/min with a priming volume of 31 mL.

Implantation of a CentriMag is less technically challenging and faster than implantation of other devices. The cannulas are inserted using techniques similar to those used for routine cannulation in cardiopulmonary bypass. Another particularly useful feature of the device is the ease of adjustment of the device speed and resulting flow. Based on the patient's clinical scenario (i.e., to increase flow during periods of sepsis and decrease flow when attempting to assess weanability from the device), the speed of the device can be increased or decreased simply by pushing a button. This system can provide isolated left ventricular support as an LVAD, isolated right ventricular support as a RVAD, or biventricular support as a full-support biventricular assist device (BiVAD).[51,52] BiVADs allow decompression of both ventricles, restore hemodynamic stability, provide enhanced peripheral perfusion, and prevent end-organ dysfunction. The CentriMag is a rescue device that can be surgically implanted in patients with acute refractory cardiogenic shock.

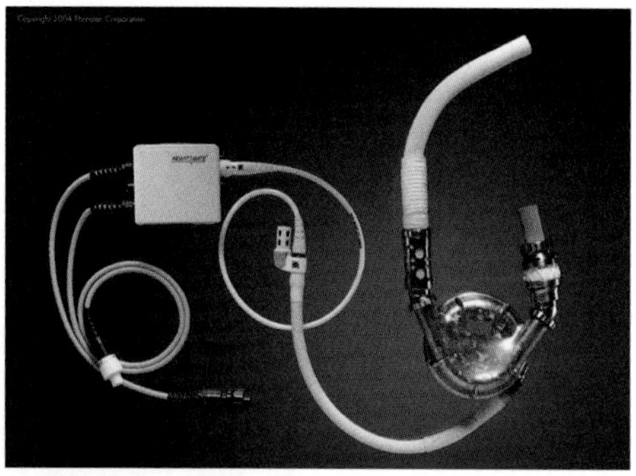

FIGURE 97-8 ■ HeartMate XVE. (Reproduced with permission from Thoratec Corp.)

Long-Term Mechanical Circulatory Support

Pulsatile Devices

Thoratec HeartMate XVE. The HeartMate XVE LVAD is FDA approved for both BTT and DT (Fig. 97-8). This device has undergone several major transformations. The older version had a pump operated by a pneumatically driven mechanism and contained a large controller console. The newer-generation device is electrically vented and contains a portable console and batteries, giving patients more mobility. Furthermore, the device produces a pulsatile flow with a stroke volume of 83 mL and a maximal flow of 10 liter/min. A large landmark trial of this device has demonstrated superior outcomes compared with optimal medical management.[1]

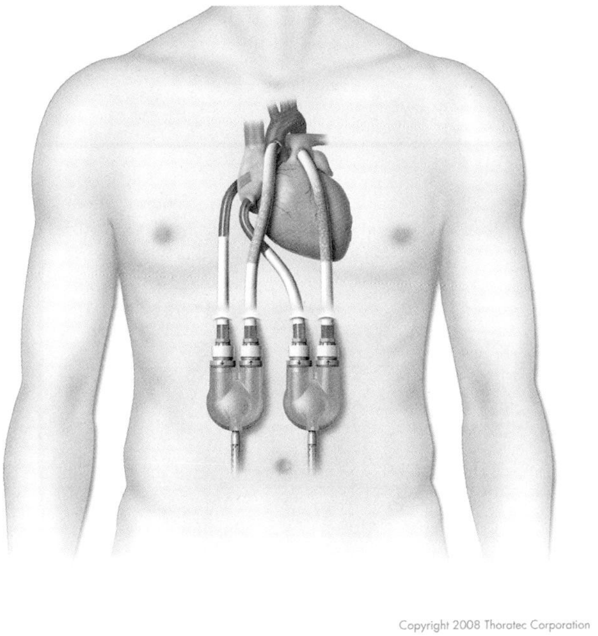

FIGURE 97-9 Thoratec PVAD (paracorporeal biventricular assist device). (Reproduced with permission from Thoratec Corp.)

However, its long-term use is limited by the high probability of device-related complications.

Thoratec Paracorporeal Ventricular Assist Device. The Thoratec paracorporeal VAD is a versatile device that has been used extensively for univentricular and biventricular support (Fig. 97-9). The paracorporeal placement of the pumping chamber allows the device to be implanted in patients with body surface areas of less than 1.5 m^2. The device consists of a polyurethane blood sac contained in a polycarbonate housing, attached to a large pneumatic console, which is used to generate a pulsatile flow with a maximal stroke volume of 65 mL. The device is capable of a flow up to 7.2 liter/min. Tilting disc mechanical valves maintain unidirectional flow. Because the device is placed paracorporeally, less dissection is required. Inflow for the LVAD is from the left atrium or LV apex, with outflow to the ascending aorta. Inflow for the RVAD is from the right atrium or right ventricle, with outflow to the pulmonary artery. The device requires systemic anticoagulation with either heparin or warfarin. With the introduction of the TLC-II portable driver, the system has become less cumbersome for patients and caregivers, improving the patients' mobility and ability to participate in rehabilitation programs.[53]

Thoratec Intracorporeal Ventricular Assist Device. The Thoratec intracorporeal VAD, like the paracorporeal VAD, is a versatile device that can provide isolated left, right, or biventricular support. Because it is implantable, it requires more dissection than the paracorporeal VAD. It is the first FDA-approved implantable VAD with biventricular capability for BTT and postcardiotomy shock. A multicenter trial including 39 patients supported with this device reported a success rate of 70% for BTT and 67% for postcardiotomy recovery, which represents an improvement over historical results for the paracorporeal VAD of 69% for BTT and 48% for postcardiotomy recovery.[54]

Axial Flow Pumps—Second-Generation Devices

Axial flow pumps are continuous flow pumps that operate with a propeller revolving at a set number of revolutions per minute (rpm). Advantages over pulsatile pumps include reduced noise levels and enhanced durability, the latter being attributed to fewer moving parts and contact bearings. The smaller size of these pumps also allows the device to be inserted with less dissection, because the size of the pocket is minimized and sometimes completely eliminated (Fig. 97-10).[3-7] Disadvantages of an axial flow pump include the lack of a mechanical backup mechanism in the event of major device malfunction, hemolysis as a result of shear forces, and the potential for creating negative intraventricular pressure, with resultant device thrombosis, air embolism, or arrhythmia. Key factors in avoiding the creation of negative intraventricular pressure include preload optimization and perfect LV apical inflow cannula placement.

Several studies have evaluated the potential adverse effects of low-pulsatile continuous flow pumps on end-organ perfusion and function. On the basis of current data, adequate end-organ perfusion and function can be maintained with low-pulsatile continuous blood flow.[55,56]

After the initial landmark trial showing a significant improvement in the quality of life and survival of patients after implantation of a continuous flow pump as compared with a pulsatile flow device (Fig. 97-11), this group of VADs has become the mainstream for BTT therapy and DT.[3,7] Since the FDA approval of the HeartMate II device for BTT therapy in 2008 and for DT in 2010, over 98% of all LVADs implanted in the United States were continuous flow pump.[6]

Thoratec HeartMate II. The Thoratec HeartMate II VAD is an axial flow rotary pump constructed of titanium (Fig. 97-12), which can generate flows up to 10 liter/min operating at pump speeds of 6000 to 15,000 rpm. Inflow is via the LV apex, and outflow is via the ascending aorta. The axial flow design eliminates the need for a blood-pumping chamber and volume compensation necessary for volume-displacement LVADs. The pump housing is implanted in the small preperitoneal space and requires only a small pocket. A small percutaneous driveline exits the skin in the right or left upper abdomen. This feature makes the device more suitable for implantation in patients with a smaller body size. Theoretical benefits over previous series of VAD system include a reduced risk of infection, greater patient comfort and quality of life, and greater device durability. Furthermore, it is substantially smaller than the HeartMate XVE and requires a less invasive operative approach. A randomized control trial demonstrated the superiority of the HeartMate II compared with the HeartMate XVE in terms of survival, quality of life, and durability.[3] The HeartMate II is approved by the FDA for both BTT therapy and DT.

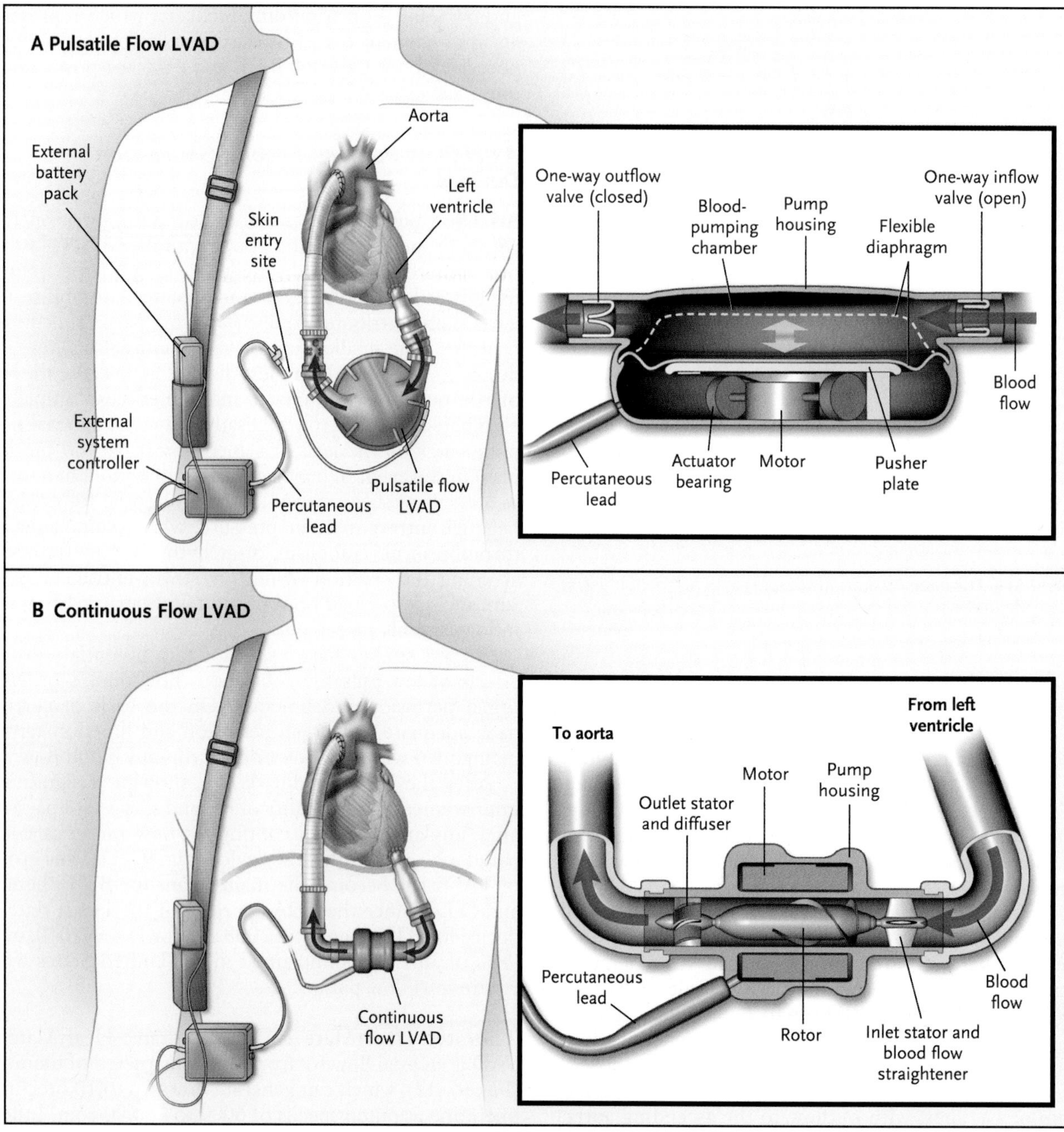

FIGURE 97-10 ■ **A,** Pulsatile flow device. **B,** Continuous flow device. *LVAD,* left ventricular assist device. (Reproduced with permission from Slaughter MS, Rogers JG, Milano CA, et al: Advanced heart failure treated with continuous flow left ventricular assist device. *New Engl J Med* 361(23):2241–2251, 2009.)

The accumulating clinical experience suggests that the pump is associated with a notable improvement in survival. The original HeartMate II BTT trial demonstrated a 1-year overall survival rate of 68%, which has improved to 85% according to more recent data.[7] In the HeartMate II DT trial, the 2-year survival rate improved from 58% in the early era to 63% in the later era.[57]

Jarvik 2000. The Jarvik 2000 (Jarvik Heart, Inc., New York, NY) is an electromagnetically actuated pump constructed of titanium, measuring 2.5 cm in diameter and weighing 90 g (Fig. 97-13), with a displacement of approximately 30 mL. The titanium impeller blades are held in place by ceramic bearings. The impeller rotates at speeds of 8000 to 12,000 rpm and can generate a flow of up to 7 liter/min. A unique feature of this device is that the pumping chamber is implanted in the left ventricle. The outflow graft is anastomosed to the descending thoracic aorta. Surgical implantation of the device is typically accomplished through a left thoracotomy.[58] The pump speed can be adjusted by an external controller dial ranging from 1 to 5. The speed setting of 1 is the slowest, driving the impeller at 8000 rpm and producing a blood flow of 1 to 2 liter/min, whereas the speed setting of 5 is the fastest, driving the impeller at 12,000 rpm and producing a blood flow of 5 to 7 liter/min.[59]

The multiple versions of the Jarvik 2000 device can be differentiated by their energy source. The percutaneous model has a single driveline that exits through the patient's anterior abdominal wall. One version contains skull-mounted pedestals used with cochlear implants: a titanium pedestal is screwed into the skull with a transcutaneous connector that attaches to the power cord. The behind-the-ear cable system may have significant quality-of-life advantages and reduced risk of infection compared with the abdominal cables. Furthermore, it enables patients to shower and bathe normally and even go swimming. This system is currently under trial for DT.[59,60]

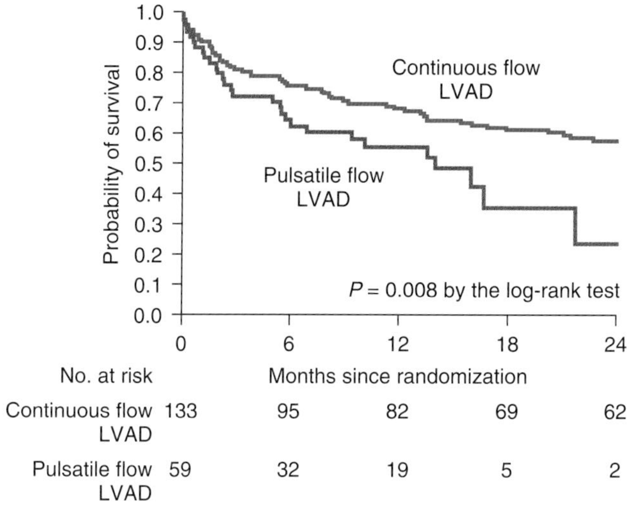

FIGURE 97-11 ■ Survival after continuous versus pulsatile flow left ventricular assist device (LVAD) implant. (Reproduced with permission from Slaughter MS, Rogers JG, Milano CA, et al: Advanced heart failure treated with continuous flow left ventricular assist device. *New Engl J Med* 361(23):2241–2251, 2009.)

MicroMed DeBakey. The MicroMed DeBakey VAD (MicroMed Cardiovascular, Inc., Houston, TX) was developed as a collaborative effort between the Baylor College of Medicine and National Aeronautics and Space Administration engineers. The pump unit for the MicroMed DeBakey VAD is made of titanium, weighs 95 g, and measures only 1.2 inches in diameter and 3 inches in length. The impeller is capable of generating flows up to 10 liter/min. A relatively high number of reports have described stroke and microemboli formation with this device.[61,62] The child version is approved by the FDA for BTT use in children aged 5 to 16 years.

Newer (Third-) Generation Pumps and Future Devices

Newer-generation devices, so-called third-generation devices, have been designed to address several shortcomings of second-generation axial flow pumps, such as thromboembolic complications and limited device durability. Many of these devices operate on the basis of magnetic levitation technology, in which the rotating propeller is magnetically suspended in a column of blood, obviating the need for contact-bearing moving parts and providing the theoretical benefit of enhanced durability. Continuous flow pumps are generally smaller, can be inserted with only a small device pocket or no pocket at all, are less traumatic, and may have a decreased risk for

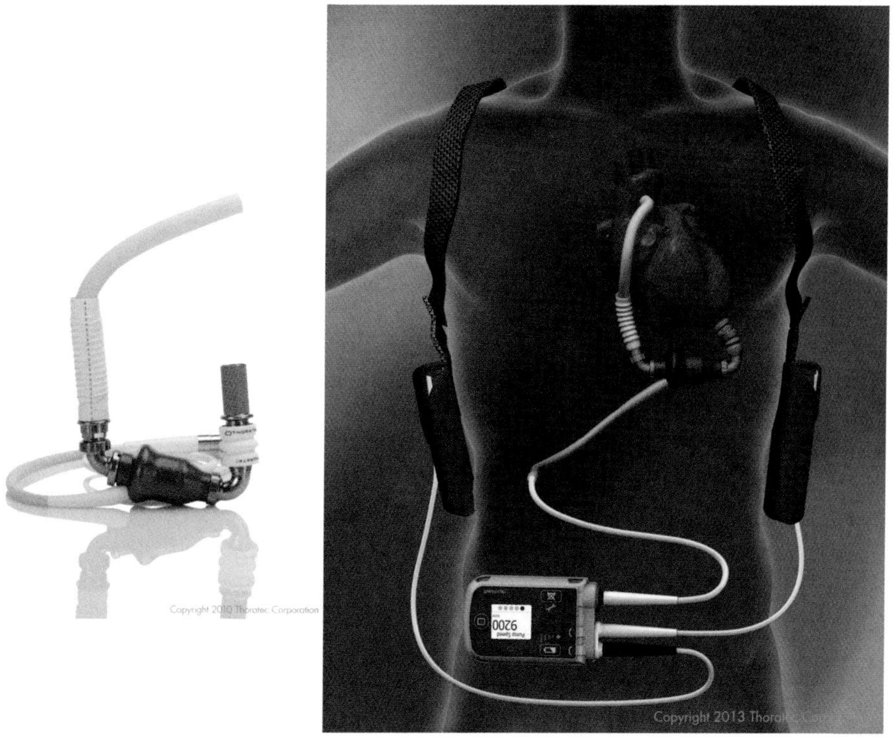

FIGURE 97-12 ■ HeartMate II. (Reproduced with permission from Thoratec Corp.)

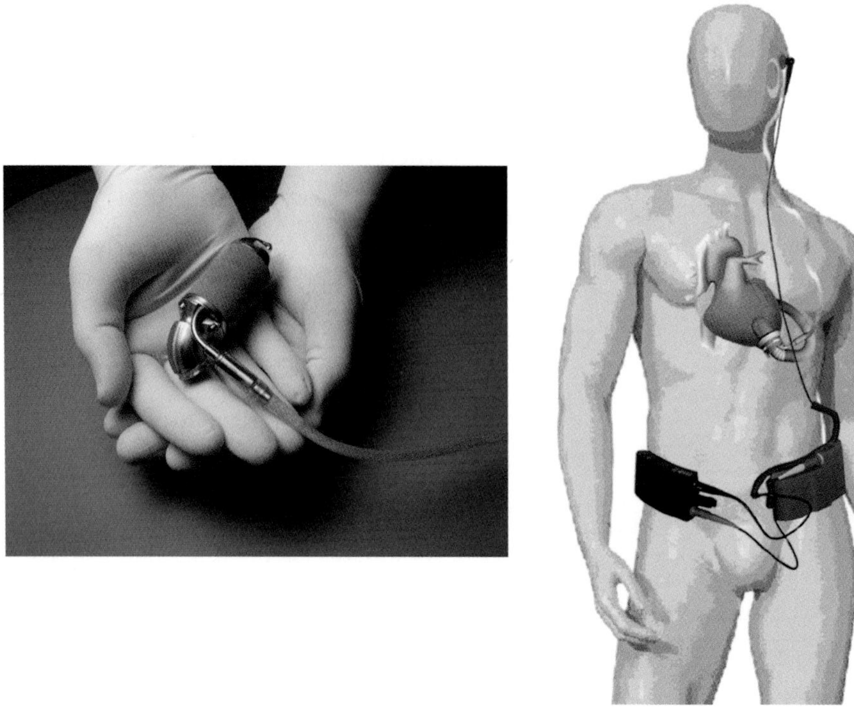

FIGURE 97-13 ■ Jarvik 2000. (Reproduced with permission from Jarvik Heart, Inc.)

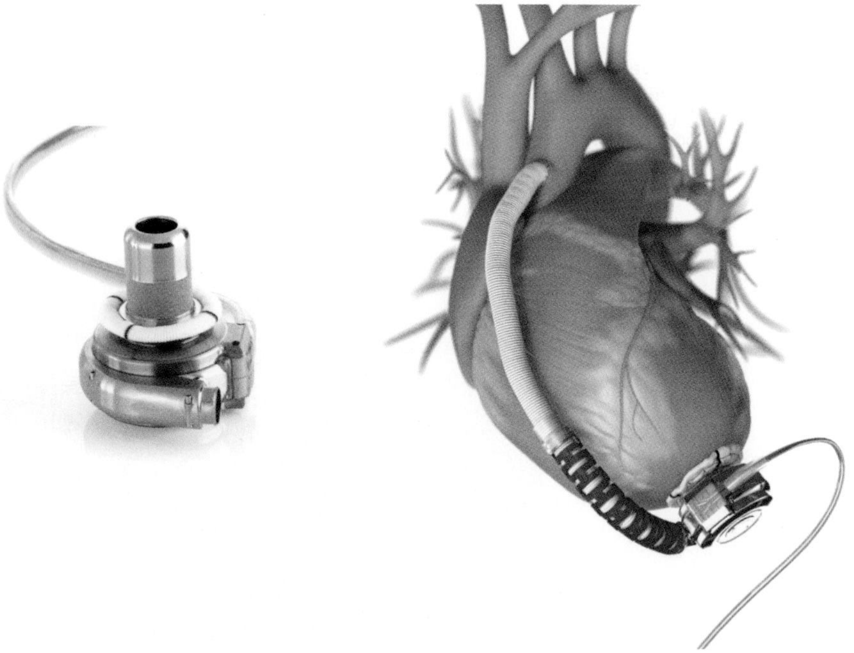

FIGURE 97-14 ■ HeartWare HVAD. (Reproduced with permission from HeartWare, Inc.)

associated infection. Some have been designed to be completely implantable with a transcutaneous energy transfer system. Along with smaller control consoles, these devices allow patients to be readily discharged from the hospital and increase their ability to ambulate. These devices will probably be associated with a significant improvement in quality of life for patients.

HeartWare HVAD. The HeartWare HVAD (HeartWare International, Inc., Framingham, MA) is a centrifugal pump with no mechanical bearings (Fig. 97-14), weighing 145 g, with a displaced stroke volume of 45 mL and a flow of up to 10 liter/min at 2000 to 3000 rpm. The inflow cannula is integrated into the left ventricle. The device is implanted in the pericardial space without the need for an abdominal incision. This miniaturized device may be used as a biventricular assist system as well as an LVAD.[63] A single, flexible driveline measuring 4.2 mm in diameter exits the anterior abdomen. The device has been tested in several centers throughout

Europe with good results.[64,65] A clinical trial of BTT demonstrated noninferior 180-day survival to contemporary LVAD registry controls in the United States.[66] In the study, 127 out of 140 patients (91%) either survived for at least 180 days on the pump or received a heart transplant within that time. The HeartWare LVAD is approved by the FDA for BTT therapy.

The HeartWare MVAD is an investigational device with a continuous axial flow pump, approximately one-third the size of the HVAD.

DuraHeart. The Terumo DuraHeart LVAD (Terumo Heart, Inc., Ann Arbor, MI) uses magnetic levitation technology.[67] The device can provide a flow of 2 to 8 liter/min at 1200 to 2400 rpm. In case of magnetic failure, the device can levitate the Impella hydrolytically. The pump weighs 540 g and has a diameter of 72 mm and a height of 45 mm. Favorable clinical outcomes as a BTT therapy have been reported in studies conducted in Europe and Japan.[68,69]

Thoratec HeartMate III. The Thoratec HeartMate III device is also a magnetically suspended centrifugal pump, powered by a magnetically levitated centrifugal impeller (Fig. 97-15). The device can provide a flow of 10 liter/min. This device has the ability to produce a pulsatile flow and has a large gap that may significantly reduce shear stress.[70] This device is not currently being tested in any clinical trials.

Synergy. The Synergy (HeartWare International, Inc., Framingham, MA) device is a partial-support LVAD that can be placed intravascularly (Fig. 97-16). An inflow cannula is placed through the subclavian vein, into the right atrium, and across the interatrial septum into the left atrium. Outflow is to the subclavian artery. Data from a European trial showed that the partial-support LVAD can provide improvements in hemodynamics and a reduction of heart failure symptoms.[71]

Total Artificial Heart

MCS options for patients requiring long-term biventricular support remain limited. TAH currently represents one long-term treatment option for patients requiring biventricular support.[72] Others include paracorporeal BiVAD and implantable BiVAD.[53,54] Thus, despite the enthusiasm of continuous flow pumps, pulsatile technology still has an important role in the treatment of biventricular failure. BiVAD provides biventricular support for the failing native heart, which is left intact. TAH completely replaces the failed ventricles and the four native valves in the orthotopic position. By replacing the failing heart, the TAH can eliminate the native heart complications such as valve dysfunction and arrhythmias.

The TAH is currently approved by the FDA only for BTT. The use of TAH is indicated in transplant candidates at risk of imminent death from nonreversible biventricular failure. Contraindications include transplant ineligibility, absence of biventricular failure, inability to have anticoagulation, and small thoracic cavity size.[72] According to INTERMACS data, only 2% of current MCS implants are TAH.[6] A recent large report of 101 patients receiving TAH demonstrated survival to transplantation rate of 68% and 1-year overall survival rate of 77% after transplant.[73] Recent retrospective data from Europe showed no difference in survival rate while on support and after transplant between TAH, paracorporeal BiVADs, and implantable BiVADs.[74] No randomized prospective clinical trials have compared TAH with BiVAD.

SynCardia

The SynCardia TAH (SynCardia Systems, Inc., Tucson, AZ) system is a pneumatic, pulsatile, biventricular device that completely replaces a patient's native ventricles and all valves, while pumping blood to both the pulmonary and the systemic circulation orthotopically (Fig. 97-17). The system consists of the implantable SynCardia TAH and an external console connected via drivelines. It weighs 160 g and displaces 400 mL of volume. It is lined

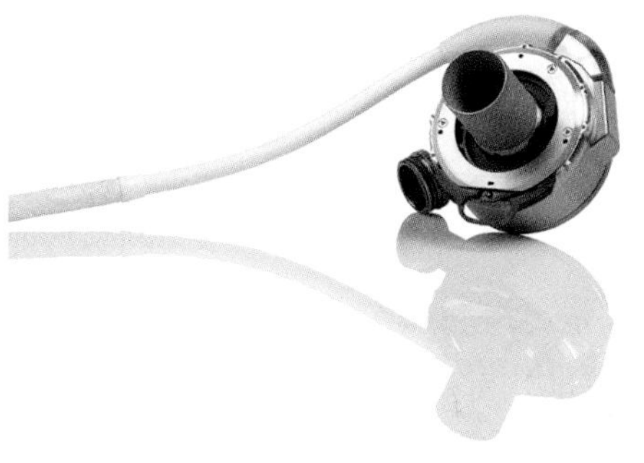

FIGURE 97-15 ■ HeartMate III. In development; not approved for clinical use. (Reproduced with permission from Thoratec Corp.)

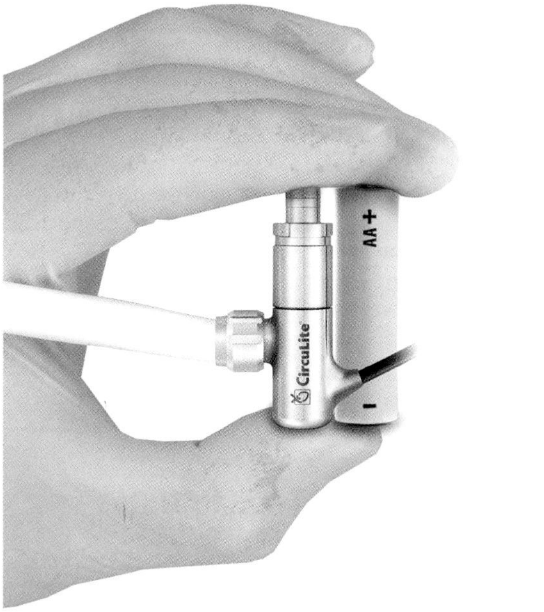

FIGURE 97-16 ■ Synergy. (Reproduced with permission from HeartWare, Inc.)

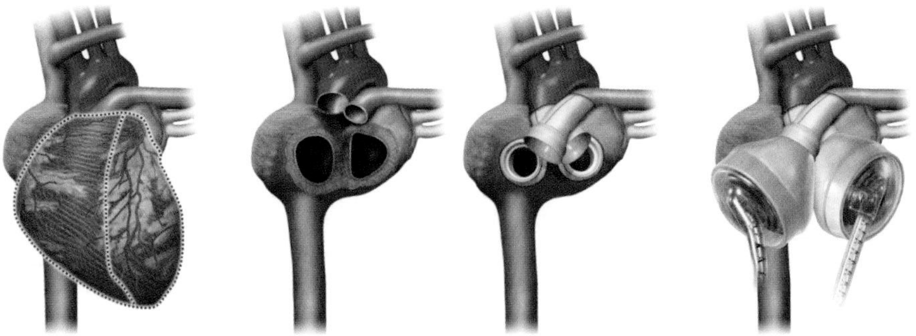

FIGURE 97-17 ■ SynCardia total artificial heart. (Reproduced with permission from SynCardia Systems, Inc.)

with polyurethane and has a four-layer, pneumatically driven diaphragm. Four mechanical Hall valves (Medtronic, Inc.) (two 27-mm inflow, two 25-mm outflow) are mounted on the housing. The diaphragm within the pump is actuated by movement of air from an external console. At maximal stroke volume (70 mL), it delivers a cardiac output of more than 9 liter/min. The artificial ventricles are connected via atrial inflow connectors to the native left and right atrium and to the native aorta and pulmonary artery by the outflow cannulas. The major drawbacks are the complexity of the implant procedure, relatively large device size (body surface area > 1.7 m^2 and thoracic diameter of at least 10 cm are required), and higher noise level compared with continuous flow pumps. This device is approved by the FDA for BTT therapy. A landmark trial including 81 patients who received SynCardia TAH demonstrated survival to transplantation rate of 79%, 1-year overall survival of 70%, and 1- and 5-year survival rates of 86% and 64% after transplantation, respectively.[72] The most common adverse events were infection and bleeding.

DEVICE SELECTION

A wide spectrum of MCS devices is available. Important factors that should be considered when selecting a device include the expected duration of support (short- versus long-term support); whether right, left, or biventricular support is required; the patient's neurologic status and overall prognosis; and whether the intent is to bridge the patient to recovery or to transplant, or if the device is to serve as DT. Other important patient-specific factors include the patient's body habitus, blood type, transplant candidacy, and contraindications to anticoagulation. Surgeon preference, level of familiarity, and device availability may also play a role in deciding which device to implant. Moreover, these issues should be raised during multidisciplinary team discussions with experienced surgeons and cardiologists

INDICATIONS FOR MECHANICAL CIRCULATORY SUPPORT

Major indications for MCS include acute cardiogenic shock after acute MI, postcardiotomy cardiogenic shock, myocarditis, refractory ventricular arrhythmias, acute on chronic heart failure, and chronic heart failure. Patients can be roughly divided into the following two categories depending on the trajectory of heart failure progression and overall clinical status: (1) patients with acute cardiogenic shock, or (2) patients with chronic advanced heart failure.

Patients in Acute Cardiogenic Shock

Implantation of durable LVADs is associated with poor outcomes in patients with acute cardiogenic shock (INTERMACS level 1) after an acute MI, myocarditis, acute on chronic heart failure, or after cardiotomy.[6] Generally, transplant eligibility is uncertain in patients with a combination of end-organ failure, uncertain neurologic status, and uncertain social support. Furthermore, the recent IABP-SHOCK II trial suggested that IABP confers no benefit in cardiogenic shock associated with acute MI.[75,76] Therefore, there is clearly a role for short-term MCS in this population to provide BTD, BTT, or recovery (Fig. 97-18). The current options include the VA-ECMO, Impella, TandemHeart, and CentriMag. Each of these devices seems to be safe, effective, and reliable.[38-42,44,50-52] They can provide optimal flow to this subset of very-high-risk patients in cardiogenic shock whose predicted mortality rate is almost 100% without mechanical support. In our program, the VA-ECMO or CentriMag BiVAD is preferably used. For patients with unclear neurologic status, profound shock, and severe coagulopathy, the less invasive VA-ECMO is selected. After resuscitation with these short-term devices, the patient's neurologic status, end-organ function, and myocardial function can be evaluated appropriately. Depending on the results, the short-term MCS device is explanted as a transition to each definitive goal (BTD). Ninety patients received either the ECMO or the CentriMag BiVAD through this algorithm for cardiogenic shock. An exchange with an implantable VAD was required in 26% of patients. Other destinations included myocardial recovery in 18% and heart transplantation in 11%. The survival to hospital discharge rate was 49%.[77]

Cardiogenic Shock after Acute Myocardial Infarction

Approximately 6% to 7% of all MI patients develop cardiogenic shock as a complication, with most of these being ST-elevation MIs.[78] When cardiogenic shock

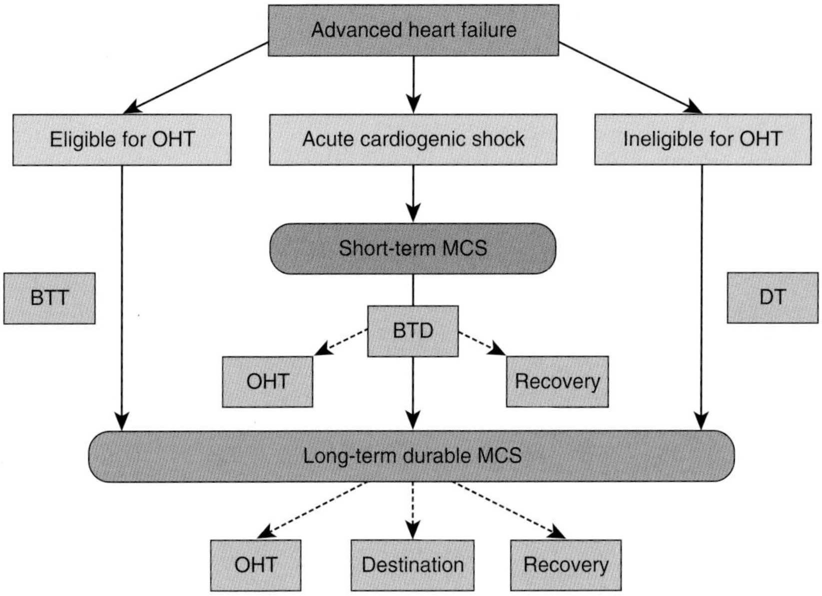

FIGURE 97-18 Patient and device selection flow chart. *BTD,* Bridge to decision; *BTT,* bridge to transplant; *DT,* destination therapy; *MCS,* mechanical circulatory support; *OHT,* orthotopic heart transplantation.

complicates an acute MI, the reported associated mortality rate has traditionally been 85% to 90%.[79] For patients with refractory cardiogenic shock despite maximal pharmacologic support, the mortality rate approaches 100%.[80] Moreover, a recent large prospective randomized trial demonstrated that additional IABP treatment did not result in a significant reduction in 30-day mortality rate compared with medical therapy alone.[75,76] Implantation of a MCS device to provide adequate circulatory support may be the only viable option for survival in these cases. By providing adequate circulatory support, MCS can reverse hypotension while maintaining vital organ perfusion and adequate coronary perfusion pressures.[42,46-48] The goal of MCS in patients with cardiogenic shock after an acute MI is to bridge the patient to a second procedure, which includes PCI, CABG, CABG plus valve, implantation of a long-term durable LVAD, and explantation of the short-term MCS devices after myocardial recovery.

Cardiogenic Shock after Cardiotomy

Patients in cardiogenic shock after cardiotomy are also best treated with a short-term MCS device. Like the goal of mechanical support in patients after an acute MI, the goal of mechanical support in patients with cardiogenic shock after cardiotomy—irrespective of which mechanical device is used—is to bridge the patient to a second procedure, which includes implantation of a long-term durable LVAD, as well as explantation of the short-term MCS after myocardial recovery.[44,81,82]

Myocarditis

Acute heart failure and cardiogenic shock from myocarditis are seen typically in a younger patient population. Because the probability of recovery is relatively high in these patients, they should receive a short-term MCS device, such as the ECMO or CentriMag.[83] In general, our preference is to implant a biventricular device in these patients. After normalization of end-organ perfusion and function, myocardial function and recovery are assessed.

Refractory Ventricular Arrhythmias

The subgroup of patients with refractory arrhythmias is heterogeneous. Some do not have significantly reduced cardiac function, whereas others have severely depressed ejection fractions.[24,25,84] Pharmacologic therapy, such as amiodarone, lidocaine, and beta blockers, failed to control their arrhythmias. Among the patients with reduced LV function, RV function can be either preserved or reduced. These patients can be candidates for both short-term and long-term MCS.

Patients with Chronic Advanced Heart Failure

A progression to chronic heart failure is characteristic of the largest subgroup of patients who receive long-term, durable LVADs. There are two definitive arms depending on transplant eligibility (BTT or DT).[1,6-8] However, the initial management plan can change over time. For example, comorbidities may improve in a DT patient who was previously ineligible for transplant, making the patient transplant-eligible after LVAD support. Alternatively, a BTT patient may become transplant-ineligible because of device-related complications or progression of comorbidities. Additionally, the INTERMACS registry data demonstrated that 42% of the durable LVAD implants were intended as a BTC.[6] Thus, in a dynamic clinical situation, it is often difficult to decide between BTT and DT.

Patients Who Are Eligible for Heart Transplantation

Heart transplantation is the optimal treatment for patients with a history of chronic congestive heart failure who may have additional chronic deterioration or an acute exacerbation. However, the constant shortage of available donors has resulted in an increasing number of patients with longer waiting times on the transplantation lists. The use of a long-term durable LVAD as a BTT has become common in patients who would otherwise not survive or who would develop progressive end-organ dysfunction before an organ becomes available.[7,31] Dependence on intravenous inotropes (INTERMACS profile level 2 or 3) is traditionally considered the threshold that accelerates consideration of durable VAD therapies in these patients. The BTT strategy is especially reasonable in patients listed for transplant who are expected to have an extended waiting time because of their blood type, large body size, or high degree of allosensitization.

Since the FDA approved the HeartMate II, placement of a continuous flow LVAD such as the HeartMate II or HeartWare has been the mainstream circulatory support therapy for these patients. They are often discharged from the hospital after their VAD is implanted and return at a later date for a transplant.[7,66] Contemporary, continuous flow, durable LVADs have favorable waiting list outcomes, unless a serious LVAD-related complication occurs.[85] In addition, the data from the UNOS registry demonstrated that posttransplant graft survival after a bridge with continuous flow durable LVADs was similar to that in patients bridged with inotropes or pulsatile flow LVADs.[86]

Patients Who Are Not Eligible for Heart Transplantation

The REMATCH trial, which randomized 129 non-transplant candidates to optimal medical therapy or mechanical support, demonstrated a 48% reduction in the risk of death from any cause in the LVAD group compared with the group of patients treated with optimal medical therapy.[1] Based on this result, the FDA approved the use of an LVAD (HeartMate XVE) as a lifelong support therapy (DT). Mortality rate increases to an almost prohibitive value with the onset of end-organ failure—such as renal failure—and in the presence of active infection. In a study of 280 patients who underwent HeartMate XVE LVAD implantation as DT in the post-REMATCH era, the most important determinants of in-hospital mortality were poor nutrition, hematologic abnormalities, markers of end-organ or RV dysfunction, and lack of inotropic support.[26] Current requirements for DT are patients with NYHA class IV end-stage ventricular heart failure who are not candidates for heart transplant and who meet all the following conditions: (1) have failed to respond to optimal medical management (including beta blockers and ACE inhibitors, if tolerated) for at least 45 of the last 60 days, or have been balloon pump dependent for 7 days, or IV inotrope dependent for 14 days; (2) have a left ventricular ejection fraction less than 25%; and (3) have demonstrated functional limitation with a peak oxygen consumption of up to 14 mL/kg/min unless balloon pump or inotrope dependent, or physically unable to perform the test.

Currently, the FDA-approved continuous flow device for DT is the HeartMate II. Since the approval of HeartMate II for DT in 2010, the number of LVADs implanted for lifelong support in transplant-ineligible patients has increased up to 10-fold.[6] The evolution from pulsatile to continuous flow technology has dramatically improved survival in these patients. A large body of data from the INTERMACS registry demonstrated a 1-year survival rate of 75% (Fig. 97-19).[87] A subset of their population with no cancer, not in cardiogenic shock, and blood urea

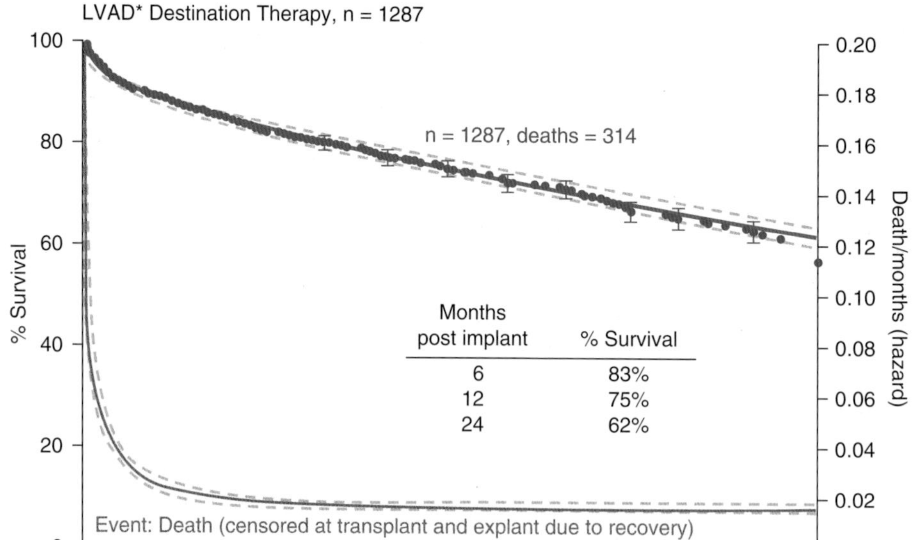

FIGURE 97-19 ■ **Survival after left ventricular assist device (LVAD) implant as a destination therapy.** (Reproduced with permission from Kirklin JK, Naftel DC, Pagani FD, et al: Long-term mechanical circulatory support [destination therapy]: on track to compete with heart transplantation? *J Thorac Cardiovasc Surg* 144(3):584–603, 2012.)

nitrogen less than 50 mg/dL experienced a 2-year survival rate of 80% or more, which is competitive with heart transplantation.

Given the improvements in technology, as well as in patient selection and care over the past decade, there is a movement to use LVAD therapy in patients who are less ill than those currently eligible for DT. The NHLBI has sponsored the Randomized Evaluation of the VAD intervention before the Inotropic Therapy (REVIVE-IT) trial to test the LVAD therapy in advanced heart failure patients with significant functional impairment who are ineligible for transplant but who have not yet manifested serious consequences of end-stage heart failure, such as end-organ dysfunction, immobility, or cardiac cachexia.[88]

SURGICAL TECHNIQUE USED FOR DURABLE LEFT VENTRICULAR ASSIST DEVICE IMPLANTATION

The technique used for durable LVAD implantation varies depending on the institution and the surgeon. However, the common steps in the operation can be summarized as follows: (1) skin incision; (2) creation of a preperitoneal pocket, if required; (3) mediastinal exposure; (4) cannulation of the aorta and venous system; (5) cardiopulmonary bypass commencement; (6) coring of the LV, placing core sutures on the LV, inserting the inflow core into the LV apex; (7) outflow graft anastomosis to the ascending aorta; (8) de-airing of the device; (9) weaning off cardiopulmonary bypass, actuating LVAD; (10) hemostasis establishment; (11) closing sternotomy.

A vertical midline incision is made beginning just below the sternal notch with variable extension below the xyphoid, depending on the type of device being implanted and the required pocket size based on the device used. A sternotomy is made. A pocket of an appropriate size is created in the preperitoneal space in the upper abdomen. Alternatively, the LVAD pocket can be created between the posterior rectus sheath and the muscle. Careful attention is given to hemostasis during this process. If applicable, a model of the device is used to confirm the appropriate size of the pocket. The driveline is tunneled, exiting the patient via the right upper quadrant. The device is then placed in the preperitoneal pocket.

The patient is fully heparinized. The distal ascending aorta is cannulated at the level of the pericardial reflection. The right atrium is cannulated—unless a tricuspid valve repair or closure of an atrial septal defect is planned, in which case the patient is bicavally cannulated with umbilical tapes and snares placed around the superior and inferior vena cava cannulas.

Cardiopulmonary bypass is then commenced, maintaining normothermia. The LV is decompressed by placing a vent through a stab wound at the LV apex. The LV apex is then cored. Care must be taken when coring to avoid deviation into the septum or the lateral wall. Any prominent trabeculation or thrombus that may impede inflow into the LVAD inflow cannula is excised. Full-thickness 2-0 Tevdek pledget sutures (Genzyme, Fall River, MA) are placed in a horizontal mattress fashion around the circumference of the LV core. For the fragile myocardium, this suture line is reinforced with a strip of Teflon felt. The sutures are placed through the sewing ring of the inflow cuff, the sewing ring is seated, and the sutures are tied. The cuff is then inserted into the inflow cannula and secured with multiple ties.

The ascending aorta is clamped with a side-biting, partial-occluding clamp. An aortotomy is made, followed by the outflow graft anastomosis using 4-0 Prolene pledget sutures, which involves placement of two mattress sutures buttressed with pledgets in the heel and toe of the graft and corresponding aorta, followed by parachuting of the graft down onto the aorta. BioGlue (CryoLife, Inc., Kennesaw, GA) is applied to the anastomosis just before the clamp is released. The anastomosis is then inspected for bleeding. The outflow graft is clamped.

The de-airing process is then commenced by allowing the heart to fill under mechanical ventilation. The device is de-aired through the outflow housing. The outflow graft is connected to the outflow housing, and a de-airing hole is made in the outflow graft. The cross-clamp is kept on the outflow graft.

With the HeartMate II, the device is started only after the de-airing is completed and the patient is off cardiopulmonary bypass. The device is started at 6000 rpm, the cross-clamp is released, and the device's speed is gradually increased to an adequate rpm level to avoid oversucking of the LV. Throughout this process, the de-airing hole in the outflow graft is kept open.

Chest tubes are inserted. A Gore-Tex pericardial membrane (Gore Medical Products, Flagstaff, AZ) or a CorMatrix (CorMatrix Cardiovascular, Inc., Alpharetta, GA) is sutured to the pericardial edges to minimize reentry injury at reoperation. The sternum is closed in the standard fashion. The abdominal portion of the incision is closed with interrupted sutures, with careful attention to obtain adequate purchase of the fascia and avoid wound dehiscence. The superficial soft tissue and skin are closed in the standard fashion.

In the event of a diffuse coagulopathy with excessive bleeding, the mediastinum is packed with long rolls of gauze and a patch is placed on the skin. The patient is brought back to the operating room after adequate resuscitation and when the coagulopathy has resolved, which generally occurs 24 hours after the initial surgery.

Concomitant Valve Surgery

Preexisting valve pathology is common in patients with heart failure. Patients frequently require concurrent valve procedures at the time of LVAD placement. Patients with mild or more severe aortic insufficiency (AI) should have their native aortic valve repaired or oversewn at the time of VAD implantation. Most cases of AI can be repaired by approximating the raphe of each leaflet.[89,90] Any patient with a mechanical valve in the aortic position should have the aortic valve oversewn with a patch or replaced with a tissue valve to prevent thromboembolism. Treatment of significant mitral regurgitation (MR) is controversial. The cause of most cases of MR in patients with advanced heart failure is annular enlargement secondary to LV dilation. In general, once the LV is unloaded with the

LVAD, MR will likely improve. However, a recent study demonstrated that approximately one third of the patients continued to have significant MR after LVAD insertion.[91] In addition, concomitant mitral valve repair may result in a greater decrement in pulmonary vascular resistance.[92] Currently, we prefer to address significant MR. Severe mitral stenosis needs to be repaired at the time of VAD implantation if it significantly interferes with inflow to the device. Moderate to severe tricuspid regurgitation should be considered for repair or replacement to optimize RV function.[93,94] This is especially important for patients with pulmonary hypertension. Tricuspid valve repair can be performed with annuloplasty repair. If the valve lesions cannot be repaired, a tissue valve is preferred because it has a lower risk of thromboembolism than does a mechanical valve.

Patients who require valve procedures are sicker and have a higher early mortality rate. Furthermore, RV dysfunction is increased in these patients.[95]

Other Concomitant Procedure

Patients with an atrial septal defect or a patent foramen ovale should have these lesions corrected at the time of VAD implantation using standard techniques. Failure to correct these lesions may result in severe hypoxia as a result of right-to-left shunting after the left ventricle is unloaded. Furthermore, any intracardiac thrombus identified in the left atrium or ventricle should be removed before LVAD implantation.

POSTOPERATIVE MANAGEMENT AFTER DURABLE LEFT VENTRICULAR ASSIST DEVICE IMPLANTATION

Early Postoperative Management

Antibiotics are administered preoperatively as prophylaxis for infection and are continued for at least 24 hours after LVAD implantation.

Major effects of a continuous flow LVAD on hemodynamics include increased diastolic pressure and flow. Because a continuous flow pump generates blood flow throughout the entire cardiac cycle, the pulse pressure is greatly reduced. The pulse pressure is influenced by LV contractility, preload, afterload, and pump speed (rpm). An increase in pump speed leads to rising of the diastolic pressure and reduced pulsatility—making it often difficult to palpate the patient's pulse. An arterial catheter is mandatory to monitor blood pressure in the early postoperative period. The mean arterial blood pressure should be maintained between 70 and 80 mm Hg with pressors, because the amount of blood flow through a continuous flow pump is greatly affected by afterload. Vasodilatory hypotension is treated with norepinephrine and arginine vasopressin.[96]

Optimization of RV function is crucial for patients receiving isolated LVAD. RV failure should be aggressively treated with milrinone, dobutamine, epinephrine, and nitric oxide.[12,13,97] If the optimization of RV function cannot be achieved by pharmacologic treatments, RVAD support should be considered.

Ventricular and atrial arrhythmias are managed with standard antiarrhythmic agents, such as amiodarone and lidocaine.

Late Postoperative Management

Late postoperative management focuses on encouraging ambulation and rehabilitation as well as patient education about the care and maintenance of the device. After discharge, patients are followed at the outpatient LVAD clinic weekly for the first month after discharge from the hospital and less frequently thereafter. Although continuous flow technology has dramatically improved survival and quality of life, readmission because of bleeding, cardiac difficulties (heart failure and arrhythmia), infections, and thrombosis is common within the first 6 months after discharge.[98] Comprehensive care from a multidisciplinary medical team, including the patient and caregivers, is mandatory for successful long-term LVAD support.

Anticoagulation

The HeartMate I XVE does not require anticoagulation with heparin or warfarin. In contrast, contemporary continuous flow LVADs such as HeartMate II and HVAD all require anticoagulation with warfarin, as well as antiplatelet therapy with aspirin—and occasionally Persantine—to prevent thromboembolic complications. Intravenous heparin is generally used until the INR reaches target range in the postoperative period. The decision as to when to start anticoagulation and antiplatelet therapies, as well as the dosage, is individualized for each patient based on the device type, risk of thromboembolism, chest tube output, coagulation profile, and treatment plan for the patient.

COMPLICATIONS

Postoperative Bleeding

Bleeding after VAD insertion can be excessive and may result from surgical causes or a diffuse coagulopathy. Significant bleeding can contribute to RV failure, infection, and numerous adverse effects related to multiple blood transfusions. Coagulopathy can result from alterations in the hemostatic system, including dilutional thrombocytopenia and exposure to long-acting antiplatelet or antithrombotic agents. For bleeding caused by a diffuse coagulopathy, platelets, fresh-frozen plasma, or cryoprecipitate may be administered. The decision as to whether to administer these products is based on the profile of INR, partial thromboplastin time, and fibrinogen. Patients with coagulopathy are often hypothermic and should be warmed with heating blankets. A bleeding patient with a rising central venous pressure, downward-trending VAD flows, increasing pressor requirements, and decreasing urine output should be presumed to be experiencing tamponade and should be taken to the operating room immediately for reexploration.

Gastrointestinal Bleeding and Epistaxis

Gastrointestinal (GI) tract bleeding and epistaxis have emerged as major sources of morbidity in patients with continuous flow LVADs.[99] The bleeding event rate after HeartMate II implantation was 0.67 events per patient-year.[100] Possible mechanisms associated with obligate device anticoagulation include acquired von Willebrand disease, GI tract arteriovenous malformations associated with reduced pulsatility, and impaired platelet aggregation.[99] The management of bleeding issues is inextricably linked to the risk of thromboembolic events. Considering the individual risks and benefits, careful reduction of anticoagulation and antiplatelet therapy is required for recurrent events.

Infection

Infection, one of the most common complications in LVAD patients, can manifest as a driveline, pocket, blood, or device endocarditis.[101] Sepsis occurs in 17% to 28% and driveline infection occurs in 14% to 27% of patients receiving contemporary continuous flow LVADs.[3-7,57,66] It is important to prophylactically begin antibiotics preoperatively, as previously described, as well as to treat infections aggressively with antibiotics when they do occur. More aggressive treatments including surgical drainage, wound vacuum-assisted closure therapy, and pump exchange may be necessary. The only way to definitively eradicate device endocarditis is to explant the device. Infection is generally not a contraindication to heart transplantation.

Multisystem Organ Failure

Despite effective restoration of adequate cardiac output for tissue perfusion, some patients progress to develop multisystem organ failure—which is related to the preoperative severity of organ dysfunction. Multisystem organ failure often results from a cascade of events, such as bleeding, sepsis, RV failure, and other events.

Thromboembolism

Thromboembolic complications are a major concern in LVAD patients because of the blood-device interface. Thromboembolic events with continuous flow LVADs have been reported to occur in 5% to 8% of cases.[3-7,57,66] The key factors associated with development of stroke after LVAD implantation are likely to include a previous history of stroke, persistent malnutrition and inflammation, increased severity of heart failure, and postoperative LVAD infections.[102] To avoid conversion to hemorrhagic stroke, anticoagulation and antiplatelet therapies may need to be discontinued.

Right Ventricular Failure

Adequate RV function is essential to achieve sufficient LVAD flow. Significant RV failure is associated with poor outcomes in LVAD recipients. The incidence of RV failure after continuous flow LVAD implantation is approximately 20%.[10-13] The proposed underlying mechanisms include intrinsic myocardial dysfunction and insufficient RV afterload reduction.[10-13] It is important to keep in mind numerous other potential complications after LVAD surgery such as renal failure, infection, and bleeding, which might predispose patients to RV failure. Additionally, patients with a continuous flow pump can develop RV failure from a significant leftward septal shift and distortion of RV geometry caused by LV oversucking. It is therefore critical to avoid setting an excessive pump speed in continuous flow LVAD recipients. Postoperative echocardiography should be performed routinely to monitor RV function, and pump speed should be adjusted to adequate speed levels (rpm).

Signs of RV failure include an elevated central venous pressure (>15 mm Hg), marginal VAD flows of up to 2.2 liter/min/m^2, low mixed venous oxygen saturation, and decreased urine output. RV failure treatment involves aggressive diuresis and starting or increasing milrinone and/or dobutamine as well as nitric oxide in some cases.[91] When RV failure is refractory to medical management, timely insertion of a RVAD is mandatory before end-organ dysfunction progresses.[12-14,103]

Arrhythmia

Cardiac arrhythmia, especially ventricular arrhythmia, is also a common issue in the early and late postoperative periods. Although such arrhythmia may not be lethal in the presence of LVAD, it could put patients at risk of RV failure. Adjustment of pump speed under echocardiography may be necessary to evaluate excessive LV unloading or contact between the inflow cannula and LV wall. In addition to implantable cardioverter–defibrillator therapy, interventions aimed at minimizing the risk of recurrent arrhythmias (e.g., antiarrhythmic medication use and catheter ablation) may also be considered.[104]

Aortic Insufficiency

The development of de novo AI during a continuous flow LVAD support has been reported. After receiving continuous flow LVAD support for 3 years, 38% of patients are expected to develop at least moderate AI.[105] Significant AI can cause the recycling of blood flow from the LVAD outflow graft into the LV, resulting in decreased forward cardiac output, inadequate ventricular unloading, and increased pump work. This may lead to clinical decompensation requiring surgical correction. Because the non-opening of the aortic valve during continuous flow LVAD support is strongly associated with de novo AI development, optimization of pump speed under echocardiography may be necessary to maintain some pulsatility with intermittent aortic valve opening.[105]

Device Malfunction

The severity of a device malfunction varies from minor to fatal. With improvement in device design and engineering, the overall incidence of serious device malfunctions has decreased significantly over time.[106] However, device replacement related to device failure is still inevitable in some patients. Of the 1128 patients implanted with the HeartMate II, serious device failure requiring pump replacement occurred in 71 (6.4%) patients for the following reasons: percutaneous lead damage (36 events, 3.0%), device thrombosis (25 events, 2.1%), infection (7 events, 0.6%), and miscellaneous other (11 events, 0.9%).[107] Most recently, an unexpected abrupt increase in the device thrombosis rate with the HeartMate II has been reported.[108] In an analysis of 382 patients who underwent implantation of the HeartWare HVAD, pump thrombosis occurred in 8.1% of the cohort.[109] Device thrombosis is caused by various mechanical or nonmechanical factors.[110] Close monitoring of lactate dehydrogenase levels and echo-guided ramp studies are useful for early detection of device thrombosis.[110,111] Pump exchange can be safely performed through a subcostal approach.[112]

SUMMARY

MCS represents the standard of care for patients with advanced heart failure from various causes. In addition, MCS may be used as a BTT or a DT and may be the only option for survival in patients with acute cardiogenic shock that is refractory to maximal medical therapy. Tremendous progress has been made over the past 10 years with respect to the evolution of devices, patient selection, surgical techniques, and postoperative management of patients. The limitations of current devices have stimulated research and innovation in an attempt to reduce device size, minimize the invasiveness of the surgical approach, increase device durability, decrease infection, reduce associated thromboembolic complications, and enhance the quality of life of patients with MCS. The outcomes can be expected to improve as the technology continues to evolve.

REFERENCES

1. Rose EA, Gelijns AC, Moskowitz AJ, et al: Randomized Evaluation of Mechanical Assistance for the Treatment of Congestive Heart Failure (REMATCH) Study Group. Long-term mechanical left ventricular assistance for end-stage heart failure. *N Engl J Med* 345(20):1435–1443, 2001.
2. Rogers JG, Butler J, Lansman SL, et al: Chronic mechanical circulatory support for inotrope-dependent heart failure patients who are not transplant candidates: results of the INTrEPID Trial. *J Am Coll Cardiol* 50(8):741–747, 2007.
3. Slaughter MS, Rogers JG, Milano CA, et al: Advanced heart failure treated with continuous-flow left ventricular assist device. *N Engl J Med* 361:2241–2251, 2009.
4. Pagani FD, Miller LW, Russell SD, et al: Extended mechanical circulatory support with a continuous-flow rotary left ventricular assist device. *J Am Coll Cardiol* 54:312–321, 2009.
5. Starling RC, Naka Y, Boyle AJ, et al: Results of the post-U.S. food and drug administration-approval study with a continuous flow left ventricular assist device as a bridge to heart transplantation: a prospective study using the INTERMACS (Interagency Registry for Mechanically Assisted Circulatory Support). *J Am Coll Cardiol* 57:8–2011, 1890.
6. Kirklin JK, Naftel DC, Kormos RL, et al: Fifth INTERMACS annual report: risk factor analysis from more than 6,000 mechanical circulatory support patients. *J Heart Lung Transplant* 32:141–156, 2013.
7. Miller LW, Pagani FD, Russell SD, et al: Use of a continuous-flow device in patients awaiting heart transplantation. *N Engl J Med* 357:885–896, 2007.
8. Peura JL, Colvin-Adams M, Francis GS, et al: Recommendations for the use of mechanical circulatory support: device strategies and patient selection: a scientific statement from the American Heart Association. *Circulation* 126:2648–2667, 2012.
9. Anand I, Maggioni A, Burton P, et al: The Seattle Heart Failure Model: prediction of survival in heart failure. *Circulation* 113(11):1424–1433, 2006.
10. Dang NC, Topkara VK, Mercando M, et al: Right heart failure after left ventricular assist device implantation in patients with chronic congestive heart failure. *J Heart Lung Transplant* 25(1):1–6, 2006.
11. Ochiai Y, McCarthy PM, Smedira NG, et al: Predictors of severe right ventricular failure after implantable left ventricular assist device insertion: analysis of 245 patients. *Circulation* 106(12 Suppl 1):I198–I202, 2002.
12. Kormos RL, Teuteberg JJ, Pagani FD, et al: Right ventricular failure in patients with the HeartMate II continuous-flow left ventricular assist device: incidence, risk factors, and effect on outcomes. *J Thorac Cardiovasc Surg* 139(5):1316–1324, 2010.
13. Takeda K, Naka Y, Yang JA, et al: Outcome of unplanned right ventricular assist device support for severe right heart failure after implantable left ventricular assist device insertion. *J Heart Lung Transplant* 33(2):141–148, 2014.
14. Fitzpatrick JR, 3rd, Frederick JR, Hiesinger W, et al: Early planned institution of biventricular mechanical circulatory support results in improved outcomes compared with delayed conversion of a left ventricular assist device to a biventricular assist device. *J Thorac Cardiovasc Surg* 137(4):971–977, 2009.
15. Zimpfer D, Zrunek P, Roethy W, et al: Left ventricular assist devices decrease fixed pulmonary hypertension in cardiac transplant candidates. *J Thorac Cardiovasc Surg* 133(3):689–695, 2007.
16. Etz CD, Welp HA, Tjan TD, et al: Medically refractory pulmonary hypertension: treatment with nonpulsatile left ventricular assist devices. *Ann Thorac Surg* 83(5):705–2007, 1697.
17. Rao V, Oz MC, Flannery MA, et al: Revised screening scale to predict survival after insertion of a left ventricular assist device. *J Thorac Cardiovasc Surg* 125:855–862, 2003.
18. Topkara VK, Dang NC, Barili F, et al: Predictors and outcomes of continuous veno-venous hemodialysis use after implantation of a left ventricular assist device. *J Heart Lung Transplant* 25(4):404–408, 2006.
19. Topkara VK, Dang NC, Martens TP, et al: Bridging to transplantation with left ventricular assist devices: outcomes in patients aged 60 years and older. *J Thorac Cardiovasc Surg* 130(3):881–882, 2005.
20. Sandner SE, Zimpfer D, Zrunek P, et al: Renal function and outcome after continuous flow left ventricular assist device implantation. *Ann Thorac Surg* 87(4):1072–1078, 2009.
21. Holman WL, Kormos RL, Naftel DC, et al: Predictors of death and transplant in patients with a mechanical circulatory support device: a multi-institutional study. *J Heart Lung Transplant* 28(1): 44–50, 2009.
22. Schulman AR, Martens TP, Christos PJ, et al: Comparisons of infection complications between continuous flow and pulsatile flow left ventricular assist devices. *J Thorac Cardiovasc Surg* 133(3):841–842, 2007.
23. Argenziano M, Catanese KA, Moazami N, et al: The influence of infection on survival and successful transplantation in patients with left ventricular assist devices. *J Heart Lung Transplant* 16:822–831, 1997.
24. Oz MC, Goldstein DJ, Pepino P, et al: Screening scale predicts patients successfully receiving long-term implantable left ventricular assist devices. *Circulation* 92:II169–II173, 1995.
25. Deng MC, Loebe M, El-Banayosy A, et al: Mechanical circulatory support for advanced heart failure: effect of patient selection on outcome. *Circulation* 103:231–237, 2001.
26. Lietz K, Long JW, Kfoury AG, et al: Outcomes of left ventricular assist device implantation as destination therapy in the post-REMATCH era: implications for patient selection. *Circulation* 116(5):497–505, 2007.
27. Cowger J, Sundareswaran K, Rogers JG, et al: Predicting survival in patients receiving continuous flow left ventricular assist devices: the HeartMate II risk score. *J Am Coll Cardiol* 61(3):313–321, 2013.
28. Yang JA, Kato TS, Shulman BP, et al: Liver dysfunction as a predictor of outcomes in patients with advanced heart failure

requiring ventricular assist device support: Use of the Model of End-stage Liver Disease (MELD) and MELD eXcluding INR (MELD-XI) scoring system. *J Heart Lung Transplant* 31(6):601–610, 2012.
29. Matthews JC, Pagani FD, Haft JW, et al: Model for end-stage liver disease score predicts left ventricular assist device operative transfusion requirements, morbidity, and mortality. *Circulation* 121(2):214–220, 2010.
30. Holdy K, Dembitsky W, Eaton LL, et al: Nutrition assessment and management of left ventricular assist device patients. *J Heart Lung Transplant* 24(10):1690–1696, 2005. 16210148.
31. Mancini D, Lietz K: Selection of cardiac transplantation candidates in 2010. *Circulation* 122(2):173–183, 2010. Review.
32. Butler J, Howser R, Portner PM, et al: Body mass index and outcomes after left ventricular assist device placement. *Ann Thorac Surg* 79(1):66–73, 2005.
33. Brewer RJ, Lanfear DE, Sai-Sudhakar CB, et al: Extremes of body mass index do not impact mid-term survival after continuous-flow left ventricular assist device implantation. *J Heart Lung Transplant* 31(2):167–172, 2012.
34. Eshelman AK, Mason S, Nemeh H, et al: LVAD destination therapy: applying what we know about psychiatric evaluation and management from cardiac failure and transplant. *Heart Fail Rev* 14(1):21–28, 2009.
35. Dietl CA, Berkheimer MD, Woods EL, et al: Efficacy and cost-effectiveness of preoperative IABP in patients with ejection fraction of 0.25 or less. *Ann Thorac Surg* 62:401–408, 1996.
36. Mueller HS: Role of intra-aortic counterpulsation in cardiogenic shock and acute myocardial infarction. *Cardiology* 84:168–174, 1994.
37. Sirbu H, Busch T, Aleksic I, et al: Ischaemic complications with intra-aortic balloon counter-pulsation: incidence and management. *Cardiovasc Surg* 8:66–71, 2000.
38. Duncan BW: Pediatric mechanical circulatory support in the United States: past, present, and future. *ASAIO J* 52(5):525–529, 2006.
39. Paden ML, Conrad SA, Rycus PT, et al: Extracorporeal Life Support Organization Registry Report 2012. *ASAIO J* 59(3):202–210, 2013.
40. Burkhoff D, Cohen H, Brunckhorst C, et al: TandemHeart Investigators Group. A randomized multicenter clinical study to evaluate the safety and efficacy of the TandemHeart percutaneous ventricular assist device versus conventional therapy with intraaortic balloon pumping for treatment of cardiogenic shock. *Am Heart J* 152(3):469, e1–8, 2006.
41. Kar B, Gregoric ID, Basra SS, et al: The percutaneous ventricular assist device in severe refractory cardiogenic shock. *J Am Coll Cardiol* 57(6):688–696, 2011.
42. Thiele H, Sick P, Boudriot E, et al: Randomized comparison of intra-aortic balloon support with a percutaneous left ventricular assist device in patients with revascularized acute myocardial infarction complicated by cardiogenic shock. *Eur Heart J* 26(13): 1276–1283, 2005.
43. Siegenthaler MP, Brehm K, Strecker T, et al: The Impella Recover microaxial left ventricular assist device reduces mortality for post-cardiotomy failure: a three-center experience. *J Thorac Cardiovasc Surg* 127(3):812–822, 2004.
44. Griffith BP, Anderson MB, Samuels LE, et al: The RECOVER I: a multicenter prospective study of Impella 5.0/LD for postcardiotomy circulatory support. *J Thorac Cardiovasc Surg* 145(2):548–554, 2013.
45. Lauten A, Engström AE, Jung C, et al: Percutaneous left-ventricular support with the Impella-2.5-assist device in acute cardiogenic shock: results of the Impella-EUROSHOCK-registry. *Circ Heart Fail* 6(1):23–30, 2013.
46. Seyfarth M, Sibbing D, Bauer I, et al: A randomized clinical trial to evaluate the safety and efficacy of a percutaneous left ventricular assist device versus intra-aortic balloon pumping for treatment of cardiogenic shock caused by myocardial infarction. *J Am Coll Cardiol* 52(19):1584–1588, 2008.
47. O'Neill WW, Kleiman NS, Moses J, et al: A prospective, randomized clinical trial of hemodynamic support with Impella 2.5 versus intra-aortic balloon pump in patients undergoing high-risk percutaneous coronary intervention: the PROTECT II study. *Circulation* 126(14):1717–1727, 2012.
48. Cheng JM, den Uil CA, Hoeks SE, et al: Percutaneous left ventricular assist devices vs. intra-aortic balloon pump counterpulsation for treatment of cardiogenic shock: a meta-analysis of controlled trials. *Eur Heart J* 30(17):2102–2108, 2009.
49. Morgan JA, Stewart AS, Lee BJ, et al: Role of the Abiomed BVS 5000 device for short-term support and bridge to transplantation. *ASAIO J* 50(4):360–363, 2004.
50. Worku B, Naka Y, Pak SW, et al: Predictors of mortality after short-term ventricular assist device placement. *Ann Thorac Surg* 92:1608–1612, discussion 1612–1613, 2011.
51. John R, Long JW, Massey HT, et al: Outcomes of a multicenter trial of the Levitronix CentriMag ventricular assist system for short-term circulatory support. *J Thorac Cardiovasc Surg* 141:932–939, 2011.
52. Worku B, Pak SW, van Patten D, et al: The CentriMag ventricular assist device in acute heart failure refractory to medical management. *J Heart Lung Transplant* 31(6):611–617, 2012.
53. Farrar DJ: The Thoratec ventricular assist device: a paracorporeal pump for treating acute and chronic heart failure. *Semin Thorac Cardiovasc Surg* 12:243–250, 2000.
54. Slaughter MS, Tsui SS, El-Banayosy A, et al: Results of a multicenter clinical trial with the Thoratec Implantable Ventricular Assist Device. *J Thorac Cardiovasc Surg* 133(6):1573–1580, 2007.
55. Hasin T, Topilsky Y, Schirger JA, et al: Changes in renal function after implantation of continuous-flow left ventricular assist devices. *J Am Coll Cardiol* 59(1):26–36, 2012.
56. Russell SD, Rogers JG, Milano CA, et al: Renal and hepatic function improve in advanced heart failure patients during continuous-flow support with the HeartMate II left ventricular assist device. *Circulation* 120(23):2352–2357, 2009.
57. Park SJ, Milano CA, Tatooles AJ, et al: Outcomes in advanced heart failure patients with left ventricular assist devices for destination therapy. *Circ Heart Fail* 5(2):241–248, 2012.
58. Frazier OH, Gregoric ID, Cohn WE: Initial experience with non-thoracic, extraperitoneal, off-pump insertion of the Jarvik 2000 Heart in patients with previous median sternotomy. *J Heart Lung Transplant* 25(5):499–503, 2006.
59. Jarvik R: Jarvik 2000 pump technology and miniaturization. *Heart Fail Clin* 10(1 Suppl):S27–S38, 2014.
60. Frazier OH, Shah NA, Myers TJ, et al: Use of the Flowmaker (Jarvik 2000) left ventricular assist device for destination therapy and bridging to transplantation. *Cardiology* 101(1–3):111–116, 2004.
61. Thoennissen NH, Schneider M, Allroggen A, et al: High level of cerebral microembolization in patients supported with the DeBakey left ventricular assist device. *J Thorac Cardiovasc Surg* 130(4):1159–1166, 2005.
62. Wilhelm MJ, Hammel D, Schmid C, et al: Long-term support of 9 patients with the DeBakey VAD for more than 200 days. *J Thorac Cardiovasc Surg* 130(4):1122–1129, 2005.
63. Krabatsch T, Potapov E, Stepanenko A, et al: Biventricular circulatory support with two miniaturized implantable assist devices. *Circulation* 124(11 Suppl):S179–S186, 2011.
64. Wood C, Maiorana A, Larbalestier R, et al: First successful bridge to myocardial recovery with a HeartWare HVAD. *J Heart Lung Transplant* 27(6):695–697, 2008.
65. Wieselthaler GM, O Driscoll G, Jansz P, et al: Initial clinical experience with a novel left ventricular assist device with a magnetically levitated rotor in a multi-institutional trial. *J Heart Lung Transplant* 29(11):1218–1225, 2010.
66. Aaronson KD, Slaughter MS, Miller LW, et al: Use of an intrapericardial, continuous-flow, centrifugal pump in patients awaiting heart transplantation. *Circulation* 125(25):3191–3200, 2012.
67. Nojiri C, Kijima T, Maekawa J, et al: Development status of Terumo implantable left ventricular assist system. *Artif Organs* 25:411–413, 2001.
68. Sakaguchi T, Matsumiya G, Yoshioka D, et al: DuraHeart™ magnetically levitated left ventricular assist device: Osaka University experience. *Circ J* 77(7):41–2013, 1736.
69. Morshuis M, El-Banayosy A, Arusoglu L, et al: European experience of DuraHeart magnetically levitated centrifugal left ventricular assist system. *Eur J Cardiothorac Surg* 35(6):1020–1027, 2009.
70. Farrar DJ, Bourque K, Dague CP, et al: Design features, developmental status, and experimental results with the Heartmate III centrifugal left ventricular assist system with a magnetically levitated rotor. *ASAIO J* 53(3):310–315, 2007.

71. Meyns B, Klotz S, Simon A, et al: Proof of concept: hemodynamic response to long-term partial ventricular support with the synergy pocket micro-pump. *J Am Coll Cardiol* 54(1):79–86, 2009.
72. Copeland JG, Smith RG, Arabia FA, et al: Cardiac replacement with a total artificial heart as a bridge to transplantation. *N Engl J Med* 351(9):859–867, 2004.
73. Copeland JG, Copeland H, Gustafson M, et al: Experience with more than 100 total artificial heart implants. *J Thorac Cardiovasc Surg* 143(3):727–734, 2012.
74. Kirsch M, Mazzucotelli JP, Roussel JC, et al: Survival after biventricular mechanical circulatory support: does the type of device matter? *J Heart Lung Transplant* 31(5):501–508, 2012.
75. Thiele H, Zeymer U, Neumann FJ, et al: Intraaortic balloon support for myocardial infarction with cardiogenic shock. *N Engl J Med* 367(14):1287–1296, 2012.
76. Thiele H, Zeymer U, Neumann FJ, et al: Intra-aortic balloon counterpulsation in acute myocardial infarction complicated by cardiogenic shock (IABP-SHOCK II): final 12 month results of a randomised, open-label trial. *Lancet* 382(9905):45–2013, 1638.
77. Takayama H, Truby L, Koekort M, et al: Clinical outcome of mechanical circulatory support for refractory cardiogenic shock in the current era. *J Heart Lung Transplant* 32(1):106–111, 2013.
78. Goldberg RJ, Gore JM, Alpert JS, et al: Cardiogenic shock after acute myocardial infarction. Incidence and mortality from a community-wide perspective, 1975 to 1988. *N Engl J Med* 325:1117–1122, 1991.
79. Goldberg RJ, Gore JM, Thompson CA, et al: Recent magnitude of and temporal trends (1994-1997) in the incidence and hospital death rates of cardiogenic shock complicating acute myocardial infarction: the second National Registry of Myocardial Infarction. *Am Heart J* 141:65–72, 2001.
80. Hochman JS, Sleeper LA, White HD, et al: One-year survival following early revascularization for cardiogenic shock. *JAMA* 285:190–192, 2001.
81. Hoy FB, Mueller DK, Geiss DM, et al: Bridge to recovery for postcardiotomy failure: is there still a role for centrifugal pumps? *Ann Thorac Surg* 70:1259–1263, 2000.
82. Akay MH, Gregoric ID, Radovancevic R, et al: Timely use of a CentriMag heart assist device improves survival in postcardiotomy cardiogenic shock. *J Card Surg* 26(5):548–552, 2011.
83. Mody KP, Takayama H, Landes E, et al: Acute mechanical circulatory support for fulminant myocarditis complicated by cardiogenic shock. *J Cardiovasc Transl Res* 7(2):156–164, 2014.
84. Farrar DJ, Hill JD, Gray LA, et al: Successful biventricular circulatory support as a bridge to cardiac transplantation during prolonged ventricular fibrillation and asystole. *Circulation* 80:III147–III151, 1989.
85. Wever-Pinzon O, Drakos SG, Kfoury AG, et al: Morbidity and mortality in heart transplant candidates supported with mechanical circulatory support: is reappraisal of the current United network for organ sharing thoracic organ allocation policy justified? *Circulation* 127(4):452–462, 2013.
86. Hong KN, Iribarne A, Yang J, et al: Do posttransplant outcomes differ in heart transplant recipients bridged with continuous and pulsatile flow left ventricular assist devices? *Ann Thorac Surg* 91(6):906–2011, 1899.
87. Kirklin JK, Naftel DC, Pagani FD, et al: Long-term mechanical circulatory support (destination therapy): on track to compete with heart transplantation? *J Thorac Cardiovasc Surg* 144(3):584–603, 2012.
88. Baldwin JT, Mann DL: NHLBI's program for VAD therapy for moderately advanced heart failure: the REVIVE-IT pilot trial. *J Card Fail* 16(11):855–858, 2011.
89. McKellar SH, Deo S, Daly RC, et al: Durability of central aortic valve closure in patients with continuous flow left ventricular assist devices. *J Thorac Cardiovasc Surg* 147(1):344–348, 2014.
90. Goda A, Takayama H, Pak SW, et al: Aortic valve procedures at the time of ventricular assist device placement. *Ann Thorac Surg* 91(3):750–754, 2011.
91. Kitada S, Kato TS, Thomas SS, et al: Pre-operative echocardiographic features associated with persistent mitral regurgitation after left ventricular assist device implantation. *J Heart Lung Transplant* 32(9):897–904, 2013.
92. Taghavi S, Hamad E, Wilson L, et al: Mitral valve repair at the time of continuous-flow left ventricular assist device implantation confers meaningful decrement in pulmonary vascular resistance. *ASAIO J* 59(5):469–473, 2013.
93. Piacentino V, 3rd, Troupes CD, Ganapathi AM, et al: Clinical impact of concomitant tricuspid valve procedures during left ventricular assist device implantation. *Ann Thorac Surg* 92(4):1414–1418, discussion 1418–1419, 2011.
94. Piacentino V, 3rd, Ganapathi AM, Stafford-Smith M, et al: Utility of concomitant tricuspid valve procedures for patients undergoing implantation of a continuous-flow left ventricular device. *J Thorac Cardiovasc Surg* 144(5):1217–1221, 2012.
95. John R, Naka Y, Park SJ, et al: Impact of concurrent surgical valve procedures in patients receiving continuous-flow devices. *J Thorac Cardiovasc Surg* 147(2):581–589, 2014 2.
96. Argenziano M, Choudhri AF, Oz MC, et al: A prospective randomized trial of arginine vasopressin in the treatment of vasodilatory shock after left ventricular assist device placement. *Circulation* 96:II90, 1997.
97. Argenziano M, Choudhri AF, Moazami N, et al: Randomized, double-blind trial of inhaled nitric oxide in LVAD recipients with pulmonary hypertension. *Ann Thorac Surg* 65(2):340–345, 1998.
98. Hasin T, Marmor Y, Kremers W, et al: Readmissions after implantation of axial flow left ventricular assist device. *J Am Coll Cardiol* 61(2):153–163, 2013.
99. Suarez J, Patel CB, Felker GM, et al: Mechanisms of bleeding and approach to patients with axial-flow left ventricular assist devices. *Circ Heart Fail* 4:779–784, 2011.
100. Boyle AJ, Jorde UP, Sun B, et al: Preoperative risk factors of bleeding and stroke during left ventricular assist device support: an analysis of more than 900 HeartMate II outpatients. *J Am Coll Cardiol* 63:880–888, 2014.
101. Topkara VK, Kondareddy S, Malik F, et al: Infectious complications in patients with left ventricular assist device: etiology and outcomes in the continuous-flow era. *Ann Thorac Surg* 90(4):1270–1277, 2010.
102. Kato TS, Schulze PC, Yang J, et al: Pre-operative and post-operative risk factors associated with neurologic complications in patients with advanced heart failure supported by a left ventricular assist device. *J Heart Lung Transplant* 31(1):1–8, 2012.
103. Takeda K, Naka Y, Yang JA, et al: Timing of temporary right ventricular assist device insertion for severe right heart failure after left ventricular assist device implantation. *ASAIO J* 59(6):564–569, 2013.
104. Garan AR, Yuzefpolskaya M, Colombo PC, et al: Ventricular arrhythmias and implantable cardioverter-defibrillator therapy in patients with continuous-flow left ventricular assist devices: need for primary prevention? *J Am Coll Cardiol* 61:2542–2550, 2013.
105. Jorde UP, Uriel N, Nahumi N, et al: Prevalence, significance, and management of aortic insufficiency in continuous flow left ventricular assist device recipients. *Circ Heart Fail* 7:310–319, 2014.
106. Holman WL, Naftel DC, Eckert CE, et al: Durability of left ventricular assist devices: Interagency Registry for Mechanically Assisted Circulatory Support (INTERMACS) 2006 to 2011. *J Thorac Cardiovasc Surg* 146(2):437–441, e1, 2013.
107. Moazami N, Milano CA, John R, et al: Pump replacement for left ventricular assist device failure can be done safely and is associated with low mortality. *Ann Thorac Surg* 95(2):500–505, 2013.
108. Starling RC, Moazami N, Silvestry SC, et al: Unexpected abrupt increase in left ventricular assist device thrombosis. *N Engl J Med* 370(1):33–40, 2014.
109. Najjar SS, Slaughter MS, Pagani FD, et al: An analysis of pump thrombus events in patients in the HeartWare ADVANCE bridge to transplant and continued access protocol trial. *J Heart Lung Transplant* 33(1):23–34, 2014.
110. Uriel N, Han J, Morrison KA, et al: Device thrombosis in HeartMate II continuous-flow left ventricular assist devices: a multifactorial phenomenon. *J Heart Lung Transplant* 33(1):51–59, 2014.
111. Uriel N, Morrison KA, Garan AR, et al: Development of a novel echocardiography ramp test for speed optimization and diagnosis of device thrombosis in continuous-flow left ventricular assist devices: the Columbia ramp study. *J Am Coll Cardiol* 60(18):75–2012, 1764.
112. Ota T, Yerebakan H, Akashi H, et al: Continuous-flow left ventricular assist device exchange: clinical outcomes. *J Heart Lung Transplant* 33(1):65–70, 2014.

CHAPTER 98

Heart Transplantation

Peter Chiu • Robert C. Robbins • Richard Ha

CHAPTER OUTLINE

In the span of 5 decades, cardiac transplantation has progressed from an experimental dream to a treatment reality for patients with heart failure.[1] According to the 2013 Registry of the International Society for Heart and Lung Transplantation, 4096 transplants were performed in 2011. The registry captures an estimated 66% of all transplants. Short- and long-term results improved until 2006, after which they remained stable.[2] Consequently, heart transplantation has continued to be the gold standard for surgical treatment of heart failure. With a rising prevalence of heart failure, it is estimated that more than 25,000 patients annually could benefit from cardiac transplantation.[3] Despite this, the limiting factor continues to be the donor organ supply. Therefore, more importance has been placed on expanding the donor pool while developing alternative medical and surgical therapies. These therapies are meant to either bridge the heart failure patient to heart transplantation or serve as a destination therapy.

This chapter reviews the current practice of cardiac transplantation. Importance is placed on donor and recipient selection, recipient management, identifying and managing complications, and long-term results.

HISTORICAL BACKGROUND

The success of heart transplantation can be traced to the 1950s to 1960s, when pioneering achievements in the laboratory eventually translated to clinical usefulness. The earliest attempts at experimental heart transplantation involved heterotopically implanting hearts in animals through vessels in the neck or abdomen. In 1905, Alexis Carrel and Charles Guthrie[4] revealed that heterotopically transplanted hearts resume spontaneous contraction for several hours. Continued inquiry into the physiologic basis of heart transplantation generated further advancement and interest. This included the important work of Vladimir Demikhov,[5] in which he implanted both heterotopic and orthotopic hearts in the thorax. The advent of hypothermia and mechanical pump oxygenators in the 1950s made orthotopic heart transplantation (OHT) a stronger possibility. In the 1960s at Stanford University, Richard Lower and Norman Shumway[6] continuously refined the technique of experimental OHT. Shumway and his team reported survival of up to 3 weeks after the procedure in dogs.[7] Concurrent with a better understanding of the principles of tissue rejection, critical immunosuppressive regimens developed. The Stanford group demonstrated long-term allograft survival in dogs when a combination of azathioprine and corticosteroids was administered after transplantation.[8]

In 1964, the first heart to be transplanted into a human recipient was performed by James Hardy[9] using a chimpanzee donor heart. In 1967, the first human-to-human heart transplant was performed by Christian Barnard in Cape Town, South Africa.[10] The patient, a 57-year-old man with ischemic heart disease, died on postoperative day 18. Soon thereafter, Shumway and the Stanford group performed the first successful cardiac transplant in the United States.[11] Additional attempts at cardiac transplantation were made without long-term success, resulting in decreased enthusiasm as the problems of acute rejection and infection became more apparent. Along with Stanford, only a handful of centers worldwide continued performing heart transplants. During this time and over the next decade, the outcomes improved as patient selection criteria were refined and postoperative care advanced. In 1973, Philip Caves and associates[12] introduced percutaneous endomyocardial biopsy, which allowed early diagnosis and treatment of acute rejection. The advancement of immunosuppression, including the use of antithymocyte globulin, offered prophylaxis and treatment for acute rejection.[13] The introduction of cyclosporine in 1980 was particularly key in the success of cardiac transplantation. Early studies in the United Kingdom by Roy Calne and associates[14] and in the United States by the Stanford group demonstrated its efficacy.[15] Ultimately, combined immunosuppression regimens consisting of cyclosporine or tacrolimus, azathioprine, and prednisone led to long-term patient survival.

The early success of cardiac transplantation played a key role in increasing the number of heart transplant programs worldwide. In turn, the number of transplant procedures performed yearly grew rapidly in the late 1980s and reached its peak by the early 1990s.[1] Ongoing advances in surgical technique, organ preservation, and immunosuppression continue to yield better outcomes in the modern era of heart transplantation.

INDICATIONS AND EVALUATION FOR HEART TRANSPLANTATION

Recipient Selection

Over the years, selection criteria have emerged to identify patients who will benefit most from heart transplantation. The early reports of long-term survival after transplantation validated the effectiveness of transplantation as a treatment for end-stage heart failure such that it is now considered the gold standard for heart failure surgical treatment. The increasing use of ventricular assist devices (VADs) accounts for the decreasing mortality rate of patients on the waiting list, specifically status 1A patients. Because outcomes have improved, recipient selection has become more liberal. The resulting increase in waiting list size has not been matched by an increase in the donor pool. Even with a corresponding liberalization of donor selection criteria, yearly donor organ allocation numbers 2400 in the United States.[2] This disparity between the growing demand for organs and a limited donor pool has led to careful reevaluation of recipient selection criteria, as well as exploration of alternative medical and surgical therapies for heart failure. It is clear that organs must be allocated in the most rational and judicious manner possible.

The process of selecting appropriate candidates for cardiac transplantation has become increasingly formalized. Instituting a recipient selection meeting has become standard. Before this meeting occurs, candidates for listing should have their clinical history carefully reviewed and a panel of laboratory and supplementary tests performed (Box 98-1). The process of selecting patients should be as objective as possible. The selection committee should include physicians, nurses, coordinators, dieticians, social workers, and physical therapists.

Common indications include New York Heart Association (NYHA) class III or IV heart failure refractory to maximal medical therapy; debilitating ischemia not amenable to interventional or surgical revascularization; or recurrent, symptomatic ventricular arrhythmias refractory to medical therapy, implantable cardioverter defibrillator (ICD) therapy, and surgical treatment.[16] Asymptomatic patients with severe left ventricular dysfunction alone or patients who are adequately managed with medical therapy should not be considered for transplantation.

For ambulatory patients, important techniques of risk stratification have been developed to identify those at low, moderate, or high risk for mortality while awaiting transplantation. Peak exercise oxygen consumption, or Vo_2, is a measure that correlates well with waiting list mortality.[17] Current International Society for Heart and Lung Transplantation (ISHLT) guidelines suggest that patients who tolerate beta blockade qualify for listing if they have a Vo_2 up to 14 mL/kg/min. Those who do not tolerate beta blockade qualify if their Vo_2 is up to 12 mL/kg/min.[18] In support of routine repeat cardiopulmonary testing were two previous studies that showed a correlation between increases in peak Vo_2 on serial exercise testing and improved survival for listed cardiac transplant patients.[19,20]

In addition to Vo_2, Aaronson and colleagues[21] at Columbia University have derived the Heart Failure Survival Score (HFSS) to risk-stratify ambulatory patients awaiting heart transplantation. The HFSS may be particularly useful in patients whose Vo_2 is ambiguous.[18] The HFSS has two components. The noninvasive component is composed of seven parameters: diagnosis of ischemic cardiomyopathy, resting heart rate, left ventricular ejection fraction (LVEF), mean blood pressure, peak Vo_2, serum sodium, and presence of intraventricular conduction delay. The invasive component is composed of eight parameters: diagnosis of ischemic cardiomyopathy, resting heart rate, LVEF, mean blood pressure, peak Vo_2, serum sodium, presence of intraventricular conduction delay, and mean pulmonary capillary wedge pressure. Both models can be used to identify a patient's pretransplant mortality risk. Koelling and colleagues[22] retrospectively reviewed a database of 524 patients undergoing heart failure evaluation and showed that the HFSS

BOX 98-1 Evaluation of Potential Cardiac Transplant Recipients

PHASE I: ASSESSMENT OF CANDIDACY

General Information

- History and physical examination
- Complete blood cell count with differential and platelet count
- Blood chemistry panel
- Liver function tests
- Renal function panel
- Prothrombin and activated partial thromboplastin time
- Urinalysis
- Chest radiograph
- Pulmonary function test

Assessment of Cardiac Function

- Electrocardiography
- Echocardiography
- Radionuclide ventriculography*
- Right-sided heart catheterization*
- Left-sided heart catheterization*
- Endomyocardial biopsy*
- Peak exercise oxygen consumption (V_{O_2}) testing

Screening Tests

- Stool guaiac (three times)*
- Mammography*
- Prostate specific antigen screening*
- Papanicolaou smear*
- Bone densitometry*
- Carotid duplex*

Infectious Disease Screening

- Hepatitis B surface antigen
- Hepatitis B and hepatitis C virus antibodies
- Human immunodeficiency virus serology
- Human T cell leukemia/lymphoma virus (HTLV-1 and HTLV-2) serology
- Cytomegalovirus IgM and IgG titers
- Toxoplasma serology
- Epstein-Barr virus serology
- Rapid plasma reagin
- Purified protein derivative testing

PHASE 2: PRETRANSPLANT DATA

- Blood type and antibody screening
- HLA-DR typing
- Panel-reactive antibody screening
- 12-hour urine collection for creatinine clearance and total protein

*Performed if indicated by history, age, or physical examination.
HLA, Human leukocyte antigen; *Ig*, immunoglobulin.

continues to provide important prognostic information in patients with heart failure with or without beta blocker therapy. In addition, the HFSS has been found to be better than V_{O_2} when applied to all genders and races.[23]

Recent advances in medical therapy for patients with heart failure have resulted in improved patient survival rates. In 2001, the Carvedilol Prospective Randomized Cumulative Survival (COPERNICUS) trial found that treating patients with severe heart failure with carvedilol reduced the 1-year mortality rate to 11% compared with a placebo mortality rate of 19%.[24] Although no randomized trials comparing heart transplantation with medical therapy have been performed, it is clear that in some cases, medical therapy yields short-term outcomes as good as or better than cardiac transplantation. However, because the greatest mortality risk associated with transplantation occurs in the first year, long-term follow-up is needed to compare late survival in medically treated cohorts with that in transplanted cohorts. Freudenberger and coworkers[25] developed a decision analytic model that simulated a randomized clinical trial comparing optimal medical therapy (OMT) with heart transplantation therapy for each individual NYHA class. The authors showed that OMT was superior to heart transplantation for NYHA classes I, II, and III. They also demonstrated life expectancy gains of 113 months, 38 months, and 6 months, respectively. However, heart transplantation was more beneficial than OMT in NYHA class IV patients, with a gain in life expectancy of 26 months.

TABLE 98-1 Underlying Diagnoses of Adult Heart Transplant Recipients 2006–6/2012

Diagnosis	Percentage of Recipients (%)
Cardiomyopathy	54
Coronary artery disease	37
Valvular disease	2.8
Retransplantation	2.5
Congenital heart disease	2.9
Other causes	0.9

From Lund LH, Edwards LB, Kucheryavaya AY, et al: The Registry of the International Society for Heart and Lung Transplantation: Thirtieth Official Adult Heart Transplant Report—2013; focus theme: age. J Heart Lung Transplant 32(10):951–964, 2013.

The most common diagnoses leading to heart transplantation in adults are idiopathic dilated cardiomyopathy and ischemic cardiomyopathy (Table 98-1). Comparison of the 2013 registry of the ISHLT data with the corresponding 2007 registry data reveals new trends. The percentage of recipients with the diagnosis of cardiomyopathy has increased from 48% to 54%. The percentage with coronary artery disease has decreased from 43% to 37%. The diagnosis of valvular, retransplant, and congenital disease has remained relatively stable at 2.8%, 2.5%, and 2.9% respectively. Importantly, survival after transplantation is related to the underlying diagnosis. Risk factors for 1-year mortality include a history of congenital heart disease, prior heart transplant, dialysis, transfusions, ventilator support, and hospitalization. Female donor to male recipient transplants had a higher risk of mortality as well. Five-year mortality risk factors are similar to that of 1-year mortality, but with the added risk of pregnancy, diabetes, and obesity. Finally, at 15 to 20 years, data regarding risk factors for mortality are limited. What is seen is an increased risk with retransplant; however, congenital recipients have better long-term survival than other diagnoses.[2]

Other studies have shown controversial results. In the United Kingdom, Aziz and colleagues[26] performed a retrospective study of 220 heart transplant recipients and compared long-term survival rates of patients with underlying diagnoses of ischemic heart disease and dilated cardiomyopathy. At 5 years, the survival rates were 96% in the dilated cardiomyopathy cohort and 47% in the ischemic heart disease cohort. At 10 years, the survival rates were 92% in the dilated cardiomyopathy cohort and only 29% in the ischemic heart disease cohort. This provocative study suggests that the benefit of transplantation may be greater in patients with dilated cardiomyopathy. The risk of retransplantation for a recipient is also not clear. In one study, cardiac retransplants performed from January 2003 to December 2006 showed improved survival outcomes compared with those in previous eras, with an 82% 1-year survival rate and 75% 3-year survival rate, both similar to rates seen in primary transplant recipients.[27] Atluri and coworkers[28] conducted a retrospective review of 709 heart transplant patients at the University of Pennsylvania, 15 of whom received retransplants. The authors demonstrated an 86% 1-year survival rate and a 71% 5-year rate for the retransplant recipients, which were similar to the primary transplant patients' survival rates of 90% and 79%, respectively.[1] Revisiting these outcomes using the ISHLT and United Network for Organ Sharing (UNOS) databases will be necessary on a periodic basis to help guide recipient listing decisions. Absolute and relative contraindications to cardiac transplantation are listed in Box 98-2.

BOX 98-2 Recipient Contraindications to Heart Transplantation

Absolute Contraindications

- Pulmonary hypertension (PVR > 6 Wood units despite maximal therapy)
- Significant irreversible renal dysfunction (e.g., creatinine clearance < 50 mg/mL/min)
- Significant irreversible hepatic dysfunction (e.g., bilirubin > 3.0 mg/dL)
- Active malignancy

Relative Contraindications

- Active infection (except in the setting of severe device complication, which is a status 1A criterion)
- Age older than 65 years
- Peripheral vascular disease not amenable to surgical or percutaneous therapy
- Diabetes mellitus with secondary organ damage
- Severe lung disease
- Uncorrected abdominal aortic aneurysm greater than 4 to 6 cm
- Systemic infection with immune suppression risk (human immunodeficiency virus, hepatitis B virus, cytomegalovirus)
- Obesity
- Osteoporosis
- Active peptic ulcer disease
- Substance abuse
- Psychiatric disorder
- Noncompliance with medical care

PVR, Pulmonary vascular resistance.

Noncardiac organ dysfunction plays a large role in recipient selection. Pulmonary hypertension continues to be an absolute contraindication to adult cardiac transplantation. Currently, a pulmonary vascular resistance (PVR) greater than 6 Woods units despite maximal vasodilator therapy is considered an absolute contraindication.[18] The increased PVR presents a large load for the donor right ventricle, which often has mild dysfunction secondary to ischemic time. Those with elevated PVRs benefit more from a combined heart-lung transplant. Further details on heart-lung transplantation can be found in Chapter 99. Renal insufficiency is associated with early mortality after heart transplant, especially if dialysis is instituted either preoperatively or postoperatively.[29,30] Analysis of the UNOS database by Schaffer and coworkers clearly shows that patients with severe renal failure benefit from heart-kidney transplantation. This benefit is especially strong for those on dialysis.[31] Hepatic failure also is associated with poor outcomes. As such, combined heart-liver transplants have been accepted as a treatment modality for these patients. Cardiac indications for heart-liver transplants at the time of transplant included restrictive cardiomyopathy (38%), congenital heart disease (21%), idiopathic dilated cardiomyopathy (17%), ischemic cardiomyopathy (8%), and hypertrophic cardiomyopathy (8%). Hepatic indications included cardiac cirrhosis (43%), amyloidosis (28%), hepatitis-induced cirrhosis (10%), metabolic disease (5%), and hemochromatosis (4%). In their analysis of the UNOS database, Schaffer and coworkers noted that the incidence of waiting list mortality was higher in heart-liver candidates, but survival was not different. Further analysis showed that undergoing a heart-liver transplant was associated with enhanced survival compared with undergoing a heart transplant alone.[32]

The consideration of heart transplantation for recipients with human immunodeficiency virus (HIV) has been controversial. However, with the advent of effective antiretroviral therapy, a 10-year survival rate of 90% can be expected.[33] To date, there have been a few case studies, the largest of which reported on seven HIV-positive patients who received a heart. The survival rate at 5 years follow-up for this group of patients was 100%.[34] Further review of outcomes for this patient population is necessary to ensure equivalent survival to HIV-negative patients. The allocation of donor hearts to recipients with known malignancy is also controversial. The ISHLT listing guidelines published in 2006 indicated that those patients with skin cancer, cancers in remission for 5 years, and low-grade cancer were acceptable for transplant candidacy.[18] Possible candidates for cardiac transplant should have appropriate screening studies performed, including prostate specific antigen, mammographic screening, colonoscopy, and Papanicolaou smear. For those with a known history of malignancy, close cooperation with oncology is required to ascertain the prognosis of the patient and adjunctive management.

Increasingly liberal acceptance of other comorbidities is expanding recipient lists. Diabetes mellitus is increasing in the general population and now constitutes 10% of patients undergoing transplantation.[33] A review of the UNOS database revealed that survival for patients with uncomplicated diabetes mellitus was similar to that of heart transplant recipients without diabetes.[35] Amyloidosis is another disease that has been a relative contraindication to heart transplantation. Our center, as well as others, has adopted protocols to determine which patients with amyloidosis would be eligible for a heart transplant. General exclusion criteria include involvement of more than two organs, creatinine that is elevated above 2.0 mg/dL, and an alkaline phosphatase level higher than 250 U/liter. Patients with significant autonomic instability also should be excluded. The results for this cohort are promising, but further review of data is needed.[33] The age requirement for transplant has also been changing. In the 2013 ISHLT report, the number of patients in the 60- to 69-year-old range and the 70 years and older range has increased in comparison with the 1996-2005 cohort. Survival with increasing age is similar in the first five years, excluding those in the older than 75 years cohort.[2] The Scientific Registry of Transplant Recipients (SRTR) database confirms that survival in older cohorts is similar to that of younger recipients.[36] Patients older than 65 years also have a decreased risk of rejection, likely because of physiologic aging of the immune system. This is reflected in the increased rate of infections and malignancy in this older group.[33]

To increase the availability of heart transplantation as an option for older patients, extended criteria cardiac transplantation (ECCT) was started at several centers, most notably by Hillel Laks and colleagues at the University of California, Los Angeles.[37] ECCT patients were offered organs that were not normally used for transplantation. The initial results were promising with similar early survival for non-ECCT recipients, but longer term data were needed.[38] Comparison between ECCT patients and destination therapy left ventricular assist device (LVAD) patients at Duke University Medical Center revealed similar 1-year survival. However, at 3 years, overall survival was better for the ECCT group.[39] A study looking at ECCT in the UNOS database revealed similar 1-year survival of 89% versus 86% for standard criteria versus ECCT. However, at 3 years, there was a significant decrease in survival (66% vs. 77%) for ECCT patients compared with standard criteria patients.[40] The data appear to argue for liberalized use of ECCT to increase the availability of heart transplantation. Other relative contraindications to transplantation include obesity (body mass index [BMI] > 32), osteoporosis, substance abuse, clear history of medical noncompliance not related to socioeconomic difficulties, and lack of dedicated social support.[41,42]

In summary, the decision to list a patient for cardiac transplantation requires examination of multiple medical, psychological, and social factors by the selection committee. Because of the scarcity of donor hearts as well as the need for lifelong medical care, the recipient candidate should be selected for optimal success in the context of increasing indications for cardiac transplantation.

Allosensitization in the Heart Transplant Recipient

ABO blood typing is performed on all candidate recipients. In addition, candidate recipients undergo screening to establish an anti–human leukocyte antigen (anti-HLA) antibody profile. This is referred to as the panel reactive antibody (PRA) test. The PRA is expressed as a percentage of the population against which the recipient has developed antibodies.[43] In some centers, a PRA greater than 10% prompts direct testing of a prospective recipient's serum against a prospective donor's lymphocytes.[44] This is referred to as a crossmatch. A PRA greater than 10% signifies allosensitization. A PRA of greater than 80% indicates a high likelihood that the recipient will have antibodies to a donor.[45] PRA should be seen as a screening test and not an actual quantitative measurement. Loh and colleagues followed cardiac transplant recipients with a PRA of greater than 25% and showed decreased survival in these patients versus recipients with a PRA of less than 25%.[46] A PRA greater than 11% was also shown to be a predictor of earlier and more clinically severe rejection when the UCLA Heart Transplant Group retrospectively reviewed pretransplant PRA screens from 311 patients.[47] Sensitized recipients have a significantly lower 3-year survival compared with those who are not sensitized. This holds true even if the recipient has a negative donor-specific crossmatch.

Newer methods of determining allosensitization in candidate recipients are coming to the forefront. In particular, calculated PRA (cPRA) has emerged as a possibility for traditional PRA calculation. It is derived from HLA frequencies in the 12,000 kidney donors in the United States. It equals the percentage of possible donors that may have one or more HLA antigens that are not compatible with a given recipient. Because it is derived from known crossmatch incompatibility, it may be more accurate than a traditional PRA screening test. Another method of determining possible allosensitization is the virtual crossmatch (VXM). Essentially, the recipient's complete HLA antibody profile is compared with the possible donor's complete HLA antigen profile to determine a match.[49] To be able to perform it correctly requires a complete identification of the recipient's antibody profile. Although some false negatives and false positives can occur, the use of a VXM strategy can increase the number of transplants for sensitized patients, especially when donors from outside the immediate region are considered. The VXM has a positive predictive value of 79% and a negative predictive value of 92%.[50] The risk of antibody-mediated rejection in negative VXM transplants is very low.[51]

The frequency of PRA testing varies from center to center. However, certain guidelines can be followed. For patients without detectable antibodies, PRA testing should be done every 6 months.[52] Patients who have demonstrated detectable antibodies should be tested every 3 months.[52] For patients who have had an infection or blood transfusion, the antibody levels should be checked within 1 to 2 weeks. Patients who have had a VAD placed should have their PRA levels checked every 1 to 2 months.[52] Outcomes for heart transplant are better associated with lower PRA levels rather than peak levels.[43]

Managing allosensitization also varies from center to center. To reduce a potential recipient's antibody load, administration of plasmapheresis, intravenous immunoglobulin (IVIG), and immunosuppressive drugs is pursued.[53-57] A study performed in 1994 first showed the effectiveness of plasmapheresis, reducing a recipient's PRA from 92% to 10%.[58] Plasmapheresis was continued for at least 2 weeks after transplantation, and the PRA level remained low. At Columbia University, the superiority of IVIG (one to three monthly courses of 2 g/kg, divided in four daily doses) over plasmapheresis (administered as one to two monthly courses, two to three times per week) was shown in terms of greater reduction in IgG anti-HLA class I.[59] The study also demonstrated that recipients who received one or two courses of IVIG (2 g/kg) had a mean duration of 3.3 months on the cardiac transplantation waiting list as opposed to 7.1 months for those not receiving IVIG therapy. The Columbia group also suggested that IVIG (2 g/kg) had a better safety profile than plasmapheresis based on the fact that plasmapheresis-treated recipients had more systemic infections and episodes of systemic anaphylaxis (defined by hypotension with pressor support requirement). IVIG has the added benefit of protecting from infection.[60] Itescu and colleagues supplemented IVIG therapy with intravenous cyclophosphamide pulse therapy before cardiac transplantation and as part of a triple immunosuppressive therapy (cyclosporine-based) regimen and demonstrated that this therapy significantly reduced immunologic markers of alloreactivity, prolonged rejection-free intervals, and decreased overall cumulative frequency of rejection.[54] The authors also concluded that cyclophosphamide was superior to mycophenolate in reducing rejection in sensitized recipients.

Leech and coworkers established that the combination of plasmapheresis and IVIG therapy in presensitized cardiac recipients reduced T cell and B cell PRA levels as well as crossmatch positivity.[61] They concluded that the combined treatment allows a successful outcome in the sensitized cardiac recipient. However, it was noted that there was an increased risk of rejection. Rituximab is increasingly being used in sensitized cardiac transplantation recipients. A chimeric anti-CD20 monoclonal antibody, rituximab decreases B cells and has no effect on plasma cells and, thus, no immediate effect on circulating antibody levels.[62] It is often used for recipients refractory to other forms of desensitization.[63] Guidelines for identification and pretreatment of sensitized patients awaiting cardiac transplantation, as well as for treatment during and after the surgery, are outlined in Box 98-3.

HLA typing of the prospective recipient may be done before transplantation. However, prospective matching of recipient and donor HLA antigens is not routinely performed because it delays the donor operating room time by 4 to 8 hours.

Recipient Management after Listing

During the time in which the patient is awaiting transplantation, optimal medical management should be continued. The patient should be seen by a cardiologist regularly. During this time, the patient should also be enrolled in cardiac rehabilitation. The better the patient's physical state heading into the transplant is, the less likely complications will occur.

As a patient's heart failure becomes more severe, oral medical therapy becomes inadequate. At this time,

BOX 98-3 Identification and Treatment of Sensitized Patients

Identification

- Detailed medical history, including history of previous transplants, blood transfusions, and pregnancies; human leukocyte antigen (HLA) typing for HLA class I (A, B) and class II (DR, DQ) within 3 months prior to listing
- Autoantibody crossmatch without dithiothreitol (DTT)
- Panel-reactive antibody (PRA) using complement-dependent cytotoxicity and solid phase assays (sensitized when PRA > 10%)
- If positive for antibodies against C, DQA, or DP loci, then also type for HLA-C, -DQA, and -DP
- If initial autoantibody results are positive, crossmatch with DTT to identify antibody isotype

Preoperative Treatment for PRA Greater than 50%

- Evaluate response to intravenous immunoglobulin (IVIG) with in vitro IVIG inhibition assay
- If patient is hospitalized, adjunctive plasmapheresis should be considered
- IVIG (1 g/kg, with a maximum of 70 g) twice monthly for up to 6 months
- Rituximab administered via central line or peripheral line—first infusion is at 50 mg/hr increasing until a maximum of 400 mg/hr is reached; subsequent infusions at 100 mg/hr increasing to 400 mg/hr as tolerated
- Success of antibody reduction monitored by HLA laboratory (levels obtained before first dose of IVIG and before and after each subsequent IVIG infusion) every 2 weeks
- Post-IVIG testing includes PRA and specificity with and without DTT on full-screen panel (T and B cells) for classes I and II

Perioperative and Postoperative Treatment of Sensitized Patients

- On bypass: one-volume plasmapheresis, reconstituting with 5% albumin (50%) and fresh-frozen plasma (50%)
- Rabbit antithymocyte globulin (1.5 mg/kg IV): first dose after hemostasis achieved in operating room (OR); repeat dosing on postoperative days (PODs) 2, 3, 5, and 7
- Methylprednisolone (10 mg/kg IV, maximum 500 mg) after hemostasis achieved in OR and 2.5 mg (maximum, 125 mg) IV every 8 hours, three times
- IVIG 2 g/kg (maximum, 140 g) divided into two doses on consecutive days in intensive care unit
- Rituximab as outlined in preoperative section
- Mycophenolate mofetil (1000 mg PO twice in POD 1)
- Oral prednisone (1 mg/kg divided into two doses, POD 2)
- Tacrolimus (0.5 mg PO twice a day, PODs 1 to 5)
- Plasmapheresis POD 7, and every other day for four treatments thereafter

institution of intravenous therapy is necessary. This includes the use of dopamine, dobutamine, or milrinone. Dopamine, a sympathomimetic catecholamine, has both alpha and beta agonist activity and should be used at dosages of less than 5 μg/kg/min; at higher dosages, its arrhythmogenic and renal vasoconstrictive effects predominate. Dobutamine, a β_1-adrenergic agonist, is most effective at dosages of less than 10 μg/kg/min. Milrinone, a phosphodiesterase inhibitor with inotropic and vasodilator effects, is effective at dosages of up to 0.5 μg/kg/min. Often, a combination of these medications is used. The use of short-term intravenous dobutamine and milrinone has been found to have an adverse effect on survival in the treatment of acute decompensated heart.[64] As such, the American College of Cardiology Foundation and American Heart Association discourage their routine use in patients with stage D heart failure and patients without evidence of shock or threatened end-organ perfusion. The institution of chronic intravenous inotropic therapy may be reasonable either for patients with cardiogenic shock awaiting definitive therapy or for patients with stage D heart failure, especially those refractory to guideline-directed medical therapy awaiting mechanical circulatory support (MCS) or heart transplantation.[65]

If patients continue to do poorly despite pharmacologic maneuvers, MCS becomes an important option to bridge to transplantation (BTT). MCS devices may be broadly categorized as either short term or long term. Short-term devices include intra-aortic balloon pump (IABP), percutaneous VAD, paracorporeal VAD, and venoarterial extracorporeal membrane oxygenation (VA-ECMO). IABP counterpulsation reduces afterload and augments diastolic coronary perfusion. For this reason, it is especially useful in patients with ischemic cardiomyopathy. These devices can be left in place only for a short period of time (usually several days) and are not effective if left ventricular ejection is severely compromised. There is a risk for infectious complications associated with IABP use, and the 1-year mortality rate is increased in heart transplant recipients who have previously been supported with an IABP.[1]

Percutaneous VADs, such as the Impella[66] and the Tandem Heart,[67] have been shown to be effective in treating severe cardiogenic shock. However, no data have shown an increase in survival with these devices as primary therapy. Severe, refractory cardiogenic shock can also be treated with VA-ECMO. By virtue of their temporary nature, all short-term devices should be a bridge to recovery, to decision, to transplantation, or to long-term device implantation. Early in the experience, temporary circulatory support was high risk, with a detrimental effect that continued into the posttransplant period. Taylor and associates reported a 238% increase in risk of mortality at 1 year in the 52 patients who underwent BTT between 2002 and 2005.[1] Even with increasing experience—163 patients between 2006 and 2011—the requirement for temporary circulatory support still imparted a 180% increase in the risk of mortality at 1-year post transplantation.[2]

With the development of improved mechanical assist devices, long-term MCS has become an invaluable tool in the management of end-stage heart failure. The results of the Randomized Evaluation of Mechanical Assistance for the Treatment of Congestive Heart Failure (REMATCH) trial, which compared 1- and 2-year survival rates of patients with heart failure who were ineligible for transplantation treated with OMT versus LVAD placement, were encouraging.[68] The investigators found a 25% 1-year survival rate and an 8% 2-year survival rate in the medical therapy group, compared with a 52% 1-year survival rate and a 23% 2-year survival rate in the LVAD group. Based on this study, it was clear that developing a VAD with fewer complications might lead to greater 2-year survival.

In 2007, the Investigation of Nontransplant-Eligible Patients Who Are Inotrope Dependent (INTrEPID) trial, a prospective nonrandomized study, further validated the survival benefit of LVAD placement versus OMT with survival rates of 46% versus 22% at 6 months and 27% versus 11% at 1 year, respectively.[69] Patients in the OMT group did not experience any improvement in NYHA functional class, whereas 85% of LVAD patients experienced either minimal or no symptoms. The authors concluded that no further randomized trials should be conducted comparing these two groups because of the overwhelming survival advantage of LVAD versus OMT seen in both REMATCH and INTrEPID trials.

As a follow-up to the REMATCH trial, Slaughter and colleagues evaluated the efficacy of the Heartmate II (Thoratec, Pleasanton, CA) and demonstrated superiority of the continuous flow LVAD as compared with the pulsatile Heartmate XVE. Survival at 2 years in the continuous flow group was 67% compared with 59% in the pulsatile group. Additionally, reoperation because of pump-related complication (device repair, replacement, or explantation including for transplantation) occurred in 24 of 66 patients (36%) receiving a pulsatile device but in only 13 of 134 (10%) of continuous flow LVAD recipients.[70]

Predictably, the effect of LVAD on waiting list survival has been profound. A preliminary study published in 2002 by Aaronson and colleagues[71] retrospectively compared the use of LVADs and high-dose inotropes as BTT in 104 patients at Columbia-Presbyterian Medical Center. Survival to transplantation was 81% in the LVAD group, compared with 64% in the inotrope group. Dardas and coworkers confirmed the benefit of LVAD implantation in an analysis of the Scientific Registry of Transplant Recipients (SRTR) between 2005 and 2010.[72] Patients who received an LVAD with elective status 1A had a significantly lower cumulative hazard of adverse events (death or delisting because of illness), at 1% within 30 days, compared with medically treated status 1A patients with or without IABP, at 6% within 30 days. Patients with an implanted LVAD who were status 1B also had reduced hazard of adverse events compared with status 1B medically treated patients. On the basis of the low risk of death or illness resulting in delisting among patients with an implantable LVAD, the authors suggested downgrading these patients to a status between 1B and 2. On the other hand, paracorporeal VADs were found to have sustained risk justifying status 1A listing indefinitely.

Wozniak and colleagues reviewed the UNOS database for patients receiving VAD BTT between 1998 and

2012.[73] Patients who received any form of ventricular support (either isolated LVAD or biventricular assist device [BiVAD] support) had similar waiting list survival compared with those requiring only inotropic support. However, in patients who received an isolated LVAD, waiting list survival was significantly improved compared with the cohort of medically treated patients including those requiring IABP placement.

Whereas the waiting list outcomes are clear, the effect of LVAD implantation on posttransplantation survival has been controversial. Between 2002 and 2005, pulsatile VAD implantation was associated with a 27% increased relative risk of mortality 1 year post transplantation.[1] This difference in mortality may be attributable to differences among devices, as Russo and colleagues determined in a multivariate analysis of the UNOS database between 2001 and 2006. Patients with extracorporeal VADs had significantly reduced risk-adjusted 90-day graft survival compared with intracorporeal and paracorporeal devices. Posttransplantation survival was similar among patients who were not bridged with a VAD and those receiving either an intracorporeal or a paracorporeal device.[74]

Posttransplant mortality at 4 years among patients bridged to transplantation with a pulsatile LVAD fell significantly as experience developed not only with the operation itself but also with the management of these patients. Those who were bridged to transplantation between 2000 and 2004 were at 30% greater risk of mortality than those who received pulsatile devices between 2004 and 2008. In the latter period, Nativi and associates reported similar outcomes between patients who underwent BTT with pulsatile and continuous-flow devices, and these were not significantly different from patients who did not receive an LVAD.[75] Contemporary registry data have confirmed this finding with no significant difference in intermediate survival up to 6 years post transplantation among patients who preoperatively had an LVAD, patients who required inotropic support, and patients requiring neither.[2]

In spite of the benefits of pretransplant implantation on waiting list outcomes and the growing evidence that modern LVADs do not necessarily affect posttransplantation outcomes, the use of LVADs is not without risk. First, patients are exposed to the potential morbidity of device complication; however, this may be acceptable given the improved survival on the waiting list. Of the potential complications that may prompt status 1A listing for heart transplantation (i.e., thromboembolism, device infection, and life-threatening arrhythmia), only infection was associated with worse survival at both 1 year and 10 years post transplantation.[76]

Another potential difficulty with LVAD implantation is the associated increase in PRA.[77] Although this increase in PRA could be attributable to transfusion of cellular blood products,[78] the avoidance of leukofiltered cellular blood products has not been shown to be of benefit.[48,79] LVAD type appears to have an impact on the development of allosensitization related to the interaction between the patient and the device as has been shown in single-institution retrospective studies.[80,81] The impact of PRA on the subsequent management of patients, including the need to reduce HLA antibodies, has been discussed previously.

BiVAD implantation is associated with significantly worse outcomes than LVAD implantation alone.[82,83] Additionally, there are patients for whom LVAD may be contraindicated (e.g., those with aortic insufficiency, acquired VSD, or right ventricular failure). The total artificial heart was thus conceived as a means to provide biventricular support. In 2004, Copeland and colleagues reported a 79% success rate in BTT, which was superior to historically matched controls.[84] However, the overall experience with the total artificial heart remains limited, and this remains an area of active investigation.

ORGAN PROCUREMENT AND PRESERVATION

Donor Selection

The selection of donors for cardiac transplantation follows the guidelines outlined in Box 98-4. The regional organ procurement organization is the first group to begin the selection process, at which time information is collected regarding cause of death, body size, ABO blood type, serologies (including human immunodeficiency virus, hepatitis B virus, and hepatitis C virus), and clinical course. A transplant physician then performs a secondary screen. This includes a review of relevant history, baseline electrocardiogram, chest radiograph, laboratory data, echocardiogram, and in some cases cardiac catheterization. The final screen is performed by the procuring surgeon at the donor hospital site.

Potential donors must meet standard requirements for brain death. Donors who died from cardiac causes, have had an acute coronary event, have intractable arrhythmias, or have deleterious structural abnormalities should be excluded.[85] In addition, donors with a history of severe chest trauma causing severe cardiac contusion with resulting cardiac depression should be excluded. The importance of left ventricular hypertrophy is being reevaluated in light of the shortage of donor organs. Previously, posterior wall (PW) and interventricular

BOX 98-4 Cardiac Donor Selection Criteria

- Age younger than 55 years
- No history of chest trauma or cardiac disease
- No prolonged hypotension or hypoxemia
- Meets hemodynamic criteria:
  - Mean arterial pressure greater than 60 mm Hg
  - Central venous pressure 6 to 10 mm Hg
- Inotropic support less than 10 mg/kg/min (dopamine or dobutamine)
- Normal electrocardiogram
- Normal echocardiogram
- Normal cardiac angiography*
- Negative hepatitis B surface antigen, hepatitis C virus, and HIV serologies

*Performed as indicated by donor age and history.

septal (IVS) thickness was expected to be less than 1.2 cm. In a study by Goland and associates, donors with a thickness of up to 1.7 cm showed no decrease in survival, arguing for more liberal use of hearts with left ventricular hypertrophy.[86] Donor age younger than 55 years is preferable, although on occasion older donors are considered. Many transplant centers, including Stanford University, have become more flexible regarding the donor age criterion. For all male donors older than 45 years and female donors older than 50 years, cardiac catheterization with coronary angiography should be performed to rule out significant coronary artery disease.[87] Relative contraindications include positive hepatitis B or C serology, sepsis, history of cancer, or prolonged hypotension or hypoxemia.

Reviewing the 2013 data from the ISHLT registry reveals important trends. The use of donors with diabetes mellitus (3.0%) and hypertension (14%) is increasing. Expansion of the donor pool has been achieved by liberalization of other criteria as well, including increasing ischemic time, mild valvular abnormality, and mild coronary disease.[88] The use of hearts that have undergone longer arrest and resuscitation has also been noted.[89] Given this recent liberalization, long-term outcomes with these organs for non-ECCT recipients have not yet been determined. In addition, some data indicate that donor characteristics, such as older age and prolonged ischemic time, may interact synergistically to increase recipient mortality risk.[90]

Donor Management

Meticulous and aggressive hemodynamic management of donors can increase the cardiac donor pool.[91,92] Because all patients have brain death, they are often hemodynamically unstable as a result of neurogenic shock, excessive fluid losses, and bradycardia.[93,94] Detailed fluid management is required, with intravascular volume replacement given to maintain a central venous pressure (CVP) between 6 and 10 mm Hg. Whereas excessive use of inotropes or vasoconstrictors is frowned on, the use of low-dose dopamine is associated with improved outcomes after heart transplant.[95] Intravenous vasopressin can be used to help control diabetes insipidus, which is common in patients with brain death. Ventilator settings should be set with the plan to offer the donor lungs for transplant. The settings should be adjusted to, at most, a fractional inspired oxygen of 40% and a positive end-expiratory pressure of 5 cm H_2O to prevent atelectasis. Although some donor organizations have begun to liberalize transfusion triggers, the outcomes are unclear. As such, a minimal hematocrit of 30% should be maintained. The blood should be cytomegalovirus-negative and leukocyte-filtered blood if possible.[96]

Serial echocardiograms should be pursued in the setting of brain injury. A single echocardiogram may provide initial information but likely is not representative of the true function of the heart. Cardiac dysfunction, as confirmed by echocardiogram, occurs in up to 42% of brain-dead patients, and the correlation between these abnormalities and actual pathologic findings is often poor.[97,98] Placement of a pulmonary artery catheter is useful in assessing initial cardiac function and the response to therapy. Typical hemodynamic goals include a mean arterial pressure of greater than 60 mm Hg, a CVP of 6 to 10 mm Hg, and a pulmonary capillary wedge pressure of less than 12 mm Hg.

The Papworth group has reported an increase in organ retrieval of 30% by using an aggressive protocol for donor management.[99,100] This included placement of a pulmonary artery catheter to guide the process of resuscitating the patient and provision of hormonal therapy, including thyroxine,[101] cortisol, antidiuretic hormone, and insulin. Using this protocol, most donors originally deemed unacceptable by strict hemodynamic criteria were converted into acceptable donors. The Crystal City Guidelines outline another management strategy for potential organ donors. The algorithm begins with conventional management; correction of acidosis, hypoxemia, and anemia; and appropriate titration of inotropes to maintain adequate organ perfusion. This is then followed by an initial echocardiogram. If the LVEF is greater than 45%, the heart is suitable for recovery. If the LVEF is less than 45%, hormonal resuscitation and hemodynamic management with a pulmonary artery catheter should be undertaken. The heart will be recovered only if appropriate hemodynamic parameters can be reached.[87]

Organ Allocation

Allocation algorithms have been developed to facilitate organ distribution. In the United States, organ allocation is governed by UNOS. The current heart algorithm takes into account medical urgency, time on the waiting list, and blood type.[102] The waiting list status categories (1A, 1B, 2, and inactive) are defined in Table 98-2. Listing can also be modified by age; for example, adolescent donor hearts are preferably allocated to pediatric recipients. Geographic location also plays an important role in the allocation. Prior to 2006, local thoracic organ allocation was performed before regional allocation. After 2006, thoracic organ allocation by UNOS changed such that regional allocation played a larger role. The policy change allowed for greater regional sharing of organs with a goal of increased allocation to status 1A patients and reduced waiting list mortality. As a result of the change in policy, Schulze and coworkers found an overall increase in waiting list time for status 1A and 1B patients of 17.8 days. However, there was a decrease in waiting list mortality after the change (13.3 vs. 7.9%; $P < 0.001$). At the same time, 2-year posttransplantation survival improved (82.7% vs. 85.4%; $P < 0.001$).[103]

Donor and Recipient Matching

Prospective recipients and donors must be ABO blood type compatible, although not necessarily ABO identical.[104] In the past, differences up to and greater than 20% could be tolerated. For recipients whose PVR remains at the upper limit of acceptable, a donor whose body size is at least equal to that of the recipient should be chosen to decrease the likelihood of acute right-sided heart failure.[105] In the case of patients with normal PVR, the lower limit of an acceptable size match is an area of active

TABLE 98-2 **UNOS Medical Urgency Status Categories**

Status Level	Category
Status 1A	The candidate is admitted to the transplant hospital that registered the candidate on the waiting list, or an affiliated Veterans Administration (VA) hospital, and the candidate also meets at least one of the requirements: 1. Has one of the following MCS devices in place: TAH, IABP, ECMO. 2. Requires continuous mechanical ventilation. 3. Requires continuous infusion of a single high-dose intravenous inotrope or multiple intravenous inotropes, and requires continuous hemodynamic monitoring of left ventricular filling pressures. 4. A candidate who is at least 18 years old at the time of registration, and may or may not be currently admitted to the transplant hospital, may be assigned adult status 1A if the candidate meets at least one of the following requirements: a. Has one of the following MCS devices in place: LVAD, RVAD, BiVAD.* b. Candidate has MCS and there is medical evidence of significant device-related complications.†
Status 1B	At least one of the following devices or therapies in place: 1. LVAD, RVAD, or BiVAD. 2. Continuous infusion of intravenous inotropes.
Status 2	All other actively listed patients.
Inactive	Temporarily unsuitable for transplant. The patient will not receive any heart offers.

*The candidate may be registered as adult status 1A for 30 days at any point after being implanted once an attending physician determines the candidate is medically stable. The 30 days do not have to be consecutive. However, if the candidate undergoes a procedure to receive another device, then the candidate qualifies for a new term of 30 days. Any 30 days granted by the new device would substitute and not supplement any time remaining from the previous adult status 1A classification.

†Thromboembolism, device infection, mechanical failure, or life-threatening ventricular arrhythmias. A candidate's sensitization is not an acceptable device-related complication to qualify as adult status 1A.

BiVAD, Biventricular assist device; *ECMO,* extracorporeal membrane oxygenation; *IABP,* intraaortic balloon pump; *LVAD,* left ventricular assist device; *MCS,* mechanical circulatory support; *RVAD,* right ventricular assist device; *TAH,* total artificial heart; *UNOS,* United Network for Organ Sharing.

From Department of Health and Human Services: Organ procurement and transplantation network: policies. Apr 10, 2014. http://optn.transplant.hrsa.gov/ContentDocuments/OPTN_Policies.pdf#nameddest=Policy_06.

debate. Jayarajan and associates demonstrated that a donor-to-recipient weight ratio as low as 0.6 may be tolerated in gender-matched patients and in male-to-female heart transplants. However, female-to-male heart transplants were found to have increased hazard of mortality and reduced median survival compared with gender-discordant size-matched individuals.[106] In rare situations, small hearts may be heterotopically transplanted into larger recipients, but the outcomes in these cases are significantly worse than size-matched OHT.[107] In patients with an elevated PRA, either a prospective or a virtual crossmatch may be performed with the potential donor.[108] A positive crossmatch portends a high likelihood of hyperacute rejection, and in such cases the donor organ cannot be accepted for that recipient.

Donor Operative Technique

Retrieval of the donor heart typically occurs as part of a multiorgan procurement. In most cases, the cardiothoracic team must work in conjunction with an abdominal team that is procuring the liver and/or kidneys. Communication between the two teams is essential to prevent unnecessary prolongation of ischemic time. This includes agreeing on a start-time for the procuring teams based on the status of the recipient teams. Delays to donor crossclamp may occur if the heart recipient requires a redo sternotomy, especially in the case of a previous LVAD patient who requires explantation. There are minor modifications to the heart procurement technique when either one lung or both lungs are being procured.

A median sternotomy is performed, and the pericardium is opened longitudinally. The heart is carefully inspected for external signs of trauma, infarction, congenital anomalies, and overall right and left ventricular function. The coronary arteries are palpated to evaluate for coronary artery disease. Significant abnormalities preclude use of the donor heart in transplantation. The ascending aorta is dissected from the pulmonary artery and encircled with an umbilical tape. The superior vena cava (SVC) is mobilized to the level of the azygos vein and is then encircled with a single heavy silk tie and snared loosely. The azygos vein is then doubly ligated, but it is not divided.

When the abdominal procurement team has completed their dissection, 30,000 units of intravenous heparin is administered to the donor. A cannula for infusion of cold cardioplegia is inserted into the ascending aorta and secured. If the lungs are being procured, a pulmonoplegia line is inserted through a purse-string stitch and into the main pulmonary artery. Any central venous lines are withdrawn high into the SVC. The SVC is then snared tightly to limit venous return to the heart. The right heart is decompressed, and the donor is exsanguinated by incising the inferior vena cava (IVC) at the diaphragm ensuring enough of a cuff for implantation of both the heart and the liver. Sufficient length on the SVC and IVC will be needed for later bicaval anastomoses. Blood and perfusate from the liver will drain into the right pleural cavity, and suction should be available to keep the field clear. The left side of the heart is decompressed by incising the left inferior pulmonary vein.

Alternatively, if the lungs are also being procured, the left side of the heart is decompressed by amputating the left atrial appendage. As the heart empties, the aortic cross-clamp is placed and cold crystalloid cardioplegia (10 mL/kg) solution is rapidly infused into the aorta ensuring diastolic arrest. It is important to continually observe the left ventricle for distention. Pulmonoplegia solution is also rapidly infused into the pulmonary artery if the lungs are being procured. While the plegia solutions are being delivered, the thoracic organs are topically cooled with several liters of ice-cold slush.

When the infusions are completed and the heart has been appropriately cooled and arrested, the chest is emptied of the cold slush. The heart is rapidly excised by dividing the four pulmonary veins, the IVC, the SVC, the aorta (as high as possible), and the pulmonary arteries. If the lungs are being procured, a short cuff of left atrial tissue may be retained with the pulmonary veins, and the pulmonary artery is divided at the bifurcation of the left and right pulmonary arteries. Once removed from the donor, the heart is examined for debris, including the possibility of an amputated central venous catheter. It is then rinsed in cold saline and sterilely bagged first in cold preservation solution and then in slush. The heart is then placed in a container filled with cold slush and transported in a cooler designated specifically for this purpose. A section of donor pericardium is additionally harvested in the event that it is needed for reconstruction.

Organ Preservation

Several strategies are used for cardiac preservation during organ retrieval and ischemic storage, including the use of hypothermia, cardioplegia, and preservation solutions.[109] Hypothermia at 4° C to 8° C markedly decelerates metabolism and is used during organ retrieval, storage, and transport.[110] Cardioplegia is used to arrest electrical activity of the heart.[111] Adequate decompression of the ventricles during organ retrieval limits injury to the heart during procurement. The heart may be stored in any of a variety of preservation solutions, which can be broadly categorized as intracellular and extracellular types, based on their ionic composition. Intracellular solutions have a moderate to high potassium concentration and little calcium or sodium, whereas extracellular solutions have a high sodium concentration and a low to moderate concentration of potassium.[112] In addition to electrolyte constituents, these solutions often contain impermeants and colloids to prevent the development of intracellular edema. Most contain glucose to prevent intracellular acidosis secondary to anaerobic metabolism. Many contain antioxidant additives to protect against reperfusion injury. The possibility of improving donor heart preservation with additives to the preservation solution is being studied, and rho-kinase inhibitor[113] and small interfering RNA[114] have been proposed. In rare cases, preservation solutions are used as alternatives to standard cardioplegia during organ procurement.

Cardiac preservation currently is limited to 4 to 6 hours of cold ischemic storage. Longer ischemic periods adversely affect recipient survival.[51] Most notably, in February 2007, the U.S. Food and Drug Administration (FDA) approved the clinical use of a system developed by TransMedics, Inc., called the Organ Care System (OCS). OCS involves perfusing donor hearts with warm, oxygenated, nutrient-rich blood while maintaining the organ in a beating, functioning state in transit, with the hope that the heart arrives in a healthier and more dynamic state. The recently completed global clinical trial PROCEED II evaluated the safety and performance of the OCS for the preservation of donor hearts during transplantation, but results have not yet been published.[115] Several cardiac transplant recipients have received donor hearts that have undergone OCS and have recovered successfully. Long-term results and the comparison between OCS and standard organ preservation methods have yet to be elucidated.

RECIPIENT OPERATIVE TECHNIQUE

Both orthotopic and heterotopic techniques for clinical heart transplantation are performed. Orthotopic transplantation is performed in most cases, whereas heterotopic transplantation is reserved for cases in which the recipient has significant pulmonary hypertension or the donor is notably smaller than the recipient.

For many years, the technique of Lower, Stofer, and Shumway, described in 1961, was the standard.[6] This technique, often referred to as the biatrial or standard technique, involves excision of the recipient heart at the mid-atrial level and sewing corresponding anastomoses between the donor and recipient left atrium, right atrium, aorta, and pulmonary artery. This technique permits short operative times and avoids potential complications that result from individual caval and pulmonary venous anastomoses, including but not limited to stenosis and thrombosis. Disadvantages of the method include distortion of atrioventricular geometry, which can result in atrial enlargement, atrioventricular valve insufficiency, impaired atrial function, atrial thrombosis, and sinoatrial node dysfunction.[116,117] Barnard[118] introduced an important modification of the technique in 1968: the incision in the donor heart's right atrium was extended from the opening of the IVC into the base of the right atrial appendage, rather than into the SVC, avoiding the region of the sinoatrial node, which may be injured because of its proximity to the right atrial suture line in the classic orthotopic standard technique.

The standard technique is declining in popularity. Newer techniques, including the "bicaval" and "total" techniques, offer the advantage of better preservation of atrial geometry.[119-121] In the bicaval technique, the native recipient's right atrium is excised, and separate SVC and IVC anastomoses are made in addition to the left atrial, aortic, and pulmonary artery anastomoses. The total technique uses separate SVC, IVC, aortic, and pulmonary artery anastomoses as with the bicaval technique. However, rather than use a single left atrial anastomosis, the total technique uses separate right and left pulmonary vein anastomoses. The left atrial remnant is divided longitudinally leaving left and right pulmonary vein cuffs, which are then anastomosed to the left and right pulmonary vein orifices in the donor heart's left atrium. Technical considerations include shortening of the IVC, kinking of the pulmonary artery, and SVC stenosis; an early series from Stanford University reported a 2.4% incidence of SVC stenosis.[122] The total technique may be associated with additional complications, including bleeding from inaccessible pulmonary vein suture lines and pulmonary vein stenosis.

The bicaval technique is now the most commonly used anastomotic method with 62.0% of recipients undergoing this operation and 34.7% undergoing biatrial anastomosis in 2007 as compared with 2.3% and 97.6% in 1997.[123,124] The bicaval technique has been increasing in popularity because of the lower incidence of permanent pacemaker implantation, improved tricuspid valve function, and improved right atrial hemodynamics. With respect to mortality benefit, Weiss and coworkers demonstrated using the UNOS database that although gross mortality was higher in patients undergoing biatrial anastomosis at 24% compared with bicaval anastomosis at 18%, this difference was eliminated after controlling for confounders. However, Davies and colleagues were able to show, in a larger cohort, favorable survival for the bicaval technique compared with both biatrial and total orthotopic techniques.[124-127]

Orthotopic Standard Technique

In the orthotopic standard technique, the recipient is positioned supine on the operating room table. The chest is entered through a median sternotomy, and the pericardium is opened longitudinally. After heparinization, cardiopulmonary bypass (CPB) is initiated via cannulas in the ascending aorta, SVC, and IVC. Snares are placed around the SVC and IVC for total CPB, and the patient is cooled to 28°C.

Once the donor heart has been brought to the operating room, the recipient heart is excised. The aorta is cross-clamped proximal to the aortic cannulation site. The right and left atrial walls, atrial septum, pulmonary artery, and aorta are divided. The pulmonary artery and aorta should be divided just above the semilunar valves (Fig. 98-1*A*).

The donor heart is prepared for implantation by excising the tissue between the orifices of the four pulmonary veins leaving a single large opening. The right atrium is then opened, beginning from the lateral aspect of the IVC and extending into the base of the right atrial appendage. The heart is carefully examined for any valvular or congenital anomalies.

In the original description of the standard technique, anastomoses were performed in the following order: left atrium, right atrium, pulmonary artery, and aorta. In an attempt to achieve earlier reperfusion, the sequence of anastomoses may be altered. For example, in the case of prolonged ischemic time, the aortic anastomosis can be performed immediately after the left atrial anastomosis allowing the aortic crossclamp to be removed. The original sequence of anastomoses is described as follows.

The anastomosis of the donor and recipient left atria is performed with a double-armed running 3-0 or 4-0 polypropylene suture. The first stitch is placed in the recipient left atrium at the level of the left superior pulmonary vein and at the base of the donor left atrial appendage. The suture line is continued around the superior and inferior borders of the left atrium and then tied along the interatrial septum. Once this suture line is complete, the left atrial appendage is cannulated with a line of cold saline to facilitate endocardial cooling. In addition, cold saline is continuously infused into the pericardial well to achieve topical cooling.

The two right atria are anastomosed with a double-armed running 4-0 or 5-0 polypropylene suture (see Fig. 98-1*B*). The first stitch is placed through the midpoint of the donor septum and through the midpoint of the suture line along the atrial septum. The suture line is continued inferiorly first, and then the superior suture line is completed. The two ends of the suture are tied along the right atrial free wall. Once the right atrial anastomosis is completed, systemic rewarming is initiated.

The donor and recipient pulmonary arteries are trimmed to an appropriate length and anastomosed with a running 4-0 polypropylene suture. The donor and recipient aortas are also trimmed and anastomosed with a running 4-0 polypropylene suture (see Fig. 98-1*D*).

The ascending aorta and pulmonary artery are cleared of air. The SVC and IVC snares are then released, followed by the aortic crossclamp. De-airing is continued as needed. Transesophageal echocardiography aids in de-airing the heart and assessing cardiac function. The line in the left atrial appendage is removed, and the hole is oversewn. Temporary atrial and ventricular wires are placed in the transplanted heart. The heart is then allowed to recover fully. Defibrillation may be necessary. After at least 30 minutes of reperfusion, the patient is gradually weaned from CPB and the cannulas are removed. Intravenous methylprednisolone (500 mg) is administered. Mediastinal drains are placed, as well as pleural chest tubes if the pleura were opened. The chest is then closed in the standard fashion.

Orthotopic Bicaval Technique

In recent years, the bicaval technique for OHT has become the preferred approach at most transplant centers. The bicaval anastomosis was reported in 1991 by Dreyfus and colleagues[119] Several modifications distinguish it from the standard approach. First, the recipient SVC is cannulated just below the innominate vein junction, and the IVC is cannulated at the diaphragm. Recipient cardiectomy is performed as a two-step procedure. In the first step, the heart is transected at the mid-atrial level, the aorta and pulmonary artery are divided, and the heart is removed. In the second step, the posterior walls of both atria are removed; on the right side, the SVC and IVC are transected at their junction with the right atrium, and on the left side, the left atrium is trimmed, leaving a cuff of tissue around the pulmonary vein orifices (Fig. 98-2*A*). The donor heart's left atrium is trimmed, leaving a single orifice where the pulmonary vein entry sites had been, and the right atrium remains intact (see Fig. 98-2*B*). In the bicaval approach, the typical sequence of anastomoses is left atria, venae cavae, pulmonary arteries, and aortas. The left atrial, pulmonary artery, and aortic anastomoses

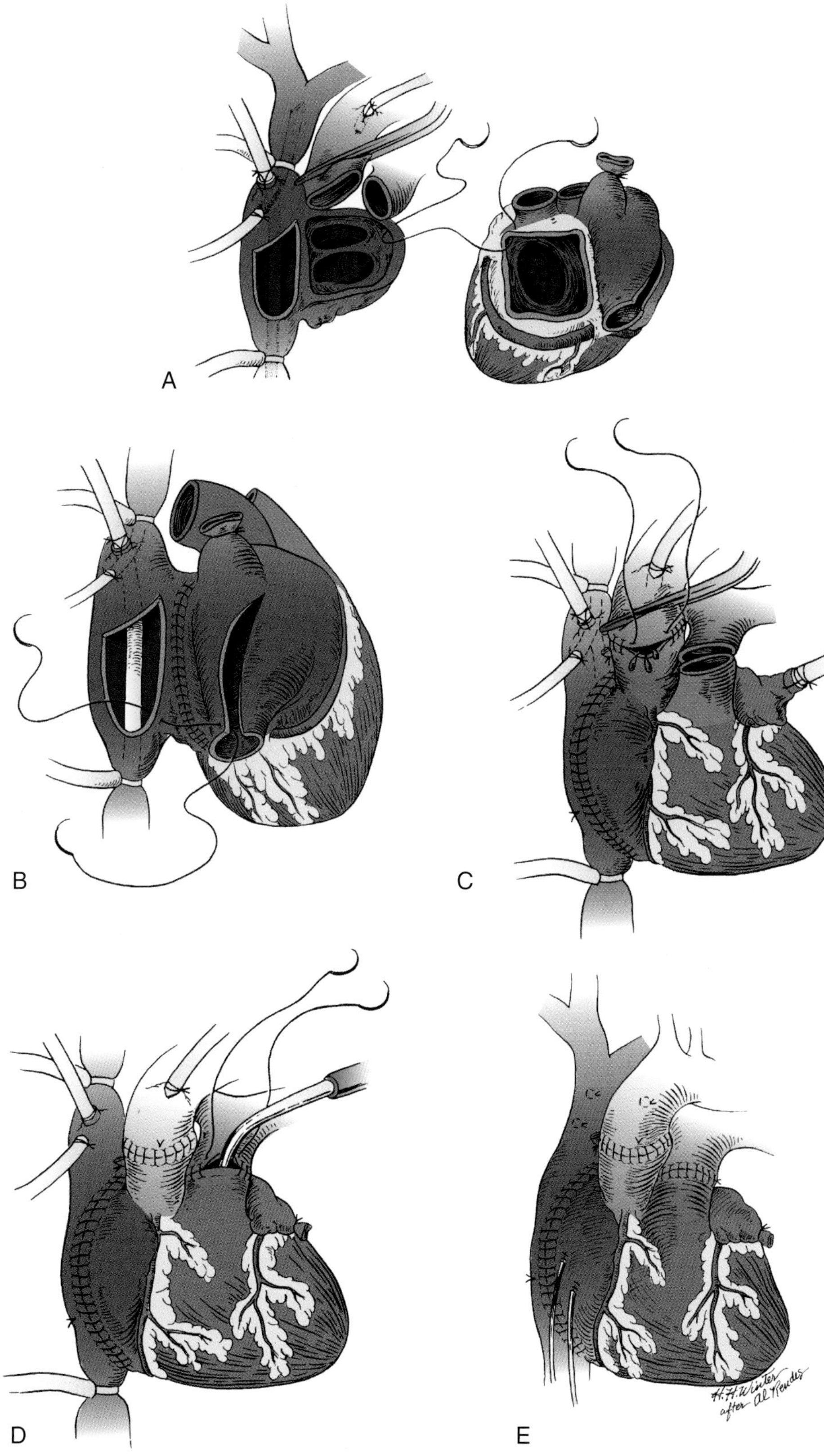

FIGURE 98-1 ■ Biatrial or "standard" technique for orthotopic heart transplantation. **A,** Cannulation technique is similar to that performed in routine cardiac procedures with central cannulation. Tapes have been placed around the superior and inferior venae cavae, and the aorta has been cross-clamped to exclude the heart from the circulation. The recipient's heart has been excised at the atrioventricular groove. The superior vena cava (SVC) of the donor's heart has been ligated, and the left atrial anastomosis has been started. **B,** The left atrial anastomosis has been completed. The incision in the right atrium of the donor heart is curved away from the SVC and the adjacent sinoatrial node. The right atrial anastomosis is begun. **C,** The right atrial, pulmonary artery, and aortic anastomoses are completed. The aortic crossclamp is removed, and the patient is weaned from cardiopulmonary bypass. **D** and **E,** When the heart is fully recovered, the bypass cannulas are removed. (From Baumgartner WA, Reitz BA, Oyer PE, et al: Cardiac homotransplantations. *Curr Probl Surg* 16:1–61, 1979.)

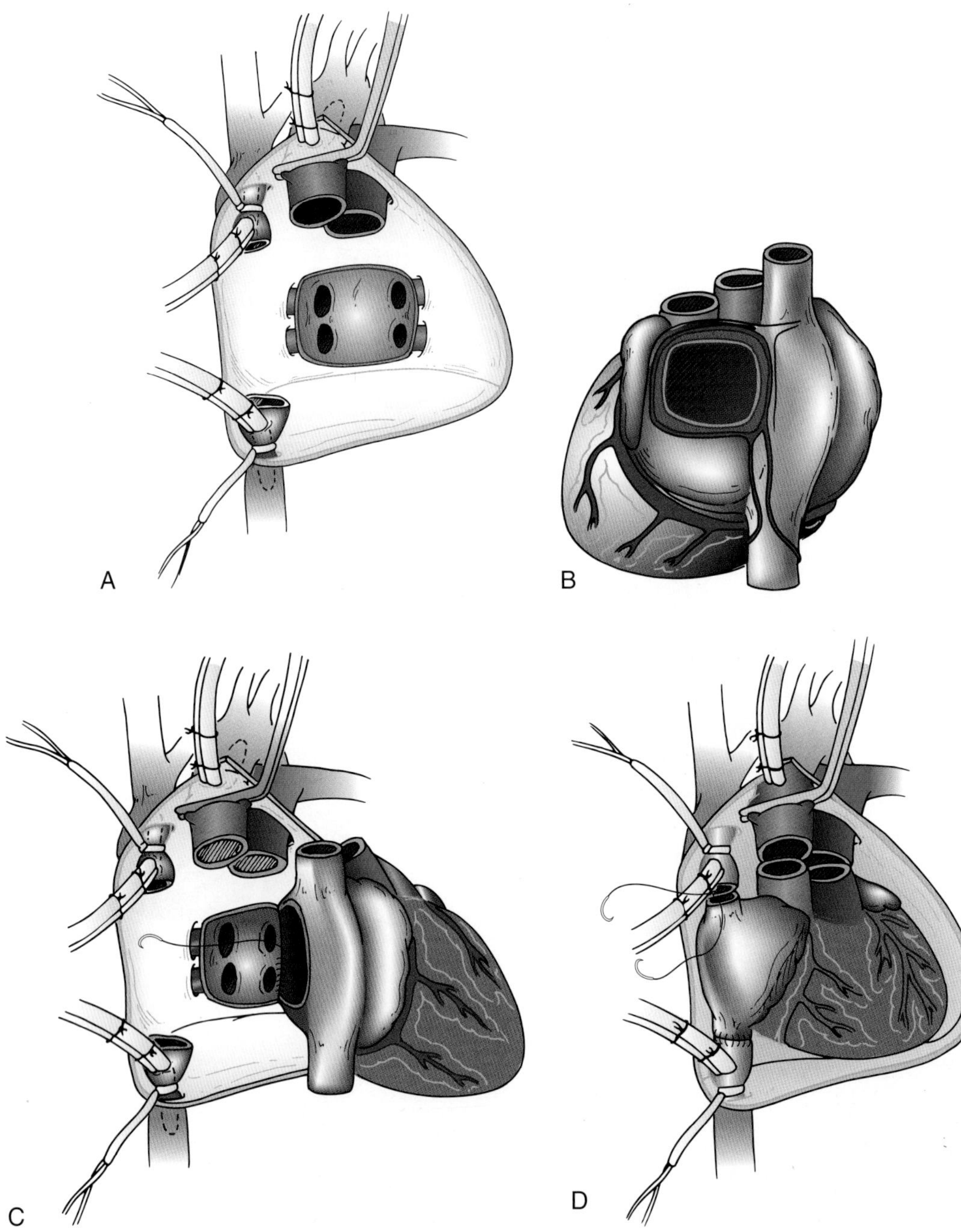

FIGURE 98-2 ■ Bicaval technique for orthotopic heart transplantation. **A,** Cardiopulmonary bypass is initiated after cannulation of the superior vena cava (SVC), inferior vena cava (IVC), and aorta. The aorta is cross-clamped, and native recipient cardiectomy is performed. A cuff of left atrial tissue is preserved around the four pulmonary vein orifices. **B,** The donor heart is prepared for transplantation. The left atrial tissue surrounding the four pulmonary vein orifices has been excised, leaving a single large orifice. **C,** The left atrial anastomosis is performed. **D,** The IVC anastomosis is completed, and the SVC anastomosis is performed. Once this is completed, the pulmonary artery and aortic anastomoses will be performed.

are performed as described earlier in the standard technique (see Fig. 98-2*C*). The SVC anastomosis is performed with a running 5-0 polypropylene suture and the IVC anastomosis with running 4-0 polypropylene suture (see Fig. 98-2*D*).

A further modification to this technique has been practiced at Stanford University by Oyer and associates since 1992, although it was first published in 2001 by Kitamura and colleagues.[128] The modified bicaval anastomosis technique for OHT leaves the posterior portion of the right atrial wall connecting both the SVC and the IVC intact. This modification makes the anastomosis technically easier with respect to proper orientation and eliminates the retraction, tension, or kinking of the venae cavae.

Orthotopic Total Technique

The orthotopic total technique is used at a small number of centers. It is similar to the bicaval approach except that during recipient cardiectomy, the left atrial cuff surrounding the pulmonary vein orifices is divided longitudinally into separate right and left pulmonary vein cuffs. Preparation of the donor heart requires separate preparation of the right and left pulmonary veins leaving two orifices on the donor heart's left atrium. Two left atrial anastomoses are fashioned, followed by the bicaval, pulmonary artery, and aortic anastomoses.

Heterotopic Technique

In the heterotopic approach, the donor IVC and right pulmonary veins are ligated, followed by anastomosis of the donor and recipient left atria, SVC, aortas, and pulmonary arteries. SVC and aortic anastomoses are performed in an end-to-side manner, and a short length of graft is used to connect the pulmonary arteries (Fig. 98-3). The heterotopic approach can be used when recipient PVR is markedly elevated given the possibility of acute right-sided heart failure in a donor right ventricle unaccustomed to the pulmonary resistance. In addition, it has been used in cases of donor and recipient size mismatch when medical urgency for transplantation is high.[107] Improvements in mechanical assist devices and a growing experience in their use as BTTs have made the indications for heterotopic heart transplantation almost obsolete.

RECIPIENT POSTOPERATIVE MANAGEMENT

Clinical Management in the Early Postoperative Period

On completion of the transplant, the patient is transported to the intensive care unit. The patient remains mechanically ventilated with continuous monitoring of electrocardiogram, arterial blood pressure, CVP, and pulse oximetry. In most cases, a pulmonary artery catheter is used to further monitor hemodynamics. Temperature, urine output, and mediastinal drain output are monitored as well.

As with other patients undergoing cardiac surgery, dysrhythmias are frequent in the early postoperative period. Junctional rhythms are particularly common after OHT. Because cardiac output of the denervated transplanted heart is primarily rate dependent, the heart rate should be maintained between 90 and 110 beats per minute during the first few postoperative days.[129] Isoproterenol infusion, theophylline, oral albuterol, and temporary pacing may be used to augment the heart rate. Another option is to place temporary atrial and ventricular pacing leads in the operating suite, allowing for postoperative heart rate adjustment. Less than 5% of patients

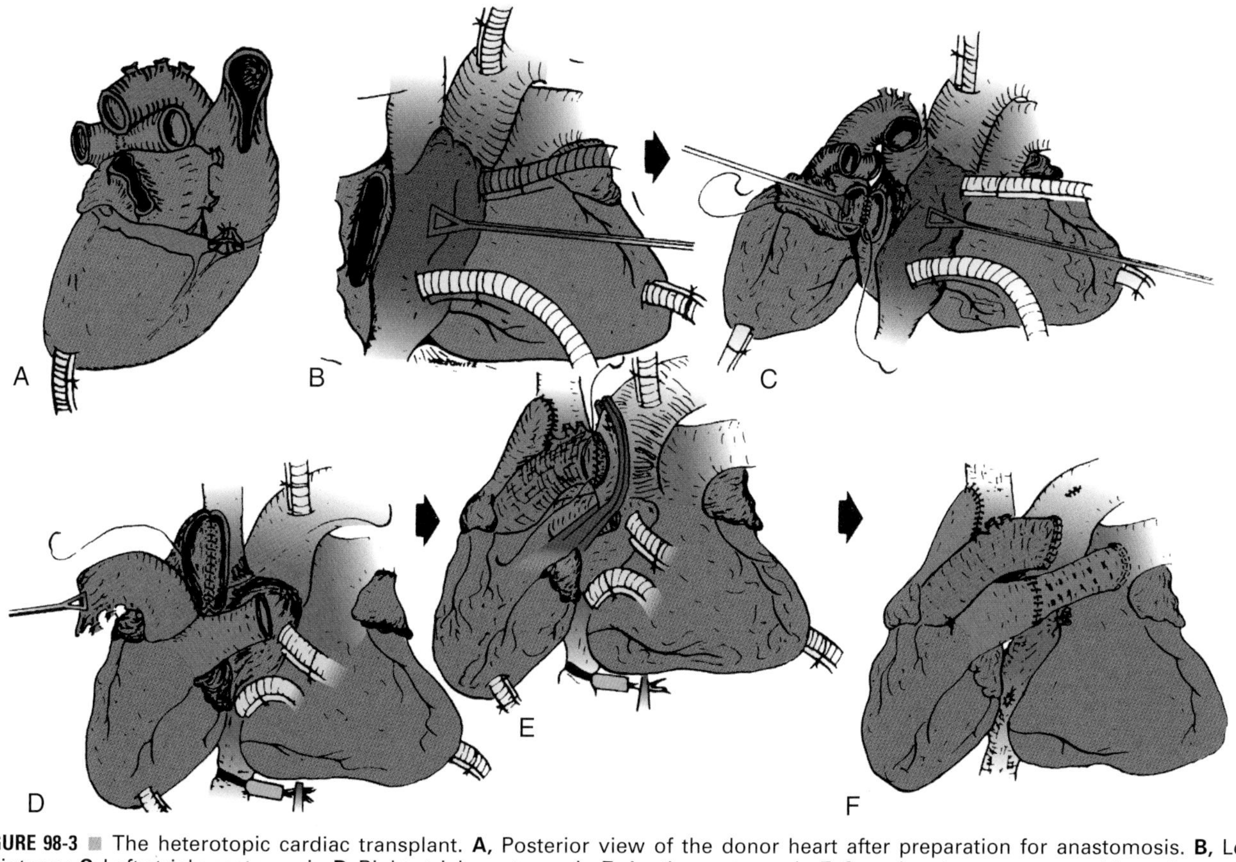

FIGURE 98-3 ■ The heterotopic cardiac transplant. **A,** Posterior view of the donor heart after preparation for anastomosis. **B,** Left atriotomy. **C,** Left atrial anastomosis. **D,** Right atrial anastomosis. **E,** Aortic anastomosis. **F,** Completed anastomoses with a pulmonary-to-pulmonary arterial graft. (**A-E** from Barnard CN, Wolpowitz A: Heterotopic versus orthotopic heart transplantation. *Transplant Proc* 11:309–312, 1979.)

have permanent sinus node dysfunction and require placement of a permanent transvenous pacemaker. The rate of sinus node dysfunction may be reduced when the bicaval technique is used.[129]

In most cases, the postoperative course after transplantation is uncomplicated. The patient is extubated when alert and hemodynamically stable, typically within 6 hours of surgery. The patient is gradually weaned from inotropic support over the first few postoperative days. Invasive catheters are removed as soon as possible to reduce the risk for sepsis, and mediastinal drains are removed when drainage has fallen to less than 200 mL/day. Temporary pacing wires are removed approximately 1 week after transplantation, provided that pacing is not required.

Early complications after transplantation include bleeding, depressed global myocardial performance, and right-sided heart failure. Significant hemorrhage may require surgical reexploration. Depressed global myocardial performance is uncommon but may occur in the setting of prolonged organ ischemia or inadequate preservation.[130] In such cases, aggressive hemodynamic and ventilatory management is necessary, and support from inotropic agents and vasopressors is needed. Hypovolemia, cardiac tamponade, sepsis, and bradycardia can result in depressed myocardial performance and should be treated expeditiously if they are present.

Right-sided heart failure can occur after transplantation, particularly in recipients who have elevated preoperative PVR.[131] In such cases, the donor right ventricle is unable to work against the elevated PVR and begins to fail within hours after transplantation. Aggressive early management may mitigate the consequences of this complication. Intraoperative transesophageal echocardiography should be performed routinely to assess right ventricular function and evaluate for technical failure such as kinking of the pulmonary artery or anastomotic stenosis. Treatment of right-sided heart failure includes correction of any technical problems, optimization of volume status, medical treatment with inotropes, implementation of pulmonary vasodilators (nitroprusside, inhaled epoprostenol, and inhaled nitric oxide), and avoidance of hypercarbia (goal CO_2, <40 mm Hg). Refractory right-sided heart failure may necessitate placement of a right ventricular assist device.

Maintenance Immunosuppression

In addition to careful monitoring of cardiac function during the immediate postoperative period, much focus is placed on institution of immunosuppression. In most cases, immunosuppression is initiated intraoperatively with intravenous methylprednisolone and continued postoperatively with a combination of intravenous and oral medications. Most centers have adopted triple drug combinations of a calcineurin inhibitor (cyclosporine or tacrolimus), an antiproliferative agent (azathioprine or mycophenolate mofetil [MMF]), and a corticosteroid. Immediately after transplantation, many of these medications are administered intravenously, although some must be delivered via nasoenteric tube. Once patients are tolerating oral intake, they can be converted to a completely oral immunosuppressive regimen. Because the risk for allograft rejection is highest in the first several months after transplantation, immunosuppression is most aggressive during this period. If patients remain free of rejection, immunosuppression is gradually decreased over time. Typical immunosuppressive dosing regimens (early and late) are demonstrated in Box 98-5.

Multidrug immunosuppression targets multiple sites in the immune cascade that lead to allograft rejection.[132] Calcineurin inhibitors block the activity of calcineurin, a calcium- and calmodulin-dependent phosphatase that is required for early T cell activation and interleukin-2 (IL-2) formation. Antiproliferative agents inhibit lymphocyte replication through a variety of mechanisms. Azathioprine inhibits the de novo and salvage pathways for purine biosynthesis. MMF inhibits the de novo synthesis of guanine nucleotides. Because activated lymphocytes use the de novo pathway predominantly, MMF is thought to have greater selectivity than azathioprine. Corticosteroids inhibit lymphocyte proliferation by inhibiting macrophage production of cytokines, including IL-1 and IL-6.

The drugs in these regimens act synergistically, permitting dosage reduction when used in combination. This helps minimize dosage-dependent toxicity to the transplant recipient. Cyclosporine can cause nephrotoxicity, neurotoxicity, hypertension, hyperlipidemia,

BOX 98-5 Immunosuppression Regimen for Heart Transplant Recipients

Perioperatively

- Corticosteroid—methylprednisolone (125 mg IV, every 8 hours for three doses, starting 8 hours after the induction dose in the operating room)

Postoperatively

Induction Therapy

- rATG (1 mg/kg, with a maximum of 125 mg, over 6 hours daily for 3 days; premedication with diphenhydramine and acetaminophen, addition of hydrocortisone premedication if timing does not coincide with prednisone or methylprednisolone)

Maintenance Therapy

- Prednisone (20 mg twice daily; taper to baseline dosage by 3 months after transplant)
- Tacrolimus (dosage according to level, with daily trough; beginning dosage, 0.5 mg daily; aim for whole blood level of 12-15 for normal renal function, 8-10 for mild renal insufficiency, 4-6 for severe renal insufficiency)
- Cellcept (1000 mg twice a day, ½ hour before or 2 hours after food)

Alternative Immunosuppressive Agents

- Azathioprine (2 mg/kg PO every night; decrease dosage by half if WBC < 5000 or in the presence of severe renal failure, then titrate for WBC count; hold dosage if WBC < 4000)
- Sirolimus (1 mg PO every day; target level, 5-7)

WBC, White blood cell count.

hirsutism, and gingival hyperplasia. Tacrolimus is also nephrotoxic and neurotoxic and has been associated with glucose intolerance and new-onset diabetes mellitus. Both cyclosporine and tacrolimus are metabolized by the liver and cause upregulation of the cytochrome P450 system. Azathioprine and MMF cause dosage-dependent bone marrow suppression. Corticosteroids are associated with myriad side effects, including poor wound healing, development of cushingoid features, hypertension, diabetes mellitus, osteoporosis, and peptic ulcer disease.

Rapamycin, or sirolimus, is an alternative immunosuppressive agent that has been used successfully in renal and liver transplantation.[133] It inhibits mTOR (mammalian target of rapamycin), thereby blocking IL-2 signaling pathways.[132,134] Rapamycin also inhibits smooth muscle proliferation and has been used in drug-eluting coronary stents to inhibit neointimal hyperplasia. Experimental animal models have shown inhibition of cardiac allograft vasculopathy (CAV) with rapamycin treatment and this has been validated in small, single-institution studies.[135-137] A randomized clinical trial performed by Keogh and associates in OHT recipients compared sirolimus with azathioprine in combination with cyclosporine and steroid immunosuppression. Those patients receiving sirolimus showed a significant decrease in acute rejection: 32.4% to 32.8% of sirolimus-treated patients versus 56.8% of azathioprine patients. Sirolimus appeared to also aid in the prevention of CAV at 6 months and up to 2 years.[138] Additionally, Topilsky and coworkers retrospectively reviewed patients transitioned from a calcineurin inhibitor–based immunosuppressive regimen to a sirolimus-based regimen. In their study, patients receiving sirolimus ended up having lower overall mortality and lower incidence of CAV-related events.[136]

The role of mTOR inhibitors, including sirolimus and everolimus, in the immunosuppressive armamentarium for OHT recipients continues to be controversial, especially regarding calcineurin inhibitor withdrawal and sirolimus conversion in patients with renal impairment. Transition from calcineurin inhibitor to sirolimus in OHT recipients with significant renal dysfunction (requiring hemodialysis) has yielded beneficial results in terms of renal improvement and number of episodes of clinical rejection at 1 year.[139] On the other hand, evidence shows that mTOR inhibitors may be associated with an increase in wound healing complications. Conflicting data were summarized by a cardiac transplant multidisciplinary committee in 2008, which concluded that calcineurin inhibitor withdrawal in OHT recipients should not be instituted until after the first year of transplantation.[140]

Despite the huge advancement of immunosuppressive drug therapy for cardiac transplantation, the specific combination of agents necessary for increased survival, safety profile, and decreased rejection has not been established. Transplant centers' immunosuppressive protocols vary widely, and most existing studies report only short-term findings. Taylor and colleagues[141] performed a small prospective randomized multicenter study comparing the efficacy of tacrolimus-based immunosuppression with that of cyclosporine-based immunosuppression. At 1-year follow-up, rejection rates were comparable in both groups, although the incidence of hypertension and hyperlipidemia was less in the tacrolimus group. A randomized multicenter trial comparing the triple drug regimens of cyclosporine–azathioprine–prednisone and cyclosporine–MMF–prednisone showed improved 1-year survival and greater freedom from rejection in the cyclosporine–MMF–prednisone group.[142] A greater increase in herpes simplex viral infection was found in the cyclosporine–MMF–prednisone group compared with that in the cyclosporine–azathioprine–prednisone group (21% vs. 15%), but no difference in other infectious complications or malignancy was found. In 2006, Kobashigawa and coworkers[143] conducted a large multicenter randomized trial consisting of 343 OHT recipients who were randomized to receive steroids and either tacrolimus–sirolimus, tacrolimus–MMF, or cyclosporine–MMF. The primary endpoint was incidence of ISHLT grade 3A or greater rejection or hemodynamic compromise requiring therapy within the first 6 months. Secondary endpoints included patient and graft survival at 1 year, rejection incidence, and safety profile. ISHLT grade 3A rejection episodes were diminished in the tacrolimus–MMF group versus the cyclosporine–MMF group at 1 year (23% vs. 36%). At 35%, the tacrolimus–sirolimus group had the lowest incidence of treated rejection episodes of any of the groups. The incidence was 42% in the tacrolimus–MMF group and 59% in the cyclosporine–MMF group. The tacrolimus–MMF group had significantly lower mean serum creatinine compared with the tacrolimus-sirolimus and cyclosporine-MMF groups: 1.3 mg/dL versus 1.5 mg/dL. The triglyceride level (126 mg/dL versus 162 mg/dL in tacrolimus–MMF and 154 mg/dL in cyclosporine–MMF) was also better for the tacrolimus-MMF group. The authors concluded that the combination of steroids, tacrolimus, and MMF may be the most beneficial immunosuppressive regimen in OHT recipients because of fewer rejection episodes and improved side effect profiles.

Along with multidrug immunosuppression regimens, many centers use cytolytic induction therapy to rapidly deplete lymphocytes in heart transplant recipients. This therapy occurs over a 3- to 10-day course, beginning immediately after transplantation. Induction immunosuppressive therapy has declined in popularity to the point that only 47% of heart transplant recipients received it in early 2012.[2] Currently available induction agents include the following: IL-2 receptor antagonists, such as daclizumab and basiliximab,[144,145] which are humanized antibodies that effect the destruction of activated T cells expressing the IL-2 receptor on their cell surface; polyclonal antilymphocytic antibodies, for example, antithymocyte globulin (ATG), which is a rabbit or equine polyclonal antibody preparation that results in rapid cytolytic depletion of T cells; and alemtuzumab, a monoclonal antibody directed at CD52.[146] Induction therapy has advantages and disadvantages. Because immunosuppression is immediate, maintenance immunosuppression with other drugs can be delayed. In cases of hemodynamic instability or questionable renal function, this can be advantageous. Initial doses of ATG may be associated with a "cytokine release syndrome," which manifests with fever, chills, hypotension, and bronchospasm. Patients receiving this induction agent should be premedicated with acetaminophen, antihistamines, and corticosteroids and should be monitored closely. Because these preparations are raised in animals, patients may develop neutralizing antibodies, making prolonged and repeated courses impossible. Induction therapy with ATG may decrease the incidence of acute rejection in some cases, but in others, it simply delays the time of onset to rejection. Both are associated with a higher incidence of infectious complications and posttransplant lymphoproliferative disorder.[132] Of note, OKT3 (muromonab-CD3), a mouse monoclonal antibody targeting the CD3 receptor on activated T cells, is no longer available because of a higher incidence of posttransplantation lymphoproliferative disease and side effect profile with no demonstrable benefit over other antibodies.[147,148]

The experience with IL-2 receptor blockade is more limited, but 1-year follow-up studies have shown a decrease in the frequency and severity of acute rejection and a decrease in development of CAV.[149,150] Kobashigawa and colleagues[151] investigated the safety profile of daclizumab with patients on triple drug therapy consisting of cyclosporine–MMF–steroids from the Scientific Registry of Transplant Recipients. They demonstrated that daclizumab-induced patients had no increased risk for death or infectious death when compared with no induction therapy. Daclizumab-treated recipients also experienced lower rates of acute rejection at 6 and 12 months, with an overall 23% reduction when compared with non-induced patients.

A Cochrane review revealed that IL-2R antagonists were associated with lower incidence of acute rejection compared with no induction therapy. However, polyclonal antibody induction may be associated with a reduced incidence of biopsy-proven severe acute rejection compared with IL-2R antagonists.[152] Long-term prospective studies are needed to determine whether induction with IL-2 receptor antagonists provides a survival benefit and to define patient populations that would benefit most from these therapies.

COMPLICATIONS

Hyperacute Rejection

Hyperacute rejection is a form of humorally mediated rejection. Preformed antibodies in the recipient recognize donor vascular endothelial antigens, resulting in activation of inflammatory and coagulation cascades. Graft vessels thrombose resulting in graft loss. ABO matching of donor and recipient has decreased the rate of hyperacute rejection. For recipients with an elevated PRA, prospective crossmatching of donor lymphocytes with recipient serum has also decreased the rate of hyperacute rejection.

Acute Rejection

The risk for acute rejection is highest during the first few months after transplantation and then persists at a low constant level. Most heart transplant patients experience at least one episode of acute rejection, and there is a small mortality risk associated with each of these episodes. According to ISHLT data, acute rejection is the cause of death in approximately 11% of patients between 1 and 3 years after transplantation.[2] In 1994, the Cardiac Transplant Research Database group identified risk factors for recurrent rejection after heart transplantation.[153] In the first year after transplantation, these risk factors include shorter interval since previous rejection episode, young age, female sex, female donor, positive cytomegalovirus serology, prior infections, and OKT3 induction. After the first year, the dominant risk factors are a greater number of rejection episodes during the first year and the presence of prior cytomegalovirus infections.

The clinical presentation of acute rejection varies widely. Patients may be asymptomatic or may have nonspecific clinical signs and symptoms, including fever, anorexia, leukocytosis, and mild hypotension. In rare cases, acute rejection manifests with severe hypotension and circulatory collapse. Because these clinical signs and symptoms lack a high degree of sensitivity or specificity in the diagnosis of acute rejection, the gold standard diagnostic test is a tissue biopsy. Percutaneous endomyocardial biopsy is performed as a part of routine surveillance protocols after heart transplantation. A bioptome is passed through a sheath in the right internal jugular vein and advanced through the tricuspid valve into the right ventricle, where tissue biopsies are taken. Clinicians should be well versed in tissue sampling, because tricuspid regurgitation, although rare, is a recognized complication. Pathologically, acute rejection can be a focal patchy process, so four to six biopsies should be taken to reduce sampling error.[154] A typical surveillance endomyocardial biopsy protocol includes weekly biopsies for the first 4 weeks after transplantation, biweekly biopsies for the next month, and then monthly biopsies through the sixth month after transplantation. If the patient is free from rejection at 6 months, the frequency of biopsies is reduced to every 3 months.

Because of the cost, invasive nature, and potential for complications associated with endomyocardial biopsy, investigators are now developing alternative noninvasive techniques to monitor cardiac allograft rejection.[155] Emerging and promising techniques include magnetic resonance imaging,[156] wall motion analysis with tissue Doppler imaging,[157] electrical event monitoring with ventricular evoked response amplitude assessment,[158] identification of peripheral blood markers of rejection (e.g., P-selectin, prothrombin fragments, B-type natriuretic peptides, troponin),[159,160] imaging for necrosis with antimyosin antibody–based scintigraphy,[161] and imaging for apoptosis with technetium 99m–labeled annexin V.[162]

Acute Cellular Rejection

The primary process leading to acute rejection is acute cellular rejection, which is T cell mediated. Donor antigen presenting cells (APCs) may be directly recognized by recipient T cells, or donor antigens may cross into the recipient to be taken up by recipient APCs.[163] The presentation of antigens to T cells via APCs causes conformational changes in the T cell receptor. In the presence of a

TABLE 98-3 **ISHLT Standardized Cardiac Biopsy Grading: Acute Cellular Rejection***

Grade	Criteria
Grade 0R†	No rejection
Grade 1R, mild	Interstitial and/or perivascular infiltrate with up to one focus of myocyte damage
Grade 2R, moderate	Two or more foci of infiltrate with associated myocyte damage
Grade 3R, severe	Diffuse infiltrate with multifocal myocyte damage ± edema ± hemorrhage ± vasculitis

*The presence or absence of acute antibody-mediated rejection (AMR) may be recorded as AMR 0 or AMR 1, as required.
†R denotes revised grade, to avoid confusion with 1990 scheme.
ISHLT, International Society for Heart and Lung Transplantation.
From Stewart S, Winters GL, Fishbein MC, et al: Revision of the 1990 working formulation for the standardization of nomenclature in the diagnosis of heart rejection. J Heart Lung Transplant 24(11):1710–1720, 2005.

costimulatory molecule, i.e., B7 (CD80 or CD86), on the APC interacting with CD28 on the T cell, promotion of T cell proliferation and cytokine production occurs.[164] Following the sensitization of effector cells, there is a migration of lymphocytes into the allograft with subsequent activation of either the FAS-FAS ligand or perforin/granulolysin pathway resulting in myocyte death.[165]

A standardized grading system for cardiac acute rejection was developed by the ISHLT Heart Rejection Study Group in 1990. This system graded acute rejection with a score of 0 to 4, with 0 being no rejection and 4 being severe acute rejection. However, with the advent of newer, more effective immunosuppressive regimens and better understanding of transplant immunobiology, a revision of the previous Working Formulation, focused mainly on grade 2 cellular rejection, was approved by the ISHLT board in December 2004.[166] Table 98-3 illustrates this revised ISHLT standardized cardiac biopsy grading system of acute cellular rejection. Briefly, 1990 ISHLT grades 1A, 1B, and 2 combined into 2004 ISHLT grade 1R; 1990 ISHLT grade 3A is now 2004 ISHLT grade 2R; and 1990 ISHLT grades 3B and 4 became 2004 ISHLT grade 3R.

Treatment of Acute Cellular Rejection

When a histologic diagnosis of rejection is made, treatment consists of augmentation of immunosuppression. The degree of augmentation depends on the grade of rejection in addition to symptomatic status (Fig. 98-4). Asymptomatic patients with low grade rejection detected on surveillance biopsy may be managed with adjustments in the patient's regimen, titration to drug levels, and follow-up biopsy. Patients with moderate to severe acute cellular rejection should be treated aggressively even in the absence of symptoms or graft dysfunction.[129] In the symptomatic patient, prompt institution of therapy is critical independent of the grade of rejection. Options for acute therapy include corticosteroids or ATG.

Modifications to a patient's long-term immunosuppressive regimen may include substituting tacrolimus for cyclosporine. Similarly, sirolimus or MMF may be substituted for azathioprine. If rejection does not respond to this treatment, an additional pulse of steroids may be given. Acute rejection is rarely refractory to these measures. In such cases, total lymphoid irradiation,[167] plasmapheresis,[168] and conversion of azathioprine to cyclophosphamide or methotrexate have been used.[169]

Antibody-Mediated Rejection

Antibody-mediated rejection (AMR), which is a process mediated by donor-specific antibodies (DSAs), has emerged as a major cause of allograft loss. This has led to intense study of evaluation, diagnosis, and treatment. Patients with AMR are more susceptible to developing CAV, and they have a significant mortality rate (17%) in the early posttransplant period.[170] Long-term survival was decreased in recipients with a diagnosis of AMR. Taylor and coworkers[171] found that in patients with AMR, allograft 3-year survival was 57%, and the risk for graft loss and dysfunction was approximately twice that in recipients with cellular rejection only.

Acute AMR is estimated to occur in 15% of cardiac recipients. Both the presence of acute AMR and cellular rejection were reported in 23% of biopsy specimens from 587 cardiac recipients. AMR manifests clinically as early as 2 to 7 days if the recipient has been presensitized with donor HLA, or as late as 1 month after transplant, and it may be associated with a rise in DSAs. [171] For patients experiencing early AMR, approximately 70% develop allograft dysfunction.[172] If AMR occurs late—several months to years—graft dysfunction is much less common, at 13%.

Generally, the incidence of AMR is increased in transplant recipients with prior sensitization to HLA antigens.[173] This is not limited to HLA; there is a growing body of evidence that non-HLA autoantibodies may also contribute to AMR.[174,175] Patients with PRA greater than 10% are at increased risk of AMR.[176] With the increasing number of cardiac retransplants and patients receiving LVAD, the proportion of potential recipients who are sensitized and on the waiting list is expanding. The causes of preformed antibodies are transfusion, previous transplantation, and pregnancy, with pregnancy being a major cause of allosensitization in women.

The development of de novo antibodies occurs in a large proportion of patients,[177] up to 35% in one report with associated decrease in 5-year survival. However, not all autoantibodies will inflict allograft injury. In a process known as "accommodation," patients may continue to have normal function in the presence of circulating antibodies against donor antigens.

In 2004, the ISHLT assembled an updated version of the grading system for AMR—the Revision of the 1990 Working Formulation for the Standardization of Nomenclature in the Diagnosis of Heart Rejection.[166] In these guidelines, allograft dysfunction and presence of DSAs were requisite criteria for diagnosis of AMR. Wu and colleagues found that patients with asymptomatic AMR developed CAV with greater frequency than did matched controls, suggesting that outcome may be affected in the absence of allograft dysfunction.[178] Moreover, patients

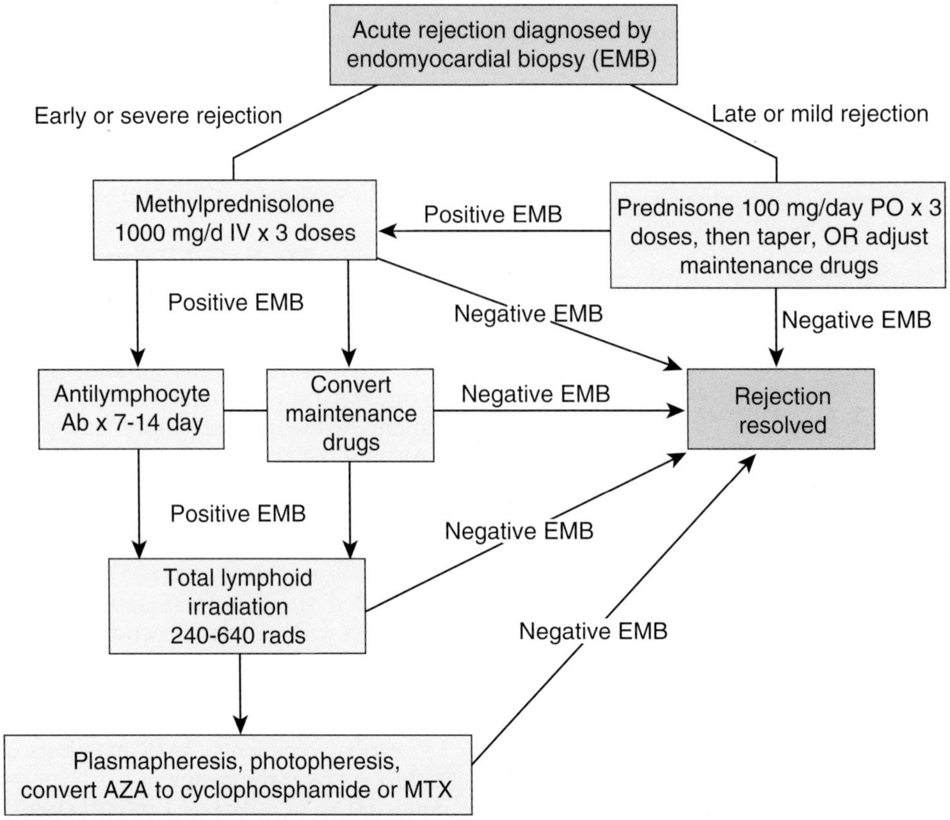

FIGURE 98-4 ■ Treatment algorithm for acute rejection in heart transplant recipients. *Ab,* Antibody; *AZA,* azathioprine; *MTX,* methotrexate.

with asymptomatic AMR may be at greater risk for cardiovascular mortality than cellular rejection.[179] Based on this evidence, a consensus conference on AMR was convened in 2010 with the recommendation that the diagnosis be based on histopathology and immunopathology rather than relying on clinical presentation and serologic studies. In 2013, the ISHLT published a statement standardizing the diagnosis of AMR incorporating the recommendations from the 2010 consensus conference[176] (Table 98-4).

Treatment of Antibody-Mediated Rejection

Although the exact treatment regimens for recipients with AMR vary between transplant centers, the principles on which it is based are the same: aggressive hemodynamic management along with augmentation of the immunosuppressive regimen to maximize the effort against circulating DSAs and lessen B cell activity. Plasmapheresis, steroid therapy, rituximab, ATG, bortezomib, and IVIG are used in a variety of combinations.[176] Figure 98-5 shows a proposed algorithm for the treatment of AMR in cardiac recipients.

Infection

An inherent complication of immunosuppression is increased risk for infection. In the first three years after transplantation, infection is the cause of death in 12% to 29% of patients.[2] The pathogens involved vary depending on the time after transplantation. Early infections in the first month after transplantation are commonly caused by bacteria and often manifest as pneumonia or urinary tract infections.[180] Typical pathogens include *Pseudomonas aeruginosa*, *Escherichia coli*, and *Staphylococcus aureus*. Whereas infectious episodes are decreasing in frequency overall, the proportion of infections caused by gram-positive organisms is increasing.[181] The use of perioperative antibiotics and early removal of invasive catheters may aid in the prevention of perioperative infections. Late infections are typically caused by opportunistic pathogens, fungi, and viruses. However, the risk of infection decreases over time as immunosuppressive therapy is generally tapered.[182] The proportion of mortality attributable to infection is only 11% to 12% greater than 3 years out from heart transplantation.[2]

Cytomegalovirus (CMV) is the most common and clinically significant viral pathogen in heart transplant recipients.[183] It may cause a variety of syndromes and has been implicated as a trigger for accelerated CAV. Heart transplant recipients are at high risk for CMV infection because cell-mediated immunity, which is necessary to combat CMV, is impaired by conventional immunosuppressive drugs. CMV infection may manifest either as primary infection or as reactivation of a latent infection. Primary CMV infection may develop in seronegative recipients receiving a heart from a CMV seropositive donor. In such cases, donor leukocytes or the allograft itself may harbor CMV and transmit it to the recipient.

TABLE 98-4 ISHLT Standardized Cardiac Biopsy Grading: Acute Antibody-Mediated Rejection (AMR)

Grade	Definition	Substrates
pAMR 0	Negative for pathologic AMR	Histologic and immunopathologic studies are both negative.
pAMR 1 (H+)	Histopathologic AMR alone	Histologic findings are present and immunopathologic findings are negative.
pAMR 1 (I+)	Immunopathologic AMR alone	Histologic findings are negative and immunopathologic findings are positive (CD68+ and/or C4d+).
pAMR 2	Pathologic AMR	Histologic and immunopathologic findings are both present.
pAMR 3	Severe pathologic AMR	Interstitial hemorrhage, capillary fragmentation, mixed inflammatory infiltrates, endothelial cell pyknosis, and/or karyorrhexis, and marked edema and immunopathologic findings are present. These cases may be associated with profound hemodynamic dysfunction and poor clinical outcomes.

ISHLT, International Society for Heart and Lung Transplantation.

From Berry GJ, Burke MM, Andersen C, et al: The 2013 International Society for Heart and Lung Transplantation working formulation for the standardization of nomenclature in the pathologic diagnosis of antibody-mediated rejection in heart transplantation. J Heart Lung Transplant 32(12):1147–1162, 2013.

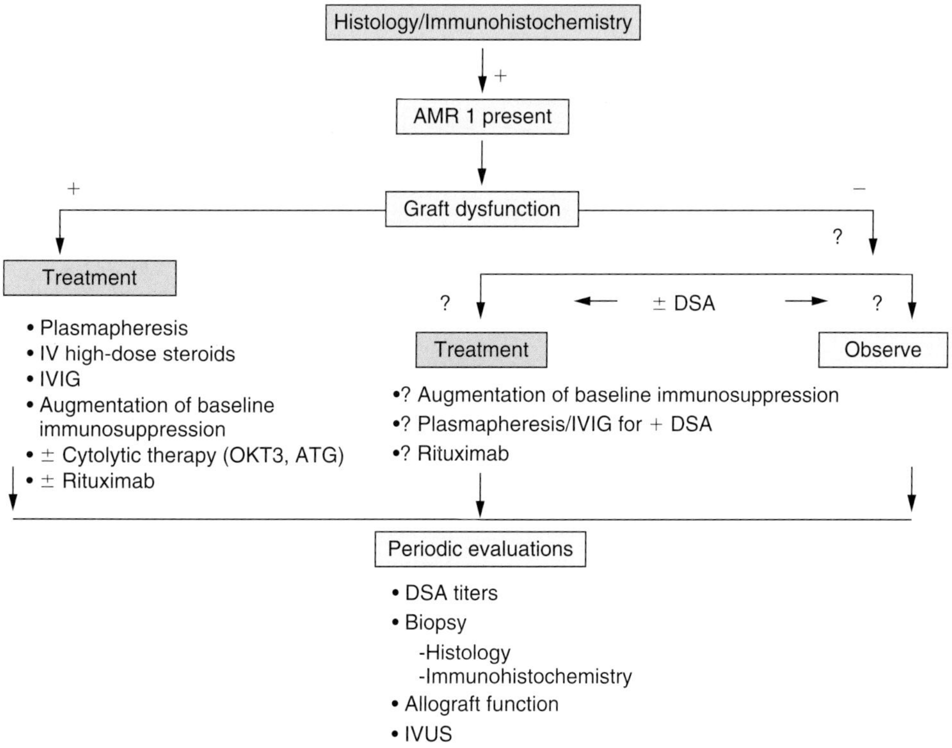

FIGURE 98-5 Algorithm for treatment of antibody-mediated rejection (AMR) in cardiac transplant recipients. *ATG,* Antithymocyte globulin; *DSA,* donor-specific antibody; *IV,* intravenous; *IVIG,* intravenous immunoglobulin; *IVUS,* intravascular ultrasound. (From Uber WE, Self SE, Van Bakel AB, et al: Acute antibody-mediated rejection following heart transplantation. *Am J Transplant* 7[9]:2064–2074, 2007.)

Reactivation of latent CMV may occur in seropositive recipients. The risk for CMV infection in different populations of cardiac transplant recipients is illustrated in Table 98-5. The seronegative recipient of a heart from a seropositive donor and those being treated for acute rejection with antilymphocyte antibody preparations are at highest risk.

CMV infection can manifest as a mononucleosis-like syndrome, or it may be tissue invasive. The most common sites for tissue invasion are the lung, liver, and gastrointestinal tract. Less common sites include the retina and skin. Diagnosis is made by measurement of viral load with either quantitative polymerase chain reaction or antigenemia assays; by direct culture of the virus from blood, urine, or tissue specimens; or by observation of characteristic histologic changes (enlarged cells containing nuclear inclusion bodies). A combination of intravenous ganciclovir and hyperimmune globulin is used to treat CMV infection.[183]

Several populations of cardiac transplant patients benefit from prophylactic treatment against CMV infection. Serologically mismatched patients (seronegative recipient of heart from seropositive donor) are treated with a combination of ganciclovir and hyperimmune globulin for weeks to months after transplantation.[183,184] Often, seropositive recipients are also treated with a

TABLE 98-5 **Risk of Cytomegalovirus (CMV) Disease in Populations of Cardiac Transplant Recipients**

Donor CMV Serotype Status	Recipient CMV Serotype Status	Antilymphocyte Antibody Therapy	Incidence of Disease (%)
Positive	Negative	—	50-75
Positive or negative	Positive	No	10-15
Positive or negative	Positive	Induction	≈25
		Antirejection	50-75
Negative	Negative	—	≈0*

*In donor negative/recipient negative transplants, CMV disease is uncommonly seen under two circumstances: transfusion of viable leukocyte containing blood products from a seropositive donor or acquisition of virus in the community through intimate person-to-person contact.

From Rubin RH: Prevention and treatment of cytomegalovirus disease in heart transplant patients. J Heart Lung Transplant 19(8):731–735, 2000.

course of ganciclovir to prevent reactivation infection. Some groups have shown that administration of intravenous ganciclovir when antilymphocyte antibody therapy is used to treat rejection reduces the risk for CMV disease to baseline levels.

Protozoal pathogens that can appear after heart transplantation include *Pneumocystis carinii* and *Toxoplasma gondii*. Pulmonary infection with *P. carinii* can be prevented by routine postoperative prophylaxis with trimethoprim sulfamethoxazole or aerosolized pentamidine (for sulfa-allergic patients). Toxoplasmosis may occur in serologically mismatched patients (e.g., *T. gondii*–seronegative recipient of heart from *T. gondii*–seropositive donor) but may be prevented by prophylaxis with atovaquone.[181,185]

Invasive fungal infections are uncommon after cardiac transplantation, but when they occur, they cause significant morbidity and mortality. Fungal pathogens include *Candida albicans* and *Aspergillus*. Treatment consists of fluconazole, itraconazole, or amphotericin B.

Cardiac Allograft Vasculopathy

The long-term success of cardiac transplantation is limited to some extent by the development of CAV. The mechanism of injury leading to CAV is poorly described. The recipient immune response to the donor heart results in endothelial injury mediated by recipient APCs and direct recognition of donor MHC.[163,186,187] The process of T cell activation produces a cascade of events that increases leukocyte adhesion to vessel walls and stimulates vascular remodeling.[50] The end result is the development of intimal fibromuscular hyperplasia, atherosclerosis, or vasculitis, which results in a histopathologic appearance similar to atherosclerotic disease in the nontransplanted patient.[43] However, CAV differs from atherosclerosis in extent and tempo. The disease process results in diffuse concentric narrowing of both epicardial and intramyocardial vessels. In addition, disease can appear within weeks of transplantation in spite of rigorous screening for coronary disease.[188]

Analyzing data in the Cardiac Transplant Research Database, Costanzo and colleagues reported that at 5 years, angiographically evident CAV was present in 42% of transplant patients with 7% having severe disease. Risk factors for the development of CAV in this study included older donor age,[189] donor history of hypertension, donor male sex, recipient male sex, and recipient black race.[190] Additional risks include recipient factors such as posttransplantation hyperlipidemia, hypertension, and diabetes, and donor factors including explosive method of death and intracranial hemorrhage.[191,192] Aziz and coworkers stratified the incidence of CAV by underlying patient diagnosis and correlated a primary diagnosis of ischemic cardiomyopathy with an increased incidence of CAV.[26]

Significant CAV results in diminished coronary artery blood flow and may lead to arrhythmias, myocardial infarction, sudden death, or impaired left ventricular function with congestive heart failure. It is unusual for patients with severe CAV to have classic anginal symptoms, because the cardiac graft is denervated. Between 10% and 12% of late deaths after heart transplantation are attributable to CAV.[2] Because of the significant morbidity and mortality associated with CAV, screening for CAV occurs at most transplant programs. Yearly coronary angiography is recommended, although it lacks sensitivity and typically underestimates the presence of disease. Dobutamine stress echocardiography also may be used for routine screening.[193] Intracoronary ultrasound, when available, is a more sensitive procedure that provides information about intimal area, lumen area, and plaque morphology.[194,195]

Treatment for CAV is limited. Because of the diffuse nature of the disease, patients are rarely candidates for coronary artery bypass grafting. Focal stenoses have been treated with angioplasty and stenting, but there is a high rate of restenosis.[196] Ultimately, severe progressive disease may require retransplantation. Because treatment options are limited, prevention of CAV is essential. Risk factor modification, including control of hyperlipidemia, hypertension, and hyperglycemia, may limit development of the disease. At-risk patients should receive routine prophylaxis against CMV.

Neoplasm

The incidence of neoplasia is higher in transplant recipients than in the general population. This is undoubtedly a consequence of chronic immunosuppression. Moreover, because immunosuppressive regimens are particularly aggressive in thoracic organ transplantation, these patients develop malignancies more often than renal and liver transplant recipients.[197] The ISHLT reports that between 28% and 32% of heart transplant recipients develop malignancies by the tenth year after transplantation.[1,2] Of these, most are skin cancers (squamous cell carcinoma and basal cell carcinoma)[198] and B cell lymphoproliferative disorders. B cell lymphoproliferative disorders cause the greatest degree of morbidity and mortality. They represent a spectrum of diseases ranging from cellular hyperplasia to true lymphomas, and more than 95% are associated with Epstein-Barr virus infection.[197] The mainstay of treatment for posttransplant lymphoproliferative disorder is reduction of immunosuppression and antiviral therapy.[199] Chemotherapy, radiotherapy, and immunotherapy have been used successfully in some cases. Other malignancies that occur at higher frequency in the transplant population include Kaposi sarcoma, carcinoma in situ of the cervix, and carcinoma of the vulva and anus. The incidence of solid organ tumors common in the general population (i.e., carcinoma of the lung, breast, colon and rectum, and prostate) is not higher in the transplant population.[200]

LONG-TERM RESULTS IN HEART TRANSPLANTATION

Long-term outcomes in heart transplantation have improved considerably in the past several decades, and median survival for all patients since 1982 is now 11 years (Fig. 98-6). Risk factors for 1-year mortality reported in the 2013 ISHLT registry include preoperative temporary circulatory support, chronic device therapy, total artificial heart, dialysis dependence, previous transfusions, gender mismatch, ventilator dependence prior to transplantation, and diagnosis.[2] Additionally, low preoperative albumin,[201] renal insufficiency not requiring dialysis,[31] race, heart failure causes,[202] and poor preoperative clinical status may contribute to poor postoperative outcomes.[203] Aside from recipient factors, annual heart transplant center volume has been shown to affect 30-day and 1-year mortality.[204] Rather than a strict reflection of procedural success, annual volume appears to be a proxy for the aggregate of human factors and health systems.

Significant risk factors for late mortality include both pretransplantation recipient and posttransplantation characteristics. Elevated PRA, HLA mismatch, ventilator dependence, temporary circulatory support,[2] recipient age younger than 55 years, recipient history of diabetes, and race all contributed to late mortality, suggesting that recipient selection continues to be a key component in the determination of posttransplantation survival.[205] After transplantation, an increasing burden of rejection episodes and more frequent infectious complications affect longevity.[206] Annual heart transplant center volume has been an area of increasing interest. Increasing transplant center volume confers a protective effect on survival at 1, 5, and 15 years post transplantation. Performing nine or more transplants per year has been shown to be a significant inflection point for the determination of long-term success.[205]

Approximately 40% of patients are hospitalized in the first year after transplant, often for treatment of rejection or infection. By the second year after transplant, only 20% are hospitalized. The vast majority, approximately 90%, report good functional status after transplantation as reflected by a Karnofsky score of 80% to 100%. However, only 35% of working-age (25 years to 60 years old) heart transplant recipients were working at 1 year and 46% at 3 years after transplantation.[2]

SUMMARY

The history of heart transplantation is a remarkable one. Its development has exemplified the paradigm of surgical translational research that drives so many new therapies today. It remains the gold standard for surgical treatment of late-stage heart failure, even in the presence of emerging and exciting technologies. Although heart transplantation is still limited by the number of donor hearts available, liberalization of donor selection criteria as well as novel methods of preservation and resuscitation of donor hearts will likely increase the donor pool. Continued improvement in developing immunosuppressive therapies as well as postoperative care is decreasing mortality, complications, and hospital length of stay. The surgical principles that define the operative course of heart transplantation will likely remain the same as future possibilities such as stem cell–derived hearts appear.

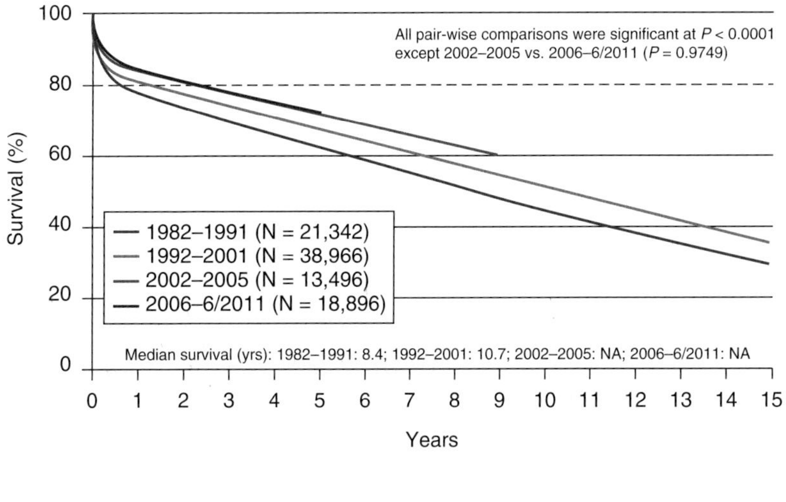

FIGURE 98-6 ■ Kaplan-Meier long-term survival by era (adult recipients). (From Lund LH, Edwards LB, Kucheryavaya AY, et al: The Registry of the International Society for Heart and Lung Transplantation: Thirtieth Official Adult Heart Transplant Report—2013; focus theme: age. *J Heart Lung Transplant* 32[10]:951–964, 2013.)

REFERENCES

1. Taylor DO, Edwards LB, Boucek MM, et al: Registry of the International Society for Heart and Lung Transplantation: twenty-fourth official adult heart transplant report–2007. *J Heart Lung Transplant* 26:769–781, 2007.
2. Lund LH, Edwards LB, Kucheryavaya AY, et al; International Society for Heart and Lung Transplantation: The Registry of the International Society for Heart and Lung Transplantation: thirtieth official adult heart transplant report–2013; focus theme: age. *J Heart Lung Transplant* 32:951–964, 2013.
3. Costanzo MR, Augustine S, Bourge R, et al: Selection and treatment of candidates for heart transplantation. A statement for health professionals from the Committee on Heart Failure and Cardiac Transplantation of the Council on Clinical Cardiology, American Heart Association. *Circulation* 92:3593–3612, 1995.
4. Carrel AG, Guthrie CC: The transplantation of veins and organs. *Am Med* 10:1101–1102, 1905.
5. Demikhov VP: *Experimental transplantation of vital organs,* trans. Basil Haigh. New York, 1962, Consultants Bureau.
6. Lower RR, Stofer RC, Shumway NE: Homovital transplantation of the heart. *J Thorac Cardiovasc Surg* 41:196–204, 1961.
7. Lower RR, Shumway NE: Studies on orthotopic homotransplantation of the canine heart. *Surg Forum* 11:18–19, 1960.
8. Lower RR, Dong E, Jr, Shumway NE: Long-term survival of cardiac homografts. *Surgery* 58:110–119, 1965.
9. Hardy JD, Kurrus FD, Chavez CM, et al: Heart transplantation in man. Developmental studies and report of a case. *JAMA* 188:1132–1140, 1964.
10. Barnard CN: The operation. A human cardiac transplant: an interim report of a successful operation performed at Groote Schuur Hospital, Cape Town. *S Afr Med J* 41:1271–1274, 1967.
11. Stinson EB, Dong E, Jr, Schroeder JS, et al: Initial clinical experience with heart transplantation. *Am J Cardiol* 22:791–803, 1968.
12. Caves PK, Stinson EB, Graham AF, et al: Percutaneous transvenous endomyocardial biopsy. *JAMA* 225:288–291, 1973.
13. Griepp RB, Stinson EB, Dong E, Jr, et al: Use of antithymocyte globulin in human heart transplantation. *Circulation* 45:I147–I153, 1972.
14. Calne RY, White DJ, Rolles K, et al: Prolonged survival of pig orthotopic heart grafts treated with cyclosporin A. *Lancet* 1:1183–1185, 1978.
15. Grattan MT, Moreno-Cabral CE, Starnes VA, et al: Eight-year results of cyclosporine-treated patients with cardiac transplants. *J Thorac Cardiovasc Surg* 99:500–509, 1990.
16. Deng MC, Smits JM, Packer M: Selecting patients for heart transplantation: which patients are too well for transplant? *Curr Opin Cardiol* 17:137–144, 2002.
17. Mancini DM, Eisen H, Kussmaul W, et al: Value of peak exercise oxygen consumption for optimal timing of cardiac transplantation in ambulatory patients with heart failure. *Circulation* 83:778–786, 1991.
18. Mehra MR, Kobashigawa J, Starling R, et al: Listing criteria for heart transplantation: International Society for Heart and Lung Transplantation guidelines for the care of cardiac transplant candidates—2006. *J Heart Lung Transplant* 25:1024–1042, 2006.
19. Florea VG, Henein MY, Anker SD, et al: Prognostic value of changes over time in exercise capacity and echocardiographic measurements in patients with chronic heart failure. *Eur Heart J* 21:146–153, 2000.
20. Stevenson LW, Steimle AE, Fonarow G, et al: Improvement in exercise capacity of candidates awaiting heart transplantation. *J Am Coll Cardiol* 25:163–170, 1995.
21. Aaronson KD, Schwartz JS, Chen TM, et al: Development and prospective validation of a clinical index to predict survival in ambulatory patients referred for cardiac transplant evaluation. *Circulation* 95:2660–2667, 1997.
22. Koelling TM, Joseph S, Aaronson KD: Heart failure survival score continues to predict clinical outcomes in patients with heart failure receiving beta-blockers. *J Heart Lung Transplant* 23:1414–1422, 2004.
23. Goda A, Lund LH, Mancini DM: Comparison across races of peak oxygen consumption and heart failure survival score for selection for cardiac transplantation. *Am J Cardiol* 105:1439–1444, 2010.
24. Packer M, Coats AJ, Fowler MB, et al; Carvedilol Prospective Randomized Cumulative Survival Study Group: Effect of carvedilol on survival in severe chronic heart failure. *N Engl J Med* 344:1651–1658, 2001.
25. Freudenberger RS, Kim J, Tawfik I, et al: Optimal medical therapy is superior to transplantation for the treatment of class I, II, and III heart failure: a decision analytic approach. *Circulation* 114:I62–I66, 2006.
26. Aziz T, Burgess M, Rahman AN, et al: Cardiac transplantation for cardiomyopathy and ischemic heart disease: differences in outcome up to 10 years. *J Heart Lung Transplant* 20:525–533, 2001.
27. Belli E, Leoni Moreno JC, Hosenpud J, et al: Preoperative risk factors predict survival following cardiac retransplantation: analysis of the United Network for Organ Sharing database. *J Thorac Cardiovasc Surg* 2014.
28. Atluri P, Hiesinger W, Gorman RC, et al: Cardiac retransplantation is an efficacious therapy for primary cardiac allograft failure. *J Cardiothorac Surg* 3:26, 2008.
29. Lietz K, Miller LW: Improved survival of patients with end-stage heart failure listed for heart transplantation: analysis of organ procurement and transplantation network/U.S. United Network of Organ Sharing data, 1990 to 2005. *J Am Coll Cardiol* 50:1282–1290, 2007.
30. Alam A, Badovinac K, Ivis F, et al: The outcome of heart transplant recipients following the development of end-stage renal disease: analysis of the Canadian Organ Replacement Register (CORR). *Am J Transplant* 7:461–465, 2007.
31. Schaffer JM, Chiu P, Singh SK, et al: Heart and combined heart-kidney transplantation in patients with concomitant renal insufficiency and end-stage heart failure. *Am J Transplant* 14:384–396, 2014.
32. Schaffer JM, Chiu P, Singh SK, et al: Combined heart-liver transplantation in the MELD era: do waitlisted patients require exception status? *Am J Transplant* 14:647–659, 2014.
33. Mancini D, Lietz K: Selection of cardiac transplantation candidates in 2010. *Circulation* 122:173–183, 2010.
34. Uriel N, Jorde UP, Cotarlan V, et al: Heart transplantation in human immunodeficiency virus-positive patients. *J Heart Lung Transplant* 28:667–669, 2009.
35. Russo MJ, Chen JM, Hong KN, et al; Columbia University Heart Transplant Outcomes Research Group: Survival after heart transplantation is not diminished among recipients with uncomplicated diabetes mellitus: an analysis of the United Network of Organ Sharing database. *Circulation* 114:2280–2287, 2006.
36. Colvin-Adams M, Smithy JM, Heubner BM, et al: OPTN/SRTR 2012 Annual Data Report: heart. *Am J Transplant* 14(Suppl 1):113–138, 2014.
37. Laks H, Marelli D: The alternate recipient list for heart transplantation: a model for expansion of the donor pool. *Adv Card Surg* 11:233–244, 1999.
38. Laks H, Marelli D, Fonarow GC, et al: Use of two recipient lists for adults requiring heart transplantation. *J Thorac Cardiovasc Surg* 125:49–59, 2003.
39. Daneshmand MA, Rajagopal K, Lima B, et al: Left ventricular assist device destination therapy versus extended criteria cardiac transplant. *Ann Thorac Surg* 89:1205–1209, discussion 1210, 2010.
40. Samsky MD, Patel CB, Owen A, et al: Ten-year experience with extended criteria cardiac transplantation. *Circ Heart Fail* 6:1230–1238, 2013.
41. Cimato TR, Jessup M: Recipient selection in cardiac transplantation: contraindications and risk factors for mortality. *J Heart Lung Transplant* 21:1161–1173, 2002.
42. Hunt SA: Who and when to consider for heart transplantation. *Cardiol Rev* 9:18–20, 2001.
43. Lu WH, Palatnik K, Fishbein GA, et al: Diverse morphologic manifestations of cardiac allograft vasculopathy: a pathologic study of 64 allograft hearts. *J Heart Lung Transplant* 30:1044–1050, 2011.
44. Betkowski AS, Graff R, Chen JJ, et al: Panel-reactive antibody screening practices prior to heart transplantation. *J Heart Lung Transplant* 21:644–650, 2002.
45. Bray RA, Nolen JD, Larsen C, et al: Transplanting the highly sensitized patient: the emory algorithm. *Am J Transplant* 6:2307–2315, 2006.

46. Loh E, Bergin JD, Couper GS, et al: Role of panel-reactive antibody cross-reactivity in predicting survival after orthotopic heart transplantation. *J Heart Lung Transplant* 13:194–201, 1994.
47. Kobashigawa JA, Sabad A, Drinkwater D, et al: Pretransplant panel reactive-antibody screens. Are they truly a marker for poor outcome after cardiac transplantation? *Circulation* 94:II294–II297, 1996.
48. Drakos SG, Stringham JC, Long JW, et al: Prevalence and risks of allosensitization in HeartMate left ventricular assist device recipients: the impact of leukofiltered cellular blood product transfusions. *J Thorac Cardiovasc Surg* 133:1612–1619, 2007.
49. Mulley WR, Kanellis J: Understanding crossmatch testing in organ transplantation: a case-based guide for the general nephrologist. *Nephrology (Carlton)* 16:125–133, 2011.
50. Zhang XP, Kelemen SE, Eisen HJ: Quantitative assessment of cell adhesion molecule gene expression in endomyocardial biopsy specimens from cardiac transplant recipients using competitive polymerase chain reaction. *Transplantation* 70:505–513, 2000.
51. Russo MJ, Chen JM, Sorabella RA, et al: The effect of ischemic time on survival after heart transplantation varies by donor age: an analysis of the United Network for Organ Sharing database. *J Thorac Cardiovasc Surg* 133:554–559, 2007.
52. Kobashigawa J, Mehra M, West L, et al: Report from a consensus conference on the sensitized patient awaiting heart transplantation. *J Heart Lung Transplant* 28:213–225, 2009.
53. De Marco T, Damon LE, Colombe B, et al: Successful immunomodulation with intravenous gamma globulin and cyclophosphamide in an alloimmunized heart transplant recipient. *J Heart Lung Transplant* 16:360–365, 1997.
54. Itescu S, Burke E, Lietz K, et al: Intravenous pulse administration of cyclophosphamide is an effective and safe treatment for sensitized cardiac allograft recipients. *Circulation* 105:1214–1219, 2002.
55. Pisani BA, Mullen GM, Malinowska K, et al: Plasmapheresis with intravenous immunoglobulin G is effective in patients with elevated panel reactive antibody prior to cardiac transplantation. *J Heart Lung Transplant* 18:701–706, 1999.
56. Ratkovec RM, Hammond EH, O'Connell JB, et al: Outcome of cardiac transplant recipients with a positive donor-specific crossmatch—preliminary results with plasmapheresis. *Transplantation* 54:651–655, 1992.
57. Schmid C, Garritsen HS, Kelsch R, et al: Suppression of panel-reactive antibodies by treatment with mycophenolate mofetil. *Thorac Cardiovasc Surg* 46:161–162, 1998.
58. Hodge EE, Klingman LL, Koo AP, et al: Pretransplant removal of anti-HLA antibodies by plasmapheresis and continued suppression on cyclosporine-based therapy after heart-kidney transplant. *Transplant Proc* 26:2750–2751, 1994.
59. John R, Lietz K, Burke E, et al: Intravenous immunoglobulin reduces anti-HLA alloreactivity and shortens waiting time to cardiac transplantation in highly sensitized left ventricular assist device recipients. *Circulation* 100:II229–II235, 1999.
60. Jordan SC, Pescovitz MD: Presensitization: the problem and its management. *Clin J Am Soc Nephrol* 1:421–432, 2006.
61. Leech SH, Lopez-Cepero M, LeFor WM, et al: Management of the sensitized cardiac recipient: the use of plasmapheresis and intravenous immunoglobulin. *Clin Transplant* 20:476–484, 2006.
62. Vo AA, Lukovsky M, Toyoda M, et al: Rituximab and intravenous immune globulin for desensitization during renal transplantation. *N Engl J Med* 359:242–251, 2008.
63. Kobashigawa JA, Patel JK, Kittleson MM, et al: The long-term outcome of treated sensitized patients who undergo heart transplantation. *Clin Transplant* 25:E61–E67, 2011.
64. Abraham WT, Adams KF, Fonarow GC, et al; Investigators and Group AS: In-hospital mortality in patients with acute decompensated heart failure requiring intravenous vasoactive medications: an analysis from the Acute Decompensated Heart Failure National Registry (ADHERE). *J Am Coll Cardiol* 46:57–64, 2005.
65. Yancy CW, Jessup M, Bozkurt B, et al: 2013 ACCF/AHA guideline for the management of heart failure: executive summary: a report of the American College of Cardiology Foundation/American Heart Association Task Force on practice guidelines. *Circulation* 128:1810–1852, 2013.
66. Seyfarth M, Sibbing D, Bauer I, et al: A randomized clinical trial to evaluate the safety and efficacy of a percutaneous left ventricular assist device versus intra-aortic balloon pumping for treatment of cardiogenic shock caused by myocardial infarction. *J Am Coll Cardiol* 52:1584–1588, 2008.
67. Burkhoff D, Cohen H, Brunckhorst C, et al; TandemHeart Investigators G: A randomized multicenter clinical study to evaluate the safety and efficacy of the TandemHeart percutaneous ventricular assist device versus conventional therapy with intraaortic balloon pumping for treatment of cardiogenic shock. *Am Heart J* 152:469 e1–469 e8, 2006.
68. Rose EA, Gelijns AC, Moskowitz AJ, et al; Randomized Evaluation of Mechanical Assistance for the Treatment of Congestive Heart Failure Study Group: Long-term use of a left ventricular assist device for end-stage heart failure. *N Engl J Med* 345:1435–1443, 2001.
69. Rogers JG, Butler J, Lansman SL, et al; Investigators IN: Chronic mechanical circulatory support for inotrope-dependent heart failure patients who are not transplant candidates: results of the INTrEPID Trial. *J Am Coll Cardiol* 50:741–747, 2007.
70. Slaughter MS, Rogers JG, Milano CA, et al; HeartMate III: Advanced heart failure treated with continuous-flow left ventricular assist device. *N Engl J Med* 361:2241–2251, 2009.
71. Aaronson KD, Eppinger MJ, Dyke DB, et al: Left ventricular assist device therapy improves utilization of donor hearts. *J Am Coll Cardiol* 39:1247–1254, 2002.
72. Dardas T, Mokadam NA, Pagani F, et al: Transplant registrants with implanted left ventricular assist devices have insufficient risk to justify elective organ procurement and transplantation network status 1A time. *J Am Coll Cardiol* 60:36–43, 2012.
73. Wozniak CJ, Stehlik J, Baird BC, et al: Ventricular assist devices or inotropic agents in status 1A patients? Survival analysis of the United Network of Organ Sharing database. *Ann Thorac Surg* 97:1364–1371, discussion 1371–1372, 2014.
74. Russo MJ, Hong KN, Davies RR, et al: Posttransplant survival is not diminished in heart transplant recipients bridged with implantable left ventricular assist devices. *J Thorac Cardiovasc Surg* 138:1425–1432, e1–3, 2009.
75. Nativi JN, Drakos SG, Kucheryavaya AY, et al: Changing outcomes in patients bridged to heart transplantation with continuous- versus pulsatile-flow ventricular assist devices: an analysis of the registry of the International Society for Heart and Lung Transplantation. *J Heart Lung Transplant* 30:854–861, 2011.
76. Healy AH, Baird BC, Drakos SG, et al: Impact of ventricular assist device complications on posttransplant survival: an analysis of the United network of organ sharing database. *Ann Thorac Surg* 95:870–875, 2013.
77. Bull DA, Reid BB, Selzman CH, et al: The impact of bridge-to-transplant ventricular assist device support on survival after cardiac transplantation. *J Thorac Cardiovasc Surg* 140:169–173, 2010.
78. Moazami N, Itescu S, Williams MR, et al: Platelet transfusions are associated with the development of anti-major histocompatibility complex class I antibodies in patients with left ventricular assist support. *J Heart Lung Transplant* 17:876–880, 1998.
79. Massad MG, Cook DJ, Schmitt SK, et al: Factors influencing HLA sensitization in implantable LVAD recipients. *Ann Thorac Surg* 64:1120–1125, 1997.
80. Drakos SG, Kfoury AG, Kotter JR, et al: Prior human leukocyte antigen-allosensitization and left ventricular assist device type affect degree of post-implantation human leukocyte antigen-allosensitization. *J Heart Lung Transplant* 28:838–842, 2009.
81. George I, Colley P, Russo MJ, et al: Association of device surface and biomaterials with immunologic sensitization after mechanical support. *J Thorac Cardiovasc Surg* 135:1372–1379, 2008.
82. Kirklin JK, Naftel DC, Stevenson LW, et al: INTERMACS database for durable devices for circulatory support: first annual report. *J Heart Lung Transplant* 27:1065–1072, 2008.
83. Cleveland JC, Jr, Naftel DC, Reece TB, et al: Survival after biventricular assist device implantation: an analysis of the Interagency Registry for Mechanically Assisted Circulatory Support database. *J Heart Lung Transplant* 30:862–869, 2011.
84. Copeland JG, Smith RG, Arabia FA, et al; CardioWest Total Artificial Heart I: Cardiac replacement with a total artificial heart as a bridge to transplantation. *N Engl J Med* 351:859–867, 2004.
85. Harringer W, Haverich A: Heart and heart-lung transplantation: standards and improvements. *World J Surg* 26:218–225, 2002.

86. Goland S, Czer LS, Kass RM, et al: Use of cardiac allografts with mild and moderate left ventricular hypertrophy can be safely used in heart transplantation to expand the donor pool. *J Am Coll Cardiol* 51:1214–1220, 2008.
87. Zaroff JG, Rosengard BR, Armstrong WF, et al: Consensus conference report: maximizing use of organs recovered from the cadaver donor: cardiac recommendations, March 28-29, 2001, Crystal City, Va. *Circulation* 106:836–841, 2002.
88. Taghavi S, Jayarajan SN, Wilson LM, et al: Cardiac transplantation can be safely performed using selected diabetic donors. *J Thorac Cardiovasc Surg* 146:442–447, 2013.
89. Southerland KW, Castleberry AW, Williams JB, et al: Impact of donor cardiac arrest on heart transplantation. *Surgery* 154:312–319, 2013.
90. Del Rizzo DF, Menkis AH, Pflugfelder PW, et al: The role of donor age and ischemic time on survival following orthotopic heart transplantation. *J Heart Lung Transplant* 18:310–319, 1999.
91. van der Hoeven JA, Molema G, Ter Horst GJ, et al: Relationship between duration of brain death and hemodynamic (in)stability on progressive dysfunction and increased immunologic activation of donor kidneys. *Kidney Int* 64:1874–1882, 2003.
92. Totsuka E, Fung JJ, Ishii T, et al: Influence of donor condition on postoperative graft survival and function in human liver transplantation. *Transplant Proc* 32:322–326, 2000.
93. Dickerson J, Valadka AB, Levert T, et al: Organ donation rates in a neurosurgical intensive care unit. *J Neurosurg* 97:811–814, 2002.
94. Nygaard CE, Townsend RN, Diamond DL: Organ donor management and organ outcome: a 6-year review from a Level I trauma center. *J Trauma* 30:728–732, 1990.
95. Benck U, Hoeger S, Brinkkoetter PT, et al: Effects of donor pre-treatment with dopamine on survival after heart transplantation: a cohort study of heart transplant recipients nested in a randomized controlled multicenter trial. *J Am Coll Cardiol* 58:1768–1777, 2011.
96. Wood KE, Becker BN, McCartney JG, et al: Care of the potential organ donor. *N Engl J Med* 351:2730–2739, 2004.
97. Dujardin KS, McCully RB, Wijdicks EF, et al: Myocardial dysfunction associated with brain death: clinical, echocardiographic, and pathologic features. *J Heart Lung Transplant* 20:350–357, 2001.
98. Venkateswaran RV, Townend JN, Wilson IC, et al: Echocardiography in the potential heart donor. *Transplantation* 89:894–901, 2010.
99. Stoica SC, Satchithananda DK, Charman S, et al: Swan-Ganz catheter assessment of donor hearts: outcome of organs with borderline hemodynamics. *J Heart Lung Transplant* 21:615–622, 2002.
100. Wheeldon DR, Potter CD, Oduro A, et al: Transforming the "unacceptable" donor: outcomes from the adoption of a standardized donor management technique. *J Heart Lung Transplant* 14:734–742, 1995.
101. Salim A, Vassiliu P, Velmahos GC, et al: The role of thyroid hormone administration in potential organ donors. *Arch Surg* 136:1377–1380, 2001.
102. Renlund DG, Taylor DO, Kfoury AG, et al: New UNOS rules: historical background and implications for transplantation management. United Network for Organ Sharing. *J Heart Lung Transplant* 18:1065–1070, 1999.
103. Schulze PC, Kitada S, Clerkin K, et al: Regional differences in recipient waitlist time and pre- and post-transplant mortality after the 2006 United Network for Organ Sharing policy changes in the donor heart allocation algorithm. *JACC Heart Fail* 2:166–177, 2014.
104. Taghavi S, Jayarajan SN, Wilson LM, et al: Cardiac transplantation with ABO-compatible donors has equivalent long-term survival. *Surgery* 154:274–281, 2013.
105. Patel ND, Weiss ES, Nwakanma LU, et al: Impact of donor-to-recipient weight ratio on survival after heart transplantation: analysis of the United Network for Organ Sharing Database. *Circulation* 118:S83–S88, 2008.
106. Jayarajan SN, Taghavi S, Komaroff E, et al: Impact of low donor to recipient weight ratios on cardiac transplantation. *J Thorac Cardiovasc Surg* 146:1538–1543, 2013.
107. Bleasdale RA, Banner NR, Anyanwu AC, et al: Determinants of outcome after heterotopic heart transplantation. *J Heart Lung Transplant* 21:867–873, 2002.
108. Yanagida R, Czer LS, Reinsmoen NL, et al: Impact of virtual cross match on waiting times for heart transplantation. *Ann Thorac Surg* 92:2104–2110, discussion 2111, 2011.
109. Jahania MS, Sanchez JA, Narayan P, et al: Heart preservation for transplantation: principles and strategies. *Ann Thorac Surg* 68:1983–1987, 1999.
110. Southard JH, Belzer FO: Organ preservation. *Annu Rev Med* 46:235–247, 1995.
111. Cannata A, Botta L, Colombo T, et al: Does the cardioplegic solution have an effect on early outcomes following heart transplantation? *Eur J Cardiothorac Surg* 41:e48–e52, discussion e52–e53, 2012.
112. Michel P, Vial R, Rodriguez C, et al: A comparative study of the most widely used solutions for cardiac graft preservation during hypothermia. *J Heart Lung Transplant* 21:1030–1039, 2002.
113. Kobayashi M, Tanoue Y, Eto M, et al: A Rho-kinase inhibitor improves cardiac function after 24-hour heart preservation. *J Thorac Cardiovasc Surg* 136:1586–1592, 2008.
114. Zheng X, Lian D, Wong A, et al: Novel small interfering RNA-containing solution protecting donor organs in heart transplantation. *Circulation* 120:1099–1107, 1 p following 1107, 2009.
115. Esmailian F, Kobashigawa JA, Naka Y, et al: The PROCEED II International Heart Transplant Trial with the Organ Care System Technology (OCS). *J Heart Lung Transplant* 32:S95–S96, 2013.
116. Angermann CE, Spes CH, Tammen A, et al: Anatomic characteristics and valvular function of the transplanted heart: transthoracic versus transesophageal echocardiographic findings. *J Heart Transplant* 9:331–338, 1990.
117. Miniati DN, Robbins RC: Techniques in orthotopic cardiac transplantation: a review. *Cardiol Rev* 9:131–136, 2001.
118. Barnard CN: What we have learned about heart transplants. *J Thorac Cardiovasc Surg* 56:457–468, 1968.
119. Dreyfus G, Jebara V, Mihaileanu S, et al: Total orthotopic heart transplantation: an alternative to the standard technique. *Ann Thorac Surg* 52:1181–1184, 1991.
120. Baumgartner WA, Traill TA, Cameron DE, et al: Unique aspects of heart and lung transplantation exhibited in the "domino-donor" operation. *JAMA* 261:3121–3125, 1989.
121. Sievers HH, Weyand M, Kraatz EG, et al: An alternative technique for orthotopic cardiac transplantation, with preservation of the normal anatomy of the right atrium. *Thorac Cardiovasc Surg* 39:70–72, 1991.
122. Sze DY, Robbins RC, Semba CP, et al: Superior vena cava syndrome after heart transplantation: percutaneous treatment of a complication of bicaval anastomoses. *J Thorac Cardiovasc Surg* 116:253–261, 1998.
123. Aziz TM, Burgess MI, El-Gamel A, et al: Orthotopic cardiac transplantation technique: a survey of current practice. *Ann Thorac Surg* 68:1242–1246, 1999.
124. Davies RR, Russo MJ, Morgan JA, et al: Standard versus bicaval techniques for orthotopic heart transplantation: an analysis of the United Network for Organ Sharing database. *J Thorac Cardiovasc Surg* 140:700–708, 708 e1–e2, 2010.
125. Sun JP, Niu J, Banbury MK, et al: Influence of different implantation techniques on long-term survival after orthotopic heart transplantation: an echocardiographic study. *J Heart Lung Transplant* 26:1243–1248, 2007.
126. Weiss ES, Nwakanma LU, Russell SB, et al: Outcomes in bicaval versus biatrial techniques in heart transplantation: an analysis of the UNOS database. *J Heart Lung Transplant* 27:178–183, 2008.
127. Schnoor M, Schafer T, Luhmann D, et al: Bicaval versus standard technique in orthotopic heart transplantation: a systematic review and meta-analysis. *J Thorac Cardiovasc Surg* 134:1322–1331, 2007.
128. Kitamura S, Nakatani T, Bando K, et al: Modification of bicaval anastomosis technique for orthotopic heart transplantation. *Ann Thorac Surg* 72:1405–1406, 2001.
129. Costanzo MR, Dipchand A, Starling R, et al: The International Society of Heart and Lung Transplantation guidelines for the care of heart transplant recipients. *J Heart Lung Transplant* 29:914–956, 2010.
130. Hauptman PJ, Aranki S, Mudge GH, Jr, et al: Early cardiac allograft failure after orthotopic heart transplantation. *Am Heart J* 127:179–186, 1994.

131. Stobierska-Dzierzek B, Awad H, Michler RE: The evolving management of acute right-sided heart failure in cardiac transplant recipients. *J Am Coll Cardiol* 38:923–931, 2001.
132. Baran DA, Galin ID, Gass AL: Current practices: immunosuppression induction, maintenance, and rejection regimens in contemporary post-heart transplant patient treatment. *Curr Opin Cardiol* 17:165–170, 2002.
133. Kreis H, Cisterne JM, Land W, et al: Sirolimus in association with mycophenolate mofetil induction for the prevention of acute graft rejection in renal allograft recipients. *Transplantation* 69:1252–1260, 2000.
134. Gambino A, Testolin L, Gerosa G, et al: New trends in heart transplantation. *Transplant Proc* 33:3536–3538, 2001.
135. Poston RS, Billingham M, Hoyt EG, et al: Rapamycin reverses chronic graft vascular disease in a novel cardiac allograft model. *Circulation* 100:67–74, 1999.
136. Topilsky Y, Hasin T, Raichlin E, et al: Sirolimus as primary immunosuppression attenuates allograft vasculopathy with improved late survival and decreased cardiac events after cardiac transplantation. *Circulation* 125:708–720, 2012.
137. Mancini D, Pinney S, Burkhoff D, et al: Use of rapamycin slows progression of cardiac transplantation vasculopathy. *Circulation* 108:48–53, 2003.
138. Keogh A, Richardson M, Ruygrok P, et al: Sirolimus in de novo heart transplant recipients reduces acute rejection and prevents coronary artery disease at 2 years: a randomized clinical trial. *Circulation* 110:2694–2700, 2004.
139. Vazquez de Prada JA, Vilchez FG, Cobo M, et al: Sirolimus in de novo heart transplant recipients with severe renal impairment. *Transpl Int* 19:245–248, 2006.
140. Zuckermann A, Manito N, Epailly E, et al: Multidisciplinary insights on clinical guidance for the use of proliferation signal inhibitors in heart transplantation. *J Heart Lung Transplant* 27:141–149, 2008.
141. Taylor DO, Barr ML, Radovancevic B, et al: A randomized, multicenter comparison of tacrolimus and cyclosporine immunosuppressive regimens in cardiac transplantation: decreased hyperlipidemia and hypertension with tacrolimus. *J Heart Lung Transplant* 18:336–345, 1999.
142. Kobashigawa J, Miller L, Renlund D, et al: A randomized active-controlled trial of mycophenolate mofetil in heart transplant recipients. Mycophenolate Mofetil Investigators. *Transplantation* 66:507–515, 1998.
143. Kobashigawa JA, Miller LW, Russell SD, et al; Study I: Tacrolimus with mycophenolate mofetil (MMF) or sirolimus vs. cyclosporine with MMF in cardiac transplant patients: 1-year report. *Am J Transplant* 6:1377–1386, 2006.
144. Mattei MF, Redonnet M, Gandjbakhch I, et al: Lower risk of infectious deaths in cardiac transplant patients receiving basiliximab versus anti-thymocyte globulin as induction therapy. *J Heart Lung Transplant* 26:693–699, 2007.
145. Carrier M, Leblanc MH, Perrault LP, et al: Basiliximab and rabbit anti-thymocyte globulin for prophylaxis of acute rejection after heart transplantation: a non-inferiority trial. *J Heart Lung Transplant* 26:258–263, 2007.
146. Teuteberg JJ, Shullo MA, Zomak R, et al: Alemtuzumab induction prior to cardiac transplantation with lower intensity maintenance immunosuppression: one-year outcomes. *Am J Transplant* 10:382–388, 2010.
147. Swinnen LJ, Costanzo-Nordin MR, Fisher SG, et al: Increased incidence of lymphoproliferative disorder after immunosuppression with the monoclonal antibody OKT3 in cardiac-transplant recipients. *N Engl J Med* 323:1723–1728, 1990.
148. Webster A, Pankhurst T, Rinaldi F, et al: Polyclonal and monoclonal antibodies for treating acute rejection episodes in kidney transplant recipients. *Cochrane Database Syst Rev* CD004756, 2006.
149. Beniaminovitz A, Itescu S, Lietz K, et al: Prevention of rejection in cardiac transplantation by blockade of the interleukin-2 receptor with a monoclonal antibody. *N Engl J Med* 342:613–619, 2000.
150. Mancini D, Beniaminovitz A, Edwards N, et al: Effect of Daclizumab induction therapy on the development of cardiac transplant vasculopathy. *J Heart Lung Transplant* 20:194, 2001.
151. Kobashigawa J, David K, Morris J, et al: Daclizumab is associated with decreased rejection and no increased mortality in cardiac transplant patients receiving MMF, cyclosporine, and corticosteroids. *Transplant Proc* 37:1333–1339, 2005.
152. Penninga L, Moller CH, Gustafsson F, et al: Immunosuppressive T-cell antibody induction for heart transplant recipients. *Cochrane Database Syst Rev* (12):CD008842, 2013.
153. Kubo SH, Naftel DC, Mills RM, Jr, et al: Risk factors for late recurrent rejection after heart transplantation: a multiinstitutional, multivariable analysis. Cardiac Transplant Research Database Group. *J Heart Lung Transplant* 14:409–418, 1995.
154. Billingham ME, Cary NR, Hammond ME, et al: A working formulation for the standardization of nomenclature in the diagnosis of heart and lung rejection: Heart Rejection Study Group. The International Society for Heart Transplantation. *J Heart Transplant* 9:587–593, 1990.
155. Mehra MR, Uber PA, Uber WE, et al: Anything but a biopsy: noninvasive monitoring for cardiac allograft rejection. *Curr Opin Cardiol* 17:131–136, 2002.
156. Wu YL, Ye Q, Sato K, et al: Noninvasive evaluation of cardiac allograft rejection by cellular and functional cardiac magnetic resonance. *JACC Cardiovasc Imaging* 2:731–741, 2009.
157. Dandel M, Hummel M, Muller J, et al: Reliability of tissue Doppler wall motion monitoring after heart transplantation for replacement of invasive routine screenings by optimally timed cardiac biopsies and catheterizations. *Circulation* 104:I184–I191, 2001.
158. Bainbridge AD, Cave M, Newell S, et al: The utility of pacemaker evoked T wave amplitude for the noninvasive diagnosis of cardiac allograft rejection. *Pacing Clin Electrophysiol* 22:942–946, 1999.
159. Masters RG, Davies RA, Veinot JP, et al: Discoordinate modulation of natriuretic peptides during acute cardiac allograft rejection in humans. *Circulation* 100:287–291, 1999.
160. Segal JB, Kasper EK, Rohde C, et al: Coagulation markers predicting cardiac transplant rejection. *Transplantation* 72:233–237, 2001.
161. Hesse B, Mortensen SA, Folke M, et al: Ability of antimyosin scintigraphy monitoring to exclude acute rejection during the first year after heart transplantation. *J Heart Lung Transplant* 14:23–31, 1995.
162. Narula J, Acio ER, Narula N, et al: Annexin-V imaging for noninvasive detection of cardiac allograft rejection. *Nat Med* 7:1347–1352, 2001.
163. Shoskes DA, Wood KJ: Indirect presentation of MHC antigens in transplantation. *Immunol Today* 15:32–38, 1994.
164. Smith-Garvin JE, Koretzky GA, Jordan MS: T cell activation. *Annu Rev Immunol* 27:591–619, 2009.
165. Parham P: *The immune system*, New York, NY, 2009, Garland Science, Taylor & Francis Group LLC.
166. Stewart S, Winters GL, Fishbein MC, et al: Revision of the 1990 working formulation for the standardization of nomenclature in the diagnosis of heart rejection. *J Heart Lung Transplant* 24:1710–1720, 2005.
167. Ross HJ, Gullestad L, Pak J, et al: Methotrexate or total lymphoid radiation for treatment of persistent or recurrent allograft cellular rejection: a comparative study. *J Heart Lung Transplant* 16:179–189, 1997.
168. Berglin E, Kjellstrom C, Mantovani V, et al: Plasmapheresis as a rescue therapy to resolve cardiac rejection with vasculitis and severe heart failure. A report of five cases. *Transpl Int* 8:382–387, 1995.
169. Chan GL, Weinstein SS, Vijayanagar RR: Treatment of recalcitrant cardiac allograft rejection with methotrexate. Cardiac Transplant Team. *Clin Transplant* 9:106–114, 1995.
170. Michaels PJ, Fishbein MC, Colvin RB: Humoral rejection of human organ transplants. *Springer Semin Immunopathol* 25:119–140, 2003.
171. Taylor DO, Yowell RL, Kfoury AG, et al: Allograft coronary artery disease: clinical correlations with circulating anti-HLA antibodies and the immunohistopathologic pattern of vascular rejection. *J Heart Lung Transplant* 19:518–521, 2000.
172. Reed EF, Demetris AJ, Hammond E, et al; International Society for H and Lung T: Acute antibody-mediated rejection of cardiac transplants. *J Heart Lung Transplant* 25:153–159, 2006.
173. Reinsmoen NL, Lai CH, Vo A, et al: Acceptable donor-specific antibody levels allowing for successful deceased and living donor

kidney transplantation after desensitization therapy. *Transplantation* 86:820–825, 2008.

174. Opelz G, Collaborative Transplant S: Non-HLA transplantation immunity revealed by lymphocytotoxic antibodies. *Lancet* 365:1570–1576, 2005.
175. Mahesh B, Leong HS, McCormack A, et al: Autoantibodies to vimentin cause accelerated rejection of cardiac allografts. *Am J Pathol* 170:1415–1427, 2007.
176. Kobashigawa J, Crespo-Leiro MG, Ensminger SM, et al; Consensus Conference Participants: report from a consensus conference on antibody-mediated rejection in heart transplantation. *J Heart Lung Transplant* 30:252–269, 2011.
177. Tambur AR, Pamboukian SV, Costanzo MR, et al: The presence of HLA-directed antibodies after heart transplantation is associated with poor allograft outcome. *Transplantation* 80:1019–1025, 2005.
178. Wu GW, Kobashigawa JA, Fishbein MC, et al: Asymptomatic antibody-mediated rejection after heart transplantation predicts poor outcomes. *J Heart Lung Transplant* 28:417–422, 2009.
179. Kfoury AG, Hammond ME, Snow GL, et al: Cardiovascular mortality among heart transplant recipients with asymptomatic antibody-mediated or stable mixed cellular and antibody-mediated rejection. *J Heart Lung Transplant* 28:781–784, 2009.
180. Montoya JG, Giraldo LF, Efron B, et al: Infectious complications among 620 consecutive heart transplant patients at Stanford University Medical Center. *Clin Infect Dis* 33:629–640, 2001.
181. Haddad F, Deuse T, Pham M, et al: Changing trends in infectious disease in heart transplantation. *J Heart Lung Transplant* 29:306–315, 2010.
182. Fishman JA: Infection in solid-organ transplant recipients. *N Engl J Med* 357:2601–2614, 2007.
183. Rubin RH: Prevention and treatment of cytomegalovirus disease in heart transplant patients. *J Heart Lung Transplant* 19:731–735, 2000.
184. Valantine HA, Luikart H, Doyle R, et al: Impact of cytomegalovirus hyperimmune globulin on outcome after cardiothoracic transplantation: a comparative study of combined prophylaxis with CMV hyperimmune globulin plus ganciclovir versus ganciclovir alone. *Transplantation* 72:1647–1652, 2001.
185. Gentry LO: Cardiac transplantation and related infections. *Semin Respir Infect* 8:199–206, 1993.
186. Ciubotariu R, Liu Z, Colovai AI, et al: Persistent allopeptide reactivity and epitope spreading in chronic rejection of organ allografts. *J Clin Invest* 101:398–405, 1998.
187. Adams DH, Wyner LR, Karnovsky MJ: Experimental graft arteriosclerosis. II. Immunocytochemical analysis of lesion development. *Transplantation* 56:794–799, 1993.
188. Rahmani M, Cruz RP, Granville DJ, et al: Allograft vasculopathy versus atherosclerosis. *Circ Res* 99:801–815, 2006.
189. Nagji AS, Hranjec T, Swenson BR, et al: Donor age is associated with chronic allograft vasculopathy after adult heart transplantation: implications for donor allocation. *Ann Thorac Surg* 90:168–175, 2010.
190. Costanzo MR, Naftel DC, Pritzker MR, et al: Heart transplant coronary artery disease detected by coronary angiography: a multiinstitutional study of preoperative donor and recipient risk factors. Cardiac Transplant Research Database. *J Heart Lung Transplant* 17:744–753, 1998.
191. Mehra MR, Uber PA, Ventura HO, et al: The impact of mode of donor brain death on cardiac allograft vasculopathy: an intravascular ultrasound study. *J Am Coll Cardiol* 43:806–810, 2004.
192. Yamani MH, Starling RC, Cook DJ, et al: Donor spontaneous intracerebral hemorrhage is associated with systemic activation of matrix metalloproteinase-2 and matrix metalloproteinase-9 and subsequent development of coronary vasculopathy in the heart transplant recipient. *Circulation* 108:1724–1728, 2003.
193. Spes CH, Klauss V, Mudra H, et al: Diagnostic and prognostic value of serial dobutamine stress echocardiography for noninvasive assessment of cardiac allograft vasculopathy: a comparison with coronary angiography and intravascular ultrasound. *Circulation* 100:509–515, 1999.
194. Gao HZ, Hunt SA, Alderman EL, et al: Relation of donor age and preexisting coronary artery disease on angiography and intracoronary ultrasound to later development of accelerated allograft coronary artery disease. *J Am Coll Cardiol* 29:623–629, 1997.
195. Raichlin E, Bae JH, Kushwaha SS, et al: Inflammatory burden of cardiac allograft coronary atherosclerotic plaque is associated with early recurrent cellular rejection and predicts a higher risk of vasculopathy progression. *J Am Coll Cardiol* 53:1279–1286, 2009.
196. Simpson L, Lee EK, Hott BJ, et al: Long-term results of angioplasty vs stenting in cardiac transplant recipients with allograft vasculopathy. *J Heart Lung Transplant* 24:1211–1217, 2005.
197. Kwok BW, Hunt SA: Neoplasia after heart transplantation. *Cardiol Rev* 8:256–259, 2000.
198. Brewer JD, Colegio OR, Phillips PK, et al: Incidence of and risk factors for skin cancer after heart transplant. *Arch Dermatol* 145:1391–1396, 2009.
199. Tsai DE, Hardy CL, Tomaszewski JE, et al: Reduction in immunosuppression as initial therapy for posttransplant lymphoproliferative disorder: analysis of prognostic variables and long-term follow-up of 42 adult patients. *Transplantation* 71:1076–1088, 2001.
200. Penn I: Incidence and treatment of neoplasia after transplantation. *J Heart Lung Transplant* 12:S328–S336, 1993.
201. Kato TS, Cheema FH, Yang J, et al: Preoperative serum albumin levels predict 1-year postoperative survival of patients undergoing heart transplantation. *Circ Heart Fail* 6:785–791, 2013.
202. Weiss ES, Allen JG, Arnaoutakis GJ, et al: Creation of a quantitative recipient risk index for mortality prediction after cardiac transplantation (IMPACT). *Ann Thorac Surg* 92:914–921, discussion 921–922, 2011.
203. Barge-Caballero E, Segovia-Cubero J, Almenar-Bonet L, et al: Preoperative INTERMACS profiles determine postoperative outcomes in critically ill patients undergoing emergency heart transplantation: analysis of the Spanish National Heart Transplant Registry. *Circ Heart Fail* 6:763–772, 2013.
204. Weiss ES, Meguid RA, Patel ND, et al: Increased mortality at low-volume orthotopic heart transplantation centers: should current standards change? *Ann Thorac Surg* 86:1250–1259, discussion 1259–1260, 2008.
205. Kilic A, Weiss ES, George TJ, et al: What predicts long-term survival after heart transplantation? An analysis of 9,400 ten-year survivors. *Ann Thorac Surg* 93:699–704, 2012.
206. Radovancevic B, Konuralp C, Vrtovec B, et al: Factors predicting 10-year survival after heart transplantation. *J Heart Lung Transplant* 24:156–159, 2005.

CHAPTER 99

HEART–LUNG TRANSPLANTATION

Steve K. Singh • Hari R. Mallidi

CHAPTER OUTLINE

The clinical realization of heart–lung transplantation evolved through much earlier experimental developments in the laboratory. Alexis Carrel[1] (Fig. 99-1) and later Demikhov[2] and Marcus and associates[3] performed experiments that explored the possibility of using heart–lung transplantation to replace diseased organs. When heart transplantation was first performed in 1968, Cooley, Lillehei, and Barnard all performed human heart–lung transplants, but patient survival time was short. Progress in the laboratory translated to the clinical application of the first successful human heart–lung transplant performed at Stanford in 1981.[4] Since the time that these initial clinical transplantations were performed, combined heart–lung transplantation and isolated lung transplantation have undergone dramatic changes in all aspects, including indications, operative technique, and postoperative management. This chapter reviews the state-of-the-art and current issues in the field of heart–lung transplantation.

INDICATIONS FOR HEART–LUNG TRANSPLANTATION

Over time, with the increased technical success of isolated single- (SLT) or double-lung transplantation (DLT), the indications for combined heart–lung transplantation have narrowed. The primary reason for heart–lung transplantation is irreversible dysfunction of both organ systems. The primary underlying defect could be cardiac in origin, such as congenital heart disease with irreversible end-stage cardiomyopathy and secondary pulmonary hypertension—also known as *Eisenmenger syndrome*. Alternatively, the primary defect could be pulmonary dysfunction, leading to irreversible heart disease over time. In general, the cardiac dysfunction is severe right-sided heart failure secondary to chronically elevated pulmonary arterial pressure—or *cor pulmonale*.

Another group of patients who have combined heart and lung disease has two separate disease processes that may not be related, such as a patient with a heavy smoking history who has severe emphysema and end-stage ischemic cardiomyopathy. These patients are rarely considered for heart–lung transplantation. However, experience with patients who have separate disease processes in the lungs and the heart has suggested that combined heart–lung transplantation is not a good treatment option and is associated with poor postoperative results and diminished long-term survival rates.

Recipient Diagnosis

The diagnostic profile of heart–lung transplant recipients reported to the Registry of the International Society for Heart and Lung Transplantation (ISHLT) from 1990 through 2007 is depicted in Figure 99-2.[5] Pulmonary hypertension secondary to congenital heart disease is the most frequent diagnosis, found in 33.9% of individuals who require heart–lung transplantation.[5] Cardiac lesions that can result in secondary pulmonary hypertension include atrial and ventricular septal defects, patent ductus arteriosus, truncus arteriosus, and other complex congenital anomalies, including univentricular heart with pulmonary atresia and hypoplastic left heart syndrome. Pulmonary hypertension secondary to congenital heart disease varies prognostically when compared with primary pulmonary hypertension (PPH). Despite comparable levels of pulmonary arterial pressures, individuals with Eisenmenger syndrome have lower right atrial pressures, a better cardiac index, and an overall better prognosis than patients with pulmonary hypertension without congenital heart disease.[6] Therefore, hemodynamic variables are less reliable in this group as an indicator for transplantation than is the presence of progressive symptoms (discussed later). Significant hemodynamic derangements in patients may be effectively managed with medical therapy, thus delaying transplantation.

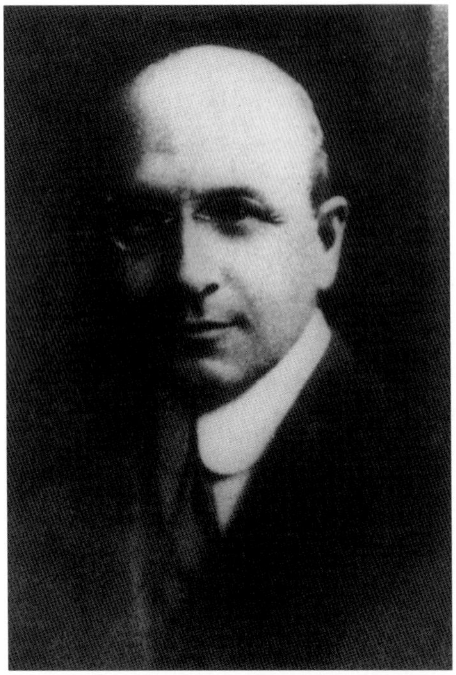

FIGURE 99-1 Alexis Carrel described the first heart–lung transplantation in a feline model in 1907. This experiment and numerous other observations predicted the eventual benefit of organ transplantation. For these outstanding accomplishments, Carrel received the Nobel Prize in 1912.

Secondary pulmonary hypertension with complex, irreparable cardiac defects must be treated with heart–lung transplantation. In a recent study, patients with Eisenmenger syndrome caused by a ventricular septal defect or multiple congenital anomalies had a highly significant survival advantage when a heart–lung transplantation was performed as opposed to cardiac repair combined with lung transplantation.[7] However, patients with simple cardiac defects, such as atrial septal defects, should be considered for repair of the cardiac defect combined with single or bilateral lung transplantation. Lung transplantation with intracardiac repair has evolved as a viable alternative to heart–lung transplantation for several reasons. First, right ventricular function improves after lung transplantation as a result of the normalization of pulmonary vascular resistance.[8] In addition, there is a shortage of donor hearts. Furthermore, denervation and graft coronary artery disease associated with cardiac transplantation is avoided.

Primary pulmonary hypertension associated with irreversible right ventricular failure is the second most

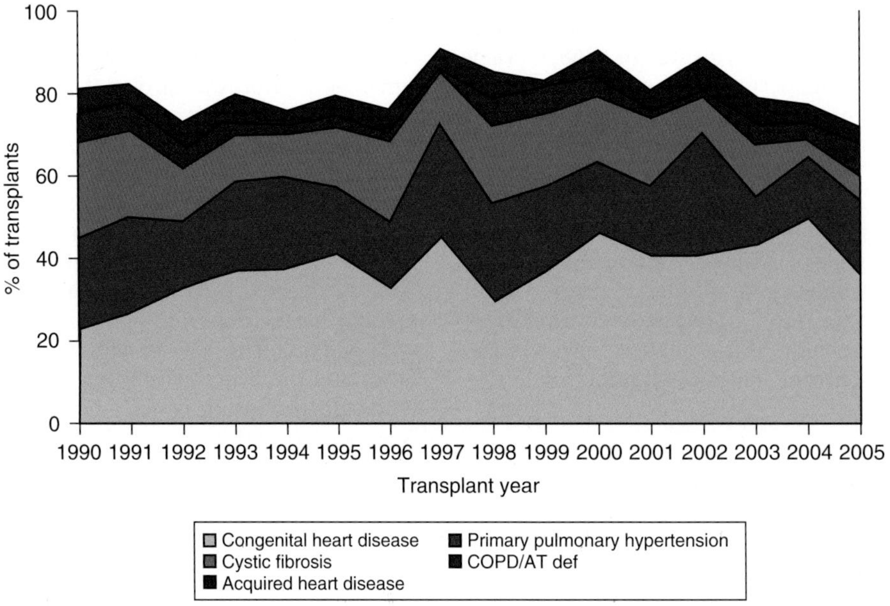

FIGURE 99-2 Indications for heart–lung transplantation from 1990 to 2005. *AT def,* Antitrypsin deficiency; *COPD,* chronic obstructive pulmonary disease. (Modified from Trulock EP, Christie JD, Edwards LB, et al: The Registry of the International Society of Heart and Lung Transplantation: Twenty-Fourth Official Adult Lung and Heart-Lung Transplant Report—2007. *J Heart Lung Transplant* 26:782–795, 2007.)

common indication for heart–lung transplantation, with 24% of recipients having this diagnosis.[5] In contrast to secondary pulmonary hypertension from congenital heart disease, abnormal hemodynamic parameters are closely related to increased mortality.[9] Therefore, patients with PPH should be promptly referred to a transplant pulmonologist for initiation of intravenous (IV) pulmonary vasodilators. If severe right ventricular failure persists despite aggressive medical therapy, heart–lung transplantation may be indicated.

The role of heart–lung transplantation in the setting of PPH has also evolved over the past several years. Individuals with pulmonary vascular disease and improved right ventricular function after initiation of medical therapy may also be treated effectively with either SLT or DLT. In the setting of PPH, DLT results in both greater hemodynamic improvement and a shorter duration of postoperative mechanical ventilation than does SLT,[10] and it is the preferred operation in most transplantation centers. Furthermore, comparable survival rates were noted in patients with PPH after heart–lung transplantation and after DLT.[11] Because DLT decreases the use of scarce donor hearts, a trend has recently emerged in favor of DLT for patients with PPH. This trend has resulted in a decrease in the number of heart–lung transplants for PPH during the past 10 years. The subsets of patients who have fixed pulmonary vascular resistance that is not responsive to vasodilators, and who have irreversible right-sided heart dysfunction, are still candidates for heart–lung transplantation.

The remainder of heart–lung transplantations are performed for a variety of disorders that result in end-stage pulmonary failure and irreversible cardiac failure. These include individuals with septic lung disease, such as cystic fibrosis and bronchiectasis; ischemic and restrictive cardiomyopathies with intercurrent end-stage lung disease; or acquired pulmonary vascular disease. Primary parenchymal lung disease, such as idiopathic pulmonary fibrosis, desquamative interstitial pneumonitis, and lymphangioleiomyomatosis, may occur with severe right-sided heart failure and may also be a reason for heart–lung transplantation.

The introduction of the "domino" transplantation procedure renewed interest in heart–lung transplantation for septic lung disease. In this procedure, the recipient of a heart–lung transplant served as a heart donor for a second recipient, thus maintaining donor organ allocation.[12,13] Recent studies have demonstrated equivalent survival rates in recipients of domino heart grafts and in recipients of cadaveric heart grafts. However, this procedure is rarely performed, and bilateral lung transplantation remains the procedure of choice for most septic or parenchymal lung disease.

The distribution of preoperative diagnoses managed with heart–lung transplantation at Stanford from 1981 to the present has been as follows: Eisenmenger syndrome, 44%; PPH, 23%; cystic fibrosis, 12%; complex congenital heart disease, 12%; α_1-antitrypsin deficiency, 2%; cardiomyopathy with pulmonary hypertension, 2%; failure of SLT, 1%; congenital bronchiectasis, less than 1%; pulmonary lymphangioleiomyomatosis, less than 1%; and other diagnoses, 3%.[14]

Recipient Selection Criteria

The selection of appropriate candidates for heart–lung transplantation is of paramount importance for success of the procedure. Any patient with end-stage cardiopulmonary disease with the capacity for full rehabilitation is a potential candidate for heart–lung transplantation. Suitable candidates should have a life expectancy of less than 2 years and generally have marked persistent functional disability, with a New York Heart Association (NYHA) class designation of III or IV. Patients must otherwise be in good general health without other serious systemic illness. The occurrence of life-threatening complications, such as severe right-sided congestive heart failure with liver dysfunction, massive hemoptysis, or multiple syncopal episodes, suggests a poor prognosis and the need to list a patient as a candidate for heart–lung transplantation.

Recipients of heart–lung transplants generally are younger than heart transplant recipients, with 44% being between the ages of 35 and 49 years, and only 15% being older than 60 years.[5] It must be determined that the patient and the family are emotionally prepared for transplantation. Each patient must be assessed for the presence of adequate emotional and psychosocial support to withstand the rigorous and intrusive medical regimen that will continue throughout their remaining life. Heart–lung transplantation has become more common as a therapeutic option for complex congenital heart disease in infants and children.[15,16] These recipients also must be carefully evaluated, and they should have an extremely strong family support network to cope with the complex regimen and the frequent medical follow-up.

The risk for mortality while a patient is on the waitlist must be balanced with the 1-year mortality risk after transplantation to determine the ideal time to activate someone on the transplant waitlist. The individual's disease process should be severe enough to warrant heart–lung transplantation, yet the patient must be well enough to survive the long wait until the transplantation occurs, and well enough to survive the surgical procedure itself.[17] The underlying disease determines the appropriate window. Survival with or without transplantation varies by disease process and by the patient's overall physical condition. Identification of a critical turning point in a patient's disease that signals an accelerated decline is the key to appropriate referral for transplantation. Pulmonary and cardiac clinical signs that can be used to gauge the appropriateness of listing include changes in the rate of decline in exercise capacity or pulmonary function, increasing frequency of infectious complications, increasing number and duration of hospitalizations, and increasing supplemental oxygen requirements. Other signs include increasing requirements for diuretics and increased hepatomegaly and bilirubin levels. Hyperbilirubinemia has been shown to be a marker for poor postoperative outcome in patients with pulmonary hypertension and right ventricular dysfunction. Patients with chronic bilirubin levels greater than 2.1 mg/dL who are undergoing heart–lung transplantation have been demonstrated to have significantly worse postoperative mortality (58%).[18] The rate of perioperative complications, including coagulopathy, hepatic encephalopathy, poor wound healing, and impaired clearance of cyclosporine with resultant nephrotoxicity, were also significantly increased after heart–lung transplantation in such patients.[19]

Heart–lung transplantation should be undertaken before multisystem organ failure and severe malnutrition ensue. Although patients await a suitable donor, many become increasingly debilitated. Every opportunity to optimize a patient's physical strength and nutritional status should be aggressively pursued.[20] Good physical performance before transplantation has been associated with improved postoperative recovery. Therefore, patients should be referred for physical therapy early in an effort to improve their functional status and optimize their recovery potential.

In the past, most centers considered conditions associated with extensive adhesions, such as previous thoracotomy or sternotomy, septic lung disease, and previous chemical or surgical pleurodesis, an absolute contraindication to heart–lung transplantation. Historically, patients with these conditions had increased morbidity and short-term mortality resulting primarily from excessive blood loss and pulmonary issues associated with massive transfusions of blood products. The introduction of antifibrinolytic therapy (aprotinin) in thoracic organ transplantation has provided improved outcomes for this group of patients.[21] However, with increasing evidence that this drug is associated with worse survival and a higher risk for renal and neurologic complications after isolated coronary artery bypass surgery, its use in North American surgical programs has diminished markedly. Heart–lung transplantation in patients with previous surgery may remain one indication for its continued use.[22] Current alternative antifibrinolytic options include aminocaproic acid and tranexamic acid. We now routinely accept patients with previous cardiac or thoracic surgery for heart–lung transplantation, and they represent a significant proportion of patients on the current waiting list.

In patients selected for transplantation, routine pretransplantation screening is performed for ABO blood group, the presence of preformed antibodies, human leukocyte antigen (HLA) and reaction of degeneration tissue types, and titers of antibodies against cytomegalovirus, herpes simplex virus, and toxoplasmosis. ABO compatibilities are strictly adhered to because isolated episodes of hyperacute rejection have been observed in patients in which transplantations were performed across ABO barriers. In addition to ABO compatibility, donor–recipient matching is also based on body size. In practice, matching donor and recipient height seems to be the most reproducible method for selecting the appropriate donor lung size. In general, the dimensions of the donor lungs should not be greater than 4 cm greater than those in the recipient. Other investigators have proposed that the simplest method of matching donor-to-recipient lung size is to use the respective predicted total lung capacity values.[23,24]

Once an appropriate donor–recipient match is made, the recipient is screened for preformed antibodies against a panel of 50 random donors. A percent reactive antibody (PRA) level greater than 25% prompts a prospective specific crossmatch between the donor and recipient. A positive crossmatch indicates the presence of anti-donor circulating antibodies in the recipient, and the organ cannot be accepted for transplantation. Despite several retrospective studies that reveal improved graft survival with HLA matching,[25-27] prospective HLA matching is not feasible given the short ischemic times tolerated. Furthermore, in a recent multicenter study, HLA matching for lung transplantation did not have a large effect on clinical outcome, including the development of obliterative bronchiolitis (OB).[28]

Recent data suggest that the presence of an elevated PRA level is associated with both early and late mortality.[29] In addition, elevated PRA levels have been shown to be associated with an increased incidence of acute rejection in both lung and heart transplantation patients, with an increased incidence of graft vascular disease in heart transplantation patients, and with an increased occurrence of accelerated bronchiolitis in lung transplantation patients.[30,31] Methods to decrease the patient's PRA level and to avoid antibody production by virtual, or, when time allows, prospective crossmatching, have decreased the negative effects of high baseline PRA levels on late survival.[32]

Many heart–lung transplant patients, especially in the pediatric population, have undergone previous cardiac surgery and are extremely sensitized when they present for heart–lung transplantation. Specific protocols using immunoglobulin, plasmapheresis, and rituximab have been shown to decrease the PRA levels in potential organ recipients. In addition, posttransplant treatment initiated in the operating room with plasma exchange, plasmapheresis, weekly immunoglobulin injections, and monitoring for the development of donor-specific antibodies has minimized the risk for hyperacute rejection in this population.[33] The current desensitization protocol being used at Stanford is shown in Box 99-1.

TREATMENT OF PATIENTS AWAITING TRANSPLANTATION

The average waiting period for a heart–lung block is greater than 18 months; therefore, treatment of recipients after they have been listed is a critical aspect of the preoperative plan. Routine medical care, including clinical surveillance, optimization of cardiopulmonary function, and management of disease-specific and age-specific issues, should be addressed during this time. General considerations in the pretransplantation period include appropriate surveillance protocols and screening for malignancies such as prostate, breast, and colon cancer. Other issues that should be addressed include appropriate prophylaxis for thromboembolism with warfarin[34] and aggressive maximization of bone density, because osteoporosis is increasingly recognized as a clinical problem for patients who are receiving long-term steroid therapy.[35] Nutrition and high-intensity pulmonary rehabilitation should be optimized. Finally, psychosocial issues need to be addressed with referral for supportive counseling, support groups, and other training means to help each patient cope with the upcoming challenges.

BOX 99-1 Treating the Highly Sensitized Heart–Lung Transplant Patient

WEEK 1

- IVIG × 2 consecutive days; each dose, 1 g/kg at 100 mL/hr

WEEK 2

- Rituximab, 375 mg/m^2 IV

WEEK 3

- Rituximab, 375 mg/m^2 IV

WEEK 4

- IVIG × 2 consecutive days; each dose, 1 g/kg dose at 100 mL/hr
- Monthly IVIG treatment thereafter until transplantation

TRANSPLANT MANAGEMENT

- PRA level > 50% and complement fixation (C1q) absent:
  - Plasmapheresis in the operating room when patient is on cardiopulmonary bypass
  - Immediate retrospective crossmatch
- PRA level > 50% and complement fixation (C1q) present:
  - Prospective crossmatch before transplantation

IV, Intravenously; *IVIG,* intravenous immune globulin; *PRA,* percent reactive antibody.

BOX 99-2 Heart–Lung Donor Selection Criteria

- Age <40 years
- Smoking history <20 pack-years
- Arterial Po_2 of 140 mm Hg on an Fio_2 of 40%, or 350 mm Hg on an FIo_2 of 100%
- Normal chest radiograph
- Sputum free of bacteria, fungus, or significant numbers of white blood cells on Gram and fungal staining
- Bronchoscopy showing absence of purulent secretions or signs of aspiration
- Absence of thoracic trauma
- Human immunodeficiency virus (HIV)–negative status

Disease-specific issues in patients awaiting heart–lung transplantation need to be addressed. These patients require optimal treatment of heart failure with standard therapeutic measures such as sodium restriction, aggressive diuresis, and vasodilators. Afterload reduction with nitrates, hydralazine, and angiotensin-converting enzyme inhibitors prolongs survival in patients awaiting transplantation.[36] In patients with PPH, supplemental oxygen is recommended to avoid hypoxic pulmonary vasoconstriction. Indications for outpatient oxygen therapy include an arterial partial pressure of oxygen (Pao_2) of 55 mm Hg or less (or arterial oxygen saturation [Sao_2] < 88% on room air) at rest, during physical exertion, or while asleep.[37] The prognosis of patients with PPH is determined by hemodynamic variables, and the following parameters are associated with a poor outcome: increased mean pulmonary artery pressure (mPAP > 85 mm Hg; median survival, 12 months), increased mean right atrial pressure (RAP > 20 mm Hg; median survival, 1 month), and decreased cardiac index (CI < 2.0 $L/min/m^2$; median survival, 17 months).[9] In addition to supplemental oxygen therapy, initiation of pulmonary vasodilator therapy improves hemodynamics and survival in patients awaiting transplantation. Epoprostenol is a short-acting prostaglandin, normally released by the endothelium, that vasodilates the pulmonary vascular bed and inhibits platelet aggregation. Continuous infusion of epoprostenol (Flolan; GlaxoSmithKline, London, UK) has been demonstrated to significantly improve pulmonary hemodynamics, exercise capacity, and survival in patients with NYHA classes III and IV heart failure.[38,39] Patients may then wait longer for transplantation. Despite improvements in pulmonary hemodynamics and survival, diseases often progress or tachyphylaxis develops. Therefore, patients need to be followed closely and returned to the active transplant list if any clinical deterioration is noted. In patients who have right ventricular failure while awaiting transplantation, the creation of an interatrial shunt to decompress the pressure-overloaded ventricle may need to be considered.[40]

Patients with cystic fibrosis awaiting heart–lung transplantation have special needs. Pulmonary hygiene is of critical importance, because greater than 80% of patients are chronically colonized with *Pseudomonas aeruginosa*.[41] Pulmonary clearance techniques, institution of bronchodilators, and initiation of antibiotics in the setting of acute infection are lifelong requirements. Prophylactic antibiotics are not routinely given because of the development of multiresistant organisms.[42] Sinus disease and lower respiratory tract infections are risks in most patients with cystic fibrosis. Bilateral maxillary sinus antrostomies performed in the pretransplantation period have resulted in fewer infectious complications in the posttransplant period.[43] In addition to infectious issues, other associated risk factors such as malnutrition secondary to malabsorption, pancreatic insufficiency, and diabetes mellitus must be properly addressed.

SELECTION AND MANAGEMENT OF DONORS

The satisfactory criteria for heart–lung blocks are similar to those for hearts and lungs separately (Box 99-2). The lungs are the most delicate solid organ, with frequent parenchymal damage and neurogenic edema occurring after brain death, as well as the increased risk for aspiration. These factors result in only 20% to 30% of multiorgan donors having lungs suitable for donation. Preliminary donor evaluation includes a detailed history, review of electrocardiogram and echocardiogram, chest radiograph, and arterial blood gas analysis. A donor age of less than 40 years is preferred. However, potential donors aged 40 to 50 years are considered at most transplant centers, provided they have normal cardiopulmonary functioning and a normal coronary arteriogram. Acceptance criteria also include no significant lung contusion or history of aspiration or sepsis. There should be no history of prior cardiac or pulmonary surgery. A donor chest radiograph must be clear with no signs of pathology. An arterial blood gas analysis should reveal an arterial oxygen tension level of greater than 350 mm Hg on a fractional inspired oxygen concentration (FiO_2) of 100%, and 100 mm Hg on an FiO_2 of 30%. Lung compliance is estimated by measuring peak inspiratory pressures, which should not exceed 30 cm H_2O. Tracheobronchial infection must be excluded with chest radiography, Gram stain of sputum, and bronchoscopy.

On arrival at the donor hospital, the retrieval team assesses the chest radiograph, recent arterial blood gas analyses, and hemodynamic parameters to confirm that there has been no deterioration in oxygenation or cardiac function. If possible, the bronchoscopic examination is repeated to ensure that there are no mucopurulent secretions suggestive of infection or aspiration, as in tracheobronchitis. The final assessment includes visual and manual intraoperative assessment of the heart and lungs, confirming normal lung parenchyma with no palpable masses or evidence of contusion.

Because of growing waiting lists and increased mortality before a transplant is received, most centers have expanded their donor acceptance criteria with the increased use of so-called marginal donors.[44] Thoracic trauma with a resultant pneumothorax is not a contraindication, provided there is not a continuous air leak. Furthermore, lungs that are mildly contused can also be used, provided ongoing bleeding is not noted on bronchoscopy and/or there is no major atelectasis. Patients with prolonged intubation and ventilation (>70 hours), once thought to be a contraindication, should also be considered. As noted previously, older donors also are being considered, provided that pulmonary functional parameters are normal and no significant coronary artery disease is detected. Donor infection with hepatitis C virus is an evolving area in cardiopulmonary transplantation. Hepatitis C–negative recipients have an increased risk for acquiring hepatitis, but the effect on patient survival remains unclear.[45] Absolute contraindications include severe coronary or structural heart disease, prolonged cardiac arrest, active malignancy (sometimes excluding primary brain cancers such as astrocytoma and skin cancers), smoking history of greater than five pack-years, and positive human immunodeficiency virus (HIV) status.

Donor management after a declaration of brain death is a critical area in which there are opportunities for significantly improving the number and quality of potential donors. Aggressive management strategies implemented by organ procurement organizations have made "unacceptable" lungs, defined as a PaO_2-to-FiO_2 ratio of less than 150, acceptable for transplant.[46] Donors with unacceptable lungs were treated with invasive monitoring, methylprednisolone, fluid restriction, inotropic agents, bronchoscopy, and diuresis. The resultant "acceptable" organs were successfully transplanted without compromise of either 30-day or 1-year graft survival.[46] The major goal in the initial management of these donors is the maintenance of hemodynamic stability and pulmonary function. Patients who have suffered an acute brain injury are usually hypovolemic, and appropriate fluid resuscitation is the initial step. Complicating factors include the development of diabetes insipidus, which should be treated with a vasopressin infusion (0.1 to 0.4 U/hr).[47] Fluid administration is guided by the central venous pressure, keeping in mind that a central venous pressure greater than 8 mm Hg has been demonstrated to be an independent risk factor for the development of lung dysfunction.[48] Inotropic agents such as dopamine or phenylephrine are instituted to maintain perfusion pressure after intravascular volume has been repleted. The donor is not hyperventilated after brain death is declared, and a pH of 7.40 is the goal, thus avoiding pulmonary vasoconstriction. Positive end-expiratory pressure of 5 is maintained to prevent atelectasis, and higher levels are avoided because of their deleterious effect on cardiac output.

The pathophysiology of brain death and its deleterious effect on the cardiovascular system have been well described.[49] The resultant endocrine and metabolic derangements are a potential area of intervention in the marginal donor with hemodynamic instability. Hormonal therapy, including triiodothyronine (T_3), cortisol, insulin, and vasopressin, has been shown to have beneficial effects on the hemodynamic profile of marginal donors.[50] Physiologic resuscitation, guided by a better understanding of the pathophysiology of brain death, ultimately leads to an increase in the number and quality of heart–lung donors.

HEART–LUNG PRESERVATION

The goal of optimal heart–lung preservation is to ameliorate the effect of ischemia-reperfusion (IR) injury on the allograft. In early heart–lung transplantations, donor transportation to the transplant center with on-site procurement was considered essential because of a lack of confidence in lung-preservation techniques. As with heart transplantation, better preservation techniques would expand the pool of available donors and would make donation more acceptable to referring hospitals and donors' families.

Minimization of IR injury ultimately results in optimization of allograft function in the posttransplantation period. Nonspecific graft failure, which most likely represents IR injury, remains a significant cause of perioperative morbidity and possibly mortality.[51] Reperfusion injury may predispose the transplant recipient to an increased risk for acute rejection secondary to the upregulation of histocompatibility class II antigens.[52] Understanding the pathophysiology of IR injury allows the implementation of strategies aimed at preserving function, minimizing injury, and prolonging allograft and patient survival.

The result of inadequate preservation is activation of the inflammatory cascade, resulting in pulmonary endothelial injury and increased capillary permeability. The resulting pulmonary interstitial and alveolar edema leads to diminished airway compliance, poor gas exchange, and increased pulmonary vascular resistance. Numerous recent studies have elucidated the role of the neutrophil and its interaction with the pulmonary endothelium in the pathogenesis of IR injury.[53-55] Reperfusion injury is caused in part by a complex interplay between leukocyte activation and the subsequent release of inflammatory mediators and cytokines, which leads to pulmonary endothelial injury.

Since the early 1980s, various methods have been developed to provide adequate heart–lung preservation. These methods have varied from simple graft excision and cold storage to sophisticated autoperfusion with donor blood and a working heart–lung preparation. Today, only two methods are actively used: (1) perfusion with pulmonoplegia solutions and cold storage and (2) perfusion with cold donor blood. Both methods include the use of pulmonary vasodilators. Pulmonary artery flush, the most widely adopted method of allograft preservation,[56] allows the rapid cooling of both lungs, resulting in a significant improvement in allograft function noted after both the infusion note (4 minutes) and total volume (60 mL/kg) are increased.[57] To counteract the reflex pulmonary vasoconstriction arising from preservation solutions, donors are pretreated with prostaglandins. These selective pulmonary vasodilators, alprostadil in North America and epoprostenol in Europe, improve the distribution of the pulmonary arterial flush and thus improve lung preservation. Recently, the role of retrograde flush through the left atrium has been advanced because of the improved distribution of the flush in a porcine model.[58,59]

The two types of crystalloid pulmonary artery flush solutions, intracellular and extracellular, are both designed to counteract the cellular swelling that results from graft ischemia and hypothermia. The intracellular solutions, Euro-Collins (EC) and University of Wisconsin, are composed of electrolytes that mimic the intracellular environment. The extracellular solutions include the Wallwork solution, which uses donor blood, and low-potassium dextran (Perfadex; XVIVO Perfusion AB, Gothenburg, Sweden). The most commonly used preservation solution is EC crystalloid solution, which has been modified with magnesium sulfate and 50% dextrose. A recent study has demonstrated that lung procurement with low-potassium dextran resulted in a significantly decreased incidence and severity of reperfusion injury with improved allograft function, as well as improved survival, when compared with EC.[60] The addition of a retrograde flush for isolated lung transplantation has resulted in improved posttransplant lung function.[61] This retrograde flush technique can be safely used in combined heart–lung transplantation by making a small left atrial incision, flushing the preservation solution retrograde via the veins, and collecting the effluent in the proximal pulmonary artery, where a separate small incision is made. In contrast, the use of Celsior solution as a lung-preservation solution resulted in lethal posttransplant outcomes in a porcine model of lung transplantation.[62]

Recent investigations in the laboratory and clinic have demonstrated improvements in allograft preservation after the modification of pulmonary arterial flush solutions. The focus has been to intervene at the level of the leukocyte–endothelial interaction in an effort to preserve the function of the pulmonary endothelial cell. The impact of toxic inflammatory mediators elaborated by the leukocyte has been reduced by techniques such as leukocyte filtration,[63] introduction of monoclonal antibodies directed against anti-intercellular adhesion molecules and selectins,[53,55,64] and vascular immunotargeting strategies.[54] Furthermore, treatments aimed at preserving pulmonary endothelial function by restoring endothelium-derived mediators, such as nitric oxide (NO) and prostacyclin, have been shown to improve allograft pulmonary function.[65-68] Instead of focusing on the preservation solutions or additives, others have focused their attention on the development of continuous organ perfusion systems. The TransMedics Organ Care System is an organ perfusion system that preserves organs by using a warm-blood perfusion of the organ during storage. The system has been approved for use in Europe for donor heart procurement and in late-stage clinical trial protocols in the United States.

OPERATIVE TECHNIQUE FOR DONOR HEART–LUNG REMOVAL

In the early days of heart–lung transplantation, the donor was transported to the recipient hospital, and in an adjacent operating room, the recipient heart–lung block was excised simultaneously with donor organ preparation. Long-distance procurement is now the rule as a result of improvements in donor selection, donor management, and preservation techniques. Numerous procurement teams work together, and optimal communication is essential.

The donor operation is performed via a median sternotomy (Fig. 99-3). The pericardium is opened vertically and laterally on the diaphragm, and a pericardial cradle is created. Both pleural spaces are then opened, followed by the inspection of both lungs and pleural spaces. In cases of trauma, cardiac and pulmonary contusions are immediately ruled out. The pulmonary ligaments are then divided inferiorly by using electrocautery. The ascending aorta and aortic arch are dissected free and encircled with tapes. The superior and inferior venae cavae are then dissected free and also encircled with tapes. The azygos and innominate veins are ligated and divided, which affords excellent exposure to the proximal trachea. The tissue overlying the proximal trachea is incised vertically and encircled with a tape. Dissection of the distal trachea is kept to a minimum to avoid injury to the peribronchial vessels at the carina.

The patient is administered 300 U/kg of IV heparin, and the aorta and pulmonary artery are cannulated. Approximately 15 minutes before applying the aortic crossclamp, prostaglandin E_1 (PGE_1) is infused IV, initially at a rate of 20 ng/kg per minute and gradually increasing to a target rate of 100 ng/kg per minute. During PGE_1 infusion, the mean arterial blood pressure should be maintained at greater than 55 mm Hg. Inflow occlusion is accomplished by ligating the superior vena cava distally to avoid damage to the sinoatrial node. The inferior vena cava is clamped with a straight Potts clamp. The heart is allowed to empty, and the aortic crossclamp is applied. Cold crystalloid cardioplegia (10 mL/kg) is

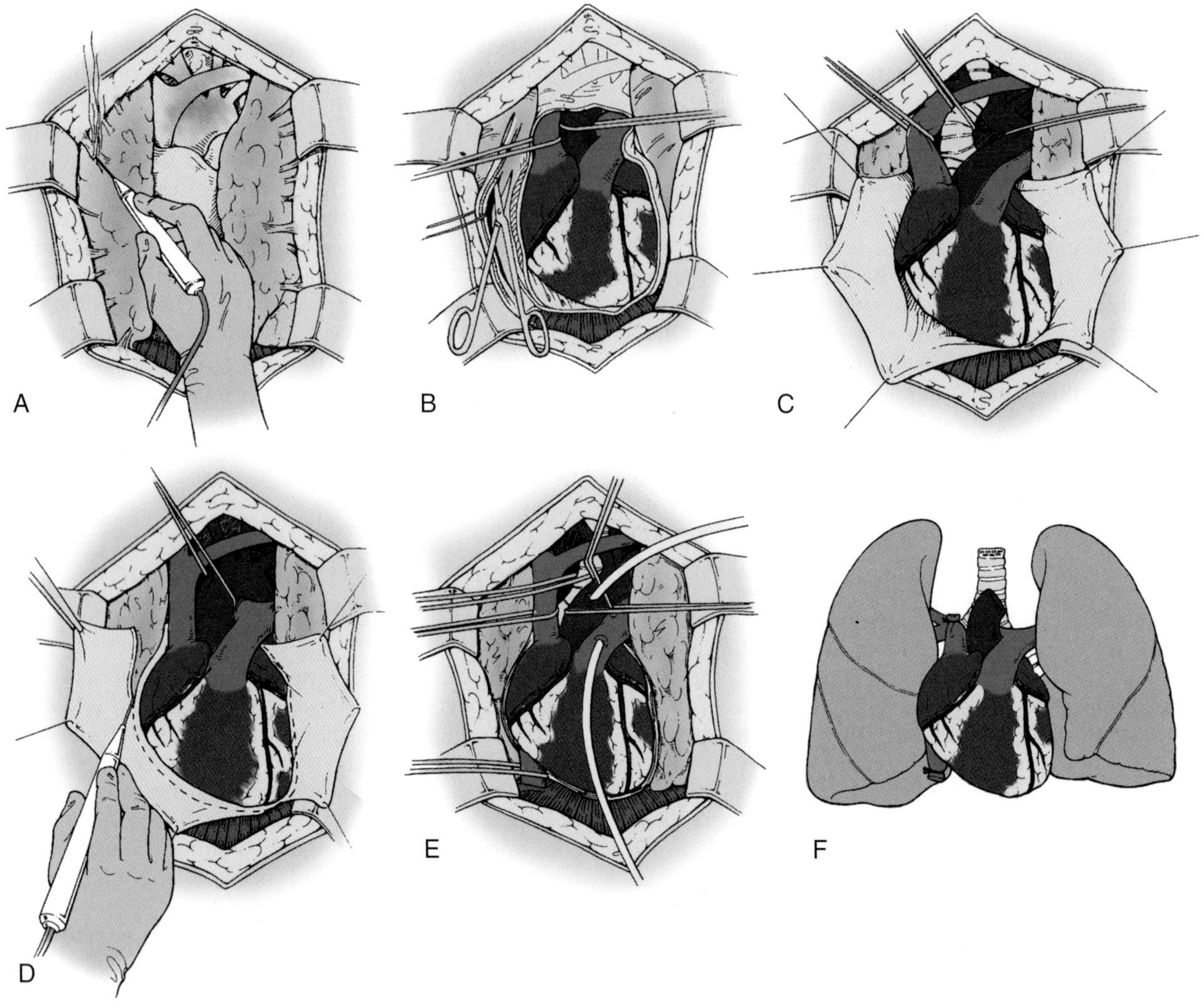

FIGURE 99-3 ■ The donor operation. **A,** Through a median sternotomy, adhesions are lysed and the pulmonary ligaments are divided inferiorly. **B,** The pericardium is opened and cradled, followed by dissection of the ascending aorta, venae cavae, pulmonary artery, and trachea. **C,** Tapes are placed around the aorta, venae cavae, and trachea. **D,** The entire anterior pericardium is excised back to each hilum. **E,** Cardioplegia and pulmonoplegia solutions are infused simultaneously into the aorta and main pulmonary artery after aortic crossclamping. Application of topical cold Physiosol follows immediately. **F,** The venae cavae and aorta are divided, and the heart–lung block is dissected free from the esophagus and posterior hilar attachments. After the trachea is stapled and divided at the highest point possible, the entire heart–lung block is removed from the chest. (From Yuh DD, Robbins RC, Reitz BA: Transplantation of the heart and lungs. In Edmunds LH, editor: *Cardiac Surgery in the Adult,* New York, 1997, McGraw-Hill, pp 1451–1475.)

administered via the aortic root. The inferior vena cava is incised, and the left atrial appendage is amputated immediately after initiating the pulmonoplegia. Adequate venting should be ensured and cardiac distention avoided. Pulmonoplegia with an EC solution at 4°C is rapidly infused at a rate of 15 mL/kg per minute for 4 minutes. During the administration of cold cardioplegia and pulmonary perfusate, copious amounts of cold topical saline are immediately poured over the heart and lungs. The lungs are ventilated with half-normal tidal volumes of room air while the dissection is completed, separating the heart–lung block from the posterior mediastinum, from inferior to superior. The lungs are inflated to a tidal volume of three-fourths normal, and the trachea is stapled with a TA-55 stapler and divided. The aorta is then divided, and the heart–lung block is removed, wrapped with sterile towels, and immersed in ice-cold saline at 4°C in preparation for transport (see Fig. 99-3). Clinically, we have used grafts preserved for up to 6 hours with successful implantation and outcome.

OPERATIVE PROCEDURE

The operation to replace the heart and lungs is one of the most fascinating and challenging procedures for cardiothoracic surgeons. The anatomy that is encountered and the areas of the thorax that are dissected are not otherwise commonly seen. Careful attention to details can simplify the procedure in even the most challenging patients.

Patients with PPH with end-stage right ventricular failure are usually the ideal candidates for heart–lung transplantation. These patients generally have not had previous cardiac or thoracic surgery and do not have large mediastinal collaterals from cyanosis. Conversely, patients with congenital heart disease and pulmonary atresia, or Eisenmenger syndrome and cyanosis, may have large mediastinal bronchial collaterals that require careful ligation. The most challenging aspect of the procedure is to remove the heart and lungs without injury to the phrenic, recurrent laryngeal, and vagus nerves. Careful attention to hemostasis is necessary before implantation of the graft, because exposure of many of the areas of dissection is difficult.

The recipient procedure for heart–lung transplantation has evolved over the past decade, with two major changes often used: the conversion from atrial cuff to bicaval anastomoses, and the positioning of the pulmonary hila anterior to the phrenic nerve pedicle. The right atrial cuff anastomosis was initially proposed in heart–lung transplantation to facilitate cannulation for cardiopulmonary bypass and eliminate the possibility of stenoses at the vena caval anastomoses. As in the transplantation of the heart alone, asynchronous contraction of both atrial cuffs is associated with an increased incidence of atrioventricular valve regurgitation. A demonstrated clinical benefit of caval anastomosis is fewer postoperative arrhythmias.[69] Because the pulmonary hila are positioned anterior to the phrenic nerve pedicle, less posterior mediastinal dissection is required, resulting in decreased rates of phrenic and vagus nerve injury.[70] Another advantage to this technique is that it allows for easier inspection of the posterior mediastinum for bleeding by rotation of the heart–lung block anteriorly and medially while the patient is still on cardiopulmonary bypass.

With careful attention to detail in the posterior mediastinal dissection and during the creation of the windows in the pericardium, the placement of the lungs posterior to the phrenic nerves can be performed safely. The primary advantage to this approach is seen in the reoperation setting. The placement of the donor lungs posterior to the phrenic nerves results in maintenance of the normal anatomic relationships, which facilitates the dissection at the time of repeat transplantation.

The patient is prepared for operation with the usual monitoring lines. After the induction of general anesthesia, the chest and both groins are prepared and draped in a sterile manner. A standard median sternotomy incision is made, and both pleural spaces are opened anteriorly (Fig. 99-4). A portion of the pericardium is removed anteriorly, avoiding the phrenic nerves. The ascending aorta and both venae cavae are dissected free and encircled with tapes. After fully heparinizing the recipient, the high ascending aorta and both venae cavae are cannulated separately, cardiopulmonary bypass is instituted, and the patient is cooled to 28° C. The aorta is cross-clamped, and a small amount of cardioplegia may be given to induce cardiac arrest.

First, the heart is excised as in heart transplantation. Next, the lungs are removed sequentially. The right and left bronchi are skeletonized, and a stapling device (TA 30, 4.8 mm) is used to occlude them. Cutting the bronchus distally allows the lung to be removed easily and avoids contamination from the open bronchus.

The native main pulmonary artery remnant is then removed. A portion of the pulmonary artery is left intact adjacent to the underside of the aorta in the region of the ligamentum arteriosum, which minimizes damage to the recurrent laryngeal nerve. The final step in preparing the recipient is to open the pericardium at the superior part of the pericardial space just anterior to the right and left bronchi, allowing dissection back to the carina. The stapled ends of the right and left bronchi are grasped, and dissection is carried up to the level of the distal trachea. In this area, it is important to stay directly on the bronchus, use electrocautery if possible, and avoid injury to the vagus nerve as it passes posterior to the bronchus and anterior to the esophagus. The vascular lymph nodes in this area may be very large, particularly in patients with cystic fibrosis. Bronchial vessels are individually identified and ligated or clipped. Patients with secondary pulmonary hypertension from congenital heart disease have large mediastinal bronchial collaterals that must be carefully ligated. Hemostasis is imperative in this area of dissection because exposure to this region is difficult after transplantation of the heart–lung block. The chest wall also is carefully inspected, and electrocautery or an argon beam coagulator is used. After absolute hemostasis is ensured, the donor heart–lung graft is prepared for implantation.

The donor heart–lung block is removed from its sterile container and brought to the operative field in a basin of cold saline solution. The donor trachea is excised several rings above the carina, and the superior tracheal segment, with the clamp attached, is then removed from the field. The tracheobronchial tree is aspirated with a sucker that is later discarded. At the same time, a sample to be cultured is taken directly from the trachea. The trachea is trimmed back so that only one complete cartilaginous ring is left just above the carina. A syringe full of normal saline is used to irrigate the bronchi and visualize them for retained secretions or any foreign body that might have been aspirated by the donor.

The heart–lung graft is then lowered into the chest with the lung hila anterior to the phrenic nerve pedicles (see Fig. 99-4). A cold saline solution and gauze pads soaked in cold saline are placed over the lung and heart to maintain hypothermia during implantation. The recipient trachea is opened one cartilaginous ring above the carina, and all the adventitial peritracheal tissue that is adjacent to the superior tracheal segment is left in place. Small bronchial vessels may require a Liga clip or suture; use of electrocautery at the cut edge of the trachea should be avoided. The tracheal anastomosis is performed with a running suture of 3-0 polypropylene, starting on the left side of the trachea and completing the posterior row from the inside. The same suture is continued anteriorly from outside the trachea. There should be a fairly close size match between donor and recipient, but any disparity can generally be accommodated by the flexible membranous part of the trachea. These bites usually go around at least one cartilaginous ring, and the donor trachea slightly invaginates the recipient trachea in most cases. When the tracheal anastomosis is complete, the chest is irrigated with several liters of ice-cold saline solution to cool the graft and to help remove any contamination from the trachea.

The recipient inferior vena cava is then anastomosed to the donor inferior vena cava by using a running 4-0

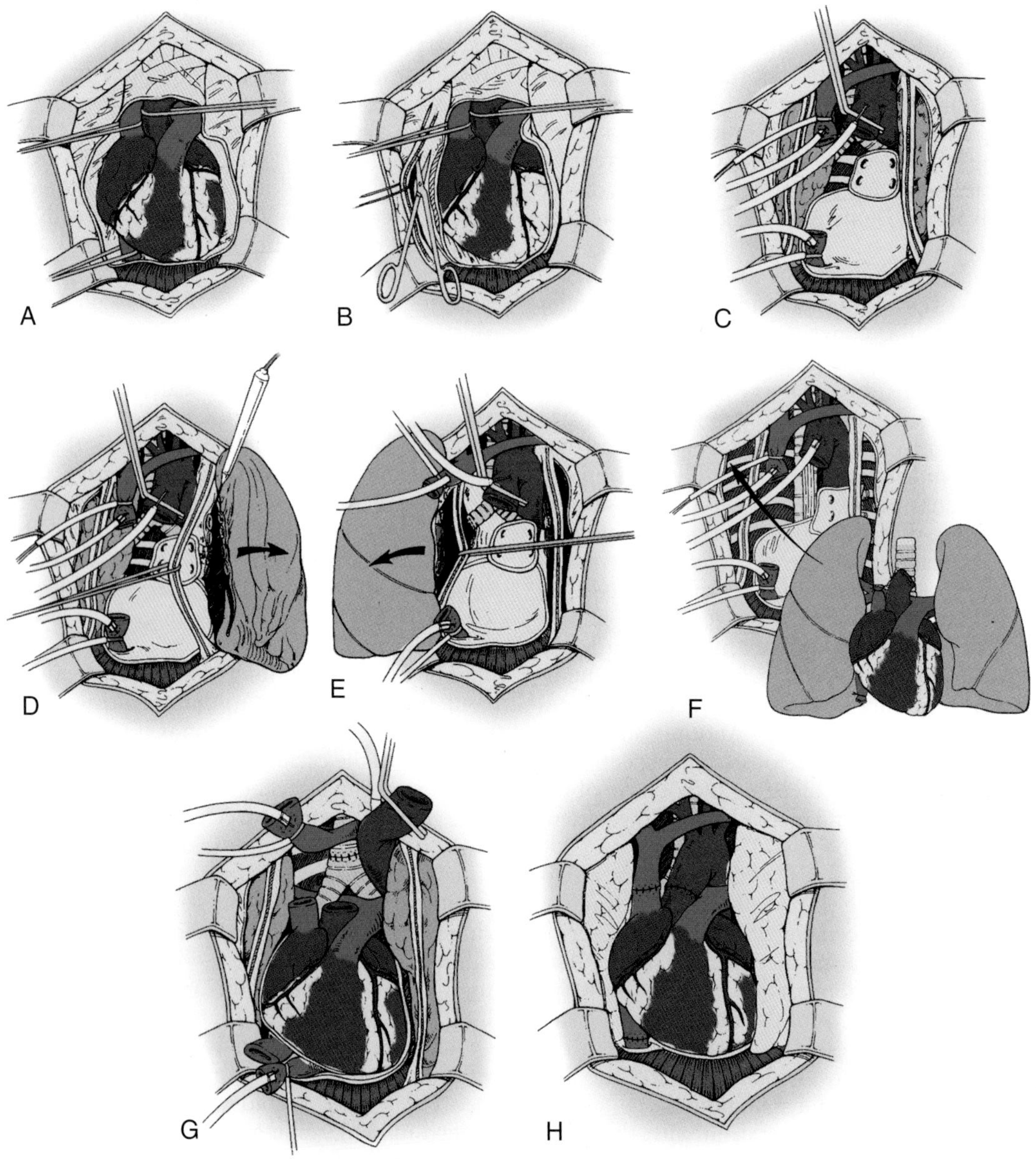

FIGURE 99-4 ■ The recipient operation. **A,** Through a median sternotomy, the anterior pericardium is partially removed, and the ascending aorta and both venae cavae are dissected and encircled with tapes. **B,** The right phrenic nerve is carefully separated from the right hilum. **C,** Cannulation for cardiopulmonary bypass consists of a cannula in the high ascending aorta and separate vena caval cannulas. Once the patient is on cardiopulmonary bypass, the native heart is excised in a manner similar to that used for standard cardiac transplantation. **D-E,** Left and right pneumonectomies are performed by dividing the respective inferior pulmonary ligament, pulmonary artery and veins, and main-stem bronchus. **F,** The heart–lung block is lowered into the chest, placing the hila anterior to each respective phrenic nerve pedicle. **G,** The tracheal anastomosis is performed with a continuous 3-0 polypropylene suture. **H,** The caval and aortic anastomoses are performed with a continuous 4-0 polypropylene suture. (From Yuh DD, Robbins RC, Reitz BA: Transplantation of the heart and lungs. In Edmunds LH, editor: *Cardiac Surgery in the Adult,* New York, 1997, McGraw-Hill, pp 1451–1475.)

polypropylene suture. At this point, the patient is rewarmed toward 37° C, and the superior vena caval and aortic anastomoses are performed in an end-to-end fashion by using a continuous 4-0 polypropylene suture (see Fig. 99-4). After completion of the aortic anastomosis, the patient is placed in a slightly head-down position, the ascending aorta and pulmonary artery are aspirated for air, and the caval tapes and the aortic crossclamp are removed. A leukocyte filter in the cardiopulmonary bypass circuit is opened 10 to 20 minutes before the aortic unclamping. The tracheal tube is aspirated by using sterile technique, and ventilation is resumed with room air. The left atrial opening at the appendage is repaired. When the patient's body temperature is almost normal and heart and lung function are satisfactory, cardiopulmonary bypass is discontinued and decannulation is performed routinely. The inspired concentration of oxygen is increased as required. Temporary pacing wires are applied to the donor right atrium and ventricle and brought out through the skin below the incision. Right-angled chest tubes are placed in the right and left pleural spaces, and a straight chest tube is placed in the mediastinum. Methylprednisolone (500 mg) is given to the recipient after heparin reversal with protamine sulfate.

The posterior mediastinum is then inspected for bleeding by carefully rotating the heart–lung block anteriorly and medially while the anesthesiologist uses hand ventilation. This maneuver is facilitated by using the most recent modification, in which the pulmonary hila are placed anterior to the phrenic nerves. Large amounts of warm saline solution at 37° C are used to irrigate both pleural spaces and the mediastinum. When hemostasis is satisfactory, the sternum is closed routinely with multiple stainless steel sternal wires.

POSTOPERATIVE MANAGEMENT

Intensive Care Unit

The immediate postoperative management of the patient undergoing heart–lung transplant is similar to that of any patient after cardiac surgery. Patients are allowed to awaken early in the postoperative course and are monitored closely for hemodynamic stability and bleeding. Endotracheal tube suctioning is performed when appropriate, and the patient is weaned from the ventilator in a routine manner. When the patient is alert and hemodynamically stable and blood gases and ventilatory mechanics are satisfactory, the patient is extubated. Strict attention is paid to fluid balance, and a vigorous diuresis is encouraged in most patients. As soon as possible, the patient is allowed to sit in a chair and begin ambulation. A physical therapist works with the patient to facilitate rapid rehabilitation.

Several points must be kept in mind when treating heart–lung transplant patients in the immediate postoperative period. Early graft dysfunction, manifested by progressive hypoxemia and hypercapnia, can be present in up to 10% to 15% of patients.[51] The proposed etiology is IR injury in the transplanted lung. This injury results in increased pulmonary capillary permeability, alveolar edema, impaired pulmonary compliance, and increased pulmonary vascular resistance with right ventricular dysfunction. Graft dysfunction can progress rapidly, and early treatment is essential. Initiation of pulmonary vasodilators such as alprostadil or inhaled NO may be necessary. Inhaled NO has been demonstrated to decrease the intrapulmonary shunt, optimizing ventilation-perfusion matching after lung transplantation.[71] In another study, inhaled NO administered in the setting of lung allograft dysfunction doubled the ratio of arterial oxygen tension to inspired oxygen fraction (Pa_{O_2} to Fi_{O_2}) within 1 hour of administration.[51] Furthermore, significant reductions in airway complications, duration of mechanical ventilation, and mortality were noted.[51] In cases of persistent, severe pulmonary graft dysfunction refractory to all intervention, extracorporeal membrane oxygenation has been used successfully to stabilize gas exchange in several patients.[72]

Immunosuppression

The immunosuppression regimen for heart–lung transfer recipients includes induction therapy with polyclonal rabbit antithymocyte globulin (RATG) and maintenance therapy with tacrolimus, mycophenolate mofetil, and prednisone. Standard protocol is depicted in Tables 99-1 and 99-2.

Induction therapy is used on the basis of data showing that it decreases the incidence of early acute rejection, chronic rejection, and OB.[73,74] Induction therapy is initiated with RATG (1.5 mg/kg IV) on postoperative days (POD) 1, 2, 3, 5, and 7 (see Table 99-1). If the patient is hemodynamically unstable or allograft function is compromised from reperfusion injury, RATG dosing is delayed for several days. From 1987 to 1993, induction therapy at some centers was switched from RATG to OKT3, the murine monoclonal antibody directed specifically against the T cell (CD3) receptor. However, the use of OKT3 was later shown to be associated with a greater incidence of acute pulmonary allograft rejection, postoperative infection, and OB when compared with RATG.[75] These findings resulted in a return to using the polyclonal anti–T cell antibody for induction therapy. More recently, there has been a switch to using the interleukin (IL)-2 receptor blocker daclizumab for induction therapy, or to using no induction therapy, especially in patients with significant posttransplant IR injury.

TABLE 99-1 Early Induction Immunosuppressive Therapy after Heart–Lung Transplantation

Immunosuppressive Agent	Dosage
Methylprednisolone	500 mg IV after administration of protamine in the OR
	125 mg IV every 8 hours for 3 doses
Rabbit antithymocyte globulin	1.5 mg/kg IV on POD 1, 2, 3, 5, and 7
Daclizumab	1 mg/kg (first dose in OR, then every 14 days on POD 14, 28, 42, and 56)

IV, Intravenously; *OR,* operating room; *POD,* postoperative days.

TABLE 99-2 Early Immunosuppression Therapy after Heart–Lung Transplantation

Immunosuppressive Agent	Dose
Tacrolimus	Start with 1 mg orally twice a day on POD 1
0-6 mo	12-15 ng/mL
7-12 mo	10-15 ng/mL
>12 mo	8-10 ng/mL
If sirolimus added	5-7 ng/mL
Mycophenolate mofetil	Start at 500 mg twice a day on POD 1; adjust to white cell count >4 and side effects
Prednisone	
Induction	Hold 8 days, then start at 0.6 mg/kg, divided doses
No induction	Start on POD 1 at 0.6 mg/kg, divided doses

POD, Postoperative day.

Methylprednisolone (500 mg IV) is administered intraoperatively and continued postoperatively at a dose of 125 mg IV every 8 hours for three doses. If induction therapy is used, maintenance prednisone is withheld for 1 week. Steroids are then restarted on POD 8 with a daily divided oral dose of 0.6 mg/kg prednisone, which is gradually tapered over the next 3 to 4 weeks to 0.1 to 0.2 mg/kg per day. The risk for airway complications after transplantation is not adversely affected by the use of postoperative steroids.[76] If induction immunotherapy is not used, then prednisone is started after the IV dosing is completed at a dose of 0.6 mg/kg per day in divided doses, with gradual tapering down to a maintenance dosage of 0.1 mg/kg per day.

In addition to steroids, maintenance immunosuppressive therapy includes mycophenolate mofetil and tacrolimus. Mycophenolate mofetil is initiated on POD 1, starting at a dosage of 500 mg twice daily. The dosage is titrated to maintain a leukocyte count greater than 4000/mm^3 and to avoid significant side effects. Tacrolimus is also initiated on POD 1 and titrated slowly based on trough levels, with the goal of achieving therapeutic levels on POD 5. This strategy avoids high serum levels and prevents nephrotoxicity. Patients who are unable to tolerate oral intake secondary to prolonged intubation or malabsorption are administered one third of the calculated total dosage IV in a continuous manner.

Although this immunosuppressive regimen has served heart–lung transplantation well, high rates of acute allograft rejection, infection, and chronic rejection, primarily manifested as OB, still exist. The quest for more efficacious and less toxic immunosuppressive regimens is a continual investigative challenge. Starting in approximately 2005, there was a shift from the use of cyclosporine to tacrolimus that was based on studies suggesting that the incidence of OB syndrome was lower with the use of tacrolimus.[77] Mycophenolate mofetil has been shown to have antiproliferative effects on T and B cells by inhibiting de novo purine biosynthesis, with improved efficacy and reduced toxicity.[78] An added advantage of using mycophenolate mofetil is the selective expansion of regulatory T cells, which may lead to better host tolerance of the transplanted organ.[79] In addition, newer T cell–inhibitory agents, such as sirolimus (rapamycin), which specifically block smooth muscle cell proliferation, can potentially prevent both acute rejection and the manifestations of chronic rejection, also with less toxic side effects.[80,81]

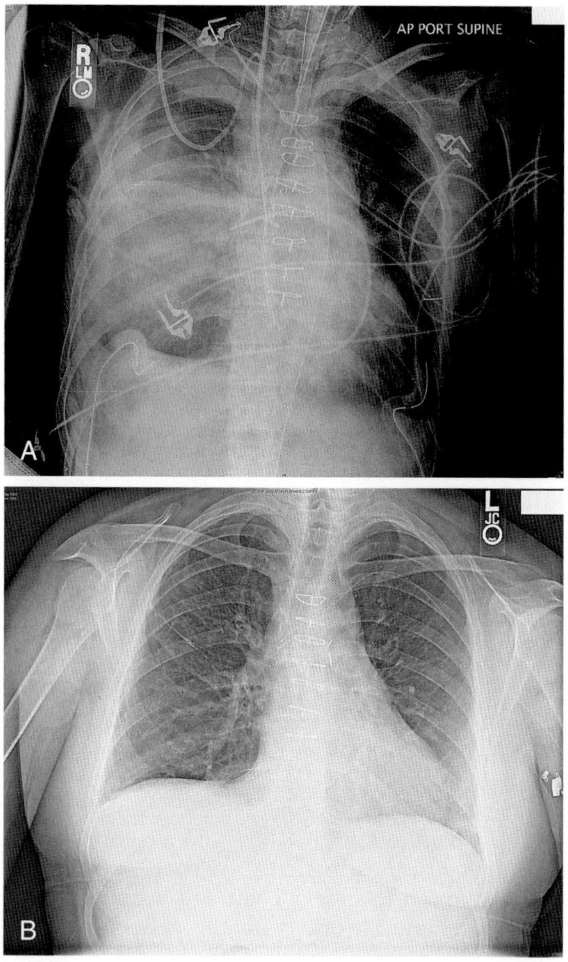

FIGURE 99-5 ■ Acute and resolving lung rejection. **A,** Chest radiograph illustrates bilateral infiltrates characteristic of acute pulmonary rejection. **B,** Follow-up chest radiograph after pulsed methylprednisolone treatment of acute rejection demonstrates resolution of infiltrates.

COMPLICATIONS

Acute Rejection

The fine balance between adequate immunosuppression and the risk for infection and rejection remains one of the most difficult problems in heart–lung transplantation, as with any lung transplantation. The detection of acute rejection is rare in the first postoperative week, and the majority of episodes occur within the first year after transplantation. The diagnosis of acute rejection in the early posttransplantation period is usually based on clinical parameters manifested by lung allograft dysfunction. Signs of acute rejection include dyspnea, low-grade fever, impaired oxygenation and ventilatory parameters (including a diminished forced expiratory volume in 1 second [FEV_1]), and diffuse interstitial infiltrates on chest radiograph (Fig. 99-5).[82] Acute cellular rejection during the first month is associated with an infiltrate seen on the chest radiograph in 75% of cases. After the first month, however, the chest film is normal or without change in 80% of patients.[83,84] The role of other modalities such as spirometry, computed tomography (CT), and bronchoscopy with transbronchial biopsy (TBB) become increasingly important.

Acute allograft rejection in the early postoperative period is the single most significant risk factor for the development of subsequent OB, so the role of surveillance modalities in detecting and treating early rejection become critical in preventing chronic rejection and improving survival rates. Spirometric surveillance has been shown to be a reasonable screening tool for acute rejection. FEV_1 and forced expiratory flow rate at 25% to 75% of vital capacity ($FEF_{25\%-75\%}$) were noted to be decreased during episodes of acute rejection, with $FEF_{25\%-75\%}$ being the best parameter to distinguish acute rejection from infection.[85] Because of some lack of sensitivity and specificity of spirometric surveillance, however, TBB remains the gold standard for the detection of rejection.

In heart–lung transplantation, the simultaneous rejection of both the heart and lung is rare,[86] and endomyocardial biopsy does not help diagnose acute lung rejection.[87] Furthermore, histologic assessment by using TBB is superior to cardiac biopsies because cardiac rejection is very rare without lung rejection, and thus the need for routine endomyocardial biopsies has been eliminated.[88] Surveillance bronchoscopy with TBB in heart–lung recipients is routinely performed at 2 and 4 weeks after transplantation, and then at 2, 3, 6, and 12 months thereafter, or as clinically indicated. At least five TBB specimens that contain lung parenchyma are necessary to obtain an adequate quantity of specimen. TBBs performed in the setting of clinical symptoms were positive for rejection or infection in 72% of cases.[86] The yield for surveillance biopsies after 1 year in asymptomatic patients, however, is very low.[89] Late postoperative biopsies are therefore guided by clinical parameters, and any deterioration in pulmonary function leads to further evaluation.

Rejection episodes occurring within the first 3 months, or those graded as moderate or severe, are treated with IV methylprednisolone at a dose of 1000 mg/day for 3 consecutive days, followed by an increased oral maintenance dose of 0.6 mg/kg per day, tapered to 0.2 mg/kg per day over 3 to 4 weeks. Both the chest radiograph appearance and clinical symptoms usually improve rapidly after the initiation of pulsed steroid therapy. In milder cases of rejection, or in cases occurring after 3 months, treatment consists of increased oral prednisone, followed by a gradually tapered dose over 3 to 4 weeks. Patients with steroid-resistant or persistent allograft rejection are treated with either monoclonal (OKT3) or polyclonal (RATG) antilymphocyte therapy. Other potential treatments in refractory and recurrent cases include switching to rapamycin, methotrexate, total lymphoid irradiation, or extracorporeal photochemotherapy.[90-93]

Infection

Infectious complications remain a significant cause of morbidity and mortality in heart–lung recipients. The spectrum of potential pathogens is extensive, yet some common patterns can be appreciated. Bacterial infections are most prevalent early in the postoperative period, with the highest incidence noted in the first month after heart–lung transplantation.[94] Bacterial infections can manifest as pneumonia, mediastinitis, line sepsis, urinary tract infections, and skin infections. Gram-negative bacilli are the most common bacterial pathogens. Late after transplant, opportunistic pathogens such as viral, fungal, and protozoal species are more common.

Cytomegalovirus (CMV) is the most common viral pathogen in heart–lung transplants. CMV has been associated with pneumonitis in as much as 50% of patients and is associated with an increased incidence of chronic rejection manifested as accelerated graft coronary artery disease and OB.[95,96] In addition to pneumonia, CMV infection can have presenting symptoms such as leukopenia and fever, gastroenteritis, hepatitis, and retinitis. CMV events occur within the first 12 months, with the majority appearing within the first 3 months. Individuals at the greatest risk for serious infections are seronegative recipients (R^-) receiving a heart–lung block from a seropositive donor (D^+). The incidence of serious infections in these patients is 90%, which falls to 10% when recipient and donor are CMV–negative. The diagnosis of CMV disease (symptomatic) or CMV infection (without symptoms) is established by several means: seroconversion from anti-CMV immunoglobulin M (IgM) negative to positive; a fourfold rise in CMV IgG antibody titers; positive viral cultures from urine, blood, or dimercaprol (bronchoalveolar lavage); or CMV inclusion bodies on transbronchial biopsy.

Most transplant centers perform transplants across CMV serologic barriers, implementing prophylactic measures in high-risk patients (D^+R^-). These patients receive prophylaxis with CMV hyperimmunoglobulin (CytoGam; CSL Behring, King of Prussia, PA) in addition to ganciclovir (DHPG).[97] This combination regimen resulted in a significant decrease in both CMV disease and CMV infection when compared with DHPG alone.[98] Standard protocol is to administer DHPG at 5 mg/kg IV twice per day for 14 days, then at 6 mg/kg once per day for 20 days. After DHPG, valganciclovir (Valcyte; Genentech, South San Francisco, CA) (900 mg) is initiated for 6 weeks after transplant. CytoGam is given at a dosage of 150 mg/kg IV within the first 72 hours after transplantation and then continued at a dosage of 100 mg/kg at 2, 4, 6, and 8 weeks, followed by 50 mg/kg at weeks 12 and 16 after transplant.

Fungal organisms are the least common pathogens, yet these infections are associated with the greatest mortality. The risk of fungal infections after lung, heart–lung, and heart transplantation can be significantly lowered by prophylaxis with aerosolized amphotericin B.[99] Inhaled treatments with amphotericin B have been shown to decrease the rate of fungal infections at 3 months from 0.8% to 0.2%, and the incidence fell twofold at 12 months when compared with a group that did not receive the inhaled treatment.[99] Bronchodilators are administered prophylactically before treatment to reduce bronchospasm. Fungal infections, diagnosed by sputum culture or CT-guided needle aspirate, are aggressively treated with intravenous amphotericin B administration.

Pneumocystis jiroveci pneumonia has been effectively prevented in heart–lung recipients since the initiation of prophylaxis with the combination of sulfamethoxazole and trimethoprim.[100] The dosages of sulfamethoxazole and trimethoprim are 800 mg and 160 mg, respectively, twice daily, 3 days per week, adjusting the dosage for renal insufficiency. If patients have a sulfur allergy or leukopenia develops, inhaled pentamidine (300 mg) is initiated once a month. *Toxoplasma gondii*–negative recipients receiving a transplant from a seropositive donor are treated with a 6-week course of pyrimethamine (25 mg) every day and leucovorin (10 mg) every day. In addition, long-term prophylaxis typically includes clotrimazole

(Mycelex Troches) for the prevention of mucosal candidal infections.

Chronic Rejection—Obliterative Bronchiolitis

The main cause of long-term morbidity and mortality after heart–lung transplantation is chronic rejection, primarily manifested as OB. The clinical diagnoses of bronchiolitis obliterans syndrome (BOS) and the pathologic diagnoses of OB were defined in the working formulation by the ISHLT.[101] BOS does not require a histologic diagnosis; it is defined as a deterioration of graft function secondary to progressive airways disease. Other potential etiologies such as acute rejection and infection must be excluded before a diagnosis of BOS is reached. The clinical manifestations of BOS include a dry cough and progressive dyspnea. Interstitial pulmonary infiltrates are seen on the chest radiograph, and an obstructive pattern is seen in pulmonary function tests. BOS can be staged on the basis of the deterioration of FEV_1.[101] OB, on the other hand, is a histologic diagnosis based on the presence of eosinophilic fibrous scarring of the membranous and respiratory bronchioles, with partial or complete obliteration of the lumen.[102]

The overall incidence of BOS or OB at 5 years after heart–lung transplantation, as reported by the ISHLT Registry, is approximately 48% (Fig. 99-6).[5] Significant risk factors associated with the development of OB include the frequency and severity of acute rejection, as well as the appearance of lymphocytic bronchiolitis on TBB.[73] Furthermore, organizing pneumonia, as well as CMV infection, significantly potentiates the effects of acute rejection.

A growing body of evidence supports the hypothesis that OB is an immunologically mediated process. In addition to its association with acute rejection, the disease is most commonly found in patients with the greatest degree of HLA mismatch.[19] Patients with OB have an increased number of mismatched major histocompatibility complex (MHC) class II antigens,[103] immunologic mediators such as IL-2 and IL-6 in bronchioalveolar lavage fluid,[104] and a predominance of $CD8^+$ cytotoxic and suppressor cells on TBB.[105] CMV infection may have a stimulatory effect on the immune system that enhances the viral injury.[106] CMV prophylaxis with ganciclovir has been demonstrated to delay the onset of OB.[107] In addition to its immunologic stimulus, CMV also has a direct stimulatory effect on the smooth muscle cells of the airways, as well as indirectly via the elaboration of growth factors and mitogenic mediators.[108] Better control of the immune response, prevention of acute rejection, and reducing CMV infection are the best therapies for preventing the incidence of BOS or OB.

For long-term surveillance, patients are provided with a portable spirometer so that expiratory flow can be checked frequently between clinic visits.[109,110] If there is any interval decrease or any signs of respiratory tract infection, the patient is instructed to contact the transplant center or primary care physician so that pulmonary function tests can be performed. Any subsequent alteration in $FEF_{25\%-75\%}$ prompts further evaluation with bronchoscopy and bronchoalveolar lavage, and TBB. After infection has been ruled out, augmentation of immunosuppression is the current mode of therapy. If acute rejection is seen with the TBB, pulsed-dose steroids are started (methylprednisolone, 1 g IV for 3 days). In the setting of augmented immunosuppression, CMV prophylaxis is begun, with ganciclovir and fungal prophylaxis combined with inhaled amphotericin B.

Despite stabilization of pulmonary function with augmented immunosuppression, relapse rates are greater than 50%, and mortality is significant.[111,112] The actuarial survival curves for heart–lung transplant patients are quite different for patients with BOS/OB and those without BOS/OB (Fig. 99-7). Markedly better survival rates were also demonstrated in patients with BOS stage 1 than in those with BOS stages 2 or 3.[111] The main cause of death is usually respiratory failure secondary to a superimposed pneumonia. Retransplantation often remains the only therapeutic option, although the results of retransplantation in patients who have developed

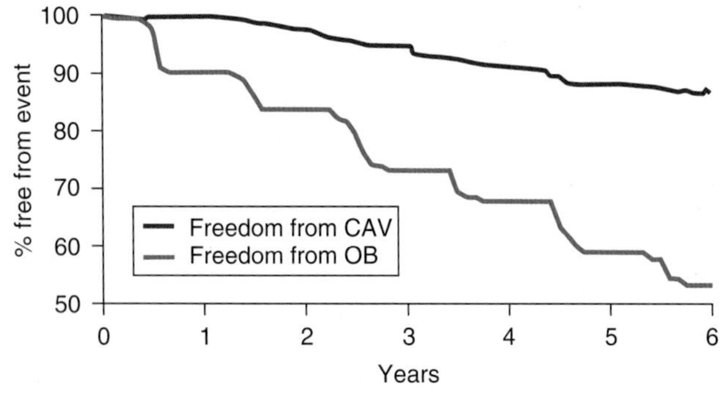

FIGURE 99-6 ■ **Freedom from obliterative bronchiolitis (OB) and cardiac allograft vasculopathy (CAV), or accelerated graft coronary disease, after heart–lung transplantation.** (Modified from Trulock EP, Christie JD, Edwards LB, et al: The Registry of the International Society of Heart and Lung Transplantation: Twenty-Fourth Official Adult Lung and Heart-Lung Transplant Report—2007. *J Heart Lung Transplant* 26:782–795, 2007.)

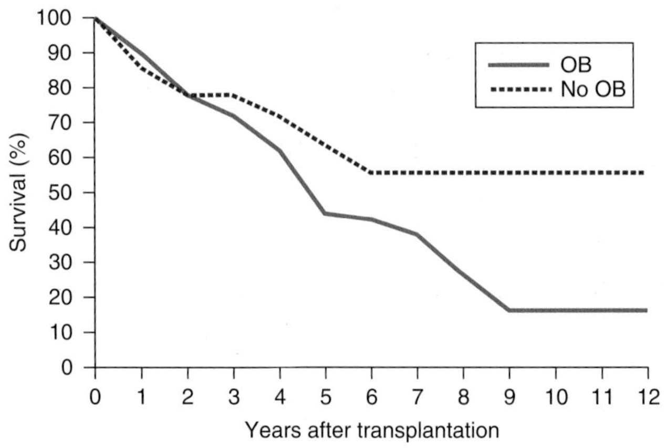

FIGURE 99-7 ■ **Effect of obliterative bronchiolitis (OB) on patient survival rate after lung and heart–lung transplantations.** (Modified from Reichenspurner H, Girgis R, Robbins RC, et al: Stanford experience with obliterative bronchiolitis after lung and heart-lung transplantation. *Ann Thorac Surg* 62:1467–1472, 1996.)

end-stage OB are poor, with an actuarial survival rate of only 25% at 1 and 3 years after transplantation.[113]

Chronic Rejection—Graft Coronary Artery Disease

Very few heart–lung recipients who survive the first year will die as a result of graft coronary artery disease.[114,115] The incidence of cardiac allograft rejection in heart–lung recipients is low.[87] The incidence of angiographically detectable coronary artery disease was only 11% at 5 years after heart–lung transplantation,[114] which is similar to the data from the ISHLT Registry (see Fig. 99-6).[5] This is in contrast to heart-only transplant recipients, of whom as many as 50% develop significant angiographic disease by 5 years; this is the major cause of mortality and retransplantation in these patients. A recent study using intracoronary ultrasonography confirmed the low incidence of transplant coronary artery disease in heart–lung recipients when compared with the heart-alone recipient group.[116] When the lungs and heart are both transplanted, the lungs are more immunologically active. This observation was confirmed in an animal model, in which hearts that were transplanted in combination with lungs or spleen displayed an impressive reduction in myocardial rejection; this phenomenon is termed the *combi-effect*.[117]

Complications of Immunosuppression

There are several side effects resulting from long-term immunosuppression. Cyclosporine causes nephrotoxicity, hypertension, hepatotoxicity, hirsutism, and gingival hyperplasia, and it is associated with an increased incidence of lymphoma. Azathioprine causes a generalized bone marrow depression manifested as leukopenia, thrombocytopenia, and anemia. Long-term use of steroids causes hypertension, diabetes, osteoporosis, and impaired wound healing. Induction therapy with either RATG or OKT3 can cause significant hemodynamic instability and respiratory compromise manifested as fever, hypotension, and bronchospasm. Patients are therefore premedicated with corticosteroids, acetaminophen, and antihistamines before the administration of immunosuppressive agents.

One of the more troubling consequences of heart–lung transplantation is the development of posttransplant lymphoproliferative disorder (PTLD).[118] This is characterized by lymphadenopathy and often a diffuse lymphocytic infiltrate on TBB.[119] The treatment is immediate reduction in the intensity of the immunosuppression. The disease has essentially two forms: malignant and nonmalignant. Early onset of PTLD (<12 months after transplantation) is typically benign and resolves rapidly after reduced immunosuppression. Conversely, late PTLD is associated with a 70% to 80% mortality rate and typically resists reduction by immunotherapy or traditional chemotherapy.[120]

Additional Complications

Airway complications have become rare after heart–lung and lung transplantation as the result of improvements in surgical technique and postoperative management. The risk for a major airway complication after heart–lung transplantation is approximately half of that after a single-lung transplantation, with a reported incidence as low as 3.8%.[121] The incidence of airway complications is unrelated to steroid use in the preoperative or postoperative period.[76] Furthermore, no significant correlation could be identified with the ischemic interval, anastomotic wrapping, or date of first rejection episode.[122]

Abdominal complications after heart–lung transplantation remain a significant source of morbidity and mortality.[123] The prevalence of symptomatic gastroparesis after heart–lung transplantation is high, probably as a result of vagotomy at the time of removal of the heart–lung block.[124] Gastroparesis with gastric distention can lead to gastroesophageal reflux with subsequent aspiration. Episodes of aspiration and the resultant inflammatory response can result in significant lung allograft dysfunction. Furthermore, whether this allograft injury predisposes the patient to an increased risk for BOS or OB remains to be determined.[125] Laparoscopic antireflux surgery should also be considered in patients with severe reflux disease after heart–lung transplantation, because pulmonary function and reflux symptoms have been shown to significantly improve with this treatment.[126]

PHYSIOLOGY OF THE TRANSPLANTED LUNG

Standard measure of pulmonary function indicates that long-term function of the transplanted heart and lungs is well maintained. Integrated cardiopulmonary function with exercise is also largely intact.[127,128] Some debate has centered on a bronchial hyper-responsiveness to a methacholine challenge.[129] There does appear to be an associated decrease in mucociliary clearance, which may be a contributing factor to the serious and repeated infections seen in heart–lung recipients.[130] In the absence of OB and severe recurrent infection, the function of the transplanted heart and lungs is conducive to an excellent quality of life.[127]

LATE RESULTS

A retrospective review of all 174 patients with end-stage cardiopulmonary disease who underwent heart–lung transplantation at Stanford University between the time of the first landmark operation in 1981 to 2000 revealed that 40% of these patients were still alive, with a 5-year actuarial survival rate of 49% (Fig. 99-8). This record compares closely with the worldwide experience with heart–lung transplantation, as reported by the ISHLT Registry, and is similar to that for patients receiving double-lung transplantation alone (Fig. 99-9).[5] A review of the experience at Stanford from 1991 to 2002 reveals improved survival when compared with the preceding decade.[14]

Causes of mortality after heart–lung transplantation differ over time after surgery. Early deaths, occurring less than 1 month after surgery, are most often the result of

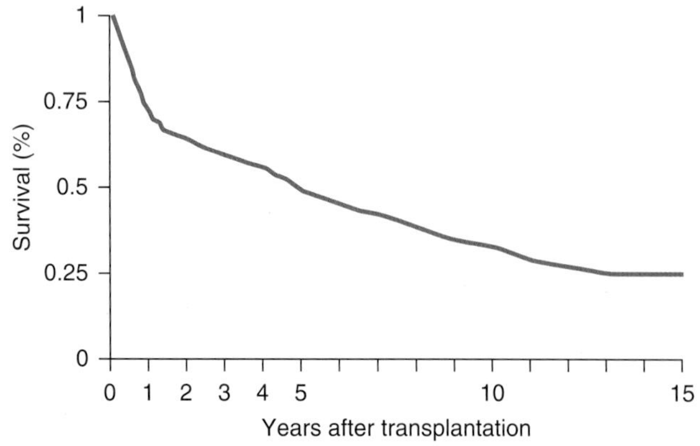

FIGURE 99-8 ■ Actuarial survival of patients who underwent heart–lung transplantation at Stanford University, 1981 to 2000.

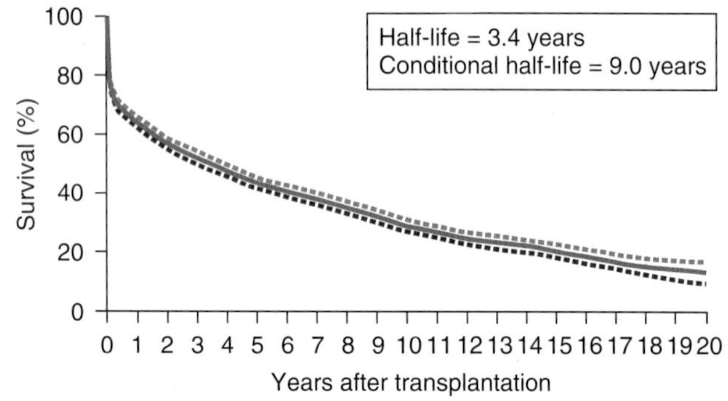

FIGURE 99-9 ■ Heart–lung transplantation actuarial survival based on data from the International Society for Heart and Lung Transplantation (ISHLT) Registry. Half-life is time to 50% survival; conditional half-life is time to 50% survival of hospital survivors. (Modified from Trulock EP, Christie JD, Edwards LB, et al: The Registry of the International Society of Heart and Lung Transplantation: Twenty-Fourth Official Adult Lung and Heart-Lung Transplant Report—2007. *J Heart Lung Transplant* 26:782–795, 2007.)

infection (36% of overall deaths), hemorrhage (8% to 20%), acute respiratory disease syndrome (4%), and nonspecific graft failure (7% to 9%).[14,114] Acute rejection of the heart–lung graft is fairly uncommon, resulting in mortality in less than 2% of patients. Almost all rejection events in these patients occur within the first 3 months, with a linearized rejection rate twice as high for the lung (0.7 events per 100 days) when compared with the heart (0.35 events per 100 days). The most common cause of death after the immediate postoperative phase is OB. The overall prevalence of OB in patients surviving heart–lung transplantation longer than 3 months was 64%, with an overall mortality greater than 70% after 5 years of follow-up.[111] Additional causes of late death include infection, malignancy, and coronary artery disease. The incidence and severity of transplant coronary artery disease are significantly less when compared with those of the heart transplantation population.[131] However, this complication remains an important cause of late death in heart–lung recipients.[114]

The long-term functional results after heart–lung transplantation are encouraging. Most recipients are able to resume an active lifestyle without the need for supplemental oxygen, and they demonstrate significant increases in exercise capacity after transplantation.[128,132] Pulmonary function as measured by spirometry is also markedly improved after heart–lung transplantation.[128] The functional benefits of heart–lung transplantation are particularly evident when considering that this subgroup of patients would otherwise have a life expectancy of less than 2 years, despite maximal medical and nontransplantation surgical therapy.

FUTURE DEVELOPMENTS

Imperfections remain in the use of heart–lung transplantation for definitive treatment of end-stage cardiopulmonary disease. Significant improvements in selective immunosuppression and the development of precise immunotolerance are required before heart–lung transplantation can restore normal heart and lung function without significant long-term morbidity and mortality. The development of new immunosuppressive agents, the use of genetic engineering to formulate new humanized monoclonal antibodies, and the field of pharmacogenomics provide continued hope for an improved outlook for heart–lung transplant recipients. Novel approaches such as ex vivo gene therapy, the induction of immunotolerance, and xenotransplantation are promising areas of continual investigation.

REFERENCES

1. Carrel A: The surgery of blood vessels. *Johns Hopkins Hosp Bull* 18:18, 1907.
2. Demikhov VP: *Experimental transplantation of vital organs*, vol 1, New York, 1962, Consultant Bureau.
3. Marcus E, Wong SNT, Luisada AA: Homologous heart grafts: transplantation of the heart in dogs. *Surg Forum* 2:212, 1951.
4. Reitz BA, Wallwork JL, Hunt SA, et al: Heart-lung transplantation: successful therapy for patients with pulmonary vascular disease. *N Engl J Med* 306:557–564, 1982.
5. Trulock EP, Christie JD, Edwards LB, et al: The Registry of the International Society of Heart and Lung Transplantation: twenty-fourth official adult lung and heart-lung transplant report—2007. *J Heart Lung Transplant* 26:782–795, 2007.
6. Hopkins WE, Ochoa LL, Richardson GW, et al: Comparison of the hemodynamics and survival of adults with severe primary pulmonary hypertension or Eisenmenger syndrome. *J Heart Lung Transplant* 15:100–105, 1996.
7. Waddell TK, Bennett L, Kennedy R, et al: Heart-lung or lung transplantation for Eisenmenger syndrome. *J Heart Lung Transplant* 21:731–737, 2002.
8. Pasque MK, Trulock EP, Cooper JD, et al: Single lung transplantation for pulmonary hypertension. Single institution experience in 34 patients. *Circulation* 92:2252–2258, 1995.
9. D'Alonzo GE, Barst RJ, Ayres SM, et al: Survival in patients with primary pulmonary hypertension. Results from a national prospective registry. *Ann Intern Med* 115:343–349, 1991.
10. Bando K, Armitage JM, Paradis IL, et al: Indications for and results of single, bilateral, and heart-lung transplantation for pulmonary hypertension. *J Thorac Cardiovasc Surg* 108:1056–1065, 1994.
11. Whyte RI, Robbins RC, Altinger J, et al: Heart-lung transplantation for primary pulmonary hypertension. *Ann Thorac Surg* 67:937–941, 1999.
12. Baumgartner WA, Traill TA, Cameron DE, et al: Unique aspects of heart and lung transplantation exhibited in the "domino-donor" operation. *JAMA* 261:3121–3125, 1989.
13. Yacoub MH, Banner NR, Khaghani A, et al: Heart-lung transplantation for cystic fibrosis and subsequent domino heart transplantation. *J Heart Transplant* 9:459–466, 1990.

14. Demers P, Robbins RC, Doyle R, et al: Twenty years of combined heart-lung transplantation at Stanford University. *J Heart Lung Transplant* 21:S77, 2003.
15. Michler RE, Rose EA: Pediatric heart and heart-lung transplantation. *Ann Thorac Surg* 52:708–709, 1991.
16. Smyth RL, Scott JP, Whitehead B, et al: Heart-lung transplantation in children. *Transplant Proc* 22:1470–1471, 1990.
17. Marshall SE, Kramer MR, Lewiston NJ, et al: Selection and evaluation of recipients for heart-lung and lung transplantation. *Chest* 98:1488–1494, 1990.
18. Kramer MR, Marshall SE, Tiroke A, et al: Clinical significance of hyperbilirubinemia in patients with pulmonary hypertension undergoing heart-lung transplantation. *J Heart Lung Transplant* 10:317–321, 1991.
19. Harjula AL, Baldwin JC, Oyer PE, et al: Recipient selection for heart-lung transplantation. *Scand J Thorac Cardiovasc Surg* 22:193–196, 1988.
20. Schwebel C, Pin I, Barnoud D, et al: Prevalence and consequences of nutritional depletion in lung transplant candidates. *Eur Respir J* 16:1050–1055, 2000.
21. Royston D: Aprotinin therapy in heart and heart-lung transplantation. *J Heart Lung Transplant* 12:S19–S25, 1993.
22. Ferguson DA, Hebert PC, Mazer CD, et al: A comparison of aprotinin and lysine analogues in high-risk cardiac surgery. *N Engl J Med* 358:2319–2331, 2008.
23. Ouwens JP, van der Mark TW, van der BW, et al: Size matching in lung transplantation using predicted total lung capacity. *Eur Respir J* 20:1419–1422, 2002.
24. Tamm M, Higenbottam TW, Dennis CM, et al: Donor and recipient predicted lung volume and lung size after heart-lung transplantation. *Am J Respir Crit Care Med* 150:403–407, 1994.
25. Harjula AL, Baldwin JC, Glanville AR, et al: Human leukocyte antigen compatibility in heart-lung transplantation. *J Heart Transplant* 6:162–166, 1987.
26. Iwaki Y, Yoshida Y, Griffith B: The HLA matching effect in lung transplantation. *Transplantation* 56:1528–1529, 1993.
27. Wisser W, Wekerle T, Zlabinger G, et al: Influence of human leukocyte antigen matching on long-term outcome after lung transplantation. *J Heart Lung Transplant* 15:1209–1216, 1996.
28. Quantz MA, Bennett LE, Meyer DM, et al: Does human leukocyte antigen matching influence the outcome of lung transplantation? An analysis of 3,549 lung transplantations. *J Heart Lung Transplant* 19:473–479, 2000.
29. Shah AS, Nwakanma L, Simpkins C, et al: Pretransplant panel reactive antibodies in human lung transplantation: an analysis of over 10,000 patients. *Ann Thorac Surg* 85:1919–1924, 2008.
30. Hadjiliadis D, Chaparro C, Gutierrez C, et al: Impact of lung transplant operation on bronchiolitis obliterans syndrome in patients with chronic obstructive pulmonary disease. *Am J Transplant* 6:183–189, 2006.
31. Grinita AL, Duquesnoy R, Yousem SA, et al: HLA-specific antibodies are risk factors for lymphocytic bronchiolitis and chronic lung allograft dysfunction. *Am J Transplant* 5:131–138, 2005.
32. Appel JZ, 3rd, Hartwig MG, Cantu E, 3rd, et al: Role of flow cytometry to define unacceptable HLA antigens in lung transplant recipients with HLA-specific antibodies. *Tansplantation* 81:1049–1057, 2006.
33. Appel JZ, 3rd, Hartwig MG, Davis RD, et al: Utility of peritransplant and rescue intravenous immunoglobulin and extracorporeal immunoadsorption in lung transplant patients sensitized to HLA antigens. *Hum Immunol* 66:378–386, 2005.
34. Fuster V, Steele PM, Edwards WD, et al: Primary pulmonary hypertension: natural history and the importance of thrombosis. *Circulation* 70:580–587, 1984.
35. Adachi JD, Bensen WG, Brown J, et al: Intermittent etidronate therapy to prevent corticosteroid-induced osteoporosis. *N Engl J Med* 337:382–387, 1997.
36. Cohn JN, Archibald DG, Ziesche S, et al: Effect of vasodilator therapy on mortality in chronic congestive heart failure. Results of a Veterans Administration Cooperative Study. *N Engl J Med* 314:1547–1552, 1986.
37. O'Donohue WJ, Jr: Home oxygen therapy. *Clin Chest Med* 18:535–545, 1997.
38. Barst RJ, Rubin LJ, Long WA, et al: A comparison of continuous intravenous epoprostenol (prostacyclin) with conventional therapy for primary pulmonary hypertension. The Primary Pulmonary Hypertension Study Group. *N Engl J Med* 334:296–302, 1996.
39. Rubin LJ: Pathology and pathophysiology of primary pulmonary hypertension. *Am J Cardiol* 75:51A–54A, 1995.
40. Kerstein D, Levy PS, Hsu DT, et al: Blade balloon atrial septostomy in patients with severe primary pulmonary hypertension. *Circulation* 91:2028–2035, 1995.
41. Fitzsimmons SC: The changing epidemiology of cystic fibrosis. *J Pediatr* 122:1–9, 1993.
42. Ramsey BW: Management of pulmonary disease in patients with cystic fibrosis. *N Engl J Med* 335:179–188, 1996.
43. Lewiston N, King V, Umetsu D, et al: Cystic fibrosis patients who have undergone heart-lung transplantation benefit from maxillary sinus antrostomy and repeated sinus lavage. *Transplant Proc* 23:1207–1208, 1991.
44. Wheeldon DR, Potter CD, Oduro A, et al: Transforming the "unacceptable" donor: outcomes from the adoption of a standardized donor management technique. *J Heart Lung Transplant* 14:734–742, 1995.
45. Pereira BJ, Wright TL, Schmid CH, et al: A controlled study of hepatitis C transmission by organ transplantation. The New England Organ Bank Hepatitis C Study Group. *Lancet* 345:484–487, 1995.
46. Straznicka M, Follette DM, Eisner MD, et al: Aggressive management of lung donors classified as unacceptable: excellent recipient survival one year after transplantation. *J Thorac Cardiovasc Surg* 124:250–258, 2002.
47. Iwai A, Sakano T, Uenishi M, et al: Effects of vasopressin and catecholamines on the maintenance of circulatory stability in brain-dead patients. *Transplantation* 48:613–617, 1989.
48. Pennefather SH, Bullock RE, Dark JH: The effect of fluid therapy on alveolar arterial oxygen gradient in brain-dead organ donors. *Transplantation* 56:1418–1422, 1993.
49. Wijnen RM, van der Linden CJ: Donor treatment after pronouncement of brain death: a neglected intensive care problem. *Transpl Int* 4:186–190, 1991.
50. Novitzky D: Donor management: state of the art. *Transplant Proc* 29:3773–3775, 1997.
51. Date H, Triantafillou AN, Trulock EP, et al: Inhaled nitric oxide reduces human lung allograft dysfunction. *J Thorac Cardiovasc Surg* 111:913–919, 1996.
52. Shackleton CR, Ettinger SL, McLoughlin MG, et al: Effect of recovery from ischemic injury on class I and class II MHC antigen expression. *Transplantation* 49:641–644, 1990.
53. Demertzis S, Langer F, Graeter T, et al: Amelioration of lung reperfusion injury by L- and E-selectin blockade. *Eur J Cardiothorac Surg* 16:174–180, 1999.
54. Kozower BD, Christofidou-Solomidou M, Sweitzer TD, et al: Immunotargeting of catalase to the pulmonary endothelium alleviates oxidative stress and reduces acute lung transplantation injury. *Nat Biotechnol* 21:392–398, 2003.
55. Levine AJ, Parkes K, Rooney SJ, et al: The effect of adhesion molecule blockade on pulmonary reperfusion injury. *Ann Thorac Surg* 73:1101–1106, 2002.
56. Baldwin JC, Frist WH, Starkey TD, et al: Distant graft procurement for combined heart and lung transplantation using pulmonary artery flush and simple topical hypothermia for graft preservation. *Ann Thorac Surg* 43:670–673, 1987.
57. Haverich A, Aziz S, Scott WC, et al: Improved lung preservation using Euro-Collins solution for flush-perfusion. *Thorac Cardiovasc Surg* 34:368–376, 1986.
58. Varela A, Montero C, Cordoba M, et al: Clinical experience with retrograde lung preservation. *Transpl Int* 9(Suppl 1):S296–S298, 1996.
59. Varela A, Montero CG, Cordoba M, et al: Improved distribution of pulmonary flush solution to the tracheobronchial wall in pulmonary transplantation. *Eur Surg Res* 29:1–4, 1997.
60. Muller C, Furst H, Reichenspurner H, et al: Lung procurement by low-potassium dextran and the effect on preservation injury. Munich Lung Transplant Group. *Transplantation* 68:1139–1143, 1999.
61. Kofidis T, Struber M, Warnecke G, et al: Antegrade versus retrograde perfusion of the donor lung: impact on the early reperfusion phase. *Transpl Int* 16:801–805, 2003.
62. Wittwer T, Franke UF, Fehrenbach A, et al: Experimental lung transplantation: impact of preservation solution and route of delivery. *J Heart Lung Transplant* 24:1081–1090, 2005.

63. Levine AJ, Parkes K, Rooney S, et al: Reduction of endothelial injury after hypothermic lung preservation by initial leukocyte-depleted reperfusion. *J Thorac Cardiovasc Surg* 120:47–54, 2000.
64. Schmid RA, Yamashita M, Boasquevisque CH, et al: Carbohydrate selectin inhibitor CY-1503 reduces neutrophil migration and reperfusion injury in canine pulmonary allografts. *J Heart Lung Transplant* 16:1054–1061, 1997.
65. Kawashima M, Bando T, Nakamura T, et al: Cytoprotective effects of nitroglycerin in ischemia-reperfusion-induced lung injury. *Am J Respir Crit Care Med* 161:935–943, 2000.
66. Nawata S, Sugi K, Ueda K, et al: Prostacyclin analog OP2507 prevents pulmonary arterial and airway constriction during lung preservation and reperfusion. *J Heart Lung Transplant* 15:470–474, 1996.
67. Schmid RA, Hillinger S, Walter R, et al: The nitric oxide synthase cofactor tetrahydrobiopterin reduces allograft ischemia-reperfusion injury after lung transplantation. *J Thorac Cardiovasc Surg* 118:726–732, 1999.
68. Vainikka T, Heikkila L, Kukkonen S, et al: L-Arginine in lung graft preservation and reperfusion. *J Heart Lung Transplant* 20:559–567, 2001.
69. Milano CA, Shah AS, Van Trigt P, et al: Evaluation of early postoperative results after bicaval versus standard cardiac transplantation and review of the literature. *Am Heart J* 140:717–721, 2000.
70. Lick SD, Copeland JG, Rosado LJ, et al: Simplified technique of heart-lung transplantation. *Ann Thorac Surg* 59:1592–1593, 1995.
71. Adatia I, Lillehei C, Arnold JH, et al: Inhaled nitric oxide in the treatment of postoperative graft dysfunction after lung transplantation. *Ann Thorac Surg* 57:1311–1318, 1994.
72. Slaughter MS, Nielsen K, Bolman RM, III: Extracorporeal membrane oxygenation after lung or heart-lung transplantation. *ASAIO J* 39:M453–M456, 1993.
73. Girgis RE, Tu I, Berry GJ, et al: Risk factors for the development of obliterative bronchiolitis after lung transplantation. *J Heart Lung Transplant* 15:1200–1208, 1996.
74. Reichenspurner H, Girgis RE, Robbins RC, et al: Obliterative bronchiolitis after lung and heart-lung transplantation. *Ann Thorac Surg* 60:1845–1853, 1995.
75. Reichenspurner H, Robbins RC, Miller J, et al: RATG-induction therapy significantly reduces incidence of acute pulmonary rejection compared to OKT3 treatment. *J Heart Lung Transplant* 15:S103, 1996.
76. Date H, Trulock EP, Arcidi JM, et al: Improved airway healing after lung transplantation. An analysis of 348 bronchial anastomoses. *J Thorac Cardiovasc Surg* 110:1424–1432, 1995.
77. Meiser BM, Uberfuhr P, Schulze C, et al: Tacrolimus (FK506) proves superior to OKT3 for treating episodes of persistent rejection following intrathoracic transplantation. *Transplant Proc* 29:605–606, 1997.
78. Ransom JT: Mechanism of action of mycophenolate mofetil. *Ther Drug Monit* 17:681–684, 1995.
79. Lim DG, Joe IY, Park YH, et al: Effect of immunosuppressants on the expansion and function of naturally occurring regulatory T cells. *Transpl Immunol* 18:94–100, 2007.
80. Hausen B, Gummert J, Berry GJ, et al: Prevention of acute allograft rejection in nonhuman primate lung transplant recipients: induction with chimeric anti-interleukin-2 receptor monoclonal antibody improves the tolerability and potentiates the immunosuppressive activity of a regimen using low doses of both microemulsion cyclosporine and 40-O-(2-hydroxyethyl)-rapamycin. *Transplantation* 69:488–496, 2000.
81. Snell GI, Levvey BJ, Chin W, et al: Sirolimus allows renal recovery in lung and heart transplant recipients with chronic renal impairment. *J Heart Lung Transplant* 21:540–546, 2002.
82. Hoeper MM, Hamm M, Schafers HJ, et al: Evaluation of lung function during pulmonary rejection and infection in heart-lung transplant patients. Hannover Lung Transplant Group. *Chest* 102:864–870, 1992.
83. Millet B, Higenbottam TW, Flower CD, et al: The radiographic appearances of infection and acute rejection of the lung after heart-lung transplantation. *Am Rev Respir Dis* 140:62–67, 1989.
84. Rajagopalan N, Maurer J, Kesten S: Bronchodilator response at low lung volumes predicts bronchiolitis obliterans in lung transplant recipients. *Chest* 109:405–407, 1996.
85. Starnes VA, Theodore J, Oyer PE, et al: Evaluation of heart-lung transplant recipients with prospective, serial transbronchial biopsies and pulmonary function studies. *J Thorac Cardiovasc Surg* 98:683–690, 1989a.
86. Starnes VA, Theodore J, Oyer PE, et al: Pulmonary infiltrates after heart-lung transplantation: evaluation by serial transbronchial biopsies. *J Thorac Cardiovasc Surg* 98:945–950, 1989b.
87. Baldwin JC, Oyer PE, Stinson EB, et al: Comparison of cardiac rejection in heart and heart-lung transplantation. *J Heart Transplant* 6:352–356, 1987.
88. Higenbottam T, Hutter JA, Stewart S, et al: Transbronchial biopsy has eliminated the need for endomyocardial biopsy in heart-lung recipients. *J Heart Transplant* 7:435–439, 1988.
89. Girgis RE, Reichenspurner H, Robbins RC, et al: The utility of annual surveillance bronchoscopy in heart-lung transplant recipients. *Transplantation* 60:1458–1461, 1995.
90. Andreu G, Achkar A, Couetil JP, et al: Extracorporeal photochemotherapy treatment for acute lung rejection episode. *J Heart Lung Transplant* 14:793–796, 1995.
91. Cahill BC, O'Rourke MK, Strasburg KA, et al: Methotrexate for lung transplant recipients with steroid-resistant acute rejection. *J Heart Lung Transplant* 15:1130–1137, 1996.
92. Ross HJ, Gullestad L, Pak J, et al: Methotrexate or total lymphoid radiation for treatment of persistent or recurrent allograft cellular rejection: a comparative study. *J Heart Lung Transplant* 16:179–189, 1997.
93. Valentine VG, Robbins RC, Wehner JH, et al: Total lymphoid irradiation for refractory acute rejection in heart-lung and lung allografts. *Chest* 109:1184–1189, 1996.
94. Kramer MR, Marshall SE, Starnes VA, et al: Infectious complications in heart-lung transplantation. Analysis of 200 episodes. *Arch Intern Med* 153:2010–2016, 1993.
95. Grattan MT, Moreno-Cabral CE, Starnes VA, et al: Cytomegalovirus infection is associated with cardiac allograft rejection and atherosclerosis. *JAMA* 261:3561–3566, 1989.
96. Soghikian MV, Valentine VG, Berry GJ, et al: Impact of ganciclovir prophylaxis on heart-lung and lung transplant recipients. *J Heart Lung Transplant* 15:881–887, 1996.
97. Wreghitt TG, Hakim M, Gray JJ, et al: Cytomegalovirus infections in heart and heart and lung transplant recipients. *J Clin Pathol* 41:660–667, 1988.
98. Valantine HA, Luikart H, Doyle R, et al: Impact of cytomegalovirus hyperimmune globulin on outcome after cardiothoracic transplantation: a comparative study of combined prophylaxis with CMV hyperimmune globulin plus ganciclovir versus ganciclovir alone. *Transplantation* 72:1647–1652, 2001.
99. Reichenspurner H, Gamberg P, Nitschke M, et al: Significant reduction in the number of fungal infections after lung-, heart-lung, and heart transplantation using aerosolized amphotericin B prophylaxis. *Transplant Proc* 29:627–628, 1997.
100. Kramer MR, Stoehr C, Lewiston NJ, et al: Trimethoprim-sulfamethoxazole prophylaxis for *Pneumocystis carinii* infections in heart-lung and lung transplantation—how effective and for how long? *Transplantation* 53:586–589, 1992.
101. Cooper JD, Billingham M, Egan T, et al: A working formulation for the standardization of nomenclature and for clinical staging of chronic dysfunction in lung allografts. International Society for Heart and Lung Transplantation. *J Heart Lung Transplant* 12:713–716, 1993.
102. Yousem SA: Lymphocytic bronchitis/bronchiolitis in lung allograft recipients. *Am J Surg Pathol* 17:491–496, 1993.
103. Yousem SA, Curley JM, Dauber J, et al: HLA-class II antigen expression in human heart-lung allografts. *Transplantation* 49:991–995, 1990.
104. Griffith BP, Paradis IL, Zeevi A, et al: Immunologically mediated disease of the airways after pulmonary transplantation. *Ann Surg* 208:371–378, 1988.
105. Milne DS, Gascoigne A, Wilkes J, et al: The immunohistopathology of obliterative bronchiolitis following lung transplantation. *Transplantation* 54:748–750, 1992.
106. Keller CA, Cagle PT, Brown RW, et al: Bronchiolitis obliterans in recipients of single, double, and heart-lung transplantation. *Chest* 107:973–980, 1995.
107. Keenan RJ, Lega ME, Dummer JS, et al: Cytomegalovirus serologic status and postoperative infection correlated with risk of

developing chronic rejection after pulmonary transplantation. *Transplantation* 51:433–438, 1991.

108. Lemstrom KB, Bruning JH, Bruggeman CA, et al: Cytomegalovirus infection enhances smooth muscle cell proliferation and intimal thickening of rat aortic allografts. *J Clin Invest* 92:549–558, 1993.
109. Otulana BA, Higenbottam T, Ferrari L, et al: The use of home spirometry in detecting acute lung rejection and infection following heart-lung transplantation. *Chest* 97:353–357, 1990.
110. Otulana BA, Higenbottam TW, Scott JP, et al: Pulmonary function monitoring allows diagnosis of rejection in heart-lung transplant recipients. *Transplant Proc* 21:2583–2584, 1989.
111. Reichenspurner H, Girgis RE, Robbins RC, et al: Stanford experience with obliterative bronchiolitis after lung and heart-lung transplantation. *Ann Thorac Surg* 62:1467–1472, 1996.
112. Valentine VG, Robbins RC, Berry GJ, et al: Actuarial survival of heart-lung and bilateral sequential lung transplant recipients with obliterative bronchiolitis. *J Heart Lung Transplant* 15:371–383, 1996.
113. Adams DH, Cochrane AD, Khaghani A, et al: Retransplantation in heart-lung recipients with obliterative bronchiolitis. *J Thorac Cardiovasc Surg* 107:450–459, 1994.
114. Sarris GE, Smith JA, Shumway NE, et al: Long-term results of combined heart-lung transplantation: the Stanford experience. *J Heart Lung Transplant* 13:940–949, 1994.
115. Valantine HA, Reichenspurner H, Girgis R, et al: CMV prophylaxis with CMV hyperimmune globulin and ganciclovir is more effective than ganciclovir alone. *J Heart Lung Transplant* 15:S57, 1996.
116. Lim TT, Botas J, Ross H, et al: Are heart-lung transplant recipients protected from developing transplant coronary artery disease? A case-matched intracoronary ultrasound study. *Circulation* 94:1573–1577, 1996.
117. Westra AL, Petersen AH, Prop J, et al: The combi-effect—reduced rejection of the heart by combined transplantation with the lung or spleen. *Transplantation* 52:952–955, 1991.
118. Yousem SA, Randhawa P, Locker J, et al: Posttransplant lymphoproliferative disorders in heart-lung transplant recipients: primary presentation in the allograft. *Hum Pathol* 20:361–369, 1989.
119. Yousem SA, Dauber JA, Keenan R, et al: Does histologic acute rejection in lung allografts predict the development of bronchiolitis obliterans? *Transplantation* 52:306–309, 1991.
120. Armitage JM, Kormos RL, Stuart RS, et al: Posttransplant lymphoproliferative disease in thoracic organ transplant patients: ten years of cyclosporine-based immunosuppression. *J Heart Lung Transplant* 10:877–886, 1991.
121. Shumway SJ, Hertz MI, Maynard R, et al: Airway complications after lung and heart-lung transplantation. *Transplant Proc* 25:1165–1166, 1993.
122. Colquhoun IW, Gascoigne AD, Au J, et al: Airway complications after pulmonary transplantation. *Ann Thorac Surg* 57:141–145, 1994.
123. Smith PC, Slaughter MS, Petty MG, et al: Abdominal complications after lung transplantation. *J Heart Lung Transplant* 14:44–51, 1995.
124. Sodhi SS, Guo JP, Maurer AH, et al: Gastroparesis after combined heart and lung transplantation. *J Clin Gastroenterol* 34:34–39, 2002.
125. Berkowitz N, Schulman LL, McGregor C, et al: Gastroparesis after lung transplantation. Potential role in postoperative respiratory complications. *Chest* 108:1602–1607, 1995.
126. Lau CL, Palmer SM, Howell DN, et al: Laparoscopic antireflux surgery in the lung transplant population. *Surg Endosc* 16:1674–1678, 2002.
127. Theodore J, Marshall S, Kramer M, et al: The "natural history" of the transplanted lung: rates of pulmonary functional change in long-term survivors of heart-lung transplantation. *Transplant Proc* 23:1165–1166, 1991.
128. Theodore J, Morris AJ, Burke CM, et al: Cardiopulmonary function at maximum tolerable constant work rate exercise following human heart-lung transplantation. *Chest* 92:433–439, 1987.
129. Herve P, Picard N, Le Roy LM, et al: Lack of bronchial hyperresponsiveness to methacholine and to isocapnic dry air hyperventilation in heart/lung and double-lung transplant recipients with normal lung histology. The Paris-Sud Lung Transplant Group. *Am Rev Respir Dis* 145:1503–1505, 1992.
130. Herve P, Silbert D, Cerrina J, et al: Impairment of bronchial mucociliary clearance in long-term survivors of heart/lung and double-lung transplantation. The Paris-Sud Lung Transplant Group. *Chest* 103:59–63, 1993.
131. Sarris GE, Moore KA, Schroeder JS, et al: Cardiac transplantation: the Stanford experience in the cyclosporine era. *J Thorac Cardiovasc Surg* 108:240–251, 1994.
132. Schwaiblmair M, Reichenspurner H, Muller C, et al: Cardiopulmonary exercise testing before and after lung and heart-lung transplantation. *Am J Respir Crit Care Med* 159:1277–1283, 1999.

CHAPTER 100

LEFT VENTRICULAR RESTORATION: SURGICAL TREATMENT OF THE FAILING HEART

Lorenzo Menicanti • Serenella Castelvecchio

In memory of Professor Marisa Di Donato.

In response to the increasing health, economic, and social impacts of heart failure, clinicians are investigating new surgical therapies that do not involve heart transplantation. Heart failure affects about 5 million patients in the United States, and more than 250,000 die annually. Nearly 70% of patients with heart failure have coronary artery disease, and nearly all have had a myocardial infarction (MI).[1] In part, the increase in the prevalence and incidence of heart failure results from improved diagnosis and treatment of cardiac disease (especially ischemic disease), but another factor is the aging of the population.[2] Despite improvements in medical treatment since the 1960s and the introduction of potent new drugs, the prognosis for patients affected by heart failure remains extremely poor.[3,4] However, with recent advances in surgical therapy for cardiac disease, new surgical options can be offered to some of these patients as an alternative to medical therapy. Some conventional drug therapies have not shown any significant improvement in the survival of patients with heart failure.[5-8]

After a diagnosis of heart failure, the 5-year mortality rate is still 60% for men and 45% for women, despite improvements in its medical management.[9] Currently, improvements in surgery technology and in surgeons' skills have broadened the indications for cardiac surgery. Historically, patients with severe congestive heart failure (CHF) were listed for heart transplantation, and although this is a very effective therapy for end-stage heart failure, the limited number of donor organs remains a crucial problem.[10] Indeed, the Registry of the International Society for Heart and Lung Transplantation shows that the number of heart transplant centers worldwide has dropped from 248 in 1995 to 201 in 2005.[11]

Until recently, surgical management was directed toward the underlying pathology of coronary disease and the secondary mitral insufficiency that evolves as the heart dilates, but surgeons do not systematically approach the ventricle. Surgical ventricular restoration (SVR), the topic of this chapter, was launched by Dor and colleagues[12] and represents a relatively novel surgical approach that aims to restore (i.e., bring back to normal) the dilated, distorted left ventricular (LV) cavity to improve function. It requires knowledge of the remodeling infrastructure, of the structural changes that lead to geometric abnormalities, and of the role of compensatory, remote muscle and stretching mechanisms that lead to electrical instabilities.[13]

SVR is more than a single procedure, because it includes coronary grafting and mitral repair when needed, and thus it has the potential to treat the three components of the disease: the ventricle, the vessels, and the valve ("triple V" as defined by Buckberg[14,15]).

PATHOPHYSIOLOGY OF HEART FAILURE

Left Ventricular Remodeling

In dilated cardiomyopathy (a common cause of heart failure), a primary determinant of the disease process is LV remodeling. The underlying causes of dilated cardiomyopathy are diverse, and the origin may be nonischemic or ischemic.

LV remodeling is a complex, dynamic, and time-dependent phenomenon that involves molecular, cellular, interstitial, and genome-expression changes that manifest clinically as changes in the size, shape, and function of the heart after cardiac injury.[16] The process can evolve slowly or rapidly after the myocardial injury, and it contributes importantly in the progression to end-stage CHF. Box 100-1 summarizes the principal changes that occur in LV remodeling. The extracellular matrix participates in the altered ventricular geometry after MI. Cardiologists and cardiac surgeons traditionally viewed the extracellular matrix as an inert collection of structural macromolecules that serve as a scaffold for cells. However, a large body of evidence supports a central role for the extracellular matrix in the control of numerous cellular functions[17] and supports the idea that the extent of LV remodeling is a critical determinant of clinical outcome after MI.

Current working models for heart failure include the cardiorenal model (excessive salt and water retention), the hemodynamic model (pump failure and excessive vasoconstriction), and the neurohormonal model (overexpression of biologically active molecules capable of exerting unfavorable effects on the heart and circulation). Each of these may be necessary but not entirely sufficient to explain all the causes of disease progression in the failing heart. After the myocardial insult and the initial decline in pumping capacity, a variety of compensatory mechanisms are evoked to restore cardiovascular function and normal homeostasis. Adrenergic, renin-angiotensin, and cytokine systems are activated systemically and locally in the myocardium in response to reduced cardiac output.[18,19] A variety of circulating and tissue proteins and peptides (e.g., norepinephrine, angiotensin II, endothelin, aldosterone, tumor necrosis factor, interleukins) are generated in an initial adapting response. However, chronic overexpression of these biologically active molecules may fundamentally alter gene expression, changing protein synthesis in both myocytes and fibroblasts.

The biomechanical model for heart failure described by Mann and Bristow helps to explain the progression of heart failure independent of the neurohormonal status of the patient.[20] In fact, current medical therapy, acting against neurohormonal activation, tends to slow progression but fails to arrest the process of remodeling. In addition, many types of neurohormonal inhibition proved to be ineffective or even harmful in patients with heart failure.[21]

To explain the failure of neurohormonal antagonism, Mann and Bristow focus on LV size and geometric abnormalities as being responsible for progression of the disease. Geometric changes lead to structural abnormalities of the myocytes and of the myocardium, which worsen cardiac function and increase neurohormonal activation; this may make the cardiovascular system less responsive to normal homeostatic control mechanisms.[20]

BOX 100-1 Left Ventricular Remodeling

MYOCARDIAL CHANGES
- Myocyte loss
- Necrosis
- Apoptosis

ALTERATIONS IN EXTRACELLULAR MATRIX
- Matrix degradation
- Replacement fibrosis

ALTERATIONS IN LV CHAMBER GEOMETRY
- LV dilation
- Increased LV sphericity
- LV wall thinning
- Mitral valve insufficiency

LV, Left ventricular.

Left Ventricular Geometric Abnormalities in Ischemic and Nonischemic Ventricles

The determinants of LV geometry are shape, volume, and cardiac mass, and these three components may be altered by cardiac disease, which can be primarily degenerative, valvular, or ischemic in origin. Ischemic cardiomyopathy leads to a sequence of structural changes to compensate for the increased load produced from the nonfunctional akinetic or dyskinetic regions.[22]

In anterior myocardial infarction, the LV apex is primarily involved, so regional changes affect the anterior, septal, and inferoseptal ventricular components. Globally, the elongation and widening of the ventricle occur proportionally to maintain a constant ratio (i.e., a constant *sphericity index*, or short ratio to long axis). However, when patients develop secondary mitral insufficiency, the sphericity index is abnormal and the ventricle is more spherical. In the absence of mitral regurgitation (MR), therefore, the sphericity index fails to detect shape abnormalities in anterior postinfarction cardiomyopathy. The *conicity index* has been proposed to assess the conical shape of the apex and its changes after MI (Fig. 100-1).[23] Another important shape change that occurs after an anterior MI is the displacement of the papillary muscles laterally and toward the apex, which produces tethering of the posterior mitral leaflet and mitral restriction.

Alternatively, shape changes after an inferior MI are different[24]: the short axis is widened more than the long axis is elongated, which leads to an increase in the sphericity index and accounts for the more frequent occurrence and the more severe degree of MR. Table 100-1 compares the geometric abnormalities that occur in anterior and inferior myocardial infarctions.[25]

Nonischemic dilated cardiomyopathy exhibits a more spherical shape than ischemic cardiomyopathy: the short axis is enlarged, MR is more frequently involved, and wall motion is severely and diffusely hypokinetic. Pump function is markedly reduced and there are apparently no regional differences in contractility. However, biopsy studies show nonhomogeneous disease in many patients, with the amount of scarring and fibrosis ranging from 4% to 60% between the free wall and the septum, which may account for the failure of some types of surgery, such as the Batista operation, to reduce the ventricular cavity in patients with nonischemic dilated cardiomyopathy.[26,27]

Rationale for Reshaping Cardiac Architecture

Figure 100-2 shows the spiral arrangement of myocardial fibers as reported in a very old anatomy atlas. Studies[28,29] established that fiber orientation was a function of transmural location, with fiber direction being predominantly longitudinal in the endocardial region, transitioning into a circumferential direction in the midwall, and becoming longitudinal again over the epicardial surface. Such an alignment of fibers in double layers (left- and right-handed from the base to the apex) forms a double helix. These layers are not aligned parallel to one another; rather, the myofiber sheets diverge within the LV wall, creating angulations with respect to the plane of the epicardial surface. These fiber angulations serve to resist deformation and to maintain the distribution of tension within normal limits at the three levels: longitudinal, radial, and circumferential. Moreover, this architecture gives to the heart a form resembling a geometric ellipsoid, which favors the direction of flow toward the aorta. When angulations are deformed by fiber disruption, fibrosis, or scarring of myocardial tissue, the shape of the ventricle loses its characteristics and its functionality (following the strict relationship between form and function). For a given fiber contractile status, the ejection fraction (EF) changes according to the shape of the ventricle, being low in a spherical ventricle (sphericity index, toward 1) and high in an elliptical shape (sphericity index, toward 0). In fact, macroscopic anatomic alterations can affect wall tension, which, according to the Laplace law, is directly proportional to LV pressure and chamber radius and inversely proportional to wall thickness. In animal models of myocardial damage or after MI in humans, ventricular remodeling alters the major determinants of wall stress,[30,31] and functional impairment has been reported in the remote zones of dilated LV with geometric abnormalities.[32] When the ischemic systolic dysfunction is superimposed on the use of preload to

TABLE 100-1 Geometric Differences According to Site of Myocardial Infarction

	Inferior	Anterior	*P* value
Diastolic diameter (mm)	69 ± 10	63 ± 9	0.009
Systolic diameter (mm)	57 ± 12	50 ± 11	0.009
Septum thickness in diastole (mm)	12.8 ± 3	10.5 ± 3	0.001
Posterior thickening (%)	16 ± 15	32 ± 23	0.008
Left ventricular mass index (gm/m^2)	217 ± 51	165 ± 39	0.000
Left atrium size (mm)	48 ± 8	44 ± 7	0.008
Mitral regurgitation present (%)	87	69	0.04
Mitral regurgitation grade	2.9 ± 1.1	2.0 ± 1.1	0.0003

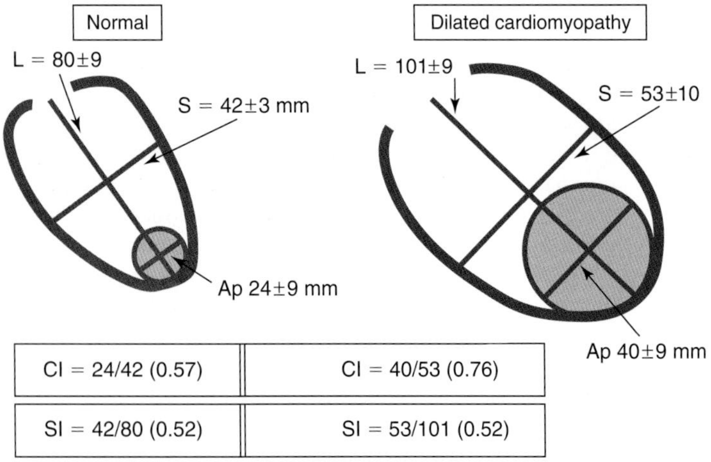

FIGURE 100-1 ■ Geometric measures in normal and dilated cardiomyopathy. Sphericity index (SI) is calculated as the short- to long-axis ratio (S/L), and conicity index (CI) as the apical to short-axis ratio (Ap/S). Apical diameter is determined by using the diameter of the sphere that best fits the apex. Note that the SI has the same value in normal subjects and in patients with dilated cardiomyopathy, because the elongation of the ventricle is proportional to the increase in width, so the ratio remains stable, whereas the CI is markedly abnormal in the patients.

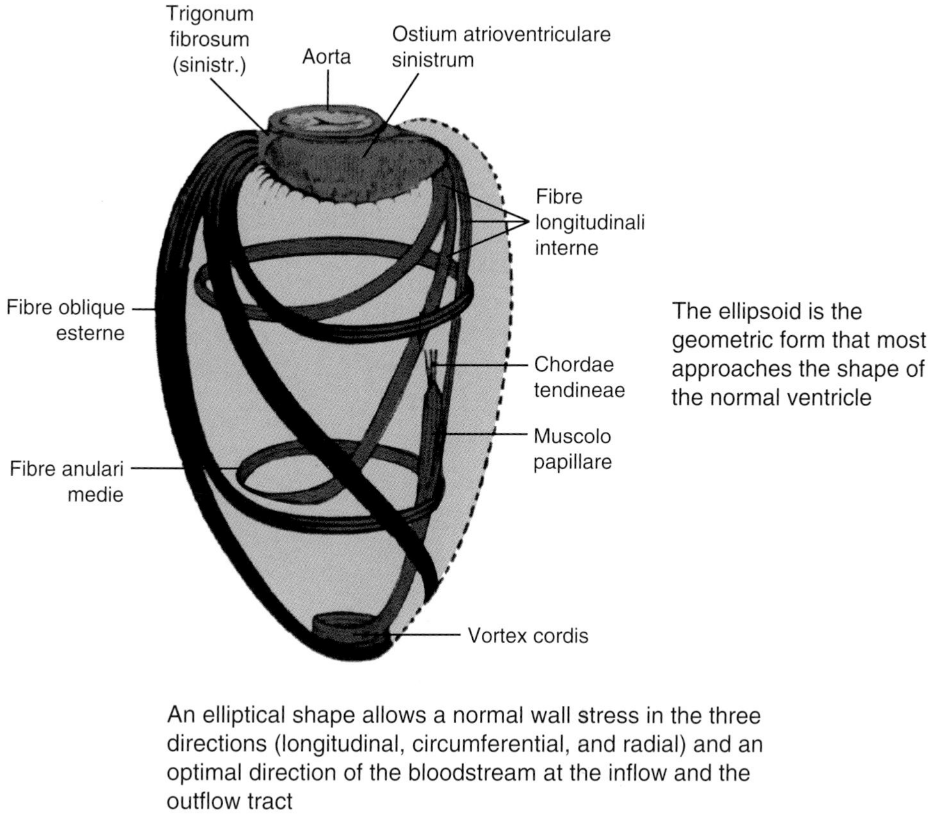

FIGURE 100-2 ■ The three-dimensional architecture of the heart. From an eighteenth-century atlas of anatomy. (From Benninghoff-Goertler: *Atlas of anatomy,* vol II, Padova, Italy, 1996, Piccin Editore.)

improve cardiac output during exercise, the ventricle can be further dilated because of its inability to eject blood, starting a cycle that further deteriorates LV function. In addition, LV end-diastolic pressure can increase in the presence of reduced myocardial compliance (resulting from tissue stiffening), which tends to resist deformation, whereas increased stiffness leads to decreased systolic function.

A further increase in end-diastolic and end-systolic volumes (ESVs) leads to an adverse prognosis.[33] As part of the GUSTO (Global Utilization of Streptokinase and t-PA for Occluded Arteries) trial, Migrino and associates[33] evaluated ESV at 90 to 180 minutes into reperfusion during acute MI. They demonstrated that in successfully reperfused patients after MI, an increase in ESV beyond 40 mL/m^2 worsens prognosis in terms of both development of heart failure and mortality. A post-MI ESV index equal to or greater than 60 mL/m^2 carries a 1-year mortality rate of up to 30%. In the SAVE (Survival and Ventricular Enlargement) trial, left ventricular size was a strong independent risk factor for mortality after 2 years.[34]

Even after coronary artery bypass surgery, patients with large ventricles have a worse prognosis. Yamaguchi and coworkers[35] identified LV ESV index greater than 100 mL/m^2 as an independent risk factor for the development of CHF in ischemic cardiomyopathy. These reports helped cardiac surgeons focus on the importance of reconstruction of the left ventricle in ischemic cardiomyopathy.

Left Ventricular Aneurysm or Ischemic Dilated Cardiomyopathy?

Left ventricular aneurysm was first described in the eighteenth century.[36] In 1816, Cruveilhier[37] attributed ventricular aneurysm to myocardial fibrosis, although its association with coronary thrombosis was not generally appreciated until a century later. It was not until Tennant and Wiggers showed paradoxical motion in acutely ischemic myocardium that the physiologic implications of ventricular injury became apparent.[38] Subsequently, Murray described systolic paradoxical expansion of acutely infarcted myocardium and correlated this with diminished cardiac output and falling blood pressure.[39] In 1967, Klein and coworkers[40] published a hemodynamic study on LV aneurysm that became a milestone in the field of mechanics and energetics of the left ventricle after an ischemic injury. Gorlin and coauthors were the first to state that when approximately 20% to 25% of left ventricular area is inactivated by any pathologic process, the degree that the myofiber must shorten to maintain stroke volume exceeds physiologic limits, and cardiac enlargement (Starling mechanism) must ensue to maintain adequate ejection of blood. With this concept, they anticipated the concept of LV remodeling and described the way MI relates to the genesis of aneurysm. Furthermore, they described that the aneurysm can be either dyskinetic (i.e., paradoxical expansion resulting during systole) or akinetic (i.e., myocardial fibrosis, calcification within the scar, thickened overlying pericardium, mural thrombosis, and endocardial thickening may rigidify the aneurysm wall and prevent its expansion).

Gorlin offered the following definition:

> *An aneurysm is identified by a left ventricular angiogram as any akinetic or dyskinetic segment of myocardium. An akinetic segment is defined as a segment that appears to have no motion during systole, whereas a dyskinetic segment appears to bulge paradoxically during systole. Intraoperatively, an aneurysm is identified as a circumscribed area of scar, which is thin, often adherent to the pericardium and which may or may not bulge paradoxically during systole. The aneurysmal segment is easily outlined by looking for the area that puckers and collapses when the left ventricle is vented.*

This cineangiographic and surgical definition of ventricular aneurysm is compatible with the pathologic definition: "A localized outpouching of the cavity of a cardiac chamber, with or without outward bulging of the external surface."[41]

Early revascularization, with either thrombolysis or primary percutaneous transluminal coronary angioplasty, has beneficial effects on infarct size and LV function and therefore has profoundly changed the picture of MI and its sequelae.[42-44] However, even with early mechanical relief of the coronary occlusion, unfavorable global LV remodeling may occur. Bolognese and coauthors demonstrated that almost 30% of patients with excellent infarct-related artery patency at 6 months continue to undergo LV remodeling.[45,46] In patients with an anterior MI, this occurs more frequently when myocardial contrast echocardiography demonstrates a higher incidence of microvascular dysfunction. Figure 100-3 shows the progression of an anterior MI toward ischemic dilated cardiomyopathy in one of our patients. Figure 100-4 shows two of the shape abnormalities that may occur after successful early recanalization for anterior MI as analyzed by the centerline method.[47-49] Thus, an acute MI, either anterior or inferior, may result in any of four types of shape abnormalities (Fig. 100-5).[50] This classification is incomplete because it does not take into account abnormalities occurring at the septum or at the lateral wall. However,

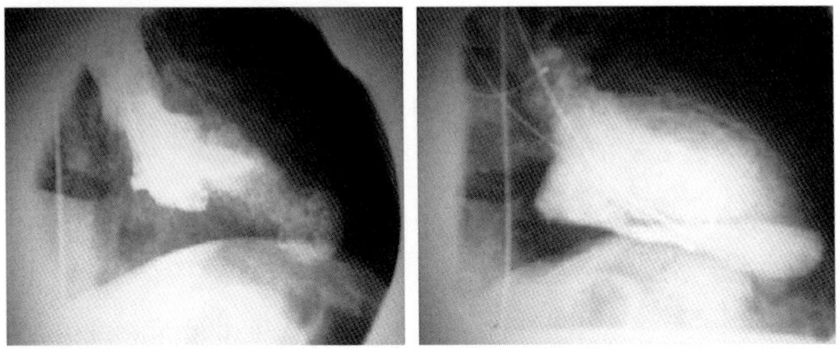

FIGURE 100-3 ■ Left ventricle (LV) angiography, 30-degree right anterior oblique projection. *Left,* Early after myocardial infarction, systolic frame. Note the small apical aneurysm. The left anterior descending artery was successfully reperfused. *Right,* The LV angiogram 1 year later showed marked end-systolic volume dilation of the ventricle, and the patient had symptoms of heart failure.

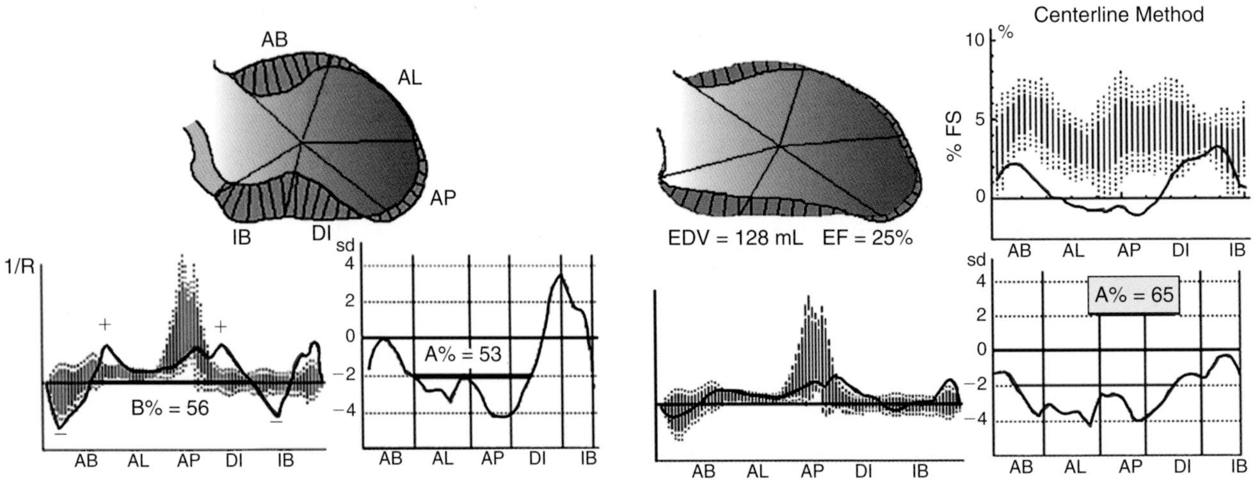

FIGURE 100-4 ■ Left ventricular (LV) curvature and regional wall motion analyses in two patients after an anterior myocardial infarction was successfully reperfused. LV shape on the left represents the true aneurysm, with the classic neck at the border between thickening and nonthickening myocardium. LV shape on the right represents the true dilated ischemic cardiomyopathy, without borders between thickening and nonthickening myocardium. Graphs below each silhouette represent the curvature analysis *(left)* and the centerline analysis *(right).* Curvature values, expressed as the reciprocal of the radius (1/R) on the ordinate, are measured from the aortic to the mitral plane around the ventricular perimeter. Shadowing indicates standard deviation of normal motion; the line indicates wall motion in the patient. The curvature of the apex is greater in the normal heart and reduced in the patient. Note the sharp variation of curvature values from negative (–) to positive (+) and from + to – in the patient on the left. Curvature values in the patient on the right are extremely reduced without variations (neither negative nor positive)—that is, the curvature is flattened all along the perimeter. Centerline analysis: regional wall motion of 45 chords around the LV perimeter is quantified. *A%,* Extent of asynergy; *AB,* anterobasal region; *AL,* anterolateral region; *AP,* apical region; *B%,* extent of curvature abnormalities; *DI,* diaphragmatic region; *EDV,* end-diastolic volume; *EF,* ejection fraction; *FS,* fractional shortening; *IB,* inferobasal. (From Baroni M, Barletta G: Digital curvature estimation for left ventricular shape analysis. *Image Vis Comp* 10:485–494, 1992; and Sheehan FH, Stewart DK, Dodge HT, et al: Variability in the measurement of regional left ventricular wall from contrast angiograms. *Circulation* 68:550–559, 1983.)

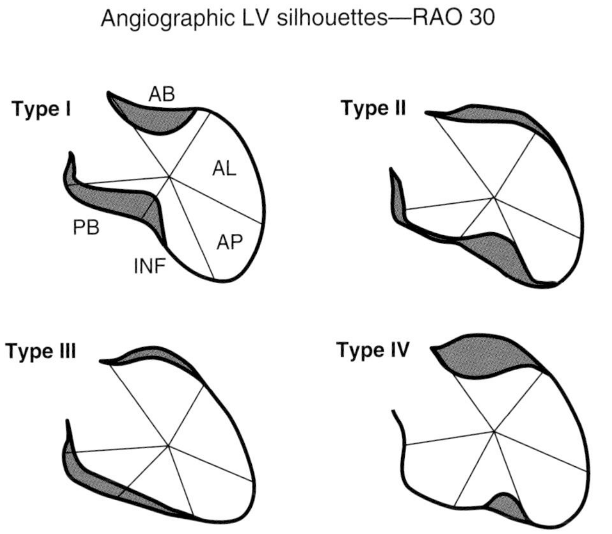

FIGURE 100-5 Silhouettes of left ventricle (LV) shape abnormalities after myocardial infarction. Diagrams represent evaluation by angiography in 30-degree right anterior oblique projection. *Type 1:* LV shape is geometrically delimited by two systolic "borders" between thickening and nonthickening myocardium; the classic neck of the true aneurysm is evident. *Type 2:* The shape is characterized by only one border between thickening and nonthickening myocardium, not two borders as in type 1. *Type 3:* LV systolic shape is without borders (i.e., the curvature is flattened along the overall perimeter of the ventricle). *Type 4:* Double-site myocardial infarction (anterior and inferior). *AB,* Anterobasal region; *AL,* anterolateral region; *AP,* apical region; *INF,* inferior; *PB,* posterobasal region; *RAO,* right anterior oblique projection.

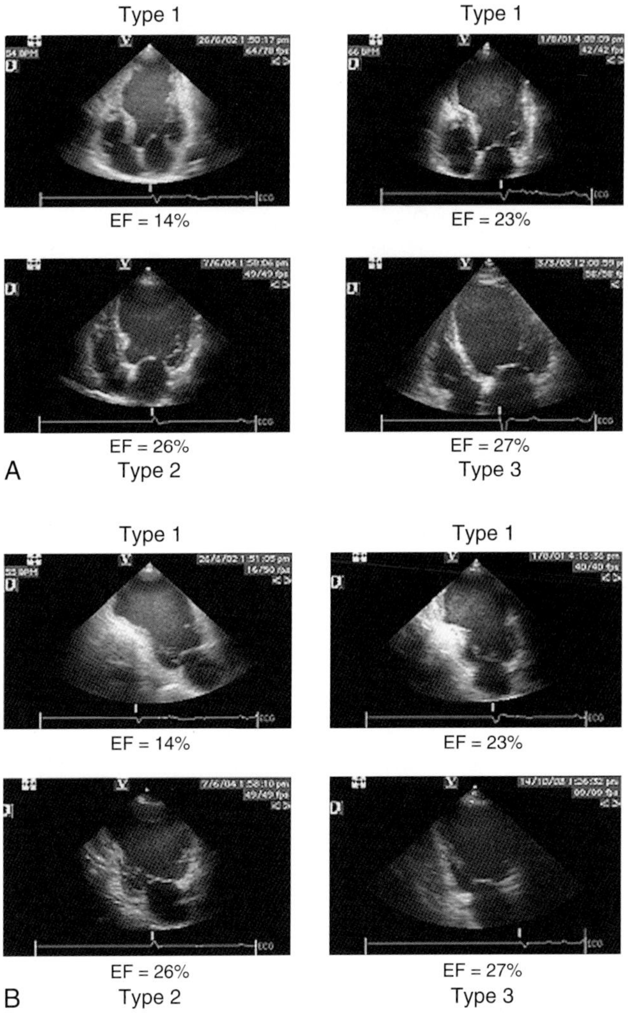

FIGURE 100-6 Echocardiographic four-chamber **(A)** and two-chamber **(B)** views are shown in four patients after an anterior myocardial infarction. All patients have marked left ventricular dilation with low ejection fraction (EF), but the shapes are definitely different. Types 1, 2, and 3 are shown.

it is useful for assessing treatment results, especially after volume reduction surgery, when the results after repair of a true aneurysm look profoundly different from the results after surgery for types 2, 3, or 4. Figure 100-6 shows an echocardiographic study from four patients with three types of shape abnormalities. Apical four-chamber and two-chamber views are shown.

Left Ventricular Aneurysmectomy

The first successful surgical correction of an LV aneurysm occurred in 1957.[51] Denton Cooley described the technique of open resection and simple closure on cardiopulmonary bypass in 1958.[52] This technique was the standard of the profession for the next 30 years. In 1968, Favaloro and colleagues[53] reported on a series of 130 patients who underwent resection for LV aneurysm, with a hospital mortality of 13%.

In 1979, Grondin and associates[54] reported on a series of 40 patients with aneurysms who were medically treated. They divided the group into those with and those without symptoms. After 10 years, survival was 90% in asymptomatic patients but only 46% in patients who were symptomatic at the time of diagnosis. The causes of death were predominantly CHF, thromboembolism, and arrhythmias. They suggested that mortality depended on aneurysm size, with large aneurysms conferring a higher risk. These reports implied that medical management resulted in improved survival, and they fostered a reluctance to use surgery to treat this disease. As recently as 1983, Cohen and coworkers[55] recommended that aneurysms be resected only after maximal medical management (for heart failure, angina pectoris, recurrent thromboembolism refractory to anticoagulation, and refractory ventricular tachycardia) had failed.

In 1985, the concept of surgical repair of the LV aneurysm was altered. Newer techniques described by Jatene[56] involved excluding the dyskinetic scar when performing a circular endoventricular suture, and Dor and colleagues[12] began using an endoventricular patch to rebuild a failing ventricle after extended endocardiectomy for ventricular tachycardia. The concept was to reduce the LV size and reconstruct a more elliptical cavity, treating the dilation in all its components (anterior, apical, and septal), as opposed to performing a linear resection[57,58] of the aneurysm, which left untouched a septal dilation and created a distortion of the residual chamber. The concept of excluding all diseased tissue from the cavity was a fundamental improvement.[12] With this change in technique, a reduction was seen in hospital mortality as well as in late mortality. Dor and coworkers demonstrated that the technique is

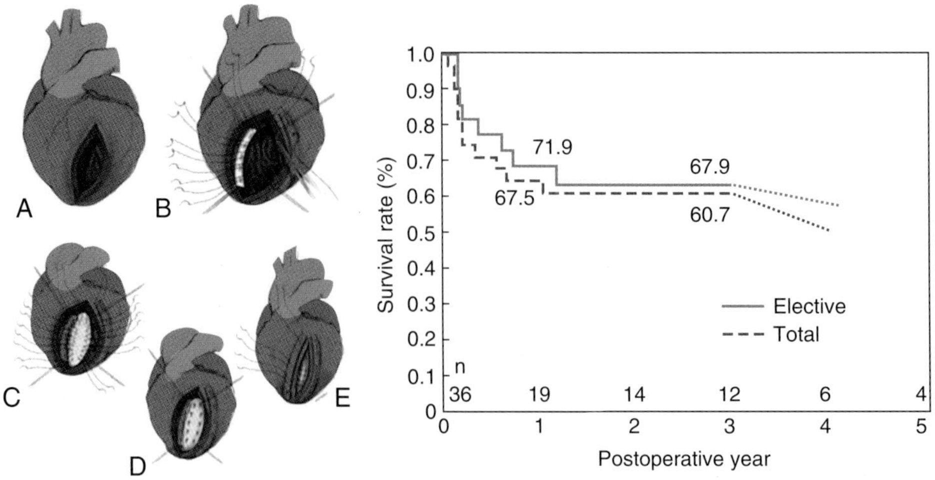

FIGURE 100-7 ■ *Left,* Septal anterior ventricular exclusion (SAVE) procedure, with steps A to E. See text for explanation. *Right,* Survival rates after the SAVE procedure were slightly higher when the surgery was elective. The number of patients (*n*) surviving at each follow-up year is shown above the abscissa. (With permission from Suma H, Isomura T, Horii T, et al: Septal anterior ventricular exclusion procedure for idiopathic dilated cardiomyopathy. *Ann Thorac Surg* 82:1344–1348, 2006.)

applicable not only to dyskinetic but also to akinetic areas. As a consequence, the indications and patient selection for volume reduction surgery have changed.[59]

DIAGNOSIS AND PATIENT SELECTION FOR SURGERY

Nonischemic Cardiomyopathy

LV reconstruction for dilated cardiomyopathy (the Batista procedure, or partial left ventriculectomy) has been abandoned, primarily because of unacceptable perioperative mortality and morbidity.[27] One reason for its failure was that the pathology of the whole chamber was assumed to be uniform and homogeneous. However, there is evidence that the disease is nonhomogeneous, and that the septal and lateral walls differ in scarring and fibrosis.[60,61] Thus, in the Batista operation, if a minimally diseased lateral wall was excised and a very fibrotic septum was retained, postoperative LV function was adversely affected, even if the left ventricle was properly downsized.

Therefore, Suma and colleagues[61] suggested an intraoperative echocardiographic evaluation to assess the regional contractile response to preload reduction, to aid site selection, and to improve surgical results. In the intraoperative echocardiography-guided volume reduction test, the initiation of partial cardiopulmonary bypass decompresses the dilated (stretched) chamber and induces functional changes of left ventricular wall motion and thickness. Identification of wall motion changes means that the most diseased region can be selected for exclusion, leaving the more viable muscle to resume function after restoration. This idea comes from experience in restoring the ischemic left ventricle, when the scar is evident and can be excluded. However, the concept of nonhomogeneity in nonischemic cardiomyopathy is new. Suma reports that if intraoperative echocardiography shows that the septum is the weakest part, the septal anterior ventricle is excluded. Septal anterior ventricular exclusion (SAVE) was introduced by Suma and colleagues[26,60,61] and called *pacopexy* by Buckberg and coauthors[62] in recognition of the contributions of Francisco (Paco) Torrent-Guasp, whose ingenious anatomic concepts defined the helical ventricular myocardial band and furthered our understanding of the relationship between structure and function.[14,63] To make an elliptical ventricle, a long and narrow endoventricular patch is placed along the septum with interrupted mattress sutures so that the septum and a part of the anterior wall are excluded (Fig. 100-7). In patients with nonischemic dilated cardiomyopathy and advanced New York Heart Association (NYHA) class, results in terms of survival rate are promising.

When intraoperative echocardiography shows that the weakest part is the lateral wall, Suma and coworkers[61] perform a partial left ventriculoplasty (Fig. 100-8).

Asynergic Areas

Appropriate candidates for LV reconstruction have suffered an MI, have a dilated left ventricle, and have an asynergic area (either dyskinetic or akinetic) of 35% or more of the ventricular perimeter. These patients have symptoms of heart failure, angina, or intractable ventricular arrhythmias.

The left ventricle should be evaluated carefully with coronary angiography (ventricular angiography in right and left anterior oblique projections), by a complete echocardiographic study (four- and two-chamber views, and parasternal long- and short-axis views), or by a magnetic resonance imaging (MRI) study. The objectives of these imaging techniques are to assess parameters for patient selection (Box 100-2), treatment planning, and follow-up.

Patients with either akinetic or dyskinetic scar may benefit from SVR, and it is the *extent* of asynergy rather than the *type* of asynergy that is related to outcome after the surgery.[64] The region to be surgically excluded should be carefully evaluated for wall motion and thickening.

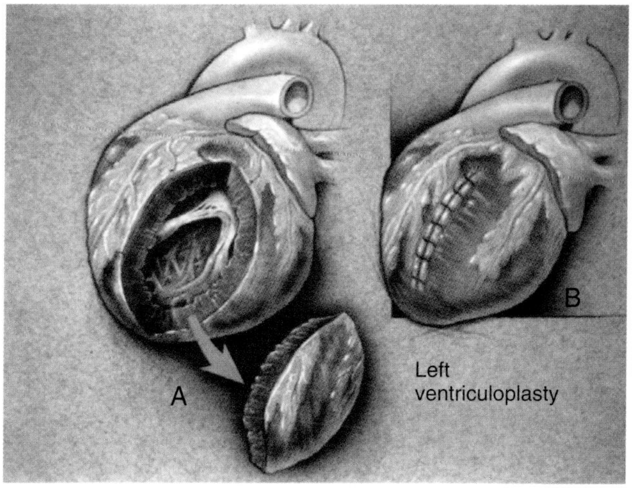

FIGURE 100-8 ■ Left ventriculoplasty, or Batista operation. **A,** Lateral partial ventriculectomy. **B,** Closure of the ventriculotomy.

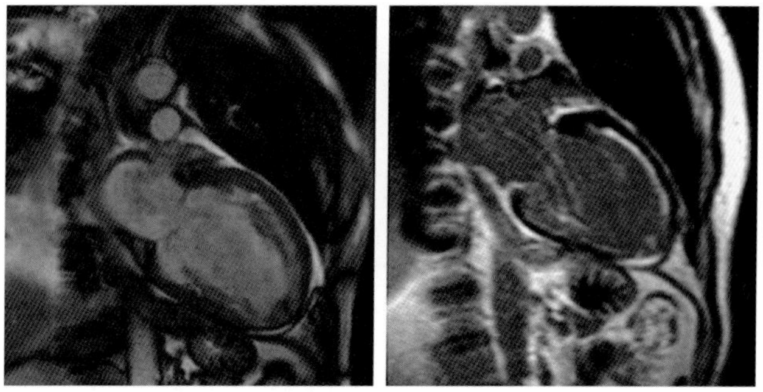

FIGURE 100-9 ■ Cardiac magnetic resonance images with late gadolinium enhancement. *Left,* Normal subject, without myocardial scar. *Right,* An example of extensive transmural myocardial scar in a patient who will undergo surgical left ventricular restoration. The two-chamber view is shown. Note the bright myocardium extending from the basal anterior region to the apex and inferoapical region.

BOX 100-2 Parameters for Patient Selection

- Internal dimensions of the ventricle
- Ventricular volumes (both in diastole and in systole)
- Ejection fraction
- Thickness and thickening of the wall
- Extent of asynergic area
- Status of the remote regions
- Presence or absence of viability
- Presence or absence of mitral regurgitation
- Mitral annulus size and left atrium size
- Right ventricular function

Wall motion assessment can be accomplished by LV angiography, echocardiography, or nuclear scintigraphy, but MRI provides a more accurate determination of LV volumes and EF, because it shows the epicardial and endocardial border from the base to the apex in a three-dimensional view.

LV angiography is a planar technique that shows at most two projections along the ventricle. It does not show the epicardial border, so it does not help in a calculation of thickening. However, application of the centerline method to LV angiography resulted in a reliable quantitative assessment of regional wall motion[49] with clear definition of asynergy. Echocardiography allows visualization of both the endocardial and the epicardial borders, so wall thickening and wall motion can be assessed. However, an echocardiographic method that precisely defines regional wall motion is not available. Therefore, wall motion is measured by the wall motion score index,[65] which results from a qualitative (thus subjective) evaluation of motion and is expressed by a number derived from the sum of the degree of asynergy at 16 different segments (normal, 1; hypokinetic, 2; akinetic, 3; dyskinetic, 4; aneurismal, 5).

Echocardiography has several other limitations: (1) the LV apex is not adequately seen when the ventricle is enlarged (e.g., in dilated cardiomyopathy); (2) the endocardial border is often not clearly seen, which accounts for intraobserver and interobserver variability in measuring LV volumes and EF; and (3) many patients have comorbidities (e.g., obstructive pulmonary disease, obesity) that make the echocardiography images suboptimal.

Nuclear scintigraphic methods display endocardial border motion in planar views (with radionuclide angiography, labeling the blood pool) or the myocardium, including endocardial and epicardial visualization with gated single-photon-emission computed tomography. However, such studies require the use of radioactive tracers and are not available in all cardiac centers. Also, cardiovascular MRI is not available everywhere, and some patients have contraindications to the study (e.g., claustrophobia, presence of implantable cardioverter-defibrillator). However, it allows a most comprehensive evaluation with highly accurate and reproducible measurements in a single session.[66] The greatest usefulness of cardiovascular MRI is in the detection of myocardial scar with late gadolinium enhancement. Myocardial scar tends to accumulate a significantly higher concentration of gadolinium than normal myocardium. Ten to 20 minutes after infusion, scarred regions appear very bright, whereas normal myocardium appears dark, at typical imaging times. Figure 100-9 shows a patient with extensive scarring in the anterior and apical territory. A predictor of myocardial viability is the ratio of the thickness of tissue exhibiting late contrast enhancement in a segment to the total LV wall thickness in that segment. Segments with nearly transmural extent of late contrast enhancement are highly unlikely to have recovery of function after revascularization.[67]

Commercially available software dedicated to LV function analysis now provides a semi-automated assessment of regional wall motion, the extent of normal and abnormal contracting myocardium, and the percentage of scarred tissue (Fig. 100-10). This allows a prediction of myocardial viability without a need for pharmacologic stress. Cardiovascular MRI also allows quantification of regional deformation by radionuclide tagging and calculation of strain and strain rate, which can be particularly useful for examining the remote regions and the apical twisting and untwisting.[68] Torsion and twisting and

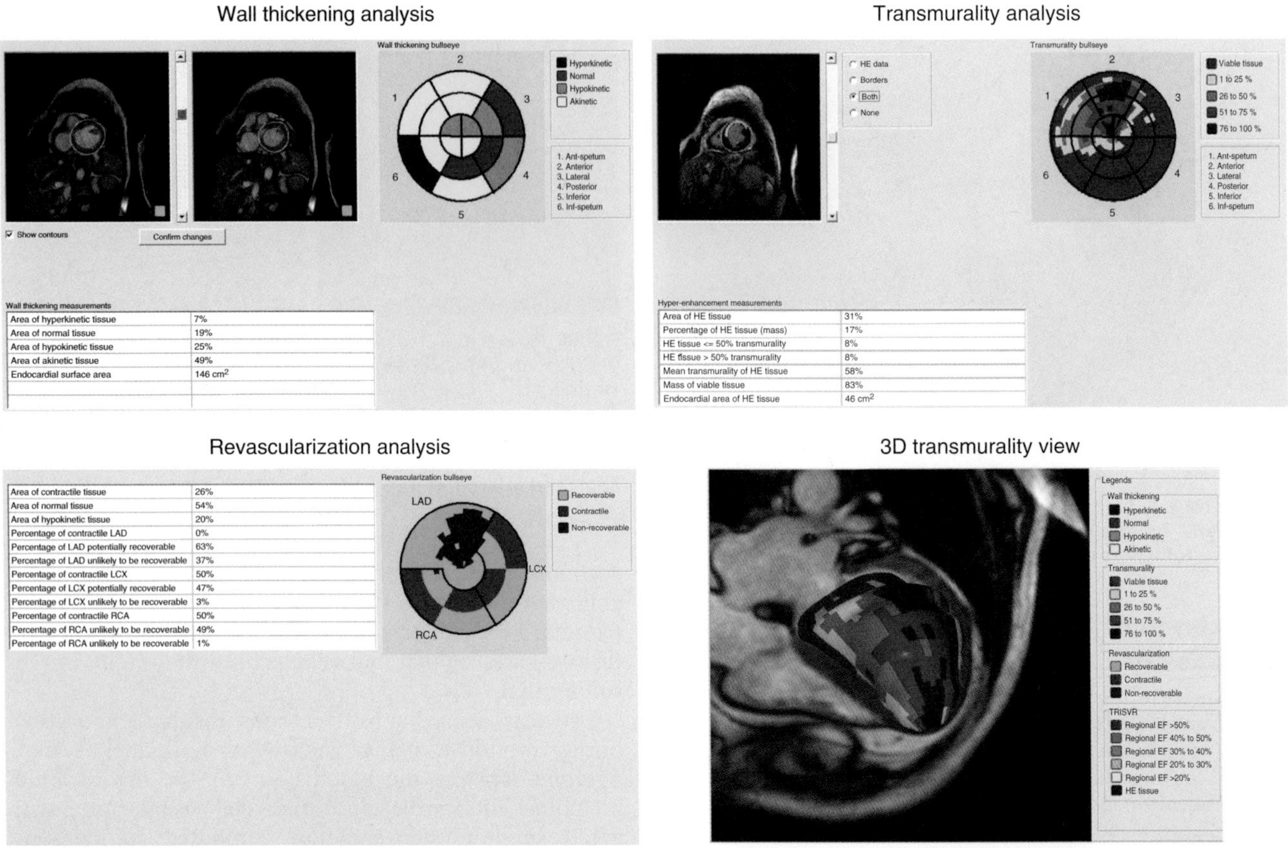

FIGURE 100-10 ■ Analysis of cardiac function using MARISA software (Magnetic Resonance Imaging System Analysis [Chase Medical, Richardson, Texas]). *Top left,* Wall motion analysis quantified as normal, hyperkinesia, hypokinesia, and akinesia. The percentage distribution of asynergy is calculated. *Top right,* Assessment of scar transmurality with late gadolinium enhancement. The extent of the transmurality from 0% to 100% is color coded, and the percentage of scarred tissue is calculated. *Bottom left,* Analysis of viability: the green area represents potentially viable myocardium that may improve with revascularization; the blue area represents the transmural, nonviable scar. *Bottom right,* Three-dimensional reconstruction of the left ventricle superimposed on the four-chamber view. The extent of the scar as evaluated by late gadolinium enhancement is shown.

untwisting movements of the apex (as opposed to the base) greatly contribute to blood ejection and to maintaining a good pump function; these mechanisms are reduced or even lost after an anterior MI, resulting in further impairment in cardiac function. Cardiovascular MRI tagging, however, is not routinely performed in clinical practice but is confined to research studies because the data analysis is laborious and time consuming and requires intensive computation. With the development of a tissue Doppler imaging technique and the two-dimensional "speckles" or endocardial border tracking analysis,[69,70] it is easier to measure systolic and diastolic deformation either longitudinally or radially. Vector direction gives the clockwise and counterclockwise directions of contraction, which is particularly useful for assessing torsional mechanics at the apical level. An analysis of untwisting also provides information on diastolic function, at least on rapid filling.

Status of Remote Regions

The quantification of remote regions is performed to determine whether a patient is a candidate for an SVR procedure, and these regions are often not evaluated by conventional imaging studies. After an anterior MI, remote regions may show hypokinesia or even akinesia resulting from critical coronary disease in the right or left circumflex coronary artery (hibernating myocardium), or remote myocardium may be dysfunctional in the absence of coronary stenosis because of the high local tension that reduces shortening. Several years ago, we demonstrated[32] that SVR induced an improvement in remote nonischemic regions in patients with anterior infarction; in that study, we excluded patients with significant stenosis in the right and left coronary arteries. Nowadays, with cardiovascular MRI, we can predict the recovery of function in ischemic, hibernating areas that will benefit from concomitant coronary artery bypass grafting (CABG), and we can also predict whether dysfunctional, nonischemic segments may recover after volume reduction. Therefore, we propose a term other than *hibernating* or *stunned* for dysfunctional nonischemic myocardium in dilated cardiomyopathy—*exhausted myocardium*—which implies recovery of function if the hemodynamic burden that imposes a high wall tension is relieved by SVR.

On the other hand, the detection of scar in remote regions by late gadolinium enhancement may predict an unsatisfactory pump improvement and a higher mortality rate after SVR. A significant scarring in a myocardial segment precludes, in fact, the likelihood of postoperative contractile recovery of that segment.

In summary, extensive preoperative imaging studies are necessary for selecting patients, planning treatment, and evaluating the results of SVR. Cardiovascular MRI is the best option, because it provides the surgeon with all the necessary information for planning an effective, comprehensive surgery tailored to the individual patient, and all the information can be obtained in a single examination taking less than 1 hour.

Finally, cardiologists, radiologists, and surgeons must collaborate to improve knowledge about patient selection and to achieve an optimal surgical outcome.

SURGICAL VENTRICULAR RESTORATION FOR ISCHEMIC CARDIOMYOPATHY

Left ventricular reconstruction by endoventricular circular patch plasty repair was described and proposed by Dor and colleagues in 1984[12] for rebuilding the left ventricle after an MI, either during the acute phase (surgical treatment of septal rupture or refractory ventricular arrhythmias according to the Harken technique[71]) or in patients with chronic MI and with LV asynergy (akinesia or dyskinesia) to exclude all the akinetic nonresectable areas (e.g., septum and posterior wall). In addition, a complete coronary revascularization is achieved and mitral repair or replacement is performed if needed.[72]

The term *surgical ventricular restoration* includes operative methods that reduce LV volume and restore ventricular elliptical shape. The concept of reducing wall stress through the surgical restoration of LV cavity size and geometry is the guiding principle behind this innovative technique.

Since the first description by Dor and colleagues,[12] the procedure has been adopted by many surgeons, but it is not widely used because surgeons have been unwilling to incise and exclude the akinetic normal-appearing segments often encountered after early reperfusion. Instead, CABG is performed, and the nonfunctioning akinetic muscle containing deeper scar is left undisturbed.[73]

The technique has not been standardized, and surgeons use essentially four variations of LV reconstruction to exclude the septum. These include a linear closure by Jatene,[56] a modified linear closure by Mickleborough,[74] a circular closure with a patch by Dor and Menicanti,[75] and a double cerclage closure without a patch by McCarthy.[76] All of these techniques involve an incision into the diseased anterior wall, an exclusion of the entire diseased segment, and a reduction in ventricular cavity size. In the majority of patients, reconstruction is done on the anterior portion of the left ventricle. However, reconstruction has also been performed on the posterior wall after circumflex or right coronary artery occlusion. Most of these patients undergo concomitant coronary artery bypass, and many also undergo mitral valve repair.

Surgical Details of Anterior Surgical Ventricular Restoration

Surgical LV restoration as performed since 2001 by our group at the San Donato Hospital in Italy is conducted on the arrested heart with antegrade crystalloid or cold-blood cardioplegia. CABG is first performed, as completely as possible, almost always on the left anterior descending coronary artery, to preserve the upper part of the septum and to guarantee complete revascularization. The ventricle is opened at the middle of the scar on the anterior wall, with an incision parallel to the left anterior descending artery, starting from the midportion and proceeding toward the apex. The internal part of the cavity is examined, and thrombi are removed if present. The mitral valve is repaired, when necessary, through the ventricular opening with a double-armed stitch at the posterior annulus, from trigone to trigone, and the mitral orifice is undersized with a 26-mm valve sizer.[77]

In July 2001, we introduced the Mannequin (Chase Medical, Richardson, TX), which we fill with 50 to 60 mL of saline per square meter of the patient's body surface area to optimize the size and shape of the new ventricle. This TRISVR technique is a refinement of the Dor technique that introduced a sizer device in 1998, which allows standardization of the procedure. The device is inserted into the LV cavity after an incision is created (Fig. 100-11) and then carefully inflated with saline when it is seated properly in the cavity, to avoid the risk of inflating the device when it is in the mitral valve. The new apex will be placed at the apex of the Mannequin, and this is the starting point for the 2/0 endoventricular circular suture. The suture is carried

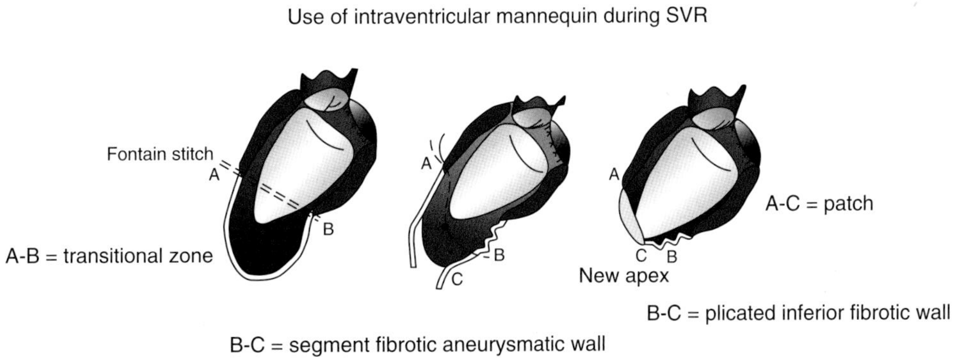

FIGURE 100-11 ■ The use of the intraventricular mannequin during surgical left ventricle reconstruction. *SVR,* Surgical ventricular restoration.

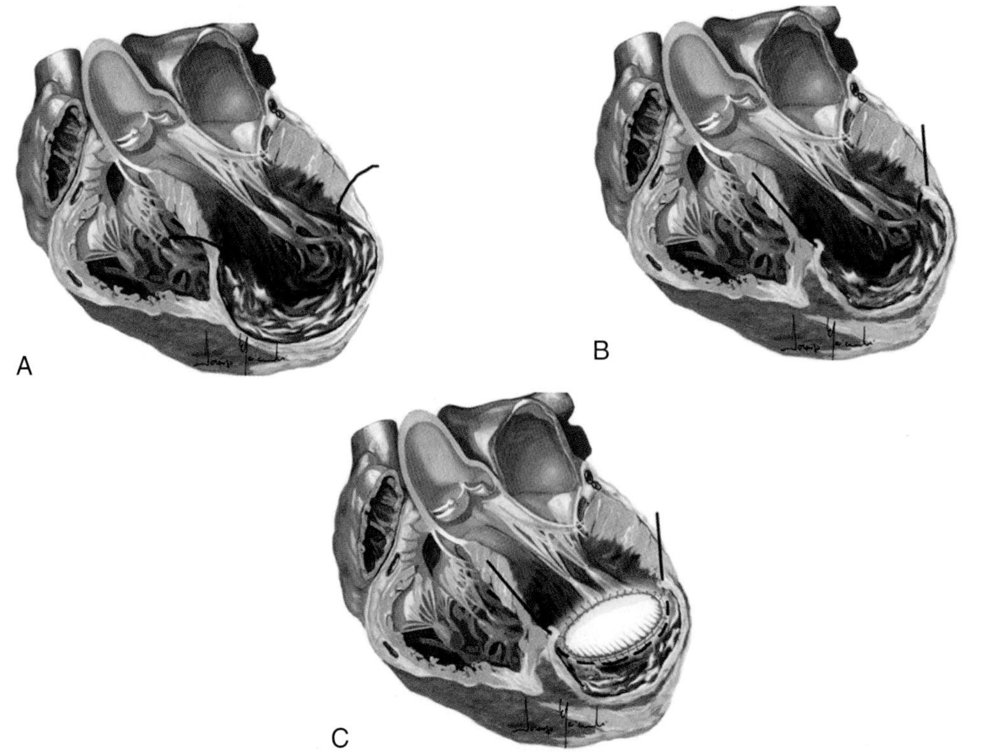

FIGURE 100-12 ■ Sequence of a suboptimal endoventricular suture. **A,** Suturing is done on a plane parallel to the mitral valve. **B,** The suture is tightened. **C,** The patch is inserted, and its resultant position is parallel to the mitral valve.

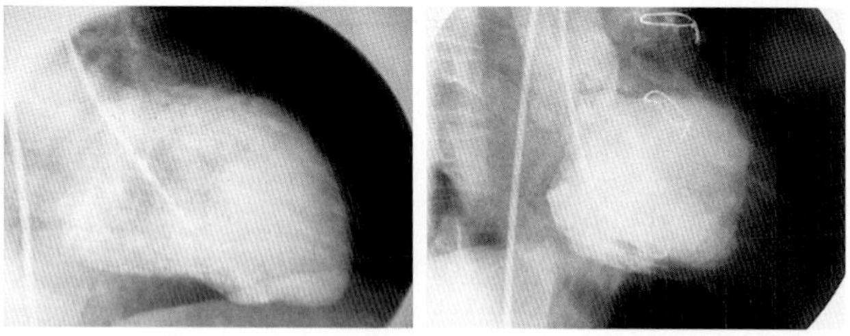

FIGURE 100-13 ■ Angiography preoperatively (Pre-op) and postoperatively after surgical left ventricular reconstruction (Post-SVR). *Left,* Before surgery. *Right,* After surgery. Note the spherical left ventricular chamber achieved after surgery.

deep toward the septum and up toward the aortic outflow tract on an oblique plane to reconstruct an elliptical shape, not a spherical chamber. The suture is then brought toward the lateral wall, and back to the apex, and tightened on the Mannequin. The plane of the closure should not be parallel to the mitral valve (Fig. 100-12). If the closure plane is parallel to the mitral valve, the result is a spherical chamber (Fig. 100-13). The shape of the device is appositely conical with a physiologic short-to-long-axis ratio to reconstruct a more physiologic, elliptical shape. After positioning the new apex, the surgeon places the circular stitches at the transitional zone (between the scarred and the sound tissue). When the ventricle is not very enlarged, the Mannequin reduces the risk of creating a residual cavity that is too small. It is also useful when the infarcted region is not clearly demarcated, as occurs in dilated cardiomyopathy (type III silhouette [see Fig. 100-5], as described by our group).[50] In this circumstance, the transitional zone between

BOX 100-3 Surgical Pitfalls

- Incorrect indications
- Incomplete revascularization
- Embolism
- Cavity dimension: too large or too small
- Cavity shape: spherical or distorted

scarred and nonscarred myocardium is not well defined, and the Mannequin allows rebuilding of the ventricle in an elliptical way with a proper residual size. Box 100-3 shows surgical pitfalls during SVR.

The use of the Mannequin is a refinement of the technique introduced by Dor in 1998 using a toy balloon. The size of the device is chosen by multiplying the body surface area of the patient by 50 or 60 mL. This choice is empirical: we prefer to leave a residual chamber with a normal volume (52 ± 13 mL/m^2 in a series of 52 normal subjects from our echocardiography laboratory).[23]

The technique used by Menicanti is shown in Figure 100-14. In some circumstances, the inferoapical region is dilated after an anterior MI because of left dominance of the anterior descending artery. When the device is in place during reconstruction, a gap between the transitional zone and the position of the new apex is evident; in such cases, we thread a direct suture from inside to reduce the inferior dilation and to lift up the new apex, bringing the lateral wall toward the septum (Fig. 100-15). Usually, this suture runs for 1 to 1.5 cm. In chronic anterior MI, the LV apex, in addition to being enlarged, is also shifted inferiorly and posteriorly (Fig. 100-16), and this alters the direction of flow toward the aorta. Thus,

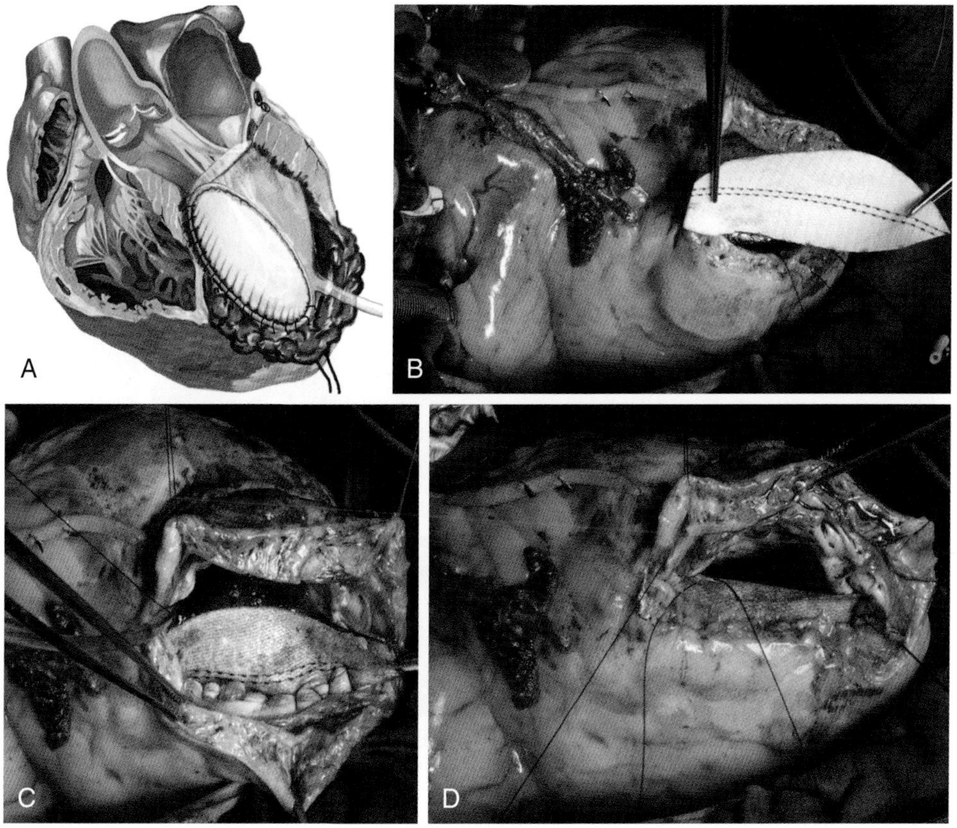

FIGURE 100-14 ■ **A,** Schematic representation of surgical left ventricular reconstruction as performed by Menicanti. The device is inserted in the correct position, and the patch is sutured when the device is in place and parallel to the septum (i.e., oblique to the aorta). In photographs from the operating room **(B-D),** mammary anastomosis to the left anterior descending artery is completed, as is the venous sequential graft. **B,** The Dacron patch is prepared with an elliptical shape and appropriate size. **C,** The patch is trimmed during the suturing. **D,** Suturing of the completed patch.

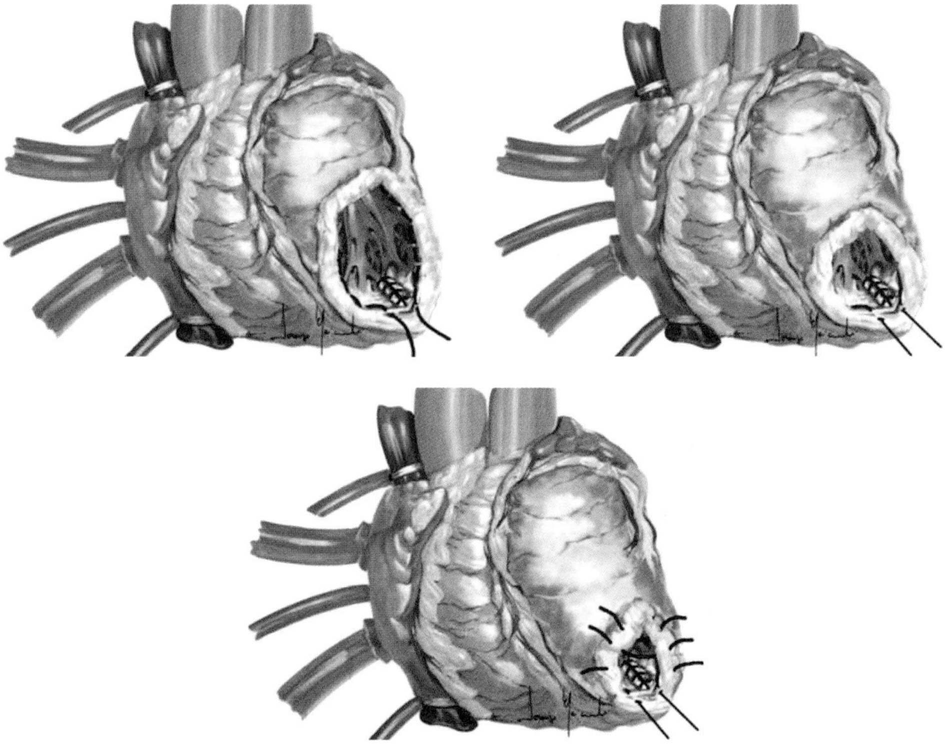

FIGURE 100-15 ■ To reduce the inferior wall dilation, a direct suture is brought from inside. In this way, the lateral wall is approximated to the septum, and the new apex is lifted up to a more anterior position.

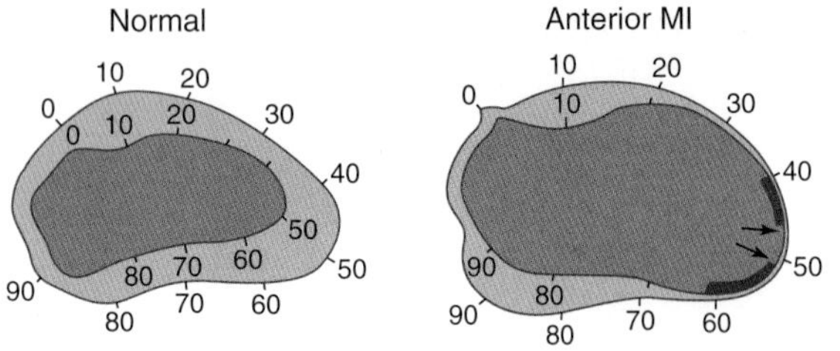

FIGURE 100-16 ■ The shape of the left ventricle, obtained by Fourier analysis of curvature as seen by 30-degree right anterior oblique angiography. Reconstructed silhouettes are averages for normal subjects and for patients with anterior myocardial infarction (MI). The apex in the patient silhouette is enlarged (less conical) and shifted downward and toward the mitral plane in both systole (inner line) and diastole (outer line). Numbers refer to the 90 chords as identified by the centerline.[49] (From Baroni M, Barletta G: Digital curvature estimation for left ventricular shape analysis. *Image Vis Comp* 10:485–494, 1992.)

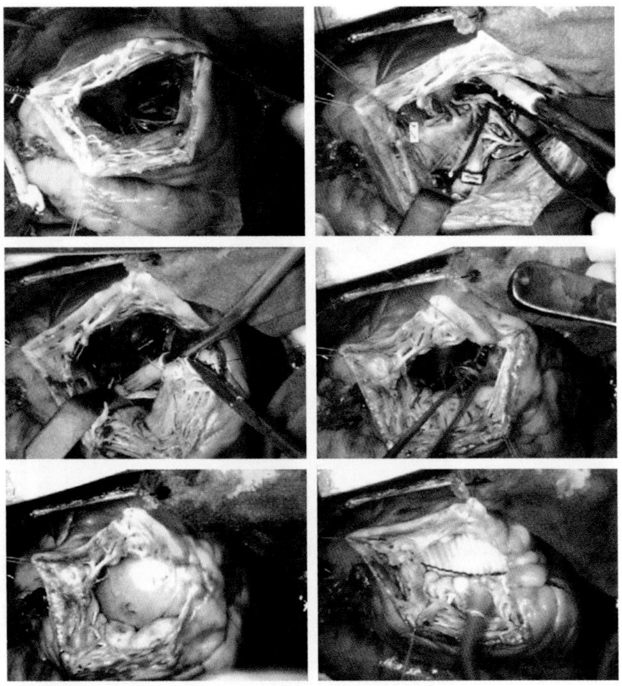

FIGURE 100-17 ■ Intraoperative mitral valve repair via the ventricular approach. Note the orientation of the patch at the end of the procedure: it is placed very deep into the septum and oblique to the aorta.

it is very important for the surgeon to give the apex a conical form in an anterior position, because this reestablishes the correct blood vortex at the apex and a more physiologic direction of flow.

The Mannequin is then removed and the opening of the ventricle is closed with a direct suture if it is less than 3 cm, or it is closed with an elliptical synthetic patch if it is greater than 3 cm. The suture attaching the patch is continuous and conducted in an everting manner, starting from the deeper septal part of the opening, going toward the apex, and then up again toward the lateral wall.

Mitral Valve Repair during Surgical Ventricular Restoration

We have adopted a new surgical technique to repair the mitral valve during SVR with CABG. Because our technique reduces the dimensions of the mitral annulus, we avoid an atrial approach to the annulus and access it through the same ventricular incision that is used to perform SVR (Figs. 100-17 and 100-18). After the LV cavity is opened, each papillary muscle head is identified, and the mitral valve leaflets and chords are evaluated. The posteromedial fibrous trigone is visualized, and a pledgeted 2/0 polyester suture is placed from the ventricular side to the atrial side. The two arms of this suture progress with a running stitch toward the anteromedial trigone, carrying it to a few millimeters from the mitral annulus with biting sutures into atrial and ventricular muscle. The suture arms pass through the anterolateral trigone, and a second pledget is inserted. The entire posterior annulus becomes completely bounded by this suture. To undersize the mitral annulus and avoid valve constriction, a 26-mm sizer is introduced into the mitral orifice, and the suture is tied against the second pledget.

We analyzed the shapes of the left ventricle in a series of patients with MR undergoing SVR and compared them with a series of patients without MR. Quantitative shape analysis showed a flattening of the inferior curvature in patients with MR (Fig. 100-19), as well as reduced regional fractional shortening by centerline analysis. Patients with MR also had a less concave systolic inferior segment. Furthermore, overall shape differed significantly, with more spherical chambers in patients with MR than in those without (Table 100-2). Between July 2001 and April 2008 at the San Donato Hospital, 116 of 458 patients undergoing SVR with CABG had an associated mitral repair. Operative cardiac mortality was 12.9% (15/116), significantly higher than the 4.7% mortality without mitral repair (16/342). Figure 100-20 shows geometric features of the mitral valve before and after surgery. We focused on anterior infarctions to avoid the changes in the submitral apparatus that occur with inferior infarction, and because LV shape changes that occur in anterior infarctions are the primary determinants of functional MR in patients with severe heart failure. Increased sphericity plays a central role in the development of functional MR, because it progressively widens the LV transverse diameter; our findings (see Table 100-2) confirm this causation.

The decision for valve repair is based on preoperative measurements of ventricular volume, annular size, and the degree of MR. Formerly, we repaired moderate or severe MR (grade 3 or 4+) and mild MR (grade 2+) if the annulus was dilated (>38 mm). In a recent series of patients with mild MR treated with SVR but without mitral repair,[78] the outcome was excellent in terms of improvement in function and survival. Thus, successful surgical treatment of functional MR depends on reestablishing normal leaflet coaptation by changing the architecture of the mitral annulus or of the ventricular wall, or both. Consequently, surgical interventions include coronary revascularization, reducing mitral annulus, and restoring LV shape to reduce tethering and ventricular volume. The mitral annulus can be reduced with a prosthetic ring via the atrial approach or by annular suture of the posterior ring via a ventricular approach.[77] Downsizing the ring is essential to optimize the extent of coaptation, as emphasized by Bolling and colleagues.[79]

Surgical Details of Posterior Surgical Ventricular Restoration

Limited data are available on surgical repair for LV dilation resulting from inferior MI.[80] Changes in LV geometry vary with the site of coronary occlusion—for example, the classic posterior aneurysm with a bulging of inferior wall and good contraction in the remaining cavity, or global dilation of the LV chamber with regional wall dysfunction at the inferior and posterobasal region. Although both conditions can lead to secondary MR, it happens more frequently in the global dilation because of the enlargement of the transverse diameter and the globular shape. Surgery for the posterior aneurysm generally involves a patch to close the neck of dilation, but the treatment of global dilation of the inferoposterior wall is more complex, especially because of the relationship between the scar and the dilation with respect to the papillary muscles.

A very short incision is made in the scar, or where a depression is evident during venting. Through this incision, the position of papillary muscles is carefully checked. After an inferior MI, there are two possibilities: (1) the dilation is mainly between the two papillary muscles or (2) the dilation is between the posteromedial papillary muscle and the septum, which is deeply involved (Fig. 100-21). We use two techniques for LV dilation after an inferior MI. The first, shown on the left in Figure 100-22, begins with opening the scarred wall at the level of the scar or at the level of the collapsed area, parallel to the posterior descending artery. A continuous 2/0 Prolene suture reapproximates the two papillary muscles

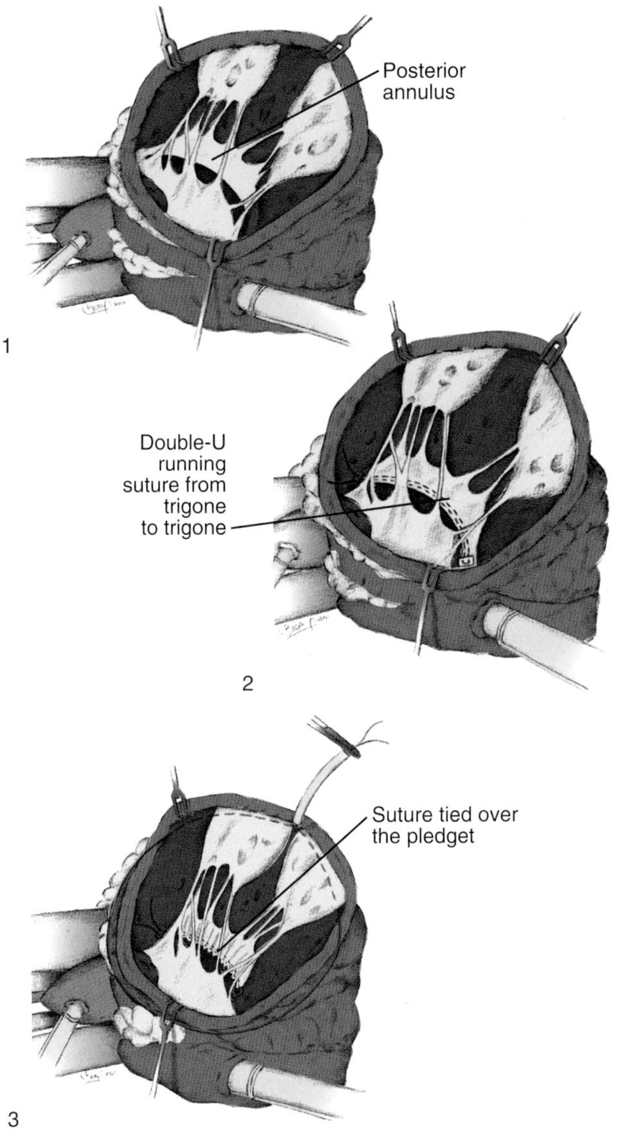

FIGURE 100-18 ■ Schematic representation of mitral repair through a ventricular opening.

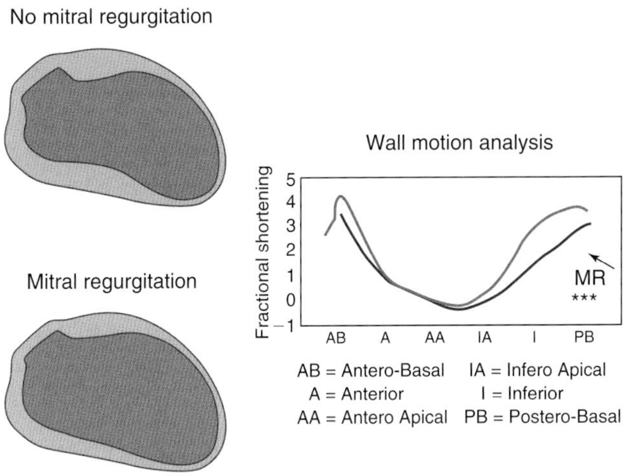

FIGURE 100-19 ■ Reconstructed left ventricle shapes by Fourier analysis. The inferior curvature is flattened in patients with mitral regurgitation (MR), and regional wall motion (as evaluated by the centerline method) is reduced in these patients at the inferior and posterobasal regions. ***P = 0.001. (From Sheehan FH, Stewart DK, Dodge HT, et al: Variability in the measurement of regional left ventricular wall from contrast angiograms. *Circulation* 68:550–559, 1983.)

TABLE 100-2 **Relationship between Left Ventricular Sphericity and Degree of Mitral Regurgitation**

	No MR	MR Grade 1 to 2+	MR Grade 3 to 4+	ANOVA
Sphericity index: diastole	0.49 ± 0.08	0.55 ± 0.09	0.60 ± 0.10	0.0001
Sphericity index: systole	0.40 ± 0.09	0.47 ± 0.11	0.54 ± 0.11	0.0001

ANOVA, Analysis of variance; *MR*, mitral regurgitation.

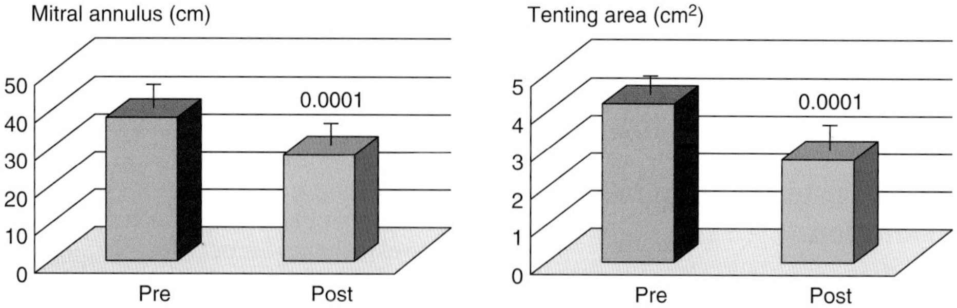

FIGURE 100-20 Improvements in mitral geometry seen after surgical left ventricular reconstruction plus mitral repair. Improvements in size of annulus and tenting area after surgery; $P = 0.0001$.

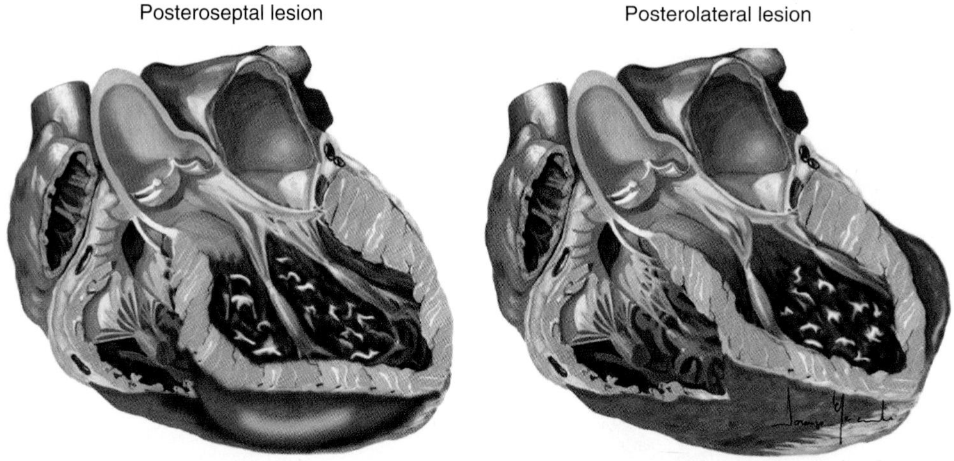

FIGURE 100-21 Two types of lesions occur after inferior myocardial infarction, as recognized by the position of the papillary muscles after the incision at the posterior scar. *Right,* The dilation is between the two papillary muscles. *Left,* The dilation is between the posteromedial papillary muscle and the septum.

and excludes the entire dilated zone. The suture is started at the beginning of the dilation (sometimes just at the mitral annulus) and continues toward the apex. In the second procedure (see Fig. 100-22, on the right), the wall is opened, and then the continuous suture is brought past the posteromedial papillary muscle, bringing the posterior wall against the septum. In this way, when MR is determined only by the displacement of the posteromedial papillary muscle, mitral insufficiency is repaired. Our results from about 125 patients who received posterior SVR show a significant decrease in end-diastolic and ESV and an improvement in EF and clinical status. Operative mortality rate is higher than in anterior SVR (7.2%) and survival rate is significantly lower.[77]

OUTCOMES

Many groups have found the results of SVR to be favorable and consistent.[15,59,81-104] In Table 100-3, a summary of the best-evidence studies, we have recorded the number of patients enrolled, the number of associated mitral procedures, the operative (30-day) mortality, and improvements in ESV and EF. Follow-up is also reported, when available.

The largest reported series (from the RESTORE group, a team of cardiologists and surgeons from 12 centers on four continents[102]) and, more recently, a single-center experience from Menicanti and associates[98] reported on SVR for 1198 and 1161 patients with anterior MI, respectively, and demonstrated that SVR improves symptoms and long-term survival in patients with ischemic cardiomyopathy and severe heart failure. The beneficial effects of SVR in improving cardiac function and in reducing LV volume, ventricular arrhythmias, and MR has been largely accepted.[59,72,85-89,92,95,97] A reduction in mechanical intraventricular dyssynchrony has also been demonstrated.[105-107]

The RESTORE group (Reconstructive Endoventricular Surgery returning Torsion, Original Radius and Elliptical shape to the left ventricle), organized by Gerald Buckberg in 1998, is the first international team to find evidence that for patients with CHF, rebuilding the heart by addressing a geometric solution (to bring back to normal the shape and size of the damaged ventricle) is an effective method to treat ischemic dilated cardiomyopathy.[108]

Data reported in the literature are in close agreement: SVR results in a significant acute improvement of systolic function, significant acute reduction of mechanical dyssynchrony, and significant reduction in wall stress. Although data are more limited for changes in diastolic function, these changes are comparable with the changes in patients with preserved LV function who undergo elective CABG.[109,110] The acute beneficial effects on systolic function are largely maintained in the long term, and

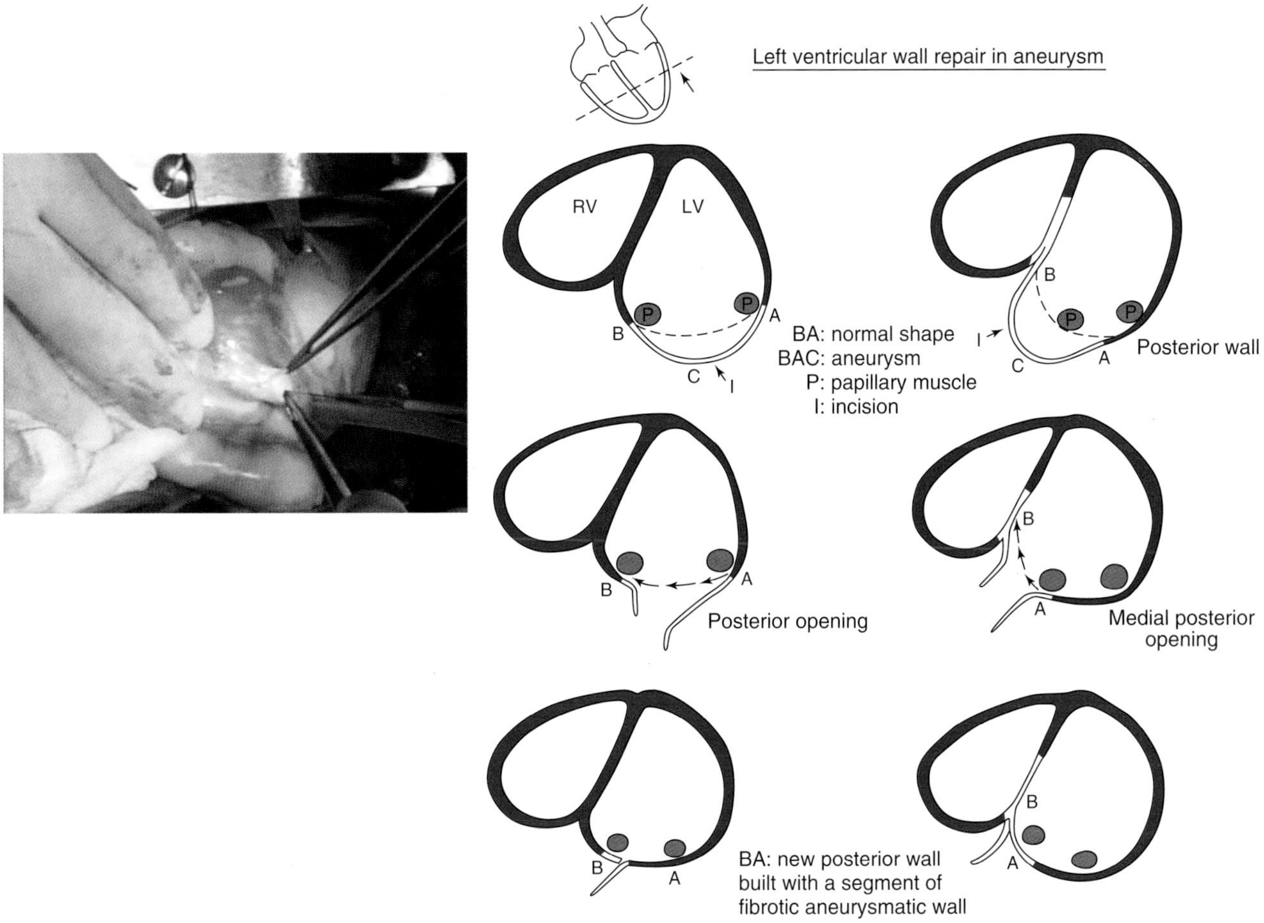

FIGURE 100-22 ■ Two techniques of posterior repair of the left ventricle of a patient with an aneurysm. The image shows the posterior wall of the ventricle. The diagrams show the two techniques, from top to bottom on the left, and from top to bottom on the right. *Left,* After the opening of the scarred wall, the base of the papillary muscles is identified, and the dilation is observed to be mainly between the two papillary muscles. A 2/0 Prolene suture is started at the beginning of the dilation (sometimes at the mitral annulus) and continues toward the apex, excluding all the damaged tissue from the cavity. *Right,* After the wall is opened, a continuous suture is threaded past the posteromedial papillary muscle, bringing the posterior wall against the septum. In this way, when mitral regurgitation results from the displacement of the posteromedial papillary muscle, mitral insufficiency is repaired. *LV,* Left ventricle; *RV,* right ventricle.

SVR induces a significant reverse-remodeling associated with clinical improvement and improved survival. Interestingly, the entity of EF improvement and of LV volume reduction is uniform in all the reported series, varying from +6 to +15 (absolute points) for EF, and from 30% to 45% reduction for LV ESV (see Table 100-3). Also, survival rates appear uniform among different studies, being an average of nearly 80% at 5 years and 60% at 10 years. Survival rates in patients with advanced NYHA functional class are particularly gratifying, being 88% at 3 years in NYHA class 3 and 68% in NYHA class 4, as reported by Williams and associates,[84] and 50% at 5 and 10 years, as reported by Menicanti and colleagues (Fig. 100-23).[98] Moreover, the rate of rehospitalization for heart failure is reported to be low.[98,102] These results are similar to those reported at 6 months after heart transplantation, and a study from Cotrufo and coworkers showed no differences in mortality, clinical improvement, and survival rate between a comparable group of patients with dilated ischemic cardiomyopathy who underwent either SVR or heart transplantation.[111]

Surgical Ventricular Restoration and Diastolic Function

Data on diastolic function after SVR are limited. Experimental studies and theoretical considerations suggest that SVR induces diastolic dysfunction.[112] The effect of SVR on diastolic function was recently the focus of two studies by Tulner and colleagues.[104,106] The effects of SVR on ventricular function and the related effects of diastolic dysfunction on outcome after SVR have not been well studied until recently. However, a study by Tulner and colleagues[106] (and see the accompanying editorial by Burkhoff and Wechsler[112]) was the first in which the diastolic pressure–volume relationship was measured in patients before and after SVR. They showed that diastolic compliance appears to be reduced early after SVR, leading to a reduction in stroke volume. These effects may result from postoperative edema, because pulmonary pressures late after SVR are significantly reduced.

The factor most likely to affect diastolic function is the size of the residual LV cavity. Excessive volume

TABLE 100-3 **Best-Evidence Studies of Surgical Left Ventricular Reconstruction**

Author	Patients (N)	Mitral Valve Procedures (N)	Early Mortality (%)	ESV (mL/m²) (Change)	EF Change (Absolute Points)	Follow-Up (% Survival)
Sartipy[95]	101	29	7.9	N/A	27 ± 9 to 33 ± 7 (+6)	120 mo (1 yr, 88%; 5 yr, 65%; 10 yr, 57%)
Maxey[85]	95 (56 with SVR vs. 39 CABG alone)	14	0	N/A	22 ± 11 to 32 ± 9 (+10)	24 mo (95%)
Mickleborough[86]	285	6 (3 replacements)	2.8	N/A	Not reported	120 mo (1 yr, 95%; 5 yr, 82%; 10 yr, 62%)
Athanasuleas[102] Multicenter Registry	1198	22% repairs 1% replacements	5.3	80 ± 51 to 57 ± 34 (−46%)	29 ± 11 to 39 ± 12 (+10)	5 yr (69%)
Dor[101]	870	61/388 (16%) not reported in the overall series	7.3	N/A	Not reported (+10 to +15)	N/A
Di Donato[87]	207	N/A	8.1	112 ± 64 to 46 ± 26	35 ± 13 to 48 ± 12	60 mo (1 yr, 98%; 5 yr, 82%)
Cirillo[99]	69	12/69 (17.3%) (1 replacement)	4.3	100 ± 35 to 68 ± 15 (−32%)	32 ± 4 to 44 ± 7 (+12)	24 mo (92%)
Menicanti[98]	1161	90/488 (18%) not reported in the overall series (2 replacements)	4.7	145 ± 64 to 88 ± 40 (mL) (−39%)	33 ± 9 to 40 ± 10 (+7)	120 mo (62% at 10 yr)
Ribeiro[100]	137 (significant MR excluded) 34 patients, CABG alone	None	2.6	107 ± 19 to 63 ± 17 (−41%)	34 ± 6 to 44 ± 5 (+10)	24 mo (95%)
Yamaguchi[81]	48 patients (CABG vs. CABG + SVR)	11/48 (23%)	?	112 ± 21 to 94 ± 28 in CABG alone 137 ± 24 to 65 ± 19 in CABG + SVR	21 ± 6 to 28 ± 7 in CABG alone 24 ± 7 to 42 ± 9 in CABG + SVR (+18)	5 yr: (53% ± 11% in CABG alone; 90 ± 10 in CABG + SVR)
O'Neill[83]	220	108/220 (49%)	1.0	120 ± 46 to 77 ± 26 (−36%)	21 ± 7 to 25 ± 9 (+4)	60 mo (1yr, 92%; 3 yr, 90%; 5 yr, 80%)
Conte[91]	78	17 repairs (22%) 6 replacements (7.7%)	7.7	116 ± 59 to 66 ± 23 (−43%)	23 ± 9 to 29 ± 10 (+6) Patients in NYHA IV	36 mo (88% NYHA III; 68% NYHA IV)
Hernandez[103] Multicenter Registry (STS)	731	Not reported	9.4	N/A	N/A	N/A

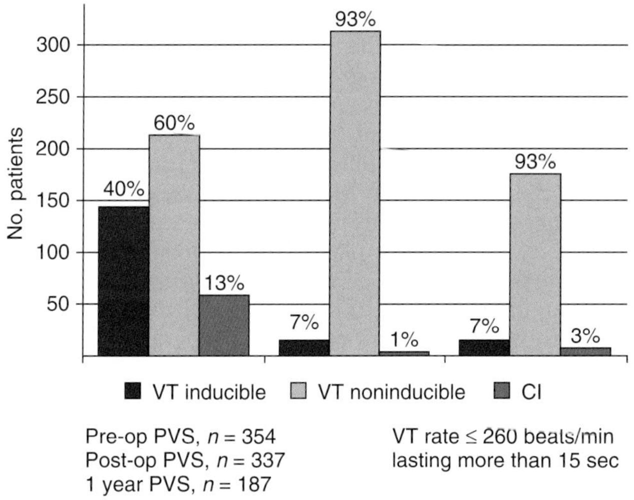

FIGURE 100-29 Inducible ventricular tachycardia (VT) at electrophysiologic study before and after surgical ventricular restoration in a large population treated at the Cardiothoracic Centre of Monaco. The electrophysiologic protocol was not aggressive (up to two extra stimuli at two different cycle lengths) and was the same at the three tests. VT is no longer inducible in a significantly high proportion of patients, both at discharge and after 1 year (only 7% are still inducible postoperatively). *CI*, Confidence interval; *PVS*, programmed ventricular stimulation.

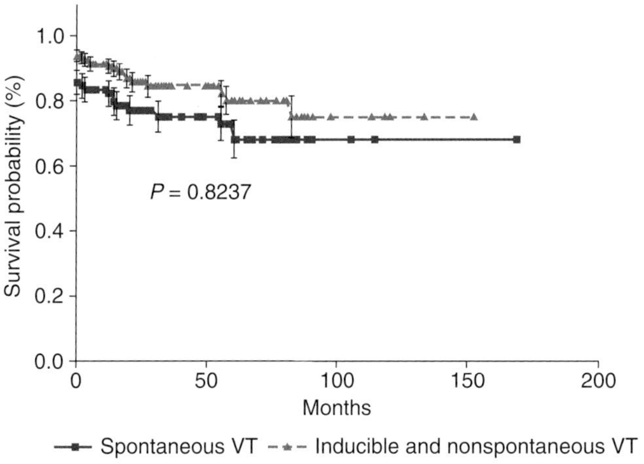

FIGURE 100-30 Kaplan-Meier survival curves in patients with spontaneous ventricular tachycardia (VT) and without ventricular arrhythmias who underwent surgical ventricular restoration. No significant difference was observed.

Coronary Artery Bypass Surgery with or without Surgical Ventricular Restoration: Insights into the STICH Trial

The STICH trial was designed to verify two hypotheses on a large population of patients affected by ischemic CHF and LV systolic dysfunction who were randomly assigned to receive medical therapy alone or combined with CABG (Hypothesis 1) and CABG alone or CABG plus SVR (Hypothesis 2).[133]

The results of Hypothesis 2 showed that SVR combined with CABG had no impact over CABG alone on mortality, heart failure hospitalizations, exercise tolerance, or quality of life.[134]

Several major limitations of the STICH trial have already been noted,[135] including: (1) patient inclusion bias (i.e., many patients whose primary surgeons considered SVR to be clinically indicated were not randomized, characterized, or studied); and (2) the average reduction of ESV in the SVR group was much smaller than planned (raising serious questions about whether the procedure was performed properly in a majority of cases). Based on that, our group analyzed the impact on survival of a residual left ventricular end-systolic volume index (LVESVI) of greater than or less than 60 mL/m^2. We showed that LVESVI after SVR affects the probability of death, being significantly higher in patients who remain with a postoperative LVESVI of greater than 60 mL/m^2.[136] We hypothesized that the lack of additional improvement in terms of survival in the SVR group observed in the STICH trial might be a result of the inadequate volume reduction, which left the patients in the two arms at identical risk. Witkowski and colleagues confirmed this observation showing that a residual postsurgical LVESVI of at least 60 mL/m^2 was independently associated with a fivefold increase of death and rehospitalization for heart failure at 2 years' follow-up after SVR.[137] Furthermore, a more recent analysis of the STICH trial data showed that SVR combined with CABG conferred a survival benefit compared with bypass alone with the achievement of a postoperative end-systolic volume index of 70 mL/m or less.[138] In the meantime, the Task Force on Myocardial Revascularization of the European Society of Cardiology (ESC) and the European Association for Cardio-Thoracic Surgery (EACTS) recognized the merit of SVR, which has been included as a surgical option combined with CABG in selected heart failure patients with a scar in the LAD territory and a baseline LVESVI greater than or equal to 60 mL/m^2 (Class of Recommendation IIb; level of evidence B).[139]

The results of Hypothesis 1 (1212 patients with an ejection fraction of 35% or less and coronary artery disease amenable to CABG randomly assigned to medical therapy alone or medical therapy plus CABG) were not far different.[140] No difference was observed in the primary end point of death for any cause; however, cardiovascular deaths were reduced compared with medical therapy alone.

It has been observed that the trial, in spite of the acronym, was a study of ischemic heart disease rather than heart failure per se. However, although it is true that only 37% of patients had severe heart failure symptoms (NYHA functional class III and IV), it should be outlined that only 4.7% had severe symptoms (Canadian Cardiovascular Society [CCS] angina class III-IV) and as much as 37% had *no* angina plus another 15% in CCS I. Therefore, the randomized population was extremely heterogeneous. Furthermore, data on LV volumes were not reported, except for the substudy on myocardial viability (601 patients) showing an LVESVI of 92 ± 39 mL/m^2. According to these baseline characteristics, the results of Hypothesis 1 were not surprising: in the literature, no benefit of any type of revascularization in patients with no angina and enlarged dysfunctional left ventricles has been reported.

Along with the results of the Hypothesis 1 group, data obtained in a substudy of patients randomized to medical therapy with or without CABG after the assessment of myocardial viability were reported.[141] There was no significant interaction between viability status (assessed using single-photon-emission computed tomography, dobutamine echocardiography, or both) and treatment assignment with respect to mortality ($P = 0.53$). These results differ markedly from results of previous retrospective studies and meta-analyses, suggesting that assessment of myocardial viability alone should not be the deciding factor in selecting the best therapy for these patients. Future prospective studies need to be designed to determine the role of cardiac imaging in clinical decision making.

Mitral Repair

Ischemic MR conveys an adverse prognosis, doubling the mortality seen in patients after an MI, in those with chronic heart failure, and after surgical or catheter revascularization.[142-147] It is common, and it increases mortality even when it is mild,[143-145] with a graded relationship between severity and reduced survival. Currently, it is not clear whether the poorer outcomes in this group depend on the valvular dysfunction or whether it is merely a surrogate marker of extensive comorbidities, particularly the amount of ventricular dysfunction.

The term *functional MR* broadly denotes abnormal function of normal leaflets in the context of impaired ventricular function; it typically occurs in globally dilated and hypokinetic ventricles or with segmental damage that affects valve closure. It occurs in roughly 20% to 25% of patients followed after MI[143,145,148,149] and in 50% of those with CHF.[150] The mechanism of MR in end-stage heart failure is multifactorial. Briefly, it is related to changes in LV geometry, with a subsequent displacement of the subvalvular apparatus, annular dilation, and restrictive leaflet motion (class IIIb according to Carpentier's classification),[151] which results in coaptation failure.

Recent advances in noninvasive Doppler echocardiography allow reliable assessment of regurgitant volume[152,153] and of the orifice of MR by combined methods.[154,155]

Since the turn of the century, laboratory and clinical studies[156] have helped to elucidate the mechanisms that underlie ischemic MR, using several different imaging modalities. These studies have demonstrated that the two key anatomic elements contributing to the development of MR are annular remodeling and disruption of the dynamic anatomic relationship between the subvalvular apparatus and the mitral annulus, which is manifested as systolic tethering of the leaflets into the LV cavity. The extent to which each of these two elements contributes to valvular incompetence varies substantially among individual patients.[157]

Although several indices of annular remodeling, including mitral annular area, intercommissural width, and septolateral annular diameter, are readily quantified by standard two-dimensional echocardiographic techniques, methods for quantifying leaflet tethering have not been standardized. Descriptive geometric indicators derived from single-plane measurements made from two-dimensional echocardiographic studies, such as tenting height and area, have been proposed.[158] Tenting is characterized by insufficient systolic leaflet body displacement toward the annulus, with coaptation limited to leaflet tips, resulting in MR. Unfortunately, these measurements are inherently inaccurate because of the high variability of scanning planes and regional variation in both mitral annular shape and leaflet tenting that develop in conjunction with postinfarction LV remodeling. Recently, three-dimensional echocardiography has been applied to the evaluation of mitral valve morphology and may play a valuable role in the assessment of patients undergoing mitral repair surgery.[159,160]

The clinical significance of functional MR is frequently underrated because of low murmur intensity and mismatch between severe symptoms and unimpressive regurgitant volume and effective regurgitant orifice. Nevertheless, functional MR is a major component of LV dysfunction, causing pulmonary hypertension and LV volume overload, which in turn potentiates LV remodeling, a major determinant of the outcome of LV dysfunction. Mild and moderate functional mitral insufficiency are also associated with significantly decreased survival in patients undergoing CABG, but whether correction of moderate functional MR at the time of CABG improves outcome has yet to be determined.

Previously, surgical treatment of MR was avoided in patients with heart failure and severe pump dysfunction because of concerns about operative risk and perioperative complications. More recently, with improvement in surgical techniques, surgical mitral annuloplasty for MR in the setting of heart failure has become a more popular treatment option. Bolling and associates have demonstrated the feasibility of mitral valve repair in patients with heart failure by downsizing the annulus using a flexible ring.[79,161] Their initial results in 48 patients who underwent restrictive mitral annuloplasty showed an early mortality rate of approximately 5% with 1- and 2-year survival rates of 82% and 71%, respectively. Several recent studies have confirmed that early mortality is low (between 5% and 7%); heart failure symptoms, LV size, and EF improve; and intermediate outcome is favorable.[162,163] However, several studies in patients treated with mitral annuloplasty demonstrated a high recurrence rate (30%) of MR after the 6-month follow-up.[164,165] In contrast to these results, Bax and coworkers[166] reported no recurrence of MR, and Szalay and associates[163] reported a recurrence rate of 3% with a mean MR grade of 0.6 at 1-year follow-up. The low recurrence rate in these latter studies may be associated with a more truly restrictive annuloplasty performed in these patients. Of note, the paper by Bax and colleagues showed reverse remodeling at follow-up, especially in patients with an LV end-diastolic diameter of less than 65 mm. However, no randomized clinical trial has yet demonstrated that surgical correction of MR by mitral annuloplasty improves survival or leads to reverse remodeling. Wu and associates demonstrated that there is no clearly demonstrable survival benefit conferred by mitral annuloplasty for significant MR in patients with chronic heart failure.[167]

Currently, the use of a stringent restrictive ring, two sizes smaller than the measured size, is advocated to achieve a better leaflet coaptation and possibly to prevent recurrence of MR and promote reverse remodeling.[161]

There are concerns that correction of MR might decrease LV systolic function as a result of afterload increase caused by closure of a low-resistance runoff into the left atrium. In addition, it has been suggested that undersizing the mitral annulus might affect LV contractility because of increased mechanical tension on the base of the heart.[168] Moreover, according to some authors, restrictive mitral repair might impair diastolic filling, but Bolling and Dion demonstrated that undersizing the annulus leads to acute beneficial geometric changes of the base of the LV, which reduces volume and stress.[79,166]

Mitral surgery is proposed in selected patients to improve cardiac function. However, often in patients with a dilated heart and severe MR, the simple correction of the mitral valve might not be sufficient to improve LV function and reverse LV remodeling. Functional MR is a ventricle disease, and a procedure on the left ventricle should be added whenever possible, especially in ischemic dilated cardiomyopathy. However, if MR is mild, SVR can be used to reduce it by improving LV function and geometry, without surgical valve correction.[78]

Different techniques were reported for reducing the mitral annulus. Kay and colleagues[169] reported mitral plasty with reduction of the posterior annulus without a ring, and Carpentier[170] used a rigid ring. A flexible ring could be also used. Menicanti and associates[77] reported that the transventricular approach for MR with LV reconstruction could be performed without a prosthetic ring, and that the results were favorable. Bolling and coworkers[79] used undersized circumferential rings to reduce the annulus in patients with severe MR associated with dilated cardiomyopathy. Isomura and coworkers used noncircumferential flexible rings initially and then changed the technique to use the circumferential semirigid rings (Carpentier-Edwards physio-ring) of a smaller size (undersized ring, 26 or 28 mm).[171]

SVR with or without an intraventricular patch is the second key component of mitral repair. Because reducing ventricular volume decreases wall stress and enhances remote regional wall motion,[32] we hypothesize that SVR-related improvement of inferior wall motion is a component of MR reduction. This enhancement, together with reduced papillary muscle width, helps reduce stress and improve remote motion.

However, although our understanding of ischemic MR evolves and the technologies used to manage these patients continue to be refined, the higher rates of recurrent MR after repair have led some to consider valve replacement instead of repair. Evidence for repair or replacement was limited until the released results from the first multicenter, randomized trial, which showed no significant difference in LV reverse remodeling or survival at 12 months between patients who underwent mitral valve repair and those who underwent mitral valve replacement.[172] Replacement provided a more durable correction of MR, but there was no significant between-group difference in clinical outcomes. A longer follow-up is needed to confirm the findings of this trial.

SUMMARY

In the current clinical practice, the choice to add SVR to CABG should be based on a careful evaluation of patients, including symptoms (heart failure symptoms should be predominant over angina); measurements of the LV volumes; careful assessment of mitral valve, including geometry and MR severity; and assessment of the transmural extent of myocardial scar tissue and viability of regions remote from the scar, and it should be performed only in centers with a high level of surgical expertise. Further clarifications of (1) ventricular properties associated with better hemodynamic effects of SVR and (2) links between hemodynamic effects and clinical outcomes could help define appropriate patient selection criteria.

REFERENCES

1. Georghiade M, Bonow RO: Chronic heart failure in the United States: a manifestation of coronary artery disease. *Circulation* 97:282–289, 1998.
2. Sharpe N, Doughty R: Epidemiology of heart failure and ventricular dysfunction. *Lancet* 352(Suppl):3–7, 1998.
3. Levy D, Kenchaiah S, Larson MG, et al: Long-term trends in the incidence of and survival with heart failure. *N Engl J Med* 347:1397–1402, 2002.
4. O'Connor CM, Gattis WA, Uretsky BF, et al: Continuous intravenous dobutamine is associated with an increased risk of death in patients with advanced heart failure: insights from the Flolan International Randomized Survival Trial (FIRST). *Am Heart J* 138:78–86, 1999.
5. Massad MG, Prasad SM, Chedrawy EG, et al: A perspective on the surgical management of congestive heart failure. *World J Surg* 32:375–380, 2008.
6. Pitt B, Zannad F, Remme WJ, et al: The effect of spironolactone on morbidity and mortality in patients with severe heart failure. Randomized Aldactone Evaluation Study Investigators. *N Engl J Med* 341:689–700, 1999.
7. Swedberg K, Kjekshus J, Snapinn S: Long-term survival in severe heart failure in patients treated with enalapril. Ten year follow-up of consensus I. *Eur Heart J* 20:136–139, 1999.
8. Packer M, Coats AJ, Fowler MB, et al: Effect of Carvedilol on survival in severe in severe chronic heart failure. *N Engl J Med* 344:1651–1658, 2001.
9. Engelfriet PM, Hoogenveen RT, Boshuizen HC, et al: To die with or from heart failure: a difference that counts: is heart failure underrepresented in national mortality statistics? *Eur J Heart Fail* 13:377–383, 2011.
10. Sheehy E, Conrad SL, Brigham LE, et al: Estimating the number of potential donors in the United States. *N Engl J Med* 349(7):667–674, 2003.
11. Taylor DO, Edwards LB, Boucek MM, et al: Registry of the International Society for Heart and Lung Transplantation: twenty-third official adult heart transplantation report-2006. *J Heart Lung Transplant* 25:869–879, 2006.
12. Dor V, Kreitmann P, Jourdan J, et al: Interest of physiological closure (circumferential plasty on contractile areas) of left ventricle after resection and endocardiectomy for aneurysm or akinetic zone. Comparison with classical technique about a series of 209 left ventricular resections. *J Cardiovasc Surg* 26:73, 1985.
13. Athanasuleas CL, Buckberg GD: Surgical restoration of the postinfarction dilated ventricle. *Heart Fail Clin* 4(3):361–370, 2008.
14. Buckberg GD, Coghlan HC, Torrent-Guasp F: The structure and function of the helical heart and its buttress wrapping. V. Anatomic and physiologic considerations in the healthy and failing heart. *Semin Thorac Cardiovasc Surg* 13(4):358–385, 2001.
15. Buckberg G: Left ventricular reconstruction for dilated ischaemic cardiomyopathy: biology, registry, randomisation and credibility. *Eur J Cardiothorac Surg* 30:753–761, 2006.

16. Cohn PF, Ferrari R, Sharpe N: Cardiac remodeling—concepts and clinical implications: a consensus paper from an international forum on cardiac remodeling. *J Am Coll Cardiol* 35:569–582, 2000.
17. Libby P, Lee R: T: Matrix matters. *Circulation* 102:1874–1876, 2000.
18. Packer M: The neurohormonal hypothesis: a theory to explain the mechanism of disease progression in heart failure. *J Am Coll Cardiol* 20:248–254, 1992.
19. Leine B, Kalman J, Mayer L, et al: Elevated circulating levels of tumor necrosis factor in severe chronic heart failure. *N Engl J Med* 323:236–241, 1990.
20. Mann DL, Bristow MR: Mechanisms and models in heart failure. The bio-mechanical model and beyond. *Circulation* 111:2837–2849, 2005.
21. Mann DL, Deswal A, Bozkurt B, et al: Therapeutics for chronic heart failure. *Annu Rev Med* 53:59–74, 2002.
22. McKay RG, Pfeffer MA, Pasternak RC, et al: Left ventricular remodelling after myocardial infarction: a corollary to infarct expansion. *Circulation* 74:693–702, 1986.
23. Di Donato M, Dabic P, Castelvecchio S, RESTORE Group, et al: left ventricular geometry in normal and post-anterior myocardial infarction patients: sphericity index and "new" conicity index comparisons. *Eur J Cardiothorac Surg* 29(Suppl 1):S225–S230, 2006.
24. Fantini F, Barletta G, Di Donato M, et al: Left ventricular shape abnormalities in inferior wall myocardial infarction. *Am J Cardiol* 70:1081–1084, 1999.
25. Di Donato M, Castellvechio S, Frigiola A: Menicanti L. Left ventricular remodeling following anterior and inferior infarction: differences in LV geometry. *Eur J Heart Fail* 7(Suppl):33, 2008.
26. Suma H: Left ventriculoplasty for non ischemic dilated cardiomyopathy. *Semin Thorac Cardiovasc Surg* 13:514–521, 2001.
27. Batista RJ, Verde J, Neri P, et al: Partial left ventriculectomy to treat end-stage heart disease. *Ann Thorac Surg* 64:634–638, 1997.
28. Streeter DD, Jr, Spotnitz HM, Patel DP, et al: Fiber orientation in the canine left ventricle during diastole and systole. *Circ Res* 24:339–347, 1969.
29. Greenbaum RA, Ho SY, Gibson DG, et al: Left ventricular fibre architecture in man. *Br Heart J* 45:248–263, 1981.
30. Anversa P, Olivetti G, Capasso JM: Cellular basis of ventricular remodeling after myocardial infarction. *Am J Cardiol* 68:7D–16D, 1991.
31. Delepine S, Furber AP, Beygui F, et al: 3-D MRI assessment of regional left ventricular systolic wall stress in patients with reperfused MI. *Am J Physiol Heart Circ Physiol* 284:H1190–H1197, 2003.
32. Di Donato M, Sabatier M, Toso A, et al: Regional myocardial performance of non-ischemic zones remote from anterior wall left ventricular aneurysm. Effects of aneurysmectomy. *Eur Heart J* 16:1285–1292, 1995.
33. Migrino RQ, Young JB, Ellis SG, et al: End-systolic volume index at 90 to 180 minutes into reperfusion therapy for acute myocardial infarction is a strong predictor of early and late mortality. *Circulation* 96:116, 1997.
34. Sutton MSJ, Pfeffer MA, Moye L, et al: Cardiovascular death and left ventricular remodeling two years after myocardial infarction. *Circulation* 96:3294, 1997.
35. Yamaguchi A, Ino T, Adachi H, et al: Left ventricular volume predicts postoperative course in patients with ischemic cardiomyopathy. *Ann Thorac Surg* 65:434, 1998.
36. Galeati DG: De bononiensi scientiarum et artium instituto atque academia commentarii. *De Morbis Duobus* 4:26, 1757.
37. Cruveilhier J: Essai sur l'anatomie pathologique en général et sur les transformations et productions organiques en particulier. *Chez l'Anteur (Paris)* 1:60, 1816.
38. Tennant R, Wiggers CJ: Effect of coronary occlusion on myocardial contraction. *Am J Physiol* 112:351, 1935.
39. Murray C: Pathophysiology of the cause of death from coronary thrombosis. *Ann Surg* 126:523, 1947.
40. Klein MD, Herman MV, Gorlin R, et al: A hemodynamic study of left ventricular aneurysm. *Circulation* 35:614–630, 1967.
41. Schlichter J, Hellerstein HK, Katz LN: Aneurysm of the heart: a correlative study of one hundred and two proved cases. *Medicine* 33:43, 1954.
42. Van der Laarse A, Kekhof PL, Vermeer F, et al: Relation between infarct size and left ventricular performance assessed in patients with first acute myocardial infarction randomized to intracoronary thrombolytic therapy or to conventional treatment. *Am J Cardiol* 61:1–7, 1988.
43. Ritchie J, Cerqueira M, Maynard C, et al: Ventricular function and infarct size: the Western Washington intravenous streptokinase in myocardial infarction trial. *J Am Coll Cardiol* 11:689–697, 1988.
44. Sheiban I, Fragasso G, Rosano GMC, et al: Time course and determinants of Left ventricular function recovery after primary angioplasty in patients with acute myocardial infarction. *J Am Coll Cardiol* 38:464–471, 2001.
45. Bolognese L, Neskovic AN, Parodi G, et al: Left ventricular remodeling after primary coronary angioplasty. Patterns of left ventricular dilation and long-term prognostic implications. *Circulation* 106:2351–2357, 2002.
46. Bolognese L, Carrabba N, Parodi G, et al: Impact of microvascular dysfunction on left ventricular remodeling and long-term clinical outcome after primary coronary angioplasty for acute myocardial infarction. *Circulation* 109:1121–1126, 2004.
47. Baroni M, Barletta G: Digital curvature estimation for left ventricular shape analysis. *Image Vis Comp* 10:485–494, 1992.
48. Fantini F, Barletta G, Baroni M, et al: Quantitative evaluation of left ventricular shape in anterior aneurysm. *Cathet Cardiovasc Diagn* 28:295–300, 1993.
49. Sheehan FH, Stewart DK, Dodge HT, et al: Variability in the measurement of regional left ventricular wall from contrast angiograms. *Circulation* 68:550–559, 1983.
50. Strobeck J, Di Donato M, Costanzo MR, et al: Importance of shape and surgically reshaping the left ventricle in ischemic cardiomyopathy. *Congest Heart Fail* 10:45–53, 2004.
51. Likoff W, Bailey CP: Ventriculoplasty: excision of myocardial aneurysm. *JAMA* 167:557, 1958.
52. Cooley DA, Collins HA, Morris GC, et al: Ventricular aneurysm after myocardial infarction. Surgical excision with the use of temporary cardiopulmonary bypass. *JAMA* 167:557, 1958.
53. Favaloro RG, Effler DB, Groves LK, et al: Ventricular aneurysm-clinical experience. *Ann Thorac Surg* 6:227, 1968.
54. Grondin P, Kretz GK, Bical O, et al: Natural history of saccular aneurysms of the left ventricle. *J Thorac Cardiovasc Surg* 77:57, 1979.
55. Cohen M, Packer M, Gorlin R: Indications for left ventricular aneurysmectomy. *Circulation* 67:717, 1983.
56. Jatene AD: Left ventricular aneurysmectomy. *J Thorac Cardiovasc Surg* 89:321, 1985.
57. Couper GS, Bunton RW, Birjiniuk V, et al: Relative risks of left ventricular aneurysmectomy in patients with akinetic scars versus true dyskinetic aneurysms. *Circulation* 82(Suppl 5):IV248–IV256, 1990.
58. Mangschau A: Akinetic versus dyskinetic left ventricular aneurysms diagnosed by gated scintigraphy: difference in surgical outcome. *Ann Thorac Surg* 47:746, 1989.
59. Dor V, Sabatier M, Di Donato M, et al: Late hemodynamic results after left ventricular patch repair associated with coronary grafting in patients with postinfarction akinetic or dyskinetic aneurysm of the left ventricle. *J Thorac Cardiovasc Surg* 110(1291):301, 1995.
60. Suma H, Isomura T, Horii T, et al: Left ventriculoplasty for non-ischemic cardiomyopathy with severe heart failure in 70 years old patients. *J Cardiol* 37(1):1–110, 2001.
61. Suma H, Horii T, Isomura T, the RESTORE Group, et al: A new concept of ventricular restoration for non-ischemic dilated cardiomyopathy. *Eur J Cardiothorac Surg* 295:S207–S212, 2006.
62. Buckberg GD, Coghlan HC, Torrent-Guasp F: The structure and function of the helical heart and its buttress wrapping. VI. Geometric concepts of heart failure and use for structural correction. *Semin Thorac Cardiovasc Surg* 13(4):386–401, 2001.
63. Torrent Guasp F, Ballester M, Buckberg GD, et al: Spatial orientation of the ventricular muscle band: physiologic contribution and surgical implications. *J Thorac Cardiovasc Surg* 122(2):389–392, 2001.
64. Di Donato M, Sabatier M, Dor V, et al: Akinetic versus dyskinetic postinfarction scar: relation to surgical outcome in patients undergoing endoventricular circular patch plasty repair. *J Am Coll Cardiol* 29:1569–1575, 1997.

65. Schiller N, Shah P, Crawford M, et al: Recommendations for quantitation of the left ventricle by two-dimensional echocardiography. American Society of Echocardiography Committee on Standards, Subcommittee on Quantitation of Two-dimensional Echocardiograms. *J Am Soc Echocardiogr* 2:358–367, 1989.
66. Lloyd GS, Buckberg GD, the RESTORE Group: Use of cardiac magnetic resonance imaging in surgical ventricular restoration. *Eur J Cardiothorac Surg* 295:S216–S224, 2006.
67. Kim RJ, Wu E, Eafael A, et al: The use of contrast-enhanced magnetic resonance imaging to identify reversible myocardial dysfunction. *N Engl J Med* 343:1445–1453, 2000.
68. Götte MJ, Germans T, Rüssel IK, et al: Myocardial strain and torsion quantified by cardiovascular magnetic resonance tissue tagging. Studies in normal and impaired left ventricular function. *J Am Coll Cardiol* 48(10):2002–2011, 2006.
69. Reisner SA, Lysyansky P, Agmon Y, et al: Global longitudinal strain: a novel index of left ventricular systolic function. *J Am Soc Echocardiogr* 17:630–633, 2004.
70. Artis NJ, Oxborough DL, Williams G, et al: Two-dimensional strain imaging: a new echocardiographic advance with research and clinical applications. *Int J Cardiol* 123:240–248, 2008.
71. Josephson ME, Harken AH, Horowitz LN: Endocardial excision: a new surgical technique for the treatment of recurrent ventricular tachycardia. *Circulation* 60:1430–1439, 1979.
72. Dor V, Sabatier M, Montiglio F, et al: Endoventricular patch reconstruction in ischemic failing ventricle. A single center with 20 years experience. Advantages of magnetic resonance imaging assessment. *Heart Fail Rev* 9:269–286, 2004.
73. Athanasuleas CL, Buckberg GD, Stanley AW, RESTORE Group, et al: Surgical ventricular restoration: the Restore Group experience. *Heart Fail Rev* 9:287–297, 2004.
74. Mickleborough LL, Carson S, Ivanov J: Repair of dyskinetic or akinetic left ventricular aneurysm: results obtained with a modified linear closure. *J Thorac Cardiovasc Surg* 121:675, 2001.
75. Menicanti L, Di Donato M: The Dor procedure: what has changed after fifteen years of clinical practice? *J Thorac Cardiovasc Surg* 124(5):886–890, 2002.
76. O'Neill JO, Starling RC, McCarthy PM, et al: The impact of left ventricular reconstruction on survival in patients with ischemic cardiomyopathy. *Eur J Cardiothorac Surg* 30(5):753–759, 2006.
77. Menicanti L, Di Donato M, Frigiola A, the RESTORE Group, et al: Ischemic mitral regurgitation: intraventricular papillary muscle imbrication without mitral ring during left ventricular restoration. *J Thorac Cardiovasc Surg* 123:1041–1050, 2002.
78. Di Donato M, Castelvecchio S, Brankovic J, et al: Effectiveness of surgical ventricular restoration in patients with dilated ischemic cardiomyopathy and unrepaired mild mitral regurgitation. *J Thorac Cardiovasc Surg* 134(6):1548–1553, 2007.
79. Bolling SF, Deeb GM, Brunsting LA, et al: Early outcome of mitral valve reconstruction in patients with end-stage cardiomyopathy. *J Thorac Cardiovasc Surg* 109:676–683, 1995.
80. Menicanti L, Dor V, Buckberg GD, the RESTORE Group, et al: Inferior wall restoration: anatomic and surgical considerations. *Semin Thorac Cardiovasc Surg* 13:504–513, 2001.
81. Yamaguchi A, Adachi H, Kawahito K, et al: Left ventricular reconstruction benefits patients with dilated ischaemic cardiomyopathy. *Ann Thorac Surg* 79(2):456–461, 2005.
82. Athanasuleas CL, Buckberg GD, Menicanti L, et al: Optimising ventricular shape in anterior restoration. *Semin Thorac Cardiovasc Surg* 13(4):459–467, 2001.
83. O'Neill JO, Starling RC, McCarthy PM, et al: The impact of left ventricular reconstruction on survival in patients with ischemic cardiomyopathy. *Eur J Cardiothorac Surg* 30:753–761, 2006.
84. Williams JA, Weiss ES, Patel ND, et al: Outcomes following surgical ventricular restoration for patients with clinically advanced congestive heart failure (New York Heart Association class IV). *J Card Fail* 13:431–436, 2007.
85. Maxey T, Reece T, Ellman P, et al: Coronary artery bypass with ventricular restoration is superior to coronary artery bypass alone in patients with ischemic cardiomyopathy. *J Thorac Cardiovasc Surg* 127:428–434, 2004.
86. Mickleborough L, Merchant N, Ivanov J, et al: Left ventricular reconstruction: early and late results. *J Thorac Cardiovasc Surg* 128:27–37, 2004.
87. Di Donato M, Toso A, Maioli M, RESTORE Group, et al: Intermediate survival and predictors of death after surgical ventricular restoration. *Semin Thorac Cardiovasc Surg* 13:468–475, 2001.
88. Di Donato M, Sabatier M, Montiglio F, et al: Outcome of left ventricular aneurysmectomy with patch repair in patients with severely depressed pump function. *Am J Cardiol* 76:557–561, 1995.
89. Dor V, Sabatier M, Di Donato M, et al: Efficacy of endoventricular patch plasty in large postinfarction akinetic scar and severe left ventricular dysfunction: comparison with a series of large dyskinetic scar. *J Thorac Cardiovasc Surg* 116:50–59, 1998.
90. Patel N, Barriero C, Williams J, et al: Surgical ventricular remodeling for patients with clinically advanced congestive heart failure and severe left ventricular dysfunction. *J Heart Lung Transplant* 24:2202–2210, 2005.
91. Conte JV: Surgical ventricular restoration: techniques and outcomes. *Congest Heart Fail* 10:248–251, 2004.
92. Di Donato M, Frigiola A, Benhamouda M, et al: Safety and efficacy of surgical ventricular restoration in unstable patients with recent anterior myocardial infarction. *Circulation* 110(II):169–173, 2004.
93. Sartipy U, Albage A, Larsson PT, et al: Changes in B-type natriuretic peptides after surgical ventricular restoration. *Eur J Cardiothorac Surg* 31:922–928, 2007.
94. Sartipy U, Albage A, Straat E, et al: Surgery for ventricular tachycardia in patients undergoing left ventricular reconstruction by the Dor procedure. *Ann Thorac Surg* 81:65–71, 2006.
95. Sartipy U, Albage A, Lindblom D: The Dor procedure for left ventricular reconstruction. Ten-year clinical experience. *Eur J Cardiothorac Surg* 27:1005–1010, 2005.
96. Sartipy U, Albåge A, Lindblom D: Improved health-related quality of life and functional status after surgical ventricular restoration. *Ann Thorac Surg* 83:1381–1388, 2007.
97. Tulner SA, Steendijk P, Klautz RJ, et al: Clinical efficacy of surgical heart failure therapy by ventricular restoration and restrictive mitral annuloplasty. *J Card Fail* 13(3):178–183, 2007.
98. Menicanti L, Castelvecchio S, Ranucci M, et al: Surgical therapy for ischemic heart failure: single-center experience with surgical anterior ventricular restoration. *J Thorac Cardiovasc Surg* 134(2): 433–441, 2007.
99. Cirillo M, Amaducci A, Brunelli F, et al: Determinants of postinfarction remodeling affect outcome and left ventricular geometry after surgical treatment of ischemic cardiomyopathy. *J Thorac Cardiovasc Surg* 127:1648–1656, 2004.
100. Ribeiro GA, da Costa CE, Lopes MM, et al: Left ventricular reconstruction benefits patients with ischemic cardiomyopathy and non-viable myocardium. *Eur J Cardiothorac Surg* 29:196–201, 2006.
101. Dor V: Left ventricular reconstruction for ischemic cardiomyopathy. *J Card Surg* 17:180–187, 2002.
102. Athanasuleas CL, Buckberg GD, Stanley AW, RESTORE Group, et al: Surgical ventricular restoration in the treatment of congestive heart failure due to post-infarction ventricular dilation. *J Am Coll Cardiol* 44(7):1439–1445, 2004.
103. Hernandez AF, Velazquez EJ, Dullum MK, et al: Contemporary performance of surgical ventricular restoration procedures: data from the Society of Thoracic Surgeons. *National Cardiac Database. Am Heart J* 152:494–499, 2006.
104. Tulner SA, Bax JJ, Bleeker GB, et al: Beneficial hemodynamic and clinical effects of surgical ventricular restoration in patients with ischemic dilated cardiomyopathy. *Ann Thorac Surg* 82:1721–1727, 2006.
105. Di Donato M, Toso Anna, Dor Vincent, the RESTORE Group, et al: Surgical ventricular restoration improves mechanical intraventricular dyssynchrony in ischemic cardiomyopathy. *Circulation* 109:2536–2543, 2004.
106. Tulner SA, Steendijk P, Klautz RJ, et al: Surgical ventricular restoration in patients with ischemic dilated cardiomyopathy: evaluation of systolic and diastolic ventricular function, wall stress, dyssynchrony, and mechanical efficiency by pressure-volume loops. *J Thorac Cardiovasc Surg* 132:610–620, 2006.
107. Schreuder JJ, Castiglioni A, Maisano F, et al: Acute decrease of left ventricular mechanical dyssynchrony and improvement of contractile state and energy efficiency after left ventricular restoration. *J Thorac Cardiovasc Surg* 129:138–145, 2005.

108. Buckberg GD: Overview: Ventricular restoration—a surgical approach to reverse ventricular remodelling. *Heart Fail Rev* 9:233–239, 2004.
109. Stendijk P, Tulner SA, Schreuder JJ, et al: Quantification of left ventricular mechanical dyssynchrony by conductance catheter in heart failure patients. *Am J Physiol Heart Circ Physiol* 286:H723–H730, 2004.
110. Tulner SAF, Klautz RJM, Engbers FHM, et al: Left ventricular function and chronotropic responses after normothermic cardiopulmonary by pass with intermittent antegrade warm blood cardioplegia in patients undergoing coronary artery by pass grafting. *Eur J Cardiothorac Surg* 27:599–605, 2005.
111. Cotrufo M, De Santo LS, Della Corte A, et al: Acute hemodynamic and functional effects of surgical ventricular restoration and heart transplantation in patients with ischemic dilated cardiomyopathy. *J Thorac Cardiovasc Surg* 135:1054–1060, 2008.
112. Burkhoff D, Wechsler AS: Surgical ventricular remodeling: a balancing act on systolic and diastolic properties. *J Thorac Cardiovasc Surg* 132:459–463, 2006.
113. Ratcliffe MB, Guy TS: The effect of preoperative diastolic dysfunction on outcome after surgical ventricular remodeling. *J Thorac Cardiovasc Surg* 134:280–283, 2007.
114. Castelvecchio S, Menicanti L, Ranucci M, et al: Impact of surgical ventricular restoration on diastolic function: implications of shape and residual ventricular size. *Ann Thorac Surg* 86(6):1849–1854, 2008.
115. Abraham WT, Fisher WG, Smith AL, et al: Cardiac resynchronization in chronic heart failure. *N Engl J Med* 346:1845–1853, 2002.
116. Auricchio A, Stellrink C, Block M, et al: Effect of pacing chamber and atrioventricular delay on acute systolic function of paced patients with congestive heart failure. The Pacing Therapy for Congestive Heart Failure Study Group. The Guidant Congestive Heart Failure Research Group. *Circulation* 99:2993–3001, 1999.
117. Anderson LJ, Miyazaki C, Sutherland GR, et al: Patient selection and echocardiographic assessment of dyssynchrony in cardiac resynchronization therapy. *Circulation* 117:2009–2023, 2008.
118. Leclercq C, Kass DA: Retiming the failing heart: principles and current clinical status of cardiac resynchronization. *J Am Coll Cardiol* 39:194–201, 2002.
119. Barold SS: What is cardiac resynchronization therapy? *Am J Med* 111:224–232, 2001.
120. Cheng A, Gupta SN, Bluemke DA, et al: Infarct tissue heterogeneity by magnetic resonance imaging identifies enhanced cardiac arrhythmia susceptibility in patients with left ventricular dysfunction. *Circulation* 115:2006–2014, 2007.
121. Zipes DP, Wellens HJ: Sudden cardiac death. *Circulation* 98:2334–2351, 1998.
122. Kim RJ, Fieno DS, Parrish TB, et al: Relationship of MRI delayed contrast enhancement to irreversible injury, infarct age, and contractile function. *Circulation* 100:1992–2002, 1999.
123. Peters NS, Wit AL: Myocardial architecture and ventricular arrhythmogenesis. *Circulation* 97:1746–1754, 1998.
124. De Bakker JM, Van Capelle FJ, Janse MJ, et al: Reentry as a cause of ventricular tachycardia in patients with chronic ischemic heart disease: electrophysiologic and anatomic correlation. *Circulation* 77:589–606, 1988.
125. Babuty D, Lab MJ: Mechanoelectric contributions to sudden cardiac death. *Cardiovasc Res* 50:270–279, 2001.
126. Di Donato M, Sabatier M, Dor V, the RESTORE Group, et al: Ventricular arrhythmias after left ventricular remodeling: surgical ventricular restoration or ICD? *Heart Fail Rev* 9:299–306, 2004.
127. Hannan EL, Kilburn H, Jr, O'Donnell JF, et al: Adult open heart surgery in New York State. An analysis of risk factors and hospital mortality rates. *JAMA* 264:2768–2774, 1990.
128. The VA Cooperative Study Group: Eighteen-year follow-up in the Veterans Affairs Cooperative Study of Coronary Artery Bypass Surgery for stable angina. *Circulation* 86:121–130, 1992.
129. Passamani E, Davis KB, Gillespie MJ, et al: A randomized trial of coronary artery bypass surgery Survival of patients with a low ejection fraction. *N Engl J Med* 312:1665–1671, 1985.
130. Sharma GV, Deupree RH, Khuri SF, et al: Coronary bypass surgery improves survival in high-risk unstable angina. Results of a Veterans Administration unstable angina cooperative study with an 8-year follow-up. Veterans Administration Unstable Angina Cooperative Study Group. *Circulation* 84:III260–III267, 1991.
131. Veenhuyzen GD, Singh SN, McAreavey D, et al: Prior coronary artery bypass surgery and risk of death among patients with ischemic left ventricular dysfunction. *Circulation* 104:1489–1493, 2001.
132. Bigger JT, for the Coronary Artery Bypass Graft (CABG) Patch Trial Investigators: Prophylactic use of implanted cardiac defibrillators in patients at high risk for ventricular arrhythmias after coronary artery bypass graft surgery. *N Engl J Med* 337:1568, 1997.
133. Velazquez EJ, Lee KL, O'Connor CM, STICH Investigators, et al: The rationale and design of the Surgical Treatment for Ischemic Heart Failure (STICH) trial. *J Thorac Cardiovasc Surg* 134:1540–1547, 2007.
134. Jones RH, Velazquez EJ, Michler RE, et al: Coronary bypass surgery with or without surgical ventricular reconstruction. *N Engl J Med* 360:1705–1717, 2009.
135. Eisen HJ: Surgical ventricular reconstruction for heart failure. *N Engl J Med* 360:1701–1704, 2009.
136. Di Donato M, Castelvecchio S, Menicanti L: End-systolic volume following surgical ventricular reconstruction impacts survival in patients with ischaemic dilated cardiomyopathy. *Eur J Heart Fail* 12:375–381, 2010.
137. Witkowski TG, ten Brinke EA, Delgado V, et al: Surgical ventricular restoration for patients with ischemic heart failure: determinants of two-year survival. *Ann Thorac Surg* 91:491–498, 2011.
138. Michler RE, Rouleau JL, Al-Khalidi HR, STICH Trial Investigators, et al: Insights from the STICH trial: change in left ventricular size after coronary artery bypass grafting with and without surgical ventricular reconstruction. *J Thorac Cardiovasc Surg* 146:1139–1145, 2013.
139. Wijns W, Kolh P, Danchin N, et al: Guidelines on myocardial revascularization: the Task Force on Myocardial Revascularization of the European Society of Cardiology (ESC) and the European Association for Cardio-Thoracic Surgery (EACTS). *Eur Heart J* 31:2501–2555, 2010.
140. Velazquez EJ, Lee KL, Deja MA, STICH Investigators, et al: Coronary-artery bypass surgery in patients with left ventricular dysfunction. *N Engl J Med* 364:1607–1616, 2011.
141. Bonow RO, Maurer G, Lee KL, STICH Trial Investigators, et al: Myocardial viability and survival in ischemic left ventricular dysfunction. *N Engl J Med* 364:1617–1625, 2011.
142. Lehmann KG, Francis CK, Dodge HT, et al: TIMI Study Group: mitral regurgitation in early myocardial infarction: incidence, clinical detection, and prognostic implications. *Ann Intern Med* 117:10–17, 1992.
143. Lamas GA, Mitchell GF, Flaker GC, et al: Survival and Ventricular Enlargement Investigators. Clinical significance of mitral regurgitation after acute myocardial infarction. *Circulation* 96:827–833, 1997.
144. Feinberg MS, Schwammenthal E, Shlizerman L, et al: Prognostic significance of mild mitral regurgitation by color Doppler echocardiography in acute myocardial infarction. *Am J Cardiol* 86:903–907, 2000.
145. Grigioni F, Enriquez-Sarano M, Zehr KJ, et al: Ischemic mitral regurgitation: long-term outcome and prognostic implications with quantitative Doppler assessment. *Circulation* 103:1759–1764, 2001.
146. Ellis SG, Whitlow PL, Raymond RE, et al: Impact of mitral regurgitation on long-term survival after percutaneous coronary intervention. *Am J Cardiol* 89:315–318, 2002.
147. Koelling TM, Aaronson KD, Cody RJ, et al: Prognostic significance of mitral regurgitation and tricuspid regurgitation in patients with left ventricular systolic dysfunction. *Am Heart J* 144:524–529, 2002.
148. Birnbaum Y, Chamoun AJ, Conti VR, et al: Mitral regurgitation following acute myocardial infarction. *Coron Artery Dis* 13:337–344, 2002.
149. Kumanohoso T, Otsuji Y, Yoshifuku S, et al: Mechanism of higher incidence of ischemic mitral regurgitation in patients with inferior myocardial infarction: quantitative analysis of left ventricular and mitral valve geometry in 103 patients with prior myocardial infarction. *J Thorac Cardiovasc Surg* 125:135–143, 2003.

150. Trichon BH, Felker GM, Shaw LK, et al: Relation of frequency and severity of mitral regurgitation to survival among patients with left ventricular systolic dysfunction and heart failure. *Am J Cardiol* 91:538–543, 2003.
151. Carpentier A: Cardiac valve surgery: the "French correction." *J Thorac Cardiovasc Surg* 86:323–337, 1983.
152. Blumlein S, Bouchard A, Schiller NB, et al: Quantitation of mitral regurgitation by Doppler echocardiography. *Circulation* 74:306–314, 1986.
153. Enriquez-Sarano M, Bailey KR, Seward JB, et al: Quantitative Doppler assessment of valvular regurgitation. *Circulation* 87:841–848, 1993.
154. Enriquez-Sarano M, Seward JB, Bailey KR, et al: Effective regurgitant orifice area: a non-invasive Doppler development of an old hemodynamic concept. *J Am Coll Cardiol* 23:443–451, 1994.
155. Enriquez-Sarano M, Miller FAJ, Hayes SN, et al: Effective mitral regurgitant orifice area: clinical use and pitfalls of the proximal isovelocity surface area method. *J Am Coll Cardiol* 25:703–709, 1995.
156. Yiu SF, Enriquez-Sarano M, Tribouilloy C, et al: Determinants of the degree of functional mitral regurgitation in patients with systolic left ventricular dysfunction: a quantitative clinical study. *Circulation* 102:1400–1406, 2000.
157. Calafiore AM, Gallina S, Di Mauro M, et al: Mitral valve procedure in dilated cardiomyopathy: repair or replacement? *Ann Thorac Surg* 71:1146–1153, 2001.
158. Di Mauro M, Di Giammarco G, Vitella G, et al: Impact of no-to-moderate mitral regurgitation on late results after isolated coronary artery bypass grafting in patients with ischemic cardiomyopathy. *Ann Thorac Surg* 81(6):2128–2134, 2006.
159. Watanabe N, Ogasawara Y, Yamaura Y, et al: Mitral annulus flattens in ischemic mitral regurgitation: geometric differences between inferior and anterior myocardial infarction. A real-time 3-dimensional echocardiographic study. *Circulation* 112(Suppl 9):I458–I462, 2005.
160. Watanabe N, Ogasawara Y, Yamaura Y, et al: Geometric differences of the mitral valve tenting between anterior and inferior myocardial infarction with significant ischemic mitral regurgitation: quantitation by novel software system with transthoracic real-time three-dimensional echocardiography. *J Am Soc Echocardiogr* 19:71–75, 2006.
161. Bolling SF, Pagani FD, Deeb GM, et al: Intermediate-term outcome of mitral reconstruction in cardiomyopathy. *J Thorac Cardiovasc Surg* 115:381–386, 1998.
162. Gummert JF, Rahmel A, Bucerius J, et al: Mitral valve repair in patients with end stage cardiomyopathy: who benefit? *Eur J Cardiothorac Surg* 23:1017–1022, 2003.
163. Szalay ZA, Civelek A, Hohe S, et al: Mitral annuloplasty in patients with ischemic versus dilated cardiomyopathy. *Eur J Cardiothorac Surg* 23:567–572, 2003.
164. McGee EC, Gillinov AM, Blackstone EH, et al: Recurrent mitral regurgitation after annuloplasty for functional ischemic mitral regurgitation. *J Thorac Cardiovasc Surg* 128:24–916, 2004.
165. Tahta SA, Oury JH, Maxwell JM, et al: Outcome after mitral valve repair for functional ischemic mitral regurgitation. *J Heart Valve Dis* 11:11–18, 2002.
166. Bax JJ, Braun J, Somer ST, et al: Restrictive annuloplasty and coronary revascularization in ischemic mitral regurgitation: results in reverse left ventricular remodeling. *Circulation* 110:II103–II108, 2004.
167. Wu AH, Aaronson KD, Bolling SF, et al: Impact of mitral valve annuloplasty on mortality risk I patients with mitral regurgitation and left ventricular systolic dysfunction. *J Am Coll Cardiol* 45:381–387, 2005.
168. Dreyfus G, Milaiheanu S: Mitral valve repair in cardiomyopathy. *J Heart Lung Transplant* 19:S73–S76, 2000.
169. Kay GL, Kay JH, Zubiate P, et al: Mitral valve repair for mitral regurgitation secondary to coronary artery disease. *Circulation* 74:88–98, 1986.
170. Carpentier A: La valvuloplastie reconstructive: une nouvelle technique de valvuloplastie mitrale. *Presse Med* 77:251–253, 1969.
171. Isomura T, Suma H, Yamaguchi A, et al: Left ventricular restoration for ischemic cardiomyopathy: comparison of presence and absence of mitral valve procedure. *Eur J Cardiothorac Surg* 23:614–619, 2003.
172. Acker MA, Parides MK, Perrault LP, CTSN, et al: Mitral-valve repair versus replacement for severe ischemic mitral regurgitation. *N Engl J Med* 370:23–32, 2014.

CHAPTER 101

Regenerative Cell-Based Therapy for the Treatment of Cardiac Disease

Nick J.R. Blackburn • Aleksandra Ostojic • Erik J. Suuronen • Frank W. Sellke • Marc Ruel

CHAPTER OUTLINE

Heart failure (HF) is a burgeoning disease. Recently published American Heart Association projections indicate that its prevalence will increase by 46% from 2012 to 2030 resulting in approximately 8 million people with HF in the United States alone.[1-4] Ischemic heart disease is the major contributor to HF and despite best practices and management strategies, many patients are left with significant disability. Events such as myocardial infarction can result in the irreparable loss of viable cardiac mass and in this and many other clinical scenarios, save for transplantation, no therapies currently exist to remedy lost myocardium. Considering the shortage of donor hearts, a rationale to develop regenerative stem cell based therapies is provided.

Thousands of clinicians and investigators worldwide are working toward harnessing the properties of adult stem or progenitor cells to treat injury in tissues and organs that have limited intrinsic capacity for repair and regeneration, such as the brain and the heart. Yet, achieving cellular cardiomyoplasty remains elusive. As a basic definition, cell therapy for regeneration is the therapeutic use of a cell population to promote growth and repair of diseased and / or damaged tissue to restore anatomy and function. The focus tends to be, typically, in settings where this does not occur appreciably such as myocardial infarction and traumatic brain or spinal cord injury. In the setting of ischemic cardiomyopathies, the goal of stem cell therapy would, preferably, be a combination of promoting the growth of new or existing blood vessels to improve tissue perfusion, and the growth of new cardiomyocytes within the damaged myocardium. Since its inception, cell therapy has achieved the most success in facilitating new blood vessel formation via either angiogenesis or vasculogenesis. Unfortunately, it has been somewhat more difficult to restore lost cardiomyocytes. Although we are likely still decades away from completely regenerating the diseased myocardium, recent evidence indicates that we are at least a little farther ahead. The aim of this chapter is to familiarize readers with the field of cell therapy for cardiac regeneration. Despite many deserving preclinical and clinical studies, unfortunately this review will not be comprehensive, because of length restrictions. Instead, only those cell types with the most promise and best available evidence will be discussed. The clinical focus will be acute MI where the loss of cardiomyocytes is a hallmark of this disorder; however, stem cell use in other clinical entities will also be briefly touched upon. Methods of administration will be covered, as well as the principal mechanisms of action that have been identified. Finally, a brief section will outline some of the current challenges facing the field and possible future directions. At the end of this chapter readers will be familiar with the field of cell therapy for cardiac repair and for those interested references are provided.

DELIVERY METHODS FOR CELL TRANSPLANTATION

Stem cell products for the injured heart can be administered through several methods—some more invasive than others—and each presenting with unique advantages and disadvantages (Table 101-1). Generally, stem cells can be infused intravenously or via patent coronary arteries supplying the ischemic region of the heart, or stem cells can be injected directly into the ventricular wall via a percutaneous transendocardial or a surgical transepicardial approach (Fig. 101-1).

TABLE 101-1 **Administration Models**

Routes	Advantages	Disadvantages
Intravenous injection	Simplest	Few migrate into the target
Intracoronary injection	Can be administered into patent artery, higher cell homing versus intravenous infusion, low risk of arrhythmia	Unsuitable for larger stem cells, hinder cellular transmigration, exacerbation of atherosclerosis
Intramyocardial injection	Most reliable under direct visualization; highest cell dose	Invasive, potential for cell "clumping"

Intravenous Infusion

Intravenous infusion is the simplest method of cell administration. Given this delivery strategy is nonspecific, it relies heavily on proper homing of the infused cells to the ischemic myocardium. Thus, the disadvantage of this method is that a low percentage of the infused cells home it to the intended target.[5] Cells can also become trapped in other organs, particularly in lymphoid tissues, so that an additional small proportion of cells enters the coronary circulation and migrates into ischemic myocardium.[6,7] This is particularly disadvantageous with pluripotent cells increasing the opportunity for off-site proliferation. In addition, with larger cell types, such as mesenchymal stem cells (MSCs) or skeletal myoblasts, microembolization can occur because these cells may be incapable of penetrating beyond a given capillary bed, making them unlikely to reach their target.

Intracoronary Infusion

Infusing stem cells via a patent coronary artery can be performed at the time of selective coronary angiography, and it is well-suited for the specific delivery of cells to the ischemic territory of the myocardium. The obvious advantage of intracoronary infusion is that cells can travel directly into myocardial regions in which nutrient-rich blood flow and oxygen supply are preserved, ensuring a favorable environment for the survival of cells, a prerequisite for stable engraftment.[8,9] Indeed, in a study performed by Hofmann and colleagues,[6] homing of unselected bone marrow cells to the infarct region was apparent only after intracoronary delivery but not after intravenous infusion. One disadvantage; however, is that high coronary flow after stem cell injection can prevent low-affinity adhesion to the myocardial capillaries, thus hindering cellular transmigration into the infarcted zone. Another disadvantage to delivering stem cells in this fashion to a potentially diseased segment of the coronary artery is that the combination of stem cells and the pro-angiogenic milieu of the plaque may serve to exacerbate macrovascular and microvascular disease. Similar to intravenous delivery, intracoronary infusion of cells might not be suitable for certain types of larger stem cells, such as skeletal myoblasts and MSCs, which can be prone to embolization. Despite some of these limitations, intracoronary injection of stem cells has been the preferred method of delivery in most clinical studies thus far.

Intramyocardial Injection

Intramyocardial injections constitute an invasive approach to delivering therapeutic cell products compared with the other methods mentioned. This approach is performed by delivering cell suspensions into target myocardial areas via direct injection during minimally invasive thoracoscopic or open procedures.[10] It can be the preferred method of delivery particularly when there is a lack of patent coronary arteries supplying the ischemic region or when the procedure is performed in tandem with mechanical revascularization. The surgical injection process is simple and can be performed under direct

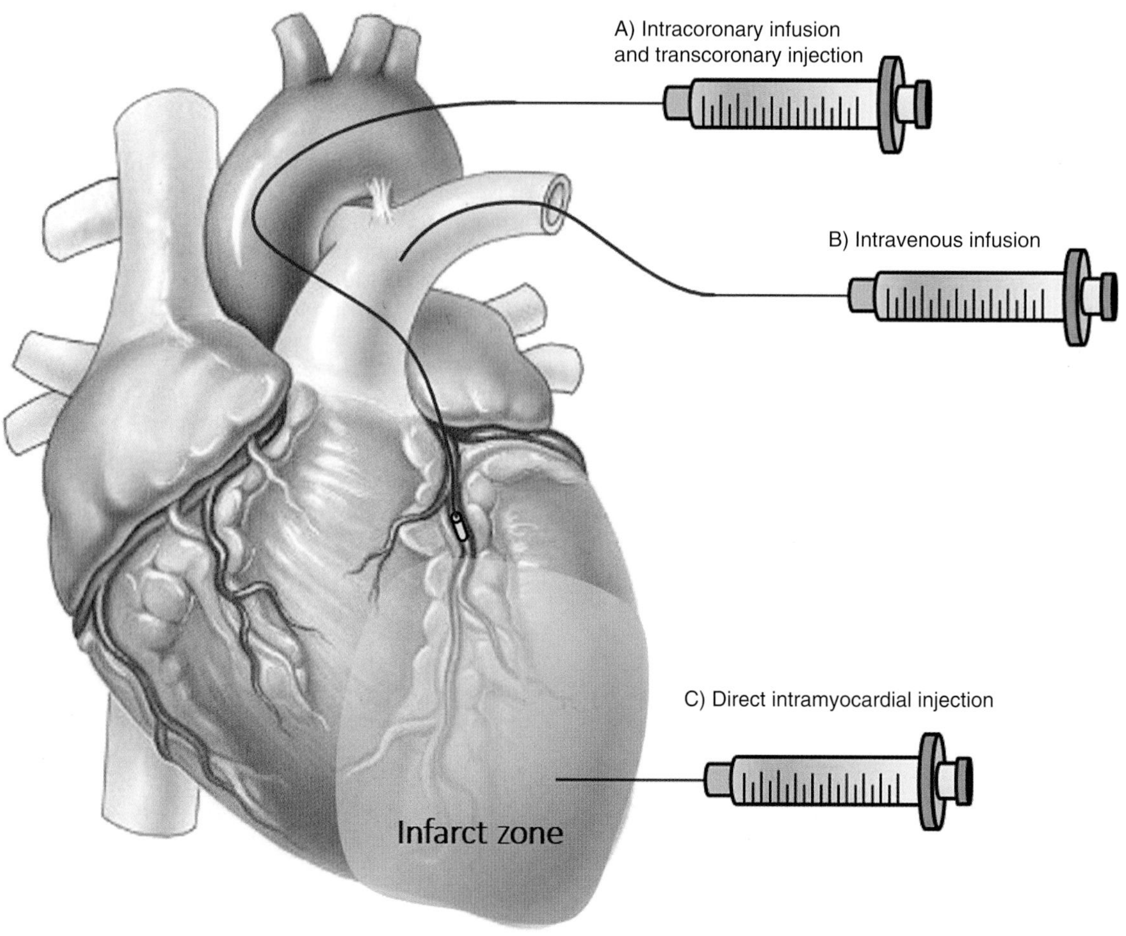

FIGURE 101-1 ■ Delivery routes for transplanted cells for the treatment of ischemic heart disease.

visualization, allowing evaluation by inspection of the potential target zones. As an alternative to user-based visualization of cell injection, electromechanical mapping (e.g., using the NOGA system) can serve to improve the reliability of surgical transepicardial injections, or assist transendocardial injections as a percutaneous procedure.[11] Multiple injections of concentrated cell suspensions at minimal volumes appear preferable to less frequent, larger volume injection. This method is feasible and potentially the most reliable in ensuring stem cells reach the intended or injured areas of the myocardium.[8] Regardless, it is still difficult to predict the survival and function of progenitor cells injected into uniformly necrotic tissue, and the ischemic or necrotic area may prove too hostile to ensure proper cell engraftment and survival.

There are disadvantages to intramyocardial injections. Some nonspecific delivery can occur often because of cell leakage during injection. Moreover, cell clumping can prevent uniform cell distribution in the target area. This method of delivering stem cells may also be inappropriate in situations of diffuse disease such as nonischemic dilated cardiomyopathy where focal deposits of directly injected cells might be poorly matched to the underlying pathophysiology.[12]

Summary

The optimal route for administering stem cells has yet to be determined, although the method of choice will likely be specific depending on a number of factors such as the cell product, patient clinical characteristics, and disease setting. In more acutely ischemic scenarios such as acute myocardial infarction (AMI), the release of chemotactic stimuli into the peripheral circulation, in response to the ischemic injury, may favor homing of intravenous or intracoronary infused cells. However, in situations in which these signals have been abated, as may be the case for chronic ischemia or old scar, injection of the cells directly into the cardiac muscle may produce a more favorable outcome.[13] To date, most trials report a low frequency of complications regardless of route of administration associated with cell base therapies supporting the safety of any of these approaches.[14]

ADULT STEM OR PROGENITOR CELLS FOR CARDIAC CELL THERAPY

A number of adult stem or progenitor cell types have been investigated for the treatment of heart disease

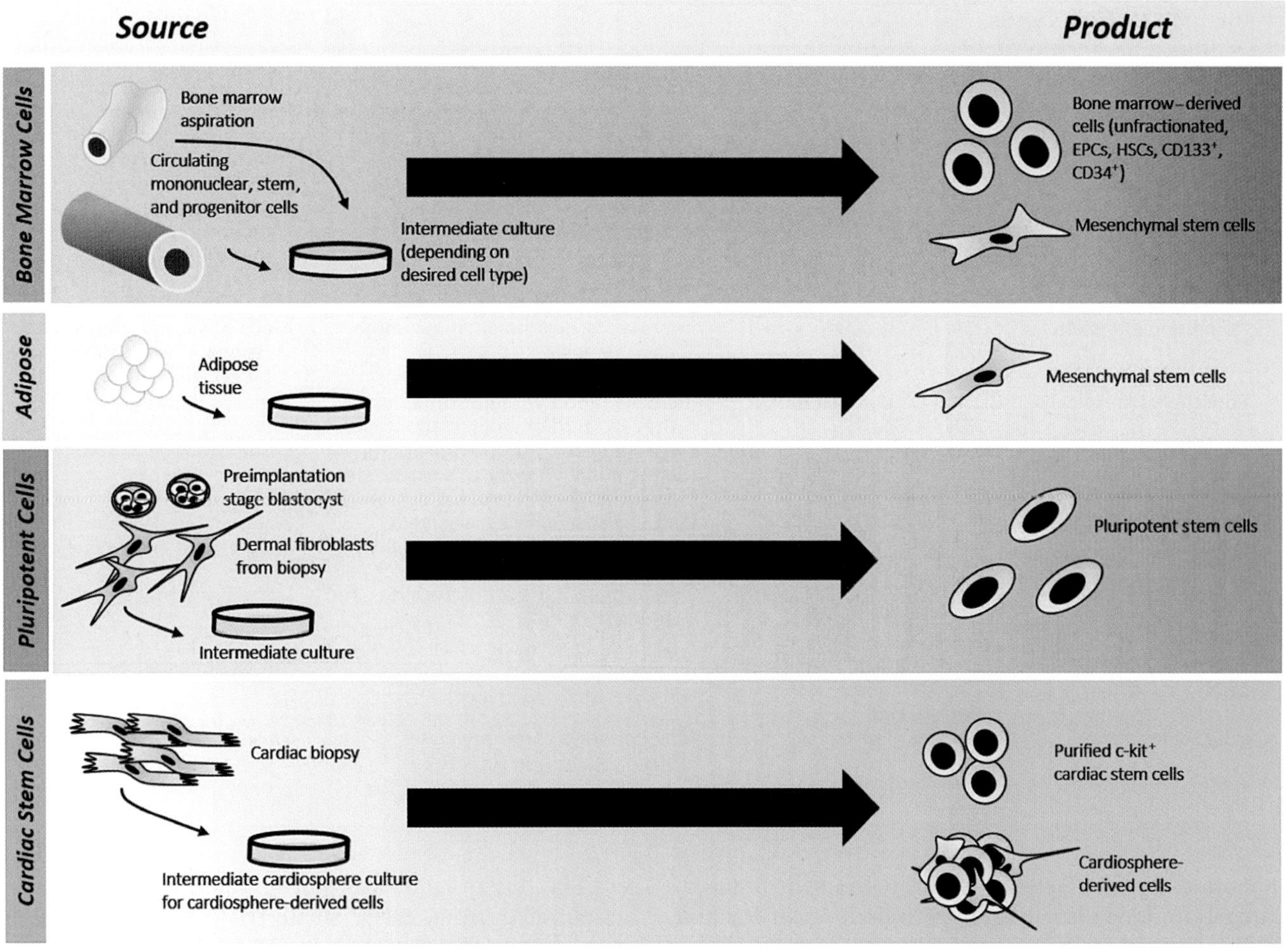

FIGURE 101-2 Cell types currently undergoing clinical trial and emerging cell types. *EPC,* Endothelial progenitor cell; *HSC,* hematopoietic stem cell.

(Fig. 101-2). They have been procured from the bone marrow (bone marrow–derived mononuclear cells [BMCs]), the peripheral circulation, adipose tissue, skeletal muscle, or cardiac muscle biopsy specimens. Pluripotent cells such as the embryonic stem cell (ESC) or the inducible pluripotent stem cell (IPSC) have also received much attention. Most have been investigated extensively in preclinical models, and some in the clinical arena. Some emerging cell types, such as the IPSC, have not yet reached clinical trial. The most pertinent cell types, either for emerging relevance or historical importance, are discussed in the following sections, and a summary is provided in Table 101-2. No consensus has been reached on the ideal cell type; however, some candidates appear more promising than others. If the ideal cell type does exist, it should fulfill most if not all the following criteria[166]:

1. Stem cells should be safe. In other words, they should not form tumors, predispose patients to fatal arrhythmias, or elicit immune reactions.
2. Stem cells should improve heart function, quality of life, and mortality.
3. Stem cell harvest and culture methods should be clinically feasible and not cost-prohibitive.
4. Stem cells should be available as a standard, "off-the-shelf" product.
5. Stem cell use should not be controversial or ethically ambiguous.

The following sections will cover the predominant cell types emphasizing clinical data. For emerging cell products that have not yet reached clinical trial, animal studies instead will be the focus. A summary of select clinical trials is provided in Table 101-3 (note that this table is not exhaustive, but is provided as an example).

Bone Marrow–Derived Cells

The bone marrow hosts a myriad of cell populations, including hematopoietic and nonhematopoietic cells and progenitors. Interest in autologous BMCs for the treatment of ischemic cardiac syndromes was first stimulated by the discovery of the putative endothelial progenitor cell (EPC) by Asahara and colleagues in 1997.[15] These EPCs, originally from the bone marrow, were found to circulate in the peripheral blood homing to sites of tissue ischemia to participate in postnatal vasculogenesis.[15] Since then, cells derived from the bone marrow have been the preferred cell type in both preclinical and clinical cardiac cell therapy studies. BMCs can be harvested via either bone marrow aspiration or peripheral blood apheresis followed by isolation of the

TABLE 101-2 **Cell Types**

Cell Type	Phenotypic Markers	Advantages	Disadvantages
Skeletal myoblasts	CD56, Desmin	Easily harvested and expanded; good survival rates; differentiate into myotubes	Poor differentiation into cardiomyocytes; high risk for arrhythmias
Embryonic stem cells	CD133, Oct 4, SSEA-3/4, Sox	Differentiate into cardiomyocytes, endothelial cells, and smooth muscle cells	Ethical challenges, tumorigenicity, ectopic differentiation, immunogenicity
Bone marrow–derived stem cells			
Hematopoietic stem cells	CD34, CD133, CD45, Sca-1, c-kit	Improve cardiac function, promote angiogenesis	Mechanistically, may only reconstitute peripheral blood leukocytes
Endothelial stem cells	CD34, CD133, VEGFR2, CD144, Sca-1	Increase blood vessel formation, prevent cardiomyocyte apoptosis	Variable efficacy
Mesenchymal stem cells	CD106, c-kit	Have reduced immunogenicity (at least initially), easy to expand and maintain ex vivo; robust secretome	Large cell type
Adipose tissue–derived cells		Less expensive, less invasive to harvest, and potentially available in great quantities	Isolation needs to be optimized for clinical use
Side population cells	CD45, CD59, CD43, CD49d, CD31, and integrin markers	Differentiate into cardiomyocytes and endothelial cells	Little if any preclinical data
Inducible pluripotent cells	Oct4, Sox2, Klf4, c-Myc, Lin28, Nanog (introduced)		Yet to be tested
Cardiac stem cells	c-kit, Sca-1, isl 1	May generate cardiomyocytes; strong paracrine repertoire	Very low numbers, isolation difficult; limited clinical experience

mononuclear cell fraction by density-gradient ultracentrifugation. Upon isolation of the mononuclear fraction, BMCs can either be kept unfractionated or be further purified to isolate subpopulations identified by specific surface antigenic expression. In some cases, depending on desired cell type, fractionated BMCs may require further ex vivo expansion in culture.[8] The subpopulations of BMCs that have been studied in the context as cardiac regenerative therapies includes hematopoietic stem cells (HSCs), EPCs, MSCs, and purified CD133$^+$ or CD34$^+$ cells (see Fig. 101-2). Bone marrow products have gained much favor from investigators mainly because of their ease of procurement and expansion in culture, and they tend to possess a relatively high concentration of adult progenitors.[8]

Unfractionated Bone Marrow Cells

The capacity for unselected or unfractionated BMCs to promote cardiac repair has been controversial,[16-18] yet they remain the most thoroughly investigated cell type in clinical trial.[19] Their popularity is driven largely by practical reasons. For example, BMCs are (1) derived from straightforward harvest protocols, (2) do not require complex or prolonged ex vivo management, and (3) contain a small niche of stem and progenitor cells despite representing a heterogeneous population.[19] BMCs have been investigated in AMI, chronic ICM, and HF, but for the sake of brevity the following section will focus on trials of AMI. Readers interested in the results of BMC therapy in other clinical settings can consult several excellent reviews.[10,19]

The safety and feasibility of BMC therapy was established from early, small trials of AMI such as the "Transplantation of Progenitor Cells and Regeneration Enhancement in Acute Myocardial Infarction" (TOPCARE-AMI).[20-22] The demonstration that cell therapy may be safe, and possibly effective, prompted further inquiry into mid-sized, double-blind, randomized trials such as the "Reinfusion of Enriched Progenitor Cells and Infarct Remodelling in Acute Myocardial Infarction" (REPAIR-AMI) and the "BOne marrow transfer to enhance ST-elevation infarct regeneration" (BOOST) trials.[23,24] Initial follow-up analysis from both the REPAIR-AMI and BOOST trials reported benefits associated with BMC therapy.[23,24] BMCs were infused 3-7 days after successful reperfusion and were associated with superior cardiac function (5.5%-6.7% improved left ventricular ejection fraction [LVEF]) compared with placebo at 6 months postintervention.[23,24] In addition, cell therapy was not associated with an increased risk for adverse clinical events.[24-26] Substudies of both trials were subsequently released by trial investigators with equally promising results. For example, patients receiving BMCs in BOOST demonstrated improvements in diastolic function,[27] whereas there was a reduction in a prespecified cumulative end-point of death, MI, or necessity for revascularization at 1-year follow-up of the REPAIR-AMI.[26] Several other trials also support the benefit of BMC therapy in patients with AMI. Trials by Assmus and colleagues,[28] Cao and colleagues,[29] Yousef and colleagues,[30] and the "FINish stem CELL study" (FINCELL) reported positive benefits associated with BMC therapy including improved global ventricular function, a reduction in

TABLE 101-3 Select Clinical Trial Results

Study	Cell Therapy Patient	Cell Type and Cell Number	Route	Follow-up	Results
TOPCARE-AMI[20,22]	AMI (n = 29) AMI (n = 30)	2.1×10^8 BMCs 1.6×10^7 CPCs	IC	1 yr	LVEF↑; perfusion↑; remodeling↓
BOOST[24,27,32,33]	AMI (n = 30)	2.4×10^9 BMCs	IC	5 yr	LVEF↑ (6 months only), no change vs. control at 5 years
Fernandez-Aviles et al[21]	AMI (n = 20)	7.8×10^7 BMCs	IC	11 mo	LVEF↑; ESV↓;
MAGIC[52]	AMI (n = 10)	1.5×10^9 G-CSF-mobilized cells	IC	6 mo	LVEF↑; ESV↓; regional perfusion↑
Choi et al[186]	AMI (n = 10)	2×10^9 G-CSF-mobilized cells	N/A	6 mo	LVEF↑
Ge et al[187]	AMI (n = 10)	4×10^7 BMC	IC	6 mo	LVEF↑; perfusion↑
Strauer et al[188]	AMI (n = 10)	2.8×10^7 BMCs	IC	3 mo	Infarct size↓; LV perfusion↑
Chen et al[189]	AMI (n = 34)	$4.8\text{-}6 \times 10^{10}$ BMCs	IC	6 mo	LVEF↑; perfusion↑; wall motion↑
REPAIR-AMI[23,26,28,190]	AMI (n = 102)	BMCs (50 mL bone marrow)	IC	1 yr	LVEF↑; infarct size↓; ↓remodeling
Janssens et al[191]	AMI (n = 33)	3×10^8 BMSCs	IC	4 mo	Infarct size↓; regional systolic function↑
Li et al[192]	AMI (n = 35)	7.3×10^7 PBSCs	IC	6 mo	LVEF↑; wall motion↑
ASTAMI[34,36-38]	AMI (n = 50)	BMCs (50 mL bone marrow)	IC	6 mo	No benefit
TOPCARE-CHD[64,193]	CMI (n = 28) CMI (n = 24)	2.1×10^8 BMCs 2.2×10^7 CPCs	IC	3 mo	Wall motion↑
Katritsis et al[194]	CMI (n = 11)	$2\text{-}4 \times 10^6$ BMCs and EPCs	IC	4 mo	Perfusion defects↓; infarct size↓
Perin et al[195]	HF (n = 14)	3×10^7 BMCs	IM	4 mo	LVEF↑; regional perfusion↑
Stamm et al[196,197]	CMI (n = 20)	5×10^6 $AC133^+$ BMCs	IM	6 mo	LVEF↑; perfusion↑
Ahmadi et al[198]	ICM (n = 19)	N/A	IM	6 mo	WMSI↓
Hendrikx et al[199]	CMI (n = 10)	6×10^7 BMCs	IM	4 mo	LVEF↑; systolic thickening↑; Defect score↓
Losordo et al[75]	RA (n = 18)	$5\text{-}50 \times 10^4$ $CD34^+$ cells/kg	IM	6 mo	Exercise tolerance↑; perfusion↑
Mocini et al[200]	ICM (n = 18)	2.9×10^8 BMCs	IM	3 mo	LVEF↑; wall motion↑
Tse et al[201]	ICM (n = 8)	BMCs (from 40 mL bone marrow)	IM	3 mo	LVEF↑; wall motion↑
G-CSF-STEMI[85]	AMI (n = 44)	G-CSF mobilized cells	N/A	1 yr	↑Perfusion 1 week and 1 month post treatment
STEMMI[86,87]	AMI (n = 78)	G-CSF mobilized cells	N/A	6 mo	No improvement, some inverse association between circulating mesenchymal cells and systolic recovery
REVIVAL-2[88]	AMI (n = 56)	G-CSF mobilized cells	N/A	4-6 mo	No improvement
FINCELL[31]	AMI (n = 40)	BMCs (360×10^6)	IC	6 mo	↑LVEF
Cao et al[29]	AMI (n = 41)	BMCs (5×10^7)	IC	4 yr	↑LVEF
Hare et al[89]	AMI (n = 53)	Allogeneic MSCs ($0.5\text{-}5 \times 10^6$ cell/kg)	IC	6 mo	↑LVEF and global symptom score in patients with anterior MI
REGENT[74]	AMI (n = 80)	BMCs or $CD34^+CXCR4^+$ selected cells (1.78×10^8 cells; 1.90×10^6 cells)	IC	6 mo	↑LVEF in patients with baseline EF < 37%
BALANCE[30]	AMI (n = 62)	BMCs (6.1×10^7 cells)	IC	5 yr	↑contractility; ↑hemodynamic status; ↑exercise capacity; ↓mortality
SCIPIO[127,132]	HF (n = 16)	c-kit+ CSCs (1×10^6 cells)	IC	1 yr	↑LVEF; ↓infarct size
HEBE[167]	AMI (n = 200)	BMCs or PBMCs ($\approx 290 \times 10^6$)	IC	4 mo	No improvements
Losordo et al[76]	RA (n = 167)	CD34+ selected BMCs ($1\text{-}5 \times 10^5$ cells/kg)	NOGA IM	1 yr	↓weekly angina frequency; ↑exercise tolerance
Quyyunmi et al[202]	AMI (n = 16)	CD34+ selected BMCs (10×10^6 cells)	IC	6 mo	↑perfusion; ↑LVEF; ↓infarct size
BONAMI et al[35]	AMI (n = 49)	BMCs (98×10^6 cells)	IC	3 mo	↑myocardial viability; ↓non-viable segments
Williams et al[203]	ICM (n = 8)	BMCs or MSCs ($100\text{-}200 \times 10^6$ cells)	IM	1 yr	↑regional contractility; ↓end-diastolic volumes; ↓infarct sizes
Chih et al[204]	RA (n = 18)	G-CSF mobilized cells	N/A	42 wk	No improvements

Continued

TABLE 101-3 **Select Clinical Trial Results—cont'd**

Study	Cell Therapy Patient	Cell Type and Cell Number	Route	Follow-up	Results
POSEIDON[90]	ICM (n = 5)	Allogeneic and autologous MSCs (20-, 100-, 200- × 10^6 cells)	IC	1 yr	↑functional capacity; ↑quality of life; ↓ventricular remodeling
TAC-HFT[205]	ICM (n = 65)	MSCs and BMCs	IC	1 yr	↓MLHFQ both cell types ↑6MWT; ↑regional function; ↓infarct sizes MSCs only
CADUCEUS[128]	AMI (n = 31)	CDCs (25 × 10^6 cells)	IC	6 mo	↓scar mass; ↑viable heart mass; ↑regional contractility; ↑regional systolic wall thickening
Perin et al[47]	HF (n = 10)	ALDH+ BMCs (2.27 × 10^6)	NOGA IM	6 mo	↓LV end-systolic volume
SWISS-AMI[42]	AMI (n = 200)	BMCs	IC	4 mo	No improvements
TIME[41]	AMI (n = 65)	BMCs (150 × 10^6 cells)	IC	1 yr	No improvements

AMI, Acute myocardial infarction; *BMC,* bone marrow–derived mononuclear cell; *CDC,* cardiosphere derived cells; *CMI,* chronic myocardial infarction; *CPC,* circulating progenitor cell; *CTO,* chronic total occlusion; *EF,* ejection fraction; *EPC,* endothelial progenitor cell; *ESV,* end-systolic volume; *G-CSF,* granulocyte colony-stimulating factor; *HF,* heart failure; *IC,* intracoronary; *IM,* intramyocardial; *LV,* left ventricular; *MSC,* mesenchymal stem cell; *RA,* refractory angina pectoris.

morbidity and mortality, and a neutral effect on severe adverse reactions, including arrhythmias and restenosis of the stented coronary artery.[28-31]

Unfortunately, despite the positive early experience with BMCs in patients, other trials have not been so promising. Moreover, follow-up from some of the earlier, positive trials were beginning to release disappointing long-term results. For example, the 2-year results of the REPAIR-AMI could not conclusively associate BMC therapy with improved morbidity and mortality[28]; in BOOST, whereas the difference in LVEF improvement between cell therapy and placebo were significant at 6-month follow-up, the effect was not sustained at 18 months.[24,32] A subgroup of patients with pronounced transmural infarcts may have benefited from cell therapy, although this was required to be tested prospectively in a randomized trial. Regardless, the lack of beneficial effects associated with BMCs in BOOST was sustained in the 5-year results.[33] Examples of results from recent trials include the "BONe marrow in Acute Myocardial Infarction" (BONAMI), which have been mixed, and those from the "Autologous Stem-Cell Transplantation in Acute Myocardial Infarction" (ASTAMI) trial, which were altogether negative.[34,35] Aside from a small improvement in exercise time, ASTAMI did not associate BMCs with improvements in global LV function, or ventricular remodelling.[34,36-38]

Before reaching clinical trial, many elements such as cell dose, frequency, or time of delivery had not been systematically determined for stem cell therapies. In some trials, such as the REPAIR-AMI, only until patients were stratified based on time of delivery after reperfused MI did some suggestion arise that timing of delivery influenced the efficacy of the therapy. This prespecified subgroup analysis associated later cell delivery (about 7 days after reperfused MI) with more pronounced benefits.[23] Thus, several recent trials including the TIME, late-TIME, and SWISS-AMI sought to test this hypothesis comparing the time of delivery between cells delivered early, mid, or late postinfarction.[39-42] Unfortunately, results from all three trials did not associate beneficial effects with BMC therapy for AMI, consistent with the BOOST and ASTAMI trials, regardless of when cells were delivered after AMI.[39-42] Results from the TIME trial may, however, require careful scrutiny as cells were procured from a novel, convenient extraction method that had not been previously validated in bioactivity assays or animals models as opposed to the already well-supported and published methods for isolation.

Establishing a concrete position on the efficacy of BMC therapy for AMI has so far been difficult and results from recent trials such as TIME, late-TIME, or SWISS-AMI have not been able to answer this question conclusively. The outlook for BMC therapy is less than optimistic. Given the conflicting evidence and emerging alternatives, favor may lean toward products with well-demonstrated capacity to produce improvements in global LV function, mortality, and quality of life. Moreover, although some cumulative evidence from recent meta-analyses suggests that BMCs are associated with modest improvements in LV function (2%-4% LVEF), the question remains of whether these improvements are clinically meaningful.[43,44] The upcoming European large, phase 3 "Effect of Intracoronary Reinfusion of Bone Marrow–derived Mononuclear Cells on All-Cause Mortality in Acute Myocardial Infarction" (BAMI) trial (NCT01569178) will probably represent the final consensus of BMCs in cardiac cell therapy in AMI.

Hematopoietic Stem Cells

Hematopoietic stem cells (HSCs) are a subset of BMCs that are multipotent and self-renewing and from which all blood cell types are derived. They are possibly the first stem cell therapeutic investigated in patients dating back from early trials of bone marrow transplantation for fatal leukemias.[45] Their use can be potentially curative for genetic blood disorders such as thalassemia and immune deficiency, or malignancies such as leukemia.[45] The prevailing hypothesis is that HSCs give rise to two lineage restricted progenitor cell types, including myeloid progenitors and lymphoid progenitors that, in turn, supply the number of lymphocytic and granulocytic cells, macrophages, platelets, and erythrocytes found in the blood. However, specific identification and classification of HSCs has been difficult largely because of the limitations of current imaging and lineage tracing methods.[46] Generally, HSCs are identified by a lack of hematopoietic or myeloid lineage (lin) markers and, depending on the report, the presence of a number of antigenic surface markers such as CD34, CD38, CD90, CD133, CD105, CD45, and c-kit (CD117) or other markers such as the presence of aldehyde dehydrogenase.[47,48] Their use as a cardiac regenerative cell product was stimulated by early studies indicating that lin$^-$, c-kit$^+$ HSCs could restore necrotic myocardium by transdifferentiating into all the major cardiac cell types (cardiomyocyte, endothelial cell, and smooth muscle cell) conferring salutary effects.[49,50] Unfortunately, this notion was met with sharp criticism and conflicting data.[16,17] Subsequent evidence instead indicates that HSCs are, in fact, not cardiomyogenic but adopt mature hematopoietic fates in ischemic myocardium.[16,17,51] Whether the benefits of HSCs are derived from an ability to restore damaged myocardium or from a separate, possibly paracrinic, mechanism remains a topic of intense debate.[50]

Consensus on what combination of surface, cytosolic, or functional markers define the HSC is lacking, thus making direct comparisons between trials difficult. Given this loose definition of HSCs, some of the trials discussed in the following section might apply equally to other BMC products, and vice versa. The MAGIC trial assessed the feasibility and efficacy of HSC infusion in patients with MI and who underwent coronary stenting.[52] Granulocyte colony-stimulating factor (G-CSF), a well-established stem-cell mobilizer, was administered to mobilize bone marrow–derived HSCs into the peripheral blood 4 days before apheresis and cell procurement.[52] This trial involved three separate arms including the HSC group, a control group (not placebo), and patients receiving G-CSF alone.[52] At 6 months after infusion, patients treated with HSCs showed significant improvements in exercise capacity (450 vs. 578 seconds), myocardial perfusion (perfusion defect, 11.6% vs. 5.3%), and systolic function (LVEF, 48.7% vs. 55.1%). Although no adverse events occurred because of cell infusion combined with G-CSF, enrollment of the G-CSF cohort was eventually discontinued because of high rates of in-stent restenosis, highlighting a potential safety concern and cautioning future trials using G-CSF administration as a strategy for endogenous stem cell mobilization.[52] Recent trials, though, such as Perin and colleagues[47] have not reported any significant adverse cardiovascular or cerebrovascular events associated with HSC infusion in similarly high-risk patient cohorts with advanced ischemic heart failure and CAD ineligible for PCI or surgical revascularization.[47] The difference, perhaps, is that Perin and colleagues[47] elected to aspirate bone marrow from the iliac crest as opposed to administering G-CSF. In their trial, HSCs were then purified based on the presence of cytosolic ADH, constituting a population of primitive Lin$^-$CD34$^+$CD38$^-$ cells. When administered to patients with advanced ischemic heart failure ADH$^+$ HSCs were associated with a significant decrease in left-ventricular end-systolic volume and a trend toward maximal oxygen consumption at 6 months.[47] It is difficult to draw meaningful conclusions given that only 20 patients were enrolled in the study. Overall, HSCs appear to be beneficial for the treatment of ischemic cardiomyopathies, but larger, randomized, controlled trials are required to confirm early results.

Endothelial Progenitor Cells

Before the characterization of a circulating EPC in 1997 by Asahara and colleagues,[15] vasculogenesis, the process of de novo blood vessel development, was believed to be limited to the embryonic development of vasculature from endothelial cell progenitors or angioblasts. Now it is understood that a subset of bone marrow cells, possibly the putative EPC, mobilizes from the bone marrow to the peripheral circulation ultimately reaching sites of tissue injury or ischemia to participate in postnatal vasculogenesis.[13,15,53,54] Circulating EPC levels have also been recognized as possibly providing clinical information on atherosclerotic burden and future cardiovascular risk.[55,56] Despite the significant attention that has been devoted to studying EPC biology, consensus on an unambiguous definition of the EPC is still lacking and, likewise, the success of many studies has been hindered by the absence of such a definition. EPCs were first characterized as a population of cells that were CD34$^+$, VEGFR2$^+$, and adherent to fibronectin (Fig. 101-3*A*).[15] Today, they are either broadly identified as the mononuclear cells adherent to fibronectin or by cell surface expression that may or may not include CD31, FLK-1 (VEGFR2), CD34, CD133 (AC133), c-kit, and other endothelial markers including VE-cadherin.[57] The criteria that distinguish an HSC from an EPC, and vice versa, may seem unclear given they seem to share many of the same surface antigenic markers.[57] As a cell therapy product, however, EPCs are distinguished from HSCs based on specific ex vivo culture requirements. Separate techniques exist to produce what can be referred to as the *early* or *late EPC*. Both early and late EPCs first require isolating the mononuclear cell fraction from the peripheral circulation, and early EPCs are generated

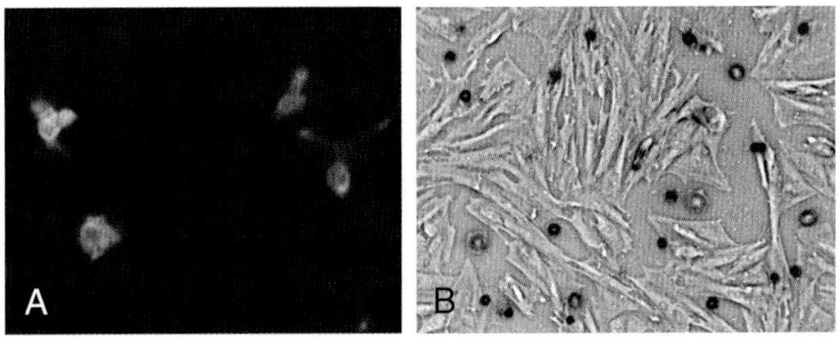

FIGURE 101-3 ■ Endothelial progenitor cells (EPCs) and mesenchymal stem cells (MSCs) in culture. **A,** EPCs from the peripheral blood mononuclear cell layer, cultured on fibronectin for 4 days. Adherent cells (CD34$^{+/-}$, VEGFR-2$^+$) typically take up the markers lectin and Dil-Oxidized Low Density Lipoprotein. **B,** MSCs cultured from human bone marrow yielding a population of adherent MSCs that characteristically express the antigens CD29 and CD44 but are negative for the hematopoietic cell marker CD45.

through subsequent culture on fibronectin for 3 to 7 days, whereas late EPCs are produced via culture for greater than 14 days on collagen type I.[55,58] For a more detailed discussion on the characterization of EPC phenotypes or potential diagnostic use of circulating EPCs, interested readers are referred to an excellent review by Fadini and colleagues.[55]

In preclinical animal models of ischemic cardiomyopathy EPC transplantation prevented cardiac myocyte apoptosis, resulted in increased blood vessel formation, decreased infarct size, and improved function.[59,60] The capacity for human EPCs to transdifferentiate into cardiomyocytes has also been reported,[61] but not all studies support this conclusion.[62] Instead, recent evidence suggests that human early EPCs may be proangiogenic, enacting their salubrious properties through paracrine mechanisms. The proangiogenic effects of late EPCs, instead, is thought to be via direct incorporation into the vasculature.[55,63]

Considering the attention EPCs have received in preclinical animal models of myocardial ischemia, there is comparatively little experience with their use in patients. This is likely owing to pragmatic considerations and investigator preference for unfractionated or sorted BMC products neither requiring ex vivo culture. EPC cell therapy has been explored in several settings, including AMI and chronic ischemic heart disease. As a therapy delivered shortly after reperfused AMI, the small TOPCARE-AMI trial reported that EPC transplant was safe, feasible, and potentially beneficial.[20] EPCs were infused approximately 4 to 5 days after MI and were associated with improved LVEF (51.6 ± 9.6% to 60.1 ± 8.6%), improved regional wall motion in the infarct zone, and profound reduction in end-systolic left-ventricular volumes at 4-month follow-up,[20] with benefits persisting in the final 1-year follow-up.[22] Indeed, contrasting results were released by the same group in a similar trial assessing EPC cell therapy for the treatment of chronic ischemic heart disease.[64] The randomized, controlled TOPCARE-CHD trial assessed the efficacy of BMC, EPC, or placebo treatment later after MI in patients who had a myocardial infarction at least 3 months before enrollment and a well-demarcated region of left ventricular dysfunction.[20] Cells were infused into the vessel supplying the most dyskinetic area of the ventricle, and the results of this study contradict those of TOPCARE-AMI, as EPC delivery was significantly inferior to BMC therapy in terms of improving global left ventricular function.[64] The absolute improvement witnessed with BMC therapy, similar to their experience in AMI, was modest. BMC therapy was associated with an increase in approximately 2.9 percentage points according to left ventricular angiography and 4.8 percentage points according to MRI.[64] The precise mechanisms underlying the benefit of BMC therapy were not investigated in the trial, and it remains unclear as to why EPCs proved inferior in this setting. A higher number of progenitors isolated from the bone marrow aspiration may account for this discrepancy. Moreover, given that patients with CHD have been shown to have pronounced EPC dysfunction, limited cell recruitment and action at the site of injury may have also contributed.[65]

Fractionated CD34⁺ Bone Marrow Cells

As an alternative to heterogeneous cell products, in recent years focus has shifted to BMCs isolated based on CD34 expression given their potent proangiogenic properties.[66] CD34 is believed to be a cell-to-cell adhesion factor expressed in some cell types, including hematopoietic cells, endothelial cells, muscle satellite cells, hair follicle stem cells, and fibrocytes.[67] The function of CD34 remains largely unknown, although in HSCs some evidence suggests that CD34 alters engraftment potential and other properties, such as cell adhesion and migration.[67,68] Peripheral blood $CD34^+$ cells have been shown to transdifferentiate into most of the major cardiac lineages,[69] including endothelial cells,[15,70] vascular smooth muscle cells,[69] and cardiomyocytes,[71] principally via cell fusion.[72] $CD34^+$ cells purified from peripheral blood BMCs have been shown to exhibit superior efficacy and safety for therapeutic neovascularization after MI compared with total mononuclear cells in rodent studies.[59,60,73] They have also been shown to exhibit superior efficacy for preserving integrity and function following MI compared with unselected mononuclear cells with an equivalent number of $CD34^+$ cells,[73] suggesting that a purified $CD34^+$ cell product might possess greater therapeutic potential than a mixed mononuclear cell population.

The REGENT trial investigated the therapeutic potential of fractionated $CD34^+$ mononuclear cells for the treatment of significant systolic dysfunction (LVEF < 37%) secondary to reperfused anterior MI.[74] Two hundred patients were randomized to intracoronary infusion of $CD34^+CXCR4^+$ purified cells, total mononuclear cells, or a control group receiving no therapy at all (no placebo) and were followed for 6 months.[74] Similar to REPAIR-MI, both the purified $CD34^+CXCR4^+$ and BMC therapies were associated with a trend in modest improvement (≈3%) in systolic function.[74] Unfortunately, the study was plagued by a high dropout rate in the control cohort, probably because of the open-label design, which may have potentially accounted for some results not reaching statistical significance. Nonetheless, for patients who received $CD34^+$ cell therapy, a clear trend for better outcomes was evident in patients with a baseline ejection fraction (EF) below the median (<37%) compared to those whose baseline EF was above the median. In addition, a low baseline EF (<37%) was an independent predictor for pronounced benefits in terms of cardiac function.[74] This pattern is consistent with the results reported in REPAIR-AMI.[23] The authors also highlighted that the use of a relatively small number of $CS34^+CXCR4^+$ cells was associated with a similar trend in functional improvement as the use of 100 times more total mononuclear cells, similar to the results published by Kawamoto and colleagues in rats.[73,74] The mechanisms that could account for these benefits were not explored, but it is unlikely that it was a result of de novo cardiomyocytes. Instead, recent laboratory evidence indicates that $CD34^+$ cells secrete exosomes that have independent angiogenic activity, potentially accounting for a significant component of the paracrinic effect of these cells.[66]

Indeed, the hallmark of ischemic cardiomyopathies, such as myocardial infarction, is the loss of myocardium.

In this scenario, cell therapy may be a futile endeavor if no meaningful restoration of myocardium can be accomplished. Moreover, the data supporting the cardiomyogenic potential of $CD34^+$ purified cells is less than convincing. However, in situations in which instead neovascularization may be preferred, $CD34^+$ cells could offer some benefit. Early evidence for the feasibility, safety, and benefit of purified $CD34^+$ cells mobilized by G-CSF administration in 24 patients with refractory angina was provided by Losordo and colleagues[75] in a pilot phase I/IIa randomized trial. Follow-up was performed in a larger double-blind, randomized phase II trial in 167 patients.[76] $CD34^+$ purified cells, or an equal volume of diluent (placebo), were injected with an electromechanical (NOGA) mapping injection catheter. Low-dose $CD34^+$ therapy improved both weekly angina frequency and exercise tolerance measures.[76] Mortality was not different between control and cell therapy cohorts at 12 months, although cell mobilization and collection procedures were associated with elevations in cardiac enzymes that will require follow-up in future studies.[76]

$CD34^+$ purified cells might represent a natural progression from unfractionated BMC therapies, and a more standard product compared with HSC- or EPC-based therapies based on their properties and preclinical results. However, cumulative evidence reviewed in a recent meta-analysis of BMC trials suggests that, overall, $CD34^+$ purified cell therapy might not offer meaningful benefits in the settings of acute MI or chronic HF, possibly because of a lack of clinically relevant cardiomyogenic potential.[43] Given their potent proangiogenic paracrinic properties, $CD34^+$ cells could offer potential in settings where neovascularization in itself could offer substantial benefits, such as refractory angina or chronic ischemic cardiomyopathy.

Mesenchymal Stem Cells

Mesenchymal stem cells are stromal cells found within the bone marrow or adipose tissue and can be expanded via ex vivo culture (see Fig. 101-3*B*).[77] Similar to other bone marrow cell types, they are loosely defined based on surface expression and culture characteristics which include adherence to plastic in cell culture and the surface antigen expression of $CD105^+/CD90^+/CD73^+/CD34^-/CD45^-/CD11b^-$ or $CD14^-/CD19^-$ or $CD79^-\alpha^-/HLA^-DR1^-$.[78] MSCs have been identified as promising candidates because of their relative ease of procurement, multilineage differentiation potential, robust secretome, antiapoptotic, immunomodulatory properties.[55,81,83,84] They have also been shown to be capable of activating resident cardiac stem cells.[51,77,79,80] Given their immune-privileged status, they may serve as ideal allograft candidates, although the long-term benefits as allogeneic products have been challenged.[81] Some authors contend that MSCs can adopt cardiomyocyte-like phenotypes when injected into both healthy and infarcted myocardium; however, these results have been scrutinized, and others attribute these observations as either MSC fusion with resident cardiomyocytes or nonexistent altogether.[79,82,83]

Purified human-derived MSCs have been shown to attenuate contractile dysfunction and to prevent adverse remodeling in rodent and swine models of myocardial infarction.[82-84] In contrast with the classical method of collecting cells and deploying via infusion or injection, initial clinical attempts at harnessing MSCs assessed pharmacologic mobilization of the cells from the bone marrow using G-CSF. Assessing G-CSF mobilized cells soon after AMI, results from the "G-CSF ST-segment Elevation Myocardial Infarction" (G-CSF STEMI), "STEM cells in Myocardial Infarction" (STEMMI), and "Regenerate Vital Myocardium by Vigorous Activation of Bone Marrow Stem Cells" (REVIVAL-2) trials showed that G-CSF administration did not result in improved systolic function compared with placebo.[85-88] A substudy of the STEMMI trial sought to describe the cells mobilized by G-CSF administration and to determine the association, if any, between plasma concentration of these cell types and changes in left ventricular systolic function.[86] The authors associated an inverse relationship between circulating MSCs and systolic functional improvement following G-CSF administration after MI.[86] This relationship was left relatively unexplored, but it could be a consequence of several mechanisms. It may be that reduced circulating MSCs is a reflection of increased homing to the infarcted myocardium, or given the large size of MSCs their increased concentration in the circulation may contribute to further microembolization and infarction.

MSCs are one of the few cell types to date that may offer a true "off-the-shelf" product given their potential immune-privileged status.[78] Hare and colleagues[89] assessed the safety of this type of allogeneic product in a double-blind, randomized, dose-ranging trial of 53 patients with reperfused MI. The primary end-point of the study was safety, whereas efficacy measured by ejection fraction and ventricular volumes constituted exploratory, secondary end-points. Safety profiles were similar between the allogeneic MSC product (Prochymal; Osiris Therapeutics Inc., Baltimore, MD) and placebo treatments.[89] Patients receiving MSCs experienced fewer episodes of ventricular tachycardia and improved pulmonary forced expiratory volumes.[89] In terms of efficacy, MSCs were associated with improved global symptom score and ejection fraction.[89] These results highlight some potential advantages of MSCs versus other BMC products. For example, the product used in this trial was a readily available allogeneic product prepared from healthy donors, circumventing any potential issues with patient clinical condition on cell potency. It also obviates the need for an invasive and highly painful bone marrow aspiration. Results from the recent POSEIDON trial reinforce some of these benefits.[90] POSEIDON was a small, randomized, pilot trial that compared the safety and efficacy of autologous or allograft MSC transendocardial delivery in patients with chronic ischemic LV dysfunction secondary to MI.[90] The primary end-point was safety measured by incidence of severe adverse reactions.[90] None of the cell products reached the predefined stopping point for incident severe adverse reactions, supporting the low immunogenicity of MSCs. In terms of secondary end-points, reflecting efficacy, the combined results appear encouraging. Autologous, but not allogeneic, therapy resulted in improvements in the

6-minute walk test and Minnesota Living with Heart Failure Questionnaire (MLHFQ) scores.[90] Moreover, both cohorts demonstrated improvements in New York Heart Association (NYHA) class.[90] Both were associated with reduced early enhancement defect, a measure of infarct size, end-systolic volumes, and sphericity.[90] In addition, patients having received allogeneic therapy demonstrated improved end-diastolic volumes.[90] Changes in EF were not apparent from the aggregate results, although a trend for an inverse dose-response relationship was observed. Increases in EF and pronounced changes in ventricular geometry were evident in patients receiving a lower dose of MSCs.[90] The results are promising but will require substantiation in several follow-up trials given the small sample size, open-label design, and lack of a placebo-controlled group.[90]

MSCs are an exciting candidate as the field of cell therapy progresses. Given their potent paracrinic properties and immune privilege, they may truly offer the potential for an off-the-shelf product. A major knowledge gap that remains before the potential for these cells can be fully realized is the mechanisms underpinning observed benefits. Nevertheless, given their purported benefits and considerable secretome, MSCs appear to be promising as cardiac cell therapy evolves.

Summary of Bone Marrow Cell–Derived Products

Establishing a firm position on the benefits of BMC-based cell therapies is challenging. Several recent meta-analyses agree that BMC cell therapy could offer modest short-term functional improvements at 6 to 12 months, with a trend indicating that these benefits may also persist long term in patients with AMI.[43,44] Some effects on left ventricular end-systolic volume, recurrent AMI, readmission for heart failure, unstable angina, or chest pain were also associated.[43,44] Given the high degree of trial variability in elements—such as the time of delivery following MI or reperfusion, cell type, cell dose, method of administration, imaging modalities to assess function, and clinical hard end-points—conclusions are difficult to draw. Moreover, many of the recent, larger trials failed to demonstrate benefits.[91] Even so, the question remains of whether modest improvements in cardiac function are clinically relevant.[43] Several of the aforementioned BMC cell types may be suitable for some clinical scenarios, although they likely do not represent the ideal candidate for regenerating lost myocardium.

Pluripotent Cells

The two cell types that may possess the most potential are the ESCs and their manmade counterparts—the inducible pluripotent stem cells (IPSCs)—although the neoplastic risk associated with pluripotent cells may preclude their use in patients. ESCs also remain a controversial cell type given their stage of harvest. ESCs are obtained from the inner cell mass of a preimplantation-stage blastocyst.[92] They were first successfully isolated in 1998,[92] and since have been differentiated into cardiomyocytes ex vivo.[93,94] Undifferentiated human ESCs express the stem cell markers Oct4, stage-specific mouse embryonic antigen (SSEA)3/4, TRA-1-60, and TRA-1-81.[95] ESC-derived cardiomyocytes exhibit proper morphology with organized sarcomeres and express cardiac specific transcription factors such as Nkx2.5, GATA-4, and MEF2C, although they lack a true, mature phenotype.[96,97,98] Transplanted ESC-derived cardiomyocytes have been shown to produce functional improvements in several rodent infarct models.[98-101] To date, only one preclinical large animal study, performed by Ménard and colleagues,[102] has been conducted to evaluate the cardiomyogenic potential of ESCs for myocardial ischemia. Ménard and colleagues[102] delivered cardiac-committed murine ESCs 2 weeks after MI into the host myocardium of immunosuppressed or immunocompetent sheep. The ESCs engrafted and functionally colonized the scar area, with new cardiomyocytes resulting in modest improvements in cardiac function.[102] ESCs represent the ultimate example of the candidate cell for cell therapy as they fulfill all the criteria of a stem cell: clonality, self-renewal, and pluripotency. However, given they can be driven to virtually any cell type they are also a significant neoplastic risk.[103] ESCs will also necessarily be allografts posing a risk for graft rejection. The benefits reported by Ménard and colleagues[102] occurred without teratoma formation or graft rejection, regardless of whether the sheep were administered immunosuppression. Others, though, have published contrasting results.[101-104] Future methodological breakthroughs may serve to significantly reduce the risk of graft rejection or neoplasticity, although it is contentious whether these risks can be eliminated completely. The modern clinical trial is a stringent and risk-adverse environment, each becoming more and more difficult to achieve regulatory approval.[5,45] Graft rejection and teratoma formation for ESC therapy, even in one patient, would constitute an unacceptable outcome. It is also doubtful that the controversy surrounding ESC use in the clinic will subside—at least anytime soon. Therefore, it is unlikely, at least for the foreseeable future, that ESCs will ever be used in the clinic.

The IPSC was the focus of the 2012 Nobel Prize in Physiology or Medicine.[105] They were first generated from adult mouse somatic cells using a collection of transcription factors known as *Yamanaka factors*, named after the senior author who led the discovery.[106] The first human IPSCs were generated in 2007 and have since successfully produced cardiomyocytes in vitro.[107-109] The IPSC has garnered significant attention in disease modeling,[110] and, unsurprisingly, many investigators agree that the IPSC holds tremendous promise for cardiac regenerative medicine.[110] At the time of writing this chapter, no clinical trials were in progress relating to IPSC use for cardiac regenerative purposes; however, several animal studies have been published offering promising early results. Canine- and porcine-derived predifferentiated IPSC-endothelial cells were shown to restore cardiac function and to reduce infarct sizes in murine models of myocardial infarction.[111,112] IPSCs could constitute a viable autologous cell therapeutic, particularly since they obviate the legal and ethical concerns traditionally associated with ESCs. Moreover, as IPSC reprogramming technology improves they may constitute the ideal cell type for personalized medicine. It may be possible one day to design patient- or disease-specific IPSCs in an effort to cater to specific clinical needs and patient characteristics. Currently, translation of IPSC based therapies into the clinic is premature. For one, similar to ESCs the methods required to produce IPSCs are known to be oncogenic.[113] New techniques have done much in addressing this issue including the use of small molecules or synthetically modified mRNA.[114,115] Predifferentiating IPSCs to the desired cell type, such as cardiomyocytes or endothelial cells, may be a possible alternative if contaminating undifferentiated IPSCs could be eliminated, or at least significantly minimized.[116] Regardless, these efforts may be futile because the process of reprogramming somatic cells can induce genetic or epigenetic aberrations that may prove irreconcilable technically and incompatible clinically.[113] Ultimately, new methods would need to be verified rigorously first to ensure the absence of a neoplastic risk before the first patient could be treated. Should the risk of tumor formation be addressed, the lack of methods to produce standardized cell products with sufficient yield is another obstacle that may also preclude their clinical use.[117] The efficiency of generating IPSCs is low, and there is significant variability in yield with current methods and technology.[113,117] Nevertheless, the results from early studies into the potential therapeutic benefits of IPSC-derived products certainly warrant further investigation.

Cardiac Stem and Progenitor Cells

The premise that the adult human heart is a postmitotic organ was the dominant view for much of the twentieth century. Observations of possible cardiomyocyte turnover in the adult human heart emerged as early as 1960, although what might constitute the most direct evidence was provided recently in 2009 by Bergman and colleagues.[118] Taking advantage of the rise in atmospheric ^{14}C from Cold War–era nuclear bomb testing that ended in 1963, they approximated that cardiomyocytes renew at 0.45% to 1% per year, gradually declining as one ages.[118] Although the actual rate of turnover remains unclear, this evidence firmly established some capacity for myocyte turnover in the heart; however, many fundamental questions persist regarding the heart's ability to self-renew.[98,119] The source of this capacity was potentially answered by Beltrami and colleagues[120] in 2003 who identified a niche of stemlike cells existing within the heart of mammals. These putative "cardiac stem cells" were negative for hematopoietic cell lineage markers and positive for stem cell marker c-kit, and they were clonogenic, could self-renew, and were multipotent.[120] They were capable of differentiating into cardiomyocytes, smooth muscle cells, and endothelial cells.[120] In addition, when injected into the ischemic rat heart, these cells or their clonal progeny were shown to develop blood carrying vessels and myocytes with features characteristic of younger cells.[120] Given these properties, the putative "cardiac stem cell" (CSC) may represent the best candidate cell type for cardiac cell therapy.

Since the results released by Beltrami and colleagues, CSC contribution to postnatal cardiomyogenesis has gained support.[121,122] However, these reports conflict with the firmly established evidence that cardiomyocyte renewal in animals that display considerable cardiac regenerative potential (e.g., amphibians, zebrafish) occurs via the proliferation of preexisting myocytes and not from the influence of stem cells.[98] Indeed, contrasting evidence was provided by Senyo and colleagues,[123] reporting that either during normal cardiac homeostasis or in response to injury cardiomyocyte renewal in mice occurs by the division of preexisting cardiomyocytes and is not mediated by a stem cell niche. Others, however, provide compelling evidence that c-kit$^+$ cardiac stem cells are necessary and sufficient for complete functional and anatomic recovery during diffuse cardiac injury with patent coronary circulation.[124] These seemingly contradictory observations may be reconciled with the hypothesis that ischemic injury depletes tissue stem cells, possibly including CSCs.[123-126]

Despite the uncertainty revolving around the cardiomyogenic potential of CSCs in situ, many researchers and clinicians have pursued using this population therapeutically. To date, several methods have been developed to isolate and expand this population ex vivo for therapeutic purposes including purified c-kit$^+$ cells, cardiosphere-derived cells (CDCs), Sca1$^+$ CSCs, side population cells, and islet-1$^+$ cells. In this review, we will focus on the CDCs and purified cardiac c-kit$^+$ cells (i.e., CSCs), which are the best studied and are the only populations in which there are ongoing clinical trials.[10,127,128]

C-kit$^+$ Cardiac Stem Cells

Cardiac stem cells isolated and purified based on c-kit surface expression are the best characterized in terms of preclinical animal models of cardiovascular disease. Human CSCs injected early after permanent coronary occlusion in immunodeficient mice and immunosuppressed rat hearts were shown to restore some contractile function to the infarcted area of the ventricle, improve ventricular performance, and alleviate some chamber dilation.[122] In addition, hearts explanted from both animal groups demonstrated chimerism and the coexistence of human and rodent cells together within the infarcted myocardium.[122] Rota and colleagues[129] assessed CSC delivery in a model of chronic HF secondary to ischemia where the isolation and injection of CSCs may be more clinically feasible and have shown that injecting CSCs into the border zone of a 20-day-old infarct in rats preserved left ventricular function, successfully replaced a portion of the myocardium, and mitigated some ventricular remodeling.[129] CSC transdifferentiation into cardiomyocytes has been offered to explain the positive effects of CSC transplantation.[129] However, others, such as Tang and colleagues,[130] report that CSC integration with the myocardium could not account completely for the benefits. In their study, GFP$^+$ CSCs only occupied 2.6% and 1.1% of the risk and noninfarcted regions, respectively[130]; therefore, a paracrine mechanism likely explains the discrepancy. The beneficial effects of CSC therapy have been replicated in large animal models as well.[131] For example, Bolli and colleagues[131] administered CSCs 3 to 4 months after reperfused MI in swine via the infarcted artery. Swine receiving CSC therapy had significantly greater LV ejection fraction, maximum LV dP/dt, and lower LV end-diastolic pressures at 1 month after treatment.[131] Together, these studies provide proof of concept that c-kit+–selected CSC transplantation may offer functional benefits and may be also capable of promoting some degree of myocardial regeneration during ischemic injury.[122]

The "Stem Cells Infusion with Patients with Ischemic cardiomyopathy" (SCIPIO) (Clinicaltrials.gov, no. NCT00474461) phase I trial is the only trial at the time of this writing assessing autologous c-kit+ lineage-negative CSC therapy for the treatment of an ischemic cardiomyopathy.[127] Results from the 2-year follow-up of SCIPIO were not available at the time of compiling this chapter, although interim results have been published.[127,132] SCIPIO is a phase I, open-label, single-center trial assessing CSCs in patients with heart failure secondary to ischemic disease. The open-label design was chosen given that blinding the control cohort would have required cardiac catheterization with placebo infusion.[127] Patient inclusion criteria included previous myocardial infarction, LVEF less than 40%, and undergoing CABG. CSCs were administered approximately 3 months after CABG being delivered to the proximal coronary artery or graft supplying the infarcted region of the ventricle. Overall, from the interim results, patients that completed the 12-month follow-up had an absolute increase in LVEF of 12.3 points, whereas no improvement was apparent in patients in the control cohort.[127] The mean LVEF of all patients before treatment was approximately 30%. In addition, the NYHA functional class decreased in all 16 patients receiving CSC treatment from a mean of 2.19 to 1.63 after 4 months and patient responses to the MLHFQ, from 46.44 to 26.69. No changes were reported in the NYHA or the MLHFQ for control patients. CSC collection in the operating room appears not to interfere with standard procedures or outcomes,[132] and harvest was successful despite the severity of disease, comorbidities, and likely feasible for most patients undergoing CABG. The procedure did not prolong cardiopulmonary bypass time, aortic cross-clamp time, or total surgical time.[132] In summary, the use of autologous c-kit+ CSCs holds much promise, likely deriving from the fact that these cells may represent a cardiac specific stem cell niche responsible for cardiomyocyte homeostasis. Thus far, phase I clinical trial results agree with the preclinical animal models, and the procedure of harvesting and CSC infusion appears to be safe warranting further study in phase II trials.

Cardiosphere-Derived Cells

Cardiosphere-derived cells represent a heterogeneous ex vivo outgrowth cell product derived from cultured cardiac biopsies.[133-135] This subpopulation was first reported by Messina and colleagues[134] in 2004. The term *cardiosphere* was coined from the observation that ventricular or atrial tissue biopsy subcultures would produce emigrating cells that formed spherical aggregates.[134] These aggregates contained, among a number of cell types, cardiac progenitors and when injected into the infarcted rat myocardium would produce functional benefits and some histological recovery.[134] Since its original description, the CDC method has been refined to include endomyocardial biopsy specimens.[135] Phenotypically, these cells express a wide array of surface antigens, including those that mark endothelial cells (KDR human; FLK1 and CD31 mouse), embryonic and stem cells (SSEA-1, abcg2, CD34, c-kit, sca-1), and mesenchymal stem cells (CD105, CD90). In rodent models, when injected shortly after experimental infarction, CDCs were associated with improved LVEF and hemodynamic parameters, as well as reduced infarct sizes and increased percentage of viable myocardium.[133-136] In swine, CDCs harvested from endomyocardial biopsy specimens infused 1 month after MI were associated with a reduction in relative infarct sizes compared with control at 8 weeks after treatment.[137] CDCs were also associated with improved hemodynamic parameters such as higher dP/dt maximum and lower dP/dt minimum, and no instances of infarction related to cell infusion was reported.[137] However, CDC infusion did not reduce final infarct size, improve LV mass, or improve contractile function of the ventricle.[137] Allogeneic CDC transplant has also been documented as being safe and relatively non-immunogenic in pre-clinical models.[136] Transplantation without immunosuppression appears safe and functional results are consistent with previous studies.[136]

The CDC method for isolating CSCs has been sharply criticized with claims that cardiospheres represent primarily a culture of fibroblasts and other cardiac cell contamination,[138] but this view is not universal as others have shown that adult cardiac stem cells can be grown directly from myocardial biopsies.[139] The promising preclinical results warranted investigation in a phase I clinical trial. To date, three clinical trials are complete or ongoing studying the use of CDCs for cardiac regeneration; these include "CArdiosphere-Derived aUtologous Stem CElls to Reverse ventricUlar dysfunction" (CADUCEUS) trial (NCT008933602), the "AutoLogous Human CArdiac-Derived Stem Cell to Treat Ischemic cArdiomyopathy" (ALCADIA; NCT00981006), and the "Allogeneic Heart Stem Cells to Achieve Myocardial Regeneration" (ALLSTAR; NCT01458405) trials. The CADUCEUS study involves the use of CDC products from septal endomyocardial biopsy specimens, the ALCADIA trial will be assessing bFGF slow release concomitant with CDC therapy, while ALLSTAR will assess allogeneic CDC transplant. At the time of this writing, both ALLSTAR and ALCADIA are in the process of recruiting patients, and results were only available for the CADUCEUS trial.[128] The CADUCEUS trial assessed CDC therapy for patients with recent myocardial infarction (≤4 weeks) and significant left ventricular dysfunction (LVEF ≥ 25%, ≤ 45%). Patients were randomly assigned to a treatment group, and those receiving CDC therapy were administered the product (≤90 days after myocardial infarction) via over-the-wire angioplasty catheter in the infarct-related artery.[128] The primary endpoint was safety 6 months after infusion, including ventricular tachycardia, fibrillation, sudden unexpected death, and MI after infusion.[128] Efficacy was assessed in terms of the NYHA class, MLHFQ, 6-min walk test, and MRI. CDC therapy did not produce complications within 24 hours of infusion. Overall, CDC therapy seems safe, with 24% of patients in the CDC group having experienced serious adverse events compared to 13% in the placebo, but conclusions are difficult to draw given the low number of patients included in the study. There were no differences reported in NYHA, or MLHFQ scores. Patients receiving CDC at 1 year increased walked distance compared with controls. No differences in LVEF were reported; however, MRI non–gadolinium-enhanced tissue in CDC patients showed reduced scar mass, increased viable heart mass, regional contractility, and regional systolic wall thickening. There were no benefits in terms of end-diastolic volume, end-systolic volume, and LVEF by 6 months. The lack of benefit in terms of global cardiac function, particularly LVEF, is consistent with the large-animal model published by Johnston and colleagues.[137]

Overall, CDCs are a heterogeneous population of cells that can be derived from several available subculture methods of atrial, ventricular, or endomyocardial biopsy specimens. Some controversy exists as to the cardiomyogenic potential of this product, but there appears to be more proponents than critics. Unfortunately, the clinical effects of CDC therapy are somewhat mixed. Results from the CADUCEUS study did not confirm meaningful effects on cardiac function or clinical status in patients treated with CDCs. Overall, CDCs represent an alternative method to the lineage-negative c-kit$^+$–purified CSC, although based on available evidence further assessment of clinical outcomes is required.

Combination Products

The clinical experience with most of the cell populations studied thus far have unarguably not met with expectations motivated by preceding preclinical results. A number of laboratories have investigated combining different cell types in the effort of taking advantage of complementary modes of action and possible synergistic effects. Some examples follow.

Early and late EPCs appear to promote neovascularization through separate modes of actions. Early-EPCs seem to be proangiogenic on account of a paracrine mechanism, whereas late EPCs tend to integrate directly within the microvasculature.[58] Given these separate yet complementary mechanisms of action, Yoon and colleagues[140] demonstrated that infusing a combination of early and late EPCs promotes a synergistic effect on neovascularization. Similarly, Latham and colleagues[141] cotransplanted CDCs with early EPCs 1 week post-MI in mice. In vitro both cell types promoted equivalent vascular networks, whereas the cell types had distinct cytokine profiles. Each offered similar functional benefits when transplanted alone, though when transplanted together offered a complementary effect on function superior to the benefits of either cell type individually.[141] In swine with reperfused MI, Williams and colleagues[142] reported that combined transplantation of MSCs and CSCs reduced infarct sizes twofold greater in combination than either cell alone, and the combination therapy restored cardiac functional parameters, such as EF, to baseline. These studies represent a growing body of evidence that begs the question as to whether the future of cell therapy will need to rely on novel strategies, such as multiple cell sources, to achieve the desired clinical outcome.[140]

POTENTIAL MECHANISMS OF ACTION FOR CELL-BASED REGENERATIVE THERAPIES

Our experience so far with cell-based regenerative therapies is that they are safe, feasible, and potentially beneficial for a number of clinical settings, including AMI, chronic ischemic cardiomyopathy, refractory angina, and heart failure. However, a major gap that persists is understanding the mechanisms underpinning their benefits. The following sections will describe our current understanding of the mechanisms of action of cell based therapeutics in cardiac regenerative medicine. A schematic representation of the major proposed mechanisms of action of transplanted cells is shown in Figure 101-4.

Transdifferentiation and Cell Fusion of Transplanted Cells

The initial hope with cell-based therapies was that it would provide a means of regenerating previously lost myocardium through transdifferentiation to cardiomyocytes. It also may appear to be the most obvious justification to explain the salutary effects of cell therapies; however, with the evidence that is available to date, it does not appear to be the major mechanism, if providing any contribution at all. For example, the transdifferentiation of bone marrow cells, including CD34$^+$ selected cells,[73,75,76,160] has equally as many critics[16,17] as there are supporters.[49,143] Instead, the concept of BMC cell-fusion with resident cardiomyocytes has been proposed, but again this has also been contested.[144,145] Initially, MSCs appeared to participate in cardiomyogenic phenomena as well, although now their benefits are believed to be derived primarily from their robust secretome.* CSCs have been reported to produce all major cardiac lineages,[120,126,129,130,149] yet some reports deem this process insufficient to account for the improvement in cardiac function.[130] The evidence supporting the cardiomyogenic potential of CDCs is somewhat less nebulous, reported as either quite minimal[150] or nonexistent altogether.[136]

It is possible that transplanted cell therapies have been able to regenerate cardiomyocytes within damaged myocardium. How much is occurring and the overall contribution to the functional effects are the questions that remain. Most reports to date agree that if any cardiomyogenesis occurs, it is certainly disproportionate with the magnitude of the benefits. Instead, other mechanisms are more likely.

Neovascularization from Transplanted Cells

Many of the cell types discussed have been demonstrated to offer some capacity to contribute to the formation of new blood vessels within the myocardium including BMCs, CSCs, MSCs, and CD34$^+$ cells (Fig. 101-5).[15,73,149,151] Neovascularization may prove beneficial in

*References 77, 78, 80, 82, 84, 146-148.

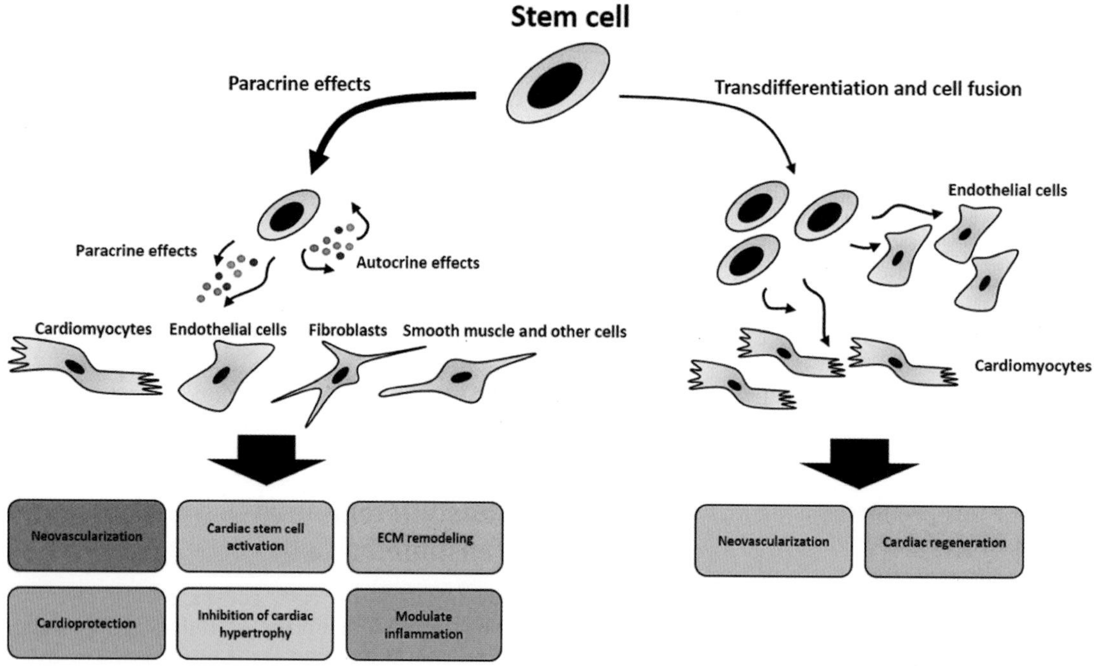

FIGURE 101-4 ■ Proposed mechanisms of action for transplanted stem cells. Transplanted stem cells were originally thought to participate in cardiac repair via direct transdifferentiation *(right side, thin arrow)*. We now understand the contribution of cell fusion and transdifferentiation of stem cells to cardiomyocytes and neovascularization to occur very minimally, if at all (denoted by *thin arrow*). Instead the predominant hypothesis is that transplanted stem cells influence the behavior and survival of resident cells through paracrine effects *(left side, thick arrow)*. Transplanted stem cells can release soluble growth factors, angiogenic cytokines, and microRNA that together serve to promote neovascularization, activate resident cardiac stem cells, favorably alter extracellular matrix (ECM) remodeling, confer cardioprotection, inhibit cardiac hypertrophy, and modulate inflammation. Intervening on these processes may ameliorate this emerging cardiac therapeutic modality.

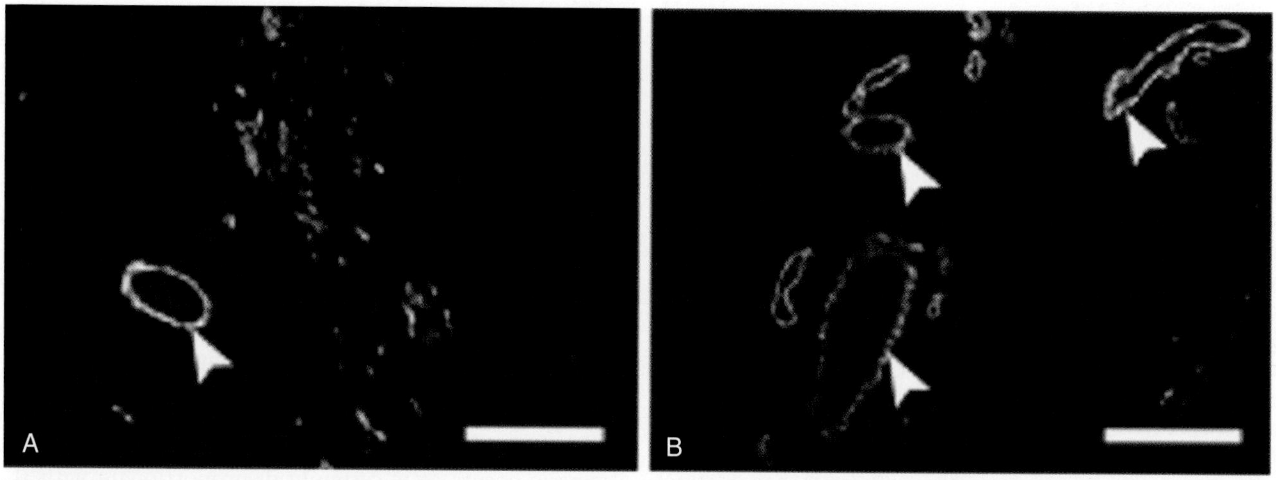

FIGURE 101-5 ■ Transplanted cell contribution to neovascularization. Transplanted endothelial progenitor cells **(A)** and mesenchymal stem cells **(B)** contributing to the formation of capillaries within muscle fibers. Arrows indicate positive α-smooth muscle acting staining in arterioles. Scale bar = 150 μm.

settings where the region of interest may constitute ischemic, but viable, myocardium. However, the benefits of increasing blood vessel density are less clear in many clinical scenarios. For example, in a scar from an old MI or during acute reperfused MI, it is hard to imagine how increased vascular density would be advantageous. Perhaps settings such as refractory angina or chronic ischemic cardiomyopathy are examples of when benefits may be potentially derived from increased vessel density, but this is not the case with all clinical scenarios.

The Paracrine Hypothesis

Paracrinic effects is the reigning hypothesis to explain the benefits associated with transplanted cells. *Paracrine* refers to the capacity of transplanted cells to release signal and growth factors (cytokines, chemokines, exosomes, microparticles, and microRNAs) into the extracellular milieu affecting the behavior and survival of neighboring cells.[146,151,152] Examples of the reparative processes associated with paracrine effects include neovascularization, cardioprotection, modulating inflammation, inhibiting remodeling, antihypertrophic responses, and activation of resident cardiac stem cells.

Neovascularization

The ability to promote neovascularization for most cell types is a result of the release of various chemokines (SDF-1a),[153,154] proteins (e.g., VEGF, bFGF, IGF-1),[155,156] and microRNAs, potentially through exosomes.[66,157,158] The cardioprotective benefits associated with c-kit$^+$ cells from the bone marrow after MI is a result of the modulation of the angiogenic cytokine milieu.[159] Reestablishing blood supply in some situations could salvage ischemic myocardium in diseases such as chronic ischemic cardiomyopathy, though as discussed, this mechanism likely does not account for benefits in patients without residual or persistent ischemia.

Cardioprotective

Paracrine-mediated cardiomyocyte salvage in an ischemic environment is an effect of transplanted cells.[146,151] For example, the functional benefits associated with MSCs appear to occur despite the lack of any evidence of their long-term engraftment within the myocardium.[84] A number of reports indicate that some of these benefits stem from antiapoptotic effects of secreted factors on cardiomyocytes and endothelial cells.[77,84,160] Cytoprotective paracrinic effects seem to underpin a number of other candidates of cell therapy, including IPSC derived endothelial cells,[112] BMCs,[60,158] EPCs,[152] and cardiac-derived stem cells.[150] The release of IGF-1 and subsequent inhibition of miR-34a processing from transplanted BMCs was recently shown to contribute to the paracrine protective effect of this cell type.[158]

Modulation of Inflammation

Chronic, unabridged inflammation is a major determinant of the severity of disease in ischemic cardiomyopathies.[161] Injected cells, such as MSCs, can act as guardians of inflammation attenuating the local inflammatory response by releasing signaling molecules within the environment.[80] Transplanted MSCs into ischemic zones have been shown to decrease proinflammatory cytokines, such as TNF-α, IL-1α, and IL-6.[146] This may be, in part, mediated by the secretion of anti-inflammatory protein TSG-6.[162] Intravenously infused MSCs after MI in mice were shown to embolize to the lungs, secrete TSG-6, and improve cardiac function and reduce infarct sizes.[162]

Extracellular Matrix Remodeling

The effect of the extracellular matrix (ECM) on proper functioning of the heart cannot be overstated. The stability and dynamic equilibrium of the ECM with cardiomyocytes ensures proper alignment and prevents overstretching of myocytes.[163] It is also equally important in secondary roles, such as ensuring proper functional and electrical behavior of the myocardium and vasomotor reactivity of coronary microvasculature.[163] In pathologic scenarios, such as myocardial infarction, impaired remodeling of the ECM plays a substantial role in LV dilation and dysfunction, and morbidity and mortality.[164] At the molecular level, an imbalance in matrix metalloproteinases (MMPs) and tissue-inhibitors of MMPs (TIMPs) production favors this impaired remodelling.[164] Paracrine factors released by transplanted cells may serve favorably to influence the outcome of ECM remodeling post-injury. For example, MSCs have been shown to decrease postinfarct fibrosis.[146] In a rat model of dilated cardiomyopathy, transplanted MSCs decreased MMP-2 and MMP-9 expression, leading to reduced fibrosis and improved function.[165] Rota and colleagues[129] demonstrated that transplanted CSCs increased MMP-2, MMP-9, and MMP-14, while decreasing TIMP-4 levels in a model of HF secondary to MI in rats.

Inhibition of Hypertrophy

Stem cells therapies have been shown to reduce the hypertrophic response of cardiomyocytes in models of ischemic heart failure.[129,130] It is uncertain, however, whether this is secondary to reduced cardiac stress and improved function or whether it constitutes a principal, paracrine function of transplanted cells.

Activation of Resident Cardiac Stem Cells

Endogenous cardiac stem cells are considered to play an important role in cardiac homeostasis, particularly in the turnover of resident cardiomyocytes.[124] Some cell types have been shown to activate endogenous CSCs. For example, Loffredo and colleagues[51] demonstrated that c-kit+ bone marrow cell stimulation of endogenous CSC cardiogenic activity was a critical mechanism of the therapy. The authors also reported that this function was limited to c-kit$^+$ BMCs and not MSCs, although others have shown similar results with MSC therapy.[82,148] The contribution of activated endogenous CSCs also has been shown to be significant with CSC-based cell therapy.[130]

CURRENT CHALLENGES AND FUTURE DIRECTIONS FOR CARDIAC REGENERATIVE MEDICINE

As we move forward in translating new cell therapies into the clinic, we must approach the next steps with careful optimism as many challenges and obstacles remain.[166] Indeed, recent successes in the laboratory and the convergence of different fields, such as tissue engineering, provides exciting opportunities as we work toward finally achieving our goal of cellular cardiomyoplasty. The early experience with stem cell therapy was largely positive, particularly with BMCs. However, since these initial pilot trials ensuing results have contradicted early reports and recent, larger trials have not been able to resolve the controversy reporting positive,[31] somewhat positive,[74] mixed,[35] and negative findings.[167,168] Other cell types have been equally controversial, and providing an explanation is difficult. Likely the answer is multifactorial and cumulative. The inconsistency in reported outcomes for stem cells may arise from clinical factors such as patient clinical characteristics and definitions of efficacy, or other elements such as the limited engraftment or survival of transplanted cells and their dysfunction.[166]

Patient Clinical Characteristics

Cumulative evidence from BMC therapy supports modest improvements in clinical parameters such as left ventricular function. These benefits appear to be comparable to current interventions such as primary PCI, mechanical revascularization, or pharmacologic therapy. Unlike BMC therapy, conventional treatments have proven survival outcomes and a well-established routine in clinical practice.[169] Thus, cell therapy may prove unnecessary and equally lack any benefit for some or most patients. In many of the discussed trials, patient cohorts comprised a relatively healthy patient population with reperfused AMI and minor dysfunction (≥50% LVEF) also treated with contemporary medical therapy. Given the comparatively minor dysfunction in these patients, it is possible that they were not those who could derive the most benefit from stem cell therapy. Interestingly, in trials in which patients were stratified based on clinical characteristics (e.g., severe cardiac dysfunction), the greatest benefits appeared to occur in the sickest patients (low baseline EF).[26,31,74] The implications for future investigations and cardiac therapy altogether are that potentially cell therapy is maximized in those who can possibly derive the greatest benefit—the very ill.

Measures of Efficacy

The prevailing surrogate marker to assess benefits derived from cell therapy has been cardiac left ventricular function, specifically LVEF. Indeed, it is possible that improvements in EF might not be best suited for our definition of efficacy, as EF can be dependent on neurohumoral influences, ventricular geometry, or load. Other metrics of improvement, such as changes in geometry, scar size, perfusion, and viable myocardium measured with modern imaging modalities (e.g., cardiac MRI or PET), may be more appropriate along with other clinically relevant metrics, such as mortality.

Transplanted Cell Dysfunction and Ex Vivo Cell Priming

Clinical trial results have obviously not been as compelling as the preclinical evidence that originally inspired their use in patients. One possible explanation is that, often, many clinical parameters are not recapitulated in animal models. For example, in contrast to preclinical rodent studies in which both donors and recipients are often healthy, young animals, patients are far from healthy and often suffer from other comorbidities. Thus, donor cells from preclinical animal studies are likely poor approximations of the clinical autologous products. For example, BMCs have been shown to be impaired functionally in the setting of diabetes, previous MI, and heart failure, and because of on-pump coronary bypass.[56,170,171] CSC function and survival, equally, appear to be impaired by diabetes.[172] In mice, recent MI impairs donor BMC therapeutic efficacy because of a high inflammatory state in the donor bone marrow.[170] As the proper functioning of autologous cells appears to depend on individual patient characteristics, several investigators have sought to use novel methods, such as priming cells ex vivo, to circumvent these potential limitations.[19] For example, our group developed a collagen I–based biomaterial matrix as a substrate to improve the potency of cultured early EPCs.[173] This culture method resulted in a higher proportion of CD34$^+$ and CD133$^+$ EPC progenitors and improved their capacity to direct de novo neovascularization compared with the traditional method of culture on fibronectin.[173] Other examples include Noiseux and colleagues,[83] who showed that over-expressing Akt in MSCs improves transplanted cell retention and engraftment. The Akt-MSCs were superior at reducing infarct sizes and improving cardiac function.[83] Overexpressing endothelial nitric oxide synthase (eNOS) in transplanted cells is an example of priming cells that is currently under clinical investigation.[19,174] Reduced eNOS expression and nitric oxide (NO) production have been implicated in both endothelial dysfunction[175] and in impaired progenitor cell function.[174,176] Pretreating BMCs ex vivo with an eNOS enhancer was demonstrated to rescue this dysfunction and improve their therapeutic efficacy in preclinical studies.[177] The Enhanced Angiogenic Cell Therapy in Acute Myocardial Infarction (ENACT-AMI; NCT00936819)[174] trial will be the first of its kind to assess transgenic, enhanced stem cells. Autologous early EPCs will be transfected with human eNOS to improve their angiogenic potency and cells will be delivered in patients with significant LV dysfunction after MI.[174] The trial is actively recruiting patients, and the first patient was treated in September 2013 in Ottawa, Canada.

Autologous versus Allogeneic Cells

The vast majority of clinical trials for cell therapy have investigated autologous products and depending on individual patient clinical features autologous cells may be suboptimal.[166] This source of cell therapy is obviously attractive as it circumvents challenges involved in allograft surgeries such as immunologic graft rejection.[166] On the other hand, allogeneic products could be advantageous as “off-the-shelf” products obviating the surgical pragmatic concerns of procuring and culturing patient-derived cells, particularly if they are to be infused soon after AMI. They could be highly standardized and produced in large numbers.[166] In turn, this could ensure the cost-efficient, timely and safe access to a cell therapy product. Immune rejection is an obvious concern, as is the potential for eventual immune tolerance. MSCs may be promising candidates as evidenced by the POSEIDON and Prochymal trials[89,90] given their purported immune-privilege.[80]

Cell Engraftment and Biomaterials

Unfortunately, whether cells have been autologous or allogeneic therapies retention and engraftment continues impede optimal performance.[178] Regardless of delivery method, cell type or method used to assess cell retention

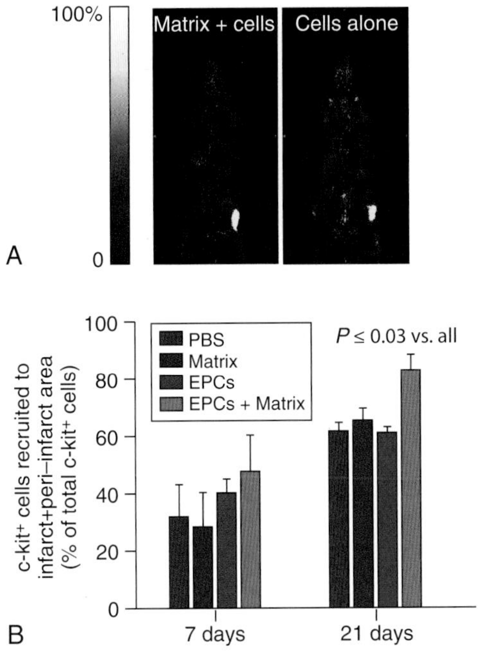

FIGURE 101-6 Stem cell therapy transplanted with collagen-based biomaterial matrix can synergize to improve cell engraftment and functional benefits. **A,** Small animal positron emission tomographic images at 150 minutes after endothelial progenitor cell (EPC) injection into the ischemic hind limb muscle. Images of transplanted ^{18}F-FDG–labeled EPCs delivered with the matrix showed significantly higher retention compared with the cells injected alone. **B,** C-kit^{+} cell recruitment is greater in EPCs + matrix–treated MI hearts at 1 and 3 weeks after treatment. *PBS,* Phosphate-buffered saline.

and survival, generally, only a small fraction of transplanted cells are retained within the myocardium over the short term.[178] Over the long term, the loss of transplanted cells is cumulative as attrition worsens.[178] Our group and others have investigated merging principles from tissue engineering and cell therapy to improve the engraftment, retention, and survival of transplanted cells.[179,180] Suuronen and colleagues[180] assessed the efficacy of CD133^{+} EPCs delivered in a collagen I–based injectable hydrogel matrix in rat ischemic hindlimb. Transplanting cells within the biomaterial improved their retention greater than twofold (Fig. 101-6*A*), and rats receiving the combined therapy had greater arteriole and capillary densities in the ischemic hind limb compared with cells delivered alone.[180,181] More recently, we demonstrated that delivering early EPCs with the hydrogel matrix improved transplanted cell engraftment and the recruitment of endogenous c-kit^{+} cells (see Fig. 101-6*B*), and synergized to improve viability, perfusion, and function of infarcted myocardium.[182] Other investigators from our institute demonstrated that CSCs encapsulated within matrix-enriched capsules delivered in a murine MI model improved the long-term retention of cells and also resulted in greater functional recovery and reduced infarct sizes.[179]

In Situ Cell Therapy

The mainstay of current cell therapies has been a workflow of cells that (1) are procured from a donor (autologous or allogeneic), (2) are or are not further purified and/or primed, and (3) are delivered either via direct injection or intravenous or intracoronary infusion. This process may still hold some clinical potential, but it is costly, labor intensive, and relatively inefficient at promoting cardiac regeneration, if at all. Emerging advances in cell reprogramming may offer new opportunities, including in situ cell therapy. Several authors demonstrated that fibroblasts migrating to and populating the infarcted region of the heart may be reprogrammed into cardiomyocyte-like cells or inducible cardiomyocyte-like cells using a technique similar to the one required to produce IPSCs.[98,183,184] The efficiency of this procedure is low, with only 7% to 15% of cardiac fibroblasts converted to cardiomyocyte-like cells, but resulted in profound reductions in scar size and improvements in cardiac function.[183,184] Optimizing the efficacy and safety of this process are obvious requirements for translating them into the clinic; nevertheless, it provides an exciting alternative to the currently accepted paradigm of ex vivo cell therapy. Other groups have investigated similar methods at promoting cardiac regeneration in situ.[185] Eulalio and colleagues[185] demonstrated that administration of select microRNAs markedly stimulated cardiomyocyte proliferation in the border zone and resulted in almost complete anatomic and functional recovery. MicroRNAs may constitute another novel method for in situ cell therapy.

SUMMARY

We are currently in an exciting phase of cardiac cell therapy. Although early forays have not exactly measured up to our initial expectations, we are definitely wiser for it. As we move forward in trying to find the optimal therapy to regenerate the injured heart several pressing issues require addressing. First, we need to return to the laboratory to further understand regenerative mechanisms and how they may be mediated up to improve the efficiency of current and future therapies. Second, an iterative and systematic process of identifying the optimal cell type, dose, and delivery method is required and needs to be substantiated by well-designed, large-multicenter trials for each clinical entity. Moreover, these effects need to be followed up with sufficient power to prove benefits as well as safety. It is possible that BMCs will likely be forgotten as alternatives emerge with proven abilities to repair injured myocardium. Further still, ex vivo cell therapy may die out and lose favor with clinicians and investigators as tissue engineering or in situ methods evolve. It is difficult to predict which cell type or technology might ultimately prevail in our pursuit of a cardiac regenerative therapy, though given that the need for such a therapy will not likely subside anytime soon, the pursuit will continue passionately until we can finally mend a broken heart.

REFERENCES

1. Yeh RW, Sidney S, Chandra M, et al: Population trends in the incidence and outcomes of acute myocardial infarction. *N Engl J Med* 362:2155–2165, 2010.
2. White HD, Chew DP: Acute myocardial infarction. *Lancet* 372:570–584, 2008.

3. Roger VL, Go AS, Lloyd-Jones DM, et al: Heart disease and stroke statistics–2012 update: a report from the American Heart Association. *Circulation* 125:e2–e220, 2012.
4. Go AS, Mozaffarian D, Roger VL, et al: Heart disease and stroke statistics–2014 update: a report from the American Heart Association. *Circulation* 129:e28–e292, 2014.
5. Menasche P: Cardiac cell therapy: lessons from clinical trials. *J Mol Cell Cardiol* 50:258–265, 2011.
6. Hofmann M, Wollert KC, Meyer GP, et al: Monitoring of bone marrow cell homing into the infarcted human myocardium. *Circulation* 111:2198–2202, 2005.
7. Kang WJ, Kang HJ, Kim HS, et al: Tissue distribution of 18F-FDG-labeled peripheral hematopoietic stem cells after intracoronary administration in patients with myocardial infarction. *J Nucl Med* 47:1295–1301, 2006.
8. Dimmeler S, Zeiher AM, Schneider MD: Unchain my heart: the scientific foundations of cardiac repair. *J Clin Invest* 115:572–583, 2005.
9. Aicher A, Brenner W, Zuhayra M, et al: Assessment of the tissue distribution of transplanted human endothelial progenitor cells by radioactive labeling. *Circulation* 107:2134–2139, 2003.
10. Sanganalmath SK, Bolli R: Cell therapy for heart failure: a comprehensive overview of experimental and clinical studies, current challenges, and future directions. *Circ Res* 113:810–834, 2013.
11. Vale PR, Losordo DW, Milliken CE, et al: Left ventricular electromechanical mapping to assess efficacy of phVEGF(165) gene transfer for therapeutic angiogenesis in chronic myocardial ischemia. *Circulation* 102:965–974, 2000.
12. Kocher AA, Schlechta B, Gasparovicova A, et al: Stem cells and cardiac regeneration. *Transpl Int* 20:731–746, 2007.
13. Perin EC, Geng YJ, Willerson JT: Adult stem cell therapy in perspective. *Circulation* 107:935–938, 2003.
14. Abdel-Latif A, Bolli R, Tleyjeh IM, et al: Adult bone marrow-derived cells for cardiac repair: a systematic review and meta-analysis. *Arch Intern Med* 167:989–997, 2007.
15. Asahara T, Murohara T, Sullivan A, et al: Isolation of putative progenitor endothelial cells for angiogenesis. *Science* 275:964–967, 1997.
16. Balsam LB, Wagers AJ, Christensen JL, et al: Haematopoietic stem cells adopt mature haematopoietic fates in ischaemic myocardium. *Nature* 428:668–673, 2004.
17. Murry CE, Soonpaa MH, Reinecke H, et al: Haematopoietic stem cells do not transdifferentiate into cardiac myocytes in myocardial infarcts. *Nature* 428:664–668, 2004.
18. Orlic D, Kajstura J, Chimenti S, et al: Bone marrow cells regenerate the infarcted myocardium. *Nature* 410:701–705, 2001.
19. Tongers J, Losordo DW, Landmesser U: Stem and progenitor cell-based therapy in ischaemic heart disease: promise, uncertainties, and challenges. *Eur Heart J* 32:1197–1206, 2011.
20. Assmus B, Schächinger V, Teupe C, et al: Transplantation of Progenitor Cells and Regeneration Enhancement in Acute Myocardial Infarction (TOPCARE-AMI). *Circulation* 106:3009–3017, 2002.
21. Fernandez-Aviles F, San Roman JA, Garcia-Frade J, et al: Experimental and clinical regenerative capability of human bone marrow cells after myocardial infarction. *Circ Res* 95:742–748, 2004.
22. Schachinger V, Assmus B, Britten MB, et al: Transplantation of progenitor cells and regeneration enhancement in acute myocardial infarction: final one-year results of the TOPCARE-AMI Trial. *J Am Coll Cardiol* 44:1690–1699, 2004.
23. Schachinger V, Erbs S, Elsasser A, et al: Intracoronary bone marrow-derived progenitor cells in acute myocardial infarction. *N Engl J Med* 355:1210–1221, 2006.
24. Wollert KC, Meyer GP, Lotz J, et al: Intracoronary autologous bone-marrow cell transfer after myocardial infarction: the BOOST randomised controlled clinical trial. *Lancet* 364:141–148, 2004.
25. Schachinger V, Erbs S, Elsasser A, et al: Intracoronary bone marrow-derived progenitor cells in acute myocardial infarction. *N Engl J Med* 355:1210–1221, 2006.
26. Schachinger V, Erbs S, Elsasser A, et al: Improved clinical outcome after intracoronary administration of bone-marrow-derived progenitor cells in acute myocardial infarction: final 1-year results of the REPAIR-AMI trial. *Eur Heart J* 27:2775–2783, 2006.
27. Schaefer A, Meyer GP, Fuchs M, et al: Impact of intracoronary bone marrow cell transfer on diastolic function in patients after acute myocardial infarction: results from the BOOST trial. *Eur Heart J* 27:929–935, 2006.
28. Assmus B, Rolf A, Erbs S, et al: Clinical outcome 2 years after intracoronary administration of bone marrow-derived progenitor cells in acute myocardial infarction. *Circ Heart Fail* 3:89–96, 2010.
29. Cao F, Sun D, Li C, et al: Long-term myocardial functional improvement after autologous bone marrow mononuclear cells transplantation in patients with ST-segment elevation myocardial infarction: 4 years follow-up. *Eur Heart J* 30:1986–1994, 2009.
30. Yousef M, Schannwell CM, Kostering M, et al: The BALANCE Study: clinical benefit and long-term outcome after intracoronary autologous bone marrow cell transplantation in patients with acute myocardial infarction. *J Am Coll Cardiol* 53:2262–2269, 2009.
31. Huikuri HV, Kervinen K, Niemela M, et al: Effects of intracoronary injection of mononuclear bone marrow cells on left ventricular function, arrhythmia risk profile, and restenosis after thrombolytic therapy of acute myocardial infarction. *Eur Heart J* 29:2723–2732, 2008.
32. Meyer GP, Wollert KC, Lotz J, et al: Intracoronary bone marrow cell transfer after myocardial infarction: eighteen months' follow-up data from the randomized, controlled BOOST (BOne marrOw transfer to enhance ST-elevation infarct regeneration) trial. *Circulation* 113:1287–1294, 2006.
33. Meyer GP, Wollert KC, Lotz J, et al: Intracoronary bone marrow cell transfer after myocardial infarction: 5-year follow-up from the randomized-controlled BOOST trial. *Eur Heart J* 30:2978–2984, 2009.
34. Lunde K, Solheim S, Aakhus S, et al: Intracoronary injection of mononuclear bone marrow cells in acute myocardial infarction. *N Engl J Med* 355:1199–1209, 2006.
35. Roncalli J, Mouquet F, Piot C, et al: Intracoronary autologous mononucleated bone marrow cell infusion for acute myocardial infarction: results of the randomized multicenter BONAMI trial. *Eur Heart J* 32:1748–1757, 2011.
36. Beitnes JO, Gjesdal O, Lunde K, et al: Left ventricular systolic and diastolic function improve after acute myocardial infarction treated with acute percutaneous coronary intervention, but are not influenced by intracoronary injection of autologous mononuclear bone marrow cells: a 3 year serial echocardiographic substudy of the randomized-controlled ASTAMI study. *Eur J Echocardiogr* 12:98–106, 2011.
37. Beitnes JO, Hopp E, Lunde K, et al: Long-term results after intracoronary injection of autologous mononuclear bone marrow cells in acute myocardial infarction: the ASTAMI randomised, controlled study. *Heart* 95:1983–1989, 2009.
38. Lunde K, Solheim S, Aakhus S, et al: Exercise capacity and quality of life after intracoronary injection of autologous mononuclear bone marrow cells in acute myocardial infarction: results from the Autologous Stem cell Transplantation in Acute Myocardial Infarction (ASTAMI) randomized controlled trial. *Am Heart J* 154(710):e1–e8, 2007.
39. Traverse JH, Henry TD, Ellis SG, et al: Effect of intracoronary delivery of autologous bone marrow mononuclear cells 2 to 3 weeks following acute myocardial infarction on left ventricular function: the LateTIME randomized trial. *JAMA* 306:2110–2119, 2011.
40. Traverse JH, Henry TD, Pepine CJ, et al: Effect of the use and timing of bone marrow mononuclear cell delivery on left ventricular function after acute myocardial infarction: the TIME randomized trial. *JAMA* 308:2380–2389, 2012.
41. Traverse JH, Henry TD, Pepine CJ, et al: One-year follow-up of intracoronary stem cell delivery on left ventricular function following ST-elevation myocardial infarction. *JAMA* 311:301–302, 2013.
42. Surder D, Manka R, Lo Cicero V, et al: Intracoronary injection of bone marrow-derived mononuclear cells early or late after acute myocardial infarction: effects on global left ventricular function. *Circulation* 127:1968–1979, 2013.
43. Jeevanantham V, Butler M, Saad A, et al: Adult bone marrow cell therapy improves survival and induces long-term improvement in cardiac parameters: a systematic review and meta-analysis. *Circulation* 126:551–568, 2012.

44. Delewi R, Andriessen A, Tijssen JG, et al: Impact of intracoronary cell therapy on left ventricular function in the setting of acute myocardial infarction: a meta-analysis of randomised controlled clinical trials. *Heart* 99:225–232, 2013.
45. Daley GQ: The promise and perils of stem cell therapeutics. *Cell Stem Cell* 10:740–749, 2012.
46. Joseph C, Quach Julie M, Walkley Carl R, et al: Deciphering hematopoietic stem cells in their niches: a critical appraisal of genetic models, lineage tracing, and imaging strategies. *Cell Stem Cell* 13:520–533, 2013.
47. Perin EC, Silva GV, Zheng Y, et al: Randomized, double-blind pilot study of transendocardial injection of autologous aldehyde dehydrogenase-bright stem cells in patients with ischemic heart failure. *Am Heart J* 163:415–421, 21 e1, 2012.
48. Wognum AW, Eaves AC, Thomas TE: Identification and isolation of hematopoietic stem cells. *Arch Med Res* 34:461–475, 2003.
49. Orlic D, Kajstura J, Chimenti S, et al: Bone marrow cells regenerate infarcted myocardium. *Nature* 410:701–705, 2001.
50. Anversa P, Kajstura J, Rota M, et al: Regenerating new heart with stem cells. *J Clin Invest* 123:62–70, 2013.
51. Loffredo FS, Steinhauser ML, Gannon J, et al: Bone marrow-derived cell therapy stimulates endogenous cardiomyocyte progenitors and promotes cardiac repair. *Cell Stem Cell* 8:389–398, 2011.
52. Kang H-J, Kim H-S, Zhang S-Y, et al: Effects of intracoronary infusion of peripheral blood stem-cells mobilised with granulocyte-colony stimulating factor on left ventricular systolic function and restenosis after coronary stenting in myocardial infarction: the MAGIC cell randomised clinical trial. *Lancet* 363:751–756, 2004.
53. Asahara T, Takahashi T, Masuda H, et al: VEGF contributes to postnatal neovascularization by mobilizing bone marrow-derived endothelial progenitor cells. *EMBO J* 18:3964–3972, 1999.
54. Takahashi T, Kalka C, Masuda H, et al: Ischemia- and cytokine-induced mobilization of bone marrow-derived endothelial progenitor cells for neovascularization. *Nat Med* 5:434–438, 1999.
55. Fadini GP, Losordo D, Dimmeler S: Critical reevaluation of endothelial progenitor cell phenotypes for therapeutic and diagnostic use. *Circ Res* 110:624–637, 2012.
56. Ruel M, Suuronen EJ, Song J, et al: Effects of off-pump versus on-pump coronary artery bypass grafting on function and viability of circulating endothelial progenitor cells. *J Thorac Cardiovasc Surg* 130:633–639, 2005.
57. Urbich C, Dimmeler S: Endothelial progenitor cells functional characterization. *Trends Cardiovasc Med* 14:318–322, 2004.
58. Hur J, Yoon CH, Kim HS, et al: Characterization of two types of endothelial progenitor cells and their different contributions to neovasculogenesis. *Arterioscl Throm Vas* 24:288–293, 2004.
59. Kawamoto A, Tkebuchava T, Yamaguchi J, et al: Intramyocardial transplantation of autologous endothelial progenitor cells for therapeutic neovascularization of myocardial ischemia. *Circulation* 107:461–468, 2003.
60. Kocher AA, Schuster MD, Szabolcs MJ, et al: Neovascularization of ischemic myocardium by human bone-marrow-derived angioblasts prevents cardiomyocyte apoptosis, reduces remodeling and improves cardiac function. *Nat Med* 7:430–436, 2001.
61. Badorff C, Brandes RP, Popp R, et al: Transdifferentiation of blood-derived human adult endothelial progenitor cells into functionally active cardiomyocytes. *Circulation* 107:1024–1032, 2003.
62. Gruh I, Beilner J, Blomer U, et al: No evidence of transdifferentiation of human endothelial progenitor cells into cardiomyocytes after coculture with neonatal rat cardiomyocytes. *Circulation* 113:1326–1334, 2006.
63. Urbich C, Aicher A, Heeschen C, et al: Soluble factors released by endothelial progenitor cells promote migration of endothelial cells and cardiac resident progenitor cells. *J Mol Cell Cardiol* 39:733–742, 2005.
64. Assmus B, Honold J, Schachinger V, et al: Transcoronary transplantation of progenitor cells after myocardial infarction. *N Engl J Med* 355:1222–1232, 2006.
65. Valgimigli M, Rigolin GM, Fucili A, et al: CD34+ and endothelial progenitor cells in patients with various degrees of congestive heart failure. *Circulation* 110:1209–1212, 2004.
66. Sahoo S, Klychko E, Thorne T, et al: Exosomes from human CD34(+) stem cells mediate their proangiogenic paracrine activity. *Circ Res* 109:724–728, 2011.
67. Faridi F, Ponnusamy K, Quagliano-Lo Coco I, et al: Aberrant epigenetic regulators control expansion of human CD34+ hematopoietic stem/progenitor cells. *Front Genet* 4:254, 2013.
68. Nielsen JS, McNagny KM: CD34 is a key regulator of hematopoietic stem cell trafficking to bone marrow and mast cell progenitor trafficking in the periphery. *Microcirculation* 16:487–496, 2009.
69. Yeh ET, Zhang S, Wu HD, et al: Transdifferentiation of human peripheral blood CD34+-enriched cell population into cardiomyocytes, endothelial cells, and smooth muscle cells in vivo. *Circulation* 108:2070–2073, 2003.
70. Quirici N, Soligo D, Caneva L, et al: Differentiation and expansion of endothelial cells from human bone marrow CD133(+) cells. *Br J Haematol* 115:186–194, 2001.
71. Zhang S, Wang D, Estrov Z, et al: Both cell fusion and transdifferentiation account for the transformation of human peripheral blood CD34-positive cells into cardiomyocytes in vivo. *Circulation* 110:3803–3807, 2004.
72. Zhang S, Shpall E, Willerson JT, et al: Fusion of human hematopoietic progenitor cells and murine cardiomyocytes is mediated by alpha 4 beta 1 integrin/vascular cell adhesion molecule-1 interaction. *Circ Res* 100:693–702, 2007.
73. Kawamoto A, Iwasaki H, Kusano K, et al: CD34-positive cells exhibit increased potency and safety for therapeutic neovascularization after myocardial infarction compared with total mononuclear cells. *Circulation* 114:2163–2169, 2006.
74. Tendera M, Wojakowski W, Ruzyllo W, et al: Intracoronary infusion of bone marrow-derived selected CD34+CXCR4+ cells and non-selected mononuclear cells in patients with acute STEMI and reduced left ventricular ejection fraction: results of randomized, multicentre Myocardial Regeneration by Intracoronary Infusion of Selected Population of Stem Cells in Acute Myocardial Infarction (REGENT) Trial. *Eur Heart J* 30:1313–1321, 2009.
75. Losordo DW, Schatz RA, White CJ, et al: Intramyocardial transplantation of autologous CD34+ stem cells for intractable angina: a phase I/IIa double-blind, randomized controlled trial. *Circulation* 115:3165–3172, 2007.
76. Losordo DW, Henry TD, Davidson C, et al: Intramyocardial, autologous CD34+ cell therapy for refractory angina. *Circ Res* 109:428–436, 2011.
77. Ranganath SH, Levy O, Inamdar MS, et al: Harnessing the mesenchymal stem cell secretome for the treatment of cardiovascular disease. *Cell Stem Cell* 10:244–258, 2012.
78. Choi YH, Kurtz A, Stamm C: Mesenchymal stem cells for cardiac cell therapy. *Hum Gene Ther* 22:3–17, 2011.
79. Pittenger MF, Martin BJ: Mesenchymal stem cells and their potential as cardiac therapeutics. *Circ Res* 95:9–20, 2004.
80. Prockop DJ, Oh JY: Mesenchymal stem/stromal cells (MSCs): role as guardians of inflammation. *Mol Ther* 20:14–20, 2012.
81. Huang XP, Sun Z, Miyagi Y, et al: Differentiation of allogeneic mesenchymal stem cells induces immunogenicity and limits their long-term benefits for myocardial repair. *Circulation* 122:2419–2429, 2010.
82. Hatzistergos KE, Quevedo H, Oskouei BN, et al: Bone marrow mesenchymal stem cells stimulate cardiac stem cell proliferation and differentiation. *Circ Res* 107:913–922, 2010.
83. Noiseux N, Gnecchi M, Lopez-Ilasaca M, et al: Mesenchymal stem cells overexpressing Akt dramatically repair infarcted myocardium and improve cardiac function despite infrequent cellular fusion or differentiation. *Mol Ther* 14:840–850, 2006.
84. Iso Y, Spees JL, Serrano C, et al: Multipotent human stromal cells improve cardiac function after myocardial infarction in mice without long-term engraftment. *Biochem Biophys Res Commun* 354:700–706, 2007.
85. Engelmann MG, Theiss HD, Hennig-Theiss C, et al: Autologous bone marrow stem cell mobilization induced by granulocyte colony-stimulating factor after subacute ST-segment elevation myocardial infarction undergoing late revascularization: final results from the G-CSF-STEMI (Granulocyte Colony-Stimulating Factor ST-Segment Elevation Myocardial Infarction) trial. *J Am Coll Cardiol* 48:1712–1721, 2006.
86. Ripa RS, Haack-Sorensen M, Wang Y, et al: Bone marrow derived mesenchymal cell mobilization by granulocyte-colony stimulating factor after acute myocardial infarction: results from the Stem Cells in Myocardial Infarction (STEMMI) trial. *Circulation* 116:I24–I30, 2007.

87. Ripa RS, Jorgensen E, Wang Y, et al: Stem cell mobilization induced by subcutaneous granulocyte-colony stimulating factor to improve cardiac regeneration after acute ST-elevation myocardial infarction: result of the double-blind, randomized, placebo-controlled stem cells in myocardial infarction (STEMMI) trial. *Circulation* 113:1983–1992, 2006.
88. Zohlnhofer D, Ott I, Mehilli J, et al: Stem cell mobilization by granulocyte colony-stimulating factor in patients with acute myocardial infarction: a randomized controlled trial. *JAMA* 295:1003–1010, 2006.
89. Hare JM, Traverse JH, Henry TD, et al: A randomized, double-blind, placebo-controlled, dose-escalation study of intravenous adult human mesenchymal stem cells (prochymal) after acute myocardial infarction. *J Am Coll Cardiol* 54:2277–2286, 2009.
90. Hare JM, Fishman JE, Gerstenblith G, et al: Comparison of allogeneic vs autologous bone marrow-derived mesenchymal stem cells delivered by transendocardial injection in patients with ischemic cardiomyopathy: the POSEIDON randomized trial. *JAMA* 308:2369–2379, 2012.
91. Delewi R, Piek JJ, Hirsch A: Letter by Delewi et al regarding article, "Adult bone marrow cell therapy improves survival and induces long-term improvement in cardiac parameters: a systematic review and meta-analysis." *Circulation* 127:e547, 2013.
92. Thomson JA, Itskovitz-Eldor J, Shapiro SS, et al: Embryonic stem cell lines derived from human blastocysts. *Science* 282:1145–1147, 1998.
93. He JQ, Ma Y, Lee Y, et al: Human embryonic stem cells develop into multiple types of cardiac myocytes: action potential characterization. *Circ Res* 93:32–39, 2003.
94. Laflamme MA, Gold J, Xu C, et al: Formation of human myocardium in the rat heart from human embryonic stem cells. *Am J Pathol* 167:663–671, 2005.
95. Lu J, Hou R, Booth CJ, et al: Defined culture conditions of human embryonic stem cells. *Proc Natl Acad Sci U S A* 103:5688–5693, 2006.
96. Xu C: Characterization and enrichment of cardiomyocytes derived from human embryonic stem cells. *Circ Res* 91:501–508, 2002.
97. Kehat I, Kenyagin-Karsenti D, Snir M, et al: Human embryonic stem cells can differentiate into myocytes with structural and functional properties of cardiomyocytes. *J Clin Invest* 108:407–414, 2001.
98. Laflamme MA, Murry CE: Heart regeneration. *Nature* 473:326–335, 2011.
99. Min JY, Yang Y, Converso KL, et al: Transplantation of embryonic stem cells improves cardiac function in postinfarcted rats. *J Appl Physiol* 92:288–296, 2002.
100. Cai J, Yi FF, Yang XC, et al: Transplantation of embryonic stem cell-derived cardiomyocytes improves cardiac function in infarcted rat hearts. *Cytotherapy* 9:283–291, 2007.
101. Caspi O, Huber I, Kehat I, et al: Transplantation of human embryonic stem cell-derived cardiomyocytes improves myocardial performance in infarcted rat hearts. *J Am Coll Cardiol* 50:1884–1893, 2007.
102. Ménard C, Hagège AA, Agbulut O, et al: Transplantation of cardiac-committed mouse embryonic stem cells to infarcted sheep myocardium: a preclinical study. *Lancet* 366:1005–1012, 2005.
103. Nussbaum J, Minami E, Laflamme MA, et al: Transplantation of undifferentiated murine embryonic stem cells in the heart: teratoma formation and immune response. *FASEB J* 21:1345–1357, 2007.
104. Wollert KC: Cell therapy for acute myocardial infarction. *Curr Opin Pharmacol* 8:202–210, 2008.
105. The 2012 Nobel Prize in Physiology or Medicine—Press Release. Nobel Media AB 2013, 2013. (Accessed November 11, 2013, at http://www.nobelprize.org/nobel_prizes/medicine/laureates/2012/press.html.)
106. Takahashi K, Yamanaka S: Induction of pluripotent stem cells from mouse embryonic and adult fibroblast cultures by defined factors. *Cell* 126:663–676, 2006.
107. Takahashi K, Tanabe K, Ohnuki M, et al: Induction of pluripotent stem cells from adult human fibroblasts by defined factors. *Cell* 131:861–872, 2007.
108. Zwi L, Caspi O, Arbel G, et al: Cardiomyocyte differentiation of human induced pluripotent stem cells. *Circulation* 120:1513–1523, 2009.
109. Zhang J, Wilson GF, Soerens AG, et al: Functional cardiomyocytes derived from human induced pluripotent stem cells. *Circ Res* 104:e30–e41, 2009.
110. Grskovic M, Javaherian A, Strulovici B, et al: Induced pluripotent stem cells–opportunities for disease modelling and drug discovery. *Nat Rev Drug Discov* 10:915–929, 2011.
111. Lee AS, Xu D, Plews JR, et al: Preclinical derivation and imaging of autologously transplanted canine induced pluripotent stem cells. *J Biol Chem* 286:32697–32704, 2011.
112. Gu M, Nguyen PK, Lee AS, et al: Microfluidic single-cell analysis shows that porcine induced pluripotent stem cell-derived endothelial cells improve myocardial function by paracrine activation. *Circ Res* 111:882–893, 2012.
113. Pera MF: Stem cells: The dark side of induced pluripotency. *Nature* 471:46–47, 2011.
114. Shi Y, Desponts C, Do JT, et al: Induction of pluripotent stem cells from mouse embryonic fibroblasts by Oct4 and Klf4 with small-molecule compounds. *Cell Stem Cell* 3:568–574, 2008.
115. Warren L, Manos PD, Ahfeldt T, et al: Highly efficient reprogramming to pluripotency and directed differentiation of human cells with synthetic modified mRNA. *Cell Stem Cell* 7:618–630, 2010.
116. Kawamura M, Miyagawa S, Miki K, et al: Feasibility, safety, and therapeutic efficacy of human induced pluripotent stem cell-derived cardiomyocyte sheets in a porcine ischemic cardiomyopathy model. *Circulation* 126:S29–S37, 2012.
117. Okano H, Nakamura M, Yoshida K, et al: Steps toward safe cell therapy using induced pluripotent stem cells. *Circ Res* 112:523–533, 2013.
118. Bergmann O, Bhardwaj RD, Bernard S, et al: Evidence for cardiomyocyte renewal in humans. *Science* 324:98–102, 2009.
119. Beltrami AP, Urbanek K, Kajstura J, et al: Evidence that human cardiac myocytes divide after myocardial infarction. *N Engl J Med* 344:1750–1757, 2001.
120. Beltrami AP, Barlucchi L, Torella D, et al: Adult cardiac stem cells are multipotent and support myocardial regeneration. *Cell* 114:763–776, 2003.
121. Hsieh PC, Segers VF, Davis ME, et al: Evidence from a genetic fate-mapping study that stem cells refresh adult mammalian cardiomyocytes after injury. *Nat Med* 13:970–974, 2007.
122. Bearzi C, Rota M, Hosoda T, et al: Human cardiac stem cells. *Proc Natl Acad Sci U S A* 104:14068–14073, 2007.
123. Senyo SE, Steinhauser ML, Pizzimenti CL, et al: Mammalian heart renewal by pre-existing cardiomyocytes. *Nature* 493:433–436, 2013.
124. Ellison GM, Vicinanza C, Smith AJ, et al: Adult c-kit(pos) cardiac stem cells are necessary and sufficient for functional cardiac regeneration and repair. *Cell* 154:827–842, 2013.
125. Leri A, Kajstura J, Anversa P: Role of cardiac stem cells in cardiac pathophysiology: a paradigm shift in human myocardial biology. *Circ Res* 109:941–961, 2011.
126. Urbanek K, Torella D, Sheikh F, et al: Myocardial regeneration by activation of multipotent cardiac stem cells in ischemic heart failure. *Proc Natl Acad Sci U S A* 102:8692–8697, 2005.
127. Bolli R, Chugh AR, D'Amario D, et al: Cardiac stem cells in patients with ischaemic cardiomyopathy (SCIPIO): initial results of a randomised phase 1 trial. *Lancet* 378:1847–1857, 2011.
128. Makkar RR, Smith RR, Cheng K, et al: Intracoronary cardiosphere-derived cells for heart regeneration after myocardial infarction (CADUCEUS): a prospective, randomised phase 1 trial. *Lancet* 379:895–904, 2012.
129. Rota M, Padin-Iruegas ME, Misao Y, et al: Local activation or implantation of cardiac progenitor cells rescues scarred infarcted myocardium improving cardiac function. *Circ Res* 103:107–116, 2008.
130. Tang XL, Rokosh G, Sanganalmath SK, et al: Intracoronary administration of cardiac progenitor cells alleviates left ventricular dysfunction in rats with a 30-day-old infarction. *Circulation* 121:293–305, 2010.
131. Bolli R, Tang XL, Sanganalmath SK, et al: Intracoronary delivery of autologous cardiac stem cells improves cardiac function in a porcine model of chronic ischemic cardiomyopathy. *Circulation* 128:122–131, 2013.
132. Chugh AR, Beache GM, Loughran JH, et al: Administration of cardiac stem cells in patients with ischemic cardiomyopathy: the

SCIPIO trial: surgical aspects and interim analysis of myocardial function and viability by magnetic resonance. *Circulation* 126:S54–S64, 2012.
133. Smith RR, Barile L, Cho HC, et al: Regenerative potential of cardiosphere-derived cells expanded from percutaneous endomyocardial biopsy specimens. *Circulation* 115:896–908, 2007.
134. Messina E, De Angelis L, Frati G, et al: Isolation and expansion of adult cardiac stem cells from human and murine heart. *Circ Res* 95:911–921, 2004.
135. Davis DR, Kizana E, Terrovitis J, et al: Isolation and expansion of functionally-competent cardiac progenitor cells directly from heart biopsies. *J Mol Cell Cardiol* 49:312–321, 2010.
136. Malliaras K, Li TS, Luthringer D, et al: Safety and efficacy of allogeneic cell therapy in infarcted rats transplanted with mismatched cardiosphere-derived cells. *Circulation* 125:100–112, 2012.
137. Johnston PV, Sasano T, Mills K, et al: Engraftment, differentiation, and functional benefits of autologous cardiosphere-derived cells in porcine ischemic cardiomyopathy. *Circulation* 120:1075–1083, 7 p following 83, 2009.
138. Andersen DC, Andersen P, Schneider M, et al: Murine "cardiospheres" are not a source of stem cells with cardiomyogenic potential. *Stem Cells* 27:1571–1581, 2009.
139. Davis DR, Ruckdeschel Smith R, Marban E: Human cardiospheres are a source of stem cells with cardiomyogenic potential. *Stem Cells* 28:903–904, 2010.
140. Yoon CH, Hur J, Park KW, et al: Synergistic neovascularization by mixed transplantation of early endothelial progenitor cells and late outgrowth endothelial cells: the role of angiogenic cytokines and matrix metalloproteinases. *Circulation* 112:1618–1627, 2005.
141. Latham N, Ye B, Jackson R, et al: Human blood and cardiac stem cells synergize to enhance cardiac repair when cotransplanted into ischemic myocardium. *Circulation* 128:S105–S112, 2013.
142. Williams AR, Hatzistergos KE, Addicott B, et al: Enhanced effect of combining human cardiac stem cells and bone marrow mesenchymal stem cells to reduce infarct size and to restore cardiac function after myocardial infarction. *Circulation* 127:213–223, 2013.
143. Fukata M, Ishikawa F, Najima Y, et al: Contribution of bone marrow-derived hematopoietic stem/progenitor cells to the generation of donor-marker(+) cardiomyocytes in vivo. *PLoS ONE* 8:e62506, 2013.
144. Rota M, Kajstura J, Hosoda T, et al: Bone marrow cells adopt the cardiomyogenic fate in vivo. *Proc Natl Acad Sci U S A* 104:17783–17788, 2007.
145. Kajstura J, Rota M, Whang B, et al: Bone marrow cells differentiate in cardiac cell lineages after infarction independently of cell fusion. *Circ Res* 96:127–137, 2005.
146. Mirotsou M, Jayawardena TM, Schmeckpeper J, et al: Paracrine mechanisms of stem cell reparative and regenerative actions in the heart. *J Mol Cell Cardiol* 50:280–289, 2011.
147. Rose RA, Jiang H, Wang X, et al: Bone marrow-derived mesenchymal stromal cells express cardiac-specific markers, retain the stromal phenotype, and do not become functional cardiomyocytes in vitro. *Stem Cells* 26:2884–2892, 2008.
148. Nakanishi C, Yamagishi M, Yamahara K, et al: Activation of cardiac progenitor cells through paracrine effects of mesenchymal stem cells. *Biochem Biophys Res Commun* 374:11–16, 2008.
149. Dawn B, Stein AB, Urbanek K, et al: Cardiac stem cells delivered intravascularly traverse the vessel barrier, regenerate infarcted myocardium, and improve cardiac function. *Proc Natl Acad Sci U S A* 102:3766–3771, 2005.
150. Chimenti I, Smith RR, Li TS, et al: Relative roles of direct regeneration versus paracrine effects of human cardiosphere-derived cells transplanted into infarcted mice. *Circ Res* 106:971–980, 2010.
151. Gnecchi M, Zhang Z, Ni A, et al: Paracrine mechanisms in adult stem cell signaling and therapy. *Circ Res* 103:1204–1219, 2008.
152. Cho HJ, Lee N, Lee JY, et al: Role of host tissues for sustained humoral effects after endothelial progenitor cell transplantation into the ischemic heart. *J Exp Med* 204:3257–3269, 2007.
153. Ceradini DJ, Kulkarni AR, Callaghan MJ, et al: Progenitor cell trafficking is regulated by hypoxic gradients through HIF-1 induction of SDF-1. *Nat Med* 10:858–864, 2004.
154. Jin DK, Shido K, Kopp HG, et al: Cytokine-mediated deployment of SDF-1 induces revascularization through recruitment of CXCR4+ hemangiocytes. *Nat Med* 12:557–567, 2006.
155. Presta M, Dell'Era P, Mitola S, et al: Fibroblast growth factor/fibroblast growth factor receptor system in angiogenesis. *Cytokine Growth Factor Rev* 16:159–178, 2005.
156. Tse HF, Siu CW, Zhu SG, et al: Paracrine effects of direct intramyocardial implantation of bone marrow derived cells to enhance neovascularization in chronic ischaemic myocardium. *Eur J Heart Fail* 9:747–753, 2007.
157. Mackie AR, Klyachko E, Thorne T, et al: Sonic hedgehog-modified human CD34+ cells preserve cardiac function after acute myocardial infarction. *Circ Res* 111:312–321, 2012.
158. Iekushi K, Seeger F, Assmus B, et al: Regulation of cardiac microRNAs by bone marrow mononuclear cell therapy in myocardial infarction. *Circulation* 125:1765–1773, S1–S7, 2012.
159. Fazel S, Cimini M, Chen L, et al: Cardioprotective c-kit+ cells are from the bone marrow and regulate the myocardial balance of angiogenic cytokines. *J Clin Invest* 116:1865–1877, 2006.
160. Nguyen BK, Maltais S, Perrault LP, et al: Improved function and myocardial repair of infarcted heart by intracoronary injection of mesenchymal stem cell-derived growth factors. *J Cardiovasc Transl Res* 3:547–558, 2010.
161. Frangogiannis NG: Regulation of the inflammatory response in cardiac repair. *Circ Res* 110:159–173, 2012.
162. Lee RH, Pulin AA, Seo MJ, et al: Intravenous hMSCs improve myocardial infarction in mice because cells embolized in lung are activated to secrete the anti-inflammatory protein TSG-6. *Cell Stem Cell* 5:54–63, 2009.
163. Weber KT, Sun Y, Bhattacharya SK, et al: Myofibroblast-mediated mechanisms of pathological remodelling of the heart. *Nat Rev Cardiol* 10:15–26, 2013.
164. Jugdutt BI: Ventricular remodeling after infarction and the extracellular collagen matrix: when is enough enough? *Circulation* 108:1395–1403, 2003.
165. Nagaya N, Kangawa K, Itoh T, et al: Transplantation of mesenchymal stem cells improves cardiac function in a rat model of dilated cardiomyopathy. *Circulation* 112:1128–1135, 2005.
166. Malliaras K, Kreke M, Marban E: The stuttering progress of cell therapy for heart disease. *Clin Pharmacol Ther* 90:532–541, 2011.
167. Hirsch A, Nijveldt R, van der Vleuten PA, et al: Intracoronary infusion of mononuclear cells from bone marrow or peripheral blood compared with standard therapy in patients after acute myocardial infarction treated by primary percutaneous coronary intervention: results of the randomized controlled HEBE trial. *Eur Heart J* 32:1736–1747, 2011.
168. Wohrle J, Merkle N, Mailander V, et al: Results of intracoronary stem cell therapy after acute myocardial infarction. *Am J Cardiol* 105:804–812, 2010.
169. Reffelmann T, Konemann S, Kloner RA: Promise of blood- and bone marrow-derived stem cell transplantation for functional cardiac repair: putting it in perspective with existing therapy. *J Am Coll Cardiol* 53:305–308, 2009.
170. Wang X, Takagawa J, Lam VC, et al: Donor myocardial infarction impairs the therapeutic potential of bone marrow cells by an interleukin-1-mediated inflammatory response. *Sci Transl Med* 3:100ra90, 2011.
171. Fadini GP, Sartore S, Schiavon M, et al: Diabetes impairs progenitor cell mobilisation after hindlimb ischaemia-reperfusion injury in rats. *Diabetologia* 49:3075–3084, 2006.
172. Katare R, Oikawa A, Cesselli D, et al: Boosting the pentose phosphate pathway restores cardiac progenitor cell availability in diabetes. *Cardiovasc Res* 97:55–65, 2013.
173. Kuraitis D, Hou C, Zhang Y, et al: Ex vivo generation of a highly potent population of circulating angiogenic cells using a collagen matrix. *J Mol Cell Cardiol* 51:187–197, 2011.
174. Taljaard M, Ward MR, Kutryk MJ, et al: Rationale and design of Enhanced Angiogenic Cell Therapy in Acute Myocardial Infarction (ENACT-AMI): the first randomized placebo-controlled trial of enhanced progenitor cell therapy for acute myocardial infarction. *Am Heart J* 159:354–360, 2010.
175. Landmesser U, Drexler H: The clinical significance of endothelial dysfunction. *Curr Opin Cardiol* 20:547–551, 2005.

176. Aicher A, Heeschen C, Mildner-Rihm C, et al: Essential role of endothelial nitric oxide synthase for mobilization of stem and progenitor cells. *Nat Med* 9:1370–1376, 2003.
177. Sasaki K, Heeschen C, Aicher A, et al: Ex vivo pretreatment of bone marrow mononuclear cells with endothelial NO synthase enhancer AVE9488 enhances their functional activity for cell therapy. *Proc Natl Acad Sci U S A* 103:14537–14541, 2006.
178. Terrovitis JV, Smith RR, Marban E: Assessment and optimization of cell engraftment after transplantation into the heart. *Circ Res* 106:479–494, 2010.
179. Mayfield AE, Tilokee EL, Latham N, et al: The effect of encapsulation of cardiac stem cells within matrix-enriched hydrogel capsules on cell survival, post-ischemic cell retention and cardiac function. *Biomaterials* 2013.
180. Suuronen EJ, Veinot JP, Wong S, et al: Tissue-engineered injectable collagen-based matrices for improved cell delivery and vascularization of ischemic tissue using CD133+ progenitors expanded from the peripheral blood. *Circulation* 114:I138–I144, 2006.
181. Zhang Y, Thorn S, DaSilva JN, et al: Collagen-based matrices improve the delivery of transplanted circulating progenitor cells: development and demonstration by ex vivo radionuclide cell labeling and in vivo tracking with positron-emission tomography. *Circ Cardiovasc Imag* 1:197–204, 2008.
182. Ahmadi A, McNeill B, Vulesevic B, et al: The role of integrin α2 in cell and matrix therapy that improves perfusion, viability and function of infarcted myocardium. *Biomaterials* 35:4749–4758, 2014.
183. Qian L, Huang Y, Spencer CI, et al: In vivo reprogramming of murine cardiac fibroblasts into induced cardiomyocytes. *Nature* 485:593–598, 2012.
184. Song K, Nam YJ, Luo X, et al: Heart repair by reprogramming non-myocytes with cardiac transcription factors. *Nature* 485:599–604, 2012.
185. Eulalio A, Mano M, Dal Ferro M, et al: Functional screening identifies miRNAs inducing cardiac regeneration. *Nature* 492:376–381, 2012.
186. Choi JH, Choi J, Lee WS, et al: Lack of additional benefit of intracoronary transplantation of autologous peripheral blood stem cell in patients with acute myocardial infarction. *Circ J* 71:486–494, 2007.
187. Ge J, Li Y, Qian J, et al: Efficacy of emergent transcatheter transplantation of stem cells for treatment of acute myocardial infarction (TCT-STAMI). *Heart* 92:1764–1767, 2006.
188. Strauer BE, Brehm M, Zeus T, et al: Repair of infarcted myocardium by autologous intracoronary mononuclear bone marrow cell transplantation in humans. *Circulation* 106:1913–1918, 2002.
189. Chen SL, Fang WW, Ye F, et al: Effect on left ventricular function of intracoronary transplantation of autologous bone marrow mesenchymal stem cell in patients with acute myocardial infarction. *Am J Cardiol* 94:92–95, 2004.
190. Schachinger V, Assmus B, Erbs S, et al: Intracoronary infusion of bone marrow-derived mononuclear cells abrogates adverse left ventricular remodelling post-acute myocardial infarction: insights from the reinfusion of enriched progenitor cells and infarct remodelling in acute myocardial infarction (REPAIR-AMI) trial. *Eur J Heart Fail* 11:973–979, 2009.
191. Janssens S, Dubois C, Bogaert J, et al: Autologous bone marrow-derived stem-cell transfer in patients with ST-segment elevation myocardial infarction: double-blind, randomised controlled trial. *Lancet* 367:113–121, 2006.
192. Li ZQ, Zhang M, Jing YZ, et al: The clinical study of autologous peripheral blood stem cell transplantation by intracoronary infusion in patients with acute myocardial infarction (AMI). *Int J Cardiol* 115:52–56, 2007.
193. Assmus B, Fischer-Rasokat U, Honold J, et al: Transcoronary transplantation of functionally competent BMCs is associated with a decrease in natriuretic peptide serum levels and improved survival of patients with chronic postinfarction heart failure: results of the TOPCARE-CHD Registry. *Circ Res* 100:1234–1241, 2007.
194. Katritsis DG, Sotiropoulou PA, Karvouni E, et al: Transcoronary transplantation of autologous mesenchymal stem cells and endothelial progenitors into infarcted human myocardium. *Catheter Cardiovasc Interv* 65:321–329, 2005.
195. Perin EC, Dohmann HF, Borojevic R, et al: Transendocardial, autologous bone marrow cell transplantation for severe, chronic ischemic heart failure. *Circulation* 107:2294–2302, 2003.
196. Stamm C, Kleine HD, Choi YH, et al: Intramyocardial delivery of CD133+ bone marrow cells and coronary artery bypass grafting for chronic ischemic heart disease: safety and efficacy studies. *J Thorac Cardiovasc Surg* 133:717–725, 2007.
197. Stamm C, Westphal B, Kleine HD, et al: Autologous bone-marrow stem-cell transplantation for myocardial regeneration. *Lancet* 361:45–46, 2003.
198. Ahmadi H, Baharvand H, Ashtiani SK, et al: Safety analysis and improved cardiac function following local autologous transplantation of CD133(+) enriched bone marrow cells after myocardial infarction. *Curr Neurovasc Res* 4:153–160, 2007.
199. Hendrikx M, Hensen K, Clijsters C, et al: Recovery of regional but not global contractile function by the direct intramyocardial autologous bone marrow transplantation: results from a randomized controlled clinical trial. *Circulation* 114:I101–I107, 2006.
200. Mocini D, Staibano M, Mele L, et al: Autologous bone marrow mononuclear cell transplantation in patients undergoing coronary artery bypass grafting. *Am Heart J* 151:192–197, 2006.
201. Tse HF, Kwong YL, Chan JK, et al: Angiogenesis in ischaemic myocardium by intramyocardial autologous bone marrow mononuclear cell implantation. *Lancet* 361:47–49, 2003.
202. Quyyumi AA, Waller EK, Murrow J, et al: CD34(+) cell infusion after ST elevation myocardial infarction is associated with improved perfusion and is dose dependent. *Am Heart J* 161:98–105, 2011.
203. Williams AR, Trachtenberg B, Velazquez DL, et al: Intramyocardial stem cell injection in patients with ischemic cardiomyopathy: functional recovery and reverse remodeling. *Circ Res* 108:792–796, 2011.
204. Chih S, Macdonald PS, McCrohon JA, et al: Granulocyte colony stimulating factor in chronic angina to stimulate neovascularisation: a placebo controlled crossover trial. *Heart* 98:282–290, 2012.
205. Heldman AW, Difede DL, Fishman JE, et al: Transendocardial mesenchymal stem cells and mononuclear bone marrow cells for ischemic cardiomyopathy: the TAC-HFT randomized trial. *JAMA* 311(1):62–73, 2014.

CHAPTER 102

SURGERY FOR PULMONARY EMBOLISM

Patricia A. Thistlethwaite • Michael Madani • Stuart W. Jamieson

CHAPTER OUTLINE

Pulmonary thromboembolism is a significant cause of morbidity and mortality in the United States and worldwide. The estimated incidence of acute pulmonary embolism is approximately 63 per 100,000 patients in the United States, based on clinical and radiographic data.[1] Acute pulmonary embolism is the cause of approximately 235,000 deaths per year based on autopsy data. Acute pulmonary embolism occurs half as often as acute myocardial infarction and is three times as common as cerebrovascular accident. It is the third most common cause of death (after heart disease and cancer).[2] Estimates of the incidence of acute pulmonary embolism, however, are generally thought to be low, because in 70% to 80% of patients in whom the primary cause of death was pulmonary embolism, the diagnosis was unsuspected premortem.[3,4]

Of patients who survive an acute pulmonary embolic event, approximately 3.8% will go on to develop chronic pulmonary hypertension (PH).[5] Once PH develops, the prognosis is poor, and this prognosis is worsened in the absence of intracardiac shunt. Patients with PH caused by pulmonary emboli fall into a higher risk category than those with Eisenmenger syndrome, and they encounter a higher mortality rate. In fact, once the mean pulmonary pressure in patients with thromboembolic disease exceeds 50 mm Hg, the 3-year mortality rate approaches 90%.[6] Despite an improved understanding of pathogenesis, diagnosis, and management, pulmonary emboli and their long-term sequelae remain frequent and often fatal disorders.

Pulmonary embolism was first described by Laennec in 1819.[7] It was he who related the condition to deep venous thrombosis, and Virchow[8] later associated the three factors predisposing to venous thrombosis as stasis, hypercoagulability, and vessel wall injury. Virchow distinguished two types of thrombus in the pulmonary arteries of such patients: the embolus that arose as thrombus in a systemic vein and the thrombus that occurred in situ within the pulmonary arteries distal to the occluding embolus as a result of the stagnant blood flow in that segment. To prove that pulmonary emboli arose from the peripheral venous circulation, Virchow inserted pieces of rubber or venous thrombi recovered from humans at autopsy into the jugular or femoral veins of dogs. When the animals were sacrificed, the foreign embolic material was found in the pulmonary arteries. Although pulmonary embolism can be caused by tumors, septic emboli, and foreign bodies, the overwhelming occurrence of pulmonary embolism is due to venous thromboembolism.[9]

ACUTE PULMONARY THROMBOEMBOLIC DISEASE

Clinical Points

The majority of pulmonary thromboembolic episodes are silent, and it is not until the amount of embolic material is substantial that the patient becomes symptomatic. After an acute, major thromboembolic episode, approximately 15% to 20% of patients die within 48 hours.[10] Most of the remaining patients resolve the emboli substantially by a variety of mechanisms. Therefore, it is in the subgroup of patients who have a sudden fatal outcome (≈100,000 annually) that invasive therapy for acute pulmonary embolism might be considered.

Although the role of surgical therapy for the PH resulting from chronic pulmonary emboli is now well established, the appropriate treatment for acute pulmonary embolism remains unclear. There are several reasons for this. Many patients die of massive pulmonary embolism in the terminal phases of another illness, which would make aggressive therapy inappropriate. For patients in whom invasive therapy is potentially indicated, there is substantial difficulty in defining which patients will respond to anticoagulation therapy for an acute massive pulmonary embolism in the limited amount of time available for diagnosis and treatment before death occurs.

The hemodynamic response to a large, sudden pulmonary embolus relates to a variety of factors, most notably the size of the embolus, the degree of obstruction that it produced in the pulmonary vascular bed, and the underlying function of the lung that remains perfused. The degree of vascular obstruction is related to the number of segmental arteries that are occluded and to prior pulmonary vascular capacitance. Thus, the hemodynamic consequences of acute pulmonary embolism are also a reflection of factors, such as the age of the patient and any possible previous thromboembolic events. The preexisting status of the right ventricle that governs the forward flow of blood is also significant in determining the hemodynamic response to pulmonary embolism. Right ventricular function is affected by factors such as the degree of right ventricular hypertrophy or dilation, tricuspid valve regurgitation, and the presence of coronary artery disease.

In addition to the mechanical factor of pulmonary artery obstruction, there are reflex and hormonal factors that can increase pulmonary vascular resistance (PVR) at the time of acute pulmonary embolism. Humoral factors, specifically serotonin, adenosine diphosphate, platelet-derived growth factor, and thromboxane, are released from platelets attached to the thrombi,[11,12] whereas platelet-activating factor and leukotrienes are secreted by neutrophils.[13] Anoxia and tissue ischemia downstream from emboli inhibit endothelium-derived relaxing factor production and enhance release of superoxide anions by activated neutrophils.[14] The combination of these humoral effects contributes to enhanced pulmonary vasoconstriction. Thus, some patients with a relatively small embolus may have an exaggerated response to the degree of pulmonary vascular obstruction.

In patients without preexisting cardiac or pulmonary disease, an obstruction of less than 20% of the pulmonary vascular bed results in minimal hemodynamic consequences. It is only when the acute pulmonary obstruction exceeds 50% to 60% of the pulmonary vascular bed that cardiac and pulmonary compensatory mechanisms are overcome and cardiac output begins to fall.[15] Right ventricular failure occurs, which is accompanied by systemic hypotension as the amount of blood reaching the left ventricle decreases. The dilated right ventricle causes a shift of the ventricular septum to the left, further compromising left ventricular filling. Although patients with chronic pulmonary artery obstruction can have high pulmonary artery pressure levels that reflect the degree of obstruction, in acute pulmonary embolism the previously normal right ventricle cannot generate these pressures. Therefore, in acute massive pulmonary embolism, pulmonary artery pressures may be normal, and a pulmonary artery systolic pressure of 30-40 mm Hg may represent severe PH.

Acute pulmonary embolism usually presents suddenly. Symptoms and signs vary with the extent of blockage, the magnitude of humoral response, and the preembolus reserve of the cardiac and pulmonary systems of the patient.[16] The clinical diagnosis is often missed or falsely made. Most pulmonary emboli occur without sufficient clinical findings to suggest the diagnosis, and in an autopsy series of proven emboli, only 16% to 38% of patients received a diagnosis while still alive.[17] The acute disease is conveniently stratified into low-risk, submassive, or massive embolism on the basis of hemodynamic stability, arterial blood gases, and lung scan or angiographic assessment of the percentage of blocked pulmonary arteries.[18,19]

For patients with minor pulmonary embolism, physical examination may reveal tachycardia, rales, low-grade fever, and sometimes a pleural rub. Heart sounds and systemic blood pressure are often normal; sometimes the pulmonary second sound is increased. Less than one third of patients with acute pulmonary embolism have concurrent evidence of clinical deep venous thrombosis.[17] Room air arterial blood gases indicate a PaO_2 between 65 and 80 torr and a normal $PaCO_2$ of approximately 35 torr.[20] Pulmonary angiograms typically show less than 30% occlusion of the pulmonary arterial vasculature. Recent studies suggest that normotensive patients who have normal biomarker levels (Brain Natriuretic peptide [BNP], N-terminal pro-BNP, Troponin I, Troponin T) and have no RV dysfunction on echocardiographic imaging have short-term mortality rates approaching 1%.[21,22,23]

Submassive pulmonary embolism is defined as an acute pulmonary embolism without systemic hypotension (sytolic blood pressure > 90 mm Hg) but with either right ventricular dysfunction or myocardial necrosis.[19] This form of embolism is associated with dyspnea, tachypnea, dull chest pain, and some degree of cardiovascular changes manifested by tachycardia, mild to moderate hypotension, and elevation of central venous pressure.[20] Some patients may have syncope rather than dyspnea or chest pain. In contrast to massive pulmonary embolism, patients with submassive embolism (at least two lobar pulmonary arteries obstructed) are usually hemodynamically stable and have adequate cardiac output.[24] Room air blood gases reveal moderate hypoxia, with a PaO_2 between 50 and 60 torr, and mild hypocarbia, with a $PaCO_2$ no more than 30 torr.[20] Echocardiograms may show right ventricular dilation. Pulmonary angiograms indicate that 30% to 50% of the pulmonary vasculature is blocked; however, in patients with preexisting cardiopulmonary disorders, a lesser degree of vascular obstruction may produce similar symptoms.

Massive pulmonary embolism is life threatening and is defined as a pulmonary embolism that causes hemodynamic instability, requiring inotropic support.[24] It is usually associated with occlusion of more than 50% of the pulmonary vasculature, but it can occur with much smaller occlusions, particularly in patients with preexisting cardiac or pulmonary disease. The diagnosis is clinical, not anatomical. Patients develop acute dyspnea, tachypnea, tachycardia, and diaphoresis and may lose consciousness. Both hypotension and low cardiac output (<1.8 L/min/m^2) are present. Cardiac arrest can occur. Neck veins are distended, central venous pressure is elevated, and a right ventricular impulse may be present. Room air blood gases show severe hypoxia (PaO_2 < 50 torr), hypocarbia ($PaCO_2$ < 30 torr), and acidosis.[20] Urine output falls, and peripheral pulses and perfusion are poor.

The clinical diagnosis of submassive or massive pulmonary embolism is unreliable and is incorrect in 70% to 80% of patients who have subsequent angiography.[25] The differentiation between submassive or massive pulmonary embolism and acute myocardial infarction, aortic dissection, septic shock, and other catastrophic states can be difficult and costly in time. Although plain chest radiography, electrocardiogram, and insertion of a bedside Swan-Ganz catheter may add confirmatory information, they will not necessarily prove the diagnosis. Routine laboratory test results are usually normal.

The most common electrocardiographic abnormalities of acute pulmonary embolism are tachycardia and nonspecific ST and T wave changes. The major value of the electrocardiogram is the exclusion of a myocardial infarction. A minority of patients with massive embolism may show evidence of cor pulmonale, right axis deviation, or right bundle branch block.[17] Chest radiography may show oligemia (Westermark sign) or linear atelectasis (Fleischner lines), both of which are nonspecific findings. Ventilation–perfusion (V/Q) scans can provide confirmatory evidence, but these studies can be unreliable because pneumonia, atelectasis, previous pulmonary emboli, and other conditions can cause a mismatch in ventilation and perfusion that mimics positive results.[26]

In general, negative V/Q scans exclude the diagnosis of clinically significant pulmonary embolism. V/Q scans are usually interpreted as high, intermediate, or low probability of pulmonary embolism to emphasize the lack of specificity but high sensitivity of the test.[27] Magnetic resonance angiography is an excellent noninvasive method for the diagnosis of pulmonary emboli, and it provides specific information regarding flow within the pulmonary vasculature.[28] Unfortunately, this method is expensive, time consuming, and not widely available. Like catheter-based pulmonary angiography, it is generally not suitable for hemodynamically unstable patients. Transthoracic echocardiography or transesophageal echocardiography with color flow Doppler mapping can provide reliable information about the presence or absence of major thrombi obstructing the main pulmonary artery; however, these techniques are usually inadequate for visualization of the lobar vessels, where the embolic material is often localized. More than 80% of patients with clinically significant pulmonary embolism have abnormalities of right ventricular volume or contractility, often associated with acute tricuspid regurgitation.[29] In a subset of patients, abnormal flow patterns can be discerned in major pulmonary arteries during transesophageal echocardiography.[30]

Prophylaxis

Although prophylactic measures should be considered and used for all patients undergoing major surgery or who have prolonged immobility, certain other patients also fall into a potentially high-risk group for pulmonary embolism. These patients include those with previous embolism, malignancy, cardiac failure, obesity, or advanced age.[31] The prevalence of deep venous thrombosis of the thigh or pelvis, its strong association with pulmonary embolism, and the identification of the associated risk factors listed earlier provide the basis and rationale for prophylactic anticoagulation for the prevention of acute pulmonary embolism. Simple measures such as compression stockings probably should be prescribed more often and should be used in most nonambulating patients in the hospital. Intermittent pneumatic compression devices are more cumbersome, but also effective. These compression devices are available for the calf or the whole leg. They can provide a range of compression pressures, inflation and deflation duration, and sequential or nonsequential inflation, although a clear difference between these variations has not been demonstrated. Both compression stockings with a compression pressure of 30 to 40 mm Hg at the ankle and pneumatic compression devices reduce the incidence of deep venous thrombosis after general surgery to approximately 40% of control patients.[32] Multiple studies have shown that low-dose subcutaneous heparin or low-molecular-weight heparin given once a day reduces the incidence of deep venous thrombosis[33,34] with a concomitant reduction in the incidence of pulmonary embolism. This reduction in thrombosis has not been associated with an excessive risk of bleeding.[33] Recent studies suggest that of patients who have deep venous thrombosis diagnosed in the hospital without pulmonary embolism, the probability of clinically diagnosed pulmonary embolism within the next 12 months is 1.7%.[35] If pulmonary embolism occurs, the probability of recurrent pulmonary embolism is 6%.[35]

Supportive and Thrombolytic Therapy

The majority of patients who die of pulmonary embolism do so within 2 hours of the initial acute event, before the diagnosis can be firmly established and before effective therapy can be instituted. Once the diagnosis is made, however, treatment will be either medical (supportive and thrombolytic therapy) or surgical (Fig. 102-1).

Oxygen should be administered to alleviate hypoxic pulmonary vasoconstriction, and it is likely that a severely affected patient will require intubation and ventilatory support. Pharmacologic agents, including cardiovascular pressors and vasoactive agents, can be used to stabilize the patient's hemodynamics. Once the circulation has been stabilized, arterial and central venous catheters are placed to monitor cardiac output and pulmonary arterial oxygen saturation. There is debate as to whether pulmonary artery catheters, although obviously helpful in management, should be used in the setting of acute pulmonary

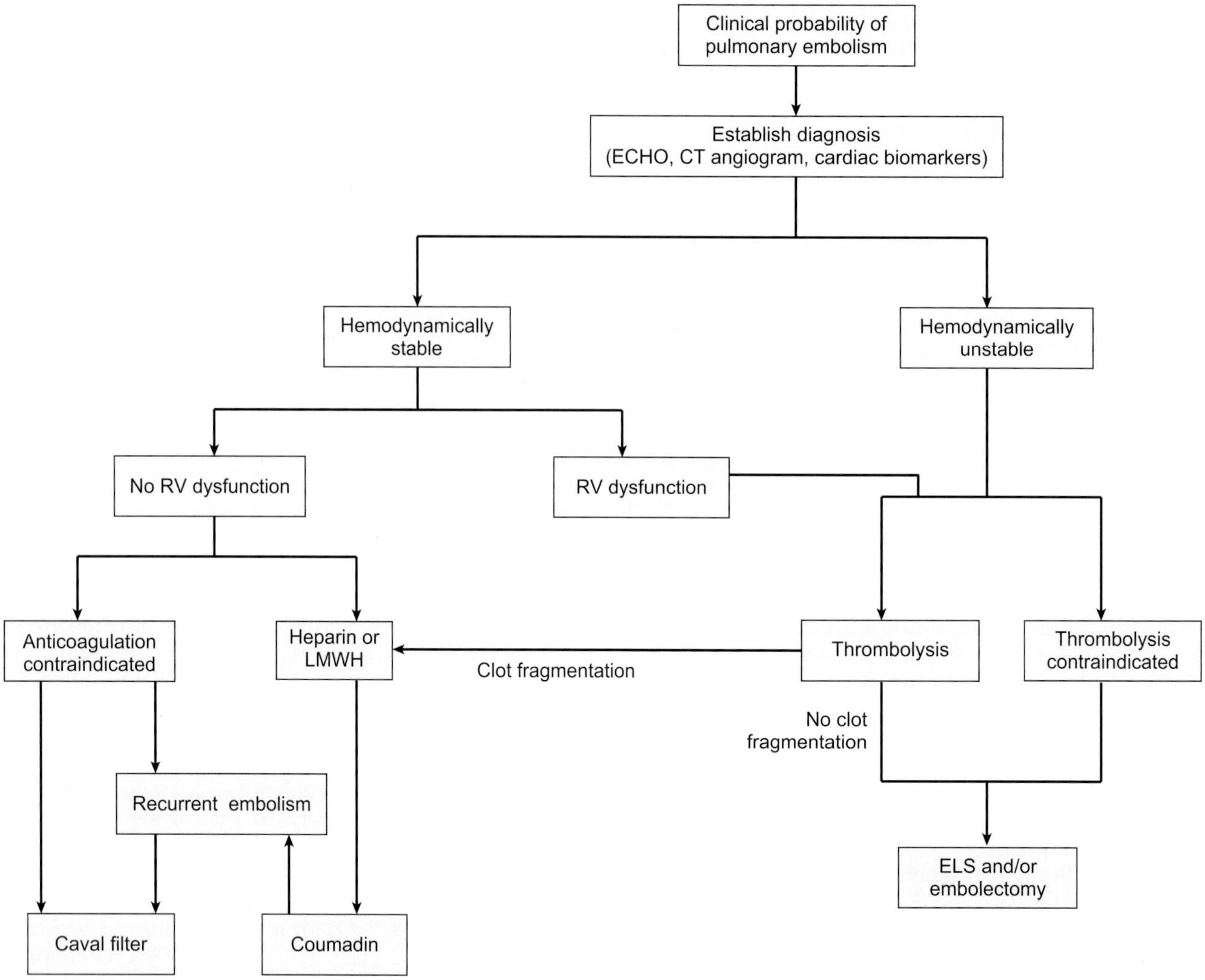

FIGURE 102-1 ■ Acute pulmonary embolism treatment scheme. *CT,* Computed tomography; *ECHO,* echocardiography; *ELS,* extracorporeal life support; *LMWH,* low-molecular-weight heparin; *RV,* right ventricle.

embolism, because of the risk of dislodging further thromboembolic material. The electrocardiogram is monitored, a Foley catheter is inserted for accurate recording of urine output, and blood gas levels are obtained. Patients with objectively confirmed pulmonary embolism and no contraindications for anticoagulation should receive prompt anticoagulant therapy with subcutaneous low-molecular-weight heparin, intravenous or subcutaneous unfractionated heparin, or subcutaneous fondaparinux (an inhibitor of activated factor Xa).[19,36] For patients with suspected or confirmed heparin-induced thrombocytopenia, a non–heparin-based anticoagulant, such as lepirudin, argatroban, or bivalirudin should be used.[37] Although each of these individual therapies prevents propagation and formation of new thromboemboli, they rarely dissolve the existing clot. In most cases, the patient's intrinsic fibrinolytic system will lyse fresh thrombi over a period of days to weeks.[38] Intravenous heparin is monitored by measurement of activated partial thromboplastin times, which are maintained between 51 and 70 seconds (roughly twice that of controls) every 6 to 8 hours. The platelet count should be measured every 2 to 3 days to detect the presence of heparin-induced thrombocytopenia. Prothrombin times are also obtained at baseline to prepare for anticoagulation with warfarin later.

Although warfarin is typically used for long-term anticoagulation after acute pulmonary embolism, several new oral anticoagulants have recently come on the market that do not require laboratory monitoring of anticoagulation (Table 102-1). They include factor Xa inhibitors, rivaroxaban (Xarelto), apixaban (Eliquis), and edoxaban (Savaysa), as well as the direct factor IIa (thrombin) inhibitor dabigatran (Pradaxa). All these drugs except edoxaban have been approved by the U.S. Food and Drug Administration (FDA) for the long-term treatment of deep venous thrombosis with or without pulmonary embolism, with edoxaban currently undergoing FDA scrutiny. To date, there are no known clinically validated reversal agents for rivaroxaban, aprixaban, edoxaban, or dabigatran. Based on the strength of available evidence and current American College of Chest Physicians Evidence-Based Guidelines, warfarin continues to be a monitorable, reversible, and effective agent in patients with venous thromboembolism and acute pulmonary embolism, and it should remain the first-line option for

TABLE 102-1 **Pharmacologic Characteristics of Direct Oral Anticoagulants**

	Dabigatran	Rivaroxaban	Apixaban	Edoxaban
Trade name	Pradaxa	Xarelto	Eliquis	Savaysa
Approved by the FDA for treatment of PE	Yes	Yes	Yes	No
Target	Factor IIa	Factor Xa	Factor Xa	Factor Xa
Onset of action	2 h	2.5-4 h	3 h	1-5 h
Half-life	12-14 h	9-13 h	8-11 h	8-10 h
Renal clearance (%)	80	60	25	35
Metabolism	P-gp	P-gp/CYP3A4	P-gp/CYP3A4	P-gp/CYP3A4
Dosing	b.i.d.	b.i.d., qd	b.i.d.	b.i.d, qd

CYP, Cytochrome P450 3A4; *PE*, pulmonary embolism; *P-gp*, P-glycoprotein.

long-term (3-6 month) treatment of pulmonary embolism.[39] However, the factor Xa inhibitors rivaroxaban and apixaban, as well as the direct thrombin inhibitor dabigatran, are each viable alternatives in patients with less than optimal INR control (targeted therapeutic range < 60%) or in whom warfarin monitoring and management is not possible.[40] Three months of warfarin anticoagulation is recommended for patients with a first-episode deep venous thrombosis related to a major reversible risk factor (i.e., recent surgery or trauma).[41,42] Six months of warfarin anticoagulation is recommended for patients who have recurrent or unprovoked deep venous thrombosis with or without pulmonary embolism as prophylaxis against recurrent disease.[43,44]

The natural history of the clot in survivors of acute embolic events is fragmentation and progressive lysis. It therefore follows that the addition of streptokinase, urokinase, or recombinant tissue plasminogen activator improves survival by increasing the rate of lysis of fresh thrombi in the pulmonary arterial tree. Thromboembolytic agents dissolve thrombi by activating plasminogen to plasmin. Plasmin, when in proximity to a thrombus, degrades fibrin to soluble peptides. Circulating plasmin also degrades soluble fibrinogen and, to variable degrees, factors II, V, and VIII. In addition, increased concentrations of fibrin and fibrinogen degradation products contribute to coagulopathy by both inhibiting the conversion of fibrinogen to fibrin and interfering with fibrin polymerization. The thromboembolytic agents currently approved by the FDA for the treatment of acute pulmonary embolism are streptokinase, urokinase, recombinant tissue plasminogen activator (alteplase), and tissue plasminogen activator.[45] Some new agents (so-called second-generation thrombolytics) such as reteplase, saruplase, staphylokinase, tenecteplase, and anistreplase are undergoing clinical testing.[46]

Although thrombolytic therapy has been shown to increase the rate of lysis of fresh pulmonary clots more than that of heparin alone,[47] there has been little difference measured in the amount of residual thrombus between the two treatments in early studies using small cohorts of patients.[48,49] However, four registries (MAPPET, ICOPER, RIETE, EMPEROR) comparing thrombolytic agents with intravenous (IV) heparin in acute pulmonary embolism have been large enough to detect a significant difference in the most important endpoint—mortality, particularly in patients with massive pulmonary embolism, presenting with hypotension.[50-55] More recent experience suggests a trend toward better results with thrombolytic therapy because of a more rapid diminution in right ventricular afterload and dysfunction.[56,57] Thus, thrombolytic therapy should also be considered in normotensive patients with evidence of severe right ventricular dysfunction on echocardiography. Compared with heparin therapy alone, thrombolytic agents carry a higher risk of bleeding problems, with up to 20% of patients experiencing a significant bleeding complication.[58,59] In general, thrombolytic therapy is contraindicated in patients with intracranial hemorrhage, fresh surgical wounds, anemia, recent stroke, peptic ulcer, or bleeding dyscrasias.

Percutaneous Treatments

Percutaneous techniques to recanalize complete and partial occlusions in the pulmonary trunk or major pulmonary arteries are potentially life saving in selected patients with massive or submassive pulmonary embolism.[60] Transcatheter procedures can be performed as an alternative to thrombolysis when there are contraindications or when emergency surgical embolectomy is unavailable or contraindicated. Catheter interventions can also be performed when thrombolysis has failed to improve hemodynamics in the acute setting. The goals of catheter-based therapy include rapidly reducing pulmonary artery pressure, increasing systemic perfusion, and facilitating RV recovery.[61-63]

There are three general categories of percutaneous intervention for removing emboli and decreasing thrombus burden: aspiration thrombectomy, thrombus fragmentation, and rheolytic thrombectomy. For aspiration thrombectomy, a device is used that consists of a small terminal cup attached to a flexible catheter.[61] Syringe suction is applied to the cup as a thrombus is engaged. The catheter and clot are removed en masse through the venotomy site, and this process can be repeated multiple times. Thrombus fragmentation has been performed with balloon angioplasty,[64] a pigtail rotational catheter,[45] or a more advanced fragmentation device (the Amplatz catheter with an impeller housed in a capsule at the tip) driven by a compact air turbine that homogenizes thrombus by maceration and fragmentation. A metal capsule protects the vessel from the rotating impellar.[65] A third technique, the rheolytic thrombectomy technique, uses a dual-lumen catheter: one small lumen for delivery of pulsatile pressurized saline and a larger effluent or exhaust lumen to drain the thrombus. High-velocity saline jets are injected toward the effluent lumen. This produces an area of low pressure at the tip of the catheter (Venturi effect), thereby fragmenting the thrombus and allowing it to be evacuated through the effluent lumen.[63,66]

Recently, a new technique of suction thrombectomy with extracorporeal venovenous support (AngioVac, Angiodynamics, Latham, NY) has been described for the removal of proximal pulmonary emboli.[67] With this technique, a drainage cannula with a balloon-actuated, expandable, funnel-shaped distal tip is introduced through a femoral or right internal jugular vein and advanced under fluoroscopy to the site of embolism. The cannula is connected in circuit with an extracorporeal circulation pump attached to a second cannula inserted into the contralateral femoral vein. Venovenous bypass is instituted, and particulate matter suctioned through the inflow cannula is trapped within filters in the circuit, allowing for reinfusion of blood that is free of gross debris. This hybrid procedure is typically performed in an operating room, with thoracic surgeon and cardiologist present.[68] Successful catheter extraction of thrombus with clinically significant reduction in pulmonary arterial pressure for each of the above methods varies between 75% and 88%, with the best results achieved for proximal and main pulmonary artery embolism.[69,70]

Acute Pulmonary Embolectomy

When contraindications preclude thrombolysis, emergency pulmonary thromboembolectomy is indicated for suitable patients with either life-threatening circulatory insufficiency from massive pulmonary embolism or submassive pulmonary embolism.[71] The decision to proceed with catheter-based versus surgical embolectomy requires interdisciplinary teamwork, discussion that involves the surgeon and interventionalist, and an assessment of the local expertise. If a patient has been taken directly to the operating room without a definitive diagnosis, transesophageal or epicardial echocardiography and color Doppler mapping can confirm or refute the diagnosis in the operating room.[72] The primary difficulty with the broad application of operative embolectomy is that it is almost impossible to determine which patients will die without intervention. An emergency pulmonary embolectomy is most feasible (because of time) and most successful in patients who ultimately may not require it, which makes it difficult to establish the efficacy of this operation. To date, no randomized trial has evaluated surgical embolectomy in patients with acute pulmonary embolism. Indications for acute surgical intervention include the following: (1) critical hemodynamic condition, with the patient deemed unlikely to survive; (2) definitive diagnosis of pulmonary embolism in the main or lobar pulmonary arteries with compromise of oxygen gas exchange; (3) unstable patients in whom thrombolytic or anticoagulation therapy is absolutely contraindicated; and (4) the presence of a large clot trapped within the right atrium or ventricle.

Acute pulmonary embolectomy was first described by Trendelenburg in 1908[73] using pulmonary artery and aortic occlusion, through a transthoracic approach. There were no surviving patients. Sharp[74] performed the first successful open embolectomy, using cardiopulmonary bypass.

For pulmonary embolectomy, a median sternotomy incision is used and cardiopulmonary bypass is instituted. The procedure is best performed on a warm, beating heart, without aortic cross-clamping, cardioplegia, or fibrillatory arrest. Occluding tapes are placed around the superior and inferior vena cavae. Two polypropylene sutures are placed in the mid–pulmonary artery for traction. A longitudinal incision is made between these sutures in the main pulmonary artery trunk 1 to 2 cm distal to the valve. If necessary, the incision can be extended directly into the left pulmonary artery. Extraction is limited to directly visible emboli, which can be accomplished to the level of the lobar and segmental arteries. Fresh clot removal from subsegmental arteries may be attempted, but is often surgically difficult because of the soft, sticky, often fragmental nature of peripheral pulmonary emboli. The emboli are extracted using forceps, suction, and balloon catheters. The right pulmonary artery also can be exposed and opened between the aorta and superior vena cava to allow better exposure in segmental vessels, if necessary. A sterile pediatric bronchoscope can be used to visualize emboli in tertiary or quaternary pulmonary vessels, so that they can be cleared with balloon embolectomy or suction. After cleaning the pulmonary arterial tree lumina, the pleural spaces can be entered, and the lungs are manually compressed to dislodge small distally lodged clots, which can then be suctioned out. The pulmonary arteriotomy is then closed with a 6-0 polypropylene suture. After restarting the heart, the patient is weaned from bypass, decannulated, and closed. The aim of this operation is to remove most of the embolic material, and no attempt is made to perform an endarterectomy.

As a corollary to this operation, some groups recommend either placement of an inferior vena caval filter or caval clipping before chest closure. Greenfield has recommended placement of an inferior vena caval filter under direct visualization before closing the chest.[75] Historically, some European surgeons clipped or plicated the intrapericardial vena cava at the end of the embolectomy to prevent migration of lower body clot into the pulmonary circulation; however, this procedure is associated with stasis in the venous system in the lower body and leg swelling.[76] In most centers that offer emergency pulmonary thromboembolectomy, no caval procedure is performed in the perioperative period, and recurrent deep venous thrombosis or pulmonary embolism are treated by anticoagulation with warfarin for 6 months.[77] Percutaneously placed filters are recommended only for patients with contraindications to anticoagulation or for patients with recurrent pulmonary embolism on therapeutic anticoagulation. The cone-shaped Greenfield filter is the most widely used permanent filter in the United States, and it is associated with a lifetime recurrent embolism rate of 5% and a lifetime patency rate of 97%.[78,79] The advent of retrievable inferior vena caval (IVC) filters appears to have lowered thresholds for IVC filter placement in the United States; however, there are few data to support or refute this claim.[19,80] Late complications of permanent and retrievable filters include recurrent deep venous thrombosis (21%), IVC thrombosis (2% to 10%), and IVC penetration (0.3%).[81] IVC filter fractures have also been reported.[82]

Extracorporeal Life Support

The wider availability of long-term mechanical perfusion (termed *extracorporeal life support* [ELS]) using peripheral vessel cannulation to stabilize the circulation offers another approach to life-threatening pulmonary embolism. Most pulmonary emboli, even those that are massive, will dissolve with time. ELS can be instituted outside the operating room setting and can be implemented with rapidity in institutions where preparation for its emergency use has been made. With a trained team, needed equipment, and associated supplies readily available, ELS can be implemented within 15 to 30 minutes.[83] For hemodynamic support during the period of a life-threatening pulmonary embolism, venoarterial extracorporeal support can be instituted and maintained for a period up to several weeks, if necessary.[84]

This procedure begins with an IV heparin bolus of 1 mg/kg, followed by percutaneous or surgical cut-down of the femoral artery and femoral or internal jugular veins. If pulses are absent or weak, a larger incision is usually faster; however, because patients need heparin and have possibly received fibrinolytic drugs, a minimal wound is preferred. The tip of the venous catheter is advanced into the right atrium to obtain a flow rate of 2.5-4.0 liters/min using an emergency pump-oxygenator circuit primed with crystalloid.[85] The perfusion circuit consists of IV or arterial access tubes, a centrifugal pump, and a membrane oxygenator.[86] An electromagnetic flowmeter is placed on the arterial line, and an arterial filter is not applied. While the patient is receiving ELS, heparin is infused to maintain the activated clotting time between 150 and 180 seconds. In the initial hours after institution of ELS, activated clotting times are measured every 30 minutes, followed by every hour thereafter until decannulation. During the period of ELS support, thrombolytic drugs may be instilled directly into the pulmonary artery via a Swan-Ganz catheter to aid in clot lysis. ELS support can provide critical support to bridge an unstable patient to surgical embolectomy.[87]

Once oxygenation has been stabilized and PVR has normalized, the patient is decannulated, and the cannulation sites are surgically closed. ELS is usually discontinued in the operating room because vessels should be sutured closed due to the need for heparin and long-term anticoagulation.

Results of Surgical Embolectomy for Acute Pulmonary Embolism

Mortality rates for emergency pulmonary embolectomy vary widely, between 0% and 62% (Table 102-2).[88-108] It is difficult to compare these retrospective studies because of the difference in time in which the operations were performed, the preoperative hemodynamic state of the patient populations, and the variation in treatment plans. In general, greater surgical mortality was encountered if a patient had a preoperative cardiac arrest or required ELS support. For example, the mortality in patients who have suffered a cardiac arrest is reported in multiple series from 27% to 64% (see Table 102-2), while the mortality in patients who have not suffered cardiac arrest is reported to be between 6% and 44%. Consequently, although some groups report low mortality rates, this may be attributable to the selection of less ill patients as candidates for surgery. In patients in whom ELS is instituted during preoperative cardiac resuscitation, subsequent operative mortality ranges between 44% and 57%.[43,85] Thus, the outcome depends largely on the

TABLE 102-2 **Surgical Pulmonary Embolectomy Series (1994-2014) with More Than 20 Patients: Comparative Mortality**

References	Date	No. of Patients *(N)*	Preoperative Cardiac Arrest	Mortality in Patients with Preoperative Cardiac Arrest	Total Mortality
Stulz[88]	1994	50	31/50 (62%)	19/31 (61%)	23/50 (46%)
Jakob[89]	1995	25	13/25 (52%)	4/13 (31%)	6/25 (24%)
Doerge[90]	1996	36	14/36 (39%)	8/14 (57%)	9/36 (25%)
Doerge[92]	1999	41	14/41 (34%)	9/14 (64%)	12/41 (29%)
Ullmann[91]	1999	40	19/40 (48%)	12/19 (63%)	14/40 (35%)
Aklog[93]	2002	29	1/29 (3%)	—	3/29 (10%)
Leacche[94]	2005	47	6/47 (11%)	2/6 (33%)	3/47 (6%)
Spagnolo[95]	2006	21	2/21 (10%)	0/2 (0%)	0/21 (0%)
Digonnet[96]	2007	21	6/21 (29%)	4/6 (67%)	13/21 (62%)
Kadner[97]	2008	25	8/25 (32%)	—	2/25 (8%)
Sádaba[98]	2008	20	—	—	2/20 (10%)
Vohra[99]	2010	21	9/21 (43%)	—	4/21 (19%)
Medvedev[101]	2011	27	—	—	0/29 (0%)
Zarrabi[100]	2011	30	3/30 (10%)	—	2/30 (7%)
Lehnert[103]	2012	33	1/33 (3%)	—	2/33 (6%)
Takahashi[104]	2012	24	11/24 (46%)	3/11 (27%)	3/24 (13%)
Taniguchi[102]	2012	32	3/32 (9%)	1/3 (33%)	6/32 (20%)
Aymard[105]	2013	28	—	—	1/28 (4%)
Wu[106]	2013	25	8/25 (32%)	4/8 (50%)	5/25 (20%)
Zarrabi[107]	2013	30	—	—	4/30 (13%)
Worku[108]	2014	20	3/20 (15%)	—	1/20 (5%)

preoperative condition of the patient. Primary causes of death include brain damage, cardiac failure, uncontrollable bleeding, and sepsis. Recurrent embolism after surgery is uncommon,[96] and approximately 80% of those who survive surgery maintain normal pulmonary artery pressures and exercise tolerance. In these patients, postoperative angiograms are normal or show obstruction in less than 10% of vessels. A minority of patients who have obstruction in more than 40% of pulmonary vessels after surgery have experienced reduced pulmonary function and exercise tolerance.[109]

CHRONIC PULMONARY THROMBOEMBOLIC DISEASE

Incidence and Natural History

The natural history of pulmonary embolism is generally total embolic resolution, or resolution leaving minimal residua, with restoration of a normal hemodynamic status. However, for unknown reasons, embolic resolution is incomplete in a small subset of patients. If the acute emboli are not lysed in 1 to 2 weeks, the embolic material becomes attached to the pulmonary arterial wall at the main pulmonary artery, lobar, segmental, or subsegmental levels.[110] With time, the initial embolic material progressively becomes converted into connective and elastic tissue filled with endothelial and smooth muscle precursor cells as well as macrophages.[111,112] Often, visualization of the pulmonary arteries by angioscopy a few weeks after unresolved pulmonary embolism reveals vessel narrowing at the site of embolic incorporation. In some patients, recanalization of some of the pulmonary arterial branches occurs, with the formation of fibrous tissue in the form of bands and webs.[113] By a mechanism that is poorly understood, this chronic obstructive disease can lead to a small vessel (precapillary) arteriolar vasculopathy characterized by excessive vascular and inflammatory cell proliferation around small arterioles in the pulmonary circulation.[114] These pulmonary microvascular changes resemble the arteriopathy observed in World Health Organization Group 1.1 or idiopathic pulmonary arterial hypertension and are gaining increased recognition as contributors to disease progression in chronic thromboembolic PH.[115] Precapillary arteriolar vasculopathy is mostly seen in the remaining open vessels, which are subjected to long exposure at high flow. Pulmonary hypertension results when the capacitance of the remaining open bed cannot absorb the cardiac output, either because of the degree of primary obstruction by thromboembolic material and adjacent remodeling or because of the combination of a proximal obstruction and secondary small-vessel vasculopathy. The importance of pulmonary arteriolar remodeling in the development of chronic thromboembolic PH is supported by the following observations: (1) there is often a lack of correlation between elevated pulmonary arterial pressure and the degree of angiographic pulmonary vascular bed obstruction, (2) PH can progress in the absence of recurrent thromboembolism, and (3) total PVR is still significantly higher in chronic thromboembolic PH patients than in acute pulmonary embolism patients with a similar degree of proximal vascular bed obstruction.[116,117]

The incidence of PH caused by chronic pulmonary embolism is even more difficult to determine than that of acute pulmonary embolism. There are more than 500,000 survivors of symptomatic episodes of acute pulmonary embolism per year.[118] The incidence of chronic thrombotic occlusion or stenosis in the population depends on which percentage of patients fails to resolve acute embolic material. One estimate is that chronic thromboembolic disease develops in only 3.8% of patients with a clinically recognized acute pulmonary embolism.[5] If these figures are correct and only patients with symptomatic acute pulmonary emboli are counted, approximately 19,000 individuals would progress to chronic thromboembolic PH in the United States each year. However, because many (if not most) patients with a diagnosis of chronic thromboembolic disease have no antecedent history of acute embolism, the true incidence of this disorder is probably much higher.

Regardless of the exact incidence, it is clear that acute embolism and its chronic relation, fixed chronic thromboembolic occlusive disease, are much more common than is generally appreciated and are seriously underdiagnosed. In 1963, Houk and colleagues[119] reviewed the literature of 240 cases of chronic thromboembolic obstruction of major pulmonary arteries, but found that only six cases were diagnosed correctly before death. Calculations extrapolated from mortality rates and the random incidence of major thrombotic occlusion found at autopsy supported the postulate that more than 100,000 people in the United States currently have PH that could be relieved by operation. An autopsy analysis of 13,216 patients showed pulmonary thromboembolism in 5.5% of autopsies and up to 31.3% in older patients.[120]

Chronic thromboembolic PH is a disease characterized by initial thromboembolism to the pulmonary arterial tree that does not resolve itself. Whether this is due to an endothelial insult, preexisting prothrombotic state, or endothelial or smooth muscle progenitor cell trapping and remodeling is the subject of debate. No clear etiology has been defined for the majority of patients who develop chronic thromboembolic PH. Lupus anticoagulant may be detected in approximately 10% of chronic thromboembolic patients,[121] and 20% carry anticardiolipin antibodies, lupus anticoagulant, or both.[122] A recent study has demonstrated that the plasma level of factor VIII, a protein that is associated with both primary and recurrent venous thromboembolism, is elevated in 39% of patients with chronic thromboembolic PH.[123] Other hematologic abnormalities observed in chronic thromboembolic PH include increased resistance to thrombolysis[124] and decreased thrombomodulin levels.[125] Analyses of plasma proteins in patients with chronic thromboembolic disease have shown that fibrin from these patients is resistant to thrombolysis in vitro.[126] In addition, in a previous pathology series, 15% of patients had an underlying autoimmune or hematologic disorder (e.g., polycythemia vera).[127] Finally, non–O blood group types are significantly more common in patients with chronic thromboembolic PH compared to patients with idiopathic pulmonary arterial hypertension[128] and compared with the general American and European populations (http://www.redcross.org).

Case reports and small series have suggested links between chronic thromboembolism and previous splenectomy, thyroid replacement therapy, permanent intravenous catheters, and ventriculoatrial shunts for the treatment of hydrocephalus or chronic inflammatory conditions, such as osteomyelitis or inflammatory bowel disease. In addition to these observations, associations with sickle cell disease, hereditary stomatocytosis, the Klippel-Trenaunay syndrome, and malignancy have been described.[129] However, the vast majority of cases of chronic thromboembolic PH are not linked with a specific coagulation defect or underlying medical condition as described earlier.

Without surgical intervention, the survival of patients with chronic thromboembolic PH is poor and is inversely related to the degree of PH at the time of diagnosis. Riedel colleagues[6] found a 5-year survival rate of 30% among patients with a mean pulmonary artery pressure greater than 40 mm Hg at the time of diagnosis and 10% in those whose pressure exceeded 50 mm Hg. In another study, a mean pulmonary artery pressure as low as 30 mm Hg was identified as a threshold for poor prognosis.[130]

Clinical Manifestations

Patients with chronic thromboembolic PH usually have subtle or nonspecific presenting symptoms. The most common symptoms are progressive exertional dyspnea and exercise intolerance.[131] These symptoms are a result of elevated dead space ventilation and a limitation in cardiac output from obstruction of the pulmonary vascular bed. As the disease progresses, additional symptoms such as edema, chest pain, lightheadedness, and syncope may develop. Early in the course of thromboembolic disease, physical findings may be limited to an accentuated P2, which can be overlooked easily during the physical examination. Nonspecific chest pains occur in approximately 50% of patients with more severe PH. Hemoptysis can occur in all forms of PH and probably results from abnormally dilated vessels distended by increased intravascular pressures. Peripheral edema, early satiety, and epigastric or right upper quadrant fullness or pain can develop as the right side of the heart fails and cor pulmonale develops.

Physical signs of PH include a jugular venous pulse that is characterized by a large A wave. As the right side of the heart fails, the V wave becomes predominant. The right ventricle is usually palpable near the lower left sternal border, and pulmonary valve closure may be audible in the second intercostal space. Patients with advanced disease may be hypoxic and cyanotic. Clubbing is an uncommon finding. As the right side of the heart fails, a right atrial gallop may be auscultated, and tricuspid insufficiency develops. Because of the large pressure gradient across the tricuspid valve in PH, the murmur is high-pitched and might not exhibit respiratory variation. These findings differ from those usually observed in tricuspid valvular disease. A murmur of pulmonic regurgitation also may be detected, and a specific auscultatory finding is a flow murmur at the back—thought to result from stenosed pulmonary vessels.[132]

Diagnostic Evaluation of Chronic Thromboembolic Pulmonary Hypertension

Pulmonary vascular disease always must be considered in the differential diagnosis of unexplained dyspnea. The diagnostic evaluation serves three purposes: to establish the presence and severity of PH; to determine its etiology; and, if thromboembolic disease is present, to determine whether it is surgically correctible (Fig. 102-2).

Chest radiography is often unrevealing in the early stages of chronic thromboembolic PH. As the disease progresses, several radiographic abnormalities may be found. These abnormalities include peripheral lung opacities suggestive of scarring from previous infarction, cardiomegaly with dilation and hypertrophy of the right-sided chambers, and dilation of the central pulmonary arteries. Pulmonary function tests are often obtained in the evaluation of dyspnea, and they serve to exclude the presence of obstructive airways or parenchymal lung disease. There are no characteristic spirometric changes that are diagnostic of chronic thromboembolic PH. Single-breath diffusing capacity for carbon monoxide (DLCO) may be moderately reduced, and it has been reported that 20% of patients have a mild to moderate restrictive defect caused by parenchymal scarring.[133] Arterial blood oxygen levels may be normal even in the setting of significant PH. Most patients, however, experience a decline in PO_2 with exertion.

Transthoracic echocardiography is the first study to provide objective evidence of the presence of PH. An estimate of pulmonary artery pressure can be provided by Doppler evaluation of the tricuspid regurgitant envelope. Additional echocardiographic findings vary depending on the stage of the disease, and they include right ventricular enlargement, leftward displacement of the interventricular septum, and encroachment of the enlarged right ventricle on the left ventricular cavity with abnormal systolic and diastolic function of the left ventricle.[134] Contrast echocardiography may demonstrate a persistent foramen ovale, which is the result of high right atrial pressures opening the previously closed intraatrial communication. Once the diagnosis of PH has been established, distinguishing between major-vessel obstruction and small-vessel pulmonary vascular disease is the next critical step.

Radioisotope ventilation-perfusion (V/Q) lung scanning is the essential test for establishing the diagnosis of unresolved pulmonary thromboembolism. A normal ventilation-perfusion scan excludes the diagnosis of chronic thromboembolic PH. The V/Q scan typically demonstrates one or more mismatched segmental defects caused by obstructive thromboembolism. This is in contrast to the normal or "mottled" perfusion scan seen in patients with primary PH or other small-vessel forms of PH.[135] It is important to note that V/Q scanning can underestimate the magnitude of perfusion defects with chronic thromboembolic PH, as partial recanalization of

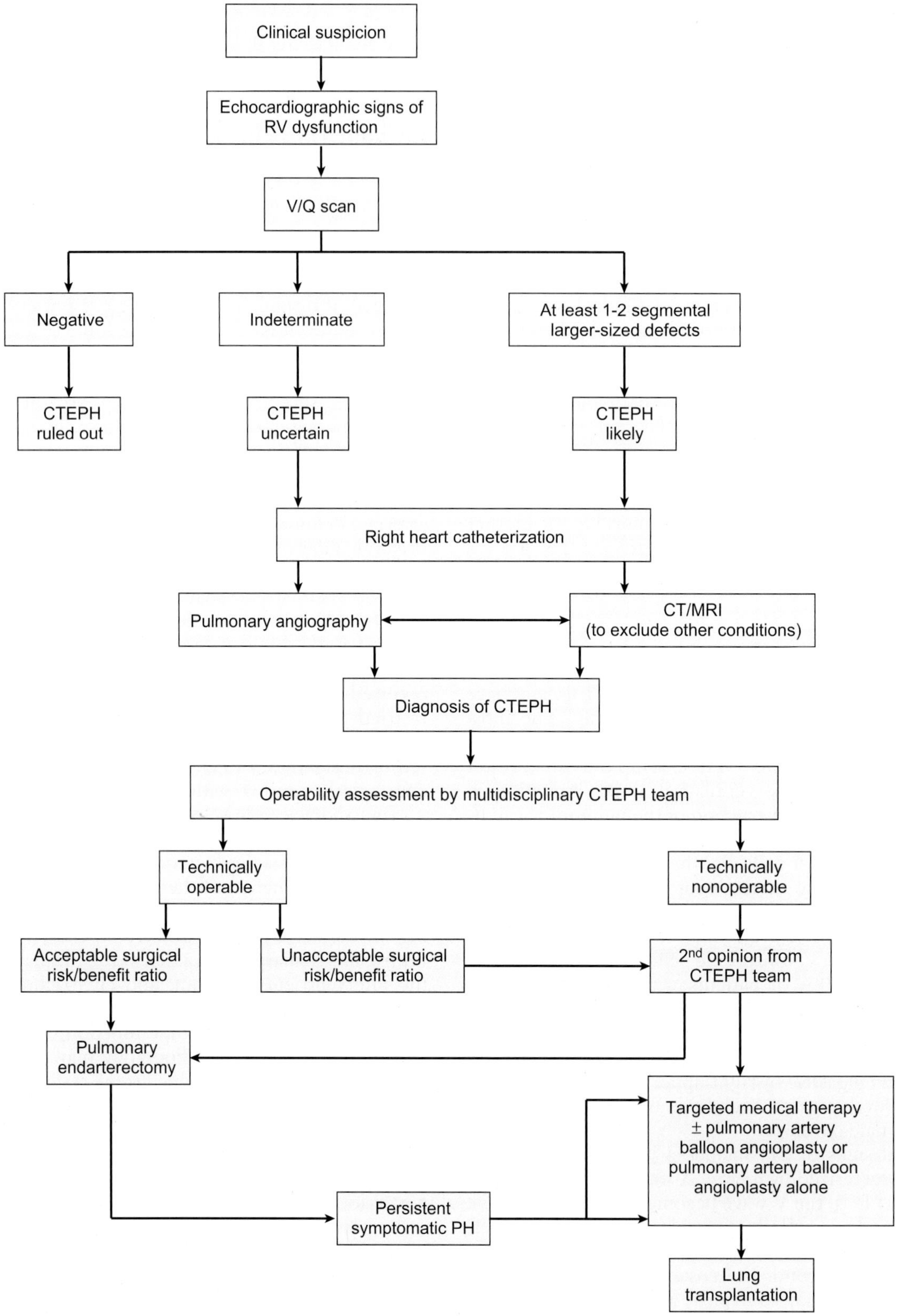

FIGURE 102-2 ■ Chronic thromboembolic pulmonary hypertension treatment scheme. *CT,* Computed tomography; *CTEPH,* chronic thromboembolic pulmonary hypertension; *MRI,* magnetic resonance imaging; *PH,* pulmonary hypertension; *RV,* right ventricular; *V/Q,* ventilation-perfusion.

the vessel lumen can occur, resulting in some perfusion though with significant obstruction to flow.[136]

Cardiac catheterization provides essential information in the evaluation of patients with suspected thromboembolic PH. Right ventricular catheterization allows for the quantification of the severity of PH and assessment of cardiac function. Measurement of oxygen saturations in the vena cava, right ventricular chambers, and the pulmonary artery may document previously undetected left-to-right shunting. Coronary angiography and left-sided heart catheterization provide additional information about patients at risk for coronary artery or valvular disease and establish baseline measurements for cardiac output and left ventricular function. This information is crucial in the preoperative risk assessment of patients deemed candidates for pulmonary endarterectomy.

Pulmonary angiography is the gold standard for defining pulmonary vascular anatomy and is performed to identify whether chronic thromboembolic obstruction is present, to determine its location and surgical accessibility, and to rule out other diagnostic possibilities. In angiographic imaging, thrombi appear as unusual filling defects, pouches, webs, or bands, or completely thrombosed vessels that may resemble congenital absence of a vessel. Organized material along a vascular wall produces a scalloped or serrated luminal edge.[137] Despite concerns regarding the safety of performing pulmonary angiography in patients with PH, with careful monitoring, pulmonary angiography can be performed safely even in patients with severe PH.[138] Biplane imaging is preferred, offering the advantage of lateral views that provide greater anatomical detail compared with the overlapped and obscured vessel images often seen with the anterior–posterior view. Maturation, organization, and recanalization of clot produces angiographic patterns of the following: (1) pouch defects, (2) webs or bands, (3) intimal irregularities, (4) abrupt narrowing of major vessels, and (5) obstruction of main, lobar, or segmental pulmonary vessels.[139]

In approximately 20% of cases, the differential diagnosis between idiopathic pulmonary arterial hypertension and distal small-vessel pulmonary thromboembolic disease is difficult to establish. In these patients, pulmonary angioscopy often may be helpful. The pulmonary angioscope is a diagnostic fiberoptic device that was developed to visualize the intima of central pulmonary arteries. It is inserted through a vascular sheath inserted in a central vein and passed through the right side of the heart into the pulmonary artery under fluoroscopic guidance. Inflation of a latex balloon affixed to the tip of the angioscope results in obstruction of blood flow in the artery and permits visualization of the arterial intima. The classic appearance of chronic pulmonary thromboembolic disease by angioscopy consists of intimal irregularity and scarring, with webbing of the vessel lumina.[140] The presence of embolic disease, occlusion of vessels, or the presence of gross thrombotic material also is diagnostic. In addition, percutaneous interventional approaches using intravascular ultrasound and optical coherence tomography have provided high-resolution, real-time imaging of vascular obstructions of chronic thromboembolic PH in vivo.[141]

More recently, multidetector computed tomography (CT) pulmonary angiography, helical CT scanning[142], single photon emission CT scanning,[143] and magnetic resonance angiography[144] have been used to screen patients with suspected thromboembolic disease. Although promising, none of these techniques yet provide the resolution of pulmonary angiography, particularly in visualizing thromboembolic disease in the segmental and subsegmental vessels. Features of chronic thromboembolic disease seen by these modalities include evidence of organized thrombus lining the pulmonary vessels in an eccentric fashion, enlargement of the right ventricle and central pulmonary arteries, variation in size of lobar arteries (relatively smaller in affected segments compared with uninvolved areas), and parenchymal changes compatible with pulmonary infarction. It is important to note that recent advances such as dual-energy CT,[145] cone-beam CT, electrocardiograph-gated 320-row area detector CT, and lung perfusion magnetic resonance imaging may change paradigms in pulmonary vascular imaging in the future.

Surgical Selection

Although previous attempts had been made, Allison and colleagues[146] performed the first successful pulmonary thromboendarterectomy through a sternotomy using surface hypothermia in a patient with a 12-day history of pulmonary embolism, but only fresh clots were removed and an endarterectomy was not performed. Since then, there have been many occasional surgical reports of the surgical treatment of chronic pulmonary thromboembolism,[147] but by far the greatest surgical experience in pulmonary endarterectomy has been at the University of California, San Diego (UCSD),[148,149] where more than 3200 operations have been performed.

The three major reasons for considering a patient for pulmonary endarterectomy are hemodynamic, respiratory, and prophylactic. The hemodynamic goal is to prevent or ameliorate right ventricular compromise caused by PH. The respiratory objective is to improve function by the removal of a large, ventilated but unperfused physiologic dead space. The prophylactic goals are to prevent progressive right ventricular dysfunction, retrograde extension of the clot, and the prevention of secondary vasculopathic changes in the remaining patent vessels. Pulmonary endarterectomy is considered in patients who are symptomatic and have evidence of hemodynamic or ventilatory impairment at rest or with exercise. Patients undergoing surgery usually exhibit a preoperative PVR greater than 300 dyn·s/cm^{-5}, typically in the range of 800 to 1200 dyn·s/cm^{-5}.[150] Although most patients have a pulmonary artery pressure that is less than systemic, the hypertrophy of the right ventricle that occurs over time makes PH possible at suprasystemic levels. Therefore, many patients have a level of PVR in excess of 1000 dyn·s/cm^{-5} and suprasystemic pulmonary artery pressures. There is no upper limit of PVR level, pulmonary artery pressure, or degree of right ventricular dysfunction that excludes patients from operation. For those with milder PH, the decision to operate is based on individual circumstances. Some patients elect to undergo surgery at this early stage of disease because of dissatisfaction with their exercise limitation or concerns about clinical deterioration in the future.

Those who choose not to pursue surgical intervention at early stages of the disease require close monitoring for progression of PH. Because of the changes that can occur, especially in the remaining patent (unaffected by clot or obstruction) pulmonary vascular bed subjected to the higher pressures and flow, pulmonary endarterectomy is usually offered to symptomatic and asymptomatic patients whenever their angiograms demonstrate significant thromboembolic disease.[139]

Guiding Principles of the Operation

There are several guiding principles of the operation: (1) the endarterectomy must be bilateral, and therefore the approach is through a median sternotomy; (2) identification of the correct dissection plan is crucial; (3) perfect visualization is essential by use of circulatory arrest, usually limited to 20 minutes for each side; and (4) a complete endarterectomy is essential. The operation must be bilateral because, for PH to be a major factor, both pulmonary arteries usually are substantially involved. The only reasonable approach to both pulmonary arteries is through a median sternotomy. Historically, there were reports of unilateral operation, and occasionally this is still performed through a thoracotomy.[151] However, the unilateral approach ignores disease on the contralateral side, subjects the patient to hemodynamic jeopardy during the clamping of the pulmonary artery, and does not allow good visibility because of the continued presence of bronchial blood flow. In addition, collateral channels develop in chronic thromboembolic PH not only through the bronchial arteries, but also from diaphragmatic, intercostal, and pleural vessels. The dissection of the lung in the pleural space via a median sternotomy, apart from bilateral access, avoids entry into the pleural cavities and allows for the ready institution of cardiopulmonary bypass.

Cardiopulmonary bypass is essential to ensure cardiovascular stability when the operation is performed and to cool the patient to allow circulatory arrest. Excellent visibility is required, in a bloodless field, to define an adequate endarterectomy plane and then follow the pulmonary endarterectomy specimen deep into the subsegmental vessels. Because of the copious bronchial blood flow usually present in these cases, periods of circulatory arrest are necessary to ensure visibility.[152] There have been recent reports of the performance of this operation without circulatory arrest.[153,154] However, it should be emphasized that although endarterectomy is possible without circulatory arrest, a complete endarterectomy is not.[155] The circulatory arrest portions of the case are limited to the most distal portion of the endarterectomy process, deep in the subsegmental vasculature, and they are usually limited to 20 minutes for each side with restoration of flow in between.

A true endarterectomy in the plane of the media must be accomplished. It is essential to appreciate that the removal of visible thrombus is largely incidental to this operation. Indeed, in many patients, no free thrombus is present; and on initial direct examination, the pulmonary vascular bed may appear normal. The early literature on this procedure indicates that thrombectomy often was performed without endarterectomy, and in these cases the pulmonary artery pressures did not improve, often resulting in death.

An IVC filter is always placed before surgery unless an obvious upper extremity or cardiac (e.g., intraventricular pacing wire, ventriculoatrial shunt) source is present. In the latter case, removal of any foreign material is undertaken, with alternative sites used, as with replacement of intravascular pacing leads with epicardial electrodes. Patients are treated with warfarin until the time of surgery, and this treatment is continued throughout the patient's life after surgery.

Pulmonary Endarterectomy: Surgical Technique

The technique for pulmonary endarterectomy has largely been developed by Dr. Stuart Jamieson at UCSD.[156] After a median sternotomy incision is made, the pericardium is incised longitudinally and attached to the wound edges. Typically the right side of the heart is enlarged, with a tense right atrium and a variable degree of tricuspid regurgitation. There is usually severe right ventricular hypertrophy, and, with critical degrees of obstruction, the patient's condition may become unstable with manipulation of the heart. Anticoagulation is achieved with the use of heparin sodium (400 U/kg, IV) administered to prolong the activated clotting time beyond 400 seconds. Full cardiopulmonary bypass is instituted with high ascending aortic cannulation and two caval cannulas. These cannulas must be inserted into the superior and inferior venae cavae sufficiently to enable subsequent opening of the right atrium. The heart is emptied on bypass, and a temporary pulmonary artery vent is placed in the midline of the main pulmonary artery, 1 cm distal to the pulmonary valve. This marks the beginning of the left pulmonary arteriotomy.

After cardiopulmonary bypass is initiated, surface cooling with both a head jacket and a cooling blanket on the operating room table is begun. The blood is cooled with the pump oxygenator. During cooling, a 10° C gradient between arterial blood and bladder or rectal temperature is maintained.[157] Cooling generally takes 45 minutes to 1 hour. When ventricular fibrillation occurs, an additional vent is placed in the left atrium through the right superior pulmonary vein. This prevents the occurrence of atrial and ventricular distention resulting from the large amount of bronchial arterial blood flow that is common with these patients. It is most convenient for the primary surgeon to stand initially on the patient's left side. During the cooling period, some preliminary dissection can be performed, with full mobilization of the right pulmonary artery from the ascending aorta. All dissection of the pulmonary arteries takes place intrapericardially, and neither pleural cavity is entered. An incision is then made in the right pulmonary artery from beneath the ascending aorta under the superior vena cava and entering the lower lobe branch of the pulmonary artery just after the takeoff of the middle lobe artery.

Any loose thrombus, if present, is removed. The endarterectomy cannot be performed in the presence of thrombus because it obscures the plane and prevents collapse of the endarterectomized specimen, hindering distal exposure. It is important to recognize that, first, an embolectomy without subsequent endarterectomy is ineffective and, second, in most patients with chronic thromboembolic hypertension, direct examination of the pulmonary vascular bed at operation generally shows no obvious embolic material. Therefore, to the inexperienced or cursory glance, the pulmonary vascular bed might appear normal, even in patients with severe chronic embolic PH. If the bronchial circulation is not excessive, the endarterectomy plane can be found during this early dissection. However, although a small amount of dissection can be performed before the initiation of circulatory arrest, it is unwise to proceed unless perfect visibility is obtained, because the development of a correct plane is essential.

When the patient's temperature reaches 20° C, the aorta is cross-clamped and a single dose of cold cardioplegic solution is administered. Additional myocardial protection is obtained with the use of a cooling jacket wrapped around the heart. The entire procedure is now performed with a single aortic cross-clamp period with no further administration of cardioplegic solution. A modified cerebellar retractor is placed between the aorta and the superior vena cava. When back bleeding from bronchial collaterals obscures direct vision of the pulmonary vascular bed, thiopental is administered (500 mg to 1 g) until the electroencephalogram becomes isoelectric. Circulatory arrest is then initiated, and the patient undergoes exsanguination. It is rare that one 20-minute period for each side is exceeded. Although retrograde cerebral perfusion has been advocated for total circulatory arrest in other procedures, it is not helpful in this operation because it does not allow a completely bloodless field, and, with the short arrest times that can be achieved, it is not necessary.

Any loose thrombotic debris encountered is removed. Next, a microtome knife is used to develop the endarterectomy plane posteriorly within the media of the vessel. Dissection in the correct plane is critical because if the plane is too deep, then the pulmonary artery may perforate, with fatal results, and if the dissection plane is not deep enough, then inadequate amounts of the partially resorbed thromboembolic material will be removed. Once the plane is correctly developed, a full-thickness layer is left in the region of the incision to ease subsequent repair. For the endarterectomy, gentle traction with forceps while sweeping the outer vessel wall layer away results in the progressive withdrawal of the endarterectomy specimen. The procedure is primarily performed with a long miniature sucker with a rounded tip.[139] As each lobar branch appears, it is grasped individually and the specimen is withdrawn until each segmental vessel branches again. Each of these subsegmental specimens is then extracted. Removal of each lobar and then segmental branch makes subsequent distal dissection easier. If a large mass of endarterectomized tissue begins to obscure visibility, it is excised. The entire specimen can thus be removed for a length of approximately 20 cm. The distal-most portion endarterectomy is performed with an eversion technique. Perforation at the level of the subsegmental vessels will become completely inaccessible later, so care must be taken to remain in the plane of the media for endarterectomy. Clear visualization in a completely bloodless field provided by circulatory arrest is therefore essential during development of the distal surgical plane. It is important that each subsegmental branch is followed and freed individually until it ends in a "tail," beyond which there is no further obstruction. Residual material should never be cut free; the entire specimen should "tail off" and come free spontaneously. Once the right-sided endarterectomy is completed, circulation is restarted and the arteriotomy is repaired with a continuous 6-0 polypropylene suture. The hemostatic nature of this closure is aided by the nature of the initial dissection, with the full thickness of the pulmonary artery being preserved immediately adjacent to the incision.

After completion of the repair of the right arteriotomy, the surgeon moves to the patient's right side. The pulmonary vent catheter is withdrawn, and an arteriotomy is made from the site of the pulmonary vent hole laterally to the pericardial reflection, avoiding entry into the left pleural space. Additional lateral dissection does not enhance intraluminal visibility, can endanger the left phrenic nerve, and makes subsequent repair of the left pulmonary artery more difficult. The left-sided dissection is virtually analogous in all respects to that accomplished on the right. The duration of circulatory arrest intervals during the performance of the left-sided dissection also is subject to the same restriction as the right. After the completion of the endarterectomy, cardiopulmonary bypass is reinstituted and warming is commenced. Methylprednisolone (500 mg IV) and mannitol (12.5 g IV) are administered, and during warming a 10° C temperature gradient is maintained between the perfusate and body temperature. If the systemic vascular resistance level is high, nitroprusside is administered to promote vasodilation and warming. The rewarming period generally takes approximately 90 minutes, but varies according to the body mass of the patient.

When the pulmonary arteriotomy has been repaired, the pulmonary artery vent is replaced at the top of the incision. The right atrium is then opened and examined unless a negative "bubble" test result before cardiopulmonary bypass reveals no persistent foramen ovale on transesophageal echocardiography. Otherwise, any intraatrial communication (present in ≈20% of patients) is closed at this point. Although tricuspid valve regurgitation is invariable in these patients and is often severe, tricuspid valve repair is not performed. Right ventricular remodeling occurs within a few days, with the return of tricuspid competence.[158] If other cardiac procedures are required, such as coronary artery or mitral or aortic valve surgery, these are conveniently performed during the systemic rewarming period.[159] Myocardial cooling is discontinued once all cardiac procedures have been concluded. The left atrial vent is removed, and the vent site is repaired. Air is evacuated from the heart, and the aortic cross-clamp is removed.

When the patient has rewarmed, cardiopulmonary bypass is discontinued. Dopamine hydrochloride is routinely administered at renal doses, and other inotropic agents and vasodilators are titrated as necessary to sustain acceptable hemodynamics. The cardiac output is generally high, with a low systemic vascular resistance. Temporary atrial and ventricular epicardial pacing wires are placed. Despite the duration of extracorporeal circulation, hemostasis is readily achieved, and the administration of platelets or coagulation factors is generally unnecessary. Wound closure is routine. A vigorous diuresis is usual for the next few hours, also the result of the previous systemic hypothermia. All patients are subjected to a maintained diuresis with the goal of reaching the patient's preoperative weight within 24 hours. Extubation is usually performed on the first postoperative day.

Thromboembolic Disease Classification and Prediction of Surgical Outcome

Four major types of pulmonary occlusive disease, based on anatomy and location of thrombus and vessel wall pathology, have been described.[139] This intraoperative classification of disease allows for the prediction of patient outcome after pulmonary endarterectomy.[160]

1. Type 1 disease (≈11% of cases of thromboembolic PH; Fig. 102-3): fresh thrombus in the main or lobar pulmonary arteries. In this situation, major vessel clot is present and visible on the opening of the pulmonary arteries. This clot usually reflects main or lobar pulmonary vessel wall disease, with stasis, and fresh propagation of clot into the major pulmonary vessels.
2. Type 2 disease (≈43% of cases; Fig. 102-4): intimal thickening and fibrosis with or without organized thrombus proximal to segmental arteries. In these cases, only thickened intima can be seen, occasionally with webs in the main or lobar arteries.
3. Type 3 disease (≈42% of cases; Fig. 102-5): fibrosis, intimal webbing, and thickening with or without organized thrombus within distal segmental and subsegmental arteries only. This type of disease presents the most challenging surgical situation. No occlusion of vessels can be seen initially. The endarterectomy plane must be raised individually in each segmental and subsegmental branch. Type 3 disease is most often associated with presumed repetitive thrombi from indwelling catheters or ventriculoatrial shunts and sometimes represents "burned out" disease, in which most of the embolic material has been reabsorbed.
4. Type 4 disease (less than 4% of cases): microscopic distal arteriolar vasculopathy without visible thromboembolic disease. Type 4 disease does not

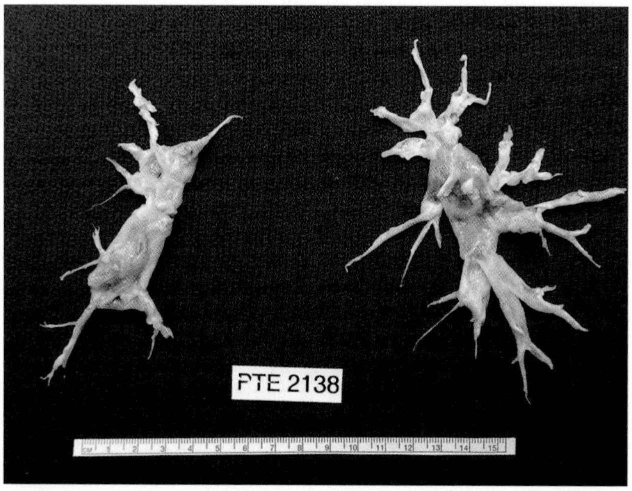

FIGURE 102-4 ■ Surgical specimen removed from the right and left pulmonary arteries indicates type 2 disease.

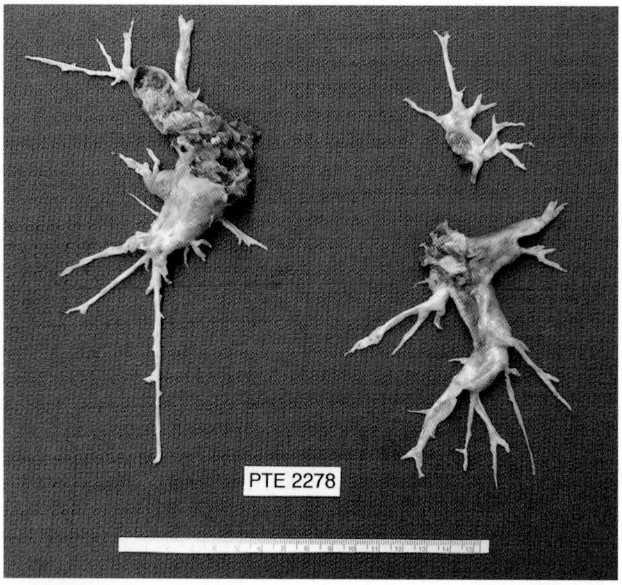

FIGURE 102-3 ■ Surgical specimen removed from right and left pulmonary arteries. Evidence of fresh thrombus indicates type 1 disease.

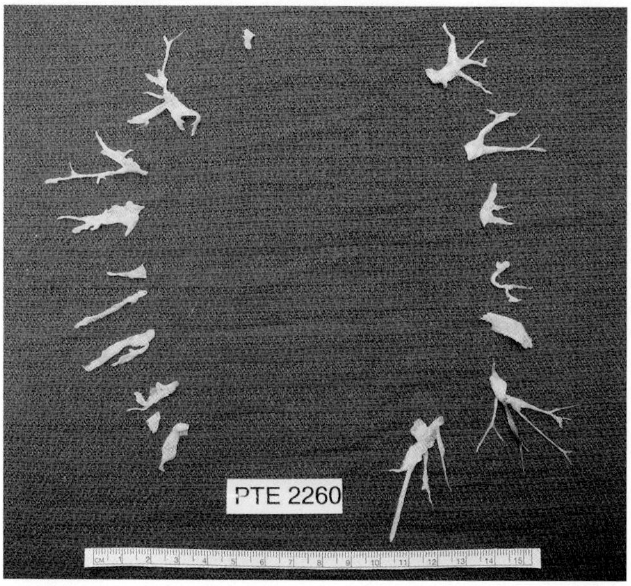

FIGURE 102-5 ■ Surgical specimen removed from right and left pulmonary arteries. In this patient with type 3 disease, the dissection plane was raised at each segmental level.

represent classic chronic thromboembolic PH and is inoperable. In this entity, there is intrinsic small-vessel disease, although secondary thrombus can occur because of stasis. Small-vessel disease may be unrelated to thromboembolic events (primary PH) or can occur in relation to thromboembolic hypertension because of a high-flow or high-pressure state in previously unaffected vessels similar to the generation of Eisenmenger syndrome.

We have noticed, in the last several hundred patients, an increase in the number of patients with type 3 disease (currently, ≈42% of cases) and a decrease in the number of patients with Type 1 (currently, ≈11% of cases) disease. Whether this reflects referral bias (i.e., difficult cases are preferentially sent to UCSD), increased recognition and diagnosis of thromboembolic PH, or a change in the presenting spectrum of disease is unclear. Nonetheless, despite seeing an increase in patients with more distal, surgically challenging disease, excellent hemodynamic and survival outcomes have been achieved at our institution.

Results of Pulmonary Endarterectomy Surgery

Although pulmonary endarterectomy is performed at several major cardiovascular centers throughout the world, the majority of experience with this operation has been at the UCSD, where the technique of this operation was pioneered and refined. More than 3200 pulmonary endarterectomy operations have been performed at UCSD since 1970, whereas the entire reported literature on this operation (exclusive of UCSD) is approximately 2000 cases; 2400 cases have been completed at UCSD since 1997. The mean patient age of the last 1000 patients undergoing operation was 51.6 years, with a range of 8.9 to 84.8 years. There is a slight male predominance, reflecting either disease predilection, surgical bias, or both. In 40% of cases, at least one additional cardiac procedure was performed at the time of operation. Most commonly, the adjunct procedure was closure of a persistent foramen ovale or atrial septal defect (18.9%) or coronary artery bypass grafting (7.9%).[159]

With this operation, a reduction in pulmonary pressures and resistance to normal levels and corresponding improvement in pulmonary blood flow and cardiac output are generally immediate and sustained.[161,162] These changes are permanent.[163] Table 102-3 lists the most current statistics for the last 1000 patients who underwent pulmonary endarterectomy at UCSD with respect to hemodynamic improvement. Table 102-4 presents results for the same patient group stratified for thromboembolic disease classification group. Whereas before the operation more than 82.6% of the patients were in New

TABLE 102-3 UCSD Pulmonary Endarterectomy Recent Hemodynamic Results*

Variable	All Patients (*N* = 1000)	PTE Patients (*n* = 882)	PTE-CABG Patients (*n* = 79)	PTE-Value Patients (*n* = 39)
Mean decrease in PAS (mm Hg)	34.7 ± 18.8	35.2 ± 18.3	35.7 ± 22.3	18.3 ± 16.9
Mean decrease in PAD (mm Hg)	10.6 ± 8.8	10.9 ± 8.8	8.7 ± 9.8	7.9 ± 7.2
Mean decrease in PVR (dyn·s/cm^{-5})	448.5 ± 345.6	455.5 ± 350.7	413.5 ± 303.3	345.5 ± 286.4
Mean increase in CO (L/min)	1.1 ± 1.5	1.1 ± 1.5	1.1 ± 1.2	1.5 ± 1.7
Mean decrease in tricuspid regurgitant velocity (m/sec)	1.2 ± 0.9	1.2 ± 0.9	1.1 ± 0.7	0.6 ± 0.9

*Data are shown as means ± standard deviation.

CABG, Coronary artery bypass grafting; *CO,* cardiac output; *PAD,* pulmonary artery diastolic pressure; *PAS,* pulmonary artery systolic pressure; *PVR,* pulmonary vascular resistance; *UCSD,* University of California, San Diego.

TABLE 102-4 UCSD Thromboembolic Disease Classification: Pulmonary Endarterectomy Hemodynamic Results*

Variable	All Patients (*N* = 1000, 100%)	Type 1 (*n* = 112, 11.2%)	Type 2 (*n* = 425, 42.5%)	Type 3 (*n* = 417, 41.7%)	Type 4 (*n* = 46, 4.6%)
PVR (dyn·sec/cm^{-5})	692 ± 382.7	832.8 ± 463.6	667.4 ± 353.8	673.2 ± 382.1	747.8 ± 367.5
	241.0 ± 131.7	226.6 ± 109.4	208.7 ± 108.2	258.8 ± 132.1	410.8 ± 200.1
CO (L/min)	4.5 ± 1.4	4.0 ± 1.4	4.5 ± 1.3	4.5 ± 1.5	4.2 ± 1.6
	5.6 ± 1.5	5.4 ± 1.2	5.8 ± 1.5	5.5 ± 1.5	4.8 ± 1.4
Systolic PA Pressure (mm Hg)	74.6 ± 20.2	76.2 ± 18.4	75.1 ± 19.8	73.7 ± 21.3	74.1 ± 17.1
	40.1 ± 13.3	38.4 ± 11.3	37.5 ± 11.6	41.7 ± 14.0	52.6 ± 15.9
Diastolic PA pressure (mm Hg)	27.0 ± 9.1	29.0 ± 8.9	27.0 ± 9.0	26.4 ± 9.2	27.1 ± 9.7
	16.3 ± 5.7	15.8 ± 4.9	15.6 ± 5.5	16.8 ± 5.7	20.5 ± 6.3
Mean PA pressure (mm Hg)	44.8 ± 11.9	46.2 ± 11.4	44.9 ± 11.6	44.2 ± 12.6	44.9 ± 10.2
	25.0 ± 7.7	24.2 ± 6.7	23.5 ± 6.9	25.9 ± 8.1	32.0 ± 8.5
Mortality (%)	15 (1.5%)	4 (3.6%)	5 (1.2%)	5 (1.2%)	1 (2.2%)

*Data are shown mean ± standard deviation or number (percentage). Upper numbers of each pair are preoperative values, and lower numbers are postoperative values obtained just prior to removal of the Swan-Ganz catheter.

CO, Cardiac output; *PA,* pulmonary artery; *PVR,* pulmonary vascular resistance.

York Heart Association (NYHA) functional class III or IV in this series, at 1 year after operation, 87.6% of patients were reclassified as NYHA functional class I or II. In addition, echocardiographic studies have demonstrated that, with the elimination of chronic pressure overload, right ventricular geometry rapidly reverts toward normal.[164,165] Right atrial and right ventricular hypertrophy and dilation regresses. Tricuspid valve function returns to normal within a few days as a result of restoration of tricuspid annular geometry after the remodeling of the right ventricle; therefore, tricuspid valve repair is not performed with this operation.[158]

Centers from around the world are now presenting results of surgical series of pulmonary endarterectomy operations. Table 102-5 summarizes the survival and hemodynamic outcome after pulmonary endarterectomy from this growing body of surgical experience.[149,153,154,163,165-187]

Severe reperfusion injury is the single most frequent complication after pulmonary endarterectomy, historically occurring in approximately 15% of patients, but now in a much smaller percentage of our patients (≈5%). Of patients with reperfusion injury, the majority resolve the problem with a short period of ventilatory support and aggressive diuresis. A minority of patients with severe lung reperfusion injury require prolonged periods of ventilatory support, whereas extreme cases require venovenous extracorporeal support for oxygenation and blood carbon dioxide removal.[188] Neurologic complications from circulatory arrest have mostly been eliminated by shorter circulatory arrest periods and the use of a direct cooling jacket placed around the head, which provides even cooling to the surface of the cranium. Stroke rates for the last 1000 pulmonary endarterectomy patients at UCSD is 0.2%. In the last 1000 pulmonary endarterectomy patients at UCSD, reexploration for bleeding occurred at a rate of 2.8%, and 33.9% of patients required intraoperative or postoperative blood transfusion. Despite an average duration of surgery of 6.2 hours, wound infection occurred in only 0.6% of patients.

The single greatest risk factor for operation remains the severity of pulmonary vascular resistance and the ability to lower it to a normal range at operation. Patients with high pulmonary vascular resistance with minimal vascular obstruction on angiogram (Type 4 small vessel vasculopathy indistinguishable from idiopathic pulmonary arterial hypertension) have the worst prognosis, and surgery does not correct PH in this population. Arteriolar-capillary vasculopathy without larger vessel thromboembolic disease was not influenced by blind endarterectomy of the proximal pulmonary arterial tree. The majority of early deaths after this operation are in this subgroup, and

TABLE 102-5 **Pulmonary Endarterectomy Series of More Than 50 patients: 2008-2014**

References	Date	Dates of Study	Patients *(N)*	Periop Deaths *(N)*	Preop Mean PA Pressure (mm Hg)	Postop Mean PA Pressure (mm Hg)	Preop Mean PVR (dyn·s/cm^{-5})	Postop Mean PVR (dyn·s/cm^{-5})
Condliffe[169]	2008	2001-2006	236	37	48	27	1091	464
Corsico[168]	2008	1994-2006	157	18	48	24	1140	327
Freed[167]	2008	1997-2006	229	0	47	25	800	244
Thistlethwaite[166]	2008	NR	1100	52	46	28	859	290
Thomson[153]	2008	2003-2006	150	22	52	29	740	336
Saouti[171]	2009	1998-2007	72	5	42	22	572	NR
Skoro-Sajer[170]	2009	1994-2006	62	NR	48	NR	746	383
Gan[173]	2010	1989-2007	360	16	81	NR	19*	NR
Kunihara[172]	2010	1995-2006	219	6	48	24	800†	300†
de Perrot[178]	2011	2005-2011	58	3	45	24	965	383
Freed[177]	2011	1997-2007	314	0	48	26	805	301
Kunihara[176]	2011	1995-2009	279	31	47	26†	872	350†
Schölzel[175]	2011	2000-2009	74	5	41	25	521	NR
Surie[165]	2011	NR	73	6	42	24	808	419
van der Plas[174]	2011	2003-2009	96	10	41	25	768	422
Ishida[163]	2012	1990-2010	77	11	47	25	868	313
Madani[149]	2012	1999-2006	1000	NR	46	29	861	294
		2006-2010	500	NR	46	26	719	253
Morsolini[154]	2012	1994-2011	347	35	45	25	999	439
Surie[179]	2012	NR	73	5	40	23	714	410
Nishimura[182]	2013	1986-2010	195	NR	43	NR	792	NR
Ross[181]	2013	1999-2012	91	NR	43	20	753	182
Sato[180]	2013	2001-2010	60	NR	49	22	998	269
Berman[187]	2014	NR	72	0	48	26	698	265
Ghio[186]	2014	1994-2012	296	0	44	23	925	303
Schölzel[185]	2014	2004-2009	52	5	40	NR	971	NR
Skoro-Sajer[184]	2014	1994-2010	110	5	NR	NR	770	368
Wietska[183]	2014	1998-2008	66	6	50	25	752	176

*Recorded as Woods units.
†Numbers were estimated from graph data in references.
NR, Not recorded; *PA,* pulmonary artery; *Periop,* perioperative; *Postop,* postoperative; *Preop,* preoperative; *PVR,* pulmonary vascular resistance.

efforts are directed at better determining who these patients are in the preoperative setting to avoid unnecessary operation.

In the UCSD experience, overall perioperative mortality was 5.4% for the entire cohort of patients, encompassing a span of more than 30 years. In the last 1000 cases, surgical mortality for pulmonary endarterectomy was 1.5%. This reflects the learning curve for safely performing this operation and the refinements in surgical technique that enhance patient outcome.

A survey of surviving patients who underwent pulmonary endarterectomy between 1970 and 1995 at UCSD has formally evaluated long-term outcome from this operation.[189] Questionnaires were mailed to 420 patients who had surgery more than 1 year prior, and responses were obtained from 308 patients. Survival, functional status, quality of life, and the subsequent use of medical assistance were assessed. Survival after pulmonary endarterectomy was found to be 75% at 6 years or more. This survival exceeds single- or double-lung transplant survival for thromboembolic PH. Ninety-three percent of the patients were found to be in NYHA class I or II, compared with approximately 95% of the patients being in NYHA class III or IV preoperatively. Of the working population, 62% of patients who were unemployed before operation returned to work. Patients who had undergone pulmonary endarterectomy scored several quality of life components slightly lower than normal individuals, but significantly higher than the patients before operation. Only 10% of patients used oxygen after surgery. In response to the question "How do you feel about the quality of your life since your surgery?" 77% replied much improved, and 20% replied improved. These data appear to confirm that pulmonary endarterectomy offers substantial improvement in survival, function, and quality of life.

Alternative Therapies for Chronic Thromboembolic Pulmonary Hypertension

There are patients with chronic thromboembolic PH who are not surgical candidates, because they are either (1) technically nonoperable, or (2) technically operable but have an unacceptable surgical risk. Determination of operable candidacy should be done by a center with expertise with pulmonary endarterectomy. Candidates that are deemed poor surgical candidates may be evaluated for the option of either balloon angioplasty of the pulmonary vasculature[190] or medical management with riociguat,[191] the only drug currently approved by the FDA for the treatment of chronic thromboembolic PH.

In 2001, Feinstein and colleagues[192] published a series of 18 patients with inoperable chronic thromboembolic PH who underwent balloon dilation of the pulmonary arteries, with variable results. More recently, Japanese investigators refined pulmonary artery balloon angioplasty by using smaller balloons, by limiting the number of balloon inflations per session to two pulmonary vascular segments, and by the use of intravascular ultrasound[193,194,195] An average of 4.8 sessions is needed per patient, and severe reperfusion edema was seen in 2% of patients. Although pulmonary artery balloon angioplasty remains largely experimental in the United States, it is rapidly gaining attention for use in nonoperable patients, such as those who have incurable malignancy or are too frail to survive operation.

Recently, riociguat, a new class of oral drug and stimulator of guanylate cyclase, met the primary and secondary endpoints (increased 6-minute walk distance, improvement in World Health Organization functional class, hemodynamics, biomarkers, and quality of life) of a phase 3, multicenter, randomized, double-blind, placebo-controlled study of 261 patients with adjudicated inoperable chronic thromboembolic PH or persistent PH after pulmonary endarterectomy.[196] This drug was approved by the FDA in October 2013 for the treatment of inoperable chronic thromboembolic PH and persistent PH following pulmonary endarterectomy. It is important to note that pulmonary endarterectomy remains the gold standard treatment of chronic thromboembolic PH, and it is curative of this disease. Only patients deemed inoperable by an experienced pulmonary endarterectomy team or those that have residual PH after pulmonary endarterectomy should be offered riociguat.

SUMMARY

Pulmonary hypertension owing to chronic pulmonary emboli is a condition that is underrecognized and carries a poor prognosis. Pulmonary endarterectomy is considered the best treatment for chronic thromboembolic PH. The only curative therapeutic alternative to pulmonary endarterectomy is lung transplantation and heart-lung transplantation. The advantages of pulmonary endarterectomy include a lower operative mortality, better long-term results with respect to survival and quality of life, and the avoidance of chronic immunosuppressive treatment and allograft rejection. Currently, mortality rates for pulmonary endarterectomy are 1.5%, and the operation allows for sustained clinical benefit. These results make it the treatment of choice over transplantation for thromboembolic disease to the lung both in the short and long term.

Although pulmonary endarterectomy is a technically demanding operation, excellent results can be achieved. Improvements in operative technique developed over the past four decades allow pulmonary endarterectomy to be offered to patients with an acceptable mortality rate and anticipation of clinical improvement. With the increasing recognition of patients who have thromboembolic PH and the realization that pulmonary endarterectomy is a safe and effective operation for this condition, it is anticipated that this will be an expanding area of surgical therapy in the future.

REFERENCES

1. DeMonaco NA, Dang Q, Kapoor WN, et al: Pulmonary embolism incidence is increasing with use of spiral computed tomography. *Am J Med* 121:611–617, 2008.
2. Goldhaber SZ, Hennekens CH, Evans DA, et al: Factors associated with correct antemortem diagnosis of major pulmonary embolism. *Am J Med* 73:822–826, 1982.

3. Lindblad B, Eriksson A, Bergqvist D: Autopsy-verified pulmonary embolism in a surgical department: analysis of the period from 1951 to 1988. *Br J Surg* 78:849–852, 1991.
4. Landefeld CS, Chren MM, Myers A, et al: Diagnostic yield of the autopsy in a university hospital and a community hospital. *N Engl J Med* 318:1249–1254, 1988.
5. Pengo V, Lensing AW, Prins MH, et al: Incidence of chronic thromboembolic pulmonary hypertension after pulmonary embolism. *N Engl J Med* 350:2257–2264, 2004.
6. Riedel M, Stanek V, Widimsky J, et al: Long-term follow-up of patients with pulmonary thromboembolism. Late prognosis and evolution of hemodynamic and respiratory data. *Chest* 81:151–158, 1982.
7. Laennec RTH: *Traite do l'auscultation mediate et des maladies des poumons et du Coeur*, Paris, 1819, Brossen et Chaude.
8. Virchow R: Uber die verstopfung der lungenarterie. *Reue Notizen auf Geb d Nature u Heilk* 37:26, 1846.
9. Ageno W, Squizzato A, Garcia D, et al: Epidemiology and risk factors of venous thromboembolism. *Semin Thromb Hemost* 32:651–658, 2006.
10. Wakefield TW, Proctor MC: Current status of pulmonary embolism and venous thrombosis prophylaxis. *Semin Vasc Surg* 13:171–181, 2000.
11. Gurewich V, Cohen ML, Thomas DP: Humoral factors in massive pulmonary embolism: an experimental study. *Am Heart J* 76:784–794, 1968.
12. Duan Q, Lv W, Wang L, et al: mRNA expression of interleukins and Th1/Th2 imbalance in patients with pulmonary embolism. *Mol Med Rep* 7:332–336, 2013.
13. Malik AB, Johnson A: Role of humoral mediators in the pulmonary vascular response to pulmonary embolism. In Weir EK, Reeves JT, editors: *Pulmonary vascular physiology and pathophysiology*, New York, 1989, Marcel Dekker, pp 445–468.
14. Wei Z, Al-Mehdi AB, Fisher AB: Signaling pathway for nitric oxide generation with simulated ischemia in flow-adapted endothelial cells. *Am J Physiol Heart Circ Physiol* 281:H2226–H2232, 2001.
15. Moser KM, Auger WR, Fedullo PF, et al: Chronic thromboembolic pulmonary hypertension: clinical picture and surgical treatment. *Eur Respir J* 5:334–342, 1992.
16. Palevsky HI: The problems of the clinical and laboratory diagnosis of pulmonary embolism. *Semin Nucl Med* 21:276–280, 1991.
17. Goldhaber SZ: Strategies for diagnosis. In Goldhaber SZ, editor: *Pulmonary embolism and deep vein thrombosis*, Philadelphia, 1985, W.B. Saunders, p 79.
18. Gelfand EV, Piazza G, Goldhaber SZ: Venous thromboembolism guidebook. *Crit Pathw Cardiol* 1:26–43, 2002.
19. Jaff MR, McMurtry MS, Archer SL, et al: Management of massive and submassive pulmonary embolism, iliofemoral deep vein thrombosis, and chronic thromboembolic pulmonary hypertension. *Circulation* 123:1788–1830, 2011.
20. Tapson VF: Acute pulmonary embolism. *N Engl J Med* 358:1037–1052, 2008.
21. Post F, Mertens D, Sinning C, et al: Decision for aggressive therapy in acute pulmonary embolism: implication of elevated troponin. *Clin Res Cardiol* 98:401–408, 2009.
22. Palmieri V, Gallotta G, Rendina D, et al: Troponin I and right ventricular dysfunction for risk assessment in patients with nonmassive pulmonary embolism in the Emergency Department in combination with clinically based risk score. *Intern Emerg Med* 3:131–138, 2008.
23. Bova C, Pesavento R, Marchiori A, et al: Risk stratification and outcomes in hemodynamically stable patients with acute pulmonary embolism: a prospective, multicentre, cohort study with 3 months of follow-up. *J Thromb Haemost* 7:938–944, 2009.
24. Hoagland PM: Massive pulmonary embolism. In Goldhaber SZ, editor: *Pulmonary embolism and deep vein thrombosis*, Philadelphia, 1986, W.B. Saunders, p 179.
25. Stein PD, Sostman HD, Bounameaux H, et al: Challenges in the diagnosis acute pulmonary embolism. *Am J Med* 121:565–571, 2008.
26. Hagen PJ, Hartmann IJ, Hoekstra OS, et al: Comparison of observer variability and accuracy of different criteria for lung scan interpretation. *J Nucl Med* 44:739–744, 2003.
27. Skarlovnik A, Hrastnik D, Fettich J, et al: Lung scintigraphy in the diagnosis of pulmonary embolism: current methods and interpretation criteria in clinical practice. *Radiol Oncol* 48:113–119, 2014.
28. Chughtai A, Kazerooni EA: CT and MRI of acute thoracic cardiovascular emergencies. *Crit Care Clin* 23:835–853, 2007.
29. Stawicki SP, Seamon MJ, Kim PK, et al: Transthoracic echocardiography for pulmonary embolism in the ICU: finding the "right" findings. *J Am Coll Surg* 206:42–47, 2008.
30. Pruszczyk P, Torbicki A, Kuch-Wocial A, et al: Diagnostic value of transoesophageal echocardiography in suspected haemodynamically significant pulmonary embolism. *Heart* 85:628–634, 2001.
31. Heit JA, Silverstein MD, Mohr DN, et al: The epidemiology of venous thromboembolism in the community. *Thromb Haemost* 86:452–463, 2001.
32. Society of American Gastrointestinal and Endoscopic Surgeons (SAGES): Guidelines for deep venous thrombosis prophylaxis during laparoscopic surgery. *Surg Endosc* 21:1007–1009, 2007.
33. Gross PL, Weitz JI: New anticoagulants for treatment of venous thromboembolism. *Arterioscler Thromb Vasc Biol* 28:380–386, 2008.
34. Lassen MR, Ageno W, Borris LC, et al: Rivaroxaban versus enoxaparin for thromboprophylaxis after total knee arthroplasty. *N Engl J Med* 358:2776–2786, 2008.
35. Poulsen SH, Noer I, Moller JE, et al: Clinical outcome of patients with suspected pulmonary embolism. A follow-up study of 588 consecutive patients. *J Intern Med* 250:137–143, 2001.
36. Simonneau G, Sors H, Charbonnier B, et al: A comparison of low-molecular-weight heparin with unfractionated heparin for acute pulmonary embolism. The THESEE Study Group. Tinzaparine ou Heparine Standard: Evaluations dans l'Embolie Pulmonaire. *N Engl J Med* 337:663–669, 1997.
37. Warkentin TE, Greinacher A, Koster A, et al: Treatment and prevention of heparin-induced thrombocytopenia: American College of Chest Physicians Evidence Based Clinical Practice Guidelines (8th ed). *Chest* 133:340S–380S, 2008.
38. Dalen JE, Banas JS, Jr, Brooks HL, et al: Resolution rate of pulmonary embolism in man. *N Engl J Med* 280:1194–1199, 1969.
39. Kearon C, Akl EA, Comerota AJ, et al: Antithrombotic Therapy for VTE Disease: Antithrombotic Therapy and Prevention of Thrombosis, 9th ed: American College of Chest Physicians Evidence-Based Clinical Practice Guidelines. *Chest* 141:e419S–e494S, 2012.
40. Rudd KM, Phillips EL: New oral anticoagulants in the treatment of pulmonary embolism: efficacy, bleeding risk, and monitoring. *Thrombosis* 2013:973710, 2013.
41. Kearon C, Ginsberg JS, Anderson DR, et al: Comparison of 1 month with 3 months of anticoagulation for a first episode of venous thromboembolism associated with a transient risk factor. *J Thromb Haemost* 2:743–749, 2004.
42. Baglin T, Luddington R, Brown K, et al: Incidence of recurrent venous thromboembolism in relation to clinical and thrombophilic risk factors: prospective cohort study. *Lancet* 362:523–526, 2003.
43. Schulman S, Rhedin AS, Lindmarker P, et al: A comparison of six weeks with six months of oral anticoagulant therapy after a first episode of venous thromboembolism. Duration of Anticoagulation Trial Study Group. *N Engl J Med* 332:1661–1665, 1995.
44. Roderick P, Ferris G, Wilson K, et al: Towards evidence-based guidelines for the prevention of venous thromboembolism: systematic reviews of mechanical methods, oral anticoagulation, dextran and regional anaesthesia as thromboprophylaxis. *Health Technol Assess* 9:1–78, 2005.
45. Stein PD: Thrombolytic therapy in acute pulmonary embolism. In Stein PD, editor: *Pulmonary embolism*, Malden, MA, 2007, Blackwell Publishing, pp 425–436.
46. Piazza G, Goldhaber SZ: Acute pulmonary embolism: part II: treatment and prophylaxis. *Circulation* 114:e42–e47, 2006.
47. Goldhaber SZ: Thrombolysis in pulmonary embolism. A large-scale trial is overdue. *Circulation* 104:2876–2878, 2001.
48. Marder VJ, Sherry S: Thrombolytic therapy: current status (2). *N Engl J Med* 318:1585–1595, 1988.
49. Goldhaber SZ, Haire WD, Feldstein ML, et al: Alteplase versus heparin in acute pulmonary embolism: randomized trial assessing

right-ventricular function and pulmonary perfusion. *Lancet* 341:507–511, 1993.
50. Kasper W, Konstantinides S, Geibel A, et al: Management strategies and determinants of outcome in acute major pulmonary embolism: results of a multicenter registry. *J Am Coll Cardiol* 30:1165–1171, 1997.
51. Goldhaber SZ, Visani L, De Rosa M: Acute pulmonary embolism: clinical outcomes in the International Cooperative Pulmonary Embolism Registry (ICOPER). *Lancet* 353:1386–1389, 1999.
52. Kucher N, Rossi E, De Rosa M, et al: Massive pulmonary embolism. *Circulation* 113:577–582, 2006.
53. Laporte S, Mismetti P, Décousus H, et al: Clinical predictors for fatal pulmonary embolism in 15,520 patients with venous thromboembolism: findings from the Registro Informatizado de la Enfermedad Trombo-Embolica venosa (RIETE) Registry. *Circulation* 117:1711–1716, 2008.
54. Lobo JL, Zorrilla V, Aizpuru F, et al: Clinical syndromes and clinical outcome in patients with pulmonary embolism: findings from the RIETE registry. *Chest* 130:1817–1822, 2006.
55. Schreiber D, Lin B, Liu G, et al: Variation in therapy and outcomes in massive pulmonary embolism from the Emergency Medicine Pulmonary Embolism in the Real World Registry (EMPEROR). *Acad Emerg Med* 16:2009.
56. Meyer G, Vicaut E, Danays T, et al: Fibrinolysis for patients with intermediate-risk pulmonary embolism. *N Engl J Med* 370:1402–1411, 2014.
57. Piazza G, Goldhaber SZ: Fibrinolysis for acute pulmonary embolism. *Vasc Med* 15:419–428, 2010.
58. Levine MN: Thrombolytic therapy for venous thromboembolism: complications and contraindications. In Tapson VF, Fulkerson WJ, Saltzman HA, editors: *Clinics in chest medicine, venous thromboembolism*, vol 16, Philadelphia, 1995, W.B. Saunders, pp 321–328.
59. Goldhaber SZ: Modern treatment of pulmonary embolism. *Eur Respir J Suppl* 35:22s–27s, 2002.
60. Kucher N: Catheter embolectomy for acute pulmonary embolism. *Chest* 132:657–663, 2007.
61. Cho KJ, Dasika NL: Catheter technique for pulmonary embolectomy or thrombofragmentation. *Semin Vasc Surg* 13:221–235, 2000.
62. Schmitz-Rode T, Janssens U, Duda SH, et al: Massive pulmonary embolism: percutaneous emergency treatment by pigtail rotation catheter. *J Am Coll Cardiol* 36:375–380, 2000.
63. Zeni PT, Blank BG, Peeler DW, et al: Use of rheolytic thrombectomy in treatment of acute massive pulmonary embolism. *J Interv Radiol* 14:1511–1515, 2003.
64. Handa K, Sasaki Y, Kiyonaga A, et al: Acute pulmonary thromboembolism treated successfully by balloon angioplasty: a case report. *Angiology* 39:775–778, 1988.
65. Fava M, Loyola S: Applications of percutaneous mechanical thrombectomy in pulmonary embolism. *Tech Vasc Interv Radiol* 6:53–58, 2003.
66. Cho KJ, Dasika NL: Catheter technique for pulmonary embolectomy or thrombofragmentation. *Semin Vasc Surg* 13:221–235, 2000.
67. Pasha AK, Elder MD, Khurram D, et al: Successful management of acute massive pulmonary embolism using Angiovac suction catheter technique in a hemodynamically unstable patient. *Cardiovasc Revasc Med* 15:240–243, 2014.
68. Donaldson CW, Baker JN, Narayan RL, et al: Thrombectomy using suction filtration and veno-venous bypass: single center experience with a novel device. *Catheter Cardiovasv Interv* 2014. [Epub ahead of print].
69. Skaf E, Beemath A, Siddiqui T, et al: Catheter-tip embolectomy in the management of acute massive pulmonary embolism. *Am J Cardiol* 99:415–420, 2007.
70. Chechi T, Vecchio S, Spaziani G, et al: Rheolytic thrombectomy in patients with massive and submassive acute pulmonary embolism. *Catheter Cardiovasc Interv* 73:506–513, 2009.
71. Sukhija R, Aronow WS, Lee J, et al: Association of right ventricular dysfunction with in-hospital mortality in patients with acute pulmonary embolism and reduction in mortality in patients with right ventricular dysfunction by pulmonary embolectomy. *Am J Cardiol* 95:695–696, 2005.
72. Zlotnick AY, Lennon PF, Goldhaber SZ, et al: Intraoperativ detection of pulmonary thromboemboli with epicardial echocardiography. *Chest* 115:1749–1751, 1999.
73. Trendelenburg F: Uber die operative behandlung der embolie der lungarterie. *Arch Klin Chir* 86:686–700, 1908.
74. Sharp EH: Pulmonary embolectomy: successful removal of a massive pulmonary embolus with the support of cardiopulmonary bypass—a case report. *Ann Surg* 156:1–4, 1962.
75. Stewart JR, Greenfield LJ: Transvenous vena caval filtration and pulmonary embolectomy. *Surg Clin North Am* 62:411–430, 1982.
76. Tapson VF, Witty LA: Massive pulmonary embolism: diagnostic and therapeutic strategies. In Tapson VF, Fulkerson WJ, Saltzman HA, editors: *Clinics in chest medicine, venous thromboembolism*, vol 16, Philadelphia, 1995, W.B. Saunders, pp 329–340.
77. Leacche M, Uric D, Goldhaber SZ, et al: Modern surgical treatment of massive pulmonary embolism: results in 47 consecutive patients after rapid diagnosis and aggressive surgical approach. *J Thorac Cardiovasc Surg* 129:1018–1023, 2005.
78. Greenfield LJ, Proctor MC: Twenty-year clinical experience with the Greenfield filter. *Cardiovasc Surg* 3:199–205, 1995.
79. Athanasoulis CA, Kaufman JA, Halpern EF, et al: Inferior vena caval filters: review of a 26-year single-center clinical experience. *Radiology* 216:54–66, 2000.
80. Kaufman JA, Rundback JH, Kee ST, et al: Development of a research agenda for inferior vena cava filers: proceedings from a multidisciplinary research consensus panel. *J Vasc Interv Radiol* 20:697–707, 2009.
81. Hann CL, Streiff MB: The role of vena caval filters in the management of venous thromboembolism. *Blood Rev* 19:179–202, 2005.
82. Chandra PA, Nwokolo C, Chuprun D, et al: Cardiac tamponade caused by fracture and migration of inferior vena cava filter. *South Med J* 101:1163–1164, 2008.
83. Kawahito K, Murata S, Adachi H, et al: Resuscitation and circulatory support using extracorporeal membrane oxygenation for fulminant pulmonary embolism. *Artif Organs* 24:427–430, 2000.
84. Bauer C, Vichova Z, French P, et al: Extracorporeal membrane oxygenation with danaparoid sodium after massive pulmonary embolism. *Anesth Analg* 106:1101–1103, 2008.
85. Maggio P, Hemmila M, Haft J, et al: Extracorporeal life support for massive pulmonary embolism. *J Trauma* 62:570–576, 2007.
86. Sung K, Lee YT, Park PW, et al: Improved survival after cardiac arrest using emergent autopriming percutaneous cardiopulmonary support. *Ann Thorac Surg* 82:651–656, 2006.
87. Doehring R, Kiss AB, Garrett A, et al: Extracorporeal membrane oxygenation as a bridge to surgical embolectomy in acute fulminant pulmonary embolism. *Am J Emerg Med* 24:879–880, 2006.
88. Stulz P, Schlapfer R, Feer R, et al: Decision making in the surgical treatment of massive pulmonary embolism. *Eur J Cardiothorac Surg* 8:188–193, 1994.
89. Jakob H, Vahl C, Lange R, et al: Modified surgical concept for fulminant pulmonary embolism. *Eur J Cardiothorac Surg* 9:557–560, 1995.
90. Doerge HC, Schoendube FA, Loeser H, et al: Pulmonary embolectomy: review of a 15-year experience and role in the age of thrombolytic therapy. *Eur J Cardiothorac Surg* 10:952–957, 1996.
91. Ullmann M, Hemmer W, Hannekum A: The urgent pulmonary embolectomy: mechanical resuscitation in the operating theatre determines the outcome. *Thorac Cardiovasc Surg* 47:5–8, 1999.
92. Doerge HC, Schoendube FA, Voss M, et al: Surgical therapy of fulminant pulmonary embolism: early and late results. *Thorac Cardiovasc Surg* 47:9–13, 1999.
93. Aklog L, Williams CS, Byrne JG, et al: Acute pulmonary embolectomy: a contemporary approach. *Circulation* 105:1416–1419, 2002.
94. Leacche M, Unic D, Goldhaber SZ, et al: Modern surgical treatment of massive pulmonary embolism: results in 47 consecutive patients after rapid diagnosis and aggressive surgical approach. *J Thorac Cardiovasc Surg* 129:1018–1023, 2005.
95. Spagnolo S, Grasso MA, Tesler UF: Retrograde pulmonary perfusion improved results in pulmonary embolectomy for massive pulmonary embolism. *Tex Heart Inst J* 33:473–476, 2006.
96. Digonnet A, Moya-Plana A, Aubert S, et al: Acute pulmonary embolism: a current surgical approach. *Interact Cardiovasc Throac Surg* 6:27–29, 2007.

97. Kadner A, Schmidli J, Schönhoof F, et al: Excellent outcome after surgical treatment of massive pulmonary embolism in critically ill patients. *J Thorac Cardiovasc Surg* 136:448–451, 2008.
98. Sádaba JR, Greco E, Alvarez LA, et al: The surgical option in the management of acute pulmonary embolism. *J Card Surg* 23:729–732, 2008.
99. Vohra HA, Whistance RN, Mattam K, et al: Early and late clinical outcomes of pulmonary embolectomy for acute massive pulmonary embolism. *Ann Throac Surg* 90:1747–1752, 2010.
100. Zarrabi K, Zolghadrasli A, Ostovan MA, et al: Short-term results of retrograde pulmonary embolectomy in massive and submassive pulmonary embolism: a single-center study of 30 patients. *Eur J Cardiothorac Surg* 40:890–893, 2011.
101. Medvedev AP, Pichugin VV, Ivanov LN, et al: Surgical management of acute pulmonary thromboembolism. *Angiol Sosud Khir* 17:78–86, 2011.
102. Taniguchi S, Fukuda W, Fukuda I, et al: Outcome of pulmonary embolectomy for acute pulmonary thromboembolism: analysis of 32 patients from a multicentre registry in Japan. *Interact Cardiovasc Thorac Surg* 14:64–67, 2012.
103. Lehnert P, Møller CH, Carlsen J, et al: Surgical treatment of acute pulmonary embolism–a 12-year retrospective analysis. *Scand Cardiovasc J* 46:172–176, 2012.
104. Takahashi H, Okada K, Matsumori M, et al: Aggressive surgical treatment of acute pulmonary embolism with circulatory collapse. *Ann Thorac Surg* 94:785–791, 2012.
105. Aymard T, Kadner A, Widmer A, et al: Massive pulmonary embolism: surgical embolectomy versus thrombolytic therapy–should surgical indications be revisited? *Eur J Cardiothorac Surg* 43:90–94, 2013.
106. Wu MY, Liu YC, Tseng YH, et al: Pulmonary embolectomy in high-risk acute pulmonary embolism: the effectiveness of a compressive therapeutic algorithm including extracorporeal life support. *Resuscitation* 84:1365–1370, 2013.
107. Zarrabi K, Zolghadrasli A, Ali Ostovan M, et al: Residual pulmonary hypertension after retrograde pulmonary embolectomy: long-term follow-up of 30 patients with massive and submassive pulmonary embolism. *Interact Cardiovasc Thorac Surg* 17:242–246, 2013.
108. Worku B, Gulkarov I, Girardi LN, et al: Pulmonary embolectomy in the treatment of submassive and massive pulmonary embolism. *Cardiology* 129:106–110, 2014.
109. Soyer R, Brunet AP, Redonnet M, et al: Follow-up of surgically treated patients with massive pulmonary embolism: with reference to 12 operated patients. *Thorac Cardiovasc Surg* 30:103–108, 1982.
110. Bernard J, Yi JS: Pulmonary thromboendarterectomy: a clinicopathologic study of 200 consecutive pulmonary thromboendarterectomy cases in one institution. *Hum Path* 38:871–877, 2007.
111. Alias S, Redwan B, Panzenbock A, et al: Defective angiogenesis delays thrombosis resolution: a potential pathogenetic mechanism underlying chronic thromboembolic pulmonary hypertension. *Arterioscler Thromb Vasc Biol* 34:810–819, 2014.
112. Zabini D, Heinemann A, Foris V, et al: Comprehensive analysis of inflammatory markers in chronic thromboembolic pulmonary hypertension. *Eur Respir J* 44:51–62, 2014.
113. Guillanta P, Peterson KL, Ben-Yehuda O: Cardiac catheterization techniques in pulmonary hypertension. *Cardiol Clin* 22:401–405, 2004.
114. Du L, Sullivan CC, Chu D, et al: Signaling molecules in nonfamilial pulmonary hypertension. *N Engl J Med* 348:500–509, 2003.
115. Galiè N, Kim NH: Pulmonary microvascular disease in chronic thromboembolic pulmonary hypertension. *Proc Am Thorac Soc* 3:571–576, 2006.
116. Azarian R, Wartski M, Collignon MA, et al: Lung perfusion scans and hemodynamics in acute and chronic pulmonary embolism. *J Nucl Med* 38:980–983, 1997.
117. Sacks RS, Remillard CV, Agange N, et al: Molecular biology of chronic thromboembolic pulmonary hypertension. *Semi Thorac Cardiovasc Surg* 18:265–276, 2006.
118. Sanchez O, Trinquart L, Colombet I, et al: Prognostic value of right ventricular dysfunction in patients with haemodynamically stable pulmonary embolism: a systematic review. *Eur Heart J* 29:1569–1577, 2008.
119. Houk VN, Hufnagel CA, McClenathan JE, et al: Chronic thrombotic obstruction of major pulmonary arteries. Report of a case successfully treated by thromboendarterectomy, and a review of the literature. *Am J Med* 35:269–282, 1963.
120. Panasiuk A, Dzieciol J, Nowak HF, et al: Pulmonary thromboembolism: random analysis of autopsy material. *Pneumonol Alergol Pol* 61:171–176, 1993.
121. Fedullo PF, Auger WR, Kerr KM, et al: Chronic thromboembolic pulmonary hypertension. *N Engl J Med* 345:1465–1472, 2001.
122. Wolf M, Boyer-Neumann C, Parent F, et al: Thrombotic risk factors in pulmonary hypertension. *Eur Respir J* 15:395–399, 2000.
123. Bonderman D, Turecek PL, Jakowitsch J, et al: High prevalence of elevated clotting factor VIII in chronic thromboembolic pulmonary hypertension. *Thromb Haemost* 90:372–376, 2003.
124. Morris TA, Marsh JJ, Chiles PG, et al: Fibrin derived from patients with chronic thromboembolic pulmonary hypertension is resistant to lysis. *Am J Respir Crit Care Med* 173:1270–1275, 2006.
125. Sakamaki F, Kyotani S, Nagaya N, et al: Increase in thrombomodulin concentrations after pulmonary thromboendarterectomy in chronic thromboembolic pulmonary hypertension. *Chest* 124:1305–1311, 2003.
126. Marsh JJ, Chiles PG, Liang NC, et al: Chronic thromboembolic pulmonary hypertension-associated dysfibrinogenemias exhibit disorganized fibrin structure. *Thromb Res* 132:729–734, 2013.
127. Blauwet LA, Edwards WD, Tazelaar HD, et al: Surgical pathology of pulmonary thromboendarterectomy: a study of 54 cases from 1990 to 2001. *Hum Pathol* 34:1290–1298, 2003.
128. Wu O, Bayoumi N, Vickers MA, et al: ABO(H) blood groups and vascular disease: a systematic review and meta-analysis. *J Thromb Haemost* 6:62–69, 2008.
129. Lang IM: Chronic thromboembolic pulmonary hypertension—not so rare after all. *N Engl J Med* 350:2236–2238, 2004.
130. Lewczuk J, Piszko P, Jagas J, et al: Prognostic factors in medically treated patients with chronic pulmonary embolism. *Chest* 119:818–823, 2001.
131. Auger WR, Kerr KM, Kim NH, et al: Evaluation of patients with chronic thromboembolic pulmonary hypertension for pulmonary endarterectomy. *Pulm Circ* 2:155–162, 2012.
132. Auger WR, Moser KM: Pulmonary flow murmurs: a distinctive physical sign found in chronic pulmonary thromboembolic disease. *Clin Res* 37:145A, 1989.
133. Morris TA, Auger WR, Ysrael MZ, et al: Parenchymal scarring is associated with restrictive spirometric defects in patients with chronic thromboembolic pulmonary hypertension. *Chest* 110:399–403, 1996.
134. D'Armini AM, Zanotti G, Ghio S, et al: Reverse right ventricular remodeling after pulmonary endarterectomy. *J Thorac Cardiovascu Surg* 133:162–168, 2007.
135. Tunariu N, Gibbs SJ, Win Z, et al: Ventilation-perfusion scintigraphy is more sensitive than multidetector CTPA in detecting chronic thromboembolic pulmonary disease as a treatable cause of pulmonary hypertension. *J Nucl Med* 48:680–684, 2007.
136. Ryan KL, Fedullo PF, Davis GB, et al: Perfusion scan findings understate the severity of angiographic and hemodynamic compromise in chronic thromboembolic pulmonary hypertension. *Chest* 93:1130–1185, 1988.
137. Coulden R: State-of-the-art imaging techniques in chronic thromboembolic pulmonary hypertension. *Proc Am Thorac Soc* 3:577–583, 2006.
138. Auger WR, Kim NH, Kerr KM, et al: Chronic thromboembolic pulmonary hypertension. *Clin Chest Med* 28:255–269, 2007.
139. Jamieson SW, Kapelanski DP: Pulmonary endarterectomy. *Curr Probl Surg* 37:165–252, 2000.
140. Pevec WC: Angioscopy in vascular surgery: the state of the art. *Ann Vasc Surg* 10:66–75, 1996.
141. Sugimura K, Fukumoto Y, Miura Y, et al: Three-dimensional-optical coherence tomography imaging of chronic thromboembolic pulmonary hypertension. *Eur Heart J* 34:2121, 2013.
142. Reichelt A, Hoeper MM, Galanski M, et al: Chronic thromboembolic pulmonary hypertension: evaluation with 64-detector row CT versus digital subtraction angiography. *Eur J Radiol* 71:49–54, 2009.
143. Soler X, Kerr KM, Marsh JJ, et al: Pilot study comparing SPECT perfusion scintigraphy with CT pulmonary angiography in chronic thromboembolic pulmonary hypertension. *Respirology* 17:180–184, 2012.

144. Marshall H, Kiely DG, Parra-Robles J, et al: Magnetic resonance imaging of ventilation and perfusion changes in response to pulmonary endarterectomy in chronic thromboembolic pulmonary hypertension. *Am J Respir Crit Care Med* 190:e18–e19, 2014.
145. Hoey ET, Mirsadraee S, Pepke-Zaba J, et al: Dual-energy CT angiography for assessment of regional pulmonary perfusion in patients with chronic thromboembolic pulmonary hypertension: initial experience. *AJR Am J Roentgenol* 196:524–532, 2011.
146. Allison PR, Dunnill MS, Marshall R: Pulmonary embolism. *Thorax* 15:273–283, 1960.
147. Chitwood WR, Jr, Sabiston DC, Jr, Wechsler AS: Surgical treatment of chronic unresolved pulmonary embolism. *Clin Chest Med* 5:507–536, 1984.
148. Jamieson SW, Sakakibara N, Manecke G, et al: Pulmonary endarterectomy: experience and lessons learned in 1500 cases. *Ann Thorac Surg* 76:1457–1462, 2003.
149. Madani MM, Auger WR, Pretorius V, et al: Pulmonary endarterectomy: recent changes in a single institution's experience of more than 2,700 patients. *Ann Thorac Surg* 94:97–103, 2012.
150. Kerr KM, Fedullo PF, Auger WR: Chronic thromboembolic pulmonary hypertension: when to suspect it, when to refer for surgery. *Adv Pulm Hyperten* 2:4–8, 2003.
151. Lambert V, Durand P, Devictor D, et al: Unilateral right pulmonary thromboendarterectomy for chronic embolism: a successful procedure in an infant. *J Thorac Cardiovasc Surg* 118:953–957, 1999.
152. Thistlethwaite PA, Madani MM, Jamieson SW: Pulmonary thromboendarterectomy surgery. *Cardiol Clin* 22:467–478, 2004.
153. Thomson B, Tsui SS, Dunning J, et al: Pulmonary endarterectomy is possible and effective without the use of complete circulatory arrest—the UK experience in over 150 patients. *Eur J Cardiothorac Surg* 33:157–163, 2008.
154. Morsolini M, Nicolardi S, Milanesi E, et al: Evolving surgical techniques for pulmonary endarterectomy according to the changing features of chronic thromboembolic pulmonary hypertension patients during 17-year single-center experience. *J Thorac Cardiovasc Surg* 144:100–107, 2012.
155. Jamieson S: Bypass, circulatory arrest, and pulmonary endarterectomy. *Lancet* 378:1359–1360, 2011.
156. Madani MM, Jamieson SW: Technical advances of pulmonary endarterectomy for chronic thromboembolic pulmonary hypertension. *Semin Thorac Cardiovasc Surg* 18:243–249, 2006.
157. Ji B, Liu J, Wu Y, et al: Perfusion techniques for pulmonary thromboendarterectomy under deep hypothermia circulatory arrest: a case series. *J Extra Corpor Technol* 38:302–306, 2006.
158. Thistlethwaite PA, Jamieson SW: Tricuspid valvular disease in the patient with chronic pulmonary thromboembolic disease. *Curr Opin Cardiol* 18:111–116, 2003.
159. Thistlethwaite PA, Auger WR, Madani MM, et al: Pulmonary thromboendarterectomy combined with other cardiac operations: indications, surgical approach, and outcome. *Ann Thorac Surg* 72:13–17, 2001.
160. Thistlethwaite PA, Mo M, Madani MM, et al: Operative classification of thromboembolic disease determines outcome after pulmonary endarterectomy. *J Thorac Cardiovasc Surg* 124:1203–1211, 2002.
161. Menzel T, Kramm T, Mohr-Kahaly S, et al: Assessment of cardiac performance using Tei indices in patients undergoing pulmonary thromboendarterectomy. *Ann Thorac Surg* 73:762–766, 2002.
162. Thistlethwaite PA, Madani MM, Jamieson SW: Outcomes of pulmonary endarterectomy surgery. *Semin Thorac Cardiovasc Surg* 18:257–264, 2006.
163. Ishida K, Masuda M, Tanabe N, et al: Long-term outcome after pulmonary endarterectomy for chronic thromboembolic pulmonary hypertension. *J Thorac Cardiovasc Surg* 144:321–326, 2012.
164. Ilino M, Dymarkowski S, Chaothawee L, et al: Time course of reversed remodeling after pulmonary endarterectomy in patients with chronic pulmonary thromboembolism. *Eur Radiol* 18:792–799, 2008.
165. Surie S, Bouma BJ, Bruin-Bon RA, et al: Time course of restoration of systolic and diastolic right ventricular function after pulmonary endarterectomy for chronic thromboembolic pulmonary hypertension. *Am Heart J* 161:1046–1052, 2011.
166. Thistlethwaite PA, Kaneko K, Madani MM, et al: Technique and outcomes of pulmonary endarterectomy surgery. *Ann Thorac Cardiovasc Surg* 14:274–282, 2008.
167. Freed DH, Thomson BM, Tsui SS, et al: Functional and haemodynamic outcome 1 year after pulmonary thromboendarterectomy. *Eur J Cardiothorac Surg* 34:525–529, 2008.
168. Corsico AG, D'Armini AM, Cerveri I, et al: Long-term outcome after pulmonary endarterectomy. *Am J Respir Crit Care Med* 178:419–424, 2008.
169. Condliffe R, Kiely DG, Gibbs SR, et al: Improved outcomes in medically and surgically treated chronic thromboembolic pulmonary hypertension. *Am J Respir Crit Care Med* 177:1122–1127, 2008.
170. Skoro-Sajer N, Hack N, Sadushi-kolici R, et al: Pulmonary vascular reactivity and prognosis in patients with chronic thromboembolic pulmonary hypertension: a pilot study. *Circulation* 119:298–305, 2009.
171. Saouti N, Morshuis WJ, Heijmen RH, et al: Long-term outcome after pulmonary endarterectomy for chronic thromboembolic pulmonary hypertension: a single institution experience. *Eur J Cardiothorac Surg* 35:947–952, 2009.
172. Kunihara T, Möller M, Langer F, et al: Angiographic predictors of hemodynamic improvement after pulmonary endarterectomy. *Ann Thorac Surg* 90:957–964, 2010.
173. Gan HL, Zhang JQ, Bo P, et al: The actuarial survival analysis of the surgical and non-surgical therapy regimen for chronic thromboembolic pulmonary hypertension. *J Thromb Thrombolysis* 29:25–31, 2010.
174. van der Plas MN, Surie S, Reesink HJ, et al: Longitudinal follow-up of six-minute walk distance after pulmonary endarterectomy. *Ann Thorac Surg* 91:1094–1099, 2011.
175. Schölzel B, Snijder R, Morshuis W, et al: clinical worsening after pulmonary endarterectomy in chronic thromboembolic pulmonary hypertension. *Neth Heart J* 19:498–503, 2011.
176. Kunihara T, Gerdts J, Groesdonk H, et al: Predictors of postoperative outcome after pulmonary endarterectomy from a 14-year experience with 279 patients. *Eur J Cadriothorac Surg* 40:154–161, 2011.
177. Freed DH, Thomson BM, Berman M, et al: Survival after pulmonary thromboendarterectomy: effect of residual pulmonary hypertension. *J Thorac Cardiovasc Surg* 141:383–387, 2011.
178. de Perrot M, McRae K, Shargall Y, et al: Pulmonary endarterectomy for chronic thromboembolic pulmonary hypertension: the Toronto experience. *Can J Cardiol* 27:692–697, 2011.
179. Surie S, Reesink HJ, van der Plas MN, et al: Plasma brain natriuretic peptide as a biomarker for haemodynamic outcome and mortality following pulmonary endarterectomy for chronic thromboembolic pulmonary hypertension. *Interact Cardiovasc Thorac Surg* 15:973–978, 2012.
180. Sato M, Ando M, Kaneko K, et al: Respiratory and hemodynamic changes in patients with chronic thromboembolic pulmonary hypertension 1 year after pulmonary endarterectomy. *Ann Vasc Dis* 6:578–582, 2013.
181. Ross RVM, Toshner MR, Soon E, et al: Decreased time constant of the pulmonary circulation in chronic thromboembolic pulmonary hypertension. *Am J Physiol Heart Circ Physiol* 305:H259–H264, 2013.
182. Nishimura R, Tanabe N, Sugiura T, et al: Improved survival in medically treated chronic thromboembolic pulmonary hypertension. *Circ J* 77:2110–2117, 2013.
183. Wieteska M, Biederman A, Kurzyna M, et al: Outcome of medically versus surgically treated patients with chronic thromboembolic pulmonary hypertension. *Clin Appl Thromb Hemost* 2014. [Epub ahead of print].
184. Skoro-Sajer N, Marta G, Gerges C, et al: Surgical specimens, haemodynamics and long-term outcomes after pulmonary endarterectomy. *Thorax* 69:116–122, 2014.
185. Schölzel BE, Post MC, van de Bruaene A, et al: Prediction of hemodynamic improvement after pulmonary endarterectomy in chronic thromboembolic pulmonary hypertension using non-invasive imaging. *Int J Cardiovasc Imaging* 31:143–150, 2015.
186. Ghio S, Morsolini M, Corsico A, et al: Pulmonary arterial compliance and exercise capacity after pulmonary endarterectomy. *Eur Respir J* 43:1403–1409, 2014.

187. Berman M, Gopalan D, Sharples L, et al: Right ventricular reverse remodeling after pulmonary endarterectomy: magnetic resonance imaging and clinical and right heart catheterization assessment. *Pulm Circ* 4:36–44, 2014.
188. Thistlethwaite PA, Madani MM, Kemp AD, et al: Venovenous extracorporeal life support after pulmonary endarterectomy: indications, techniques, and outcomes. *Ann Thorac Surg* 82:2139–2145, 2006.
189. Archibald CJ, Auger WR, Fedullo PF, et al: Long-term outcome after pulmonary thromboendarterectomy. *Am J Respir Crit Care Med* 160:523–528, 1999.
190. Tsuji A, Ogo T, Demachi J, et al: Rescue balloon pulmonary angioplasty in a rapidly deteriorating chronic thromboembolic pulmonary hypertension patient with liver failure and refractory infection. *Pulm Circ* 4:142–147, 2014.
191. Mielniczuk LM, Swiston JR, Mehta S: Riociguat: a novel therapeutic option for pulmonary arterial hypertension and chronic thromboembolic pulmonary hypertension. *Can J Cardiol* 30:1233–1240, 2014.
192. Feinstein JA, Goldhaber SZ, Lock JE, et al: Balloon pulmonary angioplasty for treatment of chronic thromboembolic pulmonary hypertension. *Circulation* 103:10–13, 2001.
193. Kataoka M, Inami T, Hayashida K, et al: Percutaneous transluminal pulmonary angioplasty for the treatment of chronic thromboembolic pulmonary hypertension. *Circ Cardiovasc Interv* 5:756–762, 2012.
194. Mizoguchi H, Ogawa A, Munemasa M, et al: Refined balloon pulmonary angioplasty for inoperable patients with chronic thromboembolic pulmonary hypertension. *Circ Cardiovasc Interv* 5:748–755, 2012.
195. Sugimura K, Fukumoto Y, Satoh K, et al: Percutaneous transluminal pulmonary angioplasty markedly improved pulmonary hemodynamics and long-term prognosis in patients with chronic thromboembolic pulmonary hypertension. *Circ J* 76:485–488, 2012.
196. Ghofrani HA, D'Armini AM, Grimminger F, et al: Riociguat for the treatment of chronic thromboembolic pulmonary hypertension. *N Engl J Med* 369:319–329, 2013.

CHAPTER 103

TUMORS OF THE HEART

Oz M. Shapira • Michael J. Reardon

CHAPTER OUTLINE

Neoplastic involvement of the heart can be divided into primary cardiac tumors arising in the heart and secondary cardiac tumors that have metastasized to the heart. Primary cardiac tumors can be further stratified into benign and malignant tumors. Secondary involvement of the heart is relatively common, with 10% to 20% of patients dying of disseminated cancer having metastatic involvement of the heart or pericardium.[1,2] Surgical resection is seldom possible or advisable for these tumors, and surgical intervention is usually limited to drainage of malignant pericardial effusions, diagnostic biopsies, or both. There are uncommon cases of metastatic disease limited to the heart for which resection is reasonable.[3]

Primary tumors of the heart are uncommon but not rare. In unselected autopsy series, the incidence of primary cardiac neoplasm ranges between 0.0017% and 0.19%.[4-8] Approximately 75% of primary cardiac tumors are benign and 25% are malignant.[2,9] Approximately 50% of the benign tumors are myxomas, and approximately 75% of the malignant tumors are sarcomas.[2,9] The clinical incidence of these tumors is approximately 1 in 500 cardiac surgical cases and, with the exception of myxomas, most surgeons will rarely encounter primary cardiac tumors. The purpose of this chapter is to summarize useful information for the evaluation and management of patients with primary and secondary cardiac tumors and to provide a reference for additional study on these subjects.

HISTORICAL BACKGROUND

Cardiac tumors were a postmortem diagnosis until the first antemortem diagnosis of a cardiac tumor was made in 1934 when Barnes diagnosed a cardiac sarcoma using electrocardiography and biopsy of a metastatic lymph node.[10] In 1936, Beck successfully resected a teratoma external to the right ventricle,[11] and Mauer removed a left ventricular lipoma in 1951.[12] Treatment of cardiac tumors was profoundly influenced by two events: the introduction of cardiopulmonary bypass in 1953 by John Gibbon allowing safe and reproducible approach to the cardiac chambers and the introduction of cardiac echocardiography allowing safe and noninvasive diagnosis of an intracardiac mass. The first echocardiographic diagnosis of an intracardiac tumor was made in 1959.[13] A large right atrial myxoma was removed by Bahnson in 1952 using caval inflow occlusion but the patient expired 24 days later.[14] Crafoord in Sweden first successfully removed a left atrial myxoma in 1954 using cardiopulmonary bypass,[15] and Kay in Los Angeles first removed a left ventricular myxoma in 1959.[16] By 1964, 60 atrial myxomas had been removed successfully with a steady increase because of increasing safety of cardiopulmonary bypass and increased use of echocardiography for detection.[17] Operations are currently routinely performed on the vast majority of patients with atrial myxoma with minimal mortality.[9,18] Primary malignant tumors, however, continue to represent a challenge.

PRIMARY BENIGN TUMORS

Myxomas

Definition, Incidence, and Prevalence

Myxomas are the most common primary cardiac tumors. They are benign. Although they have been reported in both sexes and in all age groups, they most often occur in women in the third to sixth decade of life. Myxomas are usually sporadic, but at least 7% occur as part of an autosomal dominant syndrome. In the latter situation, the myxoma is a component of a larger syndrome referred to as the *Carney complex*.[6] In the Carney complex, myxomas are associated with spotty pigmentation of the skin and endocrine hyperactivity. Myxomas that arise as part of the Carney complex affect both sexes equally and at any age. They arise as single or multiple lesions in all chambers of the heart, and tend to recur after surgical excision.[7]

Morphology

Arising from the endocardium, myxomas usually extend into a cardiac chamber. They are generally polypoid, pedunculated lesions with a smooth surface that may be covered with thrombus. The tumors range in size from 1 to 15 cm, but they are most commonly about 5 cm in diameter with a weight of approximately 70 g.[8,19-21] Myxomas are thought to arise from pluripotent mesenchymal cells. Histologically, they consist of a matrix of acid mucopolysaccharide.[22] The cells are polygonal or spindle-shaped and may form capillary-like channels that can communicate with arteries and veins located at the base of the tumor.[20]

Myxomas most commonly occur in the atria. Approximately 75% arise in the left atrium, and 15% to 20% arise in the right atrium.[20] Most left atrial myxomas are located on the border of the fossa ovalis, but they can originate from any place on the atrial wall. The remaining myxomas are located in the ventricles. Myxomas arising from cardiac valves are rare (Fig. 103-1).

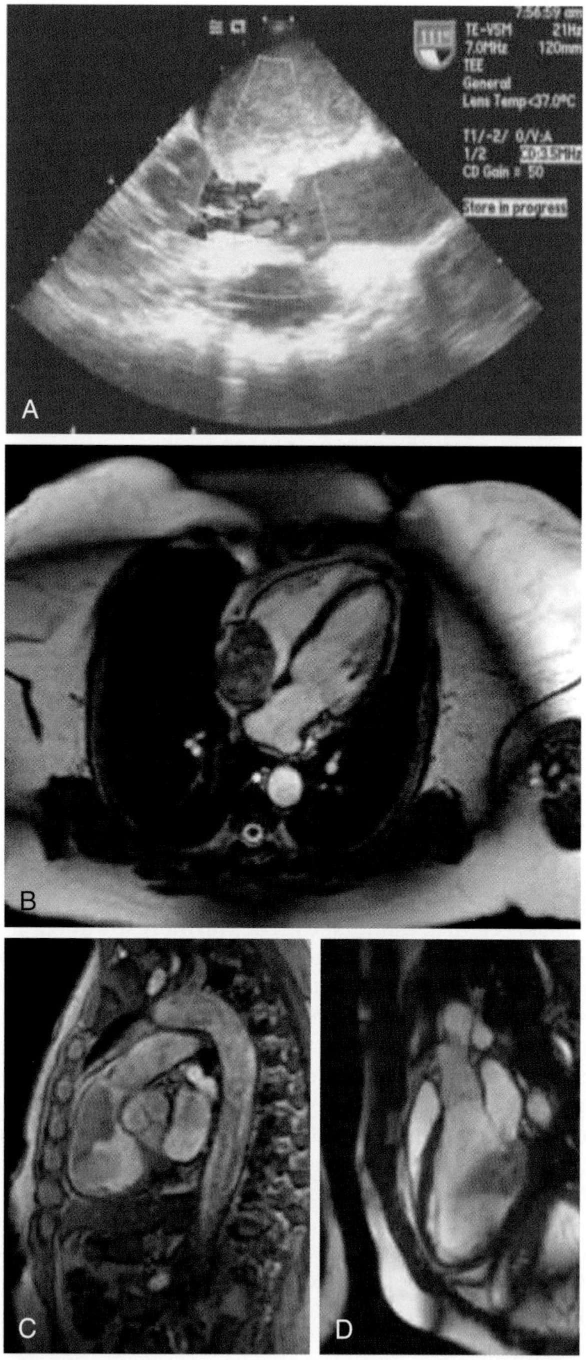

FIGURE 103-1 ■ Myxomas of the heart. **A,** Echocardiography of giant left atrial myxoma. **B,** Magnetic resonance imaging of right atrial myxoma. **C,** Magnetic resonance imaging of right ventricular myxoma. **D,** Magnetic resonance imaging of left ventricular myxoma.

Clinical Characteristics

Patients with myxomas can have a variety of symptoms. In the sporadic form, classic findings include emboli, congestive heart failure caused by obstruction of cardiac blood flow, and constitutional symptoms. These sequelae are related to the location, size, and mobility of the tumor.

Because most myxomas arise in the left atrium, systemic embolization is common, occurring in 30% to 50% of cases.[23-25] Left ventricular myxomas have an even higher propensity to embolize.[26,27] Right atrial myxomas rarely display clinical manifestations of emboli. Embolic material from myxomas can compromise blood flow to any organ, but the brain is most commonly affected. Myxoma should be included in the differential diagnosis of any systemic embolic event, and any embolic material removed should undergo histologic evaluation.

Patients with myxomas can also display signs and symptoms related to cardiac obstruction. Typically, the findings are related to the tumor's ability to impede filling of the ventricles; in such instances, signs and symptoms may mimic those of mitral or tricuspid valve stenosis. Less commonly, the tumors impede atrioventricular (AV) valve leaflet coaptation, causing valvular regurgitation. Much less frequently, ventricular tumors obstruct ventricular outflow and cause findings similar to those of aortic or pulmonic stenosis. Constitutional symptoms include fever, malaise, rash, weight loss, and myalgia. Abnormal laboratory values, including elevated erythrocyte sedimentation rate, anemia, thrombocytopenia, and an elevated C-reactive protein, are common. These constitutional symptoms and laboratory findings are not related to tumor size or location. Many patients with myxomas are however asymptomatic. The myxoma may be detected by routine screening echocardiography performed for other indications. Asymptomatic myxomas should be excised to prevent emboli, valvular dysfunction, or constitutional symptoms.

Diagnosis

Echocardiography is the imaging modality of choice for diagnosis of myxomas. Tumor location and characteristics can be delineated by two-dimensional transthoracic echocardiography. Transesophageal echo and three-dimensional echocardiography can be used to characterize the tumor further.[28,29] The echocardiographic appearance of myxomas is usually distinctive, but other causes of intracardiac masses must be included in the differential diagnosis. In cases of diagnostic uncertainty, magnetic resonance imaging (MRI) and computed tomography (CT) may be helpful. Final diagnosis is confirmed by pathologic examination.

Management

Surgical resection is the mainstay of treatment. The intracardiac mass is excised after establishing cardiopulmonary bypass and cardioplegic arrest. Bicaval cannulation is used for venous return. Great care must be taken to minimize manipulation of the heart before cross-clamping the aorta to reduce the risk of intraoperative tumor embolization. A variety of approaches are available for resection of left atrial tumors. In the absence of other cardiac disease, a minimally invasive or robotically assisted operation can be used to speed postoperative recovery. Intracardiac exposure is generally achieved through a lateral, longitudinal incision in the left atrium. When visualization is difficult, additional incisions in the right atrium and septum are made.

The tumor is resected en bloc. Tumors that arise from a relatively well-defined pedicle can be excised without full-thickness excision of a button of atrial wall. However, many surgeons prefer to excise a portion of the atrial wall, especially if the tumor arises from the interatrial septum or it is a broad-based tumor. Tumors of the ventricle may be resected without full-thickness excision of a portion of ventricular wall. Tumors arising from an AV valve can usually be resected without the need for valve replacement. Regardless of the site of origin, the AV valve in proximity to the tumor should be inspected for evidence of damage.

The results of surgical excision are good, with a low risk of morbidity and mortality (0% to 3%).[9,30,31] Recurrence of atrial myxomas is infrequent. Sporadic myxomas recur in 1% to 3% of patients at an average of 2.5 years after surgery.[32] The risk of recurrence of familial myxomas ranges from 12% to 20%.[32,33] Therefore, regular echocardiographic follow-up is recommended in the latter group. When myxomas recur, they should be resected.

Lipomas

Lipomas are well-encapsulated tumors consisting of mature fat cells that can occur anywhere in the heart, but also are found in the pericardium, subendocardium, subepicardium, or intra-atrial septum.[20] They can also occur at any age and have no sex predilection. Lipomas are slow growing and can attain considerable size before producing obstructive or arrhythmic symptoms. Many are asymptomatic and are discovered incidentally on routine chest roentgenogram, echocardiogram, or at surgery or autopsy.[34,35] Subepicardial and parietal lipomas tend to compress the heart and may be associated with pericardial effusion. Subendocardial tumors can produce chamber obstruction. The right atrium and left ventricle are sites most often affected. Lipomas lying within the myocardium or septum can produce arrhythmias or conduction abnormalities.[36] Large tumors that produce severe symptoms should be resected. Smaller, asymptomatic tumors encountered unexpectedly during cardiac operation should be removed if excision can be performed without adding risk to the primary procedure. These tumors are not known to recur.

Lipomatous Hypertrophy of the Interatrial Septum

Nonencapsulated hypertrophy of the fat within the atrial septum is known as *lipomatous hypertrophy*.[20] This abnormality is more common than cardiac lipoma and is usually encountered in older, obese, or female patients as an incidental finding during a variety of cardiac imaging procedures.[37] Various arrhythmias and conduction disturbances have been attributed to its presence.[38-40] The main problem posed is differentiation from a cardiac neoplasm when the lesion is discovered on echocardiography.[41] After the demonstration of a mass by echocardiography, the typical T1 and T2 signal intensity of fat on MRI can usually establish a diagnosis (Fig. 103-2).[42,43] Arrhythmias or heart block are considered by some as an indication for resection, but there is lack of data as to the long-term benefits from resection.[44]

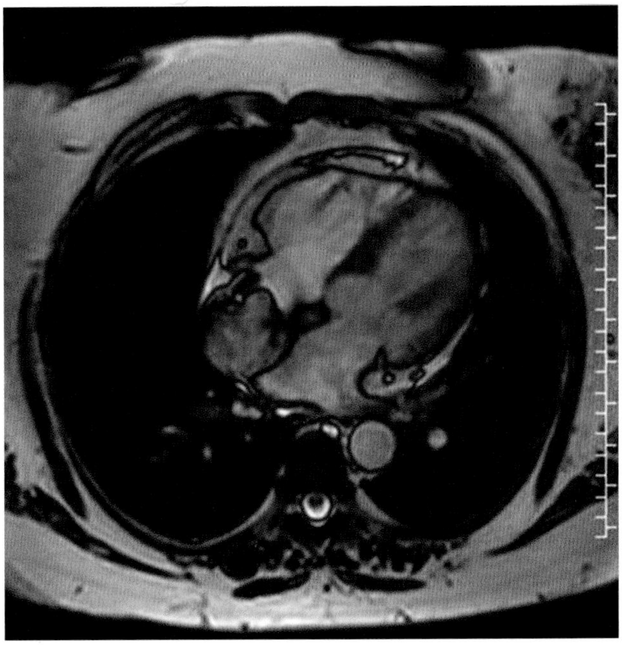

FIGURE 103-2 ■ Lipomatous hypertrophy.

Papillary Fibroelastoma of the Heart Valves

Papillary fibroelastomas are tumors that arise characteristically from the cardiac valves or adjacent endocardium.[45] Grossly, tumors are described as resembling sea anemones with frondlike projections. The AV and semilunar valves are affected with equal frequency. Ventricular fibroelastomas that occur on the left side have a high risk of stroke.[46] Papillary fibroelastomas were formerly thought to be innocuous because they were incidental findings at an autopsy. It is now known that they are capable of producing obstruction of flow, particularly coronary ostial flow, and they can embolize to the brain and produce stroke.[46,47] They are usually asymptomatic until a critical event occurs. Now they are found more often because of the more frequent use of echocardiography. Papillary fibroelastomas of the cardiac valve should be resected whenever diagnosed because of their known tendency to produce life-threatening complications. These tumors can often be resected using minimally invasive techniques (Fig. 103-3).[46] Valve repair rather than replacement should follow the resection of these benign tumors whenever technically feasible, using conservative margins of resection. Cytomegalovirus has been recovered in these tumors, suggesting the possibility of viral induction of the tumor and chronic viral endocarditis.[44]

Rhabdomyoma

Rhabdomyoma is the most frequently occurring cardiac tumor in children. It usually manifests during the first few days after birth. It is thought to be a myocardial hamartoma rather than a true neoplasm.[48] Although rhabdomyoma appears sporadically, it is associated strongly with tuberous sclerosis, a hereditary disorder characterized by hamartomas in various organs, epilepsy, mental deficiency, and sebaceous adenomas. Fifty percent of patients with tuberous sclerosis have rhabdomyoma, but more than 50% of patients with rhabdomyoma have or will develop tuberous sclerosis.[49,50] The exceptional patient is one with a solitary, single rhabdomyoma who does not have or develop tuberous sclerosis.

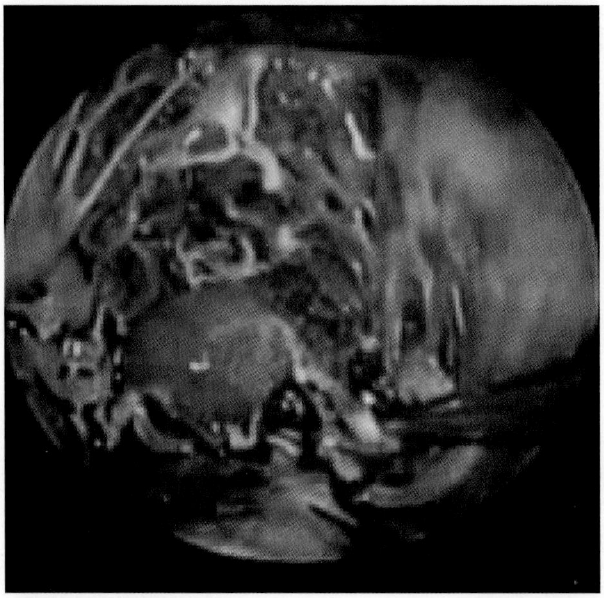

FIGURE 103-3 ■ Fibroelastoma seen through minimally invasive thoracoscopic approach.

More than 90% of rhabdomyomas are multiple and occur with approximately equal frequency in both ventricles.[51] The atrium is involved in fewer than 30% of patients. Pathologically, these tumors are firm, gray, and nodular and tend to project into the ventricular cavity. Micrographs show double normal–sized myocytes filled with glycogen and containing hyperchromatic nuclei and eosinophilic staining cytoplasmic granules.[20,49] Scattered bundles of myofibrils can be seen within cells by electron microscopy.[51]

The most common presentation is heart failure caused by tumor obstruction of cardiac chambers or valvular orifice flow. Clinical findings can mimic valvular or subvalvular stenosis. Arrhythmias, particularly ventricular tachycardia and sudden death, can be a presenting symptom.[49] Atrial tumors can produce atrial arrhythmias.[49] The diagnosis is suggested by clinical features of tuberous sclerosis and is made by echocardiography. Rarely, no intramyocardial tumor is found in a patient with ventricular arrhythmias, and the site of rhabdomyoma is located by electrophysiologic study.[49]

Early operation is recommended in patients who do not have tuberous sclerosis before 1 year of age.[50] The tumor is usually removed easily in early infancy, and some can be enucleated.[50] Unfortunately, symptomatic tumors often are both multiple and extensive, particularly in patients with tuberous sclerosis who unfortunately have a dismal long-term outlook. In such circumstances, surgery offers little benefit.

Fibroma

Fibromas are the second most common benign cardiac tumor, with over 83% occurring in children. These tumors are solitary, occur exclusively within the ventricle and the ventricular septum, and affect the sexes equally (Fig. 103-4). Fewer than 100 tumors have been reported, and most are diagnosed by the age of 2 years. These tumors are not associated with other disease, nor are they inherited. Fibromas are nonencapsulated, firm, nodular, gray-white tumors that can become bulky. They are composed of elongated fibroblasts in broad spiral bands and whirls mixed with collagen and elastin fibers. Calcium deposits or bone can occur within the tumor and occasionally are seen on radiographs.

The majority of fibromas produce symptoms through chamber obstruction, interference with contraction, or arrhythmias. Depending on size and location, such a tumor can interfere with valve function, obstruct flow paths, or cause sudden death from conduction disturbances in up to 25% of patients.[50] Intracardiac calcification on chest radiographs suggests the diagnosis, which is confirmed by echocardiogram.

Surgical excision is successful in some patients, particularly if the tumor is localized, does not involve vital

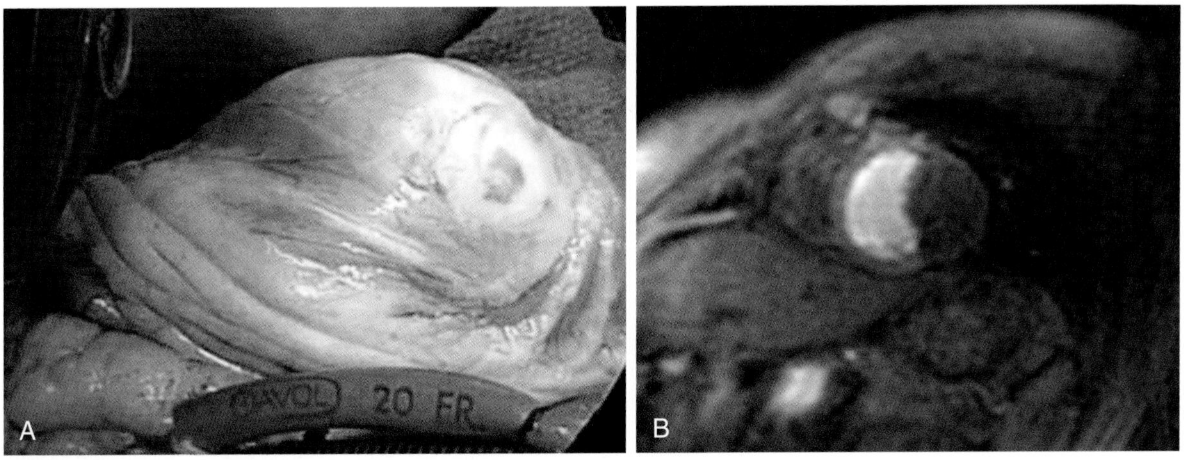

FIGURE 103-4 ■ Fibroma. **A,** Heart showing left ventricular fibroma. **B,** Cardiac magnetic resonance imaging showing left ventricular fibroma.

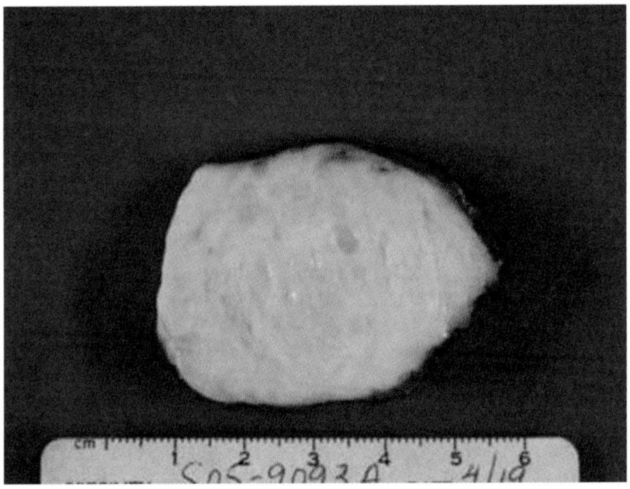

FIGURE 103-5 ■ Resected fibroma.

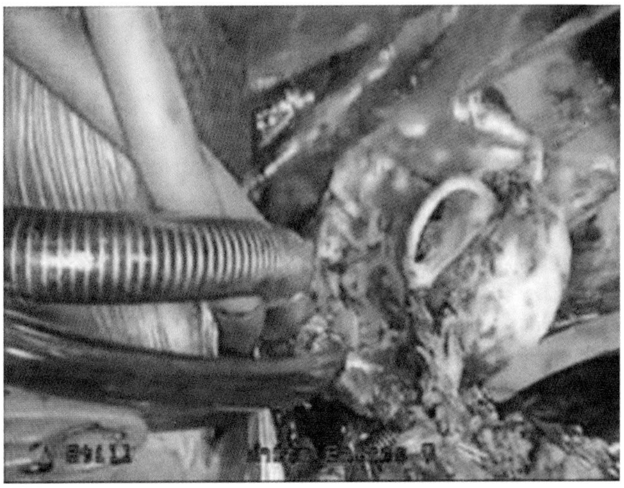

FIGURE 103-6 ■ Paraganglioma of the aortic root

structures, and can be enucleated (Fig. 103-5).[52] However, it is not always possible to completely remove the tumor, and partial removal is only palliative, although some patients have survived many years.[53,54] Operative mortality can be high in infants. Most cases involve adolescents and adults.[52] Successful, complete excision is curative.[52] Children with extensive fibromas have been treated with cardiac transplantation.[53]

Paraganglioma

Cardiac paragangliomas arise from chromaffin cells of the sympathetic nervous system and can produce excess amounts of catecholamines, particularly norepinephrine, but usually are not hormonally active. Approximately 90% of hormonally active paragangliomas are in the adrenal glands and are referred to as *pheochromocytomas*. Fewer than 2% arise in the chest and are referred to as *hormonally active cardiac paragangliomas*, with the term *pheochromocytoma* being restricted to the adrenals. Only 32 cardiac paragangliomas had been reported by 1991.[55] The tumor predominantly affects young and middle-aged adults with an equal distribution between the sexes. Approximately 60% of tumors occur in the roof of the left atrium. The remainder involve the interatrial septum or anterior surface of the heart.[56] The tumor is reddish-brown, soft, lobular, and consists of nests of chromatin cells (Fig. 103-6).

Hormonally active patients usually present with symptoms of uncontrolled hypertension or are found to have elevated urinary catecholamines. The tumor is usually located by scintigraphy using 131-I-metaiodobenzylguanidine[57,58] and CT scan or MRI.[57,58] Occasionally, cardiac catheterization with differential blood chamber sampling is necessary. Because these tumors are vascular and may be near major coronary arteries, coronary arteriograms are advisable and percutaneous biopsy should be avoided.

After the tumor is located, it should be removed, using cardiopulmonary bypass with cardioplegic arrest. Hormonally active patients require preanesthetic alpha and beta blockade, and careful intraoperative and immediate postoperative monitoring. Most tumors are extremely vascular and uncontrolled operative hemorrhage has occurred.[58] Resection may require removal of the atrial or ventricular wall, or both, or a segment of a major coronary artery.[59] Explantation of the heart to allow resection of a large left atrial paraganglioma has been attempted by Cooley and colleagues[60] and accomplished by Reardon.[59] Transplantation has been performed for nonresectable tumor. Complete excision produces cure.[59]

Hemangioma

Hemangiomas of the heart are rare (24 clinical cases reported), affect all ages, and can occur anywhere within the heart.[61-63] These vascular tumors are composed of capillaries or cavernous vascular channels. Patients usually develop dyspnea, occasional arrhythmias, or signs of right heart failure.[64] Diagnosis is difficult and chest roentgenography may be abnormal, but is not specific. Echocardiography or cardiac catheterization usually but not always establishes a diagnosis of cardiac tumor by showing an intracavity filling defect.[65] CT scan and MRI should be done. Axial T2-weighted MRI should show a high signal mass caused by vascularity.[66] Coronary angiography typically shows a tumor blush and maps the blood supply to the tumor.

The tumors can be resected in asymptomatic patients, and cardiopulmonary bypass is recommended. Meticulous ligation of feeding vessels is required to prevent postoperative residual arteriovenous fistulas or intracavity communications. Partial resections have produced long-term benefits.[61] Tumors rarely resolve spontaneously.[67]

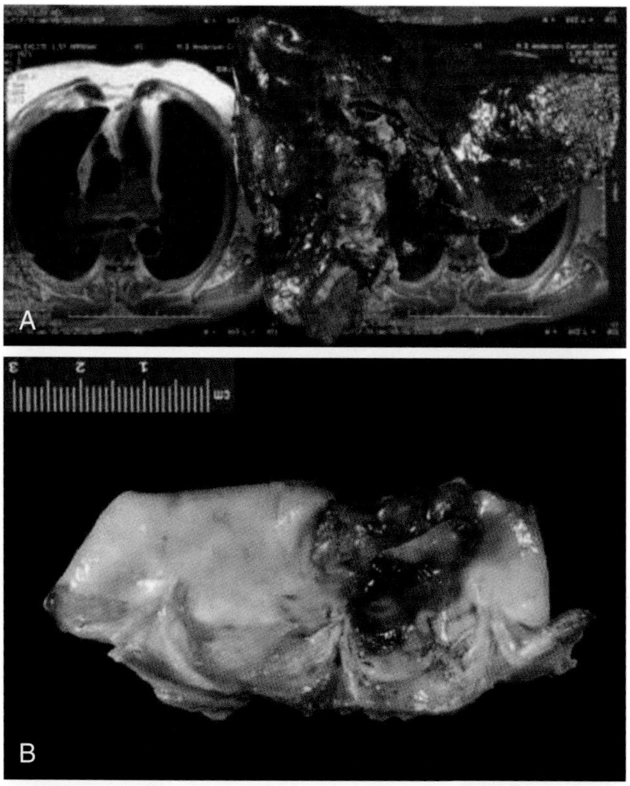

FIGURE 103-7 ■ Pulmonary artery sarcoma. **A,** Pulmonary artery sarcoma overlying computed tomographic scan. **B,** Pulmonary artery sarcoma starting at pulmonary valve.

PRIMARY MALIGNANT TUMORS

Sarcomas

Primary cardiac malignancy is uncommon, with only 21 surgically treated cases noted in a 25-year surgical experience from 1964 to 1989, combining the experience of two large institutions, the Texas Heart Institute and the M.D. Anderson Cancer Center in Houston, Texas.[68] Even in busy centers, primary cardiac malignancy continues to challenge the diagnostic ability and surgical skills of thoracic surgeons. Our current primary cardiac sarcoma database included more than 200 patients seen over 15 years, and surgical results have begun to improve.[9,69-74] Approximately 25% of primary cardiac tumors are malignant, and of these approximately 75% are sarcomas.[75] McAllister's survey of cardiac tumors found the most common to be angiosarcomas (31%), rhabdomyosarcomas (21%), malignant mesotheliomas (15%), and fibrosarcomas (11%).[20]

Primary malignant cardiac tumors arise sporadically showing no inherited linkage. Although they may span the entire age spectrum, they usually occur in adults over 40 years of age. The patients usually present with symptoms of congestive heart failure, pleuritic chest pain, malaise, anorexia, and weight loss.[76,77] The most common symptom has been dyspnea.[78] Some develop refractory arrhythmias, syncope, pericardial effusion, and tamponade.[68] The primary approach to primary cardiac sarcoma is complete surgical resection which is often a challenge. Our approach to primary cardiac sarcoma is to classify them according to location rather than cell type. Location generally determines presenting symptomatology and potential surgical approaches. We divide our cases into right heart, left heart, and pulmonary artery sarcomas.[69,79]

Pulmonary artery sarcomas often present late with pulmonary artery obstruction and can be mistaken for chronic pulmonary emboli. Cardiac MR will show tissue perfusion and allow differentiation as a tumor. These tumors arise in the dorsal pulmonary artery and often involve the valve (Fig. 103-7). Complete resection rather than endarterectomy should be performed to allow maximum survival.[72] Left heart sarcoma often presents with left heart obstruction and congestive heart failure. Surgical resection can be challenging because of the location of the posterior left atrium. We have used cardiac autotransplantation to allow full exposure, aggressive resection, and accurate reconstruction of the heart (Fig. 103-8).[70,73,75,80] Right heart sarcomas tend to be more bulky and infiltrative and less often appear with heart failure. Our experience has been that survival is markedly affected by achieving an R0 resection, which occurs in only about one third of cases. We recommend biopsy and neoadjuvant therapy to allow shrinkage of these large and bulky tumors to improve the R0 resection rate, and we are completing a protocol of this approach (Fig. 103-9).[74] These tumors are all aggressive, and we recommend postresection chemotherapy even when R0 resection is achieved. Surgical resection and overall care of these patients is complex and is best done in centers of excellence with multidisciplinary cardiac tumor teams.

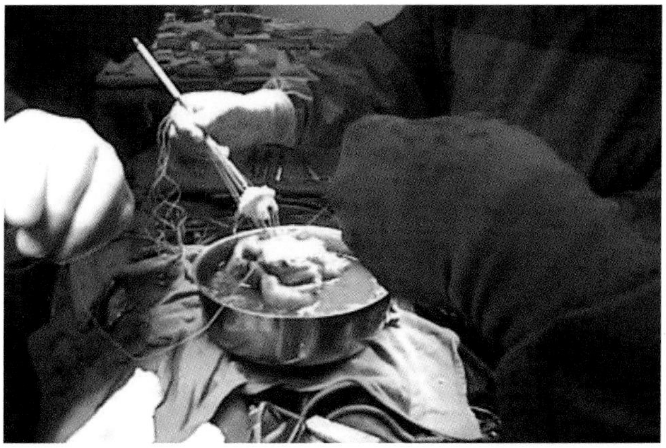

FIGURE 103-8 ■ Cardiac autotransplantation.

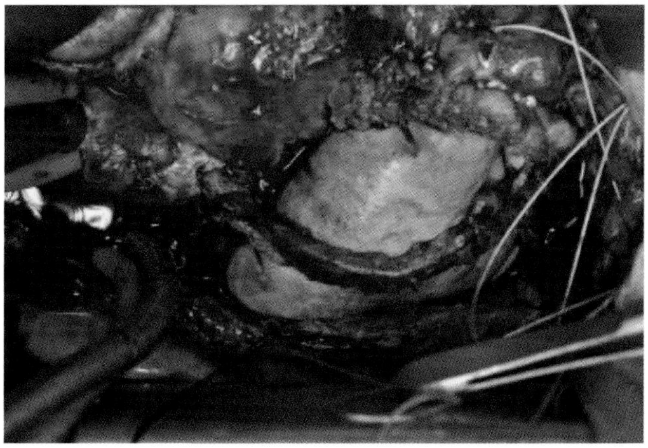

FIGURE 103-9 ■ Right atrial sarcoma resection and reconstruction.

Heart Transplantation

Malignant primary cardiac sarcomas often grow to a larger size until clinical detection. Extensive involvement may therefore make complete resection and reconstruction impossible. Because complete resection is necessary for improved results, cardiac transplantation has been considered in some cases.[74,79] Twenty-eight patients were reported to have undergone transplantation as of 2000, with 21 of the tumors being malignant. The mean survival was 12 months.[81] Transplantation has been used for sarcoma,[82-84] pheochromocytoma,[85] lymphoma,[86] fibroma,[87] and myxoma.[88] Although often technically resectable by orthotopic transplantation, most benign tumors can be removed completely by experienced teams without the need for a new heart, but malignant tumors offer several other problems. Most cardiac sarcomas involve the right or left atrium and are often in areas not routinely resected for orthotopic transplantation. This may still pose an issue with getting negative margins. Many sarcomas have metastatic disease at presentation, and using a scarce donor organ in the setting of active malignancy is generally not reasonable. There is also the mortality and morbidity inherent in transplantation. With a mean survival after transplantation for malignant primary tumors of 12 months, transplantation must be considered on a case-by-case basis by a multidisciplinary team in a center of excellence.[81]

Nonsarcomatous Primary Malignant Cardiac Tumors: Lymphomas

Lymphomas can arise from the heart, although it is rare.[89] Most of these tumors respond to radiation and chemotherapy, and we recommend biopsy of all right atrial tumors before treatment decisions if the patient's clinical condition will allow for it. Even when complete resection is not possible, and incomplete resection is performed to relieve acute obstructive systems, radiation and chemotherapy have allowed for up to 3-year survival in some patients.

SECONDARY METASTATIC TUMORS

Approximately 10% of metastatic tumors eventually reach the heart or pericardium, and almost every type of malignant tumor has been known to do so.[20,90] Secondary neoplasms are twenty to forty times more common than primary cardiac malignancies.[91] Up to 50% of patients with leukemia develop cardiac lesions. Other cancers that commonly involve the heart include breast, lung, lymphoma, melanoma, and various sarcomas.[91,92] Metastasis involving the pericardium, epicardium, myocardium, and endocardium roughly follows that order of frequency.[20,90]

The most common means of spread, particularly for melanoma, sarcoma, and bronchogenic carcinoma, is hematogenous, and ultimately via coronary arteries. In addition, metastasis can reach the heart through lymphatic channels; through direct extension from adjacent lung, breast, esophageal, and thymic tumors; and from the subdiaphragmatic vena cava. The pericardium most often is involved by direct extension of thoracic cancer; the heart is the target of hematogenous or retrograde lymphatic metastasis, or both. Cardiac metastases rarely are solitary and nearly always produce multiple microscopic nests and discrete nodules of tumor cells.[20,90] Cardiac metastases produce clinical symptoms in only about 10% of afflicted patients.[90] The most common symptom is pericardial effusion or cardiac tamponade. Occasionally, patients develop refractory arrhythmias or congestive heart failure. Chest radiographs and electrocardiograms tend to show nonspecific changes, but echocardiography is particularly useful for diagnosis of pericardial effusion, irregular pericardial thickening, or intracavity masses interfering with blood flow.

Surgical therapy is generally limited to relief of recurrent pericardial effusions or, occasionally, cardiac tamponade. In most instances, these patients have wide-spread disease with limited life expectancies. Surgical therapy is directed at providing symptomatic palliation with minimal patient discomfort and hospital stay. This is most readily accomplished via subxiphoid pericardiotomy, which can be accomplished using local anesthesia if necessary with reliable relief of symptoms, a recurrence rate of approximately 3%, and low mortality.[92] Alternatively, a large pericardial window in the left pleural space can be created using thoracoscopy, but we would recommend this only under unusual circumstances. This can be accomplished with minimal patient discomfort, but it does require general anesthesia with single-lung ventilation and may be poorly tolerated by patients with hemodynamic deterioration secondary to large effusions. There are rare cases of metastatic disease isolated to the heart in which resection can be considered, but this should be done only in the context of a center of excellence with the decision made by an experienced multidisciplinary team.[3]

REFERENCES

1. Reynen K: Frequency of primary tumors of the heart. *Am J Cardiol* 77(1):107, 1996.
2. Lam KY, Dickens P, Chan AC: Tumors of the heart. A 20-year experience with a review of 12,485 consecutive autopsies. *Arch Pathol Lab Med* 117(10):1027–1031, 1993.
3. Leja MJ, Kim M, Perryman L, et al: Metastatic melanoma to the intracavitary left ventricle treated using cardiac autotransplantation technique for resection. *Methodist Debakey Cardiovasc J* 7(4):44–46, 2011.
4. Roberts WC: Primary and secondary neoplasms of the heart. *Am J Cardiol* 80(5):671–682, 1997.
5. Shapiro LM: Cardiac tumours: diagnosis and management. *Heart* 85(2):218–222, 2001.
6. Carney JA, Hruska LS, Beauchamp GD, et al: Dominant inheritance of the complex of myxomas, spotty pigmentation, and endocrine overactivity. *Mayo Clin Proc* 61(3):165–172, 1986.
7. Vaughan CJ, Veugelers M, Basson CT: Tumors and the heart: molecular genetic advances. *Curr Opin Cardiol* 16(3):195–200, 2001.
8. Goodwin JF: Diagnosis of left atrial myxoma. *Lancet* 1(7279):464–468, 1963.
9. Bakaeen FG, Reardon MJ, Coselli JS, et al: Surgical outcome in 85 patients with primary cardiac tumors. *Am J Surg* 186(6):641–647, discussion 647, 2003.
10. Barnes AR, Beaver DC, Snell AM: Primary sarcoma of the heart: report of a case with electrocardiographic and pathologic studies. *Am Heart J* 9:480, 1934.
11. Beck C: An itrapericardial teratoma and tumor: both resected operatively. *Ann Surg* 116:161, 1942.
12. Mauer E: Successful removal of tumor of the heart. *J Thorac Surg* 3:479, 1952.
13. Goldberg HP, Glenn F, Dotter CT, et al: Myxoma of the left atrium: diagnosis made during life with operative and post mortem findings. *Circulation* 6:762–767, 1952.
14. Bahnson HT, Newman EV: Diagnosis and surgical removal of intracavitary myxoma of the right atrium. *Bull Johns Hopkins Hosp* 93:150–163, 1953.
15. Crafoord C: Panel discussion of late results of mitral commissurotomy. In Lam CR, editor: *Henry Ford Hospital international symposium on cardiovascular surgery*, Philadelphia, 1955, W.B. Saunders.
16. Kay JH, Anderson RM, Meihaus J, et al: Surgical removal of an intracavitary left ventricular myxoma. *Circulation* 20:881–886, 1959.
17. Malm JR, Bowman FO, Jr, Henry JB: Left atrial myxoma associated with an atrial septal defect. *J Thorac Cardiovasc Surg* 45:490–495, 1963.
18. Pinede L, Duhaut P, Loire R: Clinical presentation of left atrial cardiac myxoma. A series of 112 consecutive cases. *Medicine (Baltimore)* 80(3):159–172, 2001.
19. Hall RJ, Cooley DA, McAllister HA, et al: Neoplastic heart disease. In Hurst JW, editor: *The heart, arteries and veins*, ed 7, New York, 1990, McGraw Hill.
20. McAllister HA, Jr, Fenoglio JJ, Jr: Tumors of the cardiovascular system. In *Atlas of tumor pathology*, 2nd series, Washington DC, 1978, Armed Forces Institute of Pathology.
21. Prichard RW: Tumors of the heart; review of the subject and report of 150 cases. *AMA Arch Pathol* 51(1):98–128, 1951.
22. Reynen K: Cardiac myxomas. *N Engl J Med* 333(24):1610–1617, 1995.
23. Bortolotti U, Maraglino G, Rubino M, et al: Surgical excision of intracardiac myxomas: a 20-year follow-up. *Ann Thorac Surg* 49(3): 449–453, 1990.
24. Fyke FE, 3rd, Seqard JB, Edwards WD, et al: Primary cardiac tumors: experience with 30 consecutive patients since the introduction of two-dimensional echocardiography. *J Am Coll Cardiol* 5(6):1465–1473, 1985.
25. Goodwin JF: The spectrum of cardiac tumors. *Am J Cardiol* 21(3):307–314, 1968.
26. Meller J, Teichholz LE, Pichard AD, et al: Left ventricular myxoma: echocardiographic diagnosis and review of the literature. *Am J Med* 63(5):816–823, 1977.
27. Blackmon SH, Kassis ES, Ge Y, et al: Left atrial myxoma embolus to the renal artery: should a nephrectomy be advised? *Ann Thorac Surg* 90(1):289–292, 2010.
28. Mugge A, Daniel WG, Haverich A, et al: Diagnosis of noninfective cardiac mass lesions by two-dimensional echocardiography. Comparison of the transthoracic and transesophageal approaches. *Circulation* 83(1):70–78, 1991.
29. Obeid AI, Marvasti M, Parker F, et al: Comparison of transthoracic and transesophageal echocardiography in diagnosis of left atrial myxoma. *Am J Cardiol* 63(13):1006–1008, 1989.
30. Fang BR, Chiang CW, Hung JS, et al: Cardiac myxoma–clinical experience in 24 patients. *Int J Cardiol* 29(3):335–341, 1990.
31. Hanson EC, Gill CC, Razavi M, et al: The surgical treatment of atrial myxomas. Clinical experience and late results in 33 patients. *J Thorac Cardiovasc Surg* 89(2):298–303, 1985.
32. McCarthy PM, Piehler JM, Schaff HV, et al: The significance of multiple, recurrent, and "complex" cardiac myxomas. *J Thorac Cardiovasc Surg* 91(3):389–396, 1986.
33. Waller DA, Ettles DF, Saunders NR, et al: Recurrent cardiac myxoma: the surgical implications of two distinct groups of patients. *Thorac Cardiovasc Surg* 37(4):226–230, 1989.
34. Harjola PT, Ala-Kulju K, Ketonen P: Epicardial lipoma. *Scand J Thorac Cardiovasc Surg* 19(2):181–183, 1985.
35. Arciniegas E, Hakimi M, Farooki ZQ, et al: Primary cardiac tumors in children. *J Thorac Cardiovasc Surg* 79(4):582–591, 1980.
36. Edwards FH, Hale D, Cohen A, et al: Primary cardiac valve tumors. *Ann Thorac Surg* 52(5):1127–1131, 1991.
37. Grote J, Mugge A, Schfers HJ, et al: Multiplane transoesophageal echocardiography detection of a papillary fibroelastoma of the aortic valve causing myocardial infarction. *Eur Heart J* 16(3):426–429, 1995.
38. Gallas MT, Reardon MJ, Reardon PR, et al: Papillary fibroelastoma. A right atrial presentation. *Tex Heart Inst J* 20(4):293–295, 1993.
39. Di Mattia DG, Assaghi A, Mangini A, et al: Mitral valve repair for anterior leaflet papillary fibroelastoma: two case descriptions and a literature review. *Eur J Cardiothorac Surg* 15(1):103–107, 1999.
40. Grinda JM, Couetil JP, Chauvaud S, et al: Cardiac valve papillary fibroelastoma: surgical excision for revealed or potential embolization. *J Thorac Cardiovasc Surg* 117(1):106–110, 1999.
41. Wolber T, Facchini M, Huerlimann S, et al: Papillary fibroelastoma of the left atrial free wall. *Circulation* 104(17):E87–E88, 2001.
42. Shing M, Rubenson DS: Embolic stroke and cardiac papillary fibroelastoma. *Clin Cardiol* 24(4):346–347, 2001.
43. Shahian DM: Papillary fibroelastomas. *Semin Thorac Cardiovasc Surg* 12(2):101–110, 2000.
44. Grandmougin D, Fayad G, Moukassa D, et al: Cardiac valve papillary fibroelastomas: clinical, histological and immunohistochemical studies and a physiopathogenic hypothesis. *J Heart Valve Dis* 9(6):832–841, 2000.
45. Mazzucco A, Bortolotti U, Thiene G, et al: Left ventricular papillary fibroelastoma with coronary embolization. *Eur J Cardiothorac Surg* 3(5):471–473, 1989.
46. Walkes JC, Bavare C, Blackmon S, et al: Transaortic resection of an apical left ventricular fibroelastoma facilitated by a thoracoscope. *J Thorac Cardiovasc Surg* 134(3):793–794, 2007.
47. Mann J, Parker DJ: Papillary fibroelastoma of the mitral valve: a rare cause of transient neurological deficits. *Br Heart J* 71(1):6, 1994.
48. Nicks R: Hamartoma of the right ventricle. *J Thorac Cardiovasc Surg* 47:762–768, 1964.
49. Garson A, Jr, Smith RT, Jr, Moak JP, et al: Incessant ventricular tachycardia in infants: myocardial hamartomas and surgical cure. *J Am Coll Cardiol* 10(3):619–626, 1987.
50. Reece IJ, Cooley DA, Frazier OH, et al: Cardiac tumors. Clinical spectrum and prognosis of lesions other than classical benign

myxoma in 20 patients. *J Thorac Cardiovasc Surg* 88(3):439–446, 1984.
51. Fenoglio JJ, Jr, McAllister HA, Jr, Ferrans VJ: Cardiac rhabdomyoma: a clinicopathologic and electron microscopic study. *Am J Cardiol* 38(2):241–251, 1976.
52. Leja MJ, Perryman L, Reardon MJ: Resection of left ventricular fibroma with subacute papillary muscle rupture. *Tex Heart Inst J* 38(3):279–281, 2011.
53. Jamieson SW, Gaudiani VA, Reitz BA, et al: Operative treatment of an unresectable tumor of the left ventricle. *J Thorac Cardiovasc Surg* 81(5):797–799, 1981.
54. Yamaguchi M, Hosokawa Y, Ohashi H, et al: Cardiac fibroma. Long-term fate after excision. *J Thorac Cardiovasc Surg* 103(1):140–145, 1992.
55. Jebara VA, Uva MS, Farge A, et al: Cardiac pheochromocytomas. *Ann Thorac Surg* 53(2):356–361, 1992.
56. Yendamuri S, Elfar M, Walkes JC, et al: Aortic paraganglioma requiring resection and replacement of the aortic root. *Interact Cardiovasc Thorac Surg* 6(6):830–831, 2007.
57. Sisson JC, Shapiro B, Beierwaltes WH, et al: Locating pheochromocytomas by scintigraphy using 131I-metaiodobenzylguanidine. *CA Cancer J Clin* 34(2):86–92, 1984.
58. Orringer MB, Sisson JC, Glazer G, et al: Surgical treatment of cardiac pheochromocytomas. *J Thorac Cardiovasc Surg* 89(5):753–757, 1985.
59. Ramlawi B, David EA, Kim MP, et al: Contemporary surgical management of cardiac paragangliomas. *Ann Thorac Surg* 93(6):1972–1976, 2012.
60. Cooley DA, Reardon MJ, Frazier OH, et al: Human cardiac explantation and autotransplantation: application in a patient with a large cardiac pheochromocytoma. *Tex Heart Inst J* 12(2):171–176, 1985.
61. Brizard C, Latremouille C, Jebara VA, et al: Cardiac hemangiomas. *Ann Thorac Surg* 56(2):390–394, 1993.
62. Grenadier E, Margulis T, Palant A, et al: Huge cavernous hemangioma of the heart: a completely evaluated case report and review of the literature. *Am Heart J* 117(2):479–481, 1989.
63. Ramasubbu K, Wheeler TM, Reardon MJ, et al: Visceral pericardial hemangioma: unusual location for a rare cardiac tumor. *J Am Soc Echocardiogr* 18(9):981, 2005.
64. Soberman MS, Plauth WH, Winn KJ, et al: Hemangioma of the right ventricle causing outflow tract obstruction. *J Thorac Cardiovasc Surg* 96(2):307–309, 1988.
65. Weir I, Mills P, Lewis T: A case of left atrial haemangioma: echocardiographic, surgical, and morphological features. *Br Heart J* 58(6):665–668, 1987.
66. Lo LJ, Nucho RC, Allen JW, et al: Left atrial cardiac hemangioma associated with shortness of breath and palpitations. *Ann Thorac Surg* 73(3):979–981, 2002.
67. Palmer TE, Tresch DD, Bonchek LI: Spontaneous resolution of a large, cavernous hemangioma of the heart. *Am J Cardiol* 58(1):184–185, 1986.
68. Murphy MC, Sweeney MS, Putnam JB, Jr, et al: Surgical treatment of cardiac tumors: a 25-year experience. *Ann Thorac Surg* 49(4):612–617, discussion 617–618, 1990.
69. Reardon MJ, Walkes JC, Benjamin R: Therapy insight: malignant primary cardiac tumors. *Nat Clin Pract Cardiovasc Med* 3(10):548–553, 2006.
70. Blackmon SH, Patel AR, Bruckner BA, et al: Cardiac autotransplantation for malignant or complex primary left-heart tumors. *Tex Heart Inst J* 35(3):296–300, 2008.
71. Leja MJ, Shah DJ, Reardon MJ: Primary cardiac tumors. *Tex Heart Inst J* 38(3):261–262, 2011.
72. Blackmon SH, Rice DC, Correa AM, et al: Management of primary pulmonary artery sarcomas. *Ann Thorac Surg* 87(3):977–984, 2009.
73. Shapira OM, Korach A, Izhar U, et al: Radical multidisciplinary approach to primary cardiac sarcomas. *Eur J Cardiothorac Surg* 44(2):330–335, discussion 335–336, 2013.
74. Kim MP, Correa AM, Blackmon S, et al: Outcomes after right-side heart sarcoma resection. *Ann Thorac Surg* 91(3):770–776, 2011.
75. Reardon MJ, DeFelice CA, Sheinbaum R, et al: Cardiac autotransplant for surgical treatment of a malignant neoplasm. *Ann Thorac Surg* 67(6):1793–1795, 1999.
76. Bear PA, Moodie DS: Malignant primary cardiac tumors. The Cleveland Clinic experience, 1956 to 1986. *Chest* 92(5):860–862, 1987.
77. Thomas CR, Jr, Johnson GW, Jr, Stoddard MF, et al: Primary malignant cardiac tumors: update 1992. *Med Pediatr Oncol* 20(6):519–531, 1992.
78. Rettmar K, Stierle U, Sheikhzadeh A, et al: Primary angiosarcoma of the heart. Report of a case and review of the literature. *Jpn Heart J* 34(5):667–683, 1993.
79. Blackmon SH, Reardon MJ: Surgical treatment of primary cardiac sarcomas. *Tex Heart Inst J* 36(5):451–452, 2009.
80. Reardon MJ, Malaisrie SC, Walkes JC, et al: Cardiac autotransplantation for primary cardiac tumors. *Ann Thorac Surg* 82(2):645–650, 2006.
81. Gowdamarajan A, Michler RE: Therapy for primary cardiac tumors: is there a role for heart transplantation? *Curr Opin Cardiol* 15(2):121–125, 2000.
82. Goldstein DJ, Oz MC, Rose EA, et al: Experience with heart transplantation for cardiac tumors. *J Heart Lung Transplant* 14(2):382–386, 1995.
83. Baay P, Karwande SV, Kushner JP, et al: Successful treatment of a cardiac angiosarcoma with combined modality therapy. *J Heart Lung Transplant* 13(5):923–925, 1994.
84. Crespo MG, Pulpon LA, Pradas G, et al: Heart transplantation for cardiac angiosarcoma: should its indication be questioned? *J Heart Lung Transplant* 12(3):527–530, 1993.
85. Jeevanandam V, Oz MC, Shapiro B, et al: Surgical management of cardiac pheochromocytoma. Resection versus transplantation. *Ann Surg* 221(4):415–419, 1995.
86. Yuh DD, Kubo SH, Francis GS, et al: Primary cardiac lymphoma treated with orthotopic heart transplantation: a case report. *J Heart Lung Transplant* 13(3):538–542, 1994.
87. Valente M, Cocco P, Thiene G, et al: Cardiac fibroma and heart transplantation. *J Thorac Cardiovasc Surg* 106(6):1208–1212, 1993.
88. Goldstein DJ, Oz MC, Michler RE: Radical excisional therapy and total cardiac transplantation for recurrent atrial myxoma. *Ann Thorac Surg* 60(4):1105–1107, 1995.
89. Takagi M, Kugimiya T, Fujii T, et al: Extensive surgery for primary malignant lymphoma of the heart. *J Cardiovasc Surg (Torino)* 33(5):570–572, 1992.
90. Silverman NA: Primary cardiac tumors. *Ann Surg* 191(2):127–138, 1980.
91. Skhvatsabaja LV: Secondary malignant lesions of the heart and pericardium in neoplastic disease. *Oncology* 43(2):103–106, 1986.
92. Press OW, Livingston R: Management of malignant pericardial effusion and tamponade. *JAMA* 257(8):1088–1092, 1987.

SECTION 3

CONGENITAL HEART SURGERY

SECTION OUTLINE

Continued

transcription factors are required for the molecular regionalization of information in the developing heart.

CARDIAC SEPTATION OF THE ATRIA, VENTRICLES, ATRIOVENTRICULAR JUNCTION, AND OUTFLOW TRACT

Cardiac septation is a complex process that begins after looping morphogenesis has realigned the cardiac segments so that the right ventricle and left ventricle are located beside one another. Complete septation of the heart is not necessary for survival of the embryo, which may in part explain the high incidence of septation defects seen in clinical cardiology practice. Four major components must develop to divide the heart into separate systemic and pulmonary circulations: (1) the atrial septum that separates the right and left atria, (2) the atrioventricular junction that contributes to atrial and ventricular septation as well as to atrioventricular valve formation, (3) the ventricular septum that separates the right and left ventricles, and (4) outflow tract or infundibular septum that separates the pulmonary from the aortic outflow tract.

Recent studies have resulted in a newer paradigm of atrial septal development than that presented by classical embryology studies.[74-76] The atrial septum includes septum secundum (secondary atrial septum), septum primum (primary atrial septum), and contributions from the atrioventricular cushions (Fig. 104-3). Septum secundum is an infolding in the roof of the common primitive atrium. Septum primum develops from the dorsal wall of the atrium at 5 weeks' gestation, grows toward the atrioventricular cushions as a crescentic muscular septum, and closes off the ostium primum (primary atrial communication) when it fuses with the atrioventricular cushions during the sixth week of fetal development. Septum primum carries a "cap" of distinct mesenchymal tissue along its leading edge that is critical for fusion of the primary atrial septum with the atrioventricular cushions.[74] As septum primum grows toward the atrioventricular cushions and divides the atria, it develops fenestrations that coalesce into the ostium secundum (secondary foramen) and allow continued mixing of blood at the atrial level in the fetus.

Like the atrial septum, the ventricular septum is a complex structure that includes components derived from the atrioventricular cushions, the muscular ventricular septum, and the conal (infundibular) septum. In the early stages just after looping (31 to 35 days in the human), the muscular ventricular septum is a ridge of myocardium corresponding to the furrow of the primary fold on the outer curvature of the heart and separating the primitive left ventricle and primitive right ventricle.[77] In mammals, the muscular septum develops from a ridge of infolded compact myocardium.[78] As the heart grows markedly in size along the outer curvature, the muscular septum grows concordantly with the ventricles.[26] The muscular septum fuses with the endocardial cushions of the atrioventricular junction and with the outflow tract to completely separate the right and left ventricles.

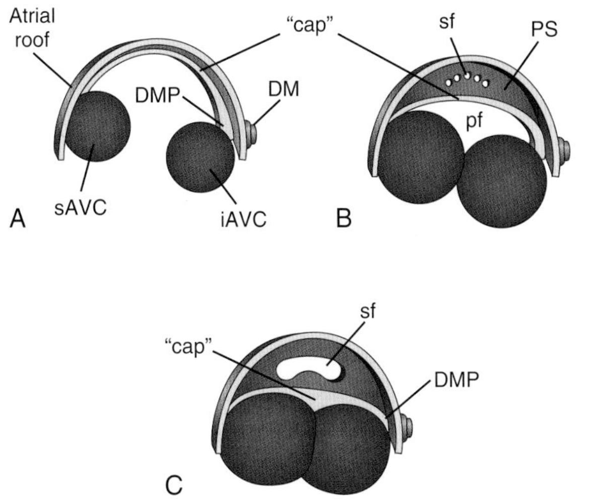

FIGURE 104-3 ■ Atrial septal development. The developing atrial septum has contributions from the septum secundum, the septum primum, and the atrioventricular (AV) cushions. **A,** Septum secundum ("atrial roof") is an infolding in the roof of the primitive common atrium. **B,** Septum primum (PS) grows from septum secundum toward the AV cushions (sAVC and iAVC), carrying with it a "cap" of mesenchymal tissue that is critical for the fusion of PS with the cushions. **C,** As PS closes off the primary interatrial communication (pf in **B**), fenestrations develop (sf in **B**) and coalesce into the foramen ovale (sf in **C**), which allows the shunting of blood at the atrial level that is necessary in the fetal circulation. *DM,* Dorsal mesocardium; *DMP,* dorsal mesenchymal protrusion. (From Wessels A, Anderson RH, Markwald RR, et al: Atrial development in the human heart: an immunohistochemical study with emphasis on the role of mesenchymal tissues. *Anat Rec* 259[3]:288–300, 2000.)

The atrioventricular junction (canal) segment of the developing heart initially connects the primitive atrium exclusively to the left ventricle (see Fig. 104-1*C*). Complex remodeling must occur to allow inflow from the atrium directly into both right and left ventricles (see Fig. 104-1*D*). In addition to establishing continuity between the right atrium and the right ventricle, the atrioventricular junction gives rise to the endocardial cushions that will form the atrioventricular valves. (Endocardial cushions also form in the outflow tract and contribute to the semilunar valves and septation of the outflow tract.) The superior and inferior atrioventricular cushions fuse in the midline to form the atrioventricular septum, with resultant separation of the inflow into mitral (left-side) and tricuspid (right-side) components. The mesenchyme of the atrioventricular junction contributes to the portion of the atrial septum just proximal to the atrioventricular valves by fusing with the primary atrial septum. In addition, the atrioventricular septum mesenchyme forms the inlet portion of the ventricular septum (between the atrioventricular valves).

The growth and maturation of the endocardial cushions has been studied at the molecular level. Cardiac cushions begin as localized thickenings of the extracellular matrix between the endocardial and myocardial layers of the primitive heart tube, termed the *cardiac jelly* (Fig. 104-4).[73] The cushions begin as acellular structures that become populated by cells that have undergone a transformation from endothelium to mesenchyme. JB3 is

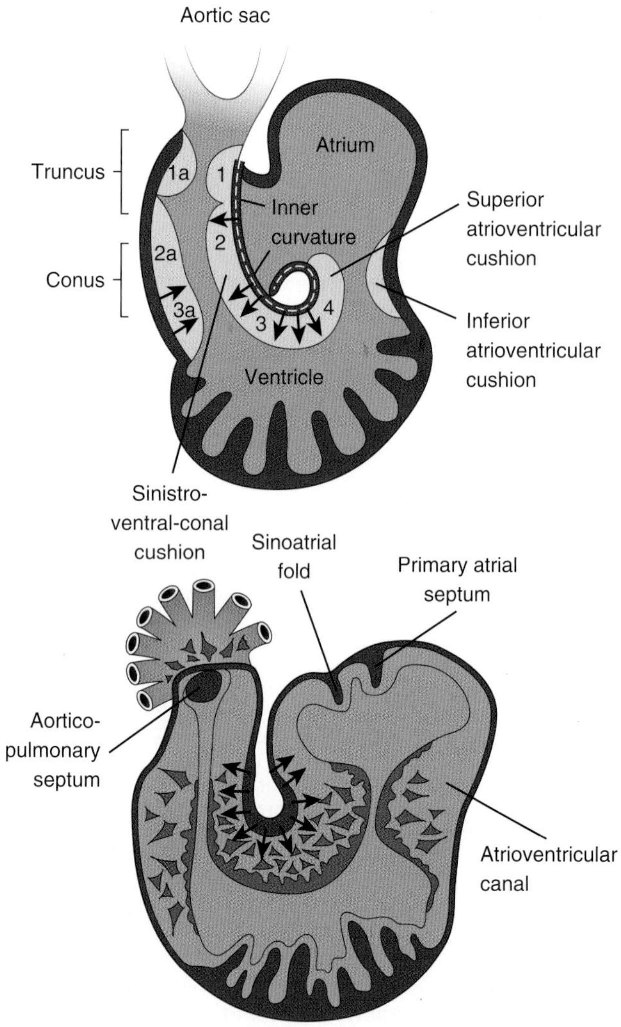

FIGURE 104-4 ■ Cushion development. The endocardial cushions appear in the atrioventricular (AV) junction (AV canal) and in the outflow tract (conus and truncus) after looping of the heart tube. The superior AV cushion (4) is contiguous with the cushions of the outflow tract (3, 3a, 2, 2a, 1, 1a) along the inner curvature of the heart. Cushion tissue contributes to the formation of the valves and also to septation of the heart. The inner curvature undergoes significant remodeling and participates in myocardialization of the cushions *(arrows).* (From Harvey RP, Rosenthal N, editors: *Heart development,* San Diego, 1999, Academic Press, p 171.)

an antibody that recognizes fibrillin-2,[79] and, in the heart, it recognizes only the subset of cells (JB3+) that have the potential to undergo the endothelium-to-mesenchyme transformation in the cushions.[80] The mesenchymal transformation is mediated by the myocardium of the atrioventricular junction via a number of molecules including BMP-2, BMP-4, and neuregulin, an epidermal growth factor–like molecule, as well as the homeobox-containing transcription factor Msx-2.[81-83] ES proteins that form complexes with fibronectin are also present in the developing cushions and appear important for the regulation of the mesenchymal transformation.[80,81]

Contributions from the endocardial cushions and the cardiac neural crest are required for outflow tract septation (Fig. 104-5). The endocardial cushions of the atrioventricular junction and the outflow tract are in physical continuity through the superior atrioventricular cushion, which extends along the inner curvature of the heart.[80] Extensive remodeling of the inner curvature occurs so as to connect the right atrium to the right ventricle and the left ventricle to the aorta.[84] Septation of the outflow tract results from the development of two structures. Below the level of the semilunar valves, the conal septum (infundibular septum or muscular outflow tract septum) develops from myocardialization of the outflow tract cushions, a process that also involves contributions from the cardiac neural crest and the epicardium.[84] Above the level of the semilunar valves, the aorticopulmonary septum grows from the aortic sac toward the heart to separate the pulmonary from the aortic outflow tracts.

The three components of the ventricular septum (the inlet and the muscular and conal septa) must join together to completely separate the ventricles. The region of the membranous ventricular septum in the adult heart is the approximate location where these three components join. This finding suggests that a defect in the development of either the inlet or the muscular or conal septa can result in a ventricular septal defect, suggesting a mechanistic rationale for the high frequency of defects at this anatomic location.

Clinical Correlates of Abnormal Chamber Septation

The term *common atrioventricular canal* (also called endocardial cushion defect or atrioventricular septal defect) refers to a spectrum of lesions that have improper development of the atrioventricular junction as the underlying developmental abnormality. In such cases, the atrioventricular junction has failed to undergo its normal septation and formation of separate atrioventricular valves, leaving a common atrioventricular valve providing inflow to both ventricles. The atrioventricular cushion contributions to atrial and ventricular septation are also abnormal, resulting in atrial septal defect of the ostium primum type and ventricular septal defect of the inlet (atrioventricular canal) type. This defect is reminiscent of the structure of the developing heart prior to atrioventricular junction septation by the developing endocardial cushions. Genes required for normal development of the atrioventricular endocardial cushions can result in common atrioventricular canal when mutated in a mouse model, as demonstrated by the ALK3 conditional receptor knockout.[85] Common atrioventricular canal can therefore be conceptualized as a developmental arrest, in which chamber septation fails to progress past the common atrioventricular junction.

Although complete common atrioventricular canal accounts for only 7.3% of all congenital malformations,[86] it is observed in approximately 40% of patients with trisomy 21 (Down syndrome).[87] The epidemiologic data suggest that a gene important for the development of the atrioventricular junction resides on chromosome 21. To date, no single gene on chromosome 21 has been implicated in the genesis of common atrioventricular canal.[88]

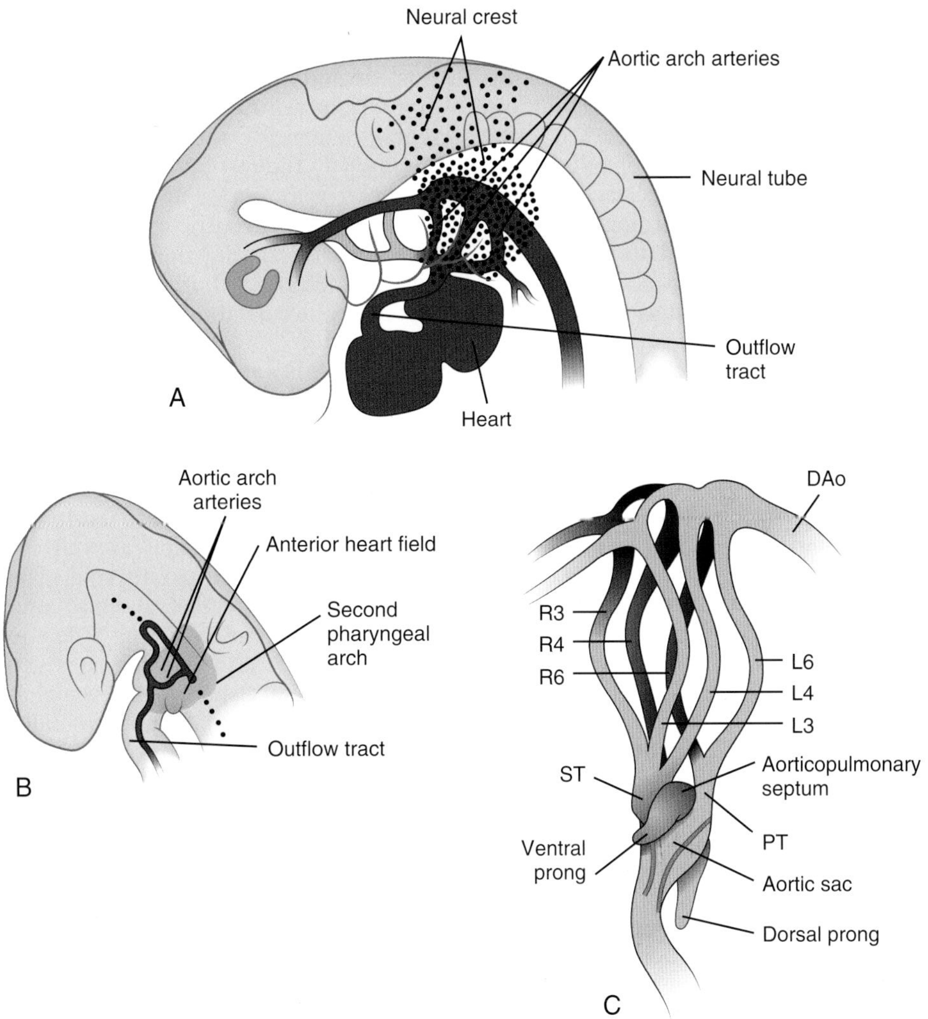

FIGURE 104-5 ■ Development of neural crest, anterior heart field, and outflow tract. **A,** The cardiac neural crest migrates into pharyngeal arches 3, 4, and 6, where it plays a crucial role in the patterning of the paired aortic arch arteries by preventing the regression of aortic arch arteries 3, 4, and 6, the precursors of the definitive great arteries. **B,** The anterior heart field is a recently described and separate migratory population of cells that originate near the second pharyngeal arch and contribute to cardiac outflow tract development. **C,** The neural crest cells condense into two prongs that insert into the endocardial cushions of the developing outflow tract. The third aortic arch arteries (L3 and R3) give rise to the right and left carotid arteries. The left fourth arch artery (L4) becomes part of the definitive aortic arch, and the right fourth arch artery (R4) contributes to the proximal right subclavian artery. The left sixth aortic arch artery (L6) forms the ductus arteriosus. *DAo,* Descending aorta; *PT,* pulmonary trunk; *ST,* systemic trunk. (**A** and **C** from Harvey RP, Rosenthal N, editors: *Heart development,* San Diego, 1999, Academic Press, pp 180, 182; **B** modified from Waldo KL, Kumiski DH, Wallis KT, et al: Conotruncal myocardium arises from a secondary heart field. *Development* 128:3179–3188, 2001.)

Isolated atrial septal defects are one of the most common congenital defects of the heart in humans. Secundum atrial septal defects result from a deficiency of septum primum in closing off the ostium secundum. Atrial septal defects are also frequently found in association with clinical syndromes. Secundum atrial septal defects are the most common structural defect resulting from the loss of one copy of the *Tbx5* gene in Holt-Oram syndrome, an autosomal dominant disorder.[89,90] Mutations in the *Nkx2.5* gene have been linked to autosomal dominant secundum atrial septal defects,[91,92] and more recently, mutations in the *GATA-4* gene have also been linked to secundum atrial septal defects.[93] The finding that *Tbx5*, *Nkx2.5*, and *GATA-4* all interact to regulate the expression of genes necessary for atrial septal development suggests that candidate genes for secundum atrial septal defects may lie downstream of these important transcription factors.

OUTFLOW TRACT DEVELOPMENT: ANTERIOR HEART FIELD AND CARDIAC NEURAL CREST

Although the vertebrate heart develops primarily from the precardiac mesoderm (the cardiac crescent), two other cell populations, the anterior heart field and the cardiac neural crest, are critical for normal outflow tract development.[20-22,94]

The existence of the anterior heart field was suspected 30 years ago, when Viragh and Challice[95] observed the transformation of epithelial cells to myocardial cells at the arterial pole of the developing mouse heart. De la Cruz and colleagues[96] used marking studies in living chick embryos to demonstrate that the distal outflow tract was a late addition to the developing heart. A series of recent studies show that a population of cells in the anterior mesoderm adjacent to the aortic sac (see Fig. 104-5*B*), distinct from both the lateral cardiogenic mesoderm and the cardiac neural crest, contribute to the myocardium of the outflow tract in both avian[21,22] and murine[20] models. In the murine model, the anterior heart field contributions extend past the outflow tract and also contribute to the developing right ventricle to the level of the interventricular septum.[28,97] This finding may ultimately help explain observed gene expression differences between the right and left ventricles.

The cardiac outflow tract is initially a tubular structure connecting the primitive right ventricle to the aortic sac, and it must undergo septation to form the pulmonary artery and the aorta. In addition, the outflow tract must gain continuity with the primitive left ventricle. This occurs by a process termed *wedging*, in which the subaortic conus is remodeled to allow the aortic valve to reach its normal adult position between the tricuspid and mitral valves. This process establishes fibrous continuity of the mitral and aortic valves.[98] The aorticopulmonary septum develops from the aortic sac mesenchyme and grows into the outflow tract, where it interacts with neural crest–derived cells in the endocardial cushions, ultimately dividing the outflow tract into the aorta and the pulmonary artery.[93]

The cardiac outflow tract receives a large contribution of cells from the neural crest, a population of migratory pluripotent cells that arise adjacent to the developing neural tube. The cardiac neural crest is a subpopulation of the neural crest that originates from between the midotic placode to the third somite (see Fig. 104-5*A*).[99] These cells migrate into the developing third, fourth, and sixth pharyngeal arches, where they interact with the third, fourth, and sixth aortic arch vessels, the progenitors of the definitive great arteries (aorta, carotid, and subclavian arteries, main pulmonary artery, and ductus arteriosus). The aortic arch vessels develop as symmetrically paired structures, but they undergo a highly specific and asymmetrical program of resorption, retaining the normal left aortic arch. The cardiac neural crest does not play a role in the formation of the aortic arch vessels but rather stabilizes the arch vessels and prevents their regression (see Fig. 104-5*C*).[100] A subpopulation of the cardiac neural crest migrates farther from the pharyngeal arches to the heart, where it forms the cardiac ganglia, participates in the septation of the outflow tract, and contributes to the formation of the semilunar valves.[101] Neural crest also interacts with the pharyngeal arch mesenchyme to form the thymus, thyroid, and parathyroid glands.

Animal models of neural crest defects have been useful in determining the cause of some congenital heart malformations. Experimental ablation of the neural crest in avian embryos[102] demonstrated abnormal development of the heart and great arteries, as well as abnormalities of the glandular derivatives of the pharyngeal arches and pouches (i.e., the thymus, thyroid, and parathyroid glands).[94] Specifically, defects of the embryonic outflow tract were observed in embryos after neural crest ablation, including persistent truncus arteriosus, double-outlet right ventricle, and tetralogy of Fallot. Ventricular septal defects of the infundibular septum were also common.[103] Interestingly, defects of the inflow portion of the heart were occasionally described as well, including double-inlet left ventricle, straddling tricuspid valve, and tricuspid atresia, and they occurred in association with outflow defects.[103] Furthermore, abnormal aortic arch patterning occurred in virtually all embryos after neural crest ablation.[103-105] The arch abnormalities demonstrated great variability and included various types of interrupted aortic arch.

Murine models with cardiac phenotypes reminiscent of neural crest ablation include the Splotch mouse, bearing a mutation in the *Pax3* homeobox gene. Splotch homozygotes demonstrate persistent truncus arteriosus and aortic arch anomalies as well as anomalies of the thymus, thyroid, and parathyroid glands. The homozygous mutation is lethal at embryonic day 14.[106] The Patch mutant mouse, bearing a deletion of a portion of chromosome 5, also demonstrates craniofacial, thymic, and outflow tract abnormalities, including arch patterning anomalies.[107] Initial efforts to understand this phenotype focused on the deletion of the gene for platelet-derived growth factor receptor (PDGFR). However, mice homozygous for a PDGFR-targeted null mutation do not consistently demonstrate cardiac anomalies, suggesting that other genes deleted in the Patch mutant must contribute to the cardiac phenotype.[107a]

Retinoic acid, the active derivative of vitamin A, has been shown to play an important role in outflow tract development. Knockouts of the retinoic acid receptor in mice produce phenotypes reminiscent of neural crest ablation. There are two families of receptors, RAR and RXR, and each family contains three isoforms. Single-isoform knockouts produce no morphologic defects; however, double mutants of RAR and RXR produce outflow tract defects (persistent truncus arteriosus, double-outlet right ventricle, and arch anomalies), as well as craniofacial, thymic, thyroid, and parathyroid anomalies.[88,107] If vitamin A is administered, the cardiac phenotype may be rescued.[108] This suggests a role for retinoic acid signaling in neural crest migration and cardiac development.

Clinical Correlates of Abnormal Outflow Tract Development: DiGeorge Syndrome and 22q11 Deletion

DiGeorge syndrome is an autosomal dominant disorder whose phenotype includes cardiac defects of the outflow tract—in particular, interrupted aortic arch, persistent truncus arteriosus, tetralogy of Fallot, and aortic arch anomalies. The syndrome also includes parathyroid hypoplasia with resultant hypocalcemia, thymic hypoplasia with resultant T cell deficit, and cleft palate and other craniofacial abnormalities. There are phenotypic similarities between DiGeorge, Takao (conotruncal anomaly face syndrome), and Shprintzen (velocardiofacial) syndromes, and, in fact, the same molecular lesion is present in all three syndromes: deletion of 22q11. *CATCH* has been proposed as an acronym for the phenotype associated with these syndromes (*c*ardiac defects, *a*bnormal facies, *T* cell deficit, *c*left palate, *h*ypocalcemia).[109,110] The phenotype demonstrates considerable variability between patients. The 22q11 deletion is the most common deletion in humans, occurring in 1 of 4000 live births[111] with an average of 30 genes removed, although smaller and larger deletions are not infrequent.[97]

A vigorous search for candidate genes residing in the commonly deleted portion of human chromosome 22 has recently yielded some success in elucidating the molecular underpinnings of the cardiac defects. Mouse models with deletions of the region of chromosome 16 syntenic to human chromosomal region 22q11 have been used to identify and test candidate genes.[107] Three independent groups have reported that haploinsufficiency of the T-box transcription factor gene *Tbx1* results in cardiac phenotypes consistent with DiGeorge syndrome.[112-114] However, not a single point mutation has been identified in any patient with DiGeorge syndrome; the phenotype in humans may require larger genetic alterations. The clinical variability seen among patients with DiGeorge syndrome has several possible sources, including variability in the size of the deletion, sensitivity to gene dosage from modifying genes (genetic background), and epigenetic factors. One study demonstrated that a targeted deletion of *Tbx1* in mice caused abnormal aortic arch patterning in 50% of embryos, implicating sensitivity to gene dosage in the variability of the DiGeorge phenotype.[114] When a larger deletion containing additional genes was studied, the mice showed parathyroid hypoplasia, thymic insufficiency, and a higher perinatal lethality, implicating deletion size. Another group demonstrated abnormal development of the fourth aortic arch in mice heterozygous for a *Tbx1* deletion.[113] Homozygous mutants were embryonic lethal with obliteration of the third, fourth and sixth arches.[113] In this model, *Tbx1* haploinsufficient animals did not display thymic, parathyroid, or facial anomalies, again suggesting that a multiple gene deletion is required for the full clinical features of DiGeorge syndrome.[113]

THE CAUSES OF CONGENITAL HEART DISEASE: ADDITIONAL FACTORS

The genetic programs underlying heart development are beginning to be elucidated, but the complexity of the developmental process has made progress painstaking. Although these genetic abnormalities in animal models do correlate to certain forms of heart disease, other experimental models use variations in blood flow to produce structural heart abnormalities. An intriguing series of experiments in chick embryos used ligation of the left atrial appendage to produce a hypoplastic left heart syndrome phenotype.[115] Subsequent work sequentially ligating the left atrial appendage and then the right atrial appendage demonstrated rescue of the hypoplastic left heart phenotype during embryonic development.[115] These studies are suggestive that fetal interventional strategies[116] and early surgical repair may positively impact heart development and chamber growth.

The interaction between genetic factors and environmental factors contributing to CHD is not yet fully understood. Observations of teratogen exposure such as thalidomide or retinoids producing congenital heart defects have been described for years.[117] Hypoplastic left heart syndrome has been demonstrated to have a genetic component,[118] but a geographic spatial analysis of cases of hypoplastic left heart cases in Baltimore, MD, demonstrated a cluster of cases near a region of industrial land with environmental exposures to solvents.[119] Complex interactions between genetic predisposition and environmental insult may contribute to the phenotypic variability of congenital heart malformations.

GENETIC ABNORMALITIES ASSOCIATED WITH CONGENITAL HEART DISEASE

In the first portion of this chapter, developmental mechanisms critical for normal heart development were reviewed. The complexity of these processes has resulted in slow painstaking progress in the understanding of specific genetic abnormalities that are associated with CHD. Table 104-1 provides a list of single gene and chromosomal region abnormalities that have a strong association with congenital heart malformations. Aneuploidy syndromes are also known to be associated with CHD. Specifically, trisomy 21 (Down syndrome) has a 40% to 50% chance of associated CHD, most commonly atrioventricular canal defects; atrial septal defect, ventricular septal defect, patent ductus arteriosus, and tetralogy of Fallot may also be seen. Turner syndrome (monosomy, 45X0) has an association of left heart obstructive lesions including coarctation, bicuspid aortic valve, and hypoplastic left heart syndrome. Trisomy 18 (Edwards syndrome) and trisomy 13 (Patau syndrome) are associated with atrial septal defect, ventricular septal defect, patent ductus arteriosus, and polyvalvular disease in 80% to 100% of patients.[120]

CONCLUSION

This chapter demonstrates some of the progress that has been made in the molecular understanding of embryonic heart development and how specific structural defects of the heart arise when the activity of single genes is interrupted. Hemodynamic and environmental factors may also contribute to malformations of the heart, and the broad range of phenotypes may be a result of complex interactions between genes, blood flow, and exposures. Details of cardiac specification and development continue to be elucidated, and it is the hope that a better understanding of the genetic mechanisms involved in heart formation will improve the care of patients with CHD.

Acknowledgment

The author would like to recognize Ivan Moskowitz, MD, PhD, for contributions to an earlier version of this chapter.

TABLE 104-1 **Genetic Abnormalities with Prominent CHD Phenotypes**

Syndrome	Locus	Gene(s)	Inheritance	Clinical Features	Most Common CHD	Percentage with CHD	OMIM
Single Gene Mutation Syndromes							
Alagille	20p12; 1p12	*JAG1; NOTCH2*	AD	Paucity of hepatic bile ducts, CHD, skeletal abnormalities, skeletal abnormalities, distinctive facies	Pulmonary artery stenosis, pulmonary valve stenosis, TOF	>90%	118450
Noonan	12q24; 12p1.21; 2p21; 3p25.2; 7q34; 15q22.31; 11p15.5; 1p13.2; 10q25.2;11q23.3; 17q11.2	*PTPN11; KRAS; SOS1; RAF1; BRAF; MEK1; HRAS; NRAS; SHOC2; CBL; NF1*	AD, AR	Distinctive facies, short stature, webbed neck, pectus deformity, cubitus valgus, CHD	PS, ASD, VSD, PDA	80%	163950
Holt-Oram	12q24	*TBX5*	AD	Upper limb deformities, CHD	ASD, VSD, PDA	85%	142900
Char	6p12	*TFAP2B*	AD	Distinctive facies, PDA, limb deformities	PDA	100% (CHD required to make diagnosis)	169100
Ellis-van Creveld	4p16	*EVC; EVC2*	AR	Skeletal dysplasia (short limbs, short ribs, polydactyly, dysplastic teeth and nails), CHD	ASD	60%	225500
Costello	11p15.5	*HRAS*	De novo, AD	Distinctive facies, short stature, failure to thrive, heart defects, developmental delay	PS, hypertrophy, arrhythmias, other structural heart disease	63%	218040
Cardiofaciocutaneous (CFC)	12p12.1; 7q34; 15q22.31; 19p13.3	*KRAS; BRAF; MAP2K1; MAP2K2*	De novo, AD	Distinctive facies, mental retardation, heart defects	PS, ASD, hypertrophy	71%	115150
CHARGE	8p12; 7q21.11	*CHD7; SEMA3E*	AD	Choanal atresia, heart disease, eye coloboma, mental retardation, genitourinary abnormalities, ear abnormalities and deafness	TOF, ASD, VSD	85%	214800
Kabuki	12q13.12	*MLL2*	De novo, AD	Mental retardation, dwarfism, distinctive facies, spine deformities, cleft palate	VSD, ASD, TOF, COA, SV, PDA	31%-55%	147920
Abnormal Chromosomal Structural Syndromes							
22q11 Deletion (DiGeorge)	22q11.2 deletion	*TBX1*	De novo, AD	Thymus hypoplasia/aplasia, parathyroid hypoplasia/aplasia, distinctive facies, CHD (particularly outflow tract abnormalities)	TOF, IAA type B, aortic arch anomalies, truncus, VSD	80%-100%	188400
Williams-Beuren	7q11.23 deletion	*ELN*	De novo, AD	Arterial stenoses, mental retardation, distinctive facies, hypercalcemia	SVAS, multiple arterial stenoses	80%-100%	194050
Cri-du-chat	5p15.2 deletion	*CTNND2*	De novo	Microcephaly, mental retardation, distinctive facies, high-pitched cry	VSD, PDA, ASD, TOF	10%-55%	123450
1p36 Deletion	1p36 deletion	*DVL1*	De novo	Microcephaly, mental retardation, distinctive facies, CHD, hearing loss, hypotonia	ASD, VSD, PDA, dilated cardiomyopathy, LV noncompaction	43%-70%	607872

AD, Autosomal dominant; *AR*, autosomal recessive; *ASD*, atrial septal defect; *CHD*, congenital heart disease; *COA*, coarctation of the aorta; *IAA*, interrupted aortic arch; *LV*, left ventricular; *OMIM*, Online Mendelian Inheritance in Man; *PDA*, patent ductus arteriosus; *PS*, pulmonary stenosis; *SV*, single ventricle; *SVAS*, supravalvular aortic stenosis; *TOF*, tetralogy of Fallot; *VSD*, ventricular septal defect.

REFERENCES

1. DeHaan RL: Morphogenesis of the vertebrate heart. In DeHaan RL, Ursprung H, editors: *Organogenesis*, New York, 1965, Holt, Rinehart and Winston, pp 377–420.
2. Sugi Y, Lough J: Anterior endoderm is a specific effector of terminal cardiac myocyte differentiation of cells from the embryonic heart forming region. *Dev Dyn* 200:155–162, 1994.
3. Schultheiss TM, Xydas S, Lassar AB: Induction of avian cardiac myogenesis by anterior endoderm. *Development* 121:4203–4214, 1995.
4. Rana MS, Christoffels VM, Moorman AFM: A molecular and genetic outline of cardiac morphogenesis. *Acta Physiologica* 207:588–615, 2013.
5. Schultheiss TM, Burch JB, Lassar AB: A role for bone morphogenetic proteins in the induction of cardiac myogenesis. *Genes Dev* 11:451–462, 1997.
6. Andree B, Duprez D, Vorbusch B, et al: BMP-2 induces ectopic expression of cardiac lineage markers and interferes with somite formation in chicken embryos. *Mech Dev* 70:119–131, 1998.
7. Reifers F, Walsh EC, Leger S, et al: Induction and differentiation of the zebrafish heart requires fibroblast growth factor 8 (fgf8/acerebellar). *Development* 127:225–235, 2000.
8. Alsan BH, Schultheiss TM: Regulation of cardiogenesis by FGF8 signalling. *Development* 129:1935–1943, 2002.
9. Pandur P, Lasche M, Eisenberg LM, et al: Wnt-11 activation of a non canonical Wnt signaling pathway is required for cardiogenesis. *Nature* 418:636–641, 2002.
10. Bergmann MW: Wnt signaling in adult cardiac hypertrophy and remodeling; lessons learned from cardiac development. *Circ Res* 107:1198–1208, 2010.
11. Tzahor E, Lassar AB: Wnt signals from the neural tube block ectopic cardiogenesis. *Genes Dev* 15:255–260, 2001.
12. Schneider VA, Mercola M: Wnt antagonism initiates cardiogenesis in *Xenopus laevis*. *Genes Dev* 15:304–315, 2001.
13. Marvin MJ, Di Rocco G, Gardiner A, et al: Inhibition of Wnt activity induces heart formation from posterior mesoderm. *Genes Dev* 15:316–327, 2001.
14. Stalsberg H, DeHaan RL: The precardiac areas and formation of the tubular heart in the chick embryo. *Dev Biol* 19:128–159, 1969.
15. DeHaan RL, Ursprung H: Morphogenesis of the vertebrate heart. In DeHaan RL, Ursprung H, editors: *Organogenesis*, Austin, Tx, 1965, Holt, Rinehart, Winston, pp 377–419.
16. Van Mierop LHS: Location of pacemaker in chick embryo heart at the time of initiation of heartbeat. *Am J Physiol* 212:407–415, 1996.
17. Inagaki T, Garcia-Martinez V, Schoenwolf GC: Regulative ability of the prospective cardiogenic and vasculogenic area of the primitive streak during avian gastrulation. *Dev Dyn* 197:57–68, 1993.
18. Tam PP, Parameswaran M, Kinder SJ, et al: The allocation of epiblast cells to the embryonic heart and other mesodermal lineages: the role of ingression and tissue movement during gastrulation. *Development* 124:1631–1642, 1997.
19. Cohen-Gould L, Mikawa T: The fate diversity of mesodermal cells within the chicken heart field during early embryogenesis. *Dev Biol* 177:265–273, 1996.
20. Kelly RG, Brown NA, Buckingham ME: The arterial pole of the mouse heart forms from Fgf10-expressing cells in pharyngeal mesoderm. *Dev Cell* 1:435–440, 2001.
21. Mjaatvedt CH, Nakaoka TH, Moreno-Rodriguez R, et al: The outflow tract of the heart is recruited from a novel heart-forming field. *Dev Biol* 238:97–109, 2001.
22. Waldo KL, Kumiski DH, Wallis KT, et al: Conotruncal myocardium arises from a secondary heart field. *Development* 128:3179–3188, 2001.
23. Patten BM: Formation of the cardiac loop in the chick. *Am J Anat* 30:373–397, 1922.
24. DeHaan RL: Regional organisation of prepacemaker cells in the cardiac primordia of the early chick embryo. *J Embryol Ex Morphol* 11:65–76, 1963.
25. Rosenquist GC, DeHaan RL: Migration of precardiac cells in the chick embryo: a radioautographic study. *Carnegie Inst Wash Contrib Embryol* 38:111–121, 1996.
26. Christoffels VM, Habets PE, Franco D, et al: Chamber formation and morphogenesis in the developing human heart. *Dev Biol* 223:266–278, 2000.
27. Redkar A, Montgomery M, Litvin J: Fate map of early avian cardiac progenitor cells. *Development* 128:2269–2279, 2001.
28. Kelly R, Buckingham M: The anterior heart-forming field: voyage to the arterial pole of the heart. *Trends Genet* 18:210–216, 2002.
29. Nonaka S, Tanaka Y, Okada Y, et al: Randomization of left right asymmetry due to loss of nodal cilia generating leftward flow of extra embryonic fluid in mice lacking KIF3B motor protein [published erratum appears in Cell 1999;99(1):117. *Cell* 95:829–837, 1998.
30. Okada Y, Nonaka S, Tanaka Y, et al: Abnormal nodal flow precedes situs inversus in iv and inv mice. *Mol Cell* 4:459–468, 1999.
31. Takeda S, Yonekawa Y, Tanaka Y, et al: Left-right asymmetry and kinesin superfamily protein KIF3A: new insights in determination of laterality and mesoderm induction by kif3a-/- mice analysis. *J Cell Biol* 145:825–836, 1999.
32. Tabin CJ, Vogan KJ: A two-cilia model for vertebrate left-right axis specification. *Genes Dev* 17:1–6, 2003.
33. Levin M, Johnson RL, Stern CD, et al: A molecular pathway determining let-right asymmetry in chick embryogenesis. *Cell* 82:803–814, 1995.
34. Pagan-Westphal SM, Tabin CJ: The transfer of left-right positional information during chick embryogenesis. *Cell* 93:25–35, 1998.
35. Rodriguez-Esteban C, Capdevila J, Economides AN, et al: The novel Cer-like protein Caronte mediates the establishment of embryonic left-right asymmetry [see comments]. *Nature* 401:243–251, 1999.
36. Yokouchi Y, Vogan KJ, Pearse RV, 2nd, et al: Antagonistic signaling by Caronte, a novel Cerberus gene, establishes left-right asymmetric gene expression. *Cell* 98:573–583, 1999.
37. Zhu L, Marvin MJ, Gardiner A, et al: Cerberus regulates left-right asymmetry of the embryonic head and heart. *Curr Biol* 9:931–938, 1999.
38. Logan M, Pagan-Westphal SM, Smith DM, et al: The transcription factor Pitx2 mediates situs-specific morphogenesis in response to left-right asymmetric signals. *Cell* 94:307–317, 1998.
39. Piedra ME, Icardo JM, Albajar M, et al: Pitx2 participates in the late phase of the pathway controlling left-right asymmetry. *Cell* 94:319–324, 1998.
40. Ryan AK, Blumberg B, Rodriguez-Esteban C, et al: Pitx2 determines left-right asymmetry of internal organs in vertebrates. *Nature* 394:545–551, 1998.
41. Yoshioka H, Meno C, Koshiba K, et al: Pitx2, a bicoid-type homeobox gene, is involved in a lefty signaling pathway in determination of left-right asymmetry. *Cell* 94:299–305, 1998.
42. Campione M, Steinbeisser H, Schweickert A, et al: The homeobox gene Pitx2: mediator of asymmetric left-right signaling in vertebrate heart and gut looping. *Development* 126:1225–1234, 1999.
43. Meno C, Saijoh Y, Fujii H, et al: Left-right asymmetric expression of the TGF beta-family member lefty in mouse embryos. *Nature* 381:151–155, 1996.
44. Collignon J, Varlet I, Robertson EJ: Relationship between asymmetric nodal expression and the direction of embryonic turning. *Nature* 381:155–158, 1996.
45. Essner JJ, Branford WW, Zhang J, et al: Mesendoderm and left-right brain, heart and gut development are differentially regulated by Pitx2 isoforms. *Development* 127:1081–1093, 2000.
46. Schweickert A, Campione M, Steinbeisser H, et al: Pitx2 isoforms: involvement of Pitx2c or Pitx2b in vertebrate left-right asymmetry. *Mech Dev* 90:41–51, 2000.
47. Kosaki R, Gebbia M, Kosaki K, et al: Left-right axis malformations associated with mutations in ACVR2B, the gene for human activin receptor type IIB. *Am J Med Genet* 82:70–76, 1999.
48. Supp DM, Witte DP, Potter SS, et al: Mutation of an axonemal dynein affects left-right asymmetry in inversus viscerum mice. *Nature* 389:963–966, 1997.
49. Supp DM, Brueckner M, Kuehn MR, et al: Targeted deletion of the ATP binding domain of left-right dynein confirms its role in specifying development of left right asymmetries. *Development* 126:5495–5504, 1999.
50. Lowe LA, Supp DM, Sampath K, et al: Conserved left-right asymmetry of nodal expression and alterations in murine situs inversus. *Nature* 381:158–161, 1996.
51. Van Praagh S, Kakou-Guikahue M, Kim H-S, et al: Atrial situs in patients with visceral heterotaxy and congenital heart disease:

conclusions based on findings in 104 postmortem cases. *Coeur* 19:483–502, 1988.
52. Tan SY, Rosenthal J, Zhao XQ, et al: Heterotaxy and complex structural heart defects in a mutant mouse model of primary ciliary dyskinesis. *J Clin Invest* 117:3742–3752, 2007.
53. Nakhleh N, Francis R, Giese RA, et al: High prevalence of respiratory ciliary dysfunction in CHD patients with heterotaxy. *Circulation* 125:2232–2242, 2012.
54. Lilly B, Zhao B, Ranganayakulu G, et al: Requirement of the MADS domain transcription factor D-MEF2 for muscle formation in Drosophila. *Science* 267:688–693, 1995.
55. Bour BA, O'Brien MA, Lockwood WL, et al: Drosophila MEF2, a transcription factor that is essential for myogenesis. *Genes Dev* 9:730–741, 1995.
56. Gajewski K, Kim Y, Lee YM, et al: D-Mef2 is a target for tinman activation during Drosophila heart development. *EMBO J* 16:515–522, 1997.
57. Gajewski K, Zhang Q, Choi CY, et al: Pannier is a transcriptional target and partner of Tinman during *Drosophila* cardiogenesis. *Dev Biol* 233:425–436, 2001.
58. Lints T, Parsons L, Hartley L, et al: Nkx-2.5: a novel murine homeobox gene expressed in early heart progenitor cells and their myogenic descendants. *Development* 119:419–431, 1993.
59. Koromuro I, Izumo S: Csx: A murine homeobox-containing gene specifically expressed in the developing heart. *Proc Natl Acad Sci USA* 90:8145–8149, 1993.
60. Liberatore CM, Searcy-Schrick RD, Vincent EB, et al: Nkx-2.5 induction in mice is mediated by a Smad consensus regulatory region. *Dev Biol* 244:243–256, 2002.
61. Cripps RM, Olson EN: Control of cardiac development by an evolutionarily conserved transcriptional network. *Dev Biol* 246:14–28, 2002.
62. Durochet D, Charron F, Warren R, et al: The cardiac transcription factors Nkx2.5 and GATA-4 are mutual cofactors. *EMBO J* 16:5687–5696, 1997.
63. Lee Y, Shioi T, Kasahara H, et al: The cardiac restricted homeobox protein Csx/Nkx2.5 physically associates with the zinc finger GATA4 and cooperatively activates atrial natriuretic factor gene expression. *Mol Cell Biol* 18:3120–3129, 1998.
64. Sepulveda JL, Belaguli N, Nigam V, et al: GATA-4 and Nkx-2.5 coactivate Nkx-2 DNA binding targets: role for regulating early cardiac gene expression. *Mol Cell Biol* 18:3405–3415, 1998.
65. Lin Q, Schwarz J, Bucana C, et al: Control of mouse cardiac morphogenesis and myogenesis by transcription factor MEF2C. *Science* 276:1404–1407, 1997.
66. Lin Q, Lu J, Yanagisawa H, et al: Requirement of the MADS-box transcription factor MEF2C for vascular development. *Development* 125:4565–4574, 1998.
67. Durochet D, Chen C-Y, Ardati A, et al: The atrial Natriuretic factor promoter is a downstream target for Nkx2.5 in the myocardium. *Mol Cell Biol* 16:4648–4655, 1996.
68. Bruneau BG, Nemer G, Schmitt JP, et al: A murine model of the Holt-Oram syndrome defines roles of the T-box transcription factor Tbx5 in cardiogenesis and disease. *Cell* 106:709–721, 2001.
69. Bao ZZ, Bruneu BG, Seidman JG, et al: Regulation of chamber specific gene expression in the developing heart by Irx4. *Science* 283:1161–1164, 1999.
70. Chen CY, Schwartz RJ: Recruitment of the *tinman* homolog Nkx-2.5 by serum response factor activates cardiac alpha-actin gene transcription. *Mol Cell Biol* 16:6372–6384, 1996.
71. Stainier DY, Fouquet B, Chen JN, et al: Mutations affecting the formation and function of the cardiovascular in the zebrafish embryo. *Development (Cambridge, UK)* 123:285–292, 1996.
72. Srivastava D, Cserjesi P, Olson EN: A subclass of bHLH proteins required for cardiac morphogenesis. *Science* 270:1995–1999, 1995.
73. Srivastava D, Thomas T, Lin Q, et al: Regulation of cardiac mesodermal and neural crest development by the bHLH transcription factor, dHAND. *Nat Genet* 16:154–160, 1997.
74. Wessels A, Anderson RH, Markwald RR, et al: Atrial development in the human heart: an immunohistochemical study with emphasis on the role of mesenchymal tissues. *Anat Rec* 259(3):288–300, 2000.
75. Kim JS, Viragh S, Moorman AFM, et al: Development of the myocardium of the atrioventricular canal and vestibular spine in the human heart. *Circ Res* 88:395–402, 2001.
76. Lamers WH, Moorman AFM: Cardiac septation: a late contribution of the embryonic primary myocardium to heart morphogenesis. *Circ Res* 91:93–103, 2002.
77. Lamers WH, Wessels A, Verbeek FJ, et al: New findings concerning ventricular septation in the human heart. *Circulation* 86:1194–1205, 1992.
78. Sedmera D, Pexieder T, Vuillemin M, et al: Developmental patterning of the myocardium. *Anat Rec* 258(4):319–337, 2000.
79. Rongish BJ, Drake CJ, Argraves WS, et al: Identification of a developmental marker, the JB3-antigen, as fibrillin-2 and its de novo organization into embryonic microfibrous arrays. *Dev Dyn* 212:461–471, 1998.
80. Mjaatvedt CH, Yamamura H, Wessels A, et al: Mechanisms of segmentation, septation, and remodeling of the tubular heart: endocardial cushion fate and cardiac looping. In Harvey RP, Rosenthal N, editors: *Heart development*, San Diego, 1999, Academic Press.
81. Eisenberg LM, Markwald RR: Molecular regulation of atrioventricular valvuloseptal morphogenesis. *Circ Res* 77(1):1–6, 1995.
82. Abdelwahid E, Rice D, Pelliniemi LJ, et al: Overlapping and differential localization of Bmp-2, Bmp-4, Msx-2 and apoptosis in the endocardial cushion and adjacent tissues of the developing mouse heart. *Cell Tissue Res* 305:67–78, 2001.
83. Srivastava D, Baldwin HS: Molecular determinants of cardiac development. In Allen HD, Gutgesell HP, Clark EB, et al, editors: *Moss and Adams' heart disease in infants children and adolescents including the fetus and young adult*, Philadelphia, 2001, Lippincott Williams and Wilkins.
84. Van den Hoff MJB, Moorman AFM, Ruijter JM, et al: Myocardialization of the cardiac outflow tract. *Dev Biol* 212:477–490, 1999.
85. Gaussin V, Van de Putte T, Mishina Y, et al: Endocardial cushion and myocardial defects after cardiac myocyte-specific conditional deletion of the bone morphogenetic protein receptor ALK3. *Proc Natl Acad Sci U S A* 99(5):2878–2883, 2002.
86. Ferencz C, Loffredo CA, Correa-Villasenor A, et al: *Genetic and environmental risk factors of major cardiovascular malformations: the Baltimore-Washington Infant Study 1981–1989*, Armonk, NY, 1997, Futura, pp 103–122.
87. Vaughan CJ, Basson CT: Molecular determinants of atrial and ventricular septal defects and patent ductus arteriosus. *Am J Med Genet* 97:304–309, 2000.
88. Pierpont MEM, Markwald RR, Lin AE: Genetic aspects of atrioventricular septal defects. *Am J Med Genet* 97:289–296, 2000.
89. Basson CT, Bachinsky DR, Lin RC, et al: Mutations in human TBX5 [corrected] cause limb and cardiac malformation in Holt-Oram syndrome. *Nat Genet* 15(1):30–35, 1997.
90. Li QY, Newbury-Ecob RA, Terrett JA, et al: Holt-Oram syndrome is caused by mutations in TBX5, a member of the Brachyury (T) gene family. *Nat Genet* 15(1):21–29, 1997.
91. Schott JJ, Benson DW, Basson CT, et al: Congenital heart disease caused by mutations in the transcription factor NKX2-5. *Science* 281(5373):108–111, 1998.
92. Benson DW, Silberbach GM, Kavanaugh-McHugh A, et al: Mutations in the cardiac transcription factor NKX2.5 affect diverse cardiac developmental pathways. *J Clin Invest* 104(11):1567–1573, 1999.
93. Garg V, Kathiriya IS, Barnes R, et al: GATA4 mutations cause human congenital heart defects and reveal an interaction with TBX5. *Nature* 424(6947):443–447, 2003.
94. Kirby ML: Contribution of neural crest to heart and vessel morphology. In Harvey RP, Rosenthal N, editors: *Heart development*, San Diego, 1999, Academic Press.
95. Viragh S, Challice CE: Origin and differentiation of cardiac muscle cells in the mouse. *J Ultrastruct Res* 42:1–24, 1973.
96. De la Cruz MV, Gomez CS, Arteaga MM, et al: Experimental study of the development of the truncus and the conus in the chick embryo. *J Anat* 123:661–686, 1977.
97. Dees E, Baldwin HS: New frontiers in molecular pediatric cardiology. *Curr Opin Pediatr* 14:627–633, 2002.
98. Kirby ML, Waldo KL: Neural crest and cardiovascular patterning. *Circ Res* 77(2):211–215, 1995.
99. Kirby ML, Turnage KL, Hays BM: Characterization of conotruncal malformations following ablation of "cardiac" neural crest. *Anat Rec* 213:87–93, 1985.

100. Waldo KL, Kumiski DH, Kirby ML: Cardiac neural crest is essential for the persistence rather than the formation of an arch artery. *Dev Dyn* 205(3):281–292, 1996.
101. Kirby ML, Hunt P, Wallis K, et al: Abnormal patterning of the aortic arch arteries does not evoke cardiac malformations. *Dev Dyn* 208:34–47, 1997.
102. Kirby ML, Gale TF, Stewart DE: Neural crest cells contribute to aorticopulmonary septation. *Science* 220:1059–1061, 1983.
103. Nishibatake M, Kirby ML, Van Mierop LHS: Pathogenesis of persistent truncus arteriosus and dextroposed aorta in the chick embryo after neural crest ablation. *Circulation* 75:255–264, 1987.
104. Tomita H, Connuck DM, Leatherbury L, et al: Relation of early hemodynamic changes to final cardiac phenotype and survival after neural crest ablation in chick embryos. *Circulation* 84:1289–1295, 1991.
105. Manner J, Seidl W, Steding G: Experimental study on the significance if abnormal cardiac looping for the development of cardiovascular abnormalities in neural crest ablated chick embryos. *Anat Embryol* 194:289–300, 1996.
106. Conway SJ, Henderson DJ, Copp AJ: Pax3 is required for cardiac neural crest migration in the mouse: evidence from the splotch mutant. *Development (Cambridge, UK)* 124:505–514, 1997.
107. Maschoff KL, Baldwin HS: Molecular determinants of neural crest migration. *Am J Med Genet* 97:280–288, 2000.
107a. Soriano P: The PDGF alpha receptor is required for neural crest cell development and for normal patterning of the somites. *Development* 124:2691–2700, 1997.
108. Wilson JG, Roth JB, Warkany J: An analysis of the syndrome of malformations induced by vitamin A deficiency: effects of restoration of vitamin A at various times during gestation. *Am J Anat* 92:189–217, 1953.
109. Wilson DI, Burn J, Scambler P, et al: DiGeorge syndrome, part of CATCH22. *J Med Genet* 30:852–856, 1993.
110. Burn J: Closing time for CATCH22. *J Med Genet* 36:737–738, 1999.
111. Burn J, Goodship J: Congenital heart disease. In Rimoin DL, Conner JM, Pyeritz RE, et al, editors: *Emery and Rimion's principles and practice of medical genetics*, London, 1996, Churchill Livingstone.
112. Jerome LA, Papaioannou VE: DiGeorge syndrome phenotype in mice mutant for the T-box gene Tbx1. *Nat Genet* 27:286–291, 2001.
113. Lindsay EA, Vitelli F, Su H, et al: Tbx1 haploinsufficiency in the DiGeorge syndrome region causes aortic arch defects in mice. *Nature* 410:97–101, 2001.
114. Merscher S, Funke B, Epstein JA, et al: Tbx1 is responsible for cardiovascular defects in velo-cardial-facial/DiGeorge syndrome. *Cell* 104:619–629, 2001.
115. DeAlmeida A, McQuinn T, Sedmera D: Increased ventricular preload is compensated by myocyte proliferation in normal and hypoplastic fetal chick left ventricle. *Circ Res* 100(9):1363–1370, 2007.
116. Makikallio K, McElhinney DB, Levine JC, et al: Fetal aortic valve stenosis and the evolution of hypoplastic left heart syndrome: patient selection for fetal intervention. *Circulation* 113(11):1401–1405, 2006.
117. Jenkins KJ, Correa A, Feinstein JA, et al: Noninherited risk factors and congenital cardiovascular defects: current knowledge. *Circulation* 115:2995–3014, 2007.
118. Hinton RB, Jr, Martin LJ, Tabangin ME, et al: Hypoplastic left heart syndrome is heritable. *J Am Coll Cardiol* 50(16):1590–1595, 2007.
119. Kuehl KS, Loffredo CA: A cluster of hypoplastic left heart malformation in Baltimore, Maryland. *Pediatr Cardiol* 27:25–31, 2006.
120. Fahed AC, Gelb BD, Seidman JG, et al: Genetics of congenital heart disease: the glass half empty. *Circ Res* 112:707–720, 2013.

CHAPTER 105

SEGMENTAL ANATOMY

Stephen P. Sanders

CHAPTER OUTLINE

The heart is a complex organ. It is difficult to understand the anatomy of the heart, particularly when abnormal, and it is even more difficult to describe it clearly and succinctly. Yet this is the goal of the diagnostician cardiologist: to understand and describe the anatomy of a defective heart in a way that colleagues will comprehend sufficiently to be able to contribute meaningfully to the care of the patient. Another objective is to learn about the behavior of the various defects: occurrence rate, natural history, response to treatment, and long-term prospects. Finally, discovery of the causes and developmental mechanisms of heart defects is of great interest. These objectives require a system of analysis and naming that facilitates data gathering and communication of information.

The system of nomenclature should have certain characteristics if it is to be useful. First, the name should be descriptive and convey a picture of the defect. Who can remember the meaning of type 1B? On the other hand, tricuspid atresia with normally related great arteries and pulmonary stenosis is clear. Second, names should be unambiguous. Each name should refer to only one defect. It is less of a problem for a defect to have more than one name, as long as they map only to the same defect. For example, it makes little difference whether one uses the terms *membranous*, *perimembranous*, or *paramembranous ventricular septal defect*. They all refer to, and can be mapped to, the same type of ventricular septal defect. A problem arises if one calls a membranous defect *muscular* or *subpulmonary*, because these names refer to other types of defects as well. This would be hopelessly confusing because one name could refer to multiple types of defects. Third, the system of names should be inclusive. There should be a name for all defects, even rare ones. A large "other" category makes it hard to find rare defects, which can be highly informative regarding cause or developmental mechanism. Finally, the system must be capable of evolution and growth while remaining consistent.

The language used to describe the heart is an integral part of the analysis process. An effective way to discuss the language of the heart is to describe a process for analyzing the heart. This process is called the "segmental approach to cardiac analysis and diagnosis."[1-3] Why a segmental approach? The task of elucidating cardiac anatomy is made simpler by analyzing the cardiac segments separately and then constructing a synthesis or comprehensive diagnosis.

The heart is one of many organs in the abdomen and thorax. Analysis of the organization of these other organs provides a context for understanding and describing heart defects.

VISCERAL SITUS

The external bilateral symmetry of the human body hides the asymmetry of most internal organs. In the usual arrangement, called *situs solitus*, the left lung is bilobed and somewhat smaller than the trilobed right lung; this is apparent from the branching pattern of the bronchi. The abdomen contains several unpaired and lateralized organs, including the right-sided liver and gall bladder and the left-sided spleen and stomach. The normal rotation of the intestine places the caecum and appendix in the right lower quadrant and the sigmoid colon on the left. Rare individuals have inverted or mirror-image organization of the thoracic and abdominal viscera called *situs inversus*, which is inversion of the usual arrangement or situs solitus. In anatomy, inversion means left-right mirror imagery with no superior-inferior (cranial-caudal) or anterior-posterior (ventral-dorsal) change.

Laterality information is transmitted to the lateral plate mesoderm, the source of the viscera including the heart, around the time of gastrulation by the action of cilia in the node at the cranial end of the primitive streak.[4] A cascade of transcription factors culminating in expression of Pitx2 induces left-sided features in derivatives of the left lateral plate. Apparently, the absence of these factors leads to right-sided features in right lateral plate derivatives. The atria are lateralized structures whose development is strongly influenced by the left-right gene regulatory networks (the left atrium, pulmonary vein, and atrial septal structures express Pitx2c, but right atrial structures do not[5]). Consequently, visceral and atrial situs are closely linked. In fact, the linkage is so tight that the term *visceroatrial situs* is often used to describe both at once.

The relationship between visceral situs and ventricular and outflow development is a little less strong. It is unknown how gene regulatory networks influence ventricular looping and development of the outflow and aortic sac derivatives.

Heterotaxy syndromes, abnormal symmetry and placement of usually asymmetrical and lateralized organs, result from defective or failed establishment of the left-right body axis. Abnormal atrial development is almost uniform in these conditions, whereas defective ventricular and outflow development is frequent but more variable. Heterotaxy syndromes are characterized by variability and unpredictability, although patterns of visceral and cardiac anatomy can be recognized. The concepts of "bilateral left sidedness" and "bilateral right sidedness" are useful mnemonic devices to help recall associations, but they should not be taken too seriously. These concepts probably apply best to the airways and lungs; symmetrical bronchi and lung lobation are frequently encountered (Fig. 105-1). The liver lobation is often symmetrical, but duplication of the gall bladder rarely occurs. The spleen might be absent or multiple, but never duplicated on opposite sides of the abdomen. Similarly, the asplenia and polysplenia syndromes are often associated with particular combinations of findings, but the watchword is variability.

LOCATION OF THE HEART

The heart can be in the left chest with the apex to the left (levocardia), in the right chest with the apex to the right (dextrocardia), or in the midline with the apex down (mesocardia; Fig. 105-2). In some cases, the heart is partially or completely outside the chest (partial or complete ectopia cordis). It can be located partially or completely outside the body through a cleft in the sternum, predominantly in the abdomen, or even the neck. If the right lung is hypoplastic, or if there is a space occupying lesion in the left chest, the heart is often positioned in the right chest, but the apex points to the left or inferiorly (Fig. 105-3). This has been called *dextroposition* or *secondary dextrocardia*, as opposed to primary dextrocardia with a rightward apex. The implications of dextroposition differ from those of dextrocardia both for imaging the

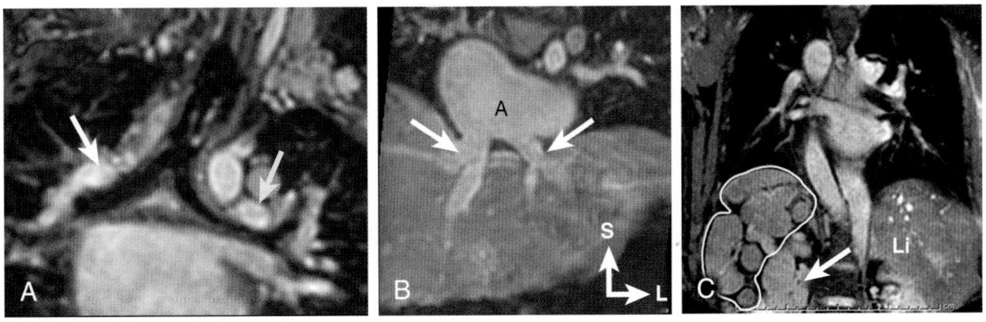

FIGURE 105-1 ■ Coronal magnetic resonance images in patients with heterotaxy syndrome. **A,** Symmetrical hyparterial bronchi, both of left-sided morphology (long bronchi with the first branch some distance from the carina), in a patient with polysplenia syndrome. The right *(white arrow)* and left *(yellow arrow)* pulmonary arteries are above the ipsilateral bronchus. **B,** Symmetrical hepatic veins *(arrows)* draining separately into the common atrium (A) in the same patient with polysplenia. (Directional marker applies to all three images.) **C,** Multiple spleens *(white outline)* on the right side of the abdomen in a patient with right-sided polysplenia. In our autopsy series, right polysplenia is slightly more frequent than left polysplenia. The right kidney *(white arrow)* is seen medial and inferior to the spleens. The liver (Li) is left-sided. *L,* Left; *S,* superior.

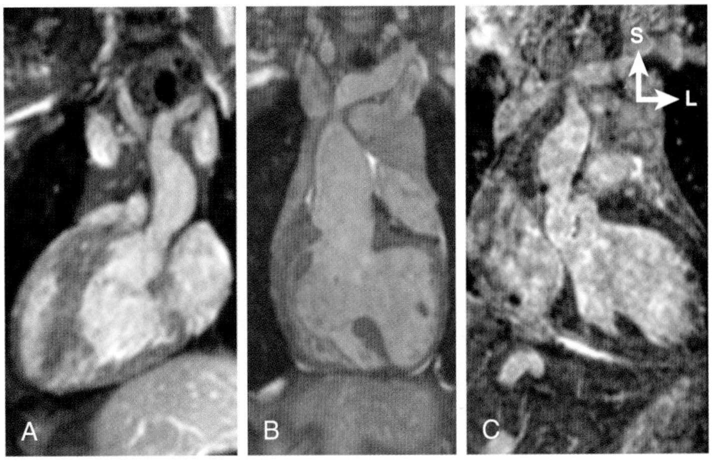

FIGURE 105-2 ■ Magnetic resonance images obtained using a steady-state free precession sequence reformatted in coronal plane showing: **A,** Dextrocardia with the apex of the heart to the right. **B,** Mesocardia with the apices of the ventricles directed inferiorly. **C,** Levocardia with the apex of the heart to the left. Directional marker applies to all three images. *L,* Left; *S,* superior.

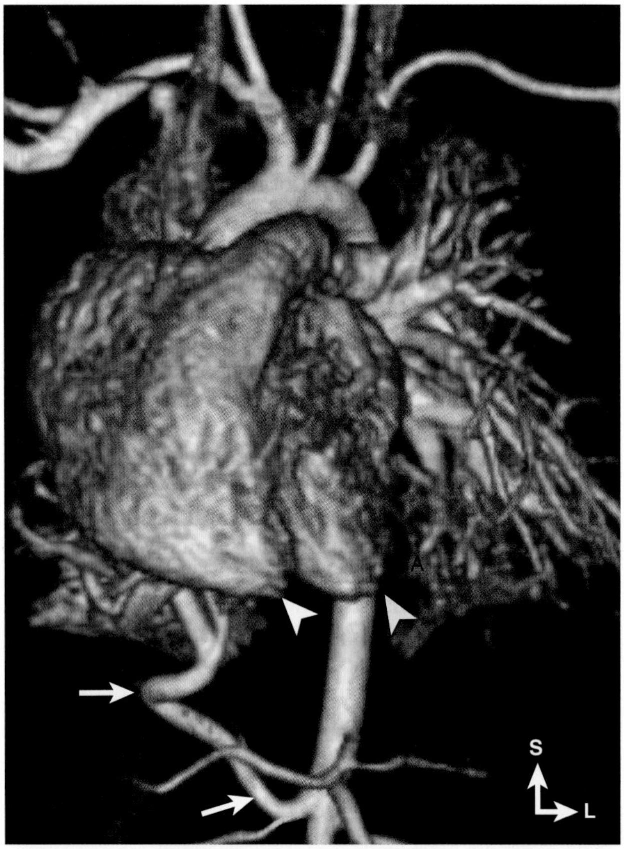

FIGURE 105-3 ■ A frontal view of a three-dimensional volumetric reconstruction of a magnetic resonance angiogram in a patient with scimitar syndrome. A portion of the hypoplastic right lung is seen below the heart, which is displaced into the right chest exposing virtually all the left lung. The apices of the right *(white arrowhead)* and left *(yellow arrowhead)* ventricles point left and inferior, indicating a nearly normal orientation of the heart. A sequestration artery *(arrows)* originates from the descending aorta and enters the base of the right lung. *L,* Left; *S,* superior.

heart and for associated diagnoses. Dextroposition or secondary dextrocardia is associated with scimitar syndrome, right lung hypoplasia, and noncardiac diagnoses such as diaphragmatic hernia. The orientation of the heart is often similar to normal, simply moved into the right chest. Consequently, imaging planes are similar to those used in levocardia but centered over the right chest. Dextrocardia and mesocardia are associated with heterotaxy syndrome and congenitally corrected transposition. The defects tend to be more complex and very different imaging planes are usually required to display the anatomy.

SEGMENTAL ANALYSIS

Once the general location of the heart is determined, one can proceed with the segmental analysis.[1,3] The heart is composed of three main segments: the atria, the ventricles, and the great arteries (Fig. 105-4). These main segments are joined—like bricks with mortar—by two connecting segments: the atrioventricular canal between

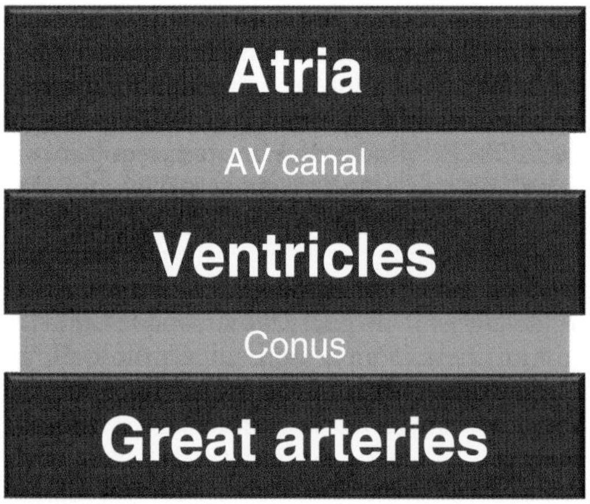

FIGURE 105-4 ■ The heart is composed of three main segments (the atria, ventricles, and great arteries) joined by two connecting segments (the atrioventricular [AV] canal and conus or infundibulum). The three main segments are not directly connected to each other. If they were, the spectrum of congenital heart defects might be more limited. The atria and ventricles are joined by the AV canal, which provides the AV valves, the membranous septum, and much of the fibrous insulating material that separates atrial and ventricular muscle (except at the AV penetrating bundle). The ventricles are joined to the great arteries by the conus or infundibulum. This connecting segment, derived from the primitive outflow, undergoes initial elongation, rotation, and subsequent shortening that usually results in normally related great arteries. If abnormal, it can be associated with one of the various anomalies of ventriculoarterial alignment and connection.

the atria and ventricles, and the conus or infundibulum between the ventricles and great arteries. The three main segments, although independent and relatively autonomous, develop harmoniously the great majority of the time. The location or situs and the internal organization of the segments are strongly correlated, but each segment can vary independently of the others.

Segmental Situs

First, the situs (location) and organization of each main segment is determined.[6] The atrial situs is either solitus or usual, inversus or the mirror image of usual, or ambiguus where the identities of the atria are unclear or ill defined. The right atrium is right-sided and the left atrium left-sided in situs solitus. In situs inversus the right atrium is left-sided and the left atrium is right-sided with opposite right-left organization (Fig. 105-5). However, the anterior-posterior and superior-inferior organization is unchanged. Consequently, the superior vena cava arises from the superior aspect of the right atrium posterior to the atrial appendage and the inferior vena cava from the inferior aspect in both cases. *Situs ambiguus* is used to describe the heterotaxy syndromes (e.g., asplenia, polysplenia syndromes), which are also called *atrial appendage isomerism syndromes*. (It should be noted that these are not identical populations or concepts.)

Criteria for identifying the right atrium (Fig. 105-6), in an approximate order of reliability, include: (1) receives the coronary sinus, (2) has pectinate muscles extending to the vestibule of the atrioventricular valve, (3) receives

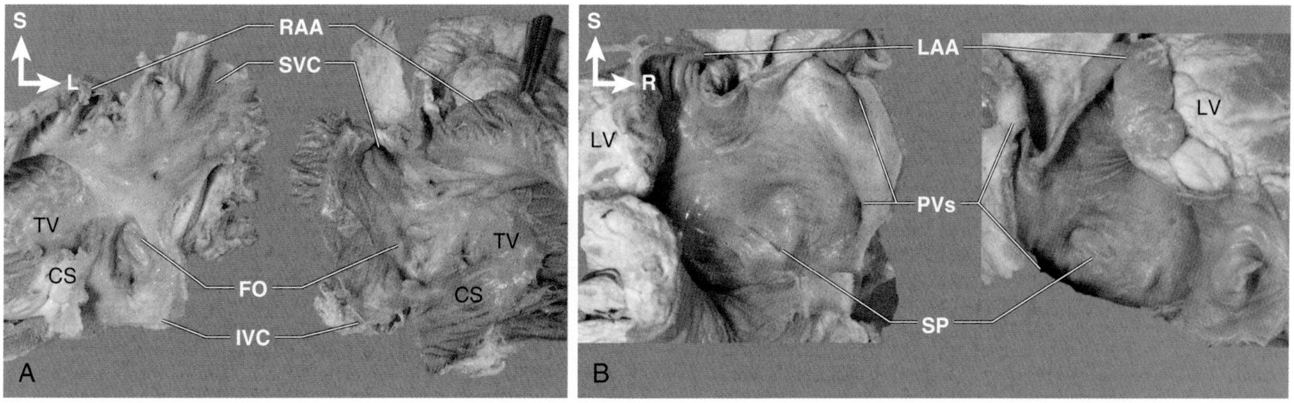

FIGURE 105-5 ■ **A,** The opened right atria of two hearts, one in situs solitus *(right)* and one in situs inversus *(left)*. The atria are mirror images: there is left-right inversion but no superior-inferior or anterior-posterior change. Using the fossa ovalis (FO) as a reference point, the superior vena cava (SVC) is directed superior and rightward in situs solitus but superior and leftward in situs inversus. The coronary sinus (CS) is leftward and inferior in situs solitus but rightward and inferior in situs inversus, and the tricuspid valve (TV) is to the left in situs solitus but to the right in situs inversus. In both cases the inferior vena cava (IVC) is inferior to the fossa, and the right atrial appendage (RAA) is anterior to the superior vena cava (imagine closing the atrium by folding the right atrial appendage in front of the plane of the image). **B,** The opened left atria of the same two hearts placed back-to-back but with the situs solitus heart to the left and the situs inversus heart to the right (opposite placement to panel **A**) for clarity of labeling. Note the mirror image organization of the atria. The pulmonary veins (PVs) adjacent to the atrial septum are posterior to septum primum (SP) in both cases, but rightward in situs solitus *(left)* and leftward in situs inversus *(right)*. The left atrial appendage (LAA) is superior to septum primum, but it points anterior and leftward in the situs solitus heart *(left)* but anterior and rightward in the situs inversus heart *(right)*. *L,* Left; *LV,* left ventricle; *R,* right; *S,* superior.

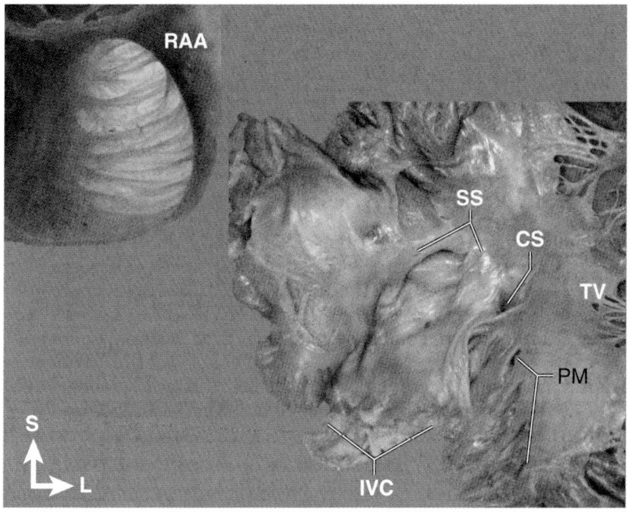

FIGURE 105-6 ■ The opened right atrium *(lower right)* and a section from a waxed, distended heart specimen *(upper left)* illustrate the characteristic right atrial features: coronary sinus (CS), pectinate muscles (PM) extending around the vestibule of the tricuspid valve (TV), inferior vena cava (IVC), septum secundum (SS) or superior limbic band on the septal surface, and large triangular appendage (RAA) with broad communication with the body of the atrium. *L,* Left; *S,* superior.

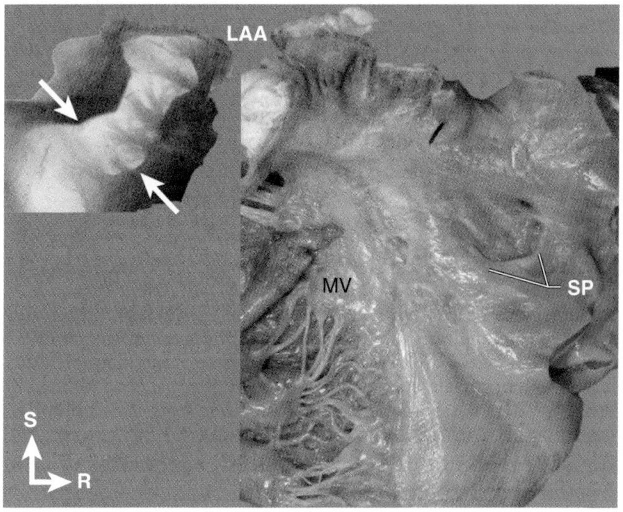

FIGURE 105-7 ■ The opened left atrium *(lower right)* and a section from a waxed, distended heart *(upper left)* illustrate the characteristic left atrial features: smooth walls with the pectinate muscles confined to the left atrial appendage (LAA), septum primum (SP) or primary atrial septum on the septal surface, and a small, finger-like appendage with a narrow junction *(arrows)* with the body of the atrium. *MV,* Mitral valve; *R,* right; *S,* superior.

the inferior vena cava, (4) has septum secundum on the septal surface, and (5) has a large, triangular appendage with a broad orifice communicating with the atrium. If the coronary sinus is present, it is an extremely reliable marker because it develops from the sinus horn contralateral to the one that forms part of the right atrium. Unfortunately, it is often absent (or unroofed) in heterotaxy syndromes, where most help is needed to identify the atria. The pectinate muscle morphology appears to be reliable as well but can be difficult to detect with current imaging technology. The inferior vena cava is a useful practical marker for the right atrium but it can also drain to the coronary sinus and is often interrupted in heterotaxy syndromes.

Criteria for the left atrium (Fig. 105-7) include (1) smooth walls with pectinate muscles confined to the atrial appendage, (2) septum primum on the septal surface, and (3) small, finger-like appendage. Practically, if one can identify the right atrium, the other atrial chamber is the left atrium. If one cannot clearly identify the right atrium, the

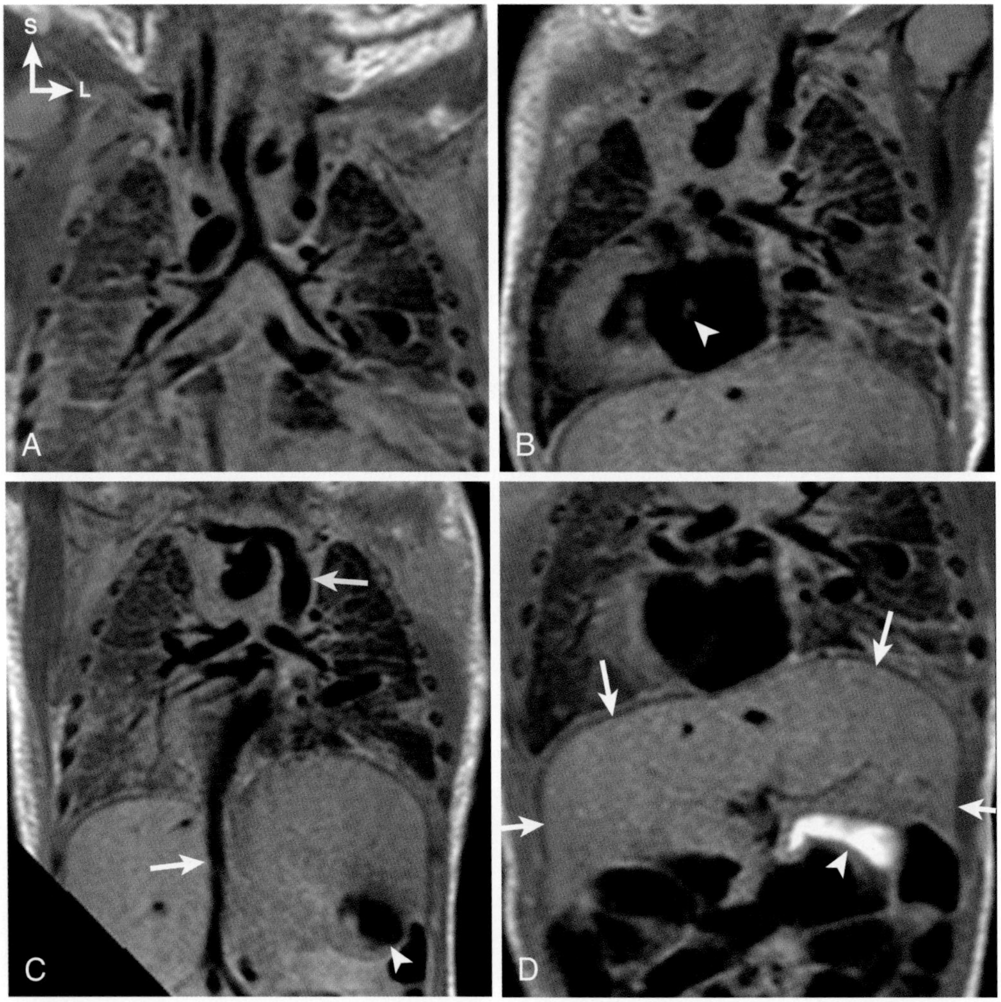

FIGURE 105-8 ■ A series of coronal sections of a black blood magnetic resonance sequence in an infant with a heterotaxy syndrome to illustrate the variability of organ symmetry and placement often seen in these syndromes. The directional indicator at the *upper left* applies to all images. **A,** Symmetrical bronchi of right-sided morphology (compare with Fig. 105-1*A*). The upper lobe bronchi arise a short distance after the carina on both sides in contrast to the long, unbranched bronchi seen in Figure 105-1*A*. **B,** Dextrocardia with near absence of atrial septum. Only a small strand of the atrial septum *(arrowhead)* remains. **C,** The inferior vena cava *(white arrow)* is right-sided, whereas the superior vena cava *(yellow arrow)* is left-sided. The stomach *(arrowhead)* is left-sided. **D,** Large, symmetrical liver *(arrows)* spans the upper abdomen. The gall bladder *(arrowhead)* is left-sided. *L,* Left; *S,* superior.

situs is likely ambiguous. The superior vena cava and pulmonary veins are not reliable markers of atrial identity.

In some hearts the atrial anatomy is difficult to discern. These are generally hearts with heterotaxy syndrome (see Figs. 105-1 and 105-8). The coronary sinus is usually absent or unroofed. The inferior vena cava often changes sides in the liver and hepatic veins enter the atrial floor separately. The atrial septum is poorly represented, with only a muscular strand of tissue remaining. The atria can exhibit similar pectinate muscle morphology, but the appendages are rarely similar in size and shape. In such cases, it is best to indicate that the atrial morphology is ambiguous and to describe the anatomy in detail.

The ventricular situs or loop is either solitus or d-loop, or inversus or l-loop. Rarely (most often in double-inlet right ventricle), it is impossible to determine the ventricular loop, which is then listed as unknown *(X)*.

The definition of the ventricular loop or situs is based on internal organization or chirality of the ventricles and not on their locations. *Left* and *right* should be considered as the names of the ventricles rather than an indication of location. Consequently, constructions such as *morphologically left ventricle* are superfluous. The analysis of chirality is most conveniently performed on the right ventricle because the inflow and outflow are separated by an angle of nearly 90 degrees, but it can be done on either ventricle. A d-loop or solitus right ventricle is organized with the inflow from the right and the outflow to the left as viewed from the free wall; an l-loop or inverted right ventricle is organized oppositely. A simple way to understand the organization of the ventricle is to imagine which hand can be used to describe the ventricle if the thumb represents the tricuspid valve, the fingers the outflow tract, and the palm is against the septal surface (Fig. 105-9*A*). Only the right hand works for a solitus or d-loop right ventricle. Only a left hand works for an inverted or l-loop right ventricle.

The left ventricle is organized oppositely (see Fig. 105-9*B*). The left hand describes a d-loop or solitus left ventricle and the right hand an inverted or l-loop left

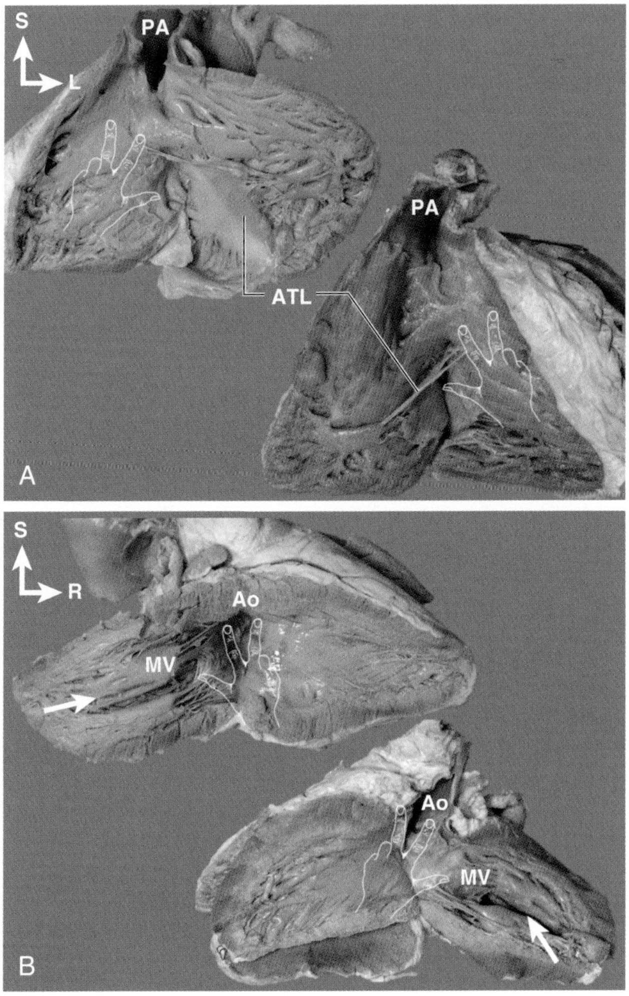

FIGURE 105-9 ■ **A,** The opened right ventricles of two hearts, one with solitus or d-loop ventricles *(lower right)* and one with inverted or l-loop ventricles *(left upper)*. The chirality or handedness of the two right ventricles is opposite, as illustrated by the hand required to describe the ventricle. A right hand describes the d-loop ventricle on the right, with the thumb in the tricuspid valve, the fingers in the outflow and the palm against the septum. The l-loop right ventricle is organized oppositely and requires a left hand to describe it. **B,** The opened left ventricles of two hearts, one with solitus or d-loop ventricles *(lower right)* and one with inverted or l-loop ventricles *(left upper)*. As for the right ventricles in the previous figure, the chirality or handedness of these left ventricles is opposite. A left hand, with the thumb in the mitral valve, the fingers in the outflow, and the palm against the septum, describes the d-loop left ventricle *(right)*, whereas a right hand is needed for the l-loop left ventricle *(left)*. Comparing this figure with the previous one shows that in both d-loop and l-loop ventricles, the left and right ventricles are organized oppositely: the d-loop right ventricle is right-handed while the d-loop left ventricle is left-handed; in l-loop ventricles the organization is opposite, the right ventricle is left-handed and the left ventricle is right-handed. *White arrow,* Papillary muscles on left ventricular free wall. *Ao,* Aorta; *ATL,* anterior tricuspid leaflet; *L,* left; *MV,* mitral valve; *PA,* pulmonary artery; *R,* right; *S,* superior.

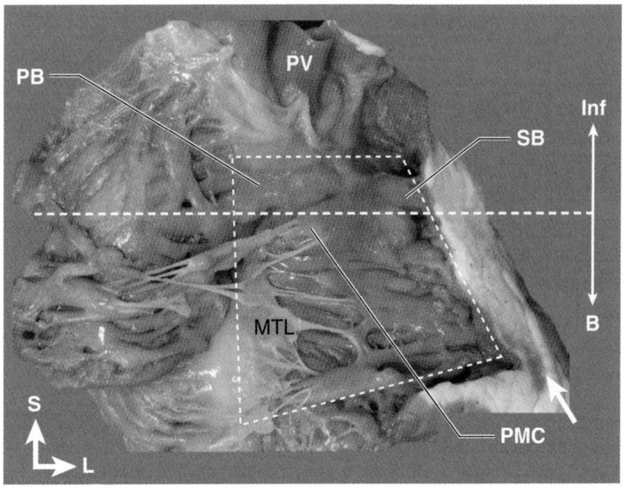

FIGURE 105-10 ■ Characteristic features of the right ventricle are illustrated in this opened specimen of a d-loop right ventricle: (1) trapezoidal shape bounded by the tricuspid annulus to the right, the diaphragmatic wall inferiorly, the apex and anterior wall to the left, and the pulmonary valve superiorly; (2) coarse trabeculations; (3) multiple attachments of the medial or septal tricuspid leaflet (MTL) to the septum; (4) division into an inflow or body (B) portion below the papillary muscle of the conus (PMC) and an outflow or infundibulum (Inf) above (the muscular crest marking the division between the two is composed of the septal band [SB], parietal band [PB], and moderator band [divided in this specimen]); and (5) discontinuity between the pulmonary valve (PV) and tricuspid valve because of intervening conal muscle (parietal band). *L,* Left; *S,* superior.

ventricle. The septal wall of the left ventricle is present and identifiable even when there is only an outflow chamber or infundibulum, and no right ventricle, present on the other side. Consequently, one can use the hand rule even in cases of double-inlet left ventricle and tricuspid atresia where there is generally only one ventricle. Conversely, in cases of double-inlet right ventricle where no left ventricle is found, it may be impossible to identify the septum.[7] In such cases, the hand rule cannot be applied and the ventricular loop cannot be determined.

The morphologic features of the normal right ventricle include (Fig. 105-10) (1) trapezoidal shape; (2) coarse trabeculations; (3) a body or sinus portion and an outflow or infundibulum demarcated by a muscular crest composed of the parietal band, septal band, and moderator band; (4) a tricuspid valve with chordal insertions on the ventricular septum; and (5) tricuspid valve–pulmonary valve discontinuity owing to intervening infundibular muscle. The characteristic features of the left ventricle include (Fig. 105-11) (1) ellipsoidal or bullet shape; (2) fine trabeculations on the free wall and apical septum, with a smooth mid and basal septum; (3) adjacent inflow and outflow tracts; (4) two well defined papillary muscle groups originating from the free wall; (5) absence of septal insertions of the mitral valve; (6) an outflow tract between the medial leaflet of the mitral valve and the ventricular septum; and (7) fibrous continuity between the mitral and aortic valves.

The great artery position or situs is a little more complicated because there are more possibilities. First, consider situations in which the great arteries are normally related—to each other and to the ventricles. This can occur in situs solitus or the usual position of the great arteries (solitus normally related great arteries), where the aorta is posterior and rightward of the pulmonary

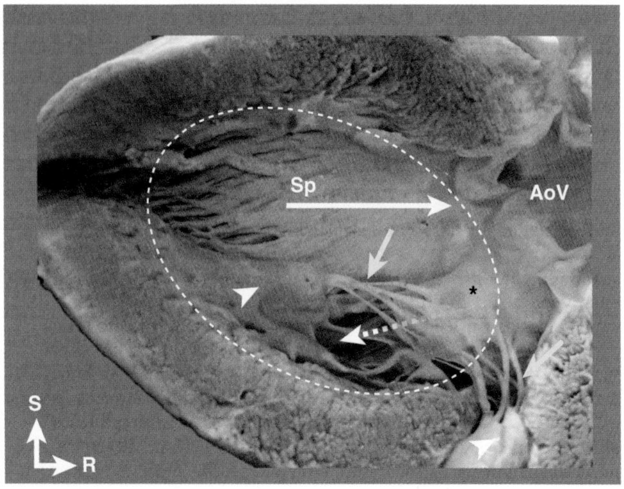

FIGURE 105-11 ■ Characteristic features of the left ventricle are shown in this specimen: ellipsoidal shape, smooth basal septal surface (Sp) with fine apical and free wall trabeculations, adjacent and nearly parallel inflow *(dashed white arrow)* and outflow *(solid white arrow)*, two free-wall papillary muscle groups *(white arrowheads)* receiving chordal insertions of the mitral valve *(yellow arrows)*, absence of septal insertions of the mitral valve, the outflow tract lying between the septum and the medial leaflet of the mitral valve (between *yellow arrows*), and fibrous continuity *(asterisk)* between the mitral and aortic (AoV) valves. *R*, Right; *S*, superior.

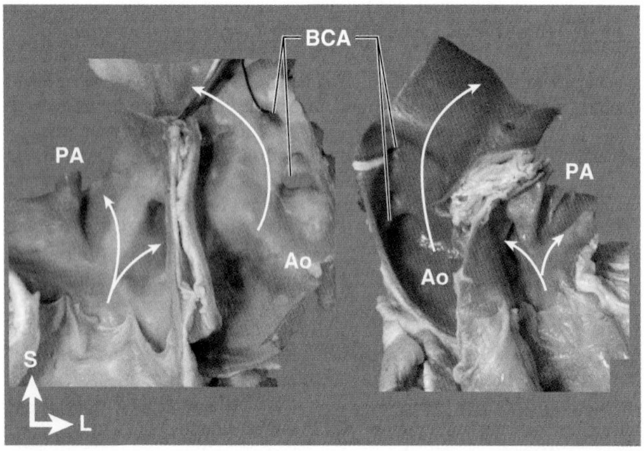

FIGURE 105-12 ■ The proximal aorta (Ao) and pulmonary artery (PA) from two hearts, one with solitus normally related great arteries *(right)* and one with inversus normally related great arteries *(left)*. In the solitus great arteries *(right)*, the aorta is rightward and posterior to the pulmonary artery and forms an arch *(curved arrow)*, whereas the pulmonary artery is anterior and leftward with the bifurcation *(bifurcating arrows)* to the left. Conversely, in inversus normally related great arteries *(left)* the aorta is posterior and leftward, whereas the pulmonary artery is anterior and rightward with the bifurcation *(bifurcating arrows)* to the right. The pulmonary branch that passes posterior to the ascending aorta is the right pulmonary artery in situs solitus but the left pulmonary artery in situs inversus. *BCA*, Brachiocephalic arteries; *L*, left; *S*, superior.

artery and aligned with the left ventricle, or in situs inversus or the mirror image of usual (inversus normally related great arteries), where the aorta is posterior and leftward of the pulmonary artery and aligned with the left ventricle (Fig. 105-12). In both cases, the pulmonary artery is aligned with the right ventricle. In situs solitus, the pulmonary artery bifurcation is to the left of the ascending aorta, whereas in situs inversus it is to the right.

Now consider situations in which the great arteries are abnormally related to each other or the ventricles. These malpositions of the great arteries are named according to the position of the aorta. If the aorta is to the right of the pulmonary artery, it is called *d-malposition* (*d* = dextro), to the left of the pulmonary artery is called *l-malposition* (*l* = levo), and directly anterior is called *a-malposition* (*a* = anterior). The term *p-malposition* has been used to describe cases in which the aorta is posterior to the pulmonary artery, mostly in rare cases of transposition of the great arteries. Malposition is a general and nonspecific term that includes all great artery arrangements, except solitus or inversus normally related great arteries.

Some hearts have only a single arterial trunk. In such cases, it makes no sense to describe its position because there is no other arterial root as a reference. An example is truncus arteriosus in which there is only the truncal root. The arterial arrangement in these hearts can be considered a form of normally related great arteries ({_,D,S} or {_,L,I}). The same approach can be used for tetralogy of Fallot with aortopulmonary collaterals and no pulmonary trunk. The truncal root or aorta overrides the septum and is in fibrous continuity with the mitral valve (and often the tricuspid valve); this is much like the aorta in tetralogy of Fallot. Consequently, it seems reasonable to consider the arterial arrangement in these hearts a form of normally related great arteries.

There are other hearts with a single arterial trunk in which this is not the case. In rare cases of truncus arteriosus, the truncal root is completely related to the right ventricle and there is a complete subtruncal conus. Clearly, this is not a variation of normally related great arteries. Similarly, some hearts have a right ventricular aorta with subaortic conus and long-segment pulmonary atresia. This is surely not normally related great arteries, but what is it? One could assign it as transposition or double-outlet right ventricle with pulmonary atresia, but this seems arbitrary because there is no pulmonary trunk. The most accurate description is a single right ventricular arterial root—either truncus or aorta. An arterial position is not assigned because there is no other root for comparison, so that the third member of the segmental set is either left blank or assigned an *X* for unknown.

Practical criteria for identifying the great arteries include: (1) the aorta forms an arch and gives rise to at least some of the brachiocephalic arteries and (2) the pulmonary artery bifurcates into right and left branches (see Fig. 105-12); however, there are significant exceptions. The aortic arch can be interrupted; one or even both branch pulmonary arteries can arise from the ascending aorta; a branch pulmonary artery can be absent; the left pulmonary artery can arise distally from the right pulmonary artery in left pulmonary artery sling syndrome.

Set notation is used to summarize the situs of the three main segments (Fig. 105-13). The first element of the set is the atrial situs: *S* for solitus, *I* for inversus, or *A* for ambiguus. The second element is the ventricular situs or

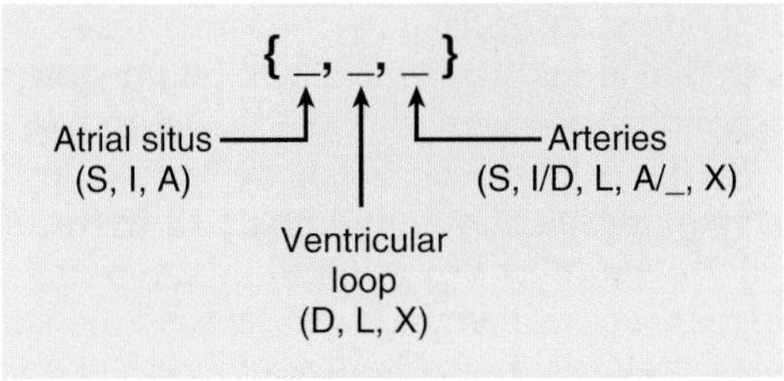

FIGURE 105-13 Segmental set notation used to describe the segmental situs of the main cardiac segments. The first member of the set is the atrial situs: solitus (S), inversus (I), or ambiguus (A). The second member is the ventricular loop or situs: dextro (D), levo (L), or unknown (X). Finally, the situs of the great arteries is the third member: S and I are used only for normally related great arteries; D, L, and A are used for malpositions of the great arteries, where the letter refers to the location of the aorta, right, left, or anterior, respectively. In cases with a right ventricular single arterial root, the third element of the set is either blank or an X, indicating that it is not possible to assign arterial position.

loop: *D* for solitus or d-loop, *L* for inversus or l-loop, or, rarely, *X* for unknown loop. The third element is the great artery position: *S* or *I* for solitus or inversus normally related great arteries, respectively; *D*, *L*, or *A* (some include *P*) for the various malpositions; or blank or *X* for hearts with a right ventricular single arterial root.

Segmental Alignments

Next, the alignments of the segments are defined based on what is aligned with or drains into what. Chambers are aligned if blood flows from one to the other (e.g., from right atrium to right ventricle in the normal heart). Alignment is concordant if the aligned segments are appropriate (e.g., right atrium aligned with right ventricle, or left ventricle aligned with aorta), or discordant if inappropriate (e.g., left atrium with right ventricle, or left ventricle with pulmonary artery). The concept of concordant and discordant alignment is useful when it works, but it is not universally applicable.[8] Is the ventriculoarterial alignment in double-outlet right ventricle concordant or discordant? It is concordant for the pulmonary artery but discordant for the aorta. What about the left ventricle? What is the atrioventricular alignment in straddling atrioventricular valve?

In fact, alignment is more complicated than simply concordance or discordance, because the blood must pass through the connecting segments before reaching the distal chamber or vessel; this adds a layer of variability and complexity. There are five basic types of atrioventricular alignment, determined by the situs of the atria and ventricles and the anatomy of the atrioventricular canal (Fig. 105-14):

1. Concordant—the atria are aligned with the appropriate ventricle through separate or a common atrioventricular (AV) valve ({S,D,_} or {I,L,_})
2. Discordant—the atria are aligned with the inappropriate ventricle through separate or a common AV valve ({S,L,_} or {I,D,_})
3. Straddling AV valve (including double-outlet atrium)—one atrium is aligned with one ventricle and the other with both ventricles
4. Double-inlet ventricle—both atria are aligned with one ventricle through two AV valves or a common AV valve, and
5. AV valve atresia—only one atrium is aligned with a ventricle and the other atrium drains across the atrial septum (Note that straddling of the remaining AV valve is possible in the context of AV valve atresia.)

There are five basic types of ventriculoarterial alignment (Fig. 105-15):

1. Concordant—both great arteries are aligned with the appropriate ventricle
2. Transposition (discordant)—the great arteries are on the opposite side of the septum from normal (i.e., aorta from right ventricle or infundibulum and pulmonary artery from left ventricle)
3. Double-outlet ventricle—both great arteries arise completely or nearly completely from one ventricle
4. Straddling single arterial trunk (sometimes considered a form of normally related great arteries and, therefore, concordant)—both ventricles are aligned with (eject into) a single arterial root, and
5. Right ventricular single arterial trunk—only the right ventricle is aligned with an arterial root and the left ventricle ejects across the ventricular septal defect

Concordant ventriculoarterial alignment includes normally related great arteries (in situs solitus and inversus), anatomically corrected malposition, isolated ventricular discordance, and isolated infundibuloarterial discordance (see Fig. 105-15*A*). In these, the sequence of blood flow is normal—from the left ventricle to the aorta and from the right ventricle to the pulmonary artery. However, the connection of the left ventricle to the aorta is abnormal in anatomically corrected malposition (see below, Segmental Connections).[9]

Transposition indicates that the great arteries arise on the opposite side of the ventricular septum from normal—the pulmonary artery from the left ventricle and the aorta from the right ventricle or outlet chamber.[10,11] Although there is a strong association between transposition and anterior placement of the aorta, this is not the meaning of the term. It is possible to have transposition with side-by-side vessels or even a posterior aorta.[12,13]

Double-outlet ventricle indicates just what the name says—both great arteries arise completely or nearly completely above one or the other ventricle. Although the "50% rule" is often used to define double-outlet ventricle,[14] its only attractive feature is that it simplifies cardiac bookkeeping. It has little or no clinical significance and is of no help in clinical decision making. Because it seems important for names of defects to be clinically meaningful, we do not use the 50% rule.

Single arterial trunk includes hearts with truncus arteriosus and pulmonary atresia. The aorta (or truncus) can be aligned with both ventricles (e.g., tetralogy of Fallot with pulmonary atresia or usual truncus) or only with the right ventricle (e.g., truncus with complete conus, pulmonary atresia with right ventricular aorta). Note that in aortic atresia, there is virtually always a hypoplastic ascending aorta and aortic root that sits above an atretic ventricular outflow tract and supplies the coronary

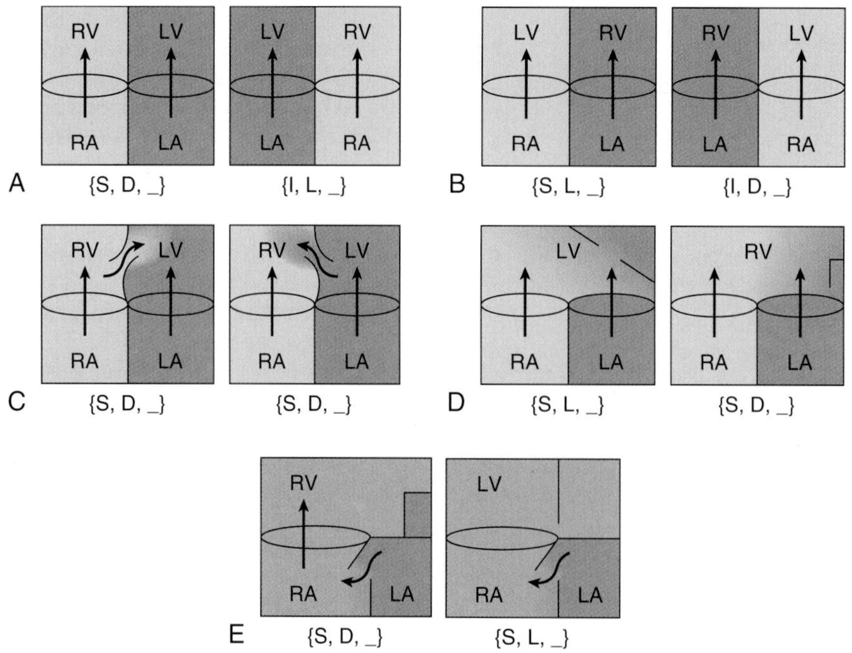

FIGURE 105-14 Examples of the five types of atrioventricular alignments.* **A,** Concordant. The left figure is the usual alignment in situs solitus (right-sided right atrium [RA] aligned with right-sided right ventricle [RV] and left-sided left atrium [LA] aligned with left-sided left ventricle [LV]), but atrioventricular alignment is concordant as well if both atria and ventricles are inverted *(right panel).* **B,** Discordant. In the *left panel,* atrioventricular alignment discordance is due to ventricular inversion in situs solitus (right-sided right atrium aligned with a right-sided [inverted] left ventricle and a left-sided left atrium aligned with a left-sided [inverted] right ventricle), which can be associated with isolated ventricular inversion {S,L,S}, anatomically corrected malposition {S,L,D}, congenitally corrected transposition {S,L,L}, superior-inferior ventricles with double-outlet right ventricle {S,L,D}, and others. Note that the mirror images of these arrangements in situs inversus also produce atrioventricular alignment discordance (e.g., isolated ventricular noninversion {I,D,I}, anatomically corrected malposition {I,D,L}, congenitally corrected transposition {I,D,D}). Isolated atrial inversion *(right panel),* such as normally related great arteries {I,D,S}, also results in atrioventricular alignment discordance. **C,** Straddling atrioventricular valve. The example shows straddling tricuspid valve *(left panel)* and straddling mitral valve *(right panel)* in atrioventricular situs concordance (as in **A**) but could be situs discordance (as in **B**) as well. Although concordance–discordance works for situs, it does not work for alignment. What is the alignment of the right atrium in the left figure or the left atrium in the right figure? It is both concordant and discordant, because the atrium with the straddling valve is aligned with both ventricles through the normal and straddling orifices of the valve. **D,** Double-inlet ventricle. In the *left panel,* there is double-inlet left ventricle with atrioventricular situs discordance {S,L,_} (solitus atria with a right-sided right atrium and left-sided left atrium, but l-loop or inverted left ventricle with the outlet chamber to the left and the left ventricle to the right). Situs concordance is possible as well (e.g., double-inlet left ventricle with normally related great arteries {S,D,S}, also known as Holmes heart, which is not shown). The *right panel* illustrates double-inlet right ventricle with atrioventricular situs concordance {S,D,_} (the right atrium is right-sided and the left atrium left sided, the ventricles are solitus or d-loop with a right-sided right ventricle and a left-sided hypoplastic left ventricle). Concordance–discordance does not work for atrioventricular alignment in this case because both atria are aligned with the same ventricle so that the alignment of one atrium is concordant and the other discordant. **E,** Atrioventricular valve atresia. The *left panel* illustrates mitral atresia in atrioventricular situs concordance {S,D,_} (solitus atria with the right atrium to the right and the left atrium to the left and d-loop or solitus ventricles with the right ventricle to the right and the hypoplastic left ventricle to the left). This could also occur in situs inversus (the mirror image of the example shown) or in atrioventricular situs discordance, such as {S,L,_} with right-sided mitral atresia. The *right panel* shows tricuspid atresia in atrioventricular situs discordance {S,L,_} (solitus atria with a right-sided right atrium and left-sided left atrium and a right-sided inverted [l-loop] left ventricle and left-sided outlet chamber). Here the right atrial alignment is discordant, but the left atrial alignment is neither concordant nor discordant because it does not drain directly into either ventricle. It drains across the atrial septum into the right atrium. This could occur in atrioventricular situs concordance as well, such as tricuspid atresia with transposition {S,D,D}. Note that it is also possible for the remaining atrioventricular valve to straddle the septum. **Although we have stressed in the text that the ventricular loop or situs is based on the chirality or handedness of the chamber and not its position in space, we have used position as a surrogate for ventricular loop or situs in this and the next figure to facilitate creating the illustrations.*

arteries. Consequently, the single arterial root is essentially never a pulmonary trunk.

Segmental Connections

Finally, the connections of the segments are described. Alignment and connection are different and both are important. As noted above, the three main segments are not connected directly to each other. Rather, they are joined by the two connecting segments. Atrioventricular connections are (1) two valves into separate ventricles, (2) common valve into two ventricles, (3) straddling AV valve, (4) two valves into one ventricle, (5) common valve into one ventricle, (6) absent AV connection, and (7) imperforate AV valve. Atrioventricular alignments and connections are closely related. For example,

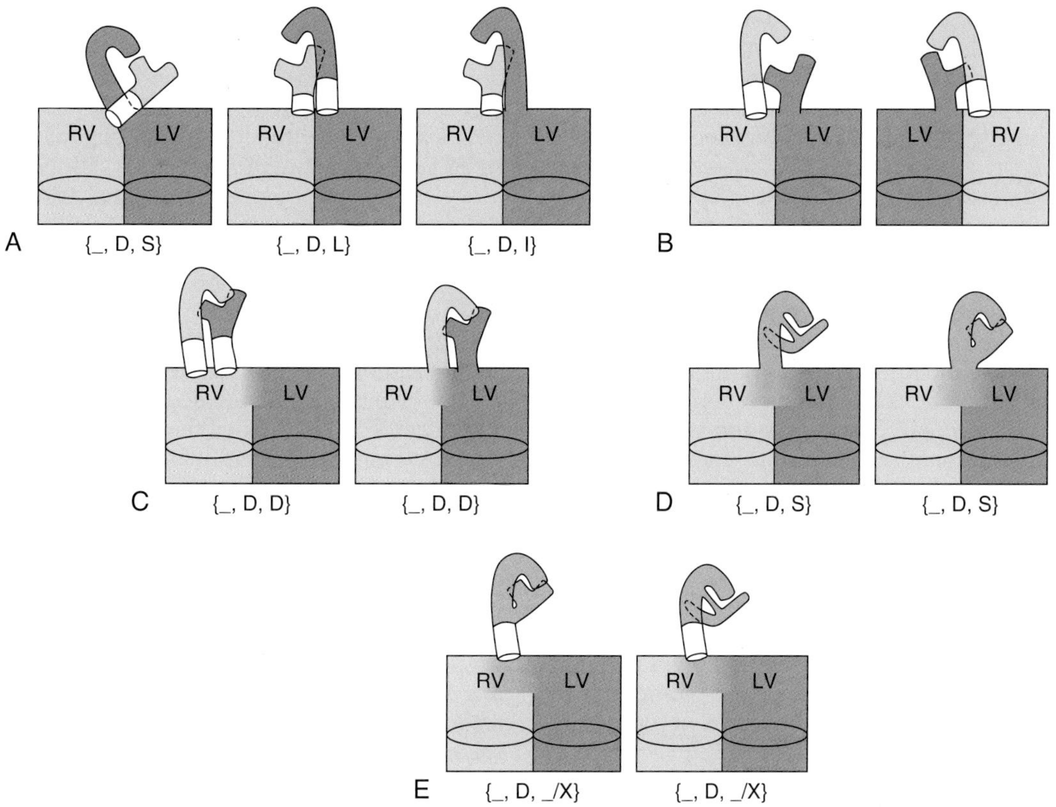

FIGURE 105-15 Examples of the five types of ventriculoarterial alignment.* **A,** Concordant. The *left panel* shows normally related great arteries in situs solitus {_,D,S} (rightward and posterior aorta aligned with the left ventricle [LV] and connected by mitral-aortic fibrous continuity and the leftward, anterior pulmonary artery aligned with the right ventricle [RV] and connected by a subpulmonary conus). Ventriculoarterial alignment is also concordant in normally related great arteries in situs inversus {_,L,I} (the mirror image of the *left panel,* not shown), anatomically corrected malposition {_,D,L} (*middle panel,* left-sided d-loop left ventricle aligned with a left-sided aorta and connected by a subaortic conus, right-sided d-loop right ventricle aligned with the right-sided pulmonary artery and connected by a [often deficient] subpulmonary conus) or {_,L,D} (the mirror image of {_,D,L}, not shown), isolated infundibuloarterial discordance {S,D,I} (*right panel,* right-sided d-loop right ventricle aligned with a right-sided and anterior pulmonary artery and connected by subpulmonary conus, and a left-sided d-loop left ventricle aligned with a leftward and posterior aorta and connected by aortic-mitral fibrous continuity) or {I,L,S}, its mirror image, and others. **B,** Discordant. The *left panel* shows common transposition of the great arteries {S,D,D} (right-sided d-loop right ventricle aligned with the right-sided aorta and connected by subaortic conus and the left-sided d-loop left ventricle aligned with the leftward pulmonary artery and connected by pulmonary-mitral fibrous continuity). The *right panel* is congenitally corrected transposition {S,L,L} (right-sided inverted or l-loop left ventricle aligned with the right-sided pulmonary artery and connected by pulmonary-mitral fibrous continuity and the left-sided inverted or l-loop right ventricle aligned with the left-sided aorta and connected by subaortic conus). **C,** Double-outlet ventricle. The *left panel* shows double-outlet right ventricle {S,D,D} (a right-sided d-loop right ventricle is aligned with both great arteries [the right-sided aorta and left-sided pulmonary artery], whereas the left-sided d-loop left ventricle is aligned with neither). The *right panel* shows double-outlet left ventricle {S,D,D} where both great arteries are aligned with the left ventricle and neither with the right ventricle. Concordance–discordance does not make sense in this context because one ventricle is aligned with both great arteries and the other with neither. In the illustration, the great arteries are connected to the right ventricle, in the case of double-outlet right ventricle, by bilateral subarterial conus and to the left ventricle, in the case of double-outlet left ventricle, by fibrous continuity between the mitral valve and both semilunar valves. Keep in mind, however, that more than one type of ventriculoarterial connection can occur with either type of double-outlet ventricle. **D,** Overriding single arterial trunk. The *left panel* shows tetralogy of Fallot with pulmonary atresia and no pulmonary trunk, considered to be a type of normally related great arteries. However, both ventricles are aligned with the overriding single aortic root, so that concordance–discordance does not really apply. The alignment is the same in typical truncus arteriosus with an overriding truncal root *(right panel).* In the great majority of such cases, there is semilunar-mitral fibrous continuity as shown in the illustration. **E,** Right ventricular single arterial trunk. In truncus arteriosus with complete subtruncal conus *(left panel)* the truncal root is completely above and aligned with the right ventricle. The left ventricle is not aligned with a great artery and ejects through the ventricular septal defect. The *right panel* demonstrates a right ventricular aorta with pulmonary atresia. The aorta is aligned with the right ventricle, but the left ventricle is not aligned with a great artery. Concordance–discordance is not useful for describing this arrangement. **Although we have stressed in the text that the ventricular loop or situs is based on the chirality or handedness of the chamber and not its position in space, we have used position as a surrogate for ventricular loop or situs in this and the previous figure to facilitate creating the illustrations. The cylinder indicates subarterial conus or infundibulum.*

double-inlet alignment can only be associated with two valves or a common valve into one ventricle. The term *AV valve atresia* has been used both for conditions with absent connection (usual tricuspid atresia) and for conditions in which valve components are present but there is no orifice (many cases of mitral atresia). This is unlikely to change, nor is such a change being proposed. However, distinguishing between these types of atrioventricular connection is likely to be informative regarding developmental mechanism and possibly outcome.

Ventriculoarterial connection and alignment are less closely related. The aorta might be connected normally to the left ventricle with fibrous continuity between the mitral and aortic valves (normally related great arteries) or abnormally by a muscular conus between the left ventricle and the aorta (anatomically corrected malposition). In both cases, the ventriculoarterial alignment is concordant; the aorta receives blood from the left ventricle and the pulmonary artery from the right ventricle. However, the ways in which the great arteries are connected to the ventricles differ. A given ventriculoarterial alignment can be associated with multiple types of connection. This has implications for associated abnormalities (e.g., the subaortic conus in anatomically corrected malposition can become obstructed) and surely for the developmental mechanisms that produce the defect.

There are four ventriculoarterial connections: subpulmonary conus only, subaortic conus only, bilateral subarterial conus, and bilaterally absent subarterial conus. A subpulmonary conus is typical of normally related great arteries, but it can occur with a rare form of transposition with a posterior aorta, with double-outlet right ventricle with mitral atresia, and with isolated infundibuloarterial discordance.[15] Subaortic conus is typical of common and congenitally corrected transposition, but it occurs in some forms of double-outlet left ventricle.[16] Bilateral conus is most often associated with double-outlet right ventricle, but it can occur with transposition[13] and anatomically corrected malposition. Bilaterally absent subarterial conus is seen in double-outlet left ventricle,[16] but it can also occur in transposition.[13] As already noted, the ventriculoarterial connection has implications for outflow obstruction, great artery size, and arterial obstruction.

Disharmony between Situs and Alignment

There is typically concordance or harmony among the atrial situs, the loop or situs of the ventricles, and the situs or position of the great arteries. When the atrial situs is solitus, there are usually d-loop ventricles and the aorta is usually to the right—either solitus normally related great arteries or some type of d-malposition of the great arteries—and conversely in situs inversus.

Situs discordance between segments is a feature of a number of heart defects. For example, in congenitally corrected transposition {S,L,L}, there is atrioventricular situs discordance (solitus atria but inverted ventricles) and alignment discordance (right atrium aligned with right-sided left ventricle and left atrium aligned with a left-sided right ventricle). The situs correctly predicts the atrioventricular alignments; this is the case in the vast majority of hearts.

However, some hearts are characterized by discrepancy or disharmony between segmental situs and segmental alignments.[4,17,18] In the vast majority of hearts, when there is situs solitus of the atria and d-loop ventricles, or situs inversus and l-loop ventricles, the right atrium is aligned with (drains into) the right ventricle and the left atrium is aligned with the left ventricle. The situs of the segments correctly predicts the alignments. There is said to be concordance or harmony between situs and alignments. It is mostly in hearts with superoinferior ventricles and crisscross hearts where one sees discordance or disharmony between situs and atrioventricular alignment: a solitus right atrium aligned with a d-loop left ventricle and a solitus left atrium aligned with a d-loop right ventricle (and the converse). Especially in these hearts, one cannot assume that situs correctly predicts atrioventricular alignments. Virtually all the hearts with situs-alignment discordance that have been reported also have right juxtaposition of the atrial appendages.[18] In other types of hearts, it seems a practical assumption that situs correctly predicts atrioventricular alignment.

Situs and ventriculoarterial alignment are less tightly linked. Often one cannot deduce the ventriculoarterial alignment from the situs of the ventricles and great arteries. For example, a heart with the cardiotype {S,D,D} could be transposition (discordant) or double-outlet ventricle (right or left). Or the cardiotype {S,D,L} could be associated with transposition (discordant), anatomically corrected malposition (concordant) or double-outlet ventricle. Sometimes this is because the concept of concordance and discordance does not apply, as in double-outlet ventricle. Other times it simply reflects the variability of arterial position. Consequently, the ventriculoarterial alignment is typically stated in the diagnosis along with the cardiotype (e.g., anatomically corrected malposition {S,D,L}).

Examples of Segmental Analysis

The following examples illustrate the use of segmental analysis.

1. Normal heart in situs solitus
   a. Segmental situs: atrial situs solitus {S,_,_}; ventricular d-loop or situs solitus {_,D,_}; solitus normally positioned and related great arteries {_,_,S}. The cardiotype, using set notation, is {S,D,S}.
   b. Segmental alignments: the atrioventricular alignment is concordant; the ventriculoarterial alignment is concordant (see Figs. 105-14*A* and 105-15*A*).
   c. Segmental connections: the atrioventricular connection is two valves into separate ventricles; the ventriculoarterial connection is subpulmonary conus only with mitral-aortic fibrous continuity.

   The normal heart in situs inversus has the cardiotype {I,L,I} (situs inversus [I]; ventricular l-loop or situs inversus [L]; inversus normally related great arteries [I]), but the alignments and connections are the same as noted previously.

   In these hearts, the location, alignments, and connections of the heart segments are all appropriate so that any hemodynamic abnormality is due to one or more of the myriad possible other defects such as a venous drainage anomaly, abnormal intracardiac communication, outflow obstruction, and so on.
2. Common transposition of the great arteries
   a. Segmental situs: atrial situs solitus {S,_,_}; ventricular d-loop or situs solitus {_,D,_};

transposition of the great arteries with the aorta anterior and rightward {_,_,D}. The cardiotype is {S,D,D}.

b. Segmental alignments: the atrioventricular alignment is concordant; the ventriculoarterial alignment is transposition (discordant; see Figs. 105-14*A* and 105-15*B*).

c. Segmental connections: the atrioventricular connection is two valves into separate ventricles; the ventriculoarterial connection is usually subaortic conus with pulmonary-mitral fibrous continuity, but, as noted, can be variable.

Here there is a single segmental alignment discordance between the ventricles and great arteries. The patient is blue because systemic venous blood from the right atrium is recycled back to the aorta through the right ventricle. Creating ventriculoarterial alignment concordance by performing an arterial switch operation corrects the abnormal blood flow pattern and places the left ventricle in the systemic circulation.

3. Double-outlet right ventricle with straddling mitral valve
   a. Segmental situs: atrial situs solitus {S,_,_}; ventricular d-loop or situs solitus {_,D,_}; double-outlet ventricle with aorta rightward {_,_,D}. The cardiotype is {S,D,D}.
   b. Segmental alignments: the atrioventricular alignment is mitral straddling. The right atrium is normally aligned with the right ventricle; the left atrium is aligned partially with both ventricles. The ventriculoarterial alignment is double-outlet ventricle (right; see Figs. 105-14*C* and 105-15*C*).
   c. Segmental connections: the atrioventricular connection is two valves into separate ventricles with straddling of the mitral valve; the ventriculoarterial connection could be subaortic conus with fibrous continuity between the pulmonary valve and the straddling part of the mitral valve or bilateral subarterial conus.

The information conveyed by the situs, alignments, and connections is essential, but other important information must be supplied before a treatment plan can be formulated, including relation of the arterial roots to the ventricular septal defect (if one is present); presence, severity, and mechanism of outflow obstruction; and ventricular hypoplasia that might preclude a biventricular repair. Details of the mitral straddling are also important for surgical planning.

4. Anatomically corrected malposition of the great arteries
   a. Segmental situs: atrial situs solitus {S,_,_}; ventricular d-loop or situs solitus {_,D,_}; anatomically corrected malposition with the aorta to the left {_,_,L}. The cardiotype is {S,D,L}.
   b. Segmental alignments: the atrioventricular alignment is concordant. The right atrium is normally aligned with the right ventricle; the left atrium is normally aligned with the left ventricle. The ventriculoarterial alignment is concordant. The left-sided aorta is aligned with the left-sided left ventricle, and the right-sided pulmonary artery is aligned with the right-sided right ventricle (see Figs. 105-14*A* and 105-15*A*).
   c. Segmental connections: the atrioventricular connection is two valves into separate ventricles; the ventriculoarterial connection is bilateral conus, although the subpulmonary conus is often deficient.

Anatomically corrected malposition {S,D,L} is the most frequent type. There is no alignment discordance here; therefore, ventricular septal defect closure might be all that is needed. This defect illustrates the difference between alignment and connection. Although the ventriculoarterial alignments are concordant (right ventricle–pulmonary artery and left ventricle–aorta), the connections are abnormal. There is typically a long subaortic conus or infundibulum connecting the aorta with the left ventricle and a deficient subpulmonary conus connecting the pulmonary artery with the right ventricle. Outflow obstruction can occur on either or both sides because of the abnormal conus or infundibulum.

There are types of anatomically corrected malposition with atrioventricular discordance (e.g., {S,L,D}). There is ventriculoarterial alignment concordance, because the right-sided left ventricle is aligned with the right-sided aorta and the left-sided right ventricle is aligned with the left-sided pulmonary artery, but the ventriculoarterial connections are abnormal as described previously. Here an atrial switch operation might be indicated to correct the segmental (atrioventricular) alignment discordance, but an arterial switch operation would not be so because there is already ventriculoarterial alignment concordance.

5. Isolated infundibuloarterial inversion
   a. Segmental situs: atrial situs solitus {S,_,_}; ventricular d-loop or situs solitus {_,D,_}; inverted normally related great arteries {_,_,I}. The cardiotype is {S,D,I}.
   b. Segmental alignment: the atrioventricular alignment is concordant; the ventriculoarterial alignment is concordant (see Figs. 105-14*A* and 105-15*A*). The posterior and leftward aorta is aligned with the left-sided left ventricle, and the anterior rightward pulmonary artery is aligned with the right-sided right ventricle.
   c. Segmental connections: the atrioventricular connection is two valves into separate ventricles; the ventriculoarterial connection is subpulmonary conus with aortic-mitral fibrous continuity.

   This is an example of segmental situs discordance ({_,D,I}) with segmental alignment concordance. Although this anomaly can occur with an otherwise essentially normal heart, it is usually associated with subvalvar and valvar pulmonary stenosis. The conotruncus is similar to inverted tetralogy of Fallot.[15] The patient is blue because of pulmonary outflow obstruction with a right-to-left shunt through the ventricular septal defect rather than to an alignment discordance. The right coronary artery arises from the left-sided aorta and passes to the right AV groove in front of the obstructed pulmonary outflow, which can complicate treating this anomaly as one might treat tetralogy of Fallot.

SUMMARY

The segmental analysis provides a comprehensive understanding of the organization of the heart and the principal diagnoses. This type of analysis indicates whether cyanosis is due to alignment discordance or some other local problem (e.g., pulmonary atresia with atrial right-to-left shunt). If alignment discordance is part of the problem, segmental analysis also indicates the type of operation needed (e.g., atrial switch for isolated atrioventricular alignment discordance, arterial switch for isolated ventriculoarterial alignment discordance, double switch for both atrioventricular and ventriculoarterial [double] alignment discordance). Specific local diagnoses (e.g., additional muscular ventricular septal defect, subaortic stenosis, persistent ductus arteriosus) are then added to the context of the segmental analysis. It is useful to think of the heart segment by segment when establishing the comprehensive diagnosis—from veins, to atria, to atrioventricular valves, to ventricles, to outflow tracts, to great arteries—to avoid missing any component. Organizing the information segmentally in the diagnostic report not only helps to avoid oversight, it also lets the reader know where to find information about any specific part of the heart.

Acknowledgment

I would like to acknowledge and thank Dr. Richard Van Praagh for being a mentor, colleague, and friend over many years and for writing the previous version of this chapter, which was extremely helpful in preparing the current version. I also acknowledge Dr. Paul Weinberg for originating or contributing to many of the concepts expressed in this chapter. I am grateful to Dr. Tal Geva for reviewing the chapter and making some excellent contributions.

REFERENCES

1. Van Praagh R: The segmental approach to diagnosis in congenital heart disease. The cardiovascular system. *Birth Defects Orig Artic Ser* 8:4–23, 1972.
2. Calcaterra G, Anderson RH, Lau KC, et al: Dextrocardia–value of segmental analysis in its categorisation. *Br Heart J* 42:497–507, 1979.
3. Van Praagh R: Diagnosis of complex congenital heart disease: morphologic anatomic method and terminology. *Cardiovasc Intervent Radiol* 7:115–120, 1984.
4. Hirokawa N, Tanaka Y, Okada Y: Cilia, KIF3 molecular motor and nodal flow. *Curr Opin Cell Biol* 24:31–39, 2012.
5. Franco D, Campione M, Kelly R, et al: Multiple transcriptional domains, with distinct left and right components, in the atrial chambers of the developing heart. *Circ Res* 87:984–991, 2000.
6. Van Praagh R: The importance of segmental situs in the diagnosis of congenital heart disease. *Semin Roentgenol* 20:254–271, 1985.
7. Saleeb SF, Juraszek A, Geva T: Anatomic, imaging, and clinical characteristics of double-inlet, double-outlet right ventricle. *Am J Cardiol* 105:542–549, 2010.
8. Van Praagh R: When concordant or discordant atrioventricular alignments predict the ventricular situs wrongly. I. Solitus atria, concordant alignments, and L-loop ventricles. II. Solitus atria, discordant alignments, and D-loop ventricles. *J Am Coll Cardiol* 10:1278–1279, 1987.
9. Van Praagh R, Durnin RE, Jockin H, et al: Anatomically corrected malposition of the great arteries (S, D, L). *Circulation* 51:20–31, 1975.
10. Van Praagh R: Transposition of the great arteries. II. Transposition clarified. *Am J Cardiol* 28:739–741, 1971.
11. Anderson RH, Weinberg PM: The clinical anatomy of transposition. *Cardiol Young* 15(Suppl 1):76–87, 2005.
12. Van Praagh R, Perez-Trevino C, Lõpez-Cuellar M, et al: Transposition of the great arteries with posterior aorta, anterior pulmonary artery, subpulmonary conus and fibrous continuity between aortic and atrioventricular valves. *Am J Cardiol* 28:621–631, 1971.
13. Pasquini L, Sanders SP, Parness IA, et al: Conal anatomy in 119 patients with d-loop transposition of the great arteries and ventricular septal defect: an echocardiographic and pathologic study. *J Am Coll Cardiol* 21:1712–1721, 1993.
14. Anderson RH, Becker AE, Wilcox BR, et al: Surgical anatomy of double-outlet right ventricle—a reappraisal. *Am J Cardiol* 52:555–559, 1983.
15. Foran RB, Belcourt C, Nanton MA, et al: Isolated infundibuloarterial inversion (S,D,I): a newly recognized form of congenital heart disease. *Am Heart J* 116(5 Pt 1):1337–1350, 1988.
16. Bharati S, Lev M, Stewart R, et al: The morphologic spectrum of double outlet left ventricle and its surgical significance. *Circulation* 58(3 Pt 1):558–565, 1978.
17. Anderson RH, Smith A, Wilkinson JL: Disharmony between atrioventricular connections and segmental combinations: unusual variants of "crisscross" hearts. *J Am Coll Cardiol* 10:1274–1277, 1987.
18. Geva T, Sanders SP, Ayres NA, et al: Two-dimensional echocardiographic anatomy of atrioventricular alignment discordance with situs concordance. *Am Heart J* 125:459–464, 1993.

CHAPTER 106

Diagnostic Imaging: Echocardiography and Magnetic Resonance Imaging

Tal Geva

CHAPTER OUTLINE

Before the advent of cardiopulmonary bypass in the mid-1950s, little attention was given to the diagnosis of congenital heart disease (CHD) because no effective treatment was available. Physical examination, auscultation, electrocardiography, and radiography were the main diagnostic tools. Progress in open-heart techniques for repair of CHD required accurate and comprehensive delineation of cardiovascular anatomy and function. During the 1960s and 1970s, cardiac catheterization and angiography were the principal tools used to diagnose CHD. Echocardiography entered the arena in the late 1970s. The diagnostic capability of M-mode echocardiography proved insufficient in patients with CHD, but the rapid evolution of two-dimensional echocardiography during the following decade transformed the field. The technologic advances in transducer design, image processing, and image display—together with development and refinement of new imaging planes and examination techniques—allowed high-quality tomographic visualization of most cardiac defects.[1] The application of Doppler ultrasound to investigate blood flow allowed comprehensive hemodynamic assessment. By the mid-1980s, much of the necessary anatomic and hemodynamic information required for patient management could be obtained noninvasively, obviating the need for a diagnostic catheterization in many patients. During the late 1990s and into the 2000s, the field of pediatric cardiac imaging experienced accelerated progress in areas such as three-dimensional echocardiography, sophisticated techniques for assessment of myocardial function, and the application of magnetic resonance imaging (MRI) to CHD. At the same time, the proportion of cardiac catheterization procedures performed solely for diagnostic purposes has drastically declined. More recently, the role of multimodality cardiac imaging for preintervention planning and for guidance of cardiovascular procedures has expanded dramatically.[2]

This chapter discusses the clinical application of the two main noninvasive diagnostic imaging modalities used for anatomic and physiologic evaluation of preoperative and postoperative CHD: echocardiography and cardiovascular MRI.

ECHOCARDIOGRAPHY AND DOPPLER ULTRASOUND

Echocardiography is an ideal diagnostic tool in pediatric cardiology because of its noninvasive nature, relatively low cost, superb spatial and temporal resolutions, and ability to image cardiovascular anatomy and to evaluate physiology in real time. In addition, modern cardiac ultrasound equipment is portable and adaptable to different environments, such as the operating room, intensive care unit, at the bedside, and in an outpatient office setting. In today's pediatric cardiology practice, echocardiography is the primary diagnostic modality used to evaluate anatomy and physiology preoperatively, intraoperatively, postoperatively, during follow-up of CHD, and prenatally.[1-3]

Description of Technique

To obtain an echocardiographic image, a burst of ultrasound energy is generated by a piezoelectric crystal and travels through the soft tissue at an average speed of approximately 1540 m/sec. When the propagating ultrasound wave encounters an interface between tissues with different acoustic properties, some of the energy is reflected back toward the transducer and some of the energy is refracted and continues to travel in the medium until it encounters the next interface. The returning ultrasound energy is captured by the piezoelectric crystal and converted into an electrical energy that goes through a series of electronic processes, including amplification, filtering, postprocessing, and display.

M-Mode Echocardiography

A narrow beam of ultrasound energy is emitted toward the heart, and structures along the beam path reflect echoes back toward the transducer. A dot is displayed on the screen in a position corresponding to its distance from the transducer. This process is repeated rapidly to create an image. The distance from the transducer is displayed on the *y*-axis and time is displayed on the *x*-axis (Fig. 106-1). This provides an anatomically one-dimensional image of the heart that is characterized by excellent temporal and axial resolutions. In today's clinical pediatric echocardiography, two-dimensional imaging has replaced M-mode for anatomic imaging of the heart and for assessment of ventricular size and function.[4] In selected circumstances, when superior temporal resolution is required, two-dimensional directed M-mode is used to assess motion of specific structures such as native and prosthetic valve leaflets.

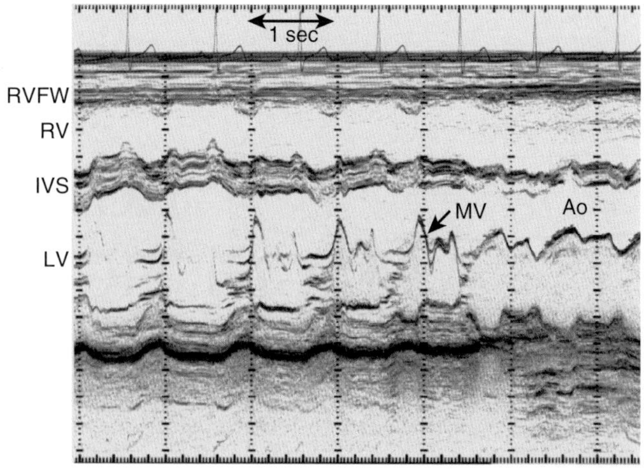

FIGURE 106-1 ■ M-mode tracing of the left ventricle and the aortic root. *Ao,* Aortic root; *IVS,* interventricular septum; *LV,* left ventricle; *MV,* mitral valve; *RV,* right ventricle; *RVFW,* right ventricular free wall.

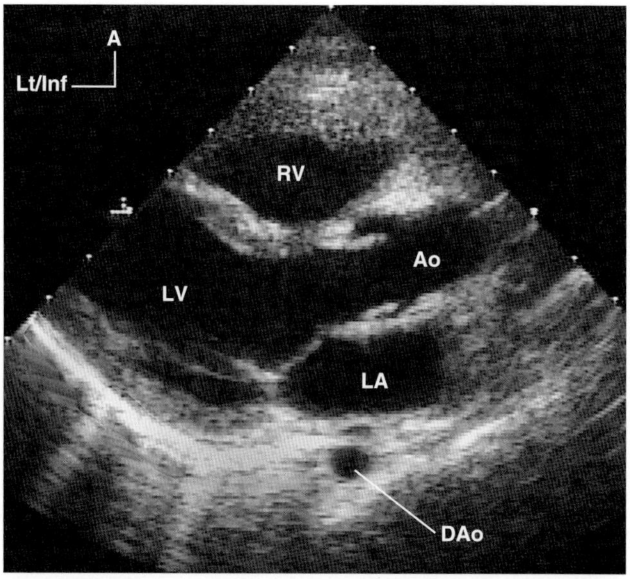

FIGURE 106-2 ■ Two-dimensional image from the parasternal long-axis view showing the left atrium (LA), left ventricle (LV), aortic root (Ao), descending aorta (DAo), and right ventricle (RV).

Two-Dimensional Echocardiography

By rapidly sweeping an ultrasound beam through an arc, multiple "M-mode lines" are placed next to each other to construct a cross-sectional two-dimensional image of the heart (Fig. 106-2). This can be accomplished by electronically sweeping the sound beam through multiple piezoelectric crystals (transducer elements), as in phased array transducers. Recent advances in transducer technology and image processing permit very high frame rates (>200 Hz), a feature that greatly enhances temporal resolution.[5]

Three-Dimensional Echocardiography

Accurate spatial perception of an object depends on recognition of its three dimensions: length, width, and depth. Although an experienced examiner can mentally construct a three-dimensional image of the heart from serial two-dimensional tomographic images obtained by sweeping the transducer across the heart, three-dimensional echocardiography offers enhanced perspective of cardiovascular structures and their interrelations. Previous approaches to obtaining three-dimensional echocardiographic images of the heart were based on computer reconstruction of contiguous two-dimensional cross-sectional images. These efforts were hampered by difficulties in accurately registering the ultrasound image data in time and space and by long processing times. Currently, three-dimensional images are generated by real-time three-dimensional echocardiography. This technology, which is based on a new generation of matrix array transducers with several thousands of simultaneously transmitting and receiving piezoelectric elements and sophisticated parallel data processing, provides real-time three-dimensional images with sufficient temporal resolution to display in cine-loop format (Fig. 106-3).[6-8] More recently, miniaturization of matrix array transducer technology has allowed development of a real-time three-dimensional transesophageal echocardiographic probe.[9] Further refinements of this technology will result in continued improvement of spatial and temporal resolutions as well as better, more intuitive, user interface. Such advances will likely contribute to the ongoing acceptance of this technology in routine practice.

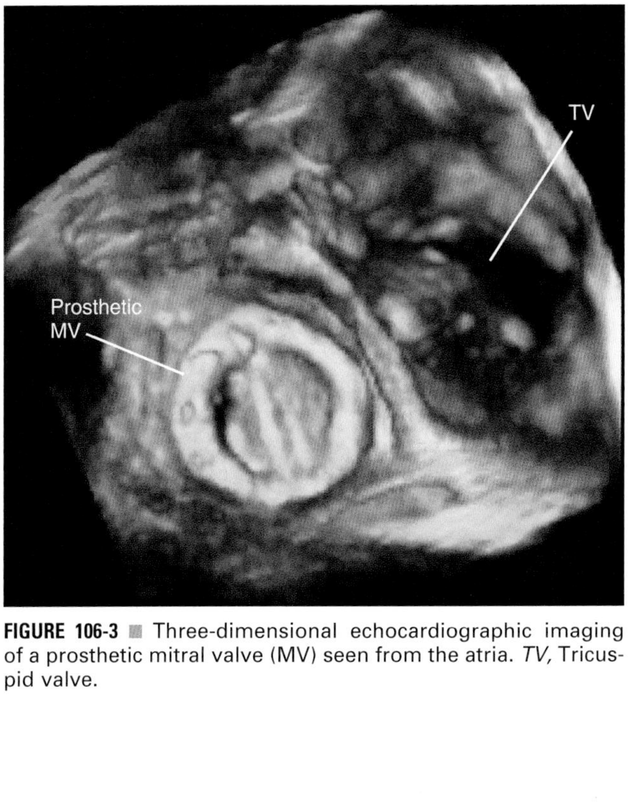

FIGURE 106-3 ■ Three-dimensional echocardiographic imaging of a prosthetic mitral valve (MV) seen from the atria. *TV*, Tricuspid valve.

Doppler Echocardiography

The use of Doppler ultrasound to assess normal and abnormal hemodynamics has become an integral part of the echocardiographic examination.[4,10] The advent of two-dimensional directed Doppler interrogation has greatly enhanced the clinical application of this technique by allowing evaluation of flow characteristics in specific regions within the heart and great vessels. In today's echocardiography, spectral and color-coded Doppler flow mapping are used extensively to measure velocity and direction of blood flow (Fig. 106-4). Calculations based on Doppler-derived measurements allow quantitative estimation of flow volume (such as cardiac output), pressure gradient across a stenotic region, cross-sectional flow area, and prediction of intracardiac pressures. Doppler echocardiography also provides qualitative and semiquantitative assessment of valve regurgitation, intra- and extracardiac shunts, as well as myocardial motion (tissue Doppler imaging). Detailed discussion of Doppler physics is beyond the scope of this text and can be found elsewhere.[11]

Speckle-Tracking Echocardiography

Speckle-tracking echocardiography (STE) is an echocardiographic technique that allows depiction and measurements of myocardial motion and function. The technique is based on frame-to-frame analysis of changes in the unique ultrasonic backscatter features (speckles) of sequential two-dimensional images while filtering out noise. STE displays local displacement of the myocardium that can be then analyzed for indices of myocardial deformation such as strain and strain rate, in any direction within the two-dimensional image (Fig. 106-5).[12] The technique, which was introduced in 2004,[13] has been validated in an animal model against sonomicrometry and in vivo against cardiac MRI tagging.[14,15] Advantages of STE over Doppler-based techniques for assessment of tissue motion include independence of angle of interrogation and insensitivity to tethering of the myocardium. More recently, three-dimensional STE has been developed and validated.[16] A review of the use of STE in CHD can be found elsewhere.[17]

Contrast Echocardiography

As early as the late 1960s, Gramiak and colleagues[18] noted that intravascular injection of almost any solution resulted in a contrast effect detectable by echocardiography. Initially, this technique was used to identify structures seen by M-mode echocardiography. Contrast echocardiography has been used to detect systemic[19] and pulmonary venous anomalies,[20] and for the detection of intracardiac and great artery level shunts.[21] In today's pediatric echocardiography, contrast studies are infrequently performed and are usually limited to detection of intracardiac shunts in patients with limited echocardiographic windows, patch or baffle leak after cardiac surgery, and in pulmonary arteriovenous malformations.[3]

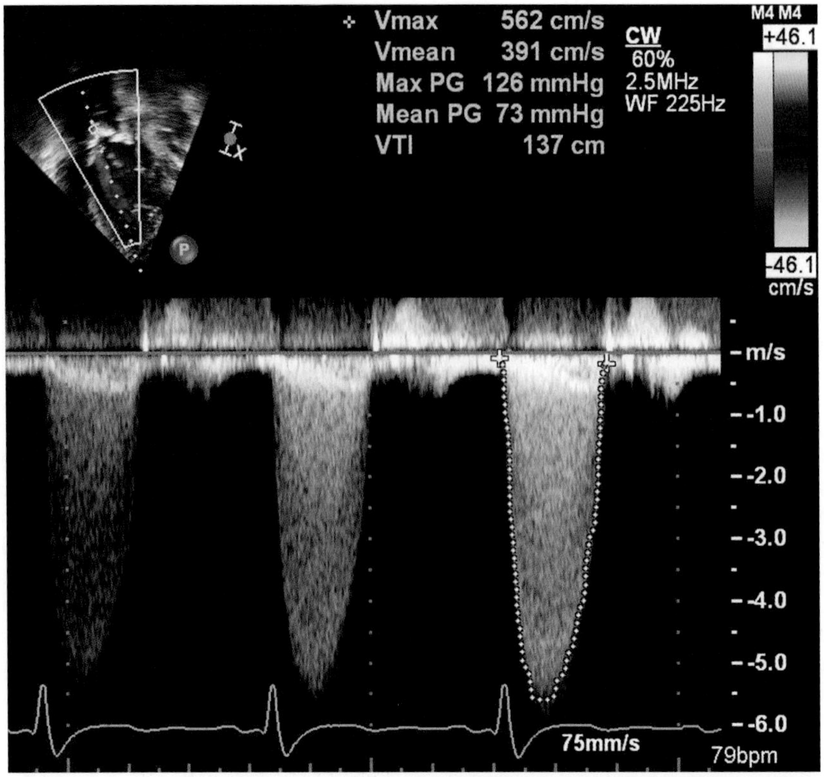

FIGURE 106-4 ■ Doppler echocardiography. Visualization of a high-velocity jet by color Doppler aids in aligning the continuous wave Doppler cursor in a patient with severe aortic valve stenosis (maximal instantaneous and mean gradients ≈126 and 73 mm Hg, respectively).

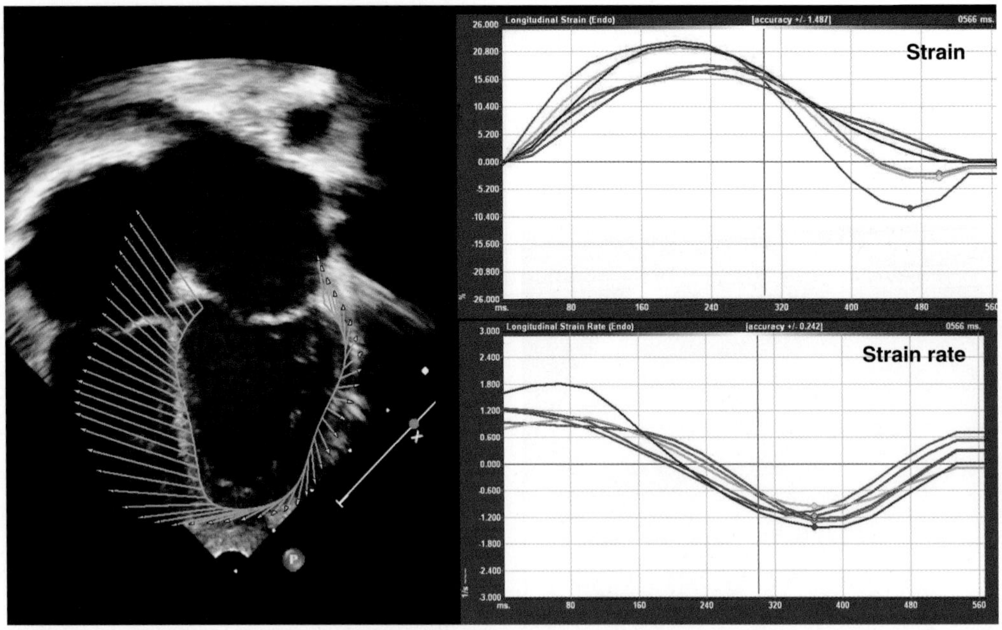

FIGURE 106-5 ■ Speckle-tracking echocardiography. Left panel: Apical four-chamber view with velocity vector mapping of the left ventricle. Right upper panel: Longitudinal strain versus time curves in six segments of the left ventricular wall. Right lower panel: Longitudinal strain rate versus time curves in the same segments.

Objectives of the Echocardiographic Examination

The objectives of the echocardiographic examination must be tailored to the individual patient. The initial evaluation should include a comprehensive survey of all anatomic elements of the central cardiovascular system.[10] Subsequent examinations are often targeted to answer specific clinical questions. It is important, however, to repeat complete echocardiograms during follow-up, even in patients who underwent a comprehensive initial examination, because of the dynamic nature of CHD. Examples include the late onset of discrete subaortic stenosis in patients with ventricular septal defect and/or coarctation of the aorta,[22] double-chambered right ventricle,[23] and supramitral stenosing ring.[24]

Examination Technique

Proper planning of the echocardiographic examination is important to ensure that all diagnostic information is obtained most efficiently. This is particularly relevant in sedated patients in whom the time available for data acquisition is limited. Ideally, a complete segmental examination of cardiovascular anatomy and function should be performed in every new patient. This includes determination of visceral situs, heart position, atrial situs, systemic and pulmonary venous connections, ventricular situs, atrioventricular and ventriculoarterial alignments and connections, and coronary and great arterial anatomy. Assessment of ventricular function, intracardiac and vessel dimensions, and flow analysis across all valves, septa, chambers, and vessels are integral parts of the examination. Echocardiographic techniques include two-dimensional and three-dimensional imaging, blood flow imaging by color Doppler, measurements of flow velocities by pulsed and continuous wave Doppler, and assessment of myocardial function by tissue Doppler or STE. In young children with suspected heart disease, the examination begins from the subxiphoid approach by determining the abdominal situs and then proceeding by scanning the heart and great vessels, using a step-by-step segmental analysis (Fig. 106-6*A* and *B*).[10,25,26] This approach is advantageous because it provides a wide-angle view of heart position and cardiovascular anatomy and function at an early stage in the examination. Subsequent two-dimensional and Doppler analyses from the apical, parasternal, and suprasternal notch views supplement and confirm findings from the subxiphoid window (see Fig. 106-6*C*-*G*). The examination strategy should be tailored to the individual patient and modified according to the clinical situation as necessary. Although the standard views just described should be obtained in almost every patient and represent the minimum acceptable examination, flexibility and improvisation are important to optimally use the full potential of echocardiography.

Anatomic Analysis

When performing and reviewing an echocardiographic examination in a patient suspected of having CHD, a stepwise segmental approach to analysis of cardiac anatomy is taken. Each component of the heart is analyzed separately according to its unique morphologic features.[25,26] The heart is composed of five segments—three main segments and two connecting segments. The three main segments are the atria, the ventricles, and the great arteries. The atrioventricular canal, which includes the mitral and tricuspid valves and the atrioventricular septum, connects the atria with the ventricles. The infundibulum (or conus) connects the ventricles with the great arteries. When analyzing cardiac anatomy, each cardiac chamber must be identified individually according to its unique anatomic-morphologic features and not according to its spatial position (right-sided or left-sided), valve of entry, or artery of exit. Throughout a systematic echocardiographic study, the examiner must go over a mental checklist of segments, their anatomic organization and position (situs), their connections and alignments with adjacent segments, and associated malformations. Using the aforementioned principles, any potential CHD can be accurately described in specific and precise terms. A detailed review of echocardiographic analysis of each cardiac segment can be found elsewhere.[10,25]

SPECIAL ECHOCARDIOGRAPHIC PROCEDURES

Transesophageal Echocardiography

Transesophageal echocardiography (TEE) was first introduced in 1976 and appeared in pediatric use in 1989. The miniaturization of probes and development of multiplanar imaging have greatly increased its role as an adjunct to transthoracic imaging, during surgical repair of CHD (intraoperative TEE), and to guide interventional catheterization procedures. Advances in transducer technology and image processing now allow real-time three-dimensional TEE.[9]

Indications and Objectives

A TEE examination is usually performed to answer specific clinical questions. It is advisable, however, to perform a comprehensive examination of the heart and blood vessels for additional unsuspected anatomic and/or hemodynamic anomalies (Fig. 106-7).[27] Miniaturization of TEE probes designed for use in young infants weighing 3 to 3.5 kg or less has greatly enhanced the scope of TEE in the pediatric age group.[28-31] Successful TEE examinations have been reported in patients weighing as little as 2.3 kg.[32,33] The role of TEE in pediatric cardiology is continuously evolving. Although the transthoracic window is adequate in most situations, TEE provides distinct advantages during cardiovascular surgery,[28,30,33] during video-assisted thoracoscopic procedures,[34] for guidance of interventional catheter procedures,[35,36] in the intensive care unit,[28,37] for detection of intracardiac thrombi and vegetations,[38] in the assessment of prosthetic valves,[39] in selected patients on mechanical assist device and extracorporeal membrane oxygenator,[40] and in selected patients with poor transthoracic windows, such as adults with CHD.[41] The usefulness of selective versus routine use of intraoperative TEE in patients with CHD deserves further study.[27,42]

Safety and Complications

Although in expert hands TEE is quite safe, complications have been reported, including oropharyngeal trauma and compression of airways and vascular structures.[43,44] TEE is contraindicated in patients with an unrepaired tracheoesophageal fistula, esophageal

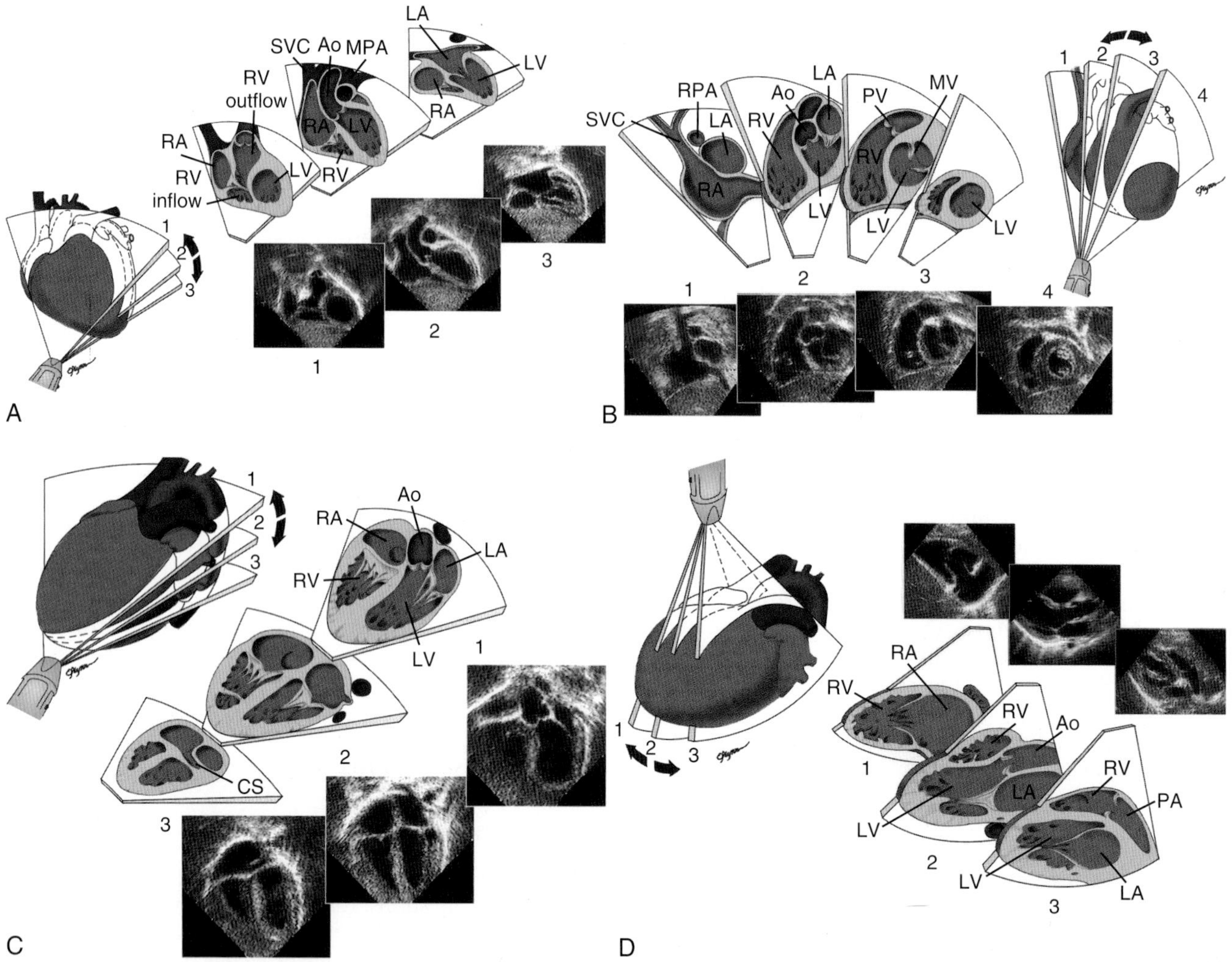

FIGURE 106-6 ■ Standard two-dimensional transthoracic imaging sweeps. **A,** Subxiphoid long-axis sweep. Slow gradual sweep starting at the level of the upper abdomen will show the connection of the inferior vena cava to the right atrium (RA). The left atrium (LA) is seen next. The connection of the pulmonary veins and the atrial septum can be demonstrated from this view. The left ventricle (LV) is seen along its long axis. Further superior angulation of the transducer depicts the left ventricular outflow tract, aortic valve, and ascending aorta (Ao). The superior vena cava (SVC) is seen to the right of the Ao and the main pulmonary artery (MPA) is seen to the left of the aorta. Further superior tilt of the transducer shows the inflow and outflow of the right ventricle (RV) and the pulmonary valve. The sweep ends with anterior free wall of the right ventricle. **B,** Subxiphoid short-axis sweep. From the subxiphoid long-axis view, the transducer is rotated clockwise approximately 90 degrees. The sweep begins at the rightward-most aspect of the heart and progresses from right to left through the cardiac apex. The superior vena cava (SVC) and inferior vena cava are seen entering the right atrium (RA). The right pulmonary artery (RPA) is seen in cross-section behind the SVC and above the left atrium (LA). The atrial septum is well seen in this plane. Sweeping the transducer leftward will show the base of the left ventricle (LV) and right ventricle (RV) and the atrioventricular valves. The aortic valve is seen in cross-section at this level. Further leftward tilt of the transducer depicts a cross-sectional view of the LV and mitral valve (MV) as well as the right ventricular outflow tract and pulmonary valve (PV). The sweep ends with imaging of the mid-muscular septum, the papillary muscles, and the apical portions of both ventricles. **C,** Apical four-chamber sweep. The transducer is positioned over the apex and angled to obtain a cross-sectional view of the atria and ventricles as shown in level 2. The transducer is then angled posteriorly to image the posterior aspect of the heart (level 3). In this plane, the coronary sinus (CS) can be viewed along the posterior left atrioventricular groove. Antero-superior tilt of the transducer will show the left ventricular outflow tract and proximal ascending aorta (Ao). **D,** Parasternal long-axis sweep. The transducer is placed over the left precordium to the left of the sternum with the index mark toward the patient's right shoulder. A rightward and inferior tilt of the transducer toward the right hip shows the right atrium (RA), tricuspid valve, and right ventricular inflow (RV) (level 1). The coronary sinus can be followed into the right atrium in this view. A leftward and superior tilt of the transducer toward the left shoulder depicts the right ventricular outflow tract (RV), pulmonary valve, and main pulmonary artery (PA) (level 3).

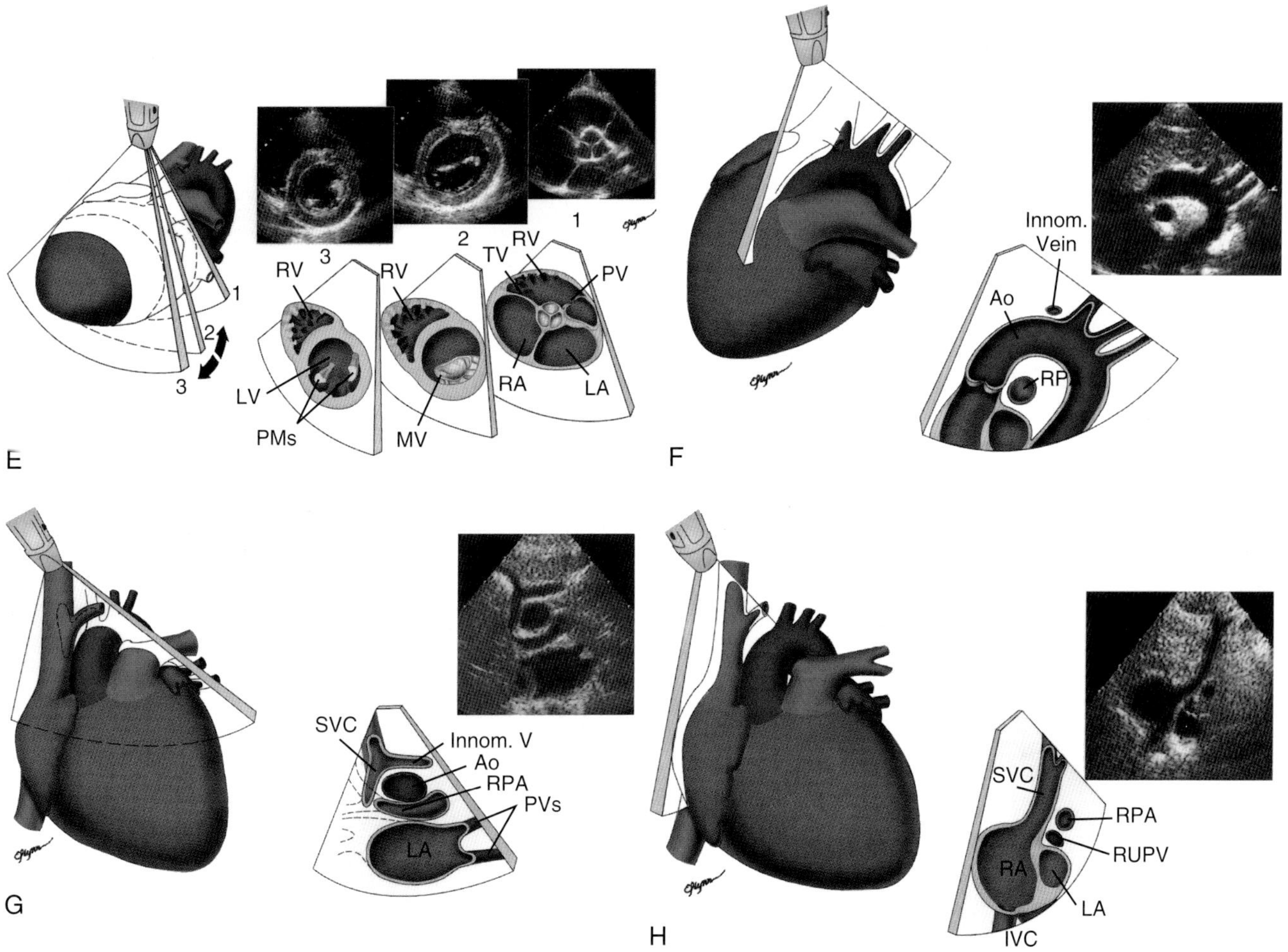

FIGURE 106-6, cont'd **E,** Parasternal short-axis sweep. From the parasternal long-axis view, the transducer is rotated clockwise approximately 90 degrees. The sweep progresses from a plane that shows the right and left atria (RA and LA), atrial septum, tricuspid valve (TV), right ventricle (RV), pulmonary valve (PV), and main pulmonary artery (level 1) toward the apex. Cross-sectional views of the right ventricle (RV), left ventricle (LV), ventricular septum, mitral valve (MV), and papillary muscles (PMs) are obtained. **F,** Aortic arch view from the suprasternal notch window. The innominate vein (Innom. Vein) is seen anterior to the innominate artery. The right pulmonary artery (RPA) is seen in cross-section behind the ascending aorta. **G,** Suprasternal notch view in the transverse plane. The left innominate vein (Innom. V) is seen draining into the superior vena cava (SVC). The distal ascending aorta (Ao) is seen superior to the right pulmonary artery (RPA), which is seen along its length above the left atrium (LA). Note the pulmonary veins entering the left atrium. **H,** High right parasternal view in the sagittal plane view showing the superior vena cava (SVC) entering the right atrium (RA). This view allows demonstration of the sinus venosus septum. *IVC,* Inferior vena cava; *RUPV,* right upper pulmonary vein.

obstruction or stricture, perforated viscus, or active gastrointestinal bleeding; in an unwilling or uncooperative patient who is inadequately sedated; or with an uncontrolled airway in a patient with respiratory or cardiac decompensation. Relative contraindications include cervical spine injury, immobility, or deformity; history of esophageal surgery; known esophageal varices or diverticulum; oropharyngeal deformities; and severe coagulopathy.[27,45,46]

Fetal Echocardiography

Examination of the human fetal cardiovascular system dates back to the late 1960s when continuous wave Doppler was used to record fetal heart rate. Although Kleinman and coworkers[47] in the late 1970s had some success in detecting CHD in the fetus by M-mode echocardiography, it was not until high-resolution two-dimensional imaging became available in the mid-1980s that accurate delineation of cardiovascular anatomy became clinically routine. Today, prenatal detection of CHD can be reliably diagnosed by 17 to 20 weeks of gestation by transabdominal imaging. Using the transvaginal window, the heart and great vessels can be imaged as early as late first trimester.[48]

Indications and Objectives

Although several studies have demonstrated a low detection rate of CHD by routine level I obstetric ultrasound,[49] cost-benefit considerations preclude universal fetal echocardiographic screening by expert pediatric echocardiographers. Alternatively, an approach based on targeting pregnancies that are at high risk for CHD is taken. Such an approach increases the yield of fetal echocardiography to approximately 30% when extracardiac anomalies are detected, to approximately 60% when level I scan detects possible CHD, and to almost 100% when a second

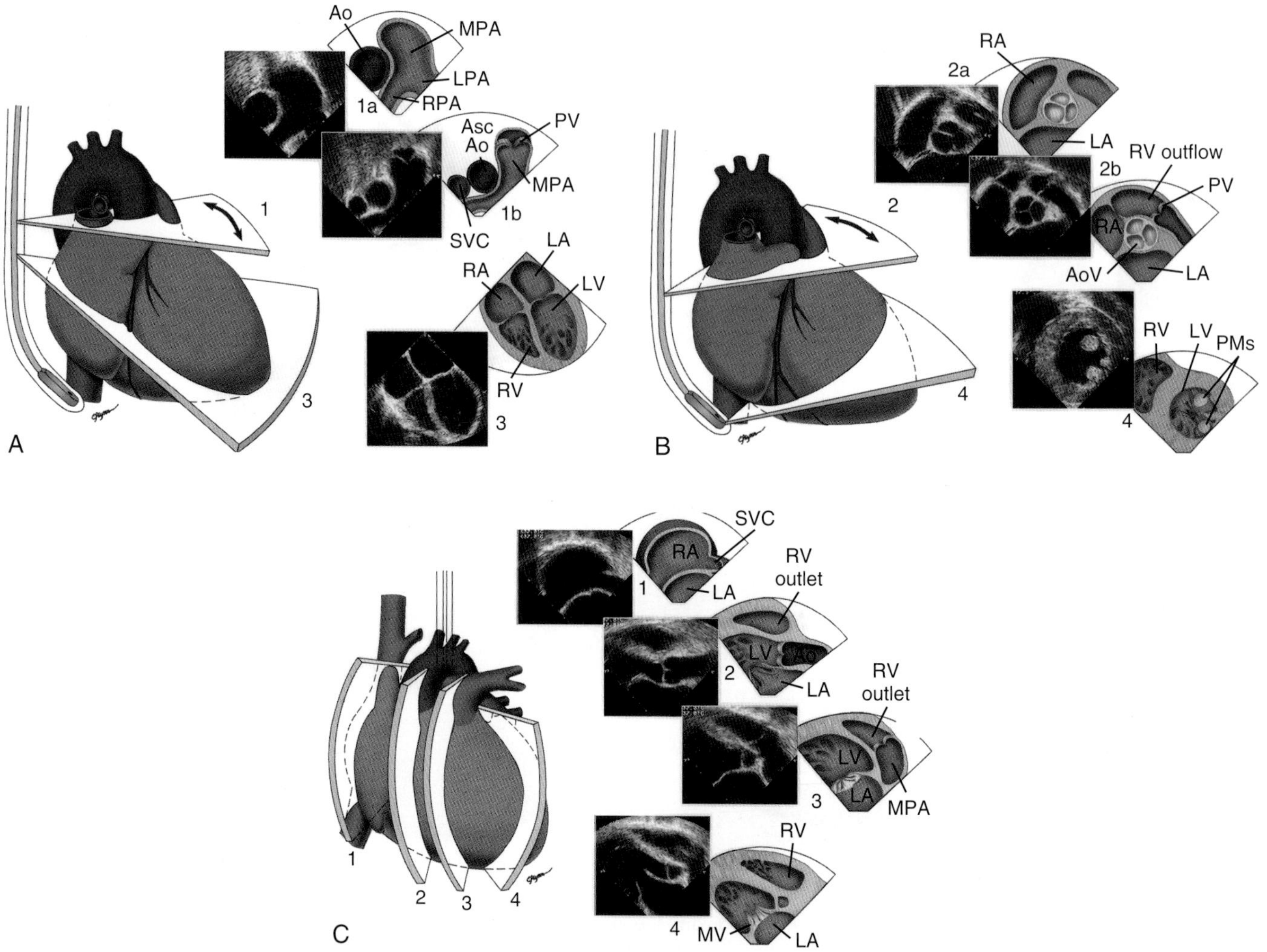

FIGURE 106-7 ■ Transesophageal imaging. **A,** Transverse plane: cross-sectional view at level 1a depicts the proximal ascending aorta (Ao), main pulmonary artery (MPA), and left and right pulmonary arteries (LPA and RPA, respectively). A rightward tilt of the transducer shows the RPA as it passes behind the superior vena cava (SVC) and ascending aorta (Asc Ao). To obtain a four-chamber view (level 3), the transducer is advanced in the esophagus with slight retroflexion of the scope. **B,** Level 2 is parallel to the transthoracic parasternal short-axis view. In level 2a, the atrial septum is imaged by a slight rightward tilt of the transducer. In level 2b, the aortic valve (AoV) is seen in cross-section in the center of the image, and the left atrium (LA), right atrium (RA), tricuspid valve, right ventricular outflow (RV outflow), pulmonary valve (PV), and the proximal main pulmonary artery are seen. By advancing the transducer into the lower esophagus and anteflexing the scope, a cross-sectional view of the left ventricle (LV), mitral valve, and papillary muscles (PMs) is obtained (level 4). Note that image orientation is the same as in transthoracic echocardiography. **C,** Vertical (longitudinal) plane: the sweep begins at a plane that crosses the superior vena cava (SVC), left atrium (LA), right atrium (RA), and atrial septum (level 1). Next, a leftward tilt of the transducer shows an image parallel to the transthoracic parasternal long-axis view of the left atrium (LA), mitral valve, left ventricle (LV), left ventricular outflow tract, and proximal aorta (Ao) (level 2). Further leftward tilt of the transducer (level 3) shows the right ventricular outflow tract (RV outlet), pulmonary valve, and main pulmonary artery (MPA). The sweep continues leftward to show the leftward aspects of the left atrium, mitral valve, and left ventricle (level 4). Further leftward tilt depicts the left atrial appendage and the left pulmonary veins (not shown). Note that image orientation is the same as in transthoracic echocardiography. *MV,* Mitral valve.

opinion is requested.[50,51] The indications for fetal echocardiography are summarized in Box 106-1.

Description of Technique

Echocardiographic examination of the cardiovascular system in the fetus is based on the same principles of the segmental approach to diagnosis of CHD that is applied after birth. The main difference between examination of the fetus and the newborn is that the operator has no control over fetal position and, consequently, over the views obtained. Once fetal position is ascertained and the spatial coordinates are determined, the examination then continues according to the principles outlined in the previous sections. Given optimal acoustic windows and favorable fetal position, even the most complex cardiovascular anomalies can be detected (Fig. 106-8).[52] Defects that remain difficult to diagnose in utero include secundum atrial septal defect, patent ductus arteriosus, small or moderate ventricular septal defect, coarctation of the aorta, and some valve and great vessel abnormalities.[53] Distinguishing between normal patency of the foramen ovale and an atrial septal defect is usually not possible in the fetus. Similarly, it is not possible to predict whether

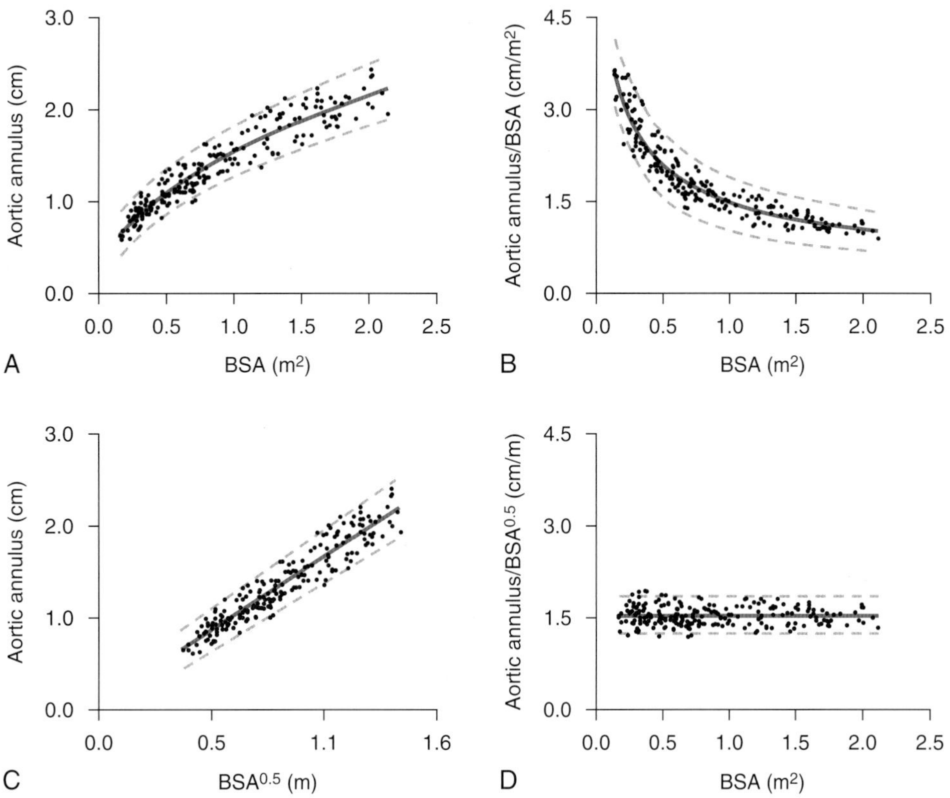

FIGURE 106-9 Rationale for indexing linear measurements to the square root of body surface area (BSA). **A,** Plot of aortic valve annulus diameter against BSA showing a nonlinear curve. **B,** Plot of aortic valve annulus diameter indexed to BSA against BSA shows that the indexed diameter decreases exponentially as BSA increases. **C,** Aortic valve annulus diameter plotted against the square root of BSA showing a linear relationship. **D,** Plot of aortic valve diameter indexed to the square root of BSA against BSA showing that the indexed aortic valve diameter is the same in children and adults with widely varying body size.

two-dimensional techniques.[8,64-68] Therefore, it is reasonable to expect that within several years three-dimensional echocardiography will replace two-dimensional methods for measurements of left and right ventricular volumes. Left ventricular myocardial volume can be measured from the two-dimensional echocardiogram by subtracting the endocardial volume from the epicardial volume. Left ventricular mass is calculated by multiplying the resultant myocardial volume by the density of muscle (1.055 g/mL). Because it is not influenced by acoustic windows and is independent of chamber geometry, MRI provides an excellent alternative to echocardiography in measuring chamber volume and mass and is considered the reference standard to which other techniques are compared (see Magnetic Resonance Imaging section, later).

Ventricular Function

Left ventricular function can be assessed at several levels. The heart may be viewed as a pump designed to maintain adequate flow to vital organs.[69] This approach focuses on the external work performed by the heart, but it ignores the internal work and the functional state of the myocardium. Measuring cardiac output and systemic and pulmonary venous blood pressures can assess the pump function of the heart. It is known, however, that cardiac output and blood pressure can remain within the normal limits despite significant myocardial dysfunction.[69]

Ejection-phase indices of ventricular function, including shortening fraction, fractional area change, ejection fraction, velocity of circumferential fiber shortening (VCF), peak dP/dt, and systolic time intervals, measure global pump function.[1,4,69] Common to these indices is their dependence on loading conditions. These indices are unable to distinguish between the effect(s) of altered loading conditions and abnormalities in myocardial contractility. Hence, abnormalities in preload and afterload can result in depressed shortening or ejection fractions leading to the erroneous interpretation that myocardial contractility is depressed. Conversely, left ventricular myocardial contractility may be depressed even in the presence of normal shortening or ejection fractions. The advantage of most of these indices is their relative simplicity and ease of acquisition. Load-independent assessment of left ventricular systolic function requires a more sophisticated analysis. The interested reader is referred to the relevant chapters in this book and to other reviews of this topic.[69]

The previously described methods of ventricular function assessment rely in part on measurements of ventricular dimensions. An alternative approach is to evaluate myocardial motion and deformation.[70] Several methods have been developed to measure myocardial velocities, strain, strain rate, displacement, and torsion (twist). One method uses Doppler to measure myocardial velocities (Doppler tissue imaging [DTI]) and to calculate strain, strain rate, and other variables of tissue deformation

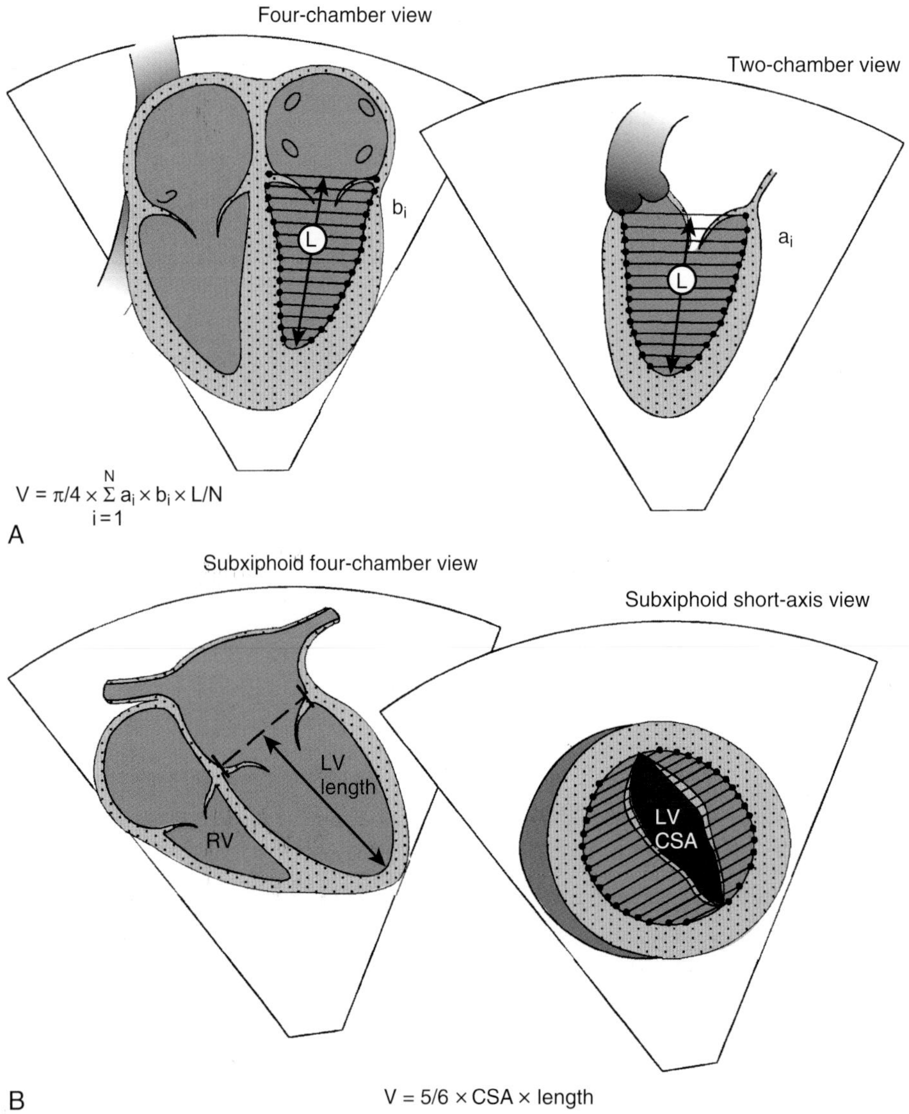

FIGURE 106-10 ■ Methods for assessment of left ventricular volume by two-dimensional echocardiography. **A,** Biplane Simpson rule for calculating left ventricular volume (see text for details). **B,** Area-length method for calculating left ventricular volume. *a_i,* Slice radius in the apical two-chamber view; *b_i,* slice radius in the apical four-chamber view; *CSA,* cross-sectional area; *L,* left ventricular length; *N,* number of slices; *V,* volume.

(Fig. 106-11*A*).[71-73] The other method, STE, analyzes the frame-to-frame changes in ultrasonic signal characteristics and uses that information to track the myocardium throughout the cardiac cycle (see Fig. 106-11*B*).[12,74] These methods are independent of ventricular geometry and provide information on systolic and diastolic function.[75-77] The reproducibility and the prognostic role of these techniques in patients with CHD are the subject of ongoing investigations.[17]

Doppler Evaluation of Pressure Gradients

Estimation of the pressure difference between adjacent compartments has been widely applied in clinical pediatric echocardiography (see Fig. 106-4).[1,4,10] Among the most common uses is estimation of pressure drop across stenotic areas and prediction of pressure in cardiac chambers. For example, the systolic pressure in the right ventricle can be predicted from the peak pressure difference between it and the right atrium derived from the peak velocity of the tricuspid regurgitation jet. Right ventricular systolic pressure can also be assessed from knowledge of left ventricular pressure (by measurement of systemic blood pressure by sphygmomanometry) and the pressure drop across a ventricular septal defect. In principle, the pressure gradient across any two compartments connected by flow can be estimated by Doppler, provided that the limitations of the technique are taken into consideration and the sources of error in the application and interpretation of the technique are eliminated.

Calculation of Pressure Gradients

The Bernoulli equation relates pressure difference (ΔP) between two points separated by a distance (s) to the

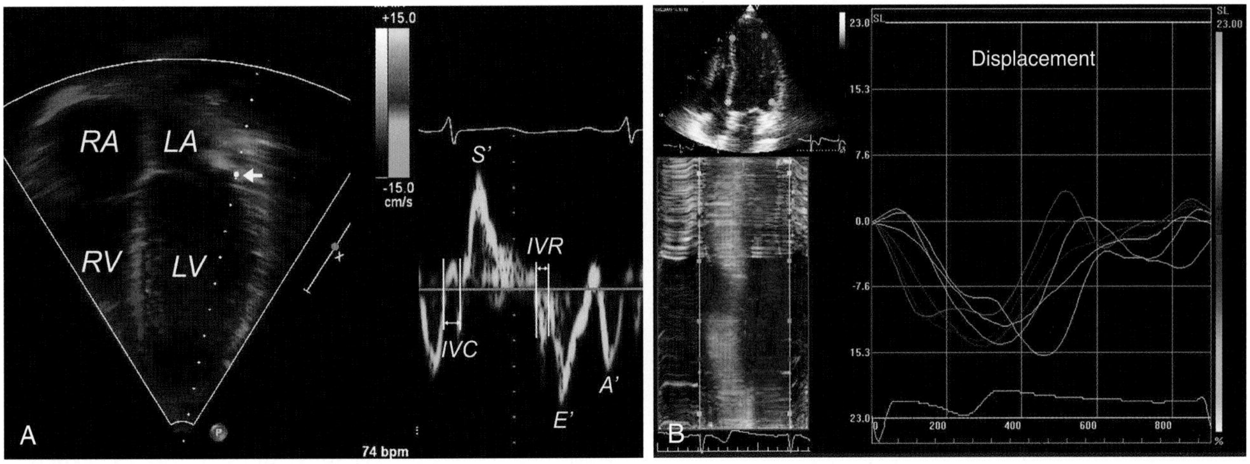

FIGURE 106-11 Evaluation of myocardial motion by echocardiography. **A,** Tissue Doppler imaging. Left ventricular myocardial velocity is sampled at the level of the mitral valve annulus *(arrow)*. The velocity-time curve shown on the right panel demonstrates myocardial velocities relative to the apex. **B,** Speckle-tracking evaluation of left ventricular wall motion evaluated from the apical four-chamber view. Displacement of the left ventricular free wall and septum is simultaneously tracked in multiple points. *A',* Late (atrial) diastolic velocity; *bpm,* beats per minute; *E',* early diastolic velocity; *IVC,* isovolumic contraction period; *IVR,* isovolumic relaxation period; *LA,* left atrium; *LV,* left ventricle; *RA,* right atrium; *RV,* right ventricle; *S',* systolic velocity.

velocities at the two points (V_1 and V_2, respectively), the fluid density (for blood, ρ = 1060 kg/liter), and the velocity-dependent viscous friction according to the following equation:

$$\Delta P = \overbrace{\frac{1}{2}\rho\left(V_2^2 - V_1^2\right)}^{\text{convective acceleration}} + \overbrace{\rho\int_1^2 \frac{d\vec{V}}{dt}d\vec{s}}^{\text{flow acceleration}} + \overbrace{R(\vec{V})}^{\text{viscous friction}}$$

For most clinical applications of the Bernoulli equation, the convective acceleration component of the formula is considered the most significant. After combining ρ for blood with conversion factors to mm Hg and velocity to m/sec, the coefficient calculates out to 3.98. In most clinical applications this factor is rounded to 4.0. The second term of the equation, flow acceleration, represents the pressure drop generated by flow acceleration. This phenomenon, however, is important only during a very brief period at the rapid acceleration phase when there is a lag between the velocity and the pressure curves. During that time period, the pressure gradient is not considered clinically important. The third term represents the force necessary to overcome viscous friction. When considering pressure drops across a discrete orifice, viscous friction becomes negligible. Hence, for most clinical applications the formula is simplified based on the following assumptions: (1) the velocity proximal to the obstruction (V_1) is assumed to be negligible compared with the velocity just distal to the obstruction (V_2); (2) in most clinical situations, peak flow acceleration occurs in early systole when the pressure gradient is irrelevant and can be ignored; and (3) viscous friction is assumed to be trivial. The Bernoulli equation can therefore be simplified: $\Delta P = 4(V_2)^2$. This formula has been shown to be valid in in vitro flow models[78] and in various clinical settings.[79] However, the assumptions that govern the use of the simplified Bernoulli equation may not always be correct. For example, in long-segment narrowing such as a Blalock-Taussig shunt, ignoring the viscous friction term of the Bernoulli equation may lead to significant underestimation of the pressure drop. The limitations and pitfalls that can potentially lead to errors in estimation of pressure gradients have been reviewed elsewhere.[1,11]

Safety and Complications

Because of the widespread use of echocardiography in the diagnosis and monitoring of children with suspected heart disease, safety of the technique is of prime importance. This is particularly relevant in fetal echocardiography where fetuses may be exposed to ultrasound energy early in gestation. To date, no reports on adverse effects from diagnostic ultrasound have been reported. Physicians involved with diagnostic ultrasound must be aware that ultrasound is a form of mechanical energy that under certain conditions can cause biological damage to exposed tissue. This damage can result from conversion of mechanical energy to heat or from creation of gaseous microcavitations. Thus far, it appears that biological damage has been observed only in nonclinical laboratory conditions. The American Institute of Ultrasound in Medicine stated that "no confirmed biologic effects on patients or instrument operator caused by exposure at intensities typical of present diagnostic ultrasound instruments have ever been reported. Although the possibility exists that such biologic effects may be identified in the future, current data indicate that the benefits to patients of the prudent use of diagnostic ultrasound outweigh the risks, if any, that may be present."[80]

MAGNETIC RESONANCE IMAGING

Cardiovascular MRI is a sophisticated noninvasive imaging modality that overcomes many of the limitations of echocardiography and cardiac catheterization. High-resolution static and dynamic images of the heart, blood vessels, and other thoracic structures are obtained regardless of body size and acoustic barriers. Moreover, cardiovascular MRI provides additional unique information that is not made available by other imaging techniques. As a result of the rapid technologic evolution in computer sciences, electronics, and engineering over the past decade, cardiovascular MRI has evolved from a technique that produced several static images in an hour-long examination to a modality capable of real-time imaging,[81,82] succinct dynamic three-dimensional visualization of cardiovascular anatomy,[83] imaging of the fetus,[84] and accurate quantification of blood flow[85] and myocardial function.[86] These capabilities have greatly expanded the role of cardiovascular MRI in preoperative and postoperative evaluation of infants, children, and adults with CHD.

Magnetic Resonance Imaging Techniques and Their Clinical Applications

In MRI, magnetic fields and radiofrequency energy are used to stimulate hydrogen nuclei in selected regions of the body to emit radiofrequency waves that are then used to construct images. As with other cardiovascular imaging modalities, a thorough understanding of the underlying imaging physics enhances the quality and interpretation of the diagnostic data. This section provides a practical introduction to cardiovascular MRI; a more detailed discussion can be found in other sources.[87,88]

To produce an image, the patient is first placed inside the scanner, which applies a static high-strength magnetic field. Most clinical scanners use static magnetic field strengths ranging from 0.5 tesla (T) to 3 T (1 tesla = 10,000 gauss [G]; the strength of earth's magnetic field at its surface is approximately 0.5 G). Higher magnetic field strengths are used mostly in research scanners. Once positioned within the scanner, a section of the patient's body is then excited using a radiofrequency pulse, and an echo is formed by means of a second radiofrequency pulse (spin echo) and/or gradient pulses (gradient echo). The signal from the echo is then processed by Fourier transformation and the data are used to fill a line of matrix from which the image is generated.

Cardiac and Respiratory Gating

The heart, blood, and blood vessels are in relatively rapid motion compared with other body structures. Although the speed of MRI continues to improve, standard techniques are too slow to image the heart in real time with adequate spatial and temporal resolution for most applications. Rather, an image at a particular point during the cardiac cycle is built up from data acquired over multiple cardiac cycles. Consequently, synchronization with the cardiac cycle is required to "return" to the same point in the cycle and effectively freeze cardiac motion. Imaging may be synchronized or "gated" with a pulse oxymetry trace (so-called peripheral gating) or, more optimally, with a high-quality electrocardiogram signal. Because images are constructed over multiple cardiac cycles, respiratory motion can degrade image quality. One approach to minimizing respiratory artifacts is to have the patient hold his or her breath during image acquisition. Although this solution is often effective, it cannot be used in patients who are too young or ill to cooperate. In such cases, respiratory motion compensation can be achieved by synchronizing image data acquisition to the respiratory as well as the cardiac cycle. Respiratory motion can be tracked either by a bellows device placed around the body or by MRI navigator echoes that concurrently image the position of the diaphragm or heart. The principal limitation of respiratory gating is that it substantially prolongs scan times because image data are accepted during only a portion of the respiratory cycle. A final strategy to minimize respiratory motion artifacts is to acquire multiple images at the same location and average them, thereby minimizing variations due to respiration. As expected, the disadvantage of this approach is again increased scan time.

This discussion highlights the need for more rapid high-quality MRI techniques that will obviate the need for cardiac gating and respiratory motion compensation. Recent advances in gradient coil performance and parallel acquisition methods have achieved this goal and have become widely available in the clinical arena.[89-93]

Cardiovascular MRI examination is performed by repeatedly selecting a pulse sequence, prescribing an imaging location, and acquiring the image data to address specific clinical questions.[94] The pulse sequence specifies how the magnetic field gradients and radiofrequency pulses are applied and read during image acquisition. Table 106-1 summarizes the features of some of the common cardiovascular MRI sequences used in clinical practice. In general, there are two major categories of pulse sequences—spin echo and gradient echo (see Table 106-1). Spin echo sequences are characterized by applying a radiofrequency pulse that tips hydrogen protons by 90 degrees, followed by a second, 180-degree pulse, and they are usually used to generate images in which flowing blood appears black. Gradient echo sequences apply radiofrequency pulses that are less than 90 degrees (usually 15 to 60 degrees), are faster than spin echo sequences, and are usually used to generate images in which flowing blood appears white. Adding preparatory pulses that alter tissue contrast can often modify a particular pulse sequence. In addition, there are numerous user-selectable imaging parameters that affect tissue contrast, image quality, and temporal and spatial resolution. The numerous imaging techniques and parameters to choose from allow the operator to adjust image contrast for optimal anatomic definition and detection of abnormal tissue. They also provide the capability for sophisticated functional assessment. The following section reviews the more common cardiovascular MRI techniques with a focus on their clinical usefulness.

Anatomic Imaging and Tissue Characteristics

Spin echo pulse sequences are usually used to produce images in which flowing blood has low signal intensity and appears dark ("black blood" imaging). Other tissues

TABLE 106-1 **Summary of MRI Techniques**

Technique	ECG Triggering	Appearance of Blood Flow	Dynamic (Cine*) vs. Static†	Clinical Application
I. Spin Echo				
Standard spin echo	Yes	Dark	Static	Anatomy, tissue characterization
Fast spin echo with double-inversion recovery	Yes	Dark	Static	Anatomy, tissue characterization, faster image acquisition relative to standard spin echo
II. Gradient Echo				
Segmented k-space fast gradient echo or steady-state free precession	Yes	Bright	Dynamic	Anatomy, ventricular function, blood flow imaging
Phase contrast	Yes	Bright	Dynamic	Flow quantification and characterization
Tagging	Yes	Bright	Dynamic	Analysis of myocardial mechanics and flow
Gadolinium-enhanced three-dimensional MRA	No	Bright	Static	Three-dimensional anatomic data set
MR fluoroscopy	No	Bright	Dynamic	Anatomy, function, guidance of interventional procedures
Delayed enhancement	Yes	Intermediate	Static	Myocardial viability

*Cine: Multiple images are obtained throughout the cardiac cycle in each anatomic location. The stacked images are then displayed on a computer screen in a cine-loop format.
†Static: A single image is obtained in each anatomic location.
ECG, Electrocardiography; *MR,* magnetic resonance; *MRA,* magnetic resonance angiography.

appear as varying shades of gray. Although cardiac-gated spin echo sequences produce only one image per location and thus provide only static anatomic information, their advantages include high spatial resolution, excellent blood-myocardium contrast, and decreased artifact from metallic biomedical implants (e.g., sternal wires, stents, prosthetic valves). Spin echo sequences are also easily modified to alter tissue contrast and characterize abnormal structures. Their clinical uses include evaluation for arrhythmogenic right ventricular cardiomyopathy,[95] cardiac tumors,[96-98] constrictive pericardial disease,[99] vessel wall abnormalities,[100] trachea and mainstem bronchi,[101] and thoracic masses (Fig. 106-12).[102] Fast (turbo) spin echo sequences allow one location to be imaged rapidly enough for the patient to breath-hold (10 to 15 seconds). A double-inversion preparatory pulse is usually applied to suppress the blood signal,[103] and an additional inversion pulse may be applied to suppress fat signal.

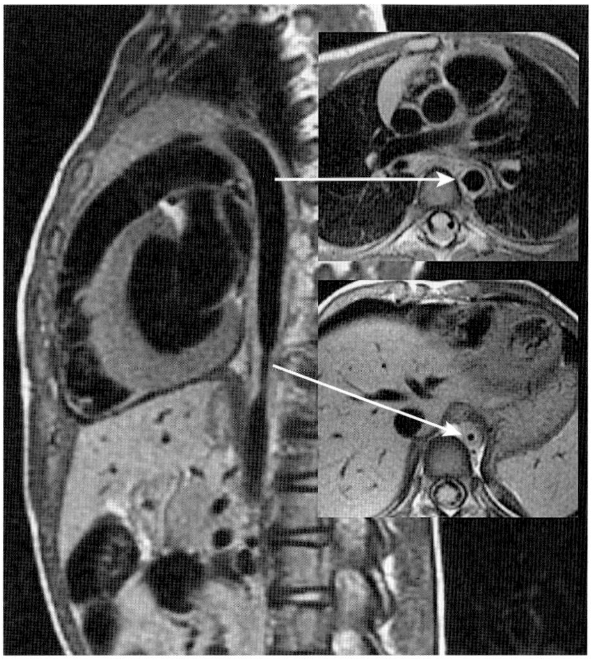

FIGURE 106-12 ■ Electrocardiographically triggered, breath-hold, proton density–weighted, fast spin echo with double-inversion recovery images showing severe coarctation of the descending aorta at the level of the diaphragm in a 5-year-old patient with Takayasu aortitis. Note the markedly thickened aortic wall with severe luminal narrowing on the axial plane image *(arrows).*

Cine Magnetic Resonance Imaging

Cardiac-gated gradient echo sequences can be used to produce multiple images over the cardiac cycle in each anatomic location. These images can then be displayed in a cine-loop format to demonstrate the motion of the heart and vasculature over the cardiac cycle. On such cine MR images, flowing blood produces a bright signal, and the myocardium and vessel wall are relatively dark ("bright-blood" imaging) (Fig. 106-13). The most commonly used cine MR technique is steady-state free precession cine MR sequences.[104,105] This technique relies on the ratio of T2-to-T1 relaxation, which results in high contrast between the blood pool (T2/T1 = 360/1200 =

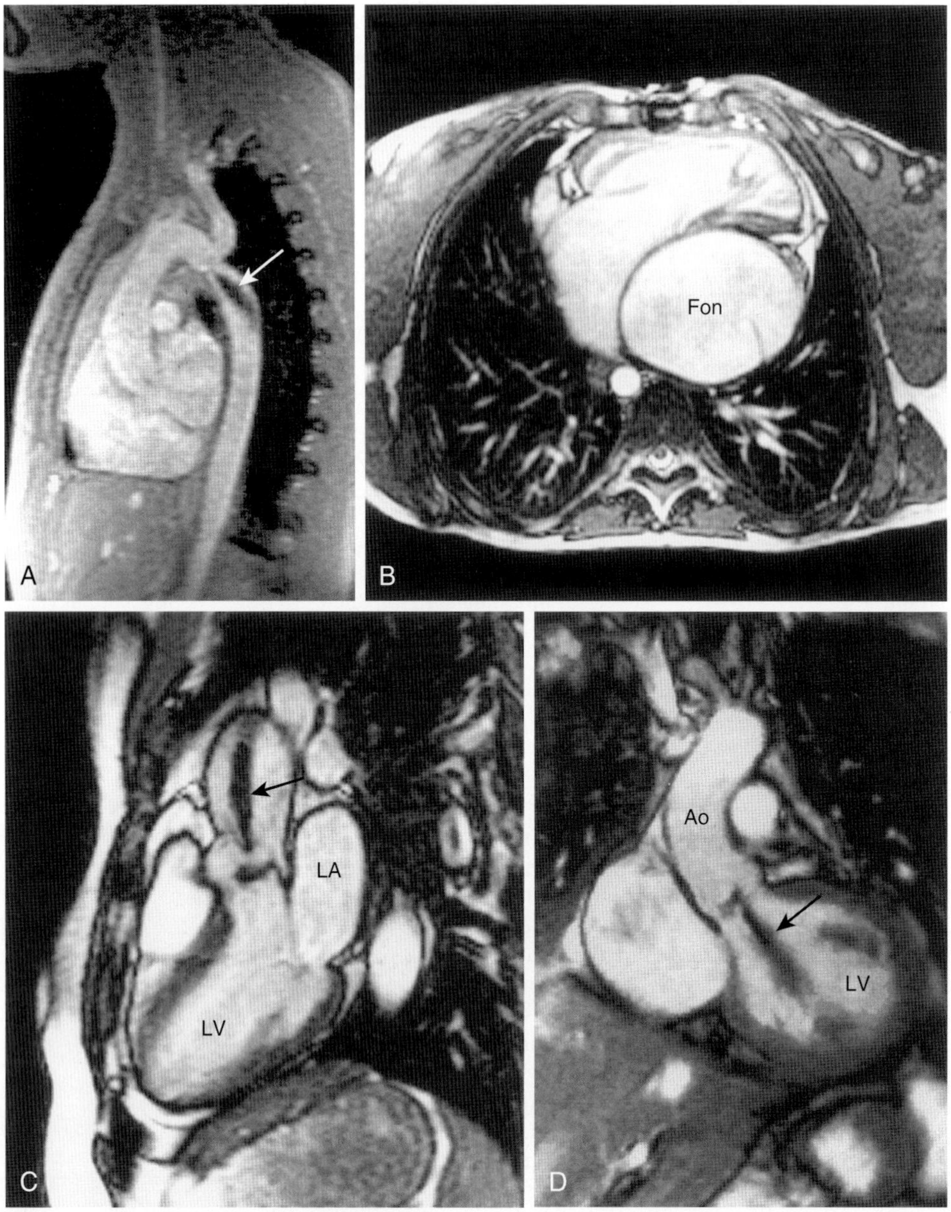

FIGURE 106-13 ■ Clinical applications of gradient echo cine magnetic resonance imaging. **A,** Electrocardiographically triggered breath-hold segmented k-space fast spoiled gradient echo multiphase sequence in a patient with severe coarctation of the aorta. The relatively long echo time allows for clear depiction of the dephasing jet in systole *(arrow)* indicating high-velocity turbulent flow. **B,** Axial plane electrocardiographically triggered steady-state free precession multiphase sequence in a patient with heterotaxy syndrome and single ventricle after a Fontan operation. Note the left-sided Fontan pathway (Fon) as well as the clear depiction of intracardiac anatomy. **C,** Systolic turbulent jet *(arrow)* in a patient with aortic valve stenosis. **D,** Diastolic turbulent jet *(arrow)* in a patient with aortic valve regurgitation. *Ao,* Aorta; *LA,* left atrium; *LV,* left ventricle.

0.3) and the myocardium (T2/T1 = 57/880 = 0.085), providing clear definition of cardiovascular structures. Image acquisition is short (4 to 10 seconds depending on heart rate) and is further shortened by parallel processing, permitting real-time magnetic resonance fluoroscopy.[84,106-108]

Cine MRI is used to delineate cardiovascular anatomy and assess ventricular function. It is helpful for evaluating the systemic and pulmonary veins,[109] atrial and ventricular septa,[110-112] intracardiac baffles and pathways (e.g., after Fontan, Mustard, Senning, and Rastelli procedures),[113] ventricular outflow tracts, ventricular-arterial conduits,[114] pulmonary arteries, and the aorta. It is also useful in identifying stenotic and regurgitant jets, which appear as dark signal voids (see Fig. 106-13). Myocardial tagging is a modification of cine MRI that allows for a sophisticated analysis of regional myocardial function (see Ventricular Function section, earlier).[86,115]

Magnetic Resonance Imaging Assessment of Ventricular Function

The principal MRI sequence used for evaluation of ventricular function is gradient echo cine MRI. An electrocardiographically triggered segmented k-space fast (also termed *turbo*) gradient recall echo sequence was used extensively during the 1990s, and its accuracy and reproducibility in measuring left and right ventricular volumes, mass, and ejection fraction have been extensively validated.[116-118] Since the early 2000s, steady-state free precession cine MR has replaced other gradient echo techniques. This sequence has been shown to provide a sharper contrast between the blood pool and the myocardium and to reduce motion-induced blurring during systole.[89,119,120]

Quantitative evaluation of ventricular function is achieved by obtaining a series of contiguous cine MRI slabs that cover the ventricles in short-axis view (Fig. 106-14).[82,86,121,122] By tracing the blood-endocardium boundary, the slab's volume is calculated as the product of its cross-sectional area and thickness (which is prescribed by the operator). Ventricular volume is then determined by summation of the volumes of all slabs. The process can be repeated for each frame in the cardiac cycle to obtain a continuous time-volume loop, or it can be performed only on a diastolic and a systolic frame to calculate diastolic and systolic volumes. From these data, left and right ventricular ejection fractions and stroke volumes can be calculated. Because the patient's heart rate at the time of image acquisition is known, left and right ventricular output can be calculated. Ventricular mass is calculated by tracing the epicardial borders, subtracting the endocardial volumes, and multiplying the resultant muscle volume by the specific gravity of the myocardium (1.05 g/mm^3). Most manufacturers of MRI scanners and some third-party companies offer software packages that automatically perform these calculations. Development of algorithms for automatic border detection has facilitated the application of these techniques, but further refinements are required to improve its accuracy.[123] Because of the accurate spatial and temporal registration of data, MRI measurements of chamber dimensions have become the accepted reference standard to which other methods are compared.[124,125] For example, Bellenger and colleagues measured left ventricular volumes in 64 patients with dilated cardiomyopathy.[126] They reported an intraobserver variability of 2.4% ± 2.5%, interobserver variability of 5.1% ± 3.7%, and interstudy variability (repeat MRI examinations) of 2.9% ± 1.2%. In patients with normal and dilated right ventricles, Mooij and coworkers reported interobserver intraclass correlation coefficients of 0.977 for right ventricular end-diastolic volume, 0.989 for left ventricular end-diastolic volume, 0.947 for right ventricular stroke volume, 0.973 for left ventricular stroke volume, and 0.789 and 0.81 for right and left ventricular ejection fraction, respectively.[127]

Steady-state free precession cine MRI is also used to evaluate regional wall motion abnormalities and segmental wall thickening.[128] Dobutamine stress MRI has been reported to be a useful test in adults with coronary artery disease,[129-131] and initial experience in pediatric patients is

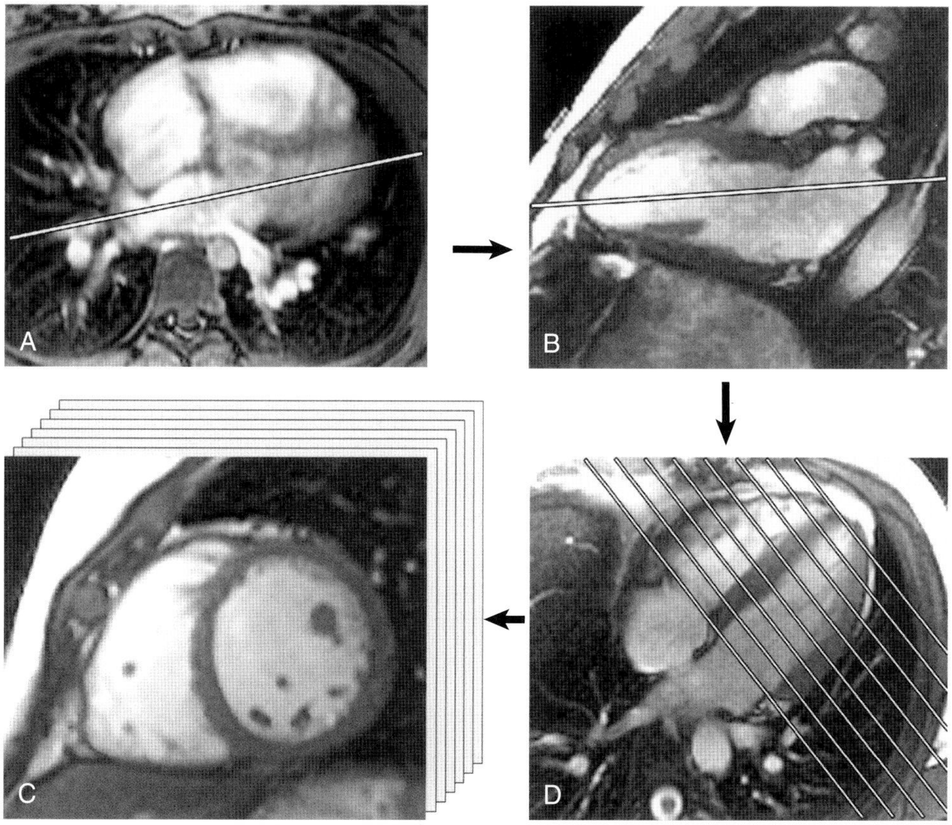

FIGURE 106-14 ■ Cine magnetic resonance imaging technique for assessment of ventricular dimensions and function. **A,** Using a localizing image in the axial plane, an imaging plane is placed parallel to the left ventricular septal surface. **B,** Two-chamber plane. **C,** Four-chamber plane. **D,** Short-axis plane. To obtain complete coverage of the ventricles, 12 contiguous imaging slabs are placed from the plane of the atrioventricular valves through the cardiac apex.

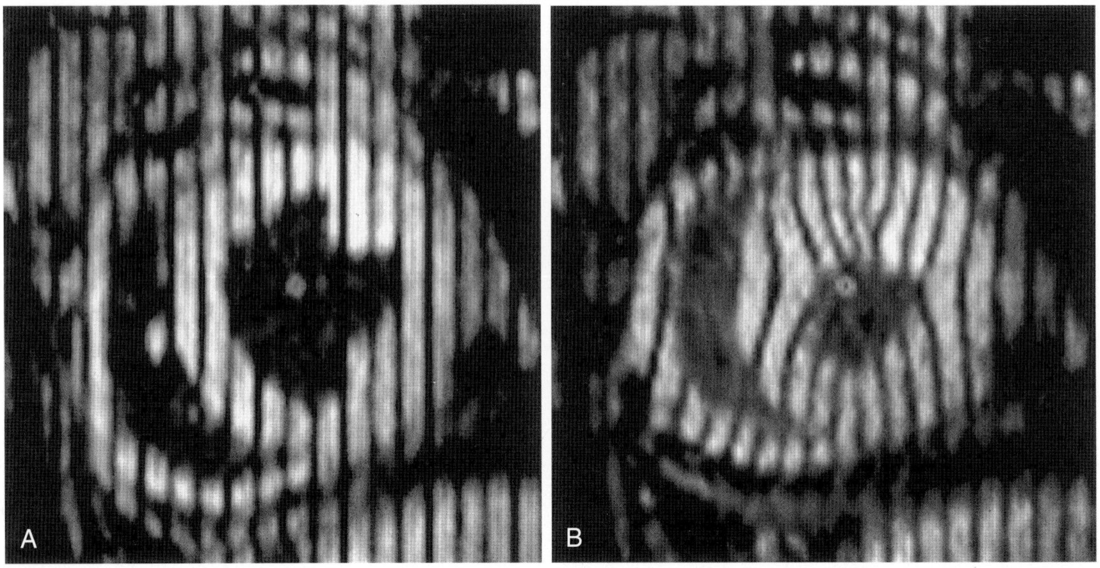

FIGURE 106-15 ■ Myocardial tagging. **A,** Diastolic frame shows the undistorted tags before the onset of systole. **B,** Systolic frame shows distortion of the myocardial tags caused by cardiac motion. Notice the undistorted tags on the chest wall and liver.

encouraging.[132] More recently, the use of an MRI-compatible supine cycle ergometer has been reported to allow assessment of ventricular function and valve regurgitation response to exercise.[133,134]

Another approach to MRI evaluation of ventricular function and myocardial mechanics is to visualize and measure myocardial motion. This can be done by myocardial tagging,[135] velocity-encoded cine MRI, or feature-tracking cardiac MRI.[136] In myocardial tagging, with the use of a preparatory radiofrequency gradient echo pulse sequence such as spatial modulation of magnetization (SPAMM), the spin of the protons in selected parts of the image volume are flipped in such a way as to render them incapable of producing a signal. This results in stripes of signal void (dark stripes) across the image (Fig. 106-15). The grid or stripes are placed at the onset of the R wave and is followed by a gradient echo cine MRI sequence. As the myocardium moves during the cardiac cycle, the tags follow it and their rotation, translation, and deformation can be tracked, allowing for calculation of myocardial strain and strain rate.[137-140] A recently described technique for the analysis of myocardial tagging data, harmonic phase imaging, shortens the analysis time because it does not require manual tracing of the tags.[141] Despite extensive research on myocardial tagging, the technique has not gained general acceptance in routine clinical practice. More recently, use of feature tracking MRI has been reported in CHD patients with promising early results (Fig. 106-16).[142,143] An advantage of feature tracking over myocardial tagging is that it can be performed on routinely acquired cine SSFP images, as opposed to the special image acquisitions required for tagging analysis.

Blood Flow Analysis

An ECG-gated velocity-encoded cine MRI (VEC MRI) sequence, a type of gradient echo sequence, can be used to measure blood flow velocity and quantify blood flow rate.[85,144] The VEC MRI technique is based on the principle that the signal from hydrogen nuclei (such as those in blood) flowing through specially designed magnetic field gradients accumulates a predictable phase shift that is proportional to its velocity. Multiple phase images are constructed across the cardiac cycle in which the voxel intensity or brightness is proportional to blood velocity within that voxel. Flow quantification is performed by placing an imaging slab across a blood vessel or through the area at question within the heart (Fig. 106-17*A*). The operator then determines whether flow velocity encoding is performed only perpendicular to the imaging plane (*z*-axis) or in other directions as well (*x*-axis and *y*-axis). The data are then analyzed off-line using specialized software. A region of interest (ROI) is defined by the operator around the lumen of the relevant vessel and the instantaneous mean velocity of each voxel is calculated (see Fig. 106-17*B* and *C*). Flow rate is calculated as the product of the mean velocities within the ROI and its cross-sectional area. Integration of the instantaneous flow rates over the cardiac cycle yields the stroke volume (see Fig. 106-17*D*). This technique has been shown by in vitro and in vivo studies to be accurate and reproducible.[144,145] Cine phase contrast has been widely applied to measure systemic and pulmonary blood flow and their ratio, as well as flow in individual pulmonary arteries, across the mitral and tricuspid valves, across an atrial septal defect, in systemic and pulmonary veins and in other individual blood vessels. This technique also allows accurate quantification of regurgitation volume and fraction across any cardiac valve.[146] An example of an important application of this technique in CHD is the quantification of pulmonary regurgitation in patients who have undergone tetralogy of Fallot repair.[147] When flow encoding is performed in three spatial directions, multidimensional flow imaging and analysis can be accomplished by resolving the flow velocities and directions into flow vectors that can be viewed in cine-loop format (Fig. 106-18). This technique allows unique

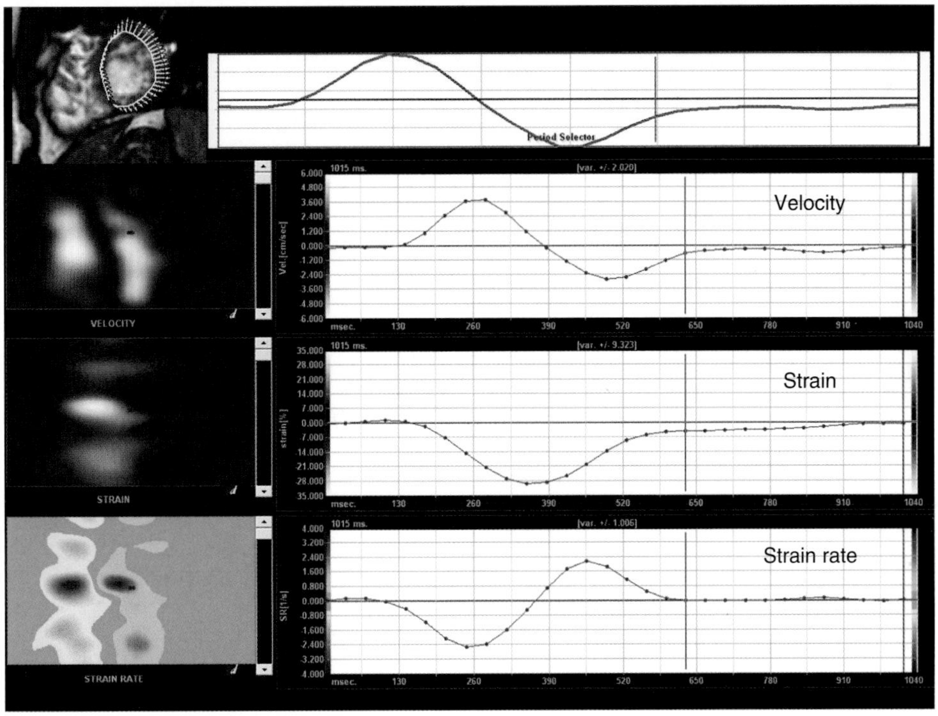

FIGURE 106-16 ■ Magnetic resonance imaging evaluation of myocardial deformation using speckle-tracking analysis. Circumferential left ventricular myocardial velocity, strain, and strain rates are shown.

imaging of blood flow in five dimensions (*x*, *y*, and *z* spatial dimensions, velocity, and time).[148] It also allows quantitative analysis of flow dynamics, including the ability to calculate the shear stress exerted by the flowing blood on the vessel wall.[149]

Contrast-Enhanced Magnetic Resonance Angiography

Another approach for improving the contrast between vascular and nonvascular structures is to administer an exogenous intravenous contrast agent, typically a gadolinium chelate, which dramatically shortens the T1 relaxation of blood, resulting in a bright signal on T1-weighted sequences. This method of angiography is less prone to flow-related artifacts than other MR techniques and has a short acquisition time. Contrast-enhanced magnetic resonance angiography (MRA) is usually performed without cardiac gating using a three-dimensional fast gradient echo acquisition lasting 15 to 30 seconds while the patient holds his or her breath.[150] The time delay between contrast administration and image acquisition determines the vascular territory illustrated, and several acquisitions can be performed. The entire procedure takes only a few minutes to perform and yields a high-contrast and high-resolution three-dimensional data set depicting all or part of the thorax. The three-dimensional data set can be navigated on dedicated workstations using various image display techniques, including rapid construction of intuitive three-dimensional models (Fig. 106-19). Unlike cine MRI, conventional contrast-enhanced MRA is not time resolved. However, with continued improvements in imaging speed, time-resolved MRA is now possible.[151] MRA is ideally suited to elucidate the anatomy of the aorta and its branches, pulmonary arteries, pulmonary veins, and systemic veins.[152,153] Although this technique is mostly used for imaging of extracardiac anatomy, we have found it useful in the evaluation of intra-atrial systemic and pulmonary baffles (such as in Mustard and Senning operations and after Fontan procedures), as well as for imaging of the outflow tracts (such as in repaired tetralogy of Fallot and the arterial switch operation). In addition, MRA clearly delineates the spatial relationships between vascular structures, the tracheobronchial tree, chest wall, spine, and other landmarks that may be useful for planning of interventional catheterization or surgical procedures.

Myocardial Ischemia and Viability

Although traditionally the diagnosis of myocardial ischemia has not been a focus of imaging in CHD, it clearly has relevance in patients who have congenital and acquired coronary abnormalities (e.g., anomalous origin of the left coronary artery, pulmonary atresia with intact ventricular septum, and Kawasaki disease). Moreover, myocardial ischemia is an important diagnostic challenge in patients postoperatively and in adults with CHD. Several MRI techniques for imaging the coronary arteries with sufficient resolution to detect stenotic lesions are now available.[154] However, the optimal approach and clinical usefulness will likely remain in evolution for the next several years. MRI techniques are also available for assessment of regional left ventricular myocardial perfusion.[155,156] Typically, after a rapid intravenous gadolinium contrast injection, ultrafast, multislice imaging with an

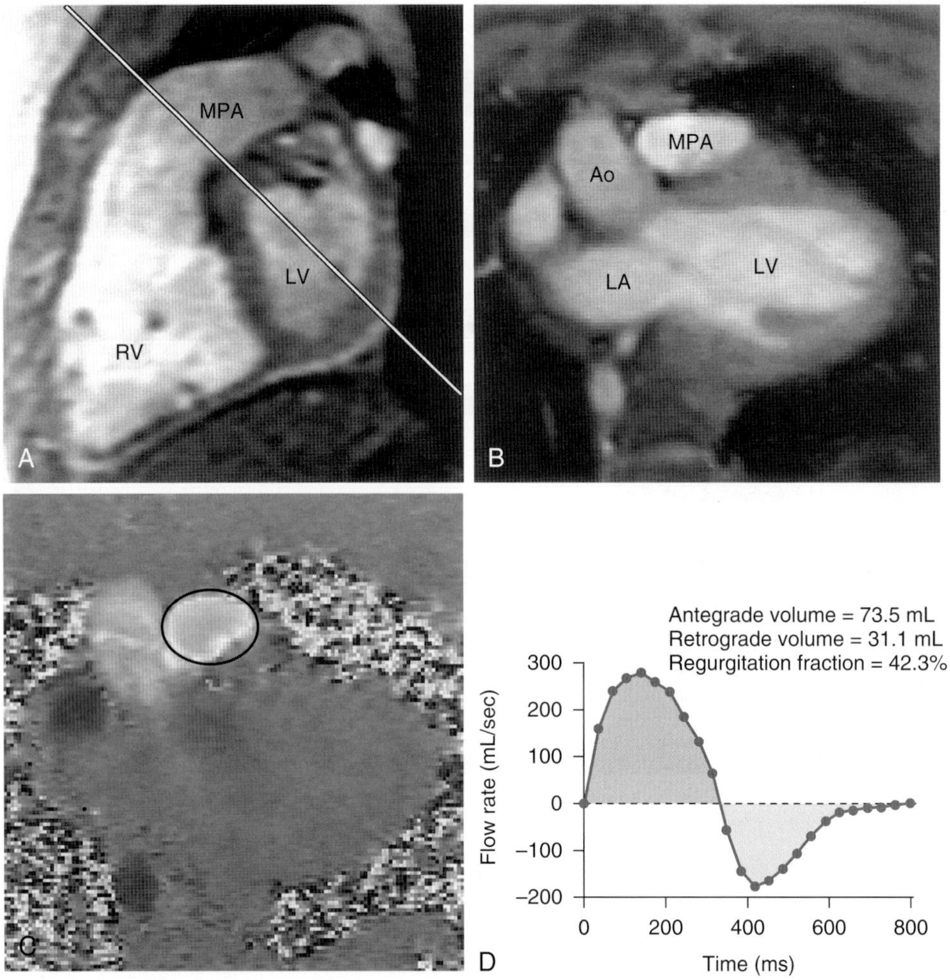

FIGURE 106-17 ■ Quantitative assessment of pulmonary regurgitation by velocity-encoded cine magnetic resonance imaging (MRI) in a 26-year-old patient with repaired tetralogy of Fallot. **A,** An imaging plane is placed across the main pulmonary artery (MPA) (multiphase gradient echo cine MR). **B,** Magnitude image showing bright signal in the proximal MPA. **C,** The corresponding phase image contains the velocity and directional data. Using a computer workstation, a region of interest *(oval)* is placed around the MPA. **D,** The systolic flow-time integral (area under the curve above the baseline) yields the antegrade flow volume, and the diastolic flow-time integral (below the baseline) corresponds to the regurgitant flow volume. Regurgitation fraction is calculated as the ratio of retrograde (regurgitant volume) to antegrade volume. *Ao,* Aorta; *LA,* left atrium; *LV,* left ventricle; *RV,* right ventricle.

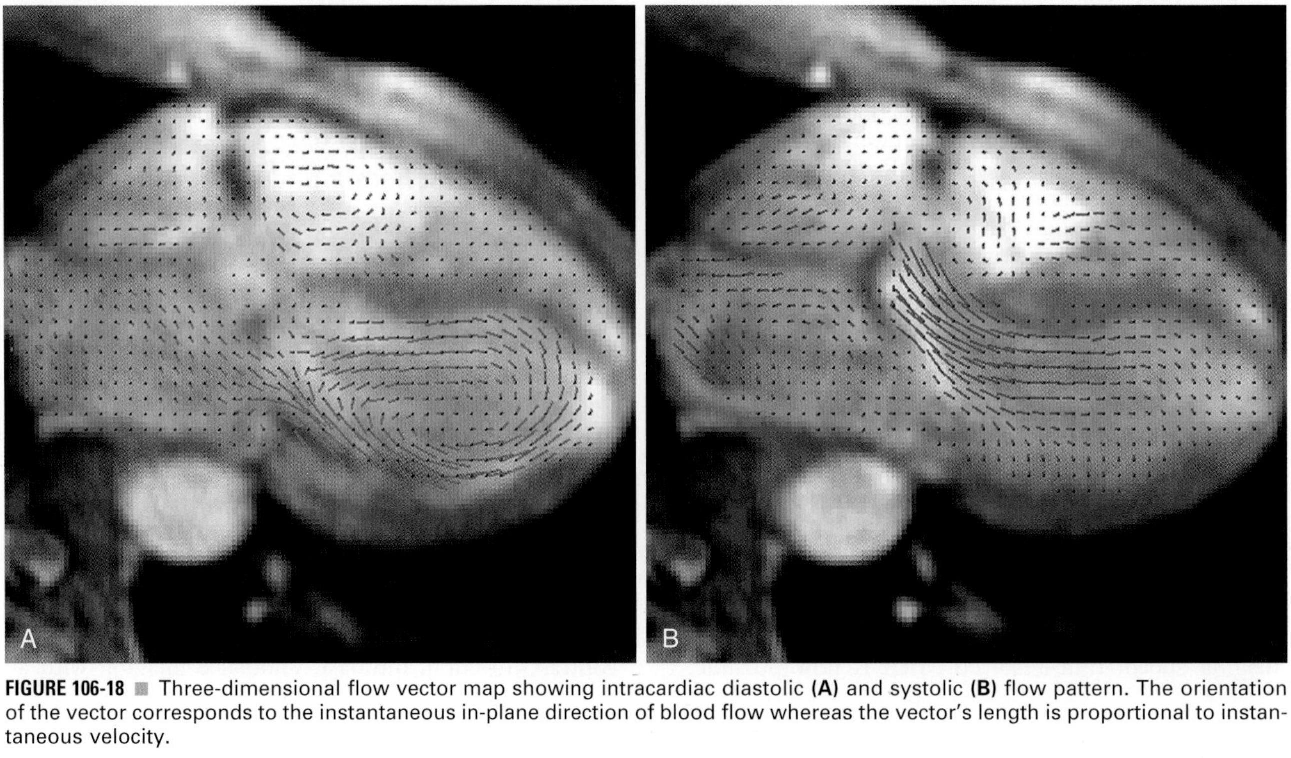

FIGURE 106-18 ■ Three-dimensional flow vector map showing intracardiac diastolic **(A)** and systolic **(B)** flow pattern. The orientation of the vector corresponds to the instantaneous in-plane direction of blood flow whereas the vector's length is proportional to instantaneous velocity.

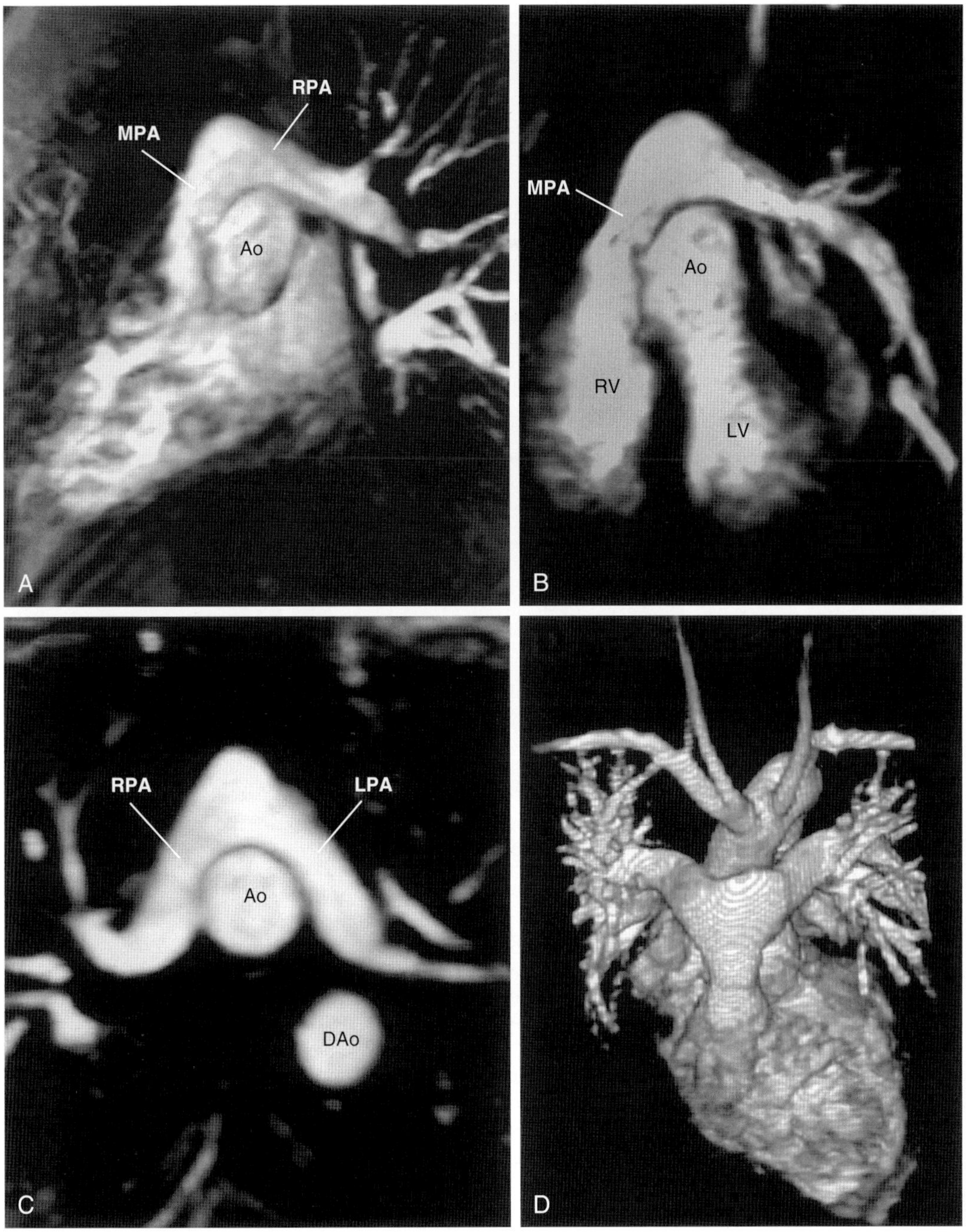

FIGURE 106-19 ■ Gadolinium-enhanced three-dimensional magnetic resonance angiography in a patient with D-loop transposition of the great arteries after an arterial switch operation. **A,** Subvolume maximum intensity projection (MIP) image in an oblique sagittal plane showing the main (MPA) and right (RPA) pulmonary arteries. **B,** Leftward angulation of the imaging plane shows the left pulmonary artery. **C,** Axial plane MIP image demonstrates the left (LPA) and right (RPA) pulmonary arteries wrapped around the ascending aorta (Ao) (Lecompte maneuver). **D,** Three-dimensional volume reconstruction provides enhanced perception of the relationships between the great vessels. *DAo,* Descending aorta; *LV,* left ventricle; *RV,* right ventricle.

echo-planar pulse sequence is performed during a 20- to 25-second breath-hold to image the first pass of contrast through the myocardium (Fig. 106-20). The procedure can be repeated after administering a coronary vasodilator (e.g., adenosine or dipyridamole). Although MR perfusion imaging offers superior spatial resolution compared with nuclear cardiology techniques without the use of ionizing radiation, its widespread application has been limited by the need for time-intensive analysis and insufficient clinical validation. Alternatively, cine MRI can be used to detect focal wall motion abnormalities with pharmacologic stress-induced ischemia. Several studies have demonstrated that for dobutamine stress studies, MRI compares favorably with transthoracic echocardiography, primarily as a result of its superior image quality.[157-159] Finally, various MRI techniques have been used to assess myocardial viability. In particular, hyperenhanced myocardial regions observed 10 to 15

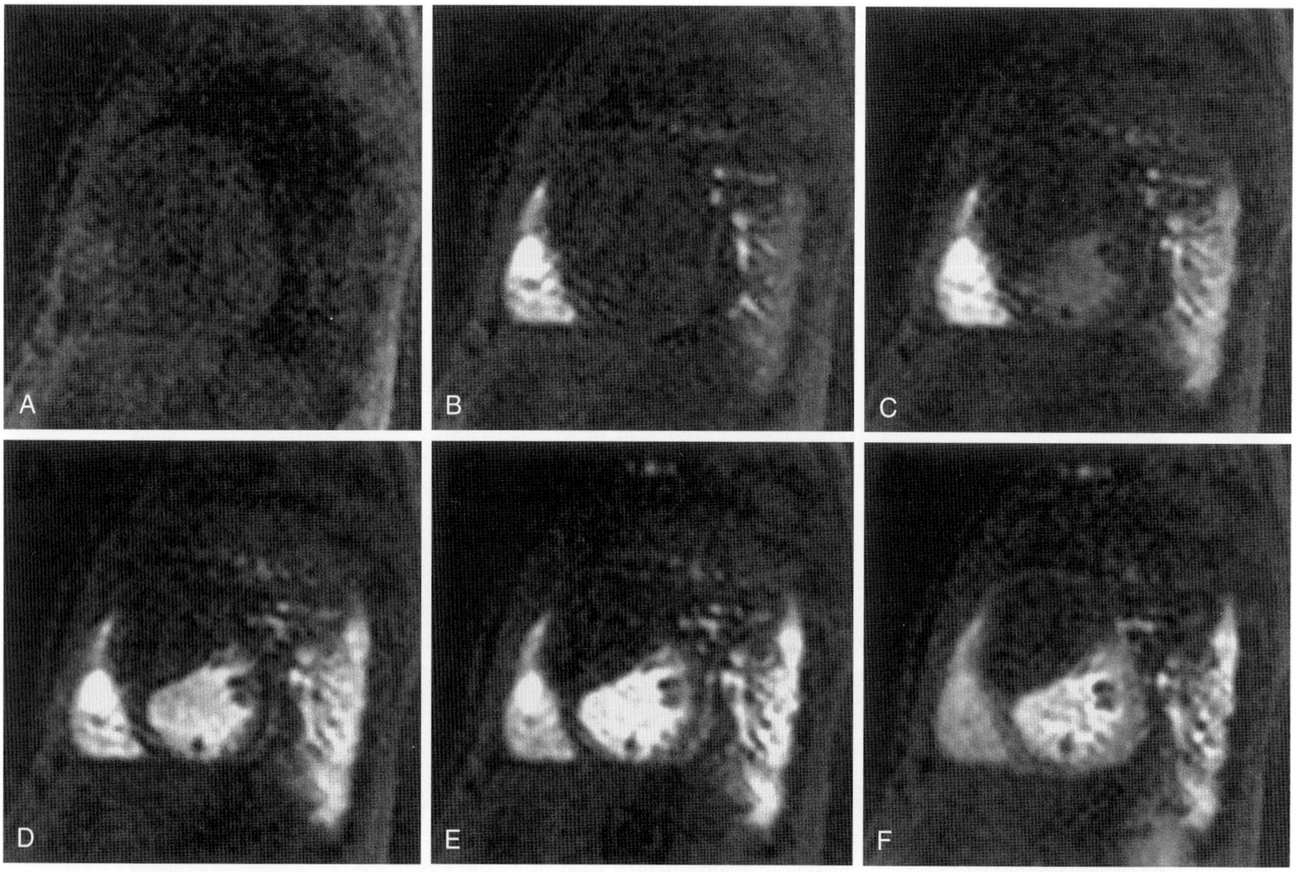

FIGURE 106-20 ■ First-pass myocardial perfusion scan in a patient with left ventricular fibroma. **A,** At onset of scan there is no contrast in the heart. **B,** Arrival of contrast in the right ventricle. **C,** Arrival of contrast in the pulmonary veins and early enhancement of left ventricular cavity. **D,** Arrival of contrast in the left ventricular cavity (notice the unenhanced left ventricular myocardium). **E,** Arrival of contrast in the left ventricular myocardium (notice the hypoperfused tumor in the anterolateral aspect of the septum). **F,** Late myocardial enhancement with hypoperfused tumor.

minutes after the administration of gadolinium contrast agents (termed *delayed myocardial enhancement*) are indicative of irreversible myocardial injury (Fig. 106-21).[160-162] Human studies assessing the usefulness of this technique have demonstrated its ability to detect scar tissue and other myocardial abnormalities in various types of acquired heart disease in adults.[159,163-167] Although experience in patients with CHD is limited, several studies have demonstrated the ability of this technique to detect scar tissue in patients with tetralogy of Fallot, systemic right ventricle, endocardial fibroelastosis, and other conditions.[156,168-171]

Indications for Cardiovascular Magnetic Resonance Imaging

The indications for cardiac MRI in patients with congenital and acquired pediatric heart disease are rapidly expanding. In general, the clinical reasons for a cardiac MRI examination may fall into one or more of the following three categories: (1) when transthoracic echocardiography is incapable of providing the required diagnostic information; (2) as an alternative to diagnostic cardiac catheterization with its associated discomfort, ionizing radiation exposure, contrast agent load, risks of morbidity and mortality, and high cost; and (3) for MRI's

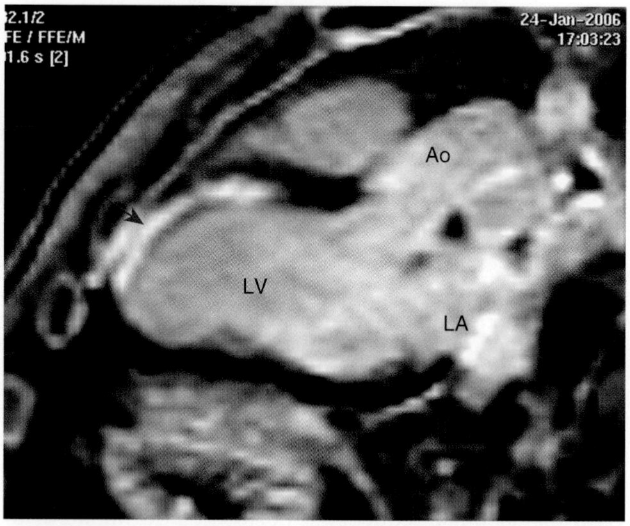

FIGURE 106-21 ■ Assessment of myocardial viability in a patient with Kawasaki disease, giant coronary artery aneurysm, and large anterior myocardial infarction extending to the apex. Nonviable myocardium produced bright signal *(arrow)* on an electrocardiographically triggered post-gadolinium, delayed-enhancement, inversion-recovery T1-weighted gradient echo sequence. Notice the dark signal from the viable left ventricular myocardium. *Ao,* Aorta; *LA,* left atrium; *LV,* left ventricle.

unique capabilities such as tissue imaging, myocardial tagging, and vessel-specific flow quantification.

General Considerations

Detailed preexamination planning is crucial given the wide array of imaging sequences available and the often complex nature of the clinical, anatomic, and functional issues in patients with CHD.[94] The importance of a careful review of the patient's medical history—including details of all cardiovascular surgical procedures, interventional catheterizations, findings of previous diagnostic tests, and current clinical status—cannot be overemphasized. As is the case with echocardiography and cardiac catheterization, cardiovascular MRI examination of CHD is an interactive diagnostic procedure that requires on-line review and interpretation of the data by the supervising physician. The unpredictable nature of the anatomy and hemodynamics often requires adjustment of the examination protocol; modification of imaging planes; adding, deleting, or changing sequences; and adjustment of imaging parameters. Reliance on standardized protocols and post hoc reading alone in these patients might result in incomplete or even erroneous interpretation.

Sedation is often required in young patients who cannot cooperate with a cardiac MRI examination. Most patients younger than 5 or 6 years require sedation, some patients between age 6 and 10 years are capable of cooperation, and most children older than 10 years can undergo a cardiac MRI study without sedation provided their mental development is age appropriate and they are not claustrophobic. Anxiolysis with oral midazolam or other medications is helpful in patients with mild or moderate claustrophobia or other forms of anxiety.[172] Screening for sedation need is part of the scheduling process for cardiac MRI, and consultation with the referring cardiologist and parents is advised. Both conscious sedation and general anesthesia have been successfully used in cardiac MRI. In our experience, advantages of general anesthesia include a better safety profile (secured airways and close monitoring by a pediatric anesthesiologist); ability to suspend respiration, leading to improved image quality and a shorter examination time; and control over duration of sedation.[173,174] Disadvantages of this approach include a higher cost and availability of skilled anesthesia personnel. Other centers have successfully used different methods of sedation.[175-177]

Safety and Complications

Standard clinical imaging scanners present no known hazards to biological materials. Three different magnetic fields are used by such magnets: the relatively large static magnetic field, smaller but rapidly varying magnetic fields secondary to the magnetic field gradients, and radiofrequency pulses. Guidelines set by the U.S. Food and Drug Administration keep the strength of these fields well below levels that could cause significant biological effects. Animal studies evaluating the influence of static magnetic fields have not demonstrated significant biological effects for fields of up to 2 T.[178] Millions of patients have undergone MRI studies without any noticeable immediate or long-term sequelae. Pregnancy is presently a relative contraindication to MRI studies, although the magnetic field levels used in clinical imagers have no known effects on the embryo. Many women have undergone MRI during all trimesters of pregnancy without reported ill effect on the mother, fetus, or resultant infant. When maternal and fetal health considerations require diagnostic studies, MRI is preferable to methods that use x-rays, such as computed tomography (CT) or angiography.

Implanted metallic objects are of particular concern, because they could potentially undergo undesirable torquing movements if the magnetic field were sufficiently strong and if they contained sufficient ferromagnetic material. Fortunately, surgical clips and sternotomy wires implanted in the chest and abdomen are typically only weakly ferromagnetic. Furthermore, these devices quickly become immobilized by surrounding fibrous tissue, so MRI can be safely performed in patients with these implants.[179] The wires and clips, however, may cause image artifact. Similarly, patients with implanted intravascular coils, stents, and occluding devices can be imaged by MRI once the implants are believed to be immobile. Many centers choose to avoid exposing these patients to MRI for an arbitrarily chosen period of time after implantation (usually for several weeks), but such practice is not supported by conclusive published data. A decision to perform MRI examination shortly after cardiac surgery or implantation of a biomedical device must weigh the risk-to-benefit ratio for the individual patient.[179,180]

A number of devices are considered either relative or absolute contraindications to MRI.[179,180] Presence of an intracranial, intraocular, or intracochlear metallic object is considered a contraindication to MRI. The presence of a cardiac pacemaker is also considered a strong relative contraindication to MRI,[181] although some reports have suggested that scanning patients who have modern pacemakers may be possible.[182-185]

Because MRI scanners attract ferromagnetic objects, extreme caution should be used in approaching magnets with objects containing iron or other ferromagnetic materials. Only specially designed MRI-compatible physiologic monitoring equipment should be used in conjunction with MRI studies. There have been several reported cases of patient burns resulting from the use of MRI-incompatible pulse oximeters and electrocardiographic monitoring devices.

SUMMARY

Accurate diagnosis of CHD can be accomplished by the judicious use of a variety of modalities. Echocardiography has assumed a leading role as the primary diagnostic tool in pediatric cardiology because of its noninvasive nature and its ability to provide comprehensive accurate diagnostic information in real time, in various clinical settings, and at a reasonable cost. Cardiovascular MRI is rapidly becoming an important diagnostic tool in pediatric cardiology because of its ability to provide anatomic and functional information that cannot be obtained by echocardiography or, in some cases, by catheterization.

REFERENCES

1. Geva T: Echocardiography and Doppler ultrasound. In Garson A, Bricker JT, Fisher DJ, et al, editors: *The science and practice of pediatric cardiology*, Baltimore, 1997, Williams & Wilkins, pp 789–843.
2. Prakash A, Powell AJ, Geva T: Multimodality noninvasive imaging for assessment of congenital heart disease. *Circ Cardiovasc Imaging* 3:112–125, 2010.
3. Silverman NH: *Pediatric echocardiography*, Baltimore, 1993, Williams & Wilkins.
4. Lopez L, Colan SD, Frommelt PC, et al: Recommendations for quantification methods during the performance of a pediatric echocardiogram: a report from the Pediatric Measurements Writing Group of the American Society of Echocardiography Pediatric and Congenital Heart Disease Council. *J Am Soc Echocardiogr* 23:465–495, quiz 576–577, 2010.
5. Rein AJ, Nadjari M, Bromiker R, et al: Detection of an obstructive membrane in the ductus arteriosus of a fetus using high frame rate echocardiography. *Fetal Diagn Ther* 13:250–252, 1998.
6. Song JM, Kim MJ, Kim YJ, et al: Three-dimensional characteristics of functional mitral regurgitation in patients with severe left ventricular dysfunction: a real-time three-dimensional colour Doppler echocardiography study. *Heart* 94:590–596, 2008.
7. Tsukiji M, Watanabe N, Yamaura Y, et al: Three-dimensional quantitation of mitral valve coaptation by a novel software system with transthoracic real-time three-dimensional echocardiography. *J Am Soc Echocardiogr* 21:43–46, 2008.
8. Soriano BD, Hoch M, Ithuralde A, et al: Matrix-array 3-dimensional echocardiographic assessment of volumes, mass, and ejection fraction in young pediatric patients with a functional single ventricle: a comparison study with cardiac magnetic resonance. *Circulation* 117:1842–1848, 2008.
9. Sugeng L, Shernan SK, Salgo IS, et al: Live 3-dimensional transesophageal echocardiography initial experience using the fully-sampled matrix array probe. *J Am Coll Cardiol* 52:446–449, 2008.
10. Lai WW, Geva T, Shirali GS, et al: Guidelines and standards for performance of a pediatric echocardiogram: a report from the task force of the Pediatric Council of the American Society of Echocardiography. *J Am Soc Echocardiogr* 19:1413–1430, 2006.
11. Colan SD: Hemodynamic measurements. In Lai WL, Mertens LL, Cohen MS, et al, editors: *Echocardiography in pediatric and congenital heart disease*, Oxford, UK, 2009, Wiley-Blackwell, pp 63–75.
12. Mor-Avi V, Lang RM, Badano LP, et al: Current and evolving echocardiographic techniques for the quantitative evaluation of cardiac mechanics: ASE/EAE consensus statement on methodology and indications endorsed by the Japanese Society of Echocardiography. *J Am Soc Echocardiogr* 24:277–313, 2011.
13. Leitman M, Lysyansky P, Sidenko S, et al: Two-dimensional strain-a novel software for real-time quantitative echocardiographic assessment of myocardial function. *J Am Soc Echocardiogr* 17:1021–1029, 2004.
14. Pirat B, Khoury DS, Hartley CJ, et al: A novel feature-tracking echocardiographic method for the quantitation of regional myocardial function: validation in an animal model of ischemia-reperfusion. *J Am Coll Cardiol* 51:651–659, 2008.
15. Amundsen BH, Helle-Valle T, Edvardsen T, et al: Noninvasive myocardial strain measurement by speckle tracking echocardiography: validation against sonomicrometry and tagged magnetic resonance imaging. *J Am Coll Cardiol* 47:789–793, 2006.
16. Altman M, Bergerot C, Aussoleil A, et al: Assessment of left ventricular systolic function by deformation imaging derived from speckle tracking: a comparison between 2D and 3D echo modalities. *Eur Heart J Cardiovasc Imaging* 15:316–323, 2013.
17. Friedberg MK, Mertens L: Deformation imaging in selected congenital heart disease: is it evolving to clinical use? *J Am Soc Echocardiogr* 25:919–931, 2012.
18. Gramiak R, Shah PM, Kramer DH: Ultrasound cardiography: contrast studies in anatomy and function. *Radiology* 92:939–948, 1969.
19. Cohen BE, Winer HE, Kronzon I: Echocardiographic findings in patients with left superior vena cava and dilated coronary sinus. *Am J Cardiol* 44:158–161, 1979.
20. Snider AR, Silverman NH, Turley K, et al: Evaluation of infradiaphragmatic total anomalous pulmonary venous connection with two-dimensional echocardiography. *Circulation* 66:1129–1132, 1982.
21. Allen HD, Sahn DJ, Goldberg SJ: New serial contrast technique for assessment of left to right shunting patent ductus arteriosus in the neonate. *Am J Cardiol* 41:288–294, 1978.
22. Kleinert S, Geva T: Echocardiographic morphometry and geometry of the left ventricular outflow tract in fixed subaortic stenosis. *J Am Coll Cardiol* 22:1501–1508, 1993.
23. Wong PC, Sanders SP, Jonas RA, et al: Pulmonary valve-moderator band distance and association with development of double-chambered right ventricle. *Am J Cardiol* 68:1681–1686, 1991.
24. Manganas C, Iliopoulos J, Chard RB, et al: Reoperation and coarctation of the aorta: the need for lifelong surveillance. *Ann Thorac Surg* 72:1222–1224, 2001.
25. Sanders S: Echocardiography and related techniques in the diagnosis of congenital heart disease. I. Veins, atria and interatrial septum. *Echocardiography* 1:185–217, 1984.
26. Geva T: Nomenclature and the segmental approach to congenital heart disease. In Taeusch WH, Ballard RA, Gleason CA, editors: *Avery's diseases of the newborn*, Philadelphia, 2004, Elsevier Saunders, pp 779–789.
27. Ayres NA, Miller-Hance W, Fyfe DA, et al: Indications and guidelines for performance of transesophageal echocardiography in the patient with pediatric acquired or congenital heart disease: report from the task force of the Pediatric Council of the American Society of Echocardiography. *J Am Soc Echocardiogr* 18:91–98, 2005.
28. Gentles TL, Rosenfeld HM, Sanders SP, et al: Pediatric biplane transesophageal echocardiography: preliminary experience. *Am Heart J* 128:1225–1233, 1994.
29. Stevenson JG, Sorensen GK, Gartman DM, et al: Transesophageal echocardiography during repair of congenital cardiac defects: identification of residual problems necessitating reoperation. *J Am Soc Echocardiogr* 6:356–365, 1993.
30. Stevenson JG: Role of intraoperative transesophageal echocardiography during repair of congenital cardiac defects. *Acta Paediatr Suppl* 410:23–33, 1995.
31. Lam J, Neirotti RA, Nijveld A, et al: Transesophageal echocardiography in pediatric patients: preliminary results. *J Am Soc Echocardiogr* 4:43–50, 1991.
32. Lam J, Neirotti RA, Hardjowijono R, et al: Transesophageal echocardiography with the use of a four-millimeter probe. *J Am Soc Echocardiogr* 10:499–504, 1997.
33. Lam J, Neirotti RA, Lubbers WJ, et al: Usefulness of biplane transesophageal echocardiography in neonates, infants and children with congenital heart disease. *Am J Cardiol* 72:699–706, 1993.
34. Lavoie J, Burrows FA, Gentles TL, et al: Transoesophageal echocardiography detects residual ductal flow during video-assisted thoracoscopic patent ductus arteriosus interruption. *Can J Anaesth* 41:310–313, 1994.
35. Van. Der Velde ME, Perry SB: Transesophageal echocardiography during interventional catheterization in congenital heart disease. *Echocardiography* 14:513–528, 1997.
36. Lai WW, al-Khatib Y, Klitzner TS, et al: Biplanar transesophageal echocardiographic direction of radiofrequency catheter ablation in children and adolescents with the Wolff-Parkinson-White syndrome. *Am J Cardiol* 71:872–874, 1993.
37. Marcus B, Wong PC, Wells WJ, et al: Transesophageal echocardiography in the postoperative child with an open sternum. *Ann Thorac Surg* 58:235–236, 1994.
38. Feltes TF, Friedman RA: Transesophageal echocardiographic detection of atrial thrombi in patients with nonfibrillation atrial tachyarrhythmias and congenital heart disease. *J Am Coll Cardiol* 24:1365–1370, 1994.
39. Daniel WG, Mugge A, Grote J, et al: Comparison of transthoracic and transesophageal echocardiography for detection of abnormalities of prosthetic and bioprosthetic valves in the mitral and aortic positions. *Am J Cardiol* 71:210–215, 1993.
40. Shanewise JS, Sadel SM: Intraoperative transesophageal echocardiography to assist the insertion and positioning of the intraaortic balloon pump. *Anesth Analg* 79:577–580, 1994.
41. Hirsch R, Kilner PJ, Connelly MS, et al: Diagnosis in adolescents and adults with congenital heart disease. Prospective assessment of individual and combined roles of magnetic resonance imaging

and transesophageal echocardiography. *Circulation* 90:2937–2951, 1994.
42. Siwik ES, Spector ML, Patel CR, et al: Costs and cost-effectiveness of routine transesophageal echocardiography in congenital heart surgery. *Am Heart J* 138:771–776, 1999.
43. Savino JS, Hanson CW, 3rd, Bigelow DC, et al: Oropharyngeal injury after transesophageal echocardiography. *J Cardiothorac Vasc Anesth* 8:76–78, 1994.
44. Frommelt PC, Stuth EA: Transesophageal echocardiographic in total anomalous pulmonary venous drainage: hypotension caused by compression of the pulmonary venous confluence during probe passage. *J Am Soc Echocardiogr* 7:652–654, 1994.
45. Fyfe DA, Ritter SB, Snider AR, et al: Guidelines for transesophageal echocardiography in children. *J Am Soc Echocardiogr* 5:640–644, 1992.
46. Stevenson JG: Incidence of complications in pediatric transesophageal echocardiography: experience in 1650 cases. *J Am Soc Echocardiogr* 12:527–532, 1999.
47. Kleinman CS, Hobbins JC, Jaffe CC, et al: Echocardiographic studies of the human fetus: prenatal diagnosis of congenital heart disease and cardiac dysrhythmias. *Pediatrics* 65:1059–1067, 1980.
48. Allan LD, Santos R, Pexieder T: Anatomical and echocardiographic correlates of normal cardiac morphology in the late first trimester fetus. *Heart* 77:68–72, 1997.
49. Buskens E, Grobbee DE, Frohn-Mulder IM, et al: Efficacy of routine fetal ultrasound screening for congenital heart disease in normal pregnancy. *Circulation* 94:67–72, 1996.
50. Kleinman C: Fetal echocardiography: diagnosing congenital heart disease in the human fetus. *ACC Educational Highlights* Summer: 10–14, 1996.
51. Buskens E, Stewart PA, Hess J, et al: Efficacy of fetal echocardiography and yield by risk category. *Obstet Gynecol* 87:423–428, 1996.
52. Rychik J, Ayres N, Cuneo B, et al: American Society of Echocardiography guidelines and standards for performance of the fetal echocardiogram. *J Am Soc Echocardiogr* 17:803–810, 2004.
53. Benacerraf BR, Pober BR, Sanders SP: Accuracy of fetal echocardiography. *Radiology* 165:847–849, 1987.
54. Hornberger LK, Sahn DJ, Kleinman CS, et al: Antenatal diagnosis of coarctation of the aorta: a multicenter experience. *J Am Coll Cardiol* 23:417–423, 1994.
55. Matsui H, Mellander M, Roughton M, et al: Morphological and physiological predictors of fetal aortic coarctation. *Circulation* 118:1793–1801, 2008.
56. Kumar RK, Newburger JW, Gauvreau K, et al: Comparison of outcome when hypoplastic left heart syndrome and transposition of the great arteries are diagnosed prenatally versus when diagnosis of these two conditions is made only postnatally. *Am J Cardiol* 83:1649–1653, 1999.
57. Tworetzky W, McElhinney DB, Reddy VM, et al: Improved surgical outcome after fetal diagnosis of hypoplastic left heart syndrome. *Circulation* 103:1269–1273, 2001.
58. Sklansky M, Tang A, Levy D, et al: Maternal psychological impact of fetal echocardiography. *J Am Soc Echocardiogr* 15:159–166, 2002.
59. Kleinman CS, Copel JA, Hobbins JC: Combined echocardiographic and Doppler assessment of fetal congenital atrioventricular block. *Br J Obstet Gynaecol* 94:967–974, 1987.
60. Rein AJ, O'Donnell C, Geva T, et al: Use of tissue velocity imaging in the diagnosis of fetal cardiac arrhythmias. *Circulation* 106:1827–1833, 2002.
61. Sluysmans T, Colan SD: Theoretical and empirical derivation of cardiovascular allometric relationships in children. *J Appl Physiol* 99:445–457, 2005.
62. Tanner J: Fallacy of per-weight and per-surface area standards, and their relation to spurious correlation. *J App Physiol* 2:1–15, 1949.
63. Gutgesell HP, Rembold CM: Growth of the human heart relative to body surface area. *Am J Cardiol* 65:662–668, 1990.
64. Kuroda T, Kinter TM, Seward JB, et al: Accuracy of three-dimensional volume measurement using biplane transesophageal echocardiographic probe: in vitro experiment. *J Am Soc Echocardiogr* 4:475–484, 1991.
65. Soliman OI, Kirschbaum SW, van Dalen BM, et al: Accuracy and reproducibility of quantitation of left ventricular function by real-time three-dimensional echocardiography versus cardiac magnetic resonance. *Am J Cardiol* 102:778–783, 2008.
66. Lu X, Nadvoretskiy V, Bu L, et al: Accuracy and reproducibility of real-time three-dimensional echocardiography for assessment of right ventricular volumes and ejection fraction in children. *J Am Soc Echocardiogr* 21:84–89, 2008.
67. Jenkins C, Bricknell K, Hanekom L, et al: Reproducibility and accuracy of echocardiographic measurements of left ventricular parameters using real-time three-dimensional echocardiography. *J Am Coll Cardiol* 44:878–886, 2004.
68. Chuang ML, Hibberd MG, Salton CJ, et al: Importance of imaging method over imaging modality in noninvasive determination of left ventricular volumes and ejection fraction: assessment by two- and three-dimensional echocardiography and magnetic resonance imaging. *J Am Coll Cardiol* 35:477–484, 2000.
69. Colan SD: Assessment of ventricular and myocardial performance. In Fyler DC, editor: *Nadas' pediatric cardiology*, Philadelphia, 1992, Hanley & Belfus, pp 225–248.
70. Amundsen BH, Crosby J, Steen PA, et al: Regional myocardial long-axis strain and strain rate measured by different tissue Doppler and speckle tracking echocardiography methods: a comparison with tagged magnetic resonance imaging. *Eur J Echocardiogr* 10:229–237, 2009.
71. D'Hooge J, Herbots L, Sutherland GR: Quantitative assessment of intrinsic regional myocardial deformation by Doppler strain rate echocardiography in humans. *Circulation* 107:e49, author reply e49, 2003.
72. Teske AJ, De Boeck BW, Olimulder M, et al: Echocardiographic assessment of regional right ventricular function: a head-to-head comparison between 2-dimensional and tissue Doppler-derived strain analysis. *J Am Soc Echocardiogr* 21:275–283, 2008.
73. Rösner A, Bijnens B, Hansen M, et al: Left ventricular size determines tissue Doppler-derived longitudinal strain and strain rate. *Eur J Echocardiogr* 10:271–277, 2009.
74. Pavlopoulos H, Nihoyannopoulos P: Strain and strain rate deformation parameters: from tissue Doppler to 2D speckle tracking. *Int J Cardiovasc Imaging* 24:479–491, 2008.
75. Opdahl A, Helle-Valle T, Remme EW, et al: Apical rotation by speckle tracking echocardiography: a simplified bedside index of left ventricular twist. *J Am Soc Echocardiogr* 21:1121–1128, 2008.
76. Takeuchi M, Nakai H, Kokumai M, et al: Age-related changes in left ventricular twist assessed by two-dimensional speckle-tracking imaging. *J Am Soc Echocardiogr* 19:1077–1084, 2006.
77. Lorch SM, Ludomirsky A, Singh GK: Maturational and growth-related changes in left ventricular longitudinal strain and strain rate measured by two-dimensional speckle tracking echocardiography in healthy pediatric population. *J Am Soc Echocardiogr* 21:1207–1215, 2008.
78. Valdes-Cruz LM, Yoganathan AP, Tamura T, et al: Studies in vitro of the relationship between ultrasound and laser Doppler velocimetry and applicability to the simplified Bernoulli relationship. *Circulation* 73:300–308, 1986.
79. Yoganathan AP, Valdes-Cruz LM, Schmidt-Dohna J, et al: Continuous-wave Doppler velocities and gradients across fixed tunnel obstructions: studies in vitro and in vivo. *Circulation* 76:657–666, 1987.
80. Bioeffects considerations for the safety of diagnostic ultrasound. American Institute of Ultrasound in Medicine. Bioeffects Committee. *J Ultrasound Med* 7:S1–S38, 1988.
81. Serfaty JM, Yang X, Aksit P, et al: Toward MRI-guided coronary catheterization: visualization of guiding catheters, guidewires, and anatomy in real time. *J Magn Reson Imaging* 12:590–594, 2000.
82. Setser RM, Fischer SE, Lorenz CH: Quantification of left ventricular function with magnetic resonance images acquired in real time. *J Magn Reson Imaging* 12:430–438, 2000.
83. Okuda S, Kikinis R, Geva T, et al: 3D-shaded surface rendering of gadolinium-enhanced MR angiography in congenital heart disease. *Pediatr Radiol* 30:540–545, 2000.
84. Moniotte S, Powell AJ, Barnewolt CE, et al: Prenatal diagnosis of thoracic ectopia cordis by real-time fetal cardiac magnetic resonance imaging and by echocardiography. *Congenit Heart Dis* 3:128–131, 2008.
85. Powell AJ, Geva T: Blood flow measurement by magnetic resonance imaging in congenital heart disease. *Pediatr Cardiol* 21:47–58, 2000.
86. Fogel MA: Assessment of cardiac function by magnetic resonance imaging. *Pediatr Cardiol* 21:59–69, 2000.

87. Mulkern RV, Chung T: From signal to image: magnetic resonance imaging physics for cardiac magnetic resonance. *Pediatr Cardiol* 21:5–17, 2000.
88. Sodickson D: Clinical cardiovascular magnetic resonance imaging techniques. In Pennel D, editor: *Cardiovascular magnetic resonance*, New York, 2002, Churchill Livingstone, pp 18–30.
89. Lee VS, Resnick D, Bundy JM, et al: Cardiac function: MR evaluation in one breath hold with real-time true fast imaging with steady-state precession. *Radiology* 222:835–842, 2002.
90. Wech T, Pickl W, Tran-Gia J, et al: Whole-heart cine MRI in a single breath-hold - a compressed sensing accelerated 3D acquisition technique for assessment of cardiac function. *Rofo* 186:37–41, 2014.
91. Hulet JP, Greiser A, Mendes JK, et al: Highly accelerated cardiac cine phase-contrast MRI using an undersampled radial acquisition and temporally constrained reconstruction. *J Magn Reson Imaging* 39:455–462, 2014.
92. Feng L, Srichai MB, Lim RP, et al: Highly accelerated real-time cardiac cine MRI using k-t sparse-sense. *Magn Reson Med* 70:64–74, 2013.
93. Bassett EC, Kholmovski EG, Wilson BD, et al: Evaluation of highly accelerated real-time cardiac cine MRI in tachycardia. *NMR Biomed* 27:175–182, 2014.
94. Geva T, Powell AJ: Magnetic resonance imaging. In Allen HD, Driscoll DJ, Feltes TF, et al, editors: *Moss & Adams' heart disease in infants, children, and adolescents*, Philadelphia, 2008, Lippincott Williams & Wilkins, pp 163–199.
95. Midiri M, Finazzo M: MR imaging of arrhythmogenic right ventricular dysplasia. *Int J Cardiovasc Imaging* 17:297–304, 2001.
96. Mackie AS, Kozakewich HP, Geva T, et al: Vascular tumors of the heart in infants and children: case series and review of the literature. *Pediatr Cardiol* 26:344–349, 2005.
97. Kiaffas MG, Powell AJ, Geva T: Magnetic resonance imaging evaluation of cardiac tumor characteristics in infants and children. *Am J Cardiol* 89:1229–1233, 2002.
98. Beroukhim RS, Prakash A, Valsangiacomo Buechel ER, et al: Characterization of cardiac tumors in children by cardiovascular magnetic resonance imaging a multicenter experience. *J Am Coll Cardiol* 58:1044–1054, 2011.
99. Frank H, Globits S: Magnetic resonance imaging evaluation of myocardial and pericardial disease. *J Magn Reson Imaging* 10:617–626, 1999.
100. Kim WY, Stuber M, Bornert P, et al: Three-dimensional black-blood cardiac magnetic resonance coronary vessel wall imaging detects positive arterial remodeling in patients with nonsignificant coronary artery disease. *Circulation* 106:296–299, 2002.
101. Myer CM, 3rd, Auringer ST, Wiatrak BJ, et al: Magnetic resonance imaging in the diagnosis of innominate artery compression of the trachea. *Arch Otolaryngol Head Neck Surg* 116:314–316, 1990.
102. Herman M, Paucek B, Raida L, et al: Comparison of magnetic resonance imaging and (67)gallium scintigraphy in the evaluation of posttherapeutic residual mediastinal mass in the patients with Hodgkin's lymphoma. *Eur J Radiol* 64:432–438, 2007.
103. Simonetti OP, Finn JP, White RD, et al: "Black blood" t2-weighted inversion-recovery MR imaging of the heart. *Radiology* 199:49–57, 1996.
104. Carr JC, Simonetti O, Bundy J, et al: Cine MR angiography of the heart with segmented true fast imaging with steady-state precession. *Radiology* 219:828–834, 2001.
105. Plein S, Bloomer TN, Ridgway JP, et al: Steady-state free precession magnetic resonance imaging of the heart: comparison with segmented k-space gradient-echo imaging. *J Magn Reson Imaging* 14:230–236, 2001.
106. Tsao J, Kozerke S, Boesiger P, et al: Optimizing spatiotemporal sampling for k-t blast and k-t sense: application to high-resolution real-time cardiac steady-state free precession. *Magn Reson Med* 53:1372–1382, 2005.
107. Raval AN, Telep JD, Guttman MA, et al: Real-time magnetic resonance imaging-guided stenting of aortic coarctation with commercially available catheter devices in swine. *Circulation* 112:699–706, 2005.
108. Raman VK, Karmarkar PV, Guttman MA, et al: Real-time magnetic resonance-guided endovascular repair of experimental abdominal aortic aneurysm in swine. *J Am Coll Cardiol* 45:2069–2077, 2005.
109. Grosse-Wortmann L, Al-Otay A, Goo HW, et al: Anatomical and functional evaluation of pulmonary veins in children by magnetic resonance imaging. *J Am Coll Cardiol* 49:993–1002, 2007.
110. Durongpisitkul K, Tang NL, Soongswang J, et al: Predictors of successful transcatheter closure of atrial septal defect by cardiac magnetic resonance imaging. *Pediatr Cardiol* 25:124–130, 2004.
111. Taylor AM, Stables RH, Poole-Wilson PA, et al: Definitive clinical assessment of atrial septal defect by magnetic resonance imaging. *J Cardiovasc Magn Reson* 1:43–47, 1999.
112. Valente AM, Sena L, Powell AJ, et al: Cardiac magnetic resonance imaging evaluation of sinus venosus defects: comparison to surgical findings. *Pediatr Cardiol* 28:51–56, 2007.
113. Fogel MA, Hubbard A, Weinberg PM: A simplified approach for assessment of intracardiac baffles and extracardiac conduits in congenital heart surgery with two- and three-dimensional magnetic resonance imaging. *Am Heart J* 142:1028–1036, 2001.
114. Takawira F, Ayer JG, Onikul E, et al: Evaluation of the extracardiac conduit modification of the fontan operation for thrombus formation using magnetic resonance imaging. *Heart Lung Circ* 17:407–410, 2008.
115. McVeigh E: Regional myocardial function. *Cardiol Clin* 16:189–206, 1998.
116. Graves MJ, Berry E, Eng AA, et al: A multicenter validation of an active contour-based left ventricular analysis technique. *J Magn Reson Imaging* 12:232–239, 2000.
117. Pattynama PM, de Roos A, Van der Velde ET, et al: Magnetic resonance imaging analysis of left ventricular pressure-volume relations: validation with the conductance method at rest and during dobutamine stress. *Magn Reson Med* 34:728–737, 1995.
118. Lamb HJ, Doornbos J, van der Velde EA, et al: Echo planar MRI of the heart on a standard system: validation of measurements of left ventricular function and mass. *J Comput Assist Tomogr* 20:942–949, 1996.
119. Thiele H, Paetsch I, Schnackenburg B, et al: Improved accuracy of quantitative assessment of left ventricular volume and ejection fraction by geometric models with steady-state free precession. *J Cardiovasc Magn Reson* 4:327–339, 2002.
120. Barkhausen J, Goyen M, Ruhm SG, et al: Assessment of ventricular function with single breath-hold real-time steady-state free precession cine mr imaging. *AJR Am J Roentgenol* 178:731–735, 2002.
121. Lorenz CH, Walker ES, Morgan VL, et al: Normal human right and left ventricular mass, systolic function, and gender differences by cine magnetic resonance imaging. *J Cardiovasc Magn Reson* 1:7–21, 1999.
122. Lorenz CH: The range of normal values of cardiovascular structures in infants, children, and adolescents measured by magnetic resonance imaging. *Pediatr Cardiol* 21:37–46, 2000.
123. Furber A, Balzer P, Cavaro-Menard C, et al: Experimental validation of an automated edge-detection method for a simultaneous determination of the endocardial and epicardial borders in short-axis cardiac mr images: application in normal volunteers. *J Magn Reson Imaging* 8:1006–1014, 1998.
124. Danias PG, Chuang ML, Parker RA, et al: Relation between the number of image planes and the accuracy of three-dimensional echocardiography for measuring left ventricular volumes and ejection fraction. *Am J Cardiol* 82:1431–1434, A1439, 1998.
125. Kuhl HP, Bucker A, Franke A, et al: Transesophageal 3-dimensional echocardiography: in vivo determination of left ventricular mass in comparison with magnetic resonance imaging. *J Am Soc Echocardiogr* 13:205–215, 2000.
126. Bellenger NG, Francis JM, Davies CL, et al: Establishment and performance of a magnetic resonance cardiac function clinic. *J Cardiovasc Magn Reson* 2:15–22, 2000.
127. Mooij CF, de Wit CJ, Graham DA, et al: Reproducibility of MRI measurements of right ventricular size and function in patients with normal and dilated ventricles. *J Magn Reson Imaging* 28:67–73, 2008.
128. Lamb HJ, Singleton RR, van der Geest RJ, et al: MR imaging of regional cardiac function: low-pass filtering of wall thickness curves. *Magn Reson Med* 34:498–502, 1995.
129. Kuijpers D, Ho KY, van Dijkman PR, et al: Dobutamine cardiovascular magnetic resonance for the detection of myocardial

ischemia with the use of myocardial tagging. *Circulation* 107:1592–1597, 2003.

130. Pennell DJ, Underwood SR, Manzara CC, et al: Magnetic resonance imaging during dobutamine stress in coronary artery disease. *Am J Cardiol* 70:34–40, 1992.
131. Nagel E, Lehmkuhl HB, Bocksch W, et al: Noninvasive diagnosis of ischemia-induced wall motion abnormalities with the use of high-dose dobutamine stress MRI: comparison with dobutamine stress echocardiography. *Circulation* 99:763–770, 1999.
132. Strigl S, Beroukhim R, Valente AM, et al: Feasibility of dobutamine stress cardiovascular magnetic resonance imaging in children. *J Magn Reson Imaging* 29:313–319, 2009.
133. Roest AA, Kunz P, Lamb HJ, et al: Biventricular response to supine physical exercise in young adults assessed with ultrafast magnetic resonance imaging. *Am J Cardiol* 87:601–605, 2001.
134. Roest AA, Helbing WA, Kunz P, et al: Exercise MR imaging in the assessment of pulmonary regurgitation and biventricular function in patients after tetralogy of Fallot repair. *Radiology* 223:204–211, 2002.
135. Bolster BD, Jr, McVeigh ER, Zerhouni EA: Myocardial tagging in polar coordinates with use of striped tags. *Radiology* 177:769–772, 1990.
136. Harrild DM, Han Y, Geva T, et al: Comparison of cardiac MRI tissue tracking and myocardial tagging for assessment of regional ventricular strain. *Int J Cardiovasc Imaging* 28:2009–2018, 2012.
137. Fischer SE, McKinnon GC, Scheidegger MB, et al: True myocardial motion tracking. *Magn Reson Med* 31:401–413, 1994.
138. Bogaert J, Rademakers FE: Regional nonuniformity of normal adult human left ventricle. *Am J Physiol Heart Circ Physiol* 280:H610–H620, 2001.
139. Klein SS, Graham TP, Jr, Lorenz CH: Noninvasive delineation of normal right ventricular contractile motion with magnetic resonance imaging myocardial tagging. *Ann Biomed Eng* 26:756–763, 1998.
140. Nagel E, Stuber M, Fleck E, et al: Myocardial tagging for the analysis of left ventricular function. *MAGMA* 6:91–93, 1998.
141. Garot J, Bluemke DA, Osman NF, et al: Fast determination of regional myocardial strain fields from tagged cardiac images using harmonic phase MRI. *Circulation* 101:981–988, 2000.
142. Ortega M, Triedman JK, Geva T, et al: Relation of left ventricular dyssynchrony measured by cardiac magnetic resonance tissue tracking in repaired tetralogy of Fallot to ventricular tachycardia and death. *Am J Cardiol* 107:1535–1540, 2011.
143. Schmidt R, Orwat S, Kempny A, et al: Value of speckle-tracking echocardiography and MRI-based feature tracking analysis in adult patients after Fontan-type palliation. *Congenit Heart Dis* 9:397–406, 2014.
144. Prakash A, Garg R, Marcus EN, et al: Faster flow quantification using sensitivity encoding for velocity-encoded cine magnetic resonance imaging: in vitro and in vivo validation. *J Magn Reson Imaging* 24:676–682, 2006.
145. Powell AJ, Maier SE, Chung T, et al: Phase-velocity cine magnetic resonance imaging measurement of pulsatile blood flow in children and young adults: in vitro and in vivo validation. *Pediatr Cardiol* 21:104–110, 2000.
146. Reid SA, Walker PG, Fisher J, et al: The quantification of pulmonary valve haemodynamics using MRI. *Int J Cardiovasc Imaging* 18:217–225, 2002.
147. Geva T: Repaired tetralogy of Fallot: the roles of cardiovascular magnetic resonance in evaluating pathophysiology and for pulmonary valve replacement decision support. *J Cardiovasc Magn Reson* 13:9, 2011.
148. Be'eri E, Maier SE, Landzberg MJ, et al: In vivo evaluation of Fontan pathway flow dynamics by multidimensional phase-velocity magnetic resonance imaging. *Circulation* 98:2873–2882, 1998.
149. Oshinski JN, Ku DN, Mukundan S, Jr, et al: Determination of wall shear stress in the aorta with the use of MR phase velocity mapping. *J Magn Reson Imaging* 5:640–647, 1995.
150. Ohno Y, Kawamitsu H, Higashino T, et al: Time-resolved contrast-enhanced pulmonary MR angiography using sensitivity encoding (sense). *J Magn Reson Imaging* 17:330–336, 2003.
151. Warmuth C, Schnorr J, Kaufels N, et al: Whole-heart coronary magnetic resonance angiography: contrast-enhanced high-resolution, time-resolved 3D imaging. *Invest Radiol* 42:550–557, 2007.
152. Geva T, Greil GF, Marshall AC, et al: Gadolinium-enhanced 3-dimensional magnetic resonance angiography of pulmonary blood supply in patients with complex pulmonary stenosis or atresia: comparison with x-ray angiography. *Circulation* 106:473–478, 2002.
153. Greil GF, Powell AJ, Gildein HP, et al: Gadolinium-enhanced three-dimensional magnetic resonance angiography of pulmonary and systemic venous anomalies. *J Am Coll Cardiol* 39:335–341, 2002.
154. Danias PG, Manning WJ: Coronary MR angiography: current status. *Herz* 25:431–439, 2000.
155. Laddis T, Manning WJ, Danias PG: Cardiac MRI for assessment of myocardial perfusion: current status and future perspectives. *J Nucl Cardiol* 8:207–214, 2001.
156. Prakash A, Powell AJ, Krishnamurthy R, et al: Magnetic resonance imaging evaluation of myocardial perfusion and viability in congenital and acquired pediatric heart disease. *Am J Cardiol* 93:657–661, 2004.
157. Dall'Armellina E, Morgan TM, Mandapaka S, et al: Prediction of cardiac events in patients with reduced left ventricular ejection fraction with dobutamine cardiovascular magnetic resonance assessment of wall motion score index. *J Am Coll Cardiol* 52:279–286, 2008.
158. Raman SV, Donnally MR, McCarthy B: Dobutamine stress cardiac magnetic resonance imaging to detect myocardial ischemia in women. *Prev Cardiol* 11:135–140, 2008.
159. Barmeyer AA, Stork A, Bansmann M, et al: Prediction of myocardial recovery by dobutamine magnetic resonance imaging and delayed enhancement early after reperfused acute myocardial infarction. *Eur Radiol* 18:110–118, 2008.
160. Kim RJ, Hillenbrand HB, Judd RM: Evaluation of myocardial viability by MRI. *Herz* 25:417–430, 2000.
161. Oshinski JN, Yang Z, Jones JR, et al: Imaging time after gd-dtpa injection is critical in using delayed enhancement to determine infarct size accurately with magnetic resonance imaging. *Circulation* 104:2838–2842, 2001.
162. Pereira RS, Prato FS, Wisenberg G, et al: The use of gd-dtpa as a marker of myocardial viability in reperfused acute myocardial infarction. *Int J Cardiovasc Imaging* 17:395–404, 2001.
163. Guillaume MD, Phoon CK, Chun AJ, et al: Delayed enhancement cardiac magnetic resonance imaging in a patient with Duchenne muscular dystrophy. *Tex Heart Inst J* 35:367–368, 2008.
164. Matoh F, Satoh H, Shiraki K, et al: The usefulness of delayed enhancement magnetic resonance imaging for diagnosis and evaluation of cardiac function in patients with cardiac sarcoidosis. *J Cardiol* 51:179–188, 2008.
165. Adabag AS, Maron BJ, Appelbaum E, et al: Occurrence and frequency of arrhythmias in hypertrophic cardiomyopathy in relation to delayed enhancement on cardiovascular magnetic resonance. *J Am Coll Cardiol* 51:1369–1374, 2008.
166. Bohl S, Wassmuth R, Abdel-Aty H, et al: Delayed enhancement cardiac magnetic resonance imaging reveals typical patterns of myocardial injury in patients with various forms of non-ischemic heart disease. *Int J Cardiovasc Imaging* 24:597–607, 2008.
167. Kim RJ, Wu E, Rafael A, et al: The use of contrast-enhanced magnetic resonance imaging to identify reversible myocardial dysfunction. *N Engl J Med* 343:1445–1453, 2000.
168. Babu-Narayan SV, Kilner PJ, Li W, et al: Ventricular fibrosis suggested by cardiovascular magnetic resonance in adults with repaired tetralogy of Fallot and its relationship to adverse markers of clinical outcome. *Circulation* 113:405–413, 2006.
169. Babu-Narayan SV, Goktekin O, Moon JC, et al: Late gadolinium enhancement cardiovascular magnetic resonance of the systemic right ventricle in adults with previous atrial redirection surgery for transposition of the great arteries. *Circulation* 111:2091–2098, 2005.
170. Tworetzky W, del Nido PJ, Powell AJ, et al: Usefulness of magnetic resonance imaging of left ventricular endocardial fibroelastosis in infants after fetal intervention for aortic valve stenosis. *Am J Cardiol* 96:1568–1570, 2005.
171. Wald RM, Haber I, Wald R, et al: Effects of regional dysfunction and late gadolinium enhancement on global right ventricular function and exercise capacity in patients with repaired tetralogy of Fallot. *Circulation* 119:1370–1377, 2009.

172. Francis JM, Pennell DJ: Treatment of claustrophobia for cardiovascular magnetic resonance: use and effectiveness of mild sedation. *J Cardiovasc Magn Reson* 2:139–141, 2000.
173. Odegard KC, DiNardo JA, Tsai-Goodman B, et al: Anaesthesia considerations for cardiac MRI in infants and small children. *Paediatr Anaesth* 14:471–476, 2004.
174. Dorfman AL, Odegard KC, Powell AJ, et al: Risk factors for adverse events during cardiovascular magnetic resonance in congenital heart disease. *J Cardiovasc Magn Reson* 9:793–798, 2007.
175. Fogel MA, Weinberg PM, Parave E, et al: Deep sedation for cardiac magnetic resonance imaging: a comparison with cardiac anesthesia. *J Pediatr* 152:534–539, 539 e531, 2008.
176. Rosenberg DR, Sweeney JA, Gillen JS, et al: Magnetic resonance imaging of children without sedation: preparation with simulation. *J Am Acad Child Adolesc Psychiatry* 36:853–859, 1997.
177. Beekman RP, Hoorntje TM, Beek FJ, et al: Sedation for children undergoing magnetic resonance imaging: efficacy and safety of rectal thiopental. *Eur J Pediatr* 155:820–822, 1996.
178. Wolff S, James TL, Young GB, et al: Magnetic resonance imaging: absence of in vitro cytogenetic damage. *Radiology* 155:163–165, 1985.
179. Levine GN, Gomes AS, Arai AE, et al: Safety of magnetic resonance imaging in patients with cardiovascular devices: an American Heart Association scientific statement from the Committee on Diagnostic and Interventional Cardiac Catheterization, Council on Clinical Cardiology, and the Council on Cardiovascular Radiology and Intervention: endorsed by the American College of Cardiology Foundation, the North American Society for Cardiac Imaging, and the Society for Cardiovascular Magnetic Resonance. *Circulation* 116:2878–2891, 2007.
180. Shellock FG: Metallic surgical instruments for interventional MRI procedures: evaluation of MR safety. *J Magn Reson Imaging* 13:152–157, 2001.
181. Rozner MA, Burton AW, Kumar A: Pacemaker complication during magnetic resonance imaging. *J Am Coll Cardiol* 45:161–162, author reply 162, 2005.
182. Mitka M: First MRI-safe pacemaker receives conditional approval from FDA. *JAMA* 305:985–986, 2011.
183. Sorrentino RA: A novel MRI-safe dual-chamber pacemaker system: its time has come. *Heart Rhythm* 8:74–75, 2011.
184. Pulver AF, Puchalski MD, Bradley DJ, et al: Safety and imaging quality of MRI in pediatric and adult congenital heart disease patients with pacemakers. *Pacing Clin Electrophysiol* 32:450–456, 2009.
185. Roguin A, Zviman MM, Meininger GR, et al: Modern pacemaker and implantable cardioverter/defibrillator systems can be magnetic resonance imaging safe: in vitro and in vivo assessment of safety and function at 1.5 T. *Circulation* 110:475–482, 2004.

CHAPTER 107

Cardiac Catheterization and Fetal Intervention

Audrey C. Marshall

CHAPTER OUTLINE

INTRODUCTION AND OVERVIEW

Catheterization in the field of congenital cardiology continues to improve understanding of disease and expand options for therapy. Diagnostic information previously obtained exclusively through catheterization is now routinely acquired through use of a host of diverse and highly sophisticated, noninvasive diagnostic imaging modalities. Invasive hemodynamic measurement and angiographic assessment, however, remain a mainstay in the comprehensive evaluation of the patient with complex heart disease. Furthermore, the interventional role of cardiac catheterization in the management of congenital heart disease continues to evolve, and in conjunction with surgical improvements, presents expanding opportunities for therapeutic intervention. Thus, the catheterization laboratory is increasingly like an operative suite, and in many cases of "hybrid" suites, it incorporates functions of a more traditional cardiac operating room.

Ongoing advances in transcatheter technology ensure that the historical border zone between transcatheter and open therapies will continue to shift and likely broaden. Thus, the team of cardiac surgeons and cardiologists who deal with congenital heart disease will benefit from a contemporary awareness of the capabilities and limitations of their partners' work. What follows is a brief summary of the basic hemodynamic and angiographic information acquired through cardiac catheterization and a rough sketch of the currently practiced procedures. The remainder of the chapter provides a survey of the current state of transcatheter therapies, from valvuloplasty to valve replacement, including angioplasty and defect closure using implantable devices. It also provides an overview of the experience to date with fetal cardiac intervention.

ROLE OF DIAGNOSTIC CATHETERIZATION

A primary role of the catheterizer, since the earliest days of invasive physiologic assessment of congenital heart disease, has been to safely obtain the data necessary to formulate a complete and accurate anatomic and hemodynamic understanding of the patient. This role as an investigator of physiology remains a defining role of the best invasive cardiologists; a thorough diagnostic catheterization constitutes a valuable part of almost all studies performed, even in the current era of intervention. An equally important role is to assist in planning management and to perform necessary transcatheter interventions as indicated, part of the integrated care of the patient with congenital disease. The ideal care of the most anatomically complex patients will likely require an orchestrated series of both open surgical and catheter-based procedures to achieve good, long-term, functional outcomes. A third, and more recent, role of the interventional cardiologist is to provide definitive therapy via a minimally invasive route, for some highly selected cardiac defects, as an alternative to surgery.

For decades, traditional biplane angiographic imaging constituted an important component of anatomic assessment of congenital heart disease. Expertise in acquisition and interpretation of these images secured the role of angiography in the preoperative investigation of patients with most major anatomic defects. The enormous volume of information provided by this modality has, fortunately, been exhaustively catalogued by Freedom and colleagues.[1] Preoperative anatomic information is now routinely and comprehensively acquired by noninvasive imaging modalities, primarily echocardiography, and increasingly, magnetic resonance imaging (MRI) or computed tomography (CT), as discussed in Chapter 106. Valvar anatomy is beautifully displayed using transesophageal or three-dimensional echocardiography; ventricular volumes and function are quantified using MRI. Vascular abnormalities, such as aortic arch anomalies, or the complex venous patterns in heterotaxy syndrome, can similarly be well rendered through CT or MRI reconstruction.[2] These modalities will no doubt continue to undergo improvements in ease of acquisition, image resolution, and post-processing capabilities, likely avoiding the need for diagnostic angiography in all but rare cases. With currently available technology, vascular beds in which angiography remains the gold standard include pulmonary vessels beyond the hilum, and the coronary arterial bed, particularly in younger and smaller patients with highly atypical variants (Fig. 107-1).[3]

With the changing, and increasingly interventional, role of catheterization, the need for integration of three-dimensional anatomic information into the procedure has driven the development of "overlay" technologies and transfer/display of non-angiographic imaging data into the catheterization laboratory. As a natural evolution, the techniques and technology to acquire three-dimensional angiographic data sets have developed and matured to the point of incorporation into clinical practice in many centers. For patients who may also have indications for direct hemodynamic measurement and are candidates for intervention, this alternative provides the advantage of giving the interventionalist highly directed, immediate, as-needed, anatomic information at the time of catheterization. This advantage obviously needs to be considered in the context of the associated radiation exposure but will certainly warrant the angiographic information in some cases. The feasibility of MRI-guided cardiac catheterization has been shown, and MRI-guided interventions have been performed in experimental settings.[4,5] To date, limitations have been posed by the availability of adequate MRI-compatible intravascular tools and by the processing speed of MRI systems, which lack the real-time feedback of fluoroscopy.

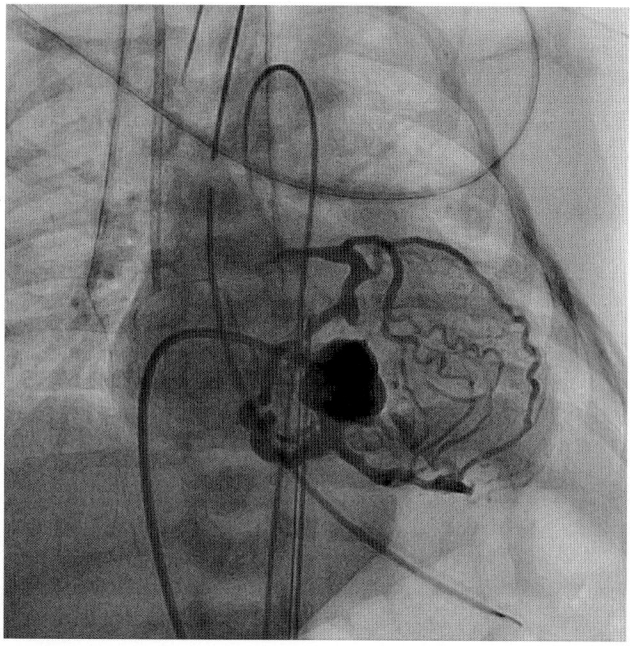

FIGURE 107-1 ■ Right ventricular angiography in a neonate with pulmonary atresia and intact ventricular septum. Injection in the right ventricle opacifies the entire coronary artery system and documents right coronary ostial atresia.

Much hemodynamic information can also be derived from echocardiography and MRI, as is discussed in great depth in Chapter 106. In some cases, there is no substitute for directly measured pressures that must be obtained invasively. When the best possible estimate of pulmonary vascular resistance is critical—as in the case of (1) pulmonary hypertension, (2) pretransplant evaluation, or (3) preoperative risk assessment for single ventricle palliation—cardiac catheterization is performed despite the availability of other methods. Similarly, even with a myriad of noninvasive indicators of diastolic function, direct measurement of the end-diastolic pressure is not infrequently an indication for catheterization. In the case of both pulmonary vascular assessment and measurement of filling pressures, the catheterization procedure also provides the opportunity to perform maneuvers to understand physiologic responses to intervention, such as administration of nitric oxide, expansion of intravascular volume, infusion of inotropes, or manipulation of pacing parameters. Fortunately for the invasive cardiologist, cardiac catheterization is a highly interactive process, and so as observations are made, hypotheses can be tested, disruptions such as test occlusions can be imposed, or interventions can be undertaken.

For surgical patients, the operating surgeon ultimately decides whether the accuracy and completeness of preoperative diagnostics is sufficient to plan and proceed with the operation with the best possible outcome expected. For patients with complex disease or those with atypical management, early and steady involvement of the surgeon in the preoperative evaluation, including the conduct of the catheterization, is invaluable. A firm grasp of the advantages and limitations of data gained through all available techniques is critical, as is the ability to resolve apparently conflicting findings and place the appropriate weight on specific measurements or interpretations.

Although a series of preoperative hemodynamic catheterizations have been a staple of management for single ventricle disease, it is increasingly argued that many of these studies may be of marginal benefit and may not warrant the risk of an invasive procedure and radiation exposure. Most clinically well patients with favorable findings of noninvasive evaluation are likely to undergo successful bidirectional Glenn operation, or even Fontan, without excess of morbidity and without the benefit of a preoperative catheterization.[6,7] The role of hemodynamic catheterization in this setting is ultimately determined by the reliability of noninvasive imaging modalities, primarily echocardiography, to screen for and accurately identify potential problems, such as pulmonary arterial distortion or arch obstruction, which should be addressed either in the catheterization laboratory or at the time of operation. Also, it is incumbent on the catheterizer to demonstrate the usefulness of some interventions that might occur at preoperative catheterization. The routine scheduling of catheterization before a Glenn or Fontan procedure is likely to receive increasing scrutiny in the future, and the added value of these studies will need to be defended.

HEMODYNAMIC ASSESSMENT

A full hemodynamic data set allows estimation of systemic and pulmonary blood flow, measurement of intracardiac and intravascular pressures with evaluation of pathologic gradients, and calculation of systemic and pulmonary vascular resistances. Two important vulnerabilities of traditional hemodynamic assessment in the catheterization laboratory are the designation of oxygen consumption, which is most often assumed, and the assumption of a steady state. Both of these limitations are more pronounced when dealing with more extreme or labile circulations. Ideally, the primary hemodynamic data can be obtained during catheterization under conditions that approximate each patient's baseline condition. The routine use of general anesthetic may pose some difficulty in this regard.

Flows

Systemic blood flow, or cardiac index, is commonly estimated either by a thermodilution technique or by using the Fick method. Calculation of flow using the Fick method is based on the principle that the total uptake (or release) of a substance by an organ is the product of blood flow to that organ and the difference between the concentrations of an indicator substance in the arteries and veins leading into and out of that organ. When calculating the systemic blood flow, the whole of the systemic tissues are considered the organ, and oxygen is considered the indicator. By measuring the hemoglobin concentration, the percent oxygen saturation of hemoglobin, and the partial pressure of oxygen in a given sample of blood, the oxygen content can be calculated. The oxygen contents of aortic and mixed systemic venous blood samples serve as the necessary concentrations of indicator, and the patient's oxygen consumption represents the total uptake of indicator in a given unit of time (1 minute). The systemic blood flow, or cardiac index (Qs), can be calculated according to the following equation:

$$Qs\,(L/min/m^2) = \frac{O_2\text{ consumption }(mL\ O_2/min/m^2)}{\text{systemic arterial} - \text{systemic venous } O_2\text{ content }(mL\ O_2/dL) \times 10}$$

Although methods exist for measuring oxygen consumption during catheterization, most catheterization laboratories assume a level of oxygen consumption based on the patient's age, sex, and heart rate.

Pulmonary blood flow can be similarly calculated by calculating the oxygen content of pulmonary arterial and venous blood. With the systemic and pulmonary blood flow rates in hand, various shunts can be calculated, and the ratio of pulmonary to systemic blood flow, or Qp : Qs, can be determined. A rapid bedside calculation of Qp : Qs can be obtained by simply using the following equation:

$$Qp : Qs = \frac{\text{aortic saturation} - \text{mixed venous saturation}}{\text{pulmonary venous} - \text{pulmonary arterial saturation}}$$

Pressures

At catheterization, pressure measurements are obtained through fluid-filled catheters, which are vulnerable to various errors, ranging from an inappropriate zero level, to catheter entrapment with waveform distortion. Ideal catheters for pressure transduction provide free communication between the environment external to the catheter tip and the lumen of the catheter. Thus, larger-bore catheters, or catheters with multiple end or side holes, yield the most accurate depiction of the intracardiac waveform. A complete set of pressure measurements includes pressure waveforms recorded in all cardiac chambers and great vessels. When the left atrium is not entered directly, a pulmonary capillary wedge tracing is recorded in lieu of a left atrial trace. Systolic and diastolic pressures are noted in arterial vessels, whereas mean pressures are commonly noted in atrial or venous tracings. In the ventricle, the systolic and end-diastolic pressures are specified. Gradients can be documented by single catheter pullback or by simultaneous recordings in adjacent chambers or vessels using multilumen catheters or multiple catheters. When interpreting pressure gradients to determine the severity of obstructive lesions, the general principle of Ohm's law as it applies to hemodynamic variables must be considered, and the gradient should be considered in the context of the flow across the lesion.

Resistances

Having measured pressures and calculated flows, the resistance across a vascular bed can be calculated by relating the mean pressure change (ΔP) across that vascular bed to its flow. In the following equation,

$$R = \frac{\Delta P}{Q}$$

will thus be applied as

$$PVR = \frac{TPG}{Qp},$$

where TPG is the transpulmonary gradient, which is equal to the mean pulmonary artery pressure minus mean pulmonary venous pressure, and PVR is pulmonary vascular resistance. The pressures are measured in millimeters of mercury (mm Hg), and flows are typically indexed and expressed in liter/min/m^2. Thus resistance is commonly expressed as mm Hg/liter/min/m^2, or indexed Wood units.

SEDATION AND ANESTHESIA

There is wide institutional variability in approaches to sedation for catheterization.[8] Stimuli associated with catheterization include local pain related to percutaneous placement of access sheaths and more visceral pain related to intracardiac or intravascular manipulation and interventions. Provoked ectopy or arrhythmia, even if hemodynamically stable, may be disturbing to awake patients. Older, cooperative children without major hemodynamic compromise can, for the most part, undergo a routine catheterization safely and comfortably with conscious sedation and a spontaneous airway. In preparation for the procedure, oral benzodiazepines can be administered as anxiolytics before placing an intravenous line. Once intravenous access is established, a combination of benzodiazepines and opioids works well for most children who undergo catheterization without general anesthesia. Bolus doses of these drugs may be administered over the course of the procedure, or a continuous infusion may be preferable, depending on the nature and duration of the case. Alternative agents that have been used successfully with appropriate oversight are ketamine in conjunction with midazolam, and propofol infusion.

In the current era, general inhalational anesthetic is administered for most pediatric cases, to minimize the potential for patient discomfort. Some interventional cases warrant general anesthetic almost regardless of the tolerance or cooperativity of the patient, because of the anticipated duration of the procedure, high-risk nature of the intervention, necessity of patient immobility, and/or the need for both airway and hemodynamic control. Most infants and young children who are likely to be undergoing interventional procedures are most safely catheterized under general anesthesia. In addition, individuals who require uncomfortable additional impositions, such as placement of a transesophageal echocardiographic probe for monitoring device closure of atrial septal defects (ASDs), or placement of internal jugular or subclavian catheters, are less likely to be distressed if under a general anesthetic.

Very rarely, the induction of general anesthesia or use of inhalational anesthetic may, in and of itself, be destabilizing, as can be the case in children with left ventricular (LV) outflow obstruction and/or coronary compromise, or those with severe restrictive physiology. Patients with severe heart failure who rely on endogenous catecholamine levels for maintenance of circulation can also be at risk with typical anesthetic induction techniques. Consultation with, and anticipatory inclusion of, members of a dedicated cardiac anesthesia team before catheterization serves the best interests of the patients and their caregivers and contributes to successful completion of the procedure.

VASCULAR ACCESS

Standard Arterial and Venous Access

For most catheterization procedures, intravascular access is established and maintained in both an artery and a vein. Even when a single venous catheter may provide access for a full hemodynamic data set, an arterial catheter is often placed for continuous intraprocedural monitoring. Placement of an arterial line in these cases should be weighed against the risk of compromised postprocedural perfusion of the extremity. Highly focused cases in stable, healthy subjects (e.g., ASD closure, pulmonary valvuloplasty) are usually performed with only a venous line, as are many pulmonary hypertension studies and routine cardiac biopsies. In some emergent clinical situations, when there is a premium on speed of intervention, the case should not be delayed while placing "elective" access, but rather the catheterizer should be creative about the most expedient access possible to complete the procedure.

Vascular access is typically established in the femoral vessels, as the consistent anatomy, superficial course, and relative sizes of these vessels allow straightforward percutaneous entry. The side-by-side placement of femoral venous and arterial lines allows the operator to stand over a well-circumscribed field that can easily be kept sterile and allows the patient to be continuously audited for catheter displacement or bleeding. Given the placement of standard anteroposterior and lateral cameras in a biplane lab, the femoral sites are also the most ergonomically favorable. Approach to the heart via the femoral vein and the inferior vena cava allows entry to almost all necessary catheter sites, including complex transseptal courses that can be difficult from a superior approach. At the conclusion of the procedure, catheter removal and control of the vessels in the groin with manual compression is relatively easy, and the procedure is well tolerated by individuals of all ages. In pediatric catheterization, manual compression is most often applied to achieve hemostasis. In larger patients, especially those who have had large caliber sheaths in the femoral vessels, the use of percutaneous site closure systems can

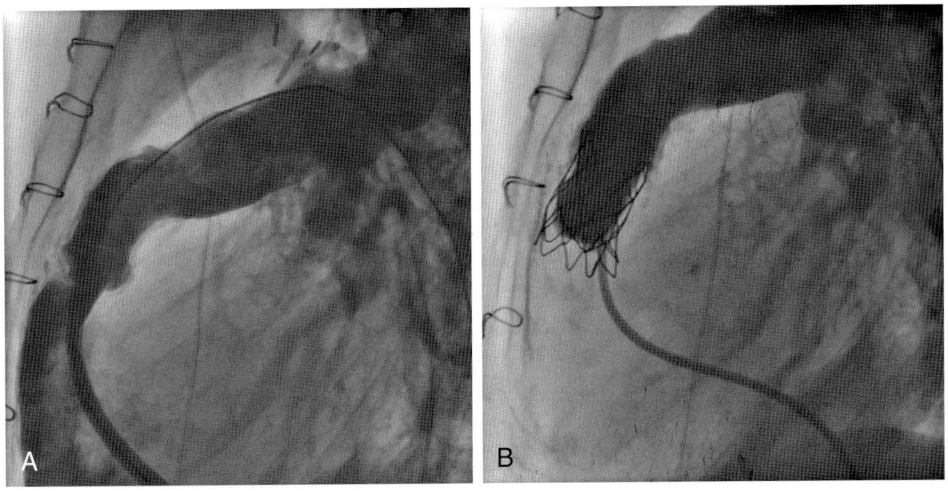

FIGURE 107-4 Right ventricular outflow tract angiography in a lateral projection. The highly obstructed and calcified conduit is seen in an immediate retrosternal position. **A,** Contrast injection in the distal conduit demonstrates antegrade flow along the wire course into the right pulmonary artery, as well as severe pulmonary regurgitation opacifying the right ventricle. **B,** After placement of a stent-mounted bovine jugular valve, the pulmonary regurgitation is abolished.

stent-based valve and percutaneous delivery system and provided a candidate population in which to advance the concept of percutaneous valve replacement. A unique convergence of conditions—(1) driving clinical interest, (2) broad interventional experience with stent delivery in RV to pulmonary artery conduits, (3) surgical experience with bioprosthetic valve materials, and (4) multiple precedents for industry collaboration in device development—allowed the process to move rapidly.

The approval of the Melody stent-based, bovine jugular vein valve in 2010 marked a major milestone in interventional catheterization, with subsequent widespread use of this device and dissemination of the procedure.[48] Although the device was approved for use in patients with dysfunctional RV to pulmonary artery conduits, patients with native outflow tracts and sufficient narrowing to seat the device have now also been treated.[49] These patients are the target population of newer devices currently under study, tailored to the highly variable anatomy of the postoperative native outflow tract. The original device, used when indicated for conduit failure, effectively relieves obstruction and decreases pulmonary regurgitation as observed angiographically, echocardiographically, and by MRI-derived pulmonary regurgitant fraction (Fig. 107-4).[50-52] These improvements are sustained in medium-term follow-up. Perhaps of greatest significance is a demonstrable improvement in New York Heart Association class and measured exercise parameters.[53] Early concerns about valve failure related to stent fracture have been addressed in part by changes in delivery technique (pre-stenting), although debate continues regarding the possibility of predisposition of the device to infection.[54,55] The concept of repeated re-replacement with serial, nested, stent-based devices offers, in theory, the potential for lifetime avoidance of reoperation. It seems likely that many patients will be managed with initial placement of a surgical bioprosthetic valve with subsequent catheter-based interventions. The off-label use of the Melody for valve replacement in other positions, including aortic and mitral, has been described.[56]

Vascular Interventions

All manner of congenital and postoperative vascular obstructions, both venous and arterial, are responsive to balloon angioplasty. Although indications and results vary, the principles of effective angioplasty are common, regardless of the target site. Effective angioplasty is achieved by creating a controlled tear in the vessel wall—ideally, a partial-thickness medial tear. The conditions under which this tear can be produced depend on the intrinsic compliance of the vessel wall and the severity of the obstruction. Mild stenoses and highly compliant lesions are particularly difficult to dilate effectively but may respond to endovascular stent placement. In contrast, severe noncompliant obstructions present significant risk for an uncontrolled transmural tear. To perform angioplasty safely, empiric guidelines around technical variables have been established based on the nature of the vessel being intervened on. Common indications for balloon angioplasty in the treatment of congenital heart disease are coarctation of the aorta and pulmonary arterial stenosis.

Coarctation of the Aorta

Restenosis occurs after surgical repair of coarctation of the aorta, and its incidence has been estimated at 10% to 20%, related to age at repair, and the degree of associated arch hypoplasia.[57] After pioneering work by Sos and colleagues[58] and Lock and coworkers[59] to test the feasibility of balloon dilation on postmortem or surgically excised specimens, Singer and colleagues[60] reported the first successful balloon dilation of recoarctation in a patient in 1982. Kan and coworkers[61] described the first seven patients in 1983, and, in 1990, the VACA Registry results showed gradient reduction to less than 20 mm Hg in 78% of patients treated.[62] In 1991, Hijazi and coworkers argued that balloon dilation should be the treatment of choice for recurrent coarctation, based on an 88% success rate and a low rate of complications.[63] The field has generally concurred, and recurrent coarctation is now largely managed in the catheterization laboratory.[64]

Native coarctation of the aorta was one early target for catheter intervention, although the observation of aneurysm formation tempered initial enthusiasm. Through the current era, the reported efficacy of balloon dilation for native coarctation has failed to support primary, nonsurgical intervention. Among infants younger than 3 months, authors have described favorable results of balloon dilation of native coarctation[32] but with restenosis occurring in more than 50% of patients.[65,66] Concern over these high restenosis rates and a 5% to 15% rate of late aneurysms has precluded widespread acceptance of angioplasty as primary therapy in unoperated infants.[67] Therefore, in these younger patients, balloon dilation is pursued primarily as a palliative procedure. Rates of iliofemoral arterial complications, which were high during the early experience with this infant population, have become lower as low-profile dilating balloon catheters have evolved.[68] In rarer, late-presenting older children and adults with unoperated coarctation, primary catheter intervention can be effective and may be considered an alternative to surgery, although there are few data to support this as a superior approach.[69] Patients with mild obstruction and potentially poorly developed collaterals may be good candidates for therapy without aortic cross-clamping.

Although the earliest discussion of stent implantation in coarctation described the treatment of severe aortic obstruction, the procedure has proven uniquely effective in treating disease at the other end of the spectrum—mild native or recurrent obstruction.[70] In this setting (peak gradient < 20 mm Hg), standard balloon angioplasty may be ineffective in the setting of a highly compliant lesion or segmental obstruction. Stent placement can allow a controlled enlargement of a mildly narrowed aorta over the length of the stent.[71] Reduction of even relatively low gradients has been associated with improvement in LV end-diastolic pressure.[72] Freedom from reintervention after stent placement for coarctation is 50% at 5 years, notably higher than in surgical series, reflecting a deliberate staged approach to transcatheter relief of some obstructions. This high rate of reintervention also reflects aggressive treatment of even mild obstruction, with 40% of reinterventions performed in patients with a gradient of 10 mm Hg or less. Overall, pathologic aortic mural injuries such as aneurysm, dissection, or rupture occurred at the time of dilation or stenting in 3 of 153 patients (2%).[73] These potentially catastrophic situations can be managed with placement of a covered stent, and this device is now available in trial. Whether covered stents will prove to be safe as a primary therapy for coarctation or should only be reserved for higher risk situations or as rescue therapy remains to be seen.

Pulmonary Artery Stenosis

As with coarctation, proximal pulmonary arterial obstructions confined to the prehilar area can often be relieved surgically, and balloon angioplasty provides an alternative to an open approach. In contrast, more distal obstructions, often inaccessible to the surgeons, are quite amenable to transcatheter therapy. These obstructions can occur in association with congenital heart disease, most commonly tetralogy of Fallot variants, or in association with arteriopathies such as Williams syndrome.[74] Although a poorly studied population before now, older patients with chronic thromboembolic disease may also benefit from transcatheter therapy for relief of distal obstructions.[75,76]

Tools for pulmonary artery dilations have improved considerably over the recent decade. Initial reports used compliant, low-pressure balloons, with perhaps predictably poor results. Since that time, high-pressure balloons, cutting balloons, and now ultra high–pressure balloons have become staples in labs treating these lesions.

Indications for balloon dilation or stenting of pulmonary arteries include elevated RV pressure, diminished distal flow, or hypertension in unaffected segments as a result of flow maldistribution. Postoperative anastomotic lesions, typically of the proximal branch pulmonary arteries, generally respond well to standard balloon dilation, as do some congenital stenoses and hypoplasia. In contrast, pulmonary arterial obstruction resulting from vessel kinking or compression often requires stent placement to achieve relief.

Using low-pressure balloons, with highly variable relative dilating diameters, the earliest pulmonary artery dilations achieved success in only 38% to 59% of cases.[58-60,77-79] Results improved as high-pressure balloons came into use; these provided relief of obstruction in up to 72% of vessels.[80] Despite the use of high-pressure balloons, a significant proportion of pulmonary arterial obstructions remained resistant to balloon angioplasty. Newer strategies to treat these lesions involve cutting balloons that are used to initiate controlled vascular injury at the site of resistant lesions.[81] By using coronary cutting balloons on small-vessel pulmonary arterial lesions resistant to high-pressure angioplasty, operators have substantially increased lumen diameter in 92% of previously refractory vessels.[82] After the introduction of larger, peripheral cutting balloons, this technology has been applied to larger-caliber vessels with good effect, although the percentage increase in lumen diameter was less dramatic in these larger vessels.[83] The most recent addition to the treatment of pulmonary artery stenosis is the ultra high–pressure balloon, developed to treat peripheral vessels or grafts in adults. These balloons, capable of achieving inflation pressure of 30 atm (relative to 4 to 8 atm of a conventional balloon) can be applied to treat highly resistant lesions, whether native vascular obstruction or previously placed stents in noncompliant segments.[84]

Balloon angioplasty of pulmonary vessels is associated with an appreciable rate of complications, some of which can be life-threatening. When obstruction to highly stenotic vessels is relieved, distal vessels may be exposed acutely to higher pressure, resulting in pulmonary edema.[85] This consequence can usually be averted by limiting relief of obstruction to create mean distal pressures not in excess of 25 mm Hg. Direct trauma to the dilation site can create obstructive intimal flaps, contained tears, and vascular rupture.[86] Strategies to manage these complications should be directed at reestablishing an unobstructed lumen (in the case of a flap), maintaining

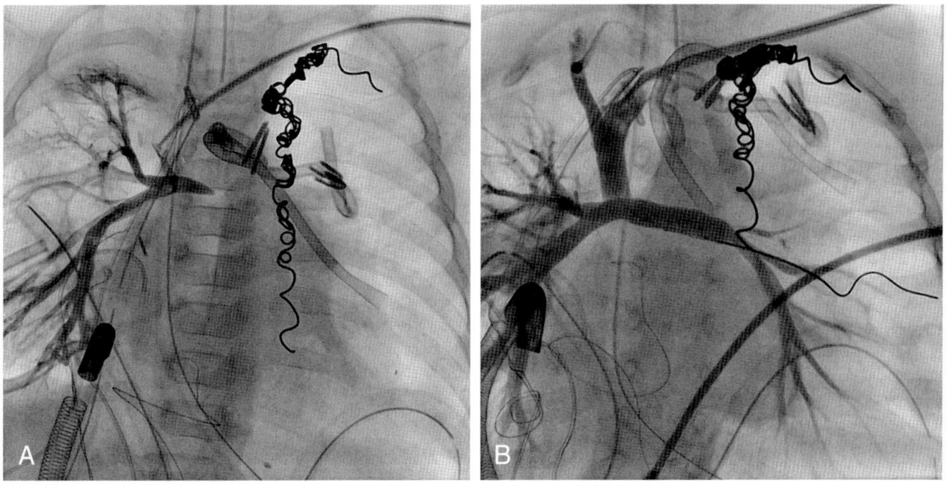

FIGURE 107-5 Early postoperative pulmonary angiography in an infant after a bidirectional Glenn operation. Flow from the superior vena cava travels exclusively into the right pulmonary artery. **A,** A "beak" is evident at the site of acquired left pulmonary artery atresia. **B,** After wire recanalization and stent placement, bilateral pulmonary flow is reestablished.

distal flow, and controlling any hemorrhage. In some cases, uncontrolled tears may be managed by temporary occlusion of upstream vessels, when this maneuver can be hemodynamically tolerated. Occasionally, feeding vessel occlusion, using a coil or other occlusion device, may be necessary.

Balloon-expandable stents have been used successfully to relieve pulmonary arterial obstruction since the early 1980s. Stents were first applied predominantly in proximal branch pulmonary artery stenoses in larger children, simply because of the size of the available stents, the size of the stent or balloon delivery system, and the risk of iatrogenic "restenosis" caused by the stent after somatic growth. After experimental evidence that endovascular stents could be safely and effectively redilated, McMahon and associates reported on mechanisms of successful redilation in a large group of patients.[87] The introduction of more flexible, smaller, and lower-profile stenting systems in the early 2000s resulted in stents being placed more frequently in distal vessels and in infants and smaller children.[88,89] Using tools such as ultra high–pressure balloons, the potential for some degree of further stent expansion at a later date can be presumed. In the case of early postoperative anastomotic obstruction, stent placement may be preferable to simple angioplasty, because vessel occlusions or stenoses can be opened without using oversize balloons and risking vessel or suture line rupture (Fig. 107-5).[90]

Conduits, Systemic and Pulmonary Veins

Transcatheter angioplasty techniques have also proved valuable in extending the life of allograft or prosthetic shunts in palliated postoperative patients, such as those with RV to pulmonary artery conduits after stage I for HLHS or those with conduits used in RV outflow tract reconstruction as in tetralogy of Fallot with pulmonary atresia. These grafts can become obstructive and require replacement because of contraction, kinking, neointimal "peel" accumulation, external compression, or simply patient growth. Standard balloon angioplasty rarely provides definitive relief, although ultra high–pressure balloons have been used with greater success.[91] Predictably, balloon expandable stent placement can effectively delay the need for surgical reintervention although at the expense of loss of competency of any existent valve.[92,93] In a single-center review of 221 patients with stents implanted in RV to pulmonary artery conduits, acute hemodynamic changes after stenting included significantly decreased RV systolic pressure and peak RV to pulmonary artery gradient. Stents could be redilated, and at subsequent catheterization, additional stents could be placed. By Kaplan-Meier analysis, median freedom from conduit surgery after stenting was almost 3 years. Younger age, smaller conduit diameter, and higher ratio of RV to aortic pressure predicted shorter freedom from surgery.[94]

Systemic venous obstruction occurs in a number of postoperative congenital cardiac settings, most notably in patients after atrial switch procedures. In both cardiac and noncardiac patient populations, systemic venous obstruction occurs with increasing frequency as a result of chronic indwelling catheters and, in some cases, cannulation for extracorporeal membrane oxygenation. Both angioplasty and stent placement have been applied successfully in the setting of superior vena cava obstruction.[95,96] Patients with extensive venous obstruction have been treated for the classical symptoms of superior vena caval syndrome but also for some less well understood indications, including respiratory insufficiency.[97] In these cases, elevated superior caval pressure is thought to contribute to impairments of pulmonary lymphatic drainage and thus lung function. The superiority of stent placement over simple balloon angioplasty with regard to gradient relief and durability of result is suspected but has not been firmly established, although stent placement should be carefully considered in the young infant with anticipation of significant superior vena cava growth over a lifetime.

Pulmonary vein stenosis that occurs either as "isolated" disease or in the context of congenital heart disease, particularly in young infants, remains one of the most challenging lesions to treat, either by surgery or with transcatheter techniques. On the basis of favorable results after balloon dilation angioplasty of congenital lesions, Driscoll and colleagues attempted pulmonary vein dilation in the early 1980s, and they observed early restenosis associated with clinical decline.[98] Endovascular stents applied to pulmonary venous obstruction almost a decade later failed to alter the course of the progressive and intractable reobstruction, which rapidly redeveloped within months of intervention.[99,100] All manner of therapies have been attempted in limited settings, including mass removal/endovascular biopsy, covered stents, drug-eluting stents, and rotational atherectomy. None of these have provided any measurable advantage in the treatment of pulmonary vein stenosis. Currently, we use standard high-pressure and cutting balloons rather than more elaborate tools, reserving stenting for multiply reobstructed vessels or those with clear kinking at the left atrial junction.[101,102] None of these therapies has consistently provided lasting relief of obstruction/favorable remodeling; thus, frequent reintervention is often necessary, sometimes as often as every 8 to 10 weeks.

Defect Occlusion

To date, transcatheter relief of obstructions, whether valvar or vascular, has been accomplished largely by applying relatively simple devices, such as angioplasty balloons or balloon-expandable stents. In contrast, the field of defect closure has been defined by the variety of devices developed. In 1987, after almost 20 years of development, Rashkind and colleagues described the use of an occluding device to treat patent ductus arteriosus (PDA).[103] Since that time, numerous catheter-based devices have been used to close defects without surgery. These devices have encompassed a range of sizes, configurations, materials, delivery systems, and release mechanisms. They not only have been implanted in patients with PDA, ASD, and ventricular septal defect (VSD) but also have been used for innovative indications, including such lesions as perivalvular leak, coronary artery fistula, and pulmonary arteriovenous malformation.[104,105]

Despite the broad range of devices produced and evaluated, only a few have been fully approved and marketed for use in patients with congenital heart disease. Perhaps the greatest evolution in the fields of pediatric interventional cardiology and device closure has been the engagement of the regulatory process by the interventional community. Only by carefully designing and carrying out intelligent, nonrandomized, multicenter trials has there been sufficient enrollment of patients and data collection to support device approval applications. Even so, the number of patients enrolled and devices implanted is typically in the range of a few hundred, and follow-up periods are relatively short. Ongoing evaluation of each approved device is the responsibility of the implanting interventional cardiology community.

Patent Ductus Arteriosus, Collaterals, and Shunts

The development and ultimate U.S. Food and Drug Administration (FDA) approval of the Amplatzer duct occluder device changed the entire approach to PDA. The history of attempts at device closure of PDA provides a useful introduction to general principles of transcatheter defect closure. In 1967, Porstmann and colleagues reported the use of foam plugs to occlude PDA via a transcatheter approach.[106] After this isolated experience, a full decade elapsed before the Rashkind PDA occluder was developed to close moderate-size PDAs. Although more effective than the previous device, a high incidence of incomplete closure made it a poor alternative to surgical closure, and it never came to market.[103,107] Ultimately, PDAs were effectively closed by catheter delivery of the Gianturco vascular occlusion coil used in an off-label fashion. This conceptually simple, inexpensive, versatile, and easy-to-use device rapidly came into widespread use. Coil occlusion of small PDAs (<3 mm) became a routine catheter procedure. Most small PDAs could be safely and effectively closed using a single coil,[108,109] and closure rates when multiple coils were available were 93%.[110,111]

Closure of larger PDAs continued to prove a challenge, often requiring multiple coils or advanced coil delivery techniques, with attendant increase in rates of embolization and residual flow. One device, essentially a sac designed to retain a large coil cluster, was approved for vascular occlusion, but the combination of a large delivery system, expense, and a complex delivery mechanism were unacceptable to most implanters.[112] The unsatisfactory results of coil-based approaches to large PDAs spurred a search for a different type of device, and the plugging concept was reexplored. In 1998, the Amplatzer duct occluder device received approval after a multicenter trial demonstrated successful closure of larger PDAs (>3.5 mm), with closure rates of 100% at the 1-year follow-up. The advantages over the existing products included ease of use, low-profile delivery, and retrievability.[113] The recently approved Nit-Occlud device, resurrecting the coil concept, further increases the likelihood that the isolated PDA in an older infant or child will rarely be encountered by the cardiac surgeon.[114] Although the hemodynamically important PDA in the premature infant has also been treated using these devices, in this population, surgical intervention remains the standard.[115]

In the setting of more complex heart disease, devices such as embolization coils and vascular occluders can be used to advantage in management of unwanted extracardiac shunts, whether biologic or prosthetic, as well as in the management of intracardiac defects. Aortopulmonary collateral vessels, commonly seen in patients with palliated single ventricle disease, may impair postoperative recovery by imposing a disadvantageous volume load on the single ventricle. Furthermore, they can inhibit efficient oxygenation by competing with caval flow for entry to the peripheral pulmonary vasculature, and they may contribute to persistent pleural effusions postoperatively.[116] Closure of these vessels to decrease unwanted return into the field at the time of operation remains controversial, as flow studies have questioned the extent of their contribution to pulmonary venous return. Recent MRI data suggest that prior reports may have underestimated the flow capacity and clinical consequences of these vessels. Using embolization coils or particles, flow may be eliminated in up to 75% of treated aortopulmonary collaterals in patients with congenital heart disease.[117,118]

Occlusion devices may also be used in occlusion of iatrogenic shunts, such as a supplementary Blalock-Taussig shunt or a stented PDA in a patient with pulmonary atresia with an intact ventricular septum (PA/IVS). In patients with pulmonary atresia who undergo RV decompression, the shunt may become superfluous as RV compliance improves. At subsequent hemodynamic assessment, if shunt occlusion is indicated, it can be performed with high rates of total occlusion and minimal risk for adverse events, sparing the patient reoperation.[117]

Atrial Septal Defect Closure

Since the first clinical report of percutaneous, device-based ASD closure by King and Mills in 1974, transcatheter closure has repeatedly been shown to be feasible, safe, and effective in both standard-risk and high-risk surgical patients.[119] This procedure is now available in most centers as an alternative to surgical closure for typical ASDs, although surgical closure may still yield the best outcome in specific cases. All catheter-based procedures for ASD closure rely on the implantation of a device that has some overlap onto surrounding septal tissue to permit device stabilization. These devices are appropriate only in secundum defects and have never been credibly applied to sinus venosus or primum-type ASDs. Furthermore, not all secundum ASDs are candidates for device closure, depending on their size and proximity to other cardiac structures (e.g., the aortic root, superior vena cava, or atrioventricular valves). Variability in septal defect size, shape, and position has thwarted efforts to design a single device that could be uniformly successful in closing ASDs (Fig. 107-6). As a result, a myriad of devices have been used, but results are difficult to compare because of inherent differences in mechanisms and timing of closure. Each device also results in unique unintended outcomes, including failure to implant, device fracture, erosion, malposition, and late embolization.

Early devices were based on the double umbrella concept, and in 1989, the clamshell device was the first to be implanted under protocol of a prospective multicenter investigational device exemption (IDE) trial. Although results were promising, difficulties with the device and the process of approval resulted in the abandonment of this device in favor of a second generation of umbrella devices. An alternative approach was pursued with the Amplatzer atrial septal occluder, which incorporated self-centering capability and retrievability into a remarkably simple and effective design. In 2002, the Amplatzer atrial septal occluder became the first device to receive FDA approval based on reports of a 100% successful implantation rate, a complete closure rate of 98%, and a low rate (2%) of complications.[120] This device was designed to close secundum ASDs up to 38 mm in diameter. Comparison with surgical closure showed comparable rates of defect closure (99%) and adverse events (8%). However, device closure offered the benefit of shorter length of stay and lower rate of major adverse events. Subsequently, a second device was approved for closure of smaller ASDs. In a multicenter trial, the Helex device (Gore and Associates, Flagstaff, AZ) was implanted in 143 patients who had an ASD less than 22 mm in diameter, with good results.[121] Closure rates using this device were comparable to surgery, although the size of the candidate defect was a limitation, and a 25% incidence of small residual leak was recognized. This device received approval in 2006, at which time development of an alternatively configured device with a somewhat simplified delivery system was already under way. The Gore Septal Occluder, marketed overseas, has yet to receive approval and is still in trial in the United States.

Ongoing evaluations of these devices have revealed late device-related complications, including malposition/embolization, thrombus formation, and erosion.[122,123] When embolization occurs, devices can often be retrieved using tools such as intravascular snares. The potential for entrapment of the device, or valvar damage, should be considered and may dictate that surgical removal is a safer solution. The incidence of thrombus formation appears to be related to device type, although whether delivery, materials, or device configuration plays a causative role remains unknown.[124] Erosion has been reported immediately after implantation, as well as several years later, and can be catastrophic. Its occurrence remains rare but disturbingly poorly predicted. It is believed to result from ongoing radial and possibly rotational forces exerted by the edge of the device on cardiac tissues.[125] Biodegradable closure devices have historically been a topic of great interest, based on the potential superiority with regard to profile and thrombogenicity. These devices have thus far failed to equal the performance of the currently available, more traditional occluders.

Although most small or moderate-sized secundum ASDs can be closed using intracardiac devices, surgery remains the primary approach for most types of VSDs requiring closure. Some exceptions exist, as in the case of very apical or anterior muscular defects, postoperative intramural defects, or extensive multiple muscular defects (i.e., the "Swiss cheese" septum).[126,127] These VSDs pose significant surgical challenges and may ultimately be most effectively managed through a combination of surgical and catheter intervention, or hybrid approach.

Ventricular Septal Defect Closure

The earliest attempts at transcatheter closure of VSDs, using a double umbrella device, were described by Lock and colleagues in 1988.[128] These authors described technical aspects and feasibility of the procedure for six patients who were not considered candidates for operative closure. Bridges and coworkers[129] added to the experience with a review of highly selected patients with muscular VSD occurring in association with complex heart lesions who underwent device closure. It was suggested that preoperative transcatheter closure could simplify subsequent surgical repair of relatively inaccessible lesions.[129] In the first large reported experience with transcatheter VSD closure, patients considered high risk for surgical VSD closure were treated with transcatheter

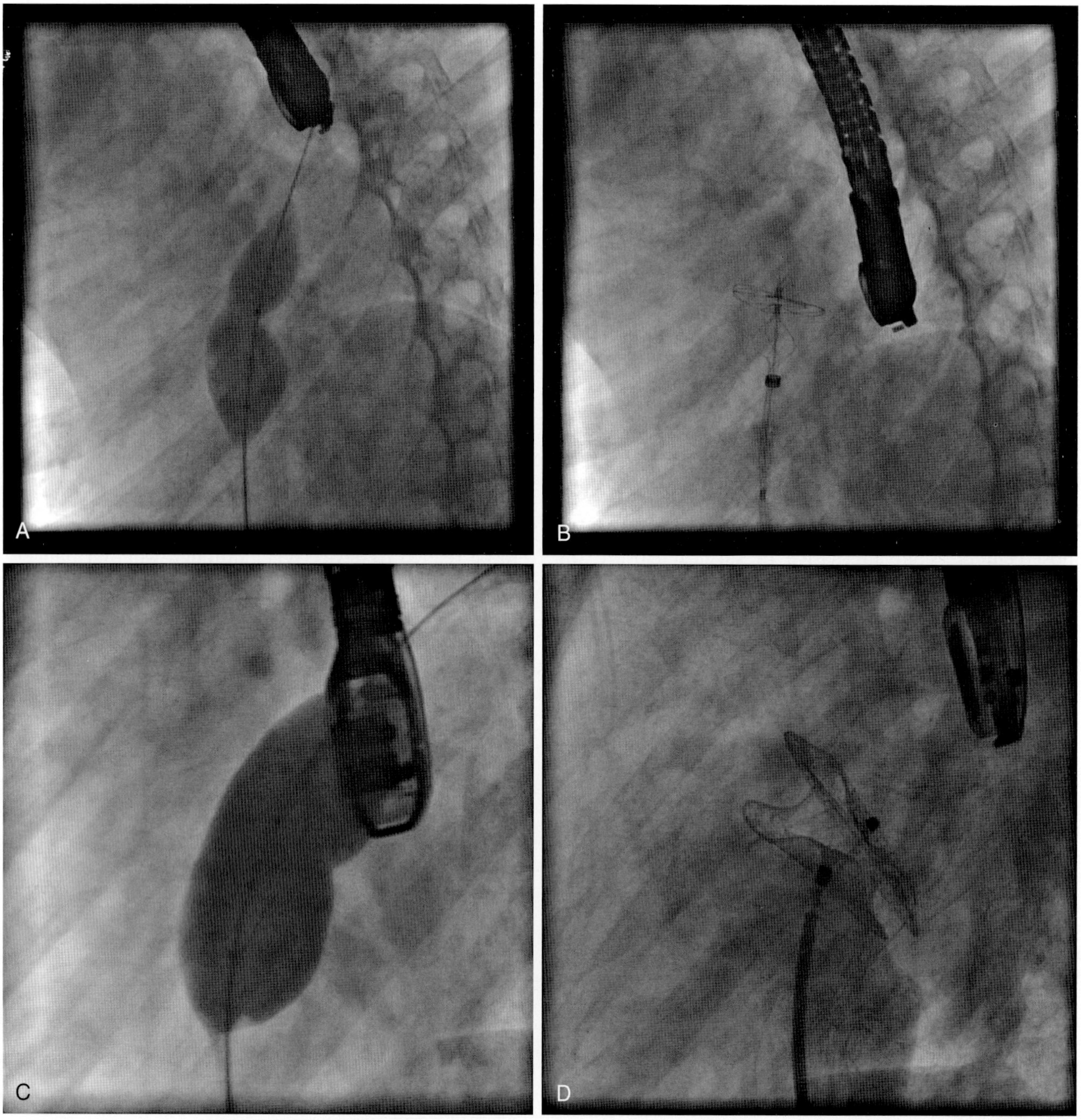

FIGURE 107-6 ■ Lateral projection images during transcatheter atrial septal defect closure with fluoroscopic and transesophageal echocardiographic imaging. **A,** Balloon sizing of a small defect. **B,** Imaging during partial deployment of the right atrial disc after complete formation of the left atrial disc, using a Helex device. **C,** Balloon sizing of a larger defect with minimal waist apparent on anterior aspect of balloon. **D,** Following left and right atrial disc deployment of an Amplatzer septal occluder, right atrial angiography aids in confirming appropriate position, particularly inferiorly.

device and showed improvement on a composite VSD size and severity scale.[127] However, the complex catheter courses, the size of the delivery system, and the vulnerable hemodynamic situation of patients resulted in a high rate of major adverse events, perhaps 45%.

Results of muscular VSD closure using the Amplatzer muscular VSD device were reported in 2004.[130] This device, similar in concept to the Amplatzer duct occluder and the Amplatzer septal occluder devices, offered the advantage of a smaller delivery system and a significantly lower adverse event rate (11%) when compared with results for prior VSD devices. The procedural success rate of only 86% reflects the fact that despite significant improvements in deliverability of devices, transcatheter VSD closure remains a technically challenging intervention. Among 75 patients treated with the Amplatzer muscular VSD device, late complete closure was achieved by echocardiographic criteria in 92%, although follow-up was incomplete. This device received FDA approval for marketing in 2004. Perventricular delivery, or even intraoperative delivery under direct visualization, has been described and should be considered as part of a surgical strategy for closure of complex, multiple muscular defects.

At this time, the feasibility of device closure of perimembranous VSD using an asymmetric device has been demonstrated and there is growing clinical experience overseas.[131] However, no membranous VSD device has yet received domestic approval. The risks of percutaneous device delivery include interference with aortic and atrioventricular valves, leading to regurgitation, and device-related conduction abnormalities, including heart block. In the context of widely available surgical therapies with excellent results, outcomes of transcatheter closure will likely have to be improved over those seen thus far to justify a primarily device-based treatment.

COMPLICATIONS

In large centers, between 55% and 75% of all catheterizations now involve intervention.[132] As with all minimally invasive techniques, effective transcatheter interventions for congenital heart disease offer the potential for treatment with lower morbidity and cost. However, the indirect nature of these catheter procedures also creates a unique set of potential complications. The overall rate of serious complications from interventional catheterization, investigated repeatedly, ranges from 3% to 7%.[133-135] Although relatively few of these complications (approximately 2%) require emergent surgery, interventional procedures should not be undertaken unless surgical backup is available. Complications requiring surgical intervention include access vessel injury, valvar disruption, cardiac perforation, and device malposition or embolization.[136] A collaborative relationship between the interventional cardiologist and the pediatric cardiac surgeon allows each to better understand the benefits and risks of the two different therapeutic modalities.

SURGICAL COLLABORATION

Although hybrid procedures, using combined surgical and catheter collaboration, have been performed for decades, the publication of results of the hybrid stage I procedure for HLHS launched an era of enthusiastic expansion of this type of approach.[137,138] The hybrid stage I was initially described as open chest placement of pulmonary artery bands, with direct main pulmonary artery access for placement of a catheter-delivered stent in the PDA and, often at a later procedure, the creation of an unrestrictive ASD. Results at selected centers that gained routine experience with this approach were as good as standard surgical stage I, and because the patients were spared cardiopulmonary bypass and circulatory arrest, postprocedural recovery was remarkably rapid. At this time, most large centers continue to routinely perform surgical stage I.

The rewards of more extensive interventionalist-surgeon collaboration and promotion of the broader hybrid concept remain compelling. These approaches will no doubt be applied more widely as devices for management of ASD, VSD, and valve failure become more sophisticated and widely available. Surgical control will allow the delivery of intravascular devices to be independent of access vessel patency or size and will also allow for stabilization of nonsecured devices. Balloons and stents, developed for percutaneous use, will increasingly become part of the surgeon's toolbox with procedures such as intraoperative stent placement or combined valve commissurotomy with annular balloon expansion. As experience with these collaborations accrues, the cross-disciplinary knowledge gained will benefit the field.

Surgeons and interventional cardiologists will also collaborate in the management of the postoperative patient. As patients with increasingly complex anatomy present for repair and can be supported with ever-improving intensive care, the opportunity to perform postoperative invasive assessment will present more frequently. Early intervention on residual postoperative lesions can be carried out safely and may shorten stays or reduce residual hemodynamic burden prolonging hospitalization.[139,140] A generally held belief that angioplasty is safer after approximately 6 weeks following surgery will likely never be proven, and, to the contrary, increasing experience with intervention on postoperative obstruction will likely prove useful in postoperative management.

As extracorporeal support and circulatory assist devices are applied to greater numbers of patients with congenital heart disease, new situations will present themselves to the interventionalist. In cases of extracorporeal membrane oxygenation support, left atrial decompression may be necessary to protect from excessive pulmonary venous hypertension and pulmonary hemorrhage. This procedure can be performed safely and can be associated with near immediate improvement in pulmonary conditions of the circulation at various levels of device support.[141]

FETAL INTERVENTION

Background

The rationale for fetal cardiac intervention, as for all fetal invasive procedures, is based on the premise that intervention in the rapidly changing and potentially highly responsive fetal environment may alter the natural history of a developmental error and possibly avert serious, even lethal, postnatal disease. For intervention to be considered, the diagnosis must be certain, the procedure must be feasible, and the risk of fetal or neonatal morbidity without intervention must be sufficient to justify the risk posed to both fetus and mother. Given the rapid sequencing of serial heart development, once developmental derangement is diagnosed, early intervention likely yields the greatest potential for significant clinical benefit.

Fetal Cardiac Interventions

Conditions for which prenatal cardiac interventions may be considered include those in which (1) the fetus is at risk for demise as a result of the condition, (2) the

TABLE 107-1 **Congenital Cardiovascular Anomalies Potentially Amenable to Prenatal Intervention**

Indication for Intervention	Condition	Intervention
Risk of fetal death	Congenital heart block	Pacemaker Maternal pharmacotherapy
	Severe congenital MR with AS and intact atrial septum	Balloon aortic valvuloplasty Creation of ASD
Risk of acute neonatal instability or death	HLHS with intact atrial septum	Creation of ASD
	Obstructed, totally anomalous pulmonary venous return	Stenting of obstructed vertical vein or ductus venosus
Risk of primary anomaly evolving into more severe condition	Fetal AS with evolving HLHS	Balloon aortic valvuloplasty
	Pulmonary atresia with evolving HRHS	Pulmonary valve perforation and dilation
	Premature closure of ductus arteriosus	Ductal stenting
	Absent pulmonary valve syndrome	Closure of pulmonary valve

AS, Aortic stenosis; *ASD,* atrial septal defect; *HLHS,* hypoplastic left heart syndrome; *HRHS,* hypoplastic right heart syndrome; *MR,* mitral regurgitation.

disorder is likely to result in acute neonatal instability or death, or (3) intervention may alter the evolution of the disease so that the postnatal morbidity is substantially reduced. Potential examples of these classes of indication are listed in Table 107-1. Of course, the ability to carry out an appropriate intervention must be taken into consideration. To illustrate this point, although fetal Ebstein anomaly and severe fetal mitral regurgitation pose risks of hydropic demise, fetal interventions to address atrioventricular disease do not exist. In contrast, fetuses with HLHS face a significant risk of neonatal mortality and lifelong morbidity, and in the cases related to aortic stenosis, a procedure can be performed to dilate the aortic valve. The clinical benefit of the procedure depends on the probability that the anatomic change imposed by the successful intervention in utero will alter the subsequent course of cardiac growth and development sufficiently to have a major impact on survival or postnatal outcome.

The mechanism through which anatomic modification of the fetal heart alters subsequent development is postulated to be through alteration in loading conditions. Although there is no conclusive evidence that abnormalities or alterations of flow or loading contribute to the development of cardiovascular malformations in the human fetus, data from various experimental animal systems support this contention. Fetal lambs exposed to chronically decreased LV preload by late partial occlusion of the left atrial cavity exhibit significant decrease in combined ventricular output and placental blood flow and a significant decrease in LV mass and volume.[142] These changes appear to be time dependent, with more marked alterations in fetuses with longer exposure to decreased LV inflow. In another model, in fetal lambs exposed to increased LV afterload by banding of the ascending aorta, there is a decrease in combined ventricular output, in conjunction with a significant decrease in LV chamber volume and an increase in LV wall thickness.[142] Initially, LV weight increases relative to the weight of the RV, but with a prolonged duration of aortic banding, the ratio of LV to RV weight decreases significantly. These studies and others demonstrate that alterations in ventricular loading or embryonic blood flow patterns in normal fetuses and embryos can be associated with cardiovascular development and function.

The potential for prenatal cardiac intervention has been realized for nearly three decades; as early as 1986 there was a reported attempt at in utero pacing for fetal complete heart block.[143] By 1991, there were reports of prenatal aortic valve dilation and prenatal pericardiocentesis in human fetuses.[144,145] Through the 1990s, there were several additional reports of human fetal cardiac intervention, mostly sporadic, primarily for aortic stenosis.[146] Also during this period, a number of animal studies were performed to investigate the pathophysiology of cardiac bypass and cardioprotection in the fetus, anticipating fetal cardiac surgery, as well as alternative approaches to transvascular fetal cardiac intervention.[147-150]

In 2000, we at Boston Children's Hospital initiated a program for fetal cardiac intervention, focusing on treatment of fetal aortic stenosis with evolving HLHS. Later, the program expanded to include procedures for established HLHS with an intact or highly restrictive atrial septum, pulmonary atresia with evolving hypoplastic right heart syndrome, and structural anomalies causing fetal hydrops.[151-156] At this time, more than 160 procedures have been carried out, numerous publications have described our experience, and the outcomes of the first 100 procedures for fetal aortic stenosis have recently been reported.[157]

General Approach to Fetal Cardiac Intervention

Common to all of the procedures that we perform is a percutaneous ultrasound-guided approach with maternal and fetal anesthesia. In an operating room environment, with the mother supine with left lateral tilt for uterine displacement, the location of the placenta and the fetal orientation are determined using conventional ultrasonographic techniques. A combination of spontaneous fetal movements and external version maneuvers are used to accomplish fetal positioning, and once an approach vector for percutaneous cardiac puncture is identified, fetal intramuscular anesthetic is administered intramuscularly. In the early experience, a limited laparotomy without externalization of the uterus was used to enable direct, manual, transuterine fetal positioning. This incision has been largely obviated by the application of more refined

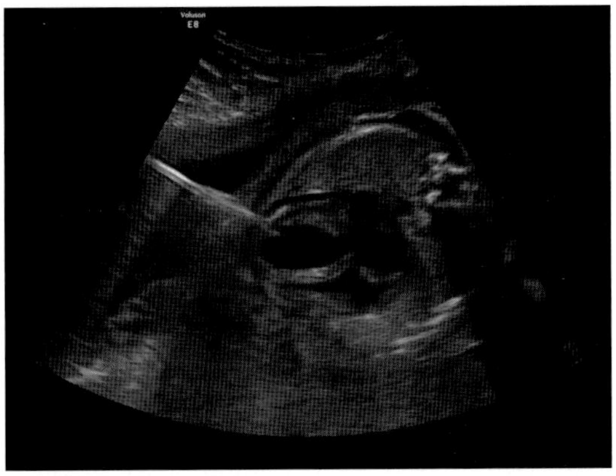

FIGURE 107-7 ■ Fetal echocardiography during prenatal intervention for critical stenosis of the fetus with evolving hypoplastic left heart syndrome. The left ventricle is dilated and dysfunctional, appearing globular, and the stainless steel needle is positioned to enter the ventricle from the apex.

maternal/fetal selection criteria and improvements in the techniques of cannula manipulation. Access to the target is achieved by direct puncture of the maternal abdomen, uterus, fetal chest wall, and the target cardiac chamber. The most commonly used cannula is a 19-gauge, 11-cm-long biopsy needle with a sharp, solid stylet and a non-beveled, dull edge, because this instrument is commercially available (Fig. 107-7). The length enables percutaneous access in most mothers between 20 and 30 weeks gestation and with a body mass index of less than 40. The inner and outer diameters of this thin-walled cannula allow for passage of most coronary artery angioplasty balloons while minimizing the potential for uterine/placental trauma and pericardial effusion.

Aortic Stenosis with Evolving HLHS

A subset of patients born with HLHS are diagnosed during the mid-second trimester with valvar aortic stenosis and a left ventricle that is normal in size or dilated but has severe dysfunction. When the left ventricle is normal in size or dilated, abnormal physiologic features associated with progression to a diagnosis of HLHS at birth include retrograde flow in the transverse aortic arch, truncated, monophasic mitral valve inflow, and left-to-right flow across the foramen ovale.[158] We refer to such mid-gestation fetuses as having severe aortic stenosis with evolving HLHS. The goal of fetal aortic valve dilation is to avert HLHS in favor of a biventricular postnatal circulation.

Predicting the evolution from aortic stenosis with a normal-size or dilated left ventricle in mid gestation to HLHS at term is complicated, and although several predictive models have attempted to predict left heart adequacy among neonates with aortic stenosis,[159-161] choosing the optimal approach in a given patient remains a challenge. Furthermore, few prenatal studies report serial data, and most include only a small number of fetuses.[162,163] Nonetheless, mid-gestation fetal aortic stenosis that does not progress to HLHS is rare, and it can be distinguished from aortic stenosis with evolving HLHS on the basis of the previously described physiologic features.[158]

Decreasing LV afterload and promoting flow through the left side of the heart by relieving aortic obstruction may help prevent progressive left heart dysfunction and growth failure over the subsequent course of gestation. Candidates with the diagnosis of aortic stenosis with evolving HLHS should be considered in light of (1) the likelihood that a technically successful procedure can be performed, and (2) the potential for salvage of the left heart—that is, the potential for LV functional recovery and growth enabling a biventricular circulation postnatally.

Fetal aortic valvuloplasty is performed according to the general practices outlined earlier. The goal is to enter the left ventricle apically but away from the interventricular septum, with a trajectory that is in line with the outflow tract. The dilating balloon size, a function of nominal balloon size and inflation pressure, is targeted to a balloon-to-annulus diameter ratio of 1.0 to 1.2. Once the cannula has been advanced to the LV cavity and the stylet removed, the coaxial guidewire and dilating balloon are introduced down its lumen, and the wire is used to probe for the orifice of the aortic valve. Once the wire is clearly visualized in the ascending aorta, the balloon is advanced across the valve and serial inflations are performed with an inflation gauge after systematic adjustment of balloon depth. When it is clear that the valve has been dilated, the entire cannula-balloon system is removed from the fetus and mother without resheathing the balloon into the cannula, and ultrasound imaging is continued. Treatment for fetal hemodynamic instability or hemopericardium is administered as necessary.[164]

We reported our initial experience with aortic valvuloplasty for fetal aortic stenosis in 2004.[153] In 2007, we reviewed outcomes of 56 fetuses with similar echocardiographic features at diagnosis, 28 of whom underwent technically successful aortic valve dilation, in an attempt to characterize a number of potentially important physiologic changes that occur after successful fetal aortic alvuloplasty.[165] On follow-up echocardiography at 32.8 ± 2.8 weeks, all control (unintervened) patients continued to have retrograde flow in the transverse aortic arch and exclusively left-to-right flow across the foramen ovale; notably, left heart structures seemed to become frozen in their anatomic size once we made the diagnosis of critical aortic stenosis with impending HLHS, and thus they became progressively more abnormal as the fetus grew.

Refinement of selection criteria has increased the percentage of infants achieving biventricular outcome after fetal aortic valve dilation, and at this time, almost 50% will not require a stage I procedure. Pediatric follow-up of these infants born after fetal aortic valvuloplasty reveals that many have significant, persistent, and sometimes refractory dysfunction of both left heart valves and myocardium. Many have significant medical and surgical burden through early childhood. With the oldest survivor just now reaching teen years, we look forward to continuing to learn what the longer-term natural history of "averted" HLHS will be. We continue to work to improve our understanding of how best to select fetuses with aortic stenosis and evolving HLHS for prenatal aortic valvuloplasty and when to intervene for optimal benefit.[157]

HLHS with Intact or Restrictive Atrial Septum

HLHS with an intact or highly restrictive atrial septum can be diagnosed on the basis of fetal imaging of the septum in conjunction with demonstration of markedly abnormal pulmonary venous flow patterns in dilated-appearing pulmonary veins.[166] Although limited pulmonary venous egress may be well tolerated in utero, neonates with major septal restriction are at substantially higher risk of death than are those without such restriction.[15,18,167] They present with profound hypoxemia after birth and often shock. Chronic pulmonary venous hypertension in utero also appears to cause pulmonary venous changes, contributing to neonatal and perioperative morbidity and mortality over the course of single ventricle palliation.

Prenatal intervention may be of benefit in fetuses with HLHS and an intact atrial septum with respect to both of the major problems posed by the restriction of pulmonary venous outflow. If the left atrium can be decompressed before birth, the profound hypoxemia and acidosis that can occur shortly after birth may be prevented and the morbidity of these metabolic insults and the risks of emergency neonatal intervention can be avoided. Also, if pulmonary venous decompression can be achieved sufficiently early in gestation, the pulmonary venous remodeling that occurs may be prevented or given an opportunity to subside or reverse. We first reported atrial septoplasty for fetuses with HLHS and intact atrial septum in 2004, and cases of prenatal atrial septoplasty for this condition have been reported by investigators from other centers as well, using various monitoring and interventional approaches.[152,168]

In theory, immediate treatment of left atrial hypertension on diagnosis would maximize the potential benefits. However, technical difficulties encountered in performing the procedure on very young fetuses have led to a shift in focus. Rather than risk fatal events in very young fetuses for the advantage of long-term preservation of pulmonary vasculature, we have prioritized early neonatal stabilization, which is dependent on a maximal ASD at the time of delivery, therefore favoring intervention later in gestation (i.e., early to mid third trimester).

The atrial septum is typically approached from the right atrial aspect. The atrial septum is perforated with a sharp instrument, either the access cannula or a smaller-gauge ultra-sharp biopsy needle, after which a dilating balloon is used to enlarge the newly created atrial defect. The largest effective balloon that can be introduced through equipment currently in use is less than 4 mm. The size of the resultant defect, as measured by intraprocedural ultrasound, is invariably smaller than the size of the dilating balloon, ranging from 1 to 3 mm. When the atrial septum appears very thick and there is an expectation that simple balloon dilation will result in septal recoil and only a very small communication, septal stent placement is feasible but exceedingly challenging.[156]

We recently reported our experience with prenatal intervention for 21 fetuses with HLHS and an intact or highly restrictive atrial septum.[169] Fetal demise occurred in two cases after the intervention, and complications, including bradycardia and pericardial or pleural effusion, occurred in eight procedures. Among neonates delivered after fetal intervention for HLHS with highly restrictive or intact atrial septum, surgical survival remains poor (58%), although in utero creation of an ASD did appear to have some benefit in terms of pre–stage I management.

Pulmonary Atresia with Intact Septum

Isolated cases of fetal pulmonary valvuloplasty in the third trimester have been reported by several groups.[170-172] It is impossible to determine from isolated cases whether prenatal intervention has the intended benefit. Since 2002, we have offered prenatal pulmonary valvuloplasty for selected mid-gestation fetuses with pulmonary atresia and evolving hypoplastic right heart, with the intent of promoting right heart growth and functional development and increasing the likelihood of a biventricular circulation after birth. Identification of potential candidates for prenatal treatment of PA/IVS has been a challenge, given the rarity of the disease, the wide spectrum of severity, and the paucity of insight about prenatal predictors of biventricular circulation.[173] Technically, the procedure presents a unique challenge because the RV (as opposed to the left ventricle in fetal aortic stenosis) is usually hypoplastic (rather than dilated) and the angle of the pulmonary valve arising off the conus can be very difficult to achieve. The effects of this strategy on right heart growth and functional development, and, ultimately, on postnatal outcome, remain to be determined.

Much remains to be learned about the benefits and potential adverse effects of prenatal cardiac intervention. Since our first procedure in 2000, referrals have grown steadily, with more than 90% of prospective and actual patients coming from outside our usual geographic catchment area. Ultimately, the value of prenatal cardiac intervention will depend on a variety of clinical and technological factors, including more frequent, earlier diagnosis of congenital heart disease in utero, characterization of prognostic features in fetuses with congenital heart disease, better understanding of the optimal gestational windows and their capacity for cardiovascular remodeling after fetal intervention, and improved and focused technology. Advances in imaging technologies and specially developed instrumentation should facilitate greater precision and effectiveness of intervention and may open the door to procedures for other, more complex indications.

REFERENCES

1. Freedom RM, Mawson JB, Yoo SJ, et al, editors: *Congenital heart disease: textbook of angiocardiography*, Armonk, NY, 1997, Futura.
2. Greil GF, Powell AJ, Gildein HP, et al: Gadolinium-enhanced three-dimensional magnetic resonance angiography of pulmonary and systemic venous anomalies. *J Am Coll Cardiol* 39(2):335–341, 2002.
3. Geva T, Greil GF, Marshall AC, et al: Gadolinium-enhanced 3-dimensional magnetic resonance angiography of pulmonary blood supply in patients with complex pulmonary stenosis or atresia: comparison with x-ray angiography. *Circulation* 106(4):473–478, 2002.
4. Ratnayaka K, Faranesh AZ, Hansen MS, et al: Real-time MRI-guided right heart catheterization in adults using passive catheters. *Eur Heart J* 34(5):380–389, 2013.

5. Raval AN, Telep JD, Guttman MA, et al: Real-time magnetic resonance imaging-guided stenting of aortic coarctation with commercially available catheter devices in Swine. *Circulation* 112(5):699–706, 2005.
6. Brown DW, Gauvreau K, Powell AJ, et al: Cardiac magnetic resonance versus routine cardiac catheterization before bidirectional glenn anastomosis in infants with functional single ventricle: a prospective randomized trial. *Circulation* 116(23):2718–2725, 2007.
7. Brown DW, Gauvreau K, Powell AJ, et al: Cardiac magnetic resonance versus routine cardiac catheterization before bidirectional Glenn anastomosis: long-term follow-up of a prospective randomized trial. *J Thorac Cardiovasc Surg* 146(5):1172–1178, 2013.
8. Cladis FP, Davis PJ, Motoyama EK: *Smith's anesthesia for infants and children*, ed 8, St. Louis, Mo., 2011, Mosby, p 1. online resource (xix, 1356 p.).
9. Shim D, Lloyd TR, Beekman RH, 3rd: Transhepatic therapeutic cardiac catheterization: a new option for the pediatric interventionalist. *Catheter Cardiovasc Interv* 47(1):41–45, 1999.
10. Ing FF, Fagan TE, Grifka RG, et al: Reconstruction of stenotic or occluded iliofemoral veins and inferior vena cava using intravascular stents: re-establishing access for future cardiac catheterization and cardiac surgery. *J Am Coll Cardiol* 37(1):251–257, 2001.
11. Rashkind WJ, Miller WW: Creation of an atrial septal defect without thoracotomy: a palliative approach to complete transposition of the great arteries. *JAMA* 196(11):991–992, 1966.
12. McQuillen PS, Hamrick SE, Perez MJ, et al: Balloon atrial septostomy is associated with preoperative stroke in neonates with transposition of the great arteries. *Circulation* 113(2):280–285, 2006.
13. Petit CJ, Rome JJ, Wernovsky G, et al: Preoperative brain injury in transposition of the great arteries is associated with oxygenation and time to surgery, not balloon atrial septostomy. *Circulation* 119(5):709–716, 2009.
14. Zellers TM, Dixon K, Moake L, et al: Bedside balloon atrial septostomy is safe, efficacious, and cost-effective compared with septostomy performed in the cardiac catheterization laboratory. *Am J Cardiol* 89(5):613–615, 2002.
15. Glatz JA, Tabbutt S, Gaynor JW, et al: Hypoplastic left heart syndrome with atrial level restriction in the era of prenatal diagnosis. *Ann Thorac Surg* 84(5):1633–1638, 2007.
16. Perry SB, Lang P, Keane JF, et al: Creation and maintenance of an adequate interatrial communication in left atrioventricular valve atresia or stenosis. *Am J Cardiol* 58(7):622–626, 1986.
17. Atz AM, Feinstein JA, Jonas RA, et al: Preoperative management of pulmonary venous hypertension in hypoplastic left heart syndrome with restrictive atrial septal defect. *Am J Cardiol* 83(8):1224–1228, 1999.
18. Vlahos AP, Lock JE, McElhinney DB, et al: Hypoplastic left heart syndrome with intact or highly restrictive atrial septum: outcome after neonatal transcatheter atrial septostomy. *Circulation* 109(19):2326–2330, 2004.
19. Vida VL, Bacha EA, Larrazabal A, et al: Hypoplastic left heart syndrome with intact or highly restrictive atrial septum: surgical experience from a single center. *Ann Thorac Surg* 84(2):581–585, 2007.
20. Kan JS, White RI, Mitchell SE, et al: Percutaneous balloon valvuloplasty: a new method for treating congenital pulmonary valve stenosis. *N Engl J Med* 307(9):540–542, 1982.
21. McCrindle BW, Kan JS: Long-term results after balloon pulmonary valvuloplasty. *Circulation* 83(6):1915–1922, 1991.
22. Stanger P, Cassidy SC, Girod DA, et al: Balloon pulmonary valvuloplasty: results of the Valvuloplasty and Angioplasty of Congenital Anomalies Registry. *Am J Cardiol* 65(11):775–783, 1990.
23. O'Connor BK, Beekman RH, Lindauer A, et al: Intermediate-term outcome after pulmonary balloon valvuloplasty: comparison with a matched surgical control group. *J Am Coll Cardiol* 20(1):169–173, 1992.
24. Harrild DM, Powell AJ, Tran TX, et al: Long-term pulmonary regurgitation following balloon valvuloplasty for pulmonary stenosis risk factors and relationship to exercise capacity and ventricular volume and function. *J Am Coll Cardiol* 55(10):1041–1047, 2010.
25. Ring JC, Kulik TJ, Burke BA, et al: Morphologic changes induced by dilation of the pulmonary valve anulus with overlarge balloons in normal newborn lambs. *Am J Cardiol* 55(1):210–214, 1985.
26. Radtke W, Keane JF, Fellows KE, et al: Percutaneous balloon valvotomy of congenital pulmonary stenosis using oversized balloons. *J Am Coll Cardiol* 8(4):909–915, 1986.
27. Colli AM, Perry SB, Lock JE, et al: Balloon dilation of critical valvar pulmonary stenosis in the first month of life. *Cathet Cardiovasc Diagn* 34(1):23–28, 1995.
28. Zeevi B, Keane JF, Fellows KE, et al: Balloon dilation of critical pulmonary stenosis in the first week of life. *J Am Coll Cardiol* 11(4):821–824, 1988.
29. Rosenthal E, Qureshi SA, Chan KC, et al: Radiofrequency-assisted balloon dilatation in patients with pulmonary valve atresia and an intact ventricular septum. *Br Heart J* 69(4):347–351, 1993.
30. Alwi M, Geetha K, Bilkis AA, et al: Pulmonary atresia with intact ventricular septum percutaneous radiofrequency-assisted valvotomy and balloon dilation versus surgical valvotomy and Blalock Taussig shunt. *J Am Coll Cardiol* 35(2):468–476, 2000.
31. Hasan BS, Bautista-Hernandez V, McElhinney DB, et al: Outcomes of transcatheter approach for initial treatment of pulmonary atresia with intact ventricular septum. *Catheter Cardiovasc Interv* 81(1):111–118, 2013.
32. Lababidi Z, Wu JR, Walls JT: Percutaneous balloon aortic valvuloplasty: results in 23 patients. *Am J Cardiol* 53(1):194–197, 1984.
33. Rocchini AP, Beekman RH, Ben Shachar G, et al: Balloon aortic valvuloplasty: results of the Valvuloplasty and Angioplasty of Congenital Anomalies Registry. *Am J Cardiol* 65(11):784–789, 1990.
34. Sholler GF, Keane JF, Perry SB, et al: Balloon dilation of congenital aortic valve stenosis. Results and influence of technical and morphological features on outcome. *Circulation* 78(2):351–360, 1988.
35. Magee AG, Nykanen D, McCrindle BW, et al: Balloon dilation of severe aortic stenosis in the neonate: comparison of anterograde and retrograde catheter approaches. *J Am Coll Cardiol* 30(4):1061–1066, 1997.
36. Demkow M, Ruzyllo W, Ksiezycka E, et al: Long-term follow-up results of balloon valvuloplasty for congenital aortic stenosis: predictors of late outcome. *J Invasive Cardiol* 11(4):220–226, 1999.
37. Hawkins JA, Minich LL, Shaddy RE, et al: Aortic valve repair and replacement after balloon aortic valvuloplasty in children. *Ann Thorac Surg* 61(5):1355–1358, 1996.
38. Satou GM, Perry SB, Lock JE, et al: Repeat balloon dilation of congenital valvar aortic stenosis: immediate results and midterm outcome. *Catheter Cardiovasc Interv* 47(1):47–51, 1999.
39. Petit CJ, Maskatia SA, Justino H, et al: Repeat balloon aortic valvuloplasty effectively delays surgical intervention in children with recurrent aortic stenosis. *Catheter Cardiovasc Interv* 82(4):549–555, 2013.
40. Han RK, Gurofsky RC, Lee KJ, et al: Outcome and growth potential of left heart structures after neonatal intervention for aortic valve stenosis. *J Am Coll Cardiol* 50(25):2406–2414, 2007.
41. McElhinney DB, Lock JE, Keane JF, et al: Left heart growth, function, and reintervention after balloon aortic valvuloplasty for neonatal aortic stenosis. *Circulation* 111(4):451–458, 2005.
42. Lock JE, Khalilullah M, Shrivastava S, et al: Percutaneous catheter commissurotomy in rheumatic mitral stenosis. *N Engl J Med* 313(24):1515–1518, 1985.
43. Spevak PJ, Bass JL, Ben Shachar G, et al: Balloon angioplasty for congenital mitral stenosis. *Am J Cardiol* 66(4):472–476, 1990.
44. Moore P, Adatia I, Spevak PJ, et al: Severe congenital mitral stenosis in infants. *Circulation* 89(5):2099–2106, 1994.
45. McElhinney DB, Sherwood MC, Keane JF, et al: Current management of severe congenital mitral stenosis: outcomes of transcatheter and surgical therapy in 108 infants and children. *Circulation* 112(5):707–714, 2005.
46. Chaturvedi RR, Redington AN: Pulmonary regurgitation in congenital heart disease. *Heart* 93(7):880–889, 2007.
47. Geva T, Gauvreau K, Powell AJ, et al: Randomized trial of pulmonary valve replacement with and without right ventricular remodeling surgery. *Circulation* 122(11 Suppl):S201–S208, 2010.
48. Bonhoeffer P, Boudjemline Y, Saliba Z, et al: Transcatheter implantation of a bovine valve in pulmonary position: a lamb study. *Circulation* 102(7):813–816, 2000.

49. Meadows JJ, Moore PM, Berman DP, et al: Use and performance of the Melody Transcatheter Pulmonary Valve in native and post-surgical, nonconduit right ventricular outflow tracts. *Circ Cardiovasc Interv* 7(3):374–380, 2014.
50. Hasan BS, Lunze FI, Chen MH, et al: Effects of transcatheter pulmonary valve replacement on the hemodynamic and ventricular response to exercise in patients with obstructed right ventricle-to-pulmonary artery conduits. *JACC Cardiovasc Interv* 7(5):530–542, 2014.
51. Zahn EM, Hellenbrand WE, Lock JE, et al: Implantation of the melody transcatheter pulmonary valve in patients with a dysfunctional right ventricular outflow tract conduit early results from the U.S. Clinical trial. *J Am Coll Cardiol* 54(18):1722–1729, 2009.
52. McElhinney DB, Hellenbrand WE, Zahn EM, et al: Short- and medium-term outcomes after transcatheter pulmonary valve placement in the expanded multicenter US melody valve trial. *Circulation* 122(5):507–516, 2010.
53. Khambadkone S, Coats L, Taylor A, et al: Percutaneous pulmonary valve implantation in humans: results in 59 consecutive patients. *Circulation* 112(8):1189–1197, 2005.
54. McElhinney DB, Benson LN, Eicken A, et al: Infective endocarditis after transcatheter pulmonary valve replacement using the Melody valve: combined results of 3 prospective North American and European studies. *Circ Cardiovasc Interv* 6(3):292–300, 2013.
55. Buber J, Bergersen L, Lock JE, et al: Bloodstream infections occurring in patients with percutaneously implanted bioprosthetic pulmonary valve: a single-center experience. *Circ Cardiovasc Interv* 6(3):301–310, 2013.
56. Lurz P, Coats L, Khambadkone S, et al: Percutaneous pulmonary valve implantation: impact of evolving technology and learning curve on clinical outcome. *Circulation* 117(15):1964–1972, 2008.
57. Rao PS, Chopra PS: Role of balloon angioplasty in the treatment of aortic coarctation. *Ann Thorac Surg* 52(3):621–631, 1991.
58. Sos T, Sniderman KW, Rettek-Sos B, et al: Percutaneous transluminal dilatation of coarctation of thoracic aorta post mortem. *Lancet* 2(8149):970–971, 1979.
59. Lock JE, Niemi T, Burke BA, et al: Transcutaneous angioplasty of experimental aortic coarctation. *Circulation* 66(6):1280–1286, 1982.
60. Singer MI, Rowen M, Dorsey TJ: Transluminal aortic balloon angioplasty for coarctation of the aorta in the newborn. *Am Heart J* 103(1):131–132, 1982.
61. Kan JS, White RI, Mitchell SE, et al: Treatment of restenosis of coarctation by percutaneous transluminal angioplasty. *Circulation* 68(5):1087–1094, 1983.
62. Hellenbrand WE, Allen HD, Golinko RJ, et al: Balloon angioplasty for aortic recoarctation: results of Valvuloplasty and Angioplasty of Congenital Anomalies Registry. *Am J Cardiol* 65(11):793–797, 1990.
63. Hijazi ZM, Fahey JT, Kleinman CS, et al: Balloon angioplasty for recurrent coarctation of aorta. Immediate and long-term results. *Circulation* 84(3):1150–1156, 1991.
64. Yetman AT, Nykanen D, McCrindle BW, et al: Balloon angioplasty of recurrent coarctation: a 12-year review. *J Am Coll Cardiol* 30(3):811–816, 1997.
65. Mendelsohn AM, Lloyd TR, Crowley DC, et al: Late follow-up of balloon angioplasty in children with a native coarctation of the aorta. *Am J Cardiol* 74(7):696–700, 1994.
66. Rao PS, Chopra PS, Koscik R, et al: Surgical versus balloon therapy for aortic coarctation in infants < or = 3 months old. *J Am Coll Cardiol* 23(6):1479–1483, 1994.
67. Tynan M, Finley JP, Fontes V, et al: Balloon angioplasty for the treatment of native coarctation: results of Valvuloplasty and Angioplasty of Congenital Anomalies Registry. *Am J Cardiol* 65(11):790–792, 1990.
68. Burrows PE, Benson LN, Williams WG, et al: Iliofemoral arterial complications of balloon angioplasty for systemic obstructions in infants and children. *Circulation* 82(5):1697–1704, 1990.
69. Harris KC, Du W, Cowley CG, et al: Congenital Cardiac Intervention Study C. A prospective observational multicenter study of balloon angioplasty for the treatment of native and recurrent coarctation of the aorta. *Catheter Cardiovasc Interv* 83(7):1116–1123, 2014.
70. O'Laughlin MP, Perry SB, Lock JE, et al: Use of endovascular stents in congenital heart disease. *Circulation* 83(6):1923–1939, 1991.
71. Forbes TJ, Kim DW, Du W, et al: Comparison of surgical, stent, and balloon angioplasty treatment of native coarctation of the aorta: an observational study by the CCISC (Congenital Cardiovascular Interventional Study Consortium). *J Am Coll Cardiol* 58(25):2664–2674, 2011.
72. Marshall AC, Perry SB, Keane JF, et al: Early results and medium-term follow-up of stent implantation for mild residual or recurrent aortic coarctation. *Am Heart J* 139(6):1054–1060, 2000.
73. Qureshi AM, McElhinney DB, Lock JE, et al: Acute and intermediate outcomes, and evaluation of injury to the aortic wall, as based on 15 years experience of implanting stents to treat aortic coarctation. *Cardiol Young* 17(3):307–318, 2007.
74. Cunningham JW, McElhinney DB, Gauvreau K, et al: Outcomes after primary transcatheter therapy in infants and young children with severe bilateral peripheral pulmonary artery stenosis. *Circ Cardiovasc Interv* 6(4):460–467, 2013.
75. Feinstein JA, Goldhaber SZ, Lock JE, et al: Balloon pulmonary angioplasty for treatment of chronic thromboembolic pulmonary hypertension. *Circulation* 103(1):10–13, 2001.
76. Mizoguchi H, Ogawa A, Munemasa M, et al: Refined balloon pulmonary angioplasty for inoperable patients with chronic thromboembolic pulmonary hypertension. *Circ Cardiovasc Interv* 5(6):748–755, 2012.
77. Rocchini AP, Kveselis D, Dick M, et al: Use of balloon angioplasty to treat peripheral pulmonary stenosis. *Am J Cardiol* 54(8):1069–1073, 1984.
78. Rothman A, Perry SB, Keane JF, et al: Early results and follow-up of balloon angioplasty for branch pulmonary artery stenoses. *J Am Coll Cardiol* 15(5):1109–1117, 1990.
79. Zeevi B, Berant M, Blieden LC: Midterm clinical impact versus procedural success of balloon angioplasty for pulmonary artery stenosis. *Pediatr Cardiol* 18(2):101–106, 1997.
80. Gentles TL, Lock JE, Perry SB: High pressure balloon angioplasty for branch pulmonary artery stenosis: early experience. *J Am Coll Cardiol* 22(3):867–872, 1993.
81. Rhodes JF, Lane GK, Mesia CI, et al: Cutting balloon angioplasty for children with small-vessel pulmonary artery stenoses. *Catheter Cardiovasc Interv* 55(1):73–77, 2002.
82. Bergersen LJ, Perry SB, Lock JE: Effect of cutting balloon angioplasty on resistant pulmonary artery stenosis. *Am J Cardiol* 91(2):185–189, 2003.
83. Sugiyama H, Veldtman GR, Norgard G, et al: Bladed balloon angioplasty for peripheral pulmonary artery stenosis. *Catheter Cardiovasc Interv* 62(1):71–77, 2004.
84. Maglione J, Bergersen L, Lock JE, et al: Ultra-high-pressure balloon angioplasty for treatment of resistant stenoses within or adjacent to previously implanted pulmonary arterial stents. *Circ Cardiovasc Interv* 2(1):52–58, 2009.
85. Arnold LW, Keane JF, Kan JS, et al: Transient unilateral pulmonary edema after successful balloon dilation of peripheral pulmonary artery stenosis. *Am J Cardiol* 62(4):327–330, 1988.
86. Baker CM, McGowan FX, Jr, Keane JF, et al: Pulmonary artery trauma due to balloon dilation: recognition, avoidance and management. *J Am Coll Cardiol* 36(5):1684–1690, 2000.
87. McMahon CJ, El Said HG, Grifka RG, et al: Redilation of endovascular stents in congenital heart disease: factors implicated in the development of restenosis and neointimal proliferation. *J Am Coll Cardiol* 38(2):521–526, 2001.
88. Forbes TJ, Rodriguez-Cruz E, Amin Z, et al: The Genesis stent: a new low-profile stent for use in infants, children, and adults with congenital heart disease. *Catheter Cardiovasc Interv* 59(3):406–414, 2003.
89. Ing FF, Khan A, Kobayashi D, et al: Pulmonary artery stents in the recent era: immediate and intermediate follow-up. *Catheter Cardiovasc Interv* 84(7):1123–1130, 2014.
90. Zahn EM, Dobrolet NC, Nykanen DG, et al: Interventional catheterization performed in the early postoperative period after congenital heart surgery in children. *J Am Coll Cardiol* 43(7):1264–1269, 2004.
91. Hainstock MR, Marshall AC, Lock JE, et al: Angioplasty of obstructed homograft conduits in the right ventricular outflow tract with ultra-noncompliant balloons: assessment of therapeutic

efficacy and conduit tears. *Circ Cardiovasc Interv* 6(6):671–679, 2013.
92. Hosking MC, Benson LN, Nakanishi T, et al: Intravascular stent prosthesis for right ventricular outflow obstruction. *J Am Coll Cardiol* 20(2):373–380, 1992.
93. Powell AJ, Lock JE, Keane JF, et al: Prolongation of RV-PA conduit life span by percutaneous stent implantation. Intermediate-term results. *Circulation* 92(11):3282–3288, 1995.
94. Peng LF, McElhinney DB, Nugent AW, et al: Endovascular stenting of obstructed right ventricle-to-pulmonary artery conduits: a 15-year experience. *Circulation* 113(22):2598–2605, 2006.
95. Tzifa A, Marshall AC, McElhinney DB, et al: Endovascular treatment for superior vena cava occlusion or obstruction in a pediatric and young adult population: a 22-year experience. *J Am Coll Cardiol* 49(9):1003–1009, 2007.
96. Frazer JR, Ing FF: Stenting of stenotic or occluded iliofemoral veins, superior and inferior vena cavae in children with congenital heart disease: acute results and intermediate follow up. *Catheter Cardiovasc Interv* 73(2):181–188, 2009.
97. Kazanci SY, McElhinney DB, Thiagarajan R, et al: Obstruction of the superior vena cava after neonatal extracorporeal membrane oxygenation: association with chylothorax and outcome of transcatheter treatment. *Pediatr Crit Care Med* 14(1):37–43, 2013.
98. Driscoll DJ, Hesslein PS, Mullins CE: Congenital stenosis of individual pulmonary veins: clinical spectrum and unsuccessful treatment by transvenous balloon dilation. *Am J Cardiol* 49(7):1767–1772, 1982.
99. Coles JG, Yemets I, Najm HK, et al: Experience with repair of congenital heart defects using adjunctive endovascular devices. *J Thorac Cardiovasc Surg* 110(5):1513–1519, 1995.
100. Mendelsohn AM, Bove EL, Lupinetti FM, et al: Intraoperative and percutaneous stenting of congenital pulmonary artery and vein stenosis. *Circulation* 88(5 Pt 2):II210–II217, 1993.
101. Balasubramanian S, Marshall AC, Gauvreau K, et al: Outcomes after stent implantation for the treatment of congenital and postoperative pulmonary vein stenosis in children. *Circ Cardiovasc Interv* 5(1):109–117, 2012.
102. Peng LF, Lock JE, Nugent AW, et al: Comparison of conventional and cutting balloon angioplasty for congenital and postoperative pulmonary vein stenosis in infants and young children. *Catheter Cardiovasc Interv* 75(7):1084–1090, 2010.
103. Rashkind WJ, Mullins CE, Hellenbrand WE, et al: Nonsurgical closure of patent ductus arteriosus: clinical application of the Rashkind PDA Occluder System. *Circulation* 75(3):583–592, 1987.
104. Shapira Y, Hirsch R, Kornowski R, et al: Percutaneous closure of perivalvular leaks with Amplatzer occluders: feasibility, safety, and shortterm results. *J Heart Valve Dis* 16(3):305–313, 2007.
105. Valente AM, Lock JE, Gauvreau K, et al: Predictors of long-term adverse outcomes in patients with congenital coronary artery fistulae. *Circ Cardiovasc Interv* 3(2):134–139, 2010.
106. Porstmann W, Wierny L, Warnke H, et al: Catheter closure of patent ductus arteriosus. 62 cases treated without thoracotomy. *Radiol Clin North Am* 9(2):203–218, 1971.
107. Rashkind WJ, Cuaso CC: Transcatheter closure of a patent ductus arteriosus: successful use in a 3.5-kg infant. *Pediatr Cardiol* 1:3–7, 1979.
108. Lloyd TR, Fedderly R, Mendelsohn AM, et al: Transcatheter occlusion of patent ductus arteriosus with Gianturco coils. *Circulation* 88(4 Pt 1):1412–1420, 1993.
109. Moore JW, George L, Kirkpatrick SE, et al: Percutaneous closure of the small patent ductus arteriosus using occluding spring coils. *J Am Coll Cardiol* 23(3):759–765, 1994.
110. Hijazi ZM, Geggel RL: Transcatheter closure of patent ductus arteriosus using coils. *Am J Cardiol* 79(9):1279–1280, 1997.
111. Patel HT, Cao QL, Rhodes J, et al: Long-term outcome of transcatheter coil closure of small to large patent ductus arteriosus. *Catheter Cardiovasc Interv* 47(4):457–461, 1999.
112. Grifka RG, Mullins CE, Gianturco C, et al: New Gianturco-Grifka vascular occlusion device. Initial studies in a canine model. *Circulation* 91(6):1840–1846, 1995.
113. Faella HJ, Hijazi ZM: Closure of the patent ductus arteriosus with the amplatzer PDA device: immediate results of the international clinical trial. *Catheter Cardiovasc Interv* 51(1):50–54, 2000.
114. Moore JW, Greene J, Palomares S, et al: Results of the Combined U.S. Multicenter Pivotal Study and the Continuing Access Study of the Nit-Occlud PDA device for percutaneous closure of patent ductus arteriosus. *JACC Cardiovasc Interv* 7(12):1430–1436, 2014.
115. Dimas VV, Takao C, Ing FF, et al: Outcomes of transcatheter occlusion of patent ductus arteriosus in infants weighing ≤ 6 kg. *JACC Cardiovasc Interv* 3(12):1295–1299, 2010.
116. Grosse-Wortmann L, Drolet C, Dragulescu A, et al: Aortopulmonary collateral flow volume affects early postoperative outcome after Fontan completion: a multimodality study. *J Thorac Cardiovasc Surg* 144(6):1329–1336, 2012.
117. Sharma S, Kothari SS, Krishnakumar R, et al: Systemic-to-pulmonary artery collateral vessels and surgical shunts in patients with cyanotic congenital heart disease: perioperative treatment by transcatheter embolization. *AJR Am J Roentgenol* 164(6):1505–1510, 1995.
118. Dori Y, Glatz AC, Hanna BD, et al: Acute effects of embolizing systemic-to-pulmonary arterial collaterals on blood flow in patients with superior cavopulmonary connections: a pilot study. *Circ Cardiovasc Interv* 6(1):101–106, 2013.
119. King TD, Mills NL: Nonoperative closure of atrial septal defects. *Surgery* 75(3):383–388, 1974.
120. Du ZD, Hijazi ZM, Kleinman CS, et al: Comparison between transcatheter and surgical closure of secundum atrial septal defect in children and adults: results of a multicenter nonrandomized trial. *J Am Coll Cardiol* 39(11):1836–1844, 2002.
121. Jones TK, Latson LA, Zahn E, et al: Results of the U.S. multicenter pivotal study of the HELEX septal occluder for percutaneous closure of secundum atrial septal defects. *J Am Coll Cardiol* 49(22):2215–2221, 2007.
122. Chessa M, Carminati M, Butera G, et al: Early and late complications associated with transcatheter occlusion of secundum atrial septal defect. *J Am Coll Cardiol* 39(6):1061–1065, 2002.
123. Divekar A, Gaamangwe T, Shaikh N, et al: Cardiac perforation after device closure of atrial septal defects with the Amplatzer septal occluder. *J Am Coll Cardiol* 45(8):1213–1218, 2005.
124. Krumsdorf U, Ostermayer S, Billinger K, et al: Incidence and clinical course of thrombus formation on atrial septal defect and patient foramen ovale closure devices in 1,000 consecutive patients. *J Am Coll Cardiol* 43(2):302–309, 2004.
125. Amin Z, Hijazi ZM, Bass JL, et al: Erosion of Amplatzer septal occluder device after closure of secundum atrial septal defects: review of registry of complications and recommendations to minimize future risk. *Catheter Cardiovasc Interv* 63(4):496–502, 2004.
126. Preminger TJ, Sanders SP, van der Velde ME, et al: "Intramural" residual interventricular defects after repair of conotruncal malformations. *Circulation* 89(1):236–242, 1994.
127. Knauth AL, Lock JE, Perry SB, et al: Transcatheter device closure of congenital and postoperative residual ventricular septal defects. *Circulation* 110(5):501–507, 2004.
128. Lock JE, Block PC, McKay RG, et al: Transcatheter closure of ventricular septal defects. *Circulation* 78(2):361–368, 1988.
129. Bridges ND, Perry SB, Keane JF, et al: Preoperative transcatheter closure of congenital muscular ventricular septal defects. *N Engl J Med* 324(19):1312–1317, 1991.
130. Holzer R, Balzer D, Cao QL, et al; Amplatzer Muscular Ventricular Septal Defect I: Device closure of muscular ventricular septal defects using the Amplatzer muscular ventricular septal defect occluder: immediate and mid-term results of a U.S. registry. *J Am Coll Cardiol* 43(7):1257–1263, 2004.
131. Thanopoulos BV, Rigby ML, Karanasios E, et al: Transcatheter closure of perimembranous ventricular septal defects in infants and children using the Amplatzer perimembranous ventricular septal defect occluder. *Am J Cardiol* 99(7):984–989, 2007.
132. Schroeder VA, Shim D, Spicer RL, et al: Surgical emergencies during pediatric interventional catheterization. *J Pediatr* 140(5):570–575, 2002.
133. Bergersen L, Gauvreau K, Foerster SR, et al: Catheterization for Congenital Heart Disease Adjustment for Risk Method (CHARM). *JACC Cardiovasc Interv* 4(9):1037–1046, 2011.
134. Cassidy SC, Schmidt KG, Van Hare GF, et al: Complications of pediatric cardiac catheterization: a 3-year study. *J Am Coll Cardiol* 19(6):1285–1293, 1992.
135. Fellows KE, Radtke W, Keane JF, et al: Acute complications of catheter therapy for congenital heart disease. *Am J Cardiol* 60(8):679–683, 1987.

136. McElhinney DB, Reddy VM, Moore P, et al: Surgical intervention for complications of transcatheter dilation procedures in congenital heart disease. *Ann Thorac Surg* 69(3):858–864, 2000.
137. Galantowicz M, Cheatham JP, Phillips A, et al: Hybrid approach for hypoplastic left heart syndrome: intermediate results after the learning curve. *Ann Thorac Surg* 85(6):2063–2070, discussion 70–1, 2008.
138. Egan MJ, Hill SL, Boettner BL, et al: Predictors of retrograde aortic arch obstruction after hybrid palliation of hypoplastic left heart syndrome. *Pediatr Cardiol* 32(1):67–75, 2011.
139. Siehr SL, Martin MH, Axelrod D, et al: Outcomes following cardiac catheterization after congenital heart surgery. *Catheter Cardiovasc Interv* 84(4):622–628, 2014.
140. Nicholson GT, Kim DW, Vincent RN, et al: Cardiac catheterization in the early post-operative period after congenital cardiac surgery. *JACC Cardiovasc Interv* 7(12):1437–1443, 2014.
141. Eastaugh LJ, Thiagarajan RR, Darst JR, et al: Percutaneous left atrial decompression in patients supported with extracorporeal membrane oxygenation for cardiac disease. *Pediatr Crit Care Med* 16:59–65, 2015.
142. Fishman NH, Hof RB, Rudolph AM, et al: Models of congenital heart disease in fetal lambs. *Circulation* 58(2):354–364, 1978.
143. Carpenter RJ, Jr, Strasburger JF, Garson A, Jr, et al: Fetal ventricular pacing for hydrops secondary to complete atrioventricular block. *J Am Coll Cardiol* 8(6):1434–1436, 1986.
144. Maxwell D, Allan L, Tynan MJ: Balloon dilatation of the aortic valve in the fetus: a report of two cases. *Br Heart J* 65(5):256–258, 1991.
145. Benatar A, Vaughan J, Nicolini U, et al: Prenatal pericardiocentesis: its role in the management of intrapericardial teratoma. *Obstet Gynecol* 79(5 Pt 2):856–859, 1992.
146. Kohl T, Sharland G, Allan LD, et al: World experience of percutaneous ultrasound-guided balloon valvuloplasty in human fetuses with severe aortic valve obstruction. *Am J Cardiol* 85(10):1230–1233, 2000.
147. Champsaur G, Parisot P, Martinot S, et al: Pulsatility improves hemodynamics during fetal bypass. Experimental comparative study of pulsatile versus steady flow. *Circulation* 90(5 Pt 2):II47–II50, 1994.
148. Kohl T, Szabo Z, Suda K, et al: Fetoscopic and open transumbilical fetal cardiac catheterization in sheep. Potential approaches for human fetal cardiac intervention. *Circulation* 95(4):1048–1053, 1997.
149. Reddy VM, Liddicoat JR, Klein JR, et al: Long-term outcome after fetal cardiac bypass: fetal survival to full term and organ abnormalities. *J Thorac Cardiovasc Surg* 111(3):536–544, 1996.
150. Fenton KN, Heinemann MK, Hickey PR, et al: Inhibition of the fetal stress response improves cardiac output and gas exchange after fetal cardiac bypass. *J Thorac Cardiovasc Surg* 107(6):1416–1422, 1994.
151. Tworetzky W, Wilkins-Haug L, Benson C, et al: Balloon dilation of severe aortic stenosis in the fetus: technical advances. *J Am Coll Cardiol* 41(Suppl A):496A, 2003.
152. Marshall AC, van der Velde ME, Tworetzky W, et al: Creation of an atrial septal defect in utero for fetuses with hypoplastic left heart syndrome and intact or highly restrictive atrial septum. *Circulation* 110(3):253–258, 2004.
153. Tworetzky W, Wilkins-Haug L, Jennings RW, et al: Balloon dilation of severe aortic stenosis in the fetus: potential for prevention of hypoplastic left heart syndrome: candidate selection, technique, and results of successful intervention. *Circulation* 110(15):2125–2131, 2004.
154. Marshall AC, Tworetzky W, Bergersen L, et al: Aortic valvuloplasty in the fetus: technical characteristics of successful balloon dilation. *J Pediatr* 147(4):535–539, 2005.
155. Mizrahi-Arnaud A, Wilkins HL, Marshall A, et al: Maternal mirror syndrome after in utero aortic valve dilation. A case report. *Fetal Diagn Ther* 21(5):439–443, 2006.
156. Kalish BT, Tworetzky W, Benson CB, et al: Technical challenges of atrial septal stent placement in fetuses with hypoplastic left heart syndrome and intact atrial septum. *Catheter Cardiovasc Interv* 84(1):77–85, 2014.
157. Freud LR, McElhinney DB, Marshall AC, et al: Fetal aortic valvuloplasty for evolving hypoplastic left heart syndrome: postnatal outcomes of the first 100 patients. *Circulation* 130(8):638–645, 2014.
158. Makikallio K, McElhinney DB, Levine JC, et al: Fetal aortic valve stenosis and the evolution of hypoplastic left heart syndrome: patient selection for fetal intervention. *Circulation* 113(11):1401–1405, 2006.
159. Lofland GK, McCrindle BW, Williams WG, et al: Critical aortic stenosis in the neonate: a multi-institutional study of management, outcomes, and risk factors. Congenital Heart Surgeons Society. *J Thorac Cardiovasc Surg* 121(1):10–27, 2001.
160. Colan SD, McElhinney DB, Crawford EC, et al: Validation and re-evaluation of a discriminant model predicting anatomic suitability for biventricular repair in neonates with aortic stenosis. *J Am Coll Cardiol* 47(9):1858–1865, 2006.
161. Rhodes LA, Colan SD, Perry SB, et al: Predictors of survival in neonates with critical aortic stenosis. *Circulation* 84(6):2325–2335, 1991.
162. Danford DA, Cronican P: Hypoplastic left heart syndrome: progression of left ventricular dilation and dysfunction to left ventricular hypoplasia in utero. *Am Heart J* 123(6):1712–1713, 1992.
163. Simpson JM, Sharland GK: Natural history and outcome of aortic stenosis diagnosed prenatally. *Heart* 77(3):205–210, 1997.
164. Mizrahi-Arnaud A, Tworetzky W, Bulich LA, et al: Pathophysiology, management, and outcomes of fetal hemodynamic instability during prenatal cardiac intervention. *Pediatr Res* 62(3):325–330, 2007.
165. Wilkins-Haug LE, Tworetzky W, Benson CB, et al: Factors affecting technical success of fetal aortic valve dilation. *Ultrasound Obstet Gynecol* 28(1):47–52, 2006.
166. Rychik J, Rome JJ, Collins MH, et al: The hypoplastic left heart syndrome with intact atrial septum: atrial morphology, pulmonary vascular histopathology and outcome. *J Am Coll Cardiol* 34(2):554–560, 1999.
167. Photiadis J, Urban AE, Sinzobahamvya N, et al: Restrictive left atrial outflow adversely affects outcome after the modified Norwood procedure. *Eur J Cardiothorac Surg* 27(6):962–967, 2005.
168. Quintero RA, Huhta J, Suh E, et al: In utero cardiac fetal surgery: laser atrial septotomy in the treatment of hypoplastic left heart syndrome with intact atrial septum. *Am J Obstet Gynecol* 193(4):1424–1428, 2005.
169. Marshall AC, Levine J, Morash D, et al: Results of in utero atrial septoplasty in fetuses with hypoplastic left heart syndrome. *Prenat Diagn* 28(11):1023–1028, 2008.
170. Tulzer G, Arzt W, Franklin RC, et al: Fetal pulmonary valvuloplasty for critical pulmonary stenosis or atresia with intact septum. *Lancet* 360(9345):1567–1568, 2002.
171. Arzt W, Tulzer G, Aigner M, et al: Invasive intrauterine treatment of pulmonary atresia/intact ventricular septum with heart failure. *Ultrasound Obstet Gynecol* 21(2):186–188, 2003.
172. Galindo A, Gutierrez-Larraya F, Velasco JM, et al: Pulmonary balloon valvuloplasty in a fetus with critical pulmonary stenosis/atresia with intact ventricular septum and heart failure. *Fetal Diagn Ther* 21(1):100–104, 2006.
173. Salvin JW, McElhinney DB, Colan SD, et al: Fetal tricuspid valve size and growth as predictors of outcome in pulmonary atresia with intact ventricular septum. *Pediatrics* 118(2):e415–e420, 2006.

CHAPTER 108

Surgical Approaches and Cardiopulmonary Bypass in Pediatric Cardiac Surgery

Luis Quinonez • Pedro J. del Nido

CHAPTER OUTLINE

Thoracic incisions traditionally used in adult cardiac and thoracic surgery have been used in children with varying success with respect to exposure, pain, and cosmetic result. Special considerations relevant to pediatric surgery are related to the lack of development and growth of soft tissue structures such as breast tissue and bony structures such as ribs and vertebra. Thus, incisions that fix growing bony structures, such as ribs in a posterior or lateral thoracotomy, may lead to scoliosis.[1] Anterior thoracic incisions may also injure underdeveloped breast tissue and pectoral muscles, resulting in chest wall deformities and sensory loss. Then again, the flexibility of the chest cage and ribs in young children permit the use of limited incisions with adequate exposure of relevant structures, whereas in adults this may not be possible without the risk of rib or sternal fracture or instability of the chest cage. Therefore, these factors should be considered when selecting the optimal approach to intrathoracic structures in children, to optimize exposure and for the safe conduct of the procedure, and to minimize pain and achieve a cosmetically acceptable result.

The child should be positioned so that the surgeon and assistant have a direct view of the relevant anatomic structures and so that the anesthesiologist has access to the airway and major access lines. Because the head size of newborns and infants is significantly larger in proportion to the chest than it is in older children and adults, a shoulder roll should be used when children are placed supine on the table, to elevate the shoulders and relieve some of the pressure from the occiput. Soft padding, such as gel-filled plastic bags, should be placed under all pressure areas. Cooling or heating blankets are used routinely in pediatric cardiac surgery, but these require relatively direct patient contact to optimize heat transfer. Perforated blankets, filled with cold or heated air that is blown through, have improved heat-transfer properties compared with water-filled blankets. Direct skin contact should be avoided, however, with either method, because injury to the skin can result in full-thickness skin loss, particularly in infants. For a lateral thoracotomy, an axillary roll is used to elevate the thorax and relieve pressure on the shoulder and potentially the brachial plexus. As with any thoracotomy incision, care must be taken not to extend the arm and shoulder under tension, even in infants, because this may cause injury to the brachial plexus.

For cosmetic purposes, the skin incision can be placed below the actual entry site into the thorax, whether the incision is a sternotomy or a lateral intercostal approach. Care must be taken, however, to minimize creation of flaps, particularly in infants, because this often leads to breakdown of subcutaneous tissue with fat necrosis, resulting in wound separation. Excessive use of cautery, particularly in the subcutaneous fat in infants, is another cause of fat necrosis and wound separation, often prolonging hospital stay and resulting in a poor cosmetic result.

APPROACHES TO CARDIAC STRUCTURES AND GREAT VESSELS FOR TRANSTHORACIC CANNULATION FOR BYPASS

Full Sternotomy

The most commonly used incision for access to the heart and anterior mediastinal structures is a sternotomy. A vertical skin incision over the sternum, staying below the manubrium, permits full division of the sternum and provides an unobstructed view of all anterior mediastinal structures and direct access from branches of the aortic arch down to the inferior vena cava (IVC) at the level of the diaphragm. This approach is necessary when the surgical procedure requires access to upper and lower mediastinal structures, such as the aortic arch and right atrium, branch pulmonary arteries, and right ventricle. Examples include a first-stage procedure for hypoplastic left heart syndrome, repair of truncus arteriosus, and pulmonary atresia with ventricular septal defect.

The incision in the pericardium is also vertical. If it is placed directly over the cardiac structures to be accessed, it can facilitate exposure, particularly when transatrial procedures to access the ventricles are being performed. By opening the pericardium to the right of midline and retracting the right side of the pericardium to the sternum, the ventricles fall away leftward, aiding exposure. Sutures to suspend the pericardium to the sternum are critical in children, and they should also be used to rotate the heart to facilitate exposure to the chamber or vessels required. When the right atrium and cavae need exposure, suspension of the right-sided pericardial edge to the periosteum of the sternum is often required to visualize the lateral wall of the right atrium and inferior cava. If the left side of the pericardium is left unsuspended and is incised along the edge of the diaphragm to the apex, the entire ventricular mass will rotate away from the surgeon, facilitating exposure of the atrioventricular valves and interventricular septum to the level of the apex. A similar approach can be used to optimize exposure of the right ventricular outflow tract for surgery to correct tetralogy of Fallot. Here, the pericardium at the level of the great vessels is suspended to the periosteum, leaving the pericardial edge at the diaphragm unsuspended, facilitating the view of the ventricular septal defect through the ventriculotomy.

Limited Sternotomy Incisions

For many procedures, a full sternotomy is not necessary to provide adequate access to all the relevant structures of the heart. This is particularly true in infants and young children because their sternum and rib cage are pliable, which permits retraction with minimal force. Preoperative planning of the procedure includes determining which mediastinal structures will need exposure for the surgical procedure and for cannulation for cardiopulmonary bypass (CPB). With the availability of thin-walled, wire-reinforced, small-diameter cannulas for use in children, cannulation for CPB can often be achieved with minimal extension of the thoracic incision beyond that needed for the repair itself. These approaches usually provide exposure sufficient to use standard techniques for myocardial protection, such as cardioplegia and left ventricular venting. A full sternotomy is unnecessary when, for example, the intracardiac repair is accomplished via a right atriotomy, such as for repair of atrial septal defect, ventricular septal defect, or complete atrioventricular canal defect, and in transatrial repair of tetralogy of Fallot and mitral valve repair.[2-4]

Trans-Xyphoid Mini-Sternotomy

With the trans-xyphoid mini-sternotomy approach, the skin incision extends from the level of the areola (mid thorax) down to the tip of the xyphoid process (Fig. 108-1). By detaching anterior diaphragm attachments to the cartilaginous segment of the rib cage anteriorly, access is gained to the anterior mediastinum. Before

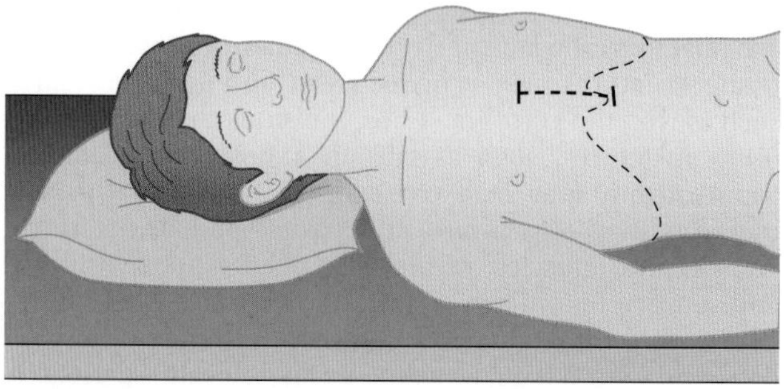

FIGURE 108-1 ■ A partial or limited sternotomy incision.

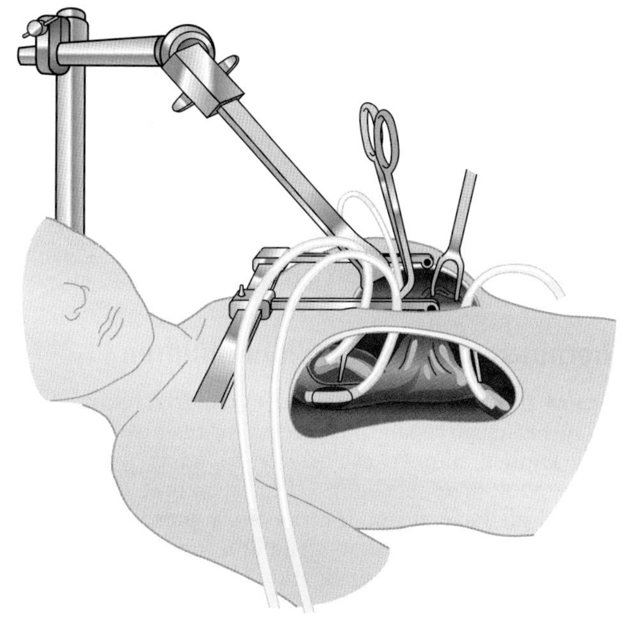

FIGURE 108-2 ■ The limited sternotomy allows cannulation of the ascending aorta and both cavae. Insertion of the inferior caval cannula through a separate skin incision keeps the cannula out of the way, and the incision can later be used for tube thoracostomy.

performing the partial sternotomy, blunt dissection is required to detach the pericardium and thymus from the sternum. A partial sternotomy can be performed with a saw, but in infants, heavy bandage scissors are sufficient for dividing the lower sternum. Once the partial sternotomy is completed, a narrow-blade retractor such as an army-navy retractor is used to lift the sternum anteriorly and cephalad to provide exposure to the ascending aorta for cannulation. The retractor should not be placed on the skin and subcutaneous tissue, because adequate exposure of the upper mediastinum will not be achieved and necrosis of the skin could occur from prolonged retraction. To expose the aorta, however, caudal and anterior traction must be placed on the pericardium. This maneuver requires that thymus attachments to the pericardium be divided, or mobility of the pericardium and aorta will be inadequate. The pericardial incision must be made to the right of midline, and the pericardium should be pinned to the right edge of the divided sternum to expose the right atrium and cavae. In most cases, cannulation of the ascending aorta and both cavae can be easily achieved with this approach. Insertion of the inferior caval cannula through a separate skin incision keeps the cannula out of the way, and the incision can later be used for tube thoracostomy (Fig. 108-2).

Midsternal Mini-Sternotomy

When the right ventricular outflow tract or aortic root must be accessed, the partial sternotomy approach may still be used, but usually the skin and sternal incisions need to be extended superiorly 1 or 2 cm above the level of the areola. In this case, traction sutures on the pericardium at the level of the pulmonary and aortic roots suspend these structures into view, permitting adequate exposure. To assist with caval cannulation, traction sutures should be placed only on the right side of the pericardium, lifting both cavae toward the right side of the sternotomy. The cardiac structures are allowed to rotate and shift leftward, enhancing exposure to the right atrium, the left atrium via the right upper pulmonary veins, and the aortic root.

Anterior or Anterolateral Thoracotomy

An anterior thoracotomy has been advocated for surgical repair of atrial septal defect and occasionally ventricular septal defects.[5,6] A meta-analysis of six case control trials found that intubation time and hospital length of stay were shorter using an anterolateral mini-thoracotomy over a median sternotomy, whereas cardiopulmonary and cross-clamp times were longer.[7] Axillary incision have also been advocated for simple heart lesions using CPB.[8,9]

For the anterolateral thoracotomy, the incision is made in the anterior fourth intercostal space (ICS), and in females great care must be taken to incise well below breast tissue. Dissection of the pericardial attachments to the sternum and thymus greatly facilitates exposure by permitting retraction of the pericardium down toward the diaphragm and bringing the ascending aorta closer into view. Direct cannulation of the ascending aorta is preferable to peripheral cannulation via the femoral or axillary artery because these vessels are small in children and stenosis at the cannulation site can result in claudication with exercise. Recently, more flexible cannulas, available in all sizes for pediatric use, have facilitated aortic cannulation. Some arterial cannulas can be introduced over a guidewire, which makes insertion easier and safer. The cavae can be cannulated directly, although the superior cava cannula is often best introduced via the right atrial appendage and directed retrograde into the superior vena cava (SVC). Aortic clamping to achieve cardiac arrest can be difficult with conventional arterial clamps, which were designed for application via a sternotomy. In small children, a bulldog clamp is sufficient for aortic occlusion, and for larger children and teenagers, flexible clamps are available. Cardioplegia can be delivered via a small flexible cannula inserted into the aortic root; some have advocated transthoracic insertion of a needle into the aortic root.

APPROACHES TO EXTRACARDIAC STRUCTURES IN INFANTS AND CHILDREN

Noncardiac thoracic surgery for the treatment of congenital cardiac defects or complications of cardiac surgery most often requires exposure to the posterior mediastinum. Exceptions include procedures to plicate the diaphragm, or for unifocalization of aortopulmonary collaterals, which requires dissection of the hilum of the lung. A posterolateral incision extending from just anterior to the tip of the scapula to the mid-posterior scapula provides access, through the fourth, fifth, or sixth ICS, to posterior mediastinal structures as well as the hilum of

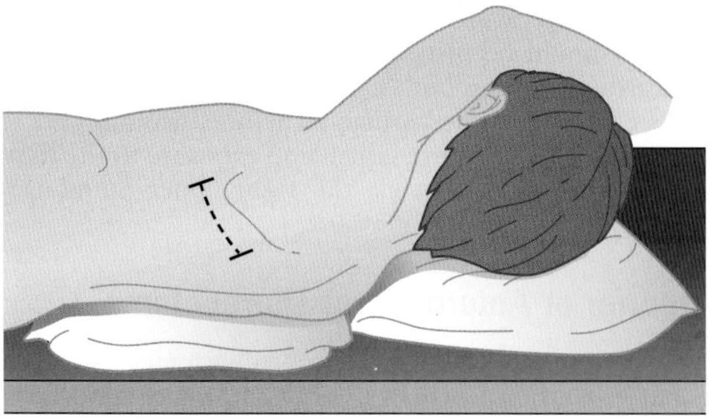

FIGURE 108-3 ■ A left posterolateral incision extending from just anterior to the tip of the scapula to the mid-posterior scapula provides access, through the fourth, fifth, or sixth intercostal spaces, to posterior mediastinal structures, as well as to the hilum of the lung, pericardium, and diaphragm.

the lung, the pericardium, and the diaphragm (Fig. 108-3). If the upper half of the mediastinum needs exposure, an incision through the fourth ICS is optimal. For access to the hilum of the lung, the fifth ICS is optimal, and, for access to the thoracic duct at the level of the diaphragm, or to the central tendon of the diaphragm, a sixth ICS incision is optimal. The most common procedures in which a thoracotomy is performed routinely are operations on the thoracic aorta or branches, such as surgery for repair of coarctation of the aorta or for ligation of the patent ductus. Care should be taken to ensure that the appropriate interspace is entered, because exposure to the upper thorax can be very difficult in small children if the fifth interspace, or lower, is entered. Although counting ribs starting at the second rib, which has attachments of the anterior scalene muscle, can be done, external landmarks can also be used. A useful landmark is the position of the areola when the arm is extended over the head. With the arm extended, the interspace below the areola is usually the fourth ICS, and this landmark can confirm a particular interspace identified by other techniques. This method for identification of interspace is particularly useful in neonates and premature infants. Extensive division of the intercostal muscle is usually unnecessary in infants and small children. Adequate exposure can be obtained by separating the ribs, which are more flexible in this age group and entail less risk for fracture.

This same approach can be used for exposure of intrapericardial structures such as the pulmonary trunk for pulmonary artery banding and even for intracardiac procedures. Exposure to the IVC for cannulation through a posterolateral thoracotomy can be difficult, however, and may require division of one rib posteriorly. Closure of the thoracotomy incision, as in adults, should be done in layers, approximating the serratus muscle and fascia separate from the latissimus dorsi muscle and subcutaneous tissue. This approach minimizes distortion of the chest wall muscles and provides the best cosmetic results as well.

A transaxillary approach has been described for ligation of the patent ductus, access to the transverse aortic arch and descending aorta, and, from the right axilla, closure of atrial septal defects. Either a transverse incision is made over the third interspace between the fold of the pectoralis muscle and scapula or, as some have described, a vertical incision is made from the axilla down to the fourth ICS. The third interspace is then entered, which provides direct access to the distal aortic arch and arterial duct. However, exposure is limited and extension of the incision, if more exposure is required, is difficult. In experienced hands, however, this approach is adequate for ductus ligation, even in small infants, with a less visible incision.

Thoracoscopic Approach in Children

Because most cardiac procedures in children require CPB and intracardiac repair, port access for reconstruction has been applied almost exclusively to adult patients or, rarely, adult-size teenagers. Thoracoscopic procedures in children have been, for the most part, confined to approaches to noncardiac structures or to the pericardium. Examples include ligation of the patent ductus, division of vascular rings, creation of a pericardial window, and, more recently, insertion of pacer leads.[10,11] More recently, total thoracoscopic approaches for repair of atrial and ventricular septal defects have been described.[12,13] Much of the instrumentation has been adapted from other surgical applications, and the thoracoscopic procedures have involved primarily dissection and ligation or division with little reconstruction or suturing. Using induced electromyography to establish the location and local course of the recurrent laryngeal nerve may be of some benefit in infants and small children undergoing patent ductus arteriosus ligation or vascular ring procedures.[14]

Positioning and location of port incisions follow the principles of thoracoscopy or thoracotomy in adults. For access to the distal transverse aortic arch and descending aorta, the patient should be in a full lateral decubitus position. For access to anterior mediastinal structures, such as the anterior pericardium or thymus, a partial decubitus position with the thorax tilted toward a supine position is optimal. Usually, four incisions are required, two for the surgeon's instruments for the dissection, one for the scope and camera, and the fourth for the assistant to introduce lung retractors or occasionally a grasper or suction. As with any thoracoscopic procedure, the central port is used for the camera and the instrument ports are to each side of the camera port, separated by sufficient distance to prevent the scope from interfering with instrument movement. When a surgical robot is used to assist, the same port position is used, but the port for the lung retractor and suction is placed at the midaxillary line at the sixth or seventh ICS (Fig. 108-4).

For the approach to anterior mediastinal structures, the same arrangement is used with respect to the camera and instrument ports. In cases such as dissection of the right lobe of the thymus for thoracoscopic innominate artery suspension to relieve tracheal compression, the central port for the scope is placed at the anterior axillary line in the fourth ICS, and the two instrument ports are placed two or three interspaces to each side and 2 to 3 cm more anterior. A fourth port can be used for lung retraction and should be placed one or two ICSs lower toward

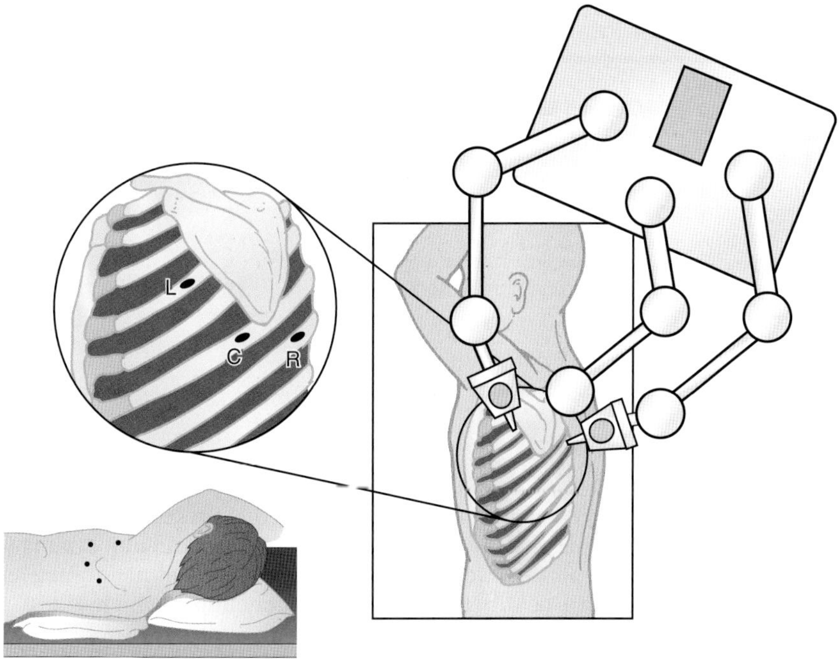

FIGURE 108-4 Port position for robot-assisted thoracoscopic division of vascular ring. The scope and camera are introduced through the central port (C), and instruments are introduced through the other two ports for the robot's left arm (L) and right arm (R). (From Mihaljevic T, Cannon JW, del Nido PJ: Robotically assisted division of a vascular ring in children. *J Thorac Cardiovasc Surg* 125:1163–1164, 2003.)

the diaphragm so as not to interfere with instrument motion. For the anterior pericardium, the three ports are placed more inferiorly on the chest using the fourth or fifth ICS for the scope and camera, and the instrument ports one or two interspaces on either side.

CARDIOPULMONARY BYPASS IN CHILDREN

History

The use of extracorporeal circulatory techniques in the repair of congenital cardiac defects began in the 1950s, shortly after the concept of CPB appeared and a heart-lung machine was constructed. Gibbon repaired an atrial septal defect using the first heart-lung machine, which required 12 to 14 units of blood prime, in 1953.[15] At approximately the same time, Lillihei and colleagues began using cross-circulation to repair a variety of defects in relatively young infants and children, including ventricular septal defects, atrioventricular canal defects, and tetralogy of Fallot, achieving a remarkable overall survival of greater than 60%.[16] Shortly thereafter, Kirklin developed a pump oxygenator derived from Gibbon's earlier efforts.[17] This device required approximately half of the original amount of fresh blood prime but also extreme care to prevent severe foaming of blood, which was lethal; nonetheless, the survival rate was 50%. These early reports prompted many subsequent investigations aimed at developing the scientific and technologic knowledge needed to successfully undertake extracorporeal circulation in infants and children. In spite of these efforts, the morbidity and mortality associated with the use of CPB remained high throughout the 1960s.

The next major advance occurred in the early 1970s, when Castaneda and colleagues[18] and Barratt-Boyes[19] described the use of deep hypothermic circulatory arrest (DHCA) in infants. These techniques relied primarily on surface cooling, with exposure to the CPB circuit limited to a brief period of core cooling and rewarming, so that total CPB time was typically kept under 20 to 30 minutes. Progressive advances in the design of circuit components and perfusion techniques for infants and small children occurred throughout the 1980s and into the early 1990s. As a result, the "toxicity" associated with the use of CPB in infants declined significantly. Currently, lengthy and complex repairs, such as the arterial switch procedure for transposition of the great arteries and primary repair of tetralogy of Fallot, can be undertaken using CPB in neonates and very young infants and result in an overall mortality rate of less than 5%. Nonetheless, the morbidity associated with the use of CPB in infants and children is still widely held to be a major limitation to completely successful outcomes.

Differences between Pediatric and Adult Cardiopulmonary Bypass

There are many significant differences in circuit technology and the physiologic effects of CPB in neonates, infants, and small children compared with adults. The surface area and volume of the CPB circuit relative to

TABLE 108-1 **Sample Scheme for Infant and Pediatric Oxygenators***

Oxygenator	Optimal Body Surface Area (m^2)†	Estimated Total Prime Volume‡ (mL)	Membrane Surface Area (m^2)	Heat Exchange Surface Area (m^2)	Manufactured Recommendation Maximal Flow Rate (mL/min)
Dideco Kids D100	<0.23	240-265	0.22	0.03	700
Terumo Baby RX	0.3-0.4	290-320	0.5	0.035	1500
Terumo RX15-30	0.5-0.7	590-655	1.5	0.14	4000
Terumo RX15-30 Small Adult/KVAD	1.0-1.3	990-1075	1.5	0.14	5000
Terumo RX25 Adult/KVAD	>1.34	1200-1275	2.5	0.2	7000

*Used under standard configuration.
†Assuming maximum 3 liter/min/m^2 flow rate.
‡Assuming use of standard configuration and usual tubing size and length for weight.
KVAD, Kinetic-assisted venous drainage.

patient size and blood volume is much greater for neonates and infants. Arterial and venous cannulas are smaller but more likely to deform or obstruct the aorta or venae cavae. The placement of these cannulas can be different and more variable than in adults—for example, separate superior and inferior vena caval cannulas or initial placement of the aortic cannula in the pulmonary artery (with retrograde systemic perfusion via the ductus arteriosus) during stage I repair of hypoplastic left heart syndrome. To minimize hemodilution, the sizes of various circuit components and tubing diameters are kept as small as possible. Nonetheless, hemodilution that is equivalent to one to two blood volumes from the circuit prime and cardioplegia is fairly common in neonates and small infants (see Table 108-1).

DHCA, although used much less frequently than even a few years ago, is still used occasionally. Overall, pump flow rates can range from no flow (i.e., circulatory arrest) to more than 200 mL/min; mean arterial pressures can vary from 10 to 20 mm Hg during low-flow CPB to more than 50 mm Hg at full or high flow. Temperatures are typically lower in CPB for infants (core temperatures of 15° to 18° C for deep hypothermia; 22° to 25° C is used by some for many other complex repairs), and different blood pH management strategies may be used (i.e., alpha-stat versus pH-stat). In part because of these differences, the magnitude of neuroendocrine stress responses and systemic inflammatory responses to CPB, as well as their consequences, are generally believed to be more profound in neonates and infants than in adults.

Patient Factors

Patient-specific variables and the diverse pathophysiology associated with specific congenital cardiac defects further complicate CPB in neonates, infants, and small children. It is likely that neonates, in general, and particularly those who are premature or weigh less than 1.8 to 2.0 kg, comprise a high-risk group because of immature organ function and coexisting diseases such as sepsis, respiratory distress syndrome, and other congenital anomalies.[20] The immature myocardium may be similarly prone to CPB-related dysfunction for several reasons, including its relatively deficient (compared with in adults) contractile protein mass and organization of contractile proteins, the presence of fetal contractile protein isoforms, immature calcium cycling (which occurs primarily via the sarcolemmal membrane as opposed to the sarcoplasmic reticulum, which is less abundant and less well organized), and fewer mitochondria.

Various aspects of congenital heart disease can mean additional complicating features. Hypertrophic and cyanotic myocardium is more likely to be injured by ischemia-reperfusion and other consequences of CPB.[21-24] Aortopulmonary collaterals, which can be particularly significant in various cyanotic lesions, may promote pulmonary dysfunction as a result of high flow on CPB, whereas steal from systemic perfusion can compromise the function of other organs, and collaterals to the coronary circulation can wash out cardioplegia and thereby hinder effective myocardial preservation. Pulmonary dysfunction after CPB may be more prevalent in infants with other routes of high pulmonary blood flow (e.g., truncus arteriosus, hypoplastic left heart syndrome, transposition of the great arteries) and in cyanotic infants.[20,25] Diffuse organ dysfunction is likely to be more common in patients who were severely cyanotic and hypoperfused at the time of delivery or who required complex surgery in the early neonatal period. In the neonate who was compromised at the time of delivery or thereafter, most centers have found it beneficial to allow a period of stabilization of the circulation and recovery of organ function prior to undertaking CPB and cardiac surgery, using lesion-appropriate interventions such as prostaglandin E1, inotropic support, ventilatory strategies to balance systemic and pulmonary blood flow, and even extracorporeal circulatory support (see later). Post-CPB organ dysfunction (e.g., kidney, liver) can also be a source of morbidity in older (i.e., adult-age) patients with various forms of congenital heart disease complicated by long-standing cyanosis, low cardiac output, or high systemic venous pressures.

Differences in the Cardiopulmonary Bypass Circuit

A summary of the components of different-sized CPB circuits is shown in Table 108-1.

Oxygenators. Oxygenator systems for infants and children must function over a wide range of pump flow rates (maximal flow rates range between 800 and 4000 mL/min, and they must be efficient over a range of flows equivalent to 0 to 250 mL/kg), temperatures (10° to 38° C), hematocrits (15% to 40%), and line pressures (because of different sizes of cannulas and tubing).

Virtually all current pediatric CPB applications use membrane-type oxygenators. The two main types are microporous (hollow-fiber or folded-membrane) and nonporous membrane oxygenators. The major advantage of microporous-type membranes is their ability to effect gas exchange with a relatively modest membrane surface area, typically in the range of 0.2 to 1.5 m^2, depending on the specific oxygenator and configuration. Major disadvantages include some blood-gas contact at the start of CPB (until protein accumulation blocks the 0.05- to 0.25-μm pores) and protein leakage across the membrane, along with the potential for gas embolization if negative pressure develops on the blood side of the artificial membrane. Nonporous oxygenator membranes, typically of the folded-sheet silicone-membrane variety, require a larger surface area to achieve gas exchange but do not accumulate or leak protein as readily and are therefore more often selected for longer-term circulatory support applications (e.g., extracorporeal membrane oxygenation).

There is a real need to minimize circuit priming volume to minimize hemodilution, blood product exposure, and the potential for fluid overload and edema.[26] Priming volume is usually defined as the volume of the membrane compartment plus the minimal amount required for the venous reservoir. Typical priming volumes of commercial membrane oxygenators range from approximately 225 to 375 mL when used in the open configuration. The Dideco Lilliput hollow-fiber membrane oxygenator (Dideco, Mirandola, Italy) is an example of one with a smaller prime volume (≈70 mL), but it is not available in an open-system configuration. More recently, oxygenators and arterial filters have been combined into one unit, further reducing priming volume (e.g., Quadrox-I Neonatal and Pediatric with integrated arterial filter, Maquet, Rastatt, Germany; or Capiox FX05, Terumo Corporation, Tokyo, Japan). Various schema for achieving low priming volume and thereby reducing or avoiding the need for blood products as a component of the priming solution have been described.[27-33]

Pumps. Most pediatric circuits use roller pumps. Pump flow rate is governed by the revolutions per minute (rpm) of the pump head, the degree of occlusion produced by the rollers, and the internal diameter of the tubing. A significant advantage is that pump flow is relatively independent of resistive and hydrostatic forces in the circuit. However, adequate flow is highly dependent on proper setting of roller head occlusion (which also affects the degree of blood trauma and hemolysis), along with accurate knowledge of pump head speed (rpm) and tubing size. Failure to accurately account for any of these variables can lead to excessive or inadequate pump flow.

Tubing. Competing considerations govern selection of tubing size for infant and pediatric CPB (Table 108-2). The internal diameter needs to be large enough to permit the required full flow rate (see later) without inordinately increasing circuit line pressures. On the other hand, the tubing should be as narrow and as short as practical, to minimize priming volume. Some neonatal circuits use ¼-inch tubing on both arterial and venous limbs, and most centers have further decreased the diameter of the arterial tubing to 3/16 inch; some use 3/16-inch tubing for both arterial and venous limbs (although vacuum-assisted venous drainage may be required in this case).[20] The pump is usually situated as close to the surgical field as possible to reduce tubing length, which is a major contributor to overall circuit volume.

TABLE 108-2 **Infant and Pediatric Cardiopulmonary Bypass Tubing**

Tubing Diameter (inch)	Tubing Volume (mL/ft)	Flow Rate (mL/revolution)
3/16	5.0	7.4
¼	9.7	13
⅜	21.7	27
½	38.6	45

Venous Drainage. As in adult circuits, venous blood usually flows from the patient to the venous reservoir of the CPB circuit by gravity. The level of blood in the venous reservoir serves as an important safety mechanism: it is a source of volume to increase arterial inflow and to assess the adequacy of venous return. If venous return and the level in the venous reservoir decline, the cause (e.g., unrecovered or lost blood in the surgical field, malpositioned venous cannulas, excessive capillary leak) can be identified, and interventions (e.g., decreasing pump flow rate, adding volume, adjusting operating table height, repositioning venous cannulas) can be performed.

Many venous reservoirs are rigid and used in a configuration that is open to the atmosphere. Advantages include ease of removing entrained venous air, free flow of venous drainage (i.e., no air lockage or buildup of pressure in the reservoir), integration of the cardiotomy reservoir (as opposed to having a separate reservoir for cardiotomy suction), and the ability to accurately measure reservoir volume via calibration lines on the side of the chamber. This last feature is a useful aid to assess the patient's intravascular volume and may therefore facilitate weaning from CPB. Major disadvantages of open, rigid venous reservoirs include the presence of a blood-air interface, which may promote blood trauma and activation of the coagulation, fibrinolytic, and inflammatory cascades (see later), and the need for a larger priming volume.

A soft, collapsible venous reservoir bag that expands and contracts in relationship to overall blood volume, venous return, and arterial inflow rate is used with increasing frequency in infant CPB. Advantages include the absence of direct blood-air contact and the fact that air is not entrained if the venous reservoir becomes empty, which collapses the bag. A major disadvantage can be the inability to accurately measure venous reservoir volume or to recognize subtle but important changes in venous return. Other relative disadvantages compared with rigid reservoirs include the need for a removal mechanism if air is entrained, the need for a separate cardiotomy suction reservoir, and the fact that venous drainage will be significantly reduced if pressure builds up as a result of overfilling of the reservoir with blood volume or air.

Vacuum-assisted venous drainage has been used for pediatric patients.[20,28,34-36] Although this has not been well studied in a controlled or prospective fashion, advantages may include the ability to reduce total circuit volume by using lower venous reservoir volume and $\frac{3}{16}$-inch venous tubing, improving operating conditions to some extent by allowing use of smaller venous cannulas, and improving venous drainage through the small cannulas and tubing. Theoretically, the improvement of venous drainage could lead to reduced tissue and organ edema and congestion, improved organ function, and reduced inflammatory activation (e.g., via endotoxin release from congested, hypoperfused intestine). A major potential complication of vacuum-assisted venous drainage is venoarterial air embolism.[37-41]

Arterial Cannulas. Issues regarding cannula size are much more significant in infants and small children than in adults. Arterial cannulas for neonates and small infants must be of sufficient size to permit appropriate arterial inflow rates at reasonable line pressures, with minimal shearing or jetting of blood flow (which can damage the vessel intima, aortic valve, or blood elements), yet small enough to fit in small aortas without obstructing aortic flow (Table 108-3). Small cannulas (i.e., 8 Fr) with a thin-walled, reinforced design that prevents cannula kinking and allows a larger luminal diameter for a given external diameter have become popular choices for infant bypass (Biomedicus, Medtronic, Minneapolis, MN). Care also needs to be taken not to kink or compress the infant's pliable aorta by the location and orientation of the aortic cannula and its tubing. As noted, the cannula itself can significantly obstruct flow in the vessel around the cannula. Location of the tip can direct blood flow toward or away from specific vessels; for example, locating and directing the tip more distally toward the transverse arch may reduce flow through the right carotid artery or favor lower body perfusion at the expense of cerebral perfusion and optimal brain cooling.[42]

Certain congenital cardiac lesions require unique aortic cannulation sites. For example, the aortic cannula is typically placed more distally in the aorta for repairs that involve extensive proximal aortic surgery, such as the arterial switch procedure for transposition of the great vessels; this distal location may alter distribution of blood flow to the carotid vessels. Repair of interrupted aortic arch requires two arterial cannulas, one in each segment of the aorta (perfusing the head and lower body, respectively). The aortic cannula is placed in the pulmonary artery at the beginning of CPB for stage I repair of hypoplastic left heart syndrome because of the typically diminutive size of the ascending aorta in this lesion. The distal pulmonary arteries are occluded with tourniquets and the aorta is perfused via the ductus arteriosus until the aortic reconstruction is completed, at which time the cannula is repositioned in the neo-aorta. The aortic cannula can also be placed into a side graft, which is anastomosed to the innominate artery, for arch reconstruction using antegrade cerebral perfusion.

Unlike in adults, femoral arterial cannulation for CPB is not usually a viable option in infants and small children (weighing less than ≈10 to 15 kg), because small vessel size precludes inserting an arterial cannula that is large enough to allow arterial inflow rates that are sufficient to completely meet metabolic needs (see later). In small infants (without recent sternotomy), the neck vessels are the preferred extrathoracic cannulation sites (see later). However, as a resuscitative measure in emergent situations (e.g., cardiopulmonary arrest in the cardiac catheterization laboratory, particularly when femoral vascular access is already in place), insertion of smaller perfusion cannulas in the femoral artery has often been life-saving in terms of facilitating rapid establishment of extracorporeal support. Femoral access is performed occasionally for older children, either electively, when there is concern that a cardiac chamber or vascular conduit lies immediately beneath the sternum, or emergently, when one of these structures is entered inadvertently during the dissection.

Venous Cannulas. Choice and location of venous cannulas can also be more complex and variable than is typically the case in adults, and variations in venous anatomy and drainage as well as the operative approach must be taken into account. Venous cannulas are available in a variety of sizes and with design features for particular indications (Table 108-4). For example, thin-walled cannulas with multiple side holes enhance venous drainage; right-angled tips are frequently used in the SVC to improve alignment (and therefore drainage) and minimize impact on the surgical field; metal-tipped, to prevent kinking; straight, short-tipped in the IVC, to limit hepatic venous obstruction.

Overall, most repairs use separate SVC and IVC cannulas to achieve maximal collection of venous return and to minimize interference with the operative field. Common variations in venous anatomy that can complicate venous cannulation and must be taken into account include left or bilateral SVCs, azygous or hemiazygous continuation of the IVC, and direct drainage of the hepatic veins into the atrium. A single atrial cannula is frequently used when DHCA is planned; in this case, the venous cannula is removed after the patient is adequately cooled, to provide a clear operative field.

TABLE 108-3 Representative Pediatric Arterial Cannulas

Weight (kg)	Standard Arterial Size (Fr)	Biomedicus Pediatric Arterial Size (Fr)
<5	10	8
5-10	12	10
10-14	14	12
14-28	16	14
28-40	18	15
40-55	20	17

TABLE 108-4 **Representative Venous Cannulas for Pediatric Cardiopulmonary Bypass**

Weight (kg)	Single Venous (Fr)	
<3.5	14	
3.5-5	14	
5-8	16	
8-12	16	
12-18	18	
18-26	20	
26-55	22	
>55	24	
	Metal-Tip, Right-Angle Venous* (Fr)	
Weight (kg)	**SVC**	**IVC**
<3	12	12
3-6	12	14
6-8	12	16
8-12	14	16
12-16	14	18
16-22	16	18
22-30	16	20
30-34	18	20
34-46	18	20-22
46-58	20	22
Weight (kg)	**Dual-Stage† (Fr)**	
<12	18/24	
12-30	20/28	
30-65	29/29	
>65	29/37*	
Weight (kg)	**Dual-Stage with Venous Assist (Fr)**	
<20	18/24	
20-45	20/28	
45-85	29/29	
>85	29/37	

*For example, the Medtronic DLP (Minneapolis, MN).
†For example, Edwards Lifesciences (Irvine, CA).
IVC, Inferior vena cava; *SVC*, superior vena cava.

Regardless of location, it is important that the cannula be appropriately sited and that it cause as little obstruction to venous drainage as possible. Poor venous drainage may be difficult to detect and is more likely to occur in patients with complicated venous anatomy. The consequences of impaired venous drainage and increased venous pressures are likely to be magnified during CPB because arterial perfusion pressure is frequently reduced. Obstruction of the SVC may promote cerebral edema and otherwise increase the risk of brain injury by decreasing cerebral blood flow (CBF) and hindering effective brain cooling. Many physicians find monitoring of SVC pressure by a catheter placed in the internal jugular vein useful to detect possible SVC obstruction in this setting. In addition, the patient's head and face should also be inspected at regular intervals during CPB for the appearance of congestion or swelling. It is likely that monitoring CBF velocity using transcranial Doppler methodology might be useful in this regard. A drop in cerebral near-infrared spectroscopy (NIRS) saturation may herald poor SVC drainage and need for cannula adjustment. IVC obstruction will increase lower body venous pressures and potentially decrease hepatic, renal, or mesenteric perfusion; isolated hepatic vein obstruction can also occur. Consequences can include hepatic dysfunction, renal dysfunction, ascites, and perhaps increased inflammatory consequences of mesenteric congestion.[43,44] IVC obstruction during CPB can be difficult to detect and should be suspected whenever there is development of ascites, decreased urine output, or impaired venous return.

Filters. Almost all applications use 0.2-μm filters in the gas inflow lines to prevent bacterial or particulate contamination. Similarly, all crystalloid prime and cardioplegia solutions are passed through 0.2-μm filters prior to final addition to the CPB circuit. A 20- or 40-μm filter is used on the cardiotomy suction return line to remove macro- and microaggregates and other debris from the blood returning from the surgical field. Exogenous blood is also filtered (typically through a 40-μm blood filter) before it is added to either the pump circuit or to cardioplegia. Specific removal of blood polymorphonuclear leukocytes using leukocyte-depleting filters placed in-line on the CPB circuit (which typically reduces circulating leukocyte counts in the patient by ≈75%) is advocated by some centers as a significant means to reduce reperfusion injury.[25,45]

Use of an arterial filter (40 μm) is somewhat more controversial. Many consider arterial filtering essential to limit the microemboli and amount of other debris from platelet and leukocyte microaggregates, traumatized blood elements, fat, and other sources, particularly because these might contribute to post-CPB neurologic injury and damage to other organ systems. Some physicians do not feel strongly about these issues and omit arterial line filters, at least in part to reduce priming volume and hemodilution.[20] As mentioned previously, there are now oxygenators with integrated arterial filters.[46]

Cardiopulmonary Bypass Prime. The priming volume of even the smallest neonatal and infant CPB circuits is usually equivalent to approximately 1.5 to 3 times the patient's blood volume. Thus, dilution of red cells, clotting factors, and other plasma constituents is potentially of far greater magnitude than in adults. Physiologic crystalloid solutions (e.g., Normosol-R, Hospira, Lake Forest, IL) are the major component of CPB priming solutions in infants and children; colloidal primes are used infrequently. Significant additions to the infant CPB prime include packed red blood cells (or occasionally whole blood), as well as fresh-frozen plasma or other colloids such as albumin.

Other agents that may be included in the pump prime include mannitol, steroids, heparin, and buffers (e.g., sodium bicarbonate or tris[hydroxymethyl]aminomethane [THAM]). Mannitol is used primarily for its osmotic properties and is intended to reduce organ and cellular edema as well as to promote diuresis and thereby contribute to renal protection. The osmotic diuresis may be particularly beneficial in some congenital cardiac operations in which a substantial amount of hemolysis from blood trauma caused by cardiotomy suction and high pump flow rates can occur. Stabilization of cellular membranes and various antioxidant properties, including radical scavenging, have also been attributed to mannitol. The significance of any of these effects has not been proven in pediatric CPB. Steroids are used to reduce inflammatory effects of CPB (see later).

The use of albumin or other colloid to prime CPB circuits is also controversial.[47-49] There is evidence that reduced plasma protein concentrations and diminished plasma oncotic pressure can reduce lymphatic flow and increase capillary leak in the lung and other vascular beds.[50-53] Although fluid balance and weight gain were favorably influenced, a recent study that randomized pediatric CPB patients to crystalloid or colloid prime did not demonstrate significant differences in mortality or in length of mechanical ventilation, intensive care unit stay, or hospital stay.[53] These results are similar to those obtained in adults, where albumin does prevent CPB-induced reductions in colloid oncotic pressure and lung water accumulation, but it appears to have little effect on overall outcome or measures of pulmonary, myocardial, or renal function. Synthetic colloids are available but have not demonstrated benefits in adults.

Hemodilution. As noted earlier, some centers have gone to substantial lengths to modify circuit design to reduce the degree of hemodilution associated with infant CPB and decrease the use of exogenous blood and other products. These modifications have included the use of the smallest possible tubing, cannulas, and oxygenators; altered orientation of the CPB circuit to decrease tubing length; vacuum-assisted venous drainage to improve return through the small cannulas and tubing; and omission of arterial filters. Resultant priming volumes in the range of 180 to 250 mL have been reported. Ultrafiltration techniques (see later) are also used to offset the hemodiluting effects of CPB and thereby reduce the requirement for donor blood and blood products. With the possible exception of ultrafiltration, there is no evidence that edema, the inflammatory response to CPB, or overall outcome is improved by these measures, and, at present, it remains difficult to avoid the use of exogenous blood or blood products in patients who weigh less than approximately 10 kg.

Both packed red cells and whole blood have been used to ensure age-, lesion-, and temperature-appropriate hematocrit during CPB. Packed red cells are readily available and are probably used by most centers to increase and maintain hematocrit during CPB. A major disadvantage of whole blood compared with packed red cells is the higher glucose load that accompanies whole blood; hyperglycemia may increase the risk of brain injury during cerebral ischemia. On the other hand, whole blood more effectively maintains plasma factor concentrations, which can be significantly reduced by CPB in these patients (see later). Questions about the actual oxygen carrying and delivery capacity of stored red blood cells have been raised.[54] Increased duration of blood cell storage has been related to postoperative morbidity.[55]

The optimal hematocrit for neonatal and infant CPB remains controversial. Perhaps the most important consideration is the temperature and flow rate that are to be used (e.g., deep hypothermia, low flow, or circulatory arrest). More profound degrees of hypothermia are used in pediatric patients to suppress metabolic demands and increase tolerance to periods of low flow (25° to 18° C) or absent flow (15° to 18° C). Although the oxygen-carrying capacity of hemoglobin increases at lower temperatures, its ability to donate oxygen to the tissues is also reduced. Moreover, the increase in blood viscosity that accompanies hypothermia is a significant impediment to microcirculatory flow and can lead to sludging and regional ischemia. The nonpulsatile flow patterns typical of most CPB applications may also decrease microcirculatory flow, particularly in the setting of increased viscosity. It is also important to note that the oxygen-carrying capacity of the non–red cell fluid component of blood (i.e., plasma) increases at decreasing temperatures because of the increased solubility of gas in the liquid phase that occurs as temperature declines; as a result, the net effect of hemodilution during hypothermia is to improve microvascular flow and oxygen delivery.

Despite these theoretical considerations, the optimal and maximal tolerable levels of hemodilution for a given degree of hypothermia are not established. Normovolemic hemodilution with hematocrit levels down to 15% is believed to be well tolerated during normothermia in terms of cerebral and myocardial function as long as blood pressure, oxygenation, and cardiac output are maintained.[56,57] Long-standing practice at many centers has been to aim for hematocrit levels in the 18% to 22% range during deep hypothermic CPB, and this is based on the aforementioned improvements in blood rheology and overall oxygen-carrying capacity that accompany the combination of hemodilution and hypothermia. Animal studies and reports of children of the Jehovah's Witnesses faith undergoing hypothermic CPB suggest no detectable effect on overall outcome or cerebral or cardiovascular morbidity at hematocrits in the range of 10% to 18% when a low temperature, perfusion pressure, and flow rate are maintained.[57-60] Hematocrits of 10% or less in infants have been associated with acidosis and other evidence of inadequate oxygen delivery.

More recent evidence has cast doubt on the safety of very low hematocrits during hypothermic CPB in infant patients. In experimental infant CPB models, higher hematocrit (in the 25% to 30% range) has been associated with enhanced preservation of brain high-energy phosphates, intracellular pH, tissue oxygenation, maintained capillary density and microvascular flow, reduced leukocyte activation, and reduced neurologic injury.[61-63] A recent clinical study that randomized infants to either a low hematocrit (mean hematocrit, 22% ± 3%) or high hematocrit (28% ± 3%) strategy at the start of low-flow hypothermic CPB found lower postoperative cardiac index, higher serum lactate, and higher total body water in the low hematocrit group. At 1 year, overall neurologic evaluations and mental development index scores were similar in the two groups, but the low hematocrit group had significantly lower psychomotor development index scores.[64] Our current practice is to aim to keep the hematocrit between approximately 25% and 30% during all types of CPB. A hematocrit level at the onset of low-flow CPB of approximately 25% was associated with higher psychomotor development index scores and reduced lactate levels.[65,66] In addition to any direct effects, it is likely that the somewhat higher hematocrit provides some degree of safety margin against other problems with perfusion, collaterals, and alterations in cerebral autoregulation and CBF.[59,65-70] However, similar variations in patient age, anatomy, collaterals, flow rate, pH strategy, and cooling, for example, make it impossible to pronounce a single optimal hematocrit for infants or children.

The optimal hematocrit for weaning from CPB is also controversial. The overall goal is adequate systemic oxygen delivery. Our current practice is to aim for hematocrits in the range of 25% to 30% during rewarming and at termination of CPB. These levels (and perhaps even somewhat lower) are likely to be well tolerated by patients who have good myocardial function, minimal or no hemodynamic lesions, and a physiologic repair with normal oxygen saturation at the conclusion of their surgery. Consideration should be given to increasing hematocrit to improve oxygen-carrying capacity and oxygen delivery in patients with reduced myocardial function or palliative or staged operations that result in cyanosis. In these cases, hematocrits of 40% or even slightly higher may be beneficial, but definitive data are lacking.

Pump Flow Rates during Pediatric Cardiopulmonary Bypass. Optimal pump flow rates for pediatric CPB are, as for adults, based on considerations of adequate systemic oxygenation, oxygen delivery, and organ perfusion at normothermia as assessed by oxygen consumption and metabolic rate, mixed venous oxygen saturation, acid-base balance, and lactate production.[71] These are typically indexed to body weight. The higher metabolic rate of neonates and infants (≈1.5- to 2.5-fold greater than that of adults) mandates proportionately higher flow rates during normothermic CPB (Table 108-5).

Heparinization. The approach to anticoagulation during pediatric CPB is similar to that for adults. Heparin is administered in a dose of approximately 4 mg/kg (400 U/kg) prior to initiation of bypass, either directly into the right atrium or into a central venous catheter; teams at some centers include a portion of the total heparin dose in the CPB pump prime. Confirmation of heparin injection by blood aspiration, as well as the adequacy of heparin effect, should be performed before beginning CPB. The activated clotting time (ACT) is the primary method of monitoring the efficacy of heparin anticoagulation (and reversal) in infants and children. Typical guidelines require an ACT of greater than 400 seconds before initiating CPB, and ACT should be maintained between 400 and 600 seconds during CPB to prevent activation of blood coagulation pathways and clot formation. Inadequate concentrations of heparin are believed to be a major contributor to excessive activation of the coagulation and fibrinolytic systems.[72] Other methods of monitoring heparin effect, anticoagulation, and clotting parameters, such as blood heparin concentration and thromboelastography, are adjunctive at present and used mainly to assess residual heparin activity and diagnose and treat coagulopathies after termination of CPB.[73] Heparin brand and formulation will affect the level of anticoagulation and even the amount of postoperative bleeding.[74,75]

TABLE 108-5 Estimated Flow Rates for Normothermic Infant and Pediatric Cardiopulmonary Bypass

Body Weight (kg)	Flow Range (mL/kg/min)	Usual Full-Flow Rate (mL/kg/min)
<3	150-200	200
3-10	125-175	150
10-15	120-150	125
13-30	80-120	100

Although substantive data are scant, there is some evidence that, generally, neonates and young infants are more sensitive to the effects of heparin administered for CPB and that the efficacy and duration of heparin-based anticoagulation is significantly more variable in neonates and young infants.[72,76-78] Potential mechanisms include the variable and generally lower levels of both procoagulant and anticoagulant factors present during the first few months of life and in some patients with congenital heart disease.[79-82] The degree of hypothermia, amount of hemodilution, and relative immaturity of drug metabolism can also contribute to an increased and prolonged heparin effect in infants. Heparin resistance, on the other hand, is seen infrequently in infants, although sporadic examples resulting from recent heparin exposure or antithrombin III deficiency do occur. Heparin-induced thrombocytopenia and thrombosis appear to be less common in infants and children than in adult heart surgery patients, but the incidence may increase as the number of children who are repeatedly exposed in the operating room, catheterization laboratory, and other sites continues to increase.[83,84] There is at present only limited and anecdotal experience with the use of heparin alternatives such as bivalirudin, hirudin, and argatroban, for anticoagulation during pediatric CPB.[85-87]

Heparin Reversal. Protamine sulfate is administered at the end of CPB to reverse the anticoagulant effects of heparin. As with heparin, there is little prospective, controlled information about the dosing of protamine in neonates and infants. Protamine dosing is usually based on body weight (3 to 4 mg/kg) or in a ratio to the heparin dose (milligrams-to-milligrams) of 1 : 1 or 1.3 : 1; in vitro titration to neutralize heparin in a patient sample is also used by some physicians. In general, the target ACT after protamine administration is within approximately 10% of the pre-CPB baseline. The first two empirical methods usually result in relative protamine excess, which is intentional because of greater heparin sensitivity and duration in infants and because of other factors that may potentiate heparinization, such as hemodilution, hypothermia, and delayed metabolic clearance. However, as with adults, there is evidence that empirical protamine dosing is associated with excess protamine administration and perhaps greater blood loss and transfusion requirements as compared with doses that directly measure blood heparin using titration or other methods.[77,78,88,89] Another argument against empiric dosing is that relatively small excesses of circulating protamine compared with heparin may have direct antiplatelet effects that can exacerbate bleeding after CPB.[90]

Typically, the drug is administered slowly over approximately 10 minutes. For unclear reasons, severe hypotensive, pulmonary vasoconstrictive, or anaphylactic/anaphylactoid reactions to protamine are uncommon in infants and children.[91] Of these, hypotension is most frequent, occurring in between approximately 1.5% and 3% of protamine administrations. It is dependent on dose and rate of administration, most likely resulting from histamine release, usually fairly mild and transient, and responsive to volume replacement or calcium administration. Severe pulmonary vasoconstriction appears to be much less common than in adults, maybe as a result of complement activation or pulmonary thromboxane release, and can be particularly troubling in patients with depressed contractile function.

Initiation of Pediatric Cardiopulmonary Bypass

CPB is initiated once the arterial and venous cannulas are correctly positioned and connected to the circuit, the absence of air in the arterial line (especially at the connection between cannula and circuit tubing) is confirmed, and adequate anticoagulation is established. Under most circumstances in neonates and infants, arterial inflow is begun slowly and then the venous line is unclamped. Rapid onset of bradycardia and loss of myocardial function can ensue when a cold prime is used. Therefore, when using either normothermic or cold pump primes, full flow is usually reached fairly rapidly in neonates and infants to ensure adequate systemic perfusion and oxygen delivery. When it is important to keep the heart beating and potentially ejecting, prime electrolyte concentrations—specifically calcium and potassium—are usually normalized, along with the temperature of the prime solution, so as to maintain myocardial function and prevent myocardial distention during the initiation of bypass. Compromised venous drainage can also distend the heart and promote myocardial damage.

Large collateral vessels arising from the arterial tree (as can be seen in many forms of cyanotic heart disease, including tetralogy of Fallot and pulmonary atresia), patent ductus arteriosus, and surgical aortopulmonary shunts can promote runoff from the systemic circulation during CPB and thereby reduce perfusion pressure, effective organ (i.e., brain, heart, kidneys) blood flow, and cooling despite seemingly adequate total pump flow. Surgical control and effective occlusion of large aortopulmonary collateral vessels, surgical shunts, and the patent ductus arteriosus is accomplished immediately before or shortly after commencing CPB. Significant aortopulmonary collateral vessels that are not important sources of pulmonary blood flow or contributors to arterial oxygenation can be coil-occluded in the cardiac catheterization laboratory before surgery, which will also decrease the volume load on the systemic ventricle.

Monitoring during Pediatric Cardiopulmonary Bypass

Circuit Monitoring

Important CPB circuit variables include arterial line pressure, pump flow rate, oxygenator gases, and temperature. Arterial line pressure is measured via a pressure transducer placed in the arterial inflow limb. Line pressure can be substantially higher than patient arterial pressure because of the driving pressure required to achieve adequate flow through small-diameter infant arterial cannulas and tubing, and it is typically in the range of 225 to 260 mm Hg at mean arterial pressures of 40 to 60 mm Hg. Excessively high arterial line pressures (>300 to 400 mm Hg) can result from tubing or cannula obstruction or cannula malposition and can result in circuit rupture. Many circuits include a sensor on the oxygenator reservoir to detect critically low volume levels and a sensor on the arterial line to detect air.

The flow output of roller pumps is governed by roller head rpm, occlusion pressure, and the internal tubing diameter. Pump flow rate on roller pumps is not measured directly but rather *calculated* by the perfusionist (or electronics on the pump) based on these variables. Because the flow output of the pump is not measured directly, incorrectly measuring or inputting rpm, tubing size, or occlusion, as well as possible shunts in the circuit, can lead to potentially harmful perfusion errors (either increased or decreased). Unexpectedly low or high mean arterial pressure for the calculated flow rate may be the first clue to these possibilities. In the case of low flow in particular, abnormal biochemical variables result if the condition is of sufficient magnitude and duration (see later).

Oxygenator gases can include oxygen, air, and carbon dioxide. Continuous in-line monitors of pH, PO_2, and PCO_2 are used frequently. The gas "sweep speed" (flow rate) and oxygen concentration delivered to the oxygenator are controlled with a flowmeter or blender and measured with appropriate electrodes. Starting sweep speeds are usually at a ratio to pump flow rate of 1:1 for membrane oxygenators. However, the variability in pump flow rates, temperatures, and blood gas management strategies leads to wide variations in gas flow and composition in pediatric patients. pH-stat management can require altered gas sweep rates and the ability to add and precisely control carbon dioxide in the sweep gas.

Thermistors measure temperatures of the water bath and heat exchanger, along with arterial and venous blood temperatures. The temperature gradient between the patient and perfusate should not exceed 10° C. This can be especially important during rewarming to prevent formation of gaseous bubbles and emboli that result from decreased gas solubility as fluid temperature increases.

Patient Monitoring

Monitoring of mean arterial pressure is required during CPB and is most often accomplished via catheters in either the radial or the femoral arteries. Arterial catheter location can occasionally be governed by considerations such as prior surgical or shunt (e.g., Blalock-Taussig) sites and the current lesion and planned operation. Femoral arterial pressure monitoring (with or without concomitant radial arterial monitoring) is preferred by some for aortic reconstructions and for increased reliability when deep hypothermia is planned, particularly in small infants. Left atrial and SVC or right atrial filling pressures are also measured routinely, depending on the surgery.

Nasopharyngeal, esophageal, and rectal temperatures are measured with appropriate thermistors. Nasopharyngeal or tympanic membrane temperatures are most often used and are probably the most accurate in terms of tracking brain temperature, although no extracranial site is truly reliable in this regard.[57] Rectal (or occasionally bladder) temperature is used to monitor core temperature. Esophageal temperature reflects aortic temperature and does not correlate well with core or brain temperatures.

Arterial and venous blood gases should be measured within 5 to 10 minutes after commencing and then at 15- to 30-minute intervals for the remainder of CPB but more frequently if there is evidence of compromised perfusion. In addition to pH, PO_2, and PCO_2, most analyzers can use the same samples to simultaneously measure hematocrit and serum electrolyte levels, including levels of sodium, potassium, and ionized calcium. Many centers favor allowing or even promoting (e.g., via the chelating effects of citrate in added blood products) reduced ionized calcium during CPB in an attempt to reduce the contribution of that cation to reperfusion injury. Ionized hypomagnesaemia, another potential contributor to ischemia-reperfusion damage and dysrhythmias, has been found after pediatric CPB, although its clinical significance is unclear.[92,93] Increasing blood lactate concentrations before and shortly after pediatric CPB have been suggested to correlate postoperative morbidity and mortality.[94]

The oxygen saturation of venous blood (SVO_2) is an important index of tissue perfusion, and it should be measured from venous blood samples at intervals as discussed in the previous paragraph and also continuously via a calibrated in-line monitor on the venous line. Optimal and minimal acceptable values for SVO_2 during CPB, particularly as temperature and flow rate decrease, are not well defined. At normothermic or near normothermic temperatures, SVO_2 can be interpreted as is done in non-CPB situations, and hence low values (less than ≈60% to 70%) should raise concern about inadequate tissue oxygen delivery (e.g., inadequate flow, low hemoglobin). The development of shunting around major vascular beds that may occur as a consequence of CPB, in addition to any preexisting collateral vessels, may increase SVO_2 in an artifactual way; in other words, some degree of organ hypoperfusion may exist despite what appear to be acceptable SVO_2 values. At deeper levels of hypothermia, dissolved oxygen contributes an increasing proportion of total oxygen delivery, and the increased affinity of hemoglobin for oxygen impairs transfer from hemoglobin to tissue.[95] As a result, the interpretation of SVO_2 during deep hypothermia becomes more problematic, and it may be prudent to require substantially higher levels of SVO_2 (>90%) when this measure is used to infer the adequacy of perfusion during deep hypothermic CPB.

Cerebral saturation measured by NIRS has been used as a surrogate for SVO_2 and, therefore, tissue perfusion. Cerebral NIRS correlates with SVC saturation.[96] Decrease in cerebral NIRS can be a warning of decreased cerebral perfusion. Periods of diminished intraoperative and perioperative cerebral saturation, as measured by NIRS, has been related to compromised neurodevelopmental outcome and abnormalities in cerebral magnetic resonance imaging.[97] Flank saturation measured with NIRS can also be used to alert to decreased tissue perfusion to the lower body during bypass.

Frequent monitoring of blood glucose and efforts to maintain it in the normoglycemic range are important during CPB in neonates, infants, and children. The major cause of hypoglycemia appears to be limited hepatic glycogen stores and gluconeogenic capability, especially in neonates, and perhaps also in cyanotic and malnourished (e.g., because of congestive heart failure) infants and young children. Failure to provide exogenous glucose can result in severe hypoglycemia and neurologic injury. The potential neurologic consequences of hypoglycemia may be exacerbated by hypocarbia, which seems to lower the threshold for hypoglycemic neuronal damage, and by patient lesions (e.g., aortopulmonary collaterals) and bypass strategies that independently reduce cerebral autoregulation or CBF (or both).[98-100]

Hyperglycemia can also be a frequent occurrence during pediatric CPB. Blood glucose may increase because of an increased supply from exogenous sources such as intravenous fluids and cardioplegia, or because of reduced glucose uptake, which is primarily caused by increases in stress hormones such as cortisol, growth hormone, and catecholamines that counter the effects of insulin.[101] Additionally, deep hypothermia can also suppress glucose-stimulated insulin secretion during hypothermic CPB and for at least a few hours thereafter. Hyperglycemia can potentiate cerebral ischemia-reperfusion injury under a variety of circumstances in infants and children[102-104] and a trend is seen toward similar results in pediatric CPB patients, although these data are largely retrospective and uncontrolled.[98,105] Proposed mechanisms of hyperglycemic-ischemic brain injury include hyperosmolar cellular swelling from glucose loading and promotion of lactic acidosis or increased intracellular acidosis caused by increased anaerobic glycolytic flux.

However, this issue remains controversial. Increased blood glucose concentration may be important for adequate brain glucose delivery when CBF and autoregulation are impaired. There was only a weak correlation between blood glucose with brain creatine kinase (CK-BB) levels and no correlation with neurodevelopmental outcome in the Boston Circulatory Arrest study, and there was some evidence that post-CPB hyperglycemia was in fact protective, particularly against seizures, which are associated with worse neurodevelopmental outcomes.[106,107] There are also substantial data in a variety of non-CPB animal models that pre-ischemic hyperglycemia may protect immature brain from hypoxia, asphyxia, or hypoxia-ischemia.[108-111] One important caveat is that these studies were conducted almost exclusively in immature rat models where circulation and ventilation were unsupported, and some of the protective effect of hyperglycemia may have resulted from better maintenance of the circulation or ventilation in hyperglycemic animals (an effect that would be largely irrelevant during CPB).

Further complicating this issue are reports suggesting that relatively modest degrees of hyperglycemia were associated with worse overall outcome in a variety of circumstances, including adult cardiac surgery and in at least some adult and pediatric patients under intensive care, and that tight glucose control could be beneficial.[112-120] Particularly in the case of adult cardiac surgery patients, at least some of the benefit appeared to be obtained in diabetic (and perhaps prediabetic) patients and to involve risks and complications not typically associated with infant congenital heart surgery.[121-123] However, additional and more recent analyses have called this conclusion into question, with a number of studies suggesting that moderate degrees of hyperglycemia are not associated with worse outcome and that tight control may in fact be detrimental.[114,117,124-126]

In 2012 the *New England Journal of Medicine* published the results of a randomized controlled trial of tight glycemic control compared with standard care after pediatric cardiac surgery. Investigators found low hypoglycemia rates but were not able to demonstrate changes in mortality, infection, or organ failure between the two groups.[127]

Hypothermia

Hypothermia continues to be the mainstay for protection of the brain and other organs during CPB. Its major and most pervasive effect is to decrease metabolic rate and consequently decrease metabolic demand for oxygen and other substrates. During ischemia, hypothermia slows consumption of high-energy phosphate compounds and also maintains them intracellularly, thereby facilitating recovery of adenosine triphosphate (ATP) and phosphocreatine during reperfusion. Hypothermia delays loss of ionic homeostasis during ischemia, particularly entry of sodium and calcium and resultant cellular edema, by energy-dependent, energy-independent, and membrane-stabilizing mechanisms.[128] Reduced amounts of free-radical generation, inflammatory cytokine production, white cell activation, and leukocyte adhesion molecule synthesis have all been associated with hypothermia or hypothermic CPB. Hypothermia suppresses release of excitatory amino acid neurotransmitters during ischemia and reperfusion, which is likely to be an important cerebral protective mechanism, especially in neonatal and immature brains.[107,128]

Low-Flow Hypothermic Cardiopulmonary Bypass

The reductions in metabolic rate produced by hypothermia allow CPB flow rates to be reduced, thereby reducing the amount of blood returning to the heart and improving surgical conditions. Most centers use values of approximately 50 mL/kg/min or 0.70 liter/min/m^2 for low-flow CPB. Studies in adults and children have suggested the relative safety, particularly in terms of cerebral protection compared with DHCA, of this range of low-flow CPB in combination with hypothermia.[57,71,129-131]

Further reductions in pump flow to one quarter or less of normal may be used at deep levels of hypothermia (<18° C). However, there is no agreement on what a safe degree of flow reduction might be for a given temperature in infants and children. Kern and colleagues[70] have suggested that the critical pump flow rate in terms of the crucial juncture at which cerebral metabolism becomes flow dependent is between approximately 30 and 35 mL/kg/min at moderate hypothermia (26° to 29° C) and between 5 and 30 mL/kg/min during deep hypothermia (18° to 22° C). The bulk of evidence suggests that cerebral autoregulation is markedly diminished or absent at temperatures below 20° C, and hence CBF becomes pressure-passive at very low temperatures during CPB in infants.[57,67,70] Burrows and Bissonnette showed that a significant percentage of neonates and infants who undergo low-flow CPB (<22% of normal pump flow) have no detectable CBF as measured by transcranial Doppler and require higher perfusion pressures to reestablish CBF.[132] Similar results have been found by others at flow rates typical during profound (14° to 20° C, nasopharyngeal temperature) hypothermic CPB, where some infants lost CBF at flow rates as high as 25% to 35% of normal.[133] Thus, it is possible that the result of low-flow CPB in at least some infants is the opposite of what is intended in terms of using low-flow to avoid DHCA—that is, low-flow hypothermic CPB may result in, rather than prevent, cerebral ischemia. The development of critical closing and opening pressures during CPB may contribute to a no-reflow phenomenon and uneven brain cooling during low-flow CPB.[57] The notion of critical closing and opening pressures in the cerebral vascular bed (and other vascular beds as well) also suggests that blood flow may be more dependent on arterial *pressure* than pump flow rate in these circumstances and that a minimum mean arterial pressure is necessary to maintain adequate flow to the brain and other organs.

Hypothermic protection of the brain during periods of low or absent flow depends on homogeneous cooling of all brain regions. There is evidence that this may not occur, based on the temperature or oxygen saturation of jugular bulb venous blood, which indicates the likelihood of ongoing cerebral metabolic activity despite low tympanic or nasopharyngeal temperatures.[42,57] These data indicate that tympanic or nasopharyngeal temperatures may not identify subsets of patients with inadequately cooled brains. Risk factors for nonhomogeneous and delayed brain cooling may include the position of the aortic cannula, vascular anomalies, and aortopulmonary and other collaterals, as well as blood gas or pH management strategy (see later), and the duration of cooling. For example, using alpha-stat pH management, the duration of core cooling prior to a period of DHCA was the intraoperative variable most closely associated with postoperative cognitive outcome. Over cooling times between 11 and 18 minutes, increasing cooling time by 5 minutes increased the development score by 26 points. It was speculated that shorter cooling times (less than ≈15 minutes) permitted ongoing metabolism in nonhomogeneously cooled regions of the brain, making them susceptible to injury during the period of DHCA.[134] Also of interest, there was a trend for worse neurodevelopmental outcome (that did not reach statistical significance) with cooling times longer than 20 minutes, perhaps because of the effects of prolonging exposure to the deleterious consequences of CPB, including microembolic events.

Deep Hypothermic Circulatory Arrest

DHCA has been used since the 1970s for the repair of congenital heart defects, primarily in neonates and small infants, and occasionally in older children. Use of DHCA can decrease the length of time the patient is on CPB. This was an important advantage during the early congenital cardiac surgical experience, when limitations in CPB equipment and techniques put the neonate and small infant at increased risk. The impetus to minimize exposure to CPB has diminished as CPB methods for infants have improved. Continuous refinement of perfusion methods for neonates and infants has led to a reduction in DHCA use in many centers. Nonetheless, DHCA offers optimal surgical exposure in a small heart and chest by allowing removal of the perfusion cannulas, and its use (or similar alternatives, such as DHCA alternated with periods of intermittent perfusion) is unavoidable for some lesions.

Both surface and core cooling are used prior to DHCA. Surface cooling is facilitated during the induction of anesthesia and surgical exposure and cannulation for CPB by lowering the room temperature as low as possible (to <20° C), placing ice-filled bags around the head and neck, and positioning the patient on a cooling/warming blanket set to approximately 10° C. Using these methods, the usual rectal temperature at the time of initiating CPB is approximately 33° C (temperature-related dysrhythmias and ventricular fibrillation are rare in neonates and small infants at core temperatures of greater than 28° to 30° C). For most cases of DHCA, an ascending aortic arterial cannula (the pulmonary artery is cannulated initially for hypoplastic left heart syndrome) and a single right atrial venous cannula are inserted. As noted, extremely rapid cooling (core temperature decreasing to 15° to 18° C in less than ≈15 minutes) is usually avoided. The efficiency of different heat exchangers can vary widely, in part because of their surface areas relative to membrane surface area and flow rates (see Table 108-1). Cooling is continued until both rectal and tympanic membrane temperatures are less than 18° C. Cardioplegia is administered, and CPB is then discontinued. Several pharmacologic adjuncts are usually given as part of DHCA. Many include an alpha blocker (such as phentolamine or phenoxybenzamine) in the pump prime to reduce vascular resistance, improve regional blood flow, and aid in homogeneous and effective cooling. High-dose methylprednisolone (30 mg/kg) is given for the reasons already discussed. Some administer sodium pentothal (5 to 10 mg/kg) just prior to the start of DHCA to reduce cerebral electrical activity and metabolism; this is based in part on experience showing that up to 20% to 30% of neonatal brains will not be electrically silent despite tympanic and core temperatures of less than 18° C. As discussed previously, a higher hematocrit than used previously (≈25% to 28% instead of 15% to 20%) is now favored by many, on the basis of evidence that it does not impair the hypothermic cerebral circulation and may be associated with improved myocardial function, less total body water accumulation, and perhaps improved performance on some neurodevelopmental tests at 1 year of age.[61,63] Finally, drainage of blood from the patient is promoted by several inflations of the lungs and manual compression of the abdomen. The venous cannula is then usually clamped and removed.

Before rewarming, initial steps are taken to remove air from the left ventricle, left atrium, and pulmonary veins. Cannulas are reinserted, and CPB is slowly resumed at 18° C.

There are different approaches to rewarming. In the oldest approach, rewarming begins immediately, maintaining a temperature differential between the warming circuit and patient's venous blood of less than 10° C and a maximum water temperature of 42° C. Because concerns about cerebral injury *after* DHCA and information about the potential protective effects of hypothermia and harmful effects of even mild hyperthermia *after* a cerebral injury have increased, many centers currently undertake a period (≈10 to 15 minutes) of 18° C perfusion on resumption of CPB after DHCA and try to limit both hyperthermic reperfusion (by keeping aortic perfusate temperatures lower) and post-CPB hyperthermia.[20,57,135,136] Prior to aortic cross-clamp removal, mannitol (0.25 to 0.5 g/kg) is frequently given. Ionized calcium, which had been allowed to decrease to approximately 0.4 to 0.8 mmol/L during cooling and early rewarming, is normalized once the heart has had a period of reperfusion and the core temperature has increased to approximately 30° to 32° C. It is probably important to keep both flow rate and mean arterial pressure at age-appropriate normal values because of the loss of cerebral autoregulation and consequent pressure-flow dependence of CBF after DHCA. Once calcium is normalized and the patient is rewarmed to approximately 34° C, pulsatile ejection is stimulated by restricting venous return, and ventilation is begun; this is another opportunity to remove any residual intracardiac air. Observations of the heart, intracardiac filling pressures, arterial blood pressure, and other available information (e.g., contractility and filling on transesophageal echocardiography) are useful at this point to estimate the degree of inotropic support required when weaning from CPB. Typically, low doses of dopamine (≈5 to 7.5 μg/kg/min) are all that is required.

Management of Arterial Blood Gases during Pediatric Cardiopulmonary Bypass

Most centers adjust oxygen delivery to the CPB circuit so that arterial PO_2 values are in the range of approximately 400 to 600 mm Hg. This hyperoxic approach is based on evidence that brain injury is greater during normoxic CPB than with hyperoxic CPB.[137] Potential explanations for this effect include that the brain mainly uses dissolved oxygen during deep hypothermic CPB, the amount of gas microemboli is decreased when nitrogen is omitted from the sweep gas, and oxygen microemboli are resorbed much faster than those containing nitrogen.[95,135] On the other hand, some centers favor significantly reducing PO_2 during CPB, to reduce oxygen radical production.[25,137] This mechanism may be especially important in cyanotic infants, in whom antioxidant reserves and scavenging enzyme systems may be downregulated.[25,137,138] The issue remains unresolved, and it is likely that the relative benefits of the two oxygenation strategies depend in part on the organ system in question. For example, reperfusing myocardium (especially cyanotic myocardium) at lower PO_2 may be quite beneficial for recovery of cardiac function, whereas it has recently been stated that the significance of hyperoxia-induced oxygen radical injury to the brain is far less important than the deleterious effects of low perfusate PO_2, especially when CBF and cerebral autoregulation are impaired, as is the case with low-flow deep hypothermic (or circulatory arrest) CPB.[135]

The optimal management strategy for pH and CO_2 during profound hypothermia, with or without DHCA, remains controversial. Both alpha-stat and pH-stat management strategies are used during pediatric CPB, and both have potential advantages and disadvantages. During hypothermia, the efficacy of the body's primary buffering systems (e.g., bicarbonate, phosphate) is markedly reduced, and amino acids become the most important intracellular buffers as temperature falls; of these, the α-imidazole ring of histidine is the most effective proton acceptor (i.e., buffer). Water is less ionized (into H^+ and OH^-) as temperature falls, and thus the pH of water (the major fluid in the body) increases with falling temperature. The neutral point of water (i.e., the pH at which $[H^+] = [OH^-]$) also rises as temperature falls. This state (the pH at which water is electrochemically neutral) is approximately pH 7.4 at 37° C and approximately pH 7.7 to 7.8 at profound hypothermic temperatures. Alpha-stat management is based on preserving electrical neutrality at reduced temperatures and therefore the buffering capability of the α-imidazole ring of the amino acid histidine. Most enzyme, receptor, and metabolic systems function best at pH 7.4; several have been shown to function more efficiently at 20° C and at a pH of approximately 7.7.[139,140] Blood from a normal patient cooled under alpha-stat methods will have a pH of approximately 7.4 and a CO_2 concentration of approximately 40 mm Hg when the sample is warmed to 37° C in the blood-gas analyzer. The alleged biochemical advantages of preserving electrochemical neutrality and intracellular buffering via alpha-stat management include better preservation of metabolism and protein and enzyme function (by preserving intracellular pH [pH_i] and preventing abnormal charge accumulation on proteins) and slowing the diffusion of key charged intermediates such as ADP and adenosine monophosphate (AMP) out of the cell, thereby promoting faster recovery of oxidative metabolism and high-energy phosphates when oxygen and substrate supply are restored.[140] Alpha-stat management is likely to be associated with better preservation of cerebral autoregulation at mild to moderate hypothermic temperatures, lower CBF, and less brain swelling. These features may have a net beneficial effect in adults, where microemboli and cerebral edema appear to be major components of the insult, as compared with the higher brain blood flow and greater microemboli load associated with pH-stat.[107,141] On the other hand, the alpha-stat strategy causes a leftward shift in the oxyhemoglobin dissociation curve. In the setting of low flow, low perfusion pressures, and low temperatures, overall oxygen delivery under alpha-stat management may be marginal to meet metabolic needs, and CBF may be inadequate to evenly and effectively cool the brain.[107,142,143]

In contrast, pH-stat uses a mathematical correction for the effects of temperature on pH and then adds CO_2 to the circuit to correct pH for the fall in temperature. pH-stat therefore attempts to normalize the patient's pH (i.e., make it ≈7.4) and PCO_2 *at the hypothermic temperature.* When this sample is analyzed at 37° C, it will be relatively acidotic (pH of ≈7.1 to 7.2) and hypercarbic (PCO_2 ≈60 to 70 mm Hg). The addition of CO_2 will theoretically lower pH_i and disrupt electrical neutrality. However, evidence suggests that pH-stat may only minimally reduce pH_i.[144,145] The increase in CBF associated with pH-stat, along with the rightward shift in the oxyhemoglobin dissociation curve, may favor even and effective brain cooling and oxygen delivery as long as perfusion pressure and flow are maintained. Hypercapnia decreases cerebral metabolic rate, energy use, glycolytic flux, and lactate production.[107,146-148] Hypercapnia and acidosis may also decrease excitatory amino acid neurotoxicity by inhibiting *N*-methyl-D-aspartate (NMDA) receptor function, glutamate release, and neuronal calcium fluxes.[107,148,149]

Based on the work of Aoki and Swain showing that cerebral pH_i becomes alkalotic during deep hypothermia even with pH-stat management, it may be that the biochemical advantages of alpha-stat are largely present during pH-stat management and are supplemented by the effects of pH-stat to increase CBF and oxygen availability as a result of its effect to shift rightward the oxyhemoglobin dissociation.[130,145,150] These effects are likely to be paramount in the neonate and infant exposed to low flow or no flow, because hypoxic and ischemic injury probably pose the greatest risk to the infant, in contrast to the adult with significant atherosclerosis and vascular disease managed at mild or moderate hypothermia, in whom minimizing microemboli and preserving autoregulation (and therefore favoring alpha-stat management) may be the primary pathophysiologic considerations.

A small retrospective study using relatively brief cooling times (<15 minutes on average) suggested that pH-stat might be preferable to alpha-stat in terms of neurodevelopmental outcome when DHCA is used for Senning correction of arterial transposition.[151] In a larger, prospective, randomized, single-center study, no consistent improvement or impairment could be related to pH management strategy during deep hypothermic CPB.[152] Overall, DHCA has been found to result in greater short-term (1 year) and long-term (8 years of age) functional neurologic and neurodevelopmental deficits compared with low-flow CPB; interestingly, both strategies were associated with increased neurodevelopmental risk.[153] By contrast, in another study of patients with hypoplastic left heart after Norwood procedure, impaired neurodevelopmental outcome was not associated with the use of DHCA and also not associated with pH strategy or hematocrit.[154]

On the basis of this information, many centers have begun to favor pH-stat management for infant and pediatric CPB when deep hypothermia, low flow, or circulatory arrest is going to be used.* Patient factors can also influence this choice. The presence of cyanosis and aortopulmonary collaterals are considered by many to be indications for pH-stat management; CO_2 increases pulmonary vascular resistance, leading to improved systemic blood flow in these patients; cerebral perfusion is directly increased by CO_2 and also by the reduction in flow through the collaterals.[128,135,155]

Bleeding after Pediatric Cardiopulmonary Bypass

Bleeding is a significant problem after many cardiac surgical procedures in neonates, infants, and children. The cause in most cases is likely to be multifactorial. In addition to the difficulties surrounding heparinization and its antagonism by protamine (see Heparin Reversal, earlier), numerous factors (related to the patient, pathophysiology of the lesion, technical aspects of the operation, and the effects of CPB) can promote blood loss. Most of the procoagulant and anticoagulant blood factors are present in reduced concentration in neonates and infants; these concentrations approach adult values at varying rates over the first 6 to 12 months of life.[79,80,82,157] Infants therefore appear to be functionally balanced albeit at a lower set-point, which enhances the effects of hemodilution by CPB. Reduced levels of both procoagulant and anticoagulant factors compared with age-matched controls have been found in many infants and children with congenital heart disease, particularly those with various forms of single-ventricle physiology.[79,80,158] The cause is unclear at present, as is whether these abnormalities are linked to any functional disturbances (either increased or decreased) in ability to clot.

Increased bleeding can occur in association with lesions that increase systemic venous pressures (e.g., Fontan physiology, Mustard or Senning atrial baffles, right ventricular dysfunction) resulting from hepatic dysfunction, development of large venous collateral vessels, and high venous pressures. Hepatic dysfunction can also occur in lesions with significant systemic hypoperfusion (large left-to-right shunt, left-sided obstructive lesion such as critical coarctation). Cardiac lesions that generate large shear forces such as aortic stenosis and ventricular septal defects can promote the degradation of active von Willebrand factor multimers to less active and inactive monomers, leading to an acquired form of von Willebrand disease. Prostaglandin E1, used to maintain ductal patency preoperatively, can impair platelet function. Changes attributed to cyanosis that increase the risk of bleeding may include reduced platelet function, increased fibrinolysis, decreased total body amount of clotting factors (resulting from polycythemia and hence decreased plasma volume), and the development of collateral vessels. Unlike most adult cardiac surgery, many congenital cardiac operations require extensive suture lines and reconstructions using tissue or prosthetic graft materials, often on high-pressure vessels (e.g., stage I operation for hypoplastic left heart syndrome, the arterial switch procedure). Reoperations also make up a substantial part of pediatric cardiac surgery.

The effects of CPB on blood activation, coagulation, and fibrinolysis are arguably greater in neonates and infants because of the greater degree of hemodilution, deeper degrees of hypothermia, higher shear forces resulting from higher flow rates, more blood trauma and greater blood-air contact (higher flows, small tubing and cannulas, more cardiotomy suction), and proportionately greater degree of blood contact with the foreign surface. CPB reduces platelet number and causes platelet dysfunction by several mechanisms, including hypothermia, contact activation from the CPB circuit, activation via coagulation mechanisms, and cleavage of platelet adhesive receptors by fibrinolytic proteases that are also activated by CPB. Platelet number in neonates and small infants is approximately halved at the end of bypass following protamine reversal, and platelet function is believed to be markedly impaired for the reasons outlined. Ongoing consumption of platelets and clotting factors resulting from bleeding at complex and pressurized anastomotic sites can add to the problem.

Neonates presenting for CPB are likely to have normal platelet counts but reduced (compared with age-matched subjects, who, as already noted, have lower clotting factor levels compared with adult values) concentrations of factors II, VII, VIII, IX, and X. A subset of neonates may also have significantly lower fibrinogen at the outset, which can then be critically low at the end of bypass and be a major contributor to post-bypass bleeding.[157] Other significant abnormalities at the end of CPB after protamine administration include further reductions and functionally low concentrations of factors V, VII, and VIII. Low post-protamine platelet counts and fibrinogen concentrations correlate with bleeding in neonates and small infants.[159]

Treatment of Bleeding after Cardiopulmonary Bypass

The treatment approach to post-CPB bleeding in pediatric patients is based on the preceding considerations, driven by both the expected coagulation abnormalities and the presence of complex reconstructions and extensive vascular suture lines. Platelets are the initial therapy after adequate heparin reversal because of the documented deficiencies in platelet count and function. One to two units of platelets are typically administered to neonates and small infants to start, and up to six to eight units are administered in larger children. One rule of thumb has it that each unit per 10 kg body weight will increase platelet count by approximately 50,000/mm^3;

*References 20, 61, 143, 151, 155, and 156.

the actual result in this setting is less, at least in part because administration is done during ongoing bleeding and consumption. Also, platelets are supplied in fluid that is essentially plasma, so a fair amount of clotting factors is supplied simultaneously. Cryoprecipitate is usually the next blood component administered after platelets, and it is chosen in part because it is a good source of fibrinogen in a relatively small volume. This sequence of platelets followed by cryoprecipitate has been shown to restore hemostasis in most pediatric patients after CPB.[159] Fresh-frozen plasma is usually reserved to replete measured factor deficiencies not amenable to cryoprecipitate, particularly because there is some evidence that it has little effect or may even be detrimental to most post-CPB infants.[159] Some pediatric cardiac centers prefer to use fresh whole blood as the primary therapy after protamine reversal. When used within 24 to 48 hours of collection, fresh whole blood contains active platelets and significant amounts of clotting factors, and it has been shown to reduce bleeding, transfusion requirements, and the use of other components in both neonates and adults.[160,161] One major limitation is the difficulty in obtaining reliable quantities within the 48-hour time frame, in part because of required blood banking procedures and testing for infectious agents. Thromboelastography may help identify coagulopathy and may help direct the treatment of bleeding after CPB, thereby reducing blood product utilization.[162,163]

Although truly accelerated fibrinolysis is probably uncommon during pediatric CPB (and largely resolves after protamine administration),[73,159] it is likely that the activation of the fibrinolytic system that accompanies surgical trauma and bleeding, and particularly in association with CPB-induced activation of coagulation and inflammatory cascades, has a significant role in consumption of clotting factors, generation of anticoagulant degradation products, and loss of adhesive receptors on platelets. For these reasons, antifibrinolytic agents such as ε-aminocaproic acid and tranexamic acid have become increasingly popular. Until recently, in many pediatric centers, aprotinin was also used frequently for neonates and for complex repairs. It is not available for clinical use at present because of reports of increased complications in adult cardiac surgery patients; these include stroke, renal failure, graft occlusion, and perhaps death. Interestingly, meta-analyses of adult aprotinin studies indicate a protective effect against neurologic injury, particularly stroke, that appeared to be at least in part the result of reduced patient reinfusion of shed blood.[164,165] Of course, the applicability of the adverse events and likely underlying mechanisms in adult patients to the pediatric population is highly questionable.[166,167] At present, there is little controlled evidence that antifibrinolytic agents are beneficial in terms of, for example, blood loss, transfusion requirement, and platelet dysfunction, in primary operations, although many centers use them for procedures such as arterial switch operations and stage I hypoplastic left heart reconstruction. A meta-analysis of randomized trials using tranexamic acid concluded that the evidence in support of its use is weak.[168] There is evidence in favor of their use for reoperations, particularly of the complex variety.[169-173] Theoretical concerns remain about potential deleterious prothrombotic consequences during low flow or DHCA and in tenuous anatomic or circulatory situations postoperatively (e.g., Fontan fenestration, coronary anastomoses, surgical shunts), although there are no direct reports of such and one retrospective study was unable to identify any role for these agents in similar problems.[169,174]

For problematic and excessive bleeding resistant to blood product treatment, administration of activated recombinant factor VII has been described as being effective.[175-177] There are concerns of the potential risk of thrombotic complications associated with factor VIIa administration. This has not been demonstrated in accumulated series.[177]

Organ Injury during Pediatric Cardiopulmonary Bypass

The damaging mechanisms of CPB include global (i.e., low-flow or DHCA) and regional (e.g., heart, lung, gastrointestinal tract) periods of ischemia and reperfusion, activation of multiple limbs of the systemic inflammatory response, and intramyocardial and systemic air and particulate microemboli. During hypothermic CPB at full flow rates, the skeletal muscle functions as a large-capacitance reservoir, and blood flow is to some extent shunted away from the vital organs. During low-flow hypothermic CPB, skeletal muscle vasculature constricts and the flow to vital organs is preserved, so oxygen delivery is able to maintain oxygen consumption despite approximately a 50% reduction in flow rate.[178] The presence of large collateral vessels, arterial obstructive lesions, cannula position, and other shunts from the systemic circulation may further compromise vital organ blood flow, as previously discussed.

Pulmonary Effects

The lungs are at significant risk for injury from CPB. This is likely to be caused by hemodilution, inflammation, and ischemia-reperfusion effects.[179,180] Infants with current (e.g., infection, congestive heart failure, pulmonary overcirculation) or prior (e.g., respiratory distress syndrome, bronchopulmonary dysplasia) disorders may be at greater risk. Manifestations of CPB-induced lung injury include loss of endothelium-dependent dilation and increased pulmonary vascular resistance, decreased compliance, decreased functional residual capacity, increased alveolar-arterial oxygen difference, leakage of fluid into the interstitial space, and reduced surfactant activity.[180-186] Hemodilution promotes fluid extravasation by reducing oncotic pressure. Activated complement, leukocytes, cytokines, and leukotrienes induce alveolar and capillary membrane damage; augment capillary leak; increase platelet and white blood cell plugging; and induce the release of additional mediators that further increase pulmonary vascular resistance and pulmonary parenchymal and vascular damage. Facilitating lung cooling by allowing a period of pulmonary blood flow on CPB during core cooling has been suggested as one means to reduce ischemic lung injury and its consequences.[187]

Renal Effects

As many as 3% to 7% of children have evidence of renal dysfunction after CPB.[188] However, estimates vary depending on the criteria used: 11% using AKIN (Acute Kidney Injury Network) criteria or 51% when using RIFLE (*r*isk, *i*njury, *f*ailure, *l*oss, and *e*nd-stage kidney disease) criteria.[189,190] Most of the acute kidney injury defined this way will resolve in 48 to 72 hours, and mild renal dysfunction may not have any bearing on postoperative outcomes.[189,190] The risk of acute kidney injury in neonates may be as high as 64%.[191] Preoperative renal dysfunction or injury and low cardiac output after CPB may be the best predictors of post-CPB renal dysfunction. Glomerular filtration rate and renal diluting and concentrating abilities are immature in neonates and very young infants. Preoperative renal injury appears to be more likely in neonates, who may in fact have multiorgan dysfunction after delivery and initial stabilization (e.g., hypoplastic left heart syndrome, arterial transposition), as well as in older patients with long-standing systemic ventricular dysfunction, chronically elevated systemic venous pressures, or cyanosis (e.g., "failing" Fontan circulations, tetralogy of Fallot with severe right or biventricular dysfunction).[192] Low flow and reduced mean arterial pressure, nonpulsatile perfusion, and hypothermia lead to the production and release of hormones such as endothelin, catecholamines, antidiuretic hormone, atrial natriuretic factor, and renin/angiotensin.[101,180,188,193] In addition to renal dysfunction, these factors may contribute to increased total body water, delayed fluid clearance after CPB, and related complications such as myocardial and pulmonary interstitial edema, delayed chest closure, and prolonged ventilatory support. Few studies have been specifically devoted to infant and pediatric heart disease patients in terms of renal protection or preventive therapies. In larger patients, vacuum-assisted venous drainage has some theoretical advantages. Several recent adult cardiac surgery studies (where, of course, much of the underlying pathophysiology may be different) suggest that relatively low doses of fenoldopam or nesiritide can reduce renal-related morbidity in at-risk patients.[194-198]

Brain Injury

Neurologic injury continues to be one of the most problematic aspects of surgery for congenital heart disease. As overall operative mortality has declined in association with improved cardiac outcomes and life expectancy, quality-of-life issues have assumed greater importance. Prevention of neurologic injury has therefore become increasingly important. Earlier retrospective series estimated the incidence of major neurologic injuries after pediatric heart surgery to be between approximately 2% and 30%.[57,199,200] Although there appears to have been a progressive decline in major complications such as seizures, persistent choreoathetosis, and severe developmental delay (for reasons that are largely unknown), more subtle but significant cognitive and neurodevelopmental delays in IQ, language and motor skills, attention, learning skills, visual and spatial skills, and working memory have recently been found in children who underwent neonatal repair of arterial transposition, as well as in some single-ventricle patients and those who underwent complicated biventricular repairs; outcomes were generally worse in those who underwent DHCA.[153,201-203] Cognitive development also appears to be lower in school-age survivors of hypoplastic left heart syndrome and patients with Fontan physiology.[204,205] Risks for lower achievement included hypoplastic left heart syndrome, use of DHCA, and reoperation within 30 days; brain magnetic resonance imaging (MRI) has been used with increasing frequency to detect abnormalities before and after infant cardiac surgery and other procedures.[206-212] Interestingly, it appears that a substantial number of infants with congenital heart disease can manifest a variety of brain MRI abnormalities before surgery as well as after interventional cardiac procedures (e.g., balloon atrial septostomy). New MRI abnormalities have been observed at equal rates in children undergoing cardiac surgery with and without CPB, although, when CPB was used, the duration of bypass was associated with increased severity of the new abnormalities; DHCA was associated with the severity of new MRI findings in infants undergoing arch surgery; and the severity of new postoperative MRI abnormalities was associated with brain maturity score and their presence before surgery.[213]

It has become apparent that preoperative, intraoperative, and postoperative factors are involved.[214] The developing infant brain may be particularly susceptible to injury by hypoxia, ischemia-reperfusion, and the systemic inflammatory response because of its relatively fragile vasculature, high metabolic activity, and the fact that it is undergoing an intensive period of neuronal migration, axonal outgrowth, target finding and arborization, synaptogenesis, myelinization, astroglial development, and selective neuronal reduction (largely via apoptosis).[107] Most if not all of these processes are under the control of biochemical factors, neurotransmitters, and gene expression pathways that are likely to be affected by CPB and its consequences (e.g., cytokine and growth factor production, generation of oxygen radical and nitroxyl radical species, and altered release and reuptake of excitotoxic amino acid neurotransmitters caused by ischemia).

A substantial number of children with congenital heart disease have genetic syndromes associated with developmental delay of various sorts, including Down syndrome and the CATCH-22 syndrome.[215] The latter is linked to microdeletions in the 22q11 region of chromosome 22, DiGeorge and velocardiofacial syndromes, developmental delays in language and speech, and mild hypotonia, and it is present in 2% to 10% of children with congenital heart disease. It seems likely that other genetic abnormalities as yet undefined result in both neurologic problems and congenital heart disease. Indeed, a sizable number of children with heart disease may have congenital brain malformations; more than 30% of infants with hypoplastic left heart syndrome have evidence of brain dysgenesis or other anomalies before surgery.[98,216,217] Low cardiac output, high venous pressures, thromboemboli, and chronic cyanosis are all likely to contribute to both gross and subtle neurocognitive lesions.[135,216,218]

Intraoperative causes of brain injury include abnormalities of cerebral autoregulation and cerebral perfusion, ischemia-reperfusion mechanisms, and emboli. Many of these factors were discussed previously. The "safe" period of DHCA remains controversial, and in part it depends on how it is defined and under what conditions of flow, pH, temperature, cooling strategy, and patient population it is assessed. Using experimental energetic depletion or the cerebral metabolic rate for oxygen as the endpoint led to estimates of 20 to 30 minutes or 40 to 65 minutes, respectively.[69,130] Clinical experience and some evidence suggest periods of DHCA as short as 20 minutes or as long as 45 minutes before major complications such as seizures or choreoathetosis begin to increase in frequency.[107] Overall, the consensus has become that the risk of neurologic injury and developmental abnormalities increase and IQ decreases in direct proportion to the duration of DHCA.[143,153,202,203,219-222]

This realization has led to evaluation of methods to avoid DHCA or reduce its duration, with the understanding that in some anatomic circumstances it cannot be avoided. The problems and potential for neurologic dysfunction with low-flow hypothermic bypass were discussed previously, and recent clinical outcome evidence supports the notion that this strategy is far from a perfect solution, although it is better than DHCA.[57,132,133,153,201] Use of selective cerebral perfusion to avoid or reduce the use of DHCA appears to be an attractive and increasingly popular option. In many centers, the flow rates and perfusion pressures used during selective cerebral or arch perfusion are guided by continuous measurement of CBF velocity or NIRS.[223-229] It is important to note, however, that these techniques have yet to be subjected to widespread and thorough appraisals or to controlled comparisons with DHCA or other low-flow techniques.[61]

The post-bypass period is also receiving increased attention as a vulnerable period for neurologic injury. As discussed, both low-flow deep hypothermic CPB and DHCA techniques can lead to compromises in CBF, autoregulation, and metabolism. Therefore, ensuring appropriate cardiac output, cerebral perfusion pressure, and oxygen delivery (i.e., appropriate hematocrit for the level of oxygen saturation and cardiac output) in the postoperative period are probably quite important. In addition to standard volume replacement and inotropic maneuvers, more novel strategies to support cardiac output in this setting include delayed sternal closure and ready use of extracorporeal membrane oxygenation.[20,230,231] Maintaining normothermic or even mildly hypothermic body temperatures in the first 24 to 48 hours postoperatively may also be beneficial.[136]

Clearly, the ability to sensitively and accurately assess and follow the status of the brain, as well as to guide and evaluate therapeutic interventions, would be advantageous. Although various forms of perioperative neurologic monitoring (e.g., electroencephalography, NIRS, cerebral Doppler blood flow velocity) are used and advocated with increasing frequency, no one technique or combination of techniques has emerged to fill this need.[229,232-236] Most centers currently use some form of NIRS monitoring of cerebral (and often somatic as well) oxygen saturation. The NIRS value reflects tissue (arterioles, venules, capillaries) oxygen saturation, and is (in a somewhat oversimplified fashion) algorithmically weighted to represent approximately 85% venous blood and 15% arterial blood. When used in the cerebral position, the NIRS value reflects frontal cortex oxygen content; the measured values most closely correlate with, in most patients, jugular bulb/jugular venous or SVC oxygen saturation; thus, in some ways, it can function as a noninvasive monitor of "mixed" venous O_2 saturations. There is some experimental data indicating that both the degree and the duration of cerebral "desaturation" may predict neurologic injury.[237-239] However, human clinical data demonstrating a correlation between NIRS and neurologic injury or outcome are minimal, and data defining when intervention based on NIRS (i.e., level of desaturation) might be indicated. How to best intervene and whether NIRS-driven interventions alter outcome remain to be generated.[239-241] There may also be a role for improved techniques to detect microemboli during CPB.[242-244]

Stress Response to Cardiopulmonary Bypass

The stress response to CPB is characterized by the release of a large number and diverse group of neurohumoral substances, including catecholamines, endothelin, various prostaglandins, cortisol, and growth hormone. The concentrations that have been measured in neonates and infants during or soon after CPB are some of the highest measured in humans, and they generally exceed those measured in adult CPB patients by 5-fold to 10-fold.[101,245] Stimuli include extensive and prolonged foreign surface contact, profound hypothermia, low flow, low perfusion pressure, and nonpulsatile perfusion. Clearance of many of these compounds by the liver, kidney, or lungs may also be delayed. Possible deleterious consequences include vasoconstriction and reduced organ perfusion, direct tissue injury, pulmonary hypertension, endothelial damage, and increased pulmonary vasoreactivity.

On the other hand, the release of many of these compounds and the response overall clearly has adaptive benefits. However, it is unclear what level, circumstances, or substances cause a net harmful response, to what extent acutely ill infants with congenital heart disease require some degree of stress response for hemodynamic stability, wound repair, and overall homeostasis, and to what degree the seemingly exaggerated response seen particularly in neonates and infants exposed to CPB is pathologic and should be attenuated. Decreased stress response hormones and possibly improved morbidity and mortality have been associated with high-dose synthetic opioid administration to infants undergoing CPB and other stressful procedures.[245,246]

Systemic Inflammatory Response to Cardiopulmonary Bypass

CPB causes a systemic inflammatory response via multiple mechanisms. These mechanisms include surgical trauma, blood contact with the CPB circuit, ischemia-reperfusion injury, and protamine administration.[179,247-254] These initiating events stimulate complex and interconnected cell- and humoral-based systems that include activation of the complement, coagulation, and fibrinolytic pathways, endotoxin release, cytokine production, endothelial activation and expression of leukocyte adhesion molecules, leukocyte and platelet activation, and production and release of oxygen radicals, nitric oxide, prostanoids, eicosanoids, and proteolytic enzymes (e.g., myeloperoxidase and superoxide from activate neutrophils). The resultant tissue and organ injury, capillary leak, increased need for inotropic and ventilatory support, and perhaps effects on infection risk are widely believed to have a major impact on duration of hospitalization and overall outcome.[255]

Complement activation occurs via both alternate (stimulated by foreign surface contact, endotoxin, and kallikrein) and classical (protamine) pathways. Significant increases in activated complement fragments occur with initiation of bypass, and further still during rewarming, and these levels have correlated with post-CPB renal, cardiac, and pulmonary dysfunction.[179,180,247,249,256] Various complement fragments cause white cell and platelet activation, white cell free-radical production and degranulation, smooth muscle constriction, and capillary leak. Terminal complement fragments and the membrane attack complex can cause direct cell lysis.

Blood concentrations of bacterial endotoxin can increase because of its almost ubiquitous presence in sterile fluids and equipment and also perhaps because of decreased intestinal perfusion, which can augment reperfusion injury independent of endotoxin.[257,258] Endotoxin can directly injure endothelial cells and cause capillary leak, and it can stimulate the production of proinflammatory cytokines such as tumor necrosis factor (TNF), interleukin (IL)-1, IL-6, and IL-8. Cytokine production can also be stimulated by foreign surface contact, complement fragments, and other cytokines. Mechanisms of cytokine-induced tissue injury are multiple.

Cytokines such as IL-1 and TNF are directly toxic to endothelial and other cells, cause wasting and edema, cause myocardial contractile dysfunction, and stimulate a number of cytotoxic and cytoprotective signaling mechanisms such as inducible (high-output and potentially cytotoxic) nitric oxide production, various proapoptotic and antiapoptotic pathways and proteins, enhanced oxygen radical injury, and induction of cellular antioxidant enzymes. Levels of TNF and IL-1 are inconsistently increased by CPB in neonates and infants. Cytokine-induced nitric oxide production can result in profound hypotension (it is the major mechanism of vascular depression in septic shock), myocardial depression, and inhibition of cellular respiration and metabolism. IL-6 has been demonstrated in some studies to be a good predictor of clinical outcome and may be related to the extent of tissue injury.[180] IL-8 is a potent neutrophil chemoattractant and also causes leukocytosis and activation of neutrophil proteases and free radical enzymes. Increased IL-8 has been found in pediatric CPB in proportion to ischemic and total bypass times.[180,183,248,259] Some children have increased levels of some cytokines preoperatively; the causes and significance of this finding are unclear, but there is some evidence that neonates with a preoperative biochemical profile consistent with inflammation (e.g., increased plasma elastase and complement fragments) are more likely to manifest a capillary leak syndrome postoperatively.[248,255]

Neutrophil activation is believed to be an important mechanism of cellular injury during and after CPB. It is produced by a wide variety of stimuli, including foreign surface contact, endotoxin, cytokines, complement, platelet-activating factor, and ischemia-reperfusion. Activated neutrophils express proadhesive molecules on their cell surface (that are complementary to ones induced on endothelial and other cell membranes), marginate into the tissue, and have increased lipoxygenase and myeloperoxidase activities (the source of superoxide and hypochlorous acid, respectively) and release neutrophil elastase. These products cause damage to lipids, proteins, and DNA. Elastase also causes endothelial damage, inactivates serine proteases in the coagulation pathway, and cleaves adhesive receptors from the platelet membrane.[107,260-262] Both myeloperoxidase and elastase, as well as evidence of neutrophil-mediated oxidant injury, have been detected after pediatric CPB.[25,180,263]

It has recently become apparent that CPB also induces a corresponding increase in anti-inflammatory cytokines such as IL-10 and IL-1 receptor antagonist (IL-1ra). C-reactive protein (CRP), an acute phase protein that is a marker of inflammation and has anti-inflammatory effects by decreasing neutrophil chemotaxis, also increases during and after pediatric CPB.[†] Transient immunosuppression mediated by these events and others such as loss of activated neutrophils and inhibition of cellular immune responses have also been found after pediatric CPB.[264]

Overall, there is substantial variability in the release pattern and plasma concentrations of cytokines in infants and children undergoing cardiac surgery compared with adults.[183,248,254,265-267] Although increased elements of the systemic inflammatory response are generally associated with increased risk of postoperative organ dysfunction and morbidity and mortality, better-designed studies with direct assays and endpoints are necessary to truly define any cause-effect relationship between systemic inflammatory response mediators and organ damage. It is also likely that the *balance* between proinflammatory and anti-inflammatory stimuli and their diverse effects on a wide range of cellular types and functions must be taken into account.[254,268] Finally, the possibility that at least some of these substances are required to regulate the overall response and in fact potentially contribute to eventual repair and resolution should not be forgotten. For example, although the deleterious effects of substances such as TNF-α and cyclooxygenase pathway derivatives have been demonstrated in numerous cellular and animal models, genetic or pharmacologic abrogation of these pathways can also lead to increased cell death and organ dysfunction under clinically relevant circumstances (e.g., ischemia-reperfusion).

Other Current Approaches to Limiting the Negative Consequences of Pediatric Cardiopulmonary Bypass

Efforts and potential targets to decrease the negative impact of CPB in infants and children that have been

[†]References 179, 180, 248, 252, 254, and 264.

discussed include modifications to reduce circuit area and volume, improve venous drainage, and define the optimal pH, hematocrit, temperature,[269] flow rate, arterial pressure, and duration of CPB and DHCA. Additional targets of intervention have included oxygen, anesthetic technique, remote ischemic preconditioning, and peritoneal dialysis.[270-273]

Steroids

Administration of relatively high doses of steroids prior to pediatric CPB (either dexamethasone or methylprednisolone) may suppress the production of proinflammatory cytokines and improve organ function.[223,274-276] Because a major effect of steroid treatment is to alter gene expression and cellular activation, maximal effect may require administration some time before bypass (up to 8 hours) and repeated dosing.[20] Improvements in body water accumulation, alveolar-arterial oxygen gradients, pulmonary artery pressure, duration of mechanical ventilation, and length of intensive care unit stay have been observed.[20,274,275] Results from more extensive investigations in adults confirm beneficial alterations in the balance of proinflammatory to anti-inflammatory mediators.[277] However, there were no significant effects on fluid balance, and there were possibly detrimental effects on pulmonary function and glucose homeostasis (hyperglycemia). Furthermore, as with the stress response, it remains unclear whether broad-spectrum suppression of the systemic inflammatory response is beneficial. These differences may be partly because steroids may be more likely to show a positive effect in neonates and infants in whom the magnitude and consequences appear to be greater. However, there is some evidence that at least more prolonged periods of corticosteroid administration may be detrimental to the developing brain. Steroids are being used not only preoperatively and intraoperatively but also postoperatively for the treatment of hemodynamic instability and around the time to extubation. Prolonged steroid exposure may suppress the adrenal gland and use may also predispose to infection. In retrospective studies, data are conflicting as to the benefit of steroids.[278-281] Thus, it would seem that caution is warranted until large randomized, prospective, placebo-controlled studies with tightly regulated perioperative management are performed in pediatric patients.

Ultrafiltration

Conventional and modified ultrafiltration techniques are being used with increasing frequency during pediatric cardiac surgery. Potential beneficial mechanisms include hemoconcentration, removal of various inflammatory mediators and vasoactive compounds in the ultrafiltrate, and decreased total body water and tissue edema. Significant clinical improvements in tissue edema, post-CPB weight gain, hematocrit, blood pressure, global left ventricular function, lung compliance, oxygenation, and duration of mechanical ventilation have been reported, along with decreased postoperative bleeding, decreased postoperative transfusion and blood product requirements, and decreased pulmonary vascular resistance; one or more of these benefits have been observed in many, but not all, studies.[252,259,282-289] Less clear are the mechanisms responsible for these effects, because significant reductions in blood concentrations of inflammatory cytokines, complement fragments, and prostanoids have not been universally identified.[252,282,290] Although ultrafiltration techniques appear to be safe for infants and children, there is theoretically valid concern about removal of protective mediators and deleterious increases in viscosity and clotting factors (i.e., hypercoagulability). A recent meta-analysis of randomized trials found that modified ultrafiltration led to higher hematocrit and higher mean arterial pressure compared with conventional ultrafiltration.[291] Future studies are needed to define the mechanisms of the ultrafiltration effect and identify patients who are most likely to benefit.

REFERENCES

1. Rosengart TK, Stark JF: Repair of atrial septal defect through a right thoracotomy. *Ann Thorac Surg* 55:1138–1140, 1993.
2. Bichell DP, Geva T, Bacha EA, et al: Minimal access approach for the repair of atrial septal defect: the initial 135 patients. *Ann Thorac Surg* 70:115–118, 2000.
3. Cherup LL, Siewers RD, Futrell JW: Breast and pectoral muscle maldevelopment after anterolateral and posterolateral thoracotomies in children. *Ann Thorac Surg* 41:492–497, 1986.
4. Laussen PC, Bichell DP, McGowan FX, et al: Postoperative recovery in children after minimum versus full-length sternotomy. *Ann Thorac Surg* 69:591–596, 2000.
5. Abdel-Rahman U, Wimmer-Greinecker G, Matheis G, et al: Correction of simple congenital heart defects in infants and children through a minithoracotomy. *Ann Thorac Surg* 72:1645–1649, 2001.
6. Nicholson IA, Bichell DP, Bacha EA, et al: Minimal sternotomy approach for congenital heart operations. *Ann Thorac Surg* 71:469–472, 2001.
7. Ding C, Wang C, Dong A, et al: Anterolateral minithoracotomy versus median sternotomy for the treatment of congenital heart defects: a meta-analysis and systematic review. *J Cardiothorac Surg* 7:43, 2012.
8. Yan L, Zhou ZC, Li HP, et al: Right vertical infra-axillary mini-incision for repair of simple congenital heart defects: a matched-pair analysis. *Eur J Cardiothorac Surg* 43:136–141, 2013.
9. Dave HH, Comber M, Solinger T, et al: Mid-term results of right axillary incision for the repair of a wide range of congenital cardiac defects. *Eur J Cardiothorac Surg* 35:864–869, 2009.
10. Burke RP, Michielon G, Wernovsky G: Video-assisted cardioscopy in congenital heart operations. *Ann Thorac Surg* 58:864–868, 1994.
11. Yoshimura N, Yamaguchi M, Oshima Y, et al: Repair of atrial septal defect through a right posterolateral thoracotomy: a cosmetic approach for female patients. *Ann Thorac Surg* 72:2103–2105, 2001.
12. Wang F, Li M, Xu X, et al: Totally thoracoscopic surgical closure of atrial septal defect in small children. *Ann Thorac Surg* 92:200–203, 2011.
13. Ma ZS, Dong MF, Yin QY, et al: Totally thoracoscopic repair of ventricular septal defect: a short-term clinical observation on safety and feasibility. *J Thorac Cardiovasc Surg* 142:850–854, 2011.
14. Odegard KC, Kirse DJ, del Nido PJ, et al: Intraoperative recurrent laryngeal nerve monitoring during video-assisted thoracoscopic surgery for patent ductus arteriosus. *J Cardiothorac Vasc Anesth* 14:562–564, 2000.
15. Gibbon JH, Jr: Application of a mechanical heart and lung apparatus to cardiac surgery. *Minn Med* 37:171–185, passim, 1954.
16. Lillehei CW, Varco RL, Cohen M, et al: The first open-heart repairs of ventricular septal defect, atrioventricular communis, and tetralogy of Fallot using extracorporeal circulation by cross-circulation: a 30-year follow-up. *Ann Thorac Surg* 41:4–21, 1986.
17. Kirklin JW: The middle 1950s and C. Walton Lillehei. *J Thorac Cardiovasc Surg* 98:822–824, 1989.

18. Castaneda AR, Lamberti J, Sade RM, et al: Open-heart surgery during the first three months of life. *J Thorac Cardiovasc Surg* 68:719–731, 1974.
19. Barratt-Boyes B: Complete correction of cardiovascular malformations in the first two years of life using profound hypothermia. In Barratt-Boyes BG, Neutze JM, Harris EA, editors: *Heart disease in infancy*, Edinburgh, 1973, Churchill Livingstone.
20. Ungerleider RM, Shen I: Optimizing response of the neonate and infant to cardiopulmonary bypass. *Semin Thorac Cardiovasc Surg Pediatr Card Surg Annu* 6:140–146, 2003.
21. del Nido PJ: Myocardial protection and cardiopulmonary bypass in neonates and infants. *Ann Thorac Surg* 64:878–879, 1997.
22. Friehs I, del Nido PJ: Increased susceptibility of hypertrophied hearts to ischemic injury. *Ann Thorac Surg* 75:S678–S684, 2003.
23. Stamm C, Friehs I, Cowan DB, et al: Inhibition of tumor necrosis factor-alpha improves postischemic recovery of hypertrophied hearts. *Circulation* 104:I350–I355, 2001.
24. del Nido PJ, Mickle DA, Wilson GJ, et al: Inadequate myocardial protection with cold cardioplegic arrest during repair of tetralogy of Fallot. *J Thorac Cardiovasc Surg* 95:223–229, 1988.
25. Allen BS: The clinical significance of the reoxygenation injury in pediatric heart surgery. *Semin Thorac Cardiovasc Surg Pediatr Card Surg Annu* 6:116–127, 2003.
26. Richmond ME, Charette K, Chen JM, et al: The effect of cardiopulmonary bypass prime volume on the need for blood transfusion after pediatric cardiac surgery. *J Thorac Cardiovasc Surg* 145:1058–1064, 2013.
27. Durandy Y: Usefulness of low prime perfusion pediatric circuit in decreasing blood transfusion. *ASAIO J* 53:659–661, 2007.
28. Durandy Y: The impact of vacuum-assisted venous drainage and miniaturized bypass circuits on blood transfusion in pediatric cardiac surgery. *ASAIO J* 55:117–120, 2009.
29. Miyaji K, Kohira S, Miyamoto T, et al: Pediatric cardiac surgery without homologous blood transfusion, using a miniaturized bypass system in infants with lower body weight. *J Thorac Cardiovasc Surg* 134:284–289, 2007.
30. Miyaji K, Miyamoto T, Kohira S, et al: Miniaturized cardiopulmonary bypass system in neonates and small infants. *Interact Cardiovasc Thorac Surg* 7:75–78, 2008.
31. Kotani Y, Honjo O, Nakakura M, et al: Single center experience with a low volume priming cardiopulmonary bypass circuit for preventing blood transfusion in infants and small children. *ASAIO J* 55:296–299, 2009.
32. Redlin M, Huebler M, Boettcher W, et al: Minimizing intraoperative hemodilution by use of a very low priming volume cardiopulmonary bypass in neonates with transposition of the great arteries. *J Thorac Cardiovasc Surg* 142:875–881, 2011.
33. Redlin M, Habazettl H, Boettcher W, et al: Effects of a comprehensive blood-sparing approach using body weight adjusted miniaturized cardiopulmonary bypass circuits on transfusion requirements in pediatric cardiac surgery. *J Thorac Cardiovasc Surg* 144:493–499, 2012.
34. Ojito JW, Hannan RL, Miyaji K, et al: Assisted venous drainage cardiopulmonary bypass in congenital heart surgery. *Ann Thorac Surg* 71:1267–1271, discussion 71–72, 2001.
35. Willcox TW: Vacuum assist: angel or demon CON. *J Extra Corpor Technol* 45:128–132, 2013.
36. Durandy Y: Vacuum-assisted venous drainage, angel or demon: PRO? *J Extra Corpor Technol* 45:122–127, 2013.
37. Davila RM, Rawles T, Mack MJ: Venoarterial air embolus: a complication of vacuum-assisted venous drainage. *Ann Thorac Surg* 71:1369–1371, 2001.
38. Wang S, Baer L, Kunselman AR, et al: Delivery of gaseous microemboli with vacuum-assisted venous drainage during pulsatile and nonpulsatile perfusion in a simulated neonatal cardiopulmonary bypass model. *ASAIO J* 54:416–422, 2008.
39. Schreiner RS, Rider AR, Myers JW, et al: Microemboli detection and classification by innovative ultrasound technology during simulated neonatal cardiopulmonary bypass at different flow rates, perfusion modes, and perfusate temperatures. *ASAIO J* 54:316–324, 2008.
40. Rider AR, Ji B, Kunselman AR, et al: A performance evaluation of eight geometrically different 10 Fr pediatric arterial cannulae under pulsatile and nonpulsatile perfusion conditions in an infant cardiopulmonary bypass model. *ASAIO J* 54:306–315, 2008.
41. Undar A: International conference on pediatric mechanical circulatory support systems and pediatric cardiopulmonary perfusion: outcomes and future directions. *ASAIO J* 54:141–146, 2008.
42. Kern FH, Jonas RA, Mayer JE, Jr, et al: Temperature monitoring during CPB in infants: does it predict efficient brain cooling? *Ann Thorac Surg* 54:749–754, 1992.
43. Friesen RH, Thieme R: Changes in anterior fontanel pressure during cardiopulmonary bypass and hypothermic circulatory arrest in infants. *Anesth Analg* 66:94–96, 1987.
44. Hickey PR, Andersen NP: Deep hypothermic circulatory arrest: a review of pathophysiology and clinical experience as a basis for anesthetic management. *J Cardiothorac Anesth* 1:137–155, 1987.
45. Chiba Y, Morioka K, Muraoka R, et al: Effects of depletion of leukocytes and platelets on cardiac dysfunction after cardiopulmonary bypass. *Ann Thorac Surg* 65:107–113, discussion 13–14, 1998.
46. Qiu F, Peng S, Kunselman A, et al: Evaluation of Capiox FX05 oxygenator with an integrated arterial filter on trapping gaseous microemboli and pressure drop with open and closed purge line. *Artif Organs* 34:1053–1057, 2010.
47. Tigchelaar I, Gallandat Huet RC, Korsten J, et al: Hemostatic effects of three colloid plasma substitutes for priming solution in cardiopulmonary bypass. *Eur J Cardiothorac Surg* 11:626–632, 1997.
48. Myers G: A comparative review of crystalloid, albumin, pentastarch, and hetastarch as perfusate for cardiopulmonary bypass. *J Extra-Corporeal Technol* 29:30–35, 1997.
49. Boks RH, van Herwerden LA, Takkenberg JJ, et al: Is the use of albumin in colloid prime solution of cardiopulmonary bypass circuit justified? *Ann Thorac Surg* 72:850–853, 2001.
50. Byrick RJ, Kay C, Noble WH: Extravascular lung water accumulation in patients following coronary artery surgery. *Can Anaesth Soc J* 24:332–345, 1977.
51. Marelli D, Paul A, Samson R, et al: Does the addition of albumin to the prime solution in cardiopulmonary bypass affect clinical outcome? A prospective randomized study. *J Thorac Cardiovasc Surg* 98:751–756, 1989.
52. Schupbach P, Pappova E, Schilt W, et al: Perfusate oncotic pressure during cardiopulmonary bypass. Optimum level as determined by metabolic acidosis, tissue edema, and renal function. *Vox Sang* 35:332–344, 1978.
53. Riegger LQ, Voepel-Lewis T, Kulik TJ, et al: Albumin versus crystalloid prime solution for cardiopulmonary bypass in young children. *Crit Care Med* 30:2649–2654, 2002.
54. Spiess BD: Blood transfusion for cardiopulmonary bypass: the need to answer a basic question. *J Cardiothorac Vasc Anesth* 16:535–538, 2002.
55. Ranucci M, Carlucci C, Isgrò G, et al: Duration of red blood cell storage and outcomes in pediatric cardiac surgery: an association found for pump prime blood. *Crit Care* 13:R207, 2009.
56. Spahn DR, Smith LR, Veronee CD, et al: Acute isovolemic hemodilution and blood transfusion. Effects on regional function and metabolism in myocardium with compromised coronary blood flow. *J Thorac Cardiovasc Surg* 105:694–704, 1993.
57. Pua HL, Bissonnette B: Cerebral physiology in paediatric cardiopulmonary bypass. *Can J Anaesth* 45:960–978, 1998.
58. Henling CE, Carmichael MJ, Keats AS, et al: Cardiac operation for congenital heart disease in children of Jehovah's Witnesses. *J Thorac Cardiovasc Surg* 89:914–920, 1985.
59. Johnston WE, Jenkins LW, Lin CY, et al: Cerebral metabolic consequences of hypotensive challenges in hemodiluted pigs with and without cardiopulmonary bypass. *Anesth Analg* 81:911–918, 1995.
60. Stein JI, Gombotz H, Rigler B, et al: Open heart surgery in children of Jehovah's Witnesses: extreme hemodilution on cardiopulmonary bypass. *Pediatr Cardiol* 12:170–174, 1991.
61. Jonas RA: Deep hypothermic circulatory arrest: current status and indications. *Semin Thorac Cardiovasc Surg Pediatr Card Surg Annu* 5:76–88, 2002.
62. Duebener LF, Hagino I, Sakamoto T, et al: Effects of pH management during deep hypothermic bypass on cerebral microcirculation: alpha-stat versus pH-stat. *Circulation* 106:I103–I108, 2002.
63. Duebener LF, Sakamoto T, Hatsuoka S, et al: Effects of hematocrit on cerebral microcirculation and tissue oxygenation during deep hypothermic bypass. *Circulation* 104:I260–I264, 2001.

64. Jonas RA, Wypij D, Roth SJ, et al: The influence of hemodilution on outcome after hypothermic cardiopulmonary bypass: results of a randomized trial in infants. *J Thorac Cardiovasc Surg* 126:1765–1774, 2003.
65. Newburger JW, Jonas RA, Soul J, et al: Randomized trial of hematocrit 25% versus 35% during hypothermic cardiopulmonary bypass in infant heart surgery. *J Thorac Cardiovasc Surg* 135(54):347–354, e1–4, 2008.
66. Wypij D, Jonas RA, Bellinger DC, et al: The effect of hematocrit during hypothermic cardiopulmonary bypass in infant heart surgery: results from the combined Boston hematocrit trials. *J Thorac Cardiovasc Surg* 135:355–360, 2008.
67. Greeley WJ, Ungerleider RM, Kern FH, et al: Effects of cardiopulmonary bypass on cerebral blood flow in neonates, infants, and children. *Circulation* 80:I209–I215, 1989.
68. Greeley WJ, Ungerleider RM: Assessing the effect of cardiopulmonary bypass on the brain. *Ann Thorac Surg* 52:417–419, 1991.
69. Greeley WJ, Kern FH, Ungerleider RM, et al: The effect of hypothermic cardiopulmonary bypass and total circulatory arrest on cerebral metabolism in neonates, infants, and children. *J Thorac Cardiovasc Surg* 101:783–794, 1991.
70. Kern FH, Ungerleider RM, Reves JG, et al: Effect of altering pump flow rate on cerebral blood flow and metabolism in infants and children. *Ann Thorac Surg* 56:1366–1372, 1993.
71. Fox LS, Blackstone EH, Kirklin JW, et al: Relationship of whole body oxygen consumption to perfusion flow rate during hypothermic cardiopulmonary bypass. *J Thorac Cardiovasc Surg* 83:239–248, 1982.
72. Chan AK, Leaker M, Burrows FA, et al: Coagulation and fibrinolytic profile of paediatric patients undergoing cardiopulmonary bypass. *Thromb Haemost* 77:270–277, 1997.
73. Miller BE, Guzzetta NA, Tosone SR, et al: Rapid evaluation of coagulopathies after cardiopulmonary bypass in children using modified thromboelastography. *Anesth Analg* 90:1324–1330, 2000.
74. Guzzetta NA, Amin SJ, Tosone AK, et al: Change in heparin potency and effects on the activated clotting time in children undergoing cardiopulmonary bypass. *Anesth Analg* 115:921–924, 2012.
75. Gruenwald CE, Manlhiot C, Abadilla AA, et al: Heparin brand is associated with postsurgical outcomes in children undergoing cardiac surgery. *Ann Thorac Surg* 93:878–882, 2012.
76. D'Errico C, Shayevitz JR, Martindale SJ: Age-related differences in heparin sensitivity and heparin-protamine interactions in cardiac surgery patients. *J Cardiothorac Vasc Anesth* 10:451–457, 1996.
77. Malviya S: Monitoring and management of anticoagulation in children requiring extracorporeal circulation. *Semin Thromb Hemost* 23:563–567, 1997.
78. Horkay F, Martin P, Rajah SM, et al: Response to heparinization in adults and children undergoing cardiac operations. *Ann Thorac Surg* 53:822–826, 1992.
79. Odegard KC, McGowan FX, Jr, DiNardo JA, et al: Coagulation abnormalities in patients with single-ventricle physiology precede the Fontan procedure. *J Thorac Cardiovasc Surg* 123:459–465, 2002.
80. Odegard KC, McGowan FX, Jr, Zurakowski D, et al: Coagulation factor abnormalities in patients with single-ventricle physiology immediately prior to the Fontan procedure. *Ann Thorac Surg* 73:1770–1777, 2002.
81. Andrew M, Paes B, Milner R, et al: Development of the human coagulation system in the full-term infant. *Blood* 70:165–172, 1987.
82. Peters M, ten Cate JW, Jansen E, et al: Coagulation and fibrinolytic factors in the first week of life in healthy infants. *J Pediatr* 106:292–295, 1985.
83. Severin T, Zieger B, Sutor AH: Anticoagulation with recombinant hirudin and danaparoid sodium in pediatric patients. *Semin Thromb Hemost* 28:447–454, 2002.
84. Newall F, Barnes C, Ignjatovic V, et al: Heparin-induced thrombocytopenia in children. *J Paediatr Child Health* 39:289–292, 2003.
85. Argueta-Morales IR, Olsen MC, DeCampli WM, et al: Alternative anticoagulation during cardiovascular procedures in pediatric patients with heparin-induced thrombocytopenia. *J Extra Corpor Technol* 44:69–74, 2012.
86. Gates R, Yost P, Parker B: The use of bivalirudin for cardiopulmonary bypass anticoagulation in pediatric heparin-induced thrombocytopenia patients. *Artif Organs* 34:667–669, 2010.
87. Dragomer D, Chalfant A, Biniwale R, et al: Novel techniques in the use of bivalirudin for cardiopulmonary bypass anticoagulation in a child with heparin-induced thrombocytopenia. *Perfusion* 26:516–518, 2011.
88. Martindale SJ, Shayevitz JR, D'Errico C: The activated coagulation time: suitability for monitoring heparin effect and neutralization during pediatric cardiac surgery. *J Cardiothorac Vasc Anesth* 10:458–463, 1996.
89. Gruenwald CE, Manlhiot C, Chan AK, et al: Randomized, controlled trial of individualized heparin and protamine management in infants undergoing cardiac surgery with cardiopulmonary bypass. *J Am Coll Cardiol* 56:1794–1802, 2010.
90. Griffin MJ, Rinder HM, Smith BR, et al: The effects of heparin, protamine, and heparin/protamine reversal on platelet function under conditions of arterial shear stress. *Anesth Analg* 93:20–27, 2001.
91. Seifert HA, Jobes DR, Ten Have T, et al: Adverse events after protamine administration following cardiopulmonary bypass in infants and children. *Anesth Analg* 97:383–389, table of contents, 2003.
92. Mencia De Lucas N, Lopez-Herce J, Munoz R, et al: Magnesium metabolism after cardiac surgery in children. *Pediatr Crit Care Med* 3:158–162, 2002.
93. Munoz R, Laussen PC, Palacio G, et al: Whole blood ionized magnesium: age-related differences in normal values and clinical implications of ionized hypomagnesemia in patients undergoing surgery for congenital cardiac disease. *J Thorac Cardiovasc Surg* 119:891–898, 2000.
94. Munoz R, Laussen PC, Palacio G, et al: Changes in whole blood lactate levels during cardiopulmonary bypass for surgery for congenital cardiac disease: an early indicator of morbidity and mortality. *J Thorac Cardiovasc Surg* 119:155–162, 2000.
95. Dexter F, Kern FH, Hindman BJ, et al: The brain uses mostly dissolved oxygen during profoundly hypothermic cardiopulmonary bypass. *Ann Thorac Surg* 63:1725–1729, 1997.
96. Ginther R, Sebastian VA, Huang R, et al: Cerebral near-infrared spectroscopy during cardiopulmonary bypass predicts superior vena cava oxygen saturation. *J Thorac Cardiovasc Surg* 142:359–365, 2011.
97. Kussman BD, Wypij D, Laussen PC, et al: Relationship of intraoperative cerebral oxygen saturation to neurodevelopmental outcome and brain magnetic resonance imaging at 1 year of age in infants undergoing biventricular repair. *Circulation* 122:245–254, 2010.
98. Glauser TA, Rorke LB, Weinberg PM, et al: Acquired neuropathologic lesions associated with the hypoplastic left heart syndrome. *Pediatrics* 85:991–1000, 1990.
99. Sieber F, Derrer SA, Saudek CD, et al: Effect of hypoglycemia on cerebral metabolism and carbon dioxide responsivity. *Am J Physiol* 156:H697–H706, 1989.
100. Siesjo BK, Ingvar M, Pelligrino D: Regional differences in vascular autoregulation in the rat brain in severe insulin-induced hypoglycemia. *J Cereb Blood Flow Metab* 3:478–485, 1983.
101. Anand KJ, Hansen DD, Hickey PR: Hormonal-metabolic stress responses in neonates undergoing cardiac surgery. *Anesthesiology* 73:661–670, 1990.
102. Lanier WL: Glucose management during cardiopulmonary bypass: cardiovascular and neurologic implications. *Anesth Analg* 72:423–427, 1991.
103. LeBlanc MH, Huang M, Patel D, et al: Glucose given after hypoxic ischemia does not affect brain injury in piglets. *Stroke* 25:1443–1447, discussion 8, 1994.
104. Michaud LJ, Rivara FP, Longstreth WT, Jr, et al: Elevated initial blood glucose levels and poor outcome following severe brain injuries in children. *J Trauma* 31:1356–1362, 1991.
105. Steward DJ, Da Silva CA, Flegel T: Elevated blood glucose levels may increase the danger of neurological deficit following profoundly hypothermic cardiac arrest. *Anesthesiology* 68:653, 1988.
106. Rappaport LA, Wypij D, Bellinger DC, et al: Relation of seizures after cardiac surgery in early infancy to neurodevelopmental outcome. Boston Circulatory Arrest Study Group. *Circulation* 97:773–779, 1998.

107. Burrows F, McGowan FX: Neurodevelopmental consequences of cardiac surgery for congenital heart disease. In Greeley W, editor: *Perioperative management of the patient with congenital heart disease*, Baltimore, 1996, Williams & Williams.
108. Callahan DJ, Engle MJ, Volpe JJ: Hypoxic injury to developing glial cells: protective effect of high glucose. *Pediatr Res* 27:186–190, 1990.
109. Hattori H, Wasterlain CG: Posthypoxic glucose supplement reduces hypoxic-ischemic brain damage in the neonatal rat. *Ann Neurol* 28:122–128, 1990.
110. Vannucci RC: Experimental biology of cerebral hypoxia-ischemia: relation to perinatal brain damage. *Pediatr Res* 27:317–326, 1990.
111. Vannucci RC, Mujsce DJ: Effect of glucose on perinatal hypoxic-ischemic brain damage. *Biol Neonate* 62:215–224, 1992.
112. Dickerson H, Cooper DS, Checchia PA, et al: Endocrinal complications associated with the treatment of patients with congenital cardiac disease: consensus definitions from the Multi-Societal Database Committee for Pediatric and Congenital Heart Disease. *Cardiol Young* 18(Suppl 2):256–264, 2008.
113. Lecomte P, Van Vlem B, Coddens J, et al: Tight perioperative glucose control is associated with a reduction in renal impairment and renal failure in non-diabetic cardiac surgical patients. *Crit Care* 12:R154, 2008.
114. Levy MM, Rhodes A: The ongoing enigma of tight glucose control. *Lancet* 373:520–521, 2009.
115. Oeyen S: Do you (still) believe in tight blood glucose control? *Crit Care Med* 36:3277–3278, 2008.
116. Patel KL: Impact of tight glucose control on postoperative infection rates and wound healing in cardiac surgery patients. *J Wound Ostomy Continence Nurs* 35:397–404, quiz 5–6, 2008.
117. Rossano JW, Taylor MD, Smith EO, et al: Glycemic profile in infants who have undergone the arterial switch operation: hyperglycemia is not associated with adverse events. *J Thorac Cardiovasc Surg* 135:739–745, 2008.
118. Van den Berghe G: Tight blood glucose control with insulin in "real-life" intensive care. *Mayo Clin Proc* 79:977–978, 2004.
119. Van den Berghe G: Does tight blood glucose control during cardiac surgery improve patient outcome? *Ann Intern Med* 146:307–308, 2007.
120. Wiener RS, Wiener DC, Larson RJ: Benefits and risks of tight glucose control in critically ill adults: a meta-analysis. *JAMA* 300:933–944, 2008.
121. Lazar HL, McDonnell M, Chipkin SR, et al: The Society of Thoracic Surgeons practice guideline series: blood glucose management during adult cardiac surgery. *Ann Thorac Surg* 87:663–669, 2009.
122. Furnary AP, Wu Y: Clinical effects of hyperglycemia in the cardiac surgery population: the Portland Diabetic Project. *Endocr Pract* 12(Suppl 3):22–26, 2006.
123. Furnary AP, Wu Y, Bookin SO: Effect of hyperglycemia and continuous intravenous insulin infusions on outcomes of cardiac surgical procedures: the Portland Diabetic Project. *Endocr Pract* 10(Suppl 2):21–33, 2004.
124. Inzucchi SE, Siegel MD: Glucose control in the ICU—how tight is too tight? *N Engl J Med* 360:1346–1349, 2009.
125. Finfer S, Chittock DR, Su SY, et al: Intensive versus conventional glucose control in critically ill patients. *N Engl J Med* 360:1283–1297, 2009.
126. Gandhi GY, Nuttall GA, Abel MD, et al: Intensive intraoperative insulin therapy versus conventional glucose management during cardiac surgery: a randomized trial. *Ann Intern Med* 146:233–243, 2007.
127. Agus MS, Steil GM, Wypij D, et al: Tight glycemic control versus standard care after pediatric cardiac surgery. *N Engl J Med* 367:1208–1219, 2012.
128. Kern FH, Shulman S, Greeley WJ: Cardiopulmonary bypass: techniques and effects. In Greeley WJ, editor: *Perioperative management of the patient with congenital heart disease*, Baltimore, 1996, Williams and Wilkins, pp 67–120.
129. Watanabe T, Orita H, Kobayashi M, et al: Brain tissue pH, oxygen tension, and carbon dioxide tension in profoundly hypothermic cardiopulmonary bypass. Comparative study of circulatory arrest, nonpulsatile low-flow perfusion, and pulsatile low-flow perfusion. *J Thorac Cardiovasc Surg* 97:396–401, 1989.
130. Swain JA, McDonald TJ, Jr, Griffith PK, et al: Low-flow hypothermic cardiopulmonary bypass protects the brain. *J Thorac Cardiovasc Surg* 102:76–83, discussion 84, 1991.
131. Miyamoto K, Kawashima Y, Matsuda H, et al: Optimal perfusion flow rate for the brain during deep hypothermic cardiopulmonary bypass at 20 degrees C. An experimental study. *J Thorac Cardiovasc Surg* 92:1065–1070, 1986.
132. Burrows FA, Bissonnette B: Cerebral blood flow velocity patterns during cardiac surgery utilizing profound hypothermia with low-flow cardiopulmonary bypass or circulatory arrest in neonates and infants. *Can J Anaesth* 40:298–307, 1993.
133. Taylor RH, Burrows FA, Bissonnette B: Cerebral pressure-flow velocity relationship during hypothermic cardiopulmonary bypass in neonates and infants. *Anesth Analg* 74:636–642, 1992.
134. Bellinger DC, Wernovsky G, Rappaport LA, et al: Cognitive development of children following early repair of transposition of the great arteries using deep hypothermic circulatory arrest. *Pediatrics* 87:701–707, 1991.
135. Scallan MJ: Brain injury in children with congenital heart disease. *Paediatr Anaesth* 13:284–293, 2003.
136. Shum-Tim D, Nagashima M, Shinoka T, et al: Postischemic hyperthermia exacerbates neurologic injury after deep hypothermic circulatory arrest. *J Thorac Cardiovasc Surg* 116:780–792, 1998.
137. Nollert G, Nagashima M, Bucerius J, et al: Oxygenation strategy and neurologic damage after deep hypothermic circulatory arrest. II. hypoxic versus free radical injury. *J Thorac Cardiovasc Surg* 117:1172–1179, 1999.
138. Cowan DB, Weisel RD, Williams WG, et al: The regulation of glutathione peroxidase gene expression by oxygen tension in cultured human cardiomyocytes. *J Mol Cell Cardiol* 24:423–433, 1992.
139. Rahn H, Reeves RB, Howell BJ: Hydrogen ion regulation, temperature, and evolution. *Am Rev Respir Dis* 112:165–172, 1975.
140. Somero G, White FN: Enzymatic consequences under alpha stat regulation. In Rahn H, Prakash O, editors: *Acid-base regulation and body temperature*, Boston, 1985, Nijhoff, pp 55–80.
141. Murkin JM, Farrar JK, Tweed WA, et al: Cerebral autoregulation and flow/metabolism coupling during cardiopulmonary bypass: the influence of PaCO2. *Anesth Analg* 66:825–832, 1987.
142. Bove EL, West HL, Paskanik AM: Hypothermic cardiopulmonary bypass: a comparison between alpha and pH stat regulation in the dog. *J Surg Res* 42:66–73, 1987.
143. Jonas RA: Hypothermia, circulatory arrest, and the pediatric brain. *J Cardiothorac Vasc Anesth* 10:66–74, 1996.
144. Aoki M, Jonas RA, Nomura F, et al: Effects of aprotinin on acute recovery of cerebral metabolism in piglets after hypothermic circulatory arrest. *Ann Thorac Surg* 58:146–153, 1994.
145. Swain JA, McDonald TJ, Jr, Robbins RC, et al: Relationship of cerebral and myocardial intracellular pH to blood pH during hypothermia. *Am J Physiol* 260:H1640–H1644, 1991.
146. Vannucci RC, Towfighi J, Heitjan DF, et al: Carbon dioxide protects the perinatal brain from hypoxic-ischemic damage: an experimental study in the immature rat. *Pediatrics* 95:868–874, 1995.
147. Miller AL, Corddry DH: Brain carbohydrate metabolism in developing rats during hypercapnia. *J Neurochem* 36:1202–1210, 1981.
148. Tombaugh GC, Sapolsky RM: Evolving concepts about the role of acidosis in ischemic neuropathology. *J Neurochem* 61:793–803, 1993.
149. Ou-Yang Y, Kristian T, Mellergard P, et al: The influence of pH on glutamate- and depolarization-induced increases of intracellular calcium concentration in cortical neurons in primary culture. *Brain Res* 646:65–72, 1994.
150. Aoki M, Nomura F, Stromski ME, et al: Effects of pH on brain energetics after hypothermic circulatory arrest. *Ann Thorac Surg* 55:1093–1103, 1993.
151. Jonas RA, Bellinger DC, Rappaport LA, et al: Relation of pH strategy and developmental outcome after hypothermic circulatory arrest. *J Thorac Cardiovasc Surg* 106:362–368, 1993.
152. Bellinger DC, Wypij D, du Plessis AJ, et al: Developmental and neurologic effects of alpha-stat versus pH-stat strategies for deep hypothermic cardiopulmonary bypass in infants. *J Thorac Cardiovasc Surg* 121:374–383, 2001.

153. Bellinger DC, Wypij D, duDuplessis AJ, et al: Neurodevelopmental status at eight years in children with dextro-transposition of the great arteries: the Boston Circulatory Arrest Trial. *J Thorac Cardiovasc Surg* 126:1385–1396, 2003.
154. Newburger JW, Sleeper LA, Bellinger DC, et al: Early developmental outcome in children with hypoplastic left heart syndrome and related anomalies: the single ventricle reconstruction trial. *Circulation* 125:2081–2091, 2012.
155. Kirshbom PM, Skaryak LA, DiBernardo LR, et al: Effects of aortopulmonary collaterals on cerebral cooling and cerebral metabolic recovery after circulatory arrest. *Circulation* 92:II490–II494, 1995.
156. Abdul Aziz KA, Meduoye A: Is pH-stat or alpha-stat the best technique to follow in patients undergoing deep hypothermic circulatory arrest? *Interact Cardiovasc Thorac Surg* 10:271–282, 2010.
157. Kern FH, Morana NJ, Sears JJ, et al: Coagulation defects in neonates during cardiopulmonary bypass. *Ann Thorac Surg* 54:541–546, 1992.
158. Odegard KC, McGowan FX, Jr, Zurakowski D, et al: Procoagulant and anticoagulant factor abnormalities following the Fontan procedure: increased factor VIII may predispose to thrombosis. *J Thorac Cardiovasc Surg* 125:1260–1267, 2003.
159. Miller BE, Mochizuki T, Levy JH, et al: Predicting and treating coagulopathies after cardiopulmonary bypass in children. *Anesth Analg* 85:1196–1202, 1997.
160. Mohr R, Martinowitz U, Lavee J, et al: The hemostatic effect of transfusing fresh whole blood versus platelet concentrates after cardiac operations. *J Thorac Cardiovasc Surg* 96:530–534, 1988.
161. Manno CS, Hedberg KW, Kim HC, et al: Comparison of the hemostatic effects of fresh whole blood, stored whole blood, and components after open heart surgery in children. *Blood* 77:930–936, 1991.
162. Niebler RA, Gill JC, Brabant CP, et al: Thromboelastography in the assessment of bleeding following surgery for congenital heart disease. *World J Pediatr Congenit Heart Surg* 3:433–438, 2012.
163. Romlin BS, Wåhlander H, Berggren H, et al: Intraoperative thromboelastometry is associated with reduced transfusion prevalence in pediatric cardiac surgery. *Anesth Analg* 112:30–36, 2011.
164. Murkin JM: Attenuation of neurologic injury during cardiac surgery. *Ann Thorac Surg* 72:S1838–S1844, 2001.
165. Smith PK, Datta SK, Muhlbaier LH, et al: Cost analysis of aprotinin for coronary artery bypass patients: analysis of the randomized trials. *Ann Thorac Surg* 77:635–642, discussion 42–43, 2004.
166. Bojan M, Vicca S, Boulat C, et al: Aprotinin, transfusions, and kidney injury in neonates and infants undergoing cardiac surgery. *Br J Anaesth* 108:830–837, 2012.
167. Wilder NS, Kavarana MN, Voepel-Lewis T, et al: Efficacy and safety of aprotinin in neonatal congenital heart operations. *Ann Thorac Surg* 92:958–963, 2011.
168. Faraoni D, Willems A, Melot C, et al: Efficacy of tranexamic acid in paediatric cardiac surgery: a systematic review and meta-analysis. *Eur J Cardiothorac Surg* 42:781–786, 2012.
169. Gruber EM, Shukla AC, Reid RW, et al: Synthetic antifibrinolytics are not associated with an increased incidence of baffle fenestration closure after the modified Fontan procedure. *J Cardiothorac Vasc Anesth* 14:257–259, 2000.
170. Reid RW, Zimmerman AA, Laussen PC, et al: The efficacy of tranexamic acid versus placebo in decreasing blood loss in pediatric patients undergoing repeat cardiac surgery. *Anesth Analg* 84:990–996, 1997.
171. Miller BE, Tosone SR, Tam VK, et al: Hematologic and economic impact of aprotinin in reoperative pediatric cardiac operations. *Ann Thorac Surg* 66:535–540, discussion 41, 1998.
172. D'Errico CC, Munro HM, Bove EL: Pro: the routine use of aprotinin during pediatric cardiac surgery is a benefit. *J Cardiothorac Vasc Anesth* 13:782–784, 1999.
173. D'Errico CC, Shayevitz JR, Martindale SJ, et al: The efficacy and cost of aprotinin in children undergoing reoperative open heart surgery. *Anesth Analg* 83:1193–1199, 1996.
174. Casta A, Gruber EM, Laussen PC, et al: Parameters associated with perioperative baffle fenestration closure in the Fontan operation. *J Cardiothorac Vasc Anesth* 14:553–556, 2000.
175. Pychyńska-Pokorska M, Pągowska-Klimek I, Krajewski W, et al: Use of recombinant activated factor VII for controlling refractory postoperative bleeding in children undergoing cardiac surgery with cardiopulmonary bypass. *J Cardiothorac Vasc Anesth* 25(6):987–994, 2011.
176. Karsies TJ, Nicol KK, Galantowicz ME, et al: Thrombotic risk of recombinant factor seven in pediatric cardiac surgery: a single institution experience. *Ann Thorac Surg* 89:570–576, 2010.
177. Okonta KE, Edwin F, Falase B: Is recombinant activated factor VII effective in the treatment of excessive bleeding after paediatric cardiac surgery? *Interact Cardiovasc Thorac Surg* 15:690–694, 2012.
178. Lazenby W, Ko W, Zelano JA, et al: Effects of temperature and flow rate on regional blood flow and metabolism during cardiopulmonary bypass. *Ann Thorac Surg* 54:449–459, 1981.
179. Seghaye MC, Duchateau J, Grabitz RG, et al: Complement activation during cardiopulmonary bypass in infants and children. Relation to postoperative multiple system organ failure. *J Thorac Cardiovasc Surg* 106:978–987, 1993.
180. Brix-Christensen V: The systemic inflammatory response after cardiac surgery with cardiopulmonary bypass in children. *Acta Anaesthesiol Scand* 45:671–679, 2001.
181. Gillinov AM, Redmond JM, Zehr KJ, et al: Inhibition of neutrophil adhesion during cardiopulmonary bypass. *Ann Thorac Surg* 57:126–133, 1994.
182. McGowan FX, Jr, Ikegami M, del Nido PJ, et al: Cardiopulmonary bypass significantly reduces surfactant activity in children. *J Thorac Cardiovasc Surg* 106:968–977, 1993.
183. Ozawa T, Yoshihara K, Koyama N, et al: Clinical efficacy of heparin-bonded bypass circuits related to cytokine responses in children. *Ann Thorac Surg* 69:584–590, 2000.
184. Morita K, Ihnken K, Buckberg GD, et al: Pulmonary vasoconstriction due to impaired nitric oxide production after cardiopulmonary bypass. *Ann Thorac Surg* 61:1775–1780, 1996.
185. Schulze-Neick I, Penny DJ, Rigby ML, et al: L-arginine and substance P reverse the pulmonary endothelial dysfunction caused by congenital heart surgery. *Circulation* 100:749–755, 1999.
186. Dreyer WJ, Michael LH, Millman EE, et al: Neutrophil sequestration and pulmonary dysfunction in a canine model of open heart surgery with cardiopulmonary bypass. Evidence for a CD18-dependent mechanism. *Circulation* 92:2276–2283, 1995.
187. Chai PJ, Williamson JA, Lodge AJ, et al: Effects of ischemia on pulmonary dysfunction after cardiopulmonary bypass. *Ann Thorac Surg* 67:731–735, 1999.
188. Picca S, Principato F, Mazzera E, et al: Risks of acute renal failure after cardiopulmonary bypass surgery in children: a retrospective 10-year case-control study. *Nephrol Dial Transplant* 10:630–636, 1995.
189. Aydin SI, Seiden HS, Blaufox AD, et al: Acute kidney injury after surgery for congenital heart disease. *Ann Thorac Surg* 94:1589–1595, 2012.
190. Taylor ML, Carmona F, Thiagarajan RR, et al: Mild postoperative acute kidney injury and outcomes after surgery for congenital heart disease. *J Thorac Cardiovasc Surg* 146:146–152, 2013.
191. Morgan CJ, Zappitelli M, Robertson CM, et al: Risk factors for and outcomes of acute kidney injury in neonates undergoing complex cardiac surgery. *J Pediatr* 162:120–127, 2013.
192. Price JF, Mott AR, Dickerson HA, et al: Worsening renal function in children hospitalized with decompensated heart failure: evidence for a pediatric cardiorenal syndrome? *Pediatr Crit Care Med* 9:279–284, 2008.
193. Anand KJ, Hickey PR: Pain and its effects in the human neonate and fetus. *N Engl J Med* 317:1321–1329, 1987.
194. Landoni G, Biondi-Zoccai GG, Marino G, et al: Fenoldopam reduces the need for renal replacement therapy and in-hospital death in cardiovascular surgery: a meta-analysis. *J Cardiothorac Vasc Anesth* 22:27–33, 2008.
195. Roasio A, Lobreglio R, Santin A, et al: Fenoldopam reduces the incidence of renal replacement therapy after cardiac surgery. *J Cardiothorac Vasc Anesth* 22:23–26, 2008.
196. Cogliati AA, Vellutini R, Nardini A, et al: Fenoldopam infusion for renal protection in high-risk cardiac surgery patients: a randomized clinical study. *J Cardiothorac Vasc Anesth* 21:847–850, 2007.
197. Chen HH, Sundt TM, Cook DJ, et al: Low dose nesiritide and the preservation of renal function in patients with renal dysfunction undergoing cardiopulmonary-bypass surgery: a double-blind placebo-controlled pilot study. *Circulation* 116:I134–I138, 2007.

198. Mentzer RM, Jr, Oz MC, Sladen RN, et al: Effects of perioperative nesiritide in patients with left ventricular dysfunction undergoing cardiac surgery: the NAPA Trial. *J Am Coll Cardiol* 49:716–726, 2007.
199. Ferry PC: Neurologic sequelae of open-heart surgery in children. An "irritating question." *Am J Dis Child* 144:369–373, 1990.
200. Menache CC, du Plessis AJ, Wessel DL, et al: Current incidence of acute neurologic complications after open-heart operations in children. *Ann Thorac Surg* 73:1752–1758, 2002.
201. Bellinger DC, Wypij D, Kuban KC, et al: Developmental and neurological status of children at 4 years of age after heart surgery with hypothermic circulatory arrest or low-flow cardiopulmonary bypass. *Circulation* 100:526–532, 1999.
202. Forbess JM, Visconti KJ, Hancock-Friesen C, et al: Neurodevelopmental outcome after congenital heart surgery: results from an institutional registry. *Circulation* 106:I95–I102, 2002.
203. Forbess JM, Visconti KJ, Bellinger DC, et al: Neurodevelopmental outcomes after biventricular repair of congenital heart defects. *J Thorac Cardiovasc Surg* 123:631–639, 2002.
204. Mahle WT, Spray TL, Wernovsky G, et al: Survival after reconstructive surgery for hypoplastic left heart syndrome: a 15-year experience from a single institution. *Circulation* 102:III136–III141, 2000.
205. Wernovsky G, Stiles KM, Gauvreau K, et al: Cognitive development after the Fontan operation. *Circulation* 102:883–889, 2000.
206. Dent CL, Spaeth JP, Jones BV, et al: Brain magnetic resonance imaging abnormalities after the Norwood procedure using regional cerebral perfusion. *J Thorac Cardiovasc Surg* 131:190–197, 2006.
207. Dent CL, Spaeth JP, Jones BV, et al: Brain magnetic resonance imaging abnormalities after the Norwood procedure using regional cerebral perfusion. *J Thorac Cardiovasc Surg* 130:1523–1530, 2005.
208. Ditsworth D, Priestley MA, Loepke AW, et al: Apoptotic neuronal death following deep hypothermic circulatory arrest in piglets. *Anesthesiology* 98:1119–1127, 2003.
209. Miller SP, McQuillen PS, Hamrick S, et al: Abnormal brain development in newborns with congenital heart disease. *N Engl J Med* 357:1928–1938, 2007.
210. McQuillen PS, Barkovich AJ, Hamrick SE, et al: Temporal and anatomic risk profile of brain injury with neonatal repair of congenital heart defects. *Stroke* 38:736–741, 2007.
211. McQuillen PS, Hamrick SE, Perez MJ, et al: Balloon atrial septostomy is associated with preoperative stroke in neonates with transposition of the great arteries. *Circulation* 113:280–285, 2006.
212. Miller SP, McQuillen PS, Vigneron DB, et al: Preoperative brain injury in newborns with transposition of the great arteries. *Ann Thorac Surg* 77:1698–1706, 2004.
213. Beca J, Gunn JK, Coleman L, et al: New white matter brain injury after infant heart surgery is associated with diagnostic group and the use of circulatory arrest. *Circulation* 127:971–979, 2013.
214. Limperopoulos C, Majnemer A, Shevell MI, et al: Neurodevelopmental status of newborns and infants with congenital heart defects before and after open heart surgery. *J Pediatr* 137:638–645, 2000.
215. Gerdes M, Solot C, Wang PP, et al: Cognitive and behavior profile of preschool children with chromosome 22q11.2 deletion. *Am J Med Genet* 85:127–133, 1999.
216. Miller G, Vogel H: Structural evidence of injury or malformation in the brains of children with congenital heart disease. *Semin Pediatr Neurol* 6:20–26, 1999.
217. Glauser TA, Rorke LB, Weinberg PM, et al: Congenital brain anomalies associated with the hypoplastic left heart syndrome. *Pediatrics* 85:984–990, 1990.
218. Kern FH, Schulman S, Greeley WJ: Cardiopulmonary bypass: techniques and effects. In Greeley WJ, editor: *Perioperative management of the patient with congenital heart disease*, Baltimore, 1996, Williams and Wilkins, pp 67–120.
219. Wells FC, Coghill S, Caplan HL, et al: Duration of circulatory arrest does influence the psychological development of children after cardiac operation in early life. *J Thorac Cardiovasc Surg* 86:823–831, 1983.
220. Wypij D, Newburger JW, Rappaport LA, et al: The effect of duration of deep hypothermic circulatory arrest in infant heart surgery on late neurodevelopment: the Boston Circulatory Arrest Trial. *J Thorac Cardiovasc Surg* 126:1397–1403, 2003.
221. du Plessis AJ, Bellinger DC, Gauvreau K, et al: Neurologic outcome of choreoathetoid encephalopathy after cardiac surgery. *Pediatr Neurol* 27:9–17, 2002.
222. Gaynor JW, Jarvik GP, Gerdes M, et al: Postoperative electroencephalographic seizures are associated with deficits in executive function and social behaviors at 4 years of age following cardiac surgery in infancy. *J Thorac Cardiovasc Surg* 146:132–137, 2013.
223. Langley SM, Chai PJ, Miller SE, et al: Intermittent perfusion protects the brain during deep hypothermic circulatory arrest. *Ann Thorac Surg* 68:4–12, 1999.
224. Pigula FA, Gandhi SK, Siewers RD, et al: Regional low-flow perfusion provides somatic circulatory support during neonatal aortic arch surgery. *Ann Thorac Surg* 72:401–406, discussion 6–7, 2001.
225. Pigula FA: Competing perfusion strategies: effect on microvascular oxygen tension. *J Thorac Cardiovasc Surg* 125:456, 2003.
226. Pigula FA: Arch reconstruction without circulatory arrest: scientific basis for continued use and application to patients with arch anomalies. *Semin Thorac Cardiovasc Surg Pediatr Card Surg Annu* 5:104–115, 2002.
227. Williams GD, Ramamoorthy C: Brain monitoring and protection during pediatric cardiac surgery. *Semin Cardiothorac Vasc Anesth* 11:23–33, 2007.
228. Fraser CD, Jr, Andropoulos DB: Principles of antegrade cerebral perfusion during arch reconstruction in newborns/infants. *Semin Thorac Cardiovasc Surg Pediatr Card Surg Annu* 61–68, 2008.
229. Khan MS, Fraser CD: Neonatal brain protection in cardiac surgery and the role of intraoperative neuromonitoring. *World J Pediatr Congenit Heart Surg* 3:114–119, 2012.
230. Duncan BW, Hraska V, Jonas RA, et al: Mechanical circulatory support in children with cardiac disease. *J Thorac Cardiovasc Surg* 117:529–542, 1999.
231. McElhinney DB, Reddy VM, Parry AJ, et al: Management and outcomes of delayed sternal closure after cardiac surgery in neonates and infants. *Crit Care Med* 28:1180–1184, 2000.
232. Ghanayem NS, Mitchell ME, Tweddell JS, et al: Monitoring the brain before, during, and after cardiac surgery to improve long-term neurodevelopmental outcomes. *Cardiol Young* 16(Suppl 3):103–109, 2006.
233. Hoffman GM: Pro: near-infrared spectroscopy should be used for all cardiopulmonary bypass. *J Cardiothorac Vasc Anesth* 20:606–612, 2006.
234. Hoffman GM: Neurologic monitoring on cardiopulmonary bypass: what are we obligated to do? *Ann Thorac Surg* 81:S2373–S2380, 2006.
235. Johnson BA, Hoffman GM, Tweddell JS, et al: Near-infrared spectroscopy in neonates before palliation of hypoplastic left heart syndrome. *Ann Thorac Surg* 87:571–577, discussion 7–9, 2009.
236. Nelson DP, Andropoulos DB, Fraser CD, Jr: Perioperative neuroprotective strategies. *Semin Thorac Cardiovasc Surg Pediatr Card Surg Annu* 49–56, 2008.
237. Kurth CD, McCann JC, Wu J, et al: Cerebral oxygen saturation-time threshold for hypoxic-ischemic injury in piglets. *Anesth Analg* 108:1268–1277, 2009.
238. Kurth CD, Levy WJ, McCann J: Near-infrared spectroscopy cerebral oxygen saturation thresholds for hypoxia-ischemia in piglets. *J Cereb Blood Flow Metab* 22:335–341, 2002.
239. Hirsch JC, Charpie JR, Ohye RG, et al: Near-infrared spectroscopy: what we know and what we need to know—a systematic review of the congenital heart disease literature. *J Thorac Cardiovasc Surg* 137:154–159, 9e1–12, 2009.
240. Kussman BD, Gauvreau K, DiNardo JA, et al: Cerebral perfusion and oxygenation after the Norwood procedure: comparison of right ventricle-pulmonary artery conduit with modified Blalock-Taussig shunt. *J Thorac Cardiovasc Surg* 133:648–655, 2007.
241. Kussman BD, Wypij D, DiNardo JA, et al: Cerebral oximetry during infant cardiac surgery: evaluation and relationship to early postoperative outcome. *Anesth Analg* 108:1122–1131, 2009.
242. Blauth CI, Arnold JV, Schulenberg WE, et al: Cerebral microembolism during cardiopulmonary bypass. Retinal microvascular studies in vivo with fluorescein angiography. *J Thorac Cardiovasc Surg* 95:668–676, 1988.

243. Win KN, Wang S, Undar A: Microemboli generation, detection and characterization during CPB procedures in neonates, infants, and small children. *ASAIO J* 54:486–490, 2008.
244. Miller A, Wang S, Myers JL, et al: Gaseous microemboli detection in a simulated pediatric CPB circuit using a novel ultrasound system. *ASAIO J* 54:504–508, 2008.
245. Anand KJ, Hickey PR: Halothane-morphine compared with high-dose sufentanil for anesthesia and postoperative analgesia in neonatal cardiac surgery. *N Engl J Med* 326:1–9, 1992.
246. Anand KJ, Sippell WG, Aynsley-Green A: Randomised trial of fentanyl anaesthesia in preterm babies undergoing surgery: effects on the stress response. *Lancet* 1:62–66, 1987.
247. Butler J, Rocker GM, Westaby S: Inflammatory response to cardiopulmonary bypass. *Ann Thorac Surg* 55:552–559, 1993.
248. Seghaye MC, Grabitz RG, Duchateau J, et al: Inflammatory reaction and capillary leak syndrome related to cardiopulmonary bypass in neonates undergoing cardiac operations. *J Thorac Cardiovasc Surg* 112:687–697, 1996.
249. Seghaye MC, Duchateau J, Grabitz RG, et al: Complement, leukocytes, and leukocyte elastase in full-term neonates undergoing cardiac operation. *J Thorac Cardiovasc Surg* 108:29–36, 1994.
250. Plotz FB, van Oeveren W, Bartlett RH, et al: Blood activation during neonatal extracorporeal life support. *J Thorac Cardiovasc Surg* 105:823–832, 1993.
251. Ashraf SS, Tian Y, Zacharrias S, et al: Effects of cardiopulmonary bypass on neonatal and paediatric inflammatory profiles. *Eur J Cardiothorac Surg* 12:862–868, 1997.
252. Chew MS, Brix-Christensen V, Ravn HB, et al: Effect of modified ultrafiltration on the inflammatory response in paediatric open-heart surgery: a prospective, randomized study. *Perfusion* 17:327–333, 2002.
253. Gessler P, Pfenninger J, Pfammatter JP, et al: Inflammatory response of neutrophil granulocytes and monocytes after cardiopulmonary bypass in pediatric cardiac surgery. *Intensive Care Med* 28:1786–1791, 2002.
254. Chew MS, Brandslund I, Brix-Christensen V, et al: Tissue injury and the inflammatory response to pediatric cardiac surgery with cardiopulmonary bypass: a descriptive study. *Anesthesiology* 94: 745–753, discussion 5A, 2001.
255. Wheeler DS, Dent CL, Manning PB, et al: Factors prolonging length of stay in the cardiac intensive care unit following the arterial switch operation. *Cardiol Young* 18:41–50, 2008.
256. Li RK, Shaikh N, Weisel RD, et al: Oxyradical-induced antioxidant and lipid changes in cultured human cardiomyocytes. *Am J Physiol* 266:H2204–H2211, 1994.
257. Moore EE, Moore FA, Franciose RJ, et al: The postischemic gut serves as a priming bed for circulating neutrophils that provoke multiple organ failure. *J Trauma* 37:881–887, 1994.
258. Koike K, Moore EE, Moore FA, et al: Gut ischemia/reperfusion produces lung injury independent of endotoxin. *Crit Care Med* 22:1438–1444, 1994.
259. Journois D, Pouard P, Greeley WJ, et al: Hemofiltration during cardiopulmonary bypass in pediatric cardiac surgery. Effects on hemostasis, cytokines, and complement components. *Anesthesiology* 81:1181–1189, discussion 26A–27A, 1994.
260. Wachtfogel YT, Pixley RA, Kucich U, et al: Purified plasma factor XIIa aggregates human neutrophils and causes degranulation. *Blood* 67:1731–1737, 1986.
261. Wachtfogel YT, Kucich U, James HL, et al: Human plasma kallikrein releases neutrophil elastase during blood coagulation. *J Clin Invest* 72:1672–1677, 1983.
262. Wachtfogel YT, Kucich U, Hack CE, et al: Aprotinin inhibits the contact, neutrophil, and platelet activation systems during simulated extracorporeal perfusion. *J Thorac Cardiovasc Surg* 106:1–9, discussion 9–10, 1993.
263. Larson DF, Bowers M, Schechner HW: Neutrophil activation during cardiopulmonary bypass in paediatric and adult patients. *Perfusion* 11:21–27, 1996.
264. Tarnok A, Schneider P: Pediatric cardiac surgery with cardiopulmonary bypass: pathways contributing to transient systemic immune suppression. *Shock* 16(Suppl 1):24–32, 2001.
265. McBride WT, Booth JV: Human cytokine responses to cardiac operations: prebypass factors. *J Thorac Cardiovasc Surg* 112:560–561, 1996.
266. McBride WT, Armstrong MA, Crockard AD, et al: Cytokine balance and immunosuppressive changes at cardiac surgery: contrasting response between patients and isolated CPB circuits. *Br J Anaesth* 75:724–733, 1995.
267. Allan CK, Newburger JW, McGrath E, et al: Relationship between inflammatory activation and clinical outcome after infant cardiopulmonary bypass. *Anesth Analg* in press.
268. Appachi E, Mossad E, Mee RB, et al: Perioperative serum interleukins in neonates with hypoplastic left-heart syndrome and transposition of the great arteries. *J Cardiothorac Vasc Anesth* 21:184–190, 2007.
269. Stocker CF, Shekerdemian LS, Horton SB, et al: The influence of bypass temperature on the systemic inflammatory response and organ injury after pediatric open surgery: a randomized trial. *J Thorac Cardiovasc Surg* 142:174–180, 2011.
270. Caputo M, Mokhtari A, Rogers CA, et al: The effects of normoxic versus hyperoxic cardiopulmonary bypass on oxidative stress and inflammatory response in cyanotic pediatric patients undergoing open cardiac surgery: a randomized controlled trial. *J Thorac Cardiovasc Surg* 138:206–214, 2009.
271. Naguib AN, Tobias JD, Hall MW, et al: The role of different anesthetic techniques in altering the stress response during cardiac surgery in children: a prospective, double-blinded, and randomized study. *Pediatr Crit Care Med* 14:481–490, 2013.
272. Jones BO, Pepe S, Sheeran FL, et al: Remote ischemic preconditioning in cyanosed neonates undergoing cardiopulmonary bypass: a randomized controlled trial. *J Thorac Cardiovasc Surg* 2013. [Epub ahead of print].
273. Sasser WC, Dabal RJ, Askenazi DJ, et al: Prophylactic peritoneal dialysis following cardiopulmonary bypass in children is associated with decreased inflammation and improved clinical outcomes. *Congenit Heart Dis* 9:106–115, 2014.
274. Bronicki RA, Backer CL, Baden HP, et al: Dexamethasone reduces the inflammatory response to cardiopulmonary bypass in children. *Ann Thorac Surg* 69:1490–1495, 2000.
275. El Azab SR, Rosseel PM, de Lange JJ, et al: Dexamethasone decreases the pro- to anti-inflammatory cytokine ratio during cardiac surgery. *Br J Anaesth* 88:496–501, 2002.
276. Shum-Tim D, Tchervenkov CI, Jamal AM, et al: Systemic steroid pretreatment improves cerebral protection after circulatory arrest. *Ann Thorac Surg* 72:1465–1471, discussion 71–72, 2001.
277. Chaney MA: Corticosteroids and cardiopulmonary bypass: a review of clinical investigations. *Chest* 121:921–931, 2002.
278. Pasquali SK, Hall M, Li JS, et al: Corticosteroids and outcome in children undergoing congenital heart surgery: analysis of the Pediatric Health Information Systems database. *Circulation* 122:2123–2130, 2010.
279. Clarizia NA, Manlhiot C, Schwartz SM, et al: Improved outcomes associated with intraoperative steroid use in high-risk pediatric cardiac surgery. *Ann Thorac Surg* 91:1222–1227, 2011.
280. Bronicki RA, Checchia PA, Stuart-Killion RB, et al: The effects of multiple doses of glucocorticoids on the inflammatory response to cardiopulmonary bypass in children. *World J Pediatr Congenit Heart Surg* 3:439–445, 2012.
281. Mastropietro CW, Barrett R, Davalos MC, et al: Cumulative corticosteroid exposure and infection risk after complex pediatric cardiac surgery. *Ann Thorac Surg* 95:2133–2139, 2013.
282. Gaynor JW: The effect of modified ultrafiltration on the postoperative course in patients with congenital heart disease. *Semin Thorac Cardiovasc Surg Pediatr Card Surg Annu* 6:128–139, 2003.
283. Gaynor JW: Use of ultrafiltration during and after cardiopulmonary bypass in children. *J Thorac Cardiovasc Surg* 122:209–211, 2001.
284. Bando K, Vijay P, Turrentine MW, et al: Dilutional and modified ultrafiltration reduces pulmonary hypertension after operations for congenital heart disease: a prospective randomized study. *J Thorac Cardiovasc Surg* 115:517–525, discussion 25–27, 1998.
285. Chaturvedi RR, Shore DF, White PA, et al: Modified ultrafiltration improves global left ventricular systolic function after open-heart surgery in infants and children. *Eur J Cardiothorac Surg* 15:742–746, 1999.
286. Hiramatsu T, Imai Y, Kurosawa H, et al: Effects of dilutional and modified ultrafiltration in plasma endothelin-1 and pulmonary vascular resistance after the Fontan procedure. *Ann Thorac Surg* 73:861–865, 2002.

287. Maluf MA, Mangia C, Silva C, et al: Conventional and conventional plus modified ultrafiltration during cardiac surgery in high-risk congenital heart disease. *J Cardiovasc Surg (Torino)* 42:465–473, 2001.
288. Friesen RH, Campbell DN, Clarke DR, et al: Modified ultrafiltration attenuates dilutional coagulopathy in pediatric open heart operations. *Ann Thorac Surg* 64:1787–1789, 1997.
289. Elliott MJ: Ultrafiltration and modified ultrafiltration in pediatric open heart operations. *Ann Thorac Surg* 56:1518–1522, 1993.
290. Huang H, Yao T, Wang W, et al: Continuous ultrafiltration attenuates the pulmonary injury that follows open heart surgery with cardiopulmonary bypass. *Ann Thorac Surg* 76:136–140, 2003.
291. Kuratani N, Bunsangjaroen P, Srimueang T, et al: Modified versus conventional ultrafiltration in pediatric cardiac surgery: a meta-analysis of randomized controlled trials comparing clinical outcome parameters. *J Thorac Cardiovasc Surg* 142:861–867, 2011.

CHAPTER 109

Surgical Approaches, Cardiopulmonary Bypass, and Mechanical Circulatory Support in Children

Francis Fynn-Thompson • Ravi R. Thiagarajan • Luis Quinonez

CHAPTER OUTLINE

For infants and children, mechanical support of the circulation has important roles in providing short-term circulatory support for reversible myocardial failure, in providing cardiopulmonary support before and after cardiac surgery, and in providing longer-term support as a potential bridge to cardiac transplantation. Mechanical circulatory support (MCS) modalities commonly available include extracorporeal membrane oxygenation (ECMO), intra-aortic balloon pump (IABP) counterpulsation, and ventricular assist devices (VADs). Although a variety of assist devices are available for adult-size patients, the need for miniaturization has delayed their application in children. ECMO therefore remains the most common form of MCS for pediatric patients. ECMO was first introduced to provide respiratory support in pediatric patients with severe lung disease failing mechanical ventilator support. Some institutions with an established ECMO program have been able to transition this methodology to provide biventricular support and oxygenation in pediatric patients with a failing circulation.[1-3] There are no established guidelines for the indications or management of cardiac ECMO support, and there is considerable inter-institutional variability with respect to use and outcomes, based on local experience and philosophy. VADs offer the potential for both short- and long-term support of circulation in patients who do not have concurrent pulmonary parenchymal or vascular disease, and there is increasing experience in developing this form of support as an effective longer-term bridge to transplantation in the pediatric patients with heart disease.

EXTRACORPOREAL MEMBRANE OXYGENATION

Overview of Uses

The use of ECMO to support children with impaired gas exchange failing to respond to mechanical ventilation as a result of acute respiratory disease is now an accepted and successful therapy. This is particularly true in neonates with a variety of parenchymal and vascular lung diseases (e.g., meconium aspiration, respiratory distress syndrome, diaphragmatic hernia, persistent hypertension of the newborn) survival outcomes are excellent with the use of ECMO.[3,4] Good ECMO outcomes in these patients depends on the early diagnosis of severe pulmonary failure, the prompt institution of ECMO, and the reversible nature of the pulmonary dysfunction.[4] However, the advent of other therapies, such as high-frequency oscillatory ventilation, surfactant therapy, permissive hypercapnia, and inhaled nitric oxide, has led to a reduction in the need for ECMO in neonates.[5-7] According to the cumulative data on 55,658 patients reported by the Extracorporeal Life Support Organization (ELSO) Registry, 75% of all neonates who have been placed on ECMO for respiratory support have survived to discharge from hospital (Table 109-1).[5] The outcome for older patients with respiratory failure is considerably lower, with the reported cumulative survival for pediatric and adult patients placed on ECMO for respiratory support being approximately 57% and 56%, respectively.

The past decade has seen a steady increase in the number of patients and institutions using ECMO to support a failing circulation, both after congenital cardiac surgery or as a bridge to transplantation.[5,8-19] Another growing indication for ECMO is its use during resuscitation from cardiac arrest. ECMO can be deployed rapidly during cardiac arrest in patients failing to respond to conventional cardiopulmonary resuscitation; however, ECMO use and efficacy in promoting survival when used for this indication is controversial.[8,10,11,20-22]

Despite the increased enthusiasm for ECMO support of the circulation, the survival to discharge as reported by the ELSO registry (40% for neonates and 49% for pediatric patients) has not changed much over the past decade (Fig. 109-1) and has lagged considerably when compared with the experience with respiratory ECMO (Table 109-2).[5] The majority of cardiac patients are given ECMO after cardiac surgery. Adverse outcomes after cardiac ECMO are primarily related to irreversible underlying cardiac disease and to the presence of significant end-organ injury before ECMO deployment. Recovery from severe myocardial dysfunction while on mechanical support can occur, provided the myocardium has only sustained a transient and reversible injury. ECMO facilitates ventricular recovery by reducing myocardial wall tension, increasing coronary perfusion

TABLE 109-1 Survival after ECMO Support

Age Group and Indication	No. of Patients	No. That Survived to Discharge
Neonates		
Respiratory	26,583	19.818 (75%)
Cardiac	5,159	2,078 (40%)
ECPR	914	358 (39%)
Pediatric Age Group		
Respiratory	5,923	3,359 (57%)
Cardiac	6,459	3,197 (49%)
ECPR	1,878	770 (41%)
Adults		
Respiratory	4,382	2,439 (56%)
Cardiac	3,401	1,349 (40%)
ECPR	969	267 (28%)
Total	55,668	33,635 (60%)

ECMO, Extracorporeal membrane oxygenation; *ECPR,* ECMO for cardiopulmonary resuscitation.
From Extracorporeal Life Support Organization: International Summary, July 2013.

TABLE 109-2 Neonatal Respiratory and Cardiac ECMO: Differences in Survival Reported by the ELSO Registry for Specific Diagnostic Groups

Diagnosis	Survival (%)
Meconium aspiration syndrome	94
Primary pulmonary hypertension	77
Sepsis	73
Air leak syndrome	73
Congenital diaphragmatic hernia	51
Cardiac disease	40

ECMO, Extracorporeal membrane oxygenation; *ELSO,* Extracorporeal Life Support Organization.
From Extracorporeal Life Support Organization: International Summary, July 2013.

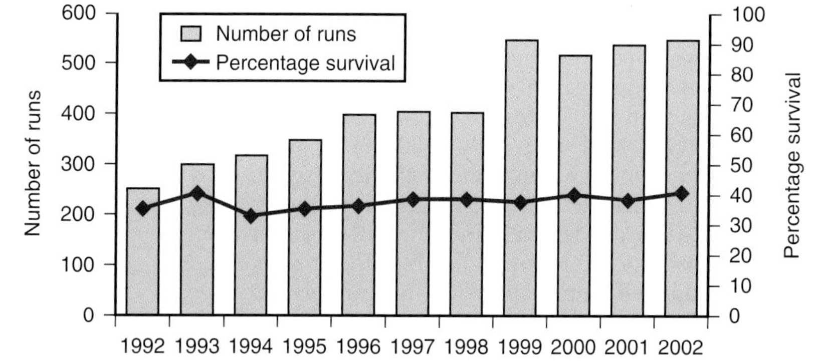

FIGURE 109-1 ■ Number of cardiac extracorporeal membrane oxygenation (ECMO) runs and survival rates for all patients receiving cardiac ECMO support reported to the Extracorporeal Life Support Organization Registry over a 10-year period.

pressure, and maintaining systemic perfusion with oxygenated blood.

In infants, in whom myocardial failure is frequently biventricular and associated with respiratory insufficiency or pulmonary hypertension, ECMO is the preferred means of mechanical support. Although there has been some support for the concept of "resting the lungs" for patients who are given ECMO for respiratory failure and lung injury,[4] in cardiac patients in who ejection is present, coronary blood flow is often from left ventricular ejection. Mechanical ventilation with increased fraction of inspired oxygen concentration in inspired air can increase oxygen content of blood returned to the left heart and thus can improve myocardial oxygen delivery and may promote recovery. The heart must regain contractile function and conduction as soon as possible to maintain a workload and to avoid involution of the myocardial mass. This requires frequent evaluation, often with echocardiography, and it is critical that overdistention of the heart be avoided.

It also is important to appreciate the differences between the ECMO circuit and management, and the routine cardiopulmonary bypass (CPB) used during cardiac surgery. The ECMO circuit is a closed circuit. It has limited ability to handle any air in the venous limb of the circuit, and careful de-airing of both the arterial and venous cannulas is essential when connecting to the ECMO circuit. The average duration for cardiac ECMO runs reported to ELSO over the past 15 years has increased slightly from approximately 4 to 5 days to about 5 to 7 days; the longest reported run is 62 days.[5] These data emphasize that ECMO should be viewed only as a relatively short-term support of the circulation; beyond 7 days of ECMO support, the chances of successful decannulation and survival decrease substantially. These data also support the need to develop longer-term mechanical support devices, particularly as a bridge to transplantation for patients on ECMO who remain suitable candidates for cardiac transplantation.

The significant time limitation associated with cardiac ECMO use indicates that, ideally, only patients with known reversible cardiac disease should be considered candidates for cardiac ECMO. However, this is often not possible when a quick decision needs to be made to place a patient on ECMO because of cardiac arrest or a severe low cardiac output state. In general, institutions with an efficient and well-established ECMO service are more likely to use this form of support for the failing circulation. However, differences in decision making regarding ECMO candidacy and timing of ECMO deployment, case type and surgical complexity, surgical technique and CPB management used, and many other confounding factors make comparison of efficacy of ECMO among institutions difficult.[23] However, one can make a case that ECMO should be readily available in any center undertaking complex congenital cardiac surgery, as it can provide effective short-term cardiac support while awaiting myocardial recovery in some patients improving their probability of survival. Establishing a structured and coordinated team approach to cannulation is a key step for any successful ECMO service.[11] In our experience at Boston Children's Hospital, the introduction of a dedicated cardiac ECMO program and development of a rapid response system for its use during active resuscitation has contributed to an increase in the survival-to-discharge rate for ECMO circulatory support, from 45% in 1995 to 59% in 2002, regardless of the diagnosis or indication for cardiac support.[21]

Indications

There is no specific cardiac procedure or diagnostic group for which ECMO is a proven therapy. Rather than trying to determine indications for cardiac ECMO according to specific diagnoses or procedures, the indications can be examined in five broad categories: preoperative resuscitation; inability to wean from cardiopulmonary bypass; postcardiotomy; cardiomyopathy, myocarditis, and bridge to transplantation; and after in-hospital cardiac arrest and cardiopulmonary resuscitation (CPR). According to the ELSO Registry report of outcomes based on broad diagnostic categories, patients given ECMO because of complications related to fulminant myocarditis have the highest survival rate (Table 109-3), although it lags behind the successful outcomes achieved with ECMO for respiratory support in neonates. The survival from cardiac ECMO to hospital discharge according to selected congenital defects is shown in Table 109-4.

TABLE 109-3 **Survival for Cardiac ECMO Runs Based on Broad Diagnostic Categories**

Diagnosis	Survival (%)
Congenital cardiac defect	39
Cardiac arrest	28
Cardiogenic shock	38
Cardiomyopathy	60
Myocarditis	50

ECMO, Extracorporeal membrane oxygenation.
From Extracorporeal Life Support Organization: International Summary, July 2013.

TABLE 109-4 **Survival for Selected Congenital Cardiac Defects by Age and Diagnosis**

Diagnosis	Neonates (%)	Infants (%)
Left-right shunt	37	43
Left obstruction	33	40
Hypoplastic left heart syndrome	32	40
Right obstruction	43	49
Cyanosis (with increased pulmonary blood flow)	34	42
Total anomalous pulmonary venous return	43	42
Cyanosis (with decreased pulmonary blood flow)	40	41
Other	45	51

From Extracorporeal Life Support Organization: International Summary, July 2013.

Preoperative Resuscitation

ECMO can be beneficial for critically ill patients awaiting cardiac surgery, enabling preoperative stabilization and optimization or prevention of end-organ dysfunction before repair. These patients represent a small group (usually newborns), and indications include severely low cardiac output states (e.g., critical aortic stenosis), pulmonary hypertension (e.g., obstructed total anomalous pulmonary venous drainage), and severe hypoxemia (e.g., transposition of the great arteries and pulmonary hypertension).[23-25]

Inability to Wean from Cardiopulmonary Bypass

The reported survival is poor for patients who are given ECMO because they were unable to wean directly from CPB in the operating room (i.e., without any period of stability off CPB).[8,9,16,23] Issues such as primary myocardial dysfunction, pulmonary hypertension, severe hypoxemia, and refractory dysrhythmias are recognized as major factors in determining successful outcome, but unrecognized residual or irreparable defects are also important.[9] Residual cardiac defects must be investigated in the operating room, using a combination of echocardiography and the careful measurement of oxygen saturations and intracardiac pressures. Ideally, only children with potentially reversible myocardial injury who cannot be weaned from CPB should be considered candidates for ECMO; however, this can be extremely difficult to determine in the operating room immediately after cardiac surgery. Additional considerations for use of ECMO in patients failing to wean from cardiopulmonary bypass after cardiac surgery include preoperative condition, intraoperative course, and the likelihood of being a transplant candidate. Severe hemorrhage is a major problem in the transition from the CPB circuit to the ECMO circuit. Although a lower activated clotting time (ACT; 160 to 180 seconds) can be used, small doses of protamine are often necessary to assist with the initial control of bleeding. We usually administer protamine in 1-mg/kg increments until a target ACT of 180 seconds is achieved. Infusions of antifibrinolytic drugs such as tranexamic acid (bolus of 100 mg/kg, followed by infusion at 10 mg/kg/hr), or ε-aminocaproic acid (bolus of 100 mg/kg, followed by infusion at 30 mg/kg/hr) should be considered. Exploration of the chest may be necessary, particularly if the bleeding persists at a rate greater than 10 mL/kg/hr and if problems with ECMO flow are encountered because of decreased venous cannula drainage from a tamponade-like effect. The large transfusion requirement can place a considerable burden on the supply of donor blood products. As an alternative, it is possible to connect a chest tube to cell-saver tubing to enable blood to be collected in the cell-saver reservoir and subsequently spun for retransfusion.

When a patient requires ECMO in the operating room, discussions with the patient's family must be clear and direct. Recovery of myocardial function should be expected within 2 to 3 days,[26] and if this is not evident, either listing for cardiac transplantation, if appropriate, or withdrawal from support must be considered.

After Cardiotomy

ECMO is an effective therapeutic option for infants and children who have had a period of relative stability after successful termination of CPB and exclusion of significant residual cardiac defects. Myocardial or respiratory failure causing a low cardiac output state, hypoxemia, or pulmonary hypertension and cardiac arrest are the major indications in this group. This group of patients is large, with reported good survival rates (60% to 70%), provided ECMO is instituted rapidly and effectively.[8-10,16,23,27]

Cardiomyopathy, Myocarditis, and Bridge to Transplantation

Patients with acute fulminant myocarditis can be managed successfully with ECMO.[5,28] Patients with fulminant myocarditis may arrive at the hospital undergoing full cardiac arrest, but more commonly they are in cardiogenic shock from an extremely low cardiac output state or they have hemodynamically significant dysrhythmias, including ventricular tachycardia or heart block. The heart is usually distended and is contracting poorly. Prompt institution of ECMO may allow sufficient resuscitation and stabilization to prevent end-organ injury and to enable the myocardium to rest while awaiting potential recovery. After ECMO is instituted, the heart must be fully decompressed, and urgent atrial septostomy or left atrial vent placement may be necessary.[4,29] The heart might not begin to eject for the first 24 to 36 hours after ECMO is started, although recovery of electrical activity within the first few hours should be expected. If recovery of ventricular ejection is not evident within 2 to 3 days, ECMO can be continued either as a bridge to heart transplantation or as a bridge to alternative longer-term support with a VAD, if feasible.[14,26,30-37] ECMO should be viewed as a short-term bridge to transplantation because of the limited donor availability and the time-related risks for complications, such as infection, bleeding, end-organ impairment, problems resulting from immobilization, and difficulties in maintaining adequate nutrition.[32,38] In our experience at Boston Children's Hospital, the median time spent on ECMO awaiting heart transplantation is currently 140 hours (range, 26 to 556 hours), and only 50% of our listed patients have been effectively bridged. In a small number of older and larger children, ECMO has been used to initially resuscitate the circulation and end-organs, and if a donor heart has not become available by day 6 or 7 of ECMO, we have successfully transitioned from ECMO to longer-term VAD. Survival for patients with acute myocarditis supported with ECMO was recently reported to be 61% using data reported to the ECMO registry of ELSO. Because ECMO can provide good survival in any patients with acute fulminant myocarditis these patients should be cared for in facilities that have an ECMO or other MCS options.

ECMO also has been used to support the failing heart after transplantation. This may be necessary immediately after transplantation because of graft failure, usually in the setting of pulmonary hypertension and acute right ventricle failure of the donor heart. ECMO also is effective in supporting the heart during periods of acute rejection.[34] The inflammation and myocardial edema are similar to that seen with fulminant myocarditis, and they lead to a similar spectrum of clinical features. ECMO allows the transplanted heart to decompress with decreased wall tension while antirejection therapy is increased. In our experience, survival to discharge for this indication is currently 64%, and the median duration of ECMO support is 4 days.

After In-Hospital Cardiac Arrest and CPR

Survival and outcome after in-hospital resuscitation of pediatric patients after a cardiac arrest continues to be extremely poor.[39-44] Even in a highly monitored and resource-intensive area such as a pediatric intensive care unit (ICU), the survival rate after cardiac arrest has been reported to be only 9% to 31%. The duration of cardiac arrest and resuscitation is also an important determinant of subsequent outcome, and a number of reports have noted a critical threshold of approximately 15 minutes.[39,40] ECMO has been successfully used to support children after prolonged periods of cardiac arrest that have been unresponsive to closed or open cardiac massage and all other usual interventions.[4,8,20,21] Again, it is important to emphasize that the underlying lesion, in conjunction with the effectiveness of CPR while instituting ECMO, is a major determinant of outcome when mechanical support is used in this setting. Although the exact place of ECMO in the CPR algorithm remains ill defined, patients with a witnessed arrest and rapid institution of effective CPR, and who have no apparent recovery of cardiac function within 5 to 10 minutes of initiating resuscitation and no contraindications, may be suitable candidates for ECMO.

Determining the relative contraindications to ECMO support during active resuscitation attempts can be difficult (Table 109-5). Although not always possible, discussions regarding the use of ECMO in certain patients should be undertaken before an event occurs. We have been able to successfully use our rapid-response ECMO system during CPR in patients with acquired and structural heart disease, and in patients with double- or single-ventricle defects. In the latter group are neonates who have had a sudden, reversible event, such as acute thrombosis and obstruction to a systemic-to-pulmonary artery shunt after a Norwood procedure, and they have been readily resuscitated with ECMO. On the other hand, patients with cavopulmonary corrections (i.e., Fontan or bidirectional Glenn anastomosis) have been difficult to resuscitate using ECMO, in part because of limitations with cannulation, and an inability to maintain adequate systemic oxygen delivery and avoid cerebral venous hypertension during CPR with chest compressions. Although we have used ECMO in the resuscitation of patients with pulmonary hypertension and patients with systemic outflow obstruction, the severe limitation to cardiac output and oxygenations during CPR in these patients has meant that their overall outcomes on ECMO have been poor because of the development of severe end-organ injury.

Historically, successes using ECMO during active resuscitation and chest compressions (E-CPR) have been reported for a small number of series.[8,20-22,45] A recent subanalysis of the ELSO Registry E-CPR data reports a 37% overall survival to discharge for patients placed on ECMO in this circumstance.[4,5] To avoid significant delays, a rapid response ECMO system has been established at some institutions.[4,21,22] The success of a rapid response system depends on a multidisciplinary approach, with equipment being immediately available, and the personnel with assigned roles being in-house, including cardiac surgery and intensive care fellows, respiratory and ECMO specialists, and trained nursing staff. At Boston Children's Hospital, a vacuum and CO_2-primed circuit using a roller pump and a 0.8- to 1.5-m^2 membrane oxygenator is available at all times and is suitable for children weighing up to approximately 15 kg. Even in older children, this circuit initially provides sufficient flow for resuscitation, stabilization, and hopefully prevention of end-organ damage, until a larger oxygenator can be spliced into the circuit. Generally, however, for older children and adults, a new circuit with a hollow-fiber membrane is used, which takes little time to de-air and

TABLE 109-5 **ECMO Support during Active Cardiopulmonary Resuscitation**

Resuscitation Event	Considerations
Indications	
Event witnessed and monitored (e.g., tamponade, arrhythmia, systemic to pulmonary artery shunt, obstruction)	In-hospital event: ICU, OR, catheterization laboratory
Immediate and effective basic life support and CPR	Effective ECMO system and resources
No response to advanced life support in 10 min	Primed circuit (vacuumed or crystalloid)
Acceptable cardiac transplant candidate (e.g., fulminant myocarditis)	Equipment and personnel immediately available
Absolute Contraindications	
Event not witnessed or monitored	Out-of-hospital arrest
Known comorbidities that preclude listing for transplantation	Other congenital or chromosomal abnormalities
	Sepsis
	Central nervous system injury
	Renal failure
Relative Contraindications	
Effective ECMO support system not established	Circuit not immediately available
Known comorbidities that preclude effective resuscitation (e.g., pulmonary hypertension, systemic in-house outflow tract obstruction, semilunar or AV valve insufficiency, hypertrophic cardiomyopathy, cavopulmonary connection)	Equipment and personnel not trained for CPR

AV, Atrioventricular; *CPR*, cardiopulmonary resuscitation; *ECMO*, extracorporeal membrane oxygenation; *ICU*, intensive care unit; *OR*, operating room.

can be established within 15 minutes. Once the patient is in stable condition with ECMO, the hollow-fiber membrane can be exchanged for a conventional membrane for longer-term support as necessary. An alternative rapid response system has been described, which uses a heparin-coated circuit, centrifugal pump, and a hollow-fiber membrane with a priming volume of only 250 mL and a priming time of only 5 minutes.

In postoperative cardiac patients, atrial and aortic cannulation via a reopened sternotomy is usually the access mode of choice. In other patients, experienced practitioners can rapidly gain access via the neck vessels. During resuscitation, the circuit is primed with crystalloid supplemented with 5% albumin. We do not wait for donor blood to be crossmatched to complete a blood prime of the circuit because of the inevitable delay. We prefer to reestablish organ perfusion as soon as possible, and once ECMO is satisfactorily established, blood products can be added or the priming crystalloid can be removed via hemofiltration. To assist with neurologic protection, where possible we maintain mild hypothermia (34° to 35° C) for the first 12 hours after administering ECMO during active resuscitation. Using the rapid response system, we can be ready to place a patient on ECMO within 15 minutes, and the main limitation is then the problems associated with cannulation. We have deployed the rapid response system during active resuscitation in more than 170 children since 1996, and we have been able to achieve a survival-to-discharge rate of 51% in this group of patients.[4]

TECHNICAL ASPECTS OF ECMO CANNULATION

Cannulation for ECMO begins with preemptive maneuvers that will ensure expedient delivery of this lifesaving measure. Prior planning is key and can ensure smooth cannulation in a situation that may be chaotic. The first step is identifying patients in unstable condition and who may require institution of ECMO. If during the evaluation of the patient by the treating team in the ICU, a patient is believed to be at risk of hemodynamic or respiratory deterioration enough to require AV or VV ECMO, then it is important to communicate with the ECMO team. This communication includes the surgeon who will be performing the procedure and the ECMO specialists who will be priming and running the circuit. This will give them time to know patient details that will help to develop a cannulation and support strategy. Heparin can be drawn up and prepared. A range of cannulas can be preselected. An appropriately sized circuit can be prepared. The blood bank can be alerted. Identifying potential ECMO patients early can also allow for calm and sober discussion about the appropriateness of the intervention.

For the cannulating surgeon, intimate knowledge of the systemic venous and arterial anatomy, especially the patency of the peripheral vessels that may be considered for access, is vital. If peripheral cannulation is to be performed, it is appropriate to have confirmatory imaging obtained beforehand. In our cardiac ICU, we maintain a sheet of paper by the bedside detailing which peripheral arterial and venous access points are patent. This sheet can prevent unnecessary delays from cutting down on a vessel that is stenosed, scarred, or not patent. For patients with congenital cardiac anomalies, it is important to know in detail the topography of the heart, the intracardiac anatomy, and systemic venous arrangement. These details can have bearing on the cannulation strategy. For example, if a patient has a single left superior vena cava (SVC), venous access should be ideally obtained in the left neck. A patient with unoperated hypoplastic left heart syndrome may occasionally need to be cannulated centrally in the duct or main pulmonary artery for arterial inflow.

Access

Cannulation access can be central or peripheral. By central cannulation, we mean access to the intrathoracic structure to cannulate. This access can be gained through a sternotomy or, less commonly, a thoracotomy. The indications for central cannulation include postcardiotomy, open chest, small neonate or infant, need for supraphysiologic flows, when peripheral access cannot sustain adequate ECMO flow, and when no other access is available. Venous drainage can be obtained via the right atrium, superior vena cava, inferior vena cava (IVC), or even the pulmonary artery. Rarely, the only access for return to the pump is from the pulmonary venous atrium. Arterial perfusion is most commonly performed into the aorta, although arch vessels can be accessed. Direct cannulation of the artery is usually performed, although if time allows, placing a graft on an arch vessel is feasible and has the advantage of minimizing the risk of occluding that vessel.

The advantages of central cannulation are that it is the easiest access after sternotomy, it provides the most reliable cannula position, it give the best venous drainage and therefore most optimal flows, it is easy to vent the left side, and it can be easily converted to cardiopulmonary bypass. The disadvantages of central cannulation are that it is labor intensive, it is better done in the operating room, it is not ideal if the chest is closed in an emergency, there may be more bleeding, and there is the risk of mediastinal infection. Central cannulation can be very difficult if a previous sternotomy was performed greater than 2 weeks prior. In this circumstance we may elect to cannulate peripherally, even in the context of recent cardiac surgery.

Peripheral cannulation is cannulation of the extra thoracic vessels. This can be performed in the neck for neonates, infants, children (including teenagers), and young adults. The subclavian and axillary vessels can be used occasionally in older patients. The other common point of access is the femoral artery and vein. Rarely, the iliac vessels, abdominal aorta, or abdominal cava may be used. The indications for peripheral cannulation include an arrest situation, a contraindication to central cannulation, and in some circumstances after cardiotomy. Contraindications to peripheral cannulation include a known small vessel and vessel stenosis or occlusion. Previous cannulation of a peripheral vessel is not an absolute contraindication to repeat access, as long as the vessels are known to be adequate in size and patent.

Access to the peripheral vasculature can be open or closed. Open technique involves a surgical cutdown to visualize the vessel directly. Indications for vessel cutdown include surgeon preference, an arrest situation, uncertainty about vessel patency, or failure of percutaneous access. The advantages of open technique include certain identification of vessels, the ability to assess the vessels, less risk of injury to the vessels and adjacent structures, and the ability to insert larger cannulas. We believe that in the context of cardiopulmonary resuscitation with ongoing cardiac massage, cutdown is the most reliable way to differentiate an artery from a vein. Both vessels may have pulsatile deoxygenated blood during cardiac massage, making needle identification unreliable. Disadvantages of the cutdown technique include the time to perform the procedure, the need for available equipment and expertise, bleeding, infection, and the potential need for secondary intervention to decannulate. Once the vessels are identified by cutdown, the cannulas can be introduced using arteriotomy and venotomy or direct Seldinger technique.

Closed access to the peripheral vessels is also referred to as *percutaneous access*. This is commonly done with the Seldinger technique. It is best performed in a patient in stable condition or during an arrest situation when the vessels have already been identified by previous vascular access. Contraindications to percutaneous access are known obstruction of the vessel, percutaneous cannulas not being available, and a small patient (neonate, infant, small child weighing < 15 kg). The advantages of closed access is that it is less technically demanding, less personnel and equipment are required, it can be faster, it is more hemostatic, and it is usually a single procedure. Disadvantages are that it is a blind technique (unless ultrasound is available); it is unreliable for distinguishing an artery from a vein with cardiac massage; it is associated with the use of smaller cannulas, which can compromise flow; it is difficult to perform in a small patient; and it makes the open technique more difficult if there is a technical failure.

Special Circumstances

Single Ventricle

Patients with single-ventricle physiology can be cannulated centrally or peripherally, depending on the circumstances. When performing the first stage of palliation, we use antegrade cerebral perfusion through a graft anastomosed end-to-side onto the innominate artery. At the end of the procedure, the graft is clipped at the base and left long. If ECMO support is needed, the graft can be cannulated for arterial inflow. It is extremely important to flush the graft to remove any debris or thrombus before placing a cannula.

Patients with a modified BT shunt may require the shunt to be clipped partially to maintain adequate perfusion pressure, while receiving ECMO. Clipping the shunt completely risks thrombosis of pulmonary arteries and lung ischemia because of unreliable bronchial circulation. Despite narrowing of the BT shunt, ECMO flows may need to be supraphysiologic to maintain adequate perfusion.

Patients with a superior cavopulmonary connection present a challenge when cannulated through the neck. Care must be taken to avoid perforating the pulmonary arteries by advancing the venous cannula too far. Obtaining sufficient venous drainage for adequate support is difficult and, therefore, additional sites for drainage may be necessary. Femoral cannulation is usually not an option when the child is small. Central cannulation may be necessary to get adequate flows.

Patients with a Fontan circulation needing ECMO may present at a wide range of ages. It is ideal to place the venous drainage cannula in the Fontan pathway. However, whether doing cervical or femoral cannulation, it may be difficult to negotiate the cannula into the pathway. Occasionally, image guidance may be necessary. The presence of aortopulmonary collaterals may require supraphysiologic flows to maintain adequate perfusion.

Femoral Cannulation

Cannulation of the femoral artery and ipsilateral vein risks ischemia of the lower extremity. One option is to cannulate the contralateral vein. If the artery and vein are cannulated on the same side, we routinely place a small distal perfusion catheter on the distal femoral artery. It may be advanced into the superficial femoral vein or the profunda femoris. An additional maneuver is to place a distal drainage cannula in the femoral vein, to avoid suffusion of the leg.

Neck Cannulation

Internal jugular venous drainage can be optimized by placement of a small catheter up toward the head for cephalic drainage. It can contribute a significant amount of venous return obviating the need for an additional cannula elsewhere. Cephalic drainage is especially important to avoid cerebral edema, if the contralateral internal jugular vein is obstructed.

Venting

It is paramount to have an adequately decompressed ventricle while receiving ECMO to maximize the chances of ventricular recovery and to avoid lung injury from left atrial hypertension. The ventricle must be able to handle the pulmonary venous return. One must always be aware that significant left atrial hypertension can occur, even in the presence of apparent ventricular contractility. However, if there is any ventricular distention by echocardiography, this should be dealt with urgently. In a child, often all that is necessary is to create or enlarge an interatrial communication, to allow left to right shunting. This can be done in the catheterization laboratory. Alternatively, a vent can be placed into the left atrium; into the ventricle across the mitral valve, or into the ventricle itself. Any of these can be done surgically during central cannulation. A vent can also be placed across an interatrial communication in the catheterization laboratory. In

TABLE 109-6 **ECMO Circuit Guidelines: Boston Children's Hospital**

	Weight (kg)					
	2-15	**16-20**	**21-35**	**36-60**	**>60**	**Stat (>15 kg)**
Circuit	Neonatal	Pediatric	Pediatric	Adult	Adult	Stat
Membrane (m^2)	0.8-1.5	2.5	3.5	4.5	4.5	Optima*
Prime						
5% albumin (mL)	50	100	100	100	100	100
Packed red blood cells (mL)	500	1000	1000	1500	1500	1000
Fresh-frozen plasma (mL)	200	400	400	500	500	400
Cryoprecipitate (U)	2	3	3	4	4	3
Platelets (U)	2	4	4	6	6	6
Medications						
Heparin (U)	500	500	500	800	800	500
THAM (mL)	100	200	300	300	300	200
Calcium gluconate (mg)	1500	3000	3000	4000	4000	3000
Flows						
Minimum (mL/min)	100	200	250	300	600	0.5
Maximum (L/min)	1.8	4.5	5.5	6.5	6.5 (ea)	8.0
Sweep gas range (L/min)	1-4.5	2-8	2-11	2-13	2-13	0.5-20
Membrane volume (mL)	174	455	575	665	1330	260
Circuit volume (mL)	580	1500	1600	2500	3200	1000

*Cobe Cardiovascular, Inc., Amada, CO.
ECMO, Extracorporeal membrane oxygenation.

children, vents are prone to thrombosis because of their small size, long length, and limited flows.

Conduct of Cannulation

ECMO cannulation is often done under emergent circumstances during a resuscitation in an ICU. It is important for the cannulating surgeon to remain calm in the face of chaos. Communication with the entire team during the procedure is key. If CPR is ongoing, it must be stopped at the request of the surgeon. Timing of heparin delivery must be communicated clearly to the ICU team by the surgeon. The surgeon communicates with the ECMO specialists regarding cannula choice and required pump flows.

The importance of adequately positioning the patient for access to the neck, chest, or groin, as necessary, cannot be overstated. Necessary equipment for the procedure must be immediately available, ideally in the ICU. A head light is invaluable, as well as operating loupes for small children. Sometimes, the surgeon will have to begin the procedure with an inexperienced assistant and without an operating room team. The surgeon must be able to direct their assistant precisely, and be very familiar with the organization of the available surgical instruments. To mitigate the stress of cannulation, simulation team training with "cannulatable" models may be helpful.

Circuit and Cannula Management

The ECMO system circuit includes a reservoir, membrane oxygenator, and heat exchanger. The ECMO and cannula guidelines used at Boston Children's Hospital are shown in Tables 109-6 and 109-7. The circuit volume can range from approximately 350 mL (in neonates) to 2 to 3 L (in adults). Before cannulation, heparin is administered and the ACT is usually maintained between 180 and 200 by continuous heparin infusion. Occasionally, the ACT is maintained at a somewhat lower level in the presence of significant bleeding. At times, large doses of drugs such as heparin, fentanyl, or midazolam may be necessary because of binding to the circuit and oxygenator, or because of dilution by bleeding. Perfusion flow rates in infants and small children typically range from 100 to 150 mL/kg/min during full circulatory support. Blood products are administered to keep the hematocrit level between 35% and 45%, typically, and the platelet count greater than 100,000/mm^3.

TABLE 109-7 **ECMO Cannula Size According to Patient Weight**

Weight (kg)	Venous (Fr)	Arterial (Fr)
2-4	8-14	8-10
5-15	15-19	12-15
16-20	19-21	15-17
21-35	21-23	17-19
35-60	23	19-21
60+	23	21

ECMO, Extracorporeal membrane oxygenation.

Arteriovenous cannulation is usually used for cardiac ECMO, although venovenous bypass can be used in patients who require ventilatory support only. In the immediate postoperative period, mediastinal cannulation, using single right atrial and ascending aortic cannulas, is often preferable because cannulation can be rapidly achieved, along with left atrial decompression if necessary. For the risk of infection to be reduced further, if possible, the skin is closed over the cannulas and the chest, or a surgical Silastic membrane is used instead. Alternatively, the internal jugular vein and carotid artery can be used, with the potential advantage of less bleeding, a more stable cannula position, and, by avoiding an open sternum, a possible reduction in the risk for infection. If neck cannulation is used, the carotid artery can be either ligated or repaired. Despite concerns about uneven cerebral blood flow, ligation seems to be surprisingly well tolerated clinically, but reconstruction requires long-term follow-up because of the increased risk of stenosis at the anastomotic site.[46,47] The femoral vessels in infants and young children might not accommodate cannulas of sufficient size to permit complete circulatory support. However, these sites have been used occasionally to provide resuscitation and stabilization in acute emergency situations (e.g., in the cardiac catheterization laboratory) or when femoral access has already been established.

Children with complex structural cardiac defects may have associated abnormalities with systemic venous damage (e.g., heterotaxy syndromes), or they may have undergone previous cardiac catheterization or interventions that have caused occlusion of femoral vessels. Therefore, their venous and arterial anatomy must be well known and well documented to prevent inappropriate cannulation attempts.

The daily management of a patient on ECMO or other forms of extracorporeal life support requires a meticulous assessment of cardiorespiratory function, end-organ perfusion and injury, evolving complications such as bleeding or sepsis, and the mechanics of the ECMO circuit.[48] If a patient fails to wean from ECMO or there is a delay in anticipated recovery of myocardial function, the possibility of a residual surgical problem must always be considered. This is usually difficult to diagnose by echocardiography alone, and cardiac catheterization (diagnostic or interventional) should be considered.

Assessing the adequacy of flow and systemic perfusion soon after initiation of ECMO is of paramount importance. Inadequate flow states or persistent hypotension despite perceived adequate flow requires immediate analysis and intervention (Table 109-8). Venous cannula malposition or inadequate size limits venous drainage if a roller pump is used, thereby contributing to circuit chatter and bladder collapse. This should be addressed immediately, and the venous cannula should be repositioned, an additional venous cannula placed, or the existing cannula upsized. When ECMO flow appears inadequate to meet the needs of the patient and limited venous drainage restricts additional flow, interpretation of arterial and atrial pressures may aid the formulation of a differential diagnosis. For example, a low atrial pressure and inadequate venous drainage may represent hypovolemia from ongoing or unrecognized bleeding. On the other hand, high atrial pressures with inadequate venous drainage may represent tamponade physiology that requires surgical exploration in a postoperative patient, or it may reflect left ventricle overdistention from inadequate decompression or aortic valve regurgitation. Elevated postmembrane pressures may reflect malposition of the arterial cannula or a cannula that is too small and needs to be revised. Elevated premembrane pressure (e.g., >350 mm Hg) at normal flows without change in postmembrane pressure, or evidence of a blood-gas leak, constitutes membrane oxygenator dysfunction and may dictate oxygenator replacement. Extensive thrombus and consumptive coagulopathy with hypofibrinogenemia and thrombocytopenia are other indications for circuit replacement.

Echocardiography, especially transesophageal (and occasionally cardiac catheterization), is used to assess cardiac structure and contractile function and to detect residual lesions and the need for left atrial decompression.[29,49] Venting the left atrium may be necessary to lower the left atrial pressure and decrease left ventricular wall stress, thereby minimizing ongoing myocardial injury. Adequate decompression can be assessed early by echocardiography and signs of pulmonary edema. Strategies to assist with decompressing the ventricle include placing a vent in the left atrium by direct placement through an open chest, a transcatheter approach in the catheterization laboratory,[29] or by creating an unrestrictive atrial septal defect via septostomy and then augmenting ventricular ejection with inotropic agents.

Once ECMO is successfully established, inotropic support is usually reduced, and vasodilators may be required to improve systemic perfusion and enable appropriate flow rates. The fraction of inspired oxygen (FiO_2) and ventilatory support also are decreased to a low respiratory rate (5 to 10 breaths/min), low peak inspiratory pressures (20 to 25 cm H_2O), and low levels of positive end-expiratory pressure to preserve lung volume and to limit inactivation of alveolar surfactant.

Considerations regarding cannulation and flow rates once the patient is receiving ECMO may be specific to the underlying cardiac defect or surgical repair. For example, the management of an aortopulmonary shunt is critical in patients with single-ventricle physiology. Systemic and pulmonary flow should be balanced by either partially clipping the shunt or using high ECMO flows. With ECMO, circuit flows up to 200 mL/kg/min (or even greater) are usually necessary to maintain adequate systemic perfusion while accounting for runoff into the

TABLE 109-8 Causes of Inadequate ECMO Flow and Perfusion

	Cannula	Anatomic	Physiologic
Inadequate venous drainage	Too small Malpositioned Air occlusion	Heterotaxy syndromes Vessel occlusion or stenosis	Hypovolemia Tamponade Nonvented, distended ventricle
Inadequate systemic perfusion	Too small (high postmembrane pressure) Malpositioned Occlusion	Aortic valve regurgitation Vessel stenosis	Systemic vasoconstriction or vasodilation

ECMO, Extracorporeal membrane oxygenation.

pulmonary circulation through the shunt. Although partial temporary narrowing of the shunt may be advisable in some circumstances, it is unwise to completely occlude the only source of pulmonary blood flow to the pulmonary endothelium. It is possible to bypass the membrane oxygenator in patients after the Norwood procedure with a modified Blalock-Taussig shunt in patients without lung disease if higher flows are maintained and the shunt is patent.[50] This maneuver simplifies the circuit and can permit the use of less of heparin. ECMO thus effectively becomes a VAD.

Problems related to cannula placement and adequacy of venous drainage may be particularly evident in patients with complex venous anatomy, such as heterotaxy syndrome, and in patients with a cavopulmonary connection. The site of cannulation is affected by vessel patency, and the underlying physiology might influence the number of venous cannulas used. For example, patients with a superior cavopulmonary anastomosis (bidirectional Glenn shunt) as the primary source of pulmonary blood flow frequently require separate venous drainage of the SVC and IVC, unless there is congenital interruption of the infrahepatic IVC with drainage of lower body blood to the azygos vein. In the latter case, a single venous cannula in the SVC might be sufficient. On the other hand, placement of a cannula in the SVC may be detrimental in patients with bidirectional Glenn shunt physiology because of the potential for reduced cerebral venous drainage and therefore decreased cerebral perfusion. This is also a concern for patients with Fontan physiology; although it may be possible to achieve adequate drainage with a venous cannula placed in the Fontan baffle, an additional SVC catheter is often necessary to achieve the desired or necessary flow rates on ECMO.[51]

Weaning from Extracorporeal Membrane Oxygenation

The strategies for weaning from cardiac ECMO are often quite different from those used to wean patients who are receiving ECMO for respiratory support. For patients with structurally normal hearts who require ECMO support for respiratory illness, the ability to wean depends on resolution of the primary pulmonary process, often with little need for support of the myocardium beyond moderate inotropic support, fluid and electrolyte management, and nutritional support. Once lung compliance and gas exchange are normalized, improvement of the lungs on the chest radiograph is apparent, and a stable circulation with sufficient negative fluid balance has been achieved, the patient is sedated, paralyzed, and fully ventilated, and the ECMO circuit is clamped.

Before weaning a patient from ECMO used for circulatory support, an understanding of the underlying cardiac physiology and cardiorespiratory interactions and an appreciation for the expected range of oxygen saturation levels are important. Because of the increased risk of complications and mortality in patients with cardiac disease when the duration of MCS extends beyond 7 days, consideration as to when and how to wean cardiac patients from ECMO should begin once circulatory stability has been established. The disease process and circumstances resulting in hemodynamic failure or cardiac arrest can influence the expected duration of mechanical support. For example, patients who fail to separate from CPB after cardiac surgery as a result of severe pulmonary hypertension usually respond to a period of 24 to 48 hours on ECMO with inhaled nitric oxide (NO) therapy and inotropic support of the right side of the heart. Similarly, patients who have a low cardiac output state or suffer cardiac arrest after cardiac surgery may have residual defects that allow rapid weaning and decannulation soon after reoperation. The likelihood of recovery of ventricular function should be decided within the first 48 to 72 hours so that cardiac transplantation status can be ascertained. ECMO instituted for catheter intervention or arrhythmia ablation procedures may be discontinued within hours of patient cannulation.[52] In contrast, patients with severe cardiomyopathies or those awaiting heart transplantation may require mechanical assistance for a much longer period. Patients with severe bronchiolitis because of respiratory syncytial virus complicating repair of congenital heart disease on CPB typically require 2 to 3 weeks of ECMO support for respiratory failure.

Patients requiring cardiovascular support with ECMO are partially weaned within the first 48 hours for assessment of myocardial function by echocardiography and hemodynamic evaluation. An acceptable PaO_2 obtained while the ECMO circuit is clamped varies substantially according to the underlying anatomy and pathophysiology. If transthoracic cannulation was used and problems with bleeding were encountered during the ECMO run, the mediastinum may require exploration before or during the weaning process. If only a short period of reconditioning of the myocardium is anticipated, the patient is frequently sedated and paralyzed, dopamine infusion is increased to 5 to 10 mg/kg/min, intravascular volume status is optimized, and ventilator settings are adjusted according to lung compliance and expected arterial O_2 saturation. ECMO flow is decreased by 25% to 50% over a period of time until the circuit is clamped. Volume is infused to achieve appropriate preload. Echocardiographic assessment of ventricular systolic function, valvular function, systemic and pulmonary outflow obstruction, and location and direction of intracardiac shunts is useful before weaning, as well as if there is a change in hemodynamics after the circuit has been clamped. Arterial blood gases, serum lactate levels, and systemic and mixed venous oxygen saturation levels are important guides to the stability of the circulation, ventilation, and adequacy of perfusion after the circuit has been clamped. Decannulation from ECMO is undertaken once the patient has maintained a stable circulation and acceptable gas exchange for a period of up to 4 hours.

INTRA-AORTIC BALLOON COUNTERPULSATION

Intra-aortic balloon pump (IABP) counterpulsation is commonly used for the treatment of myocardial failure in adults, especially in the postoperative period. When used in infants and children, however, results have been disappointing, with survival rates of less than 50%.[53-55] Many factors contribute to the reduced efficacy in children. Heart failure in pediatric patients is often caused by either right ventricular or biventricular dysfunction, conditions in which the IABP is not effective. Placement of an IABP in the pulmonary artery has been reported but is usually challenging, in part because of the small balloon size required and the increased compliance of the pulmonary artery.[56,57] The relatively rapid heart rate of infants and small children and the variable delay between aortic valve closure and the appearance of the arterial tracing on the oscilloscope make effective timing of inflation and deflation more difficult. At heart rates greater than 160 beats/min, the IABP is often reduced to a 1 : 2 or even 1 : 4 pumping frequency to facilitate cycle timing, at the same time decreasing the effectiveness to 50% to 80%.[58,59] The aorta is typically more distensible in both infants and children; therefore, both coronary flow augmentation during diastole (balloon inflation) and afterload reduction during systole (balloon deflation) are likely to be less. In addition, the effect of diastolic augmentation on normal coronaries, prevailing in the pediatric population, has been questioned.[60,61] Severe cyanotic heart disease in children can be accompanied by extensive aortopulmonary collateral vessels, which permit shunting of blood into the pulmonary circulation during balloon inflation, thus reducing augmentation of coronary blood flow.

The smallest balloon system available for children is 2.5 mL, which can be used for neonates as small as 2 kg. In general, for children weighing less than 30 kg, a balloon volume of 0.5 mL/kg is recommended. For balloon inflation, helium is preferred over CO_2, as it allows a faster pneumatic response because of its low density. Interestingly, the incidence of vascular complications, such as bleeding, emboli, or limb ischemia, correlates well with the adult population, where it is reported in 10% to 20% of cases. Other potential complications are infection, renal dysfunction, mesenteric occlusion or embolism, and cerebrovascular accidents.[62,63]

Numerous technical improvements have been made to enhance efficacy in the pediatric population. These improvements include modified pumping consoles and small-sized catheters, improved tracking at higher heart rates, more rapid inflation and deflation, and the use of M-mode echocardiography for cycle timing.[64] Further study is necessary to evaluate the importance and continued role of IABP support for pediatric patients, particularly in the face of growing availability of other modes of circulatory support.

VENTRICULAR ASSIST DEVICES

The experience with VADs in infants and children remains relatively small when compared with that in adults, but it has been growing steadily over the last 5 years. As with adult patients, VAD support is useful as a bridge to transplantation, and it allows recovery of end-organ function, elimination of edema, and improvement in nutrition, and it provides rehabilitation of critically ill patients. An important component of these benefits is the ability of the device to allow extubation and ambulation, which cannot be accomplished currently with ECMO and centrifugal VADs.

The main problem in adapting the VADs used for adult patients had been size limitations and flow requirements; the risk for thromboembolic complications increases with lower flow. In pediatric patients, the selection of pump sizes carries particular importance. A pump that is too small can result in less than adequate cardiac output, and when run at higher rates, it risks inducing significant hemolysis. However, if the pump is too large and is then run at rates too slow, it can result in increased risk of thrombus formation and can be associated with persistent systemic hypertension.

In addition to the obvious variability in size, there are other factors that provide distinct differences between adult and pediatric recipients. These factors include the anatomic variations that are encountered in complex congenital heart disease, the potential of growth, and the unique susceptibility to anticoagulation that children can exhibit. Because of these differences, VAD therapy in children imposes unique challenges that must be anticipated with its application.[65]

As with ECMO, the selection of appropriate candidates for VAD therapy is crucial, and surgical problems or residual defects should be excluded where possible. Whereas ECMO can be instituted by peripheral cannulation of neck or femoral vessels, the currently available VADs require direct cannulation of the heart through a sternotomy. The reported survival rates with VADs are similar to those achieved with cardiac ECMO,[12,26,66,67] and left VADs (LVADs), right VADs (RVADs), or dual-support VADs (biVADs) can successfully support the circulation, depending on the circumstances. The majority of reported pediatric patients have received LVADs, which have been particularly beneficial in patients with decompensated cardiomyopathy, an ischemic myocardium secondary to an anomalous origin of left coronary artery from the pulmonary artery, and for "retraining" of the poorly prepared left ventricle after an arterial switch procedure.[68-70] There are also increasing numbers of case reports describing the use of VAD support in patients with complex congenital heart disease such as single ventricles, including the Fontan circulation (Fig. 109-2).[71,72]

The advantages of the VAD circuit over ECMO are that the former is relatively simple in design, takes less time to prime, and requires little technical assistance once established. Bleeding complications and requirements for blood products and platelet transfusions are generally less in patients on VADs compared with those on ECMO.[12,47] Requirement for heparinization and maintaining a prolonged ACT is proportionately less. Because of the lower complication rate, a VAD is more suitable for long-term support as a bridge to transplantation.[11,12,73]

Another possible advantage of VADs is superior left ventricular drainage and unloading, a prerequisite for myocardial rest and potential recovery.[11,47,74] While adequate ventilation of the left atrium on ECMO is possible, it does not provide equivalent ventricular decompression when compared with a VAD. Whenever a patient is connected to a VAD, the response of the

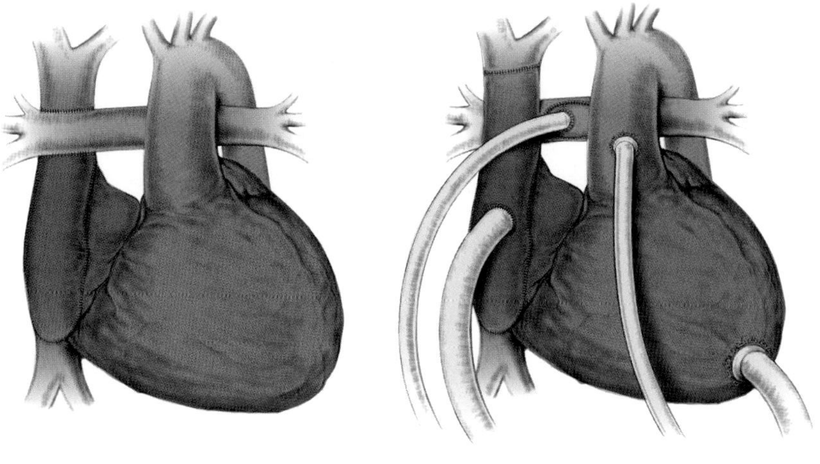

FIGURE 109-2 ■ Use of a ventricular assist device after a Fontan operation.

unsupported ventricle must be closely monitored. Ideally, the reduction in left atrial pressure during LVAD support, associated with adequate decompression of the left ventricle, reduces pulmonary venous and arterial pressures and improves right ventricular function. Unfortunately, based on adult data, right ventricular failure can still develop in up to 25% of patients, especially in LVAD-supported patients with ischemic myocardium, with preexisting anatomic defects, or after prolonged bypass procedures.[75-77]

Nonpulsatile Devices

Early in the pediatric VAD experience, most VADs for small children were nonpulsatile systems, either roller pumps or a centrifugal pump such as the Bio-Medicus circuit (Medtronic; Bio-Medicus, Minneapolis, MN). Although these pumps are now mostly of historical value, excellent results were reported using them to support infants and children (<6 kg).[42] The centrifugal pump, in which blood is entrained by creating a vortex using spinning cones, is highly sensitive to changes in preload and systemic resistance. This is useful when adapting inotropic support or afterload reduction in preparation for weaning. Furthermore, the pump is designed to create constant flow rather than pressure, so the risk of accidental line disruption is reduced. The Bio-Medicus centrifugal pump can be used in infants and older children, and because gravity is not needed to achieve venous drainage, the pump housing can be placed close to the patient and is readily portable.

In 2004, the DeBakey VAD Child (Micromed Technology, Houston, TX) became the first VAD to receive U.S. Food and Drug Administration (FDA) humanitarian device exemption approval for use in children (with a body surface area [BSA] of 0.7 to 1.5 m^2). It is a fully implantable axial flow pump that is electromechanically coupled to its power source. The inlet flow is achieved by apical ventricular cannulation with outlet cannulation of the ascending or descending aorta. Early results for the device had been mixed and the experience is still limited. Hemolysis is a concern with axial flow and roller pumps, and this possible complication needs to be monitored closely.[78,79] Other devices, such as the PediVas (Levitronix Centrimag and Maquet Rotaflow), and more minimally invasive devices (e.g., the Tandem Heart) and impeller-type pumps (e.g., the Impella VAD) are currently under evaluation in pediatric patients, mostly as temporary devices as a bridge to decision or bridge to recovery.

Pulsatile Devices

Several pulsatile devices (both paracorporeal and implantable) used in adult patients have been adapted for use in older children (BSA > 1.2 m^2) to achieve a flow rate of at least 2 L/min. Successful use of the HeartMate LVAD (Thermocardiosystems, Woburn, MA) has been reported in adolescents with a BSA ranging from 1.4 to 2.2 m^2.[80] The implantation of the paracorporeal Thoratec VAD (Thoratec Laboratories, Berkeley, CA) has been used extensively in teenagers and has been reported in children as young as 11 years.[81] Other such paracorporeal devices include the Abiomed AB 5000. In our experience at Boston Children's Hospital, the smallest patient to undergo implantation of this device had a BSA of 1.3 m^2. The reported incidence of thromboembolic events with the adult devices is higher in the pediatric population than in the adult population.

The Berlin Heart VAD (Berlin Heart AG, Berlin, Germany) and the Medos HIA-VAD (Medos Medizintechnik AG, Stolberg, Germany) are paracorporeal pneumatic devices for longer-term support in infants and small children.[73,82-85] Both are produced in various sizes. Both are pneumatically driven pumps that can deliver varying stroke volumes that can be matched to even the smallest pediatric patients. A measured amount of compressed air is delivered through a pneumatic line that then compresses the ventricular chamber or bladder, thereby enforcing ejection of blood. Diastolic pump filling is achieved with gravity or gentle suction. Because of the high resistance of the small-bore cannulas, positive systolic pressures of up to 350 mm Hg and negative suction of 100 mm Hg at pumping rates of up to 140 beats/min may be necessary, increasing the power requirements for the driving unit considerably, compared with adult devices. Polyurethane trileaflet valves with low transvalvular pressure gradients and rapid closure, as well

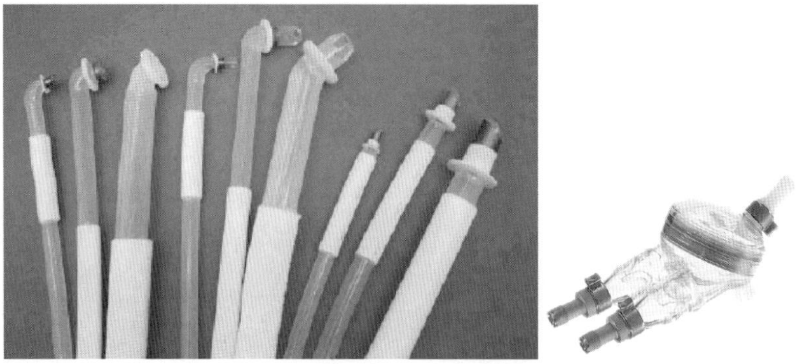

FIGURE 109-3 ■ The Berlin Heart Excor ventricular assist device.

as the use of heparin-coated (Carmeda) systems, reduce the thromboembolic risk, one of the major problems associated with VADs in children.[86]

Berlin Heart

The Berlin Heart Excor VAD (Berlin Heart AG) was the first commercially available ventricular assist system designed specifically for pediatric patients. First developed in Germany, it has been the paracorporeal device most frequently implanted in children in the United States. The Excor pediatric VAD is an extracorporeal, pneumatically driven, pulsatile VAD designed to support the right or left ventricle (or both) synchronously or asynchronously. Cannulas connect the blood pumps to the atrium or ventricle and to the great arteries, and an electropneumatic driving unit provides alternating air pressure to the blood pumps through drive lines (Fig. 109-3). The blood pump is divided into an air chamber and a blood chamber by a polyurethane membrane, and pulses of air pressure move the membrane, allowing both filling and emptying of the blood chamber. Polyurethane valves are located at the inlet and outlet positions of the blood pump, thus ensuring unidirectional blood flow. The blood pumps are available in six different sizes, with stroke volumes of 10, 25, 30, 50, and 60 mL that can be matched for all patient ages and sizes (Fig. 109-4).

Being a pulsatile and mobile support system, the Berlin Heart enables patients to be extubated from mechanical ventilation, to discontinue sedative and paralytic drugs, and to transition to enteral nutrition. A major benefit is the improvement in end-organ function, particularly renal and gut function and, in many cases, patients can be ambulatory. This benefit is particularly important because patients are able to undergo cardiac transplantation in a much better overall condition, which hastens their subsequent recovery after heart transplantation.[87]

The device was first approved in Europe in the 1990s, and experience suggests that the Berlin Heart can provide effective ventricular support for a number of months in children as small as 3 kg. The North American experience dates back to 2000, when the first implantation was performed at the University of Arizona. In early 2007, a multicenter North American trial evaluating the Berlin Heart Excor Pediatric VAD was initiated. The 12-center study, which included two Canadian centers, was designed to provide basic safety information needed to support FDA approval of the device under a formal investigational device exemption status. This clinical trial was a prospective, multicenter, single-group cohort study comparing children who had implantation of the Excor Pediatric VAD (Berlin Heart) as a bridge to transplantation, with a historical control group of children who received circulatory support with ECMO. Forty-eight Berlin Heart patients were matched with 48 patients from the ELSO Registry. The Berlin Heart patients were divided equally into two cohorts: cohort 1 with BSA < $0.7\ m^2$ and cohort 2 with BSA of 0.7 to $1.5\ m^2$. For cohort 1, the median time to death or weaning from the device with unacceptable neurologic outcome had not been reached at 174 days. By contrast, the matched ECMO group median time to death was 13 days. For cohort 2, the median time was 144 days, and the matched ECMO group was 10 days. For cohort 1, at 174 days, 88% had undergone transplantation and 12% had died or had an unacceptable neurologic outcome after device wean. In the matched ECMO group for cohort 1, 35% had died at 21 days and none were alive receiving support. For cohort 2, at 192 days, 92% had undergone transplantation or weaning from device, while 8% had died. In the matched ECMO group for cohort 2, 33% had died at 30 days and none were alive on support. Serious adverse events included major bleeding (cohort 1, 42% and cohort 2, 50%); infection (63% and 50%, respectively); and stroke (29%, in each). Although not a randomized trial, this study demonstrated that survival to transplant

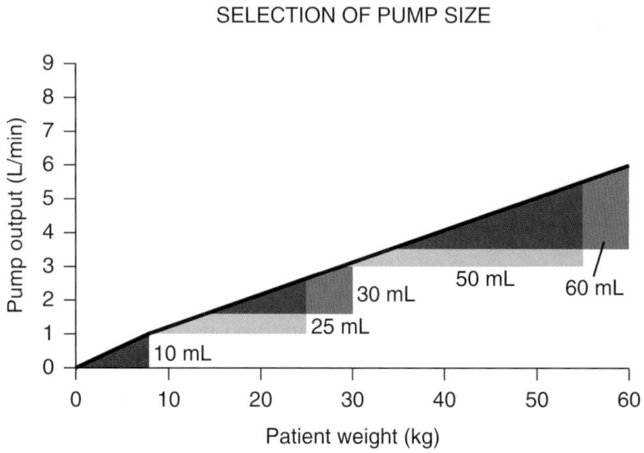

FIGURE 109-4 ■ Selection of pump size matched to patient weight for the Berlin Heart.

or recovery was better with a VAD compared with ECMO. Nevertheless, the rate of complications with the Berlin Heart was significant. Most concerning was the 29% stroke rate. The device received humanitarian device exemption approval in December 2011.

Although the Berlin Heart is currently the most widely used pediatric VAD available for longer-term support of the circulation in children, a number of alternative devices now under investigation will increase the treatment options and, it is hoped, improve outcomes for children with acute and chronic heart failure. There are also a multitude of other MCS devices that are being used in children with increasing frequency through other regulatory pathways. The FDA permits VAD implantation in children under the following pathways: (1) off-label use of an otherwise FDA-approved adult device, (2) compassionate use of investigational adult devices, (3) emergency use of investigational device on a case-by-case basis, and (4) use of a device fabricated from FDA-approved components (e.g., ECMO circuits). Once medical devices are approved for use in adults, they can then be used in children depending on how the device is labeled (i.e., whether there is a specific weight, size or age restriction listed for the device). Currently approved VADs in adults have no restriction specifically outlined for age or size; therefore, they can be used in children. Off-label use of medical devices is a common occurrence in the field of pediatric MCS. It entails the use of a device outside the population or purpose for which the device's safety and efficacy profile was originally evaluated. For short-term support (temporary MCS), the following devices have been used in children: the TandemHeart (Cardiac Assist, Inc., Pittsburgh, PA) percutaneous VAD, the Rotaflow (Maquet Medical Systems, Wayne, NJ), the Centrimag (Thoratec Corporation, Pleasanton, MA), and the Abiomed Impella 2.5/5.0 (Abiomed, Inc., Danvers, MA). For long-term support (durable MCS), the following devices have been used primarily in larger children and adolescents: the HeartMate II (Thoratec Corporation), the HeartWare HVAD (HeartWare, Inc., Framingham, MA), and the Syncardia Total Artificial Heart (TAH; Syncardia Systems, Inc., Tucson, AZ).

Recognizing that pediatric mechanical support represents an unmet need in the United States, the National Heart Lung and Blood Institute (NHLBI) under its Pediatric Circulatory Support initiative, awarded five contracts in 2004, exceeding $20 million, to support the preclinical development of innovative circulatory support devices designed specifically for infants and smaller children.[88] As a follow-up to its Pediatric Circulatory Support Program initiative, the NHLBI awarded four contracts totaling $23.6 million in January 2010 to begin preclinical testing of devices to help children with congenital heart defects or those who develop heart failure. The 4-year program is called *Pumps for Kids, Infants, and Neonates (PumpKIN)*. It includes three of the original five contractors from the previous 2004 NHLBI Pediatric Circulatory Support Program and another. As such, the PumpKIN program is the next phase of NHLBI support for the development and clinical realization of novel pediatric circulatory support devices. The program's goal is to complete the needed investigational device exemption clinical studies for some of the new investigational pediatric circulatory support devices.

EXPANDING VAD SUPPORT TO CHALLENGING PEDIATRIC POPULATIONS

Single-Ventricle Anatomy and Ventricular Assist Device Support

Improvement in preoperative, perioperative, and postoperative management of patients with congenital heart disease (CHD) has resulted in dramatic increase in long-term survival. Life expectancy for children with most types of congenital heart lesions is comparable to the general population; however, there is a subset of CHD—namely single ventricle anatomy—in which long-term mortality and morbidity into adulthood remains unacceptably high. This growing population of failed single ventricle palliations will benefit from effective mechanical support as a bridge to transplantation or even destination therapy; however, to date this endeavor has been disappointing, with higher mortality and morbidity reported in a variety of single-center experiences. The unnatural history of Fontan (total cavopulmonary connection) circulation is that of progressive systemic venous congestion with the sequelae of protein-losing enteropathy, renal, hepatic and intestinal congestion. The pathways of deterioration can vary and include systemic systolic ventricular dysfunction with low cardiac output and elevated left atrial pressures or diastolic ventricular dysfunction with elevated ventricular end-diastolic pressures resulting in elevated Fontan pressures. Pure systolic ventricular dysfunction can be managed successfully with implantation of a VAD. In situation of diastolic dysfunction or restrictive physiology in addition to decreased systolic function, a continuous-flow pump may be superior by providing continuous unloading of the pulmonary venous system.

Options to unload the systemic venous system in failed Fontan circulation include (1) revision of the Fontan pathway with creation of a larger systemic venous capacitance chamber and insertion of cannula to an extracorporeal device (Berlin Heart EXCOR or centrifugal pump), or (2) takedown of the Fontan back to Glenn (bidirectional cavopulmonary anastomosis) and implantation of systemic VAD. This last option provides better unloading of the infradiaphragmatic circulation, at the cost of lower oxygen saturations and risk of paradoxic emboli. There is also the possibility that a systemic VAD in patients with preserved systolic function but elevated end-diastolic pressures and consequently pulmonary venous congestion may be beneficial in lowering left atrial pressures and alleviating symptoms of Fontan failure. Even a marginal decrease in left atrial pressures may be sufficient to decrease Fontan pressures and improve systemic venous congestion. As device technology improves—with lower adverse event profile and better compatibility with activities of daily living—VADs may soon prove to be adjunctive therapy in protein-losing enteropathy refractory to maximal medical therapy.

Posttransplant Graft Failure and Ventricular Assist Device Support

Cardiac graft failure can manifest either early (<30 days) or late after transplantation because of variable causes. Current strategies to increase the donor pool—including the use of marginal donors[28] and desensitization with human leukocyte antigen–incompatible donor[28]—may be increasing the risk of posttransplant graft failure.

ECMO has been the mainstay of MCS strategies for graft dysfunction, providing complete respiratory and cardiac support, allowing for recovery or preservation of end-organ function. However, ECMO is limited in its duration of support to weeks and fraught with bleeding, thrombotic, and infectious complications that increase exponentially over time. As such, intermediate to long-term MCS strategies have been attempted with guarded success. The challenges of MCS in graft failure are multifaceted and include redo sternotomy, increased risk of infection and poor wound healing in the setting of continued immunosuppression, progressive biventricular dysfunction with polyvalvar involvement, and arrhythmia. Thus, standard LVAD support is generally not successful, with most patients requiring biventricular support. As such, many believe that total extraction of the graft with implantation of a total artificial heart, the Syncardia TAH (Syncardia Systems, Inc., Tucson, AZ), may be an advantageous support strategy, as it obviates the need for continued immunosuppression. Currently, the TAH is not applicable for use in most children, as the two 70-cc pneumatically driven pumps for right and left heart support require a minimum anterior-posterior chest diameter of 10 cm at the level of thoracic vertebra 10 (T10) to fit. However, a 50-cc Syncardia TAH pump has been developed with a lower size range of 1 m^2 BSA which may have a wider applicability to the pediatric population.

Destination Ventricular Assist Device Therapy in Children

Destination therapy (DT) is the use of a VAD as a primary therapeutic option when heart transplantation is contraindicated or not desired. The landmark Randomized Evaluation of Mechanical Assistance in the Treatment of Congestive Heart Failure (REMATCH) trial in adults demonstrated that the implantation of LVADs for DT was superior to standard medical therapy in patients with end-stage heart failure who were not eligible for transplantation.[32] Now, more than a decade after this trial, the use of VADs as DT in adults is an accepted therapy to improve quality of life.[33,34]

Based on the success of DT in adults, it is not surprising that this indication is now being more widely considered for children. However, the ability to offer DT remains restricted to children who are large enough to use the currently available intracorporeal devices suitable for outpatient care. Patient selection for this type of therapy will be of paramount importance, and likely an evolving process. Children who may benefit from DT include those with Duchene muscular dystrophy with cardiomyopathy, chemotoxicity induced cardiomyopathy with ongoing malignancy or unlikely long-term remission, complex palliated CHD with multiple comorbidities, retransplant graft dysfunction in the setting of noncompliance, and cardiac dysfunction in the setting of neurological impairment or uncertain neurodevelopmental outcomes. There have been reported cases of LVAD implantation for Duchene Muscular Dystrophy (MD),[35] and it is expected that this will continue to grow because of strong advocacy by the patients and their families.

Pediatric DT programs are now emerging in North America. DT VAD programs mandate the integrated services of an extensive and dedicated multidisciplinary team, with heavy involvement of psychology, social work, occupational and physiotherapy, in addition to nursing and medical support. Perhaps the most important aspect of DT is outlining the expectations of what VAD therapy may offer the patients and their families prior to device implantation. Ultimately, the goal of DT is not only to prolong life, but to improve the quality of life for the patient and family. The use of VADs for DT in children will continue to evolve as device technology improves, narrowing the gap between quality of life and survival outcomes for VADs and heart transplantation. Commensurate with the advancement in device technology, we, as a field in pediatric advanced cardiac support, will need to keep pace with the ethical implications and clinical challenges of altering the natural history of life limiting conditions by acknowledging the benefits and critically evaluating the consequences.

LONGER-TERM OUTCOMES FROM MECHANICAL SUPPORT IN CHILDREN

Formal, prospective evaluation of the longer-term outcomes for children receiving mechanical support of the circulation has not been undertaken. Despite the successful deployment of mechanical support to enable cardiac recovery and discharge from hospital, longer-term cardiac function and the functional status of patients should be determined. In addition to cardiac status, end-organ injury and residual deficits need to be evaluated, particularly neurologic outcomes.[45] The ELSO Registry data indicate a combined neurologic complication rate of 26% in all patients receiving cardiac ECMO, with seizures being the most common neurologic event (9.5%). In a recent retrospective report of outcomes for infants supported with ECMO after cardiotomy (median follow-up, 55 months), only 50% of survivors were determined to have no motor or cognitive deficit of any sort.[89] As waiting times for cardiac transplantation increase as a result of the increasing number of potential recipients, the need for device options that can provide extended durations of support is more pressing than ever. Longer-term VAD support often allows patients to be bridged more effectively to transplantation than on continuous inotropic support. A multi-institutional retrospective analysis from the Pediatric Heart Transplant Study examined the outcomes in nearly 100 children supported with a variety of

VADs while awaiting transplantation from 1993 to 2003.[90] In the study, overall, three quarters of the children survived to transplantation—a figure that improved to 85% in the more recent era and is comparable to outcomes reported in adults. Notably, the wait-list survival with mechanical support exceeded that of patients who were supported on maximal medical therapy.

Concurrently with the Pediatric Circulatory Support initiative from the NHLBI in 2004, the National Institutes of Health also sponsored the creation of the Interagency Registry for Mechanically Assisted Circulatory Support (INTERMACS). This registry is being designed to have a dedicated pediatric arm that will collect both retrospective and prospective data and will hopefully facilitate the eventual approval of pediatric devices in the United States.

As the technology and indications for mechanical support of the circulation in children continue to evolve and advance, simultaneous outcome studies will be essential to allow us to make better decisions about available mechanical support options for children.

REFERENCES

1. Duncan BW, editor: *Mechanical support for cardiac and respiratory failure in pediatric patients*, New York, 2001, Marcel Dekker.
2. Kern F, Schulman SR, Darling EM, et al: Extracorporeal circulation and circulatory assist devices in the pediatric patient. In Lake C, editor: *Pediatric cardiac anesthesia*, Stamford, Conn, 1998, Appleton & Lange, pp 219–257.
3. Zwischenberger JB, Bartlett RH, editors: *ECMO. Extracorporeal cardiopulmonary support in critical care*, Ann Arbor, MI, 1995, Extracorporeal Life Support Organization.
4. Thiagarajan RR, Laussen PC, Rycus PT, et al: Extracorporeal membrane oxygenation to aid cardiopulmonary resuscitation in Kane DA, Thiagarajan RR, Wypij D, Scheurer MA, Fynn-Thompson F, Emani S, del Nido PJ, Betit P, Laussen PC. Rapid-response extracorporeal membrane oxygenation to support cardiopulmonary resuscitation in children with cardiac disease. *Circulation* 122(11 Suppl):S241–S248, 2010.
5. Extracorporeal Life Support Organization: *ECLS registry report: international summary*, Ann Arbor, 2013, Extracorporeal Life Support Organization, pp 1–30.
6. Kennaugh JM, Kinsella JP, Abman SH, et al: Impact of new treatments for neonatal pulmonary hypertension on extracorporeal membrane oxygenation use and outcome. *J Perinatol* 17(5):366–369, 1997.
7. Wilson JM, Bower LK, Thompson JE, et al: ECMO in evolution: the impact of changing patient demographics and alternative therapies on ECMO. *J Pediatr Surg* 31(8):1116–1122, discussion 1122–1123, 1996.
8. Aharon AS, Drinkwater DC, Churchwell KB, et al: Extra-corporeal membrane oxygenation in children after repair of congenital cardiac lesions. *Ann Thorac Surg* 72:2095–2102, 2001.
9. Black MD, Coles JG, Williams WG, et al: Determinants of success in pediatric cardiac patients undergoing extracorporeal membrane oxygenation. *Ann Thorac Surg* 60(1):133–138, 1995.
10. del Nido PJ: Extracorporeal membrane oxygenation for cardiac support in children. *Ann Thorac Surg* 61:336–339, 1996.
11. Duncan BW: Mechanical circulatory support for infants and children with cardiac disease. *Ann Thorac Surg* 73:1670–1677, 2002.
12. Karl TR: Extracorporeal circulatory support in infants and children. *Semin Thorac Cardiovasc Surg* 6(3):154–160, 1994.
13. Khan A, Gazzaniga AB: Mechanical circulatory assistance in paediatric patients with cardiac failure. *Cardiovasc Surg* 4(1):43–49, 1996.
14. Kirshbom PM, Bridges ND, Myung RJ, et al: Use of extracorporeal membrane oxygenation in pediatric thoracic organ transplantation. *J Thorac Cardiovasc Surg* 123:130–136, 2002.
15. Klein MD, Shaheen KW, Wittlesby GC, et al: Extracorporeal membrane oxygenation for the circulatory support of children after repair of congenital heart disease. *J Thorac Cardiovasc Surg* 100(4):498–505, 1990.
16. Kulik TJ, Moler FW, Palmisaro JM, et al: Outcome-associated factors in pediatric patients treated with extracorporeal membrane oxygenator after cardiac surgery. *Circulation* 94(Suppl 9):II63–II68, 1996.
17. Pennington DG, Swartz MT: Circulatory support in infants and children. *Ann Thorac Surg* 55(1):233–237, 1993.
18. Raithel SC, Pennington DG, Boegner E, et al: Extracorporeal membrane oxygenation in children after cardiac surgery. *Circulation* 86(Suppl 5):II305–II310, 1992.
19. Sidiropoulos A, Hotz H, Konertz W: Pediatric circulatory support. *J Heart Lung Transplant* 17(12):1172–1176, 1998.
20. del Nido PJ, Dalton HJ, Thompson AE, et al: Extracorporeal membrane oxygenator rescue in children during cardiac arrest after cardiac surgery. *Circulation* 86(Suppl 5):II300–II304, 1992.
21. Duncan BW, Ibrahim AE, Hraska V, et al: Use of rapid-deployment extracorporeal membrane oxygenation for the resuscitation of pediatric patients with heart disease after cardiac arrest. *J Thorac Cardiovas Surg* 116(2):305–311, 1998.
22. Jacobs JP, Ojito JW, McConaghey TW, et al: Rapid cardiopulmonary support for children with complex congenital heart disease. *Ann Thorac Surg* 70:742–750, 2000.
23. Walters HL, 3rd, Hakimi M, Rice MD, et al: Pediatric cardiac surgical ECMO: multivariate analysis of risk factors for hospital death. *Ann Thorac Surg* 60(2):329–336, discussion 336–337, 1995.
24. Hunkeler NM, Center CE, Donze A, et al: Extracorporeal life support in cyanotic congenital heart disease before cardiovascular operation. *Am J Cardiol* 69(8):790–793, 1992.
25. Ishino K, Alexi-Meskishvili V, Hetzer R: Preoperative extracorporeal membrane oxygenation in newborns with total anomalous pulmonary venous connection. *Cardiovasc Surg* 7(4):473–475, 1999.
26. Duncan BW, Hraska V, Jonas RA, et al: Mechanical circulatory support in children with cardiac disease. *J Thorac Cardiovasc Surg* 117(3):529–542, 1999.
27. Rogers AJ, Trento A, Siewers RD, et al: Extracorporeal membrane oxygenation for postcardiotomy cardiogenic shock in children. *Ann Thorac Surg* 47(6):903–906, 1989.
28. Duncan BW, Bohn DJ, Atz AM, et al: Mechanical circulatory support for the treatment of children with acute fulminant myocarditis. *J Thorac Cardiovasc Surg* 122:440–448, 2001.
29. Booth KL, Roth SJ, Perry SB, et al: Cardiac catheterization of patients supported by extracorporeal membrane oxygenation. *J Am Coll Cardiol* 40:1681–1686, 2002.
30. Dalton HJ, Siewers RD, Fuhrman BP, et al: Extracorporeal membrane oxygenation for cardiac rescue in children with severe myocardial dysfunction. *Crit Care Med* 21(7):1020–1028, 1993.
31. del Nido PJ, Armitage JM, Fricker FJ, et al: Extracorporeal membrane oxygenation support as a bridge to pediatric heart transplantation. *Circulation* 90(5 Pt 2):II66–II69, 1994.
32. Delius RE: As originally published in 1990: prolonged extracorporeal life support of pediatric and adolescent cardiac transplant patients. Updated in 1998. *Ann Thorac Surg* 65(3):877–878, 1998.
33. Gajarski RJ, Mosca RS, Ohye RG, et al: Use of extracorporeal life support as a bridge to pediatric cardiac transplantation. *J Heart Lung Transplant* 22:28–34, 2003.
34. Galantowicz ME, Stolar CJ: Extracorporeal membrane oxygenation for perioperative support in pediatric heart transplantation. *J Thorac Cardiovasc Surg* 102(1):148–151, discussion 151–152, 1991.
35. Ishino K, Weng Y, Alexi-Meskishvili V, et al: Extracorporeal membrane oxygenation as a bridge to cardiac transplantation in children. *Artif Organs* 20(6):728–732, 1996.
36. Levi D, Marelli D, Plunkett M, et al: Use of assist devices and ECMO to bridge pediatric patients with cardiomyopathy to transplantation. *J Heart Lung Transplant* 21:760–770, 2002.
37. Thiagarajan RR, Roth SJ, Margossian S, et al: Extracorporeal membrane oxygenation as a bridge to cardiac transplantation in a patient with cardiomyopathy and hemophilia A. *Int Care Med* 29:985–988, 2003.
38. Sable CA, Shaddy RE, Suddaty EC, et al: Impact of prolonged waiting times of neonates awaiting heart transplantation. *J Perinatol* 17(6):481–488, 1997.

39. Parra DA, Totapally BR, Zahn E, et al: Outcome of cardiopulmonary resuscitation in a pediatric cardiac intensive care unit. *Crit Care Med* 28:3296–3300, 2000.
40. Schindler MB, Bohn D, Cox PN, et al: Outcome of out-of-hospital cardiac or respiratory arrest in children. *N Engl J Med* 335:1473–1479, 1996.
41. Slomin AD, Patel KM, Ruttimann UE, et al: Cardiopulmonary resuscitation in pediatric intensive care units. *Crit Care Med* 25:1951–1955, 1997.
42. Von Seggern K, Egar M, Fuhrman BP: Cardiopulmonary resuscitation in a pediatric ICU. *Crit Care Med* 14(4):275–277, 1986.
43. Zaritsky A: Cardiopulmonary resuscitation in children. *Clin Chest Med* 8(4):561–571, 1987.
44. Zaritsky A: Outcome following cardiopulmonary resuscitation in the pediatric intensive care unit. *Crit Care Med* 25:1997, 1937.
45. Ibrahim AE, Duncan BW, Blume ED, et al: Long-term follow-up of pediatric cardiac patients requiring mechanical circulatory support. *Ann Thorac Surg* 69:186–192, 2000.
46. Cheung PY, Vickar DB, Hallgren RA, et al: Carotid artery reconstruction in neonates receiving extracorporeal membrane oxygenation: a 4-year follow-up study. Western Canadian ECMO Follow-Up Group. *J Pediatr Surg* 32(4):560–564, 1997.
47. Karl TR, Sano S, Horton S, et al: Centrifugal pump left heart assist in pediatric cardiac operations. Indication, technique, and results. *J Thorac Cardiovasc Surg* 102(4):624–630, 1991.
48. Wessel DL, Almodovar MC, Laussen PC: Intensive care management of cardiac patients on extracorporeal membrane oxygenation. In Duncan BW, editor: *Mechanical support for cardiac and respiratory failure*, New York, 2000, Marcel Dekker, pp 75–111.
49. Marcus B, Alkinson JB, Wong PC, et al: Successful use of transesophageal echocardiography during extracorporeal membrane oxygenation in infants after cardiac operations. *J Thorac Cardiovasc Surg* 109(5):846–848, 1995.
50. Jaggers JJ, Forbess JM, Shah AS, et al: Extracorporeal membrane oxygenation for infant postcardiotomy support: significance of shunt management. *Ann Thorac Surg* 69:1476–1483, 2000.
51. Booth KL, Roth SJ, Thiagarajan RR, et al: ECMO support of Fontan and bidirectional Glenn circulation. *Ann Thorac Surg* in press.
52. Charmichael TB, Walsh EP, Roth SJ: Anticipatory use of venoarterial extracorporeal membrane oxygenation for a high-risk interventional cardiac procedure. *Resp Care* 1002–1006, 2003.
53. Akomea-Agyin C, Kejriwal NK, Franks R, et al: Intraaortic balloon pumping children. *Ann Thorac Surg* 67:1415–1420, 1999.
54. Park JK, Hsu DT, Gersony WM: Intraaortic balloon pump management of refractory congestive heart failure in children. *Pediatr Cardiol* 14(1):19–22, 1993.
55. Webster H, Veasy LG: Intra-aortic balloon pumping in children. *Heart Lung* 14(6):548–555, 1985.
56. Moran JM, Opravil M, Gorman AJ, et al: Pulmonary artery balloon counterpulsation for right ventricular failure: II. Clinical experience. *Ann Thorac Surg* 38(3):254–259, 1984.
57. Opravil M, Gorman AJ, Krejcie TC, et al: Pulmonary artery balloon counterpulsation for right ventricular failure: I. Experimental results. *Ann Thorac Surg* 38(3):242–253, 1984.
58. Cadwell CA, Quaal SJ: Intra-aortic balloon counterpulsation timing [see comments]. *Am J Crit Care* 5(4):254–261, quiz 262–263, 1996.
59. Pantalos GM, Minich LL, Tani LY, et al: Estimation of timing errors for the intraaortic balloon pump use in pediatric patients. *ASAIO J* 45(3):166–171, 1999.
60. Amsterdam EA, Awan NA, Lee G, et al: Intra-aortic balloon counterpulsation: rationale, application and results. *Cardiovasc Clin* 11(3):79–96, 1981.
61. Chatterjee S, Rosensweig J: Evaluation of intra-aortic balloon counterpulsation. *J Thorac Cardiovasc Surg* 61(3):405–410, 1971.
62. Beckman CB, Geha AS, Hammond GL, et al: Results and complications of intraaortic balloon counterpulsation. *Ann Thorac Surg* 24(6):550–559, 1977.
63. Lazar JM, Ziady GM, Dermmer SJ, et al: Outcome and complications of prolonged intraaortic balloon counterpulsation in cardiac patients. *Am J Cardiol* 69(9):955–958, 1992.
64. Minich LL, Tani LY, McGough EC, et al: A novel approach to pediatric intraaortic balloon pump timing using M-mode echocardiography. *Am J Cardiol* 80(3):367–369, 1997.
65. Reinhartz O, Stiller B, Eilers R, et al: Current clinical status of pulsatile pediatric circulatory support. *ASAIO J* 48:455–459, 2002.
66. Hetzer R, Loebe M, Potapov EV, et al: Circulatory support with pneumatic paracorporeal ventricular assist device in infants and children. *Ann Thorac Surg* 66(5):1498–1506, 1998.
67. Thuys CA, Mullaly RJ, Horton SB, et al: Centrifugal ventricular assist in children under 6 kg. *Eur J Cardiothorac Surg* 13(2):130–134, 1998.
68. del Nido PJ, Duncan BW, Mayer JE, Jr, et al: Left ventricular assist device improves survival in children with left ventricular dysfunction after repair of anomalous origin of the left coronary artery from the pulmonary artery. *Ann Thorac Surg* 67(1):169–172, 1999.
69. Karl TR, Horton SB, Mee RB: Left heart assist for ischemic postoperative ventricular dysfunction in an infant with anomalous left coronary artery. *J Card Surg* 4(4):352–354, 1989.
70. Mee RB, Harada Y: Retraining of the left ventricle with a left ventricular assist device (Bio-Medicus) after the arterial switch operation. *J Thorac Cardiovasc Surg* 101(1):171–173, letter, 1991.
71. Nathan M, Baird C, Fynn-Thompson F, et al: Successful implantation of a Berlin heart biventricular assist device in a failing single ventricle. *J Thorac Cardiovasc Surg* 131(6):1407–1408, 2006.
72. Calvaruso DF, Ocello S, Salviato N, et al: Implantation of a Berlin Heart as single ventricle by-pass on Fontan circulation in univentricular heart failure. *ASAIO J* 53(6):e1–e2, 2007.
73. Stiller B, Weng Y, Hubler M, et al: Pneumatic pulsatile ventricular assist devices in children under 1 year of age. *Eur J Cardiothoracic Surg* 28:234–239, 2005.
74. Loebe M, Muller J, Hetzer R: Ventricular assistance for recovery of cardiac failure. *Curr Opin Cardiol* 14(3):234–248, 1999.
75. Pavie A, Leger P: Physiology of univentricular versus biventricular support. *Ann Thorac Surg* 61(1):347–349, discussion 357–358, 1996.
76. Santamore WP, Austin EH, 3rd, Gray LA, Jr: Overcoming right ventricular failure with left ventricular assist devices. *J Heart Lung Transplant* 16(11):1122–1128, 1997.
77. Santamore WP, Gray LA, Jr: Left ventricular contributions to right ventricular systolic function during LVAD support. *Ann Thorac Surg* 61(1):350–356, 1996.
78. Oku T, Harasaki H, Smith W, et al: Hemolysis. A comparative study of four nonpulsatile pumps. *ASAIO Trans* 34(3):500–504, 1988.
79. Imamura M, Hale S, Johnson C, et al: The first successful DeBakey VAD child implantation as a bridge to transplant. *ASAIO J* 51:670–672, 2005.
80. Helman DN, Addonizio LJ, Morales DLS, et al: Implantable left ventricular assist devices can successfully bridge adolescent patients to transplant. *J Heart Lung Transplant* 19:121–126, 2000.
81. Korfer R, El-Banayosy A, Arusoghi L, et al: Single-center experience with the Thoratec ventricular assist device. *J Thorac Cardiovasc Surg* 119:596–600, 2000.
82. Asfour B, Weyard M, Kececioglu D, et al: A novel paracorporeal mechanical assist device for newborns and infants allows bridging to transplantation. *Transplant Proc* 29(8):3330–3332, 1997.
83. Ishino K, Loebe M, Uhlemann F, et al: Circulatory support with paracorporeal pneumatic ventricular assist device (VAD) in infants and children. *Eur J Cardiothrac Surg* 11:965–972, 1997.
84. Konertz W, Hotz H, Schneider M, et al: Clinical experience with the MEDOS HIA-VAD system in infants and children: a preliminary report. *Ann Thorac Surg* 63(4):1138–1144, 1997.
85. Shum-Tim D, Duncan BW, Hraska V, et al: Evaluation of a pulsatile pediatric ventricular assist device in an acute right heart failure model. *Ann Thorac Surg* 64(5):1374–1380, 1997.
86. Cohen G, Permut L: Decision making for mechanical cardiac assist in pediatric cardiac surgery. *Semin Thorac Cardiovasc Surg Pediatr Card Surg Ann* 8:41–50, 2005.
87. Duncan B: Pediatric mechanical circulatory support. *ASAIO J* 51:ix–xiv, 2005.
88. Baldwin T, Borovetz H, Duncan B, et al: The National Heart, Lung and Blood Institute Pediatric Circulatory Support Program. *Circulation* 113:147–155, 2006.
89. Hamrick SEG, Gremmels DB, Keet CA, et al: Neurodevelopmental outcome of infants supported with extracorporeal membrane oxygenation after cardiac surgery. *Pediatrics* 111:e671–e675, 2003.
90. Blume ED, Naftel DC, Bastardi HJ, et al: Outcomes of children bridged to heart transplantation with ventricular assist devices: a multi-institutional study. *Circulation* 113:2313–2319, 2006.

CHAPTER 110

PEDIATRIC ANESTHESIA AND CRITICAL CARE

Kirsten C. Odegard • James A. DiNardo

CHAPTER OUTLINE

The management of congenital heart disease (CHD) has progressed significantly over the past three decades. Most congenital heart lesions are now amenable to anatomic or physiologic repair early in infancy. Advances in diagnostic and interventional cardiology, the evolution of surgical techniques and conduct of cardiopulmonary bypass, and refinements in postoperative management have all contributed to a substantial decrease in morbidity and mortality associated with CHD. The approach to repairing CHD as early as possible, preferably in the neonatal period, has had significant implications for the anesthetic care of these critically ill infants during cardiac surgery. To meet this challenge, a clear understanding of neonatal respiratory and cardiac physiology, neonatal responses to anesthesia and surgery, and the pathophysiology of complex congenital heart defects is necessary.

PATHOPHYSIOLOGY

Care of the critically ill neonate requires an appreciation of the special structural and functional features of immature organs. The neonate appears to respond more quickly and extremely to physiologically stressful circumstances; this can be expressed in terms of rapid changes in, for example, pH, lactic acid, glucose, and temperature.[1]

The physiology of the preterm and full-term neonate is characterized by a high metabolic rate and O_2 demand (a twofold to threefold increase compared with adults), which may be compromised at times of stress because of limited cardiac and respiratory reserve. The myocardium in the neonate is immature, with only 30% of the myocardial mass being composed of contractile tissue, compared with 60% in mature myocardium. In addition, neonates have a lower velocity of shortening, a diminished length–tension relationship, and a reduced ability to respond to afterload stress.[2,3] Because the compliance of the myocardium is reduced, the stroke volume is relatively fixed and cardiac output is heart rate dependent; therefore, the Frank-Starling relationship is functional only within a narrow range of left ventricular end-diastolic pressure. The cytoplasmic reticulum and T-tubular system are underdeveloped, and the neonatal heart is dependent on the trans-sarcolemmal flux of extracellular calcium both to initiate and sustain contraction.

Cardiorespiratory interactions are important in neonates and infants. In simple terms, *ventricular interdependence* refers to a relative increase in ventricular end-diastolic volume and pressure, causing a shift of the ventricular septum and diminished diastolic compliance of the opposing ventricle.[4] This effect is particularly prominent in the immature myocardium. Therefore, a volume load from an intracardiac shunt or valve regurgitation, and a pressure load from ventricular outflow obstruction or increased vascular resistance, could lead to biventricular dysfunction. For example, in neonates with tetralogy of Fallot and severe outflow obstruction, hypertrophy of the ventricular septum can contribute to diastolic dysfunction of the left ventricle and an increase in end-diastolic pressure. This does not improve immediately after repair in the neonate, as it takes some weeks or months for the myocardium to remodel; therefore, an elevated left atrial pressure is not an unexpected finding after neonatal tetralogy repair. This circumstance can be exacerbated further if there is a persistent volume load to the left ventricle after surgery, such as from residual ventricle septal defects (VSDs).

The mechanical disadvantage of an increased chest wall compliance and reliance on the diaphragm as the main muscle of respiration limits ventilatory capacity in the neonate. The diaphragm and intercostal muscles have fewer type I muscle fibers (i.e., slow-contracting, high oxidative fibers for sustained activity), and this contributes to early fatigue when the work of breathing is increased. In the newborn, only 25% of fibers in the diaphragm are type I, reaching a mature proportion of 55% by 8 to 9 months of age.[5,6] Diaphragmatic function can be compromised significantly by raised intra-abdominal pressure, such as from gastric distention, hepatic congestion, or ascites.

The tidal volume of full-term neonates is 6 to 8 mL/kg and, because of the mechanical limitations just mentioned, minute ventilation is respiratory-rate dependent. The resting respiratory rate of the newborn infant is between 30 and 40 breaths per minute, which provides the optimal alveolar ventilation to overcome the work of breathing and match the compliance and resistance of the respiratory system. When the work of breathing increases, such as with parenchymal lung disease, airway obstruction, cardiac failure, or increased pulmonary blood flow, a larger proportion of total energy expenditure is required to maintain adequate ventilation. Infants therefore fatigue readily and fail to thrive.

The neonate has a reduced functional residual capacity (FRC) secondary to an increased chest wall compliance (FRC being determined by the balance between chest wall and lung compliance). Closing capacity is also increased in newborns, with airway closure occurring during normal tidal ventilation.[7] Oxygen reserve is therefore reduced, and in conjunction with an increased basal metabolic rate and oxygen consumption two to three times adult levels, neonates and infants are at risk for hypoxemia. However, atelectasis and hypoxemia do not occur in the normal neonate because FRC is maintained by dynamic factors, including tachypnea, breath stacking (early inspiration), expiratory breaking (expiratory flow interrupted before zero flow occurs), and laryngeal breaking (auto–positive end-expiratory pressure [PEEP]).

Organ immaturity of the liver and kidney may be associated with reduced protein synthesis and glomerular filtration, such that drug metabolism is altered and synthetic function is reduced. These problems can be compounded by the normally increased total body water of the neonate compared with the older patient, along with the propensity of the neonatal capillary system to leak fluid out of the intravascular space.[8] This is especially pronounced in the neonatal lung, in which the pulmonary vascular bed is almost fully recruited at rest and the lymphatic recruitment required to handle increased mean capillary pressures associated with increases in pulmonary blood flow may be unavailable.[9]

The caloric requirement for neonates, especially preterm neonates, is high (100 to 150 kcal/kg per 24 hr) because of metabolic demand. The task of supplying nutrition for growth becomes even more difficult when necessary limits are placed on the total amount of fluid that may be administrated parentally or by the enteral route. Hyperosmolar feedings have been associated with an increased risk for necrotizing enterocolitis in the preterm neonate, or to the neonate born at term who has decreased splanchnic blood flow of any cause (e.g., left-sided obstructive lesions).[10,11]

PHYSIOLOGIC APPROACH TO CONGENITAL HEART DISEASE

Specific classification of congenital heart defects is difficult because of the complex nature of many lesions. Basing identification and classification on physiology brings an organized framework to the intraoperative anesthetic management and postoperative care of children with complex CHD.

Single Ventricle Physiology

Single ventricle physiology is used to describe the situation wherein complete mixing of pulmonary venous and systemic venous blood occurs at the atrial or ventricular level and the ventricles then distribute output to both the systemic and pulmonary beds. Because of this physiology:

- Ventricular output is the sum of pulmonary blood flow (Qp) and systemic blood flow (Qs).
- Distribution of systemic and pulmonary blood flow is dependent on the relative resistances to flow (both intra- and extra-cardiac) into the two parallel circuits.
- Oxygen saturations are the same in the aorta and the pulmonary artery.

This physiology can exist in patients with one well-developed ventricle and one hypoplastic ventricle and in patients with two well-formed ventricles.

In the case of a single anatomic ventricle, there is always obstruction to either pulmonary or systemic blood flow because of complete or near complete obstruction to inflow and/or outflow from the hypoplastic ventricle. In this circumstance, there must be a source of both systemic and pulmonary blood flow to assure postnatal survival. In some instances of a single anatomic ventricle, a direct connection between the aorta and the pulmonary artery via a patent ductus arteriosus (PDA) is the sole source of systemic blood flow (hypoplastic left heart syndrome) or of pulmonary blood flow (pulmonary atresia with intact ventricular septum); this is known as *ductal dependent circulation*. In other instances of a single anatomic ventricle, intracardiac pathways provide both systemic and pulmonary blood flow without the necessity of a PDA. This is the case in tricuspid atresia with normally related great vessels, a nonrestrictive VSD, and minimal or absent pulmonary stenosis.

Single ventricle physiology can exist in the presence of two well-formed anatomic ventricles when there is complete or near complete obstruction to outflow from one on the ventricles:

- Tetralogy of Fallot (TOF) with pulmonary atresia (PA) where pulmonary blood flow is supplied via a PDA or multiple aortopulmonary collateral arteries (MAPCA)
- Truncus arteriosus
- Severe neonatal aortic stenosis and interrupted aortic arch (in both lesions a substantial portion of systemic blood flow is supplied via a PDA)
- Heterotaxy syndrome, in which there are components of systemic venous (superior vena cava, inferior vena cava, hepatic veins, azygous veins) and pulmonary venous return to both right and left sided atria, and in which atrial morphology is ambiguous

With single ventricle physiology, the arterial saturation (SaO_2) will be determined by the relative volumes and saturations of pulmonary venous and systemic venous blood flows that have mixed and reach the aorta. This is summarized in the following equation:

$$\begin{aligned}\text{Aortic saturation} = [&(\text{Systemic venous saturation})\\ &\times(\text{Total systemic venous blood flow})\\ &+(\text{Pulmonary venous saturation})\\ &\times(\text{Total pulmonary venous blood flow})]/\\ &(\text{Total systemic venous blood flow}\\ &+\text{Total pulmonary venous blood flow})\end{aligned}$$

A typical example is as follows:

$$SaO_2 = [(65)(3.3)+(98)(2.8)]/(3.3+2.8) = 80\%$$

Intercirculatory Mixing

Intercirculatory mixing is the unique situation that exists in transposition of the great vessels, in which two parallel circulations exist because of the existence of atrioventricular concordance (RA-RV, LA-LV) and ventriculoarterial discordance (RV-Ao, LV-PA). This produces a parallel rather than a normal series circulation. In this arrangement, blood flow will consist of parallel recirculation of pulmonary venous blood in the pulmonary circuit and systemic venous blood in the systemic circuit. Therefore, the physiologic shunt or the percentage of venous blood from one system that recirculates in the arterial outflow of the same system is 100% for both circuits. Unless there are one or more communications (atrial septal defect [ASD], PFO, VSD, PDA) between the parallel circuits to allow intercirculatory mixing, this lesion is incompatible with life.

An anatomic right-to-left (R-L) shunt is necessary to provide effective pulmonary blood flow, whereas an anatomic left-to-right (L-R) shunt is necessary to provide effective systemic blood flow. Effective pulmonary blood flow, effective systemic blood flow, and the volume of intercirculatory mixing must always be equal. Total systemic blood flow is the sum of recirculated systemic venous blood plus effective systemic blood flow. Likewise, total pulmonary blood flow is the sum of recirculated pulmonary venous blood plus effective pulmonary blood flow. Recirculated blood composes the largest portion of total pulmonary and total systemic blood flow, with effective blood flows contributing only a small portion of the total flows. This is particularly true in the pulmonary circuit in which the total pulmonary blood flow (Q_P) and the volume of the pulmonary circuit (LA-LV-PA) is twofold to threefold greater than the total systemic blood flow (Q_S) and the volume of the systemic circuit (RA-RV-Ao). The net result is transposition physiology, wherein the pulmonary artery oxygen saturation is greater than the aortic oxygen saturation.

Arterial saturation (SaO_2) will be determined by the relative volumes and saturations of the recirculated systemic and effective systemic venous blood flows reaching the aorta. This is summarized in the following equation:

$$\begin{aligned}\text{Aortic saturation} = [&(\text{Systemic venous saturation})\\ &\times(\text{Recirculated systemic venous blood flow})\\ &+(\text{Pulmonary venous saturation})\\ &\times(\text{Effective systemic venous blood flow})]/\\ &(\text{Total systemic venous blood flow})\end{aligned}$$

A typical example is as follows:

$$SaO_2 = [(50)(1.2)+(99)(1.1)]/2.3 = 73\%$$

Simple Shunts

Shunting is the process whereby venous return into one circulatory system is recirculated through the arterial outflow of the same circulatory system. Flow of blood from the systemic venous atrium or right atrium to the aorta produces recirculation of systemic venous blood. Flow of blood from the pulmonary venous atrium or left atrium to the pulmonary artery produces recirculation of pulmonary venous blood. Recirculation of blood produces a physiologic shunt. Recirculation of pulmonary venous blood produces a physiologic L-R, whereas recirculation of systemic venous blood produces a physiologic R-L shunt. A physiologic R-L or L-R shunt commonly is the result of an anatomic R-L or L-R shunt. In an anatomic shunt, blood moves from one circulatory system to the other via a communication at the level of the cardiac chambers or great vessels. Physiologic shunts can exist in the absence of an anatomic shunt. Transposition physiology is the primary example of this process.

Effective blood flow is the quantity of venous blood from one circulatory system reaching the arterial system of the other circulatory system. Effective pulmonary blood flow is the volume of systemic venous blood reaching the pulmonary circulation, whereas effective systemic blood flow is the volume of pulmonary venous blood reaching the systemic circulation. Effective pulmonary blood flow and effective systemic blood flows are the flows necessary to maintain life. Effective pulmonary blood flow and effective systemic blood flow are always equal, no matter how complex the lesions. Effective blood flow usually is the result of a normal pathway through the heart, but it can occur as the result of an anatomic R-L or L-R shunt.

Total pulmonary blood flow (Qp) is the sum of effective pulmonary blood flow and recirculated pulmonary blood flow. Total systemic blood flow (Qs) is the sum of effective systemic blood flow and recirculated systemic blood flow. Total pulmonary blood flow and total systemic blood flow do not have to be equal. Therefore, it is best to think of recirculated flow (physiologic shunt flow) as the extra, non-effective flow superimposed on the nutritive effective blood flow.

Shunts causing an increase in pulmonary blood flow may be simple or complex, occurring among the ventricles, atria, or great arteries, and they are described by the ratio of pulmonary blood flow (Qp) to systemic blood flow (Qs), or Qp/Qs. Patients may be acyanotic or cyanotic, have one or two ventricles, or have a single outflow trunk, yet have a significant increase in Qp/Qs and be at risk for congestive heart failure (CHF) and pulmonary hypertension (Table 110-1).

In patients with large L-R shunts and low pulmonary vascular resistance, a substantial increase in pulmonary blood flow can occur. If the increase in pulmonary blood flow and pressure continues, structural changes occur in the pulmonary vasculature until eventually pulmonary vascular resistance (PVR) becomes persistently elevated.[12,13] The time course for developing pulmonary vascular obstructive disease depends on the amount of shunting, but changes with some lesions may be evident by 4 to 6 months of age. The progression is more rapid when both the volume and pressure load to the pulmonary circulation is increased, such as with a large VSD. As PVR decreases in the first few months after birth and the hematocrit falls to its lowest physiologic value, the increased L-R shunt, and therefore volume load on the systemic ventricle, can lead to congestive cardiac failure and failure to thrive.

The end-diastolic volume is increased in patients with an increased Qp/Qs ratio, but the time course over which irreversible ventricular dysfunction develops is variable. Generally, if surgical intervention to correct the volume overload is undertaken within the first 2 years of life, residual dysfunction is uncommon.[14]

The volume load on the systemic ventricle and increased end-diastolic pressure contribute to increased lung water and pulmonary edema by increasing pulmonary venous and lymphatic pressures. Compliance of the lung is therefore decreased, and airway resistance increased secondary to small airway compression by distended vessels.[15-17] Lungs may feel stiff on hand ventilation and deflate slowly. Besides cardiomegaly on the chest radiograph, the lung fields are usually hyperinflated. Ventilation-perfusion mismatch contributes to an increased alveolar–arterial oxygen gradient, and dead-space ventilation.[18] Minute ventilation is therefore increased, primarily by an increase in respiratory rate. Pulmonary artery and left atrial enlargement may compress main-stem bronchi, causing lobar collapse. Symptoms and signs of CHF to note in neonates and infants are shown in Box 110-1.

Manipulating PVR is an important means of limiting pulmonary blood flow and pressure. During anesthesia, PVR can be maintained or increased by using a low fraction of inspired oxygen (FiO_2) and altering ventilation to achieve a normal pH and $PaCO_2$.[19] Care must be taken at induction of anesthesia, because patients may have a

TABLE 110-1 Simple Shunts: Defects and Surgical Procedures Contributing to an Increased Ratio of Pulmonary Blood Flow (Qp) to Systemic Blood Flow (Qs)

Type of Shunt	Acyanotic	Cyanotic
Two ventricles	ASD VSD CAVC DORV	D-TGA/VSD PA/VSD
Single ventricle	—	TA ± TGA HLHS DORV/MA Norwood/Sano procedure BT shunt
Aortopulmonary (AP) connection	PDA Truncus arteriosus AP window	PA/MAPCA

AP, Aortopulmonary; *ASD*, atrial septal defect; *BT*, Blalock-Taussig; *CAVC*, complete atrioventricular canal; *DORV*, double-outlet right ventricle; *D-TGA*, dextro-transposition of the great arteries; *HLHS*, hypoplastic left heart syndrome; *MA*, mitral atresia; *MAPCA*, multiple aortopulmonary collateral arteries; *PA*, pulmonary atresia; *PDA*, patent ductus arteriosus; *TA*, tricuspid atresia; *TGA*, transposition of the great arteries; *VSD*, ventral septal defect.

BOX 110-1 Symptoms and Signs of Cardiac Failure in a Neonate or Infant

POOR GROWTH

- Poor feeding
- Diaphoresis

INCREASED WORK OF BREATHING

- Tachypnea
- Grunting
- Flaring of ala nasi
- Chest wall retraction

DECREASED CARDIAC OUTPUT

- Tachycardia
- Gallop rhythm
- Cardiomegaly
- Poor extremity perfusion
- Hepatomegaly

diminished contractile reserve. Preload, contractility, and heart rate must be maintained; afterload reduction is often well tolerated and will reduce pulmonary flow and myocardial work.

Complex Shunts

In complex shunts, there is additional pulmonary or systemic outflow obstruction, and the Qp/Qs ratio is determined by the size of the orifice, the outflow gradient, and the resistance across the pulmonary or systemic vascular bed. The obstruction may be fixed as with valvular stenosis, or dynamic as in forms of TOF.

Outflow Obstruction

Severe outflow obstruction in the newborn may be associated with ventricular hypertrophy and vessel hypoplasia distal to the level of obstruction. The increased pressure load can cause ventricular failure, with mixing or shunting at the atrial or ventricular level (or both) necessary to maintain cardiac output if there is complete outflow obstruction. Maintenance of preload, afterload, and normal sinus rhythm is important to prevent a fall in cardiac output or coronary hypoperfusion. As the time to develop significant ventricular dysfunction is longer in patients with a chronic pressure load than in those with a chronic volume load, symptoms of CHF are uncommon unless the obstruction is severe and prolonged.

Pulmonary Hypertension

Pulmonary hypertension may be idiopathic. Patients with CHD typically have pulmonary hypertension secondary to increased pulmonary artery flow and pressure, pulmonary venous obstruction, or left atrial hypertension from systemic ventricular atrioventricular valve dysfunction or ventricular systolic or diastolic dysfunction. Factors that increase PVR and pulmonary pressures include light anesthesia with a poorly attenuated stress response, hypoxemia, hypoventilation with a fall in FRC and respiratory acidosis, metabolic acidosis, hypothermia, prolonged bypass with associated inflammatory response and capillary leak, and administration of protamine or blood products (e.g., platelets; Box 110-2).

After repair of defects with large L-R shunts, pulmonary artery pressures may remain elevated immediately after bypass, as the pulmonary arteries initially remain reactive to factors that increase PVR. While the patient is on bypass, factors contributing to this elevated pressure include compression and atelectasis of the lung, and pulmonary edema from inadequate venting of the left atrium or from the humoral and cellular response to bypass. Attenuation of the stress response with deep anesthesia using high-dose narcotics will prevent increases in PVR.[20] A high FiO_2 and hyperventilation to induce a respiratory alkalosis will reduce PVR, and boluses of bicarbonate may be necessary to maintain metabolic alkalosis.[21-23] Ideally, the pH should be approximately 7.45 to 7.50 and the arterial CO_2 should be 30 to 35 mm Hg. A strategy of hyperventilation to induce a respiratory alkalosis and lower PVR may have an adverse effect on central nervous system recovery by lowering cerebral blood flow. The pattern of ventilation and maintenance of lung volumes is important: atelectasis and decreases in lung compliance can cause a significant rise in PVR and pulmonary pressures. Changes in ventilation must be made cautiously and reassessed frequently.

BOX 110-2 Causes of Abnormally Elevated Pulmonary Artery Pressure

- Left-to-right shunt lesion (e.g., large ventricular septal defect or patent ductus arteriosus)
- Pulmonary arteriolar smooth muscle hypertrophy (e.g., pulmonary vascular obstructive disease)
- Increased pulmonary venous pressure
- Mechanical obstruction of the pulmonary circulation
- Anatomic defects (e.g., pulmonary vein or branch pulmonary artery stenosis)
- Pulmonary embolus
- Raised intrathoracic pressure
- Lung hyperinflation
- Lung hypoinflation and hypoplasia
- Decreased alveolar oxygen tension
- Acidemia (respiratory or metabolic)
- Inflammatory response to cardiopulmonary bypass
- Drugs: protamine
- Hyperviscosity (from polycythemia)
- Blood product administration (platelets)
- Artifactual (e.g., monitoring problems, catheter malposition)

Several intravenous vasodilators, including the nitric oxide (NO) donors nitroprusside and glycerol trinitrate, the phosphodiesterase inhibitor milrinone, the eicosanoids prostaglandin E_1 and prostaglandin I_2[24], tolazoline, and isoproterenol have been used to treat postoperative patients with elevated PVR.[25-27] The chief limitation of these pharmacologic agents is that their vasodilatory effects are not specific to the pulmonary vasculature; therefore, vasodilation of the systemic vasculature and systemic hypotension may accompany reduction of pulmonary hypertension.

Inhaled NO selectively dilates smooth muscle cells in small pulmonary vessels and lowers PVR.[28] The selective effect of inhaled NO on the pulmonary vasculature is a result of the rapid uptake and inactivation by hemoglobin as NO diffuses from alveoli to the lumen of lung capillaries. The usefulness of inhaled NO for patients with congenital heart disease and pulmonary hypertension has been documented in several populations.[29,30] After surgery, NO has been shown to reduce pulmonary artery pressure and PVR in patients with pulmonary venous obstruction, such as total anomalous pulmonary venous connection and mitral stenosis, to a lesser extent in patients with a large preexisting L-R shunt, and in those with cavopulmonary connections (Fontan physiology)[31] or pulmonary hypertensive crises related to cardiopulmonary bypass (CPB). NO has also improved both pulmonary hypertension and impaired gas exchange in patients who have undergone lung transplantation. Patients with a variety of other pulmonary vascular or parenchymal diseases, including persistent pulmonary hypertension of the newborn,[32-34] primary pulmonary hypertension, acute respiratory distress syndrome,[35] and acute chest syndrome in sickle cell disease[36] have also shown significant improvements in oxygenation from treatment with inhaled NO.

Recent therapeutic advances have significantly improved the prognosis for patients with pulmonary arterial hypertension.[24,37,38] The role of newer pulmonary vasodilating drugs such as the phosphodiesterase type V inhibitor sildenafil, and endothelin I blocking drugs, such as bosentan, have shown encouraging results.[39-42] The value of these drugs in children with CHD is yet to be established.

PREOPERATIVE EVALUATION

Patients with complex defects require frequent evaluation and often repeated cardiac operations as a staged approach to surgical repair. Previous anesthetic, bypass, or surgical problems should be noted. In general, providing continuity of care in these patients, such as by a dedicated cardiac anesthesia service, is useful to ensure consistent management practices, and it enhances the long-term relationship with patients and families.

Failure to thrive is an important indicator of cardiopulmonary compromise. Symptoms as described in Box 110-1 should be noted. Murmurs and extra heart sounds may be difficult to interpret if tachycardic, but a palpable thrill usually indicates a significant murmur. Failure to thrive, lethargy, and poor exercise tolerance are significant symptoms in older children. Orthopnea, syncope, and palpitations may also be described. Recurrent respiratory infections and wheezing are common in patients with L-R shunts. Four-limb blood pressures should be compared, and room air baseline peripheral arterial saturations should be noted along with potential airway problems. The chest radiograph should be analyzed for cardiomegaly, pulmonary congestion, airway compression, and atelectasis. Echocardiographic assessment and cardiac catheterization results provide valuable information about anatomic structure, myocardial function, intracardiac pressures, shunting, and gradients across obstructions. They should be interpreted in conjunction with the cardiologist and surgeon. Patients with cardiac failure are often stabilized on digoxin, diuretics, and oral vasodilators such as captopril. Preoperative digoxin levels and hypokalemia must be checked.

The consequences of chronic hypoxemia also need special consideration. Polycythemia increases oxygen-carrying capacity, but when the hematocrit rises to greater than 65%, the increased blood viscosity causes stasis and potential thrombosis, and it exacerbates tissue hypoxia. Dehydration must be avoided, and intravenous (IV) maintenance fluids should be begun while the patient is fasting preoperatively. Bleeding disturbances, common in cyanotic patients,[43] can result from thrombocytopenia, defective platelet aggregation, or clotting factor abnormalities.

MONITORING

The monitoring technique used for a patient should depend on the child's condition and the magnitude of the planned procedure. For elective patients, noninvasive monitoring (electrocardiography, pulse oximetry, capnography, and a noninvasive blood pressure cuff) is placed before induction of anesthesia.

Monitoring by electrocardiogram (ECG) is essential, because significant rhythm disturbances can occur before and after bypass, particularly with VSD and outflow tract surgery. Myocardial ischemia occurs in pediatric patients mostly because of anatomic and shunt-related problems rather than coronary occlusive disease. Anomalous coronary arteries are associated with a number of complex defects, such as transposition of the great vessels and pulmonary atresia. Ischemia also occurs when coronary perfusion pressure falls, such as in hypoplastic left heart syndrome, truncus arteriosus, and critical aortic stenosis. Ventricular fibrillation can occur in these settings,[44] particularly on induction of anesthesia. Ischemia after bypass can result from air embolism or complications related to surgery, such as coronary reimplantation or coronary compression from conduits.

Pulse oximetry is an important monitor before and after bypass, as peripheral arterial saturation levels provide an indicator of pulmonary blood flow. The anesthesiologist needs to know the patient's baseline, prebypass peripheral O_2 saturation (SpO_2), and the anticipated level after surgery. Causes for lower than expected SpO_2, in patients with single-ventricle physiology, include pulmonary venous desaturation and intrapulmonary shunt, reduced pulmonary blood flow, and low cardiac output. For patients who have undergone a two-ventricle repair, a lower than expected SpO_2 is usually secondary to intrapulmonary shunting, because of parenchymal lung disease (e.g., atelectasis, edema) or restrictive pulmonary defects (e.g., pleural effusion, pneumothorax). After repair of a neonatal right ventricular outflow tract, such as TOF or truncus arteriosus, a small atrial communication is an advantage as it provides a R-L atrial shunt. Although these patients may be cyanotic immediately after surgery, the R-L shunt will decrease and the SpO_2 will rise as the compliance of the right ventricle improves.

Once the patient is anesthetized, a direct arterial line is placed percutaneously or through a cutdown. The site of the arterial line placement needs careful consideration. For example, patients undergoing placement of a modified Blalock-Taussig shunt from the subclavian or innominate artery should have the radial arterial line placed in the opposite extremity. Similarly, a right radial arterial line is necessary when repair of coarctation of the aorta is planned. The arch anatomy and possible aberrant arterial vessels are additional considerations when planning arterial access. Aortic root pressure monitoring may be necessary immediately after bypass if the peripheral arterial pressure is damped from hypothermia or low output state. Alternatively, a femoral artery catheter may provide a more reliable arterial waveform after CPB, particularly in newborns and infants, and it is often preferable to a peripheral arterial catheter. Care must be taken to prevent thrombus and distal limb ischemia, and femoral lines are best removed early once the patient is in stable condition. Caution is necessary when flushing arterial catheters in neonates and infants, because retrograde flow into the carotid arteries is possible.[45]

Some centers routinely use central venous pressure monitoring for all cardiovascular surgery. Percutaneous central venous access enables titration of volume replacement and administration of vasoactive infusions before CPB, and during CPB it may provide a measure of the adequacy of cerebral venous drainage. Insertion of central venous catheters can be particularly difficult in pediatric patients, and central venous lines should be used with caution in neonates and infants because of the risk for infection and superior vena cava thrombosis, which can have significant sequelae if collateral veins are poorly developed. Transthoracic right and left atrial lines can be inserted by the surgeon for hemodynamic pressure monitoring and drug infusions after bypass.[46] They have a low complication rate. In addition, they can be left in situ for longer during postoperative recovery and then easily removed in the intensive care unit (ICU). Swan-Ganz catheters are rarely used in pediatric cardiac surgery because of anatomic limitations. Direct pulmonary artery catheters can be inserted by the surgeon to measure pulmonary saturations, to detect residual outflow tract gradients, and for thermodilution measurement of cardiac output. Oximetric catheters can be placed percutaneously for continuous measurement of mixed venous oxygen saturation (SvO_2) in the superior vena cava.[47]

Ultrasound-guided technique has been shown to increase the overall success rate and reduce the incidence of traumatic complications associated with central venous cannulation.[48,49] The anatomy of the central venous drainage should be known before attempting percutaneous cannulation. Heterotaxy syndrome and possible vein occlusions after previous catheterization are considerations, and if in doubt, ultrasound evaluation of the position and size of a central vein before cannulation is useful.

Neurologic Monitoring

Long-term neurodevelopmental impairment is common in newborns and infants undergoing repair for complex CHD. The etiologies of adverse neurologic sequelae in these patients are multifactorial and include prenatal, preoperative, intraoperative, and postoperative factors. Cerebral protection is a concern during bypass for congenital heart surgery, particularly if deep hypothermic arrest or low-flow bypass is used, and the importance of routine perioperative monitoring of the brain is increasingly recognized. Tympanic or nasopharyngeal temperature monitoring is used to assess the adequacy of cerebral cooling and rewarming. Continuous electroencephalographic monitoring,[50] transcranial Doppler,[51] and frontal lobe near-infrared spectroscopy[52-55] or cerebral oximetry can be used to evaluate cerebral blood flow velocity and perfusion, and O_2 delivery and extraction.

Intraoperative Echocardiography

Intraoperative transesophageal echocardiography (TEE) has achieved a role in intraoperative monitoring of patients undergoing repair of CHD.[56-58] The development of smaller probes has allowed transesophageal monitoring to replace epicardial echocardiographic imaging in many cases, and it is performed routinely. Placement of a transesophageal probe after the induction of anesthesia in the operating room enables reevaluation of the anatomy before surgical intervention, but, more importantly, the adequacy of surgical repair can be evaluated as soon as the patient is weaned from CPB. Interference of the probe with the airway and the effect on unstable hemodynamics before and after CPB must be evaluated carefully to avoid the complications of this monitoring.

ANESTHESIA

Risks of Anesthesia for Children with Congenital Heart Disease

The frequency of anesthesia-related cardiac arrests during general pediatric procedures has been reported to be between 1.4 and 4.6 per 10,000 anesthesia events, which is higher than that reported in adults. An American Society of Anesthesiologists (ASA) Physical Status of greater than 3 and younger age are risk factors for cardiac arrest during pediatric anesthesia, and a recent study demonstrated that patients with CHD are also at increased risk for cardiac arrest during cardiac surgery.[59] The incidence of anesthesia-related and procedure-related cardiac arrests was highest in neonates, and although it can be difficult to distinguish contributing factors in patients with underlying cardiac disease, there is a possible association between altered coronary perfusion and myocardial ischemia and cardiac arrest. Coronary perfusion can be reduced in patients who have uncontrolled or continuous runoff of blood flow from the systemic to pulmonary circulation, and therefore low aortic root diastolic pressure (e.g., patients with a diagnosis of truncus arteriosus, and patients with a ductus-dependent systemic circulation such as hypoplastic left heart syndrome and interruption of the aortic arch or coarctation with VSD). Patients with altered coronary blood flow, such as those with pulmonary atresia, an intact ventricular septum, and a right ventricle–dependent coronary circulation from fistulas, are also at increased risk for ischemia. These patients also have a limited ability to increase coronary blood flow when myocardial oxygen demand is increased, such as occurs secondary to tachycardia, increased contractility, or wall stress in response to a surgical stimulus if there is an inadequate depth of anesthesia to blunt a stress response.[20,44,60] The importance of maintaining diastolic pressure and coronary perfusion is also important in the setting of severe left ventricle hypertrophy (e.g., Williams syndrome, hypertrophic cardiomyopathy).[61]

Induction of Anesthesia

Because of the potential for rapid and dramatic hemodynamic changes in young patients with CHD, especially infants, the complete preparation of anesthetic and monitoring equipment and required drugs is essential. Adequate assistance should be immediately available during the induction of anesthesia in case problems develop.

The choice of induction technique is influenced by the response to premedications, the parent–child–anesthesiologist relationship, and the anesthetic management plan. In older patients who have minimal compromise of their cardiac reserve, the choice of induction techniques is large. Inhalation, intravenous, or intramuscular induction of anesthesia can be accomplished provided individual pathophysiologic limitations are understood. Cooperative children with an adequate cardiac reserve and difficult intravenous (IV) access or a morbid fear of needles can have anesthesia induced cautiously with inhaled anesthetics, even if the patients are cyanotic. An inhalation induction with sevoflurane is suitable for most infants and children, provided they have stable ventricular function and adequate hemodynamic reserve. This emphasizes the importance of preoperative evaluation when planning the induction technique. Inhalational induction can be used safely in patients with cyanotic heart disease, although uptake may be slower because of the R-L shunt.[62] Saturations will generally increase, provided cardiac output is maintained and airway obstruction is avoided.

An IV induction should be used for all patients with severely limited hemodynamic reserve, particularly those with severe ventricular failure or pulmonary hypertension. When hemodynamic instability during induction is likely, starting an inotropic agent such as dobutamine or dopamine before induction should be considered. Although the stress of placing an IV line may be considerable for some patients, particularly those with difficult IV access after previous procedures, the IV line is preferable to the potential myocardial depression during an inhalation induction.

A combination of fentanyl (15 to 25 μg/kg) and rocuronium (1.0 mg/kg) provides hemodynamic stability and prompt airway control, and it attenuates the stress-induced increase in PVR associated with intubation. IV ketamine (1 to 3 mg/kg) is safe and reliable, providing hemodynamic stability and minimal increases in PVR. It is particularly useful in patients with severe CHF and ventricular outflow tract obstructions. Atropine (20 μg/kg) or glycopyrrolate (10 μg/kg) is traditionally given concurrently because of increased secretions. If IV access is difficult and stressful in infants, a combination 4 mg/kg of ketamine, 10 μg/kg of glycopyrrolate, and 2 mg/kg of suxamethonium intramuscularly allows prompt induction and airway control.

Etomidate is an anesthetic induction agent with minimal cardiovascular and respiratory depression,[63] and it is frequently used to induce anesthesia in patients with limited hemodynamic reserve. An IV dosage of 0.1 to 0.3 mg/kg induces rapid loss of consciousness with a duration of action of 3 to 5 minutes. Etomidate can be used as an alternative to the synthetic opioids for induction of anesthesia in patients with limited myocardial reserve.

Barbiturates and propofol can be used in patients with normal ventricular function. The principal hemodynamic effect of propofol in children with CHD is a decrease in systemic vascular resistance (SVR) and direct myocardial depression. In children with an intracardiac L-R shunt, this can result in changes in the Qp/Qs ratio, and it can lead to a low cardiac output state.[64] Patients with a R-L intracardiac shunt may experience a faster induction and loss of consciousness, and the dosage must be carefully titrated to effect in these circumstances. Titrated dosages are suitable for short procedures, such as cardioversion or TEE. Midazolam (0.1 to 0.2 mg/kg) is also a useful adjunct during a narcotic induction, but it can cause hypotension in patients dependent on a high sympathetic drive.

Maintenance of Anesthesia

Anesthesia maintenance techniques depend on the patient's preoperative cardiorespiratory status, the pathophysiology of the underlying cardiac defect, the surgical procedure, the conduct of CPB, potential postoperative surgical problems, and the anticipated postoperative management. Once induction of anesthesia and control of the airway are accomplished and monitoring is adequate, anesthesia can be maintained with inhaled anesthetics or additional IV drugs as dictated by the response of each patient, intraoperative events, and postoperative plans.

Stress responses to pain and other noxious stimuli are profound in even the youngest neonates, regardless of postconception age.[1,65] These hormonal and metabolic stress responses can be deleterious,[66] particularly in patients with marginal hemodynamic reserve. High-dose narcotic techniques provide hemodynamic stability and are commonly used to maintain anesthesia, with the choice of agent and dosage dependent on the planned procedure, the duration of bypass, and the anticipated postoperative management. Patients with good cardiac function undergoing relatively short bypass procedures, such as ASD closure, can be extubated in the operating room or soon after surgery. Fentanyl (10 to 20 μg/kg) in combination with isoflurane or sevoflurane is suitable before bypass. During CPB, awareness is a potential problem. Methods to prevent this vary, but isoflurane (1%) can be continued on the bypass machine or doses of midazolam might be given intermittently. After bypass, inhalational agents are titrated as required according to hemodynamic responses.

Stress Response

In general terms, the stress response is a systemic reaction to injury, with hemodynamic, endocrinologic, and immunologic effects (Box 110-3). Stress and adverse postoperative outcome have been closely linked in critically ill newborns and infants, which is not surprising because of the precarious balance of limited metabolic reserve and increased resting metabolic rate. Metabolic derangements, such as altered glucose homeostasis, metabolic acidosis, salt and water retention, and a catabolic state contributing to protein breakdown and lipolysis, are commonly seen in sick neonates and infants after major stress.[67] This complex of maladaptive processes may be associated with prolonged mechanical ventilation and ICU stay, as well as increased morbidity and mortality.

The neuroendocrine stress response is activated by afferent neuronal impulses from the site of injury, traveling via sensory nerves through the dorsal root of the spinal cord to the medulla and hypothalamus. Anesthesia can therefore have a substantial modulating effect on the

BOX 110-3 Systemic Response to Injury

AUTONOMIC NERVOUS SYSTEM ACTIVATION
- Catechol release
- Hypertension, tachycardia, vasoconstriction

ENDOCRINE RESPONSE
- Anterior pituitary: ↑ ACTH, growth hormone
- Posterior pituitary: ↑ Vasopressin
- Adrenal cortex: ↑ Cortisol, aldosterone
- Pancreas: ↑ Glucagon, insulin resistance
- Thyroid: ↓/→ T_4/T_3

METABOLIC RESPONSE
- Protein catabolism
- Lipolysis
- Glycogenolysis/gluconeogenesis
- Hyperglycemia
- Salt and water retention

IMMUNOLOGIC RESPONSES
- Cytokine production
- Acute phase reaction
- Granulocytosis

ACTH, Adrenocorticotropic hormone.

neuroendocrine pathways of the stress response by virtue of providing analgesia and loss of consciousness.

It is important to distinguish between suppression of the endocrine response and attenuation of hemodynamic responses to stress. Because of their direct effects on the myocardium and vascular tone, anesthetic agents can readily suppress the hemodynamic side effects of the endocrine stress response. The same is true when inotropic and vasoactive agents are administered during anesthesia. However, the postoperative consequences of the endocrine stress response—in particular, fluid retention and increased catabolism—remain unabated. Relying on hemodynamic variables to assess the level of stress is therefore often inaccurate. Metabolic indices such as hyperglycemia and hyperlactatemia are also indirect markers of stress, particularly as they are influenced by other factors such as fluid administration and cardiac output.

The effect of surgical stress has been particularly evaluated in neonates and infants undergoing cardiac surgery.[66,68,69] A conclusion from these studies supported the notion that reducing the stress response with large-dose opioid anesthesia, and extending this into the immediate postoperative period, was important to reduce the morbidity and mortality associated with congenital heart surgery in neonates.

However, these studies were performed over a decade ago, and during the intervening period, there have been substantial changes in the perioperative management of children with heart disease as well as the management of cardiopulmonary bypass in general. With these changes, outcomes have improved considerably. In the early experience of bypass in neonates and infants, the use of high-dose opioid anesthesia to modulate the stress response was perceived to be one of the few clinical strategies available that was associated with demonstrable improvement in morbidity and mortality.[68] More recently, it has been demonstrated that opioids do not in fact modify the endocrine or metabolic stress response initiated by CPB; despite this, mortality and morbidity continue to remain low.

Although the neonate may be more labile to changes in intravascular pressures, PVR, and cardiac output than older children, in fact the neonate is highly capable of coping with the acute phase of surgical stress. It is less common nowadays to see neonates in the immediate post-bypass period with extensive peripheral edema or anasarca and, along with that, impaired ventricular function, reactive pulmonary hypertension, and substantial alterations in lung compliance and airway resistance. One example is the incidence of postoperative pulmonary hypertensive events. Pulmonary hypertensive crisis was more common a decade or more ago in infants who had been exposed to weeks or months of high pulmonary pressure and flow, such as truncus arteriosus, complete atrioventricular canal defects, and transposition of the great arteries with ventricular septal defects. High-dose opioids were an important component of management for patients at risk for pulmonary hypertensive crises, but this occurs much less frequently nowadays when patients undergo an operation at an earlier age and are therefore less likely to have significant or irreversible changes in the pulmonary vascular bed. Therefore, changes in surgical practice, and in particular the timing of surgery, have meant that the longer-term pathophysiologic consequences of various defects are less apparent than they were 10 to 20 years ago. A strategy of high-dose opioid anesthesia to blunt the stress response may therefore be a less critical determinant of outcome.

This is not to say, however, that high-dose synthetic opioids are not necessary for neonatal cardiac surgery. Synthetic opioids are potent analgesics and provide hemodynamic stability because of their lack of negative inotropic or vasoactive properties. Because of the limited physiologic reserve, the pathophysiology of underlying cardiac defects, and the clinical consequences of the systemic inflammatory response to bypass in the neonates, using an anesthetic technique that has minimal hemodynamic side effects is clearly desirable.

The main aim is to provide an anesthetic that maintains hemodynamic stability and allows the anesthesia team to concentrate on all other aspects of the surgery, bypass, and post-CPB care. Sudden changes in hemodynamics before and after bypass may develop secondary to myocardial dysfunction, residual anatomic lesions, loss of sinus rhythm, changes in preload state, variable pulmonary vascular resistance, and alterations in mechanical ventilation, to mention a few. Using a high-dose opioid anesthesia technique allows the anesthesiologist to focus on an evolving hemodynamic picture without the distraction of side effects from anesthetic drugs.

DISCONTINUATION OF CARDIOPULMONARY BYPASS

The effects of prolonged CPB are in part related to the interactions of blood components with the extracorporeal circuit, which cause a systemic inflammatory response. This is magnified in children because of the large bypass circuit surface area and priming volume relative to patient blood volume. The clinical consequences include increased interstitial fluid and generalized capillary leak, and potential multiorgan dysfunction. Total lung water is increased with an associated decrease in lung compliance and increase in the alveolar–arterial oxygen gradient. Myocardial edema results in impaired ventricular systolic and diastolic function. A secondary fall in cardiac output by 20% to 30% is common in neonates in the first 6 to 12 hours after surgery, contributing to decreased renal function and oliguria.[70] Sternal closure may need to be delayed because of mediastinal edema and associated cardiorespiratory compromise when closure is attempted. Ascites, hepatic ingestion, and bowel edema may affect mechanical ventilation, cause a prolonged ileus, and delay feeding. A coagulopathy after CPB can contribute to delayed hemostasis.

An organized approach must be taken to weaning a patient from CPB so that a smooth transition is ensured. There should be communication between the surgeon and the anesthesiologist regarding anticipated difficulties. Blood volume is assessed by direct visualization of the heart and by monitoring right or left atrial filling pressures. When filling pressures are adequate, the patient is fully warmed, acid–base status is normalized, heart rate is adequate, adequate minute ventilation is established, and sinus rhythm is achieved, the drainage from the venous cannula is retarded, flow is reduced gradually, and the patient is weaned from CPB. The need for vasopressor and inotropic support during weaning from bypass is determined by close observation of the heart during the rewarming phase.

Optimal ventricular filling pressures are estimated by referring to filling pressures from preoperative catheterization data, the appearance of the heart, and infusion of small increments of volume while watching filling and systemic arterial pressures. The direct measurement of oxygen saturations from chambers of the heart enables calculations of a residual intracardiac shunt immediately after surgery, and direct pressure measurements across systemic and pulmonary outflow tracts enables detection of significant residual obstruction. TEE can be used to evaluate ventricular function and to assess surgical repair.

After discontinuing bypass, and despite full rewarming on bypass, rebound mild hypothermia often develops in neonates and infants. Active measures to decrease radiant and evaporative losses are necessary because of the increased metabolic stress, pulmonary vasoreactivity, coagulopathy, and potential for dysrhythmias associated with hypothermia. However, hyperthermia must also be actively avoided because of the associated increase in metabolic rate and the potential for ongoing neurologic injury, particularly when myocardial function may be depressed and cerebral autoregulation impaired.[71]

Hemostasis may be difficult to obtain if bypass has been prolonged and if there are extensive, high-pressure (often concealed) suture lines. Prompt management and meticulous control of surgical bleeding is essential to prevent the complications associated with a massive transfusion. Besides hemodilution of coagulation factors and platelets, complex surgery with long bypass times increases endothelial injury and exposure to the non-endothelialized surface of the pump circuit, thereby stimulating the intrinsic pathway, and thus platelet activation and aggregation. Early transfusion of platelets and clotting factors, either as cryoprecipitate or fresh-frozen plasma, is recommended. Pharmacologic approaches to reduce bleeding and transfusion in cardiac surgical patients include the use of lysine analogue antifibrinolytics, which have been demonstrated to reduce blood loss and transfusion requirements after cardiac surgery.[72] The optimal doses and target plasma level of these agents have not been established, but typically aminocaproic acid is administered as a 75-mg/kg bolus to the patient, a 75-mg/kg bolus to the CPB pump prime, and a continuous infusion of 75 mg/kg/hr. Recently it was suggested that low plasma levels (20 μg/mL) of tranexamic acid would be obtained for children between 5 and 40 kg with a 6.4-mg/kg bolus followed by a continuous infusion of 2.0 to 3.1 mg/kg/hr (larger infusion rate in smaller patients)[73] At Boston Children's Hospital, we typically administer a 100-mg/kg bolus to the patient, a 100-mg/kg bolus to the CPB pump prime, and a continuous infusion of 10 mg/kg/hr in neonates, infants, and children weighing less than 20 kg.

The serine protease inhibitor aprotinin was effective[74] but it has been withdrawn from clinical use because of concerns for possible increase in mortality and end-organ damage after cardiac surgery in the adult.[75-78] Recombinant factor VIIa seems to effectively and immediately reduce excessive or life-threatening nonsurgical bleeding that is unresponsive to standard hemostatic therapy, but caution is required because of an increased risk for thromboembolic complications, such as graft occlusion, stroke, and myocardial infarction.[79-81] In addition, administration of rFVIIa should not halt efforts to find and remedy all sources of medical and surgical bleeding.

POSTOPERATIVE MANAGEMENT

The optimal postoperative management of patients with CHD requires a multidisciplinary approach, with a thorough understanding of the precise anatomic diagnosis, pathophysiology, and details of the surgical and CPB technique. For most patients, postoperative recovery is uncomplicated, and, in general, when the patient's clinical progress or postoperative cardiorespiratory function does not follow the expected course, myocardial function must be evaluated and possible residual defects must be investigated with echocardiography, cardiac catheterization, or both.

Analgesia

The assessment of adequate analgesia in children can be difficult, particularly when they are paralyzed and ventilated. Primarily, autonomic signs such as hypertension, tachycardia, pupillary size, and diaphoresis are used. If not paralyzed, children will grimace and withdraw from a painful stimulus, and if they are breathing spontaneously, changes in respiratory pattern may be evident, such as tachypnea, grunting, and splinting of the chest wall.

However, changes in autonomic signs reflect not only pain. Other causes include awareness as patients emerge from anesthesia and sedation, fever, hypoxemia, hypercapnia, changes in vasoactive drug infusions, and seizures. If not diagnosed correctly, patients may receive additional opioid or benzodiazepine doses when hypertensive and tachycardic, which will only contribute to tolerance and possible withdrawal symptoms later.

Sedatives

Chloral hydrate is commonly used to sedate children before medical procedures and imaging studies.[82] It can be administered orally or rectally in a dose ranging from 25 to 50 mg/kg (maximum dosage, 1 g), with an onset of action within 15 to 30 minutes and a duration of action 2 to 4 hours. Chloral hydrate should be used to promote intermittent sedation in the ICU and not be prescribed as a repetitive scheduled medication.[83] Administered intermittently, it can be used to supplement benzodiazepines and opioids, it can assist sedation during drug withdrawal, and it is useful as a nocturnal hypnotic when trying to establish normal sleep cycles.

Benzodiazepines are the most commonly used sedatives in the ICU because of their anxiolytic, hypnotic, and amnestic properties. Although they provide excellent conscious sedation, they can cause dose-dependent respiratory depression and result in significant hypotension in patients with limited hemodynamic reserve. After long-term administration, tolerance and withdrawal symptoms are common.

Opioid analgesics are the mainstay of pain management in the ICU. They can also provide sedation for patients who require mechanical ventilation and for blunt hemodynamic responses to procedures such as endotracheal tube suctioning. Intermittent dosing of opioids can provide effective analgesia and sedation after surgery, although periods of oversedation and undermedication can occur because of peaks and troughs in drug levels. A continuous infusion is therefore advantageous.

Morphine, in intermittent IV doses of 0.05 to 0.1 mg/kg or as a continuous infusion at 50 to 100 μg/kg/hr, provides excellent postoperative analgesia for most patients. The sedative property of morphine is an advantage over the synthetic opioids; however, histamine release can cause systemic vasodilation and an increase in pulmonary artery pressure.

The synthetic opioids fentanyl, sufentanil, and alfentanil have a shorter duration of action than morphine and do not cause histamine release; therefore, they produce less vasodilation and hypotension. Fentanyl is commonly prescribed after cardiac surgery. It blocks the stress response in a dose-related fashion while maintaining both systemic and pulmonary hemodynamic stability.[20,84] Chest wall rigidity is an idiosyncratic and dosage-related reaction that can occur with a rapid bolus in newborns and older children. A continuous infusion of fentanyl (5 to 10 μg/kg/hr) provides analgesia after surgery, although it often needs to be combined with a benzodiazepine to maintain sedation. High variability between children exists in fentanyl clearance, making titration of an infusion difficult. The experience with extracorporeal membrane oxygenation indicates that tolerance to and dependence on a fentanyl infusion develops rapidly, and significant increases in infusion rate may be required.

The development of tolerance is dose and time related, and it is a particular problem after cardiac surgery in patients who received a high-dose opioid technique to maintain anesthesia. Physical dependence with withdrawal symptoms (e.g., dysphoria, fussiness, crying, agitation, tachypnea, tachycardia, diaphoresis, feeding intolerance) may be seen in children and can be managed by gradually tapering the opioid dosage or administering a longer-acting opioid, such as methadone. Methadone has a potency similar to that of morphine, with the advantage of a prolonged elimination half-life of 18 to 24 hours. It can be administered IV and is absorbed well orally.

Alternative methods of opioid delivery that are often effective after cardiac surgery include patient-controlled analgesia and epidural opioids, as a bolus or by continuous infusion. Patients receiving epidural opioids must be monitored closely for potential respiratory depression, and side effects include pruritus, nausea, vomiting, and urinary retention.

Newer agents such as dexmedetomidine (an α_2-adrenergic agonist) are being used increasingly for sedation and analgesia in pediatric patients because of their favorable sedative and anxiolytic properties combined with their limited effect on respiratory function. Dexmedetomidine is used during general anesthesia or for conscious sedation, and for sedation in the critical care unit, and it also has a potential role in preventing emergence delirium and helping with narcotic withdraw.[85] Because of its adverse cardiovascular effects, including hypotension and bradycardia, it should be used with caution in children with CHD.[86]

In children who are difficult to sedate, and in those who have often received significant doses of opioids or benzodiazepines for sedation, a low-dose infusion of propofol (30 to 100 μg/mg/min) can be used. It is not approved for sedation in children in the intensive care setting, but it can be highly effective for a short period (up to 6 to 8 hours) to assist with weaning from mechanical ventilation and, in effect, with detoxification from previous sedatives to which they have become tolerant. Because of potential hemodynamic complications, propofol must be used with caution in patients with limited hemodynamic reserve, and the dosage and duration of use must be strictly limited because of the potential yet rare complication of propofol infusion syndrome.[87]

Assessment of Cardiac Output

A complete evaluation of cardiac output (CO) should be the initial focus of management in the ICU after cardiac surgery. Low CO is associated with longer duration of mechanical ventilatory support, ICU stay, and hospital stay, all of which can increase the risk for morbidity or mortality. Data from physical examination, routine laboratory testing, and bedside hemodynamic monitoring are all considered during the initial assessment.

Postoperative patients with low CO can exhibit a variety of abnormalities on physical examination or on bedside monitoring and laboratory values (Table 110-2). The mechanisms underlying low CO in a specific patient can be related to a number of factors, including residual or unrecognized anatomic cardiovascular defects, type of surgical procedure (e.g., right ventricular [RV] dysfunction after right ventriculotomy), surgical complications (e.g., compromised coronary artery perfusion), dysrhythmia (supraventricular or ventricular) or loss of atrioventricular conduction, low preload (ongoing bleeding), high afterload (e.g., systemic vasoconstriction related to CPB), metabolic derangement (e.g., hypocalcemia, hypomagnesemia), and pulmonary hypertension (primarily affecting RV function).

In neonates and infants, a fall in CO of approximately 30% within 9 to 12 hours after surgery can be anticipated even when the surgical repair is excellent. This pattern is best documented for neonates with d-transposition of the great arteries,[70] but it also occurs in neonates undergoing complete repair of TOF or truncus arteriosus. Pharmacologic support of the myocardium may be necessary and anticipated to mitigate the effects of decreased cardiac index in these patients, including an increase in inotropic support with dopamine or the use of drugs such as milrinone to lower afterload.

TABLE 110-2 Manifestations of Low Cardiac Output after Cardiac Surgery

By Examination	
	Core hyperthermia
	Tachycardia or bradycardia
	Hypotension (for age and weight)
	Narrow pulse pressure
	Decreased peripheral perfusion
	Hepatomegaly
	Ascites
	Oliguria
By Monitoring	
Arterial waveform	Blunted or dampened upstroke
	Narrow pulse pressure
RAp or CVP, LAp (decreased)	Low intravascular fluid status
	Inadequate preload
RAp or CVP, LAp (increased)	Poor ventricular function
	Residual volume load
	Residual outflow tract obstruction
	Ischemia
	Loss of normal sinus rhythm
	Atrioventricular valve regurgitation/stenosis
	Tamponade
By Laboratory and Radiographic Results	
Svo_2	Decreased with an increased arteriovenous O_2 difference (>25%-30%)
Acid–base balance	Metabolic acidosis with increased anion gap
	Increased arterial lactate
	Elevated blood urea nitrogen and creatinine
	Increased liver transaminases
Chest radiography	Cardiac enlargement
	Pulmonary edema
	Pleural effusion

CVP, Central venous pressure; *LAp*, left atrial pressure; *RAp*, right atrial pressure.

Strategies for treating the patient with a low CO state should focus on optimizing the balance between oxygen delivery and demand. In a low CO state, oxygen and metabolic demand should be minimized by maintaining an adequate depth of analgesia and sedation, including chemical paralysis to avoid movement and reduce muscle tone and oxygen debt. Strict avoidance of hyperthermia from any cause is essential, and in some circumstances mild hypothermia may be preferable, although the effect of peripheral vasoconstriction and increase in SVR could have an adverse effect on myocardial wall stress and oxygen requirement.

Oxygen delivery can be increased by optimizing O_2 content (hemoglobin and FiO_2) and by a combination of the factors contributing to CO (i.e., contractility, preload, afterload, and heart rate). Because decreased myocardial contractility occurs frequently after reparative or palliative surgery with CPB, pharmacologic enhancement of contractility is used commonly in the ICU. Before initiating treatment with an inotrope, the volume status, serum ionized Ca^{+2} level, and cardiac rhythm should be evaluated. Dopamine is often the initial treatment for hypotension; it increases contractility by elevating intracellular Ca^{+2}, from direct binding to myocyte β_1-adrenoceptors, and by increasing norepinephrine levels. At a dose of greater than 5 μg/kg/min, dopamine should be infused through a central venous catheter to avoid superficial tissue damage should extravasation occur. The dose is titrated to achieve the desired systemic blood pressure, although some patients, especially older children and adults, may develop an undesirable dose-dependent tachycardia. Dobutamine may be less effective than dopamine as a single agent in the treatment of moderate hypotension because it reduces SVR.[88]

If a patient does not respond adequately to dopamine (up to 10 μg/kg/min) and has persistent signs of a low CO state, including poor extremity perfusion, hypotension (>30% decrease in mean arterial blood pressure for age), tachycardia, elevated atrial filling pressure, oliguria, and lactic acidemia, treatment with epinephrine should be considered. Epinephrine can be added to dopamine at a starting dose of 0.05 to 0.1 μg/kg/min, with subsequent titration of the infusion to achieve the target systemic blood pressure. At high doses (i.e., ≥0.5 μg/kg/min), epinephrine can produce significant renal and peripheral vasoconstriction plus significant tachycardia, and those who require persistent doses of epinephrine greater than 0.3 to 0.5 μg/kg/min should be evaluated for the possibility of mechanical circulatory support. Norepinephrine at doses of 0.01 to 0.2 μg/kg/min can also be considered in patients with severe hypotension and low SVR (e.g., "warm" or "distributive" shock), inadequate coronary artery perfusion, or inadequate pulmonary blood flow with a systemic–to–pulmonary artery shunt. A combination of low-dose epinephrine (e.g., <0.1 μg/kg/min) or dopamine with an IV afterload-reducing agent such as milrinone is frequently beneficial to support patients with significant ventricular dysfunction accompanied by elevated afterload. There can be a decrease in responsiveness to increasing dosages of catecholamines over time, and vasopressin, at a dose of 10 to 120 mU/kg/hr, is a potent vasopressor, which could help to improve the hemodynamics in advanced shock without compromising cardiac function.[89]

Patients with the clinical features of relative adrenal insufficiency can benefit from stress steroid therapy. This insufficiency is primarily a clinical finding of poor vascular tone with persistent hypotension and volume requirement, refractory to increasing inotrope and vasopressor support. The serum cortisol level may be low or show a limited response to adrenocorticotropic hormone stimulation testing, but the ranges of normal have not been established for pediatric patients, in particular for newborns and infants after cardiac surgery, and there is no consistent correlation between serum cortisol level and low cardiac output state. Nevertheless, stress doses of hydrocortisone (50 mg/m^2/day) have been demonstrated to increase systemic blood pressure and lower inotrope scores, although they have not been definitively demonstrated to improve eventual survival.[90-92] The increased risk for infection and poor wound healing dictates that stress dosing of steroids should be for a brief period (3 to 5 days) rather than continuing with a long taper.

Hypothyroidism is another cause for persistent low cardiac output state after cardiac surgery. Triiodothyronine (T_3) levels have been demonstrated to be low after CPB, and they may remain low for up to 48 hours after surgery, particularly if a sick euthyroid state develops and there is decreased conversion of thyroxine to the active T_3 in peripheral tissues. An infusion of T_3 at a dose of 0.05 µg/kg/hr has been shown to improve blood pressure and a composite score of recovery after cardiac surgery in newborns and infants.[93,94]

If the rhythm cannot be determined with certainty from a surface 12- or 15-lead ECG, then temporary epicardial atrial pacing wires, if present, can be used with the limb leads to generate an atrial ECG.[95] Temporary epicardial atrial or ventricular pacing wires (or both) are routinely placed in most patients to allow mechanical pacing should sinus node dysfunction or heart block occur in the early postoperative period. Because atrial wires are applied directly to the atrial epicardium, the electrical signal generated by atrial depolarization is significantly larger and thus easier to distinguish than the P wave on a surface ECG. Sinus tachycardia, which is common and often secondary to medications (e.g., sympathomimetics), pain and anxiety, or diminished ventricular function, must be distinguished from a supraventricular, ventricular, or junctional tachycardia. Heart block can diminish cardiac output by producing either bradycardia or loss of atrioventricular synchrony, or both. Complete heart block may be transient in approximately a third of cases, but if it persists beyond postoperative day 9 or 10, it is unlikely to resolve, and a permanent pacemaker is indicated.[96]

Elevated afterload in both the pulmonary and systemic circulations frequently follows surgery with CPB.[97] An increase in systemic afterload from elevated SVR may significantly increase myocardial work and reduce end-organ perfusion. Treatment of elevated SVR includes recognizing and improving conditions that exacerbate vasoconstriction (e.g., pain and hypothermia) and administering a vasodilating agent such as a phosphodiesterase inhibitor milrinone or a NO donor (e.g., nitroprusside).[98-102]

Fluid Management

Fluid management in the immediate postoperative period is critical because of the inflammatory response to CPB and significant increase in total body water that often occurs. Capillary leak and interstitial fluid accumulation continue after surgery in neonates and infants, often necessitating ongoing volume replacement. A fall in cardiac output and increased antidiuretic hormone secretion contribute to delayed water clearance and potential pre-renal dysfunction. An elevated CVP will result in elevated renal venous pressure, further compromising renal perfusion particularly in the setting of diminished arterial blood pressure. During bypass, optimizing the circuit prime hematocrit and oncotic pressure, attenuating the inflammatory response with steroids, and using modified ultrafiltration techniques may help to limit interstitial fluid accumulation.[103-105] During the first 24 hours after surgery, maintenance fluids should be restricted to 50% of full maintenance, and volume replacement should be titrated to appropriate filling pressures and hemodynamic response.

Oliguria in the first 24 hours after complex surgery and CPB is common. Cardiac output should be enhanced, with volume replacement and vasoactive drug infusions if necessary, before diuretics can be effective. In addition, low-dose dopamine (3 µg/kg/min) has the advantage of redistributing renal blood flow to promote diuresis. Fenoldopam mesylate, a selective dopamine (DA_1) receptor agonist that causes smooth muscle relaxation, leading to both renal and splanchnic vasodilation, has been used to provide renal protection during periods of ischemia and hypoxia such as during hypothermic CPB.[106] At a dose of 0.1 to 0.5 µg/kg/min, it may also have a role in postoperative ICU management to enhance renal perfusion by decreasing renal vascular resistance.[107] It should be recognized that fenoldopam has a hemodynamic profile similar to sodium nitroprusside and as such the advantages of selective renal vasodilation may be offset by systemic hypotension.

Furosemide (1 to 2 mg/kg IV every 8 hours) is a commonly prescribed loop diuretic that is excreted into the renal tubular system before producing diuresis; therefore, low cardiac output reduces its efficacy. Bolus dosing may result in a significant diuresis over a short period, thereby causing changes in intravascular volume and possibly hypotension. A continuous infusion of 0.2 to 0.3 mg/kg/hr after an initial IV bolus of 1 mg/kg often provides a consistent and sustained diuresis without sudden fluid shifts. Chlorothiazide (10 mg/kg IV or orally every 12 hours) is also an effective diuretic, particularly when used in conjunction with loop diuretics.

Peritoneal dialysis, hemodialysis, and continuous venovenous hemofiltration provide alternative renal replacement therapy in patients with persistent oliguria and renal failure.[108,109] In addition to enabling water and solute clearance, nutritional support can be increased. A peritoneal dialysis catheter can be placed into the peritoneal cavity at the completion of surgery or later in the ICU. This can be done in the ICU because of the need for renal support, to reduce intra-abdominal pressure from ascites that may be compromising mechanical ventilation, and to improve fluid management to allow administration of parenteral nutrition. Drainage may be significant in the immediate postoperative period as third-space fluid losses continue, and replacement with albumin or fresh-frozen plasma (or both) may be necessary to treat hypovolemia and hypoproteinemia. To enhance fluid excretion if oliguria persists, low-volume peritoneal dialysis may be effective, although a persistent communication between the peritoneum, mediastinum, and pleural cavities after surgery will limit the effectiveness of peritoneal dialysis and is a relative contraindication.

Pulmonary Function and Mechanical Ventilation

Altered respiratory mechanics and positive-pressure ventilation may have a significant influence on hemodynamics after congenital heart surgery. Although changes in alveolar O_2 (PAO_2), $PaCO_2$, and pH significantly affect PVR, the mean airway pressure and changes in lung volume during positive-pressure ventilation also affect PVR, preload, and ventricular afterload. Therefore, the approach to mechanical ventilation should be directed not only at achieving a desired gas exchange but also at addressing the potential cardiorespiratory interactions of positive-pressure ventilation. This is particularly critical during weaning.

Altered lung mechanics and ventilation-perfusion abnormalities are common problems in the immediate postoperative period.[110,111] Besides preoperative problems resulting from increased Qp/Qs, additional considerations include the surgical incision and lung retraction, increased lung water after CPB, possible pulmonary reperfusion injury, surfactant depletion, and restrictive defects from atelectasis and pleural effusions. In general, neonates and infants, with their limited physiologic reserve, should not be weaned from mechanical ventilation until hemodynamically stable, and until factors contributing to an increase in intrapulmonary shunt and altered respiratory mechanics have improved.

An increase in mean intrathoracic pressure during positive-pressure ventilation decreases preload to both pulmonary and systemic ventricles, but it has opposing effects on afterload to the ventricles[112,113] (i.e., it decreases afterload to the systemic ventricle but increases afterload on the pulmonary ventricle). Changes in lung volume have a major effect on PVR, which is lowest at FRC, whereas hypoinflation or hyperinflation can result in a significant increase in PVR.[114] An increase in PVR increases the afterload or wall stress on the right ventricle, compromising RV function and contributing to decreased LV compliance secondary to interventricular septal shift. In addition to low cardiac output, signs of RV dysfunction (e.g., tricuspid regurgitation, hepatomegaly, ascites, pleural effusions) may be observed. An increase in mean intrathoracic pressure increases the afterload on the RV from direct compression of extra-alveolar and alveolar pulmonary vessels. Patients with normal RV compliance, and without residual volume load or pressure load on the ventricle after surgery, usually show little change in RV function from the alteration in preload and afterload that occurs with positive-pressure ventilation. However, these effects can be magnified in patients with restrictive RV physiology or poor diastolic function after congenital heart surgery, especially in neonates who have required a right ventriculotomy for repair of TOF, pulmonary atresia, or truncus arteriosus, and in patients with concentric RV hypertrophy.

The systemic arteries are under higher pressure and not exposed to radial traction effects during inflation or deflation of the lungs. Therefore, changes in lung volume will affect LV preload, but the effect on afterload depends on changes in intrathoracic pressure alone rather than changes in lung volume. Wall stress is directly proportional to the transmural LV pressure—that is, to the difference between the intracavity LV pressure and surrounding intrathoracic pressure. An increase in intrathoracic pressure, as occurs during positive-pressure ventilation, therefore reduces the transmural gradient and wall stress on the left ventricle. This is one explanation for the beneficial effect of positive-pressure ventilation and PEEP in patients with LV failure.[115] In addition, patients with LV dysfunction may have impaired pulmonary mechanics secondary to increased lung water, decreased lung compliance, and increased airway resistance. The work of breathing is increased and neonates and infants in particular can fatigue early because of limited respiratory reserve. A significant proportion of total body oxygen consumption is directed at the increased work of breathing in neonates and infants with LV dysfunction, contributing to poor feeding and failure to thrive. Therefore, positive-pressure ventilation has an additional benefit in patients with significant volume overload and systemic ventricular dysfunction by reducing the work of breathing and oxygen demand.

Weaning from positive-pressure ventilation can be difficult in patients with persistent systemic ventricular dysfunction. During spontaneous respiration, the transmural pressure across the systemic ventricle is increased, and this sudden increase in wall stress can contribute to pulmonary edema and low cardiac output state. It is therefore often beneficial to continue vasoactive support during weaning and extubation if there is concern for ventricular dysfunction.

Weaning from Mechanical Ventilation

After congenital cardiac surgery, most patients wean without difficulty if they have had no complications with repair or CPB, but some patients with borderline cardiac function and residual volume overload may require prolonged mechanical ventilation and a slower weaning process. Weaning is a dynamic process, and continued reevaluation is necessary.

The method of weaning varies among patients. Most patients can be weaned using either a volume- or pressure-limited mode by simply decreasing the intermittent mandatory ventilation rate. Guided by physical examination,

BOX 110-4 Factors Contributing to the Inability to Wean from Mechanical Ventilation after Congenital Heart Surgery

Residual Cardiac Defects
- Volume load
- Pressure load
- Ventricular dysfunction
- Dysrhythmias

Pulmonary Restrictive Defects
- Pulmonary edema
- Pleural effusion
- Atelectasis
- Ascites
- Chest wall edema
- Phrenic nerve injury

Airway
- Edema or subglottic stenosis
- Retained secretions
- Vocal cord injury
- Extrinsic compression
- Bronchomalacia

Metabolic
- Inadequate nutrition
- Diuretic therapy (contraction alkalosis)
- Sepsis

BOX 110-5 Considerations for Planned Early Extubation after Congenital Heart Surgery

Patient Factors
- Limited cardiorespiratory reserve
- Pathophysiology of specific congenital heart defects
- Timing of surgery and preoperative management

Anesthetic Factors
- Premedication
- Drug distribution and maintenance of anesthesia on cardiopulmonary bypass
- Postoperative analgesia requirements

Surgical Factors
- Extent and complexity of surgery
- Residual defects
- Risks for bleeding and protection of suture lines

Conduct of Cardiopulmonary Bypass
- Degree of hypothermia
- Level of hemodilution
- Myocardial protection
- Modulation of the inflammatory response and reperfusion injury

Postoperative Management
- Myocardial reserve
- Cardiorespiratory interactions
- Neurologic recovery
- Analgesia management

hemodynamic criteria, respiratory pattern, and arterial blood gas measurements, the mechanical ventilator rate is gradually reduced. Patients with limited hemodynamic and respiratory reserve may demonstrate tachypnea, diaphoresis, and shallow tidal volumes as they struggle to breathe spontaneously against the resistance of the endotracheal tube. The addition of pressure- or flow-triggered pressure support of 10 to 15 cm H_2O above PEEP is often beneficial in reducing the work of breathing.

Numerous factors contribute to the inability to wean from mechanical ventilation after congenital heart surgery (Box 110-4). In general, however, residual cardiac defects after surgery causing either a volume or pressure load must be excluded by echocardiography or cardiac catheterization if a patient fails to wean from ventilation as expected.

Indications for Early Tracheal Extubation

The heterogeneous nature of congenital cardiac defects and wide age range make it difficult to establish rigid protocols for cardiovascular and respiratory management after surgery. Each patient must be viewed individually and managed according to preoperative condition and stability, surgeon preference, any surgical or CPB-related complications, and postoperative cardiorespiratory status (Box 110-5). In keeping with the strategy of early surgical intervention and repair to promote improved longer-term growth and development, and with less emphasis on complete suppression of the stress response in the immediate postoperative period, it is possible to move patients expeditiously through the ICU in a safe yet efficient fashion.

Patients undergoing selected non-CPB or closed cardiac surgery and thoracic procedures are usually suitable for early tracheal extubation. This includes infants and older children undergoing procedures such as patent ductus arteriosus and vascular ring ligation. Infants and older children undergoing repair of coarctation of the aorta may benefit from early extubation to avoid the hypertension and tachycardia that often accompanies a slow wean from mechanical ventilation in the ICU after surgery. The risk for rebound hypertension and need to protect high-pressure surgical suture lines often dictates early blood pressure control with vasodilating and β-blocking drugs. In addition, mild-to-moderate hypothermia is often deliberately induced during surgery in an effort to optimize spinal cord protection while the aorta is cross-clamped, and tracheal extubation should be delayed until patients are normothermic.

In our experience, neonates and infants who require surgical modification of pulmonary blood flow, either by placement of a pulmonary artery band or creation of a systemic–to–pulmonary artery shunt, are not suitable for early extubation management protocols. We routinely continue mechanical ventilation and deep sedation for at least the first postoperative night until cardiorespiratory stability is attained.

Children undergoing relatively short bypass procedures using mild-to-moderate hypothermia, such as ASD repair, small VSD closure, and right ventricle–to–pulmonary artery conduit replacement, are often suitable for weaning and extubation in the operating room or early after ICU admission. These patients generally have a stable preoperative clinical status, demonstrate few complications related to CPB, and have an uncomplicated postoperative course.[116]

Infants who are in stable clinical condition before surgery and who are undergoing a complete repair using moderate-to-deep hypothermia on CPB, such as those undergoing closure of a large VSD, complete atrioventricular canal defect, or TOF, are often suitable for early extubation in the first 6 to 12 hours after surgery, provided they have stable cardiac output, stable gas exchange, and no surgical complications such as bleeding. Nevertheless, if there has been a large volume load on the ventricle before surgery or a labile pulmonary vascular resistance secondary to increased pulmonary blood flow, cautious management should be guided by hemodynamic and respiratory function as patients begin to emerge from sedation.

Infants and older children undergoing some types of LV outflow tract repair, including subaortic stenosis repair with the Konno operation or subaortic membrane resection, and aortic valvuloplasty or replacement, usually have well-preserved and often hyperdynamic ventricular systolic function. Hypertension and tachycardia are frequently a management concern in these patients in the immediate postoperative period. Not only will these factors increase the risk for disruption of suture lines, but the increased myocardial work can contribute to ischemia and increase the likelihood for ventricular tachyarrhythmias. This is especially a concern during emergence from anesthesia and sedation. Provided ventricular function is stable, hemostasis has been secured, and there are no concerns for ventricular tachyarrhythmias, it is often preferable for these patients to be extubated early after surgery (6 to 12 hours), rather than undergoing a more prolonged weaning process. The combination of esmolol and sodium nitroprusside is useful for controlling blood and reflex increases in contractility in patients with increased LV mass following procedures to relieve LVOTO. This combination prevents the development of tachycardia and diastolic hypotension that potentially compromises subendocardial perfusion in patients with LVH.

After creation of a cavopulmonary connection, such as a bidirectional Glenn shunt or a modified Fontan procedure, patients usually benefit from early tracheal extubation. Effective pulmonary blood flow is enhanced during spontaneous ventilation because of the lower mean intrathoracic pressure, but despite this goal, these patients should be weaned only after hemodynamic stability is achieved. After a bidirectional Glenn procedure, it is usually possible to extubate the trachea within 12 hours after surgery.

After the modified Fontan procedure, patients can also typically be weaned and extubated within 12 hours of surgery. In the current surgical era of almost routine fenestration of the right atrial baffle, the arterial oxygen saturation should be in the range of 80% to 90% after surgery. Provided the patient is well perfused, has a transpulmonary gradient of 5 to 10 mm Hg, does not have an acidosis or persistent large volume requirement, transfer from the ICU within 2 to 3 days of surgery can be accomplished.

The response to surgery and bypass can vary considerably between neonates and is often unpredictable. At Boston Children's Hospital, neonates undergoing two-ventricle repairs are usually managed with sedation or paralysis, or both, in the immediate postoperative period until hemodynamic and respiratory stability has been attained, although there are clear differences depending on diagnosis and procedure. For example, after procedures such as an uncomplicated arterial switch operation for d-transposition of the great arteries, or repair of an interrupted aortic arch with VSD closure, many neonates are sufficiently stable to start to wean from mechanical ventilation and be extubated by the first or second postoperative day.

On the other hand, neonates who have undergone a right ventriculotomy, such as after neonatal repair of TOF or truncus arteriosus, commonly demonstrate restrictive RV physiology in the immediate postoperative period. A low cardiac output state with increased right-sided filling pressure may be evident, and continuing sedation and paralysis is often necessary for the first 48 to 72 hours until diastolic function improves.

Neonates undergoing a Norwood-type or a Sano procedure for hypoplastic left heart syndrome or other forms of single ventricle with aortic arch obstruction, can pose considerable management problems in the immediate postoperative period. This is one group of patients in whom sedation and paralysis should be continued initially after surgery to minimize the stress response and any imbalance between oxygen supply and demand until a stable circulation and gas exchange has been achieved. Inotrope and vasoactive support is usually required, often combined with afterload reduction to reduce myocardial work and improve systemic perfusion. Volume replacement to maintain preload is essential, and monitoring mixed venous O_2 saturation as an indicator of cardiac output is beneficial.

Discharge

The cost of intensive care medicine is high. As the mortality and morbidity associated with congenital cardiac surgery have declined, length of ICU stay, total hospital stay, and cost effectiveness have become important outcome variables. The timing of discharge from the ICU is therefore an important management decision. For the majority of patients who have a stable hemodynamic and respiratory status, the decision to transfer out of the ICU is not difficult. The function of all organ systems should be assessed and considered in this decision, although the focus will be on cardiovascular and respiratory function. In addition to poor cardiac output and residual anatomic lesions, a variety of noncardiac problems can complicate recovery and prolong ICU stay (Box 110-6). This decision should be multidisciplinary, with particular attention paid to nursing availability and experience, and the availability of adequate monitoring.

BOX 110-6 Criteria for Intensive Care Unit Discharge

CARDIOVASCULAR

- Stable blood pressure and systemic perfusion without requiring intravenous vasoactive support
- Invasive intravascular monitoring not indicated
- Stable cardiac rhythm (usually sinus) and no need for external pacing using temporary wires

RESPIRATORY

- Adequate ventilation rate and pattern, no signs of airway obstruction, and effective cough
- Appropriate oxygenation (according to physiology after surgery)
- No restrictive pulmonary defects that would limit ventilation or oxygenation, including atelectasis, pneumothorax (after chest tube removal), or pleural effusion
- Neurologic status adequate to protect airway

FLUID AND METABOLISM

- Afebrile
- Advancing on caloric requirements with stable glucose levels
- Even fluid balance with stable diuretic management
- Stable electrolyte balance with appropriate supplementation

APPROPRIATE NURSING INTENSITY

- Minimal chest physical therapy or bronchodilator treatments required
- Established nutrition plan (enteral or parenteral)
- Controlled analgesic or sedation requirements
- Appropriate nursing staff numbers according to the intensity of care

REFERENCES

1. Anand KJ, Sippell WG, Aynsley-Green A: Randomised trial of fentanyl anaesthesia in preterm babies undergoing surgery: effects on the stress response. *Lancet* 1:62–66, 1987.
2. Baum VC, Palmisano BW: The immature heart and anesthesia. *Anesthesiology* 87:1529–1548, 1997.
3. Friedman WF: The intrinsic physiologic properties of the developing heart. *Prog Cardiovasc Dis* 15:87–111, 1972.
4. Bove AA, Santamore WP: Ventricular interdependence. *Prog Cardiovasc Dis* 23:365–388, 1981.
5. Berman W: The hemodynamics of shunts in congenital heart disease. In Johansen KM, Burggren WW, editors: *Cardiovascular shunts: phylogenetic, ontogenetic, and clinical aspects*, New York, 1985, Raven Press, pp 399–410.
6. Keens TG, Bryan AC, Levison H, et al: Developmental pattern of muscle fiber types in human ventilatory muscles. *J Appl Physiol* 44:909–913, 1978.
7. Mansell A, Bryan C, Levison H: Airway closure in children. *J Appl Physiol* 33:711–714, 1972.
8. Mills AN, Haworth SG: Greater permeability of the neonatal lung. Postnatal changes in surface charge and biochemistry of porcine pulmonary capillary endothelium. *J Thorac Cardiovasc Surg* 101:909–916, 1991.
9. Feltes TF, Hansen TN: Effects of an aorticopulmonary shunt on lung fluid balance in the young lamb. *Pediatr Res* 26:94–97, 1989.
10. Giannone PJ, Luce WA, Nankervis CA, et al: Necrotizing enterocolitis in neonates with congenital heart disease. *Life Sci* 82:341–347, 2008.
11. Pickard SS, Feinstein JA, Popat RA, et al: Short- and long-term outcomes of necrotizing enterocolitis in infants with congenital heart disease. *Pediatrics* 123:e901–e906, 2009.
12. Hoffman JI, Rudolph AM, Heymann MA: Pulmonary vascular disease with congenital heart lesions: pathologic features and causes. *Circulation* 64:873–877, 1981.
13. Rabinovitch M, Haworth SG, Castaneda AR, et al: Lung biopsy in congenital heart disease: a morphometric approach to pulmonary vascular disease. *Circulation* 58:1107–1122, 1978.
14. Graham TP, Jr: Ventricular performance in congenital heart disease. *Circulation* 84:2259–2274, 1991.
15. Bancalari E, Jesse MJ, Gelband H, et al: Lung mechanics in congenital heart disease with increased and decreased pulmonary blood flow. *J Pediatr* 90:192–195, 1977.
16. Howlett G: Lung mechanics in normal infants and infants with congenital heart disease. *Arch Dis Child* 47:707–715, 1972.
17. Lees MH, Way RC, Ross BB: Ventilation and respiratory gas transfer of infants with increased pulmonary blood flow. *Pediatrics* 40:259–271, 1967.
18. Levin AR, Ho E, Auld PA: Alveolar-arterial oxygen gradients in infants and children with left-to-right shunts. *J Pediatr* 83:979–987, 1973.
19. Rudolph AM, Yuan S: Response of the pulmonary vasculature to hypoxia and H+ ion concentration changes. *J Clin Invest* 45:399–411, 1966.
20. Hickey PR, Hansen DD, Wessel DL, et al: Blunting of stress responses in the pulmonary circulation of infants by fentanyl. *Anesth Analg* 64:1137–1142, 1985.
21. Drummond WH, Gregory GA, Heymann MA, et al: The independent effects of hyperventilation, tolazoline, and dopamine on infants with persistent pulmonary hypertension. *J Pediatr* 98:603–611, 1981.
22. Morray JP, Lynn AM, Mansfield PB: Effect of pH and PCO2 on pulmonary and systemic hemodynamics after surgery in children with congenital heart disease and pulmonary hypertension. *J Pediatr* 113:474–479, 1988.
23. Schreiber MD, Heymann MA, Soifer SJ: Increased arterial pH, not decreased PaCO2, attenuates hypoxia-induced pulmonary vasoconstriction in newborn lambs. *Pediatr Res* 20:113–117, 1986.
24. Yung D, Widlitz AC, Rosenzweig EB, et al: Outcomes in children with idiopathic pulmonary arterial hypertension. *Circulation* 110:660–665, 2004.
25. Heymann MA: Control of the pulmonary circulation in the perinatal period. *J Dev Physiol* 6:281–290, 1984.
26. Rimensberger PC, Spahr-Schopfer I, Berner M, et al: Inhaled nitric oxide versus aerosolized iloprost in secondary pulmonary hypertension in children with congenital heart disease: vasodilator capacity and cellular mechanisms. *Circulation* 103:544–548, 2001.
27. Friesen RH, Williams GD: Anesthetic management of children with pulmonary arterial hypertension. *Paediatr Anaesth* 18:208–216, 2008.
28. Pepke-Zaba J, Higenbottam TW, Dinh-Xuan AT, et al: Inhaled nitric oxide as a cause of selective pulmonary vasodilatation in pulmonary hypertension. *Lancet* 338:1173–1174, 1991.
29. Atz AM, Wessel DL: Inhaled nitric oxide in the neonate with cardiac disease. *Semin Perinatol* 21:441–455, 1997.
30. Ryan A, Tobias JD: A 5-year survey of nitric oxide use in a pediatric intensive care unit. *Am J Ther* 14:253–258, 2007.
31. Goldman AP, Delius RE, Deanfield JE, et al: Pharmacological control of pulmonary blood flow with inhaled nitric oxide after the fenestrated Fontan operation. *Circulation* 94:II44–II48, 1996.
32. Khemani E, McElhinney DB, Rhein L, et al: Pulmonary artery hypertension in formerly premature infants with bronchopulmonary dysplasia: clinical features and outcomes in the surfactant era. *Pediatrics* 120:1260–1269, 2007.
33. Roberts JD, Jr, Fineman JR, Morin FC, 3rd, et al: Inhaled nitric oxide and persistent pulmonary hypertension of the newborn. The Inhaled Nitric Oxide Study Group. *N Engl J Med* 336:605–610, 1997.
34. Neonatal Inhaled Nitric Oxide Study G: Inhaled nitric oxide in full-term and nearly full-term infants with hypoxic respiratory failure. *N Engl J Med* 336:597–604, 1997.
35. Gerlach H, Rossaint R, Pappert D, et al: Time-course and dose-response of nitric oxide inhalation for systemic oxygenation and pulmonary hypertension in patients with adult respiratory distress syndrome. *Eur J Clin Invest* 23:499–502, 1993.
36. Atz AM, Wessel DL: Inhaled nitric oxide in sickle cell disease with acute chest syndrome. *Anesthesiology* 87:988–990, 1997.

37. Ricachinevsky CP, Amantea SL: Treatment of pulmonary arterial hypertension. *J Pediatr (Rio J)* 82:S153–S165, 2006.
38. Rosenzweig EB, Barst RJ: Pulmonary arterial hypertension in children: a medical update. *Curr Opin Pediatr* 20:288–293, 2008.
39. Apostolopoulou SC, Manginas A, Cokkinos DV, et al: Long-term oral bosentan treatment in patients with pulmonary arterial hypertension related to congenital heart disease: a 2-year study. *Heart* 93:350–354, 2007.
40. Nagendran J, Archer SL, Soliman D, et al: Phosphodiesterase type 5 is highly expressed in the hypertrophied human right ventricle, and acute inhibition of phosphodiesterase type 5 improves contractility. *Circulation* 116:238–248, 2007.
41. O'Callaghan DS, Savale L, Montani D, et al: Treatment of pulmonary arterial hypertension with targeted therapies. *Nat Rev Cardiol* 8:526–538, 2011.
42. van Loon RL, Hoendermis ES, Duffels MG, et al: Long-term effect of bosentan in adults versus children with pulmonary arterial hypertension associated with systemic-to-pulmonary shunt: does the beneficial effect persist? *Am Heart J* 154:776–782, 2007.
43. Kontras SB, Sirak HD, Newton WA, Jr: Hematologic abnormalities in children with congenital heart disease. *JAMA* 195:611–615, 1966.
44. Hickey PR, Hansen DD: High-dose fentanyl reduces intraoperative ventricular fibrillation in neonates with hypoplastic left heart syndrome. *J Clin Anesth* 3:295–300, 1991.
45. Butt WW, Gow R, Whyte H, et al: Complications resulting from use of arterial catheters: retrograde flow and rapid elevation in blood pressure. *Pediatrics* 76:250–254, 1985.
46. Gold JP, Jonas RA, Lang P, et al: Transthoracic intracardiac monitoring lines in pediatric surgical patients: a ten-year experience. *Ann Thorac Surg* 42:185–191, 1986.
47. Crowley R, Sanchez E, Ho JK, et al: Prolonged central venous desaturation measured by continuous oximetry is associated with adverse outcomes in pediatric cardiac surgery. *Anesthesiology* 115:1033–1043, 2011.
48. Haas NA, Haas SA: Central venous catheter techniques in infants and children. *Curr Opin Anaesthesiol* 16:291–303, 2003.
49. Leyvi G, Taylor DG, Reith E, et al: Utility of ultrasound-guided central venous cannulation in pediatric surgical patients: a clinical series. *Paediatr Anaesth* 15:953–958, 2005.
50. Rung GW, Wickey GS, Myers JL, et al: Thiopental as an adjunct to hypothermia for EEG suppression in infants prior to circulatory arrest. *J Cardiothorac Vasc Anesth* 5:337–342, 1991.
51. Hillier SC, Burrows FA, Bissonnette B, et al: Cerebral hemodynamics in neonates and infants undergoing cardiopulmonary bypass and profound hypothermic circulatory arrest: assessment by transcranial Doppler sonography. *Anesth Analg* 72:723–728, 1991.
52. Andropoulos DB, Stayer SA, Diaz LK, et al: Neurological monitoring for congenital heart surgery. *Anesth Analg* 99:1365–1375, 2004.
53. Hoffman GM, Stuth EA, Jaquiss RD, et al: Changes in cerebral and somatic oxygenation during stage 1 palliation of hypoplastic left heart syndrome using continuous regional cerebral perfusion. *J Thorac Cardiovasc Surg* 127:223–233, 2004.
54. Kussman BD, Wypij D, DiNardo JA, et al: An evaluation of bilateral monitoring of cerebral oxygen saturation during pediatric cardiac surgery. *Anesth Analg* 101:1294–1300, 2005.
55. Kussman BD, Wypij D, DiNardo JA, et al: Cerebral oximetry during infant cardiac surgery: evaluation and relationship to early postoperative outcome. *Anesth Analg* 108:1122–1131, 2009.
56. Hsu YH, Santulli T, Jr, Wong AL, et al: Impact of intraoperative echocardiography on surgical management of congenital heart disease. *Am J Cardiol* 67:1279–1283, 1991.
57. Muhiudeen IA, Roberson DA, Silverman NH, et al: Intraoperative echocardiography for evaluation of congenital heart defects in infants and children. *Anesthesiology* 76:165–172, 1992.
58. Weintraub R, Shiota T, Elkadi T, et al: Transesophageal echocardiography in infants and children with congenital heart disease. *Circulation* 86:711–722, 1992.
59. Odegard KC, DiNardo JA, Kussman BD, et al: The frequency of anesthesia-related cardiac arrests in patients with congenital heart disease undergoing cardiac surgery. *Anesth Analg* 105:335–343, 2007.
60. Hansen DD, Hickey PR: Anesthesia for hypoplastic left heart syndrome: use of high-dose fentanyl in 30 neonates. *Anesth Analg* 65:127–132, 1986.
61. Burch TM, McGowan FX, Jr, Kussman BD, et al: Congenital supravalvular aortic stenosis and sudden death associated with anesthesia: what's the mystery? *Anesth Analg* 107:1848–1854, 2008.
62. Tanner GE, Angers DG, Barash PG, et al: Effect of left-to-right, mixed left-to-right, and right-to-left shunts on inhalational anesthetic induction in children: a computer model. *Anesth Analg* 64:101–107, 1985.
63. Sarkar M, Laussen PC, Zurakowski D, et al: Hemodynamic responses to etomidate on induction of anesthesia in pediatric patients. *Anesth Analg* 101:645–650, table of contents, 2005.
64. Williams GD, Jones TK, Hanson KA, et al: The hemodynamic effects of propofol in children with congenital heart disease. *Anesth Analg* 89:1411–1416, 1999.
65. Anand KJ, Hickey PR: Pain and its effects in the human neonate and fetus. *N Engl J Med* 317:1321–1329, 1987.
66. Anand KJ, Hansen DD, Hickey PR: Hormonal-metabolic stress responses in neonates undergoing cardiac surgery. *Anesthesiology* 73:661–670, 1990.
67. Shew SB, Jaksic T: The metabolic needs of critically ill children and neonates. *Semin Pediatr Surg* 8:131–139, 1999.
68. Anand KJ, Hickey PR: Halothane-morphine compared with high-dose sufentanil for anesthesia and postoperative analgesia in neonatal cardiac surgery. *N Engl J Med* 326:1–9, 1992.
69. Wood M, Shand DG, Wood AJ: The sympathetic response to profound hypothermia and circulatory arrest in infants. *Can Anaesth Soc J* 27:125–131, 1980.
70. Wernovsky G, Wypij D, Jonas RA, et al: Postoperative course and hemodynamic profile after the arterial switch operation in neonates and infants. A comparison of low-flow cardiopulmonary bypass and circulatory arrest. *Circulation* 92:2226–2235, 1995.
71. Shum-Tim D, Nagashima M, Shinoka T, et al: Postischemic hyperthermia exacerbates neurologic injury after deep hypothermic circulatory arrest. *J Thorac Cardiovasc Surg* 116:780–792, 1998.
72. Eaton MP: Antifibrinolytic therapy in surgery for congenital heart disease. *Anesth Analg* 106:1087–1100, 2008.
73. Grassin-Delyle S, Couturier R, Abe E, et al: A practical tranexamic acid dosing scheme based on population pharmacokinetics in children undergoing cardiac surgery. *Anesthesiology* 118:853–862, 2013.
74. Mossinger H, Dietrich W, Braun SL, et al: High-dose aprotinin reduces activation of hemostasis, allogeneic blood requirement, and duration of postoperative ventilation in pediatric cardiac surgery. *Ann Thorac Surg* 75:430–437, 2003.
75. Fergusson DA, Hebert PC, Mazer CD, et al: A comparison of aprotinin and lysine analogues in high-risk cardiac surgery. *N Engl J Med* 358:2319–2331, 2008.
76. Mangano DT, Miao Y, Vuylsteke A, et al: Mortality associated with aprotinin during 5 years following coronary artery bypass graft surgery. *JAMA* 297:471–479, 2007.
77. Mangano DT, Tudor IC, Dietzel C: The risk associated with aprotinin in cardiac surgery. *N Engl J Med* 354:353–365, 2006.
78. Mouton R, Finch D, Davies I, et al: Effect of aprotinin on renal dysfunction in patients undergoing on-pump and off-pump cardiac surgery: a retrospective observational study. *Lancet* 371:475–482, 2008.
79. Agarwal HS, Bennett JE, Churchwell KB, et al: Recombinant factor seven therapy for postoperative bleeding in neonatal and pediatric cardiac surgery. *Ann Thorac Surg* 84:161–168, 2007.
80. Dunkley S, Phillips L, McCall P, et al: Recombinant activated factor VII in cardiac surgery: experience from the Australian and New Zealand Haemostasis Registry. *Ann Thorac Surg* 85:836–844, 2008.
81. Guzzetta NA, Russell IA, Williams GD: Review of the off-label use of recombinant activated factor VII in pediatric cardiac surgery patients. *Anesth Analg* 115:364–378, 2012.
82. Cote CJ: Sedation for the pediatric patient. A review. *Pediatr Clin North Am* 41:31–58, 1994.
83. American Academy of Pediatrics Committee on Drugs: Guidelines for monitoring and management of pediatric patients during and after sedation for diagnostic and theurapeutic procedures. *Pediatrics* 89:1110–1115, 1992.

84. Hickey PR, Hansen DD, Wessel DL, et al: Pulmonary and systemic hemodynamic responses to fentanyl in infants. *Anesth Analg* 64:483–486, 1985.
85. Tobias JD: Dexmedetomidine: applications in pediatric critical care and pediatric anesthesiology. *Pediatr Crit Care Med* 8:115–131, 2007.
86. Hammer GB, Drover DR, Cao H, et al: The effects of dexmedetomidine on cardiac electrophysiology in children. *Anesth Analg* 106:79–83, 2008.
87. Kam PC, Cardone D: Propofol infusion syndrome. *Anaesthesia* 62:690–701, 2007.
88. Leier CV, Heban PT, Huss P, et al: Comparative systemic and regional hemodynamic effects of dopamine and dobutamine in patients with cardiomyopathic heart failure. *Circulation* 58:466–475, 1978.
89. Jerath N, Frndova H, McCrindle BW, et al: Clinical impact of vasopressin infusion on hemodynamics, liver and renal function in pediatric patients. *Intensive Care Med* 34:1274–1280, 2008.
90. Millar KJ, Thiagarajan RR, Laussen PC: Glucocorticoid therapy for hypotension in the cardiac intensive care unit. *Pediatr Cardiol* 28:176–182, 2007.
91. Shore S, Nelson DP, Pearl JM, et al: Usefulness of corticosteroid therapy in decreasing epinephrine requirements in critically ill infants with congenital heart disease. *Am J Cardiol* 88:591–594, 2001.
92. Suominen PK, Dickerson HA, Moffett BS, et al: Hemodynamic effects of rescue protocol hydrocortisone in neonates with low cardiac output syndrome after cardiac surgery. *Pediatr Crit Care Med* 6:655–659, 2005.
93. Bettendorf M, Schmidt KG, Grulich-Henn J, et al: Tri-iodothyronine treatment in children after cardiac surgery: a double-blind, randomised, placebo-controlled study. *Lancet* 356: 529–534, 2000.
94. Mackie AS, Booth KL, Newburger JW, et al: A randomized, double-blind, placebo-controlled pilot trial of triiodothyronine in neonatal heart surgery. *J Thorac Cardiovasc Surg* 130:810–816, 2005.
95. Perry J, Walsh EP: *Diagnosis and management of cardiac arrhythmias*, Baltimore, 1998, Williams & Wilkins.
96. Weindling SN, Saul JP, Gamble WJ, et al: Duration of complete atrioventricular block after congenital heart disease surgery. *Am J Cardiol* 82:525–527, 1998.
97. Wessel DL: Hemodynamic responses to perioperative pain and stress in infants. *Crit Care Med* 21:S361–S362, 1993.
98. Benzing G, 3rd, Helmsworth JA, Schreiber JT, et al: Nitroprusside and epinephrine for treatment of low output in children after open-heart surgery. *Ann Thorac Surg* 27:523–528, 1979.
99. Chang AC, Atz AM, Wernovsky G, et al: Milrinone: systemic and pulmonary hemodynamic effects in neonates after cardiac surgery. *Crit Care Med* 23:1907–1914, 1995.
100. Hoffman TM, Wernovsky G, Atz AM, et al: Efficacy and safety of milrinone in preventing low cardiac output syndrome in infants and children after corrective surgery for congenital heart disease. *Circulation* 107:996–1002, 2003.
101. Lawless ST, Zaritsky A, Miles M: The acute pharmacokinetics and pharmacodynamics of amrinone in pediatric patients. *J Clin Pharmacol* 31:800–803, 1991.
102. Wessel DL: Testing new drugs for heart failure in children. *Pediatr Crit Care Med* 7:493–494, 2006.
103. Booker PD: Intra-aortic balloon pumping in young children. *Paediatr Anaesth* 7:501–507, 1997.
104. Davies MJ, Nguyen K, Gaynor JW, et al: Modified ultrafiltration improves left ventricular systolic function in infants after cardiopulmonary bypass. *J Thorac Cardiovasc Surg* 115:361–369, discussion 369–370, 1998.
105. Elliott MJ: Ultrafiltration and modified ultrafiltration in pediatric open heart operations. *Ann Thorac Surg* 56:1518–1522, 1993.
106. Halpenny M, Lakshmi S, O'Donnell A, et al: Fenoldopam: renal and splanchnic effects in patients undergoing coronary artery bypass grafting. *Anaesthesia* 56:953–960, 2001.
107. Costello JM, Goodman DM, Green TP: A review of the natriuretic hormone system's diagnostic and therapeutic potential in critically ill children. *Pediatr Crit Care Med* 7:308–318, 2006.
108. Giuffre RM, Tam KH, Williams WW, et al: Acute renal failure complicating pediatric cardiac surgery: a comparison of survivors and nonsurvivors following acute peritoneal dialysis. *Pediatr Cardiol* 13:208–213, 1992.
109. Paret G, Cohen AJ, Bohn DJ, et al: Continuous arteriovenous hemofiltration after cardiac operations in infants and children. *J Thorac Cardiovasc Surg* 104:1225–1230, 1992.
110. Jenkins J, Lynn A, Edmonds J, et al: Effects of mechanical ventilation on cardiopulmonary function in children after open-heart surgery. *Crit Care Med* 13:77–80, 1985.
111. Lister G, Talner N: *Management of respiratory failure of cardiac origin*, New York, 1981, Churchill-Livingstone.
112. Pinsky MR, Summer WR, Wise RA, et al: Augmentation of cardiac function by elevation of intrathoracic pressure. *J Appl Physiol* 54:950–955, 1983.
113. Robotham JL, Lixfeld W, Holland L, et al: The effects of positive end-expiratory pressure on right and left ventricular performance. *Am Rev Respir Dis* 121:677–683, 1980.
114. West JB: *Respiratory physiology: the essentials*, Baltimore, 1974, Williams & Wilkins.
115. Michard F: Changes in arterial pressure during mechanical ventilation. *Anesthesiology* 103:419–428, quiz 449-5, 2005.
116. Singh KE, Baum VC: Pro: early extubation in the operating room following cardiac surgery in adults. *Semin Cardiothorac Vasc Anesth* 16:182–186, 2012.

CHAPTER 111

NEUROMONITORING AND NEURODEVELOPMENTAL OUTCOMES IN CONGENITAL HEART SURGERY

Christopher E. Mascio • J. William Gaynor

CHAPTER OUTLINE

HISTORY OF INTRAOPERATIVE NEUROMONITORING

Brain injury is the most common and potentially disabling complication following congenital heart surgery. With improved survival, the focus has shifted to optimizing functional outcomes. An important goal of therapy for every congenital heart surgical patient is to reduce the risk of brain injury as much as possible. Along with updated perfusion, anesthetic, and surgical strategies, techniques for neuromonitoring have been refined and adopted by many centers performing pediatric cardiothoracic surgery.

Penfield and Boldrey first reported intraoperative neurophysiologic monitoring in 1937.[1] They used direct cortical stimulation during operations for epilepsy. Recording an electroencephalogram directly from the cerebral cortex, also for epilepsy surgery, was first done in 1949 by Jasper and Marshall and Walker.[1] Routine scalp electroencephalography (EEG), used first during carotid endarterectomy, was introduced in the late 1960s.[1] Doppler ultrasound evaluation of the extracranial cerebral arteries was first reported in 1965 by Miyazaki and Kato.[2] Transcranial Doppler (TCD) was reported by Aaslid in 1982 after measuring the flow of the middle cerebral artery with a probe placed on the scalp over the temporal bone.[3] Near-infrared spectroscopy (NIRS) was introduced clinically in 1985 for monitoring cerebral oxygenation in preterm infants.[4] Spinal intraoperative monitoring, specifically somatosensory evoked potentials, was developed in the 1970s.[1] The first intraoperative neuromonitoring clinical service was established at the University of California at Los Angeles in 1979,[1] and commercial neurophysiologic monitoring equipment became available in the early 1980s.

NEURODEVELOPMENTAL OUTCOMES

Introduction

Survival after congenital heart surgery has improved, and the focus has shifted to optimizing neurodevelopmental outcomes. Survivors of repair of congenital heart disease in the neonatal period demonstrate cognitive, motor, speech, visual, and learning abnormalities.[5]

Determining causation in abnormal neurodevelopment and the occurrence of neurodevelopmental disability is a challenging endeavor. Genetic predisposition and many other nonmodifiable patient factors, including prematurity, socioeconomic status, and maternal education, have been shown to be risk factors for worse neurodevelopmental outcomes. In addition, there is increasing evidence that congenital heart disease alters fetal brain growth and development.

In addition to nonmodifiable factors, operative management factors have been implicated in altering neurodevelopmental outcome. This includes preoperative/postoperative hypoxemia and arrest, cardiopulmonary bypass and circulatory arrest strategies, hematocrit levels during cardiopulmonary bypass, and blood gas management during bypass.

Nonmodifiable Factors Associated with Adverse Neurodevelopmental Outcomes

Fetal Brain Development and Preoperative Brain Abnormalities

Beginning in the third trimester of fetal life, patients with congenital heart disease are known to have smaller gestational age- and weight-adjusted brain volumes and impaired neuroaxonal development and metabolism.[6] These abnormalities are most pronounced in patients with complex types of heart defects such as hypoplastic left heart syndrome and transposition of the great arteries.[6] Structural malformations of the brain occur at a much higher rate in patients with congenital heart disease than in the general population.[7] Microcephaly, microencephaly, and other malformations, including absence of the corpus callosum, have been documented in necropsy series of patients with hypoplastic left heart syndrome.[8] Neonates with congenital heart disease have altered cerebral hemodynamics often with lower than normal cerebral blood flow and/or oxygen delivery. There is evidence of delayed white matter development, which can lead to an increased risk of white matter injury (periventricular leukomalacia [PVL]) and microcephaly. One study of neonates with complex congenital heart disease used preoperative pulsed arterial spin-label perfusion magnetic resonance imaging (MRI) to quantitate cerebral blood flow.[9] More than half of the cohort had developmental or acquired lesions, and the cerebral blood flow was less than half of that reported in normal, term neonates.[10] The same study also examined cerebrovascular responsiveness to CO_2, and found that PVL was associated with decreased CO_2 responsiveness. Abnormal cerebrovascular reactivity to CO_2 has been associated with increased mortality and worse neurodevelopmental outcomes.[11,12] White matter injury characterized by PVL is the most common pattern of injury.[13] The mechanism of this injury is thought to be the result of effects of hypoxia and/or ischemia on pre-myelinating oligodendrocyte precursors during their most vulnerable time of 24 to 34 weeks gestation.[14] Up to 40% of neonates with congenital heart disease have PVL on preoperative MRI, and PVL has been shown to be associated with poor neurodevelopmental outcomes.[9,15,17] The incidence of PVL is highest in neonates undergoing cardiopulmonary bypass. A study by Galli and colleagues revealed a 54% incidence of PVL in neonates compared to 4% in infants.[18] PVL is the neurologic lesion associated with cerebral palsy in infants born prematurely.[19] This pattern of brain injury is seen not only in preterm newborns but also in term neonates with congenital heart disease.[20] A comparison of newborns with congenital heart disease and a control cohort without heart defects revealed that almost one third of those with congenital heart disease had white matter injury.[21] The injury pattern was not seen in those without heart defects.

Prematurity

Preterm birth, even in infants without congenital heart disease, is a powerful predictor of worse neurodevelopmental outcome. Along with low birth weight, preterm birth has been associated with long-term behavioral and learning issues. In a study of 125 very low-birth-weight preterm infants who were evaluated with the Bayley Scales of Infant and Toddler Development III at 24 months, later gestational age was associated with better neurodevelopmental outcome.[22]

Socioeconomic Factors

Other nonmodifiable patient factors that adversely affect neurodevelopmental outcomes are socioeconomic status and maternal education. In a study of neurodevelopmental outcomes after repair of total anomalous pulmonary venous connection, lower socioeconomic status was predictive of lower scores on the Mental Developmental Index (MDI) of the Bayley Scales of Infant Development II.[23] The Single Ventricle Reconstruction trial is the randomized, prospective trial comparing shunt types in the Norwood procedure. Evaluation of this cohort at 14 months demonstrated that lower maternal education was associated with lower MDI scores.[24]

Genetic Polymorphisms

Many genetic syndromes are associated with congenital heart disease, including Down syndrome,[25] Noonan syndrome,[26] Williams syndrome,[27] and DiGeorge syndrome (22q11.2 microdeletion).[28] These syndromes are associated with developmental delay, and assigning causation of neurodevelopmental delay can be challenging. For example, individuals with DiGeorge syndrome have a mean IQ in the 70s,[29] a predisposition to psychiatric disorders,[30] and an increased incidence of white matter abnormalities.[31]

There is also evidence that genetic variants that modify the brain's response to injury and subsequent recovery may also be important determinants of neurodevelopmental outcomes. The first genetic polymorphism studied in relation to congenital heart disease and operations was apolipoprotein E (APOE).[5] APOE regulates cholesterol metabolism and is the primary lipid transport vehicle in the central nervous system; there also is evidence that APOE is important for neuronal repair.[5] There are three APOE alleles (e2, e3, e4) on chromosome 19 that vary by a single amino acid. The Children's Hospital of Philadelphia evaluated the association of APOE genotype and postoperative neurodevelopmental outcome at age 1 year.[5] Neurodevelopmental outcomes were evaluated using the Bayley Scales of Infant Development II. The APOE e2 allele was associated with a significantly lower Psychomotor Developmental Index (PDI) score after adjustment for perioperative covariates, including gestational age, age at operation, sex, race, socioeconomic status, cardiac defect, and the use of circulatory arrest. Further analysis of this group revealed patient-specific factors that significantly predicted neurodevelopmental outcomes at age 1 year, including presence of genetic syndrome, low birth weight, and presence of APOE e2 allele.[33] Neurobehavioral outcomes were then evaluated in the cohort between ages 4 and 5.[34] Those with the APOE e2 allele had increased behavior problems, restricted behavior patterns, and impaired social skills. The entire cohort had a significantly higher proportion of patients considered either at risk for, or in the clinically significant range for, neurodevelopmental problems. The cohort was further evaluated for other genetic causes of poor neurodevelopmental outcomes beyond APOE genetic polymorphisms. A genome-wide association study identified single nucleotide polymorphisms (SNPs) associated with neurobehavioral abnormalities.[35] Ten SNPs reached a threshold for suggested significant associations with neurobehavioral phenotypes. These results identify additional genes—after adjusting for the effects of APOE and other genetic syndromes—that may contribute to adverse neurodevelopmental outcomes.

A study comparing the relative contribution of patient factors (gestational age, genetic syndrome, birth weight, etc.) to management factors on neurodevelopmental outcomes at 1 year of age after neonatal and infant cardiac surgery showed that patient factors explained more of the variability in the PDI (21% vs. 8%) and MDI (13% vs. 5%) than did management factors.[36] Factors such as gender, birth weight, and presence of genetic syndrome had a more significant impact on neurodevelopmental outcomes than did cardiopulmonary bypass time, circulatory arrest time, and hematocrit. Not all patients with congenital heart disease enter the operating room with the same neurodevelopmental prognosis. Interindividual variation of many nonmodifiable patient factors significantly contributes to widely disparate neurodevelopmental outcomes of different patients with the same cardiac diagnosis.

Management Factors Associated with Adverse Neurodevelopmental Outcomes

Many studies have examined the impact of different management strategies before and during congenital heart operations on neurodevelopmental outcomes. Operative management strategies and type of support (circulatory arrest versus low-flow cardiopulmonary bypass), pH strategy, target hematocrit value, and others have all been evaluated in relation to postoperative neurodevelopmental outcomes. Preoperative management can have a profound impact on neurodevelopmental outcomes. Acidosis, hypoxemia, hypotension, and cardiac arrest are all examples of preoperative management factors that contribute to neurodevelopmental outcomes.

Hypoxemia, Cardiac Arrest

Ductal-dependent cardiac lesions put patients at risk of acidosis, hypoxemia, and cardiovascular collapse if the diagnosis is not known and ductal closure occurs.[8,37] The number of prenatal diagnoses of congenital heart lesions has increased in recent years. This often results in delivery in centers equipped to care for severe forms of congenital heart disease and has permitted immediate or early infusion of prostaglandin to maintain ductal patency and avoid profound acidosis and subsequent neurologic issues.[38-40] Preoperative hypoxemia has been shown to be associated with abnormal neurodevelopmental outcomes. Neurodevelopmental testing done on a cohort of patients 5 to 10 years after repair for both cyanotic and acyanotic heart defects demonstrated more speech and language dysfunction in the group with preoperative cyanosis.[41] Cardiac arrest puts all organs at risk until circulation (spontaneous or mechanical) is restored. A recent review of extracorporeal cardiopulmonary resuscitation (ECPR) survivors identified 10 studies that examined neurologic outcomes after ECPR.[42] Overall survival of ECPR was 79%, and nine of the reports described Pediatric Cerebral Performance Category (PCPC) scores, an early test of neurologic function. Seventy-nine percent of survivors had a PCPC score of 2 or less, indicating normal or mild impairment. There are no data describing long-term neurodevelopmental outcomes after cardiac arrest and ECPR.

Many intraoperative aspects of pediatric cardiac operations have been thought to put the patient at risk for acute neurologic injury and subsequent suboptimal neurodevelopmental outcomes. As mentioned earlier, type of support (circulatory arrest versus low-flow cardiopulmonary bypass), pH strategy, and target hematocrit value have all been evaluated in relation to postoperative neurodevelopmental outcomes.

A prospective, randomized study from Boston Children's Hospital in 1988 assigned patients with transposition of the great arteries undergoing the arterial switch operation to receive either hypothermic circulatory arrest or low-flow cardiopulmonary bypass.[43] Neurodevelopmental outcomes (formal neurodevelopmental evaluation and MRI) for this cohort were reported at age 1 year. Patients randomized to circulatory arrest had a significantly lower mean score on the PDI of the Bayley Scales of Infant Development, and the score was inversely related to the duration of circulatory arrest. A longer duration of circulatory arrest was associated with an increased risk of neurologic abnormalities. The authors were unable to determine a safe threshold for circulatory arrest but noted that a period shorter than 35 minutes had minimal effect on the PDI score and that significant deficits were more prevalent in the group of children that had a circulatory arrest period greater than 45 minutes. At 4- and 8-year follow-up, the Boston study revealed worse motor and speech function in the circulatory arrest group.[44,45] However, measures of behavior were worse in subjects randomized to continuous cardiopulmonary bypass. At the 16-year evaluations, most differences between the treatment groups had disappeared, but the circulatory arrest cohort scored lower on tests of executive function and visual spatial skills.[46] Both treatment groups fared worse on tests of neurodevelopment than did population controls. Socioeconomic status explained more test variation than did treatment group assignment.

Cerebral Perfusion

A study of 57 neonates examined pre- and postoperative MRI and 1-year neurodevelopmental outcomes after receiving regional cerebral perfusion (RCP) during aortic arch reconstruction.[47] The mean RCP time was 71 minutes and the mean RCP flow was 57 mL/kg/min. New postoperative brain injury on MRI was seen in 40% of patients, which is comparable to other studies examining new postoperative MRI brain injury. The 1-year cognitive testing was at reference population norms, whereas language and motor outcomes were lower than reference population norms.

There has been increasing interest in RCP to avoid use of circulatory arrest. A study from the University of Michigan randomized 77 patients to receive either circulatory arrest or RCP during the Norwood operation.[48] They then performed neurodevelopmental testing on each cohort before the second stage operation and at age 1. The entire cohort demonstrated delayed neurodevelopment with the PDI scores being lower than the MDI scores. No statistically significant difference in MDI or PDI scores was found between the two groups, although the RCP group had lower average point estimates for both the MDI and the PDI compared with the circulatory arrest cohort.

pH strategy is an important part of the operative management of patients requiring hypothermic cardiopulmonary bypass. A recent study from the Netherlands randomized neonates to either deep hypothermic circulatory arrest or antegrade cerebral perfusion.[49] MRI was done preoperatively and 1 week postoperatively. The authors found no difference between the circulatory arrest and antegrade perfusion cohorts in terms of new cerebral injury (78% vs. 72%, respectively; $P = 0.66$). The most common type of injury was white matter injury, but infarctions of the thalamus and/or basal ganglia were seen only after antegrade cerebral perfusion. Motor and cognitive testing done at 24 months showed no difference between the two groups.

Neurodevelopmental outcomes were evaluated at 4 years of age in an observational study of the impact of *APOE* genotype for an association with the use of deep hypothermic circulatory arrest.[50] No differences in unadjusted outcomes were found between those that received circulatory arrest and those that did not. However, consistent with previously published data, nonmodifiable patient factors were significantly associated with neurodevelopmental outcomes. Presence of a genetic anomaly, lower socioeconomic status and maternal education, and younger gestational age were all associated with worse outcomes.

Blood Gas Management

Two methods of blood gas management during cardiopulmonary bypass are commonly used: alpha stat and pH stat. A prospective, randomized study comparing these two strategies demonstrated an early return of electroencephalographic activity in patients randomized to pH-stat management.[51] However, neurodevelopmental testing at 1 year of age showed no benefit or detriment associated with either strategy.[51,52]

Hematocrit

Hematocrit is a modifiable, operative management variable. It is vitally important for oxygen delivery and has been shown to affect neurodevelopmental outcomes. A prospective, randomized study done at Boston Children's Hospital assigned patients to a hypothermic bypass hematocrit of either 20% or 30%.[53] At 1 year, the lower hematocrit group had lower PDI scores. A second prospective, randomized study by the same group compared bypass hematocrits of 25% and 35%.[54] There were no differences between the groups on tests of neurodevelopment at 1 year of age. Based largely on these studies, most centers have chosen 25% as the lowest acceptable hematocrit while on cardiopulmonary bypass.

Glucose Management

Adult cardiac surgery literature has recently touted the benefits of tight glycemic control.[55] One study of glycemic control in a mixed (medical and surgical patients) pediatric intensive care unit compared tight glycemic control with standard management.[56] The cohort receiving tight glycemic control had a lower mortality rate but experienced high rates of hypoglycemia. Hypoglycemia is potentially dangerous to the developing brain. A more recent randomized, prospective trial enrolled 980 patients after cardiopulmonary bypass to receive either tight glycemic control or standard glucose management. No differences were found in infection rate, mortality, length of stay, or measures of organ failure. This trial had a low rate of hypoglycemia; but, with no obvious benefits, it seems unnecessary to institute tight glycemic control and risk deleterious effects on the developing brain with episodes of hypoglycemia.

INTRAOPERATIVE NEUROMONITORING

Introduction

Many institutions have adopted intraoperative neuromonitoring as a potential mechanism to minimize brain injury resulting from congenital heart surgery. It can be as simple as having the anesthesiologist monitor NIRS or as complex as using four modalities with a certified neuromonitoring professional in the operating room providing feedback during each case. The most common modalities used are NIRS, EEG, and TCD. Intraoperative NIRS is used at most congenital heart centers for all cardiopulmonary bypass cases. Somatosensory evoked potentials (SSEPs or SEPs) are used very little in congenital heart surgery and will not be discussed. Figure 111-1 demonstrates the appearance of a patient after placement of multimodality neuromonitoring devices. It should be noted, however, that there is a lack of prospective, randomized data showing any benefit to intraoperative neuromonitoring.

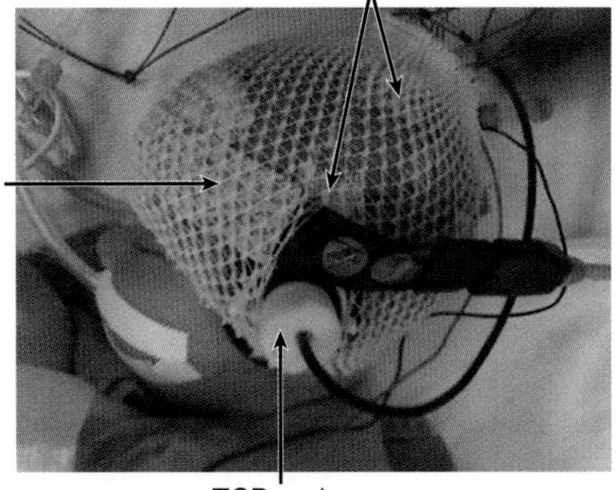

FIGURE 111-1 ■ Intraoperative photograph demonstrating the proper placement of multimodality neuromonitoring probes. *EEG,* Electroencephalography; *NIRS,* near-infrared spectroscopy; *TCD,* transcranial Doppler. (Photo used with permission and courtesy of Harvey L. Edmonds, Jr., PhD.)

Near-infrared Spectroscopy

NIRS noninvasively provides an estimate of cerebral oxygen saturation because of the different absorption spectra between oxygenated and total hemoglobin. The translucency of the skull of the pediatric patient allows probes placed on the forehead to monitor the cerebral cortex. The value obtained is predominately from blood in tissue that is mostly venous blood (75% venous blood). NIRS is the only modality capable of monitoring the brain during circulatory arrest as EEG is flat and TCD will indicate no flow. Cooling and increasing levels of anesthetics will decrease metabolism and increase an individual patient's NIRS value. It is unknown what thresholds are important in the pediatric cardiac surgery patient. Some centers use parameters derived from adult studies (a decrease in NIRS below 50% and/or a drop greater than 20% from baseline) because there are no established guidelines in pediatric patients. Many centers follow trends rather than absolute numbers because there is significant interindividual variation.

Electroencephalography

Intraoperative electroencephalography is used to detect ischemia during congenital heart surgery. In normothermic patients under anesthesia, electroencephalographic slowing indicates inadequate cerebral perfusion and/or oxygenation. To monitor the EEG, cup electrodes are placed on the scalp and shaving hair is not required. Four-channel EEG (four electrodes over each hemisphere and a ground in the middle) will measure the anterior and posterior circulations of both hemispheres. Electroencephalographic recordings demonstrate significant variability between individuals, and proper analysis requires experience and skill at pattern recognition.[57] In general, patients with adequate cerebral oxygen delivery will demonstrate low-amplitude, high-frequency EEG. Ischemia is represented by high-amplitude, low-frequency waveforms.

Increasing amounts of anesthetics reliably cause diffuse slowing.[57] Slowing is usually not focal or asymmetric unless there is previous cortical injury, cortical abnormality, or new, acute injury. Fast-frequency activities are seen with lower levels of anesthetics.[57] They can be difficult to distinguish from epileptiform waves. As with slowing, focal disparities are a sign of previous injury or new, acute ischemia or injury. New epileptiform or epileptic activity indicates cortical dysfunction usually caused by ischemia. Distinguishing concerning changes from artifact can be a challenge and requires significant experience. Artifact can be caused by pulsation (near a pulsatile vessel), electrocardiogram (ECG) interference, electrical interference (such as a headlight, operating room bed, or lower extremity compression devices), or a loose electrode.[58] Comparing the EEG abnormalities to the QRS complexes on the ECG often helps resolve cases of suspected pulsation and ECG artifact.[58] Temporarily interrupting other electrical sources in the operating room can help determine if electrical interference is present.[58] Securing electrodes and checking them will help prevent artifact caused by loose electrodes.[58]

There are times during a congenital heart operation with cardiopulmonary bypass that changes in the EEG can be expected.[59] Slowing in the EEG is often seen during cannulation of smaller patients. It is thought that the larger cannula-to-vessel ratio in small patients may cause obstruction to flow. In addition, a moderate amount of blood loss has a larger negative impact on circulating blood volume than in an adult. There is a transient depression in the EEG at the onset of cardiopulmonary bypass, likely caused by the relatively oxygen-deficient pump prime. Finally, hypotension after the release of the aortic crossclamp will cause EEG slowing. Deep hypothermic circulatory arrest causes slowing, and eventually flattening, of the EEG. One limitation of EEG monitoring is that the slowing seen with ischemia and/or hypoxia cannot be differentiated from that caused by anesthetics and/or cooling. The most important neuromonitoring change associated with cerebral ischemia is EEG slowing.[59] It provides continuous feedback on the function of the cerebral cortex. Combined with the other modalities, it can be used to help decide if a response to worsening neuromonitoring parameters is indicated.

Bispectral Index Scale (BIS) is another neuromonitoring tool that is used for intraoperative monitoring. The Food and Drug Administration approved it in 1996 as an EEG-based monitor of anesthetic effect.[60] BIS describes the continuous, varying signal of EEG as a number ranging from 100 (awake) to 0 (complete cortical suppression).[61] It is an easy-to-use, quickly applied, one-channel processed EEG.[61] In congenital heart surgery, it can be used as a marker of cortical silence when deep hypothermic circulatory arrest is used. It has also been used in conjunction with other neuromonitoring modalities to assess adequacy of cerebral perfusion.[62]

Transcranial Doppler

TCD measures the velocity of red blood cells.[59] TCD can determine both the presence and direction of blood flow. The probe is positioned over the temporal bone and monitors flow in the middle cerebral artery. Peak systolic velocity is a marker of cerebral inflow, and end-diastolic velocity is inversely related to cerebrovascular resistance. Inflow obstruction will result in a decrease in the peak systolic velocity. If accompanied by EEG slowing, an ischemic process is likely evolving.[59] Outflow obstruction (venous cannula malposition, for example) will increase the cerebrovascular resistance and decrease the end-diastolic velocity. High-intensity transient signals (HITSs) represent the presence of gaseous or particulate emboli within the blood vessel. Data from adult studies indicate that an increasing number of HITSs may predict postoperative neurobehavioral, pulmonary, and renal complications.[63] TCD is unable to differentiate between types of emboli.

Biomarkers

Various serum biomarkers have been found to be associated with neurodevelopmental outcome. In a study of infants undergoing congenital heart surgery aged 6 weeks and younger, postoperative lactic acid level correlated with survival and neurodevelopmental outcome. Adverse survivors, or those survivors with suboptimal neurodevelopmental outcomes, had a higher peak lactate concentration (7.9 vs. 6.5 mmol/liter) and a longer time to plasma lactate normalization (16 vs. 11 hours) when compared with those survivors with normal or intact neurodevelopmental outcomes.[64]

Brain type natriuretic peptide (BNP) is a serum marker of heart failure that is elevated when right and/or left heart pressures are increased. A study of single ventricle patients in the enalapril trial examined the association of BNP and height with neurodevelopmental outcomes.[65] The investigators discovered that patients with high BNP values and poor growth had worse MDI (Bayley Scales of Infant Development II) scores at 14 months.

CURRENT DATA

Optimizing long-term functional outcome for every patient is a major focus of congenital heart surgery as survival has improved. As mentioned earlier, many institutions now use one or more modalities of intraoperative neuromonitoring. However, there is a paucity of randomized, prospective trials and there remains considerable debate about the benefit, if any, that intraoperative neuromonitoring provides. Many single-institution case-control, observational, and retrospective studies have been conducted.

Surgeons at one institution discussed their approach to multimodality monitoring and reviewed available evidence.[66] Clark and colleagues use NIRS, TCD, EEG, and SEP and intervene when NIRS decreases more than 20% from baseline. However, they admit that this threshold is derived from adult studies and that a pediatric threshold has not been defined. Their use of TCD is no different than what has been reported previously; that is, they use TCD for detecting alterations in cerebral blood flow and emboli. The surgeons also describe their preference for four-channel EEG in patients younger than 2 years (eight-channel EEG for patients older than 2 years) and their routine use of SEP in patients older than 2 years. Clark and colleagues then provide a review of the available data for NIRS, TCD, EEG, SEP, and multimodality monitoring and conclude there are no data that support the routine use of these modalities in the operating room.

Another report describes an institution's attempts to decrease the risk of neurologic injury to neonates undergoing cardiac surgery through the use of intraoperative neuromonitoring.[67] Khan and Fraser review their protocol for neonatal cardiopulmonary bypass and discuss their use of bilateral NIRS and TCD to guide antegrade cerebral perfusion to minimize time of deep hypothermic circulatory arrest. They review the literature on intraoperative NIRS and TCD and describe their plans for future neuroprotection studies. The authors conclude that their cardiopulmonary bypass strategy is based on the data currently available but that further studies of long-term neurologic outcomes are warranted.

A systematic review done by a group that included pediatric cardiac surgeons, a pediatric neurologist, and a pediatric anesthesiologist concluded that data supporting the use of current neuromonitoring and neuroprotective techniques are limited.[68] The literature review encompasses 20 years (1990 to 2010) and initially identified 527 manuscripts. Review of this group of abstracts resulted in 187 potential manuscripts based on inclusion and exclusion criteria. Another review generated the final list of 162 manuscripts. The primary outcome was evidence of structural brain injury or functional disability and was demonstrated in only 43% of the manuscripts analyzed. Only 13% of the studies were randomized prospective trials. Manuscript categories analyzed included blood gas management, hematocrit, EEG, cooling, glycemic control, S-100β, TCD, NIRS, and deep hypothermic circulatory arrest/low-flow cardiopulmonary bypass/RCP. The largest groups were those of deep hypothermic circulatory arrest/low-flow cardiopulmonary bypass/RCP (n = 44 manuscripts) followed by NIRS (n = 35). Only two studies (1.3%) were graded as procedures or treatments that are recommended because the benefits clearly outweigh the risks (American College of Cardiology/American Heart Association level of evidence grade class I, level B).[68] These two studies examined the effect of hemodilution on neurodevelopmental outcomes; results suggest that severe hemodilution (probably 24% or less) is associated with adverse neurodevelopmental outcomes.[68] No category reached class I, level A—demonstration of a clear benefit and recommended as effective.[68] Since this systematic review was done, few manuscripts have been added to the literature on the subject of intraoperative neuromonitoring.

Neuroprotection

The aforementioned study that reviewed 20 years of literature on neuroprotection included examination of many aspects of neuroprotection done during the perioperative period, including some of the following: blood gas management, hematocrit, EEG, cooling, glycemic control, S-100β, TCD, NIRS, and deep hypothermic circulatory arrest/low-flow cardiopulmonary bypass/RCP. As mentioned, of the 162 manuscripts that met inclusion criteria, only two were recommended as having benefits that outweighed the risks. Both involved hemodilution and advised that the hematocrit stay at or above 24% during cardiopulmonary bypass cases. The study also reviewed the use of perioperative medications, including phenobarbital, erythropoietin, allopurinol, aprotinin, tranexamic acid, steroids, methylprednisolone, and dexamethasone. There are no studies that report a benefit to using any of these medications. Most centers have adopted protocols for neuroprotection and neuromonitoring that they feel are safe and work best at their institution. At the Children's Hospital of Philadelphia, the neuromonitoring and neuroprotection strategy currently includes the following: The cardiopulmonary bypass pump setup contains a bubble detector and continuous arterial blood gas and venous saturation monitors. The priming protocol contains Solu-Medrol. The goal hematocrit for patients younger than 1 year of age is higher than 30%. For patients older than 1 year, the goal hematocrit is higher than 25%. While on cardiopulmonary bypass, the goal mean arterial pressure is 25 to 55 mm Hg for neonates weighing 5 kg or less. This increases to 60 to 80 mm Hg for patients aged 11 years and older and weighing more than 40 kg. Alpha stat is used at normothermia and when warming. pH stat is used when cooling and when maintaining hypothermia. The arterial-to-patient temperature gradient is maintained between 8° C and 10° C when cooling. Cooling is performed for at least 15 minutes prior to circulatory arrest, and the arterial temperature is maintained higher than 15° C. Warming is also done with the arterial-to-patient temperature gradient maintained at 8° C to 10° C.

Many questions about neurodevelopmental outcomes, neuromonitoring, and neuroprotection remain unanswered. It is clear now that many patients have preoperative cerebral abnormalities. Some patients with a structurally and functionally normal brain are at higher risk of brain injury during congenital heart surgery because of a genetic predisposition. Longer-term follow-up will continue to help plan future strategies to optimize neurodevelopmental outcomes. Available modalities of intraoperative neuromonitoring include EEG, TCD, NIRS, and SSEP. Whether these techniques prevent brain injury remains to be seen. A prospective, randomized study with longer-term neurodevelopmental outcomes has not been accomplished. This study may never be accomplished because many centers have already adopted these technologies as standard without proof of benefit. The hardware used in the cardiopulmonary bypass circuit continues to evolve. However, there is still no consensus on what type of cerebral perfusion, if any, is best during deep hypothermic circulatory arrest. The best outcomes in such a heterogeneous field of congenital heart surgery are often achieved by doing what is comfortable and safe for an individual surgeon, team, and institution.

REFERENCES

1. Nuwer MR: Introduction, history, and staffing for intraoperative monitoring. In Galloway GM, Nuwer MR, Lopez JR, et al, editors: *Intraoperative neurophysiologic monitoring*, Cambridge, 2010, Cambridge University Press.
2. Miyazaki M, Kato K: Measurement of cerebral blood flow by ultrasonic Doppler technique. *Jpn Circ J* 29:375–382, 1965.
3. Aaslid R, Markwalder T-M, Nornes H: Noninvasive transcranial Doppler ultrasound recording of flow velocity in basal cerebral arteries. *J Neurosurg* 57:769–774, 1982.
4. Brazy JE, Lewis DV, Mitnick MH, et al: Noninvasive monitoring of cerebral oxygenation in preterm infants: preliminary observations. *Pediatrics* 75:217–225, 1985.
5. Gaynor JW, Gerdes M, Zackai EH, et al: Apolipoprotein E genotype and neurodevelopmental sequelae of infant cardiac surgery. *J Thorac Cardiovasc Surg* 126:1736–1745, 2003.
6. Limperopoulos C, Tworetzky W, McElhinney DB, et al: Brain volume and metabolism in fetuses with congenital heart disease: evaluation with quantitative magnetic resonance imaging and spectroscopy. *Circulation* 121(1):26–33, 2010.
7. Mahle WT, Wernovsky G: Neurodevelopmental outcomes in hypoplastic left heart syndrome. *Semin Thorac Cardiovasc Surg Pediatr Card Surg Annu* 7:39–47, 2004. Review.
8. Glauser TA, Rorke LB, Weinberg PM, et al: Congenital brain anomalies associated with the hypoplastic left heart syndrome. *Pediatrics* 85(6):984–990, 1990.
9. Licht DJ, Wang J, Silvestre DW, et al: Preoperative cerebral blood flow is diminished in neonates with severe congenital heart defects. *J Thorac Cardiovasc Surg* 128(6):841–849, 2004.
10. Chiron C, Raynaud C, Mazière B, et al: Changes in regional cerebral blood flow during brain maturation in children and adolescents. *J Nucl Med* 33(5):696–703, 1992.
11. Ashwal S, Perkin RM, Thompson JR, et al: CBF and CBF/PCO2 reactivity in childhood strangulation. *Pediatr Neurol* 7(5):369–374, 1991.
12. Ashwal S, Stringer W, Tomasi L, et al: Cerebral blood flow and carbon dioxide reactivity in children with bacterial meningitis. *J Pediatr* 117(4):523–530, 1990.
13. Kinney HC, Panigrahy A, Newburger JW, et al: Hypoxic-ischemic brain injury in infants with congenital heart disease dying after cardiac surgery. *Acta Neuropathol* 110(6):563–578, 2005.
14. Licht DJ, Shera DM, Clancy RR, et al: Brain maturation is delayed in infants with complex congenital heart defects. *J Thorac Cardiovasc Surg* 137(3):529–536, discussion 536–537, 2009.
15. Mahle WT, Tavani F, Zimmerman RA, et al: An MRI study of neurological injury before and after congenital heart surgery. *Circulation* 106(12 Suppl 1):I109–I114, 2002.
16. Reference deleted in page proofs.
17. Miller SP, Ferriero DM, Leonard C, et al: Early brain injury in premature newborns detected with magnetic resonance imaging is associated with adverse early neurodevelopmental outcome. *J Pediatr* 147(5):609–616, 2005.
18. Galli KK, Zimmerman RA, Jarvik GP, et al: Periventricular leukomalacia is common after neonatal cardiac surgery. *J Thorac Cardiovasc Surg* 127(3):692–704, 2004. Erratum in: *J Thorac Cardiovasc Surg* 128(3):498, 2004.
19. Folkerth RD: Periventricular leukomalacia: overview and recent findings. *Pediatr Dev Pathol* 9(1):3–13, 2006.
20. Dimitropoulos A, McQuillen PS, Sethi V, et al: Brain injury and development in newborns with critical congenital heart disease. *Neurology* 81(3):241–248, 2013.
21. Miller SP, McQuillen PS, Hamrick S, et al: Abnormal brain development in newborns with congenital heart disease. *N Engl J Med* 357(19):1928–1938, 2007.
22. Filipouski GR, Silveira RC, Procianoy RS: Influence of perinatal nutrition and gestational age on neurodevelopment of very low-birth-weight preterm infants. *Am J Perinatol* 30(8):673–680, 2013.
23. Alton GY, Robertson CM, Sauve R, et al: Early childhood health, growth, and neurodevelopmental outcomes after complete repair of total anomalous pulmonary venous connection at 6 weeks or younger. *J Thorac Cardiovasc Surg* 133(4):905–911, 2007.
24. Newburger JW, Sleeper LA, Bellinger DC, et al: Early developmental outcome in children with hypoplastic left heart syndrome

and related anomalies: the single ventricle reconstruction trial. *Circulation* 125(17):2081–2091, 2012.

25. Wälti U: Intelligence profile in children with trisomy 21. *Helv Paediatr Acta* 30(Suppl):38–39, 1973.
26. Wood A, Massarano A, Super M, et al: Behavioural aspects and psychiatric findings in Noonan's syndrome. *Arch Dis Child* 72(2):153–155, 1995.
27. Franceschini P, Guala A, Vardeu MP, et al: The Williams syndrome: an Italian collaborative study. *Minerva Pediatr* 48(10):421–428, 1996.
28. Swillen A, Vogels A, Devriendt K, et al: Chromosome 22q11 deletion syndrome: update and review of the clinical features, cognitive-behavioral spectrum, and psychiatric complications. *Am J Med Genet* 97(2):128–135, 2000. Review.
29. Moss EM, Batshaw ML, Solot CB, et al: Psychoeducational profile of the 22q11.2 microdeletion: a complex pattern. *J Pediatr* 134(2): 193–198, 1999.
30. van Amelsvoort T, Henry J, Morris R, et al: Cognitive deficits associated with schizophrenia in velo-cardio-facial syndrome. *Schizophr Res* 70(2–3):223–232, 2004.
31. Barnea-Goraly N, Menon V, Krasnow B, et al: Investigation of white matter structure in velocardiofacial syndrome: a diffusion tensor imaging study. *Am J Psychiatry* 160(10):1863–1869, 2003.
32. Reference deleted in page proofs.
33. Gaynor JW, Wernovsky G, Jarvik GP, et al: Patient characteristics are important determinants of neurodevelopmental outcome at one year of age after neonatal and infant cardiac surgery. *J Thorac Cardiovasc Surg* 133:1344–1353, 2007.
34. Gaynor JW, Nord AS, Wernovsky G, et al: Apolipoprotein E genotype modifies the risk behavior problems after infant cardiac surgery. *Pediatrics* 124:241–250, 2009.
35. Kim DS, Stanaway IB, Rajagopalan R, et al: Results of genome-wide analyses on neurodevelopmental phenotypes at four-year follow-up following cardiac surgery in infancy. *PLoS ONE* 7(9): e45936, 2012.
36. Gaynor JW, Jarvik GP, Bernbaum J, et al: The relationship of postoperative electrographic seizures to neurodevelopmental outcome at 1 year of age after neonatal and infant cardiac surgery. *J Thorac Cardiovasc Surg* 131(1):181–189, 2006.
37. Miller G, Eggli KD, Contant C, et al: Postoperative neurologic complications after open heart surgery on young infants. *Arch Pediatr Adolesc Med* 149(7):764–768, 1995.
38. Mahle WT, Clancy RR, McGaurn SP, et al: Impact of prenatal diagnosis on survival and early neurologic morbidity in neonates with the hypoplastic left heart syndrome. *Pediatrics* 107(6):1277–1282, 2001.
39. Satomi G, Yasukochi S, Shimizu T, et al: Has fetal echocardiography improved the prognosis of congenital heart disease? Comparison of patients with hypoplastic left heart syndrome with and without prenatal diagnosis. *Pediatr Int* 41(6):728–732, 1999.
40. Tworetzky W, McElhinney DB, Reddy VM, et al: Improved surgical outcome after fetal diagnosis of hypoplastic left heart syndrome. *Circulation* 103(9):1269–1273, 2001.
41. Hövels-Gürich HH, Bauer SB, Schnitker R, et al: Long-term outcome of speech and language in children after corrective surgery for cyanotic or acyanotic cardiac defects in infancy. *Eur J Paediatr Neurol* 12(5):378–386, 2008.
42. Joffe AR, Lequier L, Robertson CM: Pediatric outcomes after extracorporeal membrane oxygenation for cardiac disease and for cardiac arrest: a review. *ASAIO J* 58(4):297–310, 2012.
43. Bellinger DC, Jonas RA, Rappaport LA, et al: Developmental and neurologic status of children after heart surgery with hypothermic circulatory arrest or low-flow cardiopulmonary bypass. *N Engl J Med* 332:549–555, 1995.
44. Bellinger DC, Wypij D, Kuban KCK, et al: Developmental and neurologic status of children at 4 years of age after heart surgery with hypothermic circulatory arrest or low-flow cardiopulmonary bypass. *Circulation* 100:526–532, 1999.
45. Bellinger DC, Wypij D, duPlessis AJ, et al: Neurodevelopmental status at eight years in children with dextro-transposition of the great arteries: the Boston Circulatory Arrest Trial. *J Thorac Cardiovasc Surg* 126:1385–1396, 2003.
46. Bellinger DC, Wypij D, Rivkin DR, et al: Adolescents with d-transposition of the great arteries corrected with the arterial switch procedure: neuropsychological assessment and structural brain imaging. *Circulation* 124:1361–1369, 2011.
47. Andropoulos DB, Easley RB, Brady K, et al: Neurodevelopmental outcomes after regional cerebral perfusion with neuromonitoring for neonatal aortic arch reconstruction. *Ann Thorac Surg* 95(2):648–654, discussion 654–655, 2013.
48. Goldberg CS, Bove EL, Devaney EJ, et al: A randomized clinical trial of regional cerebral perfusion versus deep hypothermic circulatory arrest: outcomes for infants with functional single ventricle. *J Thorac Cardiovasc Surg* 133(4):880–887, 2007.
49. Algra SO, Jansen NJ, van der Tweel I, et al: Neurological injury after neonatal cardiac surgery: a randomized controlled trial of two perfusion techniques. *Circulation* 129:224–233, 2014.
50. Fuller S, Rajagopalan R, Jarvik GP, et al: Deep hypothermic circulatory arrest does not impair neurodevelopmental outcome in school-age children after infant cardiac surgery. *Ann Thorac Surg* 90:1985–1995, 2010.
51. du Plessis AJ, Jonas RA, Wypij D, et al: Perioperative effects of alpha-stat versus pH-stat strategies for deep hypothermic cardiopulmonary bypass in infants. *J Thorac Cardiovasc Surg* 114(6):991–1000, discussion 1000–1001, 1997.
52. Bellinger DC, Wypij D, du Plessis AJ, et al: Developmental and neurologic effects of alpha-stat versus pH-stat strategies for deep hypothermic cardiopulmonary bypass in infants. *J Thorac Cardiovasc Surg* 121(2):374–383, 2001. Erratum in: *J Thorac Cardiovasc Surg* 121(5):893, 2001.
53. Jonas RA, Wypij D, Roth SJ, et al: The influence of hemodilution on outcome after hypothermic cardiopulmonary bypass: results of a randomized trial in infants. *J Thorac Cardiovasc Surg* 126(6):1765–1774, 2003.
54. Newburger JW, Jonas RA, Soul J, et al: Randomized trial of hematocrit 25% versus 35% during hypothermic cardiopulmonary bypass in infant heart surgery. *J Thorac Cardiovasc Surg* 135(2):347–354, 354.e1–4, 2008.
55. Furnary AP, Gao G, Grunkemeier GL, et al: Continuous insulin infusion reduces mortality in patients with diabetes undergoing coronary artery bypass grafting. *J Thorac Cardiovasc Surg* 125(5):1007–1021, 2003.
56. Kavanagh BP: Glucose in the ICU–evidence, guidelines, and outcomes. *N Engl J Med* 367(13):1259–1260, 2012.
57. Simon MV: Neurophysiologic tests in the operating room. In Simon MV, editor: *Intraoperative neurophysiology: a comprehensive guide to monitoring and mapping*, New York, 2010, Demos Medical Publishing.
58. Simon MV, Gerrard JL, Eskandar EN: Electrocorticography. In Simon MV, editor: *Intraoperative neurophysiology: a comprehensive guide to monitoring and mapping*, New York, 2010, Demos Medical Publishing.
59. Edmonds HL, Jr, Rodriguez RA, Audenaert SM, et al: The role of neuromonitoring in cardiovascular surgery. *J Cardiothorac Vasc Anesth* 10(1):15–23, 1996. Review.
60. Johansen JW, Sebel PS: Development and clinical application of electroencephalographic bispectrum monitoring. *Anesthesiology* 93(5):1336–1344, 2000.
61. Fraser CD, Jr, Andropoulos DB: Neurologic monitoring for special cardiopulmonary bypass techniques. *Semin Thorac Cardiovasc Surg Pediatr Card Surg Annu* 7:125–132, 2004.
62. Toyama S, Sakai H, Ito S, et al: Cerebral hypoperfusion during pediatric cardiac surgery detected by combined bispectral index monitoring and transcranial Doppler ultrasonography. *J Clin Anesth* 23(6):498–501, 2011.
63. Clark RE, Brillman J, Davis DA, et al: Microemboli during coronary artery bypass grafting. Genesis and effect on outcome. *J Thorac Cardiovasc Surg* 109(2):249–257, discussion 257–258, 1995.
64. Cheung PY, Chui N, Joffe AR, et al: Postoperative lactate concentrations predict the outcome of infants aged 6 weeks or less after intracardiac surgery: a cohort follow-up to 18 months. *J Thorac Cardiovasc Surg* 130(3):837–843, 2005.
65. Ravishankar C, Zak V, Williams IA, et al: Association of impaired linear growth and worse neurodevelopmental outcome in infants with single ventricle physiology: a report from the pediatric heart

network infant single ventricle trial. *J Pediatr* 162(2):250–256, e2, 2013.
66. Clark JB, Barnes ML, Undar A, et al: Multimodality neuromonitoring for pediatric cardiac surgery: our approach and a critical appraisal of the available evidence. *World J Pediatr Congenit Heart Surg* 3(1):87–95, 2012.
67. Khan MS, Fraser CD: Neonatal brain protection in cardiac surgery and the role of intraoperative neuromonitoring. *World J Pediatr Congenit Heart Surg* 3(1):114–119, 2012.
68. Hirsch JC, Jacobs ML, Andropoulos D, et al: Protecting the infant brain during cardiac surgery: a systematic review. *Ann Thorac Surg* 94:1365–1373, 2012.

CHAPTER 112

Congenital Tracheal Disease

Emile A. Bacha

CHAPTER OUTLINE

HISTORY OF PEDIATRIC TRACHEAL SURGERY

In 2000, the Congenital Heart Surgery Nomenclature and Database Project classified congenital tracheal stenosis as congenital–complete tracheal rings, postintubation, traumatic, or congenital web.[1] Localized stenosis was defined as less than 50% of the tracheal length, and long-segment stenosis as greater than 50% of the tracheal length.[1] The initial classification of tracheal stenosis had been proposed by Drs. Cantrell and Guild from the University of Washington, Seattle, in 1964.[2] They classified these patients into three morphologic types: (1) generalized hypoplasia, (2) funnel-like stenosis, and (3) segmental stenosis. They also noted the frequent association of a tracheal right upper lobe bronchus that is present in 20% of these patients (Fig. 112-1). Dr. Hermes Grillo from Massachusetts General Hospital is considered to be the father of tracheal surgery. In a series of landmark publications in the 1960s, he defined the blood supply of the trachea, the surgical approach to the trachea, and tracheal release procedures for resection.[3,4] The first successful operation for congenital stenosis of the trachea was reported by Dr. Ken Kimura from Kobe Children's Hospital in Kobe, Japan, in 1982.[5] He used a costal cartilage graft to augment the tracheal lumen of a 12-month-old infant with tracheal stenosis secondary to complete tracheal rings (cartilage tracheoplasty). The use of pericardium to augment the tracheal lumen was first performed by Dr. Farouk Idriss from Children's Memorial Hospital, Chicago, in 1982.[6] The operation was facilitated by the use of cardiopulmonary bypass for respiratory support during the procedure. Slide tracheoplasty was first reported by Drs. Victor Tsang and Peter Goldstraw from Brompton Hospital in London, England, in 1989.[7] Its use in children was popularized by Dr. Grillo and his associates.[8] Drs. Claus Herberhold and Martin Elliott from Great Ormond Street Hospital, London, performed the first successful tracheal homograft to augment the lumen of a patient with a failed prior intervention for tracheal stenosis from congenital tracheal rings in 1994.[9] Drs. Carl Backer and Constantine Mavroudis reported the use of a free tracheal autograft for infants with congenital tracheal stenosis in 1998, 2 years after they performed the first operation.[10] Pulmonary artery sling repair was first performed by Dr. Willis J. Potts at Children's Memorial Hospital in 1953.[11] The left pulmonary artery was divided at its origin from the right pulmonary artery and reanastomosed anterior to the trachea.

CLINICAL PRESENTATION AND DIAGNOSTIC TECHNIQUES

The two most common congenital tracheal anomalies in infants and children are tracheomalacia and tracheal stenosis. Congenital tracheal stenosis is most commonly caused by complete cartilage tracheal rings, and it is the most common indication for surgical intervention.[12] The normal trachea has an anterior arch-shaped cartilage and a posterior membranous trachea. In children with complete tracheal rings, the cartilage ring is circumferential and the membranous trachea is absent (Fig. 112-2). In contrast, tracheomalacia is associated with a normal or sometimes broad membranous trachea. Failure of the C-shaped cartilaginous portion to maintain a minimum of rigidity to the trachea results in "floppiness," which results in functional tracheal narrowing, particularly

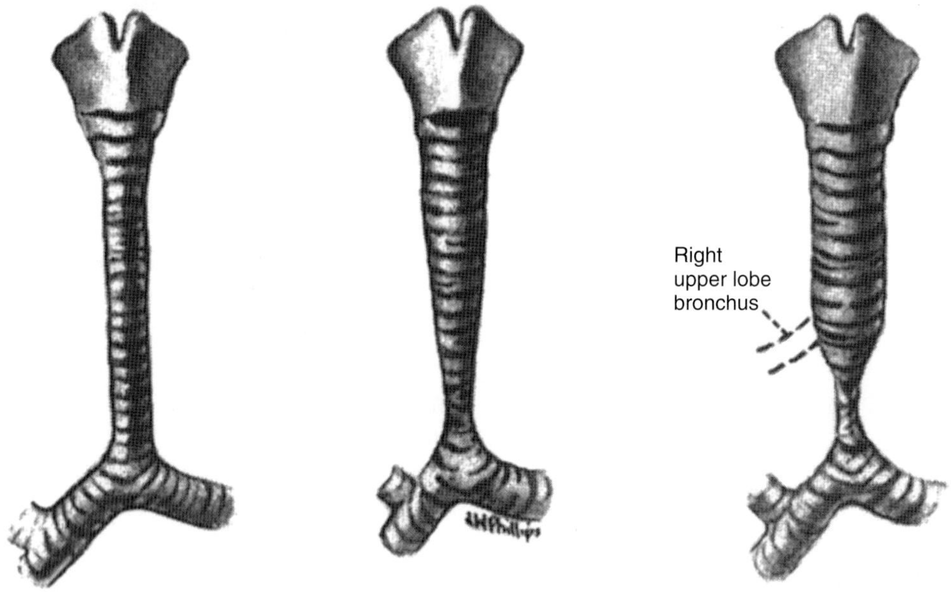

FIGURE 112-1 ■ The three morphologic variants of congenital stenosis of the trachea. *Left,* Generalized hypoplasia; *center,* funnel-like stenosis; *right,* segmental stenosis. The occurrence of an anomalous right upper lobe bronchus (or tracheal right upper lobe) *(right)* is most common in the segmental form. (From Cantrell JR, Guild HG: Congenital stenosis of the trachea. *Am J Surg* 108:297, 1964.)

during expiration. The circumference of the trachea is typically normal during inspiration, or when a patient is intubated (e.g., for a computed tomography [CT] study). Tracheomalacia is a chronic condition that infrequently requires surgical intervention. It often improves with time and growth of the child. Patients with tracheal stenosis often have associated anomalies, most commonly pulmonary artery sling and congenital cardiac anomalies.[13] Pulmonary artery sling is present in a third of patients with congenital tracheal stenosis. Major intracardiac anomalies are present in 25% of the patients with congenital tracheal stenosis.

The diagnosis of congenital tracheal stenosis should be suspected in any infant who has stridor (noisy breathing), respiratory distress, apnea, cyanosis, wheezing, retractions, or respiratory failure requiring intubation. Tracheal stenosis can result in a difficult intubation (e.g., the endotracheal tube selected for the patient's size fails to pass into a normal location in the trachea), and this traumatization of the trachea can cause future tracheal stenosis.

Patients with known or suspected tracheal problems should be evaluated with a chest radiograph, CT or magnetic resonance imaging (MRI) (or both), bronchoscopy, and echocardiography (Box 112-1). The chest radiograph often demonstrates the diminutive nature of the tracheal lumen. It reveals lung agenesis or hypoplasia. A CT scan or MRI shows the tracheal lumen in cross section and provides a measurement of the tracheal stenosis. A tracheal right upper lobe can be identified if present. Three-dimensional reconstruction can generate a very good representation of the tracheal pathology (Fig. 112-3).[14]

In our experience, CT has been more helpful than MRI because it is usually quicker (i.e., requires less sedation, or obviates the need for intubation), and there is less movement artifact. It can be performed as a dynamic expiratory CT scan—that is, in synchrony with the child's inspiration and expiration. End-inspiratory and dynamic expiratory volumetric imaging can be obtained. This type of dynamic study is helpful when evaluating children who might have tracheomalacia but do not fit a typical symptomatic pattern.[15] However, CT results in a much higher radiation burden, which should be taken into consideration if the child is likely to require repeated imaging studies. Contrast tracheobronchography, which generates high-quality images, is still used sometimes. However, CT generates such excellent images that the risks of contrast tracheograms mostly outweigh the benefits, so this technique is usually used only in conjunction with a catheterization. A pulmonary artery sling can be demonstrated by CT if the CT is performed with contrast, or by MRI. For the sick neonate who is transferred with a critically positioned endotracheal tube and congenital tracheal stenosis, transthoracic echocardiography is the diagnostic procedure of choice to demonstrate a pulmonary artery sling.[16] Echocardiography should be performed on all of these infants because of the 25% incidence of congenital heart disease found in patients with congenital tracheal stenosis.[13]

The most important diagnostic procedure in all patients is a rigid bronchoscopy. This can be performed as a separate procedure before the planned tracheal operation, or it can be done at the time of the tracheal

BOX 112-1 Diagnostic Techniques for Infants with Complete Tracheal Rings

- Chest radiography
- Computed tomography (CT) with contrast, including three-dimensional reconstruction or dynamic CT
- Rigid bronchoscopy
- Echocardiography (to rule out pulmonary artery sling, congenital cardiac anomalies)

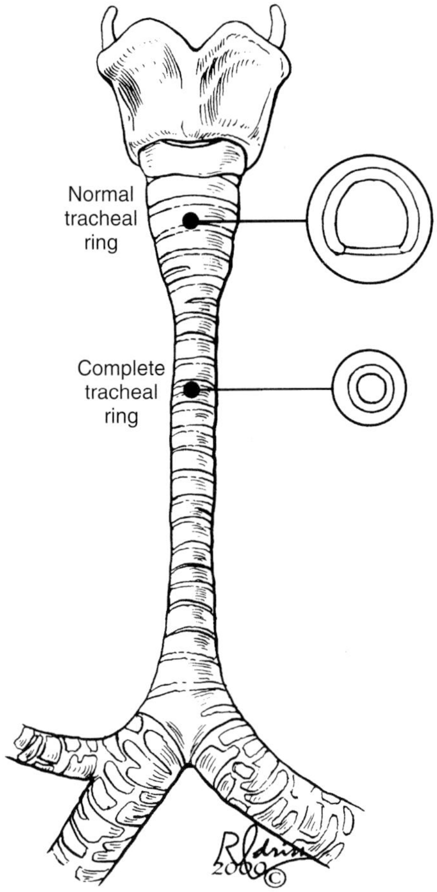

FIGURE 112-2 ■ The trachea of an infant with long-segment tracheal stenosis secondary to complete tracheal rings. There are three normal tracheal rings immediately below the cricoid. The upper cutaway shows a normal tracheal ring with the anterior cartilage and flat posterior membranous trachea. This is followed by 18 complete tracheal rings that progress almost to the carina, one of which, shown in the lower cutaway, is a complete cartilage ring with a substantially reduced tracheal lumen. The tracheal lumen in some of these infants is as small as 1.5 to 2 mm.

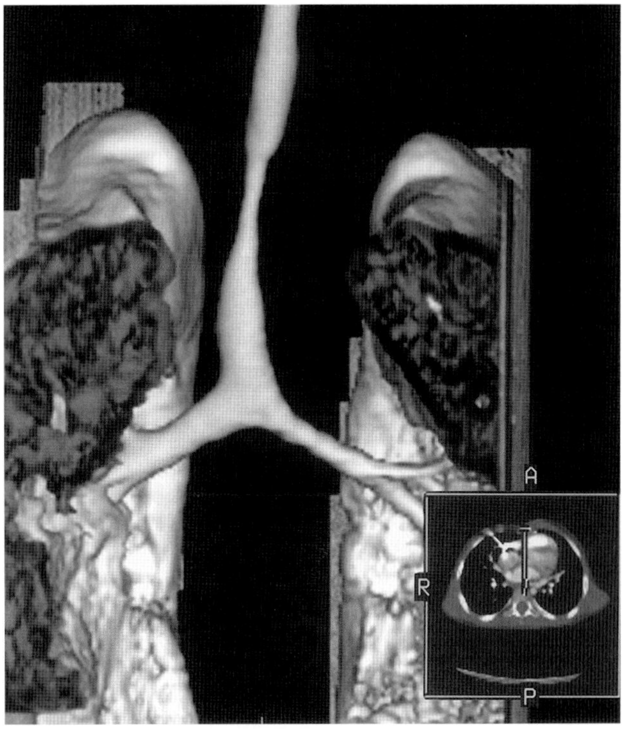

FIGURE 112-3 ■ Computed tomography (CT) *(inset)* with three-dimensional reconstruction reveals a significant tracheal stenosis in the midportion of this child's trachea. The pathology at the time of surgery was essentially identical to the pathology indicated by the CT scan. *A,* Anterior; *P,* posterior; *R,* right.

procedure. In some severe cases, distal visualization of the trachea cannot be obtained by bronchoscopy because of the risk of occluding the tracheal lumen. The child can then be placed on cardiopulmonary bypass, and bronchoscopy can be performed safely.[17]

SURGICAL TECHNIQUES

General Principles

In general, the incidence of airway complications, including anastomotic dehiscence, rises with the length or amount of trachea that is resected. Younger patients and reoperative tracheal procedures also have significantly higher complication rates.[18] Tracheal anatomy, including blood supply, should be well understood. Grillo expressed concern about devascularization in adults,[3] but this appears to be less important in children, who have an excellent mediastinal blood supply. Right and left recurrent laryngeal nerves should be protected at all cost. A good relationship with pediatric otorhinolaryngologists with special expertise in endoscopic and surgical airway management is essential.

Postoperative management differs with the age of the child. For older children, adult principles can be applied, and a "chin stitch" can be used to prevent neck extension. In all cases, a flexible bronchoscopy is performed at 5 to 7 postoperative days. Younger children can be fitted with a neck prosthesis to prevent important neck excursions, but this is rarely used. It may be best to leave neonates and young infants sedated and intubated for 5 to 7 days, and to perform flexible bronchoscopic examination before extubation.

Tracheal Resection

Cantrell and Guild published an early report of a successful tracheal resection in a child in 1964, and they also reported the three morphologic varieties of congenital tracheal stenosis.[2] The 7-year-old patient had a tracheal right upper lobe and a bridging bronchus to the carina. The bridging bronchus, which was stenotic, was excised, and the carina was brought up to the main trachea. An anastomosis was performed with interrupted sutures of braided stainless steel. The child survived the operation and was asymptomatic on follow-up.

Tracheal stenosis amenable to tracheal resection with end-to-end anastomosis was originally thought to be feasible for stenosis involving up to 50% of the total tracheal length. However, a report from Massachusetts General

Hospital has indicated that resections of more than 30% of the trachea have a substantial failure rate.[19] We believe that tracheal resection is the preferred technique if the stenosis is less than a third of the total tracheal length. This is usually six to eight complete tracheal rings.

We use the technique developed by Grillo for tracheal resection and reanastomosis (TRR).[20] In adults, most TRRs are performed via a transverse cervical ("collar") incision. The airway can be safely managed intraoperatively with careful endotracheal tube positioning. In children, especially small children and infants, control of the airway is much more precarious. As in most experienced pediatric centers, we believe that most if not all tracheal resections in younger children should be performed through a median sternotomy approach with cardiopulmonary bypass. If the tracheal stenosis extends up to the cricoid, a collar incision is made in the neck, forming a "T" with the median sternotomy incision. This incision tends to heal better than a midline extension of the median sternotomy onto the neck. The strap muscles are divided in the midline. The thymus is partially or entirely excised. The innominate artery and vein are dissected free and encircled with vessel loops. These may then be retracted superiorly or inferiorly to address the various components of the trachea. The aorta is mobilized from its pericardial attachments and retracted with a small pledgeted suture to the left. Care is taken to avoid injury to the right or left recurrent laryngeal nerves. The anterior surface of the trachea is freed from pericardial attachments so that it may be completely visualized from cricoid to carina if necessary.

The site of the stenosis is identified externally. At the site of the stenosis and up to one ring above and below the stenotic segment (at most, two rings above or below), dissection must be performed circumferentially and posteriorly to facilitate the removal of the stenotic portion of the trachea. Attention must be paid to the lateral blood supply of the tracheal wall and a decision made regarding which vessels can be preserved for an adequate blood supply to the eventual anastomosis. In most cases, the carinal attachments are freed, as are the pericardial attachments of the right and left mainstem bronchi. Cardiopulmonary bypass is initiated with a single right atrial and aortic cannula, and the aorta is retracted to the left. Cooling is not necessary, and we aim for a temperature of 32° to 34°C. The trachea is opened in the midline through the extent of the tracheal stenosis. If the stenotic portion can be identified from the outside, bronchoscopic guidance is not needed. Three-dimensional CT scan reconstruction has been used to identify the area of stenosis with enough accuracy to allow opening at the correct site. If the focal area of stenosis cannot be identified externally, intraoperative bronchoscopy, using the illuminated tip of the bronchoscope for guidance, can demonstrate the area of stenosis.

The technique of passing a 25-gauge needle through the lightest portion of the stenosis also is useful for some patients. The anterior tracheal incision is extended proximally and distally until the extent of the complete tracheal rings or stenosis has been encompassed. If this length is less than 30% of the trachea (six to eight complete tracheal rings), the segment is then simply excised.

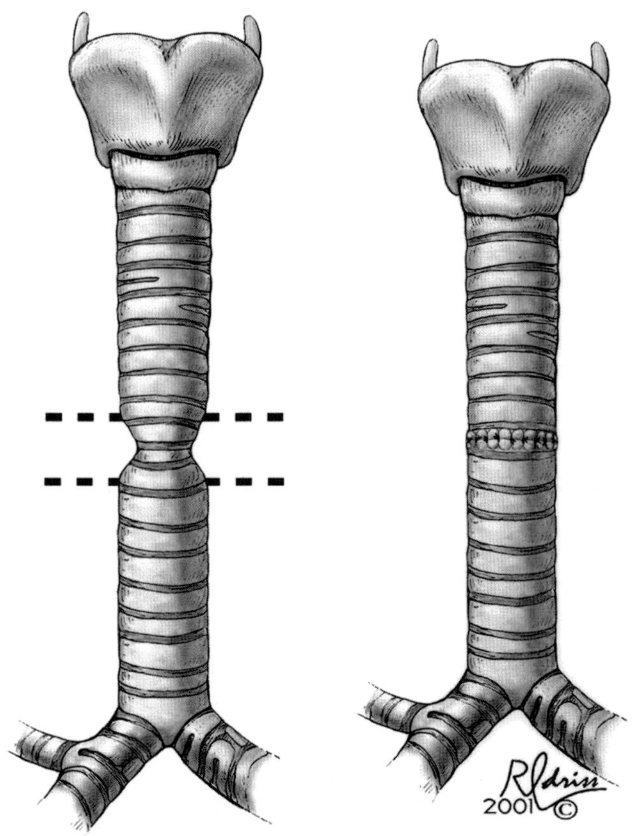

FIGURE 112-4 ■ Tracheal resection. The localized segment of tracheal stenosis is excised. The trachea is extensively mobilized, specifically in the right and left mainstem bronchi and carina. This allows the trachea to be brought together without tension for an end-to-end anastomosis using interrupted polydioxanone sutures. (From Backer CL, Mavroudis C, Holinger LD: Repair of congenital tracheal stenosis. *Semin Thorac Cardiovasc Surg Pediatr Card Surg Annu* 5:173–186, 2002.)

The two ends are brought together, and the anastomosis is performed with interrupted polydioxanone (PDS) sutures (Fig. 112-4), with the knots tied outside. If there is little tension, it is acceptable to run the posterior wall. Before the anterior sutures are tied, the trachea is suctioned free of secretions and blood with a fine plastic suction catheter. At completion, flexible bronchoscopy is always performed before leaving the operating room. A tension-free anastomosis is the key, and we liberally use the Grillo-derived lateral stay sutures, placed one ring above and one below the anastomosis, to bring the two edges together and take some of the tension away from the suture line itself.

It is important to determine before the resection of tracheal tissue (including the stenotic portion) whether a TRR or a slide tracheoplasty will be performed. In the slide tracheoplasty, the extent of tracheal resection should be minimized to use the tracheal wall as a flap. If the length of the stenosis is too long for a successful end-to-end anastomosis, the operation can be converted to the tracheal autograft technique. Results of tracheal resection in infants and children are shown in Table 112-1.[19,21-23] Complications include anastomotic leak, restenosis, and tracheomalacia.

Slide Tracheoplasty

Slide tracheoplasty is our preferred technique for long-segment narrowing, typically seen in complete tracheal rings. It was first reported by Tsang and colleagues from Brompton Hospital, London, England, in 1989.[7] The slide tracheoplasty can be performed through a cervical collar incision or through a median sternotomy approach. The procedure has been performed with and without cardiopulmonary bypass. Only the midportion of the tracheal stenosis is transected (Fig. 112-5). The two tracheal halves are then opened longitudinally, one anteriorly and the other posteriorly. The corners of the transecting tracheal incision are trimmed. Figure 112-6 shows an anterior tracheotomy inferiorly and a posterior tracheotomy superiorly. The two openings are then "slid" together and approximated with interrupted absorbable sutures (Fig. 112-7) or with a continuous absorbable suture. It is

TABLE 112-1 **Results of Tracheal Resection in Infants and Children**

Surgeon	Year	Patients *(N)*	Mortality
Ziemer[23]	1998	8	1 (12%)
Jones[22]	1999	6	1 (16%)
Grillo[19]	2002	46	2 (4%)
Backer[21]	2002	12	1 (8%)
Totals		72	5 (7%)

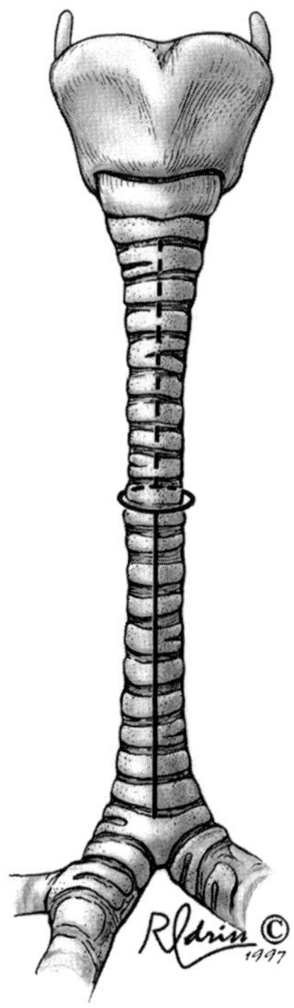

FIGURE 112-5 ■ Slide tracheoplasty. The trachea is transected at the midpoint of the long-segment congenital tracheal stenosis. The superior position of the trachea is incised posteriorly, and the inferior aspect of the trachea is incised anteriorly. (From Dayan SH, Dunham ME, Backer CL, et al: Slide tracheoplasty in the management of congenital tracheal stenosis. *Ann Otol Rhinol Laryngol* 106:914–919, 1997.)

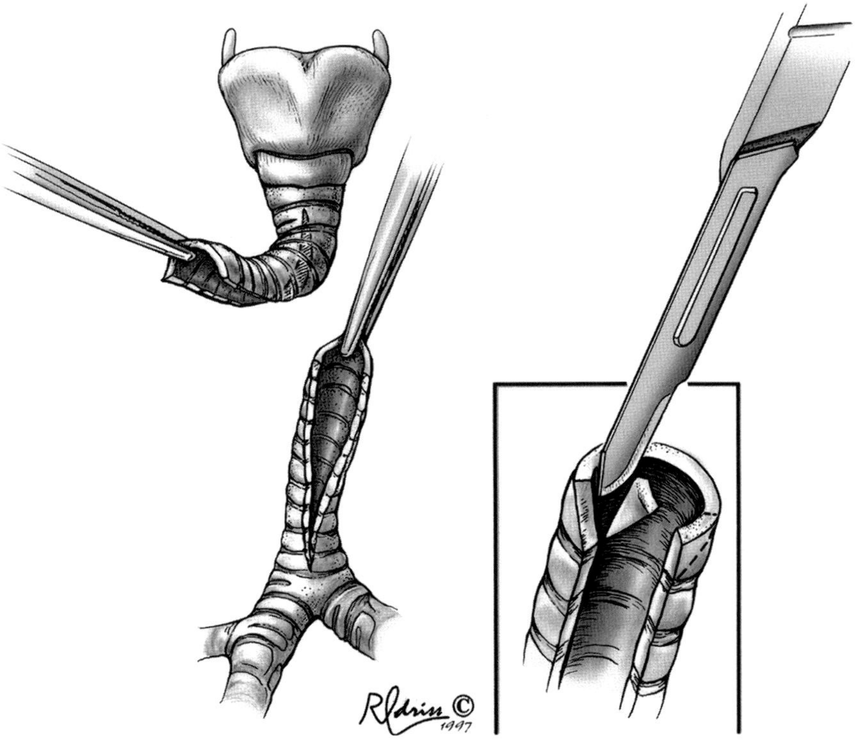

FIGURE 112-6 ■ Slide tracheoplasty. The upper trachea has been opened posteriorly, and the lower trachea has been opened anteriorly. The corners of the transected trachea are trimmed so that the leading edge will fit into the V-portion of the other component. (From Dayan SH, Dunham ME, Backer CL, et al: Slide tracheoplasty in the management of congenital tracheal stenosis. *Ann Otol Rhinol Laryngol* 106:914–919, 1997.)

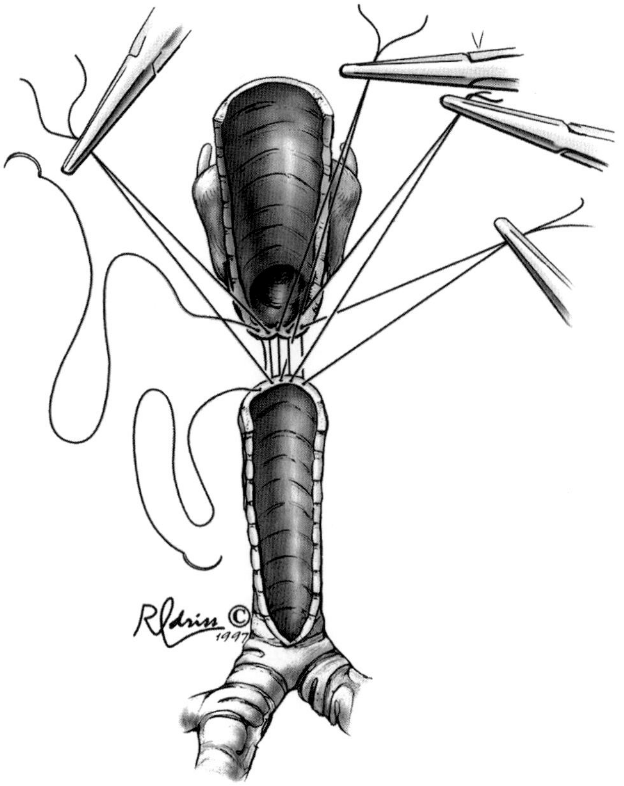

FIGURE 112-7 ■ Slide tracheoplasty. The beginning of the long anastomotic suture line is performed with an interrupted 6-0 polydioxanone suture while the patient is on cardiopulmonary bypass. (From Dayan SH, Dunham ME, Backer CL, et al: Slide tracheoplasty in the management of congenital tracheal stenosis. *Ann Otol Rhinol Laryngol* 106:914–919, 1997.)

important to carry the suture as an everting suture line; otherwise, a ledge of cartilage will protrude into the tracheal lumen. Correctly done, the result is a trachea that is half the original length with four times the internal luminal diameter, as seen in Figure 112-8, where the configuration of the anastomosis is shown in the small inset. If the tracheal stenosis extends into one of the right or left mainstem bronchi, the slide incisions can be performed laterally, so that the inferior incision extends onto the superior surface of the narrow bronchus.

The results of slide tracheoplasty are reported in Table 112-2.[7,8,11,21,24-26] The overall mortality was 12% in 33 patients. Complications include granulation tissue, a figure-eight configuration of the trachea, and recurrent stenosis.[8,11,27]

Cartilage Tracheoplasty

The first report of a successful surgical procedure for long-segment congenital tracheal stenosis described a cartilage tracheoplasty performed by Kimura and associates[5] in 1982, at Kobe Children's Hospital in Japan. They operated on a 12-month-old female infant who had had recurrent respiratory distress since birth. The entire trachea was stenotic, as seen by bronchoscopy. The left bronchus was of normal caliber, and the right lung was completely aplastic. Through a median sternotomy incision, the left bronchus was incised and cannulated for ventilation. A longitudinal incision was made through the entire length of the anterior wall of the trachea. Two separate pieces of costal cartilage were used to fill the defect in the anterior wall of the trachea. The grafts were

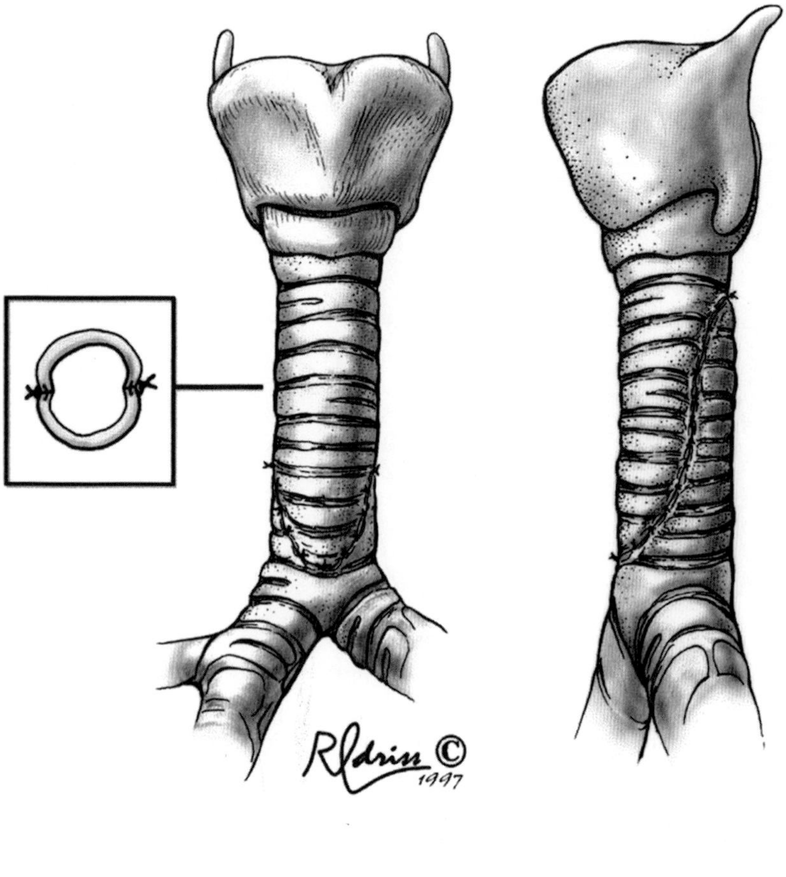

FIGURE 112-8 ■ Slide tracheoplasty. Anterior *(left)* and lateral *(right)* views of the anastomosed trachea. The tracheal length has been reduced by almost half, and the internal luminal diameter has been increased by four times. The cross-sectional appearance of the trachea is shown in the *inset*. (From Dayan SH, Dunham ME, Backer CL, et al: Slide tracheoplasty in the management of congenital tracheal stenosis. *Ann Otol Rhinol Laryngol* 106:914–919, 1997.)

TABLE 112-2 Results of Slide Tracheoplasty

Surgeon	Year	Patients *(N)*	Mortality
Tsang[7]	1989	2	1 (50%)
Lang[25]	1999	2	0
Harrison[24]	2000	3	0
Matute[26]	2001	4	0
Backer[21]	2002	3	1 (33%)
Grillo[8]	2002	8	0
Manning[11]	2003	11	2 (18%)
Totals		33	4 (12%)

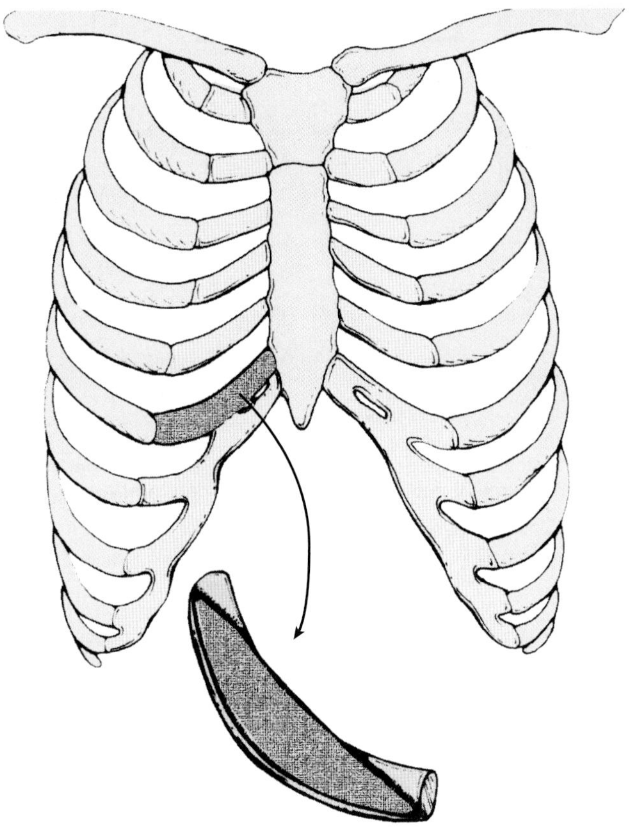

FIGURE 112-9 Cartilage tracheoplasty. Before the median sternotomy, a segment of cartilage is harvested from the sixth or seventh rib. The cartilage is then tailored to correspond to the subsequent tracheal opening. (From Jaquiss RD, Lusk RP, Spray TL, et al: Repair of long-segment tracheal stenosis in infancy. *J Thorac Cardiovasc Surg* 110:1504–1512, 1995.)

attached to the tracheal edges with interrupted 5-0 Dexon sutures. This patient required prolonged intubation and ventilation but was successfully extubated 2 months postoperatively.

For airway control in the infant, cartilage tracheoplasty for long-segment congenital tracheal stenosis is best performed via a median sternotomy with cardiopulmonary bypass. The midline incision is extended onto the neck, or (preferably) a collar incision is used for further exposure of the trachea in the neck. The cartilage graft can be harvested via the median sternotomy incision (Fig. 112-9). Median sternotomy is performed while preliminary preparation of the cartilage graft takes place. The trachea is dissected and exposed on its anterior surface.

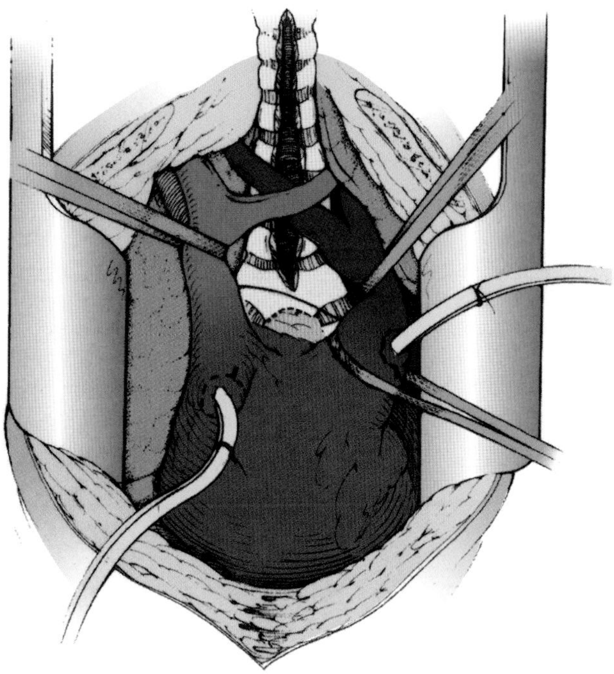

FIGURE 112-10 Cartilage tracheoplasty. Exposure of the trachea through a sternotomy is demonstrated, including the relative positions of bypass cannulas and retraction of the great vessels for optimal exposure. Tracheal incision has been performed to the carina. (From Jaquiss RD, Lusk RP, Spray TL, et al: Repair of long-segment tracheal stenosis in infancy. *J Thorac Cardiovasc Surg* 110:1504–1512, 1995.)

The patient is heparinized and cannulated for cardiopulmonary bypass via the right atrium and ascending aorta. Extracorporeal circulation is initiated, with cooling to 32° C, so the heart remains beating in normal sinus rhythm. Ventilation is stopped. The anterior wall of the stenotic trachea is opened through the extent of the stenosis (Fig. 112-10). Bronchoscopic guidance is often helpful to assess the degree of stenosis. The segment of costal cartilage is then tailored to a size and shape suitable for the anterior opening of the trachea. Care is taken to preserve the perichondrium, which is placed on the luminal surface, and the graft is secured with interrupted absorbable monofilament suture (Fig. 112-11). Intraluminal suture exposure is avoided, and the graft is seated on the tracheotomy rather than being allowed to prolapse into the lumen.

After completion of the graft suture line, the anesthesiologist inflates the lungs with air, and the suture line is confirmed to be airtight, with additional sutures placed as necessary. Bronchoscopy is performed to confirm the tracheal lumen adequacy and to clear retained secretions. The endotracheal tube is repositioned in the midportion of the cartilage graft. The patient is ventilated and weaned from cardiopulmonary bypass. The tracheal suture line can be sealed with biological glue. Hemoclips are placed in the soft tissue adjacent to the trachea to mark the location of the cartilage graft. Sternotomy is closed in the standard fashion. Patients are maintained on heavy sedation and with muscle relaxant to minimize motion of the endotracheal tube in the airway.

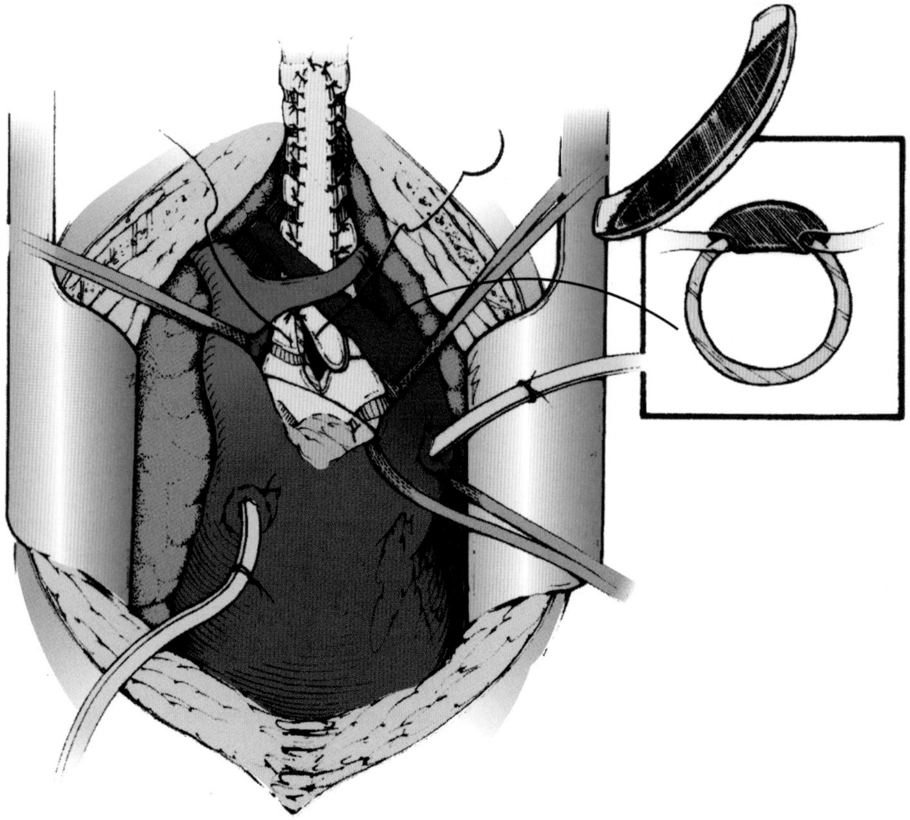

FIGURE 112-11 ■ Cartilage tracheoplasty. Placement of the cartilage graft is indicated. The graft is oriented with preserved perichondrium placed on the luminal side and secured with interrupted sutures. Intraluminal suture exposure is avoided, and the graft is seated on the tracheal opening, rather than being allowed to prolapse into the lumen. (From Jaquiss RD, Lusk RP, Spray TL, et al: Repair of long-segment tracheal stenosis in infancy. *J Thorac Cardiovasc Surg* 110:1504–1512, 1995.)

One week after the procedure, the patient is reexamined with bronchoscopy. If necessary, granulation tissue is removed and secretions are suctioned. If the airway appears to be stable and adequately healed, the patient is weaned from the ventilator over the next several days and extubated. Follow-up bronchoscopies are performed as necessary until the trachea is cleared of granulation tissue.

Long-term follow-up of these infants has shown that the graft becomes incorporated into the tracheal structure and grows with the patient. In addition, reepithelialization of the graft site with ciliated columnar epithelium occurs.[28] The most common indication for this surgery is a prior failed pericardial or slide tracheoplasty.[29]

Pericardial Tracheoplasty

Pericardial tracheoplasty was first performed by Idriss in 1984 at Children's Memorial Hospital.[6] This procedure also marked the first use of cardiopulmonary bypass for a patient undergoing an operation for complete tracheal rings. Idriss reported on five infants with long-segment tracheal stenosis, all operated on through a median sternotomy with extracorporeal circulation, and all had a pericardial patch inserted to augment the tracheal lumen. There were no deaths or infections. This technique was the procedure of choice at Children's Memorial Hospital for the next 15 years. However, it was not used often in other centers because of problems related to granulation tissue formation, the need for repeated bronchoscopies for airway clearance, and the need for repeat operations for restenosis.[29] The typical approach was through a median sternotomy, with cardiopulmonary bypass for respiratory support.

The approach is similar to that used for TRR. Once the full extent of the tracheal stenosis has been opened, a suitably shaped pericardial patch is fashioned. The patch should be oversized in both width and length, because some shrinking will occur over time. The patch is made of autologous pericardium and is not treated with glutaraldehyde but simply kept in a saline-soaked sponge during the dissection and opening of the trachea. The patch is anchored in place using interrupted or running Vicryl (Polyglactin 910; Ethicon, Somerville, NJ) or PDS sutures (Fig. 112-12).

The suturing begins in the area of the carina, which is the most critical location. This area is chosen because it is the most inferior point of the dissection, and once the lower portion of the patch is in place, less blood and fluid tend to accumulate in the tracheal lumen. A completion bronchoscopy is performed, and the endotracheal tube is replaced and repositioned under direct vision. The patient is ventilated, and the anesthesiologist inflates the lungs to a pressure of 35 or 40 cm H_2O to test the patch for air leaks, which are controlled with additional sutures. The patient is then ventilated and weaned from cardiopulmonary bypass. The heparin is reversed with

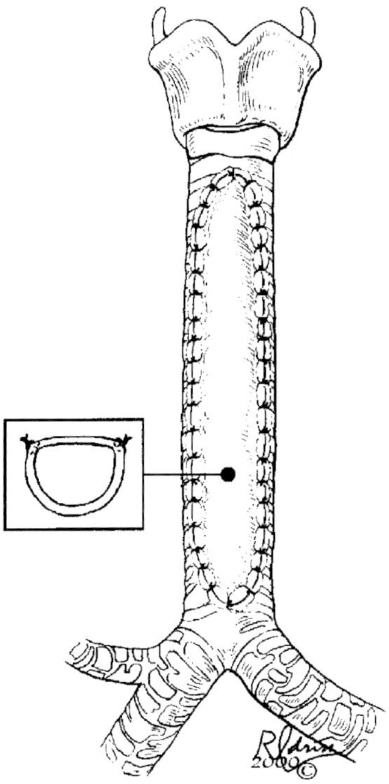

FIGURE 112-12 ■ A completed pericardial patch tracheoplasty. The pericardium is anchored with interrupted Vicryl sutures. In cross section *(inset),* the tracheal lumen is now normal in size. (From Backer CL, Mavroudis C, Gerber ME, et al: Tracheal surgery in children: an 18-year review of four techniques. *Eur J Cardiothorac Surg* 19:777–784, 2001.)

protamine. The edges of the patch are sealed with a very fine spray of biological glue. The extent of the pericardial patch is marked with small hemoclips placed in the soft tissues of the adjacent mediastinum at the superior and inferior portions of the patch. For prevention of patch tracheomalacia, fine monofilament Prolene sutures are used to take partial-thickness bites of the pericardium and fix it to the posterior wall of the ascending aorta and the innominate artery. This acts as a suspending device, holding the patch open. The patient is kept on muscle relaxants and heavily sedated for 1 week. Repeat bronchoscopy is performed.

If the repair is adequate, with a good tracheal lumen and minimal granulation tissue, the patient is then weaned from the ventilator and extubated in 5 to 7 days. Many of these patients, however, have patch tracheomalacia, necessitating a prolonged period of intubation for 1 or 2 more weeks after the first successful bronchoscopy. Repeat bronchoscopies are performed as needed to clear granulation tissue and retained secretions. Over several months, the patch becomes reepithelialized with pseudostratified columnar epithelium.[30]

As mentioned, the pericardial tracheoplasty has a low operative mortality rate, but it requires a prolonged hospitalization because patients must be kept intubated for a prolonged time. In addition, these patients require frequent bronchoscopic examinations for resection of granulation tissue, which tends to occur chiefly at the carinal area, where there is a critical junction of the pericardial patch, the carina, and the irritation from the distal end of the endotracheal tube. In addition, a significant percentage of these patients have required a repeat procedure—a tracheotomy to stent the patch, an intraluminal stenting, or other tracheal reoperations.[29] Because of all these chronic problems, we consider this procedure to be essentially obsolete. A small pericardial patch can be helpful, however, as an adjunct when tracheal tissue is lacking, for example, to complete a slide tracheoplasty.

Tracheal Autograft Technique

The principle of the tracheal autograft technique is to shorten the trachea and use the excised piece of trachea as an anterior patch (i.e., as an autograft).[10] Patients are operated on through a median sternotomy, with cardiopulmonary bypass. The trachea is incised anteriorly through the area of stenosis, and the midportion of the stenotic trachea is excised. The posterior trachea is brought together with interrupted 6.0 PDS sutures (Fig. 112-13). This leaves an anterior opening that is then augmented with the autograft.[21] The corners of the autograft are trimmed so that the autograft fits into the anastomosis. The autograft does not shrink like pericardium and therefore does not need to be oversized. The autograft is sutured in place with multiple interrupted 6-0 PDS sutures (Fig. 112-14). If the autograft is not long enough to completely augment the anterior tracheal lumen, the superior portion of the tracheal opening that remains after autograft insertion can be patched with pericardium or cartilage (Fig. 112-15). Placement of the endotracheal tube depends on the anatomy. If the autograft is low enough, we prefer to keep the tube above the anastomosis to avoid irritation of the suture line from tube friction. Alternatively, the tube can be positioned through the area of the autograft if it is in a superior location. After the patients have been ventilated and assessed for air leaks, they are weaned from cardiopulmonary bypass. The autograft is sealed with glue. If the autograft suture line ends up being compressed by the innominate artery, a cervical strap muscle can be mobilized and brought in as an interposition between the innominate artery and the tracheal autograft. The largest published series using this technique is from Children's Memorial Hospital of Chicago.[10,13,21] We have used this technique occasionally, but we prefer the slide tracheoplasty when feasible.

Homograft Tracheoplasty

The homograft tracheoplasty technique was first performed in adults by Claus Herberhold of Germany. Herberhold and Elliott first applied the technique to a child in 1994.[9] Jacobs and colleagues reported the largest series of patients undergoing this procedure.[31] Most of these patients were infants who had a prior failed operation for complete tracheal rings. Cadaveric trachea is harvested, fixed in formalin, washed in thimerosal, and stored in acetone. The operation is performed through a median sternotomy with the patient on cardiopulmonary bypass. The stenosed tracheal segment is opened to widely patent segments proximally and distally. The anterior cartilage is partially excised, and the posterior tracheal muscle or

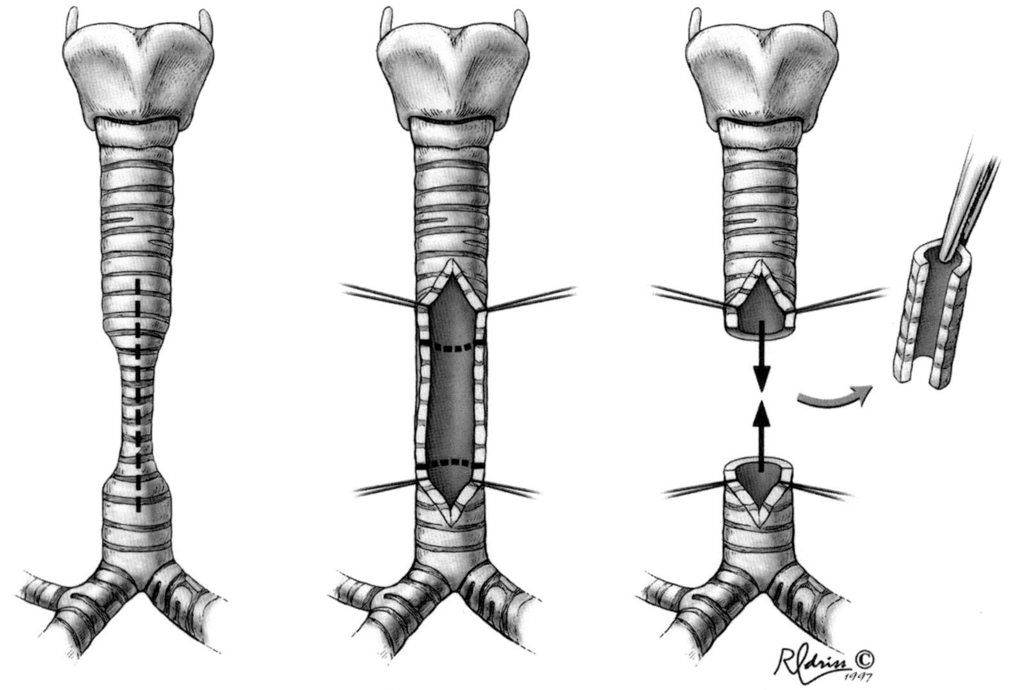

FIGURE 112-13 ■ Tracheal autograft. An anterior longitudinal incision is made through the complete extent of the tracheal rings *(left)*. The midportion of the trachea is excised *(center)* to be used as the tracheal autograft. The two remaining orifices of the trachea are reapproximated posteriorly *(right)*. (From Backer CL, Mavroudis C, Dunham ME, et al: Repair of congenital tracheal stenosis with a free tracheal autograft. *J Thorac Cardiovasc Surg* 113:869–874, 1998.)

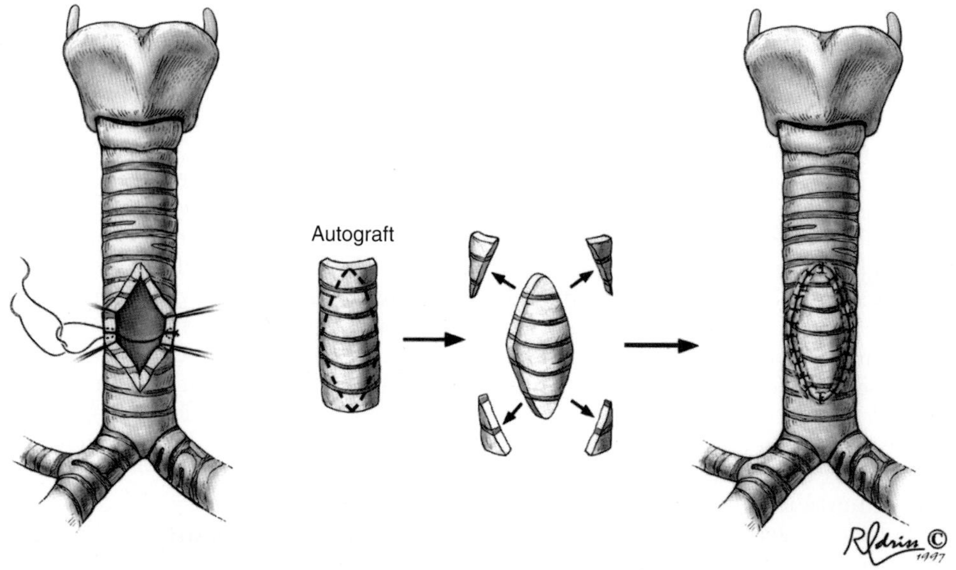

FIGURE 112-14 ■ Tracheal autograft. The posterior tracheal anastomosis is performed with interrupted 6-0 polydioxanone sutures *(left)*. The corners of the autograft are trimmed *(center)*. The autograft is sutured in place to cover the remaining opening in the anterior trachea *(right)*. (From Backer CL, Mavroudis C, Dunham ME, et al: Repair of congenital tracheal stenosis with a free tracheal autograft. *J Thorac Cardiovasc Surg* 113:869–874, 1998.)

tracheal wall remains. A temporary silicone rubber intraluminal stent is placed, and absorbable sutures secure the homograft (trimmed appropriately) in position. Regular postoperative bronchoscopic treatments are needed to clear granulation tissue. The stent is removed endoscopically after endothelialization occurs over the homograft. In Jacobs and colleagues' initial report there were 24 patients, most of whom were reoperations.[31] Four deaths occurred, for an overall mortality rate of 17%. In Jacobs and associates' more recent report of their North American experience with the homograft, there was one early death among six patients.[32] The procedure is used only as an alternative for the patient who had a failed previous primary procedure.

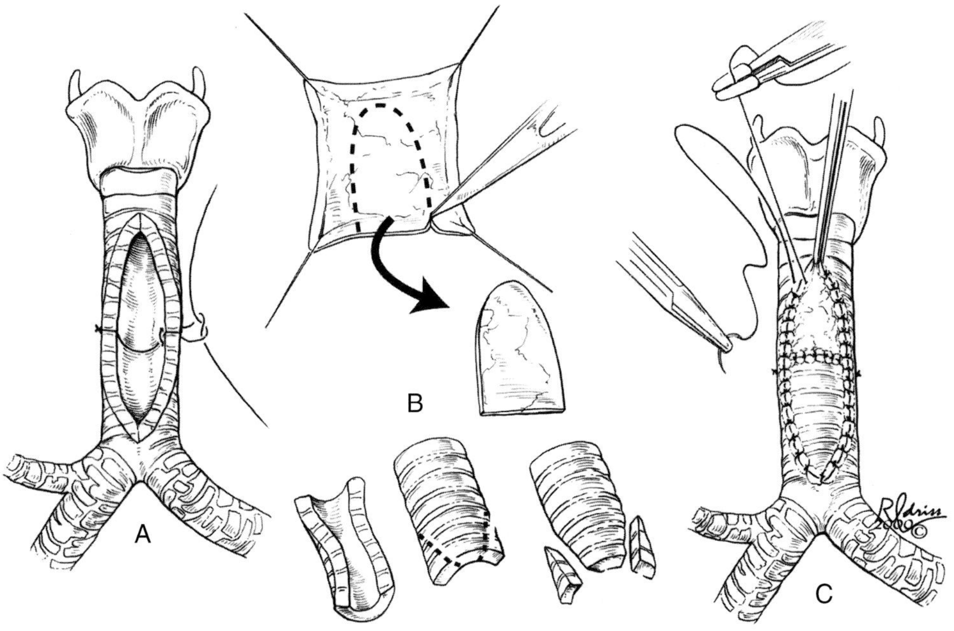

FIGURE 112-15 ■ Composite tracheal autograft. **A,** The posterior anastomosis is performed. **B,** The autograft is trimmed, cutting only the inferior corners of the autograft. A portion of pericardium is harvested and tailored. **C,** The autograft is sutured in place anteriorly, adjacent to the carina. The pericardial patch is inserted superiorly to complete the repair. (From Backer CL, Mavroudis C, Gerber ME, et al: Tracheal surgery in children: an 18-year review of four techniques. *Eur J Cardiothorac Surg* 19:777–784, 2001.)

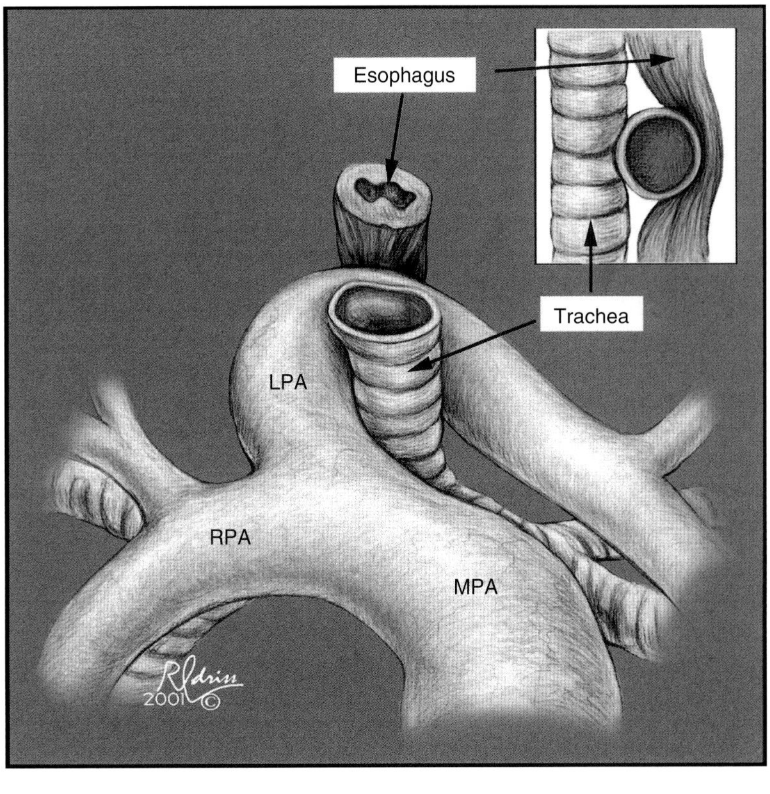

FIGURE 112-16 ■ Pulmonary artery sling. The left pulmonary artery (LPA) originates from the right pulmonary artery (RPA) and acts as a sling, pulling on and compressing the distal trachea and right main bronchus. The *inset* shows anterior compression of the esophagus by the anomalous LPA on the lateral view. *MPA,* Main pulmonary artery. (From Mavroudis C, Backer CL: Vascular rings and pulmonary artery sling. In Mavroudis C, Backer CL, editors: *Pediatric cardiac surgery,* ed 3, Philadelphia, 2003, Mosby, pp 234–250.)

PEDIATRIC TRACHEAL ANOMALIES

Pulmonary Artery Sling

A pulmonary artery sling is found in one third of patients who have tracheal stenosis.[13] The left pulmonary artery originates anomalously from the right pulmonary artery and courses craniad to the right mainstem bronchus and posteriorly to the trachea on the way to the left lung. This compresses the right main bronchus and distal trachea (Fig. 112-16). The first pulmonary artery sling repair was reported by Potts from Children's Memorial Hospital.[33] Potts operated on a 5-month-old child who had severe right bronchial compression without a known diagnosis. Potts approached the sling through a right thoracotomy. He made the intraoperative diagnosis of a pulmonary artery sling with origin of the left pulmonary artery from the right pulmonary artery. After considering several surgical alternatives, including a pneumonectomy, Potts clamped and divided the left pulmonary artery and transposed it anterior to the tracheobronchial tree. He then reanastomosed the site of origin into the right pulmonary artery. The patient survived the operation but was found, almost 25 years later, to have an occluded left pulmonary artery.[34]

Historically the next series of patients who underwent pulmonary artery sling repair were operated on through a left thoracotomy.[35] This allowed better exposure for the anastomosis. However, many of these patients continued to have significant problems with tracheal stenosis and left pulmonary artery stenosis or occlusion. This is because none of the techniques described up to that time had dealt directly with the associated tracheal stenosis that is present in roughly two thirds of patients with pulmonary artery sling. Thus, once the diagnosis of pulmonary artery sling is made, a workup of the airway must be performed in all cases. The current approach is via a median sternotomy with cardiopulmonary bypass, which allows the surgeon to approach both pathologies if necessary.[36] Mild hypothermia is used, and the heart remains beating throughout the procedure. The right, left, and main pulmonary arteries are widely mobilized to minimize the tension of the anastomosis. As it passes behind the posterior trachea, the left pulmonary artery may be closely adherent to it and must be dissected off with caution. The left pulmonary artery is divided and transposed anterior to the trachea. It is then reanastomosed to the distal main pulmonary artery, at a site selected to approximate the normal origin of the left pulmonary artery (Fig. 112-17). The anastomosis is performed with running polypropylene suture that is locked at every three to four bites. The tracheal repair is also performed while the patient is on cardiopulmonary bypass. Depending on the length of the stenosis, TRR or slide tracheoplasty is performed.

Tracheomalacia

Tracheomalacia can be a difficult entity to deal with in the infant and young child. It can be classified as primary or secondary. Causes of secondary tracheomalacia include tracheoesophageal fistula and external compression from vascular structures (i.e., the innominate artery, vascular rings), cardiac structures, congenital cysts, and neoplasms. Tracheomalacia accounts for almost half of all congenital tracheal anomalies that are seen with stridor.[37] Symptoms depend on the location, length, and severity of the pathology. Intrathoracic tracheomalacia typically produces expiratory stridor or wheezing, which mimics asthma. Symptoms also may include a harsh barking cough, hyperextension of the neck, recurrent respiratory infections, and, when associated with compression by an anomalous innominate artery, reflex apnea.

Lateral chest radiograph shows narrowing of the trachea during expiration. The diagnosis is confirmed at bronchoscopy if spontaneous respiration is maintained during bronchoscopy—the wide posterior membranous trachea is observed to collapse anteriorly during expiration. These dynamics are not observed when the child is paralyzed and ventilated with positive pressure. Dynamic CT with contrast medium is performed after bronchoscopy to define the nature of underlying suspected extrinsic compression.

Most patients with mild to moderate tracheomalacia eventually grow to the point where the tracheomalacia does not require surgical intervention. However, a small number of patients who have severe tracheomalacia require intubation, ventilation, and usually very high positive end-expiratory pressure (PEEP) to keep the airway open and allow adequate ventilation of the patient.

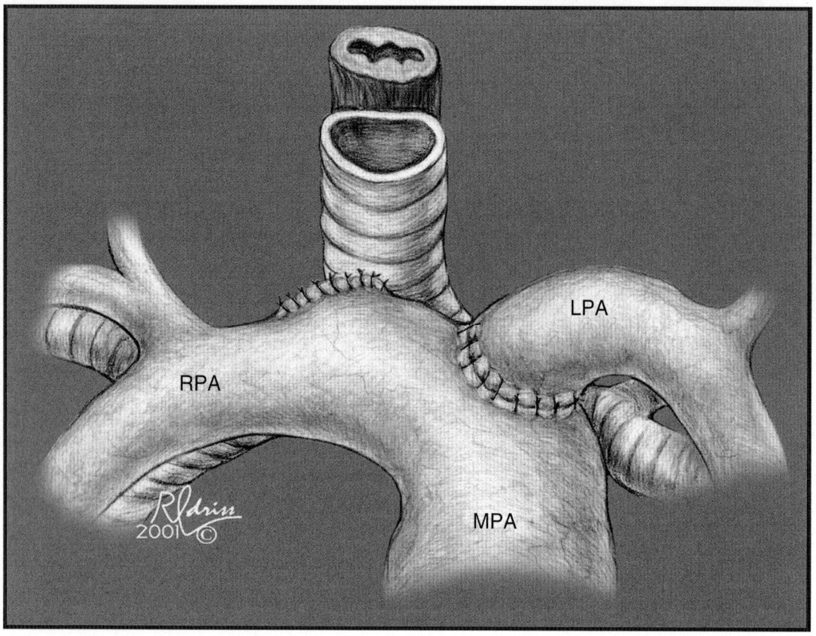

FIGURE 112-17 ■ Pulmonary artery sling repair. The right pulmonary artery (RPA) origin of the left pulmonary artery (LPA) has been oversewn with interrupted sutures (to prevent RPA stenosis). The LPA has been anastomosed to an opening created in the main pulmonary artery (MPA), again with interrupted sutures. The LPA is now anterior to the trachea.

For these severe cases of tracheomalacia, there are several surgical alternatives.

Secondary tracheomalacia is always treated by treating the offending compressing structure first—for example, by repair of a vascular ring or by fixation of an innominate artery. The trachea itself is typically left alone with the anticipation that decompression in conjunction with the growth of the child will result in a more stable airway.

For primary tracheomalacia, one option is tracheostomy. This may obviate the need for positive pressure ventilation because the tracheostomy tube holds open the trachea. With associated bronchomalacia, PEEP may be necessary. Increasingly, these patients are discharged home on ventilation. Many children's hospitals have a separate service for those who become chronically ventilator dependent for a variety of reasons. As the trachea matures and the cartilage gains more strength, these patients can eventually be weaned from their ventilators.

A second alternative is to bronchoscopically place a balloon-expandable wire stent (Fig. 112-18). Stents are usually a procedure of last resort in pediatric airway surgery. However, for severe primary tracheomalacia in patients who are usually ventilator dependent, this can be a life-saving procedure. The largest experience in infants is with the Palmaz stent (Johnson & Johnson International Systems, Warren, NJ).[38,39] The most common indications in the series from Children's Memorial in Chicago occurred after pericardial tracheoplasty or in patients with tetralogy of Fallot and absent pulmonary valve who had severe compression of the tracheobronchial tree from enlarged pulmonary arteries. These stents were effective in selected patients, but several patients had complications from significant granulation tissue formation. Again, stents are usually used as a measure of last resort in infants who have not responded to tracheostomy and positive pressure ventilation.

A surgical procedure for infants with tracheomalacia was reported by Hagl and associates from Heidelberg, Germany.[40] This operation was performed either through a thoracotomy or via a median sternotomy approach. External stabilization of the severely dysplastic distal trachea (six patients) or left main bronchus (two patients) was achieved by suspending the malacic segment in an oversized and longitudinally opened, ring-reinforced polytetrafluoroethylene prosthesis. Multiple pledgeted sutures were placed extramucosally to the dysplastic tracheal wall and the dyskinetic pars membranacea, as well as to the polytetrafluoroethylene prosthesis in a radial orientation. Guided by simultaneous video-assisted bronchoscopy, reexpansion of the collapsed segments was achieved by gentle traction on the sutures while tying (Fig. 112-19). Hagl and associates reported excellent results in six of seven patients. Long-term results are unknown.

Postintubation Stenosis

The largest series of pediatric patients undergoing tracheal surgery for a postintubation stenosis was reported from Massachusetts General Hospital.[19] Wright and colleagues reported 72 patients evaluated for postintubation

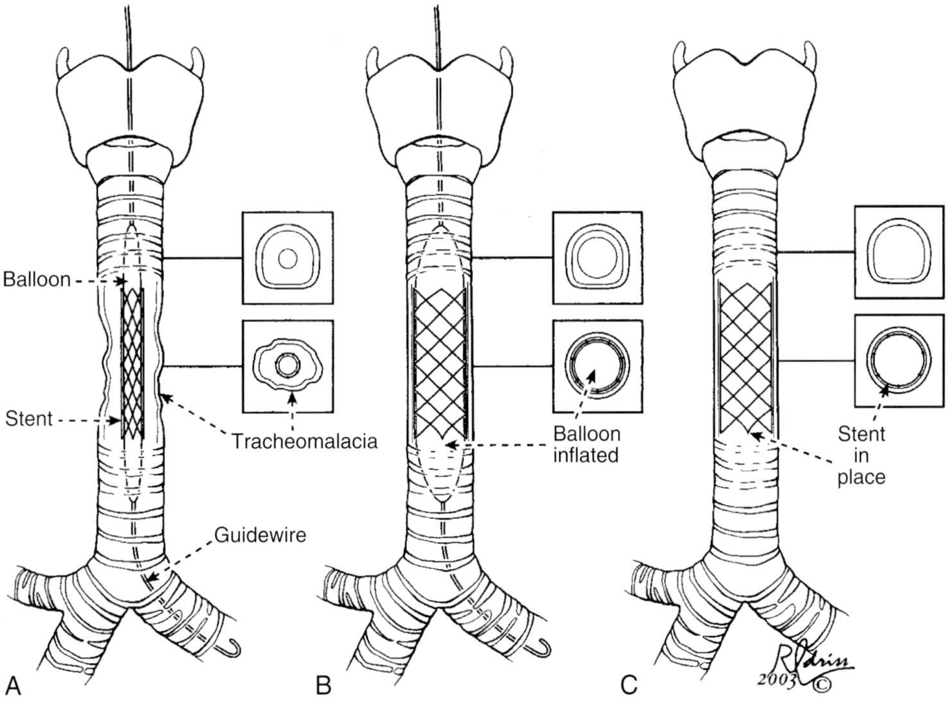

FIGURE 112-18 ■ Palmaz stent insertion in a child with severe tracheomalacia. **A,** The Palmaz stent (mounted on a balloon-tipped catheter) has been positioned in the mid trachea. Positioning of the stent is with both fluoroscopy and bronchoscopy. **B,** The balloon is inflated, compressing the stent against the tracheal wall. **C,** The balloon catheter has been removed, and the stent is now in place. The tracheal lumen is held open by the stent.

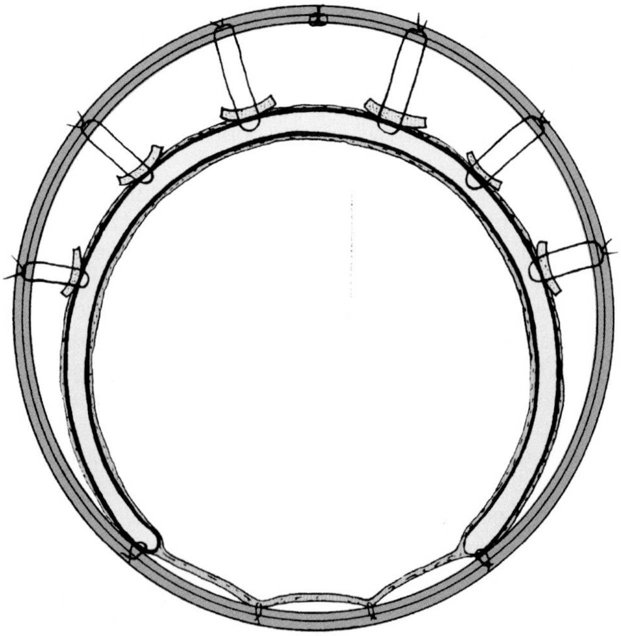

FIGURE 112-19 ■ Cross-sectional view of tracheal external stabilization with "onlay" fixation of the flaccid pars membranacea and free suspension of the malacic cartilaginous portions within an oversized polytetrafluoroethylene prosthesis. (From Hagl S, Jakob H, Sebening C, et al: External stabilization of long-segment tracheobronchomalacia guided by intraoperative bronchoscopy. *Ann Thorac Surg* 64:1412–1421, 1997.)

stenosis during an almost 25-year period. Of these patients, 31 were treated with tracheal resection and 17 were treated with laryngotracheal resection. Postintubation tracheal stenosis typically occurs from a stricture caused by scarring at the site of compression of the tracheal mucosa by the balloon from the endotracheal tube. Historically, balloons were used with low volume and high pressure. Since converting to high-volume, low-pressure balloons, the incidence of postintubation stenosis has diminished significantly. Evaluation of postintubation stenosis is chiefly with bronchoscopy. The larynx should undergo a detailed examination to identify commonly associated superglottic (arytenoid scarring and fixation), glottic (vocal cord paralysis or granulomas), or proximal subglottic pathology. Here again, the connection with a pediatric otolaryngologist is paramount. These commonly associated problems may require attention before the tracheal stenosis is repaired. The technical details of the tracheal resection for these patients are similar to those of resection for patients with congenital stenosis secondary to complete tracheal rings.

Tracheal Web

Web-like diaphragms most often occur at the subcricoid level. These webs typically do not involve a significant length of the trachea. Tracheal webs are evaluated in a fashion similar to that used for other patients with tracheal stenosis, and bronchoscopy continues to be the primary diagnostic tool. Tracheal webs have been removed or excised bronchoscopically with biopsy forceps and occasionally with the use of an insulating cauterizing electrode. Laser therapy or balloon dilation also may be successful. If this should fail, a tracheostomy done below the web may be a temporary solution, allowing the patient to grow and have a definitive resection later in life. In most cases, these webs are cared for by the pediatric otolaryngologist, with only occasional need for tracheal resection by the thoracic surgeon.

SUMMARY

The most common indication for a surgical procedure on the trachea of an infant or small child is tracheal stenosis secondary to complete tracheal rings. Close cooperation between the pediatric cardiothoracic surgeons and the otolaryngologists is essential. We approach all cases via a median sternotomy and perform the repair on beating-heart cardiopulmonary bypass. We prefer TRR for short segments (six to eight tracheal rings, one third of the trachea), and slide tracheoplasty for long-segment stenosis. If the patient has an associated pulmonary artery sling or intracardiac anomaly, that lesion should be repaired simultaneously. Bronchoscopic expertise is essential to make the diagnosis, for intraoperative management, and for postoperative airway management and clearance. The outlook for these patients has evolved significantly from the mid 1970s, when most of these patients died, to the current era—the mortality rate for complete tracheal rings is now less than 15%. The postoperative management of these patients is complex, often because of comorbid conditions, and requires extreme attention to detail and vigilance.

REFERENCES

1. Backer CL, Mavroudis C: Congenital Heart Surgery Nomenclature and Database Project. Vascular rings, tracheal stenosis, pectus excavatum. *Ann Thorac Surg* 69:S308–S318, 2000.
2. Cantrell JR, Guild HC: Congenital stenosis of the trachea. *Am J Surg* 108:297–305, 1964.
3. Grillo HC: Surgical approaches to the trachea. *Surg Gynecol Obstet* 129:347–352, 1969.
4. Salassa JR, Pearson BW, Payne WS: Gross and microscopical blood supply of the trachea. *Ann Thorac Surg* 24:100–107, 1977.
5. Kimura K, Mukohara N, Tsugawa C, et al: Tracheoplasty for congenital stenosis of the entire trachea. *J Pediatr Surg* 17:869–871, 1982.
6. Idriss FS, DeLeon SY, Ilbawi MN, et al: Tracheoplasty with pericardial patch for extensive tracheal stenosis in infants and children. *J Thorac Cardiovasc Surg* 88:527–536, 1984.
7. Tsang V, Murday A, Gillbe C, et al: Slide tracheoplasty for congenital funnel-shaped tracheal stenosis. *Ann Thorac Surg* 48:632–635, 1989.
8. Grillo HC, Wright CD, Vlahakes GJ, et al: Management of congenital tracheal stenosis by means of slide tracheoplasty or resection and reconstruction, with long-term follow-up of growth after slide tracheoplasty. *J Thorac Cardiovasc Surg* 123:145–152, 2002.
9. Elliott MJ, Haw MP, Jacobs JP, et al: Tracheal reconstruction in children using cadaveric homograft trachea. *Eur J Cardiothorac Surg* 10:707–712, 1996.
10. Backer CL, Mavroudis C, Dunham ME, et al: Repair of congenital tracheal stenosis with a free tracheal autograft. *J Thorac Cardiovasc Surg* 115:869–874, 1998.
11. Rutter MJ, Cotton RT, Azizkhan RG, et al: Slide tracheoplasty for the management of complete tracheal rings. *J Pediatr Surg* 38:928–934, 2003.
12. Benjamin B, Pitkin J, Cohen D: Congenital tracheal stenosis. *Ann Otol Rhinol Laryngol* 90:364–371, 1981.

13. Backer CL, Mavroudis C, Gerber ME, et al: Tracheal surgery in children: an 18-year review of four techniques. *Eur J Cardiothorac Surg* 19:777–784, 2001.
14. Manson D, Babyn P, Filler R, et al: Three-dimensional imaging of the pediatric trachea in congenital tracheal stenosis. *Pediatr Radiol* 24:175–179, 1994.
15. Lee KS, Sun MR, Ernst A, et al: Comparison of dynamic expiratory CT with bronchoscopy for diagnosing airway malacia: a pilot evaluation. *Chest* 131:758–764, 2007.
16. Alboliras ET, Backer CL, Holinger LD, et al: Pulmonary artery sling: diagnostic and management strategy. *Pediatrics* 98:530, 1996.
17. Nicotra JJ, Mahboubi S, Kramer SS: Three-dimensional imaging of the pediatric airway. *Int J Pediatr Otorhinolaryngol* 41:299–305, 1997.
18. Tsugawa C, Kimura K, Muraji T, et al: Congenital stenosis involving a long segment of the trachea: further experience in reconstructive surgery. *J Pediatr Surg* 23:471–475, 1988.
19. Wright CD, Graham BB, Grillo HC, et al: Pediatric tracheal surgery. *Ann Thorac Surg* 74:308–314, 2002.
20. Grillo HC: Slide tracheoplasty for long-segment congenital tracheal stenosis. *Ann Thorac Surg* 58:613–621, 1994.
21. Backer CL, Mavroudis C, Holinger LD: Repair of congenital tracheal stenosis. *Semin Thorac Cardiovasc Surg Pediatr Card Surg Annu* 5:173–186, 2002.
22. Cotter CS, Jones DT, Nuss RC, et al: Management of distal tracheal stenosis. *Arch Otolaryngol Head Neck Surg* 25:325–328, 1999.
23. Heinemann MK, Ziemer G, Sieverding L, et al: Long-segment tracheal resection in infancy utilizing extracorporeal circulation. In Imai Y, Momma K, editors: *Proceedings of the Second World Congress of Pediatric Cardiology and Cardiac Surgery*, New York, 1998, Futura, pp 711–713.
24. Acosta AC, Albanese CT, Farmer DL, et al: Tracheal stenosis: the long and the short of it. *J Pediatr Surg* 35:1612–1616, 2000.
25. Lang FJ, Hurni M, Monnier P: Long-segment congenital tracheal stenosis: treatment by slide-tracheoplasty. *J Pediatr Surg* 34:1216–1222, 1999.
26. Matute JA, Romero R, Garcia-Casillas MA, et al: Surgical approach to funnel-shaped congenital tracheal stenosis. *J Pediatr Surg* 36:320–323, 2001.
27. Dayan SH, Dunham ME, Backer CL, et al: Slide tracheoplasty in the management of congenital tracheal stenosis. *Ann Otol Rhinol Laryngol* 106:914–919, 1997.
28. Oue T, Kamata S, Usui N, et al: Histopathologic changes after tracheobronchial reconstruction with costal cartilage graft for congenital tracheal stenosis. *J Pediatr Surg* 36:329–333, 2001.
29. Backer CL, Mavroudis C, Dunham ME, et al: Reoperation after pericardial patch tracheoplasty. *J Pediatr Surg* 32:1108–1112, 1997.
30. Cheng ATL, Backer CL, Holinger LD, et al: Histopathologic changes after pericardial patch tracheoplasty. *Arch Otolaryngol Head Neck Surg* 123:1069–1072, 1997.
31. Jacobs JP, Elliott MJ, Haw MP, et al: Pediatric tracheal homograft reconstruction: a novel approach to complex tracheal stenoses in children. *J Thorac Cardiovasc Surg* 112:1549–1558, 1996.
32. Jacobs JP, Quintessenza JA, Andrews T, et al: Tracheal allograft reconstruction: the total North American and worldwide pediatric experiences. *Ann Thorac Surg* 68:1043–1051, 1999.
33. Potts WJ, Holinger PH, Rosenblum AH: Anomalous left pulmonary artery causing obstruction to right main bronchus. Report of a case. *JAMA* 155:1409–1411, 1954.
34. Campbell CD, Wernly JA, Koltip PC, et al: Aberrant left pulmonary artery (pulmonary artery sling): successful repair and 24 year follow-up report. *Am J Cardiol* 45:316–320, 1980.
35. Koopot R, Nikaidoh H, Idriss FS: Surgical management of anomalous left pulmonary artery causing tracheobronchial obstruction. Pulmonary artery sling. *J Thorac Cardiovasc Surg* 69:239–246, 1975.
36. Backer CL, Mavroudis C, Dunham ME, et al: Pulmonary artery sling: results with median sternotomy, cardiopulmonary bypass, and reimplantation. *Ann Thorac Surg* 67:1738–1744, 1999.
37. Holinger LD, Green CG, Benjamin B, et al: Tracheobronchial tree. In Holinger LD, Lusk RP, Green CG, editors: *Pediatric laryngology and bronchoesophagology*, Philadelphia, 1997, Lippincott-Raven, pp 234–250.
38. Filler RM, Forte V, Fraga JC, et al: The use of expandable metallic airway stents for tracheobronchial obstruction in children. *J Pediatr Surg* 30:1050–1056, 1995.
39. Furman RH, Backer CL, Dunham ME, et al: The use of balloon-expandable metallic stents in the treatment of pediatric tracheomalacia and bronchomalacia. *Arch Otolaryngol Head Neck Surg* 125:203–207, 1999.
40. Hagl S, Jakob H, Sebening C, et al: External stabilization of long-segment tracheobronchomalacia guided by intraoperative bronchoscopy. *Ann Thorac Surg* 64:1412–1421, 1997.

CHAPTER 113

Patent Ductus Arteriosus, Coarctation of the Aorta, and Vascular Rings

Sitaram M. Emani

CHAPTER OUTLINE

Included under the rubric of congenital heart defects are abnormalities involving the distal transverse arch and proximal descending aorta. Clinical manifestations range widely, from severe congestive heart failure or debilitating stridor to mere incidental finding on routine evaluation. The treatment of these conditions represents the first procedures performed for congenital cardiovascular malformations. The first surgical closure of a patent ductus arteriosus (PDA), performed by Dr. Robert Gross in 1938, opened the era of pediatric cardiac surgery.

PATENT DUCTUS ARTERIOSUS

Introduction

The prevalence of PDA at several days of age varies from 20% to 80% and varies inversely with gestational age and birth weight.[1] Between 1998 and 2008, the Nationwide Inpatient Sample database demonstrated increase in the prevalence of PDA in the United States from 1.9 to 2.8 per 1000 live births, likely because of increased detection and improvements in prenatal and neonatal care.[2] It is frequently associated with other heart defects ranging in severity from patent foramen ovale to complex congenital malformations. Several genetic defects have been implicated in the development of PDA, including genes that encode prostaglandin receptors and regulators of smooth muscle cell contraction.[3-5]

Pathophysiology and Natural History

Although the ductus arteriosus shunts mostly right to left in utero, expansion of the lungs shortly after birth results in a decline in the pulmonary vascular resistance and increased pulmonary blood flow and arterial oxygen tension. Ductal closure usually occurs within the first several hours after birth, and is thought to be mediated by loss of the placental source of prostaglandins, increased degradation of prostaglandins within the lungs, and increased arterial oxygen tension, which stimulate constriction of smooth muscle cells within the wall of the ductus. The prostaglandin-mediated mechanism is most active in the ductus of premature infants, whereas oxygen tension primarily promotes ductal closure in the term infant, likely because of differences in cyclooxygenase (COX) isoforms present in the ductal tissue at various stages of gestation.[6] Thus, the PDA of a term infant is generally unresponsive to COX inhibition, whereas the PDA of a premature infant frequently responds.

Spontaneous closure of the ductus within 4 days occurs in 90% to 95% of full-term infants and in 80% to 90% of premature infants at 30 to 37 weeks' gestation.[7] The rate of spontaneous closure is inversely proportional to birthweight, with only 50% spontaneous closure in extremely low-birthweight infants (500-999 g).[8] In premature infants, PDA increases the risk of prolonged ventilation and oxygen requirements, pulmonary hemorrhage, and bronchopulmonary dysplasia.[9-11] The diastolic steal is associated with renal hypoperfusion, intestinal ischemia, necrotizing enterocolitis (NEC), reduced middle cerebral artery blood flow velocity, and increased risk of intraventricular hemorrhage.[12-18] The long-term persistence of PDA is associated with development of endocarditis, congestive heart failure, and eventual development of irreversible pulmonary vascular obstructive disease. Estimated mortality without intervention is 60% by 60 years of age.[19]

Clinical Presentation

Presentation ranges from asymptomatic murmur on examination to symptoms of congestive heart failure caused by large left-to-right shunting. Manifestations of pulmonary overcirculation include hypotension, pulmonary edema, and failure to thrive in infants and children. Neonates, particularly premature neonates, may demonstrate intestinal malperfusion and renal insufficiency in addition to respiratory compromise. Cyanosis is occasionally the presenting symptom in older patients with pulmonary hypertension.

Diagnosis

Physical examination reveals the presence of a "to and fro" murmur heard best from the left upper sternal border, and leads to suspicion of PDA. Chest radiography may show cardiomegaly, signs of pulmonary congestion, and pulmonary edema. Transthoracic echocardiography is used to make the diagnosis (Fig. 113-1). Retrograde flow in the descending aorta indicates significant left-to-right shunting. The presence of a left-sided aortic arch must be confirmed if surgical therapy is contemplated, as this influences the choice of incision. Continuous left-to-right shunting through the ductus is expected, and the presence of right-to-left shunting or bidirectional shunting should raise suspicion for pulmonary hypertension. In adults, echocardiographic windows may be suboptimal, and computed tomography (CT) or magnetic resonance angiography may be necessary to establish the diagnosis. Diagnostic cardiac catheterization is only necessary if pulmonary hypertension is suspected.

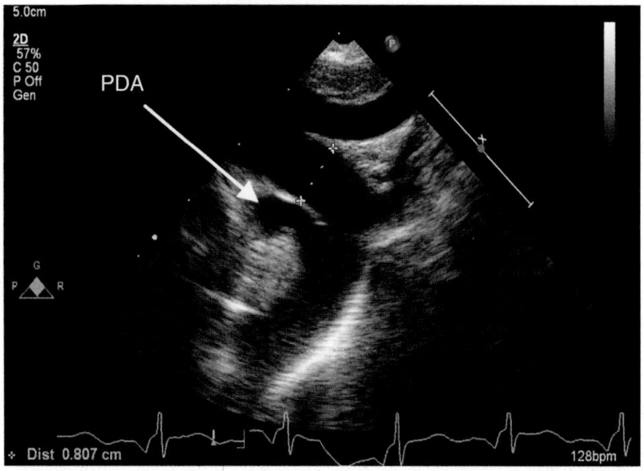

FIGURE 113-1 ■ Echocardiographic appearance of the patent ductus arteriosus (PDA). Note the insertion just distal to the takeoff of the left subclavian artery.

Treatment

Medical

Medical treatment of PDA can be separated into (1) management of heart failure and (2) pharmacologic closure in premature neonates. Management of heart failure focuses on reducing the clinical impact of left to right shunting. Diuretics are the mainstay of therapy in patients with pulmonary congestion, but afterload reduction with angiotensin-converting enzyme inhibitor may be a useful adjunct. In hospitalized patients, strategies to avoid reduction of pulmonary vascular resistance limit the degree of left-to-right shunting, and include maintenance of spontaneous ventilation and avoidance of supplemental oxygen when possible. In intubated patients, an increase in the peak end expiratory pressure can reduce left-to-right shunting.[20]

Pharmacological closure of PDA with a COX inhibitor (COXi) in premature neonates, even if asymptomatic, improves the rate of eventual ductal closure and incidence of intraventricular hemorrhage, decreases the need for surgical closure, but does not improve mortality or incidence of NEC. Early treatment of a symptomatic

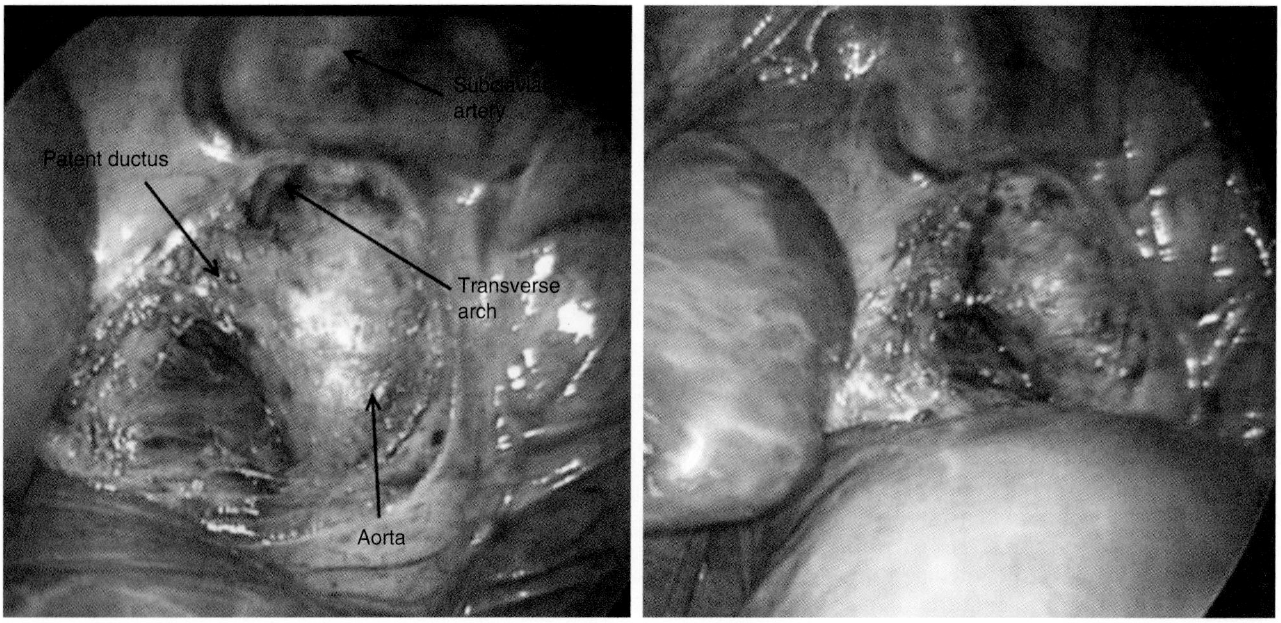

FIGURE 113-2 ■ Intraoperative view of patent ductus arteriosus before *(left)* and after *(right)* clip placement.

PDA (i.e., when clinical signs first appear) has been shown to decrease the incidence of chronic lung disease, duration of mechanical ventilation, and NEC when compared with late symptomatic treatment (i.e., after signs of congestive cardiac failure).[21] The COXi indomethacin and ibuprofen are equally effective at producing ductal closure. Closure rate between 60% and 80% is achieved with one course of indomethacin, but the success rate of each subsequent course is 40%.[22,23] A COXi is ineffective at producing ductal closure in term infants because of the lack of prostaglandin-responsive contractile smooth muscle in the ductal tissue. Complications owing to COXi include renal impairment, intestinal perforation, and NEC.[24] A randomized clinical study compared oral paracetamol with ibuprofen in preterm infants and demonstrated that paracetamol may be a medical alternative in the management of PDA.[25]

Surgical

Premature Infants. In premature infants, surgical therapy is generally reserved for failure of COXi therapy in symptomatic patients or for those who develop contraindications to COXi therapy: NEC, renal dysfunction, and intraventricular hemorrhage. This strategy of reserving surgery for failure of medical therapy can lead to a higher incidence of NEC when compared with early surgery, although no difference in mortality has been demonstrated.[26-29] Early surgical duct closure allows early institution of full oral feeding, but this does not necessarily translate into shorter hospital stay.[30] Yet controversy regarding the indications and timing for surgical therapy remains, and variability in practice patterns have been observed.[31]

Preoperative evaluation focuses on medical stabilization, including detection and appropriate treatment of pre-existing infections prior to surgery. Surgery for premature infants can be performed either in the intensive care unit or in the operating theater. Surgical ductal ligation is generally performed via left thoracotomy, although video-assisted thoracoscopic surgery (VATS) approach has been described, and the PDA is occluded by placement of an external clip (Fig. 113-2). Preoperative imaging must exclude the presence of ductal or pulmonary artery aneurysms, which may necessitate extensive resection and vascular reconstruction rather than simple ductal ligation.[32]

Full-Term Infants, Children, and Adults. Pharmacologic closure is ineffective in full-term infants, children, and adults, leaving surgical or transcatheter closure as the only options. Ductal closure is indicated in both symptomatic and asymptomatic patients to reduce the risks of endocarditis and pulmonary hypertension. Asymptomatic infants may undergo elective closure between 1 and 2 years of age to facilitate VATS or transcatheter closure, whereas symptomatic infants should undergo prompt evaluation and closure. The presence of cyanosis and bidirectional shunting through the PDA on echocardiography should prompt preoperative cardiac catheterization to measure pulmonary vascular resistance. If elevated pulmonary vascular resistance is unresponsive to oxygen or nitric oxide, closure is contraindicated.

Options for surgical closure in infants include thoracotomy or VATS (see Surgical Approaches). Children and adults are candidates for closure via the transcatheter, thoracotomy, VATS, or sternotomy approaches, depending on the morphology of the PDA. Short length and large diameter of the PDA increase the risk of device embolization during transcatheter closure and bleeding during VATS closure.[33] A severe adverse event rate of approximately 2% is seen with transcatheter closure, with younger age being a significant risk factor.[34,35] To avoid the risk of recanalization, some advocate ductal division in addition to ligation in children and adults.[36] Extensive ductal calcification increases the risk of bleeding during external ligation by VATS or thoracotomy. In these patients, median sternotomy, cardiopulmonary bypass, and closure through a pulmonary arteriotomy may be the safer alternative.

Prognosis

Operative mortality related to PDA ligation in full-term infants and children is less than 1%.[36] Premature infants with multiple comorbidities may have hospital mortality as high as 20%. Complications of surgical ligation include left recurrent laryngeal nerve injury, bleeding, postoperative chylothorax, and development of coarctation. Asymptomatic recurrent laryngeal nerve injury can be detected in up to 7% of patients by systematic endoscopy, and the major risk factor for this injury is birth weight less than 1 kg.[37] Symptomatic nerve injury manifested by aspiration of feeds is rare.

COARCTATION OF THE AORTA

Introduction

Narrowing of the thoracic aorta beyond the level of the innominate artery (discrete coarctation of the aorta or transverse arch hypoplasia) represents 4% to 8% of cases of congenital heart disease, with an incidence in the general population estimated at 0.2 per 1000 live births.[2] Bicuspid aortic valve is an associated finding in up to 50% of patients, and hypoplasia of left heart structures is relatively common. A ventricular septal defect (VSD) may be seen in 30 to 60% of patients, and it may be associated with posterior malalignment of the conal septum leading to left ventricular outflow tract obstruction. Complex congenital heart disease and associated with hypoplasia of the systemic ventricle (hypoplastic left heart syndrome, right dominant atrioventricular canal, transposition of the great arteries with hypoplastic right ventricle) may have associated coarctation that affects management. The incidence of coarctation in patients with right aortic arch is unknown, but it has been estimated to be approximately 4%.[38]

Anatomy and Pathophysiology

The location and extent of aortic obstruction can vary from patient to patient. Discrete coarctation typically occurs just below the origin of the left subclavian artery at the insertion of the ductus arteriosus (juxtaductal coarctation). More diffuse hypoplasia of the distal arch between the left carotid artery and left subclavian artery occurs more commonly in patients with bovine arterial trunk, in which the innominate artery and the right carotid artery arise within close proximity from the proximal transverse arch. An aberrant right subclavian artery arising distal to the coarctation occurs in approximately 3% of patients.

The etiology of coarctation with hypoplasia of the distal transverse arch is not well defined, but its association with hypoplasia of left heart structures suggests common genetic, hemodynamic, or environmental mechanisms.[39] Discrete coarctation of the aorta at the isthmus likely results from abnormal infiltration of ductal tissue onto the juxtaductal aorta.[40] Synchronous with ductal closure, the contractile ductal tissue within the aorta constricts, resulting in luminal narrowing of the aorta and development of a posterior shelf. It is not uncommon for the aorta to appear of adequate size in the presence of a patent ductus arteriosus, yet manifest coarctation following ductal closure.

Natural History

If the coarctation is left untreated, the prognosis varies from severe heart failure in infancy to asymptomatic hypertension in older children and adults. Collateral vessels become prominent because of increased flow within the intercostal, internal mammary, and scapular blood vessels. The increased flow within these vessels can be sufficient to reduce the blood pressure gradient between the upper and lower extremities at rest. With exercise, however, the gradient may rise significantly because of the elevated vascular impedance. Upregulation of circulating catecholamines and the renin-angiotensin system leads to systemic hypertension. Left ventricular hypertrophy is a result of elevated systemic vascular resistance. Untreated coarctation is associated with a substantially diminished long-term survival, with 75% mortality by 50 years of age.[41] Death in these patients is usually due to systemic effects of hypertension, including heart failure, intracranial hemorrhage, coronary artery disease, or aortic rupture or dissection.

Clinical Presentation

The clinical presentation varies depending on the age at presentation. Almost half of patients with coarctation will develop symptoms within the first month of life and will often have the preductal subtype of coarctation with hypoplasia of the arch. Neonates with unsuspected critical coarctation usually have systemic hypoperfusion, metabolic acidosis, and congestive heart failure manifested as tachypnea and difficulty feeding. The timing of the onset of symptoms generally correlates with constriction of the PDA, which provides systemic circulatory support for a period of time after birth. As the ductus closes, perfusion to the lower extremities and abdominal viscera becomes compromised, and end-organ failure manifests with renal dysfunction, hepatic failure, intestinal ischemia, and profound metabolic acidosis. On physical examination, prominent upper extremity and weak lower extremity pulses may be found. Neonates presenting in this manner have a high mortality without urgent intervention. With less severe degrees of coarctation, or in the presence of sufficient collateral development, symptoms may not develop until infancy or adolescence. Asymptomatic patients have a murmur or hypertension. Young adults usually demonstrate hypertension refractory to pharmacotherapy, exercise intolerance, headaches, or angina.

The classic physical findings include the presence of brachiofemoral pulse delay, diminished or absent femoral pulses, and a blood pressure gradient between the upper

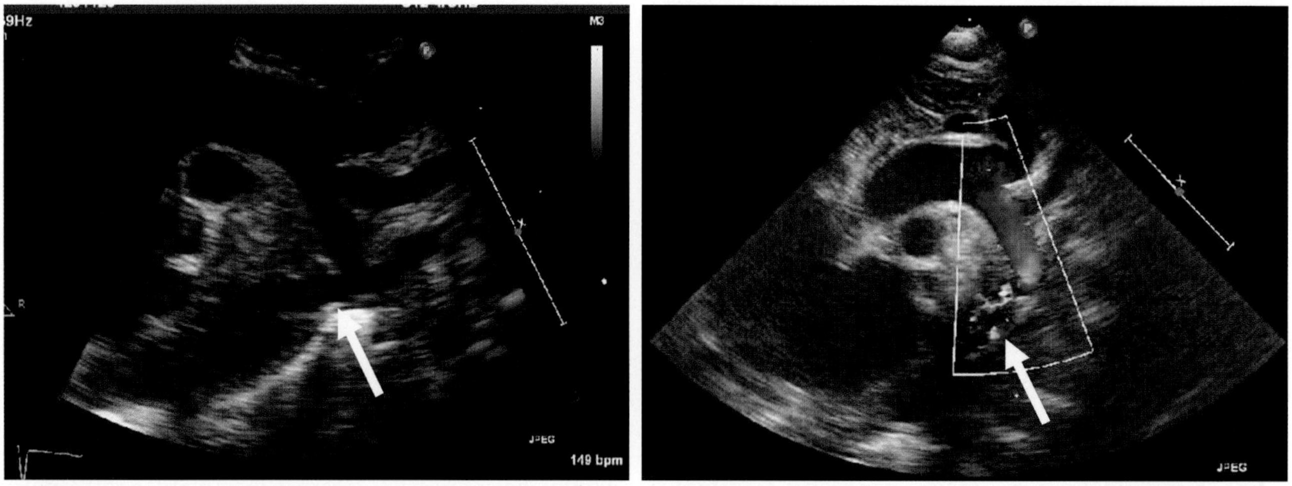

FIGURE 113-3 ■ Discrete coarctation of the aorta on two-dimensional echocardiography and color Doppler imaging. Although there appears to be mild hypoplasia of the transverse arch, color Doppler does not reveal flow acceleration across this segment.

and lower extremities. In the presence of well-developed collaterals, there might not be a significant gradient between upper and lower extremity blood pressures. A systolic ejection murmur is audible over the base of the heart and left interscapular region. The electrocardiogram may reveal evidence of left ventricular hypertrophy in older patients.

Diagnosis

Infants with severe coarctation may demonstrate radiographic signs of cardiac enlargement and pulmonary congestion. During adolescence or adulthood, the findings can include a "figure-three" configuration resulting from proximal and post-stenotic dilation of the aorta. Notching of the inferior border of the ribs from the development of intercostal collateral vessels is common by adolescence.

The segment of coarctation can usually be visualized easily in neonates and children with two-dimensional echocardiography (Fig. 113-3). Normalized measurements of the transverse aorta, aortic isthmus, and descending aorta must be obtained. In neonates, a z-score less than −2 indicates significant narrowing. In older children and adults, a greater than 50% decrease in diameter at the aortic isthmus should be considered severe coarctation. As mentioned previously, associated VSD, aortic and mitral valvular abnormalities, and ventricular hypoplasia must be ruled out. Pulsed- and continuous-wave Doppler estimates the pressure gradient directly at the area of coarctation. In the neonate, the pressure gradient measured by echocardiography may be confounded by presence of a PDA or severe ventricular dysfunction. Similarly, in the older child or adult, the pressure gradient may underestimate the severity of the narrowing because of the presence of significant collaterals. A peak gradient greater than 20 mm Hg, especially if accompanied by continuous forward flow during diastole in the descending or abdominal aorta, suggests significant aortic coarctation.

It is important to define the anatomy of the aortic arch in patients with coarctation, because hypoplasia of the transverse arch can alter surgical management. A transverse arch z-score of less than −2 often requires surgical management at the time of coarctation repair. The presence of a "bovine trunk," in which the innominate artery and left common carotid artery arise as a single trunk, should raise concerns of hypoplasia of the transverse arch between the common trunk and the left subclavian artery.

In older children and adults, the anatomy may be difficult to define with echocardiography because of poor sonographic windows. CT, CT angiography, and magnetic resonance imaging (MRI) have become valuable diagnostic tools in these patients, because they provide superior imaging of the transverse and descending aorta, as well as important information regarding the extent of collateral development. Catheterization with angiography is used to determine the diagnosis and severity of coarctation in patients with disparate clinical and echocardiographic findings. It is also used to determine the degree of coronary artery stenosis in adult patients requiring surgical repair. Transcatheter intervention is preferred for treatment of recoarctation, but its application for native coarctation remains controversial.

Treatment

Patients with significant coarctation or recoarctation are candidates for surgical or transcatheter intervention to reduce the risk of long-term complications. This includes patients with arm-to-leg systolic blood pressure difference greater than or equal to 20 mm Hg, brachiofemoral pulse delay, peak transcoarctation gradient greater than 20 mm Hg at angiography, and those with long-standing hypertension or left ventricular hypertrophy. Elective repair in asymptomatic patients should be performed before 2 years of age, because persistent hypertension following repair has been documented in patients undergoing delayed repair.

Medical Management

Severe neonatal coarctation manifests with profound acidosis from lower extremity hypoperfusion caused by ductal closure, and it can be associated with moderate to severe ventricular dysfunction. Medical stabilization before operating in these patients improves outcomes compared with emergent operation. Ventilatory and inotropic support and intravenous administration of bicarbonate are used to control the metabolic acidosis and ventricular dysfunction. Prostaglandin E_1 (0.01-0.1 μg/kg/min) is given to reestablish ductal patency, and its efficacy is monitored with serial echocardiograms. Cardiovascular collapse can be difficult to resuscitate medically, and may require extracorporeal membrane oxygenation support (ECMO). A major pitfall of preoperative ECMO support in a patient with coarctation is the inadequacy of lower-body perfusion. Neonatal ECMO cannulation is often performed through the carotid artery and jugular vein. With this approach, however, perfusion distal to the coarctation segment remains compromised, and measures to improve distal perfusion must be pursued immediately. These measures include prostaglandin E1 infusion, transcatheter intervention (balloon angioplasty), or traditional surgical resection and reanastomosis.

Surgical Repair

Surgical repair may entail anatomic repair versus extra-anatomic bypass. Anatomic repair involves reconstruction with native aortic tissue, patch augmentation, or interposition grafting, and it is the preferred strategy for primary repair and reoperative repair in children. Extra-anatomic ascending aorta to descending aortic bypass is reserved for adults with complex coarctation undergoing concomitant cardiac surgical procedures (valve replacement or coronary artery bypass grafting).

Anatomic repair in children entails resection of the coarctation segment with end-to-end anastomosis of the distal transverse arch to the descending aorta. Primary treatment for neonates and infants is extended end-to-end anastomosis in which (following coarctation resection) the descending aorta is mobilized, advanced, and anastomosed onto the undersurface of the transverse arch at the level of the left carotid artery (Fig. 113-4). Patch angioplasty or interposition grafts are typically necessary for adults and adolescents, in whom limited aortic mobility prevents a tension-free aortic anastomosis. Subclavian flap angioplasty involves division of the left subclavian artery and use of the proximal portion for aortic reconstruction. The flap is placed on the aorta distal to the subclavian artery for traditional coarctation repair, whereas a reverse flap is used to augment the transverse arch when hypoplasia between the left carotid and subclavian artery is encountered. Coarctation in patients with right aortic arch is approached with a right thoracotomy and treated by patch angioplasty rather than extended end-to-end anastamosis.[38]

Recurrent aortic arch obstruction following previous coarctation repair can be treated surgically with native arch reconstruction, patch aortoplasty, or placement of an interposition graft.[42] In rare circumstances, ascending-to-descending aortic grafts are used for repair of native or recurrent coarctation associated with significant cardiac disease that requires concomitant surgical management (coronary artery bypass grafting, aortic valve replacement).[43] Access to the descending aorta can be obtained by incising the posterior pericardium and dissecting the supradiaphragmatic aorta. Ascending to abdominal aorta bypass avoids the risk of paraplegia associated with left thoracotomy repair of recoarctation in adults.[43,44]

During thoracotomy in an older child or adult, large collateral vessels may be encountered and require meticulous hemostasis. To minimize the risk of spinal cord injury, hyperthermia should be treated aggressively, and mild hypothermia (33-35° C) is preferred. Although repair of coarctation through a left thoracotomy does not require circulatory support, partial bypass may be helpful in adolescents and adults in whom collateral vessels are underdeveloped or have been surgically interrupted. Partial left heart bypass is instituted by providing venous drainage (left atrial appendage or pulmonary vein) and arterial cannulation (femoral artery or descending aorta). Native heart ejections are maintained to provide antegrade blood flow to the upper body during the cross-clamp period.

Coarctation and Ventricular Septal Defect

The presence of a VSD can alter the management of coarctation. Elevated resistance to systemic outflow from coarctation or associated left ventricular outflow tract obstruction can drive increased pulmonary blood flow and result in profound heart failure. Factors that influence therapeutic strategy include the size and likelihood of closure of the VSD and the degree of proximal transverse arch hypoplasia. The location of the VSD is an important determinant of the probability of eventual closure, with the highest closure rates seen with muscular VSDs. Surgical options for patients with unrestrictive VSD and coarctation include single-stage and staged repair of both lesions. Single-stage repair of both coarctation and VSD through a midline sternotomy requires cardiopulmonary bypass but is preferred if transverse arch hypoplasia (z-score < -3.0) is present.[45] Staged repair of the coarctation through a left thoracotomy with or without placement of a pulmonary artery band to control left-to-right shunting avoids the use of cardiopulmonary bypass. This approach is preferable if spontaneous closure of the VSD is likely or if cardiopulmonary bypass is contraindicated.[46]

Transcatheter Intervention

Balloon angioplasty with stenting is an effective treatment for recurrent coarctation of the aorta and is the treatment of choice.[47] For native coarctation, percutaneous balloon angioplasty with or without stenting is an evolving modality of treatment.[48] Compared with surgical repair, balloon angioplasty is associated with a higher incidence of restenosis.[49,50] Acute outcomes of stenting for native coarctation are favorable, but long-term follow-up is lacking.[51,52] The use of a covered stent instead of a bare metal stent may be associated with decreased recoarctation rate, but it does not prevent aneurysm formation.[53]

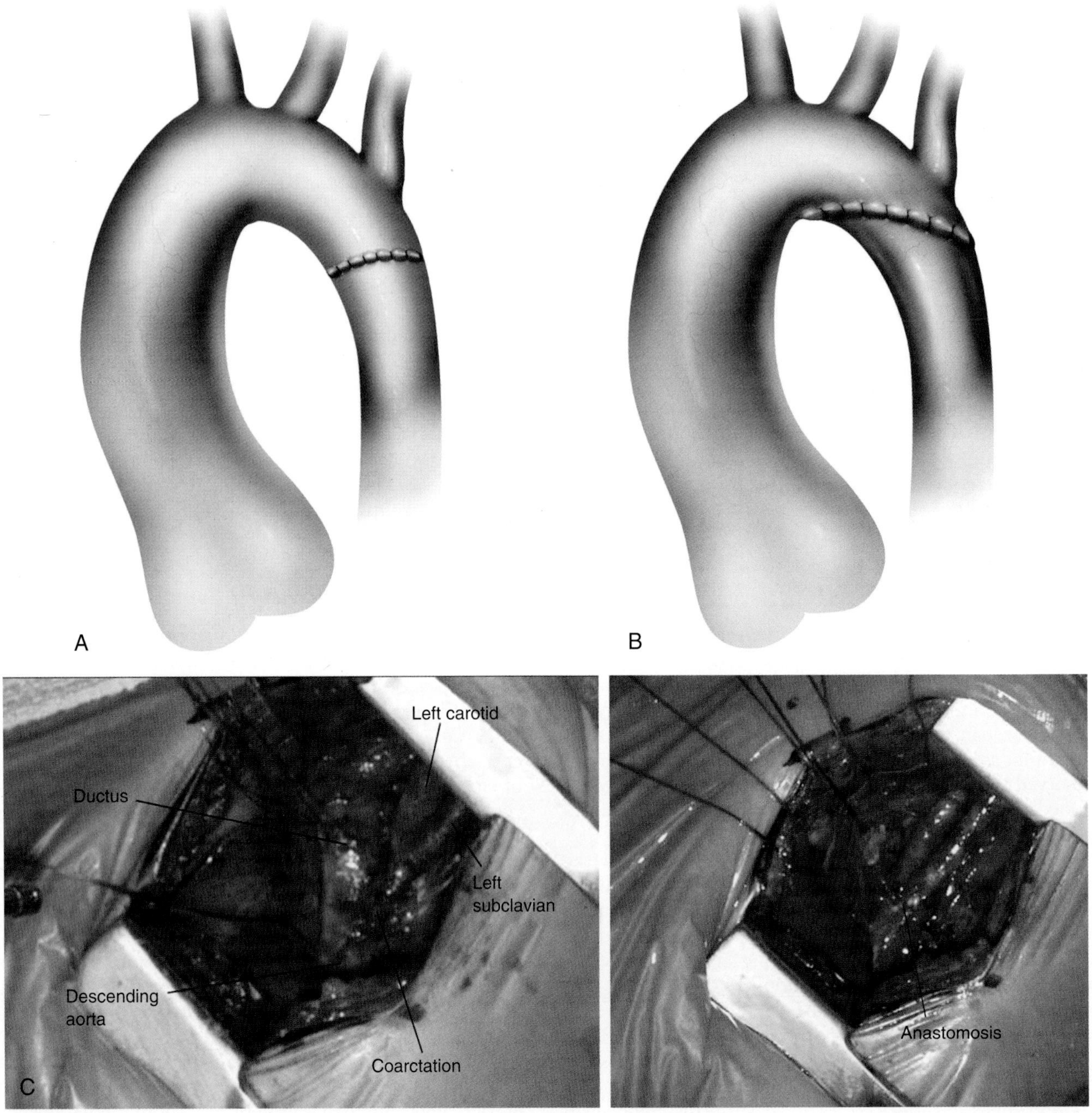

FIGURE 113-4 ■ Techniques for surgical repair of coarctation include **(A)** end-to-end anastomosis or **(B)** extended end-to-end anastomosis. **C,** Intraoperative appearance of coarctation segment *(left)* and extended end-to-end anastomosis *(right)*.

Angioplasty and stenting are alternatives to surgery in high-risk patients in whom temporary relief of discrete coarctation is desired. In adults, balloon dilation and stenting of native coarctation has resulted in aneurysm formation, rupture, and aortic dissection, and recoarctation.[54-56]

Postoperative Complications

Complications specific to coarctation repair include persistent hypertension, mesenteric arteritis, spinal cord ischemia, aneurysm formation, and recurrent coarctation. Significant hypertension can persist in the postoperative period despite a successful operation, and intravenous esmolol is effective at controlling this in the acute postoperative period.[57,58] Acute abdominal pain, thought to be secondary to mesenteric arteritis, was once a common occurrence following coarctation repair. In recent years, the reported incidence of this complication has been low, likely because of improvements in early diagnosis and intervention. Complications related to the thoracotomy and aortic dissection include pneumothorax, chylothorax, and recurrent laryngeal nerve injury. The major risk factor for persistent late hypertension is older age at time of repair, such that 70% of adult patients require ongoing long-term antihypertensive therapy.[59-61]

Prognosis

Operative mortality for neonates and infants with isolated coarctation or coarctation with VSD ranges from 1% to 5%.[62-64] Survival rates at 10 and 30 years following repair are approximately 90% and 70%, which is slightly less than the age-matched general population.[65] The incidence of recoarctation ranges from 10% to 30% in infants, with younger age being a significant risk factor for recurrence and shorter duration to reintervention.[66-70] The presence of a small transverse arch is also a risk factor for reintervention.[67]

In infants, the surgical techniques of extended end-to-end anastomosis and subclavian flap arterioplasty have been associated with the lowest risk of recoarctation in most series.[71,72] Subclavian artery ligation affects limb development, but it does not result in limitation of lifestyle.[63] In children, adolescents, and adults, patch repair of coarctation with or without luminal ridge resection has been associated with a higher incidence of late aneurysm formation when compared with end-to-end anastomosis or interposition grafting.[73,74] Extra-anatomic bypass is associated with a low rate of paraplegia and stroke in adults with complex coarctation.[75] Although low rates of recoarctation have been demonstrated following balloon angioplasty of native coarctation, these results have not been reproduced consistently.[76,77]

VASCULAR RINGS

Introduction

The term *vascular ring* refers to a vascular anomaly that leads to encirclement of the trachea and esophagus. Included in this discussion are vascular compression syndromes, in which the trachea and esophagus are compressed by vascular structures that do not form a complete ring. Symptomatic vascular rings constitute approximately 1% of all cardiovascular anomalies; however, the prevalence of asymptomatic vascular rings, which are more common than symptomatic rings, is unknown. Associated intracardiac pathology may be present in 10% to 30% of patients and includes VSDs, tetralogy of Fallot, patent ductus arteriosus, and congenitally corrected transposition of the great arteries.

Classification

The Congenital Heart Surgery Nomenclature and Database Project classifies vascular rings and compression syndromes as double aortic arch, right arch/left ligamentum, pulmonary artery sling, and innominate compression.[78] Double aortic arch and right aortic arch with left-sided ductus are examples of complete rings. Innominate artery compression and pulmonary artery sling, which do not form complete rings, lead to specific compression syndromes.

Anatomy and Pathophysiology

During normal embryologic development of the thoracic great vessels, regression of specific segments of the embryologic aortic arch results in normal development of a left-sided aorta with the typical branching pattern and a normal pulmonary artery. Both a right and left dorsal aorta are present in the embryo during the first 3 weeks of development. Dissolution of the right dorsal aorta leads to persistence of a dominant left dorsal aorta. Abnormal regression of the dorsal aortic segments leads to abnormalities of the aortic arch.

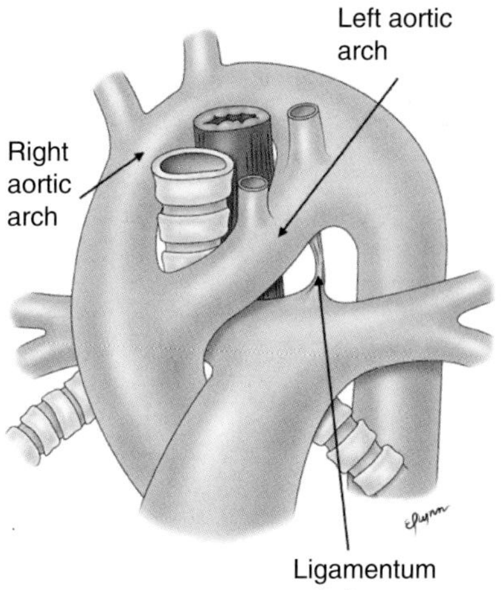

FIGURE 113-5 ■ Double aortic arch creating complete ring around aorta and esophagus. (Compliments of Andrew Powell, MD, and Emily Flynn-Thompson, Children's Hospital Boston.)

Double Aortic Arch

Failure of the regression of the right fourth arch and persistence of the left fourth arch results in development of a double aortic arch. In this abnormality, two separate arches from the distal ascending aorta travel on opposite sides of the trachea and esophagus and join the descending aorta (Fig. 113-5). The trachea and esophagus are compressed by the two arches, which are connected proximally and distally, thus forming a complete ring. In many cases, one of the arches, typically the left, is either hypoplastic or atretic. The right-sided arch is dominant in 70% to 75% of patients, the left arch is dominant in approximately 20%, and codominance is seen in the remainder. Because the complete ring is created by proximal and distal continuity of the right and left aortic arches, interruption of the ring requires division of one of the arches.

Right Aortic Arch with Left Ligamentum

Right aortic arch results from regression of the left fourth arch and persistence of the right fourth arch, with an incidence that ranges between 0.05% and 0.2% in adult patients with congenital heart disease. A complete vascular ring is formed if there is a left-sided ductus or ligamentum arteriosum. The boundaries of the complete ring are the right aortic arch posteriorly and rightward, the pulmonary artery anteriorly, and the ligamentum arteriosum or ductus arteriosus to the left (Fig. 113-6). The ligamentum arteriosum usually arises from the base of the left subclavian artery and connects to the pulmonary artery. Thus, if there is an aberrant left

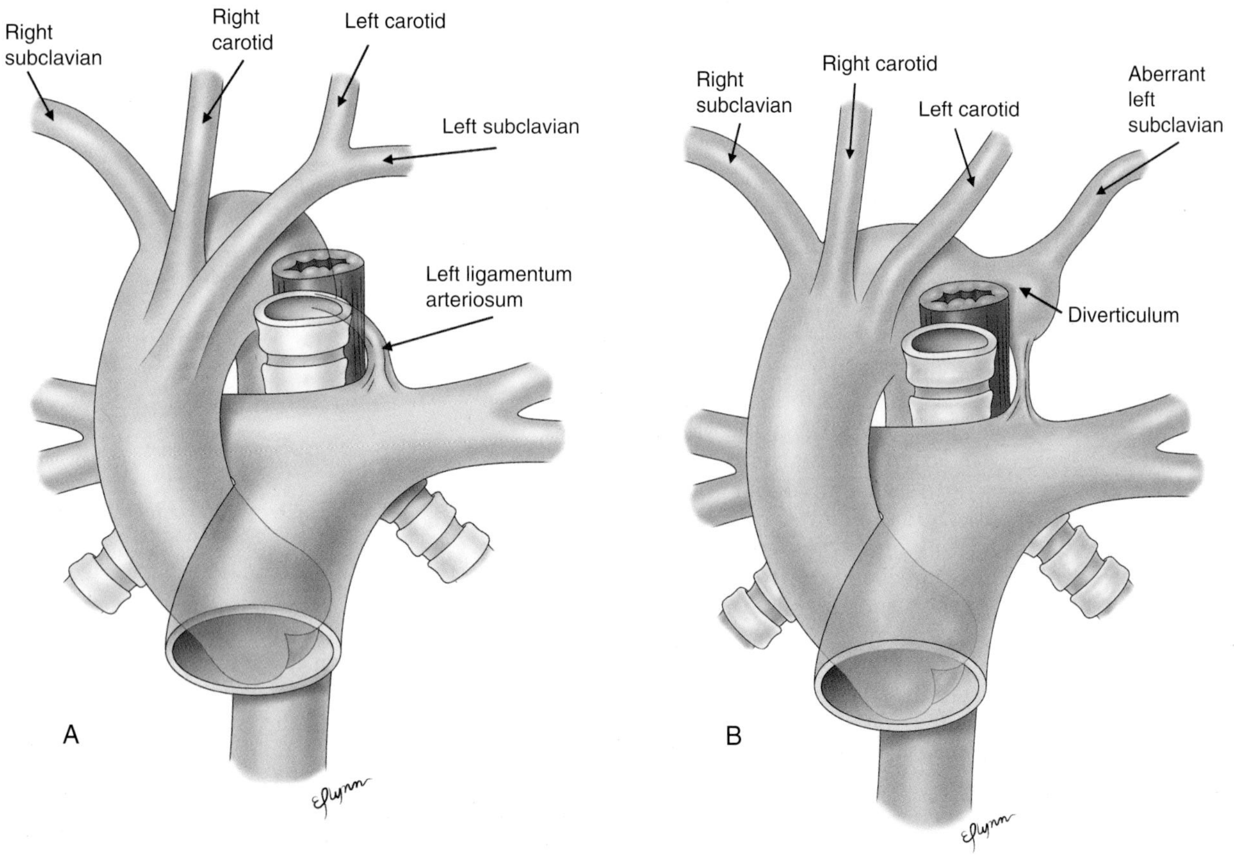

FIGURE 113-6 ■ Right aortic arch with left ligamentum arteriosum. **A,** Mirror-image branching. **B,** Aberrant right subclavian artery. (Compliments of Andrew Powell, MD, and Emily Flynn-Thompson, Children's Hospital Boston.)

subclavian artery that arises from the descending aorta, a left ligament is almost always present. Similarly, in patients with mirror-image branching (MIB), the left subclavian artery arises from the proximal ascending aorta. Because the ligament courses anterior to the airway, most patients with MIB do not experience airway compression. Occasionally, however, in a patient with MIB, the ligamentum may connect to the descending aorta (left ligamentum) and create a complete vascular ring (see Fig. 113-6). This arrangement, although uncommon, must be suspected in a patient with MIB and airway compression. In patients with right aortic arch and left ligamentum, the ligamentum may attach to a diverticular remnant of the left fourth arch, referred to as the *diverticulum of Kommerell*. Associated aneurysm of the diverticulum has been described and may contribute to symptoms by direct compression of the trachea and esophagus.[79] Interruption of the ring is most easily performed by dividing the ligamentum arteriosum or ductus arteriosus, whereas management of the diverticulum is controversial.

Circumflex Retroesophageal Aorta

A rare form of complete vascular ring is the circumflex retroesophageal aortic arch. In this anomaly, the distal transverse arch crosses the midline, posterior to the esophagus, to descend on the contralateral side, thus placing the aortic arch and the descending aorta on the opposite sides of the spine. A complete ring is formed if the ligamentum arteriosum or ductus arteriosus is present on the side contralateral to the aortic arch. Even if a complete vascular ring is not formed (in the presence of an ipsilateral ligamentum), posterior compression of the esophagus can still occur.[80] Embryologically, this malformation is a consequence of preservation of the proximal ipsilateral fourth arch (right or left aortic arch), and persistence of the contralateral sixth segment (ligamentum or ductus) and distal portion of the contralateral fourth arch (descending aorta). The two forms of this anomaly are left aortic arch (LAA) with right descending aorta (Fig. 113-7) and right aortic arch with left descending aorta. Circumflex left aortic arch is frequently associated with aberrant origin of the right subclavian artery (RSCA) from the descending aorta. Right aortic arch can be associated with either MIB or aberrant left subclavian artery (LSCA) patterns, but a complete ring only occurs in the presence of a left ligamentum. Cervical aortic arch is an associated finding in some patients consisting of superior extension of the aortic arch into the cervical region. This results from persistence of the right or left third branchial arch and regression of the fourth branchial arches.

Left Aortic Arch and Anomalous (Retroesophageal) Right Subclavian Artery

The most common arch anomaly, present in approximately 0.5% of the population, is the LAA with aberrant RSCA and left-sided ligamentum arteriosum (Fig. 113-8). Embryologically, this anomaly results from normal involution of the right fourth arch and dorsal

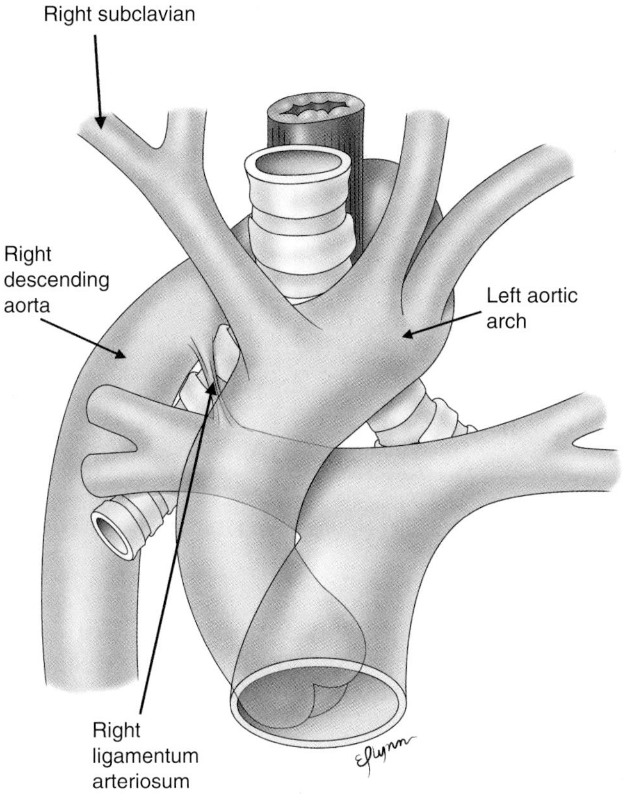

FIGURE 113-7 ■ Circumflex left aortic arch with right descending aorta and right ligamentum, creating a complete vascular ring. (Compliments of Andrew Powell, MD, and Emily Flynn-Thompson, Children's Hospital Boston.)

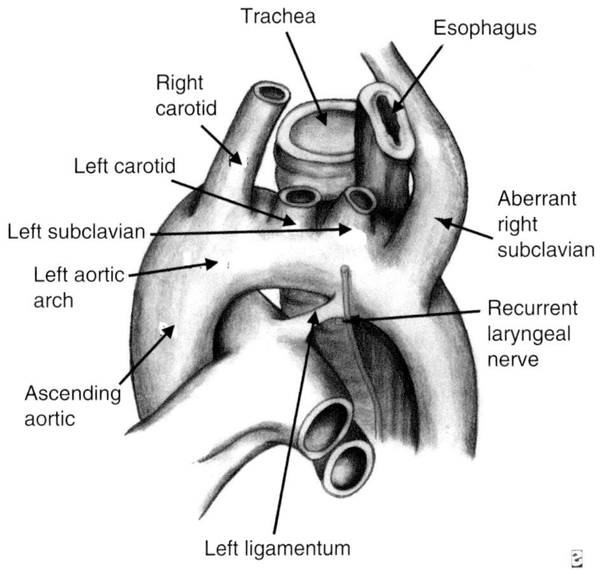

FIGURE 113-8 ■ Aberrant right subclavian artery coursing posterior to esophagus.

aorta, but persistent attachment of the right seventh intersegmental segment to the descending aorta. Most individuals with this anomaly are asymptomatic, but symptoms of dysphagia can occur if this vessel compresses the esophagus as it courses posteriorly. The presence of an aneurysm of the artery or Kommerell diverticulum at its aortic origin is more likely to produce

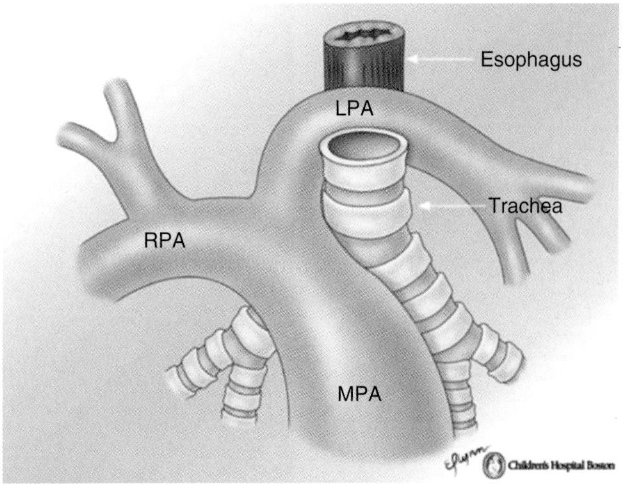

FIGURE 113-9 ■ Left pulmonary artery (LPA) sling originating from the right pulmonary artery (RPA) and coursing posterior to the trachea. *MPA,* Main pulmonary artery. (Compliments of Andrew Powell, MD, and Emily Flynn-Thompson, Children's Hospital Boston.)

symptoms from esophageal compression, but it can also result in hematemesis from arterial-esophageal fistula.[81] There have been case reports of LAA, aberrant RSCA, and right ligamentum attaching to the right subclavian artery, which creates a complete vascular ring and tracheal compression.[82]

Pulmonary Artery Sling

This vascular malformation is formed when the left pulmonary artery (LPA) arises from the right pulmonary artery (RPA), and it courses around the right mainstem bronchus toward the left lung between the airway and the esophagus (Fig. 113-9). In the developing embryo, the pulmonary artery is formed by amalgamation of the sixth branchial arch with postbranchial vessels that arise from the primitive lung bud. If the left postbranchial vessel connects to the right instead of left sixth branchial arch, then a pulmonary artery sling develops. This results in compression of the tracheobronchial tree, most commonly at the distal trachea or the right mainstem bronchus. It is associated with complete tracheal rings in approximately 50% of patients, and has been associated with agenesis of the right lung.[83]

Innominate Artery Compression Syndrome

Anterior compression of the airway can occur because of an unusual (leftward and posterior) takeoff of the innominate artery from the aorta. The presence of a prominent thymus gland and pectus deformity of the chest wall exacerbate the anterior tracheal compression. Innominate artery compression of the trachea in infants can cause severe biphasic stridor, cyanosis, and respiratory arrest, sometimes referred to as *dying spells*.

Clinical Presentation

Most common forms of presentation include respiratory distress, stridor, dysphagia or a combination of these

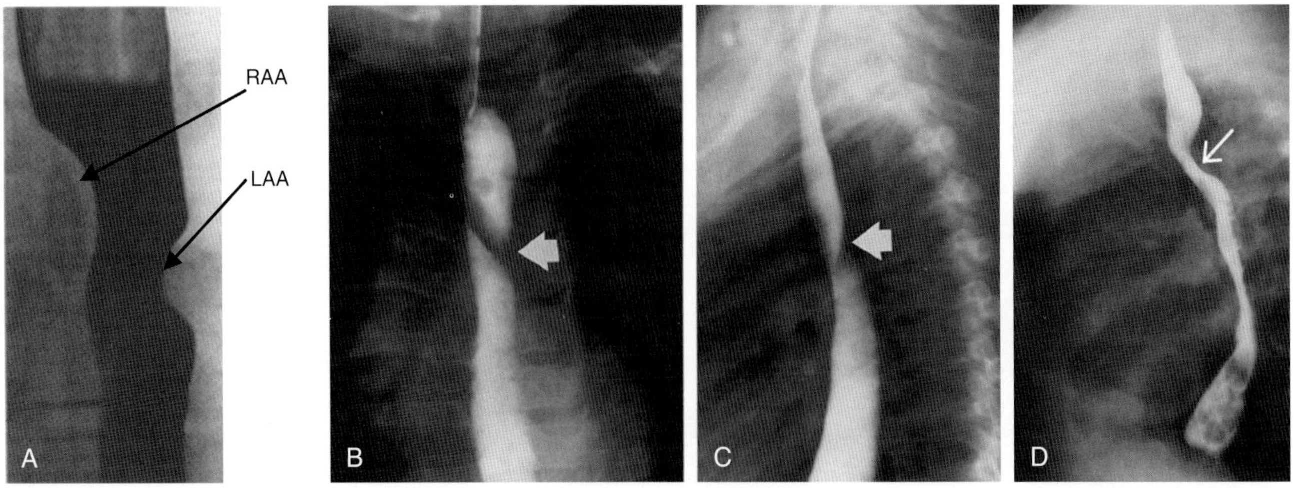

FIGURE 113-10 ■ Barium esophagograms demonstrating bilateral compression of the esophagus by a double aortic arch **(A)** and posterior compression of the esophagus by an aberrant right subclavian artery **(B, C)** and circumflex aorta **(D)**. *Arrow* in **B-D** demonstrates area of compression. *LAA,* Left aortic arch; *RAA,* right aortic arch.

symptoms, depending on the underlying lesion. Compression of the esophagus by an aberrant right subclavian artery can produce dysphagia, previously called *dysphagia lusoria* (or "dysphagia by freak of nature"). Patients with pulmonary artery sling can be in severe respiratory compromise, occasionally severe enough to require salvage by preoperative ECMO.[84] Coarctation of the aorta or hypoplasia of aortic segments can accompany arch abnormalities and manifest as a murmur, hypertension, or blood pressure gradient between extremities. On physical examination, the child may have stridulous breathing that must be differentiated from wheezing or asymmetric breath sounds from unilateral airway compression. Many patients are referred after being treated with bronchodilators for presumed asthma. A pulsatile mass in the neck suggests the presence of a cervical aorta.

Diagnosis

A diagnostic workup for vascular ring should be initiated in a child or adolescent with airway or esophageal symptoms if symptoms are not relieved by medical management. History of recurrent pneumonia, bronchoconstriction that is unresponsive to bronchodilators, and dysphagia to solid foods should raise suspicion and further workup. On chest radiography, the findings include tracheal narrowing at the level of the aortic arch and unclear delineation of the aortic knob. Unilateral hyperinflation of one lung field may suggest obstruction at the mainstem bronchial level.

CT and MRI are the primary modalities to establish the diagnosis and plan an operative procedure.[85,86] MRI with three-dimensional reconstruction is preferred in most centers to avoid exposure to ionizing radiation (Fig. 113-10).[87] Specific information that must be obtained includes the course and origin of arterial branches, arch dominance in patients with double aortic arch, location of the ligamentum arteriosum, and the degree of airway or esophageal compression. Airway compression might not be apparent in patients who are intubated and mechanically ventilated, and dynamic imaging during inspiration and expiration increases the sensitivity of detecting airway compromise. Echocardiography is helpful for delineating the arch anatomy in neonates and infants, but it cannot definitely make the diagnosis of a vascular ring unless there is a double aortic arch and both arches are patent.

Barium esophagography is a reliable initial study for workup of the patient with dysphagia. The most common appearance on esophagogram includes the presence of posterior extrinsic compression in the presence of a right aortic arch, anterior esophageal compression in the presence of a pulmonary artery sling, and extrinsic compression on anteroposterior views of the esophagus in the setting of double aortic arch (Fig. 113-11).

Bronchoscopy is helpful in the assessment of patients with vascular rings and suspected airway compression. Although routine bronchoscopy is not necessary in the setting of a complete vascular ring with clinical or imaging evidence of airway obstruction, it may be useful in situations where the diagnosis or significance of vascular anomaly is unclear. Anterior compression of the trachea by the innominate artery visualized at bronchoscopy may establish the diagnosis and severity of innominate artery compression when noninvasive imaging is equivocal, and thus guide clinical management. Under certain circumstances, bronchoscopy can reveal several separate causes of airway compromise in a patient with a vascular ring, thus altering surgical management. For example, bronchoscopy can detect the presence of associated complete tracheal rings or tracheomalacia. Immediate postprocedure intraoperative bronchoscopy allows the surgeon to assess the efficacy of the intervention. Adjunctive aortopexy or anterior tracheal suspension can be performed during the same operative procedure if persistent airway compromise is encountered.[88] Preoperative or intraoperative bronchoscopy alters management in approximately 3% to 5% of patients.[89]

Angiography is rarely indicated for patients with vascular rings, but it may be necessary if coexistent coarctation of the aorta is suggested. In patients with right or left aortic arch and contralateral ligamentum, the

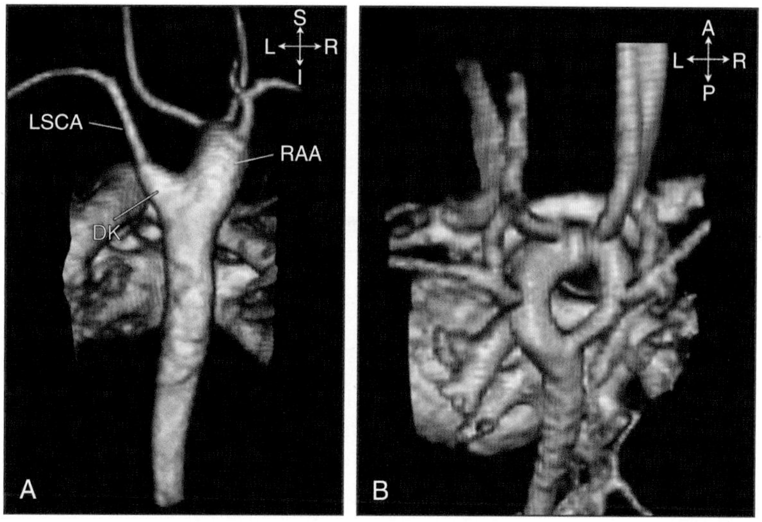

FIGURE 113-11 ■ Three-dimensional magnetic resonance imaging reconstructions demonstrating right aortic arch (RAA), aberrant left subclavian artery (LSCA) **(A)**, and double aortic arch **(B)**. *DK,* Diverticulum of Kommerell. (Compliments of Andrew Powell, MD, Children's Hospital Boston.)

presence of a ligamentum might not be demonstrated by noninvasive methods. In these cases, a rudimentary diverticulum at the insertion of the ligament into the aorta may be detected by angiography, suggesting the presence of the vascular ring.[90]

Treatment

Controversy exists regarding indications for repair of the vascular ring. The presence of airway or esophageal symptoms corresponding with anatomic narrowing on imaging should prompt surgical treatment. In the asymptomatic patient, surgical treatment should be considered in patients with evidence of significant narrowing (>50%) by imaging, whereas patients with negligible anatomic narrowing can be managed safely by observation with serial imaging. Patients with pulmonary artery sling are likely to develop tracheal narrowing with time, and early operative intervention is recommended.

The options for surgical approach to a vascular ring include sternotomy, thoracotomy, or VATS. The optimal approach depends on the morphology of the arch anomaly and associated abnormalities (coarctation or complete tracheal rings) that require intervention. Regardless of the etiology of the vascular ring or the surgical approach, an important component of ring division is lysis of residual fibrotic tissue overlying the adventitia of the esophagus and trachea.

Double Aortic Arch

More than 85% of patients with double aortic arch display right dominance with atresia or hypoplasia of the left arch. Even when balanced arches or left dominance are present, division of the LAA is possible without development of significant obstruction to flow through the remaining right-sided arch. Measurement of upper and lower extremity blood pressures during test occlusion of the left arch can be used to predict adequacy of the right arch. If the right-sided arch is significantly hypoplastic or atretic, then division of the right aortic arch becomes necessary. Regardless of which arch requires division, surgery for double aortic arch can be performed through the left pleural space, using thoracotomy or VATS. The open approach is generally required for division of the right arch and may be preferable for division of a patent left arch. A ligamentum arteriosum or PDA is divided before further dissection. If this is not performed and only the left arch is divided, a vascular ring will persist. When atresia of the nondominant arch is present, division must be performed at the atretic segment to preserve blood flow to the branch vessels. Once the vascular ring has been divided, fibrous attachments tethering the trachea and the esophagus must be divided longitudinally to ensure relief of anatomic obstruction (Fig. 113-12).

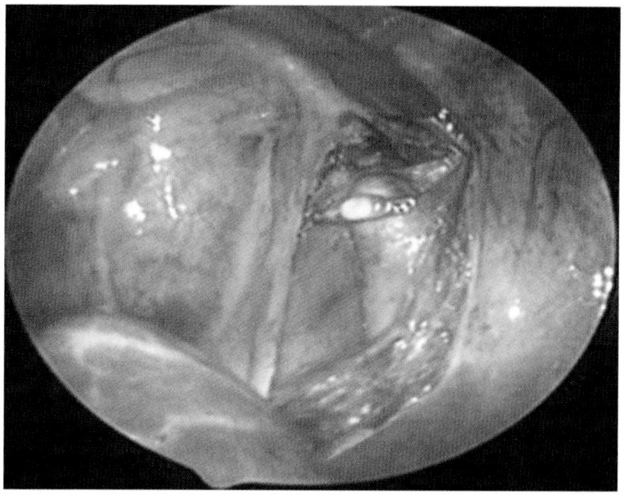

FIGURE 113-12 ■ Division of left ligamentum arteriosum in a patient with right aortic arch. Tethering attachments across the underlying esophagus must be divided to provide complete relief of obstruction in patients with double aortic arch or right aortic arch with left ligamentum.

Right Aortic Arch with Left Ligamentum Arteriosum

Division of the ligamentum arteriosum and underlying fibrous bands along the esophagus relieves tracheal and esophageal compression (see Figure 113-12). Occasionally, the left ligamentum (and aberrant LSCA, if present) will arise from a diverticulum of Kommerell. Management of this diverticulum is controversial. Diverticular resection and repeated anastomosis of the aberrant LSCA to the left carotid artery avoids the risk of further dilation of the diverticulum and recurrent tracheoesophageal compression.[91] Other options for management include plication and posterior diverticulopexy to the prevertebral fascia.

Circumflex Retroesophageal Aorta

The boundaries of the complete ring include the circumflex aorta, the pulmonary artery, and the ligamentum arteriosum or ductus arteriosus contralateral to the aortic arch, and division of the ring is simply performed by dividing the ligamentum. If the aberrant subclavian artery arises from a diverticulum, resection of the diverticulum and reimplantation of the subclavian artery is recommended. This is performed through a thoracotomy ipsilateral to the ligamentum. In some patients with circumflex aorta, simple division of the ligamentum and reimplantation of aberrant subclavian artery might not be sufficient to relieve the posterior esophageal compression. In these patients, aortic division and "uncrossing" by mobilization and rerouting of the descending aorta ipsilateral to the descending aorta relieves esophageal compression. Extra-anatomic reconstruction with division of the transverse aorta and ascending to descending prosthetic graft is another option.[92] Coarctation and hypoplasia of the circumflex aorta (particularly right circumflex aorta) can occur, and they are treated with resection with reanastomosis or interposition graft.[93,94]

Left Aortic Arch and Aberrant Right Subclavian Artery

Patients with a diagnosis of LAA and aberrant RSCA rarely experience airway compromise, and alternative causes of airway symptoms should be sought. In the rare patient with a right ligamentum, a complete vascular ring is formed, and division of the ligamentum provides relief of airway compression. For symptomatic esophageal compression, surgical treatment involves division of the subclavian artery at its origin from the aorta. This can be performed through a sternotomy or left thoracotomy approach. Reimplantation of the RSCA into the ascending aorta avoids the small risk of chronic upper extremity ischemia, but is controversial. If aneurysmal dilation of the aorta or proximal subclavian artery is encountered, one must be prepared to institute left heart or cardiopulmonary bypass and possibly hypothermic circulatory arrest during repair. Endovascular options for treatment have emerged, but the long-term results of this approach are still lacking.[95]

Pulmonary Artery Sling

The repair of this anomaly is typically performed via median sternotomy, and consists of division of the LPA from the RPA and reimplantation into the main pulmonary artery anterior to the trachea. Alternatively, the trachea can be divided and brought posterior to the pulmonary artery. The latter approach is useful if tracheal resection or reconstruction is necessary because of the presence of complete tracheal rings and tracheal stenosis. The decision to perform concomitant airway reconstruction depends on the degree of intrinsic airway abnormality, and it can be aided by performance of intraoperative bronchoscopy following release of the pulmonary artery sling. If concomitant airway surgery is required, the reconstruction with sliding tracheoplasty is the preferred procedure.[96] Cardiopulmonary bypass is essential if airway reconstruction is required. For LPA reimplantation alone, bypass is not essential but minimizes the hemodynamic burden on the right ventricle and allows unencumbered performance of the anastomosis. Immediate postoperative complications following repair of a pulmonary artery sling include persistent respiratory difficulties secondary to an abnormal airway, and long-term complications are seen in patients who require tracheal reconstruction during infancy.[97] Late stenosis of the LPA anastomosis occurs infrequently and is effectively treated with percutaneous balloon dilation.

Innominate Artery Compression

Children with suspected innominate artery compression syndrome should undergo thorough imaging and preoperative bronchoscopy to confirm anterior airway compression attributable to the innominate artery before proceeding with repair. Direct compression of the airway by the innominate artery or the aorta can be treated with thymectomy and innominate artery suspension through the right or left transpleural approach. Thymectomy is helpful when preoperative studies indicate the presence of a large thymus, which can exacerbate the posterior displacement of the innominate artery onto the anterior trachea. Innominate artery suspension can be performed through a right- or a left-sided approach, or through a partial sternotomy. The pericardial reflection at the base of the innominate artery is suspended to the posterior aspect of the sternum, thus lifting the innominate artery anteriorly. Improvements in symptoms and pulmonary function have been demonstrated following repair.[98,99]

Prognosis

Low hospital mortality is expected following division of vascular ring. The proportion of patients experiencing improvement in respiratory symptoms following surgery ranges widely from 50% to 90%.[100-102] Recurrence of symptoms may be attributed to the presence of an enlarging Kommerell diverticulum, circumflex aorta, or underlying tracheobronchial malacia.[103] Management with resection of the diverticulum and primary reanastomosis of the LSCA into the left carotid artery, aortic "uncrossing" for circumflex aorta, or aortopexy and tracheopexy for trachea-broncho-malacia.[103,104] Bronchoscopy at the time of vascular ring division or reoperation for residual compression provides feedback during surgical manipulation. The long-term results of vascular ring division are generally dependent on the degree of intrinsic airway

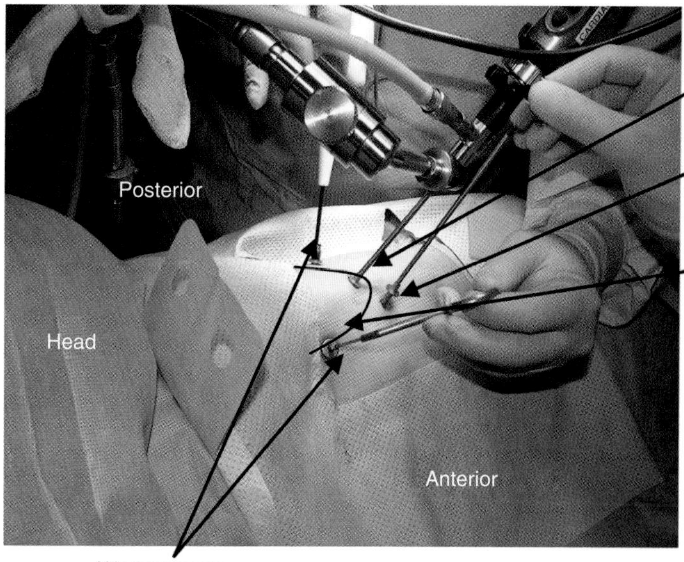

FIGURE 113-13 ■ Placement of ports in relationship to scapula during left video-assisted thoracoscopic surgery with the patient in the right decubitus position.

abnormality, such as tracheomalacia or complete tracheal rings. In one long-term analysis, follow-up surveys revealed that approximately half of the patients with preoperative breathing difficulties were symptom free at long-term follow-up, and the remaining patients described improvement in symptoms compared with preoperative status.[105] Younger age at operation and underlying genetic syndromes are risk factors for persistent symptoms. After repair of pulmonary artery sling, significant improvements in pulmonary function tests have been noted.[106]

Complications

The most common cause of in-hospital morbidity relates to underlying airway abnormalities, and adequate pulmonary toilet must be maintained in the postoperative period. Patients undergoing pulmonary artery sling repair are at the highest risk for persistent airway instability and pulmonary insufficiency. Surgical complications related to the mediastinal dissection include recurrent laryngeal nerve injury, pneumothorax, chylothorax, and esophageal leak. Chylothorax is best managed by early reoperation for ligation of the injured lymphatic vessel, although percutaneous embolization of the thoracic duct is an effective alternative.[107]

Surgical Approaches

The muscle-sparing thoracotomy, VATS, and sternotomy are the most commonly used approaches for repair of PDA, coarctation, and vascular rings. Sternotomy is the approach used if cardiopulmonary bypass is necessary (hypoplastic arch in addition to coarctation, calcified PDA in an adult). Sternotomy can provide security of cardiopulmonary bypass in case of unexpected vascular injury in a patient with unusual anatomy (PDA associated with ductal aneurysm). Although selective single-lung ventilation by means of a double-lumen endotracheal tube provides superior visualization in adults, a single-lumen endotracheal tube is sufficient to perform procedures in most patients. For left-sided aortic arch, a left chest approach is preferred. The patient is placed in a right lateral decubitus position with a roll under the axilla to avoid nerve compression injury. A blood pressure cuff on the lower extremity allows intraoperative measurement of upper-lower extremity gradient, which is a crude but useful estimate of residual aortic obstruction. In the operating room, a pulse oximeter or blood pressure cuff should be placed on a lower extremity to confirm lower body perfusion after surgical manipulation of the descending aorta. Early identification and treatment of obstruction prevents subsequent morbidity and delay in treatment.

Thoracotomy

A posterolateral thoracotomy is performed by making an infrascapular incision parallel to the course of the underlying ribs. The latissimus muscle is divided, but the serratus anterior muscle is spared. For repair of coarctation or vascular ring, the fourth intercostal space is entered, and for PDA ligation the third interspace provides direct exposure. The pleura is opened for vascular ring and coarctation surgery, whereas an extrapleural or transpleural approach can be used for PDA ligation. With either approach, the pleura overlying the aorta is mobilized, and the recurrent laryngeal is identified and dissected away from the aorta. Complications related to the thoracotomy and dissection include recurrent laryngeal nerve injury, chylothorax, pneumothorax, and surgical site infections. Musculoskeletal deformities late after thoracotomy in children have become less frequent with the adoption of muscle-sparing techniques.[108]

Video-Assisted Thoracoscopic Surgery

There are several different methods of VATS for division of vascular rings or patent ductus arteriosus. Our approach is to make four 3 mm incisions as shown in Figure 113-13. Exposure of the aorta is provided by an expandable lung retractor, and thoracoscopic instruments are used to perform the dissection, ligation, and division of atretic ligaments. Thoracoscopic division of a patent double aortic arch must be performed with a plan for vascular control (tourniquet, direct pressure, thoracotomy) should uncontrollable bleeding be encountered. Thoracoscopic division of vascular rings and PDA has not been shown to decrease operative times, postoperative pain, or hospital length of stay compared with the thoracotomy approach.[109]

REFERENCES

1. Koch J, Hensley G, Roy L, et al: Prevalence of spontaneous closure of the ductus arteriosus in neonates at a birth weight of 1000 grams or less. *Pediatrics* 117:1113–1121, 2006.
2. Egbe A, Uppu S, Lee S, et al: Temporal variation of birth prevalence of congenital heart disease in the United States. *Congenit Heart Dis* 10:43–50, 2015.
3. Huang J, Cheng L, Li J, et al: Myocardin regulates expression of contractile genes in smooth muscle cells and is required for closure of the ductus arteriosus in mice. *J Clin Invest* 118:515–525, 2008.
4. Yokoyama U, Minamisawa S, Quan H, et al: Chronic activation of the prostaglandin receptor EP4 promotes hyaluronan-mediated neointimal formation in the ductus arteriosus. *J Clin Invest* 116:3026–3034, 2006.
5. Zhu L, Bonnet D, Boussion M, et al: Investigation of the MYH11 gene in sporadic patients with an isolated persistently patent arterial duct. *Cardiol Young* 17:666–672, 2007.
6. Coceani F, Ackerley C, Seidlitz E, et al: Function of cyclo-oxygenase-1 and cyclo-oxygenase-2 in the ductus arteriosus from foetal lamb: differential development and change by oxygen and endotoxin. *Br J Pharmacol* 132:241–251, 2001.
7. Reller MD, Ziegler ML, Rice MJ, et al: Duration of ductal shunting in healthy preterm infants: an echocardiographic color flow Doppler study. *J Pediatr* 112:441–446, 1988.
8. Schmidt B, Davis P, Moddemann D, et al: Long-term effects of indomethacin prophylaxis in extremely-low-birth-weight infants. *N Engl J Med* 344:1966–1972, 2001.
9. Kluckow M, Evans N: Ductal shunting, high pulmonary blood flow, and pulmonary hemorrhage. *J Pediatr* 137:68–72, 2000.
10. Rojas MA, Gonzalez A, Bancalari E, et al: Changing trends in the epidemiology and pathogenesis of neonatal chronic lung disease. *J Pediatr* 126:605–610, 1995.
11. Brown ER: Increased risk of bronchopulmonary dysplasia in infants with patent ductus arteriosus. *J Pediatr* 95:865–866, 1979.
12. Hammerman C: Patent ductus arteriosus. Clinical relevance of prostaglandins and prostaglandin inhibitors in PDA pathophysiology and treatment. *Clin Perinatol* 22:457–479, 1995.
13. Martin CG, Snider AR, Katz SM, et al: Abnormal cerebral blood flow patterns in preterm infants with a large patent ductus arteriosus. *J Pediatr* 101:587–593, 1982.
14. Nestrud RM, Hill DE, Arrington RW, et al: Indomethacin treatment in patent ductus arteriosus. A double-blind study utilizing indomethacin plasma levels. *Dev Pharmacol Ther* 1:125–136, 1980.
15. Shimada S, Kasai T, Konishi M, et al: Effects of patent ductus arteriosus on left ventricular output and organ blood flows in preterm infants with respiratory distress syndrome treated with surfactant. *J Pediatr* 125:270–277, 1994.
16. Weir FJ, Ohlsson A, Myhr TL, et al: A patent ductus arteriosus is associated with reduced middle cerebral artery blood flow velocity. *Eur J Pediatr* 158:484–487, 1999.
17. Dudell GG, Gersony WM: Patent ductus arteriosus in neonates with severe respiratory disease. *J Pediatr* 104:915–920, 1984.
18. Osborn DA, Evans N, Kluckow M: Effect of early targeted indomethacin on the ductus arteriosus and blood flow to the upper body and brain in the preterm infant. *Arch Dis Child Fetal Neonatal Ed* 88:F477–F482, 2003.
19. Campbell M: Natural history of persistent ductus arteriosus. *Br Heart J* 30:4–13, 1968.
20. Fajardo MF, Claure N, Swaminathan S, et al: Effect of positive end-expiratory pressure on ductal shunting and systemic blood flow in preterm infants with patent ductus arteriosus. *Neonatology* 105:9–13, 2014.
21. Clyman RI: Recommendations for the postnatal use of indomethacin: an analysis of four separate treatment strategies. *J Pediatr* 128:601–607, 1996.
22. Sangem M, Asthana S, Amin S: Multiple courses of indomethacin and neonatal outcomes in premature infants. *Pediatr Cardiol* 2007.
23. Van Overmeire B, Smets K, Lecoutere D, et al: A comparison of ibuprofen and indomethacin for closure of patent ductus arteriosus. *N Engl J Med* 343:674–681, 2000.
24. Little DC, Pratt TC, Blalock SE, et al: Patent ductus arteriosus in micropreemies and full-term infants: the relative merits of surgical ligation versus indomethacin treatment. *J Pediatr Surg* 38:492–496, 2003.
25. Oncel MY, Yurttutan S, Erdeve O, et al: Oral paracetamol versus oral ibuprofen in the management of patent ductus arteriosus in preterm infants: a randomized controlled trial. *J Pediatr* 164:510–514.e1, 2014.
26. Grosfeld JL, Chaet M, Molinari F, et al: Increased risk of necrotizing enterocolitis in premature infants with patent ductus arteriosus treated with indomethacin. *Ann Surg* 224:350–355, discussion 355–357, 1996.
27. Cassady G, Crouse DT, Kirklin JW, et al: A randomized, controlled trial of very early prophylactic ligation of the ductus arteriosus in babies who weighed 1000 g or less at birth. *N Engl J Med* 320:1511–1516, 1989.
28. Fujii AM, Brown E, Mirochnick M, et al: Neonatal necrotizing enterocolitis with intestinal perforation in extremely premature infants receiving early indomethacin treatment for patent ductus arteriosus. *J Perinatol* 22:535–540, 2002.
29. Palder SB, Schwartz MZ, Tyson KR, et al: Management of patent ductus arteriosus: a comparison of operative v pharmacologic treatment. *J Pediatr Surg* 22:1171–1174, 1987.
30. Jaillard S, Larrue B, Rakza T, et al: Consequences of delayed surgical closure of patent ductus arteriosus in very premature infants. *Ann Thorac Surg* 81:231–234, 2006.
31. Wardle AJ, Osman A, Tulloh R, et al: Patent ductus arteriosus: an analysis of management. *Cardiol Young* 24:941–943, 2014.
32. Tefera E, Teodori M: Pulmonary artery aneurysm with patent arterial duct: resection of aneurysm and ductal division. *World J Pediatr Congenit Heart Surg* 4:427–429, 2013.
33. Giroud JM, Jacobs JP: Evolution of strategies for management of the patent arterial duct. *Cardiol Young* 17(Suppl 2):68–74, 2007.
34. Liem NT, Tung CV, Van Linh N, et al: Outcomes of thoracoscopic clipping versus transcatheter occlusion of patent ductus arteriosus: randomized clinical trial. *J Pediatr Surg* 49:363–366, 2014.
35. El-Said HG, Bratincsak A, Foerster SR, et al: Safety of percutaneous patent ductus arteriosus closure: an unselected multicenter population experience. *J Am Heart Assoc* 2:e000424, 2013.
36. Mavroudis C, Backer CL, Gevitz M: Forty-six years of patient ductus arteriosus division at Children's Memorial Hospital of Chicago. Standards for comparison. *Ann Surg* 220:402–409, discussion 409–410, 1994.
37. Zbar RI, Chen AH, Behrendt DM, et al: Incidence of vocal fold paralysis in infants undergoing ligation of patent ductus arteriosus. *Ann Thorac Surg* 61:814–816, 1996.
38. Ismat FA, Weinberg PM, Rychik J, et al: Right aortic arch and coarctation: a rare association. *Congenit Heart Dis* 1:217–223, 2006.
39. McBride KL, Riley MF, Zender GA, et al: NOTCH1 mutations in individuals with left ventricular outflow tract malformations reduce ligand-induced signaling. *Hum Mol Genet* 17:2886–2893, 2008.
40. Liberman L, Gersony WM, Flynn PA, et al: Effectiveness of prostaglandin E1 in relieving obstruction in coarctation of the aorta without opening the ductus arteriosus. *Pediatr Cardiol* 25:49–52, 2004.
41. Maron BJ, Humphries JO, Rowe RD, et al: Prognosis of surgically corrected coarctation of the aorta. A 20-year postoperative appraisal. *Circulation* 47:119–126, 1973.
42. Mery CM, Khan MS, Guzman-Pruneda FA, et al: Contemporary results of surgical repair of recurrent aortic arch obstruction. *Ann Thorac Surg* 98:133–140, 2014.

43. Brown ML, Burkhart HM, Connolly HM, et al: Late outcomes of reintervention on the descending aorta after repair of aortic coarctation. *Circulation* 122:S81–S84, 2010.
44. Levy Praschker BG, Mordant P, Barreda E, et al: Long-term results of ascending aorta-abdominal aorta extra-anatomic bypass for recoarctation in adults with 27-year follow-up. *Eur J Cardiothorac Surg* 2008.
45. Alsoufi B, Cai S, Coles JG, et al: Outcomes of different surgical strategies in the treatment of neonates with aortic coarctation and associated ventricular septal defects. *Ann Thorac Surg* 84:1331–1336, discussion 1336–1337, 2007.
46. Walters HL, 3rd, Ionan CE, Thomas RL, et al: Single-stage versus 2-stage repair of coarctation of the aorta with ventricular septal defect. *J Thorac Cardiovasc Surg* 135:754–761, 2008.
47. Siblini G, Rao PS, Nouri S, et al: Long-term follow-up results of balloon angioplasty of postoperative aortic recoarctation. *Am J Cardiol* 81:61–67, 1998.
48. Wong D, Benson LN, Van Arsdell GS, et al: Balloon angioplasty is preferred to surgery for aortic coarctation. *Cardiol Young* 18:79–88, 2008.
49. Hernandez-Gonzalez M, Solorio S, Conde-Carmona I, et al: Intraluminal aortoplasty vs. surgical aortic resection in congenital aortic coarctation. A clinical random study in pediatric patients. *Arch Med Res* 34:305–310, 2003.
50. Shaddy RE, Boucek MM, Sturtevant JE, et al: Comparison of angioplasty and surgery for unoperated coarctation of the aorta. *Circulation* 87:793–799, 1993.
51. Ringel RE, Vincent J, Jenkins KJ, et al: Acute outcome of stent therapy for coarctation of the aorta: results of the coarctation of the aorta stent trial. *Catheter Cardiovasc Interv* 82:503–510, 2013.
52. Butera G, Manica JL, Marini D, et al: From bare to covered: 15-year single center experience and follow-up in trans-catheter stent implantation for aortic coarctation. *Catheter Cardiovasc Interv* 83:953–963, 2014.
53. Sohrabi B, Jamshidi P, Yaghoubi A, et al: Comparison between covered and bare Cheatham-Platinum stents for endovascular treatment of patients with native post-ductal aortic coarctation: immediate and intermediate-term results. *JACC* 7:416–423, 2014.
54. Forbes TJ, Garekar S, Amin Z, et al: Procedural results and acute complications in stenting native and recurrent coarctation of the aorta in patients over 4 years of age: a multi-institutional study. *Catheter Cardiovasc Interv* 70:276–285, 2007.
55. Lee CL, Lin JF, Hsieh KS, et al: Balloon angioplasty of native coarctation and comparison of patients younger and older than 3 months. *Circ J* 71:1781–1784, 2007.
56. Rodes-Cabau J, Miro J, Dancea A, et al: Comparison of surgical and transcatheter treatment for native coarctation of the aorta in patients > or = 1 year old. The Quebec Native Coarctation of the Aorta study. *Am Heart J* 154:186–192, 2007.
57. Tabbutt S, Nicolson SC, Adamson PC, et al: The safety, efficacy, and pharmacokinetics of esmolol for blood pressure control immediately after repair of coarctation of the aorta in infants and children: a multicenter, double-blind, randomized trial. *J Thorac Cardiovasc Surg* 136:321–328, 2008.
58. Gidding SS, Rocchini AP, Beekman R, et al: Therapeutic effect of propranolol on paradoxical hypertension after repair of coarctation of the aorta. *N Engl J Med* 312:1224–1228, 1985.
59. Seirafi PA, Warner KG, Geggel RL, et al: Repair of coarctation of the aorta during infancy minimizes the risk of late hypertension. *Ann Thorac Surg* 66:1378–1382, 1998.
60. Brouwer RM, Erasmus ME, Ebels T: Influence of age on survival, late hypertension, and recoarctation in elective aortic coarctation repair. Including long-term results after elective aortic coarctation repair with a follow-up from 25 to 44 years. *J Thorac Cardiovasc Surg* 108:525–531, 1994.
61. Duara R, Theodore S, Sarma PS, et al: Correction of coarctation of aorta in adult patients–impact of corrective procedure on long-term recoarctation and systolic hypertension. *Thorac Cardiovasc Surg* 56:83–86, 2008.
62. Barreiro CJ, Ellison TA, Williams JA, et al: Subclavian flap aortoplasty: still a safe, reproducible, and effective treatment for infant coarctation. *Eur J Cardiothorac Surg* 31:649–653, 2007.
63. Pandey R, Jackson M, Ajab S, et al: Subclavian flap repair: review of 399 patients at median follow-up of fourteen years. *Ann Thorac Surg* 81:1420–1428, 2006.
64. Conte S, Lacour-Gayet F, Serraf A, et al: Surgical management of neonatal coarctation. *J Thorac Cardiovasc Surg* 109:663–674, discussion 674-665, 1995.
65. Brown ML, Burkhart HM, Connolly HM, et al: Coarctation of the aorta: lifelong surveillance is mandatory following surgical repair. *J Am Coll Cardiol* 62:1020–1025, 2013.
66. Sudarshan CD, Cochrane AD, Jun ZH, et al: Repair of coarctation of the aorta in infants weighing less than 2 kilograms. *Ann Thorac Surg* 82:158–163, 2006.
67. McElhinney DB, Yang SG, Hogarty AN, et al: Recurrent arch obstruction after repair of isolated coarctation of the aorta in neonates and young infants: is low weight a risk factor? *J Thorac Cardiovasc Surg* 122:883–890, 2001.
68. Whiteside W, Hirsch-Romano J, Yu S, et al: Outcomes associated with balloon angioplasty for recurrent coarctation in neonatal univentricular and biventricular norwood-type aortic arch reconstructions. *Catheter Cardiovasc Interv* 83:1124–1130, 2014.
69. Fiore AC, Fischer LK, Schwartz T, et al: Comparison of angioplasty and surgery for neonatal aortic coarctation. *Ann Thorac Surg* 80:1659–1664, discussion 1664–1655, 2005.
70. Corno AF, Botta U, Hurni M, et al: Surgery for aortic coarctation: a 30 years experience. *Eur J Cardiothorac Surg* 20:1202–1206, 2001.
71. Vouhe PR, Trinquet F, Lecompte Y, et al: Aortic coarctation with hypoplastic aortic arch. Results of extended end-to-end aortic arch anastomosis. *J Thorac Cardiovasc Surg* 96:557–563, 1988.
72. Dodge-Khatami A, Backer CL, Mavroudis C: Risk factors for recoarctation and results of reoperation: a 40-year review. *J Card Surg* 15:369–377, 2000.
73. Aebert H, Laas J, Bednarski P, et al: High incidence of aneurysm formation following patch plasty repair of coarctation. *Eur J Cardiothorac Surg* 7:200–204, discussion 205, 1993.
74. Walhout RJ, Lekkerkerker JC, Oron GH, et al: Comparison of polytetrafluoroethylene patch aortoplasty and end-to-end anastomosis for coarctation of the aorta. *J Thorac Cardiovasc Surg* 126:521–528, 2003.
75. Said SM, Burkhart HM, Dearani JA, et al: Ascending-to-descending aortic bypass: a simple solution to a complex problem. *Ann Thorac Surg* 97:2041–2047, 2014.
76. Walhout RJ, Lekkerkerker JC, Oron GH, et al: Comparison of surgical repair with balloon angioplasty for native coarctation in patients from 3 months to 16 years of age. *Eur J Cardiothorac Surg* 25:722–727, 2004.
77. Karl TR: Surgery is the best treatment for primary coarctation in the majority of cases. *J Cardiovasc Med (Hagerstown)* 8:50–56, 2007.
78. Backer CL, Mavroudis C: Congenital heart surgery nomenclature and database project: vascular rings, tracheal stenosis, pectus excavatum. *Ann Thorac Surg* 69:S308–S318, 2000.
79. Kouchoukos NT, Masetti P: Aberrant subclavian artery and Kommerell aneurysm: surgical treatment with a standard approach. *J Thorac Cardiovasc Surg* 133:888–892, 2007.
80. McLeary MS, Frye LL, Young LW: Magnetic resonance imaging of a left circumflex aortic arch and aberrant right subclavian artery: the other vascular ring. *Pediatr Radiol* 28:263–265, 1998.
81. Miller RG, Robie DK, Davis SL, et al: Survival after aberrant right subclavian artery-esophageal fistula: case report and literature review. *J Vasc Surg* 24:271–275, 1996.
82. Chen FL, Vick GW, Ge S: Left cervical aortic arch with right ligamentum arteriosum forming a vascular ring. *Tex Heart Inst J* 35:78–79, 2008.
83. Fiore AC, Brown JW, Weber TR, et al: Surgical treatment of pulmonary artery sling and tracheal stenosis. *Ann Thorac Surg* 79:38–46, discussion 38-46, 2005.
84. Huang SC, Wu ET, Chi NH, et al: Perioperative extracorporeal membrane oxygenation support for critical pediatric airway surgery. *Eur J Pediatr* 166:1129–1133, 2007.
85. Chen X, Qu Y, Peng ZY, et al: Clinical value of multi-slice spiral computed tomography angiography and three-dimensional reconstruction in the diagnosis of double aortic arch. *Exp Ther Med* 8:623–627, 2014.
86. Cantinotti M, Hegde S, Bell A, et al: Diagnostic role of magnetic resonance imaging in identifying aortic arch anomalies. *Congenit Heart Dis* 3:117–123, 2008.

87. Hellinger JC, Daubert M, Lee EY, et al: Congenital thoracic vascular anomalies: evaluation with state-of-the-art MR imaging and MDCT. *Radiol Clin North Am* 49:969–996, 2011.
88. Mitchell ME, Rumman N, Chun RH, et al: Anterior tracheal suspension for tracheobronchomalacia in infants and children. *Ann Thorac Surg* 98:1246–1253, 2014.
89. Backer CL, Mavroudis C, Rigsby CK, et al: Trends in vascular ring surgery. *J Thorac Cardiovasc Surg* 129:1339–1347, 2005.
90. Singh GK, Greenberg SB, Balsara RK: Diagnostic dilemma: left aortic arch with right descending aorta–a rare vascular ring. *Pediatr Cardiol* 18:45–48, 1997.
91. Backer CL, Russell HM, Wurlitzer KC, et al: Primary resection of Kommerell diverticulum and left subclavian artery transfer. *Ann Thorac Surg* 94:1612–1617, 2012.
92. Grillo HC, Wright CD: Tracheal compression with "hairpin" right aortic arch: management by aortic division and aortopexy by right thoracotomy guided by intraoperative bronchoscopy. *Ann Thorac Surg* 83:1152–1157, 2007.
93. Hilmes M, Hernandez R, Devaney E: Markedly hypoplastic circumflex retroesophageal right aortic arch: MR imaging and surgical implications. *Pediatr Radiol* 37:63–67, 2007.
94. Ahluwalia GS, Rashid AG, Griselli M, et al: Hypoplastic circumflex retroesophageal right-sided cervical aortic arch with unusual vascular arrangement and severe coarctation. *Ann Thorac Surg* 84:1014–1016, 2007.
95. Shennib H, Diethrich EB: Novel approaches for the treatment of the aberrant right subclavian artery and its aneurysms. *J Vasc Surg* 47:1066–1070, 2008.
96. Beierlein W, Elliott MJ: Variations in the technique of slide tracheoplasty to repair complex forms of long-segment congenital tracheal stenoses. *Ann Thorac Surg* 82:1540–1542, 2006.
97. Backer CL, Mavroudis C, Dunham ME, et al: Pulmonary artery sling: results with median sternotomy, cardiopulmonary bypass, and reimplantation. *Ann Thorac Surg* 67:1738–1744, discussion 1744–1735, 1999.
98. Weber TR, Keller MS, Fiore A: Aortic suspension (aortopexy) for severe tracheomalacia in infants and children. *Am J Surg* 184:573–577, discussion 577, 2002.
99. Jones DT, Jonas RA, Healy GB: Innominate artery compression of the trachea in infants. *Ann Otol Rhinol Laryngol* 103:347–350, 1994.
100. Alsenaidi K, Gurofsky R, Karamlou T, et al: Management and outcomes of double aortic arch in 81 patients. *Pediatrics* 118:e1336–e1341, 2006.
101. Backer CL, Ilbawi MN, Idriss FS, et al: Vascular anomalies causing tracheoesophageal compression. Review of experience in children. *J Thorac Cardiovasc Surg* 97:725–731, 1989.
102. Ruzmetov M, Vijay P, Rodefeld MD, et al: Follow-up of surgical correction of aortic arch anomalies causing tracheoesophageal compression: a 38-year single institution experience. *J Pediatr Surg* 44:1328–1332, 2009.
103. Backer CL, Monge MC, Russell HM, et al: Reoperation after vascular ring repair. *Semin Thorac Cardiovasc Surg Pediatr Card Surg Annu* 17:48–55, 2014.
104. Backer CL, Hillman N, Mavroudis C, et al: Resection of Kommerell's diverticulum and left subclavian artery transfer for recurrent symptoms after vascular ring division. *Eur J Cardiothorac Surg* 22:64–69, 2002.
105. Humphrey C, Duncan K, Fletcher S: Decade of experience with vascular rings at a single institution. *Pediatrics* 117:e903–e908, 2006.
106. Yu JM, Liao CP, Ge S, et al: The prevalence and clinical impact of pulmonary artery sling on school-aged children: a large-scale screening study. *Pediatr Pulmonol* 43:656–661, 2008.
107. Pamarthi V, Stecker MS, Schenker MP, et al: Thoracic duct embolization and disruption for treatment of chylous effusions: experience with 105 patients. *J Vasc Interv Radiol* 25:1398–1404, 2014.
108. Bal S, Elshershari H, Celiker R, et al: Thoracic sequels after thoracotomies in children with congenital cardiac disease. *Cardiol Young* 13:264–267, 2003.
109. Kogon BE, Forbess JM, Wulkan ML, et al: Video-assisted thoracoscopic surgery: is it a superior technique for the division of vascular rings in children? *Congenit Heart Dis* 2:130–133, 2007.

CHAPTER 114

ATRIAL SEPTAL DEFECT AND COR TRIATRIATUM

David P. Bichell • Thomas P. Doyle

CHAPTER OUTLINE

HISTORICAL CONSIDERATIONS

Ingenious and risky surgical corrections of atrial septal defect (ASD) predated cardiopulmonary bypass. The earliest closed approaches included a technique in which a straight needle with suture, guided by palpation, was passed blindly through the defect and both atria, and the free walls of the left and right atria were drawn together to obstruct the defect.[1] Bailey and colleagues described the "atrio-septo-pexy" consisting of a digital invagination of the atrial appendage through the defect with external suture attachment of the atrial tissue to the perimeter of the defect (Fig. 114-1*A*).[2] Tyge Søndergaard devised a purse-string external suture closure of ASD by a near circumferential dissection around the defect in the plane of the interatrial groove and a plication of its edges (see Fig. 114-1*B*).[3]

Semiopen techniques used before cardiopulmonary bypass became common practice included the "atrial well" technique, where a right atriotomy was formed, controlled by partial atrial clamping. A 15-cm tall, open-ended rubber cone was then attached to the atriotomy to produce an open column of blood in continuity with the beating heart. Working through the atrial well by palpation, the defect was closed by direct suture or patch. Regional intermittent heparinization prevented blood clotting within the well (see Fig. 114-1*C*).[4]

Lewis and Taufic reported the first successful open-heart ASD closure under direct visualization, using surface cooling and circulatory arrest by inflow occlusion in 1953.[5]

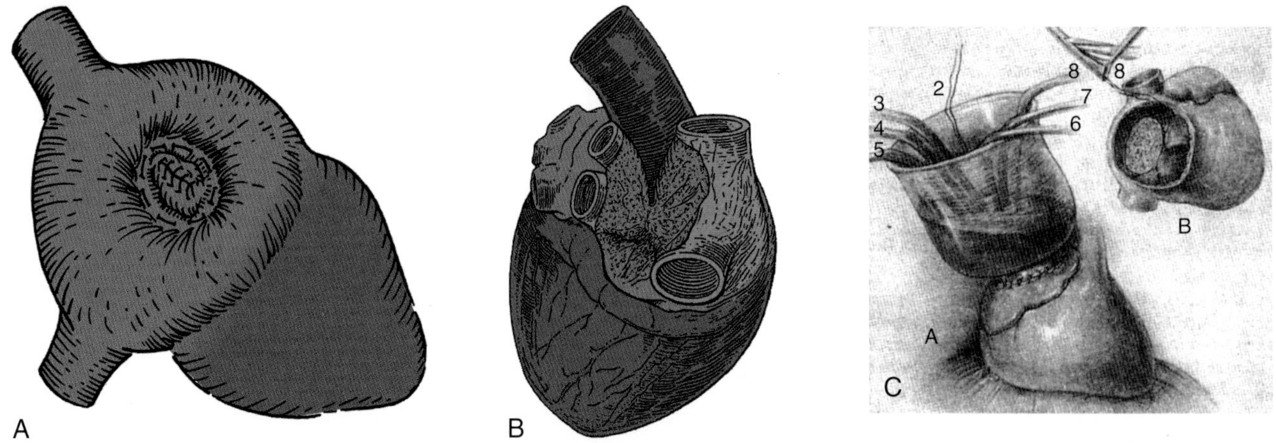

FIGURE 114-1 ■ Techniques for surgical atrial septal defect closure predating cardiopulmonary bypass. **A,** Atrio-septo-pexy. **B,** External purse-string suture closure. **C,** Atrial well technique. (**A,** From Bailey CP, Nichols HT, Bolton HE, et al: Surgical treatment of forty-six interatrial septal defects by atrio-septo-pexy. *Ann Surg* 140:805–820, 1954; **B,** from Søndergaard T: Closure of atrial septal defects; report of three cases. *Acta Chir Scand* 107:492–498, 1954; **C,** from Barratt-Boyes BG, Ellis FH Jr, Kirklin JW: Technique for repair of atrial septal defect using the atrial well. *Surg Gynecol Obstet* 103:646–649, 1956.)

Further modification of this technique to include continuous coronary perfusion improved the safety of this and other early intracardiac procedures and represented a precursor to modern myocardial protection techniques.[6]

The modern era of cardiac surgery was heralded by the introduction of the pump oxygenator in 1953, and the earliest application of this technology was for ASD closure.[7] Intracardiac repairs by inflow occlusion were not uniformly replaced by cardiopulmonary bypass techniques until 1960.

EMBRYOLOGY AND GENETICS

Formation of the Interatrial Septum

The embryonic common atrium undergoes partitioning by the formation of two parallel, overlapping septa, the septum primum and the septum secundum, starting in the fourth week of gestation.

The septum primum, emerging from the roof of the embryonic common atrium, begins the septation. The ostium primum, a gap between the septum primum and the atrial floor, almost closes by the completion of the septum primum. A de novo defect in the septum primum forms when a portion of its superior aspect resorbs, forming the ostium secundum.

The septum secundum, forming by the end of the sixth week of gestation, grows parallel to and immediately rightward of the septum primum, obliterating any remaining ostium primum, and circumscribing a central opening, the fossa ovalis.

In its final configuration, the atrial septum consists of the two layers, fused except for the overlapping, offset openings of the fossa ovalis and the ostium secundum. The free edge of the ostium secundum forms a flap valve covering the left side of the fossa ovalis, providing free right-to-left flow through the foramen ovale, until postnatal physiology closes the valve (Fig. 114-2). Conditions impairing the competence of the valve, or abnormalities in the formation of its components, lead to a persistent interatrial communication.

Simultaneous with atrial septal formation, pulmonary vein connections with the primitive left atrium are forming. During the fourth week of gestation, the common pulmonary vein orifice forms from posterior invaginations of the sinus venosus segment into the mesenchyme of the primitive lung buds. The sinus venosus segment of the posterior common atrium forms where right and left omphalomesenteric and cardinal veins drain into the left and right sinus horns. An abnormal persistence of the right-sided anlage of the common pulmonary vein might be the embryologic basis for the development of abnormal connections of pulmonary veins to the right atrium, or partial anomalous pulmonary venous connection (PAPVC).[8]

Genetics

A familial predisposition to ASD is well documented. A study that included more than 18,000 subjects with congenital heart disease from a Danish population determined a recurrence risk for isolated secundum ASD of approximately 7%, a finding similar to prior studies.[9-11]

Numerous genetic conditions and syndromes known for their extracardiac manifestations are also associated with ASD. Secundum ASD is the most common congenital cardiac defect associated with VACTERL (*v*ertebral anomalies, *a*nal atresia, *c*ardiac defects, *t*racheal anomalies, *e*sophageal atresia, *r*enal anomalies, and *l*imb anomalies). Genetic syndromes with associated ASD include Holt-Oram, Rubinstein-Taybi, Okihiro, and Townes-Brocks syndromes.[12] Trisomy 21 is associated with ASD either in isolation or as part of a constellation of endocardial cushion defects. Noonan syndrome is associated with ASD and pulmonary valve stenosis.[13] DiGeorge syndrome (22q11.4 deletion) and Ellis–Van Creveld syndromes are associated with primum ASD. Additional

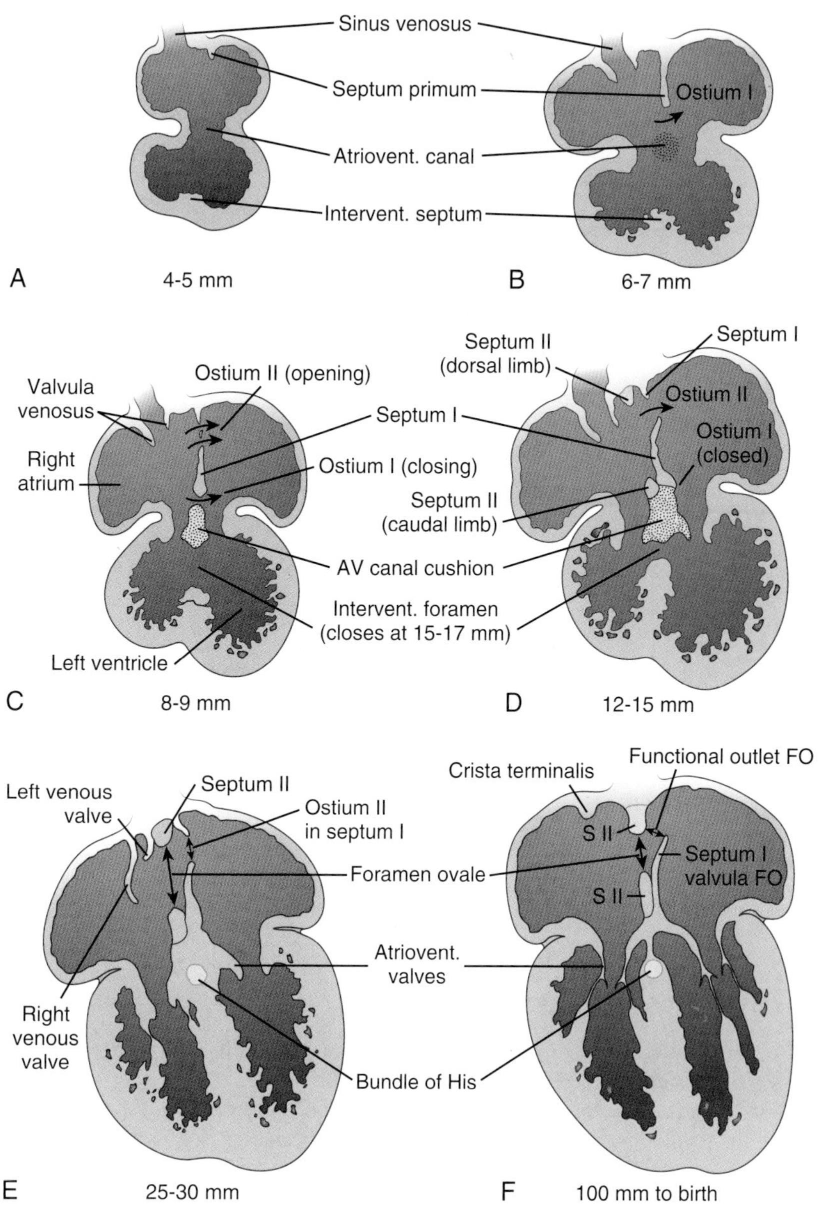

FIGURE 114-2 ■ Four-chamber sectional diagrams of the fetal heart with particular attention to the morphology of the forming interatrial septum and the foramen ovale. **A,** The early stages in the formation of the septum primum, from the superior aspect of the common atrium. **B,** As the septum primum grows toward the endocardial cushion, the ostium primum is defined. **C,** As the ostium primum closes, the ostium secundum forms by the resorption of the cephalad portions of the septum primum. **D,** The septum secundum begins to form rightward and parallel to the septum primum, obliterating the remaining ostium primum. **E** and **F,** The septum secundum circumscribes the foramen ovale, and the septum primum creates a flap valve permitting only right-to-left flow. *AV,* Atrioventricular; *FO,* foramen ovale. (Reproduced with permission from Patten BM: Developmental defects at the foramen ovale. *Am J Pathol* 14:135–161, 1938.)

specific genes implicated in familial forms of ASD include *GATA4*, *NKX2.5*,[14] alpha-cardiac actin 1 *(ACTC)*,[15] alpha-myosin heavy chain *(MYH6)*,[16] and *MSX1*.[17]

The conduction system forms concurrently with atrial septation and PR prolongation can accompany ASD, in likely association with abnormalities of the TBX5 transcription factor gene.[18]

Patent Foramen Ovale

The patent foramen ovale (PFO) denotes a failure of the septum primum and septum secundum to fuse. A failure of fusion results in either a valve-competent, "probe patent" PFO or valvular incompetence with or without an aneurysm of the septum primum component (Fig. 114-3*A*). Forces producing an enlarged foramen ovale or a deficient septum primum contribute to incompetence of the valve, a physiologically significant PFO, and transseptal shunting.

Secundum Atrial Septal Defect

The secundum defect lies within the bounds of the fossa ovalis, widely ranging in morphology from the slit-like PFO at the superior aspect of the fossa, to defects involving part or all of the remainder of the fossa, with a single or multiply fenestrated communication. Defects of various specific morphologies classified as secundum ASD can form as a result of underdevelopment of the septum secundum or a malformation of the septum primum resulting in incomplete coverage of the ostium secundum (see Fig. 114-3*B*).

Primum Atrial Septal Defect

The primum defect is a persistence of the ostium primum and is most commonly associated with an atrioventricular (AV) septal defect (see Fig. 114-3*C*). This lesion is discussed further in Chapter 116.

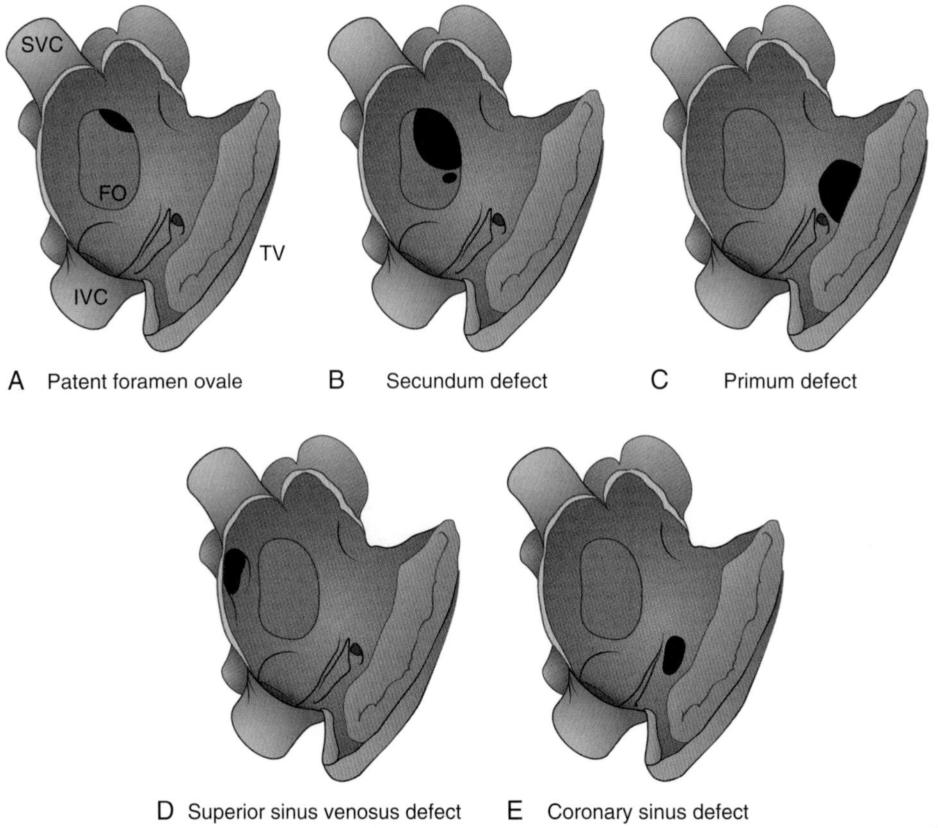

FIGURE 114-3 The morphologic classification of atrial septal defects. **A,** Patent foramen ovale. **B,** Secundum atrial septal defect. **C,** Primum atrial septal defect. **D,** Superior sinus venosus defect. **E,** Coronary sinus interatrial defect. *FO,* Foramen ovale; *IVC,* inferior vena cava; *SVC,* superior vena cava; *TV,* tricuspid valve.

Sinus Venosus Defect

The sinus venosus interatrial defect is associated with a PAPVC. Ninety percent of PAPVCs are right-sided, 7% left-sided, and 2% bilateral. The most common subtype is right upper pulmonary vein–to–superior vena cava (SVC) connection, accounting for 74% of PAPVC cases, in usual association with sinus venosus ASD.[19] The more common superior variant of sinus venosus defect is an interatrial communication lying posterior and superior to the true atrial septum, and the SVC overrides the defect. The right upper pulmonary veins, usually two or more, drain to the right atrium at the superior cavoatrial junction or enter the SVC directly (see Fig. 114-3*D*). In rare cases, they may enter the azygous vein as well. The SVC is commonly enlarged as it enters the right atrium.

The less common inferior sinus venosus defect is a communication inferior and posterior to the fossa ovalis with the right pulmonary veins entering the right atrium near the inferior cavoatrial junction. Although the sinus venosus ASD is remote from the fossa ovalis, a PFO or secundum ASD also may be present.

Atrial Septal Aneurysm

Redundant atrial septal tissue within the fossa ovalis with a respiratory excursion greater than 10 mm is termed an *atrial septal aneurysm* (ASA).[20] The ASA may occur with or without a PFO and has been implicated in the formation of paradoxic embolus. ASA is present in 2% to 4% of the normal population, and 70% of cases are associated with a PFO.[21]

Coronary Sinus–Type Atrial Septal Defect

The uncommon coronary sinus–type ASD results from a complete or partial unroofing of the coronary sinus along its course through the floor of the left atrium. A communication of the coronary sinus with the left atrium results in an interatrial communication at the level of the coronary sinus ostium, the size of which is determined by the extent of unroofing and the size of the ostium (see Fig. 114-3*E*). Concomitant cardiac lesions occurring with coronary sinus ASD include ASDs within the fossa ovalis, persistent left-sided SVC, and pulmonary or tricuspid atresia. The rarity of coronary sinus defects, their tendency to elude echo diagnosis, and the finding that many elude even intraoperative recognition, underscore the importance of maintaining suspicion for this lesion when the degree of intracardiac shunt observed is inordinate for the known defect elsewhere.

Iatrogenic and Traumatic Atrial Septal Defect

Iatrogenic ASDs are found after 87% of catheter-based transseptal pulmonary vein isolation procedures. Most are smaller than 1 mm in diameter and 96% resolve spontaneously, requiring no intervention.[22] Rare cases of traumatic ASD after blunt or penetrating trauma have been described.[23]

INCIDENCE AND NATURAL HISTORY

More than 60% of healthy full-term infants have a PFO identifiable on transthoracic echocardiogram.[24] With the postnatal fall in pulmonary resistance and rise in left ventricular end-diastolic pressure, the pressure in the left atrium exceeds that in the right atrium, and the flap valve consisting of septum primum closes the foramen ovale. Fibrous adhesions form in the first year of life to seal the interatrial communication in most cases. Spontaneous closure rates of PFO diagnosed in infancy are high—87% to 96% for those diagnosed in the first 12 months of life.[25] The overall incidence of persistent PFO in adulthood, deduced from autopsy specimens, is 27%. A PFO is present in one third of people younger than 29 years of age, one fourth of those 30 to 79 years, and one fifth of persons older than 80.[26]

Secundum ASD occurs in 1.6 out of 1000 live births, second in prevalence only to ventricular septal defect (VSD). ASD accounts for 10% to 15% of congenital heart defects in children[27] and 20% to 40% of defects discovered in adults. Women are affected twice as often as men.[28] Maternal exposures associated with ASD in offspring include alcohol, hydantoin, valproic acid, and amphetamines. Infections and additional conditions associated with ASD include cytomegalovirus or rubella infection during pregnancy, diabetes, older maternal age, multigestational birth, and obesity. Low-birth-weight and premature infants have a higher prevalence of ASD than does the general population.[29-31]

A significant number of ASDs close spontaneously within the first few years of life, but spontaneous closure after age 3 to 4 is rare.[32] The likelihood of spontaneous closure is best predicted by the initial diameter of the secundum defect. Longitudinal data demonstrate that more than half of defects diagnosed in infancy and measuring 4 to 5 mm close spontaneously. Thirty percent regress in size to smaller than 3 mm. However, none close spontaneously when the defect measures larger than 10 mm at diagnosis.[33] Defects larger than 8 mm at diagnosis usually enlarge over time. If there is aneurysmal formation, sizes diminish regardless of whether they are larger than 8 mm.[34]

In contrast to children with ASDs, most patients older than 40 years of age are symptomatic and have evidence of elevated pulmonary vascular resistance. If these patients are not treated, their average life expectancy is 40 to 50 years. Seventy-five percent die by age 50, and 90% die by 60 years of age.[35] Even the asymptomatic adult with ASD has a measurably diminished aerobic exercise capacity, which further declines with advancing age.[36] A 2008 European heart survey of 882 adults with isolated secundum ASD, including 505 unrepaired patients, demonstrated a precipitous rise in the prevalence of right ventricular dysfunction in unrepaired patients after 45 years of age. The degree of right ventricular volume overload was the best predictor of reduced exercise capacity. A steady rise in the prevalence of pulmonary hypertension was observed in unrepaired patients after age 30. Findings support the suggestion that the magnitude of the intracardiac shunt may increase over time. Hemodynamically small defects tend more to remain stable and may not require closure.[37]

Isolated ASD can predispose the patient to subacute bacterial endocarditis, although the actual incidence of endocarditis in this setting is rare. Scattered case reports describe atrial septal endocarditis in direct association with native ASD, ASD repaired by surgical or device closure, and by septal involvement of endocarditis that extends from other intracardiac structures. Risk of endocarditis from an unrepaired ASD is sufficiently low that antibiotic prophylaxis is not recommended, according to the latest American Heart Association guidelines. Incompletely repaired defects and those closed with prosthetic material or devices suspected of incomplete endothelialization are regarded as endocarditis risks, and do require antibiotic prophylaxis for dental or surgical procedures.[38]

ASSOCIATED FEATURES

Isolated ASD in infancy and childhood is seldom symptomatic, even for large defects, and symptoms of congestive failure should prompt a careful effort to rule out additional associated abnormalities. Associated lesions found in the study of infants with ASD dying in the first year of life included left-to-right shunting lesions, such as VSD or patent ductus arteriosus (PDA); right-sided obstructive lesions, such as pulmonary stenosis; and left-sided obstructive lesions, such as aortic stenosis, mitral stenosis, or coarctation of the aorta. Necropsy data show that patients with VSD had an associated ASD in 18% of cases, those with left-sided obstruction had an associated ASD in 29% of cases, and those with right-sided obstructive lesions had ASD in 31% of cases.[39] These associations support the hypothesis that some secundum ASDs are acquired, driven by remote lesions that favor persistent atrial level shunting and atrial dilation, in turn leading to valvar incompetence at the fossa ovalis.

Mitral valve abnormalities have long been recognized as associated with ASD, although their associated incidence is uncommon. Mitral stenosis with pulmonary artery dilation in association with ASD, or Lutembacher syndrome, was perhaps a more frequent association found in the era when rheumatic heart disease was more prevalent, although nonrheumatic mitral stenosis is occasionally found in association with ASD.[40] A cleft anterior mitral leaflet, mitral prolapse, or regurgitation has also been reported in uncommon association with ASD. Mitral prolapse may be a result of septal distortion by right ventricular volume overload and a secondary effect on mitral valve geometry. As evidence in favor of this hypothesis, mitral prolapse has been shown to reverse after ASD closure.[41]

Tricuspid regurgitation in association with ASD is usually caused by annular dilation from the enlarged right ventricle, and it also reverses with ASD closure. The most common additional cardiac anomalies associated with ASD include PAPVC, VSD, PDA, persistent left SVC, pulmonary valve stenosis, and branch pulmonary artery stenosis.[42]

P wave prolongation associated with ASD may predispose the patient to the eventual development of atrial fibrillation. P wave duration may be shortened by ASD closure in younger adults, suggesting that the chronicity of atrial stretch is a contributing factor.[43] Closure of ASD in older adults does not affect this electrical pathophysiology and does not shorten preexistent P wave prolongation.[44] The presence of paroxysmal atrial fibrillation prior to ASD closure results in no shortening of P wave duration by closure.[45]

HEMODYNAMICS AND PATHOPHYSIOLOGY

Left-to-Right Shunt

In early infancy, when pulmonary resistance is high, left and right ventricular compliances are similar, and net shunting through an ASD is typically slight. As the left ventricle matures, it becomes less compliant in diastole than the right, and left atrial pressure rises. This drives a left-to-right shunt at the atrial level in the presence of an ASD. With age, the disparity between systemic and pulmonary resistance, and in turn between left and right ventricular compliance, results in increased left-to-right shunting and advancing right ventricular volume loading. Over time, right ventricular volume load results in dilation and hypertrophy, eventually affecting the function of both ventricles. Atrial enlargement may contribute to the late incidence of atrial fibrillation. Right ventricular volume overload is noted to occur as a rule when ASDs are larger than 6 mm in diameter.[46]

Volume-induced hypertrophy of the right ventricle produces a loss of coronary reserve and eventual impairment of right ventricular systolic and diastolic function. Left ventricular functional reserve is diminished by adulthood in most patients with ASD. Although left ventricular systolic function may be normal at rest, the left ventricle exhibits a subnormal diastolic dimension, and a loss of functional reserve at exercise. Mechanisms that account for left ventricular dysfunction include (1) septal displacement secondary to right ventricular dilation and hypertrophy and (2) systolic anterior movement of the mitral valve. In general, the functional loss in the left and right ventricles is normalized 6 months following ASD closure in children and young adults.[47]

Pulmonary Vascular Disease

Pulmonary hypertension associated with an isolated ASD is rare in childhood, although 35% to 50% of patients with unrepaired ASD have elevated pulmonary resistance by age 40. The development of pulmonary vascular disease is not uniformly related to age or degree of shunting across the ASD. In contrast, patients with VSD predictably develop pulmonary hypertension earlier and more severely, subjected to similar left-to-right shunting and elevated pulmonary blood flow. No explanation has been found for why shunts of similar volume from ASDs or VSDs, generating similar elevations in pulmonary blood flow, produce different patterns of pulmonary hypertension. In a study of 128 patients with ASD and pulmonary hypertension (all older than 18 years), one third demonstrated an elevation in pulmonary vascular resistance (PVR) before 20 years of age, one third between 20 and 40, and the remainder after 40 years of age.[48]

Pulmonary hypertension can develop at an earlier age in premature infants and in children with Trisomy 21. Histopathologic evidence of increased preacinar and intra-acinar arterial muscularity in infants with ASD and pulmonary vascular disease suggests that the pulmonary vasculopathy is the primary disorder in the uncommon population with early pulmonary vascular disease. The ASD may be acquired as a consequence, or it may be incidentally associated.[49]

Clinical Presentation

A great majority of ASDs are asymptomatic, and palpitations, atrial fibrillation, and congestive failure are late sequelae, uncommon in patients younger than 40 years of age. Occasional dyspnea on extreme exertion is observed even in children. Recurrent respiratory infection in the presence of a large ASD is not uncommon. Chylothorax has been reported as a presenting manifestation of ASD and is cured by ASD closure.[50]

In rare cases, ASDs may be associated with cyanosis. Bidirectional shunting across the ASD without an elevation in the pulmonary resistance has been demonstrated as a source of cyanosis.[51] An alternative anatomic source for cyanosis is a streaming of desaturated inferior vena cava (IVC) blood across the ASD, caused by a persistently enlarged eustachian valve or other venous drainage anomaly that directs blood flow into the left atrium.[52] More ominously, cyanosis can develop in the setting of advanced irreversible pulmonary hypertension.

Additional clinical associations with PFO include stroke, migraine headache, high altitude pulmonary edema, and diver's decompression disease.[53]

Diagnostics and Examination

Findings consistent with ASD at physical exam largely reflect the left-to-right shunting and elevated right ventricular volume and flow. A prominent right ventricle impulse is present, with a precordial right ventricular lift, leftward displacement of the apex, and possible left chest wall prominence.

Auscultatory findings include a systolic flow murmur heard over the left upper sternal border from elevated flow across the pulmonary valve, a split S2, fixed throughout the respiratory cycle, with a prominent pulmonary valve component. An apical mid-diastolic murmur, especially at inspiration, reflects increased flow across the tricuspid valve.

The chest X-ray demonstrates cardiomegaly with prominent pulmonary vascularity and a prominent pulmonary artery bulb.

The electrocardiogram in ASD shows right ventricular hypertrophy, lengthened PR interval, incomplete right bundle branch block, and an RSR pattern in V_1. Electrocardiographic criteria for right ventricular enlargement are found in more than 50% of young patients with a large ASD. A traditional teaching is that the secundum ASD is associated with right-axis deviation and incomplete right bundle branch block (rSR' pattern in right precordial leads), whereas the primum defect exhibits left-axis deviation with incomplete right bundle branch block. A normal preoperative electrocardiogram was found in only 6% of a study population of sinus venosus ASD.[54] Although some of these electrocardiographic findings are reported as useful in children, they are not sensitive diagnostic features in adults and are seldom referenced in an era when an echocardiographic diagnosis is sensitive, specific, and readily available.[55]

Cardiac catheterization is similarly seldom used in the diagnosis of ASD, but, when performed, an SVC to right atrium O_2 saturation step-up is reflective of the left-to-right shunting at the atrial level. A pressure gradient, usually less than 25 mm Hg at peak, may be detected across the pulmonary valve that is physiologic, reflecting the elevated pulmonary blood flow. Echocardiography is the most common mode of diagnosis, capable of acquiring sufficient morphologic and physiologic data to obviate the need for catheterization in a great majority of cases.

Transthoracic echocardiography with color Doppler flow mapping is accepted as the most accurate modality of ASD diagnosis in children, capable of detecting smaller intracardiac shunts compared with two-dimensional echocardiography alone. Small defects and defects in obscure locations, such as coronary sinus defects and some sinus venosus defects, may remain difficult to image by echocardiogram. High-resolution computed tomography (CT) and cardiac magnetic resonance imaging (MRI) have been used to image some interatrial defects that have eluded adequate echocardiographic characterization. MRI is particularly useful in imaging partial anomalous pulmonary venous structures that may lie adjacent to the airways and lung, where air interface interferes with the echocardiographic image resolution (Fig. 114-4).[56]

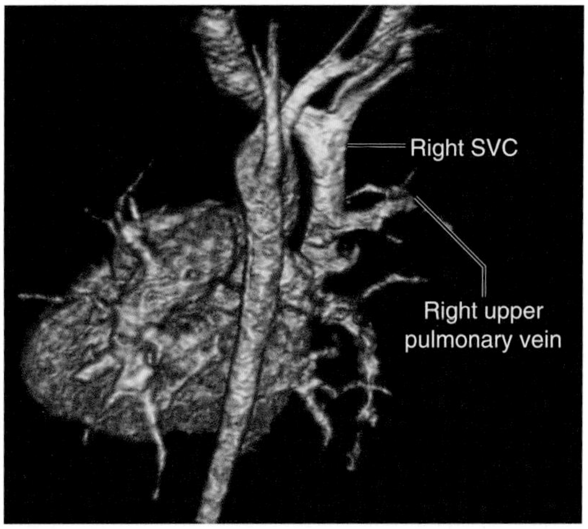

FIGURE 114-4 ■ Three-dimensional cardiac magnetic resonance image of a heart (posterior view), showing right upper pulmonary veins anomalously entering the superior vena cava (SVC), cephalad to the atriocaval junction in a patient with superior sinus venosus atrial septal defect. (Courtesy David Parra, MD, Vanderbilt Children's Heart Institute.)

MANAGEMENT OF ATRIAL SEPTAL DEFECT AND PATENT FORAMEN OVALE

Indications and Contraindications for Atrial Septal Defect Closure

The patients benefiting most from ASD closure are those at risk for developing pulmonary hypertension, but once pulmonary hypertension is present, surgical risk increases. This principle is the basis for the recommendation to close all significant ASDs.[57] Elective closure of ASD is generally recommended when the ratio of pulmonary to systemic blood flow (Qp : Qs) is 1.5:1 or greater. Ideally, ASD closure should be performed at age 2 to 5 years, before exercise capacity changes, while chest wall compliance is optimal, and before school age. An echo diagnosis of a significant defect with right ventricular volume overload is common and is a sufficient indication to close an ASD. Long-term follow-up data after surgical ASD closure show survival equal to the normal population when repair is performed early in life, with an age-related diminution in survival when closure is delayed. The 27-year survival for those repaired after 40 years of age is only 40%.[58]

A small hemodynamically insignificant ASD, without cardiomegaly, does not warrant closure. Pregnancy is a relative contraindication to closure, with closure safely delayed until after delivery. Severe left ventricular failure is a contraindication to ASD closure.

Advanced pulmonary hypertension is a contraindication to ASD closure. It is important to consider that, in a high flow state, with a large Qp : Qs, high pulmonary artery pressure may not represent fixed pulmonary hypertension. As a general guideline, irreversible pulmonary hypertension is characterized by a PVR 8 to 12 Wood unit X m^2, with Qp : Qs less than 1.2:1, despite aggressive vasodilator challenge.

Moderate pulmonary hypertension with a reactive component is not a contraindication to ASD closure, although pulmonary hypertension may progress in these patients regardless of closure. In cases of severe pulmonary hypertension, a fenestrated ASD closure may be successfully performed, depending on the degree of reversibility and PVR. Guidelines for inoperability are largely based on VSD data. Generally, the PVR must fall below 7 Wood unit X m^2 with vasodilator therapy at cardiac catheterization for ASD closure risk to be less than prohibitive.[59] Vasodilators used at cardiac catheterization to determine the reversible component of pulmonary hypertension include hyperoxia, inhaled nitric oxide, and intravenous prostacycline (Flolan). Chronic preparatory vasodilator therapy with sildenafil has been successfully used to convert inoperable pulmonary hypertension to operable.[60]

Patent Foramen Ovale Management

Indications for Patent Foramen Ovale Closure

The aggressive expansion of catheter-based therapies for PFO has resulted in a proliferation of clinical studies and case reports to reexamine indications for PFO closure. Although a subject of some continuing controversy, there are presently insufficient data to support the medical, surgical, or device treatment of the incidentally diagnosed, hemodynamically insignificant PFO. Adverse events attributed to the presence of a PFO or associated ASA include embolic stroke or peripheral embolus, brain abscess, gas embolization in diver's decompression illness, platypnea-orthodeoxia syndrome, migraine headache, and exacerbated hypoxia in settings of pulmonary embolus or elevated right heart pressures following a right ventricle infarct.[61] Indications for PFO closure in these settings are also controversial and are discussed later.

Patent Foramen Ovale and Stroke

The associations of PFO with stroke are complicated, age dependent, and not fully resolved. When discussing the risk of stroke, it is important to distinguish first ischemic stroke from cryptogenic stroke (stroke with no known underlying causal condition) and from recurrent stroke.

An association between PFO and cryptogenic stroke is accepted in the younger population, an age group for whom stroke is rare in general. An association between cryptogenic stroke and the presence of PFO is strong for patients younger than 55 years of age, and the association is even stronger if ASA, with or without PFO, is present.[62] Prospective studies corroborate this trend but with no statistical significance, leaving some room for controversy.[53]

Causality after 55 years of age is less clear, complicated by various other sources for ischemic stroke that occur concurrently in the older population. Although the association is not as strong as that of the younger population, PFO independently remains associated with cryptogenic stroke in older patients.[63]

There appears to be no relationship between size of interatrial shunt and risk of recurrent stroke.[62,64]

Although there is a convincing association between cryptogenic stroke and PFO, the presence of PFO as predictor of first or recurrent stroke is less well established. Whereas the presence of untreated PFO predicts a 2.3% risk of recurrent cerebrovascular event by 4 years after the initial event, the presence of ASA with PFO predicts a 15.2% recurrence risk at 4 years.[65] Antiplatelet therapy following stroke mitigates the risk for recurrent stroke. For stroke victims with PFO and no ASA younger than 55 years of age, the annual risk of recurrent stroke while taking aspirin is only 1% to 2%.

Strategies for treatment of PFO after an ischemic event include PFO closure or medical management with aspirin or Coumadin. Various reports support the superiority of either anticoagulation therapy or mechanical closure of PFO for patients who have suffered cryptogenic stroke.

Obstacles remain to fully understanding the relationship of PFO to stroke and to determining the optimum treatment strategy. Antiplatelet therapy routinely applied after device closure further confuses the distinction between the effects of mechanical versus medical treatment. Systematic review fails to demonstrate advantages of closure versus anticoagulant therapy for the prevention of recurrent cryptogenic stroke in the presence of PFO, although there are data to suggest that the benefit of device closure may be device specific and that treatment may need to be individualized.[66-68]

Generally accepted practice guidelines suggest a treatment strategy as follows:

1. Aspirin alone for any asymptomatic patients with PFO or ASA. Risk of stroke in this population is 1%/yr or less.
2. Coumadin for patients with PFO and a hypercoagulable state, history of stroke, transient ischemic attack (TIA) or deep vein thrombosis (DVT) preceding stroke. Coumadin imposes a 2.2%/yr risk of bleeding complication, 0.2% fatal. PFO closure for this population may be indicated.
3. PFO closure for patients younger than 60 years old who have suffered cryptogenic stroke if the PFO is associated with ASA (4%/yr risk of stroke, even on aspirin), with DVT before stroke, or with TIA or stroke while on antithrombotic therapy.[69]

Patent Foramen Ovale and Migraine

Although PFO may be present in more migraine sufferers than in the general population, especially for those with migraine accompanied by an aura, a clear association is not well established. Migraine cure or improvement has been reported in many patients undergoing closure of PFO, but the association of PFO closure and migraine improvement may be affected by placebo effect, periprocedural anticoagulation therapy, short follow-up, and device complications. The only randomized clinical trial of PFO closure for severe migraine has failed to demonstrate a positive effect.[70] Closure of PFO cannot firmly be recommended for the treatment of migraine at present, although additional randomized clinical trials are under way.[53,71]

Patent Foramen Ovale and Diver's Decompression Illness

Bubbles in the left heart are documented by echocardiogram to demonstrate diver's decompression illness in association with PFO. Underwater pressure and its effects on ventilation elevate the pulmonary resistance, reducing left ventricular preload while increasing right-sided pressures, and favoring right-to-left shunting across the PFO. The overall risk of diver's decompression illness with PFO is low, with 5 events per 10,000 divers, but these odds are fivefold above the odds for those without PFO.

In a prospective, nonrandomized, controlled trial of PFO closure among divers with PFO, long-term follow-up demonstrated an apparent advantage to PFO closure in preventing symptomatic decompression injury and asymptomatic neurologic findings on MRI.[72] These findings suggest consideration of PFO closure for frequent divers, although firm evidence to support screening or prophylactic PFO closure is lacking.[53]

Catheter-Based Treatment

King and Mills reported the first catheter-delivered ASD closure in 1976, using a double umbrella device and a 23 Fr delivery catheter. The large-delivery catheter and complex delivery method prevented widespread use.[73] In 1983, Rashkind introduced a self-expanding patch device that attached to the septum with small barbed hooks. The device was unfortunately hindered by the inability for repositioning and its risk of inadvertent attachment to other structures within the heart.[74] The concept of a self-expanding patch led to the development of the Lock Clamshell device—a double disc, self-expanding device that could be delivered through an 11 Fr delivery sheath. First reported in 1990, this was the first device to receive widespread use.[75] Device arm fracture resulted in its eventual redesign. In 1993, Das reported the use of the Angel Wings device—a self-expanding, double patch device with a conjoint central ring acting as a waist. Although its use was limited by its rigid frame, its sharp edges, and difficulty with its retrieval, its circular central waist demonstrated the benefit of a self-centering device.[76] Over the subsequent 20 years, numerous devices have been designed and investigated for the treatment of secundum ASDs. The two devices currently approved by the Food and Drug Administration (FDA) in the United States are the Amplatzer septal occluder (St. Jude Medical, St. Paul, MN)[77] and the Helex septal occluder (Gore & Associates, Flagstaff, AZ).[76] Devices currently available outside the United States include the Gore septal occluder (W.L. Gore & Associates, Flagstaff, AZ)[78]; the Ultrasept ASD occluder, which is a modification of the Atriasept device (Cardia, Inc., Eagan, MN)[79]; Occlutech Figulla ASD occluder (Occlutech, Jena, Germany)[80]; the Cardi-O-Fix (CSO) ASD occluder (Starway Medical Technology, Inc., Beijing, China)[81]; and the Cera ASD occluder (Lifetech Scientific Co., Ltd., Shenzhen, China).[82]

Most ASDs today are closed by catheter-based devices. The Amplatzer and Helex occluders are the most commonly used approved devices at this time. A national sampling of community hospital practices found a 58-fold increase in the annual number of devices placed from 2002 to 2004, whereas surgical closure rates remained constant.[83] The success rate and morbidity are almost equal when comparing device closure with surgical closure. Current published studies comparing the two approaches with anatomically similar defects show a device success rate of 80% to 95.7% and a surgical closure success rate of 95% to 100%, although the success of device closures continues to evolve. Complications requiring treatment (defined to include anemia, arrhythmia requiring minor treatment, post pericardotomy syndrome, pericardial or pleural effusion, transfusion, fever, wound complication) occur in up to 8% of device closures and 23% to 24% of surgical closures, and mean length of hospital stay is 1 day in the device group versus 3.4 days in the surgical group.[84,85] Continual advances in the hardware and experience with device closures are improving the success rate of these catheter-based approaches.

Anatomic determinants that prohibit device closure remain the major indications for surgical ASD closure in the current era. Defects unsuitable for device closure include those that have failed attempted device closure, common atria or those without sufficient septal rim to engage the device, and sinus venosus defects for which device closure would threaten obstruction of pulmonary veins, IVC, or SVC. Anterior-inferior septal deficiency can result in device interference with the tricuspid valve, mitral valve, or coronary sinus. Individual deficient septal rims, although originally constituting contraindication to device closure, no longer are absolute contraindications but may reduce success rates.[86] The largest Amplatzer septal occlusion device presently available in the United States is 38 mm, and defects exceeding this size require surgical closure. Multiple defects can be closed with multiple devices, although the cost of multiple device closures may exceed the cost of surgery. Determinants of the limitations to device closure are under evolution as devices and their delivery systems continue to undergo refinements.

Pooled data from multiple sources estimate that major complications of device closure of ASD and PFO occur in 1.4% of cases and minor complications in 1.4%.[87] Early major procedural complications of device closure include device embolization; cardiac tamponade; stroke or TIA; retroperitoneal hematoma; thrombosis; device erosion; obstruction of the IVC, coronary sinus, or pulmonary vein; and tricuspid or mitral insufficiency. Noncardiac complications include iliac vein dissection, retroperitoneal or groin hematoma, and leg ischemia. Minor complications include minor vascular complications, arrhythmia, transient ST-segment elevation, percutaneously retrieved device embolization, pericardial effusion, device malposition not requiring surgery, and pulmonary edema. Late complications include device-related death, cerebrovascular events, device thrombosis or malposition, embolization, erosion, aortoatrial fistula, arrhythmia, device fracture, pericardial effusion, endocarditis, and nickel toxicity.[87]

As experience with devices matures, their indications and limits are better defined. Evidence suggests that a higher incidence of complications is expected for patients who weigh less than 15 kg and that waiting for somatic growth may be preferable.[88] A fluoroscopically guided catheter-based approach raises concern for radiation exposure; this consideration is eliminated when echo-guided ASD closure is used.[89,90] A large defect or a large device is a risk factor for AV block.[91] Careful avoidance of device oversizing, especially in patients with a deficient aortic rim, may prevent erosion or perforation.[92,93] Absent posterior-inferior rims may increase risk of dislodgement, and patients with this anatomy might more safely be served by surgery.[94]

A recent 20-year outcome comparison of device versus surgical treatment of comparable ASDs shows no significant differences in survival, functional capacity, arrhythmia, or late embolic stroke between methods of closure, supporting a transcatheter approach for defects amenable to device closure.[95]

Surgical Treatment

Secundum Atrial Septal Defect and Patent Foramen Ovale

The standard surgical incision for the repair of ASD is partial or complete median sternotomy. A portion of the anterior pericardium is preserved for use as a patch. Various other materials have been used as a patch, including bovine pericardium and polytetrafluoroethylene (PTFE), but autologous pericardium is a compliant, durable, and cost-efficacious choice. Bicaval venous cannulation, mild hypothermia, and antegrade cardioplegia are used to provide a still, blood-free field through which to expose the interatrial septum via right atriotomy. A careful examination of the interatrial septum ensures the correct identification of the margins of the defect. The SVC and IVC are identified, with special attention to any structures that might represent partial anomalous pulmonary venous return (PAPVR) to the right atrium or vena cavae. The eustachian valve is identified to avoid the error of baffling the IVC to the left atrium. The coronary sinus is identified and protected from inclusion in the suture line. A determination is made to close the defect primarily where there is sufficient septum primum tissue, or with a patch. Care is exercised to place sutures firmly into surrounding tissue but without interfering with the adjacent noncoronary sinus of the aorta superiorly, the tricuspid or mitral valves anteriorly, the coronary sinus and AV node inferoanteriorly, the IVC and right lower pulmonary vein orifice inferiorly and posteriorly, or the right upper pulmonary vein and SVC superoposteriorly (Fig. 114-5). When the defect is closed primarily, adequate redundant tissue must be present to ensure that no tension will be placed on the repair once the heart is filled and beating.

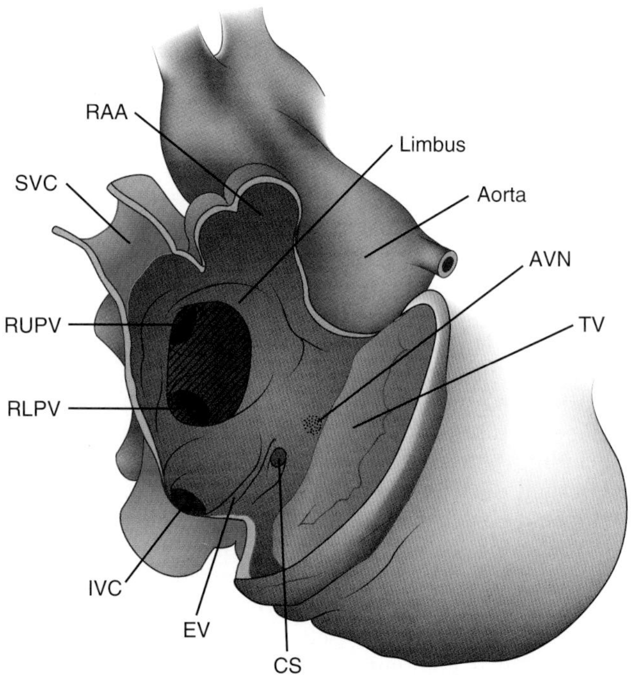

FIGURE 114-5 ■ Surgical anatomy of the interatrial septum with atrial septal defect. *AVN,* Atrioventricular node; *CS,* coronary sinus; *EV,* eustachian valve; *IVC,* inferior vena cava; *RAA,* right atrial appendage; *RLPV,* right lower pulmonary vein; *RUPV,* right upper pulmonary vein; *SVC,* superior vena cava; *TV,* tricuspid valve.

Sinus Venosus Atrial Septal Defect with Partial Anomalous Pulmonary Venous Return

The most common variant of sinus venosus ASD is the superior, when the right upper pulmonary vein drains anomalously to the right atrium or SVC. A single intra-atrial patch can be positioned to baffle the pulmonary vein through the septal defect into the left atrium in many cases. Care is exercised to place the SVC incision remote from the sinoatrial node. The single-patch technique may predispose to SVC narrowing, as the baffle occupies space within the SVC lumen.[96] A two-patch approach enlarges the SVC to accommodate the baffle.

When one or more pulmonary veins connect to the SVC too cephalad to permit simple baffling, an adjunctive patch plasty of the lateral SVC must be carried out. Anticipating such geometry, an atriotomy can be planned at the lateral base of the SVC, so that septal and caval patch plasties can be placed through a single atriotomy, extended as far as necessary onto the SVC (Fig. 114-6). ASD enlargement may also be needed to ensure an unobstructed baffle.

The Warden procedure, described in 1984,[97] consists of transection of the SVC cephalad to the connection of the anomalous pulmonary vein, thereby committing the atriocaval junction to pulmonary venous blood flow exclusively. An intra-atrial patch baffles the atriocaval junction to the left atrium, through a preexistent or created ASD. The transected SVC is then reimplanted into the right atrial appendage by direct anastomosis (Fig. 114-7). A tensionless SVC anastomosis is imperative to the success of the SVC reimplantation, and patch augmentation is sometimes necessary. Special care must be taken to resect all trabecular muscle in the atrial appendage that might impair SVC flow through the reimplantation site.

A retrospective examination of 54 patients with superior sinus venosus ASD and PAPVR treated at Children's Memorial Hospital showed a 55% incidence of the loss of sinus rhythm. These patients had a low atrial or junctional rhythm that did not increase normally with exercise. These data support consideration of the Warden procedure for the correction of all superior sinus venosus ASDs when the right upper pulmonary veins enter the SVC.[98]

Primum Atrial Septal Defect

Characterized by the absence of any septal tissue between the AV valves, the primum ASD closure requires that the patch be sutured directly to mitral or tricuspid tissue, avoiding the subjacent ventricular septum and the His bundle, and sometimes leaving the coronary sinus on the left atrial side to avoid the AV node. An examination of the mitral valve and closure of the associated cleft is

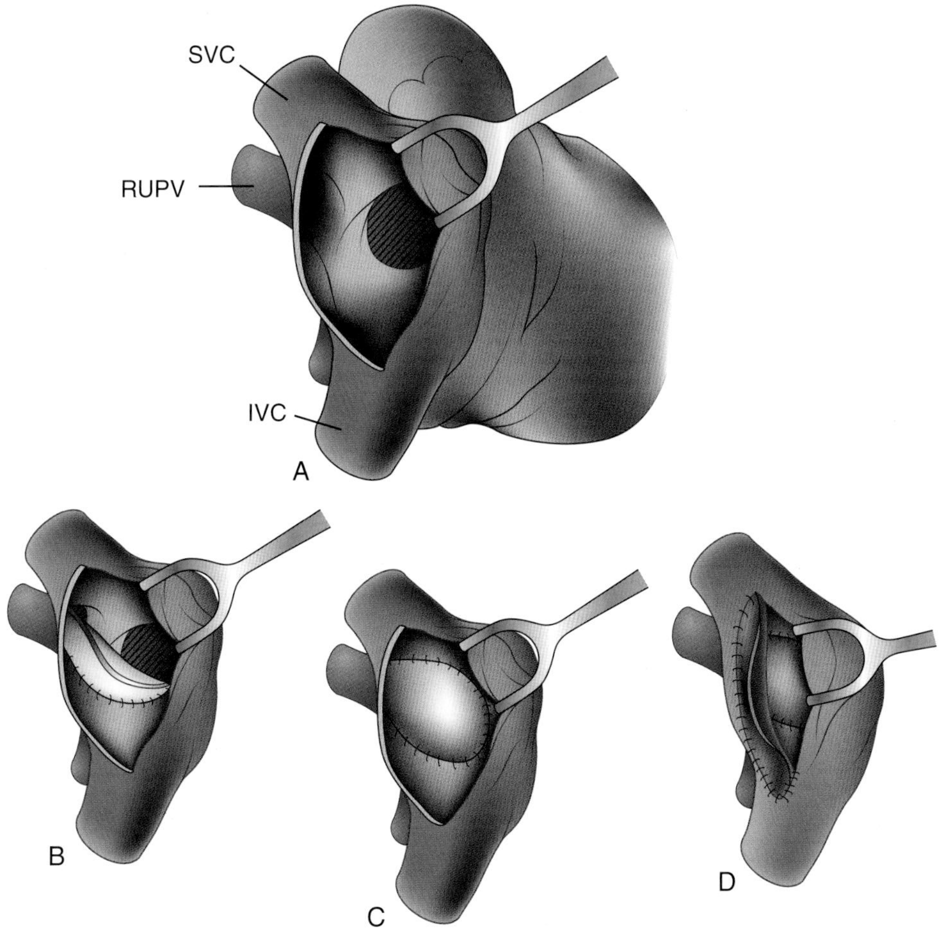

FIGURE 114-6 ■ Repair of superior sinus venosus atrial septal defect. **A,** A lateral atriotomy provides exposure to the anomalous right upper pulmonary vein. **B,** A pericardial baffle is constructed to direct right upper pulmonary vein flow to the left atrium, through a created or enlarged secundum defect. **C,** Completed intra-atrial baffle. **D,** A patch plasty of the atriotomy extends sufficiently cephalad on the superior vena cava to avert caval obstruction. *IVC,* Inferior vena cava; *RUPV,* right upper pulmonary vein(s); *SVC,* superior vena cava.

indicated, even in the absence of mitral regurgitation. Care is taken to avoid creating mitral stenosis. The primum defect is discussed fully with AV septal defects.

Minimally Invasive Approaches

Various alternatives to the median sternotomy have been described for the repair of ASD. An inframammary or axillary incision with thoracotomy provides exposure of the right atrium with a scar that is more easily concealed than the full median sternotomy. The subxiphoid "ministernotomy" or partial lower sternotomy can be performed through small vertical or transverse inframammary incisions, and cannulation through the incision rather than peripherally.[99] Experience continues to expand with methods that use even smaller incisions, femoral cannulation, and video or robotic assistance.[100-102] These alternative approaches may confer a cosmetic advantage over the standard midline incision and median sternotomy, although to date it has been difficult to demonstrate objective advantages in cardiac physiology, pulmonary physiology, pain, length of anesthesia, length of hospital stay, or cost.[103]

Complications of Surgery

Early complications following the surgical closure of ASD include patch dehiscence, thromboembolism, and arrhythmia such as heart block, sinus node dysfunction, and atrial fibrillation or flutter. Early postoperative arrhythmia following ASD repair may predict an eventual need for pacemaker.[104] The incidence of residual shunt after surgical closure is negligibly small.[84] Residual right-to-left shunting can occur with incomplete closure, with undiagnosed additional defects, and when ASD closure mistakenly engages the eustachian valve, baffling the IVC inadvertently to the left atrium and resulting in cyanosis. In the setting of pulmonary hypertension, ASD closure can result in systemic venous hypertension, right ventricular failure, or low cardiac output and can require a return to cardiopulmonary bypass to fenestrate the closure.

An examination of late outcome 27 to 32 years after surgical repair of ASD showed that age at the time of repair is an independent risk factor for late complications. Late cardiac failure, stroke, and atrial fibrillation are more frequent when the patient's age at repair is older

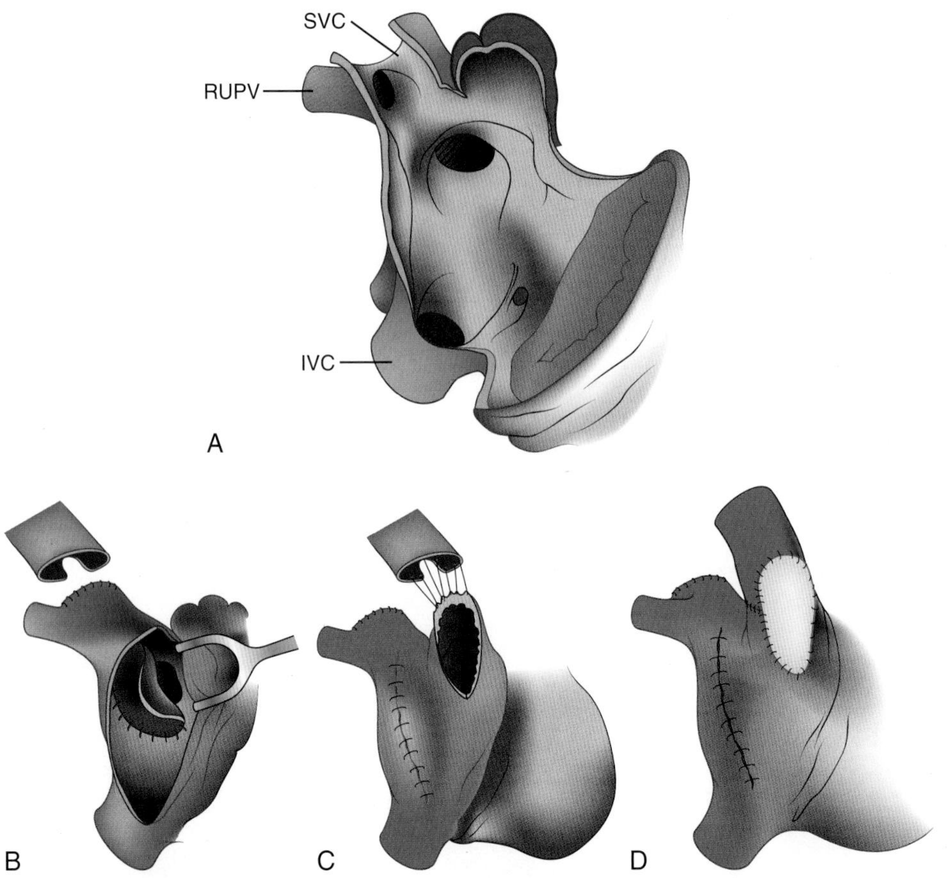

FIGURE 114-7 ■ The Warden procedure. **A,** Cutaway view of the right atrium, showing the relationship of the displaced right upper pulmonary vein (RUPV) and its distance from the atrial septal defect and left atrium. **B,** Superior vena cava (SVC) transected above the abnormal pulmonary vein. The RUPV with the SVC orifice is baffled to the left atrium. **C,** The transected SVC is anastomosed directly to the right atrial appendage. **D,** Patch augmentation of the anastomosis averts cavoatrial obstruction. *IVC,* Inferior vena cava.

than 25 years.[58] Independent risk factors for the development of atrial fibrillation with ASD, repaired or not, include age older than 25 years, left atrial enlargement, and mitral or tricuspid regurgitation.[105] Thirty to forty percent of patients older than 40 who exhibit atrial fibrillation after ASD repair may have an embolic event within 10 years of ASD repair, and systemic anticoagulation is a consideration in this group.[106]

Reported complications of thoracotomy approaches include phrenic nerve palsy, lung herniation, cardiac herniation, scoliosis, and breast or chest muscle deformity.[107,108]

OUTCOME

Physiology of Atrial Septal Defect Closure

Subtle changes in exercise performance in ASD patients can be measured even in childhood. An abnormal ventilatory threshold during submaximal exercise returns to normal by 6 months after repair of ASD in patients younger than 5 years of age but remains subnormal for patients repaired older than 5 years.[109] Most patients older than 5 years old at the time of repair have at least some residual right ventricle dilation and abnormal septal wall motion after ASD closure, not predicted by preoperative shunt or ASD size.[110] The clinical significance of this finding is unclear. These data may further support a strategy of ASD closure before school age.

Adults

Although the adult with ASD benefits by improvement in exercise physiology and reduction of right ventricle dilation after closure of ASD, the improvements are less pronounced with advancing age.[57,111] There is a clear survival advantage and a reduction in the incidence of cardiovascular events for ASD closure in patients younger than 40, when compared with expectant management.[112] Some controversy remains as to the best treatment strategy in the older adult population.

Regardless of the presence of symptoms, the incidence of right heart enlargement in adults decreases after surgical or device closure of ASD, although right atrial enlargement may persist, proportional to the age at repair.[113-115] Although younger adults demonstrate an improved VO_{2max} within months of ASD closure, patients older than 40 years who undergo repair may take years to show improvement. A low preoperative peak oxygen uptake has been demonstrated in adults with ASD, increasing by 4 months after repair, fully normalizing by 10 years after surgical ASD repair.[113,116] Prior to ASD closure, more than 60% of patients older than 40 years of age are New York Heart Association (NYHA) class III to IV, whereas after ASD closure, more than 80% are NYHA class I to II.[117] Patients older than 60 show functional class improvement, immediate and late reduction in pulmonary artery pressure, and improved 5- and 10-year survival after ASD closure in comparison with expectant management.[118,119] These data support a strategy of ASD closure regardless of age for most patients. Independent risk factors for prolonged hospital stay in adults after ASD closure include preoperative atrial fibrillation, larger ASD, older age at operation, and longer cardiopulmonary bypass time.[120] A higher incidence of postclosure acute left ventricular failure and pulmonary congestion occurs with larger ASDs and with older age at repair.[121]

Arrhythmia

If ASD closure is performed in childhood, the incidence of early or late atrial tachyarrhythmia or sinus node dysfunction is rare.[122] The prevalence of atrial flutter or fibrillation may already be rising in the unrepaired young teenager, and prevalence is clearly increased after age 40.[14,44,58]

A significant incidence of postoperative atrial fibrillation in the adult has given consideration to performing a Cox-Maze arrhythmia ablation procedure concurrent with ASD closure for patients older than 40 years of age. No randomized data support performing a Cox-Maze procedure, but observational studies show benefit in adult patients undergoing ASD closure who have preoperative atrial fibrillation or flutter.[123] A right atrial Maze procedure alone may be ineffective in restoring and maintaining sinus rhythm after ASD closure, and higher success is achieved by performing a biatrial Maze procedure.[124]

COR TRIATRIATUM

Cor triatriatum sinistrum, one of the rarest cardiac anomalies, comprises 0.1% of congenital heart defects. In the classic form, described by Church in 1868, cor triatriatum is a separation of the pulmonary veins from the left atrium by a fibromuscular membrane. The anatomic elements of the left atrium, including the atrial appendage, are all ventral to the membrane, and the communication between pulmonary veins and left atrium is restricted to an orifice in the membrane.[125] The membrane can contain single or multiple fenestrations and can also communicate with the right atrium directly through an ASD, or indirectly, through an ascending or descending vertical vein. A variety of classifications have been devised to characterize the various drainage patterns of the pulmonary venous chamber into the heart (Fig. 114-8).

A subdivided right atrium, sometimes referred to as cor triatriatum dexter, is a membranous division of the right atrium, unrelated to cor triatriatum sinistrum. Cor triatriatum dexter forms from a persistence of the right sinus venosus valve, which normally regresses by 12 weeks of embryonic age.[126] The subdividing right atrial membrane can take on a variety of forms, ranging from a prominent Chiari network to a full septation that subdivides the right atrium or prolapses through the tricuspid valve, even to the extent that right ventricular outflow is obstructed.[127]

Embryology

The cor triatriatum sinistrum membrane contains elements of the embryonic common pulmonary vein and the wall of the left atrium. Van Praagh suggests that the dorsal chamber is the embryonic common pulmonary vein and that entrapment of the left atrial ostium of the common pulmonary vein by sinus venosus tissue results in a failure of the normal course of incorporation into the ventral left atrial chamber during the fifth embryonic week.[128] Van Praagh's explanation is the most widely accepted. Other theories postulate a malformation of the septum primum or an incomplete incorporation of the common pulmonary vein into the left atrium.[129-131]

The partially obstructed pulmonary venous chamber of cor triatriatum may form an ascending or descending vertical vein decompressing it into the systemic venous circulation at the IVC or SVC, similar to that of supracardiac or infracardiac total anomalous pulmonary venous connection. The degree of connectedness between the chambers determines the degree of obstruction.

Associated Abnormalities

Combinations of cor triatriatum and partial anomalous pulmonary venous drainage have been described, with normally draining left- or right-sided veins to the proper left atrium and contralateral veins connecting to a dorsal venous chamber. Associated partial anomalous pulmonary venous drainage to a vertical vein or to the coronary sinus has been described.[132] Cor triatriatum has a high association with the presence of a left SVC, an association theorized to be involved in the pathogenesis of cor triatriatum.[131]

Other intracardiac anomalies associated with cor triatriatum sinister include pulmonary stenosis, Ebstein anomaly, tricuspid anomalies, VSD, tetralogy of Fallot, AV septal defect, and hypoplastic left heart.[133,134]

Clinical Presentation

The clinical presentation of cor triatriatum is usually in infancy and is manifested by symptoms and signs of pulmonary venous congestion and pulmonary hypertension. Poor growth, episodic exacerbations of pulmonary edema, and frequent pulmonary infections are common. The severity of the presentation is dependent on the degree of pulmonary venous obstruction. Those patients with a communication to the right atrium generally have a milder progression of symptoms, as the pulmonary venous chamber decompresses into the right atrium. Patients presenting later in life may additionally have syncope, hemoptysis, atrial fibrillation, embolic

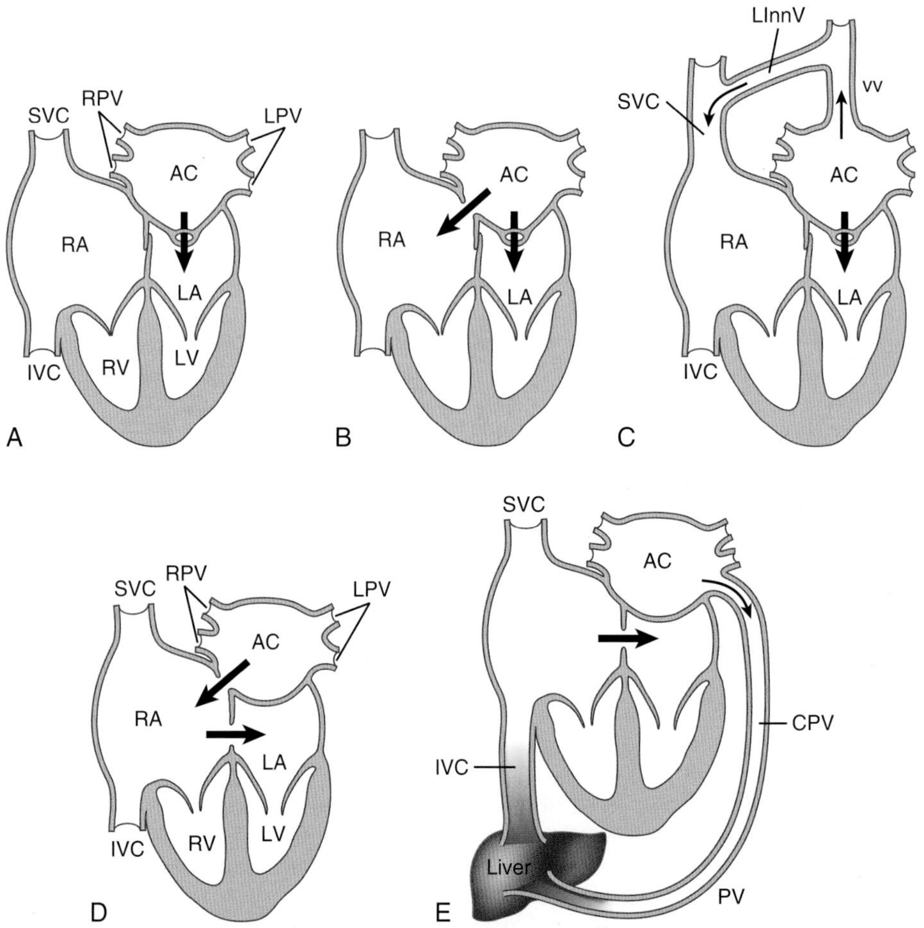

FIGURE 114-8 ■ The subtypes of cor triatriatum. **A,** The classic cor triatriatum, with the common pulmonary chamber draining through a restrictive membrane perforation, into the true left atrium. **B,** Communications between the common pulmonary venous chamber and both right and left atria. **C,** A vertical decompressing vein from the common pulmonary venous chamber to the innominate vein. **D,** Pulmonary venous effluent entering the right atrium through a direct communication, and the left atrium through a secundum atrial septal defect. **E,** An infracardiac vertical decompressing vein from the pulmonary venous chamber to the systemic venous system. *AC,* Accessory chamber; *CPV,* common pulmonary vein; *IVC,* inferior vena cava; *LA,* left atrium; *LInnV,* left innominate vein; *LPV,* left pulmonary vein; *LV,* left ventricle; *PV,* pulmonary vein; *RA,* right atrium; *RPV,* right pulmonary vein; *RV,* right ventricle; *SVC,* superior vena cava; *vv,* vertical vein. (Reproduced with permission from Hammon JW, Bender HW: Major anomalies of pulmonary and thoracic systemic veins. In Sabiston DC, Spencer FC, editors: *Surgery of the chest,* ed 6, Philadelphia, 1995, WB Saunders, p 1422.)

complications, and right heart failure.[135] The progression of symptoms in the adult with cor triatriatum may be the result of the development of mitral regurgitation. Calcification of the membrane is found in adults and can account for a narrowing of the perforation in the membrane, with a resultant exacerbation of symptoms. In a study of 31 necropsy specimens from untreated patients prior to 1960, the mean age at death was 3.3 months if the ostial diameter was smaller than 3 mm and 16 years for an ostial diameter larger than 3 mm.[136] Patients presenting as adults may exhibit progressive dyspnea and palpitations as presenting symptoms.

The physical exam is remarkable for congested lungs and a prominent second pulmonary sound on auscultation. Findings in patients presenting late with long-standing pulmonary hypertension and right heart failure include liver enlargement and jugular venous distention with a V wave. A systolic murmur at the left sternal border may be present.

The electrocardiogram demonstrates peaked P waves, suggesting right atrial enlargement. Right-axis deviation and voltage are consistent with right ventricular enlargement.

The chest radiograph shows cardiomegaly consistent with right ventricular enlargement, prominent pulmonary artery, and vascular markings.

The diagnosis of cor triatriatum is typically made by echocardiogram, and cardiac catheterization is seldom necessary. Findings at cardiac catheterization include a gradient from pulmonary capillary wedge pressure to left atrium, pulmonary hypertension, venous phase angiographic imaging of an upper chamber, prolonged pulmonary transit time, differential opacification of upper chamber and left atrium, and an occasional linear definition of the membrane. In rare cases, thrombus may occur proximal to the membrane and present as a left atrial mass.

Pathophysiology

In the anatomic subtype in which the orifice of the membrane communicates exclusively with the left atrium, the physiology of cor triatriatum is similar to that of mitral stenosis, with pulmonary congestion and/or edema depending on the degree of restriction at the membrane. For the subtypes with communication to the right atrium, a convoluted pathway of pulmonary venous flow delivers pulmonary venous effluent to the right atrium and then back to the left atrium through an interatrial communication below the membrane. Restricted filling of the left heart, low cardiac output, and pulmonary edema result, dependent on the degree of restriction along the pathway to the left atrium.

Pulmonary vein obstruction from cor triatriatum has been demonstrated to produce progressive medial thickening and intimal fibrosis in pulmonary veins and arteries, and lymphangiectasia, although neither as early nor as severe as is the progression of pulmonary vascular disease in VSD. The cellular intimal proliferation and advanced irreversible vascular changes characteristic of VSD or other left-to-right shunting lesions are not seen with pulmonary venous obstruction, and reversibility is the rule.[137]

When an interatrial communication exists between the proximal chamber and the right atrium, a left-to-right shunt exists. When a communication exists between the right atrium and the underfilled left atrial chamber, a right-to-left shunt can occur.

Treatment and Outcome

The surgical repair of cor triatriatum is performed with bicaval venous cannulation, moderate hypothermia, and cardioplegic arrest. An examination of the surface anatomy of the heart often confirms the presence of a dilated pulmonary venous chamber behind the heart. The repair is typically performed through a right atriotomy and a subsequent incision into the left atrium across the interatrial septum. Caution is exercised to identify the mitral valve and protect it from injury during the resection of the membrane. Time taken to fully define the membrane prevents injury to adjacent structures, notably the mitral valve. The membrane is widely excised, so as to leave no flow gradient from the pulmonary vein orifices to the mitral inflow region of the left atrium. A careful external examination of the heart exposes any ascending or descending venous structures for ligation.

Cor triatriatum repair has excellent outcomes, with expected mortality of less than 2% of cases. Reintervention for recurrent obstruction is rare.[133]

A concomitant Maze procedure has been described for the treatment of adults with cor triatriatum and atrial fibrillation.[138]

Although the standard approach includes a complete surgical resection of the obstructing membrane, a percutaneous balloon dilation of cor triatriatum membranes by a transseptal approach has been reported.[139]

REFERENCES

1. Murray G: Closure of defects in cardiac septa. *Ann Surg* 128(4):843–852, 1948.
2. Bailey CP, Nichols HT, Bolton HE, et al: Surgical treatment of forty-six interatrial septal defects by atrio-septo-pexy. *Ann Surg* 140(6):805–820, 1954.
3. Søndergaard T: Closure of atrial septal defects; report of three cases. *Acta Chir Scand* 107(5):492–498, 1954.
4. Gross RE, Pomeranz AA, Watkins E, Jr, et al: Surgical closure of defects of the interauricular septum by use of an Atrial well. *N Engl J Med* 247(13):455–460, 1952.
5. Lewis FJ, Taufic M: Closure of atrial septal defects with the aid of hypothermia; experimental accomplishments and the report of one successful case. *Surgery* 33(1):52–59, 1953.
6. Spencer FC, Bahnson HT: Intracardiac surgery employing hypothermia and coronary perfusion performed on 100 patients. *Surgery* 46:987–995, 1959.
7. Gibbon JH: Application of a mechanical heart and lung apparatus to cardiac surgery. *Minn Med* 37(3):171–185, passim, 1954.
8. Männer J, Merkel N: Early morphogenesis of the sinuatrial region of the chick heart: a contribution to the understanding of the pathogenesis of direct pulmonary venous connections to the right atrium and atrial septal defects in hearts with right isomerism of the atrial appendages. *Anat Rec* 290(2):168–180, 2007.
9. Caputo S: Familial recurrence of congenital heart disease in patients with ostium secundum atrial septal defect. *Eur Heart J* 26(20):2179–2184, 2005.
10. Øyen N, Poulsen G, Wohlfahrt J, et al: Recurrence of discordant congenital heart defects in families. *Circ Cardiovasc Genet* 3(2):122–128, 2010.
11. Burn J, Brennan P, Little J, et al: Recurrence risks in offspring of adults with major heart defects: results from first cohort of British collaborative study. *Lancet* 351(9099):311–316, 1998.
12. Weismann CG, Gelb BD: The genetics of congenital heart disease: a review of recent developments. *Curr Opin Cardiol* 22(3):200–206, 2007.
13. Sznajer Y, Keren B, Baumann C, et al: The spectrum of cardiac anomalies in Noonan syndrome as a result of mutations in the PTPN11 gene. *Pediatrics* 119(6):e1325–e1331, 2007.
14. Webb G, Gatzoulis MA: Atrial septal defects in the adult: recent progress and overview. *Circulation* 114(15):1645–1653, 2006.
15. Matsson H, Eason J, Bookwalter CS, et al: Alpha-cardiac actin mutations produce atrial septal defects. *Hum Mol Genet* 17(2):256–265, 2007.
16. Ching Y-H, Ghosh TK, Cross SJ, et al: Mutation in myosin heavy chain 6 causes atrial septal defect. *Nat Genet* 37(4):423–428, 2005.
17. Cordell HJ, Bentham J, Topf A, et al: Genome-wide association study of multiple congenital heart disease phenotypes identifies a susceptibility locus for atrial septal defect at chromosome 4p16. *Nat Genet* 45(7):822–824, 2013.
18. Basson CT, Cowley GS, Solomon SD, et al: The clinical and genetic spectrum of the Holt-Oram syndrome (heart-hand syndrome). *N Engl J Med* 330(13):885–891, 1994.
19. Alsoufi B, Cai S, van Arsdell GS, et al: Outcomes after surgical treatment of children with partial anomalous pulmonary venous connection. *Ann Thorac Surg* 84(6):2020 2026, 2007.
20. Pearson AC, Nagelhout D, Castello R, et al: Atrial septal aneurysm and stroke: a transesophageal echocardiographic study. *J Am Coll Cardiol* 18(5):1223–1229, 1991.
21. Olivares-Reyes A, Chan S, Lazar EJ, et al: Atrial septal aneurysm: a new classification in two hundred five adults. *J Am Soc Echocardiogr* 10(6):644–656, 1997.
22. Rillig A, Meyerfeldt U, Birkemeyer R, et al: Persistent iatrogenic atrial septal defect after pulmonary vein isolation. *J Interv Card Electrophysiol* 22(3):177–181, 2008.
23. Thors A, Guarneri R, Costantini EN, et al: Atrial septal rupture, flail tricuspid valve, and complete heart block due to nonpenetrating chest trauma. *Ann Thorac Surg* 83(6):2207–2210, 2007.
24. Connuck D, Sun JP, Super DM, et al: Incidence of patent ductus arteriosus and patent foramen ovale in normal infants. *Am J Cardiol* 89(2):244–247, 2002.
25. Radzik D, Davignon A, van Doesburg N, et al: Predictive factors for spontaneous closure of atrial septal defects diagnosed in the first 3 months of life. *J Am Coll Cardiol* 22(3):851–853, 1993.
26. Hagen PT, Scholz DG, Edwards WD: Incidence and size of patent foramen ovale during the first 10 decades of life: an autopsy study of 965 normal hearts. *Mayo Clin Proc* 59(1):17–20, 1984.
27. van der Linde D, Konings EEM, Slager MA, et al: Birth prevalence of congenital heart disease worldwide a systematic review and meta-analysis. *J Am Coll Cardiol* 58(21):2241–2247, 2011.

28. Brickner ME, Hillis LD, Lange RA: Congenital heart disease in adults. *N Engl J Med* 342(4):256–263, 2000.
29. Reller MD, Strickland MJ, Riehle-Colarusso T, et al: Prevalence of congenital heart defects in metropolitan Atlanta, 1998-2005. *J Pediatr* 153(6):807–813, 2008.
30. Jenkins KJ, Correa A, Feinstein JA, et al: Noninherited risk factors and congenital cardiovascular defects: current knowledge. *Circulation* 115:2995–3014, 2007.
31. Tikkanen J, Heinonen OP: Risk factors for atrial septal defect. *Eur J Epidemiol* 8(4):509–515, 1992.
32. Ghisla RP, Hannon DW, Meyer RA, et al: Spontaneous closure of isolated secundum atrial septal defects in infants: an echocardiographic study. *Am Heart J* 109(6):1327–1333, 1985.
33. Hanslik A, Pospisil U, Salzer-Muhar U, et al: Predictors of spontaneous closure of isolated secundum atrial septal defect in children: a longitudinal study. *Pediatrics* 118(4):1560–1565, 2006.
34. Demir T, Öztunç F, Eroğlu AG, et al: Outcome for patients with isolated atrial septal defects in the oval fossa diagnosed in infancy. *Cardiol Young* 18(01):75–78, 2008.
35. Dalen JE, Haynes FW, Dexter L: Life expectancy with atrial septal defect. Influence of complicating pulmonary vascular disease. *JAMA* 200(6):442–446, 1967.
36. Fredriksen PM, Veldtman G, Hechter S, et al: Aerobic capacity in adults with various congenital heart diseases. *Am J Cardiol* 87(3):310–314, 2001.
37. Engelfriet P, Meijboom F, Boersma E, et al: Repaired and open atrial septal defects type II in adulthood: an epidemiological study of a large European cohort. *Int J Cardiol* 126(3):379–385, 2008.
38. Wilson W, Taubert KA, Gewitz M, et al: Prevention of infective endocarditis: guidelines from the American Heart Association. *Circulation* 116(15):1736–1754, 2007.
39. Tandon R, Edwards JE: Clinicopathologic correlations. Atrial septal defect in infancy: common association with other anomalies. *Circulation* 49(5):1005–1010, 1974.
40. Lutembacher R: De la stenose mitrale avec communication interauriculaire. *Arch Mal Coeur* 9:237–260, 1916.
41. Schreiber TL, Feigenbaum H, Weyman AE: Effect of atrial septal defect repair on left ventricular geometry and degree of mitral valve prolapse. *Circulation* 61(5):888–896, 1980.
42. Keith JD, Rowe RD, Vlad P: *Heart disease in infancy and childhood*, New York, 1978, Macmillan.
43. Morton JB: Effect of chronic right atrial stretch on atrial electrical remodeling in patients with an atrial septal defect. *Circulation* 107(13):1775–1782, 2003.
44. Gatzoulis MA, Freeman MA, Siu SC, et al: Atrial arrhythmia after surgical closure of atrial septal defects in adults. *N Engl J Med* 340(11):839–846, 1999.
45. Guray U, Guray Y, Mecit B, et al: Maximum p wave duration and p wave dispersion in adult patients with secundum atrial septal defect: the impact of surgical repair. *Ann Noninvasive Electrocardiol* 9(2):136–141, 2004.
46. McMahon CJ: Natural history of growth of secundum atrial septal defects and implications for transcatheter closure. *Heart* 87(3):256–259, 2002.
47. Bonow RO, Borer JS, Rosing DR, et al: Left ventricular functional reserve in adult patients with atrial septal defect: pre- and postoperative studies. *Circulation* 63(6):1315–1322, 1981.
48. Craig RJ, Selzer A: Natural history and prognosis of atrial septal defect. *Circulation* 37(5):805–815, 1968.
49. Haworth SG: Pulmonary vascular disease in secundum atrial septal defect in childhood. *Am J Cardiol* 51(2):265–272, 1983.
50. Mignosa C, Duca V, Ferlazzo G, et al: Chylothorax: an unusual manifestation of a large atrial septal defect. *J Thorac Cardiovasc Surg* 122(6):1252–1253, 2001.
51. Galve E, Angel J, Evangelista A, et al: Bidirectional shunt in uncomplicated atrial septal defect. *Br Heart J* 51(5):480–484, 1984.
52. Morrison JG, Merrill WH, Friesinger GC, et al: Cyanosis, interatrial communication, and normal pulmonary vascular resistance in adults. *Am J Cardiol* 58(11):1128–1129, 1986.
53. Leong MC, Uebing A, Gatzoulis MA: Percutaneous patent foramen ovale occlusion: current evidence and evolving clinical practice. *Int J Cardiol* 169(4):238–243, 2013.
54. Attenhofer Jost CH, Connolly HM, Danielson GK, et al: Sinus venosus atrial septal defect: long-term postoperative outcome for 115 patients. *Circulation* 112(13):1953–1958, 2005.
55. Arrington CB, Tani LY, Minich LL, et al: An assessment of the electrocardiogram as a screening test for large atrial septal defects in children. *J Electrocardiol* 40(6):484–488, 2007.
56. Valente AM, Sena L, Powell AJ, et al: Cardiac magnetic resonance imaging evaluation of sinus venosus defects. *Pediatr Cardiol* 28(1):51–56, 2007.
57. Ghosh S, Chatterjee S, Black E, et al: Surgical closure of atrial septal defects in adults: effect of age at operation on outcome. *Heart* 88(5):485–487, 2002.
58. Murphy JG, Gersh BJ, McGoon MD, et al: Long-term outcome after surgical repair of isolated atrial septal defect. Follow-up at 27 to 32 years. *N Engl J Med* 323(24):1645–1650, 1990.
59. Neutze JM, Ishikawa T, Clarkson PM, et al: Assessment and follow-up of patients with ventricular septal defect and elevated pulmonary vascular resistance. *Am J Cardiol* 63(5):327–331, 1989.
60. Lim ZS, Salmon AP, Vettukattil JJ, et al: Sildenafil therapy for pulmonary arterial hypertension associated with atrial septal defects. *Int J Cardiol* 118(2):178–182, 2007.
61. Kerut EK, Norfleet WT, Plotnick GD, et al: Patent foramen ovale: a review of associated conditions and the impact of physiological size. *J Am Coll Cardiol* 38(3):613–623, 2001.
62. Overell JR, Bone I, Lees KR: Interatrial septal abnormalities and stroke: a meta-analysis of case-control studies. *Neurology* 55(8): 1172–1179, 2000.
63. Handke M, Harloff A, Olschewski M, et al: Patent foramen ovale and cryptogenic stroke in older patients. *N Engl J Med* 357(22):2262–2268, 2007.
64. Serena J, Marti-Fàbregas J, Santamarina E, et al: Recurrent stroke and massive right-to-left shunt. *Stroke* 39(12):3131–3136, 2008.
65. Mas J-L, Arquizan C, Lamy C, et al: Recurrent cerebrovascular events associated with patent foramen ovale, atrial septal aneurysm, or both. *N Engl J Med* 345(24):1740–1746, 2001.
66. Hernandez J, Moreno R: Percutaneous closure of patent foramen ovale: "closed" door after the last randomized trials? *World J Cardiol* 6(1):1–3, 2014.
67. Rizvi AA, Margey R: PFO and ASD closure in adulthood: where do we stand? *Curr Treat Options Cardiovasc Med* 16:295–310, 2014.
68. Kitsios GD, Dahabreh IJ, Abu Dabrh AM, et al: Patent foramen ovale closure and medical treatments for secondary stroke prevention: a systematic review of observational and randomized evidence. *Stroke* 43(2):422–431, 2012.
69. Amarenco P: Patent foramen ovale and the risk of stroke: smoking gun guilty by association? *Heart* 91(4):441–443, 2005.
70. Dowson A, Mullen MJ, Peatfield R, et al: Migraine Intervention with STARFlex Technology (MIST) Trial: a prospective, multicenter, double-blind, sham-controlled trial to evaluate the effectiveness of patent foramen ovale closure with STARFlex septal repair implant to resolve refractory migraine headache. *Circulation* 117:1397–1404, 2008.
71. Rundek T, Elkind MSV, Di Tullio MR, et al: Patent foramen ovale and migraine: a cross-sectional study from the Northern Manhattan Study (NOMAS). *Circulation* 118(14):1419–1424, 2008.
72. Billinger M, Zbinden R, Mordasini R, et al: Patent foramen ovale closure in recreational divers: effect on decompression illness and ischaemic brain lesions during long-term follow-up. *Heart* 97(23): 1932–1937, 2011.
73. King TD: Secundum atrial septal defect nonoperative closure during cardiac catheterization. *JAMA* 235(23):2506–2509, 1976.
74. Rashkind WJ: Transcatheter treatment of congenital heart disease. *Circulation* 67:711–716, 1983.
75. Rome JJ, Keane JF, Perry SB, et al: Double-umbrella closure of atrial defects. Initial clinical applications. *Circulation* 82(3):751–758, 1990.
76. Das GS, Voss G, Jarvis G, et al: Experimental atrial septal defect closure with a new, transcatheter, self-centering device. *Circulation* 88(4 Pt 1):1754–1764, 1993.
77. Masura J, Gavora P, Formanek A, et al: Transcatheter closure of secundum atrial septal defects using the new self-centering amplatzer septal occluder: initial human experience. *Cathet Cardiovasc Diagn* 42(4):388–393, 1997.
78. Kozlik-Feldmann R, Dalla Pozza R, Römer U, et al: First experience with the 2005 modified Gore Helex ASD occluder system. *Clin Res Cardiol* 95(9):468–473, 2006.
79. Stolt VS, Chessa M, Aubry P, et al: Closure of ostium secundum atrial septum defect with the Atriasept occluder: early European experience. *Catheter Cardiovasc Interv* 75(7):1091–1095, 2010.

80. Pac A, Polat TB, Cetlin I, et al: Figulla ASD Occluder versus Amplatzer Septal Occluder: a comparative study on validation of a novel device for percutaneous closure of atrial septal defects. *J Interv Cardiol* 22(6):489–495, 2009.
81. Saritas T, Kaya MG, Lam YY, et al: A comparative study of Cardi-O-Fix septal occluder versus Amplatzer septal occluder in percutaneous closure of secundum atrial septal defects. *Catheter Cardiovasc Interv* 82(1):116–121, 2013.
82. Zhang D, Zhang Z, Zi Z, et al: Fabrication of graded TiN coatings on nitinol occluders and effects on in vivo nickel release. *Biomed Mater Eng* 18(6):387–393, 2008.
83. Opotowsky AR, Landzberg MJ, Kimmel SE, et al: Trends in the use of percutaneous closure of patent foramen ovale and atrial septal defect in adults, 1998-2004. *JAMA* 299(5):521–522, 2008.
84. Du ZD, Hijazi ZM, Kleinman CS, et al: Comparison between transcatheter and surgical closure of secundum atrial septal defect in children and adults: results of a multicenter nonrandomized trial. *J Am Coll Cardiol* 39(11):1836–1844, 2002.
85. Cowley CG, Lloyd TR, Bove EL, et al: Comparison of results of closure of secundum atrial septal defect by surgery versus Amplatzer septal occluder. *Am J Cardiol* 88(5):589–591, 2001.
86. Du Z-D, Koenig P, Cao QI-L, et al: Comparison of transcatheter closure of secundum atrial septal defect using the Amplatzer septal occluder associated with deficient versus sufficient rims. *Am J Cardiol* 90(8):865–869, 2002.
87. Abaci A, Unlu S, Alsancak Y, et al: Short and long term complications of device closure of atrial septal defect and patent foramen ovale: meta-analysis of 28,142 patients from 203 studies. *Catheter Cardiovasc Interv* 82(7):1123–1138, 2013.
88. Bartakian S, Fagan TE, Schaffer MS, et al: Device closure of secundum atrial septal defects in children. *JACC Cardiovasc Interv* 5(11):1178–1184, 2012.
89. Wagdi P, Ritter M: Patient radiation dose during percutaneous interventional closure of interatrial communications. *J Cardiol* 53(3):368–373, 2009.
90. Schubert S, Kainz S, Peters B, et al: Interventional closure of atrial septal defects without fluoroscopy in adult and pediatric patients. *Clin Res Cardiol* 101(9):691–700, 2012.
91. Wang Y, Hua Y, Li L, et al: Risk factors and prognosis of atrioventricular block after atrial septum defect closure using the amplatzer device. *Pediatr Cardiol* 35(3):550–555, 2014.
92. Amin Z, Hijazi ZM, Bass JL, et al: Erosion of Amplatzer septal occluder device after closure of secundum atrial septal defects: review of registry of complications and recommendations to minimize future risk. *Catheter Cardiovasc Interv* 63(4):496–502, 2004.
93. Crawford GB, Brindis RG, Krucoff MW, et al: Percutaneous atrial septal occluder devices and cardiac erosion: a review of the literature. *Catheter Cardiovasc Interv* 80(2):157–167, 2012.
94. Mathewson JW, Bichell D, Rothman A, et al: Absent posteroinferior and anterosuperior atrial septal defect rims: factors affecting nonsurgical closure of large secundum defects using the Amplatzer occluder. *J Am Soc Echocardiogr* 17(1):62–69, 2004.
95. Kutty S, Hazeem AA, Brown K, et al: Long-term (5-to 20-year) outcomes after transcatheter or surgical treatment of hemodynamically significant isolated secundum atrial septal defect. *Am J Cardiol* 109(9):1348–1352, 2012.
96. Iyer AP, Somanrema K, Pathak S, et al: Comparative study of single- and double-patch techniques for sinus venosus atrial septal defect with partial anomalous pulmonary venous connection. *J Thorac Cardiovasc Surg* 133(3):656–659, 2007.
97. Warden HE, Gustafson RA, Tarnay TJ, et al: An alternative method for repair of partial anomalous pulmonary venous connection to the superior vena cava. *Ann Thorac Surg* 38(6):601–605, 1984.
98. Stewart RD, Bailliard F, Kelle AM, et al: Evolving surgical strategy for sinus venosus atrial septal defect: effect on sinus node function and late venous obstruction. *Ann Thorac Surg* 84(5):1651–1655, 2007.
99. del Nido PJ, Bichell DP: Minimal-access surgery for congenital heart defects. *Semin Thorac Cardiovasc Surg Pediatr Card Surg Annu* 1:75–80, 1998.
100. Yao DK, Chen H, Ma LL, et al: Totally endoscopic atrial septal repair with or without robotic assistance: a systematic review and meta-analysis of case series. *Heart Lung Circ* 22(6):433–440, 2013.
101. Wang F, Li M, Xu X, et al: Totally thoracoscopic surgical closure of atrial septal defect in small children. *Ann Thorac Surg* 92(1):200–203, 2011.
102. Argenziano M, Oz MC, Kohmoto T, et al: Totally endoscopic atrial septal defect repair with robotic assistance. *Circulation* 108(Suppl 1):II191–II194, 2003.
103. Morgan JA, Peacock JC, Kohmoto T, et al: Robotic techniques improve quality of life in patients undergoing atrial septal defect repair. *Ann Thorac Surg* 77(4):1328–1333, 2004.
104. Cuypers JAAE, Opic P, Menting ME, et al: The unnatural history of an atrial septal defect: longitudinal 35 year follow up after surgical closure at young age. *Heart* 99(18):1346–1352, 2013.
105. Oliver JM, Gallego P, González A, et al: Predisposing conditions for atrial fibrillation in atrial septal defect with and without operative closure. *Am J Cardiol* 89(1):39–43, 2002.
106. Hawe A, Rastelli GC, Brandenburg RO, et al: Embolic complications following repair of atrial septal defects. *Circulation* 39(5 Suppl 1):I185–I191, 1969.
107. Sasidharan B, Moideen I, Warrier G, et al: Cardiac herniation following closure of atrial septal defect through limited posterior thoracotomy. *Interact Cardiovasc Thorac Surg* 5:272–274, 2006.
108. Cherup LL, Siewers RD, Futrell JW: Breast and pectoral muscle maldevelopment after anterolateral and posterolateral thoracotomies in children. *Ann Thorac Surg* 41(5):492–497, 1986.
109. Reybrouck T, Bisschop A, Dumoulin M, et al: Cardiorespiratory exercise capacity after surgical closure of atrial septal defect is influenced by the age at surgery. *Am Heart J* 122(4):1073–1078, 1991.
110. Pearlman AS, Borer JS, Clark CE, et al: Abnormal right ventricular size and ventricular septal motion after atrial septal defect closure: etiology and functional significance. *Am J Cardiol* 41(2):295–301, 1978.
111. Brochu M-C, Baril J-F, Dore A, et al: Improvement in exercise capacity in asymptomatic and mildly symptomatic adults after atrial septal defect percutaneous closure. *Circulation* 106(14):1821–1826, 2002.
112. Konstantinides S, Geibel A, Olschewski M, et al: A comparison of surgical and medical therapy for atrial septal defect in adults. *N Engl J Med* 333(8):469–473, 1995.
113. Takaya Y, Taniguchi M, Akagi T, et al: Long-term effects of transcatheter closure of atrial septal defect on cardiac remodeling and exercise capacity in patients older than 40 years with a reduction in cardiopulmonary function. *J Interv Cardiol* 26(2):195–199, 2012.
114. Du ZD, Cao QL, Koenig P, et al: Speed of normalization of right ventricular volume overload after transcatheter closure of atrial septal defect in children and adults. *Am J Cardiol* 88(12):1450–1453, 2001.
115. Kort HW, Balzer DT, Johnson MC: Resolution of right heart enlargement after closure of secundum atrial septal defect with transcatheter technique1. *J Am Coll Cardiol* 38(5):1528 1532, 2001.
116. Helber U, Baumann R, Seboldt H, et al: Atrial septal defect in adults: cardiopulmonary exercise capacity before and 4 months and 10 years after defect closure. *J Am Coll Cardiol* 29(6):1345–1350, 1997.
117. Jemielity M: Do patients over 40 years of age benefit from surgical closure of atrial septal defects? *Heart* 85(3):300–303, 2001.
118. de Lezo JS, Medina A, Romero M, et al: Effectiveness of percutaneous device occlusion for atrial septal defect in adult patients with pulmonary hypertension. *Am Heart J* 144(5):877–880, 2002.
119. John Sutton MG, Tajik AJ, McGoon DC: Atrial septal defect in patients ages 60 years or older: operative results and long-term postoperative follow-up. *Circulation* 64(2):402–409, 1981.
120. Hörer J, Eicken A, Müller S, et al: Risk factors for prolonged intensive care treatment following atrial septal defect closure in adults. *Int J Cardiol* 125(1):57–61, 2008.
121. Masutani S, Senzaki H: Left ventricular function in adult patients with atrial septal defect: implication for development of heart failure after transcatheter closure. *J Card Fail* 17(11):957–963, 2011.
122. Roos-Hesselink JW, Meijboom FJ, Spitaels SEC, et al: Excellent survival and low incidence of arrhythmias, stroke and heart failure long-term after surgical ASD closure at young age. *Eur Heart J* 24:190–197, 2003.

123. Giamberti A, Chessa M, Foresti S, et al: Combined atrial septal defect surgical closure and irrigated radiofrequency ablation in adult patients. *Ann Thorac Surg* 82(4):1327–1331, 2006.
124. Im Y-M, Kim JB, Yun S-C, et al: Arrhythmia surgery for atrial fibrillation associated with atrial septal defect: right-sided maze versus biatrial maze. *J Thorac Cardiovasc Surg* 145(3):648–655, e1, 2013.
125. Church WS: Congenital malformation of heart: abnormal septum in left auricle. *Trans Path Soz* 19:188–190, 1868.
126. Hansing CE, Young WP, Rowe GG: Cor triatriatum dexter. Persistent right sinus venosus valve. *Am J Cardiol* 30(5):559–564, 1972.
127. Trento A, Zuberbuhler JR, Anderson RH: Divided right atrium (prominence of the eustacian and thebesian valves). *J Thorac Cardiovasc Surg* 96(3):457–463, 1988.
128. Van Praagh R, Corsini I: Cor triatriatum: pathologic anatomy and a consideration of morphogenesis based on 13 postmortem cases and a study of normal development of the pulmonary vein and atrial septum in 83 human embryos. *Am Heart J* 78(3):379–405, 1969.
129. Parsons CG: Cor Triatriatum. Concerning the nature of an anomalous septum in the left auricle. *Br Heart J* 12(4):327, 1950.
130. Fowler JK: Fowler: membranous band in the left auricle. *Tran Pathol Soc Lond* 33:77–94, 1881.
131. Gharagozloo F, Bulkley BH, Hutchins GM: A proposed pathogenesis of cor triatriatum: impingement of the left superior vena cava on the developing left atrium. *Am Heart J* 94(5):618–626, 1977.
132. Geggel RL, Fulton DR, Chernoff HL, et al: Cor triatriatum associated with partial anomalous pulmonary venous connection to the coronary sinus: echocardiographic and angiocardiographic features. *Pediatr Cardiol* 8(4):279–283, 1987.
133. Yaroglu Kazanci S, Emani S, McElhinney DB: Outcome after repair of cor triatriatum. *Am J Cardiol* 109(3):412–416, 2012.
134. Marín-García J, Tandon R, Lucas RV, Jr, et al: Cor triatriatum: study of 20 cases. *Am J Cardiol* 35(1):59–66, 1975.
135. Nagatsu M: Clinical classification and surgical treatment of cor triatriatum. *Nihon Kyobu Geka Gakkai Zasshi* 40(4):473–484, 1992.
136. Niwayma G: Cor triatriatum. *Am Heart J* 59(2):291–317, 1960.
137. Endo M, Yamaki S, Ohmi M, et al: Pulmonary vascular changes induced by congenital obstruction of pulmonary venous return. *Ann Thorac Surg* 69(1):193–197, 2000.
138. Nakajima H, Kobayashi J, Kurita T, et al: Maze procedure and cor triatriatum repair. *Ann Thorac Surg* 74(1):251–253, 2002.
139. Huang T-C, Lee C-L, Lin C-C, et al: Use of Inoue balloon dilatation method for treatment of Cor triatriatum stenosis in a child. *Catheter Cardiovasc Interv* 57(2):252–256, 2002.

CHAPTER 115

SURGICAL CONSIDERATIONS IN PULMONARY VEIN ANOMALIES

Mauro Lo Rito • Osami Honjo • Christopher A. Caldarone

CHAPTER OUTLINE

ETIOLOGY

Normal embryologic development of the pulmonary venous system involves creation of a connection between the left atrium and the pulmonary venous plexus, and subsequent regression of systemic-to-pulmonary venous connections. Inappropriate connection of the pulmonary venous system to the systemic venous system is termed *anomalous pulmonary venous drainage*.

As part of normal embryologic development, the lungs are derived from buds arising from the primitive foregut. During the initial stages of pulmonary development (25 to 27 days' gestation), the pulmonary venous drainage is through the cardinal and umbilical-vitelline venous system (systemic veins). During the later stages of development (27 to 29 days' gestation), an outpouching of the common atrium forms to the leftward of the developing septal primum.[1] The structure, termed the common pulmonary vein, primordial pulmonary vein, or pulmonary pit, extends and bifurcates into the pulmonary venous plexus and establishes venous drainage of the developing lung buds at 28 to 30 days' gestation (Fig. 115-1). Thereafter, the connection between the lung buds and the systemic venous system regresses, leaving the developing lungs with direct drainage to the left atrium.

Human genetic studies of kindreds with total anomalous pulmonary venous drainage showed an autosomal-dominant inheritance with incomplete penetrance and variable expression with involvement of genetic loci located in the human chromosome 4q12.[2] During heart morphogenesis, an avascular zone forms between the caudal primitive vascular structures (that will become part of the systemic vein circulation) and the pulmonary vein plexus, which arises from the lung.[3] Disruption of this avascular zone and of the patterning of the pulmonary vein may be the primary developmental anomaly in the genesis of total anomalous pulmonary connection. In mice, a secreted repellent guidance molecule, semaphorin 3d, is located in the avascular zone and plays a key role in the correct patterning of the pulmonary vein connection to the left atrium (Fig. 115-2). Deficiency of

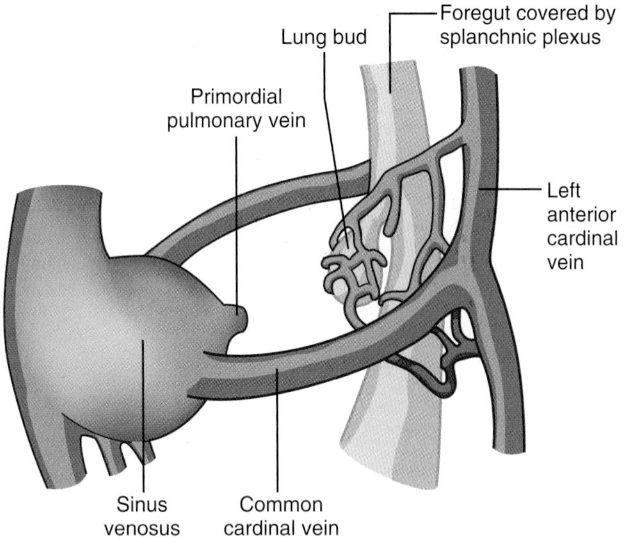

FIGURE 115-1 ■ Lung buds arise from the primitive foregut with systemic venous drainage during early embryologic development. At later stages, an outpouching from the common atrium extends and bifurcates into the pulmonary venous plexus to establish drainage to the atrium, followed by regression of the systemic venous drainage. (Modified from Jonas RA, Smolinsky A, Mayer JE, et al: Obstructed pulmonary venous drainage with total anomalous pulmonary venous connection to the coronary sinus. *Am J Cardiol* 59:431–435, 1987.)

semaphorin 3d is associated with anomalous connection of pulmonary veins with both atria or the coronary sinus. The mechanism suggested is based on the lack of repulsion guidance that leads to a broad domain of abnormal endothelial sprouts from the lung buds which may persist when blood flow through the connection begins (Fig. 115-3). In preliminary studies in humans with anomalous pulmonary venous connection, specific mutations in the gene sequence for semaphorin 3d have been identified.[4]

Anomalous pulmonary venous drainage can result from failure of fusion between the left atrial outpouching and the pulmonary venous plexus, or from malposition of the relationship between the atrial outpouching and the development of the atrial septum. If all the pulmonary veins maintain an anomalous connection to a single systemic venous site, the lesion is termed *total anomalous pulmonary venous drainage*. If all the pulmonary veins drain anomalously to multiple discrete systemic veins, the lesion is called *mixed total anomalous pulmonary venous drainage*. If one to three pulmonary veins drain via an anomalous pathway and at least one pulmonary vein drains to the left atrium, the lesion is termed *partial anomalous pulmonary venous drainage*.

PARTIAL ANOMALOUS PULMONARY VENOUS DRAINAGE

Anatomy

Partial anomalous pulmonary venous drainage is characterized by a failure of one to three of the pulmonary veins to connect with the left atrium during fetal development. Typically, the pulmonary vein has an abnormal connection to the superior vena cava near the cavoatrial junction. More than 80% of patients have associated congenital heart defects, the most common of which is an atrial septal defect. A minority of patients (18%) have an intact atrial septum.[5] Most commonly, a combination of right upper and middle lobe pulmonary veins drain to the superior vena caval–right atrial junction (Fig. 115-4). Less commonly, isolated anomalous right upper lobe venous drainage is present. Least commonly, the entire right lung drains via an anomalous vein into the right atrium.[5] Other less common sites of anomalous venous drainage include the inferior vena cava (e.g., as part of the scimitar syndrome), the left-sided superior vena cava, and the innominate vein. The left pulmonary veins rarely can also have an anomalous drainage to the systemic venous circulation as isolated disease.[6]

Presentation

Patients are often asymptomatic and display a murmur noted on routine examination that is caused by increased flow across the pulmonary valve. A split and prominent second heart sound is also present. Symptomatic patients display the sequelae of a left-to-right shunt, including decreased exercise tolerance and poor growth. Patients are not cyanotic unless they have developed pulmonary hypertension as a late manifestation of a large left-to-right shunt. In such patients, Eisenmenger syndrome is characterized by the reversal of the shunt from right to left in association with an atrial septal defect.

Pathophysiology

The dominant hemodynamic abnormality is related to the left-to-right shunt imposed by pulmonary venous drainage into the right atrium. In the absence of an atrial septal defect, the left-to-right shunt is limited by the amount of flow in the anomalous pulmonary vein. In contrast, an associated atrial septal defect adds potential for increased left-to-right shunting at the atrial level. Increased right-sided flow can lead to right ventricular dilation, tricuspid insufficiency, and supraventricular arrhythmias.

Surgical Repair

The goal of surgical therapy is to divert the anomalous pulmonary venous effluent to the left atrium in an unobstructed fashion. In the presence of a sinus venosus atrial septal defect and anomalous right upper pulmonary veins, the flow is diverted with a baffle constructed along the edge of the sinus venosus atrial septal defect. The defect may have to be enlarged to create an unobstructed pathway to the left atrium. In the absence of an atrial septal defect (i.e., the atrial septum is intact), an atrial septal defect must be created in the region of the fossa ovalis with extension in the region of the limbus and a similar baffle constructed to divert flow from the anomalous pulmonary vein to the newly created atrial septal defect.

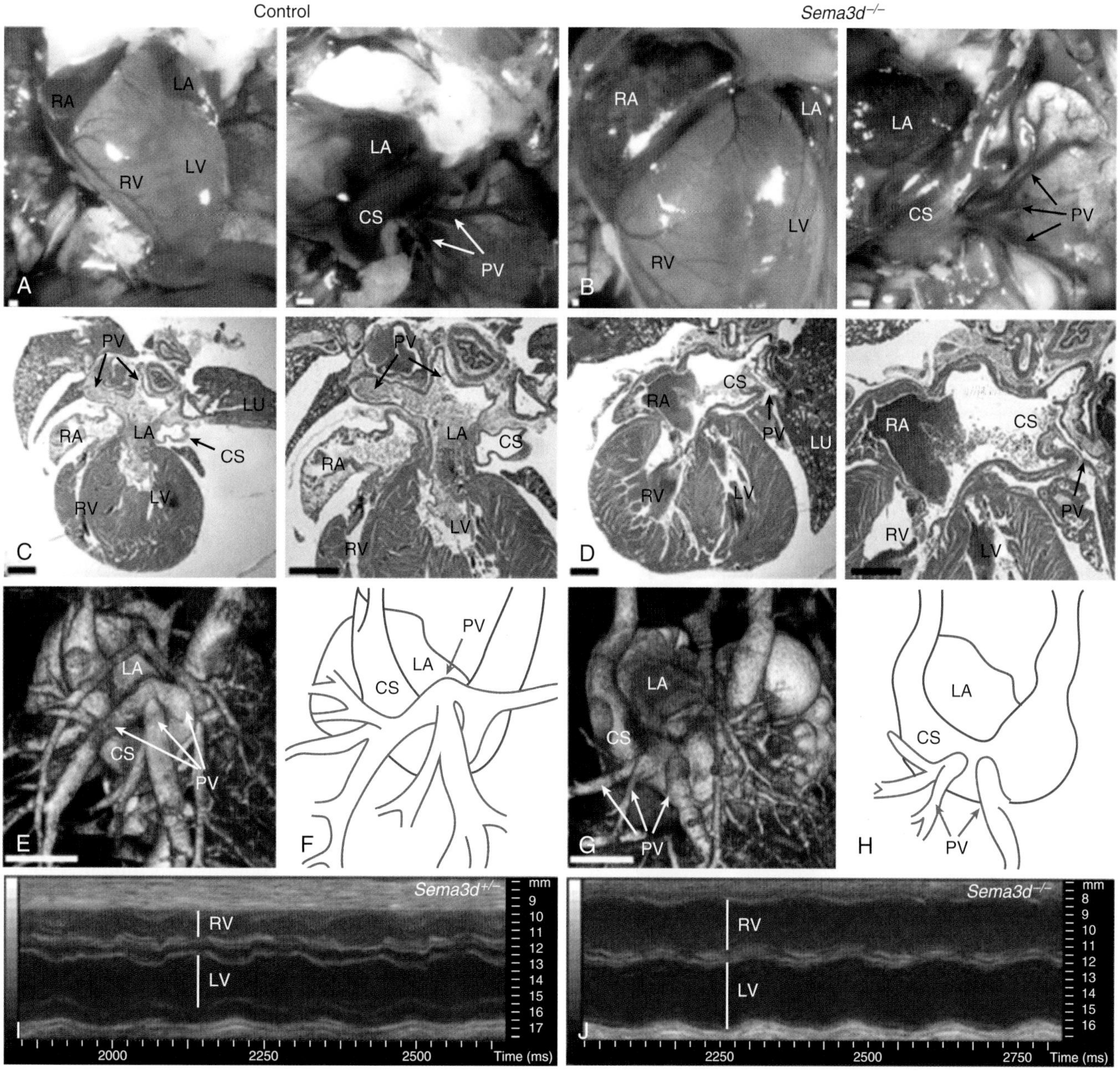

FIGURE 115-2 Mice heart comparison between Semaphorin3d–/– type and control. Anterior views of **(A)** adult control and **(B)** Sema3d–/– hearts. Severe cardiomegaly is showed the mutants **(B)** because of right atrial (RA) and right ventricular (RV) dilation. In mutant mouse pulmonary veins (PV) enter the coronary sinus (CS; in **B**, left image). In control mice **(A)**, pulmonary veins (PV) enter the left atrium (LA) as normal. **C** and **D**, Photomicrographs of hematoxylin and eosin–stained sections showing a normal connection of the pulmonary veins to the left atrium in Sema3d+/– mice **(C)** and anomalous pulmonary venous connections to the coronary sinus in Sema3d–/– mice **(D)**. **E–H**, Volume-rendered micro–computed tomography images (dorsal view) showing the pulmonary veins entering the posterior left atrium in a newborn wild type mouse **(E)** and entering the coronary sinus in a newborn mutant mouse **(G)**. **F** and **H**, The diagrams of the microCT images in **E** and **G**, respectively. **I** and **J**, M-mode echocardiograms through the ventricles of a Sema3d+/– **(I)** and a Sema3d–/– **(J)** heart showing the relative dilation of the right ventricle in an adult Sema3d–/– mouse and paradoxical septal wall motion indicative of right-sided volume overload. Scale bars (in panels A-E and G) = 1 mm. *LU,* Lung; *LV,* left ventricle. (Modified from Degenhardt K, Singh MK, Aghajanian H, et al: Semaphorin 3d signaling defects are associated with anomalous pulmonary venous connections. *Nat Med* 19:760–765, 2013.)

Planning the Superior Vena Caval Cannulation

Careful review of the anatomy by preoperative echocardiography, computed tomography, or magnetic resonance imaging[7] is the single most important component in developing an operative plan. Definition of the pulmonary venous anatomy and associated defects allows assessment of options for cannulation techniques and surgical approaches. This is especially important in preparation for partial anomalous pulmonary venous drainage, because the location of the anomalous pulmonary venous

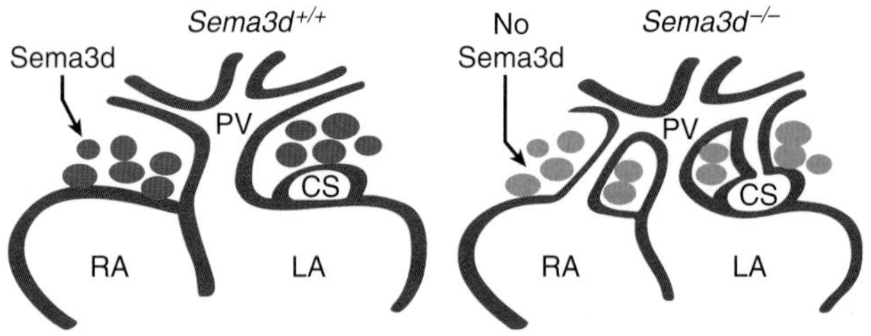

FIGURE 115-3 ■ Model showing the role of Sema3d in pulmonary vein patterning. Normally *(left)* Sema3d is expressed between the heart and the developing pulmonary vasculature where it repels endothelial cells to prevent the formation of anomalous connections. Deficiency of Sema3d *(right)* allows endothelial cells to enter this region and form anomalous vascular connections. *CS,* Coronary sinus; *LA,* left atrium; *PV,* pulmonary veins; *RA;* right atrium. (Modified from Degenhardt K, Singh MK, Aghajanian H, et al: Semaphorin 3d signaling defects are associated with anomalous pulmonary venous connections. *Nat Med* 19:760–765, 2013.)

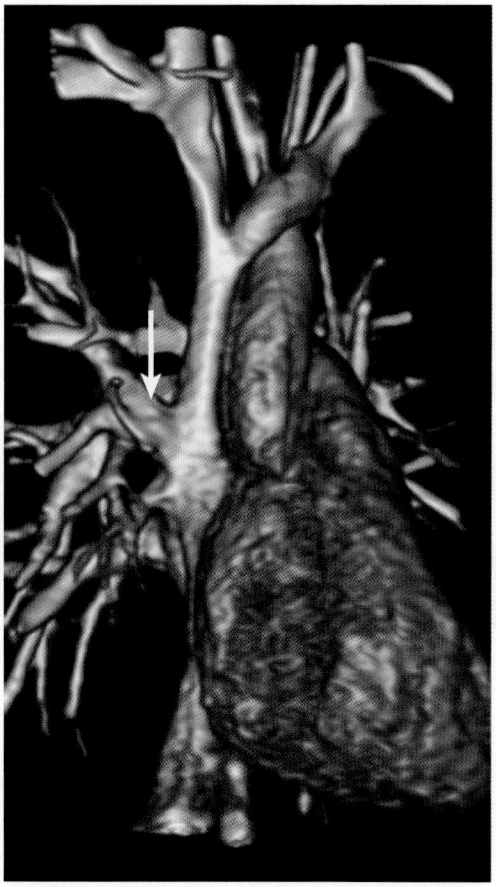

FIGURE 115-4 ■ A contrast-enhanced magnetic resonance three-dimensional angiogram seen from right anterior projection shows an anomalous connection of the right upper and middle pulmonary vein draining into the superior vena cava *(arrow).* The right lower pulmonary vein normally drains into the left atrium. (Modified from Vyas HV, Greenberg SB, Krishnamurthy R: MR imaging and CT evaluation of congenital pulmonary vein abnormalities in neonates and infants. *Radiographics* 32:87–98, 2012.)

drainage determines the feasibility of a minimally invasive approach and placement of venous cannulas. A common clinical scenario involves an anomalous right upper pulmonary vein inserting high into the superior vena cava, at or above the level of the pulmonary artery. Options for control of the superior vena cava include a high cannulation of the superior vena cava, cannulation of the innominate vein, or percutaneous cannulation via the internal jugular vein with vacuum-assisted venous drainage. A minimally invasive approach through a lower midline partial sternal split can be difficult when a high insertion of an anomalous pulmonary vein is present. In this case a right posterior lateral minithoracotomy can be used as a minimally invasive approach to achieve better access to the high pulmonary veins. The cannulation strategy for this approach includes percutaneous cannulation of the internal jugular vein and direct surgical cannulation of the right femoral vein and artery. The use of peripheral cannulation augmented with vacuum assisted venous drainage is helpful.[8] Limitations to the use of this approach are: patient's weight less than 20 kg and femoral vein or artery anomalies. During cardiopulmonary bypass, monitoring of right leg near-infrared spectroscopy is suggested. Near-infrared spectroscopy saturations less than 30% suggest that distal leg perfusion is insufficient. In patients with small femoral arteries, the use of a graft sewn to the femoral artery in end-to-side fashion can be helpful to avoid problems with distal leg perfusion.[9]

A final technique to consider is the use of a straight venous cannula in the right atrial appendage, which can be directed into the superior vena cava. After snaring the cava around the cannula (cephalad to the anomalous pulmonary vein insertion), an atrial incision allows access to the origin of the anomalous pulmonary vein from within the atrium. Although this technique is easily accomplished with a minimally invasive lower midline partial sternal split, working around the cannula through the right atrial–superior vena caval junction can be challenging.

Before initiation of cardiopulmonary bypass (CPB), the location of the pulmonary veins is confirmed. Drainage to the superior vena cava requires dissection of the lateral margin of the superior vena cava to identify all pulmonary vein branches. During dissection of the superior vena cava and right pulmonary veins particular attention is needed to avoid injury to the right phrenic nerve. Frequently, multiple branches drain into the vena cava through a large confluence. The source of the veins is not always clear, and any systemic veins draining into the region must be identified. When the source of the pulmonary venous drainage is not clearly defined, needle aspiration can be used to determine the oxygen saturation of the effluent, and then the systemic veins can be distinguished from the pulmonary veins.

After heparinization, cannulation, and initiation of normothermic CPB, the aorta is clamped and blood cardioplegic arrest is obtained. It is often helpful to place a vent into the left atrium for later de-airing. A lateral right atriotomy is made and the atrium is explored to identify any additional anomalies (Fig. 115-5). If the atrial septum is intact, an atrial septal defect is created by incising the region of the foramen ovale and extending the incision

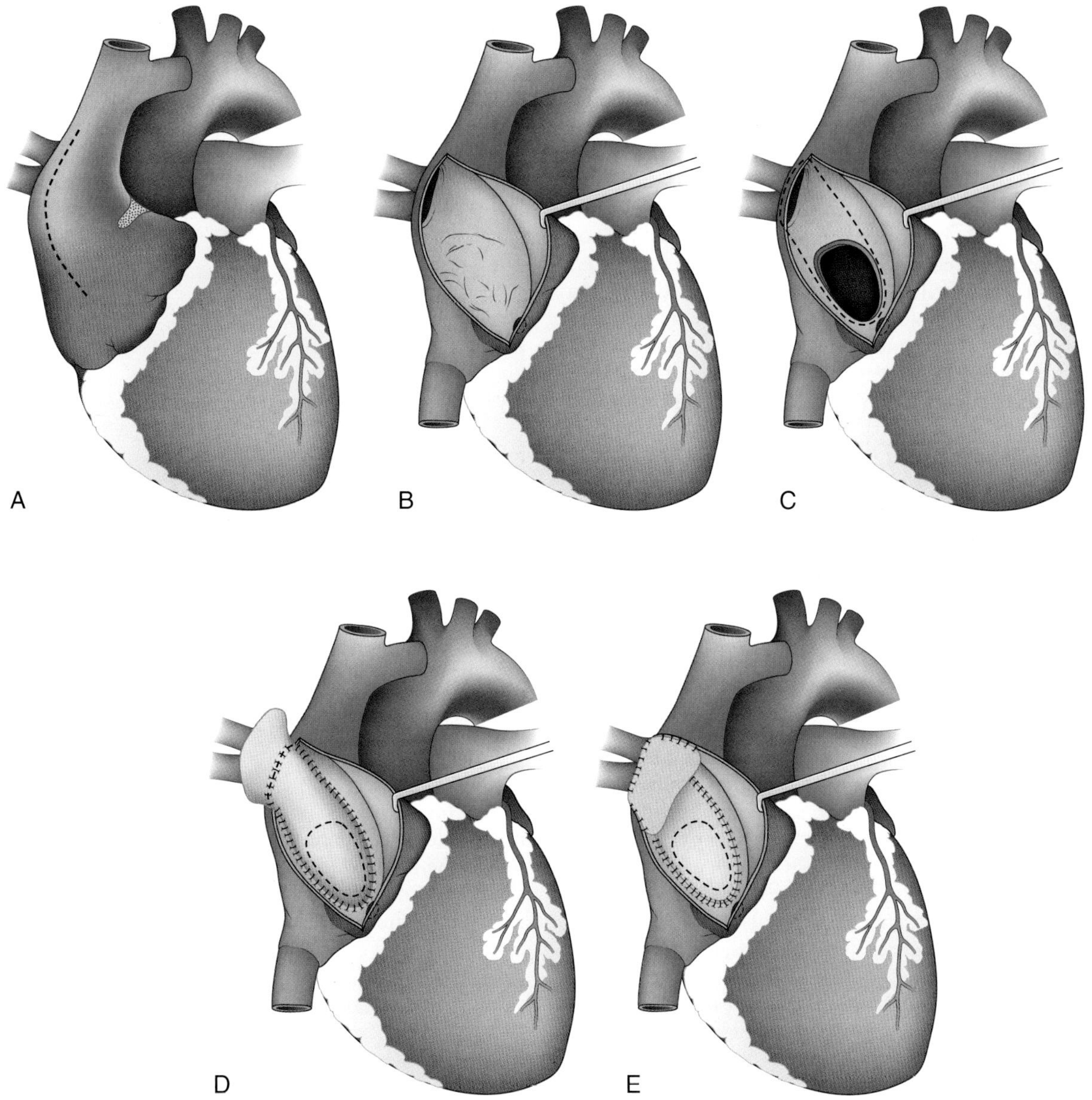

FIGURE 115-5 ■ **A,** After initiation of cardiopulmonary bypass and cardioplegic arrest, a lateral right atrial incision is made *(dashed line)*. The *stippled area* represents the approximate location of the sinoatrial node. **B,** The orifice of the anomalous pulmonary veins and the intact atrial septum are exposed. A secundum atrial septal defect is created by excising the septum primum in the region of the limbus, with care taken to avoid potential injury to the conduction system by keeping clear of the triangle of Koch. **C,** The limbus can be resected cephalad to increase the diameter of the atrial septal orifice. **D,** A glutaraldehyde-treated autologous pericardial patch is sutured in place along the rim of the newly created defect, thereby creating a tunnel from the pulmonary vein orifice to the left atrium. **E,** The patch is deliberately longer than necessary to reach the pulmonary vein orifice, and the redundant portion is left unattached as the suture line is extended across the edge of the divided pulmonary vein–atrial edge. The redundant portion of the patch is then folded anteriorly to augment the diameter of the superior cavoatrial junction, thereby preventing obstruction of the superior vena cava.

across the limbus in the direction of the anomalous pulmonary vein. Resection in the region of the limbus allows enlargement of the newly created atrial septal defect. Injury to the sinus node artery can occur when creating the atrial septal defect in patients whose artery courses through the superior portion of the intra-atrial septum. Enlargement of the sinus venosus defect might be necessary if it is too small to divert the anomalous pulmonary veins to the left atrium. Typically, a glutaraldehyde-treated pericardial patch can be used to create a baffle, so that pulmonary venous blood flows beneath the baffle and through the atrial septal defect into the left atrium.

Systemic venous blood from the superior vena cava must pass to the right atrium over the pulmonary vein–to–left atrial baffle without obstruction. If the origin of the pulmonary vein was high in the superior vena cava, the baffle must be constructed carefully to avoid obstruction to flow on either side of the baffle. A longitudinal incision in the lateral aspect of the superior vena cava allows the baffle construction to be better visualized. Placement of the incision on the lateral aspect of the superior vena cava is important to diminish the risk of injury to the sinus node. Closure of the superior vena cava incision with a generous patch to augment the superior vena cava diameter can be used to prevent stenosis of the superior cavoatrial junction.

Alternatively, a new anastomosis between the superior vena cava and the right atrial appendage is established by dividing the superior vena cava cephalad to the anomalous pulmonary venous entry and translocating the cephalad end of the superior vena cava to the right atrial appendage (Warden technique). The divided cardiac end of the superior vena cava (bearing the anomalous pulmonary venous connection) is closed, and a baffle is created from the orifice of the superior vena cava to the newly created atrial septal defect.[5,10] By creating a new superior vena caval–right atrial junction, this procedure eliminates the need to partition the superior vena cava with a baffle dividing the systemic and pulmonary venous flow paths. This approach can be particularly helpful in infants and small children with a high insertion of an anomalous pulmonary vein into the superior vena cava.

Results

Early and long-term outcomes for patients after repair are excellent. In children, closure of an associated atrial septal defect almost eliminates the risk of late development of atrial arrhythmias. However, in adults, closure of the atrial septal defect is associated with persistent risk of development of atrial arrhythmias.[11] Although extrapolation of these data for atrial septal defect closure to patients with partial anomalous pulmonary venous drainage and intact atrial septum has not been specifically validated, it seems reasonable to conclude that early removal of a left-to-right shunt associated with right ventricular overload is appropriate. In fact, surgical closure of the sinus venosus atrial septal defect at an older age is associated with increased risk of mortality, adverse events, and poor functional outcomes.[12]

Pertinent complications after repair of partial anomalous pulmonary venous drainage include stenosis of the superior vena cava or the anomalous pulmonary vein,[13] residual atrial septal defects, and atrial arrhythmias or sinus node dysfunction (or both).[14] Failure to include all pulmonary veins in the newly constructed baffle to the left atrium can result in a residual left-to-right shunt. However, incorporation of a systemic vein into the newly constructed baffle results in a residual right-to-left shunt. Finally, injury to the sinus node or sinus node artery can lead to the requirement for pacemaker insertion in patients with severe sinus node dysfunction.[14]

SCIMITAR SYNDROME

Scimitar syndrome is an unusual congenital anomaly that is manifested by partial anomalous pulmonary venous drainage of the right lung to the inferior vena cava; it is often associated with hypoplasia of the right lung, dextrocardia, systemic pulmonary arterial supply from the abdominal aorta to the lower lobe of the right lung, and bronchial abnormalities. Other commonly associated anomalies include atrial septal defect, aortic coarctation, and a left-sided superior vena cava.[15,16] The morphology of the anomalous pulmonary venous drainage to the right lower lobe creates a characteristic appearance to the right-sided heart border suggestive of a Turkish sword, hence the term *scimitar syndrome* (Fig. 115-6). The right-sided pulmonary veins drain to the inferior portions of the right atrium, the inferior vena caval–right atrial junction, or, more commonly, the inferior vena cava below the diaphragm. Stenosis can occur in 10% to 20% of scimitar veins at their junction to the inferior vena cava.[16,17]

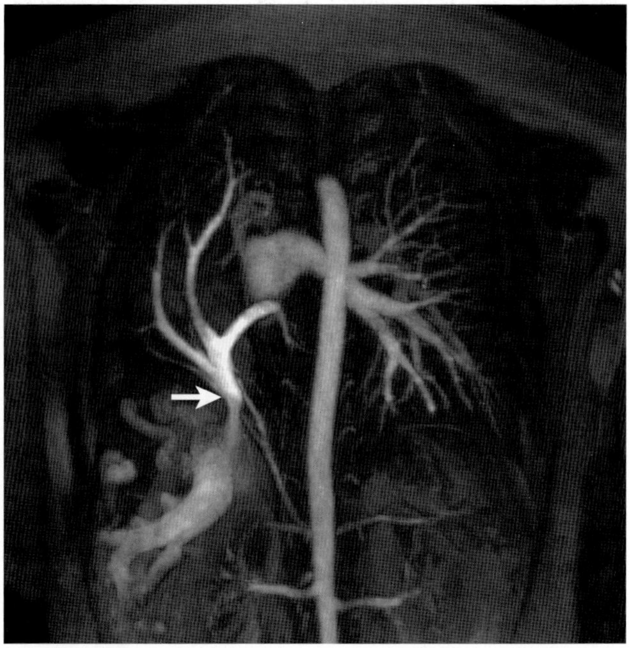

FIGURE 115-6 ■ Contrast-enhanced magnetic resonance angiogram shows the scimitar vein draining most of the right pulmonary venous blood flow into the inferior vena cava *(arrow)*. The scimitar vein has severe stenosis at its junction with the inferior vena cava.

The presentation of patients with scimitar syndrome can be variable and depends on the severity of the associated lesions. There are generally two forms of clinical presentation in scimitar syndrome: (1) an infantile form with significant symptoms, morbidity, and mortality and (2) a form with mild symptoms seen in children or adults. At the most benign end of the spectrum, patients can display an asymptomatic flow murmur on physical examination as a result of increased pulmonary blood flow secondary to the left-to-right shunt caused by the anomalous pulmonary venous drainage to the inferior vena cava. At the most severe end of the spectrum, infants can exhibit symptoms of severe congestive heart failure, failure to thrive, tachypnea, and occasionally cyanosis. Infantile pulmonary artery pressures are often elevated (e.g., >40% of the systemic pressure), with a ratio of pulmonary blood flow (Qp) to systemic blood flow (Qs), or Qp/Qs, of up to 2:1.[15]

Surgical Management

The management strategy for patients with scimitar syndrome is determined by the degree of right lung hypoplasia, the presence of aortopulmonary sources of blood flow to the right lung, and the location and pattern of the right-sided pulmonary venous drainage. The degree of right lung hypoplasia is an important determinant of the likelihood of salvaging a functional right lung, and in cases of severe hypoplasia, a right pneumonectomy has been advocated.[18] In cases with less severe hypoplasia, attention is turned to correction of the pulmonary venous drainage patterns, control of aortopulmonary sources of blood flow, and correction of associated anomalies. Control of the aortopulmonary sources of blood flow can be achieved with coil embolization in the catheterization laboratory or with ligation in the operating room.[19]

Surgical repair of the pulmonary venous drainage is designed to create unobstructed flow from the anomalous pulmonary vein to the left atrium. To accomplish this repair, a direct surgical approach is to place a long baffle in the lumen of the inferior vena cava to channel the anomalous pulmonary vein effluent to the right atrium, and then through an atrial septal defect to the left atrium (originally described by Zubiate and Kay in 1962).[20] It can be challenging to create an unobstructed baffle when the anomalous pulmonary venous connection is relatively caudad in the inferior vena cava. To construct a partitioning baffle, a period of circulatory arrest is typically necessary to secure a baffle between the pulmonary vein orifice and left atrium that allows unobstructed pulmonary vein flow without restricting flow in the inferior vena cava or in nearby hepatic veins.

When partitioning the inferior vena cava between the systemic and pulmonary venous flow paths, a right atrial incision can be carried down to the level of the anomalous pulmonary vein orifice, and the orifice is augmented with a patch of autologous pericardium if stenosis is present. The baffle is then constructed in the lumen of the inferior vena cava, and, if necessary, the inferior vena cava diameter can be augmented with a patch to ensure that there is no residual obstruction in the vena cava. This technique has a relatively high incidence of late stenosis, presumably because of the length of the intracaval baffle and because the blood must pass through a nearly 180-degree turn as it travels caudad toward the inferior vena cava and then cephalad up through the baffle to the atrial septal defect.[16,18]

A second approach is to divide the anomalous pulmonary vein and reimplant it at a convenient location in the right atrium and then create a baffle to divert flow to the left atrium through an atrial septal incision or atrial septal defect if present.[16,21] This approach provides a shorter, more direct pathway for the pulmonary venous effluent. It is difficult to use this approach, however, when the anomalous pulmonary vein courses in the posterior portion of the lung and necessitates a great deal of augmentation to create an anastomosis with the atrium. When the pulmonary vein passes through the posterior mediastinum and the right lung is relatively hypoplastic, Huddleston and associates[18] recommend pneumonectomy because of the high incidence of late stenosis with reimplantation techniques. As further justification of pneumonectomy in this setting, Huddleston and colleagues point out that the left lung has typically undergone some compensatory growth. Furthermore, perfusion scans typically demonstrate diminished pulmonary blood flow to the right lung in patients with scimitar syndrome.[15] Calhoun and Mee[22] described an alternative surgical approach for this entity, in which the inferior vena cava is transected under deep hypothermic circulatory arrest and divided into posterior (the anomalous pulmonary vein channel) and anterior (inferior vena cava and hepatic vein) compartments with a pericardial patch. An incision is made on the inferior aspect of the left atrium and carried to the atrial septum. The posterior compartment of the inferior vena cava is sutured to the left atriotomy, and the pericardial patch is used to close the atrial septal defect. The anterior compartment of the inferior vena cava is anastomosed to the right atrium. This approach connects the anomalous pulmonary vein to the left atrium at a relatively gentle angle. Brown and coworkers[17] reported favorable results with direct anastomosis of the anomalous pulmonary vein to the left atrium via right thoracotomy without the use of CPB.

Results and Complications

Survival after complete repair (embolization or ligation of anomalous pulmonary arterial flow with correction of the anomalous pulmonary venous return) is anticipated in older children and adults. In recent series, 5-year survival rates have reached 100%, although a significant incidence of late pulmonary vein obstruction remains. In the infantile form of the lesion, however, hospital mortality is higher and depends on the degree of lung hypoplasia and the presence of pulmonary hypertension.[15] Even with a technically perfect repair, blood flow to the right lung often remains diminished. The left-to-right shunt, however, is eliminated. Pulmonary venous obstruction is a prevalent late finding in many series and may be related to the surgical techniques used. Long pulmonary venous pathways through the inferior vena cava with acute angulation may predispose to stenosis. Recent reports using direct reimplantation techniques have demonstrated minimal rates of postoperative stenosis in small series of patients.[17] Pneumonectomy remains an option in patients with persistently compromised pulmonary blood flow resulting from pulmonary hypertension or pulmonary venous obstruction.[18]

TOTAL ANOMALOUS PULMONARY VENOUS DRAINAGE

Total anomalous pulmonary venous drainage is a condition in which all the pulmonary venous effluent from the lungs drains to the systemic venous system, creating a large left-to-right shunt. This entity accounts for 1% to 3% of all congenital heart malformations, with an incidence of 7.1 per 100,000 live births.[23] A right-to-left shunt must be present to allow blood to reach the left ventricle and thereby contribute to systemic cardiac output. Commonly, this shunt is at the atrial level as an atrial septal defect or patent foramen ovale. Less commonly, the shunt may be present as a ventricular septal defect. The absence of a shunt is incompatible with survival, and the magnitude of the shunt determines the systemic cardiac output.

Anatomy

Although well palliated in utero, infants with total anomalous pulmonary venous drainage have abnormalities in the pulmonary vascular system. There is often hypertrophy of the media of the pulmonary veins and arteries, intimal fibrous thickening of the pulmonary veins, and lymphangiectasia. These findings are accentuated in patients with pulmonary hypertension and evidence of pulmonary venous obstruction.[24] The various types of total anomalous pulmonary venous drainage are classified by the site of connection to the systemic venous system.

Supracardiac Anatomy

Supracardiac drainage is the most common anatomic variant, occurring in 45% to 55% of patients with total anomalous pulmonary venous drainage.[23,25] The venous connection is typically through a pulmonary venous confluence behind the left atrium to a connecting vein (often termed a vertical vein) to the innominate vein. Other sites of pulmonary–systemic connection can be to a left- or right-sided superior vena cava.[23]

Cardiac Anatomy

The pulmonary–systemic venous connection can be present at the cardiac level in 15% to 20% of patients.[23,25] In this setting, the pulmonary veins typically drain to a pulmonary venous confluence behind the left atrium. The confluence then drains into the coronary sinus or, less commonly, to the right atrium. In some patients, the right- and left-sided pulmonary veins converge into a short vertical vein before draining into the coronary sinus. The latter variant may be more susceptible to late obstruction.[25,26]

Infracardiac Anatomy

The systemic–pulmonary venous connection is present at the infracardiac level in 15% to 26% of patients.[23,25] In this setting, the pulmonary veins drain to a confluence behind the left atrium, which drains via a descending vertical vein to the portal vein, to the ductus venosus (Fig. 115-7) or directly to the inferior vena cava. This subset displays obstruction in the pulmonary venous circuit in the majority of patients.

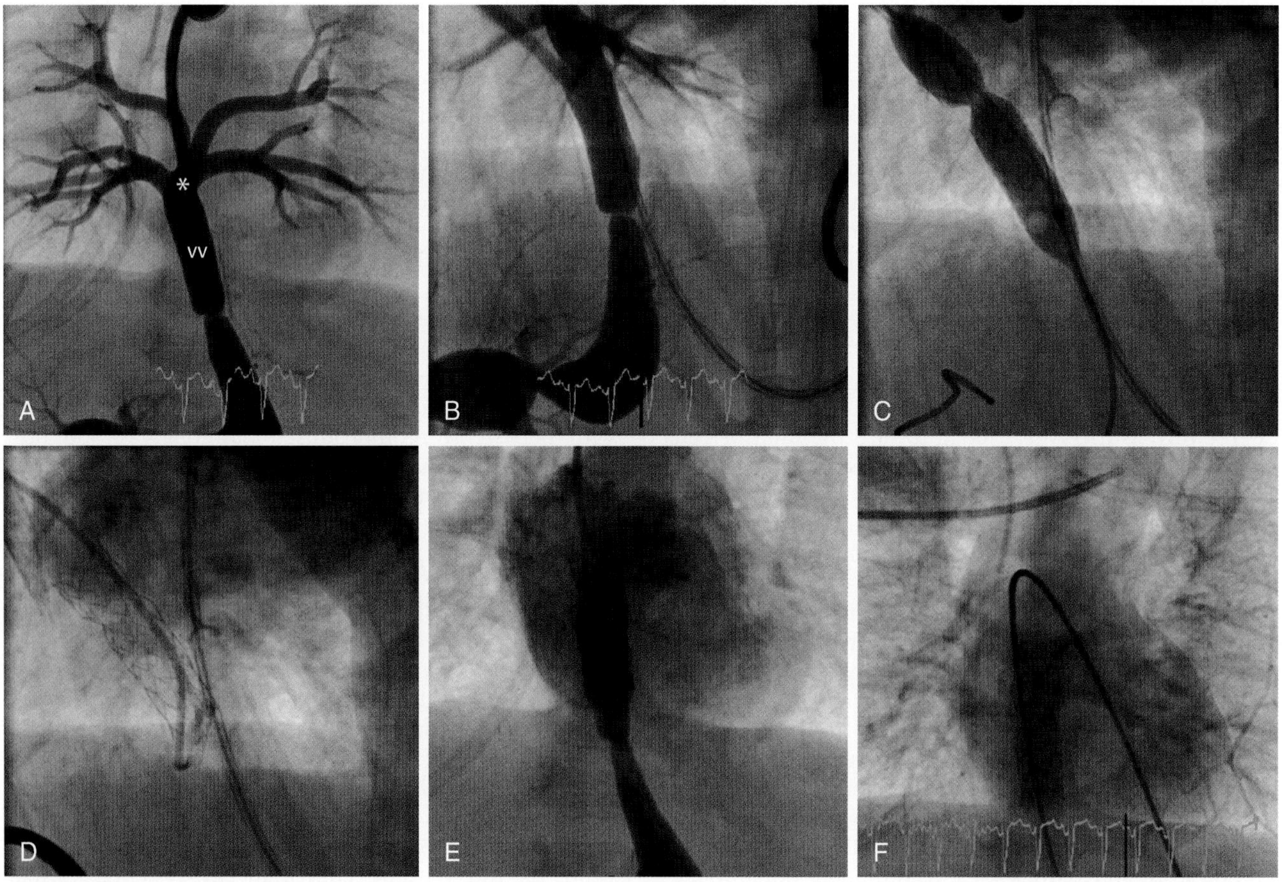

FIGURE 115-7 ■ **A** and **B,** Angiogram shows the infracardiac total anomalous pulmonary venous drainage *(asterisk)* draining in a stenotic vertical vein (VV). **C,** Stent deployment in the stenotic vertical vein during balloon inflation. **D** and **E,** Different projection of the stent implanted. **F,** Final result shows no obstructed flow returning from the pulmonary veins to the vertical vein. (Modified from Chaturvedi RR, Van Arsdell GS, Jacques F, et al: Delayed repair of right atrial isomerism with obstructed total anomalous pulmonary venous drainage by hybrid stent insertion between the left-sided atrium and pulmonary venous confluence. *J Thorac Cardiovasc Surg* 144:271–273, 2012.)

Mixed Anatomy

Mixed-type total anomalous pulmonary venous drainage accounts for 5% to 10% of patients.[23,25] The most common mode (46%) of mixed-type total anomalous pulmonary venous drainage consists of bilateral and asymmetrical connections, with three pulmonary veins typically draining to a common site and one pulmonary vein to a remote site.[27] The second most common mode (29%) is bilateral and symmetrical connections, with separate anomalous connections of all veins from each lung forming confluences and then connecting to the systemic veins at separate sites. The third group, which accounts for 18%, has a common confluence to which all pulmonary veins drain, and then the confluence itself drains to the systemic veins at separate sites. Sites of connection can be at the supracardiac, cardiac, and infracardiac levels.

Presentation

Patients without significant pulmonary venous obstruction present in infancy or early childhood with signs and symptoms related to the presence of a large left-to-right shunt. These patients have dyspnea, poor feeding, and poor growth. They may have cyanosis on examination, but this manifestation is usually mild. Other findings include a second heart sound that is split and a systolic flow murmur caused by increased flow across the pulmonary valve.

Patients with high-grade pulmonary venous obstruction present in the neonatal period with cyanosis, respiratory distress, and poor growth. On examination, the infant is tachypneic and cyanotic and has poor systemic perfusion. The second heart sound is prominent and split as a result of pulmonary arterial hypertension. Obstruction in the pulmonary venous pathway in patients with total anomalous pulmonary venous drainage constitutes a surgical emergency. Medical measures to stabilize and resuscitate the patient include intubation, ventilation with 100% oxygen, hyperventilation, correction of pH, and inotropic support. These medical measures are minimally effective. Administration of prostaglandin E_1 has been reported to open the ductus venosus in an attempt to decompress the pulmonary veins in patients with infracardiac total anomalous pulmonary venous drainage and obstruction.[28] Catheter-based techniques to place a stent in the obstructed pulmonary venous confluence have been reported to relieve obstruction and to allow resuscitation of the patient in preparation for surgical repair.[29]

Pathophysiology

The hemodynamic abnormality, in patients with total anomalous pulmonary venous drainage, is related to the complete diversion of pulmonary venous blood away from the left atrium to a systemic vein. Consequently, the most important anatomic factors in determining the clinical status of the patient include the presence and location of a right-to-left shunt, and the presence or absence of obstruction in the pulmonary venous circuit.

Because pulmonary venous blood is diverted from the left atrium, blood cannot reach the left ventricle in the absence of a right-to-left shunt. Therefore, to sustain life, a right-to-left shunt must be present. Most commonly, a patent foramen ovale or atrial septal defect is present to allow entry of blood into the left atrium and then to the left ventricle for systemic output. The cardiac output of the patient is therefore limited by the amount of blood that can cross the atrial septum. Thus, the characteristics of the obligatory right-to-left shunt determine the systemic cardiac output.

A second important anatomic factor determining the clinical status of the patient is the presence or absence of obstruction in the pulmonary venous pathway. When obstruction is present, egress of blood from the lungs is limited, resulting in pulmonary venous congestion and impairment of oxygenation. This can lead to life-threatening cyanosis in neonates. In addition to deficits in oxygenation and pulmonary blood flow, restriction at the level of the atrial septal defect reduces systemic cardiac output and further exacerbates the patient's precarious clinical status.

In patients with supracardiac anomalous pulmonary venous drainage, obstruction can occur in the ascending vertical vein connecting the pulmonary venous confluence to the innominate vein. In this situation, the passage of the vertical vein between the left pulmonary artery and the left bronchus can cause compression in the vertical vein. As the egress of blood from the lungs is restricted, the pulmonary artery pressure rises, causing further distention of the pulmonary artery and further compression of the vertical vein. This can create a repeating cycle of progressive pulmonary venous obstruction. Obstruction also can occur at the site of the connection between the pulmonary venous confluence and the systemic vein. This is a common feature of infracardiac total anomalous pulmonary venous drainage.

Diagnostic Techniques

Arterial blood gas sampling is useful in resuscitation of a neonate with obstruction and total anomalous pulmonary venous drainage. Often, severe metabolic acidosis and mild hypoxemia are seen.

Chest Radiography

The appearance of the lung fields on chest radiographs is determined by the presence or absence of obstruction to pulmonary venous drainage. In patients without obstruction, pulmonary vascularity is increased because of the large left-to-right shunt created by drainage of pulmonary venous return into the right side of the heart. In patients with obstruction, the lung fields may be extremely congested because of the obstruction of blood egress from the pulmonary veins and the left-to-right shunt. A prominence of the pulmonary artery shadow and the right atrium silhouette often exists. In supracardiac drainage, the prominence of the upper mediastinal silhouette can create the classic "snowman" or figure-eight appearance.

Echocardiography

Echocardiography is the study of choice in diagnosing total anomalous pulmonary venous drainage. The pulmonary venous confluence, pulmonary veins, and connection to the systemic venous system can typically be defined, allowing an expeditious and noninvasive diagnosis in critically ill infants, as well as in asymptomatic children. Consequently, echocardiography has largely replaced angiography as the principal diagnostic study in patients with total anomalous pulmonary venous drainage. Echocardiography also can offer important prognostic data. Jenkins and colleagues[30] correlated operative survival to the size of the pulmonary venous confluence and the sum of the pulmonary venous diameters (Fig. 115-8).

Fetal echocardiography can diagnose total anomalous pulmonary venous drainage and potential obstruction of the pulmonary venous pathways.[31] Fetal diagnosis of total anomalous pulmonary venous drainage is of particular importance if the patient has prominent obstruction in the pulmonary venous pathway, because the patient requires immediate medical and surgical intervention after birth. The sensitivity of fetal echocardiography, however, is uncertain, and the impact of fetal diagnosis of total anomalous pulmonary venous drainage on clinical outcomes is yet to be fully clarified.

Echocardiography is also helpful in monitoring pulmonary veins for obstruction during preoperative and long-term postoperative follow-up. The demonstration of turbulence in the pulmonary veins can be used as a sensitive marker for the presence of obstruction in the pulmonary venous circuit. Because obstruction in the pulmonary veins late after surgical repair can progress in a clinically silent fashion, the sensitivity of the echocardiogram to detect the presence of turbulence in the pulmonary vein may allow early detection and correction of pulmonary vein stenosis after repair.

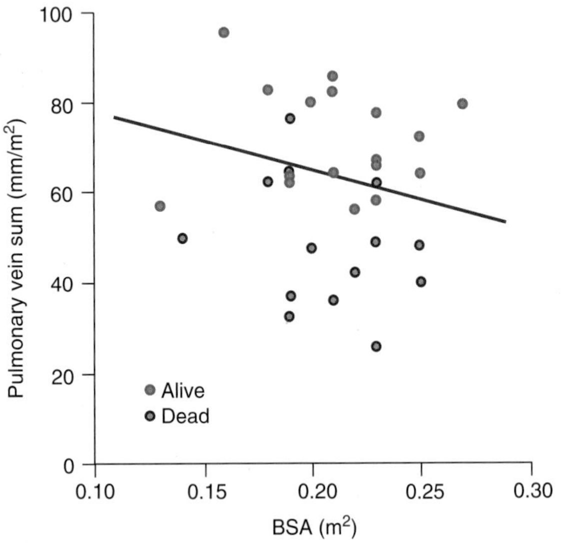

FIGURE 115-8 ■ Graph showing the distribution between operative survival and the pulmonary veins diameters sum at the confluence indexed to body surface area (BSA). The *straight line* is the regression line for indexed pulmonary vein sum and BSA derived from normal data. (From Jenkins KJ, Sanders SP, Orav EJ, et al: Individual pulmonary vein size and survival in infants with totally anomalous pulmonary venous connection. *J Am Coll Cardiol* 22:201–206, 1993.)

Cardiac Catheterization

Cardiac catheterization is used infrequently for diagnosis of routine total or partial anomalous pulmonary venous drainage. Cardiac catheterization is helpful when echocardiographic findings are ambiguous or when the patient has other complex defects. A classic finding at catheterization associated with total anomalous pulmonary venous drainage is identical oxygen saturations in all chambers of the heart. This occurs because of upstream mixing of oxygenated pulmonary venous effluent and deoxygenated systemic venous blood, and subsequent delivery of partially saturated blood to the right side of the heart, as well as to the left side of the heart through the atrial septal defect. Catheterization is also helpful in defining the anatomy of pulmonary vein stenosis, which can develop after repair of total anomalous pulmonary venous drainage.

Catheterization is helpful when the patient needs catheter-based intervention to stabilize the clinical status. Balloon atrial septostomy may be helpful in hemodynamic stabilization before surgical repair in patients with obstruction of pulmonary venous return at the level of a restrictive atrial septal defect. In this situation, the relief of an obstruction at the atrial septal defect allows increased right-to-left shunting and improved systemic cardiac output. Stent placement in the obstructed vertical vein in a patient with infracardiac total anomalous pulmonary venous drainage has been reported (see Fig. 115-7).[29,32] These procedures may temporarily stabilize critically ill patients with obstructive anomalous pulmonary venous drainage, allowing time to recover from multiorgan dysfunction before definitive surgical repair.

Magnetic Resonance Imaging

Recently, magnetic resonance imaging has emerged as an important diagnostic tool in evaluating total anomalous pulmonary venous drainage. It offers complete visualization of all pulmonary veins, with precise delineation of stenotic segments. In addition, it offers hemodynamic evaluation, including measurement of segmental blood flow and blood flow velocity of the pulmonary veins, calculation of the pulmonary-to-systemic blood flow ratio (Qp/Qs) and the possibility of three-dimensional reconstruction.[7]

Computed Tomography Angiography

Computed tomography angiography can be used to define the anatomy of the total anomalous pulmonary venous return because of its superior spatial definition and its shorter examination duration compared with magnetic resonance imaging. Computed tomography also allows the creation of three-dimensional reconstruction of the cardiac structures. The disadvantages are related mainly to exposure to ionizing radiation, more nephrotoxic contrast used and due to the fact that computed tomography does not provide any hemodynamic measurement. Computed tomography can be used in cases in which magnetic resonance imaging cannot be performed or is contraindicated.[33]

Surgical Repair

The goal of surgical intervention is to create unobstructed egress of blood from the pulmonary veins into the left atrium. Aorto-bicaval cannulation offers the flexibility to repair all forms of total anomalous pulmonary venous drainage. In some centers, deep hypothermic circulatory arrest is preferred to allow improved visualization of the pulmonary veins in a bloodless field. Continuous perfusion techniques require the use of cardiotomy suction devices in the pulmonary veins to allow visualization during the repair. For this reason, systemic hypothermia is used to allow the safe decrease of perfusion flow rates during the critical portions of the anastomosis.

After initiation of CPB, ductus arteriosus ligation, and systemic cooling to 18° to 20° C, the aorta is cross-clamped, and cold antegrade blood cardioplegia is administered. The vertical vein is ligated. The pulmonary venous confluence is seen in the posterior pericardium by retracting the heart anteriorly and to the right. Because of the lack of pulmonary vein attachments to the left atrium, the heart is usually mobile, and retraction of the heart out of the mediastinum offers excellent exposure of the pulmonary venous confluence. A longitudinal incision is created in the pulmonary venous confluence to match a corresponding incision in the posterior left atrium, extended out towards the left atrial appendage. With care to avoid distortion, a left-atrial-to-pulmonary-confluence anastomosis is made using fine sutures. Controversy exists regarding the use of absorbable versus nonabsorbable sutures, as well as interrupted versus continuous techniques.[34,35] With all techniques, the primary goal is to create a large, unobstructed anastomosis, and the superiority of any one of these techniques has not been convincingly demonstrated. A short period of low-flow CPB may be needed to improve visualization during construction of a meticulous anastomosis.

The use of the approach described in the preceding paragraph is applicable to all types of total anomalous pulmonary venous drainage. It can be challenging, however, to orient the left atrial and pulmonary vein confluence incisions while simultaneously retracting the heart. Furthermore, the retraction required to visualize the anastomosis can place tension on the developing suture line during construction of the anastomosis. Finally, the left atrium tends to be small in patients with total anomalous pulmonary venous drainage and, consequently, the limitation to rightward extension of the anastomosis by the atrial septum can limit the size of the anastomosis. The limitation imposed by the location of the atrial septum is a greater issue in patients in whom the pulmonary venous confluence is oriented rightward with respect to the left atrium.

An alternative approach is to create the anastomosis through a generous atriotomy extended transversely across the right atrium and then across the atrial septum (Fig. 115-9). This approach allows visualization of the posterior wall of the left atrium, which allows the surgeon to place the left atrial incision precisely over the area corresponding to the incision in the pulmonary venous confluence. Furthermore, in patients with a small left atrium and rightward displacement of the pulmonary vein confluence, the approach allows patch augmentation of the left atrium when reconstructing the atrial septum and right atrial incision.

A third operative approach to construction of a pulmonary-vein-to-left-atrial anastomosis is between the

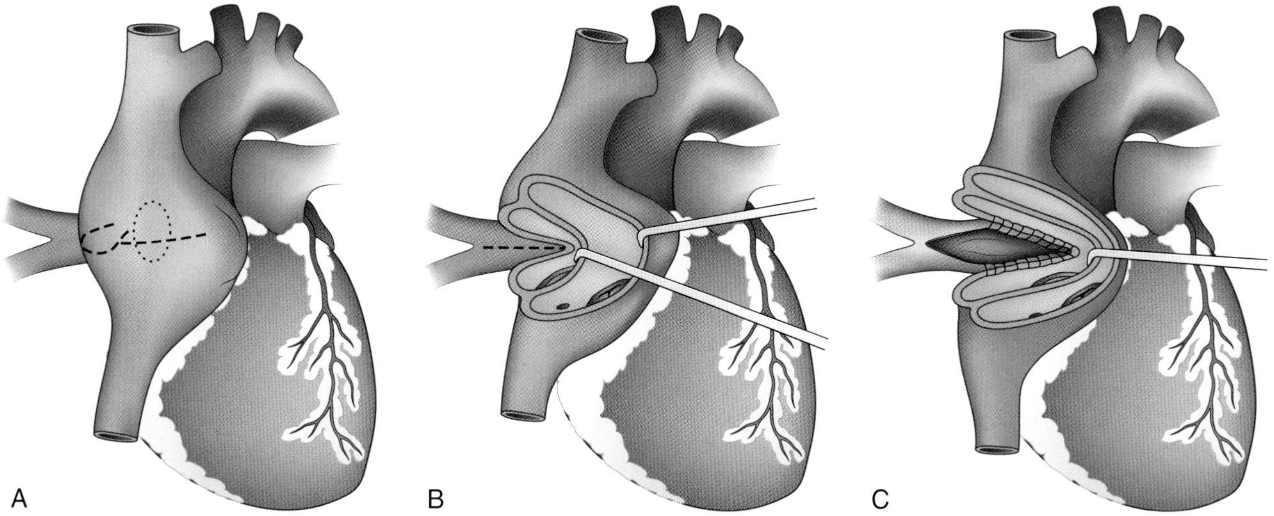

FIGURE 115-9 ■ Repair of total anomalous pulmonary venous drainage under hypothermic cardiopulmonary bypass and cardioplegic cardiac arrest. **A,** A right atrial incision is made from the midportion of the right atrium and extends posteriorly to the pulmonary venous confluence *(dashed line)*. The incision is carried leftward across the atrial septum to the secundum atrial septal defect *(dotted line)* and posterior across the back of the left atrial wall in the direction of the left atrial appendage. **B,** Retraction of the atrium to the left exposes the pulmonary venous confluence, which is incised as widely as possible *(dashed line)*. **C,** A direct anastomosis is constructed between the divided pulmonary veins and the left atrial wall. If the left atrium is small, or if the pulmonary venous confluence is rightward, the left atrial size can be augmented with a patch along the rightward edge of the anastomosis.

aorta and the superior vena cava. Using this technique, the aorta and the superior vena cava are retracted laterally, exposing the dome of the left atrium and the pulmonary vein confluence. This approach is especially helpful in patients with supracardiac variants of total anomalous pulmonary venous drainage. Further exposure can be obtained easily by dividing the aorta.[36]

Repair of the intracardiac type of total anomalous pulmonary venous drainage is performed using moderate hypothermia and standard cannulation techniques. If obstruction in the individual pulmonary veins is suggested, deep hypothermic CPB is considered for possible circulatory arrest. A transverse right atriotomy is made, and the atrial septum is exposed. If the pulmonary vein confluence enters the coronary sinus, the atrial septum between the patent foramen ovale and the coronary sinus is incised (Fig. 115-10*A*). The superior aspect of the coronary sinus is unroofed until the left atrial wall and coronary sinus becomes a common chamber without any separating ridge (see Fig. 115-10*B*). Care must be taken that the incision and resection are not too close to the mitral valve or to individual pulmonary veins. Any connecting vein between the pulmonary venous confluence and the coronary sinus must be completely incised so that there is no residual circumferential connecting vein. If completely unroofed, the pulmonary vein ostia should be easily visualized through the unroofed coronary sinus. A glutaraldehyde-treated or fresh autologous pericardial patch is used to reconstruct the atrial septum, leaving the pulmonary venous drainage to flow through the unroofed coronary sinus into the left atrium (see Fig. 115-10*C*). Concern has been expressed that this unroofing technique may have a higher risk of late stenosis in patients who have a short segment of venous confluence interposed between the pulmonary venous confluence and the coronary sinus.[26] As an alternative, direct anastomosis of the pulmonary veins to the left atrial wall can be performed.

In patients with infracardiac pulmonary venous connections, the pulmonary venous confluence tends to be oriented more vertically, creating a Y-shaped confluence that drains through a vertical vein to the portal system. Consequently, the incision into the left atrium is more vertical or Y-shaped to maximize the size of the newly created left atrium. Some surgeons leave the vertical vein intact to provide a pressure relief "pop-off" if left atrial pressure is high in the early postoperative period because of small left atrial size or poor ventricular compliance.[37,38]

Poor hemodynamics in the early postoperative period should raise concerns for potential obstruction at the site of the venous anastomosis and for pulmonary hypertensive crisis. Any suspicion of residual postoperative pulmonary venous obstruction should prompt echocardiographic examination to interrogate the pulmonary venous anastomosis. In patients with preoperative pulmonary venous obstruction, chest radiographic findings of pulmonary vascular obstruction persist for several days despite normal hemodynamics. Therefore, the presence of congestion on a chest radiograph is not sufficient to make the diagnosis of postoperative pulmonary venous obstruction. Pulmonary hypertensive crises are a common feature in the postoperative management of infants after repair of total anomalous pulmonary venous drainage. In many centers, routine postoperative pulmonary artery or right ventricular pressure monitoring allows early detection and treatment of pulmonary hypertensive crises with deep sedation, controlled ventilation, and inotropic support for right-sided heart failure. Inhaled nitric oxide also can be used for postoperative pulmonary arterial hypertension, although it can create paradoxic pulmonary venous hypertension by rapidly increasing the

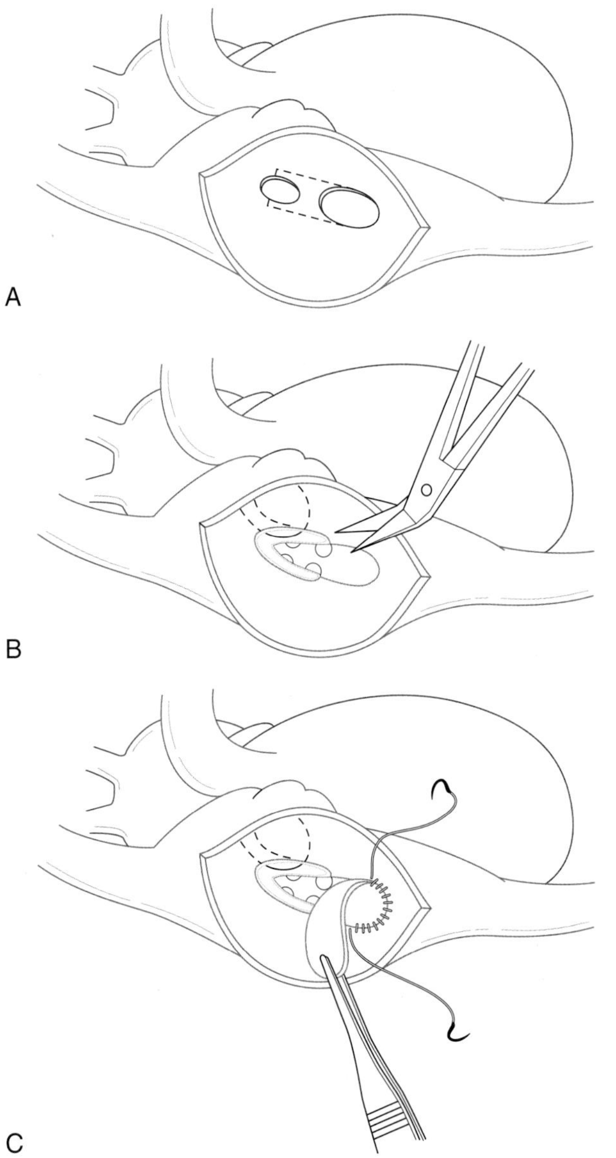

FIGURE 115-10 ■ Repair of intracardiac-type total anomalous pulmonary venous drainage. **A,** The atrial septum between the patent foramen ovale and coronary sinus is incised, and the septal tissue surrounded by the *dotted lines* is resected. **B,** The superior aspect of the coronary sinus is incised until close to the mitral valve, creating a common chamber including the left atrium and the dilated coronary sinus. The surgeon must identify all four pulmonary vein orifices. **C,** A large defect created by resection of the tissue between the foramen ovale and the coronary sinus is patched with a glutaraldehyde-treated or fresh autologous pericardial patch, redirecting the coronary sinus drainage to the left atrium.

left ventricular preload in patients with noncompliant or small left ventricles.[39]

In patients with a small pulmonary venous confluence and small pulmonary veins, direct anastomosis of the divided edge of the pulmonary veins to the left atrial wall can lead to geometric distortion of the pulmonary vein anastomosis, local trauma from handling the delicate pulmonary vein, and local reaction from suture-related ischemia. In patients with small pulmonary vein confluences, the preferred anastomotic technique at the Hospital for Sick Children in Toronto has evolved into a "sutureless" anastomosis.[40,41] This technique includes a longitudinal incision in the posterior pericardium and the underlying pulmonary venous confluence. A corresponding incision is made in the overlying portion of the left atrium (Fig. 115-11*A*). In contrast to direct suture techniques, however, the left atrium is not sutured directly to the divided edge of the pulmonary veins. Instead, the left atrial edge is sutured to the pericardium circumferentially around the pericardial incision, avoiding direct suturing to the pulmonary veins (see Fig. 115-11*B*). A "neo-atrium" is thereby created, into which the pulmonary veins bleed in a controlled fashion into the remainder of the left atrium and the left ventricle.

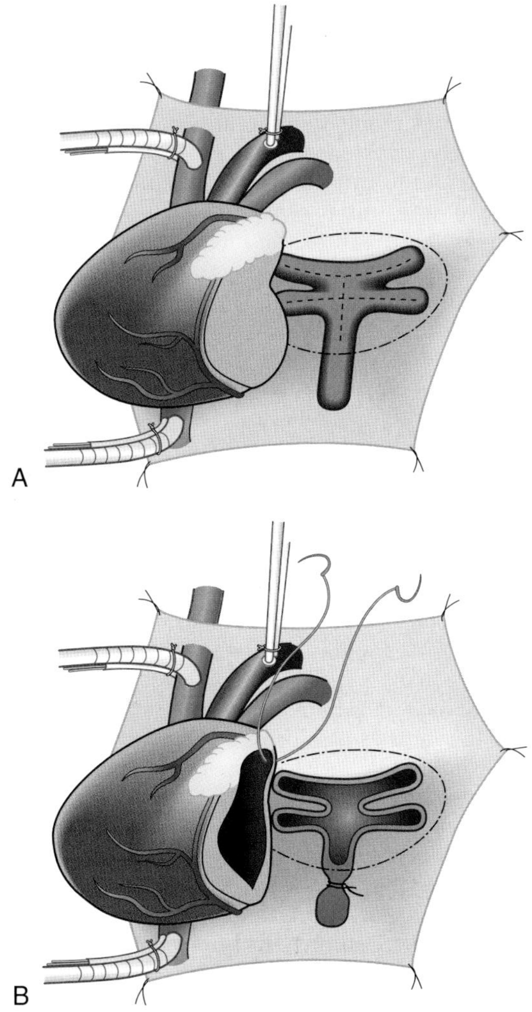

FIGURE 115-11 ■ Primary repair of infracardiac total anomalous pulmonary venous drainage using a "sutureless" technique. **A,** The heart is retracted anteriorly and rightward, exposing the pulmonary venous confluence. **B,** The vertical vein is ligated, and the divided edges of the left atrial wall are sutured to the posterior pericardium using a suture line that is remote from the incised pulmonary venous confluence.

Results

Operative survival for patients with total anomalous pulmonary venous drainage has markedly improved in the most recent decade, with survival rates of more than 90% reported in the current era.[23,25] Long-term prognosis for patients after repair of total anomalous pulmonary venous drainage is also favorable, with relatively few late deaths.[23,25] Approximately 10% to 17% of patients have some evidence of late pulmonary vein obstruction; therefore, long-term surveillance is important.[42] Recent studies raise concerns about neurologic development after repair of total anomalous pulmonary venous drainage—concerns associated with the use of deep hypothermic circulatory arrest and metabolic instability at the early postoperative period.[43]

SPECIAL CONSIDERATIONS

Total Anomalous Pulmonary Venous Drainage in Heterotaxy

Visceral heterotaxy is characterized by abnormalities of multiple organ systems, including the heart, lungs, liver, spleen, and systemic veins. In the subset of patients with asplenia, or right atrial isomerism, cardiac anomalies include a common atrium, common atrioventricular valves, pulmonary outflow tract obstruction, and hypoplastic left or right ventricles resulting in functional single ventricles. Total anomalous pulmonary venous drainage is present in approximately 90% of patients.[44]

Patients with the common combination of total anomalous pulmonary venous drainage and functional single ventricles typically present within the first month of life for palliation.[44] The type of palliation required is determined by the presence of uncontrolled pulmonary blood flow (e.g., a functional single ventricle with unrestrictive pulmonary valve) or restricted pulmonary blood flow (e.g., pulmonary stenosis or atresia). Superimposed on the alterations of pulmonary arterial flow is the frequent presence of pulmonary venous obstruction, which may be present in up to 30% of patients.[44] The presence of obstruction, however, may not be readily apparent until after augmentation of pulmonary blood flow (e.g., systemic-to-pulmonary shunt) in patients initially displaying pulmonary stenosis or atresia.[45] The majority of these patients have increased muscularity of the pulmonary arteries and "arterialization" of the pulmonary veins.

Patients requiring palliation in the neonatal period often have a complex combination of physiologic problems because pulmonary venous obstruction may coexist with either an unrestricted source of pulmonary blood flow or a restricted source of pulmonary blood flow. Thus, the patient might require repair of obstructed total anomalous pulmonary venous drainage in combination with pulmonary artery banding or a systemic to pulmonary artery shunt—with a poor prognosis.[44,45] Recent reports suggest that aggressive repair of total anomalous pulmonary venous drainage repair for right atrial isomerism is associated with improved survival in the more recent era. The sutureless repair is associated with a trend for improved survival but so far has not shown statistical significance for this patient subset.[46]

Pulmonary Vein Stenosis After Repair

Development of stenosis after repair of total anomalous pulmonary venous drainage occurs in 5% to 17.5% of patients after initial repair,[23,42,47,48] and the patients typically present within the first year after initial repair. The obstruction can occur in one of three general patterns. The simplest form involves a ring of fibrosis limited to the site of the anastomotic suture line. The second form is more complex, involving the distal pulmonary veins in a localized region of intimal proliferation. The most complex form involves diffuse retrograde pulmonary vein stenosis extending far into the distal pulmonary veins. These types of obstruction can occur in a unilateral fashion, progressing to complete occlusion of the pulmonary venous drainage of the involved lung.[47] Patients with unilateral pulmonary vein stenosis have better survival than patients with bilateral stenosis.[47,48] Diffuse pulmonary vein stenosis after repair is associated with a high mortality rate.

Pulmonary vein obstruction after repair is associated with pulmonary vascular congestion on chest radiographs. On echocardiogram, the principal diagnostic criterion is the presence of turbulence at the pulmonary venous anastomosis.[49] Angiography can add information to the echocardiographic findings. Because the echocardiographic window can be limited in postoperative patients, angiography can be helpful in defining the status of the pulmonary veins further upstream in the lung—outside the echocardiographic window. Angiography, however, is an invasive procedure and requires the use of ionizing radiation. Contrast-enhanced magnetic resonance angiography is an extremely useful diagnostic modality for pulmonary vein stenosis.[7] Contrast-enhanced magnetic resonance angiography provides anatomically detailed analysis of the stenotic pulmonary veins at the site of anastomosis and, importantly, in the lung.[7] The presence or absence of a distal dilated portion of pulmonary vein is a crucial determination in evaluating a patient with pulmonary vein stenosis after repair. Absence of dilation in the intrapulmonary portion of the pulmonary vein precludes the rationale for surgical attempts to decompress the pulmonary veins.

The presence of turbulence at the site of the anastomosis has been postulated to create a cycle of local injury leading to hyperplasia and increasing turbulence, thereby perpetuating a process of diffuse pulmonary vein stenosis. The progression of pulmonary vein stenosis retrograde (upstream) into the lung parenchyma is associated with a poor prognosis. In an animal model, upstream pulmonary vein stenosis is associated with transforming growth factor β1 expression and progressive obstruction of the pulmonary veins through a process consistent with endothelial to mesenchymal transition.[50] Identification of the mediators of progressive upstream pulmonary venous obstruction can lead to pharmacologic therapies as adjuncts to surgical or stent-based decompression at the left atrial-pulmonary venous junction.

Surgical revision of the pulmonary venous anastomosis, lung transplantation[51] and pulmonary vein stenting[52] are the most commonly prescribed therapies for pulmonary vein stenosis after repair. Pulmonary vein stenting represents a useful approach on acute relief of stenosis, but it is still associated with high reintervention rate and in stent stenosis.[52] The diameter of the stent correlates with the risk of re-stenosis, and stent diameters larger than 6 mm are associated with more prolonged patency rates.[52] Drug-eluting stents and stents delivering local doses of radiation or chemotherapy may offer benefit in the future but have not yet been demonstrated to be efficacious.

Surgical Techniques for Pulmonary Vein Stenosis After Repair of Total Anomalous Pulmonary Venous Return

Some surgeons emphasize the importance of prevention of pulmonary vein stenosis after repair by reducing surgical trauma on the endocardium of the pulmonary vein at the time of the initial repair, thereby minimizing the stimulus for ingrowth of the intimal tissue.[53] Nevertheless, approximately 10% to 17% of patients develop pulmonary vein stenosis after repair.

If the obstruction is exclusively at the anastomotic site, the surgical revision can be accomplished by resection of the ingrowth tissue obstructing the anastomotic site or by patch enlargement of the left atrial anastomosis. A polytetrafluoroethylene or pericardial patch is commonly used for enlargement. Other conventional approaches for individual pulmonary vein stenosis include endarterectomy and patch venoplasty. These approaches are associated with a high risk of recurrence ranging from 60% to 90%.[47,48]

Recent reports have described the use of sutureless techniques to treat pulmonary vein stenosis after repair.[53] Cardiopulmonary bypass is established with ascending aortic and bicaval cannulation. Patients are cooled for possible low-flow bypass or circulatory arrest to attain a bloodless field. The heart is retracted cephalad, and the posterior aspect of the left atrium is incised in the region of the previous anastomosis. The stenotic pulmonary vein tissue is incised longitudinally leftward and rightward to the level of the pericardial reflection until nonstenotic segments of pulmonary vein are reached, possibly requiring the incision of veins into secondary or tertiary branches in the pulmonary hilum or parenchyma. Stenotic areas in the mediastinum can be resected circumferentially. The left atrial incision is extended to the left atrial appendage, creating a widely open incision. The left atrial edge is then sutured to the pericardium using 6-0 or 7-0 nonabsorbable polypropylene suture extending around the site of pulmonary vein resection or incision. Midterm outcomes with sutureless techniques have

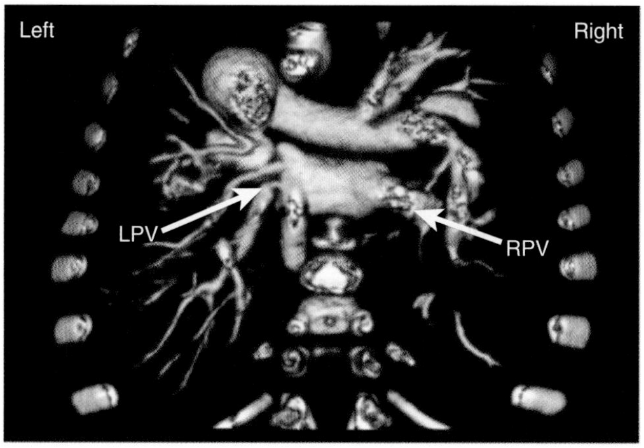

FIGURE 115-12 CT reconstruction of congenital pulmonary vein stenosis: from a posterior view of the chest the reconstruction shows diffuse stenosis of the left pulmonary veins (LPV; *arrow*) upper compared to unobstructed right lower pulmonary vein (RPV; *arrow*). Right upper pulmonary severe stenosis is not visualized in this projection.

been reported to be superior to conventional surgical techniques.[40,41,47,54]

Congenital (Primary) Pulmonary Vein Stenosis

Congenital pulmonary vein stenosis is the syndrome of primary endoluminal stenosis of one or multiple individual pulmonary veins (Fig. 115-12), which is not associated with previous surgery or catheter intervention. Pathogenesis of this entity has been postulated as being an abnormal incorporation of the common pulmonary vein into the left atrium in the later stage of cardiac development.[55] This anomaly is frequently associated with other congenital heart malformation, ranging from 30% to 80%.[56,57] Congenital pulmonary stenosis can be discrete stenosis caused by the intimal shelf or diffuse hypoplasia of the pulmonary veins. Pathologic studies have demonstrated the presence of proliferative myofibroblastic cells in the fibrotic tissue.[50]

Clinical presentation of children with congenital pulmonary vein stenosis depends on the number of pulmonary veins involved and on the severity of stenosis in the individual pulmonary veins. Most patients present in the first months to years of life with respiratory symptoms, including tachypnea, and recurrent respiratory infection. Patients with severe pulmonary venous obstruction have signs of pulmonary hypertension.

Prognosis of progressive congenital pulmonary vein stenosis is extremely poor, and it is strongly related to the number of pulmonary veins involved. Breinholt and colleagues[58] reported 13 patients with congenital pulmonary vein stenosis; 83% of the patients with three or four pulmonary vein stenosis died, whereas all patients with stenosis limited to one or two pulmonary veins survived. Conventional scar excision techniques appear to be associated with less favorable outcomes than sutureless techniques. Survival rates after sutureless repair for pulmonary vein stenosis, as reported by Viola and collagues,[59] were 64%, 47%, and 31% at 1, 5, and 10 years, respectively, and are directly related to the preoperative severity of the stenosis. Sutureless technique reduces in the postoperative period the grade of stenosis and provides a lower incidence of reoperation in the long term but does not prevent intraparenchymal lung disease progression.

In conclusion, the prognosis for these patients is poor with either technique.[54,59] Pneumonectomy may be necessary for refractory hemoptysis. Lung transplant can be considered as a viable treatment for patients with recurrent stenosis after primary repair or diffuse disease.[51] Encouraging results with bilateral sequential lung transplantation for this entity have been reported by Bharat and colleagues.[51] Catheter intervention for congenital pulmonary vein stenosis had negligible benefits.[60] The efficacy of new therapies such as sonotherapy or chemotherapy remains uncertain.

REFERENCES

1. Webb S, Brown NA, Wessels A, et al: Development of the murine pulmonary vein and its relationship to the embryonic venous sinus. *Anat Rec* 250(3):325–334, 1998.
2. Bleyl SB, Botto LD, Carey JC, et al: Analysis of a Scottish founder effect narrows the TAPVR-1 gene interval to chromosome 4q12. *Am J Med Genet A* 140(21):2368–2373, 2006.
3. van den Berg G, Moorman AFM: Development of the pulmonary vein and the systemic venous sinus: an interactive 3D overview. *PLoS ONE* 6(7):e22055, 2011.
4. Degenhardt K, Singh MK, Aghajanian H, et al: Semaphorin 3d signaling defects are associated with anomalous pulmonary venous connections. *Nat Med* 19(6):760–765, 2013.
5. Gustafson RA, Warden HE, Murray GF, et al: Partial anomalous pulmonary venous connection to the right side of the heart. *J Thorac Cardiovasc Surg* 98(5 Pt 2):861–868, 1989.
6. Kotani Y, Chetan D, Zhu J, et al: The natural and surgically modified history of anomalous pulmonary veins from the left lung. *Ann Thorac Surg* 96:1711–1718, discussion 1718–1720, 2013.
7. Grosse-Wortmann L, Al-Otay A, Goo HW, et al: Anatomical and functional evaluation of pulmonary veins in children by magnetic resonance imaging. *J Am Coll Cardiol* 49(9):993–1002, 2007.
8. Vida VL, Padalino MA, Bhattarai A, et al: Right posterior-lateral minithoracotomy access for treating congenital heart disease. *Ann Thorac Surg* 92(6):2278–2280, 2011.
9. Vida VL, Padalino MA, Boccuzzo G, et al: Near-infrared spectroscopy for monitoring leg perfusion during minimally invasive surgery for patients with congenital heart defects. *J Thorac Cardiovasc Surg* 143(3):756–757, 2012.
10. Shahriari A, Rodefeld MD, Turrentine MW, et al: Caval division technique for sinus venosus atrial septal defect with partial anomalous pulmonary venous connection. *Ann Thorac Surg* 81(1):224–230, 2006.
11. Gatzoulis MA, Freeman MA, Siu SC, et al: Atrial arrhythmia after surgical closure of atrial septal defects in adults. *N Engl J Med* 340(11):839–846, 1999.
12. Luciani GB, Viscardi F, Pilati M, et al: Age at repair affects the very long-term outcome of sinus venosus defect. *Ann Thorac Surg* 86(1):153–159, 2008.
13. Alsoufi B, Cai S, Van Arsdell GS, et al: Outcomes after surgical treatment of children with partial anomalous pulmonary venous connection. *Ann Thorac Surg* 84(6):2020–2026, discussion 6, 2007.
14. Attenhofer Jost CH, Connolly HM, Danielson GK, et al: Sinus venosus atrial septal defect: long-term postoperative outcome for 115 patients. *Circulation* 112(13):1953–1958, 2005.
15. Najm HK, Williams WG, Coles JG, et al: Scimitar syndrome: twenty years' experience and results of repair. *J Thorac Cardiovasc Surg* 112(5):1161–1168, 1996.
16. Vida VL, Padalino MA, Boccuzzo G, et al: Scimitar syndrome: a European Congenital Heart Surgeons Association (ECHSA) multicentric study. *Circulation* 122(12):1159–1166, 2010.
17. Brown JW, Ruzmetov M, Minnich DJ, et al: Surgical management of scimitar syndrome: an alternative approach. *J Thorac Cardiovasc Surg* 125(2):238–245, 2003.

18. Huddleston CB, Exil V, Canter CE, et al: Scimitar syndrome presenting in infancy. *Ann Thorac Surg* 67(1):154–159, discussion 60, 1999.
19. Uthaman B, Abushaban L, Al-Qbandi M, et al: The impact of interruption of anomalous systemic arterial supply on scimitar syndrome presenting during infancy. *Catheter Cardiovasc Interv* 71(5):671–678, 2008.
20. Zubiate P, Kay JH: Surgical correction of anomalous pulmonary venous connection. *Ann Surg* 156(2):234–250, 1962.
21. Shumacker HB, Jr, Judd D: Partial anomalous pulmonary venous return with reference to drainage into the inferior vena cava and to an intact atrial septum. *J Cardiovasc Surg (Torino)* 5:271–278, 1964.
22. Calhoun RF, Mee RB: A novel operative approach to scimitar syndrome. *Ann Thorac Surg* 76(1):301–303, 2003.
23. Seale AN, Uemura H, Webber SA, et al: British Congenital Cardiac Association. Total anomalous pulmonary venous connection: morphology and outcome from an international population-based study. *Circulation* 122(25):2718–2726, 2010.
24. Yamaki S, Tsunemoto M, Shimada M, et al: Quantitative analysis of pulmonary vascular disease in total anomalous pulmonary venous connection in sixty infants. *J Thorac Cardiovasc Surg* 104(3):728–735, 1992.
25. Karamlou T, Gurofsky R, Al Sukhni E, et al: Factors associated with mortality and reoperation in 377 children with total anomalous pulmonary venous connection. *Circulation* 115(12):1591–1598, 2007.
26. Jonas RA, Smolinsky A, Mayer JE, et al: Obstructed pulmonary venous drainage with total anomalous pulmonary venous connection to the coronary sinus. *Am J Cardiol* 59(5):431–435, 1987.
27. Chowdhury UK, Malhotra A, Kothari SS, et al: A suggested new surgical classification for mixed totally anomalous pulmonary venous connection. *Cardiol Young* 17(4):342–353, 2007.
28. Serraf A, Bruniaux J, Lacour-Gayet F, et al: Obstructed total anomalous pulmonary venous return. Toward neutralization of a major risk factor. *J Thorac Cardiovasc Surg* 101(4):601–606, 1991.
29. Wong DT, Yoo SJ, Lee KJ: Implantation of drug-eluting stents for relief of obstructed infra-cardiac totally anomalous pulmonary venous connection in isomerism of the right atrial appendages. *Cardiol Young* 18(6):628–630, 2008.
30. Jenkins KJ, Sanders SP, Orav EJ, et al: Individual pulmonary vein size and survival in infants with totally anomalous pulmonary venous connection. *J Am Coll Cardiol* 22(1):201–206, 1993.
31. Valsangiacomo ER, Hornberger LK, Barrea C, et al: Partial and total anomalous pulmonary venous connection in the fetus: two-dimensional and Doppler echocardiographic findings. *Ultrasound Obstet Gynecol* 22(3):257–263, 2003.
32. Meadows J, Marshall AC, Lock JE, et al: A hybrid approach to stabilization and repair of obstructed total anomalous pulmonary venous connection in a critically ill newborn infant. *J Thorac Cardiovasc Surg* 131(4):e1–e2, 2006.
33. Vyas HV, Greenberg SB, Krishnamurthy R: MR imaging and CT evaluation of congenital pulmonary vein abnormalities in neonates and infants. *Radiographics* 32(1):87–98, 2012.
34. Hawkins JA, Minich LL, Tani LY, et al: Absorbable polydioxanone suture and results in total anomalous pulmonary venous connection. *Ann Thorac Surg* 60(1):55–59, 1995.
35. Ricci M, Elliott M, Cohen GA, et al: Management of pulmonary venous obstruction after correction of TAPVC: risk factors for adverse outcome. *Eur J Cardiothorac Surg* 24(1):28–36, 2003.
36. Serraf A, Belli E, Roux D, et al: Modified superior approach for repair of supracardiac and mixed total anomalous pulmonary venous drainage. *Ann Thorac Surg* 65(5):1391–1393, 1998.
37. Cope JT, Banks D, McDaniel NL, et al: Is vertical vein ligation necessary in repair of total anomalous pulmonary venous connection? *Ann Thorac Surg* 64(1):23–28, discussion 9, 1997.
38. Caspi J, Pettitt TW, Fontenot EE, et al: The beneficial hemodynamic effects of selective patent vertical vein following repair of obstructed total anomalous pulmonary venous drainage in infants. *Eur J Cardiothorac Surg* 20(4):830–834, 2001.
39. Rosales AM, Bolivar J, Burke RP, et al: Adverse hemodynamic effects observed with inhaled nitric oxide after surgical repair of total anomalous pulmonary venous return. *Pediatr Cardiol* 20(3):224–226, 1999.
40. Yanagawa B, Alghamdi AA, Dragulescu A, et al: Primary sutureless repair for "simple" total anomalous pulmonary venous connection: midterm results in a single institution. *J Thorac Cardiovasc Surg* 141(6):1346–1354, 2011.
41. Honjo O, Atlin CR, Hamilton BC, et al: Primary sutureless repair for infants with mixed total anomalous pulmonary venous drainage. *Ann Thorac Surg* 90(3):862–868, 2010.
42. Seale AN, Uemura H, Webber SA, et al: British Congenital Cardiac Association. Total anomalous pulmonary venous connection: outcome of postoperative pulmonary venous obstruction. *J Thorac Cardiovasc Surg* 145(5):1255–1262, 2013.
43. Alton GY, Robertson CM, Sauve R, et al: Early childhood health, growth, and neurodevelopmental outcomes after complete repair of total anomalous pulmonary venous connection at 6 weeks or younger. *J Thorac Cardiovasc Surg* 133(4):905–911, 2007.
44. Hashmi A, Abu-Sulaiman R, McCrindle BW, et al: Management and outcomes of right atrial isomerism: a 26-year experience. *J Am Coll Cardiol* 31(5):1120–1126, 1998.
45. Caldarone CA, Najm HK, Kadletz M, et al: Surgical management of total anomalous pulmonary venous drainage: impact of coexisting cardiac anomalies. *Ann Thorac Surg* 66(5):1521–1526, 1998.
46. Yun TJ, Al-Radi OO, Adatia I, et al: Contemporary management of right atrial isomerism: effect of evolving therapeutic strategies. *J Thorac Cardiovasc Surg* 131(5):1108–1113, 2006.
47. Caldarone CA, Najm HK, Kadletz M, et al: Relentless pulmonary vein stenosis after repair of total anomalous pulmonary venous drainage. *Ann Thorac Surg* 66(5):1514–1520, 1998.
48. Lacour-Gayet F, Zoghbi J, Serraf AE, et al: Surgical management of progressive pulmonary venous obstruction after repair of total anomalous pulmonary venous connection. *J Thorac Cardiovasc Surg* 117(4):679–687, 1999.
49. Smallhorn JF, Burrows P, Wilson G, et al: Two-dimensional and pulsed Doppler echocardiography in the postoperative evaluation of total anomalous pulmonary venous connection. *Circulation* 76(2):298–305, 1987.
50. Kato H, Fu YY, Zhu J, et al: Pulmonary vein stenosis and the pathophysiology of "upstream" pulmonary veins. *J Thorac Cardiovasc Surg* 148:245–253, 2014.
51. Bharat A, Epstein DJ, Grady M, et al: Lung transplant is a viable treatment option for patients with congenital and acquired pulmonary vein stenosis. *J Heart Lung Transplant* 32(6):621–625, 2013.
52. Balasubramanian S, Marshall AC, Gauvreau K, et al: Outcomes after stent implantation for the treatment of congenital and postoperative pulmonary vein stenosis in children. *Circ Cardiovasc Interv* 5(1):109–117, 2012.
53. Lacour-Gayet F: Surgery for pulmonary venous obstruction after repair of total anomalous pulmonary venous return. *Semin Thorac Cardiovasc Surg Pediatr Card Surg Annu* 45–50:2006.
54. Yun TJ, Coles JG, Konstantinov IE, et al: Conventional and sutureless techniques for management of the pulmonary veins: evolution of indications from postrepair pulmonary vein stenosis to primary pulmonary vein anomalies. *J Thorac Cardiovasc Surg* 129(1):167–174, 2005.
55. Latson LA, Prieto LR: Congenital and acquired pulmonary vein stenosis. *Circulation* 115(1):103–108, 2007.
56. Fong LV, Anderson RH, Park SC, et al: Morphologic features of stenosis of the pulmonary veins. *Am J Cardiol* 62(16):1136–1138, 1988.
57. Bini RM, Cleveland DC, Ceballos R, et al: Congenital pulmonary vein stenosis. *Am J Cardiol* 54(3):369–375, 1984.
58. Breinholt JP, Hawkins JA, Minich LA, et al: Pulmonary vein stenosis with normal connection: associated cardiac abnormalities and variable outcome. *Ann Thorac Surg* 68(1):164–168, 1999.
59. Viola N, Alghamdi AA, Perrin DG, et al: Primary pulmonary vein stenosis: the impact of sutureless repair on survival. *J Thorac Cardiovasc Surg* 142(2):344–350, 2011.
60. Driscoll DJ, Hesslein PS, Mullins CE: Congenital stenosis of individual pulmonary veins: clinical spectrum and unsuccessful treatment by transvenous balloon dilation. *Am J Cardiol* 49(7):1767–1772, 1982.

CHAPTER 116

ATRIOVENTRICULAR CANAL DEFECTS

Aditya K. Kaza • Pedro J. del Nido

CHAPTER OUTLINE

Atrioventricular (AV) canal defects include a spectrum of lesions in which the common etiology appears to be abnormal development of the endocardial cushions, resulting in a defect in the AV septum and AV valves. This group of lesions forms approximately 3% of all major congenital cardiac defects, and approximately half of the patients have Down syndrome.[1] In children with Down syndrome, AV canal defects are seen in 20% to 25%—a 1000-fold increased risk when compared with the incidence in the general population.[2]

Although AV canal defects constitute a continuum of related anatomic lesions, it is useful to divide them into two main groups[3]—partial and complete AV canal defects—on the basis of the extent of the interventricular communication.

Partial AV canal defects consist of a large ostium primum atrial septal defect (ASD) and a cleft between the left superior and inferior bridging leaflets. In most cases, there is no interventricular communication. However, when the cleft extends to the crest of the interventricular septum, a small shunt can occur at this location between the two ventricles. There are generally two distinct AV valve orifices, corresponding to the mitral and tricuspid valves. Leaflet tissue joins the left superior and inferior leaflets together at the crest of the interventricular septum, eliminating the interventricular communication. In general, partial AV canal defects constitute approximately 5% to 10% of all ASDs.

Complete AV canal defects constitute the other end of the spectrum and are the most common form of AV canal defects. There is generally an ostium primum ASD and a nonrestrictive ventricular septal defect (VSD) in the inlet portion of the interventricular septum. One common AV valve orifice is present, with left and right components. An inlet-septal VSD alone does not fall under the heading of AV canal defects, because the AV septum is intact in these malformations and the AV valves usually form normally. On the other hand, some patients have an inlet-septal VSD and a cleft mitral valve with a restrictive or absent interatrial communication; these should be considered to be in the spectrum of AV canal defects.

In this chapter, we describe the principal anatomic features relevant to the preoperative evaluation and surgical management of defects amenable to a two-ventricle repair, and we briefly discuss the features that may preclude such an approach. Surgical techniques with early and late results are described. Various associated cardiac lesions are discussed, in addition to the management of recurrent mitral regurgitation. We will not discuss the management of AV canal defects associated with heterotaxy syndrome, because the AV canal defect is not the primary pathophysiologic abnormality, and because the anatomy of the AV valve and leaflet configuration are quite different from those of AV canal defects.

ANATOMY

The anatomic malformation that is common to all forms of AV canal defects is a deficiency in the AV septum caused by incomplete embryonic development of superior and inferior endocardial cushion tissue. The common AV canal is normally present during the early tubular stage of fetal life and constitutes the sole connection between the primitive common atrium and the primitive common ventricle. After cardiac looping, the valves of the heart develop in the embryo from precursor structures, called *endocardial cushions*. These endocardial swellings become populated by valve precursor cells formed by a transformation from endothelial to mesenchymal tissue, and they undergo directed growth and remodeling to form the valvular structures and the membranous septa of the mature heart (Fig. 116-1). Abnormal differentiation and remodeling of the cushion mesenchyme into valvuloseptal tissue is thought to be a mechanism for the development of AV canal defects.[4] The resultant anatomic defect involves the abnormal development of AV valves and the persistence of interatrial and interventricular communications.[5]

The wide variability in the degree of development of the endocardial cushions explains the variability in size and extent of the septal defects and the degree of involvement of the AV valves. Nevertheless, several anatomic features are shared between all types of AV canal defects. These include the following:

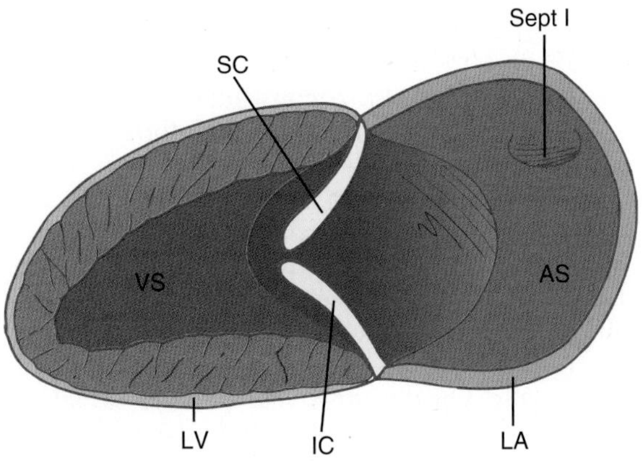

FIGURE 116-1 ■ Schematic of complete atrioventricular (AV) canal defect during morphogenesis, with the AV canal region shown in *dark gray*. Projections from the superior and inferior endocardial cushions normally differentiate into the AV valves and AV septum. *AS,* Atrial septum; *IC,* inferior endocardial cushion; *LA,* left atrium; *LV,* left ventricle; *SC,* superior endocardial cushion; *Sept 1,* septum primum; *VS,* ventricular septum. (Modified from Van Praagh R, Litovsky S: Pathology and embryology of common atrioventricular canal. *Prog Pediatr Cardiol* 10:115–127, 1999.)

- Shortened dimension of the inlet septum-to-ventricular apex, giving the interventricular septum a "scooped-out" appearance. This deficiency in the inlet septum is typically deeper in complete AV canal defects than in partial AV canal defects.
- Lengthened dimension of the outlet septum-to-ventricular apex, resulting in a goose-neck appearance and anterior displacement of the left ventricular (LV) outflow tract. Although the LV outflow tract appears narrow, true LV outflow tract obstruction (LVOTO) is rare in the absence of accessory chordal attachments of the AV valve leaflets to the outflow tract. In the normal heart, the inlet-septum-to-ventricular-apex length and the outlet-septum-to-ventricular-apex length are equal.
- Absence of the usual wedged position of the aortic valve between the AV valves, caused by maldevelopment of the endocardial cushions. This results in elevation and anterior deviation of the aortic valve.
- Decreased contribution of the left lateral leaflet to AV valve circumference. In the normal situation, the posterior mitral leaflet forms two thirds of the mitral valve circumference. In AV canal defects, the left lateral leaflet, which corresponds to the posterior mitral leaflet in the normal heart, forms only a third or less of the circumference of the AV valve.
- Inferior displacement of the AV node and coronary sinus. The bundle of His is also displaced inferiorly, coursing at the inferior rim of the scooped-out basal portion of the interventricular septum.

In addition to these fundamental concepts, anatomic features of significance to the surgeon include the following:

- Size and extent of the interventricular and interatrial communications
- Valve leaflet morphology, including papillary muscle anatomy, valve regurgitation, and presence of chordal attachments to the septum
- Relative balance of the common AV valve orifice over the two ventricles
- Other major associated cardiac and noncardiac defects

The AV valve in a canal defect has an area of apposition of leaflets that, unlike a normal commissure, is not supported by a papillary muscle. This area of apposition is called a *cleft*, and it is the apposition of the superior and inferior bridging leaflets. This cleft is not a commissure,[6] as was once thought,[7-9] for two reasons. First, a commissure is generally supported by chordae on either side of the defect, whereas a cleft is unsupported, with paucity of chordae at the edges. Second, the chordae that arise from the two adjacent leaflets in a commissure usually attach to a single papillary muscle, which promotes coaptation and prevents regurgitation. The chordae that arise from the left superior and inferior leaflets attach to two different papillary muscles; this increases the distracting force during ventricular systole and predisposes to regurgitation through the cleft. The extent of regurgitation is generally mild to moderate, although severe regurgitation can be present.

In 1966, Rastelli and colleagues[10] described a classification of complete AV canal defect based on the extent

echocardiography. One notable exception is the unoperated patient older than 1 year in whom measurement of pulmonary vascular resistance is needed to determine operative risk. Another exception is the postoperative patient in whom quantification of residual postoperative lesions, such as residual VSDs and LVOTO, are required to assess the need for reoperation.

SURGICAL TECHNIQUE

Median sternotomy, either partial or complete, has been the standard technique for exposing the heart and great vessels. Some have advocated a right anterior thoracotomy for partial AV canal defects in older female children to improve cosmesis. More recently, however, techniques to minimize surgical trauma by limiting the extent of the sternotomy have been used, such as a lower mini-sternotomy (Fig. 116-4).[38] This approach can be applied to infants and children of all ages and may be helpful in decreasing postoperative pain and development of chest wall deformities, such as pectus carinatum. We are now using this mini-sternotomy approach for nearly all AV canal defects, except when there are major associated cardiac lesions such as aortic coarctation, TOF, or TGA, where a full sternotomy is required for optimal exposure.

Cardiopulmonary bypass with moderate hypothermia and bicaval cannulation is used in nearly all cases; deep hypothermic circulatory arrest is rarely required. Aortic cross-clamping and cardioplegia are used in all cases to facilitate repair, particularly during the attachment of the septal patches near the AV node and coronary sinus.

In the setting of a large ostium primum ASD, both AV valves and intraventricular anatomy can be readily visualized. If a small or absent interatrial communication is present, then an incision in the septum primum provides access to the left AV valve for valve testing and cleft closure. This also aids in securing the VSD patch to the crest of the interventricular septum.

Complete Atrioventricular Canal

In complete AV canal defects, there is usually a large ostium primum defect and a moderate to large nonrestrictive VSD under the superior and inferior bridging leaflets (Fig. 116-5). There may be chordal attachments of either bridging leaflet, or both, to the crest of the septum, and these leaflets may be partitioned into right and left components or may form a single bridging leaflet over the crest of the septum. Two surgical approaches have been developed and are commonly used in this setting. A double-patch technique involves the placement of two separate patches, one to close the VSD and the other to close the ASD. Alternatively, a single-patch technique with autologous pericardium is used to close the VSD and ASD components, often with division of the superior bridging leaflet. More recently, a modified single-patch technique has been introduced, where the VSD is obliterated by suturing the bridging leaflets to the crest of the interventricular septum; a single pericardial patch is then used to close the ASD. Although there are advantages and disadvantages to each technique, excellent results have been reported with all three methods.

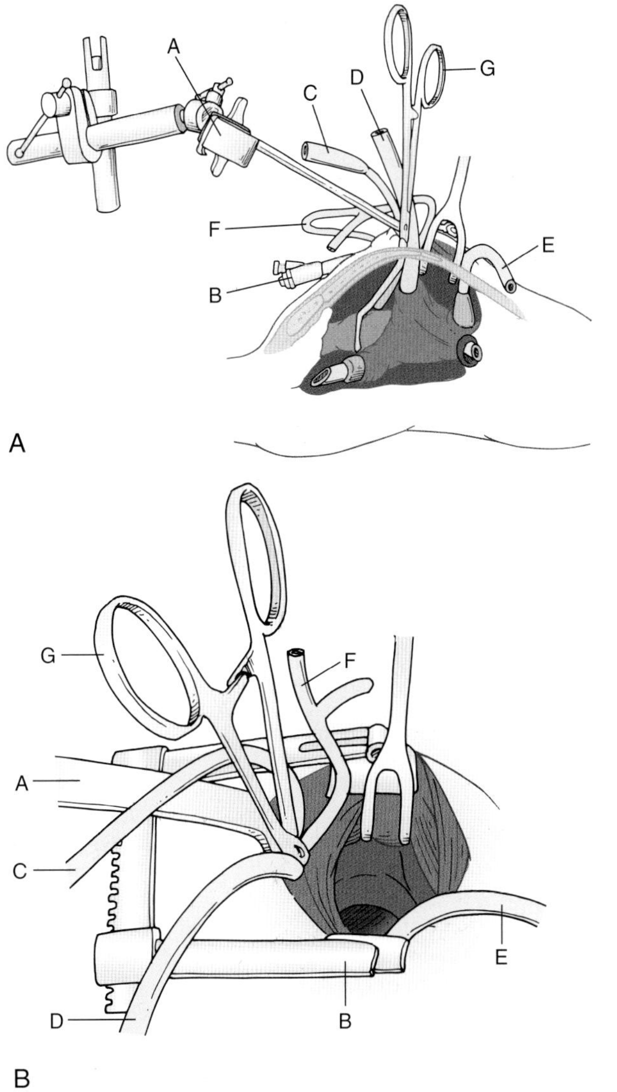

FIGURE 116-4 ■ Mini-sternotomy setup for repair of atrioventricular (AV) canal defects. **A,** Representative parasagittal cross-section with bicaval cannulation and aortic cross-clamping. **B,** Surgeon's view of the operative field. The inside of the atrium is well visualized for AV canal repair. *A,* Bookwalter retractor arm connected to an army-navy retractor; *B,* pediatric sternal retractor; *C,* aortic cannula; *D,* superior vena cava cannula via the right atrium, although direct cannulation is preferred for complete AV canal repair; *E,* inferior vena cava cannula; *F,* cardioplegia cannula; *G,* aortic crossclamp. (Modified from del Nido PJ, Bichell DP: Minimal-access surgery for congenital heart defects. *Semin Thorac Cardiovasc Surg Pediatr Card Surg Annu* 1:75–80, 1998.)

Double-Patch Technique

In the double-patch technique, separate patches are used for closure of the ventricular and atrial septal defects. The ventricular patch is made of synthetic material, such as Dacron, or glutaraldehyde-treated pericardium. The atrial patch is usually autologous pericardium, either untreated or treated with glutaraldehyde. The use of a

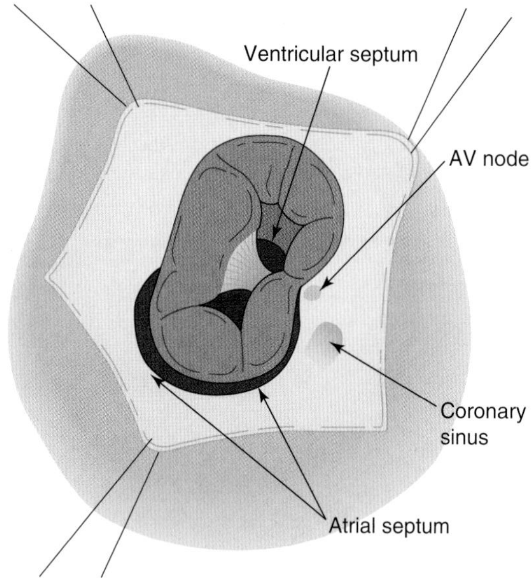

FIGURE 116-5 ■ Surgeon's view of complete atrioventricular (AV) canal defect. The superior bridging leaflet *(left)* is undivided and unattached to the underlying crest of the interventricular septum, as in a Rastelli type C defect. The AV node and coronary sinus ostium are displaced inferiorly. There is a cleft between the left superior and inferior leaflets. A large ostium primum defect is present, allowing good visualization into the left atrium.

synthetic atrial patch should be avoided, because hemolysis can result when a left AV valve regurgitant jet strikes the patch.

Initial inspection of the AV valve and filling of the left ventricle with cold saline facilitates the delineation of the point of coaptation of the left superior and inferior bridging leaflets. This permits measurement of the base-to-apex dimension of the VSD at the point of leaflet coaptation, corresponding to the height of the VSD patch. The distance between the two junction points of the interventricular septum and the AV valve annulus, at the aortic valve cephalad and the AV node caudad, should also be determined. This is helpful in determining the width of the VSD patch.

The patch shape is that of a crescent rather than a half circle because of the apical displacement of the point of coaptation of the superior and inferior bridging leaflets (Fig. 116-6*A*). The VSD patch is attached to the right of the crest of the interventricular septum using running or horizontal mattress interrupted pledgeted sutures. Care should be taken to avoid distortion of valve chordae that attach to the septum. As the suture line approaches the AV node area, the patch is attached more to the right of the septum, fixed 3 to 4 mm away from the junction of the interventricular septum and the AV valve.

The superior and inferior leaflets are then draped over the edge of the VSD patch. The pericardial patch is cut to an appropriate width, made narrower than the true distance between the aortic valve and the AV node to perform an annuloplasty of the AV valve, thereby decreasing the incidence of MR. A running horizontal suture line is performed to sandwich the AV valve leaflets between the VSD and ASD patches. These sutures pass through the pericardial patch, the left AV valve leaflets, the VSD

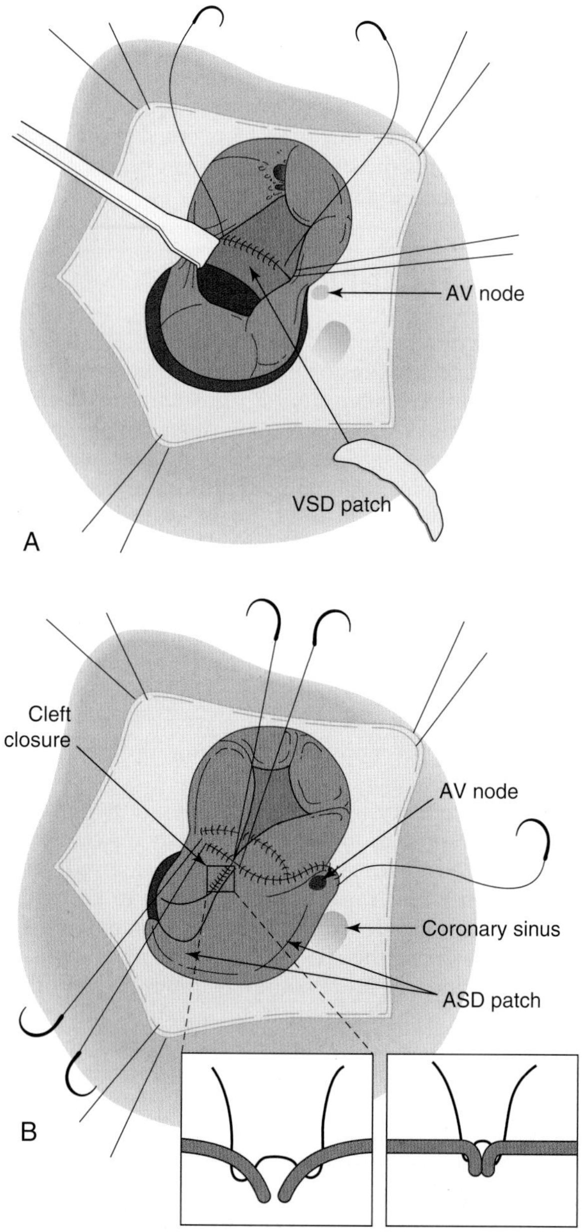

FIGURE 116-6 ■ The double-patch technique for repair of complete atrioventricular (AV) canal defects. **A,** Placement of the crescent-shaped ventricular septal defect (VSD) patch, showing suturing to the crest of the interventricular septum. The superior leaflet is retracted cephalad to allow accurate suturing without entrapment of chordae. Similar retraction is used at the inferior leaflet, where the patch is sewn to the right of the crest of the interventricular septum to avoid iatrogenic injury to the AV node. **B,** Completion of the double-patch repair is achieved by inserting the atrial septal defect (ASD) patch. Sutures are passed through the VSD patch, valve leaflets, and ASD patch, thereby sandwiching the valve between the two patches. In this example, the ASD patch is sewn to the right of the AV node and to the left of the coronary sinus. If a secundum defect or patent foramen is present, the ASD patch can be extended to cover both defects. Cleft closure is usually completed once the valve leaflets are attached to the ASD and VSD patches. *Inset,* Apposition of the cleft edges during systole.

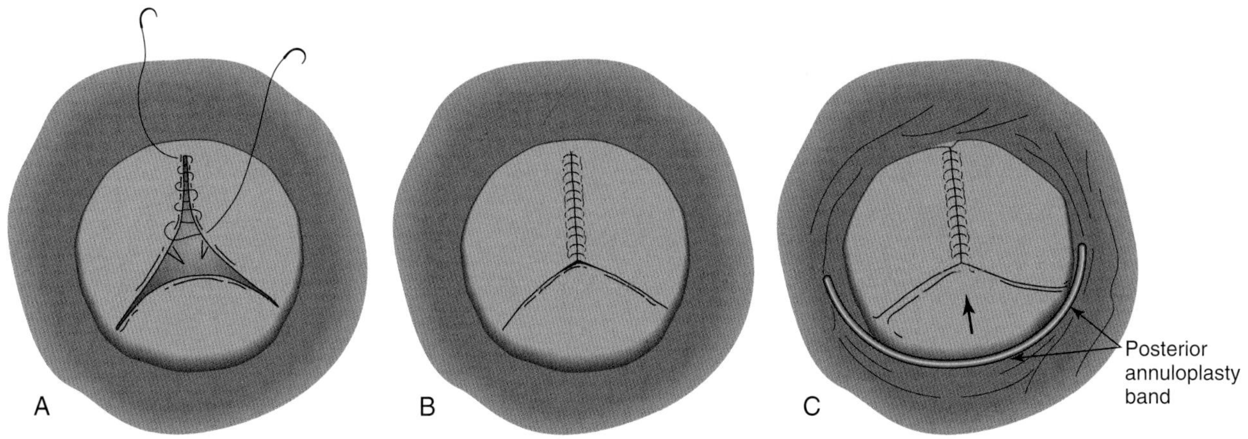

FIGURE 116-7 ■ Closure of the left atrioventricular (AV) valve cleft. Once the leaflets are attached to the ventricular septal defect and atrial septal defect patches, the zone of apposition of the superior and inferior bridging leaflets is usually well aligned. The cleft is then closed in two layers. **A,** The first layer is a running mattress suture, apposing the edges of the leaflets. **B,** The second running simple suture line ensures apposition of the leaflet edges. **C,** When there is significant annular dilation, a posterior annuloplasty is performed by inserting a flexible partial ring from the anterior fibrous continuity with the aortic valve to just posterior to the interatrial septum. The latter should remain 3 to 4 mm posterior to the junction between atrial septum and AV valve annulus to avoid injury to conduction tissue.

Dacron patch, and the right AV valve leaflets (see Fig. 116-6*B*).

The mitral valve cleft, created by coaptation of the superior and inferior bridging leaflets, is then closed, using either running or interrupted horizontal mattress sutures (Fig. 116-7*A*, *B*). Our preferred technique is the double-layer cleft closure. The first layer is a horizontal mattress layer, and the second layer is a simple running over-and-over suture, which is not tightened but left loose enough to help the pliability of the unified leaflet. The extent of cleft closure is determined in great part by the position of the papillary muscles and the size of the left lateral leaflet. Because closure of the cleft limits mobility of the superior and inferior leaflets, the greater the valve orifice area that is covered by these two leaflets, the greater the chance for creating valve stenosis. When the papillary muscles are close together or a single papillary muscle is present, closure of the cleft creates a slit-like orifice of the mitral valve, resulting in significant stenosis. In these cases, the cleft must be left at least partially open to facilitate leaflet mobility. Frequently, the edges of the leaflets creating the cleft are rolled and coapt over a small surface area. Care must be taken to preserve this degree of coaptation in closing the cleft and not to unroll the leaflet edges, because leaflet coaptation adds strength to the cleft closure, particularly during systole, thereby minimizing MR (see Fig. 116-6B).

The degree of MR is determined by injecting cold normal saline into the LV cavity. If significant regurgitation is present after cleft closure, then central regurgitation from poor leaflet coaptation is the usual culprit. This is managed by narrowing the commissure between the LSL and the left lateral leaflet and the LIL and lateral leaflet with placation sutures. When there is annular dilation, placing a posterior intra-annular absorbable suture from LIL to LSL suspends the entire lateral leaflet. This brings the left lateral leaflet closer to the interventricular septum and improves central leaflet coaptation. An additional maneuver that we have used when the left lateral leaflet does not coapt well with the sutured anterior leaflet is a posterior suture annuloplasty. We perform this maneuver using an absorbable monofilament suture, placing the suture in the annulus and then tying the suture over an appropriate sound to avoid valve stenosis. Commercially available posterior annuloplasty bands made of absorbable material can also be useful in cases of recurrent AV valve regurgitation (see Fig. 116-7*C*).

The ASD patch is then sutured to the remnants of the interatrial septum. The two surgical options available for avoiding injury to the AV node are attachment of the patch to the right or to the left of the AV node. Attaching the ASD patch to the right of the AV node involves suturing to the *right* inferior leaflet, where superficial bites are taken. The suturing continues to the right of the coronary sinus orifice, leaving the coronary sinus draining into the left atrium (Fig. 116-8*A*). Alternatively, the suturing can be extended to the edge of the coronary sinus orifice, leaving the orifice on the right atrial side (see Fig. 116-8*B*). The advantage of placing the patch to the right of the coronary sinus ostium is that the suture line remains far from conduction tissue. The disadvantage is that the coronary sinus is left draining to the left atrium. This can cause variable degrees of obstruction to coronary sinus drainage unless the coronary sinus is surgically unroofed. The arterial saturation is typically minimally affected. In a variant of this latter technique, the ASD patch can be attached to the *left* inferior leaflet, gradually returning to the edge of the interatrial septum, as initially advocated by McGoon and colleagues.[25] This leaves the coronary sinus draining into the right atrium. The disadvantage of this technique is that sutures must be placed through the LIL; in small infants, these sutures can tear through the delicate leaflet tissue or distort the leaflet enough to cause significant MR. In patients with complete AV canal and a left superior vena cava draining to the coronary sinus, the patch should be to the right of

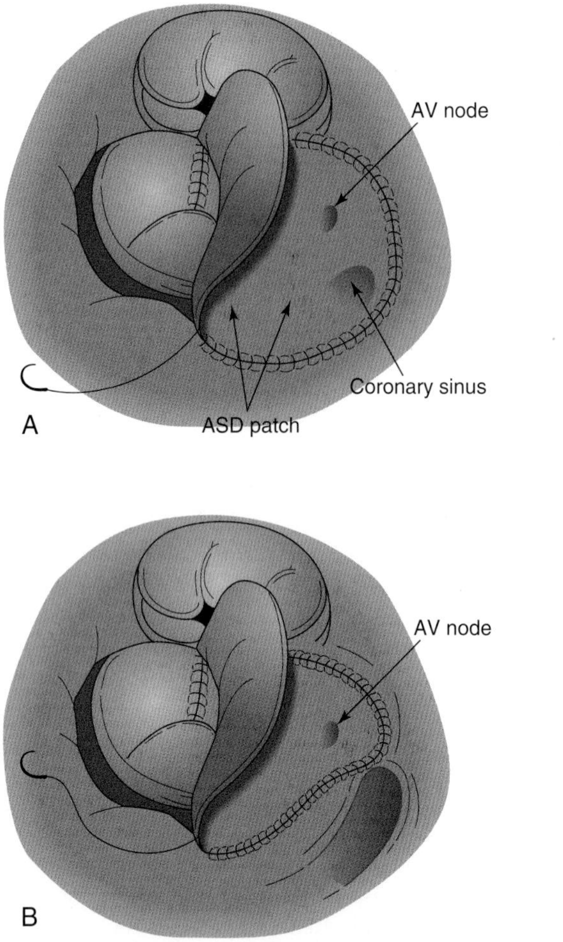

FIGURE 116-8 ■ Placement of the atrial septal defect (ASD) patch. **A,** The ASD patch can be placed entirely to the right of the atrioventricular (AV) node and coronary sinus, leaving the coronary sinus on the left atrial side of the newly constructed septum. **B,** Alternatively, the patch can be placed to the right of the AV node, but by turning the suture line back to the left of the coronary sinus, the sinus is left on the right atrial side.

the AV node and sutured to the edge of the coronary sinus ostium, leaving the ostium draining into the right atrium (see Fig. 116-8*B*).

Classic Single-Patch Technique

In the classic single-patch technique, the same patch of autologous pericardium, usually treated with glutaraldehyde, is used to cover both ventricular and atrial septal defects (Fig. 116-9).[39] It is critically important to determine the position of the mitral cleft and superior bridging leaflet with respect to the crest of the interventricular septum. When the right and left components of the AV valve are already partitioned with chordal attachments to the crest of the septum, only the position of the mitral valve cleft needs to be determined. Often, incisions must be made in the superior and inferior bridging leaflets parallel to and to the right of the interventricular septum to permit proper positioning of the single patch. The extent of leaflet division depends on the extent of the underlying VSD. Because the VSD under the superior bridging leaflet often extends to the AV valve annulus, the leaflet incision has to extend to the AV annulus as well. This is often not the case for the inferior bridging leaflet, especially in the Rastelli A subtype, where the underlying VSD may not extend to the AV valve annulus because of variable fibrous fusion between the LIL and the crest of the interventricular septum. The leaflet incision in that case is only partial, without extension to the AV valve annulus. This protects the conduction tissue and AV node from iatrogenic injury. When the VSD under the inferior bridging leaflet extends to the AV valve annulus, the division of the leaflet should be to the right of the crest of the interventricular septum. This allows placement of the patch toward the right, thereby avoiding injury to the underlying conduction tissue at the crest of the interventricular septum.

As with the double-patch technique, precise measurement of the width of the patch with respect to the width of the AV canal defect is necessary to prevent MR caused by distortion of valve leaflets. If the patch is too wide, then the AV valve annulus size will increase, particularly over the interventricular septum; the superior and inferior bridging leaflet tissue available might not be sufficient to cover the orifice, resulting in MR.

Once the AV valve is partitioned into the right and left components, the VSD patch is attached to the right of the crest of the interventricular septum using running or interrupted pledgeted sutures. As with the double-patch technique, the suture line is placed to the right of the crest of the interventricular septum to avoid injury to the bundle of His. Once the patch is attached to the ventricular septum, the AV valve leaflets must be reattached to the patch. This maneuver is greatly facilitated by prior placement of a suture marking the coaptation point of the LSL and LIL at the base of the cleft at the crest of the interventricular septum. The valve leaflets should not be reattached too far to the atrial side of the patch, because this would tether the leaflets and limit coaptation, resulting in MR. Attachment of valve leaflets to the patch is done with pledgeted sutures because these valve leaflets are thin and friable, particularly in infants, predisposing to tearing if attached with nonpledgeted sutures.

The mitral cleft is closed next. The same considerations regarding cleft closure as described for the double-patch technique are applicable here. Similarly, individual commissuroplasty sutures can be placed for the treatment of central left AV valve regurgitation. The patch is then sutured to close the interatrial communication. As discussed earlier for double-patch repair, the coronary sinus may be left draining into the right or left atrium.

Modified Single-Patch Technique

The original description of complete AV canal repair by Dr. Lillehei involved attaching the AV valve leaflets to the crest of the interventricular septum primarily, because patch material was not readily available at the time; the ASD was also closed primarily.[23] Wilcox and colleagues[30] reintroduced this method of repair for patients with small VSDs. Nicholson and colleagues[29] broadened

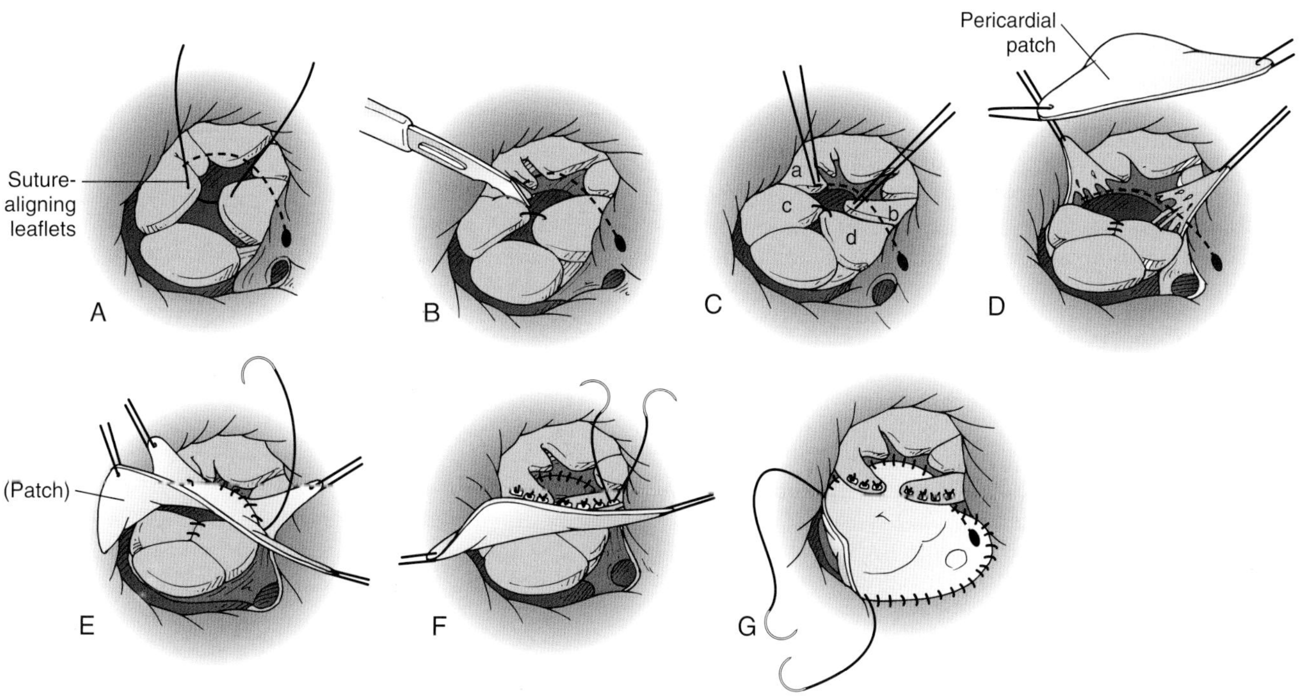

FIGURE 116-9 ■ Classic single-patch technique for repair of complete atrioventricular (AV) canal defects. **A,** Alignment sutures placed through the left superior leaflet and left inferior leaflet at the crest of the interventricular septum. **B,** The superior bridging leaflet is incised. **C,** Two portions of the superior bridging leaflet *(a* and *c)* and two portions of the inferior bridging leaflet *(b* and *d)* are shown after division of the corresponding leaflets. The division of the inferior bridging leaflet need not extend beyond the underlying interventricular communication. **D,** The left-sided cleft is closed. **E,** The pericardial patch is sewn to the crest of the interventricular septum. **F,** The right and left AV valve leaflets are suspended onto the pericardial patch. **G,** Completion of the repair by closure of the atrial septal defect. The AV node and coronary sinus ostium are shown draining on the left atrial side. (Modified from Castaneda AR, Jonas RA, Meyer JE Jr, et al: Atrioventricular canal defect. In Castaneda AR, Jonas RA, Mayer JE Jr, et al, editors: *Cardiac surgery of the neonate and infant,* Philadelphia, 1994, WB Saunders, p 179.)

the indications to patients with moderate and large VSDs. Other reports have confirmed their findings.[40,41]

In this technique, several pledgeted horizontal mattress sutures are brought through the crest of the interventricular septum, the AV valve leaflets, the autologous pericardial patch, and a narrow strip of Dacron, in that order (Fig. 116-10). Care should be taken to avoid damage to the bundle of His by keeping the sutures to the right of the crest of the interventricular septum, especially inferiorly. Suturing through the AV valve leaflets effectively partitions the bridging superior and inferior leaflets into right and left components. The strip of Dacron acts as an annuloplasty because its superior-inferior dimension is approximately 80% of the superior-inferior dimension of the AV canal defect, thereby bringing the left-sided AV valve leaflets into closer apposition and minimizing MR. Some have advocated avoiding the use of a strip of Dacron because of concerns about the effect of fixation of the mitral annulus on its long-term growth potential. One potential disadvantage of this technique is the development of LVOTO because the interventricular communication is closed primarily, without patch material. So far, although follow-up is limited, this has not been seen. The amount of MR appears similar to that seen with the classic single-patch and double-patch methods, although long-term follow-up is not yet available.

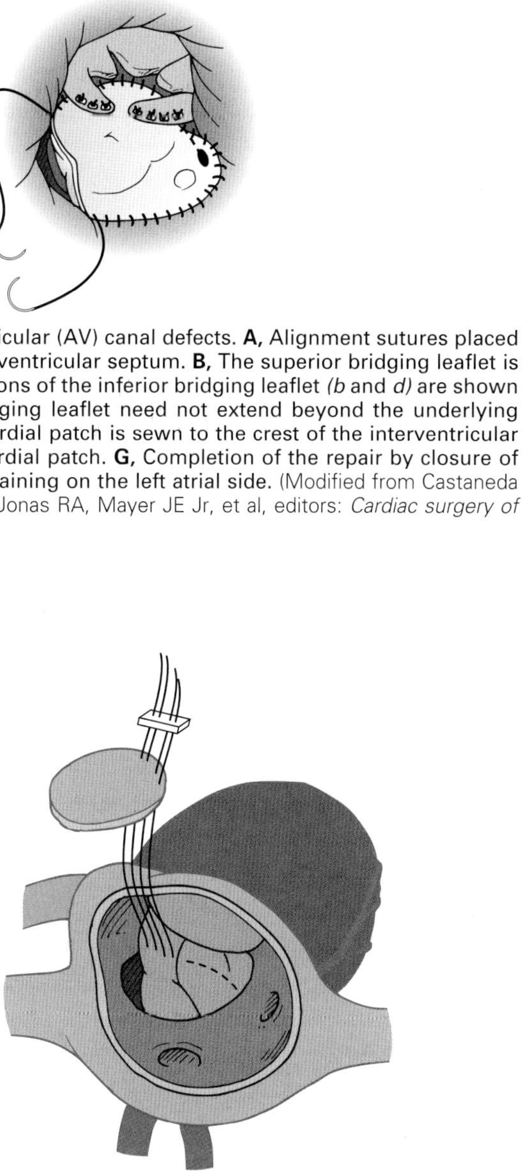

FIGURE 116-10 ■ Modified single-patch technique for repair of complete atrioventricular (AV) canal defects. Horizontal mattress pledgeted sutures are passed through the crest of the interventricular septum, the AV valve leaflets, and the pericardial patch, and then through a Dacron strip annuloplasty. (Modified from Nicholson IA, Nunn GR, Sholler GF, et al: Simplified single patch technique for the repair of atrioventricular septal defect. *J Thorac Cardiovasc Surg* 118:642–646, 1999.)

Transitional Atrioventricular Canal

In this form of AV canal defect, the VSD is restrictive and usually centrally located, formed by incomplete fusion of the point of coaptation between the LSL and LIL over the crest of the septum. There is usually a large ostium primum defect and a cleft mitral valve. The bridging leaflets are fused to the crest of the septum except for the central portion, and small VSDs may be found under the superior or inferior leaflets when the leaflets have not completely fused to the crest of the interventricular septum. When the VSDs are small, they can be difficult to identify intraoperatively. Retraction of the right superior leaflet can provide adequate access to these small defects, and a small (1- to 2-mm) probe can be used to identify residual interventricular communications.

These small VSDs can usually be closed primarily with sutures. Closure of the central VSD is usually done with the same suture that is used to close the cleft, but starting at the crest of the interventricular septum. Closure of the interatrial communication is done in a manner similar to ostium primum defects (Fig. 116-11).

Partial Atrioventricular Canal or Ostium Primum Defects

As with repair of complete AV canal, initial inspection and testing of the mitral valve is done. The presence of a partial or complete cleft is noted; in the majority of cases, the cleft extends to the interventricular septum. The technique for cleft closure is the same as that described earlier, with emphasis on maintaining leaflet coaptation. The ostium primum ASD is closed using autologous pericardium, because this tissue is more pliable than synthetic material and is less likely to distort valve leaflets. A secundum ASD or patent foramen ovale, if present, is closed either separately or with the same patch (see Fig. 116-11).

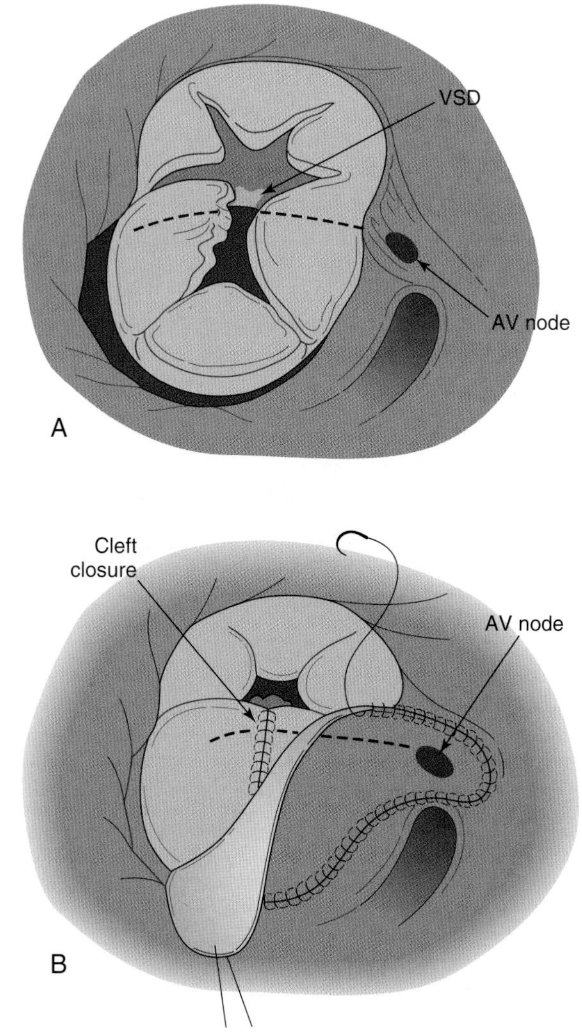

FIGURE 116-11 ■ Repair of transitional atrioventricular (AV) canal defect. **A,** The bridging leaflets are usually attached to the crest of the septum *(dashed line)* except for the central area of coaptation where there is a small ventricular septal defect (VSD). **B,** Closure of the VSD is accomplished using the same suture line as was used for cleft closure. Closure of the mitral cleft in this case is done first, then pericardial patch closure of the ostium primum defect is done. The patch is sutured to the right inferior leaflet tissue and then heads down toward the coronary sinus. An alternative technique (not shown) is suturing to the left inferior leaflet tissue, at the rim of the ostium primum defect.

ASSOCIATED CARDIAC LESIONS

Associated cardiovascular lesions are not uncommon, particularly with complete AV canal defects. Extracardiac defects such as patent ductus arteriosus and aortic coarctation are usually treated during the operative procedure for repair of the AV canal defect. The surgical techniques for repair of associated defects are usually not different in the presence of an AV canal defect from when the lesions are isolated defects. Exceptions to this include the presence of secundum ASDs or additional muscular VSDs that are close to the AV canal defect; these can be repaired by extension of the septal patch to cover both lesions. Lesions that include conotruncal abnormalities such as TOF require significant modifications to the surgical approach and are discussed separately.

Tetralogy of Fallot

Tetralogy of Fallot is a complication in approximately 5% of patients with complete AV canal defects. The LSL is typically free floating over the interventricular crest of the septum, as in a Rastelli type C defect, resulting in a large VSD with outlet extension. In contrast to the heart failure symptoms seen in the majority of patients with isolated complete AV canal defects, the main symptom in the combined lesion is cyanosis. This occurs because of right-to-left intracardiac shunting, which depends primarily on the degree of RV outflow tract obstruction. In a minority of patients, the degree of RV outflow tract obstruction is minimal; these patients display heart failure symptoms in early infancy that are similar to the symptoms in patients with isolated complete AV canal defects.

The operative management of complete AV canal defects associated with TOF requires modification of the VSD patch, because it has to extend to cover the conoventricular, anteriorly malaligned VSD. As with most forms of TOF, there is frequently infundibular obstruction, along with pulmonary valvar hypoplasia and stenosis requiring augmentation of the entire RV outflow tract. Because of the anterior position of the aortic valve annulus in this defect, visualization of the anterosuperior edge of the VSD is best accomplished through a right infundibulotomy. As with cases of uncomplicated AV canal defects, the width of the VSD patch at the AV valve annulus level must be chosen carefully to prevent enlarging the AV valve annulus and resulting in MR.

When the single-patch technique is used to repair complete AV canal in association with TOF, an incision in the superior bridging leaflet is usually needed and is particularly critical. This incision should be farther toward the right of the crest of the interventricular septum, toward the right AV valve, to accommodate the underlying anterior deviation of the conal septum. This prevents the development of subaortic obstruction and LVOTO, seen when the patch is placed too far to the left of the interventricular septum. This is less an issue with the double-patch method of repair, although correct positioning of the VSD patch under the superior leaflet is still required. The shape of the VSD patch for the combined lesion resembles a teardrop rather than the typical crescent shape in isolated complete AV canal defect. The modified single-patch technique as originally described is not applicable to canal defects with TOF, because the large malalignment defect precludes direct suturing of the LSL to the crest of the interventricular septum.

Repair of the RV outflow tract obstruction is managed in a manner similar to that of isolated TOF, often with an incision in the RV outflow tract. The major difference in the combined lesion is that MR can result in left atrial hypertension with subsequent pulmonary arterial hypertension. If a transannular patch is used, the regurgitant fraction across the enlarged RV outflow tract is increased, leading to RV distention and dysfunction. The right ventriculotomy combined with division of RV muscle bundles in the outflow tract further exacerbates RV dysfunction. In such cases, consideration should be given to the creation of a temporary single-leaflet valve made from autologous pericardium. Careful testing of the tricuspid valve should be undertaken to rule out the presence of significant tricuspid regurgitation. If present, this can often be repaired by closure of the cleft between the right superior and inferior leaflets while avoiding the underlying conduction tissue.

Some have advocated the placement of a systemic-to-pulmonary shunt (e.g., a right modified Blalock-Taussig shunt) in the neonatal period in patients with severe cyanosis, with subsequent repair at 1 to 3 years of age, which potentially decreases the need for a transannular patch.[42] We have usually undertaken complete repair in infants to avoid the episodes of hypercyanosis seen in tetralogy physiology. As with management of tetralogy, a small atrial septal communication is left to permit some right-to-left shunting because of RV diastolic dysfunction early after surgery.

Double-Outlet Right Ventricle

An anatomic scenario that can be similar to TOF is DORV, which is differentiated from TOF by the degree of aortic override. When more than 50% of the aortic valve is located over the right ventricle, the lesion is defined as DORV rather than TOF. DORV is present in approximately 1% to 2% of patients with complete AV canal defects.[43] Typically, DORV in this setting is associated with heterotaxy syndrome and unbalanced AV canal defects, increasing the likelihood of univentricular palliation.

Two-ventricle repair of DORV and complete AV canal defects parallels the repair of the two separate lesions. If the VSD is in the subaortic position, the repair is similar to TOF with complete AV canal defect. The patch is more complex, because the left ventricle has to be baffled through the VSD to the aortic valve.

Coarctation of the Aorta

If aortic coarctation is present, the left-sided cardiac structures need to be studied carefully to ensure that they are of adequate size and to rule out unbalanced AV canal with RV dominance. Aortic coarctation has been associated with a mild degree of LV outflow obstruction for valvar or subvalvar stenosis. Often, these patients have closely spaced papillary muscles in the left ventricle or, in extreme cases, a parachute mitral valve with a single papillary muscle.

If significant MR is present after repair of complete AV canal defects, an exhaustive search should be performed to rule out the presence of residual LVOTO or aortic coarctation. If present, this increases LV afterload, which increases the distracting pressure on the thin and friable mitral leaflets and worsens the degree of MR. Repair of aortic coarctation in this setting often decreases the degree of MR.

Left Ventricular Outflow Tract Obstruction

Hemodynamically significant LVOTO is relatively rare in the setting of AV canal defects. Interestingly, LVOTO is rare in the presence of Down syndrome.[44] It is more common in partial AV canal defects than in complete AV canal defects,[45] unless ventricular imbalance is present. This may be due to the modification of the LV outflow tract in complete AV canal repair through the insertion of a VSD patch, whereas no such patch is needed during partial AV canal repair because no VSD is present. LVOTO results in an increased left-to-right shunt with accelerated development of heart failure symptoms. LVOTO appears to be more commonly associated with the Rastelli A subtype of complete AV canal.[46] The development of LVOTO can be acquired, progressive, or recurrent.[47]

The normal LV outflow tract has an angle of almost 90 degrees between the plane of the crest of the interventricular septum and the plane of the outlet septum. This angle is significantly decreased in AV canal defects, measuring 22 degrees in one study.[46] In the Rastelli C subtype, the angle is nearly normal after repair of complete AV canal, accounting for the decreased incidence of LVOTO in this setting.

The mechanism and severity of LVOTO usually can be delineated with two-dimensional echocardiography.

Cardiac catheterization is reserved to confirm the degree of obstruction, particularly in patients presenting late after AV canal repair.

The surgical treatment is usually determined by the mechanism of obstruction. Obstructing primary AV valve chordal attachments can be divided off the crest of the septum if they are secondary chordae. If the cleft is directed to the LV outflow, division of the chords and closure of the cleft usually treats the outflow obstruction. In tunnel-like LVOTO, more extensive enlargement of the LV outflow tract is required, such as a modified Konno procedure. Unlike the more common forms of tunnel-like LVOTO, in AV canal defects the conduction tissue is farther away from the area of enlargement, and injury to the AV node is rare. Subaortic obstruction may be recurrent. In one study of 19 patients with subaortic stenosis associated with AV canal defects,[16] operations for LVOTO were performed.[46] The most common procedure was fibrous resection of a subaortic membrane with myectomy. Mean time to reoperation for recurrent LVOTO was 4.9 years, with a median follow-up period of 5.6 years. This resulted in a 6-year actuarial freedom from reoperation of 66%. To decrease the incidence of reoperation, leaflet augmentation with pericardium and fibromyectomy have been suggested.

Transposition of the Great Arteries

Management of TGA associated with complete AV canal defect is similar to the surgical treatment of each isolated defect. The AV canal defect is repaired, and an arterial switch procedure is performed. The AV canal repair is more challenging because valve leaflets are very friable in the first week of life compared with the first few months of life. All heart structures are smaller as well, which increases the technical complexity of the procedure. We recommend reinforcement of all sutures through AV valve leaflets with autologous pericardial pledgets, especially those placed for cleft closure. If the superior bridging leaflet is undivided, we recommend avoiding the classic single-patch technique because leaflet division is necessary. Resuspension of the leaflets onto the single patch may gather too much precious leaflet tissue, predisposing to the development of MR.

Double-Orifice Mitral Valve

Another unusual abnormality of the left-sided AV valve is double-orifice mitral valve, present in approximately 5% of cases. A second accessory orifice is present, usually on the inferior aspect of the left lateral leaflet, which can vary substantially in size. If the second orifice is small, it may be left open without consequence.

If large, the papillary muscles need to be examined because one papillary muscle may be related to each orifice, resulting in a parachute mitral valve of the major orifice. In these situations the cleft should be closed only partially, because postoperative mitral stenosis results with complete cleft closure. Splitting the bridging leaflet tissue between the two orifices is not advised; this can result in significant MR because the leaflet tissue becomes unsupported. In some cases, when regurgitation is present at the accessory orifice, addition of a triangular patch made from glutaraldehyde-treated autologous pericardium has been advocated in an attempt to extend the width of the leaflets and improve coaptation.

Parachute Mitral Valve

A single papillary muscle is present in 5% of cases of complete AV canal defect. The presence of two closely spaced papillary muscles or a single papillary muscle can result in all chordal structures attaching to a single point, referred to as *parachute mitral valve*. Closure of the cleft between the LSL and LIL frequently results in postoperative mitral stenosis in this setting. We elect to leave the cleft either partially or fully open, depending on the degree of separation of the papillary muscles, the thickness of the chordae, and the width of the interchordal spaces. Rarely, this still results in significant regurgitation at initial operation. Techniques to split the papillary muscle improve leaflet mobility by separating the chordae. Similarly, when there are two separate but closely spaced papillary muscles, mobilizing the papillary muscles away from one another may be effective in improving the effective orifice of the mitral valve.

Unbalanced Atrioventricular Canal

Bharati and colleagues[48] pointed out that the AV junction may be committed primarily to one ventricle in some cases of complete AV canal defects, resulting in associated hypoplasia of the contralateral ventricular cavity and outflow structures. This occurs in approximately 5% to 7% of patients with complete AV canal defects. In the more common right ventricle–dominant form, there is significant hypoplasia of the left ventricle, aortic valve, ascending aorta, and aortic arch. Conversely, in the left ventricle–dominant type, hypoplasia of the right ventricle is seen.

Management decisions regarding the potential use of the hypoplastic chamber as part of a two-ventricle repair should be based on objective criteria quantifying absolute ventricular volumes indexed to body surface area. Measurement of relative ventricular cavity volume to compare RV and LV volumes is frequently unreliable. Absolute ventricular volumes with values of 15 mL/m^2 or greater are felt to be sufficient criteria for successful two-ventricle repair. Three-dimensional echocardiography has significantly improved ventricular volume measurements.

If the canal is only mildly unbalanced, then a two-ventricle repair can often be performed. If the canal is grossly unbalanced with severe hypoplasia of one ventricular cavity, then a single-ventricle approach may be followed. However, there is a growing experience with two-stage repair of unbalanced defects, with partial closure of the interatrial communication performed in the first stage to encourage ventricular growth. At the second stage, VSD closure is performed. Traditionally, criteria have been developed to decide between two-ventricle and single-ventricle management. They involve a determination of relative ventricular size, AV valve architecture and function, outflow tract size and position, and the presence of associated cardiac lesions:

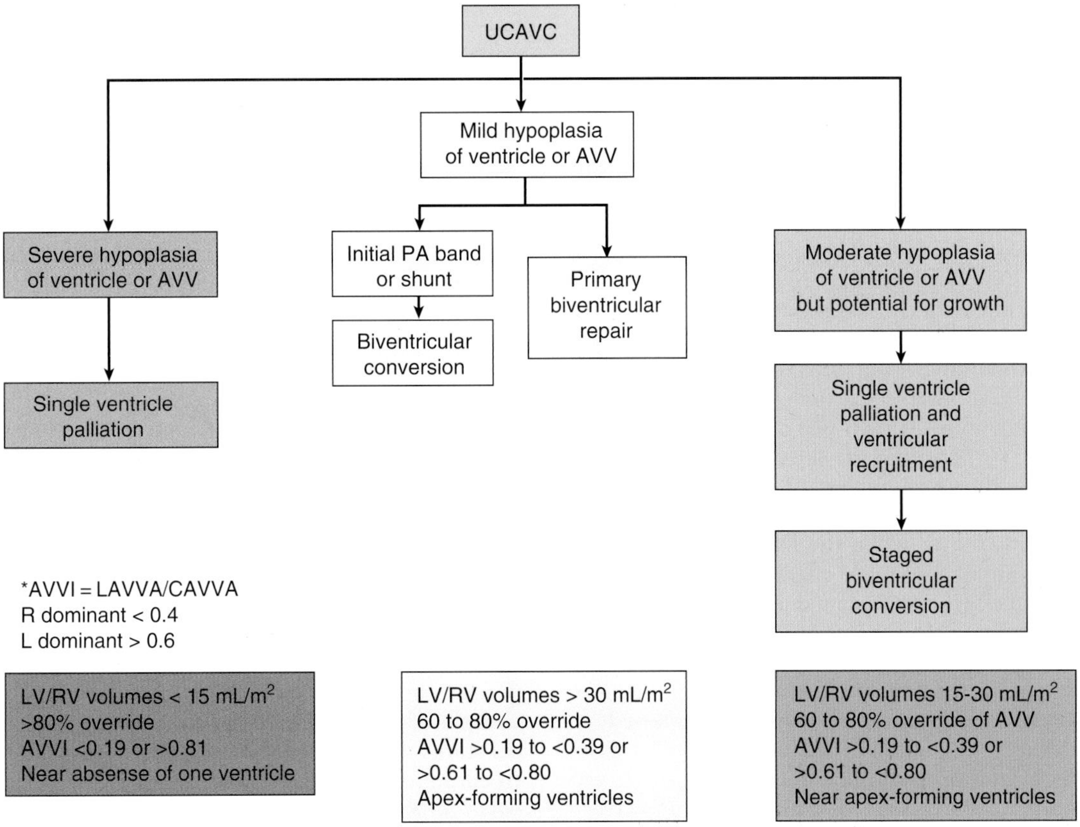

FIGURE 116-12 ■ Proposed algorithm for management of unbalanced complete atrioventricular canal defects. *AVV,* Atrioventricular valve; *AVVI,* atrioventricular valve index; *CAVVA,* common atrioventricular valve area; *L,* left; *LAVVA,* left atrioventricular valve area; *LV,* left ventricle, *PA,* pulmonary artery; *R,* right; *RV,* right ventricle; *UCAVC,* unbalanced complete atrioventricular canal. (Adapted from Nathan M, Liu H, Pigula FA, et al: Biventricular conversion after single-ventricle palliation in unbalanced atrioventricular canal defects. *Ann Thorac Surg* 95:2086–2096, 2013.)

- The left ventricle reaches the apex or near the apex.
- The calculated postoperative LV volume is 15 mL/m2 or greater.
- The calculated postoperative mitral valve annulus z-score is −2 or greater.
- Two papillary muscles are present, although a single papillary muscle is not an absolute contraindication for two-ventricle repair.
- AV valve chordae attaching to the conal septum, which is a substrate for LVOTO, are absent. Associated aortic coarctation is often present.
- Heterotaxy syndrome is absent, although rarely a patient with polysplenia has two well-balanced ventricles that are amenable to two-ventricle repair.

These criteria, however, do not account for the growth potential that exists, particularly in very young infants. Recent reports have described growth of the LV cavity after closure of interatrial communications by forcing blood flow across the left AV valve.[49] A study from Boston analyzed biventricular conversions after initial single ventricle palliation in 16 patients with unbalanced complete AV canal defects.[50] All patients had either unequal distribution of the common AV valve or hypoplastic ventricle. Eight patients were right dominant with median LV end-diastolic volume of 32 mL/m^2, and eight were left dominant with RV end-diastolic volume of 42 mL/m^2. Biventricular conversion was achieved in these patients with two patient deaths and eight patient reinterventions in the study follow-up period. The algorithm proposed by these authors for management of unbalanced complete AV canal defect patients is shown in Figure 116-12.

Heterotaxy Syndrome

There is a distinct group of patients with heterotaxy and AV canal defects. These patients are challenging to manage. The criteria for biventricular repair outlined here still apply to these patients. However, consideration needs to be given to septation of systemic and pulmonary venous return as well as repair of the common AV valve. Patients with complex anatomy may benefit from early single ventricle palliation and conversion to biventricular repair at older age.

Single Ventricle

When more complex malformations are present, such as severely unbalanced AV canal defects, consideration should be given to managing these patients along a single-ventricle pathway. In patients with complete AV canal defects and heterotaxy syndrome, associated conotruncal anomalies such as transposition and pulmonary stenosis or atresia are often treated with single-ventricle management.[51]

Recurrent Mitral Regurgitation

Significant postoperative MR requiring reoperation is present in 4% to 15% of patients after repair of AV canal defects.[52,53] In our experience, those at highest risk had at least moderate MR early postoperatively.[19] Other factors associated with progressive late postoperative MR include parachute mitral valve,[54] double-orifice mitral valve,[19,55,56] absence of Down syndrome,[28] no closure of the cleft at primary repair,[28,56,57] and preoperative MR.[53,55] Although mild deterioration is fairly common after complete AV canal repair, serious deterioration is rare, especially after the first 30 postoperative months, as reported in one study of 39 patients.[58] Another study followed two groups of patients, one in whom the cleft was closed at the time of initial AV canal surgery, and the other in whom the cleft was deliberately left open as part of a trifoliate repair.[57] Overall survival and freedom from reoperation for MR were significantly better when the mitral valve cleft was closed at the time of initial AV canal surgery. One confounding variable was the earlier date of surgery in the group in whom the cleft was left open; improvements in myocardial preservation and postoperative care could have contributed to the improved results seen in the more recent group of patients in whom the cleft was closed.

The mechanism of late MR in the majority of cases has been regurgitation through the cleft, because it was either left open initially or reopened after complete or partial closure. Annular dilation with central regurgitation is frequently an associated finding. Worsening MR leads to worsening LV volume overload and eccentric LV hypertrophy, ultimately leading to LV dysfunction and failure. One study looked at the echocardiographic changes associated with left AV valve after complete AV canal repair, this study showed that a potential mechanism for recurrent MR could be due to annular dilation which occurs posteriorly toward the free wall.[59] This mechanism points to the beneficial effect of posterior annuloplasty performed at the time of original repair to lift the left lateral leaflet toward the septum and potentially to prevent development of MR.

Preoperative echocardiographic studies should delineate the mechanism of regurgitation and the location of the regurgitant jet (either centrally or through the cleft or both). A direct measurement of the diameter of the mitral annulus should be performed and compared with the expected annular diameter for the patient's age, corresponding to a z-score of 0.

Reoperative mitral valve repair depends on the underlying anatomic abnormality. If the regurgitation is through a cleft, then closure of the cleft, along with reduction of the mitral annular diameter to an appropriate size (z-score between −2 and +2), is often effective. More complex mechanisms such as immobile, thickened, or retracted mitral leaflets are more difficult to repair and frequently require leaflet augmentation with autologous pericardium, along with reduction of the annular diameter. The presence of MR thickens the leaflets, allowing closure of the tear either primarily or with a small pericardial patch. In the older child, a flexible partial annuloplasty ring should be implanted to provide support for the repaired valve, especially during ventricular systole.

In rare cases, mitral repair is not possible, and mitral valve replacement becomes necessary, typically using a mechanical prosthesis. Because the native left AV valve encroaches on the LV outflow tract, valve replacement can result in significant LVOTO. This can be avoided by first suturing a rectangular Dacron patch to the left AV valve annulus in the subaortic region. The mitral prosthesis can then be attached to the Dacron patch superiorly.[60] The conduction tissue is located at the anteroinferior aspect of the left AV valve annulus. The native AV valve leaflet tissue should be preserved in that location and not excised. Sutures can be passed through these native leaflets rather than through the mitral annulus in that location to minimize the incidence of heart block. Care should also be taken to avoid injury to the left circumflex coronary artery, which can be surprisingly close in small patients.

Outcomes after surgical management of recurrent MR are inferior to those reported after initial AV canal defects. In a study from our institution representing the largest series to date, 46 patients underwent reoperation between 1988 and 1998 for recurrent hemodynamically significant MR.[49] Survival at 10 years was 86.6%. Three of nine patients undergoing mitral valve replacement developed complete heart block. Significant improvements in clinical status were present after mitral valve surgery. Overall freedom from reoperation at 5 years was 78.5% for mitral valve repair and 85.7% for mitral valve replacement.

POSTOPERATIVE CARE

Postoperative management of patients after repair of complete AV canal defects is similar to the management of other patients after complex cardiac surgery. Intraoperative confirmation of complete closure of the VSD and ASD should be obtained. Our preference is to use measurements of right atrial and pulmonary artery oxygen saturations to detect residual left-to-right shunts. An increase in oxygen saturation greater than 10 mm Hg or an absolute pulmonary artery oxygen saturation greater than 80% while on 50% inspired oxygen suggests the presence of a hemodynamically significant residual VSD (i.e., ratio of pulmonary blood flow [Qp] to systemic blood flow [Qs], or $Qp/Qs > 1.5$). This should prompt intraoperative confirmation by echocardiography before a return to cardiopulmonary bypass and closure of the residual VSD.

Intraoperative transesophageal echocardiogram (TEE) is highly recommended for patients weighing more than 5 kg. TEE can be performed in patients as small as 2.5 kg, albeit with a higher risk of esophageal trauma and perforation coupled with a higher probability of left atrial compression by the posteriorly positioned TEE probe, which raises left atrial pressure. TEE is especially useful in evaluating AV valve function, particularly if significant MR is suspected. Monitoring left atrial and pulmonary artery pressures aids in the postoperative care of these patients, especially when preoperative pulmonary hypertension is present.

Low cardiac output state should be judiciously managed by aggressive use of inotropic support rather than volume resuscitation, because excessive volume infusion can lead to ventricular distention and valvar dilation, resulting in worsening MR. The atrial filling pressures should be kept low, not significantly higher than 10 mm Hg, especially in the first 24 hours postoperatively. Use of afterload reduction, particularly with phosphodiesterase inhibitors such as milrinone, is particularly valuable in the early postoperative period. An aggressive search should be undertaken to exclude anatomic causes of low cardiac output syndrome.

Early postoperative pulmonary hypertension can be seen in patients with complete AV canal defects, and it is more prevalent with increasing age at the time of definitive repair and correlates with surgical mortality. Patients with Down syndrome usually have increased pulmonary artery pressure and increased pulmonary vascular resistance in the perioperative period.[61] The insertion of a pulmonary artery line at the time of surgery aids in making the diagnosis. Anatomic causes that mimic pulmonary hypertension need to be excluded, such as severe MR, severe mitral stenosis, and residual VSD. Echocardiography is helpful in differentiating anatomic from nonanatomic causes of postoperative pulmonary hypertension.

OUTCOMES

Between January 1990 and December 1998, 365 patients with various forms of AV canal defects underwent two-ventricle repair at Children's Hospital Boston.[62] Of these, 191 had a complete AV canal defect in which the VSD was deemed at least moderate in size and required patch closure. Among these 365 patients, 19 had associated TOF (5%) and 140 had either an ostium primum ASD alone or a transitional AV canal defect. Five patients had associated coarctation of the aorta, and seven had preoperative LVOTO. Trivial to mild AV valve regurgitation was present preoperatively in 159 patients (83%), and 26 (13%) had moderate to severe AV valve regurgitation. Of the patients with complete AV canal defects, 11% had at least moderate hypoplasia of one ventricle, 4% had a dominant left ventricle, and 7% had a dominant right ventricle.

The classic one-patch technique was used in 83% of the children with complete AV canal defects; the remaining 16% were repaired using the two-patch technique, depending on surgeon preference. The median age at repair was 4.6 months, and median weight was 4.5 kg.

In the 191 patients with complete AV canal defects undergoing biventricular repair, there were three early deaths, for an operative mortality of 1.5%. Three patients had complete heart block postoperatively, which required pacemaker insertion during the initial hospitalization. Trivial to mild MR was present on postoperative echocardiographic follow-up in 66% of the patients, whereas 10% had at least moderate MR at the time of discharge. There was no correlation between the presence of MR preoperatively and its presence postoperatively.

A review of 215 patients from the Pediatric Heart Network study examined outcomes and risk factors for development of MR across the various types of AV canal repairs.[63] This study included 60 patients with partial AV canal, 27 with transitional AV canal, 120 with complete AV canal, and 8 with canal-type VSD. Independent risk factors for moderate to severe MR at 6 months after surgery included older age at repair and presence of moderate or greater MR on the immediate postoperative echo. This study did not show any significant benefits of annuloplasty performed at time of original repair.

Complete Atrioventricular Canal Defect

Several factors have contributed to decreasing mortality for repair of complete AV canal defects over the past two decades. Mortality ranges between 0.5% and 13% in various studies.[27,64,65] Risk factors that affect overall survival and the need for reoperation include the following:

- *Earlier era of operation:* This has been a consistent risk factor for both early death and late reoperation in a variety of studies.[19,65-67] Improvements in myocardial preservation, intraoperative anesthetic management, perfusion methods, intraoperative TEE, postoperative care, and better understanding of lesion anatomy, along with better surgical techniques, have contributed to decreasing mortality over time.
- *Older age at surgery:* Repair beyond age 3 to 4 months has been correlated with increased perioperative mortality.[31,55] This may be related to the higher incidence of pulmonary hypertensive crises seen with increasing patient age at the time of definitive surgery.[68] Postoperative pulmonary hypertensive crises have been correlated with increased operative mortality and need for reoperation.[27,66] Increasing age as a risk factor for mortality has not been shown to be the case in all studies.[67,69] In fact, in one study of 274 patients, repair at less than 6 months of age was an incremental risk factor for perioperative mortality.[67]
- *Postoperative left AV valve regurgitation:* This has been identified in most series to be a key risk factor for the subsequent need for reoperation[56,66,70,71] and death.[19,66] The overall incidence of significant postoperative MR has slowly decreased over the years as surgical techniques have improved and a better understanding of the underlying anatomy has evolved. A review from our institution revealed a reoperation rate of 7% in recent years.[19] Other contemporary series have noted an incidence of 16% for at least moderate postoperative MR.[72]
- *Preoperative AV valve regurgitation:* A higher incidence of postoperative MR is seen in patients with higher degrees of preoperative AV valve regurgitation.[72] Leaflet division may exacerbate this association.[72] This has not been a consistent finding, with one recent study of 115 patients reporting that moderate to severe preoperative left AV valve regurgitation, present in 21 patients, was not a risk factor for operative mortality.[65] In the same study, moderate or severe late MR was present in 17% of patients with mild or less preoperative left AV valve regurgitation compared with 33% of patients with

moderate or severe preoperative left AV valve regurgitation, although this difference was not statistically significant. An earlier study of 62 infants operated on before 1987 also failed to show the correlation between preoperative and postoperative MR.[28]

- *Double-orifice mitral valve:* This adversely affects both survival and freedom from reoperation. It may be associated with unbalanced AV canal with RV dominance, a single papillary muscle, LVOTO, and aortic coarctation. If the cleft is closed completely, postoperative mitral stenosis can result. Some have recommended leaving a fenestration in the interatrial septum to allow decompression of the left atrium as needed.[56]

Partial Atrioventricular Canal Defect

The operative mortality for partial AV canal defects is low—less than 1% in most series. A small subset of patients display heart failure symptoms and several left-sided obstructive lesions within the first year of life.[33] These patients represent a higher-risk subgroup. In a study of 180 patients repaired between 1982 and 1996,[53] early mortality was 1.6%. The mean age at repair was 4.6 years; repair at less than 1 year of age was a significant risk factor for mortality. With a mean follow-up period of 6 years, 10-year actuarial survival was 98%. Important long-term sequelae were the development of late MR and subaortic obstruction.

Similar findings were reported in 2000 in the largest series to date of patients with ostium primum ASD.[73] A total of 334 patients who underwent repair over a 40-year period between 1955 and 1995 were studied, with a median follow-up period of 19 years. The 30-day perioperative mortality was 2%, whereas 20- and 40-year survival rates were 87% and 76%, respectively. Although this long-term survival was good, it was lower than that for the general population. Reoperation occurred in 11% of patients, most commonly for mitral stenosis or MR. LVOTO occurred in 11% of patients ($n = 36$), although only seven patients required reoperation. Postoperative supraventricular arrhythmias were common, especially in older patients. Although the study was descriptive, with important limitations with respect to data collection and analysis, it does provide long-term insight regarding outcomes in these patients.

Late MR, although rare, correlates with late morbidity, similar to the situation for complete AV canal defects. In partial AV canal defects, the incidence of significant MR requiring reoperation ranges between 7% and 10%, depending on the study and the length of follow-up.[74] This may be correlated with a more frequent need for valve replacement than in complete AV canal defects,[74,75] possibly related to the fixation of the superior leaflet to the crest of the interventricular septum and the association of subvalvar abnormalities.

SUMMARY

Atrioventricular canal defects represent a continuum of lesions with varying degrees of AV valvar abnormalities and interatrial and interventricular communications. In complete AV canal defects, complete elective repair should be performed early in infancy, preferably between 2 and 4 months of age. Equivalent results have been obtained with the three standard techniques of repair. Surgical intervention results in low mortality and morbidity, in both the short and the long term. When congestive heart failure or moderate to severe MR is present, complete repair should be undertaken at the time of presentation, because further delay or use of palliative procedures only increases the risks of subsequent definitive surgical therapy.

Surgical management of transitional and partial AV canal defects should include elective repair in early childhood. When left AV valve regurgitation is significant, repair should be undertaken earlier to prevent further deterioration of valve function and LV dilation and dysfunction.

Associated cardiac surgical lesions should be repaired at the time of complete AV canal repair. A remaining management dilemma is the patient with unbalanced AV canal defect, where surgical options include biventricular correction versus univentricular palliation.

Outcomes of patients with complete AV canal defects have improved steadily over the years. This reflects not only better intraoperative management, but also improved preoperative and postoperative care and follow-up in these patients.

REFERENCES

1. Fyler DC, Buckley LP, Hellenbrand WE, et al: Report of the New England Regional Infant Cardiac Program. *Pediatrics* 65:375–461, 1980.
2. Torfs CP, Christianson RE: Anomalies in Down syndrome individuals in a large population-based registry. *Am J Med Genet* 77:431–438, 1998.
3. Jacobs JP, Burke RP, Quintessenza JA, et al: Congenital Heart Surgery Nomenclature and Database Project: atrioventricular canal defect. *Ann Thorac Surg* 69:S36–S43, 2000.
4. Eisenberg LM, Markwald RR: Molecular regulation of atrioventricular valvuloseptal morphogenesis. *Circ Res* 77:1–6, 1995.
5. Van Praagh R, Litovsky S: Pathology and embryology of common atrioventricular canal. *Prog Pediatr Cardiol* 10:115–127, 1999.
6. Yilmaz AT, Arslan M, Kuralay E, et al: Repair of the left AV valve in atrioventricular septal defect in adults. *J Card Surg* 11(5):363–367, 1996.
7. Anderson RH, Zuberbuhler JR, Penkoske PA, et al: Of clefts, commissures, and things. *J Thorac Cardiovasc Surg* 90:605–610, 1985.
8. Carpentier A: Surgical anatomy and management of the mitral component of the atrioventricular canal defects. In Anderson RH, Shinebourne EA, editors: *Pediatric cardiology*, London, 1979, Churchill Livingstone, pp 466–490.
9. Ugarte M, Enriquez de Salamanca F, Quero M: Endocardial cushion defects: an anatomical study of 54 specimens. *Br Heart J* 38:674–682, 1976.
10. Rastelli G, Kirklin JW, Titus JL: Anatomic observations on complete form of persistent common atrioventricular canal with special reference to atrioventricular valves. *Mayo Clin Proc* 41:296–308, 1966.
11. Lev M: The architecture of the conduction system in congenital heart disease. I. Common atrioventricular orifice. *Arch Pathol* 65:174, 1958.
12. Feldt RH, DuShane JW, Titus JL: The atrioventricular conduction system in persistent common atrioventricular canal defect: correlations with electrocardiogram. *Circulation* 42:437–444, 1970.
13. Kertesz NJ: The conduction system and arrhythmias in common atrioventricular canal. *Prog Pediatr Cardiol* 10:153–159, 1999.

14. Tennant SN, Jr, Hammon JW, Jr, Bender HW, et al: Familial clustering of atrioventricular canal defects. *Am Heart J* 108:175–177, 1984.
15. Burn J, Brennan P, Little J, et al: Recurrence risks in offspring of adults with major heart defects: results from first cohort of British collaborative study. *Lancet* 351:311–316, 1998.
16. Emanuel R, Somerville J, Inns A, et al: Evidence of congenital heart disease in the offspring of parents with atrioventricular defects. *Br Heart J* 49:144–147, 1983.
17. Hynes JK, Tajik AJ, Seward JB, et al: Partial atrioventricular canal defect in adults. *Circulation* 66:284–287, 1982.
18. Chin AJ, Keane JF, Norwood WI, et al: Repair of complete common atrioventricular canal in infancy. *J Thorac Cardiovasc Surg* 84:437–445, 1982.
19. Hanley FL, Fenton KN, Jonas RA, et al: Surgical repair of complete atrioventricular canal defects in infancy. Twenty-year trends. *J Thorac Cardiovasc Surg* 106:387–397, 1993.
20. Newfeld EA, Sher M, Paul MH, et al: Pulmonary vascular disease in complete atrioventricular canal defect. *Am J Cardiol* 39:721–726, 1977.
21. Clapp S, Perry BL, Farooki ZQ, et al: Down's syndrome, complete atrioventricular canal, and pulmonary vascular obstructive disease. *J Thorac Cardiovasc Surg* 100:115–121, 1990.
22. Bull C, Rigby ML, Shinebourne EA: Should management of complete atrioventricular canal defect be influenced by coexistent Down syndrome? *Lancet* 1:1147–1149, 1985.
23. Lillehei C, Cohen M, Warden H, et al: The direct-vision intracardiac correction of congenital anomalies by controlled cross-circulation. *Surgery* 38:11–29, 1955.
24. Kirklin JW, Daugherty GW, Burchell HB, et al: Repair of the partial form of persistent common atrioventricular canal: ventricular communication. *Ann Surg* 142:858, 1955.
25. Rastelli GC, Ongley PA, McGoon DC: Surgical repair of complete atrioventricular canal with anterior common leaflet undivided and unattached to ventricular septum. *Mayo Clin Proc* 44:335–341, 1969.
26. Mills NL, Ochsner JL, King TD: Correction of type C complete atrioventricular canal. Surgical considerations. *J Thorac Cardiovasc Surg* 71:20–28, 1976.
27. Alexi-Meskishvili V, Ishino K, Dahnert I, et al: Correction of complete atrioventricular septal defects with the double-patch technique and cleft closure. *Ann Thorac Surg* 62:519–524, 1996.
28. Weintraub RG, Brawn WJ, Venables AW, et al: Two-patch repair of complete atrioventricular septal defect in the first year of life: results and sequential assessment of atrioventricular valve function. *J Thorac Cardiovasc Surg* 99:320–326, 1990.
29. Nicholson IA, Nunn GR, Sholler GF, et al: Simplified single patch technique for the repair of atrioventricular septal defect. *J Thorac Cardiovasc Surg* 118:642–646, 1999.
30. Wilcox BR, Jones DR, Frantz EG, et al: Anatomically sound, simplified approach to repair of "complete" atrioventricular septal defect. *Ann Thorac Surg* 64(2):487–493, discussion 493–494, 1997.
31. Stellin G, Vida VL, Milanesi O, et al: Surgical treatment of complete A-V canal defects in children before 3 months of age. *Eur J Cardiothorac Surg* 23:187–193, 2003.
32. Sommerville J: Ostium primum defect: factors causing deterioration in the natural history. *Br Heart J* 27:413–419, 1965.
33. Manning PB, Jr, Mayer JE, Sanders SP, et al: Unique features and prognosis of primum ASD presenting in the first year of life. *Circulation* 90:II30–II35, 1994.
34. Giamberti A, Marino B, di Carlo D, et al: Partial atrioventricular canal with congestive heart failure in the first year of life: surgical options. *Ann Thorac Surg* 62:151–154, 1996.
35. Levine JC, Geva T: Echocardiographic assessment of common atrioventricular canal. *Prog Pediatr Cardiol* 10:137–151, 1999.
36. van den Bosch AE, Ten Harkel OJ, Mc Ghie JS, et al: Surgical validation of real-time transthoracic 3D echocardiographic assessment of atrioventricular septal defects. *Int J Cardiol* 112(2):213–1518, 2006.
37. Cohen MS, Jacobs ML, Weinberg PM, et al: Morphometric analysis of unbalanced common atrioventricular canal using two-dimensional echocardiography. *J Am Coll Cardiol* 28:1017–1023, 1996.
38. Nicholson IA, Bichell DP, Bacha EA, et al: Minimal sternotomy approach for congenital heart operations. *Ann Thorac Surg* 71:469–472, 2001.
39. Castaneda AR, Jonas RA, Jr, Mayer JE, et al: Atrioventricular canal defect. In Castaneda AR, Jonas RA, Jr, Mayer JE, et al, editors: *Cardiac surgery of the neonate and infant*, Philadelphia, 1994, WB Saunders, pp 167–180.
40. Anil Kumar D, Suresh Kumar RN, Rao PN, et al: Complete atrioventricular septal defect repair: simplified single patch technique. *Ind J Thorac Cardiovasc Surg* 19:102–107, 2003.
41. Backer CL, Stewart RD, Bailliard F, et al: Complete atrioventricular canal: comparison of modified single-patch technique with two-patch technique. *Ann Thorac Surg* 84:2038–2046, 2007.
42. Karl TR: Atrioventricular septal defect with tetralogy of Fallot or double-outlet right ventricle: surgical considerations. *Semin Thorac Cardiovasc Surg* 9:26–34, 1997.
43. Studer M, Blackstone EH, Kirklin JW, et al: Determinants of early and late results of repair of atrioventricular septal (canal) defects. *J Thorac Cardiovasc Surg* 84:523–542, 1982.
44. De Biase L, Di Ciommo V, Ballerini L, et al: Prevalence of left-sided obstructive lesions in patients with atrioventricular canal without Down's syndrome. *J Thorac Cardiovasc Surg* 91:467–469, 1986.
45. Gurbuz AT, Novick WM, Pierce CA, et al. Left ventricular outflow tract obstruction after partial atrioventricular septal defect repair. *Ann Thorac Surg* 68:1723–1726, 1999.
46. Van Arsdell GS, Williams WG, Boutin C, et al: Subaortic stenosis in the spectrum of atrioventricular septal defects: solutions may be complex and palliative. *J Thorac Cardiovasc Surg* 110:1534–1541, 1995.
47. Reeder GS, Danielson GK, Seward JB, et al: Fixed subaortic stenosis in atrioventricular canal defect: a Doppler echocardiographic study. *J Am Coll Cardiol* 20:386–394, 1992.
48. Bharati S, Lev M, Jr, McAllister HA, et al: Surgical anatomy of the atrioventricular valve in the intermediate type of common atrioventricular orifice. *J Thorac Cardiovasc Surg* 79:884–889, 1980.
49. Foker JE, Berry J, Steinberger J: Ventricular growth stimulation to achieve two-ventricle repair in unbalanced common atrioventricular canal. *Prog Pediatr Cardiol* 10:173–186, 1999.
50. Nathan M, Liu H, Pigula FA, et al: Biventricular conversion after single-ventricle palliation in unbalanced atrioventricular canal defects. *Ann Thorac Surg* 95:2086–2096, 2013.
51. Oshima Y, Yamaguchi M, Yoshimura N, et al: Anatomically corrective repair of complete atrioventricular septal defects and major cardiac anomalies. *Ann Thorac Surg* 72:424–429, 2001.
52. Moran AM, Daebritz S, Keane JF, et al: Surgical management of mitral regurgitation after repair of endocardial cushion defects: early and midterm results. *Circulation* 102:III160–III165, 2000.
53. Najm HK, Williams WG, Chuaratanaphong S, et al: Primum atrial septal defect in children: early results, risk factors, and freedom from reoperation. *Ann Thorac Surg* 66:829–835, 1998.
54. Baufreton C, Journois D, Leca F, et al: Ten-year experience with surgical treatment of partial atrioventricular septal defect: risk factors in the early postoperative period. *J Thorac Cardiovasc Surg* 112:14–20, 1996.
55. Michielon G, Stellin G, Rizzoli G, et al: Repair of complete common atrioventricular canal defects in patients younger than four months of age. *Circulation* 96:II316–II322, 1997.
56. Najm HK, Coles JG, Endo M, et al: Complete atrioventricular septal defects: results of repair, risk factors, and freedom from reoperation. *Circulation* 96(Suppl II):II311–II315, 1997.
57. Wetter J, Sinzobahamvya N, Blaschczok C, et al: Closure of the zone of apposition at correction of complete atrioventricular septal defect improves outcome. *Eur J Cardiothorac Surg* 17(2):146–153, 2000.
58. Rhodes J, Warner KG, Fulton DR, et al: Fate of mitral regurgitation following repair of atrioventricular septal defect. *Am J Cardiol* 80:1194–1197, 1997.
59. Kaza E, Marx GR, Kaza AK, et al: Changes in left atrioventricular valve geometry after surgical repair of complete atrioventricular canal. *J Thorac Cardiovasc Surg* 143:1117–1124, 2012.
60. McGrath LB, Kirklin JW, Soto B, et al: Secondary left atrioventricular valve replacement in atrioventricular septal (AV canal) defect: a method to avoid left ventricular outflow tract obstruction. *J Thorac Cardiovasc Surg* 89:632–635, 1985.
61. Morris CD, Magilke D, Reller M: Down's syndrome affects results of surgical correction of complete atrioventricular canal. *Pediatr Cardiol* 13:80–84, 1992.

62. Daebritz S, del Nido PJ: Surgical management of common atrioventricular canal. *Prog Pediatr Cardiol* 10:161–171, 1999.
63. Kaza AK, Colan SD, Jaggers J, et al: Surgical interventions for atrioventricular septal defect subtypes: the pediatric heart network experience. *Ann Thorac Surg* 92:1468–1475, 2011.
64. Thies WR, Breymann T, Matthies W, et al: Primary repair of complete atrioventricular septal defect in infancy. *Eur J Cardiothorac Surg* 5:571–574, 1991.
65. Tweddell JS, Litwin SB, Berger S, et al: Twenty-year experience with repair of complete atrioventricular septal defects. *Ann Thorac Surg* 62:419–424, 1996.
66. Bando K, Turrentine MW, Sun K, et al: Surgical management of complete atrioventricular septal defects. A twenty-year experience. *J Thorac Cardiovasc Surg* 110:1543–1554, 1995.
67. Gunther T, Mazzitelli D, Haehnel CJ, et al: Long-term results after repair of complete atrioventricular septal defects: analysis of risk factors. *Ann Thorac Surg* 65:754–759, 1998.
68. Bando K, Turrentine MW, Sharp TG, et al: Pulmonary hypertension after operations for congenital heart disease: analysis of risk factors and management. *J Thorac Cardiovasc Surg* 112:1600–1607, 1996.
69. Al-Hay AA, MacNeill SJ, Yacoub M, et al: Complete atrioventricular septal defect, Down syndrome, and surgical outcome: risk factors. *Ann Thorac Surg* 75:412–421, 2003.
70. Capouya ER, Laks H, Jr, Drinkwater DC, et al: Management of the left atrioventricular valve in the repair of complete atrioventricular septal defects. *J Thorac Cardiovasc Surg* 104:196–201, 1992.
71. McGrath LB, Gonzalez-Lavin L: Actuarial survival, freedom from reoperation, and other events after repair of atrioventricular septal defects. *J Thorac Cardiovasc Surg* 94:582–590, 1987.
72. Fortuna RS, Ashburn DA, Carias De Oliveira N, et al: Atrioventricular septal defects: effect of bridging leaflet division on early valve function. *Ann Thorac Surg* 77:895–902, 2004.
73. El-Najdawi EK, Driscoll DJ, Puga FJ, et al: Operation for partial atrioventricular septal defect: a forty-year review. *J Thorac Cardiovasc Surg* 119:880–889, 2000.
74. Permut LC, Mehta V: Late results and reoperation after repair of complete and partial atrioventricular canal defect. *Semin Thorac Cardiovasc Surg* 9:44–54, 1997.
75. Abbruzzese PA, Napoleone A, Bini RM, et al: Late left atrioventricular valve insufficiency after repair of partial atrioventricular septal defects: anatomical and surgical determinants. *Ann Thorac Surg* 49:111–114, 1990.

CHAPTER 117

VENTRICULAR SEPTAL DEFECT AND DOUBLE-OUTLET RIGHT VENTRICLE

Emile A. Bacha

CHAPTER OUTLINE

VENTRICULAR SEPTAL DEFECT

A ventricular septal defect (VSD) is a hole between the left and right ventricles. A VSD may occur as an isolated anomaly or with a wide variety of intracardiac anomalies, such as tetralogy of Fallot or transposition of the great arteries. This chapter discusses isolated VSD.

Banding of the pulmonary artery as a palliative maneuver was first described in 1952.[1] This decreased left-to-right shunting and as a consequence prevented the development of pulmonary vascular obstructive disease and left-sided volume overload. Until the mid-1960s when primary VSD closure became safer, pulmonary artery banding was the procedure of choice in managing VSDs. The first VSD closure was performed in 1955 by Lillehei and associates[2] at the University of Minnesota, using controlled cross-circulation between the child and parent. Nineteen of the 27 patients who underwent this procedure survived. In 1957, Kirklin and associates[3] at the Mayo Clinic closed a VSD using a heart-lung machine. In 1957, transatrial VSD closure was performed,[4] followed in 1971 by the popularization of primary repair in symptomatic infants by Barratt-Boyes and associates[5] using cardiopulmonary bypass, deep hypothermia, and circulatory arrest.

Anatomy

Anatomy of the Tricuspid Valve, Right Ventricular Septum, and Conduction System

Surgeons planning VSD surgery must have intimate knowledge of the tricuspid valve, the right ventricular septal anatomy, and the conduction system.

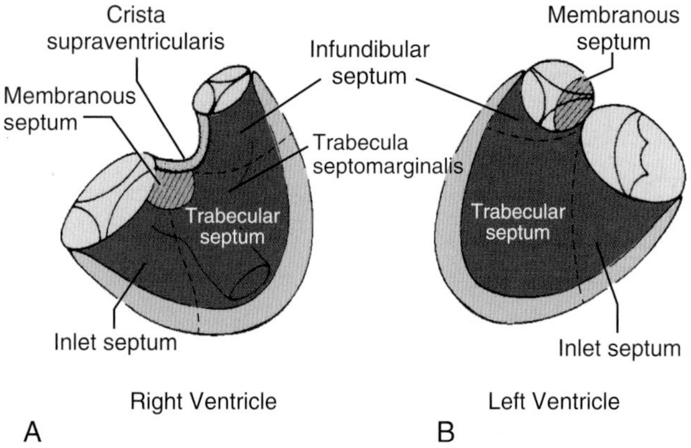

FIGURE 117-1 ■ The components of the ventricular septum as seen from the right ventricle **(A)** and the left ventricle **(B)**. (Modified from Soto B, Becker AE, Moulaert AJ, et al: Classification of ventricular septal defects. *Br Heart J* 43:332–343, 1980.)

The tricuspid valve has three leaflets: anterior, septal, and posterior. The anterior leaflet is connected via the chordae tendineae cordis to the anterior papillary muscle (located on the anterior right ventricular free wall) and to the septal papillary muscle (sometimes called muscle of Lancisi). The septal papillary muscle is itself part of the septal band of the septomarginal trabecula. The posterior leaflet is attached to the anterior and posterior papillary muscles, and the septal leaflet attaches to the posterior and septal papillary muscles.

The right ventricular septum has five components (Fig. 117-1):

1. The membranous septum
2. The atrioventricular (AV) canal or inlet septum
3. The muscular septum (apical trabecular septum or sinus septum)
4. The trabecula septomarginalis (septal band and moderator band)
5. The conal septum (infundibular septum and parietal band)

Unlike the left ventricular septum, which is free of any papillary muscle attachment (the mitral valve can be called "septophobic," whereas the tricuspid valve can be called "septophilic"), the right ventricular septum is where the septal (sometimes called medial) papillary muscle and part of the posterior papillary muscle originate. The septal papillary muscle is a portion of the septal band, which runs along the septum (hence its name). The septal band is a portion of the septomarginal trabecula, which also includes the moderator band. The moderator band links the septum to the anterior papillary muscle (called moderator band because it was erroneously thought to "moderate" the right ventricular free wall—that is, keep in sync with the rest of the ventricle). The membranous septum is the only fibrous component of the septum. It is wedged between the aortic valve, the tricuspid valve, and the mitral valve. Because the tricuspid valve is normally apically displaced vis-à-vis the mitral valve, a portion of membranous septum ends up between the right atrium and the left ventricle, called the AV part of the membranous septum. The portion of membranous septum located between both ventricles is called the interventricular part.

Knowledge of the conduction system of the heart also is critical when approaching VSDs so as to avoid damaging it (Fig. 117-2). The various atrial conduction tracts all converge toward the AV node of Aschoff-Tawara. The AV node is located in the inferior-posterior portion of the membranous septum, just inferior to the anteroseptal commissure of the tricuspid valve. A different description of its location is that it occupies the apex of the triangle of Koch, which is limited by the ligament of Todaro posteriorly, the orifice of the coronary sinus inferiorly, and the tricuspid valve annulus superiorly (see Fig. 117-2). From the AV node, the common AV bundle of His descends within the interventricular part of the membranous septum (or, in the case of a membranous VSD, the posteroinferior rim of the VSD), traverses the septum, and then courses along the left ventricular aspect of the septum. It then separates into a right bundle branch, which travels back to the right ventricular surface, as well as a left bundle branch. At the anteroinferior border at the level of the muscle of Lancisi, the right bundle branch descends toward the right ventricular apex.

Anatomic Classification of Ventricular Septal Defects

A useful surgical classification of VSDs was initially developed in 1980 by Soto and associates[6] (Fig. 117-3) and then further modified by Van Praagh and associates (Fig. 117-4).[7] Variations of this classification are used in most pediatric cardiac centers. VSDs can be classified as follows:

- Conoventricular (or membranous) defects
- Conal (or outlet) VSDs
- Inlet (or AV canal type) VSDs
- Muscular VSDs (single or multiple)

Conoventricular (or Membranous) Defects. Conoventricular defects are located between the conal septum and the ventricular septum. They are centered around the membranous septum and comprise 80% of all VSDs. They may be located exclusively in the membranous septum, or they can extend beyond the boundaries of the membranous septum in the inferior, posterior, or anterior direction and are then sometimes called perimembranous or paramembranous VSDs. The prefix *peri-*, appearing in loan words from the Greek, means "surrounding" (e.g., perimeter). Thus, a truly perimembranous VSD would surround the membranous septum. In contrast, the prefix *para-*, also from the Greek, means "adjacent to" or "beside" and more accurately reflects the notion of a defect adjacent to the membranous septum. Neither *perimembranous* nor *paramembranous* correctly describes the typical defect involving the membranous septum and extending into the adjacent septum. The current recommendation is to call these defects either membranous VSDs or conoventricular defects. Malalignment of the conal septal plane vis-à-vis the ventricular septal plane results in the typical conoventricular defect. The malalignment can be anterior, as seen in tetralogy of Fallot, for example, or posterior, as seen in interrupted aortic arch. In addition to resulting in a VSD, anterior conal septal malalignment also results in right

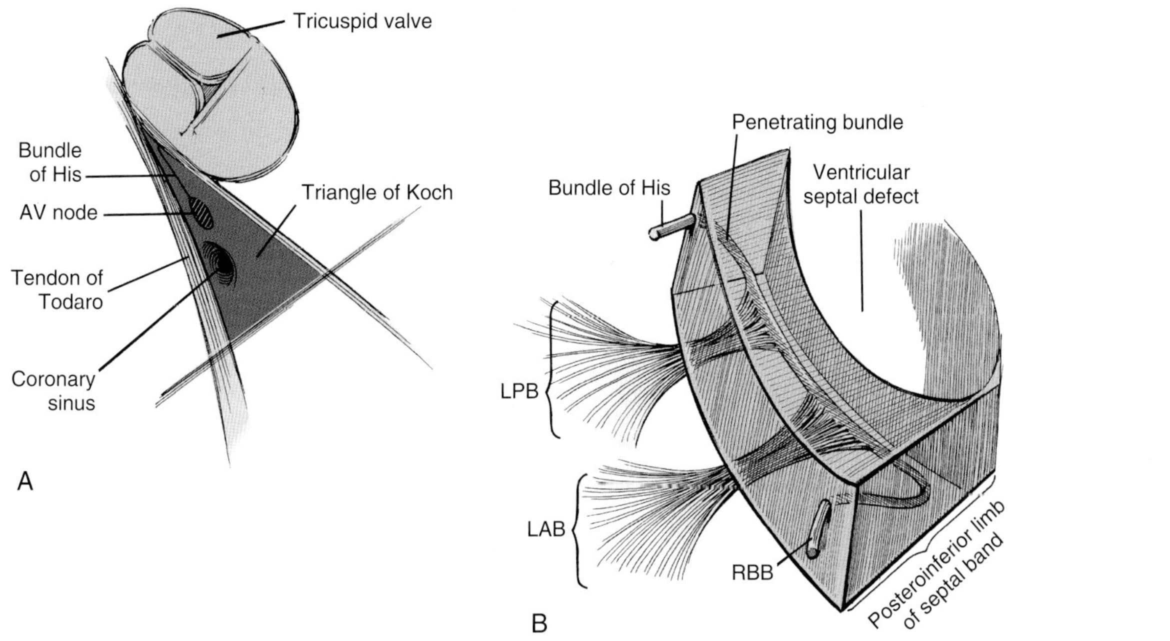

FIGURE 117-2 ■ Schematic representation of the conduction system. **A,** The atrioventricular (AV) node lies embedded within the triangle of Koch, close to the orifice of the coronary sinus and between the annulus of the tricuspid valve and the tendon of Todaro. The bundle of His originates from the AV node, extends toward the commissure between the septal and anterior leaflets of the tricuspid valve, and penetrates along the posteroinferior margin of the membranous septum and across the muscular ventricular septum. **B,** The bundle of His gives rise to the left posterior branch (LPB) and the left anterior branch (LAB). The right bundle branch (RBB) then travels back along the ventricular septum toward the right ventricular septal surface. At the level of the muscle of Lancisi, the right bundle branch descends toward the right ventricular apex. (Modified from Castaneda AR, Jonas RA, Mayer JE Jr, et al: Double outlet right ventricle. In Castaneda AR, Jonas RA, Mayer JE Jr, et al, editors: *Cardiac surgery of the neonate and infant,* Philadelphia, 1994, WB Saunders, pp 445–449.)

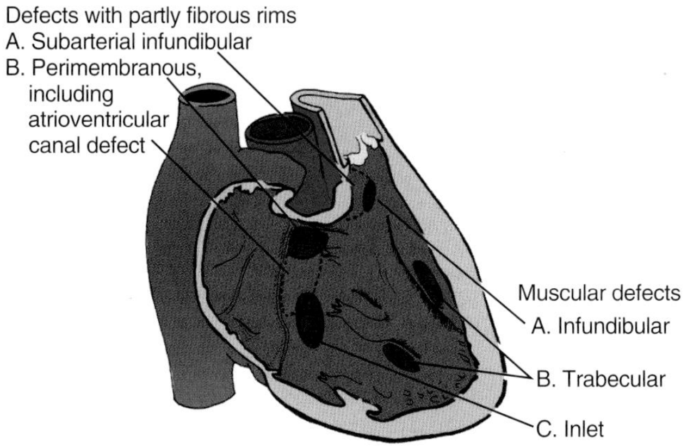

FIGURE 117-3 ■ Classification of ventricular septal defects according to their location in the septum. (Modified from Soto B, Becker AE, Moulaert AJ, et al: Classification of ventricular septal defects. *Br Heart J* 43:332–343, 1980.)

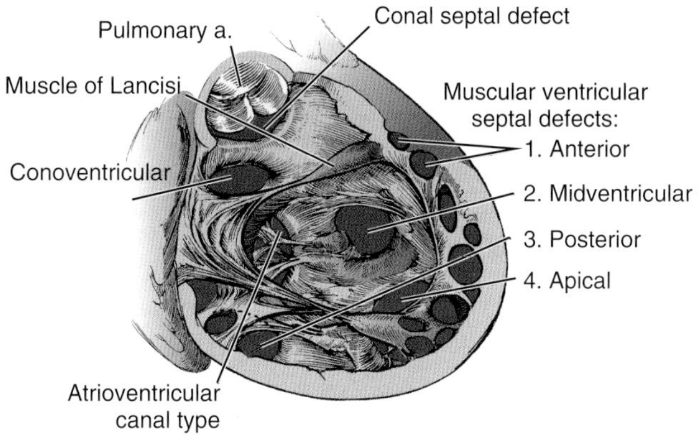

FIGURE 117-4 ■ Classification of ventricular septal defects (VSDs): atrioventricular canal type; muscular VSDs (anterior [1], midventricular [2], posterior [3], and apical [4]); conoventricular septal defect, which includes paramembranous and malalignment conoventricular septal defects; and conal septal defects. (Modified from Castaneda AR, Jonas RA, Mayer JE Jr, et al: Double outlet right ventricle. In Castaneda AR, Jonas RA, Mayer JE Jr, et al, editors: *Cardiac surgery of the neonate and infant,* Philadelphia, 1994, WB Saunders, pp 445–449.)

ventricular outflow tract obstruction, whereas posterior malalignment of the conal septum results in left ventricular outflow tract obstruction. Important landmarks in conoventricular septal defects are the anteroseptal commissure of the tricuspid valve inferiorly and the noncoronary cusp of the aortic valve. When the ventricular portion of the membranous septum is entirely absent, the VSD extends to the base of the aortic valve (sometimes called subaortic VSD). The medial papillary muscle (muscle of Lancisi) located at the inferoposterior border of the defect is also an important landmark. Both the septal and the anterior tricuspid valve leaflets are attached to it.

Conal Ventricular Septal Defects. Approximately 8% of VSDs are located in the conal (infundibulum or outlet) septum. They also are called supracristal VSDs. They are either entirely surrounded by muscle (muscular conal VSDs) or limited upstream by the aortic or pulmonary annuli (sometimes called subarterial VSDs).

Inlet (or Atrioventricular Canal Type) Ventricular Septal Defects. Inlet VSDs are characterized by the absence of part or all of the AV canal (inlet) septum. These VSDs are located immediately underneath the septal leaflet of the tricuspid valve, with no tissue in between. Approximately 6% of all VSDs are inlet-type VSDs.

Muscular Ventricular Septal Defects. Muscular VSDs (10% of all VSDs) are entirely surrounded by muscle. They can occur anywhere in the trabecular portion of the septum and can be isolated or multiple. They are described by their location—that is, anterior, midventricular (between the muscular septum and the septal band), posterior, or apical. When inspected through the left side of the septum, what appeared to be multiple muscular defects often converge into either a single hole or two separate holes.

Commonly Associated Defects

VSDs are an intrinsic portion of many, if not most, complex cardiac malformations. These VSDs are discussed separately with their respective entities (see other chapters). Almost half of patients who undergo surgical treatment of primary VSD have an associated lesion.

A large patent ductus arteriosus (PDA) is present in approximately 25% of symptomatic neonates and infants with VSDs.[5] This is important to know because preoperative echocardiography may fail to show a PDA in the presence of a large amount of left-to-right shunting. Furthermore, intraoperative transesophageal echocardiography (TEE) is notoriously unreliable in excluding PDAs. Therefore the possibility of a PDA should be kept in mind when approaching a VSD, and if there is any doubt, or if there is a large amount of backflow through the pulmonary arteries on cardiopulmonary bypass, the PDA should be ligated or clipped.

A hemodynamically significant aortic coarctation is present in approximately 10% of cases. Because of the unique pathophysiology of aortic coarctation (more left-to-right shunting across the VSD because of increased afterload caused by the coarctation), these patients usually have presenting symptoms before 3 months of age.[8]

Congenital valvar or subvalvar aortic stenosis, resulting in left ventricular outflow tract obstruction, is seen in approximately 4% of patients requiring an operation for a VSD.[9] The most common type of subaortic stenosis associated with VSDs involves the discrete fibromuscular membrane of the VSD that is located inferior or upstream to it. Congenital mitral valve stenosis is rare and occurs in approximately 2% of patients.

Other significant anomalies include large atrial septal defects (ASDs), right ventricular outflow tract obstruction, vascular ring, and persistent left superior vena cava.

Pathophysiology

Shunt Direction and Magnitude

The magnitude and direction of the shunt across a VSD depend on the size of the defect and the pressure gradient across it during the various phases of the cardiac cycle. Large VSDs offer little or no resistance to blood flow and are therefore called nonrestrictive. The right ventricular pressure equals the left ventricular pressure, and the ratio of pulmonary to systemic flow (Qp/Qs) (or shunt) is dependent on the ratio of pulmonary vascular resistance (PVR) to systemic vascular resistance (SVR). On the other hand, small VSDs offer resistance to flow across the defect and are therefore termed restrictive VSDs. The Qp/Qs rarely exceeds 1.5. Moderate-sized VSDs fall between these two categories and the Qp/Qs usually ranges between 2.5 and 3. To a lesser degree, further determinants of shunt magnitude also include the relative compliance of both ventricles and the pressure relationships during the various phases of the cardiac cycle. The size of the VSD—in particular, of muscular VSDs—also may vary during various phases of the cardiac cycle. Because the PVR is elevated during the first few weeks of life, it is unusual to have to close an isolated VSD. As the PVR falls with increasing age, left-to-right shunting increases, necessitating treatment.

Sequelae of Left-to-Right Shunting

Left-to-right shunting at the ventricular level implies increased pulmonary blood flow. Therefore, left ventricular preload is similarly increased, resulting in increased workload for both left and right ventricles. The left atrium is enlarged, and the left atrial pressure is elevated. The left ventricle dilates. The raised left atrial pressure causes many infants with VSD to have an increased accumulation of interstitial fluid in the lungs, resulting sometimes in repeated pulmonary infections. The work of breathing is increased as the lung compliance is decreased. This increases energy expenditure, which, along with the relatively low systemic blood flow, causes these infants to have striking failure to thrive. When pulmonary resistance rises as a result of the development of pulmonary vascular disease, pulmonary blood flow is reduced and the child appears to improve. Unfortunately, further increases in PVR occur, and the classic Eisenmenger complex results. These patients are characterized by fixed pulmonary hypertension, bidirectional shunting, right ventricular hypertrophy, and a normal-sized left ventricle. They are often inoperable and require heart-lung transplantation for further survival.

Pulmonary Vascular Disease

The classic description of the pathology of hypertensive pulmonary vascular disease is that of Heath and Edwards.[10] They correlated the PVR of patients with large VSDs with the histologic severity of pulmonary vascular changes. Grade 1 changes were defined as medial hypertrophy without intimal proliferation; grade 2 as medial hypertrophy with cellular intimal reaction; grade 3 as intimal fibrosis and medial hypertrophy; grade 4 as generalized vascular dilation, an area of vascular occlusion by intimal fibrosis, and plexiform lesions; grade 5 as other "dilation lesions" such as cavernous and angiomatoid lesions; and grade 6 as necrotizing arteritis. It is assumed that Heath-Edwards grade 3 or greater is not reversible. The importance of lung biopsies has decreased over the years, with catheterization-based data increasing in importance in terms of suitability for repair.

Natural History and Indications for Surgery

Approximately 30% of infants with severe symptoms such as intractable congestive heart failure or failure to thrive require surgery within the first year of life.[11] The remainder can usually be managed medically, because the natural history of VSDs is well known.[12] Aggressive medical management is indicated because most membranous and muscular VSDs tend to close spontaneously.[12] Malalignment conoventricular VSDs or inlet-type VSDs are unlikely to close spontaneously, and therefore closure at the time of diagnosis is recommended, regardless of age or weight. Asymptomatic children with isolated small restrictive VSDs can be followed safely with serial echocardiograms.

The development of pulmonary vascular disease is a tragedy that can be prevented with virtually no mortality by VSD closure. If in doubt, cardiac catheterization and measurement of PVR-to-SVR ratio should help with decision making. In addition, pulmonary artery (PA) pressures greater than one half the systemic pressure in a child older than 1 year indicate the need for surgery. If PA pressures are greater than one half the systemic, the response of the pulmonary vasculature to inhaled nitric oxide and 100% inspired oxygen should be studied during catheterization. Even children who have significant pulmonary hypertension with a reversible component to it can become operative candidates.

During the first decade of life, a small proportion (5%) of patients with membranous or outlet VSDs develop prolapse of an aortic cusp into the VSD. This usually results in a gradual decrease of the effective orifice and shunt flow and also in increasing aortic regurgitation. Increasing aortic cusp prolapse and regurgitation are an indication to operate.

Diagnosis and Workup

Results of the physical examination, chest radiograph, and electrocardiogram (ECG) depend on the underlying pathophysiology. Patients with large VSDs and increased pulmonary blood flow usually have symptoms such as tachypnea, growth failure, profuse sweating during feeding, a bulging precordium, a pansystolic murmur, an enlarged liver, and thready pulses. The chest film shows a large central and peripheral PA and enlarged left atrium and ventricles (Fig. 117-5). ECG shows signs of biventricular enlargement. In contrast, patients with small VSDs and small left-to-right shunts have only a systolic murmur. The chest radiograph and ECG may be entirely normal (Fig. 117-6). Two-dimensional echocardiography and color flow Doppler studies have essentially replaced cardiac catheterization in most patients with isolated VSDs. Cardiac catheterization is needed only when PVR and PA pressure need to be measured.

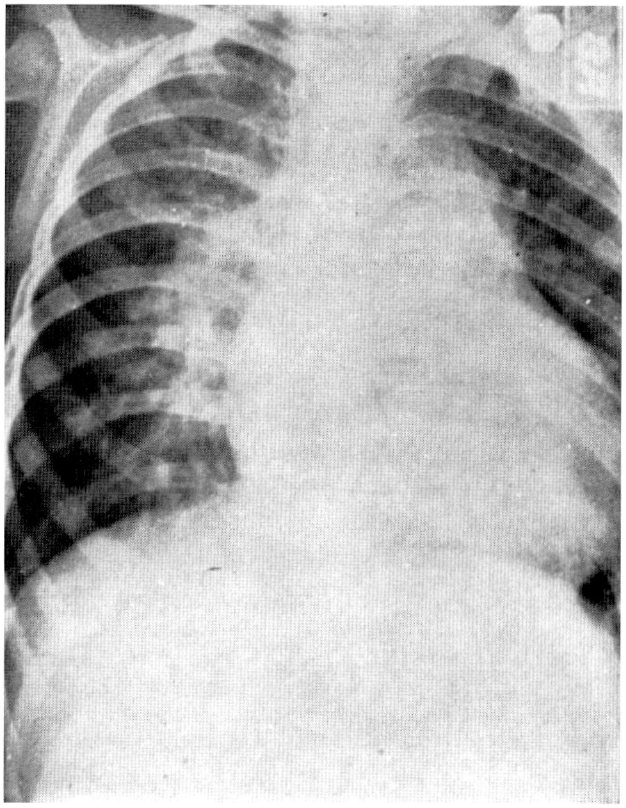

FIGURE 117-5 Chest radiograph of a child with a large ventricular septal defect, large pulmonary blood flow, and pulmonary hypertension, but only mildly elevated pulmonary vascular resistance, as indicated by left and right ventricular enlargement, enlargement of the main pulmonary artery, and a sharp increase in pulmonary vascular pattern.

Surgical Technique

For closure of conoventricular septal defects, the PDA is routinely dissected and ligated as soon as cardiopulmonary bypass is instituted. The left branch PA and distal aortic arch should be positively identified before ligation. Moderate hypothermia (rectal temperature, 28° C to 32° C) is usually sufficient. Small infants weighing less than 2.5 kg may require lower temperatures (18° C to 25° C) to safely institute low-flow bypass. Deep hypothermic circulatory arrest is rarely used for closure of VSDs. After cross-clamping the aorta and delivering the cardioplegia solution, the caval tapes are tightened. A right atriotomy approach is preferred for most VSDs. The atrium is opened obliquely (Fig. 117-7) to avoid the area of the sinus node. The atrial septum is inspected first, and if a patent foramen ovale (PFO) is present, a left atrial vent sucker can be placed. Retraction of the septal and anterior leaflets of the tricuspid valve usually provides adequate exposure. The area located behind the anteroseptal commissure of the tricuspid valve often is the most difficult to expose. If the tricuspid valve attachments are in

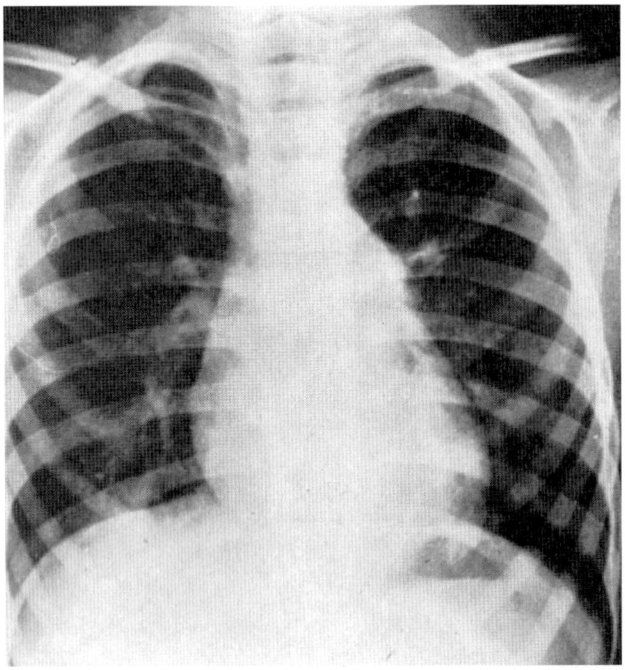

FIGURE 117-6 ■ In contrast to the heart shown in Figure 117-5, the heart in this chest radiograph is not enlarged overall. The main pulmonary artery is enlarged, but there is no evidence of increased pulmonary blood flow. This patient has a large ventricular septal defect, pulmonary hypertension, severe elevation of pulmonary vascular resistance, and pulmonary blood flow that is less than systemic blood flow. The condition is inoperable and usually requires a heart-lung transplant or a lung transplantation with concomitant intracardiac repair. (Modified from Dushane JW, Kirklin JW: Selection for surgery of patients with ventricular septal defects and pulmonary hypertension. *Circulation* 21:13, 1960; with permission of the American Heart Association, Inc.)

the way, the surgeon can detach the septal or anterior leaflet by making an incision that parallels the tricuspid annulus (see Fig. 117-7). Some surgeons perform this maneuver routinely. If VSD exposure remains poor despite rearranging the field, an infundibular incision is the usual fallback option for exposure. Interrupted mattressed or running nonabsorbable sutures are used. Teflon pledgets are very useful in neonates and infants, in whom the myocardium is friable. The first suture is usually placed into the midportion of the defect, approximately 3 mm from the rim of the defect. When the inferior margin is reached (at approximately the level of the muscle of Lancisi), sutures should be placed farther away from the edge and become more superficial. At the tricuspid annulus, sutures are passed through its fibrous tissue. Because conduction tissue is composed of specialized muscle cells, fibrous tissue offers a safe area to place sutures. There is usually very little tissue separating the aortic valve from the posterosuperior margin of the defect. Therefore, several sutures are usually placed from the right atrial side through the tricuspid valve annulus to avoid damage to the aortic valve cusp. Infusion of cardioplegic solution fills the aortic root and allows accurate delineation of the insertion of the aortic valve cusps. All sutures are then passed through an appropriately tailored patch (Dacron, Gore-Tex, or pericardium) and tied in place. The tricuspid valve should be routinely inspected and passively inflated with saline to ensure that no significant tricuspid valve regurgitation has been inadvertently created.

For closure of an AV canal type of VSD (Fig. 117-8), exposure is usually straightforward. A continuous suture technique is often preferred, because it allows weaving in and out between the various chordae and papillary muscles that usually crowd the edge of these defects. To avoid damage to the bundle of His and the right bundle branch that course along the posteroinferior edge, stitches in that area are placed farther away from the edge of the VSD.

For closure of conal VSDs (Fig. 117-9), exposure is obtained through the infundibulum, the pulmonary artery, or the aorta. Often no muscle lies between the superior edge of the defect and the pulmonary valve. Again, it can be useful to fill the aortic root with cardioplegic solution to determine the exact position of the cusps. The initial sutures are placed either within the fibrous rim separating the two semilunar valves or within the left and right pulmonary sinuses of Valsalva. The remaining sutures can be placed with no fear of injury to the conduction tissue as it travels farther caudally between the infundibular and trabecular ventricular septum.

The approach used in closure of muscular VSDs depends on their location. Mid-muscular defects are preferably closed through a right atriotomy. A single patch can cover several separate defects. Posterior muscular defects are hidden behind the posterior leaflet of the tricuspid valve. Anterior muscular defects are often difficult to find, because they are hidden behind the septal band and hypertrophied trabeculae of the right ventricular free wall. It is important to divide the muscle bundles that bind the septal band to the septum to adequately expose the true margins of the VSD. A patch is used, and the surgeon must pay close attention to avoid distortion of the left anterior descending coronary artery. Apical defects can also be difficult to expose. The coarse trabeculations located in the right ventricular apex make the exact determination of the true margins difficult. An apical right ventriculotomy is extremely helpful and virtually always allows good exposure of the apical muscular septum. Left ventricular apical incisions are essentially obsolete because of the high prevalence of left ventricular dyskinesia and apical aneurysms after this incision. Percutaneous transcatheter closure of muscular VSDs with occluding devices is another approach for patients with apical VSDs or multiple muscular VSDs. When the percutaneous approach is not possible, intraoperative deployment of a device on the beating heart via a right ventricular puncture can be used.[13]

Surgical Management of Ventricular Septal Defect with Associated Anomalies

The vast majority of patients who have VSD with coarctation of the aorta are young infants. The traditional approach has been to simultaneously repair the coarctation and band the pulmonary artery. This evolved into aortic coarctation repair followed by VSD repair during the same hospitalization, if symptoms of heart failure persisted, in the form of failure to extubate, for example.

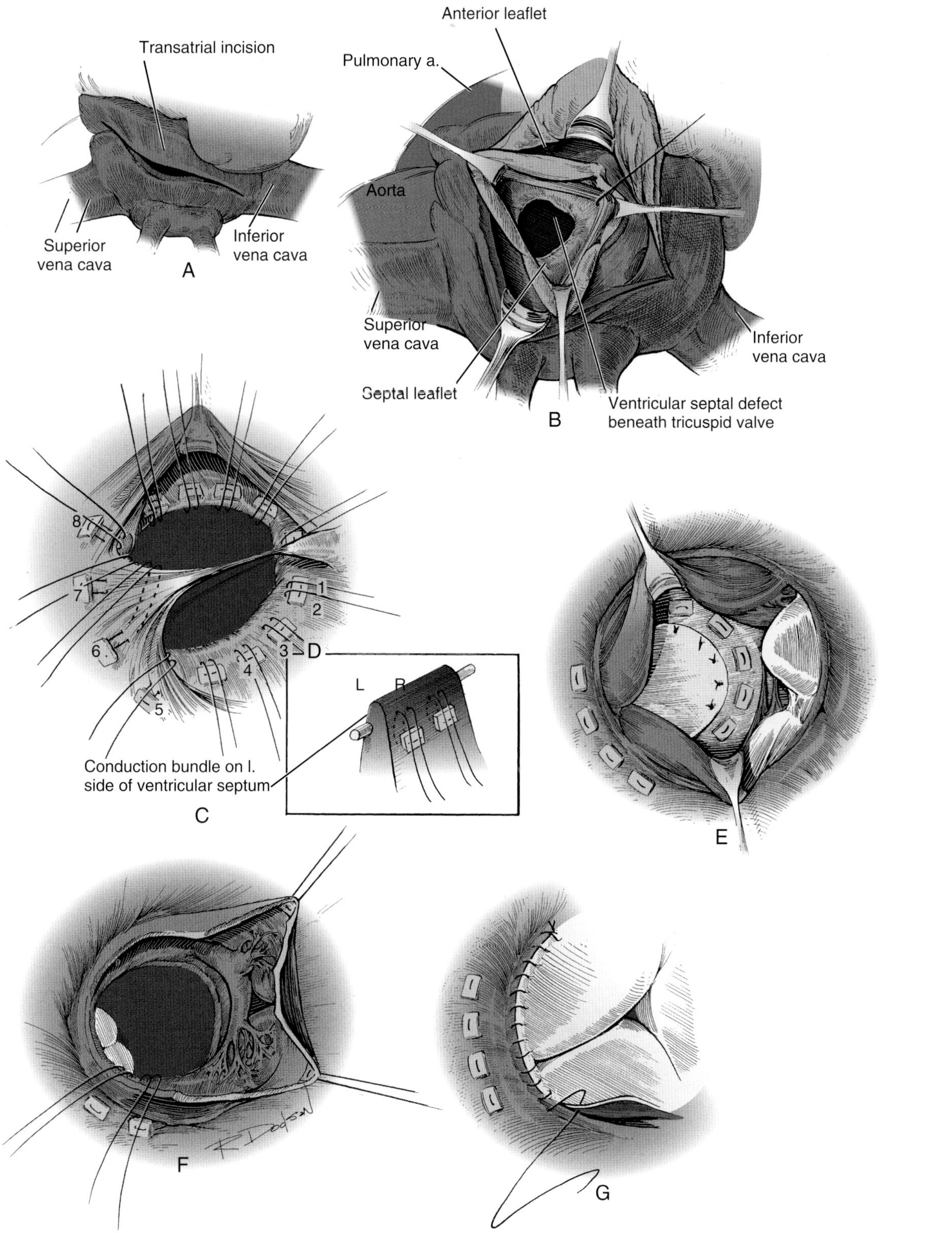

FIGURE 117-7 ■ Trans–right atrial exposure of conoventricular ventricular septal defect (VSD). **A,** Incision in the right atrium. **B,** Exposure of conoventricular VSD with retraction of the anterior and septal leaflets of the tricuspid valve. **C,** Sutures 1, 2, 3, and 4 are placed in the ventricular septal wall, approximately 3 mm from the rim of the defect. **D,** Suture 5 is placed where the leaflet fuses with the crest of the VSD, and sutures 6, 7, and 8 are passed from the right atrial side through the tricuspid annulus; the rest of the sutures are placed in the anterosuperior rim of the VSD. **E,** Completed closure of the VSD with a Dacron patch and pledgeted sutures. **F,** If chordae and papillary muscles obliterate the view of the VSD, the septal and anterior leaflets of the tricuspid valve are incised along the base, permitting complete exposure of the VSD. **G,** Septal and anterior leaflets of the tricuspid valve are resutured after closure of the VSD with a patch. (Modified from Castaneda AR, Jonas RA, Mayer JE Jr, et al: Double outlet right ventricle. In Castaneda AR, Jonas RA, Mayer JE Jr, et al, editors: *Cardiac surgery of the neonate and infant,* Philadelphia, 1994, WB Saunders, pp 445–449.)

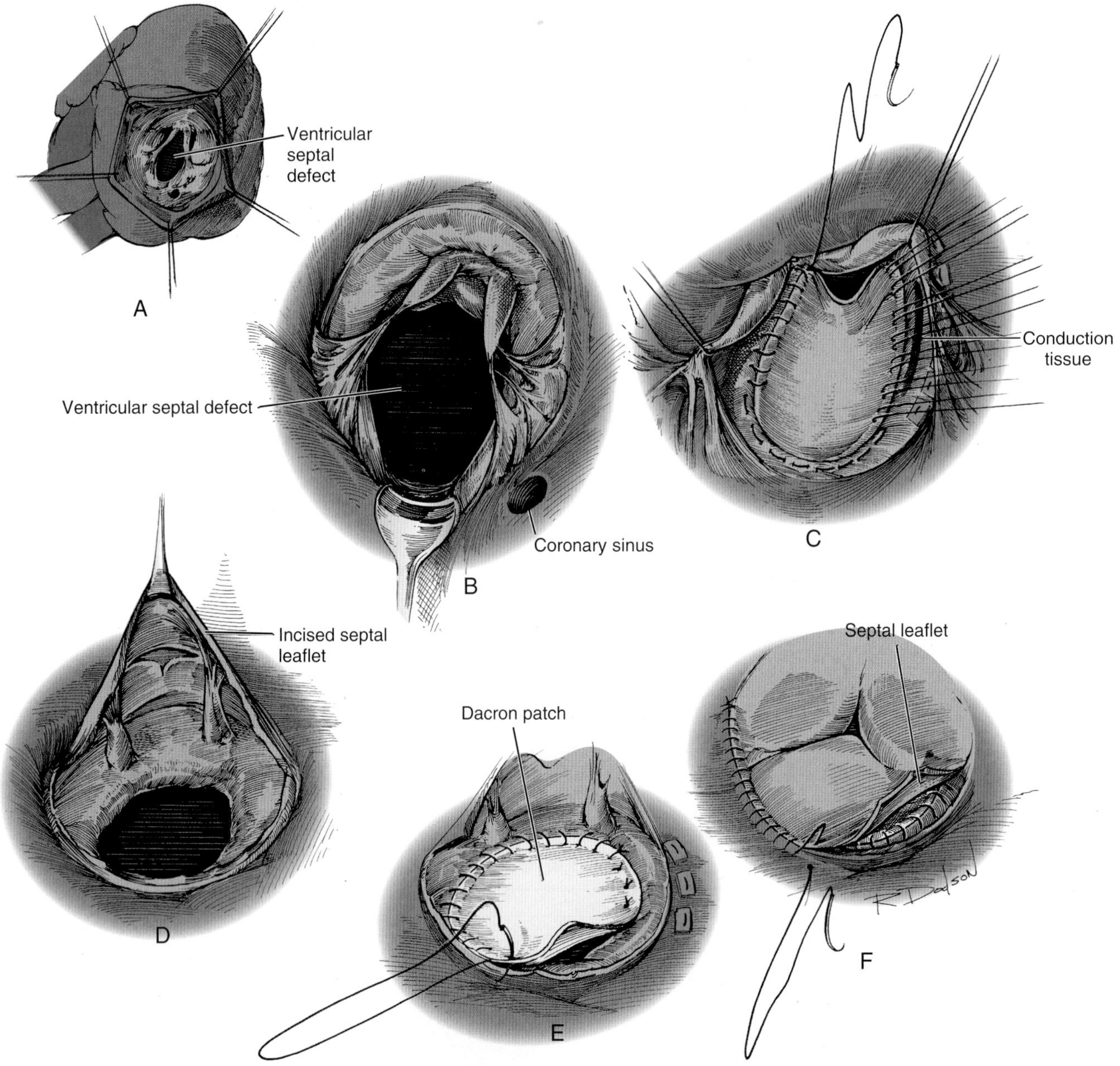

FIGURE 117-8 ■ Closure of atrioventricular (AV) canal type of ventricular septal defect (VSD). **A,** Transatrial view of AV canal type of VSD. **B,** Retraction of the septal leaflet of the tricuspid valve exposes the defect to the tricuspid valve annulus. **C,** Closure of AV canal defect with the continuous suture technique. (Note the continuous horizontal mattress suture with the septal leaflet tissue and also the interrupted horizontal mattress sutures along the posteroinferior portion of the VSD, placed approximately 4 mm from the VSD to avoid damage of the conduction bundle.) **D,** If dense chordae obstruct the view of the defect, the septal leaflet of the tricuspid valve is incised along its base, providing exposure of the entire circumference of the AV canal type of VSD. **E,** Patch closure of the AV canal type of VSD. **F,** The incised leaflet is reattached with continuous suture. (Modified from Castaneda AR, Jonas RA, Mayer JE Jr, et al: Double outlet right ventricle. In Castaneda AR, Jonas RA, Mayer JE Jr, et al, editors: *Cardiac surgery of the neonate and infant,* Philadelphia, 1994, WB Saunders, pp 445–449.)

As techniques for complex neonatal repairs matured and results improved, many centers have come to favor a single-stage method of simultaneously repairing the coarctation and the VSD via a midline approach.[8] Of course, this is done only if the VSD is judged not likely to close spontaneously, whether by size or location.

Patients who have VSD with aortic insufficiency are usually older children. The right or noncoronary cusp is prolapsing into the VSD secondary to the Bernoulli effect. When there is mild to mild-moderate aortic regurgitation with little scarring or fibrosis of the cusps, VSD closure alone is required. Patients with more than moderate aortic incompetence and cusp retraction usually require commissural resuspension of the affected cusp via an aortotomy (see Chapter 123).

Patients with VSD with prior banding are most often those with multiple muscular VSDs. The resulting right ventricular hypertrophy makes the intraoperative identification of these VSDs even more difficult. Intraoperative device closure via right ventricular puncture has been

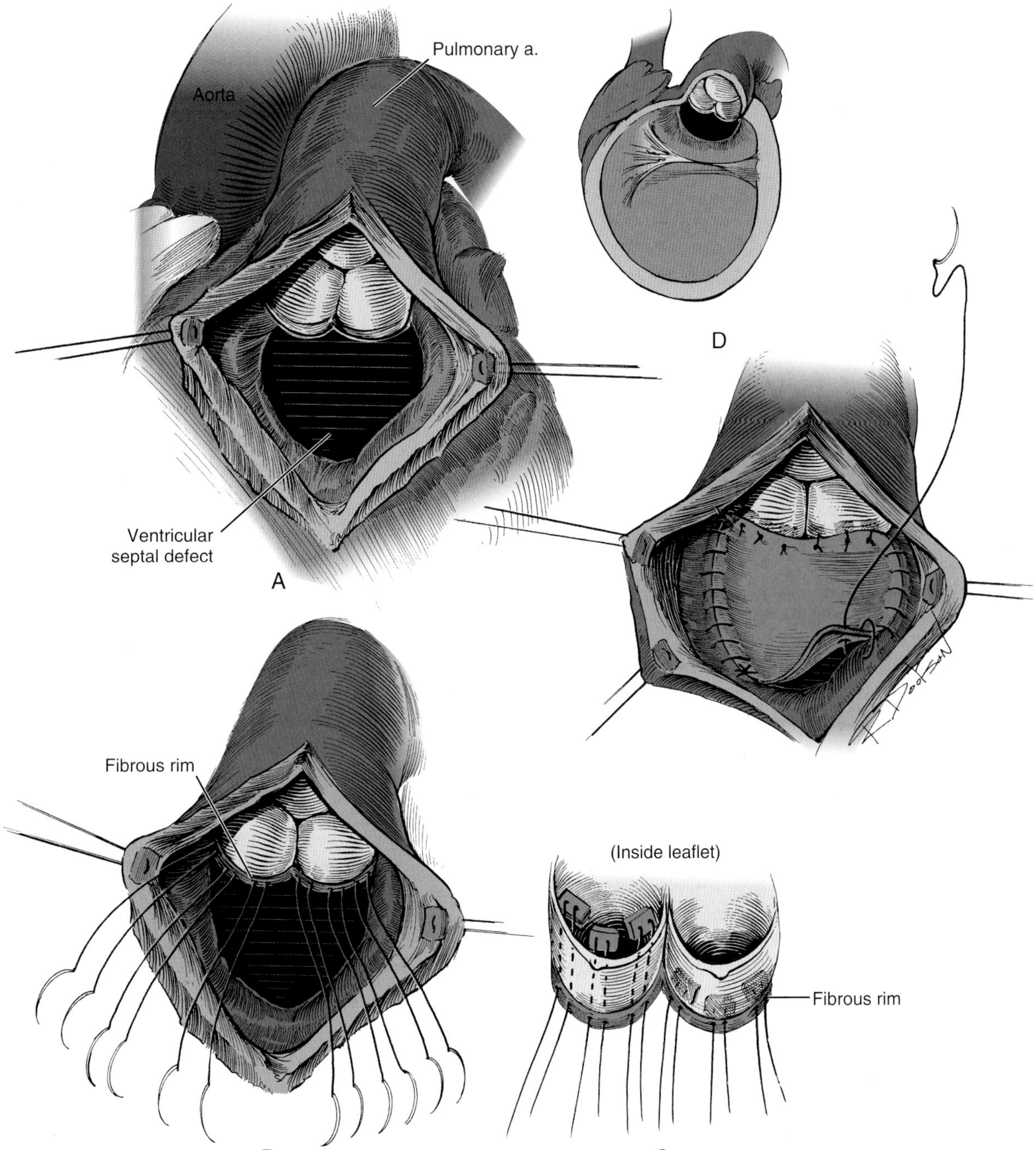

FIGURE 117-9 Transventricular approach to closure of conal ventricular septal defect. **A,** Commonly there is no intervening muscle between the superior edge of the defect and the pulmonary valve. **B,** Initial sutures placed in the fibrous rim separating the two semilunar valves. **C,** If the area between the aorta and the pulmonary cusps is tenuous, interrupted pledgeted mattress sutures are passed within the right and left pulmonary sinuses. **D,** The Dacron patch is anchored to the remainder of the ventricular septal defect with a continuous suture. (Modified from Castaneda AR, Jonas RA, Mayer JE Jr, et al: Double outlet right ventricle. In Castaneda AR, Jonas RA, Mayer JE Jr, et al, editors: *Cardiac surgery of the neonate and infant,* Philadelphia, 1994, WB Saunders, pp 445–449.)

used successfully, along with removal of the PA band and PA plasty in one setting.[13]

Postoperative Care

Most infants convalesce normally after VSD repair, and special treatment is usually not required. Patients are generally extubated within 24 hours of surgery and recover rapidly. In the unusual case of low cardiac output after surgery despite the usual supportive treatment, it is the surgeon's responsibility to prove that there are no technical issues causing the unusual postoperative course. Problems could include a large residual VSD, injury to the aortic cusp that occurred during suture placement, or tricuspid regurgitation. Bedside echocardiography usually quickly diagnoses these problems. If complete AV dissociation occurs after cardiopulmonary bypass, temporary pacing wires are used until sinus rhythm reappears. AV block can last up to 10 to 14 days, beyond which time it is usually permanent and a permanent pacemaker should be placed.

Pulmonary hypertensive crisis is a severe postoperative complication that can occur in older patients with a reactive pulmonary vasculature. If the patient is at risk, then, in the operating room, a pulmonary arterial line should be placed, introduced either via an infundibular puncture or under direct vision via the right atrium. A pulmonary hypertensive crisis can occur without a precipitating factor; however, tracheal suctioning, respiratory or metabolic acidosis, hypoxemia, and high-dose inotropes can be precipitating factors. Patients benefit from increased sedation, muscular paralysis, and hyperventilation with a high level of inspired oxygen. Inhaled nitric oxide, at dosages ranging from 5 to 40 ppm, is the preferred agent in managing pulmonary hypertension. Ideally, it is started prophylactically in the operating room as soon as ventilation resumes, while the patient is still on cardiopulmonary bypass.[14]

Results of Surgical Treatment

Early Results. Because of improvements in intraoperative and postoperative management and minimization of human error, the hospital mortality rate for repair of isolated VSD now approaches 0% in most experienced pediatric cardiac centers. Since the late 1980s, along with marked improvement in survival after complex neonatal cardiac surgery, very low-weight or very young infants with isolated VSDs also have a mortality rate of less than 5%.[15] Prematurity, significant preexisting respiratory problems such as bronchopulmonary dysplasia, or unrecognized respiratory syncytial virus infection increases morbidity and mortality slightly but not significantly. In an operable patient, elevated PVR is a risk factor for complications or prolonged hospital stay, but it is not a determinant of hospital mortality. Unrecognized additional cardiac lesions can lead to significant problems if reoperation is required. Although complete AV dissociation is uncommon after isolated VSD repair, it remains a complication that occurs in 0.5% to 3% of patients after VSD closure. Right bundle branch block occurs in most patients after VSD closure and is usually very well tolerated. Its implications in the long term are unclear. Significant residual postoperative left-to-right shunting is uncommon when proper techniques are used. Most frequently it results from suture dehiscence, seen most often in small infants with friable myocardium. When it is hemodynamically significant, reoperation should be performed expeditiously. When the patient is asymptomatic and progressing well during the postoperative course, the leak is usually smaller, and the surgeon may elect to observe the patient with serial echocardiograms for a period of several weeks. Most small residual VSDs (<3 mm) close spontaneously over a period of months because of scar formation at the edge of the patch.

Late Results. Repair of VSD in the first year or two of life cures most patients and results in full functional activity and normal or almost normal life expectancy. Normal or near-normal long-term growth and cardiac function are expected in most patients.[16] Late deaths virtually never occur in patients with normal or near-normal PVR. Detailed studies of PA pressure and PVR were performed in infants undergoing VSD closure at the Boston Children's Hospital, where 96% of infants had a mean PA pressure of greater than 40 mm Hg, and 51% continued to have elevated PA pressures at 24 hours postoperatively. Postoperative catheterization studies done 1 year later showed that PA pressure in this group had decreased to a mean of 14 mm Hg.[17,18] Severe pulmonary hypertension postoperatively can increase with time and cause premature death, usually within 3 to 10 years after the operation. Other patients with pulmonary hypertension have a stabilization of their pulmonary vascular process, with neither increase nor decrease of the PVR. They usually have limitations in their exercise tolerance. In a study of 296 surviving patients after VSD closure followed for 30 to 35 years postoperatively, higher mortality was observed in those who underwent surgery after the age of 5 years, in those with PVR greater than 7 U/m^2, and in those with transient or permanent complete heart block.[19]

DOUBLE-OUTLET RIGHT VENTRICLE WITH NORMALLY RELATED GREAT ARTERIES

Simply defined, double-outlet right ventricle (DORV) refers to a heterogeneous group of cardiac malformations in which both great arteries arise from the right ventricle.[4,7] Although the term DORV can be correctly applied to single-ventricle hearts or hearts with AV discordance (e.g., congenitally corrected transposition of the great arteries), for simplicity of discussion, only hearts with AV concordance and two adequate ventricles are discussed in this chapter. Furthermore, the management of DORV with transposition of the great arteries is discussed in greater detail in Chapter 126. Two definitions, not mutually exclusive and best used concurrently, are as follows[17,20]: The 50% rule states that a heart is termed DORV if, in addition to the PA, more than 50% of the aorta (or the PA, in DORV with transposition) arises from the right ventricle. The other definition is that a double conus (subaortic and subpulmonary conal tube, also called infundibulum) is present. This means that there should be no aorta-to-mitral valve continuity.

Classification of DORV by VSD Location and Other Anatomic Determinants of Physiology

DORV is virtually always associated with a VSD. The physiology of DORV encompasses a spectrum that extends from a tetralogy type of DORV to a transposition type of DORV (Fig. 117-10). The classic pathologic classification of DORV centers on the location of the VSD[20] (Fig. 117-11) and differentiates between subaortic,

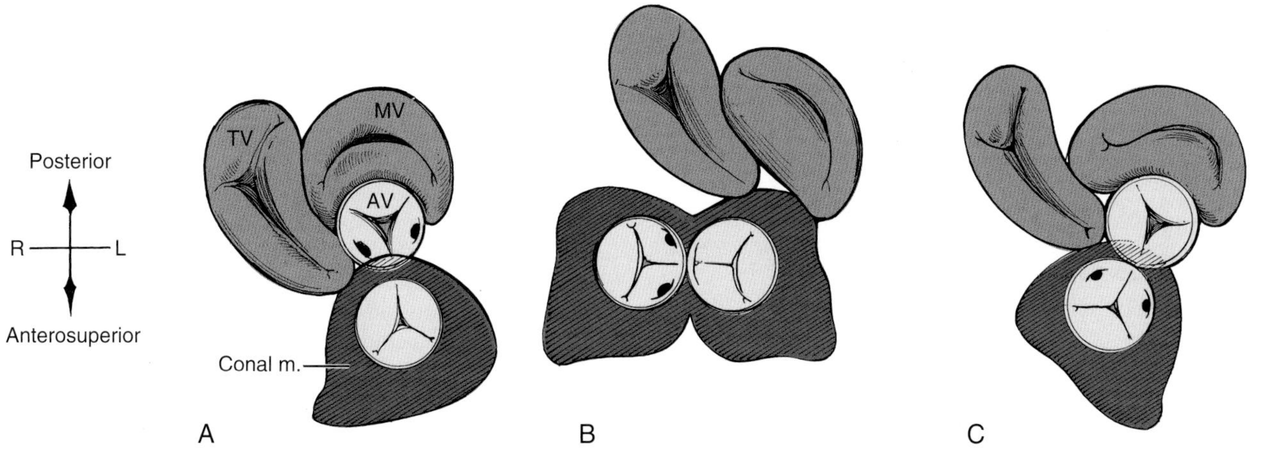

FIGURE 117-10 The spectrum of conus development between the tetralogy and transposition ends of the double-outlet right ventricle (DORV). **A,** Tetralogy of Fallot. There is a subpulmonary conus with fibrous continuity between the aortic and mitral valve. **B,** The middle of the DORV spectrum. There are both subpulmonary and subaortic coni. **C,** Transposition of the great arteries. There is a subaortic conus with fibrous continuity between the pulmonary and mitral valves. In all diaphragms, the aortic valve is indicated by the coronary ostia, the tricuspid valve by three leaflets, and the mitral valve by two leaflets; *hatching* indicates conal myocardium. *AV,* Aortic valve; *MV,* mitral valve; *TV,* tricuspid valve. (Modified from Castaneda AR, Jonas RA, Mayer JE Jr, et al: Double outlet right ventricle. In Castaneda AR, Jonas RA, Mayer JE Jr, et al, editors: *Cardiac surgery of the neonate and infant,* Philadelphia, 1994, WB Saunders, pp 445–449.)

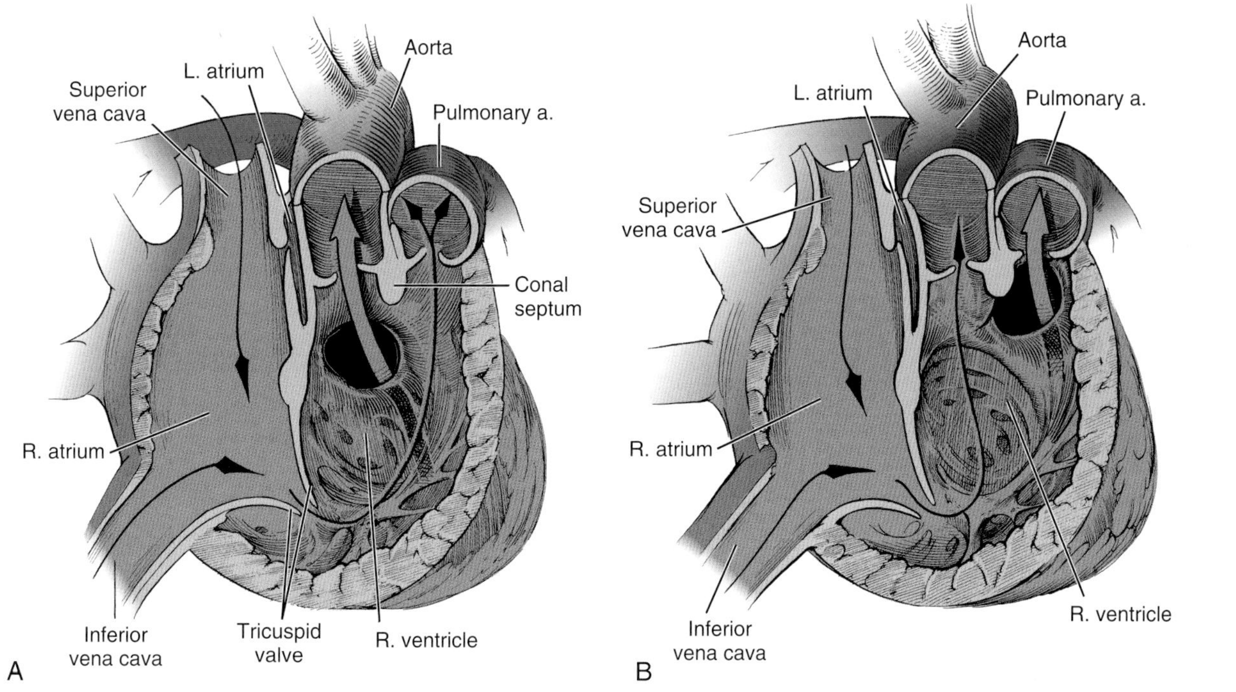

FIGURE 117-11 **A,** Double-outlet right ventricle (DORV) with a subaortic ventricular septal defect (VSD). Flow from the left ventricle preferentially enters the aorta. This is similar to what occurs in tetralogy of Fallot. **B,** DORV with a subpulmonary VSD. Left ventricular blood preferentially enters the pulmonary artery, resulting in physiology similar to that seen in transposition of the great arteries. (Modified from Castaneda AR, Jonas RA, Mayer JE Jr, et al: Double outlet right ventricle. In Castaneda AR, Jonas RA, Mayer JE Jr, et al, editors: *Cardiac surgery of the neonate and infant,* Philadelphia, 1994, WB Saunders, pp 445–449.)

subpulmonic, doubly committed, and noncommitted types of VSD. VSD location alone, although important, neither defines the physiology nor is enough information on which to base a decision of the optimal method of repair. The presence or absence of right ventricular outflow tract obstruction is critical to the physiology and clinical presentation (Table 117-1). Furthermore, the great artery relationship, the distance between the pulmonary and tricuspid valves, the prominence of the conal septum, and the coronary artery anatomy are all important factors that help determine what type of repair should be performed.[21]

DORV with subaortic VSD (see Fig. 117-11) is the most common type of DORV, comprising approximately 50% of all patients with DORV.[21] With right ventricular outflow tract obstruction, the presentation is similar to tetralogy of Fallot, where a subaortic anterior malalignment VSD is also present. However, tetralogy of Fallot

TABLE 117-1 Pathophysiology of Double-Outlet Right Ventricle

Location of VSD	Right Ventricular Outflow Tract Obstruction	Clinical Presentation
Subaortic	Absent	VSD
Subaortic	Present	TOF
Subpulmonary	Absent	TGA/VSD
Subpulmonary/ TGA	Present (subaortic stenosis)	Ductal-dependent lesion
Doubly or noncommitted	Absent	VSD
Doubly or noncommitted	Present	TOF

TGA, Transposition of the great arteries; *TOF,* tetralogy of Fallot; *VSD,* ventricular septal defect.

patients will not have a subaortic conus. The presentation and physiology without pulmonary stenosis is similar to that of a child with a large VSD.

DORV with subpulmonary VSD (see Fig. 117-11) is the second most common type of DORV, occurring in 30% of patients.[21] Because of the location of the VSD, oxygenated left ventricular blood preferentially streams through the VSD into the pulmonary artery while desaturated right ventricular blood streams into the aorta, thereby resulting in a transposition type of physiology. Association with subaortic stenosis, aortic coarctation, or interrupted aortic arch is common. The term *Taussig-Bing heart* is usually applied for hearts with subaortic and subpulmonary coni, side-by-side great arteries, and a subpulmonary VSD.[21]

The doubly committed VSD is immediately beneath both the PA and the aorta. The conal septum is absent or hypoplastic. Clinical presentation is usually similar to that of a subaortic VSD with or without pulmonary stenosis.

The noncommitted VSD type includes any VSD that is located below the conal septum or the junction of conal and muscular interventricular septa. These VSDs are likely to be so remote from the semilunar valves that it is very difficult to create a baffle that directs left ventricular blood flow into the aortic valve. These VSDs are frequently located in the inlet septum (AV canal type), or they can be mid-muscular or apical. Clinical presentation is similar to that of DORV with subaortic VSD and depends on the presence or absence of pulmonary stenosis.[22]

Other Important Anatomic Features and Impact on the Type of Repair

Distance between Tricuspid and Pulmonary Valve

The judgment as to which type of repair is best in a specific anatomic situation constitutes the fundamental complexity of the surgical management of DORV. An intraventricular repair denotes a baffle that is entirely in the right ventricle. The baffle is constructed around the VSD and creates a pathway from the left ventricle to the aorta. The right ventricular outflow thus curves around the left ventricular baffle. When the aorta is pushed away from the left ventricle by a very prominent subaortic conus or if the VSD is remote, a longer tunnel must be created. This often results in D-malposition of the aorta, where the aortic valve moves superior and anterior to the tricuspid valve, allowing the pulmonary valve to move closer to the tricuspid valve. Because the baffle must pass between the tricuspid and pulmonary valves, there is a point when this is no longer possible without either creating baffle obstruction (subaortic stenosis) or occluding the pulmonary valve, thus creating the need for a right ventricle-to-PA conduit. Thus, when planning an intraventricular repair, the distance between the tricuspid valve and the pulmonary valve must be carefully studied on multiple views obtained with echocardiography and angiography (ventriculogram).

Conal Septum

A prominent conal septum also may be in the way of a successful intraventricular baffle. The length of the conal septum is determined by the development of the subaortic and subpulmonary coni. The conal septum may be resected if there are no important AV valve chordae attached to it (Fig. 117-12). A long conal septum may be associated with a closer proximity between the tricuspid valve and the pulmonary valve. It also may be a substrate for the development of future subaortic stenosis, which in turn can be associated with aortic arch hypoplasia.[23]

Pulmonary Outflow Tract Obstruction

The presence of pulmonary outflow tract obstruction also needs to be carefully managed during surgery. Intraventricular repair must include relief of any subpulmonary stenosis, usually by means of division of hypertrophied muscle bands and placement of an infundibular outflow patch. Even in mild forms of subpulmonary stenosis, an infundibular patch may be needed because, by definition, an intraventricular baffle protrudes to some extent into the right ventricular outflow tract, thus crowding the right ventricular outflow. An infundibular patch thus prevents the creation of iatrogenic subpulmonary stenosis. Pulmonary stenosis is dealt with as it is during tetralogy surgery, by transannular patch or by valvuloplasty. A Rastelli type of repair is sometimes required when the space between the tricuspid valve and the pulmonary annulus is not sufficient and there is significant pulmonary annular hypoplasia. It is best to then incorporate the entire pulmonary annulus into the baffle, thus creating a generous subaortic passage; divide the main PA; and place a conduit (usually a homograft) between the right ventricle and distal main PA. If the pulmonary annulus is of normal size but an intraventricular baffle is not possible for the reasons cited previously, an arterial switch operation with baffling of the VSD to the pulmonary valve should be performed.[24]

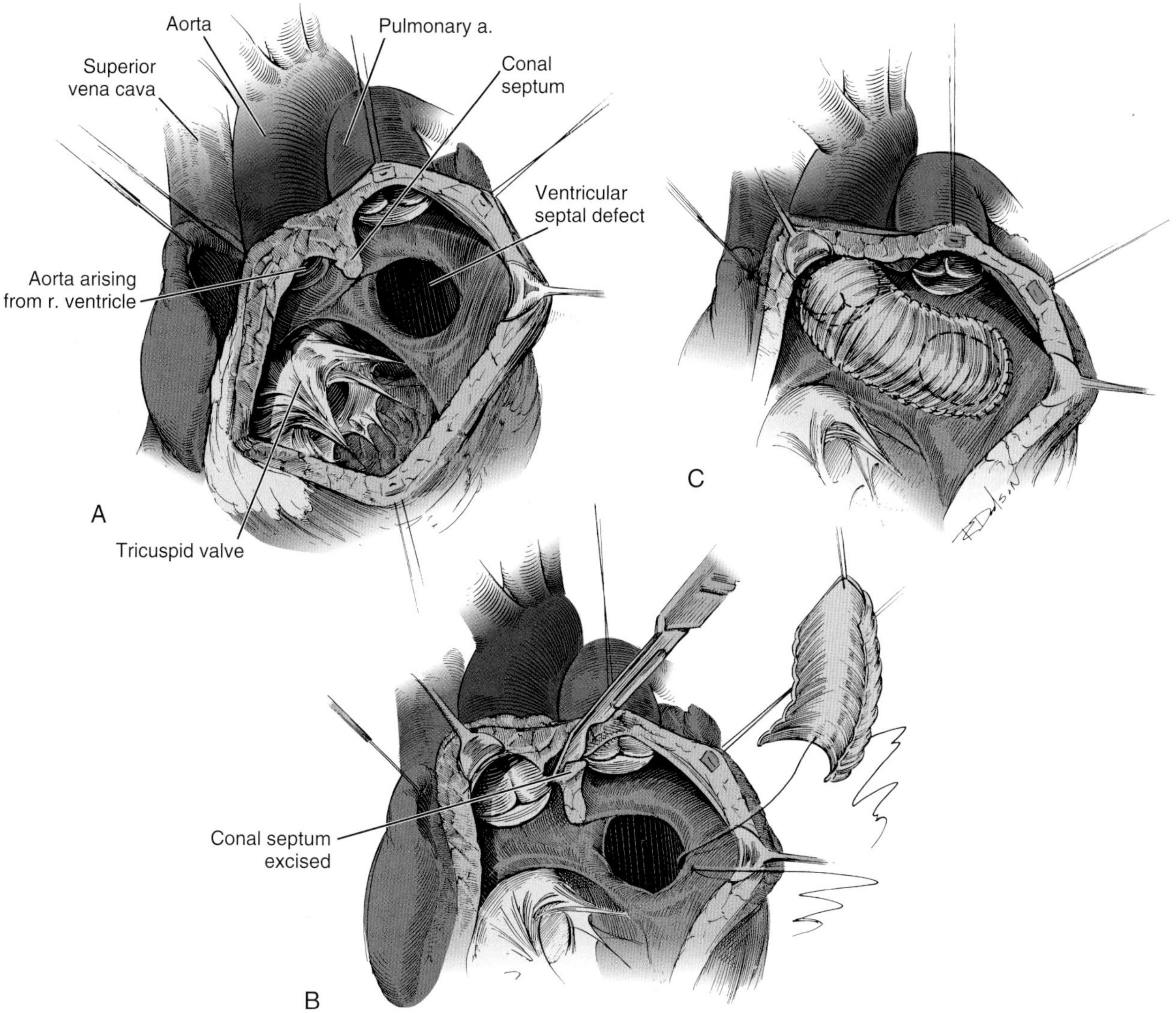

FIGURE 117-12 ■ **A,** Prominent conal septum can project into the intraventricular baffle pathway. **B,** Resection of the conal septum may be necessary to prevent subaortic stenosis. **C,** Completion of intraventricular repair with a baffle. (Modified from Castaneda AR, Jonas RA, Mayer JE Jr, et al: Double outlet right ventricle. In Castaneda AR, Jonas RA, Mayer JE Jr, et al, editors: *Cardiac surgery of the neonate and infant,* Philadelphia, 1994, WB Saunders, pp 445–449.)

Coronary Artery Anatomy

Knowledge of the coronary artery anatomy is also critical to successful management of DORV, because a left anterior descending coronary artery passing anterior to the right ventricular outflow in the tetralogy end of the spectrum excludes an intraventricular repair and requires a conduit. Complex coronary artery anatomy, frequently seen in Taussig-Bing hearts, renders an arterial switch operation more challenging.

Great Artery Relationship

Most hearts with DORV have normally related great arteries spiraling around each other, with the aorta posterior and to the right of the pulmonary artery. The VSD is usually subaortic. When the great arteries are parallel to each other without a spiral, the aorta can be found side by side with and rightward of the pulmonary artery (D-malposition), anterior to the PA, or side by side and leftward (L-malposition). The VSD is usually subpulmonary, but it can also be noncommitted.[25] Great artery relationship gives an indication of VSD location, but the two can also be independent of one another.[21]

Preoperative Evaluation

The age of the patient and the patient's symptoms are mostly determined by the degree of pulmonary stenosis. Most cases are diagnosed during the neonatal period. Echocardiography is the test of choice for neonates and young infants and is usually sufficient. At the transposition end of the spectrum, a balloon atrial septostomy may be needed to improve mixing. Catheterization also may be necessary in older children to exclude pulmonary vascular disease. To plan (or exclude) a potential intraventricular baffle, a left ventricular injection is helpful so that the dye can be followed as it is ejected by the left ventricle (preferentially into the aorta or pulmonary artery). Important echocardiographic details include the annular sizes of all

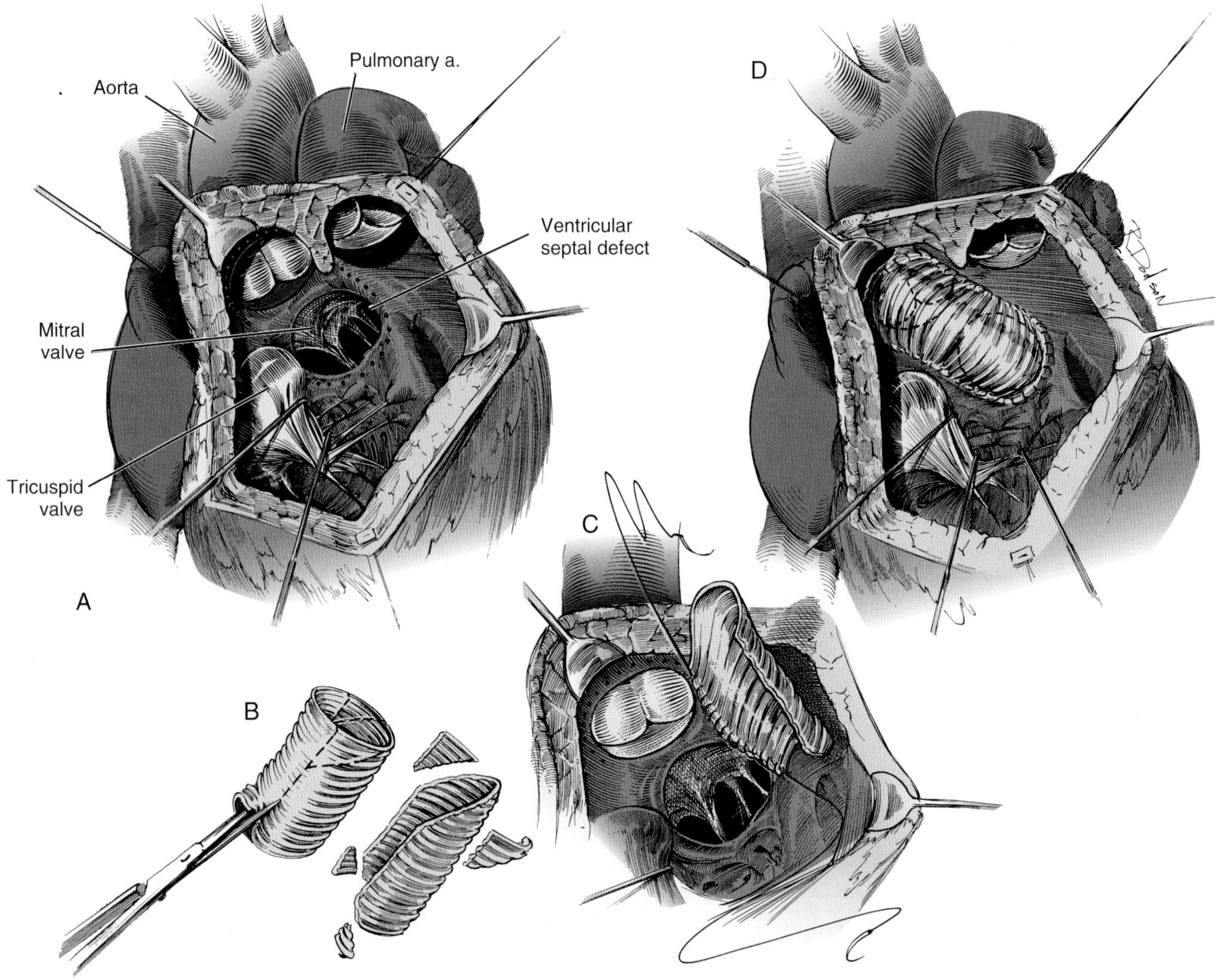

FIGURE 117-13 ■ The long synthetic baffle used to direct left ventricular blood to the aorta is best constructed from a partial tube graft. **A,** The suture line is indicated by a *dotted line.* **B,** Tailoring of the baffle from a tube graft. **C,** A continuous suture technique may be necessary for a very long baffle. **D,** Completion of intraventricular baffle repair of tetralogy of Fallot type of double-outlet right ventricle. (Modified from Castaneda AR, Jonas RA, Mayer JE Jr, et al: Double outlet right ventricle. In Castaneda AR, Jonas RA, Mayer JE Jr, et al, editors: *Cardiac surgery of the neonate and infant,* Philadelphia, 1994, WB Saunders, pp 445–449.)

valves; the size of the left and right ventricles; the relative positions of the great arteries to one another; the degree of development of the conal septum; the chordal attachment to the conal septum; the level and degree of subpulmonary or pulmonary stenosis; the position of the VSD; and the status of the remainder of the septum, the coronary artery anatomy, and the aortic arch anatomy.

Surgical Management

Management of DORV is always surgical. Medical management may be indicated in relatively asymptomatic neonates with tetralogy-type physiology until they are a few months old. Because of markedly improved results with neonatal repairs, surgical palliation in the form of pulmonary artery banding in VSD-type physiology or aortopulmonary shunting in tetralogy-type physiology is rarely performed. Routine cardiopulmonary bypass with bicaval cannulation is usually used.

Intraventricular Repair of DORV with Subaortic VSD or Doubly Committed VSD without Pulmonary Stenosis

Patients without pulmonary stenosis can generally be managed by placement of a patch baffle around the VSD, thus connecting the left ventricle to the aorta. The relationship of the aortic valve annulus to the VSD rims and to the conal septum must be carefully studied. If there appears to be a need for a larger subaortic circumference, a portion of a synthetic tube graft can be used rather than a flat patch, thus giving the baffle more of a tunnel appearance (Fig. 117-13).[17] If the VSD appears restrictive, it should be enlarged by making an incision anterosuperiorly, by resecting a wedge of the conal septum, or by doing both.

Intraventricular Repair of DORV with Subaortic VSD or Doubly Committed VSD with Pulmonary Stenosis

Techniques of repair are generally similar to those described for repair of tetralogy of Fallot. However, the VSD is closed by creation of a tunnel rather than a straight patch. Performing an infundibulotomy is generally recommended because subpulmonary stenosis is almost always present. The site of the infundibulotomy has to be carefully planned, staying away from any major coronary arteries. In case of an anomalous coronary artery crossing the right ventricular outflow tract, a conduit is sometimes necessary. Division of parietal and septal bands is always performed, along with placement of an infundibular outflow patch. Stenoses at the level of the pulmonary annulus, pulmonary valve, or branch pulmonary arteries can be handled as in tetralogy of Fallot (see Chapter 119).

Repair of DORV with Noncommitted VSD

The VSD is generally of the inlet type. Intraventricular (and thus biventricular) repair is difficult, but it can sometimes be accomplished by creating a tunnel from the left ventricle to the aorta. Anatomic variations generally considered to contraindicate a biventricular repair are multiple muscular VSDs, straddling AV valve tissue, or an inability to reliably channel the remote VSD to the aorta. If it is easier to baffle left ventricular blood to the pulmonary valve, or if the pulmonary valve is in the pathway of the baffle and there is no pulmonary stenosis, consideration should be given to performing an arterial switch procedure along with the intraventricular repair.[24] It is virtually always necessary to enlarge the VSD superoanteriorly. If the tunnel obstructs the right ventricular outflow tract, an infundibular patch or transannular patch should be placed. If there are significant tricuspid valve attachments to the anterior and superior edge of the VSD, or if a straddling tricuspid or mitral valve is present, attempting an intraventricular repair is generally contraindicated. However, there have been reports of successful division and reimplantation of the tricuspid chordae on the patch.

In the long term, the problem of subaortic stenosis with these complex baffles is real. A double-patch technique has been described that may mitigate this problem.[26] A noncommitted muscular trabecular defect can also sometimes be enlarged anteriorly and inferiorly, because the conduction system courses on the superior-posterior aspect of the defect. However, these baffles are often bulky, do not grow with the child, and are generally not very satisfactory. With the improving medium-term outcome for the single-ventricle approach in recent years, it is generally preferable to perform a straightforward single-ventricle repair with preservation of excellent ventricular function rather than a less-than-satisfactory higher-risk biventricular repair, after which multiple and usually complex reoperations will be necessary.[21] This approach might also be extended to patients who are at increased operative risk with a conventional biventricular repair.

Repair of DORV with Subpulmonary VSD

At the transposition end of the DORV spectrum, an arterial switch operation is usually preferred. A Taussig-Bing type of DORV can be repaired by an arterial switch operation (the most commonly used type of repair), a Rastelli procedure with Damus-Kaye-Stansel anastomosis, a Nikaidoh procedure, or a REV (réparation à l'étage ventriculaire) procedure. Surgical management of DORV transposition of the great arteries is discussed in Chapter 126.

Results of Surgical Treatment

The early mortality rate is low among patients with noncomplex forms of DORV, but it is higher in patients with complicating anatomic features.[27] Most complications are mechanical and should be routinely sought with the use of TEE before the patient leaves the operating room. As with VSD surgery, complete heart block and residual VSDs can occur. Inadequate enlargement of VSD or poor baffle configuration can result in subaortic obstruction. Direct measurements in the operating room can help elucidate cases in which TEE is not definitive. Residual muscular obstruction can often be resected through the aortic valve, and an aortotomy is generally a good first approach when approaching this problem. A separate patch also can be placed inside the original patch if it is too narrowing or if there is a waist created by a tortuous course. In cases of DORV with noncommitted VSD, it sometimes may be necessary to convert an acutely failed biventricular repair to a single-ventricle strategy. Significant right ventricular outflow tract obstruction can occur and should be managed as for tetralogy of Fallot. Patients with preoperative pulmonary hypertension are usually better served with implantation of a pulmonary valve. Because of the prolonged myocardial ischemic times needed for these complex repairs, myocardial protection should be carefully attended to; myocardial dysfunction can be a significant problem. Delayed sternal closure and mechanical assistance are important fallback measures that can be lifesaving.

REFERENCES

1. Muller WH, Jr, Damman JF, Jr: The treatment of certain congenital malformations of the heart by the creation of pulmonary stenosis to reduce pulmonary hypertension and excessive pulmonary blood flow: a preliminary report. *Surg Gynecol Obstet* 95:213–216, 1952.
2. Lillehei CW, Corden M, Warden HE, et al: The results of direct vision closure of ventricular septal defects in eight patients by means of controlled cross circulation. *Surg Gynecol Obstet* 101:446–450, 1955.
3. Kirklin JW, Harshbarger HG, Donald DE, et al: Surgical correction of ventricular septal defect: anatomic and technical considerations. *J Thorac Surg* 33:45–53, 1957.
4. Stirling GR, Stanley PH, Lillehei CW: The effects of cardiac bypass and ventriculotomy upon right ventricular function with report of successful closure of ventricular septal defect by use of atriotomy. *Surg Forum* 8:433–438, 1957.

5. Barratt-Boyes BG, Simpson M, Neutze JM: Intracardiac surgery in neonates and infants using deep hypothermia with surface cooling and limited cardiopulmonary bypass. *Circulation* 43(Suppl I):25–31, 1971.
6. Soto B, Becker AE, Moulaert AJ, et al: Classification of ventricular septal defects. *Br Heart J* 43:332–337, 1980.
7. Van Praagh R, Geva T, Kreutzer J: Ventricular septal defects: how shall we describe, name and classify them? *J Am Coll Cardiol* 14:1298–1303, 1989.
8. Gaynor JW: Management strategies for infants with coarctation and an associated ventricular septal defect. *J Thorac Cardiovasc Surg* 122:424–426, 2001.
9. Lauer RM, Dushane JW, Edwards JE: Obstruction of the left ventricular outlet in association with ventricular septal defect. *Circulation* 22:110–117, 1960.
10. Heath D, Edwards JE: The pathology of hypertensive pulmonary vascular disease: a description of 6 grades of structural changes in the pulmonary arteries with special reference to congenital cardiac septal defects. *Circulation* 18:533–543, 1958.
11. Collins G, Calder L, Rose V, et al: Ventricular septal defect: clinical and hemodynamic changes in the first five years of life. *Am Heart J* 84:695–701, 1972.
12. Hoffman JIE, Rudolph AM: The natural history of ventricular septal defects in infancy. *Am J Cardiol* 16:634–638, 1965.
13. Bacha EA, Cao QL, Starr J, et al: Periventricular device closure of muscular ventricular septal defects on the beating heart: technique and results. *J Thorac Cardiovasc Surg* 126:1718–1723, 2003.
14. Berner M, Behetti M, Ricou B, et al: Relief of severe pulmonary hypertension after closure of a large ventricular septal defect using low dose inhaled nitric oxide. *Intensive Care Med* 19:75–79, 1993.
15. Yeager SB, Freed MD, Keane JF, et al: Primary surgical closure of ventricular septal defect in the first year of life: results in 128 infants. *J Am Coll Cardiol* 3:1269–1273, 1984.
16. Weintraub RG, Menahem S: Early surgical closure of a large ventricular septal defect: influence on long-term growth. *J Am Coll Cardiol* 18:552–557, 1991.
17. Castaneda AR, Jonas RA, Mayer JE, Jr, et al: Double outlet right ventricle. In Castaneda AR, Jonas RA, Mayer JE, Jr, et al, editors: *Cardiac surgery of the neonate and infant*, Philadelphia, 1994, WB Saunders, pp 445–449.
18. Rein JG, Freed MD, Norwood WI, et al: Early and late results of closure of ventricular septal defect in infancy. *Ann Thorac Surg* 24:19–26, 1977.
19. Moller JH, Patton C, Varco RL, et al: Late results (30 to 35 years) after operative closure of isolated ventricular septal defect from 1954 to 1960. *Am J Cardiol* 68:1491–1496, 1991.
20. Lev M, Bharati S, Meng CCL, et al: A concept of double outlet right ventricle. *J Thorac Cardiovasc Surg* 64:271–279, 1972.
21. Walters HL, Mavroudis C, Tchervenkov CI, et al: Congenital heart surgery nomenclature and database project: double outlet right ventricle. *Ann Thorac Surg* 69:249–263, 2000.
22. Brown JW, Ruzmetov M, Okada Y, et al: Surgical results in patients with double outlet right ventricle: a 20-year experience. *Ann Thorac Surg* 72:1630–1635, 2001.
23. Sondheimer HM, Freedom RM, Olley PM: Double outlet right ventricle: clinical spectrum and prognosis. *Am J Cardiol* 709:39–45, 1977.
24. Lacour-Gayet F, Haun C, Ntalakoura K, et al: Biventricular repair of double-outlet-right ventricle with non committed ventricular septal defect by VSD rerouting to the pulmonary artery and arterial switch. *Eur J Cardiothorac Surg* 21:1042–1048, 2002.
25. Anderson RH, Pickering D, Brown R: Double outlet right ventricle with L-malposition and noncommitted ventricular septal defect. *Eur J Cardiol* 32:133–138, 1975.
26. Barbero-Marcial M, Tanamati C, Atik E, et al: Intraventricular repair of double-outlet right ventricle with non-committed ventricular septal defect: advantages of multiple patches. *J Thorac Cardiovasc Surg* 118:1056–1067, 1999.
27. Aoki M, Forbess JM, Jonas RA, et al: Results of biventricular repair for double-outlet right ventricle. *J Thorac Cardiovasc Surg* 107:338–350, 1994.

PULMONARY ATRESIA WITH INTACT VENTRICULAR SEPTUM

Erle H. Austin, III • Deborah J. Kozik

CHAPTER OUTLINE

Pulmonary atresia with intact ventricular septum (PA/IVS) is a rare congenital heart defect occurring at a rate of 4 to 10 per 100,000 live births.[1,2] This malformation is characterized by a variably sized right ventricle that has no exit, failing to provide pulmonary blood flow and unable to decompress itself through the interventricular septum. Blood flow through the ductus arteriosus permits survival at birth, but within hours hypoxemia progresses to death as the ductus closes. Thus, without early diagnosis and treatment, PA/IVS is uniformly fatal. Before 1970, reported survival to 3 years of age was less than 3%.[3] By the early 1990s, improvements in diagnosis and management resulted in a 3-year survival rate greater than 60%.[4] More recent reports indicate that careful initial evaluation and selective management of these patients can achieve survival rates in excess of 90%.[5]

Because this anomaly is rare and its morphology is heterogeneous, most reports and recommendations have been derived from small series with variable morphologic compositions. Although a great deal has been learned from the experiences of individual centers,[6-9] much more has been learned from a prospective multi-institutional study initiated by the Congenital Heart Surgeons Society in 1987[4,10,11] and from more recent, population-based studies from the United Kingdom and Ireland[1,12] and from Sweden.[2] Data acquired from these studies have provided important new insights into the spectrum of morphology and about outcomes of surgical treatment of this malformation.

PA/IVS has been described by other monikers in the past, including pulmonary atresia with normal aortic root and hypoplasia of the right heart. The first description of pulmonary atresia with an intact ventricular septum was in 1784 by Hunter.[13] Connections between the right ventricle and the coronary arteries were described by Grant in 1926 after examining the heart of a 14-month-old girl.[14] Lauer and colleagues in 1964 were the first to angiographically demonstrate intramyocardial sinusoids.[13] Freedom and colleagues postulated in 1974 that the connections between the right ventricle and the coronary arteries could possibly be related to myocardial ischemia.[13] The first successful surgical repair of a patient with PA/IVS involved a transventricular valvotomy and was reported by Weinberg and associates in 1962.[15]

ANATOMY

Characteristically, PA/IVS occurs in hearts with situs solitus and atrioventricular and ventriculoarterial concordance. The aortic arch is usually left-sided, and a left-sided ductus arteriosus is typical. The essential feature of this lesion is an absent communication between the right ventricle and the pulmonary trunk (Fig. 118-1). The character of the atretic segment ranges from a thin imperforate membrane to a long section of infundibular muscle without a definable lumen. In contrast to pulmonary atresia with ventricular septal defect, in PA/IVS the pulmonary trunk and branch pulmonary arteries are usually near normal in size and configuration. The size and morphology of the right ventricle varies significantly in this condition, and in most patients, the right ventricular cavity is reduced in size. There is a continuum from tiny "unipartite" chambers that have only an inlet component to larger-than-normal "tripartite" ventricles that have well-defined inlet, trabecular, and infundibular portions. The rare patients with enlarged right ventricular cavities also may have Ebstein anomaly with severe tricuspid regurgitation. More typically, the cavity is small, and marked hypertrophy of the right ventricular wall is present, often contributing to obliteration of the outflow (infundibular) portion of the cavity. The tricuspid valve is usually small with thickened leaflets and abnormal chordae. The diameter of the tricuspid valve correlates with the size of the right ventricular cavity and provides a useful index of right ventricular size. The right atrium is enlarged, and an interatrial communication, usually a patent foramen ovale, is present. At birth, the ductus arteriosus is patent, providing the only blood flow to the lungs. Significant aortopulmonary collateral arteries are uncommon.

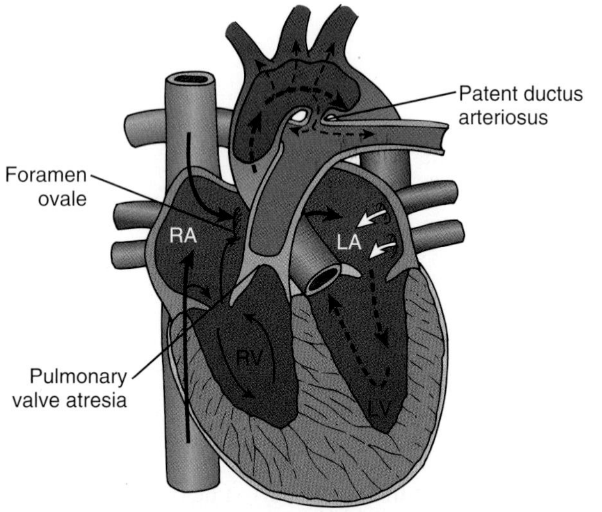

FIGURE 118-1 Schematic representation of blood flow in patients with pulmonary atresia with intact ventricular septum. An obligatory right-to-left shunt occurs at the atrial level. Peripheral oxygenation depends on flow through the ductus arteriosus. (*Black arrows,* deoxygenated blood; *white arrows,* oxygenated blood; *dashed arrows,* mixed blood; *larger arrows,* larger amount of blood flow.) *LA,* Left atrium; *LV,* left ventricle; *RA,* right atrium; *RV,* right ventricle.

An important anatomic feature of PA/IVS is the presence in some patients of connections between the right ventricle and the coronary circulation (Figs. 118-2 and 118-3). Sinusoids or "intermuscular spaces" in the right ventricular myocardium occur in approximately 50% of patients.[4] In 90% of these patients, the sinusoids communicate with the coronary arteries. The smaller the tricuspid valve (and thus the right ventricular cavity) is, the more likely it is that right ventricle–coronary arterial fistulas are present. In 15% of patients with these fistulas, significant proximal coronary artery stenoses exist, making myocardial blood flow dependent on blood from the right ventricle (see Table 118-2).[10] Knowledge of the presence of right ventricle–dependent coronary circulation (RVDCC) is important in deciding on surgical therapy, because in these cases, decompression of the right ventricle may cause myocardial ischemia or infarction.[16]

PATHOPHYSIOLOGY

In PA/IVS, desaturated systemic venous blood is obliged to cross the interatrial septum to mix with saturated pulmonary venous blood in the left atrium (see Fig. 118-1). The resultant admixture is ejected into the systemic arterial circulation, and the systemic arterial saturation depends on adequate pulmonary blood flow. Closure of the ductus arteriosus soon after birth markedly reduces pulmonary blood flow, and progressive hypoxemia and tissue acidosis leads to death. Expeditious administration of prostaglandin E_1 can temporarily reverse ductal closure

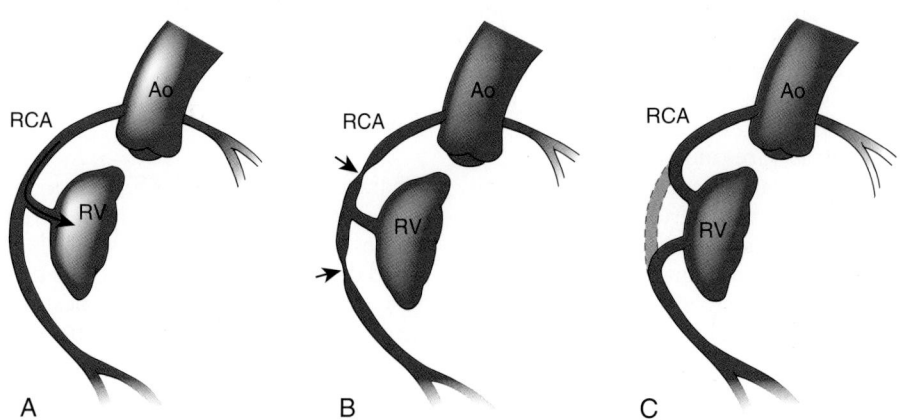

FIGURE 118-2 Right ventricle–to–coronary artery fistulas in pulmonary atresia with intact ventricular septum. **A,** Without coronary stenosis: potential right ventricular steal phenomenon. **B,** With proximal or distal coronary stenosis: potential steal or ischemia. **C,** With coronary occlusion or atresia: potential isolation and myocardial infarction. *Ao,* Aorta; *RCA,* right coronary artery; *RV,* right ventricle. (Modified from Giglia TM, Mandell VS, Connor AR, et al: Diagnosis and management of right ventricle-dependent coronary circulation in pulmonary atresia with intact ventricular septum. *Circulation* 86:1516–1528, 1992.)

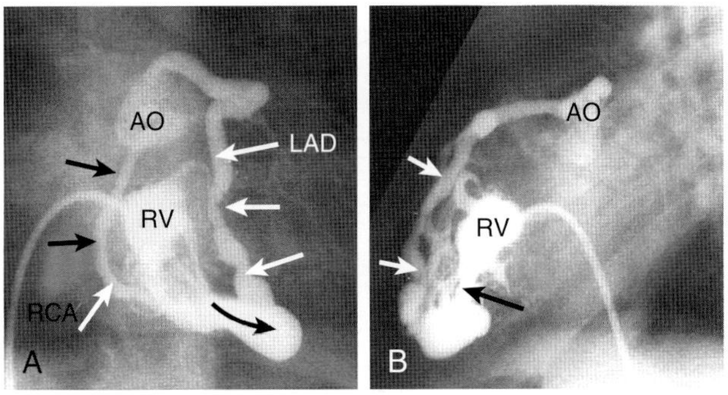

FIGURE 118-3 ■ Right ventriculogram in patient with pulmonary atresia and intact ventricular septum and ventriculocoronary connections. **A,** Frontal right ventriculogram showing severe hypoplasia of the right ventricular cavity. The right ventricle (RV) connects to the left anterior descending artery (LAD) through a ventriculocoronary connection *(curved arrow).* **B,** Lateral right ventriculogram showing ectasia and narrowing of the LAD *(white arrows),* and the connection between the RV and the coronary circulation *(black arrows). AO,* Aorta; *RCA,* right coronary artery. (Modified from Freedom RM, Anderson RH, Perrin D: The significance of ventriculo-coronary arterial connections in the setting of pulmonary atresia with an intact ventricular septum. *Cardiol Young* 15[5]:447–468, 2005.)

until a surgical procedure to increase pulmonary blood flow can be performed.

INITIAL CLINICAL PRESENTATION AND MANAGEMENT

Infants with PA/IVS are typically full-term, well-developed infants without other anomalies. Delivery is usually uncomplicated, but cyanosis develops on the first day of life and rapidly progresses to respiratory distress and metabolic acidosis. A murmur is unusual unless significant tricuspid regurgitation exists. There is no splitting of the second heart sound. Chest radiography demonstrates clear lung fields with decreased vascular markings. The electrocardiogram is often normal, although the typical neonatal pattern of right ventricular hypertrophy may be absent. Definitive diagnosis is made using two-dimensional echocardiography, which reveals the right ventricular outflow obstruction and the size of the right ventricle and tricuspid valve and, combined with color flow Doppler techniques, can identify right ventricle–coronary artery fistulas.[17,18]

As soon as the diagnosis of PA/IVS is suspected, an infusion of prostaglandin E_1 is begun. Elective intubation and controlled ventilation may be advisable, especially if the infant is to be transported to a tertiary treatment center, because apnea is a common complication of prostaglandin E_1 infusion. Cardiac catheterization and cineangiography are recommended for most of these patients, especially for those with moderate or severe right ventricular hypoplasia. Right ventriculography, aortography, and, when indicated, selective coronary angiography are performed to determine the presence and extent of right ventricle–to–coronary artery fistulas and the presence of coronary artery obstructions (see Figs. 118-2 and 118-3).[16,19] At catheterization, an adequate atrial communication must be ensured. If echocardiography and catheterization indicate that right ventricle–to–pulmonary artery decompression cannot be performed and a flow gradient exists between the right and left atrium, a balloon atrial septostomy is performed at this catheterization.

SURGICAL MANAGEMENT

The ideal long-term outcome for all infants with PA/IVS would be to achieve a two-ventricle circulation with the right ventricle providing all blood flow to the lungs at a low filling pressure without residual right-to-left shunt. The anatomic heterogeneity of this group of patients, however, prevents the achievement of this goal in all patients. In fact, this ideal is achieved in only one third of patients surviving infancy (see Fig. 118-10).[10] A more realistic outcome for the remaining patients is the elimination of cyanosis by separating the systemic and pulmonary circulations without limiting cardiac output or inducing excessively elevated systemic venous pressures. Such an outcome can be achieved with a one-ventricle repair (the Fontan operation) for hearts whose right ventricle cannot contribute to pulmonary blood flow, or with a one-and-one-half-ventricle repair for hearts whose right ventricle can provide a portion of pulmonary blood flow. Careful assessment of right ventricular size and coronary artery anatomy is crucial to selecting the appropriate strategy for each patient.

In neonates, it is useful to classify right ventricular hypoplasia into mild, moderate, and severe degrees (Table 118-1). Echocardiographic measurement of the diameter of the tricuspid valve with conversion to a z-value provides a quantitative measurement to facilitate classification.[20] A website (www.parameterz.com) is available for rapid and easy determination of z-scores. Patients with mild right ventricular hypoplasia have tricuspid valve z-values of −2 or greater. Tricuspid z-values between −4 and −2 indicate moderate right ventricular hypoplasia, and z-values of −4 or less are seen in patients with severe right ventricular hypoplasia. Tripartite right ventricles with a well-developed right ventricular outflow tract fall into the mild group, whereas unipartite right ventricles without a definable infundibular or trabecular portion are classified as severe.[21] Patients with mild right ventricular hypoplasia have definite potential for conversion to a two-ventricle system at the time of definitive repair, whereas those with severe right ventricular hypoplasia can achieve only separation of systemic and pulmonary circulations with a one-ventricle repair (a Fontan operation). Patients with moderate right ventricular hypoplasia are also potential candidates for two-ventricle or one-and-one-half-ventricle repair, provided they do not have RVDCC.

Initial Palliation

The surgical management of PA/IVS is typically undertaken in two or more stages, the first for palliation and subsequent procedures directed at definitive repair. To

TABLE 118-1 **Effect of Degree of Right Ventricular Hypoplasia on Management of Pulmonary Atresia with Intact Ventricular Septum**

	Degree of Right Ventricular Hypoplasia		
Parameter/ Management	**Mild**	**Moderate**	**Severe**
Tricuspid z-value	>–2	–2 to –4	<–4
Right ventricular morphology	Tripartite	Bipartite	Unipartite
Infundibular cavity	Present	Intermediate	Absent
Right ventricle–dependent coronary circulation	Rare	Possible	Common
Initial palliation	Transannular patch ± shunt. Consider transcatheter valvotomy or hybrid procedure	Transannular patch + shunt. Consider hybrid procedure (no right ventricular decompression if right ventricle–dependent coronary circulation)	Shunt only
Definitive operation	Two-ventricle repair	Two-ventricle repair; one-and-one-half-ventricle repair; Fontan if right ventricle–dependent coronary circulation	Fontan

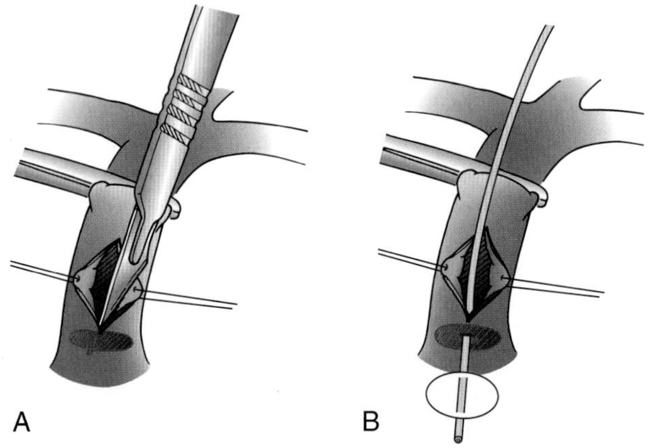

FIGURE 118-4 ■ Open pulmonary valvotomy without cardiopulmonary bypass can be performed via a median sternotomy or a left thoracotomy. **A,** After clamping the pulmonary trunk just proximal to the bifurcation, the pulmonary artery is opened and the atretic pulmonary valve is opened sharply. **B,** A Fogarty catheter positioned in the infundibulum provides hemostasis as the atretic valve is excised. (Modified from Kanter KR, Pennington DG, Nouri S, et al: Concomitant valvotomy and subclavian-main pulmonary artery shunt in neonates with pulmonary atresia and intact ventricular septum. *Ann Thorac Surg* 43:490–494, 1987.)

ensure early survival, pulmonary blood flow must be maintained after ductal closure. Although the creation of a systemic-to-pulmonary shunt can ensure continued pulmonary blood flow, the right ventricle must be assessed for its potential recruitment into the circulation. When possible, decompressing the right ventricle into the pulmonary artery permits right ventricular growth such that a two-ventricle repair may become feasible. Failure to decompress the right ventricle at initial palliation essentially eliminates the possibility of ever achieving a definitive two-ventricle repair.[22]

Thus, neonates with mild to moderate right ventricular hypoplasia are best served by relieving the right ventricle–to–pulmonary artery obstruction. This may be accomplished with or without cardiopulmonary bypass. Without bypass, a pulmonary valvotomy can be performed blindly, with a transventricular dilator,[23] or under direct vision through the main pulmonary artery (Fig. 118-4).[24] Interventional catheter and hybrid techniques are now being applied at some centers for this purpose (see Trends and Controversies, later). The use of cardiopulmonary bypass allows more controlled access into the right ventricular outflow tract so that obstructing infundibular muscle can be excised under direct vision and a transannular outflow patch can be placed (Fig. 118-5). By maximizing unobstructed forward flow, transannular patching provides the greatest possibility for right ventricular growth.[4,25] Because early postoperative right ventricular failure may cause increased right-to-left shunting across the patent foramen ovale, and antegrade flow from the right ventricle may be limited, a systemic-to-pulmonary artery shunt (a 3- or 3.5-mm polytetrafluoroethylene [PTFE] tube graft) also should be placed to prevent life-threatening hypoxia. Initial results from the Congenital Heart Surgeons Society's study suggest that concomitant insertion of a transannular patch and placement of a systemic-to-pulmonary artery shunt is the optimal initial treatment for neonates with tricuspid valve z-values between –1.5 and –4 (Fig. 118-6).[4] In that study, when a valvotomy or transannular patch was performed without a concomitant systemic-to-pulmonary artery shunt, approximately 50% of the patients required shunt placement within the first 4 weeks after the initial procedure. In addition, approximately 40% of patients treated initially with pulmonary valvotomy required a transannular patch at a subsequent operation.[4] On the other hand, any form of right ventricular decompression is contraindicated if RVDCC exists.

Neonates with severe right ventricular hypoplasia or RVDCC (or both) are best placed on a definitive one-ventricle (Fontan) pathway. Thus, initial surgical therapy should be limited to a systemic-to-pulmonary artery shunt (see Fig. 118-6).[4] A 3.5-mm PTFE tube graft placed via a median sternotomy or a right thoracotomy from the innominate or right subclavian artery to the right pulmonary artery provides adequate pulmonary blood flow and facilitates shunt access at the time of definitive one-ventricle repair. Shunts greater than 4 mm should be avoided because they may result in excessive pulmonary blood flow and low diastolic arterial blood pressure, causing life-threatening myocardial ischemia.

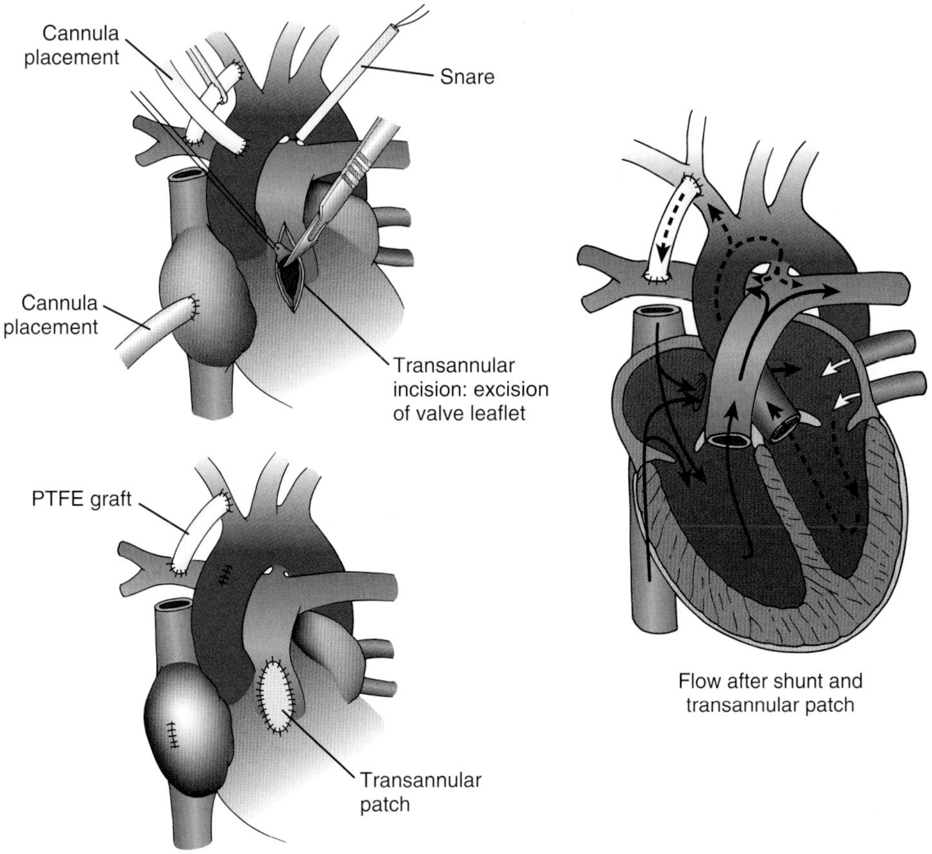

FIGURE 118-5 Placement of a transannular patch and a systemic-to-pulmonary artery shunt. A 3- or 3.5-mm polytetrafluoroethylene (PTFE) tube graft is placed from the innominate artery to the right pulmonary artery. Cardiopulmonary bypass is established and the shunt and ductus are temporarily occluded. A pulmonary artery incision is extended into the right ventricular outflow tract. Obstructing tissue is excised, and a pericardial patch is sewn in place. Separation from bypass is done with the shunt open and the ductus occluded. If peripheral oxygen saturations exceed 80%, the ductus is ligated. If peripheral oxygen saturations are less than 80%, the ductus is unsnared as demonstrated at right. (*Black arrows,* deoxygenated blood; *white arrows,* oxygenated blood; *dashed arrows,* mixed blood).

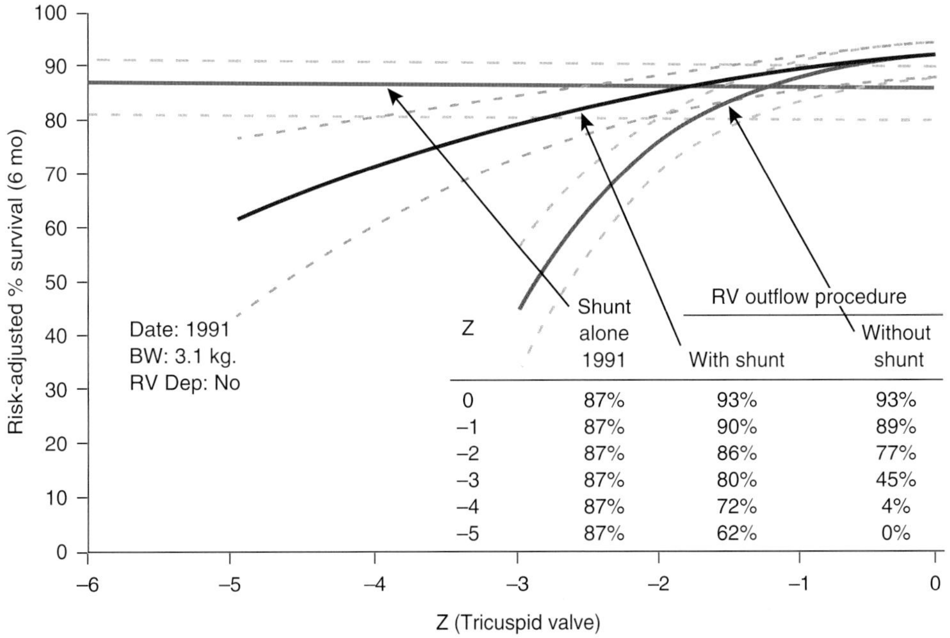

FIGURE 118-6 The effect of tricuspid valve diameter (z-value) and type of initial procedure on 6-month survival in neonates with pulmonary atresia and intact septum. This nomogram was derived after analyzing 171 neonates and solving a multivariable equation setting birth weight (BW) at "3.1 kg," right ventricle (RV)–dependent circulation at "no," and date of shunt operation at "1991." RV outflow procedure includes valvotomy and transannular patch. (Modified from Hanley FL, Sade RM, Blackstone EH, et al: Outcomes in neonatal pulmonary atresia with intact ventricular septum. A multiinstitutional study. *J Thorac Cardiovasc Surg* 105:406–423, 1993.)

Definitive Procedures

Two-Ventricle Repair

Patients selected at initial palliation for a two-ventricle strategy should have echocardiographic evidence of satisfactory right ventricular decompression with estimated right ventricular pressure less than or equal to one half of systemic arterial pressure. Those infants treated originally with valvotomy rather than transannular patching are especially vulnerable to residual or recurrent right ventricular outflow tract obstruction,[4,22] which should be relieved by a second right ventricular outflow tract procedure (a transannular patch) before considering conversion to a two-ventricle circulation. Follow-up cardiac catheterization should be performed between 6 and 12 months of age. At catheterization, the systemic-to-pulmonary artery shunt is temporarily occluded. If arterial saturations remain high, the atrial septal defect (patent foramen ovale) is occluded as well. If right atrial pressure remains below 15 mm Hg and cardiac output is adequate, the shunt and atrial communication can be closed permanently and a two-ventricle circulation achieved. At some centers, the shunt and atrial defect can be closed during the catheterization using percutaneous techniques.[26,27]

One-and-One-Half Ventricle Repair

Patients studied at 6 to 12 months who do not tolerate temporary occlusion of the systemic-to-pulmonary artery shunt are receiving too little pulmonary blood flow from the right ventricle to achieve success from a two-ventricle repair. Assuming there is no significant residual right ventricular outflow obstruction, these patients should be considered candidates for a one-and-one-half-ventricle repair. This repair involves takedown of the arterial systemic-to-pulmonary shunt and the creation of a bidirectional superior cavopulmonary anastomosis (a bidirectional Glenn procedure), which relieves the right ventricle of the superior vena caval blood flow. Ideally, the atrial septal communication is closed at the same operation. However, if the right atrial pressure exceeds 15 mm Hg, a small (4-mm) fenestration can be left. Catheter closure of the fenestration can usually be performed within months of the surgical procedure.[27] Alternatively, a purse-string suture and an adjustable snare can permit incremental closure of the atrial septal defect in the postoperative period (Fig. 118-7).[28] Patients with tricuspid z-values as small as −6 may be definitively managed with the one-and-one-half-ventricle strategy.[29]

One-Ventricle Repair

Infants with severe right ventricular hypoplasia or RVDCC (or both) are typically designated for a one-ventricle strategy at initial palliation. At 4 to 6 months of age, these patients undergo takedown of the systemic-to-pulmonary shunt and the creation of a bidirectional cavopulmonary anastomosis. At 2 to 4 years of age, they are considered candidates for the Fontan operation. Before the Fontan operation, cardiac catheterization is essential to ensure adequate left ventricular function and low pulmonary vascular resistance. Poor left ventricular function would leave cardiac transplantation as the only alternative therapy. Heart-lung transplantation is the only alternative if pulmonary vascular resistance is elevated. Fortunately, the early creation of a bidirectional cavopulmonary anastomosis appears to help preserve ventricular function and prevent the development of pulmonary vascular disease so that those drastic measures are rarely necessary. When performing the bidirectional Glenn procedure on cardiopulmonary bypass in patients with RVDCC, the surgeon must avoid low right ventricular preload to avoid poor coronary perfusion. The right ventricle should remain filled and ejecting, because myocardial perfusion occurs only during systole. Patients with RVDCC who sustain cardiac arrest may not respond well to resuscitation with extracorporeal membrane oxygenation (ECMO). ECMO will empty the right heart and significantly hinder coronary perfusion.[30] After the superior cavopulmonary anastomosis, the saturations in the right ventricular cavity are significantly increased, and this is likely beneficial for patients with RVDCC.[31]

When the Fontan procedure is performed, inferior vena caval blood flow is directed to the pulmonary arteries. This can be performed with a lateral atrial tunnel technique, wherein a baffle of PTFE is placed inside the right atrium (Fig. 118-8),[32] or with an extracardiac conduit.[33] Many surgeons prefer to place a small fenestration in the baffle to permit some right-to-left shunting

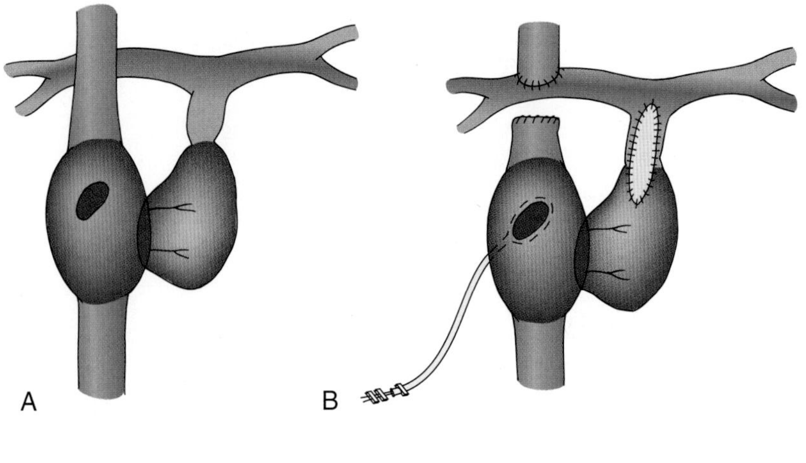

FIGURE 118-7 ■ Creation of a one-and-one-half-ventricle circulation. **A,** Small right ventricle unable to support two-ventricle repair. **B,** Superior vena caval flow is directed to the right pulmonary artery with a bidirectional cavopulmonary anastomosis. Residual right ventricular outflow tract stenosis is relieved with a transannular patch. Placement of an adjustable snare around the atrial septal defect permits incremental closure in the postoperative period. (Modified from Billingsley AM, Laks H, Boyce SW, et al: Definitive repair in patients with pulmonary atresia and intact ventricular septum. *J Thorac Cardiovasc Surg* 97:746–754, 1989.)

to maintain cardiac output in the perioperative period, when pulmonary vascular resistance may be elevated.[34] Routine fenestration, however, may not be necessary when an extracardiac conduit is used.[35] It also may be preferable to avoid fenestration when RVDCC is present. Enlarging the atrial septal defect and unroofing the coronary sinus to ensure that the blood entering the right ventricle is well oxygenated has also been recommended for RVDCC (see Fig. 118-8).

RESULTS

Early and Midterm Outcomes

The reports from the Congenital Heart Surgeons Society (CHSS) continue to provide the best overall perspective of outcomes in neonates with PA/IVS.[4,10,11] This prospective multi-institutional study involves 31 institutions and enrolled 408 unselected neonates with this diagnosis within a 10-year period (1987-1997). The initial right ventricular morphology and tricuspid valve size (z-value) were known for all patients, and follow-up through 2002 was 91% complete. Techniques for surgical management were not randomized but left to the discretion of each institution. The overall survival was 60% at 5 years and 58% at 15 years (Fig. 118-9). At 15 years, 33% had undergone a two-ventricle repair, 20% a Fontan repair, and 5% a one-and-one-half-ventricle repair, and 38% died before reaching definitive repair (Fig. 118-10). In this unselected group, 49% of patients were found to have severe right ventricular hypoplasia (z-score ≤–4), and 36% had moderate right ventricular hypoplasia (z-score –2 or –3) (Table 118-2). Additionally, 6% of the cohort had RVDCC (none with a z-score ≥–2), and 38% had right ventricle–coronary artery fistulas. Increasing tricuspid valve z-score, larger right ventricle size, higher birth weight, and a lesser degree of right ventricle–to–coronary artery fistulas were all found to be significant determinants of achieving a two-ventricle repair. Also, tricuspid valve morphology was found to be an important determinant of successful two-ventricle repair, as Ebstein malformation was associated with an increased risk of death. The 2004 CHSS report highlighted the importance of morphology-specific repair.[10] The most favorable outcomes were achieved by institutions that applied the Fontan operation for patients with severe morphology, and a two-ventricle repair for patients with favorable morphology (Fig. 118-11).

The 2005 report from the United Kingdom and Ireland Collaborative Study of Pulmonary Atresia with Intact Ventricular Septum identified three variables as independent predictors of death—these variables are birth weight, right ventricular dilation, and the partite status of the right ventricle.[36] Only one third of patients born at less than 2 kg survived, and each additional kilogram of weight was associated with a 44% reduction in the risk of death. Eighty percent of those undergoing operation with a significantly dilated right ventricle died. The 1- and 5-year survival rates for those with a tripartite right ventricle were 78% and 74%, respectively (Fig. 118-12). This is significantly better than the 44% and 22% seen for those with unipartite right ventricle anatomy. At this 9-year follow-up report, 29% had achieved a biventricular repair, 3% a one-and-a-half-ventricle repair, and 10.5% a univentricular repair, and 41% had died.

Using information derived from the CHSS study, Boston Children's Hospital applied a policy of routine coronary angiography, right ventricular decompression with transannular patching for patients without RVDCC, and a systemic-to-pulmonary shunt in virtually all patients. In a consecutive group of 47 patients from 1991 to 1998, this institution achieved an actuarial survival rate

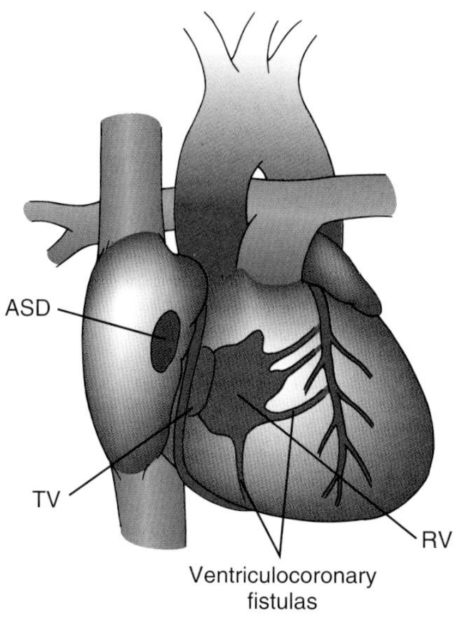

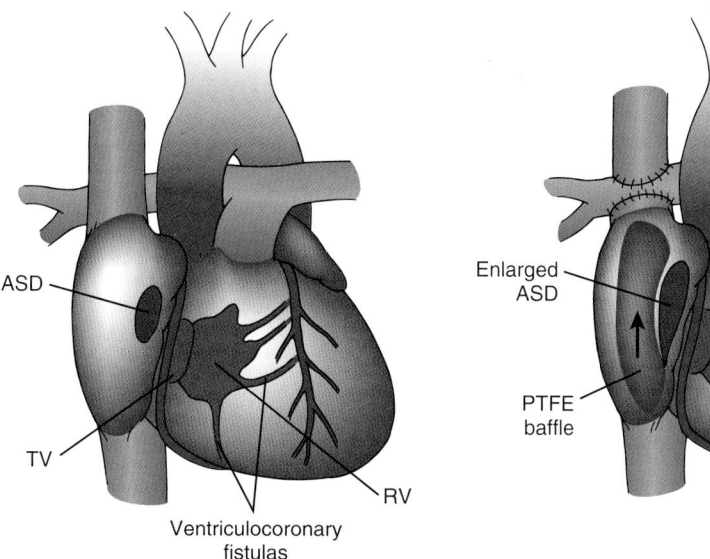

FIGURE 118-8 Lateral-tunnel Fontan procedure in a patient with right ventricle–dependent coronary circulation. Inferior vena caval flow is directed to superior vena cava by polytetrafluoroethylene (PTFE) baffle. Atrial septal defect (ASD) is enlarged, allowing fully saturated pulmonary venous blood to enter the right ventricle (RV). *TV,* Tricuspid valve. (Modified from Pearl JM, Laks H, Stein DG, et al: Total cavopulmonary anastomosis versus conventional modified Fontan procedure. *Ann Thorac Surg* 52:189–196, 1991.)

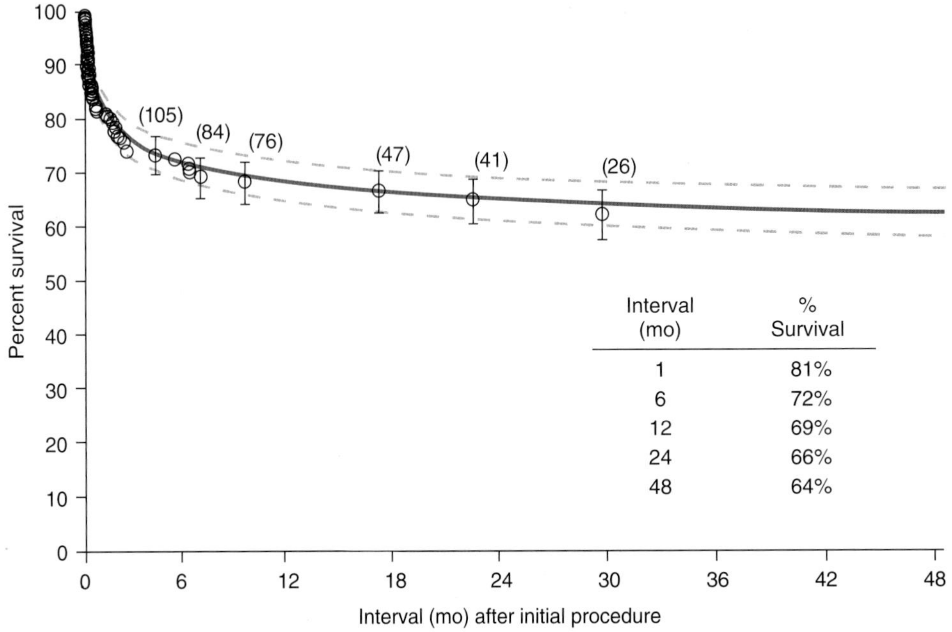

FIGURE 118-9 ■ Survival (derived from life-table and parametric methods) after the initial procedure performed on neonates with pulmonary atresia and intact ventricular septum. *Circles* represent individual deaths. *Vertical bars* and *dashed lines* represent 70% confidence intervals. (Modified from Hanley FL, Sade RM, Blackstone EH, et al: Outcomes in neonatal pulmonary atresia with intact ventricular septum. A multiinstitutional study. *J Thorac Cardiovasc Surg* 105:406–423, 1993.)

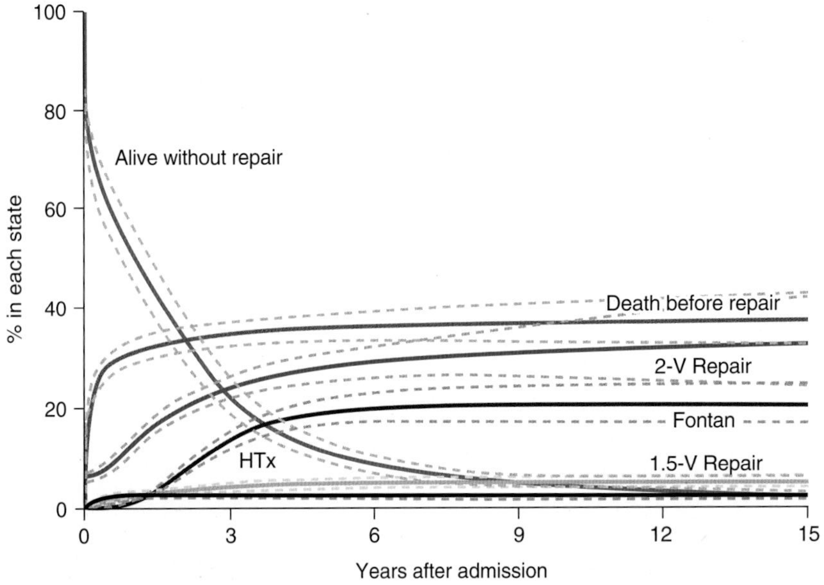

FIGURE 118-10 ■ Proportion of children reaching each end state over time after initial hospital admission. All patients begin alive at the time of initial admission (time = 0) and thereafter migrate to an end state at a time-dependent rate defined by the hazard functions. At any point in time, the sum of the proportion of children in each state is 100%. *HTx,* Heart transplantation; *V,* ventricle. (Modified from Ashburn DA, Blackstone EH, Wells WJ, et al; Congenital Heart Surgeons Study members: Determinants of mortality and type of repair in neonates with pulmonary atresia and intact ventricular septum. *J Thorac Cardiovasc Surg* 127[4]:1000–1007, 2004; discussion 1007–1008.)

of 98% at 1 year, 5 years, and 7.5 years.[5] To achieve this excellent survival rate, a one-ventricle or a one-and-one-half-ventricle repair was required in most patients. On the other hand, in patients with RVDCC, survival is not nearly as good. In another report from the same institution, patients with RVDCC had an overall mortality of almost 19%. Also, patients with aortocoronary atresia had 100% mortality.[30] Green Lane Hospital in New Zealand also had an extremely high mortality rate (91%) among patients with aortocoronary atresia.[37]

Late Follow-up

The Congenital Heart Surgeons Society recently evaluated surviving patients from its original multi-institutional study to determine if biventricular repair was associated

TABLE 118-2 **Morphologic Characteristics in 334 Neonates for Whom an RV Size Score Was Assigned**

			Tricuspid Value Z-Score				
RV Size	**Patients *(n)***	**% of 334**	**Median**	**Range***	**25th Percentile**	**RV-CA Fistulas**	**RVDCC**
−5 (severe hypoplasia)	62	19	−2.3	−5.4 to 4.8	−3.3	35 (56%)	5 (8%)
−4	100	30	−2.3	−5.3 to 0.6	−3.1	55 (55%)	10 (10%)
−3	79	24	−1.1	−5.2 to 5.0	−1.9	28 (35%)	4 (14%)
−2	40	12	−0.3	−3.1 to 3.2	−1.0	5 (13%)	0
−1	22	7	0.4	−2.9 to 2.9	−1.2	3 (14%)	0
0 (normal for age)	16	5	1.5	−1.6 to 5.0	0.6	0	0
≥1 (enlarged)	15	4	2.4	−1.0 to 6.0	0.4	0	0

*High upper limits of tricuspid valve z-score in neonates with a diminutive right ventricle are attributable to associated Ebstein malformation.
CA, Coronary artery; *RV,* right ventricle; *RVDCC,* right ventricle–dependent coronary circulation.

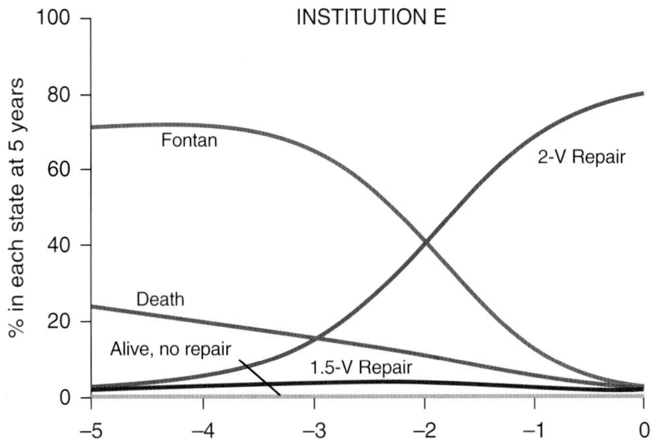

FIGURE 118-11 Results at an institution favoring both two-ventricle (2-V) and Fontan pathways. Patients with severe morphologies undergo the Fontan operation, and patients with favorable morphologies undergo two-ventricle repair. The mortality rate is low, and most children have had a definitive repair by 5 years. (Modified from Ashburn DA, Blackstone EH, Wells WJ, et al; Congenital Heart Surgeons Study members: Determinants of mortality and type of repair in neonates with pulmonary atresia and intact ventricular septum. *J Thorac Cardiovasc Surg* 127[4]:1000–1007, 2004; discussion 1007–1008.)

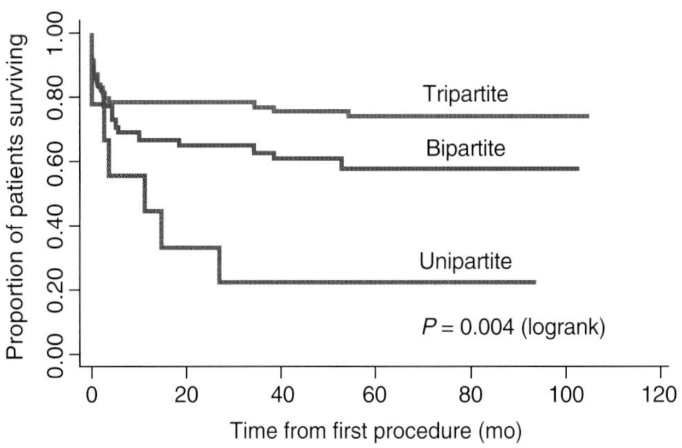

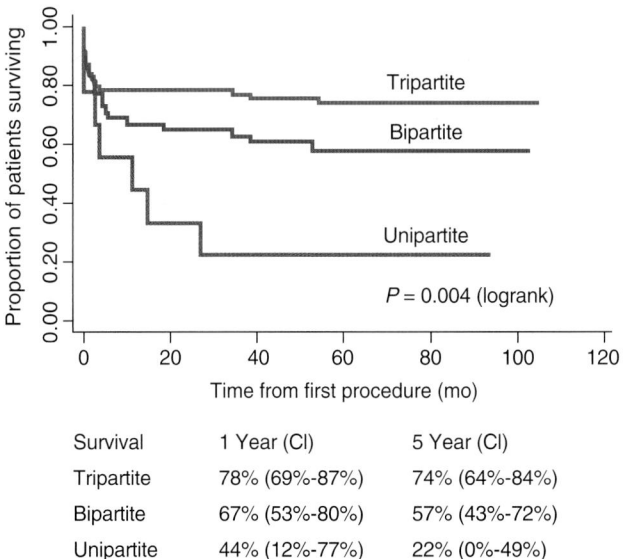

Survival	1 Year (CI)	5 Year (CI)
Tripartite	78% (69%-87%)	74% (64%-84%)
Bipartite	67% (53%-80%)	57% (43%-72%)
Unipartite	44% (12%-77%)	22% (0%-49%)

FIGURE 118-12 Survival curve for all patients undergoing operative procedures, grouped by so-called partite status of the right ventricle (N = 168). *CI,* 95% confidence interval. (Modified from Daubeney PE, Wang D, Delany DJ, et al; UK and Ireland Collaborative Study of Pulmonary Atresia with Intact Ventricular Septum: Pulmonary atresia with intact ventricular septum: predictors of early and medium-term outcome in a population-based study. *J Thorac Cardiovasc Surg* 130[4]:1071, 2005.)

with late (≥10 years) benefit in terms of functional health status and exercise capacity relative to a univentricular or one-and-one-half-ventricle repair.[11] Of 271 current survivors of the original cohort, 106 participated in the cross-sectional study. In this report, patient-perceived physical functional health status and measured exercise capacity were reduced, regardless of repair pathway. Peak oxygen consumption was low across all groups and was positively correlated with larger initial tricuspid valve z-score. The peak VO_2 in the biventricular repair group with low tricuspid valve z-scores tended to be lower than peak VO_2 in the one-and-one-half-ventricle group with comparable tricuspid valve z-scores. These findings suggest that patients with more severe degrees of right heart hypoplasia who are forced down a biventricular pathway may be at greater risk of late deficits in aerobic capacity.

Another study, from the Mayo Clinic, looked at clinical outcomes in adult survivors with PA/IVS.[38] Of 20 patients, 5 died during the 10-year study period at a median age of 32 years. All patients in this cohort required surgical or catheter reinterventions in adulthood, regardless of type of repair, and 80% developed atrial arrhythmias. Thus, despite survival into adulthood, the risk of morbidity and mortality continues for these patients.

TRENDS AND CONTROVERSIES

Transcatheter Pulmonary Valvotomy

Advances in interventional techniques now make it possible for some infants with PA/IVS to undergo antegrade decompression of the right ventricle without surgery, while still in the catheterization laboratory. Using mechanical, laser, or radiofrequency energy at the tip of a catheter, the membranous atresia can be perforated and the resulting communication dilated with percutaneous balloon technique.[39-41] As experience with this procedure increases, it is being considered as first-line treatment in place of surgical intervention at some centers.[42] Right ventricular growth and a definitive two-ventricle circulation have been achieved with this technique in some patients.[41,43] Use of this approach, however, requires careful selection of patients and is essentially limited to infants with a patent infundibulum and a right ventricle large enough to support the pulmonary circulation without a systemic-to-pulmonary shunt. This approach may not adequately address the small pulmonary annulus or significant subpulmonary obstruction. Accordingly, after catheter valvotomy, some patients have required prolonged hospitalization for continued administration of prostaglandin E_1 or surgery (or both) to place a systemic-to-pulmonary shunt.[40]

In one recent series, 88% of those undergoing transcatheter pulmonary valvotomy required surgical intervention within 2 weeks of the initial interventional procedure.[44] In that series, most operations (87%) involved a procedure directed at the right ventricular outflow tract in addition to shunt placement. In another single-institution review, 64% of those initially receiving catheter-based therapy required surgical intervention before discharge.[45] A more recent report from Boston Children's Hospital confirms a similar rate (62%) of surgery prior to discharge.[46] In this study all but one patient required a systemic to pulmonary shunt to augment pulmonary blood flow.

Stenting of the arterial duct has become an alternative technique for ensuring adequate pulmonary blood flow in selected patients while right ventricular function is being established. Ductal stenting can be performed within days after catheter-based valvotomy if the infant cannot be weaned from prostaglandin[47] or concomitantly with the valvotomy.[48] The risk factors determining the need for an additional source of pulmonary blood flow (shunt or ductal stent) continue to be defined for these patients. As expected, smaller tricuspid valve z-scores correlate with a greater need for adding pulmonary blood flow.[46,49] In one study 80% of patients with a bipartite right ventricle required an additional source of pulmonary blood flow.[47] Another case series looked at 143 patients with PA/IVS, 37 of whom had a bipartite right ventricle.[48] All 37 patients underwent radiofrequency valvotomy and stenting of the ductus as the initial procedure. Forty-eight percent of these patients went on to achieve a biventricular circulation, and 26% underwent one-and-one-half-ventricle repair. A large multicenter study that examined ductal stenting over an 18-year period reported a 94% success rate in patients with PA/IVS.[50] The long-term impact of ductal stenting on future operations and pulmonary artery anatomy is not clear. In one study, major late complications of patent ductus arteriosus stenting were not encountered, and the stented patent ductus arteriosus did not pose a major surgical challenge at the time of bidirectional Glenn surgery.[48]

Catheter-based therapy for PA/IVS patients is becoming the preferred approach at most centers when the anatomy is favorable. Moller's analysis of more than 1000 PA/IVS patients from the multi-institutional Pediatric Cardiac Care Consortium from 1982 to 2006 revealed a steady increase in the frequency of balloon pulmonary valvotomy along with a corresponding decrease in surgical pulmonary valvotomy (Table 118-3).[51]

Hybrid Procedures

Despite the increasing preference for catheter-based therapy in select neonates with PA/IVS, the percutaneous approach is associated with significant rates of procedural failure and serious complications. Many neonates have required surgical intervention in the neonatal period, either to augment pulmonary blood flow or to repair a complication associated with the percutaneous approach. An alternative hybrid approach integrating a sternotomy with transventricular perforation of the atretic pulmonary membrane and balloon pulmonary valvotomy was first described in 2007.[52] This approach also allows for radiofrequency perforation of the valve membrane.[53] Potential advantages of the hybrid approach include avoidance of neonatal cardiopulmonary bypass, mitigation of the technical failure rate of the percutaneous approach (due to direct access to the right ventricular outflow tract), and a lower complication rate.

A recent study prospectively enrolled 10 neonates with PA/IVS to undergo a hybrid procedure.[54] All patients had a successful balloon valvotomy, one patient required reopening of the patent ductus arteriosus, and one required a concomitant Blalock-Taussig (BT) shunt. Of note, all patients had a tricuspid valve z-score of −2 to 2, suggesting mild right ventricular hypoplasia. The investigators also reported mild complications in three patients and no mortality. Another single-center report compared patients who underwent surgical right ventricular decompression with a hybrid cohort.[55] The researchers found

TABLE 118-3 **Frequency of Procedures in Neonates with PA/IVS by Time Periods**

Time Period	1982-1989	1990-1995	1996-2001	2002-2006
Number of neonates	199	287	298	255
Systemic-pulmonary shunt	170 (85%)	243 (85%)	255 (86%)	206 (81%)
Pulmonary valvotomy	81 (41%)	71 (25%)	57 (19%)	22 (10%)
Balloon pulmonary valvuloplasty	0	15 (5%)	46 (15%)	81 (32%)

PA/IVS, Pulmonary atresia with intact ventricular septum.

Modified from Moller JH: Operative and interventional procedures in 1039 neonates with pulmonary valve atresia and intact ventricular septum. A multi-institutional study. Prog Pediatr Cardiol 29:15–18, 2010.

no difference between the surgical and hybrid cohorts in terms of maximum vasoactive-inotropic score, duration of mechanical ventilation, intensive care unit length of stay, or overall hospital length of stay. Overall complication rates were also similar. All surgical patients received a BT shunt, whereas only 71% of the hybrid patients received a BT shunt.

Decompression of the Right Ventricle in the Presence of Right Ventricle to Coronary Connections

Antegrade right ventricular decompression is required to recruit the right ventricle for an ultimate two-ventricle or one-and-one-half-ventricle circulation. When significant communications (fistulas) between the right ventricle and the coronary circulation are present, controversy exists regarding the advisability and technique of right ventricular decompression. Virtually all authors agree that when proximal coronary obstructions are also present that make the coronary circulation dependent on the right ventricle, decompression of the right ventricle is contraindicated. Consensus is not uniform, however, when significant right ventricle–to–coronary circulation connections are present without proximal coronary artery obstructions. Some authors advise against decompression in these cases for fear that decreasing right ventricular pressure will result in a steal phenomenon, with compromised blood flow to portions of myocardium (see Fig. 118-2*A*).[56-58] Other authors express concern that failure to decompress the right ventricle will allow these fistulas to persist, resulting in ischemia and progressive myocardial fibrosis.[23,59] To encourage regression of these connections, these authors recommend antegrade decompression if an infundibular cavity is present, or retrograde decompression by tricuspid valve excision if there is no infundibulum.[23] Other authors recommend tricuspid valve closure[60] or right ventricular thromboexclusion[59] to prevent deoxygenated blood from entering the coronary circulation. It was recently reported that thromboexclusion may increase the left ventricular shortening fraction.[61]

In a study of patients with PA/IVS who have right ventricle–to–coronary artery connections and a spectrum of coronary artery abnormalities, Giglia and associates[16] found that antegrade right ventricular decompression could be performed without jeopardizing left ventricular function when coronary stenoses were absent or when stenosis involved only a single coronary artery. At present, therefore, most centers attempt right ventricular decompression in the presence of right ventricle–to–coronary artery connections when RVDCC has been ruled out and antegrade decompression is possible.[5] When antegrade decompression is not possible, the approach to right ventricular decompression remains controversial and continues to be institution specific.[5,23,59,60,62]

Indications for Transplantation

Because early mortality continues to occur despite appropriate surgical management,[1,2] cardiac transplantation has been considered a suitable therapy for a small subset of patients with PA/IVS.[62] In the 2004 CHSS report (408 patients), only 2% of patients underwent cardiac transplantation.[10] Among patients with PA/IVS who should be considered for heart transplantation are those with RVDCC and aortocoronary atresia. The few reports of this subset indicate that other methods of treatment have resulted in almost uniform mortality.[30,37] Also, patients with PA/IVS who have severe tricuspid regurgitation and a massively dilated right ventricle ("wall-to-wall" heart) have an extremely poor prognosis and should be considered for primary heart transplantation.[63] The presence of RVDCC alone is not an absolute indication for cardiac transplantation unless there is poor left ventricular function. Some centers, however, have recommended that infants with RVDCC and satisfactory left ventricular function be considered appropriate candidates because of the high early mortality in this group, even when right ventricular decompression is avoided.[56,64] Such a policy remains controversial, however, because other centers have had satisfactory results using a single-ventricle approach with these patients,[5,59] including Powell and associates,[65] who reported a 5-year survival of 83% in these patients. Such survival exceeds the 65% to 70% that is currently being achieved for infant heart transplantation.[66] Nevertheless, for a specific infant with signs of ischemia or left ventricular dysfunction (or both), transplantation may be the best strategy.

REFERENCES

1. Daubeney PE, Webber SA: The UK and Eire collaborative study of pulmonary atresia with intact ventricular septum. In Redington AN, Brawn WJ, Deanfield JE, et al, editors: *The right heart in congenital heart disease*, London, 1998, Greenwich Medical Media, pp 35–40.
2. Ekman Joelsson BM, Sunnegardh J, Hanseus K, et al: The outcome of children born with pulmonary atresia and intact ventricular septum in Sweden from 1980 to 1999. *Scand Cardiovasc J* 35:192–198, 2001.
3. Gersony WM, Bernhard WF, Nadas AS, et al: Diagnosis and surgical treatment of infants with critical pulmonary outflow obstruction: study of 34 infants with pulmonary stenosis or atresia, and intact ventricular septum. *Circulation* 35:765, 1967.
4. Hanley FL, Sade RM, Blackstone EH, et al: Outcomes in neonatal pulmonary atresia with intact ventricular septum. A multiinstitutional study. *J Thorac Cardiovasc Surg* 105:406–423, 1993.
5. Jahangiri M, Zurakowski D, Bichell D, et al: Improved results with selective management in pulmonary atresia with intact ventricular septum. *J Thorac Cardiovasc Surg* 118:1046–1055, 1999.
6. Coles JG, Freedom RM, Lightfoot NE, et al: Long-term results in neonates with pulmonary atresia and intact ventricular septum. *Ann Thorac Surg* 47:213–217, 1989.
7. Mainwaring RD, Lamberti JJ: Pulmonary atresia with intact ventricular septum. Surgical approach based on ventricular size and coronary anatomy. *J Thorac Cardiovasc Surg* 106:733–738, 1993.
8. Pawade A, Capuani A, Penny DJ, et al: Pulmonary atresia with intact ventricular septum: surgical management based on right ventricular infundibulum. *J Card Surg* 8:371–383, 1993.
9. Steinberger J, Berry JM, Bass JL, et al: Results of a right ventricular outflow patch for pulmonary atresia with intact ventricular septum. *Circulation* 86:II167–II175, 1992.
10. Ashburn DA, Blackstone EH, Wells WJ, et al: Congenital Heart Surgeons Study members: determinants of mortality and type of repair in neonates with pulmonary atresia and intact ventricular septum. *J Thorac Cardiovasc Surg* 127(4):1000–1007, discussion 1007–1008, 2004.
11. Karamlou T, Poynter J, Walters H, et al: Long-term functional health status and exercise test variables for patients with pulmonary

atresia with intact ventricular septum: a Congenital Heart Surgeons Society study. *J Thorac Cardiovasc Surg* 145:1018–1027, 2012.
12. Daubeney PE, Delany DJ, Anderson RH, et al: Pulmonary atresia with intact ventricular septum: range of morphology in a population-based study. *J Am Coll Cardiol* 39:1670–1679, 2002.
13. Freedom RM, Anderson RH, Perrin D: The significance of ventriculo-coronary arterial connections in the setting of pulmonary atresia with an intact ventricular septum. *Cardiol Young* 15(5):447–468, review, 2005.
14. Grant RT: An unusual anomaly of the coronary vessels in the malformed heart of a child. *Heart* 13:273–483, 1926.
15. Weinberg M, Jr, Bicoff JP, Bucheleres HG, et al: Pulmonary valvulotomy and infundibulotomy in infants. *J Thorac Cardiovasc Surg* 44:433–442, 1962.
16. Giglia TM, Mandell VS, Connor AR, et al: Diagnosis and management of right ventricle-dependent coronary circulation in pulmonary atresia with intact ventricular septum. *Circulation* 86:1516–1528, 1992.
17. Leung MP, Mok C, Hue P: Echocardiographic assessment of neonates with pulmonary atresia and intact ventricular septum. *J Am Coll Cardiol* 12:719, 1988.
18. Sanders SP, Parness IA, Colan SD: Recognition of abnormal connections of coronary arteries with the use of Doppler color-flow mapping. *J Am Coll Cardiol* 13:922, 1989.
19. Burrows PE, Freedom RM, Benson LN, et al: Coronary angiographic abnormalities in infants and children with pulmonary atresia, hypoplastic right ventricle, and ventriculo-coronary communications. *Am J Radiol* 154:789–795, 1990.
20. Kirklin JW, Barratt-Boyes BG: Anatomy, dimensions, and terminology. In Kirklin JW, Barratt-Boyes BG, editors: *Cardiac surgery*, New York, 1993, Churchill Livingstone, pp 3–60.
21. Bull C, de Leval MR, Mercanti C, et al: Pulmonary atresia and intact ventricular septum: a revised classification. *Circulation* 66:266–272, 1982.
22. Bull C, Kostelka M, Sorensen K, et al: Outcome measures for the neonatal management of pulmonary atresia with intact ventricular septum. *J Thorac Cardiovasc Surg* 107:359–366, 1994.
23. Hawkins JA, Thorne JK, Boucek MM, et al: Early and late results in pulmonary atresia and intact ventricular septum. *J Thorac Cardiovasc Surg* 100:492–497, 1990.
24. Kanter KR, Pennington DG, Nouri S, et al: Concomitant valvotomy and subclavian-main pulmonary artery shunt in neonates with pulmonary atresia and intact ventricular septum. *Ann Thorac Surg* 43:490–494, 1987.
25. Foker JE, Braunlin EA, St Cyr JA, et al: Management of pulmonary atresia with intact ventricular septum. *J Thorac Cardiovasc Surg* 92:706–715, 1986.
26. Moore JM, Ing FF, Drummond D, et al: Transcatheter closure of surgical shunts in patients with congenital heart disease. *Am J Cardiol* 85:636–640, 2000.
27. Rao PS: Summary and comparison of atrial septal defect closure devices. *Curr Interv Cardiol Rep* 2:367–376, 2000.
28. Billingsley AM, Laks H, Boyce SW, et al: Definitive repair in patients with pulmonary atresia and intact ventricular septum. *J Thorac Cardiovasc Surg* 97:746–754, 1989.
29. VanArsdell GS: One and one half ventricle repairs. *Semin Thorac Cardiovasc Surg Pediatr Card Surg Ann* 3:173–178, 2000.
30. Guleserian KJ, Armsby LB, Thiagarajan RR, et al: Natural history of pulmonary atresia with intact ventricular septum and right-ventricle-dependent coronary circulation managed by the single-ventricle approach. *Ann Thorac Surg* 81(6):2250–2257, discussion 2258, 2006.
31. Miyaji K, Murakami A, Takasaki T, et al: Does a bidirectional Glenn shunt improve the oxygenation of right ventricle-dependent coronary circulation in pulmonary atresia with intact ventricular septum? *J Thorac Cardiovasc Surg* 130(4):1050–1053, 2005.
32. Pearl JM, Laks H, Stein DG, et al: Total cavopulmonary anastomosis versus conventional modified Fontan procedure. *Ann Thorac Surg* 52:189–195, 1991.
33. Marcelletti CF, Iorio FS, Abella RF: Late results of extracardiac Fontan repair. *Semin Thorac Cardiovasc Surg Pediatr Card Surg Annu*2: 131–142, 1999.
34. Bridges ND, Mayer JE, Lock JE, et al: Effect of baffle fenestration on outcome of the modified Fontan operation. *Circulation* 86:1762–1769, 1992.
35. Thompson LD, Petrossian E, McElhinney DB, et al: Is it necessary to routinely fenestrate an extracardiac Fontan? *J Am Coll Cardiol* 34:539–544, 1999.
36. Daubeney PE, Wang D, Delany DJ, et al; UK and Ireland Collaborative Study of Pulmonary Atresia with Intact Ventricular Septum: Pulmonary atresia with intact ventricular septum: predictors of early and medium-term outcome in a population-based study. *J Thorac Cardiovasc Surg* 130(4):1071, 2005.
37. Calder AL, Peebles CR, Occleshaw CJ: The prevalence of coronary arterial abnormalities in pulmonary atresia with intact ventricular septum and their influence on surgical results. *Cardiol Young* 17(4):387–396, 2007. [Epub 2007 Jun 18].
38. John A, Warnes C: Clinical outcomes of adult survivors of pulmonary atresia with intact ventricular septum. *Int J Cardiol* 161:13–17, 2012.
39. Fedderly RT, Lloyd TR, Mendelsohn AM, et al: Determinants of successful balloon valvotomy in infants with critical pulmonary stenosis or membranous pulmonary atresia with intact ventricular septum. *J Am Coll Cardiol* 25:460–465, 1995.
40. Justo RN, Nykanen DG, Williams WG, et al: Transcatheter perforation of the right ventricular outflow tract as initial therapy for pulmonary valve atresia and intact ventricular septum in the newborn. *Cathet Cardiovasc Diagn* 40:408–413, 1997.
41. Ovaert C, Qureshi SA, Rosenthal E, et al: Growth of the right ventricle after successful transcatheter pulmonary valvotomy in neonates and infants with pulmonary atresia and intact ventricular septum. *J Thorac Cardiovasc Surg* 115:1055–1062, 1998.
42. Gibbs JL, Blackburn ME, Uzun O, et al: Laser valvotomy with balloon valvoplasty for pulmonary atresia with intact ventricular septum: five years' experience. *Heart* 77:225–228, 1997.
43. Wang JK, Wu MH, Chang CI, et al: Outcomes of transcatheter valvotomy in patients with pulmonary atresia and intact ventricular septum. *Am J Cardiol* 84:1055–1060, 1999.
44. Hirata Y, Chen JM, Quaegebeur JM, et al: Pulmonary atresia with intact ventricular septum: limitations of catheter-based intervention. *Ann Thorac Surg* 84(2):574–579, discussion 579–580, 2007.
45. McLean KM, Pearl JM: Pulmonary atresia with intact ventricular septum: initial management. *Ann Thorac Surg* 82(6):2214–2219, discussion 2219–2220, 2006.
46. Hassan BS, Bautista-Hernandez V, McElhinney DB, et al: Outcomes of transcatheter approach for initial treatment of pulmonary atresia with intact ventricular septum. *Catheter Cardiovasc Interv* 81:111–118, 2013.
47. Cho M, Ban K, Kim M, et al: Catheter-based treatment in patients with critical pulmonary stenosis or pulmonary atresia with intact ventricular septum: a single institute experience with comparison between patients with and without additional procedure for pulmonary flow. *Congenit Heart Dis* 8:440–449, 2013.
48. Alwi M, Choo K, Radzi N, et al: Concomitant stenting of the patent ductus arteriosus and radiofrequency valvotomy in pulmonary atresia with intact ventricular septum and intermediate right ventricle: early in-hospital and medium-term outcomes. *J Thorac Cardiovasc Surg* 141:1355–1361, 2011.
49. Schwartz MC, Glatz AC, Dori Y, et al: Outcomes and predictors of reintervention in patients with pulmonary atresia and intact ventricular septum treated with radiofrequency perforation and balloon pulmonary valvuloplasty. *Pediatr Cardiol* 35(1):22–29, 2014.
50. Udink ten Cate F, Sreeram N, Hamza H, et al: Stenting the arterial duct in neonates and infants with congenital heart disease and duct-dependent pulmonary blood flow: a multicenter experience of an evolving therapy over 18 years. *Catheter Cardiovasc Interv* 82:E233–E243, 2013.
51. Moller JH: Operative and interventional procedures in 1039 neonates with pulmonary valve atresia and intact ventricular septum. A multi-institutional study. *Prog Pediatr Cardiol* 29:15–18, 2010.
52. Zhang H, Li SJ, Li YQ, et al: Hybrid procedure for the neonatal management of pulmonary atresia with intact ventricular septum. *J Thorac Cardiovasc Surg* 133(6):1654–1656, 2007.
53. Burke RP, Hannan RL, Zabinsky JA, et al: Hybrid ventricular decompression in pulmonary atresia with intact septum. *Ann Thorac Surg* 88:688–689, 2009.
54. Li Q, Cao H, Chen Q, et al: Balloon Valvuloplasty through the right ventricle: another treatment of pulmonary atresia with intact ventricular septum. *Ann Thorac Surg* 95:1670–1674, 2013.

55. Zampi JD, Hirsch-Romano JC, Goldstein BH, et al: Hybrid approach for pulmonary atresia with intact ventricular septum: early single center results and comparison to the standard surgical approach. *Catheter Cardiovasc Interv* 83(5):753–761, 2014.
56. Akagi T, Benson LN, Williams WG, et al: Ventriculo-coronary arterial connections in pulmonary atresia with intact ventricular septum, and their influences on ventricular performance and clinical course. *Am J Cardiol* 72:586–590, 1993.
57. Gittenberger-de Groot AC, Sauer U, Bindl L, et al: Competition of coronary arteries and ventriculo-coronary arterial communications in pulmonary atresia with intact ventricular septum. *Int J Cardiol* 18:243–258, 1988.
58. O'Connor WN, Cottrill CM, Johnson GL, et al: Pulmonary atresia with intact ventricular septum and ventriculocoronary communications: surgical significance. *Circulation* 65:805–809, 1982.
59. Waldman JD, Karp RB, Lamberti JJ, et al: Tricuspid valve closure in pulmonary atresia and important RV-to-coronary artery connections. *Ann Thorac Surg* 59:933–940, 1995.
60. Najm HK, Williams WG, Coles JG, et al: Pulmonary atresia with intact ventricular septum: results of the Fontan procedure. *Ann Thorac Surg* 63:669–675, 1997.
61. Yang JH, Jun TG, Park PW, et al: Exclusion of the non functioning right ventricle in children with pulmonary atresia and intact ventricular septum. *Eur J Cardiothorac Surg* 33(2):251–256, 2008. [Epub 2007 Dec 27].
62. Rychik J, Levy H, Gaynor JW, et al: Outcome after operations for pulmonary atresia with intact ventricular septum. *J Thorac Cardiovasc Surg* 116:924–931, 1998.
63. Freedom RM, Jaeggi E, Perrin D, et al: The "wall-to-wall" heart in the patient with pulmonary atresia and intact ventricular septum. *Cardiol Young* 16(1):18–29, 2006.
64. L'Ecuyer TJ, Poulik JM, Vincent JA: Myocardial infarction due to coronary abnormalities in pulmonary atresia with intact ventricular septum. *Pediatr Cardiol* 22:68–70, 2001.
65. Powell AJ, Mayer JE, Lang P, et al: Outcome in infants with pulmonary atresia, intact ventricular septum, and right ventricle-dependent coronary circulation. *Am J Cardiol* 86:1272–1274, 2000.
66. Dipchand AI, Kirk R, Edwards LB, et al: Registry of the International Society for Heart and Lung Transplantation: sixteenth official pediatric heart transplantation report—2013. *J Heart Lung Transplant* 32(10):979–989, 2013.

CHAPTER 119

TETRALOGY OF FALLOT WITH PULMONARY STENOSIS

Giovanni Stellin • Vladimiro Vida • Massimo Padalino

HISTORY

Stensen, in 1672, described for the first time the anatomic features of what is now termed *tetralogy of Fallot* (TOF).[1] In 1888, Etienne-Louis Arthur Fallot published his findings describing the four features of the congenital cardiac anomaly that bears his name[2]: infundibular pulmonic stenosis, ventricular septal defect (VSD), dextroposition of the aorta, and right ventricular (RV) hypertrophy.

More than 50 years later, the first successful palliative surgical therapy for TOF was performed by Alfred Blalock and Helen Taussig in 1944 at the Johns Hopkins University, following the experience of Vivien Thomas, who in Blalock's laboratory was producing an animal model of pulmonary hypertension by anastomosing end-to-side the subclavian artery to the pulmonary artery in dogs.[3] Other operative operations to augment the pulmonary blood flow were soon developed by Potts, Waterston, and others.[4-7] The first successful repair of this condition was performed by Lillehei and Varco at the University of Minnesota in 1954 using "controlled cross circulation," with either father or mother serving as the oxygenator and blood reservoir.[8,9] Kirklin reported the first repair of TOF using a pump oxygenator at the Mayo Clinic in 1955.[10,11] Barrett-Boyes and Neutze[12] and Castaneda[13] opened the avenue of the new era of TOF repair by demonstrating the feasibility and the advantages of one-stage repair compared with a two-stage approach. The literature reveals excellent operative results and a low mortality rate. Nevertheless, the results of repair over decades have shown that chronic pulmonary valve (PV) regurgitation, together with a RV geometries distortion secondary to ventricular patching, leads to chronic RV failure.[14-15] Therefore, one is now focusing on techniques aimed to preserve the long-term RV function.

PREVALENCE

Tetralogy of Fallot is the most common cyanotic congenital heart defect in all age groups, constituting approximately 8% of all congenital heart defects. It occurs in nearly 0.19 to 0.26 in 1000 live births, with a prevalence of about 3.9 per 10,000 live births in the United States.[16-20] Furthermore, TOF is one of the most common congenital heart lesions requiring intervention in the first year of life and occurs equally in males and females.[16-18] Mutations in several human genes have thus far been identified in TOF. The deletion of human *TBX1* appears to be the basis for the 15% of TOF attributable to chromosome 22q11.2 microdeletion, although *TBX1* mutations in nondeleted TOF patients remain to be identified.[21-23] Other identified mutations included the *NKX2.5*, which accounts for 4% of TOF[24] and the mutation *JAG1* in Alagille syndrome in which the incidence of TOF is high.[25,26] The gene or genes causing TOF in trisomy 21, 18, and 13, which together account for 10% of TOF cases,[27] are as yet unidentified. Thus, in approximately 70% of TOF patients, a genetic etiology remains to be determined.

ANATOMY AND PHYSIOLOGY

The original concept of four coexisting defects described by Fallot in 1888, was revisited by Richard Van Praagh in 1970,[28] who introduced the concept that TOF is actually a "monology" resulting essentially from the underdevelopment and malalignment of the RV infundibulum or conus. According to Anderson and colleagues,[29] however, the right ventricular outflow tract (RVOT) in TOF results from the deviation of the infundibular septum cephalad and anterior. This anomaly of the infundibular septum narrows the RVOT, leading to a subpulmonary obstruction of variable degree, the more severe creating an atretic infundibulum and/or valve. Prominent muscle bands originating from the septal region of the infundibular septum to extend the RV free wall contribute to the RVOT obstruction. Displacement of the infundibular septum away from the anterior and posterior limbs of the trabecula septomarginalis (septomarginalis trabeculation, septal band) results in a typical anterior malalignment VSD. The aortic valve is located directly behind the infundibular septum because of the anterior displacement of this structure; therefore, the aortic valve overrides the ventricular septum by various degrees. In those cases in which the aortic valve remains aligned predominantly to the RV, particularly when a mitral-aortic valve discontinuity (subaortic conus) is present, such a malformation is termed *double outlet right ventricle*, TOF-type.[30]

The foramen ovale is mostly open in young infants. If left open during correction, it allows decompression of the right ventricle, when failing during the early postoperative period.

Pulmonary Valve and Pulmonary Valve Annulus

The pulmonary valve is stenotic in 75% of cases because of a hypoplasia of the annulus and fusion of leaflets, supravalvar tethering, or a combination of these factors.[29,31,32] Tethering of the leaflets often distorts the main pulmonary artery at the sinotubular junction, forming a ridge that can be obstructive, producing supravalvar stenosis. The leaflets themselves are often thickened and dysplastic with fusion at their commissural attachment, further reducing the effective annulus size. The pulmonary valve annulus is invariably smaller than the aorta (the opposite of normal); however, it is not necessarily significantly obstructive.

A recent unpublished combined study of the University of Padua, Italy, and the Cardiac Registry at the Children's Hospital, Boston, have analyzed 101 heart specimens (67 belonging to Children's Hospital in Boston and 34 to the University of Padua) with TOF, focusing specially on the PV anatomic features. The PV proved to be predominantly bicuspid in 65 specimens (65%), less frequently tricuspid (n = 23 [23%]) and rarely unicuspid (n = 12 [12%]) and quadricuspid in 1 case (1%). In 53 specimens (53%) of all cases, the PV cusps were normal. This is an important finding, in view of recent new surgical techniques aimed at preserving the native PV during repair (Figs. 119-1 and 119-2).

Ventricular Septal Defect

The VSD is typically large and subaortic, and it reflects in its very nature the deviation of the infundibular septum.[29] The VSD is located between the deviated infundibular septum (conus) and the two limbs of the trabecula septomarginalis (septal band). Its posterosuperior margin is limited by the ventriculo-infundibular fold and the aortic valve (which is visible by the surgeon during repair), superiorly by the infundibular septum, anteriorly by the anterosuperior limb, and inferiorly by the posteroinferior limb of the septal band and the muscular septum (Figs. 119-3 through 119-6). In 20% of cases, there is a well-developed posterior limb, essentially forming a continuous muscular border, where the His bundle penetrates and crosses the ventricular septum deeply embedded within this muscle. In the majority of anatomic variants, however, the posteroinferior rim of the VSD is wrapped by a rim formed by the confluence

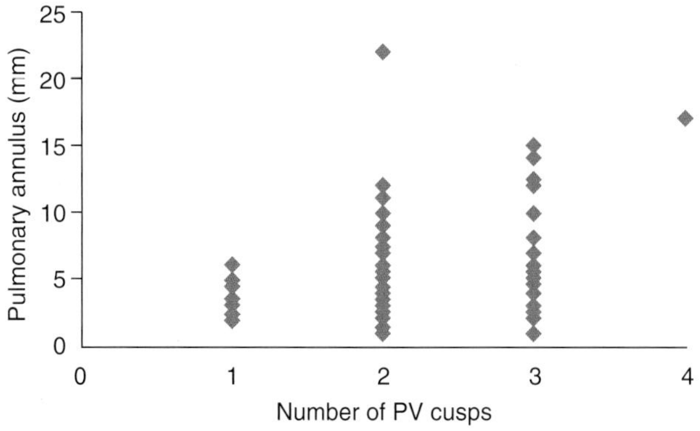

FIGURE 119-1 ■ Graph showing unpublished data on pulmonary valve (PV) anatomy of 101 heart specimens with tetralogy of Fallot (67 belonging to Children's Hospital in Boston and 34 to the University of Padua). The PV was bicuspid in 65 specimens (65%), tricuspid in 23 (23%), unicuspid in 12 (12%), and quadricuspid in 1 (1%).

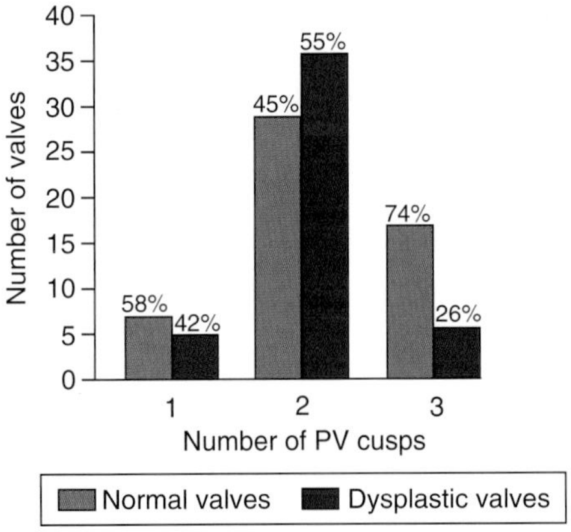

FIGURE 119-2 ■ Graph showing unpublished data on pulmonary valve (PV) anatomy of 101 heart specimens with tetralogy of Fallot (67 belonging to Children's Hospital in Boston, and 34 to the University of Padua). The PV cusps were normal in 53 specimens (53% of all cases).

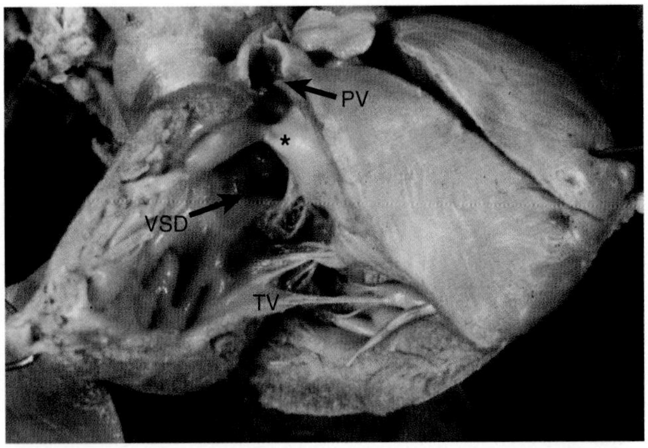

FIGURE 119-3 ■ Anatomic image of a specimen with tetralogy of Fallot showing the inflow and the outflow tracts of the right ventricle, including the infundibular septum *(asterisk),* malalignment ventricular septal defect (VSD), pulmonary valve (PV), and tricuspid valve (TV). (Courtesy Professor Gaetano Thiene.)

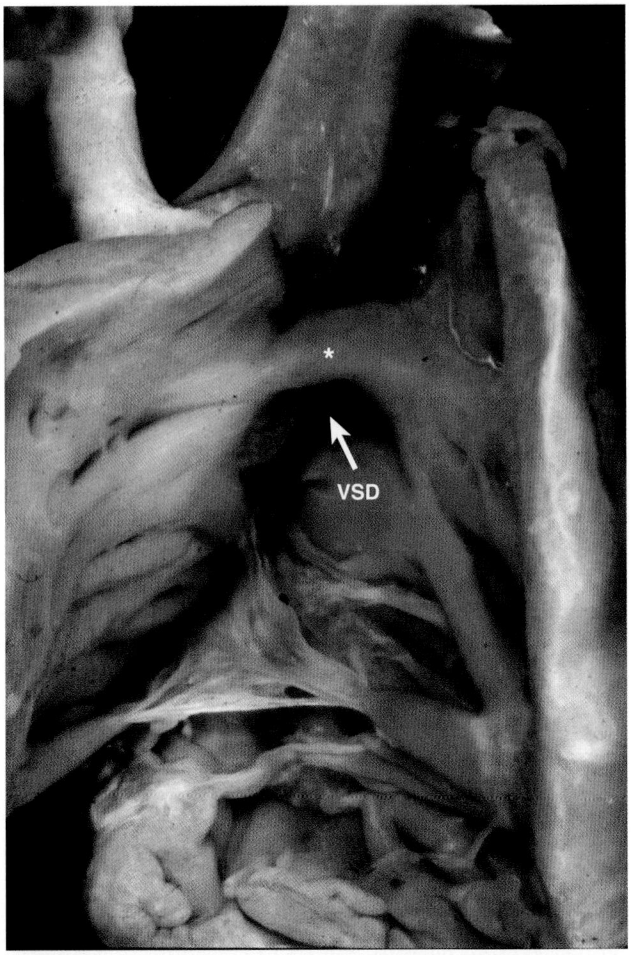

FIGURE 119-4 ■ Anatomic image of a specimen with tetralogy of Fallot showing in detail the anterior deviation of the infundibular septum *(asterisk)* and the malalignment ventricular septal defect (VSD). (Courtesy Professor Gaetano Thiene.)

of the membranous septum, attachment of the tricuspid valve, and the aortic valve annulus (perimembranous malalignment VSD).[29,33-35] The posteroinferior limb of the septal band is hypoplastic and therefore does not extend to the posteroinferior border. In this case, the His bundle penetrates and traverses the septum near the fibrous posteroinferior rim of the VSD, being at risk of injury during VSD closure, particularly when the anterior and septal TV leaflets are scarcely developed.

In a small subset of patients, the infundibular septum is extremely hypoplastic or even macroscopically absent. Consequently, the aortic and pulmonary valves are in anatomic fibrous continuity, and the VSD is positioned mostly within the subpulmonary area.

Up to 15% of patients have additional VSDs, which are usually single and muscular, residing mostly within the anterior portion of the ventricular septum.[36-37] In rare cases, an additional VSD exists in the inlet portion of the septum. Since the His bundle is within the bridge of muscular tissue separating the two VSDs, closure of such defects can be at risk for conduction disturbances.

Main Pulmonary Artery and Branch Pulmonary Arteries

The main pulmonary artery (MPA) and its right and left branches are smaller caliber than normal; localized stenosis is most often confined to the origin of the left branch, believed to be due to ductal tissue constriction or iatrogenic located at the level of previous systemic/pulmonary arteries shunts anastomosis.[34,36] In TOF and pulmonary stenosis, the pulmonary trunk and branches are rarely in discontinuity and arborization abnormalities of either left or right pulmonary artery branches are equally rare. It must be emphasized that, in the absence of major aortopulmonary collateral arteries, the pulmonary artery (PA) branches in TOF are almost never prohibitively hypoplastic, even in the presence of severe narrowing of the RVOT, and therefore remain candidates for complete repair.

Coronary Arteries

Coronary arteries anomalies are present in 5% to 12% of patients with TOF.[37-41] Most frequently, the left

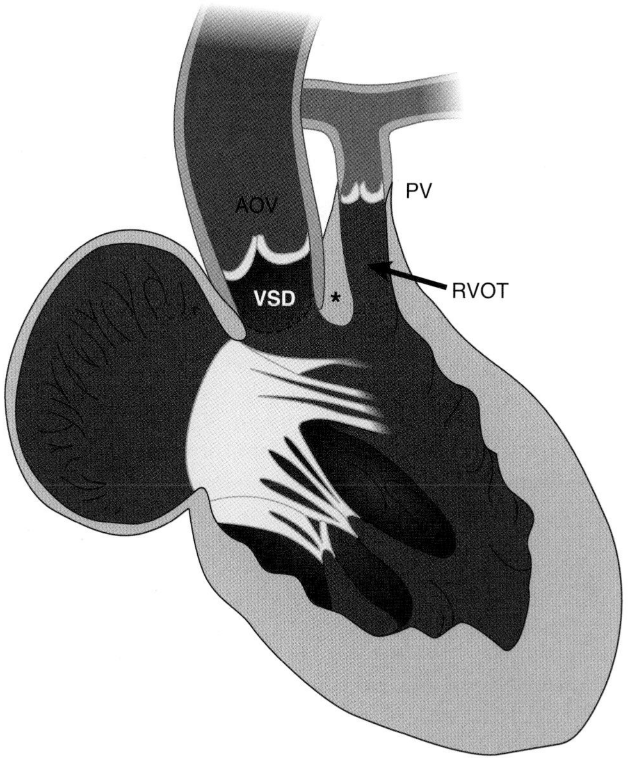

FIGURE 119-5 ■ The deviated infundibular septum *(asterisk)* and the narrow right ventricular outflow tract (RVOT). *AOV,* Aortic valve; *PV,* pulmonary valve; *VSD,* ventricular septal defect.

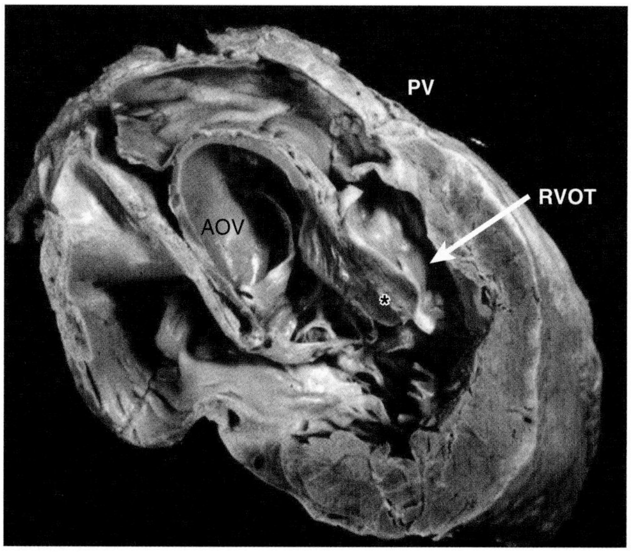

FIGURE 119-6 ■ Anatomic image of a specimen with tetralogy of Fallot showing the deviated infundibular septum *(asterisk)* and the narrow right ventricular outflow tract (RVOT). *AOV,* Aortic valve; *PV,* pulmonary valve. (Courtesy Professor Gaetano Thiene.)

anterior descending coronary artery (LAD) arises from the right coronary artery (RCA) and traverses the RVOT at various distances from the PV annulus. This anomaly is of great importance for the surgeon to avoid transaction or distortion during repair. A transannular incision is at risk under this circumstance. Other coronary artery anomalies encountered in TOF include: origin of RCA from the left coronary artery; left coronary artery from the MPA; a single coronary artery originating from the left coronary sinus; and an accessory LAD from the RCA.[37] Rarely, significant LAD coronary artery branches from the RCA cross the RVOT within the infundibular muscle and are therefore not visible on the epicardial surface, making injury of these arteries possible at the time of repair.

These coronary artery anomalies are more likely to occur in severe forms of TOF, such as coexisting with severe MPA hypoplasia and anterior and lateral rotation of the aorta.[41]

Significant coronaries abnormalities can be frequently detected preoperatively with two-dimensional echocardiography, and surgical management can be modified during repair to avoid injuring these vessels.[37]

PHYSICAL EXAMINATION

When children are admitted electively, during early infancy, they usually exhibit a good clinical state, with no or mild cyanosis (transcutaneous oxygen saturation is often greater than 80%). Cyanosis can be more than mild in the very severe forms or in older children who are presenting late with a progressive myocardial compensatory hypertrophy and significant arterial collateral vessels.

On examination of the heart, the second heart sound is often single and accentuated because of anteriorization of the aortic root. A moderate intensity midsystolic ejection murmur is heard loudest in the second and third intercostal space. Rarely in the less severe forms, TOF can present with signs of increased pulmonary blood flow.

Blood sampling to determine the presence of deletion on the long arm of chromosome 22q11 is part of the routine workup to provide the opportunity for genetic counseling and to identify other organ systems that are frequently involved, as summarized by the acronym CATCH-22 (cardiac disease, abnormal face, thymic hypoplasia, cleft palate, and hypocalcemia).

MEDICAL MANAGMENT

Since the introduction of early repair of TOF, the preoperative medical management has lost its important role in treating cyanotic children with TOF. Children are usually asymptomatic for the first 2 to 3 months after birth. Cyanosis usually progresses with spells in older children. A cornerstone of the preoperative management is maintaining these infants in well-hydrated state and to avoid contacts to protect them from viral infections. Beta blockers can be used to treat or prevent cyanotic spells. Nevertheless, early repair can avoid most of these complications by restoring a "normal" circulation. Balloon angioplasty and stenting of the RVOT has been recently developed as a palliative procedure for insuring adequate pulmonary blood flow, particularly in those centers where surgical correction in neonates and young infants is postponed (see Palliations).

DIAGNOSTIC STUDIES

Cardiac catheterization is seldom necessary for assessing the surgical anatomy, except to rule out the presence of major aortopulmonary collateral vessels, often suspected in children who are relatively pink, despite a severe obstruction of the RVOT[42] or to confirm the echocardiographic diagnosis of coronary artery anomalies (Figs. 119-7 and 119-8).

Two-dimensional echocardiography has become the gold standard to define most details required for surgical correction. A prenatal echo diagnosis is nowadays often available and it is usually reconfirmed, soon after birth.[43-51] Two-dimensional echocardiography and Doppler in TOF is routinely used for delineating the important features of the malformation and for supplying the surgeons all relevant information essential for achieving a proper repair.

In the long-axis view, the degree of overriding of the aortic valve across the VSD is assessed (Fig. 119-9). The anterior muscular septum is also interrogated to rule out any additional muscular anterior VSDs.

In the parasternal short-axis view, the degree of displacement and length of the infundibular septum is well seen together with all the pertinent anatomy related to the RVOT obstruction, including level of obstruction, type, and severity (Figs. 119-10 and 119-11). In this projection, the PV annulus, MPA, and branches are visualized and measured (see Figs. 119-10 and 119-11). Pulmonary arteries discontinuity or stenosis (particularly at the LPA origin) are usually well identified in this projection. In the absence of localized stenosis, hypoplastic pulmonary arteries very rarely contraindicate total repair (see Anatomy and Physiology).

Excellent anatomic images are also obtained from a right or oblique subcostal view. This projection is important for gathering additional information concerning the anatomy and degree and level of RVOT obstruction. Pulmonary valve anatomy, MPA and its branches are also clearly visible and measurable using this projection (Fig. 119-12).

In an apical four-chamber view, the VSD is also well visualized and sized. The muscular septum is screened to rule out any additional VSD. Through a short parasternal axis view, at the base of the heart, both coronary arteries are visualized to exclude any anomaly in origin of the LAD and of major branches of the RCA, including crossing of the RV infundibulum.

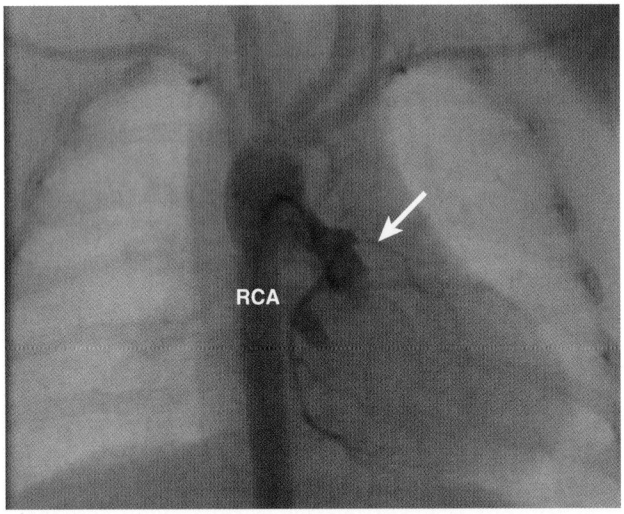

FIGURE 119-7 ■ Preoperative angiographic image showing a large conal coronary artery branch *(arrow)* originating from the right coronary artery (RCA) and crossing the right ventricular infundibulum. (Courtesy Professor Ornella Milanesi.)

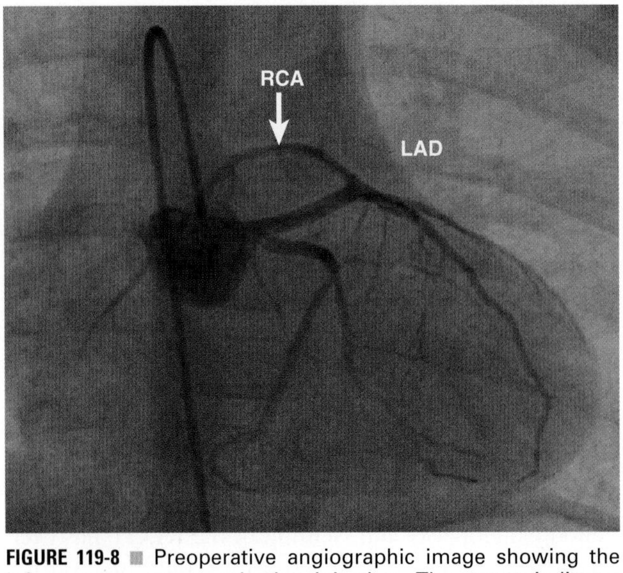

FIGURE 119-8 ■ Preoperative angiographic image showing the left coronary artery selective injection. The *arrow* indicates the anomalous origin of the right coronary artery (RCA) from the left anterior descending coronary artery (LAD) crossing the right ventricular infundibulum.

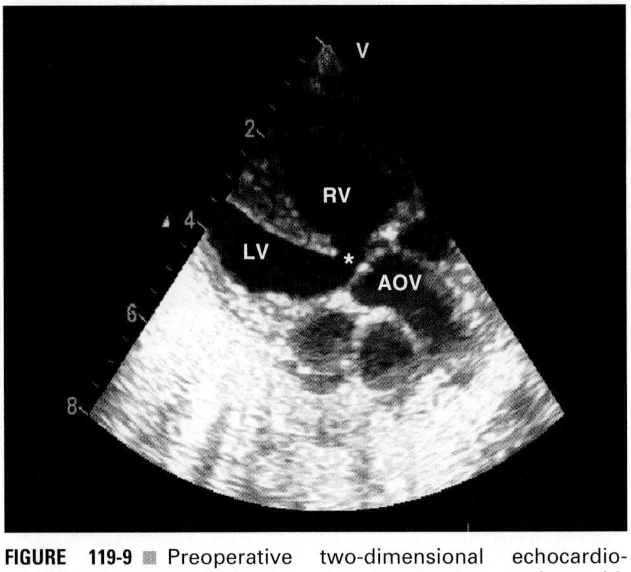

FIGURE 119-9 ■ Preoperative two-dimensional echocardiographic image, long-axis view, showing the degree of overriding of the aortic valve across the ventricular septal defect *(asterisk)*. *AOV,* Aortic valve; *LV,* left ventricle; *RV,* right ventricle. (Courtesy Professor Ornella Milanesi.)

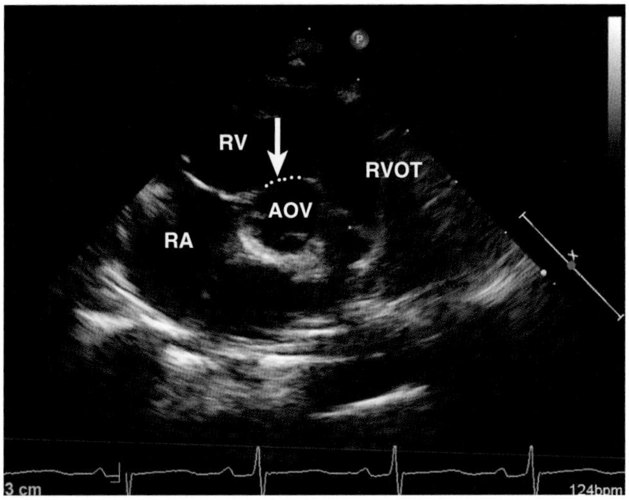

FIGURE 119-10 ■ Preoperative two-dimensional echocardiographic image, short-axis view, showing the deviation of the infundibular septum creating the interventricular communication *(white dots)* and the obstruction at the right ventricular outflow tract (RVOT). *AOV,* Aortic valve; *RA,* right atrium; *RV,* right ventricle. (Courtesy Professor Ornella Milanesi.)

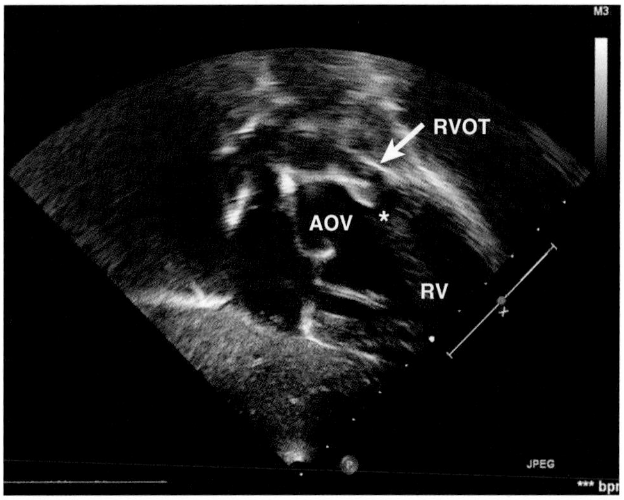

FIGURE 119-12 ■ Preoperative two-dimensional echocardiographic image, oblique subcostal view, showing the right ventricular outflow tract (RVOT) and the deviated infundibular septum *(asterisk)*. *AOV,* Aortic valve; *RV,* right ventricle. (Courtesy Professor Ornella Milanesi.)

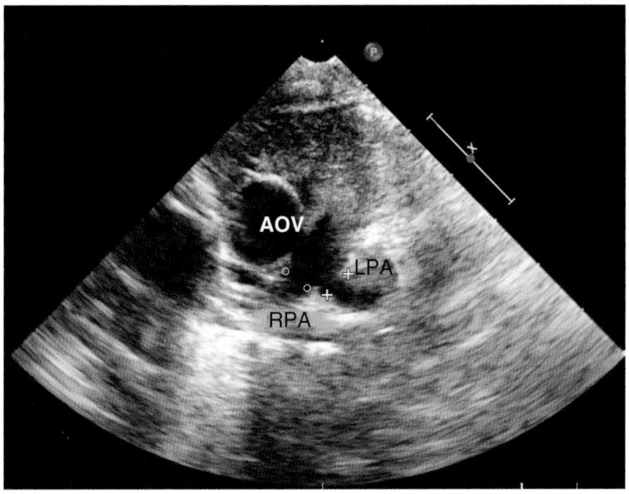

FIGURE 119-11 ■ Preoperative two-dimensional echocardiographic image, short-axis view, showing the origin of the right pulmonary artery (RPA; *empty dots*) and left pulmonary artery (LPA; *asterisks*) branches. *AOV,* Aortic valve. (Courtesy Professor Ornella Milanesi.)

The presence of abnormal coronary origin or course (see anatomy) is detected with two-dimensional echocardiography and Doppler, particularly for young infants and neonates, when coronary arteries are readily visible.[52]

SURGICAL TREATMENT

Palliations

A modified Blalock-Taussig (B-T) shunt is still the preferred palliation, in many centers, in the presence of contraindications for primary repair, which are usually dictated by local preferences and experiences. The approach is through a right or left thoracotomy, for interposing a tubular graft between the right subclavian artery (or innominate artery) or left subclavian artery, and the ipsilateral PA branch. There is a recent trend in approaching these structures through a midline sternotomy, with cardiopulmonary bypass (CPB) on standby (for achieving a total exposure of both PA branches and for better controlling episodes of hemodynamic instability).

Another palliative shunt can also be achieved by interposing a short segment of a tubular graft connecting the ascending aorta and the main pulmonary artery, with the aim of avoiding any distortion to the small and fragile PA branches.

Other palliative alternatives have been introduced by interventional cardiologists, such as stenting of the RVOT.[53,54] This procedure can be effective for delaying complete repair and for limiting increasing cyanosis and spells. Stenting of the RVOT, however, will inevitably trigger the formation of scar tissue and possibly distortion of PV, rendering the RVOT anatomy more difficult at the time of definite repair.[55]

A patent ductus arteriosus is rarely present in the absence of PV atresia. However its patency can also be maintained with transcatheter stenting when repair is to be delayed.

Repair

The timing of complete repair is still controversial and varies from center to center. Nevertheless the worldwide trend favors early repair, just as for many other complex congenital heart lesions.[56-61]

Complete early repair has been advocated to avoid:

1. Chronic cyanosis and spells
2. Systemic-to-pulmonary artery shunts and their consequences
3. Chronic RV pressure overload and myocardial compensatory hypertrophy (which requires a more extensive resection, at the time of the repair)

4. Hospital costs and offering patients one instead of two operations

Early repair will also establish a permanent physiological circulation, including a normal O^2 saturation, which will avoid the negative effects of cyanosis (and possible cyanotic spells) upon the cerebral nervous system and other developing organs.[13]

Techniques of Complete Repair

Anesthetic Management

Anesthetic management is critical for avoiding cyanotic spells during preparation and induction. A transesophageal or epicardial two- or three-dimensional echocardiogram and Doppler can be used to recall the preoperative images to the surgeon,[58] and for monitoring the heart performance before and after repair. At the end of CPB, detection of possible residual lesions and then immediate repair are of paramount importance, before transferring patients to the intensive care unit.

Surgical Access

Repair is performed via a median sternotomy. A partial division of the sternum can also be used, particularly in the less severe forms or for bigger children, according to the surgeon's preference. A large segment of anterior pericardium is harvested and treated with the glutaraldehyde used for VSD patch closure, RVOT reconstruction, MPA or branch enlargement, or PV leaflets extension. Total CPB is established by aorta and double caval cannulation. A left ventricular vent is usually placed through the interatrial sulcus, guided into the LV, placed on suction to achieve a bloodless field. Moderate hypothermia is usually induced, according to center or surgeon preference. During the cooling phase, the MPA is dissected from the aorta and its branches are explored. Right pulmonary artery and left pulmonary artery branches are then occluded distally with a Silastic double loop, to avoid blood return from the bronchial arteries which can be disturbing, particularly in very cyanotic children. On a beating heart, the MPA is incised longitudinally. The PA branches are explored and sized. The PV is inspected and sized to assess the effective PV orifice diameter. The heart is then stopped by aorta cross-clamping and by injecting cardioplegia into the aortic root. The right atrium (RA) is incised above the tenia sagittalis, parallel to the atrioventricular groove, and the whole anatomy of the RA cavity is visualized. The fossa ovalis is inspected and the presence of a foramen ovale (or an atrial septal defect) is assessed. The tricuspid valve (TV) is then retracted and the whole RV anatomy is carefully inspected, with particular attention to the size and type of the VSD (malalignment muscular, malalignment perimembranous) and the whole RVOT up to the PV annulus. The subpulmonary fibromuscular obstructions are then resected through the TV. Particular care is taken to remove any subpulmonary muscular obstruction up to the subannular level.

Further resection of the distal part of the RVOT can be achieved through the PV annulus, aiming to enlarge the whole RV outlet, up to the PV hinges. The VSD is then patch closed with continuous suture or interrupted stitches, according to the surgeon's preference. Particular care must be taken not to damage the aortic valve (the aortic valve can be better visualized through the VSD and protected by delivering short injections of cardioplegia). To facilitate the VSD closure, significant TV chordae crossing the VSD can be detached at their base, and then reattached in the same position, at the end of the VSD patch closure. The TV is then hydrodynamically tested by gentle injection of cold saline solution into the RV cavity. Any possible TV distortion must be repaired, with the aim of preserving long-term TV performance and RV functional integrity.

The foramen ovale, when present, can be left open to reduce the RV preload by allowing right-to-left shunting during the early postoperative period, when the RA pressure is not uncommonly higher than the left atrial (LA) pressure. Before RA closure, cold saline solution is injected through the foramen ovale into the LA and left ventricle (LV), for clearing the LV of air through the cardioplegia needle in the ascending aorta. During the re-warming phase, the PV valve is again inspected. This maneuver can be achieved on a beating heart during re-warming. When a transannular patch is needed, PV competence can be obtained by adding a "new cusp" of biological or prosthetic material. We have used in small children a RVOT patch bearing a valve cusp that is obtained by a divided adult size pulmonary homograft. An LA line is preferably inserted via the previous LA vent purse string. Temporary ventricular and atrial pacing wires are placed on the epicardium, and the patient is weaned from CBPB transesophageal (or epicardial) echocardiography monitoring before decannulation is routinely performed for detecting any possible residual lesions and for assessing the RV and LV performance. Right ventricular pressure can be directly measured by RV puncture, and compared with the LV pressure. Residual dynamic mild obstruction can be predicted to decrease within the 24 to 48 hours following repair.

SPECIAL TOPICS IN SURGICAL MANAGEMENT

Anomalous Coronary Patterns

Conventional repair is complicated by the occurrence of the LAD coronary artery originating totally or in part (dual LAD coronary pattern) from the RCA with the arterial supply from the right coronary artery crossing the RVOT.[62-68] Achieving adequate relief of the RVOT obstruction while maintaining the integrity of the coronary supply requires an understanding of different surgical options and flexibility in their application. Conduit reconstruction of the RVOT with origin from a ventriculotomy placed below the anomalous coronary has given reliable results but ultimately necessitates reoperation for conduit replacement. Translocation of the pulmonary artery to a distal ventriculotomy and use of the native pulmonary artery as a composite conduit to create a double outflow from the right ventricle have also been used successfully.[64-67] The transatrial transpulmonary approach has been especially successful in dealing with this difficult anatomy.[65,66] Brizard and coworkers[65] reported on Duncan's approach in 36 patients, which allowed a conduit to be avoided in all but two cases. Twenty-five patients required a limited transannular patch that was slightly deviated, when necessary, to avoid injuring the anomalous coronary artery. There were no perioperative or long-term deaths, and postoperative right ventricular pressures were low and equivalent to those obtained in contemporaneous patients undergoing TOF repair without coronary anomalies. There was also no difference in reoperation rates for patients with or without anomalous coronaries.[65] A more recent report provided evidence that adequate relief of RVOT obstruction can usually be performed with a relatively straightforward approach to patch reconstruction without the need for conduits or translocation of the coronary artery.[68]

Use of a Monocusp Valve in Reconstruction of the Right Ventricular Outflow Tract

Monocusp reconstruction of the RVOT (Fig. 119-13) can be achieved by sawing a triangular shape of tissue from the distal part of the ventriculotomy, up to the margin of the natural PV leaflets, using either autologous pericardium or heterologous tissue or prosthetic material (polytetrafluoroethylene [PTFE]). Reports vary regarding the usefulness of monocusp valve reconstruction for the RVOT.[69-74] Augmentation plasty of the PV leaflets, by adding an additional cusp can avoid PV regurgitation, early postoperatively, improving the short-term clinical outcome. Nonetheless, when a cusp needs to be added, leaflet function often deteriorates over time, resulting in a progressive PV regurgitation. When pericardium or PTFE are used to create a monocusp, the valve function is probably limited to the first weeks to months after repair, but the mode of valve failure (adherence of the monocusp to the RVOT patch) is never obstructive.[69,71] Our unpublished experience with adding a prosthetic cusp material shows that a better short and mid-term performance is achieved with a "built-in" cusp obtained from an adult size pulmonary homograft when compared with other biological added material.

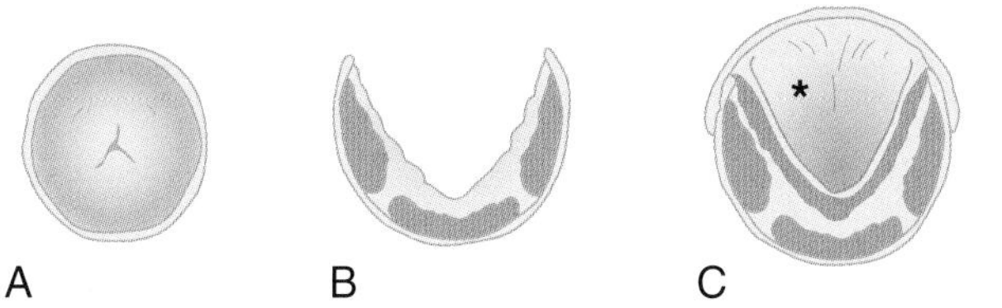

FIGURE 119-13 ■ **A,** The native hypoplastic pulmonary valve in a patient with tetralogy of Fallot. **B,** The native pulmonary valve after transannular incision. **C,** The monocusp-patch augmentation *(asterisk)* of the right ventricular outflow tract.

Preservation of the Pulmonary Valve

The use of a transannular patch, necessary in some cases, often results in pulmonary insufficiency with chronic RV volume overload, leading inevitably to progressive RV dilation and dysfunction which is associated with impaired functional capacity. The interest in preserving PV function has stimulated surgeons to devise valve-sparing techniques for TOF repair. During the last few years, some centers have combined the routine correction of TOF with intraoperative balloon dilation of the hypoplastic pulmonary annulus[75-79] in selected cases. At the time of repair, the PV is usually inspected and sized to assess the effective PV orifice diameter. In the presence of a stenotic PV, a valvar commissurotomy is performed at each commissure, down to the sinotubular junction. After this maneuver, the valve is again sized to measure the true annular diameter.

Particular care is taken to remove any possible RVOT obstruction up to the subannular level by combining transatrial, transtricuspid muscle band resection and a further transpulmonary residual muscle band excision through the PV annulus, before and after balloon dilation.

Only after a satisfactory muscle bundle resection is achieved, a high pressure, appropriate size, valvuloplasty balloon catheter is introduced through the TV across the PV orifice and inflated under direct vision,[77,78] while securing its tip, until the inner pressure reaches 10 atm (Fig. 119-14). We use short (2 cm), high-pressure (>10 atm), noncompliant balloons sized according to the calculated size of the PV orifice relative to the body surface area of the patient. When the PV effective orifice is particularly narrow (z-score < –3), we use an "in-series

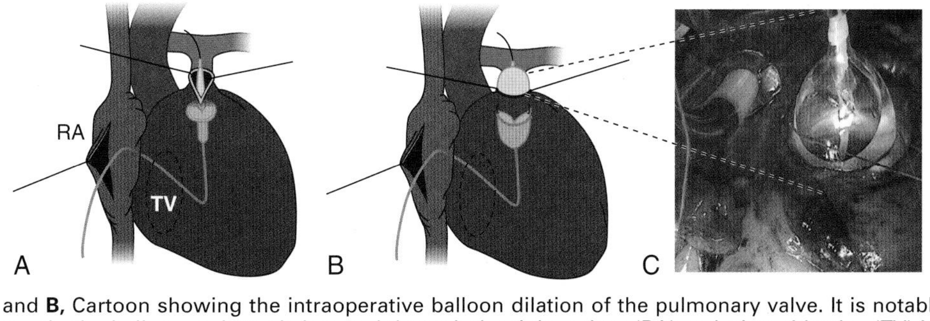

FIGURE 119-14 ■ **A** and **B,** Cartoon showing the intraoperative balloon dilation of the pulmonary valve. It is notable that, because of the transatrial approach, the balloon catheter is inserted through the right atrium (RA) and tricuspid valve (TV) into the pulmonary valve annulus. **C,** Intraoperative details of the balloon catheter through the pulmonary valve.

balloon dilation strategy" by using increasing diameters of balloons for allowing a progressive stretching and dilation of the PV annulus up to the ideal size according to body surface area. While dealing with a highly hypoplastic PV annulus (z-score range, –3 to –4), the PV leaflets, which are often separated by the balloon dilation at the commissure level, are then reconstructed by carefully delaminating them with a fine scalpel at the PV hinge point and down to the RV epicardium, thus extending the leaflets cooptation area (Figs. 119-15 through 119-17). Subsequently, the extended leaflets are "re-suspended" either directly or after further augmentation with small prosthetic (biologic) patch material. An appropriate Hegar dilator for PV size (PV z-score = 0) is passed through the new PV annulus. The MPA is eventually patch enlarged, when needed, with an autologous pericardial patch that is anchored proximally below the PV annulus, onto the RVOT epicardium, with the aim of avoiding any potential early or late constriction over the reconstructed PV apparatus (Fig. 119-18). In case the PV anatomic integrity cannot be preserved, a transannular incision is performed into the distal part of the RVOT.

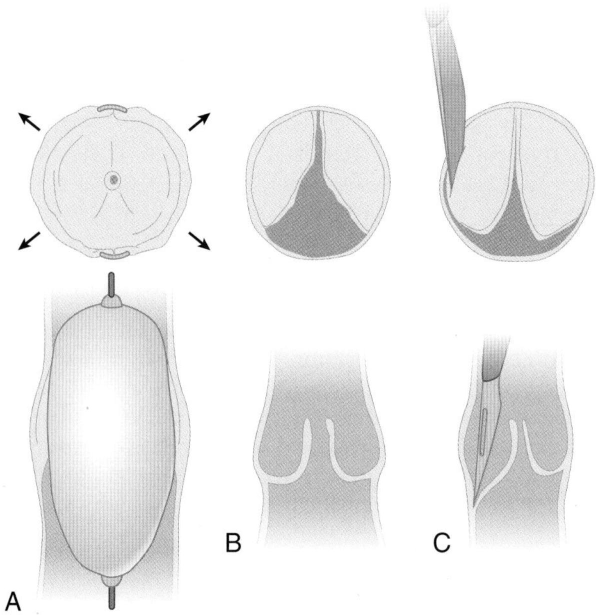

FIGURE 119-15 ■ The intraoperative delamination of the pulmonary valve leaflets to increase its coaptation area **(B** and **C)** after balloon dilation **(A)**.

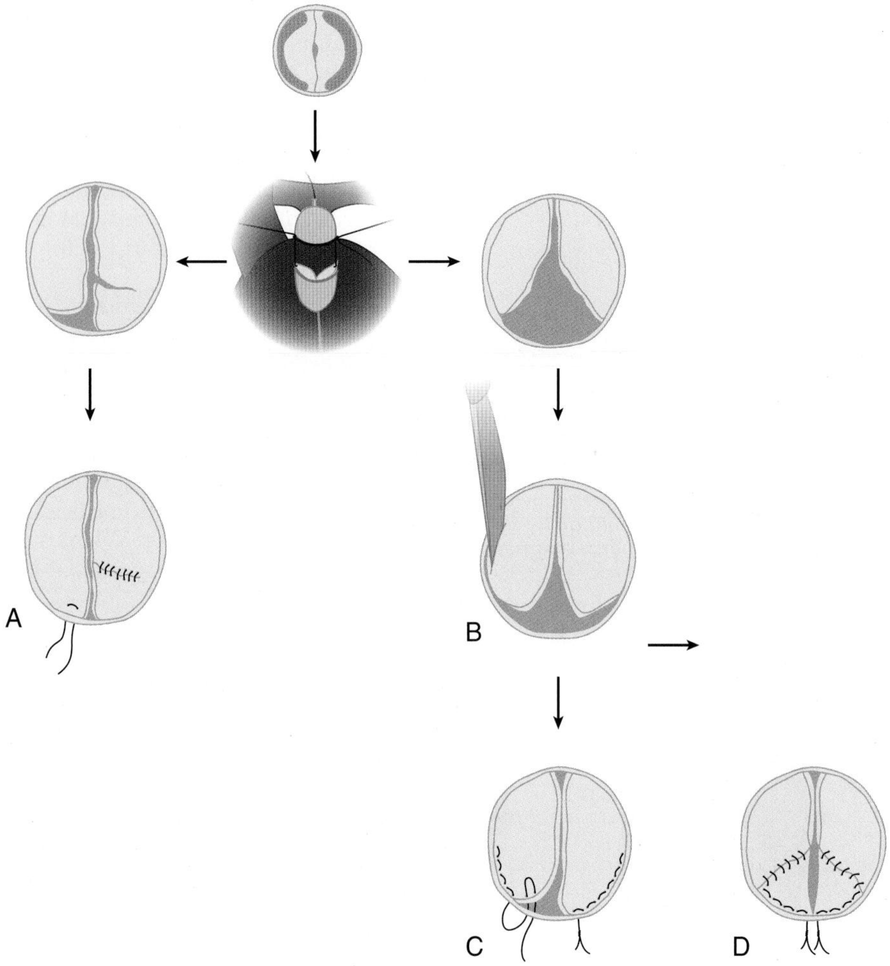

FIGURE 119-16 ■ Cartoon showing the different additional surgical maneuvers on the pulmonary valve after balloon dilation. **A,** Leaflet repair. **B,** Leaflet delamination. **C,** Leaflet resuspension. **D,** Leaflet patch augmentation and resuspension.

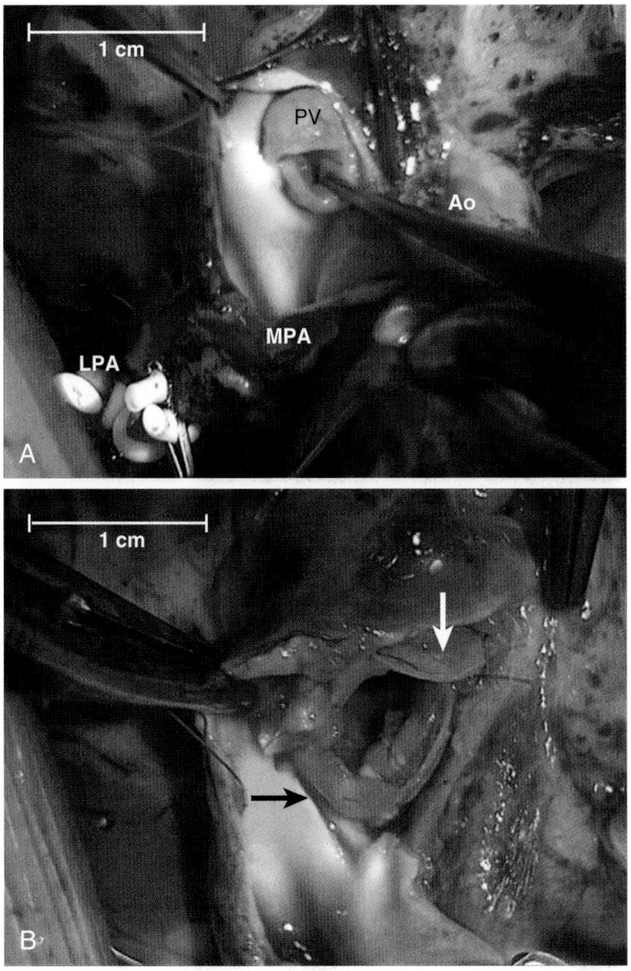

FIGURE 119-17 ■ Intraoperative images of a 3.5-month-old boy with tetralogy of Fallot showing the **(A)** initial (4 mm) and **(B)** final (10 mm) diameters of the pulmonary valve after pulmonary valve preservation technique. *Arrows* indicate the pulmonary valve leaflets. *Ao,* Ascending aorta; *LPA,* left pulmonary artery; *MPA,* main pulmonary artery; *PV,* pulmonary valve.

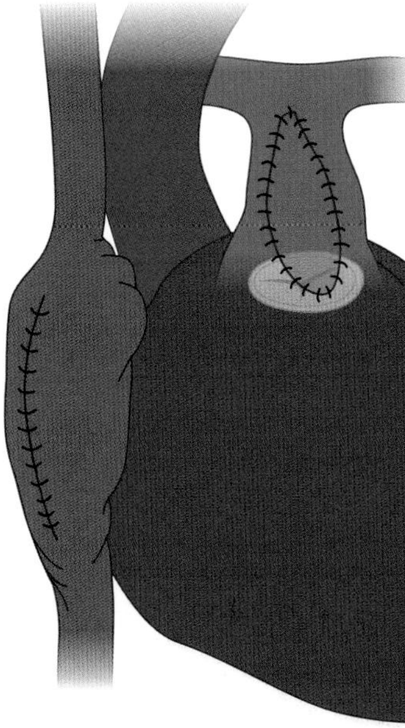

FIGURE 119-18 ■ Patch augmentation of the main pulmonary artery after pulmonary valve preservation.

CONTROVERSIES IN SURGICAL MANAGEMENT

Ventriculotomy versus Transatrial-Transpulmonary Approach

Excellent exposure of the VSD and obstructive muscle bundles in the RVOT can be achieved through either a right ventriculotomy or through an incision in the right atrium.[11,13] An approach through a right ventriculotomy (Fig. 119-19) is still preferred, in many centers.[80-86] Access to the VSD, and to obstructing muscle bundles of the RVOT is more easily achieved by incising longitudinally the RV infundibulum. After muscle bundle resection, the VSD is patch closed either with interrupted stitches or continuous suture. In light of the long-term results that reveal a chronic RV dysfunction after "pioneristic" TOF repair, which was routinely achieved by means of a "generous" ventriculotomy, there is now a common trend in limiting the right ventriculotomy for, as much as possible, limiting in this way the RV geometry distortion. In addition, some groups have reported a lower incidence of recurrent RVOT obstruction in lesions corrected through the RV ventriculotomy.[87-89]

Approach through a RA incision (Fig. 119-20) and, when necessary, a combined incision in the pulmonary artery avoids a ventriculotomy and may help to avoid RV dysfunction after repair, especially in the immediate postoperative period and in the very young heart.[90-100] Miura and coauthors[92] demonstrated better preservation of right ventricular function at baseline and in response to catecholamine infusion in patients who had undergone a transatrial transpulmonary approach than in those with a right ventriculotomy. In 1995 Stellin and colleagues[58] demonstrated a trend toward a reduced RV volume and a better ejection fraction in the long term after transatrial repair, when compared with a classic transventricular repair. If a transannular patch is required, a limited right ventriculotomy extending only a few millimeters below the pulmonary annulus is possible.[58,101] Minimizing or eliminating a right ventriculotomy altogether by using a transatrial or combined transatrial transpulmonary approach may also reduce the substrate for ventricular arrhythmias arising from incisions in the right ventricle.

Timing of Operation

The predominant trend in the timing of surgical intervention has been toward earlier intervention with elective repair in the first 4 to 6 months of life.[56-60,102-115] There is less consensus regarding the best treatment for patients who become symptomatic early in infancy or in the neonatal age. Some advocate primary repair in symptomatic infants regardless of age.[114,115] Whereas some centers have adopted a policy of elective repair for all infants at the time of presentation, even for neonates.[96,104,107,116,117] Advocates of early primary repair note that this approach limits the duration of exposure of these children to cyanosis and its attendant cumulative complications. In addition, initial complete repair avoids the attrition that can

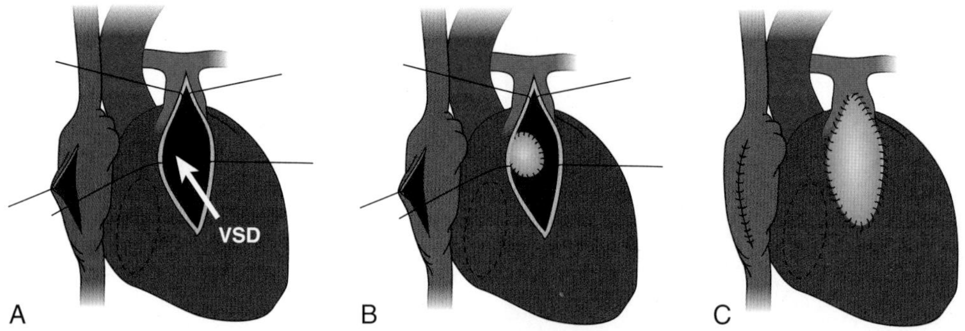

FIGURE 119-19 ■ The intraoperative phases of the transventricular tetralogy of Fallot repair. **A** and **B,** The ventricular septal defect (VSD) is visualized and closed through the right ventriculotomy. **C,** The right ventricular outflow tract and the main pulmonary artery are eventually patch augmented.

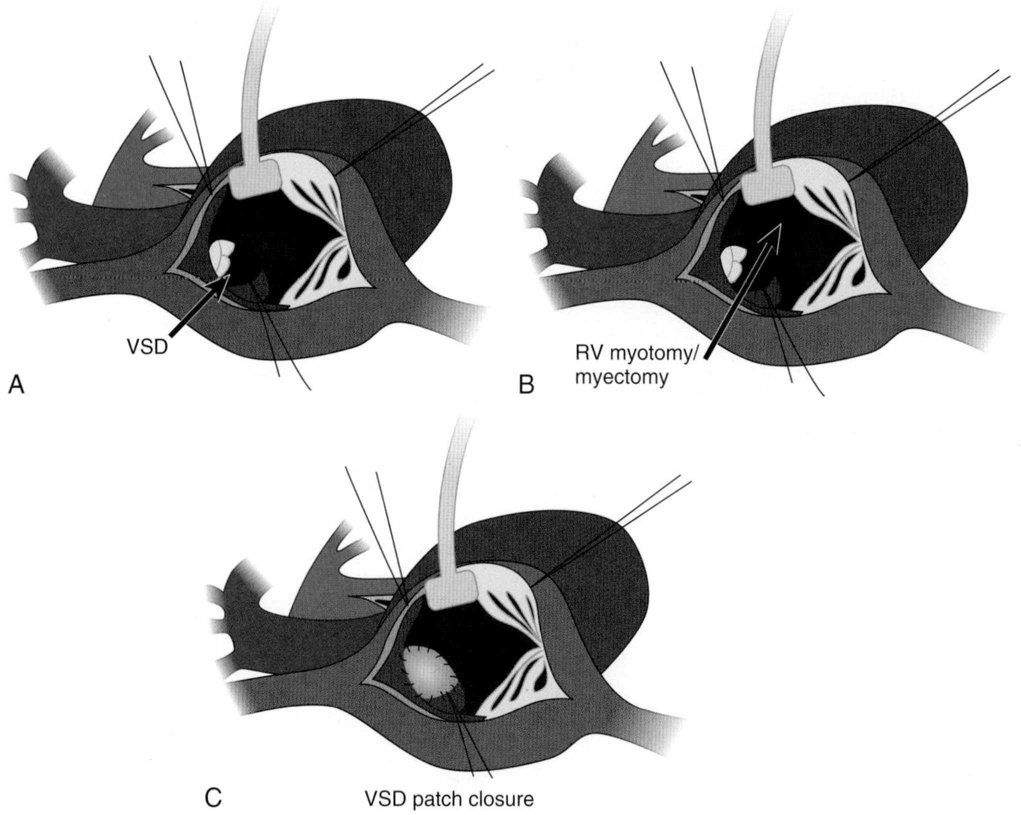

FIGURE 119-20 ■ The intraoperative phases of the transatrial tetralogy of Fallot repair. **A–C,** The ventricular septal defect (VSD) is visualized and closed through the right atrium after **(B)** a combined transatrial/transpulmonary myotomy and myectomy of the right ventricular (RV) outflow tract.

occur during the time between initial placement of a systemic-to-pulmonary arterial shunt and full repair in patients who undergo a staged approach. Furthermore, it has been postulated that ongoing pressure loading of the RV, in combination with chronic hypoxia, creates a substrate in the RV myocardium that predisposes to arrhythmia and diastolic dysfunction in patients who undergo later complete repair.[108] Some authors have reported primary repair of TOF in early infancy with mortality rates as low as 3%.[80] Nevertheless, primary repair in early infancy has been shown to require transannular patch placement as part of the repair in a higher percentage of patients and to require longer stays in the intensive care unit.[113-115] Excellent results have also been achieved with approaches that selectively use systemic-to-pulmonary arterial shunting as initial palliation for symptomatic neonates and young infants.[1,90,94] Proponents of this approach cite that mortality and morbidity are higher in the youngest infants in many series that report success with early primary repair. The neonatal myocardium may be less capable of handling the RV volume overload that follows VSD closure in a cyanotic patient, and this can be exacerbated by the additional RV volume loading from pulmonary incompetence and possible tricuspid valve

(TV) incompetence in a heart that has undergone the ischemic period required for surgical repair. Well-executed shunting in early infancy for TOF carries a very low risk of pulmonary artery distortion or early or interval mortality.[94,96,118] Fraser and colleagues[96] reported on selective application of primary repair for patients larger than 4 kg, with initial shunting of smaller patients who required earlier attention because of symptoms or anatomy. Although the majority of patients had TOF with pulmonic stenosis, this series also included patients with TOF and pulmonary atresia and patients with TOF and an AV septal defect. A single-shunted patient with TOF and a complete AV septal defect died in the interval before primary repair, but there were no perioperative deaths at the time of complete repair. Patch reconstruction of the RVOT either with a fenestrated VSD patch or without any attempt to close the VSD can be performed as an alternative to systemic-to-pulmonary arterial shunting in symptomatic patients with TOF and diminutive pulmonary arteries.[119,120]

POSTOPERATIVE MANAGEMENT

The majority of patients have a relatively uncomplicated postoperative course. Inotropic support is usually provided with low doses of dopamine, and extubation is generally possible during the first 12 to 48 hours after surgery. Right ventricular dysfunction as a cause of low cardiac output in the immediate postoperative period is rarely seen, especially when the PV integrity is preserved.[121] Significant diastolic dysfunction of the RV after TOF repair can produce a "restrictive physiology" in which the stiff RV demonstrates inadequate filling and can behave almost like a passive conduit for pulmonary blood flow.[108,122,123] The causes of RV dysfunction include PV, the presence of a right ventriculotomy, and residual lesions such as a hemodynamically significant VSD or RVOT obstruction. Right ventricular dysfunction is apparent by elevation in the RA pressure along with the accompanying clinical manifestations of liver enlargement, edema, and effusions in a patient with evidence of low cardiac output (decreased cutaneous temperature, elevated lactate levels, decreased urine output). Right ventricular dysfunction after TOF repair is usually transient and responds to increased inotropic support and diuretics. A patent foramen ovale (or a calibrated atrial septal defect) allows right-to-left shunting at the atrial level with decompression of the right heart chambers at the expense of a slight arterial oxygen desaturation. A progressive increase in the oxygen arterial saturation can be interpreted as an improvement in the RV performance in the early postoperative period. Junctional ectopic tachycardia (JET) can occur after TOF repair, especially in the first few hours after surgery.[58,78,86] When it does occur, postoperative JET is characterized by atrioventricular dissociation with rapid junctional rates of up to 230 beats per minute. In a recent report, JET occurred in 22% of patients who had undergone TOF repair,[124,125] with resection rather than simple transection of muscle bundles within the RVOT, a higher bypass temperature, and a transatrial approach to VSD closure were all associated with a higher incidence of postoperative JET. The authors concluded that avoidance of excessive muscle resection in the RVOT and traction during VSD exposure should reduce the incidence of postoperative JET. Treatment of JET includes core cooling (34-35° C), reduction in inotrope dosages, atrial pacing above the junctional rate, and the administration of antiarrhythmic agents.[126,128] Also loading with amiodarone over 2 to 4 hours, followed by continuous infusion, is a useful pharmacologic approach to JET after TOF repair.[126,128] We have found that an induced surface hypothermia (rectal temperature of 34-35° C) is a useful tool for treating a low output syndrome, particularly when in combination with arrhythmias.

Residual lesions after TOF repair include residual VSDs and significant RVOT obstruction. Even small residual VSDs (3-4 mm) that would be well tolerated in patients with repaired large left-to-right shunts (VSD, truncus arteriosus) may be poorly tolerated after TOF repair. Poor tolerance of residual left-to-right shunts after TOF repair can result from a combination of factors including coexisting pulmonic regurgitation, noncompliant ventricles, and sudden volume loading of the left ventricle, particularly in neonates and young infants.[121-123,129] The presence of a residual VSD should be ruled out using intraoperative transesophageal or epicardial echocardiography. Patients with significant VSDs will demonstrate a higher than expected LA pressure. If a pulmonary artery catheter is in place, an oxygen saturation of greater than 80% in pulmonary arterial blood is predictive of a hemodynamically significant residual VSD.[121,129] Significant residual RVOT obstruction is usually tolerated in the immediate postoperative period, but late problems including ventricular tachyarrhythmias and the need for late reoperation occur more commonly.[130] Hemodynamic instability arising from residual VSDs or RVOT obstruction may also be attributed to postoperative RV dysfunction alone, therefore residual lesions should be aggressively ruled out in patients with poor postoperative hemodynamics. An accurate intraoperative echocardiographic assessment is essential for ruling out any important residual lesion, before transferring the patient to the intensive care unit.

LONG-TERM FOLLOW-UP

Currently, surgery for TOF repair has reached excellent early and late outcomes in either neonates or children.[130] Decisions made at the time of surgery have a definite effect on the performance of TOF repair in the long-term follow-up. Despite institutional differences in surgical approach, timing of surgery, and many other aspects of management, long-term outcomes in survivors of TOF repair are uniformly favorable. Alexiou and colleagues[103] reported a 20-year survival of 98% after TOF repair, with 99% of survivors in New York Heart Association (NYHA) functional class I. Knott-Craig and coworkers[131] reported a 20-year survival of 98% with 86% freedom from reintervention on the RVOT after 20 years of follow-up. Katz and coauthors[132] demonstrated an 8-year actuarial survival of 96% after TOF repair, with

98% freedom from reoperation. In this study, older age at surgery, an increased ratio of RV to LV pressure, and the use of a preceding Potts shunt were all risk factors for late events. The use of a transannular patch during repair or a Blalock-Taussig shunt before repair were not associated with adverse late events. Murphy and associates[133] found a 32-year actuarial survival of 86%, which was less than the expected rate of 96% in age-matched controls. In this report, the authors also found that age at operation beyond 12 years and an elevated ratio of RV/LV pressure is associated with late mortality, whereas the presence of a transannular patch or a Blalock-Taussig shunt was not a significant risk factor for late mortality. Mimic and associates[134] from Great Ormond Street, have recently reported their experience with TOF repair, confirming that age at repair was not linked to early clinical outcome or reoperation/reintervention rate, and that palliative procedures postponed the timing of complete repair, but did not increase the reintervention rate. Kobayashi and coworkers[135] reported that 85% of patients had no more than mild TV regurgitation during a mean follow-up of 7 years after repair and that the development of moderate to severe TV regurgitation was independent of the operative approach used (transatrial versus transventricular) but was associated with significant pulmonary regurgitation and elevated right ventricular pressure. As a result of these improved results, currently there are an increasing number of patients with repaired TOF who reach adult age.[133,136] Thus, new problems have recently arisen other than survival to surgery: RV dysfunction and exercise intolerance, arrhythmias and sudden death, and importantly, pulmonary valve regurgitation requiring replacement.

Right Ventricular Performance and Functional Status

Right ventricular dysfunction can occur in the long term as a result of pulmonary regurgitation, a large right ventriculotomy, and eventual residual lesions.[137] In the hope of decreasing long-term complications of conventional transventricular repair, a transatrial/transpulmonary approach with limited (<1 cm) transannular right ventriculotomy has been adopted by many centers.[58,60,138] Nevertheless, benefits of this technique on RV performance in the long term are still not clearly demonstrated. Van den Berg and colleagues[98] have studied using magnetic resonance imaging (MRI), electrocardiography, and stress test in a cohort of 59 patients treated for TOF with a transatrial transpulmonary approach. At a mean follow-up time of 14 years, when compared with current data on healthy controls, TOF patients had significantly larger RV end-diastolic and end-systolic volumes and smaller RV and LV ejection fraction. In addition, maximum oxygen consumption was 97% ± 17% and maximum workload 89% ± 13% of predicted. Despite well-preserved clinical conditions, these patients exhibited RV dilation and dysfunction associated with impaired functional capacity. Sfyridis and colleagues[138] analyzed early and late results of transatrial/transpulmonary TOF repair over almost 14 years, with the aim of assessing the long-term RV function. Among 245 consecutive patients

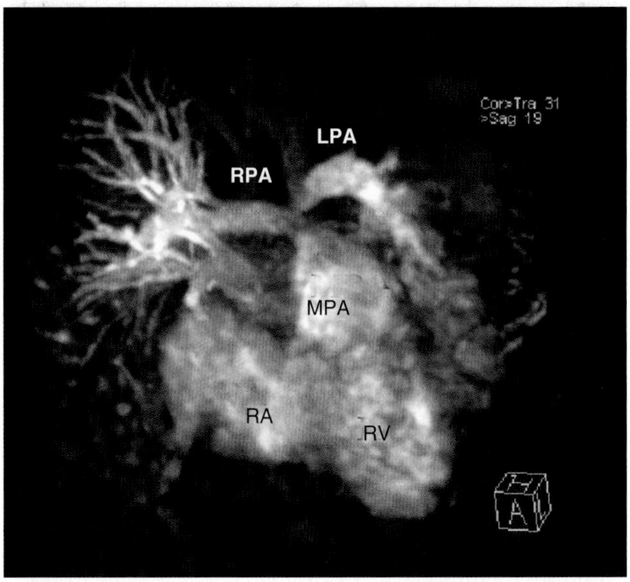

FIGURE 119-21 ■ Magnetic resonance imaging at follow-up. Three-dimensional reconstruction shows the dilated right ventricle (RV) and main pulmonary artery (MPA). Note the proximal stenosis at the left pulmonary artery branch (LPA) origin. *RA,* Right atrium; *RPA,* right pulmonary artery. (Courtesy Dr. Martina Perazzolo Marra.)

with repaired TOF (median age, 1.6 years), at a median follow-up of 8.5 years, there were no operative deaths, and only three early reoperations. Actuarial survival at 14 years was 98.8%, but 25 patients required late reoperation (mostly for pulmonary valve implantation). All survivors were asymptomatic at follow-up, and right ventricular function was reported within normal limits in most patients. Cheul and associates[139] have recently reported results from MRI (Fig. 119-21) comparing patients after a transatrial versus a transventricular TOF repair, with the aim of demonstrating whether a transatrial approach would result in less RV dilation and dysfunction, in the long term. Although the two groups differed significantly in follow-up time (12.7 ± 3.8 years vs. 17.2 ± 4.7 years; $P < 0.001$), pulmonary regurgitation fraction, indexed RV volumes and RV ejection fraction were not significantly different.

The importance of preserving the pulmonary valve function to permit a better RV late outcome has been investigated by different authors.[75-78,140,141] Recently, our institution has reported[77-78] the midterm results of 39 patients after early transatrial repair and an attempt of pulmonary valve preservation by intra-operative balloon dilation of the pulmonary valve annulus. Of these, 34 underwent a successful preservation of the pulmonary valve, at a median age of 3.8 months. Pulmonary regurgitation was absent or mild in 88% at discharge. At a median follow-up time of 1.2 years (range, 0.5-5.3 years) the integrity of the PV seemed to achieve improved RV function in comparison to patients who underwent a classical transannular patch.[78]

The performance of TOF repaired patients during exercise testing is also well maintained as reported by several authors.[141] Mahle and colleagues[142] reported that the mean maximal VO_2 of patients after conventional TOF repair was 95% of the predicted mean value for a control population, and the mean maximal work rate was 98% of predicted. In this study, the age of repair (<1 year of age versus >1 year of age) showed no effect on exercise performance, which is an important finding for decisions regarding timing of repair. Kondo and colleagues[143] found that cardiac output was normal at rest and during exercise in patients after repair, but that the incremental increase in left ventricular ejection fraction during exercise was reduced. The authors hypothesized that RV enlargement with pathologic changes in the septum (e.g., fibrosis) causes latent left ventricular dysfunction during exercise in these patients. Mueler and associates[144] investigated health-related quality of life (QOL) in children after TOF repair, and they compared the self-reported physical ability with objective exercise performance. This study included 168 patients, aged 8 to 16 years. Health-related QOL and cardiopulmonary exercise capacity were compared with those of an age-matched standard population, and correlations of health-related QOL with self-estimated physical rating and cardiopulmonary exercise capacity were analyzed. Despite health-related QOL in children and adolescents after TOF repair, results indicated no limitations; objective exercise capacity was actually impaired when compared with the standard population. Thus, the self-estimated physical functioning result was significantly overestimated compared with actual exercise capacity.

Arrhythmias and Sudden Death

Supraventricular and ventricular arrhythmias are not uncommon late after TOF repair; however, they can occur with increasing frequency as the duration of follow-up increases.[145-155] Various studies have reported that in patients followed for more than 20 years after TOF repair incidence of arrhythmias requiring treatment was 2% to 4% for atrial fibrillation or flutter, 3% to 4% for sustained ventricular tachycardia, and 2% to 4% for sudden cardiac death.[148,152,153,155] Holter monitoring detected a higher percentage of arrhythmias, with one report demonstrating that 19% of patients had sustained ventricular tachycardia and 23% of patients had atrial fibrillation or flutter on 24-hour Holter monitoring.[149] After TOF repair, the occurrence of arrhythmias is associated with elevated RV volumes and pressure, decreased right and left ventricular ejection fractions, pulmonic regurgitation, and other pathology of the RVOT such as aneurysm or significant stenosis.[127,150-154,156] Gatzoulis and associates found that PV regurgitation was associated with ventricular tachycardia and sudden death, whereas TV regurgitation was associated with atrial fibrillation or flutter.[148] In addition, they demonstrated that a substantially widened QRS complex on ECG is a prognostic marker of ventricular tachycardia and sudden cardiac death, with a QRS duration greater than 180 msec sensitively predicting the occurrence of life-threatening ventricular ectopy.[148,155] Dietl and coauthors[127] found that the type of operative approach for TOF repair was associated with significant ventricular ectopy after surgery. In fact, they reported that 39% of patients had significant ventricular ectopy after a ventricular approach to TOF repair, whereas only 2.8% had significant ventricular ectopy after a transatrial approach. In this report, the incidence of moderate to severe pulmonary regurgitation was nearly twice as high in the ventricular repair group (25.9%) as in the transatrial repair group (12.5%). Therrien and colleagues[153] found that PV replacement, when performed in the presence of important regurgitation and RV enlargement, was associated with a substantial decrease in arrhythmias and stabilization of the QRS duration. These authors used intraoperative electrophysiologic mapping and cryoablation in addition to pulmonary valve replacement in selected cases. In this series, atrial arrhythmias decreased from 17% to 12% postoperatively, and ventricular tachyarrhythmias decreased from 22% to 9%. In the 15 patients who underwent intraoperative cryoablation, there were no postoperative recurrences of significant arrhythmia.

All these studies emphasize that residual hemodynamic abnormalities drive postoperative arrhythmias after TOF repair and that all efforts should be made at the time of repair to provide the anatomic substrate to minimize long-term hemodynamic problems.

In a recent report,[156] atrial reentrant tachycardia is reported to be expected in more than 30% of patients, and high-grade ventricular arrhythmias in about 10%. The overall incidence of sudden cardiac death is estimated at 0.2% per year. Placement of an implantable cardioverter-defibrillator, despite high complications and inappropriate discharges, is often recommended for patients at higher risk. The Mayo clinic group reports that patients with TOF represent up to 40% of candidates for implantable cardioverter-defibrillator therapy.[157] Ongoing surveillance of RV function is a critical component of clinical assessment. Once RV dysfunction occurs, there are no medical therapies that have been shown to be effective, except for resynchronization with biventricular pacing in selected cases.

Late Pulmonary Valve Implantation

Currently, PV implantation is a common procedure during follow-up of patients after TOF repair, that can be done either surgically or percutaneously.[158-160] Timing and indicators for late PV implantation for PV regurgitation after TOF repair are not yet clearly defined and universally accepted.[36,161-164] MRI has been used increasingly to evaluate RV volumes and function. In most cases, PV implantation can be expected to reduce RV volumes; however, there is a point of RV enlargement beyond which normalization of RV size is unlikely to occur. Several reports support this concept of RV size reduction without normalization when pulmonary valve implantation is performed when RV end-diastolic volume is above 160 to 170 mL/m2[163-164] or even less.[165] Beyond its impact on RV dimensions, PV implantation reduces tricuspid regurgitation and clinical symptoms, and it often results in improved RV function.[145,166] The effects of pulmonary valve implantation on QRS duration and the incidence of RV arrhythmia are less well established.[146,166,167] Based on existing literature, an argument can be made to consider

PV implantation when there is documentation of progressive RV enlargement (>150 mL/m^2) and RV dysfunction, particularly in the presence of progressive TV regurgitation or decreased exercise tolerance.[168,169] A number of reports have detailed various clinical aspects of PV implantation in patients after TOF repair.[145,146,161-164,166-179] In addition to the standard surgical approach, percutaneous valve implantation has been used increasingly.[158-160] Discigil and coauthors[172] reported on 42 patients who underwent surgical pulmonary valve implantation approximately 11 years after TOF repair. Decreased exercise tolerance (58%), right heart failure (21%), arrhythmias (14%), syncope (10%), and RV dilation (7%) were the main indications for PV implantation. Ninety-eight percent of patients were hospital survivors with 5- and 10-year survival rates of 95% and 76%, respectively. Before surgery, 27% of patients were in NYHA class I or II, and after PV implantation, 97% were in NYHA class I or II. Significant atrial arrhythmias were present in 14% preoperatively and 2% postoperatively. Freedom from repeat PV implantation was 93% at 5 years and 70% at 10 years. Vliegen and coworkers[176] used MRI to evaluate patients before and after PV implantation and found that RV end-diastolic volume and RV end-systolic volume decreased, and RV ejection fraction increased, after PV implantation. As a functional correlate, NYHA class was also found to improve substantially after PV implantation. Despite improvement in RV volumes and functional status after PV implantation, a number of studies demonstrated improvement only if valve implantation was performed appropriately early.[173,174,177] De Ruijter reported an incidence of severe PV regurgitation of 31% at an average of nearly 10 years after TOF repair, with significant RV dilation in 38%.[174] For patients treated with pulmonary valve implantation, only 44% had normalization of RV size and symptomatic relief. Therrien and coworkers[173] reported no improvement in RV volumes after PV implantation. In addition, RV ejection fraction remained depressed (<0.4) in 87% of patients in whom preimplantation RV ejection was less than 0.4, whereas 50% of patients with preimplantation RV ejection fraction greater than 0.4 maintained postimplantation RV ejection fractions greater than 0.4. In light of these results, they concluded that late PV implantation failed to normalize RV volumes, and that the best chance of restoring a normal RV function was to perform PV implantation before significant RV dysfunction had occurred. Controversial results were reported by Quail and associates,[14] who studied TOF repaired patients with PV regurgitation. They compared the group of patients treated with PV implantation with matched untreated patients who were eligible for PV implantation based on hemodynamic status. Among 87 patients recruited, 51 underwent surgery while 36 were managed conservatively. Comparing 25 patients from each group using propensity score matching, they found that at 1.8 years of follow-up in patients with intermediate RV dilation, there was a very low risk of significant deterioration in RV or LV volumes and function. They concluded that slow deterioration can guide the interval for repeat imaging studies and determine the appropriate timing for PV implantation. Finally, a recent meta-analysis[180] has concluded that after PV implantation, there is an improvement of RV volumes and function and of LV function, a reduction of QRS duration, and improvement of symptoms. However, the preoperative RV geometry was capable of modulating the effect of PV implantation. In conclusion, despite important heterogeneity of the effects among the different studies, PV implantation is currently recommended as a reasonable approach to the problem even if surgical timing remains to be further defined and controversies still remain.

Finally, homografts or bioprosthetic valves are usually preferred in the PV position in patients with congenital heart disease.[161-165] However, unsatisfactory long-term results have reawakened interest in the use of mechanical valves in the pulmonary position. Waterbolk and associates[181] report excellent early and late outcomes of mechanical valve implantation in the pulmonary position in 27 of 79 patients indicated for PV replacement. Tetralogy of Fallot was the most common basic lesion. Thirty-day hospital mortality was 1 of 28 (3.6%), because of a cerebrovascular accident. One patient died late (2.8 years postoperatively). Median age was 33 years, and the median interval between primary repair and insertion of the prosthesis was 26 years. Freedom from reoperation at 1 year was 100%. No thromboembolic events were observed. Recently, Shin and colleagues[182] have investigated the long-term outcomes of mechanical valves implanted in the pulmonic position in 37 patients (median age, 13.5 years; range, 7 months to 23 years) who had undergone 38 mechanical pulmonary valve implantations. Most patients (n = 23) had TOF, and the median valve size was 23 mm (range, 17-27 mm). At a median follow-up of 24.6 months (range, 1.3 months to 22.5 years), survival rates were 97%, 97%, and 97%, at 1, 5, and 10 years, respectively. Freedom from thromboembolism or bleeding events was 92%, 92%, and 78.8%, at 1, 5 and 10 years, respectively. Freedom from reoperation was 100%, 100%, and 85.7%, at 1, 5, and 10 years, respectively. Thus they conclude that in growing patients who have undergone prior sternotomies requiring a pulmonary valve replacement, a mechanical valve could be an attractive option. Although life-long anticoagulation therapy is indicated for mechanical prostheses, the chance of subsequent reoperations can be expected to be low.

Further study is necessary for developing an ideal long-standing biological valve in the pulmonary position. Preliminary studies with decellularized pulmonary homograft are promising.[183-184] A European multicenter ongoing trial will soon report on the use of such a prosthesis, on a larger scale.

Such a new type of tissue engineered valve will certainly show, in the near future, the advantage of treating chronic PV regurgitation in an increasing population after TOF repair in comparison to conventional valve substitutes that are implanted surgically or transcutaneously.

ATRIOVENTRICULAR CANAL AND TETRALOGY OF FALLOT

A common AV valve, an ostium primum atrial septal defect, and a nonrestrictive inlet ventricular septal defect occur in combination with an anterior malalignment VSD and RVOT obstruction typical of TOF in approximately 2% of all cases of TOF.[36,185] Repair can be accomplished with a single- or double-patch technique, depending on institutional habits. In addition, transventricular or transatrial transpulmonary approaches can be used successfully.[185-193] Usually, most or all VSDs can be closed through the right atrium, as is standard for repair of an AV septal defect, but the VSD patch must be shaped appropriately for the peculiarity of this defect; in fact, it has to be elongated and wide enough anteriorly so as to close the anterior extension of the VSD without causing subaortic obstruction. Closure of the cleft in the left-sided AV valve and closure of the ostium primum ASD is performed in a standard fashion, and relief of the RV outflow tract obstruction is performed as would normally be done for TOF. In a recent retrospective analysis from Kotani and colleagues from Sick Children's Hospital in Toronto,[194] of 41 patients who underwent repair for TOF with AV septal defect, only 3 died early. The RV outflow tract was reconstructed, with pulmonary valve sparing in 56%. There was no late death, and survival was 92.1% at 15 years. During a median follow-up period of 5.9 years, freedom from all reinterventions at 15 years was 52.8%; approximately half of those procedures were related to the RV outflow tract revision, whereas only a minority had AV valve dysfunction. Freedom from RV outflow tract–related reintervention and atrioventricular valve/LV outflow tract–related reintervention were comparable between the TOF with atrioventricular septal defect and matched control groups (TOF with atrioventricular septal defect, 95.2% and 88.6% versus atrioventricular septal defect alone, 86.0% and 83.9% at 5 years, respectively; P value not significant). Thus, in the current era, the surgically modified history of TOF with atrioventricular septal defect is not significantly different from that of isolated TOF.[185,187-189,191]

TETRALOGY OF FALLOT WITH ABSENT PULMONARY VALVE

The anatomic features of TOF with absent pulmonary valve include massively enlarged pulmonary arteries, anterior malalignment VSD, absent (aplasia) or rudimentary development of the PV, a relatively small PV annulus, and usually absence of the ductus arteriosus. The etiology of the aneurysmal enlargement of the pulmonary arteries may be related to the effects of regurgitation throughout fetal development, or to abnormalities in the vessel wall. Massive enlargement of the pulmonary arteries frequently causes obstruction of the central bronchi and also alveoli. The degree of airway obstruction dictates the clinical course observed in affected patients. Presentation varies from no clinically significant airway obstruction in asymptomatic patients, to severe bronchioalveolar obstruction requiring mechanical ventilation and surgical repair in the newborn period. Operative repair requires intracardiac correction typical of simple TOF on cardiopulmonary bypass, with surgical reduction in the size of the dilated main and branch pulmonary arteries, that can be performed by different techniques.[195-210] In most cases, both the MPA and branches are massively enlarged and must be reduced surgically. Stellin and colleagues[203] advocated surgical intervention to relieve the bronchial obstruction by plicating the pulmonary artery and its branches under deep hypothermia and circulatory arrest. Alternatively, it can be transected with a portion excised posteriorly, which effectively pulls the pulmonary arteries anteriorly away from the tracheobronchial tree. The branch pulmonary arteries are reduced in diameter by resecting portions of the anterior wall, often with plication of the posterior wall.[197,198,201,202] In most cases, a transannular incision is necessary; reconstruction of the RV outflow tract can then be performed with a homograft valve insertion.[201,204,206,209] However, RV outflow tract reconstruction can also be performed with a monocusp or, often, without any valve implantation.[197,198,202,208] McDonnell and coworkers reported an experience with surgical management for 28 patients with TOF and absent pulmonary valve,[197] in which 13 patients (46%) required preoperative intubation and mechanical ventilation. There was a 21% in-hospital mortality, and rates of freedom from death or reintervention at 1 and 10 years were 68% and 52%, respectively. The requirement for preoperative mechanical ventilation was the only risk factor for mortality in this series. Hraska and associates[196,210] have reported a novel approach to this problem that includes transection and removal of a wedge-shaped portion of the ascending aorta so as to bring the aorta caudally and to the left. A LeCompte maneuver bringing the pulmonary arteries anterior to the aorta is then performed with or without concomitant plication of the branch pulmonary arteries. This approach pulls the pulmonary arteries off the tracheobronchial tree without requiring extensive suture lines, and the method of resection of the aorta creates a space for the new location of the pulmonary arteries while minimizing the risk of compression of the RCA. In a retrospective review of 62 consecutive patients following repair of TOF and absent pulmonary valve, Alsoufi and coworkers[206] reported three perioperative deaths in neonates and five late deaths. Five- and ten-year survival was 93% ± 4% and 87% ± 5%. On multivariable analysis, significant factors associated with prolonged ventilation were neonatal age ($P < 0.0001$) and preoperative mechanical ventilation ($P = 0.088$). Eight airway reinterventions were needed in seven infants with persistent postoperative airway compromise, pulmonary artery suspension ($n = 4$), innominate artery suspension ($n = 2$), and lobectomy ($n = 2$). Freedom from RV outflow tract reoperation was 89% ± 5% and 59% ± 9% at 5 and 10 years, respectively. In conclusion, TOF with absent pulmonary valve remains a complex congenital heart defect, with a perioperative mortality mainly related to a preoperatively compromised bronchial tree, and a higher rate of reintervention in follow-up when compared with classic TOF.

Acknowledgment

We would like to thank Dr. Aldo Castaneda for reviewing and improving the value of this chapter.

REFERENCES

1. Stensen N, quoted by Goldstein HI. *Bull Hist Med* 29:526, 1945.
2. Fallot ELA: Contribution a l'anatomie pathologique de la maladie bleue (cyanose cardiaque). *Marseilles Med* 25(77):138, 207, 270, 341, 403, 1888.
3. Blalock A, Taussig HB: The surgical treatment of malformations of the heart in which there is pulmonary stenosis or pulmonary atresia. *JAMA* 128:189–202, 1945.
4. Potts WJ, Smith S, Gibson S: Anastomosis of the aorta to a pulmonary artery. *JAMA* 132:627, 1946.
5. Waterston DJ: Treatment of Fallot's tetralogy in children under one year of age. *Rozhl Chir* 41:181, 1962.
6. Laks H, Castaneda AR: Subclavian arterioplasty for the ipsilateral Blaolock-Taussig shunt. *Ann Thorac Surg* 19:319, 1975.
7. Davidson JS: Anastomosi between the ascending aorta and the main pulmonary artery in the tetralogy of Fallot. *Thorax* 10:348, 1955.
8. Lillehei CW, Varco RL, Cohen M: The first open-heart repairs of ventricular septal defect, atrioventricular communis, and tetralogy of Fallot using extracorporeal circulation by cross-circulation: a thirty-year follow-up. *Ann Thorac Surg* 41:4, 1986.
9. Lillehei CW, Cohen M, Warden HE, et al: The direct-vision intracardiac correction of congenital anomalies by controlled cross-circulation: results in 32 patients with ventricular septal defects, tetralogy of Fallot, and atrioventricular communis defects. *Surgery* 38:11, 1955.
10. Kirklin JW, Dushane JW, Patrick RT, et al: Intracardiac surgery with the aid of a mechanical pump-oxygenator (Gibbon type): report of eight cases. *Mayo Clin Proc* 30:201, 1955.
11. Kirklin JW, Ellis FH, McGoon DC, et al: Surgical treatment for the treatment of tetralogy of Fallot by open intracardiac repair. *J Thorac Surg* 37:22, 1959.
12. Barrett-Boyes BG, Neutze JM: Primary repair of tetralogy of Fallot in infancy using profound hypothermia with circulatory arrest and limited cardiopulmonary bypass: a comparison with conventional two-stage management. *Ann Surg* 178:406, 1973.
13. Castaneda AR: Tetralogy of Fallot. In Castaneda AR, Jonas RA, Mayer JE, et al, editors: *Cardiac surgery of the neonate and infant*, Philadelphia, 1995, WB Saunders Company, pp 215–235.
14. Quail MA, Frigiola A, Giardini A, et al: Impact of pulmonary valve replacement in tetralogy of Fallot with pulmonary regurgitation: a comparison of intervention and nonintervention. *Ann Thorac Surg* 94(5):1619–1626, 2012.
15. Karamlou T, Silber I, Lao R, et al: Outcomes after late reoperation in patients with repaired tetralogy of Fallot: the impact of arrhythmia and arrhythmia surgery. *Ann Thorac Surg* 81(5):1786–1793, discussion 1793, 2006.
16. Report of the New England Regional Infant Cardiac Program. *Pediatrics* 65:375, 1980.
17. Perloff JK: *The clinical recognition of congenital heart disease*, ed 4, Philadelphia, 1994, WB Saunders.
18. Breitbart RE, Fyler DC: Tetralogy of Fallot, Chapter 32. In Keane JF, Lock JE, Fyler DC, editors: *Nadas' pediatric cardiology*, ed 2, Philadelphia, 2006, Saunders Elsevier Inc, p 559.
19. Ferencz C, Rubin JD, McCarter RJ, et al: Congenital heart disease: prevalence at livebirth. The Baltimore-Washington Infant Study. *Am J Epidemiol* 121:31, 1985.
20. Loffredo CA: Epidemiology of cardiovascular malformations: prevalence and risk factors. *Am J Med Genet* 97:319, 2000.
21. Merscher S, Funke B, Epstein JA, et al: TBX1 is responsible for cardiovascular defects in velo-cardio-facial/DiGeorge syndrome. *Cell* 104:619, 2001.
22. Jerome LA, Papaioannou VE: DiGeorge syndrome phenotype in mice mutant for the T-box gene, Tbx1. *Nat Genet* 27:286, 2001.
23. Gong W, Gottlieb S, Collins J, et al: Mutation analysis of TBX1 in non-deleted patients with features of DGS/VCFS or isolated cardiovascular defects. *J Med Genet* 38:E45, 2001.
24. Goldmuntz E, Geiger E, Benson DW: NKX2.5 mutations in patients with tetralogy of Fallot. *Circulation* 104:2565, 2001.
25. Krantz ID, Smith R, Colliton RP, et al: Jagged1 mutations in patients ascertained with isolated congenital heart defects. *Am J Med Genet* 84:56, 1999.
26. McElhinney DB, Krantz ID, Bason L, et al: Analysis of cardiovascular phenotype and genotypephenotype correlation in individuals with a JAG1 mutation and/or Alagille syndrome. *Circulation* 106:2567, 2002.
27. Ferencz C, Loffredo CA, Correa-Villasenor A, et al: *Genetic and environmental risk factors of major cardiovascular malformations: the Baltimore-Washington infant study 1981-1989*, Armonk, NY, 1997, Futura.
28. Van Praagh R, Van Praagh S, Nebesar RA, et al: Tetralogy of Fallot: underdevelopment of the pulmonary infundibulum and its sequelae. *Am J Cardiol* 26(1):25–33, 1970.
29. Anderson RH, Allwork SP, Ho SY, et al: Surgical anatomy of tetralogy of Fallot. *J Thorac Cardiovasc Surg* 81(6):887–896, 1981.
30. Walters HL, III, Mavroudis C, Tchervenkiv CI, et al: Congenital heart surgery nomenclature and database project: double outlet right ventricle. *Ann Thorac Surg* 69:s249–s263, 2000.
31. Kawashima Y, Kitamura S, Nakano S, et al: Corrective surgery for tetralogy of Fallot without or with minimal ventriculotomy. *Circulation* 64(Suppl II):147–153, 1981.
32. Howell CE, Ho SY, Anderson RH, et al: Variations within the fibrous skeleton and ventricular outflow tracts in tetralogy of Fallot. *Ann Thorac Surg* 50:450–457, 1990.
33. Johnson RJ, Haworth SG: Pulmonary vascular and alveolar development in tetralogy of Fallot: a recommendation for early correction. *Thorax* 37:893, 1982.
34. Hislop A, Reid L: Structural changes in the pulmonary arteries and veins in tetralogy of Fallot. *Br Heart J* 35:1178, 1973.
35. Kurosawa H, Imai Y, Becker AE: Surgical anatomy of the atrioventricular conduction bundle in tetralogy of Fallot. *J Thorac Cardiovasc Surg* 95:586–591, 1988.
36. Kirklin JW, Barrat-Boyes BG: Ventricular defect and pulmonary stenosis or atresia. In Kirklin JW, Barrat-Boyes BG, editors: *Cardiac surgery*, ed 2, New York, 1993, Churchill Livingstone, p 861.
37. Karl TR: Tetralogy of Fallot: a surgical perspective. *Korean J Thorac Cardiovasc Surg*. 45(4):213–224, 2012.
38. Meng CCL, Eckner FA, Lev M: Coronary artery distribution in tetralogy of Fallot. *Arch Surg* 90:363–366, 1965.
39. Need LR, Powell AJ, del Nido P, et al: Coronary echocardiography in tetralogy of Fallot: diagnostic accuracy, resource utilization and surgical implications over 13 years. *J Am Coll Cardiol* 36(4):1371–1377, 2000.
40. Gupta D, Saxena A, Kothari SS, et al: Detection of coronary artery anomalies in tetralogy of Fallot using a specific angiographic protocol. *Am J Cardiol* 87(2):241–244, 2001.
41. Chiu IS, Wu CS, Wang JK, et al: Influence of aortopulmonary rotation on the anomalous coronary artery pattern in tetralogy of Fallot. *Am J Cardiol* 85(6):780–784, 2000.
42. Tworetzky W, McElhinney DB, Brook MM, et al: Echocardiographic diagnosis alone for the complete repair of major congenital heart defects. *J Am Coll Cardiol* 33(1):228–233, 1999.
43. Yoo SJ, Lee YH, Kim ES, et al: Tetralogy of Fallot in the fetus: findings at targeted sonography. *Ultrasound Obstet Gynecol* 14(1):29–37, 1999.
44. Tometzki AJ, Suda K, Kohl T, et al: Accuracy of prenatal echocardiographic diagnosis and prognosis of fetuses with conotruncal anomalies. *J Am Coll Cardiol* 33(6):1696–1701, 1999.
45. Lee W, Smith RS, Comstock CH, et al: Tetralogy of Fallot: prenatal diagnosis and postnatal survival. *Obstet Gynecol* 86(4 Pt 1):583–588, 1995.
46. Kirk JS, Comstock CH, Lee W, et al: Sonographic screening to detect fetal cardiac anomalies: a 5-year experience with 111 abnormal cases. *Obstet Gynecol* 89(2):227–232, 1997.
47. Kaguelidou F, Fermont L, Boudjemline Y, et al: Fœtal echocardiographic assessment of tetralogy of Fallot and post-natal outcome. *Eur Heart J* 29(11):1432–1438, 2008.
48. Poon LC, Huggon IC, Zidere V, et al: Tetralogy of Fallot in the fetus in the current era. *Ultrasound Obstet Gynecol* 29(6):625–627, 2007.
49. Fuchs IB, Muller H, Abdul-Khaliq H, et al: Immediate and long-term outcomes in children with prenatal diagnosis of selected isolated congenital heart defects. *Ultrasound Obstet Gynecol* 29(1):38–43, 2007.
50. Chew C, Halliday JL, Riley MM, et al: Population-based study of antenatal detection of congenital heart disease by ultrasound examination. *Ultrasound Obstet Gynecol* 29(6):619–624, 2007.

CHAPTER 120

Pulmonary Atresia with Ventricular Septal Defect and Right Ventricle–to–Pulmonary Artery Conduits

Sitaram M. Emani

CHAPTER OUTLINE

PULMONARY ATRESIA WITH VENTRICULAR SEPTAL DEFECT

Pulmonary atresia with ventricular septal defect (PA/VSD) is a congenital cardiac malformation characterized by discontinuity of blood flow from the right ventricle to the pulmonary arteries, a ventricular septal defect (VSD) resulting from anterior deviation of the infundibular (conal) septum, and an overriding aorta. Because it shares many attributes of tetralogy of Fallot, it is also referred to as tetralogy of Fallot with pulmonary atresia. Incidence of PA/VSD is estimated to be 1 in 10,000 live births.[1] A right aortic arch may be seen in up to 45% of patients.[2] PA/VSD is also associated with major aortopulmonary collateral arteries (MAPCAs) that, in some cases, are the sole supply of pulmonary blood flow. The morphology of the pulmonary circulation, which varies significantly among patients, determines the management and prognosis of this malformation. PA/VSD may also be associated with other intracardiac defects, such as tricuspid atresia or stenosis, complete atrioventricular canal,

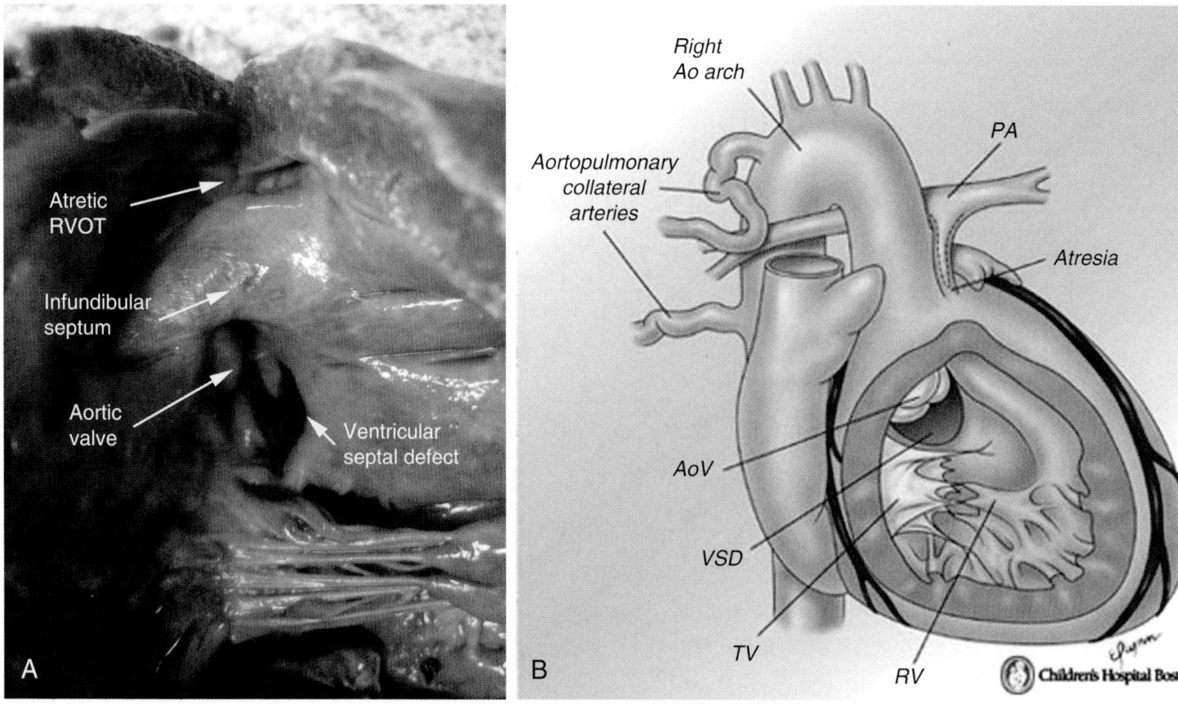

FIGURE 120-1 ■ Anatomic specimen and schematic demonstrating the features of pulmonary atresia with ventricular septal defect. *Ao,* Aortic; *AoV,* aortic valve; *PA,* pulmonary artery; *RV,* right ventricle; *RVOT,* right ventricular outflow tract; *TV,* tricuspid valve; *VSD,* ventricular septal defect. (Courtesy Children's Hospital Boston.)

complete or corrected transposition of the great arteries, left superior vena cava, anomalies of the coronary sinus, dextrocardia, and asplenia or polysplenia syndrome. These more complex forms of PA/VSD are not discussed in this chapter. The most common associated genetic defect is 22Q11 microdeletion, which is found in up to 34% of patients, and up to 65% of patients with MAPCAs are found to have this abnormality.[3] Other phenotypic abnormalities with the 22Q11 microdeletion include submucosal cleft palate, abnormal facies, delayed development, and mental retardation. Neonates with trisomy 13 or 18 may have PA/VSD as well, and the prognosis is extremely poor for these children.

Anatomy and Pathophysiology

As in tetralogy of Fallot, PA/VSD is associated with anterior deviation of the infundibular septum, a conoventricular VSD, and the resulting aortic override (Fig. 120-1). The spectrum of pulmonary atresia varies from purely valvular or subvalvular atresia (with intact main and branch pulmonary arteries) to complete absence of central pulmonary arteries. Pulmonary blood flow is dependent on the presence of an aortopulmonary communication, which may exist in the form of a patent ductus arteriosus (PDA), other major nonductal collaterals arising from the descending aorta that connect to the central native pulmonary arteries, or MAPCAs that directly enter the hilum and join the segmental pulmonary arteries. In utero, the pulmonary parenchyma is perfused by branches from the dorsal aorta as well as by the sixth aortic arch, which forms the basis for the central pulmonary arteries. Abnormal development of the central pulmonary arteries leads to persistence of the dorsal aortic branches, which ultimately develop into MAPCAs.

The lungs may be supplied by the native pulmonary arteries, by MAPCAs, or by both. If confluent central pulmonary arteries are present, the blood supply to the lung may arise from a PDA, a central "ductlike" collateral, or a MAPCA. The behaviors of these three sources of pulmonary blood flow differ in their predisposition to constrict over time, which has implications for the stability of pulmonary blood flow. Whereas MAPCAs or ductlike collaterals might remain patent beyond the neonatal period, the PDA is likely to constrict postnatally because of the presence of prostaglandin-responsive ductal tissue. Although the distinction may be difficult to establish by preoperative imaging studies, the location on the aorta from which the collateral originates is suggestive. A solitary collateral that arises just distal to the left subclavian artery (if left aortic arch) and travels to a central pulmonary confluence is likely to be a PDA, whereas a collateral that arises from any other location off the aorta and supplies a central confluence is termed a ductlike collateral. A vessel that exits the descending aorta and travels directly to the pulmonary parenchyma is likely a MAPCA. There may be heterogeneity in the sources of pulmonary blood flow within any given patient, such that one segment of lung may be supplied by the native pulmonary artery whereas another segment may be supplied by a MAPCA. Some segments may have a dual supply (Fig. 120-2). Patients with confluent central pulmonary arteries that are supplied by a PDA are less likely to have significant MAPCAs, and those with nonconfluent central pulmonary arteries depend on MAPCAs for pulmonary blood flow.

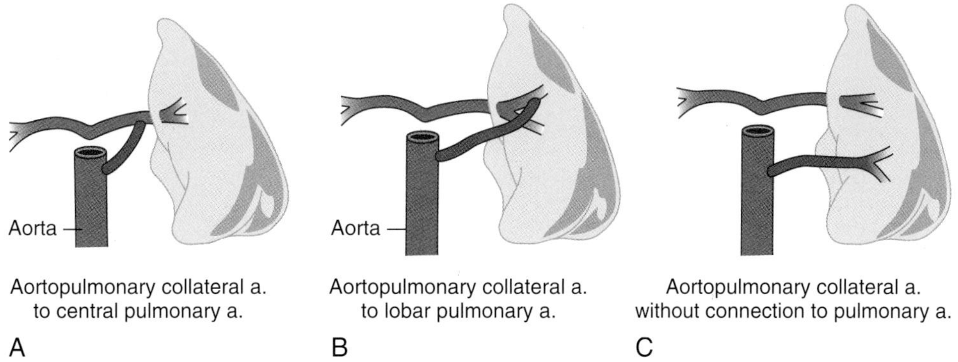

FIGURE 120-2 ■ Variations in aortopulmonary collateral morphology in pulmonary atresia with ventricular septal defect.

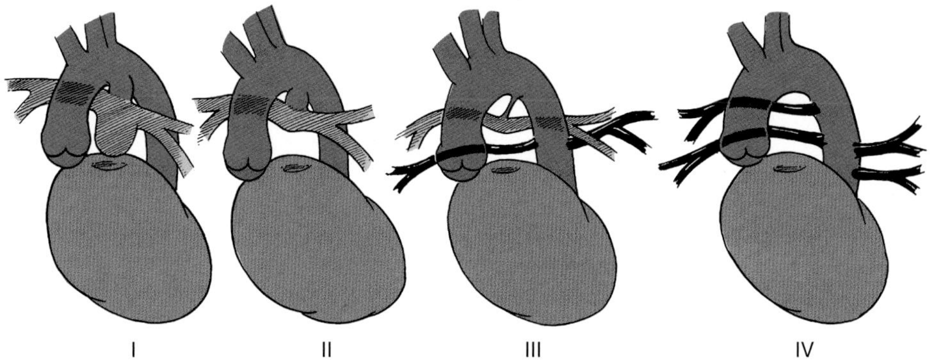

FIGURE 120-3 ■ Variations in pulmonary supply from native pulmonary arteries *(hatched gray)* and major aortopulmonary collateral arteries *(solid black)* encountered in patients with pulmonary atresia with ventricular septal defect.

Classification

There is no standard classification system for PA/VSD; however, several have been purported. Most classification schemes focus on the patterns of pulmonary blood flow. The classification system adopted by the Congenital Heart Surgery Nomenclature Project broadly divides pulmonary artery anatomy according to the following: central pulmonary arteries without MAPCAs, confluent central pulmonary arteries and dual supply with MAPCA, nonconfluent or absent central pulmonary arteries with MAPCA.[4]

Another classification scheme divides patients further according to specific patterns of pulmonary artery anatomy that are most commonly encountered (Fig. 120-3):

I. Valvar pulmonary atresia with a decent-sized main pulmonary artery and confluent central pulmonary arteries. This variant is associated with a PDA and therefore not associated with MAPCAs.
II. Absent main pulmonary artery with confluent, decent-sized or mildly hypoplastic central pulmonary arteries supplied by a PDA, without MAPCAs.
III. Confluent central pulmonary arteries with MAPCAs but no PDA.
   a. Central pulmonary artery z-score > −2.5
   b. Central pulmonary artery z-score < −2.5
IV. Nonconfluent or absent central pulmonary arteries with MAPCAs.
V. Nonconfluent central pulmonary artery with PDA and MAPCAs.

Natural History

The natural history of PA/VSD varies significantly depending on the pulmonary artery morphology. Patients presenting with PA/VSD that has ductal dependent pulmonary blood flow will experience profound fatal cyanosis in the neonatal period as the ductus begins to close. On the other hand, patients with MAPCAs with mild stenosis of collateral vessels and balanced pulmonary blood flow exhibit mild cyanosis and may survive into adolescence or adulthood without repair. Progressive development of ostial stenosis within the collateral leads to progressive cyanosis. Alternatively, excessive pulmonary blood flow from an unrestrictive collateral results in congestive heart failure. The presence of long-standing unrestrictive blood flow within a MAPCA may result in irreversible elevation of pulmonary vascular resistance within that segment. Pulmonary hypertension within a segment of the lung is seen commonly in patients who present at later age. Heterogeneity in pulmonary vascular resistance within a lung segment results in $\dot{V}/\dot{Q}$ mismatch. Without timely intervention, the overall mortality rate is approximately 60% by 30 years of age, with most of the mortality occurring within the first year of life.[1,5]

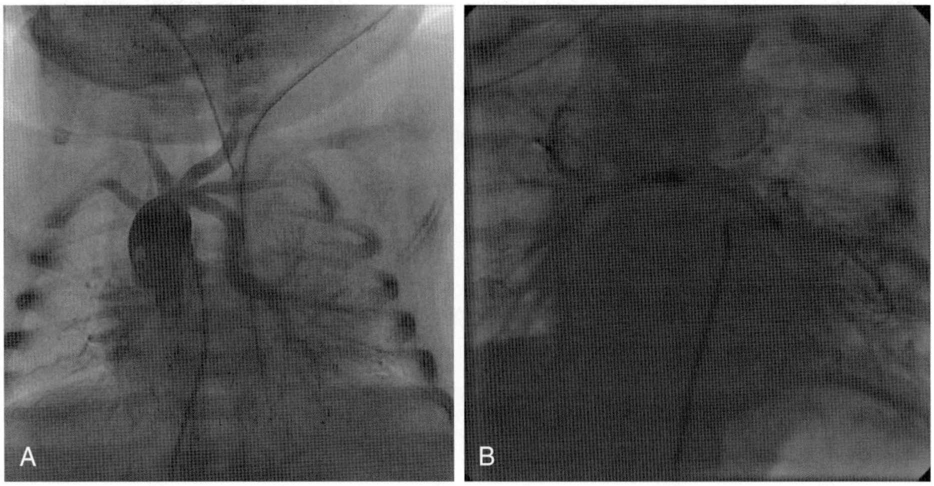

FIGURE 120-4 Angiograms demonstrating major aortopulmonary collateral artery to left lung **(A)** and redundant collateral to left lung also supplied by hypoplastic native pulmonary arteries **(B)**.

Clinical Presentation

The clinical presentation varies according to pulmonary artery morphology. Patients with ductal-dependent pulmonary circulation present with profound cyanosis during the first several weeks of life as the ductus begins to close. Children with progressively restrictive aortopulmonary collaterals may present in childhood with cyanosis, whereas patients with large, unrestrictive collaterals may present with heart failure symptoms such as failure to thrive, tachypnea, or feeding intolerance. Among infants presenting during infancy, 50% present with cyanosis and 25% present with heart failure symptoms.[5] Rarely, in a child with balanced pulmonary blood flow, symptoms may not manifest until adolescence or adulthood.

Diagnostic Studies

Initial Studies

In the current era, prenatal diagnosis is frequently established by fetal ultrasound and echocardiography by the demonstration of absence of antegrade pulmonary artery blood flow. A neonate presenting with cyanosis following ductal closure may demonstrate hypovascular lung fields by chest radiography, whereas an infant presenting with excessive pulmonary blood flow and congestive heart failure may demonstrate interstitial edema and prominent hilar vessels. A right-sided aortic arch may be demonstrated by the position of the aortic knob by chest x-ray, and the diminutive main pulmonary artery results in an exaggerated sabot shape of the cardiac silhouette. By electrocardiography, rightward deviated QRS axis and evidence of right atrial and ventricular hypertrophy are frequently seen.

Echocardiography is the primary modality for diagnosis of this defect, and it provides a significant portion of the anatomic information needed for initial decision making in neonates and infants. The data to be obtained by echocardiography include location, size, and direction of flow in the ventricular and atrial septal defects; size and confluence of the central pulmonary vessels; and presence of a PDA or other collaterals. Color flow Doppler may suggest the presence of a collateral arising from the descending aorta, but it is not reliable at delineating the entire course. Retrograde flow in the descending aorta suggests significant pulmonary flow through the collateral or PDA. Coronary artery anatomy should be delineated, particularly to exclude the presence of a left anterior descending coronary artery arising from the right coronary artery, because this impacts surgical management.

Cardiac Catheterization

Cardiac catheterization is indicated in patients with PA/VSD who have nonconfluent or hypoplastic central pulmonary arteries in whom MAPCAs are suspected (Fig. 120-4). The goal of catheterization in these patients is surgical planning by evaluating the anatomy, size, degree of stenosis, and the presence of dual supply from native pulmonary arteries or collaterals. Vascular supply to all segments must be clearly determined. Native pulmonary arteries may require visualization by pulmonary venous wedge injection if no antegrade flow to the native pulmonary arteries can be identified. Relationship of collaterals to the airway (seen best on the lateral view) is important in guiding surgical approach (sternotomy vs. thoracotomy). In older children and adults, measurements of individual pulmonary artery pressures are obtained to determine the risk of development of pulmonary hypertension in high-pressure collaterals. The pulmonary-to-systemic blood flow ratio (Qp/Qs) can be estimated by the Fick method if all pulmonary flow arises from collaterals (i.e., if there is no previous right ventricle–to–pulmonary artery [RV-to-PA] conduit). Interventions that may be performed at catheterization include balloon dilation of native pulmonary vessels, stenting of highly restrictive MAPCAs, or coiling of redundant dual-supply collaterals.

Cardiac catheterization is rarely indicated for types I or II PA/VSD with normal-sized central confluent pulmonary arteries demonstrated by echocardiogram, because the risk of collaterals is low and surgical

(ascending aorta–to-pulmonary artery graft) and Melbourne shunt (direct end-to-side anastomosis of pulmonary artery to ascending aorta).[32]

The modified Blalock-Taussig shunt may be performed through a sternotomy or thoracotomy incision. The size of shunt used depends on the size of the child and morphology of the pulmonary artery. A 3.5-mm shunt supplies adequate flow to both lungs in a neonate, whereas 3.5- to 4-mm shunt is used to provide flow to each vascular bed for an infant undergoing thoracotomy for staged unifocalization. Thrombosis prophylaxis with the platelet inhibitor aspirin is the standard of care; the addition of clopidogrel may or may not provide further advantage.[33,34] The shunt is divided once continuity is established between the right ventricle and the unifocalized confluence.

Single-Stage Unifocalization

Through a sternotomy incision, MAPCAs, as they arise from the descending aorta, are identified in the posterior mediastinum by dissecting the infracarinal and paratracheal space. On institution of cardiopulmonary bypass, all MAPCAs must be controlled to avoid significant runoff into the pulmonary vasculature. MAPCAs are identified, divided, and incorporated into a central confluence. Functional assessment of pulmonary resistance may be performed at this time to guide the decision regarding VSD closure. One-stage complete repair entails VSD closure and an RV-to-PA conduit at the time of unifocalization. After cardioplegic arrest, an infundibular right ventriculotomy is performed, through which the VSD is closed with or without a fenestration. If adequacy of the pulmonary vasculature is questionable, it is safe to leave a fenestration because suprasystemic right ventricular pressures are not as well tolerated as a small residual left-to-right shunt. The unifocalized confluence is sewn to the distal end of the conduit. The proximal portion of the conduit is anastomosed to the right ventriculotomy incision, generally with a hood of pericardium to avoid distortion and tension at the proximal anastomosis.

Multiple-Stage Unifocalization

The decision regarding order of MAPCA unifocalization (right vs. left vessels) depends on the degree of compromise of vascular supply. The side with the most severe MAPCA restrictions is generally unifocalized first because these are at highest risk for progressive occlusion, and ligation of these collaterals at the time of the procedure is less likely to result in significant systemic desaturation. Through a thoracotomy, all MAPCAs are identified and ligated proximally. The distal pulmonary vessels are exposed and correlated with preoperative images to ensure that all essential vessels are unifocalized. Hilar dissection may be necessary to expose segmental vessels. A vascular graft (homograft, pericardial tube, or prosthetic) is anastomosed to all essential branch vessels. The proximal end of this vascular graft is placed anteriorly in the pleural space to facilitate eventual access through sternotomy at the time of complete repair. A shunt is placed between the subclavian artery and the conduit to provide antegrade pulmonary blood flow. This process is repeated in the contralateral thoracic cavity during a separate operation, although staged unifocalization at a single procedure has been performed.

Postoperative Assessment and Management

The success of repair for PA/VSD depends primarily on the anatomic result of pulmonary artery unifocalization or reconstruction. If a low-impedance pulmonary vascular system is achieved, closure of VSD may be performed with low right ventricular pressures. Right ventricular pressures of less than two-thirds systemic are generally felt to be well tolerated long term, whereas suprasystemic pressures are poorly tolerated in the short or long term.

Right ventricular pressure can be assessed following closure of the VSD in the operating room by direct measurement after separation from bypass. Right ventricular pressures greater than 80% of systemic arterial pressures often indicate inadequate pulmonary vascular bed. Because elevated right ventricular pressures are poorly tolerated long term, fenestration of the VSD patch must be performed if suprasystemic right ventricular pressures are encountered.

Postoperative echocardiography and lung perfusion scanning are noninvasive modalities used to follow up on the results of repair and guide further management. Lung perfusion scanning detects perfusion defects within various pulmonary segments and indicates pulmonary artery or MAPCA occlusion. Echocardiography is used to assess right ventricular pressures, intracardiac shunts, RVOT obstruction, and conduit regurgitation. The direction of flow across any residual VSD helps determine the degree of RVOT obstruction in patients undergoing staged palliation. The presence of primarily right-to-left shunting indicates inadequate pulmonary bed and warrants further pulmonary vascular rehabilitation or recruitment prior to VSD closure.

If progressive vascular disease is suspected by echocardiogram or perfusion scanning, cardiac catheterization is indicated. If multistage repair strategy has been undertaken, catheterization is performed before each stage. At cardiac catheterization, pulmonary artery pressures and Qp/Qs are measured. The Qp/Qs measurement by the Fick method may be inaccurate if dual sources of blood supply (MAPCA and right ventricle) are present. Cardiac catheterization also reveals pulmonary artery arborization pattern and size and allows intervention for pulmonary vascular rehabilitation. Transcatheter closure of fenestration in the VSD patch or PFO is possible if favorable conditions are present.

Results

Hospital survival for the initial procedures is greater than 90% in most series. Risk factors for poor outcome (mortality, reoperation, or failure of repair) following complete repair of PA/VSD and MAPCAs that have been identified include pulmonary artery morphology, 22Q11 microdeletion, and older age at palliation.[3,35,36]

Long-term results of repair for patients with hypoplastic or absent central pulmonary artery with MAPCAs are highly variable.[17,18,20,21,37-40] Approximately 80% of infants presenting with this anatomy may be amenable to single-stage unifocalization, and up to 50% of these patients are candidates for simultaneous complete repair. The operative mortality rate for single-stage unifocalization ranges from 2% to 15%. Survival rate at 5 years with either single- or multiple-stage unifocalization is 85% with eventual complete repair achieved in 70% to 90% of patients. In patients who undergo complete repair, elevated right ventricular pressures may be encountered in up to 50% of patients. Mean right ventricular to left ventricular pressure ratio reported in the literature at mid-term follow-up ranges from 0.4 to 0.6.[35,39] More than half of septated patients will require catheter intervention within 10 years following complete repair.[41] Reoperation following complete repair for conduit replacement is inevitable when complete repair is performed in neonates and infants.

Conclusion

PA/VSD encompasses a wide spectrum of lesions that are distinguished primarily by the pulmonary vascular morphology. The preoperative evaluation must delineate the source, size, and adequacy of pulmonary blood flow. Therapeutic strategy and timing are tailored according to the pulmonary vascular morphology, with the ultimate goal being establishment of a low-resistance pulmonary vascular bed, RV-to-PA continuity, elimination of intracardiac and extracardiac shunts, and resultant low right ventricular pressure. Surgical options include single-stage complete repair or staged palliation followed by complete repair, depending on the pulmonary artery morphology. Following complete repair, reintervention for pulmonary artery balloon dilation or conduit replacement is common. Long-term outcomes are dependent on the morphology of the pulmonary vasculature and the surgeon's ability to recruit a low-resistance vascular bed.

RIGHT VENTRICLE–TO–PULMONARY ARTERY CONDUITS

Introduction

Prosthetic valves and conduits are used to establish continuity between the pulmonary ventricle (morphologic right ventricle or left ventricle) and the pulmonary arteries as a part of complete repair or palliative reconstruction. Examples of defects with pulmonary obstruction that may require conduit placement include tetralogy of Fallot, pulmonary atresia (with intact ventricular septum or VSD), truncus arteriosus, D-transposition of the great arteries (TGA)/VSD or double-outlet right ventricle with pulmonary stenosis (as a part of Rastelli or Nikaidoh operations), and L-TGA/VSD with pulmonary stenosis. Conduits are also used concomitantly during procedures for left ventricular outflow tract (LVOT) obstruction that use the normal native pulmonary valve for the LVOT reconstruction. The Ross procedure, in which the pulmonary autograft is harvested and placed into the LVOT position, uses a conduit to reestablish RV-to-PA continuity. Similarly, the operation described by Yasui and colleagues[41a] for repair of interrupted aortic arch/VSD/ severe LVOT obstruction uses the normal pulmonary valve for LVOT reconstruction and requires placement of an RV-to-PA conduit.

Choice of Conduit

Options for ventricle–to–pulmonary artery continuity include synthetic, allograft, xenograft, and autologous tissue conduits. Unfortunately, none of the currently available conduits is ideal, and each is associated with specific advantages and disadvantages. None of the currently available conduits demonstrates growth potential, and conduit stenosis develops as the child grows. Factors to consider in the choice of a conduit include the pulmonary vascular resistance, age and size of the patient, and nature of the concomitant operation (complete repair versus palliation). For example, in the presence of elevated pulmonary vascular resistance, placement of a valved conduit (as opposed to nonvalved conduit) may be preferred to mitigate the effects of pulmonary regurgitation. Age and size of the patient are important because each type of conduit has a specific size limitation (Table 120-1). The type of operation influences the type and size of conduit to be implanted. Thus, if a conduit is required as a part of a palliative operation in which the VSD is left open, a restrictive conduit may be desirable to prevent excessive pulmonary blood flow. If reoperation is planned within a short time interval as a part of staged repair strategy, implantation of a low-cost but less durable conduit may be acceptable.

Allograft

Cryopreserved aortic and pulmonary allografts (or homografts) may be used for ventricle–to–pulmonary artery reconstruction. Advantages of allografts include availability in a wide range of sizes and favorable handling characteristics during implantation. Bifurcating pulmonary grafts or aortic branch vessels can be directly anastomosed to branch pulmonary arteries in the absence of adequate central pulmonary arteries. Major disadvantages include limited supply of the smaller sizes necessary for neonatal repair, the limited shelf life of each allograft (approximately 2 years), and high cost.

Choice of allograft characteristics and size depend on the age of patient and operative indication. For infants and small children who undergo conduit placement, use of conduit other than pulmonary allograft (synthetic, porcine xenografts, aortic homograft) has been shown to be a predictor of early reintervention, suggesting superiority of the pulmonary allograft for RVOT reconstruction.[42-46] Several studies have demonstrated superior longevity of pulmonary allografts compared with aortic allografts, partly because of the accelerated calcification seen in the latter.[42,45,47,48] However, aortic

TABLE 120-1 **Conduit Choices for Patients Based on Age**

Conduit Type	Sizes Available	Typical Patient Age Range	Commercial Name (U.S. Manufacturers)
Allograft			
Aortic	6-25 mm	All ages	CryoLife, LifeNet
Pulmonary	8-29 mm	All ages	CryoLife, LifeNet
Xenograft			
Bovine jugular vein	12-22 mm	<5 yr	Contegra (Medtronic)
Bovine jugular vein (stent-mounted)	18 mm	6 mo to 5 yr	Melody (Medtronic)
Porcine aortic root	19-29 mm	>5 yr	Freestyle (Medtronic) Prima Plus (Edwards)
Synthetic			
Composite porcine aortic valve within fabric conduit	12-30 mm	All ages	Hancock valved conduit (Medtronic) Carpentier-Edwards bioprosthetic valved conduit (Edwards)
Polyester Tube Graft			
Nonvalved + implanted bioprosthetic valve (>19 mm)	>4 mm 20-30 mm	<12 mo >5 yr	Hemashield (Atrium) Gelweave (Vascutek) Ultramax (Atrium)
PTFE Tube Graft			
Nonvalved + implanted bioprosthetic valve	>3 mm 20-24 mm	<12 mo >5 yr	Gore-Tex (Gore) Impra (Bard) Advanta (Atrium)

PTFE, Polytetrafluoroethylene.

homograft is chosen if elevated pulmonary artery pressures are anticipated (palliative conduit following unifocalization), as pulmonary allografts are associated with an increased risk of pseudoaneurysm formation in this setting.[49,50] The choice of size for a neonate may be influenced by limited availability of small-sized conduits. Modification of an allograft by excision of one leaflet and creation of a smaller "bicuspid" allograft allows use of larger-sized allografts in smaller patients when the appropriate-sized smaller allografts are unavailable.[51] The practice of implanting an oversized allograft into neonates and small children to improve conduit longevity may be associated with early development of conduit regurgitation in children.[52,53]

Whereas short-term competence of the homograft valve is acceptable, long-term freedom from regurgitation and stenosis is highly variable. Freedom from reintervention rates reported in the literature range widely from 30% to over 80% at 10 years.[8,44,48,54,55]

Smaller conduit size, or younger age at operation, has been consistently shown in multiple series to be a risk factor for allograft conduit failure with freedom from reoperation at 10 years being less than 50% for homografts less than 19 mm in diameter.[54] In adolescents, freedom from valvar dysfunction and conduit reintervention at 10 years is approximately 50% and 70%, respectively.[56] Other risk factors include use of aortic homografts, residual branch pulmonary artery stenosis, ABO or HLA mismatch, and non-Ross operation (particularly operation for truncus arteriosus).[48,52,57,58] The reason for the discrepancy in durability between Ross and non-Ross patients is unclear but may be related to orthotopic position of the conduit in the former; it is placed more anteriorly in Rastelli, Yasui, and truncus repairs, which may predispose to compression from the sternum.

Xenograft

Currently available xenograft conduits include bovine jugular vein and porcine aortic root. Advantages of xenograft conduits include abundant supply, low cost, wide range of sizes, and favorable suturing characteristics. The list of commercially available xenograft conduits and size ranges are listed in Table 120-1. Choice of xenograft conduit depends primarily on size and age of patient.

An alternative to allograft in a neonate or infant is the Medtronic Contegra graft, obtained from bovine jugular vein with similar short-term durability between Contegra and pulmonary allografts.[46,55,57,59] Although short-term durability is acceptable, long-term data are highly variable. Freedom from reintervention ranges from 66% at 3 years to 90% at 7 years.[57,59-61] Young age at implantation is a risk factor for reintervention and distal conduit stenosis.[62] In patients with elevated right ventricular pressure or pulmonary hypertension, the Contegra has been associated with graft dilation and decreased durability, raising concern for its use in these patients.[60,62,63] Surgical implantation of the externally stented bovine jugular vein graft (Melody valve) may limit graft dilation and improve long-term durability.

The porcine aortic root has been used for RVOT reconstruction in older children and adults and is available in sizes ranging from 19 to 29 mm.[64] These grafts appear to have excellent durability at short-term follow-up, but long-term data are still lacking.[65,66] This is an alternative to allograft or synthetic conduit in adolescents and adults.

Autologous Tissue

Autologous pericardium can be fashioned into a valved or valveless conduit and used for RV-to-PA reconstruction.[67] Monocusp and bicuspid valved conduits have been constructed by sewing autologous pericardial leaflets within a tubular pericardial conduit. Although there have been a few reports describing acceptable durability and even increase in the size of some conduits over time in certain cases, experience with this technique is limited.[68] Smaller conduit size is associated with increased risk of failure and limits its use in neonatal applications. Lack of access to commercially available conduits (in developing countries) may be an indication for its use.

Synthetic Conduits

Nonvalved. Valveless conduits are used in several settings. A palliative synthetic tube graft from an RV-to-PA conduit may be used in patients with PA/VSD and confluent but hypoplastic central pulmonary arteries in whom pulmonary artery growth is desired. In these patients, the VSD is left open and exposes the pulmonary arteries to elevated pressure. Nonvalved PTFE tube grafts are also used for the RV-to-PA conduit in the stage 1 reconstruction of hypoplastic left heart syndrome. Transmural insertion of a ring-reinforced RV-to-PA PTFE conduit reduces the risk of proximal obstruction compared with epicardial suture technique.[69] In patients undergoing complete repair with VSD closure, selective use of nonvalved conduits is acceptable but should be avoided in patients with elevated pulmonary vascular resistance, unrepaired tricuspid valve regurgitation, or right ventricular failure.[70,71]

Valved. Composite conduits made of polyester or PTFE tube grafts with bioprosthetic or mechanical valves are available commercially or can be assembled at the time of the operation (see Table 120-1). Manually constructed composite conduits use a low profile valve secured within the synthetic conduit. Bioprosthetic valves are almost exclusively used because anticoagulation is necessary for mechanical valves, and transcatheter valve replacement is feasible only for the bioprosthetic valves.[72] Advantages of the synthetic valved conduits include excellent longevity and virtually unlimited shelf life, which makes them readily available. The enclosed bioprosthetic valves have a rigid annulus that is resistant to distortion or compression by external structures (sternum).

A major disadvantage of composite polyester conduits less than 19 mm is accelerated stenosis compared with homografts, which has limited their application in neonates and infants.[61,73,74] Manually constructed conduits are limited by size availability (the smallest bioprosthetic valve is 19 mm) and are commonly used for replacement of obstructed conduits in older children and young adults. Unlike tissue conduits, these conduits are not amenable to catheter-based enlargement if a child were to outgrow the conduit; thus, implantation of a graft between 24 and 28 mm is optimal. Previous studies suggested inferior durability of these conduits compared with allografts, but recent studies have demonstrated freedom from reintervention of greater than 90% at 5 years.[75-78] For larger-sized conduits (>19 mm), durability of porcine-valved polyester or PTFE conduit appears to be equivalent, and perhaps superior, to that of allografts.[56,71,79,80]

Results

Short- and long-term mortality rates following implantation of an RV-to-PA conduit depend primarily on the underlying cardiac diagnosis and hemodynamic result of the operation. In most recent series, the hospital mortality rate among patients who underwent RV-to-PA conduit implantation has ranged from 1% to 10%, depending on the complexity of the underlying cardiac disease.[71] Risk factors for late mortality have included older age at primary operation and elevated right ventricular to left ventricular pressure ratio.[60] Conduit freedom from reintervention (surgical or catheter-based) varies significantly depending on conduit or patient type. The strongest risk factor for early reintervention in most of these series has been younger age at operation or use of smaller-sized conduits.[81]

Conduit Replacement or Reconstruction

Conduit failure may present in the form of either obstruction or valvular incompetence. The decision to intervene on a conduit hinges on the deleterious effects of conduit failure on right ventricular function. Intervention on the conduit may come in the form of catheter-based balloon dilation and stenting for conduit stenosis or endovascular implantation of pulmonary valve for conduit regurgitation. Surgical reconstruction includes patch augmentation of stenotic conduit and implantation of a prosthetic valve within the in situ conduit. Conduit replacement refers to removal of the conduit and the insertion of a new conduit.

Although there are no established guidelines for conduit replacement, common indications for conduit reintervention include symptoms of right heart failure as well as evidence of right ventricular deterioration in an asymptomatic patient. In the presence of conduit stenosis, the development of right ventricular hypertension (>3/4 systemic) or right ventricular dysfunction should prompt consideration of intervention. Isolated conduit regurgitation, even if severe, can be well tolerated for many years. Data regarding indications for PVR following transannular patch repair of tetralogy of Fallot have been extrapolated to guide management of conduit dysfunction.[82] Symptoms of exercise intolerance, peripheral edema, and arrhythmias are considered indications for surgery. In an asymptomatic patient, right ventricular dilation (>150 mL/m^2), progressive tricuspid regurgitation, QRS prolongation, and ventricular dysfunction are relative indications.[82-85]

Frequently, catheter-based intervention is successful at relieving conduit obstruction. Greater than 90% of patients presenting with conduit stenosis are amenable to such intervention, and an immediate reduction in right ventricular pressures by approximately 20% can be expected.[86,87] Although conduit stenting has been shown to delay the need for surgical intervention, smaller conduit sizes (less than 10 mm), use of a homograft conduit, and younger age are associated with shorter freedom from surgery.[87] Experience with percutaneous transcatheter implantation of Melody valve within previous RVOT conduit is encouraging. Freedom from valvular dysfunction of 93% at 1 year and greater than 70% at 5 years has been demonstrated.[88,89] Use of this transcatheter valve has increased dramatically over the past 5 years but is limited to patients in whom conduit internal diameter can be expanded to 22 mm, which is the optimal external diameter of the Melody valve. Patients with conduit internal diameter greater than 24 mm are not candidates, because the valve cannot be sealed within the RVOT.

Options for surgical intervention on dysfunctional conduit include replacement and reconstruction. Conduit reconstruction is performed by incising the anterior portion of the conduit, implantation of a prosthetic valve, and placement of a prosthetic roof over the remaining fibrous bed of the explanted conduit. This type of reconstruction is a durable alternative to conduit replacement, with 90% freedom from reoperation at 10 years.[90] Alternatively, conduit replacement may be performed with an appropriately sized graft.

Increasing experience with transcatheter valves has prompted interest in hybrid techniques for valve insertion in patients with high surgical risk but enlarged RVOT (hence not candidates for transcatheter replacement). Techniques include transapical or transfemoral delivery with fixation in the pulmonary artery without the use of cardiopulmonary bypass.

Technical Considerations

It is important to evaluate the position of the conduit relative to the sternum on the available preoperative imaging (lateral chest x-ray, catheterization, MRI, or CT scan).[91] Fusion of calcified conduit to the posterior table of the sternum may warrant cannulation of the femoral vessels and institution of cardiopulmonary bypass prior to sternal entry.[91,92] The presence of residual intracardiac shunts (PFO or VSD) should be determined preoperatively because the decision to close any residual defects guides the intraoperative cannulation and bypass strategy. Air entrainment during cardiopulmonary bypass can be associated with stroke, and the use of cardioplegic arrest or fibrillation with left ventricular venting is preferable to empty, beating heart.

If atrial or ventricular arrhythmias are present, preoperative evaluation by electrophysiologic mapping and ablation are appropriate. Surgical cryoablation is recommended for patients with atrial or monomorphic ventricular arrhythmias in whom preoperative ablation is not performed or is unsuccessful.[93]

Results

The operative mortality rate of conduit replacement or reconstruction is 5% to 10%, and long-term results (mortality, freedom from reoperation) after reoperation for conduit replacement or reconstruction are equivalent to those of primary conduit placement.[58,94]

REFERENCES

1. Leonard H, Derrick G, O'Sullivan J, et al: Natural and unnatural history of pulmonary atresia. *Heart* 84:499–503, 2000.
2. Cantinotti M, Hegde S, Bell A, et al: Diagnostic role of magnetic resonance imaging in identifying aortic arch anomalies. *Congenit Heart Dis* 3:117–123, 2008.
3. Mahle WT, Crisalli J, Coleman K, et al: Deletion of chromosome 22q11.2 and outcome in patients with pulmonary atresia and ventricular septal defect. *Ann Thorac Surg* 76:567–571, 2003.
4. Tchervenkov CI, Roy N: Congenital Heart Surgery Nomenclature and Database Project: pulmonary atresia–ventricular septal defect. *Ann Thorac Surg* 69:S97–S105, 2000.
5. Bull K, Somerville J, Ty E, et al: Presentation and attrition in complex pulmonary atresia. *J Am Coll Cardiol* 25:491–499, 1995.
6. Geva T, Greil GF, Marshall AC, et al: Gadolinium-enhanced 3-dimensional magnetic resonance angiography of pulmonary blood supply in patients with complex pulmonary stenosis or atresia: comparison with x-ray angiography. *Circulation* 106:473–478, 2002.
7. Dowdle SC, Human DG, Mann MD: Pulmonary ventilation and perfusion abnormalities and ventilation perfusion imbalance in children with pulmonary atresia or extreme tetralogy of Fallot. *J Nucl Med* 31:1276–1279, 1990.
8. Kaza AK, Lim HG, Dibardino DJ, et al: Long-term results of right ventricular outflow tract reconstruction in neonatal cardiac surgery: options and outcomes. *J Thorac Cardiovasc Surg* 138:911–916, 2009.
9. Gerelli S, van Steenberghe M, Murtuza B, et al: Neonatal right ventricle to pulmonary connection as a palliative procedure for pulmonary atresia with ventricular septal defect or severe tetralogy of Fallot. *Eur J Cardiothorac Surg* 45:278–288, discussion 288, 2014.
10. Mumtaz MA, Rosenthal G, Qureshi A, et al: Melbourne shunt promotes growth of diminutive central pulmonary arteries in patients with pulmonary atresia, ventricular septal defect, and systemic-to-pulmonary collateral arteries. *Ann Thorac Surg* 85:2079–2083, discussion 2083–2084, 2008.
11. Amark KM, Karamlou T, O'Carroll A, et al: Independent factors associated with mortality, reintervention, and achievement of complete repair in children with pulmonary atresia with ventricular septal defect. *J Am Coll Cardiol* 47:1448–1456, 2006.
12. Gladman G, McCrindle BW, Williams WG, et al: The modified Blalock-Taussig shunt: clinical impact and morbidity in Fallot's tetralogy in the current era. *J Thorac Cardiovasc Surg* 114:25–30, 1997.
13. Walsh MA, Lee KJ, Chaturvedi R, et al: Radiofrequency perforation of the right ventricular outflow tract as a palliative strategy for pulmonary atresia with ventricular septal defect. *Catheter Cardiovasc Interv* 69:1015–1020, 2007.
14. Santoro G, Capozzi G, Caianiello G, et al: Pulmonary artery growth after palliation of congenital heart disease with duct-dependent pulmonary circulation: arterial duct stenting versus surgical shunt. *J Am Coll Cardiol* 54:2180–2186, 2009.
15. Alwi M, Choo KK, Latiff HA, et al: Initial results and medium-term follow-up of stent implantation of patent ductus arteriosus in duct-dependent pulmonary circulation. *J Am Coll Cardiol* 44:438–445, 2004.
16. Zheng S, Yang K, Li K, et al: Establishment of right ventricle-pulmonary artery continuity as the first-stage palliation in older infants with pulmonary atresia with ventricular septal defect may be preferable to use of an arterial shunt. *Interact Cardiovasc Thorac Surg* 19:88–94, 2014.
17. Carotti A, Albanese SB, Filippelli S, et al: Determinants of outcome after surgical treatment of pulmonary atresia with ventricular septal defect and major aortopulmonary collateral arteries. *J Thorac Cardiovasc Surg* 140:1092–1103, 2010.
18. Liava'a M, Brizard CP, Konstantinov IE, et al: Pulmonary atresia, ventricular septal defect, and major aortopulmonary collaterals: neonatal pulmonary artery rehabilitation without unifocalization. *Ann Thorac Surg* 93:185–191, 2012.
19. d'Udekem Y, Alphonso N, Norgaard MA, et al: Pulmonary atresia with ventricular septal defects and major aortopulmonary collateral

arteries: unifocalization brings no long-term benefits. *J Thorac Cardiovasc Surg* 130:1496–1502, 2005.
20. Watanabe N, Mainwaring RD, Reddy VM, et al: Early complete repair of pulmonary atresia with ventricular septal defect and major aortopulmonary collaterals. *Ann Thorac Surg* 97:909–915, discussion 914–915, 2014.
21. Cho JM, Puga FJ, Danielson GK, et al: Early and long-term results of the surgical treatment of tetralogy of Fallot with pulmonary atresia, with or without major aortopulmonary collateral arteries. *J Thorac Cardiovasc Surg* 124:70–81, 2002.
22. Carotti A, Di Donato RM, Squitieri C, et al: Total repair of pulmonary atresia with ventricular septal defect and major aortopulmonary collaterals: an integrated approach. *J Thorac Cardiovasc Surg* 116:914–923, 1998.
23. Honjo O, Al-Radi OO, MacDonald C, et al: The functional intraoperative pulmonary blood flow study is a more sensitive predictor than preoperative anatomy for right ventricular pressure and physiologic tolerance of ventricular septal defect closure after complete unifocalization in patients with pulmonary atresia, ventricular septal defect, and major aortopulmonary collaterals. *Circulation* 120:S46–S52, 2009.
24. Carotti A, Albanese SB, Minniti G, et al: Increasing experience with integrated approach to pulmonary atresia with ventricular septal defect and major aortopulmonary collateral arteries. *Eur J Cardiothorac Surg* 23:719–726, discussion 726–727, 2003.
25. Grosse-Wortmann L, Yoo SJ, van Arsdell G, et al: Preoperative total pulmonary blood flow predicts right ventricular pressure in patients early after complete repair of tetralogy of Fallot and pulmonary atresia with major aortopulmonary collateral arteries. *J Thorac Cardiovasc Surg* 146:1185–1190, 2013.
26. Luciani GB, Wells WJ, Khong A, et al: The clamshell incision for bilateral pulmonary artery reconstruction in tetralogy of Fallot with pulmonary atresia. *J Thorac Cardiovasc Surg* 113:443–452, 1997.
27. Goerler H, Simon A, Gohrbandt B, et al: Heart-lung and lung transplantation in grown-up congenital heart disease: long-term single centre experience. *Eur J Cardiothorac Surg* 32:926–931, 2007.
28. Brown JW, Ruzmetov M, Vijay P, et al: Right ventricular outflow tract reconstruction with a polytetrafluoroethylene monocusp valve: a twelve-year experience. *J Thorac Cardiovasc Surg* 133:1336–1343, 2007.
29. Yang JH, Jun TG, Park PW, et al: Factors related to the durability of a homograft monocusp valve inserted during repair of tetralogy of Fallot as based on the mid- to long-term outcomes. *Cardiol Young* 18:141–146, 2008.
30. Knott-Craig CJ, Elkins RC, Lane MM, et al: A 26-year experience with surgical management of tetralogy of Fallot: risk analysis for mortality or late reintervention. *Ann Thorac Surg* 66:506–511, 1998.
31. Zahorec M, Hrubsova Z, Skrak P, et al: A comparison of Blalock-Taussig shunts with and without closure of the ductus arteriosus in neonates with pulmonary atresia. *Ann Thorac Surg* 92:653–658, 2011.
32. Kim H, Sung SC, Choi KH, et al: A central shunt to rehabilitate diminutive pulmonary arteries in patients with pulmonary atresia with ventricular septal defect. *J Thorac Cardiovasc Surg* 149(2):515–520, 2015.
33. Heidari-Bateni G, Norouzi S, Hall M, et al: Defining the best practice patterns for the neonatal systemic-to-pulmonary artery shunt procedure. *J Thorac Cardiovasc Surg* 147:869–873.e3, 2014.
34. Wessel DL, Berger F, Li JS, et al: Clopidogrel in infants with systemic-to-pulmonary-artery shunts. *N Engl J Med* 368:2377–2384, 2013.
35. Ishibashi N, Shin'oka T, Ishiyama M, et al: Clinical results of staged repair with complete unifocalization for pulmonary atresia with ventricular septal defect and major aortopulmonary collateral arteries. *Eur J Cardiothorac Surg* 32:202–208, 2007.
36. Griselli M, McGuirk SP, Winlaw DS, et al: The influence of pulmonary artery morphology on the results of operations for major aortopulmonary collateral arteries and complex congenital heart defects. *J Thorac Cardiovasc Surg* 127:251–258, 2004.
37. Malhotra SP, Hanley FL: Surgical management of pulmonary atresia with ventricular septal defect and major aortopulmonary collaterals: a protocol-based approach. *Semin Thorac Cardiovasc Surg* 145–151, 2009.
38. Fouilloux V, Bonello B, Kammache I, et al: Management of patients with pulmonary atresia, ventricular septal defect, hypoplastic pulmonary arteries and major aorto-pulmonary collaterals: focus on the strategy of rehabilitation of the native pulmonary arteries. *Arch Cardiovasc Dis* 105:666–675, 2012.
39. Mainwaring RD, Reddy VM, Peng L, et al: Hemodynamic assessment after complete repair of pulmonary atresia with major aortopulmonary collaterals. *Ann Thorac Surg* 95:1397–1402, 2013.
40. Davies B, Mussa S, Davies P, et al: Unifocalization of major aortopulmonary collateral arteries in pulmonary atresia with ventricular septal defect is essential to achieve excellent outcomes irrespective of native pulmonary artery morphology. *J Thorac Cardiovasc Surg* 138:1269–1275.e1, 2009.
41. Duncan BW, Mee RB, Prieto LR, et al: Staged repair of tetralogy of Fallot with pulmonary atresia and major aortopulmonary collateral arteries. *J Thorac Cardiovasc Surg* 126:694–702, 2003.
41a. Yasui H, Kado H, Nakano E, et al: Primary repair of interrupted aortic arch and severe aortic stenosis in neonates. *J Thorac Cardiovasc Surg* 93(4):539–545, 1987.
42. Niemantsverdriet MB, Ottenkamp J, Gauvreau K, et al: Determinants of right ventricular outflow tract conduit longevity: a multinational analysis. *Congenit Heart Dis* 3:176–184, 2008.
43. Reddy VM, Rajasinghe HA, McElhinney DB, et al: Performance of right ventricle to pulmonary artery conduits after repair of truncus arteriosus: a comparison of Dacron-housed porcine valves and cryopreserved allografts. *Semin Thorac Cardiovasc Surg* 7:133–138, 1995.
44. Niwaya K, Knott-Craig CJ, Lane MM, et al: Cryopreserved homograft valves in the pulmonary position: risk analysis for intermediate-term failure. *J Thorac Cardiovasc Surg* 117:141–146, discussion 46–47, 1999.
45. Bando K, Danielson GK, Schaff HV, et al: Outcome of pulmonary and aortic homografts for right ventricular outflow tract reconstruction. *J Thorac Cardiovasc Surg* 109:509–517, discussion 517–518, 1995.
46. Boethig D, Thies WR, Hecker H, et al: Mid term course after pediatric right ventricular outflow tract reconstruction: a comparison of homografts, porcine xenografts and Contegras. *Eur J Cardiothorac Surg* 27:58–66, 2005.
47. Albert JD, Bishop DA, Fullerton DA, et al: Conduit reconstruction of the right ventricular outflow tract. Lessons learned in a twelve-year experience. *J Thorac Cardiovasc Surg* 106:228–235, discussion 235–236, 1993.
48. Tweddell JS, Pelech AN, Frommelt PC, et al: Factors affecting longevity of homograft valves used in right ventricular outflow tract reconstruction for congenital heart disease. *Circulation* 102:III130–III135, 2000.
49. DeLeon SY, Tuchek JM, Bell TJ, et al: Early pulmonary homograft failure from dilatation due to distal pulmonary artery stenosis. *Ann Thorac Surg* 61:234–236, discussion 236–237, 1996.
50. Levine JC, Mayer JE, Jr, Keane JF, et al: Anastomotic pseudoaneurysm of the ventricle after homograft placement in children. *Ann Thorac Surg* 59:60–66, 1995.
51. McMullan DM, Oppido G, Alphonso N, et al: Evaluation of downsized homograft conduits for right ventricle-to-pulmonary artery reconstruction. *J Thorac Cardiovasc Surg* 132:66–71, 2006.
52. Askovich B, Hawkins JA, Sower CT, et al: Right ventricle-to-pulmonary artery conduit longevity: is it related to allograft size? *Ann Thorac Surg* 84:907–911, discussion 911–912, 2007.
53. Karamlou T, Ungerleider RM, Alsoufi B, et al: Oversizing pulmonary homograft conduits does not significantly decrease allograft failure in children. *Eur J Cardiothorac Surg* 27:548–553, 2005.
54. Boethig D, Goerler H, Westhoff-Bleck M, et al: Evaluation of 188 consecutive homografts implanted in pulmonary position after 20 years. *Eur J Cardiothorac Surg* 32:133–142, 2007.
55. Meyns B, Jashari R, Gewillig M, et al: Factors influencing the survival of cryopreserved homografts. The second homograft performs as well as the first. *Eur J Cardiothorac Surg* 28:211–216, discussion 216, 2005.
56. Batlivala SP, Emani S, Mayer JE, et al: Pulmonary valve replacement function in adolescents: a comparison of bioprosthetic valves and homograft conduits. *Ann Thorac Surg* 93:2007–2016, 2012.
57. Sierra J, Christenson JT, Lahlaidi NH, et al: Right ventricular outflow tract reconstruction: what conduit to use? Homograft or Contegra? *Ann Thorac Surg* 84:606–610, discussion 610–611, 2007.

58. Rodefeld MD, Ruzmetov M, Turrentine MW, et al: Reoperative right ventricular outflow tract conduit reconstruction: risk analyses at follow up. *J Heart Valve Dis* 17:119–126, discussion 126, 2008.
59. Brown JW, Ruzmetov M, Rodefeld MD, et al: Valved bovine jugular vein conduits for right ventricular outflow tract reconstruction in children: an attractive alternative to pulmonary homograft. *Ann Thorac Surg* 82:909–916, 2006.
60. Shebani SO, McGuirk S, Baghai M, et al: Right ventricular outflow tract reconstruction using Contegra valved conduit: natural history and conduit performance under pressure. *Eur J Cardiothorac Surg* 29:397–405, 2006.
61. Vitanova K, Cleuziou J, Horer J, et al: Which type of conduit to choose for right ventricular outflow tract reconstruction in patients below 1 year of age? *Eur J Cardiothorac Surg* 46:961–966, discussion 966, 2014.
62. Sekarski N, van Meir H, Rijlaarsdam ME, et al: Right ventricular outflow tract reconstruction with the bovine jugular vein graft: 5 years' experience with 133 patients. *Ann Thorac Surg* 84:599–605, 2007.
63. Bautista-Hernandez V, Kaza AK, Benavidez OJ, et al: True aneurysmal dilatation of a contegra conduit after right ventricular outflow tract reconstruction: a novel mechanism of conduit failure. *Ann Thorac Surg* 86:1976–1977, 2008.
64. Hartz RS, Deleon SY, Lane J, et al: Medtronic freestyle valves in right ventricular outflow tract reconstruction. *Ann Thorac Surg* 76:1896–1900, 2003.
65. Erez E, Tam VK, Doublin NA, et al: Repeat right ventricular outflow tract reconstruction using the Medtronic Freestyle porcine aortic root. *J Heart Valve Dis* 15:92–96, 2006.
66. Kanter KR, Fyfe DA, Mahle WT, et al: Results with the freestyle porcine aortic root for right ventricular outflow tract reconstruction in children. *Ann Thorac Surg* 76:1889–1894, discussion 1894–1895, 2003.
67. Isomatsu Y, Shin'oka T, Aoki M, et al: Establishing right ventricle-pulmonary artery continuity by autologous tissue: an alternative approach for prosthetic conduit repair. *Ann Thorac Surg* 78:173–180, 2004.
68. Schlichter AJ, Kreutzer C, Mayorquim RC, et al: Five- to fifteen-year follow-up of fresh autologous pericardial valved conduits. *J Thorac Cardiovasc Surg* 119:869–879, 2000.
69. Baird CW, Myers PO, Borisuk M, et al: Ring-reinforced Sano conduit at Norwood stage I reduces proximal conduit obstruction. *Ann Thorac Surg* 99(1):171–179, 2015.
70. Downing TP, Danielson GK, Schaff HV, et al: Replacement of obstructed right ventricular-pulmonary arterial valved conduits with nonvalved conduits in children. *Circulation* 72:II84–II87, 1985.
71. Dearani JA, Danielson GK, Puga FJ, et al: Late follow-up of 1095 patients undergoing operation for complex congenital heart disease utilizing pulmonary ventricle to pulmonary artery conduits. *Ann Thorac Surg* 75:399–410, discussion 410–411, 2003.
72. Haas F, Schreiber C, Horer J, et al: Is there a role for mechanical valved conduits in the pulmonary position? *Ann Thorac Surg* 79:1662–1667, discussion 1667–1668, 2005.
73. Belli E, Salihoglu E, Leobon B, et al: The performance of Hancock porcine-valved Dacron conduit for right ventricular outflow tract reconstruction. *Ann Thorac Surg* 89:152–157, discussion 157–158, 2010.
74. Schiralli MP, Cholette JM, Swartz MF, et al: Carpentier Edwards porcine valved conduit for right ventricular outflow tract reconstruction. *J Card Surg* 26:643–649, 2011.
75. Chen PC, Sager MS, Zurakowski D, et al: Younger age and valve oversizing are predictors of structural valve deterioration after pulmonary valve replacement in patients with tetralogy of Fallot. *J Thorac Cardiovasc Surg* 143:352–360, 2012.
76. Homann M, Haehnel JC, Mendler N, et al: Reconstruction of the RVOT with valved biological conduits: 25 years experience with allografts and xenografts. *Eur J Cardiothorac Surg* 17:624–630, 2000.
77. Kobayashi J, Backer CL, Zales VR, et al: Failure of the Hemashield extension in right ventricle-to-pulmonary artery conduits. *Ann Thorac Surg* 56:277–281, 1993.
78. Agarwal KC, Edwards WD, Feldt RH, et al: Pathogenesis of nonobstructive fibrous peels in right-sided porcine-valved extracardiac conduits. *J Thorac Cardiovasc Surg* 83:584–589, 1982.
79. Razzouk AJ, Williams WG, Cleveland DC, et al: Surgical connections from ventricle to pulmonary artery. Comparison of four types of valved implants. *Circulation* 86:II154–II158, 1992.
80. Allen BS, El-Zein C, Cuneo B, et al: Pericardial tissue valves and Gore-Tex conduits as an alternative for right ventricular outflow tract replacement in children. *Ann Thorac Surg* 74:771–777, 2002.
81. Forbess JM, Shah AS, St Louis JD, et al: Cryopreserved homografts in the pulmonary position: determinants of durability. *Ann Thorac Surg* 71:54–59, discussion 59–60, 2001.
82. Geva T: Indications and timing of pulmonary valve replacement after tetralogy of Fallot repair. *Semin Thorac Cardiovasc Surg* 11–22, 2006.
83. Vliegen HW, van Straten A, de Roos A, et al: Magnetic resonance imaging to assess the hemodynamic effects of pulmonary valve replacement in adults late after repair of tetralogy of fallot. *Circulation* 106:1703–1707, 2002.
84. Therrien J, Provost Y, Merchant N, et al: Optimal timing for pulmonary valve replacement in adults after tetralogy of Fallot repair. *Am J Cardiol* 95:779–782, 2005.
85. Ammash NM, Dearani JA, Burkhart HM, et al: Pulmonary regurgitation after tetralogy of Fallot repair: clinical features, sequelae, and timing of pulmonary valve replacement. *Congenit Heart Dis* 2:386–403, 2007.
86. Aggarwal S, Garekar S, Forbes TJ, et al: Is stent placement effective for palliation of right ventricle to pulmonary artery conduit stenosis? *J Am Coll Cardiol* 49:480–484, 2007.
87. Peng LF, McElhinney DB, Nugent AW, et al: Endovascular stenting of obstructed right ventricle-to-pulmonary artery conduits: a 15-year experience. *Circulation* 113:2598–2605, 2006.
88. McElhinney DB, Hellenbrand WE, Zahn EM, et al: Short- and medium-term outcomes after transcatheter pulmonary valve placement in the expanded multicenter US melody valve trial. *Circulation* 122:507–516, 2010.
89. Lurz P, Gaudin R, Taylor AM, et al: Percutaneous pulmonary valve implantation. *Semin Thorac Cardiovasc Surg* 112–117, 2009.
90. Bermudez CA, Dearani JA, Puga FJ, et al: Late results of the peel operation for replacement of failing extracardiac conduits. *Ann Thorac Surg* 77:881–887, discussion 888, 2004.
91. Kogon BE, Daniel W, Fay K, et al: Is the liberal use of preoperative 3-dimensional imaging and presternotomy femoral cutdown beneficial in reoperative adult congenital heart surgery? *J Thorac Cardiovasc Surg* 147:1799–1804, 2014.
92. Kirshbom PM, Myung RJ, Simsic JM, et al: One thousand repeat sternotomies for congenital cardiac surgery: risk factors for reentry injury. *Ann Thorac Surg* 88:158–161, 2009.
93. Therrien J, Siu SC, Harris L, et al: Impact of pulmonary valve replacement on arrhythmia propensity late after repair of tetralogy of Fallot. *Circulation* 103:2489–2494, 2001.
94. Bielefeld MR, Bishop DA, Campbell DN, et al: Reoperative homograft right ventricular outflow tract reconstruction. *Ann Thorac Surg* 71:482–487, discussion 487–488, 2001.

CHAPTER 121

TRUNCUS ARTERIOSUS AND AORTOPULMONARY WINDOW

Jennifer C. Hirsch-Romano • Richard G. Ohye • Ming-Sing Si • Edward L. Bove

CHAPTER OUTLINE

TRUNCUS ARTERIOSUS

Truncus arteriosus is a relatively rare congenital heart defect with a single vascular trunk arising from the heart, giving origin to the true pulmonary arteries, aorta, coronary arteries, and brachiocephalic vessels. The lesion accounts for approximately 0.4% to 4.0% of all congenital heart lesions.[1-3] Truncus arteriosus was first described by Wilson[4] in 1798. In 1942, Lev and Saphir[5] defined the anatomy currently associated with truncus arteriosus.

Embryology

During the fifth week of gestation, paired lateral ridges appear in the cephalic portion of the truncus. These truncal swellings ultimately form the aorticopulmonary septum. The right superior truncus swelling, located on the right superior wall of the truncus, grows distally and leftward, whereas the left inferior truncus swelling, located on the left inferior wall, moves distally and rightward. The opposing movements of the swellings as they grow toward the aortic sac result in the spiraling of the aorticopulmonary septum. The most proximal portions of the swellings form parts of the infundibular or conal septum. Hence, variable deficiency of these truncal swellings results in the various forms of truncus arteriosus and the commonly present ventricular septal defect (VSD).

Pluripotent neural crest cells play an important role in the development of the conotruncus and aortic arch. Deletion of Cdc42 (cell division cycle 42), a GTP-binding protein that regulates cytoskeleton remodeling and is essential for neural crest cell migration, results in persistent truncus arteriosus and interrupted aortic arches in murine models.[6] Selective ablation of neural crest cells in chick embryos before migration results in a number of congenital heart defects.[7] These anomalies include truncus arteriosus and interrupted aortic arch, explaining their coexistence in approximately 10% to 20% of patients with truncus arteriosus.[8,9]

Animal models provide further insight into the genetic basis for truncus arteriosus. The mouse mutant *Splotch*, which has a mutation in the homeobox gene *Pax3*, has a phenotype with truncus arteriosus and aortic arch abnormalities.[10] In humans, monoallelic microdeletion of chromosome 22q11 is associated with multiple defects of neural crest origin, including typical facies, cleft palate, thyroid and parathyroid gland aplasia, and conotruncal and aortic arch abnormalities. The resulting phenotypic syndromes include DiGeorge, velocardiofacial, and Shprintzen syndromes, which are associated with truncus arteriosus. One candidate gene identified in the area of the microdeletion is *HIRA*. *HIRA* interacts with *Pax3*, and thus may be integral to *Pax3* regulation of neural crest cells.[11] Environmental risk factors for the development of truncus arteriosus include maternal diabetes and exposure to retinoic acid.

Anatomy

In truncus arteriosus, there is generally situs solitus and D-looping of the ventricles. A single great vessel arises from the base of the heart, giving origin to the pulmonary, systemic, and coronary arteries. Classifications of truncus arteriosus were proposed by Collett and Edwards[12] in 1949 and by Van Praagh and Van Praagh[13] in 1965 (Fig. 121-1). The system described by Collett and Edwards (Table 121-1) is based on the site of origin of the pulmonary arteries, whereas the Van Praagh classification (Table 121-2) is based on the degree of septation of the trunk and the presence or absence of a VSD. The Van Praagh scheme also requires that at least one of the pulmonary arteries arise from the common trunk. This stipulation appropriately relegates Collett-Edwards type IV, or *pseudotruncus*, to the spectrum of pulmonary atresia with aortopulmonary collaterals. The Van Praagh classification also provides for the inclusion of the relatively common association of hypoplastic or interrupted aortic arch. The term *hemitruncus* is frequently encountered in the literature to describe the anomalous origin of the right pulmonary artery from the ascending aorta with a normal origin of the left pulmonary artery from the main pulmonary artery, usually in the absence of a VSD. This lesion is distinct from Van Praagh type B3 and should not be considered a form of truncus arteriosus.

A VSD is nearly always present. It results from the deficiency of the infundibular septum and is generally

TABLE 121-1 Collett and Edwards Classification

Type	Description
I	Branch pulmonary arteries arise from a segment of the main pulmonary artery off the common trunk.
II	Branch pulmonary arteries arise in close proximity from the posterior aspect of the common trunk.
III	Branch pulmonary arteries arise from separate, widely spaced origins.
IV	Absent "true" branch pulmonary arteries with aortopulmonary collaterals

TABLE 121-2 Van Praagh and Van Praagh Classification

Classification	Description
Type A	Ventricular septal defect present
Type B	Ventricular septal defect absent
1	Partial development of the aorticopulmonary septum
2	Absence of the aorticopulmonary septum
3	Absence of one of the branch pulmonary arteries
4	Coarctation, hypoplasia, or interruption of the aortic arch with a patent ductus arteriosus

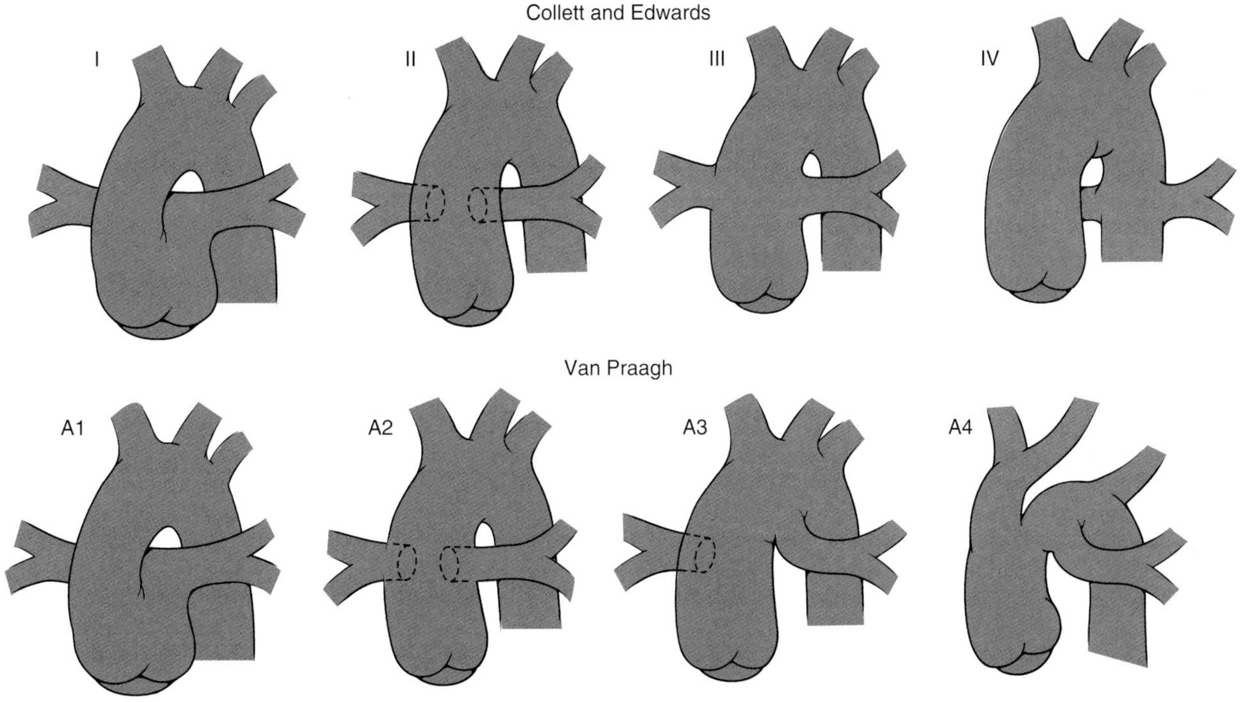

FIGURE 121-1 Comparison of the Collett and Edwards and the Van Praagh and Van Praagh classifications of truncus arteriosus.

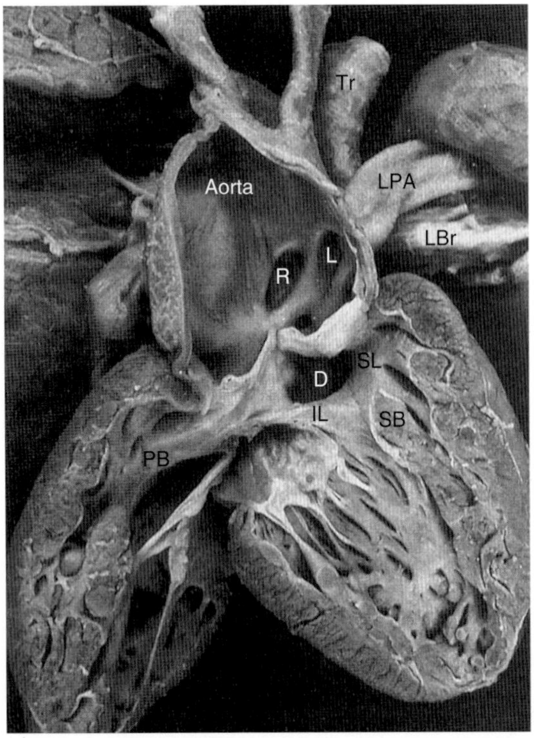

FIGURE 121-2 ■ Right ventricular view of the pathologic anatomy of truncus arteriosus. The truncal origins of the aorta and left (L) and right (R) pulmonary arteries are apparent. The ventricular septal defect (D) is cradled between the inferior (IL) and superior (SL) limbs of the septal band (SB). Insertion of the IL into the parietal band (PB) provides muscular discontinuity between the tricuspid and truncal valves. *LBr,* Left bronchus; *LPA,* left pulmonary artery; *Tr,* trachea. (Reprinted with permission from Mair DD, Edwards WD, Julsrud PR, et al: Truncus arteriosus. In Allen HD, Gutgesell HP, Clark EB, Driscoll DJ, editors: *Moss and Adams' heart disease in infants, children and adolescents,* Philadelphia, 2001, Lippincott Williams & Wilkins, p 505.)

nonrestrictive. The VSD is cradled by the two limbs of the septal band and bounded superiorly by the truncal valve (Fig. 121-2). The posterior (inferior) limb of the septal band usually inserts into the parietal band, resulting in discontinuity of the tricuspid and truncal valves, maintaining a muscular rim between the conduction system and the VSD. When there is failure of insertion, the VSD extends into the membranous septum, with the conduction system running along the posterior-inferior rim of the defect.

The truncal valve can be tricuspid (69%), quadricuspid (22%), bicuspid (9%), or, rarely, unicuspid or pentacuspid.[14] The valve is usually in continuity with the mitral valve and infrequently with the tricuspid valve. The truncus equally overrides both ventricles in 68% to 83% of cases, is deviated over the right ventricle in 11% to 29%, and is deviated to the left in 4% to 6%.[7,15] The valve may be stenotic or regurgitant, which can complicate management of the patient with truncus arteriosus. A moderate or greater degree of truncal insufficiency is present in 20% to 26% of patients.[16,17] Mild stenosis is generally detected on preoperative evaluation because of the increased flow across the truncal valve. Significant stenosis is present in only 4% to 7% of patients.[16,17] Gradients of greater than 30 mm Hg are concerning for residual stenosis after complete repair.[18]

The branch pulmonary arteries generally originate from the left posterolateral aspect of the truncus, just distal to the truncal valve. They are usually of good size without ostial or branch stenosis. Collett and Edwards type I is most frequently encountered, occurring in 48% to 68% of cases, followed by type II (29% to 48%) and type III (6% to 10%).[7,15] In practice, most cases seem to fall into a category of "type 1½," with the branch pulmonary arteries arising not from a main pulmonary artery but in proximity from the posterior aspect of the truncus. Origin of one pulmonary artery from a systemic artery other than the truncus (Van Praagh type A3/B3) is relatively rare, with an incidence of 2% to 5%.[16,19]

Associated Anomalies

An interrupted aortic arch, most commonly type B, is present in association with truncus arteriosus (Van Praagh type A4/B4) in approximately 10% to 20% of patients.[8,9] The arch is rightward, generally with mirror image branching, in 21% to 36% of patients.[8,20] Aberrant origins of the brachiocephalic vessels are reported, most commonly an aberrant right subclavian artery in 4% to 10%.[15,20]

Coronary variations are common in truncus arteriosus and are of potential importance in the surgical repair of the lesion. The left anterior descending artery is often small, with prominent conal branches from the right coronary artery supplying the right ventricular infundibulum.[21] The left anterior descending artery can originate from the right coronary artery, which has clear surgical ramifications for the right ventricular infundibulotomy. There is left coronary dominance in 27%, which is approximately threefold the incidence found in the general population.[22] Coronary ostial abnormalities are of particular surgical significance and occur in 37% to 49% of cases.[22] The usual arrangement, regardless of the number of cusps, is for the left coronary artery to arise from the left posterolateral cusp and for the right coronary artery to originate from the right anterolateral cusp. Coronaries can arise from a single orifice or from two ostia in a single cusp.[8] There may be ostial stenosis, often described as a slitlike orifice, or obstruction from abnormal valve tissue. The left coronary artery is frequently noted to have a high origin, not uncommonly near the takeoff of the pulmonary arteries. Rarely, the left coronary artery can originate from the main pulmonary trunk or a branch pulmonary artery.[15]

Other cardiac anomalies are common, and a patent foramen ovale (PFO) is usually present. A true atrial septal defect is found in 9% to 20%, a persistent left superior vena cava in 4% to 9%, and mild tricuspid valve stenosis in 6%.[15,20] Mitral valve abnormalities are reported in 5% to 10% of patients. Tricuspid atresia, complete atrioventricular septal defect, anomalies of pulmonary venous return, mitral atresia, hypoplastic left ventricle, ventricular inversion, and heterotaxy syndrome have all been reported in association with truncus arteriosus.

Extracardiac anomalies are reported in approximately 28% of patients with truncus arteriosus.[17] Described abnormalities include skeletal, genitourinary, and gastrointestinal deformities. As mentioned earlier, monoallelic microdeletion of chromosome 22q11 is common, and DiGeorge syndrome is diagnosed in at least 11%.[17] These patients are at increased risk for more complicated operative courses, longer hospital stays, and greater resource utilization.[23]

Pathophysiology

The pathophysiology of truncus arteriosus is one of a total admixture lesion, with mixing occurring at the level of the VSD and proximal truncus. Although there is cyanosis, systemic oxygen saturations are frequently 85% to 90% in the newborn period because of elevated pulmonary blood flow. In the absence of pulmonary artery stenosis or systemic outflow obstruction, the amount of pulmonary blood flow is mainly affected by the pulmonary vascular resistance (PVR). In the first few days of life, PVR remains relatively high, limiting pulmonary blood flow. As PVR decreases, the amount of pulmonary blood flow increases, leading to pulmonary overcirculation and signs and symptoms of congestive heart failure. The unrestricted left-to-right shunt results in both pressure and volume overload to the pulmonary circuit. In addition, truncus arteriosus is distinguished from other left-to-right shunt lesions by both systolic and diastolic shunting. These factors lead to the early development of irreversible pulmonary vascular occlusive disease in patients with truncus arteriosus.

Truncal valve regurgitation and, less frequently, stenosis can exacerbate the hemodynamic stresses placed on the heart in truncus arteriosus. Regurgitation adds an additional volume overload to the ventricles, worsening the signs and symptoms of congestive heart failure. The diastolic runoff, which occurs not only because of the insufficient valve but also as a result of the low-resistance pulmonary vascular bed, can lead to poor systemic perfusion, most notably to the coronary arteries. Stenosis increases the afterload on the ventricles and thereby increases myocardial oxygen demand. Significant truncal valve stenosis can limit systemic perfusion, again compounded by the runoff into the pulmonary circuit.

Diagnosis

Clinical Features

The diagnosis of truncus arteriosus is generally made in early infancy, often during the neonatal period. The lesion can also be recognized antenatally on fetal echocardiography. The degree of cyanosis or congestive heart failure depends on the PVR and the resultant volume of pulmonary blood flow. The clinical manifestations can be exacerbated by associated lesions, such as truncal valve insufficiency or interrupted aortic arch, or ameliorated by pulmonary artery stenosis.

Physical findings depend on the amount of pulmonary blood flow and the degree of truncal valve insufficiency. In general, the neonate with truncus arteriosus shows only mild cyanosis at the time of birth. As the PVR falls and pulmonary blood flow increases, signs of congestive heart failure become manifest and cyanosis decreases. Truncal regurgitation accelerates the onset and increases the severity of congestive heart failure. The infant shows the typical findings of tachypnea, tachycardia, diaphoresis, and poor feeding. The precordium is hyperactive, and a thrill may be palpable over the left sternal border. There is a normal S1 and a single loud S2, which may be associated with an opening click. An S3 is not uncommon as the degree of failure progresses. A pansystolic murmur is common at the left sternal border. A low-pitched diastolic murmur at the apex, representing increased flow across the mitral valve, may be present. A high-pitched diastolic murmur along the left sternal border is indicative of truncal valve regurgitation. In the absence of the rarely encountered pulmonary artery stenosis, a continuous murmur is distinctly uncommon. The detection of a continuous murmur is consistent with other diagnoses, notably pulmonary atresia with a patent ductus or aortopulmonary collaterals. The peripheral pulse pressure is widened because of the diastolic runoff into the pulmonary bed and is further widened by truncal insufficiency.

Diagnostic Studies

The chest radiograph generally shows moderate cardiomegaly with increased pulmonary vascular markings. The arch is rightward in approximately one third of patients, and the thymus gland may be absent in those with 22q11 microdeletion. The combination of a right arch and increased pulmonary vascular markings is strongly suggestive of truncus arteriosus. The two-dimensional and Doppler echocardiography examinations are the diagnostic modalities of choice. The echocardiogram can define the anatomy of truncus arteriosus at birth or in utero. Prenatal echocardiography is increasingly identifying congenital heart anomalies; however, because of the challenges of imaging the branch pulmonary arteries, truncus arteriosus remains one of the more commonly misdiagnosed heart defects (78.6% accuracy).[24,25] A parasternal long-axis view will demonstrate the large truncal valve overriding the VSD (Fig. 121-3*A*). The addition of Doppler interrogation will reveal truncal valve stenosis or regurgitation (see Fig. 121-3*B*). Suprasternal notch views can further define the anatomy of the pulmonary arteries and aortic arch (Fig. 121-4). Cardiac catheterization is generally reserved for the delineation of the anatomy in complex forms of truncus arteriosus, such as truncus arteriosus with a single pulmonary artery (Van Praagh type A3/B3). Cardiac catheterization is also indicated to assess PVR in the patient presenting late with truncus arteriosus. Magnetic resonance imaging (MRI) is a useful alternative or adjunct to cardiac catheterization for defining the anatomy of complex truncus arteriosus. MRI increasingly plays a role in the postoperative assessment of these patients in evaluating ventricular function as well as conduit and branch pulmonary artery anatomy.[26]

Natural History

The typical natural history of truncus arteriosus is characterized by early demise because of congestive heart

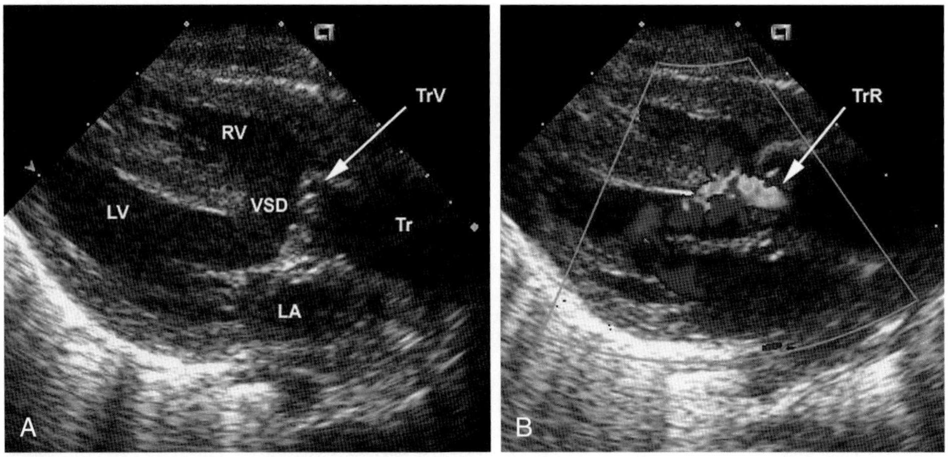

FIGURE 121-3 ■ Parasternal long-axis view of a patient with truncus arteriosus. **A,** The large truncus (Tr) overriding the ventricular septal defect (VSD) is demonstrated. **B,** The addition of Doppler reveals a jet of truncal regurgitation (TrR). *LA,* Left atrium; *LV,* left ventricle; *RV,* right ventricle; *TrV,* truncal valve.

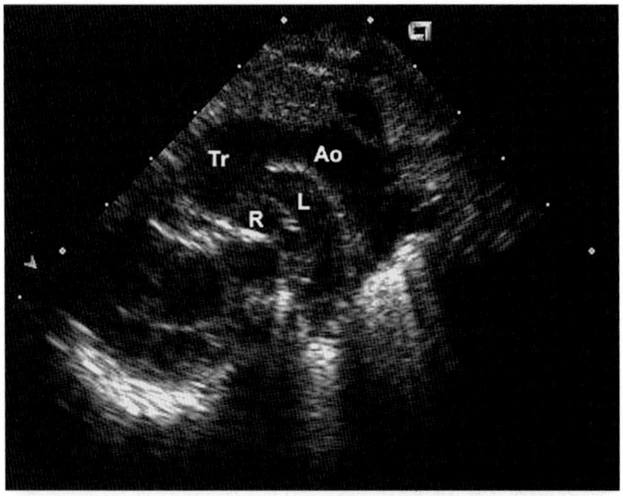

FIGURE 121-4 ■ Suprasternal notch view demonstrating close but separate origins of the right (R) and left (L) pulmonary arteries from the truncus (Tr) with continuation as the aorta (Ao).

failure. Death rates are approximately 40% at 1 month, 70% at 3 months, and 90% at 1 year.[27] Patients who survive infancy generally succumb by childhood or early adolescence because of congestive heart failure or, more commonly, pulmonary vascular obstructive disease. Rarely, patients survive infancy without developing pulmonary vascular obstructive disease, although those who do so are estimated to be less than 5% of all patients.[27]

Treatment

Because of the inherent high early mortality, truncus arteriosus warrants early intervention. Initially, the surgical treatment of truncus arteriosus was limited to the banding of one or both of the branch pulmonary arteries. The first successful intracardiac repair was accomplished by Sloan's group at the University of Michigan in 1962 using an unvalved polytetrafluoroethylene (PTFE) conduit for the pulmonary reconstruction.[28] In 1967, McGoon and colleagues[29] performed the first valved conduit repair, using an aortic allograft. During this period, complete repair was often undertaken as a staged procedure after initial pulmonary artery banding. However, complications of pulmonary artery banding, including pulmonary artery distortion, band migration, and failure to prevent the development of pulmonary vascular obstructive disease, resulted in a continued high mortality with this strategy. Ebert and coworkers[30] published the first series of patients undergoing repair of truncus arteriosus in infancy in 1984. With continued improvements in neonatal operative techniques, as well as perioperative care, management has evolved to earlier complete repair. After the early reports of neonatal repair from the University of Michigan[18] and the Children's Hospital of Boston,[31] neonatal repair has become the treatment of choice for truncus arteriosus.

Surgical Technique

The repair is performed using a standard median sternotomy. Although deep hypothermia with circulatory arrest or low-flow bypass has been advocated by some authors, the repair of simple forms of truncus arteriosus is performed easily on full-flow bypass with moderate hypothermia. More complex forms, such as Van Praagh type A3/B3 (one pulmonary artery absent) or A4/B4 (with interrupted aortic arch), may require periods of deep hypothermic circulatory arrest. The arterial cannula is placed distally in the ascending aorta at the base of the innominate artery. Bicaval cannulation is used for venous return, with an additional left ventricular vent placed through the right upper pulmonary vein. The pulmonary arteries are mobilized and snared to direct cardiopulmonary bypass flow to the systemic circulation.

The heart is arrested with antegrade cardioplegia, with the aortic crossclamp placed as distally as possible. Significant truncal valve regurgitation may necessitate the use of retrograde cardioplegia. Once the cardioplegia is delivered, the pulmonary arteries are removed. If the coronary arteries can be positively identified and the exposure is adequate, the pulmonary arteries can be removed directly from the posterior aspect of the truncus,

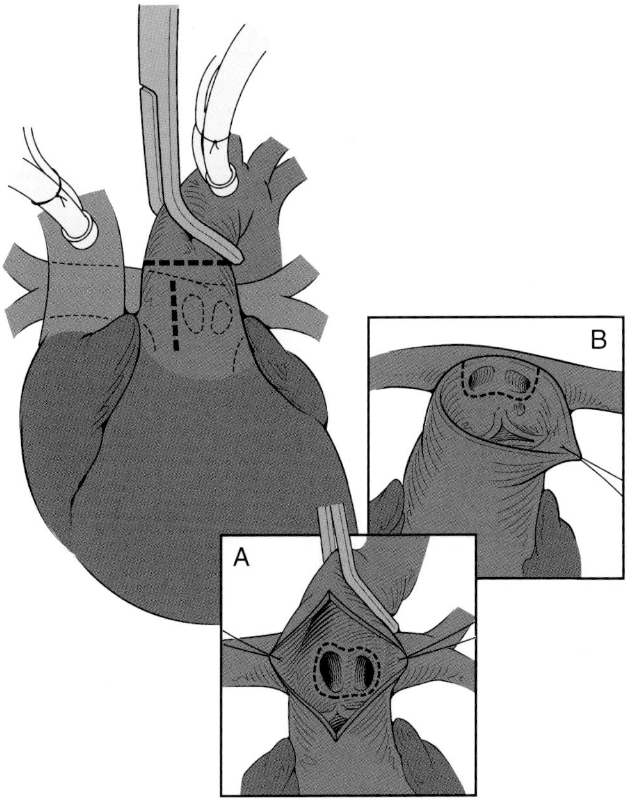

FIGURE 121-5 ■ Repair of truncus arteriosus. Removal of the pulmonary arteries from the truncus is facilitated by an anterior longitudinal aortotomy **(A)** or by transecting the aorta **(B)**.

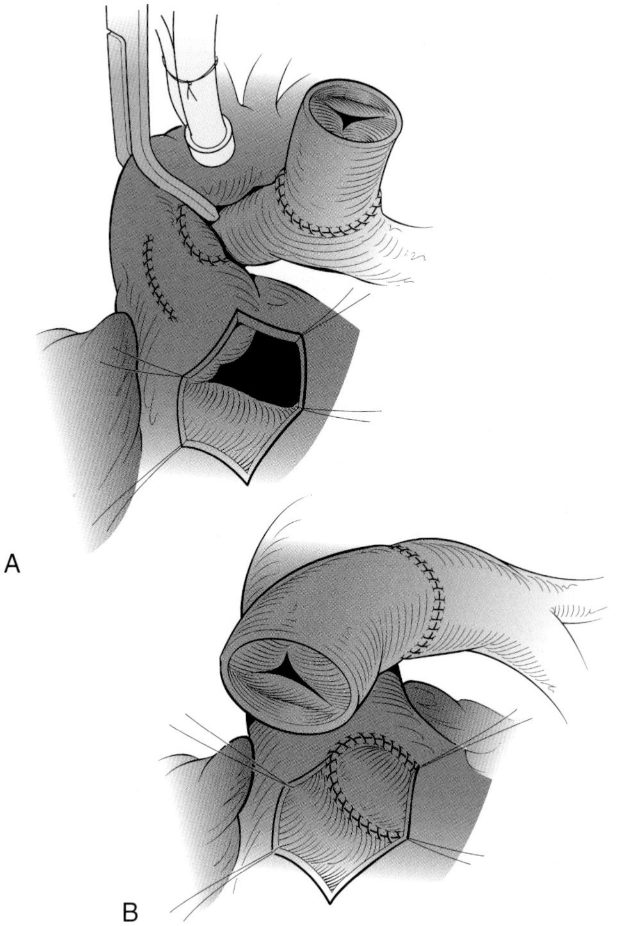

FIGURE 121-6 ■ Repair of truncus arteriosus. **A,** The ventricular septal defect (VSD) is exposed through a right infundibulotomy. **B,** The VSD patch is transitioned to the epicardium at the superior-most portion of the infundibulotomy. The posterior aspect of the pulmonary allograft is sewn directly to the superior portion of the infundibulotomy.

particularly for Collett and Edwards type I truncus arteriosus. The ostia of the coronary arteries can originate high in the sinuses or have an intramural course.[32] Direct assessment of the coronary anatomy in the aortic root is crucial if there is any uncertainty. Often, it is helpful to open the aorta anteriorly to aid in the removal of the pulmonary arteries and to identify the origins of the coronary arteries (Fig. 121-5*A*). Transection of the aorta just distal to the origins of the branch pulmonary arteries is another useful technique to facilitate pulmonary artery and coronary exposure (see Fig. 121-5*B*). The pulmonary arteries are removed, together with a small rim of adjacent truncal wall. Care is taken to avoid injuring the left coronary artery or truncal valve, which are often in close proximity to the pulmonary arteries. The truncal defect is then repaired primarily or with a patch of PTFE. At this point, additional doses of cardioplegia can be given at intervals, depending on surgeon's preference.

The heart is inspected for the presence of any large conal branches, the location of the left anterior descending artery, and the possibility of aberrant coronary arteries. A right infundibulotomy is then made in an avascular area of the right ventricular outflow tract. The infundibulotomy is carried cranially toward the truncal valve and is limited to the size necessary to allow unobstructed output from the right ventricle through the anticipated conduit (Fig. 121-6*A*). Through the infundibulotomy, the VSD is closed with a patch of PTFE. We use a running suture technique, although an interrupted technique can be used as well. When there is membranous or inlet extension of the VSD, care is taken not to injure the conduction tissue in the posteroinferior aspect of the VSD. It is helpful to transition from the endocardium of the right ventricular outflow tract to the epicardium in the anterosuperior-most portion of the infundibulotomy, to avoid injuring the truncal valve and to ensure a widely patent left ventricular outflow tract (see Fig. 121-6*B*). If present, the atrial septal defect is then closed. A small PFO can be left as a "popoff valve" to aid in postoperative management.

Once the VSD is closed, the remainder of the procedure can be performed with the crossclamp removed and the heart beating. We prefer to use cryopreserved pulmonary or aortic allografts for reconstruction of the pulmonary outflow tract, although either bovine jugular vein grafts or heterograft valved conduit are viable alternatives. The distal anastomosis of the allograft is performed to the confluence of the native branch pulmonary arteries. The posterior aspect of the allograft is then approximated to the superior portion of the right infundibulotomy. Anteriorly, the conduit is augmented with a patch of PTFE or additional allograft material (Fig. 121-7). A

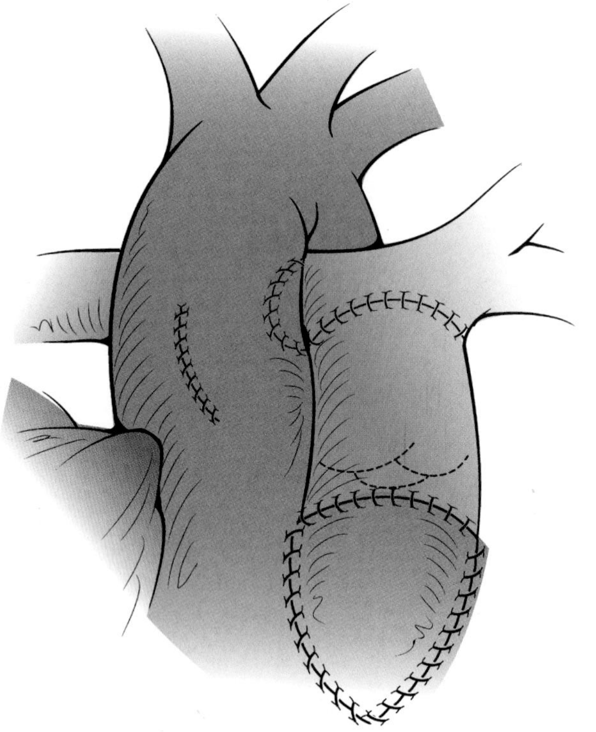

FIGURE 121-7 ■ Repair of truncus arteriosus. Right ventricle–to–pulmonary artery continuity is then completed with a hood of polytetrafluoroethylene.

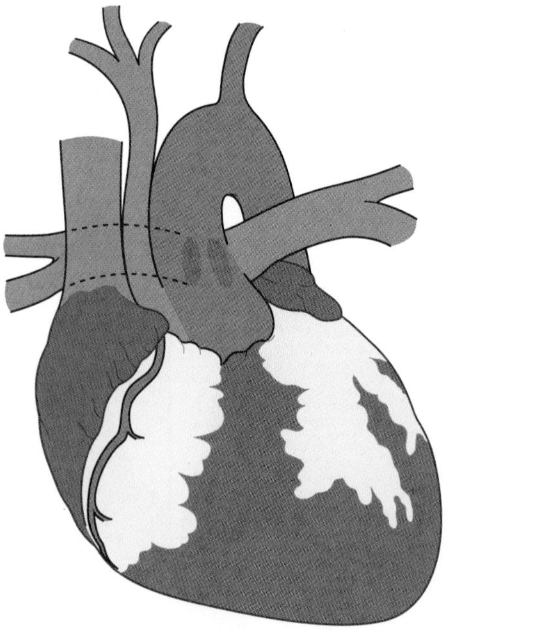

FIGURE 121-8 ■ Truncus arteriosus (Collett and Edwards type II) with a type B interrupted aortic arch.

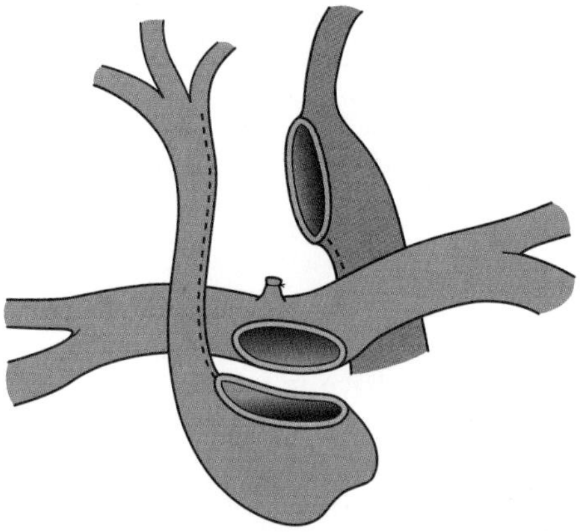

FIGURE 121-9 ■ Repair of truncus arteriosus with interrupted aortic arch. The ductus arteriosus has been ligated and divided, and the pulmonary arteries have been removed from the truncus. The areas for spatulation on the ascending aorta and proximal descending aorta are indicated *(dashed lines)*.

benefit of the bovine jugular vein grafts is the proximal extension of tissue, which can be used to patch the right infundibulotomy without additional patch material.

Other Surgical Considerations

Interrupted Aortic Arch

The surgical repair of truncus arteriosus with interrupted aortic arch (Fig. 121-8) requires several modifications to the basic operative procedure. The aortic cannulation is performed proximally at the base of the innominate artery to perfuse all of the brachiocephalic vessels, and distally in the ductus arteriosus to perfuse the distal aorta. Bicaval cannulation is used for venous return, with a left ventricular vent placed through the right upper pulmonary vein. The patient is placed on cardiopulmonary bypass and cooled to 18° C for a minimum of 20 minutes. The pulmonary arteries are snared to prevent pulmonary overcirculation. During cooling, the ascending aorta, arch, proximal descending aorta, brachiocephalic vessels, and pulmonary arteries are mobilized. The arch repair can be performed under deep hypothermic circulatory arrest. Alternatively, regional cerebral perfusion, as described by Pigula and coworkers[33] and others, can be performed by anastomosing a PTFE tube graft to the innominate artery or by directly cannulating the aorta at the base of the innominate artery and advancing the cannula into the innominate. After adequate cooling, the head vessels are snared, bypass is discontinued, and regional cerebral perfusion is initiated, if desired. The ductus arteriosus is ligated just distal to the origin of the pulmonary arteries and divided. All residual ductal tissue is resected from the proximal descending aorta. The ascending aorta and proximal descending aorta are spatulated (Fig. 121-9). The back walls of the distal ascending aorta and proximal descending aorta are approximated, and the repair is augmented with a patch of cryopreserved pulmonary allograft (Fig. 121-10). Once the arch reconstruction is completed, the aorta can be recannulated and de-aired, an aortic crossclamp can be placed, and cardiopulmonary bypass can be resumed. Additional doses of cardioplegia can be administered and rewarming can begin. The remainder of the repair, including VSD closure and pulmonary outflow tract reconstruction, is similar to the simple truncus arteriosus surgical procedure.

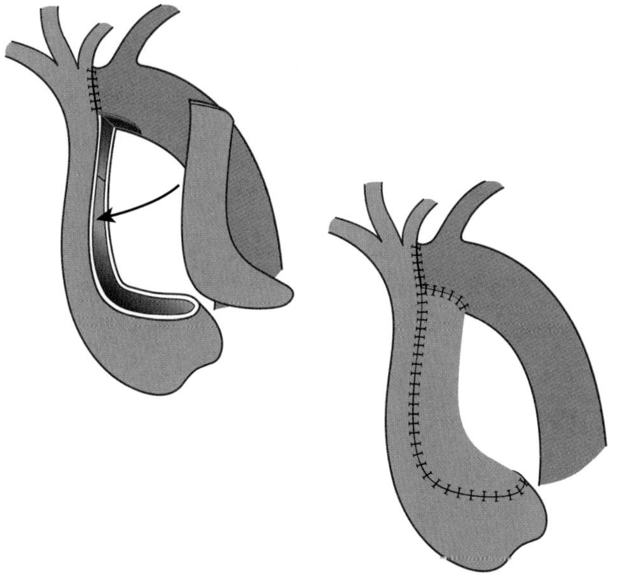

FIGURE 121-10 ■ Repair of truncus arteriosus with interrupted aortic arch. The distal ascending and proximal descending aorta are reapproximated and augmented with cryopreserved pulmonary allograft.

Truncal Valve Regurgitation or Stenosis

Significant truncal valve regurgitation, or, less frequently, stenosis, can complicate the operative management of truncus arteriosus in approximately a quarter of cases. A conservative approach is warranted, as frequently both regurgitation and stenosis improve after corrective surgery and relief of the volume overload. Gradients of less than 30 mm Hg generally do not require intervention.[18] In addition, even moderate degrees of truncal regurgitation are well tolerated, and delay of valve repair or replacement can often be accomplished. A recent analysis of the Society of Thoracic Surgeons Congenital Heart Surgery database from 2000-2009 demonstrated that concomitant truncal valve surgery at the time of truncus arteriosus is associate with a significantly higher operative mortality compared with repair of the truncus arteriosus in isolation (30% vs. 10%; $P = 0.0002$). This mortality risk increases to 60% when the truncal valve surgery is combined with repair of an interrupted aortic arch—the caveat being that patients who did not have an initial truncal valve surgery, but subsequently required surgical intervention during their index hospital admission, had a 100% mortality.[34] Hence, appropriate patient selection is essential in terms of timing of truncal valve intervention. Many patients with severe truncal regurgitation do not survive to operation. For the patients who do survive, the presence of moderate to severe truncal regurgitation after the initial operation is a risk factor for late truncal valve reintervention but not early mortality.[35] At the time of truncal valve intervention, truncal valve repair is preferred if the valve is amenable with other options, including root replacement with cryopreserved aortic allograft or mechanical valve replacement. Truncal valve replacement can be facilitated by enlargement of the valve annulus by the VSD patch. For truncal valve repair, several techniques have been described in small series of patients with reasonable survivals. These techniques include annuloplasty, resection of cusps, closure of commissures, resuspension of cusps, and cusp repair.[36,37] Backer and Mavroudis[38,39] have reported that truncal valve remodeling by leaflet excision or reduction annuloplasty is the most effective and durable method of truncal valve repair. In long-term follow-up, this group demonstrated that durable results can be achieved with valve morphology as the key determinant of success, with 75% of patients having a quadricuspid valve requiring leaflet excision and tricuspidization of the valve, with only two patients proceeding to valve replacement 9 and 10 years after repair.[40] Risk factors for reoperation following truncal valve repair include neonatal repair (hazard ratio 4.1; $P = 0.03$) and performance of leaflet thinning (hazard ratio 22.5; $P = 0.002$).[41] Older children and adults have a greater number of options for valve replacement, including aortic allograft, stented or stentless tissue valves, and mechanical valves. Repair is also an option in this population if the anatomy is amenable to a durable repair.

Pulmonary Outflow Tract Reconstruction

Although the majority of surgeons use valved heterograft or allograft conduits, several other techniques have been described. These other techniques include the use of unvalved conduits, fresh autologous pericardial valved conduits, monocusps, and various methods for achieving native tissue apposition between the right ventricle and the pulmonary artery.

Unvalved tube grafts have been used in the past with good results, but they have been largely abandoned with the development of appropriately sized valved conduits.[42] Advantages include availability and lower risk of stenosis related to valve dysfunction or calcification. The clear disadvantage is the lack of a valve in the immediate postoperative period, with free regurgitation into a right ventricle compromised by a ventriculotomy and periods of ischemia and cardiopulmonary bypass. In addition, a valve may be advantageous in neonates with labile PVR or in older patients with pulmonary vascular obstructive disease. One study analyzing neonatal repair with unvalved conduits found that patients with truncus arteriosus had the highest rate of reintervention for conduit failure compared with other diagnostic groups.[43,44]

Options for valved conduits include composite heterografts, allografts, and bovine jugular vein grafts. Porcine heterografts in Dacron tube grafts are available in sizes as small as 12 mm. Advantages include ready availability. Disadvantages are primarily related to the stiff Dacron tube graft, which is less hemostatic and less forgiving, with a greater risk of distortion of the branch pulmonary arteries. Dacron also tends to form a neointimal peel, potentially leading to stenosis. In addition, the rigid metal ring of the heterograft valve can be compressed beneath the sternum, obstructing the left anterior descending artery. Bovine jugular vein grafts have increased in popularity. They are readily available in small sizes, down to 12 mm. These grafts have excellent handling characteristics, are hemostatic, and minimize branch pulmonary artery distortion. They are available with or without supporting rings to minimize distortion from sternal compression. The bovine jugular vein grafts have similar durability to traditional allografts, however enthusiasm has been tempered by increased risk of distal stenosis especially in patients younger than 2 years.[45,46,47] Another larger series has shown the Contegra conduit and size less than 20 mm to be independent risk factors for need for graft replacement when compared with allografts.[48]

Cryopreserved pulmonary allografts have the advantages of excellent tissue handling characteristics and ease of implantation. Aortic allografts can also be used, although they appear to be less durable than their pulmonary counterparts.[17,49] The disadvantage of these conduits is primarily related to the limited availability in the very small sizes, although allografts in the range of 12 to 16 mm can generally be placed in neonates without difficulty. A larger pulmonary allograft can be downsized by removal of one of the cusps, creating a bicuspid valve. Our group and others[50-52] have successfully used this technique when appropriately sized allografts are unavailable.

Whether heterografts or allografts have superior longevity remains controversial. Several published studies, including our own experience, have shown that pulmonary allografts are the optimal conduit in neonates and infants.[17,53] Our results for the placement of a right ventricle–to–pulmonary artery conduit in a series of 155 infants demonstrated a significantly greater 5-year freedom from reoperation for cryopreserved pulmonary allograft (50%) compared with aortic allograft (24%; $P = 0.02$) and heterograft (26%; $P = 0.05$).[39] It has been shown that optimizing allograft size (z-score within +1 to +3) is important to conduit longevity, with no additional benefit from oversizing conduits.[45,54] Others have found no significant difference in longevity between heterografts and allografts for the repair of truncus arteriosus.[55]

In an effort to decrease the need for reoperation, several groups have suggested methods for achieving native tissue apposition in the right ventricular outflow tract to allow for growth. In 1990, Barbero-Marcial and associates[56] introduced a technique for anastomosing the pulmonary bifurcation directly to the superior margin of the infundibulotomy. The anterior aspect of the anastomosis is then augmented with a patch, which includes a monocusp. Late follow-up of 45 patients by Barbero-Marcial and Tanamati[57] demonstrated that this technique resulted in a reintervention rate of 12% over a mean follow-up of 47 months, with an 11.4-year actuarial survival rate of 67.5%. In addition, 44.4% had moderate to severe pulmonary regurgitation and 23.3% had pulmonary stenosis. Lacour-Gayet and colleagues[16] reported their experience with 56 consecutive patients undergoing repair for truncus arteriosus using a number of different techniques for pulmonary outflow tract reconstruction. They found equivalent rates of reintervention for heterograft and direct anastomosis of approximately 80%. Danton and associates[58] published a series of 61 patients with truncus arteriosus, 38 repaired with a conduit and 23 with direct anastomosis. Although mortality was not influenced, 10-year actuarial freedom from reoperation was 89% in the direct anastomosis group, compared with 56% in the conduit group ($P = 0.023$).

Right ventricular outflow tract reconstruction using fresh autologous pericardial valved conduits has been described by Kreutzer and associates.[59] Their series of 86 patients undergoing this technique included 23 cases of truncus arteriosus. Operative mortality for the patients with truncus arteriosus was 26%. Among the entire group, moderate to severe conduit regurgitation was present immediately after surgery in 12.7%. By 6 months after surgery, no valve tissue could be identified in any patient, either by echocardiography or by visual inspection in those patients requiring reoperation. For the entire cohort, the need for conduit-related reintervention was 83% at 5 years and 60% at 10 years for conduits less than 16 mm at the time of implantation. By contrast, in the report by Lacour-Gayet and coworkers,[16] freedom from reoperation or angioplasty at 7 years was 100% for patients receiving a pericardial conduit in the repair of truncus arteriosus. However, the authors also found the use of direct anastomosis or pericardial conduit to be a significant risk factor for operative mortality (43%), when compared with a heterograft or allograft (7.1%; $P = 0.015$).

Postoperative Management

Most patients require low doses of inotropic support with standard postoperative care techniques. The placement of a left atrial transthoracic monitoring line is helpful, as the central venous pressure may not accurately reflect left-sided filling pressures because of right ventricular dysfunction. Early operation has virtually eliminated the postoperative pulmonary hypertensive crises seen in earlier studies. For older patients in whom pulmonary vascular hypertensive crisis or pulmonary vascular obstructive disease can be anticipated, the placement of a transthoracic pulmonary artery line can aid in postoperative management. Avoiding acidosis, hypercarbia, and hypoxia can minimize PVR. Sedation and paralysis are also used to minimize fluctuations in PVR. The use of nitric oxide and sildenafil can induce pulmonary vascular smooth muscle relaxation and can be particularly useful in older patients with reversible pulmonary vascular obstructive disease.

Results

Since the first large series of truncus arteriosus repair in infants by Ebert and colleagues[30] in 1984, the management has evolved to earlier neonatal repair, with a continual improvement in survival. Hospital mortality for the neonatal repair of truncus arteriosus from the Society of Thoracic Surgeons Congenital database from 2005 to 2009 was 10.9% (range, 0%-100%).[60] The majority of deaths occur in patients with complex truncus arteriosus or truncus arteriosus associated severe truncal valve regurgitation.[16-19,32,61] More complex forms of truncus arteriosus are also associated with increased hospital morbidity and prolonged length of stay.[62] Risk factors for poor outcome identified in various studies include significant truncal regurgitation, need for truncal valve replacement, birth weight less than 2.5 kg, presence of interrupted aortic arch or coronary artery anomalies, pulmonary reconstruction with a technique other than valved heterograft or allograft, and age greater than 100 days.[16-19,31,55,61] Some single-center studies have demonstrated that interrupted aortic arch is not a risk factor.[18,19] However, a recent Congenital Heart Surgeons' Society study and a single-center study have again shown a high early mortality rate of 42% to 56% for truncus arteriosus associated with interrupted aortic arch.[63,64]

Long-term survival for patients with truncus arteriosus is also encouraging with actuarial survivals of 90% at 5 years, 85% at 10 years, and 83% at 15 years, with the majority of survivors (97%) in New York Heart Association class I or II.[20,55] Examination of the Kaplan-Meier survival curves reveals that the majority of mortality is associated with the initial operation. Late follow-up has demonstrated that although the greatest need for intervention or hospitalization is in the first year of life, patients with truncus arteriosus have significantly impaired exercise capacity and diminished physical health status and health-related quality of life compared to normative standards.[65] An issue for patients with a variety of conotruncal abnormalities is the finding of a dilated ascending aorta in adolescents and adults and the question of whether this requires intervention. The majority of patients have been found to have an aorta z-score of ≥2; however, the risk of dissection is believed to be rare and therefore conservative management with close observation is the recommended approach at this time.[66,67]

AORTOPULMONARY WINDOW

Aortopulmonary window is an uncommon malformation characterized by an anomalous communication between the adjacent portions of the ascending aorta and the main pulmonary artery. Distinctively, the aortic and pulmonary semilunar valves are both present, and the ventricular septum is typically intact. This lesion represents between 0.2% and 0.3% of all congenital heart lesions.[68,69] Aortopulmonary window was first described by Eliotson in a clinicopathologic discussion given at St. Thomas' Hospital in London in 1830.[70]

Embryology

Descriptions of cardiac embryology can be confusing because of varying terminology used by different authors. For the purpose of this discussion, the embryonic cardiac outflow tract can be considered as the portion of the primitive heart tube that connects the ventricles with the aortic arch vessels. This outflow tract comprises the conus, the truncus, and the aortic sac. Histologically, the conotruncus has an external muscle layer and internal cardiac jelly (which is cellular), whereas the aortic sac has a wall consisting of endothelium surrounded by loose mesenchyme. Septation of the outflow tract seems to occur in a craniocaudal direction by two mechanisms.[71] Initial septation occurs by an ingrowth of mesenchyme (principally neural crest tissue), which separates the aortic sac into the definitive aorta and the pulmonary artery. This aorticopulmonary septum then extends caudally to divide the distal truncus. Meanwhile, in the proximal conotruncus, paired ridges (consisting of both neural crest and non–neural crest tissue) bulge into the lumen and meet. The caudal portion of the aorticopulmonary septum ultimately fuses with the cranial extent of the conotruncal ridges to complete septation. This entire process occurs in human embryos beginning when the crown–rump length is 6 mm, and it is completed by the 9-mm stage over a period of approximately 5 days.[72]

The embryologic defect in aortopulmonary window is presumed to be related to nonfusion of the aorticopulmonary septum with the conotruncal septum, malalignment of the two septa, or complete absence of the aorticopulmonary septum.[69] The defects leading to truncus arteriosus and aortopulmonary window are thought to be distinct. Although a number of gene mutations that lead to a phenotype of truncus arteriosus have been identified, none of these has resulted in isolated aortopulmonary window. In addition, isolated aortopulmonary window is generally not seen in the constellation of conotruncal abnormalities that occur in conjunction with DiGeorge syndrome.

Anatomy

The defect in aortopulmonary window is usually oval and solitary, although its precise location can vary. Many classification schemes have been proposed to describe the variation in morphology of this anomaly. One widely used classification, proposed by Richardson and colleagues, describes three variants.[73] Type I defects represent the classic proximal window involving the posteromedial wall of the ascending aorta just above the left sinus of Valsalva and the adjacent wall of the main pulmonary artery. The inferior extent of the proximal defect may be close to the origin of the left coronary artery. Type II defects are more distal communications occurring near the origin of the right pulmonary artery. Distal windows can be associated with a variable degree of "unroofing" of the right pulmonary artery, which can lead to the apparent origin of this vessel from the posterolateral aspect of the ascending aorta. Finally, type III defects describe anomalous origin of the right pulmonary artery from the posterolateral wall of the ascending aorta (without an associated window). The type III defect has also been called *hemitruncus*, although the use of this term has been discouraged in favor of the more descriptive "anomalous origin of the right pulmonary artery from the aorta."

A more useful scheme was advanced by Mori and associates.[74] In the Mori classification, type I and II defects are analogous to their counterparts in the Richardson classification, with type I (proximal) defects occurring between the adjacent portions of the proximal ascending aorta and main pulmonary artery, and type II (distal) defects located more distally near the origin of the right pulmonary artery. Mori type III (total) defects are large defects representing a combination of types I and II.

Recently, Jacobs and members of the Congenital Heart Surgery Nomenclature and Database Project proposed general use of the Mori classification (proximal, distal, and total), with the addition of a fourth type termed intermediate and representing a window similar to the total defect but slightly smaller, with well-defined

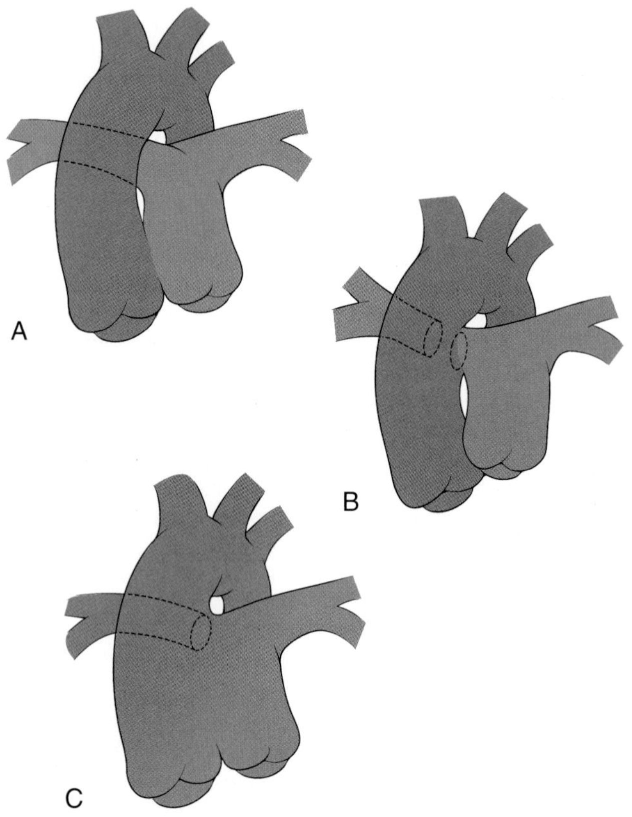

FIGURE 121-11 ■ Anatomy and classification of aortopulmonary window as recommended by the Congenital Heart Surgery Nomenclature and Database Project. **A,** Type I (proximal) defects occur between adjacent portions of the proximal ascending aorta and the main pulmonary artery. **B,** Type II (distal) defects are located more distally, near the origin of the right pulmonary artery. **C,** Type III (total) defects are large defects with poorly defined margins representing a combination of types I and II. Intermediate defects (not illustrated) are similar to total defects but are slightly smaller and have well-defined superior and inferior rims.

superior and inferior rims.[75] The remainder of this chapter will adhere to this terminology. Figure 121-11 illustrates the anatomic subtypes of aortopulmonary window.

Associated Anomalies

Associated anomalies can occur in 25% to 65% of cases of aortopulmonary window.[69,76-79] These associated defects may be considered minor or major.[80] Common minor defects include right aortic arch, patent ductus arteriosus, atrial septal defect, and PFO. Major defects commonly seen with aortopulmonary window include interrupted aortic arch (usually type A), tetralogy of Fallot, VSD, anomalous coronary artery, coarctation of the aorta, and univentricular heart lesions. Berry and colleagues[81] described a syndrome characterized by a distal aortopulmonary window, aortic origin of the right pulmonary artery, intact ventricular septum, patent ductus arteriosus, and interruption or coarctation of the aortic isthmus. Braunlin and coworkers[82] emphasized the frequency of arch obstruction in patients with an aortopulmonary window, reporting interrupted aortic arch in 43% and coarctation in 14%. The presence of an aortopulmonary window must always be excluded in infants with an interrupted aortic arch and an intact ventricular septum. A high index of suspicion for an aortopulmonary window is also warranted in cases of unexplained pulmonary artery hypertension or cardiac dilation.[83]

Pathophysiology

An aortopulmonary window invariably leads to excessive pulmonary blood flow secondary to a large-volume left-to-right shunt that occurs during systole and diastole. The degree of shunting is, of course, determined by the size of the window and the ratio of systemic to pulmonary vascular resistance. The window is usually nonrestrictive in nature, thereby leading to equalization of pressures in the aorta and pulmonary arteries. As PVR decreases after birth, shunt volume increases. The result is left ventricular volume overload, as well as a pressure load on the right ventricle. Excessive pulmonary blood flow can lead acutely to the development of interstitial pulmonary edema. Over time, pulmonary overcirculation can lead to the development of pulmonary vascular obstructive disease.

The presence of associated defects can affect the physiology of this condition. Most importantly, the presence of aortic arch obstruction exacerbates left-to-right shunting across the aortopulmonary window. In cases of severe coarctation or arch interruption, in which systemic perfusion is ductal dependent, closure of the ductus will precipitate severe systemic malperfusion and divert even more blood flow to the lungs.

Diagnosis

Clinical Features

As with truncus arteriosus, the diagnosis of aortopulmonary window is generally made during infancy. A loud continuous murmur with systolic accentuation is heard best at the left upper sternal border and may be confused with the murmur associated with a patent ductus arteriosus. The second heart sound may be accentuated and narrowly split. The diastolic blood pressure is usually reduced, with a concomitant widened pulse pressure and, on occasion, a water-hammer pulse. Patients typically present with symptoms of congestive heart failure (tachypnea, diaphoresis, failure to thrive, or recurrent respiratory infections).

The differential diagnosis of aortopulmonary window includes patent ductus arteriosus, truncus arteriosus, VSD with aortic insufficiency, and ruptured sinus of Valsalva aneurysm.

Diagnostic Studies

A chest radiograph demonstrates moderate cardiomegaly and increased pulmonary vascular markings. A right aortic arch may be present.

Echocardiography is generally diagnostic and has replaced angiography as the gold standard.[84-88] The margins of the window can be imaged with two-dimensional echocardiography, and Doppler color-flow

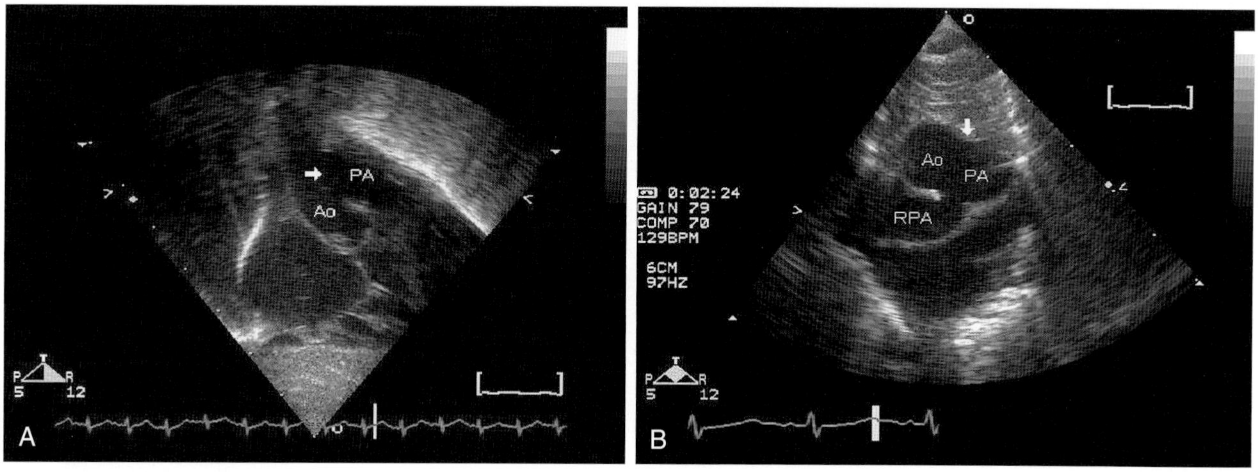

FIGURE 121-12 ■ Echocardiographic views in a patient with a large (total-type) aortopulmonary window (as well as a type A interrupted aortic arch). **A,** Subcostal coronal view shows the large communication *(arrow)* between the ascending aorta (Ao) and the main pulmonary artery (PA). **B,** Parasternal short-axis view demonstrates that the distal extent of the aortopulmonary window involves the origin of the right pulmonary artery (RPA). The anterior border of the window is identified by the *arrow.*

mapping can confirm flow across the communication. The most useful echocardiographic views to delineate the margins of the window include the suprasternal long axis, the subcostal coronal plane through the pulmonary trunk, and the high parasternal short plane cephalad to the aortic valve (Fig. 121-12). Additional echocardiographic findings include left atrial and left ventricular enlargement, which are usually in proportion to the degree of volume overload. Continuous forward flow in the distal main or branch pulmonary arteries is evident. When a jet of tricuspid or pulmonary insufficiency is present, pulmonary hypertension can be confirmed. The diagnosis of aortopulmonary window can also be made during fetal echocardiography.[89] MRI is an emerging technique that is capable of clarifying anatomy with great detail.[90,91]

Cardiac catheterization is rarely necessary unless clarification of associated defects is needed or if the coronary anatomy cannot be imaged well by echocardiography. In patients who present beyond infancy, catheterization allows the calculation of PVR to determine surgical candidacy.

Natural History

Patients with large aortopulmonary windows generally do not survive beyond childhood. Of untreated patients, 40% die within the first year of life.[92] Untreated patients generally develop pulmonary vascular obstructive disease. Because of the poor prognosis associated with this condition, it is recommended that all patients with aortopulmonary window undergo repair.

Treatment

The initial repair of aortopulmonary window involved, of necessity, closed techniques. Robert Gross performed the first surgical closure of an aortopulmonary window in 1948.[93] The patient was a 4-year-old girl who was explored via a left thoracotomy for a presumptive patent ductus arteriosus. The correct diagnosis was made at operation. Gross successfully ligated the window but acknowledged the potential risks and limitations of this technique. Scott and Sabiston[94] developed an animal model for aortopulmonary window and then devised techniques for closed division and suture closure using partial occluding clamps; they subsequently applied these techniques clinically in 1951. These closed techniques, however, were associated with several major limitations. First, dissection of the window was fairly risky because of potential bleeding complications. Second, division and primary closure of the window could lead to significant narrowing of both the aorta and the pulmonary artery and potential distortion of the semilunar valves. Third, the closed approach did not allow visualization of the coronary ostia, so coronary perfusion might be compromised after repair.

The introduction of cardiopulmonary bypass brought a greater margin of safety to the closed approach, but, more importantly, cardiopulmonary bypass permitted the development of open techniques that could be applied to the repair of all types of aortopulmonary window defects and their associated defects. Cooley and colleagues were the first to use cardiopulmonary bypass to facilitate division and oversewing of an aortopulmonary window in 1956.[95] Since that time, most published reports have emphasized the adjunctive use of cardiopulmonary bypass. In 1966, Putnam and Gross suggested a transpulmonary approach to repair, whereby the defect could be sutured closed from within the lumen of the main pulmonary artery using a longitudinal arteriotomy.[96] Although most early repairs were performed in older children, Cordell and associates reported the first closure of an aortopulmonary window in an infant (6 months of age) in 1967.[97] Wright and coworkers[98] described suture closure of the defect via a transaortic approach. This approach provided excellent exposure of the margins of the defect and the origins of the left coronary artery and right pulmonary artery. In 1969, Deverall and colleagues[99] reported their experience using a transaortic approach with closure of the defect using a Dacron patch. The advantages of patching the defect with a transaortic approach were emphasized in a report from Clarke and Richardson.[100] This became the early standard approach for most cases of aortopulmonary window. Operative mortality was significantly reduced with this change in operative strategy.[76] Studies in the early twenty-first century have demonstrated that early repair, preferably in infancy, along with concomitant repair of associated anomalies is imperative for optimal outcomes.[101-103]

The preoperative care of patients with aortopulmonary window primarily involves the management of associated congestive heart failure using standard techniques. Patients with significant aortic arch obstruction require infusion of prostaglandin E_1.

All symptomatic patients should undergo prompt repair, once the diagnosis is confirmed. Asymptomatic patients should undergo repair by 3 to 4 months of age to avoid the development of pulmonary vascular obstructive disease, which can occur in some patients at as early as 6 months of age. Older patients should undergo preoperative catheterization to assess PVR and its response to oxygen and nitric oxide. A ratio of pulmonary vascular resistance (Rp) to systemic vascular resistance (Rs) of greater than 0.4 has been shown to be a risk factor for perioperative death.[104] A PVR greater than 8 to 10 and an Rp/Rs greater than 0.7 probably represent absolute contraindications for repair.

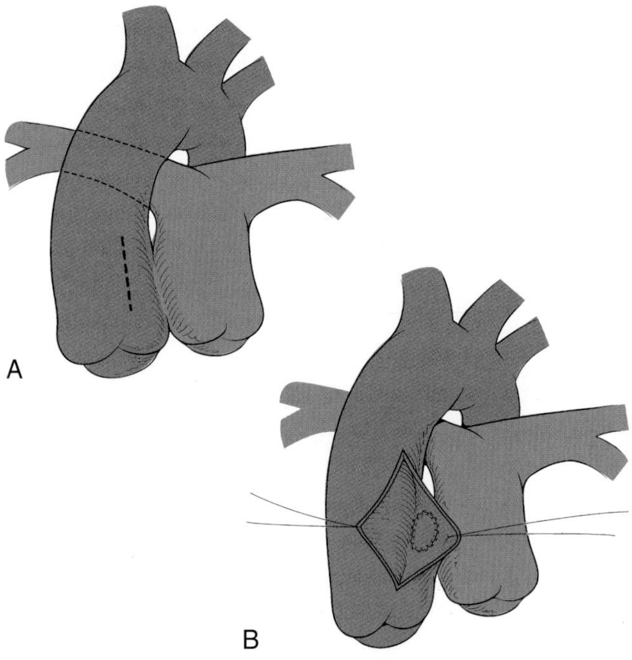

FIGURE 121-13 ■ Transaortic patch repair of a proximal aortopulmonary window. **A,** A vertical aortotomy in the proximal ascending aorta provides excellent exposure. **B,** Patch closure of the defect. Care must be taken to identify and protect the origin of the left coronary artery.

Surgical Technique

The repair is performed using standard median sternotomy. Bicaval venous and distal aortic cannulation is recommended. Snares are placed around both branch pulmonary arteries. Cardiopulmonary bypass with moderate hypothermia is initiated, and pulmonary arterial snares are tightened. After aortic cross-clamping, standard cardioplegia is delivered via the aortic root. Subsequent doses of cardioplegia (if necessary) are readily given by retrograde or direct antegrade approach.

Many centers continue to use the transaortic approach for the repair of aortopulmonary window. A longitudinal aortotomy is made in the ascending aorta. For simple proximal (type I) defects, closure is readily accomplished using a PTFE patch (Fig. 121-13). Care must be taken to identify the left coronary orifice. For distal (type II) defects, a more extensive patch must be fashioned (Fig. 121-14). When there is considerable unroofing of the right pulmonary artery, the creation of an intra-aortic baffle can result in aortic obstruction; this can be alleviated by simply closing the aortotomy with an elliptical patch (Fig. 121-15). Total (type III) and intermediate-type defects are repaired using analogous techniques (Fig. 121-16).

Johansson and colleagues[85] described a transwindow approach (also called a *sandwich-type repair*), which has gained wide acceptance as the optimal approach for the repair of aortopulmonary window. In this technique (Fig. 121-17), an incision is made in the anterior wall of the communication between the aorta and the pulmonary trunk. A patch is then sutured to the posterior wall of the defect. The suture line is subsequently carried anteriorly to incorporate the patch in the closure of the arteriotomy.

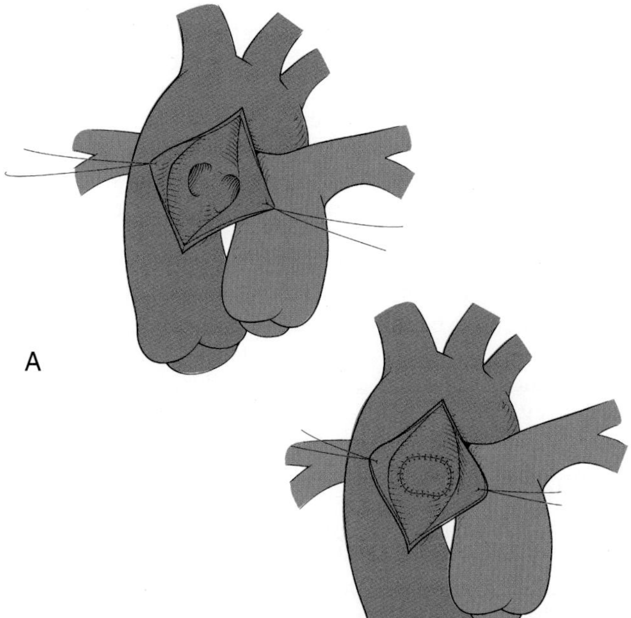

FIGURE 121-14 ■ Repair of a distal aortopulmonary window. **A,** A more distal aortotomy exposes the defect that is related to the origin of the right pulmonary artery. **B,** Use of a generous patch avoids stenosis of the origin of the right pulmonary artery.

This approach has the advantage of being slightly quicker to perform, as there is no need to close a separate aortotomy.

Several authors have used a pulmonary flap technique to avoid the use of prosthetic patch material to

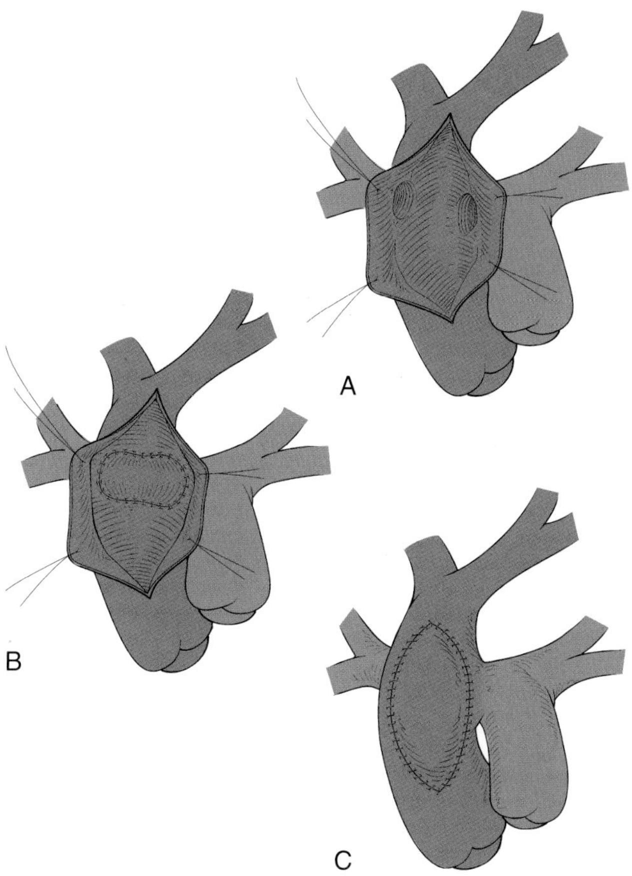

FIGURE 121-15 ■ Repair of a distal aortopulmonary window with extensive unroofing of the right pulmonary artery. **A,** Extensive unroofing leads to the appearance of anomalous origin of the right pulmonary artery from the ascending aorta. **B,** An extensive intra-aortic baffle created to join the window to the origin of the right pulmonary artery. **C,** Obstruction of the lumen of the ascending aorta can be obviated by closing the aortotomy with an elliptical patch.

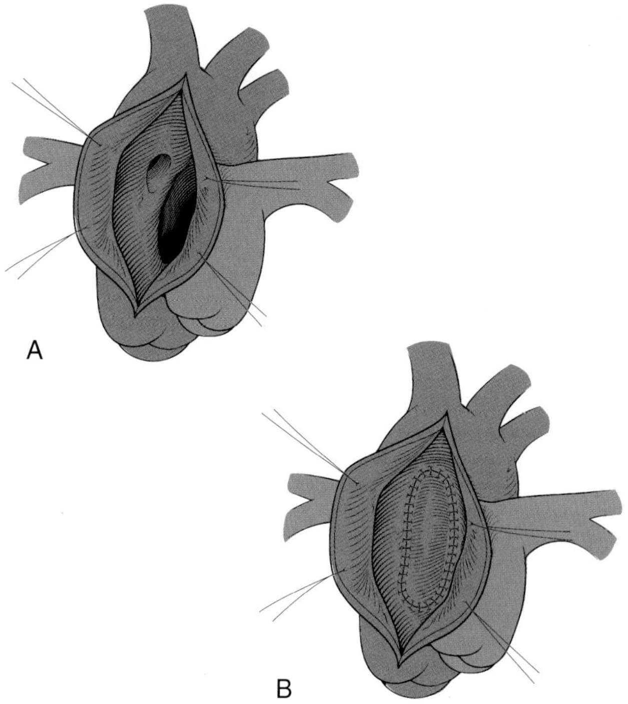

FIGURE 121-16 ■ Repair of a total-type (or intermediate-type) aortopulmonary window. **A,** Exposure is achieved with an extensive aortotomy. **B,** A large patch is used to close the defect.

reconstruct the ascending aorta.[105-108] In this approach, an anterior flap of pulmonary artery is incised in continuity with the aorta along the anterior border of the window. The anterior flap is then sewn to the posterior margin of the aortopulmonary window, thereby closing the defect in the aorta. The resultant defect in the pulmonary artery is then closed with a patch (autologous or heterologous).

Kitagawa and associates[109] reported an alternative technique to repair a distal aortopulmonary window with extensive unroofing of the right pulmonary artery. In this approach, the ascending aorta is transected at the distal extent of the window, and the right pulmonary artery is excised along with a strip of posterior aorta in continuity with the window and pulmonary trunk. The defect in the pulmonary artery is then repaired either primarily or using a patch, and the aorta is reconnected primarily. This technique has the advantage of avoiding any potential problems resulting from an intra-aortic baffle.

Other Surgical Considerations

Associated defects are generally repaired concurrently. Special consideration should be given to the repair of

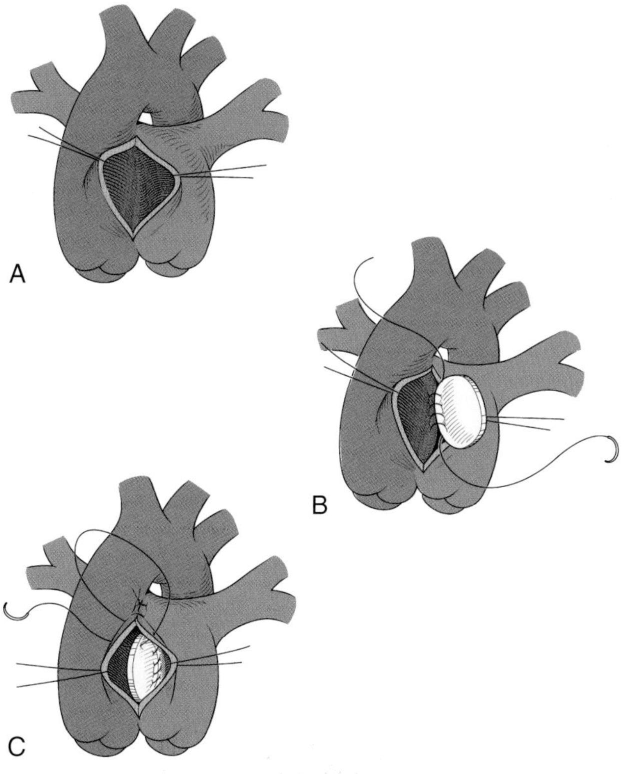

FIGURE 121-17 ■ Transwindow (sandwich) repair of aortopulmonary window. **A,** An incision is made in the anterior wall of the window. **B,** A patch is then sewn to the posterior border of the defect. **C,** Finally, the anterior portion of the defect is closed by incorporating the patch in the closure of the aortotomy.

defects associated with arch interruption, as this is associated with increased mortality and the need for late reintervention.[110,111] Because of the presence of the window, single arterial cannulation of the ascending aorta is sufficient. Cardiopulmonary bypass with deep hypothermia is used (with occlusion of the branch pulmonary arteries). The repair is typically performed under circulatory arrest or with adjunctive regional cerebral perfusion. The ductus is ligated proximally, and ductal tissue is resected distally. Two operative strategies can then be considered. Using a conventional approach, the arch interruption can be repaired first (using standard techniques), followed by repair of the window (transaortic patch or sandwich-type repair). Alternatively, the ascending aorta can be separated from the pulmonary artery at the level of the window, leaving defects in both vessels. The aortic arch is then reconstructed with patching of the defect in the ascending aorta, if necessary. Finally, the defect in the pulmonary artery is repaired with a patch.

Interventional Techniques

On rare occasions, a native aortopulmonary window or residual aortopulmonary defect after surgical closure may be small enough to allow an interventional approach. Several groups have reported success using percutaneously placed devices to close such defects.[112-116] With improved devices and experience, even large, nonrestrictive aortopulmonary windows in infants have been closed with a transcatheter approach when the anatomy is appropriate.[117,118] Following device closure, patients need to be followed for the development of aortic regurgitation at the time of the procedure as well as long-term.[119] For now, however, surgical closure remains the standard of care.

Postoperative Management

Currently, because the diagnosis and treatment of aortopulmonary window are accomplished in early infancy, pulmonary hypertensive crises are rare. However, in patients presenting later in life, management of pulmonary hypertension is the most critical aspect of postoperative care of patients undergoing repair of aortopulmonary window. A pulmonary arterial catheter can be placed with a pursestring in the right ventricular infundibulum in selected patients. Conventional methods for the control and prevention of pulmonary hypertension include the use of inhaled nitric oxide, administration of other pulmonary vasodilators, liberal use of fentanyl and muscle relaxants, and mild hyperventilation.

Results

Early mortality following the repair of simple aortopulmonary window should approach 0% in the contemporary era with excellent long-term outcomes. Even with associated arch obstruction, overall mortality has improved significantly over time. Tkebuchava and colleagues reported a 92% operative survival and an actuarial survival of 90% at the 10-year follow-up.[92] In one of the largest series, Hew and colleagues[78] observed an early survival of 92% and an actuarial survival of 88% at 10 years. Reviewing a series of 19 patients who underwent repair from 1953 to 1990, van Son and colleagues reported an overall early mortality of 21%.[104] The authors noted that all deaths occurred in patients who underwent repair before 1962. They also observed that the long-term outcome after repair depended on the PVR at the time of closure of the defect. Backer and Mavroudis reported a similar improvement in results.[77] They reported an operative mortality of 33% when the repair was performed using the technique of closed division of the window. Since changing the operative technique to the transaortic approach, they have seen no mortality. Patients need to be followed for the late development of pulmonary artery stenosis.

REFERENCES

1. Tandon R, Hauck AJ, Nadas AS: Persistent truncus arteriosus. A clinical, hemodynamic, and autopsy study of nineteen cases. *Circulation* 28:1050–1060, 1963.
2. Calder L, Van Praagh R, Van Praagh S, et al: Truncus arteriosus communis. Clinical, angiocardiographic, and pathologic findings in 100 patients. *Am Heart J* 92:23–38, 1976.
3. Rowe RD, Freedom RM, Mehrizi A, et al: The neonate with congenital heart disease. *Major Probl Clin Pediatr* 5:3–716, 1981.
4. Wilson J: A description of a very unusual malformation of the human heart. *Phil Trans R Soc London* 18:346, 1798.
5. Lev M, Saphir O: Truncus arteriosus communis persistens. *J Pediatr* 20:74, 1943.
6. Liu Y, Jim Y, Li J, et al: Inactivation of Cdc42 in neural crest cells causes craniofacial and cardiovascular morphogenesis defects. *Dev Biol* 383(2):239–252, 2013.
7. Kirby ML, Waldo KL: Role of neural crest in congenital heart disease. *Circulation* 82:332–340, 1990.
8. Butto F, Lucas RV, Jr, Edwards JE: Persistent truncus arteriosus: pathologic anatomy in 54 cases. *Pediatr Cardiol* 7:95–101, 1986.
9. Nath PH, Zollikofer C, Castaneda-Zuniga W, et al: Persistent truncus arteriosus associated with interruption of the aortic arch. *Br J Radiol* 53:853–859, 1980.
10. Epstein DJ, Vogan KJ, Trasler DG, et al: A mutation within intron 3 of the Pax-3 gene produces aberrantly spliced mRNA transcripts in the splotch (Sp) mouse mutant. *Proc Natl Acad Sci U S A* 90:532–536, 1993.
11. Farrell MJ, Stadt H, Wallis KT, et al: HIRA, a DiGeorge syndrome candidate gene, is required for cardiac outflow tract septation. *Circ Res* 84:127–135, 1999.
12. Collett RW, Edwards JE: Persistent truncus arteriosus; a classification according to anatomic types. *Surg Clin North Am* 29:1245–1270, 1949.
13. Van Praagh R, Van Praagh S: The anatomy of common aorticopulmonary trunk (truncus arteriosus communis) and its embryologic implications. A study of 57 necropsy cases. *Am J Cardiol* 16:406–425, 1965.
14. Fuglestad SJ, Puga FJ, Danielson GK, et al: Surgical pathology of the truncal valve: a study of 12 cases. *Am J Cardiovasc Pathol* 2:39–47, 1988.
15. Bharati S, McAllister HA, Jr, Rosenquist GC, et al: The surgical anatomy of truncus arteriosus communis. *J Thorac Cardiovasc Surg* 67:501–510, 1974.
16. Lacour-Gayet F, Serraf A, Komiya T, et al: Truncus arteriosus repair: influence of techniques of right ventricular outflow tract reconstruction. *J Thorac Cardiovasc Surg* 111:849–856, 1996.
17. Urban AE, Sinzobahamvya N, Brecher AM, et al: Truncus arteriosus: ten-year experience with homograft repair in neonates and infants. *Ann Thorac Surg* 66:S183–S188, 1998.
18. Bove EL, Lupinetti FM, Pridjian AK, et al: Results of a policy of primary repair of truncus arteriosus in the neonate. *J Thorac Cardiovasc Surg* 105:1057–1065, discussion 1065–1066, 1993.
19. Thompson LD, McElhinney DB, Reddy M, et al: Neonatal repair of truncus arteriosus: continuing improvement in outcomes. *Ann Thorac Surg* 72:391–395, 2001.

20. Marcelletti C, McGoon DC, Danielson GK, et al: Early and late results of surgical repair of truncus arteriosus. *Circulation* 55:636–641, 1977.
21. de la Cruz MV, Cayre R, Angelini P, et al: Coronary arteries in truncus arteriosus. *Am J Cardiol* 66:1482–1486, 1990.
22. Shrivastava S, Edwards JE: Coronary arterial origin in persistent truncus arteriosus. *Circulation* 55:551–554, 1977.
23. O'Byrne ML, Yang W, Mercer-Rosa L, et al: 22q11.2 Deletion syndrome is associated with increased perioperative events and more complicated postoperative course in infants undergoing infant operative correction of truncus arteriosus communis or interrupted aortic arch. *J Thorac Cardiovasc Surg* 2014. [epub].
24. Galindo A, Mendoza A, Arbues J, et al: Conotruncal anomalies in fetal life: accuracy of diagnosis, associated defects and outcome. *Eur J Obstet Gynecol Reprod Biol* 146(1):55–60, 2009.
25. Trivedi N, Levy D, Tarsa M, et al: Congenital cardiac anomalies: prenatal readings verus neonatal outcomes. *J Ultrasound Med* 31:389–399, 2012.
26. Dorfman AL, Geva T: Magnetic resonance imaging evaluation of congenital heart disease: conotruncal anomalies. *J Cardiovasc Magn Reson* 8:645–659, 2006.
27. Kirklin J, Barrat-Boyes B: *Truncus arteriosus. Cardiac surgery*, New York, 1993, Churchill Livingstone.
28. Behrendt DM, Kirsh MM, Stern A, et al: The surgical therapy for pulmonary artery—right ventricular discontinuity. *Ann Thorac Surg* 18:122–137, 1974.
29. McGoon DC, Rastelli GC, Ongley PA: An operation for the correction of truncus arteriosus. *JAMA* 205:69–73, 1968.
30. Ebert PA, Turley K, Stanger P, et al: Surgical treatment of truncus arteriosus in the first 6 months of life. *Ann Surg* 200:451–456, 1984.
31. Hanley FL, Heinemann MK, Jonas RA, et al: Repair of truncus arteriosus in the neonate. *J Thorac Cardiovasc Surg* 105:1047–1056, 1993.
32. Rodefeld MD, Hanley FL: Neonatal truncus arteriosus repair: surgical techniques and clinical management. *Semin Thorac Cardiovasc Surg Pediatr Card Surg Annu* 5:212–217, 2002.
33. Pigula FA, Nemoto EM, Griffith BP, et al: Regional low-flow perfusion provides cerebral circulatory support during neonatal aortic arch reconstruction. *J Thorac Cardiovasc Surg* 119:331–339, 2000.
34. Russell HM, Pasquali SK, Jacobs JP, et al: Outcomes of repair of common arterial trunk with truncal valve surgery: a review of the society of thoracic surgeons congenital heart surgery database. *Ann Thorac Surg* 93(1):164–169, 2012.
35. Henaine R, Azarnoush K, Belli E, et al: Fate of the truncal valve in truncus arteriosus. *Ann Thorac Surg* 85:172–178, 2008.
36. Black MD, Adatia I, Freedom RM: Truncal valve repair: initial experience in neonates. *Ann Thorac Surg* 65:1737–1740, 1998.
37. Elami A, Laks H, Pearl JM: Truncal valve repair: initial experience with infants and children. *Ann Thorac Surg* 57:397–401, discussion 402, 1994.
38. Backer CL: Techniques for repairing the aortic and truncal valves. *Cardiol Young* 15(Suppl 1):125–131, 2005.
39. Mavroudis C, Backer CL: Surgical management of severe truncal insufficiency: experience with truncal valve remodeling techniques. *Ann Thorac Surg* 72:396–400, 2001.
40. Russell HM, Mavroudis CD, Backer CL, et al: Long-term follow-up after truncal valve repair. *Cardiol Young* 22:718–723, 2012.
41. Myers PO, Bautista-Hernandez V, del Nido PJ, et al: Surgical repair of truncal valve regurgitation. *Eur J Cardiothorac Surg* 44(5):813–820, 2013.
42. Spicer RL, Behrendt D, Crowley DC, et al: Repair of truncus arteriosus in neonates with the use of a valveless conduit. *Circulation* 70:I26–I29, 1984.
43. Derby CD, Kolcz J, Gidding S, et al: Outcomes following non-valved autologous reconstruction of the right ventricular outflow tract in neonates and infants. *Eur J Cardiothorac Surg* 34:726–731, 2008.
44. Kaza AK, Lim HG, Dibardino DJ, et al: Long-term results of right ventricular outflow tract reconstruction in neonatal cardiac surgery: options and outcomes. *J Thorac Cardiovasc Surg* 138(4):911–916, 2009.
45. Hickey EJ, McCrindle BW, Blackstone EH, et al: Jugular venous valved conduit (Contegra) matches allograft performance in infant truncus arteriosus repair. *Eur J Cardiothorac Surg* 33:890–898, 2008.
46. Sinzobahamvya N, Asfour B, Boscheinen M, et al: Compared fate of small-diameter Contegras and homografts in the pulmonary position. *Eur J Cardiothorac Surg* 32:209–214, 2007.
47. Boethig D, Schreiber C, Hazekamp M, et al: Risk factors for distal Contegra stenosis: results of a prospective European multicenter study. *Thorac Cardiovasc Surg* 60(3):195–204, 2012.
48. Urso S, Rega F, Meuris B, et al: The Contegra conduit in the right ventricular outflow tract is an independent risk factor for graft replacement. *Eur J Cardiothorac Surg* 40(3):603–609, 2011.
49. Hirsch J, Sasson L, Ohye R, et al: *Long-term outcome of right ventricle to pulmonary artery conduits for the repair of congenital heart defects in infants. Midwest Pediatric Cardiology Society 25th Annual Meeting*, Nebraska, 2001, Omaha.
50. Koirala B, Merklinger SL, Van Arsdell GS, et al: Extending the usable size range of homografts in the pulmonary circulation: outcome of bicuspid homografts. *Ann Thorac Surg* 73:866–869, discussion 869–870, 2002.
51. McMullan DM, Oppido G, Alphonso N, et al: Evaluation of downsized homograft conduits for right ventricle-to-pulmonary artery reconstruction. *J Thorac Cardiovasc Surg* 132:66–71, 2006.
52. Shih T, Gurney JG, Bove EL, et al: Performance of bicuspidized pulmonary allografts compared with standard trileaflet allografts. *Ann Thorac Surg* 90(2):610–613, 2010.
53. Reddy VM, Rajasinghe HA, McElhinney DB, et al: Performance of right ventricle to pulmonary artery conduits after repair of truncus arteriosus: a comparison of Dacron-housed porcine valves and cryopreserved allografts. *Semin Thorac Cardiovasc Surg* 7:133–138, 1995.
54. Karamlou T, Ungerleider RM, Alsoufi B, et al: Oversizing pulmonary homograft conduits does not significantly decrease allograft failure in children. *Eur J Cardiothorac Surg* 27:548–553, 2005.
55. Rajasinghe HA, McElhinney DB, Reddy VM, et al: Long-term follow-up of truncus arteriosus repaired in infancy: a twenty-year experience. *J Thorac Cardiovasc Surg* 113:869–878, discussion 878–879, 1997.
56. Barbero-Marcial M, Riso A, Atik E, et al: A technique for correction of truncus arteriosus types I and II without extracardiac conduits. *J Thorac Cardiovasc Surg* 99:364–369, 1990.
57. Barbero-Marcial ML, Tanamati C: Repair of truncus arteriosus. *Adv Card Surg* 10:43–73, 1998.
58. Danton MH, Barron DJ, Stumper O, et al: Repair of truncus arteriosus: a considered approach to right ventricular outflow tract reconstruction. *Eur J Cardiothorac Surg* 20:95–103, discussion 103–104, 2001.
59. Kreutzer C, Kreutzer GO, De CMR, et al: Early and late results of fresh autologous pericardial valved conduits. *Semin Thorac Cardiovasc Surg Pediatr Card Surg Annu* 2:65–76, 1999.
60. Jacobs JP, O'Brien SM, Pasquali SK, et al: Variation in outcomes for benchmark operations: an analysis of the society of thoracic surgeons congenital heart surgery database. *Ann Thorac Surg* 92(6):2184–2191, 2011.
61. Brown JW, Ruzmetov M, Okada Y, et al: Truncus arteriosus repair: outcomes, risk factors, reoperation and management. *Eur J Cardiothorac Surg* 20:221–227, 2001.
62. Hawkins JA, Kaza AK, Burch PT, et al: Simple versus complex truncus arteriosus: neutralization of risk but with increased resource utilization. *World J Pediatr Congenit Heart Surg* 1(3):285–291, 2010.
63. Sinzobahamvya N, Boscheinen M, Blaschczok HC, et al: Survival and reintervention after neonatal repair of truncus arteriosus with valved conduit. *Eur J Cardiothorac Surg* 34:732–737, 2008.
64. Konstantinov IE, Karamlou T, Blackstone EH, et al: Truncus arteriosus associated with interrupted aortic arch in 50 neonates: a congenital heart surgeons society study. *Ann Thorac Surg* 81:214–222, 2006.
65. O'Byrne ML, Mercer-Rosa L, Zhao H, et al: Morbidity in children an adolescents after surgical correction of truncus arteriosus communis. *Am Heart J* 166(3):512–518, 2013.

66. Stulak JM, Dearani JA, Burkhart HM, et al: Does the dilated ascending aorta in an adult with congenital heart disease require intervention? *J Thorac Cardiovasc Surg* 140(6):S52–S57, 2010.
67. Carlo WF, McKenzie ED, Slesnick TC: Root dilation in patients with truncus arteriosus. *Congenit Heart Dis* 6(3):228–233, 2011.
68. Report of the New England Regional Infant Cardiac Program. *Pediatrics* 65:375–461, 1980.
69. Kutsche LM, Van Mierop LH: Anatomy and pathogenesis of aorticopulmonary septal defect. *Am J Cardiol* 59:443–447, 1987.
70. Eliotson J: Case of malformation of the pulmonary artery and aorta. *Lancet* 1:247–248, 1830.
71. Waldo K, Miyagawa-Tomita S, Kumiski D, et al: Cardiac neural crest cells provide new insight into septation of the cardiac outflow tract: aortic sac to ventricular septal closure. *Dev Biol* 196:129–144, 1998.
72. Orts-Llorca F, Puerta Fonolla J, Sobrado J: The formation, septation and fate of the truncus arteriosus in man. *J Anat* 134:41–56, 1982.
73. Richardson JV, Doty DB, Rossi NP, et al: The spectrum of anomalies of aortopulmonary septation. *J Thorac Cardiovasc Surg* 78:21–27, 1979.
74. Mori K, Ando M, Takao A, et al: Distal type of aortopulmonary window. Report of 4 cases. *Br Heart J* 40:681–689, 1978.
75. Jacobs JP, Quintessenza JA, Gaynor JW, et al: Congenital Heart Surgery Nomenclature and Database Project: aortopulmonary window. *Ann Thorac Surg* 69:S44–S49, 2000.
76. Backer CL, Mavroudis C: Surgical management of aortopulmonary window: a 40-year experience. *Eur J Cardiothorac Surg* 21:773–779, 2002.
77. Faulkner SL, Oldham RR, Atwood GF, et al: Aortopulmonary window, ventricular septal defect, and membranous pulmonary atresia with a diagnosis of truncus arteriosus. *Chest* 65:351–353, 1974.
78. Hew CC, Bacha EA, Zurakowski D, et al: Optimal surgical approach for repair of aortopulmonary window. *Cardiol Young* 11:385–390, 2001.
79. Neufeld HN, Lester RG, Adams P, Jr, et al: Aorticopulmonary septal defect. *Am J Cardiol* 9:12–25, 1962.
80. McElhinney DB, Reddy VM, Tworetzky W, et al: Early and late results after repair of aortopulmonary septal defect and associated anomalies in infants <6 months of age. *Am J Cardiol* 81:195–201, 1998.
81. Berry TE, Bharati S, Muster AJ, et al: Distal aortopulmonary septal defect, aortic origin of the right pulmonary artery, intact ventricular septum, patent ductus arteriosus and hypoplasia of the aortic isthmus: a newly recognized syndrome. *Am J Cardiol* 49:108–116, 1982.
82. Braunlin E, Peoples WM, Freedom RM, et al: Interruption of the aortic arch with aorticopulmonary septal defect. An anatomic review. *Pediatr Cardiol* 3:329–335, 1982.
83. Kiran VS, Singh MK, Shah S, et al: Lessons learned from a series of patients with missed aortopulmonary windows. *Cardiol Young* 18:480–484, 2008.
84. Balaji S, Burch M, Sullivan ID: Accuracy of cross-sectional echocardiography in diagnosis of aortopulmonary window. *Am J Cardiol* 67:650–653, 1991.
85. Johansson L, Michaelsson M, Westerholm CJ, et al: Aortopulmonary window: a new operative approach. *Ann Thorac Surg* 25:564–567, 1978.
86. Rice MJ, Seward JB, Hagler DJ, et al: Visualization of aortopulmonary window by two-dimensional echocardiography. *Mayo Clin Proc* 57:482–487, 1982.
87. Satomi G, Nakamura K, Imai Y, et al: Two-dimensional echocardiographic diagnosis of aorticopulmonary window. *Br Heart J* 43:351–356, 1980.
88. Smallhorn JF, Anderson RH, Macartney FJ: Two dimensional echocardiographic assessment of communications between ascending aorta and pulmonary trunk or individual pulmonary arteries. *Br Heart J* 47:563–572, 1982.
89. Valsangiacomo ER, Smallhorn JF: Images in cardiovascular medicine. Prenatal diagnosis of aortopulmonary window by fetal echocardiography. *Circulation* 105:E192, 2002.
90. Garver KA, Hernandez RJ, Vermilion RP, et al: Images in cardiovascular medicine. Correlative imaging of aortopulmonary window: demonstration with echocardiography, angiography, and MRI. *Circulation* 96:1036–1037, 1997.
91. Incesu L, Baysal K, Kalayci AG, et al: Magnetic resonance imaging of proximal aortopulmonary window. *Clin Imaging* 22:23–25, 1998.
92. Tkebuchava T, von Segesser LK, Vogt PR, et al: Congenital aortopulmonary window: diagnosis, surgical technique and long-term results. *Eur J Cardiothorac Surg* 11:293–297, 1997.
93. Gross RE: Surgical closure of an aortic septal defect. *Circulation* 5:858–863, 1952.
94. Scott HW, Jr, Sabiston DC, Jr: Surgical treatment for congenital aorticopulmonary fistula; experimental and clinical aspects. *J Thorac Surg* 25:26–39, 1953.
95. Cooley DA, McNamara DG, Latson JR: Aorticopulmonary septal defect: diagnosis and surgical treatment. *Surgery* 42:101–120, discussion 120, 1957.
96. Putnam TC, Gross RE: Surgical management of aortopulmonary fenestration. *Surgery* 59:727–735, 1966.
97. Cordell AR, McKone RC, Wilson HV: Management of aorticopulmonary septal defect in early infancy. *Am Surg* 33:962–964, 1967.
98. Wright JS, Freeman R, Johnston JB: Aorto-pulmonary fenestration. A technique of surgical management. *J Thorac Cardiovasc Surg* 55:280–283, 1968.
99. Deverall PB, Lincoln JC, Aberdeen E, et al: Aortopulmonary window. *J Thorac Cardiovasc Surg* 57:479–486, 1969.
100. Clarke CP, Richardson JP: The management of aortopulmonary window: advantages of transaortic closure with a Dacron patch. *J Thorac Cardiovasc Surg* 72:48–51, 1976.
101. Jansen C, Hruda J, Rammeloo L, et al: Surgical repair of aortopulmonary window: thirty-seven years of experience. *Pediatr Cardiol* 27:552–556, 2006.
102. Erez E, Dagan O, Georghiou GP, et al: Surgical management of aortopulmonary window and associated lesions. *Ann Thorac Surg* 77:484–487, 2004.
103. Mert M, Paker T, Akcevin A, et al: Diagnosis, management, and results of treatment for aortopulmonary window. *Cardiol Young* 14:506–511, 2004.
104. van Son JA, Puga FJ, Danielson GK, et al: Aortopulmonary window: factors associated with early and late success after surgical treatment. *Mayo Clin Proc* 68:128–133, 1993.
105. Matsuki O, Yagihara T, Yamamoto F, et al: New surgical technique for total-defect aortopulmonary window. *Ann Thorac Surg* 54:991–992, 1992.
106. Matsuki O, Yagihara T, Yamamoto F, et al: As originally published in 1992: new surgical technique for total-defect aortopulmonary window. Updated in 1999. *Ann Thorac Surg* 67:891, 1999.
107. Messmer BJ: Pulmonary artery flap for closure of aortopulmonary window. *Ann Thorac Surg* 57:498–501, 1994.
108. van Son JA, Hambsch J, Mohr FW: Anatomical reconstruction of aorta and pulmonary trunk in patients with an aortopulmonary window. *Ann Thorac Surg* 70:674–675, discussion 676, 2000.
109. Kitagawa T, Katoh I, Taki H, et al: New operative method for distal aortopulmonary septal defect. *Ann Thorac Surg* 51:680–682, 1991.
110. Konstantinov IE, Karamlou T, Williams WG, et al: Surgical management of aortopulmonary window associated with interrupted aortic arch: a Congenital Heart Surgeons Society study. *J Thorac Cardiovasc Surg* 131:1136–1141:e1132, 2006.
111. Bagtharia R, Trivedi KR, Burkhart HM, et al: Outcomes for patients with an aortopulmonary window, and the impact of associated cardiovascular lesions. *Cardiol Young* 14:473–480, 2004.
112. Jureidini SB, Spadaro JJ, Rao PS: Successful transcatheter closure with the buttoned device of aortopulmonary window in an adult. *Am J Cardiol* 81:371–372, 1998.
113. Richens T, Wilson N: Amplatzer device closure of a residual aortopulmonary window. *Catheter Cardiovasc Interv* 50:431–433, 2000.
114. Stamato T, Benson LN, Smallhorn JF, et al: Transcatheter closure of an aortopulmonary window with a modified double umbrella occluder system. *Cathet Cardiovasc Diagn* 35:165–167, 1995.
115. Tulloh RM, Rigby ML: Transcatheter umbrella closure of aortopulmonary window. *Heart* 77:479–480, 1997.

116. Noonan PM, Desai T, Degiovanni JV: Closure of an aortopulmonary window using the Amplatzer Duct Occluder II. *Pediatr Cardiol* 34(3):712–714, 2013.
117. Trehan V, Nigam A, Tyagi S: Percutaneous closure of nonrestrictive aortopulmonary window in three infants. *Catheter Cardiovasc Interv* 71:405–411, 2008.
118. Sivakumar K, Francis E: Transcatheter closure of distal aortopulmonary window using Amplatzer device. *Congenit Heart Dis* 1:321–323, 2006.
119. Bhalgat PS, Kerkar PG: Aortic regurgitation following transcatheter closure of aortopulmonary window. *J Invasive Cardiol* 23(10):E235–E236, 2011.

CHAPTER 122

INTERRUPTED AORTIC ARCH

Marshall L. Jacobs • Jeffrey P. Jacobs • Alvin J. Chin

CHAPTER OUTLINE

Interrupted aortic arch (IAA) is a rare genetic disorder of the cardiovascular system, present in approximately two cases per 100,000 live births and comprising 1.5% of all cases of congenital heart disease. Its hallmark feature is a lack of luminal continuity between the ascending aorta and the descending aorta. In the absence of surgical repair, mortality approaches 75% in the first month of life and 90% by 1 year. Despite tremendous recent progress in the management of complex congenital heart malformations in neonates and infants, the mortality and morbidity associated with surgical management of IAA and the spectrum of associated anomalies remain substantial. Areas of controversy include the choice of single-stage versus multistage repair, the assessment and management of associated obstruction or hypoplasia of the left ventricular outflow tract, and the intraoperative management of cardiopulmonary bypass with or without periods of hypothermic circulatory arrest. Important late-phase events after repair of IAA are related to the potential for development or recurrence of systemic ventricular outflow tract obstruction or aortic arch obstruction, and presurgical and postsurgical abnormalities of neurodevelopmental outcome and their impact on functional status.

HISTORICAL NOTES

The first description of an IAA is attributed to Steidele in 1778.[1] That case involved absence of the aortic isthmus. Absence of the aortic arch segment between the left common carotid artery and the left subclavian artery was described by Seidel in 1818.[2] Absence of the aortic segment between the innominate artery and the left common carotid artery was described by Weisman and Kesten in 1948.[3] In 1955, Samson and colleagues[4] performed the first successful surgical repair of IAA in a 3-year-old child. The anatomy included absence of the aortic isthmus, the presence of a patent ductus arteriosus, and two ventricular septal defects (VSDs). In the initial operation, the ductus was divided, and then it was joined to the underside of the proximal left subclavian artery, creating luminal continuity between the ascending aorta and the descending aorta. The VSDs were closed 4 years later. Case reports in the 1960s described interposition of prosthetic grafts to bridge the gap between aortic segments. The first use of turned-down aortic arch branches (left subclavian or left common carotid artery) to achieve end-to-end anastomosis to the descending thoracic aorta was described by Sirak and coworkers in 1968.[5] One of Sirak's three patients was the first neonate to survive operation. In 1970, Litwin and associates[6] palliated a neonate with arch interruption and VSD by interposition of a prosthetic tube graft between the proximal main pulmonary artery and the descending thoracic aorta, with banding of the distal main pulmonary artery.

In 1970, Barratt-Boyes and colleagues[7] described successful repair of IAA and simultaneous correction of intracardiac lesions (VSD and total anomalous pulmonary venous connection). Through a left thoracotomy incision, a 12-mm prosthetic tube graft was connected to the descending thoracic aorta. Next, through a median sternotomy, the proximal end of the conduit was connected to the ascending aorta. Hypothermic circulatory arrest facilitated this anastomosis and the repair of the intracardiac lesions. In 1975, Trusler and Izukawa[8] were the first to accomplish direct anastomosis of the descending aorta to the ascending aorta and transverse arch (with excision of all ductal tissue and with no interposition graft), together with VSD closure. The operation was accomplished through a median sternotomy approach, using cardiopulmonary bypass and deep hypothermic circulatory arrest. Primary repair via median sternotomy using continuous cardiopulmonary bypass (without a period of circulatory arrest) was reported by Asou and colleagues in 1996.[9]

In the mid-1960s, Angelo DiGeorge, a pediatric endocrinologist, described the association of hypoparathyroidism (with hypocalcemia), thymic aplasia, cleft lip and palate, and altered immunity (eventually recognized to be the consequence of a T cell abnormality). Several of the patients with this constellation had cardiac anomalies—the most prevalent among DiGeorge's patients was IAA. DiGeorge syndrome and the closely related velocardiofacial syndrome were subsequently found, in the majority of instances, to be related to a chromosomal deletion in the region of 22q11.2.[10-13] In a prospective evaluation of 251 patients with conotruncal defects who were screened for the presence of a 22q11 deletion, 50% (12 of 24) of patients with IAA were found to have a 22q11 deletion at locus D22S75 (N25).[10]

ANATOMY AND NOMENCLATURE

The definition of *interrupted aortic arch* adopted in 2000 by the International Congenital Heart Surgery Nomenclature and Database Project is "loss of luminal continuity between the ascending and descending aorta."[14] *Absence* of luminal continuity would also be an acceptable description. As a congenital defect, IAA represents a developmental abnormality of the embryologic arch elements. In the instance of left-sided aortic arch, the proximal arch (between the normally positioned innominate artery and the left common carotid artery) is derived from the aortic sac. The distal arch (between the left common carotid artery and the left subclavian artery) is derived from the left fourth embryonic arch, and the isthmus (between the left subclavian artery and the descending thoracic aorta) from the junction of the left sixth embryonic arch (ductus arteriosus) with the left dorsal aorta and the left fourth embryonic arch. It is therefore not surprising that many anatomic variants of IAA are observed, with respect to the site of discontinuity and the sites of origin of the brachiocephalic vessels.

Aberrant origin of the right subclavian artery from the descending thoracic aorta is encountered frequently in some forms of IAA, and rarely in others.[15] It is generally associated with hypoplasia or obstruction of the left ventricular outflow tract (LVOT), as there is less antegrade flow from the left ventricle. Rarely, the site of origin of the right subclavian artery is a persistent right-sided ductus. Interrupted arch can occur with a right aortic arch, with persistence of a right-sided ductus (or bilateral ducts).

In nearly 100% of cases, loss or absence of luminal continuity reflects complete absence of one element of the aortic arch. In rare instances, a fibrous strand connects the ascending aorta and associated arch elements with the descending aorta. By convention, these rare cases can be referred to as *interrupted aortic arch*, although some would make a distinction and refer to such cases as *atresia* of a particular portion of the arch. Celoria and Patton originally described the most widely accepted classification for IAA in 1959.[16] They divided interrupted arch anomalies into three varieties, based on the site of aortic arch interruption (Fig. 122-1). In the common circumstance of left-sided aortic arch, type A refers to interruption that is distal to the left subclavian artery. In type B, the interruption is between the left common carotid and the left subclavian artery. Finally, in type C, the interruption is between the innominate and left carotid arteries. In a multi-institutional outcome study of 472 patients with IAA by the Congenital Heart Surgeons' Society (CHSS), McCrindle and associates[17] reported that type A was observed in 28% of patients, type B was by far the most common in 70%, and type C was the rarest, seen in only 1%. An aberrant right subclavian artery, originating from the descending aorta and taking a retroesophageal course, is frequently seen in patients with IAA, particularly type B.[15] In other uncommon variations, the aberrant right subclavian artery can originate instead from the right pulmonary artery via a persistent right-sided patent ductus arteriosus (isolated subclavian artery), or the right pulmonary artery can be the vessel that is isolated. These variations have been reported and analyzed, and attempts have been made to expand on the classification system of Celoria to include a description of the origin of the right subclavian artery. The classification system reported by Dische and coworkers in 1975[18] added the subscript 2 to the letter A, B, or C from the Celoria classification when the aberrant right subclavian artery originated from the descending aorta distal to the interruption. Thus, in the system described by Dische, in type A_2 the interruption is distal to the left subclavian artery, and the only major arch vessel taking origin from the aorta distal to the interruption is the aberrant right subclavian artery. Similarly, in type B_2, both carotid arteries arise from the aortic arch proximal to the interruption and both subclavian arteries arise from the aorta distal to the interruption. In 1982, the nomenclature system of Oppenheimer-Dekker and colleagues[19] offered an alternative subclassification also based on the system of Celoria and Patton. This system also includes subdivisions based on the presence of an aberrant right subclavian artery, but here nine types of IAA are classified. Types A, B, and C are determined based on the system of Celoria. No subscript number is used if the right subclavian artery has a normal origin, a subscript 1 is used when the aberrant right subclavian artery originates from the descending aorta, and a subscript 2 is used when the aberrant right subclavian artery arises from the right pulmonary artery via ductal tissue. Most common usage involves the A-B-C system of Celoria together with a specific verbal description of abnormalities of the origin of brachiocephalic vessels, branch pulmonary arteries, or patent ductus arteriosus.

The following is the classification of IAA used in the Diagnostic Long List of the version of the International Paediatric and Congenital Cardiac Code derived from the nomenclature of the International Congenital Heart

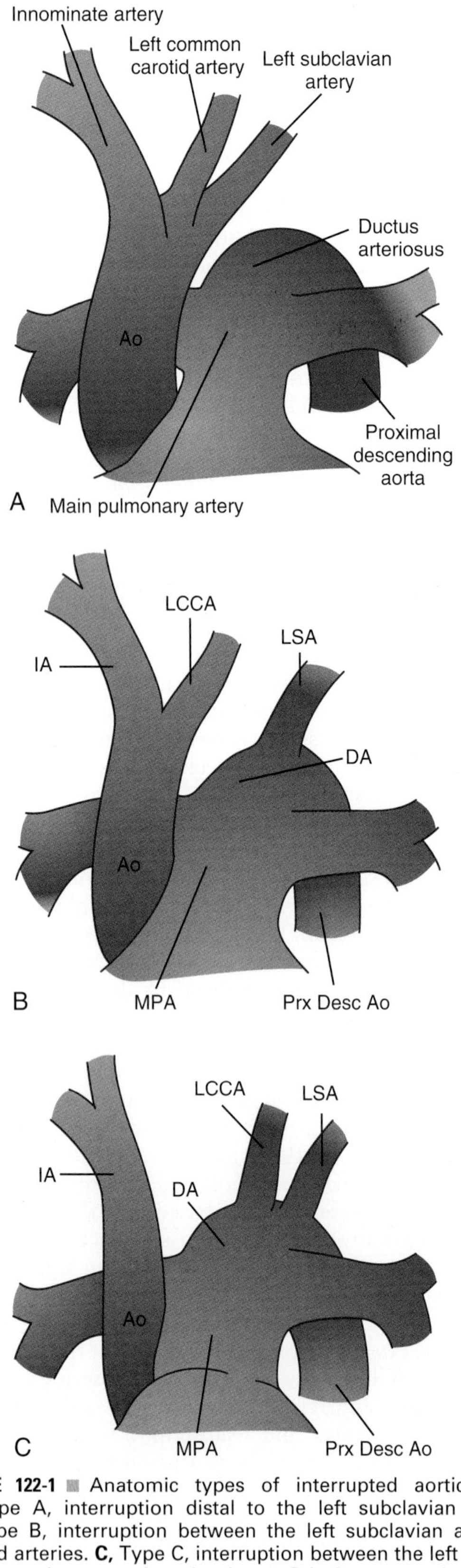

FIGURE 122-1 ■ Anatomic types of interrupted aortic arch. **A,** Type A, interruption distal to the left subclavian artery. **B,** Type B, interruption between the left subclavian and left carotid arteries. **C,** Type C, interruption between the left carotid and innominate arteries. *Ao,* Aorta; *DA,* ductus arteriosus; *IA,* innominate artery; *LCCA,* left common carotid artery; *LSA,* left subclavian artery; *MPA,* main pulmonary artery; *Prx Desc Ao,* proximal descending aorta. (From Jonas RA: Interrupted aortic arch. In Mavroudis C, Backer CL, editors: *Pediatric cardiac surgery,* ed 3, Philadelphia, 2003, Mosby.)

Surgery Nomenclature and Database Project of the European Association for Cardio-Thoracic Surgery and the Society of Thoracic Surgeons[20]:

1. IAA
2. IAA, type A (interruption distal to the subclavian artery)
3. IAA, type A2 (interruption distal to one subclavian artery, with the only major arch vessel taking origin from the aorta distal to the interruption being an aberrant subclavian artery)
4. IAA, type B (interruption between the carotid and subclavian arteries)
5. IAA, type B2 (interruption between the carotid and subclavian arteries, with both subclavian arteries arising from the aorta distal to the interruption)
6. IAA, type C (interruption between the carotid arteries)
7. IAA, type C2 (interruption between the carotid arteries, with both subclavian arteries arising from the aorta distal to the interruption)

Interrupted aortic arch complexes nearly always have a large VSD (the exception being cases of IAA with aortopulmonary window, of which a majority have an intact ventricular septum). In the setting of IAA with VSD, the VSD can be of any type. Most commonly, it is of the malalignment type. In this circumstance, the conal (outlet) septum is malaligned posteriorly and leftward with respect to the true trabecular septum.[21,22] The malalignment of the conal septum is associated with varying degrees of subaortic obstruction.[23-25] When a malalignment-type VSD is present, the conal septum may be not only misplaced but also hypoplastic. In an echocardiographic study of 53 patients with IAA with VSD, Chin and Jacobs[26] found that 43 of 45 patients with type B IAA had VSDs involving maldevelopment of the outflow region. In type A IAA, only four of eight had this type of VSD.[26] In the complex of the left side of the heart and the aorta (the left heart–aorta complex), other levels of obstruction that are often associated with IAA include a prominent and obstructive anterolateral muscle of the left ventricle (muscle of Moulaert), aortic valvar stenosis with or without aortic annular hypoplasia, and fibrous or fibromuscular subaortic stenosis.[27] IAA can coexist with a wide variety of cardiac lesions, as evidenced by the first report from the CHSS in 1994. Jonas and associates[15] reported that among 250 cases of IAA at participating centers, associated cardiac anomalies included VSD (183 [73%]), truncus arteriosus (25 [10%]), aortopulmonary window (10 [4%]), univentricular atrioventricular connection (9 [4%]), transposition of the great arteries with VSD (8 [3%]), double-outlet right ventricle (5 [2%]), Taussig-Bing anomaly (4 [2%]), complete atrioventricular canal defect (1 [0.4%]), and congenitally corrected transposition of the great arteries (1 [0.4%]). Isolated IAA (without VSD or associated anomalies) was present in only 4 of 250 patients [2%]). More unusual associations have been the subject of individual case reports, including several cases of aortic atresia with IAA and VSD, in which flow to the ascending aorta and thus the coronary arteries depended on flow either through the circle of Willis or through a patent right-sided ductus arteriosus.

PRESENTATION AND PREOPERATIVE MANAGEMENT

During fetal development, the left ventricular output supplies the arterial circulation proximal to the interruption, and right ventricular output supplies arterial circulation distal to the interruption via the left ductus arteriosus. Postnatally, this arrangement continues, with the addition of the pulmonary blood flow to the volume load of the left ventricle. The postnatal pathophysiology of virtually all IAA complexes is predicated on ductal dependency of a portion of the systemic circulation (distal to the interruption), and on a usually large but variable ratio of pulmonary to systemic blood flow (Qp/Qs). This ratio is influenced by the anatomic substrate for left-to-right shunting. That may be a VSD alone or a variety of other lesions such as common arterial trunk or aortopulmonary window. In addition, the physiology is influenced by the presence of other obstructive lesions in the left heart–aorta complex. Obstructive or hypoplastic elements of the left heart–aorta complex, alone or in combination with left ventricular dysfunction, may contribute to left-to-right shunting at the atrial level, through either an atrial septal defect or a stretched patent foramen ovale.

Despite the markedly abnormal circulatory arrangement, manifestations of the abnormal physiology may be subtle in the early neonatal period. If ductal patency persists, typical signs of congestive heart failure may emerge in the first few weeks of life, as the pulmonary vascular resistance begins to fall and pulmonary blood flow increases. More typically, and importantly, constriction of the ductus arteriosus can begin and progress any time in the first days or weeks of life. This may be manifest as a mottled or gray appearance of the lower body, and it is accompanied by signs of congestive heart failure (tachypnea, tachycardia, hepatomegaly, and poor feeding) and then of circulatory insufficiency (irritability progressing to lethargy, oliguria, and then metabolic acidosis and profound shock with multiple organ dysfunction and coagulopathy). Early visual evidence of the difference in oxygen saturation between the upper and lower body may be present. Neither this nor differential blood pressure between upper and lower extremities is a constant or particularly useful finding, as either may be influenced by the dynamic variability of the Qp/Qs, by diminished cardiac performance, and by abnormal anatomy, including aberrant origin of the right subclavian artery (which, in the setting of IAA type B or type C, results in all four extremities having postductal blood pressures). In the absence of a prenatal diagnosis, approximately half of patients present during the first day of life, and nearly all do within the first 2 weeks of life. In rare instances, persistent patency of the ductus arteriosus is associated with a later presentation.

Echocardiography with color flow mapping is the primary diagnostic study in virtually all cases. When the diagnosis is suspected or established, evaluation as an inpatient in an intensive care setting is advised. Intravenous prostaglandin E_1 should be administered promptly to maintain patency of the ductus arteriosus.[28] The need for an arterial line and assisted ventilation can be judged best from the initial arterial blood gas measurement. Unless a period of shock has accompanied ductal constriction, pharmacologic support with catecholamine infusions is rarely indicated. In recent years, the use of milrinone, a phosphodiesterase-3 inhibitor, as a continuous infusion has achieved wide acceptance. It probably contributes to the improvement of myocardial performance that generally occurs with correction of acidosis, and it has the added effect of reducing systemic vascular resistance. Assessment of the presence and degree of secondary organ dysfunction includes laboratory evaluation of metabolic status, serum indicators of renal and hepatic function, and a coagulation profile. Hypocalcemia, a frequent finding, may indicate the presence of DiGeorge syndrome, including the hypoparathyroidism phenotype. Fluorescent in situ hybridization can reveal the typical hemizygous 22q11.2 deletion seen in 85% to 95% of patients with DiGeorge syndrome.[10]

In most cases, the key features of the anatomy are revealed by a detailed echocardiographic evaluation. A complete study should clarify the site of aortic interruption and the sites of origin of the arch branches. Additional essential information includes the presence and nature of atrial and VSDs, and a detailed assessment of the LVOT. This includes measurement of the dimensions of the subaortic region (including a description of the outlet or conal septum, which may be either thickened or hypoplastic, and which may be posteriorly malaligned, thus narrowing the caliber of the subaortic LVOT), as well as the aortic valve annulus and orifice, and the sinotubular junction and ascending aorta.[29] The mitral valve is assessed, including the size of its orifice, its competence, and the nature of the subvalvar apparatus. The size of the left ventricle is measured, and a determination is made regarding whether it extends to the apex of the ventricular mass. Important associated diagnoses to consider include truncus arteriosus communis,[30] aortopulmonary window,[31,32] transposition of the great arteries, and various forms of univentricular atrioventricular connection. A general visual or quantitative assessment of myocardial contractility is made. Although color flow mapping with Doppler studies can be helpful in evaluating some intracardiac obstructive lesions, the definitive echocardiographic assessment is most often made in the setting of a widely patent ductus (and, in most cases, a nonrestrictive interventricular communication). As a result, quantitation of the degree of LVOT obstruction by estimation of a gradient in that region can be misleading.

In some cases, cardiac catheterization with angiography provides important additional information. In particular, it may be helpful in clarifying instances of discontinuous branch pulmonary arteries, anomalous pulmonary venous connections, or transposition of the great arteries (in which case, balloon atrial septotomy may be beneficial). In cases with coexistent aortic atresia, it may help to define the source of coronary blood flow. Another indication for cardiac catheterization is the need to restore and/or maintain patency of the arterial duct. Until recently, maintenance of ductal patency by means of deployment of an intravascular stent was reserved for unusual circumstances. An example would be the case of late presentation of an infant with IAA type A with VSD, who had a restrictive duct and respiratory syncytial virus pneumonia. Ductal dilation and stenting provided temporary palliation, making it possible to defer arch repair and VSD closure for several weeks to allow resolution of airway inflammation and improvement of pulmonary function. The recent emergence and increasingly widespread adoption of so-called hybrid strategies for initial management of numerous forms of critical heart disease in neonates that share the common feature of ductal dependency of the systemic circulation has added to the surgical armamentarium and increased the therapeutic options for patients with IAA. When such a strategy is applied to neonates with IAA, maintenance of ductal patency (either by stent deployment or by continuous administration of prostaglandin E1) is generally accompanied by bilateral application of pulmonary artery bands to the proximal branch pulmonary arteries to limit pulmonary blood flow.

Increasingly, both computed tomography (CT) and magnetic resonance imaging (MRI) are being used to further clarify the anatomy of complex cardiac anomalies in neonates and infants.[33] Each technology lends itself to three-dimensional reconstruction, which can be helpful in clarifying anatomic details, with particular attention to spatial relationships. CT has the advantage of rapid data acquisition, and in some instances it can be accomplished without general anesthesia. It has the disadvantage of radiation exposure. MRI does not involve radiation exposure, but it generally requires the patient to be anesthetized for the study.

SURGICAL MANAGEMENT

Indications and Timing of Surgery

Interrupted aortic arch is incompatible with life without patency of the ductus arteriosus or an alternative pathway for perfusion of the lower body. Before the availability of prostaglandins, the diagnosis of IAA was a surgical emergency. Most often, neonates were in poor condition, with a closing ductus, and resuscitative measures had little efficacy. Patients had to be taken to surgery in poor condition. Emergent palliative operations were performed under less than ideal conditions, and they often yielded less than optimal outcomes. In the current era, restoration of ductal patency after infusion of prostaglandin E_1 is generally accomplished, facilitating resuscitation in an intensive care unit.[28] Recovery of renal and hepatic function usually follows correction of acidosis and optimization of respiratory parameters and fluid and metabolic status. This then facilitates stabilization and assessment of neurologic status, and recovery or correction of coagulation disorders. Genetic evaluation can be initiated, and meaningful family education and counseling can occur before surgery is undertaken. An operation is usually indicated as soon as these preliminary objectives have been achieved, as there is no definitive medical therapy for IAA.

Operative Management

As noted, the history of surgery for IAA began during an era when the use of cardiopulmonary bypass to accomplish repair of intracardiac defects in infants and neonates was a theoretical goal for the future rather than a therapeutic reality. As a result, most early arch repairs were closed-heart (i.e., nonbypass) procedures.[6,34] Arch repair was accomplished using an interposition graft or a brachiocephalic vessel turndown, either in isolation or in combination with banding of the pulmonary artery. In most instances, repair of the VSD (with removal of the pulmonary artery band) would be undertaken some months later. Even after the introduction and successful achievement of one-stage repair of IAA and VSD closure, both via median sternotomy with cardiopulmonary bypass and hypothermic circulatory arrest, there persisted at many centers a bias favoring a staged approach to IAA with VSD or other more complex cardiac anatomy.[35] In 1997, Mainwaring and Lamberti reported on their 10-year experience with a two-stage approach to repair IAA type B with VSD.[36] Twenty-six of 27 patients survived stage 1 (arch repair with interposition graft). Twenty-two of 25 patients who underwent subsequent VSD closure were long-term survivors. Freedom from reoperation for arch graft enlargement was 86% at 3 years and 55% at 5 years.

In 1994, the CHSS published a report of their first multi-institutional outcome study of patients with IAA and VSD.[15] Patients were enrolled as neonates between 1987 and 1992, and 173 patients underwent reparative surgery. The initial procedure consisted of arch repair and VSD closure (one stage) in 116 (67%), arch repair and banding of the pulmonary trunk in 40, and only repair of the arch interruption in 17. Thus, one-stage repair was chosen in 67% of cases, with intent to undertake two-stage repair in 33%. In the past two decades, single-stage repair of IAA and intracardiac defects has gained wide acceptance. At most centers, it is the usual or routine technique used, with a two-stage approach being reserved for specific uncommon circumstances.[37-41]

Techniques of Arch Repair

An optimal method of arch repair would be one that could be performed safely and reproducibly in neonates, with minimal likelihood of stenosis in the short or long term. Thus, it would result in normal growth of all aortic segments including the anastomotic area. Ideally, it would not require use or division of any of the principal brachiocephalic vessels. In the traditional multistage approach, a synthetic tube graft was interposed between the proximal (ascending) and distal (descending) aortic elements. Although this can generally be accomplished without cardiopulmonary bypass support through either a lateral or an anterior approach, the certainty that the graft will not grow with the patient ensures an absolute requirement for arch reintervention in all survivors.[42-44] That reintervention can consist of graft replacement in situ, augmentation in situ, or extra-anatomic placement of an additional graft. An alternative technique that has been used in both one-stage and two-stage strategies is the use of a turned-down brachiocephalic artery (carotid or subclavian artery) that is anastomosed to the descending aorta. Monro and colleagues[45] published a small series demonstrating satisfactory growth of the arch elements and anastomotic region in the majority of patients at follow-up of 8 to 19 years. More recently, John Brown and associates[46] reviewed their experience with 47 patients who underwent repair of IAA by means of left carotid artery turndown. Approximately one third of patients underwent subsequent reinterventions on the arch. The authors claimed as advantages the reduced exposure to circulatory arrest and cardiopulmonary bypass in the newborn period and low incidence of bronchial compression by the reconstructed arch.

In the current era, the approach most often used is a one-stage approach entailing direct anastomosis between the ascending aorta and the descending aorta. This approach involves extensive mobilization of both proximal and distal elements. Several centers have reported excellent early outcomes with the technique of end-to-side anastomosis of the descending thoracic aorta either to the ascending aorta or to the ascending aorta and the underside of the proximal aortic arch.[41,47-49] Patch augmentation of the anastomosis of the proximal and distal aortic segments was described by Norwood in 1990, and intermediate-term results were reported by Jacobs and Norwood in 1995.[50] This technique is intended to reduce tension on the anastomosis, to enlarge the connection between segments, and to address hypoplasia of the ascending aorta, which is particularly common in IAA types B and C.[22,25] In addition, the use of patch augmentation generally obviates the need to divide either the left subclavian artery or an anomalous right subclavian artery to bring the elements of the arch together. It also lessens the likelihood of left bronchial compression, which can complicate some repairs of IAA.[51] We have used cryopreserved pulmonary artery homograft tissue for the patch material. Successful use of other patch materials has been reported, including pulmonary artery autograft tissue.[52]

The 1994 CHSS report of outcomes in patients with IAA and VSD included an important observation concerning the potential benefit of patch augmentation of the amalgamation of the ascending and descending aorta in patients with additional levels of obstruction or hypoplasia in the left heart–aorta complex.[15] Multivariable analysis identified subaortic or annular narrowing as incremental risk factors for death after repair (Fig. 122-2). The report by Jonas and associates[15] concluded, "In the 20% of patients in whom obstruction existed elsewhere in the left heart-aorta complex, the percent survival was highest among those undergoing ascending aorta/arch augmentation." More recently, in a CHSS analysis of intermediate- and long-term outcomes of an expanded cohort of 472 neonates with IAA, McCrindle and associates[17] reported that reintervention was more likely for those who had IAA repair by a method other than direct anastomosis with patch augmentation. In a single institution study from Marie Lannelongue Hospital in 2002, Roussin and associates[53] described excellent results with the incorporation of a pulmonary artery autograft patch into the aortic arch reconstruction. Among 20 patients who underwent repair of IAA with pulmonary autograft patch aortoplasty, actuarial freedom from interventions for recurrent arch obstruction was 100% at median follow-up of 29 months.

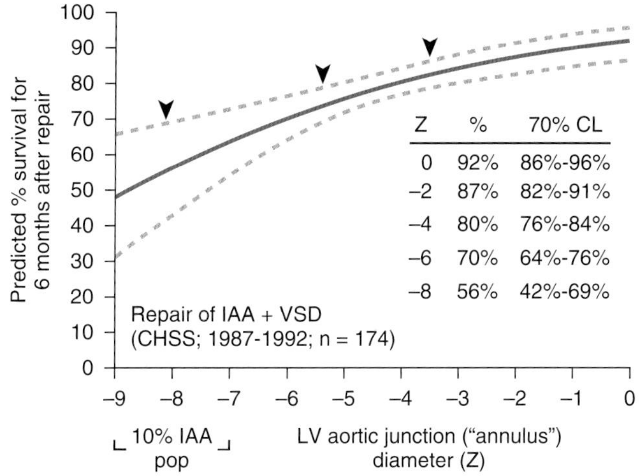

FIGURE 122-2 Data from the Congenital Heart Surgeons' Society (CHSS) study of outcomes in neonates with interrupted aortic arch (IAA) and ventricular septal defect (VSD). Nomogram of a specific solution of a multivariable equation demonstrating the risk-adjusted effect of the measured diameter of the left ventricular (LV)–aortic junction. The value of 3.1 kg was entered for the birth weight, 7 days for age at repair, type B for IAA, and conoventricular for the VSD. *Arrowheads* indicate points of evident difference, from *right* to *left*. *CL,* Confidence limits. (From Jonas RA, Quaegebeur JM, Kirklin JW, et al: Outcomes in patients with interrupted aortic arch and ventricular septal defect. A multiinstitutional study. Congenital Heart Surgeons Society. *J Thorac Cardiovasc Surg* 107:1099–1109, 1994.)

Left Ventricular Outflow Tract Obstruction

Estimates of the incidence of occurrence of important LVOT obstruction in the setting of IAA vary considerably[24,34,54-59] because of the inability to measure an outflow tract gradient accurately in the setting of a large VSD and a patent ductus, and also because there currently is no consensus on the morphologic criteria or threshold measurements that should be used to assign such a diagnosis. Narrowing of the subaortic region can be mild to severe as a consequence of deviation of the conal septum into the LVOT in the setting of IAA with malalignment-type VSD. In addition, as mentioned, posterior deviation of the conal septum can contribute to LVOT obstruction even when the conal septum is hypoplastic and entirely fibrous. In these cases, there is generally hypoplasia of the aortic annulus. As there is no option of resecting muscle to enlarge the subaortic region, the need to anchor the top of the VSD patch to this fibrous rim not only results in a narrow subaortic region; it can also result in fixation of a portion of the aortic annulus, preventing subsequent normal growth. In the 1994 report of the first multi-institutional study of IAA by the CHSS, subaortic or annular narrowing was predictive of mortality after repair.[15] The techniques used by participating surgeons to address subaortic narrowing included partial resection of obstructing muscle in the LVOT (myotomy or myectomy) and techniques to bypass the narrowed systemic ventricular outflow tract. In the analysis, these were combined together as Damus-Kaye-Stansel procedures. The analysis led to an interesting but unsatisfying conclusion. Investigators reported, "Procedural risk factors for death after repair were (1) repair without concomitant procedures in patients with other important levels of obstruction in the left heart-aorta complex, (2) a Damus-Kaye-Stansel anastomosis, and (3) subaortic myotomy or myectomy in the face of subaortic narrowing. One-stage repair plus ascending aorta/arch augmentation had the highest predicted time-related survival in the 20% of patients with IAA and one or more coexisting levels of obstruction in the left heart-aorta complex, as did initial repair without or with aorta/arch augmentation in the 80% without these." The troubling inference, of course, was that the presence of obstructing lesions in the left heart–aorta complex was associated with an increased likelihood of death after repair, but that specific procedures directed at these obstructions (other than patch augmentation of the arch repair) did not (in this study) reduce the risk of mortality.

It is important to recognize that not all procedures to bypass subaortic obstruction are the same. The first report of such a procedure was by Yasui and colleagues in 1987.[60] The operation consisted of ligation of the patent ductus arteriosus, restoration of aortic continuity with an 8-mm polytetrafluoroethylene graft, placement of an internal patch to tunnel all left ventricular blood from the left ventricle through the VSD into the pulmonary artery, transection of the main pulmonary artery, anastomosis between the proximal pulmonary artery and the ascending aorta, and interposition of a valved conduit between the right ventricle and the distal pulmonary artery. Others adapted the type of aortopulmonary amalgamation with arch augmentation developed by Norwood to cases of IAA with severe LVOT obstruction. Jacobs and Norwood[50] reported a series of nine patients treated with arch repair, aortopulmonary amalgamation, and homograft patch augmentation of the entire aortic reconstruction (Fig. 122-3). Seven patients received aortopulmonary shunts, and two patients underwent one-stage biventricular repair with tunneling of left ventricular outflow through the VSD to the pulmonary valve, and establishment of continuity between the right ventricle and the confluence of branch pulmonary arteries using a valved homograft. There was one hospital mortality.

As part of the aforementioned study by Jacobs and associates,[50] Chin undertook a detailed retrospective analysis of all of the preoperative echocardiography studies. One important observation was that when the dimensions of the subaortic region were measured in images obtained from four standard echocardiographic windows, the values for a given patient varied considerably from one view to another. In most instances, the smallest dimensions were measured using the subcostal left anterior oblique window. Another observation was that nearly half of the patients in this series with narrowing of the subaortic region also had a bicuspid aortic valve. Investigators from other centers have also reported encouraging surgical results using a technical approach that combines features of the Norwood procedure with the Rastelli operation. In 2001, Erez and associates[61] reported a series of 12 patients with IAA and LVOT obstruction treated initially with a Norwood procedure. The mean z-value for the subaortic diameter was -5 ± 1.7. There were no hospital deaths. At the time of the report, six patients had gone on to successful biventricular repair. Therefore, Norwood's technique of aortopulmonary amalgamation, modified to include augmentation of the reconstructed aortic arch, can be applied to patients with IAA and LVOT obstruction to accomplish biventricular repair in one stage at the time of initial arch repair, or as part of a staged approach leading either to biventricular repair or to univentricular palliation.

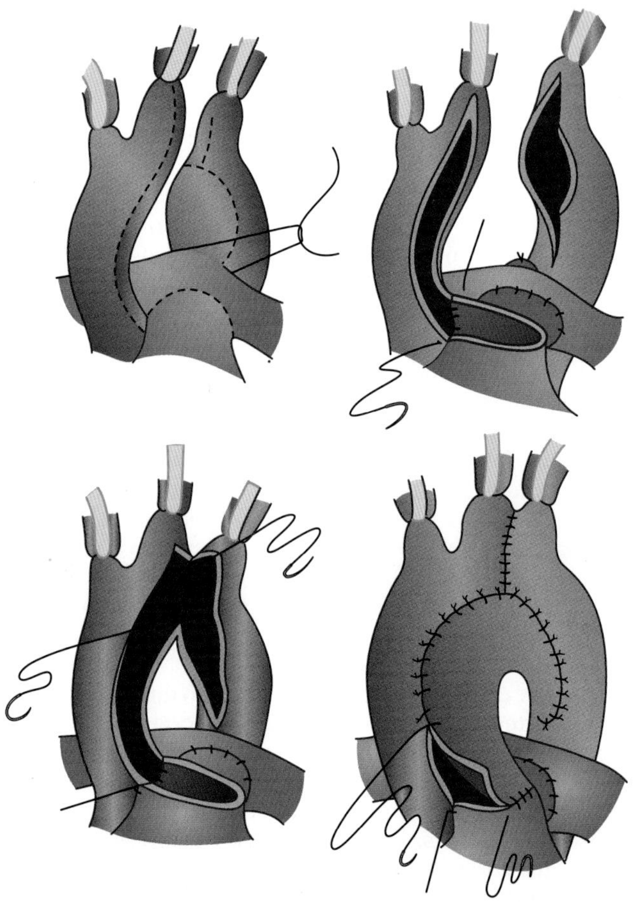

FIGURE 122-3 ■ A technique for repair of interrupted aortic arch with a severe degree of left ventricular outflow obstruction. The repair incorporates transection of the main pulmonary artery, proximal main pulmonary artery–ascending aortic amalgamation, anastomosis of proximal and distal aortic elements, and pulmonary homograft patch augmentation of the reconstructed arch. (From Jacobs ML, Chin AJ, Rychik J, et al: Interrupted aortic arch. Impact of subaortic stenosis on management and outcome. *Circulation* 92[9 suppl]:II128–II131, 1995.)

Others have reported success with less radical procedures for management of IAA with LVOT obstruction. In 1993, Bove and associates[54] described an approach to LVOT enlargement in patients with IAA and LVOT obstruction. At operation, the posteriorly displaced infundibular septum was partially removed through a right atrial approach by resecting the superior margin of the VSD up to the aortic annulus. The resulting enlarged VSD was then closed with a patch to widen the subaortic

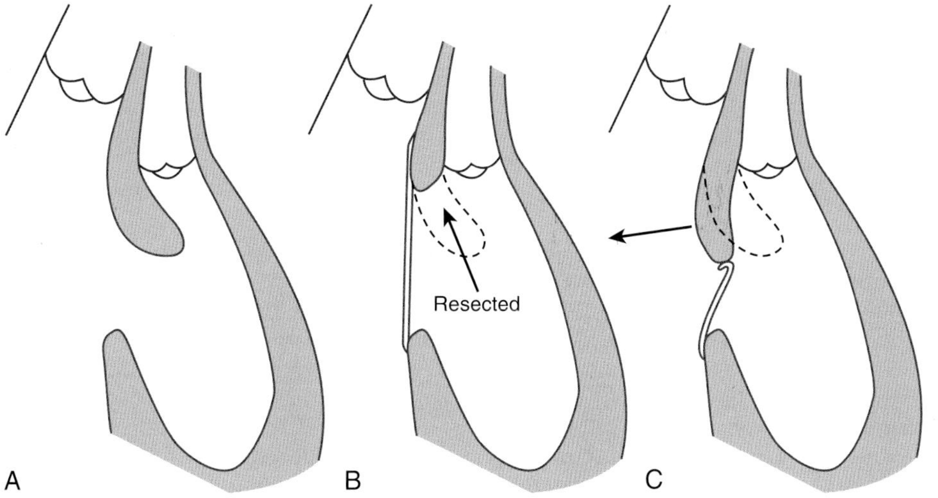

FIGURE 122-4 Alternative techniques for closure of the ventricular septal defect (VSD) in the setting of interrupted aortic arch with malalignment type VSD. **A,** Preoperative anatomy, showing displacement of the malaligned conal septum into the left ventricular outflow tract. **B,** Patch closure of the VSD after partial resection of the conal septum. **C,** Patch closure of the VSD as advocated by Luciani and associates.[63] The upper end of the VSD patch is placed on the left side of the septum to deflect the conal septum anteriorly and away from the subaortic area. (From Tchervenkov CI, Jacobs JP, Sharma K, et al: Interrupted aortic arch: surgical decision making. *Semin Thorac Cardiovasc Surg Pediatr Card Surg Annu* 92–102, 2005.)

area. In each patient, the aortic arch was repaired by direct anastomosis. All three patients survived operation. More recently, investigators from the same center analyzed a group of 27 patients with IAA and malalignment type VSD.[62] Fifteen patients with the smallest subaortic areas underwent myectomy or myotomy of the infundibular septum concomitant with IAA and VSD repair. Two hospital deaths occurred in this group. No late deaths occurred. Six patients required nine reoperations for LVOT obstruction. Five patients underwent resection of a new subaortic membrane. Only one patient had recurrent muscular LVOT obstruction. Three patients required a second reoperation, primarily related to aortic valve stenosis. The authors concluded that this approach to subaortic narrowing was effective at preventing or prolonging the interval to reinterventions for recurrent LVOT obstruction.

In 1997, Luciani and associates[63] described a novel approach to one-stage repair of IAA, VSD, and subaortic obstruction. In nine neonates, the VSD was closed with either a transpulmonary (seven patients) or transatrial (two patients) approach. Without resection of the conal septum, the upper end of the ventricular septal patch was placed on the left side of the septum to deflect the conal septum anteriorly and away from the subaortic area. The authors emphasized the importance of not oversizing the VSD patch, so as to keep it from bulging into the LVOT (Fig. 122-4). It is noteworthy that the degree of severity of subaortic stenosis according to preoperative echocardiography (mean ratio of subaortic to descending aortic diameter, 0.63 ± 0.08) was somewhat less in patients in this series than in those judged to have significant LVOT obstruction in some other series.

Schreiber and associates[40] recently reported a single institution's 20-year experience with 94 patients diagnosed with IAA. Thirteen patients were considered to have significant LVOT obstruction. Procedures directed at subaortic obstruction included myomectomy, homograft aortic root replacement, and the Norwood procedure. A preoperative diagnosis of LVOT obstruction was found to be a significant predictor of early and late mortality. More recently, several groups have described success with Ross-Konno procedures for IAA with LVOT obstruction either as a primary repair or, more frequently, as a reintervention in the setting of recurrent LVOT obstruction.[64-66]

Not all investigators agree that LVOT obstruction is a risk factor for mortality after repair or for the need for reoperation. In 1999, Fulton and associates reported outcomes of a series of 72 patients who underwent repair of IAA between 1985 and 1997.[55] Thirty-six patients (50%) had LVOT obstruction by one or more of the authors' multiple criteria: (1) dimensions of the LVOT smaller than the mean value minus 1 standard deviation (indexed to body surface area), (2) presence of a gradient of greater than 10 mm Hg across the LVOT, measured by Doppler echocardiography or at cardiac catheterization, (3) posterior deviation of the conal septum into the LVOT, and (4) presence of obstructing tissue in the subaortic area. Patients with LVOT obstruction had comparable survival rates to those without obstruction. At 10 years, the difference in freedom from reoperation did not significantly differ between groups. However, of 36 patients judged to have LVOT obstruction, only 15 (42%) were believed to have obstruction that was severe enough to require surgical treatment at the initial operation. This is an example of the difficulty encountered in interpreting various investigators' recommendations in regard to LVOT obstruction in the setting of IAA. There is no consensus definition, and the criteria vary from one study to another. Unlike Fulton and associates, authors of many outcome studies include in the LVOT obstruction group only those patients for whom the initial operative approach is altered to address the problem specifically.

Tchervenkov and associates[67] recently undertook a review of published experiences with management of

IAA with LVOT obstruction and offered the following guidelines:

- If the diameter of the LVOT is smaller in millimeters than the baby's weight in kilograms, then survival with a conservative approach is unlikely. For example, for a 3-kg baby, survival is unlikely if the LVOT is smaller than 3 mm and the LVOT is not addressed.
- If the LVOT diameter is greater than the baby's weight (in kilograms) plus 2 mm (e.g., if weight is 3 kg, then diameter greater than 5 mm), survival without significant LVOT obstruction is likely.
- Between these two numbers is a gray zone, where, although survival may be possible, it is likely that significant residual LVOT obstruction will exist.

These general guidelines were based on impressions drawn by Tchervenkov and his coauthors[67] from their review of other surgeons' series and from personal experience. It is important to recognize that they are not derived from a statistical analysis of any actual data set.

The foregoing discussion addresses the questions of the potential effects of LVOT obstruction on survival after repair, and the primary surgical approaches to the management of moderate to severe LVOT obstruction. Important information is also available regarding the effects of LVOT obstruction on the need for subsequent interventions and long-term survival after repair. Geva and associates[68] undertook a retrospective study of 37 patients who had undergone repair of IAA, and they investigated the relationship between preoperative morphology and postoperative development of LVOT obstruction. They found a correlation between a preoperative indexed LVOT cross-sectional area of less than 0.7 cm^2/m^2 and subsequent development of LVOT obstruction. They used a threshold value of a gradient of 20 mm Hg to define the presence of LVOT obstruction. This value is lower than has been applied by some others. Apfel and associates[69] used a gradient of 40 mm Hg as their definition of postoperative LVOT obstruction. They reviewed the preoperative echocardiograms and the postoperative clinical course and echocardiograms of 23 consecutive patients who underwent primary repair of IAA without a surgical modification aimed at widening of the subaortic region. Nine patients (39%) went on to develop significant LVOT obstruction (seven of them by 1 month, eight by 2 months, and all nine by 1 year). On retrospective analysis of the preoperative echocardiograms, the indexed cross-sectional area of the LVOT, the subaortic diameter index, and the subaortic diameter z-score were all significantly smaller in those requiring re-intervention ($P < 0.04$, $P < 0.05$, $P < 0.05$, respectively). Indexed cross-sectional area had the least reproducibility, and subaortic diameter index had the most. The authors concluded that most patients who develop significant LVOT obstruction after repair of IAA do so early after operation. Although subaortic indexed cross-sectional area was the most sensitive predictor of LVOT obstruction after primary repair, other, simpler standardized measurements of the subaortic diameter were comparably predictive and had better reproducibility.

In 2010, Hirata and associates[70] reported an analysis of outcomes of 38 patients who underwent single-stage complete repair at Morgan Stanley Children's Hospital of New York. Using a minor modification of the criteria described by Tchervenkov,[67] they classified patients into two groups. If the aortic annulus was greater than the patient's weight (in kilograms) plus 1.5 mm, the patient was included in group "large," and if the aortic annulus was equal to or smaller than the patient's weight plus 1.5 mm, the patient was included in group "small." The average follow-up was 7.9 ± 4.2 years. Among the patients with small aortic annulus ($n = 12$), there was one hospital death and six reoperations for LVOT obstruction, and one late death. There was only one reoperation for LVOT obstruction among the patients with larger aortic annulus ($n = 26$; $P < 0.001$).

In 2013, Chen and associates[71] at Boston Children's Hospital reported their analysis of predictors of reintervention following neonatal repair of IAA with VSD. Retrospective data were collected on neonates with IAA with VSD who underwent single-stage repair from 1995 to 2009. Sixteen patients (23%) required surgical or percutaneous reintervention for clinically significant postoperative LVOT obstruction. By univariate analysis, LVOT cross-sectional area, LVOT diameter, and aortic root size (all from two-dimensional echocardiography before neonatal repair) were predictors of reintervention. On multivariable linear regression model, aortic root size (from the parasternal long-axis view in end systole) was identified as an independent predictor of reintervention. In identifying an aortic root size inflection point, patients with an aortic root size less than 6.5 mm were at greater risk for reintervention compared with patients with a root size greater than 6.5 mm (reintervention rate 44% and 12%, respectively).

The procedures used to address residual or recurrent LVOT obstruction after initial repair of IAA are numerous, and the choice depends on the specific morphology encountered. Fibrous or fibromembranous subaortic stenosis can generally be approached through the aortic valve. Enucleation of fibrous tissue from the LVOT may need to be preceded by aortic valvotomy (if valvar stenosis is present) and accompanied by myotomy and myectomy of obstructing muscle in the LVOT. Long-segment fibromuscular subaortic stenosis, if present, is best managed with extended ventricular septoplasty (the modified Konno procedure). Working through a right ventricular infundibular incision, an incision is made in the ventricular septum, generally through the area of the previously closed VSD. This incision is carefully monitored by periodic visualization through an aortotomy, looking down through the aortic valve. From the right ventricular approach, the septal incision is extended into the LVOT and is carried up to within a few millimeters of the aortic valve annulus. A patch is then placed on the right ventricular aspect of the surgically enlarged VSD. The infundibulotomy is closed either directly or with a patch. If significant aortic annular hypoplasia is an element of complex LVOT obstruction, then a conventional Konno procedure (with aortic valve prosthesis) or a Ross-Konno procedure is performed. The latter involves an anterior incision through the aortic annulus and into the ventricular septum, and pulmonary autograft replacement of the aortic valve, with the use of a patch or of infundibular muscle attached to the autograft to enlarge the LVOT.[65] Finally, the placement of a valved conduit from the left ventricular apex to the descending thoracic aorta remains an option,[44] although it is rarely used.

Conduct of Surgery and Cardiopulmonary Bypass Support

The availability of prostaglandin and the resultant opportunity to stabilize the condition of most patients before surgery, together with refinements in the technology and conduct of cardiopulmonary bypass and the use of deep hypothermia with circulatory arrest, led to the widespread acceptance and performance of one-stage repair of IAA and associated intracardiac defects. Operative strategies based on preliminary surface cooling and core cooling on cardiopulmonary bypass, followed by a period of circulatory arrest and then reperfusion and rewarming on bypass, remain in widespread use today. Essential features include perfusion inflow through the main pulmonary trunk, with temporary tourniquet occlusion of the branch pulmonary arteries. Although adequate cooling of the brain (as reflected by appropriately falling nasopharyngeal and tympanic temperature) can generally be accomplished in this fashion, many surgeons routinely place an additional small (6- or 8-French) inflow cannula in the ascending aorta. The two perfusion cannulas are set up in advance, joined by a Y-connector. Cannulation of the ascending aorta must be undertaken with great care, as the vessel is particularly small in the setting of IAA type B or C (Fig. 122-5). The purse-string suture through which the aortic perfusion cannula will be inserted should be placed so that it will be just opposite the anastomosis that will be made; it is generally slightly more than half-way between the aortic valve and the origin of the first branch vessel (innominate or right common carotid artery) and toward the right side of the ascending aorta. Alternatively, the need for an aortic perfusion cannula can be assessed by addition of cerebral monitoring with near infrared spectroscopy to supplement temperature monitoring.

Regardless of perfusion technique, all repairs of IAA are facilitated by extensive mobilization of the ascending aorta and each of its branches, as well as the descending aorta and its branches. In general, this can be accomplished during the initial cooling phase of cardiopulmonary bypass. Extensive manipulation and dissection before the initiation of bypass can sometimes upset the already fragile hemodynamic state. If hypothermic circulatory arrest is anticipated, suture tourniquets are loosely placed around each of the aortic arch branches; they are not snugged down and occluded until immediately before circulatory arrest. Venous return to the pump oxygenator is either by single cannula in the right atrium (in which case, closure of a VSD is accomplished either during the period of circulatory arrest or by a transpulmonary approach while on cardiopulmonary bypass) or by means of bicaval cannulation (in which case, the intracardiac portion of the repair can be accomplished on bypass, either before or after the arch repair). If single cannulation of the right atrium with transpulmonary closure of the VSD is planned, intracardiac visualization can be

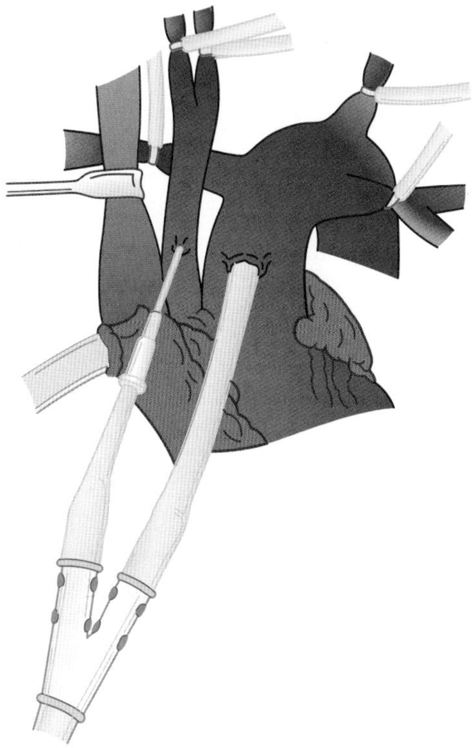

FIGURE 122-5 ■ Systemic perfusion via cannulation of both the main pulmonary trunk and the diminutive ascending aorta. Tourniquets are used to occlude the right and left branch pulmonary arteries during perfusion, and to occlude the aortic arch branches only during a period of hypothermic circulatory arrest. (From Luciani GB, Ackerman RJ, Chang AC, et al: One-stage repair of interrupted aortic arch, ventricular septal defect, and subaortic obstruction in the neonate: A novel approach. *J Thorac Cardiovasc Surg* 111:348–358, 1996.)

enhanced with the use of vacuum-assisted venous drainage. Although a single dose of antegrade cardioplegia suffices in most cases, this can be replaced or supplemented with single or multiple doses of retrograde cardioplegia via the coronary sinus. If the total duration of hypothermic circulatory arrest is anticipated to exceed 35 to 40 minutes, a brief period of hypothermic reperfusion can be accomplished immediately after completion of the arch reconstruction, with the remainder of the repair being accomplished during a second period of circulatory arrest.

Many surgeons have been pleased with the results of direct end-to-side anastomosis of the descending aorta to the left lateral aspect of the ascending aorta (Fig. 122-6), or to the left side of the distal ascending aorta and the underside of the proximal arch (in IAA type A). We and others[72] have generally preferred to create an anastomosis that is augmented with a gusset of homograft vascular patch material (Fig. 122-7). To accomplish this, an incision is made in the left lateral aspect of the ascending aorta beginning a few millimeters above the sinotubular junction. The incision is carried onto the left side of the most distal arch branch associated with the ascending aorta. (To facilitate this, the occluding suture tourniquet must be placed as far distally as possible.) After ligation of the pulmonary artery end of the ductus, the ductus is divided, and all ductal tissue associated with the

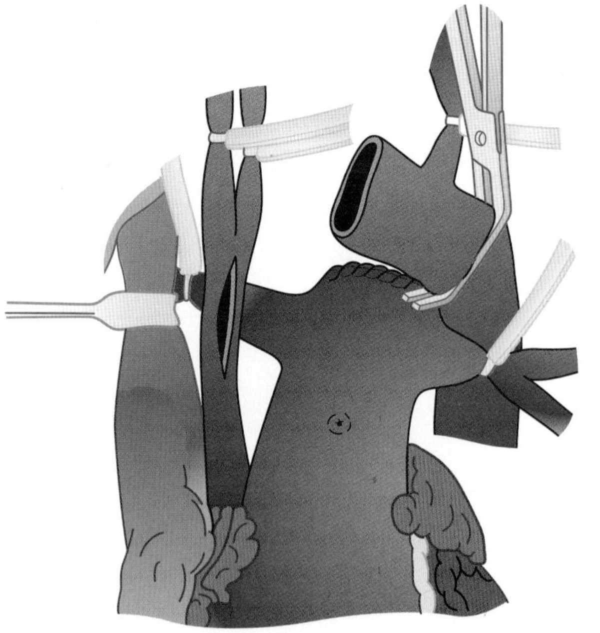

FIGURE 122-6 ■ Direct end-to-side anastomosis of the descending aorta to the left lateral aspect of the ascending aorta. A vascular clamp is applied across the descending thoracic aorta to facilitate positioning of this segment for the anastomosis. (From Luciani GB, Ackerman RJ, Chang AC, et al: One-stage repair of interrupted aortic arch, ventricular septal defect, and subaortic obstruction in the neonate: A novel approach. *J Thorac Cardiovasc Surg* 111:348–358, 1996.)

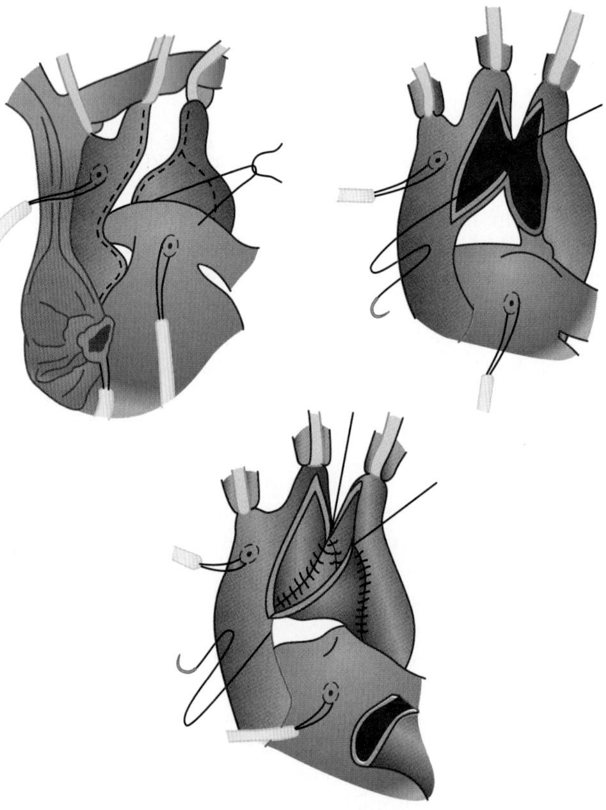

FIGURE 122-7 ■ Our preferred technique for interrupted aortic arch repair with homograft vascular patch augmentation of the aortic anastomosis. (From Jacobs ML, Chin AJ, Rychik J, et al: Interrupted aortic arch. Impact of subaortic stenosis on management and outcome. *Circulation* 92[9 suppl]:II128–II131, 1995.)

descending thoracic aorta is excised. The resulting opening into the descending aorta is extended a few millimeters along the right side of the first branch associated with the descending aorta (in IAA type B, this is the left subclavian artery). An incision is also carried down from the opening into the descending aorta, along the medial aspect of the aorta, to a point approximately 1 cm below the opening of the ductus into the aorta, as is done in a stage I Norwood procedure. Direct anastomosis of the proximal and distal aortic elements along their greater curvature is accomplished, including side-to-side amalgamation of the last aortic branch associated with the proximal segment and the first branch associated with the distal segment. The entire aortic arch is then augmented along its lesser curvature with a homograft vascular patch, beginning distally on the descending thoracic aorta. Once the arch reconstruction has been completed, the aorta is cannulated through a pursestring suture that, ideally, is situated on the right side of the augmented ascending aorta, several millimeters distal to the most proximal extent of the homograft patch. This minimizes the likelihood of aortic narrowing resulting when tying down the pursestring suture after decannulation. Perfusion can be resumed at this time, or alternatively the VSD can be closed before resumption of cardiopulmonary bypass. The technique of homograft patch augmentation of the aortic anastomosis has proved particularly useful in the setting of repair of truncus arteriosus with IAA.[73]

These methods have yielded satisfactory outcomes, and they remain in use at many centers. Recently, however, techniques allowing continuous cerebral perfusion have gained favor, because they minimize the use or duration of hypothermic circulatory arrest.[9,74,75] Clinical studies comparing neurodevelopmental outcomes in patients undergoing arch repair with continuous cerebral perfusion to those with hypothermic circulatory arrest have, for the most part, been in the setting of stage I Norwood procedures, and the results at 1 year are similar between groups. Issues pertaining to optimal temperature, rates of flow, and pH strategy remain to be resolved. Nonetheless, the idea of continuous cerebral perfusion is appealing to many surgeons, and its use is increasing steadily.

Continuous antegrade cerebral perfusion is accomplished either by advancing a small aortic perfusion cannula into the right common carotid artery[75] or by direct cannulation of the innominate artery (with a 6 or 8 Fr cannula),[74] or by anastomosis of a 4- or 5-mm polytetrafluoroethylene graft to the innominate artery, into which a perfusion cannula is placed with care to exclude air. A second perfusion cannula is placed in the main pulmonary artery (Fig. 122-8). After hypothermic bypass is established and the target core temperature is reached, the perfusion cannula in the pulmonary artery is clamped and removed. Flow is reduced and maintained at a level of 40 to 70 mL/kg/min. The ductus is suture-ligated at the pulmonary artery end. A small vascular clamp is placed on the descending aorta approximately 1 cm distal to the point of insertion of the ductus. The left subclavian artery (and an aberrant right subclavian artery if present) is occluded temporarily with a small removable neurovascular clip. The ductus is divided, and

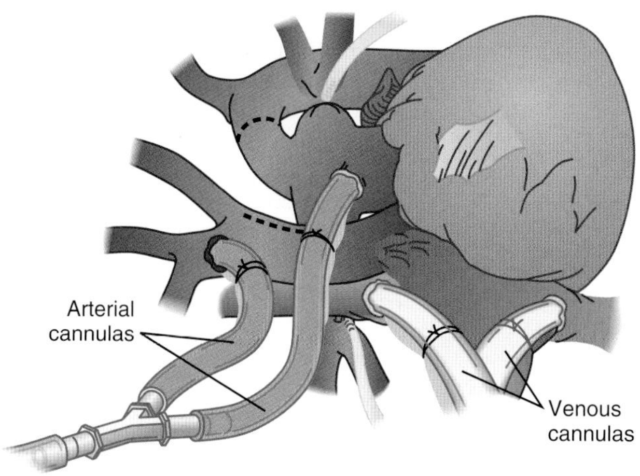

FIGURE 122-8 ■ A perfusion arrangement for interrupted aortic arch repair that facilitates arch anastomosis during a period of selective antegrade cerebral perfusion. This arrangement, used by Malhotra and Hanley[74] and others, includes direct cannulation of the innominate artery and the main pulmonary trunk. The *dotted line* indicates proposed sites for incision in the ascending aorta and for transection of the ductus arteriosus. (From Coarctation of the aorta and interrupted aortic arch. In Kouchoukos NT, Blackstone EH, Doty DB, Hanley FH, Karp RB, editors: *Kirklin and Barratt-Boyes' cardiac surgery,* ed 3, Philadelphia, 2003, Churchill Livingstone, pp 1315–1375.)

any ductal tissue associated with the descending thoracic aorta is excised. The vascular clamp on the descending aorta is required in this circumstance to prevent backbleeding, but it is also useful under conditions of circulatory arrest to aid in manipulation of the distal aortic segment. If direct end-to-side anastomosis of the descending aorta to the ascending aorta is planned, a small straight vascular clamp is placed across the arch of the aorta at the base of the innominate artery and the left common carotid artery (Fig. 122-9), maintaining luminal continuity and facilitating perfusion of both branches.[74] The end-to-side anastomosis is accomplished proximal to this point (Fig. 122-10). Cardioplegia solution is administered in antegrade fashion into the ascending aorta. If patch augmentation of the anastomosis is planned, the straight vascular clamp is applied proximal to the perfusion cannula at the base of the innominate artery. The left common carotid (in addition to any more distal branches associated with the ascending aorta) is gently occluded somewhat distally, with either a suture tourniquet or a neurovascular clip. In this way, the anastomosis of the proximal and distal aortic segments can include side-to-side amalgamation of most proximal portions of the last aortic branch associated with the ascending aorta, and the first branch associated with the descending aorta. The anastomosis is augmented along its lesser curvature with a gusset of cryopreserved homograft vascular patch material. When this technique is used, it is rarely necessary to ligate and divide a left or an aberrant right subclavian artery. All tourniquets and other occluding devices are removed from the aorta and its branches. Full flow (or systemic perfusion at a level appropriate to the core temperature) is resumed. An additional dose of antegrade cardioplegia is given if so desired, and the intracardiac repair is undertaken. The VSD is closed using a

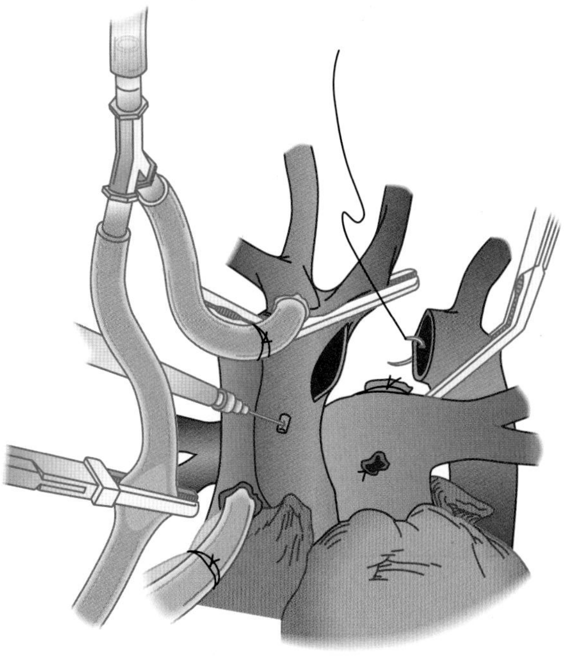

FIGURE 122-9 ■ The operation shown in Figure 122-8, here showing the placement of a small vascular clamp across the arch of the aorta at the base of the innominate artery and left common carotid artery, maintaining luminal continuity and facilitating continuous perfusion of both branches. (From Coarctation of the aorta and interrupted aortic arch. In Kouchoukos NT, Blackstone EH, Doty DB, Hanley FH, Karp RB, editors: *Kirklin and Barratt-Boyes' cardiac surgery,* ed 3, Philadelphia, 2003, Churchill Livingstone, pp 1315–1375.)

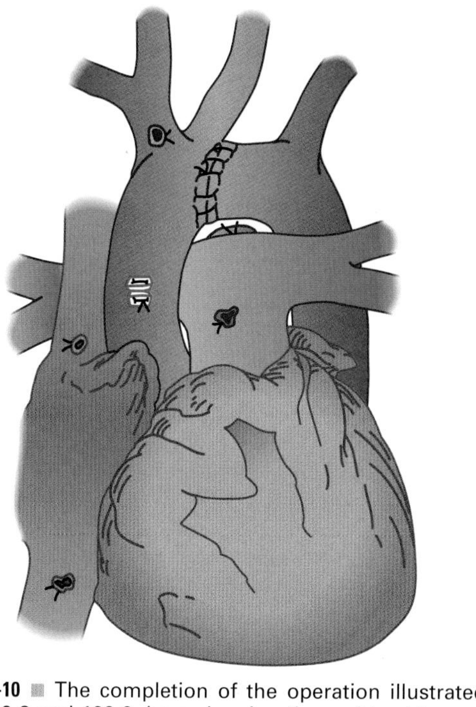

FIGURE 122-10 ■ The completion of the operation illustrated in Figures 122-8 and 122-9, here showing the end-to-side anastomosis of the descending aorta to the ascending aorta. Also shown are the oversewn cannulation sites for arterial perfusion, venous drainage, and cardioplegia administration. (From Coarctation of the aorta and interrupted aortic arch. In Kouchoukos NT, Blackstone EH, Doty DB, Hanley FH, Karp RB, editors: *Kirklin and Barratt-Boyes' cardiac surgery,* ed 3, Philadelphia, 2003, Churchill Livingstone, pp 1315–1375.)

transpulmonary or transatrial approach, and an atrial septal defect or stretched foramen is approached through the right atrium. After rewarming, separation from bypass is accomplished.

Hybrid Palliation

In selected cases, a decision may be made to delay definitive repair of the interrupted arch and associated intracardiac defects, in favor of a course of treatment based on initial stabilization of the circulation by a combination of maneuvers that restore and maintain patency of the arterial duct and that limit pulmonary blood flow. Based on the same principles as the so-called hybrid strategy for initial palliation of hypoplastic left heart syndrome, this generally involves a median sternotomy approach for bilateral application of bands to the right and left branch pulmonary arteries and either prolonged continuous infusion of prostaglandin E1 or transpulmonary artery deployment of an intravascular stent in the arterial duct.[76,77] This alternative strategy is generally reserved for instances of rescue therapy for neonates with shock and secondary organ dysfunction in the setting of ductal constriction or with significant infection. It can also be used when temporary delay of definitive repair requiring cardiopulmonary bypass is judged to be advantageous, which might include instances of extreme prematurity or of neurologic complications such as intraventricular hemorrhage.

RESULTS: SURVIVAL, COMPLICATIONS, AND LATE EVENTS

In general, single-institution series describing results of surgical management of IAA reflect the challenge and complexity of this group of lesions, but they offer encouraging results that in the aggregate suggest that a good deal of progress has been made over the past 2 decades.[41,42,46,55] Several institutions describe operative survival on the order of 90%. In individual series, the incidence of reintervention during follow-up varies from as little as 10% to greater than 50%.* In the Congenital Heart Surgery Database of the Society of Thoracic Surgeons,[79] the mortality at discharge from hospital after IAA repair in the 4-year interval from 2004 through 2007 is 8.9% (32/359).

Multi-institutional outcome studies provide a broader overview of experience and offer the opportunity to undertake risk analysis on a large set. The CHSS initiated its first prospective multi-institutional outcome study of patients with IAA in 1987, with patient enrollment at 30 participating institutions. In 1994, the first CHSS report, by Jonas and associates,[15] analyzed the outcomes from management of 183 neonates with IAA and VSD entering the study between 1987 and 1992. Nine patients died without any surgery. Among the remaining 174, survival rates at 1 month and 1, 3, and 4 years after repair were 73%, 65%, 63%, and 63%, respectively. The risk factors for death were low birth weight, younger age at repair, interrupted arch type B, outlet and trabecular VSDs, smaller size of the VSD, and subaortic narrowing.

Echocardiographically measured dimensions at all levels of the left heart–aorta complex were small. As previously noted, procedural risk factors for death after repair were (1) repair without concomitant procedures in patients with other important levels of obstruction in the left heart–aorta complex, (2) a Damus-Kaye-Stansel anastomosis, and (3) subaortic myotomy or myectomy in the face of subaortic narrowing. One-stage repair plus ascending aorta or arch augmentation had the highest predicted time-related survival in the 20% of patients with IAA and one or more coexisting levels of obstruction in the left heart–aorta complex, as did initial repair without or with aorta or arch augmentation in the 80% without these. Only 26% of patients in whom a lateral thoracotomy was used (as in most initial repairs in which the VSD was not closed) had a direct anastomosis, in contrast to 92% of those in whom a median sternotomy with a one-stage repair was performed. Among the 57 patients who did not have the VSD closed at the initial procedure, essentially all who survived had it closed within 36 months of the initial repair. The peak rate of VSD closure by a subsequent procedure was highest during the first month after the initial procedure, suggesting that the untreated VSD was not being well tolerated and that a one-stage repair at the initial procedure might have been preferable. By the time the analysis was undertaken, 20 patients had undergone reintervention for arch obstruction. In nine patients, the procedure was percutaneous balloon dilation. The peak of the hazard function for this reintervention was approximately 4 months after the initial repair. Fifteen of the 116 patients undergoing one-stage repair had a first reintervention for one or more coexisting obstructive lesions in the left heart–aorta complex (e.g., LVOT obstruction). Freedom from such reinterventions was only 77% at 3 years. This unique multi-institutional study revealed that optimal management of coexisting obstructive left heart lesions in association with IAA remained an unresolved challenge at the time. It also pointed out the ongoing risks of recurrent arch obstruction and LVOT obstruction in survivors of neonatal repair. These findings encouraged the CHSS to enlarge the patient cohort through further enrollment, and to continue the analysis of these late-phase events.

A more recent CHSS multi-institutional study on IAA reported in 2005 by McCrindle and associates[17] evaluated an expanded cohort of 472 patients (including the patients previously reported by Jonas and associates). Additional insights concerning the significance and management of LVOT obstruction became apparent, at least in part because of the large size of the study population. Of the 472 patients with IAA, 143 underwent a variety of interventions to address LVOT obstruction, of which 52 took place some time after the initial IAA repair. Subaortic resection was performed in 75 of these patients, and 51 underwent LVOT bypass procedures (Norwood or Yasui). Two patients required cardiac transplantation. Competing risks analysis revealed that at 16 years after initial admission, 38% were alive without a LVOT procedure,

*References 15, 41-43, 55, 58, 59, 62, 73, and 78.

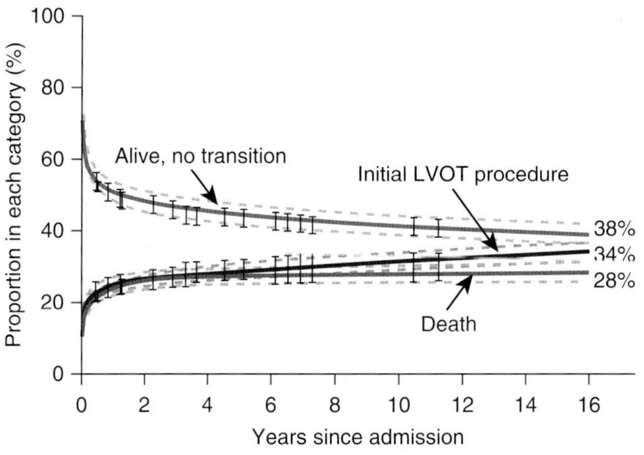

FIGURE 122-11 ■ Graphic representation from the 2005 Congenital Heart Surgeons' Society (CHSS) study of interrupted aortic arch (IAA) competing risks analysis for initial procedure aimed at addressing potential or actual left ventricular outflow tract (LVOT) obstruction. All patients began at the time of initial admission to a CHSS member institution (N = 472) and could transition to either death or initial procedure aimed at addressing potential or actual LVOT obstruction. *Solid lines,* parametric point estimates; *dashed lines,* limits of 70% confidence intervals; *circles with error bars,* nonparametric estimates; *y-axis,* proportion of patients (expressed as percentage of total) in each of three categories at any given time after IAA repair. (From McCrindle BW, Tchervenkov CI, Konstantinov IE, et al; Congenital Heart Surgeons Society: Risk factors associated with mortality and interventions in 472 neonates with interrupted aortic arch: a Congenital Heart Surgeons Society study. *J Thorac Cardiovasc Surg* 129:343–350, 2005.)

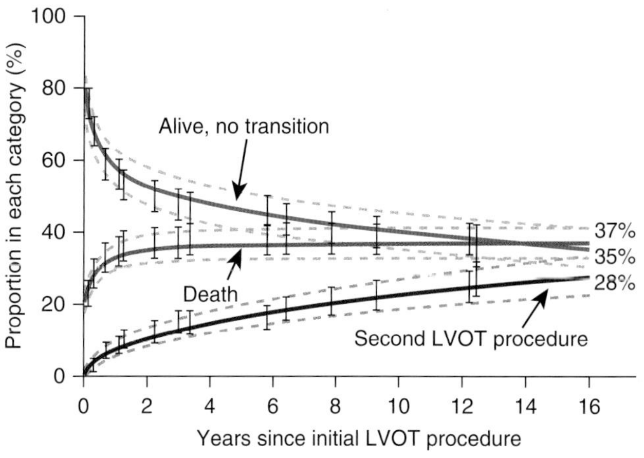

FIGURE 122-12 ■ Graphic representation from the 2005 Congenital Heart Surgeons' Society study of interrupted aortic arch (IAA) competing risks analysis for subsequent procedure aimed at addressing residual or recurrent left ventricular outflow tract (LVOT) obstruction. All patients began at the time of the initial procedure aimed at addressing potential or actual LVOT obstruction (N = 143) and could transition to either death or similar subsequent procedure. *Solid lines,* parametric point estimates; *dashed lines,* limits of 70% confidence intervals; *circles with error bars,* nonparametric estimates; *y-axis,* proportion of patients (expressed as percentage of total) in each of three categories at any given time after IAA repair. (From McCrindle BW, Tchervenkov CI, Konstantinov IE, et al; Congenital Heart Surgeons Society: Risk factors associated with mortality and interventions in 472 neonates with interrupted aortic arch: a Congenital Heart Surgeons Society study. *J Thorac Cardiovasc Surg* 129:343–350, 2005.)

whereas 34% had undergone an initial LVOT procedure (Fig. 122-11). For the 143 patients who had an initial LVOT procedure, there was a high risk of early death and a nearly constant risk of a second procedure. At 16 years after the initial LVOT procedure, 35% were alive without a second procedure, and 28% required a second LVOT procedure. Of the patients who had an initial LVOT procedure, 37% had died by 16 years (Fig. 122-12). Risk factors for a second LVOT procedure were absence of a large VSD and initial balloon dilation of the LVOT. These observations certainly emphasize the significance of the problem of LVOT obstruction in IAA and its negative effects on survival and reoperation-free survival. Regarding the fate of the initial arch repair, reintervention for arch obstruction occurred in 109 cases. Of these, 52 were by transcatheter balloon dilation and 57 were surgical. The time-related hazard function for survival to an arch repair intervention showed two phases: an early phase accounting for 89 events and a smaller constant hazard phase accounting for 20 events. The time-related hazard function for death without an IAA repair intervention was characterized by an early phase only. The competing risks for the two events showed that 16 years after IAA repair, 33% had died without an IAA repair intervention, 29% were surviving to an IAA repair intervention, and 38% remained alive without an IAA repair intervention (Fig. 122-13). Finally, with respect to overall mortality, improving outcomes were evident for patients born later in the study enrollment period (Fig. 122-14). This

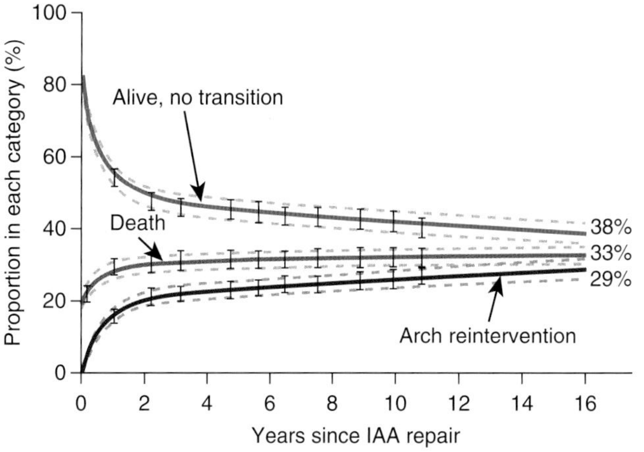

FIGURE 122-13 ■ Graphic representation from the 2005 Congenital Heart Surgeons' Society study of interrupted aortic arch (IAA) competing risks analysis for subsequent intervention for residual or recurrent obstruction at IAA repair site. All patients began at the time of repair of IAA (N = 453) and could transition to either death or subsequent intervention for residual or recurrent obstruction at the arch repair site. *Solid lines,* parametric point estimates; *dashed lines,* limits of 70% confidence intervals; *circles with error bars,* nonparametric estimates; *y-axis,* proportion of patients (expressed as percentage of total) in each of three categories at any given time after IAA repair. (From McCrindle BW, Tchervenkov CI, Konstantinov IE, et al; Congenital Heart Surgeons Society: Risk factors associated with mortality and interventions in 472 neonates with interrupted aortic arch: a Congenital Heart Surgeons Society study. *J Thorac Cardiovasc Surg* 129:343–350, 2005.)

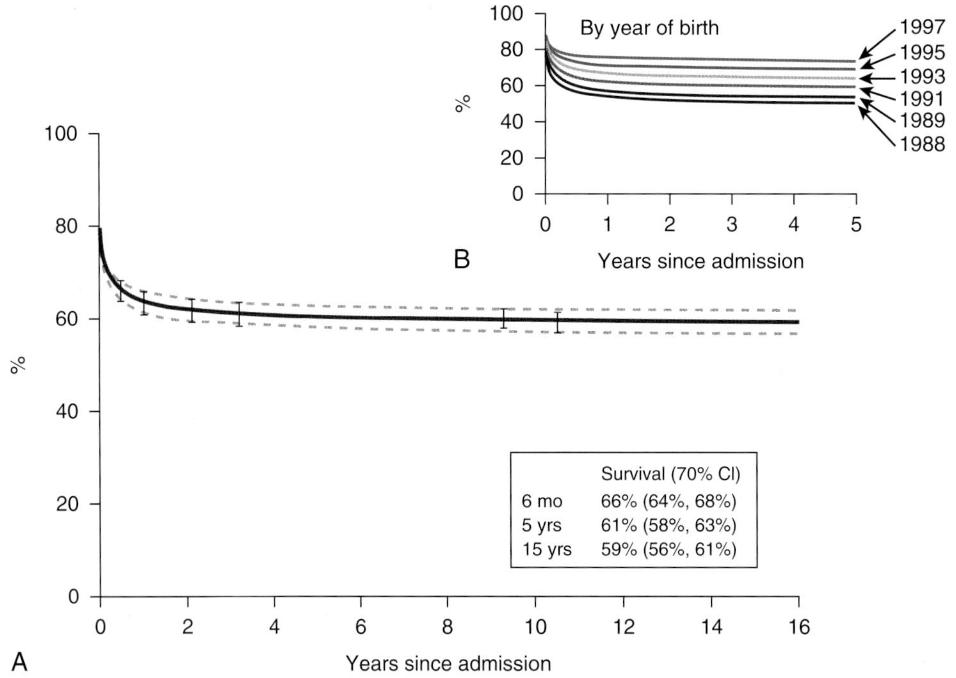

FIGURE 122-14 ■ Graphic representation from the 2005 Congenital Heart Surgeons' Society (CHSS) study of interrupted aortic arch (IAA) depicting overall time-related survival of 472 neonates with IAA. All patients began at the time of initial admission to a CHSS member institution. **A,** Overall survival. **B,** Predicted overall survival for first 5 years after admission, stratified by patient date of birth. *Solid lines,* Parametric point estimates; *dashed lines,* limits of 70% confidence intervals (CI). (From McCrindle BW, Tchervenkov CI, Konstantinov IE, et al; Congenital Heart Surgeons Society: Risk factors associated with mortality and interventions in 472 neonates with interrupted aortic arch: a Congenital Heart Surgeons Society study. *J Thorac Cardiovasc Surg* 129:343–350, 2005.)

positive message regarding steadily improving rates of overall survival over the period of patient enrollment (1987 to 1997) is tempered by the sobering data concerning the significant requirement for late re-interventions. It should also be noted that, while the initial CHSS report was restricted to patients with IAA and VSD, the 2005 report by McCrindle and associates also included patients with complex lesions, including IAA with truncus arteriosus, with an aortopulmonary window, and with a single ventricle.

The most recent report on the CHSS cohort by Jegatheeswaran and associates[80] clearly reinforced the impression that IAA is a chronic disease, with many repaired patients requiring multiple subsequent procedures. Among 447 patients with IAA enrolled from 1987 to 1997 at 33 institutions, there were 158 subsequent arch interventions and 100 left ventricular outflow tract procedures. Overall freedom from death at 21 years was 60%. The risk of additional subsequent arch procedures decreased after the first subsequent arch procedure in the acute phase, but did not significantly change in the chronic phase. The risk of additional subsequent left ventricular outflow tract procedures increased after the first subsequent left ventricular outflow tract procedure in the chronic phase. These results indicate the need for practitioners, patients, and their families to understand the concept that IAA is a chronic disorder and not a structural anomaly definitively treated in the newborn period.

This concept is further amplified by a recent single-center follow-up study undertaken at the Children's Hospital of Philadelphia. Intermediate term status of children and adolescents who had undergone repair of IAA as neonates was evaluated by O'Byrne and associates.[81] A cross-sectional study of patients age 8 to 18 years included genetic testing, cardiac magnetic resonance imaging, cardiopulmonary exercise testing, and assessment of health status and health-related quality of life. A concurrent retrospective study reviewed their postoperative use of medical care, including operative and transcatheter reinterventions, noncardiac surgeries, and hospitalizations. Twenty-one subjects with a median age of 9 years were studied. Reintervention rates were 38% for left-ventricular outflow tract, 33% for aortic arch, and 24% for both. Rates of reintervention were highest in the first year of life. Left-ventricular ejection fraction was preserved (72% ± 6%). Maximal oxygen consumption, maximal work, and forced vital capacity were significantly decreased from age and sex norms ($P < 0.0001$). Health status and quality of life were both severely decreased.

An uncommon but important complication that can occur after IAA repair is compression of the left mainstem bronchus. This problem has been reported after repair of IAA with VSD and with truncus arteriosus. Signs of this complication may be present or appear early after initial repair; they can cause failure to liberate from mechanical ventilation. While the patient is receiving positive-pressure ventilation, the compression can manifest as air trapping and hyperinflation. Without mechanical support and positive pressure, it can give the opposite picture—that of total atelectasis of the left lung.

and treatment of congenital aortic valve disease may present unique anatomic and physiologic considerations. Although aortic insufficiency can afflict congenitally abnormal valves later in life, it is an uncommon lesion during infancy and early childhood. When present in these age groups, it is usually an iatrogenic consequence of a procedure designed to relieve congenital aortic stenosis. This chapter will address these considerations and the related challenges encountered in the surgical treatment of congenital aortic valve disease.

SURGICAL ANATOMY OF THE AORTIC VALVE AND ROOT

The aortic valve and root span the transition from the left ventricular chamber and the systemic circulation, and they include the subaortic LVOT, the aortic valve, and the aortic wall up to the level of the sinotubular junction. Congenital heart disease can involve one or more levels of the aortoventricular complex. A thorough understanding and appreciation of these inconspicuous anatomic relationships form the basis of successful surgical treatment of congenital aortic valve disease, and these relationships will be referred to throughout this chapter.[1]

The normal aortic valve sits wedged into the LVOT. In addition to supporting the coronary circulation, this central location places the aortic valve at the nexus of several critical intracardiac structures. Among these structures are the anterior leaflet of the mitral valve, the membranous interventricular septum, and the conduction apparatus. Because multiple levels of the aortoventricular complex can be involved in congenital heart disease, it is helpful to consider the normal anatomy to consist of subvalvular, valvular, and supravalvular components.

The subvalvular anatomy is dominated by the anatomic relationships among the aortic valve, interventricular septum, membranous septum, mitral valve, and conduction apparatus (Fig. 123-1). Parts of the aortic

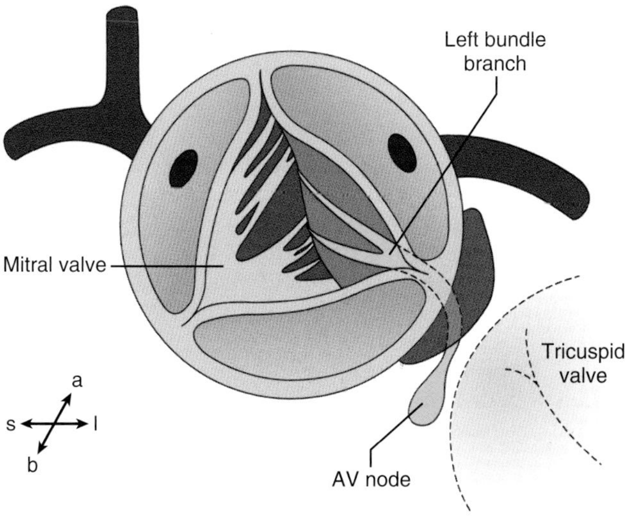

FIGURE 123-1 Anatomic relationships within the aortic valve. *AV,* Atrioventricular.

leaflets are in fibrous continuity with the anterior leaflet of the mitral valve as well as the tricuspid valve (via the membranous septum). These structures contribute to the central supporting structure of the heart, the fibrous skeleton. In addition to providing points of fixation for the atrioventricular valves, the fibrous skeleton also provides electrical insulation between the atria and the ventricles, restricting impulse conduction to the bundle of His. After arising from the atrioventricular node, the bundle of His penetrates the membranous septum, emerging on the surface of the left ventricular septum immediately below the aortic annulus. Looking through the aortic valve, the bundle will lie beneath the annulus, just below the commissure between the noncoronary and right coronary leaflet. From the surgeon's perspective, important radiations of the bundle reach to the nadir of the right coronary leaflet as they fall away, toward the apex of the heart.

Valvular anatomy is dominated by the semilunar leaflets, commissures, and sinuses of Valsalva. The leaflets and their sinuses are identified by the associated coronary artery. The right coronary artery ostium is found in the right coronary sinus, which is almost directly anterior as viewed by the surgeon. The left coronary artery emerges posteriorly from the left coronary sinus. The leaflets themselves are composed of a fibrous core lined by endothelium. The commissures, along with the free-edge coaptation provided by the leaflets themselves, provide the strength necessary to provide a competent valve.

The aortic sinuses are dilations of the aortic wall above distal to the insertion of the semilunar leaflets, and they are well suited to support the coronary ostia. While the leaflets retract during systole, eddy currents developing within the sinuses prevent occlusion of the coronary ostia by the retracted aortic leaflets. Their presence is probably important to the long-term function of the aortic valve leaflets.[2-4]

Finally, the supravalvular area denotes the transition from the left ventricle–aorta complex to the aorta proper. For practical purposes, this area includes the sinotubular junction, the area just distal to the tips of the commissural posts, and the dilations of the aortic sinuses. Abnormalities at any level can be expected in congenital heart disease, and a discussion of the various forms of congenital aortic valve pathology will be categorized by its level: valvular, subvalvular, or supravalvular.

AORTIC STENOSIS

Valvular Aortic Stenosis

Prevalence

Congenital aortic stenosis has been reported to be present in between 3% and 6% of children with congenital heart disease.[5] Males are affected more commonly than females with an incidence of 3 : 1.[6]

Clinical Characteristics

The clinical presentation varies with the severity of the lesion and the age at presentation. In the neonate, critical aortic stenosis may present rapidly and dramatically, with abrupt hemodynamic deterioration, cardiovascular collapse, and shock. The cardiogram may reveal left ventricular hypertrophy with S-T and T wave abnormalities. On chest radiography, there may be cardiomegaly and pulmonary edema. Transthoracic echocardiogram will rapidly establish the diagnosis, and it is useful to determine the presence of associated abnormalities of the left ventricle, mitral valve, or aortic arch. Aggressive resuscitation with inotropes and prostaglandin is required to support the circulation.

Older children may be asymptomatic, and aortic stenosis may be suggested by physical examination results. Chest pain and exercise intolerance is possible but uncommon. Like the neonate, the diagnosis can be confirmed with echocardiography.

Diagnosis

Physical examination results may be suggestive of the diagnosis of congenital aortic valve disease. There may be a harsh crescendo-decrescendo murmur heard best at the right second interspace, with transmission into the neck. A thrill will be present in the suprasternal notch, and over the right second intercostal spaces in severe aortic stenosis. Because ventricular systole is prolonged in the setting of aortic stenosis, the second heart sound may be prolonged, resulting in narrowly split second heart sound. An associated diastolic murmur would suggest an element of aortic insufficiency.

Electrocardiographic changes are consistent with ventricular hypertrophy, as evidenced by increased left-sided R wave voltage. Changes in S-T segment and T wave in the left precordial leads may denote LV strain. Except in the situation of obvious congestive heart failure, the chest radiograph is usually unremarkable.

Echocardiography. Echocardiography is the mainstay for contemporary diagnosis of congenital aortic valve disease. This noninvasive test provides important anatomic and physiologic information, such as the number and anatomy of the aortic leaflets, the size of the aortic annulus and ascending aorta, the location of the coronary arteries, the adequacy of the subaortic LVOT, and the site of the hemodynamic stenosis. The peak instantaneous gradient can be estimated by measuring the velocity of blood flow across the stenosis, and using a modification of the Bernoulli equation (velocity $[m/sec]^2 \times 4$).[7]

Recent developments in imaging include the availability of three-dimensional echocardiographic technology. Ventricular mass and volume measurements obtained with three-dimensional echocardiography compare well with those obtained with cardiac magnetic resonance imaging, and their utility in determining the etiology of congenital aortic valvular disease is currently under investigation.[8]

Stress Testing. Stress testing may be helpful in older patients with mild to moderate aortic stenosis in whom symptoms may be vague or suspicious and are not clearly related to the aortic valve disease. Stress-related changes in the S-T segment or T wave morphology would suggest important stenosis with myocardium at jeopardy. In these instances, relief of the stenosis should be seriously considered, despite mild to moderate resting peak gradients.

Cardiac Catheterization. Currently, the major roles of cardiac catheterization include diagnostic and therapeutic options. Diagnostically, catheterization may be helpful to assess left ventricular diastolic function, pulmonary artery pressure, and associated vascular lesions. Therapeutically, balloon valvotomy can be used in patients with isolated aortic valvular stenosis or occasionally in patients with complex multilevel LVOT obstruction.

Natural History

Critical "valvular" aortic stenosis in the neonate often presents as an "emergent" situation, and without prompt treatment these children may succumb from cardiovascular collapse. By contrast, older children with aortic stenosis are often asymptomatic. Given the important considerations pertaining to pediatric aortic valve repair and replacement, the timing of the operation becomes an important consideration, and understanding the natural history and progression of asymptomatic children is useful.

Aortic valve disease in children tends to be a progressive disease. Valvar aortic stenosis can be classified as mild, moderate, or severe. Categorized by Hossack and colleagues,[9] mild stenosis includes those patients with normal pulse volumes with a resting peak systolic gradient (measured at catheterization) between the left ventricle and aorta of less than 40 mm Hg. Patients are considered to have moderate aortic stenosis when they exhibit diminished pulse volumes by palpation and resting peak systolic gradients of 40 to 75 mm Hg at rest. Patients are considered to have severe stenosis when they present with abnormal pulse volumes and a resting peak systolic pressure gradient in excess of 75 mm Hg.

It should be noted that these gradient criteria were obtained at catheterization by direct pullback measurements. Currently, gradients across the LVOT are frequently obtained with echocardiography, and in most cases Doppler-derived peak instantaneous gradient correlates well with catheter-derived data; however, at lower gradients, Doppler echocardiography can result in an overestimation.[10,11]

Because aortic valve disease in children is a progressive disease, the natural history of this progression is of some interest. Among children with nonobstructive aortic lesions, Mills and colleagues[12] reported that 7% progressed to mild obstruction after 7 to 15 years. When mild stenosis was present upon the initial evaluation, progression was rapid.[12] Twenty percent of patients developed moderate or severe stenosis within 10 years, with 45% progressing within 20 years. Finally, approximately 60% of patients presenting with moderate stenosis will progress to severe stenosis within 10 years.[9]

Treatment

Catheter versus Surgical Relief of Aortic Stenosis in the Neonate. Aortic stenosis presenting in the neonatal

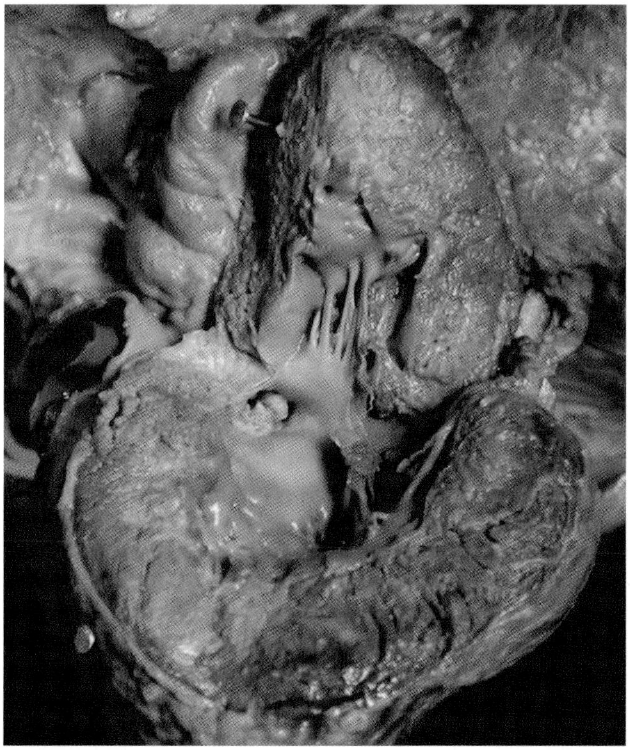

FIGURE 123-2 ■ Pathologic specimen showing aortic stenosis in the neonatal heart.

period can be a severe hemodynamic lesion that is life threatening (Fig. 123-2). These children often present in shock as a consequence of ductal closure in the setting of left heart structures that are inadequate to support the systemic circulation; their systemic circulation is "ductal dependent." These children require urgent medical stabilization, including assisted ventilation and inotropic support. Prostaglandin E1 is administered to reopen the duct and to maintain ductal patency. Once stabilized, a thorough echocardiographic examination of the left-sided structures is required to determine their suitability to support the systemic circulation.

When approaching critical aortic stenosis in neonates, the single most important decision regarding treatment is to decide which patients will benefit from biventricular repair, and which are better suited to a single ventricle approach. The importance of proper treatment selection is reflected by the high mortality in older, unstratified series of neonates undergoing valvotomy for critical aortic stenosis.[13] An accurate determination of which patients will benefit from a single ventricle treatment pathway (Stage I/Norwood operation) is critical, and it has been the impetus for the study sponsored by the Congenital Heart Surgeons Society (CHSS) and designed to accomplish this.[14] An estimate of survival benefit for specific left heart morphology can be obtained at the CHSS website (www.chssdc.org). The management of these patients has been detailed elsewhere. This discussion will focus on patients with aortic stenosis as the dominant lesion in the setting of two adequate ventricles.

For patients with anatomy deemed suitable to support a two-ventricle circulation, aortic valvotomy provides effective relief of aortic stenosis. Two techniques of aortic valvotomy have been developed: balloon dilation of the stenotic valve and surgical valvotomy (open and closed). While balloon valvotomy is the favored technique at many institutions, surgical valvotomy remains preferred by some. Proponents of balloon valvotomy cite avoidance of potential surgical morbidity, while advocates of surgical valvotomy maintain that a more accurate valvotomy is possible under direct vision.

Although there are no prospective randomized studies directly comparing these two techniques, some data are available. McCrindle and colleagues[15] reported a CHSS-sponsored multi-institutional review of 110 neonates undergoing either surgical (28) or balloon (82) valvotomy for critical aortic valve stenosis in the neonatal period. Survival was similar between the two procedures (82% at 1 month, 72% at 5 years).[15] Balloon valvotomy was more effective at relieving stenosis (mean residual gradient 20 vs. 36 mm Hg), but it was accomplished at the expense of a higher incidence of important aortic insufficiency (18% after balloon valvotomy versus 3% after surgical valvotomy). Despite these differences, the outcome data between the two techniques is comparable. Overall freedom from reintervention was similar for both groups (91% at 1 month, 48% at 5 years). The need for subsequent procedures, regardless of technique, emphasizes the palliative nature of valvotomy for critical aortic stenosis.

McElhinney and colleagues[16] reported medium- and long-term follow-up of 113 patients (age ≤ 60 days) from Children's Hospital Boston performed between 1985 and 2002. They reported a normalization of aortic annular and left ventricular end-diastolic dimensions within 1 to 2 years. Freedom from moderate or severe aortic regurgitation was 65%, with a reintervention free survival of 48% at 5 years. These data suggest that early relief of the LVOT obstruction allows for catch-up growth without neonatal surgery.

Although balloon valvotomy has assumed a prominent role in the treatment of congenital aortic stenosis in many institutions, its role vis-à-vis surgical valvotomy remains controversial. Hawkins and colleagues[17] have estimated the incidence of aortic valve operation after balloon valvotomy to be 5% to 7% per year. Others have reported the risk of surgery to be lower, but the incidence of reintervention, including subsequent balloon dilation, remains high (60% at 8 years).[18] It may be, however, that specific aortic valvular substrates lend themselves to one treatment or the other. In a group of 54 infants (57% neonates) undergoing surgical aortic valvotomy, Bhabra and colleagues[19] reported significant differences in the long-term outcomes based on leaflet morphology. When valvotomy resulted in a trileaflet structure, patients did significantly better than when only a bileaflet valve was achieved. At 10 years, the actuarial freedom from reintervention was 92% among trileaflet valves, but only 33% among bileaflet valves ($P = 0.01$). Similar differences were reported for freedom from aortic valve reoperation ($P = 0.04$). Freedom from aortic valve replacement (AVR) was 100% in trileaflet valves and 57% in bileaflet valves. However, by echocardiogram, the authors were only able to retrospectively identify 14 of 28 bileaflet valves, whereas 7 of 8 valves with trileaflet potential could be identified (88% sensitivity, 50% specificity). These results have yet to be confirmed, but closer examination of the anatomic subtypes of aortic valve stenosis may be justified before selecting the appropriate technique.

Currently there appears to be little if any role for surgical transventricular (closed) aortic valvotomy.

Catheter versus Surgical Relief of Aortic Stenosis in Infancy. A few studies have compared balloon aortic valvotomy to surgical valvotomy in older children. McCrindle and colleagues[20] reported their analysis of 630 balloon valvotomies on 606 patients from 23 institutions, with a median age of 6.8 years (range, 1 day to 18 years). The procedure was abandoned 4.1% of the time because of technical issues, and procedural mortality was 1.9%. A suboptimal result (including failure to complete procedure, residual gradient >60 mm Hg, left ventricle aortic pressure ≥1.6) or major morbidity or mortality were reported in 17% of patients. Independent risk factors for poor outcomes were age less than 3 months, earlier procedure date, higher preoperative gradient, unrepaired aortic coarctation, and the use of undersized balloons.

Other groups have reported similar results with balloon valvotomy in non-neonates. Moore and colleagues reported successful dilation in 87% of patients (129/148), with a very low procedural mortality (0.7%) and good long-term survival (95% at 8 years).[18] Freedom from reintervention at 8 years was 50%, a figure that is consistent with other studies.[21]

In these patients, the risk of repeated intervention was related to the degree of regurgitation and to residual gradients after initial balloon valvotomy. Reminiscent of the report by Bhabra and colleagues,[19] they reported differential results based on angiographic morphology of the stenotic aortic valve; however, as in neonates, it is difficult to demonstrate clearly the superiority of balloon or surgical aortic valvotomy. Chartrand and colleagues[22] reported their experience with 67 children (age > 6 months) undergoing surgical valvotomy during 1960 to 1992. There was no operative mortality, and the 20-year freedom from death, reoperation, and AVR was 94%, 63%, and 73%, respectively. The authors concluded that surgical valvuloplasty is a safe and effective procedure with durable results.

In summary, as in neonates, aortic valve morphology appears to influence the response to intervention in infants, and further characterization may be justified. Currently there appear to be institutional preferences for balloon or surgical valvotomy that can be defended on the basis of experience.

Aortic Stenosis in the Older Child. In contrast to clinical presentation of the neonate with critical aortic stenosis, older children are commonly asymptomatic. For them, durable preservation of left ventricular function becomes the primary goal of treatment. The etiology of aortic stenosis in the older child (>1 year of age) is most commonly due to valvular aortic stenosis (79%), followed by subvalvular aortic stenosis (7%) and supravalvular stenosis (6%) being much less common.[6] Aortic regurgitation is often associated with congenital aortic stenosis and may be the result of previous interventions for the relief of stenosis.

Older children with aortic stenosis generally enjoy normal growth and development. When present, symptoms such as chest pain, exercise intolerance, or syncope constitute clear surgical indications. For asymptomatic patients, the indications for intervention are subtler. For patients with severe stenosis in whom the left ventricle to aortic (LV-Ao) gradient is greater than 75 mm Hg, operation is recommended. For children thought to have moderate stenosis (40-75 mm Hg LV-Ao gradient), more information may be needed before a recommendation can be made. In this setting, electrocardiographic changes (ST-T wave changes consistent with left ventricular strain, left ventricular hypertrophy) or a positive stress test result would be indications for operation. For these asymptomatic patients, somatic growth, surgical options, and timing of intervention become important concerns.

Because of the progressive nature of the disease, older children thought to have mild aortic stenosis (gradient < 40 mm Hg) should be followed with periodic examinations and echocardiograms. It should be remembered that the gradient depends on the cardiac output and in a severely dysfunctional left ventricle the gradient may be unimpressive.

The management options for older children depend on the context of their disease. Older children newly diagnosed with important aortic stenosis with minimal insufficiency may be well served by balloon valvotomy. The more common scenario is several years of excellent palliation following an initial valvotomy, during which time the child grows and develops normally. However, with time or repeated interventions, or both, many patients will develop important aortic insufficiency (see Aortic Regurgitation section). Any residual valvular stenosis can be magnified by the resulting volume load, and the combinations of these lesions conspire to threaten left ventricular function. However, by virtue of their older age and larger size, these children are better candidates for durable surgical palliation, usually including valve replacement.

SUBVALVULAR AORTIC STENOSIS

Congenital subvalvular aortic stenosis is an obstruction below the aortic valve secondary to a discrete or short, localized fibrous or fibromuscular ridge or a longer diffuse fibromuscular tunnel (Fig. 123-3). It is important to note that there is a spectrum between discrete and tunnel-like subaortic stenosis, which has contributed the variable difference in the reported prevalence. In addition, it is often difficult to distinguish hypertrophic obstructive cardiomyopathy from tunnel-like subaortic stenosis (see Hypertrophic Obstructive Cardiomyopathy).

Subaortic Membrane

Subaortic membrane is found in association with other congenital lesions in 60% to 70% of cases, with ventral septal defect being the most common (35%).[23]

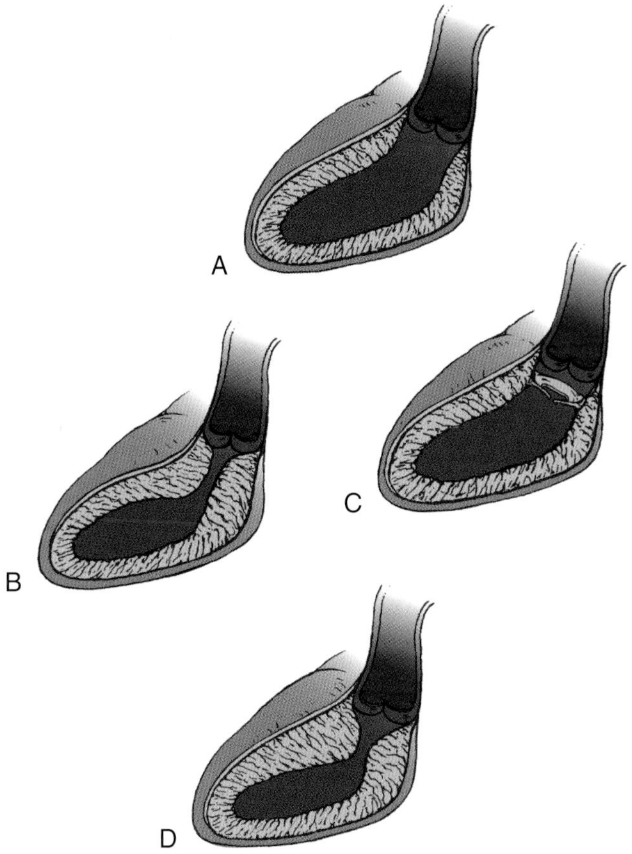

FIGURE 123-3 ■ Examples of forms of **(A)** fixed aortic stenosis, **(B)** discrete membrane, **(C)** tunnel-like stenosis, and **(D)** muscular obstruction.

Membranous subaortic stenosis results from the proliferation of fibrous tissue just beneath the leaflets of the aortic valve. This tissue may be very thin and tough, and is often circumferential, involving the underside of the anterior leaflet of the mitral valve. In fact, careful review of the echocardiogram may suggest a hinge point representing tethering on the leaflet by the membrane.[24,25] Although the etiology of this form of aortic pathology is not known, studies have implicated shear stress, precipitated by abnormal angles between the ventricular septum and the aortic barrel, as playing an important role. The addition of a ventral septal defect adds to the generation of shear stress in this setting.[26]

Natural History and Surgical Indications

In general, the surgical indications for membranous subaortic stenosis adhere to the general recommendations for aortic stenosis. However, citing a lower incidence of recurrence, some centers advocate earlier surgical resection for subaortic stenosis. Brauner and colleagues[27] reported that the recurrence rate of subaortic stenosis (predominately composed of membranous, but with a few tunnel-like stenoses) was related to a preoperative gradient of 40 mm Hg or greater and suggested that surgical resection at lower gradients was justified. Others have advocated repair at the time of diagnosis, irrespective of the gradient.[28,29] However, the advantages of early intervention have not been confirmed, as other investigators have reported no benefit of early surgery on recurrence.[30]

Because the timing of surgery remains controversial, it is helpful to examine the natural history of membranous subaortic stenosis. There are data suggesting that some children with mild subaortic stenosis (peak systolic gradient < 40 mm Hg) might not require surgery for several years. A large representative study of the rate of progression of subvalvular aortic stenosis was reported by Rohlicek and colleagues[31] studying children from several centers in Eastern Canada. To document the natural history and surgical outcomes, they followed 92 children from the time of diagnosis. There were slightly more males (1.6 : 1), and the mean age at diagnosis was 5.3 years. Thirteen patients had bicuspid aortic valves. At a mean follow-up of four years, 42 of these children ultimately came to surgery an average of 2.2 ± 0.4 years after diagnosis; 44 were followed medically and never came to operation. Children ultimately requiring surgery presented with higher initial gradients (40 ± 5 mm Hg vs. 21 ± 2 mm Hg) and were more likely to present with aortic insufficiency at diagnosis (35% vs. 13%). Analysis showed the echo gradient at diagnosis to be predictive of subsequent gradient progression as well as the appearance of aortic insufficiency. Eight children undergoing surgery required reoperation for recurrent subaortic stenosis at an average of 4.9 ± 0.9 years after initial resection. These patients initially presented with significantly higher gradients (66 ± 10 mm Hg).

In contrast to a more aggressive approach of aggressive surgical resection of membranous subaortic stenosis at time of diagnosis, these data suggest that a significant proportion of these patients will have stable or at least slowly progressive gradients. The management approach to patients remains variable, but it seems reasonable to pursue surgical resection for peak systolic gradients of 40 mm Hg or greater (obtained by echocardiography). The new onset of aortic insufficiency should be considered an important indication for surgery, regardless of the gradient. While these authors did not discern any improvement in aortic insufficiency following operation, it has been the experience of others that careful débridement of fibrous tissue encroaching on the aortic leaflets often results in significant improvement in aortic insufficiency.[32]

Surgical Approach

The surgical approach to this lesion requires cardiopulmonary bypass. A single right atrial venous cannula is usually adequate. The aortic valve is exposed through a transverse aortotomy, which can be carried down into the noncoronary sinus if needed. Careful retraction of the aortic leaflets will reveal the subaortic membrane. The distance between the aortic valve and the membrane may vary slightly, but can usually be well visualized. The membrane is incised in the safe zone of the ventricular septum, just leftward of the nadir of the right coronary sinus. In many instances, the membrane can be peeled or endarterectomized from the endocardium anteriorly and rightward, and from the anterior leaflet of the mitral valve posteriorly. In severe cases, this membrane may encroach upon and even involve the belly of the aortic valve leaflets. In this instance, the leaflets require careful débridement of the thick, fibrous tissue.

Surgical Results

Membranous subaortic stenosis has been the subject of intense scrutiny for its incidence and its propensity for recurrence after seemingly adequate surgical resection. The recurrence rate for membranous subaortic stenosis has been reported to be between 0% and 55%, with most reports documenting a recurrence rate of 15% to 21%.[30,33-37]

Independent predictors of reoperation for recurrent subaortic stenosis include proximity of the membrane to the aortic valve (<6 mm), and a peak gradient greater than 60 mm Hg. Adherence of the membrane to the aortic or mitral valve identified at surgery was also a predictor for recurrence.[38] Septal myotomy, in addition to membrane resection, has been reported to reduce the incidence of recurrence. Lupinetti and colleagues[39] reported a recurrence rate of 4% when a septal myomectomy was performed in addition to membrane resection; however, this finding has not been confirmed by others.[27,40]

Other surgeons advocate an even more aggressive approach. Yacoub and colleagues[33] have suggested that an important pathologic feature of membranous subaortic stenosis is fibrous tissue ingrowth at the point of insertion of the anterior leaflet of the mitral valve into the left ventricular myocardium (Fig. 123-4). This ingrowth interferes with dynamic widening of the outflow tract, including posterior displacement of the mitral apparatus, during systole. Adding resection of the fibrous tissue from the mitral valve trigones to membrane resection and septal myomectomy, Yacoub and colleagues[33] reported excellent relief of LVOT gradient (mean, 8 mm Hg) in 57 patients. Over an average follow-up of 15 years, seven patients had mild to moderate aortic regurgitation, but importantly, no patient required reoperation for recurrent stenosis.

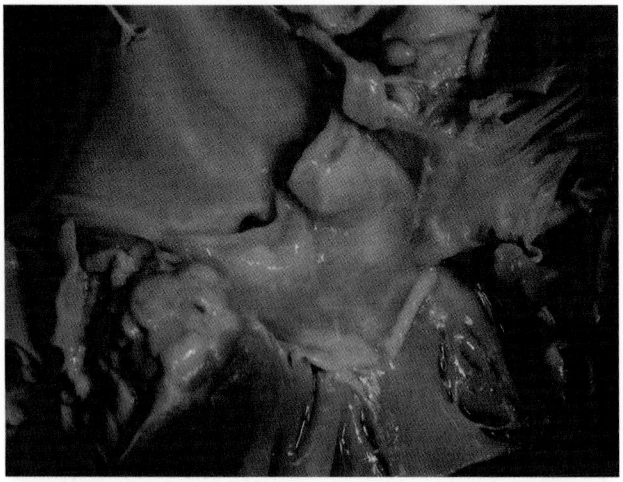

FIGURE 123-4 ■ Pathologic specimen showing fibrous tissue in growth at the insertion of the anterior leaflet of the mitral valve into the left ventricle.

While periodic attempts at balloon dilation in these patients have been performed, the resulting gradients are generally high (≈30 mm Hg), and subsequent surgery is required in a majority. Among 13 patients undergoing dilation, Moskowitz and colleagues[41] reported that 9 required subsequent surgery. Suarez de Lezo and colleagues[42,43] reported a 50% recurrence rate within 3 years. At this time, balloon dilation should not be considered a primary treatment of discrete subaortic stenosis.

Tunnel-Like Subaortic Stenosis

Long segment or tunnel-like stenosis has been defined as a muscular or fibromuscular subaortic stenosis, the length of which was more than one third the aortic diameter.[44] While tunnel-like stenosis may be associated with other lesions, such as interrupted aortic arch and atrioventricular septal defect, this discussion will confine itself to diffuse, long segment, or tunnel-like stenosis in the setting of concordant atrioventricular and ventriculoarterial connections with an intact ventricular septum. The indications for operation for subaortic tunnel are similar to those described for membranous subaortic obstruction.

Surgical Treatment Options

Modified Konno Operation

Surgical Indications. The indications for the modified Konno operation in the relief of subaortic obstruction are evolving. Roughneen and others described their experience with the modified Konno operation in 16 children.[45,46] Indications for operation were recurrent subaortic stenosis (3), hypertrophic subaortic stenosis (3), tunnel stenosis of the LVOT (2), and subaortic stenosis following atrioventricular septal defect (2), or ventricular septal defect (VSD) (5). Long-term follow-up will be important for these patients, as it is likely a large number of these patients will have recurrent sub AS.

Surgical Approach. The degree of hypoplasia encountered in tunnel-like subaortic stenosis does not lend itself to transaortic resection, as might be performed for membranous subaortic stenosis. The surgical treatment of tunnel-like stenosis requires a more extensive procedure. In the presence of a suitable aortic valve, the modified Konno operation has become a favored option when approaching tunnel-like subaortic stenosis. It has the great appeal of enlarging the LVOT while preserving the native aortic valve. Excellent technical reviews of this technique are available.[45,47,48]

Briefly, under moderate hypothermia with bicaval cannulation, an aortotomy is performed, and the aortic valve and subaortic area is examined. Only if the aortic valve is satisfactory should the valve-sparing modified Konno operation be performed. If the valve is inadequate, a more extensive procedure designed to enlarge the LVOT and replace the aortic valve will be necessary, such as the Konno-Rastan (discussed later) or Ross-Konno operation.

After inspection of the aortic valve, the infundibulum of the right ventricle is incised in a transverse fashion. Visualization of the ventricular septum from these two perspectives (through the aortic valve and through the infundibulum) allows an accurate incision through the ventricular septum (Fig. 123-5). Indentation of the safe area of ventricular septum (leftward of the nadir of the right coronary leaflet) with a right-angled clamp placed through the aortic valve allows an accurate incision through the septum via the infundibulotomy. Alternatively, a stitch can be placed from the LVOT to the right ventricular outflow tract (RVOT) to pull up and help guide this incision. It is important that the trajectory of this incision be directed toward the apex of the left ventricle, which from the surgeon's perspective is almost directly leftward, and carried as distally as necessary to relieve the obstruction. Proximally the incision can be carried up to, and if necessary into, the commissure between the right and left aortic leaflets. Septal tissue can be débrided from the left ventricle side of the septum, but this should be on the leftward portion of the incision, to spare the left-sided conduction apparatus as it courses down the ventricular septum. The resulting VSD is then closed with a generous patch (Dacron or polytetrafluoroethylene) augmenting the LVOT. The aortic valve is carefully débrided of any fibrous tissue, and the incision is closed.

Surgical Results. The modified Konno operation is highly effective in reducing the LVOT gradient, and it can be achieved without damage to the conduction tissue. In the series by Jahangiri and colleagues,[45] 15 of 46 patients with tunnel-like sub AS underwent a modified Konno procedure with excellent relief of LVOT obstruction and minimal incidence of aortic regurgitation and heart block.[45] Caldarone and colleagues[49] reported similar results among 18 patients. Although the technique is highly effective in relieving subaortic stenosis resulting from a variety of lesions, complications can occur. In general, operative mortality among published reports has been negligible. However, right bundle branch block has been commonly noted following the modified Konno operation. This is significant in the setting of preexisting left bundle branch blocks, as may exist following transaortic resection of subaortic stenosis, and complete heart block has been noted in up to 12.5% of cases. Although the aortic valve is at risk and residual VSDs can occur, these complications are uncommon with careful technique. Given these results, some surgeons have advocated this operation for recurrent membranous subaortic stenosis. While the modified Konno certainly alters the geometry of the LVOT, thought to contribute to the genesis of membrane, its effect on additional recurrences is unknown.

Konno-Rastan Aortoventriculoplasty

Surgical Approach. The Konno-Rastan operation, described independently by Konno and Rastan in 1975

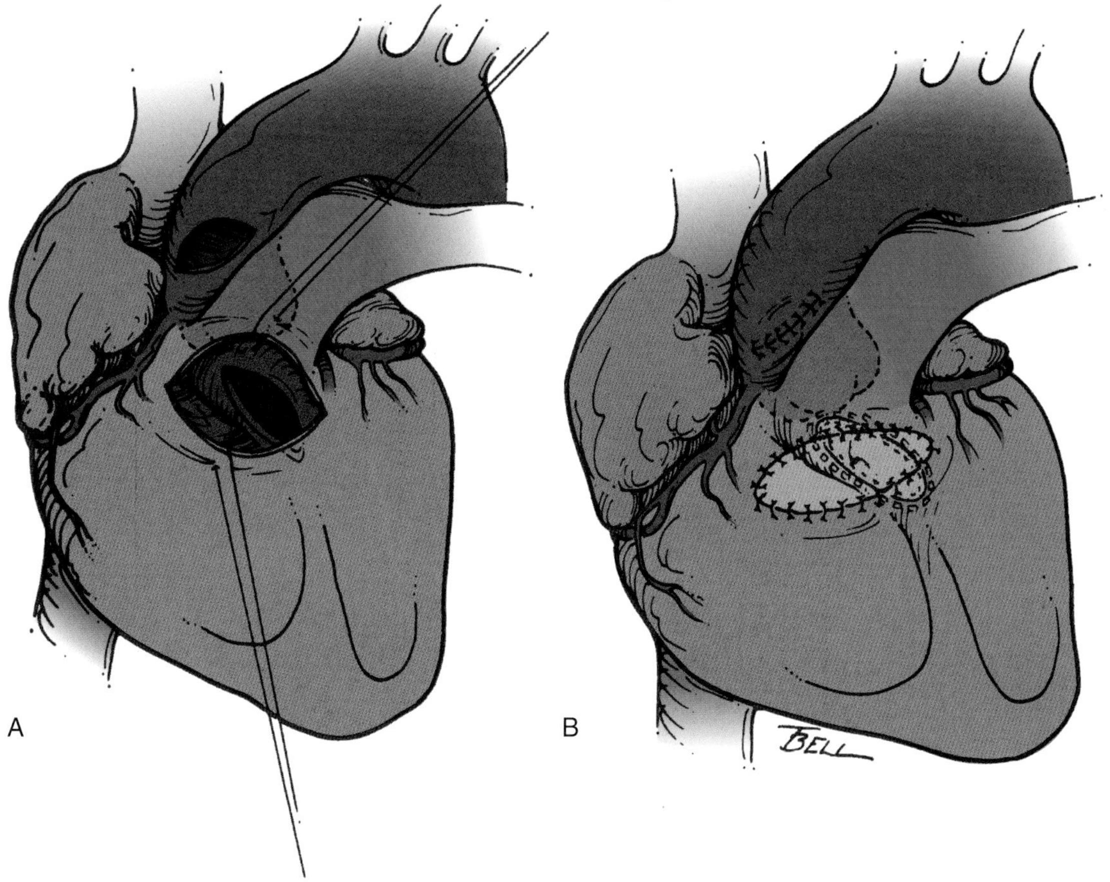

FIGURE 123-5 ■ Modified Konno operation. **A,** Transverse incision of the infundibulum showing the perspective of the ventricle septum through the aortic valve and the infundibulum. **B,** Superimposed patches of the ventricular septum and the infundibulum, respectively.

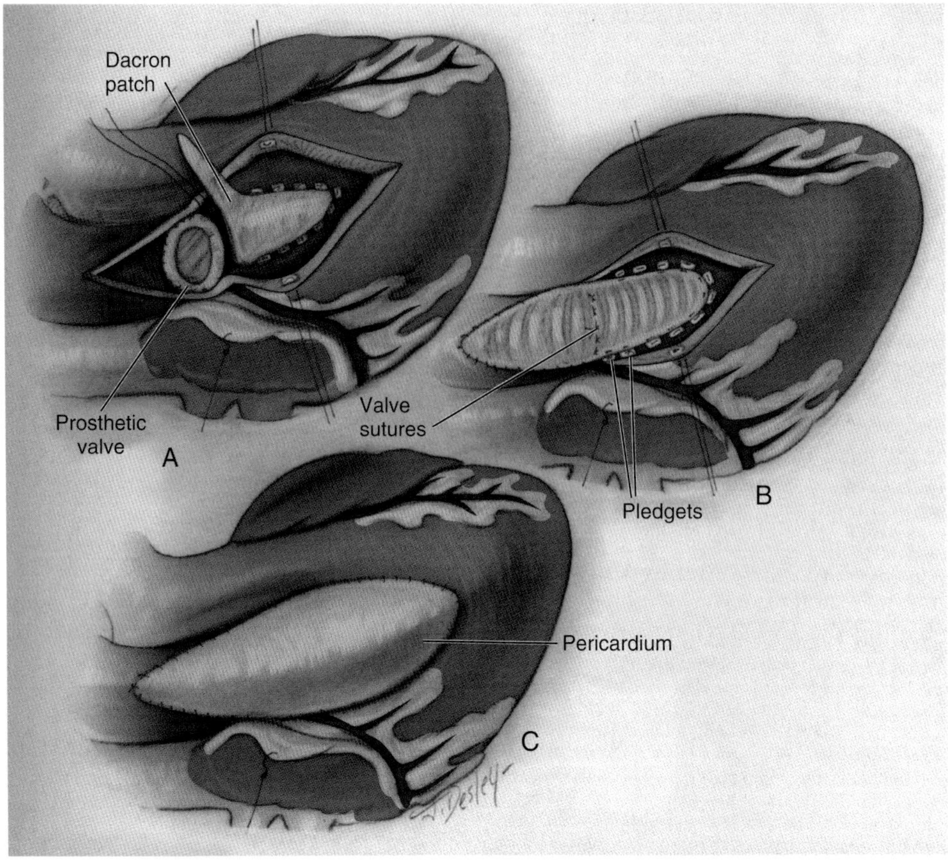

FIGURE 123-6 ■ Konno-Rastan aortoventriculoplasty. **A,** Atrioventriculoplasty with valve insertion. **B,** Closure of ventricular septal defect; aorta with Dacron patch. **C,** Closure of right ventricular outflow tract.

and 1976,[50,51] is required when tunnel-like subaortic stenosis coexists with significant aortic valve pathology. Incision of the ventricular septum, as performed in the modified Konno operation through the aortic annulus, and the ascending aorta, provides effective relief of all levels of obstruction. This operation requires bicaval cannulation. A vertical aortotomy is made leftward of the right coronary artery. At this point, an incision in the infundibulum of the right ventricle is helpful in guiding the septal incision. The annulus of the aortic valve is incised leftward of the nadir of the right coronary leaflet, and extended into the interventricular septum, relieving the subaortic stenosis. The aortic annulus is débrided, and an appropriately sized mechanical (or biological) prosthesis is inserted and fixed into the posterior annulus. A patch of Dacron or polytetrafluoroethylene is fashioned such that it enlarges the LVOT, and it is sutured into place up to the aortic annulus enlarging the subaortic dimensions. Sutures are then passed through the valve sewing ring and patch, reestablishing annular continuity. The patch is then carried distally, enlarging and closing the ascending aorta (Fig. 123-6). The enlargement or width of the Dacron patch has to be considered carefully because the right coronary artery anatomy can be altered. Figure 123-7 is an example of a distorted right coronary artery following aortic root enlargement. If the aortic root is extremely hypoplastic, a Nicks-type incision in the contralateral sinus may allow a more uniform aortic root enlargement. The RVOT is repaired, allowing adequate clearance for the underlying augmented LVOT. Treated bovine pericardium works well for this application.

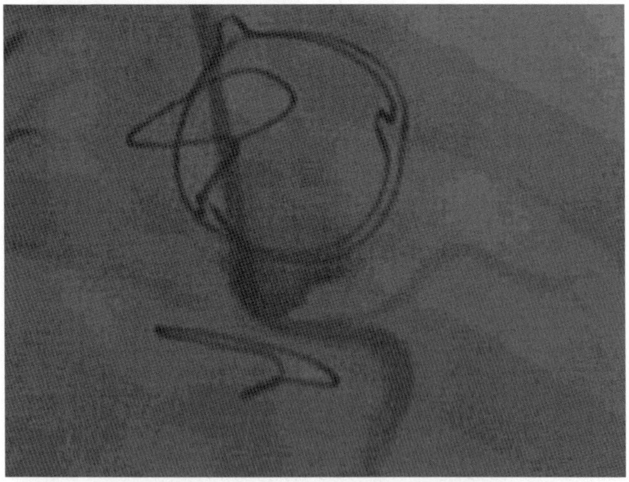

FIGURE 123-7 ■ Cardiac catheterization showing a distorted right coronary artery after Konno-Rastan aortoventriculoplasty.

Surgical Results. The results of the Konno operation have improved since its introduction in 1975. Erez and colleagues[52] reported their experience with the Konno operation in 60 pediatric patients between 1982 and 2000. Forty-two received mechanical valves, nine received homografts, six received xenografts, and fifteen received

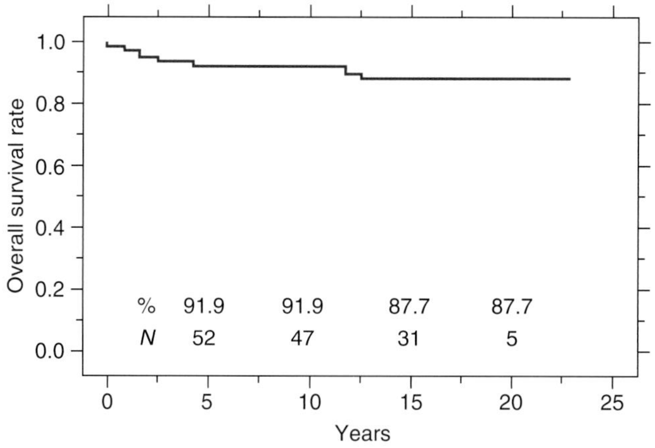

FIGURE 123-8 ■ Overall survival rate. The actuarial survival rates calculated with the Kaplan-Meier curves were 91.9% at 10 years and 87.7% at 15 years. (From Sakamoto T, Matsumura G, Kosaka Y, et al: Long-term results of Konno procedure for complex left ventricular outflow tract obstruction. *Eur J Cardiothorac Surg* 34:37–41, 2008.)

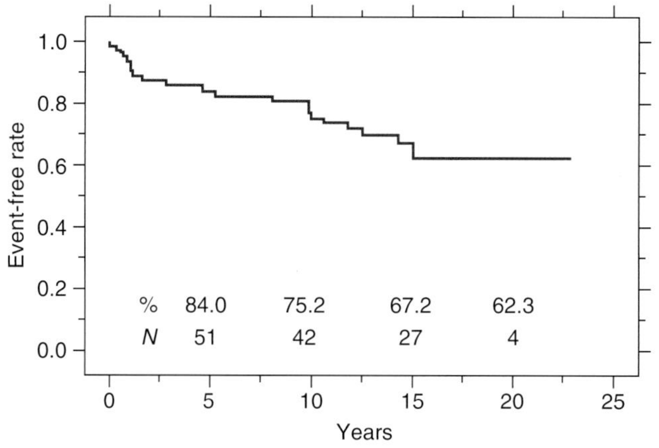

FIGURE 123-9 ■ Freedom from all events. Event-free rates including all mortality, reoperation, catheter intervention, and significant complications were 75.2% at 10 years and 67.2% at 15 years. (From Sakamoto T, Matsumura G, Kosaka Y, et al: Long-term results of Konno procedure for complex left ventricular outflow tract obstruction. *Eur J Cardiothorac Surg* 34:37–41, 2008.)

autografts. Operative mortality declined from 25% early in the experience to approximately 10%, which is comparable to other contemporary pediatric series.[53-55] Similar recent results were reported in 63 patients by Sakamoto and colleagues[56] undergoing the Konno operation using a mechanical valve (Figs. 123-8 and 123-9). Although mortality has continued to decline, complications remain common. Sixteen percent of patients with a Konno operation or prosthetic valve required surgical reexploration for bleeding, whereas only 6.8% (1 of 15) of patients undergoing Ross-Konno operation required reoperation for bleeding. Heart block occurred in 8.8% of Konno or prosthetic valve operations and in 6.7% of Ross-Konno operations. Long-term survival for the Konno operation has been related to the underlying pathology and recurrent or residual LVOT obstruction that might require complex reoperations.

The freedom from reoperation following the Konno operation has not been satisfactory. Among patients

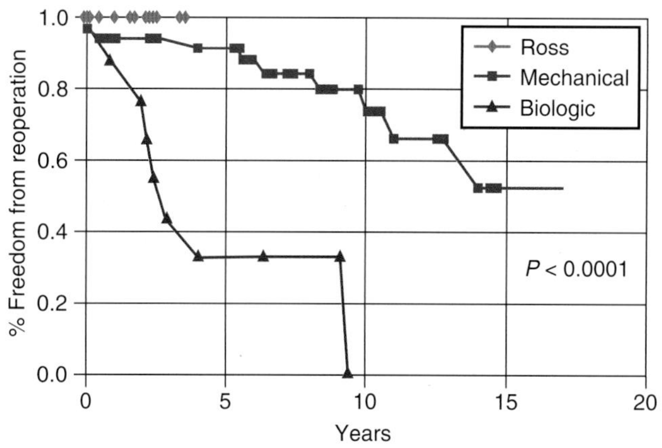

FIGURE 123-10 ■ Comparison of failure rate percentage of Ross, mechanical, and biological procedures and time to reoperation.

receiving biologic valves (homograft or xenografts), freedom from reoperation at 10 years was 0% (Fig. 123-10). Reoperation was primarily for valve failure. The patients with mechanical valves primarily required reoperation for valve outgrowth (6) and endocarditis (3).

Ross-Konno Operation. There is limited long-term follow-up on patients undergoing neonatal or infant Ross-Konno operation. Among the 15 patients undergoing the Ross-Konno operation between 1997 and 2000, there was one operative death (6.7%) and two late deaths in syndromic children. While the authors concluded that the Ross-Konno operation was less morbid, the durability of the autograft in the aortic position remains a concern, especially in the very young.[49] Ohye and colleagues[57] have reported their neonatal and infant experience in 10 patients with the Ross-Konno operation. At a median follow-up of 48 months, they reported no reoperations on the autograft, although two patients have developed significant autograft insufficiency, and there was no operative mortality. More recently, Brown and colleagues[58] reported their experience in 14 patients with a mean follow-up of 5.7 years and an actuarial survival at 10 years of 86%. Freedom from RVOT and autograft reoperation at 10 years was 77% and 92%, respectively. Oka and colleagues[59] reported their experience in patients undergoing Ross-Konno and associated mitral valve procedures. Patients undergoing concomitant mitral valve operation had significantly more morbidity and mortality; actuarial survival at 5 years was 44% versus 92%.[59] Despite concerns about the durability of the autograft, the Ross-Konno probably presents the best available option for relief of complex LVOT obstruction in small children (Fig. 123-11).

Aortoapical Conduit. The aortoapical conduit is largely of historic interest. Brown and colleagues reported their experience in 22 children with tunnel-like stenosis between 1978 and 1992.[34] They reported one early death and six late deaths, for an overall mortality of 32%. The ACC is associated with a high rate of reoperation and poor long-term durability.[60] This technique has largely been abandoned in favor of surgical alternatives, such as

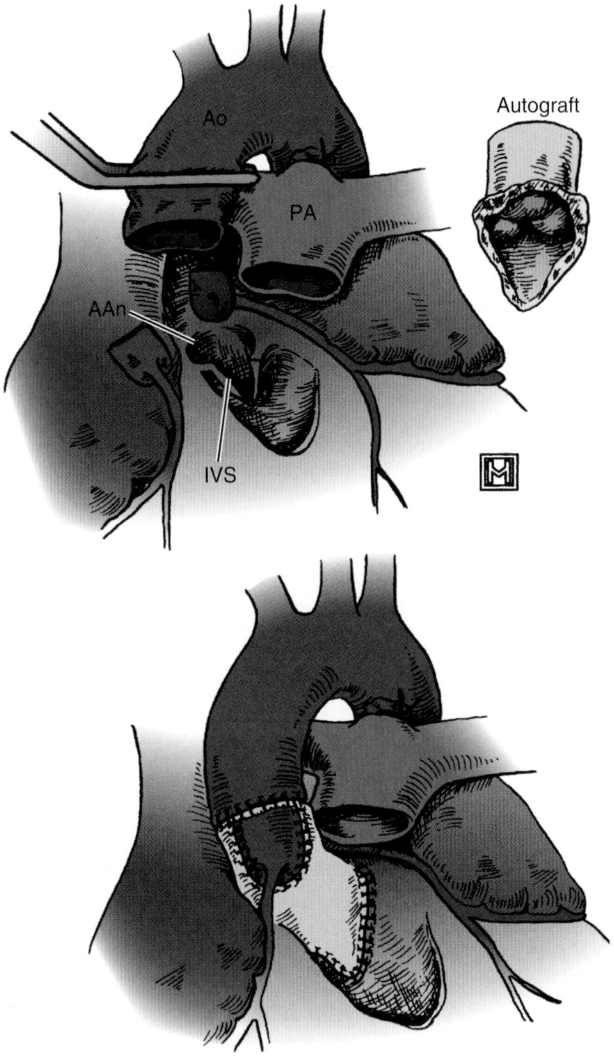

FIGURE 123-11 ■ Ross-Konno operation for complex left ventricular outflow tract obstruction in a small child. *AAn,* Aortic annulus; *Ao,* aorta; *IVS,* interventricular septum; *PA,* pulmonary artery.

the modified Konno, Konno-Rastan, and Ross-Konno procedures.

Hypertrophic Obstructive Cardiomyopathy

Hypertrophic obstructive cardiomyopathy (HOCM) is an autosomal dominant disease with limited information on children.[61] Some of these patients develop a dynamic form of subaortic LVOT obstruction that results from myocardial hypertrophy prominently affecting the interventricular septum, but also can affect the mid-ventricle and LV apex. A variety of treatments, including calcium channel blockers, beta blockers, and dual-chamber pacing have met with mixed success.[62-65]

Surgical relief can be accomplished by transaortic septal myotomy designed to relieve the subaortic septal muscular obstruction. First described by Morrow and colleagues,[66] septal myotomy provides effective hemodynamic relief of the obstruction and can be expected to provide both symptomatic relief and improvement in New York Heart Association class. Improvement in survival, however, has been more difficult to document. Despite an operative mortality of 1% to 2%, the subsequent annual mortality rate approaches 2%, comparable to that reported in patients treated nonsurgically.[67] Recently, the modified Konno operation has also been applied successfully to HOCM.

Surgical Indications

Surgical indications for this condition remain controversial.[68] In general, operation has been advocated for symptomatic patients (New York Heart Association class III-IV) with peak instantaneous gradients exceeding 50 mm Hg, or asymptomatic patients with gradients exceeding 100 mm Hg, despite medical management.[69,70]

More recently, attenuation of the interventricular septum has been induced by the injection of absolute ethanol into the proximal septal coronary artery.[71] This technique has been successful in lowering the outflow tract gradient by 60% to 80%, but 11% to 29% of these patients develop complete heart block.[72,73] Although alcohol ablation holds promise, it represents a selective alternative to surgical therapy, and currently it has no place in the treatment of young children. Currently, septal myomectomy remains the gold standard for medically refractory symptomatic patients with high-grade LVOT obstruction.[74]

Preoperative Assessment

In the preoperative assessment, it is important to establish the extent of the hypertrophy and the mechanism of any associated mitral regurgitation (MR). Most patients with HOCM with have some MR, and it is generally related to systolic anterior motion (SAM) of the mitral valve. The typical posteriorly directed MR that occurs after the SAM of the mitral valve is generally alleviated with septal myectomy alone; however, if the MR precedes the SAM, the MR will likely persist after myectomy. Caution is warranted if placing a ring annuloplasty, because it increases the risk of SAM. In older patients, one must rule out coronary disease or any associated myocardial bridges.[75]

Surgical Approach

Standard cardiopulmonary bypass with mild hypothermia is initiated. Because of the extreme hypertrophy, myocardial protection is critically important. Topical cooling and cold blood cardioplegia are used. Once the heart is arrested, vented, and cooled, an oblique hockey-stick incision is used to expose the aortic root. Looking into the subaortic area, the papillary muscles and chordae are obscured by the septum. An index finger in the LVOT and a thumb anterior to the RVOT confirms the septal thickness. The landmarks for the myectomy incisions are the area immediately below the middle of the right coronary cusp and the leftward muscle bar that extends to the mitral valve. The left bundle branch of the conduction system is under the commissure between the right and noncoronary cusp, and it extends leftward. After resection, the Doppler gradient should remain less than 15 to 20 mm Hg. On occasion there will be inconsequential fistulous connections from the divided septal coronary arteries.[76,77]

Surgical Results

Ommen and colleagues[78] reported a multi-institutional experience analyzing the effect of surgical myectomy on long-term survival in hypertrophic cardiomyopathy. Operative mortality was 0.8%, and 1-, 5-, and 10-year overall survival was 98%, 96%, and 83%, respectively. When comparing operated with nonoperated HOCM, operated myectomy patients experienced significantly improved survival ($P < 0.001$).[78] More recently, Swistel and colleagues[79] reported on 16 patients with complete follow-up at 2.5 years and no deaths, reoperations, or other adverse consequences. The mean preoperative, postoperative, and late LVOT gradients were 137 ± 45, 10 ± 17, and 6 ± 14 mm Hg.[79] Altarabsheh and colleagues[80] reported a large series of 127 children (12.9 ± 5.9 years) who underwent septal myectomy for HOCM. Preoperative mean gradient was 89 mm Hg and 95% had MR related to SAM. Mean follow-up was 8.3 years; there were no early deaths and four late deaths. Overall survival was 91%, 88%, 79%, and 73% at 1-, 5-, 10-, 15-, and 20 years, respectively. Six patients underwent repeated septal myectomy. The authors' data support improved late survival with myectomy compared with previous reports in patients with untreated HOCM.[80]

Supravalvular Stenosis

Supravalvular aortic stenosis (SVAS) is the least common form of aortic stenosis, accounting for 6% to 7% of aortic outflow abnormalities. First described by Mencarelli in 1930,[81] supravalvular aortic stenosis is the result of narrowing of the aorta beginning just above the aortic valve, usually at the level of the sinotubular junction. The gender incidence is more equitable than most forms of aortic stenosis with an approximately 1 : 1 male-to-female ratio. In 1961, Williams and colleagues[82] described the common association of several other features, including characteristic facial features (elfin facies), mental retardation, and, infrequently, hypercalcemia.[82] Soon afterwards, an association with Williams syndrome and peripheral pulmonary artery stenosis was identified.[83,84]

In addition to its association with Williams syndrome, SVAS occurs in a familial form transmitted by autosomal dominant inheritance, and in a sporadic form. Microdeletion of chromosome 7q11.23 has been identified in patients suffering from all three forms of supravalvular stenosis.[44,85] Affected individuals express only about 50% of the normal amount of tropoelastin, resulting in reduced elastin deposition and fiber disorganization within the arterial wall.

Clinical Presentation

Williams syndrome may be suggested on the basis of characteristic facies, and all patients with possible Williams syndrome should be evaluated for supravalvular aortic stenosis. Any asymptomatic patient with a familial history should be evaluated, and the presence of a cardiac murmur or thrill should undergo echocardiography.

Other, nonaortic vascular lesions are commonly present and should be sought. These lesions include pulmonary artery stenosis (30%), renal artery stenosis (5%), and coarctation of the aorta (15%).[86] The degree of involvement in the aorta can vary from localized disease at the sinotubular junction with or without left main coronary ostial involvement, to diffuse involvement of the aortic arch and brachiocephalic vessels. Thus, patients with supravalvular aortic stenosis should undergo catheterization to fully delineate the extent of vascular involvement (Fig. 123-12).

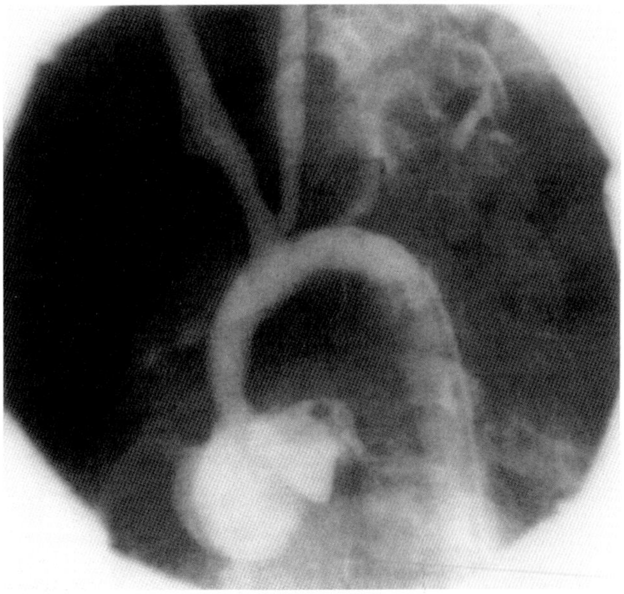

FIGURE 123-12 ■ Extent of supravalvular aortic stenosis determined by catheterization.

Surgical Indications

Like the other forms of aortic obstruction, supravalvular aortic stenosis tends to be a progressive lesion. Indications for operation are generally consistent with those in other forms of aortic stenosis (symptoms, gradient >40-50 mm Hg). Syncope or chest pain may represent cusp adherence to the sinotubular junction and episodic coronary ischemia, and it is a clear indication for surgery.[87]

Significant pulmonary artery stenosis is often present in patients requiring relief of supravalvular aortic stenosis. Surgery should not be delayed in these patients, as the natural history of associated pulmonary stenosis is generally indolent, with regression of these lesions over time. However, a few patients will have severe central or branch pulmonary artery stenosis, or both, and in the presence of markedly elevated right ventricular pressures, relief of the pulmonary artery stenosis should also be performed if the lesions are surgically accessible.

Surgical Approach

The surgical treatment of SVAS is determined by the extent of the stenosis. A variety of techniques have been used to relieve localized SVAS. In 1961 at the Mayo

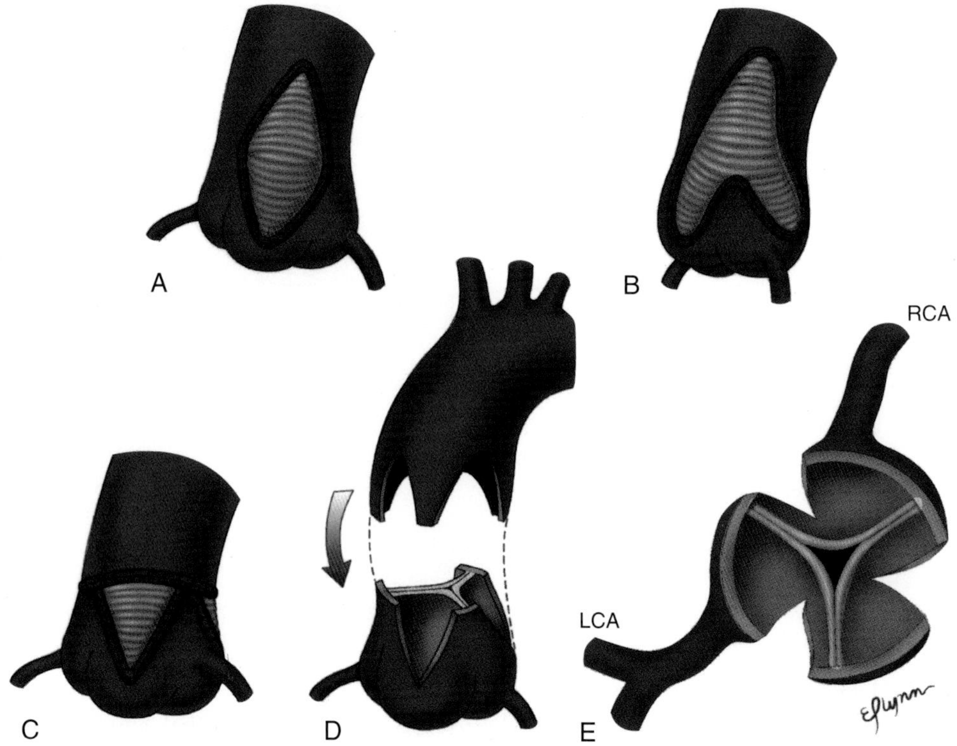

FIGURE 123-13 ■ Surgical treatment of supravalvular aortic stenosis. **A,** Single-patch technique into noncoronary sinus. **B,** Two-sinus augmentation technique (Doty). **C,** Three-patch (modified Brom). **D,** Autologous interdigitating technique. **E,** Cranial view of aortic sinus incisions. *LCA,* Left coronary artery; *RCA,* right coronary artery.

clinic, McGoon and colleagues[88] initially described a single-patch technique, with the placement of a teardrop or diamond-shaped patch across the sinotubular junction, extending between the bases of the noncoronary sinus into the ascending aorta. Doty and colleagues[89] extended the aortoplasty by fashioning a bifurcated, pantaloon shaped patch that straddled the commissure between the right-noncoronary leaflet, enlarging both the noncoronary and right coronary sinuses (Fig. 123-13). Concern about an untreated left coronary sinus, as well as the functional effect of an asymmetric augmentation on the aortic valve led Brom to propose a three-sinus repair.[90] A modification of this technique, proposed by Myers and colleagues[91] accomplishes a three-sinus augmentation by placing counter incisions into the ascending aorta, enlarging the sinuses without prosthetic tissue.

Approximately 30% of patients will have diffuse stenosis involving the ascending aorta, sometimes with extension into the transverse arch.[92] The diffuse form of supravalvular aortic stenosis has been shown to be an independent risk factor for death and reoperation.[93] When the lesion is limited to the ascending aorta, patch enlargement is usually possible using cardiopulmonary bypass. When the stenosis involves the transverse arch, deep hypothermic circulatory arrest is used to extend the patch across the entire transverse arch. Patients with lesions in the origins of the brachiocephalic vessels may require patch augmentation of these vessels as well.[94,95]

Supravalvular aortic stenosis can also involve the coronary ostia, possibly in the form of restricted coronary inflow secondary to leaflet fusion along the narrowed and exaggerated sinotubular ridge, or less commonly because of the encroachment on the ostial lumen by the disease. Although relief of the supravalvular stenosis treats the former, true ostial involvement may require specific attention. Modest encroachment on the coronary ostium by sinus tissue may be amenable to simple débridement, whereas severe cases may require patching of the ostium or bypass grafting.[96-98]

Surgical Results

There has been a gradual evolution from the single patch to the double patch, and ultimately to the three-sinus repair for the relief of discrete supravalvular aortic stenosis. In a review of 75 patients with supravalvular aortic stenosis, Stamm and colleagues[93] reviewed the effects of surgical technique on long-term outcomes. Comparison of the single versus multiple sinus augmentations (inverted bifurcated aortoplasty, $n = 35$; three sinus technique, $n = 6$) showed that patients undergoing single sinus augmentation had significantly higher mean gradients (20 vs. 10 mm Hg; $P = 0.008$) at a mean late follow-up of 12.8 years. Similar results have been reported by others.[34] Analysis has shown that single sinus augmentation is an independent risk factor for death and reoperation. These findings were independent from the year of operation (Fig. 123-14). The authors concluded that multiple sinus augmentation was superior to single sinus augmentation. It seems reasonable to expect that augmentation of all three sinuses, using techniques developed by Brom, Myers, and others may provide additional long-term advantages by allowing a more complete restoration of aortic root geometry.[90,91]

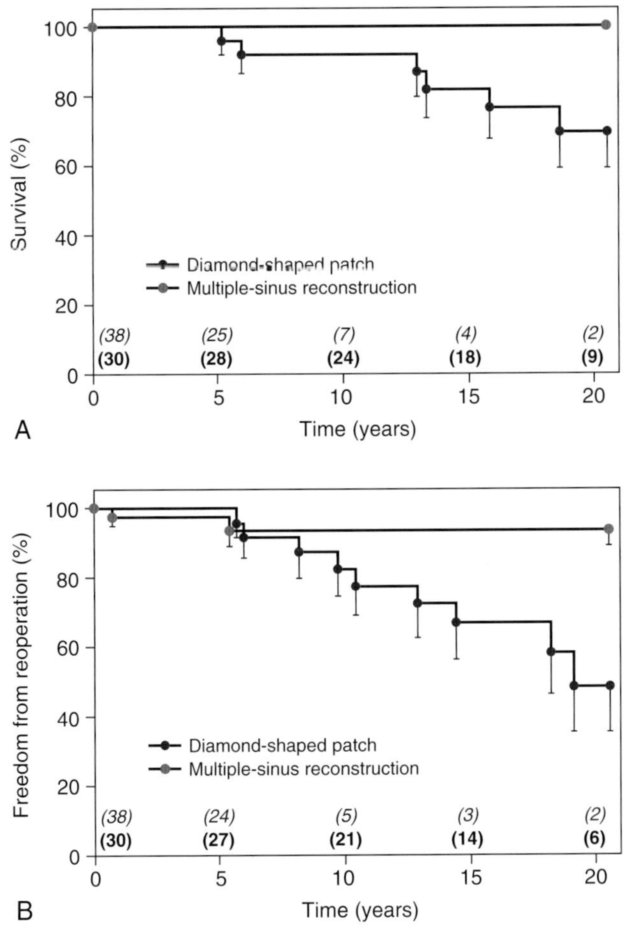

FIGURE 123-14 ■ **A,** Comparison of long-term survival in patients with single or multiple reconstructions. **B,** Freedom from reoperation percentage by type of operation and length of time to first reoperation.

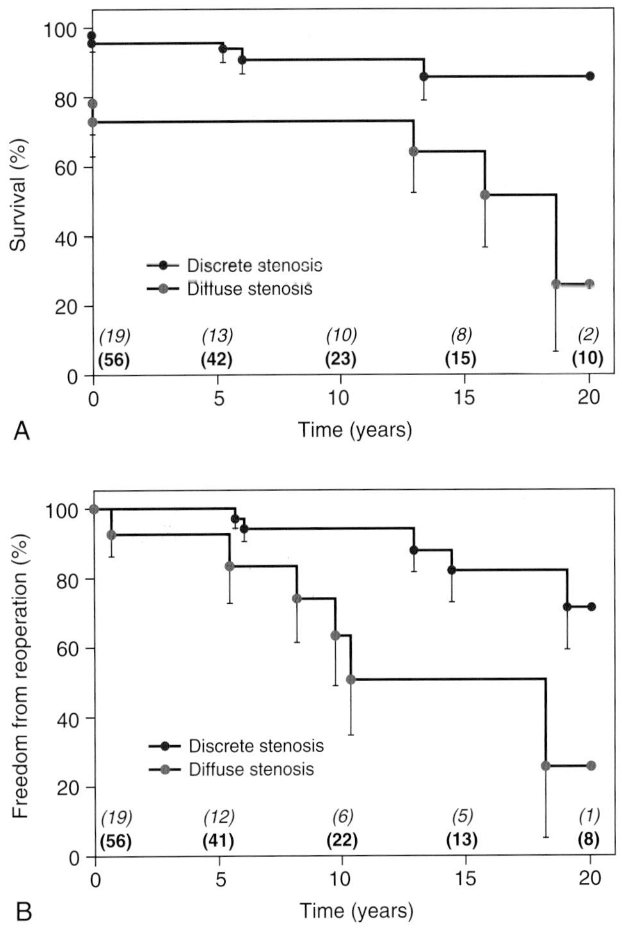

FIGURE 123-15 ■ **A,** Survival rate comparison of discrete and diffuse stenosis, in years. **B,** Freedom from reoperation of discrete and diffuse stenosis, in years.

The prognosis of diffuse supravalvular aortic stenosis appears to be worse than for the discreet variant, and it has been identified as an independent risk factor for reoperation and death (Fig. 123-15).

AORTIC REGURGITATION

Isolated congenital aortic regurgitation (AR) is a rare primary lesion, and it is usually secondary to another underlying congenital lesion.[99] Most commonly, AR is the consequence of efforts designed to relieve congenital aortic stenosis.[100]

Primary Congenital Aortic Valve Regurgitation

Primary congenital AR is rare, but it most commonly occurs in patients with a congenitally bicuspid aortic valve.[101] In this scenario, the anterior or right coronary leaflet is often deficient or incompletely fused to one of the adjacent leaflets. Over time, the progressive AR leads to increased thickening of the leaflet edges. Another rare but important association with primary AR is a quadricuspid aortic or truncal valve.[102] Myers and colleagues[103] have reported on 36 patients who underwent valve repair for significant truncal valve regurgitation. A quadricuspid valve had worse freedom from reoperation and tricuspidization tended to improve freedom from reoperation. Neonatal repair and leaflet thinning were independent predictors of reoperation.[103]

Aortic Regurgitation Associated with a Ventral Septal Defect

Aortic regurgitation can be associated with perimembranous or subarterial VSDs. It is less common that a perimembranous VSD has associated aortic regurgitation, because the defect is generally under the commissure between the right and noncoronary leaflets. In the case of subpulmonic VSD, right coronary leaflet prolapse is more common because it is not supported with a commissure.

In the setting of a perimembranous or subarterial VSD, associated aortic valve prolapse is an indication for surgery. Eroglu and colleagues[104] reported that 38% of these patients with prolapse developed aortic insufficiency within 1 year. Once present, the progression of aortic insufficiency was relatively rapid, with 31% of patients progressing from mild to moderate insufficiency

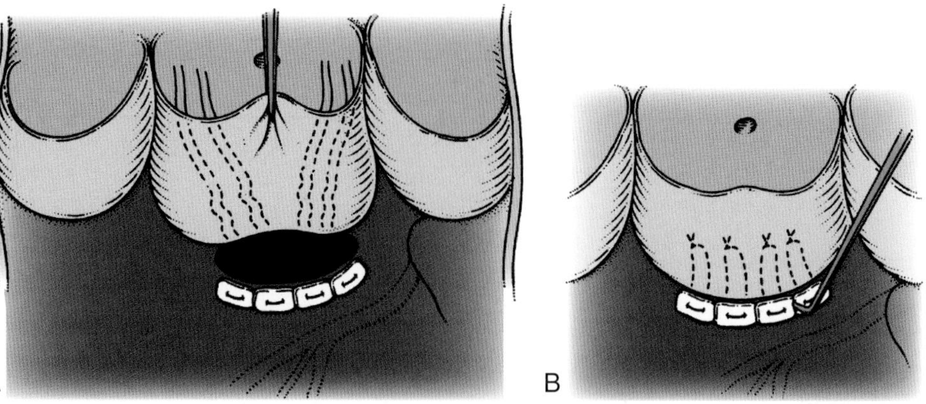

FIGURE 123-16 ■ Repair of the aortic valve including plication of the aortic sinus.

within 1.1 years. VSD closure in the setting of severe aortic insufficiency is less successful than with mild or moderate aortic insufficiency. Freedom from reoperation was 64% versus 77% at 10 years ($P < 0.05$).[105] Thus, repair of perimembranous or subarterial VSDs presenting with aortic valve prolapse is justified, even in the setting of hemodynamically small defects.

Simple VSD closure in the face of severe prolapse and aortic insufficiency may be inadequate. In these instances, repair of the aortic valve, including plication of the aortic sinus, may be effective (Fig. 123-16). Yacoub and colleagues[106] reported their results in 46 such patients, with an average follow-up of 8.4 years. Under these circumstances, VSD closure with aortic sinus plication is effective and durable.

Aortic Regurgitation following Balloon Dilation for Aortic Stenosis

Aortic regurgitation is most commonly associated with catheter-based balloon dilation in patients with congenital aortic stenosis. The most common lesion is tearing of the anterior leaflet at the anterior commissure (or raphe) in a patient with a bicuspid aortic valve. Bacha and colleagues[107] reported the Boston Children's Hospital experience in which 20 of 21 patients had right coronary cusp involvement.

Efforts to relieve aortic stenosis early in life come at the expense of introducing AR. These patients may present acutely with severe AR or years later with ventricular dysfunction in the setting of mixed aortic valve pathology. Determining the appropriate timing for operation in these often-asymptomatic patients can be difficult, and it should be noted that there might be different guidelines depending on the surgical approach. For example, expertise in aortic valve repair may persuade one toward earlier surgical intervention at a younger age.

Cheung and colleagues[108] have addressed the timing of operation for AR in children. They studied a group of 21 asymptomatic young patients (median age, 13 years) with AR undergoing the Ross operation. Eighteen of these patients had previously undergone aortic valvotomy (surgical or balloon) for aortic stenosis. In their experience, the z-score of the preoperative left ventricular end-diastolic dimension was the most sensitive predictor of postoperative left ventricular performance. Postoperative left ventricular performance was significantly impaired in patients with a preoperative z-score of 4 or greater, and the authors recommended AVR in asymptomatic patients when the left ventricular end-diastolic z-score exceeded 3.[108] Accepted guidelines for aortic valve intervention in the adolescent and young adult include the appearance of symptoms, asymptomatic left ventricular systolic dysfunction, or asymptomatic progressive left ventricular enlargement with z-scores greater than 4.[109]

Aortic Regurgitation Associated with a Dilated Aortic Root

Aortic root dilation can be seen in connective tissue disorders such as Marfan and Ehlers-Danlos syndromes, conotruncal abnormalities including tetralogy of Fallot and pulmonary atresia, and in patients having undergone a Damus-Kaye-Stansel procedure with a neoaortic valve. The regurgitation in these patients often begins central as the commissural posts at the sinotubular junction dilate with resultant leaflet stretching and prolapse.

Marfan syndrome is a systemic collagen vascular disorder that can affect the aortic valve early in life. Van Karnebeck and colleagues reported the natural history of Marfan syndrome in 52 pediatric patients (25 male) with a mean age at presentation of 7.9 years (range, 1-16 years) with median follow-up of 7.7 years (range, 2-15 years).[110] Sixty-three percent represented familial cases, and 33% were sporadic. Aortic dilation was present in 80% of patients, and aortic regurgitation developed in 13 (25%); 10 of 13 (77%) patients required aortic operation. The authors concluded that childhood and adolescence are crucial periods in the development of the cardiovascular manifestations associated with Marfan syndrome. When the syndrome is diagnosed in the newborn period, cardiac mortality is high (33% 1-year mortality) and is reported to result from multivalve disease.[111,112]

With the potential for aortic dissection in older patients with Marfan syndrome, attempts have been made to identify patients that would benefit from preemptive surgery. Leggett and others reported that an aortic ratio (normalized for age and body surface area) of 1.3 or greater, or a rate of progression exceeding 5% per year, indicates patients at increased risk for aortic root complications.[113] Cameron and colleagues[114] have suggested that indications for aortic root replacement in children with Marfan syndrome include aneurysm diameter measuring 5 cm or greater, aneurysm diameter increasing more than 1 cm/yr, and progressive aortic valve insufficiency.[114] Indications for surgery in young children (<12 years) include a "giant" aneurysm that meets adult criteria for intervention, and rapid interval enlargement with progressive valvar insufficiency.[115] Using these criteria, this group reported their experience with valve-sparing aortic root replacement in 51 patients (34 with Marfan syndrome) with aortic root aneurysm and competent aortic valves. There were no deaths, and valve function remained stable during follow-up.[116]

Myers and colleagues[117] recently reported the Boston Children's Hospital experience of a combined valve-sparing and valve reconstruction approach over a 12-year period. Thirty-four patients were included with seven having documented connective tissue disorders, with a mean age of 15.4 ± 8.7 years. The surgery consisted of reimplantation technique in 13 patients and remodeling in 21 patients. Valve repair consisted of leaflet procedures in 25 patients and subannular reduction in 15 patients. During a mean follow-up of 14.4 ± 2.8 months, there were five reoperations for AVR because of aortic regurgitation, and two patients exhibited moderate regurgitation. Freedom from structural valve deterioration (SVD) was 75.9% ± 9.4% at 6 months, 70.1% ± 10.3% at 1 year, and remained stable thereafter, although it was significantly worse in the reimplantation group ($P = 0.028$). A more severe degree of aortic regurgitation ($P = 0.001$) and smaller graft–to–aortic annulus ratio ($P = 0.003$) were the only predictors of SVD.

AORTIC VALVE RECONSTRUCTIVE TECHNIQUES

Aortic valve reconstruction is particularly attractive for children with limited valve replacement options. The effectiveness of reconstructive techniques for aortic insufficiency has been variable, and it is related to the etiology of the underlying aortic valve disease. In some specific instances, such as in association with a VSD, repair can be successful and durable as noted previously. However, there are other situations in which there is complex aortic valve disease, and results have been variable.

Aortic Valve Leaflet Prolapse

There have been several techniques described for aortic valve leaflet prolapse. In addition to the original leaflet resuspension techniques described by Trussler,[117a] Cosgrove and colleagues[118] described a central triangular shaped wedge resection of the prolapsed leaflet, and Boodhwani and colleagues[119] recently reported on plication of the free edge of the prolapsing leaflet.

When there is associated leaflet prolapse with a VSD, the Yacoub technique is often used. The defect can be approached through an aortotomy, and then interrupted nonabsorbable sutures are supported with pledgets and inserted through the rightward crest of the septum, through the annulus of the aortic valve, through the redundant portion of right coronary sinus of Valsalva to achieve plication, and then through the media of the aorta.[106]

Aortic Valve Leaflet Extensions

When aortic insufficiency results from lack of central leaflet coaptation, reparative techniques often use some variant of leaflet extension. Fixed pericardium, either bovine or autologous, has been used to extend the diseased leaflets, thereby increasing the area of coaptation. Myers and colleagues[103] compared untreated autologous, glutaraldehyde-treated bovine and PhotoFix-bovine pericardium in 78 children with rheumatic aortic valve disease. During a median follow-up of 10.7 years, 15 patients required reoperation, and fresh autologous and PhotoFix pericardium trended toward better durability than glutaraldehyde-fixed bovine pericardium did.[103]

The results of aortic valve repair using leaflet extensions has been used increasingly and reported by a number of centers with acceptable early results in patients with primary congenital aortic valve disease and rheumatic disease. Polimenakos and colleagues[120] recently reported a large experience with 142 pediatric patients with primary congenital aortic valve disease undergoing pericardial aortic cusp extension valvuloplasty with a median follow-up of 14.4 years. Sixty-four patients underwent aortic valve reintervention and freedom from reoperative aortic cusp extension valvuloplasty or AVR at 18 years was 82.1% ± 4.2% and 60% ± 7.2%, respectively. A review by Bacha and colleagues[107] reported on 81 pediatric patients undergoing surgical aortic valvuloplasty, including 65 undergoing aortic leaflet augmentation with pericardium. While freedom from aortic valve reintervention was only 63% at 5 years, this technique can be valuable when valve replacement options are considered unsuitable.

Others have reported results in patients primarily with rheumatic aortic valve disease. Duran and Gometza[121] reported their experience with leaflet extension in 72 patients. Over a limited follow-up (≤5 years) there were two late deaths (2.8%) and four (5.5%) reoperations between 4 and 38 months postoperatively. Similar results have been reported by Grinda and colleagues.[122] Among 89 patients (mean age, 16 years) undergoing leaflet extension, the 5-year survival and freedom from reoperation was 96% and 92%, respectively.

AORTIC VALVE REPLACEMENT

Aortic valve substitutes include biologic, bioprosthetic, and mechanical valves. The available options for biologic valve replacement include xenografts, homografts, and autografts. The choice of valve substitute in the pediatric population must balance several competing factors including durability, size, growth potential, and the need for anticoagulation.

Aortic Valve Replacement with Bioprosthetic Aortic Valves

Bioprosthetic valves have been used for several decades in adult patients. Experience has been accumulating in pediatric patients, but currently there are limited reports. There are several contributing factors that are clearly important to the limited longevity of bioprosthetic valves in younger patients, including patient–prosthesis mismatch (PPM) and the propensity to calcify. Flameng and colleagues[123] reported that PPM predicts structural valve degeneration in bioprosthetic heart valves. Additional confounding valve related factors were also found to be important, such as valve design (stented or stentless), tissue type (porcine aortic valve or bovine pericardium), and anticalcification treatments to mitigate calcification. In a large follow-up study including 648 adult patients, the absence of antimineralization treatment and PPM were independent predictors of SVD. Freedom from SVD at 10 years was significantly worse in patients receiving a nontreated (70% ± 4.3%) versus treated (90% ± 3.6%) valve ($P < 0.0001$), and in patients with PPM and nontreated valves (59.8% ± 7.0%) versus those with PPM and treated valves (88.7 ± 3.6%; $P < 0.0001$).[124] Based on this series and others, longer-term outcomes on bioprosthetic heart valves in children are needed.

Aortic Valve Replacement: Comparing Mechanical and Biologic Valves

The surgeon is faced with several options for AVR in the pediatric patient. Each option presents a unique profile of advantages, disadvantages, and performance characteristics that will be reviewed.

A major decision point in valve selection for pediatric AVR is between mechanical versus biologic (xenograft, homograft, and autograft). The early mortality of mechanical AVR is 0% to 13%, and the late mortality is 0% to 11%. The incidence of reoperation on these valves is 6% to 16%.[125-127] Patients receiving xenografts appear to have a lower mortality (early and late mortality, 0%), but a higher risk of reoperation, as approximately 50% will require repeat AVR within 6 years. In general, homografts and autografts have superior resistance to postoperative endocarditis compared with mechanical valves. Mechanical valves demonstrated a higher risk of prosthesis endocarditis in the early postoperative period that declines within 1 year, approximating the low level hazard of biologic valves.[128] The risk of endocarditis in the autograft and homograft appear comparable, and they are preferred over other prostheses in the setting of active endocarditis.

Because of their tendency to degenerate, xenograft valves have generally been avoided among pediatric patients. Turrentine and colleagues[129] compared the results of mechanical versus biological valves (autograft, homograft, and xenograft) in the aortic position. They reported a lower incidence of valve-related complications in the autograft group as compared with all other valve options. The homograft and xenograft performed particularly poorly in terms of freedom from reoperation, with 70% (7/10) xenografts and 50% (1/2) homografts requiring replacement for deterioration within 9 years (Fig. 123-17). While efforts to develop xenografts suitable for the pediatric population continues, follow-up remains short.[130] Thus, in the absence of compelling indications for their use, homografts and xenografts in the aortic position in children should probably be avoided.

Comparisons between the autograft (Ross operation) and mechanical AVR have also been reported. Following the Ross operation, Elkins has reported an 89% freedom from reoperation or death at 6 years, as compared with only 49% among children receiving a mechanical AVR.[131] However, these populations were from different time periods, with the mechanical AVR being performed before 1986. A more contemporary study reported by Alexiou and colleagues[132] reported results more consistent with those obtained with the Ross operation. They performed mechanical AVR on 56 children between 1972

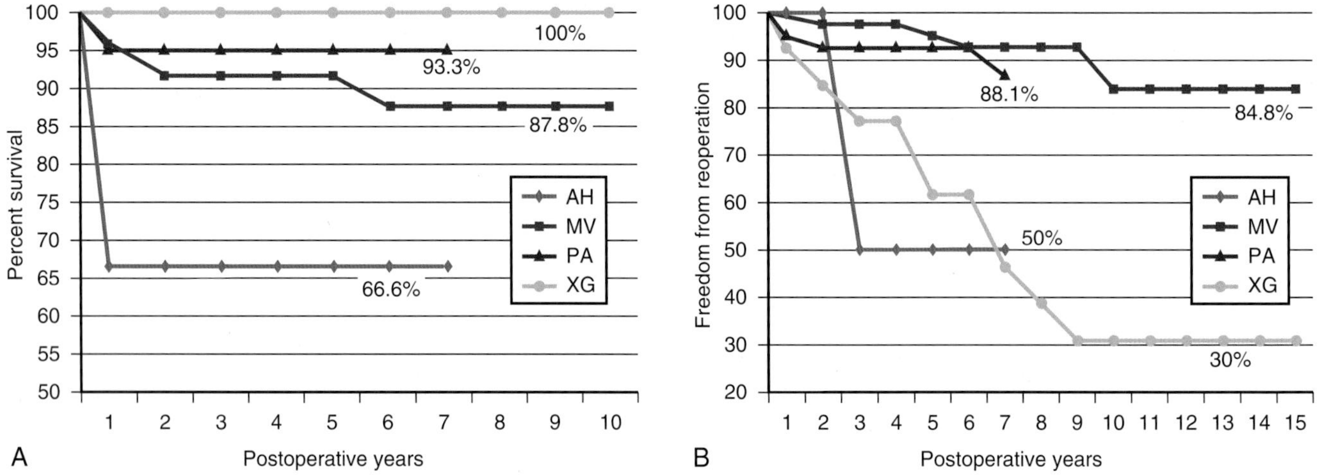

FIGURE 123-17 ■ Survival **(A)** and freedom from reoperation **(B)** rates comparing mechanical and biological valve replacements in postoperative years. *AH,* Aortic homograft; *MV,* mechanical valves; *PA,* pulmonary autograft; *XG,* xenograft tissue valves.

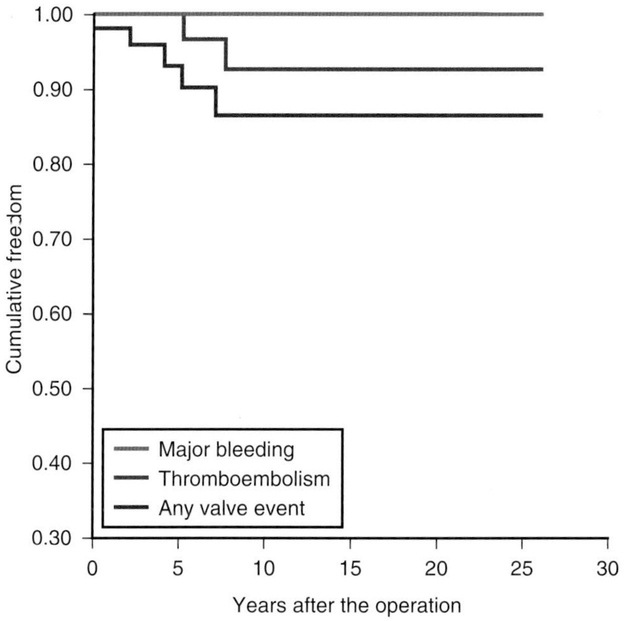

FIGURE 123-18 Freedom from late events in mechanical aortic valve replacements.

and 1999. Freedom from late events, including thrombosis, hemorrhage, and reoperation, was approximately 90% at 6 years (Fig. 123-18). This group presented excellent results with pediatric AVR, but it should be noted that the majority of these patients were older than 10 years, and 50% underwent aortic root enlargement at the time of valve insertion. There were two major (valve thrombosis, stroke) and four minor (nose bleeds) complications related to anticoagulation. Interestingly, a recent review of 45 pediatric patients receiving bileaflet mechanical aortic valves reported a 6% incidence of repeat valve replacement at 10 years, similar to that reported in many Ross operation series.[133]

The indications for valve replacement can also affect outcomes. Lubiszewska and colleagues[134] found mechanical valves in the aortic position to be satisfactory substitutes, especially for aortic insufficiency. These children often have a normal or enlarged aortic annulus, and adult sized valves are readily accepted.

In a review of 51 patients undergoing AVR (25 mechanical, 19 autografts, 6 homografts), Lupinetti and colleagues[135] reported a significantly higher incidence of late complications in those receiving a mechanical valve. The most common long-term complication reported in this group was the development of subaortic stenosis because of pannus ingrowth. Others have also reported significant numbers of anticoagulation related complications. Cabalka and colleagues[136] reported six serious complications among 36 patients undergoing isolated AVR between 1982 and 1994, with all occurring in the setting of supratherapeutic prothrombin times. Freedom from anticoagulation-related bleeding for isolated AVR was approximately 80% at 4 years.

We recently reviewed our experience at Boston Children's Hospital from 2004 to 2013, during which time 38 patients underwent AVR with the On-X prosthetic valve (On-X Life Technologies, Inc., Austin, TX). During a median follow-up of 4.3 years, there was no evidence of structural valve failure or deterioration, no patients had greater than mild prosthetic valve regurgitation, and one patient had moderate stenosis. No patients had evidence of valve thrombosis, embolism, or other bleeding complications. Survival was 98% ± 1.9% at 1 year and 91.3% ± 5% at 5 and 8 years, and it was significantly better in patients with isolated AVR ($P < 0.001$).

Aortic Valve Replacement: Comparing Autografts and Homografts

Homografts share some of the advantages provided by the autograft, but they also present serious disadvantages. Besides a lack of growth potential, early degeneration requiring replacement has been documented, especially among young patients, and some authors have reported inferior hemodynamics as compared with autograft.[137,138] This has led some investigators to compare outcomes of the Ross procedure with its most comparable alternative, the homograft.

In the earliest and largest series comparing the autograft to homografts in young patients, Gerosa and colleagues[139] compared the results of 103 young patients receiving a homograft in the aortic position to 43 receiving an autograft. The 15-year freedom from reoperation was 54% ± 8% versus 68% ± 11%, freedom from endocarditis was 97% ± 2% versus 75% ± 10%, and freedom from any complication was 41% ± 7% versus 50% ± 10%. Primary tissue failure was identified in 19 homografts, but in none of the autografts.

Aklog and colleagues[140] examined the performance of these two options in a prospective randomized trial. A total of 182 patients were randomized, with a mean age of 37 years (range, 2-64 years). Ninety-seven patients received a pulmonary autograft, and 85 patients received a homograft. Thirty-day mortality was 1% for autografts and 4% for homografts, and actuarial survival was 97.8% and 95.3% at 48 months, respectively. There were no autograft-related reoperations. Freedom from reoperation was slightly higher in the autograft group (94.2% vs. 87.7%; $P = \text{NS}$). Regarding the pediatric age group, they reported that 2 of 6 (33%) children required reoperation on the homograft, compared with 0 of 10 in the autograft group. Furthermore, there was echocardiographic evidence of progressive, subclinical deterioration in the homograft group that was absent in the autograft group. The authors concluded that the autograft appeared to be superior in the pediatric population, and they suggested that longer follow-up will reveal a continued durability advantage.

Lupinetti and colleagues[141] examined the comparative effects of autografts and homografts on left ventricular remodeling in the pediatric population. While the authors reported that initial LVOT gradients and left ventricular wall thickness (surrogates for hemodynamic efficiency) were comparable among 78 children undergoing the Ross operation and 25 receiving a homograft, a divergence was noted over time. Whereas peak LVOT velocities decreased over time after the Ross operation, they increased significantly over a similar time period in the homograft group. The decrease in left ventricular wall thickness seen in those undergoing the Ross operation was absent in the homograft group. This effect may be most important in young patients in whom significant somatic growth can be expected.

Thus, while the homograft may provide acceptable palliation among older patients, its lack of durability appears to be a serious disadvantage, especially among younger children. Under these circumstances, its use should probably be relegated to an option for children deemed unsuitable for the autograft or a mechanical valve.

Aortic Valve Replacement with the Pulmonary Autograft (Ross Operation)

The transplantation of the pulmonary valve to the aortic position, introduced by Donald Ross in 1967, has several potential advantages over other valve replacement options in pediatric patients.[142] Most notably among children, the growth potential of the autograft is a unique feature, especially in the infant population in which small caliber homografts are the only alternative. In addition, superior hemodynamics are obtainable, and there is no need for systemic anticoagulation.

The autograft may be inserted into the aortic position using a variety of techniques, including the subcoronary technique, the root inclusion technique, or the root replacement technique. Excellent reviews of each technique are available.[143,144] The autograft root replacement is usually performed with bicaval cannulation. The aortic valve is inspected and if irreparable, the pulmonary artery is opened at the bifurcation. The pulmonary valve is inspected, and valves with important anatomic abnormalities (bicuspid valve, significant leaflet fenestrations) are not suitable for use in the aortic position, and an alternative valve replacement is chosen. Small leaflet fenestrations, particularly near the valve commissures, are probably acceptable.

The autograft is excised with a rim of infundibular muscle. Posteriorly, care must be taken to avoid the first septal perforator, because significant ventricular dysfunction may accompany its injury. After débridement of the aortic annulus, the autograft is oriented anatomically and sutured into the aortic position. The coronary arteries are inserted into the appropriate sinus, and the distal anastomosis between the autograft and the ascending aorta is performed. The RVOT is reconstructed with the aid of a cryopreserved homograft. Although some groups have advocated direct approximation of the pulmonary arteries to the right ventricle (similar to the REV technique), oversized homografts provide excellent durability and are probably a superior option.[145] Disadvantages of the Ross operation include increased technical complexity, homograft reconstruction of the RVOT, and potential autograft failure.

Elkins has reported his midterm and late results with the Ross operation between 1986 and 2001.[146] Operative mortality was 4.5%, with a 12-year actuarial survival of 92% ± 3%. Actuarial freedom from autograft replacement and from RV homograft replacement was 93% ± 3% and 90% ± 4% at 12 years, respectively. Most contemporary series place the operative mortality between 0% and 4%.[147-150] Because of the low mortality and effectiveness of the Ross operation, it has become the procedure of choice at some institutions.

In a recent large series reported by Pessotto and colleagues,[148] 67 children underwent the Ross operation. Two neonates (2/67, 3%) undergoing a Ross-Konno procedure after a failed attempt at balloon dilation for critical aortic stenosis died of multisystem organ failure. Two patients (2/67, 3%) have required reoperation for progressive autograft insufficiency; in one patient, annular reduction was successful in salvaging the autograft.

The question of durability is a concern that continues to be examined. The longest follow-up to date has been reported by Chambers and Ross,[151] who described the experience of the 131 hospital survivors undergoing the Ross operation between 1967 and 1984. Of the survivors, they reported that the freedom from autograft replacement was 88% at 10 years and 75% at 20 years. Interestingly, this was similar to freedom from reoperation on the RVOT (89% and 80%). Of the 30 autografts explanted, only three showed histologic signs of focal degenerative changes. All others showed evidence of transmural cellular viability.

In a recent pediatric series, conflicting information has been emerging. While Brown and colleagues[152] have reported a low incidence of autograft failure requiring replacement at 10 years (4%), others have reported autograft failure rates as high as 31% at 13 years.[153] While the long-term fate and patient selection criteria remain an area of investigation, the Ross operation remains an important option for the pediatric patient with severe aortic valve disease.

Contraindications to the Pulmonary Autograft (Ross Operation)

The Ross operation requires careful patient selection. Systemic collagen vascular disorders and anatomic abnormalities of the pulmonary valve constitute a clear contraindication to the Ross operation. Others have also suggested that the Ross operation should be avoided in the setting of systemic inflammatory conditions, such as rheumatoid arthritis, lupus, and rheumatic heart disease.[154-156] There have been mixed results in patients with bicuspid aortic valve disease.

Al-Halees and colleagues[157] reviewed their results with 78 patients undergoing the Ross operation in the Middle East. Eighty percent of these patients suffered from rheumatic disease of the aortic valve, and 28% had significant mitral regurgitation. Five (8%) of these patients have required reoperation between 20 and 26 months postoperatively—four for autograft failure and one for recurrent mitral regurgitation. One autograft demonstrated histologic evidence of valvulitis consistent with rheumatic disease. Choudhary and colleagues[158] performed the Ross operation in 75 patients suffering from rheumatic aortic valve disease. Two patients required reoperation for autograft failure, and 13 showed evidence of moderate or severe autograft insufficiency, with leaflet thickening, generally between 12 and 24 months after operation. Autograft function was significantly inferior in rheumatic patients.

Bicuspid aortic valve disease is considered to be contraindication for the Ross procedure by some; however, the data remain controversial. Examining the pulmonary trunk in patients with bicuspid aortic valve disease, de Sa and colleagues[159] reported histologic evidence of cystic medial necrosis, elastic fragmentation, and smooth muscle cell abnormalities. They suggested that these findings manifest themselves as subsequent autograft dilation; however, conflicting results have also been reported. Luciani and colleagues[160] have reported no histopathology of the pulmonary trunk in the setting of bicuspid aortic valve disease, and they noted no greater tendency for autografts in this setting to dilate. Likewise, in a large pediatric experience, Elkins and colleagues[161,162] reported that preoperative aortic regurgitation, but not valve morphology, was associated with autograft degeneration.

PROSTHETIC MECHANICAL VALVES, ANTICOAGULATION, AND PREGNANCY

Prosthetic valves, systemic anticoagulation, and pregnancy are important issues for young women with aortic valve disease. Edmunds reported that women with mechanical valves were at risk for thrombotic complications if anticoagulation were interrupted.[163] However, it has been suggested that up to 30% of fetuses exposed to warfarin between the sixth and ninth weeks of gestation will develop warfarin embryopathy (nasal hypoplasia, stippled epiphyses).[164] Warfarin exposure during the second trimester has been implicated in central nervous system abnormalities in approximately 3% of fetuses.[165] In 1994, major European centers were queried about the clinical approach to anticoagulation, prosthetic valves, and pregnancy.[166] There were 214 pregnancies in 182 women, 151 pregnancies in 133 women with mechanical valves, and 63 pregnancies in 45 women with bioprosthetic valves. Including abortions (spontaneous and therapeutic), 83% of pregnancies among women with bioprosthetic valves, and 73% of pregnancies among women with mechanical prosthesis, resulted in healthy children, consistent with other reports.[167]

Anticoagulation was administered in 150 of the 151 pregnancies among 133 women with mechanical valves. Thirty-four women received subcutaneous heparin throughout the pregnancy, 50 received warfarin for the duration of gestation, and 66 received subcutaneous heparin for the first trimester and warfarin thereafter. Warfarin was discontinued, and subcutaneous heparin was restarted 2 to 4 weeks before the estimated date of confinement. No cases of warfarin embryopathies were reported. There were 13 mechanical valve thromboses; 12 of these were in the mitral position, and 10 were taking heparin ($P < 0.05$). The single woman suffering aortic valve thrombosis refused all anticoagulation and died from valve thrombosis. Of the seven major bleeding complications, five occurred in women taking heparin and two were in women taking warfarin ($P < 0.05$). The incidence of spontaneous abortions did not differ between the two groups (10% and 12%). Among the 45 women with bioprosthetic valves, pregnancy tended to accelerate deterioration of these valves. Thirty-one percent of these women required replacement during pregnancy or shortly thereafter.

More recent series reporting on large numbers of pregnancies in women receiving warfarin for prosthetic valves suggest that the risk of warfarin embryopathy may be overstated, and the incidence of spontaneous abortion, thromboembolic episodes, or bleeding have been shown to be similar to those among women treated with heparin during the first trimester.[168,169] However, warfarin dosages, but not the international normalized ratio [INR], were found to influence fetal outcomes.[170]

In conclusion, these authors suggested that mechanical valves were preferable in women of childbearing potential and that oral warfarin therapy for the duration (except the last 2 weeks) was appropriate.

Potential discrepancies between these two bodies of data may be related to techniques used for monitoring warfarin anticoagulation. In the early 1990s, the United States adopted the INR (patient's prothrombin time divided by the control time using the thromboplastin standard of the World Health Organization). Before the adoption of INR, the use of thromboplastins of low responsiveness may have contributed to over-anticoagulation, equivalent to INRs of up to 9 in some preparations.[171,172] Warfarin embryopathy is thought to be a dose-related phenomenon, and may have been exacerbated by these discrepancies.

Finally, the Ross operation has been proposed as an excellent option for young women anticipating future motherhood. In a retrospective review of pregnancy in 8 women following the Ross operation, there were 14 uncomplicated pregnancies and no deterioration in autograft function during or after the pregnancies.[173]

SUMMARY

Congenital aortic valve disease is a progressive, lifelong condition that can be palliated, but not cured. The surgical management of congenital disease of the aortic valve and root remains challenging. In general, there has been a movement away from indirect surgical therapies (e.g., apical-aortic conduits) toward more direct surgical procedures designed to address the pathology directly (e.g., valve repair, Konno-Rastan, modified Konno, Ross operation). Despite the development of techniques designed to relieve stenosis at all levels, the ultimate success of palliation will often depend on the suitability of associated left heart structures.

Areas such as patient selection (particularly in the neonatal population), evolving aortic valve repair techniques, and the long-term results of procedures such as the Ross operation remain areas of investigation. The development of catheter-based interventions designed to treat specific forms of aortic root and valve pathology will continue. Lifelong surveillance is mandatory to provide long-lasting preservation of left ventricular function.

REFERENCES

1. Becker AE: Surgical and pathological anatomy of the aortic valve and root. *Oper Tech Thorac Cardiovasc Surg* 1:3–14, 1996.

2. Leyh RG, Schmidtke C, Sievers HH, et al: Opening and closing characteristics of the aortic valve after different types of valve-preserving surgery. *Circulation* 100:2153–2160, 1999.
3. Grande-Allen KJ, Cochran RP, Reinhall PG, et al: Re-creation of sinuses is important for sparing the aortic valve: a finite element study. *J Thorac Cardiovasc Surg* 119:753–763, 2000.
4. Thubrikar M, Nolan SP, Bosher LP: The cyclic changes and structure of the base of the aortic valve. *Am Heart J* 99:217–224, 1980.
5. Kitchiner DJ, Jackson M, Walsh K, et al: Incidence and prognosis of congenital aortic valve stenosis in Liverpool (1960–1990). *Br Heart J* 69:71–79, 1993.
6. Walsh EP, Berul CI, Triedman JK: Cardiac arrhythmias. In Fyler DC, editor: *Nadas' pediatric cardiology*, Philadelphia, 1992, Hanley & Belfus, Inc., pp 494–495.
7. Requarth JA, Goldberg SJ, Vasko SD, et al: In vitro verification of Doppler prediction of transvalve pressure gradient and orifice area in stenosis. *Am J Cardiol* 53:1369–1373, 1984.
8. Soriano BD, Hoch M, Ithuralde A, et al: Matrix-array 3-dimensional echocardiographic assessment of volumes, mass, and ejection fraction in young pediatric patients with a functional single ventricle: a comparison study with cardiac magnetic resonance. *Circulation* 117:1842–1848, 2008.
9. Hossack KF, Neutze JM, Lowe JB, et al: Congenital aortic valvar stenosis. Natural history and assessment for operation. *Br Heart J* 43:561–573, 1980.
10. Scholler GF, Colan SD, Sanders SP, et al: Noninvasive estimation of the left ventricular pressure waveform throughout ejection in young patients with aortic stenosis. *J Am Coll Cardiol* 12:492–497, 1998.
11. Barker PC, Ensing G, Ludomirsky A, et al: Comparison of simultaneous invasive and noninvasive measurements of pressure gradients in congenital aortic stenosis. *J Am Soc Echocardiogr* 15:1496–1502, 2002.
12. Mills P, Leech G, Davies M, et al: The natural history of a non-stenotic bicuspid aortic valve. *Br Heart J* 40:951, 1978.
13. Gaynor JW, Bull C, Sullivan UID, et al: Late outcome of survivors of intervention for neonatal aortic valve stenosis. *Ann Thorac Surg* 60:122–125, 1995.
14. Lofland GK, McCrindle BW, Williams WG, et al: Critical aortic stenosis in the neonate: a multi-institutional study of management, outcomes and risk factors. *J Thorac Cardiovasc Surg* 121:10–27, 2001.
15. McCrindle BW, Blackstone EH, Williams WG, et al: Are outcomes of surgical versus transcatheter balloon valvotomy equivalent in neonatal critical aortic stenosis. *Circulation* 104:I–152, 2001.
16. McElhinney DB, Lock JE, Keane JF, et al: Left heart growth, function, and reintervention after balloon aortic valvuloplasty for neonatal aortic stenosis. *Circulation* 111:451–458, 2005.
17. Hawkins JA, Minich LL, Shaddy RE, et al: Aortic valve repair and replacement after balloon aortic valvuloplasty in children. *Ann Thorac Surg* 61:1355–1358, 1996.
18. Moore P, Egito E, Mowrey H, et al: Midterm results of balloon dilatation of congenital aortic stenosis: predictors of success. *J Am Coll Cardiol* 27:1257–1263, 1996.
19. Bhabra MS, Dhillon R, Bhudia S, et al: Surgical aortic valvotomy in infancy: impact of leaflet morphology on long-term outcomes. *Ann Thorac Surg* 76:1412–1416, 2003.
20. McCrindle BW: Independent predictors of immediate results of percutaneous balloon aortic valvotomy in children. Valvuloplasty and angioplasty on congenital anomalies (VACA) registry investigators. *Am J Cardiol* 77:286–293, 1996.
21. Echigo S: Balloon valvuloplasty for congenital heart disease: immediate and long-term results of multi-institutional study. *Ped Int* 43:542–547, 2001.
22. Chartrand CC, Saro-Servando E, Vobecky JS: Long-term results of surgical valvuloplasty for congenital valvar aortic stenosis in children. *Ann Thorac Surg* 68:1356–1359, 1999.
23. Newfield EA, Muster AJ, Paul MH, et al: Discrete subvalvar aortic stenosis in childhood. *Am J Cardiol* 38:53–61, 1976.
24. Choi JY, Sullivan ID: Fixed subaortic stenosis; anatomical spectrum and nature of progression. *Br Heart J* 65:280–286, 1991.
25. Orie JD, Beerman LB, Ettedgui JA, et al: Discrete subaortic stenosis in children: natural and unnatural history[abstract]. *J Am Coll Cardiol* 23:119A, 1994.
26. Cape EG, Vanauker MD, Sigfusson G, et al: Potential role of shear stress in the etiology of pediatric heart disease: septal shear stress in subaortic stenosis. *J Am Coll Cardiol* 30:247–254, 1997.
27. Brauner R, Laks H, Drinkwater DC, et al: Benefits of early surgical repair in fixed subaortic stenosis. *J Am Coll Cardiol* 30:1835–1842, 1997.
28. Stellin G, Mazzucco A, Bartolotti U, et al: Late results after resection of discrete and tunnel subaortic stenosis. *Eur J Cardiothorac Surg* 3:325–340, 1989.
29. Rizzoli G, Tiso E, Mazzucco A, et al: Discrete subaortic stenosis; operative age and gradient as predictors of late aortic valve incompetence. *J Thorac Cardiovasc Surg* 106:95–104, 1993.
30. DeVries AG, Hess J, Witsengurg M, et al: Management of fixed subaortic stenosis: a retrospective study of 57 cases. *J Am Coll Cardiol* 19:1013–1017, 1992.
31. Rohlicek CV, Font del Pino S, Hosking M, et al: Natural history and surgical outcomes for isolated discrete subaortic stenosis in children. *Heart* 82:708–713, 1999.
32. Parry AJ, Kovalchin JP, Suda K, et al: Resection of subaortic stenosis; can a more aggressive approach be justified? *Eur J Cardiothorac Surg* 15:631–638, 1999.
33. Yacoub M, Onuzo O, Riedel B, et al: Mobilization of the left and right fibrous trigones for relief of severe left ventricular outflow obstruction. *J Thorac Cardiovasc Surg* 117:126–133, 1999.
34. Brown JW, Ruzmetov M, Palaniswamy V, et al: Surgery for aortic stenosis in children: a 40-year experience. *Ann Thorac Surg* 76:1398–1411, 2003.
35. Frommelt MA, Snider R, Bove EL, et al: Echocardiographic assessment of subvalvular aortic stenosis before and after operation. *J Am Coll Cardiol* 19:1018–1023, 1992.
36. Hazenkamp MG, Hardjowijono FM, Quagebeur JM, et al: Surgery for membranous subaortic stenosis: long-term follow-up. *Eur J Casrdiothorac Surg* 7:356–359, 1993.
37. Jaumin P, Rubay J, Lintermans J, et al: Surgical treatment of subvalvular aortic stenosis: long-term results. *J Cardiovasc Surg* 31:31–35, 1990.
38. Geva A, McMahon CJ, Gauvreau K, et al: Risk factors for reoperation after repair of discrete subaortic stenosis in children. *J Am Coll Cardiol* 50:1498–1504, 2007.
39. Lupinetti FM, Pridjian AK, Callow MB, et al: Optimum treatment of discrete subaortic stenosis. *Ann Thorac Surg* 54:467–471, 1992.
40. Coleman DM, Smallhorn JF, McCrindle BW, et al: Postoperative follow-up of fibromuscular subaortic stenosis. *J Am Coll Cardiol* 24:1558–1564, 1992.
41. Moskowitz WB, Schieken RM: Balloon dilation of discrete subaortic stenosis associated with other cardiac defects in children. *J Invasive Cardiol* 11:116–120, 1999.
42. Saurez de Loze J, Pan M, Sancho M, et al: Percutaneous transluminal balloon dilatation. For discrete subaortic stenosis. *Am J Cardiol* 58:619–621, 1986.
43. Saurez de Lezo J, Pan M, Medina A, et al: Immediate and follow-up results of transluminal balloon dilatation for discrete subaortic stenosis. *J Am Coll Cardiol* 18:1309–1315, 1991.
44. Feigl A, Feigl D, Lucas RV, Jr, et al: Involvement of the aortic valve cusps in discrete subaortic stenosis. *Pediatr Cardio* 5:185–190, 1984.
45. Jahangiri M, Nicholson IA, del Nido PJ, et al: Surgical management of complex and tunnel-like subaortic stenosis. *Eur J Cardiothorac Surg* 17:637–642, 2000.
46. Roughneen PT, DeLeon SY, Cetta F, et al: Modified Konno-Rastan procedure for subaortic stenosis: indications operative techniques and results. *Ann Thor Surg* 65:1368–1375, 1998.
47. Caldarone CA: Left ventricular outflow tract obstruction: the role of the modified Konno procedure. *Semin Thorac Cardiovasc Surg Pediatr Card Surg Annul* 6:98–107, 2003.
48. Jonas RA: Modified Konno procedure for tunnel subaortic stenosis. *Oper Tech Thorac Cardiovasc Surg* 7:176–180, 2003.
49. Caldarone CA, Van Natta TL, Frazer JR, et al: The modified Konno procedure for complex left ventricular outflow tract obstruction. *Ann Thorac Surg* 75:147–151, 2003.
50. Konno S, Imai Y, Iida Y, et al: A new method for prosthetic valve replacement in congenital aortic stenosis associated with hypoplasia of the aortic valve ring. *J Thorac Cardiovasc Surg* 70:909–917, 1975.

51. Rastan H, Koncz J: Aortoventriculoplasty: a new technique for the treatment of left ventricular outflow tract obstruction. *J Thorac Cardiovasc Surg* 71:920–927, 1976.
52. Erez E, Kanter KR, Tam VK, et al: Konno aortoventriculoplasty in children and adolescents: from prosthetic valves to the Ross operation. *Ann Thorac Surg* 74:122–126, 2002.
53. Frommelt PC, Lupinetti FM, Bove EL: Aortoventriculoplasty in infants and children. *Circulation* 86(Suppl II):176–180, 1992.
54. Ross DB, Trusler GA, Coles JG, et al: Small aortic root in childhood: surgical options. *Ann Thorac Surg* 58:1617–1624, 1994.
55. Cobanoglu A, Thyagarajan GK, Dobbs J: Konno-aortoventriculoplasty with a mechanical prosthesis in dealing with small aortic root: a good surgical option. *Eur J Cardiothorac Surg* 12:766–770, 1997.
56. Sakamoto T, Matsumura G, Kosaka Y, et al: Long-term results of Konno procedure for complex left ventricular outflow tract obstruction. *Eur J Cardiothoracic Surg* 34:37–41, 2008.
57. Ohye RG, Gomez CA, Ohye BJ, et al: The Ross/Konno procedure in neonates and infants: intermediate—term survival and autograft function. *Ann Thorac Surg* 72:823–830, 2001.
58. Brown JW, Ruzmetov M, Vijay P, et al: The Ross-Konno procedure in children: outcomes, autograft and allograft function, and reoperations. *Ann Thorac Surg* 82:1301–1306, 2006.
59. Oka N, Al-Radi O, Alghamdi AA: Ross-Konno procedure with mitral valve surgery. *Annal Thorac Surg* 89:1366–1370, 2010.
60. Brown JW, Ruzmetov M, Palaniswamy V, et al: Long-term results of apical aortic conduits in children with complex left ventricular outflow tract obstruction. *Ann Thorac Surg* 80:2301–2308, 2005.
61. Nugent AW, Daubeney PE, Chondros P, et al: Clinical features and outcomes of childhood hypertrophic cardiomyopathy: results from a national population-based study. *Circulation* 112:1332–1338, 2005.
62. Rosing DR, Kent KN, Borer JS, et al: Verapamil therapy: a new approach to the pharmacologic treatment of hypertrophic cardiomyopathy I. Hemodynamic effects. *Circulation* 60:1201–1207, 1979.
63. Stenson RE, Flamm MD, Jr, Harrison DC, et al: Hypertrophic subaortic stenosis. Clinical and henmodynamic effects of long-term propranololtherapy. *Am J Cardiol* 31:763–773, 1973.
64. Sherrid M, Delia E, Dwyer E: Oral disopyramide therapy for obstructive hypertrophic cardiomyopathy. *Am J Cardiol* 62:1085–1088, 1988.
65. Maron BJ, Nishimura RA, McKenna WJ, et al: Assessment of permanent dual-chamber pacing as a treatment for drug-refractory symptomatic patients with obstructive hypertrophic cardiomyopathy. A randomized, double blind, cross-overstudy n(M-PATHY). *Circulation* 99:2927–2933, 1999.
66. Morrow AG, Reitz BA, Epstein SE, et al: Operative treatment in hypertrophic subaortic stenosis. Techniques and the results of pre and postoperative assessments in 83 patients. *Circulation* 52:88–102, 1975.
67. McKenna W, Deabfield J, Faruqui A, et al: Prognosis in hypertrophic cardiomyopathy: role of age and clinical, echocardiographic and hemodynamic features. *Am J Cardiol* 47:532–538, 1981.
68. Maron BJ, McKenna WJ, Danielson GK, et al: American College of Cardiology/European Society of Cardiology clinical expert consensus document on hypertrophic cardiomyopathy. A report of the American College of Cardiology Foundation Task Force on Clinical Expert Consensus Documents and the European Society of Cardiology Committee for Practice Guidelines. *J Am Coll Cardiol* 42:1687–1713, 2003.
69. Mohr R, Schaff HV, Danielson GK, et al: The outcome of surgical treatment of hypertrophic obstructive cardiomyopathy. Experience over 15 years. *J Thorac Cardiovasc Surg* 97:666–674, 1989.
70. Morrow AG, Koch JP, Maron BJ, et al: Left ventricular myotomy and myomectomy in patients with obstructive hypertrophic cardiomyopathy and previous cardiac arrest. *Am J Cardiol* 46:313, 1980.
71. Kuhn H, Gietzen F, Leuner C, et al: Induction of subaortic septal ischemia to reduce obstruction in hypertrophic obstructive cardiomyopathy. Studies to develop a new catheter-based concept of treatment. *Eur Heart J* 18:846–851, 1997.
72. Chojnowska L, Ruzyllo W, Witkowski A, et al: Early and long-term results of non-surgical septal reduction in patients with hypertrophic cardiomyopathy. *Kardiol Pol* 59:269–282, 2003.
73. Faber L, Seggewiss H, Gleichman U: Percutaneous transluminal septal myocardial ablation in hypertrophic obstructive cardiomyopathy: results with respect to intraprocedural myocardial contrast echocardiography. *Circulation* 98:2415–2421, 1998.
74. Maron BJ, McKenna WJ, Danielson GK, et al: American College of Cardiology/European Society of Cardiology Clinical Expert Consensus Document on Hypertrophic Cardiomyopathy. *J Am Coll Cardiol* 42:1687–1713, 2003.
75. Yetman AT, McCrindle BW, MacDonald C, et al: Myocardial bridging in children with hypertrophic cardiomyopathy—a risk factor for sudden death. *N Engl J Med* 339:1201–1209, 1998.
76. Williams WG, Konstantinov IE: Subaortic Myectomy for Patients with HOCM. *Operative Techniques in Thor and CV Surgery* 9:254–260, 2004.
77. Dearani JA, Danielson GK: Septal myectomy for obstructive hypertrophic cardiomyopathy. *Semin Thorac Cardiovasc Surg Pediatr Card Surg Annu* 86–91, 2005.
78. Ommen SR, Maron BJ, Olivotto I, et al: Long-term effects of surgical septal myectomy on survival in patients with obstructive hypertrophic cardiomyopathy. *J Am Coll Cardiol* 46:470–476, 2005.
79. Swistel DG, deRose JJ, Sherrid MV: Management of patients with complex hypertrophic cardiomyopathy: resection/plication/release. *Oper Tech Thorac Cardiovasc Surg* 10:261–267, 2010.
80. Altarabsheh SE, Dearani JA, Burkhart HM, et al: Outcome of septal myectomy for obstructive hypertrophic cardiomyopathy in children and young adults. *Ann Thorac Surg* 95:663–669, 2013.
81. Mencarelli L: Stenosis sopravalvolare aortica and ancello. *Arch Ital Anat Istol Patol* 1:829, 1930.
82. Williams JCP, Barrat-Boyes BG, Lowe JB: Supravalvular aortic stenosis. *Circulation* 24:1311–1318, 1961.
83. Beuren AJ, Schulze C, Eberle P, et al: The syndrome of supravalvular aortic stenosis, peripheral pulmonary stenosis, mental retardation and facial appearance. *Am J Cardiol* 13:471–483, 1964.
84. Bourassa MG, Campeau L: Combined supravalvular aortic and pulmonic stenosis. *Circulation* 28:572–581, 1963.
85. Ewart AK, Morris CA, Ensing CA, et al: A human vascular disorder, supravalvular aortic stenosis, maps to chromosome 7. *Proc Natl Acad Sci USA* 90:3226–3230, 1993.
86. Walsh EP, Berul CI, Triedman JK: Cardiac arrhythmias. In Fyler DC, editor: *Nadas' pediatric cardiology*, Philadelphia, 1992, Hanley & Belfus, Inc., p 506.
87. Sun CC, Jacot J, Brenner JI: Sudden death in supravalvular aortic stenosis: fusion of coronary leaflet to the sinus ridge, dysplasia and stenosis of aortic and pulmonary leaflets. *Pediatr Pathol* 12:751–759, 1992.
88. McGoon DC, Mankin HT, Vlad P, et al: The surgical treatment of supravalvular aortic stenosis. *J Thorac Cardiovasc Surg* 41:125–133, 1961.
89. Doty DB, Polansky DB, Jenson CB: Supravalvular aortic stenosis. Repair by extended aortoplasty. *J Thorac Cardiovasc Surg* 74:362–371, 1977.
90. Brom AG. In Khonsari S, editor: *Cardiac surgery; safeguards and pitfalls in operative technique*. Rockville, MD, 1988, Aspen, pp 276–280.
91. Myers JL, Waldhausen JA, Cyran SE, et al: Results of surgical repair of congenital supravalvular aortic stenosis. *J Thorac Cardiovasc Surg* 105:281–288, 1993.
92. Wessel A, Pankau R, Kececioglu D, et al: Three decades of follow-up of aortic and pulmonary vascular lesions in the Williams-Beuren syndrome. *Am J Med Genet* 52:297–301, 1994.
93. Stamm C, Kreutzer C, Zurakowski D, et al: Forty-one years of surgical experience with congenital supravalvular aortic stenosis. *Thorac Cardiovasc Surg* 118:874–885, 1999.
94. Petre R, Arbenz U, Vogt PR, et al: Application of successive principles to correct supravalvular aortic stenosis. *Ann Thorac Surg* 67:1167–1169, 1999.
95. van Son JAM, Danielson GK, Puga FJ, et al: Supravalvular aortic stenosis; long-term results of surgical treatment. *J Cardiovasc Thorac Surg* 107:103–115, 1994.
96. Martin MM, Lemmer JH, Shaffer E, et al: Obstruction to the left coronary artery blood flow secondary to obliteration of the coronary ostium in supravalvular aortic stenosis. *Ann Thorac Surg* 45:16–20, 1988.
97. Matsuda H, Miyamoto Y, Takahashi T, et al: Extended aortic and left main coronary angioplasty with a single pericardial patch in a

patient with Williams syndrome. *Ann Thorac Surg* 52:1331–1333, 1991.

98. Shin H, Katogi T, Yozu R, et al: Surgical angioplasty of left main coronary stenosis complicating supravalvular aortic stenosis. *Ann Thorac Surg* 67:1147–1148, 1999.
99. Olson J, Subramanian R, Edwards D: Surgical pathology of pure aortic insufficiency: a study of 225 cases. *Mayo Clin Proc* 59:835–841, 1984.
100. Donofrio MT, Engle MA, O'Loughlin JE, et al: Congenital aortic regurgitation: natural history and management. *J Am Coll Cardiol* 20:366–372, 1992.
101. Roberts WC, Morrow AG, McIntosh CL, et al: Congenitally bicuspid aortic valve causing severe, pure aortic regurgitation without superimposed infective endocarditis. Analysis of 13 patients requiring aortic valve replacement. *Am J Cardiol* 47:206–209, 1981.
102. Iglesias A, Oliver J, Muñoz JE, et al: Quadricuspid aortic valve associated with fibromuscular subaortic stenosis and aortic regurgitation treated by conservative surgery. *Chest* 80:327–328, 1981.
103. Myers PO, Bautista-Hernandez V, del Nido PJ, et al: Surgical repair of truncal valve regurgitation. *Eur J Cardiothorac Surg* 44:813–820, 2013.
104. Eroglu AG, Oztunc F, Saltik L, et al: Aortic valve prolapse and aortic regurgitation in patients with ventricular septal defect. *Pediatr Cardio* 24:36–39, 2003.
105. Hisatomi K, Isomura T, Sato T, et al: Long-term results after conservative aortic valve repair for aortic regurgitation with ventricular septal defect. *J Cardiovasc Surg* 36:541–544, 1995.
106. Yacoub MH, Khan H, Stavri G, et al: Anatomic correction of the sinus of prolapsing right coronary aortic cusp, dilatation of the sinus of Valsalva, and ventricular septal defect. *J Thorac Cardiovas Surg* 113:253–261, 1997.
107. Bacha EA, McElhinney DB, Guleserian KJ, et al: Surgical aortic valvuloplasty in children and adolescents with aortic regurgitation: acute and intermediate effects on aortic valve function and left ventricular dimensions. *J Thorac Cardiovasc Surg* 135:552–559, 2008.
108. Cheung MMH, Sullivan ID, de Leval MR, et al: Optimal timing of the Ross procedure in the management of chronic aortic incompetence in the young. *Cardiol Young* 13:253–257, 2003.
109. Bonow RO, Carabello B, de Leon AC, Jr, et al: Guidelines for the management of patients with valvular heart disease; executive summary. A report of the American College of Cardiology/American Heart Association Task Force on Practice Guidelines (Committee on Management of Patients with Valvular Heart Disease). *Circulation* 98:1949–1984, 1998.
110. Van Karnebeck CDM, Naeff MSJ, Mulder BJM, et al: Natural history of cardiovascular manifestations in Marfan syndrome. *Arch Dis Child* 84:129–137, 2001.
111. Abdel-Massih T, Goldenberg A, Vouhe P, et al: Marfan syndrome in the newborn and infants less than 4 months: a series on 9 patients. *Arch Mal Coeur Vaiss* 95:469–472, 2002.
112. Tsang VT, Pawade A, Karl TR, et al: Surgical management of Marfan syndrome in children. *J Card Surg* 9:50–54, 1994.
113. Legget ME, Unger TA, O'Sullivan CK, et al: Aortic root complications in Marfan's syndrome: identification of a lower risk group. *Heart* 75:389–395, 1996.
114. Cameron DE, Vricella LA: Valve-sparing aortic root replacement in Marfan Syndrome. *Semin Thorac Cardiovasc Surg Pediatr Card Surg Ann* 8:103–111, 2005.
115. Gillinov AM, Zehr KJ, Redmond JM, et al: Cardiac operations in children with Marfan's syndrome. *Ann Thorac Surg* 64:1140–1145, 1997.
116. Patel ND, Williams JA, Barreiro CJ, et al: Valve-sparing aortic root replacement; Early experience with the De Paulis Valsalva graft in 51 patients. *Ann Thorac Surg* 82:548–553, 2006.
117. Myers PO, Tissot C, Christenson JT, et al: Aortic valve repair by cusp extension for rheumatic aortic insufficiency in children: long-term results and impact of extension material. *J Thorac Cardiovasc Surg* 140:836–844, 2010.

117a. Trusler GA, Moes CA, Kidd BS: Repair of ventricular septal defect with aortic insufficiency. *J Thorac Cardiovasc Surg* 66:394–403, 1973.

118. Cosgrove DM, Rosenkranz ER, Hendren WG, et al: Valvuloplasty for aortic insufficiency. *J Thorac Cardiovasc Surg* 102:571–576, 1991.
119. Boodhwani M, de Kerchove L, Glineur D, et al: A simple method for the quantification and correction of aortic cusp prolapse by means of free margin plication. *J Thorac Cardiovasc Surg* 139:1075–1077, 2010.
120. Polimenakos AC, Sathanandam S, Elzein C, et al: Aortic cusp extension valvuloplasty with or without tricuspidization in children and adolescents: long-term results and freedom from aortic valve replacement. *J Thorac Cardiovasc Surg* 139:933–941, 2009.
121. Duran CMG, Gometza B: Aortic valve reconstruction in the young. *J Card Surg* 9(Suppl 2):204–208, 1994.
122. Grinda JM, Latremouille C, Berrebi AJ, et al: Aortic cusp extension for rheumatic aortic valve disease: midterm results. *Ann Thorac Surg* 74:438–443, 2002.
123. Flameng W, Herregods MC, Vercalsteren M, et al: Prosthesis-patient mismatch predicts structural valve degeneration in bioprosthetic heart valves. *Circulation* 121:2123–2129, 2010.
124. Flameng W, Rega F, Vercalsteren M, et al: Antimineralization treatment and patient-prosthesis mismatch are major determinants of the onset and incidence of structural valve degeneration in bioprosthetic heart valves. *J Thorac Cardiovasc Surg* 147:1219–1224, 2014.
125. Mazzitelli DF, Guenther T, Schreiber C, et al: Aortic valve replacement in children: are we on the right track? *Eur J Cardiothorac Surg* 13:565–571, 1998.
126. Champsaur G, Robin J, Tronc F, et al: Mechanical valve in aortic position is a valid option in children and adolescents. *Eur J Cardiothorac Surg* 11:117–122, 1997.
127. Lupinetti FM, Warner J, Jones TK, et al: Comparison of human tissues and mechanical prostheses for aortic valve replacement in children. *Circulation* 96:321–325, 1997.
128. Kirklin JW, Barratt-Boyes BG: Aortic valve disease. In Kirklin JW, Barratt-Boyes BG, editors: *Cardiac surgery* (vol 1), ed 2, New York, 1993, Churchill Livingston, p 546.
129. Turrentine MW, Ruzmetov M, Vijay P, et al: Biological versus mechanical aortic valve replacement in children. *Ann Thorac Surg* 71:356–360, 2001.
130. Berrebi AC, Carpentier SM, Phan P, et al: Results of up to 9 years of high-temperature-fixed valvular bioprosthesis in a young population. *Ann Thorac Surg* 71:S353–S355, 2001.
131. Elkins RC: Congenital aortic valve disease: evolving management. *Ann Thorac Surg* 59:269–274, 1995.
132. Alexiou C, McDonald A, Langley SM, et al: Aortic valve replacement in children: are mechanical prosthesis a good option? *Eur J Cardiothorac Surg* 17:125–133, 2000.
133. Masuda M, Kado H, Ando Y, et al: Intermediate-term results after the aortic valve replacement using bileaflet mechanical prosthetic valve replacement in children. *Eur J Cardiothorac Surg* 34:42–47, 2008.
134. Lubiszewska B, Rozanski J, Szufladowicz M, et al: Mechanical valve replacement in congenital heart disease in children. *J Heart Valve Dis* 8:74–77, 1999.
135. Lupinetti FM, Marner J, Jones TK, et al: Comparison of human and mechanical prostheses for aortic valve replacement in children. *Circulation* 96:321–325, 1997.
136. Cabalka AK, Emery RW, Petersen RJ, et al: Long-term follow-up of the St. Jude medical prosthesis in pediatric patients. *Ann Thorac Surg* 60:S618–S623, 1995.
137. Clarke DR, Campbell DN, Hayward AR, et al: Degeneration of aortic valve allografts in young recipients. *J Thorac Cardiovasc Surg* 103:934–941, 1992.
138. Ng SK, O'Brien MF, Harrocks S, et al: Influence of patient age and implantation technique on the probability of re-replacement of the homograft aortic valve. *J Heart Valve Dis* 11:217–223, 2002.
139. Gerosa G, McKay R, Davies J, et al: Comparison of the aortic homograft and the pulmonary autograft for aortic valve or root replacement in children. *J Thorac Cardiovasc Surg* 102:51–61, 1991.
140. Aklog L, Carr-White GS, Birks EJ, et al: Pulmonary autograft versus aortic homograft for aortic valve replacement: interim results from a prospective randomized trial. *J Heart Valve Dis* 9:176–189, 2000.
141. Lupinetti FM, Duncan BW, Lewin M, et al: Comparison of autograft and allograft aortic valve replacement in children. *J Thorac Cardiovasc Surg* 126:240–246, 2003.
142. Ross DN: Replacement of the aortic and mitral valves with a pulmonary autograft. *Lancet* 11:956–958, 1967.

143. Spray TL: Technique of pulmonary autograft aortic valve replacement in children (the Ross procedure). *Semin Thorac Cardiovasc Surg Pediatr Card Surg Annu* 165–178, 1998.
144. Elkins RC: The Ross operation: applications to children. *Semin Thorac Cardiovasc Surg* 8:345–349, 1995.
145. Couetil JP, Berrebi A, Ferdinand FD, et al: New approach for reconstruction of the pulmonary outflow tract during the Ross procedure. *Circulation* 98(19 Suppl):II368–II371, 1998.
146. Elkins RC, Lane MM, McCue C: Ross operation in children: late results. *J Heart Valve Dis* 10:736–741, 2001.
147. Hokken RB, Cromme-Dijkhuis AH, Bogers AJ, et al: Clinical outcome and left ventricular function after pulmonary autograft implantation in children. *Ann Thorac Surg* 63:1713–1717, 1997.
148. Pessotto R, Wells WJ, Baker CJ, et al: Midterm results of the Ross procedure. *Ann Thorac Surg* 71:S336–S339, 2001.
149. Pigula FA, Paolillo J, McGrath M, et al: Aortopulmonary size discrepancy is not a contraindication to the pediatric Ross operation. *Ann Thorac Surg* 72:1610–1614, 2001.
150. Khwaja S, Nigro JJ, Starnes VA: The Ross operation is an ideal aortic valve replacement operation for the teen patient. *Semin Thorac Cardiovasc Surg Pediatr Card Surg Annu* 173–175, 2005.
151. Chambers JC, Somerville J, Stone S, et al: Pulmonary autograft procedure for aortic valve disease: long-term results of the pioneer series. *Circulation* 96:2206–2214, 1997.
152. Brown JW, Ruzmetov M, Fukui T, et al: Fate of the autograft and homograft following Ross aortic valve replacement: reoperative frequency. Outcome and management. *J Heart Valve Dis* 15:253–259, 2006.
153. Klieverik LM, Takkenberg JJ, Bekkers JA, et al: The Ross operation: a Trojan horse? *Eur Heart J* 28:1993–2000, 2007.
154. van Suylen RJ, Schoof PH, Bos E, et al: Pulmonary autograft failure after aortic root replacement in a patient with juvenile rheumatoid arthritis. *Eur J Cardiothorac Surg* 6:571–572, 1992.
155. de Vries H, Bogers AJ, Schoof PH, et al: Pulmonary autograft failure caused by a relapse of rheumatic fever. *Ann Thorac Surg* 57:750–751, 1994.
156. Pieters F, Al-Halees Z, Zwann F, et al: Autograft failure after the Ross operation in a rheumatic population: pre- and postoperative echocardiographic observation. *J Heart Valve Dis* 5:404–409, 1996.
157. Al-Halees Z, Kumar N, Gallo R, et al: Pulmonary autograft for aortic valve replacement in rheumatic disease: a caveat. *Ann Thorac Surg* 60:S172–S176, 1995.
158. Choudhary SK, Mathur A, Sharma R, et al: Pulmonary autograft: should it be used in young patients with rheumatic disease? *J Thorac Cardiovasc Surg* 118:483–490, 1999.
159. de Sa M, Moshkovitz Y, Butany J, et al: Histologic abnormalities of the ascending aorta and pulmonary trunk in patients with bicuspid aortic valve disease: clinical relevance to the Ross procedure. *J Thorac Cardiovasc Surg* 118:588–594, 1999.
160. Luciani GB, Barozzi L, Tomezzoli A, et al: Bicuspid aortic valve disease and pulmonary autograft root dilatation after the Ross procedure: a clinicopathologic study. *J Thorac Cardiovasc Surg* 122:74–79, 2001.
161. Elkins RC, Lane MM, McCue C, et al: Ross operation and aneurysm or dilatation of the ascending aorta. *Sem in Thorac Cardiovasc Surg* 11(Suppl I):50–54, 1999.
162. Elkins RC, Lane MM, McCue C: Ross operation in children: late results. *J Heart Valve Dis* 10:736–741, 2001.
163. Edmunds LH, Jr: Thrombotic and bleeding complications of prosthetic heart valves. *Ann Thorac Surg* 44:430–445, 1987.
164. Iturbe-Alessio I, Fonseca M, Mutchinik O, et al: Risks of anticoagulant therapy in pregnant women with artificial heart valves. *N Engl J Med* 315:1390–1393, 1986.
165. Hall JG, Pauli RM, Wilson KM: Maternal and fetal sequelae of anticoagulation during pregnancy. *Am J Med* 68:122–140, 1980.
166. Sbarouni E, Oakley CM: Outcomes of pregnancy in women with valve prostheses. *Br Heart J* 71:196–201, 1994.
167. Larrea JL, Nunez L, Reque JA, et al: Pregnancy and mechanical valve prosthesis: a high-risk situation for the mother and the fetus. *Ann Thorac Surg* 36:459–463, 1983.
168. Geelani MA, Singh S, Verma A, et al: Anticoagulation in patients with mechanical valves during pregnancy. *Asian Cardiovasc Thorac Surg* 13:30–33, 2005.
169. Al-Lawati AA, Venkitramen M, Al-Delaime T, et al: Pregnancy and mechanical heart valves replacement; dilemma of anticoagulation. *Eur J Cardio thorac Surg* 22:223–227, 2002.
170. Khamooshi AJ, Kashfi F, Hoseini S, et al: Anticoagulation for prosthetic heart valves in pregnancy. Is there an answer? *Asian Cardiovasc Thorac Ann* 15:493–496, 2007.
171. Hirsh J, Deykin D, Poller L: Therapeutic range for oral anticoagulant therapy. *Chest* 89(2 Suppl):S11–S15, 1986.
172. Hirsh J: Is the dose of warfarin prescribed by American physicians unnecessarily high? *Arch Int Med* 147:769–771, 1987.
173. Dore A, Somerville J: Pregnancy in patients with pulmonary autograft valve replacement. *Eur Heart J* 18:1659–1661, 1997.

CHAPTER 124

Surgery for Congenital Anomalies of the Coronary Arteries

Julie A. Brothers • J. William Gaynor

CHAPTER OUTLINE

This chapter discusses the management of coronary artery anomalies in patients without other congenital heart defects. Most coronary artery anomalies in number, origin, and distribution are of intellectual interest only. However, a few are clinically significant because they may result in myocardial ischemia, left ventricular dysfunction, and sudden death. Anomalies discussed in this chapter include anomalous origin of a coronary artery from the pulmonary artery, anomalous coronary artery that courses between the aorta and pulmonary artery, coronary artery fistula, and congenital atresia of the left main coronary artery.

In normal coronary anatomy, two coronary arteries arise from separate ostia in the right and left aortic sinuses of Valsalva. The left main coronary artery (LMCA) originates from the left aortic sinus and usually bifurcates into the left anterior descending coronary artery (LAD) and the left circumflex coronary artery. The LAD runs in the anterior interventricular groove, and the left circumflex coronary artery courses in the left atrioventricular groove. The right coronary artery (RCA) originates anteriorly from the right aortic sinus, runs along the right atrioventricular groove, and usually gives rise to the posterior descending artery at its terminus.

In most individuals, each coronary artery ostium is located centrally in the appropriate sinus of Valsalva. In some patients, the ostium may be eccentrically located, and in others a coronary artery may arise close to a valve

BOX 124-1 Origin of Both Coronary Arteries from One Sinus

1. Left main coronary artery originates from right sinus of Valsalva (either from right coronary artery or separate ostia).
   Left main coronary artery courses anterior to pulmonary artery.
   Left main coronary artery courses through interventricular septum.
   Left main coronary artery courses between aorta and pulmonary artery.
   Left main coronary artery courses posterior to aorta.
   In rare cases, the left anterior descending coronary or left circumflex coronary artery alone may originate from the right sinus.
2. Single left main coronary artery arises from the left sinus and bifurcates into the left anterior descending coronary and left circumflex coronary arteries. The left circumflex coronary artery crosses the crux and continues as the right coronary artery.
3. Single right coronary artery from sinus, which crosses crux, continues as left anterior descending coronary and left circumflex coronary artery.
4. Right coronary artery originates from left sinus of Valsalva (either from left main coronary artery or as separate ostium).
   Right coronary artery courses posterior to aorta.
   Right coronary artery courses interior anterior to pulmonary artery.
   Right coronary artery courses between aorta and pulmonary artery.

commissure. One or both coronary ostia may arise from the tubular aorta above the sinotubular junction, which is usually a benign finding. However, this high take-off of the coronary artery becomes significant if an aortotomy is necessary for aortic valve replacement or for another indication; if not recognized, the coronary artery could be transected. Another anomaly is when both coronary arteries arise from the same aortic sinus with either a single ostium or two separate ostia (Box 124-1). This is generally not clinically significant if the aberrant vessel courses posterior to the aorta or anterior to the pulmonary artery, but it becomes important if either the aberrant LMCA or RCA courses between the two great vessels, because this may lead to myocardial ischemia and sudden death.

ANOMALOUS ORIGIN OF A CORONARY ARTERY FROM THE PULMONARY ARTERY

Anomalous origin of a coronary artery from the pulmonary artery is a rare congenital anomaly that is almost always fatal if not diagnosed and treated.[1,2] Although anomalous origin of the LMCA from the pulmonary artery (ALCAPA) is the most common, other coronary arteries may rarely also arise from the pulmonary artery. The RCA arises from the pulmonary artery approximately 10 times less frequently than ALCAPA but is also associated with ischemia and sudden cardiac death. The LAD, the circumflex, or both the left and right coronary arteries may arise from the pulmonary artery; these variants are extremely rare and are almost uniformly fatal.

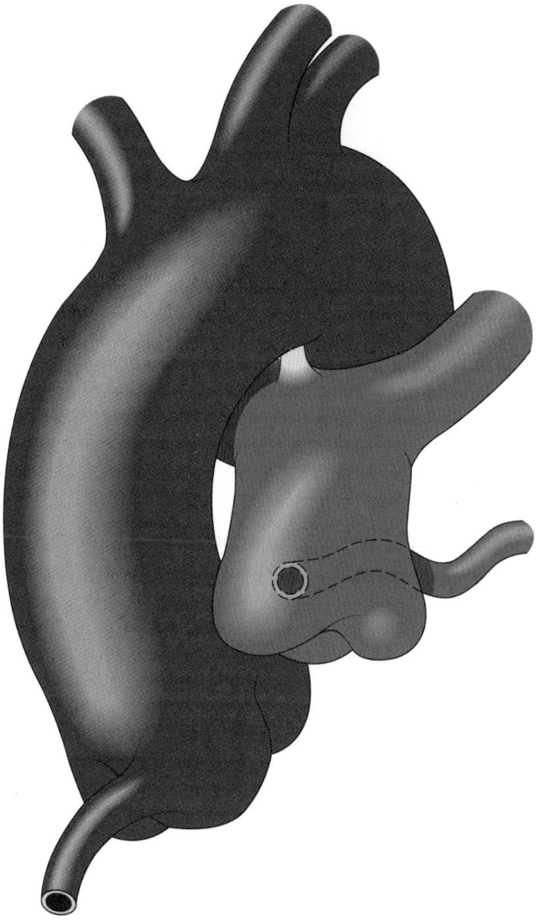

FIGURE 124-1 The aorta and pulmonary artery showing anomalous origin of the left main coronary artery from the posterior-facing sinus of the pulmonary artery with the anomalous artery coursing behind the pulmonary artery. (Reprinted with permission from Gaynor JW: Coronary artery anomalies in children. In Kaiser LR, Kron IL, Spray TL, editors: *Mastery of cardiothoracic surgery*, Philadelphia, 1998, Lippincott-Raven, p 881.)

ALCAPA is the most important congenital coronary artery anomaly in this class. The incidence of ALCAPA ranges from 1 in 30,000 to 1 in 300,000 people. It is the most common cause of myocardial infarction in childhood. If not diagnosed and treated, the mortality rate is 90% by age 1 year. ALCAPA is otherwise known as the Bland-White-Garland syndrome, after Bland and colleagues reported on both clinical and autopsy findings in an infant with this anomaly in 1933.[3]

Anatomy

In ALCAPA, the LMCA usually arises from the main pulmonary artery (MPA); occasionally, it arises from the right pulmonary artery. It usually originates from the rightward aspect of the posterior (facing) sinus of the MPA (Figs. 124-1 and 124-2), but it may also originate from the leftward aspect of the posterior (facing) and, in rare cases, from the anterior (nonfacing) sinus of

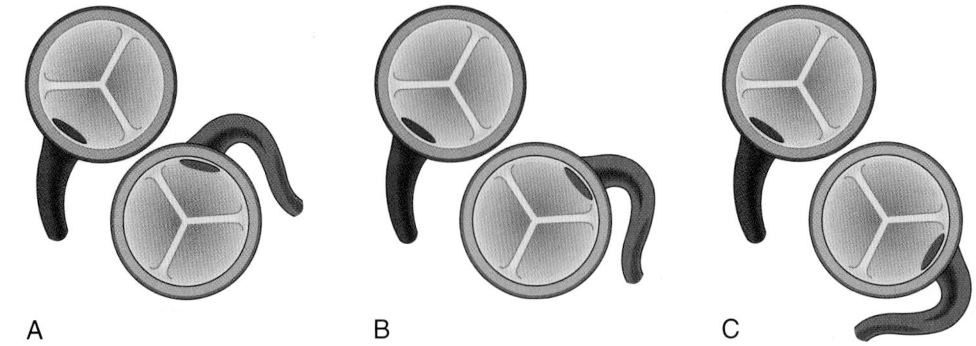

FIGURE 124-2 ■ **A,** Anomalous origin of the left main coronary artery from the rightward aspect of the posterior-facing sinus of the pulmonary artery. **B,** Anomalous origin of the left main coronary artery from the leftward aspect of the posterior-facing sinus. **C,** Anomalous origin of the left main coronary artery from the nonfacing sinus of the pulmonary artery. (Reprinted with permission from Gaynor JW: Coronary artery anomalies in children. In Kaiser LR, Kron IL, Spray TL, editors: *Mastery of cardiothoracic surgery,* Philadelphia, 1998, Lippincott-Raven, p 882.)

the MPA (see Fig. 124-2). An anomalous RCA most commonly originates from the anterior portion of the pulmonary artery.

Although ALCAPA usually occurs in isolation, other associated cardiac defects include patent ductus arteriosus (PDA), ventricular septal defect (VSD), coarctation of the aorta, and tetralogy of Fallot.

Pathophysiology

Children with ALCAPA usually develop symptoms after closure of the ductus arteriosus and the subsequent fall in pulmonary vascular resistance. During fetal life, the systemic and pulmonary circulation pressures are similar, and myocardial perfusion remains intact because the pulmonary arterial pressure is systemic. After birth but before ductal closure, the pulmonary artery pressure remains elevated, thereby maintaining perfusion of the anomalous coronary artery. This explains why children are rarely diagnosed with ALCAPA in the first few days of life. The clinical course after ductal closure is largely determined by the presence or absence of collaterals from the RCA to the left coronary system. If there is inadequate collateral circulation, myocardial ischemia and ventricular dysfunction result from insufficient myocardial perfusion.[4] This occurs because of subsystemic pulmonary artery pressure, and the left ventricle is thus perfused with desaturated blood at a low pressure. However, if the pulmonary artery pressure remains elevated because of the presence of another cardiac defect, such as PDA or VSD, left ventricular perfusion pressure may be adequate to prevent ischemia. If this coronary anomaly is unknown before the catheter or surgical closure of these defects, it will become apparent shortly after closure because of the subsequent drop in pulmonary arterial pressure—usually with a fatal outcome.

Alternatively, if there is adequate collateralization, perfusion of the left coronary system is maintained. As the pulmonary vascular resistance falls, however, a left-to-right shunt develops from the RCA to the pulmonary artery. There is progressive dilation of the RCA and left coronary artery systems, with reversal of flow in the left coronary leading to a pulmonary-coronary steal. Although the shunt is relatively small compared with overall cardiac output, it is significant with regard to coronary blood flow. Children with extensive collaterals may survive past infancy; however, there is usually progressive left ventricular dysfunction.[5] In a small percentage of cases, the collateral vessels are enough to maintain adequate myocardial perfusion at rest and sometimes even during exertion, and these patients may not come to clinical attention until adulthood.[6] In most children, however, severe mitral regurgitation is present secondary to papillary muscle dysfunction and ventricular dilation.

Clinical Presentation

Infants frequently present between 4 and 6 weeks of age after the pulmonary vascular resistance has dropped.[7] However, infants may not be diagnosed until 2 to 3 months of age, when symptoms have increased in severity. Infants usually show signs and symptoms of congestive heart failure, including sweating and discomfort with feeding, tachypnea, poor weight gain, and pallor. The discomfort with feeding most likely represents myocardial ischemia. Children who do not present when they are infants may be diagnosed in later infancy as a result of the loud murmur of mitral regurgitation. Older children, adolescents, and adults may remain asymptomatic, whereas others may come to clinical attention because of exertional chest pain, pre-syncope, or syncope. There have been reports of sudden death with exercise in these older patients. The symptoms associated with anomalous origin of the RCA from the pulmonary artery are less severe, but myocardial ischemia and death can still occur.

Physical examination of the infant with ALCAPA may reveal signs of congestive heart failure, including tachypnea, tachycardia, and hepatomegaly. Left ventricular dysfunction caused by ALCAPA can be difficult to distinguish from a dilated cardiomyopathy. The left heart is usually enlarged, often with associated mitral regurgitation, and a gallop rhythm also may be present. If left heart failure has resulted in pulmonary hypertension, then there may also be evidence of right heart enlargement and an accentuated pulmonary component of the second heart sound on examination.

Infants with ALCAPA generally have an enlarged cardiac silhouette on chest radiograph, resulting mainly from the enlarged left atrium and left ventricle. In infants with congestive heart failure, the electrocardiogram (ECG) can provide a useful diagnostic clue because there are classic findings of Q waves and ST-segment elevation in leads I, aVL, and V4-V6 as a result of lateral or anterolateral wall infarction. Although this pattern can be found in other causes of myocardial infarction or cardiomyopathy, if these electrocardiographic abnormalities are seen in an infant with congestive heart failure, the diagnosis of ALCAPA needs to be strongly considered. Certainly, any infant diagnosed with dilated cardiomyopathy must be extensively evaluated for ALCAPA. This diagnosis should also be considered in older children and adolescents with a dilated cardiomyopathy, because occasional patients survive past infancy.

Diagnostic Imaging

Echocardiography with color flow Doppler usually demonstrates a dilated left ventricle with severe mitral regurgitation. The mitral regurgitation commonly seen with ALCAPA is caused by infarction of the posterior leaflet of the mitral valve and subsequent poor movement of the leaflet; fibrosis and fibroelastosis of the papillary muscle also can be present. Imaging of the coronary arteries, including origin and course, has become possible as a result of improved echocardiographic techniques, but it can still be challenging. An enlarged RCA is almost always present and should raise suspicion of this diagnosis. Careful attention should be paid to the origins of both coronary arteries, including the abnormal origin of the LMCA to the pulmonary artery. If visualization of the anomalous vessel is unclear, color flow Doppler may reveal retrograde flow from the coronary artery to the pulmonary artery. However, underdiagnosis by echocardiography is relatively common; thus, if any question remains about visualization of both coronary ostia, then cardiac catheterization is mandatory to rule out ALCAPA.

Cardiac catheterization with angiography remains the gold standard in the diagnosis of ALCAPA. Cardiac catheterization demonstrates elevated filling and pulmonary arterial pressures and a low cardiac output. In older asymptomatic patients, it may show only mildly elevated pulmonary arterial pressures but normal filling pressures and cardiac output. A small left-to-right shunt may be present. An aortogram will demonstrate a single, dilated RCA arising normally from the aorta. If significant collaterals are present, aortic root angiography will show the collaterals providing late, retrograde filling of the left coronary artery with a blush of contrast subsequently filling the MPA. If there is a large left-to-right shunt from the collaterals, a step-up in oxygen saturation may be noted in the MPA. If doubt remains regarding the diagnosis, a main pulmonary arteriogram with distal balloon occlusion should demonstrate the anomalous left coronary artery.[8]

Magnetic resonance imaging (MRI) has emerged as a useful noninvasive diagnostic tool for delineating congenital coronary anomalies.[9,10] Although there have been case reports of using this method in diagnosing ALCAPA, no case series with this anomaly have been reported. However, studies have shown that magnetic resonance angiography has a similar sensitivity and specificity when compared with coronary angiography and may be especially helpful in delineating the proximal course of anomalous coronary arteries. Computed tomography (CT) has been used extensively for coronary artery delineation in adults. Advantages of this technique include rapid acquisition time and high resolution, but the disadvantages include radiation exposure and the need for a slower heart rate with ECG gating, precluding its use in infants.

Surgical Management

Indications for Surgery

Surgical repair is indicated in all patients with ALCAPA. In infants with congestive heart failure, surgery should occur within the first few days of diagnosis because risk of continuing myocardial ischemia and death is very high.[11] In older patients who present without symptoms, surgery is necessary but can be performed electively. In an infant who presents in severe heart failure secondary to myocardial infarction, surgery will probably need to be delayed for at least 24 hours to stabilize the patient using mechanical ventilation, inotropic support, and vasodilators, when necessary. Del Nido and colleagues reported that even in the sickest infants, a two-vessel surgical repair is possible if left ventricular assist devices (LVADs) are used postoperatively.[12] Others may need extracorporeal membrane oxygenation (ECMO). Because infants requiring surgery are often quite ill, it is important that centers performing ALCAPA surgery have these options available, or else the child should be transferred to a hospital with these capabilities.

The goal of surgery is restoration of a two-coronary system; therefore, simple ligation of the anomalous coronary should not be performed.[13] Severe left ventricular dysfunction and mitral insufficiency are not contraindications to revascularization in infants, because significant recovery of function usually occurs. Because the severity of mitral regurgitation almost always decreases after revascularization, left ventricular aneurysmectomy and mitral valve repair or replacement are rarely indicated at the time of initial procedure, even if severe mitral regurgitation is present.

Surgical Techniques

The first successful operation for correction of ALCAPA was simple ligation of the anomalous artery at the pulmonary artery. Ligating the anomalous vessel prevents the left-to-right shunt, thereby allowing perfusion of the left ventricle through collaterals from the RCA. Because of the early mortality rates and increased risk of late sudden death with this procedure, a variety of techniques have been developed to create a dual coronary artery system, including coronary artery bypass grafting, aortopulmonary window, and direct reimplantation.

Bypass grafts were accomplished using the left subclavian artery, the internal mammary artery (IMA), and the saphenous vein. Meyer and colleagues reported the first successful left subclavian artery–to–left coronary artery bypass in 1968.[14] The results of bypass grafting, especially with saphenous vein grafts, have been disappointing. Takeuchi and associates were the first to describe the creation of an aortopulmonary window and intrapulmonary artery baffle using a pulmonary artery flap to direct blood flow from the aorta to the anomalous coronary artery.[15] Finally, the procedure of choice in many institutions has become direct reimplantation of the anomalous coronary onto the aorta, as experience with the arterial switch operation for transposition of the great vessels has increased.[16,17]

Coronary Artery Bypass Grafting. Coronary artery bypass grafting is rarely used in patients with ALCAPA. In the current era, it is usually used to create a dual coronary artery system after previous ligation or because of stenosis or occlusion after a previous attempt at repair. The IMA is the conduit of choice and can be used successfully, even in neonates and infants; in addition, there is some evidence for growth of the IMA after bypass grafting.[18-20] The saphenous vein should not be used unless it is the only conduit available, because of the risk of occlusion and poor long-term results.[21] Similarly, left subclavian–to–left coronary artery anastomosis is infrequently used because of the risk of anastomotic stenosis or occlusion.[22,23]

Direct Reimplantation. In most patients with ALCAPA, direct reimplantation of the anomalous coronary artery onto the aorta can be performed (Fig. 124-3).[24,25] When the anomalous coronary ostium is in the posterior-facing sinus, the procedure is fairly straightforward. Direct implantation is possible even if the ostium is located in the nonfacing sinus by excising a large button of pulmonary artery to extend the coronary artery.

After induction of anesthesia and placement of monitoring lines, a median sternotomy is performed. The thymus is resected. The pericardium is opened and suspended in stay sutures. Because of the likelihood of myocardial ischemia and left ventricular dysfunction, there is a risk of ventricular fibrillation, so contact with the myocardium should be kept at a minimum until the patient is placed on cardiopulmonary bypass. This operation may be performed using either continuous low-flow bypass with moderate hypothermia (25° to 28° C) or deep hypothermic circulatory arrest (18° C) in very small infants. Before cannulation, an aortic purse-string suture is placed distally near the innominate artery, and another is placed in the right atrial appendage for a single venous cannula. Heparin is administered, the aortic and right atrial cannulas are inserted, and cardiopulmonary bypass is established. The left ventricle should be decompressed by placing a left ventricular vent via the right superior pulmonary vein. The pulmonary artery and epicardial course of the left coronary artery are visualized. If the anomalous left coronary artery originates far leftward in the posterior-facing sinus or on the anterior nonfacing sinus, direct reimplantation may not be possible.

The aorta and both pulmonary arteries are fully mobilized. To improve mobility of the pulmonary artery, the ductus (or ligamentum) arteriosus is ligated. Tourniquets are placed around both the right and the left branch pulmonary arteries to occlude the branch pulmonary

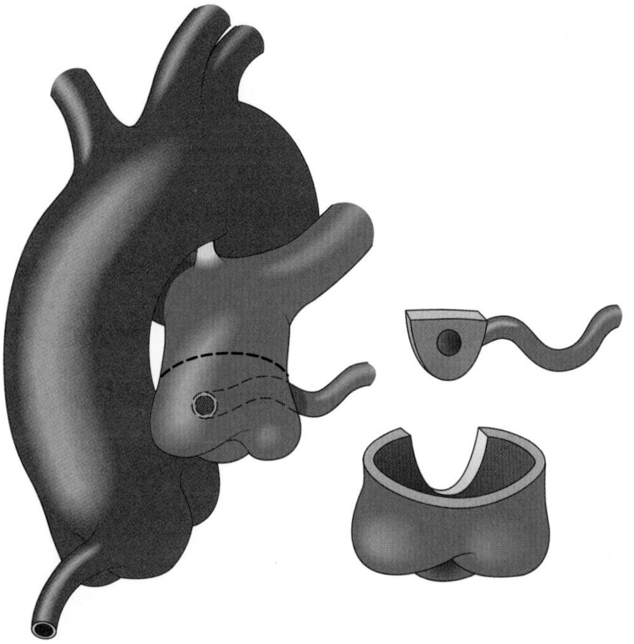

FIGURE 124-3 ■ After institution of cardiopulmonary bypass and induction of cardioplegia, the pulmonary artery is transected above the sinotubular junction, and the anomalous coronary ostium is excised with a generous button of pulmonary artery wall. (Reprinted with permission from Gaynor JW: Coronary artery anomalies in children. In Kaiser LR, Kron IL, Spray TL, editors: *Mastery of cardiothoracic surgery,* Philadelphia, 1998, Lippincott-Raven, p 883.)

arteries and prevent runoff of cardioplegia solution into the lungs. Another option to prevent runoff is to compress the origin of the coronary artery from the pulmonary artery during administration of cardioplegia solution. A cannula is inserted in the ascending aorta for administration of cardioplegia solution, the aorta is cross-clamped, and cold cardioplegia is administered via the aortic root. If circulatory arrest is used, the head vessels are then occluded with tourniquets after adequate cooling, the circulation is arrested, venous blood is drained into the reservoir, and the cannulas are removed. After adequate arrest, the pulmonary artery is transversely opened just above the sinotubular junction (see Fig. 124-3). The anomalous coronary orifice is identified. The pulmonary artery is divided and the coronary ostium is excised from the pulmonary artery with a generous button of arterial wall, as in the procedure used for the arterial switch operation. The segment of the pulmonary wall that is excised extends the proximal end of the coronary artery, thus allowing the aortic anastomosis to be accomplished without tension. To excise the coronary button, the pulmonary commissure may need to be taken down if the coronary ostium is located near a commissure. An alternative technique that can be used if the coronary arises anteriorly from the pulmonary artery or from a branch pulmonary artery involves extension of the coronary artery with a tube constructed from pulmonary artery wall to allow reimplantation (Fig. 124-4). The proximal portion of the coronary artery is mobilized with cautery, using caution to avoid any small branches. As in the arterial switch operation, the aorta is then opened transversely immediately above the sinotubular junction, and

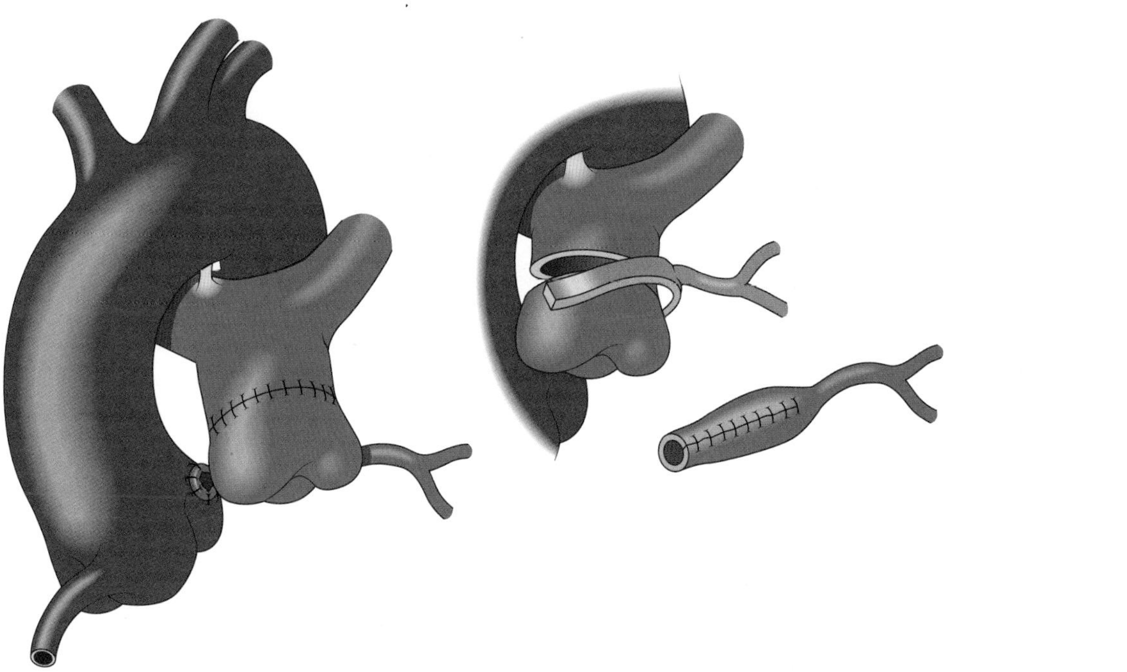

FIGURE 124-4 ■ Occasionally when the coronary artery arises from the leftward or anterior aspect of the pulmonary artery, direct reimplantation may not be possible. In these situations, a tube can be constructed from a segment of pulmonary artery to lengthen the coronary and allow reimplantation on the aorta. (Reprinted with permission from Gaynor JW: Coronary artery anomalies in children. In Kaiser LR, Kron IL, Spray TL, editors: *Mastery of cardiothoracic surgery,* Philadelphia, 1998, Lippincott-Raven, p 883.)

the incision is carried posteriorly above the left posterior sinus (Fig. 124-5). The sinus is then incised vertically to accept the coronary button. The coronary button is carefully aligned with the aortic incision to avoid twisting or kinking. A continuous suture of 7-0 polypropylene (Prolene) is used to start the anastomosis at the most inferior aspect of the coronary button, which is attached to the most inferior aspect of the incision in the sinus. The suture line is carried to the top of the incision anteriorly and posteriorly. The aorta is closed with a continuous suture of 7-0 Prolene, which is tied to the coronary button suture as the anastomosis is completed (see Fig. 124-5). Once the aorta has been closed, cardioplegia solution is administered and the anastomotic site is inspected for adequate filling of the coronary and for hemostasis. Occasionally, the anomalous artery may arise from the right pulmonary artery and run along or within the aortic wall to the sinus. If there is a common wall with the aorta, mobilization may not be possible. In this case, unroofing of the intra-mural segment should be performed.[26]

In some cases, the pulmonary artery can be repaired primarily with a continuous suture of 7-0 Prolene (Fig. 124-6). The ductus should be divided to improve mobility of the pulmonary artery confluence, thus allowing reconstruction without tension. However, more often, the pulmonary artery is repaired with a patch of autologous pericardium (see Fig. 124-6). If a commissure was taken down during excision of the coronary button, the pulmonary artery should be reconstructed with pericardium and the commissure resuspended.

The patient is rewarmed and the aortic cross-clamp is removed. The cross-clamp may be removed before the pulmonary artery reconstruction to minimize ischemia

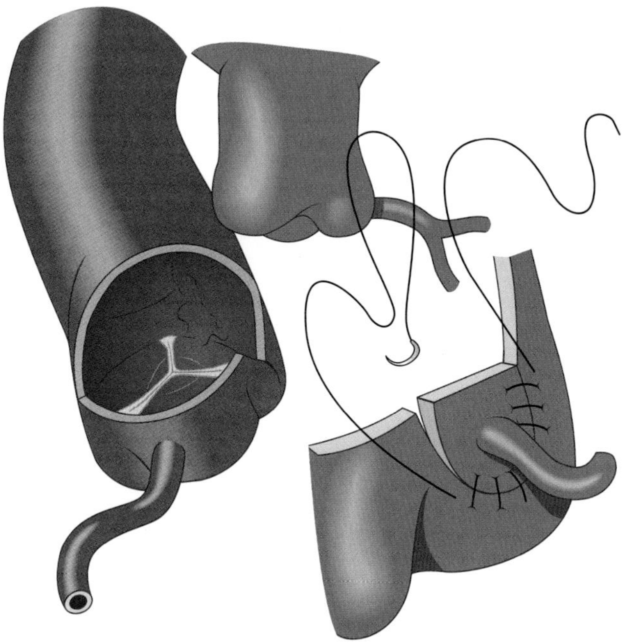

FIGURE 124-5 ■ After the anomalous coronary artery is mobilized, the aorta is opened transversely above the sinotubular junction and a vertical incision is made in the left posterior sinus to accept the reimplanted coronary. (Reprinted with permission from Gaynor JW: Coronary artery anomalies in children. In Kaiser LR, Kron IL, Spray TL, editors: *Mastery of cardiothoracic surgery,* Philadelphia, 1998, Lippincott-Raven, p 884.)

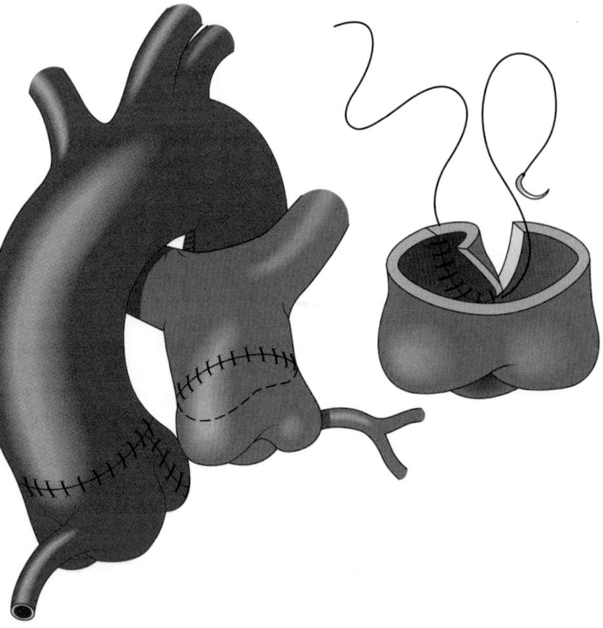

FIGURE 124-6 ■ After the coronary is reimplanted, the aorta is closed primarily. The pulmonary artery may often be closed primarily. Ligation and division of the ligamentum arteriosus improves mobility of pulmonary artery. Occasionally, patch repair of the defect in the pulmonary artery with autologous pericardium may be necessary *(inset).* (Reprinted with permission from Gaynor JW: Coronary artery anomalies in children. In Kaiser LR, Kron IL, Spray TL, editors: *Mastery of cardiothoracic surgery,* Philadelphia, 1998, Lippincott-Raven, p 884.)

time. The left ventricle is inspected to assess for adequate perfusion and function, and suture lines are inspected for hemostasis. Right and left atrial lines are placed to adequately monitor pressure and for drug administration. Atrial and ventricular pacing wires are also placed. The patient is separated from cardiopulmonary bypass after complete rewarming. Attention should be paid to the ECG during reperfusion and after separation from bypass for evidence of ischemia. Inotropic support may be necessary temporarily if there was left ventricular dysfunction preoperatively.

Modified Takeuchi Operation. The Takeuchi operation, or intrapulmonary artery tunnel, is an alternative surgical strategy for repair of ALCAPA. Originally, Takeuchi and colleagues described the creation of an aortopulmonary window using a portion of anterior pulmonary artery wall to form a baffle that would direct blood from the aorta to the ostium of the anomalous coronary artery.[15] In the modified repair, the baffle is constructed using a polytetrafluoroethylene (PTFE) (Gore-Tex) patch. Creating a baffle may not be possible if the ostium is located near a commissure or arises from a branch pulmonary artery. The procedure may be performed with either continuous low-flow cardiopulmonary bypass (25° C to 28° C) or deep hypothermic circulatory arrest (18° C). Cannulation is performed as for direct reimplantation.

After induction of cardioplegia, a longitudinal incision is made in the anterior portion of the pulmonary artery (Fig. 124-7), and the ostium of the anomalous coronary

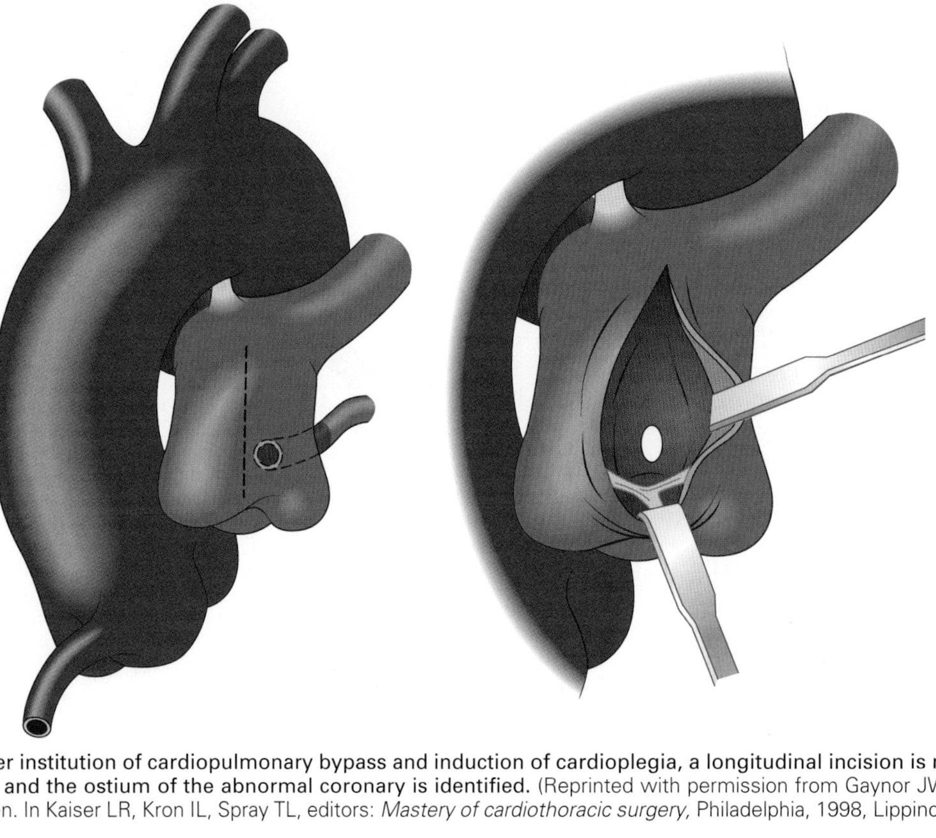

FIGURE 124-7 ■ After institution of cardiopulmonary bypass and induction of cardioplegia, a longitudinal incision is made in the main pulmonary artery, and the ostium of the abnormal coronary is identified. (Reprinted with permission from Gaynor JW: Coronary artery anomalies in children. In Kaiser LR, Kron IL, Spray TL, editors: *Mastery of cardiothoracic surgery,* Philadelphia, 1998, Lippincott-Raven, p 885.)

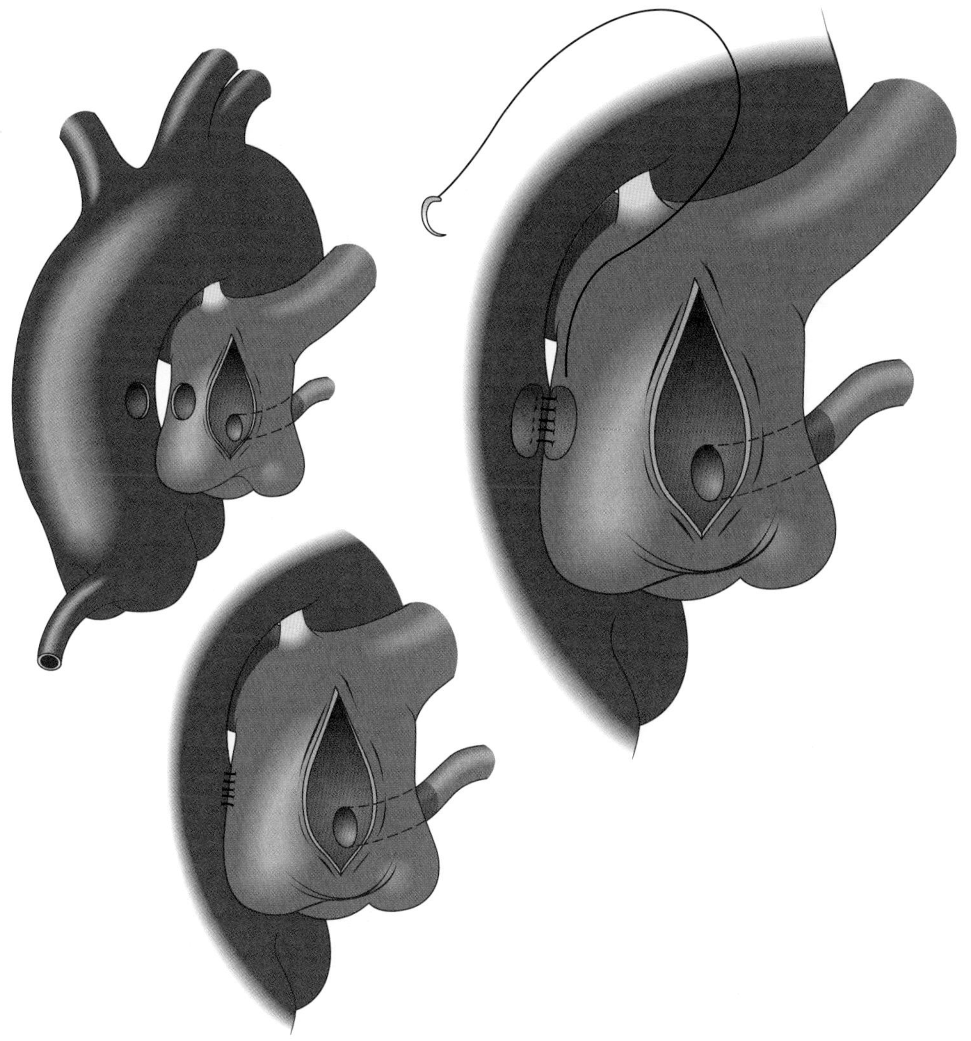

FIGURE 124-8 ■ Using a punch, a 5-mm opening is made in the aorta on the leftward aspect above the sinotubular junction. A similar opening is made in the pulmonary artery at the same level, and these are anastomosed to create an aortopulmonary window. (Reprinted with permission from Gaynor JW: Coronary artery anomalies in children. In Kaiser LR, Kron IL, Spray TL, editors: *Mastery of cardiothoracic surgery,* Philadelphia, 1998, Lippincott-Raven, p 885.)

is identified. Using a punch, a 5-mm diameter opening is made on the leftward aspect of the aorta above the sinotubular junction (Fig. 124-8). An anterior aortotomy should be performed if there is any question about placement of the aortic opening, and the incision should be directly visualized to avoid damage to the aortic valve. Creating the aortopulmonary window above the sinotubular junction allows a downward angle of the baffle into the sinus if the ostium is located deep in a sinus. After a similar incision is made in the pulmonary artery directly opposite the opening in the aorta, these are anastomosed using a continuous suture of 7-0 Prolene and creating an aortopulmonary window (see Fig. 124-8). A 4-mm PTFE tube graft is split longitudinally and customized to an appropriate length (Fig. 124-9). This graft acts as an intrapulmonary artery tunnel, baffling blood from the aortopulmonary window to the anomalous coronary ostium. The suture line starts at the anomalous coronary and is continued inferiorly along the pulmonary artery wall to the aortopulmonary window. The suture line is completed by returning to the coronary artery and completing the superior aspect of the baffle. After the baffle is created, repair of the pulmonary artery can be accomplished using a prosthetic patch or autologous pericardium to avoid supravalvar pulmonary artery obstruction (Fig. 124-10). The main complications of the modified Takeuchi operation include baffle leak, baffle occlusion, and supravalvar pulmonary artery obstruction.

Postoperative Management

Regardless of the surgical technique used, the most common postoperative issues are those related to the infant's preoperative state: low cardiac output, left ventricular dysfunction, and hypotension. Optimizing the patient's hemoglobin, electrolytes, acid-base status, and fluid status and providing adequate inotropic support are extremely important. In infants and children with severe preoperative cardiac dysfunction, temporary support with an LVAD or ECMO may be necessary in

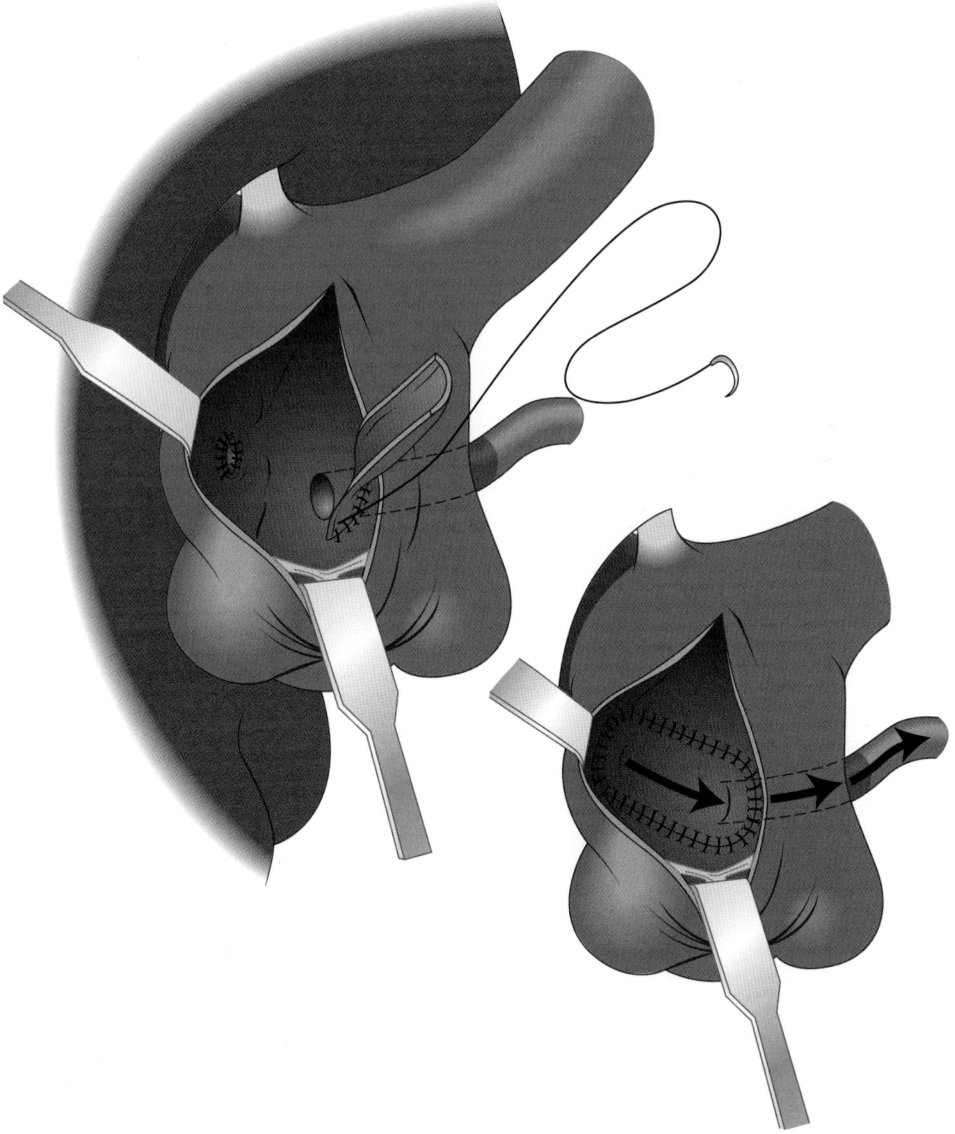

FIGURE 124-9 ■ A segment of 4-mm polytetrafluoroethylene (Gore-Tex) graft is opened longitudinally and used to fashion a baffle that directs blood flow from the aortopulmonary window to the anomalous coronary ostium. (Reprinted with permission from Gaynor JW: Coronary artery anomalies in children. In Kaiser LR, Kron IL, Spray TL, editors: *Mastery of cardiothoracic surgery,* Philadelphia, 1998, Lippincott-Raven, p 886.)

the postoperative period. Bleeding is also common postoperatively and is more frequently encountered in small infants and those who require mechanical support. Platelets and fresh-frozen plasma should be used aggressively to replace ongoing loss. Patients with low cardiac output or bleeding issues may require delayed sternal closure (2 to 3 days).

Results

Simple ligation of ALCAPA has been shown to have unacceptable early and late mortality rates. In general, survival after establishment of a dual coronary system is excellent.[13,27] In 1987, Bunton and colleagues from Boston reported on 24 patients with ALCAPA.[28] From among these 24 patients, 11 received coronary ligation or ostial closure, 11 had a Takeuchi repair, and 2 underwent other procedures. Of the patients who underwent coronary ligation or ostial closure, there was a 27% early mortality and a 25% late mortality over an average 10.5-year follow-up period. In those who underwent a Takeuchi procedure, there were no early or late deaths in over an 18.5-month follow-up period. After Takeuchi repair, two patients developed right ventricular outflow tract obstruction (one required a second operation), and one patient was found to have baffle occlusion.

Backer and colleagues reported the follow-up surgical results of 20 patients with ALCAPA who underwent different procedures.[29] There were two early deaths and one late death among nine patients who underwent ligation. In contrast, there were no deaths among the 10 patients who underwent creation of a dual coronary artery system

arteriovenous fistulas are those that end in right-sided structures, such as the right atrium, right ventricle, or pulmonary artery, whereas those that terminate in left-sided structures are called arterio-arterial fistulas.

Coronary artery fistulas are usually congenital, comprising 0.2% to 0.4% of congenital heart defects, but they make up almost half of all congenital coronary anomalies. They can be found in isolation or in association with other congenital heart disease. Acquired fistulas are the result of cardiac surgery, cardiac catheterization, or a complication from Kawasaki disease.[70]

Anatomy

Coronary artery fistulas may arise from either the right or the left coronary artery; occasionally, both coronary arteries are affected.[71] Most fistulas arise from a coronary artery with an otherwise normal distribution. The fistulous connection may occur in the midportion of the coronary artery with a normal vessel continuing beyond the fistula origin, or as an end artery at the termination of the vessel. The coronary is dilated and elongated in the portion of the vessel proximal to the fistula, usually in proportion to the size of the shunt across the fistulous connection. The portion of the vessel distal to the fistula usually returns to a small diameter.

The right ventricle and right atrium are the most common sites of termination. Fernandes and colleagues reported on 93 patients with coronary artery fistulas.[72] A single fistula was present in 83 patients, and the other 10 had multiple fistulas. The RCA was the most common site of origin and the right ventricle was the most common drainage site. Fifty-six patients had isolated coronary fistulas, and the others had additional cardiac lesions. Lowe and colleagues reviewed 286 patients and found the RCA to be the site of origin in just over half of the patients, and the left coronary artery system the origin site in approximately one third.[73] The right ventricle was the most common site of drainage (39%), with the right atrium (including the coronary sinus and superior vena cava) and the pulmonary artery as the drainage sites in 33% and 20%, respectively. The site of drainage was the left atrium or left ventricle in the remaining 8%.

Pathophysiology

Coronary fistulas result in a left-to-right or left-to-left shunt. When a fistula drains to the right side of the circulation, there is usually a small- to moderate-sized shunt. However, when it drains into a left-sided chamber (i.e., left-to-left shunt), an aortic runoff develops, with physiology similar to that of aortic regurgitation. The effects of the shunt are related to the amount of blood flow from the fistula to the chamber and into which chamber the fistula drains. It can also be affected by myocardial ischemia resulting from coronary circulation steal.

Clinical Presentation

Patients with a coronary artery fistula are usually asymptomatic; they rarely present in infancy and are often diagnosed in adulthood. Many patients are diagnosed during a murmur evaluation. When symptomatic, the most common complaints are shortness of breath with exercise and fatigue. Even though there may be coronary steal, angina is uncommon. Ventricular dysfunction and congestive heart failure are occasionally present and are much more common in the adult. Atrial fibrillation in an older patient may result from right atrial enlargement caused by a coronary artery fistula to the right atrium.

On examination of a patient with a coronary artery fistula, a continuous murmur is often auscultated. The murmur may be suggestive of a PDA, but it is heard lower on the sternal border, which is an atypical location for a PDA. As is the case with aortic regurgitation, large left-to-left shunts may cause a wide pulse pressure.

Natural History

In patients with congenital coronary arterial fistulas, most likely the fistula was present early in life and gradually increased in size over several years. Despite progressive enlargement of the coronary arteries, spontaneous rupture is rare and usually results from aneurysmal dilation and weakening of the vessel wall as a result of a congenital defect or atherosclerosis. Bacterial endocarditis can occur secondary to turbulent flow. Spontaneous closure of small fistulas has been reported.

Diagnostic Imaging

Depending on the size of the fistula, the ECG may be normal, or it may show evidence of ventricular volume overload. Atrial fibrillation may be noted in older adult patients who have a right atrial fistulous connection. If coronary steal is present, evidence of myocardial ischemia in the affected region may be noted. Chest films are usually normal but may show cardiomegaly or evidence of congestive heart failure. Giant aneurysms of the involved coronary artery can sometimes be noted. Two-dimensional echocardiography can demonstrate the enlarged coronary artery, the origin of the fistula, the chamber into which it drains, and any cardiac chamber enlargement or hypertrophy. The actual fistula may be demonstrated best by color Doppler. MRI is a promising additional noninvasive imaging technique used to diagnose and provide detailed anatomy of the coronary arterial fistula and may take the place of cardiac catheterization, but now it is used as an adjunctive imaging modality.

Coronary catheterization with selective coronary angiography remains the gold standard to accurately define the coronary anatomy and the hemodynamic significance of the fistula. Often, an experienced interventional cardiologist can successfully coil-embolize the coronary artery fistula without the morbidities associated with cardiopulmonary bypass and sternotomy.[74] However, the indications for coil embolization have not been defined; therefore, most patients undergo surgical closure as the preferred therapy.[75]

Surgical Management

Indications for Surgery

All patients with symptomatic fistulas should undergo closure. Patients with very small fistulas may not require

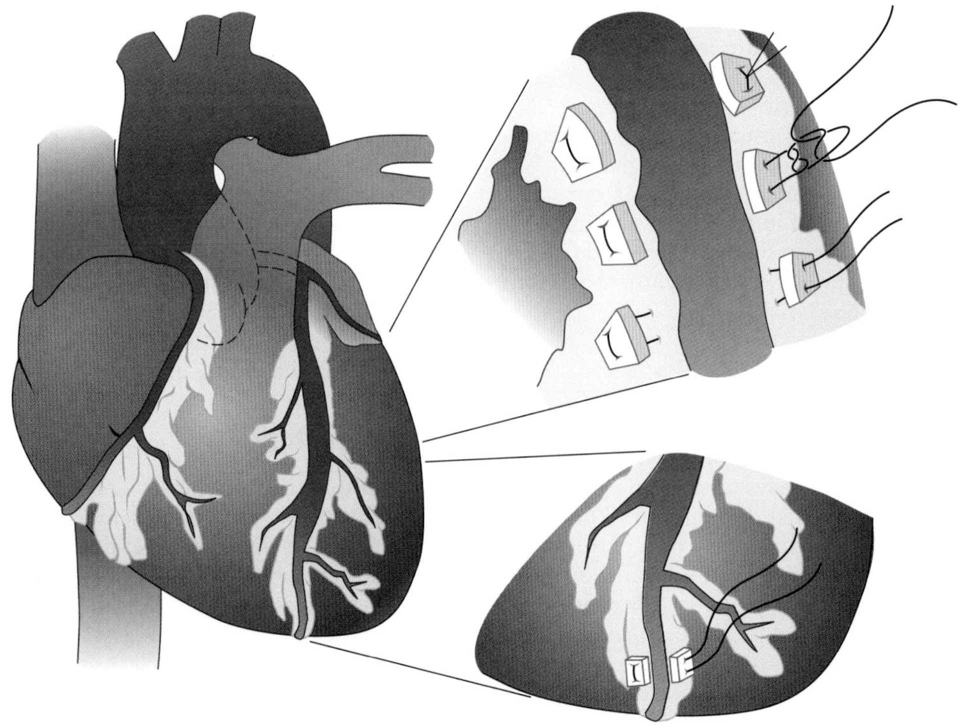

FIGURE 124-15 ■ If the termination site of the fistula is at the distal aspect of the coronary and no significant myocardium is in jeopardy, the coronary may be ligated proximal to the termination site. If the fistula terminates in the midportion of the left anterior descending coronary artery, the fistulous communication may be closed with multiple pledgeted sutures placed underneath the coronary artery so as not to impair distal perfusion. (Reprinted with permission from Gaynor JW: Coronary artery anomalies in children. In Kaiser LR, Kron IL, Spray TL, editors: *Mastery of cardiothoracic surgery,* Philadelphia, 1998, Lippincott-Raven, p 888.)

surgical closure; however, because the natural progression of a fistula is to enlarge, these patients should be closely followed.[76] Asymptomatic patients with moderate to large fistulas should undergo surgical closure electively.

Surgical Techniques

Coronary artery anatomy must be clearly defined by coronary angiography before surgical closure. Each operation should be individualized on the basis of anatomy. Often, the fistula can be ligated or oversewn at its origin or termination without the use of cardiopulmonary bypass; however, cardiopulmonary bypass should always be available.

Through a median sternotomy, the coronary anatomy is visualized and carefully inspected, and the site of the enlarged vessel is noted. The fistula can be ligated without the use of cardiopulmonary bypass when it is located at the distal end of the coronary artery and there is no viable myocardium distal to the fistula (Fig. 124-15). This is performed by placing a ligature around the coronary artery immediately proximal to the fistula, thereby temporarily occluding the fistula. The heart is observed for signs of ischemia, and the ECG is monitored closely. If there are no signs of ischemia and there is adequate myocardial perfusion, the ligature is tied. To ensure complete closure, a second suture ligature should also be placed. Intraoperative transesophageal echocardiography can be used to verify that the fistula is closed.

Cardiopulmonary bypass is indicated if the fistula arises from the middle of a coronary artery, if the fistula is inaccessible, if another cardiac lesion needs to be repaired simultaneously, or if the complete coronary course cannot be completely defined. The aorta and both cavae are cannulated and bypass is initiated. If cardioplegic arrest is necessary, the fistula should be temporarily compressed during administration of the cardioplegia to prevent runoff through the fistula into the heart. If adequate arrest is not possible because of flow through the fistula, retrograde administration of cardioplegia solution may be necessary.

A variety of techniques can be used to close the fistula. If it ends in the midportion of the LAD, the fistulous communication can be closed by placing multiple pledgeted sutures beneath the coronary artery, taking care to avoid compromising distal perfusion (see Fig. 124-15). However, if distal perfusion of the coronary bed is affected after closure of the fistula, coronary bypass grafting may be necessary. Another technique that can be used when the fistula arises from the midportion of the coronary is to open the coronary longitudinally on the epicardial surface and oversew the origin of the fistula from within the coronary artery (Fig. 124-16). The coronary artery can then be closed primarily.

If the fistula terminates in the right atrium or right ventricle, the fistula may be closed directly from within the cardiac chamber (Fig. 124-17). A right atriotomy is performed after cardiopulmonary bypass, and the termination site of the fistula is identified from within the

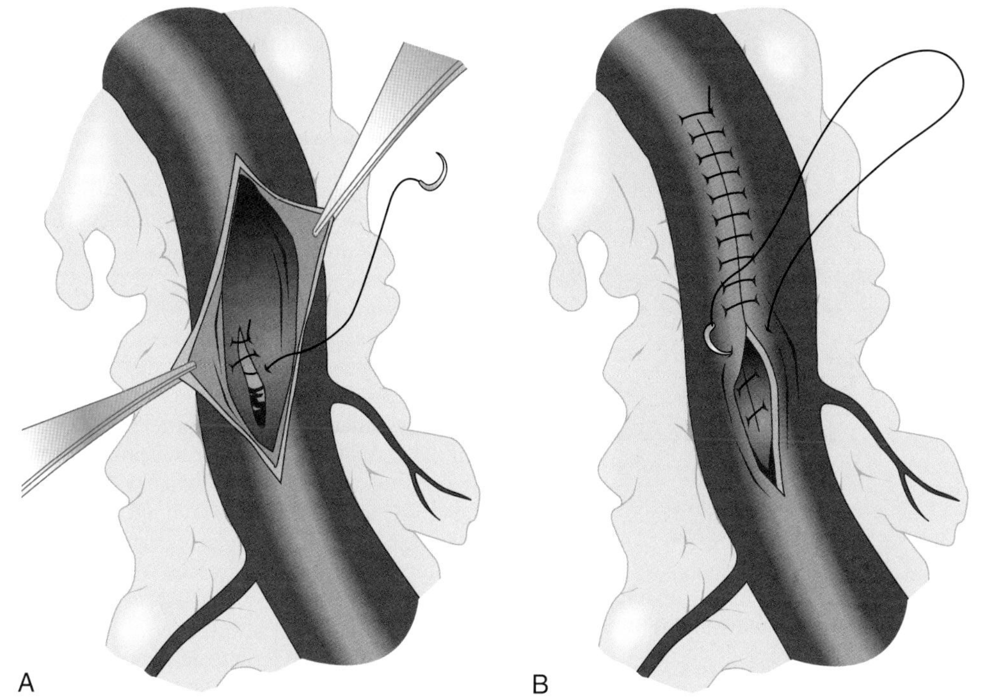

FIGURE 124-16 ■ **A,** When the fistulous communication arises from the midportion of the dilated coronary, the coronary may be opened longitudinally and the origin of the fistula oversewn from within the coronary. **B,** The coronary artery is closed primarily. (Reprinted with permission from Gaynor JW: Coronary artery anomalies in children. In Kaiser LR, Kron IL, Spray TL, editors: *Mastery of cardiothoracic surgery,* Philadelphia, 1998, Lippincott-Raven, p 889.)

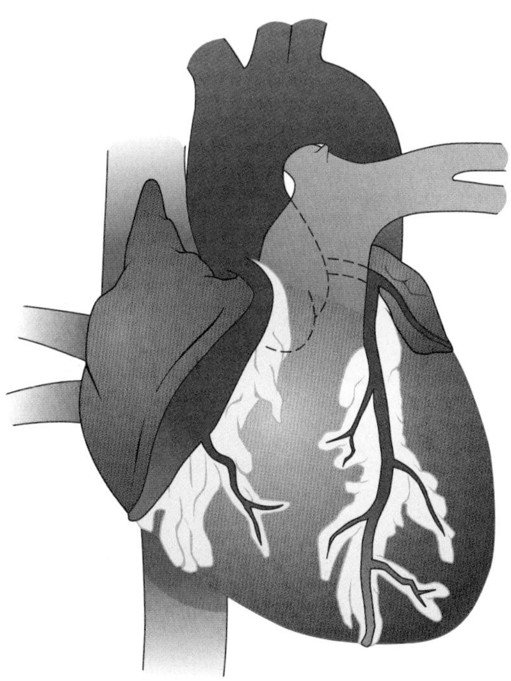

FIGURE 124-17 ■ A coronary arterial venous fistula arising from the midportion of the right coronary artery and terminating in the right atrium. (Reprinted with permission from Gaynor JW: Coronary artery anomalies in children. In Kaiser LR, Kron IL, Spray TL, editors: *Mastery of cardiothoracic surgery,* Philadelphia, 1998, Lippincott-Raven, p 890.)

chamber. Using cardioplegia may be helpful for localization. The termination site can be closed primarily or with a pericardial patch (Fig. 124-18).

Surgical Results

The operative mortality rate for coronary artery fistula repair is very low, and late results are outstanding with very few patients experiencing a recurrence of the fistula.[71,77] Lowe and colleagues reported on 22 patients after surgical closure of coronary artery fistulas.[73] In 14 patients, the fistula was closed using sutures without cardiopulmonary bypass. The termination of a fistula within a cardiac chamber was closed using cardiopulmonary bypass in six patients. In the remaining two patients, saphenous vein bypass grafts were necessary to maintain distal perfusion after fistula closure. The operative mortality rate was zero, as was the long-term rate at an average follow-up of 10 years. Although a small residual fistula remained in one patient, there were no recurrences. Fernandes and colleagues reported on 56 patients who had coronary artery fistula closure.[72] There was no early or late mortality, but two patients had perioperative myocardial infarctions. Finally, Mavroudis and colleagues reported on 17 pediatric patients with an average age of 5.5 years.[75] Eight underwent fistula closure using cardiopulmonary bypass, and one of these patients needed distal IMA bypass graft. There was complete closure in all patients, and there were no recurrences and no operative or late deaths.

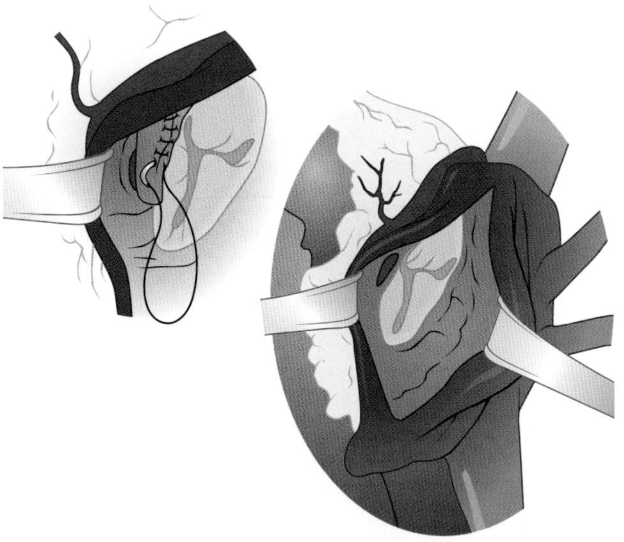

FIGURE 124-18 ■ After institution of cardiopulmonary bypass and induction of cardioplegia, the right atrium is opened, and the termination site of the fistula is identified from within the right atrium. This may be done primarily or with a patch of pericardium. (Reprinted with permission from Gaynor JW: Coronary artery anomalies in children. In Kaiser LR, Kron IL, Spray TL, editors: *Mastery of cardiothoracic surgery,* Philadelphia, 1998, Lippincott-Raven, p 890.)

CONGENITAL OSTIAL ATRESIA OF THE LEFT MAIN CORONARY ARTERY

Anatomy

Congenital atresia of the LMCA ostium is a congenital coronary anomaly that is quite rare, with fewer than 50 reported cases in the literature. In this coronary anomaly, there is no LMCA ostium; rather, the correctly positioned LAD and circumflex coronary arteries have a blind ending and they receive blood flow retrograde through the RCA via at least one collateral vessel.[78] On the inner aortic surface in the left sinus of Valsalva, there may be a dimple, a blind pouch, or no marking at all. This lesion should be differentiated from a single RCA where blood flow occurs in a centrifugal, or antegrade, manner. Most patients with a single RCA remain asymptomatic, except in the setting of atherosclerosis or other congenital heart defects. The congenital atresia of the LMCA ostium usually occurs in the absence of other structural heart disease; however, associations have been noted with supravalvar aortic stenosis, VSD with pulmonic stenosis, right coronary ostial stenosis, and PDA and aortic regurgitation.[78,79]

Pathophysiology

The main pathophysiology from congenital left main ostial atresia is inadequate collateral vessel flow from the RCA. Blood flows from the RCA to the left coronary artery system through collateral vessels, which are smaller in size than the left-sided coronary arteries; thus, there is inadequate blood flow through these smaller vessels to perfuse the myocardium. This leads to myocardial ischemia and the potential for sudden death and causes these patients to be almost universally symptomatic.

Clinical Presentation

The timing of when these patients present with symptoms can occur at different ages, with some presenting during infancy and others in adolescence or adulthood. Despite age at presentation, almost every patient reported in the literature was symptomatic at diagnosis, although the signs and symptoms were different. The infants and toddlers generally present with heart failure symptoms, including feeding difficulty, failure to thrive, emesis, and dyspnea.[78,80] Their clinical picture is similar to that of ALCAPA or dilated cardiomyopathy, both of which would need to be ruled out as well. The youngest patients also are more likely to have an associated cardiac defect, suggesting that there are earlier ischemic events from other congenital lesions that may increase the myocardial oxygen demand. School-age children and adolescents may be diagnosed after experiencing syncope, dyspnea, angina, and ventricular tachyarrhythmias, whereas adults are likely to have dyspnea and angina. Indeed, for any age, sudden death may be the first presentation.

Diagnostic Imaging

Accurate diagnostic imaging is essential in this diagnosis because symptoms are nonspecific and can be caused by other diseases. In young children, cardiomegaly with pulmonary congestion as a result of heart failure may be evident on chest radiograph, whereas in adults, the radiograph may be normal. The 12-lead ECG may be normal or may show a variety of abnormalities, including anterolateral Q waves, lateral T wave inversion, right bundle branch block, or ventricular tachycardia. The initial imaging procedure should be transthoracic echocardiography. This is likely to show a dilated left ventricle with poor function and mitral regurgitation, a finding also seen with ALCAPA and dilated cardiomyopathy. Delineation of the coronary artery ostia is essential. The use of Doppler color flow is helpful to demonstrate flow from the RCA retrograde to the left coronary artery system without evidence of blood flowing to the pulmonary artery. Although echocardiographic techniques have improved over the past several years, delineating coronary anatomy and blood flow can be difficult in some cases. Because of this, cardiac catheterization with coronary angiography remains the gold standard and should be performed on any patient who may have either ALCAPA or congenital atresia of the left main coronary ostium. The direction of flow from the RCA to the left coronary system and whether the PA is filled retrograde should be delineated. If any question remains regarding the diagnosis, selective RCA angiography should be performed.

Surgical Management

Once diagnosed, surgery should occur expeditiously because of the high risk of sudden death with this anomaly.

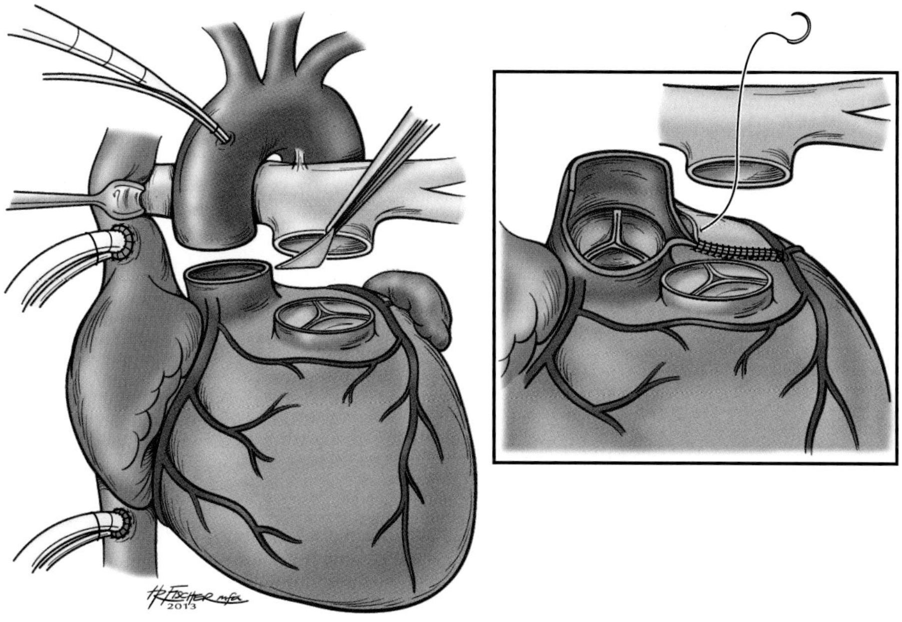

FIGURE 124-19 ■ Technique for ostioplasty of the left coronary ostium with homograft patch. Left coronary ostial atresia before intervention *(main illustration)* and with homograft patch augmentation of the ostium and left main coronary artery *(inset)*. (Reprinted with permission from Kaczorowski DJ, Sathanandam S, Ravishankar C, et al: Coronary ostioplasty for congenital atresia of the left main coronary artery ostium. *Ann Thorac Surg* 94:1307–1310, 2012, Fig. 2.)

The literature mainly reports the use of coronary artery bypass grafting (CABG) for all ages.[78,81,82] Some reports have described the creation of a dual coronary artery system for these patients, with the belief that, similar to ALCAPA, long-term outcomes may be improved.[80,83,84] This type of surgical revascularization has important implications for children and young adults in whom the bypass graft longevity is of concern.

For the creation of a dual coronary artery system, there have been a few somewhat different surgical techniques described. Varghese and colleagues described the use of an autologous pericardial patch to attain surgical revascularization in a single case of left main coronary ostial atresia.[83] The aorta is transected under cardiopulmonary bypass to find the dimple from where the left coronary normally would be located. An incision is made vertically in the aorta to the location of the ostium and then extended down the LMCA; the incision should end prior to the LAD and circumflex coronary artery bifurcation. An atretic membrane, if present, should be removed. An autologous pericardial patch is then used to reconstruct the LMCA ostium that is atretic.

Bonnet and colleagues described surgical revascularization of the left main coronary arteries and included two of the patients with LMCA atresia.[84] To help attain myocardial preservation, after standard cardiopulmonary bypass, first hot-induction blood cardioplegia, followed by cold blood cardioplegia, and subsequent warm reperfusion are used. The MPA is then transected so that the aortic root and left coronary artery system can be visualized. The aortic incision starts on the anterior portion of the aortic root, continues toward the coronary orifice, and extends beyond the atretic portion. The aortic and coronary incisions are then connected together using an onlay patch, which is obtained from saphenous vein, autologous pericardium, or PTFE. The creation of this patch enlarges not only the LMCA but also the section of the aorta that was incised, now creating a "funnel-shaped" neo-ostium.

A third revascularization procedure, as described by Kaczorowski and colleagues, is homograft patch ostioplasty in the treatment of LMCA ostial atresia (Fig. 124-19).[80] Bicaval cannulation is used and cardiopulmonary bypass established. Two of the three children in the report were initially diagnosed with ALCAPA; therefore, their pulmonary artery was opened to evaluate for a coronary ostium. When there was not one identified, an aortotomy was performed. No left main coronary ostium was identified in the aorta. After the blind-ending LMCA was located on the cardiac surface, in two patients, an incision was made in the aortic wall that was directed inferiorly to the aortic sinus. A second incision was made in the LMCA until its division into LAD and circumflex coronary arteries. Using a pulmonary homograft patch, the ostium was enlarged and also joined the aortic sinus to the proximal LMCA. In the third patient, the blind-ending LMCA was sewn onto the posterior aortic wall with anterior augmentation. To help confirm coronary patency, coronary probes should be used as well as noting evidence of back bleeding. The aortotomy is subsequently closed and the patient is removed from bypass.

Surgical Results

Postoperative morbidity and mortality, at least in the short-term, appear to be related to amount of myocardial damage at the time of diagnosis and operation. If LMCA ostial atresia is recognized early and the patient has enough collateral vessels, then short-term results are encouraging after surgical revascularization, notably with those procedures that establish a dual coronary system. However, long-term outcome data are lacking in this population. Long-term results from CABG used for other coronary arterial abnormalities (e.g., ALCAPA) remain somewhat uncertain, although some reports using IMA grafts have shown good results.

OUTCOMES

Surgical outcomes after repair of anomalous coronary artery arising from the pulmonary arteries have significantly improved over the past several years, even in the high-risk patients who present with significant left ventricular dysfunction and mitral regurgitation. Overall survival is now greater than 90%. Mitral valve repair is rarely needed, even in patients with severe preoperative mitral regurgitation. Long-term outcome data are limited, particularly with regard to left ventricular function and late mortality. The data suggest that establishing a dual coronary system is associated with overall improved survival and left ventricular function when compared with simple ligation of the anomalous artery.[85]

Similarly, there are limited data on long-term morbidity and mortality after surgical repair of anomalous aortic origin of a coronary artery coursing between the aorta and the pulmonary artery.[13,60,65,86] Surgical mortality appears to be rare. It is unknown whether these surgical techniques truly reduce the incidence of myocardial ischemia and sudden cardiac death. After surgical closure of coronary artery fistulae, mortality is minimal with a low recurrence rate and excellent long-term outcome.[72,75] No long-term data are currently available for operative mortality after LMCA ostial atresia repair. Short-term results are encouraging when there is early recognition of the anomaly, the patient has adequate collateral vessels, and surgical revascularization consists of establishing a dual coronary artery system.[80,83,84]

REFERENCES

1. Brooks HSJ: Two cases of an abnormal coronary artery of the heart, arising from the pulmonary artery; with some remarks upon the effect of this anomaly in producing cirsoid dilatation of the vessels. *J Anat Physiol* 20:26–29, 1885.
2. Smith A, Arnold R, Anderson RH, et al: Anomalous origin of the left coronary artery from the pulmonary trunk. *J Thorac Cardiovasc Surg* 98:16–24, 1989.
3. Bland EF, White PD, Garland J: Congenital anomalies of the coronary arteries: report of an unusual case associated with cardiac hypertrophy. *Am Heart J* 8:787–801, 1933.
4. Berdjis F, Takahashi M, Wells WJ, et al: Anomalous left coronary artery from the pulmonary artery. Significance of intercoronary collaterals. *J Thorac Cardiovasc Surg* 108:17–20, 1994.
5. Shivalkar B, Borgers M, Daenen W, et al: ALCAPA syndrome: an example of chronic myocardial hypoperfusion. *J Am Coll Cardiol* 23:772–778, 1994.
6. Schwerzmann M, Salehian O, Elliot T, et al: Anomalous origin of the left coronary artery from the main pulmonary artery in adults: coronary collateralization at its best. *Circulation* 110:e511–e513, 2004.
7. Wesselhoeft H, Fawcett JS, Johnson AL: Anomalous origin of the left coronary artery from the pulmonary trunk. Its clinical spectrum, pathology, and pathophysiology, based on a review of 140 cases with seven further cases. *Circulation* 68:403–425, 1968.
8. Piechaud JF, Shalaby L, Kachaner J, et al: Pulmonary artery "stop-flow" angiography to visualize the anomalous origin of the left coronary artery from the pulmonary artery in infants. *Pediatr Cardiol* 8:11–15, 1987.
9. Douard H, Barat JL, Laurent F, et al: Magnetic resonance imaging of an anomalous origin of the left coronary artery from the pulmonary artery. *Eur Heart J* 9:1356–1360, 1988.
10. Molinari G, Balbi M, Bertero G, et al: Magnetic resonance imaging in Bland-White-Garland syndrome. *Am Heart J* 129:1040–1042, 1995.
11. Cohcrane AD, Austin C, Goh TH, et al: Incipient left ventricular rupture complicating anomalous left coronary artery. *Ann Thorac Surg* 67:254–256, 1999.
12. Del Nido PJ, Duncan BW, Mayer JE, Jr, et al: Left ventricular assist device improves survival in children with left ventricular dysfunction after repair of anomalous origin of the left coronary artery from the pulmonary artery. *Ann Thorac Surg* 67:169–172, 1999.
13. Dua R, Smith JA, Wilkinson JL, et al: Long-term follow-up after two coronary repair of anomalous left coronary artery from the pulmonary artery. *J Card Surg* 8:384–390, 1993.
14. Meyer BW, Stefanik G, Stiles QR, et al: A method of definitive surgical treatment of anomalous origin of left coronary artery. *J Thorac Cardiovasc Surg* 56:104–107, 1968.
15. Takeuchi S, Imamura H, Katsumoto K, et al: New surgical method for repair of anomalous left coronary artery from pulmonary artery. *J Thorac Cardiovasc Surg* 78:7–11, 1979.
16. Alexi-Meskishvili V, Hetzer R, Weng Y, et al: Anomalous origin of the left coronary artery from the pulmonary artery. Early results with direct aortic reimplantation. *J Thorac Cardiovasc Surg* 108:354–362, 1994.
17. Bonhoeffer P, Bonnet D, Piechaud JF, et al: Coronary artery obstruction after the arterial switch operation for transposition of the great arteries in newborns. *J Am Coll Cardiol* 29:202–206, 1997.
18. Chan RK, Hare DL, Buxton BF: Anomalous left main coronary artery arising from the pulmonary artery in an adult: treatment by internal mammary artery grafting. *J Thorac Cardiovasc Surg* 109:393–394, 1995.
19. Kitamura S, Kawachi K, Nishii T, et al: Internal thoracic artery grafting for congenital coronary malformations. *Ann Thorac Surg* 53:513–516, 1992.
20. Kitamura S, Seki T, Kawachi K, et al: Excellent patency and growth potential of internal mammary artery grafts in pediatric coronary artery bypass surgery: new evidence for a "live" conduit. *Circulation* 78(3 Pt 2):I129–I139, 1988.
21. El-Said GM, Ruzyllo W, Williams RL, et al: Early and late result of saphenous vein graft for anomalous origin of left coronary artery from pulmonary artery. *Circulation* 48(III):2–6, 1973.
22. Kesler KA, Pennington DG, Nouri S, et al: Left subclavian-left coronary artery anastomosis for anomalous origin of the left coronary artery. *J Thorac Cardiovasc Surg* 98:25–29, 1989.
23. Montigny M, Stanley P, Chartrand C, et al: Postoperative evaluation after end-to-end subclavian-left coronary artery anastomosis in anomalous left coronary artery. *J Thorac Cardiovasc Surg* 100:270–273, 1990.
24. Laks H, Ardehali A, Grant PW, et al: Aortic implantation of anomalous left coronary artery. Improved surgical approach. *J Thorac Cardiovasc Surg* 109:519–523, 1995.
25. Turley K, Szarnick RJ, Flachsbart KD, et al: Aortic implantation is possible in all cases of anomalous origin of the left coronary artery from the pulmonary artery. *Ann Thorac Surg* 60:84–89, 1995.
26. Adachi I, Kagisaki K, Yagihara T, et al: Unroofing aortic intramural left coronary artery arising from right pulmonary artery. *Ann Thorac Surg* 85:675–677, 2008.
27. Sauer D, Stem H, Meisner H, et al: Risk factors for perioperative mortality in children with anomalous origin of the left coronary artery from the pulmonary artery. *J Thorac Cardiovasc Surg* 104:696–705, 1992.
28. Bunton R, Jonas RA, Lang P, et al: Anomalous origin of left coronary artery from pulmonary artery. *J Thorac Cardiovasc Surg* 93:103–108, 1987.
29. Backer CL, Stout MJ, Zales VR, et al: Anomalous origin of the left coronary artery. A twenty-year review of surgical management. *J Thorac Cardiovasc Surg* 103:1049–1057, 1992.
30. Vouhe PR, Tamisier D, Sidi D, et al: Anomalous left coronary artery from the pulmonary artery: results of isolated aortic reimplantation. *Ann Thorac Surg* 54:621–626, 1992.

31. Lange R, Vogt M, Horer J, et al: Long-term results of repair of anomalous origin of the left coronary artery from the pulmonary artery. *Ann Thorac Surg* 83:1463–1471, 2007.
32. Yam MC, Menahem S: Mitral valve replacement for severe mitral regurgitation in infants with anomalous left coronary artery from the pulmonary artery. *Pediatr Cardiol* 17:271–274, 1996.
33. Isomatsu Y, Imai Y, Shin'oka T, et al: Surgical intervention for anomalous origin of the left coronary artery from the pulmonary artery: the Tokyo experience. *J Thorac Cardiovasc Surg* 121:792–797, 2001.
34. Virmani R, Chun PKC, Goldstein RE, et al: Acute takeoffs of the coronary arteries along the aortic wall and congenital coronary ostial valve-like ridges: association with sudden death. *J Am Coll Cardiol* 3:766–771, 1984.
35. Roberts WC: Major anomalies of coronary arterial origin seen in adulthood. *Am Heart J* 111:941–963, 1986.
36. Roberts WC, Shirani J: The four subtypes of anomalous origin of the left main coronary artery from the right aortic sinus (or from the right coronary artery). *Am J Cardiol* 70:119–121, 1992.
37. Roynard JL, Cattan S, Artigou JY, et al: Anomalous course of the left anterior descending coronary artery between the aorta and pulmonary trunk: a rare cause of myocardial ischaemia at rest. *Br Heart J* 72:397–399, 1994.
38. Shirani K, Roberts WC: Solitary coronary ostium in the aorta in the absence of other major congenital cardiovascular anomalies. *J Am Coll Cardiol* 21:137–143, 1993.
39. Barth CW, Robert WC: Left main coronary artery originating from the right sinus of Valsalva and coursing between the aorta and pulmonary trunk. *J Am Coll Cardiol* 7:366–373, 1986.
40. Basso C, Maron BJ, Corrado D, et al: Clinical profile of congenital coronary artery anomalies with origin from the wrong aortic sinus leading to sudden death in young competitive athletes. *J Am Coll Cardiol* 35:1493–1501, 2000.
41. Cheitlin MD, DeCastro CM, McAllister HA: Sudden death as a complication of anomalous left coronary origin from the anterior sinus of Valsalva: a not-so-minor congenital anomaly. *Circulation* 50:780–787, 1974.
42. Liberthson RR, Dinsmore RE, Fallon JT: Aberrant coronary artery origin from the aorta: report of 18 patients, review of literature and delineation of natural history and management. *Circulation* 59:748–754, 1979.
43. Maron BJ, Shirani J, Poliac LC, et al: Sudden death in young competitive athletes: clinical, demographic and pathological profiles. *JAMA* 276:199–204, 1996.
44. Mustafa I, Gula G, Radley-Smith R, et al: Anomalous origin of the left coronary artery from the anterior aortic sinus: a potential cause of sudden death. *J Thorac Cardiovasc Surg* 82:297–300, 1981.
45. Taylor AJ, Rogan KM, Virmani R: Sudden cardiac death associated with isolated congenital coronary artery anomalies. *J Am Coll Cardiol* 20:640–647, 1992.
46. Frescura C, Basso C, Thiene G, et al: Anomalous origin of coronary arteries and risk of sudden death: a study based on an autopsy population of congenital heart disease. *Hum Pathol* 29:689–695, 1998.
47. Kragel AH, Roberts WC: Anomalous origin of either the right or left main coronary artery from the aorta with subsequent coursing between aorta and pulmonary trunk: analysis of 32 necropsy cases. *Am J Cardiol* 62:771–779, 1988.
48. Roberts WC, Kragel AH: Anomalous origin of either the right or left main coronary artery from the aorta without coursing of the anomalously arising artery between aorta and pulmonary trunk: analysis of 32 necropsy cases. *Am J Cardiol* 62:1263–1267, 1988.
49. Davis JA, Cecchin F, Jones TK, et al: Major coronary artery anomalies in a pediatric population: incidence and clinical importance. *J Am Coll Cardiol* 37:593–597, 2001.
50. Zeppilli P, dello Russo A, Santini C, et al: In vivo detection of coronary artery anomalies in asymptomatic athletes by echocardiographic screening. *Chest* 114:89–93, 1998.
51. Brothers JA, McBride MG, Seliem MA, et al: Evaluation of myocardial ischemia following surgical repair of anomalous aortic origin of a coronary artery in a series of pediatric patients. *J Am Coll Cardiol* 50:2078–2082, 2007.
52. Brothers JA, Stephens P, Gaynor JW, et al: Anomalous aortic origin of a coronary artery with an interarterial course: should family screening be routine? *J Am Coll Cardiol* 51:2062–2064, 2008.
53. Frommelt PC, Frommelt MA, Tweddell JS, et al: Prospective echocardiographic diagnosis and surgical repair of anomalous origin of a coronary artery from the opposite sinus with an interarterial course. *J Am Coll Cardiol* 42:148–154, 2003.
54. Romp RL, Herlong R, Landolfo CK, et al: Outcome of unroofing procedure for repair of anomalous aortic origin of left or right coronary artery. *Ann Thorac Surg* 76:589–596, 2003.
55. Towbin JA: Myocardial infarction in childhood. In Garson A, Bricker JT, McNamara DG, editors: *The science and practice of pediatric cardiology*, Philadelphia, 1990, Lea & Febiger, p 1684.
56. Frommelt PC, Berger S, Pelech AN, et al: Prospective identification of anomalous origin of left coronary artery from the right sinus of Valsalva using transthoracic echocardiography: importance of color Doppler flow mapping. *Pediatr Cardiol* 22:327–332, 2001.
57. Post JC, van Rossum AC, Bonzwaer JGF, et al: Magnetic resonance angiography of anomalous coronary arteries. A new gold standard for delineating the proximal course? *Circulation* 92:3163–3171, 1995.
58. Taylor AM, Thorne SA, Rubens P, et al: Coronary artery imaging in grown up congenital heart disease: complementary role of magnetic resonance and x-ray coronary angiography. *Circulation* 101:1670–1678, 2000.
59. Yamanaka O, Hobbs RE: Coronary artery anomalies in 126,595 patients undergoing coronary arteriography. *Cathet Cardiovasc Diagn* 21:28–40, 1990.
60. Brothers J, Carter C, McBride M, et al: Anomalous left coronary artery origin from the opposite sinus of Valsalva: evidence of intermittent ischemia. *J Thorac Cardiovasc Surg* 140:e27–e29, 2010.
61. Erez E, Tam VKH, Doublin NA, et al: Anomalous coronary artery with aortic origin and course between the great arteries: improved diagnosis, anatomic findings, and surgical treatment. *Ann Thorac Surg* 82:973–977, 2006.
62. Gulati R, Reddy VM, Culbertson C, et al: Surgical management of coronary artery arising from the wrong coronary sinus, using standard and novel approaches. *J Thorac Cardiovasc Surg* 134:1171–1178, 2007.
63. Rodefeld MD, Casey B, Culbertson CB, et al: Pulmonary artery translocation: a surgical option for complex anomalous coronary artery anatomy. *Ann Thorac Surg* 72:2150–2152, 2001.
64. Alphonso N, Anagnostopoulos PV, Nolke L, et al: Anomalous coronary artery from the wrong sinus of Valsalva: a physiologic repair strategy. *Ann Thorac Surg* 83:1472–1476, 2007.
65. Wittlieb-Weber CA, Paridon SM, Gaynor JW, et al: Medium-term outcome after anomalous aortic origin of a coronary artery repair in a pediatric cohort. *J Thorac Cardiovasc Surg* 147:1580–1586, 2014.
66. Rinaldi RG, Carballido J, Giles R, et al: Right coronary artery with anomalous origin and slit ostium. *Ann Thorac Surg* 58:828–832, 1994.
67. Pedra SR, Pedra CA, Abizaid AA, et al: Intracoronary ultrasound assessment late after the arterial switch operation for transposition of the great arteries. *J Am Coll Cardiol* 45:2061–2068, 2005.
68. Liberthson RR, Sagar K, Berkoben JP, et al: Congenital coronary arteriovenous fistula. Report of 13 patients, review of the literature and delineation of management. *Circulation* 59:849–854, 1979.
69. McNamara JJ, Gross RE: Congenital coronary artery fistula. *Surgery* 65:59–69, 1969.
70. Koenig PR, Kimball TR, Schwartz DC: Coronary artery fistula complicating the evaluation of Kawasaki disease. *Pediatr Cardiol* 14:179–180, 1993.
71. Davis JT, Allen HD, Wheller JJ, et al: Coronary artery fistula in the pediatric age group: a 19-year institutional experience. *Ann Thorac Surg* 58:760–763, 1994.
72. Fernandes ED, Kadivar H, Hallman GL, et al: Congenital malformations of the coronary arteries: the Texas Heart Institute experience. *Ann Thorac Surg* 54:732–740, 1992.
73. Lowe JE, Oldham HN, Sabiston DC: Surgical management of congenital coronary artery fistulas. *Ann Surg* 194:373–380, 1981.
74. Reidy JF, Anjos RT, Qureshi SA, et al: Transcatheter embolization in the treatment of coronary artery fistulas. *J Am Coll Cardiol* 18:187–192, 1991.
75. Mavroudis C, Backer CL, Rocchini AP, et al: Coronary artery fistulas in infants and children: a surgical review and discussion of coil embolization. *Ann Thorac Surg* 63:1235–1242, 1997.

76. Farooki ZQ, Nowlen T, Hakimi M, et al: Congenital coronary artery fistulae: a review of 18 cases with special emphasis on spontaneous closure. *Pediatr Cardiol* 14:208–213, 1993.
77. Blanche C, Chaux A: Long-term results of surgery for coronary artery fistulas. *Int Surg* 75:238–239, 1990.
78. Musiani A, Cernigliaro C, Sansa M, et al: Left main coronary artery atresia: literature review and therapeutical considerations. *Eur J Cardiothorac Surg* 11:505–514, 1997.
79. Chou HH, Chan CH, Tsai KT, et al: Congenital atresia of the left main coronary artery associated with patent ductus arteriosus and aortic regurgitation. *Circ J* 73:1163–1166, 2009.
80. Kaczorowski DJ, Sathanandam S, Ravishankar C, et al: Coronary ostioplasty for congenital atresia of the left main coronary artery ostium. *Ann Thorac Surg* 94:1307–1310, 2012.
81. Amaral F, Tanamati C, Granzotti JA, et al: Congenital atresia of the ostium of the left coronary artery: diagnostic difficulty and successful surgical revascularization in two patients. *Arq Bras Cardiol* 74:339–342, 2000.
82. Shen TC, Chou HH, Tsai KT: Ectopic and atretic ostium of the left main coronary artery: from interleaflet triangle between left and noncoronary cusps. *Tex Heart Inst J* 39:60–62, 2012.
83. Varghese P, Leanage RU, Peek GJ: Congenital atresia of the ostium of the left main coronary artery: a rare coronary anomaly, diagnostic difficult and successful surgical revascularization. *Congenit Heart Dis* 2:347–350, 2007.
84. Bonnet D, Bonhoeffer P, Sidi D, et al: Surgical angioplasty of the main coronary arteries in children. *J Thorac Cardiovasc Surg* 117:352–357, 1999.
85. Imamura M, Dossey AM, Jaquiss RDB: Reoperation and mechanical circulatory support after repair of anomalous origin of the left coronary artery from the pulmonary artery: a twenty-year experience. *Ann Thorac Surg* 92:167–173, 2011.
86. Mainwaring RD, Redd VM, Reinhartz O, et al: Anomalous aortic origin of a coronary artery: medium-term results after surgical repair in 50 patients. *Ann Thorac Surg* 92:691–697, 2011.

CHAPTER 125

TRANSPOSITION OF THE GREAT ARTERIES: SIMPLE AND COMPLEX FORMS

Frank A. Pigula • Pedro J. del Nido

CHAPTER OUTLINE

HISTORY

Transposition of the great arteries (TGA) was first recognized and described more than 2 centuries ago. Although reference was made to malposition of the aorta and pulmonary artery by Steno in 1672 and Morgagni in 1761, the anatomic description of TGA is credited to Baillie in 1797.[1] It was Farre in 1814 who introduced the term *transposition of aorta and pulmonary artery*, meaning that the aorta and pulmonary artery are displaced across the ventricular septum.[2] An attempt to classify the various types of transposition was reported by von Rokitansky, and the first clinical recognition of TGA in life was noted by Fanconi in 1932.[3,4] In 1938, Taussig described the pathologic anatomy and hemodynamic and clinical characteristics of the cardiac defect.[5]

With the development of cardiac surgery in the 1950s, effective therapy for this disease is relatively new. Initial treatments were palliative and included atrial septectomy, first described by Blalock and Hanlon.[6] The first successful attempts to reroute the circulations were at the atrial level. These attempts were followed later by successful arterial level repair and correction of TGA and ventricular septal defect (VSD). These developments are further described in this chapter.

EPIDEMIOLOGY

Today TGA is known to be relatively common, accounting for 9.9% of infants with congenital heart disease, or 0.206 of 1000 live births, in one New England study.[7] The 2 : 1 male-to-female ratio increases to 3.3 : 1 when the ventricular septum is intact.[8] In complex forms of transposition, gender predominance has not been noted. If TGA is not treated, 90% of children with D-TGA (see Classification and Embryology section for explanation of D-TGA) and intact septum will die by 1 year of age.

CLASSIFICATION AND EMBRYOLOGY

TGA is generally classified as a type of conotruncal abnormality, a group of abnormalities that has a common theme of deranged development of the cardiac outflow tract. In this disease, there is ventriculoarterial discordance—the aorta arises from the right ventricle and the pulmonary artery from the left ventricle. The more common form of the disease is associated with otherwise normal cardiac structural relationships, including normal ventricular (D) looping. There is atrioventricular concordance but ventriculoarterial discordance {S,D,D}. This set of relationships is commonly referred to as D-transposition (D-TGA). In this form of TGA, the aorta is, by definition, anterior and to the right of the pulmonary artery. This pattern results in the systemic and pulmonary circulations performing in parallel rather than in series. As a consequence, deoxygenated blood is continuously pumped to the body and never passes through the lungs, and oxygenated blood is recirculated through the lungs and does not supply the rest of the body. For the patient to survive, there must be an obligatory shunt elsewhere, usually at the level of the atrial septum, that allows mixing of oxygenated and deoxygenated blood.

Although some have used the term *transposition* to describe a discordant ventriculoarterial connection, other authors have used this term to describe any heart in which the aorta is anterior to the pulmonary artery. The term *TGA* has also been used to describe some patients with double-inlet ventricle or absent atrioventricular connection and patients with nonlateralized atrial arrangements (some heterotaxy syndromes). *D-TGA* has been used to describe a concordant atrioventricular and discordant ventriculoarterial arrangement, but this nomenclature does not adequately describe patients in whom the aorta is anterior and to the left of the pulmonary artery. Thus, in this chapter, complete TGA is defined as normal atrial situs, atrioventricular concordance, and ventriculoarterial discordance.

Several theories have been advanced regarding the morphogenesis of the abnormal relationship between the great arteries and the ventricles in patients with TGA. It has been suggested that the subaortic conus persists and develops during normal looping of the ventricles while the subpulmonary conus undergoes absorption and thus establishes eventual fibrous continuity between the mitral and pulmonary valves, the reverse of the normal situation.[9] In the normal heart, the subaortic conus does not grow, and dominant growth of the pulmonary conus forces the pulmonary valve anterior, superior, and to the left. In transposition, differential growth of the subaortic conus pushes the aorta anteriorly and disrupts aortic to mitral valve continuity. If the subpulmonary conus fails to develop, the pulmonary artery will maintain a posterior location and pulmonary to mitral valve continuity will occur. As a consequence of this relationship, the aortic valve becomes anterior to the pulmonary valve, permitting both semilunar valves to connect with the distal great vessels without the rotation that is hypothesized to occur in normal cardiac development. Because conal development determines rotation of the truncus arteriosus, the great arteries are similar in relationship at the semilunar valves as they are at the arch, resulting in no twist in the great arteries.

Some debate also exists about the relationship between the various conotruncal abnormalities, which include tetralogy of Fallot and double-outlet right ventricle. Recent evidence suggests that TGA may be unique in that it is not seen in the spectrum of conotruncal abnormalities generated from the most common experimental model of these disorders.[10] A new animal model, which is the most reliable to date for producing isolated D-TGA, suggests that TGA may be the result of abnormal migration of neural crest cells during a critical phase of outflow tract development.[11]

ANATOMY

Anatomic variations in TGA can increase the surgical complexity of repair, described later in this chapter. Normal atrial situs occurs in 95% of patients, whereas left-to-right juxtaposition of the atrial appendages signals the presence of other intracardiac anomalies. Although a true ostium secundum atrial septal defect (ASD) is present in 10% to 20% of cases, most atrial communications are through a patent foramen ovale. Right aortic arch is present in 4% of patients with intact ventricular septum and up to 16% of those with VSD.[12] Up to 50% of patients with TGA have an associated VSD, many of which spontaneously close.[13] The VSDs are commonly perimembranous, although they may be found anywhere in the ventricular septum. Pulmonary stenosis or atresia, overriding or straddling atrioventricular valves, coarctation of the aorta, and interruption of the aortic arch have all been noted in association with transposition and VSD.

The spatial relationship of the great vessels is variable; however, the aorta is most frequently to the right and anterior to the pulmonary artery. In almost all cases, the sinuses of Valsalva and the coronary artery ostia face the corresponding pulmonary arterial sinuses. This situation is favorable for transfer of the coronary arteries with the arterial switch operation, although the origin of a coronary artery from a nonfacing sinus poses a problem for arterial switch in only a small number of patients. Many

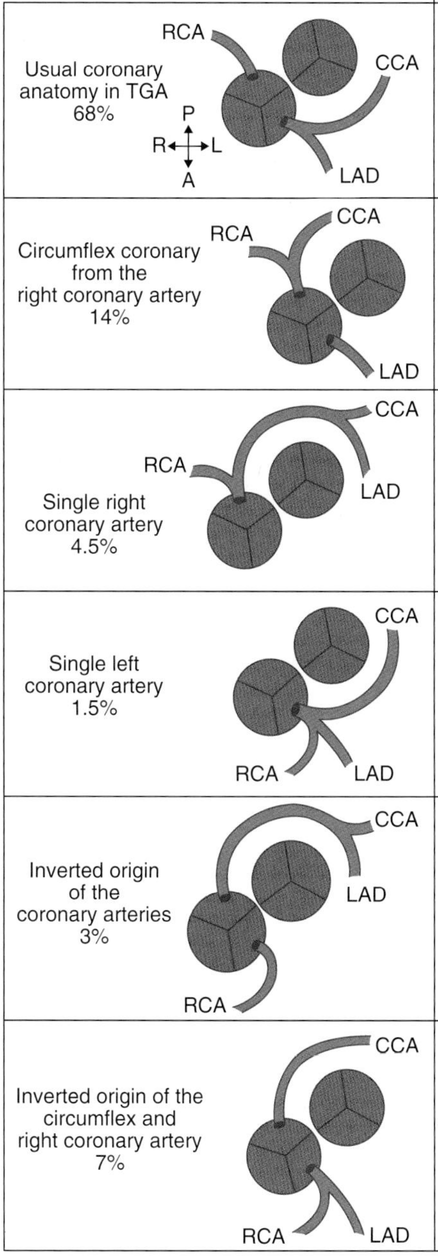

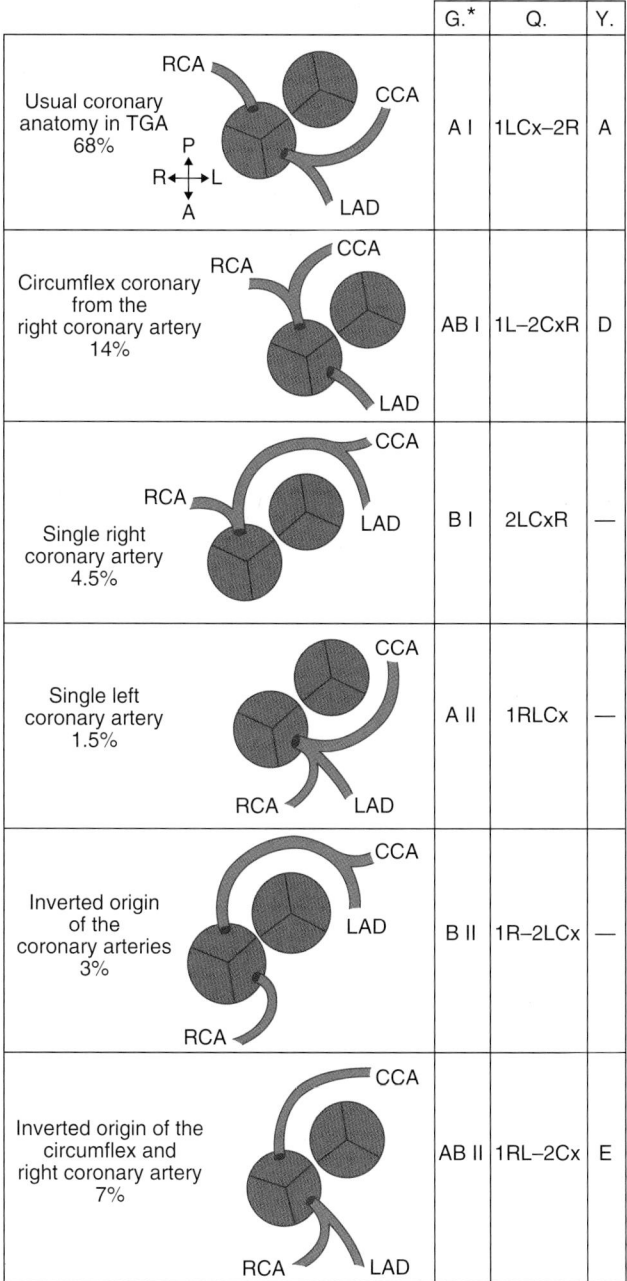

	G.*	Q.	Y.
Usual coronary anatomy in TGA 68%	A I	1LCx–2R	A
Circumflex coronary from the right coronary artery 14%	AB I	1L–2CxR	D
Single right coronary artery 4.5%	B I	2LCxR	—
Single left coronary artery 1.5%	A II	1RLCx	—
Inverted origin of the coronary arteries 3%	B II	1R–2LCx	—
Inverted origin of the circumflex and right coronary artery 7%	AB II	1RL–2Cx	E

*G., Gittenberger-de-Groot; Q., Quaegebeur; Y., Yacoub

FIGURE 125-1 The six most common types of coronary artery anatomy in transposition of the great arteries (TGA). Descriptive classification is on the left, and three simplified classification codes are on the right. *CCA,* Circumflex coronary artery; *LAD,* left anterior descending artery; *RCA,* right coronary artery.

classification systems have been used to describe the coronary anatomy in TGA. The most widely accepted scheme within the surgical community is the Leiden classification system, which is depicted with the other common systems of classification in Figure 125-1. The most common coronary pattern in D-TGA (68%) consists of the left main coronary arising from the leftward coronary sinus, giving rise to the left anterior descending and circumflex coronary arteries.[14] The right coronary artery arises as a separate ostium from the rightward posterior-facing sinus. Occasionally, there is no true circumflex coronary artery, but separate branches arise from the left coronary to supply the corresponding portion of the left ventricle. In up to 20% of cases, the circumflex coronary arises from the right coronary artery off the rightward posterior-facing sinus and passes behind the pulmonary artery. The left anterior descending artery then arises from a separate coronary ostium off the left coronary sinus. More rare coronary patterns involve a single right coronary artery from the rightward posterior sinus (4.5%) or a single left coronary artery from the leftward coronary sinus (1.5%).[15] Intramural coronary arteries that proceed in the aortic wall for a distance before exiting to the epicardial surface have been described and commonly occur at the commissural attachment of the semilunar valve.[16] A single coronary ostium or separate ostia close together arising from a single sinus have also been described. Abnormal coronary anatomy is more commonly seen in transposition with VSD than in the intact septum variety. Abnormal coronary patterns have also been found to be more common when the relationship of the great arterial trunks is not usual (aorta anterior and to the right).[17]

CLINICAL FEATURES

In complete TGA, the pulmonary and systemic circulations exist in parallel instead of in series. This results in nonoxygenated venous blood passing through the right ventricle to the aorta while the oxygenated pulmonary venous blood passes through the left ventricle back to the pulmonary arterial circulation. Mixing between the pulmonary and systemic circulations through a patent foramen ovale or ASD, a VSD, or a patent ductus arteriosus (PDA) is mandatory for survival. Patients with TGA and an intact ventricular septum survive initially because of aortopulmonary flow through a PDA. After birth, both ventricles are relatively noncompliant, and infants with TGA often have an increased pulmonary blood flow, which causes enlargement of the left atrium and functional incompetence of the foramen ovale, resulting in atrial-level mixing of oxygenated and nonoxygenated blood. Inadequacy of this mixing, however, may result in only marginal tissue oxygenation, which does not improve with oxygen administration.

Patients with TGA and significant VSD often have higher oxygen saturations by virtue of greater pulmonary blood flow and greater mixing at both atrial and ventricular levels. In children with high pulmonary blood flow, pulmonary resistance may progressively increase throughout infancy. Ferencz has observed significant histologic changes in children older than 2 years of age with TGA, and children as young as 1 month of age have had intimal fibrosis noted in the pulmonary arteries.[18] This early development of severe pulmonary vascular disease in children with TGA is exacerbated in patients with associated VSD, but early important pulmonary vascular disease can occur in patients with TGA regardless of the presence of a VSD as demonstrated by Ferguson in 1960 and Ferencz in 1966.[18,19] The rapidity of development of pulmonary obstructive disease may be related to

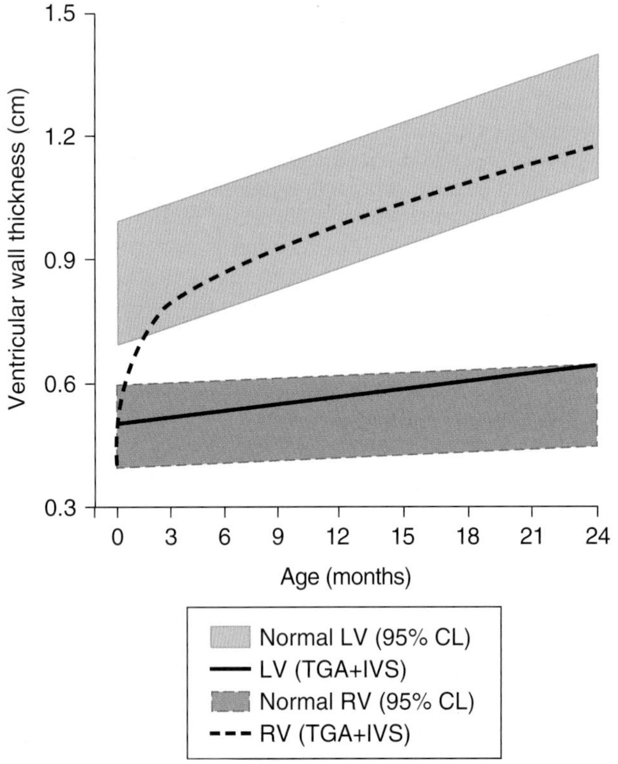

FIGURE 125-2 ■ The normal left ventricular (LV) wall thickness in transposition of the great arteries (TGA) after birth. The *solid line* shows the decreased development of LV mass in TGA that results from a rapid decrease in pulmonary vascular resistance and drop in LV pressure. The *upper bar* shows an increase in LV thickness with normally related great arteries. The *dashed line* shows the similar increase in right ventricular (RV) muscle mass over time in TGA. *CL*, Confidence limits; *IVS*, intact ventricular septum.

hypoxemia associated with increased sympathetic activity and in association with excessive pulmonary blood flow.[20]

Although neonatal pulmonary vascular resistance is normal in infants with TGA, the resistance falls progressively during the neonatal period with associated changes in the pulmonary and systemic ventricular compliance. Shortly after birth in the normal infant, there is an increase in the left ventricular volume load and pressure load and a decrease in right ventricular volume and pressure load. These physiologic changes result in a rapid increase in the left ventricular myocardial mass.[21] This normal development of the left ventricle is lost in infants with D-TGA where the left ventricle ejects to the lower resistance pulmonary vascular bed (Fig. 125-2). Thus, the left ventricle does not increase muscle mass relative to the right ventricle, and within a few weeks it loses the ability to maintain adequate cardiac output against significant afterload. This change occurs despite the fact that the left ventricle still maintains a volume load in patients with transposition and an intact ventricular septum. When, however, a VSD or large PDA is present, both volume and pressure overload of the left ventricle is maintained, and in D-TGA with left ventricular outflow tract (LVOT) obstruction without a VSD, a ventricular pressure load is imposed without a significant volume load. These physiologic changes in the neonatal heart are important for the consideration of surgical approaches because after a few weeks to months of postuterine life, the left ventricle in D-TGA with intact ventricular septum takes on the characteristics and wall thickness of a pulmonary ventricle and may not be adequate to support the systemic circulation.

The most common clinical finding in the infant with TGA is cyanosis (arterial PO_2 of 25 to 40 mm Hg), which will vary in degree depending on associated anomalies. Typically, the cyanosis is more pronounced when the ventricular septum is intact and is often present at birth. The development of cyanosis later in infancy is usually associated with the presence of a significant VSD. Congestive heart failure may be the predominant clinical finding in patients with a large VSD or PDA, and the combination of cyanosis and increased pulmonary blood flow is almost pathognomonic of TGA in the infant. Symptoms of cardiac failure rarely present in the first week of life but commonly appear by 1 month of age as pulmonary vascular resistance decreases and pulmonary blood flow becomes excessive, even in the patient with an intact ventricular septum.

DIAGNOSIS

Physical Examination

Cardiac examination typically reveals a mildly overactive precordium, and 75% of patients with TGA and an intact ventricular septum have a soft systolic murmur. The second heart sound is typically single and loud because of the proximity of the aorta to the anterior chest wall, which may make assessment of pulmonary vascular resistance difficult.[20] End-diastolic gallop rhythms are often noted in patients with associated VSD. In the presence of a large PDA, the femoral pulses are often bounding. The liver may be enlarged in patients with a large systemic-to-pulmonary shunt and may be associated with tachypnea, intercostal retractions, and inability to successfully nurse. Children with significant valvular or subvalvular pulmonary stenosis often have a crescendo-decrescendo cardiac murmur along the left sternal border transmitted to the right clavicular area.

Diagnostic Studies

The electrocardiogram may be normal at birth but over time shows signs of increasing right ventricular or biventricular hypertrophy. Chest x-ray findings in D-TGA include an egg-shaped cardiac configuration, narrow superior mediastinum, and increased pulmonary markings with cardiomegaly.

The widespread use of fetal ultrasound techniques has resulted in the common antenatal diagnosis of TGA. This fact and the fact that most children with TGA are cyanotic in the first week of life have led to the initiation of treatment at a very early age. Whereas in the past, cardiac catheterization was generally necessary to confirm the diagnosis of TGA and to demonstrate the position of the cardiac chambers and the associated lesions, echocardiography is now usually all that is necessary in most cases. Echocardiographic views confirming a posterior

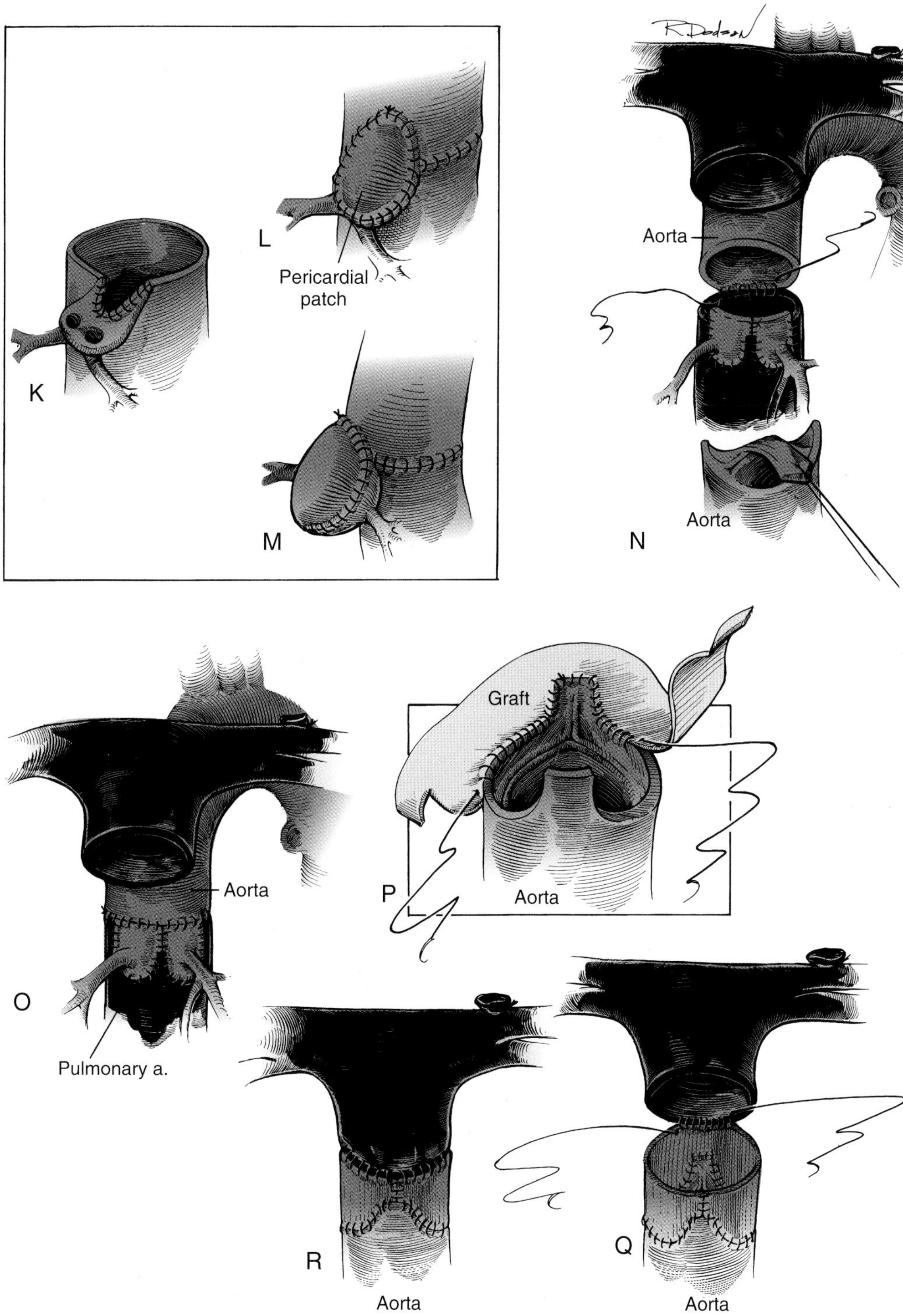

FIGURE 125-5, cont'd ■ **K,** If right and left intramural coronary arteries are present, the aortic coronary flap is left in place and sutured along the cephalic border to an incision in the anterior neoaorta. **L** and **M,** A pericardial patch is then used to provide unrestricted entrance of blood into the coronary ostia. **N,** After completion of the coronary transfer, the distal aorta is anastomosed to the neoaorta. **O,** The pulmonary bifurcation is brought anterior to the aorta in the Lecompte maneuver. **P,** The defect in the aorta from which the coronary arteries have been excised is augmented with a pantaloon-shaped patch of pericardium. **Q,** The pulmonary bifurcation is then anastomosed to the augmented aorta. In most cases, pericardium is not sutured completely around the aorta to create a complete pericardial tube. **R,** Completed anastomosis of the pulmonary artery anterior to the new aorta.

In most series, reoperation is most commonly indicated for right ventricular outflow tract (RVOT) lesions, which may occur in up to approximately 10% of patients.[53,54] However, technical modifications to the procedure are thought to be responsible for a reduction in reoperation for RVOT obstruction to less than 2% to 3%. More long-term follow-up data are now available on children undergoing neonatal arterial switch. Prifti and colleagues reported the results of a large series of patients with a mean follow-up of 3.5 years. The early mortality rate was 12.7% but significantly lower (5.7%) for those children with isolated TGA. Actuarial survival rates were 98%, 93%, and 91.5% at 1, 3, and 5 years, respectively, after surgery. Freedom from reoperation was 95%, 90.5%, and 83% at the same time points. The presence of a VSD adversely affected survival. Predictors of reintervention included VSD, coronary anomalies, aortic coarctation, and LVOT obstruction or moderate pulmonary stenosis.[55] Another series of 181 patients with a mean follow-up of 5.8 years revealed a 5.5% early mortality rate and 92% survival rate at 5 and 10 years. VSD was a risk factor for early and late death.[56] The largest series in the literature with long-term follow-up was reported in 2001 and included data on 1095 patients from a single institution. Mean follow-up was approximately 5 years. Early mortality was 8.6%. Survival was 89% at 1 year and 88% at 10 and 15 years (including those patients who died early). Simple TGA was found to be associated with improved survival (92% vs. 80% for complex TGA). Freedom from reintervention was 90%, 83%, and 82% at 5, 10, and 15 years, respectively, of follow-up.[57]

Although the early mortality rate seems high in some of the larger series that include earlier results, the current operative mortality rate is approximately 2% to 3%.[58-60] Analysis of large series found complex anatomy (large VSD, multiple VSDs, Taussig-Bing anomaly but not aortic coarctation), coronary anomalies, previous operation, and prolonged bypass time to be risk factors for early death.[58] Another study identified female gender and preoperative instability as risk factors for operative mortality and suggested that in the current era, abnormal coronary patterns were less of a factor. A recent review of contemporary data (1999-2005) reported that coronary anatomy was not a factor affecting survival and that factors affecting mortality included gestational age less than 36 weeks and bypass time less than 150 minutes.[61]

Although this seems to be true, a single coronary ostium and intramural coronary course are still risk factors for mortality in some studies.[62] Coronary artery–related problems are the most common cause of early death, followed by right ventricular failure and pulmonary hypertension.[60] It has been suggested that risk factors for late death include an unusual relationship of the great vessels, single coronary ostium, prolonged bypass time, and coarctation of the aorta, although none of these proved to be significant in a multivariate analysis.[58]

Cardiac rhythm abnormalities are unusual after arterial switch operation with over 90% of patients in normal sinus rhythm. Left ventricular function is generally normal. Most patients (>95%) are in NYHA functional class I at long-term follow-up.[59] Aortic stenosis is very rare, and mild aortic insufficiency is seen in approximately 10% of patients. Although there was initial concern that the neoaortic root dilated disproportionately, raising the concern of progressive aortic insufficiency, longitudinal analysis has shown that the neoaorta undergoes dilation during the first year of life but then tends toward the normal size as further growth occurs.[63] Pulmonary stenosis is seen slightly more frequently.[56] Very few patients are taking cardiac medications at midterm follow-up.[60,64] Late coronary artery problems are rare.

Late Follow-up. A recent review of long-term outcomes compared those of the arterial switch operation to those of the Mustard and Senning atrial switch operations.[65] It was reported that the change from the atrial to the arterial switch in 1983 has led to improved long-term survival (Fig. 125-6) but that reoperation rates are similar. Interestingly, the reoperations performed following the arterial switch operation were predominately targeting RVOT lesions, but approximately 2% of patients required aortic valve replacement. Importantly, systemic ventricular dysfunction occurred in 9.1% of patients after atrial switch but only 0.4% of patients after the arterial switch.

Whereas early and long-term survival favors the arterial switch operation, the late neurologic outcome has been investigated. Despite evidence of neurologic impairment 3 to 4 years after arterial switch operation, these effects showed moderation at later follow-up.[66] More long-term longitudinal follow-up of patients entered into the Boston circulatory arrest study has shown a gradual moderation in developmental disabilities manifest in early childhood.[67,68] Although this group shows that behavioral dysfunction (attention and executive functions) persists among these patients, few differences were found to be attributable to the method of operative treatment. This underscores the increasing awareness that children treated for congenital heart disease are at increased risk for behavioral and neuropsychiatric disabilities well into their childhood.[69]

In summary, outcomes after arterial switch are generally very good. Follow-ups to date suggest that, as expected, the results are superior to atrial switch operations in terms of late ventricular function, freedom from arrhythmias, and functional status. The rapidly decreasing mortality for arterial switch operations has resulted in this surgical approach becoming the standard corrective surgical procedure at the present time and results in both an anatomic and a physiologic reconstruction of this cardiac defect.

Fate of the Neoaortic Valve and Late Coronary Lesions. The arterial switch operation is generally considered a corrective operation because no future operations are planned. However, several longitudinal studies are reporting a significant rate of reoperation. Reoperation on the RVOT is generally the most common indication and is related to inadequate growth at the neopulmonary anastomotic site. However, progressive neoaortic dilation and late coronary artery lesions are also being recognized as potential surgical problems.

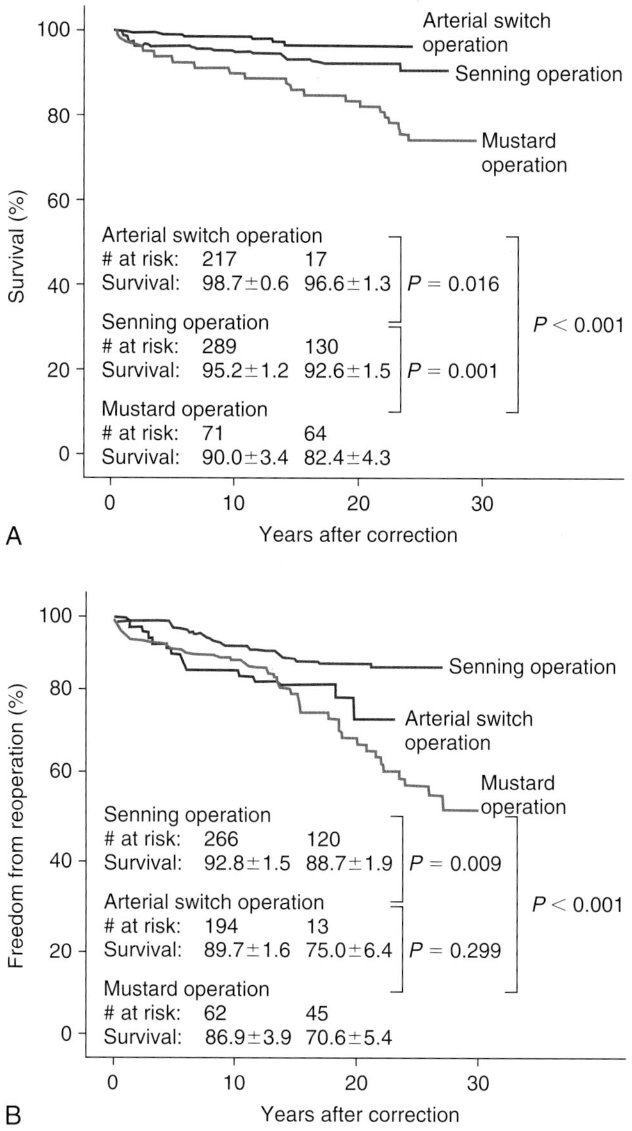

FIGURE 125-6 ■ **A,** Estimated survival among 929 hospital survivors after correction, stratified by type of operation: Senning versus Mustard versus arterial switch. **B,** Estimated freedom from reoperation among survivors, stratified by type of operation: Senning versus Mustard versus arterial switch. (From Horer, J, Schreiber C, Cleuziou J, et al: Improvement in long-term survival after hospital discharge but not in freedom from reoperation after the change from atrial to arterial switch for transposition of the great arteries. *Thorac Cardiovasc Surg* 137:347–354, 2009.)

In a recent review, Schwartz and coworkers reported that aortic root dilation (z-score > 3) is common after arterial switch operation, affecting approximately 50% of survivors at 10 years. Root dilation did not necessarily translate into aortic insufficiency—only approximately 7% of patients demonstrated significant aortic insufficiency (moderate or greater). However, approximately 5% of patients required neoaortic valve or root surgery at 10 years. The authors reported that older age at the time of repair, VSD, and a previous pulmonary artery band were independent risk factors for aortic insufficiency in these patients.[70] Longer-term follow-up has similarly shown that aortic root dilation is present in 66% of patients 20 years after arterial switch operation but that surgery on the neoaortic root or valve remains uncommon. It is important to note that left ventricular function is preserved in these patients.[71]

A recent review of a European center's experience reported an incidence of aortic insufficiency that increased with time, with 2% of patients requiring aortic valve replacement an average of 11 years after the arterial switch operation. Independent risk factors identified for late aortic valve replacement were the presence of LVOT obstruction and aortic insufficiency at 1 year.[72]

Although coronary issues are thought to be rare among hospital survivors after the arterial switch operation, Raisky and colleagues found that coronary lesions were detectable in 12% of survivors undergoing coronary angiography an average of 33 months after arterial switch. Forty-five percent of angiographically documented coronary lesions were observed in the absence of ischemia as assessed clinically and by myocardial perfusion imaging. Of the 55% of patients undergoing revascularization, 17 of 19 revascularized lesions resided within the left coronary system. Whereas 16 of 19 patients were treatable with angioplasty, 3 underwent surgical revascularization without any mortality.[73]

Because of the excellent results obtained with the neonatal arterial switch operation, this has become the standard of care. However, there are occasions when the diagnosis of TGA with intact ventricular septum might be delayed, or when no surgery is immediately available, and late arterial switch operation is considered. In general, primary arterial switch operation within 3 weeks of life is noncontroversial. However, because of progressive deconditioning of the postnatal pulmonary left ventricle, primary arterial switch operation has been considered high risk, and rapid two-stage arterial switch operation has been advocated by some. However, several groups have reported that the rapid two-stage arterial switch operation results in impaired left ventricular contractility in up to 25% of patients, an increased incidence of neoaortic insufficiency, and RVOT obstruction. Bisoi and associates reported the combined early mortality rate of the rapid two-stage arterial switch operation is higher than that for the late primary arterial switch operation (55% vs. 14%).[74-77]

These results have prompted groups to perform primary arterial switch operation on children presenting later in infancy. When Kang and colleagues reported their outcomes for 105 patients undergoing late primary arterial switch operation (older than 3 weeks), they found no difference in hospital mortality (3.8% vs. 5.5%) or ECMO (5.7% vs. 3.6%) when compared to early primary arterial switch operation.[78]

Similar results have been published by Edwin and coworkers, who reported no mortality (two ECMO) in six patients undergoing primary arterial switch operation between the ages of 31 and 66 days.[79]

These experiences suggest that the rapid two-stage arterial switch operation may be unnecessary for most patients presenting well into infancy and that primary arterial switch operation, with ECMO backup, is justifiable.

COMPLEX TRANSPOSITION

Anatomic Variants of Transposition of the Great Arteries

Although discordant relationship between the ventricles and great vessels is an integral component of transposition, associated defects often dominate the clinical presentation and management of these infants. The term *complex transposition* refers to those defects in which there are conotruncal anomalies in addition to TGA. The associated conotruncal defects include malalignment or deviation of the conal septum into either the LVOT or RVOT or persistence of a conus over the left ventricle separating the mitral valve from the semilunar valve, also called the Taussig-Bing anomaly. Together these complex forms account for 10% to 15% of all transposition cases.[80]

Conal Septum

The conal septum separates the two semilunar valves and forms part of the septation of the common arterial trunk, present early in fetal cardiac development, into the aorta and the pulmonary trunk. Although abnormal development of the conus with regression of the subpulmonary component rather than the subaortic component has been proposed as the cause of transposition, the position, orientation, and size of the conal septum may vary independent of ventriculoarterial connection.[81] Thus, a prominent conal septum that deviates posteriorly can cause left ventricular outflow obstruction; similarly, anterior deviation of the conal septum can result in right ventricular outflow obstruction. In hearts with normally related great arteries, when the conal deviation is associated with a conoventricular septal defect, the downstream consequences of the ventricular outflow obstruction are hypoplasia or atresia of the affected great artery as seen in interrupted aortic arch (left ventricular outflow obstruction) and tetralogy of Fallot (right ventricular outflow obstruction). In transposition, however, the affected downstream circulation is the inverse with left ventricular outflow obstruction resulting in decreased pulmonary trunk blood flow and right ventricular outflow obstruction resulting in aortic arch hypoplasia, interruption, or both.[82,83]

Transposition and Left Ventricular Outflow Tract Obstruction

LVOT obstruction in an infant with TGA can occur in the presence or absence of a VSD. In patients with an intact ventricular septum, most often the pressure gradient measured across the outflow tract is a result of dynamic displacement of the interventricular septum posteriorly as a result of the pressure difference between the right (systemic) and left (pulmonary) ventricles, with the latter functioning at lower pressures.

Once the left ventricle assumes the systemic circulation following an arterial switch, the septum usually bows toward the right ventricle and the pressure gradient disappears. A fixed obstruction from a prominent conal septum deviated posteriorly or a fibrous ridge or muscle bundle is uncommon in the absence of a conoventricular septal defect and, in most cases, can be resected and does not preclude an arterial switch operation.

LVOT obstruction in the presence of a conoventricular septal defect most often results from posterior deviation of the conal septum. In long-standing obstruction, a fibrous ridge or even fibromuscular tunnel can develop, further increasing the degree of obstruction. The obstruction is usually subvalvar but can be associated with pulmonary valve hypoplasia or dysplasia (bicuspid valve and/or thickened leaflets) precluding the use of this valve for an arterial switch procedure. The degree of obstruction in LVOT obstruction with a VSD is often more severe than in TGA with intact septum, and the obstruction often progresses early in infancy during the first few months of life requiring surgical intervention because of progressive cyanosis.

Transposition and Right Ventricular Outflow Tract Obstruction

Similar to LVOT obstruction, deviation of the conal septum, in this case anteriorly into the RVOT, is the most common cause of obstruction to flow into the systemic circulation. In transposition, RVOT obstruction is almost always associated with a malalignment-type conoventricular septal defect and is also frequently associated with double-outlet right ventricle, also called Taussig-Bing anomaly. In this latter defect, there is persistence of a conus or infundibulum under the pulmonary trunk, resulting in muscular separation between the mitral and pulmonary valve annulus. This complex lesion accounts for 5% to 7% of transposition cases based on autopsy series.[84] Associated defects include downstream hypoplasia of the aortic valve and aortic arch with coarctation. In some infants, the degree of aortic valve and arch hypoplasia is severe, requiring maintenance of a patent arterial duct to achieve adequate systemic perfusion. Hypoplasia of the right ventricle and tricuspid valve has also been described in this complex to a degree that a two-ventricle repair was not possible.[85] Often enlargement of the RVOT is necessary in conjunction with an arterial switch operation to prevent the development of subpulmonary obstruction. Hypoplasia of the aortic valve annulus in transposition can vary in degree and in severe forms requires a transannular patch along with an arterial switch to relieve right ventricular outflow obstruction.

In most cases of RVOT obstruction and transposition, there is a significant mismatch in diameter between the pulmonary trunk and the ascending aorta. This fact complicates the arterial switch procedure because enlargement of the ascending aorta and, if aortic arch hypoplasia is present, enlargement of the entire transverse arch and isthmus are required to achieve a hemodynamically satisfactory result.

Double-Outlet Right Ventricle with Transposition

Double-outlet right ventricle with TGA is often termed *double-outlet right ventricle with subpulmonary VSD* to

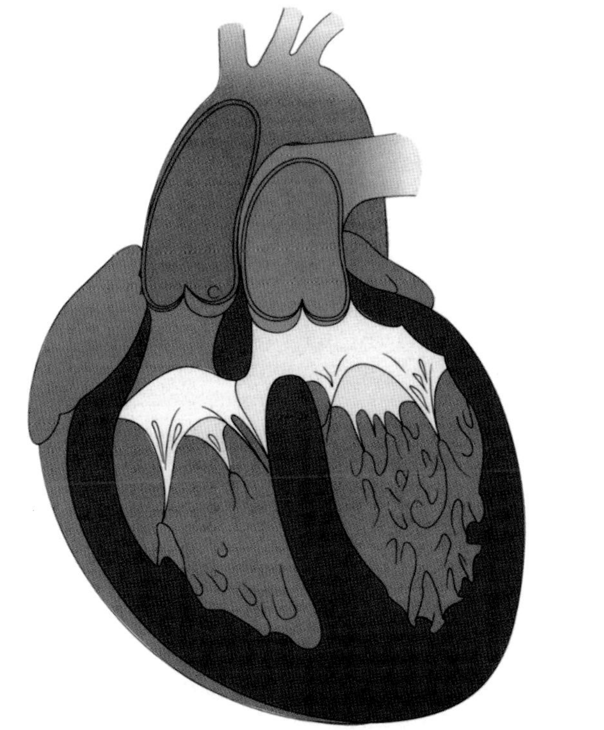

FIGURE 125-7 ■ Transposition with double-outlet right ventricle. The conal septum is positioned over the right ventricle. In cases in which there is deviation of the conal septum from this neutral position, the outflow semilunar valve and great artery often are hypoplastic.

describe the great vessel relationship to the right ventricle and to the VSD. Unlike double-outlet right ventricle with normally related great arteries, the vessel closest to the VSD in this case is the pulmonary trunk and determines the method of anatomic repair required for correction. Subpulmonary or subaortic obstruction can be associated with transposition and double-outlet right ventricle, usually resulting in hypoplasia of the downstream semilunar valve and great vessel. The relationship of the great vessels to each other often is that of a side-by-side arrangement with the aorta most commonly to the right of the pulmonary valve.

The VSD is described as a malalignment type because the conal septum does not meet the septomarginal trabecula, similar to double-outlet right ventricle with normally related great vessels (Fig. 125-7). The VSD can extend to the annulus of the tricuspid valve, and in these cases, the conduction tissue runs on the edge of the VSD in the posterocaudal margin of the defect starting at the junction with the tricuspid valve annulus.[86] In some cases, the VSD can extend to the inlet septum; this complicates the repair because the defect is partially covered by the septal leaflet of the tricuspid valve. In such cases, chordae from the tricuspid valve can attach to the crest of the septum and even straddle into the left ventricle. In most cases, however, the degree of straddling is limited and does not preclude a two-ventricle repair. Rarely, additional septal defects are present in the muscular septum or apical trabecular area, and these can be difficult to identify and close, particularly in the apical posterior septum.

Coronary Artery Anatomy

Coronary artery anatomy can also be variable with complex forms of transposition. Transposition and double-outlet right ventricle in particular is associated with unusual patterns of coronary artery anatomy, including a relatively high incidence of a single coronary artery giving rise to branches to both ventricles. The high association between side-by-side great vessels and unusual coronary artery pattern has been emphasized previously. In a detailed pathologic study, Uemura and associates found that a single coronary artery was present in 27% of hearts with a side-by-side great artery relationship.[87]

Gordillo and colleagues have also described a higher incidence of unusual coronary artery pattern in double-outlet right ventricle with a subpulmonary VSD.[88] Coronary anatomy continues to be an important factor in anatomic repair of transposition, however, only when an arterial switch is contemplated as part of the repair. Although in most larger centers coronary artery pattern is no longer a significant risk factor for death, it can complicate the surgical procedure and may result in a higher rate of complications.

Aortic Arch Anatomy

Aortic arch anomalies occur in 7% to 10% of infants with transposition and VSD. This association is more common when the pulmonary valve overrides the ventricular septum, particularly in double-outlet right ventricle and transposition. A wide spectrum of arch obstruction exists from discrete coarctation at the level of the ductus to hypoplasia of the distal arch and even aortic arch interruption. The degree of severity of arch hypoplasia is thought to be associated with the degree of subaortic obstruction, usually from anterior deviation of the outlet or conal septum into the right ventricular outflow. Additionally, there can be relative hypoplasia of the tricuspid valve in comparison with the mitral valve, and in extreme cases, the degree of hypoplasia of the tricuspid valve can preclude a two-ventricle repair. It is important to recognize this association. Preoperative measurements of the atrioventricular valves normalized to body surface area can be most helpful in deciding surgical management.

Diagnosis and Preoperative Management

Echocardiography is usually the initial diagnostic study performed when complex congenital heart defects are detected because it provides not only the anatomic detail required to plan surgical repair but also physiologic information on valve function, presence, location, and severity of obstructions to flow, particularly in the outflow tracts of the ventricles as well as the pulmonary arteries and arch vessels. As with all echocardiographic studies, a systematic evaluation of chambers, connections, inflow and outflow valves, and ventricular size and function is imperative, particularly with difficult defects such as complex transposition. In addition, specific anatomic details—such as the relationship of the pulmonary root to the VSD, conal septal position, coronary artery pattern, and chordal attachments of the atrioventricular valves with respect to the septum—are important for the development of a plan for surgical correction.

Cardiac catheterization is not required in most cases of complex transposition because echocardiography is usually sufficient to detail the anatomy and important physiologic features. Cardiac catheterization and angiography are therefore used to resolve specific questions where accurate pressure measurements are required, such as pulmonary artery pressures for calculation of pulmonary vascular resistance, or to measure the pressure gradient across a potentially restrictive VSD. Also, in cases in which a palliative procedure has been performed, catheterization and angiography are needed to identify potential anatomic distortion from the previous surgical interventions such as systemic-to-pulmonary shunts. Rarely is interventional catheterization required in infants unless there is a restrictive interatrial communication and inadequate mixing of blood from the pulmonary and systemic circuits, a situation more common in transposition with intact septum.

Transposition of the Great Arteries with Left Ventricular Outflow Tract Obstruction

Palliative Procedures. The pathophysiology of transposition results in cyanosis that often is unresponsive to oxygen therapy. When transposition is complicated by obstruction to the LVOT, cyanosis can be more severe, frequently worsening in the first few months of life. In the extreme, when there is atresia of the LVOT, pulmonary blood flow is entirely dependent on a patent arterial duct and/or systemic-to-pulmonary collaterals. In these cases, repair of this defect can be delayed by placing a systemic-to-pulmonary shunt and ligating collaterals or the arterial duct. The corrective procedure can then be deferred several months. In cases in which cyanosis is not severe, a systemic-to-pulmonary shunt is not indicated, and if delayed repair is contemplated, this can usually be deferred several weeks or months. The most common reason for delaying the corrective procedure is when resection of the left ventricular outflow is not feasible and a conduit will be required to establish right ventricle to pulmonary artery continuity (see Rastelli Operation section). The institutional philosophy at Children's Hospital Boston, however, is to achieve anatomic and physiologic correction of the cardiac defect as early in life as possible.

Surgical Technique. The preferred shunt procedure for TGA with LVOT obstruction is a modified Blalock shunt with an expanded polytetrafluoroethylene (PTFE) tube graft. In infants with a left aortic arch, the origin of the shunt is the base of the right subclavian artery, and the distal end connects to the right pulmonary artery. The surgical approach for a shunt is usually through a median sternotomy that provides access to the arch vessels and branch pulmonary arteries. The thymus gland is mobilized, and the innominate vein is freed from attachments to the pericardium and aorta. Because the course of the shunt will be parallel to the superior vena cava, tissue between the ascending aorta and superior cava must be cleared. Once the innominate artery and right subclavian origin are dissected, the right pulmonary artery is mobilized from its origin to the bifurcation of the upper lobe. Heparin (50 U/kg) is administered to prevent thrombus formation in the vessels or the graft during insertion. The caudal side of the innominate-subclavian artery junction is identified for the anastomosis, and a curved vascular clamp is used for occlusion. The anastomosis is done with fine monofilament sutures (7-0 polypropylene), and care is taken not to damage the fragile intima of the innominate artery. The distal end is sewn to the cephalad side of the pulmonary artery, also with fine monofilament sutures. De-airing of the graft is performed, and brisk flow through the graft should be confirmed prior to completing the distal anastomosis. The graft is usually 3.5 mm in diameter for neonates and young infants and provides adequate pulmonary blood flow for several months until corrective surgery is performed. In some centers, a larger shunt (4.0 mm) is chosen in an effort to gain more time with palliation. This approach, although effective, runs the risk of producing pulmonary overcirculation in the early period after shunt insertion with complications such as inadequate renal perfusion and renal insufficiency or necrotizing enterocolitis. If a larger shunt is used, great care must be taken in the early postoperative period to maintain adequate systemic perfusion to avoid these complications.

Once the shunt is unclamped, the oxygen saturations should rise within seconds confirming adequate shunt flow. An additional indicator is a modest fall in diastolic pressure. The ductus arteriosus is typically ligated. Once stable, a single chest drain is left in the pericardial space and the sternum is closed. Low-dose heparin (10 to 20 U/kg/hr) can be continued in the postoperative period once mediastinal bleeding has subsided.

Corrective Procedures. Management of the LVOT obstruction in transposition depends on the severity and location of the obstruction. In cases in which the obstruction appears dynamic from leftward deviation of the interventricular septum because of systemic pressure in the right ventricle, an arterial switch procedure with closure of a VSD, when present, is the preferred method of correction. In these cases, the pulmonary valve annulus is within the normal range for the child's size, and instantaneous gradient across the left ventricular outflow, as estimated by echo Doppler, is less than 35 to 40 mm Hg in the presence of a small or closed arterial duct.

Transposition of the Great Arteries with Posterior Deviation of Conal Septum

In most cases in which the conal septum is the major source of left ventricular outflow obstruction and the pulmonary valve is adequate (z-score of −2.5 or better), the resection of the conal septum with closure of the VSD (when present) and an arterial switch procedure is the best option. This approach establishes anatomic repair and avoids the use of conduits, although there is a small but present risk of developing more severe LVOT obstruction later. Resection of the subpulmonary obstruction is most often possible through the pulmonary trunk, by retracting the pulmonary valve leaflets. This approach also ensures adequate visualization of the hinge points of the leaflets because these can attach to the conal septum directly. The left ventricular outflow can also be seen through the mitral valve, although this approach is rarely better than through the pulmonary artery.

When the obstruction to the left ventricular outflow cannot be resected or is associated with pulmonary valve hypoplasia or severe dysplasia, the pulmonary root cannot be used to achieve a two-ventricle repair. In these cases, the aortic root arising from the right ventricular conus must be used for systemic flow and a conduit used to establish right ventricle to pulmonary artery continuity. There are two options to achieve this result: (1) the Rastelli operation, in which the aortic root is left attached to the right ventricle and left ventricular blood flow is diverted through the VSD to the aorta by means of a baffle, and (2) mobilization of the aortic root off the right ventricle, similar to a pulmonary autograft in normally related great vessels, and reimplantation of it into the opened left ventricular outflow, patch enlarging the left ventricular outflow and reimplanting the coronary arteries (autograft translocation and arterial switch operation). In both cases, a conduit is used to connect the right ventricle to the pulmonary artery bifurcation.

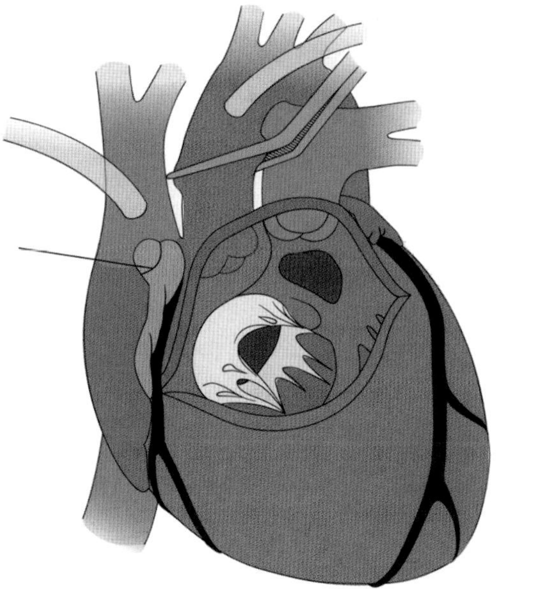

FIGURE 125-8 ■ Rastelli procedure. Right ventriculotomy to expose the ventricular septal defect and aortic valve.

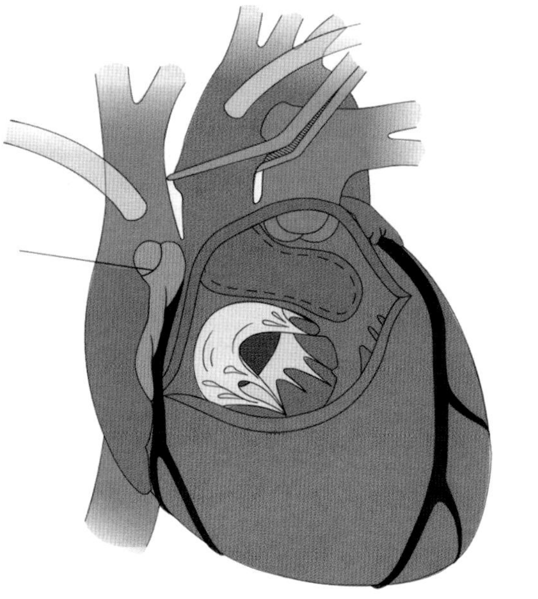

FIGURE 125-9 ■ Rastelli procedure. Baffle of left ventricular outflow through the ventricular septal defect to the rightward aorta.

Rastelli Operation. For cases in which a large conoventricular VSD is present, Rastelli and colleagues described a procedure in which a synthetic semicircular patch is sewn to the edge of the VSD inferiorly and around the aortic annulus, diverting left ventricular flow through the VSD to the aorta.[89] The pulmonary root is closed, and a conduit is inserted between the right ventricle and the pulmonary artery. Frequently the VSD must be enlarged to prevent subaortic obstruction, and as described by Rastelli, the conal septum should be resected. The approach is via a sternotomy harvesting a patch of pericardium to be treated with glutaraldehyde (0.6% for 10 to 15 minutes), which may be required for pulmonary artery augmentation or for the gusset connecting the right ventricle to the conduit anteriorly. The main pulmonary artery and branches are dissected and mobilized to the level of the upper lobe bifurcation, similar to an arterial switch. Arterial cannulation at or near the level of innominate artery facilitates retraction of the ascending aorta, and bicaval cannulation permits continuous bypass without the need for circulatory arrest. Because the aorta is frequently anterior and the VSD is conoventricular, an infundibular incision in the right ventricle provides access to the VSD for baffling and then becomes the proximal site for connection of the right ventricle to pulmonary artery conduit. The ventriculotomy should be oblique, aiming toward the leftward and superior corner of the right ventricular infundibulum (Fig. 125-8). Care must be taken to avoid opening too close to the left coronary artery because this vessel usually arises from the left-facing sinus of the aorta. The advantage gained by placing the ventriculotomy as leftward as possible is that the right ventricle to pulmonary artery conduit can then be placed to the left of midline, avoiding compression by the sternum. The VSD and conal septum can be seen easily through the ventriculotomy, and assessment is made regarding the need to enlarge the VSD. In conoventricular VSDs, conduction tissue runs on the inferior border of the VSD. Therefore, resection of the conal septum is safe, and the incision can be extended anteriorly to enlarge the VSD further if required. A tunnel-shaped synthetic patch (Dacron) is used to construct the baffle between the VSD and aortic annulus (Fig. 125-9). The pulmonary root can be closed through the ventriculotomy from the inside or from above once the pulmonary trunk is transected. The confluence of the pulmonary arteries should be mobilized to the left of the aorta as much as possible to facilitate connection with the right ventricle to pulmonary artery conduit and avoid right pulmonary artery compression by the large aortic root. Once the distal anastomosis is created, the posterior portion of the conduit is sewn to the distal edge of the ventriculotomy. The anterior portion of the connection is created with homograft patch if the distal segment of the graft is available or the treated pericardium harvested at the beginning of the procedure can be used. Once the patient is off bypass, careful evaluation must be made of the adequacy of the left ventricular outflow by intraoperative echocardiography or by direct pressure measurement through needle puncture of the left ventricular cavity pressure and ascending aorta. A gradient higher than 10 to 15 mm Hg should be addressed surgically because this will likely progress over time. The most common place for residual obstruction is at the midportion of the VSD patch because this area requires the widest diameter of the semicircular patch. Placement of an additional patch can be done without removing the original baffle in cases in which the residual obstruction is at the level of the baffle.

Alternative techniques to avoid the use of conduits for right ventricle to pulmonary artery connection have been described by Lecompte and Vouhé in which the pulmonary arteries are mobilized and placed anterior to the aorta and a primary connection is made between the transected pulmonary trunk and the ventriculotomy. This connection is augmented with autologous pericardium, avoiding the use of a prosthetic conduit or homograft that will require replacement with growth.[90,91]

Aortic Autograft Translocation and Arterial Switch. The potential long-term complications of the Rastelli operation are conduit obstruction, frequently caused by compression by the sternum because of the location of the conduit, or subaortic obstruction from a restrictive VSD or inadequate growth of the subaortic segment between the VSD and aortic annulus. To avoid these complications, an alternative procedure is to remove the aortic root from the infundibulum of the right ventricle, similar to a pulmonary autograft in normally related vessels (Fig. 125-10). Because this autograft is the

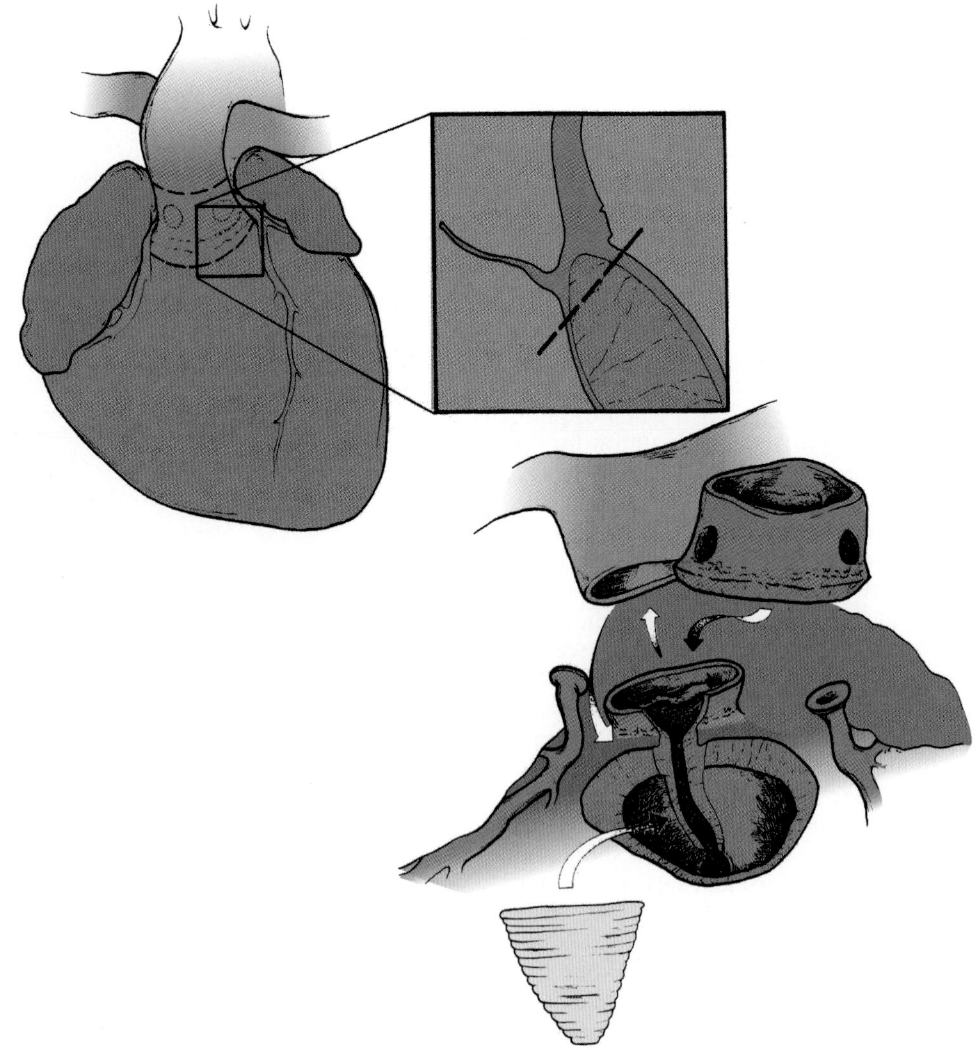

FIGURE 125-10 ■ Aortic root autograft. The aortic root is removed from the right ventricle in a manner similar to the method used for pulmonary root harvest for a pulmonary autograft procedure *(upper panel)*. Enlargement of the left ventricular outflow tract and closure of ventricular septal defect *(lower panel)*.

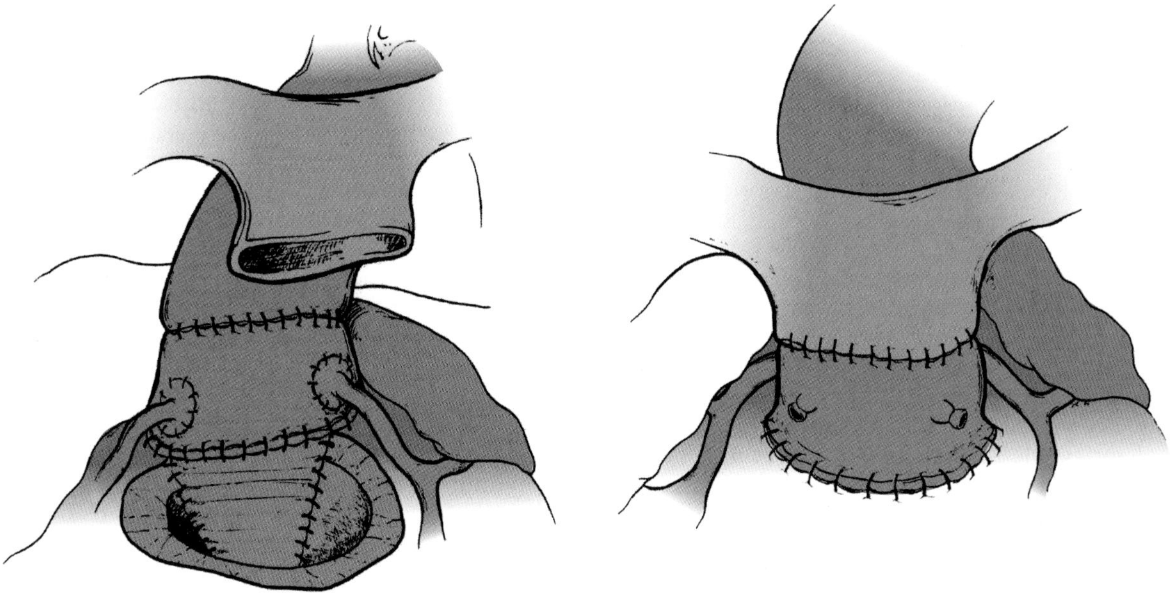

FIGURE 125-11 ■ Aortic root autograft. Right ventricle to pulmonary conduit, with the pulmonary arteries brought anterior to the aorta.

native aorta, the coronary arteries must be excised as circular buttons from the aortic root and mobilized away prior to resecting the aortic root. The left ventricular outflow can then be enlarged by incising across the conal septum into the existing VSD, or in cases in which there is no VSD or only a small restrictive defect, the incision is extended beyond the conal septum into the body of the left ventricle, similar to a Konno procedure.[92] The aortic root autograft is then sewn to the native left ventricular outflow posteriorly, and a triangular-shaped synthetic patch is used to close the VSD up to the level of the aortic autograft. The coronary arteries are then reimplanted into the aortic root in their new location posteriorly, similar to an arterial switch procedure. A homograft conduit is then inserted between the right ventricular infundibulum and the central pulmonary arteries to establish right ventricle to pulmonary artery continuity. The pulmonary arteries can be mobilized and placed anterior to the aorta, as in the Lecompte operation, or in cases where the great vessel relationship is more side-by-side, the conduit can be placed to one side of the aorta (Fig. 125-11). The advantages of the aortic root translocation and arterial switch procedure are that the LVOT is by necessity enlarged to the size of the aortic root, the position of the aortic root with relation to the left ventricular outflow is more anatomic and therefore less tortuous, and the right ventricle to pulmonary artery conduit is in the anatomic position with respect to the right ventricle and therefore less susceptible to compression by the sternum.

Transposition of the Great Arteries with Double-Outlet Right Ventricle

Subpulmonary Ventricular Septal Defect. Double-outlet right ventricle with a subpulmonary VSD is an uncommon form of transposition that is frequently associated with unusual coronary artery anatomy or aortic arch hypoplasia and coarctation. Subaortic stenosis from anterior deviation of the conal septum can also coexist with arch hypoplasia and at times requires a transannular patch to relieve the right ventricular outflow obstruction. When there is separation between the pulmonary valve and the mitral valve in double-outlet right ventricle and TGA, this combination is called the Taussig-Bing anomaly. In cases in which the VSD is conoventricular, two surgical options exist for anatomic repair. An intracardiac baffle technique has been described in which the left ventricular flow through the VSD is directed to the aorta that is usually rightward of the pulmonary valve, leaving room for right ventricular flow to go over the VSD patch to the pulmonary arteries.[93] The ability to baffle the VSD to the aorta without obstruction and while retaining the potential for growth is determined by the distance between the tricuspid valve annulus and the pulmonary root. In cases where the aorta is more posterior than the pulmonary valve, the pathway from VSD to aorta is more likely to be adequate. If this pathway is inadequate, there is a significant risk for late development of left ventricular outflow obstruction with growth of the child. The right ventricular outflow may also need to be enlarged with a patch in cases in which the left ventricle to aorta baffle occupies too much of the right ventricular outflow.

The more common method of achieving anatomic repair of TGA and double-outlet right ventricle is by a combination of closing the VSD to the pulmonary root, because it is closer, and then performing an arterial switch. This approach decreases the risk of late development of left ventricular outflow obstruction. However, because of the frequent association with single coronary artery and aortic arch hypoplasia, this operative approach is more technically demanding, and experience with complex coronary artery transfer is required. The surgical technique is similar to that of an arterial switch with mobilization of the pulmonary artery and branches, and in cases with arch hypoplasia, dissection of the entire arch and branches is required. A single arterial cannula usually is sufficient except in severe arch obstruction or arch interruption in which a second arterial cannula through the arterial duct provides flow to the descending aorta. The VSD is best approached through an infundibular incision in the RVOT directly below the aortic root. A transatrial approach can be used, but because of the frequent extension of the VSD leftward and superior in the septum, adequate visualization of the most leftward extension of the VSD can be difficult with this approach. The frequent association of this form of TGA with a small or even hypoplastic tricuspid valve further complicates this approach. With the VSD closed, an arterial switch procedure is performed with similar techniques as described for simple transposition. In cases in which a coarctation or aortic arch hypoplasia is present, resection of the coarctation with patch augmentation of the aortic arch is required.

Noncommitted Ventricular Septal Defect. In rare cases, the VSD in double-outlet right ventricle is remote from the great vessels, either in the muscular septum or in the atrioventricular canal area. In these cases, enlargement of the VSD into the conoventricular area may be possible but likely requires extensive resection and may interfere with atrioventricular valve attachments or risk injury to conduction tissue. Although techniques have been described to achieve repair without VSD enlargement, the risk of late left ventricular outflow obstruction remains a significant concern.[94] For most of these children, management as single ventricle is likely to result in lower overall morbidity and mortality and is the preferred method in most centers.

Transposition of the Great Arteries with Aortic Arch Obstruction

TGA can be associated with coarctation of the aorta or aortic arch hypoplasia and can exist in the absence of a VSD although more commonly, a VSD is present along with other anomalies such as double-outlet right ventricle and "subaortic" obstruction.[95] An important aspect in the surgical management of neonates with the combination of TGA, VSD, and aortic arch hypoplasia is the recognition that other associated intracardiac anomalies, such as right ventricular outflow obstruction and right ventricular hypoplasia, often complicate repair.

The approach to repair of these lesions is similar to that for TGA with VSD with the additional need to mobilize the entire aortic arch and enough of the descending aorta to permit complete resection of ductal tissue and end-to-end anastomosis with or without patch augmentation. If the coarctation involves only the isthmus and junction with the arterial duct, then a simple resection with end-to-end anastomosis is sufficient. Frequently in infants with double-outlet right ventricle, the transverse arch is hypoplastic to varying degrees and requires patch augmentation.

Furthermore, there is almost always a significant size discrepancy between the ascending aorta and pulmonary trunk, with the latter being substantially larger. In these cases, patch augmentation of the entire ascending aorta and arch, similar to the augmentation done for hypoplastic left heart syndrome, facilitates the arterial switch by eliminating the size discrepancy with the neoaorta.

In cases in which the right ventricle is hypoplastic, careful evaluation of tricuspid valve annulus size and right ventricular volume should be done prior to surgery. In cases in which the tricuspid valve z-score is less than approximately 2.5 or the right ventricular volume is less than 15 mL/m^2, single ventricle management is probably a better option than an attempt at two-ventricle repair. If the right ventricle is borderline in size or there is concern that the combination of a mildly hypoplastic right ventricle and/or the infundibular incision will result in diminished right ventricular diastolic compliance, then leaving a small (≈3 to 4 mm) interatrial communication will permit right-to-left shunting, preserving systemic flow at the expense of mild cyanosis similar to repair of tetralogy of Fallot in infants.

Results

Transposition of the Great Arteries with Left Ventricular Outflow Tract Obstruction

Surgical repair of complex forms of transposition carries a significantly higher risk for morbidity and mortality than repair of simpler forms. Nevertheless, improvement in results with complex forms parallels those of simple transposition over the past 2 decades. In some respects, this improvement may be attributable to the recognition that the anatomic morphology of TGA with LVOT obstruction is heterogenous, and the choice of operation becomes important. For example, the Rastelli operation, the aortic translocation, and arterial switch operation with resection of the obstructing LVOT tissue are three procedures that are designed to address the patient with TGA and LVOT obstruction. Thus, selection of the most appropriate operation that will meet the needs of the specific anatomy is important. Emani and colleagues reported their experience with 88 patients undergoing surgery for TGA with LVOT obstruction. Patients undergoing the Rastelli operation or aortic translocation were more likely to be older and to present with multilevel LVOT obstruction. Although all procedures can be performed with very low mortality, those undergoing the Rastelli operation were at highest risk for subsequent LVOT reintervention, whereas patients undergoing arterial switch operation with or without LVOT intervention or aortic translocation had a very low incidence of subsequent LVOT obstruction.[96] Long-term outcomes for the aortic translocation and primary arterial switch operation with LVOT resection are unavailable but will eventually be compared with results of the Rastelli experience. In a review of the 25-year experience with the Rastelli operation, Kreutzer and associates reported an overall mortality rate of 7% with no deaths in the most recent 7-year period.[97] On late follow-up, freedom from death or transplantation rates were 82%, 80%, 68%, and 52% at 5, 10, 15, and 20 years, respectively. Arrhythmias and sudden death accounted for almost one third of the late deaths and left ventricular dysfunction accounted for another third. Freedom from death or reintervention rates were 53%, 24%, and 21% at 5, 10, and 15 years of follow-up, respectively. The most common indication for reintervention was conduit obstruction, but LVOT obstruction was also prevalent throughout the follow-up period.

Results with the Lecompte procedure (REV [réparation à l'étage ventriculaire] procedure) for TGA and LVOT obstruction are similar to those of the Rastelli procedure with respect to early mortality, with 3 of 42 patients dying early.[98] On late follow-up, however, there were no late deaths with a median follow-up of 5.4 years. Freedom from reoperation rates were 86% ± 8% and 51% ± 22% at 5 and 10 years, respectively, with the indication for reintervention being right ventricular outflow obstruction in all patients.

Transposition of the Great Arteries with Double-Outlet Right Ventricle

Transposition with double-outlet right ventricle, or the Taussig-Bing anomaly, still represents a significant surgical challenge with respect to early morbidity and mortality. In a 2001 review, Takeuchi and colleagues reported a 20% early mortality with side-by-side great vessel relationship and associated single coronary as a significant risk factor for death.[99] In the same report, infants that were managed as single ventricle with initial Glenn connection followed by Fontan had no operative deaths and no late deaths. Of the children undergoing an arterial switch, three required reoperation late—two for subaortic stenosis and one for supravalvar pulmonary stenosis. There were no late deaths in either group at an average follow-up of 24 months. Mavroudis and coworkers reported a series of 20 infants with Taussig-Bing anomaly comparing the arterial switch procedure with intracardiac tunneling technique described by Kawashima.[100] The operative mortality rate was 6% for the arterial switch group, and among the four children undergoing intracardiac baffle, there were no deaths. Of importance, however, was the fact that the average age at operation in these patients was 1.4 years, with most requiring at least one palliative procedure prior to repair. There was a high incidence of reoperation in the arterial switch group with aortic valve regurgitation a frequent complication late, likely reflecting the effects of pulmonary artery banding as a preswitch palliation resulting in distortion of the neoaortic root.

Transposition of the Great Arteries with Aortic Arch Obstruction

In recent reports, aortic arch hypoplasia or discrete coarctation have not been associated with increased mortality when the arterial switch and arch repair are undertaken together. Blume and associates reported a significant increase in overall mortality in children who had arch repair prior to arterial switch although the reasons for this were unclear.[101] Tchervenkov and colleagues have reported no operative deaths in 12 patients undergoing arterial switch procedure for TGA with aortic arch obstruction and no late deaths after a mean follow-up time of 42 months.[95] Other centers have reported a small but present incidence of aortic arch obstruction requiring reintervention with balloon dilation late.[102]

Arterial Switch after Left Ventricular Retraining

There are two situations when left ventricular "retraining" might be necessary prior to arterial switch operation: (1) in patients with TGA and intact ventricular septum who present late, and (2) in patients that present with right ventricular dysfunction after atrial switch that is refractory to medical management. Surgical options to address the latter issue include tricuspid valve repair or replacement if there is significant tricuspid regurgitation, which has not had encouraging results, and heart transplantation, which is limited by donor availability and long-term complications. Perhaps the best option for these patients is conversion to an arterial switch. In this case, the left ventricle must be retrained to handle the systemic afterload in order for arterial switch to be successful. This is accomplished by "training" the left ventricle, imposing an afterload on the deconditioned left ventricle with the application of a pulmonary artery band. This can be performed via sternotomy without the use of CPB and is a long-term strategy, because one to three bandings over many months are typically required to adequately prepare the left ventricle.[103] The status of the left ventricle during banding must be closely assessed by echocardiography, magnetic resonance imaging, and cardiac catheterization, and various criteria have been developed to assess for adequate preparation of the ventricle. These include left ventricular mass index and left ventricle/right ventricle pressure ratio.

These procedures are significant undertakings, with substantial intensive care unit and hospital stays but when accomplished successfully can offer good long-term outcomes. Poirier and Mee reported a series of 84 patients who underwent arterial from atrial switch conversion with an 85% overall survival. Normal late left ventricular function and right ventricular function were seen in approximately 90% of these patients. The best results were obtained in patients undergoing conversion prior to adolescence, with less predictable results and higher mortality rates observed in older patients.[103]

In unoperated infants who present after the early neonatal period, preliminary pulmonary artery banding followed closely by arterial switch operation (rapid two-stage switch) banding has been performed. However, the data from more recent experiences suggest that this approach is seldom required; pulmonary artery banding for left ventricular retraining following atrial switch often takes much longer, averaging 19 months in some reports.

SUMMARY

The treatment of TGA has evolved rapidly. Current results with the arterial switch operation are excellent and make this procedure the standard of care for neonates with this diagnosis. Experience is being gained with complex forms of transposition, allowing safe anatomic repair for these patients as well. Continued surveillance of patients following repair is necessary to detect and deal with potential long-term complications in these patients.

REFERENCES

1. Bailey CP, Cookson BA, Downing DF, et al: Cardiac surgery under hypothermia. *J Thorac Cardiovasc Surg* 27:73–91, 1954.
2. Farre JR: *Pathological researches. Essay 1: On malformations of the human heart*, London, 1814, Longman, Hurst, Rees, Orme, Brown, p 28.
3. von Rokitansky C: *Die Defekte der Scheidewände des Herzens*, Vienna, 1875, Braumuller.
4. Fanconi G: Die Transposition der grossen Gefuse (das Charakteristische Rontgenbild). *Arch Kinderheilkd* 95:202, 1932.
5. Taussig HB: Complete transposition of the great vessels. *Am Heart J* 16:728, 1938.
6. Blalock A, Hanlon CR: The surgical treatment of complete transposition of the aorta and pulmonary artery. *Surg Gynecol Obstet* 90:1–15, 1950.
7. Fyler DC, Buckley LP, Hellenbrand WE: Report of the New England Regional Infant Cardiac Program. *Pediatrics* 65(Suppl):377–461, 1980.
8. Liebman J, Cullum L, Belloc NB: Natural history of transposition of the great arteries: anatomy and birth and death characteristics. *Circulation* 40:237–262, 1969.
9. Van Praagh R, Van Praagh S: Isolated ventricular inversion: a consideration of the morphogenesis, definition and diagnosis of nontransposed and transposed great arteries. *Am J Cardiol* 17:395–406, 1966.
10. Kirby M: Embryogenesis of transposition of the great arteries: a lesson from the heart. *Circ Res* 91:87–89, 2002.
11. Costell M, Carmona R, Gustafsson E, et al: Hyperplastic conotruncal endocardial cushions and transposition of great arteries in perlecan-null mice. *Circ Res* 91:158–164, 2002.
12. Lillehei CW, Varco RL: The significance of right aortic arch in d-transposition of the great arteries. *Am Heart J* 87:314, 1974.
13. Moene RJ, Oppenheimer-Dekker A, Wenink ACG, et al: Morphology of ventricular septal defect in complete transposition of the great arteries. *Am J Cardiol* 55:1566–1570, 1985.
14. Gittenberger-de Groot AC, Sauer U, Oppenheimer-Dekker A, et al: Coronary arterial anatomy in transposition of the great arteries: a morphological study. *Pediatr Cardiol* 4(Suppl):1983.
15. DiDonato RM, Castañeda AR: Anatomic correction of transposition of the great arteries at the arterial level. In Sabiston DC, Jr, Spencer FC, editors: *Surgery of the chest*, ed 5, Philadelphia, 1990, WB Saunders, pp 1435–1451.
16. Kurasawa H, Imai Y, Kawada M: Coronary arterial anatomy in regard to the arterial switch procedure. *Cardiol Young* 1:54–62, 1991.
17. Massoudy P, Baltalarli A, de Leval MR, et al: Anatomic variability in coronary arterial distribution with regard to the arterial switch procedure. *Circulation* 106:1980–1984, 2002.
18. Ferencz C: Transposition of the great vessels: pathophysiologic considerations based upon a study of the lungs. *Circulation* 33:232, 1966.
19. Ferguson DJ, Adams P, Watson D: Pulmonary arteriosclerosis in transposition of the great vessels. *Am J Dis Child* 99:653, 1960.
20. Ebert PA: Transposition of the great arteries. In Sabiston DC, Jr, editor: *Textbook of surgery*, ed 14, Philadelphia, 1986, WB Saunders, pp 2249–2259.
21. Bano-Rodrigo A, Quero-Jiminez M, Moreno-Granado F: Wall thickness of ventricular chambers in transposition of the great arteries: surgical implications. *J Thorac Cardiovasc Surg* 79:592–597, 1980.
22. Rashkind WJ, Miller WW: Creation of an atrial septal defect without thoracotomy: a palliative approach to complete transposition of the great arteries. *JAMA* 96:991, 1966.
23. Mustard WT, Chute AL, Keith JD, et al: A surgical approach to transposition of the great vessels with extracorporeal circuit. *Surgery* 36:31–54, 1954.
24. Lillehei CW, Varco RL: Certain physiologic, pathologic and surgical features of complete transposition of the great vessels. *Surgery* 34:376–400, 1953.
25. Baffes TG: A new method for surgical correction of transposition of the aorta and pulmonary artery. *Surg Gynecol Obstet* 102:227–233, 1956.
26. Albert HM: Surgical correction of transposition of the great arteries. *Surg Forum* 5:74–77, 1955.
27. Senning A: Surgical correction of transposition of the great vessels. *Surgery* 45:966–980, 1959.
28. Mustard WT: Successful two-stage correction of transposition of the great vessels. *Surgery* 55:469–472, 1964.
29. Carrel T, Pfammatter JP: Complete transposition of the great arteries: surgical concepts for patients with systemic right ventricular failure following intraatrial repair. *Thorac Cardiovasc Surg* 48:224–227, 2000.
30. Pacifico AD: Concordant transposition: Senning operation. In Stark J, DeLeval M, editors: *Surgery for congenital heart defects*, New York, 1983, Grune & Stratton, pp 345–361.
31. Trusler GA, Williams WG, Duncan KF, et al: Results with the Mustard operation in simple transposition of the great arteries. *Ann Surg* 206:251–260, 1987.
32. Oechslin E, Jenni R: 40 years after the first atrial switch procedure in patients with transposition of the great arteries: long-term results in Toronto and Zurich. *Thorac Cardiovasc Surg* 48:233–237, 2000.
33. Derrick GP, Josen M, Vogel M, et al: Abnormalities of right ventricular long axis function after atrial repair of transposition of the great arteries. *Heart* 86:203–206, 2001.
34. Millane T, Bernard EJ, Jaeggi E, et al: Role of ischemia and infarction in late right ventricular dysfunction after atrial repair of transposition of the great arteries. *J Am Coll Cardiol* 35:1661–1668, 2000.
35. Hornung TS, Kilner PJ, Davlouros PA, et al: Excessive right ventricular hypertrophic response in adults with the Mustard procedure for transposition of the great arteries. *Am J Cardiol* 90:800–803, 2002.
36. Singh TP, Wolfe RR, Sullivan NM, et al: Assessment of progressive changes in exercise performance in patients with a systemic right ventricle following the atrial switch repair. *Pediatr Cardiol* 22:210–214, 2001.
37. Fredriksen PM, Veldtman G, Hechter S, et al: Aerobic capacity in adults with various congenital heart diseases. *Am J Cardiol* 87:310–314, 2001.
38. Roest AAW, Kunz P, Helbing WA, et al: Prolonged cardiac recovery from exercise in asymptomatic adults late after atrial correction of transposition of the great arteries: evaluation with magnetic resonance flow mapping. *Am J Cardiol* 88:1011–1017, 2001.
39. Derrick GP, Narang I, White PA, et al: Failure of stroke volume augmentation during exercise and dobutamine stress is unrelated to load-independent indexes of right ventricular performance after the Mustard operation. *Circulation* 102(Suppl III):154–159, 2000.
40. Gatzoulis MA, Walters J, McLaughlin PR, et al: Late arrhythmia in adults with the Mustard procedure for transposition of the great arteries: a surrogate marker for right ventricular dysfunction? *Heart* 84:409–415, 2000.
41. Ebenroth ES, Hurwitz RA: Functional outcome of patients operated for d-transposition of the great arteries with the Mustard procedure. *Am J Cardiol* 89:353–356, 2002.
42. Hechter SJ, Fredriksen PM, Liu P, et al: Angiotensin-converting enzyme inhibitors in adults after the Mustard procedure. *Am J Cardiol* 87:660–663, 2001.
43. Jatene A, Fontes VF, Paulista PP, et al: Anatomic correction of transposition of the great vessels. *J Thorac Cardiovasc Surg* 72:364–370, 1976.
44. Yacoub MH, Radley-Smith R, Hilton CJ: Anatomical correction of complete transposition of the great arteries and ventricular septal defect in infancy. *Br Med J* 1:1112, 1976.
45. Yacoub MH, Radley-Smith R, MacLaurin R: Two-stage operation for anatomical correction of transposition of the great arteries with intact interventricular septum. *Lancet* 1:1275–1278, 1977.
46. Brawn WJ, Mee RBB: Early results for anatomic correction of transposition of the great arteries and for double-outlet right ventricle with subpulmonary ventricular septal defect. *J Thorac Cardiovasc Surg* 95:230–238, 1988.
47. Castañeda AR, Trusler GA, Paul MH, et al: Congenital Heart Surgeons Society: the early results of treatment of simple

transposition in the current era. *J Thorac Cardiovasc Surg* 95:14–28, 1988.
48. Quaegebeur JM, Rohmer J, Ottenkamp J, et al: The arterial switch operation. *J Thorac Cardiovasc Surg* 92:361–364, 1986.
49. Imura H, Modi P, Pawade A, et al: Cardiac Troponin I in neonates undergoing the arterial switch operation. *Ann Thorac Surg* 74:1998–2002, 2002.
50. Scott WA, Fixler DE: Effect of center volume on outcome of ventricular septal defect closure and arterial switch operation. *Am J Cardiol* 88:1259–1263, 2001.
51. Wernovsky G, Mayer JE, Jonas RA, et al: Factors influencing early and late outcome of the arterial switch operation for transposition of the great arteries. *J Thorac Cardiovasc Surg* 109:289–302, 1995.
52. Angeli E, Raisky O, Bonnet D, et al: Late reoperations after neonatal arterial switch operation for transposition of the great arteries. *Eur J Cardiothorac Surg* 34:32–36, 2008.
53. Haas F, Wottke M, Poppert H, et al: Long-term survival and functional follow up in patients after the arterial switch operation. *Ann Thorac Surg* 68:1692–1697, 1999.
54. Nogi S, McCrindle BW, Boutin C, et al: Fate of the neopulmonary valve after the arterial switch operation in neonates. *J Thorac Cardiovasc Surg* 115:557–562, 1998.
55. Prifti E, Crucean A, Bonacchi M, et al: Early and long term outcome of the arterial switch operation for transposition of the great arteries: predictors and functional evaluation. *Eur J Cardiothor Surg* 22:864–873, 2002.
56. Von Bernuth G: 25 years after the first arterial switch procedure: mid-term results. *Thorac Cardiovasc Surg* 48:228–232, 2000.
57. Losay J, Touchot A, Serraf A, et al: Late outcome after arterial switch operation for transposition of the great arteries. *Circulation* 104(Suppl I):121–126, 2001.
58. Daebritz SH, Nollert G, Sachweh JS, et al: Anatomical risk factors for mortality and cardiac morbidity after arterial switch operation. *Ann Thorac Surg* 69:1880–1886, 2000.
59. Hutter PA, Kreb DL, Mantel SF, et al: Twenty-five years' experience with the arterial switch operation. *J Thorac Cardiovasc Surg* 124:790–797, 2002.
60. Pretre R, Tamisier D, Bonhoeffer P, et al: Results of the arterial switch operation in neonates with transposed great arteries. *Lancet* 357:1826–1830, 2001.
61. Qamar ZA, Goldberg CS, Devaney EJ: Current risk factors and outcomes for the arterial switch operation. *Ann Thorac Surg* 84:871–879, 2007.
62. Pasquali SK, Hasselblad V, Li JS, et al: Coronary artery pattern and outcome of arterial switch operation for transposition of the great arteries: a meta-analysis. *Circulation* 106:2575–2580, 2002.
63. Hutter PA, Thomeer BJM, Jansen P, et al: Fate of the aortic root after arterial switch operation. *Eur J Cardiothor Surg* 20:82–88, 2001.
64. Hovels-Gurich HH, Seghaye MC, Dabritz S, et al: Cardiological and general health status in preschool and school-age children after neonatal arterial switch operation. *Eur J Cardiothorac Surg* 12:593–601, 1997.
65. Horer J, Schreiber C, Cleuziou J, et al: Improvement in long-term survival after hospital dischage but not in freedom from reoperation after the change from atrial to arterial switch for transposition of the great arteries. *J Thorac Cardiovas Surg* 137: 347–354, 2009.
66. Hovels-Gurich HH, Seghaye M-C, Sigler M, et al: Neurodevelopmental outcome related to cerebral risk factors in children after neonatal arterial switch operation. *Ann Thorac Surg* 71:881–888, 2001.
67. Bellinger DC, Wypij D, Kuban KCK, et al: Developmental and neurologic status at four years of age after heart surgery with hypothermic circulatory arrest or low-flow cardiopulmonary bypass. *Circulation* 100:526–532, 1999.
68. Bellinger DC, Wypij D, duPlessis AL, et al: Neurodevelopmental status at eight years in children with dexto-transposition of the great arteries. The Boston Circulatiry Arrest Trial. *J Thorac Cardiovasc Surg* 126:1385–1396, 2003.
69. Bellinger DC, Newburger JW, Wypij D, et al: Behavior at eight years in children with surgically corrected transposition: the Boston Circulatory Arrest Trial. *Cardiol Young* 19:86–97, 2009.
70. Schwartz ML, Gauvreau K, del Nido P, et al: Long-term predictors of aortic root dilation and aortic regurgitation after arterial switch operation. *Circulation* 110(Suppl II):II128–II132, 2004.
71. Vandekerckhhove K, Blom NA, Lalezari S, et al: Long-term follow-up of arterial switch operation with emphasis on functin and dimensions of left ventricle and aorta. *Eur J Cardiothorac Surg* 35:582–588, 2009.
72. Lange R, Cleuziou J, Horer J, et al: Risk factors for aortic insufficiency and aortic valve replacement after the arterial switch operation. *Eur J Cardiothorac Surg* 34:711–717, 2008.
73. Raisky O, Bergoend E, Agnoletti G, et al: Late coronary artery lesions after neonatal arterial switch operation: results of surgical coronary revascularization. *Eur J Cardiothorac Surg* 31:894–898, 2007.
74. Bisoi AK, Chauhan S, Khanzode SD, et al: D-Transposition of the great vessels with intact ventricular septum presenting at 3-8 weeks: should all go for rapid two stage arterial switch or primary arterial switch? *IJTCVS* 22:5–9, 2006.
75. Boutin C, Wernovsky G, Sanders SP, et al: Rapid two-stage arterial switch operation. Evaluation of left ventricular systolic mechanics late after an acute pressure overload stimulus in infancy. *Circulation* 90:1294–1303, 1994.
76. Colan SD, Boutin C, Canteneda AR, et al: Status of the left ventricle after arterial switch operation for transposition of the great arteries. Hemodynamic and echocardiographic evaluation. *JTCVS* 109:311–321, 1995.
77. Wernovsky G, Mayer JE, Jr, Jonas RA, et al: Factors influencing early and late outcome of the arterial switch operation for transposition of the great arteries. *JTCVS* 109:289–301, 1995.
78. Kang N, de Leval MR, Elliott M, et al: Extending the boundaries of the primary arterial switch operation in patients with transposition of the great arteries and intact ventricular septum. *Circulation* 110(Suppl II):II-123–II-127, 2004.
79. Edwin F, Kinsley RH, Brink J, et al: Late primary arterial switch for transposition of the great arteries with intact ventricular septum in an African population. *World J Pediatr Congenit Heart Surg* 2(2):237–242, 2011.
80. Fyler DC: Report of the New England regional infant cardiac program. *Pediatrics* 65:375, 1980.
81. Pasquini L, Sanders SP, Parness IA, et al: Conal anatomy in 119 patients with d-loop transposition of the great arteries and ventricular septal defect: an echocardiographic and pathologic study. *J Am Coll Cardiol* 21:1712–1721, 1993.
82. Milanesi O, Ho SY, Thiene G, et al: The ventricular septal defect in complete transposition of the great arteries: pathologic anatomy in 57 cases with emphasis on subaortic, subpulmonary, and aortic arch obstruction. *Hum Pathol* 18:392–396, 1987.
83. Pocar M, Villa E, Degandt A, et al: Long-term results after primary one-stage repair of transposition of the great arteries and aortic arch obstruction. *J Am Coll Cardiol* 46:1331–1338, 2005.
84. Pigott JD, Chin AJ, Weinberg PM, et al: Transposition of the great arteries with aortic arch obstruction. Anatomical review and report of surgical management. *J Thorac Cardiovasc Surg* 94:82–86, 1987.
85. Vogel M, Freedom RM, Smallhorn JF, et al: Complete transposition of the great arteries and coarctation of the aorta. *Am J Cardiol* 53:1627–1632, 1984.
86. Hoyer MH, Zuberbuhler JR, Anderson RH, et al: Morphology of ventricular septal defects in complete transposition. Surgical implications. *J Thorac Cardiovasc Surg* 104:1203–1211, 1992.
87. Uemura H, Yagihara T, Kawashima Y, et al: Coronary arterial anatomy in double-outlet right ventricle with subpulmonary VSD. *Ann Thorac Surg* 59:591–597, 1995.
88. Gordillo L, Faye-Petersen O, de la Cruz MV, et al: Coronary arterial patterns in double-outlet right ventricle. *Am J Cardiol* 71:1108–1110, 1993.
89. Rastelli GC, MaGoon DC, Wallace RB: Anatomic correction of transposition of the great arteries with ventricular septal defect and subpulmonary stenosis. *J Thorac Cardiovasc Surg* 58:545–552, 1969.
90. Lecompte Y, Neveux JY, Leca F, et al: Reconstruction of the pulmonary outflow tract without a prosthetic conduit. *J Thorac Cardiovasc Surg* 84:727–733, 1982.
91. Vouhé PR, Tamisier D, Leca F, et al: Transposition of the great arteries, ventricular septal defect, and pulmonary outflow tract

obstruction: rastelli or Lecompte procedure? *J Thorac Cardiovasc Surg* 103:428–436, 1992.
92. Konno S, Imai Y, Iida Y, et al: A new method for prosthetic valve replacement in congenital aortic stenosis associated with hypoplasia of the aortic valve ring. *J Thorac Cardiovasc Surg* 70:909–917, 1975.
93. McGoon DC: Intraventricular repair of transposition of the great arteries. *J Thorac Cardiovasc Surg* 64:430–434, 1972.
94. Barbero-Marcial M, Tamanati C, Jatene MB, et al: Double-outlet right ventricle with nonrelated ventricular septal defect: surgical results using the multiple patches technique. *Heart Surg Forum* 1:125–129, 1998.
95. Tchervenkov CI, Korkola SJ: Transposition complexes with systemic obstruction. *Semin Thorac Cardiovasc Surg Pediatr Card Surg Annu* 4:71–82, 2001.
96. Emani SE, Beroukhim R, Zurakowski D, et al: Outcomes after anatomic repair for d-transposition of the great arteries with left ventricular outflow tract obstruction. *Circulation* 120(Suppl 1): S53–S58, 2009.
97. Kreutzer C, De Vive J, Oppido G, et al: Twenty-five-year experience with Rastelli repair for transposition of the great arteries. *J Thorac Cardiovasc Surg* 120:211–223, 2000.
98. Petre R, Gendron G, Tamisier D, et al: Results of the Lecompte procedure in malposition of the great arteries and pulmonary obstruction. *Eur J Cardiothorac Surg* 19:283–289, 2001.
99. Takeuchi K, McGowan FX, Jr, Moran AM, et al: Surgical outcome of double-outlet right ventricle with subpulmonary VSD. *Ann Thorac Surg* 71:49–52, 2001.
100. Mavroudis C, Backer CL, Muster AJ, et al: Taussig-Bing anomaly: arterial switch versus Kawashima intraventricular repair. *Ann Thorac Surg* 61:1330–1338, 1996.
101. Blume ED, Altmann K, Mayer JE, et al: Evolution of risk factors influencing early mortality of the arterial switch operation. *J Am Coll Cardiol* 33:1702–1709, 1999.
102. Gandhi SK, Pigula FA, Siewers RD: Successful late reintervention after the arterial switch procedure. *Ann Thorac Surg* 73:88–93, 2002.
103. Poirier NC, Mee RB: Left ventricular reconditioning and anatomical correction for systemic right ventricular dysfunction. *Semin Thorac Cardiovasc Surg Pediatr Card Surg Annu* 3:198–215, 2000.

CHAPTER 126

Surgery for Congenitally Corrected Transposition of the Great Arteries

William J. Brawn • David J. Barron

CHAPTER OUTLINE

Congenitally corrected transposition of the great arteries (ccTGA) is a rare defect, seen in approximately 0.5% of patients with congenital heart defects.[1,2] It entails discordance of the atrioventricular (AV) connections and discordance of the ventricular arterial connections, so there is double discordance. The morphology of the heart is distinctly abnormal, but the circulatory system is physiologically normal. Commonly, ccTGA is associated with ventricular septal defects (VSDs), pulmonary stenosis, dysplasia of the tricuspid valve, and conduction abnormalities (e.g., heart block usually develops).[3-5] Although this condition can be compatible with a normal life span,[6,7] the majority of patients require surgery to repair the associated cardiac anomalies, and many develop heart failure because of systemic morphologic right ventricular (mRV) dysfunction, usually with tricuspid valve regurgitation.[8-11] Historically, surgery was directed toward managing the associated cardiac anomalies, closing the VSD, relieving pulmonary stenosis, repairing or replacing the tricuspid valve, and placing pacemakers to manage the conduction abnormalities. This so-called classical or conventional (physiologic) repair maintains the mRV as the systemic ventricle. More recently, the morphologic left ventricle (mLV) has been restored to the systemic circulation by an atrial switch (Senning or Mustard procedure) and an arterial switch or Rastelli procedure to connect the aorta to the mLV.[12-15] This is referred to as *anatomic repair*, and it is the preferred technique for symptomatic patients.

GENERAL DESCRIPTION AND MORPHOLOGY

In the usual situs solitus arrangement with normal systemic and pulmonary venous drainage, the ventricular apex of the heart usually points to the left side of the patient, but mesocardia and dextrocardia are common, occurring in up to 20% of cases.[4,16] Malposition of the ventricular mass so that it comes to lie in front of the atria and venous drainage to the heart can make surgical access to these structures difficult. In situs inversus, which occurs in approximately 5% of cases, mesocardia and levocardia can occur. It seems that extreme malposition of the ventricular mass is commonly associated with severe pulmonary stenosis or pulmonary atresia in association with a large VSD.[16] Characteristically, the aorta is anterior and to the left side of the more deeply placed pulmonary artery—hence the older term for this condition, L-transposition. However, the aorta can be more anterior to the pulmonary artery and even on the right side. Likewise, the mLV is usually to the right and slightly inferior to the mRV; however, the position of the ventricles relative to each other can show great variability.[3] The ascending aorta is often short and well over to the left side of the mediastinum in situs solitus, again making surgical access difficult. In the rarer form of situs inversus, the aorta lies anterior and to the right of the posterior pulmonary artery and is usually more accessible.

In ccTGA without associated cardiac anomalies (sometimes referred to as *isolated ccTGA*), the circulation is physiologically normal, with systemic venous return passing through the right atrium, through the mitral valve, and then into the mLV. Here, the mLV pumps blood through the pulmonary arteries into the lungs, from whence it returns to the pulmonary veins and to the left atrium. The blood flow continues through the tricuspid valve and into the mRV, where it is pumped around the systemic circulation via the aorta (Fig. 126-1). Without other cardiac anomalies, patients with congenitally corrected transposition can survive well into adult life without symptoms. It is the associated anomalies—VSD, pulmonary stenosis, abnormalities of the tricuspid valve, and development of arrhythmias or complete heart block—that predispose the patient to the development of cardiac failure early in life. However, even patients with isolated ccTGA can develop systemic ventricular (i.e., the mRV) dysfunction leading to congestive cardiac failure in childhood or early adult life, but predicting which patients will do so is one of the many challenges in managing the condition.

Ventricular Septal Defect

Ventricular septal defect occurs in approximately 70% of cases.[4] It is usually isolated and in the perimembranous region. Isolated VSDs can also occur in the infundibular region, and they may be multiple. When associated with severe pulmonary stenosis or pulmonary atresia, the VSD is usually subaortic and large, extending from the perimembranous region to beneath the aortic valve. This is important, because it allows the VSD to be tunneled to the aorta when the mLV is committed to the aorta as a systemic ventricle.

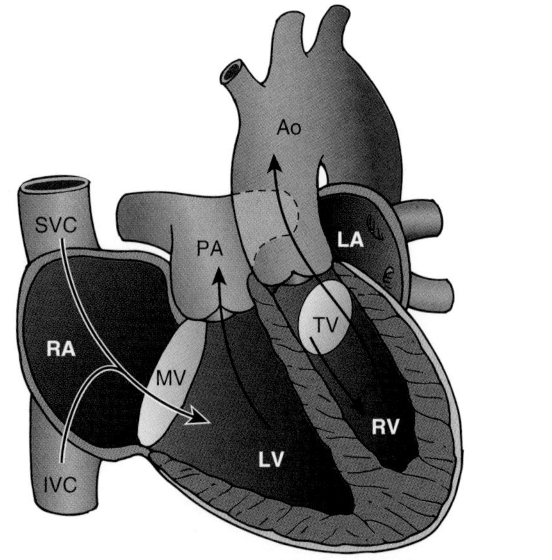

FIGURE 126-1 ■ Diagram of congenitally corrected transposition of the great arteries. *Ao,* Aorta; *IVC,* inferior vena cava; *LA,* left atrium; *LV,* left ventricle; *MV,* mitral valve; *PA,* pulmonary artery; *RA,* right atrium; *RV,* right ventricle; *SVC,* superior vena cava; *TV,* tricuspid valve.

Pulmonary Outflow Tract Obstruction (Morphologic Left Ventricular Outflow Tract Obstruction)

Obstruction to the pulmonary artery from the LV is common in congenitally corrected transposition, occurring in probably up to 50% of cases.[4,17] This is partly because the pulmonary artery is between the mitral and tricuspid valves, deep toward the crux of the heart. A potential exists for hypoplasia of the subpulmonary outflow tract. When hypoplasia occurs in association with a VSD, there may be accessory tissue around the VSD, which can balloon into the pulmonary valve. Accessory tissue tags can prolapse into the outflow tract from the mitral or the tricuspid valves, and over time fibrous tissue can be deposited in the subpulmonary area of the mLV outflow tract. Accessory attachments of the mitral or tricuspid mitral valve through the VSD can cause obstruction beneath the pulmonary valve. In the majority of these cases, the pulmonary valve and annulus are stenotic, and the morphology falls into the spectrum of requiring a Rastelli-type procedure to commit the mLV to the aorta. However, each case needs careful assessment because those with a normal-sized pulmonary valve and accessory tissue in the outflow tract may be more suitable for arterial switch and resection of tissue in the LVOT.

Mitral and Tricuspid Valves

The mitral valve is usually normal in congenitally corrected transposition. There are usually two well-formed papillary muscles on the lateral wall of the LV.

applicable to situations in which a Rastelli-Senning repair is not possible because of the position of the VSD.

Finally a Fontan-type procedure may have to be considered if it is not possible by virtue of position of the heart, location of the VSD, and hypoplasia of a ventricle to perform a septation; however, this is uncommon.

RESULTS

Physiologic Repair

Results from many centers throughout the world are now available.[9-11,19,30,32] Although the early mortality is low (5% to 10%), all groups have highlighted the long-term failure of the mRV associated with tricuspid regurgitation. The Toronto group[35] in particular highlighted this long-term problem, and the Mavroudis group,[53] in their article comparing physiologic and anatomic repair, stated the problem clearly. Thus, survival in these patients is 75% at 5 years and 50% at 20 years. In addition, 56% require reoperation in the 20 years of follow-up.

Anatomic Repair

Anatomic repair has grown in popularity because of the poor long-term outcome of physiologic repair. Early results for anatomic repair are available from centers in North America, Japan, and Europe and have reported encouraging results with early mortality in the region of 0% to 5%.*

Longer-term follow-up is now becoming available. In our series of 113 patients, the early mortality was 4.4%, and actuarial survival in the double-switch group was 84% at both 5 and 10 years versus 92% and 77% in the Rastelli-Senning group (log-rank, $P = 0.98$).[24] Within this group of patients, we have identified a subgroup of high-risk patients in the neonatal or infant age-group with severe congestive cardiac failure requiring ventilation and inotropic support. All these patients were in the double-switch group. As expected, the early mortality was high in this group (3/17, 17%) but the corollary is that the early mortality in the remaining "elective" cases was lower (2%). Freedom from reoperation for all patients was 94% at 1 year, 85% at 5 years, and 76% at 9 years. There were no reoperations for tricuspid valve regurgitation; in fact, preoperative tricuspid regurgitation was universally improved. The reoperations, as expected, were for conduit change in the Rastelli group, and this will be a continuing necessity.

As longer follow-up results are reported, there is a concern over the incidence of late mLV dysfunction occurring in 15% to 20% of patients at 20 years postoperatively. This has been reported by both ourselves and the Boston and Stanford groups with similar findings.[15,24,37,40] The etiology appears to be multifactorial and related to the development of aortic regurgitation, later age at repair (>10 years), and the need for preoperative mLV retraining with a pulmonary artery band. Aortic regurgitation is specific to the double-switch group, in which the old pulmonary valve becomes the new aortic valve. All our patients had some mild degree of aortic valve insufficiency. In four patients, it was moderately severe, and it required aortic valve replacement in two patients. Similar results have been reported in other series.[33,53]

A few centers performing the atrial-arterial switch procedure have commented that the mLV retrained by application of the pulmonary artery band may have more problems with LV dysfunction in the postoperative period. We have noted this also, as have others, but the relationship is by no means consistent.[54,55] The Boston group have shown a greater risk of late mLV dysfunction in patients who were initially banded at older than 2 years, whereas there was no incidence of late dysfunction in patients banded at younger than 2 years.[41] This group of retrained mLVs will certainly require careful follow-up. These findings add to the interest in the controversial approach of early prophylactic pulmonary artery banding in symptomless infants discussed earlier,[42] which might protect the mLV in these patients from late failure.

It has also been noted that LV dysfunction is associated with a high incidence of patients requiring pacing and of patients who have a prolonged QRS interval.[56] Resynchronization with biventricular pacing has improved mLV function in these patients, with some individual cases of dramatic improvement.[24,40] This may be of value in patients requiring pacemaker insertion after a double-switch procedure.

Despite these concerns, the outcomes of anatomic repair remain substantially better than both the natural history and for traditional physiologic repair, with more than 75% of patients sustaining good mLV function at 20 years. It is also important to note that the group of high-risk patients with severe cardiac failure have done particularly well, with no incidence of late mLV failure. Thus, with new operations, new problems arise. Only longer-term follow-up will show whether the good early results are maintained.

SUMMARY

The algorithm in Figure 126-4 summarizes our current management for these patients. We believe that the LV in the systemic circulation will be of benefit for the majority of patients with this condition; therefore, our preferred management pathways are highlighted with red arrows. Longer-term studies will show whether the problems of new aortic regurgitation, LV dysfunction, and the need for conduit change will increase over time. The problem of RV dysfunction and tricuspid regurgitation has been solved, however. An anatomic repair should be suitable for the majority of patients. Development of heart failure in the older patient may still require tricuspid valve surgery or cardiac transplantation. At this time, it is not possible to retrain the LV in older patients.[39] Debanding and closure of the VSD is *not* our preferred option.

When only physiologic repair is possible because of the position of the VSD, or because of the age of an older

*References 12, 13, 15, 18, 24, 37, 40, and 53.

patient, we would agree with Mavroudis and colleagues[52] that the mLV pressure should be maintained at approximately 50% of systemic pressures to maintain ventricular septal alignment. This can prevent development of tricuspid regurgitation and deterioration of RV function. When there is hypoplasia of one of the ventricles, or complex AV valve morphology with straddling, the only option may be to use Fontan palliation; however, this applies to a minority of patients.

Longer-term follow-up of this rare group of patients is now being reported. Although we believe that the initial enthusiasm for anatomic repair is justified, some centers have reported that there is no statistical difference in long-term survival rates between some patients undergoing physiologic repair and others undergoing anatomic repair.[57] Certainly, there is no real cure for ccTGA. There are surgical options, each of which has complications that will require management in the future. Continued surveillance is most definitely necessary.

REFERENCES

1. Ferencz C, Rubin JD, McCarter RJ, et al: Congenital heart disease: prevalence at live birth. The Baltimore-Washington Infant Study. *Ann J Epidemiol* 121:31–36, 1985.
2. Fyler DC: Report of the New England Regional Infant Cardiac Programme. *Pediatr* 65(Suppl):376–461, 1980.
3. Becker AE, Anderson RH, editors: *Atrioventricular discordance in pathology of congenital heart disease*, London, 1981, Butterworths, pp 225–240.
4. Losekoot TG, Becker AE: Discordant atrioventricular connexion and congenitally corrected transposition. In Anderson RH, MacCartney FJ, Shinebourne EA, et al, editors: *Paediatric cardiology*, Edinburgh, 1987, Churchill Livingstone, pp 867–888.
5. Van Praagh R: What is congenitally corrected transposition (editorial). *N Engl J Med* 282:1097–1098, 1970.
6. Beauchesne LM, Warnes CA, Connolly HM, et al: Outcome of the unoperated adult who presents with congenitally corrected transposition of the great arteries. *J Am Coll Cardiol* 40:285–290, 2002.
7. Presbitero P, Somerville J, Rabajoli F, et al: Corrected transposition of the great arteries without associated defects in adult patients: clinical profile and follow up. *Br Heart J* 74:57–59, 1995.
8. Connelly M, Liu PP, Williams WG, et al: Congenitally corrected transposition of the great arteries in the adult: functional status and complications. *J Am Coll Cardiol* 27:1238–1243, 1996.
9. Sano T, Riesenfeld T, Karl TR, et al: Intermediate-term outcome after intracardiac repair of associated cardiac defects in patients with atrioventricular and ventriculoarterial discordance. *Circulation* 92:II272–II278, 1995.
10. Termignon JL, Leca F, Vouhé PR, et al: "Classic" repair of congenitally corrected transposition and ventricular septal defect. *Ann Thorac Surg* 62:199–206, 1996.
11. Yeh TJ, Connelly MS, Coles JG, et al: Atrioventricular discordance: results of repair in 127 patients. *J Thorac Cardiovasc Surg* 117:1190–1203, 1999.
12. Di Donato RM, Troconis CJ, Marino B, et al: Combined Mustard and Rastelli operations. An alternative approach for repair of associated anomalies in congenitally corrected transposition in situs inversus (IDD). *J Thorac Cardiovasc Surg* 104:1246–1248, 1992.
13. Ilbawi MN, Deleon SY, Backer CL, et al: An alternative approach to the surgical management of physiologically corrected transposition with ventricular septal defect and pulmonary stenosis or atresia. *J Thorac Cardiovasc Surg* 100:410–415, 1990.
14. Stumper O, Wright JG, DeGiovanni JV, et al: Combined atrial and arterial switch procedure for congenitally corrected transposition with ventricular septal defect. *Br Heart J* 73:479–482, 1995.
15. Yagihara T, Kishimoto H, Isobe F, et al: Double Switch operation in cardiac anomalies with atrioventricular and ventriculoarterial discordance. *J Thorac Cardiovasc Surg* 107:351–358, 1994.
16. Carey LS, Ruttenberg HD: Roentgenographic features of congenitally corrected transposition of the great vessels. *Ann J Roentgenol* 92:623, 1964.
17. Freedom RM, Benson LN, Smallhorn JF: Congenitally transposition of the great arteries. In Moller JH, Neal WA, editors: *Fetal, neonatal and infant cardiac disease*, Norwalk, CT, 1989, Appleton and Lange, pp 555–570.
18. Langley SM, Winlaw DS, Stumper O, et al: Midterm results after restoration of the morphologically left ventricle to the systemic circulation in patients with congenitally corrected transposition of the great arteries. *J Thorac Cardovasc Surg* 125:1229–1241, 2003.
19. Acar P, Sidi D, Bonnet D, et al: Maintaining tricuspid valve competence in double discordance: a challenge for the paediatric cardiologist. *Heart* 80:479–483, 1998.
20. Anderson KR, Danielson GK, McGoon DW, et al: Ebstein's anomaly of the left-sided tricuspid valve. Pathological anatomy of the valvular malformation. *Circulation* 58:87–91, 1978.
21. Becker AE, Ho SY, Caruso G, et al: Straddling right atrioventricular valves in atrioventricular discordance. *Circulation* 61:1133, 1980.
22. Erath HG, Graham PT, Hammon JW, et al: Hypoplasia of the systemic ventricle in congenitally corrected transposition of the great arteries. *J Thorac Cardiovasc Surg* 79:770–775, 1980.
23. Morell VO, Jacobs JP, Quintessenza JA: Aortic translocation in the management of transposition of the great arteries with ventricular septal defect and pulmonary stenosis: results and follow-up. *Ann Thorac Surg* 79:2089–2092, 2005.
24. Murtuza B, Barron DJ, Stumper O, et al: Anatomic repair for congenitally corrected transposition of the great arteries: a single-institution 19-year experience. *J Thorac Cardiovasc Surg* 142(6):1348–1357, 2011.
25. Anderson RH, Becker AE, Arnold R, et al: The conducting tissues in congenitally corrected transposition. *Circulation* 50:911–924, 1974.
26. Daliento L, Corrado D, Buja G, et al: Rhythm and conduction disturbances in isolated, congenitally corrected transposition of the great arteries. *Am J Cardiol* 58:314–318, 1986.
27. Kurosawa H, Becker AE: *Atrioventricular conduction in congenital heart disease*, London, 1987, Springer-Verlag, pp 225–252.
28. Wilkinson JL, Smith A, Lincoln C, et al: Conducting tissues in congenitally corrected transposition with situs inversus. *Br Heart J* 40:41–48, 1978.
29. De Leval MR, Basto P, Stark J, et al: Surgical technique to reduce the risks of heart block following closure of ventricular septal defect in atrioventricular discordance. *J Thorac Cardiovasc Surg* 78:515–526, 1979.
30. Graham TP, Jr, Bernard YD, Mellen BG, et al: Long term outcome in congenitally corrected transposition of the great arteries. A multi-institutional study. *J Am Coll Cardiol* 36:255–261, 2000.
31. Mavroudis C, Backer CL: Physiologic versus anatomic repair of congenitally corrected transposition of the great arteries. *Pediatr Cardiac Surge Ann Semin Thorac Cardiovasc* 6:16–26, 2003.
32. Van Son JA, Danielson GK, Huhta JC, et al: Late results of systemic atrioventricular valve replacement in corrected transposition. *J Thorac Cardiovasc Surg* 109:642–653, 1995.
33. Imai Y: The Double Switch operation for congenitally corrected transposition. *Adv Cardiac Surg* 9:65–86, 1997.
34. Tulevski II, Zijta FM, Smeijers AS, et al: Regional and global right ventricular dysfunction in asymptomatic or minimally symptomatic patients with congenitally corrected transposition. *Cardiol Young* 14:168–173, 2004.
35. Shih WJ, Noonan JA, Mazzoleni A: Life-long follow-up in congenitally corrected transposition. *Cardiol Young* 17:681–684, 2007.
36. Espinola-Zavaleta N, Erick Alexanderson E, Attié F, et al: Right ventricular function and ventricular perfusion defects in adults with congenitally corrected transposition: correlation of echocardiography and nuclear medicine. *Cardiol Young* 14:174–181, 2004.
37. Imamura M, Drummond-Webb JJ, Murphy DJ, Jr, et al: Results of the Double Switch operations in the current era. *Ann Thorac Surg* 70:100–105, 2000.
38. Mee RBB: Severe right ventricular failure after Mustard or Senning operation two stage repair: pulmonary artery banding and switch. *J Thorac Cardiovasc Surg* 92:385–390, 1986.
39. Poirier NC, Mee RBB: Left ventricular reconditioning and anatomical correction for systemic right ventricular dysfunction. *Semin Thorac Cardiovasc Pediatr Cardiac Surg Ann* 3:198–215, 2000.
40. Bautista-Hernandez V, Myers PO, Cecchin F, et al: Late left ventricular dysfunction after anatomic repair of congenitally corrected transposition of the great arteries. *J Thorac Cardiovasc Surg* 148:254–258, 2014.

41. Myers PO, del Nido PJ, Geva T, et al: Impact of age and duration of banding on left ventricular preparation before anatomic repair for congenitally corrected transposition of the great arteries. *Ann Thorac Surg* 96(2):603–610, 2013.
42. Metton O, Gaudin R, Ou P, et al: Early prophylactic pulmonary artery banding in isolated congenitally corrected transposition of the great arteries. *Eur J Cardiothorac Surg* 38(6):728–734, 2010.
43. Jonas RA, Mee RB, Sutherland HD: Reintroduction of the Senning operation for transposition of the great arteries. *Med J Aust* 2:260–262, 1980.
44. Brawn WJ, Mee RBB: Early results for anatomic correction of transposition of the great arteries and double outlet right ventricle (50 cases). *J Thorac Cardiovasc Surg* 95:230–238, 1988.
45. Senning A: Surgical correction of transposition of the great vessels. *Surgery* 45:966–980, 1959.
46. Brawn WJ, Barron DJ: Technical aspects of the Rastelli and atrial switch procedure for congenitally corrected transposition of the great arteries with ventricular septal defect and pulmonary stenosis or atresia: results of therapy. *Semin Thorac Cardiovasc Surg Pediatr Card Surg Ann* 6:4–8, review, 2003.
47. Davies B, Oppido G, Wilkinson JL, et al: Aortic translocation, Senning procedure and right ventricular outflow tract augmentation for congenitally corrected transposition, ventricular septal defect and pulmonary stenosis. *Eur J Cardio thorac Surg* 33:934–936, 2008.
48. Nikaidoh H: Aortic translocation and biventricular outflow tract reconstruction. A new surgical repair for transposition of the great arteries associated with ventricular septal defect and pulmonary stenosis. *J Thorac Cardiovasc Surgery* 88:365–372, 1984.
49. Shumacker HB, Jr: A new operation for transposition of the great vessels. *Surgery* 50:773–777, 1961.
50. Malhotra SP, Reddy VM, Qiu M, et al: The hemi-Mustard/bidirectional Glenn atrial switch procedure in the double-switch operation for congenitally corrected transposition of the great arteries: rationale and midterm results. *J Thorac Cardiovasc Surg* 141(1):162–170, 2011.
51. Sojak V, Kuipers I, Koolbergen D, et al: Mid-term results of bidirectional cavopulmonary anastomosis and hemi-Mustard procedure in anatomical correction of congenitally corrected transposition of the great arteries. *Eur J Cardiothorac Surg* 42(4):680–684, 2012.
52. Mavroudis C, Backer CL, Kohr LM, et al: Bidirectional Glenn shunt in association with congenital heart repairs: the 1(1/2) ventricular repair. *Ann Thorac Surg* 68:976–981, 1999.
53. Karl TR, Weintraub RG, Brizard CP, et al: Senning plus arterial switch operation for discordant (congenitally corrected) transposition. *Ann Thorac Surg* 64:495–502, 1997.
54. Bove EL, Ohye RG, Devaney EJ, et al: Anatomic correction of congenitally corrected transposition and its close cousins. *Cardiol Young* 16:85–90, 2006.
55. Quinn DW, McGuirk SP, Metha C, et al: The morphologic left ventricle that requires training by means of pulmonary artery banding before the double-switch procedure for congenitally corrected transposition of the great arteries is at risk of late dysfunction. *J Thorac Cardiovasc Surg* 135(5):1137–1144, 1144.e1–1144.e2, 2008.
56. Bautista-Hernandez V, Marx G, Gauvreau K, et al: Determinants of left ventricular dysfunction after anatomic repair of congenitally corrected transposition of the great arteries. *Ann Thorac Surg* 82:2059–2066, 2006.
57. Shin'oka T, Kurosawa H, Imai Y, et al: Outcomes of definitive surgical repair for congenitally corrected transposition of the great arteries or double outlet right ventricle with discordant atrioventricular connection: risk analyses in 189 patients. *J Thorac Cardiovasc Surg* 133:1318–1328, 2007.

CHAPTER 127

CONGENITAL ANOMALIES OF THE MITRAL VALVE

Christian P. Brizard

CHAPTER OUTLINE

This chapter treats only the congenital anomalies of the mitral valve to the exclusion of the mitral valve in atrioventricular (AV) discordance, the mitral valve in univentricular hearts, and the mitral valve of the hypoplastic left heart syndrome. It also excludes all acquired mitral valve disease, including the mitral valve insufficiency secondary to myocardial infarction or stunning as seen in anomalous origin of the left coronary artery from the pulmonary artery. Because repair of secondary or recurrent left AV valve regurgitation is often found in studies of the congenital mitral valve, it is included here. Although the division between congenital valve stenosis and congenital mitral valve insufficiency is classical and seemingly practical, we shall try to avoid it. Congenital valve stenosis and congenital mitral valve insufficiency generate different pathophysiologies and mechanisms of adaptation from the cardiovascular system, but they do have similar pathologies and associated lesions, they are often combined, and they require similar surgical techniques for treatment. Mitral valve anomalies associated with congenital connective tissue disorders, in which the embryology of the mitral valve itself is normal, are also covered in this chapter.

EMBRYOLOGY OF THE MITRAL VALVE

The embryology of the mitral valve is complex. The understanding of the formation of the leaflets and suspension apparatus has evolved,[1] and the current approach is based on immunohistochemistry, in vivo labeling of cushion tissue, and scanning electron micrograph of human and chick embryos.[2] In humans, the mitral valve develops between the 5th and the 15th weeks of embryonic life. The leaflet and chordal tissue derive from the endocardial cushion tissue lying on the inner surface of the AV junction. The separation between atrial and ventricular myocardium is dependent on the sulcus tissue located on the epicardial side of the junction. As the cushion tissue elongates and grows toward the ventricular cavity, it becomes progressively delaminated from the underlying myocardium, and the leaflet transitions into a funnel-like structure completely attached to the myocardium. Then, perforations into the valve leaflet appear. The perforations grow and form the chordae tendineae. The atrial aspect of the cushion generates the spongy atrial layer, and the ventricular layer generates the fibrous part of the mitral valve and the chords. The development of the papillary muscle takes place at the same time and is originated from the myocardium. A horseshoe-shaped ridge lies in the left ventricle. Progressively, the anterior and posterior parts of the ridge lose contact with the ventricular wall. They will form the papillary muscles, and as they increase in size, they stay in contact with the cushion tissue at the tip of the papillary muscle. The midportion of the muscular ridge will be incorporated into the apical trabeculations of the left ventricle.[3]

Several AV cushions participate to form the final mitral valve. The most important are the superior and inferior cushions. However, there is no symmetry in the role of these two cushions. The superior cushion tissue generates most of the anterior leaflet of the mitral valve, whereas the inferior cushion generates most of the septal leaflet of the tricuspid valve. Smaller cushions are involved in the formation of the mural leaflet of the mitral valve. The wedging of the aortic root into the superior bridging leaflet, which originated primarily from the superior cushion, separates the developing mitral valve from its septal attachments.

PATHOLOGIC FEATURES

Supravalvar Mitral Ring

Often considered a congenital anomaly of the mitral valve, the supravalvar mitral ring is a fibrous construction attached to the posterior annulus of the mitral valve; it runs from both commissures to the mid height of the anterior leaflet. The lesion is stenotic, often to a greater extent than might be suggested by the extension of the ring. This is more a result of the limitation of the opening of the anterior leaflet than of the actual diaphragm effect of the ring (Fig. 127-1). Strictly attached to the mitral valve annulus, it is to be differentiated from the cor triatriatum. Like the subaortic membrane in the left ventricular outflow tract, the supravalvar mitral ring is an acquired lesion resulting from turbulent flow through the mitral orifice. The primary lesion of the mitral valve responsible for the turbulent flow can be obvious, stenotic, and regurgitant, or it can be discrete or mild and difficult to identify. It can be related to a prominent coronary sinus, as found in the left superior vena cava draining into the coronary sinus.[4,5] It is perhaps for these reasons that the supravalvar mitral ring is prone to reoccur after surgical resection, unless the underlying anatomic anomaly has been identified and corrected.

Cleft Mitral Valve

The cleft mitral valve is often isolated and can be easily differentiated from a left AV valve in a partial AV septal defect.[6,7] It is an actual cleft with no suspension apparatus on the edges of the defect. The cleft is centered on the aortic commissure between the noncoronary and left coronary cusps.[6] Each half of the anterior leaflet at the midportion bears the attachment of the strut chordae. With time, the cleft mitral valve regurgitation will generate secondary lesions at the edges of the cleft, such as thickening, rolling up, and retraction. The defect is never stenotic and may generate only little regurgitation for a long time.

Lesions Associated with Lack of Valvar Tissue

Three major anatomic types of lesions are almost always associated with a lack of valvar tissue to various degrees and are worth characterizing: parachute mitral valve, papillary muscle to commissure fusion, and hammock or arcade valve. There is, however, a continuum between these three types and with the normal anatomy. The functional lesion can be either predominantly regurgitant or predominantly stenotic, or it can be both stenotic and regurgitant. In rare cases, the valve functions normally.

Parachute Mitral Valve

The parachute mitral valve can be found in isolation. It is, however, almost always associated with another cardiac anomaly, such as atrial septal defect (ASD), ventricular septal defect (VSD), or coarctation,[8] and it is often integrated in Shone syndrome.[9,10] It can also be seen in hypoplasia of the left ventricle, resulting in the need for univentricular palliation. The gross pathology shows a

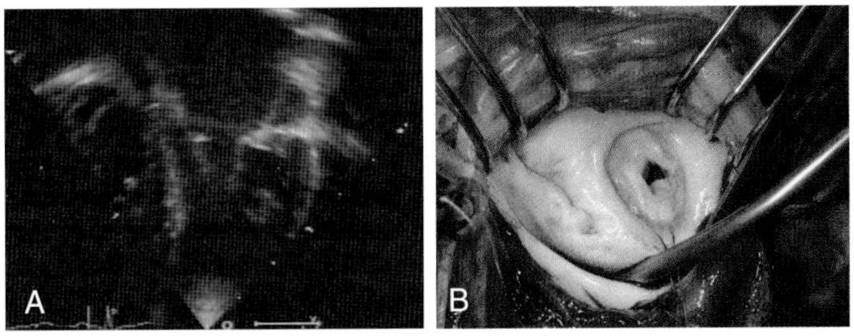

FIGURE 127-1 ■ **A,** Two-dimensional echocardiogram of supravalvar mitral ring, apical view. The membrane attached at mid height of the anterior leaflet is characteristic. The posterior part of the membrane is only suggested by the hyperechogenicity of the posterior annulus. **B,** Intraoperative photograph of a supravalvar mitral ring. Note the implantation of the supravalvar mitral ring high close to the annulus on the posterior leaflet side *(inferior side of the picture)* and at the mid level of the anterior leaflet *(left side of the picture).*

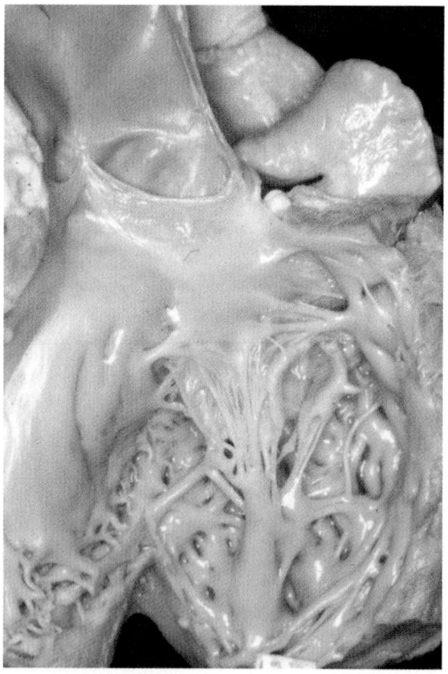

FIGURE 127-2 ■ Macroscopic view of a parachute mitral valve. A large predominant papillary muscle distributes anomalous chords to both commissures. A small diminutive papillary muscle is seen to the right of the valve.

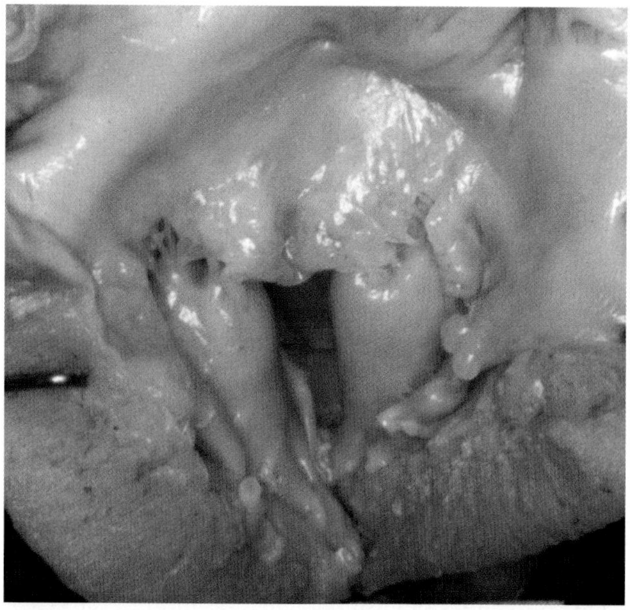

FIGURE 127-3 ■ Macroscopic view of a mitral valve with papillary muscle to commissure fusion. Extremely short chords are distributed to the anterior commissure *(left)*. The posterior papillary muscle is almost fused to the posterior commissure *(right)*.

predominant single papillary muscle, with the orifice of the mitral valve overriding the tip of the papillary muscle. The spectrum of lesions for the suspension apparatus starts with complete fusion of the tip of the papillary muscle to the free edge of the valve.[9] At the other end of the spectrum are chords that are relatively normal appearing, with good mobility of the leaflet (Fig. 127-2). The accessory papillary muscle is usually small and devoted to a short segment of the free edge, or even to the undersurface of the leaflet tissue, as would be seen if it were a larger-than-normal secondary chord. The leaflet tissue can be intact or perforated.

The functional class depends on the interaction between the amount of tissue and the mobility of the leaflet; presence and size of the fenestrations; and presence, length, and quality of the chords.[10] The parachute mitral valve almost always has a stenotic component, because the gradient is fixed but the valve grows. These patients may not require a valve operation.[11]

Double-orifice mitral valve, in which the lesser papillary muscle supports a complete orifice, is an exceedingly rare variation of the parachute mitral valve. It should be differentiated from the left AV valve, where an accessory orifice is often found when there is a diminutive or absent left lateral leaflet (mural leaflet).

Papillary Muscle to Commissure Fusion

Fusion of papillary muscle to the commissure,[12] also called short chordae syndrome, is defined by the presence of short chords and a papillary muscle tip that is attached or fused to the commissural area of the free edge (Fig. 127-3). In the most extreme form, the chords are completely absent. The papillary muscles can be of normal size and volume. The valve is then generally more regurgitant than restrictive, which is because of the lack of valvar tissue and the restriction of the leaflet motion. When the papillary muscles are hypertrophied, the bulk of their mass is generally responsible for a predominantly restrictive valve.

Hammock or Arcade Valve

In patients with hammock or arcade valve, the suspension apparatus may have lost all resemblance to the normal anatomy. The papillary muscles are not identifiable, or there are multiple small papillary muscles behind the posterior leaflet. The leaflets are suspended directly by a network of chords directly attached to the posterior wall of the ventricle. This attachment is generally displaced toward the base of the heart, with excess tension on the anterior leaflet and extreme limitation of posterior leaflet motion. The valve is most often predominantly regurgitant.

Isolated Mitral Leaflet Hypoplasia

This rare condition is almost restricted to the middle scallop of the posterior leaflet.[12,13]

Isolated Dilation of the Mitral Valve Annulus and Isolated Elongation of the Chords and Papillary Muscle

When the anatomy of the mitral valve is otherwise normal, it is difficult to ascertain the congenital origin of dilation of the mitral valve annulus and elongation of the suspension apparatus, but they are included in most studies of congenital anomalies of the mitral valve[14] and account for 15% to 40% of the patients in published studies of congenital mitral valve regurgitation.[10,15,16] However, there is no evidence of their congenital origin. Elongation of papillary muscles can be found at birth in the mitral or the tricuspid apparatus, but the muscles usually have an ischemic, beige aspect. Sometimes, the ischemic origin is demonstrated by acute rupture at or shortly after birth. Isolated dilation of the annulus is not found at birth.

Both dilation of the annulus and elongation of the suspension apparatus are usually associated with significant volume loading of the left ventricle (e.g., with a large VSD or large patent ductus arteriosus). The pathophysiology is of initial dilation of the posterior annulus under the effect of the volume loading, followed by elongation of the marginal chords and prolapse of the free edge of the anterior leaflet. In rare cases, minor anomalies of the valvar tissue or the papillary muscles indicate a true congenital origin. When a patient older than 4 years has an isolated mitral regurgitation combining anterior leaflet prolapse and various degrees of posterior leaflet retraction, especially if the latter is thickened, a rheumatic origin should be ruled out when the patient originates from a geographical area of high prevalence.

Functional mitral regurgitations secondary to cardiomyopathies are not discussed here.

Accessory Mitral Valve Tissue

The interchordal spaces are filled with a dense network of valve tissue. When there is continuity between the anterior and the posterior leaflet, the accessory valvar tissue may generate a gradient directly related to the size of the perforations in the accessory tissue (Fig. 127-4).[17] When the accessory valve tissue is entrapped in the left ventricular outflow tract, the mitral valve may become regurgitant because of the traction exerted by the accessory valvar tissue on the anterior leaflet, which results in the valve's opening at mid systole[18]; however, in that case, the left ventricular outflow tract obstruction is the predominant hemodynamic lesion and is usually responsible for the diagnosis.[19] Often, the accessory mitral valve tissue does not generate significant gradient or insufficiency.

Mitral Valve Disease with Excess of Leaflet Tissue, and Mitral Valve Prolapse

It is debatable whether the mitral valve prolapse syndrome—in its most common form, limited to the middle scallop of the posterior defect—is congenital. In a large population of neonates,[20] and using strict criteria, the incidence of mild bulging of the anterior leaflet was negligible and no prolapses were detected. This tends to prove that mitral valve prolapse is an acquired disease. In its common form, it is the exception when encountered in neonates and infants. In adults, the histologic anomalies are limited to the middle scallop of the posterior leaflet, with predominant elastic fiber alteration and myxomatous tissue proliferation.[21]

The more extensive form of mitral valve prolapse is, however, seen in neonates and infants. In this form, an excess of tissue is distributed to both the anterior and posterior leaflets, and histologic examination reveals extensive infiltration of the spongiosa with myxomatous tissue. The histologic anomalies are identical to those found in patients with Marfan syndrome,[21,22] Ehlers-Danlos syndrome, and osteogenesis imperfecta. Marfan syndrome is an autosomal dominant disorder with varying penetrance. The mutation is found on the fibrillin gene. Ehlers-Danlos syndrome is represented by a

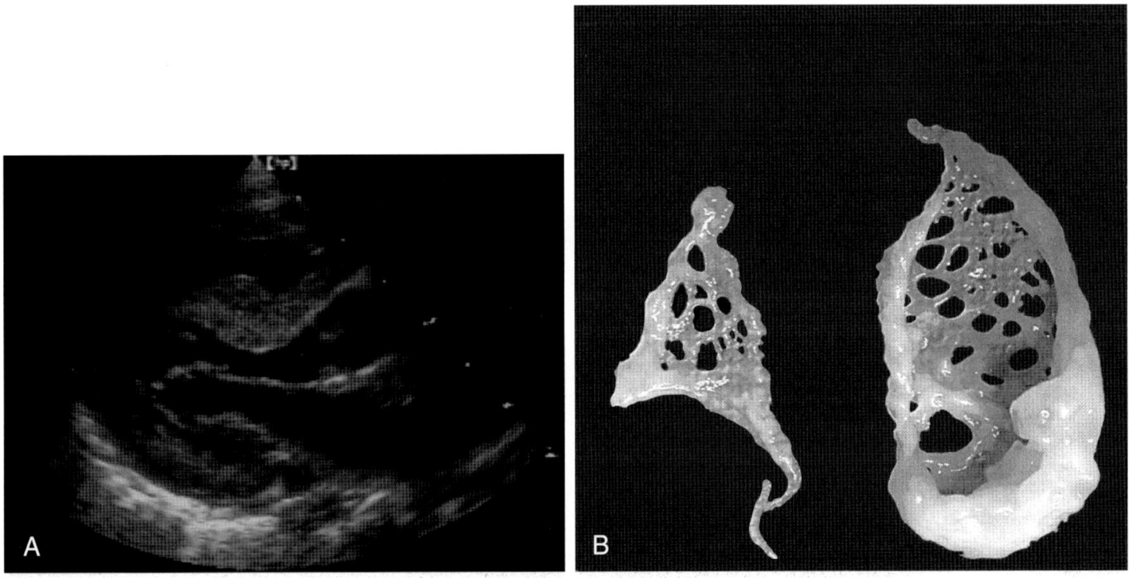

FIGURE 127-4 ■ Accessory mitral valve tissue. **A,** Long-axis view. The accessory mitral valve tissue is attached to the anterior and posterior leaflets of the mitral valve and blown like a windsock. **B,** Macroscopic view of the same tissue after surgical resection is characteristic of accessory mitral valve tissue attached to the suspension apparatus.

constellation of mutations linked to different subtypes.[23] The extensive form of the mitral valve prolapse syndrome is encountered in sporadic cases or in familial forms demonstrating autosomal dominant and X-linked inheritance. Three different loci, on chromosomes 16, 11, and 13, have been found to be linked to mitral valve prolapse, but no specific gene has been described.[24]

Recurrent Left Atrioventricular Valve Regurgitation

After repair of complete or partial atrioventricular septal defect (AVSD), there are two main mechanisms for regurgitation in valves with a normally developed left lateral leaflet (LLL).[25] The cleft may be open because the cleft closure performed in the initial surgery has ruptured or because it was never done. In this case, the regurgitation occurs through the cleft directly. On color Doppler examination, the regurgitation jet is oriented vertically through the cleft.

Alternatively, when the cleft was completely closed and has remained so, the predominant mechanism for the regurgitation is the absence of a coaptation surface in front of the tip of the LLL. In the unrepaired AVSD, the small size of the zone of apposition is an inherent feature of these parts of the superior and inferior bridging leaflets. The direct closure of the cleft does not create a larger coaptation surface; in fact, the little coaptation surface that exists can be reduced and distorted by the cleft closure. This is even more so when the cleft closure has ruptured or is stretching the free edge of the valve. On color Doppler examination, the regurgitation jet oriented posteriorly hugging the posterior wall of the left atrium is characteristic of this mechanism (Fig. 127-5).

If the regurgitation is a long-standing condition, the secondary lesions or dysplastic lesions on the edges of the cleft are severe, with thickening and retraction of the leaflet tissue, and sometimes even calcification. On the other hand, the LLL is usually thin and pliable, with no secondary or dysplastic lesion. There is no restriction of the LLL motion and no prolapse.

In the presence of hypoplastic or absent LLL, the cleft cannot be closed at the time of the primary repair without generating inflow restriction. The residual or recurrent regurgitation occurs through the cleft. On an echocardiographic study, the anatomy is suspected when a strong asymmetry of the papillary muscles can be seen on the short-axis view of the left ventricle. The predominant papillary muscle, usually the anterior one, is connected to both superior and inferior bridging leaflets. The presence of a double orifice is also a strong indicator. It is usually directly suspended to a diminutive posterior papillary muscle and in the body of the inferior bridging leaflet. On Doppler examination, the regurgitation jet is oriented vertically through the cleft.

FUNCTIONAL CLASSIFICATION OF MITRAL VALVE ANOMALIES

Carpentier's functional classification of mitral valve anomalies describes leaflet motion, regardless of the anatomy and the cause.[26] It is an essential tool for mitral valve repair and should be studied on echocardiography preoperatively.[27] It can also give significant clues to the lesions that will eventually be found during surgery.

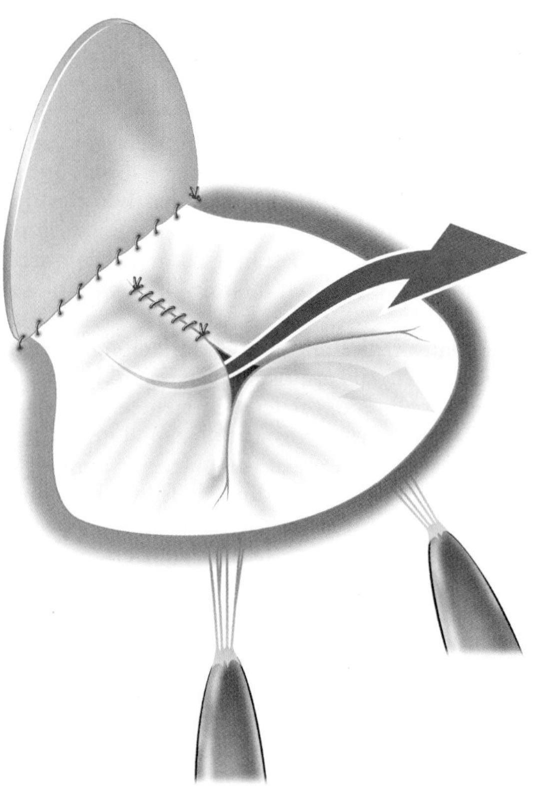

FIGURE 127-5 ■ Mechanism for the regurgitation in the absence of a zone of apposition facing the tip of the left lateral leaflet. The direction of the jet is posterior and hugging the posterior wall of the left atrium.

Type I. Normal leaflet motion. The anomaly can be either a perforation or a defect of one or two leaflets, or an annular dilation. Annular dilation associated with a type II anomaly of the anterior leaflet is most likely functional.

Type II. Enhanced leaflet motion. Most pediatric mitral valve regurgitations with a predominant type II anomaly started as functional and progressively elongated the suspension apparatus of the anterior leaflet.

Type III. Restricted leaflet motion. The valve may be stenotic or regurgitant, or both. Most patients with congenital anomalies of the mitral valve belong to this type.

Table 127-1 shows the association between functional classification and the morphologic findings adapted from Carpentier and Brizard[10] and Chauvaud and colleagues.[28]

DIAGNOSIS

The diagnosis of a congenital mitral valve anomaly relies on the clinical findings, the chest radiograph, the electrocardiogram (ECG), and, most importantly, the echocardiographic study.[27] A positive diagnosis of an isolated mitral valve anomaly can often be made before the

TABLE 127-1 **Functional Classification of Mitral Valve Anomalies**

Functional Type	Anatomic Pathology	Surgical Technique
Type I	Posterior leaflet defect	Posterior annulus plication
	Cleft mitral valve	Direct suture Patch enlargement
	Annular dilation	Adult-size annulus: remodeling annuloplasty with or without leaflet enlargement Less-than-adult-size annulus: posterior annuloplasty, leaflet enlargement
Type II	Elongated chords	PTFE chords, chordal shortening, chordal transfer Wedge resection, sliding plasty
	Absent chords	PTFE chords Chordal transfer
	Elongated papillary muscle	Sliding plasty Papillary muscle shortening
	Excess tissue	Chordal shortening Leaflet resection (techniques vary with patient age: triangular, quadrangular, central body of the leaflet)
Type III	Lack of valvar tissue	Posterior leaflet detachment and enlargement Anterior leaflet enlargement
	Papillary muscle to commissure fusion	Fenestration of papillary muscle Commissurotomy
	Parachute mitral valve	Fenestration of papillary muscle Splitting of papillary muscle Commissurotomy Posterior leaflet detachment and enlargement
	Hammock mitral valve	Mobilization of suspension apparatus, separation from posterior wall Anterior leaflet enlargement Posterior annuloplasty

PTFE, Polytetrafluoroethylene.

echocardiographic examination. However, when there are associated cardiac anomalies, the clinical investigation may only raise the index of suspicion of a mitral valve disease, or it may be missed completely. Echocardiography is part of the initial evaluation of all pediatric patients with cardiac signs, but when there are associated lesions, it is essential to the diagnosis of a congenital mitral valve anomaly. In most patients, the echocardiography shows the congenital nature of the anomaly by demonstrating the variance with the normal anatomy. The functional evaluation of the mitral valve and the impact of the lesion on the cardiovascular system are best made by echocardiographic study. Neither a catheter study nor a ventriculogram has any value in the diagnosis of or preoperative assessment for mitral valve disease, although the catheter study and angiography may be helpful for associated lesions (e.g., complex VSDs and some arch anomalies).

Clinical Examination

Patients rarely present with mitral stenosis during the neonatal period, but when they do, the associated lesions may predominate. Beyond the neonatal period, symptoms may include failure to thrive, dyspnea on exertion, pallor, hypotrophy, and a history of repeated chest infections. Signs of low cardiac output can be found, such as pallor and cold extremities, tachycardia, and dyspnea. Signs of pulmonary hypertension are present, with exacerbated second heart sound and palpation of the right ventricular impulse. A diminished first heart sound suggests thick leaflets of limited excursion. A low-intensity mid-diastolic murmur is the only direct auscultation sign, and it can be absent in a low-output situation.

Patients presenting with mitral regurgitation in the neonatal period are rare. At all ages, patients with mitral regurgitation present with various degrees of failure to thrive and with dyspnea on feeding or exertion. An enlarged left ventricular impulse may be present, and a high-frequency, high-intensity holosystolic murmur is heard at the apex extending into the axillae.

Electrocardiography and Chest Radiography

The ECG shows left atrial and left ventricular enlargement in patients with mitral regurgitation. Right atrial and right ventricular enlargements are seen when pulmonary hypertension is present. In the pediatric population, there is almost always sinus rhythm.

Chest radiography demonstrates double density of the left atrial enlargement and various degrees of pulmonary plethora with an enlarged main pulmonary artery. Left ventricular enlargement in the presence of mitral valve regurgitation is evident.

Echocardiography

The echocardiographic study is essential. Systematically conducted, it provides all the information necessary for the diagnosis of the mitral anomaly, its severity, and its impact on the physiology.[29] The anatomic lesion can usually be strongly suspected. Echocardiography provides indications for surgery and gives assistance to the surgeon in the repair.[15]

The four-chamber view obtained with the transthoracic echocardiographic study is best to provide an accurate transvalvar gradient and define the precise amplitude of any prolapse or restriction. The short-axis view of the mitral valve (en face view) gives a direct vision of the area of the mitral orifice and allows good localization of the origin of the regurgitant jet. It allows a precise analysis of the papillary muscles (presence, size, location, and symmetry). Transesophageal echocardiography is superior for anatomic details of the suspension apparatus and evaluation of the functional classification. The probe can be moved up and down in the esophagus, providing precise localization of the area of prolapse along the free edge of the anterior leaflet, using the anterior commissure (probe up) and the posterior commissure (probe down) as benchmarks.

For mitral stenosis, the peak instantaneous and mean gradients across the valve have to be interpreted according to the quality of the diastolic function of the heart and the associated lesions. The overall impact of the gradient on the indication for surgery has to be weighed with the pulmonary artery pressure, and even more with clinical tolerance.

Three-dimensional echocardiography is progressing rapidly with the exponential increase of computer power and miniaturization of the probes. However, the information generated is of little use in small patients because the spatial and temporal resolutions are still insufficient. Generally, in patients larger than 30 kg, the most obvious benefit of three-dimensional echocardiography is the ability to locate very precisely on the three-dimensional en face view image the site of a two-dimensional cut. It is then only on the two-dimensional cut that the degree of prolapse or restriction can be quantified precisely.

Other Investigation Techniques

Whatever imaging technique is used, there are limitations in small patients, in whom spatial and temporal resolutions are critical. Neither magnetic resonance imaging (MRI) nor computed tomography has enough spatial resolution for the valvar tissue or the suspension apparatus in small children.

MRI allows precise calculation of the ventricular volumes irrespective of the septal geometry; this may aid in making decisions about treating patients with small left ventricle in mitral valve stenosis.[31] The regurgitation fraction is measured accurately. Gradients and flows are demonstrated with MRI. In small patients, MRI does not help with the analysis of the valve anatomy. On the other hand, MRI can provide useful functional and morphologic information preoperatively.[32]

MEDICAL TREATMENT

Medical therapy should be vigorous when the annulus is too small to receive a mechanical prosthesis in the anatomic position. When mitral regurgitation is predominant, the treatment should include an angiotensin-converting enzyme (ACE) inhibitor, diuretics, and, if necessary, red blood cell transfusion.[33] In patients with mitral stenosis, afterload reduction is contraindicated.

SURGICAL TREATMENT

Indications for surgical intervention in infants differ from those in adults, but the difference is related more to the size of the mitral valve annulus than to the age of the patient. When the annulus is close to an adult size, the timing of the surgical intervention is directly related to the probability of successful repair of the valve. One can now say that in patients older than 1 year of age, using a wide range of mitral valve repair techniques, repair of virtually all valves is an accessible goal. Valves with great probability of repair should be operated on as soon as the regurgitation is severe, regardless of symptom severity—especially valves that usually do not need annular stabilization. The timing is then related to the experience of the surgical team. Conversely, in patients with small annuli, an important multi-institutional retrospective study[4] has demonstrated very strong risk association when there is a mismatch between the prosthetic size and the diameter of the recipient annulus.

In neonates and infants a repair can be technically challenging, and replacement is often possible only with mechanical prostheses in supra-annular position associated with significant mortality.[34] Therefore, surgery should be deferred as long as the patient can be managed medically. New techniques have been described recently to allow mitral valve replacement in annular position in small annuli, including in neonates.[35,36] These techniques should allow for a slightly more acceptable rescue strategy and hence a more aggressive approach for severely symptomatic neonates or infants; they do not, however, represent a dramatic change in the treatment paradigm.

In pediatric patients, long-term ventricular function returns to normal in severely symptomatic patients when the operation is successful,[37,38] which is different from the adult population and allows to wait longer for technical need. Recent retrospective series of mechanical valve replacements in patients younger than 24 months demonstrate favorable results. They describe patients who belong to the recent era with appropriate anticoagulation therapy and with prosthesis implanted in annular position.[39-41] An important multi-institutional retrospective study[42] has demonstrated very strong risk association when there is a mismatch between the prosthetic size and the diameter of the recipient annulus (i.e., a ratio of prosthesis size to body weight of greater than 3).

On the other hand, repair of virtually all mitral valves for patients older than 1 year, using a wide range of techniques, is an accessible goal.[15,28] In small mitral annuli, the repair is difficult, but replacement generates high mortality.[34,43] The surgery should be delayed whenever possible, but it should be conducted without hesitation when it cannot be delayed,[15,44] and associated cardiac lesions should be treated at the same time. For large mitral annuli, repair is possible most of the time, and mitral valve replacement, when necessary, can now be done with very good long-term outcomes. Results of earlier series were less satisfactory.

Mitral Valve Replacement

Mitral valve replacement in the supra-annular position in infants should be avoided at all cost. This type of implantation is responsible for most or all of the perioperative and long-term deaths in units with experience of these patients.[45] Mitral valve repair in these cases is often a palliation, for the long or short term, but it allows annular growth and eventual replacement in patients who are in better condition technically.[15]

Mitral valve replacement in larger annuli is possible now, with excellent long-term results. Only mechanical valves should be implanted. Low-profile aortic valves have proved to be useful for pediatric mitral valve replacement. The valve must be removed from the valve holder and implanted with the opening toward the ventricular cavity. The bioprostheses have been associated with early degeneration and reoperation, and they should not be used in the pediatric age group.[46]

Replacement of mechanical prostheses is not uncommon in pediatric units. The indication is usually the appearance of a gradient with pulmonary hypertension, at rest (on Doppler study or catheter study) or on exertion (on Doppler study).[47] A larger size can usually be implanted, and in exceptional cases, it may be more than two sizes greater than the prosthesis it replaces.[48] This is one of the most important motivations behind the policy of initial repair and postponement of the first replacement as much as possible. Technically, the replacement of a pediatric mechanical prosthesis differs significantly from replacement in the adult. Great care must be taken to remove all cuff tissue and pledgets. Everting mattress sutures, especially with pledgets, should be avoided, as they reduce the size of the annulus. Simple interrupted sutures or running polypropylene sutures are preferable. The mechanical valves implanted are designed for an adult flow at high velocity. When implanted in the mitral position in infants, they are submitted to approximately one fifth of the flow they are designed for and at low velocity. The target international normalized ratio (INR) has to be increased accordingly.

Two mitral valve replacement techniques[35,36] in annular position have been recently described for neonates and infants. Both use the same glutaraldehyde bovine jugular valve available commercially either in a stented version (Melody, Medtronic, Minneapolis, MN) or an unstented version (Contegra, Medtronic) (Fig. 127-6).

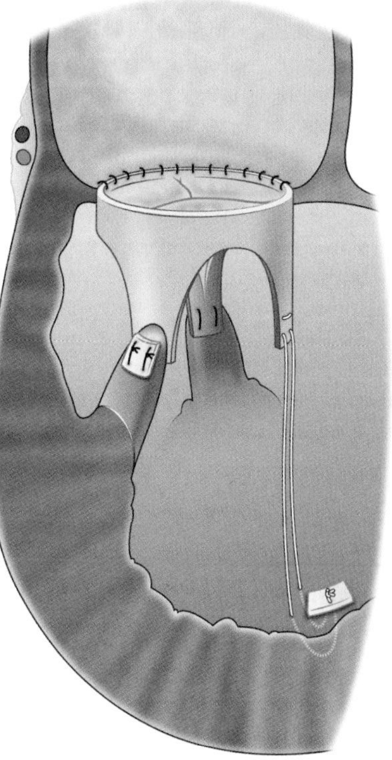

FIGURE 127-6 ■ Implantation of a Contegra valve in annular position. Note that the commissure suspended with the artificial chordae is toward the ventricular cavity (as opposed to facing the posterior wall).

Mitral Valve Repair

The techniques for mitral valve repair are described by Carpentier[26] for adult surgery, with modifications for pediatric patients and small congenital mitral valves.[15,28] Cardiopulmonary bypass in Melbourne is conducted with moderate hypothermia 32° C, hemoglobin 10 g/dL, and a pump flow of 150 to 200 mL/min/kg or 1 liter/min/m^2. Warm-blood cardioplegia, administered every 20 to 30 minutes, provides myocardial protection. Venous cannulation should allow as much room into the AV groove. The superior vena cava is cannulated directly, at a distance from the cavoatrial junction and the inferior vena cava immediately at the origin. Limited dissection of the groove is performed. After cross-clamping, the left atrium is entered via the AV groove. The exposure is enhanced with mattress sutures, inserted into the posterior annulus, that pull the valve upward and toward the operator. The snugger on the inferior vena cava pulls upward and to the left. A self-retaining retractor for mitral surgery must be adapted to the size of the patient.

Alternative approaches are less satisfactory. The transatrial septal approach does not provide an edge for the retractor blades to anchor and it exposes the conduction tissue to more pressure. It also takes time to reconstruct.

During the preparation for bypass, the mandatory preoperative transesophageal echocardiographic study is performed. Once the mitral valve is satisfactorily exposed, it is systematically analyzed, integrating preoperative information. The functional class is confirmed, whereas the extension of mitral valve prolapse or restriction is based on echocardiographic studies only. The location (A1 to 3, P1 to 3) is eventually confirmed intraoperatively. Then, the morphologic and anatomic examination is performed, which includes the following elements: a supravalvar ring is confirmed or eliminated, and determinations are made of (1) the annular diameter; (2) the texture, aspect, and size of the mitral valve leaflets; (3) the number, aspect, and distribution of the chords; (4) the presence of commissural tissue and dedicated suspension apparatus; and (5) the presence, size, location, and morphology of the papillary muscles. The examination finishes with a careful check for accessory mitral valve tissue in the interchordal spaces. The measured diameters of the annulus and of the mitral valve opening are compared with that calculated for the patient's body surface area. In Melbourne, we use a modification of the sizes provided by Kirklin and Barratt-Boyes.[49]

The treatment is adapted to the predominant functional class. A correlation between functional class, anatomic pathology, and surgical treatment is shown in Table 127-1. The techniques included in the table are identical to those used in adult mitral valve repair surgery.[26] Few modifications are dictated by the size of the pediatric patients.[15]

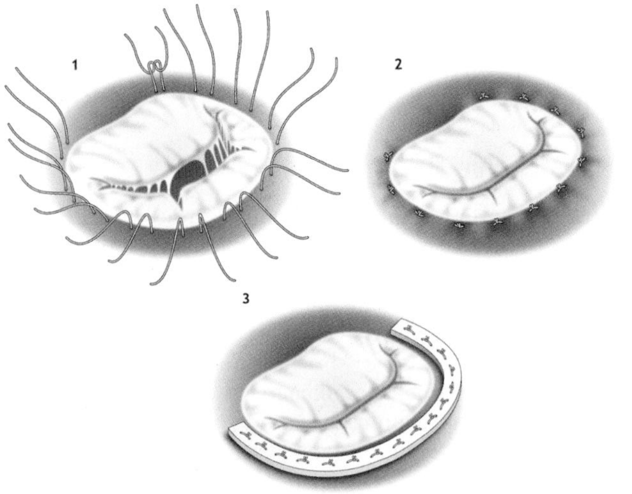

FIGURE 127-7 ■ Posterior annuloplasty made with a band of two or three layers of an expanded polytetrafluoroethylene sheet. Best results are obtained when the posterior annuloplasty is kept continuous. Alternately, the annuloplasty can be achieved by tying the mattress sutures over themselves (compression sutures).

Correction of Type I: Remodeling Annuloplasty

The annuloplasty is mandatory in all operations for mitral valve insufficiency, except in some patients with an isolated type I mitral valve anomaly without annular dilation, mostly cleft mitral valves. The purpose of the annuloplasty is to adapt the area of the mitral valve orifice (in systole) to the leaflet tissue available. Attempts to perform mitral valve repair without annuloplasty have resulted in recurrence.[28] A remodeling annuloplasty involves inserting a rigid adult-size ring (or a size larger than would be indicated by the area of the anterior leaflet). To achieve an adult-size ring in children or teenagers, the leaflet tissue must be enlarged—usually the posterior leaflet, less often the anterior leaflet, or both.[50,51] In patients with a type III mitral valve anomaly, the detachment of the posterior leaflet to gain access to the suspension apparatus is used for the leaflet enlargement.[15] When no device is available for the size of the patient, or when the device is thought to be too small, the annuloplasty is limited to the posterior annulus. The annuloplasty must incorporate both trigones. Experience with our own patients[15] suggests that the greater stability of the annuloplasty is achieved with either a continuous strip of polytetrafluoroethylene (PTFE) or a row of compression mattress sutures tied over themselves (Fig. 127-7; also see Figs. 127-1, 127-2, and 127-3). We use a sheet of expanded PTFE folded two or three times, to avoid corrugating. Mattress sutures should not be tied too tightly.

Correction of Type II

Correction of type II mitral valve anomalies is rarely necessary in patients with congenital mitral regurgitation. Type II is mostly a secondary lesion, or it is seen with associated lesions (mostly large volume loading of the left ventricle), but correction is always required in patients with a connective tissue disorder and mitral valve prolapse. Multiple techniques are available to correct the enhanced leaflet motion.[15] Whether techniques should be used in isolation or in combination depends on the extension in width of the prolapsus (i.e., localized or extended to the whole width of the free edge). It is the height of the prolapsus (based on the preoperative echocardiographic study) that will dictate the choice of the technique.

All techniques are efficient and reliable, providing that the correction restores a large surface of apposition between anterior and posterior leaflets. Overcorrection, however, generates stress directly on the repaired area and negates the stress relief provided by the surface apposition. All overcorrections eventually fail.

Artificial chords are used when chords of appropriate strength and quality are not available in the area of the prolapse. The insertion requires rigorous technique to avoid overcorrection and large knots at the free edge (Fig. 127-8). Artificial chords are safe for pediatric patients and allow adequate growth of the repair from the papillary muscle and the leaflet tissue.[52]

Chordal shortening requires thin and flexible chords. The correction generates significant shortening of the chords and is performed only when high and localized prolapse is considered (Fig. 127-9).

Chordal transfer between secondary chords and the free edge is preferred to chordal transfer from posterior leaflet to anterior leaflet, because the length is naturally adapted for the correction of localized prolapse (Fig. 127-10). The chord should be detached from the body of the anterior leaflet with a minimal amount of valvar tissue. It is then attached to the free edge directly at the required length with a small running suture.

Wedge resection and sliding plasty generate different degrees of correction of prolapsus to multiple chords. They are well adapted to prolapsus extended to a large segment of the anterior leaflet free edge (Figs. 127-11 and 127-12).

Papillary muscle shortening is essentially used in Marfan and mitral valve prolapse for the correction of combined anterior and posterior type II (Fig. 127-13).

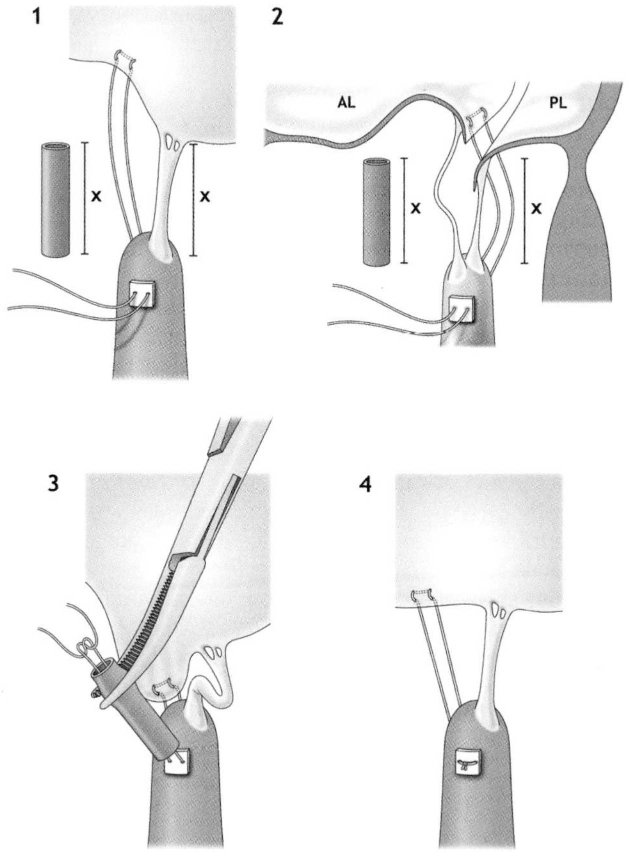

FIGURE 127-8 ■ Artificial chords of expanded polytetrafluoroethylene. Rigorous technique is necessary to avoid overcorrection and large knots at the free edge. *1,* A template is made from a short plastic tube cut at the required length and slid over the distal part of the stitch. *2,* This template can be taken from the facing posterior leaflet edge. *3,* The free edge of the leaflet is lowered to the contact of the papillary muscle. The artificial chorda is tied while the template is clamped. *4,* The template is removed and the mattress suture is pulled to bring the knot in contact of the papillary muscle. *AL,* Anterior leaflet; *PL,* posterior leaflet.

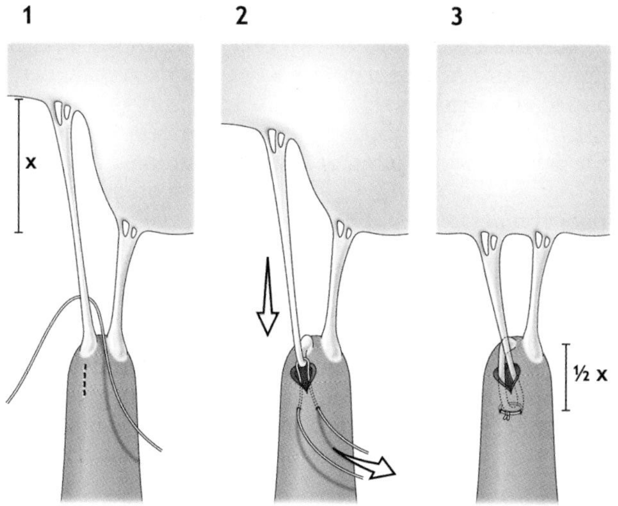

FIGURE 127-9 ■ Chordal shortening. Note the extent of the shortening achieved.

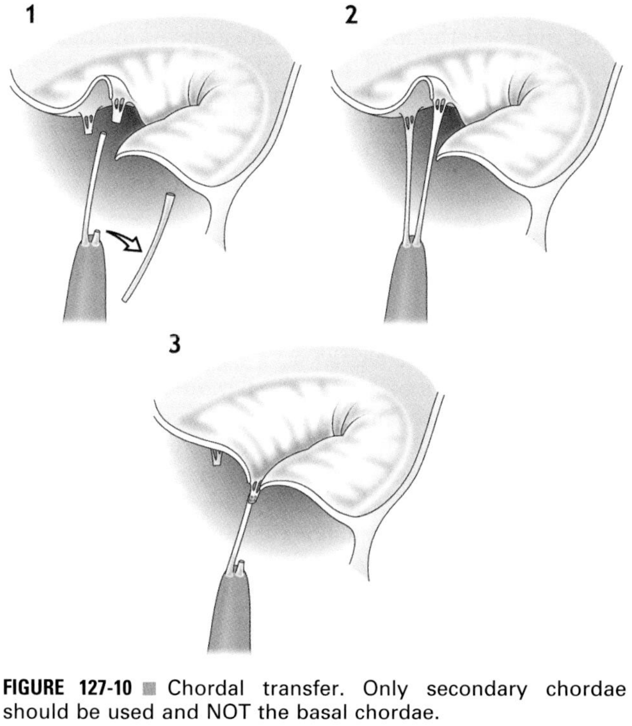

FIGURE 127-10 ■ Chordal transfer. Only secondary chordae should be used and NOT the basal chordae.

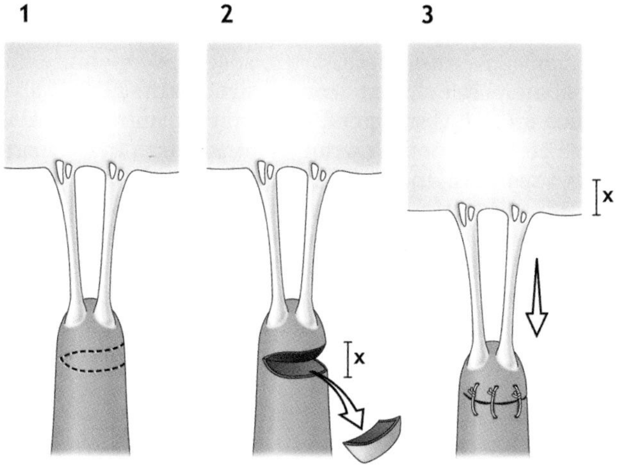

FIGURE 127-11 ■ Wedge resection. Achieves limited shortening distributed to several chordae.

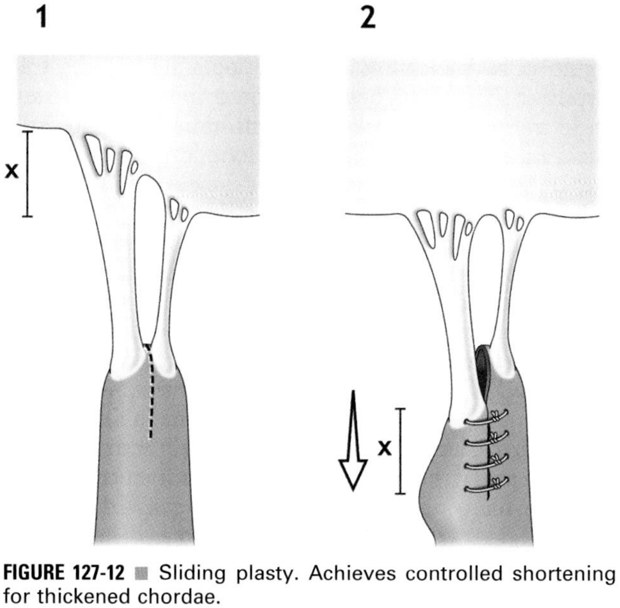

FIGURE 127-12 ■ Sliding plasty. Achieves controlled shortening for thickened chordae.

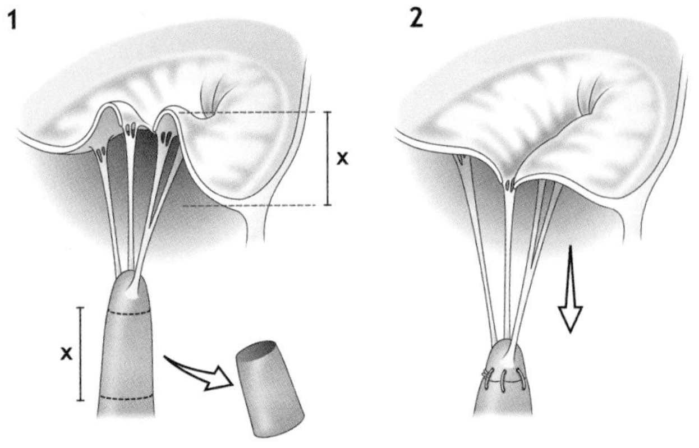

FIGURE 127-13 ■ Papillary muscle shortening.

Correction of Type III

Type III congenital mitral anomalies consist primarily of restricted leaflet motion and insufficient leaflet tissue, and their successful correction is essential, especially in the first year of life.

Mobilization of Papillary Muscles. Access to the suspension apparatus is necessary to adequately mobilize the papillary muscles. Access can be through the mitral valve orifice when it is sufficient, but often the mitral orifice is small and does not allow sufficient access to the suspension apparatus. In these situations, detachment of the posterior leaflet can provide good exposure to the papillary muscles. Adequate thinning, mobilization from the posterior wall, and splitting and fenestration of the papillary muscles can then be performed safely. The posterior leaflet is later reconstructed with enlargement of the leaflet tissue (Fig. 127-14).[15]

Enlargement of Valvar Leaflet with Pericardium Patch. Augmentation of the leaflet tissue is the only way to treat a lack of valvar tissue.[15] The anterior leaflet, the posterior leaflet, or both can be extended. Extension of the posterior leaflet should be limited to less than half of the height of the leaflet; it can be limited to the area of the middle scallop. Alternatively, when the detachment is extended from one commissure to another, the extension should reproduce a shape with three scallops and two commissures to allow a large opening in diastole. Crescent-shaped patches with a short inner edge are stenotic and the stenosis worsens with time. The extension of the anterior leaflet should be done in the body of the leaflet, leaving a strip of valvar tissue close to the hinge point to avoid mechanical stress at this level. The height of the extension should not be greater than two fifths of the height of the leaflet, leaving the area close to the free edge intact to allow a supple and effective surface of coaptation. If possible, it should be symmetrical from trigone to trigone. Since the early 1980s, the best default material has been autologous pericardium treated intraoperatively with 0.625% glutaraldehyde. Long-term results have been somehow unpredictable. Animal studies have suggested that new treatment to bovine pericardium may provide a better alternative.[53] Long-term results in clinical valvar setting are not yet available.

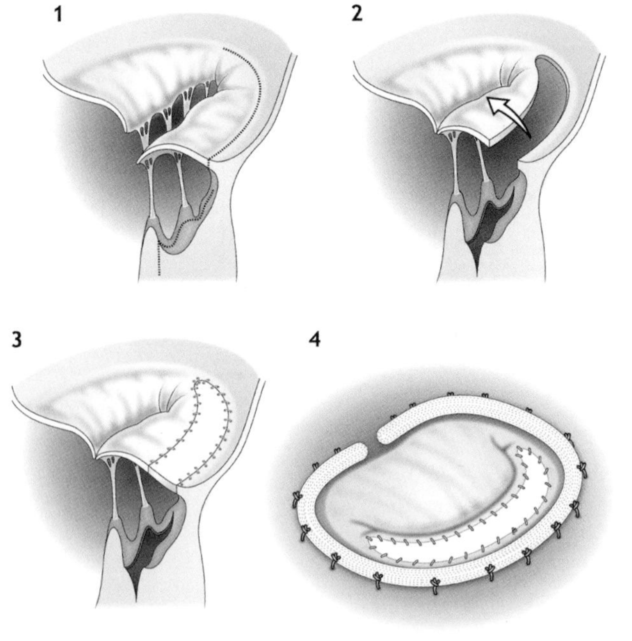

FIGURE 127-14 ■ Detachment of the posterior leaflet. *1,* Hammock or papillary commissure fusion. Access to the suspension apparatus is limited through the natural mitral orifice. *2,* After detachment of the posterior leaflet, mobilization and splitting of the suspension apparatus can be performed easily, even in the smallest valves. *3,* After repair. *4,* With annuloplasty.

Resection of Supravalvar Rings and Accessory Mitral Valve Tissue. Resection of supravalvar tissue requires an excellent exposure of the leaflet tissue. The supravalvar tissue can sometimes be peeled off the valvar tissue. More often, careful blunt dissection is needed. If perforation of the anterior leaflet occurs, it should be closed with simple figure-eight sutures (Fig. 127-15).

Resection of accessory mitral valve tissue requires similarly rigorous surgical technique. A good exposure of the subvalvar apparatus is needed to perfectly delineate the mitral valve chords from what can be resected without compromising the integrity of the suspension apparatus (Fig. 127-16). Various approaches to the suspension apparatus may have to be combined, such as through the mitral valve orifice and the aortic valve, and via detachment of the posterior leaflet.

Repair of Recurrent Left Atrioventricular Valve Regurgitation. Two separate anatomies leading to different surgical techniques have to be identified according to the size of the LLL.[25] The most common one is the normally developed LLL. The least common is the absent or diminutive LLL.

In the presence of a normal LLL, in some cases, the AV valve can be repaired by suturing or resuturing the cleft. To achieve a stable long-term result with simple suturing, the cleft should be thin and pliable and there should be redundant leaflet tissue to avoid putting suture under stress and to allow for a large zone of apposition facing the tip of the LLL. When the cleft has not ruptured or when there is significant retraction of the edges of the cleft, the valve should be repaired with adjunction of valvar tissue and pericardial patch should be used. The

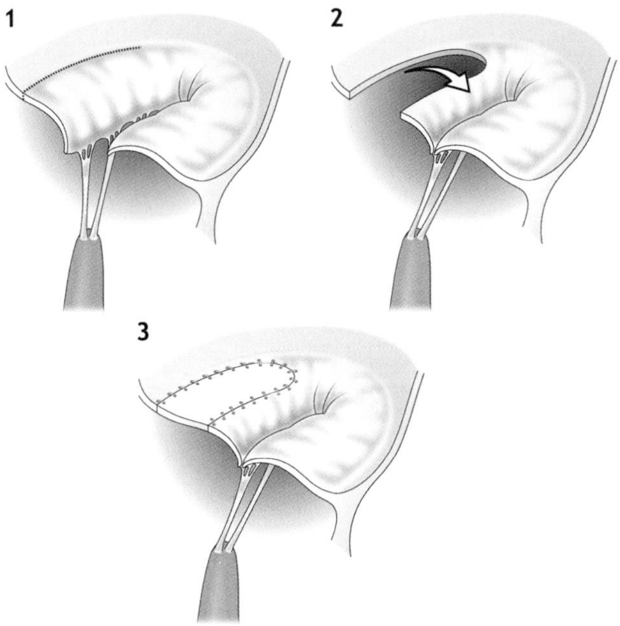

FIGURE 127-15 ■ Patch enlargement of the anterior leaflet to treat the lack of tissue in congenital valve or the retraction of the rheumatic leaflet.

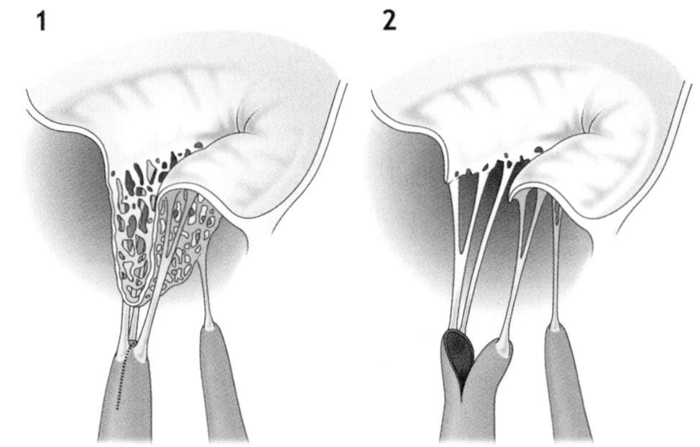

FIGURE 127-16 ■ Excision of extravalvar tissue within a parachute mitral valve. Great care must be taken to preserve the suspension apparatus.

area of the combined superior and inferior bridging leaflet can be augmented at the septal end of the leaflets.[54] At Royal Children's Hospital in Melbourne, we prefer creating a coaptation surface in front of the LLL using the cleft patch augmentation technique.[25]

The area of the cleft closure is débrided of all secondary lesions around the regurgitation zone. Sufficient resection is performed to reach pliable leaflet tissue. The area of the cleft is then closed with a long and narrow patch. The patch extends into the ventricular cavity so as to create a coaptation surface to face the tip of the LLL (Fig. 127-17).

In the case of absent or hypoplastic LLL, the cleft is reopened where it had been partially closed, and a surface of coaptation is constructed on both edges of the cleft. In this anatomy, at Royal Children's Hospital, three different techniques are used, according to the difficulty and

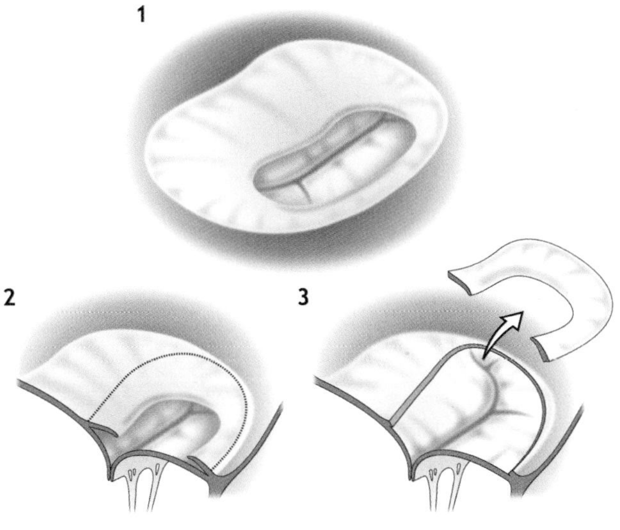

FIGURE 127-17 ■ Excision of supravalvar mitral ring.

the anatomy; most commonly, the edges of the cleft can be directly suspended using expanded PTFE chords (Fig. 127-18). A patch may be necessary to increase the surface area of the superior bridging leaflet and favor the creation of a large coaptation surface between native valvar tissue. Alternatively, we have used a partial mitral valve homograft of adapted size to reproduce the zone of apposition. This technique has demonstrated very good immediate and intermediate results in our experience and should allow sufficient palliation time to wait until an adult-size prosthesis can be used.

The double orifice should not be closed, because it is never regurgitant and can produce a valuable area of valve opening.

RESULTS

Mitral Valve Stenosis and Predominant Stenotic Valves

Between 1996 and 2014, 42 patients, 21 of whom were younger than 1 year, were operated on for congenital mitral stenosis. The most common pathologies were supramitral mitral ring (as predominant mechanism) (n = 15), papillary muscle to commissure fusion (n = 12), and parachute mitral valve (n = 6). Fourteen patients had Shone syndrome. There were three deaths, all Shone syndrome patients and all eventually after secondary mitral valve replacement. There were 10 reoperations and 4 mitral valve replacements (2 mechanical and 2 Contegra).

Mitral Valve Insufficiency and Predominant Regurgitant Valves

Ninety-eight patients were operated on for predominant congenital mitral regurgitation. There were 33 patients with mitral cleft. All are alive; one needed a reoperation, and all but two have no or mild residual regurgitation.

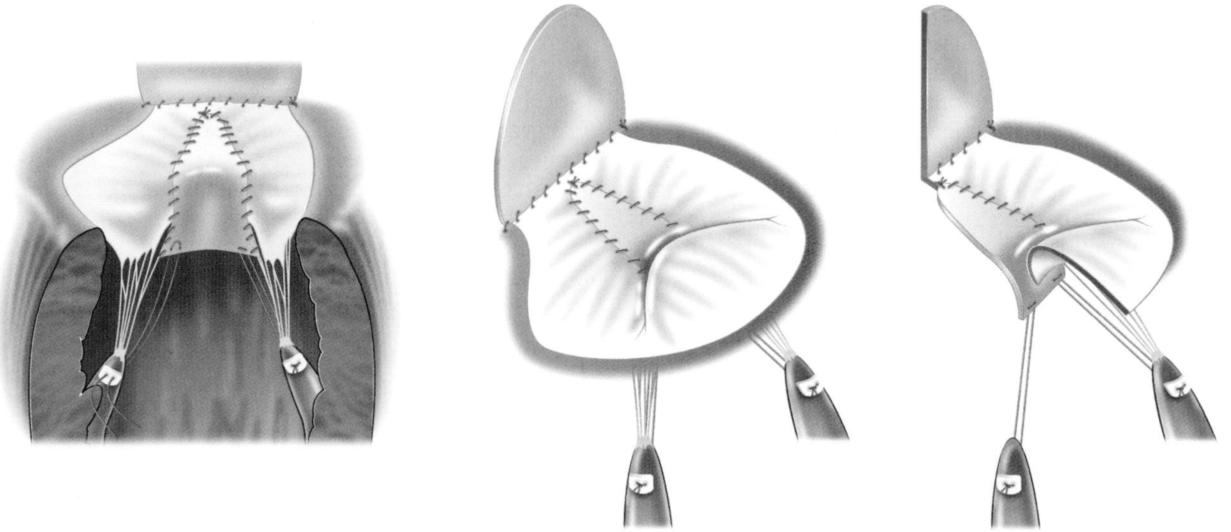

FIGURE 127-18 ■ Re-do left atrioventricular valve repair. Most common anatomy with large left lateral leaflet and two papillary muscles. A narrow pericardial patch is sutured to the edges of the cleft and extended into the inflow of the valve to enlarge the zone of apposition facing the tip of the left lateral leaflet. Suspension to the free edge of the patch is done with artificial chords.

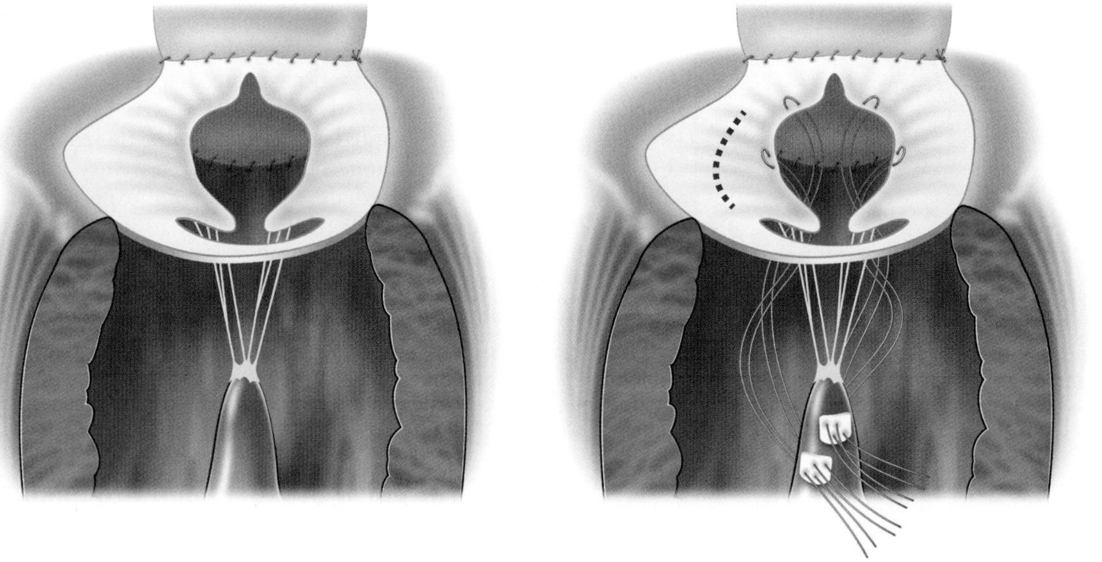

FIGURE 127-19 ■ Re-do left atrioventricular valve repair. Rare anatomy with absent left lateral leaflet. Suspension of the free edges of the superior and inferior bridging leaflet with artificial chords and posterior annuloplasty. Suitable when the edges of the cleft are flexible.

There were 65 patients with causes other than a mitral cleft, and in this group, 30 patients were younger than 1 year. This whole group had 13 reoperations and 5 deaths. The freedom from reoperation at 5 years for patients younger than 1 year of age compared with patients older than 1 year is significantly different: 59% versus 95.7% ($P = 0.007$). Two patients have had a mechanical replacement and one had a Contegra; all are alive.

Recurrent Left Atrioventricular Valve Regurgitation

Since 1978, more than 700 patients were operated on at Royal Children's Hospital in Melbourne for complete or partial AVSD. From 1996 to 2008, 42 patients were reoperated on for recurrent severe mitral regurgitation with the technique described in this chapter.[25] Five patients had a diminutive or absent LLL, and 37 had a normally developed LLL. The 42 patients had one to four (2.36 ± 1.1) left AV valve repairs, not including valve replacement. The actuarial risk for needing a second reoperation in the normal LLL group was 41% (6% to 63%; 95% CI) in the direct cleft closure group as opposed to 8% (up to 82%) in the cleft patch augmentation group ($P = 0.04$). In the diminutive or absent LLL group (Fig. 127-19), three out of five patients eventually required valve replacement at 1, 10, and 12 years postoperatively.

REFERENCES

1. Oosthoek PW, Wenink AC, Vrolijk BC, et al: Development of the atrioventricular valve tension apparatus in the human heart. *Anat Embryol (Berl)* 198(4):317–329, 1998.
2. Wessels A, Markman MW, Vermeulen JL, et al: The development of the atrioventricular junction in the human heart. *Circ Res* 78(1):110–117, 1996.
3. Oosthoek PW, Wenink AC, Wisse LJ, et al: Development of the papillary muscles of the mitral valve: morphogenetic background of parachute-like asymmetric mitral valves and other mitral valve anomalies. *J Thorac Cardiovasc Surg* 116(1):36–46, 1998.
4. Binet JP, Piot C, Losay J, et al: [A new anatomo-clinical entity? The left superior vena cava obstructing the interior of the left atrium in association with a left-right shunt. Apropos of 2 cases]. *Arch Mal Coeur Vaiss* 71(1):104–111, 1978.
5. Cochrane AD, Marath A, Mee RB: Can a dilated coronary sinus produce left ventricular inflow obstruction? An unrecognized entity. *Ann Thorac Surg* 58(4):1114–1116, 1994.
6. Kohl T, Silverman NH: Comparison of cleft and papillary muscle position in cleft mitral valve and atrioventricular septal defect. *Am J Cardiol* 77(2):164–169, 1996.
7. Tamura M, Menahem S, Brizard C: Clinical features and management of isolated cleft mitral valve in childhood. *J Am Coll Cardiol* 35(3):764–770, 2000.
8. Schaverien MV, Freedom RM, McCrindle BW: Independent factors associated with outcomes of parachute mitral valve in 84 patients. *Circulation* 109(19):2309–2313, 2004.
9. Oosthoek PW, Wenink AC, Macedo AJ, et al: The parachute-like asymmetric mitral valve and its two papillary muscles. *J Thorac Cardiovasc Surg* 114(1):9–15, 1997.
10. Carpentier A, Brizard C: Congenital malformations of the mitral valve. In Strak J, de Leval M, Tsang V, editors: *Surgery for congenital heart defects*, ed 3, Chichester, 2006, Wiley, pp 573–590.
11. Marino BS, Kruge LE, Cho CJ, et al: Parachute mitral valve: morphologic descriptors, associated lesions, and outcomes after biventricular repair. *J Thorac Cardiovasc Surg* 137(2):385–393.e4, 2009.
12. Carpentier A, Branchini B, Cour JC, et al: Congenital malformations of the mitral valve in children. Pathology and surgical treatment. *J Thorac Cardiovasc Surg* 72(6):854–866, 1976.
13. Caciolli S, Gelsomino S, Fradella G, et al: Severe hypoplasia of the posterior mitral leaflet. *Ann Thorac Surg* 86(6):1978–1979, 2008.
14. Chauvaud S, Fuzellier JF, Berrebi A, et al: Long-term (29 years) results of reconstructive surgery in rheumatic mitral valve insufficiency. *Circulation* 104(12 Suppl 1):I12–I15, 2001.
15. Oppido G, Davies B, McMullan DM, et al: Surgical treatment of congenital mitral valve disease: midterm results of a repair-oriented policy. *J Thorac Cardiovasc Surg* 135(6):1313–1320, discussion 1320–1321, 2008.
16. Stellin G, Padalino MA, Vida VL, et al: Surgical repair of congenital mitral valve malformations in infancy and childhood: a single-center 36-year experience. *J Thorac Cardiovasc Surg* 140(6):1238–1244, 2010.
17. Yoshimura N, Yamaguchi M, Oshima Y, et al: Clinical and pathological features of accessory valve tissue. *Ann Thorac Surg* 69(4):1205–1208, 2000.
18. Prifti E, Frati G, Bonacchi M, et al: Accessory mitral valve tissue causing left ventricular outflow tract obstruction: case reports and literature review. *J Heart Valve Dis* 10(6):774–778, 2001.
19. Schmid AC, Zund G, Vogt P, et al: Congenital subaortic stenosis by accessory mitral valve tissue, recognition and management. *Eur J Cardiothorac Surg* 15(4):542–544, 1999.
20. Nascimento R, Freitas A, Teixeira F, et al: Is mitral valve prolapse a congenital or acquired disease? *Am J Cardiol* 79(2):226–227, 1997.
21. Fuzellier JF, Chauvaud SM, Fornes P, et al: Surgical management of mitral regurgitation associated with Marfan's syndrome. *ATS* 66(1):68–72, 1998.
22. van Karnebeek CD, Naeff MS, Mulder BJ, et al: Natural history of cardiovascular manifestations in Marfan syndrome. *Arch Dis Child* 84(2):129–137, 2001.
23. Pepin M, Schwarze U, Superti-Furga A, et al: Clinical and genetic features of Ehlers–Danlos syndrome type IV, the vascular type. *N Engl J Med* 342(10):673–680, 2000.
24. Grau JB, Pirelli L, Yu P-J, et al: The genetics of mitral valve prolapse. *Clin Genet* 72(4):288–295, 2007.
25. Sughimoto K, d'Udekem Y, Konstantinov IE, et al: Mid-term outcome with pericardial patch augmentation for redo left atrioventricular valve repair in atrioventricular septal defect. *Eur J Cardiothorac Surg* 2015. [Epub ahead of print].
26. Carpentier A: Cardiac valve surgery—the "French correction." *J Thorac Cardiovasc Surg* 86(3):323–337, 1983.
27. Monin J-L, Dehant P, Roiron C, et al: Functional assessment of mitral regurgitation by transthoracic echocardiography using standardized imaging planes diagnostic accuracy and outcome implications. *JAC* 46(2):302–309, 2005.
28. Chauvaud S, Fuzellier JF, Houel R, et al: Reconstructive surgery in congenital mitral valve insufficiency (Carpentier's techniques): long-term results. *J Thorac Cardiovasc Surg* 115(1):84–92, discussion 92–93, 1998.
29. Banerjee A, Kohl T, Silverman NH: Echocardiographic evaluation of congenital mitral valve anomalies in children. *Am J Cardiol* 76(17):1284–1291, 1995.
30. Kutty S, Colen TM, Smallhorn JF: Three-dimensional echocardiography in the assessment of congenital mitral valve disease. *J Am Soc Echocardiogr* 27(2):142–154, 2014.
31. Grosse-Wortmann L, Yun T-J, Al-Radi O, et al: Borderline hypoplasia of the left ventricle in neonates: insights for decision-making from functional assessment with magnetic resonance imaging. *J Thorac Cardiovasc Surg* 136(6):1429–1436, 2008.
32. Cawley PJ, Maki JH, Otto CM: Cardiovascular magnetic resonance imaging for valvular heart disease: technique and validation. *Circulation* 119(3):468–478, 2009.
33. Lister G, Hellenbrand WE, Kleinman CS, et al: Physiologic effects of increasing hemoglobin concentration in left-to-right shunting in infants with ventricular septal defects. *N Engl J Med* 306(9):502–506, 1982.
34. Selamet Tierney ES, Pigula FA, Berul CI, et al: Mitral valve replacement in infants and children 5 years of age or younger: evolution in practice and outcome over three decades with a focus on supra-annular prosthesis implantation. *J Thorac Cardiovasc Surg* 136(4):954–961, 961.e1–3, 2008.
35. Abdullah I, Ramirez FB, McElhinney DB, et al: Modification of a stented bovine jugular vein conduit (melody valve) for surgical mitral valve replacement. *ATS* 94(4):e97–e98, 2012.
36. Brizard CP, d'Udekem Y, Eastaugh LJ, et al: Intra-annular mitral valve replacement in neonates and infants. *J Thorac Cardiovasc Surg* 149(1):390–392.e1, 2015.
37. Krishnan US, Gersony WM, Berman-Rosenzweig E, et al: Late left ventricular function after surgery for children with chronic symptomatic mitral regurgitation. *Circulation* 96(12):4280–4285, 1997.
38. Murakami T, Nakazawa M, Nakanishi T, et al: Prediction of postoperative left ventricular pump function in congenital mitral regurgitation. *Pediatr Cardiol* 20(6):418–421, 1999.
39. Daou L, Sidi D, Mauriat P, et al: Mitral valve replacement with mechanical valves in children under two years of age. *J Thorac Cardiovasc Surg* 121(5):994–996, 2001.
40. Henaine R, Nloga J, Wautot F, et al: Long-term outcome after annular mechanical mitral valve replacement in children aged less than five years. *Ann Thorac Surg* 90(5):1570–1576, 2010.
41. Rafii DY, Davies RR, Carroll SJ, et al: Age less than two years is not a risk factor for mortality after mitral valve replacement in children. *Ann Thorac Surg* 91(4):1228–1234, 2011.
42. Caldarone CA, Raghuveer G, Hills CB, et al: Long-term survival after mitral valve replacement in children aged. *Circulation* 104(12 Suppl 1):I143–I147, 2001.
43. Sachweh JS, Tiete AR, Mühler EG, et al: Mechanical aortic and mitral valve replacement in infants and children. *Thorac Cardiovasc Surg* 55(3):156–162, 2007.
44. Serraf A, Zoghbi J, Belli E, et al: Congenital mitral stenosis with or without associated defects: an evolving surgical strategy. *Circulation* 102(19 Suppl 3):III166–III171, 2000.
45. Selamet Tierney ES, Wald RM, McElhinney DB, et al: Changes in left heart hemodynamics after technically successful in-utero aortic valvuloplasty. *Ultrasound Obstet Gynecol* 30(5):715–720, 2007.
46. Antunes MJ: Bioprosthetic valve replacement in children–long-term follow-up of 135 isolated mitral valve implantations. *Eur Heart J* 5(11):913–918, 1984.
47. Masuda M, Kado H, Tatewaki H, et al: Late results after mitral valve replacement with bileaflet mechanical prosthesis in children:

evaluation of prosthesis-patient mismatch. *Ann Thorac Surg* 77(3):913–917, 2004.
48. Kanter KR, Forbess JM, Kirshbom PM: Redo mitral valve replacement in children. *Ann Thorac Surg* 80(2):642–645, discussion 645–646, 2005.
49. Kirklin J, Barratt-Boyes B: Anatomy, dimension and terminology. In *Cardiac surgery*, ed 2, London, 1993, Churchill Livingstone, pp 3–60.
50. Shomura Y, Okada Y, Nasu M, et al: Late results of mitral valve repair with glutaraldehyde-treated autologous pericardium. *Ann Thorac Surg* 95(6):2000–2005, 2013.
51. Chauvaud S, Jebara V, Chachques JC, et al: Valve extension with glutaraldehyde-preserved autologous pericardium. Results in mitral valve repair. *J Thorac Cardiovasc Surg* 102(2):171–177, 1991.
52. Oda S, Nakano T, Tatewaki H, et al: A 17-year experience with mitral valve repair with artificial chordae in infants and children. *Eur J Cardiothorac Surg* 44(1):e40–e45, 2013.
53. Brizard CP, Brink J, Horton SB, et al: New engineering treatment of bovine pericardium confers outstanding resistance to calcification in mitral and pulmonary implantations in a juvenile sheep model. *J Thorac Cardiovasc Surg* 148(6):3194–3201, 2014.
54. Poirier NC, Williams WG, Van Arsdell GS, et al: A novel repair for patients with atrioventricular septal defect requiring reoperation for left atrioventricular valve regurgitation. *Eur J Cardiothorac Surg* 18(1):54–61, 2000.

CHAPTER 128

Hypoplastic Left Heart Syndrome

Bret A. Mettler • Frank A. Pigula

CHAPTER OUTLINE

Hypoplastic left heart syndrome (HLHS) is characterized by a generalized underdevelopment of the left ventricle and its dependent structures: the mitral valve, the aortic valve, and the preductal and ductal aorta. Because the anatomic severity of HLHS constitutes a spectrum of disease, the value of a consistent, defined nomenclature has been recognized. Such a nomenclature has been proposed by the Congenital Heart Surgery Nomenclature and Database Project.[1] The project has proposed an operative definition for hypoplastic left heart syndrome as "a spectrum of cardiac malformations, characterized by a severe underdevelopment of the left heart–aorta complex, consisting of aortic and/or mitral atresia, stenosis, or hypoplasia with marked hypoplasia or absence of the left ventricle, and hypoplasia of the ascending aorta and the aortic arch."

The treatment of HLHS has dramatically changed over the past 2 decades. With little to offer prior to Norwood's introduction of stage I palliation in 1983, treatment has developed into a three-stage progression to the Fontan operation. Although the 1-month mortality rate for untreated patients is 95%, the current 1-month survival rate among specialized centers approaches 80% to 90%.

This chapter discusses the anatomic and physiologic challenges posed by these patients, as well as the management schemes devised to meet them.

DEMOGRAPHICS AND INCIDENCE

Two large epidemiologic reports have estimated the prevalence of HLHS to be 0.16 to 0.18 out of 1000 live births.[2,3] Males account for 57% to 67% of new cases, and the risk of sibling recurrence has been reported to be 0.5%.[4,5] No environmental risk factors associated with the diagnosis of HLHS have been identified.[6]

CLINICAL PRESENTATION

On physical examination, children with HLHS may appear entirely normal at birth. Within hours to days, however, tachypnea and pallor may become apparent with nonspecific chest radiographic and electrocardiographic findings.[7,8] Depending on the adequacy of the ductal and atrial communications, there may be rapid progress to acidosis, cyanosis, and cardiopulmonary collapse. An exception to this usual sequence occurs in neonates presenting with a restrictive atrial septum; these children will present immediately after birth in severe respiratory distress, respiratory acidosis, and cyanosis that is unresponsive to medical management.

Other congenital lesions should be sought. Natowicz and colleagues[9] reported that 28% of patients with HLHS suffered from a genetic disorder, a major noncardiac abnormality, or both. Looking specifically at the central nervous system among infants with HLHS, Glauser and colleagues[10] documented anomalies in 29% and microcephaly in 27%. Blood flow pattern in the fetus with HLHS may have important implications for brain development. Shillingford and coworkers[11] reported a correlation between microcephaly and the size of the ascending aorta. Dent and colleagues,[12] using magnetic resonance imaging (MRI) postnatally, identified ischemic lesions in 23% of patients. Thus, the preoperative evaluation of these neonates should also include genetic and neurologic evaluations.

DIAGNOSIS

Echocardiography has become the diagnostic procedure of choice in patients with HLHS. Details such as aortic valve size and status (atretic versus patent), aortic dimensions, origin of the coronary arteries, brachiocephalic branching, status of the atrial septum, function of the tricuspid and pulmonary valves, and presence of systemic or pulmonary venous anomalies should be sought. Coronary anomalies, although rare, are more likely encountered in the setting of mitral stenosis and aortic atresia and can take the form of coronary-ventricular fistulas, hypoplasia, tortuosity, or single coronary arteries (e.g., anomalous left coronary from the pulmonary artery).[12-18] Coronary abnormalities may be more frequent in mitral stenosis–aortic atresia (MS/AA) variants of HLHS, and these patients undergo additional scrutiny (discussed in further detail, later).

Cardiac Catheterization

Cardiac catheterization in patients with HLHS should be reserved for those with equivocal anatomy who may be candidates for biventricular repair, for those in whom coronary anomalies are suspected, or to delineate abnormal pulmonary venous return.

Fetal Diagnosis

Improvements in fetal echocardiography have led to an increasing frequency of antenatal diagnoses of HLHS. Tworetzky and colleagues[19] reported that prenatal diagnosis was associated with improved preoperative clinical condition as well as improved survival after the Norwood operation. Unfortunately, improved survival following Norwood palliation in children with a prenatal diagnosis has not been consistently demonstrated.[20] Mahle and others[21] have reported that although antenatal diagnosis improves these patients' preoperative clinical condition and may reduce the incidence of neurologic injury, an impact on surgical survival has not been shown.

PATHOPHYSIOLOGY

In HLHS, the right ventricle must support both the systemic and the pulmonary circulation. Pulmonary venous return must have access to the right atrium, via an atrial septal defect, via a patent foramen ovale, or, in rare cases, via anomalous pulmonary venous connections to the systemic veins. Systemic output, delivered via the ductus arteriosus, is entirely dependent on ductal patency (Fig. 128-1). Ductal involution may be a rapid process, restricting right ventricle–dependent systemic blood flow and leading to progressive metabolic acidosis, tachypnea, and irritability before cardiopulmonary collapse.

The functional size of the interatrial communication is an important physiologic determinant in these patients. In the presence of an unrestrictive atrial communication,

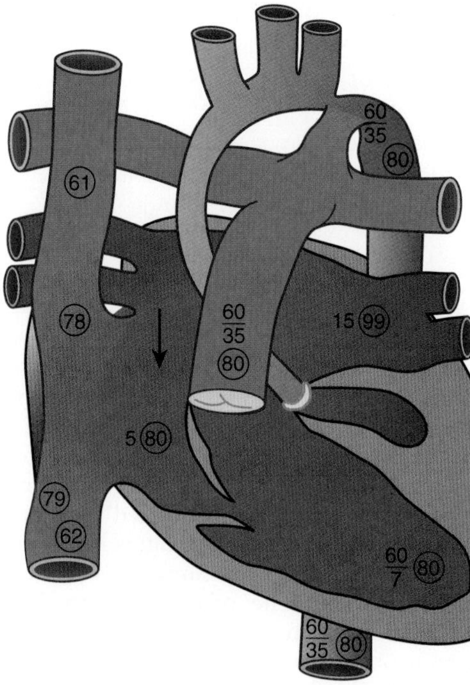

FIGURE 128-1 ■ Hemodynamics and oxygen saturations *(in circles)* of hypoplastic left heart syndrome in the unoperated state. Pulmonary venous return must cross the atrial septum *(arrow)*, where there is mixing with systemic venous return in the right atrium. Systemic cardiac output is dependent on a patent ductus arteriosus. (Reprinted with permission from Jacobs ML: Hypoplastic left heart syndrome. In Kaiser LR, Kron IL, Spray TL, editors: *Mastery of cardiothoracic surgery*, Philadelphia, 1998, Lippincott-Raven, p 859.)

pulmonary blood flow quickly becomes excessive and the signs and symptoms of congestive heart failure predominate.

A subset of neonates are born with a mildly restrictive interatrial septum (gradient of 2 to 5 mm Hg), such that pulmonary resistance is modestly elevated. This often serves to balance systemic and pulmonary blood flow, and these children may be physiologically stable, requiring little intervention before surgery. Whenever possible, allowing spontaneous respirations in an awake child often allows for the neonate to regulate the balance of pulmonary to systemic blood flows, attaining a stable circulation that greatly simplifies their preoperative management.

Finally, a few children present with severe restriction of the atrial communication. These neonates suffer from a prompt and profound hypoxemia at birth, leading rapidly to a metabolic acidosis. This variant, the functional equivalent of obstructed total anomalous pulmonary venous return (TAPVR), represents a true hemodynamic emergency requiring immediate relief. As with obstructed TAPVR, medical management of patients with this variant is uniformly unsuccessful. Interventions designed to enlarge and maintain the atrial communication have been successfully applied, such as balloon atrial septostomy and stenting.[22]

CAUSES

HLHS can be experimentally created in the chick embryo by left atrial ligation.[23] These experimental findings were anticipated clinically by Remmell-Dow and colleagues,[24] who suggested that abnormal development of the atrial septum, including underdevelopment of the eustachian valve and limbus, reduced right-to-left shunting at the atrial level, resulting in hypoplasia of the left heart structures. Premature closure of the foramen ovale has similarly been implicated, as have primary abnormalities of the aortic valve.[25-27]

Although identifiable genetic sequences have been reported to be associated with HLHS, their relevance remains unclear.[28] An understanding of the developmental factors leading to HLHS assumes new relevance as intervention during the process of cardiac morphogenesis itself (i.e., fetal surgery) is pursued.

SURGICAL TRIAGE

Patients satisfying all facets of the definition of HLHS are clearly destined for single-ventricle palliation. However, there are patients for which the decision between the pursuit of single-ventricle palliation and biventricular repair is not so clear. Once pursued, the ability to cross over to the competing treatment is difficult, and efforts to stratify patients with equivocal anatomy have been made. Rhodes and colleagues[29] combined four factors (body surface area, indexed aortic root dimension, left ventricle length, and indexed mitral valve area) to predict death after biventricular repair for critical aortic stenosis in the neonate. However, application of these criteria to hypoplastic, but nonstenotic, left heart structures using Rhodes's criteria has proven unsatisfying, as these criteria appear to be too stringent in this setting.[30] Recognizing this, the Congenital Heart Surgeons Society (CHSS) sponsored a multi-institutional study to delineate the outcomes and risk factors of critical aortic stenosis in the neonate.[31]

Presented by Lofland and colleagues,[31] this study identified multiple morphologic and functional factors that can be used to predict which surgical approach, single-ventricle palliation or biventricular repair, is more likely to result in the survival of any particular patient. This study determined that solution of a multivariable equation using these factors can predict a patient's survival. This equation, which can be found on the CHSS website (www.chssdc.org) is as follows:

Survival benefit = intercept + (age at entry)
+ (z-score of aortic valve at the sinuses)
+ (grade of EFE [endocardial fibroelastosis])
+ (ascending aortic diameter)
+ (presence of moderate or severe tricuspid regurgitation)
+ (z-score of the left ventricular length)

The prediction model was tested and refined by Hickey and the CHSS.[32] They reported that the consequences of inappropriate pursuit of a repair strategy (biventricular versus single ventricle), as predicted by the model, was minimal for single-ventricle palliation but was very significant among patients undergoing biventricular repair. This report underscores the importance of the initial decisions made when assessing and triaging neonates with borderline left heart structures to a treatment strategy.

MANAGEMENT

The natural history of HLHS is dismal: 95% of untreated patients die within 1 month.[33] Medical treatment modifies the natural history, primarily by delaying the demise.[34]

The surgical management of HLHS represents the paradigm from which a generalized approach to the shunted single ventricle has evolved. Simply stated, the cardiovascular system in HLHS consists of a single pumping chamber supporting two parallel circulations. These parallel circulations can be considered to be in competition with each other for blood flow. For any given cardiac output, the flow apportioned to each circulation is inversely proportional to the resistance of that circulation (i.e., high pulmonary vascular resistance, low pulmonary blood flow). Thus, efforts to control the circulation have focused on controlling the competing vascular resistances. These efforts have generally involved manipulation of the pulmonary vascular resistance using inspired gasses (oxygen, carbon dioxide [CO_2], and nitrous oxide) and pressures.[35-38]

More recently, an alternative approach that targets manipulation of the systemic vascular resistance to maintain the balance between the pulmonary and systemic circulations has been shown to be effective.

Manipulation of the Pulmonary Vascular Resistance

Carbon Dioxide

Inspired CO_2 has been suggested to improve the hemodynamic status after the Norwood operation.[35] Tabbutt and colleagues[39] compared the use of hypoxia (17% fraction of inspired oxygen [FiO_2]) to CO_2 in 10 neonates with HLHS prior to the Norwood operation under the conditions of fixed minute ventilation, anesthesia, and paralysis. Although both strategies reduced the ratio of pulmonary to systemic blood flow (Qp/Qs), CO_2 increased both superior vena cava co-oximetry and cerebral oximetry, whereas hypoxia reduced these indices of oxygen delivery. Bradley and coworkers[40] reported similar results among postoperative patients. It is important to note, however, that these benefits were only realized when the *minute ventilation* remained constant.

Although thought by some physicians to reflect a direct effect, there is evidence showing that the increase in pulmonary vascular resistance is reversed by alkalinization, suggesting that the effect is mediated by [H^+] and pH.[41]

Oxygen

Because the neonatal pulmonary vasculature is also sensitive to the concentration of inspired oxygen, hypoxic mixtures incorporating nitrogen have also been used to control the circulation in patients with HLHS. Animal models have shown that nitrogen-induced hypoxic mixtures increase the pulmonary vascular resistance and increase systemic blood flow. However, the prolonged use of hypoxic mixtures has been shown to quickly induce anatomic changes in the pulmonary vasculature. In animals, changes in arterial wall thickness and muscularity can be seen within 24 hours, and fewer intra-acinar arteries are recruited into the circulation.[42-44]

Day and colleagues[45] reported their clinical experience using hypoxia to manipulate the pulmonary vascular resistance in 20 neonates with single-ventricle, duct-dependent circulation awaiting heart transplant. Of these 20 patients, 8 survived; of the 10 patients who underwent lung biopsy or autopsy, 9 showed medial hypertrophy in distal arterioles, and 7 of these 9 patients died. Although the outcome cannot be completely ascribed to hypoxic management, this strategy suggests that prolonged supportive care of the neonatal single ventricle may expose these patients to significant risks.

Systemic Vascular Resistance

Manipulation of the systemic vascular resistance is a demonstrated means of controlling the shunted circulation. In fact, our ability to pharmacologically control the systemic vascular resistance probably exceeds our current ability to selectively manage the pulmonary vascular resistance. This clinical approach usually uses an irreversible α-adrenergic antagonist, phenoxybenzamine, to achieve systemic vasodilation. The desired systemic vascular resistance, defined as that which optimizes the Qp/Qs and systemic oxygen delivery, is then obtained by titrating an α-adrenergic agonist, usually norepinephrine. Specifics of this approach have been reported in the literature.[43-45]

A review of this strategy identified the use of phenoxybenzamine, continuous systemic venous oxygen monitoring, and the reduction of deep hypothermic circulatory arrest (DHCA) time as factors favoring survival to the bidirectional Glenn operation.[46] To date, no studies directly comparing outcomes for these two fundamentally different management schemes have been performed.

OPERATIVE PROCEDURE STAGE I

The anatomic goals of the stage I or Norwood operation for HLHS is threefold: (1) to provide unobstructed blood flow from the systemic right ventricle to the systemic circulation, (2) to ensure an unobstructed connection between the pulmonary venous return and the systemic right ventricle, and (3) to establish a reliable source of pulmonary blood flow. Although these goals are unchanged from those originally articulated by Norwood and colleagues in 1980, the methods by which these goals are achieved continue to evolve.

Standard Norwood Operation

The "standard" Norwood operation is performed through a median sternotomy. The branch pulmonary arteries are dissected and controlled. We routinely anastomose a 3.5-mm stretch Gore-Tex graft to the underside of the innominate artery. The graft may later serve as the right modified Blalock-Taussig shunt and is left long while it is used as the primary arterial cannulation site. Venous cannulation is performed in the right atrial appendage, through a purse-string suture large enough to allow subsequent atrial septectomy. The patient is cooled to 18° C and put on bypass, the ductus is divided, and the brachiocephalic vessels are mobilized and loosely snared. The main pulmonary artery is divided and the branch bifurcation is closed, primarily or with a patch. After at least 20 minutes of cooling and at a rectal temperature of 18° C, the brachiocephalic vessels are snared and the descending aorta is clamped. For truly diminutive aortas (<2 mm), cardioplegia is administered via a side arm into the arterial cannula, and direct needle insufflation is used in the larger aorta. We perform the Norwood operation during continuous regional low-flow perfusion, as previously described.[47-49]

The atrial septectomy is performed through a right atrial purse-string suture during a period of low-flow sucker bypass. The ductal remnant is amputated from the aorta, and the aorta is filleted open distally beyond the site of coarctation and proximally to a point adjacent to the lip of the transected pulmonary valve. The ductal insertion site is circumferentially resected, and the back wall of the aorta is sewn together, either directly or using an interdigitating technique. Proximally, a side-to-side anastomosis between the aorta and pulmonary valve is performed, and the arch is augmented using a piece of

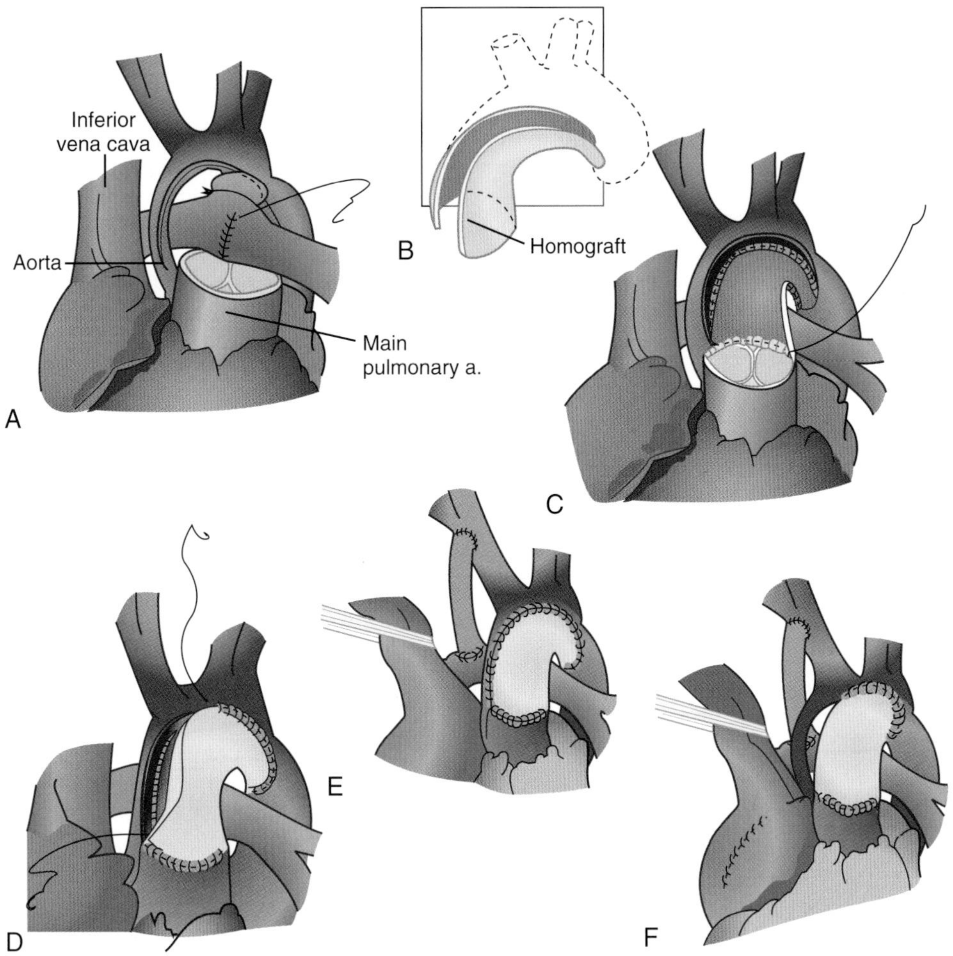

FIGURE 128-2 Technique of the Norwood operation. **A,** The pulmonary artery is transected and the bifurcation closed. The hypoplastic aorta is incised and ductal tissue excised. **B** and **C,** Graft material, usually pulmonary homograft, is cut to the appropriate size and shape for arch reconstruction. **D,** Inclusion of the pulmonary valve into the systemic circulation, with completion of the arch augmentation. **E,** Pulmonary blood flow is provided by the right modified Blalock-Taussig shunt. **F,** Anastomosis of the pulmonary artery to the arch; bypassing the diminutive ascending aorta is not recommended. Proximity of the very small ascending aorta to the shunt allows potential coronary steal and myocardial ischemia. In these cases, arch reconstruction should proceed as illustrated in **A,** or alternatively implanted into the side of the neoaorta. (Reprinted with permission from Castañeda AR: Hypoplastic left heart syndrome. In Castañeda AR, Jonas R, Mayer JE, et al, editors: *Cardiac surgery of the neonate and infant,* Philadelphia, 1994, WB Saunders, p 371.)

pulmonary homograft or fixed autologous pericardium (Fig. 128-2). Central bypass is resumed after cannulation of the reconstructed aorta, and the pulmonary anastomosis of the shunt is completed.

Results of Norwood Operation

With experience and with advances in surgical, anesthetic, and critical care management, current survival of the Norwood operation approaches 90% at specialized centers.[50,51] In one of the largest single-center series ever reported, Mahle and colleagues[52] reported their 15-year (1984-1999) experience with the Norwood operation for 840 patients with HLHS. Of these 840 patients, 65% were male and 35% female, a gender ratio similar to that reported elsewhere. The 1-, 2-, 5-, 10-, and 15-year survival rates for the group were 51%, 43%, 40%, 39%, and 39%, respectively. Risk factors identified for death were earlier era of operation, age older than 14 days, and weight less than 2.5 kg. Neither anatomic subtype nor heterotaxy was associated with mortality.

Because of the continuing evolution occurring among surgical and medical management techniques applied to HLHS, contemporary experience is important. Tweddell and colleagues[51] reported their experience with 115 consecutive patients with HLHS who underwent the Norwood operation between 1992 and 2001. They reported that, with the introduction of new management techniques in 1996, they were able to obtain a 93% hospital survival rate for neonates undergoing the Norwood operation for HLHS. These strategies included the use of phenoxybenzamine, continuous systemic venous oxygen monitoring, aprotinin, modified ultrafiltration, and, most recently, continuous cerebral perfusion. This report is also of interest because it attempts to quantify the influence of anatomic and operative variables on survival to stage II palliation rather than on operative survival. Only duration of DHCA was associated with survival to stage II palliation; no other anatomic or physiologic variable, including weight, was predictive.

A more recent review of the surgical experience of 237 patients undergoing stage I palliation at Children's Hospital Boston between 2001 and 2006 reported a hospital survival rate of 88.6%.[50] An arteriopulmonary shunt was used in 157 patients, and a right ventricle to pulmonary artery (RV-PA) conduit in 80 patients. Although the source of pulmonary blood flow did not impact hospital survival, the RV-PA conduit imparted a significant survival advantage during the interstage period (Fig. 128-3).

Anatomic Subtypes

Whereas previous studies[16,17] reported a trend toward higher mortality rates among patients with aortic valve atresia, the Children's Hospital Boston review identified patients with aortic atresia *and* mitral stenosis to be a group at higher risk than other anatomic subtypes (Fig. 128-4). Thirty-eight of 165 (23%) patients with HLHS had MS/AA. Hospital mortality and need for transplant for patients with MS/AA was significantly higher than for other anatomic subgroups (29% vs. 7.8%, $P = 0.006$; Fig. 128-5). Recently, we identified the presence of significant left ventricle to epicardial coronary artery fistula in these patients and, in one case, autopsy-proven aortocoronary atresia. A retrospective review of these patients identified echocardiographic evidence of coronary artery fistulas in 20 patients (53%) with MS/AA. The presence of suggestive echocardiographic findings was associated with a greater hospital mortality (50% vs. 6%, $P = 0.04$; Fig. 128-6). It is among this cohort of patients that the increased risk seems to be isolated; patients with MS/AA without evidence of fistulas demonstrated survival similar (94%) to other anatomic subtypes (aortic atresia–mitral atresia [AA/MA], 8.6%, and aortic stenosis–mitral stenosis [AS/MS], 7.2%; $P = 0.9$). Although these findings were originally interpreted as small muscular ventricular septal defects, cardiac catheterization has

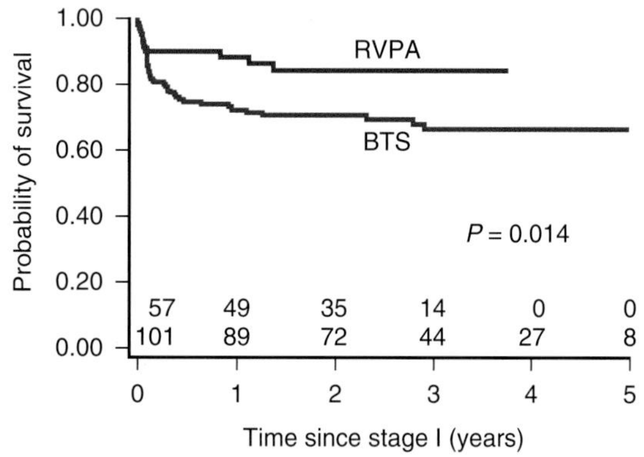

FIGURE 128-3 ■ Conditional survival based on the source of pulmonary blood flow after stage I palliation. There was no perioperative difference in survival between the arteriopulmonary (Blalock-Taussig) shunt (BTS) or the right ventricle to pulmonary artery conduit (RVPA). However, the RVPA showed a significant survival advantage during the interstage period (interstage mortality: BTS 15% vs. RVPA 0%; $P = 0.014$).

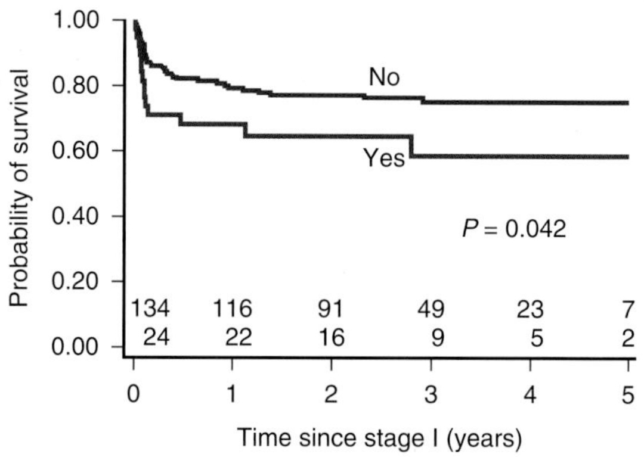

FIGURE 128-5 ■ Likelihood of survival for patients with aortic atresia with mitral stenosis (AA/MS) variant as compared with other subtypes of hypoplastic left heart syndrome. Overall survival is significantly worse for AA/MS ($P = 0.042$).

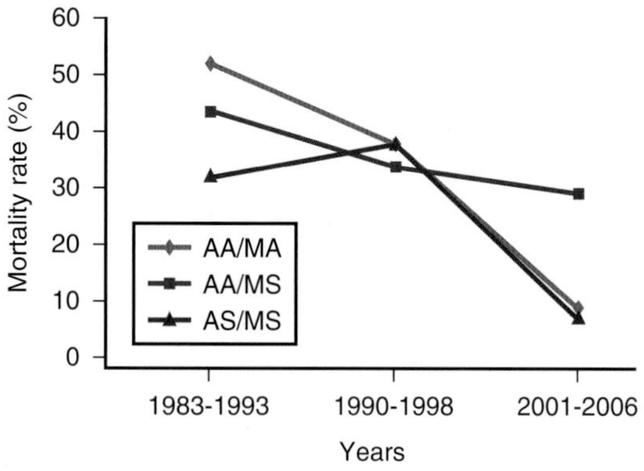

FIGURE 128-4 ■ Era effect for mortality among hypoplastic left heart syndrome anatomic subtypes aortic atresia with mitral atresia (AA/MA), aortic atresia with mitral stenosis (AA/MS), and aortic stenosis with mitral stenosis (AS/MS). Although anatomic subtypes AA/MA and AS/MS have shown improved survival, subtype AA/MS lags behind.

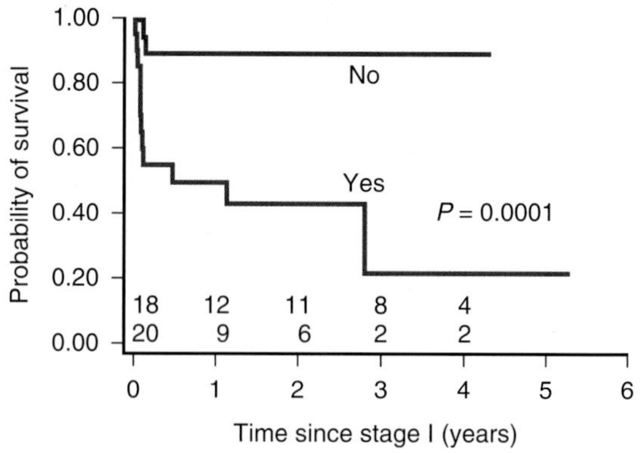

FIGURE 128-6 ■ Hypoplastic left heart syndrome (HLHS), anatomic subtype aortic atresia with mitral stenosis (AA/MS). Analysis (echocardiographic of angiographic) showed left ventricle to coronary artery fistulas to be a highly significant risk factor for death after stage I palliation for HLHS. Risk appears to reside in this subgroup (mortality, 50%) because mortality for patients with AA/MS without fistulas is similar to that for other anatomic subtypes (approximately 6%, $P = 0.0001$).

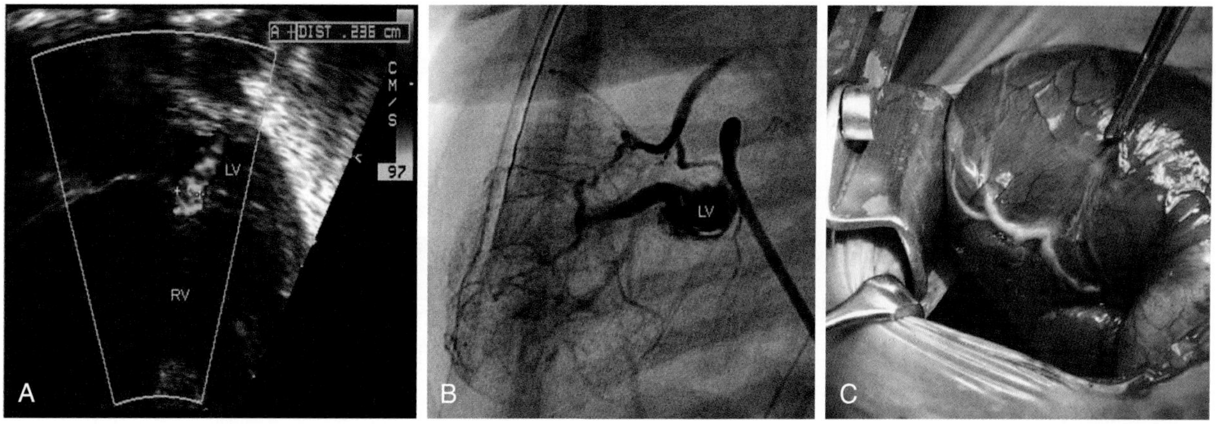

FIGURE 128-7 ■ Diagnosis of left ventricle to coronary artery fistulas. **A,** Echocardiographic examinations often reveal flow "across" the interventricular septum and have been considered to represent ventricular septal defects. **B,** Angiographic demonstration of left ventricle to coronary artery fistulas with retrograde filling of the ascending aorta in addition to the right coronary artery system. **C,** Intraoperative examination has consistently revealed a small "duvet" or "pucker" in the myocardium, presumably at the site of the fistulas, with a thickened and corkscrew appearance of the epicardial coronary artery.

clearly identified left ventricle to coronary artery fistulas in these patients (Fig. 128-7). No advantage to the arteriopulmonary shunt or the Sano modification has been identified for these patients. The exact mechanisms for the increased failure of stage I palliation in patients with AA/MS and fistulas is still unclear. We hypothesize that the presence of fistulas may contribute to dysfunction of the interventricular septum in these marginal patients. However, this remains to be proven.

Based on this experience, we have changed our institutional policy regarding the preoperative evaluation of these patients. Patients identified as being in the AA/MA subtype undergo preoperative angiography to confirm and define the incidence of left ventricle to coronary artery fistulas. In the past, many of these patients were diagnosed, by echocardiogram, with small ventricular septal defects, but in fact these echocardiographic findings most likely represent a left ventricle to coronary artery fistula. If these patients are confirmed as a high-risk group, alternative treatment pathways, such as the hybrid stage I palliation or primary transplantation, may be considered.

Source of Pulmonary Blood Flow

Surgeon experience and institutional preference have been cited as reasons for choosing the source of pulmonary blood flow after the Norwood procedure.[53-55] A prospective, multi-institutional randomized study was performed with the primary outcome death or cardiac transplantation 12 months after randomization.[56] Transplant-free survival at 12 months was greater in the patients who underwent an RV-PA conduit; however, this group had more unintended interventions and complications. Right ventricular size and function were similar within both cohorts. At 12 months of age to study completion, there was no difference in survival or transplant-free survival between the groups. Mid-term analysis of these data is currently being performed to identify if these conclusions remain true.

Interstage and Mid-term Survival

Of the 188 survivors discharged from the hospital after stage I palliation, 20 (10.6%) died in the interstage period. The median age at interstage mortality was 75 days, and it occurred exclusively in patients with an arteriopulmonary shunt (see Fig. 128-3). The cumulative pre-Glenn mortality (hospital + interstage) rate was 19.8% (47 of 237).

Low Birth Weight, Older Age

Low birth weight (<2.5 kg), consistently identified as a risk factor, was the subject of a subanalysis performed by Weinstein and colleagues.[57] They reported a 47% survival rate among 67 patients weighing less than 2.5 kg who underwent the Norwood operation between 1990 and 1997. Although lower than the institution's overall survival rate of 74%, these results are very similar to those reported by Bove and Lloyd, Forbess and colleagues, and others.[58-60] Although the patients were higher risk, there was no appreciable weight gain in neonates awaiting surgery, and the authors concluded that delaying surgery in the hope of somatic growth is unwarranted.

Whereas some reports have demonstrated poorer survival when Norwood palliation is performed after 2 to 4 weeks of life, recent reports suggest otherwise. Duncan and colleagues[61] reported 100% survival among 9 patients, aged 36 to 108 days, who underwent palliation for single-ventricle variants. Reviewing their experience with the Norwood operation for HLHS, Rossi and others[62] reported a 90% survival rate among patients older than 2 weeks of age; 100% (4 of 4) of those older than 4 weeks survived.

Norwood Operation for Hypoplastic Left Heart Syndrome Variants

Although the Norwood operation was devised specifically to treat HLHS, it has been widely applied to various

BOX 128-1 Anatomic Variants of the Great Vessels, for Which the Norwood Operation Is Performed

Normally Related Great Vessels

- Mitral atresia with ventricular septal defect (VSD)
- Mitral atresia and aortic stenosis with VSD and small left ventricle
- Interrupted aortic arch with severe subaortic obstructions
- Unbalanced atrioventricular septal defect

Abnormally Related Great Vessels

- Double-inlet left ventricle with D-transposition of the great arteries
- Tricuspid atresia, VSD, transposition
- Complex double-outlet right ventricle with arch hypoplasia

forms of congenital heart disease that show systemic outflow tract obstruction and a duct-dependent systemic circulation. Because of the impact of great vessel relationships on arch reconstruction, it is useful to define these variants as those that present with normal versus abnormal relationships between the great arteries (i.e. transposition complexes) (Box 128-1).

Surgical Results for Hypoplastic Left Heart Syndrome Variants

Whereas some groups have identified the presence of a well-developed morphologic left ventricle as being protective, others have not.[63,64] A recent comparison of the Norwood operation performed for HLHS (102 patients, 70 with aortic atresia) and other diagnoses (56 patients) between 1998 and 2001 by Gaynor and colleagues[65] identified no difference in survival between the Norwood operation for HLHS versus other anatomic diagnoses (78% vs. 75%).

Although the presence of abnormally related great arteries has not been identified as a risk factor for mortality, they may render the constructed neoaorta susceptible to twists or kinks, and modifications may be required (Figs. 128-8 and 128-9).[66]

Extracorporeal Membrane Oxygenation for Hypoplastic Left Heart Syndrome

Once thought to be futile, perioperative support with extracorporeal membrane oxygenation (ECMO) may salvage a significant proportion of infants with postcardiotomy failure following the Norwood operation. Pizarro and colleagues[67] reported that 50% (6 of 12) of patients requiring ECMO support following Norwood operation were discharged home in good condition. Prematurity, renal dysfunction, and the initiation of ECMO outside of the operating room were risk factors for death. In the setting of a shunt-dependent circulation, Jaggers and colleagues[68] have reported improved survival when the shunt is left open during ECMO support.

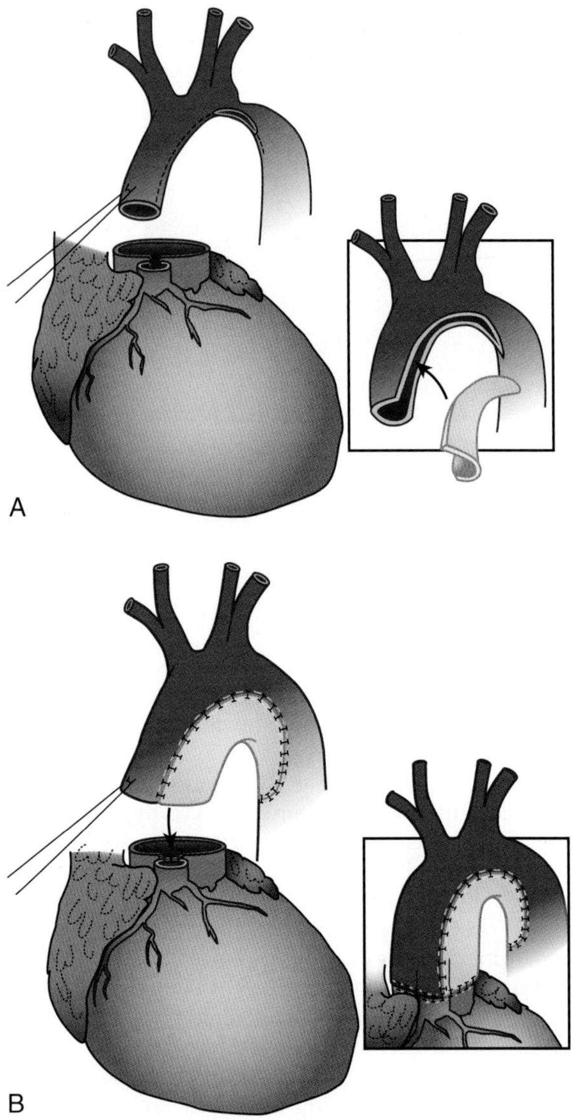

FIGURE 128-8 **A,** Single left ventricle with ventriculoarterial discordance and a rightward and anterior aorta. The atrial septum is excised, and both great vessels are transected just about at the sinotubular junction. Augmentation of the arch is accomplished with pulmonary homograft. **B,** A side-to-side anastomosis between the aorta and pulmonary artery is fashioned. The reconstructed aorta is then anastomosed to both great vessels in an end-to-end fashion. (Reprinted with permission from Mosca RS, Hennein HA, Kulik TJ, et al: Modified Norwood operation for single left ventricle and ventriculoarterial discordance: an improved surgical technique. *Ann Thorac Surg* 64:1126–1132, 1997.)

Modifications

The gradual improvement in survival for the Norwood operation is the result of continuous reappraisal of our surgical and management techniques. Bartram and colleagues[69] performed a systematic review of the causes of surgical mortality of 122 patients undergoing the Norwood operation between 1980 and 1995. Although this review is historical in nature, it deserves attention because it identifies the weaknesses of this operation.

Bartram and colleagues[69] reported that inappropriate pulmonary blood flow (too much or too little) was responsible for 36% of the deaths. The second most

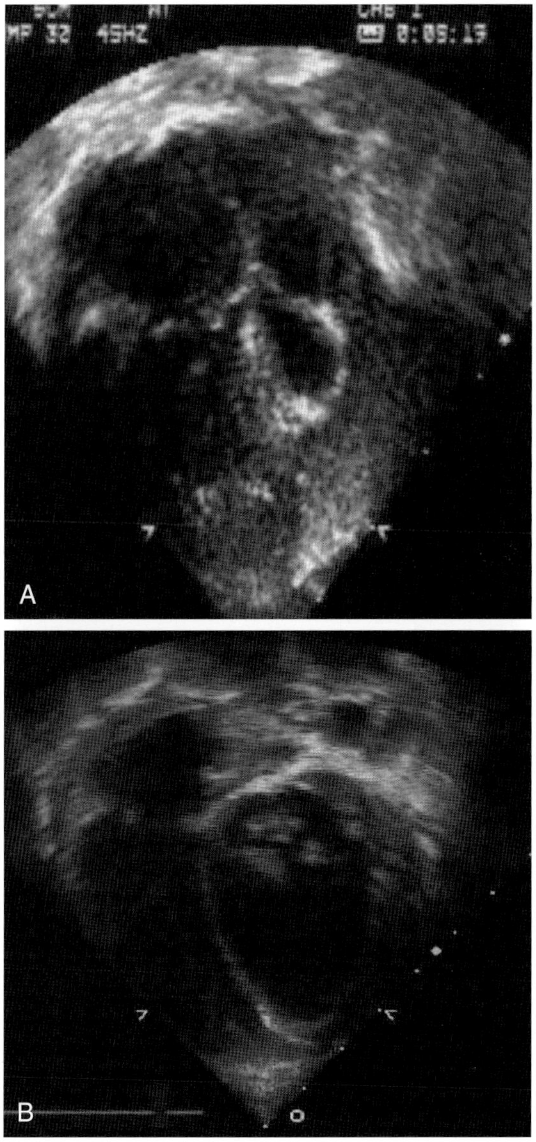

FIGURE 128-14 ■ Anatomic recruitment of the hypoplastic left ventricle into the systemic circulation. Staged intervention suggests that the postnatal left ventricle retains some capacity for growth. **A,** Echocardiogram of newborn with hypoplastic left heart syndrome, showing a hypoplastic left ventricle and thickened endocardium, consistent with endocardial fibroelastosis (EFE). **B,** Echocardiogram of the same child at age 22 months. The child was treated with stage I palliation, including EFE resection, followed by bidirectional Glenn operation with further EFE resection before subsequently undergoing successful biventricular repair at age 22 months.

REFERENCES

1. Tchervenkov CI, Jacobs ML, Tahta SA: Congenital Heart Surgery Nomenclature and Database Project: hypoplastic left heart syndrome. *Ann Thorac Surg* 69(4 Suppl):S170–S179, 2000.
2. Fyler DC, Buckley LP, Hellenbrand WE, et al: Report of the new England regional infant cardiac program. *Pediatrics* 65(Suppl):377–461, 1980.
3. Laursen HB: Some epidemiologic aspects of congenital heart disease in Denmark. *Acta Paediatr Scand* 69:619–624, 1980.
4. Bridges ND, Mayer JE, Jr, Lock JE, et al: Effect of baffle fenestration on outcome of the modified Fontan operation. *Circulation* 86:1762–1769, 1992.
5. Nora JJ, Nora AH: *Genetics and counseling in cardiovascular diseases*. Springfield, IL, 1978, Charles C Thomas, p 181.
6. Tikkanen J, Heinonen OP: Risk factors for hypoplastic left heart syndrome. *Teratology* 50:112–117, 1994.
7. Roberts WC, Perry LW, Chandra RS, et al: Aortic valve atresia: a new classification system based on necropsy study of 73 cases. *Am J Cardiol* 37:753–756, 1976.
8. Sinha SN, Rusnak SL, Sommers HM, et al: Hypoplastic left ventricle syndrome. Analysis of thirty autopsy cases in infants with surgical considerations. *Am J Cardiol* 21:166–173, 1968.
9. Natowicz M, Chatten J, Clancy RR, et al: Genetic disorders and major extracardiac anomalies associated with hypoplastic left heart syndrome. *Pediatrics* 82:698–706, 1988.
10. Glauser TA, Rorke LB, Weinberg PM, et al: Congenital brain abnormalities associated with the hypoplastic left heart syndrome. *Pediatrics* 84:984–990, 1990.
11. Shillingford AJ, Ittenbach RF, Marino BS, et al: Aortic morphometry and microcephaly in hypoplastic left heart syndrome. *Cardiol Young* 17:189–195, 2007.
12. Dent CL, Spaeth JP, Jones BV, et al: Brain magnetic resonance imaging abnormalities after the norwood procedure using regional perfusion. *J Thorac Cardiovasc Surg* 130:1523–1530, 2005.
13. Baffa JM, Chen SL, Guttenberg ME, et al: Coronary artery abnormalities and right ventricular histology in hypoplastic left heart syndrome. *J Am Coll Cardiol* 20:350–358, 1992.
14. DeRose JJ, Corda R, Dische R, et al: Isolated left ventricular ischemia after Norwood procedure. *Ann Thorac Surg* 73:657–659, 2002.
15. Ito T, Nuno M, Isiukawa J, et al: Hypoplastic left heart syndrome with a single coronary artery originating from the pulmonary artery. *Acta Pediatr Jpn* 37:60–63, 1995.
16. Malec E, Mroczek T, Pajak J, et al: Hypoplastic left heart syndrome with an anomalous origin of the left coronary artery. *Ann Thorac Surg* 72:2129–2130, 2001.
17. O'Connor WN, Ash JB, Cottrill CM, et al: Ventriculo-coronary connections in hypoplastic left hearts: an autopsy microscopic study. *Circulation* 66:1078–1086, 1982.
18. Sarris GE, Drummond-Webb JJ, Ebeid MR, et al: Anomalous origin of left coronary artery from right pulmonary artery in hypoplastic left heart syndrome. *Ann Thorac Surg* 64:836–838, 1997.
19. Tworetzky W, McElhinney DB, Reddy VM, et al: Improved surgical outcome after fetal diagnosis for hypoplastic left heart syndrome. *Circulation* 103:1269–1273, 2001.
20. Kumar RK, Newburger JW, Gauvreau K, et al: Comparison of outcome when hypoplastic left heart syndrome and transposition of the great arteries are diagnosed prenatally versus when diagnosis of these two conditions is made only postnatally. *Am J Cardiol* 83:1649–1653, 1999.
21. Mahle WT, Clancy RR, McGaurn SP, et al: Impact of prenatal diagnosis on survival and early neurologic morbidity in neonates with hypoplastic left heart syndrome. *Pediatrics* 107:1277–1282, 2001.
22. Atz AM, Feinstein JA, Jonas RA, et al: Preoperative management of pulmonary venous hypertension in hypoplastic left heart syndrome with restrictive atrial septum. *Am J Cardiol* 83:1224–1228, 1999.
23. Sedmera D, Hu N, Weiss KM, et al: Cellular changes in experimental left heart hypoplasia. *Anat Rec* 267:137–456, 2002.
24. Remmell-Dow DR, Bharati S, Davis JT, et al: Hypoplasia of the eustachian valve and abnormal orientation of the limbus of the foramen ovale in hypoplastic left heart syndrome. *Am Heart J* 130:148–152, 1995.
25. Schall SA, Dalldorf FG: Premature closure of the foramen ovale and hypoplasia of the left heart. *Int J Cardiol* 5:103–107, 1984.
26. Lev M, Arcilla R, Rimoldi HJ, et al: Premature narrowing or closure of the foramen ovale. *Am Heart J* 65:638–647, 1963.
27. Sharland GK, Chita SK, Fagg NL, et al: Left ventricular dysfunction in the fetus: relation to aortic valve anomalies and endocardial fibroelastosis. *Br Heart J* 66:419–424, 1991.
28. Phillips HM, Renforth GL, Spalluto C, et al: Narrowing of the critical region within 11q24-qter for hypoplastic left heart and identification of a candidate gene, JAM3, expressed during cardiogenesis. *Genomics* 79:475–478, 2002.
29. Rhodes LA, Colan DS, Perry S, et al: Predictors of survival in neonates with critical aortic stenosis. *Circulation* 84:2325–2335, 1991.

30. Tani LY, Minnich LL, Pagotto LT, et al: Left heart hypoplasia and neonatal aortic arch obstruction: is the Rhodes left ventricular adequacy score applicable? *J Thorac Cardiovasc Surg* 118:81–86, 1999.
31. Lofland GK, McCrindle BW, Williams WG, et al: Critical aortic stenosis in the neonate: a multi-institutional study of management, outcomes, and risk factors. *J Thorac Cardiovasc Surg* 121:10–27, 2001.
32. Hickey EJ, Calderone CA, Blackstone EH, et al: Critical left ventricular outflow tract obstruction: the disproportionate impact of biventricular repair in borderline cases. *J Thorac Cardiovasc Surg* 134:1429–1437, 2007.
33. Fyler DC, Rothman KJ, Buckley LP, et al: The determinants of 5 year survival of infants with critical congenital heart disease. In Engle MA, editor: *Pediatric Cardiovascular Disease.(Cardiovascular Clinics)*, Philadelphia, 1981, F.A. Davis, pp 393–405.
34. Hoshino K, Ogawa K, Hishitani T, et al: Hypoplastic left heart syndrome: duration of survival without surgical intervention. *Am Heart J* 137:535–542, 1999.
35. Jobes DR, Nicholson SC, Stevens JM, et al: Carbon dioxide prevents pulmonary overcirculation in hypoplastic left heart syndrome. *Ann Thorac Surg* 54:150–151, 1992.
36. Riordan CJ, Randsbaek F, Storey JH, et al: Effect of oxygen, positive end-expiratory pressure, and carbon dioxide on oxygen delivery in an animal model of the univentricular heart. *J Thorac Cardiovasc Surg* 112:644–654, 1996.
37. Mora GA, Pizzaro C, Jacobs ML, et al: Experimental model of single ventricle: influence of Carbon Dioxide on Pulmonary vascular Dynamics. *Circulation* 90(Pt 2):II43–II46, 1994.
38. Maegawa Y, Mizobe T, Yamagishi M, et al: The use of nitrogen and nitric oxide to control pulmonary blood flow in the Norwood operation. *J Cardiothorac Vasc Anesthes* 16:264–266, 2002.
39. Tabbutt S, Ramamoorthy C, Montenegro LM, et al: Impact of inspired gas mixtures on preoperative infants with hypoplastic left heart syndrome (HLHS) during controlled ventilation. *Circulation* 102(12 Suppl 1):I159–I164, 2000.
40. Bradley SM, Simsic JM, Atz AM: Hemodynamic effects of inspired carbon dioxide after the Norwood procedure. *Ann Thorac Surg* 72:2088–2094, 2001.
41. Chang AC, Zucker HA, Hickey PR, et al: Pulmonary vascular resistance in infants after cardiac surgery: role of carbon dioxide and hydrogen ion. *Crit Care Med* 23:568–574, 1995.
42. Hislop A, Reid L: New findings in pulmonary arteries of rat with hypoxia induced pulmonary hypertension. *Br J Exp Path* 57:542–554, 1976.
43. Meyrick B, Reid L: The effect of continued hypoxia on rat pulmonary arterial circulation. *Lab Invest* 38:188–200, 1978.
44. Haworth SG, Hislop AA: Effect of hypoxia on adaptation on the pulmonary circulation in the pig. *Cardiovasc Research* 16:293–303, 1982.
45. Day RW, Barton AJ, Pysher TJ, et al: Pulmonary vascular resistance of children treated with nitrogen during early infancy. *Ann Thorac Surg* 65:1400–1404, 1998.
46. Tweddell JS, Hoffman GM, Federly RT, et al: Phenoxybenzamine improves systemic oxygen delivery after the Norwood procedure. *Ann Thorac Surg* 67:161–168, 1999.
47. Pigula FA, Siewers RD, Nemoto EM: Regional perfusion of the brain during neonatal aortic arch reconstruction. *J Thorac Cardiovasc Surg* 117:1023–1024, 1999.
48. Pigula FA, Nomoto EM, Griffith BP, et al: Regional low-flow perfusion provides cerebral circulatory support during neonatal aortic arch reconstruction. *J Thorac Cardiovasc Surg* 119:331–339, 2000.
49. Pigula FA, Gandhi SK, Siewers RD, et al: Regional low-flow perfusion provides systemic circulatory support during neonatal aortic arch surgery. *Ann Thorac Surg* 72:401–407, 2001.
50. Pigula FA, Vida V, del Nido PJ, et al: Contemporary results and current strategies in the management of hypoplastic left heart syndrome. *Semin Thorac Cardiovasc Surg* 19:238–244, 2007.
51. Tweddell JS, Hoffman GM, Mussatto KA, et al: Improved survival of patients undergoing palliation of hypoplastic left heart syndrome: lessons learned from 115 consecutive patients. *Circulation* 106(Suppl 1):I82–I89, 2002.
52. Mahle WT, Spray TL, Wernovsky G, et al: Survival after reconstructive surgery for hypoplastic left heart syndrome: a fifteen-year experience from a single institution. *Circulation* 102(Suppl III):III136–III141, 2000.
53. Tabbutt S, Domingues TE, Ravishan-kar C, et al: Outcomes after stage I reconstruction comparing the right ventricular to pulmonary artery conduit with the modified Blalock Taussig Shunt. *Ann Thorac Surg* 80:1582–1590, 2005.
54. Sano S, Ishino K, Kado H, et al: Outcome of right ventricle-to-pulmonary artery shunt in first-stage palliation of hypoplastic left heart syndrome: a multi-institutional study. *Ann Thorac Surg* 78:1951–1957, 2004.
55. Tweddell JS, Hoffman GM, Fedderly RT, et al: Patients at risk for low systemic oxygen delivery after the Norwood procedure. *Ann Thorac Surg* 69:1893–1899, 2000.
56. Ohye RG, Sleeper LA, Mahony L, et al: Comparison of shunt types in the Norwood procedure for single-ventricle lesions. *N Eng J Med* 362:1980–1992, 2010.
57. Weinstein S, Gaynor JW, Bridges ND, et al: Early survival of infants weighing 2.5 kilograms or less undergoing first-stage reconstruction for hypoplastic left heart syndrome. *Circulation* 100(Suppl II):II167–II170, 1999.
58. Bove EL, Lloyd TR: Staged reconstruction for hypoplastic left heart syndrome. *Ann Surg* 224:387–395, 1996.
59. Forbess JM, Cook N, Roth SJ, et al: Ten-year institutional experience with palliative surgery for hypoplastic left heart syndrome; risk factors related to stage I mortality. *Circulation* 92(Suppl II):II262–II266, 1995.
60. Rossi AF, Seiden HS, Sadeghi AM, et al: The outcome of cardiac operations in infants weighing two kilograms or less. *J Thorac Cardiovasc Surg* 116:28–35, 1998.
61. Duncan BW, Rosenthal GL, Jones TK, et al: First-stage palliation of complex univentricular anomalies in older infants. *Ann Thor Surg* 72:2077–2080, 2001.
62. Rossi AF, Sommer RJ, Steinberg LG, et al: Effect of older age on outcome for stage one palliation of hypoplastic left heart syndrome. *Am J Cardiol* 77:319–321, 1996.
63. Daebritz SH, Nolert GD, Zurakowski D, et al: Results of Norwood stage I operation: comparison of hypoplastic left heart syndrome with other malformations. *J Thorac Cardiovasc Surg* 119:358–367, 2000.
64. Jacobs ML, Rychik J, Murphy JD, et al: Results of Norwood's operation for lesions other than hypoplastic left heart syndrome. *J Thorac Cardiovasc Surg* 110:1555–1562, 1995.
65. Gaynor JW, Mahle WT, Cohen MI, et al: Risk factors for mortality after the Norwood procedure. *Eur J Cardiothorac Surg* 22:82–89, 2002.
66. Mosca RS, Hennien HA, Kulik TJ, et al: Modified Norwood operation for single left ventricle and ventriculoarterial discordance: an improved surgical technique. *Ann Thorac Surg* 64:1126–1132, 1997.
67. Pizarro C, Davis DA, Healy RM, et al: Is there a role for extracorporeal life support after stage I Norwood? *Eur J Cardiothor Surg* 19:294–301, 2001.
68. Jaggers JJ, Forbess JM, Shah AS, et al: Extracorporeal membrane oxygenation for infant postcardiotomy support: significance of shunt management. *Ann Thor Surg* 69:1476–1483, 2000.
69. Bartram U, Grunenfelder J, Van Praagh R: Causes of death after the modified Norwood procedure: a study of 122 postmortem cases. *Ann Thorac Surg* 64:1795–1802, 1997.
70. Hoffman GM, Ghanayem NS, Kampine JM, et al: Venous saturation and the anaerobic threshold in neonates after the Norwood procedure for hypoplastic left heart syndrome. *Ann Thorac Surg* 70:1515–1521, 2000.
71. Fogel MA, Rychk JK, Vetter J, et al: Effect of volume unloading surgery on coronary flow dynamics in patients with aortic atresia. *J Thorac Cardiovasc Surg* 113:1795–1802, 1997.
72. Imoto Y, Kado H, Shiokawa Y, et al: Experience with the Norwood procedure without circulatory arrest. *J Thorac Cardiovasc Surg* 122:879–882, 2001.
73. Murakami A, Takamoto S, Takaoka T, et al: Saphenous vein homograft containing a valve as a right ventricle-pulmonary artery conduit in the modified Norwood operation. *J Thorac Cardiovasc Surg* 124:1041–1042, 2002.
74. Malec E, Januszewska K, Kolcz J, et al: Right ventricle to pulmonary artery shunt (RV-PA) versus modified Blalock Taussig shunt (BTS) in the Norwood procedure for hypoplastic left heart

syndrome—influence on early and late hemodynamic status. *Eur J Cardiothorac Surg* 23:728–733, 2003.
75. Pizzarro C, Malec E, Maher KO, et al: Right ventricle to pulmonary artery shunt has a favorable impact on postoperative physiology after stage I Norwood for hypoplastic left heart syndrome. *Circulation* 108(Suppl 1):II155–II160, 2003.
76. Fraisse A, Colan SD, Jonas RA, et al: Accuracy of echocardiography for detection of aortic arch obstruction after stage I Norwood procedure. *Am Heart J* 135:230–236, 1998.
77. Tworetzky W, Mcelhinney DB, Burch GH, et al: Balloon arterioplasty of recurrent coarctation after the modified Norwood procedure in infants. *Cathet Cardiovasc Intervent* 50:54–58, 2000.
78. Azakie A, Merklinger SL, McCrindle BW, et al: Evolving strategies and improving outcomes of the modified Norwood procedure: a 10-year single institution experience. *Ann Thorac Surg* 72:1349–1353, 2001.
79. Machii M, Becker AE: Nature of coarctation in hypoplastic left heart syndrome. *Ann Thorac Surg* 59:1491–1494, 1995.
80. Fraser CD, Mee RBB: Modified Norwood Procedure for hypoplastic left heart syndrome. *Ann Thorac Surg* 60:S546–S549, 1995.
81. Poirer NC, Drummon-Webb JJ, Hisamochi K, et al: Modified Norwood procedure with a high-flow cardiopulmonary bypass strategy results in low mortality without late arch obstruction. *J Thorac Cardiovasc Surg* 120:875–884, 2000.
82. Ishino K, Stumper O, De Giovanni JJV, et al: The modified Norwood procedure for hypoplastic left heart syndrome: early to intermediate results of 120 patients with particular reference to aortic arch repair. *J Thorac Cardiovasc Surg* 117:920–930, 1999.
83. Bautista-Hernandez V, Marx GR, Gauvreau K, et al: Coarctectomy reduces neoaortic arch obstruction in hypoplastic left heart syndrome. *J Thorac Cardiovasc Surg* 133:1540–1546, 2007.
84. Soongswang J, McCrindle BW, Jones TK, et al: Outcomes of transcatheter balloon angioplasty of obstruction in the neo-aortic arch after Norwood operation. *Cardiol Young* 11:54–61, 2001.
85. Clancy RR, McGaurn SA, Wernovsky G, et al: Preoperative risk-of death prediction model in heart surgery with deep hypothermic circulatory arrest in the neonate. *J Thorac Cardiovasc Surg* 119:347–357, 2000.
86. Visconti KJ, Rimmer D, Gauvreau K, et al: Regional low-flow perfusion versus circulatory arrest; one year neurodevelopmental outcome. *Ann Thorac Surg* 82:2207–2211, 2006.
87. Goldberg CS, Bove EL, Devaney EJ, et al: A randomized clinical trial of regional cerebral perfusion versus DHCA: outcomes for infants with functional single ventricle. *J Thorac Cardiovasc Surg* 133:880–887, 2007.
88. Mahle WT, Spray TL, Gaynor JW, et al: Unexpected death after reconstructive surgery for hypoplastic left heart syndrome. *Ann Thorac Surg* 71:61–65, 2001.
89. Reddy VM, McElhinney DB, Moore P, et al: Outcomes after bidirectional cavopulmonary shunt in infants less than 6 months old. *J Am Coll Cardiol* 29:1365–1370, 1997.
90. Forbess JM, Cook N, Serraf A, et al: An institutional experience with second—and third-stage palliative procedures for hypoplastic left heart syndrome: the impact of the bidirectional cavopulmonary shunt. *J Am Coll Cardiol* 29:665–670, 1997.
91. Jacobs ML, Norwood WI: Hypoplastic left heart syndrome. In Norwood WI, editor: *Pediatric cardiac surgery: current issues*, Stoneham, 1992, Butterworth, p 182.
92. Bove EL: Current status of staged reconstruction for hypoplastic left heart syndrome. *Pediatr Cardiol* 19:308–315, 1998.
93. Mosca RS, Kulik TJ, Goldberg CS, et al: Early results of the Fontan procedure in one hundred consecutive patients with hypoplastic left heart syndrome. *J Thorac Cardiovasc Surg* 119:1110–1118, 2000.
94. Jacobs ML: Hypoplastic left heart syndrome. In Kaiser LR, Kron IL, Spray TL, editors: *Mastery of cardiothoracic surgery*, Philadelphia-New York, 1998, Lippencott and Raven, pp 862–863.
95. Bromberg BI, Schuessler RB, Gandhi SK, et al: A canine model of atrial flutter following the intra-atrial lateral tunnel Fontan operation. *J Electrocardiol* 30(Suppl):85–93, 1998.
96. Cohen MI, Bridges ND, Gaynor JW, et al: Modifications to the cavopulmonary anastomosis do not eliminate early sinus node dysfunction. *J Thorac Cardiovasc Surg* 120:891–901, 2000.
97. Fontan F, Baudet E: Surgical repair of tricuspid atresia. *Thorax* 26:240–248, 1971.
98. Gentles TL, Mayer JE, Gauvreau K, et al: Fontan operation in five hundred consecutive patients: factors influencing early and late outcome. *J Thorac Cardiovasc Surg* 114:376–379, 1997.
99. Joshi VM, Carey A, Simpson P, et al: Exercise performance following repair of hypoplastic left heart syndrome: a comparison with other types of Fontan patients. *Pediatr Cardiol* 18:357–360, 1997.
100. Lardo AC, Webber SA, Friehs I, et al: Fluid dynamic comparison of intra-atrial and extracardiac total cavopulmonary connections. *J Thorac and Cardiovasc Surg* 117:697–704, 1999.
101. Vricella LA, Razzouk AJ, del Rio M, et al: Heart transplantation for hypoplastic left heart syndrome: modified technique for reducing circulatory arrest time. *J Heart and Lung Transplant* 17:1167–1171, 1998.
102. Ovroutski S, Dahnert I, Alexi-meskishvili V, et al: Preliminary analysis of arrhythmias after the Fontan operation with extracardiac conduit compared with intra atrial lateral tunnel. *J Thorac Cardiovasc Surg* 49:334–337, 2001.
103. Pigula FA: Heart transplantation: surgical technique. In Tejani AH, Harmon WE, Fine RN, editors: *Pediatric solid organ transplantation*, Copenhagen, 2000, Munksgaard, pp 359–370.
104. Bailey LL, Zuppan CW, Chinnock RE, et al: Graft vasculopathy among recipients of heart transplantation during the first twelve years of life. *Transplant Proc* 27:1921–1925, 1995.
105. Jenkins PC, Flanagan MF, Jenkins KJ, et al: Survival analysis and risk factors for mortality in transplantation and staged surgery for hypoplastic left heart syndrome. *J Am Coll Cardiol* 36:1178–1185, 2000.
106. Jenkins PC, Flanagan MF, Sargent JD, et al: A comparison of treatment strategies for hypoplastic left heart syndrome using decision analysis. *J Am Coll Cardiol* 38:1181–1187, 2001.
107. Razzouk AJ, Chinnock RE, Gundry SR, et al: Transplantation as a primary treatment for hypoplastic left heart syndrome: intermediate term results. *Ann Thorac Surg* 62:1–8, 1996.
108. Pahl E, Zales VR, Fricker FJ, et al: Posttransplant coronary artery disease in children: a multicenter national survey. *Circulation* 90(Pt 2):II56–II160, 1994.
109. Dearani JA, Razzouk AJ, Gundry SR, et al: Pediatric cardiac retransplantation: intermediate-term results. *Ann Thorac Surg* 71:66–70, 2001.
110. Bellinger DC, Jonas RA, Rappaport LA, et al: Developmental and Neurologic Status of children after heart surgery with hypothermic circulatory arrest of low flow cardiopulmonary bypass. *N Engl J Med* 332:549–555, 1995.
111. Kern JH, Hinton VJ, Nereo NE, et al: Early developmental outcome after the Norwood procedure for hypoplastic left heart syndrome. *Pediatrics* 102:1148–1152, 1998.
112. Mahle WT, Clancy RR, Moss EM, et al: Neurodevelopmental outcome and lifestyle assessment in school-aged and adolescent children with hypoplastic left heart syndrome. *Pediatrics* 105:1082–1089, 2000.
113. Goldberg CS, Schwartz EM, Brunberg JA, et al: Neurodevelopmental outcome of patients after the Fontan operation: a comparison between children with hypoplastic left heart syndrome and other functional single ventricle lesions. *J Pediatr* 137:646–652, 2000.
114. Gibbs JL, Wren C, Watterson KG, et al: Stenting of the arterial duct combined with banding of the pulmonary arteries and atrial septostomy: a new approach to palliation for hypoplastic left heart syndrome. *Br Heart J* 69:551–555, 1993.
115. Galantowicz ME, Cheatham JP: Lessons learned from the development of a new hybrid stage for the management of hypoplastic left heart syndrome. *Pediatr Cardiol* 26:190–199, 2005.
116. Galantowicz M, Cheatham JP, Philips A, et al: Hybrid approach for hypoplastic left heart syndrome: intermediate results after the learning curve. *Ann Thorac Surg* 85(6):2062–2070, 2008.
117. Caldarone CA, Benson L, Holtby H, et al: Initial experience with hybrid palliation for neonates with single-ventricle physiology. *Ann Thorac Surg* 84(4):1294–1300, 2007.
118. Bresiaca AA, Jureidini S, Danon S, et al: Hybrid versus Norwood procedure for hypoplastic left heart syndrome: contemporary series from a single center. *J Thorac Cardiovasc Surg* 147:1777–1782, 2014.

119. Stoica SC, Philips AB, Egan M, et al: The retrograde aortic arch in the hybrid approach to hypoplastic left heart syndrome. *Ann Thorac Surg* 88(6):1939–1946, 2009.
120. Dave H, Rosser B, Knirsch W, et al: Hybrid approach for hypoplastic left heart syndrome and its variants: the fate of the pulmonary arteries. *Eur J Cardiothorac Surg* 46:14–19, 2014.
121. Davies RR, Radtke WE, Klenk D, et al: Bilateral pulmonary arterial banding results in an increased need for subsequent pulmonary artery interventions. *J Thorac Cardiovasc Surg* 147(2):706–712, 2014.
122. Holzer RJ, Sisk M, Chisolm JL, et al: Completion angiography after cardiac surgery for congenital heart disease: complementing the intraoperative imaging modalities. *Pediatr Cardiol* 30(8):1075–1082, 2009.
123. Chetan D, Kotani Y, Jacques F, et al: Surgical palliation strategy does not affect interstage ventricular dysfunction or atrioventricular valve regurgitation in children with hypoplastic left heart syndrome and variants. *Circulation* 128(11 Suppl 1):S205–S212, 2013.
124. Davies RR, Carver SW, Schmidt R, et al: Gastrointestinal complications after stage I Norwood versus hybrid procedures. *Ann Thorac Surg* 95(1):189–195, 2013.
125. Weiss SL, Gossett JG, Kaushal S, et al: Comparison of gastrointestinal morbidity after Norwood and hybrid palliation for complex heart defects. *Pediatr Cardiol* 32(4):391–398, 2011.
126. Makikallio K, McElhinney DB, Levine JC, et al: Fetal aortic valve stenosis and the evolution of hypoplastic left heart syndrome: patient selection for fetal intervention. *Circulation* 113:1401–1405, 2006.
127. Tworetzky W, Wilkins-Haug L, Jennings RW, et al: Balloon dilation if severe aortic stenosis in the fetus: potential for prevention of hypoplastic left heart syndrome: candidate selection, technique, and results of successful intervention. *Circulation* 12:2125–2131, 2004.
128. Marshall AC, Tworetzky W, Bergersen L, et al: Aortic valvuloplasty in the fetus: technical characteristics of successful balloon dilation. *J Pediatr* 17:535–539, 2005.

CHAPTER 129

Management of Single Ventricle and Cavopulmonary Connections

Kirk R. Kanter

CHAPTER OUTLINE

Single-ventricle circulation is a generic term that covers a wide range of structural cardiac abnormalities. It is widely accepted that the definitive surgical palliation for these hearts is the Fontan circulation, whereby the pulmonary and systemic blood flows are in series with the single ventricle connected to the systemic circulation. To optimize clinical outcomes with the Fontan, many patients need prior interventions to adjust the pulmonary or systemic circulation. Because of the changing physiology in the early years of life, a series of operations is often necessary.

TERMINOLOGY AND ANATOMY

In this chapter, the term *single ventricle* refers to congenital cardiac malformations that lack two completely well-developed ventricles in which functionally there is only a single ventricular chamber that supports both the pulmonary and systemic circulations. A truly morphologic univentricular heart is rare; more often there is an additional rudimentary chamber. Over the years, numerous classifications and terms for these hearts have emerged. The Congenital Heart Surgery Nomenclature and Database Project minimum data set categorized single ventricles into seven broad categories[1]: hearts with common inlet atrioventricular connection (double-inlet right ventricle and double-inlet left ventricle), hearts with absence of one atrioventricular connection (tricuspid atresia and mitral atresia), hearts with common atrioventricular valve and only one well-developed ventricle (unbalanced common atrioventricular canal defect), hearts with only one fully developed ventricle and heterotaxia syndrome (single-ventricle heterotaxia syndrome), and other rare forms of univentricular hearts that do not fit in one of these categories. A more comprehensive classification of the Congenital Heart Surgery Nomenclature and Database Project subclassifies these categories of single ventricle into four hierarchies spanning more than three printed pages.[2] Tricuspid atresia is the most common type of single ventricle, with an incidence of 1% to 3% of all congenital heart lesions.

In addition, there are some cardiac abnormalities in which, in the presence of two well-developed ventricles, the anatomy precludes biventricular repair. Examples include hearts with major straddling of the atrioventricular valve and double-outlet right ventricle with remote ventricular septal defect. Treatment strategies for these nonseptatable hearts are the same as those applied to univentricular hearts.

The management of hypoplastic left heart syndrome, a common form of univentricular heart with a dominant right ventricle and rudimentary left ventricle is not discussed in this chapter. Chapter 128 is dedicated to this topic.

NATURAL HISTORY

Patients born with a single functional ventricle generally have a dismal long-term prognosis without eventual surgical intervention. Current results of the Fontan procedure as the final palliative surgical procedure for these patients are generally good, but it must be recognized that management of these patients begins at birth if they are to be satisfactory candidates for the Fontan procedure. The natural history of single-ventricle circulations is greatly influenced by the degree of pulmonary blood flow and associated lesions, such as coarctation of the aorta, systemic outflow tract obstruction, and anomalies of pulmonary or systemic venous return. In addition, noncardiac abnormalities may be present.

Severe obstruction to pulmonary blood flow at birth is an important determinant for early death. Patients with unobstructed pulmonary flow can develop congestive heart failure in infancy or later, and, if unoperated, can develop pulmonary vascular disease. The clinical course may be worsened by the presence of left-sided obstructive lesions such as coarctation of the aorta. In a small subset of patients, the pulmonary and systemic circulations are well balanced because of unrestricted systemic blood flow and sufficient pulmonary obstruction to control pulmonary blood flow. These patients have a more favorable life expectancy. The aim of surgical intervention is to improve the natural history by balancing blood flow between the pulmonary and systemic circulations and ultimately separating these circulations. In addition, other significant hemodynamic abnormalities should be corrected.

CLINICAL PRESENTATION AND PREOPERATIVE EVALUATION

Clinical presentation is determined by the amount of pulmonary blood flow and the associated cardiac lesions. Patients with restricted pulmonary blood flow will exhibit cyanosis. Some may have a duct-dependent pulmonary circulation and will become rapidly cyanosed as the ductus arteriosus closes after birth. In the case of a large left-to-right shunt, the patient will present with congestive heart failure. Symptoms will deteriorate with falling pulmonary resistance in the first weeks after birth. Although in most single ventricles there is mixing of circulations, streaming may occur, particularly in complex hearts, resulting in differential saturations in the great arteries.

A precise anatomic diagnosis is essential to allow proper planning of the surgical procedures. In particular, information on the size and course of the pulmonary arteries, degree of pulmonary blood flow, and presence of accessory lesions is required, as well as an assessment of cardiac function. History, clinical presentation, chest x-ray, and electrocardiogram offer important but nonspecific information. Echocardiography provides detailed information on the structure and function of the heart and has the advantage that it is a noninvasive investigation that can be performed at the bedside. In particular, in infants who have excellent echocardiographic windows, enough information often can be gathered to proceed to operation. Cardiac catheterization is uncommonly needed to evaluate pulmonary vascular resistance or accessory sources of pulmonary blood flow. Interventional procedures, such as balloon atrial septostomy for restrictive atrial communication in hearts without two well-formed atrioventricular valves, can be carried out to supplement, or sometimes replace, surgical treatment.

SURGICAL PREPARATION FOR THE FONTAN CIRCULATION

Because the ultimate success of the Fontan operation depends on a suitably low pulmonary vascular resistance and adequate pulmonary artery architecture, it is critical to commence the preparation for a Fontan procedure in the newborn period by appropriately regulating pulmonary blood flow. There is a wide variation in the distribution of pulmonary and systemic blood flow in patients with single-ventricle circulation. Some patients have restricted pulmonary blood flow, others have unrestricted pulmonary flow, and a few have a naturally balanced circulation. Most patients, therefore, require palliative procedures leading up to the Fontan circulation, either to restrict or to augment pulmonary blood flow. The choice of procedure is guided by the underlying anatomy and pulmonary vascular resistance, both of which are subject to change over time. It should always be borne in mind that improper palliative procedures can result in the loss of Fontan candidacy. The ultimate goal of surgical procedures leading up to the Fontan circulation are to (1) improve clinical symptoms, (2) provide optimal pulmonary artery architecture and low pulmonary vascular resistance, (3) preserve systolic and diastolic ventricular function, (4) preserve atrioventricular valve function, (5) relieve systemic ventricular outflow tract obstruction, and (6) provide anatomic setup for a definitive Fontan repair.

Inadequate Pulmonary Blood Flow

In the neonatal and early infantile period, when pulmonary vascular resistance is still high, if the child is ductal dependent or has inadequate systemic oxygen saturations, a systemic to pulmonary artery shunt, usually a modified Blalock-Taussig shunt, is performed.[3] Although this was classically performed through a thoracotomy approach, a sternotomy is now commonly used because it allows for concomitant ductal ligation and correction of stenosis of the proximal left pulmonary artery if present.[4,5] Despite decades of experience with the modified Blalock-Taussig shunt, there remains a persistent early and intermediate morbidity and mortality with this procedure.[6]

Excessive Pulmonary Blood Flow

In the case of excessive pulmonary blood flow, it is imperative to limit the pulmonary blood flow to protect the patient from developing pulmonary vascular disease and ventricular dysfunction as a result of chronic volume overload.[7] Adequate tightness of a pulmonary artery band can be difficult to achieve, and a band that is too loose initially can result in unprotected pulmonary arteries until the child grows into the band. The resultant pulmonary vascular disease may affect the ultimate suitability of the child for the Fontan procedure. Other complications of pulmonary artery banding include distortion of the pulmonary arteries, especially if the band migrates, and erosion of the band. Because of the fixed diameter of the pulmonary band, as the child grows, pulmonary blood flow will eventually be inadequate and cyanosis will result, necessitating further surgical intervention. Often in infants with unobstructed pulmonary blood flow and single-ventricle anatomy, a concomitant coarctation will need to be repaired at the time of pulmonary artery banding.

To avoid the complications of pulmonary artery banding in the neonate or infant with excessive pulmonary blood flow and single-ventricle physiology, Bradley and colleagues suggested the strategy of pulmonary artery division with placement of a systemic to pulmonary artery shunt; this strategy has yielded excellent clinical results.[8]

Systemic Outflow Obstruction (Subaortic Stenosis)

Some children with single ventricles can present in infancy with systemic ventricular outflow tract obstruction (subaortic stenosis), which may also develop later. The resultant myocardial hypertrophy can adversely affect the eventual suitability for a Fontan procedure. Patients at risk are those in whom the aorta arises above a small outlet chamber, such as in tricuspid atresia or double-inlet left ventricle with a rudimentary right ventricle and transposition of the great arteries, particularly if the ventricular septal defect (sometimes referred to as a bulboventricular foramen) is small or if there is coexisting aortic arch obstruction.[9] A modified Damus-Kaye-Stansel procedure can be performed to establish unobstructed systemic arterial outflow. This involves transection of both great arteries, anastomosis of the facing aortic and pulmonary walls, and connection of the distal aorta to the perimeter of the reconstructed proximal great artery. Depending on the pulmonary vascular status, blood flow to the central pulmonary arteries can be reestablished via a systemic to pulmonary shunt, a bidirectional cavopulmonary anastomosis, or the Fontan operation.[10] The Damus-Kaye-Stansel can be performed as a primary procedure[11] or after a previous pulmonary artery band.[7,12,13] Alternatively, a Norwood strategy can be followed in these patients[14,15] (see Chapter 128). Some have advocated direct relief of the systemic outflow obstruction by surgical enlargement of the ventricular septal defect (bulboventricular foramen) or resection of subaortic stenosis.[7,16,17]

Obstructed Pulmonary Venous Return

A particularly unfavorable subset of patients with single ventricles is those with total anomalous pulmonary venous connection.[18-20] Even with successful correction of the pulmonary venous return, these patients can have persistent pulmonary artery hypertension, probably related to fetal pulmonary vein and artery abnormalities,[20] which precludes the application of the Fontan procedure. To a lesser extent, children with a restrictive atrial communication and an abnormal left atrioventricular valve (as in mitral atresia) are at risk for the development of pulmonary artery hypertension.[21] Opening of the atrial septum by percutaneous atrial septostomy or stent placement in the catheterization laboratory or surgical atrial septectomy should be performed once this condition has been recognized.

BIDIRECTIONAL CAVOPULMONARY ANASTOMOSIS

The original cavopulmonary shunt was the Glenn procedure (anastomosis of the divided right pulmonary artery to the superior vena cava with ligation of the proximal superior vena cava).[22] The advantages of a venous over an arterial shunt in the palliation of cyanotic heart disease are twofold. First, the venous blood that enters the pulmonary artery is much more desaturated, and therefore a higher take-up of oxygen per milliliter of blood is possible. Second, systemic venous return is diverted to the lungs, thus reducing the volume load on the single ventricle. The original Glenn anastomosis fell into disfavor; it could not be used in neonates because of elevated pulmonary vascular resistance.[23] There were also reports of the development of ipsilateral pulmonary arteriovenous malformations.[24] However, it was noted that patients with a previous classical Glenn anastomosis fared better with a subsequent Fontan procedure.[25] For patients considered high risk for the Fontan procedure, a bidirectional cavopulmonary anastomosis (the divided superior vena cava anastomosed to the pulmonary arteries supplying both lungs) could be used successfully as an alternative to the Fontan or as a staging procedure for the Fontan[26,27] (Fig. 129-1). The hemi-Fontan modification of the cavopulmonary shunt involves patch augmentation of the central pulmonary arteries and a connection between the

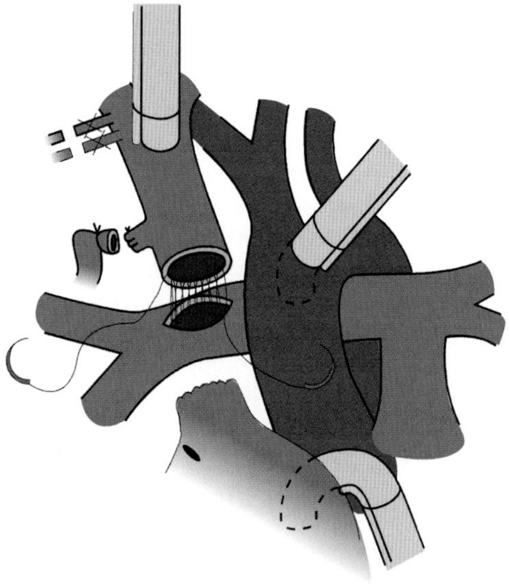

FIGURE 129-1 ■ Bidirectional cavopulmonary shunt. The superior vena cava is fully mobilized, including the junction with the innominate vein. The azygos vein and small venous branches near the innominate vein junction are ligated to prevent runoff into the inferior vena cava territory. The main and right pulmonary arteries and a right systemic to pulmonary artery shunt, if present, are mobilized. Cardiopulmonary bypass is instituted with venous drainage from a cannula in the right atrial appendage and a further cannula in the superior vena cava near the innominate junction with return via the ascending aorta. The operation is performed on a beating heart with moderate hypothermia (28°C to 32°C), but a period of aortic cross-clamping may be required for correction of other cardiac anomalies. Any right-sided systemic aortopulmonary shunt is occluded and subsequently taken down. The right and main pulmonary arteries are mobilized. The superior vena cava is snugged down. A vascular clamp is applied just above the cavoatrial junction, taking care not to damage the sinus node. The superior vena cava is divided immediately above the clamp, the cardiac end is oversewn, and the clamp is released. The upper margin of the right pulmonary artery is incised. The superior vena cava is anastomosed in an end-to-side manner with the upper margin of the right pulmonary artery. The suture is interrupted in several places to help avoid a purse-string effect and narrowing of the anastomosis. Additional sources of pulmonary blood supply, such as forward flow over a stenosed pulmonary outflow tract or left-sided arterial pulmonary shunt, are usually left in place.

right atrial–superior vena cava junction and pulmonary arteries. Norwood and Jacobs reported improved survival with the Fontan operation in children with hypoplastic left heart syndrome who had undergone an intermediate hemi-Fontan procedure.[28] Subsequent studies showed significantly improved outcomes in patients with a Fontan procedure who were staged with a bidirectional cavopulmonary anastomosis compared with those who were not staged.[21,29] The bidirectional cavopulmonary anastomosis can be performed safely in children younger than 6 months[30] and is now routinely performed electively between 4 and 6 months of age, even in children without prior surgical palliation.

Additional Sources of Pulmonary Blood Flow

Whether an additional source of pulmonary blood flow (such as a patent ductus arteriosus, patent right ventricular outflow tract or a tight pulmonary artery band, or systemic to pulmonary artery shunt) should be eliminated at the time of the cavopulmonary anastomosis remains open to discussion. Comparisons of patients with and without sources of additional pulmonary blood flow after a bidirectional cavopulmonary anastomosis have shown no deleterious effect at the time of the eventual Fontan procedure.[31-33] Evidence shows that leaving an additional source of pulmonary blood flow after the bidirectional cavopulmonary anastomosis can enhance pulmonary arterial growth.[32,34] Some patients do not tolerate this increased pulmonary blood flow, which manifests as pleural effusions and superior vena cava syndrome. These patients can be managed by catheter-based techniques to occlude the sources of additional pulmonary blood flow.[35]

Some have argued that a bidirectional Glenn anastomosis with an additional source of pulmonary blood flow can serve as definitive palliation without a subsequent Fontan procedure, especially in high-risk cases.[36,37] A multi-institutional paper from Italy reviewed 246 patients with a mean age 4.7 ± 6.2 years (range, 12 months to 30 years) who underwent a bidirectional cavopulmonary anastomosis leaving intact antegrade accessory pulmonary blood flow.[31] On intermediate follow-up of 4.2 ± 2.8 years, 173 patients (70.3%) did not require a completion Fontan procedure and had a mean resting arterial oxygen saturation of 87% ± 4%. The actuarial freedom from a Fontan procedure at 7 years was 70.2% for the entire cohort. These results suggest that this strategy provided sustained palliation for selected patients with a single-ventricle circulation and may indicate that the Fontan route is not necessarily the universal palliation for all single-ventricle circulations.

Bilateral Bidirectional Cavopulmonary Anastomoses

Approximately 15% of children with single ventricles undergoing a bidirectional cavopulmonary anastomosis will have a persistent left superior vena cava draining to the coronary sinus.[38,39] Although an earlier report from the Hospital for Sick Children in Toronto suggested that the presence of a second superior vena cava was a risk factor for thrombosis and failure to progress to the Fontan procedure,[39] a report from our institution did not identify any adverse clinical outcomes in patients undergoing bilateral bidirectional cavopulmonary anastomoses compared with those undergoing a unilateral bidirectional cavopulmonary anastomosis.[38]

Kawashima Operation and Pulmonary Arteriovenous Malformations

Some children with single-ventricle anatomy, particularly those with heterotaxy syndrome, have an interrupted inferior vena cava with azygos continuation to the right superior vena cava or hemiazygos continuation to a persistent left superior vena cava. After initial palliation in infancy, as necessary, with pulmonary artery banding or a systemic to pulmonary artery shunt determined by the status of the pulmonary blood flow, definitive palliation can be accomplished with a Kawashima operation.[40] This consists of a bidirectional cavopulmonary anastomosis (bilateral in the case of a persistent left superior vena cava) without the division of the azygos (hemiazygos) continuation. In effect, this routes all of the systemic venous return except hepatic and mesenteric flow to the pulmonary arteries. A significant percentage of these patients will develop pulmonary arteriovenous malformations (AVMs) in both lungs with resultant cyanosis. This is analogous to the ipsilateral pulmonary AVMs observed with the classical Glenn anastomosis.[24] There seems to be some factor in the hepatic venous effluent that, if not circulated to the lung, results in the development of these AVMs.[41] Rerouting the hepatic and mesenteric venous blood flow to the pulmonary arteries by completing the Fontan procedure has been shown to resolve this problem in most patients.[42-44]

Glenn Anastomosis versus Hemi-Fontan Procedure

As an intermediate stage to the Fontan procedure, either a bidirectional Glenn anastomosis or a hemi-Fontan procedure can be performed. Although there are advocates for both operations, there are few studies comparing the two operations in similar groups of patients. The hemi-Fontan procedure, as described initially by Norwood and Jacobs,[28] involves patch augmentation of the central pulmonary arteries and a connection between the right atrial–superior vena cava junction and pulmonary arteries with elimination of alternative sources of pulmonary blood flow. Although it is a more extensive operation, it simplifies the eventual Fontan procedure, particularly if a lateral tunnel Fontan is planned.[45] It also has the potential advantage of allowing nonsurgical completion of the Fontan circulation in the cardiac catheterization laboratory,[46] although this nonoperative Fontan completion can also be used with the bidirectional Glenn anastomosis.[47] Sinus node dysfunction appears to be more common early after the hemi-Fontan procedure compared with the bidirectional Glenn anastomosis, but this was no longer significant at time of hospital discharge.[48] Based on magnetic resonance imaging (MRI) reconstructions and computational and experimental fluid dynamics methodologies, it appears that the bidirectional Glenn anastomosis is more energy efficient than the hemi-Fontan procedure.[49]

ONE AND ONE-HALF VENTRICLE REPAIR

In children with a marginal pulmonary ventricle, the standard surgical options are a Fontan procedure or a high-risk biventricular repair, as is commonly seen in patients with pulmonary atresia and intact ventricular septum.[50] To reduce the risk of biventricular repair and to combat the long-term attrition related to the "Fontan state," Billingsley and colleagues proposed recruiting the hypoplastic pulmonary ventricle to manage part of the systemic venous return by closing the atrial communication, enlarging the right ventricular outflow tract, and adding a cavopulmonary anastomosis so that the small right ventricle is tasked with pumping only the venous return from the inferior vena cava and not the entire cardiac output.[51] The concept of a one and one-half ventricle repair has since been extended to other abnormalities,[52-54] such as unbalanced atrioventricular septal defects and straddling atrioventricular valves, and as an adjunct to the repair of Ebstein anomaly.[55] Strict criteria to distinguish which patients would benefit from a one and one-half ventricle repair as opposed to a biventricular repair or a Fontan procedure are not well defined.[56] Similar physiology can be achieved by only partially closing the atrial communication without performing a cavopulmonary anastomosis. This allows decompression of the smaller right-sided ventricle through this atrial communication with the disadvantage of some systemic arterial desaturation. The advantage of this modification of the one and one-half ventricle repair is that, if the pulmonary ventricle grows sufficiently to handle the complete cardiac output, the atrial communication easily can be closed in the catheterization laboratory at a later date, thus allowing for complete separation of the pulmonary and systemic circulations.

SELECTION CRITERIA FOR THE FONTAN PROCEDURE

The initial selection criteria for the procedure described by Fontan and colleagues for patients with tricuspid atresia, known as the "ten commandments," were stringent (Box 129-1).[57] With increasing experience, these criteria have been relaxed; however, because of the unique physiology that accompanies the Fontan circulation, proper patient selection remains crucial.

The age of patients undergoing the Fontan operation has been progressively lowered as experience has been gained. Increased pressure and volume load of the single ventricle, such as occurs after systemic to pulmonary artery shunts, is a risk factor for subsequent failure of the Fontan operation; therefore, early ventricular unloading with a bidirectional Glenn anastomosis has been advocated. In short-term studies, regression of ventricular mass was observed in children younger than 3 years who underwent a bidirectional Glenn anastomosis but not in children 10 years or older who underwent the same procedure.[58] Similarly, younger age at the time of

BOX 129-1 The "Ten Commandments" for Selection of Patients with Tricuspid Atresia for the Fontan Procedure

1. Minimum age 4 years
2. Sinus rhythm
3. Normal caval drainage
4. Right atrium of normal volume
5. Mean pulmonary artery pressure ≤15 mm Hg
6. Pulmonary arterial resistance <4 U/m^2
7. Pulmonary artery to aorta diameter ratio ≥0.75
8. Normal ventricular functions (ejection fraction >0.6)
9. Competent left atrioventricular valve
10. No impairing effects of previous shunts

bidirectional Glenn shunt or Fontan operation was also associated with superior exercise performance compared with those in whom surgery was delayed until a later age.[59] In contrast to Fontan's initial restriction of minimum age older than 4 years, recent data show that for patients with a dominant left ventricle (e.g., tricuspid atresia), with an average follow-up of more than 7.5 years, postoperative exercise capacity, cardiac index, and ventricular ejection fraction were significantly better in children who had their Fontan completion when they were younger than 3 years compared with a group who were older than 3 years.[60] A multivariable analysis of risk factors after the Fontan operation in 406 patients did not identify young age as a risk factor for unfavorable outcome.[61] Pizarro and colleagues demonstrated in 107 children that Fontan completion can be performed safely in children at a median age of 13 months.[62] It remains to be seen if a very early Fontan procedure has a better long-term outcome than one performed at a later age, particularly in patients with well-balanced circulations. It is certain that current strategies of early unloading of the single ventricle with an intermediate bidirectional cavopulmonary anastomosis or hemi-Fontan procedure has allowed for successful Fontan completion at a younger age.

Preoperative sinus rhythm is not an absolute requirement for a successful Fontan procedure,[63,64] although patients without preoperative sinus rhythm are more likely to have heterotaxy syndrome, which is a predictor of post-Fontan rhythm disturbances.[65,66] The requirement in Fontan's "ten commandments" for normal right atrial volume or normal caval drainage no longer seems to be of concern. On the other hand, unobstructed pulmonary venous drainage is an absolute necessity (see Obstructed Pulmonary Venous Return section).

The pulmonary vasculature and ventricular function remains the most important selection criteria for successful outcome after the Fontan operation.[61] Pulmonary arteriolar resistance (<4 U/m^2)[67] and mean pulmonary artery pressure (<15 mm Hg) should be low.[61,66] Assessment of the pulmonary vascular bed can be difficult, in particular in the presence of accessory sources of pulmonary blood flow such as aortopulmonary collateral vessels or surgical shunts.

Small size of the central pulmonary arteries has been considered a predictor of poor outcome after the Fontan procedure (death or takedown). Various attempts have been made to standardize these measurements. The McGoon ratio, originally used in patients with pulmonary atresia and ventricular septal defect,[68] is obtained from the sum of the diameters of the immediately prebranching portion of the left and right pulmonary arteries divided by the diameter of the descending aorta just above the diaphragm. In a retrospective study, Fontan and colleagues[69] found that the risk of early death or Fontan takedown rose sharply when the McGoon ratio was less than 1.8. The Nakata pulmonary artery index[70] is derived from the sum of the diameter of the left and right pulmonary arteries (measured just before the origin of the upper lobe branches) divided by the body surface area. Patients with unfavorable outcome after a modified Fontan for tricuspid atresia were shown to have a lower pulmonary artery index than those with good results (185 ± 47 versus 276 ± 83 mm^2/m^2),[71] but this was not confirmed by others.[72,73] The usefulness of these indices has been questioned because they do not take into account the compliance and maturity of the pulmonary vascular system, the peripheral and intraparenchymal pulmonary arteries, or any distortion of the central pulmonary arteries that may have occurred because of previous shunts or bands. Furthermore, many of these studies implicating small pulmonary artery size as a risk factor for poor Fontan outcomes were performed before current strategies of earlier staged Fontans using total cavopulmonary connections.[72]

Adequate ventricular function remains a prime determinant for a successful Fontan circulation.[61] The incidence of common causes of impaired systemic ventricular performance seen in the past can be reduced. For example, early elimination of volume overload by an intermediate bidirectional cavopulmonary connection or hemi-Fontan procedure can preserve ventricular function.[45,74] Also, aggressive treatment of systemic ventricular outflow obstruction (see Systemic Outflow Obstruction section) can reduce deleterious ventricular hypertrophy in these patients with resultant improved ventricular function at the time of the Fontan procedure. Also, some feel that the presence of systemic to pulmonary collateral artery connections can increase the volume load of the single ventricle with resultant impaired ventricular function or increased workload on the heart.[75-78] The impact of these collaterals can be reduced in the cardiac catheterization laboratory by coil occlusion, although some groups question its usefulness.[79-82]

Atrioventricular valve insufficiency remains a risk factor for the Fontan procedure,[83] particularly in children with heterotaxy syndrome.[18,66] Because this can cause volume overload of the single ventricle with the potential for impaired ventricular function, it is important to address this surgically when possible. Repair of the incompetent systemic atrioventricular valve can be performed reliably at the time of the bidirectional cavopulmonary anastomosis or at the time of the Fontan.[84-86] If necessary, atrioventricular valve replacement is an option.[87]

SURGICAL EVOLUTION OF THE FONTAN PROCEDURE

The Fontan procedure was first applied in 1968 for tricuspid atresia based on the principle that the right atrium could be used as a pumping chamber for the pulmonary circulation.[88] The original description of the atriopulmonary connection included the insertion of an aortic or pulmonary homograft valve at both the inflow and the outflow of the right atrium as well as a classical Glenn anastomosis of the superior vena cava to the right pulmonary artery. Kreutzer and colleagues described the use of the patient's native pulmonary valve between the right atrium and pulmonary artery.[89] Bjork and coworkers were worried about the long-term durability of conduits and valve prostheses and devised a valveless atrioventricular anastomosis whereby the right atrial appendix is

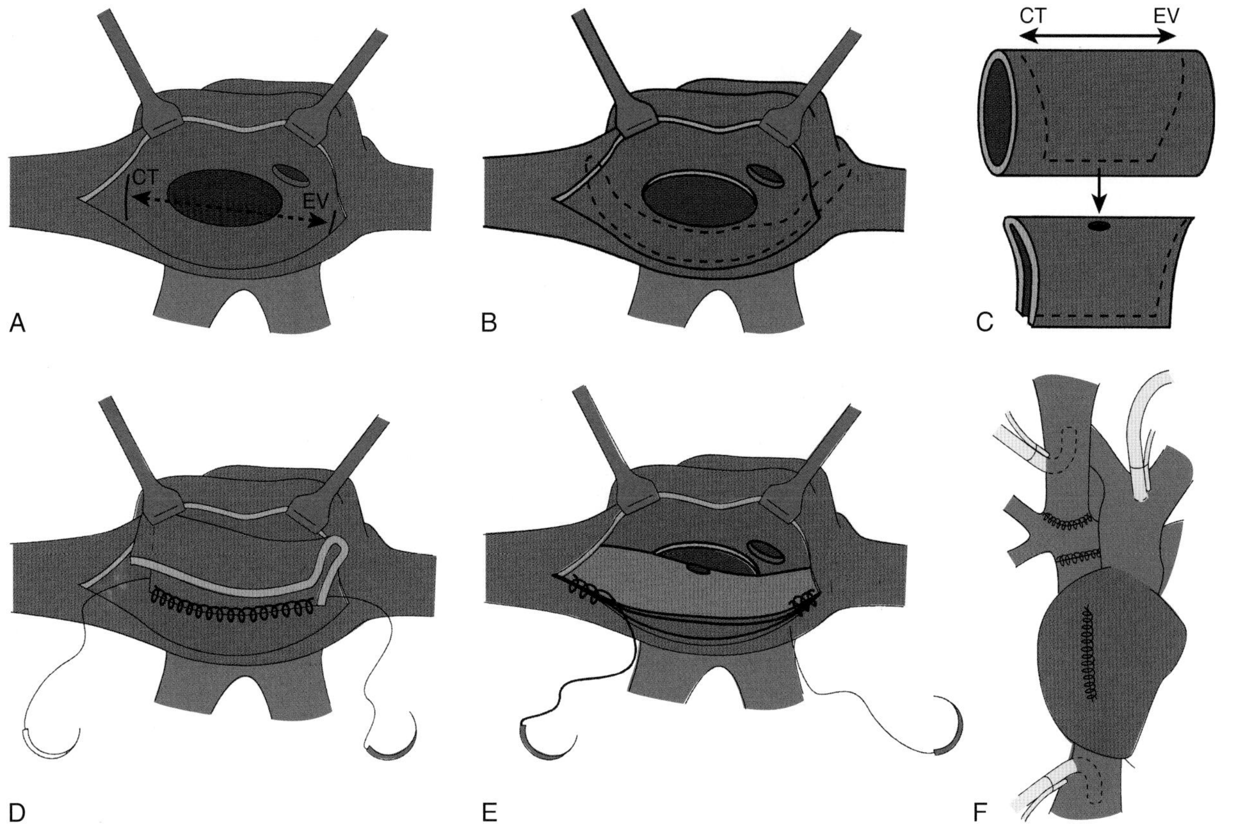

FIGURE 129-2 ■ Lateral tunnel Fontan. The beginning of the operation may involve performing a bidirectional cavopulmonary anastomosis (see Fig. 129-1), or this may already be in place. For cardiopulmonary bypass, a venous cannula is placed low down on the inferior vena cava and a further cannula high up in the superior vena cava near the junction with the innominate vein. The ascending aorta is cannulated. The operation is performed using moderate hypothermia. Any existing systemic to pulmonary artery shunts are taken down. The aorta is cross-clamped, and cold blood cardioplegia is infused. A needle vent is placed in the ascending aorta. The main pulmonary artery is transected. To prevent bleeding or aneurysm formation after closure of the proximal pulmonary artery stump, the suture line is reinforced with two small Teflon felt strips and the pulmonary valve leaflets are included in the suture line. The distal main pulmonary artery is closed, taking care not to distort or narrow the branch pulmonary arteries. **A,** The right atrium is opened along the crest of the septum. The atrial septal defect is enlarged if necessary, and the size of the intra-atrial baffle is measured between the eustachian valve (EV) and crista terminalis (CT). **B,** Future site of baffle between the superior vena cava and inferior vena cava. **C,** A Gore-Tex tube of at least 16-mm diameter is cut to size and opened longitudinally, and if required, a 4- to 5-mm fenestration is cut. **D** and **E,** The prosthetic baffle is sewn halfway around the junction of the inferior vena cava with the right atrium, along the posterior wall of the atrial septum, along the CT, and halfway around the junction with the superior vena cava. Care is taken to avoid injury to the sinus node. **F,** The cardiac end of the transected superior vena cava is anastomosed in an end-to-side manner with the undersurface of the right pulmonary artery.

anastomosed to the right ventricle with the aid of an autologous pericardial patch.[90] It soon became apparent that neither valves nor the rudimentary right ventricle needed to be incorporated into the Fontan connection, so the Fontan procedure evolved into a direct atriopulmonary connection with closure of the atrial communication for tricuspid atresia.

Lateral Tunnel Fontan (Total Cavopulmonary Connection)

Studies in hydrodynamic models by de Leval and colleagues revealed that the atriopulmonary connection performed poorly in terms of flow energetics because of turbulence that was further exaggerated by pulsation.[91] In contrast, a cavopulmonary connection had mainly laminar flow patterns. In this design, the superior vena cava blood drains directly into the pulmonary artery, and inferior vena cava blood is baffled through a straight intra-atrial conduit to the pulmonary artery (Fig. 129-2). Additional theoretical advantages are a reduced risk of thrombosis because of less blood stasis and exposure of only a limited portion of the right atrium to high venous pressures, thus reducing the risk of arrhythmias. In addition, because the coronary sinus remains in the lower pressure pulmonary venous atrium, myocardial venous drainage is unobstructed. This introduction of total cavopulmonary connection, coupled with an intermediate stage of a bidirectional Glenn anastomosis[26] or a hemi-Fontan procedure,[28] greatly improved clinical results with the Fontan procedure.[74]

Fontan Fenestration

Another important clinical improvement was the creation of a fenestration in the Fontan baffle,[92] which allows systemic venous blood to shunt to the pulmonary venous atrium, achieving better preload for the systemic

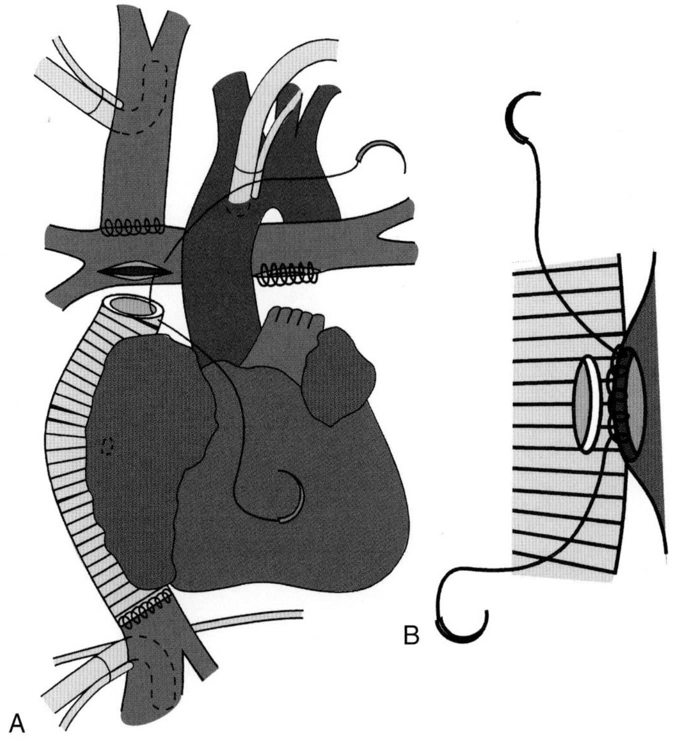

FIGURE 129-3 Construction of extracardiac Fontan on cardiopulmonary bypass. Cannulation for cardiopulmonary bypass is as described for the lateral tunnel Fontan operation (see Fig. 129-2). It is particularly important that the inferior vena cava is cannulated low down. Any systemic to pulmonary artery shunts are taken down. Transection and closure of the main pulmonary artery can be facilitated by a short period of cardioplegic arrest. A needle vent is placed in the ascending aorta. The space between the right lower pulmonary vein and the inferior vena cava is dissected. The cannula in the inferior vena cava is snared, and a clamp is placed across the cavoatrial junction, taking care to avoid occluding the coronary sinus. **A,** The cavopulmonary junction is transected on the clamp, and the cardiac end is oversewn. A Gore-Tex tube of at least 16-mm diameter (22-mm diameter in adults) is anastomosed in an end-to-end manner to the transected inferior vena cava. The conduit is gently curved around the atrium toward the right pulmonary artery. The cavopulmonary shunt is temporarily occluded, and the inferior surface of the right pulmonary artery is incised. The top end of the prosthesis is anastomosed in an end-to-side manner to the pulmonary artery. If a fenestration is required, a side-biting clamp is placed on the free wall of the right atrium and a further clamp opposite on the prosthesis. A 5-mm fenestration is cut in the prosthesis, and a slightly larger hole is cut in the opposite right atrial wall. **B,** To avoid obstruction of the fenestration by atrial tissue, the anastomotic suture line is placed a few millimeters away from the hole in the prosthesis.

ventricle at the cost of some systemic arterial desaturation. Thus, cardiac output is maintained and systemic venous pressure is reduced. The fenestration can be closed later by a transcatheter approach. A retrospective study by Bridges and associates showed a significant decrease in pleural effusions and hospital stay compared with nonfenestrated patients.[93] Consequently, the fenestrated Fontan circuit has become the procedure of choice for the high-risk population.

Baffle fenestration remains controversial in standard-risk patients, with a number of retrospective studies showing no benefit from fenestration,[61,94,95] whereas other studies showed a decreased rate of Fontan failure and lower incidence of significant pleural effusions.[96] A prospective randomized trial by Lemler and colleagues showed improved clinical outcome with less pleural drainage, shorter hospital stay, and less need for additional postoperative procedures in patients with a fenestration.[97] Fontan fenestration has also been shown to have a beneficial effect on late outcome.[98]

Apart from those patients in whom low saturations are a clinical indication for closure of the fenestration, it is not known whether fenestrations should be closed and, if so, when. A quarter or more of fenestrations will close spontaneously.[96] The remainder can be relatively easily occluded by catheter intervention. A follow-up of patients with a mean of 3.4 years following device closure showed improved oxygen saturation with an average increase of 9.4%, reduced need for anticongestive treatment, and improved somatic growth. However, 12% of patients developed new arrhythmias.[99]

Lateral Tunnel versus Extracardiac Conduit

Another modification in the design of the Fontan pathway involves the use of an extracardiac interposition graft between the transected inferior vena cava and pulmonary artery (Fig. 129-3).[100] The extracardiac conduit initially was designed to avoid pulmonary and systemic venous obstruction in patients with a small atrium. Its use has the additional advantage that it avoids extensive atrial suture lines that are potentially arrhythmogenic. Thrombogenicity and lack of growth of the prosthetic conduit remain potential late problems.

The hemodynamic superiority of cavopulmonary connections with total right heart bypass over atriopulmonary connections is generally accepted, and most surgeons now create some form of cavopulmonary connection with complete exclusion of the right heart. The lateral tunnel Fontan optimizes flow dynamics in the pulmonary artery, leaves the coronary sinus in the low pressure atrium, and has a low risk of damage to the atrioventricular node. The same advantages can be attributed to the extracardiac Fontan procedure. Computational flow dynamics show no significant differences in energetics or geometry between the two types of cavopulmonary connections, with the cross-sectional area of the pulmonary arteries having a far more significant impact on hemodynamics than the type of Fontan connection.[101,102] The extracardiac Fontan procedure has the additional advantage that no intra-atrial access is required and thus can be done without aortic cross-clamping and, in suitable cases, also without the use of cardiopulmonary bypass.[103-106]

A theoretical advantage of the extracardiac Fontan operation over the lateral tunnel Fontan is thought to be the absence of arrhythmogenic suture lines, but bradyarrhythmias have been observed with the extracardiac Fontan.[107] Although some reports have shown more postoperative arrhythmias with the lateral tunnel Fontan,[108,109] other studies have shown no difference in postoperative arrhythmias comparing the two surgical techniques.[48,110,111] One study from the Medical University of South Carolina found an increased incidence of sinus node dysfunction in a contemporaneous extracardiac group.[112]

Drawbacks of the extracardiac Fontan operation include the thrombogenicity of the prosthetic conduit and lack of conduit growth, in particular with the current tendency for surgery in small children. At the age of 2 to 4 years and body weight of 12 to 15 kg, the inferior vena cava diameter and inferior vena cava to pulmonary artery distance are approximately 60% to 80% of adult values. Oversizing the conduit may be tempting, but this has been shown to result in unfavorable Fontan hemodynamics and conduit thrombosis.[113] Intermediate follow-up of about 3 years of children with an extracardiac Fontan has shown an average reduction in conduit cross-sectional area of 14%.[114] Clearly, these extracardiac conduits need careful observation over time.

Nonoperative Fontan

The concept of completing the Fontan procedure in the cardiac catheterization laboratory was introduced with promising results from studies with laboratory animals[115] and children.[46,47] This technique requires modification of the operative technique for the bidirectional Glenn anastomosis or the hemi-Fontan procedure to allow for the percutaneous seating of a covered stent as an intra-atrial conduit. Although this procedure currently uses experimental stents and innovative techniques, it is promising and bears careful study and follow-up.

Fontan for Biventricular Hearts

Certain cardiac defects with two well-formed ventricles are better served with a Fontan procedure than with a high-risk biventricular repair. A typical group of patients have double-outlet right ventricle with a remote ventricular septal defect or a straddling atrioventricular valve, which would make a biventricular repair problematic. Results with the Fontan procedure in these patients are good.[67,116,117] Other anatomic substrates in which the Fontan procedure might be more desirable than a biventricular repair are congenitally corrected transposition of the great arteries (with difficult anatomy for a double-switch procedure) or unbalanced atrioventricular septal defects.

OUTCOME AFTER THE FONTAN PROCEDURE

Early Mortality and Morbidity

Approximately 40 years after the introduction of the Fontan operation, the early mortality after the Fontan procedure, which historically was in excess of 20%,[118] has steadily come down to less than 5%.[112,119-122] This is in spite of liberalizing the original patient selection criteria and extending the procedure to many forms of complex single ventricle. Multiple factors have contributed to this improved early outcome. Certainly, volume unloading of the single ventricle by an early bidirectional cavopulmonary anastomosis or a hemi-Fontan procedure has markedly improved the suitability for a subsequent Fontan operation,[21,28,29,74] although some physicians argue that staging with an intermediate bidirectional cavopulmonary anastomosis is unnecessary.[95] The introduction of the total cavopulmonary connection with its more energy-efficient circulation, with the use of either a lateral tunnel[91] or an extracardiac conduit,[123] has clearly been a huge advance in the improved outcome of the Fontan operation. Other factors potentially responsible for the improvement in the early results with the Fontan operation (identified by some but disputed by others) are the use of an atrial fenestration[61,94,96,97] and preoperative occlusion of aortopulmonary collaterals.[75,78,81]

Patients with a single ventricle and heterotaxy syndrome always have been a particularly high-risk population for the Fontan procedure because of multiple associated cardiovascular abnormalities, including variable anatomy of the sinus node and conduction system, potential for pulmonary venous obstruction, and atrioventricular valve regurgitation. Some reports have shown improved outcomes with these patients after the Fontan procedure, although early mortality and the incidence of postoperative rhythm disturbances and atrioventricular valve regurgitation are higher in the heterotaxy patients compared with the nonheterotaxy patients.[18,63,65,66]

Pleural and pericardial effusions constitute the most common early morbidity after the Fontan operation. Prolonged chest tube drainage has been associated with longer cardiopulmonary bypass times.[109,121] It is interesting to note that effusions are reduced in patients having Fontan completion without cardiopulmonary bypass[103] or nonoperative Fontan completion by catheter techniques.[47] The use of a baffle fenestration has been reported to reduce the duration of postoperative chest tube drainage.[96,97]

Sinus node dysfunction and atrial arrhythmias occur frequently after the Fontan procedure, particularly in patients with heterotaxy syndrome.[18] It has been proposed that an extracardiac conduit will result in fewer atrial arrhythmias compared with a lateral tunnel Fontan procedure. Although some authors have found this to be true,[108,109] others have found no difference in arrhythmias comparing the two techniques,[110,111] and there is even one report of a higher incidence of sinus node dysfunction with the extracardiac Fontan.[112]

The incidence of early Fontan takedown is generally 1% to 3% in many series and is thought to be related to improper patient selection or to unrecognized or uncorrected anatomic problems, such as outflow tract obstruction or pulmonary or systemic venous pathway obstruction.[61,98,119,122] Although Fontan takedown has a high mortality, some of these patients can be candidates for a subsequent successful Fontan after correction of underlying treatable abnormalities.[124]

An uncommon but serious complication after the Fontan procedure is hemidiaphragmatic paralysis as a result of phrenic nerve injury. Patients with a paralyzed hemidiaphragm have longer hospital stays and a higher incidence of prolonged pleural effusions and ascites.[125,126] There is evidence that subdiaphragmatic venous hemodynamics are abnormal, even after diaphragm plication.[127]

Late Outcomes

With improving operative survival, late outcome after the Fontan operation is becoming increasingly important. In 1990, 2 decades after the introduction of the procedure, Fontan reported that the "Fontan state" was associated with a premature decline in functional status and survival.[118] Even when atriopulmonary and atrioventricular Fontan procedures were performed under perfect conditions, there was a gradual attrition with a predicted survival of 86%, 81%, and 73% at 5, 10, and 15 years, respectively, after the operation. More current series with follow-up of patients undergoing total cavopulmonary connection show overall actuarial survival of 91% at 10 years with the lateral tunnel Fontan[122] and 93.6% at 10 years[128] and 85% at 15 years[129] with the extracardiac Fontan. A study from Children's Hospital Boston showed that for operative survivors, there was no difference in freedom from death or transplantation after 20 years between patients with an atriopulmonary connection and those with a total cavopulmonary connection.[130]

In addition to ongoing late mortality with the Fontan operation, these survivors have impairment of exercise function. In a large multicenter study examining 546 patients, despite a normal ejection fraction in 73% of patients, only 28% had a normal diastolic grade.[74] Peak oxygen consumption on exercise was only 65% of normal for age; this finding has been corroborated by others.[131,132] It is worrisome that age-adjusted exercise capacity tended to worsen with age.[74,133]

The exact reasons for the late attrition after the Fontan operation are unknown but no doubt are complex and multifactorial. Serial angiographic measurement of pulmonary artery size in Fontan patients shows that pulmonary artery growth lags behind somatic growth[134] or even fails to grow at all, resulting in a decreasing pulmonary artery index with time.[135] A correlation can be made between low pulmonary artery index and length of follow-up as well as with an unfavorable outcome.[135]

Atrial Arrhythmias

With the widespread adoption of the total cavopulmonary connection (either lateral tunnel or extracardiac Fontan) rather than atriopulmonary connections, the incidence of late atrial arrhythmias and the need for pacemakers have greatly diminished.[122,128] Patients with the older atriopulmonary connection are more prone to significant atrial arrhythmias (see Fontan Conversion section for a discussion on management of these patients). Children with heterotaxy syndrome remain at risk for late arrhythmias after the Fontan operation, even with the newer total cavopulmonary connection techniques.[18,65,66]

Venovenous Collaterals

After the Fontan operation, significant venovenous collateral channels can develop, which result in significant right-to-left shunting with resultant hypoxemia and cyanosis. These abnormal venous channels can be between the systemic veins and the pulmonary veins or pulmonary venous atrium. Once recognized, they can usually be interrupted by interventional catheterization techniques and less commonly require surgical intervention.[136,137] In patients with progressive cyanosis after the Fontan operation, an aggressive search for collateral vessels should be made using cardiac catheterization and angiography followed by interruption of significant collateral channels.

Thromboembolism and Prophylactic Anticoagulation

Thromboembolic complications occur both early and late after the Fontan procedure. The true incidence of thromboembolism is not known, but various studies have shown an incidence of "silent" intracardiac thrombus ranging from 9% to 33%,[107,138-140] with a higher rate found when transesophageal echocardiography is used. Cerebrovascular events, including thromboembolic strokes, occur in 2% to 9% of Fontan patients.[141,142] The presence of a fenestration may increase this risk,[142] whereas the use of aspirin may ameliorate it.[141] Many factors contribute to the risk for thrombus formation, including suboptimal flow patterns, arrhythmias, cyanosis, presence of foreign material in the circulation, preexistent coagulopathies, and liver dysfunction.

Information on the prevention of thromboembolic complications after the Fontan procedure is inconsistent. Some centers recommend aspirin alone as prophylaxis,[143,144] whereas others recommend anticoagulation with warfarin.[140,145] It is well known that anticoagulant therapy is not without risk. Anticoagulant-related bleeding is a cause for concern, particularly in active children. In the presence of cyanosis or heart failure, anticoagulation control can be difficult. Reviews of the need for and type of anticoagulation after the Fontan operation have emphasized the lack of a uniform consensus and have underscored the need for prospective clinical studies.[146-148]

Protein-Losing Enteropathy

Protein-losing enteropathy is a relatively rare but debilitating complication with a reported incidence of up to 15%. The condition involves the loss of protein within the gastrointestinal tract and can occur from weeks to years after the Fontan operation, with 50% mortality at 5 years following diagnosis.[149] The precise reasons for its occurrence are not known, but it has been suggested that it may be related to abnormal mesenteric blood flow.[150] Clinical manifestations are related to the degree of hypoproteinemia; the nonselective loss of proteins can result in peripheral edema, ascites and effusions, immunodeficiency, and coagulopathy. A detailed investigation of the cardiovascular system should take place and hemodynamics optimized if possible. Symptomatic treatment is with diuretics, diet supplements, and intermittent albumin infusions. Steroids[151] and heparin therapy[152] have been shown to improve symptoms and to reduce protein loss in some patients. It is postulated that they act through stabilizing the intestinal mucosal membrane, thus reducing the protein leak. Other treatment modalities that have shown some success are sildenafil use,[153] atrial pacing,[154] and creation of a surgical fenestration.[155] Ultimately, patients with protein-losing enteropathy may require cardiac transplantation with expected resolution of the enteropathy.[156]

Plastic Bronchitis

Plastic bronchitis is another poorly understood and unusual complication after the Fontan procedure. Noninflammatory mucin-containing casts are formed in the trachea and bronchus. Symptomatic treatment is by bronchoscopic clearance. Small series and case reports have advocated different treatment options, including Fontan baffle fenestration,[157] thoracic duct ligation,[158] and aerosolized tissue plasminogen activator.[159,160]

MANAGEMENT OF THE FAILING FONTAN

Even with current improvements in surgical strategies for management of children with a single ventricle, there continues to be a seemingly irreducible incidence of late failure, defined as Fontan takedown, need for transplantation, or death.[29,119,120] Preservation of ventricular function is of paramount importance for successful long-term outcome in patients with univentricular hearts.[61] Methods to preserve ventricular function include volume unloading of the heart with a bidirectional cavopulmonary anastomosis at an early age,[29] aggressive relief of systemic ventricular outflow tract obstruction to prevent myocardial hypertrophy and diastolic noncompliance, and repair of atrioventricular valve regurgitation. Although not universally accepted, elimination of systemic to pulmonary collateral blood flow can help preserve ventricular function as well.[75] Sometimes dysfunction of the Fontan circulation may be related to atrial arrhythmias or conduction abnormalities, which may respond to conventional pacing techniques[161,162] or resynchronization pacing.[163]

Fontan Conversion

Conversion of the failing classical atriopulmonary Fontan with refractory arrhythmias to a total cavopulmonary connection with concomitant arrhythmia surgery and correction of hemodynamically significant lesions was introduced by Mavroudis and colleagues in 1998.[164] The operation consists of defined cryoablation lesion sets in the atrium, repair of residual defects such as atrioventricular valve regurgitation, conversion to an extracardiac Fontan connection, and pacemaker placement. An update of their Fontan conversion series in 111 patients[165] reported 1 early death, 6 late deaths, and 6 subsequent transplants, with good rhythm control in over 85% of patients. Other centers have reported similarly good results with this challenging group of patients with low mortality rates and good rhythm control.[100,166] Conversion to a total cavopulmonary connection with either a lateral tunnel approach or an extracardiac conduit appear equally efficacious.[167,168]

Heart Transplantation

For patients with a failing Fontan in whom heart failure is the dominant feature or with protein-losing enteropathy refractory to more conventional therapies, cardiac transplantation offers the only solution. Although some series have reported early mortality with transplantation in patients with Fontan procedures in excess of 50%,[169,170] others have reported 1-year survival rates ranging from 71% to 86%.[15,156,171,172] Importantly, hospital survivors show uniform resolution of protein-losing enteropathy after transplantation.[156,171] Of course, there is an incidence of death on the waiting list before heart transplantation[156] as well as the need for chronic immunosuppression and concerns for post-transplant infection, rejection, and late graft failure.

Mechanical Circulatory Support

Mechanical support of the failing Fontan is problematic because of the single functional ventricle. Case reports have described the use of the Berlin Heart as a successful bridge to transplant as a left ventricular assist device (systemic ventricular apical cannulation for pump inflow with ascending aortic cannulation for pump outflow)[173] and as a "right ventricular" assist device (Fontan systemic venous pathway cannulation for pump inflow with pulmonary artery cannulation for pump outflow).[174] Designs for indwelling axial flow pumps for support of the failing Fontan circulation as a bridge to recovery or as a bridge to transplant have also been tested.[175,176] Because of the ongoing shortage of suitable donor hearts for transplantation and the seemingly inevitable incidence of Fontan failure with time, it is hoped that mechanical devices will be designed and tested in the future to successfully

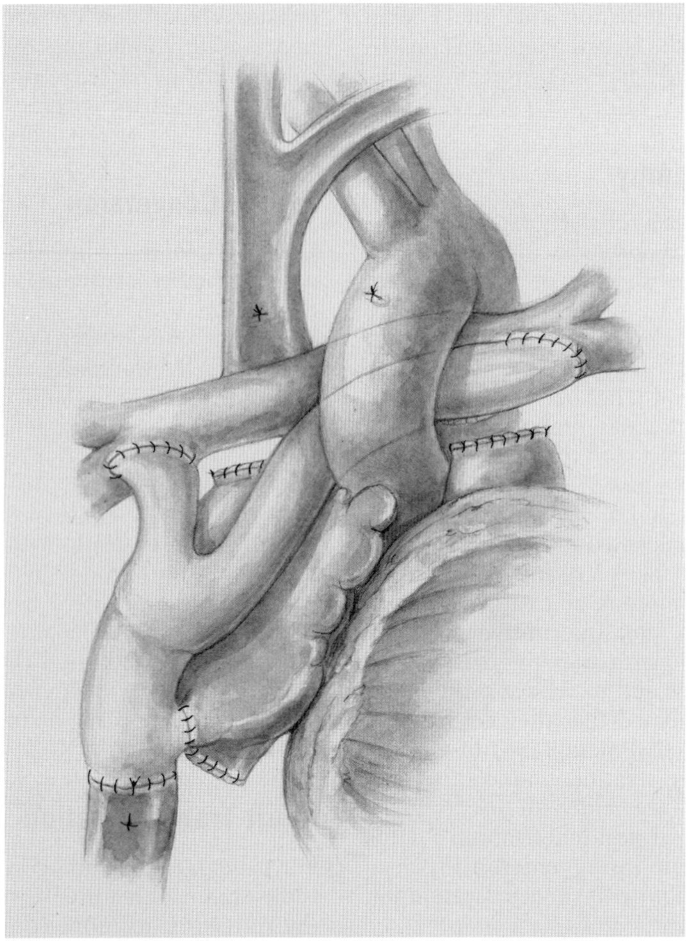

FIGURE 129-4 ■ A completed Y-graft Fontan is shown, emphasizing the importance of anastomosing the right and left limbs of the Y-graft away from the Glenn anastomosis. The fenestration to the right atrium is also depicted.

support the patient with a failing Fontan circulation indefinitely, without the need for transplantation.

COMPUTER MODELING TO OPTIMIZE FONTAN ENERGETICS

Computational fluid dynamics[177] have demonstrated designs of the total cavopulmonary connection that can cause flow disturbances and energy dissipation. Optimizing flow and diminishing power loss in the Fontan circuit presumably can improve hemodynamic efficiency and potentially improve long-term outcomes. In vitro and computational fluid dynamics studies have shown reduced energy losses with caval offset[178] and with flaring of the cavopulmonary anastomosis,[179] thus prompting modification of the total cavopulmonary connection surgical procedure.

Using computational fluid dynamics, an optimized total cavopulmonary connection using a bifurcated Y-graft for the superior vena cava to pulmonary artery connection and another bifurcated Y-graft for the inferior vena cava to pulmonary artery connection was proposed[180] (U.S. Patent No. 7811244). Although this "Optiflo" connection had superior flow characteristics predicted by flow modeling, the optimized design from a surgical standpoint was cumbersome. Subsequent studies developing surgical designs to balance hepatic blood flow distribution to the right and left pulmonary arteries in children with acquired pulmonary AVMs showed favorable results with a bifurcated Y-graft connection from the inferior vena cava to the branch pulmonary arteries.[181] Comparison of the Y-graft Fontan connection with more conventional Fontan connections using computational fluid dynamics have demonstrated improved flow characteristics, reduced energy losses, and balanced hepatic flow distribution to the pulmonary arteries.[182,183] Based on these improvements in flow dynamics predicted by computerized modeling, the Y-graft Fontan concept has been used clinically[184-187] (Fig. 129-4).

A novel computer-based surgical planning framework that enables one to virtually perform multiple surgical scenarios and determine the one that will yield the best hemodynamic performance before even entering the operating room has been proposed.[188] Such a surgical planning platform offers a unique solution for cases in which hemodynamics (and in particular hepatic flow distribution) are vital to the operation but in which the small patient population and large number of anatomic variations pose a severe obstacle to the establishment of surgical guidelines from clinical studies alone.

REFERENCES

1. Mavroudis C, Jacobs JP: Congenital Heart Surgery Nomenclature and Database Project: overview and minimum dataset. *Ann Thorac Surg* 69:S2–S17, 2000.
2. Jacobs ML, Mayer JE, Jr: Congenital Heart Surgery Nomenclature and Database Project: single ventricle. *Ann Thorac Surg* 69:S197–S204, 2000.
3. de Leval MR, McKay R, Jones M, et al: Modified Blalock-Taussig shunt. Use of subclavian artery orifice as flow regulator in prosthetic systemic-pulmonary artery shunts. *J Thorac Cardiovasc Surg* 81:112–119, 1981.
4. Alkhulaifi AM, Lacour-Gayet F, Serraf A, et al: Systemic pulmonary shunts in neonates: early clinical outcome and choice of surgical approach. *Ann Thorac Surg* 69:1499–1504, 2000.
5. Odim J, Portzky M, Zurakowski D, et al: Sternotomy approach for the modified Blalock-Taussig shunt. *Circulation* 92:II256–II261, 1995.
6. Mohammadi S, Benhameid O, Campbell A, et al: Could we still improve early and interim outcome after prosthetic systemic-pulmonary shunt? A risk factors analysis. *Eur J Cardiothorac Surg* 34:545–549, 2008.
7. Rodefeld MD, Ruzmetov M, Schamberger MS, et al: Staged surgical repair of functional single ventricle in infants with unobstructed pulmonary blood flow. *Eur J Cardiothorac Surg* 27:949–955, 2005.
8. Bradley SM, Simsic JM, Atz AM, et al: The infant with single ventricle and excessive pulmonary blood flow: results of a strategy of pulmonary artery division and shunt. *Ann Thorac Surg* 74:805–810, 2002.
9. Clarke AJ, Kasahara S, Andrews DR, et al: Mid-term results for double inlet left ventricle and similar morphologies: timing of Damus-Kaye-Stansel. *Ann Thorac Surg* 78:650–657, 2004.
10. Fiore AC, Rodefeld M, Vijay P, et al: Subaortic obstruction in univentricular heart: results using the double barrel Damus-Kaye Stansel operation. *Eur J Cardiothorac Surg* 35:141–146, 2009.
11. McElhinney DB, Reddy VM, Silverman NH, et al: Modified Damus-Kaye-Stansel procedure for single ventricle, subaortic stenosis, and arch obstruction in neonates and infants: midterm results and techniques for avoiding circulatory arrest. *J Thorac Cardiovasc Surg* 114:718–725, 1997.
12. Miura T, Kishimoto H, Kawata H, et al: Management of univentricular heart with systemic ventricular outflow obstruction by pulmonary artery banding and Damus-Kaye-Stansel operation. *Ann Thorac Surg* 77:23–28, 2004.
13. Hiramatsu T, Imai Y, Kurosawa H, et al: Midterm results of surgical treatment of systemic ventricular outflow obstruction in Fontan patients. *Ann Thorac Surg* 73:855–860, 2002.
14. Tchervenkov CI, Shum-Tim D, Beland MJ, et al: Single ventricle with systemic obstruction in early life: comparison of initial pulmonary artery banding versus the Norwood operation. *Eur J Cardiothorac Surg* 19:671–677, 2001.
15. Kanter KR, Miller BE, Cuadrado AG, et al: Successful application of the Norwood procedure for infants without hypoplastic left heart syndrome. *Ann Thorac Surg* 59:301–304, 1995.
16. Cerillo AG, Murzi B, Giusti S, et al: Pulmonary artery banding and ventricular septal defect enlargement in patients with univentricular atrioventricular connection and the aorta originating from an incomplete ventricle. *Eur J Cardiothorac Surg* 22:192–199, 2002.
17. Jahangiri M, Shinebourne EA, Ross DB, et al: Long-term results of relief of subaortic stenosis in univentricular atrioventricular connection with discordant ventriculoarterial connections. *Ann Thorac Surg* 71:907–910, 2001.
18. Anagnostopoulos PV, Pearl JM, Octave C, et al: Improved current era outcomes in patients with heterotaxy syndromes. *Eur J Cardiothorac Surg* 35:871–878, 2009.
19. Lodge AJ, Rychik J, Nicolson SC, et al: Improving outcomes in functional single ventricle and total anomalous pulmonary venous connection. *Ann Thorac Surg* 78:1688–1695, 2004.
20. Gaynor JW, Collins MH, Rychik J, et al: Long-term outcome of infants with single ventricle and total anomalous pulmonary venous connection. *J Thorac Cardiovasc Surg* 117:506–513, 1999.
21. Lee JR, Choi JS, Kang CH, et al: Surgical results of patients with a functional single ventricle. *Eur J Cardiothorac Surg* 24:716–722, 2003.
22. GLENN WW: Circulatory bypass of the right side of the heart. IV. Shunt between superior vena cava and distal right pulmonary artery; report of clinical application. *N Engl J Med* 259:117–120, 1958.
23. Robicsek F: An epitaph for cavopulmonary anastomosis. *Ann Thorac Surg* 34:208–220, 1982.
24. McFaul RC, Tajik AJ, Mair DD, et al: Development of pulmonary arteriovenous shunt after superior vena cava-right pulmonary artery (Glenn) anastomosis. Report of four cases. *Circulation* 55:212–216, 1977.
25. Pennington DG, Nouri S, Ho J, et al: Glenn shunt: long-term results and current role in congenital heart operations. *Ann Thorac Surg* 31:532–539, 1981.
26. Bridges ND, Jonas RA, Mayer JE, et al: Bidirectional cavopulmonary anastomosis as interim palliation for high-risk Fontan candidates. Early results. *Circulation* 82:IV170–IV176, 1990.
27. Mazzera E, Corno A, Picardo S, et al: Bidirectional cavopulmonary shunts: clinical applications as staged or definitive palliation. *Ann Thorac Surg* 47:415–420, 1989.
28. Norwood WI, Jacobs ML: Fontan's procedure in two stages. *Am J Surg* 166:548–551, 1993.
29. Alphonso N, Baghai M, Sundar P, et al: Intermediate-term outcome following the Fontan operation: a survival, functional and risk-factor analysis. *Eur J Cardiothorac Surg* 28:529–535, 2005.
30. Cleuziou J, Schreiber C, Cornelsen JK, et al: Bidirectional cavopulmonary connection without additional pulmonary blood flow in patients below the age of 6 months. *Eur J Cardiothorac Surg* 34:556–561, 2008.
31. Calvaruso DF, Rubino A, Ocello S, et al: Bidirectional Glenn and antegrade pulmonary blood flow: temporary or definitive palliation? *Ann Thorac Surg* 85:1389–1395, 2008.
32. Gray RG, Altmann K, Mosca RS, et al: Persistent antegrade pulmonary blood flow post-glenn does not alter early post-Fontan outcomes in single-ventricle patients. *Ann Thorac Surg* 84:888–893, 2007.
33. Berdat PA, Belli E, Lacour-Gayet F, et al: Additional pulmonary blood flow has no adverse effect on outcome after bidirectional cavopulmonary anastomosis. *Ann Thorac Surg* 79:29–36, 2005.
34. Yoshida M, Yamaguchi M, Yoshimura N, et al: Appropriate additional pulmonary blood flow at the bidirectional Glenn procedure is useful for completion of total cavopulmonary connection. *Ann Thorac Surg* 80:976–981, 2005.
35. Torres A, Gray R, Pass RH: Transcatheter occlusion of antegrade pulmonary flow in children after cavopulmonary anastomosis. *Catheter Cardiovasc Interv* 72:988–993, 2008.
36. Gatzoulis MA, Munk MD, Williams WG, et al: Definitive palliation with cavopulmonary or aortopulmonary shunts for adults with single ventricle physiology. *Heart* 83:51–57, 2000.
37. Yamada K, Roques X, Elia N, et al: The short- and mid-term results of bidirectional cavopulmonary shunt with additional source of pulmonary blood flow as definitive palliation for the functional single ventricular heart. *Eur J Cardiothorac Surg* 18:683–689, 2000.
38. Kogon BE, Plattner C, Leong T, et al: The bidirectional Glenn operation: a risk factor analysis for morbidity and mortality. *J Thorac Cardiovasc Surg* 136:1237–1242, 2008.
39. Iyer GK, Van Arsdell GS, Dicke FP, et al: Are bilateral superior vena cavae a risk factor for single ventricle palliation? *Ann Thorac Surg* 70:711–716, 2000.
40. Kawashima Y, Kitamura S, Matsuda H, et al: Total cavopulmonary shunt operation in complex cardiac anomalies. A new operation. *J Thorac Cardiovasc Surg* 87:74–81, 1984.
41. Duncan BW, Desai S: Pulmonary arteriovenous malformations after cavopulmonary anastomosis. *Ann Thorac Surg* 76:1759–1766, 2003.
42. Kim SJ, Bae EJ, Lee JY, et al: Inclusion of hepatic venous drainage in patients with pulmonary arteriovenous fistulas. *Ann Thorac Surg* 87:548–553, 2009.
43. Brown JW, Ruzmetov M, Vijay P, et al: Pulmonary arteriovenous malformations in children after the Kawashima operation. *Ann Thorac Surg* 80:1592–1596, 2005.
44. McElhinney DB, Kreutzer J, Lang P, et al: Incorporation of the hepatic veins into the cavopulmonary circulation in patients with heterotaxy and pulmonary arteriovenous malformations after a Kawashima procedure. *Ann Thorac Surg* 80:1597–1603, 2005.

45. Douglas WI, Goldberg CS, Mosca RS, et al: Hemi-Fontan procedure for hypoplastic left heart syndrome: outcome and suitability for Fontan. *Ann Thorac Surg* 68:1361–1367, 1999.
46. Galantowicz M, Cheatham JP: Fontan completion without surgery. *Semin Thorac Cardiovasc Surg Pediatr Card Surg Annu* 7:48–55, 2004.
47. Sallehuddin A, Mesned A, Barakati M, et al: Fontan completion without surgery. *Eur J Cardiothorac Surg* 32:195–200, 2007.
48. Cohen MI, Bridges ND, Gaynor JW, et al: Modifications to the cavopulmonary anastomosis do not eliminate early sinus node dysfunction. *J Thorac Cardiovasc Surg* 120:891–900, 2000.
49. Pekkan K, Dasi LP, de Zélicourt D, et al: Hemodynamic performance of stage-2 univentricular reconstruction: Glenn vs. hemi-Fontan templates. *Ann Biomed Eng* 37:50–63, 2009.
50. Ashburn DA, Blackstone EH, Wells WJ, et al: Determinants of mortality and type of repair in neonates with pulmonary atresia and intact ventricular septum. *J Thorac Cardiovasc Surg* 127:1000–1007, 2004.
51. Billingsley AM, Laks H, Boyce SW, et al: Definitive repair in patients with pulmonary atresia and intact ventricular septum. *J Thorac Cardiovasc Surg* 97:746–754, 1989.
52. Chowdhury UK, Airan B, Talwar S, et al: One and one-half ventricle repair: results and concerns. *Ann Thorac Surg* 80:2293–2300, 2005.
53. Stellin G, Vida VL, Milanesi O, et al: Surgical treatment of complex cardiac anomalies: the "one and one half ventricle repair." *Eur J Cardiothorac Surg* 22:1043–1049, 2002.
54. Van Arsdell GS: One and one half ventricle repairs. *Semin Thorac Cardiovasc Surg Pediatr Card Surg Annu* 3:173–178, 2000.
55. Quinonez LG, Dearani JA, Puga FJ, et al: Results of the 1.5-ventricle repair for Ebstein anomaly and the failing right ventricle. *J Thorac Cardiovasc Surg* 133:1303–1310, 2007.
56. Hanley FL: The one and a half ventricle repair-we can do it, but should we do it? *J Thorac Cardiovasc Surg* 117:659–661, 1999.
57. Choussat A, Fontan F, Besse P, et al: Selection criteria for Fontan's procedure. In Anderson RH, Shinebourne EA, editors: *Pediatric cardiology, 1977*, Edinburgh, 1978, Churchill Livingstone, pp 559–566.
58. Forbes TJ, Gajarski R, Johnson GL, et al: Influence of age on the effect of bidirectional cavopulmonary anastomosis on left ventricular volume, mass and ejection fraction. *J Am Coll Cardiol* 28:1301–1307, 1996.
59. Mahle WT, Wernovsky G, Bridges ND, et al: Impact of early ventricular unloading on exercise performance in preadolescents with single ventricle Fontan physiology. *J Am Coll Cardiol* 34:1637–1643, 1999.
60. Shiraishi S, Yagihara T, Kagisaki K, et al: Impact of age at Fontan completion on postoperative hemodynamics and long-term aerobic exercise capacity in patients with dominant left ventricle. *Ann Thorac Surg* 87:555–560, 2009.
61. Hosein RB, Clarke AJ, McGuirk SP, et al: Factors influencing early and late outcome following the Fontan procedure in the current era. The "Two Commandments"? *Eur J Cardiothorac Surg* 31:344–352, 2007.
62. Pizarro C, Mroczek T, Gidding SS, et al: Fontan completion in infants. *Ann Thorac Surg* 81:2243–2248, 2006.
63. Azakie A, Merklinger SL, Williams WG, et al: Improving outcomes of the Fontan operation in children with atrial isomerism and heterotaxy syndromes. *Ann Thorac Surg* 72:1636–1640, 2001.
64. Alboliras ET, Porter CB, Danielson GK, et al: Results of the modified Fontan operation for congenital heart lesions in patients without preoperative sinus rhythm. *J Am Coll Cardiol* 6:228–233, 1985.
65. Atz AM, Cohen MS, Sleeper LA, et al: Functional state of patients with heterotaxy syndrome following the Fontan operation. *Cardiol Young* 17(Suppl 2):44–53, 2007.
66. Kim SJ, Kim WH, Lim HG, et al: Improving results of the Fontan procedure in patients with heterotaxy syndrome. *Ann Thorac Surg* 82:1245–1251, 2006.
67. Ruzmetov M, Rodefeld MD, Turrentine MW, et al: Rational approach to surgical management of complex forms of double outlet right ventricle with modified Fontan operation. *Congenit Heart Dis* 3:397–403, 2008.
68. Piehler JM, Danielson GK, McGoon DC, et al: Management of pulmonary atresia with ventricular septal defect and hypoplastic pulmonary arteries by right ventricular outflow construction. *J Thorac Cardiovasc Surg* 80:552–567, 1980.
69. Fontan F, Fernandez G, Costa F, et al: The size of the pulmonary arteries and the results of the Fontan operation. *J Thorac Cardiovasc Surg* 98:711–719, 1989.
70. Nakata S, Imai Y, Takanashi Y, et al: A new method for the quantitative standardization of cross-sectional areas of the pulmonary arteries in congenital heart diseases with decreased pulmonary blood flow. *J Thorac Cardiovasc Surg* 88:610–619, 1984.
71. Knott-Craig CJ, Julsrud PR, Schaff HV, et al: Pulmonary artery size and clinical outcome after the modified Fontan operation. *Ann Thorac Surg* 55:646–651, 1993.
72. Adachi I, Yagihara T, Kagisaki K, et al: Preoperative small pulmonary artery did not affect the midterm results of Fontan operation. *Eur J Cardiothorac Surg* 32:156–162, 2007.
73. Reddy VM, McElhinney DB, Moore P, et al: Pulmonary artery growth after bidirectional cavopulmonary shunt: is there a cause for concern? *J Thorac Cardiovasc Surg* 112:1180–1190, 1996.
74. Anderson PA, Sleeper LA, Mahony L, et al: Contemporary outcomes after the Fontan procedure: a Pediatric Heart Network multicenter study. *J Am Coll Cardiol* 52:85–98, 2008.
75. Vogt KN, Manlhiot C, Van Arsdell G, et al: Somatic growth in children with single ventricle physiology impact of physiologic state. *J Am Coll Cardiol* 50:1876–1883, 2007.
76. Ascuitto RJ, Ross-Ascuitto NT: Systematic-to-pulmonary collaterals: a source of flow energy loss in Fontan physiology. *Pediatr Cardiol* 25:472–481, 2004.
77. Kanter KR, Vincent RN: Management of aortopulmonary collateral arteries in Fontan patients: occlusion improves clinical outcome. *Semin Thorac Cardiovasc Surg Pediatr Card Surg Annu* 5:48–54, 2002.
78. Kanter KR, Vincent RN, Raviele AA: Importance of acquired systemic-to-pulmonary collaterals in the Fontan operation. *Ann Thorac Surg* 68:969–974, 1999.
79. Lim DS, Graziano JN, Rocchini AP, et al: Transcatheter occlusion of aortopulmonary shunts during single-ventricle surgical palliation. *Catheter Cardiovasc Interv* 65:427–433, 2005.
80. Bradley SM: Management of aortopulmonary collateral arteries in Fontan patients: routine occlusion is not warranted. *Semin Thorac Cardiovasc Surg Pediatr Card Surg Annu* 5:55–67, 2002.
81. Bradley SM, McCall MM, Sistino JJ, et al: Aortopulmonary collateral flow in the Fontan patient: does it matter? *Ann Thorac Surg* 72:408–415, 2001.
82. McElhinney DB, Reddy VM, Tworetzky W, et al: Incidence and implications of systemic to pulmonary collaterals after bidirectional cavopulmonary anastomosis. *Ann Thorac Surg* 69:1222–1228, 2000.
83. Scheurer MA, Hill EG, Vasuki N, et al: Survival after bidirectional cavopulmonary anastomosis: analysis of preoperative risk factors. *J Thorac Cardiovasc Surg* 134:82–89, 89, 2007.
84. Ando M, Takahashi Y: Edge-to-edge repair of common atrioventricular or tricuspid valve in patients with functionally single ventricle. *Ann Thorac Surg* 84:1571–1576, 2007.
85. Hancock Friesen CL, Sherwood MC, Gauvreau K, et al: Intermediate outcomes of atrioventricular valvuloplasty in lateral tunnel Fontan patients. *J Heart Valve Dis* 13:962–971, 2004.
86. Kanter KR, Forbess JM, Fyfe DA, et al: De Vega tricuspid annuloplasty for systemic tricuspid regurgitation in children with univentricular physiology. *J Heart Valve Dis* 13:86–90, 2004.
87. Mahle WT, Gaynor JW, Spray TL: Atrioventricular valve replacement in patients with a single ventricle. *Ann Thorac Surg* 72:182–186, 2001.
88. Fontan F, Baudet E: Surgical repair of tricuspid atresia. *Thorax* 26:240–248, 1971.
89. Kreutzer G, Galindez E, Bono H, et al: An operation for the correction of tricuspid atresia. *J Thorac Cardiovasc Surg* 66:613–621, 1973.
90. Bjork VO, Olin CL, Bjarke BB, et al: Right atrial-right ventricular anastomosis for correction of tricuspid atresia. *J Thorac Cardiovasc Surg* 77:452–458, 1979.
91. de Leval MR, Kilner P, Gewillig M, et al: Total cavopulmonary connection: a logical alternative to atriopulmonary connection for complex Fontan operations. Experimental studies and early clinical experience. *J Thorac Cardiovasc Surg* 96:682–695, 1988.

malformation can range from only minimal displacement of the septal and inferior leaflets to an imperforate membrane or muscular shelf between the inlet and trabecular zones of the RV. The range of variability is infinite, and the most important pathologic finding is "failure of delamination" of the leaflets. There often is marked dilation of the true TV annulus, which is not displaced, and a large chamber separating the true annulus from the functional RV is the "atrialized" portion of the RV (aRV).

Right Ventricle

The RV is divided into two regions: the area involved with the malformation (i.e., the inlet portion or the aRV) that is functionally integrated with the right atrium (RA), and the area that is not involved by the malformation and consists of the other two components of the RV—the trabecular and outlet portions, which constitute the functional RV. The "atrialized" portion of the RV can become disproportionately dilated and may account for more than half of the RV volume. The majority (>⅔) of hearts with Ebstein malformation have RV dilation. Dilation often involves not only the atrialized inlet portion of the RV but also the functional RV apex and outflow tract. In some cases, RV dilation is so marked that the ventricular septum is deviated leftward, compressing the left ventricular (LV) chamber. In such cases, the short-axis view demonstrates a circular RV and a D-shaped LV.

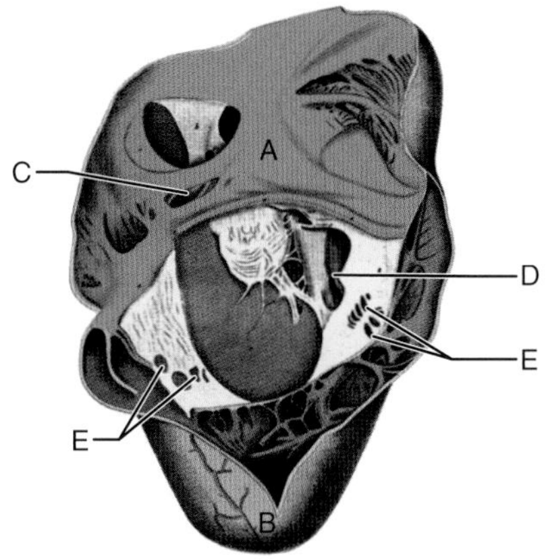

FIGURE 130-1 ■ Figure from the original Ebstein anomaly case report. The right atrium and right ventricle are shown opened along the right border beginning at the superior vena cava. *A,* Right atrium; *B,* right ventricle; *C,* rudimentary septal leaflet of tricuspid valve with its chordae tendineae, which insert on the endocardium of the ventricular septum; *D,* opening through which one can get into the right conus arteriosus, and in the opposite direction, one can get into the sac that is formed by membrane; *E,* fenestrations seen in the tricuspid leaflets. (From Said SM, Dearani JA: Ebstein anomaly, congenital tricuspid valve regurgitation and dysplasia. In Allen HD, Driscolle DJ, Shaddy RE, Feltes TF, editors: *Moss and Adams' heart disease in infants, children, and adolescents,* ed 8, Philadelphia, 2013, Lippincott Williams & Wilkins, Figure 39-1.)

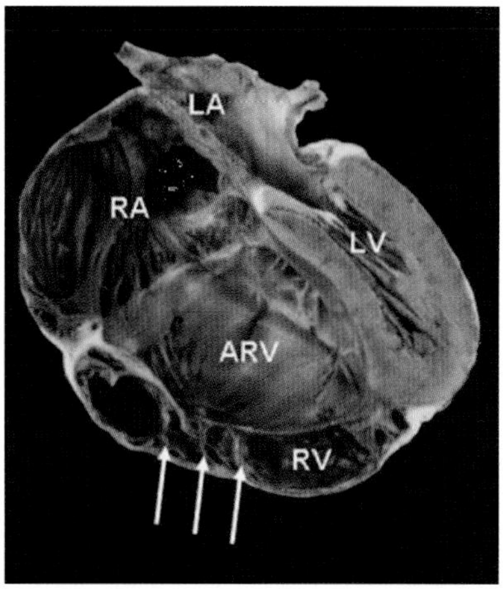

FIGURE 130-2 ■ Severe Ebstein malformation of tricuspid valve (four-chamber view) showing marked downward displacement of shelflike posterior leaflet with attachment to underlying free wall by numerous muscular stumps *(arrows),* markedly dilated atrialized portion of right ventricle (ARV), small functional portion of right ventricle (RV), leftward bowing of ventricular septum, and marked dilation of right atrium (RA). *LA,* Left atrium; *LV,* left ventricle. (From Said SM, Dearani JA: Ebstein anomaly, congenital tricuspid valve regurgitation and dysplasia. In Allen HD, Driscolle DJ, Shaddy RE, Feltes TF, editors: *Moss and Adams' heart disease in infants, children, and adolescents,* ed 8, Philadelphia, 2013, Lippincott Williams & Wilkins, Figure 39-5.)

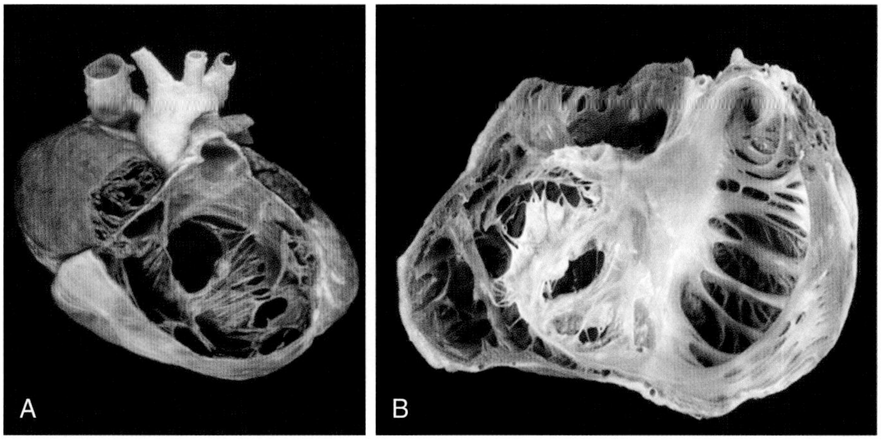

FIGURE 130-3 ■ **A and B, Ebstein heart: marked fenestrations and tethering of the tricuspid valve anterior leaflet.** (From Said SM, Dearani JA: Ebstein anomaly, congenital tricuspid valve regurgitation and dysplasia. In Allen HD, Driscolle DJ, Shaddy RE, Feltes TF, editors: *Moss and Adams' heart disease in infants, children, and adolescents,* ed 8, Philadelphia, 2013, Lippincott Williams & Wilkins, Figure 39-2.)

Associated Cardiac Defects

The most common associated cardiac defects include[5,6]:

- Atrial septal defect (ASD): either patent foramen ovale or an ASD, mostly secundum, is present in 80% to 94% of the patients
- Ventricular septal defect with or without pulmonary atresia
- RV outflow tract obstruction: this can occur secondary to structural abnormalities (pulmonary valve stenosis or pulmonary atresia), branch pulmonary artery stenosis, and rarely the displaced TV
- Patent ductus arteriosus
- Coarctation of the aorta
- Accessory conduction pathways (Wolff-Parkinson-White [WPW] syndrome) are present in up to 15% to 20% of patients and may predispose patients to arrhythmias. The majority of these pathways are located around the orifice of the malformed TV.
- Left-sided lesions (uncommon)
  - Mitral valve prolapse
  - Accessory mitral valve tissue
  - Subaortic stenosis
  - Bicuspid or atretic aortic valve
  - Muscle bands in the LV cavity
  - Myocardial changes resembling LV noncompaction[7]
- Congenitally corrected transposition of the great arteries (cc-TGA): In patients with cc-TGA, an abnormal systemic atrioventricular valve (morphologic TV) that fulfills the criteria of Ebstein valve is present in 15% to 50% of cases. This Ebsteinoid displacement of the TV into the morphologic RV is different from the classic right-sided Ebstein malformation in that there is usually lack of atrialization of the RV free wall.[8]

CLASSIFICATIONS OF EBSTEIN MALFORMATION

Several classifications have been proposed for Ebstein malformation. In general, classification systems of Ebstein malformation are difficult since there are infinite variations in the anatomy and no two hearts are alike.

Carpentier in 1988 proposed the following[9]:

Type A: the volume of the true RV is adequate

Type B: a large atrialized component of the RV exists, but the anterior leaflet of the TV moves freely

Type C: severe restriction of the anterior leaflet movement that can cause significant RV outflow tract obstruction

Type D: near complete atrialization of the ventricle except for a small infundibular component

Another classification proposed four types of Ebstein malformation based on valve analysis during surgery.[10] This is our preferred approach, which is to describe the exact anatomy of each of the involved structures of the heart as visualized at the time of surgery (Table 130-1). This includes comment about the extent of failure of delamination of each leaflet, status of the leading edges of the leaflets, degree of displacement of the septal leaflet, description of the aRV, and size of the RA and RV.

GENETIC FACTORS

Genetic factors in Ebstein malformation are heterogeneous. Most cases are sporadic and familial Ebstein is rare. Rare cases of cardiac transcription factor NKX2.5 mutations, 10p13-p14 deletion, and 1p34.3-p36.11 deletion have been described in association with Ebstein malformation.[11,12] The results of a mutational analysis in a cohort of 141 unrelated probands with Ebstein malformation has been reported;[13] eight were found to have a mutation in the gene *MYH7*, and six of the eight patients also had LV noncompaction. This result may warrant genetic testing and family evaluation in this subset of patients.

PATHOPHYSIOLOGY

The functional impairment of the RV and the incompetence of the deformed TV retard forward flow of blood through the right side of the heart into the lungs.

TABLE 130-1 **Types of Ebstein Valve Based on the Anatomic Findings during Surgery**

	Anterior Leaflet				
Type	Size	Mobility	Posterior Leaflet	Septal Leaflet	Atrialized RV Chamber Size
I	Larger	Mobile	Apically displaced, dysplastic, or absent		Varies from relatively small to large
II	Relatively small and displaced in a spiral fashion toward the apex				Moderately large
III		Restricted motion; shortened, fused, and tethered chordae; direct insertion of papillary muscles into the anterior leaflet is frequently present	Displaced, dysplastic, and usually not reconstructible		Large
IV		Severely deformed; displaced into the RVOT; few or no chordae; direct insertion of the papillary muscles into the leading edge of the valve is common	Typically dysplastic or absent	Represented by a ridge of fibrous material descending apically from the membranous septum	Nearly the entire RV cavity is atrialized; TV tissue is displaced into the RVOT and may cause obstruction of blood flow (functional tricuspid stenosis)

RV, Right ventricle; *RVOT*, right ventricular outflow tract; *TV*, tricuspid valve.

Moreover, during contraction of the atrium, the atrialized portion of the RV (which is adjacent to and in continuity with the RA) balloons out (if very thin) or acts as a passive reservoir, thus decreasing the volume to be ejected. During ventricular systole, the atrialized RV contracts, creating a pressure wave that impedes venous filling of the RA, which is in the diastolic phase. In most cases, there is a communication between the left and right atria, resulting from either patency of the foramen ovale or a distinct secundum ASD. The shunt of blood through the septal opening is generally from right to left, but may be bidirectional in some patients. The overall effect of these structural abnormalities on the RA is to produce gross dilation, which may reach enormous proportions, even in infants. This dilation leads to further incompetence of the TV and further widening of the interatrial communication.[14]

As a consequence of atrial dilation, atrial tachyarrhythmias are common and become more likely as time goes on. In addition, approximately 15% of patients will have one or more accessory conduction pathways associated with WPW syndrome, and 1% to 2% of patients will have atrioventricular nodal reentrant tachycardia (AVNRT).[15,16] In end-stage heart failure, ventricular arrhythmias can be present.

CLINICAL PRESENTATIONS

Clinical presentations vary widely, because they depend on the anatomic severity and can range from a severely symptomatic neonate to an asymptomatic octogenarian.[17]

The most common presentation varies with age at presentation[18]:

- Fetuses: an abnormal routine prenatal scan (86%)
- Neonates: cyanosis (74%)
- Infants: heart failure (43%)
- Children: an incidental murmur (63%)
- Adolescents and adults: arrhythmia (42%), decreased exercise tolerance, fatigue, or right-sided heart failure

Symptoms

Cyanosis and Heart Failure

- Secondary to significant tricuspid regurgitation
- Can appear soon after birth, because of high pulmonary vascular resistance
- Often improves as pulmonary vascular resistance decreases

Exertional Dyspnea, Fatigue, Cyanosis, and Palpitations

- Can occur at a later age
- Can recur and can be insidious in onset

Palpitations

- Secondary to atrial tachyarrhythmia (atrial flutter and fibrillation most common)
- May be present in 20% to 30% of cases
- Some of these arrhythmias are due to WPW syndrome

Paradoxic Embolization

- In the presence of an interatrial communication, patients with Ebstein malformation are at risk for paradoxic embolization, brain abscesses, and sudden death.

Physical Examination

Findings vary with the severity of pathology and the magnitude of right-to-left interatrial shunting.[19]

- Murmur and click; commonly mistaken for mitral valve prolapse
- Cyanosis
  - Can be severe in infants
  - Usually milder in older children
  - Digital clubbing will depend on the degree and duration of cyanosis
- Prominent "a" wave in the distended jugular veins
- Hepatomegaly
  - Represents passive hepatic congestion resulting from tricuspid regurgitation and elevated RA pressure
  - Becomes pulsatile because of systolic expansion of the liver
- Palpable, prominent diffuse apical impulse
- Systolic thrill at the left lower sternal border
- Widely split first and second heart sounds, resulting from right bundle branch block
- Prominent S3 or a loud S4 give the impression of multiple heart sounds (triple or quadruple gallop)
- Systolic murmur
  - Secondary to tricuspid regurgitation
  - Increases in intensity with inspiration and may be associated with a mid-diastolic murmur owing to high diastolic flow volume across the tricuspid annulus
  - Can be extremely soft or absent in adults because the low velocity of to-and-fro flow and rapid equalization of pressure across the TV does not result in blood flow turbulence
- Jugular venous pulse rarely showing a large V wave despite severe regurgitation of the TV because the large RA engulfs the increased volume

DIAGNOSTIC WORK-UP

Chest Radiography

The cardiac silhouette varies from almost normal to a markedly enlarged globe-shaped heart with a narrow waist similar to that seen with pericardial effusion (Fig. 130-4). The vascular pedicle is narrow because the pulmonary trunk is not border forming and the ascending aorta, with rare exception, is often small and inconspicuous or absent. Symptomatic neonates can have massive

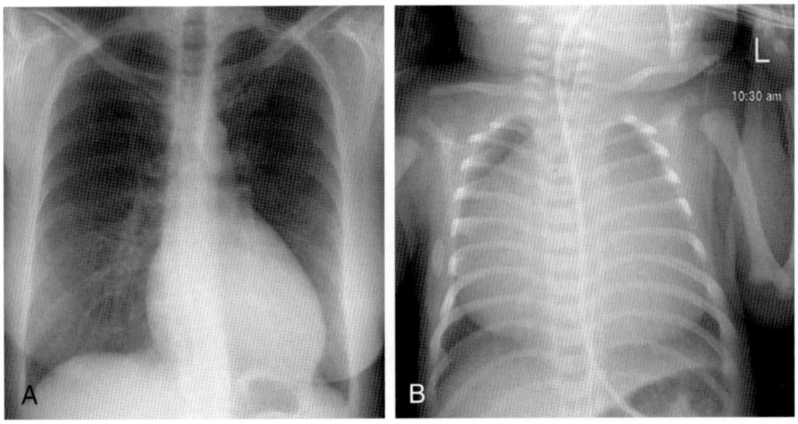

FIGURE 130-4 ■ **A,** Chest radiograph of a patient with Ebstein malformation with severe tricuspid regurgitation and a small atrial septal defect before tricuspid valve surgery. **B,** Cardiomegaly, a narrow waist, and a cardiothoracic ratio of 0.56 in a neonate with Ebstein malformation showing massive cardiomegaly ("wall-to-wall" heart). (From Said SM, Dearani JA: Ebstein anomaly, congenital tricuspid valve regurgitation and dysplasia. In Allen HD, Driscolle DJ, Shaddy RE, Feltes TF, editors: *Moss and Adams' heart disease in infants, children, and adolescents,* ed 8, Philadelphia, 2013, Lippincott Williams & Wilkins, Figures 39-11 and 39-12.)

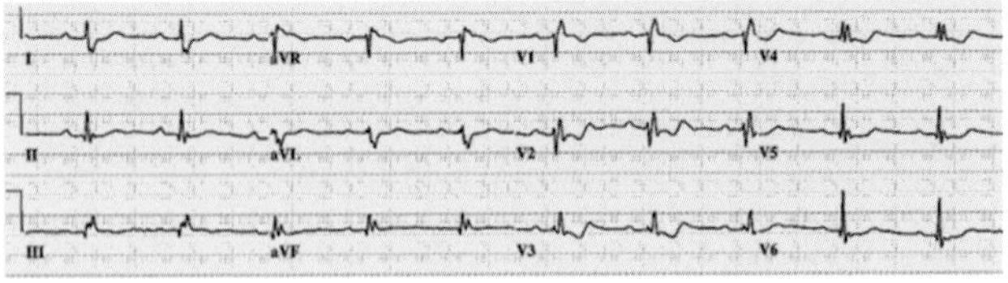

FIGURE 130-5 ■ Electrocardiogram of a patient with severe Ebstein malformation showing the typical changes, with prolongation of the PR interval (226 ms), right bundle-branch block, and somewhat bizarre configuration of the QRS complex. (From Said SM, Dearani JA: Ebstein anomaly, congenital tricuspid valve regurgitation and dysplasia. In Allen HD, Driscolle DJ, Shaddy RE, Feltes TF, editors: *Moss and Adams' heart disease in infants, children, and adolescents,* ed 8, Philadelphia, 2013, Lippincott Williams & Wilkins, Figure 39-13.)

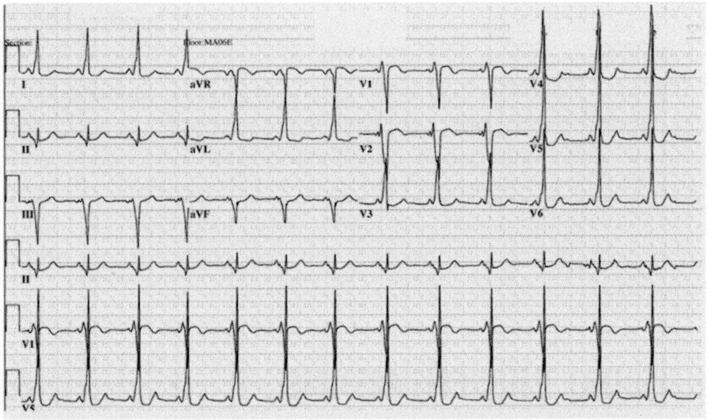

FIGURE 130-6 ■ Electrocardiogram of a patient with severe Ebstein malformation, showing sinus rhythm with preexcitation (Wolf-Parkinson-White syndrome). A delta wave is noted in the ascending limb of the QRS complex. (From Said SM, Dearani JA: Ebstein anomaly, congenital tricuspid valve regurgitation and dysplasia. In Allen HD, Driscolle DJ, Shaddy RE, Feltes TF, editors: *Moss and Adams' heart disease in infants, children, and adolescents,* ed 8, Philadelphia, 2013, Lippincott Williams & Wilkins, Figure 39-14.)

heart size and outcome is poor if the cardiothoracic ratio is greater than 0.65.

The most consistent and dramatic feature is the enlarged RA silhouette; this is seldom normal, even if the cardiac silhouette is otherwise normal. Lung fields may be normal or decreased because of hypoplasia from severe cardiomegaly (often seen in neonates).

Electrocardiography

Ebstein malformation can be diagnosed using the electrocardiogram, which is rarely normal even with a mild malformation (Fig. 130-5).

The major electrophysiologic changes include the following[20]:

- Intra-atrial conduction disturbance including PR interval prolongation and tall P waves
- Right bundle branch block
- WPW preexcitation
- Supraventricular tachycardia
- Atrial flutter or fibrillation
- Arrhythmogenic atrialized RV
- Deep Q waves in leads V1–4 and in inferior leads

Complete heart block is rare, but first-degree heart block occurs in 42% of patients because of RA enlargement and the structural abnormalities of the atrioventricular (AV) conduction system.

The AV node may be compressed but is in the normal location. Apical displacement of the septal leaflet is associated with discontinuity of the central fibrous body and the septal AV ring with direct muscular connections, creating a substrate for accessory pathways and preexcitation (Fig. 130-6).

More than one accessory pathway is present in 6% to 36% of cases; most of them are located around the orifice of the malformed TV. In addition, wide QRS tachycardia over a septal accessory AV pathway, ventricular tachycardia, as well as ectopic atrial tachycardia, atrial flutter, and atrial fibrillation, can occur.

Echocardiography

Two-dimensional echocardiography is the diagnostic test of choice (Fig. 130-7). More recently, three-dimensional echocardiography is also being used as an adjunct for additional details about TV anatomy. It accurately evaluates the TV and the size and function of different cardiac chambers.

Apical displacement of the septal leaflet by at least 8 mm/m^2 body surface area is considered a diagnostic feature of Ebstein malformation. The presence of at least three accessory attachments of the leaflet to the ventricular wall confirms leaflet tethering that causes restricted motion of the leaflet.[21] Marked enlargement of the RA and atrialized RV is present. When the combined area of the RA and atrialized RV is larger than the combined area of the functional RV, left atrium (LA), and LV in the

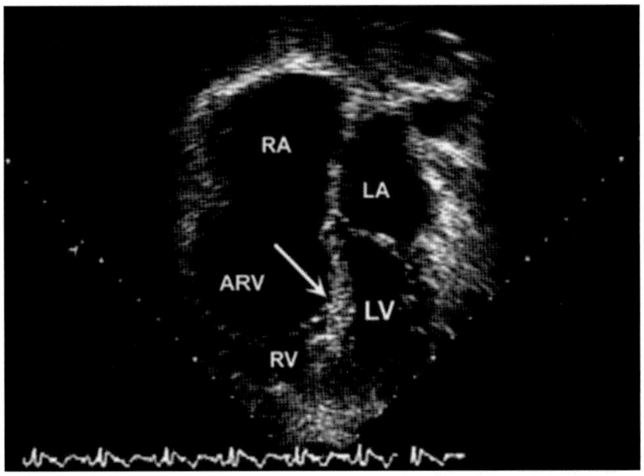

FIGURE 130-7 ■ Example of an echocardiogram (four-chamber view, apex down) of a patient with severe Ebstein malformation showing a grossly displaced septal leaflet *(arrow)*. The anterior leaflet is severely tethered ("failure of delamination") and nearly immobile. The atrialized right ventricle (ARV) is large and the functional right ventricle (RV) is small. *LA,* Left atrium; *LV,* left ventricle; *RA,* right atrium. (From Said SM, Dearani JA: Ebstein anomaly, congenital tricuspid valve regurgitation and dysplasia. In Allen HD, Driscolle DJ, Shaddy RE, Feltes TF, editors: *Moss and Adams' heart disease in infants, children, and adolescents,* ed 8, Philadelphia, 2013, Lippincott Williams & Wilkins, Figure 39-15.)

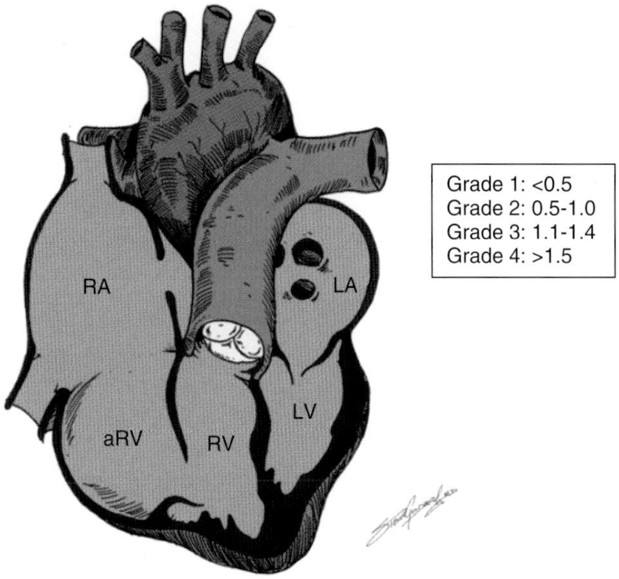

$$\frac{\text{Area of } (RA + aRV)}{\text{Area of } (RV + LV + LA)}$$

FIGURE 130-8 ■ Great Ormond Street echocardiography (GOSE) score. *aRV,* Atrialized RV; *LA,* left atrium; *LV,* left ventricle; *RA,* right atrium; *RV,* right ventricle. (From Knott-Craig CJ, Goldberg SP: Management of neonatal Ebstein's anomaly. *Semin Thorac Cardiovasc Surg Pediatr Card Surg Annu* 112–116, 2007, Figure 1.)

apical four-chamber view at end diastole, the risk of mortality is increased.

Echocardiography allows assessment of the site and degree of TV regurgitation and the feasibility of valve repair. Ebstein malformation can be diagnosed in utero using fetal echocardiography in as early as the eighteenth week of pregnancy.[22] Fetal echocardiography remains a challenge because of the small size of the heart, and it may be difficult to distinguish Ebstein malformation from pulmonary atresia or other causes of TR. Important features that can be determined echocardiographically and that can predict outcome in neonates with Ebstein malformation include the patency of the RV outflow tract and the Great Ormond Street echocardiography (GOSE) score.[23] The GOSE score, as described by Celermajer and colleagues,[23] is calculated in the four-chamber view to create a ratio of the combined areas of the RA and atrialized RV compared with the functional RV, LA, and the LV areas (Fig. 130-8). Patients with the most severe GOSE score (grades 3 and 4) have a poor prognosis (Table 130-2).

Cardiac Catheterization

Cardiac catheterization is rarely necessary, apart from preoperative coronary angiography in older patients. Pulmonary artery pressures are usually normal, although the RV end-diastolic pressure may be elevated. Despite severe TV regurgitation, the RA pressure may be normal, especially with marked RA dilation. Hemodynamic catheterization can also be performed in certain situations when there is LV dysfunction or when there is suspicion of elevated pulmonary artery pressure or elevated LV end-diastolic pressure. This is particularly important if a bidirectional cavopulmonary anastomosis is being considered.

TABLE 130-2 Mortality Risk by GOSE Score

GOSE score*	Ratio	Mortality
1-2	<1.0	8%
3 (acyanotic)	1.1-1.4	10% early, 45% late
3 (cyanotic)	1.1-1.4	100%
4	>1.5	100%

*GOSE 1, <0.5; GOSE 2, 0.5-1.0; GOSE 3, 1.1-1.4; GOSE 4, >1.5.
GOSE, Great Ormond Street echocardiography.

Magnetic Resonance Imaging

Recently, cardiac magnetic resonance imaging has emerged as another tool for evaluation of patients with Ebstein malformation. It provides quantitative measurement of RA and RV size and systolic function, even in the presence of significant distortion of RV anatomy[24] (Fig. 130-9). It also provides additional imaging of TV anatomy.

Axial imaging provides a more reliable analysis of disease severity, such as the atrialized RV volume. The ability to create three-dimensional images may provide greater delineation of disease severity. In general, echocardiographic imaging provides detailed valve anatomy and cardiac magnetic resonance imaging provides detailed ventricular anatomy.

NATURAL HISTORY

The prognosis of Ebstein malformation when diagnosed prenatally is poor. In a study of fetuses with Ebstein

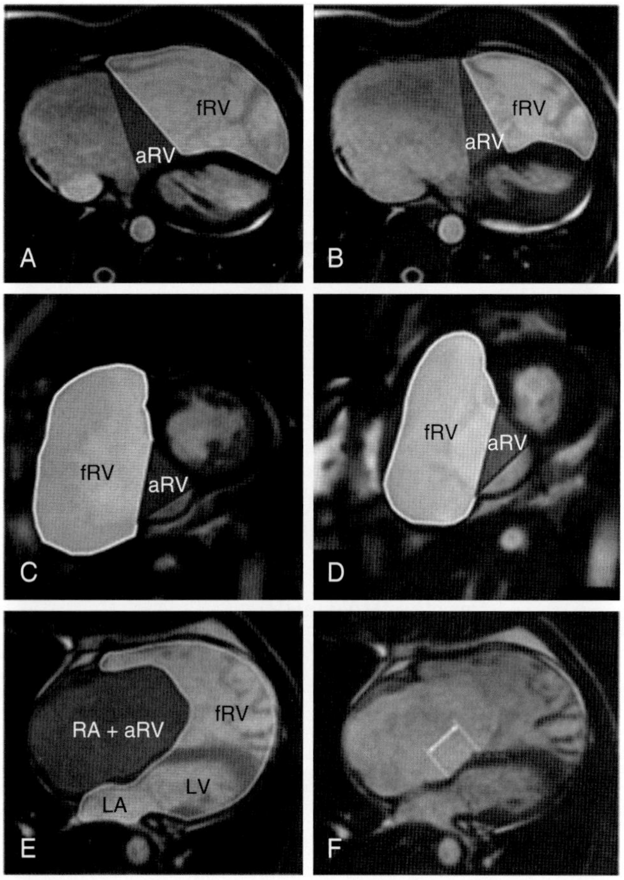

FIGURE 130-9 ■ Cardiac magnetic resonance imaging showing systolic and diastolic contours of functional right ventricle and atrialized portion of the right ventricle in (**A** and **B**) axial and (**C** and **D**) short-axis views. **E,** Severity index representing the ratio of areas of the right atrium and atrialized right ventricle in numerator and summation of functional right ventricle and left atrium and left ventricular areas in denominator (i.e., Severity index = [Right atrial area + Atrialized right ventricular area] / [Functional right ventricular area + Left atrial area + Left ventricular area]). **F,** Degree of apical displacement of septal leaflet of tricuspid valve (in millimeters) measured in ventricular diastole. *aRV,* Atrialized right ventricle; *fRV,* functional right ventricle; *LA,* left atrium; *LV,* left ventricle; *RA,* right atrium. (**A-D** from Yalonetsky S, Tobler D, Greutmann M, et al: Cardiac magnetic resonance imaging and the assessment of Ebstein anomaly in adults. *Am J Cardiol* 107:767–773, 2011, Figure 2.)

malformation or TV dysplasia from Children's Hospital Boston, eight (24% of 33) pregnancies were terminated, nine (27%) fetuses died in utero, and 16 (49%) fetuses survived to birth. Only seven (21% of 33) prenatally diagnosed patients survived beyond the neonatal period.[25] Survival was related to the severity of Ebstein malformation and the presence of RV or LV dysfunction. Elective early delivery may be needed in fetuses that exhibit signs of distress.

It is not uncommon for Ebstein malformation to be undiagnosed until adulthood. The oldest patient in the Mayo surgical series was 79 years old at time of diagnosis and subsequent surgery. However, late diagnosis is also associated with reduced survival. The mean age of diagnosis in a study of the natural history of 72 unoperated patients was 23.9 ± 10.4 years. In this group of patients, arrhythmias were the most common clinical presentation (51%).[26] The estimated cumulative overall survival rates were 89%, 76%, 53%, and 41% at 1, 10, 15, and 20 years of follow-up, respectively. Predictors of cardiac-related death on univariate analysis included (1) cardiothoracic ratio of 0.65 or greater, (2) increasing severity of TV displacement on echocardiography, (3) New York Heart Association (NYHA) class III or IV, (4) cyanosis, (5) severe TR, and (6) younger age at diagnosis. However, in a multivariate model, younger age at diagnosis, male sex, cardiothoracic ratio of 0.65 or greater, and the severity of TV leaflet displacement on echocardiography were predictors of late cardiac mortality.

MANAGEMENT

Neonates and Infants

Indications for Operation

In neonates or infants who remain in congestive heart failure or are profoundly cyanotic, operative therapy is required. In the newborn period, three pathways can be considered: the biventricular repair (Knott-Craig approach),[27] single-ventricle repair (i.e., RV exclusion technique, or Starnes approach), and cardiac transplantation.

Biventricular Repair (Knott-Craig Approach). In this approach, the TV is repaired and the ASD is partially closed. This is a monocusp type of valve repair based on a satisfactory anterior leaflet.[28] The subtotal closure of the ASD allows right-to-left shunting, which may be necessary in the early postoperative period when there is a high risk of RV dysfunction or elevated pulmonary vascular resistance. RA reduction is performed routinely and is important to reduce the size of the markedly enlarged heart to allow room for the lungs (Fig. 130-10).

The postoperative care of a newborn after a biventricular repair can be challenging. Delayed sternal closure is used liberally. Tolerance of early low peripheral oxygenation is common, and inhaled nitric oxide may be necessary to decrease pulmonary vascular resistance. Prophylactic use of a peritoneal dialysis catheter can also be used to ensure complete decompression of the abdomen.

Although early mortality for this operation is high (25%-30%), the intermediate outcome with the biventricular approach appears to be promising. In 2007, Knott-Craig and colleagues[29] published their experience with 27 neonates and young infants. These patients had concomitant anatomic or functional pulmonary atresia (n = 18), ventricular septal defect (n = 3), small LV (n = 3), and hypoplastic branch pulmonary arteries (n = 3). Twenty-five patients received a biventricular repair, with TV repair in twenty-three and valve replacement in two. Survival to hospital dismissal was 74%; risk was greater when there was anatomic pulmonary atresia. There were no late deaths (median follow-up, 5.4 years; maximum, 12 years). All patients were in functional NYHA class I. Although these early results for repair of Ebstein malformation during the neonatal period are poor compared with many other neonatal anomalies corrected in the first

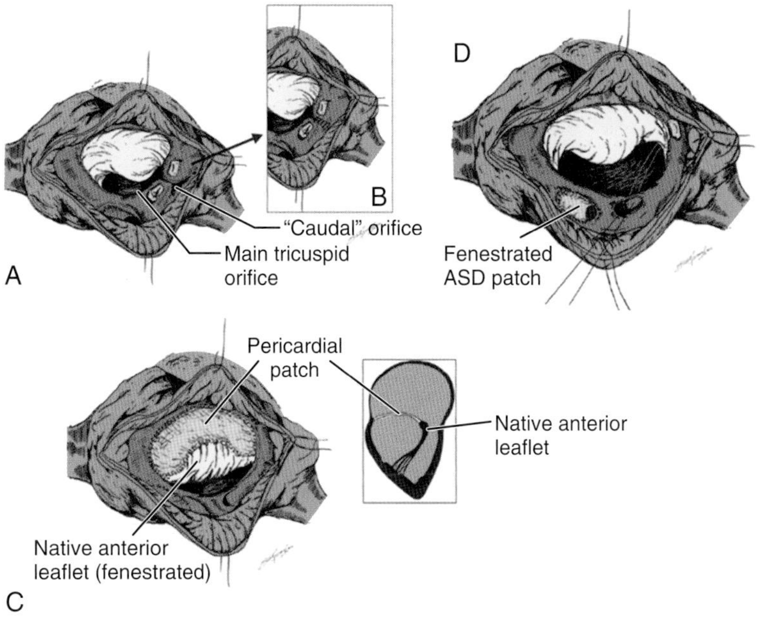

FIGURE 130-10 Biventricular repair of neonatal Ebstein (Knott-Craig). **A,** Partition of the tricuspid valve orifice into two openings by approximation of the annuloplasty stitch. **B,** Once the valve is judged to be competent, the "caudal" orifice is closed, thereby plicating the atrialized portion of the right ventricle. **C,** Creation of a competent monocuspid valve by taking down the anterior leaflet from the annulus, fenestrating it, and augmenting it with a pericardial patch. **D,** The atrial septal defect (ASD) is closed with a fenestrated patch, and an annuloplasty stitch is placed with one pledgeted end in the coronary sinus and the other pledgeted end at the location of the commissure between anterior and posterior leaflets. (From Knott-Craig CJ, Goldberg SP: Management of neonatal Ebstein's anomaly. *Semin Thorac Cardiovasc Surg Pediatr Card Surg Annu* 112–116, 2007, Figures 4, 5, and 6.)

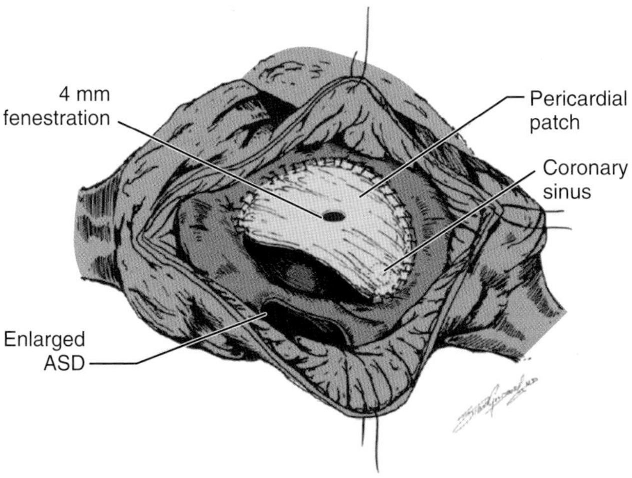

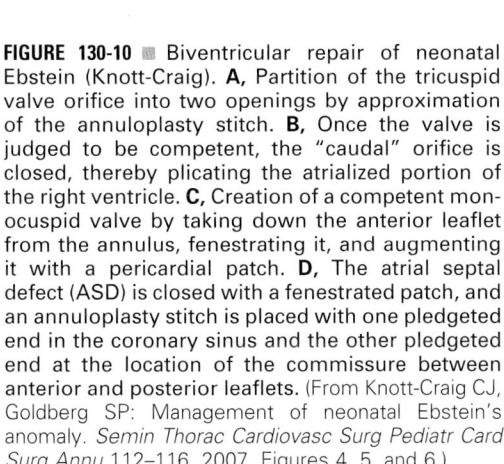

FIGURE 130-11 Starnes repair of neonatal Ebstein malformation. *ASD,* Atrial septal defect. (From Knott-Craig CJ, Goldberg SP: Management of neonatal Ebstein's anomaly. *Semin Thorac Cardiovasc Surg Pediatr Card Surg Annu* 112–116, 2007, Figure 2.)

month of life (e.g., arterial switch procedure, Norwood stage I), they have become a benchmark for this difficult patient population.

Right Ventricular Exclusion (Starnes Approach). Alternatively, the RV exclusion approach, pioneered by Starnes and colleagues,[30] involves fenestrated patch closure of the TV orifice, enlarging the interatrial connection, and placing a systemic-to-pulmonary artery shunt (Fig. 130-11). This approach is particularly appealing in patients who also have anatomic pulmonary atresia or other important RV outflow tract obstruction. A small fenestration (using a 4- to 5-mm punch) is placed in the TV patch to allow RV decompression as it passively fills with blood from the thebesian veins.[31] This also allows progressive involution of the enlarged dysfunctional RV, which is helpful in the long term when preparing for the eventual Fontan procedure.[32] In patients who have a patent RV outflow tract, a competent pulmonary valve is required to prevent blood from entering the RV, resulting in RV distention. If patients have an incompetent pulmonary valve, the main pulmonary artery should be ligated or the incompetent pulmonary valve should be closed. These issues must be considered because significant dilation of a poorly functioning RV eventually results in compression and impairment of LV function. Similar to the biventricular approach, RA reduction is routinely performed to allow space for the lungs.

Modified Starnes Approach (Total Ventricular Exclusion). A modification to the Starnes single-ventricle approach, total RV exclusion, has been advocated by Sano and associates,[33] in which the free wall of the RV is resected and closed primarily or with a polytetrafluoroethylene patch. This procedure acts like a large RV plication and RV volume reduction procedure (Fig. 130-12). This adaptation of the Starnes method may improve LV filling and provide additional space for the lungs and decompression of the LV.

Postoperative care is similar to that of any shunt-palliated patient with a univentricular heart. Optimizing systemic perfusion and obtaining adequate oxygenation is the primary goal. Delayed sternal closure and peritoneal drainage are also beneficial. As with other patients with a shunt-dependent pulmonary circulation, careful surveillance is required between the first operation and the second-stage procedure (bidirectional cavopulmonary shunt), which is usually performed at 3 to 6 months of age.

Results of the single-ventricle pathway have been reported by Reemtsen and colleagues.[34] Of 16 neonates, two patients had TV repair, one patient had heart transplant, 10 patients had a RV exclusion procedure with a fenestrated TV patch, and three patients had a RV exclusion procedure with a nonfenestrated TV patch. The

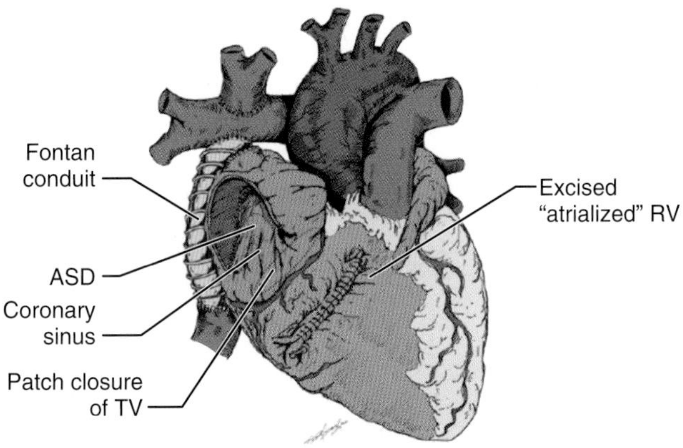

FIGURE 130-12 ■ Sano "RV exclusion" procedure. *ASD,* Atrial septal defect; *RV,* right ventricle; *TV,* tricuspid valve. (From Knott-Craig CJ, Goldberg SP: Management of neonatal Ebstein's anomaly. *Semin Thorac Cardiovasc Surg Pediatr Card Surg Annu* 112–116, 2007, Figure 3.)

operative survival was 80% (8 of 10) in patients with a fenestration, and 33% in patients with no fenestration, leading the authors to recommend fenestration of the TV patch. Among the nine hospital survivors of RV exclusion, three underwent completion of the Fontan, and all nine have had a successful bidirectional cavopulmonary shunt (second stage).

Heart Transplantation. Heart transplantation remains an option in the most severe cases of Ebstein malformation, but it is rarely necessary in the current era because of the improved results with the Knott-Craig and Starnes approaches. Limitations of heart transplantation include the scarcity of donor organs in the neonatal age group and the side effects of long-term immunosuppression and its associated complications in the transplant recipient. Finally, the development of smaller ventricular assist devices and advances in extracorporeal membrane oxygenation has provided mechanical support options in the perioperative period for these infants.

Children and Adults

Indications for Operation

Although medical management, including diuretics and antiarrhythmic drugs, can be used to manage some of the symptoms of heart failure and arrhythmias, eventually most patients require operation. Observation alone is usually advised for asymptomatic patients with no right-to-left shunting, mild cardiomegaly, and normal exercise tolerance. Most patients in NYHA class I or II can be managed medically. Operation is offered when symptoms are present (fatigue most common), increasing cyanosis becomes evident, or if paradoxical embolism occurs. Operation is also advised if there is objective evidence of deterioration, such as decreasing exercise performance by exercise testing, progressive increase in heart size on chest radiography, progressive RV dilation or reduction of systolic RV function by echocardiography, or appearance of atrial or ventricular arrhythmias. In borderline situations, the echocardiographic determination of high probability of TV repair makes the decision to proceed with operation easier. In our practice, we advise operation between 2 and 5 years of age because of our ability to successfully perform an anatomic (cone-type) repair in 95% to 98% of children. Once symptoms develop and patients progress to NYHA class III or IV, medical management has little to offer; operation then becomes the only chance for improvement.

A biventricular repair is possible for the vast majority of patients. In some circumstances, a 1.5-ventricle repair (adding a bidirectional cavopulmonary shunt) is advantageous when there is significant RV dilation or dysfunction, or if the resultant TV repair has a small effective orifice (uncommon). The bidirectional cavopulmonary shunt can also reduce hemodynamic stress on a more complex TV repair, because the volume of the RV is decreased by 35% to 45%, depending on the patient's age. Cardiac transplantation is rarely indicated and is reserved for patients with severe biventricular dysfunction.

Operative Management

Our operative management of patients with Ebstein malformation consists of (1) closure of any atrial septal communications (except during infancy); (2) correction of associated anomalies (e.g., closure of ventricular septal defect); (3) performance of any indicated antiarrhythmia procedures, such as the maze procedure (cryoablation or radiofrequency ablation), surgical division of accessory conduction pathways, or cryoablation of AVNRT; (4) internal plication (apex to base) of the atrialized portion of the RV; (5) repair of the TV; and (6) right reduction atrioplasty. In the current era, intraoperative electrophysiologic mapping for localization of accessory conduction pathways in patients with ventricular preexcitation is rarely required. When preexcitation is present, preoperative mapping and ablation is performed in the catheterization laboratory. Intraoperative transesophageal echocardiography is used routinely.

Anatomic Cone Repair. Anatomic variability of EM continues to be a challenge for the surgeon since the earliest repair techniques in 1958.[35,36] Most repair techniques address the abnormal TV in a manner that focuses on the concept of monocusp repair.[37] Monocusp repair depends on an adequate anterior leaflet with a freely mobile leading edge that allows coaptation with the ventricular septum. Significant degrees of RV or annular dilation or significant tethering of the anterior leaflet can preclude a successful monocusp repair.

The early Mayo Clinic experience focused on the Danielson monocusp repair, and the use of the Sebening stitch (suture attachment of the anterior papillary muscle to the ventricular septum) was common. The French experience (Carpentier)[38] focused on mobilization (surgical delamination) of the anterior leaflet with annular reattachment, resulting in an anterior leaflet monocusp repair. The Brazilian experience (da Silva) was an extension of the French technique. The difference was surgical delamination of all available leaflet tissue, with approximated circumferential leaflets anchored at the true annulus resulting in a "cone" of leaflet tissue. The

Brazilian experience with cone repair in 52 patients has been reported.[39,40] Mean age was 18.5 ± 13.8 years, and mean follow-up was 57 ± 45 months. There were two early deaths (3.8%) and two late deaths. The Brazilian group also reported an increase in the indexed RV functional area in the early preoperative period; however, that remained unchanged at intermediate follow-up. The reduction of TR was maintained at intermediate follow-up.

Operation for EM is performed through sternotomy using cardiopulmonary bypass, aortic and bicaval cannulation with cross-clamping, and cold blood cardioplegia. The principle of cone repair (CR) is complete surgical delamination and recruitment of all undelaminated leaflet tissue, which is reanchored at the true right AV junction, creating a 360-degree "leaflet cone." Leaflet-to-leaflet approximation is generally done with interrupted monofilament sutures to avoid a pursestring effect that can decrease the height of the reconstructed leaflet (Fig. 130-13). The atrialized, inferior RV (i.e., smooth and not trabeculated) is plicated internally from "apex to annulus." The plication typically crosses the true annulus to partially reduce the size of the dilated annulus (Fig. 130-14). Care is taken to avoid distortion or

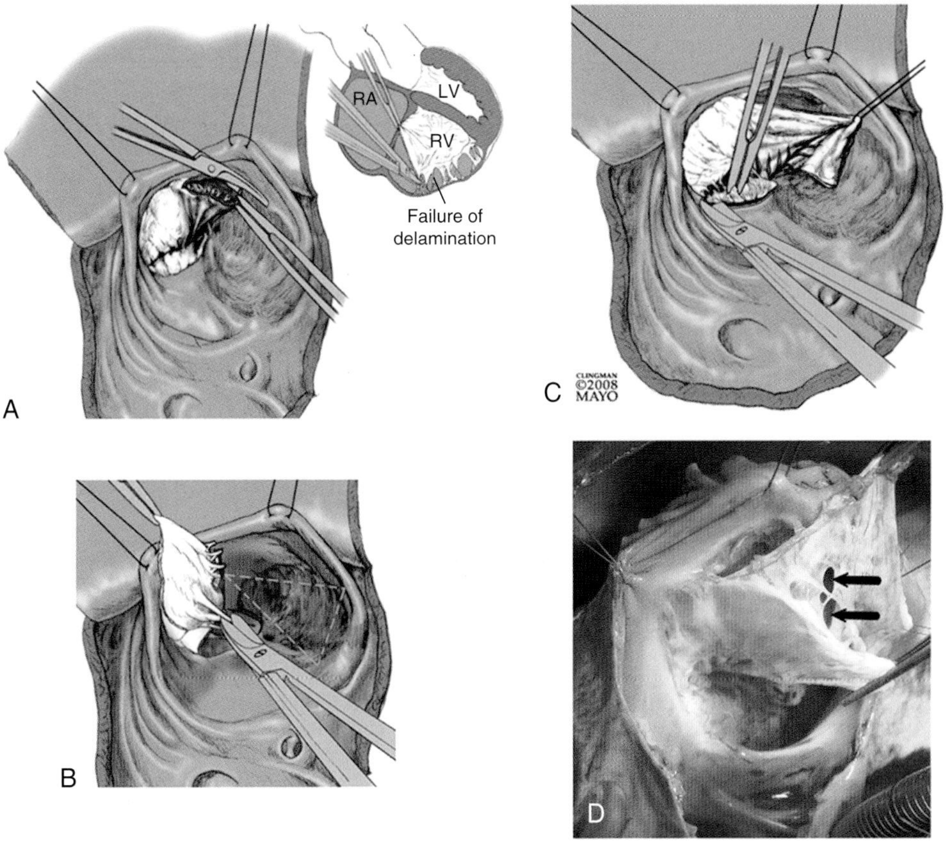

FIGURE 130-13 ■ Operative steps for the da Silva technique for Ebstein anomaly repair. **A,** The first incision is made with a no. 15 blade in the anterior leaflet at the twelve-o'clock position; the incision is a few millimeters away from the true annulus. The incision is then extended rightward in a clockwise fashion using a scissors. It is common for there to be a true space between the anterior leaflet and the right ventricle in this region (i.e., normally delaminated leaflet). However, when the transition is met between the anterior and inferior (posterior) leaflets, it is common for there to be failure of delamination *(inset)* resulting in fibrous and muscular attachments between the leaflet and myocardium. The diagram demonstrates the scissors approaching the area where there is some adherence of leaflet tissue to the underlying myocardium. Dissection continues such that a portion of distal anterior leaflet and some inferior leaflet tissue is surgically delaminated. The most important aspect of this surgical delamination is to incise all fibrous and muscular attachments between the body of the leaflet and the right ventricular myocardium, but to maintain intact all fibrous (and occasionally muscular) attachments of the leading edge of the leaflet to the underlying myocardium. Importantly, do not disrupt chordal attachments to the leading edge of any leaflet. **B,** As the anterior and surgically delaminated inferior leaflet is reflected away from the right ventricular myocardium, all fibrous and muscular attachments into the body of the underside of the leaflet are incised as shown with the scissors. It is important to keep all attachments of the leading edge of the leaflet intact. If the edge is linearly attached, then surgical fenestrations are created as depicted earlier. The *dotted triangle* represents the atrialized right ventricle. **C,** Dissection is continued with a scissors, with the goal of taking down all attachments between the septal leaflet and myocardium but preserving all attachments of the leading edge to the endocardium as described above. The dissection should proceed medially to the anteroseptal commissure. The leaflet tissue is typically fragile and thin in this area. There can be marked variability in the status of the leading edge of the septal leaflet, as was described for the anterior and inferior leaflets. If there is a linear attachment, then surgically created fenestrations are also made in this leaflet (not shown). **D,** The mobilized anterior and inferior (posterior) leaflets. Natural fenestrations are shown at the junction of the anterior and inferior leaflets *(arrows)*. *LV,* Left ventricle; *RA,* right atrium; *RV,* right ventricle. (From Said SM, Dearani JA: Ebstein anomaly, congenital tricuspid valve regurgitation and dysplasia. In Allen HD, Driscolle DJ, Shaddy RE, Feltes TF, editors: *Moss and Adams' heart disease in infants, children, and adolescents,* ed 8, Philadelphia, 2013, Lippincott Williams & Wilkins, Figure 39-22AD.)

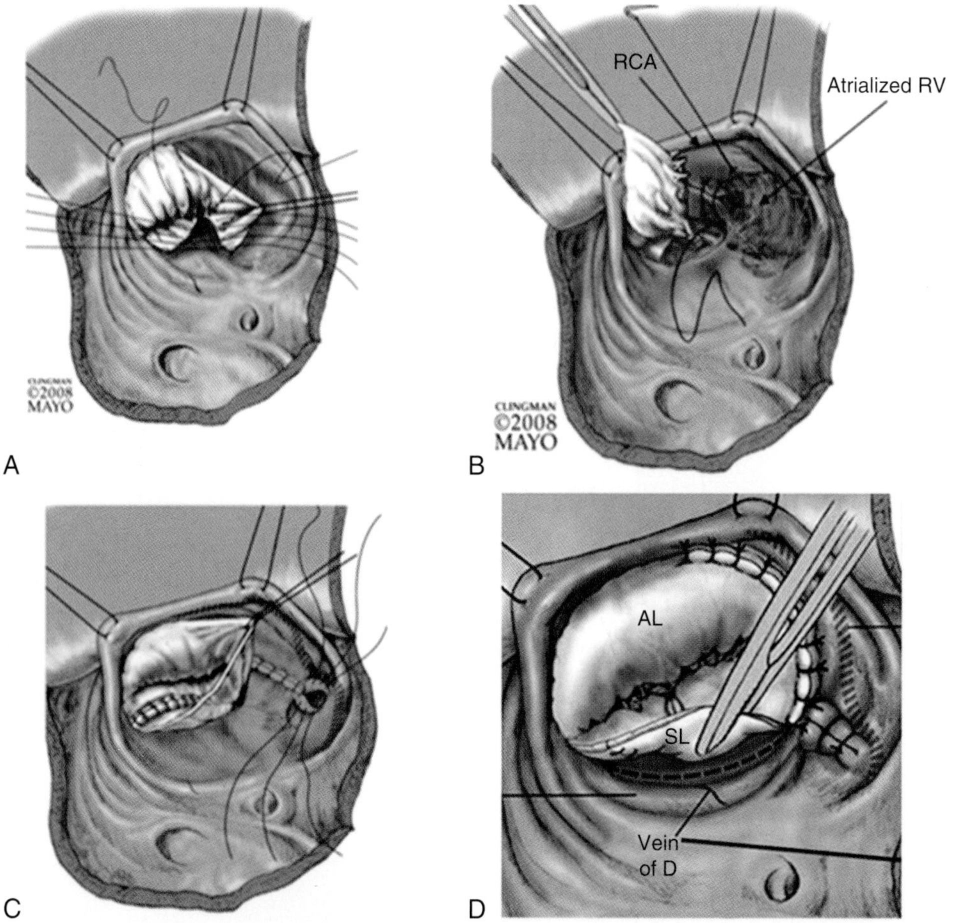

FIGURE 130-14 ■ **A,** After the anterior, inferior, and septal leaflets are completely mobilized, the cut edge of the inferior leaflet is rotated clockwise to meet the proximal edge that has been prepared on the mobilized septal leaflet. The two leaflets are approximated with interrupted fine monofilament sutures completing the cone reconstruction. This results in 360 degrees of leaflet tissue that will compose the new tricuspid valve orifice. **B,** After the cone reconstruction is completed, the atrialized right ventricle (RV) is examined to determine whether plication is necessary. Note the position of the right coronary artery (RCA) in the true tricuspid valve annulus and that the main RCA or the posterior descending coronary artery can be compromised. This figure demonstrates the technique for internal plication of the atrialized right ventricle from apex to base. Monofilament suture is used; the suture is begun distally toward the apex of the right ventricle. It is important to conduct frequent examinations of the outside of the inferior wall of the right ventricle to ensure that inadvertent compromise of the right coronary artery is avoided. **C,** The suture line is advanced toward the base of the heart (i.e., toward the atrioventricular groove). As the dotted lines of the triangle are effectively approximated, the atrialized RV is excluded. The suture line sometimes crosses the atrioventricular groove to reduce the size of the dilated annulus. After the sides of the triangle are approximated, the entrance into the excluded atrialized segment of the right ventricle is then closed to eliminate the "blind pouch." **D,** After the plication is completed, the newly constructed tricuspid valve is then reattached at the level of the true tricuspid annulus. Because the neotricuspid valve will have an orifice that is smaller than the original dilated atrioventricular junction, a plication of the inferior annulus is usually necessary to meet the size of the smaller neotricuspid valve. Reattachment of the septal leaflet should be done to the ventricular septum and to the ventricular side of the conduction tissue, which is usually marked by a small vein (Vein of D). *AL,* Anterior leaflet; *SL,* septal leaflet. (**A, C,** and **D** from Said SM, Dearani JA: Ebstein anomaly, congenital tricuspid valve regurgitation and dysplasia. In Allen HD, Driscolle DJ, Shaddy RE, Feltes TF, editors: *Moss and Adams' heart disease in infants, children, and adolescents,* ed 8, Philadelphia, 2013, Lippincott Williams & Wilkins, Figure 39-22. **B** from Dearani JA, Said SM, O'Leary PW, et al: Anatomic repair of Ebstein's malformation: lessons learned with cone reconstruction. *Ann Thorac Surg* 95:220–226, discussion 226–228, 2013, Figure 3A.)

compromise of the right coronary artery that is located in the AV groove. Additional inferior annular plication is done as needed to reduce annular size to match the size of the neo-tricuspid valve (neoTV; Fig. 130-15*A*); this area also requires reinforcement with pledgeted mattress sutures. When there is a marked size discrepancy between the neoTV and true annulus, annular plication is performed at multiple sites around the anterior and inferior annuli to avoid an exaggerated plication in one location that could compromise the right coronary artery (see Fig. 130-15*B*). Reattachment of the neoTV to the true annulus is done with interrupted or continuous suture; continuous suture does pursestring the annulus, causing further reduction in annular size, which may be desired when significant annular reduction is needed.

A flexible annuloplasty band—anteroseptal commissure clockwise to inferoseptal commissure with anchoring in the coronary sinus—is used to stabilize the repair as the tricuspid annulus is usually dilated (Fig. 130-16*A*). The normal adult TV annular size is 20 to 24 mm; the adult ring size is most often a 26- or 28-mm ring. The use of a 26- or 28-mm ring is usually possible in many

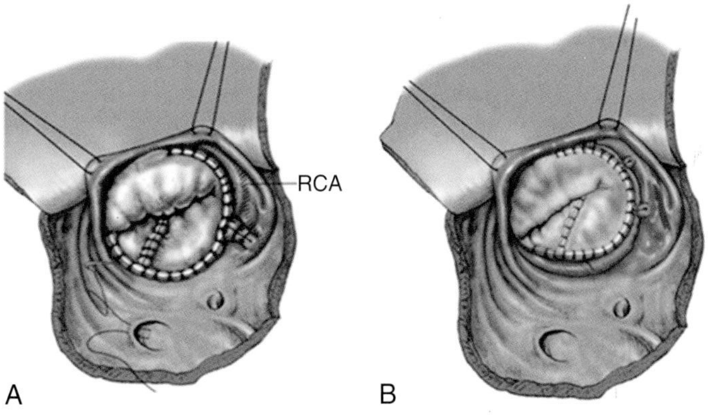

FIGURE 130-15 ■ Technique of tricuspid annular plication. This can be performed in a single inferior (A) or multiple (B) anterior and inferior sites of the annulus. Multiple plication sites help to avoid an exaggerated plication in one location that could compromise the right coronary artery (RCA). (From Dearani JA, Said SM, O'Leary PW, et al: Anatomic repair of Ebstein's malformation: lessons learned with cone reconstruction. *Ann Thorac Surg* 95:220–226, discussion 226–228, 2013, Figure 1AB.)

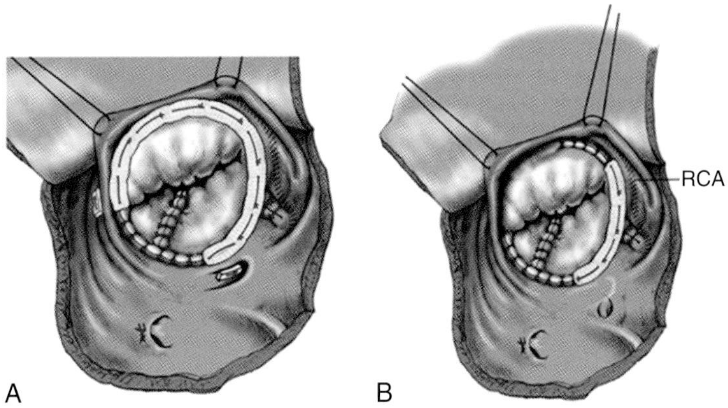

FIGURE 130-16 ■ A, The tricuspid annulus is usually dilated, and a flexible annuloplasty ring is typically used when somatic growth is complete. B, In younger patients when somatic growth is not complete, an eccentric ring confined to the inferior annulus (anteroinferior to inferoseptal commissures) can be used. *RCA,* Right coronary artery. (From Dearani JA, Said SM, O'Leary PW, et al: Anatomic repair of Ebstein's malformation: lessons learned with cone reconstruction. *Ann Thorac Surg* 95:220–226, discussion 226–228, 2013, Figure 2AB.)

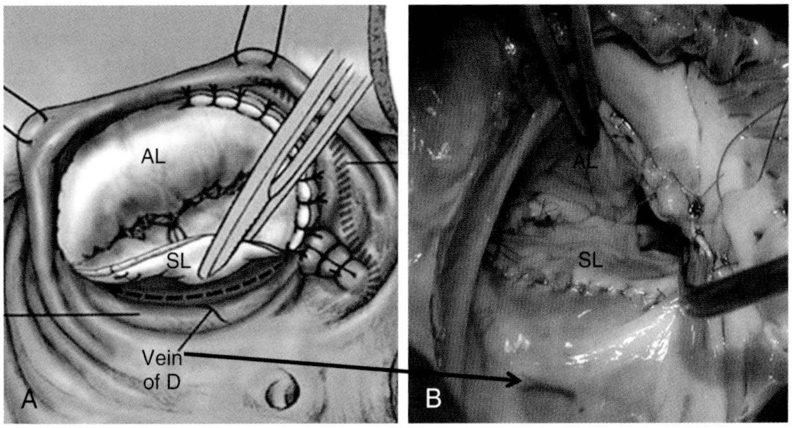

FIGURE 130-17 ■ A, Reattachment of the septal leaflet (SL) should be done to the ventricular side of the conduction tissue *(dotted line arrow),* which is usually marked by a small vein (Vein of D). B, Intraoperative photograph showing the reattachment of the completely mobilized tricuspid valve leaflets. *AL,* Anterior leaflet. (From Dearani JA, Said SM, O'Leary PW, et al: Anatomic repair of Ebstein's malformation: lessons learned with cone reconstruction. *Ann Thorac Surg* 95:220–226, discussion 226–228, 2013, Figure 3AB.)

younger patients (≈6 years old) because the starting size of the annulus is often much larger. When somatic growth is a concern, eccentric partial ring support from anteroinferior to inferoseptal commissure (down to coronary sinus) is used, because this is the area most vulnerable to annular dilation (see Fig. 130-16*B*). The septal leaflet reattachment is performed to the ventricular side of the conduction tissue. All suture lines are done twice for reinforcement. The reanchoring of the neoTV of circumferential leaflet tissue surrounding the tricuspid orifice with its hinge point at the AV groove mimics normal TV anatomy—namely, an anatomic repair (Fig. 130-17).

Adjuncts to Cone Repair. In addition to ring placement, other modifications that we applied selectively to CR to optimize a successful repair include:

1. Leaflet augmentation with Cor Matrix membrane (Cor Matrix Cardiovascular, Santa Cruz, CA) or autologous pericardium to increase leaflet height (Fig. 130-18)
2. Cone augmentation with a small triangular patch to avoid tricuspid stenosis (Fig. 130-19)
3. Leaflet plication to increase leaflet height
4. Surgical fenestrations to create autologous neochordae when a linear attachment is present (Fig. 130-20)

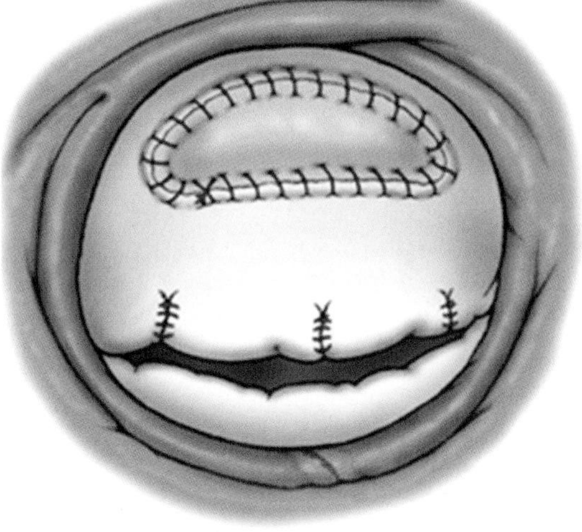

FIGURE 130-18 ■ **Tricuspid valve anterior leaflet augmentation can be performed using Cor Matrix membrane or autologous pericardium to increase the leaflet height and to improve surface area coaptation. Several small plications along the annular free edge of the leaflet can also be performed to increase the leaflet height.** (From Dearani JA, Said SM, O'Leary PW, et al: Anatomic repair of Ebstein's malformation: lessons learned with cone reconstruction. *Ann Thorac Surg* 95:220–226, discussion 226–228, 2013, Figure 4.)

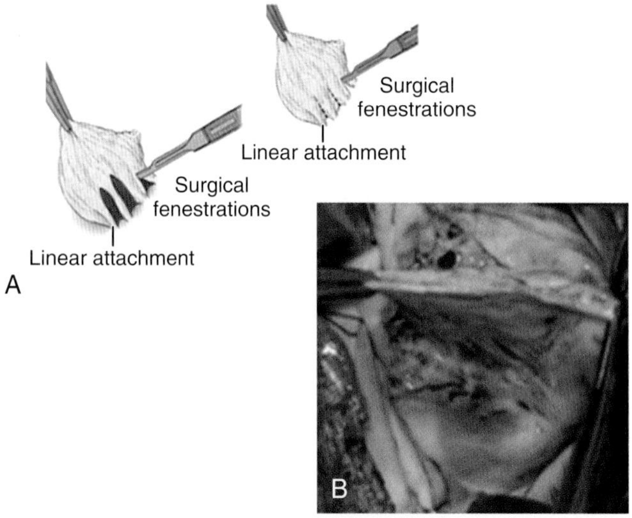

FIGURE 130-20 ■ **A and B, In the presence of a linear attachment where the leading edge is completely adherent, surgical neochordae are created by making several fenestrations apically in the distal portion of the leaflet to allow unrestricted forward blood flow into the ventricle.** (From Dearani JA, Said SM, O'Leary PW, et al: Anatomic repair of Ebstein's malformation: lessons learned with cone reconstruction. *Ann Thorac Surg* 95:220–226, discussion 226–228, 2013, Figure 6AB.)

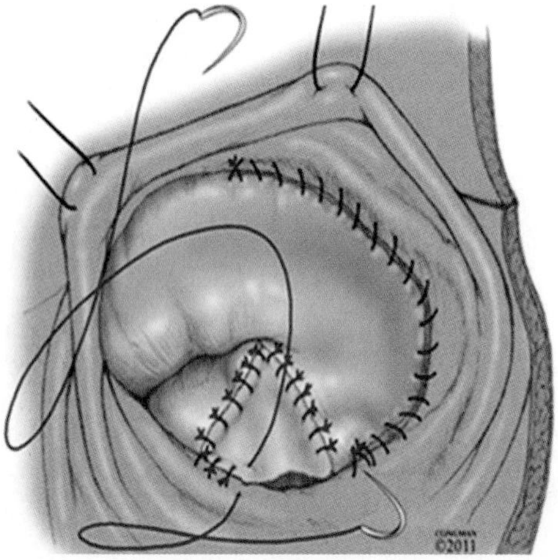

FIGURE 130-19 ■ **A triangular patch is used to augment the reconstructed cone to avoid tricuspid valve stenosis when there is a paucity of septal leaflet tissue and absent inferior leaflet.** (From Dearani JA, Said SM, O'Leary PW, et al: Anatomic repair of Ebstein's malformation: lessons learned with cone reconstruction. *Ann Thorac Surg* 95:220–226, discussion 226–228, 2013, Figure 5.)

5. The Sebening stitch, which involves approximation of the mobilized "base-intact" anterior papillary muscle to the ventricular septum (Fig. 130-21*B*)
6. Modified Sebening stitch that involves approximation of the head of the mobilized "base-intact" RV free wall papillary muscle to a corresponding head of a papillary muscle arising from the ventricular septum supporting the septal leaflet (as opposed to anterior papillary muscle approximation to the ventricular septum; see Fig. 130-21*A*)
7. Artificial Gore-Tex (WL Gore, Flagstaff, AZ) chordae

Leaflet augmentation is applied when the height of the anterior leaflet is shallow or when the rotated cone will result in a smaller than normal orifice. Importantly, when leaflet augmentation is used, the patch is placed between the mid leaflet and annulus and should never involve the leading edge. Importantly, the patch is kept as small as possible.

Relative contraindications to the cone reconstruction include older age (>60 years), moderate pulmonary hypertension, significant LV dysfunction (ejection fraction < 30%), absent septal leaflet, poor delamination or poor quality of the anterior leaflet (i.e., <50% delamination of the anterior leaflet), and severe muscularization of the anterior leaflet not amenable to sufficient debulking to obtain a pliable leaflet. Severe RV enlargement and severe dilation of the right AV junction (true tricuspid annulus) can also make successful CR challenging because there is significant stress on the many suture lines necessary to perform the CR.

In 2007, Dr. da Silva published his series of 40 patients who underwent the cone reconstruction.[39] In this series, the operative mortality was one patient (2.5%). After a mean follow-up of 4 years (range, 3 months to 12 years), only one patient died and two patients required late TV re-repair. The cone technique has the potential to cause TV stenosis, particularly when there is a paucity of leaflet tissue, although no patients in this initial cohort experienced this complication. Additional follow-up is required to determine whether this method of repair has long-term durability.

Tricuspid Valve Re-Repair. Although challenging, TV re-repair is still possible in Ebstein malformation. We have reported our experience with TV re-repair for Ebstein malformation previously.[41] This has been

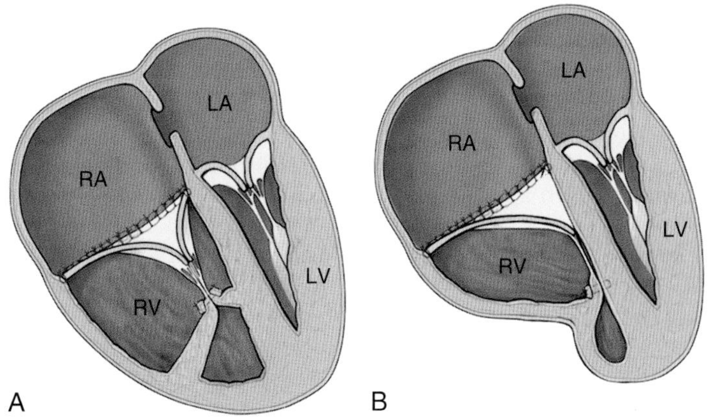

FIGURE 130-21 ■ **A,** The modified Sebening stitch in which the head of the mobilized right ventricular free wall papillary muscle is approximated to the corresponding smaller head of a septal papillary muscle (as opposed to approximation to the ventricular septum in the original Sebening stitch). **B,** It is important to avoid dimpling of the right ventricular free wall, as this indicates excessive tension. *LA,* Left atrium; *LV,* left ventricle; *RA,* right atrium; *RV,* right ventricle. (From Dearani JA, Said SM, Burkhart HM, et al: Strategies for tricuspid re-repair in Ebstein malformation using the cone technique. *Ann Thorac Surg* 96:202–208, discussion 208–210, 2013, Figure 5AB.)

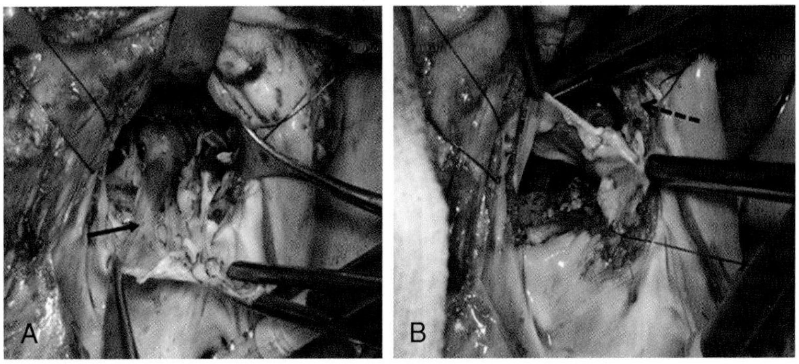

FIGURE 130-22 ■ A surgeon's view into the right atrium; the patient's head is to the left. **A,** The anterior leaflet has been detached from the annulus. There is a linear attachment of the leading edge of the anterior leaflet with a direct papillary muscle insertion *(black arrow).* **B,** The anterior leaflet was mobilized and is being prepared to be reattached to the anterior annulus. The *dotted line arrow* identifies the previous ring, which was the only repair maneuver at the initial operation. (From Dearani JA, Said SM, Burkhart HM, et al: Strategies for tricuspid re-repair in Ebstein malformation using the cone technique. *Ann Thorac Surg* 96:202–208, discussion 208–210, 2013, Figure 1AB.)

performed in 32 patients to date; our previous report of 20 patients demonstrated a median age of 15 years (range, 4 to 68 years). Four patients (20%) had prior bidirectional cavopulmonary anastomosis. Preoperative heart failure was present in eight patients (40%). Recurrent tricuspid regurgitation was due to incomplete leaflet coaptation with tethered anterior leaflet in all patients; and 10 patients (50%) had diminutive septal leaflet. This was possible because prior repair techniques focused on annuloplasty maneuvers in all patients with no or incomplete surgical delamination of leaflet tissue (Fig. 130-22). Re-repair strategies followed the previously mentioned cone reconstruction principles with complete 360 degree mobilization and recruitment of all available leaflet tissues.

There have been no early or late deaths in this group. Mean follow-up was 7.7 ± 10.7 months; during follow-up, 18 patients had no or mild TR and 2 patients had moderate TR.

Tricuspid Valve Replacement. Tricuspid valve replacement remains a reasonable option in those patients who cannot undergo valve repair. In our experience, the most common reason for the inability to obtain a satisfactory CR is significant muscularization of the anterior leaflet not amenable to debulking or resection, or absent septal leaflet; this is determined intraoperatively. Other indications to consider valve replacement include relative older age (>60 years) or massive RV or annular dilation; this is also ultimately determined intraoperatively. We have previously reported good durability with porcine bioprostheses in patients with EM. However, our preference is always to repair the TV whenever possible, and with our larger experience we have learned that it is feasible for almost all patients.

Bioprosthetic (porcine) valve replacement, as opposed to mechanical valve replacement, is generally preferred because of relative good durability of the porcine bioprosthesis in the tricuspid position and the lack of need for warfarin anticoagulation.[42] Bioprosthetic valves do not have the thromboembolic complications of mechanical valves, but they require warfarin anticoagulation for the first 3 to 6 months postoperatively. Mechanical valves in the tricuspid position are sometimes associated with a higher frequency of valve malfunction and thrombotic complications compared with mechanical valves in other cardiac positions, particularly when RV function is poor[43] and discs do not open and close properly.

When the TV cannot be reconstructed and replacement is necessary, the suture line is deviated to the atrial side of the AV node and membranous septum to avoid injury to the conduction mechanism. A small vein crossing the tricuspid annulus adjacent to the membranous septum typically marks the AV node. To avoid injury to the right coronary artery, the anterior suture line is deviated toward the atrial side of the TV annulus anteriorly (where the smooth and trabeculated portions of the RA meet each other) and posterolaterally where the tissues are frequently thin. The coronary sinus can be left to drain into the RA if there is sufficient room between it and the AV node; if the distance is short, the coronary sinus can be left to drain into the RV so that heart block can be avoided. The struts of the porcine bioprosthesis are oriented so that they straddle the area of the membranous septum and conduction tissue. The valve sutures are tied with the heart beating (after intracardiac communications are closed) to detect any disturbances in AV conduction. Tricuspid replacement also has the advantage of a short cross-clamp time (after ASD closure), which may be preferred when mild or moderate LV dysfunction is present or when there is surgeon inexperience or low confidence with a difficult tricuspid repair that might result in a prolonged cardiac ischemic time.

The 1.5-Ventricle Repair. We use the bidirectional cavopulmonary shunt selectively; it is applied in approximately 20% of patients undergoing operation. The bidirectional cavopulmonary shunt is helpful when the RV is severely dilated and functioning poorly. Although uncommon, it can also be applied when a successful TV repair has resulted in an effective valve orifice that has mild to moderate stenosis (mean gradient > 6 mm Hg). Because concomitant LV dysfunction may be present in advanced stages, it is important to document by direct pressure measurements that the pulmonary arterial and LA pressures are low; otherwise, the bidirectional cavopulmonary shunt will not be feasible. If the LV end-diastolic pressure is less than 12 mm Hg, the transpulmonary gradient is less than 10 mm Hg, and the mean pulmonary arterial pressures are less than 18 mm Hg, a bidirectional cavopulmonary shunt is permissible. Even in the presence of moderate LV dysfunction (an ejection fraction of 35% to 40%), it is usually feasible to perform a bidirectional cavopulmonary shunt in the setting of Ebstein malformation.

Others have suggested that the construction of a bidirectional cavopulmonary shunt may allow for less than perfect TV repairs, because LV filling is not completely dependent on forward flow through the RV.[44] In addition, the shunt may allow patients to tolerate longer intervals between repeated TV operations for progressive tricuspid regurgitation or failing TV prostheses. This may be due to the smaller regurgitant volume and therefore a decreased volume load to the RV.

Chavaud and colleagues[45] and Quiñonez and coworkers[46] have proposed that the use of a bidirectional cavopulmonary shunt can decrease operative mortality and facilitate the postoperative management when there is severe RV dysfunction. The literature suggests that the frequency of bidirectional cavopulmonary shunt application in patients with Ebstein malformation is increasing: in a series of 150 patients in a European registry, almost 26% underwent a 1.5-ventricle repair. Although the early results appear to be improved, late results of a bidirectional cavopulmonary shunt in patients with Ebstein malformation are unknown.

Disadvantages of the bidirectional cavopulmonary shunt include pulsations of the head and neck veins, facial swelling, and the development of arteriovenous fistulae in the pulmonary vasculature. In addition, the placement of this shunt compromises access to the heart from the internal jugular approach for electrophysiologic studies and for pacemaker lead placement. The bidirectional cavopulmonary shunt has promising applications in the management of patients with Ebstein malformation, particularly those with RV failure, but it is our belief that it should be reserved for these selected patients until the late outcomes are well described.

Surgical Treatment of Arrhythmias. The most common atrial tachyarrhythmias in Ebstein malformation are atrial fibrillation and flutter. We have successfully used the right-sided cut-and-sew lesions of Cox-Maze III procedure in the early era of maze surgery and now use the modified RA maze lesions when arrhythmia surgery is applied. With the availability of newer devices, such as radiofrequency or cryoablation, the procedure time for maze procedure is shortened significantly. Consequently, our current preference is to perform a biatrial maze procedure when there is chronic atrial fibrillation, LA dilation, or concomitant mitral regurgitation. We follow the lesions in both atria that have been described previously.[47,48] In the presence of atrial flutter, we prefer to add a "cavotricuspid isthmus" lesion, which is the posterolateral TV annulus to the coronary sinus to the inferior vena cava. We also make an effort to close the LA appendage.

In patients with AV nodal reentrant tachycardia who underwent unsuccessful ablation in the electrophysiologic laboratory preoperatively, we perform perinodal cryoablation on cardiopulmonary bypass after opening the RA and closure of the intracardiac shunt. This involves multiple applications of the cryoprobe around and in the os of the coronary sinus, which is then carried anteriorly toward the proximal AV node until temporary complete heart block is noted, at which time the rewarming is begun; normal AV conduction returns shortly thereafter. In case of accessory conduction pathway as in WPW syndrome, mapping and ablation is performed preoperatively. Intraoperative mapping and ablation is rarely performed in the current era.

Heart Transplantation. Transplantation is an option in patients with Ebstein malformation with severe biventricular dysfunction (i.e., LV ejection fraction < 25%). In our experience, patients with severe RV dysfunction and normal or mild to moderately depressed LV function can be managed with a conventional operation, which can include placement of a bidirectional cavopulmonary shunt at the time of tricuspid repair or replacement. Other patients with Ebstein malformation who should be considered for transplantation are those with significant LV dilation and dysfunction or those with severe nonstructural mitral regurgitation with significant LV dysfunction. Hemodynamic cardiac catheterization to ascertain left-sided filling pressures and pulmonary artery pressures is also helpful in this group of patients when trying to determine feasibility of conventional operation versus transplantation.

POSTOPERATIVE CARE

Early postoperative management begins in the operating room. Discontinuation of bypass is accomplished with epinephrine and milrinone. To minimize RV dilation, higher heart rates (100 to 120 beats/min) are preferred and are obtained with temporary atrial pacing if needed. Low-dose vasopressin can be helpful with right-sided heart failure because systemic vasoplegia is not uncommon in this group of patients. This may be due to the use preoperative afterload reducing agents, liver congestion, or humoral factors from atrial natriuretic peptide secondary to atrial dilation.

Volume administration should be done cautiously to avoid RV distention; RA pressures less than 10 to 12 mm Hg are preferred. This strategy can result in mild metabolic acidosis in the early postoperative period but is tolerated as long as urine output is satisfactory and peripheral perfusion is normal. Extubation is performed after metabolic parameters have normalized (≈12 hours). Nitric oxide can be helpful to offset the pulmonary vasoconstrictive effects of inotropic support, thereby reducing afterload to the dysfunctional RV.

Medical therapy at hospital discharge includes beta blocker or angiotensin-converting enzyme inhibitor, or both, and selective use of sildenafil for 6 to 8 weeks for patients who have mildly elevated pulmonary artery pressures or for patients who live at high altitude. Importantly, amiodarone therapy is used for 2 to 3 months when there are documented arrhythmias and frequently when RV plication has been performed. Long-term arrhythmia surveillance with appropriate exercise testing is essential with this diagnosis.

OUTCOMES

Our experience with surgery for Ebstein malformation now approaches 1000 patients. Analysis of various groups of patients within this large cohort has been published previously.[49] We have performed 170 cone repairs to date; our initial experience was published recently.[50] Between June 2007 and December 2011, 89 patients (47 female; 53%) underwent cone reconstruction (median age, 19 years; range, 19 days to 68 years). The indications for operation were progressive cardiomegaly in 43 (48%), cyanosis in 29 (33%), and heart failure in 13 (15%). Prior TV repair was performed in 12 patients (13%). Severe tricuspid regurgitation (TR) was present in 75 patients (84%). All patients underwent cone reconstruction. Modifications included ringed annuloplasty in 57 patients (64%), leaflet augmentation in 28 patients (31%), and autologous chordae in 17 patients (19%). Bidirectional cavopulmonary anastomosis was performed in 21 patients (24%). Early mortality occurred in 1 patient (1%). Early reoperation for recurrent TR occurred in 12 patients (13%); re-repair was performed in 6 patients (50%), and 6 (50%) required replacement. Mean follow-up was 19.7 ± 24.7 months. There was no late mortality or reoperation. At follow-up, 72 patients (87%) had no or mild TR, 9 patients (11%) had moderate TR, and 2 patients (2%) had severe TR. Ringed annuloplasty was associated with less than moderate TR at dismissal ($P = 0.01$).

Most of the literature focuses on survival and reoperation, with little discussion about the functional outcome for patients with Ebstein malformation after surgery. We reported our experience of 539 patients with Ebstein malformation (pre–cone era) who underwent 604 cardiac operations.[51] The mean age at the initial operation was 24 years (range, 8 days to 79 years) and 53% were female. Survival at 5, 10, 15, and 20 years was 94%, 90%, 86%, and 76%, respectively. Survival free of late reoperation was 86%, 74%, 62%, and 46% at 5, 10, 15, and 20 years, respectively. Two hundred and thirty-seven (83%) patients were in NYHA functional class I or II, and 34% were taking no cardiac medication. The reported exercise tolerance was comparable to that of the patients' peers. In a small subset of these patients, formal exercise testing was conducted. There was improvement in exercise tolerance after operation, but this improvement was believed to be a result of the elimination of the right-to-left shunt at the atrial level rather than improvement in ventricular function. Late reoperation, rehospitalization, and atrial tachyarrhythmias continue to be a problem, with a rate of freedom from rehospitalization (for cardiac causes including reoperation) of 91%, 79%, 68%, 53%, and 35% at 1, 5, 10, 15, and 20 years, respectively. Thus, further improvement in the durability of TV repair and replacement, as well as improved control of atrial arrhythmias, could lead to improved quality of life in patients with Ebstein malformation.

REFERENCES

1. Ebstein W: Ueber einen sehr seltenen Fall von Insuffi cienz der Valvula tricuspidalis, bedingt durch eine angeborene hochgradige Missbildung derselben. *Arch Anat Physiol* 238–254, 1866.
2. Lamers WH, Viragh S, Wessels A, et al: Formation of the tricuspid valve in the human heart. *Circulation* 91:111–121, 1995.
3. Edwards WD: Embryology and pathologic features of Ebstein's anomaly. *Prog Pediatr Cardiol* 2:5–15, 1993.
4. Anderson KR, Zuberbuhler JR, Anderson RH, et al: Morphologic spectrum of Ebstein's anomaly of the heart: a review. *Mayo Clin Proc* 54:174–180, 1979.
5. Attenhofer Jost CH, Connolly HM, O'Leary PW, et al: Left heart lesions in patients with Ebstein anomaly. *Mayo Clin Proc* 80:361–368, 2005.
6. Sumner RG, Jacoby WJ, Jr, Tucker DH: Ebstein's anomaly associated with cardiomyopathy and pulmonary hypertension. *Circulation* 30:578–587, 1964.
7. Attenhofer Jost CH, Connolly HM, Warnes CA, et al: Noncompacted myocardium in Ebstein's anomaly: initial description in three patients. *J Am Soc Echocardiogr* 17:677–680, 2004.
8. Said SM, Burkhart HM, Schaff HV, et al: Congenitally corrected transposition of great arteries: surgical options for the failing right ventricle and/or severe tricuspid regurgitation. *World J Pediatr Congenit Heart Surg* 2:64–79, 2011.
9. Carpentier A, Chauvaud S, Mace L, et al: A new reconstructive operation for Ebstein's anomaly of the tricuspid valve. *J Thorac Cardiovasc Surg* 96:92–101, 1988.
10. Dearani JA, Danielson GK: Congenital heart surgery nomenclature and database project: Ebstein's anomaly and tricuspid valve disease. *Ann Thorac Surg* 69:S106–S117, 2000.
11. Benson DW, Silberbach GM, Kavanaugh-McHugh A, et al: Mutations in the cardiac transcription factor NKX2.5 affect diverse cardiac developmental pathways. *J Clin Invest* 104:1567–1573, 1999.
12. Yatsenko SA, Yatsenko AN, Szigeti K, et al: Interstitial deletion of 10p and atrial septal defect in DiGeorge 2 syndrome. *Clin Genet* 66:128–136, 2004.
13. Postma AV, van Engelen K, van de Meerakker J, et al: Mutations in the sarcomere gene MYH7 in Ebstein anomaly. *Circ Cardiovasc Genet* 4:43–50, 2011.
14. Said SM, Dearani JA: Ebstein's anomaly, congenital tricuspid valve regurgitation, and dysplasia. In Allen HD, Driscoll DJ, Shaddy RE, et al, editors: *Moss and Adams' heart disease in infants, children, and adolescents including the fetus and young adult*, vol 39, ed 8, Philadelphia, 2013, Lippincott Williams and Wilkins, Wolters Kluwer, pp 889–912.
15. Khositseth A, Danielson GK, Dearani JA, et al: Supraventricular tachyarrhythmias in Ebstein anomaly: management and outcome. *J Thorac Cardiovasc Surg* 128:826–833, 2004.
16. Greason KL, Dearani JA, Theodoro DA, et al: Surgical management of atrial tachyarrhythmias associated with congenital cardiac

anomalies: Mayo Clinic experience. *Semin Thorac Cardiovasc Surg Pediatr Card Surg Annu* 6:59–71, 2003.
17. Adams JC, Hudson R: A case of Ebstein's anomaly surviving to the age of 79. *Br Heart J* 18:129–132, 1956.
18. Celermajer DS, Bull C, Till JA, et al: Ebstein's anomaly: presentation and outcome from fetus to adult. *J Am Coll Cardiol* 23:170–176, 1994.
19. Giuliani ER, Fuster V, Brandenburg RO, et al: Ebstein's anomaly: the clinical features and natural history of Ebstein's anomaly of the tricuspid valve. *Mayo Clin Proc* 54:163–173, 1979.
20. Perloff JK: Ebstein's anomaly of the tricuspid valve. In Perloff JK, editor: *Clinical recognition of congenital heart disease*, ed 5, Philadelphia, 2003, Saunders, pp 194–215.
21. Giuliani ER, Fuster V, Brandenburg RO, et al: Ebstein's anomaly: the clinical features and natural history of Ebstein's anomaly of the tricuspid valve. *Mayo Clin Proc* 54:163–173, 1979.
22. Hornberger LK, Sahn DJ, Kleinman CS, et al: Tricuspid valve disease with significant tricuspid insufficiency in the fetus: diagnosis and outcome. *J Am Coll Cardiol* 17:167–173, 1992.
23. Celermajer DS, Cullen S, Sullivan ID, et al: Outcome in neonates with Ebstein's anomaly. *J Am Coll Cardiol* 19:1041–1046, 1992.
24. Yalonetsky S, Tobler D, Greutmann M, et al: Cardiac magnetic resonance imaging and the assessment of Ebstein anomaly in adults. *Am J Cardiol* 107:767–773, 2011.
25. McElhinney DB, Salvin JW, Colan SD, et al: Improving outcomes in fetuses and neonates with congenital displacement (Ebstein's malformation) or dysplasia of the tricuspid valve. *Am J Cardiol* 96:582–586, 2005.
26. Attie F, Rosas M, Rijlaarsdam M, et al: The adult patient with Ebstein anomaly. Outcome in 72 unoperated patients. *Medicine (Baltimore)* 79:27–36, 2000.
27. Knott-Craig CJ, Overholt ED, Ward KE, et al: Repair of Ebstein's anomaly in the symptomatic neonate: an evolution of technique with 7-year followup. *Ann Thorac Surg* 73:1786–1793, 2002.
28. Knott-Craig CJ: Management of neonatal Ebstein's anomaly. *Oper Tech* 13:101–108, 2008.
29. Knott-Craig CJ, Goldberg SP, Overholt ED, et al: Repair of neonates and young infants with Ebstein's anomaly and related disorders. *Ann Thorac Surg* 84:587–593, 2007.
30. Starnes VA, Pitlick PT, Bernstein D, et al: Ebstein's anomaly appearing in the neonate. A new surgical approach. *J Thorac Cardiovasc Surg* 101:1082–1087, 1991.
31. Reemtsen BL, Starnes VA: Fenestrated right ventricular exclusion (Starnes' procedure) for severe neonatal Ebstein's anomaly. *Oper Tech* 13:91–100, 2008.
32. Reemtsen BL, Polimenakos AC, Fagan BT, et al: Fate of the right ventricle after fenestrated right ventricular exclusion for severe neonatal Ebstein anomaly. *J Thorac Cardiovasc Surg* 134:1406–1412, 2007.
33. Sano S, Ishino K, Kawada M, et al: Total right ventricular exclusion procedure: an operation for isolated congestive right ventricular failure. *J Thorac Cardiovasc Surg* 123:640–647, 2002.
34. Reemtsen BL, Fagan BT, Wells WJ, et al: Current surgical therapy for Ebstein anomaly in neonates. *J Thorac Cardiovasc Surg* 132:1285–1290, 2006.
35. Hunter SW, Lillehei CW: Ebstein malformation of the TV. Study of a case together with suggestions of a new form of surgical therapy. *Dis Chest* 33:297–304, 1958.
36. Hardy KL, May IA, Webster CA, et al: Ebstein's anomaly: a functional concept and successful definitive repair. *J Thorac Cardiovasc Surg* 48:927–940, 1964.
37. Danielson GK, Driscoll DJ, Mair DD, et al: Operative treatment of Ebstein anomaly. *J Thorac Cardiovasc Surg* 104:1195–1202, 1992.
38. Chauvaud S: Ebstein's malformation. Surgical treatment and results. *Thorac Cardiovasc Surg* 48:220–223, 2000.
39. da Silva JP, Baumgratz FJ, Fonseca L, et al: The cone reconstruction of the tricuspid valve in Ebstein's anomaly. The operation: early and midterm results. *J Thorac Cardiovasc Surg* 133:215–223, 2007.
40. da Silva JP, da Silva LF, Moreira LF, et al: Cone reconstruction in Ebstein's anomaly repair: early and longterm results. *Arq Bras Cardiol* 97:199–208, 2011.
41. Dearani JA, Said SM, Burkhart HM, et al: Strategies for tricuspid re-repair in Ebstein malformation using the cone technique. *Ann Thorac Surg* 96(1):202–208, discussion 208–210, 2013.
42. Kiziltan HT, Theodoro DA, Warnes CA, et al: Late results of bioprosthetic tricuspid valve replacement in Ebstein's anomaly. *Ann Thorac Surg* 66:1539–1545, 1998.
43. Said SM, Burkhart HM, Schaff HV, et al: When should a mechanical tricuspid valve replacement be considered? *J Thorac Cardiovasc Surg* 148:603–608, 2014.
44. Marianeschi SM, McElhinney DB, Reddy VM, et al: Alternative approach to the repair of Ebstein's malformation: intracardiac repair with ventricular unloading. *Ann Thorac Surg* 66:1546–1550, 1998.
45. Chauvaud S, Fuzellier JF, Berrebi A, et al: Bi-directional cavopulmonary shunt associated with ventriculo and valvuloplasty in Ebstein's anomaly: benefits in high risk patients. *Eur J Cardiothorac Surg* 13:514–519, 1998.
46. Quiñonez LG, Dearani JA, Puga FJ, et al: Results of the 1.5-ventricle repair for Ebstein anomaly and the failing right ventricle. *J Thorac Cardiovasc Surg* 133:1303–1310, 2007.
47. Mavroudis C, Deal BJ, Back CL, et al: Arrhythmia surgery in patients with and without congenital heart disease. *Ann Thorac Surg* 86:857–868, 2008.
48. Cox JL, Jaquiss RD, Schuessler RB, et al: Modification of the maze procedure for atrial flutter and atrial fibrillation. II. Surgical technique of the maze III procedure. *J Thorac Cardiovasc Surg* 110:485–495, 1995.
49. Boston US, Dearani JA, O'Leary PW, et al: Tricuspid valve repair for Ebstein's anomaly in young children: a 30-year experience. *Ann Thorac Surg* 81:690–695, 2006.
50. Dearani JA, Said SM, O'Leary PW, et al: Anatomic repair of Ebstein's malformation: lessons learned with cone reconstruction. *Ann Thorac Surg* 95(1):220–226, discussion 226–228, 2013.
51. Brown ML, Dearani JA, Danielson GK, et al: Functional status after operation for Ebstein anomaly: the Mayo Clinic experience. *J Am Coll Cardiol* 52:460–466, 2008.

CHAPTER 131

Adult Congenital Cardiac Surgery

Anne Marie Valente • Sitaram M. Emani • Michael J. Landzberg • Emile A. Bacha

CHAPTER OUTLINE

Patients with congenital heart disease require lifelong surveillance. The number of adults living with congenital heart disease continues to grow, in part because of advances in the diagnosis and treatment of congenital heart lesions.[1,2] There are more than 1 million adults with congenital heart disease in the United States; this population grows by approximately 5% each year.[3,4]

The challenges of caring for adults with congenital heart disease were underscored in the medical literature by Dr. Joseph Perloff beginning in the 1970s, when he described the pediatric congenital cardiac patient becoming a postoperative adult.[5] However, it was not until 1990 at the 22nd Bethesda Conference of the American College of Cardiology (ACC) that the care of adults with congenital heart disease was formally recognized as a subspecialty of cardiology care.[6] In 2001, the 32nd Bethesda Conference attempted to address the changing profile of adults living with congenital heart disease by developing guidelines for resource allocation.[2]

There is a paucity of literature related to the surgical care of adults with congenital heart disease. Many patients are considered for additional surgery after initial palliations earlier in life. Other patients present with previously undiscovered congenital heart disease requiring surgical intervention. This chapter discusses the expanding adults with congenital heart disease (ACHD) population and its unique challenges. Important aspects of preoperative evaluation and perioperative management are highlighted, and several of the most common lesions encountered by surgeons caring for adults with congenital heart disease are discussed.

EPIDEMIOLOGY

There are more adults than children living with congenital heart disease, and the population continues to grow. The prevalence of adults with congenital heart disease in Quebec, Canada, was 6.12 per 1000 for the year 2010, which was a 57% increase compared with 2000. This compares with an only 10% increase in the prevalence of children with congenital heart disease during the same time period.[7] This presents several unique challenges to the health care providers that care for these patients.

In 2001, the 32nd Bethesda Conference developed guidelines for resource allocation and program development directed at adults with congenital heart disease. The model for delivery of care focuses on classification of congenital heart defects into different levels of anatomic complexity (Box 131-1), with referral to specialized adult congenital disease centers for increasing levels of such classification. More than half of the ACHD population is believed to be at increased risk for sudden cardiac death, need for reoperation, and other severe complications. This report estimated that 15% of the ACHD population have anatomically complex disease and require regular follow-up at a specialized center for adult congenital heart disease, and an additional 38% have moderate anatomic complexity of disease requiring periodic follow-up in a specialized center.[2] The British Cardiac Society Working Party published a similar document addressing the care for the GUCH (grown-up congenital heart) population.[8] The consensus of both documents is

BOX 131-1 Adult Congenital Heart Disease Lesions by Severity

Simple Complexity

- Isolated congenital aortic valve disease
- Isolated congenital mitral valve disease (except parachute valve, cleft leaflet)
- Isolated patent foramen ovale or small atrial septal defect
- Isolated small ventricular septal defect (no associated lesions)
- Mild pulmonic stenosis
- Previously ligated or occluded ductus arteriosus
- Repaired secundum or sinus venosus defect without residua
- Repaired ventricular septal defect without residua

Moderate Complexity

- Aortic to left ventricular fistula
- Anomalous pulmonary venous drainage, partial or total
- Atrioventricular canal defects (partial or complete)
- Coarctation of the aorta
- Ebstein anomaly
- Infundibular right ventricular outflow obstruction of significance
- Ostium primum atrial septal defect
- Patent ductus arteriosus (not closed)
- Pulmonary valve regurgitation (moderate to severe)
- Pulmonic valve stenosis (moderate to severe)
- Sinus of Valsalva fistula/aneurysm
- Sinus venosus defect
- Subvalvar or supravalvar aortic stenosis (except hypertrophic cardiomyopathy)
- Tetralogy of Fallot
- Ventricular septal defect with
  - Absent valve or valves
  - Aortic regurgitation
  - Coarctation of the aorta
  - Mitral disease
  - Right ventricular outflow tract obstruction
  - Straddling tricuspid/mitral valve
  - Subaortic stenosis

Severe Complexity

- Conduits, valved or nonvalved
- Cyanotic congenital heart (all forms)
- Double-outlet ventricle
- Eisenmenger syndrome
- Fontan procedure
- Mitral atresia
- Single ventricle (also called double inlet or outlet, common, or primitive)
- Pulmonary atresia (all forms)
- Pulmonary vascular obstructive diseases
- Transposition of the great arteries
- Tricuspid atresia
- Truncus arteriosus/hemitruncus
- Other abnormalities of atrioventricular or ventriculoarterial connection not included above (e.g., crisscross heart, isomerism, heterotaxy syndromes, ventricular inversion)

Adapted from Warnes CA, Liberthson R, Danielson GK, et al: Task force 1: the changing profile of congenital heart disease in adult life. J Am Coll Cardiol 37:1170–1175, 2001.

that all patients (with the exception of those with simple heart lesions) should receive lifelong specialized ACHD care.

STRUCTURED ACHD PROGRAMS

Over the past decade, there has been an increase in the number of centers with specialized multidisciplinary teams committed to the lifelong care of ACHD patients. Many challenges are involved in creating and maintaining a successful team of specialized ACHD providers. Health care providers who specialize in the care of these patients have various levels of experience in ACHD diagnosis and management. Although they are committed to the care of their patients, they may not have had the benefit of training in this subspecialty.[9] Programs that specialize in ACHD care excel in multidisciplinary collaboration with specialists in not only congenital cardiac disease but also reproductive and obstetric care, nephrology, hepatology, hematology, pulmonary, rheumatology, psychiatric support, palliative care, and transition education. From a cardiac perspective, it is essential to have experienced clinicians with expertise in imaging, electrophysiology, interventional catheterization, congenital cardiac surgery, cardiac anesthesia, critical care, advanced heart failure management, and transplant medicine. The organizational structure should be regionally coordinated, so that regional centers caring for adults with congenital heart disease can easily consult and refer to the specialized programs.[10]

Lapse in medical care in adults with congenital heart disease results in adverse outcomes. In a study of 158 adult patients referred to one ACHD center, lapse of medical care, defined as an interval of more than 2 years, occurred for 99 patients (63%). The median duration of lapse of care was 10 years. Patients with lapse of care were 3.1 times more likely to require urgent cardiac interventions ($P = 0.003$).[11] In a multicenter study of 922 patients at 12 ACHD centers, 42% experienced a gap in cardiology care that lasted longer than 3 years, and 8% had a gap longer than a decade. The mean age at the first gap was 19.9 years. The most common reasons for gaps included feeling well, being unaware that follow-up was required, and complete absence from medical care. Disease complexity was predictive of a gap in care among 59% of mild, 42% of moderate, and 26% of severe disease patients reporting gaps ($P < 0.0001$).[12]

Emergencies in the ACHD patient are of particular concern. In one multicenter study of hospital admissions of adults with congenital heart disease, 63% of emergent admissions required cooperation with another specialized department.[13] An additional challenge that faces the ACHD population is lack of insurance coverage. Congenital heart disease patients without private insurance and older than 17 years are at higher risk of being admitted via the emergency room.[14]

A critical volume of patients is needed to maintain expertise in the various disciplines required in the care of ACHD patients. Adult congenital heart surgery should be performed only by surgeons who are experienced in all aspects of congenital heart surgery.[15] In an analysis of the Nationwide Inpatient Sample, early mortality and length of stay were lower for patients who underwent ACHD procedures performed by surgeons with expertise in congenital heart disease.[16] The choice of location for surgery should depend on not only the surgeon but also the multidisciplinary team's support for management of adult comorbidities. The optimal surgical location may be center dependent. Certain factors place adults with congenital heart disease at higher risk of death when surgery is performed at freestanding pediatric hospitals. These risk factors include older age, male sex, government-sponsored insurance, and greater surgical complexity.[17] Additionally, greater surgical complexity, government-sponsored insurance, DiGeorge syndrome, weekend admissions, and depression result in higher resource use in ACHD surgical admissions.[18] Analysis of the Nationwide Inpatient Sample examining ACHD surgical admissions to adult hospitals identified nonelective admissions, government-sponsored insurance, surgical complexity, heart failure, renal failure, and complications as risk factors for higher resource utilization.[19]

SURGICAL INDICATIONS IN ACHD PATIENTS

The ACC and American Heart Association (AHA) have developed guidelines for management of adults with congenital heart disease, which include recommendations for surgical interventions.[20] It is important to recognize the decision to proceed with surgery in the ACHD patient is multifactorial. The goals of prolonging survival and improving quality of life are paramount. The use of previously established measures of physical functioning (such as New York Heart Association [NYHA] class) is difficult to assess in the ACHD patient. Many patients, having lived with the sequelae of cardiac disease since birth, do not perceive themselves as "limited" in the setting of markedly diminished objective exercise capacity.[21] There is a common misconception that surgical palliation of a congenital heart defect in infancy or childhood is "curative." Therefore, by the time that patients are formally evaluated, ventricular dysfunction may be severe and irreversible.[22] Despite this, NYHA class of III or higher has been associated with increased operative mortality, major adverse events, and greater length of stay in ACHD patients undergoing surgery.[23]

Pediatric surgical risk scoring systems, such as Aristotle or STAT, may offer some prognostic value in ACHD patients but have limitations in their applicability. For example, high-risk surgeries often include procedures primarily done in infants (such as the Norwood operation or interrupted aortic arch repair), and the distribution of procedures in ACHD patients is skewed toward those classified as lower risk. Furthermore, patient comorbidities that may influence surgical outcome in the pediatric population (such as those in the Aristotle Comprehensive Scoring system, including low birth weight, prematurity, and noncardiac congenital anomalies) may not be as applicable in the adult population, whereas diabetes, hypertension, vascular disease, markers of hepatic disease, and NYHA class may be more meaningful.[24, 25] In a multicenter study of 2012 ACHD patients requiring surgery from 13 European countries, preoperative cyanosis, arrhythmias, and NYHA class of III or higher were risk factors for hospital mortality.[26]

A subset of ACHD patients are referred for primary surgical correction. The principle reason for this is late diagnosis, for example, patients with atrial septal defects or aortic coarctation. Patients may also be referred as adults for a condition that was previously considered inoperable, or because they are from a geographic region without local surgical congenital heart expertise, or because they have anatomically complex lesions but balanced systemic and pulmonary blood flows. Patients with unrepaired tetralogy of Fallot and pulmonary atresia have a poor prognosis; survival beyond the fifth decade is rare.[27]

PREOPERATIVE EVALUATION

The evaluation of an ACHD patient who is being considered for surgery is extensive. It begins with a thorough review of the underlying anatomy and physiology. This must include retrieval of any previous surgical reports, if possible, so that any unusual features or complications are known and can be anticipated. A further understanding of the current cardiac anatomy can be gained by the use of specific imaging modalities. Imaging should not only focus on cardiac function but also examine for any residua of previous surgery that should be addressed. The imager must be aware of the various potential residual sequelae to evaluate for, such as branch pulmonary artery stenosis at the insertion site of previously taken down systemic to pulmonary artery shunts. Three-dimensional echocardiography is particular useful for understanding valvular morphology and mechanisms that contribute to valvular dysfunction.

Cardiovascular magnetic resonance imaging (CMR) is increasingly used to quantify ventricular volumes, function, and vascular anatomy.[28,29] Gadolinium-enhanced contrast CMR can also evaluate myocardial viability. Cardiac computed tomography (CT) is an alternative for patients who have contraindications to CMR, and it provides excellent coronary imaging.[30]

Imaging can also be helpful to determine the anatomic relationships of certain vascular structures, particularly the relationship of the aorta to the sternum (Fig. 131-1). This is particularly important for repeat sternotomy, which may be associated with inadvertent aortic entry. Preoperative duplex ultrasonography of the femoral and iliac arteries and veins shows the status of the patency of these vessels in ACHD patients who have undergone previous interventions. This is essential in the case of those patients who may need urgent peripheral cannulation for cardiopulmonary bypass.

Cardiac catheterization is often required to determine the cardiac hemodynamics and to determine if there are any associated lesions that should be addressed in the catheterization laboratory.[31] Coronary angiography should be considered based on the presence of risk factors, presence of angina, noninvasive evidence of ischemia, reduced systemic ventricular function, history of myocardial infarction, or for those patients with prior

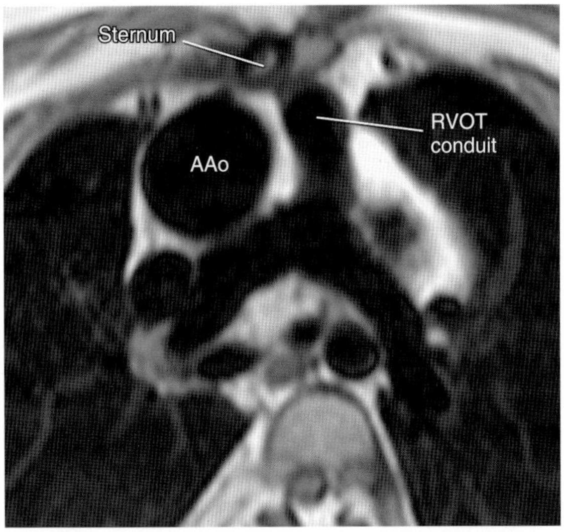

FIGURE 131-1 ■ Turbo-spin echocardiographic magnetic resonance image in the axial plane demonstrates the ascending aorta (AAo) and right ventricular outflow tract (RVOT) conduit closely adherent to the posterior table of the sternum.

coronary or great artery surgery. This includes adults with transposition of the great arteries who have undergone an arterial switch procedure with coronary translocation.[32] There is a consensus that selective coronary angiography should be performed in men older than 40 years who have congenital heart disease and have been referred for surgery and in similar postmenopausal women.[20,33] As many as 33% of selected ACHD patients may have an asymptomatic coronary artery anomaly that is discovered with coronary angiography; this is an important preoperative finding.[34] Exercise capacity should be examined with objective exercise testing.[35]

An intensive electrophysiologic evaluation of the preoperative ACHD patient is essential. The incidence of arrhythmias is highest in those patients with moderate or severe ACHD complexity. For example, as many as one third of adults with repaired tetralogy of Fallot develop symptomatic atrial tachycardia,[36] approximately 10% develop high-grade ventricular arrhythmias,[37] and approximately 5% require permanent pacemaker placement for sinus node dysfunction or atrioventricular block. Additionally, an increasing number of adults with repaired tetralogy of Fallot are receiving implantable cardioverter defibrillators for treatment of ventricular tachyarrhythmia.[38]

The importance of a multisystem approach to the ACHD patient during the preoperative evaluation cannot be overemphasized. In a retrospective analysis of more than 1100 ACHD patients, 9% had moderate or severe renal dysfunction with a reported threefold increase in mortality.[39] Lung function can be significantly diminished in the ACHD patient as a result of previous thoracotomy and resultant scoliosis and restrictive lung disease. ACHD patients with cyanosis are at risk for multisystem derangement, including abnormal hematologic indices, coagulopathy, nephropathy, and hepatic dysfunction.[40] Heart failure should be identified and medical therapies maximized to achieve critical predictors of improved outcomes.[19]

ACHD patients and their families should be educated on the potential benefits and possible risks of the surgical procedure. Some adults with congenital heart disease have emotional problems from previous childhood interventions, and their concerns must be addressed preoperatively. Additionally, patients may have a deleterious body image based on previous surgical scars.[41] A dedicated discussion to the options regarding surgical entry, including possible techniques to minimize further scarring, is often helpful.

PERIOPERATIVE MANAGEMENT

The physiology of the ACHD patient is often complex, and an experienced cardiac anesthetist must be responsible for the care of the patient from the preinduction period through the postoperative management. The experienced anesthetist is essential in managing shifts in the vascular resistance of both the systemic and pulmonary circulations, dynamics of intracardiac shunting, and intravascular volume status. Possible harmful hemodynamic effects related to each anesthetic agent must be considered.[42] For example, spinal anesthesia can result in a reduction in preload and decrease in pulmonary blood flow. It can also result in a drop in the systemic vascular resistance and an increase in pulmonary to systemic shunting, thus worsening hypoxemia. Narcotics may contribute to an acute reduction in systemic vascular resistance during induction.

Coordination of the operating room team in planning and completing successful sternal reentry is essential. Most surgeries performed on ACHD patients are reoperations. Reoperations are associated with a higher risk, particularly in those patients with cyanosis, transposed great arteries (anterior aorta), pulmonary atresia, or poor ventricular function.[43] In one report, early mortality for reoperation approached 10% for those ACHD patients who underwent five sternotomies.[44] The surgeon must recognize the relationships of cardiac structures in the ACHD patient, many of whom have greatly distorted anatomy, particularly when pericardial integrity has been lost as a result of prior surgical interventions. CMR or CT provides excellent visualization of the relationship of cardiac structures to the sternum (see Fig. 131-1).[24] In some patients, there is no discernible space between the posterior table of the sternum and a cardiac structure.

Dilated or hypertensive right heart structures are at particular risk during repeat sternotomy. For example, patients with a systemic right ventricle, such as those with complete transposition of the great arteries who have undergone atrial switch repair (Mustard, Senning), have an enlarged anterior right ventricle that may be adherent to the posterior shelf of the sternum. Aneurysmal, thin-walled right ventricular outflow tract patches and dilated ascending aortas may also be closely related to the sternum. The surgeon must be aware of the location of previously placed extracardiac conduits or shunts to avoid possible injury on sternal reentry. Another example includes a massively dilated and thinned-out right atrium in a classic Fontan. It typically crosses the midline and abuts the sternum, and injury to this structure can propagate because the wall is typically very thin. Additionally, preoperative knowledge of the coronary anatomy is helpful to avoid inadvertent coronary injury. Certain congenital diagnoses have a higher incidence of anomalous coronary origins and courses, such as tetralogy of Fallot, where the left anterior descending coronary artery crosses the right ventricular outflow tract in at least 5% of cases.[45]

Sternal Reentry Protocol

When there is a high possibility of risk to cardiac structures, femoral cannulation may be required. Femoral-to-femoral cardiopulmonary bypass can be established quickly; it allows blood salvage and control of systemic blood flow and pressure and lowers central venous pressure. Venous filling pressure must be controlled above zero to avoid entraining air into the circulation. Once this is established, retrosternal dissection can safely proceed. In some high-risk cases, it is important to dissect out the groin vessels prior to sternotomy.

Management of Bleeding during Resternotomy

Inadvertent injury to cardiac structures can result in life-threatening venous or arterial bleeding. Determining the source of bleeding is critical in the management of hemorrhage. Sources of venous bleeding include the right atrium, right ventricle, innominate vein, and/or pulmonary conduit. Venous bleeding not only causes blood loss but also allows air into the circulation, resulting in paradoxical air embolism. Therefore, positive venous pressure is needed when there is significant venous bleeding to prevent air embolism in those patients with intracardiac shunting. Additional efforts to minimize air entrainment into the circulation include placing the patient in the Trendelenburg position and rotating the table to the patient's left side.

Major arterial bleeding demands immediate control, even if temporary with a clamp, a suture, or direct compression of the bleeding site. Urgent peripheral femoral cannulation and initiation of cardiopulmonary bypass are typically needed. Once bypass is initiated, systemic cooling is performed so that flows can be lowered to control the bleeding site. Low-flow bypass is often sufficient to complete the dissection and repair any aortic injury. If the heart fibrillated, it is crucial to avoid distention, especially if aortic regurgitation is present. Manual compression of the heart may decrease distention until it begins ejecting, and left ventricular vent placement is crucial.

Unique factors that are important in the ACHD surgical patient include the systemic effects of chronic cyanosis, arrhythmia burden, presence of aortopulmonary collaterals, and ventricular dysfunction. Long-standing cyanosis results in intrinsic hemostatic abnormalities, and postoperative hemostasis may be difficult to achieve. ACHD patients with chronic cyanosis often have multiple collateral vessels that are friable and difficult to coagulate. The difficulty in achieving perioperative hemostasis is exacerbated by extensive suture lines and long cardiopulmonary bypass times, which lead to a decrease in platelet number and activity through consumption coagulopathy and fibrinolysis.

Several strategies to minimize occurrence and effects of postoperative blood loss include the following:

- Preoperative phlebotomy with postoperative autologous blood transfusion
- Preoperative stimulation of bone marrow production with iron repletion in the iron-deficient patient or with erythropoietin
- Extensive and precise hemostasis during sternotomy and dissection
- Ultrafiltration during cardiopulmonary bypass to raise the hematocrit, and administration of a cell saver device
- Administration of antifibrinolytic agents
- Administration of platelets, fresh-frozen plasma, or cryoprecipitate
- Direct application of surgical glue to suture lines

ACHD patients who have depressed ventricular function or abnormal diastolic function and limited cardiac reserve do not tolerate large volume shifts well, and meticulous attempts must be made to achieve postoperative hemostasis. Patients with decreased ventricular function may need mechanical ventricular support (e.g., ventricular assist device, extracorporeal membrane oxygenation) for a limited time in the immediate postoperative period, and appropriate devices should be available during the surgical procedure so that they can be used if a patient fails to wean from cardiopulmonary bypass.

Efforts must be made to provide optimal myocardial protection during the surgery. Almost all ACHD patients are at risk for perioperative myocardial injury by several mechanisms, depending on the underlying physiology. These include washout of cardioplegia as a result of acquired collateral vessels that involve the coronary circulation, increased pulmonary venous return causing ventricular distention, and inadequate myocardial preservation as a result of extensive ventricular hypertrophy.

Strategies to improve myocardial protection include the following:

- More frequent administration of cardioplegia
- Venting of the heart to prevent overdistention
- In selected cases, the use of low-flow hypothermic cardiopulmonary bypass

A low cardiac output state can occur immediately postoperatively for a variety of reasons. Volume management is critical and depends on adequate hemostasis. Many ACHD patients have poorly compliant ventricles, because of either hypertrophy or restrictive ventricular physiology, and this may contribute to a low output state. Postoperative arrhythmias can cause an acute change in the cardiac output. Any arrhythmia must be recognized and treated immediately.

Low systemic perfusion with accompanying low systemic vascular resistance can occur postoperatively as well. It occurs most often in patients with preoperative heart failure and congestion of systemic venous pressure, those with known presurgical liver disease, or in patients with established risk factors for postoperative systemic inflammatory response syndrome (SIRS).

Additional surgical consideration for adult patients with history of long-standing congenital heart disease or prior congenital heart surgery include propensity for calcification of cardiac structures and patch material, which can alter the surgical treatment. For example, patients with circumferential calcification of patent ductus arteriosus are at risk for fracture and bleeding with simple ligation using the traditional thoracotomy approach, and sternotomy with patch closure through the pulmonary artery may be the preferred approach. Similarly, treatment of a residual patch margin ventricular septal defect is complicated by the presence of calcification, which may prevent simple patch closure and necessitate excision of the calcified portion of the patch. Preoperative imaging must be carefully examined for evidence of calcification in the operative field.

POSTOPERATIVE MANAGEMENT

ACHD surgical care must be performed in a setting with a structured ACHD program that has a multidisciplinary team approach, and this is evident postoperatively. Intensivist and nursing staff should be skilled in working with ACHD patients. The physiology of the lesion often dictates postoperative care. Avoidance of acidosis and maintenance of adequate oxygenation and systemic perfusion are paramount. Postoperative bleeding should be anticipated and controlled. Patients should be reexplored if bleeding is excessive after the first several postoperative hours. Recognition and treatment of arrhythmias must be prompt and successful to avoid hemodynamic instability. Most ACHD patients return from the operating room with both atrial and ventricular temporary pacing wires, which may be used in determining the type of arrhythmia so as to direct therapy. Monitoring lines may be very useful: a transthoracic left atrial line, right atrial line, or pulmonary artery line may be left in the patient. The intensive care outcomes on adults operated on for congenital heart disease are favorable.[46] The early mortality for 2851 adult congenital patients operated on at the Mayo Clinic from 1993 to 2006 was 2.4%.[44]

Most ACHD patients have residual cardiac issues after repeat surgery, and they must be educated regarding the need for lifelong follow-up. Several organizations are dedicated to improving the care of adults with congenital heart disease. The International Society for Adult Congenital Heart Disease (ISACHD) was founded in 1994 with a mission to promote, maintain, and pursue excellence in the care of adults with congenital heart disease (www.isachd.org). The Adult Congenital Heart Association (ACHA), a national nonprofit organization founded in 1988 by a group of ACHD survivors and their families, is dedicated to improving the quality of life and extending the lives of adults with congenital heart defects. More than 60 specialized clinics for adults with congenital heart disease are listed on the ACHA website (www.achaheart.org).

SPECIFIC LESIONS

To provide successful care to congenital heart patients in adulthood, adult congenital heart surgeons should be experienced in all aspects of congenital heart disease that are encountered in childhood. Although a thorough review of specific lesions is beyond the scope of this chapter, the management of several more common lesions encountered in adulthood is discussed here. As mentioned earlier, the surgical indications for most congenital heart lesions encountered in adulthood are sparse. However, the ACC/AHA guidelines for the management of adults with congenital heart disease is an excellent summary of the current data.[20] Another set of guidelines was published by an international team of experts in 2001.[33,47]

Atrial Septal Defect

Atrial septal defect (ASD) is one of the most common congenital heart defects. The clinical presentation of left-to-right shunting across an ASD is right ventricular volume overload and pulmonary overcirculation. ASDs that are large may develop during childhood; however, many are not discovered until adult life when patients develop exercise intolerance, atrial arrhythmias, or dyspnea.[48,49] The indications for closure of an ASD include otherwise unexplained right atrial or right ventricular enlargement, regardless of symptoms. Additionally, patients with ASDs and evidence of established paradoxical embolism, the recurrence of which cannot be otherwise controlled, should be referred for closure, even in the absence of right heart overload. The long-term prognosis after closure for patients younger than 25 years is comparable to that of the general population. Patients corrected at an older age, particularly those older than 40 years, may have decreased long-term survival and experience higher rates of sequelae, including atrial arrhythmias, pulmonary hypertension, and right heart failure.[49] Therefore, some have questioned the benefit to repairing ASDs in later life, although general consensus and experience suggest improvement in symptomatic patients regardless of age at presentation, extending far into the older adult population.[50] Among the several types of ASDs, the most common is a secundum ASD—a defect in the region of the fossa ovalis. Surgical repair of secundum ASD has been performed since 1954. Secundum ASDs can often be closed with occluder devices placed percutaneously.[51] However, certain anatomic determinants make percutaneous closure less favorable, including large defects, inadequate tissue rims, and anomalous draining pulmonary veins. Surgical closure is required for primum ASDs, sinus venosus defects (Fig. 131-2), and coronary sinus septal defects.

It is important to recognize the possibility of pulmonary arterial hypertension in the older patient with unrepaired ASD, although it is much more prevalent in patients with large unrepaired ventricular septal defects, complete atrioventricular canal, or patent ductus arteriosus. When pulmonary arterial hypertension is present, pulmonary vascular resistance can increase, compromising potential benefits of ASD closure. Greatest extreme and potential for pathology is noted with reversal of intracardiac shunting and systemic oxygen desaturation, resulting in Eisenmenger physiology. Patients with ASD and Eisenmenger syndrome have a reduced life

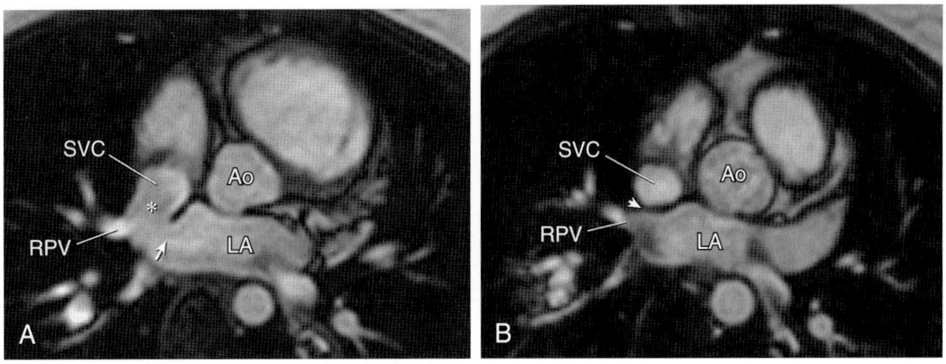

FIGURE 131-2 ■ Previously healthy 33-year-old woman with increasing shortness of breath with exertion. **A,** Cine magnetic resonance image in the axial plane demonstrates a sinus venosus defect *(*)* in the wall that separates the superior vena cava (SVC) and the right upper pulmonary vein (RPV). The *arrow* indicates the orifice of the RPV through which blood can flow between the left atrium (LA) and the SVC. **B,** Repeat imaging in the same patient performed 1 year after surgery confirms closure of the sinus venosus defect *(arrow)*. *Ao,* Aorta.

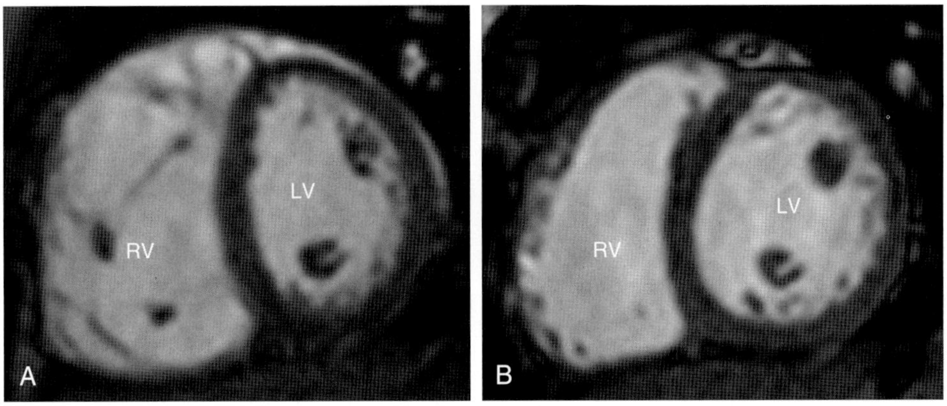

FIGURE 131-3 ■ **A,** Cine magnetic resonance image in the short-axis plane in the same patient as shown in Figure 131-2 demonstrates severe right ventricular (RV) dilation with a preoperative RV end-diastolic volume of 150 mL/m^2. **B,** Repeat imaging in the same patient performed 1 year after surgical closure demonstrates decreased RV end-diastolic volume to normal at 80 mL/m^2. *LV,* Left ventricle.

expectancy.[52] For patients with ASD and pulmonary arterial hypertension, surgery is not recommended unless the pulmonary vascular resistance is demonstrated to be sufficiently low. In patients with evidence of elevated pulmonary vascular resistance, invasive testing with oxygen or vasodilators such as nitric oxide may be useful in determining appropriateness for surgical candidacy. Patients with ASDs with measured pulmonary vascular resistance greater than 8 Wood units are unlikely to improve with surgery (and repair may shorten survival); current recommendations suggest that when resistance is as high as 4 Wood units, decision regarding surgical repair should include consultation with clinicians with expertise in the assessment and care of pulmonary vascular disease.

The closure of ASDs can sometimes be performed via a transxiphoid or mini-sternotomy approach, conferring a satisfactory cosmetic result without compromising the safety or accuracy of the repair.[53] In some select cases, closure of an ASD can be performed safely and effectively via an endoscopic approach, which further minimizes the degree of invasiveness and hastens postoperative recovery.[54]

The operative mortality for surgical closure of ASD should be less than 1%. Most symptomatic adults experience clinical improvement.[55] In one report, cardiopulmonary performance in adult patients with surgically repaired ASD was improved at 4 months postoperatively compared with preoperative assessment, and complete restitution to normal was documented 10 years after shunt closure.[56] The right ventricular volumes begin to decrease immediately after ASD closure (Fig. 131-3) and are significantly reduced as early as 3 months after closure.[57]

The long-term outcomes after ASD closure are generally excellent; however, the benefits are related to the timing of closure. Murphy and colleagues reported that patients repaired before the age of 25 years had 27-year survival rates similar to those of normal controls. However, the 27-year survival rate for patients between the ages of 25 and 40 years of age was 84%, and the survival rate was decreased to 40% for those patients older than 41 years.[49] The presence of arrhythmias preoperatively is a risk factor for postoperative rhythm disturbance, which occurs in approximately 60% of patients. Additional risk factors for recurrent arrhythmias after closure include age older than 40 years (some series have extended this to older than 60 years) and postoperative onset of atrial fibrillation, atrial flutter, or junctional rhythm.[58] Therefore, patients referred for ASD closure with existing arrhythmias and patients older than 40 (or

60) years should be considered for ablation at the time of repair.

Sinus Venosus Defect

In a retrospective review of 108 patients at the Mayo Clinic who had undergone sinus venosus defect repair over a 24-year period, symptomatic improvement was noted in 77%. Early mortality was less than 1%. Postoperative mortality was related to older age at repair and poor NYHA class preoperatively. Long-term complications from repair included sinus node dysfunction in 6% and atrial fibrillation in 14%. The presence of atrial fibrillation was related to older age at time of repair.[59]

The choice of surgical technique for repair of sinus venosus defect depends on the patient's particular anatomy, such as size of defect and distance of the anomalous draining pulmonary veins from the superior vena cava (SVC) and right atrium. A single patch repair was used in most of the patients in the Mayo series. A double patch technique consisting of pericardial patch closure of the ASD with rerouting of the pulmonary veins to the left atrium and enlargement of the SVC with a second pericardial patch has been shown in select centers to be associated with less residual vessel stenosis and arrhythmia.[60] Sinus node injury is prevented by placement of the SVC incision just anterior to the entry of the pulmonary veins into the SVC. The Warden procedure is an alternative technique, which involves division of the SVC above the insertion of the anomalous pulmonary veins with placement of a pericardial patch on the cardiac end of the SVC. The right atrial appendage is opened and anastomosed to the cut end of the SVC.[61]

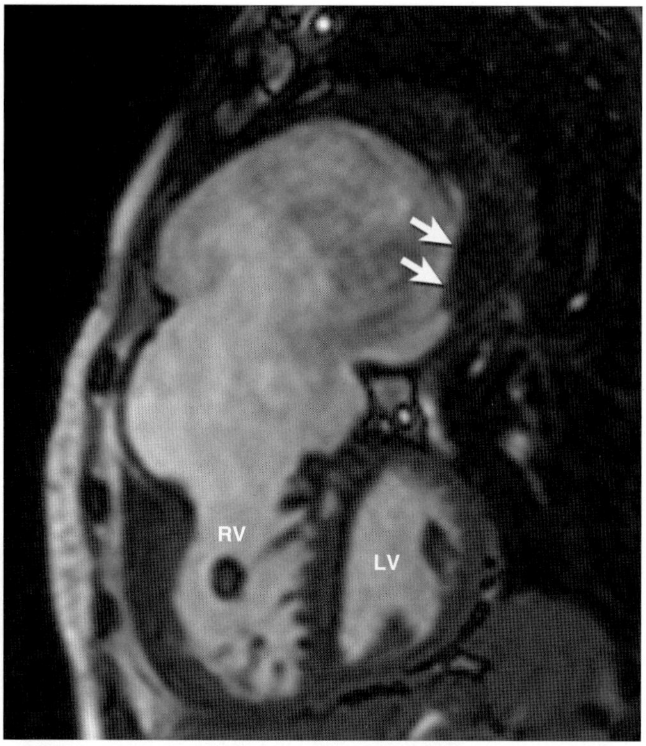

FIGURE 131-4 ■ Woman, 26 years old, with tetralogy of Fallot with pulmonary atresia who had undergone right ventricular conduit in infancy. Cine magnetic resonance image demonstrates a giant right ventricular (RV) outflow tract aneurysm measuring 13 cm × 8 cm × 8 cm. A large hemispherical thrombus *(arrows)* occupies the posterior aspect of the aneurysm. *LV,* Left ventricle. (From Valente A: Adult congenital heart disease. In Libby P, editor: *Essential atlas of cardiovascular disease,* Philadelphia, 2009, Springer/Current Medicine Group.)

Tetralogy of Fallot

Most adults with tetralogy of Fallot (TOF) underwent repair in childhood. These patients, when referred for surgical consideration in adulthood, often have multiple residual lesions that may need to be surgically addressed, on average 2.9 procedures per patient per reoperation.[62] TOF is the most common form of cyanotic congenital heart disease. The principal pathologic abnormality involves varying degrees of hypoplasia of the infundibulum, often with anterior, superior, and leftward deviation of the conal septum. As a result, TOF is characterized by right ventricular outflow tract obstruction, right ventricular hypertrophy, a large conoventricular septal defect, and an aorta that overrides the ventricular septum.

Lillehei is attributed with performing the first surgical repair of TOF in 1954; the 30-year survival rate from reoperations for the first 106 patients undergoing surgical repair was 91%.[63] The 20-year survival rate of patients treated from the late 1950s to 1972 was approximately 90%.[64,65] Patients with TOF born prior to the early 1970s were often palliated with systemic artery to pulmonary artery shunts to increase pulmonary blood flow prior to the definitive repair. Most adult survivors with TOF underwent "definitive" repair much later in life than is currently the standard of care, which is younger than 1 year. Definitive surgical repair typically involves patch closure of the ventricular septal defect and an infundibular or transannular right ventricular outflow tract patch to relieve the obstruction. However, adults who underwent definitive repair several decades ago were likely to have undergone a generous right ventricular incision and, compared with current technique, less attention to the preservation of the pulmonary valve. Right ventricular outflow tract aneurysms in the ACHD patient are common (Fig. 131-4), and they contribute to right ventricular dysfunction.[66] Surgical remodeling techniques can be used to reduce the size of the akinetic portion of the right ventricular outflow tract.

Surgical repair of TOF commonly results in anatomic and functional abnormalities in the ACHD population. Common sequelae include right ventricular dilation from pulmonary regurgitation, residual ventricular septal defects (often at the patch margin), tricuspid regurgitation, right ventricular outflow patch aneurysms, and branch pulmonary artery stenoses (commonly at the insertion site of previously taken down systemic to pulmonary artery shunts). The hemodynamic burden of these residua is often well tolerated in childhood. However, the prevalence of exercise intolerance, arrhythmias, heart failure, and death (Fig. 131-5) increase during adulthood.[67,68] The factors that may contribute to worsening clinic status are demonstrated in Figure 131-6. Gatzoulis and colleagues reported risk factors for sudden death in 793 patients with repaired TOF from six centers

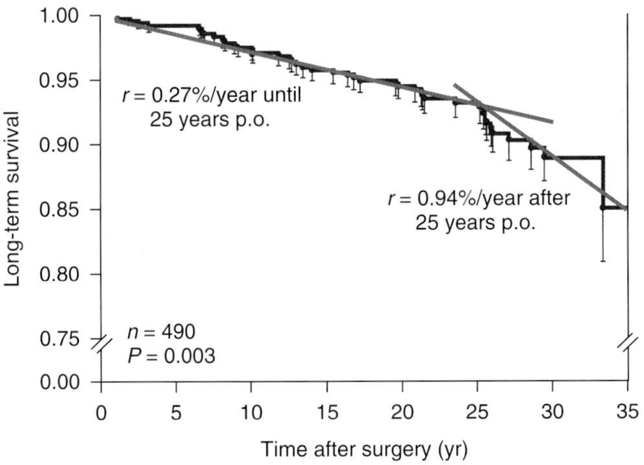

FIGURE 131-5 ■ Long-term survival curve after correction of tetralogy of Fallot. (Adapted from Nollert G, Fischlein T, Bouterwek S, et al: Long-term survival in patients with repair of tetralogy of Fallot: 36-year follow-up of 490 survivors of the first year after surgical repair. *J Am Coll Cardiol* 30[5]:1374–1383, 1997.)

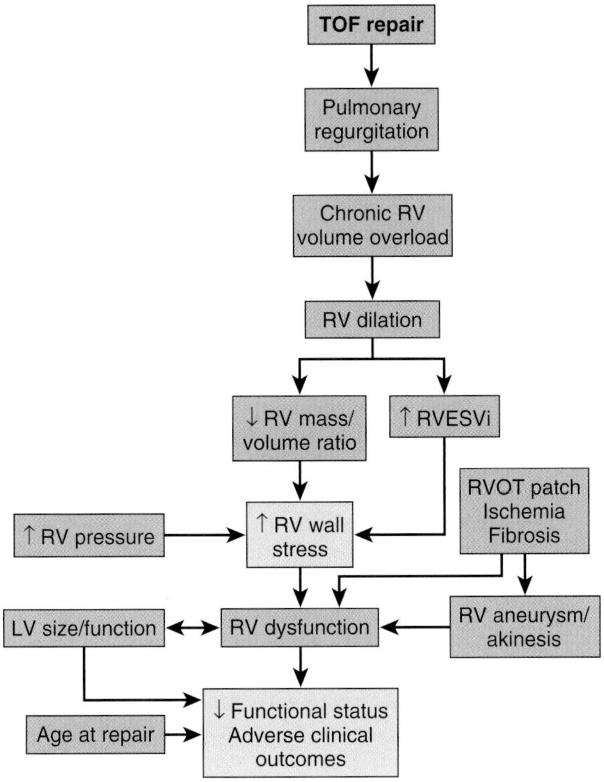

FIGURE 131-6 ■ Factors influencing right ventricular (RV) dysfunction and impaired clinical status after tetralogy of Fallot (TOF) repair. *LV,* Left ventricle; *RVESVi,* right ventricular end-systolic volume index; *RVOT,* right ventricular outflow tract. (Adapted from Geva T: Indications and timing of pulmonary valve replacement after tetralogy of Fallot repair. *Semin Thorac Cardiovasc Surg Pediatr Card Surg Annu* 11–22, 2006.)

in the United Kingdom and found that older age of repair and QRS duration 180 ms were independent predictors of sudden death. The major hemodynamic abnormality in these patients was the presence of at least moderate pulmonary regurgitation.[69] Chronic right ventricular volume overload can also dilate the tricuspid valve annulus with resultant tricuspid valve regurgitation. Progressive tricuspid valve regurgitation can accelerate right ventricular contractile failure and right atrial dilation, which is associated with increased prevalence of atrial arrhythmias.[69] Adults with repaired TOF commonly have cardiac issues that are not present in childhood, such as progressive aortic root dilation, which is present in at least 15% of adults with repaired TOF. This aortic root dilation may lead to aortic insufficiency.[70] Left ventricular dysfunction is associated with impaired clinical status and increased risk of sudden cardiac death.[67,71] Additionally, multiple other organ systems may be affected, and it is not uncommon for ACHD patients with repaired TOF to have renal, hepatic, and pulmonary comorbidities.

In considering an ACHD TOF patient for further surgery, investigation into any heart rhythm disturbances is critical. Programmed ventricular stimulation provides reasonably good predictive information on the risk of future clinical ventricular tachycardia.[72] A positive study may prompt either catheter ablation of the ventricular tachycardia circuit or implantable cardioverter defibrillator placement. Myocardial fibrosis, as demonstrated by gadolinium-enhanced CMR, has been significantly associated with clinical arrhythmia in adults with repaired TOF.[73] Rarely, adults with repaired TOF may have intra-atrial reentrant tachycardia (atrial flutter) or atrial fibrillation from chronic atrial dilation. Definitive elimination can often be achieved with a combined right and left atrial maze procedure, which can be performed during a surgery that is addressing residual hemodynamic issues.

An important question in the care of ACHD patients is the timing of pulmonary valve replacement (PVR) after TOF repair. Multiple factors can contribute to the progression of pulmonary regurgitation, including increasing capacitance of the pulmonary artery, right ventricular dilation, and increased right ventricular compliance.[74]

The decision regarding timing of PVR after TOF repair should involve consideration of the benefit of right ventricular volume reduction prior to irreversible dysfunction and the risk of subsequent valve failure and need for repeat intervention. Although there are few controlled or randomized data suggesting optimal timing of PVR for residual pulmonary regurgitation after repair of TOF, Geva has proposed the following clinical criteria in combination with CMR criteria to use in the decision making of PVR in the asymptomatic patient with repaired TOF.[75]

Repaired TOF with at least 25% pulmonary regurgitation fraction as measured by CMR and two or more of the following criteria:

1. Right ventricular (RV) end-diastolic volume index > 150 mL/m² (z-score > 4); in patients whose body surface area falls outside published normal data, RV/left ventricular (LV) end-diastolic volume ratio > 2
2. RV end-systolic volume index ≥ 80 mL/m²
3. LV ejection fraction < 55%
4. RV ejection fraction < 47%
5. Large RV outflow tract (RVOT) aneurysm
6. QRS duration > 140 ms
7. Sustained tachyarrhythmia related to right heart volume load

8. Other hemodynamically significant lesions such as RVOT obstruction with RV systolic pressure > 2/3 systemic, severe branch PA stenosis, moderate to severe tricuspid regurgitation, residual atrial or ventricular septal defects with a Qp/Qs > 1.5, and severe aortic dilation or regurgitation

The operative mortality for PVR after TOF repair is low (about 1%).[76] However, a continued low risk of death remains after PVR. Of 70 adults with TOF, Therrien reported a survival rate of 92% at 5 years and 86% at 10 years, after PVR.[77] The longevity of the valve must also be considered, because there is a wide variation in the rates of freedom from valve failure and reoperation, depending on type of valve and patient age.

Patients with TOF who undergo PVR generally have symptomatic improvement with a decrease in right ventricular end-diastolic and end-systolic volumes without significant change in the right ventricular ejection fraction.[78-80] Additionally, there is evidence that exercise performance tends to improve after PVR.[81]

Ebstein Anomaly

Ebstein anomaly is a congenital malformation of the tricuspid valve and right ventricular sinus. It is a rare disorder, accounting for about 1% of all congenital heart defects.[82] It was first described in 1866 in a 19-year-old laborer with severe tricuspid regurgitation caused by a severely malformed tricuspid valve. Ebstein anomaly is characterized by several morphologic features, which have varying degrees of severity. The pathogenesis involves failure of delamination of the septal and posterior leaflets of the tricuspid valve, resulting in adherence of the tricuspid valve leaflets to the ventricular myocardium. This results in apical displacement of the functional tricuspid valve annulus and dilation of the "atrialized" portion of the right ventricle. There are varying degrees of hypertrophy and thinning of the right ventricular wall, dilation of the true tricuspid valve annulus, and often fenestrations, redundancy, and tethering of the anterior leaflet. These abnormalities result in varying degrees of tricuspid regurgitation and ventricular dysfunction. Although patients with Ebstein anomaly share common features, no two cases are identical, and there is a great deal of variability in morphology.[83] This must be taken into consideration whenever surgical intervention is considered.

The tricuspid valve leaflets are often markedly dysplastic in severe cases. The incomplete fibrous transformation of leaflets results in a downward displacement of the hinge point of the posterior and septal leaflets in a spiral fashion below the true valve annulus. The valve leaflets may be tethered by short chordae and papillary muscles or attached to the myocardium directly or by muscular bands. Fenestrations of the leaflets are common, and chordae may be sparse or absent. In the most severe cases, the septal leaflet is a ridge of fibrous tissue that is directed toward the ventricular apex, the posterior leaflet consists of a few remnants of leaflet tissue near the apex, and the anterior leaflet may be displaced into the right ventricular outflow tract. The anterior leaflet leading edge is particularly important in determining the feasibility of tricuspid valve repair. The leading edge may be free and mobile, have hyphenated attachments (focal, segmental direct attachments to the underlying myocardium), or have linear direct attachments (entire leading edge attached to the endocardium). Varying degrees of right atrial and ventricular dilation may be present. With severe right ventricular dilation, the ventricular septum is displaced and the left ventricle may be compressed with resultant left ventricular dysfunction.[84]

Associated cardiac lesions include interatrial shunts, patent foramen ovale or ASDs, pulmonary valve stenosis or atresia, and, rarely, ventricular noncompaction. Interatrial shunts are often associated with right-to-left shunting and arterial desaturation. There is a risk of paradoxical embolism and stroke in this setting. Additionally, up to 20% of patients with Ebstein anomaly may have Wolff-Parkinson-White syndrome.[85] The accessory pathway is typically located along the posterior and septal aspect of the tricuspid ring. As many as half of these patients have more than one accessory pathway.

Ebstein anomaly of the left-sided atrioventricular valve is commonly seen in patients with physiologically corrected transposition of the great arteries. The systemic (morphologically tricuspid) atrioventricular valve is associated with the left-sided systemic morphologic right ventricle. The nature of the displacement of this valve is similar to right-sided Ebstein anomaly, but the anterior leaflet is often smaller. The functional right ventricle and tricuspid valve annulus are very rarely severely dilated.

The diagnosis of Ebstein anomaly is confirmed by two-dimensional echocardiography with the septal leaflet at the crux of the heart demonstrating apical displacement of 0.8 cm/m^2 or greater. Three-dimensional echocardiography can be particularly helpful in examining the morphology of the tricuspid valve leaflets (Fig. 131-7). CMR is useful for determining ventricular volumes and function, as well as visualization of the position of the tricuspid valve[86] (Fig. 131-8). The technique of delayed enhancement CMR can identify ventricular fibrosis[87] in these patients, which has been reported in both right and left ventricular myocardium of patients with Ebstein anomaly.

Patients with mild Ebstein anomaly may live normal life spans, and asymptomatic patients without right-to-left shunting or significant cardiomegaly may be managed medically and may not require surgical intervention. However, many adults living with congenital heart disease do not recognize their limited exercise capacity and may not report their limitations. In a study of 21 adults with Ebstein anomaly, exercise capacity was significantly reduced compared with controls (peak oxygen consumption 21.9 ± 5.4 versus 33.6 ± 8.3 mL/kg/min; P = 0.000001). All of these adults considered themselves to be in NYHA class I (71%) or class II (29%); however, objective cardiopulmonary stress testing indicated considerable reduction in the exercise performance of this group.[88]

Several factors should promote consideration of surgery. These include increasing symptoms with decreasing exercise tolerance, cyanosis, documented paradoxical embolism, progressive cardiomegaly, right ventricular dilation or dysfunction, and progression of atrial or ventricular arrhythmias. A biventricular repair is usually possible; however, in cases of severe right ventricular

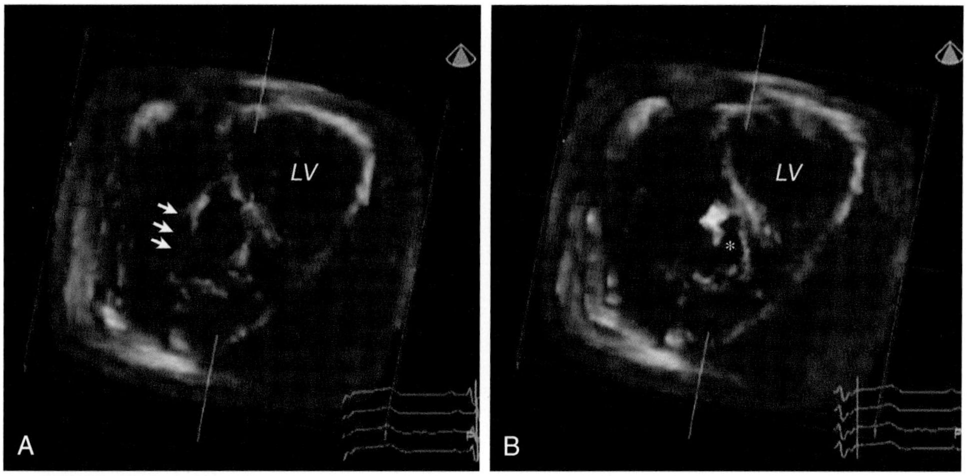

FIGURE 131-7 ■ **A,** Three-dimensional echocardiographic image of Ebstein anomaly in diastole demonstrates the redundant anterior leaflet of the tricuspid valve *(arrows)* with diminutive septal leaflet. **B,** Three-dimensional echocardiogram in systole illustrates failure of tricuspid valve coaptation *(*)*. *LV,* Left ventricle. (From Valente A: Adult congenital heart disease. In Libby P, editor: *Essential atlas of cardiovascular disease,* Philadelphia, 2009, Springer/Current Medicine Group.)

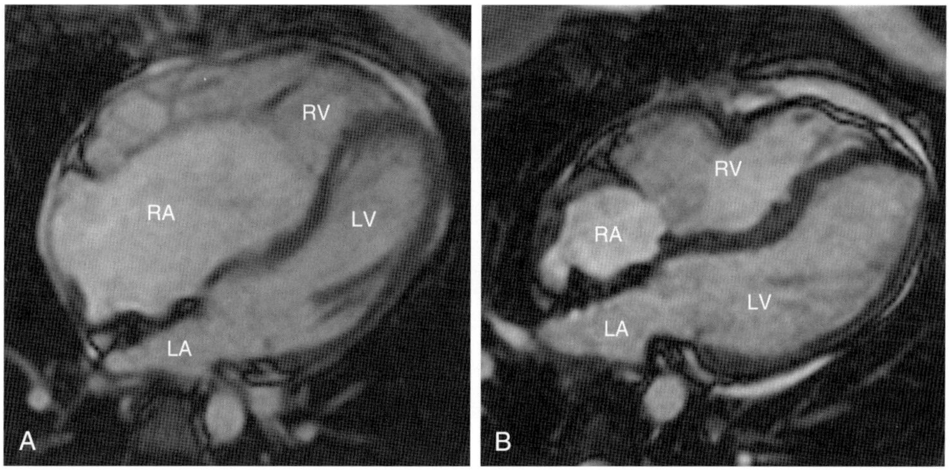

FIGURE 131-8 ■ Woman, 42 years old, with Ebstein anomaly and previous closure of an atrial septal defect with a CardioSEAL device. **A,** Cine magnetic resonance imaging (MRI) four-chamber view demonstrates how failure of delamination of the tricuspid valve septal leaflet results in apical displacement of its hinge point. **B,** Cine MRI in the four-chamber view in the same patient performed 1 year after tricuspid valvuloplasty. There is marked improvement in the right heart dilation. *LA,* Left atrium; *LV,* left ventricle; *RA,* right atrium; *RV,* right ventricle.

dysfunction with preserved left ventricular function, a bidirectional cavopulmonary shunt may be considered.[89] Cardiac transplantation is a rare option usually reserved for cases with severe left ventricular dysfunction.

Surgical repair most often involves tricuspid valve repair or replacement. Factors that are favorable for a valve repair include a large, mobile anterior leaflet with a free leading edge. The presence of leaflet tethering, presence of tricuspid valve leaflet tissue in the right ventricular outflow tract or direct insertion of the papillary muscle head into the leading edge of the anterior leaflet makes repair more difficult. Leaflets that have extensive hyphenated attachments or linear attachment of the leading edge to the underlying endocardium are not appropriate for repair. The Mayo Clinic authors reported that if more than 50% of the anterior leaflet has failure of delamination, valve replacement is preferred.[83]

Many modifications have been made to the original valvuloplasty described by Hunter and Lillehei.[90] The original repairs created a monocuspid valve, and whereas subsequent adaptations focused on trying to create a two-or-three leaflet valve, most recent technical modifications have focused on monocusp creation with "cone" repair. The principle underlying the cone repair is redistribution of redundant anterior and posterior leaflet to re-create a septal leaflet that is attached to the true annulus, along with annular reduction. Compared with conventional repair techniques, cone repair is associated with more significant reduction in tricuspid regurgitation.[91] When the valve cannot be adequately repaired, a bioprosthetic valve is implanted. Care must be taken to avoid damage to the conduction system, and the suture line is deviated away from the atrioventricular node and membranous septum. The suture line may be deviated cephalad to the tricuspid valve annulus to avoid injury to the right coronary artery.

Considerations should also include closure of any interatrial communications, correction of other associated anomalies (e.g., pulmonary stenosis), possible plication of the atrialized portion of the right ventricle, and right atrial reduction. A right-sided maze procedure is usually performed, with or without cryoablation of the right atrial isthmus. A left-sided maze is completed in the setting of left atrial enlargement or atrial fibrillation. Occasionally, surgical treatment of accessory conduction pathways is performed. Patients with Ebstein anomaly and arrhythmia show substantial improvement after surgical intervention; however, arrhythmias are not totally abolished. In a study of 45 adults with preoperative arrhythmias who had undergone Ebstein surgery, 39% of the surviving cohort continued to have arrhythmias.[92]

The largest experience of surgical outcomes in patients with Ebstein anomaly has been reported from the Mayo Clinic. The mean age at the time of initial operation at the Mayo Clinic was 24 years, and 26.5% of the patients had undergone a prior cardiac procedure. Late survival was 84.7% at 10 years and 71.2% at 20 years. Risk factors for poor outcome included right and/or left ventricular systolic dysfunction, increased hemoglobin levels, male sex, hypoplastic pulmonary arteries, and right ventricular outflow tract obstruction.[93] Hospitalizations were common even after surgical intervention, with the arrhythmias being the most common admitting diagnosis (≈39%). One third of patients continued to report fatigue and shortness of breath.[94]

Single-Ventricle Physiology and Fontan Surgery

Univentricular hearts are rare congenital anomalies, comprising approximately 1% of all congenital heart defects at birth.[95] The prognosis without surgical intervention in childhood is poor, although, in rare cases, patients with well-balanced circulations survive with reasonable functional capacity into adulthood.[96]

The physiology in infancy depends on several factors, including obstruction to ventricular inflow and outflow, flow across the interatrial septum, systemic and pulmonary venous return, and atrioventricular valve regurgitation. Surgical repair in childhood often involves several staged procedures. An initial palliation with a shunt may be performed, with the ultimate goal of a Fontan physiology.

The Fontan operation was developed in 1971 for palliation of tricuspid valve atresia.[97] Since that time, several modifications have been performed with the goal of directing systemic venous return directly to the pulmonary arteries without an interposing ventricle. The classic Fontan operation consisted of a valved conduit between the right atrium and main pulmonary artery.[97] Many of the current adults with single-ventricle physiology have a modified classic Fontan, which involves a direct anastomosis of the right atrium to the pulmonary artery. The next major modification, often referred to as a lateral tunnel, involved creation of an end-to-side anastomosis of the SVC to the undivided right pulmonary artery with an intra-atrial tunnel completed with a patch that tunnels the inferior vena caval blood through the tunnel to the transected SVC.[98] More recently, extracardiac conduits have been performed.[99]

At the time of Fontan surgery, an ASD may be created in the baffle to "fenestrate" the baffle to allow some right-to-left shunting in the case of elevated systemic venous pressure.[100] This fenestration can often be closed percutaneously later in life to eliminate this residual cause for cyanosis.[101] In an analysis of 261 patients with Fontan physiology with a mean age at follow-up of 25 years, actuarial event-free survival rates were 74.8% at 10 years, 68.3% at 20 years, and 53.6% at 25 years. The causes of death were determined to be thromboembolic, heart failure related, and sudden death.[102]

The potential complications that arise in the adult patient with previous Fontan surgery are multiple. Patients with the "older style" Fontans are particularly at risk for right atrial dilation (Fig. 131-9) with thrombus formation and atrial arrhythmias.[103] These two problems may lead to diminished cardiac output, reduced exercise capacity, and diminished quality of life. The strategy of Fontan conversion was introduced in the early 1990s in an effort to improve outcomes of adult survivors of atriopulmonary Fontan procedures.[104] The addition of intraoperative ablation has decreased arrhythmia recurrence [105] with the knowledge that as many as 50% of Fontan patients experience atrial tachycardia by 20 years of follow-up.[103] The goals of Fontan conversion are to excise a portion of the massively dilated right atrium and eliminate underlying atrial arrhythmias. The Fontan anatomy is reconstructed with a lateral tunnel or extracardiac conduit.[106]

Surgical considerations when evaluating a patient for possible Fontan conversion are multiple. These patients usually have undergone several previous sternotomies. They are often in a chronically low cardiac output state, and their output drops further with occurrence of atrial arrhythmias. Multisystem dysfunction involvement is common, including hepatic dysfunction,[107,108] renal dysfunction, and coagulation abnormalities. High central venous pressure leads to increased bleeding during sternal reentry. The electrophysiologic issues may be multiple, and coordination with an experienced electrophysiologist is crucial to success.[106] Risk factors for death, transplant, or dialysis include ventricular dysfunction, ischemic time greater than 100 minutes, age older than 25 years, more than mild atrioventricular valve regurgitation, cardiopulmonary bypass time greater than 240 minutes, and dominant right or indeterminate ventricular morphology.[106]

Deal and colleagues reported their experience with Fontan conversion surgery and 117 patients. Late mortality was 5.9% and attributed to intractable heart failure, coronary artery disease, discontinuation from renal dialysis, injury following motor vehicle accident, and sudden death after sedation administration. The overall arrhythmia recurrence was 12.8% during a mean follow-up of 56 months.[109]

SUMMARY

Adult congenital heart surgery is a growing discipline with increasing clinical relevance. Many ACHD patients are at risk for poor outcomes because of the natural progression of uncorrected defects and/or

leads required, and once implanted, leads could stretch as the child grows, increasing the risk that the leads will later dislodge or fracture. A review of indications and techniques for optimal surgical placement of electrophysiologic devices in the pediatric population is presented.

Pacemakers

The recommendations for permanent pacing in children and patients with CHD are updated regularly. The last update was a practice guideline published in 2012 jointly by the American Heart Association (AHA), the American College of Cardiology Foundation (ACCF), and the Heart Rhythm Society (HRS), and its recommendations are listed in Box 132-1.[2] A class I indication for pacing exists for atrioventricular (AV) block that persists for more than 7 days after cardiac surgery. (The 7-day cutoff is the starting point, with longer waits for very small or unstable patients who have adequate backup temporary pacing.) The recommendations put special emphasis on age-appropriate heart rates and the presence of CHD or ventricular dysfunction to guide treatment decisions.

Additional indications for permanent pacing may not be as obvious as those listed in the AHA/ACCF/HRS guidelines. If a child with a congenital heart defect requires surgery, it may be prudent to preemptively implant a pulse generator or epicardial leads during the surgery. This can benefit children with preoperative rhythm abnormalities who do not meet the indications listed in Box 132-1, but for whom pacing will be needed postoperatively based on the known natural history of a particular cardiac anomaly or type of surgery. For example, an infant with L-transposition of the great arteries (L-TGA) undergoing ventricular septal defect closure is at risk for complete AV block, even without cardiac surgery, and may benefit from prophylactic epicardial lead placement. Such placement can also assist children undergoing Fontan revision surgery in conjunction with an atrial maze procedure that is likely to result in sinus node dysfunction.[3] Careful preoperative screening with 24-hour Holter monitors and electrocardiography (ECG) can help to select the patients who would benefit from prophylactic epicardial lead placement.

BOX 132-1 Recommendations for Permanent Pacing in Children, Adolescents, and Patients with Congenital Heart Disease

Class I

1. Advanced second- or third-degree AV block associated with symptomatic bradycardia, ventricular dysfunction, or low cardiac output. (Level of evidence: C)
2. Sinus node dysfunction with correlation of symptoms during age-inappropriate bradycardia. The definition of bradycardia varies with the patient's age and expected heart rate. (Level of evidence: B)
3. Postoperative advanced second- or third-degree AV block that is not expected to resolve or that persists at least 7 days after cardiac surgery. (Level of evidence: B)
4. Congenital third-degree AV block with a wide QRS escape rhythm, complex ventricular ectopy, or ventricular dysfunction. (Level of evidence: B)
5. Congenital third-degree AV block in the infant with a ventricular rate less than 55 beats/min or with congenital heart disease and a ventricular rate less than 70 beats/min. (Level of evidence: C)

Class IIa

1. Congenital heart disease and sinus bradycardia for the prevention of recurrent episodes of intra-atrial reentrant tachycardia; sinus node dysfunction may be intrinsic or secondary to antiarrhythmic treatment. (Level of evidence: C)
2. Congenital third-degree AV block beyond the first year of life with an average heart rate less than 50 beats/min, abrupt pauses in ventricular rate that are two or three times the basic cycle length, or associated with symptoms resulting from chronotropic incompetence. (Level of evidence: B)
3. Sinus bradycardia with complex congenital heart disease with a resting heart rate less than 40 beats/min or pauses in ventricular rate longer than 3 seconds. (Level of evidence: C)
4. Congenital heart disease and impaired hemodynamics because of sinus bradycardia or loss of AV synchrony. (Level of evidence: C)
5. Unexplained syncope in the patient with prior congenital heart surgery complicated by transient complete heart block with residual fascicular block after a careful evaluation to exclude other causes of syncope. (Level of evidence: B)

Class IIb

1. Transient postoperative third-degree AV block that reverts to sinus rhythm with residual bifascicular block. (Level of evidence: C)
2. Congenital third-degree AV block in asymptomatic children or adolescents with an acceptable rate, a narrow QRS complex, and normal ventricular function. (Level of evidence: B)
3. Asymptomatic sinus bradycardia after biventricular repair of congenital heart disease with a resting heart rate less than 40 beats/min or pauses in ventricular rate longer than 3 seconds. (Level of evidence: C)

Class III

1. Transient postoperative AV block with return of normal AV conduction in the otherwise asymptomatic patient. (Level of evidence: B)
2. Asymptomatic bifascicular block with or without first-degree AV block after surgery for congenital heart disease in the absence of prior transient complete AV block. (Level of evidence: C)
3. Asymptomatic type I second-degree AV block. (Level of evidence: C)
4. Asymptomatic sinus bradycardia with the longest relative risk interval less than 3 seconds and a minimum heart rate greater than 40 beats/min. (Level of evidence: C)

AV, Atrioventricular.

Epicardial pacing, the predominant method of pediatric pacing until relatively recently, is now used mainly for patients in whom transvenous pacing is contraindicated or who are undergoing concomitant heart surgery. Some of the contraindications to transvenous pacing include prosthetic tricuspid valves, right-to-left intracardiac shunts, CHD or surgery precluding transvenous access to the cardiac chambers, and small patient size.[4] Although there are no absolute technical limitations to a transvenous route except in premature infants, venous capacitance and lead failure resulting from growth are important considerations. Although each institution should make individual decisions on the basis of local procedural capabilities and experience, we generally consider transvenous pacemaker implants in children weighing more than 10 kg.

Epicardial leads are available with sutureless (screw-on) or suture-on methods of fixation. Alternatively, a standard transvenous lead can be used in postoperative CHD patients with epicardial scarring. The transvenous lead can be placed using a transmural technique, with the lead passed through the myocardial wall and attached to the endocardium.[5] The steroid-eluting suture-on epicardial leads are our preferred lead, because the steroid can suppress the subacute threshold rise resulting from tissue inflammatory response. Several studies have shown that these steroid-eluting leads have good intermediate-term performance, with stable acute and chronic pacing and sensing thresholds and longevity similar to transvenous leads.[6-9] However, screw-on leads may be preferable for patients who have undergone prior heart surgery, as the depth of scarring can hinder suture-on techniques.

Bipolar pacing is particularly advantageous in patients with abdominal muscle stimulation, those at risk for phrenic nerve stimulation, and those with oversensing problems. Bipolar steroid-eluting suture-on epicardial leads are available, or two unipolar sutureless leads can be joined together into a bipolar pulse generator.

The surgical access can be from a midline sternotomy, a left thoracotomy, or a subxiphoid approach or via video-assisted thoracoscopy.[10] Each method has advantages, but the aim is to allow implantation of the proper number of leads in an individual patient. Finding an optimal site for maintenance of acceptable long-term pacing and sensing thresholds can be difficult because of bleeding, limited myocardial access, myocardial scarring, and pericardial adhesions. In patients with prior extensive right atrial (RA) surgery, left atrial pacing sites and the Bachmann bundle in general have better chronic pacing and sensing thresholds than do right lateral or anterior atrial sites.[11] A left thoracotomy can be used for implantation of left atrial epicardial leads in children with CHD.[12] In small infants, short leads (15-25 cm) should be used because long leads left in the pericardial space can ensnare the heart, as noted in several case reports of cardiac strangulation or constriction of a great vessel by pacing leads.[13,14]

The site of pacing is being recognized as an important determinant of ventricular performance. The systemic ventricle is the chamber of choice to pace and best if it is performed in an apical location.[15] Annular and high outflow tract locations produce worse dyssynchrony. The effects of pacing site on ventricular performance depend on baseline ventricular function. If ventricular dysfunction is present, it is better to expand the surgical entry access than to pace at a site known to produce ventricular dysfunction.

Once the leads are placed and tested, the pacemaker is typically set in a subrectus pocket, but in very small infants (<3 kg), the generator and leads can be left in the pleural cavity. Although uncommon, the abdominal-positioned generators can migrate into the pericardium,[16] peritoneum,[17] or pelvic space—a complication most often seen in very small infants.

Cardiac Resynchronization Therapy

Biventricular pacing is a treatment used in patients with symptomatic drug-refractory heart failure secondary to dilated cardiomyopathy and associated interventricular conduction delay or dyssynchrony. The aim of cardiac resynchronization therapy (CRT) treatment is to correct AV asynchrony, nonuniformity of ventricular activation, contraction, and relaxation sequences, while providing sequences that are as homogeneous as possible. The data in children for this therapy consist of retrospective reviews rather than the randomized trials seen in adults.

Indications for CRT are well established for adults with normal cardiac anatomy, but not for children and patients with CHD.[18,19] The standard adult indication for CRT is a QRS duration of greater than 120 msec, an ejection fraction less than 35%, and class II heart failure. Unfortunately, this combination rarely occurs in children. Although 90% of adults meeting these criteria have left bundle branch block, it is more common in patients with CHD such as tetralogy of Fallot to have right bundle branch block and right ventricular (RV) dysfunction. Thus standard criteria for CRT rarely are applicable in the CHD population. CRT in CHD is thus used mainly in cases of poor ventricular function and increased QRS duration (>120 msec) regardless of the QRS morphology.

Types of CRT available are biventricular, dual site, multisite, and temporary. In biventricular pacing, two distinct ventricles are present, with a pacing lead on each ventricle. If two sites on the same ventricle are paced, then it is called *dual-site pacing*. When the systemic ventricle is a single ventricle, then dyssynchrony can be decreased by pacing two widely separate sites on the same ventricle, a maneuver called *multisided pacing*. For children, temporary CRT has been used to improve cardiac output in the early postoperative setting.[20,21]

Implantable Cardioverter-Defibrillators

Indications for implantable cardioverter-defibrillator (ICD) implantation are listed in Box 132-2. The majority of ICDs are implanted via the transvenous route, but this might not be possible in small patients or those with anatomic constraints. Because ICD leads are larger and prone to fibrosis at the coils, patient size limitations for a transvenous system are different from those for a pacemaker. We try to limit transvenous ICD implantation to children who weigh more than 30 kg.

BOX 132-2 Recommendations for ICD Therapy in Children, Adolescents, and Patients with Congenital Heart Disease

Class I

1. ICD implantation is indicated in the survivor of cardiac arrest after evaluation to define the cause of the event and to exclude any reversible causes. (Level of evidence: B)
2. ICD implantation is indicated for patients with symptomatic sustained VT in association with congenital heart disease who have undergone hemodynamic and electrophysiologic evaluation.

Catheter ablation or surgical repair may offer possible alternatives in carefully selected patients. (Level of evidence: C)

Class IIa

1. ICD implantation is reasonable for patients with congenital heart disease with recurrent syncope of undetermined origin in the presence of either ventricular dysfunction or inducible ventricular arrhythmias at electrophysiologic study. (Level of evidence: B)

Class IIb

1. ICD implantation may be considered for patients with recurrent syncope associated with complex congenital heart disease and advanced systemic ventricular dysfunction when thorough invasive and noninvasive investigations have failed to define a cause. (Level of evidence: C)

Class III

1. ICD therapy is not indicated for patients who do not have a reasonable expectation of survival with an acceptable functional status for at least 1 year, even if they meet ICD implantation criteria specified in the class I, IIa, and IIb recommendations above. (Level of evidence: C)
2. ICD therapy is not indicated for patients with incessant VT or VF. (Level of evidence: C)
3. ICD therapy is not indicated in patients with significant psychiatric illnesses that may be aggravated by device implantation or that may preclude systematic follow-up. (Level of evidence: C)
4. ICD therapy is not indicated for NYHA class IV patients with drug-refractory congestive heart failure who are not candidates for cardiac transplantation or CRT-D. (Level of evidence: C)
5. ICD therapy is not indicated for syncope of undetermined cause in a patient without inducible ventricular tachyarrhythmias and without structural heart disease. (Level of evidence: C)
6. ICD therapy is not indicated when VF or VT is amenable to surgical or catheter ablation (e.g., atrial arrhythmias associated with the Wolff-Parkinson-White syndrome, right or left ventricular outflow tract VT, idiopathic VT, or fascicular VT in the absence of structural heart disease). (Level of evidence: C)
7. ICD therapy is not indicated for patients with ventricular tachyarrhythmias because of a completely reversible disorder in the absence of structural heart disease (e.g., electrolyte imbalance, drugs, or trauma). (Level of evidence: B)

CRT-D, Cardiac resynchronization therapy with defibrillator; *ICD*, implantable cardioverter-defibrillator; *NYHA*, New York Heart Association; *VF*, ventricular fibrillation; *VT*, ventricular tachycardia.

Epicardial patches were once used regularly, but they were prone to breakage, infection, and pericardial restriction. Newer techniques use coils placed in subcutaneous or pericardial positions.[22] The implantation can be performed as a hybrid procedure using a epicardial or transvenous sensing lead or as a completely subcutaneous system using a far-field electrogram for sensing. The three coil types currently available for hybrid procedures are the subcutaneous coil, superior vena cava (SVC) coil, and standard transvenous lead. The completely subcutaneous system is best used in patients with large body habitus and normal cardiac situs or those without transvenous access to the heart.[23] In young children, there have been issues of both ventricular oversensing and undersensing in addition to pocket erosion.[24]

Because of the smaller surface area of the coils and the thoracic structure interference, proper can and lead placement is essential to obtain adequate defibrillation thresholds. To achieve the lowest defibrillation energy requirements, it is best if the center of the ventricular mass is between the coil and the can. The coil should not enter the pacemaker pocket, because this can result in a short circuit and device failure.

The two basic approaches used for nontransvenous ICD implantation are a minimally invasive approach and a full exposure via sternotomy or thoracotomy. The minimally invasive approach is preferred for patients with no prior heart surgery.

In the basic implantation sequence, a bipolar epicardial pacing lead is first placed, followed by a coil in the pericardial or pleural cavity. When a minimally invasive procedure is used, an active fixation transvenous lead is placed blindly into the posterior pericardial space, followed by extension of the screw to hold the coil in a stable position. The pace or sense connector is then capped. Intraoperative fluoroscopy or portable chest radiography is used to confirm proper lead position. If full exposure of the heart is available, a 5-cm SVC coil can be sutured directly in position. In levocardia, the best configuration is a high left lateral lead and right subrectus pocket (Fig. 132-1). Finally, defibrillation testing is performed, and if the defibrillation threshold is inadequate, then a second coil (length, 25 or 5 cm) is placed in a subcutaneous or pericardial location on the opposite side.

Cardiac Sympathetic Denervation

Left cardiac sympathetic denervation (LCSD), also known as *left cervical stellate ganglionectomy*, was first described in 1971.[24a] Although LCSD is considered a highly effective method of surgical antiadrenergic therapy, its clinical use has been limited to a narrow set of indications. The procedure has been used primarily at a few centers for patients affected by the long QT syndrome (LQTS), and who are suboptimally controlled with standard medical therapy, usually consisting of beta-adrenergic

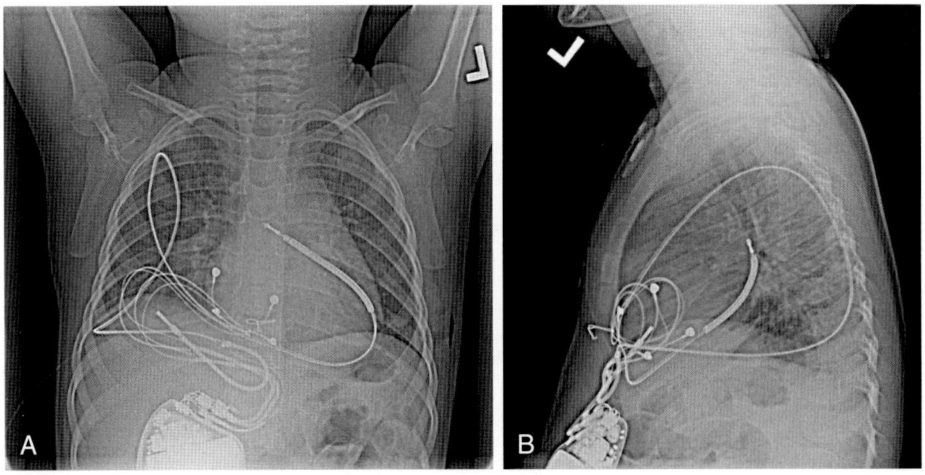

FIGURE 132-1 ■ Chest radiographs of an infant who underwent a minimally invasive nontransvenous cardioverter-defibrillator implantation. **A,** Anteroposterior view. **B,** Lateral view. Note the use of a standard transvenous lead in the pericardial cavity.

blocking medications. A recent multicenter report on a series of LQTS patients having undergone LCSD documented the efficacy of this intervention.[24b] It reported on 147 patients having undergone LCSD, with 99% having been symptomatic and 48% having suffered an aborted cardiac arrest before the operation. On a mean follow-up of 7.8 years after LCSD, 46% were asymptomatic and ICD shocks decreased by 95%.

A more recent and emerging indication is in patients with catecholaminergic polymorphic ventricular tachycardia (CPVT), a disorder of abnormal myocardial calcium homeostasis,[25] characterized by life-threatening ventricular arrhythmias triggered during states of high sympathetic output. Patients with CPVT typically have structurally and functionally normal hearts and a normal baseline electrocardiogram, including a normal QTc measurement.

The surgical technique used in performing the LCSD varies among centers.[24] Li and colleagues[26] reported the first small series of LQTS patients undergoing LCSD using the video-assisted thoracoscopic surgery (VATS) approach. We recently reported our experience[27,28] with 24 young pediatric patients who underwent high left thoracic sympathetic denervation using VATS, of whom 13 were diagnosed with LQTS, nine had CPVT, and two had idiopathic medically refractory ventricular tachycardia (VT). The LCSD procedure on all patients was performed by means of a left-sided VATS approach. After left lung isolation with a double-lumen endotracheal tube or the use of a bronchial blocker, the patient was positioned in a partial right lateral decubitus position. Three small stab incisions were made in the left side of the chest along the midaxillary line, with one incision at the level of the third intercostal space, one at the fourth, and one at the fifth. The first incision was used for the camera, the second for a grasper (or lung retractor if needed), and the third for the electrocautery hook dissector (Fig. 132-2*B*). After identifying the structures in the apex of the posterior chest wall and the heads of the ribs, the pleura was incised medial to the heads of the ribs, and the sympathetic chain was identified from the level of about T1 to T5 (see Fig. 132-2*A*). Using electrocautery, the sympathectomy involved transection of the left sympathetic chain at the level of T1, sparing the superior aspect of the stellate ganglion, and then at T5, as well as transection of the associated lateral nerves of Kuntz between those levels.

No severe complications were related to the procedure. Minor and transient postoperative complications occurred in only three patients. Only one patient experienced recurrent but transient arrhythmia in the immediate postoperative period. Longer-term follow-up was available in 22 of 24 patients at a median follow-up of 28 months (range, 4-131 months). Sixteen (73%) of the 22 patients experienced a marked reduction in their arrhythmia burden, with 12 (55%) becoming completely arrhythmia free after sympathectomy. Six (27%) of the patients were nonresponsive to treatment; each had persistent symptoms at follow-up.

This emerging early experience supports the use of cardiac sympathectomy as an effective adjunctive therapy that may be particularly useful for patients who are refractory or intolerant to medical therapy, as well as for patients who receive excessive ICD shocks. LCSD using VATS provides a minimally invasive approach that appears effective and safe, although longer-term follow-up is still required.

ARRHYTHMIA THERAPY IN ADULTS WITH CONGENITAL HEART DISEASE

The number of adult patients with CHD continues to increase. It is estimated that there are currently2 more than 1 million adults with CHD in the U.S., more than 100,000 in Canada, and 1.8 million in Europe.[28a,29] Many of these patients bear the weight of many decades of long-standing alterations in the volume- and pressure-loading conditions that result from their heterogeneous and often palliated anatomic arrangements. Approximately 50% are classified as having moderate or severe disease (e.g., tetralogy of Fallot, Ebstein anomaly,

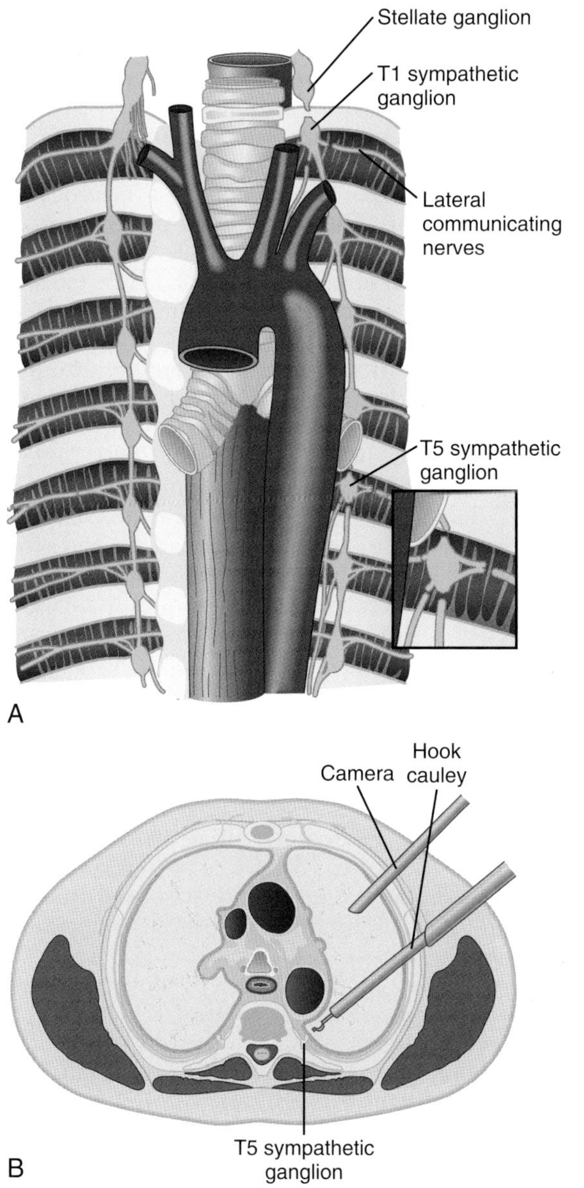

FIGURE 132-2 High left thoracic sympathetic denervation. **A,** The parietal pleura is scored with electrocautery at the T5 level, revealing the underlying left sympathetic chain, which runs along the posterior chest wall just medial to the heads of the ribs. **B,** The parietal pleural incision is carried up to the T1 level with electrocautery, and the sympathetic chain is divided at the T1 and the T5 level and then isolated by division of all lateral branches.

single-ventricle palliations). Although arrhythmias can develop with even mild disease, the incidence is highest for patients in the moderate and severe categories. As a result of the substantial and cumulative disease burden, cardiac arrhythmias late in life are a substantial source of morbidity, hospital admissions, and mortality for adults with CHD.[29] They exhibit the full spectrum of arrhythmia issues, and their complex management presents challenges that are often considerable and shared equally by cardiologist and cardiac surgeon.

Electrophysiologic Substrates in Congenital Heart Disease

Intra-atrial Reentrant Tachycardia (Atrial Flutter)

The most common mechanism for symptomatic tachycardia in the adult CHD population is macroreentry in atrial muscle.[30] The terms *intra-atrial reentrant tachycardia* (IART) and *incisional tachycardia* have become common labels for this arrhythmia, to distinguish it from the typical variety of atrial flutter that occurs in structurally normal hearts.[31-33] Generally, IART tends to be slower than typical flutter, with atrial rates in the range of 150 to 250 beats per minute. In the setting of a healthy AV node, such rates frequently conduct in a rapid 1 : 1 atrial-to-ventricular pattern that can result in hypotension, syncope, or possibly cardiac arrest.[34,35] Even if the ventricular response rate is safely titrated, sustained IART can cause debilitating symptoms in some patients from loss of AV synchrony, and it may contribute to thromboembolic complications[36] when the duration is protracted. Usually, IART appears many years after operations that involved an atriotomy or other surgical manipulation of RA tissue. It can follow simple procedures such as closure of an atrial septal defect on occasion, but the incidence is higher among patients with advanced dilation, thickening, and scarring of the right atrium.[37,38] Other risk factors for IART include concomitant sinus node dysfunction ("tachy-brady" syndrome) and older age at time of heart surgery.[39]

Thus, IART is a particular problem for older patients who have undergone the Mustard, Senning, or older-style Fontan operations, in which extensive suture lines and long-term hemodynamic stress result in markedly abnormal atrial myocardium. The route of propagation for an IART circuit varies according to the anatomic defect and type of surgical repair.[40] It is usually restricted to RA tissue (regardless of the surgical destination of this tissue) and is modulated by regions of fibrosis from suture lines or patches, which function in combination with natural conduction barriers (crista terminalis, valve orifices, and the superior and inferior caval orifices) to channel the wave front along a macro-reentrant loop.[41,42] If a tricuspid valve is present, the isthmus between the valve ring and the inferior vena cava is a common component of such circuits, but when the tricuspid valve is absent or otherwise deformed, the circuits follow less predictable paths that can be deciphered only by formal electrophysiologic mapping. Frequently, multiple IART circuits are present in the same patient.[43] Once recognized, IART can be terminated with electrical cardioversion, overdrive pacing maneuvers,[44] or administration of certain class I or III antiarrhythmic drugs.

The far more difficult task is prevention of recurrence. Multiple strategies have been developed for IART prevention, all of which can have value in certain patients, but none of which represents a universal solution. If the episodes are infrequent, well tolerated, and recognized promptly, it may be sufficient to rely on periodic cardioversion before embarking on more involved therapy. However, if IART episodes become frequent, cause significant symptoms, or are associated with atrial thrombus formation, aggressive treatment is indicated. The therapeutic options for IART include (1) antiarrhythmic drugs, (2) pacemaker implantation to correct bradycardia or provide automatic atrial antitachycardia pacing, (3) catheter ablation, and (4) surgical intervention with a modified atrial maze operation. The choice must be tailored to the hemodynamic and electrophysiologic status of the individual patient. Chronic antiarrhythmic drugs are still prescribed in some cases, but the broad experience with pharmacologic therapy for this condition has been discouraging,[34,45] even when potent agents such as amiodarone are used. Pacemaker implantation may be reasonable for patients with a picture of tachy-brady syndrome.[35] Pacemakers with advanced programming features that incorporate atrial tachycardia detection and automatic burst pacing to interrupt reentry may also be beneficial in select cases.[35,46] Catheter ablation is now used at many centers as an early intervention for IART.[47] The technique has evolved rapidly since the introduction of three-dimensional mapping for improved circuit localization.[31,48] When these technologies are combined with good anatomic definition and traditional electrophysiologic mapping maneuvers, short-term success rates of nearly 90% can be achieved.

Unfortunately, later tachycardia recurrence is still disappointingly common. The recurrence risk is particularly high (nearly 40%) among Fontan patients, who tend to have the largest number of IART circuits and the thickest or largest atrial dimensions. Although far from perfect, ablation outcomes for IART are likely to improve with continued experience and even now are far superior to the degree of control obtained with medications alone. Furthermore, even if IART episodes are not eliminated entirely by ablation, the procedure can often provide substantial improvement by reducing the frequency of episodes and eliminating the need for ongoing drug therapy.[48] If these measures fail to prevent IART, or if the patient is returning to the operating room for hemodynamic reasons, consideration should be given to surgical ablation during an RA maze operation. This procedure is used most often for the Fontan population with the most refractory variety of IART, and it is usually combined with revision of the Fontan connection from an older atriopulmonary anastomosis to a modern cavopulmonary connection in the same setting.[49]

The Fontan operation for patients with a single ventricle results in extensive suture lines and abnormal hemodynamics that predispose patients to atrial tachycardias and sinus node dysfunction. Up to 50% of patients with a single ventricle who have undergone older-style Fontan operations develop atrial tachycardia within a decade of surgery. Fontan conversion has been proposed for patients suffering from a variety of late sequelae, including conduit and vascular obstruction, atrial arrhythmias, protein-losing enteropathy, and thrombotic complications. However, documented benefits have been limited to a small number of centers and over short follow-up periods, compared with the relatively extensive data available on initial Fontan procedures.[50,51] Fontan conversion can provide symptomatic improvement in patients with late complications associated with this circulation, including atrial tachycardias.[52-54] Criteria for optimal patient selection and anticipated clinical outcomes remain controversial. Conversion alone does not appear to protect against recurrent atrial tachycardias,[55-57] whereas concomitant maze surgery can suppress postoperative tachycardia.[58-60] Several different surgical approaches have been reported in this heterogeneous patient population. The most recent series from eight centers that have reported outcomes on 10 or more patients have noted variable conversion failure rates, with an aggregate rate of death or transplantation of 8.4% in follow-up of a total of 203 patients.[53,54,61-67] Significant long-term morbidities, such as renal failure, thrombotic events, and arrhythmia, have likewise been reported.

At Children's Hospital Boston, 40 patients underwent Fontan conversion between 1990 and 2006, 21 (53%) with and 19 (48%) without concomitant arrhythmia surgery.[68] Table 132-1 summarizes baseline characteristics and surgical considerations in all patients and according to whether they had arrhythmia surgery. Clinical indications for conversion included surgically correctable anatomic lesions (n = 28), thrombi (n = 4), intracardiac right-to-left shunting (n = 4), and medically refractory atrial tachyarrhythmia (n = 29), with 16 patients having more than one indication. Four patients had protein-losing enteropathy. In the 39 patients with preoperative catheterization, the ventricular end-diastolic pressure was 9.8 (1.0-22.0) mm Hg, with four having values greater than 12 mm Hg. Preexisting atrial arrhythmias were present in 29 (73%) patients; 10 had macro-reentrant atrial tachyarrhythmia, and 19 had atrial fibrillation (paroxysmal in 12; persistent in 7). Surgical characteristics are summarized in Table 132-1. Twenty-two patients (55%) had a 4-mm fenestration at the time of conversion. Resection of a large portion of the anterior RA wall was performed on 20 patients (50%). All patients with a biatrial maze procedure had a preoperative history of atrial fibrillation. Of 19 patients with a history of AF, 10 underwent a full maze and four had a limited RA maze procedure. Eighteen patients (45%) had concomitant pacemaker implantation (including six with previously implanted devices), and six additional patients required pacemaker placement postoperatively. Perioperative complications, including bleeding, thrombosis, seizures, and renal dysfunction requiring peritoneal dialysis, were observed (Table 132-2).

Six failed conversions (five perioperative deaths, one transplantation) were seen during follow-up, for an overall rate of 15%. Survival was 84% at 3 years postoperatively. Probability of survival did not differ between the two groups, between operative eras, or by whether an extracardiac conduit or a lateral tunnel revision was performed. Univariate predictors for late postoperative arrhythmia are shown in Table 132-3. Arrhythmia interventions including RA debulking, maze procedure, and pacemaker implantation were associated with reduced risk for late postoperative arrhythmias and lower postoperative atrial tachyarrhythmia severity scores. No independent predictors of improved arrhythmia outcomes were identified.

Our experience, concordant with other reports, suggests that survivors of Fontan conversion experience an

TABLE 132-1 **Baseline Characteristics and Surgical Considerations**

Characteristic	All Conversions (*N* = 40)	Concomitant Arrhythmia Surgery Yes: Group 1 (*N* = 21)	Concomitant Arrhythmia Surgery No: Group 2 (*N* =19)	*P* Value
Age at Fontan conversion (yr)*	19.0 (13.0, 25.0)	22.0 (16.6, 31.0)	16.6 (11.3, 23.3)	0.005
Anatomic diagnosis, *N* (%)				NS
Tricuspid atresia	24 (60)	15 (71)	9 (47)	
Single left ventricle	7 (18)	1 (5)	6 (32)	
Other	9 (23)	5 (24)	4 (21)	
Type of original Fontan, *N* (%)				0.01
APC	26 (65)	14 (67)	12 (63)	
RA-RV	11 (28)	7 (33)	4 (21)	
LT	2 (5)	0	2 (11)	
ECC	1 (3)	0	1 (5)	
NYHA class before conversion, *N* (%)				NS
Class I	3 (8)	2 (10)	1 (5)	
Class II	23 (58)	12 (57)	11 (58)	
Class III	14 (35)	7 (33)	7 (37)	
Time from Fontan to conversion (yr)*	14.8 (2.8, 27.6)	16.8 (15.1, 20.3)	10.1 (5.2, 12.3)	<0.0001
Type of Fontan conversion, *N* (%)				0.01
LT	22 (55)	7 (33)	15 (79)	
ECC	16 (40)	14 (67)	2 (11)	
RA-RV	2 (5)	0 (0)	2 (11)	
Prior atrial tachycardia, *N* (%)	29 (73)	20 (95)	9 (47)	<0.001
Prior atrial fibrillation, *N* (%)	19 (48)	14 (67)	5 (26)	0.01
Prior catheter ablation, *N* (%)	13 (33)	13 (32)	0	<0.0001
Preoperative AT severity score	5.3 ± 3.7	7.3 ± 2.6	3.2 ± 3.6	0.0002
Class III anti-arrhythmic drug, *N* (%)	14 (35)	14 (67)	0	<0.0001
Concomitant arrhythmia surgery, *N* (%)				—
Limited RA maze	10 (25)	10 (48)	0	
Full maze	10 (25)	10 (48)	0	
Isthmus cryoablation alone	1 (3)	1 (5)	0	
Pacemaker implantation, *N* (%)	24 (58)	20 (95)	4 (21)	<0.001
Total bypass time, min	189 ± 76	217 ± 64	159 ± 79	0.02
Aortic cross-clamp time, min	57 ± 36	59 ± 36	55 ± 42	NS

*Non-normally distributed continuous variables are expressed as median (25th and 75th percentiles).
APC, Atriopulmonary connection; *AT,* atrial tachycardia; *ECC,* extracardiac connection; *LT,* lateral tunnel; *NS,* nonsignificant; *NYHA,* New York Heart Association; *RA,* right atrium; *RV,* right ventricle.

TABLE 132-2 **Perioperative Major Complications and Arrhythmia Status in 35 Early Operative Survivors**

	All Early Survivors (*N* = 35)	Concomitant Arrhythmia Surgery Yes: Group 1 (*N* = 18)	Concomitant Arrhythmia Surgery No: Group 2 (*N* = 17)	*P* Value
Major complication, *N* (%)	9 (26)	7 (39)	2 (12)	0.07
Intracranial hemorrhage	2 (6)	2 (11)	0	
Extensive bleeding	1 (3)	1 (6)	0	
Cerebrovascular event/seizure	3 (9)	3 (17)	0	
Thrombus	2 (6)	0	2 (12)	
Renal dysfunction	1 (3)	1 (6)	0	
Maximum serum creatinine (mg/dL)	1.2 ± 0.8	1.4 ± 1.0	1.0 ± 0.7	NS
Late atrial arrhythmia, *N* (%)	14 (40)	5 (28)	9 (53)	0.13
Atrial tachyarrhythmia severity score	3.5 ± 2.9	3.3 ± 3.0	3.7 ± 3.2	NS
Cardioversion, *N* (%)	8 (23)	4 (22)	4 (24)	NS
Subsequent catheter ablation, *N* (%)	3 (9)	1 (6)	2 (4)	NS
Antiarrhythmic drug (class III)	10 (29)	6 (33)	4 (24)	NS

improvement in functional status. However, it is our belief that this cannot be explained by overt hemodynamic improvement, because changes on postoperative catheterizations were often minimal and consistent with the effects of fenestration and, in some patients, simple relief of conduit obstruction. In patients with preoperative arrhythmia who undergo the maze procedure, decrease in tachycardia occurrence and relief from symptoms is substantial, but it is not universal. In addition, significant morbidities and mortality occur primarily in

TABLE 132-3 **Univariate Predictors for Late Postoperative Arrhythmia Status**

	Late Atrial Arrhythmia			Improvement of AT Severity Score		
	OR	95% CI	P Value	OR	95% CI	P Value
Preoperative						
Atrial fibrillation	1.1	0.3, 4.4	0.88	0.6	0.1, 2.2	0.41
Interval AT onset to conversion (yr)	1.00	1.00, 1.00	0.20	1.00	1.00, 1.00	0.48
Age at conversion (yr)	0.98	0.90, 1.06	0.72	0.98	0.89, 1.07	0.64
Time to conversion (yr)	1.00	1.00, 1,00	0.34	1.00	1.00, 1.00	0.93
Operative						
Right atrial debulking	0.3	0.1, 1.2	0.09	4.2	1.0, 18.1	0.05
Fenestration	2.0	0.5, 8.3	0.34	1.1	0.3, 4.3	0.89
Maze procedure	0.3	0.1, 1.1	0.07	3.6	0.9, 14.9	0.03
Full maze procedure	0.1	0.0, 1.0	0.05	1.5	0.3, 7.2	0.64
Pacemaker placement	0.2	0.0, 0.7	0.02	5.8	1.3, 25.4	0.02
Follow-up (yr)	1.00	1.00, 1.00	0.02	1.00	1.00, 1.00	0.03

AT, Atrial tachycardia; *CI,* confidence interval; *OR,* odds ratio.

the perioperative period and are more frequent in our series than in most other reported series. Finally, other than the unfavorable effect of older age at conversion, strong preoperative and procedural predictors of morbidity and mortality were not identified. In particular, the performance of a maze procedure was not associated with a greater risk, and it provided significant benefit to those patients with preoperative arrhythmia. Overall, our findings suggest that, although electrophysiologic and symptomatic improvement can be obtained with Fontan conversion, it is still unclear whether overall survival is favored by Fontan conversion.

Atrial Fibrillation

The principal hemodynamic derangement and site of surgical scarring in CHD tends to involve right heart structures, so that IART arising from the right atrium is by far the most common form of atrial tachycardia. However, chronic hemodynamic stress is directed toward the left atrium in a subset of CHD patients, and atrial fibrillation can occur as a result. The CHD lesions commonly associated with atrial fibrillation include aortic stenosis, mitral valve deformities, and unrepaired single ventricle.[69] Management principles are similar to those for atrial fibrillation encountered in other forms of adult heart disease, beginning with medical therapy for anticoagulation and ventricular rate control, followed by electrical or medical cardioversion. As with IART, terminating an isolated atrial fibrillation episode in CHD is not difficult, but prevention of recurrence remains a challenge. Antiarrhythmic drugs can offer long-term protection against recurrence for some patients, but as with IART, pharmacologic therapy has been only marginally successful for this purpose. Pacemaker implantation can reduce atrial fibrillation recurrences in patients with sinus node dysfunction when fibrillation is part of the tachy-brady syndrome. Definitive elimination of atrial fibrillation can be achieved with a combined right and left atrial maze operation, which should be considered if a patient requires surgery to address other hemodynamic issues.[70]

Accessory Pathways

The embryologic milieu responsible for congenital heart defects can have a direct effect on development of the conduction system. Sometimes this takes the form of simple displacement of the AV node and His bundle away from the usual septal position in the Koch triangle,[30] but occasionally the malformation results in accessory or duplicated AV connections with the potential for reentrant tachyarrhythmias. The most familiar example involves Ebstein anomaly of the tricuspid valve, which is complicated by Wolff-Parkinson-White syndrome in approximately 20% of cases.[71] The accessory pathways in Ebstein anomaly are typically located along the posterior and septal aspect of the tricuspid ring where the valve leaflets are most abnormal,[32] and nearly half of these patients are found to have multiple accessory pathways.[33,72] The same observations hold true for patients with L-TGA, who not infrequently have Ebstein malformation in association with accessory pathways along their left-side tricuspid valve. Tachycardia events for patients with Ebstein anomaly become increasingly problematic in adolescent and adult years, when atrial dilation increases the likelihood of recurrent atrial flutter or atrial fibrillation with potentially rapid anterograde conduction over the accessory pathways. Definitive therapy with catheter ablation is currently viewed as the standard of care for patients with Ebstein anomaly and Wolff-Parkinson-White syndrome. However, compared with ablation for simple accessory pathways in a structurally normal heart, the short-term success rate appears lower, and the risk of recurrence higher, with Ebstein anomaly.[37,38]

Ventricular Tachycardia

Serious ventricular arrhythmias are rare among CHD patients during their first decade or two of life, but once adulthood is reached, the potential for VT and sudden death becomes a looming concern in certain cases. Patients at greatest risk for developing VT appear to be those who have undergone a ventriculotomy or patching for certain types of ventricular septal defects. In this scenario, the mechanism for VT is reminiscent of the macroreentrant circuits described earlier for IART, involving narrow conduction corridors defined by regions of surgical scar[73,74] in conjunction with natural conduction barriers, such as the rim of a septal defect or the edge of a valve annulus. Less commonly, ventricular arrhythmias can develop independently of direct surgical scarring whenever a long-standing hemodynamic overload causes advanced degrees of ventricle dysfunction or hypertrophy. Examples of CHD lesions that can eventually lead to this myopathic variety of VT include (1) aortic valve disease,[75,76] (2) L-TGA when the right ventricle has been recruited as the systemic ventricle,[77] (3) severe Ebstein anomaly, (4) certain forms of single ventricle, (5) Eisenmenger syndrome, and (6) unrepaired tetralogy of Fallot.[78]

The bulk of literature and clinical experience regarding VT in CHD has centered on tetralogy of Fallot. The prevalence of VT after tetralogy repair has been estimated to be between 3% and 14% in several large clinical series.[46,79-83] Some patients with slow VT may be hemodynamically stable at presentation, but VT tends to be rapid for the majority, causing syncope or cardiac arrest to be the presenting symptom. Although rare cases of abrupt AV block or rapidly conducted IART have been linked to catastrophic outcomes in patients with tetralogy,[84] sustained VT appears to be the single biggest contributor to the incidence (2% per decade) of sudden cardiac death.[46,81,85-87]

Predicting VT events in patients with tetralogy has been a topic of intense investigation for nearly 30 years. To date, no perfect risk-stratification scheme has emerged, although several clinical variables with modest prognostic value have been identified, including (1) older age at time of definitive surgery, (2) history of palliative shunts, (3) high-grade ventricular ectopy, (4) inducible VT at electrophysiologic study, (5) abnormal RV hemodynamics, and (6) wide QRS width (180 msec). The correlation between QRS duration and VT[46,82] is not surprising when one considers that the most dramatic degree of QRS prolongation tends to be seen among tetralogy patients with highly dysfunctional and dilated right ventricles. A recent cohort of 873 patients with tetralogy of Fallot from four large centers identified the following factors to be associated with death and sustained VT: RV mass-to-volume ratio ≥ 0.3 g/mL, left ventricle ejection fraction z-score < −2.0, history of atrial tachyarrhythmia and elevated RV systolic pressure.[87a]

When viewed in the aggregate, this long list of variables helps to define a clinical profile for the tetralogy patient at risk, but no single item can be viewed as completely independent, and none provides perfect predictive accuracy. To compensate for lack of specificity, the practical approach to VT risk stratification in older patients with tetralogy usually incorporates attention to symptom status. Certainly, any patient who has survived a cardiac arrest or sustained VT is treated aggressively, usually with an ICD.[88,89] However, in the absence of a serious clinical event, a careful inquiry for more subtle symptoms is often required to determine whether additional testing or treatment is needed.

At most centers, tetralogy patients who report concerning symptoms of palpitations, dizziness, or syncope usually undergo invasive evaluation with hemodynamic catheterization and an electrophysiology study. Programmed ventricular stimulation provides reasonably good predictive information on the risk of future clinical VT events.[90,91] A positive study may prompt implantation of a primary-prevention ICD,[80] or, if monomorphic VT can be induced and is tolerated long enough to permit mapping, catheter ablation of the VT circuit might be considered.[92-95] An electrophysiology study might also uncover IART as a contributing or confounding factor for a patient's symptoms, which could be addressed with ablation at the same time. Correctable hemodynamic issues could also be identified at catheterization and could shift therapy toward a surgical solution, such as relief of valve regurgitation combined with formal intraoperative VT mapping and ablation.[96]

The proper approach to an entirely asymptomatic adult with repaired tetralogy remains unsettled. Most clinicians rely on a yearly evaluation with history and ECG, supplemented regularly with Holter monitoring or exercise testing to screen for high-grade ventricular ectopy, along with periodic echocardiography or magnetic resonance imaging to monitor the status of the right ventricle. Should nonsustained VT be detected on surveillance monitoring in an asymptomatic patient, or should RV function appear to be deteriorating, opinions still vary widely as to the appropriate response. Some clinicians advocate an electrophysiologic study to refine the arrhythmia risk, some recommend pulmonary valve replacement, some prescribe antiarrhythmic drugs, some implant a primary prevention ICD, and some might refrain from any treatment as long as the patient remains symptom free. Therapy continues to be individualized for asymptomatic patients depending largely on institutional experience and philosophy. With few exceptions,[46,90] studies have been limited to single-center investigations with limited statistical power. Furthermore, because the event rate for sustained VT and sudden death in patients with CHD is low compared with conditions such as ischemic heart disease, the duration of prospective follow-up necessary to answer questions in the CHD field would probably have to extend beyond 10 years. Now that the population of adults with CHD at risk for VT has reached such a substantial size, the opportunity may finally have arrived for an organized assessment of VT management.

Sinoatrial Node Dysfunction in Patients with Congenital Heart Disease

Developmental defects involving the caval–atrial junction can be associated with atypical anatomy and function for the sinoatrial node. This issue is most relevant to complex forms of heterotaxy syndrome in patients with a single ventricle. In the asplenia variety of heterotaxy, bilateral superior caval veins often exist, each with its own sinoatrial node, which results in an interesting ECG pattern of fluctuation between two discrete P waves at physiologic rates. Apart from the unusual ECG, the coexistence of two sinus nodes is of minimal clinical consequence. In contrast, patients with the polysplenia type of heterotaxy may lack a true sinus node altogether, which makes atrial depolarization dependent on slower atrial or junctional escape rhythms.[56] Most patients with this rare condition will ultimately require pacemaker implantation. A more common cause of sinus bradycardia in adults with CHD is surgical trauma to the sinoatrial node or its artery, as can occur during the Mustard, Senning, Glenn, and Fontan operations.[30,39,97,98] Chronotropic incompetence is poorly tolerated in CHD patients with compromised hemodynamics, especially those with a single ventricle or AV valve regurgitation. The likelihood of a patient developing IART or atrial fibrillation is also increased significantly in this setting.[39] Implantation of a single- or dual-chamber pacing system is currently recommended[99] as a class I indication for any patient with CHD and sinoatrial node dysfunction who has symptoms directly attributable to slow heart rate. Pacemaker implantation is also advised as a class IIb indication for CHD patients with resting rates of 40 beats/min or sinus pauses in excess of 3 seconds, even in the absence of symptoms.

Atrioventricular Block in Congenital Heart Disease

The AV conduction tissues may be congenitally abnormal in terms of both location and function in specific forms of CHD, most notably L-TGA and endocardial cushion defects.[100-102] In the former condition, the AV node and His bundle are displaced in an anterior direction away from the usual position in the Koch triangle, whereas in the latter, the AV node and His bundle are displaced posterior to the Koch triangle. The functional properties of these displaced conduction systems are often abnormal. With L-TGA, it is estimated that 3% to 5% of patients will have complete AV block at birth, and an additional 20% will develop spontaneous complete block by adulthood.[103,104] Even when intrinsic conduction appears normal, these patients appear to be more susceptible to traumatic AV block during surgical or catheter procedures. Surgical repair of certain forms of CHD can result in direct trauma to the AV conduction tissues. Although improved knowledge of the precise location for the AV node and His bundle in various forms of CHD[30,61,101,105] has reduced the occurrence, closure of some ventricular septal defects, surgery for left-heart outflow obstruction, and replacement or repair of an AV valve may still be complicated by AV block. Fortunately, in more than half of cases, this injury is a transient affair related to myocardial stretch or edema rather than to the physical severing of the conduction tissues, and AV conduction recovers within 7 days of operation.[106] However, for any patient with postoperative AV block that is not expected to resolve or that persists at least 7 days after cardiac surgery, permanent pacemaker implantation is advised[99] as a class I indication. A pacemaker may be considered by some as a class IIb indication when surgical AV block recovers but the patient is left with permanent bifascicular block.[84]

Pacemaker and Cardioverter-Defibrillator Implantation in Adults with Congenital Heart Disease

Standard transvenous systems are often contraindicated or difficult in CHD patients because of complexities of venous anatomy or because of the presence of significant intracardiac shunting that creates a thromboembolic risk from intravascular leads. Epicardial implantation is often indicated in these circumstances, although the surgery is more involved, and long-term lead performance may be inferior to transvenous systems. Epicardial lead placement in an older patient with CHD who has undergone multiple prior cardiac operations presents the surgeon with a highly scarred mediastinum; dissection down to the myocardial surface must be performed carefully and deliberately to uncover sites with good sensing and pacing function. Careful preoperative planning is often critical, and it is imperative for the surgeon to review all the imaging studies available including chest radiographs, angiograms, and echocardiograms. Many older patients also have chest computed tomography images or magnetic resonance images that are particularly helpful in providing a roadmap for the anatomic relationships and ventricular geometry. After reviewing these studies, a surgeon can often tailor the surgical approach to minimize the need for a large reoperative procedure by using a partial lower median sternotomy incision or a carefully placed limited thoracotomy incision.

If a patient with CHD is undergoing cardiac surgery for other hemodynamic reasons and it appears highly likely that epicardial pacing might be needed at some distant date, the surgeon may want to take advantage of wide intraoperative exposure to place leads for future use and tunnel them under either subcostal region for later easy access. Fortunately, 86% of leads placed at the time of cardiac surgery are found to function well when retrieved at a mean of 252 days after the operation.[107] The indications for ICD implantation in CHD patients are still evolving, but in general they follow guidelines that are similar to those for other varieties of adult heart disease. The most common type of CHD that requires ICD implantation is tetralogy of Fallot, followed by L-TGA and left-sided obstructive diseases.[88,91] The experience with biventricular resynchronization pacing in CHD patients with depressed ventricular function is limited but promising.[108] Clinical studies are currently underway to refine selection criteria and to investigate the clinical merits of RV resynchronization to offset right bundle branch block after surgical closure of ventricular septal defects and tetralogy repair.

Whether a transvenous or an epicardial approach is being considered, careful preprocedural planning is essential for successful pacemaker or ICD implantation in adults with CHD. Some of these patients have anomalies of systemic venous return and the coronary veins. If pacing in the coronary sinus is needed for cardiac resynchronization or any other purpose, anomalies of the coronary sinus need to be considered, including ostial atresia,[109] unroofed coronary sinus, and extreme dilation caused by persistent left SVC. Venous occlusion is a recognized complication of permanent transvenous pacing

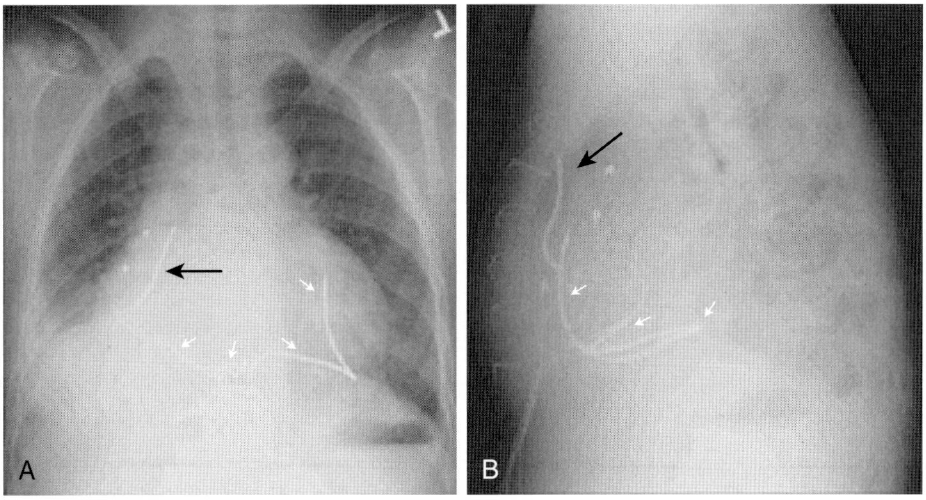

FIGURE 132-3 ■ Chest radiograph of an epicardial implantable cardioverter-defibrillator system in an adult in whom a Kawashima-type Fontan operation was performed for heterotaxy and double-outlet right ventricle. **A,** Posteroanterior projection. **B,** Lateral projection. Defibrillation was obtained via two coils placed in the pericardial space. A short (5-cm) coil is present *(large arrow),* typically used in the superior vena cava and now placed in the pericardial space along the right side of the spine. The second long (25-cm) coil *(small arrows),* normally implanted subcutaneously, lies under the heart and then ascends to the right of the spine.

leads.[110,111] Venous occlusion is therefore common in adult patients with CHD and long-term pacing, who may have multiple leads in place for several decades. If venous access is needed in the setting of a complete venous occlusion, a variety of techniques for recanalization and venous dilation are now available.[112]

Transvenous chamber access can be an issue if complicated atrial baffling has been used to redirect venous return. One major challenge in this regard occurs when ventricular pacing is needed after a Fontan repair. An epicardial approach is used in most of these cases, but successful transvenous ventricular lead implantation after the Fontan operation has now been reported.[113-115] Combined challenges of surgical obstacles, chamber access, and unusual ventricular geometry are present in patients with L-TGA after an atrial switch (Mustard or Senning) procedure.[10] Extensive atrial baffling limits sites of atrial capture to small regions in the left atrial appendage (where phrenic nerve stimulation may be hard to avoid), anterior left atrial roof, or SVC to right atrium junction. Baffle obstruction is fairly common in these patients and may require endovascular stent placement before lead placement. In addition, the ventricular lead must be placed in a morphologic left ventricle that is thin and nontrabeculated, which requires close attention to lead-tip fixation and sensing parameters. Intracardiac shunts can lead to embolic stroke via right-to-left shunting or inadvertent lead placement in the systemic circulation.[116] Trivial shunts that are predominately left to right are probably not absolute contraindications to transvenous leads, but larger shunts, particularly if right to left, need to be evaluated carefully by angiography or echocardiography before a final decision is made on the route for lead implantation. If transvenous leads are strongly preferred in such cases, shunt closure can be attempted beforehand with interventional techniques such as septal occluders, covered stents, or even surgery.[117,118] If intracardiac shunting cannot be eliminated satisfactorily, epicardial lead placement is probably the wisest alternative. Transvenous ICD lead implantation requires a thorough understanding of the ventricular anatomy and chamber positions to anchor the lead tip securely and ensure a suitable vector for defibrillation. When epicardial ICD leads are required, there has been a shift away from traditional patches to novel configurations involving coils (Fig. 132-3) placed in a subcutaneous or pericardial position.[119] This can often be accomplished through a limited subxiphoid approach or a left mini-thoracotomy to provide access to the posterior pericardial space. The experience with this approach is limited, but it appears to offer increased flexibility that can accommodate a wide variety of ventricular geometries and heart sizes.

SUMMARY

Despite the evolution of the management of arrhythmias associated with CHD away from cardiac surgeons, definitive surgical arrhythmia therapy still plays an important role, but one that has been redefined in the current era. Given the success of transcatheter approaches to treat most forms of arrhythmias, only a small number of patients will require primary surgical ablation. However, with a growing population of adults with CHD, their specific arrhythmia challenges will necessitate the continued collaboration of cardiologist and cardiac surgeon to provide novel and often hybrid solutions. In the future, advances in device technology, implant techniques, and tissue engineering will further reshape arrhythmia therapy in children. Computer-enhanced telemanipulation and advances in lead technology will facilitate more minimally invasive surgical approaches to epicardial lead placement. In addition, resynchronization and multisite pacing will become more important tools in the management of heart failure associated with congenital heart disease.

REFERENCES

1. Brockman SK, Webb RC, Bahnson HT: Monopolar ventricular stimulation for the control of acute surgically produced heart block. *Surgery* 44:910–918, 1958.
2. Epstein AE, DiMarco JP, Ellenbogen KA, et al: 2012 ACCF/AHA/HRS focused update incorporated into the ACCF/AHA/HRS 2008 guidelines for device-based therapy of cardiac rhythm abnormalities: a report of the American College of Cardiology Foundation/American Heart Association Task Force on Practice Guidelines and the Heart Rhythm Society. *Circulation* 127(3):e283–e352, 2013.
3. Setty SP, Finucane K, Skinner JR, et al: Extracardiac conduit with a limited maze procedure for the failing Fontan with atrial tachycardias. *Ann Thorac Surg* 74(6):1992–1997, 2002.
4. Ohmi M, Tofukuji M, Sato K, et al: Permanent pacemaker implantation in premature infants less than 2000 grams of body weight. *Ann Thorac Surg* 64:880–881, 1997.
5. Johnsrude CL, Backer CL, Deal BJ, et al: Transmural atrial pacing in patients with postoperative congenital heart disease. *J Cardiovasc Electrophysiol* 10(3):351–357, 1999.
6. Cohen MI, Bush DM, Vetter VL, et al: Permanent epicardial pacing in pediatric patients: seventeen years of experience and 1200 outpatient visits. *Circulation* 103(21):2585–2590, 2001.
7. Beaufort-Krol GC, Mulder H, Nagelkerke D, et al: Comparison of longevity, pacing, and sensing characteristics of steroid-eluting epicardial versus conventional endocardial pacing leads in children. *J Thorac Cardiovasc Surg* 117(3):523–528, 1991.
8. Sachweh JS, Vazquez-Jimenez JF, Schöndube FA, et al: Twenty years experience with pediatric pacing: epicardial and transvenous stimulation. *Eur J Cardiothorac Surg* 17(4):455–461, 2000.
9. Fortescue EB, Berul CI, Cecchin F, et al: Comparison of modern steroid-eluting epicardial and thin transvenous pacemaker leads in pediatric and congenital heart disease patients. *J Interv Card Electrophysiol* 14(1):27–36, 2005.
10. Warner KG, Halpin DP, Berul CI, et al: Placement of a permanent epicardial pacemaker in children using a subcostal approach. *Ann Thorac Surg* 68(1):173–175, 1999.
11. Ramesh V, Gaynor JW, Shah MJ, et al: Comparison of left and right atrial epicardial pacing in patients with congenital heart disease. *Ann Thorac Surg* 68(6):2314–2319, 1999.
12. Kucharczuk JC, Cohen MI, Rhodes LA, et al: Epicardial atrial pacemaker lead placement after multiple cardiac operations. *Ann Thorac Surg* 71(6):2057–2058, 2001.
13. Eyskens B, Mertens L, Moerman P, et al: Cardiac strangulation, a rare complication of epicardial pacemaker leads during growth. *Heart* 77:288–289, 1997.
14. Perry JC, Nihill MR, Ludomirsky A, et al: The pulmonary artery lasso: epicardial pacing lead causing right ventricular outflow obstruction. *Pacing Clin Electrophysiol* 14(6):1018–1023, 1991.
15. Janousek J, Gebauer RA: Cardiac resynchronization therapy in pediatric and congenital heart disease. *Pacing Clin Electrophysiol* 31(Suppl 1):S21–S23, 2008.
16. VanHare GF, Witherell C, Merrick SM: Migration of an epicardial pacemaker to the pericardial space of an infant. *Pacing Clin Electrophysiol* 17:1808–1810, 1994.
17. Gomez C, Dick M, Hernandez R, et al: Peritoneal migration of an abdominally implanted epicardial pacemaker: a cause of intestinal obstruction. *Pacing Clin Electrophysiol* 18:2231–2232, 1995.
18. Khairy P, Fournier A, Thibault B, et al: Cardiac resynchronization therapy in congenital heart disease. *Int J Cardiol* 109(2):160–168, 2006.
19. Cecchin F, Frangini PA, Brown DW, et al: Cardiac resynchronization therapy (and multisite pacing) in pediatrics and congenital heart disease: five years experience in a single institution. *J Cardiovasc Electrophysiol* 20(1):58–65, 2009.
20. Janousek J, Vojtovic P, Hucin B, et al: Resynchronization pacing is a useful adjunct to the management of acute heart failure after surgery for congenital heart defects. *Am J Cardiol* 88(2):145–152, 2001.
21. Dubin AM, Feinstein JA, Reddy M, et al: Electrical resynchronization: a novel therapy for the failing right ventricle. *Circulation* 107:2287–2289, 2003.
22. Stephenson EA, Batra AS, Knilans TK, et al: A multicenter experience with novel implantable cardioverter defibrillator configurations in the pediatric and congenital heart disease population. *J Cardiovasc Electrophysiol* 17(1):41–46, 2006.
23. Kowalski M, Nicolato P, Kalahasty G, et al: An alternative technique of implanting a nontransvenous implantable cardioverter-defibrillator system in adults with no or limited venous access to the heart. *Heart Rhythm* 7(11):1572–1577, 2010.
24. Jarman JW, Lascelles K, Wong T, et al: Clinical experience of entirely subcutaneous implantable cardioverter-defibrillators in children and adults: cause for caution. *Eur Heart J* 33(11):1351–1359, 2012.

24a. Moss AJ, McDonald J: Unilateral cervicothoracic sympathetic ganglionectomy for the treatment of long QT interval syndrome. *N Engl J Med* 285:903–904, 1971.

24b. Schwartz PJ, Priori SG, Cerrone M, et al: Left cardiac sympathetic denervation in the management of high-risk patients affected by the long-QT syndrome. *Circulation* 109:1826–1833, 2004.

25. Napolitano C, Priori SG: Diagnosis and treatment of catecholaminergic polymorphic ventricular tachycardia. *Heart Rhythm* 4:675–678, 2007.
26. Li J, Wang L, Wang J: Video-assisted thoracoscopic sympathectomy for congenital long QT syndromes. *Pacing Clin Electrophysiol* 26:870–873, 2003.
27. Atallah J, Fynn-Thompson F, Cecchin F, et al: Video-assisted thoracoscopic cardiac denervation: a potential novel therapeutic option for children with intractable ventricular arrhythmias. *Ann Thorac Surg* 86(5):1620–1625, 2008.
28. Hofferberth SC, Cecchin F, Loberman D, et al: Left thoracoscopic sympathectomy for cardiac denervation in patients with life-threatening ventricular arrhythmias. *J Thorac Cardiovasc Surg* 147(1):404–409, 2014.

28a. Walsh EP, Cecchin F: Arrhythmias in adult patients with congenital heart disease. *Circulation* 115:534–545, 2007.

29. Warnes CA, Liberthson R, Danielson GK, et al: Task force 1: the changing profile of congenital heart disease in adult life. *J Am Coll Cardiol* 37:1170–1175, 2001.
30. Ghai A, Harris L, Harrison DA, et al: Outcomes of late atrial tachyarrhythmias in adults after the Fontan operation. *J Am Coll Cardiol* 37:585–592, 2001.
31. Nakagawa H, Shah N, Matsudaira K, et al: Characterization of reentrant circuit in macroreentrant right atrial tachycardia after surgical repair of congenital heart disease: isolated channels between scars allow "focal" ablation. *Circulation* 103:699–709, 2001.
32. Kalman JK, Van Hare GF, Olgin JE, et al: Ablation of "incisional" reentrant atrial tachycardia complicating surgery for congenital heart disease. *Circulation* 93:502–512, 1996.
33. Triedman JK, Jenkins KJ, Colan SD, et al: Intra-atrial reentrant tachycardia after palliation of congenital heart disease: characterization of multiple macroreentrant circuits using fluoroscopically based three-dimensional endocardial mapping. *J Cardiovasc Electrophysiol* 8:259–270, 1997.
34. Garson A, Bink-Boelkens MTE, Hesslein PS, et al: Atrial flutter in the young: a collaborative study of 380 cases. *J Am Coll Cardiol* 6:871–878, 1985.
35. Rhodes LA, Walsh EP, Gamble WJ, et al: Benefits and potential risks of atrial antitachycardia pacing after repair of congenital heart disease. *Pacing Clin Electrophysiol* 18:1005–1016, 1995.
36. Anderson RH, Ho SY: The disposition of the conduction tissues in congenitally malformed hearts with reference to their embryological development. *J Perinat Med* 19:201–206, 1991.
37. Li W, Somerville J: Atrial flutter in grown-up congenital heart (GUCH) patients: clinical characteristics of affected population. *Int J Cardiol* 75:129–137, 2000.
38. Wong T, Davlouros PA, Li W, et al: Mechano-electrical interaction late after Fontan operation: relation between P-wave duration and dispersion, right atrial size, and atrial arrhythmias. *Circulation* 109:2319–2325, 2004.
39. Fishberger SB, Wernovsky G, Gentles TL, et al: Factors that influence the development of atrial flutter after the Fontan operation. *J Thorac Cardiovasc Surg* 113:80–86, 1997.
40. Collins KK, Love BA, Walsh EP, et al: Location of acutely successful radiofrequency catheter ablation of intraatrial reentrant tachycardia in patients with congenital heart disease. *Am J Cardiol* 86:969–974, 2000.

41. Triedman JK, Alexander ME, Berul CI, et al: Electroanatomic mapping of entrained and exit zones in patients with repaired congenital heart disease and intra-atrial reentrant tachycardia. *Circulation* 103:2060–2065, 2001.
42. Mandapati R, Walsh EP, Triedman JK: Pericaval and periannular intraatrial reentrant tachycardias in patients with congenital heart disease. *J Cardiovasc Electrophysiol* 14:112–119, 2003.
43. Delacretaz E, Ganz LI, Friedman PL, et al: Multiple atrial macro-reentry circuits in adults with repaired congenital heart disease: entrainment mapping combined with three dimensional electro-anatomic mapping. *J Am Coll Cardiol* 37:1665–1676, 2001.
44. Rhodes LA, Walsh EP, Saul JP: Conversion of atrial flutter in pediatric patients using transesophageal atrial pacing: a safe, effective, and minimally invasive technique. *Am Heart J* 130:323–327, 1995.
45. Triedman JK: Atrial reentrant tachycardias. In Walsh EP, Saul JP, Triedman JK, editors: *Cardiac arrhythmias in children and young adults with congenital heart disease*, Philadelphia, 2001, Lippincott Williams & Wilkins, pp 137–160.
46. Gatzoulis MA, Balaji S, Webber SA, et al: Risk factors for arrhythmia and sudden cardiac death late after repair of tetralogy of Fallot: a multicentre study. *Lancet* 356:975–981, 2000.
47. Triedman JK, Bergau DM, Saul JP, et al: Efficacy of radiofrequency ablation for control of intraatrial reentrant tachycardia in patients with congenital heart disease. *J Am Coll Cardiol* 30:1032–1038, 1997.
48. Triedman JK, Alexander MA, Love BA, et al: Influence of patient factors and ablative technologies on outcomes of radiofrequency ablation of intra-atrial tachycardia in patients with congenital heart disease. *J Am Coll Cardiol* 39:1827–1835, 2002.
49. Mavroudis C, Backer CL, Deal BJ, et al: Total cavopulmonary conversion and maze procedure for patients with failure of the Fontan operation. *J Thorac Cardiovasc Surg* 122:863–871, 2001.
50. Gentles TL, Mayer JE, Jr, Gauvreau K, et al: Fontan operation in five hundred consecutive patients: factors influencing early and late outcome. *J Thorac Cardiovasc Surg* 114:376–391, 1997.
51. Khairy P, Fernandes SM, Mayer JE, Jr, et al: Long-term survival, modes of death, and predictors of mortality in patients with Fontan surgery. *Circulation* 117:2008.
52. Mavroudis C, Backer CL, Deal BJ, et al: Total cavopulmonary conversion and maze procedure for patients with failure of the Fontan operation. *J Thorac Cardiovasc Surg* 122:863–871, 2001.
53. Agnoletti G, Borghi A, Vignati G, et al: Fontan conversion to total cavopulmonary connection and arrhythmia ablation: clinical and functional results. *Heart* 89:193–198, 2003.
54. Morales DL, Dibardino DJ, Braud BE, et al: Salvaging the failing Fontan: lateral tunnel versus extracardiac conduit. *Ann Thorac Surg* 80:1445–1451, 2005.
55. Kao JM, Alejos JC, Grant PW, et al: Conversion of atriopulmonary to cavopulmonary anastomosis in management of late arrhythmias and atrial thrombosis. *Ann Thorac Surg* 58:1510–1514, 1994.
56. McElhinney DF, Reddy VM, Moore P, et al: Revision of previous Fontan connections to extracardiac or intraatrial conduit cavopulmonary anastomosis. *Ann Thorac Surg* 62:1276–1283, 1996.
57. Kreutzer J, Keane JF, Lock JE, et al: Conversion of modified Fontan procedure to lateral atrial tunnel cavopulmonary anastomosis. *J Thorac Cardiovasc Surg* 111:1169–1176, 1996.
58. Mavroudis C, Backer CL, Deal BJ, et al: Fontan conversion to cavopulmonary connection and arrhythmia circuit cryoblation. *J Thorac Cardiovasc Surg* 115:547–556, 1998.
59. Marcelletti CF, Hanley FL, Mavroudis C, et al: Revision of previous Fontan connections to total extracardiac cavopulmonary anastomosis: a multicenter experience. *J Thorac Cardiovasc Surg* 119:340–346, 2000.
60. Deal BJ, Mavroudis C, Backer CL, et al: Comparison of anatomic isthmus block with the modified right atrial maze procedure for late atrial tachycardia in Fontan patients. *Circulation* 106:575–579, 2002.
61. Weinstein S, Cua C, Chan D, et al: Outcome of symptomatic patients undergoing extracardiac Fontan conversion and cryoablation. *J Thorac Cardiovasc Surg* 126:529–536, 2003.
62. Sheikh AM, Tang AT, Roman K, et al: The failing Fontan circulation: successful conversion of atriopulmonary connections. *J Thorac Cardiovasc Surg* 128:60–66, 2004.
63. Backer CL, Deal BJ, Mavroudis C, et al: Conversion of the failed Fontan circulation. *Cardiol Young* 16(Suppl 1):85–91, 2006.
64. Koh M, Yagihara T, Uemura H, et al: Optimal timing of the Fontan conversion: change in the P-wave characteristics precedes the onset of atrial tachyarrhythmias in patients with atriopulmonary connection. *J Thorac Cardiovasc Surg* 133:1295–1302, 2007.
65. Kim WH, Lim HG, Lee JR, et al: Fontan conversion with arrhythmia surgery. *Eur J Cardiothorac Surg* 27:250–257, 2005.
66. Shemin RJ, Cox JL, Gillinov AM, et al: Guidelines for reporting data and outcomes for the surgical treatment of atrial fibrillation. *Ann Thorac Surg* 83:1225–1230, 2007.
67. Triedman JK, Alexander ME, Love BA, et al: Influence of patient factors and ablative technologies on outcomes of radiofrequency ablation of intra-atrial re-entrant tachycardia in patients with congenital heart disease. *J Am Coll Cardiol* 39:1827–1835, 2002.
68. Takahashi K, Fynn-Thompson F, Cecchin F, et al: Clinical outcomes of Fontan conversion surgery with and without associated arrhythmia intervention. *Int J Cardiol* 2008.
69. Kirsh JA, Walsh EP, Triedman JK: Prevalence of and risk factors for atrial fibrillation and intraatrial reentrant tachycardia among patients with congenital heart disease. *Am J Cardiol* 90:338–340, 2002.
70. Deal BJ, Mavroudis C, Backer CL: Beyond Fontan conversion: surgical therapy of arrhythmias including patients with associated complex congenital heart disease. *Ann Thorac Surg* 76:542–553, 2003.
71. Attenhofer Jost CH, Connolly HM, Edwards WD, et al: Ebstein's anomaly: review of a multifaceted congenital cardiac condition. *Swiss Med Wkly* 135:269–281, 2005.
72. Smith WM, Gallagher JJ, Kerr CR, et al: The electrophysiologic basis and management of symptomatic recurrent tachycardia in patients with Ebstein's anomaly of the tricuspid valve. *Am J Cardiol* 49:1223–1234, 1982.
73. Horowitz LN, Vetter VL, Harken AH, et al: Electrophysiologic characteristics of sustained ventricular tachycardia occurring after repair of tetralogy of Fallot. *Am J Cardiol* 46:446–452, 1980.
74. Downar E, Harris L, Kimber S, et al: Ventricular tachycardia after surgical repair of tetralogy of Fallot: results of intraoperative mapping studies. *J Am Coll Cardiol* 20:648–655, 1992.
75. Wolfe RR, Driscoll DJ, Gersony WM, et al: Arrhythmias in patients with valvar aortic stenosis, valvar pulmonary stenosis, and ventricular septal defect: results of 24-hour ECG monitoring. *Circulation* 87(Suppl):I-89–I-101, 1993.
76. Keane JF, Driscoll DJ, Gersony WM, et al: Second natural history study of congenital heart defects: results of treatment of patients with aortic valvar stenosis. *Circulation* 87(Suppl):I-16–I-27, 1993.
77. Gatzoulis MA, Walters J, McLaughlin PR, et al: Late arrhythmia in adults with the mustard procedure for transposition of great arteries: a surrogate marker for right ventricular dysfunction? *Heart* 84:409–415, 2000.
78. Deanfield JE, McKenna WJ, Presbitero P, et al: Ventricular arrhythmia in unrepaired and repaired tetralogy of Fallot: relation to age, timing of repair, and haemodynamic status. *Br Heart J* 52:77–81, 1984.
79. Roos-Hesselink J, Perlroth MG, McGhie J, et al: Atrial arrhythmias in adults after repair of tetralogy of Fallot: correlations with clinical, exercise, and echocardiographic findings. *Circulation* 91:2214–2219, 1995.
80. Harrison DA, Harris L, Siu SC, et al: Sustained ventricular tachycardia in adult patients late after repair of tetralogy of Fallot. *J Am Coll Cardiol* 30:1368–1373, 1997.
81. Murphy JG, Gersh BJ, Mair DD, et al: Long-term outcome in patients undergoing surgical repair of tetralogy of Fallot. *N Engl J Med* 329:593–599, 1993.
82. Gatzoulis MA, Till JA, Somerville J, et al: Mechanoelectrical interaction in tetralogy of Fallot: QRS prolongation relates to right ventricular size and predicts malignant ventricular arrhythmias and sudden death. *Circulation* 92:231–237, 1995.
83. Valente AM, Gauvreau K, Assenza GE, et al: Contemporary predictors of death and sustained ventricular tachycardia in patients with repaired tetralogy of Fallot enrolled in the INDICATOR cohort. *Heart* 100(3):247–253, 2014.
84. Wolff GS, Rowland TW, Ellison RC: Surgically induced right bundle branch block with left anterior hemiblock: an ominous

sign in postoperative tetralogy of Fallot. *Circulation* 46:587–594, 1972.
85. Nollert G, Fischlein T, Bouterwek S, et al: Long-term survival in patients with repair of tetralogy of Fallot: 36-year follow-up of 490 survivors of the first year after surgical repair. *J Am Coll Cardiol* 30:1374–1383, 1997.
86. Silka MJ, Hardy BG, Menashe VD, et al: A population-based prospective evaluation of risk of sudden cardiac death after operation for common congenital heart defects. *J Am Coll Cardiol* 32:245–251, 1998.
87. Norgaard MA, Lauridsen P, Helvind M, et al: Twenty-to-thirty-seven-year follow-up after repair for tetralogy of Fallot. *Eur J Cardiothorac Surg* 16:125–130, 1999.
87a. Berul CI, Hill SL, Geggel RL, et al: Electrocardiographic markers of late sudden death risk in postoperative tetralogy of Fallot children. *J Cardiovasc Electrophysiol* 8:1349–1356, 1997.
88. Alexander ME, Cecchin F, Walsh EP, et al: Implications of implantable defibrillator therapy in congenital heart disease and pediatrics. *J Cardiovasc Electrophysiol* 15:72–76, 1504.
89. Dore A, Santagata P, Dubuc M, et al: Implantable cardioverter defibrillators in adults with congenital heart disease: a single center experience. *Pacing Clin Electrophysiol* 27:47–51, 2004.
90. Khairy P, Landzberg MJ, Gatzoulis MA, et al: Prognostic significance of electrophysiologic testing post tetralogy of Fallot repair: a multicenter study. *Circulation* 109:1994–2000, 2004.
91. Alexander ME, Walsh EP, Saul JP, et al: Value of programmed ventricular stimulation in patients with congenital heart disease. *J Cardiovasc Electrophysiol* 10:1033–1044, 1999.
92. Goldner BG, Cooper R, Blau W, et al: Radiofrequency catheter ablation as a primary therapy for treatment of ventricular tachycardia in a patient after repair of tetralogy of Fallot. *Pacing Clin Electrophysiol* 17:1441–1446, 1994.
93. Burton ME, Leon AR: Radiofrequency catheter ablation of right ventricular outflow tract tachycardia late after complete repair of tetralogy of Fallot using the pace mapping technique. *Pacing Clin Electrophysiol* 16:2319–2325, 1993.
94. Gonska BD, Cao K, Raab J, et al: Radiofrequency catheter ablation of right ventricular tachycardia late after repair of congenital heart defects. *Circulation* 94:1902–1908, 1996.
95. Morwood JG, Triedman JK, Berul CI, et al: Radiofrequency catheter ablation of ventricular tachycardia in children, and in young adults with congenital heart disease. *Heart Rhythm* 1:301–308, 2004.
96. Therrien J, Siu SC, Harris L, et al: Impact of pulmonary valve replacement on arrhythmia propensity late after repair of tetralogy of Fallot. *Circulation* 103:2489–2494, 2001.
97. Flinn CJ, Wolff GS, Dick M, et al: Cardiac rhythm after the Mustard operation for complete transposition of the great arteries. *N Engl J Med* 3310:1635–1638, 1984.
98. Manning PB, Mayer JE, Wernovsky G, et al: Staged operation to Fontan increases the incidence of sinoatrial node dysfunction. *J Thorac Cardiovasc Surg* 111:833–840, 1996.
99. Gregoratos G, Abrams J, Epstein AE, et al: ACC/AHA/NASPE 2002 guideline update for implantation of cardiac pacemakers and antiarrhythmia devices. *J Am Coll Cardiol* 40:1703–1719, 2002.
100. VanPraagh R, Papagiannis J, Grunenfelder J, et al: Pathologic anatomy of corrected transposition of the great arteries: medical and surgical implications. *Am Heart J* 135:772–785, 1998.
101. Anderson RH, Becker AE, Arnold R, et al: The conducting tissues in congenitally corrected transposition. *Circulation* 50:911–923, 1974.
102. Thiene G, Wenick ACG, Frescura C, et al: Surgical anatomy and pathology of the conduction tissues in atrioventricular defects. *J Thorac Cardiovasc Surg* 82:928–937, 1981.
103. Huhta JC, Maloney JD, Ritter DG, et al: Complete atrioventricular block in patients with atrioventricular discordance. *Circulation* 67:1374–1377, 1983.
104. Connelly MS, Liu PP, Williams WG, et al: Congenitally corrected transposition of the great arteries in the adult: functional status and complications. *J Am Coll Cardiol* 27:1238–1243, 1996.
105. Dick M, Norwood WI, Chipman C, et al: Intraoperative recording of specialized atrioventricular conduction tissue electrograms in 47 patients. *Circulation* 59:150–160, 1979.
106. Weindling SN, Gamble WJ, Mayer JE, et al: Duration of complete atrioventricular block after congenital heart disease surgery. *Am J Cardiol* 82:525–527, 1998.
107. Cohen MI, Rhodes LA, Spray TL, et al: Efficacy of prophylactic epicardial pacing leads in children and young adults. *Ann Thorac Surg* 1:197–202, 2004.
108. Dubin AM, Janousek J, Rhee E, et al: Resynchronization therapy in pediatric and congenital heart disease patients: an international multicenter study. *J Am Coll Cardiol* 46:2277–2283, 2005.
109. Khairy P, Triedman JK, Juraszek A, et al: Inability to cannulate the coronary sinus in patients with supraventricular arrhythmias: congenital and acquired coronary sinus atresia. *J Interv Card Electrophysiol* 2:123–127, 2005.
110. Spittell PC, Hayes DL: Venous complications after insertion of a transvenous pacemaker. *Mayo Clin Proc* 67:258–265, 1992.
111. Bracke F, Meijer A, van Gelder B: Venous occlusion of the access vein in patients referred for lead extraction: influence of patient and lead characteristics. *Pacing Clin Electrophysiol* 26:1649–1652, 2003.
112. McCotter CJ, Angle JF, Prudente LA, et al: Placement of transvenous pacemaker and ICD leads across total chronic occlusions. *Pacing Clin Electrophysiol* 28:921–925, 2005.
113. Shah MJ, Nehgme R, Carboni M, et al: Endocardial atrial pacing lead implantation and midterm follow-up in young patients with sinus node dysfunction after the Fontan procedure. *Pacing Clin Electrophysiol* 27:949–954, 2004.
114. Hansky B, Blanz U, Peuster M, et al: Endocardial pacing after Fontan-type procedures. *Pacing Clin Electrophysiol* 28:140–148, 2005.
115. Adwani SS, Sreeram N, DeGiovanni JV: Percutaneous transhepatic dual chamber pacing in children with Fontan circulation. *Heart* 77:574–575, 1997.
116. Van Gelder BM, Bracke FA, Oto A, et al: Diagnosis and management of inadvertently placed pacing and ICD leads in the left ventricle: a multicenter experience and review of the literature. *Pacing Clin Electrophysiol* 23:877–883, 2000.
117. Knauth AL, Lock JE, Perry SB, et al: Transcatheter device closure of congenital and postoperative residual ventricular septal defects. *Circulation* 110:501–507, 2004.
118. Khairy P, O'Donnell CP, Landzberg MJ: Transcatheter closure versus medical therapy of patent foramen ovale and presumed paradoxical thromboemboli: a systematic review. *Ann Intern Med* 139:753–760, 2003.
119. Stephenson EA, Batra AS, Knilans TK, et al: A multicenter experience with novel implantable cardioverter defibrillator configurations in the pediatric and congenital heart disease population. *J Cardiovasc Electrophysiol* 17:41–46, 2006.

CHAPTER 133

QUALITY IMPROVEMENT FOR THE TREATMENT OF PATIENTS WITH PEDIATRIC AND CONGENITAL CARDIAC DISEASE: THE ROLE OF THE CLINICAL DATABASE

Jeffrey P. Jacobs

CHAPTER OUTLINE

Although significant progress has been made in the care of patients with pediatric and congenital cardiac disease, complications and death still occur. As a result, optimization of outcomes remains a constant goal. Substantial effort has been devoted to advancing the science of assessing the outcomes and improving the quality of care associated with the treatment of patients with pediatric and congenital cardiac disease.[1-227] The importance of these efforts is supported by the fact that congenital heart defects are the most common birth anomalies, with moderate to severe variants occurring in approximately 6 per 1000 live births.[228]

To perform meaningful, multi-institutional outcomes analyses and quality improvement, any database must incorporate the following seven essential elements:

1. A common language and nomenclature*
2. A database with an established uniform core dataset for collection of information†
3. A mechanism for evaluating case complexity‡
4. A mechanism to ensure and verify the completeness and accuracy of the data collected§
5. Collaboration between medical and surgical subspecialties‖
6. Standardized protocols for life-long follow-up¶
7. Strategies for quality assessment and quality improvement**

The foundation of these seven elements is the use of a common language and nomenclature. The remaining six elements are all dependent on this nomenclature; therefore, quality improvement in the domain of congenital cardiac disease depends on a solid understanding of cardiac morphology and nomenclature.

*References 1-55, 62-64, 66-71, 75, 77, 79, 81, 82, 87, 88, 93, 94, 96, 100, 103, 104, 110-112, 114-116, 128-140, 148, 152, 155, 162, 167-169, 171, 172, 178, 179, 188, 191, 200-202, 209, 210, 213, 216, 218, 221.

†References 1-23, 55, 58-60, 62-64, 71, 77, 79, 80-82, 87, 88, 90, 93, 95, 98, 100, 104-106, 110-113, 115, 117-123, 145, 146, 148, 152-155, 161, 163, 164, 171, 172, 174, 178, 179, 185, 188, 189, 204, 207, 210, 212, 214, 216, 220-227.

‡References 56, 57, 61, 65, 72-74, 76-79, 81-84, 88-91, 97-102, 104, 106, 107, 110-112, 124, 125, 141, 142, 147, 148-150, 152, 178, 179, 188, 204, 215-217, 221.

§References 77, 81, 85, 86, 88, 100, 104, 110-112, 126, 148, 152, 178, 179, 188, 216, 221.

‖References 81, 100, 104, 110-140, 148, 152, 178, 179, 188, 216, 221.

¶References 104, 109-112, 127, 145, 146, 152, 164, 173, 178, 179, 184, 188, 189, 214, 216, 221.

**References 108, 110, 115, 143-148, 151, 152, 154, 156-160, 164-167, 170, 175, 176, 177-183, 186-188, 190, 192-199, 203, 205, 206, 208, 210, 211, 216, 219, 221, 222.

NOMENCLATURE

Substantial effort has been devoted to the standardization of nomenclature and definitions related to surgery for pediatric and congenital cardiac disease. During the 1990s, both the European Association for Cardio-Thoracic Surgery (EACTS) and the Society of Thoracic Surgeons (STS) created databases to assess the outcomes of congenital cardiac surgery. Beginning in 1998, these two organizations collaborated to create the International Congenital Heart Surgery Nomenclature and Database Project. By 2000, a common nomenclature and a common core minimal dataset were adopted by EACTS and STS and published in the *Annals of Thoracic Surgery*.[21-54,114] In 2000, the International Nomenclature Committee for Pediatric and Congenital Heart Disease was established. This committee eventually evolved into the International Society for Nomenclature of Paediatric and Congenital Heart Disease (ISNPCHD). By 2005, members of the ISNPCHD cross-mapped the nomenclature of the International Congenital Heart Surgery Nomenclature and Database Project of the EACTS and STS with the European Paediatric Cardiac Code (EPCC) of the Association for European Paediatric Cardiology (AEPC), and therefore created the International Paediatric and Congenital Cardiac Code (IPCCC),[112] which is available for free download at http://www.ipccc.net.

Most international databases of patients with pediatric and congenital cardiac disease use the IPCCC as their foundation. Two versions of the IPCCC are used in the overwhelming majority of multi-institutional databases throughout the world:

1. The version of the IPCCC derived from the nomenclature of the International Congenital Heart Surgery Nomenclature and Database Project of the EACTS and the STS
2. The version of the IPCCC derived from the nomenclature of the EPCC of the AEPC

These two versions of the IPCCC are also often cited with the following abbreviated short names:

1. EACTS-STS–derived version of the IPCCC
2. AEPC-derived version of the IPCCC

The STS Congenital Heart Surgery Database, the EACTS Congenital Heart Surgery Database, and the Japan Congenital Cardiovascular Surgery Database (JCCVSD) all use the EACTS-STS–derived version of the IPCCC.

The ISNPCHD has published review articles that provide a unified and comprehensive classification, with definitions, for several complex congenital cardiac malformations: the functionally univentricular heart,[92] hypoplastic left heart syndrome,[94] discordant atrioventricular connections,[96] and cardiac structures in the setting of heterotaxy.[103] These review articles include definitions and a complete listing of the relevant codes and terms in both versions of the IPCCC.

In collaboration with the World Health Organization (WHO), the ISNPCHD is developing the pediatric and congenital cardiac nomenclature that will be used in the eleventh version of the International Classification of Diseases (ICD-11). With a grant funded by the Children's Heart Foundation (www.childrensheartfoundation.org), the ISNPCHD has also linked images and videos to the IPCCC. These images and videos are acquired from cardiac morphologic specimens and imaging modalities such as echocardiography, angiography, computerized axial tomography, and magnetic resonance imaging, as well as intraoperative images and videos.[††] These images and videos are available for free download from the internet at (http://www.IPCCC-awg.NET). The IPCCC itself is available for free download from the internet at (http://www.IPCCC.NET).

The EACTS-STS–derived version of the IPCCC,[110,112,114] and the common minimum database data set created by the International Congenital Heart Surgery Nomenclature and Database Project,[21] are currently used by the STS Congenital Heart Surgery Database, the EACTS Congenital Heart Surgery Database, and the JCCVSD. Between 1998 and January 1, 2014 inclusive, this nomenclature and database was used by STS, EACTS, and JCCVSD to analyze the outcomes of 479,000 operations.

DATABASE

The STS Congenital Heart Surgery Database is the largest database in North America cataloging congenital cardiac malformations.[117,152] It has grown annually since its inception, both in terms of the number of participating centers submitting data and the number of operations analyzed (Figs. 133-1, 133-2, and 133-3). As of January 1, 2014, the STS Congenital Heart Surgery Database currently had 111 participating centers, representing 120 hospitals performing pediatric and congenital cardiac surgery in North America: 117 of an estimated 125 centers from the United States of America that perform pediatric and congenital heart surgery and 3 of 8 centers from Canada that perform pediatric and congenital heart surgery.[95,174] (The Report of the 2005 STS Congenital Heart Surgery Practice and Manpower Survey, undertaken by the STS Workforce on Congenital Heart Surgery, estimated that 122 centers in the United States of America perform pediatric and congenital heart surgery and 8 centers in Canada perform pediatric and congenital heart surgery.[95] The Report of the 2010 STS Congenital Heart Surgery Practice and Manpower Survey, undertaken by the STS Workforce on Congenital Heart Surgery, estimated that 125 centers in the United States of America perform pediatric and congenital heart surgery and 8 centers in Canada perform pediatric and congenital heart surgery.[174])

As of January 1, 2014, the STS Congenital Heart Surgery Database therefore contained data from an estimated 93.6% of hospitals (117 of 125) performing pediatric cardiac surgery in the United States. With penetrance of greater than 90%, the data in the STS Congenital Heart Surgery Database is representative of pediatric and congenital heart surgery in the United States. As of January 1, 2014, the number of cumulative total operations in the STS Congenital Heart Surgery Database was

††References 162, 191, 200-202, 209, 213, 218.

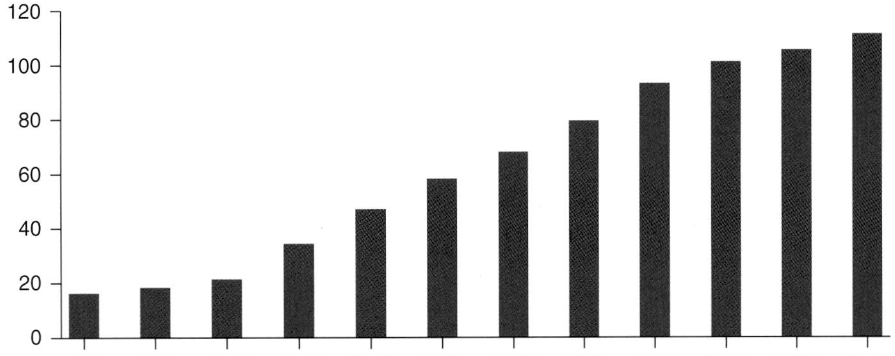

	2002	2003	2004	2005	2006	2007	2008	2009	2010	2011	2012	2013
Participating centers	16	18	21	34	47	58	68	79	93	101	105	111

FIGURE 133-1 ■ The annual growth of the Society of Thoracic Surgeons Congenital Heart Surgery Database by number of participating centers submitting data. The aggregate report from the Fall 2013 Harvest of the Society of Thoracic Surgeons Congenital Heart Surgery Database[19] includes data from 111 North American Congenital Database Participants representing 120 Congenital Heart Surgery hospitals in North America—117 in the United States and 3 in Canada.

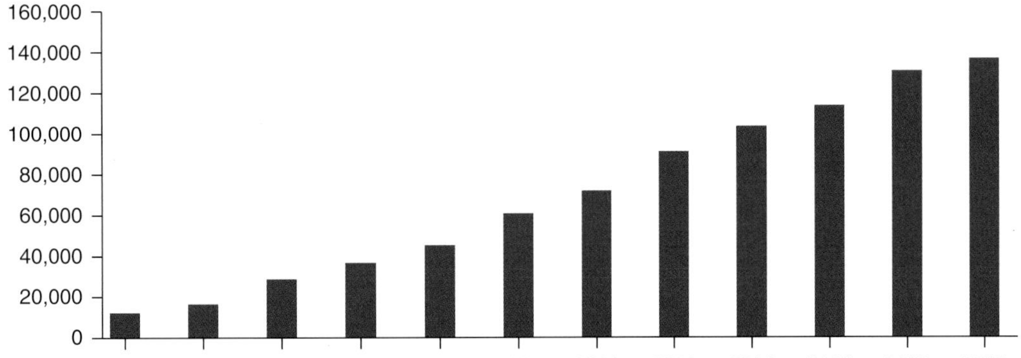

	2002	2003	2004	2005	2006	2007	2008	2009	2010	2011	2012	2013
Operations	12,787	16,481	28,351	37,093	45,635	61,014	72,002	91,639	103,664	114,041	130,823	136,617

FIGURE 133-2 ■ The annual growth of the Society of Thoracic Surgeons (STS) Congenital Heart Surgery Database by the number of operations per averaged 4-year data collection cycle. The aggregate report from the Fall 2013 Harvest of the STS Congenital Heart Surgery Database[19] includes 136,617 operations performed in the 4-year period of July 1, 2009, to June 30, 2013, inclusive, submitted from 120 hospitals in North America—117 in the United States and 3 in Canada.

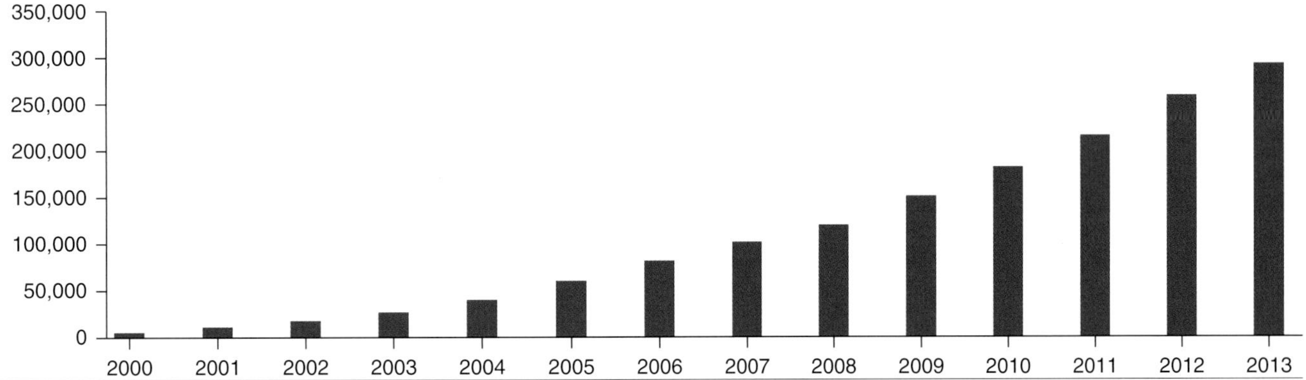

	2000	2001	2002	2003	2004	2005	2006	2007	2008	2009	2010	2011	2012	2013
Cumulative operations	4,237	9,747	16,537	26,404	39,988	58,181	73,399	98,406	119,266	148,110	179,697	213,416	257,932	292,828

FIGURE 133-3 ■ The annual growth of the Society of Thoracic Surgeons (STS) Congenital Heart Surgery Database by the cumulative number of operations over time. As of January 1, 2014, the number of cumulative total operations in the STS Congenital Heart Surgery Database is 292,828. The aggregate report from the Fall 2013 Harvest of the STS Congenital Heart Surgery Database[19] includes 136,617 operations performed in the 4-year period of July 1, 2009, to June 30, 2013, inclusive, submitted from 120 hospitals in North America—117 in the United States and 3 in Canada.

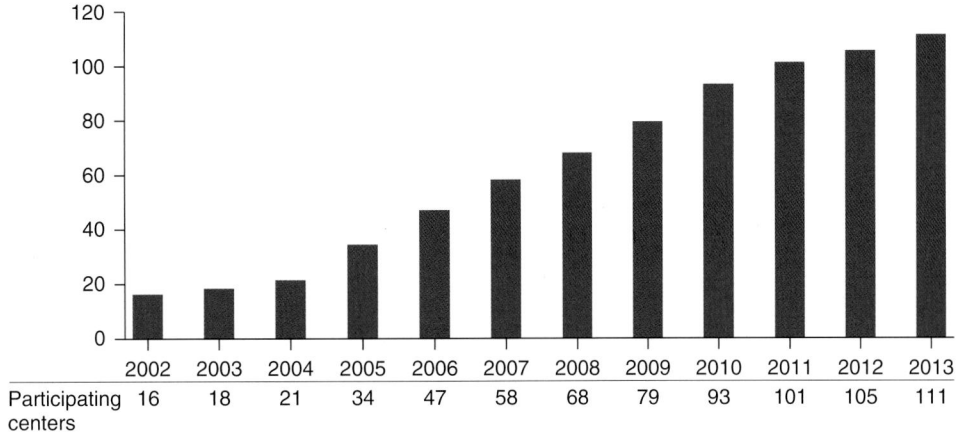

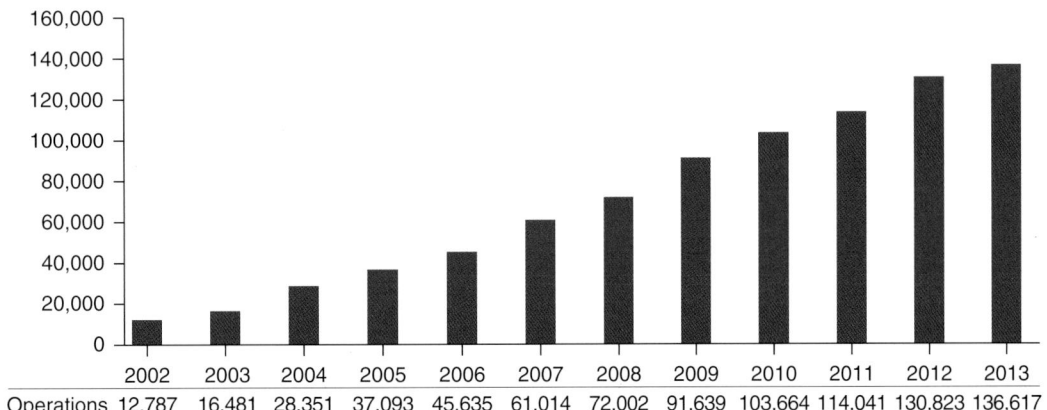

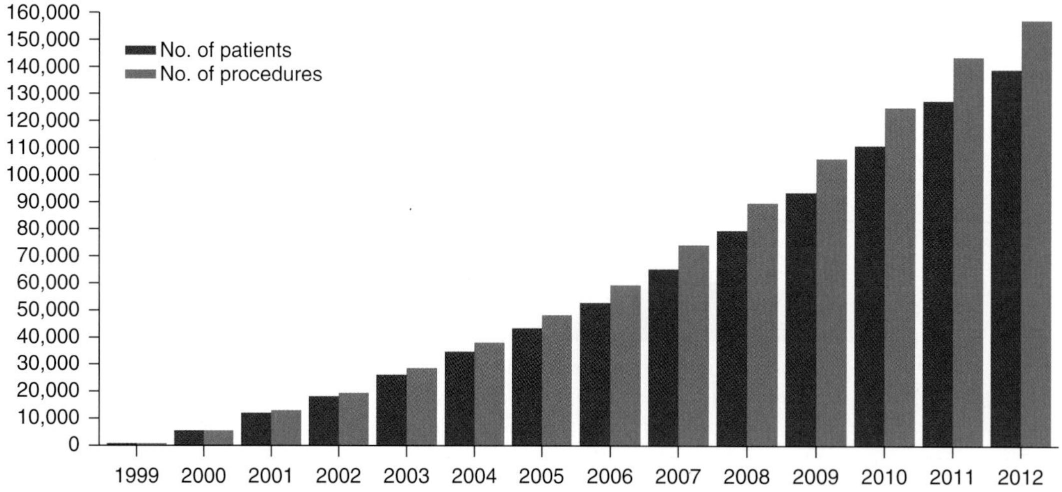

FIGURE 133-4 ■ The annual growth in the European Association for Cardio-Thoracic Surgery (EACTS) Congenital Database by both number of patients and number of operations. As of May 2013, the EACTS Congenital Heart Surgery Database contained 157,772 operations performed in 130,534 patients. As of May, 2013, the EACTS Congenital Heart Surgery Database had 348 centers from 76 countries registered, with 173 active centers from 46 countries submitting data. (Data courtesy Bohdan Maruszewski of the Children's Memorial Health Institute in Warsaw, Poland, Director of the European Association for Cardio-Thoracic Surgery Congenital Database, and Past-President of the European Congenital Heart Surgeons Association.)

292,828.[19] The aggregate Participant Feedback Report from the Fall 2013 Harvest of the STS Congenital Heart Surgery Database includes 136,617 operations performed in the 4-year analytic window of July 1, 2009 to June 30, 2013, inclusive, submitted from 120 hospitals in North America—117 in the United States and 3 in Canada. In collaboration with EACTS, the STS has developed standardized methodology for tracking mortality and morbidity associated with the treatment of patients with congenital and pediatric cardiac disease.[93,105,212]

The EACTS Congenital Heart Surgery Database is the largest database in Europe dealing with congenital cardiac malformations (Fig. 133-4).[112,117] As of May 2013, the EACTS Congenital Heart Surgery Database contained 157,772 operations performed in 130,534 patients. As of May 2013, the EACTS Congenital Heart Surgery Database had 348 centers from 76 countries registered, with 173 active centers from 46 countries submitting data.

The JCCVSD has recently been operationalized based on nomenclature and database standards identical to those used by EACTS and STS.[117] The JCCVSD began enrolling patients in 2008. By December 2011, more than 100 hospitals were submitting data, and by April 2013, more than 29,000 operations were entered into the JCCVSD, in just under 5 years of data collection (Fig. 133-5). In Japan, it is mandatory for specialists to enroll in this benchmarking project to examine their own performance objectively and to make efforts for continuous improvement. In the future, certification is to be performed solely on the basis of empirical data registered by the project. The developers of the JCCVSD hope to collaborate with their colleagues across Asia to create an Asian Congenital Heart Surgery Database.

In the United Kingdom, the United Kingdom Central Cardiac Audit Database (UKCCAD) uses the AEPC-derived version of the IPCCC as the basis for its national, comprehensive, validated, and benchmark-driven audit of all pediatric surgical and transcatheter procedures undertaken since 2000.[152] All 13 tertiary centers in the United Kingdom performing cardiac surgery or therapeutic cardiac catheterization in children with congenital cardiac disease submit data to the UKCCAD. Data about mortality are obtained from both results volunteered from the hospital databases, and by independently validated records of deaths obtained by the Office for National Statistics, using the patient's unique National Health Service number, or the general register offices of Scotland and Northern Ireland. Efforts are underway to link the UKCCAD to the EACTS Congenital Heart Surgery Database. Linkage of the UKCCAD to the EACTS Congenital Heart Surgery Database will require use of the cross-map of the AEPC-derived version of the IPCCC (used by the UKCCAD) to the EACTS-STS–derived version of the IPCCC (used by the EACTS, STS, and JCCVSD).

As of January 1, 2014, the STS Congenital Heart Surgery Database contains data from 292,828 operations, the EACTS Congenital Heart Surgery Database contains data from more than 157,772 operations, and the JCCVSD contains data from more than 29,000 operations. Therefore, the combined dataset of the STS Congenital Heart Surgery Database, the EACTS Congenital Heart Surgery Database, and JCCVSD contains data from more than 479,000 operations, all coded with the EACTS-STS–derived version of the IPCCC,[100,110,112,114] and all coded with identical data specifications.[21]

COMPLEXITY STRATIFICATION

The importance of measuring complexity derives from the fact that analysis of outcomes using raw measurements of mortality, without adjustment for complexity, is inadequate. The mix of cases can vary greatly from

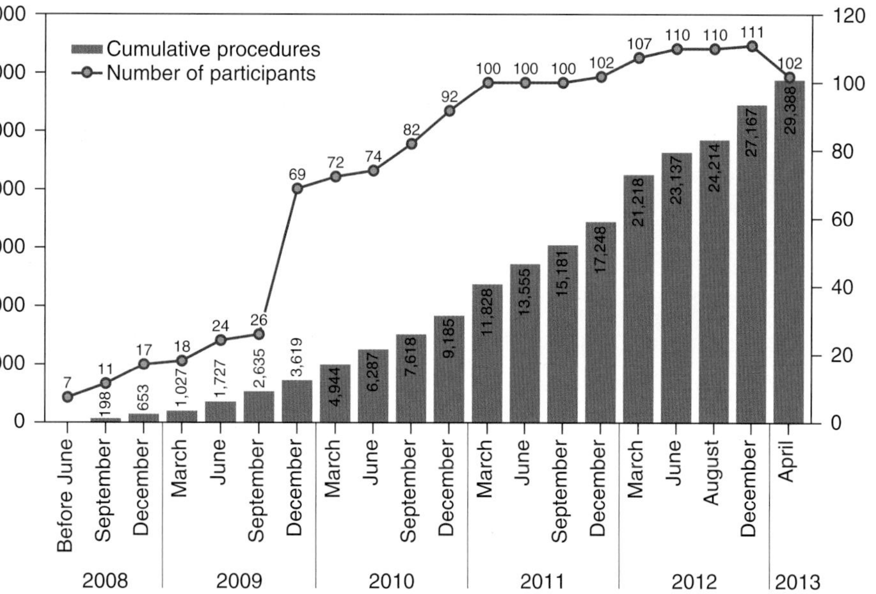

FIGURE 133-5 The initial growth of the Japan Congenital Cardiovascular Surgery Database (JCCVSD). The JCCVSD has recently been operationalized based on identical nomenclature and database standards as that used by the European Association for Cardio-Thoracic Surgery and the Society of Thoracic Surgeons. The JCCVSD began enrolling patients in 2008. By December 2011, more than 100 hospitals were submitting data, and by April 2013, more than 29,000 operations were entered into the JCCVSD, in just under 5 years of data collection. The developers of the JCCVSD hope to collaborate with their colleagues across Asia to create an Asian Congenital Heart Surgery Database. (Data courtesy Arata Murakami, MD, The University of Tokyo, Tokyo, Japan.)

program to program. Without stratification of complexity, the analysis of outcomes will be flawed.[‡‡]

The analysis of outcomes after surgery requires a reliable method of estimating the risk of adverse events. However, formal risk modeling is challenging for rare operations. Complexity stratification provides an alternative methodology that can facilitate the analysis of outcomes of rare operations. Complexity stratification is a method of analysis in which the data are divided into relatively homogeneous groups (called *strata*). The data are analyzed within each stratum.

Three major multi-institutional efforts have attempted to measure the complexity of congenital cardiac surgical operations:

1. ***R***isk ***A***djustment in ***C***ongenital ***H***eart ***S***urgery-1 methodology (RACHS-1 method)[56,73,149]
2. ***A***ristotle ***B***asic ***C***omplexity Score (ABC Score)[§§]
3. ***ST***S-***EAC***T***S*** Congenital Heart Surgery Mortality Categories (STS-EACTS Mortality Categories, or STAT Mortality Categories)[150]

RACHS-1 and the ABC Score were developed at a time when limited multi-institutional clinical data were available and were therefore based largely on subjective probability (i.e., expert opinion). The STAT Mortality Categories are a tool for complexity stratification that was developed from an analysis of 77,294 operations entered into the EACTS Congenital Heart Surgery Database (33,360 operations) and the STS Congenital Heart Surgery Database (43,934 patients) between 2002 and 2007. Procedure-specific mortality rate estimates were calculated using a Bayesian model that adjusted for small denominators. Operations were sorted by increasing risk and were grouped into five categories (the STS-EACTS Congenital Heart Surgery Mortality Categories) that were designed to be optimal with respect to minimizing within-category variation and maximizing between-category variation.

Table 133-1 compares RACHS-1, the ABC Score, and the STS-EACTS Mortality Categories. Table 133-2 shows the application in the STS Congenital Heart Surgery Database of the STAT Congenital Heart Surgery Mortality Categories.[198] STS has transitioned from the primary use of Aristotle and RACHS-1 to the primary use of the STAT Mortality Categories for three reasons:

1. STAT Score was developed primarily based on objective data, whereas RACHS-1 and Aristotle were developed primarily on subjective probability (i.e., expert opinion).
2. STAT Score allows for classification of more operations than RACHS-1 or Aristotle.
3. STAT Score has a higher c-statistic than RACHS-1 or Aristotle do.

Meaningful evaluation and comparison of outcomes require consideration of both mortality and morbidity, but the latter is much harder to measure. The STAT Mortality Categories provide an empirically based tool for analyzing mortality associated with operations for congenital heart disease.[150] STS has developed the STAT Morbidity Categories[215] on the basis of major postoperative complications and postoperative length of stay. Both major postoperative complications and postoperative length of stay were used, because models that assume a perfect one-to-one relationship between postoperative complications and postoperative length of stay are not likely to fit the data well. The incorporation of both

[‡‡]References 56, 61, 73, 74, 76, 82, 106, 149, 150.
[§§]References 61, 74, 76, 82, 106, 149.

TABLE 133-1 **Results of Comparing the STS-EACTS Categories (2009) to the RACHS-1 Categories and the Aristotle Basic Complexity Score***

Method of Modeling Procedures	Model without Patient Covariates	Model with Patient Covariates	Percent of Operations That Can Be Classified
STS-EACTS Congenital Heart Surgery Mortality Categories (2009)	C = 0.778	C = 0.812	99%
RACHS-1 Categories	C = 0.745	C = 0.802	86%
Aristotle Basic Complexity Score	C = 0.687	C = 0.795	94%

*Using an independent validation sample of 27,700 operations performed in 2007 and 2008. In the subset of procedures for which STS-EACTS Category (STAT Mortality Category), RACHS-1 Category, and Aristotle Basic Complexity Score are defined, discrimination was highest for the STS-EACTS categories (C-index = 0.778), followed by RACHS-1 categories (C-index = 0.745), and Aristotle Basic Complexity scores (C-index = 0.687).

RACHS-1, Risk Adjustment in Congenital Heart Surgery-1; *STS-EACTS,* Society of Thoracic Surgeons–European Association for Cardio-Thoracic Surgery.

TABLE 133-2 **Discharge Mortality in Patients in the STS Congenital Heart Surgery Database***

STAT Mortality Category	Total Number of Operations	Discharge Mortality (%)
1	15,441	0.55
2	17,994	1.7
3	8,989	2.6
4	13,375	8.0
5	2,707	18.4

*Patients who underwent surgery between January 1, 2005, and December 31, 2009, inclusive,[198] stratified by STAT Mortality Categories (Society of Thoracic Surgeons–European Association for Cardio-Thoracic Surgery Congenital Heart Surgery Mortality Categories).

STS, Society of Thoracic Surgeons.

major postoperative complications and postoperative length of stay allows for the creation of a much more informative model. The STAT Morbidity Categories provide an empirically based tool for analyzing morbidity associated with operations for congenital heart disease.[215]

DATA VERIFICATION

Collaborative efforts involving EACTS and STS aim to enhance mechanisms to verify the completeness and accuracy of the data in the databases.[21,126] A combination of three strategies may ultimately be required to allow for optimal verification of data:

1. Intrinsic data verification (designed to rectify inconsistencies of data and missing elements of data)
2. Site visits with "source data verification" (i.e., verification of the data at the primary source of the data)
3. External verification of the data from independent databases or registries (e.g., governmental death registries)

SUBSPECIALTY COLLABORATION

Under the leadership of the MultiSocietal Database Committee for Pediatric and Congenital Heart Disease,[110-112] further collaborative efforts are ongoing between congenital and pediatric cardiac surgeons and other subspecialties, including:

1. Pediatric cardiac anesthesiologists, via the Congenital Cardiac Anesthesia Society[105,119,139,207]
2. Pediatric cardiac intensivists, via the Pediatric Cardiac Intensive Care Society,[190] and
3. Pediatric cardiologists, via the Joint Council on Congenital Heart Disease, the American College of Cardiology (ACC), and the Association for European Paediatric Cardiology.[118]

Strategies have been developed to link databases together.[‖] By linking different databases, it is possible to capitalize on the strengths and mitigate some of the weaknesses of these databases and therefore perform analyses not possible with either dataset alone. Linked databases have facilitated both comparative effectiveness research[193,194,219] and longitudinal follow-up.[145,146,173,214] Under the leadership of the MultiSocietal Database Committee for Pediatric and Congenital Heart Disease,[110-140] additional collaborative efforts are ongoing among congenital and pediatric cardiac surgeons and other subspecialties.

LONGITUDINAL FOLLOW-UP

The transformation of the STS Database to a platform for longitudinal follow-up will ultimately result in higher quality of care for all cardiothoracic surgical patients by facilitating longitudinal comparative effectiveness research on a national level.[127,173,184,214] Several potential strategies will allow longitudinal follow-up with the STS Database, including the development of clinical longitudinal follow-up modules within the STS Database itself, and linking the STS Database to other clinical registries, administrative databases, and national death registries:

1. Using probabilistic matching with shared indirect identifiers, the STS Database can be linked to administrative claims databases (such as the CMS Medicare Database[145,146] and the Pediatric Health Information System [PHIS] database[¶¶]) and become a valuable source of information about long-term

‖References 109, 164, 189, 193, 194, 210, 219.

¶¶References 109, 164, 189, 193, 194, 210, 219.

mortality, rates of rehospitalization, long-term morbidity, and cost.[208]

2. Using deterministic matching with shared unique direct identifiers, the STS Database can be linked to national death registries, such as the Social Security Death Master File (SSDMF) and the National Death Index (NDI), to verify life status over time.[127,173,184,214]
3. Through either probabilistic matching or deterministic matching,[184] the STS Database can link to multiple other clinical registries, such as the National Cardiovascular Data Registry (NCDR) of the ACC, to provide enhanced clinical follow-up.
4. The STS Database can develop clinical longitudinal follow-up modules of its own to provide detailed clinical follow-up.[109,127,173,184,214]

QUALITY ASSESSMENT AND QUALITY IMPROVEMENT

The STS Database is being used increasingly to document variation in outcomes[182,198] and to measure quality.[179,186] Funnel plots can be used to demonstrate this variation in outcome and to facilitate the identification of centers that are outliers in performance (Fig. 133-6). Quality improvement initiatives can be initiated in low-performing centers, and best practices can be obtained from high-performing centers.

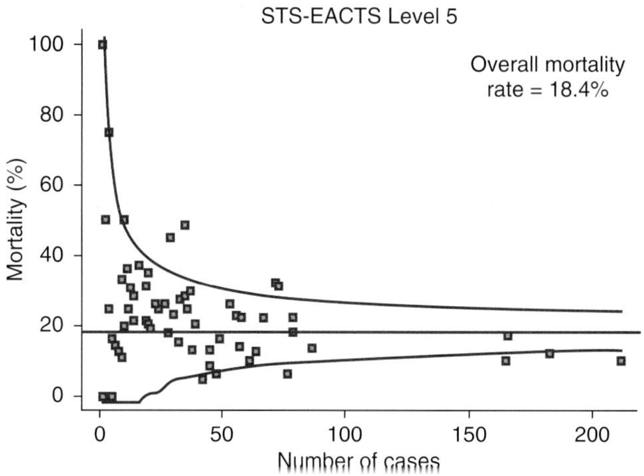

FIGURE 133-6 Mortality data displayed as a funnel plot for STAT Category 5 operations.[198] The *horizontal line* depicts aggregate Society of Thoracic Surgeons (STS) mortality before discharge. *Curved lines* depicting exact 95% binomial prediction limits were overlaid to make a funnel plot. Squares represent the number of cases and mortality before discharge for individual STS Congenital Heart Surgery Database participants (centers). This analysis includes patients undergoing surgery during the 5-year analytic window of 2005 to 2009, inclusive, and includes 70 STS centers in the STS Congenital Heart Surgery Database and 2707 operations. Centers that were identified as outliers represented 18.6% of participating centers (13 of 70): 10% (7 of 70) were "high-performing outliers" and 8.6% (6 out of 70) were "low-performing outliers." Quality improvement initiatives can be initiated in low-performing centers, and best practices can be obtained from high-performing centers. *EACTS,* European Association for Cardio-Thoracic Surgery.

STS has collaborated with the Congenital Heart Surgeons' Society (CHSS) to develop and endorse metrics to assess the quality of care delivered to patients with pediatric and congenital cardiac disease.[186] Box 133-1 and Tables 133-3 and 133-4 present 21 "Quality Measures for Congenital and Pediatric Cardiac Surgery" that were developed and approved by the STS and endorsed by the CHSS. These quality measures are organized according to Donabedian's Triad of Structure, Process, and Outcome.[229] It is hoped that these quality measures can aid in congenital and pediatric cardiac surgical quality

Text continued on p. 2392

BOX 133-1 Quality Measures for Congenital and Pediatric Cardiac Surgery

1. Participation in a national database for pediatric and congenital heart surgery
2. Multidisciplinary rounds involving multiple members of the health care team
3. Availability of institutional pediatric extracorporeal life support program
4. Surgical volume for pediatric and congenital heart surgery: total programmatic volume and programmatic volume stratified by the five STS-EACTS mortality categories
5. Surgical volume for eight pediatric and congenital heart benchmark operations
6. Multidisciplinary preoperative planning conference to plan pediatric and congenital heart surgery operations
7. Regularly scheduled quality assurance and quality improvement cardiac care conference, to occur no less frequently than once every two months
8. Availability of intraoperative transesophageal echocardiography and epicardial echocardiography
9. Timing of antibiotic administration for pediatric and congenital cardiac surgery patients
10. Selection of appropriate prophylactic antibiotics and weight-appropriate dosage for pediatric and congenital cardiac surgery patients
11. Use of an expanded preprocedural and post-procedural "time-out"
12. Occurrence of new postoperative renal failure requiring dialysis
13. Occurrence of new postoperative neurologic deficit persisting at discharge
14. Occurrence of arrhythmia necessitating permanent pacemaker insertion
15. Occurrence of paralyzed diaphragm (possible phrenic nerve injury)
16. Occurrence of need for postoperative mechanical circulatory support (IABP, VAD, ECMO, or CPS)
17. Occurrence of unplanned reoperation and/or interventional cardiovascular catheterization procedure
18. Operative mortality stratified by the five STS-EACTS mortality levels
19. Operative mortality for eight benchmark operations
20. Index Cardiac Operations free of mortality and major complication
21. Operative survivors free of major complication

CPS, Mechanical CardioPulmonary Support; *ECMO,* extracorporeal membrane oxygenation; *IABP,* intra-aortic balloon pump; *STS-EACTS,* Society of Thoracic Surgeons–European Association for Cardio-Thoracic Surgery; *VAD,* ventricular assist device.

TABLE 133-3 **Definitions of Quality Measures for Congenital and Pediatric Cardiac Surgery**

Number	Type	Title of Indicator	Description
S-1	Structure	Participation in a national database for pediatric and congenital heart surgery	Participation in at least one multicenter, standardized data collection and feedback program that provides regularly scheduled reports of the individual center's data relative to national multicenter aggregates and that uses process and outcome measures.
S-2	Structure	Multidisciplinary rounds involving multiple members of the health care team	Occurrence of daily multidisciplinary rounds on pediatric and congenital cardiac surgery patients involving multiple members of the health care team, with recommended participation including but not limited to: cardiac surgery, cardiology, critical care, primary caregiver, family, nurses, pharmacist, and respiratory therapist; involvement of the family is encouraged.
S-3	Structure	Availability of institutional pediatric extracorporeal life support program	Availability of an institutional pediatric extracorporeal life support program for pediatric and congenital cardiac surgery patients; measure is satisfied by the availability of ECMO equipment and support staff, but also applies to ventricular assist devices (including extracorporeal, paracorporeal, and implantable).
S-4	Structure	Surgical volume for pediatric and congenital heart surgery: total programmatic volume and programmatic volume stratified by the five STS-EACTS mortality categories	Surgical volume for pediatric and congenital heart surgery: STS version 2.5: All Index Cardiac Operations* STS version 3.0: Same Surgical volume for pediatric and congenital heart surgery stratified by the five STS-EACTS mortality levels, a multi-institutional validated complexity stratification tool. See O'Brien and colleagues[150] (Table 1, pp 1140-1146).
S-5	Structure	Surgical volume for eight pediatric and congenital heart benchmark operations	Surgical volume for eight benchmark pediatric and congenital heart operations: These eight benchmark pediatric and congenital heart operations are tracked when they are the primary procedure of an index cardiac operation.*

Procedure type	Abbreviation	STS-CHSDB Diagnostic and Procedural Inclusionary and Exclusionary Criteria
VSD repair	VSD	**Procedural inclusionary criteria:** 100 = VSD repair, Primary closure 110 = VSD repair, Patch 120 = VSD repair, Device† **Diagnostic inclusionary criteria:** 71 = VSD, Type 1 (Subarterial) (Supracristal) (Conal septal defect) (Infundibular) 73 = VSD, Type 2 (Perimembranous) (Paramembranous) (Conoventricular) 75 = VSD, Type 3 (Inlet) (AV canal type) 77 = VSD, Type 4 (Muscular) 79 = VSD, Type: Gerbode type (LV-RA communication) **Diagnostic exclusionary criteria:** 80 = VSD, Multiple
TOF repair	TOF	**Procedural inclusionary criteria:** 350 = TOF repair, No ventriculotomy 360 = TOF repair, Ventriculotomy, Nontransanular patch 370 = TOF repair, Ventriculotomy, Transanular patch 380 = TOF repair, RV-PA conduit **Diagnostic inclusionary criteria:** 290 = TOF 2140 = TOF, Pulmonary stenosis **Diagnostic exclusionary criteria:** 300 = TOF, AVC (AVSD) 310 = TOF, Absent pulmonary valve 320 = Pulmonary atresia 330 = Pulmonary atresia, IVS 340 = Pulmonary atresia, VSD (Including TOF, PA) 350 = Pulmonary atresia, VSD-MAPCA (pseudotruncus) 360 = MAPCA(s) (major aortopulmonary collateral[s]) (without PA-VSD)

			Complete AV canal repair	AVC	**Procedural inclusionary criteria:** 170 = AVC (AVSD) repair, Complete (CAVSD) **Diagnostic inclusionary criteria:** 100 = AVC (AVSD), Complete (CAVSD) **Diagnostic exclusionary criteria:** 110 = AVC (AVSD), Intermediate (transitional) 120 = AVC (AVSD), Partial (incomplete) (PAVSD) (ASD, primum) 300 = TOF, AVC (AVSD)
			Arterial switch	ASO	**Procedural inclusionary criteria:** 1110 = Arterial switch operation (ASO) **Procedural exclusionary criteria:** 1120 = Arterial switch operation (ASO) and VSD repair 1123 = Arterial switch procedure + Aortic arch repair 1125 = Arterial switch procedure and VSD repair + Aortic arch repair 1050 = Congenitally corrected TGA repair, Atrial switch and ASO (double switch)
			Arterial switch + VSD repair	ASO+VSD	**Procedural inclusionary criteria:** 1120 = Arterial switch operation (ASO) and VSD repair **Procedural exclusionary criteria:** 1110 = Arterial switch operation (ASO) 1123 = Arterial switch procedure + Aortic arch repair 1125 = Arterial switch procedure and VSD repair + Aortic arch repair 1050 = Congenitally corrected TGA repair, Atrial switch and ASO (double switch)
			Fontan	Fontan	**Procedural inclusionary criteria:** 950 = Fontan, Atrio-pulmonary connection 960 = Fontan, Atrio-ventricular connection 970 = Fontan, TCPC, Lateral tunnel, Fenestrated 980 = Fontan, TCPC, Lateral tunnel, Nonfenestrated 1000 = Fontan, TCPC, External conduit, Fenestrated 1010 = Fontan, TCPC, External conduit, Nonfenestrated 1030 = Fontan, Other 2340 = Fontan + Atrioventricular valvuloplasty **Procedural exclusionary criteria:** Exclude patients age ≥ 7 years 1025 = Fontan revision or conversion (Re-do Fontan)
			Truncus repair	Truncus	**Procedural inclusionary criteria:** Primary procedure must be: 230 = Truncus arteriosus repair **Procedural exclusionary criteria:** Exclude any operation if any of the component procedures is: 240 = Valvuloplasty, Truncal valve 2290 = Valvuloplasty converted to valve replacement in the same operation, Truncal valve 250 = Valve replacement, Truncal valve 2220 = Truncus + Interrupted aortic arch repair (IAA) repair
			Norwood	Norwood	**Procedural inclusionary criteria:** 870 = Norwood procedure
P-1	Process	Multidisciplinary preoperative planning conference to plan pediatric and congenital heart surgery operations	Occurrence of a preoperative multidisciplinary planning conference to plan pediatric and congenital heart surgery cases. This conference will involve multiple members of the health care team, with recommended participation including but not limited to: cardiology, cardiac surgery, anesthesia, and critical care. This measure will be coded on a per operation basis. Reporting of compliance will be as a fraction of all cardiac operations.*		

Continued

TABLE 133-3 **Definitions of Quality Measures for Congenital and Pediatric Cardiac Surgery—cont'd**

Number	Type	Title of Indicator	Description
P-2	Process	Regularly scheduled quality assurance and quality improvement cardiac care conference, to occur no less frequently than once every 2 months	Occurrence of a regularly scheduled quality assurance and quality improvement cardiac care conference to discuss care provided to patients who have undergone pediatric and congenital cardiac surgery operations, including reporting and discussion of all major complications and mortalities, and discussion of opportunities for improvement. Reporting of compliance will be by reporting the date of occurrence. Annual compliance of 100% equals no fewer than six conferences per year.
P-3	Process	Availability of intraoperative TEE and epicardial echocardiography	Availability of intraoperative TEE and appropriate physician and sonographer support for pediatric and congenital cardiac operations. Epicardial echocardiography and appropriate physician and sonographer support should be readily available for those patients in whom TEE is contraindicated or less informative. Availability means presence and availability of equipment and staff. This measure will be coded on a per operation basis. Reporting of compliance will be as the fraction of all cardiac operations with availability (as opposed to use) of TEE, epicardial echocardiography, or both.*
P-4	Process	Timing of antibiotic administration for pediatric and congenital cardiac surgery patients	Measure is satisfied for each cardiac operation when there is documentation that the patient has received prophylactic antibiotics within the hour immediately preceding surgical incision (2 hours if receiving vancomycin).*
P-5	Process	Selection of appropriate prophylactic antibiotics and weight-appropriate dosage for pediatric and congenital cardiac surgery patients	Measure is satisfied for each cardiac operation when there is documentation that the patient received body weight appropriate prophylactic antibiotics as recommended for the operation.*
P-6	Process	Use of an expanded pre-procedural and post-procedural "time-out"	Measure is satisfied for each cardiac operation* when there is documentation of performance and completion of an expanded preprocedural and postprocedural "time-out" that includes the following four elements: 1. The conventional pre-procedural "time-out," which includes identification of patient, operative site, procedure, and history of any allergies. 2. A preprocedural briefing wherein the surgeon shares with all members of the operating room team the essential elements of the operative plan, including diagnosis, planned procedure, outline of essentials of anesthesia and bypass strategies, antibiotic prophylaxis, availability of blood products, anticipated or planned implants or device applications, and anticipated challenges. 3. A postprocedural debriefing wherein the surgeon succinctly reviews with all members of the operating room team the essential elements of the operative plan, identifying both the successful components and the opportunities for improvement. This debriefing should take place *before the patient leaves the operating room or its equivalent* and may be followed by a more in-depth dialogue involving team members at a later time. (The actual debriefing in the operating room is intentionally and importantly brief, in recognition of the fact that periods of transition may be times of instability or vulnerability for the patient.) 4. A briefing and execution of a hand-off protocol at the time of transfer (arrival) to the intensive care unit at the end of the operation, involving the anesthesiologist, surgeon, physician staff of the intensive care unit (including critical care and cardiology) and nursing.
O-1	Outcome	Occurrence of new postoperative renal failure requiring dialysis	For each surgical admission (index cardiac operation*), code whether the complication occurred during the time interval beginning at admission to operating room and ending 30 days postoperatively or at the time of hospital discharge, whichever is longer. **STS version 2.5:** 220 = Acute renal failure requiring temporary dialysis 230 = Acute renal failure requiring permanent dialysis **STS version 3.0:** 230 = Renal failure—acute renal failure requiring dialysis at the time of hospital discharge 223 = Renal failure—acute renal failure requiring temporary dialysis with the need for dialysis not present at hospital discharge 224 = Renal failure—acute renal failure requiring temporary hemofiltration with the need for dialysis not present at hospital discharge

			Unless a patient requires dialysis before surgery, renal failure that requires dialysis after surgery constitutes an operative complication, despite the fact that preoperative diminished renal perfusion may have contributed to the development of this complication. This measure will be reported as percentage of all Index Cardiac Operations. This measure will also be reported stratified by the five STS-EACTS congenital heart surgery mortality categories. (STS is developing Congenital Heart Surgery Morbidity Categories. When these categories are published and available, this metric will be stratified by the STS Congenital Heart Surgery Morbidity Categories instead of the STS Congenital Heart Surgery Mortality Categories.)
O-2	Outcome	Occurrence of new postoperative neurologic deficit persisting at discharge	For each surgical admission (index cardiac operation*), code whether the complication occurred during the time interval beginning at admission to operating room and ending 30 days postoperatively or at the time of hospital discharge, whichever is longer. 320 = Neurologic deficit, neurologic deficit persisting at discharge This measure tracks "new postoperative neurologic deficits" that (1) occur during the time interval beginning at admission to operating room and ending at the time of hospital discharge and (2) persist at discharge. Such new postoperative neurologic deficits may or may not be related to a stroke. If the new postoperative neurologic deficit is the result of a stroke (that occurs during the time interval beginning at admission to operating room and ending at the time of hospital discharge) and the neurologic deficit persists at discharge, then the following two complications should both be selected: 320 = Neurologic deficit, neurologic deficit persisting at discharge 420 = Stroke Thus, this complication (320 = neurologic deficit, neurologic deficit persisting at discharge) should be coded when a patient has had a stroke (during the time interval beginning at admission to operating room and ending at the time of hospital discharge) and the neurologic deficit persists at discharge. This measure does not include a neurologic deficit (which may or may not be related to a stroke) that does not persist at discharge. NOTE: This complication (320 = Neurologic deficit, neurologic deficit persisting at discharge) should be coded even when the patient has a neurologic deficit that is present before admission to operating room and this neurologic deficit worsens (or a new neurologic deficit develops) during the time interval beginning at admission to operating room and ending at the time of hospital discharge. This measure will be reported as a percentage of all Index Cardiac Operations. This measure will also be reported stratified by the five STS-EACTS congenital heart surgery mortality categories. (STS is developing congenital heart surgery morbidity categories. When these categories are published and available, this metric will be stratified by the STS Congenital Heart Surgery Morbidity Categories instead of the STS Congenital Heart Surgery Mortality Categories.)
O-3	Outcome	Occurrence of arrhythmia necessitating permanent pacemaker insertion	For each surgical admission (Index Cardiac Operation*), code whether the complication occurred during the time interval beginning at admission to operating room and ending 30 days postoperatively or at the time of hospital discharge, whichever is longer. **STS version 2.5:** 60 = Postoperative AV block requiring permanent pacemaker **STS version 3.0:** 74 = Arrhythmia necessitating pacemaker, permanent pacemaker This measure will be reported as percentage of all Index Cardiac Operations. This measure will also be reported stratified by the five STS-EACTS congenital heart surgery mortality categories. (STS is developing Congenital Heart Surgery Morbidity Categories. When these categories are published and available, this metric will be stratified by the STS Congenital Heart Surgery Morbidity Categories instead of the STS Congenital Heart Surgery Mortality Categories.)
O-4	Outcome	Occurrence of paralyzed diaphragm (possible phrenic nerve injury)	For each surgical admission (index cardiac operation*), code whether the complication occurred during the time interval beginning at admission to operating room and ending 30 days postoperatively or at the time of hospital discharge, whichever is longer. **STS version 2.5:** 300 = Phrenic nerve injury/paralyzed diaphragm **STS version 3.0:** 300 = Paralyzed diaphragm (possible phrenic nerve injury) This measure will be reported as percentage of all Index Cardiac Operations. This measure will also be reported stratified by the five STS-EACTS Congenital Heart Surgery Mortality Categories. (STS is developing Congenital Heart Surgery Morbidity Categories. When these categories are published and available, this metric will be stratified by the STS Congenital Heart Surgery Morbidity Categories instead of the STS Congenital Heart Surgery Mortality Categories.)

Continued

TABLE 133-3 **Definitions of Quality Measures for Congenital and Pediatric Cardiac Surgery—cont'd**

Number	Type	Title of Indicator	Description
O-5	Outcome	Occurrence of need for postoperative mechanical circulatory support (IABP, VAD, ECMO, or CPS)	For each surgical admission (index cardiac operation*), code whether the complication occurred during the time interval beginning at admission to operating room and ending 30 days postoperatively or at the time of hospital discharge, whichever is longer. **STS version 2.5:** 40 = Postoperative mechanical circulatory support (IABP, VAD, ECMO, or CPS) **STS version 3.0:** 40 = Postoperative or Postprocedural mechanical circulatory support (IABP, VAD, ECMO, or CPS) This complication should be coded even when the patient had preoperative mechanical circulatory support if the patient has mechanical circulatory support postoperatively at any time until 30 days postoperatively or the time of hospital discharge, whichever is longer. This measure will be reported as percentage of all Index Cardiac Operations. This measure will also be reported stratified by the five STS-EACTS congenital heart surgery mortality categories. (STS is developing Congenital Heart Surgery Morbidity Categories. When these categories are published and available, this metric will be stratified by the STS Congenital Heart Surgery Morbidity Categories instead of the STS Congenital Heart Surgery Mortality Categories.)
O-6	Outcome	Occurrence of unplanned reoperation and/or interventional cardiovascular catheterization procedure	For each surgical admission (index cardiac operation*), code whether the complication occurred during the time interval beginning at admission to operating room and ending 30 days postoperatively or at the time of hospital discharge, whichever is longer. **STS version 2.5:** 20 = Reoperation during this admission (unplanned reoperation) 240 = Bleeding requiring reoperation **STS version 3.0:** 22 = Unplanned cardiac reoperation during the postoperative or postprocedural time period 24 = Unplanned interventional cardiovascular catheterization procedure during the postoperative or postprocedural time period 26 = Unplanned noncardiac reoperation during the postoperative or postprocedural time period 240 = Bleeding, requiring reoperation *n.b. does not include delayed sternal closure* This measure will be reported as percentage of all Index Cardiac Operations. This measure will also be reported stratified by the five STS-EACTS congenital heart surgery mortality categories. (STS is developing Congenital Heart Surgery Morbidity Categories. When these categories are published and available, this metric will be stratified by the STS Congenital Heart Surgery Morbidity Categories instead of the STS Congenital Heart Surgery Mortality Categories.) This measure counts all patients who require any additional unplanned cardiac or noncardiac operation and/or interventional cardiovascular catheterization procedure occurring (1) within 30 days after surgery or intervention in or out of the hospital, or (2) after 30 days during the same hospitalization subsequent to the operation or intervention.* The following operations will always be coded as "planned reoperation": (1) delayed sternal closure, (2) ECMO decannulation, (3) VAD decannulation, (4) removal of Broviac catheter. The following operations will always be coded as "Unplanned Reoperation": (1) reoperation for bleeding, (2) reoperation for infection, (3) reoperation for hemodynamic instability, (4) reoperation for initiation of ECMO or VAD, (5) reoperation for residual or recurrent lesion.
O-7	Outcome	Operative mortality stratified by the five STS-EACTS mortality levels	Operative mortality stratified by the five STS-EACTS mortality levels, a multi-institutional validated complexity stratification tool. See O'Brien and colleagues[150] (Table 1, pp 1140-1146).
O-8	Outcome	Operative mortality for eight benchmark operations	Operative mortality for eight benchmark pediatric and congenital heart operations: These eight benchmark pediatric and congenital heart operations are tracked when they are the primary procedure of an index cardiac operation,* and they are listed and described in this table in Measure Number S-5.

O-9	Outcome	Index Cardiac Operations free of mortality and major complication	"Index Cardiac Operations free of mortality and major complication" is defined as the percent of pediatric and congenital heart surgery Index Cardiac Operations free of the following: (1) operative mortality, (2) any one or more of the following major complications occurring or diagnosed during the time interval beginning at admission to operating room and ending 30 days postoperatively or at the time of hospital discharge, whichever is longer: (a) ***Renal failure*—acute renal failure requiring temporary or permanent dialysis (220, 230, 223, 224)** STS version 2.5: 220 = Acute renal failure requiring temporary dialysis 230 = Acute renal failure requiring permanent dialysis STS version 3.0: 230 = Renal failure—acute renal failure requiring dialysis at the time of hospital discharge 223 = Renal failure—acute renal failure requiring temporary dialysis with the need for dialysis not present at hospital discharge 224 = Renal failure—acute renal failure requiring temporary hemofiltration with the need for dialysis not present at hospital discharge (b) ***Neurologic deficit, neurologic deficit persisting at discharge*** STS version 2.5: 320 = Postoperative neurologic deficit persisting at discharge STS version 3.0: 320 = Neurologic deficit, neurologic deficit persisting at discharge (c) ***Arrhythmia necessitating pacemaker, permanent pacemaker* (60, 74)** STS version 2.5: 60 = Postoperative AV block requiring permanent pacemaker STS version 3.0: 74 = Arrhythmia necessitating pacemaker, permanent pacemaker (d) ***ECMO/VAD:* postoperative mechanical circulatory support (IABP, VAD, ECMO or CPS) (40)** STS version 2.5: 40 = Postoperative mechanical circulatory support (IABP, VAD, ECMO, or CPS) STS version 3.0: 40 = Postoperative or postprocedural mechanical circulatory support (IABP, VAD, ECMO, or CPS) (e) ***Paralyzed diaphragm (possible phrenic nerve injury)*** STS version 2.5: 300 = Phrenic nerve injury/paralyzed diaphragm STS version 3.0: 300 = Paralyzed diaphragm (possible phrenic nerve injury) (f) ***Unplanned reoperation* (20, 22, 26 or 240)** STS version 2.5: 20 = Reoperation during this admission (unplanned reoperation) 240 = Bleeding requiring reoperation STS version 3.0: 22 = Unplanned cardiac reoperation during the postoperative or postprocedural time period, exclusive of reoperation for bleeding 24 = Unplanned interventional cardiovascular catheterization procedure during the postoperative or postprocedural time period 26 = Unplanned noncardiac reoperation during the postoperative or postprocedural time period 240 = Bleeding, requiring reoperation This measure will be reported as percentage of all Index Cardiac Operations.* This measure will also be reported stratified by the five STS-EACTS congenital heart surgery mortality categories. (STS is developing congenital heart surgery morbidity categories. When these categories are published and available, this metric will be stratified by the STS Congenital Heart Surgery Morbidity Categories instead of the STS Congenital Heart Surgery Mortality Categories.)

Continued

TABLE 133-3 **Definitions of Quality Measures for Congenital and Pediatric Cardiac Surgery—cont'd**

Number	Type	Title of Indicator	Description
O-10	Outcome	Operative survivors free of major complication	"Operative survivors free of major complication" is defined as the percent of all surviving (live at discharge and 30 days postoperatively) pediatric and congenital heart surgery index operations free of all the following itemized major complications: (a) ***Renal failure*—acute renal failure requiring temporary or permanent dialysis (220, 230, 223, 224)** STS version 2.5: 220 = Acute renal failure requiring temporary dialysis 230 = Acute renal failure requiring permanent dialysis STS version 3.0: 230 = Acute renal failure requiring dialysis at the time of hospital discharge 223 = Acute renal failure requiring temporary dialysis with the need for dialysis not present at hospital discharge 224 = Acute renal failure requiring temporary hemofiltration with the need for dialysis not present at hospital discharge (b) ***Neurologic deficit, neurologic deficit persisting at discharge*** STS version 2.5: 320 = Postoperative neurologic deficit persisting at discharge STS version 3.0: 320 = Neurologic deficit, neurologic deficit persisting at discharge (c) ***Arrhythmia necessitating pacemaker, permanent pacemaker* (60, 74)** STS version 2.5: 60 = Postoperative AV block requiring permanent pacemaker STS version 3.0: 74 = Arrhythmia necessitating pacemaker, permanent pacemaker (d) ***ECMO/VAD*—postoperative mechanical circulatory support (IABP, VAD, ECMO or CPS) (40)** STS version 2.5: 40 = Postoperative mechanical circulatory support (IABP, VAD, ECMO, or CPS) STS version 3.0: 40 = Postoperative or postprocedural mechanical circulatory support (IABP, VAD, ECMO, or CPS) (e) ***Paralyzed diaphragm (possible phrenic nerve injury)*** STS version 2.5: 300 = Phrenic nerve injury, paralyzed diaphragm STS version 3.0: 300 = Paralyzed diaphragm (possible phrenic nerve injury) (f) ***Unplanned reoperation* (20, 22, 26, or 240)** STS version 2.5: 20 = Reoperation during this admission (unplanned reoperation) 240 = Bleeding requiring reoperation STS version 3.0: 22 = Unplanned cardiac reoperation during the postoperative or postprocedural time period, exclusive of reoperation for bleeding 24 = Unplanned interventional cardiovascular catheterization procedure during the postoperative or postprocedural time period 26 = Unplanned non-cardiac reoperation during the postoperative or postprocedural time period 240 = Bleeding, Requiring reoperation This measure will be reported as percentage of all Index Cardiac Operations. This measure will also be reported stratified by the five STS-EACTS congenital heart surgery mortality categories. (STS is developing Congenital Heart Surgery Morbidity Categories. When these categories are published and available, this metric will be stratified by the STS Congenital Heart Surgery Morbidity Categories instead of the STS Congenital Heart Surgery Mortality Categories.)

*A *cardiac operation* is defined as an operation of operation type "CPB" or "No CPB Cardiovascular."

†This measure is applicable when one or more septal occluder devices are implanted in the course of a surgical operation for which the primary procedure of an index cardiac operation is VSD repair. A VSD device that is placed as a purely transcatheter technique, and not as a component of a cardiac operation, is classified as an *interventional cardiology procedure* and is not tracked as part of this measure.

ASD, Atrial septal defect; *ASO,* atrial switch operation; *AV,* atrioventricular; *AVC,* atrioventricular canal; *AVSD,* atrioventricular septal defect; *CAVSD,* complete atrioventricular septal defect; *CHSDB,* Congenital Heart Surgery Databases; *CPB,* cardiopulmonary bypass; *CPS,* mechanical CardioPulmonary Support; *EACTS,* European Association for Cardio-Thoracic Surgery; *ECMO,* extracorporeal membrane oxygenation; *IAA,* interrupted aortic arch; *IABP,* intra-aortic balloon pump; *IVS,* intact ventricular septum; *LV,* left ventricle; *MAPCA,* major aortopulmonary collateral; *PA,* pulmonary artery; *PA-VSD,* pulmonary atresia with ventricular septal defect; *PAVSD,* partial ventricular septal defect; *RA,* right atrium; *STS,* Society of Thoracic Surgeons; *TCPC,* Total CavoPulmonary Connection; *TGA,* transposition of the great arteries; *TEE,* transesophageal echocardiography; *TOF,* tetralogy of Fallot; *VAD,* ventricular assist device; *VSD,* ventricular septal defect.

TABLE 133-4 **Consensus Definitions of the Morbidities**

Measure	Organ System	Complication	Definitions
12	Renal	Acute renal failure requiring dialysis at the time of hospital discharge	Acute renal failure* with a new postoperative or postprocedural requirement for dialysis, including peritoneal dialysis or hemodialysis. Code this complication if the patient requires dialysis at the time of hospital discharge or death in the hospital. (This complication should be chosen only if the dialysis was associated with acute renal failure.)
12	Renal	Acute renal failure requiring temporary dialysis with the need for dialysis not present at hospital discharge	Acute renal failure with a new postoperative or postprocedural requirement for temporary dialysis, including peritoneal dialysis and/or hemodialysis. Code this complication if the patient does not require dialysis at the time of hospital discharge or death in the hospital. (This complication should be chosen only if the dialysis was associated with acute renal failure.)
12	Renal	Acute renal failure requiring temporary hemofiltration with the need for dialysis not present at hospital discharge	Acute renal failure with a new postoperative or postprocedural requirement for temporary hemofiltration. Code this complication if the patient does not require dialysis at the time of hospital discharge or death in the hospital. (This complication should be chosen only if the hemofiltration was associated with acute renal failure.)
13	Neurologic	Neurologic deficit, neurologic deficit persisting at discharge	Newly recognized or newly acquired deficit of neurologic function leading to inpatient referral, therapy, or intervention not otherwise practiced for a similar unaffected inpatient, with a persisting neurologic deficit present at hospital discharge. In other words, new (onset intraoperatively, postoperatively, intraprocedurally, or postprocedurally) neurologic deficit persisting and present at discharge from hospital.
13	Neurologic	Stroke	Any confirmed neurologic deficit of abrupt onset caused by a disturbance in blood flow to the brain, when the neurologic deficit does not resolve within 24 hours.
13	Neurologic	Spinal cord injury, neurologic deficit persisting at discharge	Spinal cord injury with a persisting neurologic deficit present at hospital discharge; newly acquired or newly recognized deficit of spinal cord function indicated by physical examination findings, imaging studies, or both.
13	Neurologic	Peripheral nerve injury, neurologic deficit persisting at discharge	Peripheral nerve injury with a persisting neurologic deficit present at hospital discharge; newly acquired or newly recognized deficit of unilateral or bilateral peripheral nerve function indicated by physical examination findings, imaging studies, or both.
14	Arrhythmia necessitating pacemaker	Arrhythmia necessitating pacemaker, permanent pacemaker	Implantation and use of a permanent pacemaker for treatment of any arrhythmia including heart block (atrioventricular heart block).
15	Neurologic	Paralyzed diaphragm (possible phrenic nerve injury)	Presence of elevated hemidiaphragm on chest radiograph in conjunction with evidence of weak, immobile, or paradoxic movement assessed by ultrasound or fluoroscopy.
16	Mechanical support utilization	Postoperative or postprocedural mechanical circulatory support (IABP, VAD, ECMO, or CPS)	Use of postoperative or postprocedural mechanical support, of any type (IABP, VAD, ECMO, or CPS), for resuscitation or support during the postoperative or postprocedural time period. Code this complication if it occurs (1) within 30 days after surgery or intervention regardless of the date of hospital discharge, or (2) after 30 days during the same hospitalization subsequent to the operation or intervention.
17	Operative, procedural	Unplanned cardiac reoperation during the postoperative or postprocedural time period, exclusive of reoperation for bleeding	Any additional unplanned cardiac operation occurring (1) within 30 days after surgery or intervention in or out of the hospital, or (2) after 30 days during the same hospitalization subsequent to the operation or intervention. A *cardiac operation* is defined as any operation that is of the operation type of "CPB" or "No CPB Cardiovascular." The following operations will always be coded as "Planned Reoperation": (1) delayed sternal closure, (2) ECMO decannulation, (3) VAD decannulation, (4) removal of Broviac catheter. The following operations will always be coded as "Unplanned Reoperation": (1) reoperation for bleeding, (2) reoperation for infection, (3) reoperation for hemodynamic instability, (4) reoperation for initiation of ECMO or VAD, (5) reoperation for residual or recurrent lesion.
17	Operative, procedural	Unplanned interventional cardiovascular catheterization procedure during the postoperative or postprocedural period	Any unplanned interventional cardiovascular catheterization procedure occurring (1) within 30 days after surgery or intervention in or out of the hospital, or (2) after 30 days during the same hospitalization subsequent to the operation or intervention.

Continued

TABLE 133-4 **Consensus Definitions of the Morbidities—cont'd**

Measure	Organ System	Complication	Definitions
17	Operative, procedural	Unplanned noncardiac reoperation during the postoperative or postprocedural time period	Any additional unplanned noncardiac operation occurring (1) within 30 days after surgery or intervention in or out of the hospital, or (2) after 30 days during the same hospitalization subsequent to the operation or intervention.

**Acute renal failure* is defined as new onset oliguria with sustained urine output < 0.5 mL/kg/hr for 24 hours and/or a rise in creatinine > 1.5 times upper limits of normal for age (or twice the most recent preoperative/preprocedural values if these are available), with eventual need for dialysis (including peritoneal dialysis and/or hemodialysis) or hemofiltration. Acute renal failure that will be counted as an operative or procedural complication must occur prior to hospital discharge or after hospital discharge but within 30 days of the procedure. (An operative or procedural complication is any complication, regardless of cause, occurring (1) within 30 days after surgery or intervention in or out of the hospital, or (2) after 30 days during the same hospitalization subsequent to the operation or intervention. Operative and procedural complications include both intraoperative/intraprocedural complications and postoperative/postprocedural complications in this time interval.) The complication is to be coded even if the patient required dialysis, but the treatment was not instituted due to patient or family refusal.

CPB, Cardiopulmonary bypass; *CPS,* mechanical CardioPulmonary Support; *ECMO,* extracorporeal membrane oxygenation; *IABP,* intra-aortic balloon pump; *VAD,* ventricular assist device.

assessment and quality improvement initiatives. These initiatives will take on added importance as the public reporting of cardiac surgical performance becomes more common.[143,176,177]

SUMMARY: BRIDGING THE GAP FROM ANALYSIS OF OUTCOMES TO IMPROVEMENT OF QUALITY

Clinical registries represent a foundational tool in the following interrelated process:

1. Measuring the outcomes of medical and surgical practices
2. Developing evidence for best medical and surgical practices,
3. Providing actionable feedback to clinicians, and
4. Improving quality of care and outcomes

Clinical registries are the best tool for measuring the outcomes of the processes of care.[220,221] As described in this chapter, the ability to measure clinical outcomes properly requires using standardized clinical nomenclature, uniform standards for defining elements of data and collecting these data, strategies to adjust for the complexity of patients, techniques to verify the completeness and accuracy of data, and collaboration across medical and surgical subspecialties. All these elements exist in the ideal clinical registry.

Clinical registries can be used as a platform for developing evidence for best medical practices and performing comparative effectiveness research. The linkage of the STS Congenital Heart Surgery Database to the PHIS Database (funded by the National Institutes of Health [NIH]) exemplifies this approach.*** This linkage of clinical and administrative data facilitated comparative effectiveness research in the domains of perioperative methylprednisolone and outcome in neonates undergoing heart surgery[193] and antifibrinolytic medications in pediatric heart surgery.[194] Similarly, the NIH-funded ASCERT trial (American College of Cardiology Foundation—Society of Thoracic Surgeons Collaboration on the Comparative Effectiveness of Revascularization Strategies trial) also used linked clinical and administrative data to compare surgical and transcatheter strategies of coronary revascularization.[230,231] Although randomized trials have been considered by many to be the gold standard of comparative effectiveness research, recent efforts have examined the possibility of using a clinical registry as a platform for randomized trials,[232,233] potentially accomplishing the dual objectives of decreasing the cost of the trial and increasing the generalizability of the patients enrolled.

Clinical registries can provide actionable feedback to clinicians and therefore aid in initiatives to improve quality. Clinical registries can provide practitioners with accurate and timely feedback of their own outcomes and can benchmark these outcomes to regional, national, or even international aggregate data.[182,198,234,235,236]

The ultimate goal of clinical registries is to improve quality of care and outcomes. Clinical registries have been used to create standardized measures of quality that have been endorsed by multiple professional medical societies and the National Quality Forum.[186,237] Compliance with these measures and the public reporting of these measures should lead to improvements in the overall quality of care delivered to our patients.[143,176,177]

***References 164, 189, 193, 194, 210, 219.

REFERENCES

1. Mavroudis C (Chairman), Congenital Database Subcommittee: Backer CL, Bove E, Burke RP, Cameron D, Drinkwater DC, Edwards FH, Grover FL, Hammon JW Jr, Jacobs JP, Kron IL, Mayer JE, Myers JL, Ring WS, Siewers RD, Szarnicki RJ, Watson DC Jr: *Data Analyses of the Society of Thoracic Surgeons National Congenital Cardiac Surgery Database, 1994-1997,* Minnetonka, MN, September 1998, Summit Medical.
2. Jacobs JP, Jacobs ML, Mavroudis C, et al: Executive Summary: The Society of Thoracic Surgeons Congenital Heart Surgery Database—Second Harvest—(1998-2001) Beta Site Test. The Society of Thoracic Surgeons (STS) and Duke Clinical Research Institute (DCRI), Duke University Medical Center, Durham, North Carolina, United States, Fall 2002 Harvest.
3. Jacobs JP, Jacobs ML, Mavroudis C, et al: Executive Summary: The Society of Thoracic Surgeons Congenital Heart Surgery Database—Third Harvest—(1998-2002). The Society of Thoracic Surgeons (STS) and Duke Clinical Research Institute

(DCRI), Duke University Medical Center, Durham, North Carolina, United States, Spring 2003 Harvest.
4. Jacobs JP, Jacobs ML, Mavroudis C, et al: Executive Summary: The Society of Thoracic Surgeons Congenital Heart Surgery Database—Fourth Harvest—(2002-2003). The Society of Thoracic Surgeons (STS) and Duke Clinical Research Institute (DCRI), Duke University Medical Center, Durham, North Carolina, United States, Spring 2004 Harvest.
5. Jacobs JP, Jacobs ML, Mavroudis C, et al: Executive Summary: The Society of Thoracic Surgeons Congenital Heart Surgery Database—Fifth Harvest—(2002-2004). The Society of Thoracic Surgeons (STS) and Duke Clinical Research Institute (DCRI), Duke University Medical Center, Durham, North Carolina, United States, Spring 2005 Harvest.
6. Jacobs JP, Jacobs ML, Mavroudis C, et al: Executive Summary: The Society of Thoracic Surgeons Congenital Heart Surgery Database—Sixth Harvest—(2002-2005). The Society of Thoracic Surgeons (STS) and Duke Clinical Research Institute (DCRI), Duke University Medical Center, Durham, North Carolina, United States, Spring 2006 Harvest.
7. Jacobs JP, Jacobs ML, Mavroudis C, et al: Executive Summary: The Society of Thoracic Surgeons Congenital Heart Surgery Database—Seventh Harvest—(2003-2006). The Society of Thoracic Surgeons (STS) and Duke Clinical Research Institute (DCRI), Duke University Medical Center, Durham, North Carolina, United States, Spring 2007 Harvest.
8. Jacobs JP, Jacobs ML, Mavroudis C, et al: Executive Summary: The Society of Thoracic Surgeons Congenital Heart Surgery Database—Eighth Harvest—(January 1, 2004–December 31, 2007). The Society of Thoracic Surgeons (STS) and Duke Clinical Research Institute (DCRI), Duke University Medical Center, Durham, North Carolina, United States, Spring 2008 Harvest.
9. Jacobs JP, Jacobs ML, Mavroudis C, et al: Executive Summary: The Society of Thoracic Surgeons Congenital Heart Surgery Database—Ninth Harvest—(July 1, 2004–June 30, 2008). The Society of Thoracic Surgeons (STS) and Duke Clinical Research Institute (DCRI), Duke University Medical Center, Durham, North Carolina, United States, Fall 2008 Harvest.
10. Jacobs JP, Jacobs ML, Mavroudis C, et al: Executive Summary: The Society of Thoracic Surgeons Congenital Heart Surgery Database—Tenth Harvest—(January 1, 2005–December 31, 2008). The Society of Thoracic Surgeons (STS) and Duke Clinical Research Institute (DCRI), Duke University Medical Center, Durham, North Carolina, United States, Spring 2009 Harvest.
11. Jacobs JP, Jacobs ML, Mavroudis C, et al: Executive Summary: The Society of Thoracic Surgeons Congenital Heart Surgery Database—Eleventh Harvest—(July 1, 2005–June 30, 2009). The Society of Thoracic Surgeons (STS) and Duke Clinical Research Institute (DCRI), Duke University Medical Center, Durham, North Carolina, United States, Fall 2009 Harvest.
12. Jacobs JP, Jacobs ML, Mavroudis C, et al: Executive Summary: The Society of Thoracic Surgeons Congenital Heart Surgery Database—Twelfth Harvest—(January 1, 2006–December 31, 2009). The Society of Thoracic Surgeons (STS) and Duke Clinical Research Institute (DCRI), Duke University Medical Center, Durham, North Carolina, United States, Spring 2010 Harvest.
13. Jacobs JP, Jacobs ML, Mavroudis C, et al: Executive Summary: The Society of Thoracic Surgeons Congenital Heart Surgery Database—Thirteenth Harvest—(July 1, 2006–June 30, 2010). The Society of Thoracic Surgeons (STS) and Duke Clinical Research Institute (DCRI), Duke University Medical Center, Durham, North Carolina, United States, Fall 2010 Harvest.
14. Jacobs JP, Jacobs ML, Mavroudis C, et al: Executive Summary: The Society of Thoracic Surgeons Congenital Heart Surgery Database—Fourteenth Harvest—(January 1, 2007–December 31, 2010). The Society of Thoracic Surgeons (STS) and Duke Clinical Research Institute (DCRI), Duke University Medical Center, Durham, North Carolina, United States, Spring 2011 Harvest.
15. Jacobs JP, Jacobs ML, Mavroudis C, et al: Executive Summary: The Society of Thoracic Surgeons Congenital Heart Surgery Database—Fifteenth Harvest—(July 1, 2007–June 30, 2011). The Society of Thoracic Surgeons (STS) and Duke Clinical Research Institute (DCRI), Duke University Medical Center, Durham, North Carolina, United States, Fall 2011 Harvest.
16. Jacobs JP, Jacobs ML, Mavroudis C, et al: Executive Summary: The Society of Thoracic Surgeons Congenital Heart Surgery Database—Sixteenth Harvest—(January 1, 2008–December 31, 2011). The Society of Thoracic Surgeons (STS) and Duke Clinical Research Institute (DCRI), Duke University Medical Center, Durham, North Carolina, United States, Spring 2012 Harvest.
17. Jacobs JP, Jacobs ML, Mavroudis C, et al: Executive Summary: The Society of Thoracic Surgeons Congenital Heart Surgery Database—Seventeenth Harvest—(July 1, 2008–June 30, 2012). The Society of Thoracic Surgeons (STS) and Duke Clinical Research Institute (DCRI), Duke University Medical Center, Durham, North Carolina, United States, Fall 2012 Harvest.
18. Jacobs JP, Jacobs ML, Mavroudis C, et al: Executive Summary: The Society of Thoracic Surgeons Congenital Heart Surgery Database—Eighteenth Harvest—(January 1, 2009–December 31, 2012). The Society of Thoracic Surgeons (STS) and Duke Clinical Research Institute (DCRI), Duke University Medical Center, Durham, North Carolina, United States, Spring 2013 Harvest.
19. Jacobs JP, Jacobs ML, Mavroudis C, et al: Executive Summary: The Society of Thoracic Surgeons Congenital Heart Surgery Database—Nineteenth Harvest—(July 1, 2008–June 30, 2013). The Society of Thoracic Surgeons (STS) and Duke Clinical Research Institute (DCRI), Duke University Medical Center, Durham, North Carolina, United States, Fall 2013 Harvest.
20. Mavroudis C, Gevitz M, Ring WS, et al: The Society of Thoracic Surgeons National Congenital Cardiac Surgery Database. *Ann Thorac Surg* 68:601–624, 1999.
21. Mavroudis C, Jacobs JP: The international congenital heart surgery nomenclature and database project. *Ann Thorac Surg* (Suppl):S1–S372, April 2000.
22. Mavroudis C, Jacobs JP: Congenital heart surgery nomenclature and database project: introduction. In: The Annals of Thoracic Surgery April 2000 Supplement: The International Congenital Heart Surgery Nomenclature and Database Project, Constantine Mavroudis and Jeffrey P. Jacobs, MD (editors). *Annals Thorac Surg* (Suppl):S1, 2000.
23. Mavroudis C, Jacobs JP: Congenital heart surgery nomenclature and database project: overview and minimum dataset. In: The Annals of Thoracic Surgery April 2000 Supplement: The International Congenital Heart Surgery Nomenclature and Database Project, Constantine Mavroudis and Jeffrey P. Jacobs, MD (editors). *Ann Thorac Surg* (Suppl):S2–S17, 2000.
24. Jacobs JP, Quintessenza JA, Burke RP, et al: Congenital heart surgery nomenclature and database project: atrial septal defect. In: The Annals of Thoracic Surgery April 2000 Supplement: The International Congenital Heart Surgery Nomenclature and Database Project, Constantine Mavroudis and Jeffrey P. Jacobs, MD (editors). *Ann Thorac Surg* (Suppl):S18–S24, 2000.
25. Jacobs JP, Burke RP, Quintessenza JA, et al: Congenital heart surgery nomenclature and database project: ventricular septal defect. In: The Annals of Thoracic Surgery April 2000 Supplement: The International Congenital Heart Surgery Nomenclature and Database Project, Constantine Mavroudis and Jeffrey P. Jacobs, MD (editors). *Ann Thorac Surg* (Suppl):S25–S35, 2000.
26. Jacobs JP, Burke RP, Quintessenza JA, et al: Congenital heart surgery nomenclature and database project: atrioventricular canal defect. In: The Annals of Thoracic Surgery April 2000 Supplement: The International Congenital Heart Surgery Nomenclature and Database Project, Constantine Mavroudis and Jeffrey P. Jacobs, MD (editors). *Ann Thorac Surg* (Suppl):S36–S43, 2000.
27. Jacobs JP, Quintessenza JA, Gaynor JW, et al: Congenital heart surgery nomenclature and database project: aortopulmonary window. In: The Annals of Thoracic Surgery April 2000 Supplement: The International Congenital Heart Surgery Nomenclature and Database Project, Constantine Mavroudis and Jeffrey P. Jacobs, MD (editors). *Ann Thorac Surg* (Suppl):S44–S49, 2000.
28. Jacobs M: Congenital heart surgery nomenclature and database project: truncus arteriosus. In: The Annals of Thoracic Surgery April 2000 Supplement: The International Congenital Heart Surgery Nomenclature and Database Project, Constantine Mavroudis and Jeffrey P. Jacobs, MD (editors). *Ann Thorac Surg* (Suppl):S50–S55, 2000.
29. Herlong JR, Jaggers JJ, Ungerleider RM: Congenital heart surgery nomenclature and database project: pulmonary venous

anomalies. In: The Annals of Thoracic Surgery April 2000 Supplement: The International Congenital Heart Surgery Nomenclature and Database Project, Constantine Mavroudis and Jeffrey P. Jacobs, MD (editors). *Ann Thorac Surg* (Suppl):S56–S69, 2000.
30. Gaynor JW, Weinberg P, Spray T: Congenital heart surgery nomenclature and database project: systemic venous anomalies. In: The Annals of Thoracic Surgery April 2000 Supplement: The International Congenital Heart Surgery Nomenclature and Database Project, Constantine Mavroudis and Jeffrey P. Jacobs, MD (editors). *Ann Thorac Surg* (Suppl):S70–S76, 2000.
31. Jacobs M: Congenital heart surgery nomenclature and database project: tetralogy of fallot. In: The Annals of Thoracic Surgery April 2000 Supplement: The International Congenital Heart Surgery Nomenclature and Database Project, Constantine Mavroudis and Jeffrey P. Jacobs, MD (editors). *Ann Thorac Surg* (Suppl):S77–S82, 2000.
32. Lacour-Gayet F: Congenital heart surgery nomenclature and database project: right ventricular outflow tract obstruction—intact ventricular septum. In: The Annals of Thoracic Surgery April 2000 Supplement: The International Congenital Heart Surgery Nomenclature and Database Project, Constantine Mavroudis and Jeffrey P. Jacobs, MD (editors). *Ann Thorac Surg* (Suppl):S83–S96, 2000.
33. Tchervenkov CI, Roy N: Congenital heart surgery nomenclature and database project: pulmonary atresia—ventricular septal defect. In: The Annals of Thoracic Surgery April 2000 Supplement: The International Congenital Heart Surgery Nomenclature and Database Project, Constantine Mavroudis and Jeffrey P. Jacobs, MD (editors). *Ann Thorac Surg* (Suppl):S97–S105, 2000.
34. Dearani JA, Danielson GK: Congenital heart surgery nomenclature and database project: Ebstein's anomaly and tricuspid valve disease. In: The Annals of Thoracic Surgery April 2000 Supplement: The International Congenital Heart Surgery Nomenclature and Database Project, Constantine Mavroudis and Jeffrey P. Jacobs, MD (editors). *Ann Thorac Surg* (Suppl):S106–S117, 2000.
35. Nguyen KH: Congenital heart surgery nomenclature and database project: aortic valve disease. In: The Annals of Thoracic Surgery April 2000 Supplement: The International Congenital Heart Surgery Nomenclature and Database Project, Constantine Mavroudis and Jeffrey P. Jacobs, MD (editors). *Ann Thorac Surg* (Suppl):S118–S131, 2000.
36. Mitruka SN, Lamberti JJ: Congenital heart surgery nomenclature and database project: mitral valve disease. In: The Annals of Thoracic Surgery April 2000 Supplement: The International Congenital Heart Surgery Nomenclature and Database Project, Constantine Mavroudis and Jeffrey P. Jacobs, MD (editors). *Ann Thorac Surg* (Suppl):S132–S146, 2000.
37. Ring WS: Congenital heart surgery nomenclature and database project: aortic aneurysm, sinus of valsalva aneurysm, and aortic dissection. In: The Annals of Thoracic Surgery April 2000 Supplement: The International Congenital Heart Surgery Nomenclature and Database Project, Constantine Mavroudis and Jeffrey P. Jacobs, MD (editors). *Ann Thorac Surg* (Suppl):S147–S163, 2000.
38. Myers JL, Mehta SM: Congenital heart surgery nomenclature and database project: aortico-left ventricular tunnel. In: The Annals of Thoracic Surgery April 2000 Supplement: The International Congenital Heart Surgery Nomenclature and Database Project, Constantine Mavroudis and Jeffrey P. Jacobs, MD (editors). *Ann Thorac Surg* (Suppl):S164–S169, 2000.
39. Tchervenkov CI, Jacobs M, Tahta SA: Congenital heart surgery nomenclature and database project: hypoplastic left heart syndrome. In: The Annals of Thoracic Surgery April 2000 Supplement: The International Congenital Heart Surgery Nomenclature and Database Project, Constantine Mavroudis and Jeffrey P. Jacobs, MD (editors). *Ann Thorac Surg* (Suppl):S170–S179, 2000.
40. Delius RE: Congenital heart surgery nomenclature and database project: pediatric cardiomyopathies and end-stage congenital heart disease. In: The Annals of Thoracic Surgery April 2000 Supplement: The International Congenital Heart Surgery Nomenclature and Database Project, Constantine Mavroudis and Jeffrey P. Jacobs, MD (editors). *Ann Thorac Surg* (Suppl):S180–S190, 2000.
41. Myers JL, Mehta SM: Congenital heart surgery nomenclature and database project: diseases of the pericardium. In: The Annals of Thoracic Surgery April 2000 Supplement: The International Congenital Heart Surgery Nomenclature and Database Project, Constantine Mavroudis and Jeffrey P. Jacobs, MD (editors). *Ann Thorac Surg* (Suppl):S191–S196, 2000.
42. Jacobs M, Mayer JE: Congenital heart surgery nomenclature and database project: single ventricle. In: The Annals of Thoracic Surgery April 2000 Supplement: The International Congenital Heart Surgery Nomenclature and Database Project, Constantine Mavroudis and Jeffrey P. Jacobs, MD (editors). *Ann Thorac Surg* (Suppl):S197–S204, 2000.
43. Jaggers JJ, Cameron DE, Herlong JR, et al: Congenital heart surgery nomenclature and database project: transposition of the great arteries. In: The Annals of Thoracic Surgery April 2000 Supplement: The International Congenital Heart Surgery Nomenclature and Database Project, Constantine Mavroudis and Jeffrey P. Jacobs, MD (editors). *Ann Thorac Surg* (Suppl):S205–S235, 2000.
44. Wilkinson JL, Cochrane AD, Karl TR: Congenital heart surgery nomenclature and database project: corrected (discordant) transposition of the great arteries (and related malformations). In: The Annals of Thoracic Surgery April 2000 Supplement: The International Congenital Heart Surgery Nomenclature and Database Project, Constantine Mavroudis and Jeffrey P. Jacobs, MD (editors). *Ann Thorac Surg* (Suppl):S236–S248, 2000.
45. Walters HW, III, Mavroudis C, Tchervenkov CI, et al: Congenital heart surgery nomenclature and database project: double outlet right ventricle. In: The Annals of Thoracic Surgery April 2000 Supplement: The International Congenital Heart Surgery Nomenclature and Database Project, Constantine Mavroudis and Jeffrey P. Jacobs, MD (editors). *Ann Thorac Surg* (Suppl):S249–S263, 2000.
46. Tchervenkov CI, Walters HW, III, Chu VF: Congenital heart surgery nomenclature and database project: double outlet left ventricle. In: The Annals of Thoracic Surgery April 2000 Supplement: The International Congenital Heart Surgery Nomenclature and Database Project, Constantine Mavroudis and Jeffrey P. Jacobs, MD (editors). *Ann Thorac Surg* (Suppl):S264–S269, 2000.
47. Dodge-Khatami A, Mavroudis C, Backer CL: Congenital heart surgery nomenclature and database project: anomalies of the coronary arteries. In: The Annals of Thoracic Surgery April 2000 Supplement: The International Congenital Heart Surgery Nomenclature and Database Project, Constantine Mavroudis and Jeffrey P. Jacobs, MD (editors). *Ann Thorac Surg* (Suppl):S270–S297, 2000.
48. Backer CL, Mavroudis C: Congenital heart surgery nomenclature and database project: patent ductus arteriosus, coarctation of the aorta, and interrupted aortic arch. In: The Annals of Thoracic Surgery April 2000 Supplement: The International Congenital Heart Surgery Nomenclature and Database Project, Constantine Mavroudis and Jeffrey P. Jacobs, MD (editors). *Ann Thorac Surg* (Suppl):S298–S307, 2000.
49. Backer CL, Mavroudis C: Congenital heart surgery nomenclature and database project: vascular rings, tracheal stenosis, and pectus excavatum. In: The Annals of Thoracic Surgery April 2000 Supplement: The International Congenital Heart Surgery Nomenclature and Database Project, Constantine Mavroudis and Jeffrey P. Jacobs, MD (editors). *Ann Thorac Surg* (Suppl):S308–S318, 2000.
50. Deal BJ, Jacobs JP, Mavroudis C: Congenital heart surgery nomenclature and database project: arrhythmias. In: The Annals of Thoracic Surgery April 2000 Supplement: The International Congenital Heart Surgery Nomenclature and Database Project, Constantine Mavroudis and Jeffrey P. Jacobs, MD (editors). *Ann Thorac Surg* (Suppl):S319–S331, 2000.
51. Rocchini AP: Congenital heart surgery nomenclature and database project: therapeutic cardiac catheter interventions. In: The Annals of Thoracic Surgery April 2000 Supplement: The International Congenital Heart Surgery Nomenclature and Database Project, Constantine Mavroudis and Jeffrey P. Jacobs, MD (editors). *Ann Thorac Surg* (Suppl):S332–S342, 2000.
52. Gaynor JW, Bridges ND, Spray T: Congenital heart surgery nomenclature and database project: end-stage lung disease. In: The Annals of Thoracic Surgery April 2000 Supplement: The International Congenital Heart Surgery Nomenclature and Database Project, Constantine Mavroudis and Jeffrey P. Jacobs, MD (editors). *Ann Thorac Surg* (Suppl):S343–S357, 2000.

53. Mehta SM, Myers JL: Congenital heart surgery nomenclature and database project: cardiac tumors. In: The Annals of Thoracic Surgery April 2000 Supplement: The International Congenital Heart Surgery Nomenclature and Database Project, Constantine Mavroudis and Jeffrey P. Jacobs, MD (editors). *Ann Thorac Surg* (Suppl):S358–S368, 2000.
54. Joffs C, Sade RM: Congenital heart surgery nomenclature and database project: palliation, correction, or repair. In: The Annals of Thoracic Surgery April 2000 Supplement: The International Congenital Heart Surgery Nomenclature and Database Project, Constantine Mavroudis and Jeffrey P. Jacobs, MD (editors). *Ann Thorac Surg* (Suppl):S369–S372, 2000.
55. Lacour-Gayet F, Maruszewski B, Mavroudis C, et al: Presentation of the international nomenclature for congenital heart surgery—the long way from nomenclature to collection of validated data at the eacts. *Eur J Cardiothorac Surg* 18(2):128–135, 2000.
56. Jenkins KJ, Gauvreau K, Newburger JW, et al: Consensus-based method for risk adjustment for surgery for congenital heart disease. *J Thorac Cardiovasc Surg* 123:110–118, 2002.
57. Mavroudis C, Jacobs JP: Congenital heart disease outcome analysis: methodology and rationale. *J Thorac Cardiovasc Surg* 123(1):6–7, 2002.
58. Mavroudis C, Gevitz M, Elliott MJ, et al: Virtues of a worldwide congenital heart surgery database. *Semin Thoracic Cardiovasc Surg Pediatr Card Surg Annu* 5(1):126–131, 2002.
59. Williams WG, McCrindle BW: Practical experience with databases for congenital heart disease: a registry versus an academic database. *Semin Thoracic Cardiovasc Surg Pediatr Card Surg Annu* 5(1):132–142, 2002.
60. Maruszewski B, Tobota Z: The European congenital heart defects surgery database experience: pediatric European cardiothoracic surgical registry of the European Association for Cardio-thoracic Surgery. *Semin Thoracic Cardiovasc Surg Pediatr Card Surg Annu* 5(1):143–147, 2002.
61. Lacour-Gayet F: Risk stratification theme for congenital heart surgery. *Semin Thoracic Cardiovasc Surg Pediatr Card Surg Annu* 5(1):148–152, 2002.
62. Jacobs JP: Software development, nomenclature schemes, and mapping strategies for an international pediatric cardiac surgery database system. *Semin Thoracic Cardiovasc Surg Pediatr Card Surg Annu* 5(1):153–162, 2002.
63. Maruszewski B, Lacour-Gayet F, Elliott MJ, et al: Congenital heart surgery nomenclature and database project: update and proposed data harvest. *Eur J Cardiothorac Surg* 21(1):47–49, 2002.
64. Gaynor JW, Jacobs JP, Jacobs ML, et al: Congenital heart surgery nomenclature and database project: update and proposed data harvest. *Ann Thorac Surg* 73(3):1016–1018, 2002.
65. Jenkins KJ, Gauvreau K: Center-specific differences in mortality: preliminary analyses using the Risk Adjustment in Congenital Heart Surgery (RACHS-1) method. *J Thorac Cardiovasc Surg* 124:97–104, 2002.
66. Franklin RCG, Jacobs JP, Tchervenkov CI, et al: Report from the executive of the international working group for mapping and coding of nomenclatures for paediatric and congenital heart disease: bidirectional crossmap of the short lists of the European paediatric cardiac code and the international congenital heart surgery nomenclature and database project. *Cardiol Young* (Suppl II):18–22, 2002.
67. Franklin RCG, Jacobs JP, Tchervenkov CI, et al: European paediatric cardiac code short list crossmapped to STS/EACTS short list with ICD-9 & ICD-10 crossmapping. *Cardiol Young* (Suppl II):23–49, 2002.
68. Franklin RCG, Jacobs JP, Tchervenkov CI, et al: STS/EACTS short list mapping to European paediatric cardiac code short list with ICD-9 & ICD-10 crossmapping. *Cardiol Young* (Suppl II):50–62, 2002.
69. Béland M, Jacobs JP, Tchervenkov CI, et al: The international nomenclature project for paediatric and congenital heart disease: report from the executive of the international working group for mapping and coding of nomenclatures for paediatric and congenital heart disease. *Cardiol Young* 12:425–430, 2002.
70. Franklin RCG, Jacobs JP, Tchervenkov CI, et al: The international nomenclature project for pediatric and congenital heart disease: bidirectional crossmap of the short lists of the European paediatric cardiac code and the international congenital heart surgery nomenclature and database project. *Cardiol Young* 12:431–435, 2002.
71. Kurosawa H, Gaynor JW, Jacobs JP, et al: Congenital heart surgery nomenclature and database project: update and proposed data harvest. *Jpn J Thorac Cardiovasc Surg* 50(11):498–501, 2002.
72. Allen SW, Gauvreau K, Bloom BT, et al: Evidence-based referral results in significantly reduced mortality after congenital heart surgery. *Pediatrics* 112(1 Pt 1):24–28, 2003.
73. Jenkins KJ: Risk adjustment for congenital heart surgery: the RACHS-1 method. *Semin Thorac Cardiovasc Surg Pediatr Card Surg Ann* 7:180–184, 2004.
74. Lacour-Gayet FG, Clarke D, Jacobs JP, et al: The Aristotle score for congenital heart surgery. *Semin Thorac Cardiovasc Surg Pediatr Card Surg Ann* 7:185–191, 2004.
75. Béland MJ, Franklin RCG, Jacobs JP, et al: Update from the international working group for mapping and coding of nomenclatures for paediatric and congenital heart disease. *Cardiol Young* 14(2):225–229, 2004.
76. Lacour-Gayet FG, Clarke D, Jacobs JP, et al: The Aristotle score: a complexity-adjusted method to evaluate surgical results. *Eur J Cardiothorac Surg* 25(6):911–924, 2004.
77. Jacobs JP, Mavroudis C, Jacobs ML, et al: Lessons learned from the data analysis of the second harvest (1998-2001) of the Society of Thoracic Surgeons (STS) Congenital Heart Surgery Database. *Eur J Cardiothorac Surg* 26(1):18–37, 2004.
78. Boethig D, Jenkins KJ, Hecker H, et al: The RACHS-1 risk categories reflect mortality and length of hospital stay in a large German pediatric cardiac surgery population. *Eur J Cardiothorac Surg* 26:12–17, 2004.
79. Welke KF, Jacobs JP, Jenkins KJ: Evaluation of quality of care for congenital heart disease. *Semin Thorac Cardiovasc Surg Pediatr Card Surg Annu* 8:157–167, 2005.
80. Jacobs JP, Elliott MJ, Anderson RH, et al: Creating a database with cardioscopy and intra-operative imaging. In 2005 Supplement to Cardiology in the Young: Controversies of the Ventriculo-Arterial Junctions and Other Topics, Jacobs JP, Wernovsky G, Gaynor JW, and Anderson RH (editors). *Cardiol Young* 15(Suppl 1):184–189, 2005.
81. Jacobs JP, Maruszewski B, Tchervenkov CI, et al: The current status and future directions of efforts to create a global database for the outcomes of therapy for congenital heart disease. In 2005 Supplement to Cardiology in the Young: Controversies of the Ventriculo-Arterial Junctions and Other Topics, Jacobs JP, Wernovsky G, Gaynor JW, and Anderson RH (editors). *Cardiol Young* 15(Suppl 1):190–198, 2005.
82. Jacobs JP, Lacour-Gayet FG, Jacobs ML, et al: Initial application in the STS congenital database of complexity adjustment to evaluate surgical case mix and results. *Ann Thorac Surg* 79(5):1635–1649, discussion 1635–1649, 2005.
83. Lacour-Gayet F, Clarke DR, Aristotle Committee: The Aristotle method: a new concept to evaluate quality of care based on complexity. *Curr Opin Pediatr* 17(3):412–417, 2005.
84. Lacour-Gayet F, Jacobs JP, Clarke DR, et al: Performance of surgery for congenital heart disease: shall we wait a generation or look for different statistics? *J Thorac Cardiovasc Surg* 130(1):234–235, 2005.
85. Maruszewski B, Lacour-Gayet F, Monro JL, et al: An attempt at data verification in the EACTS Congenital Database. *Eur J Cardiothorac Surg* 28(3):400–404, discussion 405–406, 2005.
86. Jacobs ML: Editorial comment. *Eur J Cardiothorac Surg* 28(3):405–406, 2005.
87. Jacobs JP, Maruszewski B, the European Association for Cardio-Thoracic Surgery (EACTS) and The Society of Thoracic Surgeons (STS) Joint Congenital Heart Surgery Nomenclature and Database Committee: computerized outcomes analysis for congenital heart disease. *Curr Opin Pediatr* 17(5):586–591, 2005.
88. Jacobs JP, Jacobs ML, Maruszewski B, et al: Current status of the European Association for Cardio-thoracic Surgery and the Society of Thoracic Surgeons Congenital Heart Surgery Database. *Ann Thorac Surg* 80(6):2278–2283, discussion 2283–2284, 2005.
89. Larsen SH, Pedersen J, Jacobsen J, et al: The RACHS-1 risk categories reflect mortality and length of stay in a Danish population of children operated for congenital heart disease. *Eur J Cardiothrac Surg* 28:877–881, 2005.
90. Miyamoto T, Sinzobahamvya N, Kumpikaite D, et al: Repair of truncus arteriosus and aortic arch interruption: outcome analysis. *Ann Thorac Surg* 79:2077–2082, 2005.

91. Maruszewski B, Tobota Z, Kansy A, et al: The Aristotle Score methodology for evaluation of outcomes in congenital heart surgery. *Standard Med Pediatr* (7 Suppl 22):29–33, 2005.
92. Jacobs JP, Franklin RCG, Jacobs ML, et al: Classification of the functionally univentricular heart: unity from mapped codes. In 2006 Supplement to Cardiology in the Young: Controversies and Challenges in the Management of the Functionally Univentricular Heart, Jacobs JP, Wernovsky G, Gaynor JW, and Anderson RH (editors). *Cardiol Young* 16(Suppl 1):9–21, 2006.
93. Jacobs JP, Mavroudis C, Jacobs ML, et al: What is operative mortality? Defining death in a surgical registry database: a report from the STS Congenital Database Task Force and the Joint EACTS-STS Congenital Database Committee. *Ann Thorac Surg* 81(5):1937–1941, 2006.
94. Tchervenkov CI, Jacobs JP, Weinberg PM, et al: The nomenclature, definition and classification of hypoplastic left heart syndrome. *Cardiol Young* 16(4):339–368, 2006.
95. Jacobs ML, Mavroudis C, Jacobs JP, et al: Report of the 2005 STS congenital heart surgery practice and manpower survey: a report from the STS Work Force on congenital heart surgery. *Ann Thorac Surg* 82(3):1152–1158, 1159e1–e5; discussion 1158–1159, 2006.
96. Jacobs JP, Franklin RCG, Wilkinson JL, et al: The nomenclature, definition and classification of discordant atrioventricular connections. In 2006 Supplement to Cardiology in the Young: Controversies and Challenges of the Atrioventricular Junctions and Other Challenges Facing Paediatric Cardiovascular Practitioners and their Patients, Jacobs JP, Wernovsky G, Gaynor JW, and Anderson RH (editors). *Cardiol Young* 16(Suppl 3):72–84, 2006.
97. Sinzobahamvya N, Photiadis J, Kumpikaite D, et al: Comprehensive Aristotle score: implications for the Norwood procedure. *Ann Thorac Surg* 81:1794–1800, 2006.
98. Atrip JH, Campbell DN, Ivy DD, et al: Birth weight and complexity are significant factors for the management of hypoplastic left heart syndrome. *Ann Thorac Surg* 82:1252–1257, discussion 1258–1259, 2006.
99. Al-Radi OO, Harrell FE, Jr, Caldarone CA, et al: Case complexity scores in congenital heart surgery: a comparative study of the Aristotle Basic Complexity score and the Risk Adjustment in Congenital Heart Surgery (RACHS-1) system. *J Thorac Cardiovasc Surg* 133(4):865–875, 2007. [Epub 2007 Mar 2].
100. Jacobs JP, Mavroudis C, Jacobs ML, et al: Nomenclature and databases—the past, the present, and the future: a primer for the congenital heart surgeon. *Pediatr Cardiol* 28(2):105–115, 2007.
101. Lacour-Gayet F, Jacobs ML, Jacobs JP, et al: The need for an objective evaluation of morbidity in congenital heart surgery. *Ann Thorac Surg* 84(1):1–2, 2007.
102. Lacour-Gayet FG, Jacobs JP, Clarke DR, et al: Evaluation of quality of care in congenital heart surgery: contribution of the Aristotle complexity score. *Adv Pediatr* 54:67–83, 2007.
103. Jacobs JP, Anderson RH, Weinberg P, et al: The nomenclature, definition and classification of cardiac structures in the setting of heterotaxy. In 2007 Supplement to Cardiology in the Young: Controversies and Challenges Facing Paediatric Cardiovascular Practitioners and their Patients, Anderson RH, Jacobs JP, and Wernovsky G (editors). *Cardiol Young* 17(Suppl 2):1–28, 2007.
104. Jacobs JP, Wernovsky G, Elliott MJ: Analysis of outcomes for congenital cardiac disease: can we do better? In 2007 Supplement to Cardiology in the Young: Controversies and Challenges Facing Paediatric Cardiovascular Practitioners and their Patients, Jacobs JP, Wernovsky G, Gaynor JW, and Anderson RH (editors). *Cardiol Young* 17(Suppl 2):145–158, 2007.
105. Jacobs JP, Jacobs ML, Mavroudis C, et al: What is operative morbidity? Defining complications in a surgical registry database: a report from the STS Congenital Database Task Force and the Joint EACTS-STS Congenital Database Committee. *Ann Thorac Surg* 84:1416–1421, 2007.
106. O'Brien SM, Jacobs JP, Clarke DR, et al: Accuracy of the Aristotle Basic Complexity Score for classifying the mortality and morbidity potential of congenital heart surgery operations. *Ann Thorac Surg* 84(6):2027–2037, 2007.
107. Derby CD, Kolcz J, Kerins PJ, et al: Aristotle score predicts outcome in patients requiring extracorporeal circulatory support following repair of congenital heart disease. *ASAIO J* 53:82–86, 2007.
108. Curzon CL, Milford-Beland S, Li JS, et al: Cardiac surgery in infants with low birth weight is associated with increased mortality: analysis of the Society of Thoracic Surgeons Congenital Heart Database. *J Thorac Cardiovasc Surg* 135(3):546–551, 2008.
109. Jacobs JP, Haan CK, Edwards FH, et al: The rationale for incorporation of HIPAA compliant unique patient, surgeon, and hospital identifier fields in the STS database. *Ann Thorac Surg* 86(3):695–698, 2008.
110. Jacobs JP (Editor): 2008 Cardiology in the young supplement: databases and the assessment of complications associated with the treatment of patients with congenital cardiac disease, prepared by: the Multi-Societal Database Committee for Pediatric and Congenital Heart Disease. *Cardiol Young* 18(Suppl S2):1–530, 2008.
111. Jacobs JP: Introduction—Databases and the assessment of complications associated with the treatment of patients with congenital cardiac disease. In: 2008 Cardiology in the Young Supplement: Databases and the Assessment of Complications Associated with the Treatment of Patients with Congenital Cardiac Disease, Prepared by: The Multi-Societal Database Committee for Pediatric and Congenital Heart Disease, Jeffrey P. Jacobs, MD (editor). *Cardiol Young* 18(Suppl 2):1–37, 2008.
112. Jacobs JP, Jacobs ML, Mavroudis C, et al: Nomenclature and databases for the surgical treatment of congenital cardiac disease—an updated primer and an analysis of opportunities for improvement. *Cardiol Young* 18(Suppl 2):38–62, 2008.
113. Tchervenkov CI, Jacobs JP, Bernier P-L, et al: The improvement of care for paediatric and congenital cardiac disease across the World: a challenge for the World Society for Pediatric and Congenital Heart Surgery. *Cardiol Young* 18(Suppl 2):63–69, 2008.
114. Franklin RCG, Jacobs JP, Krogmann ON, et al: Nomenclature for congenital and paediatric cardiac disease: historical perspectives and the international pediatric and congenital cardiac code. *Cardiol Young* 18(Suppl 2):70–80, 2008.
115. Jacobs JP, Benavidez OJ, Bacha EA, et al: The nomenclature of safety and quality of care for patients with congenital cardiac disease: a report of the Society of Thoracic Surgeons Congenital Database Taskforce Subcommittee on Patient Safety. *Cardiol Young* 18(Suppl 2):81–91, 2008.
116. Strickland MJ, Riehle-Colarusso TJ, Jacobs JP, et al: The importance of nomenclature for congenital cardiac disease: implications for research and evaluation. *Cardiol Young* 18(Suppl 2):92–100, 2008.
117. Jacobs ML, Jacobs JP, Franklin RCG, et al: Databases for assessing the outcomes of the treatment of patients with congenital and paediatric cardiac disease—the perspective of cardiac surgery. *Cardiol Young* 18(Suppl 2):101–115, 2008.
118. Jenkins KJ, Beekman RH, III, Bergersen LJ, et al: Databases for assessing the outcomes of the treatment of patients with congenital and paediatric cardiac disease—the perspective of cardiology. *Cardiol Young* 18(Suppl 2):116–123, 2008.
119. Vener DF, Jacobs JP, Schindler E, et al: Databases for assessing the outcomes of the treatment of patients with congenital and paediatric cardiac disease—the perspective of anaesthesia. *Cardiol Young* 18(Suppl 2):124–129, 2008.
120. LaRovere JM, Jeffries HE, Sachdeva RC, et al: Databases for assessing the outcomes of the treatment of patients with congenital and paediatric cardiac disease—the perspective of critical care. *Cardiol Young* 18(Suppl 2):130–136, 2008.
121. Welke KF, Karamlou T, Diggs BS: Databases for assessing the outcomes of the treatment of patients with congenital and paediatric cardiac disease—a comparison of administrative and clinical data. *Cardiol Young* 18(Suppl 2):137–144, 2008.
122. O'Brien SM, Gauvreau K: Statistical issues in the analysis and interpretation of outcomes for congenital cardiac surgery. *Cardiol Young* 18(Suppl 2):145–151, 2008.
123. Hickey EJ, McCrindle BW, Caldarone CA, et al: Making sense of congenital cardiac disease with a research database: the Congenital Heart Surgeons' Society Data Center. *Cardiol Young* 18(Suppl 2):152–162, 2008.
124. Jacobs ML, Jacobs JP, Jenkins KJ, et al: Stratification of complexity: the Risk Adjustment for Congenital Heart Surgery-1 Method and the Aristotle Complexity Score—past, present, and future. *Cardiol Young* 18(Suppl 2):163–168, 2008.
125. Clarke DR, Lacour-Gayet F, Jacobs JP, et al: The assessment of complexity in congenital cardiac surgery based on objective data. *Cardiol Young* 18(Suppl 2):169–176, 2008.

126. Clarke DR, Breen LS, Jacobs ML, et al: Verification of data in congenital cardiac surgery. *Cardiol Young* 18(Suppl 2):177–187, 2008.
127. Morales DLS, McClellan AJ, Jacobs JP: Empowering a database with national long-term data about mortality: the use of national death registries. *Cardiol Young* 18(Suppl 2):188–195, 2008.
128. Bacha EA, Cooper D, Thiagarajan R, et al: Cardiac complications associated with the treatment of patients with congenital cardiac disease: consensus definitions from the Multi-Societal Database Committee for Pediatric and Congenital Heart Disease. *Cardiol Young* 18(Suppl 2):196–201, 2008.
129. Deal BJ, Mavroudis C, Jacobs JP, et al: Arrhythmic complications associated with the treatment of patients with congenital cardiac disease: consensus definitions from the Multi-Societal Database Committee for Pediatric and Congenital Heart Disease. *Cardiol Young* 18(Suppl 2):202–205, 2008.
130. Shann KG, Giacomuzzi CR, Harness L, et al, on behalf of the International Consortium for Evidence-Based Perfusion: Complications relating to perfusion and extracorporeal circulation associated with the treatment of patients with congenital cardiac disease: consensus definitions from the Multi-Societal Database Committee for Pediatric and Congenital Heart Disease. *Cardiol Young* 18(Suppl 2):206–214, 2008.
131. Cooper DS, Jacobs JP, Chai PJ, et al: Pulmonary complications associated with the treatment of patients with congenital cardiac disease: consensus definitions from the Multi-Societal Database Committee for Pediatric and Congenital Heart Disease. *Cardiol Young* 18(Suppl 2):215–221, 2008.
132. Welke KW, Dearani JA, Ghanayem NS, et al: Renal complications associated with the treatment of patients with congenital cardiac disease: consensus definitions from the Multi-Societal Database Committee for Pediatric and Congenital Heart Disease. *Cardiol Young* 18(Suppl 2):222–225, 2008.
133. Checchia PA, Karamlou T, Maruszewski B, et al: Haematological and infectious complications associated with the treatment of patients with congenital cardiac disease: consensus definitions from the Multi-Societal Database Committee for Pediatric and Congenital Heart Disease. *Cardiol Young* 18(Suppl 2):226–233, 2008.
134. Bird GL, Jeffries HE, Licht DJ, et al: Neurological complications associated with the treatment of patients with congenital cardiac disease: consensus definitions from the Multi-Societal Database Committee for Pediatric and Congenital Heart Disease. *Cardiol Young* 18(Suppl 2):234–239, 2008.
135. Ghanayem NS, Dearani JA, Welke KF, et al: Gastrointestinal complications associated with the treatment of patients with congenital cardiac disease: consensus definitions from the Multi-Societal Database Committee for Pediatric and Congenital Heart Disease. *Cardiol Young* 18(Suppl 2):240–244, 2008.
136. Walters HL, 3rd, Jeffries HE, Cohen GA, et al: Congenital cardiac surgical complications of the integument, vascular system, vascular-line(s), and wounds: consensus definitions from the Multi-Societal Database Committee for Pediatric and Congenital Heart Disease. *Cardiol Young* 18(Suppl 2):245–255, 2008.
137. Dickerson H, Cooper DS, Checchia PA, et al: Endocrinal complications associated with the treatment of patients with congenital cardiac disease: consensus definitions from the Multi-Societal Database Committee for Pediatric and Congenital Heart Disease. *Cardiol Young* 18(Suppl 2):256–264, 2008.
138. Jeffries H, Bird G, Law Y, et al: Complications related to the transplantation of thoracic organs: consensus definitions from the Multi-Societal Database Committee for Pediatric and Congenital Heart Disease. *Cardiol Young* 18(Suppl 2):265–270, 2008.
139. Vener DV, Tirotta CF, Andropoulos D, et al: Anaesthetic complications associated with the treatment of patients with congenital cardiac disease: consensus definitions from the Multi-Societal Database Committee for Pediatric and Congenital Heart Disease. *Cardiol Young* 18(Suppl 2):265–270, 2008.
140. The Multi-Societal Database Committee for Pediatric and Congenital Heart Disease: Part IV—the dictionary of definitions of complications associated with the treatment of patients with congenital cardiac disease. *Cardiol Young* 18(Suppl 2):282–530, 2008.
141. Tsang VT, Brown KL, Synnergren MJ, et al: Monitoring risk-adjusted outcomes in congenital heart surgery: does the appropriateness of a risk model change with time? *Ann Thorac Surg* 87(2):584–587, 2009.
142. Jacobs JP, Shahian DM, Jacobs ML, et al: Invited commentary of "Monitoring risk-adjusted outcomes in congenital heart surgery: does the appropriateness of a risk model change with time?" by Tsang VT, Brown KL, Synnergren MJ, Kang N, de Leval MR, Gallivan S, Utley M. *Ann Thorac Surg* 87(2):587–588, 2009.
143. Jacobs JP, Cerfolio RJ, Sade RM: The ethics of transparency: publication of cardiothoracic surgical outcomes in the lay press. *Ann Thorac Surg* 87(3):679–686, 2009.
144. Welke KF, O'Brien SM, Peterson ED, et al: The complex relationship between pediatric cardiac surgical case volumes and mortality rates in a national clinical database. *J Thorac Cardiovasc Surg* 137(5):1133–1140, 2009.
145. Dokholyan RS, Muhlbaier LH, Falletta J, et al: Regulatory and ethical considerations for linking clinical and administrative databases. *Am Heart J* 157(6):971–982, 2009.
146. Hammill BG, Hernandez AF, Peterson ED, et al: Linking inpatient clinical registry data to Medicare claims data using indirect identifiers. *Am Heart J* 157(6):995–1000, 2009.
147. DeCampli WM, Burke RP: Interinstitutional comparison of risk-adjusted mortality and length of stay in congenital heart surgery. *Ann Thorac Surg* 88(1):151–156, 2009.
148. Jacobs JP, Quintessenza JA, Burke RP, et al: Regional congenital cardiac surgery of outcomes in Florida using the Society of Thoracic Surgeons Congenital Heart Surgery Database. *Cardiol Young* 19:360–369, 2009.
149. Jacobs JP, Jacobs ML, Lacour-Gayet FG, et al: Stratification of complexity improves the utility and accuracy of outcomes analysis in a Multi-Institutional Congenital Heart Surgery Database: application of the Risk Adjustment in Congenital Heart Surgery (RACHS-1) and Aristotle Systems in the Society of Thoracic Surgeons (STS) Congenital Heart Surgery Database. *Pediatr Cardiol* 30:1117–1130, 2009.
150. O'Brien SM, Clarke DR, Jacobs JP, et al: An empirically based tool for analyzing mortality associated with congenital heart surgery. *J Thorac Cardiovasc Surg* 138(5):1139–1153, 2009.
151. Barker GM, O'Brien SM, Welke KF, et al: Major infection after pediatric cardiac surgery: a risk estimation model. *Ann Thorac Surg* 89(3):843–850, 2010.
152. Jacobs JP, Maruszewski B, Kurosawa H, et al: Congenital heart surgery databases around the world: do we need a global database? *Semin Thorac Cardiovasc Surg Pediatr Card Surg Annu* 13(1):3–19, 2010.
153. Jacobs JP, Jacobs ML, Mavroudis C, et al: A correction to an analysis from the EACTS and STS Congenital Heart Surgery Databases. *Ann Thorac Surg* 89(4):1339, 2010.
154. Burstein DS, Rossi AF, Jacobs JP, et al: Variation in models of care delivery for children undergoing congenital heart surgery in the United States. *World J Pediatr Congenit Heart Surg* 1:8–14, 2010.
155. Shann KG, Giacomuzzi CR, Jacobs JP, et al: Rationale and use of perfusion variables in the 2010 update of the Society of Thoracic Surgeons Congenital Heart Surgery Database. *World J Pediatr Congenit Heart Surg* 1:34–43, 2010.
156. Jacobs JP, Jacobs ML, Mavroudis C, et al: Atrioventricular septal defects: lessons learned about patterns of practice and outcomes from the congenital heart surgery database of the Society of Thoracic Surgeons. *World J Pediatr Congenit Heart Surg* 1:68–77, 2010.
157. Johnson JN, Jaggers J, Li S, et al: Center variation and outcomes associated with delayed sternal closure after stage 1 palliation for hypoplastic left heart syndrome. *J Thorac Cardiovasc Surg* 139(5):1205–1210, 2010.
158. Patel A, Hickey E, Mavroudis C, et al: Impact of noncardiac congenital and genetic abnormalities on outcomes in hypoplastic left heart syndrome. *Ann Thorac Surg* 89(6):1805–1813, discussion 1813–1814, 2010.
159. Fudge JC, Jr, Li S, Jaggers J, et al: Congenital heart surgery outcomes in Down syndrome: analysis of a national clinical database. *Pediatrics* 126(2):315–322, 2010.
160. Al Habib HF, Jacobs JP, Mavroudis C, et al: Contemporary patterns of management of tetralogy of Fallot: data from the Society of Thoracic Surgeons Database. *Ann Thorac Surg* 90(3):813–819, discussion 819–820, 2010.
161. Jonas RA, Jacobs JP, Jacobs ML, et al: Letter to the editor: reporting of mortality associated with pediatric and congenital cardiac surgery. *J Thorac Cardiovasc Surg* 140(3):726, author reply 726–727, 2010.

162. Giroud JM, Jacobs JP, Spicer D, et al: Report from the International Society for Nomenclature of Paediatric and Congenital Heart Disease: creation of a visual encyclopedia illustrating the terms and definitions of the International Pediatric and Congenital Cardiac Code. *World J Pediatr Congenit Heart Surg* 1:300–313, 2010.
163. Shahian DM, Edwards F, Grover FL, et al: The Society of Thoracic Surgeons National Adult Cardiac Database: a continuing commitment to excellence. *J Thorac Cardiovasc Surg* 140(5):955–959, 2010.
164. Pasquali SK, Jacobs JP, Shook GJ, et al: Linking clinical registry data with administrative data using indirect identifiers: implementation and validation in the congenital heart surgery population. *Am Heart J* 160:1099–1104, 2010.
165. Jacobs JP, Jacobs ML, Mavroudis C, et al: Transposition of the great arteries: lessons learned about patterns of practice and outcomes from the congenital heart surgery database of the Society of Thoracic Surgeons. *World J Pediatr Congenit Heart Surg* 2(1):19–31, 2011.
166. Jacobs JP, Pasquali SK, Morales DLS, et al: Heterotaxy: lessons learned about patterns of practice and outcomes from the congenital heart surgery database of the Society of Thoracic Surgeons. *World J Pediatr Congenit Heart Surg* 2(2):278–286, 2011.
167. Wallace MC, Jaggers J, Li JS, et al: Center variation in patient age and weight at Fontan operation and impact on postoperative outcomes. *Ann Thorac Surg* 91(5):1445–1452, 2011.
168. Bergersen L, Everett AD, Giroud JM, et al: Report from the International Society for Nomenclature of Paediatric and Congenital Heart Disease: cardiovascular catheterisation for congenital and paediatric cardiac disease (Part 1—procedural nomenclature). *Cardiol Young* 21(3):252–259, 2011.
169. Bergersen L, Giroud JM, Jacobs JP, et al: Report from the International Society for Nomenclature of Paediatric and Congenital Heart Disease: cardiovascular catheterisation for congenital and paediatric cardiac disease (Part 2—nomenclature of complications associated with interventional cardiology). *Cardiol Young* 21(3):260–265, 2011.
170. Burstein DS, Jacobs JP, Li JS, et al: Care models and associated outcomes in congenital heart surgery. *Pediatrics* 127(6):e1482–e1489, 2011.
171. Weintraub WS, Karlsberg RP, Tcheng JE, et al: ACCF/AHA 2011 key data elements and definitions of a base cardiovascular vocabulary for electronic health records: a report of the American College of Cardiology Foundation/American Heart Association Task Force on Clinical Data Standards. *Circulation* 124:103–123, 2011.
172. Weintraub WS, Karlsberg RP, Tcheng JE, et al: ACCF/AHA 2011 key data elements and definitions of a base cardiovascular vocabulary for electronic health records: a report of the American College of Cardiology Foundation/American Heart Association Task Force on Clinical Data Standards. *J Am Coll Cardiol* 58(2):202–222, 2011.
173. Jacobs JP, Edwards FH, Shahian DM, et al: Successful linking of the Society of Thoracic Surgeons database to social security data to examine survival after cardiac operations. *Ann Thorac Surg* 92(1):32–39, 2011.
174. Jacobs ML, Daniel M, Mavroudis C, et al: Report of the 2010 Society of Thoracic Surgeons congenital heart surgery practice and manpower survey. *Ann Thorac Surg* 92:762–769, 2011.
175. Petrucci O, O'Brien SM, Jacobs ML, et al: Risk factors for mortality and morbidity after the neonatal Blalock-Taussig shunt procedure. *Ann Thorac Surg* 92(2):642–651, discussion 651–652, 2011.
176. Shahian DM, Edwards FH, Jacobs JP, et al: Public reporting of cardiac surgery performance: Part 1—history, rationale, consequences. *Ann Thorac Surg* 92(3 Suppl):S2–S11, 2011.
177. Shahian DM, Edwards FH, Jacobs JP, et al: Public reporting of cardiac surgery performance: Part 2—implementation. *Ann Thorac Surg* 92(3 Suppl):S12–S23, 2011.
178. Jacobs JP, Pasquali SK, Gaynor JW: Invited commentary: the assessment of outcomes and the improvement of quality of the treatment of patients with congenital and pediatric cardiac disease. *World J Pediatr Congenit Heart Surg* 2(4):597–602, 2011.
179. Jacobs JP, Pasquali SK, Jeffries H, et al: Outcomes analysis and quality improvement for the treatment of patients with pediatric and congenital cardiac disease. *World J Pediatr Congenit Heart Surg* 2(4):620–633, 2011.
180. Hornik CP, He X, Jacobs JP, et al: Complications after the Norwood operation: an analysis of the Society of Thoracic Surgeons Congenital Heart Surgery Database. *Ann Thorac Surg* 92(5):1734–1740, 2011.
181. Mascio CE, Pasquali SK, Jacobs JP, et al: Outcomes in adult congenital heart surgery: analysis of the Society of Thoracic Surgeons Database. *J Thorac Cardiovasc Surg* 142(5):1090–1097, 2011.
182. Jacobs JP, O'Brien SM, Pasquali SK, et al: Clark paper: variation in outcomes for benchmark operations: an analysis of the Society of Thoracic Surgeons Congenital Heart Surgery Database. Richard clark award recipient for best use of the STS Congenital Heart Surgery Database. *Ann Thorac Surg* 92(6):2184–2192, 2011.
183. Barach PR, Jacobs JP, Laussen PC, et al: Outcomes analysis, quality improvement, and patient safety for pediatric and congenital cardiac care: theory, implementation, and applications. *Prog Pediatr Cardiol* 32:65–67, 2011.
184. Jacobs JP, Morales DLS: Strategies for longitudinal follow-up of patients with pediatric and congenital cardiac disease. *Prog Pediatr Cardiol* 32:97–102, 2011.
185. Winlaw DS, Large MM, Jacobs JP, et al: Leadership, surgeon well-being and non-technical competencies of pediatric cardiac surgery. *Prog Pediatr Cardiol* 32:129–133, 2011.
186. Jacobs JP, Jacobs ML, Austin EH, et al: Quality measures for congenital and pediatric cardiac surgery. *World J Pediatr Congenit Heart Surg* 3(1):32–47, 2012.
187. Russell HM, Pasquali SK, Jacobs JP, et al: Outcomes of repair of common arterial trunk with truncal valve surgery: a review of the Society of Thoracic Surgeons Congenital Heart Surgery Database. *Ann Thorac Surg* 93(1):164–169, 2012.
188. Barach PR, Jacobs JP, Laussen PC, et al: Outcomes analysis, quality improvement, and patient safety for pediatric and congenital cardiac care: theory, implementation, and applications part 2. *Prog Pediatr Cardiol* 33(1):1–3, 2012.
189. Pasquali SK, Li JS, Jacobs ML, et al: Opportunities and challenges in linking information across databases in pediatric cardiovascular medicine. *Prog Pediatr Cardiol* 33(1):21–24, 2012.
190. Gaies MG, Jeffries HE, Jacobs JP, et al: Measuring quality and outcomes in pediatric cardiac critical care. *Prog Pediatr Cardiol* 33(1):33–36, 2012.
191. Giroud JM, Jacobs JP, Fricker FJ, et al: Proposal for a web based "Global Virtual Museum of Congenital Cardiac Pathology." *Prog Pediatr Cardiol* 33(1):91–97, 2012.
192. Pasquali SK, Li JS, Burstein DS, et al: Association of center volume with mortality and complications in pediatric heart surgery. *Pediatrics* 129(2):e370–e376, 2012.
193. Pasquali SK, Li JS, He X, et al: Perioperative methylprednisolone and outcome in neonates undergoing heart surgery. *Pediatrics* 129(2):e385–e391, 2012.
194. Pasquali SK, Li JS, He X, et al: Comparative analysis of antifibrinolytic medications in pediatric heart surgery. *J Thorac Cardiovasc Surg* 143(3):550–557, 2012.
195. Stewart RD, Pasquali SK, Jacobs JP, et al: Contemporary Fontan operation: association between early outcome and type of cavopulmonary connection. Winner of the 2011 Clifford Van Meter President's Award for the best scientific paper presented at the 2011 STSA 58th Annual Meeting in San Antonio. *Ann Thorac Surg* 93(4):1254–1261, 2012.
196. Pasquali SK, Jacobs JP, He X, et al: The complex relationship between center volume and outcome in patients undergoing the Norwood operation. *Ann Thorac Surg* 93(5):1556–1562, 2012.
197. Hornik CP, He X, Jacobs JP, et al: Relative impact of surgeon and center volume on early mortality after the Norwood operation. *Ann Thorac Surg* 93(6):1992–1997, 2012.
198. Jacobs JP, O'Brien SM, Pasquali SK, et al: Variation in outcomes for risk-stratified pediatric cardiac surgical operations: an analysis of the STS Congenital Heart Surgery Database. *Ann Thorac Surg* 94(2):564–572, 2012.
199. Pasquali SK, He X, Jacobs JP, et al: Evaluation of failure to rescue as a quality metric in pediatric heart surgery: an analysis of the STS Congenital Heart Surgery Database. *Ann Thorac Surg* 94(2):573–580, 2012.
200. Giroud JM, Aiello VD, Spicer DE, et al: The Archiving Working Group of the International Society for Nomenclature of Paediatric and Congenital Heart Disease: a visual encyclopedia illustrating the terms and definitions of the international paediatric and

congenital cardiac code. *Congenital Cardiology Today* 10(8):8–10, 2012.

201. Aiello VD, Anderson RH, Giroud JM, et al: Image of the month (aortic valve pathology, bicuspid and pulmonary valve pathology, bicuspid)—August 2012—presented by the Archiving Working Group. *Congenital Cardiology Today* 10(8):14–15, 2012.
202. Anderson RH, Aiello VD, Spicer DE, et al: Image of the month #2 (interrupted aortic arch [IAA], type B2 [interruption between the carotid and subclavian arteries with both subclavian arteries arising from the aorta distal to the interruption])—October 2012—presented by the Archiving Working Group. *Congenital Cardiology Today* 10(10):20–21, 2012.
203. Woods RK, Pasquali SK, Jacobs ML, et al: Aortic valve replacement in neonates and infants: an analysis of the Society of Thoracic Surgeons Congenital Heart Surgery Database. *J Thorac Cardiovasc Surg* 144(5):1084–1090, 2012.
204. Jacobs JP, Jacobs ML, Maruszewski B, et al: Initial application in the EACTS and STS Congenital Heart Surgery Databases of an empirically derived methodology of complexity adjustment to evaluate surgical case mix and results. *Eur J Cardiothorac Surg* 42(5):775–780, 2012.
205. Dibardino DJ, Pasquali SK, Hirsch JC, et al: Clark Paper: effect of sex and race on outcome in patients undergoing congenital heart surgery: an analysis of the Society of Thoracic Surgeons Congenital Heart Surgery Database. Richard Clark Award recipient for best use of the STS Congenital Heart Surgery Database. *Ann Thorac Surg* 94(6):2054–2060, 2012.
206. Kansy A, Jacobs JP, Pastuszko A, et al: Major infection after pediatric cardiac surgery: external validation of risk estimation model. *Ann Thorac Surg* 94(6):2091–2095, 2012.
207. Vener DF, Guzzetta N, Jacobs JP, et al: Development and implementation of a new data registry in congenital cardiac anesthesia. *Ann Thorac Surg* 94(6):2159–2165, 2012.
208. Pasquali SK, Gaies MG, Jacobs JP, et al: Centre variation in cost and outcomes for congenital heart surgery. *Cardiol Young* 22(6):796–799, 2012.
209. Aiello VD, Spicer DE, Jacobs JP, et al: Image of the month #3 (total anomalous pulmonary venous connection [TAPVC], type 4 [mixed])—December 2012—presented by the Archiving Working Group. *Congenital Cardiology Today* 10(12):8–9, 2012.
210. Pasquali SK, Peterson ED, Jacobs JP, et al: Differential case ascertainment in clinical registry versus administrative data and impact on outcomes assessment for pediatric cardiac operations. *Ann Thorac Surg* 95(1):197–203, 2013.
211. Ungerleider RM, Pasquali SK, Welke KF, et al: Contemporary patterns of surgery and outcomes for aortic coarctation: an analysis of the Society of Thoracic Surgeons Congenital Heart Surgery Database. *J Thorac Cardiovasc Surg* 145(1):150–158, 2013.
212. Overman D, Jacobs JP, Prager RL, et al: Report from the Society of Thoracic Surgeons National Database Work Force: clarifying the definition of operative mortality. *World J Pediatr Congenit Heart Surg* 4(1):10–12, 2013.
213. Spicer DE, Jacobs JP, Giroud JM, et al: Image of the month #4 (single ventricle, DILV)—February 2013—presented by the Archiving Working Group. *Congenital Cardiology Today* 11(2):13–14, 2013.
214. Jacobs JP, O'Brien SM, Shahian DM, et al: Successful linking of the Society of Thoracic Surgeons Database to Social Security data to examine the accuracy of Society of Thoracic Surgeons mortality data. *J Thorac Cardiovasc Surg* 145(4):976–983, 2013.
215. Jacobs ML, O'Brien SM, Jacobs JP, et al: An empirically based tool for analyzing morbidity associated with operations for congenital heart disease. *J Thorac Cardiovasc Surg* 145(4):1046–1057. e1, 2013.
216. Pasquali SK, Jacobs JP: The role of databases in improving the quality of care for congenital heart disease. *World J Pediatr Congenit Heart Surg* 4(2):139–141, 2013.
217. Kansy A, Maruszewski B, Jacobs JP, et al: Application of four complexity stratification tools (Aristotle Basic Score, RACHS-1, STAT Mortality Score, and STAT Mortality Categories) to evaluate early congenital heart surgery outcomes over 16 years at a single institution. *Kardiochirurgia i Torakochirurgia Polska* 10(2):115–119, 2013.
218. Jacobs JP, Giroud JM, Anderson RH, et al: Image of the month #5 (VSD, type 2 [perimembranous] [paramembranous])—May 2013—presented by the Archiving Working Group. *Congenital Cardiology Today* 11(5):8–9, 2013.
219. Pasquali SK, He X, Jacobs ML, et al: Hospital variation in postoperative infection and outcome after congenital heart surgery. *Ann Thorac Surg* 96(2):657–663, 2013.
220. Shahian DM, He X, Jacobs JP, et al: Issues in quality measurement: target population, risk adjustment, and ratings. *Ann Thorac Surg* 96(2):718–726, 2013.
221. Shahian DM, Jacobs JP, Edwards FH, et al: The Society of Thoracic Surgeons National Database. *Heart* 99(20):1494–1501, 2013.
222. Jacobs JP, Maruszewski M: Functionally univentricular heart and the Fontan operation: lessons learned about patterns of practice and outcomes from the Congenital Heart Surgery Databases of the European Association for Cardio-Thoracic Surgery and the Society of Thoracic Surgeons. *World J Pediatr Congenit Heart Surg* 4:349–355, 2013.
223. Mascio CE, Austin EH, 3rd, Jacobs JP, et al: Perioperative mechanical circulatory support in children: an analysis of the Society of Thoracic Surgeons Congenital Heart Surgery Database. *J Thorac Cardiovasc Surg* 147:658–664, 2014.
224. Hendel RC, Bozkurt B, Smith EE, et al: ACC/AHA 2013 methodology for developing clinical data standards: a report of the American College of Cardiology/American Heart Association Task Force on Clinical Data Standards. *J Am Coll Cardiol* 63:2323–2334, 2014.
225. Hendel RC, Bozkurt B, Fonarow GC, et al: ACC/AHA 2013 methodology for developing clinical data standards: a report of the American College of Cardiology/American Heart Association Task Force on Clinical Data Standards. *Circulation* 129:2346–2357, 2014.
226. Jacobs JP, Pasquali SK, Austin E, et al: Linking the congenital heart surgery databases of the Society of Thoracic Surgeons (STS) and the Congenital Heart Surgeons' Society (CHSS): Part 1—rationale and methodology. *World J Pediatr Congenit Heart Surg* 5:256–271, 2014.
227. Jacobs JP, Pasquali SK, Austin E, et al: Linking the congenital heart surgery databases of the Society of Thoracic Surgeons (STS) and the Congenital Heart Surgeons' Society (CHSS): Part 2—lessons learned and implications. *World J Pediatr Congenit Heart Surg* 5:272–282, 2014.
228. Hoffman JI, Kaplan S: The incidence of congenital heart disease. *J Am Coll Cardiol* 39:1890–1900, 2002.
229. Donabedian A: Evaluating the quality of medical care. *Milbank Mem Fund Q* 44(3):Suppl:166–206, 1966.
230. Shahian DM, O'Brien SM, Sheng S, et al: Predictors of long-term survival following coronary artery bypass grafting surgery: results from the Society of Thoracic Surgeons Adult Cardiac Surgery Database (the ASCERT Study). *Circulation* 125(12):1491–1500, 2012.
231. Weintraub WS, Grau-Sepulveda MV, Weiss JM, et al: Comparative effectiveness of revascularization strategies. *N Engl J Med* 366(16):1467–1476, 2012.
232. Fröbert O, Lagerqvist B, Olivecrona GK, et al: Thrombus aspiration during ST-segment elevation myocardial infarction. *N Engl J Med* 369(17):1587–1597, 2013.
233. Lauer MS, D'Agostino RB, Sr: The randomized registry trial–the next disruptive technology in clinical research? *N Engl J Med* 369(17):1579–1581, 2013.
234. Shahian DM, O'Brien SM, Filardo G, et al, for the Society of Thoracic Surgeons Quality Measurement Task Force: The Society of Thoracic Surgeons 2008 cardiac surgery risk models: Part 1—coronary artery bypass grafting surgery. *Ann Thorac Surg* 88(Suppl):2–22, 2009.
235. O'Brien SM, Shahian DM, Filardo G, et al, for the Society of Thoracic Surgeons Quality Measurement Task Force: The Society of Thoracic Surgeons 2008 cardiac surgery risk models: Part 2—isolated valve surgery. *Ann Thorac Surg* 88(Suppl):23–42, 2009.
236. Shahian DM, O'Brien SM, Filardo G, et al, for the Society of Thoracic Surgeons Quality Measurement Task Force: The Society of Thoracic Surgeons 2008 cardiac surgery risk models: Part 3—valve plus coronary artery bypass grafting surgery. *Ann Thorac Surg* 88(Suppl):43–62, 2009.
237. The National Quality Forum website: http://www.qualityforum.org/. Accessed December 23, 2013.

CHAPTER 134

QUALITY IMPROVEMENT: SURGICAL PERFORMANCE

Meena Nathan • John M. Karamichalis

CHAPTER OUTLINE

BACKGROUND

According to the Centers for Disease Control and Prevention (CDC),[1] congenital heart disease (CHD) is the most common type of birth defect, affecting 1% of the population (40,000 births/year). CHD is the leading cause of illness and death associated with birth defects. Fifteen percent of all patients with CHD have associated genetic conditions, and 20% to 30% have physical, developmental, or cognitive problems.[2-5] In 2004, the health care cost for hospitalization of individuals with CHD was approximately $1.4 billion.[1] It is now feasible to offer surgical correction or palliation to most of these patients. In 2011, 33,733 congenital cardiac procedures were reported to the Society of Thoracic Surgeons (STS).[6] Between 1999 and 2006, CHD was listed as the primary cause of death in 27,960 people. Among these, 48% were infants, often following complex interventions and prolonged ICU stay. Despite recent advances in surgical management, CHD has a significant societal impact in terms of morbidity, mortality, and health care resource utilization. Thus, this patient population presents an enormous challenge to the health care environment where optimal care can greatly influence not only short-term but also long-term physical, intellectual, and psychosocial outcomes.

Outcomes in congenital cardiac surgery are multifactorial and may be affected by (1) preoperative status, such as patient factors (e.g., birth weight, gestational age, complexity of CHD), hemodynamic stability, adequacy of diagnostic evaluation, and appropriateness of the surgical plan; (2) intraoperative factors, such as conduct of anesthesia and cardiopulmonary bypass, surgical technique, and early post-bypass hemodynamic management; and (3) postoperative course, such as serious adverse events and complications. Among these many factors, technical adequacy of repair is likely a significant determinant of successful outcome. Indeed, the degree to which a congenital heart operation achieves its intended result may be the single most important factor determining long-term medical outcomes and costs.

Until recently, hospital mortality, often in the form of cumulative sum (CUSUM) analysis, had been used as a surrogate measure of technical performance in congenital heart surgery.[7-9] Raw mortality data, however, do not correct for case complexity or other associated factors that can affect outcomes. One alternative, the hospital standardized mortality ratio (HSMR), is intended as an overall measure of in-hospital deaths, a proportion of which are preventable. High ratios may thus suggest potential problems with quality of care.[10] The HSMR is a complex but inexpensive and relatively easy method to calculate, from national or other benchmark data, the patients' predicted risk of death. However, there are a number of methodological challenges in HMSR's construction and interpretation, largely because they are based on administrative databases.[11] Although risk-adjusted in-hospital death rates may be a reasonable measure of institutional performance, this measure is inadequate to assess the performance of individual physicians because many additional factors outside the control of an individual surgeon (e.g., the contribution and impact of other team members) must also be considered. This is especially problematic for high-risk operations, which require a complex multidepartmental microsystem of dedicated teams composed of many individuals and specialties.

The technical performance score (TPS), developed to address the lack of systematic methods for evaluating operative technical adequacy across diagnoses and centers, is a novel tool for assessing technical competency based on widely available clinical and echocardiographic characteristics.

DEVELOPMENT OF THE TECHNICAL PERFORMANCE SCORE

TPS was developed at Boston Children's Hospital to assess the adequacy of anatomic repair. The technical steps toward an adequate anatomic repair of a lesion are mostly under the control of the surgeon. Intraoperative technical excellence is one of the key factors in determining outcomes, especially in high-acuity operations.[12-14] A deficit in tools available to measure technical adequacy of a surgical procedure was key to the development of the TPS. This tool was designed to be used for peer and self-assessment and was initially piloted in selected surgical procedures, including repairs of ventricular septal defect, tetralogy of Fallot, complete common atrioventricular canal, arterial switch, and, later, the stage I Norwood procedure.[15,16] The use was then expanded to include more than 90% of congenital cardiac surgery operations.[17]

The score was created by dividing the surgical procedure into individual subcomponents or subprocedures, based on specific anatomic regions intervened on surgically. TPS is then assessed based on echocardiographic criteria that are designed to capture the individual components of specific operations, as well as unplanned surgical or catheter-based re-interventions prior to discharge in the anatomic areas relevant to the surgical procedure. The components of the score were defined and piloted by a modified consensus process of cardiologists and cardiac surgeons at our center. Based on these prespecified components (subprocedures) that were particular to each operation, each discharge echocardiogram could be classified into one of three categories (class 1 = optimal, class 2 = adequate, or class 3 = inadequate). If all subprocedures have a class 1 optimal score, the overall score for the entire procedure will be class 1 (optimal). If any individual subprocedure is scored as class 1 or 2, the overall TPS for the procedure will be class 2 (adequate). If any subprocedure is scored as class 3 (inadequate), or if the patient undergoes at least one surgical or catheter-based re-intervention in the anatomic area of interest prior to discharge, the TPS will be class 3. Certain specific procedures that result in an unexpected implantation of a permanent pacemaker will also result in the procedure being scored as inadequate (class 3).

PILOTING THE TECHNICAL PERFORMANCE SCORE

Initial validation was performed in four procedural groups—ventricular septal defect, tetralogy of Fallot, complete common atrioventricular canal, and arterial switch operation—using data from 2004.[15] Despite significant diversity and complexity among procedures, technical adequacy of repair could be successfully determined in this group of congenital cardiac procedures using the TPS tool.

TABLE 134-1 Association between Technical Performance Score and Outcomes in the Norwood Population

	Optimal	Adequate	Inadequate	*P* Value
Hospital LOS median (range)	18 (2-96)	19 (4-141)	33 (1-125)	0.02
Hospital mortality	4 (5%)	2 (11%)	3 (27%)	0.02
ECMO	6 (8%)	2 (11%)	8 (53%)	<0.001

ECMO, Extracorporeal membrane oxygenation; *LOS*, length of stay.

The TPS tool was then validated for the stage I procedure by a retrospective analysis of 110 patients from January 2004 to December 2006. There were 77 (70%) in the optimal group, 18 (16%) in the adequate group, and 15 (14%) in the inadequate group. Inadequate technical performance was significantly associated with greater early mortality, occurrence of adverse events (such as need for extracorporeal membrane oxygenation), and length of stay (Table 134-1).[16]

A subgroup analysis of TPS in the Norwood population showed that optimal technical performance attenuated the effects of preoperative physiologic status and case complexity with reduced hospital mortality.[12]

STANDARDIZATION OF METHODOLOGY

As part of standardization of the tool for use among multiple institutions, we developed standardized echo protocols for echo acquisition and developed anatomic modules that could be used to standardize the images obtained by the echocardiographer performing the discharge echocardiogram. These anatomic modules (Appendix 134-1) also enable the clinician finalizing the TPS to be able to accurately score all components adequately.

VALIDATION OF TECHNICAL PERFORMANCE SCORE

In subsequent studies we were able to show that TPS was useful in predicting both short- and mid-term outcomes.[13,18-21] Specifically, to define the relationship between TPS and major postoperative adverse events, we performed a prospective study[13] that included intraoperative observations of operations in risk adjustment for congenital heart surgery (RACHS-1)[22,23] categories 2 through 6 in 166 infants younger than 6 months. For the entire cohort, optimal TPS resulted in lower postoperative adverse events, lower postoperative pediatric risk of mortality (PRISM)[24] score, lower length of intensive care unit (ICU) stay and hospital stay, and shorter ventilation time ($P < 0.001$). Optimal TPS also resulted in low postoperative adverse events independent of RACHS-1 category, or preoperative PRISM (Fig. 134-1). In multivariable logistic regression, the strongest independent predictors of postoperative major adverse events were TPS, RACHS-1 category, and preoperative PRISM. In a prospective follow-up study of our cohort of neonates and infants from index surgery for a minimum of 1 year, 7 of the 166 patients had early mortality.[18] Among the remaining 159 patients, late death occurred in 13, and late unplanned interventions (in the anatomic area operated on at index surgery) were performed in 55. Using univariate analysis, inadequate TPS was associated with postdischarge mortality ($P < 0.0001$) and re-intervention ($P = 0.034$). However, on multivariable modeling, inadequate TPS was an independent predictor of only postdischarge mortality ($P = 0.017$) (Fig. 134-2). To expand the number of patients available for analysis and thereby to improve power, we performed a retrospective study of 725 patients who were followed for a minimum of 4 years[21]; TPS was an independent predictor in multivariable analysis of both late postdischarge mortality and unplanned re-interventions (Fig. 134-3).

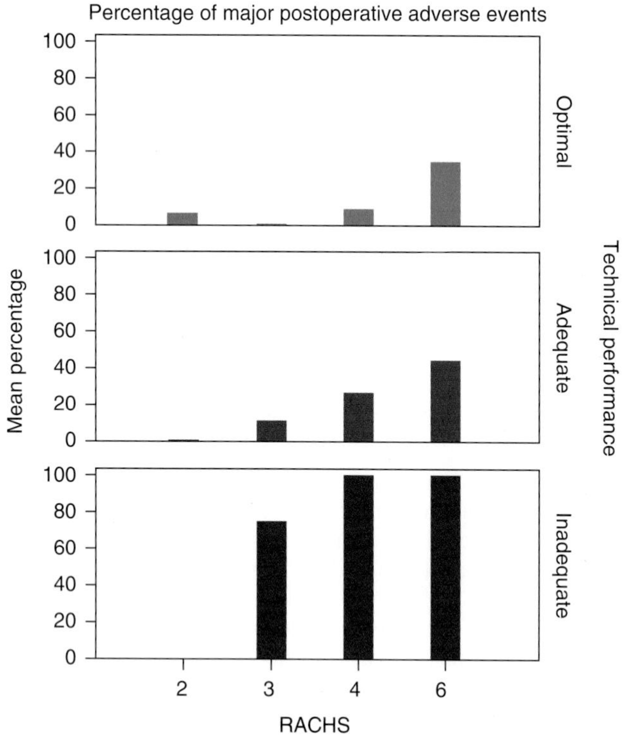

FIGURE 134-1 ■ Major postoperative adverse events as predicted by technical performance score and risk adjustment for congenital heart surgery (RACHS-1) risk categories in a prospective cohort of 166 infants younger than 6 months of age.

We also studied the association of TPS with neurodevelopmental outcomes using the Bayley Scale of Infant Development (BSID) III scores in a group of 140 children who underwent their initial cardiac operation in the first year of life.[19] Inadequate TPS was an independent predictor of poor neurodevelopmental outcomes after adjusting for other significant patient-related factors (Table 134-2).

To enhance the simplicity and reproducibility of TPS assessment, we subsequently modified the TPS to exclude intraoperative revisions (the initial five modules included such revisions as a criterion by which TPS automatically fell to class 2 [adequate]). We created 30 procedural modules and then validated these modules by prospectively assigning TPS to all discharged patients undergoing operations for CHD at our center. All patients who were discharged between January 1, 2011, and April 30, 2013, were included in this study.[20] TPS was optimal in 956 (50%), adequate in 584 (30%), inadequate in 226 (12%), and indeterminate in 160 patients (8%). There were 51 (2.6%) early deaths and 111 (5.7%) major adverse events (Fig. 134-4). In univariate analyses, mortality and occurrence of adverse events were significantly associated with age, RACHS-1 categories, and TPS. In multivariable regression analyses, inadequate TPS was a strong independent predictor of mortality ($P < 0.001$; OR [odds ratio], 16.9; 95% confidence interval [CI], 6.7-42.9), adverse events ($P < 0.001$; OR, 6.9; 95% CI, 4.1-11.6), and ICU length of stay ($P < 0.001$; coefficient, 2.3; 95% CI, 2.0-2.6).

We subsequently analyzed hospital cost data in this group of patients and found that class 3 (inadequate) TPS was associated with a significantly higher hospital cost after adjusting for other significant variables such as RACHS-1 risk category, age, prematurity, genetic syndromes, presence of extracardiac nonchromosomal anomalies, weekend admissions, and the need for multiple procedures at index surgery (Table 134-3; Fig. 134-5).[24a] TPS was an independent predictor of increased total hospital cost with the percentage of variance explained (R^2) increasing from 42% to 53% when TPS was added to the

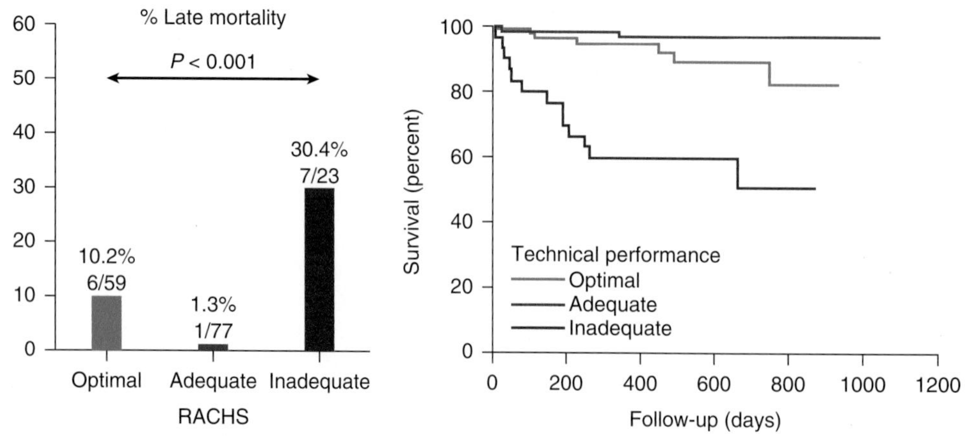

FIGURE 134-2 ■ Association between technical performance score and postdischarge mortality in a prospective cohort of 166 infants younger than 6 months of age. *RACHS,* Risk adjustment for congenital heart surgery.

TABLE 134-2 Multivariable Analysis of Bayley Scale of Infant Development (BSID) Cognitive Composite Score Adjusting for Preoperative Factors (Total R^2 = 14.6%)

	Regression Coefficient (SE)	*P* Value	Regression Coefficient (SE)	*P* Value	Partial R^2
Chromosomal anomalies	−15.1 (5.3)	0.005	−14.4 (5.2)	0.007	5.4%
Nonchromosomal anomalies	−10.4 (4.2)	0.02	−10.2 (4.2)	0.02	4.2%
RACHS-1 category 6	−11.4 (5.0)	0.03	−7.7 (5.3)	0.15	1.5%
TPS (vs. optimal)					
Adequate	—		−2.4 (3.1)	0.45	3.9%
Inadequate	—		−12.5 (5.1)	0.02	

The model on the left includes all presurgical and surgical risk factors significant at the 0.10 level. The model on the right adds in TPS. Inadequate TPS was significantly associated with a lower score after adjusting for chromosomal and nonchromosomal anomalies and RACHS-1 category.
RACHS-1, Risk adjustment for congenital heart surgery; *TPS*, technical performance score.

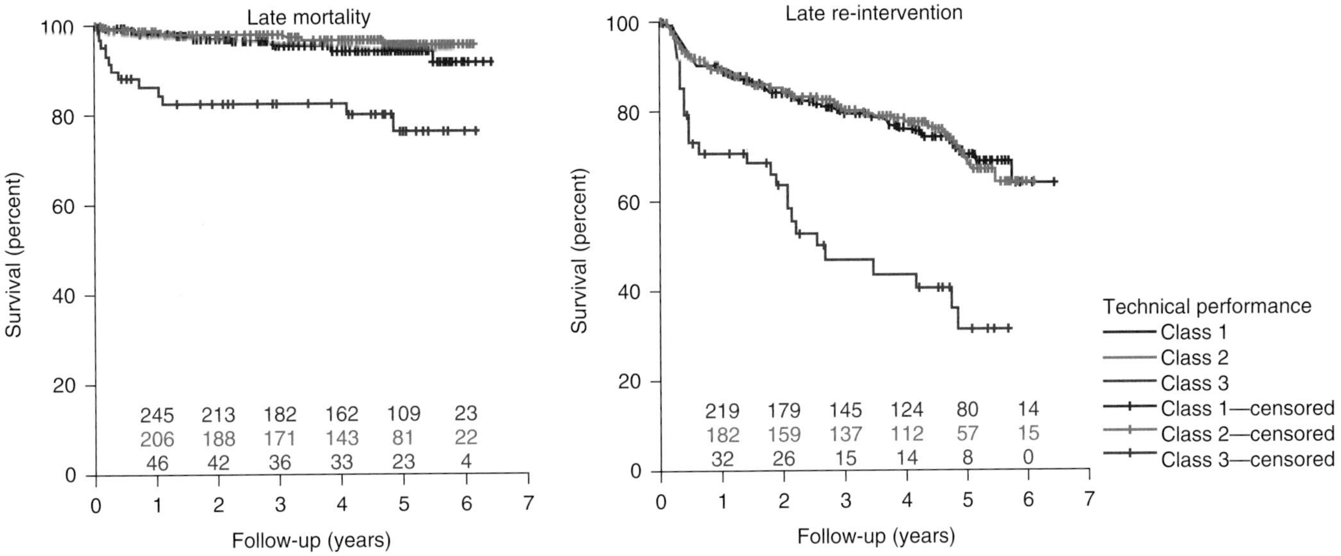

FIGURE 134-3 Association between technical performance score and postdischarge mortality and postdischarge unplanned re-intervention in a cohort of 725 patients followed for 4 years.

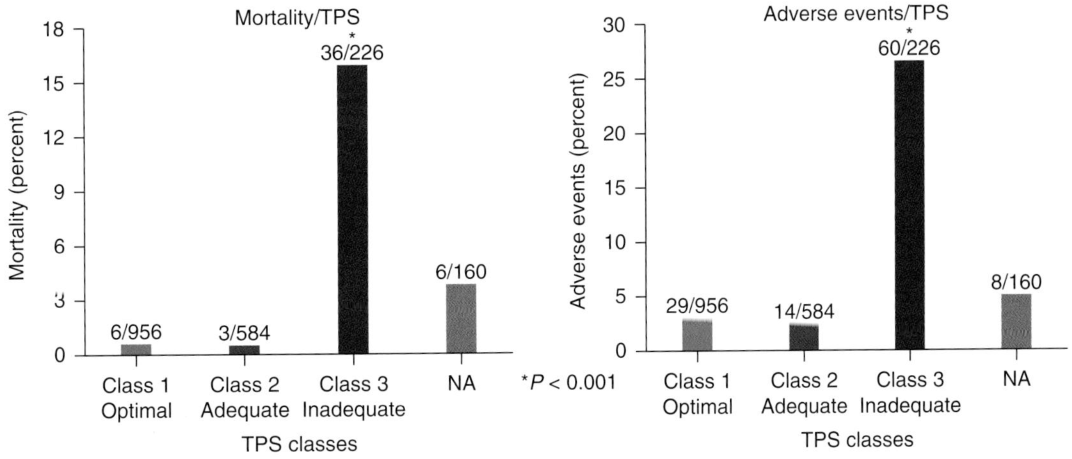

FIGURE 134-4 Mortality and adverse events based on technical performance score in a prospective cohort of 1926 patients. *NA*, TPS could not be assigned; *TPS*, technical performance score.

model, indicating that TPS explained a large additional fraction of variability in total hospital cost.

To explore the predictive validity of TPS within the multicenter environment of the Pediatric Heart Network, we recently performed a secondary analysis using the database of the Single Ventricle Reconstruction (SVR) trial. Specifically, in this 15-center study, we demonstrated that inadequate TPS was an independent predictor of longer time to extubation, higher early mortality, longer Norwood hospital length of stay (Fig. 134-6), greater

TABLE 134-3 **Multivariable Analysis of Total Hospital Costs (n = 1762)***

Variable	n	Coefficient	Confidence Interval	P Value
RACHS-1 category				<0.001 all
1	179	Ref	—	
2	474	1.31	(1.18, 1.44)	
3	532	1.89	(1.71, 2.09)	
4	166	2.35	(2.07, 2.67)	
6	60	2.78	(2.32, 3.33)	
NA < 18 yr	143	2.64	(2.32, 3.00)	
Adults	208	1.87	(1.67, 2.09)	
Age				<0.001 all
Neonate	315	1.76	(1.62, 1.92)	
Infant	427	1.29	(1.21, 1.38)	
Children	779	Ref	—	
Prematurity				<0.001
Yes	63	1.47	(1.28, 1.69)	
Genetic syndromes				<0.001
Yes	93	1.24	(1.11, 1.39)	
Extracardiac anomalies				<0.001
Yes	116	1.36	(1.22, 1.50)	
Weekend admission				<0.001
Yes	98	1.34	(1.20, 1.51)	
Multiple procedures at index surgery				<0.001
Yes	250	1.31	(1.21, 1.41)	
Technical performance score				
Optimal	879	Ref	—	0.036
Adequate	544	1.07	(1.00, 1.13)	<0.001
Inadequate	198	2.01	(1.84, 2.20)	<0.001
Not scorable	141	0.61	(0.55, 0.67)	

*Inadequate TPS was associated with higher costs after adjusting for all variables known to be associated with higher hospital costs.

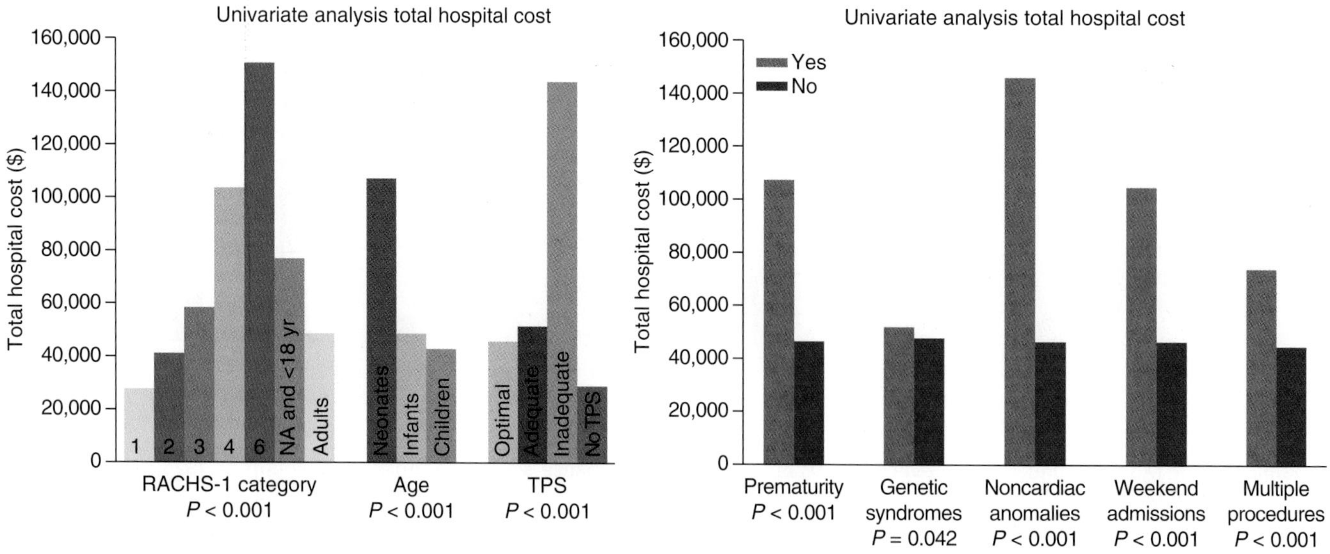

FIGURE 134-5 ■ Inadequate technical performance score (TPS) is associated with higher hospital costs. *NA*, Noncategorizable in RACHS-1 category; *RACHS*, risk adjustment for congenital heart surgery.

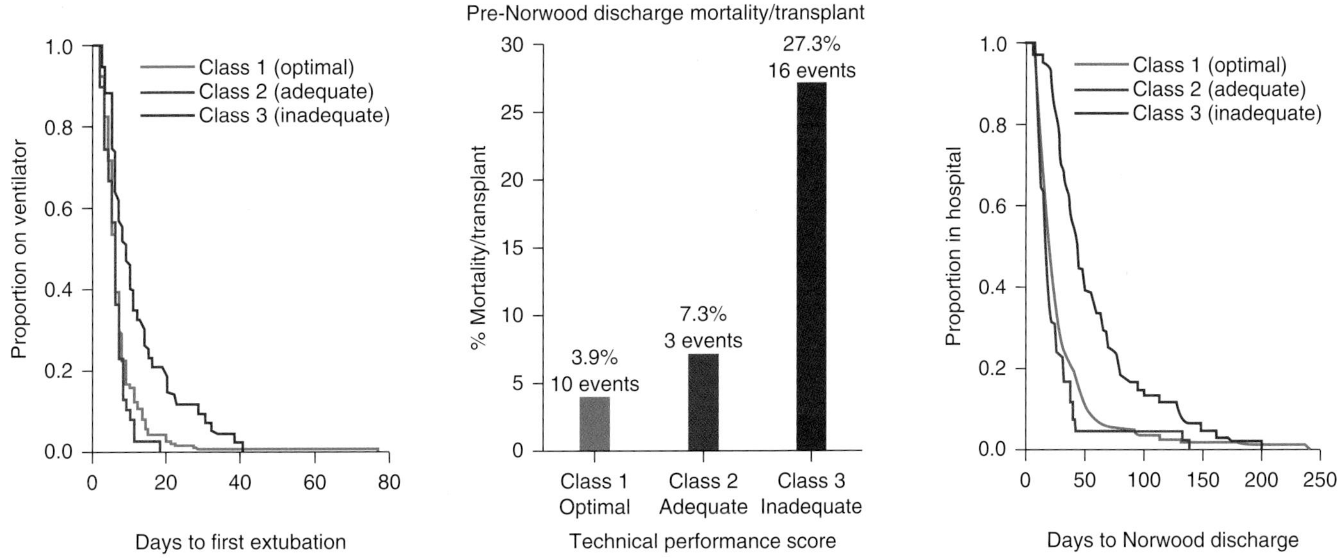

FIGURE 134-6 Inadequate technical performance score is associated with longer time to extubation, higher mortality, and longer Norwood hospital length of stay in the Single Ventricle Reconstruction trial cohort.

proportion of pre–stage II re-interventions and lower Psychomotor Development Index scores at 14 months after adjusting for important preoperative factors.[25]

FUTURE DIRECTION

Mortality and adverse events are no longer considered to be major outcome measures of quality of care. With current advances in surgical and other related technologies, attention is being turned to more subtle measures such as neurodevelopmental outcomes, resource utilization in the form of length of stay, readmissions, and unplanned postdischarge re-intervention. Although the role of human factors in outcomes after surgery has been well described,[26-28] technical adequacy of the repair may still be the single most important factor in determining these more subtle outcomes; this has been demonstrated in other surgical fields.[29-31] Models of surgical skills assessment, including video recordings of skill tests and other methods, have been developed as part of surgical training programs.[32-35] However, the use of a routine test (i.e., a test that is clinically indicated) as a tool for assessment of technical adequacy has not been described.

Our studies have shown that technical adequacy of the repair, as measured by TPS, has emerged as an important predictor of outcomes in congenital surgery. We describe a "technical imperative," defined as an absolute rule whereby it is imperative to leave the operating room with a good or, better yet, an optimal technical result, even if this requires surgical revision and going back on bypass.[12-14,16] Thus, a focus on the intraoperative assessment of the adequacy of the anatomic repair, primarily by echocardiography but also by pressure measurements and even intraoperative angiography, is paramount. Increasing intraoperative vigilance so as to detect and immediately repair significant residual lesions remains of prime importance. Our studies also indicate that residual defects repaired in a timely fashion, which usually means immediately in the operating room or within 24 hours of surgery, result in no significant impact on patient outcome, even in highly complex cases.

The development and implementation of a system for measuring technical performance in congenital cardiac surgery operations can be used not only as an outcomes measurement tool but also as a tool for surgeons' self and peer assessments. It can help determine how much of the interinstitutional variation can be attributed to adequacy of surgical repair versus other contributory factors, such as patient- and institution-related factors. The use of the TPS in conjunction with a risk adjustment method, such as RACHS-1, Aristotle, or STS-EACTS,[22,23,36-38] allows for quality improvement for specific risk populations and enables a structured approach to management based on procedural complexity. TPS need not be limited to congenital cardiac procedures but may be applied to adult cardiac operations and, in fact, could potentially be expanded across all surgical specialties. This system may also be applicable to noncardiac procedures, such as interventional cardiac catheterization, electrophysiologic ablations, and radiologic interventions.

Prospective multicenter validation of this tool will allow for further refinement of the score, particularly for procedures such as valve repairs and prosthetic valve replacement. Accrual of data on sufficiently large numbers in each procedural group will allow us to determine the relative importance of the various components of each procedure and will lead to the development of a weighted scale for the components of each procedure. This will then enable us to determine which patient with a TPS of class 2 or class 3 would warrant closer follow-up and perhaps earlier intervention to optimize outcomes, thus improving quality of life while minimizing resource utilization and indirectly having a positive impact on health care costs. Development of TPS for intraoperative post-bypass transesophageal echocardiograms and epicardial echocardiograms would allow for timely correction of residual defects and lead to significant improvements in physical, psychosocial, and fiscal costs.

APPENDIX 134-1: BOSTON CHILDREN'S HOSPITAL TECHNICAL PERFORMANCE SCORE

Subprocedures	1	2	3	Other Modules
Aortic Arch, Descending Aorta				
Descending aorta	No or trivial gradient Peak gradient < 20 mm Hg	Mild gradient Peak gradient 20-40 mm Hg	Moderate to severe gradient Peak gradient > 40 mm Hg	
Aortic arch	No or trivial gradient Peak gradient < 20 mm Hg No apparent narrowing by imaging or color Doppler jet width	Mild gradient Peak gradient 20-40 mm Hg or < 30% narrowing by imaging or color Doppler jet width	Moderate to severe gradient Peak gradient > 40 mm Hg or > 30% narrowing by imaging or color Doppler jet width	
Aortic Valve/Truncal Valve (Repair)				
Aortic valve repair Truncal valve repair	No or trivial stenosis Peak gradient < 20 mm Hg No or trivial regurgitation VC < 1 mm if < 10 kg VC < 2 mm if > 10 kg	Mild stenosis Peak gradient 20-40 mm Hg Mild regurgitation VC 1-2 mm if < 10 kg VC 2-4 mm if > 10 kg	Moderate to severe stenosis Peak gradient > 40 mm Hg Moderate to severe regurgitation VC > 2 mm if < 10 kg VC > 4 mm if > 10 kg	LVOT Supra-aortic anastomosis/repair
Aortic Valve/Truncal Valve Replacement				
Prosthetic valve implantation	Trivial or no stenosis Peak velocity < 2.5 m/sec Trivial to no regurgitation	Mild stenosis Peak velocity < 3.5 m/sec Minor paravalvular leak (VC < 2 mm)	Moderate or severe stenosis Peak velocity > 3.5 m/sec Significant paravalvular leak (VC > 2 mm)	LVOT Supra-aortic anastomosis
Autograft implantation	No aortic valvar regurgitation or stenosis VC < 2 mm	Trivial to mild regurgitation or stenosis VC 2-4 mm Peak gradient < 30 mm	Moderate or severe stenosis Peak gradient > 30 mm Moderate or severe regurgitation VC > 4 mm	LVOT Supra-aortic anastomosis
Atrial Septum/Atrial Septectomy				
Atrial septectomy	No or trivial gradient Mean gradient < 2 mm Hg (Restrictive atrial septum left on purpose; higher gradient acceptable)	Mild residual obstruction Mean gradient 2-4 mm Hg (unless intended)	Moderate to severe residual obstruction Mean gradient > 4 mm Hg (unless intended)	
ASD Repair, Patch/Primary, Common Atrium/Sinus Venosus				
ASD repair	No or trivial residual shunt <2 mm if > 10 kg <1 mm if < 10 kg	Small residual shunt 2-3 mm if > 10 kg 1-2 mm if < 10 kg	Residual shunt >3 mm if > 10 kg >2 mm if > 10 kg	
SVC (for superior sinus venosus defect) IVC (for inferior sinus venosus defect)	No SVC obstruction Mean gradient < 2 mm Hg No IVC obstruction Mean gradient < 2 mm Hg	Trivial to mild SVC obstruction Mean gradient 2-4 mm Hg Trivial to mild IVC obstruction Mean gradient 2-4 mm Hg	Mild or greater SVC obstruction Mean gradient > 4 mm Hg Mild or greater IVC obstruction Mean gradient > 4 mm Hg	

Subprocedures	1	2	3	Other Modules
AVV Plasty				
Left AV valve plasty (subaortic AV valve)	No or trivial stenosis Mean gradient < 3 mm Hg No or trivial regurgitation VC < 1 mm if < 10 kg VC < 2 mm if > 10 kg	Mild stenosis Mean gradient 3-6 mm Hg Mild regurgitation VC 1-2 mm if < 10 kg VC 2-4 mm if > 10 kg	Moderate or severe stenosis Mean gradient > 6 mm Hg Moderate or severe regurgitation VC > 2 mm if < 10 kg VC > 4 mm if > 10 kg	
Right AV valve plasty (subpulmonary AV valve)	No or trivial stenosis Mean gradient < 3 mm Hg No or trivial regurgitation VC < 3 mm if < 10 kg VC < 4 mm if > 10 kg	Mild stenosis Mean gradient 3-6 mm Hg) Mild regurgitation VC 3-5 mm if < 10 kg VC 4-6 mm if > 10 kg	Moderate or severe stenosis Mean gradient > 6 mm Hg Moderate or severe regurgitation VC > 5 mm if < 10 kg VC > 6 mm if > 10 kg	
Tricuspid valve annulus plication (cone)	No anatomic disruption of plication No coronary injury	No anatomic disruption of plication No coronary injury	Dehiscence of plication Coronary artery injury	
RV/RA plication/ excision (cone)	No anatomic disruption of plication No coronary injury	No anatomic disruption of plication No coronary injury	Dehiscence of plication Coronary artery injury	
AVV Replacement				
Mitral valve implantation	Trivial or no stenosis Mean velocity < 1.5 m/sec No paravalvar leak (follow manufacturer's guidelines for stenosis for prosthetic valve)	Mild stenosis Mean velocity 1.5-2.5 m/sec Minor paravalvular leak (VC < 2 mm)	Moderate or severe stenosis Mean velocity > 2.5 m/sec Significant paravalvular leak (VC > 2 mm)	Coronary
Tricuspid valve implantation	Trivial or no stenosis Mean velocity < 1.5 m/sec No paravalvar leak (follow manufacturer's guidelines for stenosis if prosthetic valve)	Mild stenosis Mean velocity 1.5-2.5 m/sec Minor paravalvular leak (VC < 2 mm)	Moderate or severe stenosis Mean velocity > 2.5 m/sec Significant paravalvular leak (VC > 2 mm)	Coronary
Branch Pulmonary Artery Reconstruction				
Branch pulmonary artery reconstruction	No residual stenosis Peak gradient < 20 mm Hg No discrete narrowing by imaging or color Doppler jet width	Mild residual stenosis Peak gradient 20-40 mm Hg or < 30% narrowing by imaging or color Doppler jet width	Moderate to severe residual stenosis Peak gradient > 40 mm Hg or > 30% narrowing by imaging or color Doppler jet width	
BT/Sano/Other Systemic to Pulmonary Artery Shunts, Including Unifocalization				
BT/Sano/other systemic to pulmonary artery shunts	Patent	Patent	Partial or complete occlusion, distortion of branch pulmonary arteries	
Cavopulmonary Anastomosis				
SVC-PA anastomosis Main pulmonary artery patch plasty	No obstruction No pulmonary artery distortion Mean gradient < 2 mm	Mild distortion or obstruction Mean gradient 2-4 mm Hg	Moderate to severe obstruction Mean gradient > 4 mm Hg	
IVC inflow	No or trivial obstruction Mean gradient < 2 mm Hg	Mild obstruction Mean gradient 2-4 mm Hg	Moderate to severe obstruction Mean gradient > 4 mm Hg	
Tunnel/conduit–pulmonary artery anastomosis	No or trivial obstruction Mean gradient < 2 mm Hg	Mild distortion or obstruction Mean gradient 2-4 mm Hg	Moderate to severe obstruction Mean gradient > 4 mm Hg	
Fenestration (if present)	Patent	Patent	Fenestration not patent	
Coronary Reimplantation/Unroofing				
Coronaries reimplantation/ unroofing/baffle	No obstruction to coronary flow	No obstruction to coronary flow	Coronary flow compromise, ischemia/ infarction, with echo and/or ECG findings	Aortic valve Supra-aortic anastomosis

Continued

Subprocedures	1	2	3	Other Modules
LVOT/Sub-Aortic Stenosis Resection				
LVOT	Trivial LVOT obstruction (MIG < 20 mm Hg)	Mild LVOT obstruction (MIG 20-40 mm Hg)	Moderate or severe LVOT obstruction (MIG > 40 mm Hg)	Aortic valve Supra-aortic anastomosis
PDA Ligation/Division				
PDA closure	No residual PDA	Residual PDA ≤ 1 mm	Re-intervention *or* Residual PDA > 1 mm	Arch and descending aorta Branch pulmonary arteries
Pulmonary Valve Intervention				
Pulmonary valve reconstruction Valve sparing	No residual obstruction RVOT peak gradient < 20 mm Hg No or mild pulmonary valve regurgitation VC < 3 mm if < 10 kg VC < 5 mm if > 10 kg	Mild residual obstruction RVOT peak gradient 20-40 mm Hg Mild PR VC 3-5 mm if < 10 kg VC 5-8 mm if > 10 kg	Moderate to severe residual obstruction RVOT peak gradient > 40 mm Hg Moderate to severe PR VC > 5 mm if < 10 kg VC > 8 mm if > 10 kg	Suprapulmonary anastomosis Main pulmonary artery Branch pulmonary arteries
Transannular patch	No residual obstruction RVOT peak gradient < 20 mm Hg PR—no consequence	Mild residual obstruction RVOT peak gradient 20-40 mm Hg PR—no consequence	Moderate to severe residual obstruction RVOT peak gradient > 40 mm Hg PR—no consequence	Suprapulmonary anastomosis Main pulmonary artery Branch pulmonary arteries
Pulmonary Valve Replacement				
Pulmonary valve replacement	Trivial or no stenosis Peak velocity < 2.5 m/sec No paravalvular leak (follow manufacturer's guidelines for stenosis if prosthetic valve)	Mild stenosis Peak velocity 2.5-3.5 m/sec Minor paravalvular leak (VC < 2 mm)	Moderate or severe stenosis Peak velocity > 3.5 m/sec Significant paravalvular leak (VC > 2 mm)	Suprapulmonary anastomosis Main pulmonary artery Branch pulmonary arteries Subpulmonary outflow
Pulmonary Veins				
Pulmonary vein confluence or baffle	No or trivial obstruction Mean gradient < 2 mm Hg	Mild obstruction Mean gradient 2-4 mm Hg	Moderate or severe obstruction Mean gradient > 4 mm Hg	
Scimitar vein baffle to left atrium	No or trivial obstruction Mean gradient < 2 mm Hg	Mild obstruction Mean gradient 2-4 mm Hg	Moderate or severe obstruction Mean gradient > 4 mm Hg	
Unroofing of coronary sinus	No obstruction Mean gradient < 2 mm Hg	Mild obstruction Mean gradient 2-4 mm Hg	Moderate or severe obstruction Mean gradient > 4 mm Hg	
RVOT Reconstruction/Sub-Pulmonary Stenosis Resection				
Relief of RVOT obstruction	No or trivial residual obstruction Peak gradient < 20 mm Hg	Mild residual obstruction Peak gradient 20-40 mm Hg	Moderate or severe residual obstruction Peak gradient > 40 mm Hg	Pulmonary valve Suprapulmonary Branch pulmonary arteries
RV-PA Conduit				
RV-PA conduit	Trivial to no valvar stenosis Peak gradient < 20 mm Hg Trivial to no valvar regurgitation VC < 3 mm	Mild stenosis Peak gradient 20-40 mm Hg Mild regurgitation VC 3-5 mm	Moderate or severe stenosis Peak gradient > 40 mm Hg Moderate or severe regurgitation VC > 5 mm	Subpulmonary Suprapulmonary Branch pulmonary arteries

Subprocedures	1	2	3	Other Modules
Supra-aortic Anastomosis/Repair				
Ascending aortic reconstruction Supra-aortic anastomosis	No residual gradient or narrowing Peak gradient < 10 mm Hg	Mild narrowing or mild residual gradient Peak gradient 10-20 mm Hg	Moderate or severe residual stenosis Peak gradient > 20 mm Hg	Aortic valve Aortic arch
Suprapulmonary Anastomosis/Repair				
Main pulmonary artery reconstruction Suprapulmonary anastomosis	No residual gradient or narrowing Peak gradient < 10 mm Hg	Mild narrowing or mild residual Peak gradient 10-20 mm Hg	Moderate or severe residual stenosis Peak gradient > 20 mm Hg	Pulmonary valve Branch pulmonary arteries
Systemic Venous Baffle				
Systemic venous baffle	No or trivial obstruction Mean gradient < 2 mm Hg	Mild obstruction Mean gradient 2-4 mm Hg	Moderate to severe obstruction Mean gradient > 4 mm Hg	
Transplant				
Left atrium anastomosis	No or trivial obstruction Mean gradient < 2 mm Hg	Mild obstruction Mean gradient 2-4 mm Hg	Moderate or severe obstruction Mean gradient > 4 mm Hg	
Aortic anastomosis	No obstruction Peak gradient < 10 mm	Mild obstruction Peak gradient 10-20 mm Hg	Moderate or severe obstruction Peak gradient > 20 mm Hg	
Pulmonary artery anastomosis	No obstruction Peak gradient < 10 mm Hg	Mild obstruction Peak gradient 10-20 mm Hg	Moderate or severe obstruction Peak gradient > 20 mm Hg	
SVC/IVC anastomosis	No or trivial obstruction Mean gradient < 2 mm Hg	Mild obstruction Mean gradient 2-4 mm Hg	Moderate or severe obstruction Mean gradient > 4 mm Hg	
PFO closure	No or trivial residual shunt <2 mm if > 10 kg <1 mm if < 10 kg	Small residual shunt 2-3 mm if > 10 kg 1-2 mm if < 10 kg	Residual shunt >3 mm if > 10 kg >2 mm if > 10 kg	
Ventricular Assist Devices				
Left ventricular/left atrial cannula	No obstruction to flow	Mild obstruction	Moderate or severe obstruction	
Ascending aortic cannula	No obstruction Peak gradient < 10 mm Hg	Mild obstruction Peak gradient 10-20 mm Hg	Moderate or severe obstruction Peak gradient > 20 mm Hg	
Pulmonary artery anastomosis	No obstruction Peak gradient < 10 mm Hg	Mild obstruction Peak gradient 10-20 mm Hg	Moderate or severe obstruction Peak gradient > 20 mm Hg	
Right atrial cannula	No obstruction	Mild obstruction	Moderate or severe obstruction	
VSD Repair				
VSD repair	No or trivial residual shunt <2 mm if > 10 kg <1 mm if < 10 kg	Residual defect 2-3 mm if > 10 kg 1-2 mm if < 10 kg	Residual defect >3 mm if > 10 kg >2 mm if < 10 kg	Aortic valve Tricuspid valve

If PFO was left open, fenestrated ASD closure was performed, or fenestrated VSD closure was performed, then ASD and VSD were not scored. Additional muscular VSDs not intervened on at time of surgery also were not scored.

ASD, Atrial septal defect; *AV,* atrioventricular; *AVV,* atrioventricular valve; *BT,* Blalock-Taussig; *ECG,* electrocardiogram; *IVC,* inferior vena cava; *LVOT,* left ventricular outflow tract; *MIG,* maximum instantaneous gradient; *PFO,* patent foramen ovale; *PR,* pulmonary regurgitation; *RVOT,* right ventricular outflow tract; *RV-PA,* right ventricle to pulmonary artery; *SVC,* superior vena cava; *SVC-PA,* superior vena cava to pulmonary artery; *VC,* vena contracta; *VSD,* ventricular septal defect.

REFERENCES

1. Center for Disease Control and Prevention: Congenital heart defects (CHD): data and statistics (last updated July 9, 2014). http://www.cdc.gov/ncbddd/heartdefects/data.html.
2. Fuller S, Nord AS, Gerdes M, et al: Predictors of impaired neurodevelopmental outcomes at one year of age after infant cardiac surgery. *Eur J Cardiothorac Surg* 36:40–47, 2009.
3. Mahle WT: Neurologic and cognitive outcomes in children with congenital heart disease. *Curr Opin Pediatr* 13:482–486, 2001.
4. Newburger JW, Sleeper LA, Bellinger DC, et al: Early developmental outcome in children with hypoplastic left heart syndrome and related anomalies. The single ventricle reconstruction trial. *Circulation* 125:2081–2091, 2012.
5. Marino BS, Lipkin PH, Newburger JW, et al: Neurodevelopmental outcomes in children with congenital heart disease: evaluation and management: a scientific statement from the American Heart Association. *Circulation* 126:1143–1172, 2012.
6. Data Analysis of The Society of Thoracic Surgeons Congenital Heart Surgery Database, Period ending 6/30/2011. Duke Clinical Research Institute, Duke University Medical Center. Available at https://outcomes.dcri.duke.edu/registry/. Accessed January 28, 2013.
7. Stark JF, Gallivan S, Davis K, et al: Assessment of mortality rates for congenital heart defects and surgeons' performance. *Ann Thorac Surg* 72:169–175, 2001.
8. Welke KF, Karamlou T, Ungerleider RM, et al: Mortality rate is not a valid indicator of quality differences between pediatric cardiac surgical programs. *Ann Thorac Surg* 89(1):139–144, discussion 145–146, 2010.
9. Welke KF, Diggs BS, Karamlou T, et al: The relationship between hospital surgical case volumes and mortality rates in pediatric cardiac surgery: a national sample, 1988-2005. *Ann Thorac Surg* 86(3):889–896, Discussion 889–896, 2008.
10. Jarman B, Gault S, Alves B, et al: Explaining differences in English hospital death rates using routinely collected data. *BMJ* 318:1515–1520, 1999.
11. Mohammed MA, Deeks JJ, Girling A, et al: Evidence of methodological bias in hospital standardised mortality ratios: retrospective database study of English hospitals. *BMJ* 338:b780, 2009.
12. Karamichalis JM, Thiagarajan RR, Liu H, et al: Norwood: optimal technical performance improves outcomes irrespective of preoperative physiologic status or case-complexity. *J Thorac Cardiovasc Surg* 139:962–968, 2010.
13. Nathan M, Karamichalis J, Liu H, et al: Intra-operative adverse events can be compensated in infants after cardiac surgery: a prospective study. *J Thorac Cardiovasc Surg* 142:1098–1107, 2011.
14. Karamichalis JM, del Nido PJ, Thiagarajan RR, et al: Early postoperative severity of illness predicts outcomes following the stage I Norwood procedure. *Ann Thorac Surg* 92:660–665, 2011.
15. Larrazabal LA, del Nido PJ, Jenkins KJ, et al: Measurement of technical performance in congenital heart surgery: a pilot study. *Ann Thorac Surg* 83:179–184, 2007.
16. Bacha EA, Larrazabal LA, Pigula FA, et al: Measurement of technical performance in surgery for congenital heart disease: the stage I Norwood procedure. *J Thorac Cardiovasc Surg* 136:993–997, 2008.
17. Karamichalis JM, Colan SD, Nathan M, et al: Technical performance scores in congenital cardiac surgery: a quality assessment initiative. *Ann Thorac Surg* 94:1317–1323, 2012.
18. Nathan M, Karamichalis JM, Colan S, et al: Surgical technical performance scores are predictors for late mortality and unplanned reinterventions in infants after cardiac surgery. *J Thorac Cardiovasc Surg* 144:1095–1101, 2012.
19. Nathan M, Sadhwani A, Gauvreau K, et al: Association between technical performance scores and neurodevelopmental outcomes after congenital cardiac surgery. *J Thorac Cardiovasc Surg* 148:232–237, 2014.
20. Nathan M, Karamichalis J, Liu H, et al: Technical performance scores are strongly associated with early mortality, postoperative adverse events and ICU length of stay—analysis of consecutive discharges over 2 years. *J Thorac Cardiovasc Surg* 147:389–394, 2014.
21. Nathan M, Pigula FA, Colan S, et al: Inadequate technical performance scores are associated with late mortality and need for late re-intervention in a 13 month cohort of patients followed for 4 years. *Ann Thorac Surg* 96:664–669, 2013.
22. Jenkins KJ, Gauvreau K, Newburger JW, et al: Consensus based method for risk adjustment for surgery for congenital heart disease. *J Thorac Cardiovasc Surg* 123:110–118, 2002.
23. Jenkins KJ: Risk adjustment for congenital heart surgery: the RACHS-1 method. *Semin Thorac Cardiovasc Surg Pediatr Card Surg Annu* 7:180–184, 2004.
24. Pollack MM, Patel KM, Ruttimann UE: PRISM III: an updated pediatric risk of mortality score. *Crit Care Med* 24:743–752, 1996.
24a. Nathan M, Gauvreau K, Liu H, et al: Technical performance score predicts resource utilization in congenital cardiac procedures: analysis of 27 consecutive months data. Accepted for presentation at the STS 50th Annual Meeting, Orlando, Florida, January 25-29, 2014. (PMC in process).
25. Nathan M, Sleeper L, Ohye R, et al on behalf of the PHN investigators: Technical performance score is strongly associated with outcomes after Norwood procedure: analysis of the Single Ventricle Reconstruction Trial Cohort. Accepted for presentation at the STS 50th Annual Meeting, Orlando, Florida, January 25-29, 2014. (PMC in process).
26. de Leval MR, Carthey J, Wright DJ, et al: Human factors and cardiac surgery: a multicenter study. *J Thorac Cardiovasc Surg* 119:661–672, 2000.
27. Barach P, Johnson JK, Ahmad A, et al: A prospective observational study of human factors, adverse events and patient outcomes in surgery for pediatric cardiac disease. *J Thorac Cardiovasc Surg* 136:1422–1428, 2008.
28. Schraagen JM, Schouten T, Smit M, et al: A prospective study of paediatric cardiac surgical microsystems: assessing the relationships between non routine events, team work and patient outcomes. *BMJ Qual Saf* 2011.
29. Birkmeyer JD, Finks JF, O'Reilly A, et al: Surgical skill and complications after bariatric surgery. *N Engl J Med* 369:1434–1442, 2013.
30. Zevin B, Bonrath EM, Aggarwal R, et al on behalf of the ATLAS group: Development, feasibility, validity, and reliability of a scale for objective assessment of operative performance in laparoscopic gastric bypass surgery. *J Am Coll Surg* 216:955, 2013.
31. Carty MJ, Chan R, Huckman R, et al: A detailed analysis of the reduction mammaplasty learning curve: a statistical process model for approaching surgical performance improvement. *Plast Reconstr Surg* 124:706–714, 2009.
32. Martin JA, Regehr G, Reznick R, et al: Objective Structured Assessment of Technical Skill (OSATS) for surgical residents. *Br J Surg* 84:273–278, 1997.
33. Macrae HM: Objective assessment of technical skill. *Surgeon* S23–S25, 2011.
34. Gofton WT, Dudek NL, Wood TJ, et al: The Ottawa Surgical Competency Operating Room Evaluation (O-SCORE): a tool to assess surgical competence. *Acad Med* 87:1401–1407, 2012.
35. Faurie C, Khadra M: Technical competence in surgeons. *ANZ J Surg* 82:682–690, 2012.
36. Jacobs JP, Jacobs ML, Mavroudis C: What is operative morbidity? Defining complications in a surgical registry database: a report from the STS Congenital Database Taskforce and the Joint EACTS-STS Congenital Database Committee. *Ann Thorac Surg* 84:1416–1421, 2007.
37. O'Brien SM, Clarke DR, Jacobs JP: An empirically based tool for analyzing mortality associated with congenital heart surgery. *J Thorac Cardiovasc Surg* 138(5):1139–1153, 2009.
38. Jacobs ML, Jacobs JP, Jenkins KJ, et al: Stratification of complexity: the Risk Adjustment for Congenital Heart Surgery-1 method and the Aristotle Complexity Score—past, present, and future. *Cardiol Young* 18(Suppl 2):163–168, 2008.

INDEX

Note: Page numbers followed by *f* indicate figures; *b*, boxes; *t*, tables.

C

D

E

F

G

N

Q

R

U

V

W